Textbook *of* FAMILY PRACTICE

Textbook *of* FAMILY PRACTICE

5th EDITION

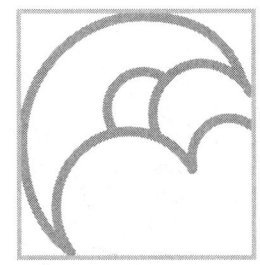
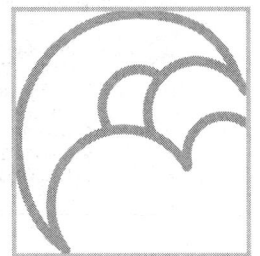
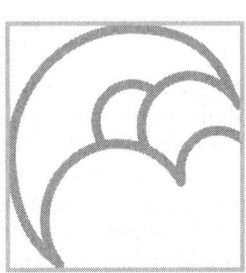
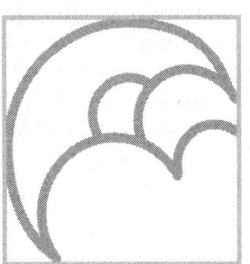
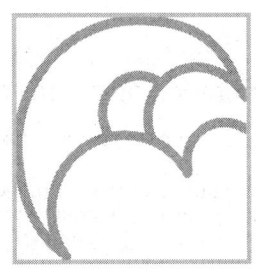

ROBERT E. RAKEL, M.D.

Chairman, Department of Family Medicine
Associate Dean for Academic and Clinical Affairs
Baylor College of Medicine
Houston, Texas

W.B. Saunders Company
A Division of Harcourt Brace & Company
Philadelphia London Toronto Montreal Sydney Tokyo

W. B. SAUNDERS COMPANY
A Division of Harcourt Brace & Company

The Curtis Center
Independence Square West
Philadelphia, PA 19106

Library of Congress Cataloging-in-Publication Data

Textbook of family practice / [edited by] Robert E. Rakel.—5th ed.
        p.   cm.
    Includes bibliographical references and index.
    ISBN 0-7216-4053-2
    1. Family medicine.   I. Rakel, Robert E.
    [DNLM: 1. Family Practice.   WB 110 T355 1995]
    RC46.T327 1995
    610—dc20
    DNLM/DLC   95-6537

Medicine is an ever-changing field. Standard safety precautions must be followed, but as new research and clinical experience broaden our knowledge, changes in treatment and drug therapy become necessary or appropriate. The editors of this work have carefully checked the generic and trade drug names and verified drug dosages to ensure that the dosage information in this work is accurate and in accord with the standards accepted at the time of publication. Readers are advised, however, to check the product information currently provided by the manufacturer of each drug to be administered to be certain that changes have not been made in the recommended dose or in the contraindications for administration. This is of particular importance in regard to new or infrequently used drugs. It is the responsibility of the treating physician, relying on experience and knowledge of the patient, to determine dosages and the best treatment for the patient. The editors cannot be responsible for misuse or misapplication of the material in this work.

THE PUBLISHER

International Edition ISBN 0–7216–6772–4

TEXTBOOK OF FAMILY PRACTICE   ISBN 0-7216-4053-2

Printed in the United States of America.

Last digit is the print number: 9   8   7   6   5   4   3

To Peggy
and our children and their families

CONTRIBUTORS

BYRON J. BAILEY, M.D.
Wiess Professor and Chairman, University of Texas Medical Branch, Galveston, Texas
Otolaryngology

RENALDO N. BATTISTA, M.D., Sc.D.
Professor, Faculty of Medicine, McGill University; Physician, Montreal General Hospital, President, Conseil d'evaluation des technologies de la sante de Quebec, Montreal, Quebec, Canada
Periodic Health Examination

ALEXANDER BERGER, M.D.
Professor of Family and Community Medicine, Eastern Virginia Medical School, Norfolk, Virginia
Ophthalmology

S. LANE BICKNELL, M.D.
Clinical Associate Professor of Urology, University of Tennessee Center for Health Sciences, Memphis; Clinical Associate Professor of Family Practice, Jackson, Tennessee
Urinary Tract Disorders

F. MARIAN BISHOP, Ph.D., M.S.P.H.
Chairman, Department of Family and Preventive Medicine, University of Utah School of Medicine, Salt Lake City, Utah
Interviewing Techniques

ALAN BLUM, M.D.
Associate Professor, Baylor College of Medicine, Houston, Texas
Nicotine Addiction

EDWARD T. BOPE, M.D.
Clinical Associate Professor, The Ohio State University; Residency Director—Family Practice, Riverside Methodist Hospitals, Columbus, Ohio
Cardiovascular Disease

WILLIAM Z. BORER, M.D.
Associate Professor, Department of Pathology and Cell Biology, Thomas Jefferson University; Director, Clinical Chemistry Section, Thomas Jefferson University Hospital, Philadelphia, Pennsylvania
Appendix I—Reference Values for the Interpretation of Laboratory Tests

JAMES H. BRAY, Ph.D.
Associate Professor of Family Medicine, Baylor College of Medicine; The Methodist Hospital; St. Luke's Episcopal Hospital, Houston, Texas
Impact of Divorce and Remarriage on the Family

JOSEPH BRODERICK, M.D.
Associate Professor, University of Cincinnati College of Medicine; Staff Neurologist, University of Cincinnati Hospitals, Cincinnati, Ohio
Neurology in Family Practice

BARUCH A. BRODY, Ph.D.
Professor of Biomedical Ethics, Baylor College of Medicine, Houston, Texas
Ethics in Family Practice

ERICH E. BRUESCHKE, B.S.E.E., M.D.
Professor of Family Medicine, Rush Medical College; Senior Attending/Vice President, Medical Affairs, Rush-Presbyterian St. Luke's Medical Center, Chicago, Illinois
Somatic Patient

SANDRA K. BURGE, Ph.D.
Associate Professor, Department of Family Practice, University of Texas Health Science Center at San Antonio, San Antonio, Texas
Spouse Abuse; Adult Victims of Sexual Assault; A Footnote about Violence Prevention

WILLIAM CAHILL, M.D.
Assistant Professor, University of Cincinnati College of Medicine; Staff Neurologist, University of Cincinnati Hospitals; Chief, Department of Neurology, Veterans' Administration Medical Center, Cincinnati, Ohio
Neurology in Family Practice

DAVID C. CAMPBELL, M.D., M.Ed.
Associate Chair and Associate Professor, Department of Community and Family Medicine, St. Louis University School of Medicine; Program Director and Chief of Family Medicine, Deaconess Hospital-Central Campus, St. Louis, Missouri
Sports Medicine

THOMAS L. CAMPBELL, M.D.
Associate Professor of Medicine and Psychiatry, University of Rochester School of Medicine and Dentistry; Family Medicine Attending, Highland Hospital, Rochester, New York
Family Stress

LAUREL CAREY, M.A.
Behavioral Science Faculty, St. Joseph Medical Center, Stamford, Connecticut
Crisis Intervention in Office Practice

M. BASEM CHAKER, M.D.
Assistant Professor, Dermatology and Dermatopathology, The University of Texas Southwestern Medical Center; Staff Dermatologist, Dalls VA Medical Center, Dallas, Texas
Evaluation of Skin Lesions

CHRISTOPHER V. CHAMBERS, M.D.
Clinical Associate Professor of Family Medicine, Fellowship Director, Jefferson Medical College, Thomas Jefferson University, Philadelphia, Pennsylvania
Childhood and Adolescence

CYNTHIA L. CHAPPELL, Ph.D.
Associate Professor of Parasitology, University of Texas School of Public Health; Adjunct Assistant Professor, Baylor College of Medicine, Houston, Texas
Parasitology

JOHN R. COLEMAN, Ph.D.
PCA Solutions, Inc. Longwood, Florida
Managed Health Care

JOSEPH V. CONNELLY, M.D.
Clinical Assistant Professor, New York Medical College, Valhalla, New York; Assistant Clinical Professor, University of Connecticut School of Medicine, Storrs, Connecticut; Adjunct Assistant Professor of Medicine, Columbia, University, New York, New York; Director, St. Joseph Family Medicine Residency Program, St. Joseph Medical Center, Stamford, Connecticut
Infectious Diseases

GEORGE S. CONOMIKES, M.A., B.A.
Conomikes Associates, Inc.
Los Angeles, California
Personnel and Time Management

JANE E. CORBOY, M.D.
Assistant Professor, Family Medicine, Baylor College of Medicine; Director, Park Plaza Family Practice Center and Residency Track, Park Plaza Hospital, Houston, Texas
Travel Medicine

JAMES C. COYNE, Ph.D.
Professor, Departments of Family Practice and Psychiatry, University of Michigan Medical Center, Ann Arbor, Michigan
Depression

SYDNEY H. CROOG, Ph.D.
Professor of Behavioral Sciences and Community Health, University of Connecticut Health Center, Farmington, Connecticut
Assessment of Functional Health Status

EARL R. CROUCH, Jr., M.D.
Professor and Chairman of Ophthalmology, Associate Professor of Pediatrics, Eastern Virginia Medical School; Surgical Director of Ophthalmology, Children's Hospital of the King's Daughters, Norfolk, Virginia
Ophthalmology

MICHAEL A. CROUCH, M.D., M.S.P.H.
Associate Professor of Clinical Family Medicine; Director, Family Medicine Residency Program, Baylor College of Medicine; Staff Physician, St. Luke's Episcopal Hospital, The Methodist Hospital; Courtesy Staff, Texas Children's Hospital, Houston, Texas
Clinical Genetics and Genetic Counseling

MEL P. DALY, M.B., B.Ch.
Associate Professor of Family Medicine and Internal Medicine, University of Maryland School of Medicine; Director, Division of Geriatrics, Department of Family Medicine, University of Maryland, Baltimore, Maryland
Care of the Elderly

ALAN K. DAVID, M.D.
Professor of Family Medicine, University of Cincinnati College of Medicine; Professor and Director, Department of Family Medicine, University of Cincinnati University Hospital, Cincinnati, Ohio
Hematology

JENNIFER LYNN DINGLE, B.Sc., B.Ed., M.B.A.
Co-ordinator, Canadian Task Force on the Periodic Health Examination, Department of Pediatrics, Dalhousie University, Halifax, Nova Scotia, Canada
Periodic Health Examination

CHARLES E. DRISCOLL, M.D.
Family Physician, Mercy Hospital, Iowa City, Iowa
Sexual Health Care by the Family Physician

DAVID V. ESPINO, M.D.
Associate Professor and Chief, Division of Geriatrics, Department of Family Practice, University of Texas Health Science Center at San Antonio; Active Staff, Medical Center Hospital, Audie L. Murphy Veterans Administration Medical Center, San Antonio, Texas
Elder Abuse

C. EDWARD EVANS, M.B.
Professor, Department of Family Medicine, McMaster University; Active Staff, McMaster University Medical Center, Hamilton, Ontario, Canada
Patient Compliance

DONNA R. FALVO, R.N., PH.D.
Professor, Rehabilitation Counseling, Rehabilitation Institute; Department of Family and Community Medicine, Southern Illinois University School of Medicine, Carbondale, Illinois
Patient Education

LORRAINE FAY, M.D.
Associate Professor of Clinical Pediatrics, Medical College of Ohio, Toledo, Ohio
Growth and Development

JOHN W. FEIGHTNER, M.D., M.SC.
Professor, Department of Family Medicine, McMaster University; Active Staff, Chedoke-McMaster Hospital, Hamilton, Ontario, Canada
Periodic Health Examination

ROBERT E. FEINSTEIN, M.D.
Director, Behavioral Science, St. Joseph Medical Center, Stamford, Connecticut; Assistant Clinical Professor of Psychiatry, Columbia University College of Physicians and Surgeons, New York, New York
Crisis Intervention in Office Practice; Personality Disorders in Office Practice

EUGENE A. FELMAR, M.D.
Clinical Professor of Family Medicine, University of California, Los Angeles, Los Angeles, California; Director, Family Practice Residency Program, Santa Monica Hospital Medical Center, Santa Monica, California
Nutrition and Family Medicine

RICHARD E. FINLAYSON, M.D.
Associate Professor of Psychiatry, Mayo Medical School; Consultant in Adult Psychiatry, Medical Director Inpatient Addiction Program, Mayo Clinic, Rochester, Minnesota
Dementia

PAUL M. FISCHER, M.D.
Private Practice, University Hospital, Augusta, Georgia
Interpreting Laboratory Tests

JOHN G. FORT, M.D., M.B.A.
Associate Professor of Medicine, Jefferson Medical College, Philadelphia, Pennsylvania
Rheumatic Disease

ROBERT E. FROELICH, M.D.
Professor of Psychiatry, University of Utah School of Medicine, Salt Lake City, Utah
Interviewing Techniques

WILLIAM FULCHER, M.D., M.ED.
Assistant Professor and Director of Education, Department of Family and Community Medicine, University of Alabama at Birmingham, Birmingham, Alabama
Poisoning; Bites, Stings, and Other Envenomation; Thermal and Environmental Injuries

JOHN P. GEYMAN, M.D.
Professor Emeritus, Department of Family Medicine, University of Washington, Seattle, Washington; Family Physician, Inter Island Medical Center, Friday Harbor, Washington
Diagnosis and Treatment of Anxiety Disorders

LARRY A. GREEN, M.D.
The Woodward-Chisholm Chairman of Family Medicine, University of Colorado Health Sciences Center, Department of Family Medicine, Denver, Colorado
Community-Oriented Primary Care

R. BRIAN HAYNES, M.D.
Professor, Department of Clinical Epidemiology and Biostatistics; Professor, Department of Medicine, McMaster University Faculty of Health Sciences; Active Staff, Chedoke-McMaster Hospital, Hamilton, Ontario, Canada
Patient Compliance

WARREN A. HEFFRON, M.D.
Professor, Department of Family and Community Medicine, University of New Mexico School of Medicine; University of New Mexico Hospital, Albuquerque, New Mexico
Preventive Health Care

JOE E. HIMES, M.D.
Associate Clinical Professor, St. Louis University; Fellowship Director, Deaconess Family Medicine; Director of Sports Medicine, Deaconess Hospital-Central Campus, St. Louis, Missouri
Sports Medicine

WARREN L. HOLLEMAN, PH.D.
Assistant Professor, Department of Family Medicine and The Center for Ethics, Medicine and Public Issues, Baylor College of Medicine, Houston, Texas
Ethics in Family Practice

O. MAX JARDON, M.D.
Associate Professor, Orthopaedic Surgery, University of Nebraska Medical Center, Omaha, Nebraska
Orthopedics

RUTH G. JENKINS, M.S.
Department of Family Medicine, Medical University of South Carolina, Charleston, South Carolina
Computer Applications in Office Practice

GLEN R. JOHNSON, M.D.
Senior Vice President for Medical Affairs, Physician Corporation of America, Miami, Florida
Managed Health Care

E. STANLEY KARDATZKE, M.D.
Founder, Chairman of the Board, and Chief Executive Office, Physician Corporation of America, Miami, Florida
Managed Health Care

WAYNE KATON, M.D.
Professor of Psychiatry, Adjunct Professor of Family Medicine, University of Washington Medical School; Chief of Division of Consultation Liaison Psychiatry, University of Washington Medical School, Seattle, Washington
Diagnosis and Treatment of Anxiety Disorders

NANCY D. KELLOGG, M.D.
Assistant Professor of Pediatrics, University of Texas Health Science Center at San Antonio; Consulting and Admitting Privileges at University Hospital and Santa Rosa Children's Hospital; Consulting Privileges at Methodist Hospital; Medical Director, Alamo Children's Advocacy Center, San Antonio, Texas
Child Abuse

ROBERT B. KELLY, M.D.
Associate Professor and Chairperson, MetroHealth Campus, Department of Family Medicine, Case Western Reserve University School of Medicine; Chairperson, Department of Family Practice, MetroHealth Medical Center, Cleveland, Ohio
Patient Education

SANFORD R. KIMMEL, M.D.
Associate Professor of Clinical Family Medicine, Medical College of Ohio; Associate Residency Director, Medical College of Ohio/St. Vincent Medical Center, Family Practice Residency, Toledo, Ohio
Growth and Development

STEPHANIE H. KONG, M.D.
Executive Vice President and Chief Operating Officer, PCA Health Plans of Georgia, Inc., Atlanta, Georgia
Managed Health Care

ROBERT E. KYNERD, M.D.
Family Physician, Highland Family Health Center, Birmingham, Alabama
Trauma

GREG L. LEDGERWOOD, M.D.
Clinical Associate Professor, Department of Family Medicine, University of Washington School of Medicine, Seattle, Washington; Private Practice, Omak, Washington
Allergy

JOSEPH A. LIEBERMAN, III, M.D., M.P.H.
Clinical Professor of Family Medicine, Jefferson Medical College, Thomas Jefferson University, Philadelphia, Pennsylvania; Chairman, Department of Family and Community Medicine, Medical Center of Delaware, Wilmington, Delaware
Practicing Biopsychosocial Medicine

JOHN L. LYMAN, M.D.
Associate Clinical Professor, Department of Emergency Medicine, Wright State University, Dayton, Ohio; Associate Regional Medical Director, EMSA, Plantation, Florida
Introduction to Emergency Medicine

MONTY S. MATHEWS, M.D.
Assistant Professor, Department of Family Practice; Staff Physician; University of Nebraska Medical Center, Omaha, Nebraska
Orthopedics

CHRISTINE C. MATSON, M.D.
Vice Chair for Education, Department of Family and Community Medicine; Associate Professor, Departments of Family and Community Medicine and Pediatrics, Eastern Virginia Medical School; Courtesy Staff, Sentara Norfolk General Hospital; Children's Hospital of the King's Daughters, Norfolk, Virginia
Gynecology

OSCAR McCALLUM, M.D.
Associate Professor of Family Practice, University of Tennessee Family Practice Center, Jackson, Tennessee
Urinary Tract Disorders

KATHLEEN McINTYRE-SELTMAN, M.D.
Associate Professor, Obstetrics and Gynecology; Director, Residency Program; Director, Benign Gynecology, Eastern Virginia Medical School, Norfolk, Virginia
Gynecology

I. R. McWHINNEY, M.D.
Professor Emeritus, University of Western Ontario, London, Ontario, Canada
Clinical Problem Solving in Family Practice

SUSAN M. MILLER, M.D., M.P.H.
Assistant Professor, Department of Medicine, Baylor College of Medicine; Medical Director, Thomas Street Clinic, Harris County Hospital District/Baylor College of Medicine, Houston, Texas
Care of the Adult HIV-1—Infected Patient

R. MICHAEL MORSE, M.D.
Professor and Vice Chair, Department of Family Medicine; Medical Director, Institute for Quality Health, University of Virginia School of Medicine; Director, Virginia Center for the Advancement of Generalist Medicine, Charlottesville, Virginia
Preventive Health Care

HAROLD C. NEU, M.D.
Professor of Medicine and Pharmacology, Columbia University College of Physicians and Surgeons; Hospital Epidemiologist, Presbyterian Hospital in the City of New York, New York, New York
Infectious Diseases

KENNETH L. NOLLER, M.D.
Professor and Chair, Department of Obstetrics and Gynecology, University of Massachusetts Medical School; Chair, Department of Obstetrics and Gynecology, The Medical Center of Central Massachusetts, Worcester, Massachusetts
Obstetrics

PAUL A. NUTTING, M.D., M.S.P.H.
Professor, Department of Family Medicine, University of Colorado, Denver, Colorado
Community-Oriented Primary Care

PATRICK J. O'CONNOR, M.D., M.P.H.
Attending Physician, St. Paul Ramsey Medical Center, St. Paul, Minnesota; Health Partners Research, Minneapolis, Minnesota
Assessment of Functional Health Status

ALICE ANNE O'DONELL, M.D.
Professor, Departments of Family Medicine, Pediatrics, and Preventive Medicine and Community Health, University of Texas Medical Branch; Attending Physician, John Sealy Hospital, and St. Mary's Hospital, Galveston, Texas
Behavioral Problems in Children and Adolescents

STEVEN M. ORNSTEIN, M.D.
Associate Professor, Medical University of South Carolina, Department of Family Medicine, Charleston, South Carolina
Computer Applications in Office Practice

AMIT G. PANDYA, M.D.
Assistant Professor, Department of Dermatology, University of Texas Southwestern Medical Center, Dallas, Texas
Evaluation of Skin Lesions

MICHAEL F. PARRY, M.D.
Associate Clinical Professor of Medicine, Columbia University College of Physicians and Surgeons, New York, New York; Vice President, Medical Affairs, Director of Infectious Diseases and Microbiology, The Stamford Hospital, Stamford, Connecticut
Infectious Diseases

RICHARD PAZDUR, M.D.
Assistant Vice President for Academic Affairs, The University of Texas M.D. Anderson Cancer Center, Houston, Texas
Oncology

ROBERT L. PERKEL, M.D.
Associate Professor of Family Medicine, Jefferson Medical College, Philadelphia, Pennsylvania
Rheumatic Disease

JOHN G. PRICHARD, M.D., M.H.S.
Associate Professor, University of California, Los Angeles, School of Medicine, Los Angeles, California; Chief, Medical Service and Director of Clinical Affairs, Ventura County Medical Center, Ventura, California
Pulmonary Medicine

JOHN QUINLAN, M.D.
Associate Professor, Department of Neurology; Director, Residency Training Program-Neurology; Director, Undergraduate Medical Education-Neurology; University of Cincinnati College of Medicine; Staff Neurologist, University of Cincinnati Hospitals, Cincinnati, Ohio
Neurology in Family Practice

ROBERT E. RAKEL, M.D.
Richard M. Kleberg Senior Professor and Chairman, Department of Family Medicine, Associate Dean for Academic and Clinical Affairs, Baylor College of Medicine; Chief of Family Medicine Service, St. Luke's Episcopal Hospital, The Methodist Hospital, Houston, Texas
The Family Physician; The Family Genogram; Care of the Dying Patient; Use of Consultants; Establishing Rapport; Nicotine Addiction; The Problem-Oriented Medical Record

JANET P. REALINI, M.D., M.P.H.
Residency Program Director, University of Texas Health Science Center, San Antonio, Texas
Contraception

VIRGINIA RHODES, M.D.
Junior Faculty Associate, Department of Medical Oncology, University of Texas M.D. Anderson Cancer Center, Houston, Texas
Oncology

SHELLEY P. ROATEN, Jr., M.D.
Professor and Chairman, Department of Family Practice and Community Medicine, University of Texas Southwestern Medical Center; Chief of Service, Zale Lipshy University Hospital and Parkland Memorial Hospital, Dallas, Texas
Evaluation of Skin Lesions

RICHARD G. ROBERTS, M.D., J.D.

Professor, Department of Family Medicine, University of Wisconsin Medical School, Madison, Wisconsin

Malpractice and Risk Management

Wм. MacMILLAN RODNEY, M.D.

Professor and Chairman, Department of Family Medicine, The University of Tennessee; Director of GI Endoscopy for Family Physicians; Baptist Memorial Hospital; NME/AMI Saint Francis Hospital, Memphis, Tennessee

Gastroenterology

JOHN C. ROGERS, M.D., M.P.H.

Professor of Family Medicine, Baylor College of Medicine, Houston, Texas

Reading and Interpreting Genograms

JOSEPH E. RONAGHAN, M.D.

Regional Chairman, Department of Surgery, Texas Tech University Health Sciences Center, Amarillo, Texas

Office Surgery

DAVID R. RUDY, M.D., M.P.H.

Professor and Chairman, Department of Family Medicine, Finch University of Health Sciences/The Chicago Medical School, North Chicago, Illinois

Endocrinology

FREDERICK SAMAHA, M.D.

Professor, Department of Neurology, University of Cincinnati College of Medicine; Chairman, Department of Neurology, Staff Neurologist, University of Cincinnati Hospitals, Cincinnati, Ohio

Neurology in Family Practice

MARC A. SCHUCKIT, M.D.

Professor of Psychiatry, University of California San Diego School of Medicine; Director, Alcohol Research Center and Alcohol and Drug Treatment Program, Veterans Affairs Medical Center, San Diego, California

Alcohol Abuse

THOMAS L. SCHWENK, M.D.

Professor and Chair, Department of Family Practice, University of Michigan Medical Center, Ann Arbor, Michigan

Depression

STUART K. SHAPIRA, M.D., Ph.D.

Assistant Professor, Department of Molecular and Human Genetics, Baylor College of Medicine, Houston, Texas

Clinical Genetics and Genetic Counseling

KEVIN M. SHERIN, M.D., M.P.H.

Visiting Associate Professor, Department of Family Medicine, University of Illinois College of Medicine, Chicago, Illinois; Family Practice Residency Program Director, UIC-Christ Family Practice Residency Program, Christ Hospital and Medical Center (Advocate), Oak Lawn, Illinois

Abuse of Controlled Substances

JEFFREY SHUREN, M.D.

Assistant Professor, University of Cincinnati College of Medicine; Staff Neurologist, University of Cincinnati Hospitals, Cincinnati, Ohio

Neurology in Family Practice

GABRIEL SMILKSTEIN, M.D.

Professor, Department of Family Practice, University of California, Davis; Director, Division of Medical Education, University of California, Davis, Medical Center, Sacramento, California; Sutter-Davis Hospital, Davis, California

Psychosocial Influences on Health

CHARLES W. SMITH, Jr., M.D.

Executive Associate Director for Clinical Affairs, University of Arkansas for Medical Sciences, Little Rock, Arkansas

Otolaryngology

ROBERT SMITH, M.D.

Professor and Director Emeritus, Department of Family Medicine, University of Cincinnati College of Medicine; Medical Director, Cincinnati Headache Institute, Drake Center, Cincinnati, Ohio

Neurology in Family Practice

SUSAN J. SPEER, M.S., R.D.

Instructor, Clinical Nutrition, Santa Monica Family Practice Residency Program, Santa Monica, California

Nutrition and Family Medicine

ROBERT HUNT SPRINKLE, M.D., Ph.D.

Assistant Professor of Community and Family Medicine, and Public Policy Studies, and Senior Fellow in the Center for Applied Ethics, Duke University, Durham, North Carolina

Care of the Newborn

PORTER STOREY, M.D.

Clinical Assistant Professor of Medicine and Family Medicine, Baylor College of Medicine; Consultant in Neuro-Oncology and Adjunct Assistant Professor of Medicine, University of Texas, M.D. Anderson Cancer Center; Medical Director, The Hospice at the Texas Medical Center, Houston, Texas

Care of the Dying Patient

CHESTER L. STRUNK, M.D.

Clinical Assistant Professor of Otolaryngology-Head and Neck Surgery, University of Texas Medical Branch; Consulting Staff, University of Texas Medical Branch Hospitals, Galveston, Texas; Active Staff, Clear Lake Regional Medical Center, Webster, Texas; Active Staff, St. John Hospital, Nassau Bay, Texas

Otolaryngology

MARIAN R. STUART, Ph.D.

Clinical Associate Professor of Family Medicine, Clinical Associate Professor of Psychiatry, UMDNJ-Robert Wood Johnson Medical School; Independent Practitioner in Psychology, Department of Family Practice, St. Peter's Medical Center, New Brunswick, New Jersey

Practicing Biopsychosocial Medicine

GEORGE A. TALER, M.D.

Assistant Professor, University of Maryland School of Medicine; Assistant Professor, Division of Geriatric Medicine, Department of Family Medicine, University of Maryland School of Medicine, Baltimore, Maryland

Care of the Elderly

LAWRENCE M. TIERNEY, Jr., M.D.

Professor of Medicine, University of California, San Francisco, School of Medicine; Assistant Chief, Medical Service, University of California Service, Veterans Administration Medical Center, San Francisco, California

Pulmonary Medicine

DOROTHY B. TREVINO, M.S.W., Ph.D.

Assistant Professor, Department of Family Medicine, University of Texas Medical Branch, Galveston, Texas

Behavioral Problems in Children and Adolescents

MANUEL TZAGOURNIS, M.D.

Professor of Internal Medicine, Division of Endocrinology, Vice President for Health Sciences, The Ohio State University College of Medicine, Columbus, Ohio

Endocrinology

ANDREW G. URY, M.D.

Physician Micro Systems, Inc., Seattle, Washington

Computer Applications in Office Practice

JACK VALANCY, M.B.A.

Senior Clinical Instructor, Department of Family Medicine, Case Western Reserve University School of Medicine, Cleveland, Ohio; Principal, Jack Valancy Consulting, Consulting, Cleveland Heights, Ohio

Accounting Systems

CARLOS VALLBONA, M.D.

Distinguished Service Professor, Professor of Rehabilitation; Professor and Chairman, Department of Community Medicine; Professor of Family Medicine, Baylor College of Medicine, Houston, Texas; Adjunct Professor of Preventive Medicine, Family Practice and Community Medicine, Preventive Medicine, The University of Texas Medical School, Houston, Texas; Chief of Staff,

Community Health Program, Harris City Hospital District; Active Staff, Texas Children's Hospital, St. Luke's Hospital, The Institute for Rehabilitation and Research; Consultant Staff, VA Hospital, Houston, Texas

Interpretation of the Electrocardiogram; Diagnosis and Treatment of Arrhythmias

PAUL P. VanARSDEL, Jr., M.D.

Deceased

Allergy

SUSAN VANDERBERG, M.D.

Department of Family Practice, Rush Medical Center, Chicago Illinois

Personality Disorders in Office Practice

RANDY WERTHEIMER, M.D.

Associate Professor of Family and Community Medicine, University of Massachusetts School of Medicine; Vice Chair, Department of Family Medicine, The Medical Center of Central Massachusetts, Worcester, Massachusetts

Obstetrics

LORI A. WHITTAKER, M.D., Ph.D.

Assistant Professor, Department of Family Medicine, Baylor College of Medicine, Houston, Texas

Oncology

CHARLES V. WRIGHT, Jr., M.D.

Regional Chair/Associate Professor, Department of Family Medicine, Texas Tech University Health Science Center Amarillo, Amarillo, Texas

Office Surgery

LUCIUS F. WRIGHT, M.D.

Clinical Associate Professor of Medicine, University of Tennessee Center for Health Science, Memphis, Tennessee; Medical Director, The Jackson Clinic Professional Association, Jackson, Tennessee

Urinary Tract Disorders

STEVEN J. YAKUBOV, M.D.

Attending Cardiologist, Riverside Methodist Hospital, Columbus, Ohio

Cardiovascular Disease

ROBERT E. ZITTER, Ph.D.

Assistant Professor, Departments of Family Practice and Social Sciences, Rush Medical College, Chicago, Illinois; Director, Behavioral Science Family Practice Residency, Christ Hospital, Oak Lawn, Florida

Somatic Patient

PREFACE

Recognition of the vital role that cost-effective primary care plays in an efficient health care system is placing greater emphasis on the importance of well trained family physicians. While a great deal of attention is paid to correcting the shortage of family physicians, it is important that the training of these physicians be based on current medical knowledge in the breadth of areas covered by our discipline. This textbook is designed to be a resource in the training of family physicians and other primary care physicians, and to help the practicing family physician remain current with recent medical advances. It is also a resource for the physician trained in a non-primary care discipline who is being increasingly called upon to provide primary care but who may feel inadequately prepared to manage some of the problems encountered.

This edition is more concise than the last to make it more manageable and economical. The focus is on material that is practical and clinically relevant. Every attempt has been made to keep the information as current as possible. Special attention has been given to the use of tables and illustrations to present a maximum amount of information in a concise manner. There are more than 1000 tables and figures (over 500 figures and EKG tracings, and almost 600 tables).

As in previous editions, most of the authors are family physicians. Of the 118 authors, 60 are new. We have continued the policy established in the first edition in 1973 of using co-authors for most chapters, usually combining an authority in the field with an experienced family physician so that the information is current and relevant to family practice.

All 66 chapters contain fresh material since those that are not written by new authors are revised and updated. New chapters this edition are: Practicing Biopsychosocial Medicine by Lieberman and Stuart patterned after their successful book *The Fifteen Minute Hour* describing the BATHE technique; Domestic Violence, which condenses material in the previous edition on child and spouse abuse and sexual abuse; and two chapters that expand the material on psychiatric disorders, Crisis Intervention in Office Practice; and Personality Disorders in Office Practice.

A new edition of the *Saunders Review of Family Practice* by Bope et al. is being published to accompany this edition to assist the family physician preparing for certification or recertification by the American Board of Family Practice.

Producing a text of this size requires the skills of many people who often go unrecognized. My special thanks to Jeanne Ullian, my editorial assistant who organizes the material and keeps me on schedule, and to Ray Kersey and the staff at W.B. Saunders for their consistently high standards and insistence on quality.

Robert E. Rakel, M.D.

CONTENTS

Part I

PRINCIPLES OF FAMILY PRACTICE

CHAPTER 1

THE FAMILY PHYSICIAN

ROBERT E. RAKEL

The family physician provides continuing, comprehensive care in a personalized manner to patients of all ages and to their families, regardless of the presence of disease or the nature of the presenting complaint. Family physicians accept responsibility for managing an individual's total health needs while maintaining an intimate, confidential relationship with the patient. The family physician personally takes care of 95 per cent of the patient's health needs; for the remainder of the patient's problems, the physician selects appropriate consulting physicians or other health professionals to assist in care (see Chapter 12). The efforts of all health professionals are coordinated by the family physician, who has ongoing responsibility for the patient's care.

Family medicine is the body of knowledge and the skills that constitute the medical discipline; when applied to the care of patients and their families, that discipline becomes the specialty of family practice. Family medicine emphasizes responsibility for total health care—from the first contact and initial assessment through the ongoing care of chronic problems. Prevention and early recognition of disease are essential features of the discipline. Coordination and integration of all necessary health services with the least amount of fragmentation, and the skills to manage most medical problems, allow family physicians to provide cost-effective health care.

Family practice is a specialty that shares many areas of content with other clinical disciplines, incorporating this shared knowledge and using it uniquely to deliver primary medical care. In addition to sharing content with other medical specialties, family practice emphasizes knowledge from areas such as family dynamics, interpersonal relations, counseling, and psychotherapy. The specialty's foundation, however, remains clinical, with the primary focus on the medical care of people who are ill.

Devotion to continuing, comprehensive, personalized care; to early detection and management of illness; to the prevention of disease and maintenance of health; and to the ongoing management of patients in a community setting uniquely qualify the family physician to deliver primary care.

The curriculum for training family physicians is designed to represent realistically the skills and body of knowledge that they will require in practice. This curriculum relies heavily on an accurate analysis of the problems seen and the skills used by family physicians in their practices. Unfortunately, the content of residency training programs for the primary care specialties has not always been appropriately directed toward solving the problems most commonly encountered by physicians practicing in these specialties. The situation is changing, however, and in the future training programs should be more appropriately designed to meet the needs of the practicing physician. The almost randomly educated primary physician of previous years is being replaced by one specifically prepared to address the kinds of problems likely to be encountered in practice. For this reason, the "model office" is an essential component of all family practice residency programs.

DEVELOPMENT OF THE SPECIALTY

About 1923, Francis Peabody commented that the swing of the pendulum toward specialization had reached its apex and that modern medicine had fragmented the health care delivery system to too great a degree. He called for a rapid return of the generalist physician who would give comprehensive, personalized care.

Dr. Peabody's declaration proved premature; society and the medical establishment were not ready for such a proclamation. The trend toward specialization gained momentum through the 1950s, and fewer physicians entered general practice. In the early 1960s, leaders in the field of general practice began advocating a seemingly paradoxical solution to reverse the trend and correct the scarcity of general practitioners—the creation of still another specialty. However, the physicians envisioned a specialty that embodied the knowledge, skills, and ideals they knew as primary care. In 1966, the concept of a new specialty in primary care received official recognition in two separate reports published 1 month apart. The first of these was the report of the Citizens' Commission on Graduate Medical Education of the American Medical Association, also known as the Millis

Commission Report. The second report came from the Ad Hoc Committee on Education for Family Practice of the Council of Medical Education of the American Medical Association, also called the Willard Committee. Three years later, in 1969, the American Board of Family Practice (ABFP) came into being as the 20th medical specialty board, thus giving birth to the specialty of family practice.

Much of the impetus for the Millis and Willard reports came from the American Academy of General Practice, which was renamed the American Academy of Family Physicians (AAFP) in 1971. The name change reflected a desire to increase emphasis on family-oriented health care and to gain academic acceptance for the new specialty of family practice.

The ABFP has distinguished itself by being the first specialty board to require recertification (every 6 years) to ensure the ongoing competence of its members. Among basic requirements for certification and recertification, the ABFP has included continuing education—the foundation on which the American Academy of General Practice had been built when organized in 1947. A member of the ABFP must participate in 50 hours of acceptable continuing education activity each year (300 hours in 6 years) to be eligible for recertification. Once eligible, a candidate's competence is examined by cognitive testing and performance evaluation. The ABFP's emphasis on quality of education, knowledge, and performance has facilitated the rapid increase in prestige for the family physician in our health care system. The obvious logic of the ABFP's emphasis on continuing education to maintain required knowledge and skills has been adopted by other specialties and state medical societies. Now, most specialty boards are committed to the concept of recertification to ensure that their diplomates remain current with advances in medicine.

DEFINITIONS

Family Practice

Family practice is the medical specialty that provides continuing and comprehensive health care for the individual and the family. It is the specialty in breadth that integrates the biologic, clinical, and behavioral sciences. The scope of family practice encompasses all ages, both sexes, each organ system, and every disease entity. The specialty of family practice is the result of the evolved and enhanced expression of general medical practice and is defined uniquely within the family context (AAFP, 1993).

Family Physician

The family physician is a physician who is educated and trained in the discipline of family prac-

tice—a broadly encompassing medical specialty. Family physicians possess unique attitudes, skills, and knowledge that qualify them to provide continuing and comprehensive medical care, health maintenance, and preventive services to each member of the family regardless of sex, age, or type of problem, be it biologic, behavioral, or social. These specialists, because of their background and interactions with the family, are best qualified to serve as each patient's advocate in all health-related matters, including the appropriate use of consultants, health services, and community resources (AAFP, 1993).

The World Organization of Family Doctors (WONCA—World Organization of National Colleges, Academies, and Academic Associations of General Practitioners/Family Physicians) defines the family doctor in part as

the physician who is primarily responsible for providing comprehensive health care to every individual seeking medical care, and arranging for other health personnel to provide services when necessary. The family physician functions as a generalist who accepts everyone seeking care whereas other health providers limit access to their services on the basis of age, sex, and/or diagnosis. (WONCA, 1991, p. 2)

Primary Care

Primary care is that care provided by physicians specifically trained for and skilled in comprehensive first contact and continuing care for persons with any undiagnosed sign, symptom, or health concern (the "undifferentiated" patient) not limited by problem origin (biologic, behavioral, or social), organ system, gender, or diagnosis. Primary care includes health promotion, disease prevention, health maintenance, counseling, patient education, diagnosis, and treatment of acute and chronic illnesses in a variety of health care settings (e.g., office, inpatient, critical care, long-term care, home care, day care). Primary care is performed and managed by a personal physician, utilizing other health professionals for consultation or referral as appropriate.

Primary care provides patient advocacy in the health care system to accomplish cost-effective care by coordination of health care services. Primary care promotes effective doctor–patient communication and encourages the role of the patient as a partner in health care (AAFP, 1994a).

Because many physicians deliver primary care in different ways and with varying degrees of preparation, the staff of the ABFP has further clarified the definition:

Primary care is a form of delivery of medical care that encompasses the following functions:

1. It is "first-contact" care, serving as a point-of-entry for the patient into the health care system;

2. It includes continuity by virtue of caring for patients over a period of time, both in sickness and in health;

3. It is comprehensive care, drawing from all the traditional major disciplines for its functional content;

4. It serves a coordinative function for all the health-care needs of the patient;

5. It assumes continuing responsibility for individual patient follow-up and community health problems; and

6. It is a highly personalized type of care.

Primary Care Physician

A primary care physician is a generalist physician who provides definitive care to the undifferentiated patient at the point of first contact and takes continuing responsibility for providing the patient's care. Such a physician must be trained specifically to provide primary care services.

Primary care physicians devote the majority of their practice to providing primary care services to a defined population of patients. The style of primary care practice is such that the personal primary care physician serves as the entry point for substantially all of the patient's medical and health care needs—not limited by problem origin, organ system, gender, or diagnosis. Primary care physicians are advocates for the patient in coordinating the use of the entire health care system to benefit the patient (AAFP, 1994a).

The ABFP and the American Board of Internal Medicine have agreed on a definition of the generalist physician and that "providing optimal generalist care requires broad and comprehensive training that cannot be gained in brief and uncoordinated educational experiences (Kimball and Young, 1994, p. 316). They define the generalist physician as one "who provides continuing, comprehensive, and coordinated medical care to a population undifferentiated by gender, disease, or organ system" (p. 315).

Physicians who provide primary care should be trained specifically to manage the problems encountered in a primary care practice. Rivo and associates (1994) identified the common conditions and diagnoses that generalist physicians should be competent to manage in a primary care practice and compared these to the training of the various "generalist" specialties. They recommended that the training of generalist physicians should include at least 90 per cent of the key diagnoses. By comparing the content of residency programs, they found that this goal was met by family practice (95 per cent), internal medicine (91 per cent), and pediatrics (91 per cent), but that obstetrics and gynecology (47 per cent) and emergency medicine (42 per cent) fell far short of this goal.

PERSONALIZED CARE

It is much more important to know what sort of patient has a disease than what sort of disease a patient has.

Sir William Osler (1904)

Family physicians do not just treat patients, they care for people. This caring function of family medicine emphasizes the personalized approach to understanding the patient as a person, respecting the person as an individual, and showing compassion for his or her discomfort. Compassion means co-suffering and reflects the physician's willingness somehow to share the patient's anguish and understand what the sickness means to that person. Compassion is an attempt to "feel" along with the patient. Pellegrino (1979) stated that "we can never *feel* with another person when we pass judgment as a superior, only when we see our own frailties as well as his." Pellegrino goes on to comment that a compassionate authority figure is effective only when others can receive the "orders" without being humiliated. The physician must not "put down" the patients, but must be ever ready, in Galileo's words, *"to pronounce that wise, ingenuous, and modest statement—'I don't know'."* Compassion, practiced in these terms in each patient encounter, obtunds the inherent dehumanizing tendencies of today's highly institutionalized and technologically oriented patterns of patient care.

Physicians engaged primarily in hospital-based medicine must make a stronger effort to maintain personalized care because of the added exposure to and the necessary use of devices and techniques directed toward specific diseases. The physician should guard against thinking in terms of diseases and instead think in terms of patients who have problems needing attention. The whole-person approach to patient care is hampered by focusing primarily on the disease; specific diseases require specific treatments and tend to direct the physician's attention away from other needs of the whole patient.

Peabody (1930) noted that "The treatment of a disease may be entirely impersonal; the care of a patient must be completely personal." If an intimate relationship with patients remains our primary concern as physicians, high-quality medical care will persist, regardless of the way it is organized and financed. For this reason, family practice emphasizes consideration of the individual patient in the full context of his or her life, rather than the episodic care of a presenting complaint. The Millis Commission Report stresses that the family physician "focuses not upon individual organs and systems but upon the whole man who lives in a complex social setting, and knows that diagnosis or treatment of a part often overlooks major causative factors and therapeutic opportunities" (1966, p. 35).

It is generally recognized that medicine has become depersonalized, owing to the rapid rise of superspecialization and technology. In 1960, Theodore F. Fox wrote:

Nobody is going to persuade me that a nice receptionist, some good notes, and an internist keeping office hours adds up to a personal doctor who knows me and my home. Even if you throw in a psychiatric social worker, I still feel that I am being put off with a plastic substitute for the real thing. (p. 752).

Indeed, as Fox predicted, personalized care is returning to medicine, largely because of the advent of the specialty that provides family physicians who know patients in their home environment and who assess the psychosocial factors that exist within the family setting, as well as the individual's problems.

Family physicians assess the illnesses and complaints presented to them, dealing personally with the majority and arranging special assistance for a few. The family physician serves as the patients' advocate, explaining the causes and implications of illness to the patients and their families, and serves as an advisor and confidant to the family—both individually and collectively. The family physician receives many intellectual satisfactions from this practice, but the greatest reward arises from the depth of human understanding and personal satisfaction inherent in family practice.

Patients have adjusted somewhat to a more impersonal form of health care delivery and frequently look to institutions rather than to individuals for their health care; yet, their need for personalized concern and compassion remains. Tumulty (1970) found that patients consider a good physician to be one who (1) shows genuine interest in them; (2) thoroughly evaluates their problem; (3) demonstrates compassion, understanding, and warmth; and (4) provides clear insight into what is wrong and what must be done to correct it.

The family physician's relationship with each patient should reflect compassion, understanding, and patience, combined with a high degree of intellectual honesty. The physician must be thorough in approaching problems, but also possess a keen sense of humor. He or she must be capable of encouraging in each patient optimism, courage, insight, and the self-discipline necessary for recovery.

CHARACTERISTICS AND FUNCTIONS OF THE FAMILY PHYSICIAN

Attributes of the Family Physician

The following characteristics are certainly desirable for all physicians, but they are of greatest importance for the physician in family practice:

1. A strong sense of responsibility for the total, ongoing care of the individual and the family during health, illness, and rehabilitation.
2. Compassion and empathy, with a sincere interest in the patient and the family.
3. A curious and constantly inquisitive attitude.
4. Enthusiasm for the undifferentiated medical problem and its resolution.

5. An interest in the broad spectrum of clinical medicine.
6. The ability to deal comfortably with multiple problems occurring simultaneously in one patient.
7. A desire for frequent and varied intellectual and technical challenges.
8. The ability to support children during growth and development and during their adjustment to family and society.
9. The ability to assist patients in coping with everyday problems and in maintaining stability in the family and community.
10. The capacity to act as coordinator of all health resources needed in the care of a patient.
11. A continuing enthusiasm for learning and for the satisfaction that comes from maintaining current medical knowledge through continuing medical education.
12. The ability to maintain composure in times of stress and to respond quickly with logic, effectiveness, and compassion.
13. A desire to identify problems at the earliest possible stage (or to prevent disease entirely).
14. A strong wish to maintain maximum patient satisfaction, recognizing the need for continuing patient rapport.
15. The skills necessary to manage chronic illness and to ensure maximal rehabilitation following acute illness.
16. An appreciation for the complex mix of physical, emotional, and social elements in holistic and personalized patient care.
17. A feeling of personal satisfaction derived from intimate relationships with patients that naturally develop over long periods of continuous care, as opposed to the short-term pleasures gained from treating episodic illnesses.
18. A skill for and commitment to educating patients and families about disease processes and the principles of good health.

The ideal family physician is an explorer, driven by a persistent curiosity and the desire to know more. He is part theologian, as was Paracelsus; part politician, as was Benjamin Rush; and part humorist, as was Oliver Wendell Holmes. At all times, however, the care of the patient—the whole patient—is the primary goal.

Continuing Responsibility

One of the essential functions of the family physician is the willingness to accept ongoing responsibility for managing a patient's medical care. Once a patient or a family has been accepted into the physician's practice, responsibility for care is both total and continuing. The Millis Commission chose the term "primary physician" to emphasize the concept of primary responsibility for the patient's welfare; however the term "primary care physician" is more popular and refers to any physician who provides first-contact care.

The family physician's commitment to patients does not cease at the end of illness, but is a continuing responsibility, regardless of the patient's state of health or the disease process. There is no need to identify the beginning or end point of treatment, because care of a problem can be reopened at any time—even though a later visit may be primarily for another problem. This prevents the family physician from focusing too narrowly on one problem and helps maintain a perspective on the total patient in his environment. Peabody (1930) believed that much patient dissatisfaction results from the physician's neglecting to assume personal responsibility for supervision of the patient's care: "For some reason or other, no one physician has seen the case through from beginning to end, and the patient may be suffering from the very multitude of his counselors" (p. 8).

The greater the degree of continuing involvement with a patient, the more capable the physician is in detecting early signs and symptoms of organic disease and differentiating it from a functional problem. Patients with problems arising from emotional and social conflicts can be managed most effectively by a physician who has intimate knowledge of the individual and of his or her family and community background. This knowledge comes only from insight gained by observing the patient's long-term patterns of behavior and responses to changing stressful situations. This longitudinal view is particularly useful in the care of children and allows the physician to be more effective in assisting children to reach their full potential. The closeness that develops between physicians and young patients increases a physician's ability to aid the patient with problems that occur during later periods in life—such as adjustment to puberty, problems with marriage or employment, and changing social pressures. As the family physician maintains this continuing involvement with successive generations within a family, the ability to manage intercurrent problems increases with knowledge of the total family background.

By virtue of this ongoing involvement and intimate association with the family, the family physician develops a perceptive awareness of a family's nature and style of operation. This ability to observe families over time allows valuable insight that improves the quality of medical care provided to an individual patient. One of the greatest challenges in family medicine is the need to be alert to the changing stresses, transitions, and expectations of family members over time and to the effect that these and other family interactions have on the health of individuals.

Although the family is the family physician's primary concern, his or her skills are equally applicable to the individual living alone or to people in other varieties of family living. Individuals with alternative forms of family living interact with others who have a significant effect on their lives. The principles of group dynamics and interpersonal relationships that affect health are equally applicable to everyone.

The family physician must assess an individual's personality so that presenting symptoms can be appropriately evaluated and given the proper degree of attention and emphasis. A complaint of abdominal pain may be treated lightly in one patient who frequently presents with minor problems, but the same complaint would be investigated immediately and in depth in another individual who has a more stoic personality. The decision regarding which studies to perform and when is influenced by knowledge of the patient's life style, personality, and previous response pattern. The greater the degree of knowledge and insight into the patient's background, which is gained through years of ongoing contact, the more capable the physician is in making an appropriate early and rapid assessment of the presenting complaint. The less background information the physician has to rely on, the greater is the need to depend on costly laboratory studies and the more likely is overreaction to the presenting symptom. Families receiving continuing comprehensive care have fewer incidences of hospitalization, fewer operations, and fewer physician visits for illnesses compared with those having no regular physician. This is due, at least in part, to the physician's knowledge of the patients, seeing them earlier for acute problems and thus preventing complications that would require hospitalization, being available by telephone, and seeing them more frequently in the office for health supervision. Care is also less expensive since there is less need to rely on radiographic and laboratory procedures and visits to emergency rooms.

Collusion of Anonymity

The need for a primary physician who accepts continuing responsibility for patient care is emphasized by Michael Balint (1965) in his concept of "collusion of anonymity." In this situation, the patient is seen by a variety of physicians, not one of whom is willing to accept total management of the problem. Important decisions are made—some good, some bad—but without anyone's feeling fully responsible for them.

Francis Peabody (1930) examined the futility of a patient's making the rounds from one specialist to another without finding relief because he

. . . lacked the guidance of a sound general practitioner who understood his physical condition, his nervous temperament and knew the details of his daily life. And many a patient who on his own initiative has sought out specialists, has had minor defects accentuated so that they assume a needless importance, and has even undergone operations that might well have been avoided. Those who are particularly blessed with this world's goods, who want the best regardless of the cost and imagine that they are getting it because they can afford to consult as many renowned specialists as they wish, are often pathetically tragic figures as they veer from one course of treatment to another. Like ships that lack a guiding hand upon the helm, they swing from tack to tack with each new gust of wind but get no nearer to the Port of Health because there is no pilot to set the general direction of their course. (pp. 21–22).

Chronic Illness

The family physician also must be committed to managing the common chronic illnesses that have no known cure but for which continuing management by a personal physician is all the more necessary to maintain an optimal state of health for the patient. It is a difficult and often trying job to manage these continuing, unresolvable, and progressively crippling problems, control of which requires a remodeling of the life style of the entire family.

Quality of Care

Primary care provided by physicians specifically trained to care for the problems presenting to personal physicians, who know their patients over a span of time, is of higher quality than that provided by other physicians. This has been confirmed by a variety of studies comparing the care given by physicians in different specialties.

Following a review of the literature on quality and cost of care, Boex and associates (1993) noted that

the quality of clinical outcomes of primary care practitioners is comparable to that of specialists or subspecialists in similar, clinically appropriate situations. . . . Practitioners working within their domains of practice have higher quality outcomes than those working outside their regular domains. . . . Physicians and advance practice nurse generalists trained in and practicing generalist competencies provide a higher quality of primary care to their patients than those whose domains of practice are by definition restricted to specialized areas.

McGann and Bowman (1990) compared the morbidity and mortality of patients hospitalized by family physicians and internists. They found that, even though the family physicians' patients were older and more severely ill, there was no significant difference in morbidity and mortality. In addition, the total charges for their hospital care was lower.

The quality of our health care system is being eroded by physicians' being extensively trained at great expense to practice in one area and instead practicing in another, such as anesthesiologists practicing in emergency rooms and surgeons practicing as generalists. Primary care, to be done well, requires extensive training specifically tailored to problems frequently seen in primary care. These include the early detection, diagnosis, and treatment of depression; the early diagnosis of cancer (especially of the breast and the colon); the management of gynecologic problems; and the care of those with chronic and terminal illnesses.

Cost-Effective Care

The physician who is well acquainted with the patient not only provides more personal and humane medical care but does so more economically than the physician involved only in episodic care. The physician who knows his or her patients well can assess the nature of their problems more rapidly and accurately. Because of the intimate, ongoing relationship, the family physician is under less pressure to exclude diagnostic possibilities by use of expensive laboratory and radiologic procedures than is the physician who is unfamiliar with the patient.

The United States has the most expensive health care system in the world, with more than 14 per cent of the gross national product devoted to health care. Schroeder (1984) believes this situation will continue as long as the system accepts a high concentration of specialists, fee-for-service payment, patient self-referral directly to specialists, practice of specialities by physicians who have not gone through the speciality certification process, and a high dependency on specialists for primary care.

Clearly, the increasing complexity of our health care system multiplies expense and wastefulness when a patient self-diagnoses his or her problems or selects his or her own specialist rather than developing a firm and ongoing relationship with a family physician. The most efficient and cost-effective system involves a single personal physician, who ensures the most logical and economical management of a problem.

Medical care should be available to patients in the precise degree needed—neither too extensive nor too limited. This ensures that simple problems will not be magnified out of proportion. The more complex and involved a diagnostic process is, the more costly it becomes, and the greater is the potential for error. Specialists generally treat their patients more resource intensively than generalists, resulting in increased cost of care. Cherkin and associates (1987) showed that internists were 1.7 times more likely to hospitalize patients than family physicians and 1.3 times more likely to refer.

Family physicians order fewer tests than do specialists, perhaps because they know their patients well. MacLean (1993) compared the hospital care given by family physicians with that of all other specialties for patients with gastrointestinal bleeding, nonsurgical back pain, and nutritional, metabolic, or dehydration disorders. He found that the effectiveness of the care was comparable but the cost of care provided by family physicians was less.

Comprehensive Care

The term "comprehensive medical care" spans the entire spectrum of medicine. The effectiveness with which a physician delivers primary care depends on the degree of involvement attained during training and practice. The family physician must be trained comprehensively to acquire all the medical skills necessary to care for the majority of patient problems. The greater the number of skills omitted from the family physician's training and practice, the more frequent is the need to refer minor problems to another physician. A truly comprehensive primary care physician adequately manages acute infections, biopsies skin and other lesions, repairs lacerations, treats musculoskeletal sprains and minor fractures, removes foreign bodies, treats vaginitis, provides obstetric care and care for the newborn infant, gives supportive psychotherapy, and supervises diagnostic procedures. The needs of a family physician's patient will range from a routine physical examination, when the patient feels well and wishes to identify potential risk factors, to a problem that calls for referral to one or more narrowly specialized physicians with highly developed technical skills. The family physician must be aware of the variety and complexity of skills and facilities available to help manage patients and must match these to the individual's specific needs, giving full consideration to the patient's personality and expectations.

Management of an illness involves much more than a diagnosis and an outline for treatment. It also requires an awareness of all the factors that may aid or hinder an individual's recovery from illness. This requires consideration of religious beliefs; social, economic, or cultural problems; personal expectations; and heredity. The outstanding clinician recognizes the effects that spiritual, intellectual, emotional, social, and economic factors have on a patient's illness.

Family practice is a comprehensive specialty involving varying depths of knowledge in many disciplines. A primary care physician requires knowledge and skills of varying degrees in each specialty area, depending on the prevalence of problems encountered in everyday practice and the degree of skills needed to become an excellent diagnostician. A physician specializing in only one discipline, however, will have a much shallower base in comprehensive medicine and a much greater depth in the chosen discipline. The subspecialist is an excellent consultant, but is not trained and cannot function effectively as a primary generalist. The distribution of his or her knowledge and skills is no more appropriate to that task than is the comprehensive physician's competence in the esoteric nuances of a limited discipline.

The family physician's ability to confront relatively large numbers of unselected patients with undifferentiated conditions and carry on a therapeutic relationship over time is a unique primary care skill. The skilled family physician will have a higher level of tolerance for the uncertain than will his or her consultant colleague.

Society will benefit more from a surgeon who has a sufficient volume of surgery to maintain proficiency through frequent use of well-honed skills than from one who has a low volume and serves also as a primary care physician. The early identification of disease while it is in its undifferentiated stage requires specific training and is not a skill that automatically can be assumed by someone whose training has been mostly in hospital intensive care units. It is unfortunate that, when the number of procedures is inadequate to fully occupy specialists skilled in complex technical procedures, their remaining time is spent providing care (frequently primary care) in areas where training was limited and often deficient. John Fry (1977) has said that

working in general practice broadens the mind and humbles the soul. It is very different from the sheltered world of hospital practice. It is as though we, in general practice, work in the natural habitat of the jungle, seeking and stalking our prey in its own environment, whereas our hospital colleagues have to function behind the bars of a zoo, dealing with patients and diseases in highly artificial situation. (p. 11)

Gonnella and Veloski (1982) studied the impact that 1 year of graduate training in different specialties has on performance in Part III of the National Board Examination, which is designed to measure general clinical knowledge. After just 1 year of a 3- or 4-year residency, the performance of physicians in all specialties *except family practice* deteriorated when compared to scores on Part II taken 1 year earlier. Only physicians in family practice training programs improved, increasing an average of 8 points. The most dramatic change was among physicians in pathology training programs, in which the mean score was 95 points *lower* than on Part II. Part III is designed to measure the essential diagnostic and therapeutic skills that the medical profession and society expect all physicians to have; therefore, academic medicine is being asked whether or not it is appropriately preparing physicians. Many physicians eventually enter a type of practice different from what their residency prepared them for; the question remains whether many, especially those entering primary care, will undergo the difficult and costly retraining necessary to do the job well.

The World Health Organization, United Nations, and other organizations sponsored a World Conference on Medical Education in Edinburgh, Scotland, in 1988, addressing the need for reform in medical education. The meeting made a number of recommendations to medical schools in its "Edinburgh Declaration":

1. Enlarge the range of settings in which educational programs are conducted, to include all health resources of the community, not hospitals alone.

2. Ensure that curriculum content reflects national health priorities and the availability of affordable resources.

3. Ensure continuity of learning throughout life, shifting emphasis from the passive methods so widespread now to more active learning, including self-directed and independent study as well as tutorial methods.

4. Build both curriculum and examination systems to ensure the achievement of professional competence and social values, not merely the retention and recall of information.

5. Train teachers as educators, not solely as experts in content, and reward education excellence as fully as excellence in biomedical research or clinical practice.

6. Complement instruction about the management of patients with increased emphasis on promotion of health and prevention of diseases.

7. Pursue integration of education in science and education in practice, also using problem-solving in clinical and community settings as a base for learning.

8. Employ selection methods for medical students that go beyond intellectual ability and academic achievement, to include evaluation of personal qualities.

9. Encourage and facilitate cooperation between the Ministries of Health, Ministries of Education, community health services and other relevant bodies in joint policy development, program planning, implementation, and review.

10. Ensure admission policies that match the numbers of students trained with national needs for doctors.

11. Increase the opportunity for joint learning, research, and service with other health and health-related professions, as part of the training for teamwork.

12. Clarify responsibility and allocate resources for continuing medical education.

Interpersonal Skills

One of the foremost skills of the family physician is the ability to utilize effectively the knowledge of interpersonal relations in the management of patients. This powerful element of clinical medicine is perhaps the specialty's most useful tool. Modern society considers the medical care system inadequate in those situations in which understanding and compassion are important to the patient's comfort and recovery from illness. Physicians too often are seen as lacking this personal concern and as being unskilled in understanding personal anxiety and feelings. There is an obvious need to nourish the seed of compassion and concern for sick people with which students enter medical school.

Family practice emphasizes the integration of compassion, empathy, and personalized concern to a greater degree than does a more technical or task-oriented specialty. Some of the earnest solicitude of the old country doctor and his untiring compassion for people must be incorporated as the effective yet impersonal modern medical procedures are applied. The patient should be viewed compassionately as a person in distress who needs to be treated with concern, dignity, and personal consideration. He or she has a right to be given some insight into his or her problems; a reasonable appraisal of the potential outcome; and a realistic picture of the emotional, financial, and occupational expenses involved in his or her care.

To relate well to patients, a physician must develop compassion and courtesy, the ability to establish rapport and to communicate effectively, the ability to gather information rapidly and to organize it logically, the skills required to identify all significant patient problems and to manage these problems appropriately, the ability to listen, the skills necessary to motivate people, and the ability to observe and detect nonverbal clues.

Much of the family physician's effectiveness in interpersonal relationships depends on his or her charisma. Charisma is a personal magic of leadership, a magnetic charm or appeal that arouses special loyalty or enthusiasm. The charismatic physician is most likely to engender maximal patient compliance and satisfaction. The physicians must be aware of his or her own feelings, however, and their effect on the patient. Charisma can be a useful therapeutic tool, but one must learn how and when to use it effectively, because it also can rebound with unfavorable consequences. The physician should be aware that the patient's needs are paramount. The temptation to take an "ego trip" is frequent and hazardous.

Accessibility

Just as charisma is therapeutic, so too is the mere *availability* of the physician. The feeling of security that the patient gains just by knowing he or she can "touch" the physician, either in person or by phone, is in itself therapeutic and has a comforting and calming influence. Accessibility is an essential feature of primary care. Services must be available when needed and should be within geographic proximity. When primary care is not available, many individuals turn to hospital emergency departments. Emergency room care is, of course, fine for emergencies, but it is no substitute for the personalized, long-term, comprehensive care a family physician can provide.

Diagnostic Skills—Undifferentiated Problems

The family physician, above all, must be an outstanding diagnostician. Skills in this area must be honed to perfection, because problems usually are seen in their early, undifferentiated state and without the degree of resolution that usually is present by the time patients are referred to consulting specialists. This is a unique feature of family practice, because symptoms seen at this stage are often vague and nondescript, with signs being either minimal or absent. Unlike the consulting specialist, the family physician does not evaluate the case after it has been preselected by another physician, and the diagnostic procedures used by the family physician must be selected from the entire spectrum of medicine.

At this stage of disease, there are often only subtle differences between the early symptoms of serious disease and those of self-limiting, minor ailments. To the inexperienced person, the clinical pictures may appear identical, but to the astute and experienced family physician, one symptom will be more suspicious than another because of the greater probability that signals a potentially serious illness. Diagnoses frequently are made on the basis of probability, and the likelihood that a specific disease is present frequently depends on the incidence of the disease relative to the symptom seen in the physician's community during a given time of year. Approximately one fourth of all patients seen will never be assigned a final, definitive diagnosis, because the resolution of a presenting symptom or a complaint will come before a specific diagnosis can be made. Pragmatically, this is an efficient method that is less costly and achieves high patient satisfaction—even though it may be disquieting to the purist physician who believes a thorough work-up and specific diagnosis always should be obtained. Similarly, family physicians are more likely to use a therapeutic trial to confirm the diagnosis.

The family physician is an expert in the rapid assessment of a problem presented for the first time. He or she evaluates its potential significance, often making a diagnosis by exclusion rather than by inclusion, after making certain the symptoms are not those of a serious problem. Once assured, some time is allowed to elapse. Time is used as an efficient diagnostic aid. Follow-up visits are scheduled at appropriate intervals to watch for subtle changes in the presenting symptoms. The physician usually identifies the symptom that has the greatest discriminatory value and watches it more closely than others. The most significant clue to the true nature of the illness may depend on subtle changes in this key symptom. The family physician's effectiveness often is determined by his or her knack for perceiving the hidden or subtle dimensions of illness and following them closely.

The maxim that an accurate history is the most important factor in arriving at an accurate diagnosis is especially appropriate to family medicine, because symptoms may be the only obvious feature of an illness at the time it is presented to the family physician. Further inquiry into the nature of the symptoms, time of onset, extenuating factors, and other unique subjective features may provide the only diagnostic clues available at such an early stage. Above all, the family physician must be a skilled clinician with the ability to evaluate symptoms, verbal and nonverbal communication, and early signs of illness in order to choose those diagnostic tests that are of greatest value in diagnosing a problem early.

The family physician attempts to minimize the degree of morbidity resulting from illness. For example, he or she pays close attention to the complete eradication of a urinary tract infection in an effort to prevent permanent damage that could result in renal failure, requiring expensive and incapacitating renal dialysis or a kidney transplant. Similar examples include the early identification of carcinoma in situ of the cervix to prevent the lethal spread of uterine carcinoma, as well as the early identification of a dysplastic hip, which, if undetected could result in a permanent deformity.

The family physician must be a perceptive humanist, alert to early identification of new problems. Arriving at an early diagnosis may, in fact, be of less importance than determining the real reason the patient came to the physician. The symptoms may be due to a self-limiting or acute problem, but anxiety or fear may be the true precipitating factor. Although the symptom may be hoarseness that has resulted from postnasal drainage accompanying an upper respiratory tract infection, the patient may fear it is caused by a laryngeal carcinoma similar to that recently found in a friend. Clinical evaluation must rule out the possibility of laryngeal carcinoma, but the patient's fears and apprehension regarding this possibility also must be allayed. Similarly, a 42-year-old man with influenza and pleuritic chest pain may be anxious and apprehensive because his father died at age 45 of an acute myocardial infarction. (In fact, a frequent reason for a patient's requesting a complete checkup and electrocardiogram is the recent heart attack of an acquaintance at work.) Mild thrombophlebitis in a 35-year-old woman could bring her to the physician in a more anxious state than is warranted because her mother died from a pulmonary embolus, or a housewife's anxiety about breast cancer may well stem from a friend's recent breast surgery.

Every physical problem has an emotional component, and although this factor is usually minimal, it can be extremely significant. A patient's personality, fears, and anxieties all play a role in every illness and are important factors in all primary care.

The Family Physician as Coordinator

Francis Peabody, Professor of Medicine at Harvard Medical School from 1921 to 1927, was a man ahead of his time; his comments remain appropriate today:

Never was the public in need of wise, broadly trained advisors so much as it needs them today to guide them through the complicated maze of modern medicine. The extraordinary development of medical science, with its consequent diversity of medical specialism and the increasing limitations in the extent of special fields—the very factors, indeed, which are creating specialists, in themselves create a new demand, not for men who are experts along narrow lines, but for men who are in touch with many lines. (1930, p. 20).

The family physician, by virtue of his or her breadth of training in a wide variety of medical disciplines, has unique insights into the skills possessed by physicians in the more limited specialties. The family physician is best prepared to select specialists whose skills can be applied most appropriately to a given case, as well as to coordinate the activities of each, so that they are not counterproductive.

As medicine becomes more specialized and complex, the family physician's role as the integrator of health services becomes increasingly important. The family physician not only facilitates the patient's access to the whole health care system but also interprets the activities of this system to the patient, explaining the nature of the illness, the implication of the treatment, and the effect of both on the patient's way of life. The following statement from the Millis Commission Report concerning expectations of the patient is especially appropriate:

The patient wants, and should have, someone of high competence and good judgment to take charge of the total situation, someone who can serve as coordinator of all the medical resources that can help solve his problem. He wants a company president who will make proper use of his skills and knowledge of more specialized members of the firm. He wants a quarterback who will diagnose the constantly changing situation, coordinate the whole team, and call on each member for the particular contributions that he is best able to make to the team effort. (1966, p. 39)

Such breadth of vision is important for a coordinating physician. He or she must have a realistic overview of the problem and an awareness of the many alternative routes in order to select the one that is most appropriate. A physician familiar with one form of treatment tends to rely on it excessively, whereas the family physician can select the best approach from all possible alternatives. As Pellegrino (1966) has stated:

It should be clear, too, that no simple addition of specialties can equal the generalist function. To build a wall one needs more than the aimless piling up of bricks, one needs an architect. Every operation which analyzes some part of the human mechanism requires to be balanced by another which synthesizes and coordinates. (p. 542)

The complexity of modern medicine frequently involves a variety of health professionals, each with highly developed skills in a particular area. In planning the patient's care, the family physician, having established rapport with a patient and family and having knowledge of the patient's background, personality, fears, and expectations, is best able to select and coordinate the activities of appropriate individuals from the large variety of medical disciplines. He or she can maintain effective communication among those involved, as well as function as the patient's advocate and interpret to the patient and family the many unfamiliar and complicated procedures being used. This prevents any one consulting physician, unfamiliar with the concepts or actions of all others involved, from ordering a test or medication that would conflict with other treatment. Dunphy (1964) has described the value of the surgeon and the family physician working closely as a team:

It is impossible to provide high quality surgical care without that knowledge of the whole patient which only a family physician can supply. When their mutual decisions . . . bring hope, comfort and ultimately, health to a gravely ill human being, the total experience is the essence and the joy of medicine. (p. 12)

The ability to orchestrate the knowledge and skills of diverse professionals is a skill to be learned during training and cultivated in practice. It is not an automatic attribute of all physicians or merely the result of exposure to a large number of professionals. These coordinator skills extend beyond the traditional medical disciplines into the many community agencies and allied health professions as well. Because of his or her close involvement with the community, the family physician is ideally suited to be the integrator of the patient's care, coordinating the skills of consultants when appropriate and involving community nurses, social agencies, the clergy, or other family members when needed. A knowledge of community health resources and a personal involvement with the community can be used to maximum benefit, not only for diagnostic and therapeutic purposes but also to achieve the best possible level of rehabilitation.

The family physician synthesizes the opinions and skills of a multitude of medical consultants with the individual patient's personal needs and the community agencies available. These must be matched to the patient's expectations and to his or her ability to respond to appropriate changes in life style. The recommended changes in life style, however, must be realistic and based on consideration of the patient's ability to comply. For example, treatment of a newly diagnosed diabetic patient recovering from ketoacidosis and who is married to a woman whose main satisfaction in life is cooking for her family requires a significant amount of tact and skill by the family physician to help both the patient and his wife readjust their life styles.

THE FAMILY PHYSICIAN IN PRACTICE

The advent of family medicine has led to a renaissance in medical education involving a reassessment of the traditional medical education environment in a teaching hospital. It is now considered more realistic to train a physician in a community atmosphere, providing exposure to the diseases and problems most closely approximating those he or she will encounter during practice. The ambulatory care skills and knowledge that most medical graduates will need cannot be taught totally within the teritary medical center. The specialty of family practice emphasizes training in ambulatory care skills in an appropriately realistic environment, using patients representing a cross section of a community and incorporating those problems most frequently encountered by physicians practicing primary care.

The lack of relevance in the referral medical center also applies to the hospitalized patient. Figure 1–1, which is derived from data accumulated in the United States and Great Britain, places the health problems of an average community in perspective. In an adult population of 1000 people age 16 years or older, 750 will experience at least one illness or injury during an average month. Most of these people will be managed by self-treatment, but 250 patients will consult a physician. Of these, five patients will be referred for consultation to another physician and nine will be hospitalized—eight of them in a community hospital and one in a university medical center. It is obvious that patients seen in the medical center (the majority of cases used for teaching) represent atypical samples of illness occurring within the community. Students exposed to patients only in this manner develop an unrealistic concept of the kinds of medical problems prevalent in society and, particularly, those comprising primary care. It focuses their training on knowledge and skills of limited usefulness in later practice.

In a typical family practice that cares for 1500 to 3000 individuals, two thirds will be seen at least once each year. Many practicing family physicians and most family practice residency programs are recording the type and frequency of problems seen. Undergraduate and graduate curricula now are being revised to address more closely the problems that will be encountered in practice.

Family physicians who admit to hospitals average 16 hospital visits a week. Those in rural practice average more hospital visits per week (20.3) than their colleagues in an urban setting (14.4) (AAFP, 1994b).

Computers are contributing significantly to cost-effective and quality care in family practice (see Chapter 65). In 1993, an estimated 67 per cent of office-based family physicians had a computer physically located in their office, using them primarily for billing, accounting, electronic claims processing, word processing, and appointment scheduling (AAFP, 1994b).

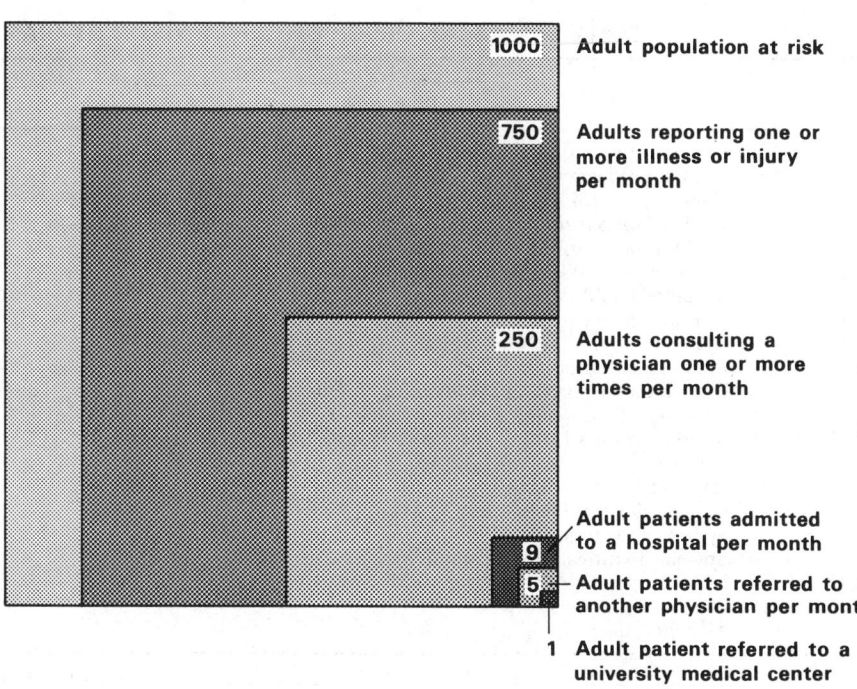

FIGURE 1–1. Number of persons experiencing illness or injury during an average month, per 1000 adult population. (From White KL, Williams F, Greenberg B: Ecology of medical care. N Engl J Med 265: 885, 1961, with permission.)

1000 **Adult population at risk**

750 **Adults reporting one or more illness or injury per month**

250 **Adults consulting a physician one or more times per month**

9 **Adult patients admitted to a hospital per month**

5 **Adult patients referred to another physician per month**

1 **Adult patient referred to a university medical center per month**

TABLE 1–1. THE TWENTY MOST COMMON PRINCIPAL REASONS FOR OFFICE VISITS IN THE UNITED STATES (1991)*

Rank	Principal Reason for Visit	Number of Visits (in thousands)	Per Cent	Cumulative Per Cent
1	General medical examination	29,720	4.4	4.4
2	Cough	24,263	3.6	8.0
3	Routine prenatal examination	19,675	2.9	10.9
4	Symptoms referable to the throat	17,882	2.7	13.6
5	Postoperative visit	16,308	2.4	16.0
6	Earache or ear infection	13,404	2.0	18.0
7	Well-baby examination	13,276	2.0	20.0
8	Back symptoms	12,977	1.9	21.9
9	Skin rash	12,119	1.8	23.7
10	Stomach pain, cramps, and spasms	11,106	1.7	25.4
11	Fever	10,318	1.5	26.9
12	Headache, pain in head	10,128	1.5	28.4
13	Vision dysfunctions	10,011	1.5	29.9
14	Knee symptoms	9,522	1.4	31.3
15	Nasal congestion	8,444	1.3	32.6
16	Blood pressure test	7,645	1.1	33.7
17	Head cold, upper respiratory infection (coryza)	7,616	1.1	34.8
18	Neck symptoms	7,193	1.1	35.9
19	Depression	7,060	1.1	37.0
20	Low back symptoms	7,051	1.1	38.1
	TOTALS	**255,718**	**38.1**	**38.1**
	All other reasons	413,971	61.8	

* Total number of visits in thousands: 669,689.

From National Center for Health Statistics (Schappert SM): 1991 summary: National Ambulatory Medical Care Survey. Advance Data Vital Health Stat no. 230, 1993.

Practice Content

The National Ambulatory Medical Care Survey conducted by the National Center for Health Statistics (NCHS) of the U.S. Department of Health and Human Services has, since 1975, annually reported the problems seen by office-based physicians (in all specialties) in the United States. A symptom classification was developed to document the complaints presented by patients to physicians in their offices. The National Ambulatory Medical Care Survey reverses the previous trend of evaluating the prevalence of disease after the fact (measuring causes of death or diagnosis upon

TABLE 1–2. RANK ORDER OF OFFICE VISITS BY DIAGNOSIS (1991)

Rank	Diagnosis	Per Cent	Cumulative Per Cent
1	Essential hypertension	3.5	3.5
2	Normal pregnancy	3.1	6.6
3	General medical examination	2.7	9.3
4	Health supervision of infant or child	2.6	11.9
5	Acute upper respiratory infections of multiple or unspecified sites	2.5	14.4
6	Suppurative and unspecified otitis media	2.4	16.8
7	Diabetes mellitus	1.9	18.7
8	Chronic sinusitis	1.7	20.4
9	Glaucoma	1.6	22.0
10	Acute pharyngitis	1.6	23.6
11	Bronchitis, not specified as acute or chronic	1.5	25.1
12	Diseases of sebaceous glands	1.4	26.5
13	Allergic rhinitis	1.4	27.9
14	Asthma	1.3	29.2
15	Cataract	1.1	30.3
16	Contact dermatitis and other eczema	1.1	31.4
17	Sprains and strains of other and unspecified parts of back	1.0	32.4
18	Special investigations and examinations	0.9	33.3
19	Neurotic disorders	0.9	34.2
20	General symptoms	0.9	35.1
	All other diagnoses	64.8	

From National Center for Health Statistics (Schappert SM): 1991 summary: National Ambulatory Medical Care Survey. Advance Data Vital Health Stat no. 230, 1993.

TABLE 1–3.   TWENTY DRUGS MOST FREQUENTLY PRESCRIBED AT OFFICE VISITS (1991)

Entry Name of Drug	Per Cent Distribution	Therapeutic Classification
Amoxicillin	2.2	Penicillins
Amoxil	1.2	Penicillins
Lasix	1.2	Diuretics
Ceclor	1.1	Cephalosporins
Allergy relief or shots	1.0	Diagnostics, nonradioactive and radiopaque
Prednisone	1.0	Adrenal corticosteroids
Synthroid	0.9	Agents used to treat thyroid disease
Lanoxin	0.9	Cardiac glycosides
Zantac	0.9	Agents used in disorders of upper GI tract
Motrin	0.9	Antiarthritics
Naprosyn	0.9	Antiarthritics
Diphtheria, pertussis, and tetanus toxoids	0.9	Vaccines and antiserums
Premarin	0.9	Estrogens and progestins
Vasotec	0.8	Antihypertensive agents
Cardizem	0.8	Antianginal agents
Tylenol	0.8	General analgesics
Seldane	0.7	Antihistamines
Poliomyelitis vaccine	0.7	Vaccines and antiserums
Proventil	0.7	Bronchodilators, antiasthmatics
Keflex	0.7	Cephalosporins

From National Center for Health Statistics (Schappert SM): 1991 summary: National Ambulatory Medical Care Survey. Advance Data Vital Health Stat no. 230, 1993.

discharge from a hospital) by evaluating the presenting complaints or symptoms at the onset of the illness. The 20 most common symptoms or reasons prompting office visits in 1991 are shown in Table 1–1. The principal diagnoses resulting from these visits are also documented by the participating physicians in Table 1–2. Table 1–3 shows the 20 drugs and their therapeutic classification most frequently prescribed by all physicians in office practice. In 1991, 12.7 per cent of patients of all ages were seen for high blood pressure and almost as many were seen for depression (6.1 per cent) as for hypercholesterolemia (6.9 per cent) (NCHS, 1993).

Office Visits

Available data concerning primary care indicate that more people use this type of medical service than any other kind, and that, contrary to popular opinion, sophisticated medical technology is not normally either required or overused in basic primary care encounters. Indeed, most primary care visits arise from patients requesting care for relatively uncomplicated problems, many of which are self-limiting but which cause them concern or discomfort. Treatment is often symptomatic, consisting of pain relief or anxiety reduction rather than a "cure." The greatest cost efficiency results when these patients' needs are satisfied, while the self-limiting course of the disease is recognized without incurring unnecessary costs for additional tests.

Each year 75 per cent of people in the United States make at least one visit to a physician. In 1991 the average was 2.7 office visits per person. Females accounted for 59.8 per cent of all visits (3.1 visits per person per year), and males had 2.2 visits per person per year. The annual visit rate ranged from 1.8 visits per person per year for young adults 15 to 24 years of age to 6.0 visits for patients 75 years of age and older. Approximately 25 per cent of all visits were to family physicians. Only 0.9 per cent of all physician visits made during 1991 ended in hospital admission, and only 3.3 per cent of office visits resulted in referral to another physician (NCHS, 1993).

House Calls

Although the number of house calls being made by family physicians has declined significantly, they are again on the increase because of the increasing need resulting from shortened hospital stay; increased home care involving intravenous fluids, chemotherapy, and respiratory care previously requiring hospitalization; and an increase in the number of homebound elderly. Adelman and associates (1994) surveyed primary care physicians and found that 63 per cent of family physicians made house calls, compared to 47 per cent of general internists and 15 per cent of general pediatricians. Those who made house calls shared the belief that house calls are important for good comprehensive patient care, and are satisfying for the physician as well as the patient.

The house call continues to be a valuable tool used by family physicians to develop a thorough understanding of patients and their environment, and family practice residencies encourage house calls in their training programs. Family physicians who make house calls report an average of 1.6 per week (AAFP, 1994b).

The cost containment pressures that arose in the 1980s with the advent of diagnosis-related groups and professional review organizations have led to a resurgence of home care. More patients with acute as well as chronic illnesses are being managed at home, and the home care industry has grown at a rate of 20 per cent a year, whereas the availability of nursing home beds has increased only 2 per cent annually (Kavesh, 1986).

Elderly patients, especially the frail elderly, often have considerable difficulty getting to and from the physician's office. The patient is more comfortable and under less stress at home and more problems can be identified, leading to improved care. Ramsdell and coworkers (1989) have shown that home visit assessments reveal two new problems and up to eight new treatment recommendations when home visits follow physician office-based assessments. Home visits may be the only way to identify some environmental hazards and to evaluate functional status accurately.

Home visits are more considerate of patients who have impaired mobility, and these patients respond better and may improve more rapidly when cared for at home by health professionals and family members (Kavesh, 1986). Only 15 per cent of patients who need long-term supportive care in the home turn to available community resources; 85 per cent receive care entirely from family and friends.

Cauthen (1981) has described eight different types of house calls: the emergency house call, the acute illness house call, the chronic illness house call, the dying patient house call, the house call to pronounce death, the grief house call, the home management–versus-hospitalization house call, and the home visit house call. Although the chronic illness house call is by far the most common, the home visit can be especially rewarding in a family practice. Some family physicians routinely visit patients in the home after a mother returns from the hospital with her new baby or after a patient is discharged following a serious illness.

Dr. Nicholas T. Grace, a family physician in California, makes a home visit whenever he enrolls a new family into his practice (*Family Practice News*, Aug. 15, 1977) because a personal visit to the family's home is an excellent way to begin a long-term relationship and is valuable in establishing good relations, not to mention the insight gained by the physician.

Group or Solo Practice

The majority of graduating family practice residents enter partnership or group practice: 40.6 per cent enter family practice groups, 11.3 per cent join multispecialty groups, and 8.9 per cent form two-person practices (partnerships). Only 6.2 per cent of graduates now enter solo practice (AAFP, 1994c).

Many graduates are attracted to group practice because of the opportunity to share calls. Such an arrangement allows physicians more time with their families and time to remain current with medical advances through continuing education. Many also select group practice because of the professional stimulation of working with colleagues. Group practices allow for overhead to be shared, and the cost of expensive equipment such as x-ray machines and flexible sigmoidoscopes can be spread over a wider financial base. Employment of paramedical personnel such as a nutritionist, clinical pharmacist, or marriage and family counselor is another luxury more easily borne by groups.

Group practice does, however, involve sacrificing some privacy and individuality, because each physician must adhere to the will of the majority. Solo practice, with the individual freedom it provides, is still alive and well in the United States. Solo physicians sacrifice the financial advantage of shared office space and more elaborate equipment for the privilege of being their own boss and making decisions unencumbered by the hassles and delays of group decision-making.

Group practices are more likely to draw physicians into rural and inner-city areas, where solo physicians are unlikely to want to practice "in isolation." Approximately 46 per cent of family physicians are located in towns of 25,000 population or less (Table 1–4).

PHYSICIAN SUPPLY

As the percentage of Americans who receive care from managed care networks continues to increase, the mix of specialties employed by those networks increasingly will indicate the number of positions likely to be available to medical graduates. Weiner (1994) projects that, by the year 2000, the number of primary care physicians needed will be about right, but specialists will exceed the need by more than 60 per cent (165,000 more than are needed). "The issue is not so much a primary care provider shortage as a specialty care surplus" (Weiner, 1994, p. 229). Table 1–5 compares the number of physicians in different specialties that are employed by 16 HMO plans with the number that currently are practicing in the United States. It is clear that, when the availability of most jobs is dictated by managed care plans, that physicians in the oversupplied specialties such as cardiology, anesthesiology, radiology, general surgery, pathology, neurology, and ophthalmology will have a difficult time finding employment. Many question whether physicians in these specialties can be retrained adequately to provide quality primary care.

The 1988 report of the American Medical Associ-

TABLE 1–4. DISTRIBUTION OF PRIMARY OFFICES OF FAMILY PHYSICIANS BY COMMUNITY SIZE (MAY 1993)*

Population of Community	Percentage (N = 1,765)
Population under 5,000, not within 25 miles of a major city	10.5
Population under 5,000, within 25 miles of a major city	4.4
Population 5,000–10,000, not within 25 miles of a major city	7.9
Population 5,000–10,000, within 25 miles of a major city	4.5
Population 10,000–25,000, not within 25 miles of a major city	10.4
Population 10,000–25,000, within 25 miles of a major city	8.4
Population 25,000–100,000	22.1
Population 100,000–500,000	18.1
Population over 500,000	12.8
Not reported	0.9

* Includes only active member respondents of the American Academy of Family Physicians.
From American Academy of Family Physicians: Facts About: Family Practice. Kansas City, MO, American Academy of Family Physicians, 1994, with permission.

TABLE 1–5. COMPARISON OF SELECTED HMOs' SPECIALTY-SPECIFIC PHYSICIAN STAFFING PATTERNS WITH NATIONAL SUPPLY LEVELS*

Specialty	Staffing of 16 HMOs	1992 U.S. Supply
Total	105.7	180.1
Primary care	49.6	65.7
Family/general practice	10.5	29.3
General internal medicine	25.0	23.3
Pediatrics	13.2	13.1
(% Primary care)	(46.8)	(36.0)
Medical subspecialties	12.5	17.8
Allergy	1.3	1.1
Cardiology	2.2	4.9
Dermatology	2.2	2.5
Endocrinology	0.8	0.8
Gastroenterology	1.5	2.4
Hematology/oncology	1.8	1.9
Infectious disease	0.6	0.6
Nephrology	0.7	1.1
Pulmonary disease	1.0	1.8
Rheumatology	0.6	0.9
Surgical specialties	29.7	43.8
Obstetrics/gynecology	10.4	11.4
General surgery	5.7	10.8
Neurosurgery	0.4	1.4
Ophthalmology	3.1	5.6
Orthopedics	4.2	6.5
Otolaryngology	2.5	2.7
Plastic surgery	0.5	1.7
Thoracic surgery	0.1	0.7
Urology	2.4	3.1
Hospital-based specialties	—	22.0
Radiology	5.3	8.6
Anesthesiology	4.4	9.2
Pathology	1.9	4.2
Other	—	—
Psychiatry	3.9	12.0
Emergency medicine	5.1	5.6
Neurology	1.5	2.7

* All figures represent full-time equivalent physicians per 100,000 population. Totals and subtotals may include some subspecialties not listed. HMO indicates health maintenance organization.
From Weiner JP: Forecasting the effects of health reform on US physician workforce requirement: Evidence from HMO staffing patterns. JAMA 272:224, 1994, with permission. Copyright 1994, American Medical Association.

ation's Council on Long Range Planning and Development notes that, although the number of family physicians will increase by 9 per cent by the year 2000, the U.S. population will increase by 12.3 per cent. Also, the increased demands that managed care will place on the need for family physicians will decrease even further the number a available to some rural areas. The total physician supply however, continues to grow 1.5 times faster than the U.S. population.

The Graduate Medical Education National Advisory Committee in 1980 projected a surplus of 150,000 physicians in the United States by the year 2020, with the greatest need in primary care. Mulhausen and McGee (1989) projected an even greater demand for primary care physicians than was estimated by Graduate Medical Education National Advisory Committee.

Another federally convened group, the Council on Graduate Medical Education (COGME), projects that, if no changes occur in the present situation by the year 2000, there will be a shortage of 35,000 generalists and a surplus of 115,000 specialists, increasing to 80,000 and 120,000, respectively, by the year 2020 (COGME, 1993). The COGME appropriately believes that the medical profession has a responsibility to produce a physician workforce that meets the nation's needs. Until recently, academic health centers have not accepted this responsibility, and many remain slow to change. If the number of generalists being produced is to increase, residency positions must be based on societal and educational needs and not on hospital service needs, as in the past. In addition, disincentives must be removed and "the practice income of generalists would have to exceed that of specialists in order to overcome the specializing influences upon medical students of the educational milieu" (COGME, 1993, p. 11). The COGME considers the family physician, general internist, and general pediatrician as the generalist specialists because these are the only physicians "trained to function as comprehensive primary care physicians for the undifferentiated problems of their patients" (COGME, 1993, p. 9).

If the growth in physician supply continues, American Medical Association analysts warn that "soon some physicians might not have enough work to stay proficient, and the status of the profession might decline" (*American Medical News*, Jan. 6, 1989, p. 31). Similarly, the quality of primary care will decline as physicians trained in a surplus subspecialty practice primary care without retraining. Rhee and associates (1981) showed that, when physicians practice outside their specialty areas, the relative quality of their performance declines.

As much-needed changes in the American medical system are implemented, it would be wise to keep some perspective on the situation regarding physician distribution. Beeson (1974) has commented,

I have no doubt at all that a good family doctor can deal with the great majority of medical episodes quickly and competently. A specialist, on the other hand, feels that he must be thorough, not only because of his training but also because he has a reputation to protect. He, therefore, spends more time with each patient and orders more laboratory work. The result is a waste of doctors' time and patients' money. This not only inflates the national health bill, but also creates an illusion of doctor shortage when the only real need is to have the existing doctors doing the right things. (p. 48)

REFERENCES

Adelman AM, Fredman L, Knight AL: House call practices: A comparison by specialty. J Fam Pract 38:39, 1994.

Ad Hoc Committee on Education for Family Practice, Council on Medical Education of the American Medical Association (Willard Committee): Meeting the Challenge of Family Practice (Report). Chicago, American Medical Association, 1966.

American Academy of Family Physicians: Congress Reporter, Congress Adopts Revised Definitions Concerning Family Physician, Oct. 5–7, 1993, pp 4–5.

American Academy of Family Physicians: Directors' Newsletter, AAFP Revises Primary Care Definition and Exhibit 1, Feb. 4, 1994a, p. 1.

American Academy of Family Physicians: Facts about: Family Practice. Kansas City, MO, American Academy of Family Physicians, 1994b.

American Academy of Family Physicians: Report on Survey of 1994 Graduating Family Practice Residents (Reprint no. 155T). City, American Academy of Family Physicians, 1994c.

Balint M: The Doctor, His Patient and the Illness. New York, Pitman, 1965.

Beeson PB: Some good features of the British National Health Service. J Med Educ 49:43, 1974.

Boex JR, Edwards J, Garg M, et al: Generalist and specialist practitioner: Analyses of quality and costs of care. Report to the W. K. Kellogg Foundation, October 7, 1993.

Cauthen DB: The house call in current medical practice. J Fam Pract 13:209, 1981.

Cherkin DC, Rosenblatt RA, Hart LG, et al: The use of medical resources by residency-trained family physicians and general internists: Is there a difference? Med Care 25:455, 1987.

Citizens' Commission on Graduate Medical Education, American Medical Association (Millis Commission): The Graduate Education of Physicians (Report). Chicago, American Medical Association, 1966.

Council on Graduate Medical Education, Bureau of Health Professions: The Third Report of the Council. Washington, DC, U.S. Department of Health and Human Services, Public Health Services, 1992.

Council on Long Range Planning and Development, American Medical Association: The Future of Family Practice. Chicago, American Medical Association, 1988.

Dunphy JE: Responsibility and authority in American surgery. Bull Am Coll Surg 49:9, 1964.

Fry J: Common sense and uncommon sensibility. J R Coll Gen Pract 27:9, 1977.

Gonnella JS, Veloski JJ: The impact of early specialization on the clinical competence of residents. N Engl J Med 306:275, 1982.

Graduate Medical Education National Advisory Committee: Final Report Vol. 1. (DHHS Publication no. [HRA] 81-651). Hyattsville, MD, Health Resources Administration, 1980.

Kavesh WN: Home care: Process, outcome, cost. Annu Rev Gerontol Geriatr 6:135, 1986.

Kimball HR, Young PR: A statement on the generalist physician from the American boards of family practice and internal medicine. JAMA 271:315, 1994.

MacLean DS: Outcome and cost of family physicians' care: Pilot study of three diagnosis-related groups in elderly inpatients. J Am Board Fam Pract 6:588, 1993.

McGann KP, Bowman MA: A comparison of morbidity and mortality for family physicians' and internists' admissions. J Fam Pract 31:541, 1990.

Mulhausen R, McGee J: Physician need: An alternative projection from a study of large, prepaid group practices. JAMA 261:1930, 1989.

National Center for Health Statistics (Schappert SM): 1991 summary: National Ambulatory Medical Care Survey. Advance Data Vital Health Stat no. 230, 1993.

Osler W: Aequanimitas, and Other Addresses. Philadelphia, Blakiston, 1904.

Peabody FW: Doctor and Patient. New York, Macmillan, 1930.

Pellegrino ED: The generalist function in medicine. JAMA 198:541, 1966.

Pellegrino ED: Humanism and the Physician. Knoxville, University of Tennessee Press, 1979.

Ramsdell JW, Swart JA, Jackson JE, Renvall M: The yield of a home visit in the assessment of geriatric patients. J Am Geriatr Soc 37(1):17, 1989.

Rhee S, Luke R, Lyons T, Payne B: Domain of practice and the quality of physician performance. Med Care 19:14, 1981.

Rivo ML, Saultz JW, Wartman SA, DeWitt TG: Defining the generalist physician's training. JAMA 271:1499, 1994.

Schroeder SA: Western European responses to physician oversupply. JAMA 252:373, 1984.

Tumulty PA: What is a clinician and what does he do? N Engl J Med 283:20, 1970.

Weiner JP: Forecasting the effects of health reform on US physician workforce requirement: Evidence from HMO staffing patterns. JAMA 272:222, 1994.

World Conference on Medical Education, World Federation for Medical Education. The Edinburgh Declaration. Edinburgh, Scotland, World Federation for Medical Education, 1988.

World Organization of National Colleges, Academies and Academic Associations of General Practitioners/Family Physicians: The Role of the General Practitioner/Family Physician in Health Care Systems. Victoria, Australia, World Organization, 1991.

SUGGESTED READINGS

Bertakis KD: Cost-effectiveness of care by family physicians. J Am Board Fam Pract 6:609, 1993.

Darley W: We need a new specialty: Family practice. New Med Materia 4(3):29, 1962.

Dunphy JE: Role of the family physician in the medical care of the future. New Physician 13:331, 1964.

Family practice, a concept or a reality? JAMA 185:208, 1963.

Fox TF: The personal doctor and his relation to the hospital. Lancet 1:743, 1960.

Geyman JP: Family Practice: Foundation of Changing Health Care. New York, Appleton-Century-Crofts, 1980.

Halsted JA: Personal care in medicine of the future. N Engl J Med 267:1233, 1962.

James G: The general practitioner of the future. N Engl J Med 270:1286, 1964.

Marsland DW, Wood M, Mayo F: Content of family practice. A Statewide Study in Virginia with Its Clinical, Educational, and Research Implications. J Fam Pract 3:23, 1976.

McWhinney IR: An Introduction to Family Medicine. New York, Oxford University Press, 1981.

National Center for Health Statistics: National Ambulatory Medical Care Survey: United States, 1975–1981 and 1985 Trends. Vital Health Stat [13], no. 93, 1988.

Steinwachs DM, Levine DM, Elzinga J, et al: Changing patterns of graduate medical education. N Engl J Med 306:10, 1982.

Surgeon-General's Consultant Group on Medical Education: Physicians for a Growing America (Bane Report). (PHS Publication no. 709). Washington, DC, U.S. Government Printing Office, 1959.

Tumulty PA: The Effective Clinician: His Methods and Approach to Diagnosis and Care. Philadelphia, WB Saunders Company, 1973.

CHAPTER **2**

THE FAMILY GENOGRAM

Standard Genogram Structure

ROBERT E. RAKEL

The family genogram is a tool used by physicians to summarize on one page a large amount of information relating to the family. It includes a family's hereditary background and the risk this places on current members, along with other major medical, social, and interactional influences. The genogram also is referred to as the family pedigree, family tree, or genealogic chart.

The genogram should indicate those conditions in the family that have hereditary significance, but it also can be used to depict problems of a less well-defined hereditary nature that appear to have a high incidence in a family. Even if these problems are not purely genetic, they may be related to social or environmental factors or to family traits or habits that predispose future family members to the likelihood of that problem developing. The genogram also can demonstrate problems of unknown etiology that are common in a family. Regardless of the cause of the problem, demonstrating its trend throughout succeeding generations of a family is valuable, because it gives offspring some idea of whether they might develop the condition. Thus, charting the incidence of cancer, heart disease, or asthma in a family alerts the individual patient to factors that should be watched for closely.

The genogram supplements the problem list, giving the physician an overview of the main problems affecting the family over three or more generations. "Genograms make it easier for a clinician to keep in mind family members, patterns, and events that may have recurring significance in a family's ongoing care" (McGoldrick and Gerson, 1985), p. 2). The greatest barrier to the universal adoption of the genogram by practicing physicians is the time required to develop one. The search for methods that require less physician and office staff time continues. Jolly and colleagues (1980) found that the average time required to complete a genogram (using pretrained patients) was 16 minutes, with a range of 9 to 30 minutes.

Physicians who use the genogram in their practice feel it is time well spent. Especially when patients are new to the practice, the process helps build rapport and enchances the doctor–patient relationship.

A clinician may find that a genogram sheds new light on a difficult case or that, in routine application, it turns up clinically significant material that otherwise would have been overlooked. Another clinician may find that doing a nonthreatening genogram dissolves resistance to exploring a patient's personal life and transforms the physician-patient relationship. (Rogers and Rohrbaugh, 1991, (p. 325)

The information obtained is of therapeutic as well as diagnostic value because patients feel the physician is truly interested in them and their family.

Genograms need not be used routinely with every patient. They are most effective when applied selectively.

FAMILY HISTORY

Family background and family influences are not merely incidental items to be considered briefly during the care of an individual; they are essential to the continuing and comprehensive care of that individual and family. The family history long has been a major component of the medical record, because information concerning family background is a potential source of valuable diagnostic information. Too often, however, family data are treated superficially when the physician asks questions regarding the frequency of hereditary or transmissible problems within the family. This ritualistic inquiry is often no more than a recitation by the physician of diseases, such as tuberculosis and diabetes, for which a yes or no answer is requested and that yields data of only limited usefulness. The astute diagnostician delves into the patient's background more thoroughly, attempting to uncover subtle trends or relationships between significant past events and the present problem. The family physician usually accumulates a complete family history over a period of time, gradually adding items to the picture during a series of patient visits. In this way the patient, by asking other family members for additional data and clarification, is able to add more information at subsequent visits. Families usually enjoy developing a family genogram and cooperate in constructing one that not only reflects their lineage but also remains a dynamic picture that can be of medical value to future generations.

The family history can be obtained on a standard questionnaire that becomes a permanent part of the record, such as the Baylor Health History Questionnaire (Fig. 2–1). A primary objective is to search for problems in the family's background that are possible threats to the health of present family members and their future offspring. The degree of susceptibility of any individual can be identified by noting the frequency of occurrence in previous family members. The amount of family data that can be collected in this manner is limited, however, and much more information is available when history forms of this type are supplemented by a genogram.

One example of an important hereditary influence is inborn errors of metabolism. Although these are rare and normally occur at a rate of only 1 in every 10,000 births, the carriers of these diseases experience a rate of 1 per every 100 births or less. The probability of one carrier marrying another is sufficiently high to cause concern, and because many of these disorders can be prevented or managed if diagnosed early, the identification of these affected individuals, or carriers, assumes greater importance. Over 1000 genetic abnormalities caused by single mutant genes in humans have been identified.

Studies in Northern Ireland and British Columbia show that up to 6 per cent of persons born in those areas are affected by a serious genetic disease at some time in their lives. Someone born in those regions and relocating to another area may not be identified as potentially transmitting a problem inherent in the previous region unless a complete family history and genogram are obtained.

BASIC DESIGN OF THE GENOGRAM

The purpose of the family genogram is to develop a realistic overview of the family's background and potential health problems. The techniques and symbols used should be those that physicians consider most meaningful in their practice and with which they feel most comfortable. Because the objective is to provide this information at a glance, the chart should be kept simple and brief. The more complicated the symbols and the more cluttered the design, the more time and effort it takes to construct the chart and to retrieve the information. (In a few instances, however, such increased detail may be worth the time.) Symbols requiring the least possible amount of explanation should be selected to represent specific problems.

The standard family genogram chart consists of three or more generations, representing all members of both spouses' families. The first-born members of each generation are the farthest to the left, with siblings following to the right in order of birth. A single generation is represented on the same line, and symbols should all be the same size. In generation I, it is traditional to place the husband's symbol on the left. The children of that marriage are indicated on the next generation line. In later generations, the first pregnancy (or first-born child) is placed to the left. The family name is placed above each major family unit, and the given names are placed below each symbol (Fig. 2–2A). An indication of either the patient's age or birthdate with each symbol is also useful. When ages are shown, it is important to indicate the date on which the chart was developed so that these ages can be adjusted over time. The other method is to show the dates of birth, as in Figure 2–2B.

There is often one member of the family who is of greater medical significance because of a chronic disease or an overwhelming problem. If such an individual is the major reason for developing a genogram, this person is called the index person (similar to the proband) and is identified by an arrow, double square, or double circle (Fig. 2–3).

The components of a genogram include the following:

1. Three or more generations
2. The names of all family members
3. Age or year of birth of all family members
4. Any deaths, including age at or date of death and cause
5. Significant diseases or problems of family members
6. Indication of members living together in the same household
7. Dates of marriages and divorces
8. A listing of first-born of each family to the left, with siblings listed sequentially to the right
9. A key depicting all symbols used
10. Symbols selected for simplicity and maximum visibility.

Familiarity with the standard symbols (Fig. 2–3) allows for more rapid retrieval of information. These standard symbols should be used whenever possible, but variations easily can be developed to provide more accurate or useful information. Examples of unconventional or individually designed symbols are shown in Figure 2–4. These symbols are of greatest value to the physician who designs them, and the symbols chosen by the physician depend entirely on his or her personal preference.

Standard symbols that maintain simplicity and avoid competition can be used with most family genograms, because only a few conditions normally require representation. When a variety of problems are represented in one genogram, the selection of symbols should be made with special care to assure that they are noncompetitive. Clut-

Baylor Family Practice Center
Health History Questionnaire

Today's Date _____

Single _____
Married _____
Divorced _____
Widowed _____
Separated _____

Name _____ Occupation _____

All previous occupations _____

Education: Years in high school _____ Years college _____ Degrees _____

Birthplace _____ Date of Birth _____

NOTE: This is a confidential record of your medical history and will be kept in this office. Information contained here will not be released to any person except when you have authorized us to do so.

Family History	If Living Age	If Living Health	Age at Death	If Deceased Cause	Has any blood relative or husband or wife ever had:	Check if Yes	Relationship if Yes
Father					Allergies		
					Asthma		
Mother					Arthritis		
(Circle) 1. Brother/Sister					Glaucoma		
					Cancer		
2. Brother/Sister					Tuberculosis		
					Diabetes		
3. Brother/Sister					Heart Trouble		
4. Brother/Sister					High Blood Pressure		
					Stroke		
Spouse					Epilepsy/Seizures		
(Circle) 1. Son/Daughter					Substance Abuse		
					Depression/Emotional Prob		
2. Son/Daughter					Suicide		
					Kidney Trouble		
3. Son/Daughter					Birth Defects		
					Sickle Cell Anemia		
4. Son/Daughter					Mental Retardation		

PERSONAL HISTORY: Please complete blanks in sections below

Date of last physical examination: _____ Physician _____

HOSPITALIZATIONS: List all, for illness or surgery, beginning with the most recent:

Date	Reason	Hospital	Physician

CURRENT MEDICATIONS: Circle those you use.

Laxatives   Birth Control Pills
Aspirin   Decongestants
Vitamins   Nasal Sprays
Tranquilizers   Cortisone
Hormones   Diet Pills
Antacids   Diuretics/Water Pills
                   Cold/Allergy Pills

LIST ANY ADDITIONAL MEDICATIONS YOU TAKE:

DATE OF LAST:

Pap Smear _____ EKG (or treadmill) _____
Mammogram _____ Stool test (blood) _____
Cholesterol _____ Sigmoidoscopy _____

HAVE YOU HAD X-RAYS OF: Date Result

Chest
Stomach (Upper GI)
Colon (Barium Enema)
Others: _____

WEIGHT: Now _____
1 yr. ago _____
Desired _____

ALCOHOLIC BEVERAGES:
Never _____ Less than
6 drinks/week _____
7-24 drinks/week _____
Over 24/week _____
Ever treated for alcoholism? _____

RECREATIONAL DRUGS:
Marijuana _____
Cocaine _____
Heroin _____
Other _____
Ever treated for drug dependency?
_____

HABITS: Use seat belts? _____
TOBACCO: Never _____
Cigarettes _____ (_____ packs/day)
Cigars _____ Pipe _____
Age started smoking _____
Age stopped smoking _____
Snuff _____ Chewing tobacco _____
ANY SPECIAL DIET? _____
Type: _____
_____

EXERCISE? Type: _____

Frequency, distance or amount:
_____
_____
_____
_____

PLEASE TURN OVER

MR-2, 4-88

FIGURE 2–1. Baylor College of Medicine Health History Questionnaire. *Illustration continued on opposite page*

Measles (10 day)

German Measles (3 day)

Mumps

Chicken pox

Whooping Cough

Scarlet fever/Scarlatina

Diphtheria

Pneumonia

Influenza

Pleurisy

Any eye disease, injury, impaired sight

Any ear disease, injury, impaired hearing

Any troubles with nose, sinuses, mouth, throat

Problems with your teeth

Rheumatic fever

Rheumatism

Any bone or joint disease

Neuritis or neuralgia

Bursitis, sciatica or lumbago

Stiff, swollen or painful joints

Polio or meningitis

Bladder or kidney infection or stones

Gonorrhea, syphilis, or herpes

Chlamydia, Venereal warts

Anemia

Yellow jaundice or hepatitis

Tuberculosis

Mononucleosis

Diabetes

Hypoglycemia

High blood pressure

Low blood pressure

Cancer

Food, chemical or drug poisoning

Received blood or plasma transfusions

Broken or cracked bones

Concussion or head injury

Knocked unconscious

Dislocations

Severe lacerations

Recent sprains

Frequent infections or boils

Hay fever or asthma

Hives

Eczema

Fainting spells

Convulsions or seizures

Frequent or severe headaches

Dizziness

Anxiety/tension

Difficulty remembering or concentrating

Difficulty sleeping

Frequent crying spells

Work or family problems

Thoughts about committing suicide

Nervous breakdown

Paralysis or numbness

Enlarged thyroid or goiter

Enlarged glands

Skin problems

Recent change in appetite or eating habits

Chest pain or angina pectoris

Spitting up of blood

Night sweats

Shortness of breath

Palpitation or fluttering heart

Heart murmur

Swelling of hands, feet or ankles

Extreme tiredness or weakness

Varicose veins

Albumin, sugar, blood or pus in urine

Difficulty urinating

Get up at night to urinate

Abnormal thirst

Stomach trouble or ulcer

Colitis or other bowel disease

Liver or gall bladder disease

Hemorrhoids

Rectal bleeding

Constipation or diarrhea

Black bowel movements

Change in bowel or bladder habits

Indigestion or difficulty swallowing

Change in a wart or mole

Hoarseness or cough

Non-healing sores

Lumps in breasts or elsewhere

Unusual bleeding or discharge

Tubal infections

Sex is not satisfactory

MEN ONLY: Have you ever had swellings of or lumps on testicles?

          Yes   No

Do you do regular testicular self-exam?   Yes   No

WOMEN ONLY: Do you do regular breast self-exam?   Yes   No

Menstrual History

Age at onset_____ Date of last period_____

Cycle (from start to start) _____ days

Usual duration of flow _____ days.

Flow is _____ Heavy _____ Medium _____ Light

Pain or cramps _____ Periods irregular _____

Have had vaginal infections or frequent discharge _____

Have taken birth control pills or used an IUD _____

Have had abnormal PAP _____ Date of last PAP _____

Pregnancies: Total number _____

How many children born alive _____

How many stillbirths _____

How many premature _____

How many Cesarean sections _____

How many miscarriages _____

How many abortions _____

IMMUNIZATIONS: List year of most recent immunization

Rubella _____

Measles and mumps_____

Tetanus_____

Polio _____

Diphtheria _____

Influenza _____

Hemophilus influenza _____

Pneumonia (Pneumovax) _____

Hepatitis _____

EXPOSURES: Have you been exposed to

Lead _____

DES _____

Asbestos_____

Others (Chemicals, Noise, etc.) _____

ALLERGIES: Are you allergic to

Penicillin, sulfa, other antibiotics _____

Aspirin, codeine or morphine _____

Any other medicines? _____

Insect bites or stings _____

Any foods? _____

_____

Physician's Signature   Date Reviewed

FIGURE 2–1. *Continued*

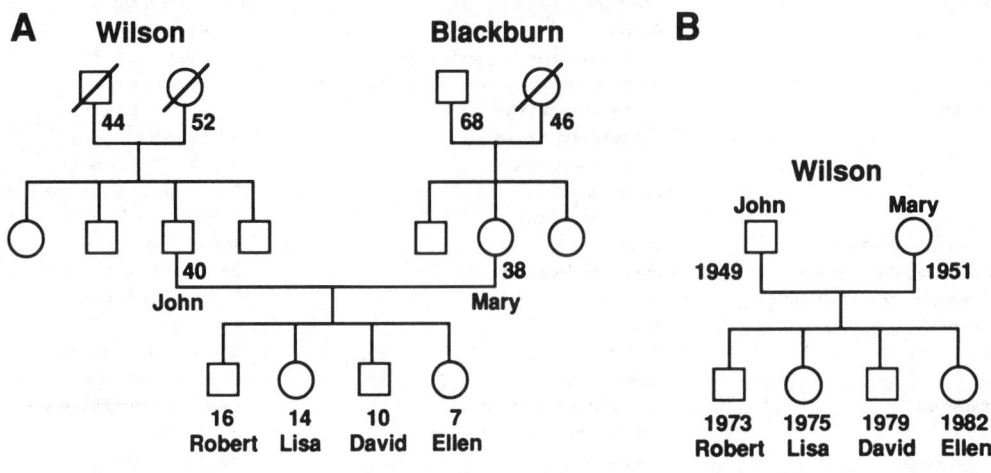

Date Prepared 8/20/89

FIGURE 2–2. Basic genogram containing family names, first names, and ages (*A*) or birthdates (*B*).

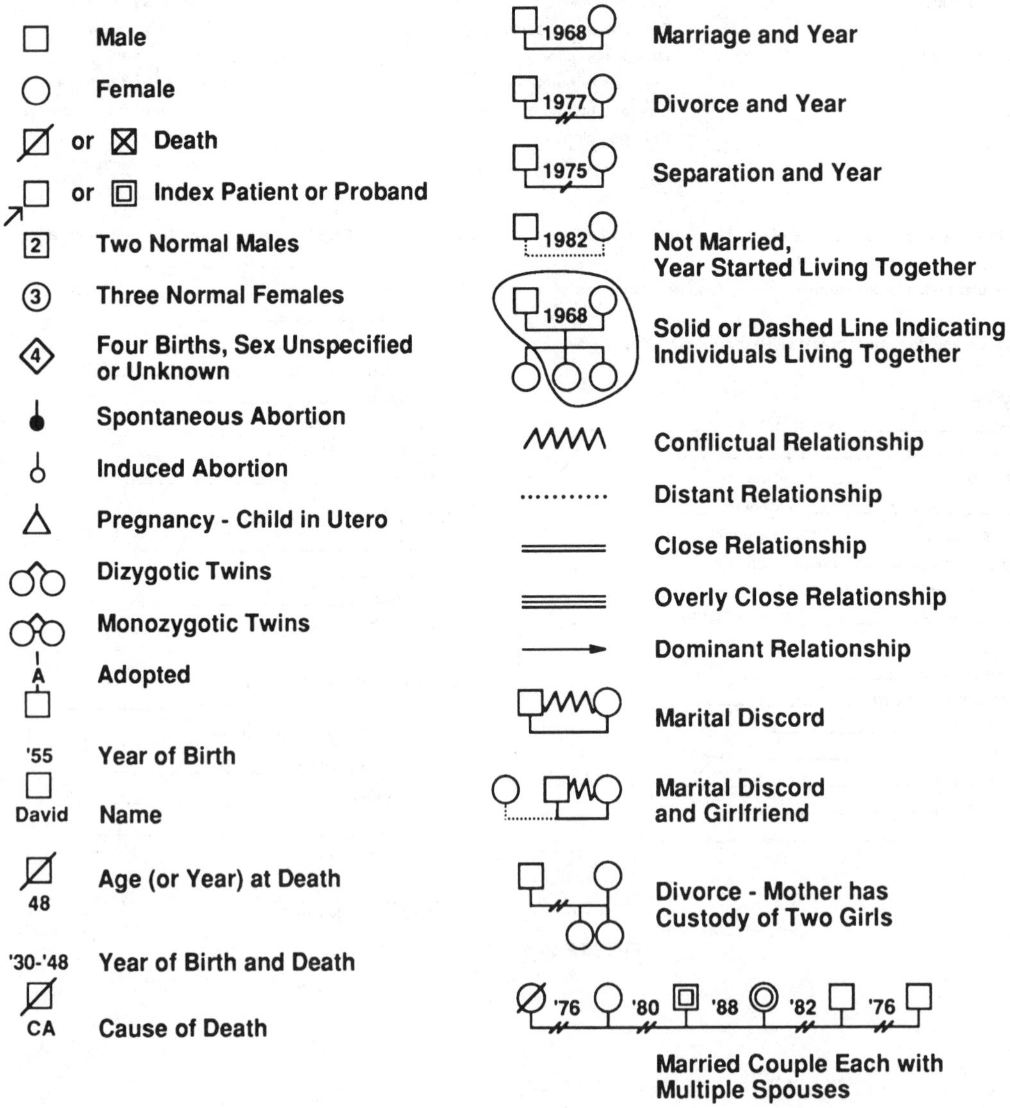

☐	Male	
○	Female	
⊘ or ⊠	Death	
☐ or ▣	Index Patient or Proband	
②	Two Normal Males	
③	Three Normal Females	
◇4	Four Births, Sex Unspecified or Unknown	
	Spontaneous Abortion	
	Induced Abortion	
△	Pregnancy - Child in Utero	
○○	Dizygotic Twins	
○○	Monozygotic Twins	
☐	Adopted	
'55 ☐	Year of Birth	
☐ David	Name	
⊘ 48	Age (or Year) at Death	
'30-'48 ⊘ CA	Year of Birth and Death / Cause of Death	

☐1968○	Marriage and Year
☐1977○	Divorce and Year
☐1975○	Separation and Year
☐1982○	Not Married, Year Started Living Together
☐1968○	Solid or Dashed Line Indicating Individuals Living Together
ᴧᴧᴧᴧ	Conflictual Relationship
··········	Distant Relationship
═══	Close Relationship
≡≡≡	Overly Close Relationship
⟶	Dominant Relationship
☐ᴧᴧ○	Marital Discord
○ ☐ᴧ○	Marital Discord and Girlfriend
☐○	Divorce - Mother has Custody of Two Girls
⊘'76 ○'80 ▣'88 ◎'82 ☐'76 ☐	Married Couple Each with Multiple Spouses

FIGURE 2–3. Standard genogram symbols.

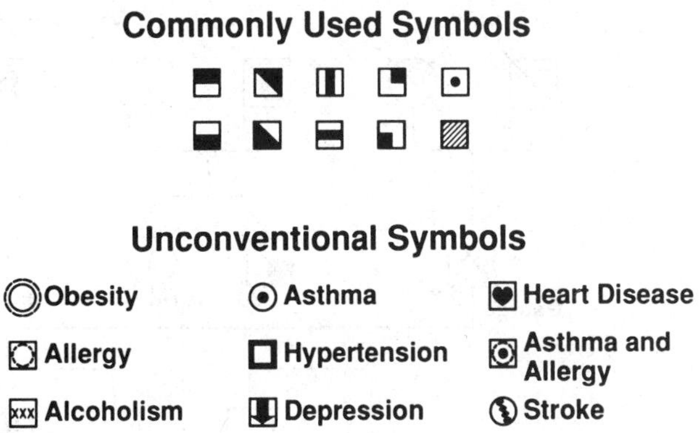

Commonly Used Symbols

Unconventional Symbols

◯ Obesity   ⊙ Asthma   ♥ Heart Disease

▢ Allergy   ☐ Hypertension   ◉ Asthma and Allergy

xxx Alcoholism   ⬇ Depression   Ⓢ Stroke

FIGURE 2–4. Individually designed (or selected) symbols and common abbreviations.

Commonly Used Abbreviations

ALC	Alcoholic
ALL	Allergy
ARTH	Arthritis
CA	Cancer
CAD	Coronary Artery Disease
CVA	Cerebrovascular Accident
DEP	Depression
DM	Diabetes Mellitus
GI	GI Tract Disease
HBP or HT	Hypertension
MI	Myocardial Infarction
MVP	Mitral Valve Prolapse
PUD	Peptic Ulcer Disease
SLE	Systemic Lupus Erythematosis
TB	Tuberculosis

tered symbols are more difficult to interpret and may defeat the chart's primary purpose. Additional notations on selected individuals regarding their occupation, level of education, general state of health, or other medical problems usually can be listed beneath the symbol or beneath the chart to give a more complete picture of that individual (Fig. 2–5).

When family members assist in constructing a genogram, they may gain additional insight into risks inherent in the family system and an increased awareness of the importance of some problems. For example, if repeated suicides occur, increased attention can be given to recognizing the early signs of depression.

It may be useful to highlight critical medical information on the genogram, using a yellow highlighter or colored pen. In this way, significant problems can be recognized immediately by anyone working with the family. This technique may be useful in educating family members about the importance of these items. For example, if cancer or heart disease is highlighted, the family can be told about the particular risk of continuing cigarette smoking.

The genogram shown in Figure 2–6 was developed by a family practice resident investigating the frequency of manic depression in a family and its relationship to alcoholism (Geron, 1976). An apparent X-linked inheritance was noted. Of medical significance to the family is the fact that the af-

fected individuals in generation III first developed symptoms at ages 22 and 32. The predictive significance for generation IV is obvious. Prompt recognition and treatment of symptoms will be possible when the problems first occur rather than later, after significant hardship has been experienced, as is so often the case.

USES OF THE GENOGRAM

The following uses of the genogram are adapted from Crouch and Davis (1987):

1.   Allowing the family physician to review quickly the family situation, such as a second marriage or two children in the home from a previous marriage.

2.   Allowing other physicians, nurses, and others to assess and understand the family quickly, thereby improving continuing comprehensive care.

3.   Building rapport by using the first names of family members and knowing who is living in the home.

4.   Identifying at a glance significant risk factors in family members, such as a family history of diabetes mellitus and overweight or a family history of coronary heart disease when several members have elevated serum cholesterol.

5.   Recognizing the need for screening in patients who are at high risk (e.g., the need for mam-

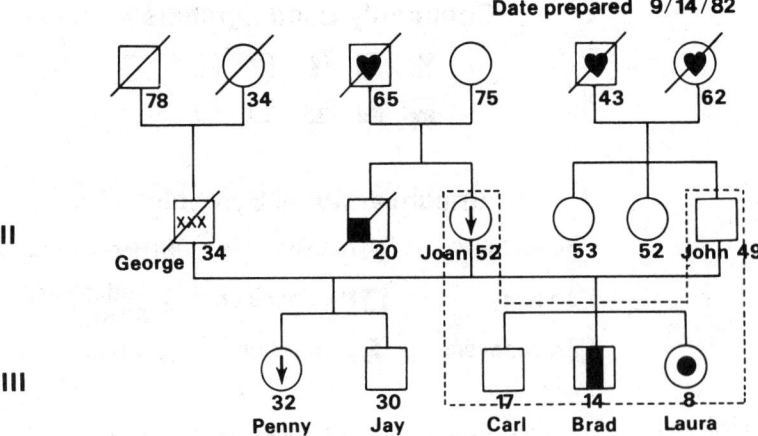

Date prepared 9/14/82

II

George 34

Joan 52

53 52 John 49

III

32 30 -17- -14- 8
Penny Jay Carl Brad Laura

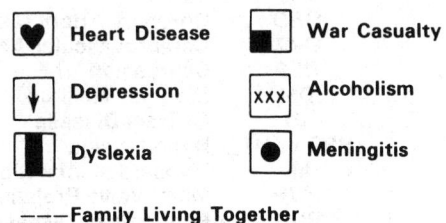

♥ Heart Disease   ■ War Casualty

↓ Depression   xxx Alcoholism

▌ Dyslexia   ● Meningitis

----Family Living Together

FIGURE 2–5. Family genogram with additional information on each individual at bottom of chart.

Joan (52)	Penny (32)	Jay (30)
Back Injury	Schoolteacher	Sailor
Rectal fissure	Migraine headaches	2 children
		Divorced
		Abdominal pain
		after father's death

Carl (17)	Brad (14)	Laura (8)
Hives	Premature birth	Meningococcal
Allergy to dust	Hyperkinetic—on Ritalin	meningitis
Undescended testicle	Inferiority complex	Wears corrective
		shoes

mograms more frequently if there is a history of breast cancer in the family).

6. Promoting lifestyle changes and placing greater emphasis on patient education (e.g., persistently encouraging smoking cessation if there is a family history of lung cancer or coronary artery disease).

7. Demonstrating that family relationships are a concern of the family physician and important to the health of each family member.

FUNCTIONAL CHARTING

An additional dimension can be added to the genogram by including the functional components shown in Figure 2–3. In this way, the social and interpersonal influences that operate within a family can be shown in addition to hereditary influences. Such a picture, which includes evidence of

the emotional relationships between individuals living together, gives a more dynamic image of the family and allows for greater insight into patterns of behavior. This visualization of family roles and interpersonal relationships allows one to judge the totality of the family unit—its strengths and weaknesses, its degree of solidarity, and its ability to withstand future stressful situations. The varying strengths of emotional bonds between individuals can be shown, as can marital discord and dominant personalties.

FAMILY CIRCLE

The family circle (Fig. 2–7) is a way to illustrate the emotional relationships of a family as depicted by one member (arrow). The size of the circle indicates importance; the distance from others reflects the degree of emotional attachment or closeness.

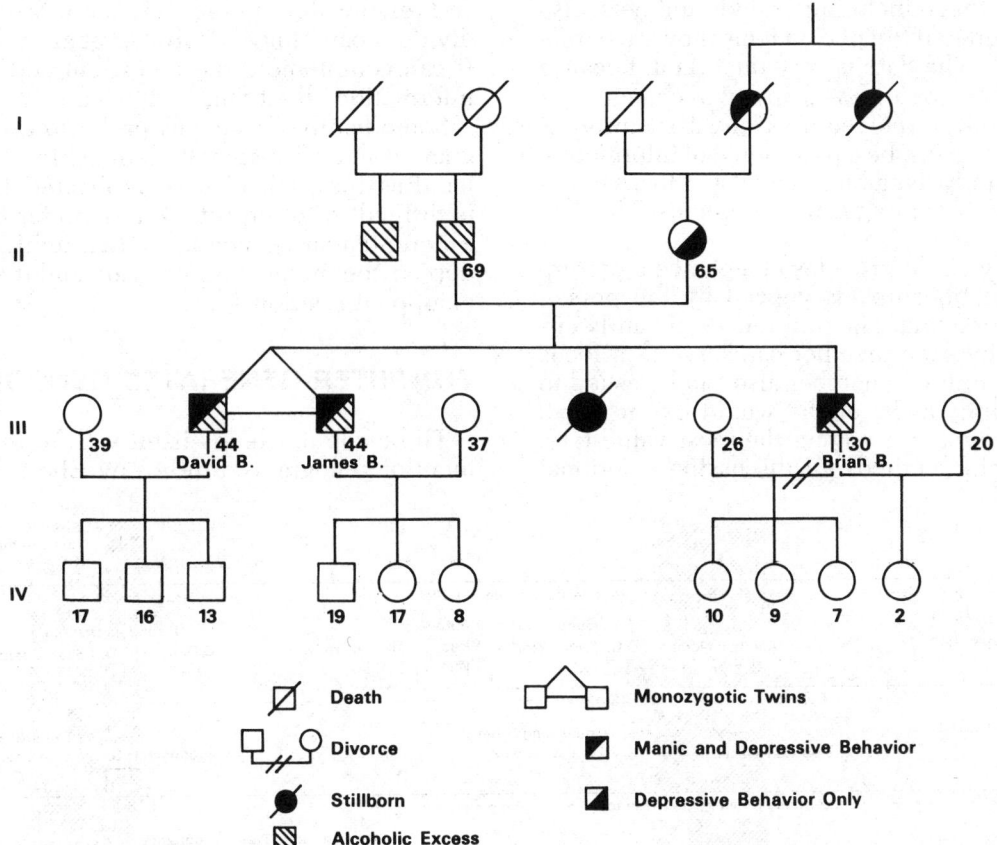

FIGURE 2–6. Family genogram with bipolar affective disorder. (From Rakel RE: Principles of Family Medicine. Philadelphia, WB Saunders Company, 1977, p 489, with permission.)

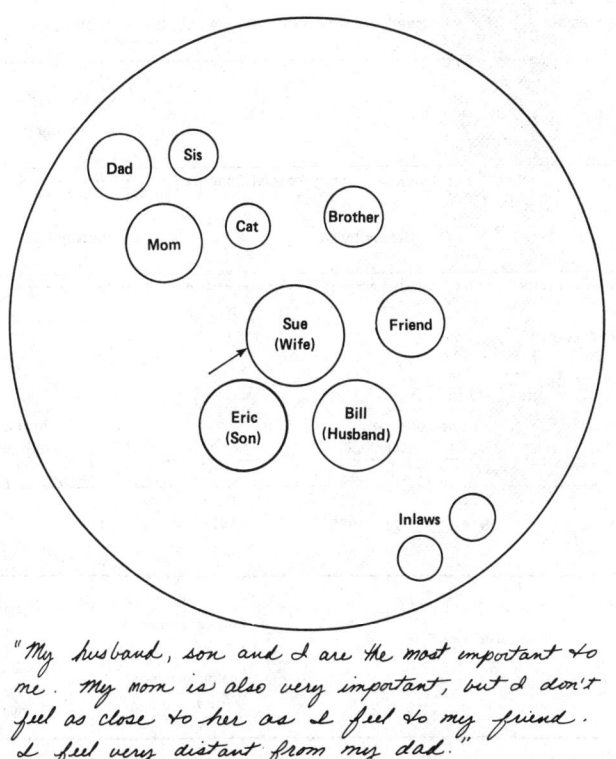

"My husband, son and I are the most important to me. My mom is also very important, but I don't feel as close to her as I feel to my friend. I feel very distant from my dad."

FIGURE 2–7. Family circle chart. (From Kertesz J: Urban family mapping. *In* Birrer RB, [ed]: Urban Family Medicine. New York, Springer-Verlag, 1987, p 74, with permission.)

Significant others, including friends and pets, also may be included if the person feels they are part of the "family." The date is very important, because these relationships almost always will change over time. The family circle requires only 2 or 3 minutes to complete and can be a rich source of information regarding family dynamics as well as a focus of opportunity for discussing family problems (Thrower et al., 1982).

The family circle provides at a glance a picture of family relationships as viewed by the person making the drawing. The differences in family circles drawn by each member can serve as a focus for discussion. Each member also can be asked to draw the family as he or she would like it to be. The family circle "is among the most value-free, nonjudgmental methods for discussing emotional and relationship problems without focusing on individual pathology" (Thrower et al., 1982, p. 457). It can complement the genogram and add useful information about family dynamics.

Some family physicians prefer to use the genogram to show functional relationships, but in some families this can lead to a complicated diagram that is difficult to interpret. Others prefer to combine a more standard genogram with a family circle; one depicts the medical information and the other, the emotional relationships.

COMPUTER-GENERATED GENOGRAM

The computer lends itself well to the development of genograms. Studies by Ebell and Heaton

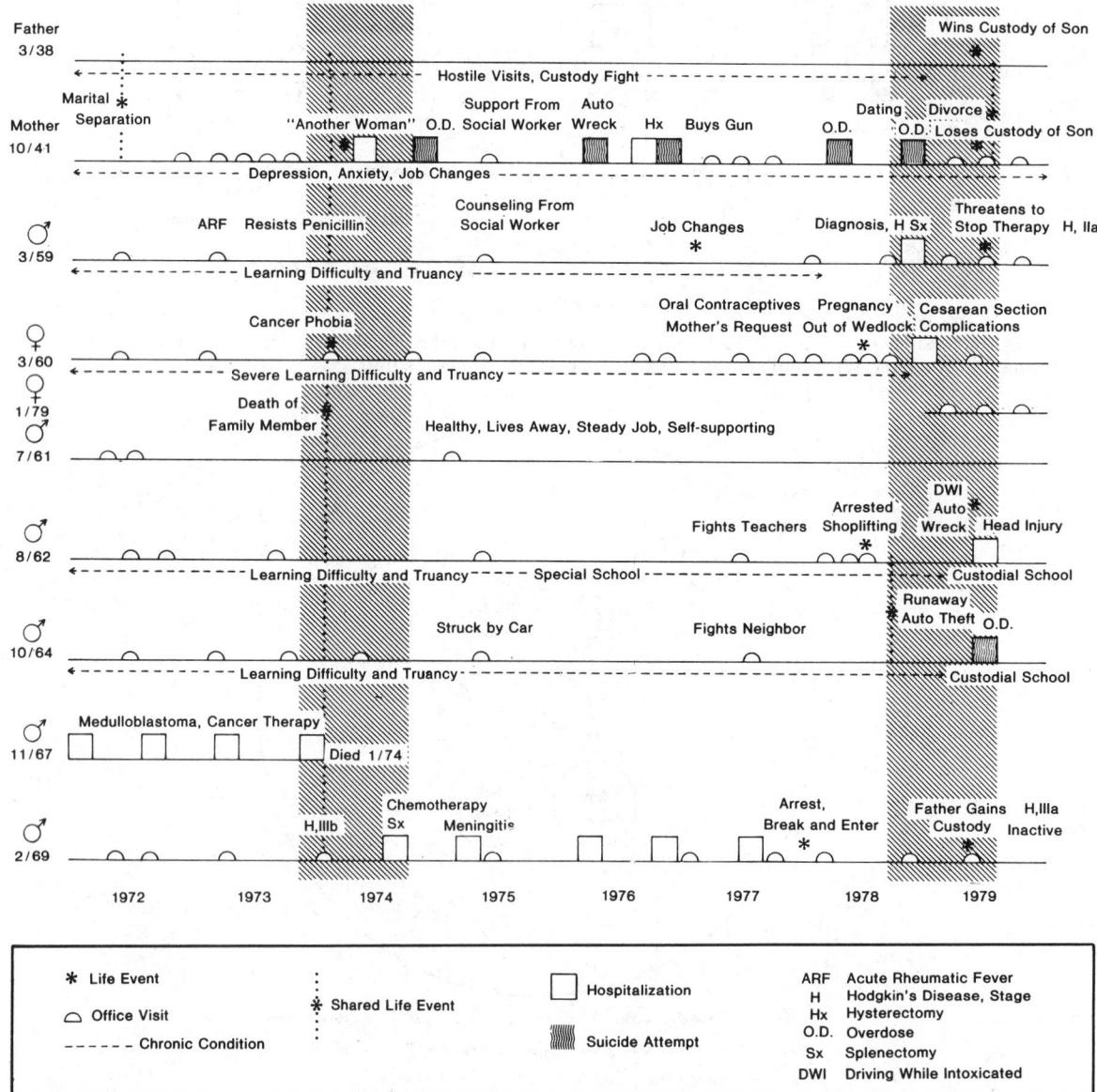

FIGURE 2–8. Flow chart of biomedical and sociomedical events that are interrelated. (From Rainsford GL, Schuman SH: The family circle in crises. JAMA 246:60, 1981, with permission. Copyright 1981, American Medical Association.)

(1988) show that familiarity with the computer is not necessary; nonusers of computers found the experience to be as pleasant and satisfying as did frequent computer users. Ninety-four per cent of the patients found creation of a computerized genogram to be a pleasant experience, even though only 15 per cent of them owned a computer, and it took an average of 19 minutes to complete the program. Ebell and Heaton also noted that patient acceptance was not affected by age or educational level.

The computer also has the advantage of collecting and standardizing a large amount of useful patient information at minimal cost of physician time.

CHARTS SHOWING CHANGES OVER TIME

An individual's or family's significant medical events over a period of time can be condensed into a single composite picture, using a variety of charting techniques. These methods conceptualize significant stresses that occur in an individual or family over time and involve the sequencing of noteworthy events within the family that may have a causal relationship. A family that remains intact in spite of a very cluttered or heavily involved flow chart demonstrates a high degree of cohesiveness.

Figure 2–8 is a time flow chart that shows significant biomedical and sociomedical events in a troubled family over 7 1/2 years. It illustrates the impact of illnesses and life events on family members and their family physician. In this family, cancer developed in three of the seven children, the mother made five suicide attempts, and the only daughter had a pregnancy out of wedlock. The two periods of severe family dysfunction from 1973 to 1974 and 1978 to 1979 are shown with vertical shading. A flow chart of this type not only provides a sequential analysis of an individual's life events but, when the vertical portion is reviewed, also shows how the same event can affect various family members. Chronically crisis-ridden families such as this need to be recognized early by the family physician.

Critical events in a family's history also can be shown on the genogram, either in the margin or at the bottom, or they may be listed chronologically on a separate page.

REFERENCES

Birrer RB (ed): Urban Family Medicine. New York, Springer-Verlag, 1987.
Crouch MA, Davis T: Using the genogram (family tree) clinically. In Crouch MA, Roberts L (eds): The Family in Medical Practice: A Family Systems Primer. New York, Springer-Verlag, 1987, pp 174–192.
Ebell MH, Heaton CJ: Development and evaluation of a computer genogram. J Fam Pract 27:536, 1988.
Geron M: Genetics of bipolar affective disorder and its application in family practice. Paper presented at the Annual Research Symposium, Department of Family Practice, Iowa City, University of Iowa, June 26, 1976.

Jolly W, Froom J, Rosen M: The genogram. J Fam Pract 10: 251, 1980.
McGoldrick M, Gerson R: Genogram in Family Assessment. New York, WW Norton, 1985.
Rainsford GL, Schuman SH: The family in crisis. JAMA 246: 60, 1981.
Rogers J, Rohrbaugh M: The SAGE-PAGE trial: Do family genograms make a difference? J Am Board Fam Pract 4:319, 1991.
Thrower SM, Bruce WE, Walton RF: The family circle method for integrating family systems concepts in family medicine. J Fam Pract 15:451, 1982.

Reading and Interpreting Genograms

JOHN C. ROGERS

READING GENOGRAMS

Experienced family physicians and family therapists can scan and interpret genograms within moments. Inexperienced learners, such as students and residents, should be taught a step-by-step, systematic approach to reading this clinical tool.

The four components of the family genogram are structure, demographics, events, and problems.

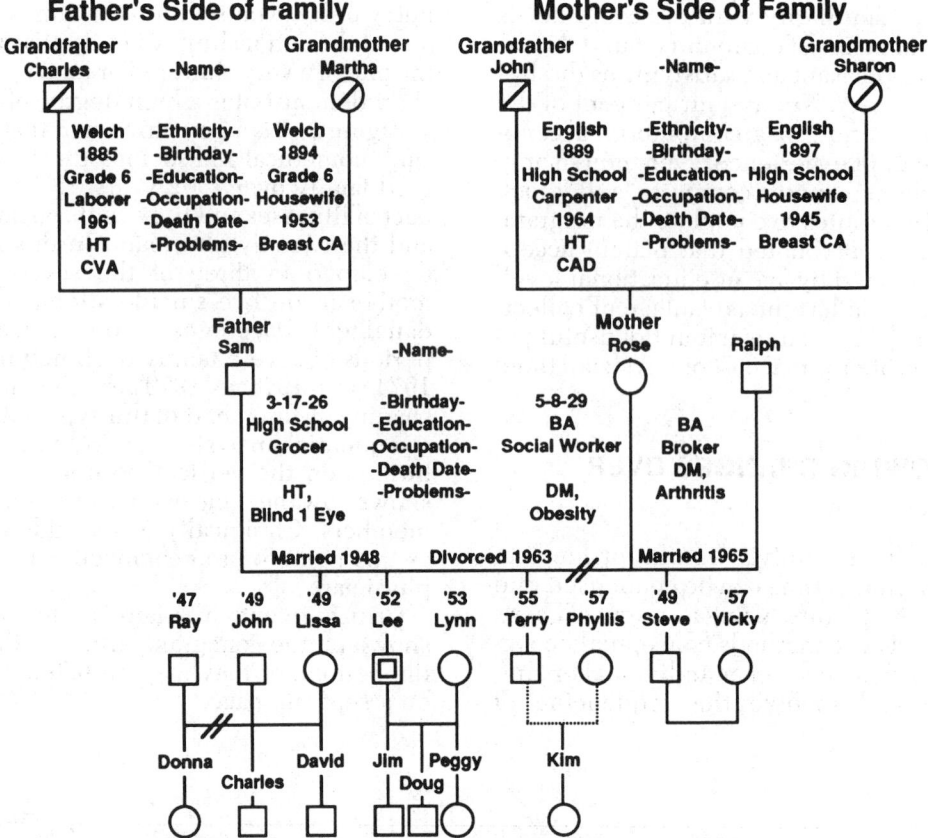

FIGURE 2–9.   Example of completed self-administered genogram (SAGE).

Structure

This refers to the composition of the index patient's current family unit and is a function of marital status (single, married, separated, divorced, widowed) and parental status (no children or natural, foster, or adopted children or stepchildren). The genogram in Figure 2–9 displays a number of different types of structure: single adult, single parent, childless couple, nuclear family, and blended family. These are the most frequent family structures recorded on genograms, but others may be encountered, especially if there are more than two generations living together, other long-term relationships, or individuals living together without legal bonds.

Family Demographic Information

This includes ethnicity, education, and occupation. Specific information about each of these three factors, as well as the consistency or lack of consistency for the items among the family members, may be important. Hence, the clinician reading this part of the genogram notes the ethnicity, education, and occupation of the index patient and

how those compare with the demographics of other members of the family.

Family Life Events

A number of major life events are recorded on genograms, including marriage, separation, and divorce; birth and death; and major social or health problems. Life events related to beginning or ending education, changes in occupational status, or leaving home often can be inferred from information on the genogram. The clinician reading the genogram notes what events have occurred, the time sequence, and whether there has been a confluence or pileup of events.

Social and Health Problems

Here the genogram reader notes the type and number of problems and their consistency among family members.

INTERPRETATION

The four-step protocol for reading the genogram extracts relevant information but does not deal with the meaning or implications of the family information—that requires interpretation. The full interpretation of the information depends on the type of clinical decisions that must be made. There is no such thing as a "normal genogram," so the interpretation of the reading clearly is dependent on the clinical situation to which the family information is being applied.

Family information is used predominantly in three types of situation: (1) evaluating a somatic complaint by testing biopsychosocial hypotheses about what caused the condition, (2) assessing a patient's risk for biomedical and mental disorders in order to implement appropriate primary and secondary prevention efforts, and (3) planning management of a patient's therapy by considering how family factors may facilitate or complicate it.

At first, the interpretation of genograms may seem to be complex, encompassing four data points (structure, demographics, events, and problems) and three possible decisions (diagnosis, prevention, and management). However, there are principles and theories that can simplify and guide the interpretative process. The first guide is the set of basic principles and methods of epidemiology. From this perspective, each of the four genogram components of structure, demographics, events, and problems is seen as a potential risk factor that may or may not be related to the biopsychosocial hypothesis under consideration, the preventable disease of concern, or the success or failure of the management option being considered. The simplest expression of these relationships is the ratio indicating the association between the family factor and the outcome of interest (relative risk and odds, mortality, and morbidity ratios). Specifically, the particular family structure, demographics, events, or problems may either increase or decrease the likelihood of a specific hypothesis, preventable disease, or success rate of a particular therapy.

This straightforward approach to interpreting genogram information requires the clinician to consider four types of family information (structure, demographics, events, and problems) and to ask the questions that are relevant to the clinical situation: Do the family's structure, demographic profile, life events, or health problems increase or decrease the likelihood of a specific biopsychosocial hypothesis? Do they increase or decrease the patient's risk of developing a specific preventable condition? Do they increase or decrease the success rate of a particular management option?

For example, the family structure variable of marital status has been studied in relation to a number of health outcomes. It is well documented that nonmarried persons have increased death rates for all major causes of death: cardiovascular diseases, infectious diseases, malignancies, accidents, homicides, and suicides. The age-specific death rates for widowed or divorced individuals are from two to four times higher than those of their married peers (Lynch, 1977). The demographic variable of education also has been related to mortality ratios; individuals with the lowest levels of education have the highest death rates for malignant neoplasms, cardiovascular and renal diseases, diabetes, tuberculosis, influenza, cirrhosis of the liver, accidents, and suicides. Breast cancer is the exception to this trend; in this situation, women with higher education have a higher death rate than those with lower education (Syme and Berkman, 1976). Mortality ratios also have been studied for the family life event of a spouse's death, with death rates as high as 12 times normal noted during the first year after the death of a spouse (Campbell, 1986). The epidemiologic concepts of risks and ratios also have been applied to a number of diseases that appear to run in families, such as breast cancer and maturity-onset diabetes mellitus.

Although this epidemiologic approach to interpreting genograms may be useful, it does not provide any explanations as to how or why the family factors are related to the outcomes of interest, nor does it provide any guidance for interventions aimed at the family factors themselves. There are four theories that are relevant to the genogram that also may be of assistance in addressing these two issues: (1) life cycle theory, (2) stress–social support theory, (3) genetic theory, and (4) family systems theory.

Life cycle or developmental theory describes how the structure and function of a family changes as it moves through the predictable phases of marriage: childbearing and rearing, child launching, and death of a spouse. This theory specifies the developmental tasks that each individual has at each phase as well as the key issues during transition from one stage to another (Ramsey, 1984). Because family members are dependent on one another for successful completion of their individual stage and transitional tasks, a condition or problem that seems to affect only one member can have ramifications for the family. This theory is useful for preventive care because it helps the clinician anticipate key transitions and educate family members about the upcoming change. It is also useful for testing hypotheses about exacerbations of chronic problems, such as diabetes or asthma; frequency of acute illnesses; or onset of apparently psychosomatic problems, such as headache, backache, fatigue, or abdominal pain.

Whereas family life cycle theory uses both family structure and some information about family events for interpreting the genogram, the *stress–social support theory* uses all four categories of genogram information. This theory asserts that stressful life events can cause illness unless buffered by social support. In addition, social support itself may have an independent beneficial effect on health, regardless of the presence or absence of stressful events (Medalie, 1978;

Smilkstein, 1978). The four categories of genogram information provide the data by which the stress and support can be determined. Clearly the genogram does not include all things that may be stressors or all sources of support, and these other areas may need to be explored by the clinician using this theoretical framework to interpret the genogram.

Genetic theory dominates most attempts to understand how health problems are transmitted from one family generation to another. This theory includes Mendelian transmission of autosomal dominant, autosomal recessive, sex-linked recessive, and intermediate inheritance as well as the issue of genetic susceptibility. The last requires information about environmental factors as well as familial tendencies (Warrell, 1987). This theory is relevant to the diagnosis and prevention of specific biologic diseases as well as some mental disorders and can be used to generate risk predictions for first- and second-degree relatives of those afflicted with particular conditions (Pauls et al., 1979; Smeraldi et al., 1981; Warrell, 1987).

Family systems theory is a rubric that includes several family function constructs and theories developed by a number of experts (Bray, 1987). Bowen's Intergenerational Family Systems Theory is the framework most closely associated with the use of the genogram by family therapists in their clinical work. A discussion of that theory is beyond the scope of this chapter because it requires a level of abstraction about family processes that is not pertinent to the practices of most family physicians.

Once the clinician has completed the four-step protocol for reading the genogram, epidemiologic principles and life cycle, stress–social support, and genetic theories can be used to guide the interpretation. Following this two-part procedure ensures a systematic reading and interpretation of the genogram and allows for effective use of routine family information in clinical decision making. The theoretical principles used for the interpretation of the genogram also can guide the clinician as additional family information is gathered or therapeutic interventions are designed and implemented.

CLINICAL EXAMPLES

This chapter attempts to show that the family genogram, when accurately derived and correctly interpreted, can help family physicians make more efficient use of basic family information as they make their daily decisions. The assumption is that knowing more about the entire family allows the clinician to be more effective. The genogram can guide the physician into more in-depth psychological assessments of the family and help him or her explore subtle problems that may have originated from the family situation, as illustrated in the following cases.

Case I: Kathryn

Kathryn is a 2-year-old child who is seen 2 days after her second birthday complaining that her stomach burns. Functional abdominal pain may be one of the biopychosocial hypotheses to be considered. The genogram in Figure 2–10 may be useful in testing this hypothesis. The genogram is read as follows:

Family structure:	Single-parent family with one child at home
Family demographics:	High school-educated parents, mother employed; status consistent with that of other family members
Family life events:	Divorce of patient's parents 1 year prior to visit; patient's birthday 2 days prior to visit
Family problems:	Patient's father has emotional and work problems; this also appears to be a pattern among his siblings.

Interpretation

From an individual and family life cycle perspective, the patient may not be progressing adequately in her development because of the absence of her father. Normal family development has been disrupted by the divorce and, depending on the father's visitation privileges, the patient may be having inadequate contact with a male parental figure. From a stress–social support perspective, the divorce of the parents within the last year is a major life event, as is the child's second birthday 2 days before the visit. The impact of these events on the child may need to be explored further. In addition, there are the daily problems of attending day care while the mother works and the fact that only a single parent is home during evenings and weekends.

The interpretation of this genogram suggests that there is the necessary and sufficient information to support a functional abdominal pain hypothesis. A standard biomedical evaluation is of course indicated to evaluate the clinical hypotheses, and more focused family information may need to be gathered to further test the psychosocial hypothesis. The genogram reading and interpretation provide a guide to help the clinician efficiently gather the most relevant additional family data.

Case II: Robert

Although the index patient was an adopted child brought in for a well-baby checkup, the physician also was concerned about the mother's health and the man-

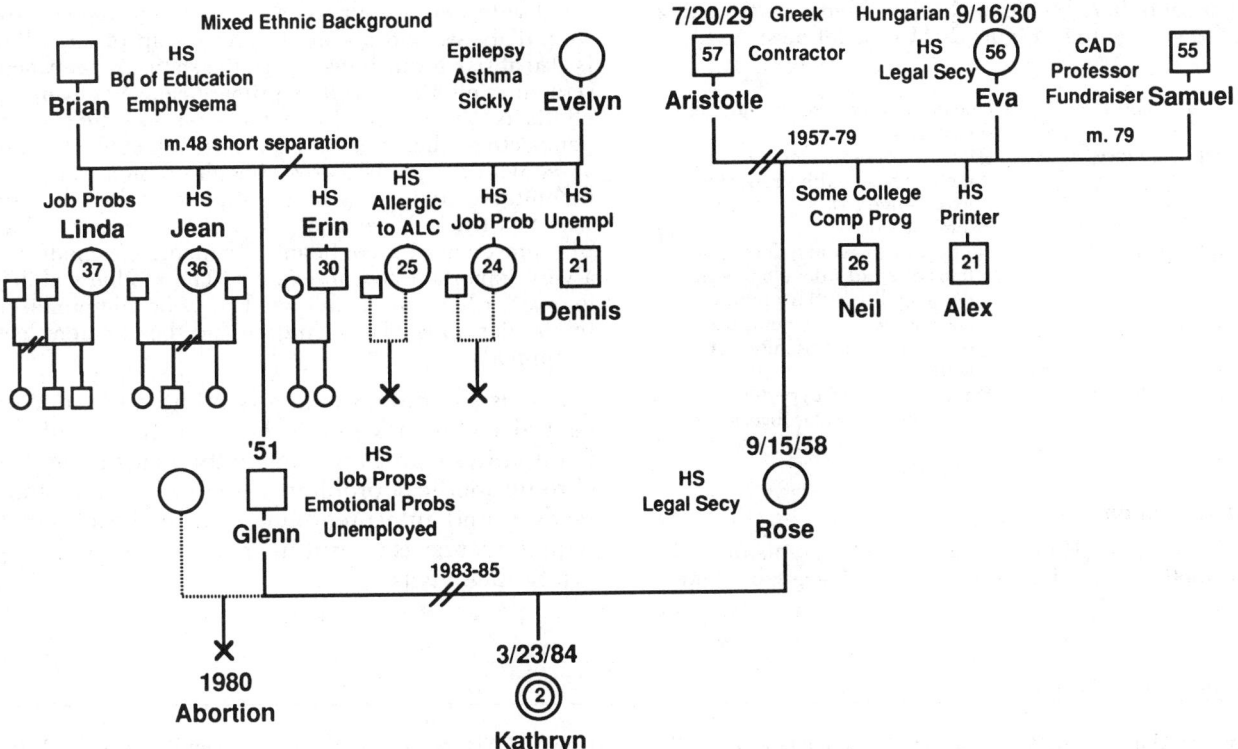

FIGURE 2–10. Case example: Kathryn.

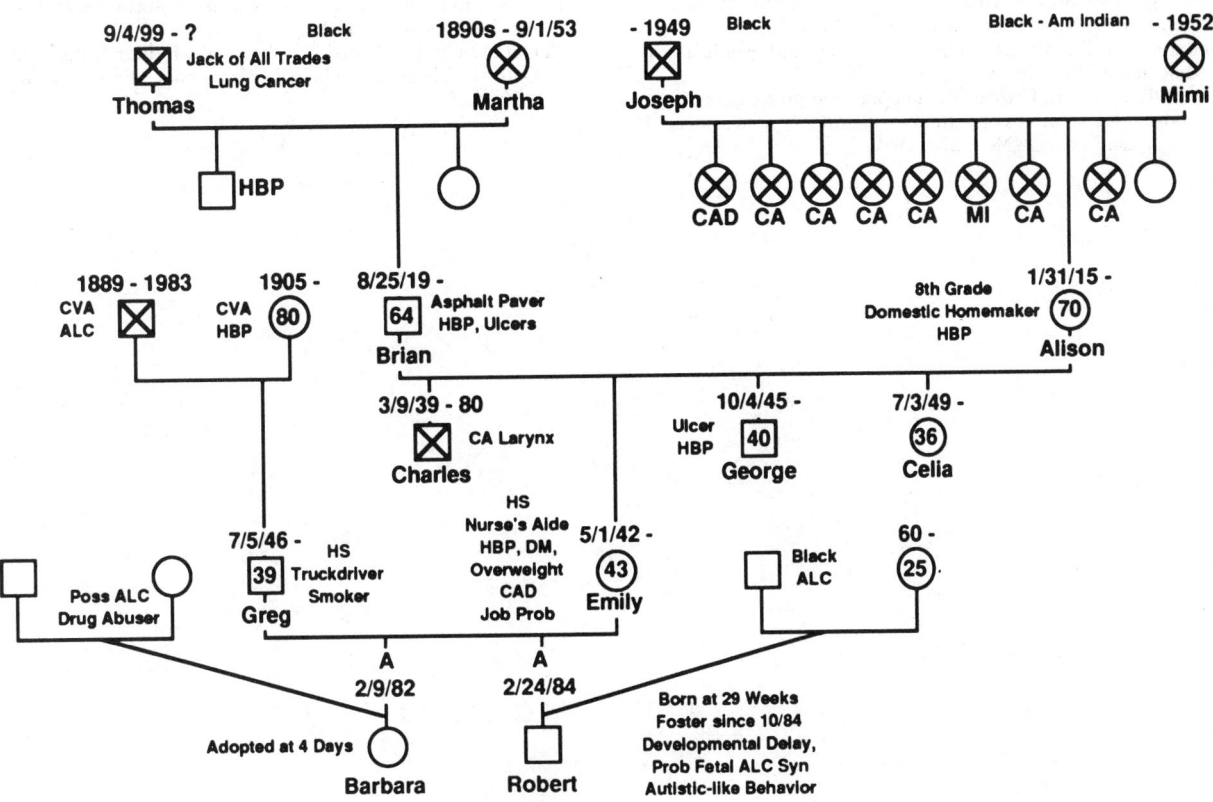

FIGURE 2–11. Case example: Robert.

agement of her chronic medical problems. The reading of the genogram in Figure 2–11 is as follows:

Family structure:	Nuclear family with two adopted children
Family demographics:	High school–educated parents; mother has health profession experience but current problems at work
Family life events:	No major life events; daily problems of child's developmental delay and behavior problems and mother's chronic health problems and difficulties at work
Family problems:	Family history of hypertension and cardiovascular disease and a very strong family history of cancer.

Interpretation

From the epidemiologic and genetic points of view, the mother's risk for cardiovascular disease has inter-acted with her current risk factors of high blood pressure, diabetes, and obesity to cause heart disease. She is also at risk for malignancy, so the status of her cancer screening efforts as well as primary cancer prevention efforts is of concern. From the stress–social support perspective, the stresses of young, adopted children along with the mother's own health problems may not be buffered adequately by the support of the husband, who is a truck driver and is out of town a great deal. The presence of a confidant to support the mother is a very important area to explore. The mother's ability to care for her own health needs may be compromised by the demands of her children and the apparent lack of support.

In this situation, the family information may be central to the preventive health activities of the family physician as well as to the management of chronic medical problems. Again, the genogram reading and interpretation provide the clinician with guidance as to fruitful areas to explore during brief office visits.

REFERENCES

Bray JH, Harvey DM, Williamson DS: Intergenerational family relationships: An evaluation of theory and measurement. Psychotherapy 24:516, 1987.

Campbell TL: Family's Impact on Health: A Critical Review and Annotated Bibliography. National Institute of Mental Health Series no. 6. Department of Health and Human Services publication no. (ADM) 86-1461. Washington, DC: U.S. Department of Health and Human Services, 1986.

Lynch JJ: The Broken Heart: The Medical Consequences of Loneliness. New York, Basic Books, 1977.

Medalie JH: Family Medicine Principles and Applications. Baltimore, Williams & Wilkins, 1978.

Pauls DL, Noyes R, Crowe RR: The familial prevalence in second-degree relatives of patients with anxiety neurosis (panic disorder). J Affect Dis 1:279, 1979.

Ramsey CN: Developmental theory of families: The family life cycle. *In* Rakel RE (ed): Textbook of Family Practice. Philadelphia, WB Saunders Company, 1984, pp 41–49.

Smeraldi E, Negri F, Hembuch RC, Kidd KK: Familial patterns and possible modes of inheritance of primary affective disorders. J Affect Dis 3:173, 1981.

Smilkstein G: The cycle of family function: A conceptual model for family medicine. J Fam Pract 6:1231, 1978.

Syme SL, Berkman L: Social class, susceptibility, and sickness. Am J Epidemiol 104:1, 1976.

Warrell DA (ed): Oxford Textbook of Medicine, 2nd edition, Oxford, England, Oxford University Press, 1987, pp 4.10–4.36.

CHAPTER 3

THE FAMILY'S INFLUENCE ON HEALTH

Family Stress

THOMAS L. CAMPBELL

Family physicians are the only health care providers whose primary mission is to care for families as well as individuals. A family orientation is a core characteristic that distinguishes family physicians from other medical specialists and from general practitioners. Most family practice residency programs provide trainees with the basic skills for working with families of all ages. Research on family stress and family support has demonstrated the powerful influence of the family in health and illness (Campbell, 1986). Family physicians have a unique opportunity to detect family stresses and problems, help patients cope effectively with them, and bolster family supports.

FAMILY STRESS AND ILLNESS

Despite significant advances in our understanding of health and illness, little is known about why some people become ill while others remain healthy when exposed to the same pathogens and risk factors. Research on psychosocial factors in health has demonstrated that stress and social support can affect an individual's susceptibility to disease. This research also has shown that the family is often the most important source of both stress and social support in patients' lives (Doherty and Campbell, 1988).

Stress has become widely accepted by patients and health care professionals as influencing health. Patients often explain to their physicians that they are "under a lot of stress" and that their ulcer, back pain, or headache is "acting up." Yet, stress is difficult to define and study. One successful method for studying stress and health has been to examine the relationship of stressful life events to illness. Holmes and Rahe (1967) developed a life event scale by asking a random sample of the population to rank how stressful they perceived each of 43

common life events to be. Many retrospective and prospective studies have used this scale and shown that an increase in stressful life events precedes the development of a wide range of different diseases.

Most of the events on the Holmes and Rahe scale occur within the family, and 10 of the 15 most stressful events are family events. Because children are likely to be affected by this stress, several studies have looked at the relationship of family life events and child health. Meyer and Haggerty (1962) found that chronic stress was associated with higher rates of streptococcal pharyngitis, and that 30 per cent of the strep infections were preceded by a stressful family event. A prospective study of over 1000 preschoolers found that family life events were strongly correlated with subsequent visits to the physician and hospital admissions for a wide range of conditions. Children from families experiencing more than 12 life events during the 4-year study period were six times more likely to be hospitalized (Beautrais et al., 1982).

The death of a spouse is the most stressful common life event, and the health consequences of bereavement have been extensively studied. Census data and cross-sectional studies consistently have shown that widowers have much higher death rates from all causes than do married individuals. In prospective studies of bereavement, widowers consistently have a higher death rate when compared to matched controls, particularly during the first 6 months after the death of their wives. Widowers who remarry have lower death rates than those who do not, suggesting a protective effect of marriage on health. The effects of bereavement on women are less consistent or predictable.

Divorce or marital separation is also an extremely stressful event and is ranked second on the Holmes and Rahe scale. Several cross-sectional studies have shown that divorcées have a higher death rate from all diseases than single, widowed, or married persons. However, chronic physical illness has an adverse effect on marital satisfaction and may eventually lead to divorce. Prospective studies of divorce and health are needed to determine cause-and-effect relationships.

Recent research in psychoimmunology has suggested one of several possible biologic mechanisms for the adverse health effects of bereavement and divorce. Studies in animals and humans reveal that stress can lead to immunosuppression and an increase in illness (Kiecolt-Glaser and Glaser, 1992). Bereavement is associated with a decrease in cellular immunity (T-lymphocyte stimulation), especially in those who are clinically depressed. Divorced or separated women have significantly poorer immune function than sociodemographically matched married women (Kiecolt-Glaser et al., 1987). Among married women, poor marital quality correlates with both depression and decreased immunity. Immune function also is impaired in major depression, and researchers have suggested that changes occurring in the central nervous system during depression may be a final common pathway.

Although family stress can have harmful effects on health, family support can be beneficial. Social support can be defined as the emotional, instrumental, and financial aid that is obtained from one's social network. An extensive body of research has shown that social networks and supports can improve health directly, as well as buffer the adverse effects of stress (Cohen and Syme, 1985; Rosengren et al., 1993). Also, the family has been found to be the most important source of social support.

In a seminal study of over 6000 adults, Berkman and Syme (1979) showed that social networks were a major predictor of mortality over a 9-year period, independent of socioeconomic status, previous health status, or health practices. The most socially isolated adults had more than twice the death rate of the least isolated group. Marital status and contacts with relatives and friends were the most powerful predictors of health. Many similar studies have confirmed these results, both for healthy populations and for patients with chronic illnesses.

Studies of social supports in the elderly have shown that the relative importance of different aspects of family support may change over the life span. Older persons with impaired social supports have two to three times the death rate of those with good supports (Berkman et al., 1992). Unlike younger populations, marital status was not associated with mortality in the elderly. The presence and number of living children are the most powerful predictors of survival. This finding suggests that adult children become the most important source of social support in the elderly.

In an article in the journal *Science*, sociologist James House and his colleagues (1988) reviewed the research on social support and health and concluded:

The evidence regarding social relationships and health increasingly approximates the evidence in the 1964 Surgeon General's report that established cigarette smoking as a cause or risk factor for mortality and morbidity from a range of diseases. The age-adjusted relative risk ratios are stronger than the relative risks for all cause mortality reported for cigarette smoking. (p. 543)

Thus, social relationships deserve the same attention and study by physicians as smoking now receives.

These lines of research clearly demonstrate that family support and family stress, especially bereavement, can have a powerful influence on overall mortality. An understanding of the family and their potential sources of stress and support can provide physicians with ways to reduce family stress, bolster family supports, and improve health.

CLINICAL IMPLICATIONS

The research on family stress and health has important implications for the assessment and treatment of patients and their families. Many patients present with physical symptoms or health problems that are related to stress experienced within the family context. However, patients seldom identify family stress as a source of these symptoms. The family physician's challenge is to determine the importance of family stress during the patient's visits and to develop appropriate interventions (McDaniel et al., 1990).

To assess and treat family stress adequately, the physician must use a biopsychosocial approach and understand the family context of each patient visit. Physical symptoms or illness may result from or be exacerbated by stress. Family physicians often know the families or the family context of their patients and are aware of potential sources of family stress.

The family tree or genogram is an especially useful tool for gathering and recording information about the patient's family, including the family structure, relationship patterns, and life cycle issues, as well as the family history of genetic disorders (McGoldrick and Gerson, 1986; Chapter 2). It furnishes a visual record of the family and can provide clues to sources of family stress and dysfunction. The genogram can be particularly helpful in caring for difficult and frustrating patients with complex biomedical and psychosocial problems. For some patients, the genogram can help the patient and doctor begin a gradual shift from narrowly focusing on physical symptoms to taking a broader view of the patient's life.

Another useful approach to detecting family stress is for the physician to be alert for "red flags" that signal the need to assess psychosocial factors in more detail (Doherty and Baird, 1983). Common stress-related symptoms, such as chronic headaches, back pain, or fatigue, and unexplained or inconsistent physical signs or symptoms are often red flags. The patient's affect, the manner in which the clinical history is presented, or the family member who accompanies the patient to the visit also may be clues to the physician that there may be underlying psychosocial issues.

To manage family stresses effectively, the family physician needs to maintain a positive relationship or alliance with each family member and avoid taking sides in a family problem or conflict. Whenever families experience major stress, there is a tendency to blame one person as having the problem and to try to get others, especially the physician, to support that view. Thus patients often complain to their physician about another family member (e.g., "My daughter is using drugs," "My wife won't listen to me," or "My mother drinks too much"), hoping to get the physician's support and advice for how the family member should change. The challenge to the family physician is to acknowledge the difficulty the patient is experiencing without validating his or her view of the problem. It is easy to side inadvertently with one family member against another. Meeting with the patient and the other relevant family members can help the physician avoid taking sides in a family problem and maintain positive relationships with everyone involved.

Although many family stresses can be handled during regular visits, it is often helpful to meet with the patient and other family members, or to convene the entire family to discuss a family problem. This can be as simple as inviting a family member who has accompanied the patient into the exam room. When there are serious marital or family problems, a 30- to 45-minute family meeting is usually necessary to evaluate the situation. In these situations, either the patient or one or more other family members may be reluctant to attend a family meeting. The patient may not want the physician to hear the "other side" of the story, and the other family members may worry about being blamed by the physician for the problem. It is often helpful for the physician to discuss with the patient how to invite other family members to the office, and sometimes necessary to call the family members directly.

When meeting with a family about a problem or stressor, it is important to have a specific plan for conducting the session (McDaniel et al., 1990). Open-ended and unstructured discussions are likely to disintegrate into unproductive arguments. At the beginning of a family meeting, the physician should greet and briefly socialize with each family member, so that they feel ready to work collaboratively with the physician. Negotiating clear goals for the meeting is important early in the session. The physician needs actively to gather information

TABLE 3–1. WHEN TO REFER FAMILY PROBLEMS TO A FAMILY THERAPIST OR OTHER MENTAL HEALTH PROFESSIONAL

Problems Commonly Managed by Family Physicians Alone	Problems Commonly Referred to Mental Health Professionals
Adjustment to the diagnosis of a new illness	Suicidal or homicidal ideation or behavior
Other adjustment or situational disorders	Psychotic behavior
Child behavior problems	Sexual or physical abuse
Mild to moderate anxiety and depression	Substance abuse
Uncomplicated grief reactions	Severe depression or anxiety
	Chronic or severe marital and sexual problems

Adapted from McDaniel SH, Campbell TL, Seaburn D: Family-Oriented Primary Care: A Manual for Medical Providers. New York, Springer-Verlag, 1990, with permission.

about the problem from each person present and to facilitate discussion while blocking unproductive arguments. When there are serious family stresses and conflicts, there is a tendency to focus on problems and pathology. The physician should take an active role in identifying family strengths, resources, and previous successes that can be drawn on to deal with the current problem.

During a family meeting, the physician should work with the family members to develop a plan to address the identified problem. During this period, the physician must decide whether the problem can be managed with primary care family counseling or whether the family should be referred to a family therapist. Part of this decision will depend on the interests, expertise, and time availability of the physician. Table 3–1 lists the common problems that often can be managed solely by the family physician and those that usually are handled best by a family therapist or other mental health professional.

To care effectively for families, the family physician must establish a collaborative relationship with one or more family therapists to use as consultants. Many family problems are too complex or time-consuming for most family physicians to treat. Therapy is more likely to be successful if the physician knows the therapist well, and they can work together and communicate regularly, both at the time of referral and during treatment.

CONCLUSION

Research demonstrates that family stress and family supports have a powerful influence on the health of patients. Clinical experience shows that many physical symptoms and health problems result from stress or are exacerbated by family problems. The family physician is uniquely qualified to recognize and address the family stresses that affect patients' health. Using a biopsychosocial approach, the family physician can bridge the mind–body dualism and deal with the interactions between psychosocial and biologic processes. By evaluating the family context of each patient visit, the family physician can identify family problems and develop family interventions.

REFERENCES

Beautrais AL, Fergusson DM, Shannon FT: Life events and childhood morbidity: A prospective study. Pediatrics 70:935, 1982.

Berkman LF, Leo-Summers L, Horwitz RI: Emotional support and survival after myocardial infarction: A prospective, population-based study of the elderly. Ann Intern Med 117:1003, 1992.

Berkman LF, Syme SL: Social networks, host resistance and mortality: A nine year follow-up study of Alameda County residents. Am J Epidemiol 109:186, 1979.

Campbell TL: Family's impact on health: A critical review and annotated bibliography. Fam Syst Med 4(2&3):135, 1986.

Cohen S, Syme SL (eds): Social Support and Health. Orlando, FL, Academic Press, 1985.

Doherty WJ, Baird MA: Family Therapy and Family Medicine: Toward the Primary Care of Families. New York, Guilford Press, 1983.

Doherty WJ, Campbell TL: Families and Health (Sage Family Studies Series). Beverly Hills, CA, Sage Publications, 1988.

Holmes TH, Rahe RH: The Social Readjustment Scale. J Psychosom Res 39:413, 1967.

House JS, Landis KR, Umberson D: Social relationships and health. Science 241:540, 1988.

Kiecolt-Glaser JK, Fisher LD, Ogrockl P, et al: Marital quality, marital disruption, and immune function. Psychosom Med 49:13, 1987.

Kiecolt-Glaser JK, Glaser R: Psychoimmunity: Can psychological interventions modulate immunity? J Consult Clin Psychol 60:569, 1992.

McDaniel S, Campbell T, Seaburn D: Family-Oriented Primary Care: A Manual for Medical Providers. New York, Springer-Verlag, 1990.

McGoldrick M, Gerson S: Genograms in Family Assessment. New York, WW Norton, 1986.

Meyer RJ, Haggerty RJ: Streptococcal infections in families: Factors altering individual susceptibility. Pediatrics 29:539, 1962.

Rosengren A, Orth-Gomer K, Wedel H, Wilhelmsen L: Stressful life events, social support, and mortality in men born in 1933. BMJ 307:1102, 1993.

Impact of Divorce and Remarriage on the Family

JAMES H. BRAY

The health and well-being of all family members is greatly influenced by the process of separation, divorce, and remarriage. Marital separation and divorce are not single events, but represent a series of transitions that continue for many years. Millions of children and adults are impacted directly by the many stresses and changes caused by their families' marital transitions (Bray and Hetherington, 1993). Many families will be involved in even more changes because of multiple divorces and remarriages.

Divorce and remarriage involve a complex series of changes that often affect every aspect of family functioning. Divorce and remarriage affect parent–child relationships, parenting practices and effectiveness, family conflict, family income and residence, extended family relationships, and peer and social relationships. These changes may produce both short-term crises and long-term effects on individual family members (Bray and Hetherington, 1993).

DIVORCE

Individuals within a family may have very different *experiences* of a divorce, and these differences are important for understanding and helping them through this process. For example, a woman may be very unhappy in a marriage and psychologically divorcing her husband for years. Yet, the husband may be generally satisfied with the marriage and "shocked and surprised" when his wife tells him she wants a divorce. The children each may have different reactions and align with the mother or father during the process. Thus, by the time of the actual legal divorce, the wife may have resolved much of her grief and negative feelings, but the husband and/or some of the children may be in the middle of the emotional turmoil of the divorce process. The family physician must understand these differences to treat individual family members most effectively during these transitions.

Divorce is not necessarily "bad" for family members. Staying together in an unhappy, conflictual marriage for the "children's sake" or any other reason may not be in their best interests. Children actually adjust better in a stable divorced home than in an unhappy, highly conflictual intact home (Hetherington et al., 1978). Hetherington et al. (1978) stated that, "Our study and previous research show that a conflict-ridden intact family is more deleterious to family members than a stable home situation in which parents are divorced. Divorce is often a positive solution to destructive family functioning" (p. 34). This is not to say that divorce is always good or that it is always recommended. In fact, most research indicates that, in general, being married is associated with better outcomes and fewer health problems than being divorced or single (Kitson and Morgan, 1990).

Process of Separation and Divorce

The decision for adults to separate and ultimately divorce results in a high degree of emotional distress. During the deliberation period, prior to the separation, partners often quarrel, confront their partners with their unhappiness, and seek outside assistance from friends, ministers, primary care physicians, and marital counselors (Kelly, 1988). Many families turn to their family physician for support and assistance because the family physician is seen as someone who has unique knowledge about families. The physician's role is to decrease the psychological risks to patients, to promote healthy methods of coping with stress, to teach parents ways of relating to their children that maximize their coping, and to make appropriate referrals for additional help.

During the early stages of marital distress, patients may present with anxiety, depression, impotence, ulcers, migraines, or other psychosomatic symptoms related to the stress of living in an unhappy relationship. Common feelings include disillusionment, alienation, anger, and general dissatisfaction. Conflict may escalate between the spouses, and children may become involved as a way of deflecting the marital conflict. Later, there is likely to be withdrawal, both emotional and physical, and a "yo-yo" effect in which partners may attempt alternately to deny problems and to win the other back. Physicians should be prepared to recommend marriage counseling if patients present evidence of marital distress. In its early stages, deterioration of the relationship may be reversible, because a substantial number of couples who file for divorce do not complete the process (Bray, 1991). Early assessment, intervention, and, if necessary, referral for marriage counseling can short circuit the difficulty of a marital separation and help save the marriage. If reconciliation is not possible, counseling may allow the couple to negotiate the separation process with less distress to themselves and any children involved.

Post Divorce Families

Following the legal divorce, the family enters a phase in which they attempt to achieve a new equilibrium and stability. There are two basic child custody arrangements following a divorce, sole custody and joint custody (Bray, 1991). Sole custody is by far the most common custodial arrangement following a divorce. In the sole custody arrangement, the custodial parent retains custody of the children and the noncustodial parent has visitation with the children. There are many types of joint custody. In discussing this area, it is important to distinguish between joint legal custody and joint physical custody. The common element of the two types is that both parents retain the legal rights of a parent and have equal power and authority over their children's general welfare, education, and upbringing. With joint physical custody, both parents retain the rights, privileges, and duties of a parent and the children live with both parents on a shared basis. It is important to note that usually the custodial parent has the exclusive right to seek medical treatment for the children. This means that, without the permission of the custodial parent, the noncustodial parent can only seek medical treatment under emergency situations.

Adults' Reactions to Divorce

The first year after divorce is highly stressful for adults. Both men and women report decreases in self-esteem and feelings of loss of control, loneliness, and isolation. Adults come to physicians with complaints of fatigue and depression and general somatic complaints. These are signs that the person is having difficulty coping with the family changes.

Marital disruption is the single most powerful sociodemographic predictor of stress-related physical illness (Somers, 1979). Separated individuals have 30 per cent more acute illness and physician visits than married adults (Somers, 1979). Separated and divorced adults have the highest rates of acute medical problems, chronic medical conditions that interfere with social activity, and disability—even when age, race, and income are controlled (Verbrugge, 1979). Divorced men have increased rates of suicide and admissions to mental hospitals, increased vulnerability to minor and major physical illness, and increased risk of being victims of violence (Kitson and Morgan, 1990). Marital separation is associated with reduced qualitative and quantitative immune functioning in men and women compared with married controls (Kiecolt-Glaser et al., 1987, 1988), which may explain their increased risk of illness.

Within approximately 2 years after the divorce, most adults have adjusted to the marital breakup and have developed a new stability in their lives (Bray and Hetherington, 1993). Many people expect to recover from the effects of divorce much faster than is realistic. The physician can advise the patient to set goals for recovery that are achievable rather than overwhelming. With time, feelings of well-being increase, and most adults experience more internal control and satisfaction in life.

Effects of Divorce on Children

The process of divorce has wide-reaching influences on children. The effects vary depending on a number of factors that include sex of the child, age of the child, length of time since the divorce, postdivorce family relationships, and socioeconomic factors (Amato and Keith, 1991; Bray and Hetherington, 1993; Wallerstein and Kelly, 1980). Many studies have found that divorce is more difficult and traumatic for boys than for girls, and boys have more severe and enduring negative reactions to divorce than girls. Boys tend to develop more behavior, sex-role adjustment, and academic problems than girls, and these problems often persist for 4 to 7 years after the divorce, particularly if the custodial mother remains single. However, recent studies indicate that many of the problems exhibited by children after divorce may be present prior to the marital separation (Block et al., 1986).

Children's ages at the time of the divorce are related to the type and quality of their reactions (Bray, 1991). Table 3–2 presents children's reactions based on age groups found by various studies. It is important to point out that an individual child may have a wide range of reactions that include some or all of those problems listed in Table 3–2.

Very young children, 3 years old or less, are likely to regress in their behavior (e.g., bed wetting) and experience developmental delays (e.g., difficulty in toilet training). They are also likely to experience intensified separation anxiety when leaving the custodial parent or primary caregiver. Children at this age are highly influenced by their custodial parent and may respond to their parents' anxiety and fear by becoming upset and anxious, particularly when left at day care centers and when the noncustodial parent visits.

Preschool children, ages 4 to 6, are also likely to exhibit regressive behavior and have some developmental delays. They may be whiny and clinging. They will be more aware of and upset by the absence of a parent. Children's anxiety is influenced by their parent's feelings and they often will respond to the parents' distress rather than other situational factors. Parents often will assume the child's distress is caused by visitation of the noncustodial parent, but if the child calms down rapidly (5 to 10 minutes) after the transition from one parent to the other, then the child is most likely responding to the parents' tension and anxiety about the transition.

School-age children, ages 6 to 11, are likely to respond to the divorce with sadness, anxiety, and distress. Younger children, ages 6 to 8, usually are unable to understand the divorce process completely or separate themselves psychologically from their parents' influence and wishes. Thus, they may feel responsible for the divorce and blame themselves for the breakup of the family. Older children, ages 9 to 11, can understand more about the divorce process. Children at these ages often report frequent reconciliation fantasies. Boys are likely to have increased behavioral problems and adjustment difficulties, while girls are likely to internalize their feelings and be depressed and withdrawn. However, girls also may have an increase in behavioral problems as well.

Adolescents, ages 12 to 18, usually are able to separate themselves from their parents' divorce and not blame themselves for the breakup of the family. Anger, resentment, and hostility are common reactions to the divorce. Both boys and girls are likely to have more behavioral problems and adjustment difficulties.

It takes about 2 years for the postdivorce family to stabilize and readjust to the disruption caused by divorce. This is a time of great change, upheaval, and opportunity for the family. The first year after the divorce is characterized as a crisis period in which the family undergoes major changes and restructuring. Parenting practices change and children respond differently to their parents as the family struggles to find a new equilibrium. Parenting methods that worked prior to the divorce may not be effective after the divorce. Children, especially boys, are less compliant to their parents' discipline and parenting. Parents are less effective in their discipline, particularly custodial mothers with their sons. This decrease in effectiveness occurs for many reasons, including changes in parenting practices, parental guilt over the divorce, less structure and routine for the family, trouble coping with feelings over the divorce, and role overload. During the second year after divorce, the family usually settles down and becomes stabilized in new patterns and roles. Parenting often improves and children respond more to their custodial parent's discipline. The family phy-

TABLE 3–2. CHILDREN'S REACTIONS TO DIVORCE*

Age of Child	Reaction of Child	Expected Problems	Risk Factors	Advice to Parents
Infancy (0–3)	Perceives loss of parent	Regression and developmental delays Problems with feeding, sleeping, and toileting Irritability, excessive crying Apathy, withdrawal	Loss of caregiver Diminished capacity of custodial parent Psychological disturbance of custodial parent	Maintain predictable routines Expect normal separation anxiety to be exaggerated Support for parent caring for herself and baby Substitute care for infant if parent is seriously depressed
Preschool (3–5)	Fears of abandonment Fears loss of custodial parent Confusion	Whining, clinging, and fearful behavior Regression and developmental delays Nightmares, bewilderment, confusion, aggression Sadness, neediness, low self-esteem Denial, perfect behavior	Persistent or severe regression, nightmares, or separation anxiety Persistent encopresis with smearing Refusal of nonresident parent to visit or of resident parent to allow visits Inability of parent to enforce discipline	Both parents should tell children about divorce and what is occurring Establish daily routine Maintain consistent discipline Emphasize that children are not responsible for divorce Encourage involvement of both parents in children's lives
Early school age (6–8)	Guilt, self-blame for divorce Sense of loss Feels betrayed, rejected Confusion	Sadness, crying, depression Longing for absent parent Anger, tantrums, acting out Asks for reconciliation Increased behavior problems	Developmental arrest, no new learning Loss of interest in peers and activities Other losses—friends, pet, relatives Changes in school or teacher	Regular frequent visits by noncustodial parent Shielding from parental hostility Involvement of both parents in child's care Consistent discipline Regular school attendance
Older school age (9–11)	Can view divorce as parents' problem but needs to find blame or reason Feels shame, rejection, resentment, loneliness	Conflicting loyalties between parents Worry about custody Hostility toward one or both parents Dependency School problems Increased behavior problems	Ongoing hostility between parents Complete rejection of one parent Parents pressure child to take sides Decrease in school performance	Involvement of both parents Parents avoid blaming each other Parental honesty Defuse child's anger
Adolescence (12–18)	Concern about loss of family life Concern about own future Feels responsible for family members Anger, hostility	Immature behavior Early or late development of independence Overcloseness or competition with same-sex parent Worry about own role as sexual or marital partner	Persistent academic failure Depression and suicide threats Delinquency or promiscuity Substance abuse	Maintain parent role with child Limit involvement in parent worries Child needs peer support Maintain consistent discipline Be aware of emotional ups and downs of adolescence—may be aggravated by stress of divorce

* Adapted from Anstett and Lewis (1986), Hetherington and Camara (1984), Rae-Grant and Robson (1988), Rhyne (1986), and Wallerstein and Kelly (1980).

sician can help with a number of potential problem areas that may remain for the binuclear family.

Role of the Family Physician

The concerned physician can offer a great deal to divorcing families in the form of support and counseling. To accomplish this, physicians need a general understanding of the situation and an understanding of its particular significance to the individual patient. As noted before, people can have dramatically different *experiences* of a divorce process. Patients may not volunteer the information that they are contemplating or are involved in a divorce. They may wish to avoid embarrassment or protect their privacy, or assume such information is irrelevant to their care. Inquiry by the physician opens the door and makes it clear that such changes are important to the ongoing care of the patient. Open-ended inquiry such as, "How have things been since our last appointment?" or "How are things going at home?" are good ways to elicit information about such psychosocial changes. Once divorce has been identified, it should be noted in the chart either in the problem list or in the family genogram. If a patient presents who is already a single parent, it is important to ascertain if the patient is a single parent by choice and whether this came about by divorce, death, or other means (Anstett and Lewis, 1986). It is also important to know if the patient sees the transition to single parenthood as a positive or negative one. Questions such as "People have many reactions to a divorce; what has it been like for you and your children?" provide a way to elicit information without making biased assumptions about individual experiences.

Adults may seek medical evaluation at the time of separation and want medication for their anxiety, depression, or sleep difficulties. Physicians can assist patients going through this process by considering the role of stress and grief in their physical problems and by making patients aware of their vulnerability during this time. Educating them about the effects of stress and negative life events can normalize their experiences and help them cope with some of the physical and emotional effects of divorce.

Anstett and Lewis (1986) found that single parents unanimously agreed that physicians gave advice *without* first learning about single parenthood, and frequently *ignored* the problem altogether. The majority of single parents in their practice preferred that the physician just listen empathically, rather than give advice concerning the problems of single parenthood. Most advice was seen as superficial and not really responsive to the particular needs of the individual. A more effective approach is to be an empathic listener and to reassure patients that their feelings are a normal part of a grief process and that this process is temporary and *will change* over time.

Children may be brought to the family physician for behavior and academic problems and stress-related somatic complaints. Parents may or may not recognize the possibility that divorce-related stress is involved. The family physician has the opportunity here to act as the child's advocate. As with other family members, it is important to determine each child's unique perception of events. How each child has been informed about the divorce and what it means is critical. Wallerstein and Kelly (1980) noted that less than 10 per cent of children had any adult talk to them about the divorce. Parents may even present unrealistic stories about why one parent has left the household. Physicians should ask parents how the divorce has been presented to the children. This will also give informa-

tion about how the parents are handling it themselves.

Ideally, both parents should tell the children about the divorce and where the departing parent will be living in terms the children can understand. It should be emphasized that the parents are divorcing each other, not the children. All children need reassurance that they are not the cause of the divorce. Books about divorce are helpful for both older and younger children. Reassurances about continuity of parent–child relationships and blamelessness of the children should be reiterated throughout the divorce process.

The physician needs to be alert to signs that a child is at risk for emotional and developmental damage. Suspicion should be aroused by depression, anxiety, vague somatic complaints, fatigue and boredom, a drop in school performance, irritability, and withdrawal from parents, friends, and usual social activities. More severe problems, such as running away, promiscuity, and alcohol and drug abuse, also may indicate problems adjusting to divorce that need professional intervention (Price et al., 1983).

The physician can assist in prevention and management of problems by suggesting ways for parents to deal with their children during and after the divorce. Consistent parenting, maintaining discipline, and allowing children to express feelings should be encouraged. It should be acknowledged that effective parenting and emotional support of children may be difficult to achieve when parents feel emotionally overwhelmed and drained, because role overload is a major stress. Supportive encouragement always should include praise for the parents' concern and efforts. Patterns of behavior that suggest blurring of generational boundaries or inappropriate dependency between parent and children should be identified and discouraged. Both parents should be urged to stay involved with monitoring the children's well-being and planning for the future. The physician should discourage actions that force children to take sides between parents or require children to be message bearers between parents.

The physician can assist the child directly during office visits. The child should be allowed to express his or her feelings and perceptions about the divorce. This process can be assisted by asking how the child feels about his or her parents' divorce, and how life has changed. If misperceptions and fears are revealed, the physician can act as the child's advocate and help the parents interpret the divorce more appropriately to the child (Musty, 1983).

If the child becomes seriously ill during the divorce, the physician should encourage both parents to provide support to the child (Musty, 1983). Divorced parents of hospitalized children have been shown to need more reassurance from the hospital staff because they often feel that they or the divorce contributed to the child's illness or accident (Ahrons and Arrn, 1981). Divorced couples may carry their interpersonal hostility into the hospital to the detriment of the child's interests. The physician may have to take responsibility for coordinating communication between the parents, and encourage them to acknowledge their feelings so that they do not subvert efforts to care for the child.

Children also can develop physical and emotional problems as a way to keep their parents together. If the custodial parent constantly relies on the assistance of the noncustodial parent because he or she cannot handle the child's problems, this reinforces the child to be sick or misbehave. This indicates a lack of emotional divorce for the family. The family physician has a unique opportunity and authority to promote change in these situations through direct intervention.

STEPFAMILIES

A stepfamily is formed when an adult with children from a previous relationship remarries. Stepfamilies are quite diverse in their structure and membership. The adult with children may have been divorced, widowed, or never married. The new spouse or stepparent may or may not have been previously married and may or may not have children. The term *step* comes from the Anglo-Saxon term *steop*, which means to make an orphan or bereave (Bray and Berger, 1992). Prior to the turn of the century, most children entered a stepfamily as a result of the death of a parent (usually their mother), whereas most children now enter a stepfamily as a result of the breakup of their parents' marriage. Thus, most stepfamilies are born from a failed marriage, and they are also "instantly formed families" because of the presence of children from the beginning of the marriage.

Stepfamilies also grow through a process with predictable and unpredictable changes and stresses. Three major tasks are required for stepfamilies during the first years of remarriage: (1) integrating the stepparent into the new family and negotiating parenting of the children, (2) developing a good marital bond and relationship, and (3) integrating the noncustodial parent and his or her kinship system into the stepfamily (Bray and Berger, 1992). Parenting stepchildren is a major task and stress for couples in new stepfamilies. It is usually best if the stepparent plays a secondary parental role and supports the biological parent in disciplining the children, rather than trying to move in and take over the parental and disciplinary functions early in the remarriage. It may take from 2 to 4 years for the stepparent to be accepted as a parental figure by the children in a stepfamily. This is likely to occur faster with younger children than with older children and adolescents. Boys seem to accept a stepfather faster and more easily than girls.

Girls often have more conflict with their stepparent and have more negative relationships with their stepfathers.

It is important to understand that stepfamilies are much more complex, have more change, and are fundamentally different than first-marriage families. Accepting this continuing change, much of which is unpredictable, is one of the most difficult developmental tasks for stepfamilies (Visher and Visher, 1988). For example, it is common for remarried couples to have their weekend plans disrupted because the noncustodial parent does not pick the children up for a visitation. This constant change is a reminder that a stepfamily is not a first-marriage family, and trying to mold a stepfamily into a first-marriage family is like trying to "force a square peg into a round hole"—it just does not fit.

Effects of Remarriage on Adults and Children

During early remarriage, there is considerable stress for parents and female children (Bray and Berger, 1992). The stresses are both positive and negative. The remarriage starts a series of changes for family members. For example, positive stresses often include moving to a new and better home, having more income, and having two adults to help with the children and household. However, moves are often negatively stressful; they require developing new friends, going to new schools, and losing old friends and familiar surroundings for children. There is often conflict over parenting and deciding on household routines. The stress appears to decrease after 2 years as the family integrates and develops their own routines.

Children in stepfamilies have more behavioral problems and adjustment difficulties than children in first-marriage families. These problems vary with the age of the child. It appears that both boys and girls below the age of 9 have increased behavioral problems and that these problems decrease after about 2 years of remarriage (Hetherington, 1987). Children between the ages of 9 and 13 in stepfamilies also intially have more behavioral problems than children in first-marriage families, but girls have the most difficult time adjusting and their problems persist for longer periods after remarriage (Bray and Hetherington, 1993). The problems are somewhat different after a remarriage than after a divorce. Children tend to "act out," having more behavioral problems and conflicts with parents after a remarriage.

Role of the Family Physician

Family physicians can provide help to stepfamilies by anticipating problems and providing preventive guidance and counseling. Producing a genogram is a good way for the physician to understand the new family relationships and will contribute to a thorough history (Wood and Poole, 1983; Chapter 2). The physician should inquire about behavioral changes and symptoms for each family member, including their temporal relationship to family transitions. Because remarriage entails more change for the family, including further alteration of social and lifestyle patterns, previous adjustment problems may re-emerge or intensify after the remarriage. Family members, especially children, may experience new grief because the new marriage underscores the permanence of the divorce (Visher and Visher, 1988).

As in the case of divorce, the physician can provide support and guidance to ease the impact of these stressors. An important aspect of this guidance is to dispel some of the myths about stepfamily formation that cause families distress (Visher and Visher, 1988; Wood and Poole, 1983). These include the belief that formation of a stepfamily will bring an immediate increase in stability. Families also may believe that affection, respect, and love will occur instantly between new members, resulting in guilt, anger, and confusion when this does not occur.

The family physician also can recommend activities that will ease the transition into the new family and encourage the formation of appropriate bonds between its members. Validating and normalizing conflicting feelings will help families accept that they may feel grief, sadness, and anxiety in addition to positive feelings like hope, joy, and excitement at the new opportunities. Helping parents negotiate parenting and household responsibilities and helping the family develop their own rituals and rules can greatly facilitate adjustment within the stepfamily. The physician should encourage open communication between family members about these feelings with patients during office visits.

New emotional bonds can be supported by having the family identify common interests and shared goals or values (Wood and Poole, 1983). New and old sources of social support should be fostered by adults and children. Younger children may need help from their parents to achieve this. The physician also can provide important assistance by attending to the often-overlooked marriage bond. The new marriage is the basis of the new family, and its importance can become overshadowed by the stresses of family formation. Couples should be encouraged to take time for themselves without the children in order to renew their commitment to each other.

In the case of severe or longstanding adjustment problems, the family physician may choose to refer the family to a professional counselor. Wood and Poole (1983) recommend that physicians make a referral if there are multiple problems in the family, if there has been marital separation or family violence, if a child has repeatedly run away, or if any family members feel that the situation is hopeless. It is important to refer to a counselor who has specific experience with the problems encountered by stepfamilies.

CONCLUSION

The process of separation, divorce, and remarriage is replete with potential pitfalls, stresses, problems, *and opportunities* to make positive changes in family members' lives. Understanding the unique experiences of each family member, providing an empathic listening ear, and acknowledging the stresses and problems they are experiencing can contribute greatly to helping family members cope with these life transitions. The family physician plays an important role in this process by helping family members focus on the opportunities and options available to make a positive difference in their current lives and for their future health and well-being.

REFERENCES

Ahrons CR, Arrn S: When children from divorced families are hospitalized: Issues for staff. Health Soc Work 6:21, 1981.

Amato PR, Keith B: Parental divorce and the well-being of children: A meta-analysis. Psychol Bull 110:26, 1991.

Anstett R, Lewis B: The single parent family: How an understanding physician can help. Postgrad Med 80:137, 1986.

Block JH, Block J, Gjerde PF: The personality of children prior to divorce: A prospective study. Child Dev 57:827, 1986.

Bray JH: Psychosocial factors affecting custodial and visitation arrangements. Behav Sci Law 9:419, 1991.

Bray JH, Berger SH: Stepfamilies. *In* Procidano ME, Fisher CB (eds): Contemporary Families: A Handbook for School Professionals. New York, Teachers College Press, 1992, pp 57–79.

Bray JH, Hetherington EM: Families in transition: Introduction and overview. J Fam Psychol 7:3, 1993.

Hetherington EM: Family relations six years after divorce. *In* Pasley K, Ihinger-Tallman M (eds): Remarriage and Stepparenting Today: Current Research and Theory. New York, Guilford Press, 1987, pp 185–205.

Hetherington EM, Camara K: Families in transition: The processes of dissolution and reconstitution. *In* Parke RD (ed): Review of Child Development Research, Vol. 7: The Family. Chicago, University of Chicago Press, 1984, pp 398–439.

Hetherington EM, Cox M, Cox R: The aftermath of divorce. *In* Stevens JH, Mathews M (eds): Mother-Child, Father-Child Relations. Washington, DC: NAEYC, 1978, pp 30–45.

Kelly JB: Longer-term adjustment in children of divorce. J Fam Psychol 2:119, 1988.

Kiecolt-Glaser JK, Fisher LD, Ogrocki P, et al: Marital quality, marital disruption, and immune function. Psychosom Med 49:13, 1987.

Kiecolt-Glaser JK, Kennedy S, Malkoff S, et al: Marital discord and immunity in males. Psychosom Med 50:213, 1988.

Kitson GC, Morgan LA: The multiple consequences of divorce: A decade review. J Marriage Fam 52:913, 1990.

Musty TA: Divorce in medical practice: Helping patients through the process. Ariz Med 6:392, 1983.

Price WA, Shorokey JJ, Enyeart JJ: Children of divorce: Counseling guidelines for the primary care physician. Postgrad Med 74:93, 1983.

Rae-Grant Q, Robson BE: Moderating the morbidity of divorce. Can J Psychiatry 33:443, 1988.

Rhyne MC: Understanding and supporting families in the process of divorce. Nurse Pract 11(12):37, 1986.

Somers AR: Marital status, health, and the use of health services. JAMA 241:1818, 1979.

Verbrugge LM: Marital status and health. J Marriage Fam 41:267, 1979.

Visher EB, Visher JS: Old Loyalties, New Ties: Therapeutic Strategies with Stepfamilies. New York, Brunner/Mazel, 1988.

Wallerstein JS, Kelly J: Surviving the Break-Up: How Children and Parents Cope with Divorce. New York, Basic Books, 1980.

Wood LE, Poole SR: Stepfamilies in family practice. J Fam Pract 16:739, 1983.

CHAPTER 4

PSYCHOSOCIAL INFLUENCES ON HEALTH

GABRIEL SMILKSTEIN

The earliest texts known to medical historians postulate psychosocial influences on health. In the three mainstreams of ancient medical practice, Chinese, South Asian, and Mediterranean, references are made to the negative influences on health of envy, fear, anger, grief, and other emotions (Caudill, 1976; Gould, 1972; Leslie, 1976). It was not until the 20th century, however, that scientific scrutiny was applied to the effects of emotions on health outcome.

Dunbar (1954), who coined the label "psychosomatic," identified a number of disease states she related to life's stressors. Empirical studies of other investigators in the field of psychosomatics confirmed Dunbar's findings. Associations were established between anxiety-like emotional states and such diseases as colitis (Wolf and Wolff, 1947) cardiovascular disease (Wolff, 1950), asthma (Ziegler and Elliott, 1926), and dermatitis (Bernstein, 1938). However, in the absence of knowledge of the physiological mechanisms by which emotional responses could be translated into physical pathology, acceptance of psychosomatic theory remained limited.

Although Cannon (1928) and Selye (1946; Selye and Fortier, 1950) published seminal research on the relationship of emotions to the neuroendocrine system, it was not until the second half of the 20th century that the sciences of psychoneuroimmunology and psychoneuroendocrinology truly flourished. Ader et al. (1991) collated studies that support the hypothesis that life's stressors generate emotional responses that trigger hypothalamic and pituitary mediators that initiate endocrinological and immunological mechanisms that alter physiologic homeostasis.

Many animal and human studies now indicate that stressor-induced anxiety has significant impact on an individual's endocrine and immune systems (Ader, 1992; Ader et al., 1991; Azad et al., 1991; Borysenko and Borysenko, 1982; Calabrese et al., 1987; Coe, 1993; Cunnick et al., 1992; Dorian and Garfinkel, 1987; Hall, 1989; Locke, 1982; O'Donnell et al., 1987; Schliefer et al., 1983). Individuals so affected will be more likely to experience adverse health outcomes with such problems

as heart disease (Brodsky et al., 1987; Gorbin et al., 1993; Medalie and Goldbort, 1976; Ruberman, 1992; Siltanen, 1987), infectious disease (Dorian and Garfinkel, 1987; Loria and Padgett, 1992; Schmidt and Schmidt, 1991; Sternberg et al., 1992), cancer (Baltrusch et al., 1992; Riley, 1981; Zonderman et al., 1989), and asthma (Lehrer et al., 1993; Sibbald et al., 1988).

The clinical application of knowledge of psychosocial influences on health is captured in the biopsychosocial model (Engel, 1977, 1980). This model is structured on historical and scientific evidence that suggests that every health problem should be assessed on the basis of both biomedical and psychosocial risks (Girard et al., 1985; Levi, 1979). Pragmatic constraints, however, limit a physician to the data that will most appropriately address a patient's health problem. Thus, although a physician must be alert to the cues and clues that suggest both biomedical and psychosocial risk factors, success in the use of the biopsychosocial model requires weighing of the evidence obtained in a clinical encounter. The physician who is sensitive to biomedical and psychosocial risks as factors in health outcome will choose a balanced assessment and therapy approach that will best meet the needs of the patient and physician.

According to Engel (1980), a physician's understanding of the stabilizing and destabilizing events and relationships in the life of a patient is central to the successful application of the biopsychosocial model in health care. In this chapter, stabilizing and destabilizing forces are equated with social support resources and emotional stressors, respectively (Smilkstein, 1983). This chapter acknowledges the relationship, but the focus will be on giving the reader an understanding of psychosocial risk—how it is assessed, and how it is managed in a primary care setting.

A CYCLE OF PSYCHOSOCIAL RISK: AN ASSESSMENT MODEL

A model is needed that forms into a cohesive unit the components that contribute to psychoso-

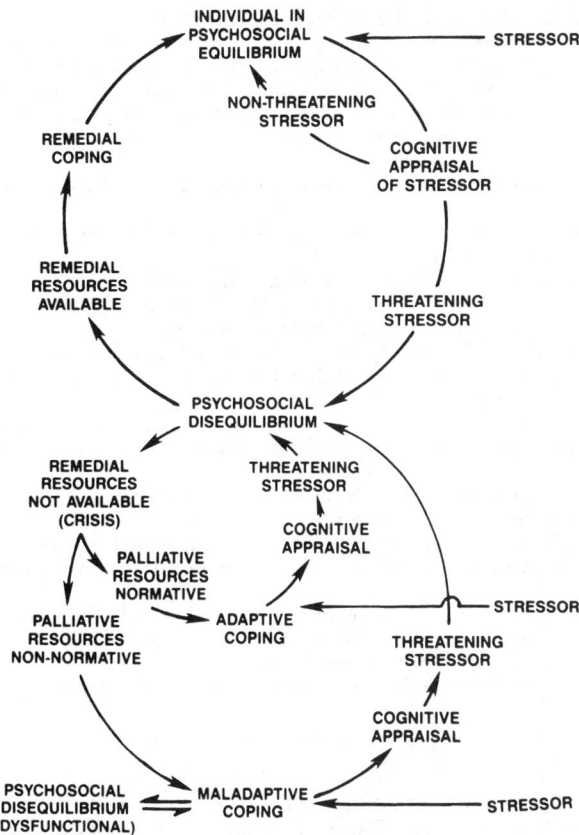

FIGURE 4–1. Cycle of psychosocial risk.

coping strategies. A definition of terms used in the cycle is given in Table 4–1.

The Upper Cycle: Stressor Resolution

Multiple stressors impact on an individual's psyche each day (Dohrenwend and Dohrenwend, 1984; Hinkle, 1973). These stressors are received and processed, and a response is generated that reflects the individual's cognitive appraisal of the stressor (Lazarus and Folkman, 1984). Cognitive appraisal is influenced by many factors. Among these factors are the individual's psychosocial equilibrium at the time the stressor is received, the individual's past experience with similar stressors, the number and intensity of other stressors being processed by the individual, and the perceived threat to relationships and self-esteem (Lazarus et al., 1974).

Not all stressors stimulate an alarm reaction. Cognitive appraisal may result in a view of the stressor as nonthreatening. This response usually occurs when past experience with the stressor has been favorable, and when resources are deemed to be available. Nonstressful experiences will not alter psychosocial equilibrium significantly (Holmes and Rahe, 1967; Masuda and Holmes, 1978).

However, if the stressors are perceived as threatening (based on past experience or knowledge that needed resources may not be available), the individual moves into a state of psychosocial disequilibrium (Cassel, 1974; Pearlin et al., 1981). Because of the "dis-ease" associated with psychosocial disequilibrium, resources are sought to neutralize or buffer the stressor (Cobb, 1976). A number of psychosocial resource categories have been identified—social, cultural, religious, educational, economic, environmental, and medical (Smilkstein, 1983). Of these, social support from family members, friends, and work supervisors appears to be the most influential in altering psychosocial risk (Cassel, 1976; Cohen et al., 1986). If resources are available and remedial coping strategies are employed, the individual usually will experience stressor resolution and a return to psychosocial equilibrium.

The Lower Cycle: Unresolved Stressors

The downward spiral in the cycle occurs when individuals experience threatening psychosocial stressors and find their resources or coping mechanisms inadequate for stressor resolution (Shonkoff, 1985; Thoits, 1986). An inability to identify or utilize the resources needed to solve a problem results in a crisis state (Baldwin, 1978). Crisis is usually associated with anxiety (Spielberger, 1972). This concept of anxiety as an outcome of crisis or

cial risk. A cyclic model of psychosocial risk will be presented that displays emotional responses reported to occur when an individual perceives a life experience as a stressor (Fig. 4–1). The purpose of the model is to facilitate an understanding of the forces that influence the relationship between psychosocial risk and health.

The fundamental structure of this model is drawn from the Cycle of Family Function, which offers a conceptual framework for viewing the responses of a family when it experiences a stressful life event (Smilkstein, 1980). Although the Cycle of Family Function was built on the contributions of many social scientists, Hill's (1965) studies of families under stress were seminal for this paper. Hill's ABCX formula offered the following conceptual framework: "A (the event); interacting with B (the family's crisis-meeting resources); interacting with C (the definition the family makes of the event); produces X (the crisis)." In this paper, Hill's formula is interpreted as a stressor–resources interaction (modified by idiosyncratic coping mechanisms), producing a qualitatively predictable alteration in an individual's emotional homeostasis.

This model focuses on an individual's response to life stressors and demonstrates how an individual's psychosocial equilibrium may be influenced by an interaction of stressors, social support, and

TABLE 4–1. DEFINITION OF TERMS FROM THE CYCLE OF PSYCHOSOCIAL RISK

Stressors	A stressor is a life experience that may disrupt or endanger an individual's personal and social values and relationships. (This definition is in accordance with Selye's language of stress, in which the noxious stimulating condition or stressor has the potential for producing emotional disequilibrium or stress.) Stressors are divided into two categories: (1) life change events and (2) role strains or chronic life situations.
Psychosocial equilibrium	A state of psychologic homeostasis in which resources are available to meet the routine challenges of life's stressors.
Cognitive appraisal	The process by which an individual evaluates a life event or role strain in terms of the impact of the experience on his or her emotional and social integrity.
Threatening stressor	A life event or role strain that represents a danger or challenge to a relationship or self-esteem.
Psychosocial disequilibrium	A state of impaired emotional and social functioning that occurs when an individual's resources are inadequate or unavailable to meet an intense stressor or an accumulation of stressors.
Resources, social support	Those assets that serve to nurture an individual and that supply the means for solving stressor-induced problems. Resources fall into the general categories of social, cultural, religious, economic, educational, environmental, and medical support systems.
Remedial coping	The process by which an individual uses resources and adaptive strategies to maintain some degree of psychosocial function when resources are inadequate or not available to solve a stressor-induced problem.
Crisis	A state of emotional disequilibrium, usually becoming manifest by anxiety that results from the failure of an individual to identify or use resources to resolve a stressor-induced problem.
Maladaptive coping	The use of pathologic defense mechanisms to escape from an unresolved crisis, resulting in a state of impaired emotional and social functioning. In a medical setting, the most commonly seen pathologic defenses are projection and somatization.
Chronic psychosocial disequilibrium	A state of emotional and social dysfunction, usually becoming manifest by an individual's inability to cope with life's responsibilities, such as work, home, or school. The dysfunctional state is characterized by responses such as depression, panic attacks, and disabling somatization.

emotional disequilibrium is of central importance, because studies have shown that anxiety is the primary emotional mediator of neuroendocrinologic and neuroimmunologic system changes that alter health outcome (Ader and Cohen, 1975; Borysenko and Borysenko, 1982; Stein et al., 1976).

In the absence of problem-solving resources, individuals choose some form of palliative coping to obtain relief from anxiety and to maintain ongoing function. Some individuals temporize and gain release from the emotional tensions induced by an unresolved stressor through activities such as taking time out, physical exercise, and relaxation through behavior modification (Kobosa et al., 1982; Martin and Coates, 1987). These palliative coping techniques permit transient equilibrium and modified function in the face of an unresolved stressor. A host of psychological defense mechanisms may be used on a short-term basis to bide time while seeking resources to manage the stressor. Avoidance, denial, projection, and somatization are examples of psychological defense mechanisms that may be employed to gain relief from the pressure of an unresolved, anxiety-producing stressor.

Not all stressors are resolvable. For example, after the death of a spouse, there is a period of bereavement with its concomitant psychological disequilibrium and dysfunction, yet individuals find it necessary to get on with life. In general, those who return to psychological equilibrium the soonest are those who have social support and use "mature" coping strategies (Walker et al., 1977). Some of the "mature" strategies used for both remedial and palliative coping are altruism, anticipa-

tion, humor, resource sharing, role adjustment, sublimation, and time out (Smilkstein, 1985).

Knowledge of a patient's social support, coping strategies, and stressors will enhance the physician's ability to understand an individual's psychosocial risk, but the idiosyncratic effect of personal resources also must be considered when assessing the quality of a patient's ability to manage stressors. Kobosa and colleagues (1982) applied the term "hardiness" to the subjects in their studies who demonstrated a low incidence of illness in the face of high stress. The developmental history of hardiness has not been elaborated; however, individuals so labeled have been characterized as having (1) a greater sense of control over what occurs in their lives, (2) a feeling of commitment to the various activities in which they are engaged, (3) a view of change as a challenge rather than a threat, and (4) a sense of a meaningfulness to their lives. It is likely that hardiness reflects past successes in employing resources to overcome life stressors. A postulate that needs examination is that hardiness will erode if an individual experiences a series of coping failures as a result of unresolvable stressors and the loss of social support.

The Lower Cycle: Long-Term Maladaptive Psychosocial Equilibrium

When stressors present an overwhelming threat or become chronic, individuals seek long-term defense strategies to modify anxiety. That is, individuals use strategies that permit them to retain self-esteem and maintain relationships, even though their function in assigned roles may be impaired (Bowden, 1983).

The strategies chosen to address anxiety-provoking stressors may be consciously planned, initiated with only partial awareness, or generated from an unconscious level. Although many psychological defense mechanisms may be seen in a health care setting, the ones with somatic manifestations attract the most interest. Two of the more frequently encountered are projection and somatization (Ford, 1983).

Projection is most commonly seen in families. A child with a health problem may become the identified patient onto whom the unresolved family problems are transferred. The greater the number and intensity of the family stressors, the more likely the child is to appear in the clinic and hospital (Beautrais et al., 1982). In contrast, families rated as functionally intact have significantly fewer visits to health care professionals (Pratt, 1976; Smilkstein, 1984).

Somatization occurs when an individual consciously or unconsciously employs physical symptoms to address the anxiety of an unresolved stressor. The physical symptoms usually are associated with an existing health problem, but they also may be related to a past personal or family experience with illness or physical disability (Mechanic, 1972; Rosen et al., 1982). Somatization in one of its many forms (such as chronic low back pain) is among the most common problems seen by physicians (Nachemson, 1984). Somatization is an expedient defense mechanism because it places individuals in the sick role, and individuals who are granted the sick role usually are released from responsibilities associated with work, school, and home. Furthermore, they also are permitted to be cared for by others (Parsons, 1958).

A DYNAMIC MODEL

The Cycle of Psychosocial Risk represents pathways that may be followed as an individual strives for emotional homeostasis. The dynamic nature of the cycle reflects the ever-changing pressures of unresolved stressors and the impact of new stressors, and changes in the quality, quantity, and availability of resources.

If and when new resources for coping are discovered, the individual can be expected to cycle upward to a higher level of functional equilibrium. At other times, when the number and intensity of stressors increase, a resource-poor person may move from long-term maladaptive coping into the dysfunctional state of chronic disequilibrium. Those who move into this category usually are unable to carry on tasks of daily living. Major therapeutic intervention usually is required to bring individuals out of chronic disequilibrium and into the emotional homeostasis that is required for positive functioning both as an individual and with family, friends, and community.

CLINICAL APPLICATIONS

The physician who is receptive to psychosocial cues and willing to intervene should establish dual therapeutic goals. The first should be to offer short-term symptomatic relief from the disabling anxiety that usually is associated with psychosocial disequilibrium. Such relief from anxiety may be obtained with the use of palliative coping techniques. These include supportive interventions such as the ancient art of listening to the patient as well as instructing the patient in health-promoting activities (exercise, regular sleep, and balanced diet) (Fordyce, 1976). Because the impact of stressors on the patient may be buffered by social support, the patient should be counseled to seek aid from family and friends, but assessment of the quality of the patient's social support also is needed. Although family and friends usually are recognized as the first line of social support, the quality of these resources must be investigated, because family and friends also may be the source of stress for the patient. In addition, psychotropic medication should be prescribed when needed to augment the above program.

A companion therapeutic goal should be long-term problem resolution or remedial coping. This activity requires the identification and assessment of stressors such as life change events and role strains (chronic life situations) (Pearlin and Johnson, 1977).

To help the patient achieve an adequate level of remedial coping ability, the physician's challenge is to determine the resources that will help the patient manage stressors. Figure 4–2 is a biopsychosocial computational model that can be used to make an empirical determination of health outcome. The psychosocial risk portion of the equation demonstrates an interactive relationship between stressors and resources (Sarason et al., 1985). For example, psychosocial risk is heightened when there is an increase in stressors (numerator) and a decrease in resources (denominator). This simple arithmetic model can be applied in routine practice situations. Support for application

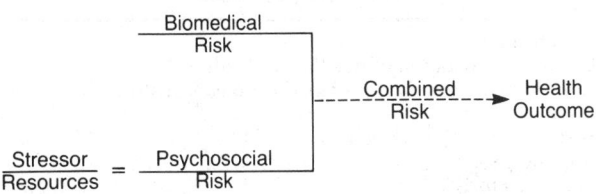

FIGURE 4–2. A biopsychosocial model for predicting health outcome.

TABLE 4–2. EXAMPLES OF OVERT CUES OF PSYCHOSOCIAL DISEQUILIBRIUM OR MALADAPTATION

Depression	Family member abuse
Panic attacks	(child, spouse, elder)
History of alcohol or substance	Delinquency
abuse	Running away
Sexual dysfunction	School behavior problem
Divorce/separation	School failure
Incest	

of this model can be found in health outcome studies that have examined such health problems as complications of pregnancy (Pagel et al., 1990; Reeb et al., 1987; Smilkstein et al., 1984) and cardiovascular disease (Haynes et al., 1980; Medalie and Goldbourt, 1976).

How does a physician identify the patient whose health problem indicates that assessment of psychosocial risk is appropriate? Because, in this cyclic model, psychosocial risk relates primarily to emotional disequilibrium caused by a rise in stressor intensity or a loss of social support, or both, a physician must be attitudinally prepared to recognize emotional disequilibrium. To do this, the physician must be able to receive cues from patients that reflect psychosocial risk. Tables 4–2 and 4–3 list examples of overt and covert cues that suggest significant disturbances in the patient's psychosocial equilibrium.

Application of the Biopsychosocial Model

When the patient presents with both biomedical and psychosocial risks, rational responses are necessary. The medical, economic, and temporal resources of the patient, physician, and health system must be used appropriately and frugally if the biopsychosocial approach to health care is to be accepted. Present medical training and practice highlight biomedical factors so strongly that iatrogenic reinforcement of a patient's somatization frequently occurs. This problem, which has been labeled as "somatic fixation" (Van Eijk et al., 1983),

TABLE 4–3. EXAMPLES OF COVERT CUES OF PSYCHOSOCIAL DISEQUILIBRIUM OR MALADAPTATION

Somatization
Excessive utilization of health care facilities
Noncompliance with use of medications or instructions for self-care
History of multiple surgeries
Chronic pain
Failure to thrive
Recurrent childhood poisonings
Shopping for different physicians

is the process by which a patient becomes locked into a physical problem with the support of a physician who pursues a patient's persistent or exaggerated physical symptoms through an escalation of laboratory tests, office visits, and consultations. It is true that good medical practice requires a relevant pursuit of persistent or exaggerated physical symptoms with follow-up visits, objective studies, and second opinions. A study of physicians involved in "somatic fixation," however, suggests that their patients would have experienced emotional and economic benefits if psychosocial risks had been examined along with biomedical risk.

Case Discussion

Figure 4–3 illustrates psychosocial risk assessment applied to a case study using the Cycle of Psychosocial Risk. The psychosocial risk assessment was carried out in harmony with biomedical studies. The dynamically interrelated components revealed by this assessment can be observed by following the Cycle of Psychosocial Risk pathways.

The patient initially reported anxiety due to chest pain. He admitted to a fear that chest pain was associated with heart problems and death. The physician also learned that within the last year the patient had experienced a series of stressful life events that challenged his emotional homeostasis—a major move, a painful divorce, and a new job. The job was a daily hassle because of conflicts with the boss and the patient's concern regarding the adequacy of his job performance.

Life change events, such as those experienced by the patient in this case study, have been studied extensively over the past 30 years. This research has established that life change events are significantly associated with adverse health outcomes such as cardiovascular disease (Ostfeld et al., 1985). Such findings emphasize the value of a biopsychosocial approach, especially when anxiety is expressed along with the presenting complaint.

Although all life events have an impact on a patient's psychosocial equilibrium, negative life experiences seem to cause the most intense responses (Sarason et al., 1978). These include loss of relationships (especially of family members and friends), loss of self-esteem, loss of or decrease in body function, major economic reversals, and change of home site (Masuda and Holmes, 1978). Identification of high-impact stressors is important, but the physician also should seek to identify other life change events that may be troubling the patient, because in some patients it will be a "pile-up" of life change events that causes emotional disequilibrium (Patterson, 1988).

The second category of stressors that contributes to psychosocial risk includes role strains or chronic life situations associated with an individual's position as a parent, friend, patient, employee, student, or member of a family or group (Pearlin and John-

CASE HISTORY: A 35-year-old, white, divorced, male computer scientist, who recently moved to a new city, reported to his physician the recent onset of chest pain and anxiety. Psychosocial assessment is shown below following the pathways of the Cycle of Psychosocial Risk. Biomedical assessment, which was also completed by his physician, did not reveal any organic pathology.

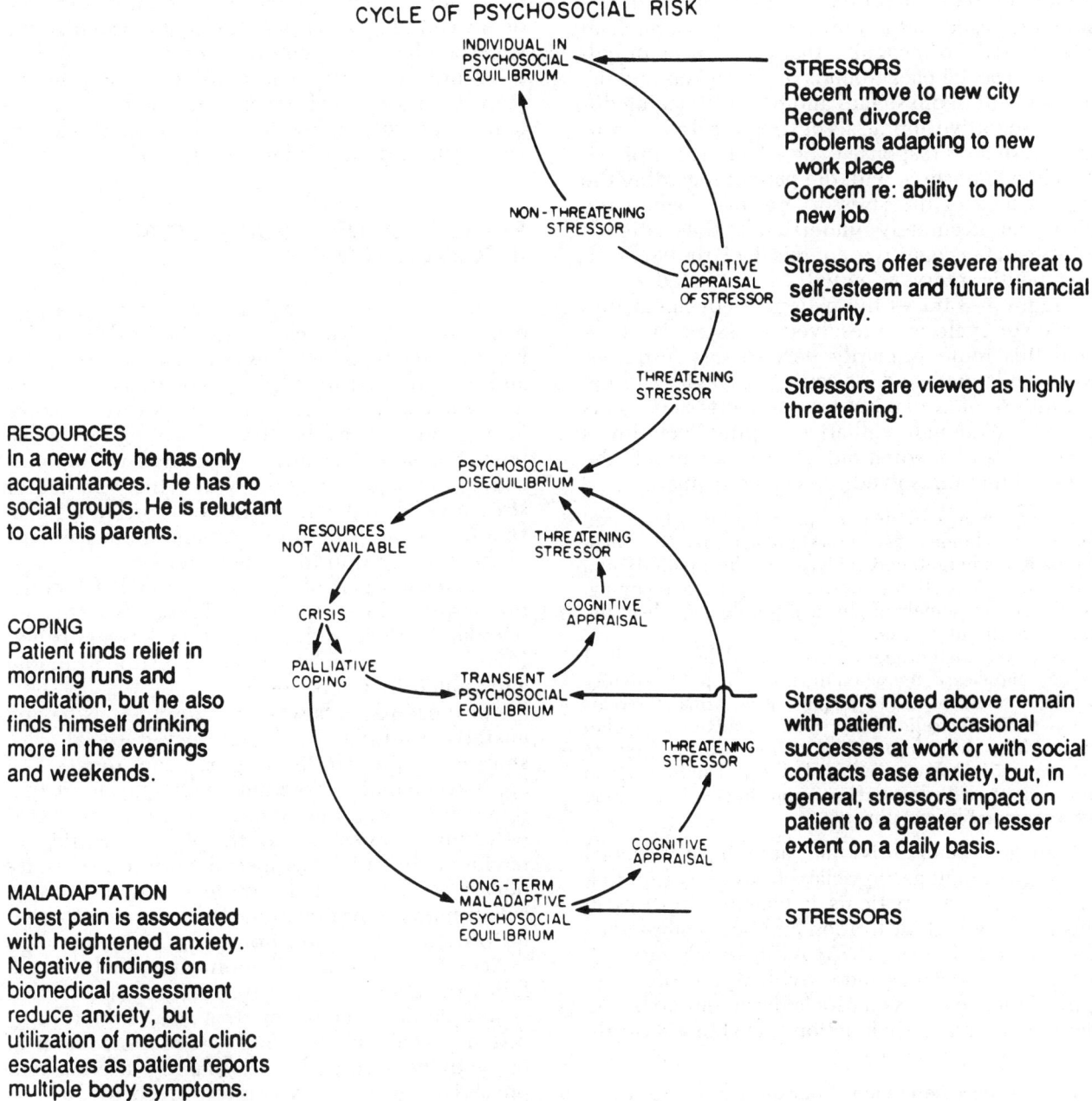

CYCLE OF PSYCHOSOCIAL RISK

INDIVIDUAL IN PSYCHOSOCIAL EQUILIBRIUM

STRESSORS
Recent move to new city
Recent divorce
Problems adapting to new work place
Concern re: ability to hold new job

NON-THREATENING STRESSOR

COGNITIVE APPRAISAL OF STRESSOR

Stressors offer severe threat to self-esteem and future financial security.

THREATENING STRESSOR

Stressors are viewed as highly threatening.

RESOURCES
In a new city he has only acquaintances. He has no social groups. He is reluctant to call his parents.

PSYCHOSOCIAL DISEQUILIBRIUM

RESOURCES NOT AVAILABLE

THREATENING STRESSOR

CRISIS

COGNITIVE APPRAISAL

COPING
Patient finds relief in morning runs and meditation, but he also finds himself drinking more in the evenings and weekends.

PALLIATIVE COPING

TRANSIENT PSYCHOSOCIAL EQUILIBRIUM

THREATENING STRESSOR

Stressors noted above remain with patient. Occasional successes at work or with social contacts ease anxiety, but, in general, stressors impact on patient to a greater or lesser extent on a daily basis.

COGNITIVE APPRAISAL

MALADAPTATION
Chest pain is associated with heightened anxiety. Negative findings on biomedical assessment reduce anxiety, but utilization of medical clinic escalates as patient reports multiple body symptoms.

LONG-TERM MALADAPTIVE PSYCHOSOCIAL EQUILIBRIUM

STRESSORS

FIGURE 4–3. Psychosocial stressors and resources are given empiric values so that psychosocial risk may be calculated. The interactive effect of biomedical and psychosocial risk yields a combined risk. Knowledge of a combined risk enhances the physician's ability to predict health outcome.

son, 1977). Conflicts in role relationships, such as with one's boss, may challenge an individual's psychosocial equilibrium severely and have a negative impact on health (Hamburg and Killilea, 1979).

The physician who is able to identify role strains and stressful life events that contribute to a patient's maladaptive behavior is in a position to combine biomedical and psychosocial interventions to the patient's advantage. In all psychosocial risk studies, however, it is not enough to identify stressors. The physician also must assess the significance of stressors to the patient (Eisenberg and Kleinman, 1981; Kleinman and Smilkstein, 1980). This is perhaps the most problematic aspect of psychosocial assessment because physicians often assume they understand the intensity of a patient's stressors based on their own experiences. Such an attitude fails to recognize that differences in cultural and social backgrounds of physicians and patients result in physicians and patients making different cognitive appraisals of stressors. In order for the physician's response to be effective, the physician need not agree with the patient regarding the significance of the stressor; however, when the physician accurately understands the patient's idiosyncratic cognitive appraisal of the stressor, therapeutic intervention will be facilitated.

Figure 4–3 traces the patient's movement into the lower cycle of unresolved stressors. He traveled this route primarily because his resources were inadequate and his coping strategies did not permit use of available social support, such as his parents. Although palliative coping techniques (exercise and meditation) gave some relief, the strain of the unresolved stressors remained.

The appearance of the chest pain significantly altered the patient's homeostasis. As a somatic representation of the patient's heightened anxiety, the chest pain denied the patient the option of exercise for palliative coping. However, the perceived physical problem did lead the patient to the physician.

The physician thoroughly investigated the biomedical aspects of the case, but when the physical and laboratory findings were reported to the patient as normal, the reassurance did not relieve the patient's anxiety. Psychotropic drugs were prescribed to relieve this anxiety; however, the physician's records showed an increase in office visits, with the patient reporting early morning wakening and loss of appetite.

Management of individuals at high psychosocial risk is challenging. Physicians frequently find that the care of these patients is characterized, as in this case, by high utilization and poor compliance (Becker and Maiman, 1975). As stress takes its toll, depression becomes more evident and often requires intense biopsychosocial intervention by the physician to maintain function and, at times, to prevent suicide.

When it became evident from the psychosocial risk assessment that this patient's anxiety and depression were a major problem, interventions based on the cyclic model were designed. These included interventions that specifically addressed components of the cyclic model, such as regular scheduled office visits to the physician, listening time by the physician to identify work and home problems, reassurance regarding the patient's heart status, and counseling to encourage use of support from family and friends.

After the biopsychosocial therapeutic interventions were initiated by the physician, changes were observed in the patient that suggested improvement. He identi-fied a few individuals in the community with whom he shared common interests. He realistically examined his stressors to determine whether they were resolvable, and he voluntarily discontinued his psychotropic drugs and decreased the number of his office visits.

In general, as clarified by the cyclic model, movement toward psychosocial equilibrium can be measured by a patient's ability to recognize the stressors that are jeopardizing emotional stability, to identify resources and employ them appropriately, to move away from drug and physician assistance, and to employ coping strategies that advance physical and emotional health.

PRINCIPLES OF PSYCHOSOCIAL INTERVENTION

The physician who wishes to identify the psychosocial risks that may influence health care or health outcome must assess the patient's stressors and resources (Hinkle, 1987). The process is initiated when a cue suggests overt or covert evidence for psychosocial dysfunction. A willingness to listen to the patient usually will facilitate the identification of major stressors. Once the stressor or stressors have been identified, the physician should ask the patient to estimate the importance of the stressor(s) in his or her life.

The second part of the psychosocial risk equation requires the assessment of resources. It is not enough to establish that the patient has family and friends. The resource person(s) must be available and valued by the patient.

For those patients who are identified as having anxiety resulting from high psychosocial risk, short-term intervention requires consideration of appropriate medications and techniques for palliative coping (e.g., time out, aerobic exercises, and behavior modification). In the office or clinic, behavior modification has special merit. If continuity of care can be effected, wellness activities can be substituted for dysfunctional behavior such as high utilization and somatization.

An outline of behavior modification includes the following agenda: physical activity is chosen that is acceptable to the patient (e.g., walking); time or distance goals, or both, are set; reinforcement of the activity is carried out by family, friends, and physician; and the activity is rehearsed, monitored, and shaped to advance the patient's performance and improve the patient's self-esteem. Central to the success of behavior modification is the identification of appropriate goals and the encouragement given by the patient's social support system (Martin and Coates, 1987).

The quality of social support may be the single most important assessment in the evaluation of psychosocial risk in an individual who is experiencing life's stressors. Much has been written about the significant role social support plays in relation to an individual's health (Dean and Lin, 1977; Sarason et al., 1985). For example, Ruberman et al. (1984) reported that patients who are socially isolated and having a high degree of life stressors had four times the risk of death as those with good social support. Impaired social support also has been related to cardiovascular disease morbidity (Bland et al., 1991; Helgeson, 1991; Medalie and Goldbourt, 1976; Orth-Gomer et al., 1993).

Social support may be ascertained in a clinical encounter by asking the patient, "When you have a personal problem, to whom do you turn for help?" The question regarding social support usually will follow a patient's report of a life stressor. In this situation, another question that might follow is, "With whom can you discuss your problem?" The patient's response usually will indicate to the clinician the availability and quality of social support.

Whenever possible, remedial coping should be the long-range goal of the physician–patient partnership. This long-term intervention requires identification of resources that may be directed toward the management of anxiety-producing stressors (e.g., social support person(s), use of counseling, educational programs, social agencies, and psychotherapy).

Physicians should recognize that they are major resources in the treatment of patients at psychosocial risk. Even with optimal physician assistance, high-risk patients with poor social support, whose lives are characterized by an accumulation of high-intensity stressors, frequently experience an accentuation of physical and emotional health problems. The most effective treatment for such patients may be long-term, supportive therapy. This therapy involves three strategies: (1) offering regular appointments at which time positive feedback is given to bolster self-esteem (usually focusing on behavior modification); (2) addressing stressors as contributors to illness problems; and (3) searching for new resources at each patient encounter.

REFERENCES

Ader R: On the clinical relevence of psychneuroimmunology. Clin Immunol Immunopathol 64:6, 1992.

Ader R, and Cohen N: Behaviorally conditioned immunosuppression. Psychosom Med 37:333, 1975.

Ader R, Felton DL, Cohen N (eds): Psychoneuroimmunology, 2nd edition. San Diego, Academic Press, 1991.

Azad N, Agrawal L, Emanuele MA, et al: Neuroimmunoendocrinology: Current trends. Am J Reprod Immunol 26:160, 1991.

Baldwin BA: A paradigm for the classification of emotional crisis: Implications for crisis intervention. Am J Orthopsychiatry, 48:438, 1978.

Baltrusch HJF, Gehde E, Titze I, Heinze HJ: Early socialization and development of cancer in later life: Biopsychosocial and psychoneuroimmunologic aspects. Ann N Y Acad Sci 650:355, 1992.

Beautrais AL, Fergusson BA, and Shannon FT: Life events and childhood morbidity: A prospective study. Pediatrics 70:935, 1982.

Becker MH, and Maiman LA: Sociobehavioral determinations of compliance with health care recommendations. Med Care 13:10–14, 1975. Bernstein ET: Skin disease from an emotional standpoint. Int Clin 1:155, 1938.

Bland SH, Krogh V, Winkelstein W, Trevisan M: Social network and blood pressure: A population study. Psychosom Med 53:598, 1991.

Borysenko M, Borysenko J: Stress, behavior and immunity: Animal models and mediating mechanisms. Gen Hosp Psychiatry 4:49, 1982.

Bowden CL: Anxiety defenses and adaptation. *In* Bowden CL, Burstein AG (eds): Psychosocial Basis of Health Care, 3rd edition. Baltimore, Williams & Wilkins, 1983.

Brodsky MA, Sato AA, Iseri LT, et al: Ventricular tachyarrhythmia associated with psychological stress: The role of the sympathetic nervous system. JAMA 257:2064, 1987.

Calabrese JR, Kling MA, Gold PW: Alterations in immunocompetence during stress, bereavement and depression: Focus on neuroendocrine regulation. Am J Psychiatry 144:1123, 1987.

Cannon WB: The mechanism of emotional disturbance of bodily functions. N Engl J Med 198:877, 1928.

Cassel JC: Psychosocial processes and stress: A theoretical formulation. Int Health Serv 3:471, 1974.

Cassel J: The contributions of social environments to host resistance. Am J Epidemiol 104:107, 1976.

Caudill W: The cultural and interpersonal context of everyday health and illness in Japan and America. *In* Leslie C (ed): Asian Medical Systems: A Comparative Study. Berkeley, University of California Press, 1976, p 161.

Cobb S: Social support as a moderator of life stress. Psychosom Med 38:300, 1976.

Coe CL: Psychosocial factors and immunity in nonhuman primates: A review. Psychosom Med 55:298, 1993.

Cohen S, Sherrod DR, Clark MS: Social skills and the stress-protection role of social support. J Pers Soc Psychol 50:963, 1986.

Cunnick JE, Lysle DT, Kucinski BJ, Rabin BS: Stress-induced alterations in immune function: Diversity of effects and mechanisms. Ann NY Acad Sci 650:283, 1992.

Dean A, Lin N: The stress-buffering role of social support. J Nerv Ment Dis 165:403, 1977.

Dohrenwend BS, Dohrenwend, BP: Stressful Life Events and Their Contexts. New Brunswick, NJ, Rutgers University Press, 1984.

Dorian B, Garfinkel PE: Stress, immunity and illness—a review. Psychol Med 17:393, 1987.

Dunbar F (ed): Emotions and Bodily Changes, 4th edition. New York, Columbia University Press, 1954.

Eisenberg L, Kleinman A (eds): The Relevance of Social Science for Medicine. Boston, D. Reidel, 1981, p 12.

Engel GL: The need for a new medical model: A challenge for biomedicine. Science 196:129, 1977.

Engel GL: The clinical application of the bio-psychosocial model. Am J Psychol 137:535, 1980.

Ford CV: The Somatizing Disorders: Illness as a Way of Life. New York, Elsevier Biomedical, 1983.

Fordyce WE: Behavioral Methods for Chronic Pain and Illness. St. Louis, CV Mosby, 1976.

Girard DE, Arthur RJ, Reler JB: Psychosocial events and subsequent illness: A review. West J Med 142:358, 1985.

Gorbin L, Schron EB, Brooks MM, et al: Psychosocial predictors of mortality in Cardiac Arrhythmia Suppression Trial-1 (CAST-1). Am J Cardiol 71:263, 1993.

Gould GP (ed): Hippocrates, Vol. 1. Cambridge, MA, Fletcher and Sons, 1972, p 289.

Hall SS: A molecular code links emotions, mind and health. Smithsonian, (June): 62, 1989.

Hamburg BA, Killilea M: Relation of social support, stress, illness and use of health services. *In* The Surgeon General's Report/Institute of Medicine. Washington, DC, National Institute of Medicine, 1979, pp 253–276.

Helgeson VS: The effects of masculinity and social support on recovery from myocardial infarction. Psychosom Med 53:621, 1991.

Hill R: Generic features of families under stress. *In* Parad HJ (ed): Crisis Intervention: Selected Readings. New York, Family Service Association of America, 1965, pp 32–52.

Hinkle LE, Jr: The concepts of stress in the biologic and social sciences. Sci Med Man 1:31, 1973.

Hinkle, LE, Jr: Stress and disease: The concept after 50 years. Soc Sci Med 25:561, 1987.

Holmes TH, Rahe RH: The Social Readjustment Rating Scale. J Psychosom Res 11:213, 1967.

Kleinman A, Smilkstein G: Psychosocial issues. *In* Rosen GM, Geyman JP, Layton RH (eds): Behavioral Science in Family Practice. New York, Appleton-Century-Crofts, 1980.

Kobosa SC, Maddi SR, Kahn S: Hardiness and health: A prospective study. J Pers Soc Psychol 42:168, 1982.

Lazarus RS, Averill JR, Opton EM, Jr: The psychology of coping: Issues of research and assessment. *In* Coelho GV, Hamburg DA, Adams JE (eds): Coping and Adaptation. New York, Basic Books, 1974, p 264.

Lazarus RS, Folkman S: Stress, Appraisal and Coping. New York, Springer, 1984, pp 266–270.

Lehrer PM, Isenberg S, Hochren SM: Asthma and emotions: A review. J Asthma 30:5, 1993.

Leslie C (ed): Asian Medical Systems: A Comparative Study. Berkeley, University of California Press, 1976, pp 1, 2.

Levi L: Psychosocial factors in preventive medicine. *In* The Surgeon General's Report/Institute of Medicine: Healthy People. Washington, DC, National Institute of Medicine, 1979, pp 207–252.

Locke SE: Stress, adaptation, and immunity. Gen Hosp Psychiatry 4:49, 1982.

Loria RM, Padgett DA: Mobilization of cutaneous immunity for systemic protection against infections. Ann NY Acad Sci 650:363, 1992.

Martin AR, Coates TJ: A clinician's guide to helping patients change behavior. West J Med 146:751, 1987.

Masuda M, Holmes TH: Life events: Perceptions and frequencies. Psychosom Med 40:236, 1978.

Mechanic D: Social psychologic factors affecting the presentation of bodily complaints. N Engl J Med 286:1132, 1972.

Medalie JA, Goldbourt U: Angina pectoris among 10,000 men: II. Psychosocial and other risk factors as evidenced by a multivariate analysis of a five year incidence study. Am J Med 60:910, 1976.

Nachemson A: Prevention of chronic back pain: The orthopedic challenge for the '80's. Bull Hosp Dis Orthop Inst 44:1, 1984.

O'Donnell L, O'Meara N, Owens D, et al: Plasma catecholemines and lipoproteins in chronic psychological stress. J R Soc Med 80:339, 1987.

Orth-Gomer K, Rosengren A, Wilhelmsen L: Lack of social support and coronary heart disease in middle-aged Swedish men. Psychosom Med 55:37, 1993.

Ostfeld AM, Berkman LF, Kahn RL, et al: Social support and social networks. *In* Ostfeld AM, Eaker ED (eds.): Measuring Psychosocial Variables in Epidemiologic Studies of Cardiovascular Disease. NIH Publication no. 85-2270, Washington, DC, National Institutes of Health, 1985, pp 49–101.

Pagel MD, Smilkstein G, Regen H, Montano D: Psychosocial influences on newborn outcomes: A controlled prospective study. Soc Sci Med 30:597, 1990.

Parsons T: Definitions of health and illness in the light of American values and social structure. *In* Jaco EG (ed): Patients, Physicians, and Illness. Glencoe, IL, Free Press, 1958.

Patterson JM: Families experiencing stress. Fam Syst Med 6:202, 1988.

Pearlin LI, Johnson JS: Marital status, life-strains and depression. Am Soc Rev 42:704, 1977.

Pearlin L, Menaghan E, Lieberman M, Mullan JT: The stress process. J Health Soc Behav 22:237, 1981.

Pratt L: Family Structure and Effective Health Behavior: The Energized Family. Boston, Houghton Mifflin, 1976.

Reeb K, Graham A, Zyzanski S, Kitson G: Predicting low birthweight and complicated labor in urban black women: A biopsychosocial perspective. Soc Sci Med 25:1321, 1987.

Riley V: Psychoneuroendocrine influences on immunocompetence and neoplasia. Science 212:1100, 1981.

Rosen G, Kleinman A, Katon W: Somatization in family practice: A biopsychosocial approach. J Fam Pract 14:493, 1982.

Ruberman W: Psychosocial influences on mortality of patients with coronary heart disease [Editorial]. JAMA 267:559, 1992.

Ruberman W, Weinblatt AB, Goldberg JD, Chaudhary BS: Psychosocial influences on mortality after myocardial infarction. N Engl J Med 311:552, 1984.

Sarason IG, Johnson J, Siegel J: Assessing the impact of life changes: Development of the Life Experiences Survey. J Consult Clin Psychol 46:932, 1978.

Sarason IG, Sarason BR, Potter EH III, Antoni MH: Life events, social support, and illness. Psychosom Med 47:156, 1985.

Schleifer SJ, Keller SE, Camarino M, et al: Suppression of lymphocyte stimulation following bereavement. JAMA 250:374, 1983.

Schmidt DD, Schmidt PM: Family systems, stress and infectious disease. Adv J Mind-Body Health 7:7, 1991.

Selye H: The general adaptation syndrome and the disease of adaptation. J Clin Endocrinol 6:117, 1946.

Selye H, Fortier C: Adaptive reactions to stress. Proc Assoc Res Nerv Ment Dis 29:3, 1950.

Shonkoff JP: Social support and vulnerability to stress: A pediatric perspective. Pediatr Ann 14:550, 1985.

Sibbald B, White P, Pharoah C, et al: Relationship between psychosocial factors and asthma morbidity. Fam Pract 5:12, 1988.

Siltanen P: Stress, coronary disease and coronary death. Am Clin Res 19:96, 1987.

Smilkstein G: The cycle of family function: A conceptual model for family medicine. J Fam Pract 11:223, 1980.

Smilkstein G: The unity of biomedical and psychosocial issues in individual and family health care. *In* Carr JE, Dengerink HA (eds): Behavioral Science in the Practice of Medicine. New York, Elsevier Biomedical, 1983, pp 168–183.

Smilkstein G: The physician and family function assessment. Fam Syst Med 2:263, 1984.

Smilkstein G: Family assessment tools. *In* Henao S, Grose NP (eds): Principles of Family Systems in Family Medicine. New York, Brunner/Mazel, 1985, pp 372–389.

Smilkstein G, Helsper-Lucas A, Ashworth C, et al: Prediction of pregnancy complications: An application of the biopsychosocial model. Soc Sci Med 18:315, 1984.

Spielberger CD: Anxiety: Current Trends in Theory and Research. New York, Academic Press, 1972, pp 23–49.

Stein M, Schiavi RC, Camerino M: Influence of brain and behavior on the immune system. Science 191:435, 1976.

Sternberg EM, Chrousos GP, Wilder RL, Gold PW: The stress response and the regulation of inflammatory disease. Ann Intern Med 117:854, 1992.

Thoits PS: Social support as coping assistance. J Consult Clin Psychol 54:416, 1986.

Van Eijk JTM, Grol RPTM, Hugen FJA, et al: The family doctor and the prevention of somatic fixation. Fam Syst Med 2:5, 1983.

Walker KN, MacBride A, Vachon MSS: Social support networks and the crisis of bereavement. Soc Sci Med 11:35, 1977.

Wolf S, Wolff HG: An experimental study of changes in gastric function in response to varied life experiences. Rev Gastroenterol 14:419, 1947.

Wolff HG: Life stress and cardiovascular disease. Circulation 1:187, 1950.

Ziegler LH, Elliott DC: The effect of emotions on certain cases of asthma. Am J Med Sci 172:860, 1926.

Zonderman AB, Costa PT, McCrae RR: Depression as a risk for cancer morbidity in a nationally representative sample. JAMA 262:1191, 1989.

CHAPTER 5

PRACTICING BIOPSYCHOSOCIAL MEDICINE

JOSEPH A. LIEBERMAN, III, and MARIAN R. STUART

Treating each patient as a unique human being, with an individual history, educational level, behavioral style, cultural heritage, health belief system, and vulnerabilities, living in a particular community, and presenting with a specific problem can present a formidable challenge. It is not a challenge that traditional medical education has adequately prepared the practitioner to meet.

SHIFTING PARADIGMS

Medical education in the United States has undergone one major paradigm shift and is about to undergo another. The first of these occurred shortly after the turn of the century. Prior to 1910, physicians in this country were trained almost exclusively in an apprenticeship experience. Typically the aspiring doctor would be taken under the wing and tutelage of an established clinician and then, on the recommendation of that clinician, would be examined by a sanctioned organization such as the State Medical Society, and awarded an MD degree if the organization found this individual ready to embark on a medical career (Starr, 1984). After 1910, and spurred on by the famous Flexner (1910) report, the American medical education community adopted the "university model," thereby bringing medical schools into the more traditional higher education graduate school format. In this mode, medical investigators engaged in scholarly inquiry as dictated by the tenets of the scientific method. In many ways this led to standardization of the body of medical knowledge, with an emphasis on science and the utilization of reductionistic methodology in areas of scholarly exploration.

Applying the scientific method to medical education and to medical inquiry has led to spectacular discoveries in biomedicine and has pushed back the frontiers of our understanding of physiology and of pathology. Daily, we are learning more and more about the functioning of the human organism at the cellular level, and the exploration of the biochemistry of health and disease is a major activity of the American medical education and research communities (Jolly and Hudley, 1993). However, this approach, which is ideally suited to scientific investigation, has created an inappropriately dichotomous situation with regard to patients. That is, patients are considered either to have or not to have a given disease. Diseases are treated as independent entities amenable to categorization and presumed to have a specific cause. The physician's task is to diagnose and prescribe a cure that will alter the natural course of disease. In this process, however, there is a loss of many of those human qualities that comprise the patient's total being, or, as George Engel (1980) has so eloquently stated:

The crippling flaw of the model is that it does not include the patient and his attributes as a person, as a human being. The biomedical model can make provision neither for the person as a whole nor for data of a psychological or social nature, for the reductionism and mind-body dualism on which the model is predicated requires that these must first be reduced to physio-chemical terms before they can have meaning. Hence, the very essence of medical practice perforce remains "art" and beyond the reach of science. (p. 536)

It is not only medical scholars, such as Dr. Engel, who are questioning the system. Patients also are expressing dissatisfaction with this one-dimensional (biomedical) approach to multidimensional problems (Bertakis et al., 1991). This public dissatisfaction is emerging simultaneously with a body of knowledge that would indicate that a more rational way to both investigate and deliver health care services requires the re-engagement of the psyche and soma. A recent study linked depression to a fivefold increased risk of mortality following myocardial infarction (Frasure-Smith et al., 1993). Great strides also are being made in disciplines such as psychoneuroimmunology, which are scientifically investigating the relationships between the patient, his or her environment, stress, and the development of specific diseases (Ader et al., 1991; Cohen et al., 1991; Spiegel et al., 1989). This activity is a welcome departure from inquiry that previously had been directed only at the cellular level.

The physicians on the cutting edge of both the delivery of these broader based services and their investigation are family physicians, who have had to deal with the vaguaries of an undifferentiated patient population as their daily bill of fare. Working at the interface of the biomedical, behavioral, and social sciences, these physicians must be facile in the reductionistic approach to delving into the biomedical nature of a patient's problems but also must integrate an understanding of the multiple influences that work on a patient to produce a biomedical dysfunction. On the micro level, we deal with patients and their biomedical problems, but on a macro level, we also deal with patients and their complex relationships with others, their communities, and the world community. A failure to comprehend this dualistic role has the potential to flaw fatally any practitioner's best clinical efforts.

Thus we come to the second major paradigm shift in American medicine. It derives from the notion that the contemporary physician has multiple responsibilities, including an understanding of the biomedical coupled with the integration of the behavioral and social into the comprehensive management of any patient and his or her problems. This reorientation already is well underway and will rival the shift in emphasis in medical education that resulted from Flexner's 1910 report.

UBIQUITY OF STRESS

Regardless of the origin of a patient's dysfunction, whether it is a mechanical failure of the biomedical system or a physical manifestation of some other problem, the ultimate result is that a patient presents to a family physician with symptoms and a diminished ability to deal with the "hand fate has dealt." A consistent companion of the patient in this process is stress. This stress may be generated by a biomedical dysfunction or the biomedical dysfunction may be generated by the patient's reaction to stress. It is the patient's lack of tolerance for the symptoms or the anxiety about the symptoms that frequently triggers the visit to the physician. How that patient deals with the stress associated with his or her problem will, in many ways, determine the patient's ultimate outcome. In order to treat the patient effectively, the physician must be aware of, and understand, the impact of stress on the overall problem presented by the patient.

Today stress is endemic. Consider the ease with which startling information is instantaneously transmitted to our population. We are literally the eyewitnesses to death and destruction around the globe to a degree unimagined only a few decades ago. During World War II, Lowell Thomas's descriptions of a burning London during the blitz were "state of the art" and had a frightening quality never before experienced by an American citizen. Only 50 short years later, cameras and reporters

are transmitting the visual horrors that go along with equally catastrophic events in a real-time fashion to a much larger population that has access to the means of viewing the carnage in all of its grizzly detail. This capacity to transmit information has a tremendous potential to be constructive, but the dark side of the human condition tends to revel in the sensationalism of violence and man's inhumanity to man rather than spending equal time delighting in the many accomplishments of a Mother Theresa.

All of these influences working collectively produce a level of stress heretofore unencountered in society at large, which has had an unmeasured and untenable impact. Many people feel overwhelmed, overstimulated, and out of control. Others turn off all feelings and develop somatic complaints. These new problems, in concert with many of the biomedical maladies that have been with us throughout the history of the species, have resulted in compounding the difficulties for practitioners of the art and science of medicine, and called for a revisiting of some of the basic tenets of medical practice if the practitioner is to accommodate to the needs of a contemporary society.

POSITIVE POWER OF PHYSICIANS

One may legitimately ask what would enable a physician to deal effectively with this dizzying array of variables and influences. If one were to pause, however, and take inventory of the physician's social powers in our society, one could make a compelling case that the physician is indeed *best* positioned to deal with these problems. Social scientists have identified an array of social powers, but five of the most predominant of these powers are possessed by physicians. This singularly qualifies them among all the professions to influence the behavior of their patients and bring constructive forces to bear at a time when patients are surviving in a destructive environment. These powers are as follows:

1. *Reward power*—society has given physicians the authority to reward certain types of patient behavior. Physicians have the power to prescribe medications that relieve symptoms, sign forms that provide reimbursement, and certify to patients' illnesses. Physicians control many resources that patients require. A physician's certification of "a clean bill of health" is highly rewarding to the patient.

2. *Coercive power*—physicians also are given the authority to coerce good behavior and compliance from a patient. This coercion can take a variety of forms but is mainly an attempt to influence the patient's behavior by exerting the threat of a negative outcome. For example, patient lack of compliance with a medical regimen or diet can re-

sult in a hospitalization or other onerous entity, which is the option of the physician and the bane of the patient.

3. *Expert power*—patients still view physicians as being the proprietors of a unique body of knowledge, and they most frequently will defer to the physician application of this body of knowledge related to all aspects of the human body, mind, and social interaction.

4. *Referent power*—patients regularly and routinely use a relationship with their physicians as a means of substantiating and supporting their own sense of self. The words "my doctor says" are part of the lexicon and carry with them the bonding of the expert authority figure to the patient and for the patient.

5. *Legitimate power*—government has conferred on the physician the ability to direct the activities of other members of the society. A physician can prohibit someone from driving an automobile, place someone in the protective custody of a psychiatric hospital, or absent someone from work and a variety of other activities when, in the best judgement of the physician, such actions are to the patient's benefit. By consulting the physician, the patient accepts the doctor's legitimate power.

These are but a few examples of the social powers possessed by physicians. Although some have a highly refined understanding of these issues, most physicians are unaware of their considerable ability to influence the thinking and behavior of their patients. Many physicians do not realize that their specific use of words is a procedure that not only can make patients feel supported but actually can alter patients' views of themselves and their options.

LISTENING TO AND HELPING PATIENTS EDIT THEIR STORIES

With this array of social powers at a physician's disposal, one of the most constructive things he or she can do for patients is to guide patients as they work their way through solving their problems, whether they be biological, psychological, social, or, most likely, a combination. Patients have a unique and distinct view of the world and, although no one can precisely know someone else's view of the world, physicians are uniquely positioned to enable their patients to cope more effectively, regardless of the nature of the patients' problems. Skillfully employed, this professional attribute alone can decrease patients' stress and empower them to deal more effectively with the factors contributing to their misery.

When restoring the patient's power to cope, the physician is being highly therapeutic. Looking generically at the common elements found in all schools of psychotherapy, we can reduce them to five major components. (Refreshingly, reductionism of this sort enhances our understanding.) These elements are as follows:

1. *The expectation of receiving help*—in the overwhelming majority of cases patients enter into a relationship with the physician believing that the physician is going to be able to help them with their symptoms. Feelings of distress, helplessness, and hopelessness precipitate the visit to the doctor's office. The patient's faith in the physician's ability to relieve suffering restores the patient's confidence.

2. *The therapeutic relationship*—physicians and patients bond to foster the well-being of the patient. This bonding produces a contract for caring and concern that is the core of therapy. It is the quality of the therapeutic relationship that makes the patient feel accepted and valued. This is also the essence of social support, which reduces the patient's perceived stress.

3. *Obtaining an external perspective*—patients expect the wise and knowledgeable physician to assist them in formulating their thought processes and improving their problem-resolution skills. By listening to the patient's story objectively and commenting briefly, physicians allow patients to check their narrow or inaccurate perceptions of their situations. This provides an invaluable assist for the patient struggling with issues of self-doubt, recrimination, or any overwhelming situation. When stressed, it is hard to see options or engage in creative problem solving. Here the physician's involvement is crucial.

4. *Encouraging a corrective experience*—within this dimension of psychotherapeutic technique, the physician provides the external motivation for patients to change the way in which they function, react, and/or respond. This is a positive attribute of the psychotherapeutic relationship that will help patients translate insights into actions that are more productive and beneficial. The physician is the facilitator and the cheerleader.

5. *The opportunity to test reality repeatedly*—in this capacity the physician is the patient's "port in a storm." Patients frequently may have to "dock" as they attempt to wade their way through unchartered and stormy seas. It is the physician's responsibility to provide that perspective for that patient as an assist to his or her voyage.

In all of these activities, the physician is the supportive listener and occasional commentator as the patient works through the process of problem resolution and self-actualization.

EXPANDING, NOT SHRINKING

In its reductionist approach to problem solving, the American medical educational and delivery systems have reduced the process of diagnosis to an "all-or-none" phenomenon. A patient either has or does not have mental illness, and any emotional disturbance is treated as either the presence or absence of a psychiatric disorder. This dichotomous approach fails to accommodate the vast number of patients whose responses to the stress in their lives leads to temporary dysfunction and some degree of pain but who are clearly not mentally ill.

Even patients with the most "purely biomedical" problem are likely to have stress associated with their condition and will respond accordingly. In the majority of cases they do not need a psychiatrist; rather, they need a physician equipped with the tools to expand their behavioral repertoire to help them deal with the stressful components of their illnesses or the stress that is in fact producing their illnesses. It is the responsibility of the physician to address each and every component of a patient's illness, be it organic or psychological, or related to their social environment. In our experience, the ability of most physicians to deal with the biomedical is quite highly refined, the psychological not so nearly well defined, and the social frequently beyond the capabilities or interest of physicians. These last two areas hold the greatest promise for the physician to integrate the biomedical, psychological, and social and, in the process, expand the patient's behavioral repertoire and sense of personal power. A reasonable expectation is that the physician will restore the patient's premorbid level of functioning and enhance his or her sense of self-esteem.

BATHING THE PATIENT

As with all skills in medicine, the ability to incorporate thoughtfully appropriate questions regarding a patient's psychosocial situation is an acquired skilled. To get to the core of problems in this area succinctly and expediently, in the context of a busy office practice, requires a systematic approach that is well within the repertoire of most physicians but highly organized in very few. In *The Fifteen Minute Hour*, Stuart and Lieberman (1986), first introduced the acronym BATHE as a supplement to the widely accepted SOAP format of medical records keeping. At some point during the encounter with the patient, ideally right after exploring the presenting problem, the physician can employ the BATHE technique to obtain the necessary information to assess the patient's psychosocial situation and then react accordingly. The acronym BATHE triggers four questions and an appropriate response, as follows:

B *Stands for Background.* A simple question, "What is going on in your life?" will elicit the context of the patient's visit.
A *Stands for Affect (the feeling state).* Questions such as "How do you feel about that?" or what is your mood? allow the patient to report the current feeling state.
T *Stands for Trouble.* The question, "What about the situation troubles you the most?" helps both the physician and the patient focus on the situation's subjective meaning.
H *Stands for Handling.* The answer to, "How are you handling that?" gives an assessment of functioning.
E *Stands for Empathy.* The statement, "That must be very difficult for you," legitimizes the patient's reaction. (Stuart and Lieberman, 1993, p. 97)

Although not the only technique a clinician can employ, busy practitioners have found that BATHE tends to bring order out of what is frequently a chaotic approach to a psychosocial assessment. In the process, it helps tie the biomedical to the psychosocial in a way that is meaningful for both physicians and patients. By asking pointed, focused questions, which lend themselves to a brief but reasonably comprehensive answer, the physician is able to incorporate this very necessary form of assessment and treatment into a format that is both effective and efficient. It will not interfere with the physician's ability to see large numbers of patients in a given day.

For patients, being led through an organized exploration of their problems is highly therapeutic. First, patients begin to recognize that the stress in their lives is contributing to their physical state. Then, the physician's inquiry about their feelings is highly gratifying and often elicits important reactions. The inquiry about what is most troubling about the situation brings out the symbolic meaning of the event for the patient. Often this is surprising. At this point, it is important for both the physician and the patient to assess how the patient is handling the situation. Finally, the physician's empathic response provides closure and allows return to other aspects of the interview. This brief intervention can help the patient feel more competent to deal with his or her situation as well as feeling very supported by the physician.

Physicians have a responsibility to provide comprehensive health care services to each patient, but also a responsibility to the community at large to care for a number of patients. The proper blending of these two responsibilities can be facilitated by the use of this technique.

OWNERSHIP

The physician's inquiry into the patient's psychosocial status is designed to produce an enhanced comprehension on the part of the physician of the overall dimensions of a patient's presenting problem. The physician does not assume responsibility for the patient's particular situation, but rather assesses the patient's circumstances in order to make therapeutic suggestions that enable the patient to deal with his or her problem more effectively. The patient continues to own his or her problem, but the physician is better able to assist that patient in the resolution of the problem because the physician has a complete and comprehensive understanding of its derivation. This is true whether the problem is predominantly biomedical or psychosocial because these aspects are ingrained in the patient's overall situation. Ownership of the problem remains with the patient, who now understands that the physician is there to help. The physician's ability to intervene effectively is enhanced by the psychosocial assessment, revealing the array of influences working on a given patient.

OTHER FORMS OF THERAPEUTIC TALK

BATHEing the patient creates a highly therapeutic relationship and often elicits evidence of anxiety or depression connected with psychosocial problems. The physician is now in a position to treat these conditions with therapeutic talk, along with medication, if appropriate.

Giving Advice

Although patients ask for advice, focusing them on their own resources, with some guidance for developing alternatives, is always more effective. When the physician gives advice or directly solves a problem, the patient is not empowered. It is better to make patients aware of their own strengths and their ability to assess and exercise their own options. However, there are certain suggestions that the physician can make that focus primarily on the *process* of dealing with problems. Patients should be instructed to focus in the here-and-now, to look at their options, and to apply tincture of time. Along with the physician's support and the opportunity to return to discuss the situation further, this is often enough to trigger a significant positive change in the patient's affective response. Using the BATHE technique to structure subsequent visits is highly effective. There are also other brief interventions that the physician can employ.

Distinguishing between Thoughts, Feelings, and Behavior

Patients must learn to differentiate between thoughts, feelings, and behavior. *Thoughts* are related to our beliefs and the stories that we tell ourselves about the world, other people, and ourselves. They are the judgments, expectations, generalizations, and unfounded prognostications we all make. Physicians must acknowledge patients' views before being able to challenge them.

Feelings are emotional responses to a situation based on thoughts and judgments. Feelings must be expressed and accepted. In this process, feelings change. Feelings also change when irrational thoughts and unrealistic expectations are altered. *Behavior* consists of the actions we take. Our behavior is the only thing in this life that we can control. A depressed patient should be encouraged to express thoughts and feelings related to being defeated and discouraged, but given instructions to take daily walks, regardless of whether the activity holds any enjoyment.

Assuming That There Are Options

When patients are overwhelmed by the circumstances of their lives, they lose sight of the fact that they still have choices. The physician's suggestion that there are always options and that the patient needs to explore them cues the patient in a positive direction. It is not the physician's task to generate these options; rather, it is the patient's. The physician communicates the expectation that the patient can and will do this and return to report the results. This therapeutic intervention helps patients be more open to possibilities, look at their world, including themselves, in a new way, and become aware of having choices.

Changing the Story

It is also useful to encourage patients to reinterpret their situations. Every trying circumstance can be seen as an opportunity to learn a necessary lesson or develop an essential skill. This is called reframing. Physicians can point out that there are four healthy options for handling a bad situation:

1. Leaving it; this dictates exploring the *best* and *worst* possible outcomes that might result.
2. Changing it; this requires an investigation of what is possible and what additional resources must be brought to bear.
3. Accepting it as it is; recognizing that, if it *could* be different, it would be different.
4. Reframing it; finding a way to interpret the situation as a positive.

Therapeutic talk is that direct conversation that focuses the patient on his or her strengths and choices. It changes the "story" that the patient is "inadequate and that no one cares." Instead, it makes patients feel competent to deal with the circumstances of their lives and makes them feel good about themselves and their relationship with their physician.

DEALING WITH DIFFICULT PATIENTS

Groves (1978) developed four stereotypes of hateful patients, which he labeled dependent clingers, manipulative help-rejectors, entitled demanders, and self-destructive deniers. These patients consistently trigger negative feelings in physicians, who cannot satisfy their endless demands and complaints. Every family physician has his or her own panel of difficult patients. Our approach to maintaining physician mental health while treating these patients is to recognize that each of these individuals is trying desperately to get his or her needs met in the only way they see possible at this time. Because they experience little success, they become more frustrated and more difficult. It is important for the physician to acknowledge their suffering.

Except when there is an immediate threat to life, physicians must limit the time they spend with patients that arouse negative emotions to less than 15 minutes, regardless of the complexity of the problems or number of complaints. Part of the time should be spent integrating medical and psychosocial concerns. If all problems cannot be addressed in one visit, the patient can be brought back the following week, demonstrating the physician's interest and concern. With frequent brief sessions, these patients often feel less rejected. Also, they organize the details of their stories to fit into abbreviated time slots once convinced that the physician listens attentively and responds appropriately. Ultimately, this will result in fewer frustrating sessions of miscommunication and better utilization of the physician's time.

The Hypochondriacal Patient

The hypochondriacal patient, whose preoccupation with every symptom triggers anxiety about real or imagined illness, can try the patience of any physician. Barsky and colleagues (1993) concluded that hypochondriacs believe "good health" to be relatively "symptom free," and suggest that this accounts for their numerous somatic complains and resistance to reassurance. These patients focus their attention on their physical symptoms, actually suffer from anxiety and depression while being unsuccessful in finding anyone to cure them. Hypochondriacs benefit from regular visits at predetermined intervals. It is wise to start by seeing them as often as biweekly and then lengthening the time between visits.

When seeing these patients, the physician must acknowledge seriously their concerns about their current symptoms and reflect with empathy that "It must be awful not to ever feel well." Then, it is essential to follow with the BATHE protocol. Even these patients ultimately will realize that the number and intensity of their somatic symptoms are correlated with their levels of stress and anxiety.

The Chronic Complainer

There are real differences between hypochondriacs, who are concerned about the state of their health (the "worried well"), and chronic complainers (Rittelmeyer, 1985), who have multiple complaints, demand to be seen frequently, rarely get better, and never appreciate the physician's efforts on their behalf. Here, again, the best treatment is to acknowledge their suffering and to recognize the futility of trying to alleviate it. These patients seem to need their disease in order to function at all.

The Depressed Patient

It is depressing to acknowledge that depression *not* diagnosed or treated by the primary care physician often results in long-lasting symptomatology, decreased quality of life, and suicide (Murphy et al., 1986). Even mild to moderate depression affects peoples' lives negatively. BATHEing the patient results in the diagnosis, after which depression can be treated effectively using brief sessions with or without medication. Specific suggestions for a variety of brief and effective interventions for managing patients suffering from depression, anxiety, and other emotional upheavals can be found in *The Fifteen Minute Hour* (Stuart and Lieberman, 1993).

PHYSICIAN, TREAT THYSELF

Incorporating the psychosocial aspects of medicine into daily practice can be challenging but extremely gratifying provided that the physician observes a number of basic rules for survival. Of the dozen rules Stuart and Lieberman (1993) prescribe, the most important are: (1) not to take responsibility for things you cannot control; (2) to take care of yourself, or you cannot take care of anyone else; and (3) to recognize that you have to start where the patient is, which means that it is crucial to do a psychosocial assessment along with a biomedical one. Applying these principles is the essence of practicing biopsychosocial medicine.

REFERENCES

Ader R, Felton DL, Cohen N (eds): Psychoneuroimmunology, 2nd edition. San Diego, CA, Academic Press, 1991.

Barsky AJ, Coeytaux RR, Sarnie MK, et al: Hypochondriacal patients' beliefs about good health. Am J. Psychiatry 150(7): 1085–9, 1993.

Bertakis KD, Roter D, Putnam SM: The relationship of physician medical interview style to patient satisfaction. J Fam Pract 32:175, 1991.

Cohen SC, Tyrrell DAJ, Smith AP: Psychological stress and susceptibility to the common cold. N Engl J Med 325:606, 1991.

Engel GL: The Clinical application of the biopsychosocial model. Am J Psychiatry 137:536, 1980.

Flexner A: Medical Education in the United States and Canada. New York, Carnegie Foundation for the Advancement of Teaching, 1910.

Frasure-Smith N, Lesperance F, Talajic M: Depression following myocardial infarction. JAMA 270:1819, 1993.

Groves JE: Taking care of the hateful patient. N Engl J Med 298:883, 1978.

Jolly P, Hudley D: AAMC Data Book: Statistical Information Related to Medical Education. Washington, DC, Association of American Medical Colleges, 1993.

Murphy JM, Olivier DC, Sobol AM, et al: Diagnosis and outcome: Depression and anxiety in a general population. Psychol Med 16:117, 1986.

Rittelmeyer LF Jr: Coping with the chronic complainer. Am Fam Physician 31:211, 1985.

Spiegel D, Bloom J, Kraemer HC, Gottheil E: Effect of psychosocial treatment on survival of patients with metastatic breast cancer. Lancet 2:888, 1989.

Starr P: The Social Transformation of American Medicine. New York, Basic Books, 1984.

Stuart MR, Lieberman JA III: The Fifteen Minute Hour: Applied Psychotherapy for the Primary Care Physician. New York, Praeger, 1986.

Stuart MR, Lieberman JA III: The Fifteen Minute Hour: Applied Psychotherapy for the Primary Care Physician, 2nd edition. Westport, CT, Praeger, 1993.

CHAPTER 6

DOMESTIC VIOLENCE

Child Abuse

NANCY D. KELLOGG

Any professional who cares for children will encounter child abuse at some point in his or her career. Although child abuse has been documented throughout recorded history, public and medical awareness and concern has emerged only in the last 30 years. In 1962, Henry Kempe's description of the "battered child syndrome" established child abuse and neglect as a condition that must be recognized, reported, and treated.

DEFINITION OF TERMS

Physical abuse is any intentional injury resulting in tissue damage. Tissue damage includes bruises, burns, lacerations, and organ rupture. Corporal punishment that involves the use of an instrument or that requires medical attention is outside the range of normal punishment (Bross et al., 1988). Corporal punishment has been outlawed in more than 19 states (Fleischman, 1990). In addition to the abuser, a person who does not make a reasonable effort to stop or prevent physical abuse injuries or sexual abuse is also subject to penalty.

Sexual abuse is "the involvement of dependent, developmentally immature children and adolescents in sexual activities they do not fully comprehend, to which they are unable to give informed consent, or that violate social taboos of family roles" (CH Kempe, 1980). In contrast to physical abuse, tissue damage is not an essential part of the sexual abuse definition; sexual abuse may not involve bodily contact (such as sexual conduct intentionally performed in a child's presence).

PREVALENCE AND INCIDENCE

In 1992, almost 3 million children were reported to Child Protective Services as alleged victims of child maltreatment. Of this total, approximately 800,000 were alleged victims of physical abuse and 500,000 were alleged victims of sexual abuse (McCurdy and Daro, 1993); over 10 per cent are victims of more than one type of abuse. The numbers continue to increase each year, a fact attributed primarily to enhanced public awareness leading to more reporting of cases.

While the reported numbers are alarming, estimates of unreported and undetected cases are much higher. Child abuse is said to affect an estimated 10 per cent of all children under the age of 5 who present to emergency rooms with traumatic injuries (Holter and Friedman, 1968). Based on retrospective studies, approximately 38 per cent of females will have been sexually abused by the time they reach their 18th birthday (Russel, 1983); for males, the estimated incidence is 10 per cent (Shearer and Herbert, 1987). Child abuse is largely a hidden epidemic.

Morbidity and mortality are high: Repeat physical abuse occurs in more than 20 per cent of children (Kottmeier, 1987), while incidents of child sexual abuse or assaults recur in over 65 per cent of victims (ND Kellogg, R Huston, J Parra, J Legler, J Hons, and M Roman, unpublished data). In the United States, more than three children die each day as a result of maltreatment (McCurdy and Daro, 1993).

ETIOLOGY/RISK FACTORS

Although recognition and treatment of child abuse is a recent phenomenon, examples of child abuse and neglect have been documented for thousands of years. In ancient times, the infant's right to live was not recognized until this right was ritually bestowed, usually by the father (Radbill, 1980). Sexual abuse of children has been recorded in Greek and Roman history. For hundreds of years, physical and sexual violence against children has not been considered "abuse."

Child abuse occurs through the interaction of

three factors: the adult abuser, the child, and a triggering event or situation. Economic stress and substance abuse are important risk factors in today's society (McCurdy and Daro, 1993). When an individual becomes unemployed and is forced to spend more time at home, his children may bear the violent consequences of this stress. Substance abuse, including alcoholism, may provide disinhibition of violent or sexual impulses. Social isolation, marital discord, and other minor stressors also may trigger abusive acts. Stressors alone do not cause child abuse; most people bear mild to severe stress on a daily basis yet do not abuse children. Stressors serve as a catalyst between the potential abuser and the child at risk.

ABUSERS

As with elder and spouse abuse, there is no stereotypical profile of a child abuser. Although lower socioeconomic status has been cited as a risk factor for abuse, abusers represent all levels of income, education, and intelligence. Over 90 per cent of abusers are well known to the child (Behrman and Vaughan, 1983). Although there is no sex predilection among those who physically abuse children, the majority of child sexual abusers are men.

Based on the approach to the child victim, there are different types of abusers. In most cases of physical abuse and approximately 20 per cent of sexual abuse cases (Groth, 1978), the abuser is one who views the child negatively, uses coercion, and intentionally inflicts pain. In contrast, the molester uses deception and enticement to lure the child into a sexually abusive situation. This type of abuser wants the child to participate in and to enjoy the experience. At least 80 per cent of individuals who sexually abuse children use this latter approach (Groth, 1978). Whereas visible evidence is more likely in cases of physical abuse and rape, evidence of tissue damage typically is not seen in cases of molestation.

Finkelhor (1985) has described four preconditions necessary for sexual abuse to occur: (1) *motivation,* which includes emotional congruence, sexual arousal by children, and inability to form satisfactory relationships with appropriate adults; (2) *overcoming of internal inhibitions,* such as moral and religious beliefs; (3) *removal of external inhibitors,* such as parents or witnesses; and (4) *overcoming resistance in the child.* Resistance can be overcome with physical force, or, more commonly, through a careful, deliberate, and long process that begins with obtaining trust and accessibility to the child. The abuse usually begins with "accidentally-on-purpose" touching, followed by mutual fondling, with more penetrating acts of abuse occurring months, even years, later. Molesters strive for cooperation and participation from their victim, further compounding the child's con-

fusion and feelings of guilt. Abusers exploit these feelings to secure secrecy: "All daddies do this to their little girls"; "If you tell I'll say you wanted it"; "If you do this I'll give you money." Commonly threats are used to further secure silence: "If you tell I'll hurt your mother"; "If you tell, Mom will be mad and I'll have to go to jail"; "If you tell they'll put you in a foster home." The child is thus instilled with a paradoxical responsibility for keeping his or her family intact and secure.

Many abusers were abused as children. This is especially true of physical abuse, because excessive corporal punishment traditionally has been viewed not as child abuse but rather as a parent's undeniable right. Most adolescent sexual offenders were sexually abused as children (Sauzier and Mitkus, 1986).

VICTIMS

With respect to physical abuse, the "child at risk" is one who requires more time, money, effort, or attention. Typically this will be the child with a physical or mental handicap, but it also includes premature infants and hyperactive children. Children who are not handicapped are also at risk for physical abuse during certain developmental stages: periods of colic during infancy, toilet training and the "terrible twos," and independence-seeking behaviors during adolescence are classic examples. These stages tax the patience of caregivers who are at risk for becoming abusers.

In a clinical setting, most physical abuse victims are very young, usually under the age of 4. These young victims tend to require medical attention because they are less able to defend themselves. However, over 40 per cent of physical abuse victims are adolescents (U.S. Department of Health and Human Services, 1980), many of whom do not actively seek medical assistance. Community and protective services for adolescents are few because of the societal view that older children are better able to defend and speak up for themselves. Most reported cases of sexual abuse involve females, although male victims are thought to be largely underreported. Fear of homosexuality and societal expectations that males will withstand any hardship are proposed reasons for this underreporting (Finkelhor et al., 1990). Although the average age of sexual abuse victims is about 10, a bimodal distribution with one peak around 2 to 4 years and another at puberty or 12 to 14 years has been observed. Toddlers, when they first connect genital touching with pleasure, unequivocally trust adults for guidance and are naive to any wrongdoing that may result. Similarly, children entering puberty frequently are bewildered by the rapid physical and emotional changes, and thereby are susceptible to the false reassurances of an abusive adult. In general, victims of sexual abuse tend to be more reserved, quieter, unsure, and lonely. They are attracted to accepting, generous, and self-confident adults and may even welcome the abuse as a form of attention and affection. With intrafamilial abuse, one female child (especially if she is a stepchild) typically is singled out as a victim, although it is not uncommon for all the female children to be abused.

CONSEQUENCES OF ABUSE

There are physical and psychological, short- and long-term consequences of child abuse.

Physical Consequences

Injuries to the skin and subcutaneous tissues are seen in 90 per cent of physically abused children (Kessler and Hyden, 1991). Although the location and pattern of such injuries may suggest abuse, the most important consideration is whether the explanation offered is consistent with the characteristics of the injury(s). Most soft tissue injuries of childhood are undoubtedly accidental. However, those that occur on the buttocks, abdomen, inner thighs, genitalia, lower back, and sides of the face/head are not typically a result of normal childhood play. Patterned and symmetrical or bilateral bruises are suspicious for abuse. Patterned bruises resemble the object used to inflict injury: slap marks, particularly on the face; welt marks caused by a belt, cord, switch, or board; binding bruises/friction burns resulting in a circumferential pattern at the wrists or ankles; gag marks at the corners of the mouth. Over 50 per cent of physical abuse injuries involve the orofacial area (Sperber, 1980). Inflicted burns may be patterned when hot objects such as curling irons and cigarette butts are used. Intentional water immersion burns may produce a stocking-glove pattern of burning on the hands or feet/ankles. In cases of trunk/lower body immersion, an irregular burn pattern may be seen as the child draws his or her legs up protectively, thereby sparing the popliteal, inguinal, and parts of the posterior thigh and calf areas. Third-degree water burns are rarely accidental (Kessler and Hyden, 1991).

Child abuse fractures also tend to occur in specific sites with characteristic configurations. For example, metaphyseal injuries of the long bones, typically caused by violent shaking or pulling of the extremity, are considered diagnostic of physical abuse (Kessler and Hyden, 1991). Such fractures present primarily as bucket-handle or chip fractures. Spiral fractures involving the shaft of long bones also may result from violent twisting or pulling of an extremity. Posterior and lateral rib fractures are produced when a small child or infant is squeezed around the thorax. In the absence of

a history for significant trauma (such as falling from a height of more than 5 feet), skull fractures in infants are rarely accidental.

Head injuries are the most common cause of death in child abuse (Kessler and Hyden, 1991). Any intracranial hemorrhage in a young child without a history for extreme trauma should be considered nonaccidental until proven otherwise. Shaking an infant may produce such an injury, although some researchers (Bruce and Zimmerman, 1989) argue that impact is also necessary to rupture the vessels involved. Approximately half of the patients with intracranial hemorrhages will have no externally visible signs of trauma (Kessler and Hyden, 1991). The presence of retinal hemorrhages helps make the diagnosis of abuse initially, but these are not always present.

Abdominal injuries are second to head injuries as causes of death from abuse (Touloukian, 1968). A penetrating blow to the abdomen may cause rupture of organs (especially liver) and intestinal lacerations or hematomas, typically within the duodenum or proximal jejunum. Bruising is rarely observed because the impact does not crush soft tissue against bone. As a result, children often present with nonspecific signs of abdominal distention and obstruction, so that the diagnosis of abuse is made intraoperatively or on autopsy.

Physical injuries resulting from child or adolescent sexual abuse or assault are seen only occasionally. In an article that summarizes the findings of several studies (Paradise, 1990), an average of 52.5 per cent of all examinations were normal. While a proportion of the remaining cases may have "suggestive evidence" (worrisome but not specific for abuse), a much smaller proportion of cases (about 10 per cent) will have "definite evidence." The reasons for this are threefold. First, most victims of sexual abuse are not seen in a clinical setting within hours or minutes of an assault. One study (Kellogg et al., unpublished data) found that victims wait an average of 2.3 years to disclose abuse. Significant injuries resulting from sexual abuse or assault can heal completely in as little as 1 to 12 days (Finkel, 1989; McCann and Voris, 1993). Second, not all types of abusive acts result in physical evidence. Fondling, oral–genital contact, anal penetration, digital vaginal penetration, and vulvar/vestibular penetration are examples of acts that rarely result in specific physical findings. Even vaginal penile penetration may not produce observable evidence. Third, although many child and adolescent victims may *describe* penetration of the vagina or anus ("yes, he put it *inside*"), they may in fact be experiencing vulvar or vestibular penetration, not penetration past the hymen into the vagina. The size of the hymenal opening in a school-age child is about one-half inch, making *vaginal* penetration difficult. Both vaginal and vulvar penetration are experienced as painful by the child victim, who may be unable to differentiate between the two acts.

Examples of acute injuries caused by sexual assault include lacerations or hemorrhages of the hymen, posterior vestibule, and/or anus and anal sphincter muscle spasm. Nonacute findings indicative of chronic abuse include scarring of the hymen, vestibule, and anus and dilation of the hymenal and anal openings. Physical evidence of anal penetration is rarely seen except in cases of chronic, repeated abuse over several months (remember that children pass very large stools without injury). Sexually transmitted diseases, especially chlamydia and gonorrhea, are additional indicators of abuse. Teenage pregnancy is highly associated with sexual abuse, either as a direct result of abuse or as a means of escaping abuse.

Short-Term Psychological Consequences

Most victims of child abuse experience some degree of fear and guilt. Although the fear of being physically or sexually hurt is considerable, many children have a greater fear of the consequences that may result from exposing "the family secret." Similarly, guilt stems more from fear of consequences should abuse be discovered. Abused children frequently feel that they somehow deserve to be abused—because adults are always "right." Many children offer partial disclosures of abuse and then recant once the consequences of disclosure become more threatening than the abuse. With long-term abuse, children may learn to be helpless and to accommodate the abuse, sometimes developing elaborate mechanisms of coping.

Efforts to cope often result in observable behavior changes. Two general classes of behavioral responses have been described: internalizing and externalizing responses (Koverola, 1992). Internalizing behaviors include depression, anxiety, blocking, and somatization. Externalizing responses include physical or sexual acting out, delinquency, promiscuity, and hyperactivity. Blocking, or dissociation of the physical act from psychological acknowledgment of the act, is a very effective manner of coping for many children. These children may describe themselves as "going to sleep" or "forgetting" what happened. This should not be confused with the child who recants by saying "I forgot what happened."

Long-Term Psychological Consequences

The extent of symptomatology in child abuse victims depends on a number of factors: the length of abuse, the type of abuse, the number of abusers, whether the abuse was intra- or extrafamilial, the child's individual coping abilities, and the family's response once abuse is uncovered. Many victims suffer from poor self-esteem, a limited ability to relate to others, social isolation with superficial yet dependent and unstable relationships, and poor problem-solving skills (RS Kempe, 1980). Inability to form appropriate intimate bonds with others—whether it be a partner or child—is an especially significant effect of long-term abuse. As Shearer and Herbert so aptly stated: "Difficulties in interpersonal relationships frequently result from poor resolution of conflict between the trust necessary for intimacy and the mistrust necessary for self-protection" (Shearer and Herbert, 1987). It is this instability that predisposes abused children to become abusive adults and to seek out exploitative abusive relationships when they become adults.

FAMILY PRACTICE INTERVENTIONS

Family practice interventions may occur on three levels: (1) detection, (2) treatment, and (3) prevention.

Detection

All professionals working with children should be aware of the prevalence and the sometimes masked clinical presentations of child abuse. Victims rarely present with classic examples of abusive injuries; diagnosis depends on the clinician's index of suspicion and a comprehensive assessment of the risk factors, characteristics of the injury(s), explanations offered by the child and caregivers, and the social factors involved.

If abuse is suspected, the family physician should attempt to interview the child in private. In general, indirect rather than direct statements are less threatening and more likely to elicit disclosure. Several messages can be related to the child in this manner. The following is a sample dialogue with a school-age child who has injuries highly suspicious for sexual abuse:

"Susie, I often have to talk to lots of boys and girls [*message:* you are not alone] about things that happen to their bodies that make them feel uncomfortable, funny, bad, or sometimes good [*message:* not all sexual abuse is experienced as "bad" by the child]. Lots of children feel scared talking about these kinds of touches because they think they or someone else might get in trouble. Lots of times the person doing the touching is someone they love or like a whole lot. You know, when this happens, it is never the child's fault [*message:* it's not your fault]. It is always best to tell another grown-up about what happened. Did you know that when a grown-up touches a child like this that he or she needs help too? [Many children are surprised to hear this.] It's a bit like being on drugs—they can't stop the touching unless they get help. Also, grown-ups who do this do it to more than one child [surprise #2 for children], so you can help other children by telling if this happens to you. If you ever need to talk to me about something that's happened to you or someone else, please call me [*message:* I will believe you]."

Some child victims may "process" this information and disclose at a later time. It is critical not to make promises ("It will never happen to you again") that cannot be guaranteed because this will jeopardize the child's trust in you.

Treatment

All 50 states in the United States have laws that mandate reporting whenever child abuse is suspected. It is *not* the professional's responsibility to *prove* abuse occurred; that is left to Child Protective Services and the legal system. Whenever a child's safety is in question, hospitalization should be considered.

Treatment also entails the necessary medical treatment for injuries as well as providing for crisis intervention counseling. Many hospitals and communities have specialized programs to meet these needs. Child Protective Services may provide the necessary services and referrals for your area.

Prevention

Family physicians are uniquely qualified to employ preventative measures on several levels: for the child, for the parent, and for the adult abused as a child. A dialogue such as that described under "Detection" can be used in the course of well-child checkups *whether or not* abuse is suspected. Additional points important to cover include a "safety plan": "Try to think of three people you would tell if this happens to you. It doesn't always have to be Mom or Dad because sometimes it's very hard to tell them and to see them get upset. Let's think of three people together." Similarly, a parent can be encouraged to undertake the same kind of dialogue with his or her child.

New parents need assurance that the stress and fatigue of having a new baby are normal. It is also normal sometimes to feel tempted to take out frustrations on a relentlessly crying infant. Acknowledge these feelings, then explore stress-relieving methods with the parents. Agencies such as Parents Anonymous also can provide assistance anonymously to parents who call.

Finally, the adult patient who manifests symptoms and behaviors suspicious for prior abuse, or who confides about prior abuse, can be encouraged to seek out counseling. Sometimes suggesting that counseling *now* can impact future relationships with partners and children may provide the impetus the patient needs to seek out help. On all levels, it is important for the clinician first to acknowledge the patient's feelings, as varied and unpredictable as they may be, and then to move forward with a plan of action or prevention.

REFERENCES

Behrman RE, Vaughan VC: Nelson Textbook of Pediatrics. Philadelphia, WB Saunders Company, 1983.
Bross DC, Krugman RD, Lenherr MR, et al: The New Child Protection Team Handbook. New York, Garland Publishing, 1988.
Bruce DA, Zimmerman RA: Shaken impact syndrome. Pediatr Ann 18:482, 1989.
Finkel MA: Anogenital trauma in sexually abused children. Pediatrics 84:317, 1989.
Finkelhor D: Child Sexual Abuse: New Theory and Research. New York, Free Press, 1985.
Finkelhor D, Hotaling G, Lewis IA: Sexual abuse in a national survey of adult men and women: Prevalence, characteristics and risk factors. Child Abuse Negl 14:19, 1990.
Fleischman D: Advocates join forces to abolish corporal punishment. Am Acad Pediatr News (September):4, 1990.
Groth N: Sexual Assault of Children and Adolescents. Lexington, MA, Lexington Books, 1978.
Holter JC, Friedman SB: Child abuse: Early case findings in the emergency department. Pediatrics 42:128, 1968.
Kempe CH, Silverman FN, Steele BF, et al: The battered child syndrome. JAMA 181:17, 1962.
Kempe CH: Incest and other forms of sexual abuse. *In* Kempe CH, Helfer RE (eds): The Battered Child, 3rd edition. Chicago, University of Chicago Press, 1980, p 286.
Kempe RS: A developmental approach to the treatment of the abused child. *In* Kempe CH, Helfer RE (eds): The Battered

Child, 3rd Edition. Chicago, University of Chicago Press, 1980, p 17.
Kessler DB, Hyden P: Physical, sexual, and emotional abuse of children. Clin Symp 43:1, 1991.
Kottmeier PK: The battered child. Pediatr Ann 16:343, 1987.
Koverola C: Psychological effects of child sexual abuse. *In* Heger A, Emans SJ (eds): Evaluation of the Sexually Abused Child. New York, Oxford University Press, 1992.
McCann J, Voris J: Perianal injuries resulting from sexual abuse: a longitudinal study. Pediatrics 91:390, 1993.
McCurdy K, Daro D: Current trends in child abuse reporting and fatalities: The results of the 1992 annual fifty state survey. Chicago, National Committee for the Prevention of Child Abuse, 1993.
Paradise JE: The medical evaluation of the sexually abused child. Pediatr Clin North Am 37:839, 1990.
Radbill SX: Children in a world of violence: A history of child abuse. *In* Kempe CH, Helfer RE (eds): The Battered Child, 3rd edition. Chicago, University of Chicago Press, 1980, p. 4.
Russel DEH: The incidence and prevalence of intrafamilial and extrafamilial sexual abuse of female children. Child Abuse Negl 7:133, 1983.
Sauzier M, Mitkus C: Emergencies II: Sexual abuse and rape in childhood. *In* Robinson KS (ed): Manual of Clinical Child Psychiatry. Washington, DC: American Psychiatric Press, 1986.

Shearer SL, Herbert CA: Long-term effects of unresolved sexual trauma. Am Fam Physician 36:169, 1987.

Sperber N: The dual responsibility of dentists in child abuse. Can Dent Assoc J (March):31, 1980.

Touloukian RJ: Abdominal visceral injuries in battered children. Pediatrics 42:642, 1968.

U.S. Department of Health and Human Services: Recognition and Reporting of Child Maltreatment: Findings from the National Study of the Incidence and Prevalence of Child Abuse and Neglect. Washington, DC: U.S. Department of Health and Human Services, 1980.

Elder Abuse

DAVID V. ESPINO

Current awareness of the potential for violence within families, combined with the increasing numbers of frail elderly in our population (and the demands for caregiving that their presence signifies) has led researchers and clinicians to a recent focus on elder abuse and neglect.

Elder abuse lacks uniform classifications. The broadest area of agreement recognizes that elder abuse is characterized by fiscal, material, psychological, and physical abuse and/or neglect (Trilling et al. 1987). Fiscal abuse entails misuse of the victim's financial resources, as in fraud and embezzlement. Material abuse involves the violation of the victim's material possessions, involving (for example) theft or misuse of property. Psychological abuse includes environmental deprivation, verbal abuse, or a denial of rights. Physical abuse may include assault, rape, burns, starvation, or bondage. While our society's most common image of "abuse" results from such intentional physical violence, several scholars have noted that the most common form of elder abuse is neglect (Taler and Ansello, 1985). Neglect is characterized by inattention to or isolation of the elderly individual; for those who are dependent on others to provide daily necessities, this passive form of abuse can be very serious.

PREVALENCE

The difficulties with definition and reporting of elder abuse have led to a paucity of accurate data. Current estimates of the numbers of elderly who are maltreated vary from 0.5 to 2.5 million persons (Salond et al., 1984). Recent reports indicate that cognitively impaired adults may be at higher risk for physical abuse than for other age-associated illnesses Coyne et al., 1993; Paveza et al., 1992).

ETIOLOGY

The causes of elder abuse in the family, like other forms of violence, are multifactorial and, undoubtably, interrelated. Risk factors that have been proposed include: (1) development of a depending relationship (and consequent vulnerability of the elder person), (2) lack of close family ties, (3) history of family violence, (4) lack of financial resources, (5) psychopathology of the abuser/caregiver, and (6) a lack of community support (Hickey and Douglass, 1981; Kimsey et al., 1981). Predictive characteristics of violent feelings on the part of the caregivers may include physical aggression by the care recipient, disruptive behaviors by the care recipient, and shared living situation (Pillemer, 1992).

VICTIM AND ABUSER

The typical abused elder is in poor health and is living with another person or persons (Steinmetz and Amsden, 1983; Wolf et al., 1984). Most have been subjected to a combination of the abuses described above (Sengstock and Barnett, 1986). Approximately equal numbers of males and females in the population are abused; however, Pillemer and Finkelhor (1988) reported that abused women suffer more physical and psychological consequences from the violence than do the men.

Most often, the abuser of the elder is a relative of the victim and has taken care of that person for a number of years. In many cases, the caregiver burden overwhelms abusers to such an extent that they feel they are in an inextricable situation. Feeling "stuck" further increases the burden of caregiving, predisposing the individual to violent reactions. Other factors that may be associated with elder abuse include the caregiver's age, use of alcohol, and poor-quality relationships (Homer and Gilleard, 1990; Pillemer, 1992).

A predominant image, reinforced by the lay press and media, is that abuse is committed by ungrateful children toward their unreasonable aging parents (Sengstock and Hwalek, 1987). This image recently has been challenged, however, with findings indicating that the more common perpetrator of elder abuse is the spouse (Pillemer and Finkelhor, 1988; Wolf et al., 1984). This suggests that elder abuse is often a form of spouse abuse, indicating that clinical approaches to spouse abuse are appropriate for many elderly victims.

AFTERMATH OF VIOLENCE

The abused elder may exhibit various indicators that, although not pathognomonic, should alert the practitioner to possible abuse or neglect. Common behavioral indicators of abuse, such as generalized fear, may be misinterpreted as paranoia related to dementia or a latent psychosis (Council on Scientific Affairs, 1987). Physical indicators of elder abuse are similar to those of spouse abuse, with bruises, lacerations, multiple fractures to ribs or long bones, and rope burns being part of the initial presentation.

FAMILY PRACTICE INTERVENTIONS

The successful identification of abused elders and the development of effective prevention plans has been difficult to achieve. Unfavorable societal attitudes toward older persons, in combination with a culture-wide denial of the existence of abuse, means that many professionals will fail to identify elder abuse when it is presented. The lack of uniform definitions of elder abuse further hinders efforts to identify it. Finally, inconsistent federal, state, and local approaches of reporting elder abuse and enforcing legal protection of the abused has slowed prevention efforts.

To identify elder abuse, a high index of suspicion is recommended for the following findings: older persons with physical findings inconsistent with the medical history; caregivers with an absence of assisting behaviors; observation of angry, hostile, or abusive behavior on the part of the caregiver; and observation of a caregiver obsessed with control, showing excessive concern, or harping on the burdens of caregiving (Taler and Ansello, 1985). Because research in this area is still rudimentary and inconclusive, physicians are directed to assume that the likelihood for abuse is equal in males and females, in dependent and independent individuals, and in those who live alone as well as those who live with others. Whenever the diagnosis is in doubt, impartial third-party cooperation is necessary.

Family physicians are in an ideal position to take the lead in developing a management plan for abused elders; however, it is important to utilize a multidisciplinary approach. Physicians should become familiar with the local services available to the aged (Trilling et al., 1987). Social workers, mental health professionals, and other area agency professionals (such as legal aid, Meals-on-Wheels, or local adult protection agencies) can help assure adequate continuity of care and proper utilization of community resources.

REFERENCES

Council on Scientific Affairs: Elder abuse and neglect. JAMA 257:966, 1987.

Coyne AC, Reichman WE, Berbig LJ: The relationship of dementia and elder abuse. Am J Psychiatry 150:643, 1993.

Hickey T, Douglass RL: Mistreatment of the elderly in the domestic setting: An exploratory study. Am J Public Health 71:500, 1981.

Homer AC, Gilleard C: Abuse of elderly people by their carers. BMJ 301:1359, 1990.

Kimsey LR, Tarbon AR, Bragg DF: Abuse of the elder—the hidden agenda. I. The caretakers and the categories of abuse. J Am Geriatr Soc 29:465, 1981.

Paveza GJ, Cohen D, Eisdorfer C, et al: Severe family violence and Alzheimer's disease: Prevalence and risk factors. Gerontologist 32:493, 1992.

Pillemer K, Suitor JJ: Violence and violent feelings: What causes them among family caregivers? J Gerontol 47:S165, 1992.

Pillemer K, Finkelhor D: The prevalence of elder abuse: A random sample survey. Gerontologist 28:51, 1988.

Salond E, Kane RA, Satz M, Pynoos J: Elder abuse reporting: Limitations of statutes. Gerontologist 24:61, 1984.

Sengstock MC, Barnett S: Elderly victims of family abuse, neglect, and maltreatment: Can legal assistance help? J Gerontol Soc Work 9:43, 1986.

Sengstock MC, Hwalek M: A review and analysis of measures for the identification of elder abuse. J Gerontol Soc Work 10:21, 1987.

Steinmetz S, Amsden DJ: Dependent elders, family stress, and abuse. *In* Brubaker TH (ed): Family Relationships in Later Life. Beverly Hills, CA, Sage Publications, 1983.

Taler G, Ansello EF: Elder Abuse. Am Fam Physician 32:107, 1985.

Trilling JS, Greenblatt L, Shepard C: Elder abuse and utilization of support services for elderly patients. J Fam Pract 24:581, 1987.

Wolf R, Godkin M, Pillemer K: Elder Abuse and Neglect: Report from Three Model Projects. Worcester, University of Massachusetts Medical Center, 1984.

Spouse Abuse

SANDRA K. BURGE

"Spouse abuse" is a term that refers to intentional physical abuse by one's spouse or significant other that causes pain or injury (Pagelow, 1981). In two landmark studies of family violence, Straus and Gelles (1986) found that many husbands and wives reported violent behaviors toward each other (see also Cascardi et al., 1992). However, while wives sometimes strike out at their husbands, the husbands inflict far more injuries (Straus et al., 1980). In Cascardi et al.'s study (1992), wives were ten times more likely to receive broken bones or teeth as a result of domestic violence than husbands. Browne (1987) noted that 91 to 95 per cent of all violent crimes between spouses are victimizations of wives by husbands. Given the far greater likelihood that wives will be injured and/or traumatized by husbands, the remainder of this discussion will focus specifically on "wife abuse" to describe this phenomenon.

PREVALENCE AND INCIDENCE

Straus and Gelles' (1986) national probability survey indicated a husband-to-wife violence rate of 11.3 per cent per year. The violent behavior included slapping, pushing, and throwing objects, as well as more severe behavior such as punching, kicking, and using weapons. Three per cent of the wives in this study had been subjected to severe violence; this translates into 1.6 million severely abused wives per year. Assuming substantial underreporting by subjects, the investigators estimated that the actual incidence of wife abuse could be two times higher.

Two studies conducted with female patients in family practice settings found even higher rates of wife abuse (Rath et al., 1989; Hamberger et al., 1992); The prevalence of at least minor physical violence (slapping) was 44 and 38 per cent, respectively. Rath et al. noted that 28 per cent reported severe abuse. Hamberger et al. also inquired about 1-year incidence; 22.7 per cent of their sample reported at least minor violence within the past year, and 14.8 per cent had injuries resulting from their abuse.

ETIOLOGY

Women who are chronically battered do not choose to be so. Most men do not hit women during courtship; instead, violence begins after both partners have a deep emotional investment in each other. The first violent incident comes as complete surprise to the victim, and is not recognized as a precursor to a violent pattern. However, the nature of aggression is such that it escalates over time (Browne, 1987). Thus, earlier injuries may be minor and the woman's commitment to her husband may outweigh the harm done to her. Later, as the violence increases in frequency and severity, the emotional investment may decrease, but fear of further violence if she leaves, in combination with little help from social institutions, will keep a woman trapped in an abusive marriage. Beyond the current marriage, violence tends to cycle into future generations. Male children of violent husbands are likely to become violent husbands themselves; female children of violent husbands tend to become battered wives (Huesmann et al., 1984; Jaffe et al., 1990).

Why does violent behavior occur? Violence has been attributed to the psychopathology of the abuser, examined as a behavior learned from one's family of origin, and explained as a phenomenon that serves a function in our society (Gelles and Straus, 1979). Certainly several influences impact the problem of wife abuse. Gelles (1983) proposed a multifactorial theory that suggested people will use violence when the costs of being violent do not outweigh the rewards. He stated that men abuse their wives "because they can" (p. 157), and it works. Campbell (1993) described aggression in men as "instrumental," used to impose control over people, establishing a specific hierarchy. Men's anger erupts when "inferiors" challenge or question their authority. A man's violence is rewarded when it stops an emotional argument (and he wins), when he gets his wishes granted, and when he is able to vent his frustrations without fear of retaliation (Browne, 1987). For men, the costs of being violent to family members are low. Most wives are unable to retaliate, either physically or economically, and interference on the part of public agencies (e.g., legal authorities) is severely limited by our society's belief that what goes on inside a family is private business.

ABUSER AND VICTIM

Research has uncovered no "typical" battered woman (Browne, 1987; Walker, (1983). Expecting to find a "victim-prone" personality among battered women, Walker (1983) instead discovered that abused wives perceived themselves to be stronger, more independent, less traditional, and more sensitive than other women. Hotaling and Sugarman (1986), in a systematic review of 52 studies pertaining to husband-to-wife violence, looked at risk markers such as socioeconomic variables, psychopathology, self-esteem, substance abuse, economic dependency, traditional sex roles, and family history of violence. They found that the only consistent risk marker of being an abused wife was witnessing violence as a child, significant in 11 out of 15 studies. A second variable was worth noting: Experiencing violence as a child was significantly related to being an abused wife in 9 out of 13 studies.

In contrast, batterers present a more consistent profile. Hotaling and Sugarman (1986) identified the following consistent risk markers in abusing husbands: sexual aggression toward their partner, violence toward their children, witnessing violence as a child, alcohol use, lack of assertiveness, low-status jobs, lower income, and lower educational level. These men might be described as people with high economic stress, violent role models, and destructive ways of coping, expressing their distress through violence and drinking. Qualitative studies have noted additional personality characteristics in men who batter, such as: low self-esteem, extreme controlling behavior and beliefs of entitlement, pathological jealousy, traditional sex-role attitudes, and other-directed blame (Browne, 1987; Pagelow, 1981).

To summarize, it may be easier to identify a man at risk for abusive behavior than a woman at risk for victimization. To screen for victimization of a woman, one might begin with a discussion about the quality of her relationships and the nature of her parents' relationship when she was growing up. The most direct approach, asking about hitting in her current relationship, is also very appropriate.

AFTERMATH OF VIOLENCE

Victimized women demonstrate higher health care utilization than other women. Physician visits are twice as frequent, and health care costs are 2.5 times higher (Koss et al., 1991). Acutely, the injuries of battered women look different than the injuries of accident victims. Battered women are more likely to have facial injuries, and 13 times more likely to have injuries on the chest, breasts, and abdomen (Stark et al., 1979). Additionally, they are more likely to present with multiple injuries than are accident victims. Evidence of old and new injuries in the same location is common. Because of the repetitive, escalating pattern of violence that perpetrators tend to display, battered women's visits to physicians are repeated with increasingly severe injuries (Health Care Systems Committee of Tulsa, 1984).

In addition to acute injuries, abused women have a higher prevalence of chronic health problems and often turn to their family physicians for relief from vague but unremitting symptoms (Koss and Heslet, 1992). Common complaints include somatic symptoms such as insomnia, fatigue, gastrointestinal symptoms, premenstrual symptoms, chronic pain, and anemia (Haber and Roos, 1985; Kerouac et al., 1986; Koss and Heslet, 1992). In pregnancy, risk for abuse increases for many women; battered women experience more negative pregnancy outcomes, including miscarriages, stillbirths, and low-birth-weight newborns (Helton et al., 1987). Finally, victimization may be associated with negative health behaviors, such as eating disorders, substance abuse, and risk for sexually transmitted diseases and human immunodeficiency virus (Koss and Heslet, 1992).

Battered women's psychological reactions to violence are like other victims' reactions to catastrophe or threat (Browne, 1987). During the violence, the individual's focus is primarily on self-protection and survival. Reactions of shock, denial, disbelief, withdrawal, confusion, and fear are common. Long-term reactions include fear, confusion, and anger (Rosewater, 1988). Some remain withdrawn and passive, and exhibit symptoms of depression and listlessness. Chronic fatigue and tension, intense startle reactions, sleeping and eating disturbances, and nightmares may be noted (Browne, 1987). Psychological reactions can be severe and sometimes are misdiagnosed as schizophrenia or borderline personality disorder. Rosewater (1988) advocated the avoidance of psychiatric labels and directed professionals to explore and treat the source of the problem (the battering) instead of the symptoms.

The impact of violence in marriages extends beyond the battered wife. Jaffe and colleagues (1990) reviewed an extensive literature on the effect of wife abuse on children. They noted that children of battered women have poorer adjustment than children in nonviolent families. Infants who witness violence often are characterized by poor health, poor sleeping habits, and excessive screaming. Preschoolers show signs of terror, exhibited as yelling, irritable behavior, hiding, shaking, and stuttering. School-age children experience more somatic complaints and regress to earlier stages of functioning. Adolescents may use aggression as a predominant form of problem solving, may project blame onto others, and may exhibit a high degree of anxiety (e.g., bite nails, pull hair, somatize feelings).

FAMILY PRACTICE INTERVENTIONS

The impact of continuing violence on a woman's health and on the family's health demands a response from physicians that addresses more than the treatment of acute injuries. Family physicians who offer continuing, whole-person, family-oriented health care are in an ideal position to assist battered women. Effective intervention requires an accepting, collaborative attitude, in addition to the following actions.

The very most important service a physician can offer to battered women is to ask about the violence: "Is anyone at home hitting you?" (Finkelhor and Yllo, 1985). Focusing one's language on specific behaviors (like hitting or hurting) will elicit a more accurate response from patients; many battered women do not define their experiences as "abuse," "battery," or "victimization" (Koss and Heslet, 1992). A physician who asks about "hitting" communicates to the patient that: (1) this problem is not too shameful/deviant/insignificant/irrelevant to talk about; (2) the patient's discomfort with and reactions to her husband's violence are understandable and rational; and (3) the situation is changeable, not hopeless.

The second step involves assessing the patient's current level of safety and collaboratively developing a concrete "safe plan" that will allow her and her children to escape or avoid future violence. Discussion should address options relating to: decisions about leaving; if she leaves, where to stay; how to arrange transportation; how long to stay; getting legal protection; and so forth. Many women have resources that allow some respite and protection (such as a relative who will temporarily shelter them), but others will need public assistance, such as that provided by battered women's shelters.

Third, a physician must provide battered women with appropriate referrals. In a study of women who "beat" wife-beating (Bowker, 1983), subjects recommended contacting social service agencies, women's self-help groups, and women's shelters. Such agencies guide women to basic resources (food, shelter, jobs, legal assistance) and offer emotional support for the wives and interventions for violent husbands.

Finally, follow-up is necessary. Options discussed in the physician's office (such as legal intervention or psychotherapy for the husband) require contemplation, planning, and time on the part of the patient. One discussion generally does not "cure" violence in a family, but continuing communication, support, and exploration of options will empower women to make changes that eliminate violence from their lives.

REFERENCES

Bowker LH: Beating Wife-Beating. Lexington, MA, Lexington Books, 1983.

Browne A: When Battered Women Kill. New York, Free Press, 1987.

Campbell A: Men, Women and Aggression. New York, Basic Books, 1993.

Cascardi M, Langhinrichsen J, Vivian D: Marital aggression: Impact, injury, and health correlates for husbands and wives. Arch Intern Med 152:1178, 1992.

Finkelhor D, Yllo K: License to Rape: Sexual Abuse of Wives. New York, Free Press, 1985.

Gelles RJ: An exchange/social control theory. *In* Finkelhor D, et al. (eds): The Dark Side of Families: Current Family Violence Research. Beverly Hills, CA, Sage Publications, 1983, pp 151–165.

Gelles RJ, Straus MA: Determinants of violence in the family: Toward a theoretical integration. *In* Burr WR, et al. (eds): Contemporary Theories about the Family, Vol. I. New York, Free Press, 1979, pp 549–581.

Haber JD, Roos C: Effects of spouse abuse and/or sexual abuse in the development and maintenance of chronic pain in women. Adv Pain Res Ther 9:889, 1985.

Hamberger LK, Saunders DG, Hovey M: Prevalence of domestic violence in community practice and rate of physician inquiry. Fam Med 24:283, 1992.

Health Care Systems Committee of Tulsa, Oklahoma: Adult Abuse and Neglect: Handbook for Medical Personnel. Tulsa, Health Care Systems Committee, 1984.

Helton A, McFarland J, Anderson E: Battered and pregnant: A prevalence study. Am J Public Health 77:1337, 1987.

Hotaling GR, Sugarman DB: An analysis of risk markers in husband to wife violence: The current state of knowledge. Violence Victims 1(2):101, 1986.

Huesmann LR, Eron LD, Lefkowitz MM, Walder LO: Stability of aggression over time and generations. Dev Psychol 20:1120, 1984.

Jaffe PG, Wolfe DA, Wilson SK: Children of Battered Women. Newbury Park, CA, Sage Publications, 1990.

Kerouac S, Taggart ME, Lescop J, Fortin MF: Dimensions of health in violent families. Health Care Women Int 7:413, 1986.

Koss MP, Heslet L: Somatic consequences of violence against women. Arch Fam Med 1:53, 1992.

Koss MP, Koss PG, Woodruff WJ: Deleterious effects of criminal victimization on women's health and medical utilization. Arch Intern Med 151:342, 1991.

Pagelow MD: Woman-Battering: Victims and Their Experiences. Beverly Hills, CA, Sage Publications, 1981.

Rath GD, Jarratt LG, Leonardson G: Rates of domestic violence against adult women by men partners. J Am Board Fam Pract 2:227, 1989.

Rosewater LB: Battered or schizophrenic? Psychological tests can't tell. *In* Yllo K, Bograd M (eds): Feminist Perspectives on Wife Abuse. Newbury Park, CA, Sage Publications, 1988, pp 200–216.

Stark E, Flitcraft A, Frazier W: Medicine and patriarchal violence: The social construction of a "private" event. Int J Health Serv 9:461, 1979.

Straus MA, Gelles RJ: Societal change and change in family

violence from 1975 to 1985 as revealed by two national surveys. J Marriage Fam 48:465, 1986.
Straus MA, Gelles RJ, Steinmetz SK: Behind Closed Doors: Violence in the American Family. Garden City, NY, Anchor Press, 1980.

Walker LE: The battered woman syndrome study. *In* Finkelhor D, et al. (eds): The Dark Side of Families: Current Family Violence Research. Beverly Hills, CA, Sage Publications, 1983, pp 31–48.

Adult Victims of Sexual Assault

SANDRA K. BURGE

When hearing the word "rapist," the usual image that leaps to mind is the boogeyman, a sinister sociopath who lurks in the shadows, waiting for hapless young strangers to stroll innocently by. Why include a discussion of stranger violence in a chapter about domestic violence? In fact, the definition of sexual assault is not limited to rapes by strangers. Among adults, sexual assault can be perpetrated by spouses, lovers, dates, relatives, and acquaintances as well as strangers. The truth about sexual assault is that it is most often perpetrated by someone known to the victim.

The definition of sexual assault, simply stated, is "sex without consent, obtained by force or threat." The Texas penal code (Vernon's Texas Codes Annotated, Section 22.011) defines sexual assault as:

(a) A person commits an offense [of sexual assault] if the person:
  (1) intentionally or knowingly:
   (a) causes the penetration of the anus or female sexual organ of another person . . . by any means, without that person's consent
   (b) causes the penetration of the mouth of another person . . . by the sexual organ of the actor without that person's consent or
   (c) causes the sexual organ of another person . . . , without that person's consent, to contact or penetrate the mouth, anus, or sexual organ of another person, including the actor.

According to this code, "without consent" is defined as: (1) "compel[ling] the other person to submit or participate by the use of physical force or violence" (2) causing them to submit by "threatening to use force or violence" or (3) "the person has not consented and the actor knows the other person is [physically or mentally] unable to resist." It is noteworthy that, in Texas, sexual assault between spouses who live together is undefined; that is, a cohabiting husband is legally allowed to force his wife to have sex. This is not true in every state in the United States, and is a principle that is disputed by many, especially feminists and social scientists who study sexual assault. Some husbands do rape wives, with consequences to their victims that are parallel to those who are raped by the boogeyman.

EPIDEMIOLOGY

According to the Federal Bureau of Investigation, (FBI), 92,486 women in the United States reported being a victim of rape in 1988. However, these figures are based on police reports, and others estimate that the actual incidence of rape ranges from 4 to 20 times higher. In Russell's (1982) prevalence study of rape in the San Francisco area, nearly 3 per cent of the sample population had been victims of rape or attempted rape during the previous year. These findings were 40 times greater than the FBI's estimates from the same population during 1980. Of Russell's subjects, 44 per cent had been victims of rape or attempted rape in their lifetimes; one half of these women had been assaulted more than once. Only 25 per cent of the victimized women had been assaulted by strangers; 8 per cent had been assaulted by their husbands.

Koss and colleagues (1987) studied sexual aggression and victimization in a nationwide sample of 6159 college and university students. Among the women, 53.7 per cent indicated some form of sexual victimization since age 14; 27.5 per cent reported experiences that met the legal definitions for rape or attempted rape. Of those assaulted, 84 per cent knew the offender; 57 per cent of the offenders were dates. The incidence of victimization by rape or attempted rape for these women students in the previous year was 8.3 per cent.

Men can be sexually assaulted too, and their perpetrators are nearly always other men. The prevalence of victimization is less clear; most men who are assaulted do not report it. In my own setting, the Medical Center Hospital in San Antonio, the incidence of adult male sexual victimization is small. In 1992, out of 362 adults who presented to the Emergency Department for a forensic examination related to sexual assault, only 16 (4.4 per cent) were men (SK Burge, unpublished data). The prevalence of male sexual victimization during childhood is probably greater than during adulthood. In a study in our Family Health Center, 142 young adults (18 to 22 years old; 60 per cent females) were asked about "unwanted sexual experiences" (ND Kellogg, unpublished data). Of the males, 16 per cent reported such experiences, compared to 39 per cent of the females.

ETIOLOGY

As for any complex human behavior, theorists have posed several explanations for sexual assault. First, a psychopathological explanation of rape assumes that men who rape are psychologically maladjusted and different from other men. However, few elevations in psychiatric symptomatology among rapists are known. A physiological explanation regards rape as the expression of a male's uncontrollable desire for sex. This perspective assumes that sexual repression or a lack of sexual outlets will contribute to sexually aggressive acts. However, this theory does not explain nonaggressive sexual men in our society. Third, a sociocultural perspective notes that rape occurs in cultures characterized by male dominance, low female status and power, high rates of crime and violence, and adversarial sexual relations. In such a society, rape is regarded as a logical extension of a dominant ideology that degrades women and justifies coercive sexuality (Lottes, 1988). Why, then, do some men in our society not rape?

Most acknowledge that several factors contribute to the occurrence of sexual aggression in our society. Hall and Hirschman (1991) described four components that interact to cause sexual aggression in men: (1) physiological sexual arousal (especially when arousal is linked with aggression); (2) cognitions that justify sexual aggression (based on society-wide beliefs about men's and women's sexuality); (3) affective dyscontrol (especially anger or hostility); and (4) underlying personality problems (such as antisocial behavior). Among men who rape, one of these four components may dominate, acting as a motivational precursor that will increase the probability of sexually aggressive behavior, and also determine the way the aggression is perpetrated.

In our society, even though rape is illegal, sexual aggression is encouraged in men in subtle and not-so-subtle ways: by idealizing aggression as a desirable and necessary male trait; by failing to enforce laws prohibiting sexual assault; by attributing fault to the victim (rather than the assailant); and by justifying assault under most conditions. Feminists note how rape functions as a social control for women's behavior; fear of rape limits women's freedom and keeps them dependent on men for protection. All men, even nonrapists, can claim this advantage (Epstein, 1988).

PERPETRATORS

Perpetrators of sexual assault tend to be young men; 47 per cent of all rapists who are arrested are under 25 (Koss, 1988). However, those arrested represent a tiny proportion of sexual aggressors. In Koss et al.'s (1987) study of rape on college campuses, investigators queried men about their involvement as sexual aggressors; 25.1 per cent of men revealed some involvement in sexual aggression, with 7.7 per cent reporting behaviors that met the legal definition for rape or attempted rape. Most—88 per cent—were adamant that their behavior was not rape. Only 2 per cent of those who perpetrated sexual assault claimed that the police had been notified.

As noted above, perpetrators are more likely to be acquaintances than strangers. Koss et al. (1988) studied differences between stranger and acquaintance rape among college students. They found that perpetrators who were acquainted with the victims were more likely to act alone and to assault the victim multiple times. Strangers, in contrast, were more aggressive, and were more likely to use threats, hitting and slapping, and weapons. Both strangers and acquaintances were equally likely to use arm twisting, holding down, or beating. Men who rape men may be more likely to assault in groups. One study examined medical records of 28 male victims and noted that the mean number of assailants was 2.8 (Hillman et al., 1991).

VICTIMS

The typical adult victim of sexual assault is a young middle-class woman. Koss (1988) noted that the highest victimization rates for women occur in the 16- to 24-year age group. Winfield et al. (1990) found that college-educated women were more likely to report experience with sexual assault victimization than women with less education. Among women raped by husbands, Russell (1982) found that most came from upper-middle-class backgrounds. While these categories reflect the characteristics of those most frequently assaulted, physicians must be aware that victimization by sexual assault cuts across all ages, socioeconomic levels, and ethnic and racial groups.

It should be noted that few victims of sexual assault identify their experiences as "assault." In Koss et al.'s (1987) study, only 27 per cent of women whose experience met legal definitions of rape labeled themselves as rape victims. Women who were assaulted by strangers (and thus fit the boogeyman stereotype of rape) were more likely to view their experience as rape. Most did not consider their experience as ANY kind of crime (Koss et al., 1987, 1988). While most women readily admit that these experiences are extremely distressing, a woman is more likely to label the aggressor as a "creep" than an "assailant," especially if he is someone she knows. Only 5 per cent of victims in Koss et al.'s (1987) study contacted the police; in Russell's (1982) study, only 9.5 per cent of sexual assault victims contacted the police.

CONSEQUENCES TO THE VICTIM

A victim's acute psychological reaction to sexual assault typically includes shock, numbness, withdrawal, and denial (Burgess and Holmstrom, 1974). Those who are assaulted by strangers may be extremely fearful of repeat attacks; those who are assaulted by acquaintances experience an abrupt violation of trust and intense feelings of vulnerability, doubting their ability to protect themselves from danger. Self-blame often occurs, but is usually focused on situational factors ("I shouldn't have gone to that party") rather than the victim's character ("I am the victim type") (Frazier, 1990). For most victims, the overriding emotion is fear, and they may display phobic behavior and severe startle reactions, especially when exposed to reminders of the assault (Burgess and Holmstrom, 1974).

Long-term psychological reactions to rape include chronic anxiety and feelings of vulnerability, loss of control, alcohol abuse, and depression (Winfield et al., 1990). Long-term reactions may not be affected by stranger versus acquaintance assaults (Koss et al., 1988), but often are associated with the perceived dangerousness of the assault. Many victims will display symptoms of post-traumatic stress disorder (PTSD), with both depressive and anxious features (Bownes et al., 1991). The diagnostic criteria for PTSD, listed in the *Diagnostic and Statistical Manual IIIR* (American Psychiatric Association, 1987) are that the victim must have experienced an event outside the range of normal human experience and have symptoms lasting for longer than 1 month in each of the following categories: intrusive re-experiencing of the trauma; persistent avoidance of stimuli associated with the trauma, or numbing of general responsiveness; and persistent autonomic signs of anxiety. PTSD has

been seen more frequently in women who were assaulted by strangers, who were subjected to physical force and threats with weapons, and who sustained injuries (Bownes et al., 1991; Resnick et al., 1992).

Koss and Heslet (1992) provide a thorough discussion of medical and somatic sequelae to victimization experiences in women. They note that 40 per cent of rape victims will present acutely with physical injuries, with abrasions or contusions most likely to involve the head, neck, and face. Severe injuries are equally likely to include multiple traumas, major fractures, and major lacerations. Half of rape victims seen in trauma centers have vaginal and perineal trauma, including vulvar contusions and hymenal and vaginal lacerations. Symptoms of skeletal muscle tension or gastrointestinal irritability, as reactions to the stress of victimization, also may be manifested. Sexually transmitted diseases (STDs) occur in 3.6 to 30 per cent of rape victims, and approximately 5 per cent become pregnant as a result of rape.

In addition to acute problems, rape victims are more likely than nonvictims to display long-term somatic problems such as chronic pelvic pain and other chronic pain, premenstrual syndrome, gastrointestinal symptoms, eating disorders, and chemical dependency (Koss and Heslet, 1992). Following an assault, rape victims view their health more poorly than nonvictims, and increase their utilization of health care services (Koss et al., 1990).

ACUTE CARE OF THE ADULT SEXUAL ASSAULT VICTIM

Victims who report their assaults to the police, regardless of the level of injuries, will be asked to undergo a medical exam to search for evidence that can be used in court to support their claim. Most emergency departments have a standardized protocol to guide this forensic exam. The purpose of this protocol is to respond to typical arguments used in court to defend sexual assault perpetrators: mistaken identity or consent versus force. If identity is a question, the forensic exam can provide a link in identifying the assailant; if consent is a question, the exam can establish evidence of harm.

Occasionally, victims may assert their preference to be examined by a known, trusted physician, and will ask their family doctor to conduct the forensic exam. In most communities this is acceptable, as long as it is timely, the standardized protocol is followed, and the chain of custody of evidence is not broken. However, the more likely scenario is that victims will refuse to report the assault to the police, and will present acutely to their family physician for the purpose of treating injuries or preventing STDs. Under this circumstance, it is appropriate to offer the victims (in addition to the care requested) the option of a forensic exam, in case they may decide to go to the police at a later date. Unless the victim is a child, or the injuries are severe (as in knife or gunshot wounds), there is no legal mandate for the physician to report the assault to legal authorities.

Although the forensic exam has specific, perhaps nonmedical, goals, the physician's overriding concern should be the safety and comfort of the victim. The standardized protocol generally includes the following (adapted from the protocol from Medical Center Hospital, San Antonio):

1. A history of the assault (time and location of assault, number of assailants, sites of penetration, ejaculation if known, violent contact) and activities following the assault (such as bathing, douching, urinating, drinking, other sexual contact) is necessary to guide the exam. The physician should adopt a patient, respectful, empathic attitude, using open-ended questions and an attentive listening posture.

2. If the victim is wearing the same clothing and underclothing as during the assault, it is collected to assess for blood or semen stains.

3. A thorough physical exam is conducted to assess for injuries as well as evidence such as blood, semen, or hair from the assailant. Beginning "at the top" is less threatening than beginning with the genital exam. The appropriate use of gowns and drapes allows the victim to maintain a sense of modesty and dignity, and will decrease feelings of vulnerability.

4. Pubic hair samples are collected, first by combing the pubic hairs to obtain any loose fibers or hairs that are foreign to the victim, and next by cutting 10 to 12 pubic hairs at the skin line for standards for comparison. Standards do not have to be plucked.

5. Fingernail scrapings or cuttings may be done, to assess for skin, blood, or fibers from the assailant.

6. Two slides per site penetrated are prepared to assess for sperm. Slides should be air dried.

7. Two swabs per site penetrated are prepared, using small amounts of tap water to facilitate sampling. Swabs are air dried and sealed in tubes; extra water or saline should NOT be used in the tube. These samples are assessed for semen, acid phosphatase, and other prostatic fluid enzymes.

8. Wet prep slides are used to look for sperm and motility. Visualization of sperm is positive proof of a sexual encounter; however, nonvisualization should be considered INCONCLUSIVE, not negative.

9. Blood samples are drawn on victims as standards for comparison. Even if no other evidence is indicated, collect blood; blood may appear on evidence the physician does not see.

10. Other lab tests are conducted both for forensic and treatment purposes: sensitive urine pregnancy test; cultures for gonorrhea and chlamydia; serology for syphilis and human immunodeficiency virus.

11. Document findings. Medical records may be admissible as evidence and may be subpoenaed. Trials tend to occur long after the assault, so the record must be legible, descriptive, and specific. Standard medical nomenclature for conditions, impressions, and terms are acceptable. Schematic drawings are useful. Avoid vague terms such as "within normal limits" or "appropriate affect." Legal jargon such as "alleged assault" is not necessary, but physicians are advised to use the patient's own words when referring to details of the assault (e.g., "he hit me with his fist" is preferable to "the patient was assaulted") (American Medical Association, 1992).

Acute treatment generally addresses injuries, STDs, and pregnancy. Provide any necessary treatment for injuries. Provide tetanus prophylaxis if indicated by history. Prophylactic antibiotic treatment for STDs, specifically gonorrhea, infection with chlamydia, and incubating syphilis, is recommended. A follow-up exam and serologic tests should be done 4 weeks after the assault. If the patient is at risk for pregnancy as a result of the assault, and is not already pregnant, discuss postcoital contraception (PCC). PCC is not recommended if there has been previous unprotected intercourse during this menstrual cycle, if the patient is already pregnant, or if follow-up with the patient is uncertain. PCC is considered to be an abortifacient and may be an unacceptable option to some women. Careful discussion of ethical issues, side effects, and other options is warranted.

LONG-TERM CARE: FAMILY PRACTICE INTERVENTIONS

Koss et al. (1991) noted that victims of crime, particularly sexual assault, have an unusually high rate of medical utilization for years following the assault. Sexual assault victims are far more likely to seek help from physicians than from legal personnel, mental health professionals, or victim advocates. Furthermore, sexual assault is associated with many psychiatric and somatic complaints that patients bring to physicians. Thus, physicians, more than any other professionals in our society, are in the best position to identify and intervene with victims of sexual assault. The American Medical Association Council on Scientific Affairs recommends (1992):

1. *Routine screening.* Trauma history should be included in the social history part of a routine medical history. Questions such as, "Has anyone ever tried to hurt you or force you to do something you didn't want to do?" and "Tell me about stressful experiences in your life" may elicit victimiza-

tion experiences, even when patients have not labeled them as "abuse" or "assault." If the patient screens positive, ask about the impact the event(s) had, identify how the patient copes with reactions to the event(s), and assess the potential for further danger, especially immediate danger.

2. *Validation of the experience.* When a patient discloses a victimization experience, the physician's response should validate and normalize the patient's perspective on the problem. The physician can tell the patient that many people have sexual assault experiences, that most are afraid to tell anyone about it, that memories about the experience can be very painful, and that the fear of future assaults is a reasonable fear. Acknowledging that the experience was painful and disturbing and that

stress reactions are normal is a very powerful and therapeutic act.

3. *Record keeping.* In addition to noting a trauma history, physicians should document symptoms that may be linked to the victimization and referrals made. These items can provide a basis for later review of treatment plans, and are useful to assess progress or to indicate the need for more intensive interventions.

4. *Referral.* After disclosure of victimization, referrals to "trauma-specific" resources, such as rape crisis centers, should be made as quickly as possible. Physicians should become familiar with these resources in their communities in order to provide ready access to their patients who are recovering from sexual assault trauma.

REFERENCES

American Medical Association: Diagnostic and Treatment Guidelines on Domestic Violence. Chicago, American Medical Association, 1992.

American Psychiatric Association: Diagnostic and Statistical Manual of Mental Disorders, 3rd edition (revised). Washington, DC, American Psychiatric Press, 1987.

Bownes IT, O'Gorman EC, Sayers A: Assault characteristics and posttraumatic stress disorder in rape victims. Acta Psychiatr Scand 83:27, 1991.

Burgess AW, Holmstrom LL: Rape trauma syndrome. Am J Psychiatry 131:981, 1974.

Council on Scientific Affairs, American Medical Association: Violence against women: Relevance for medical practitioners. JAMA 267:3184, 1992.

Epstein CF: Deceptive Distinctions: Sex, Gender, and the Social Order. New York, Russell Sage Foundation, 1988.

Frazier PA: Victim attributions and post-rape trauma. J Pers Soc Psychol 59:298, 1990.

Hall GCN, Hirschman R: Toward a theory of sexual aggression: A quadripartite model. J Consult Clin Psychol 59:662, 1991.

Hillman R, O'Mara N, Tomlinson D, Harris JR: Adult male victims of sexual assault: An underdiagnosed condition. Int J STD & AIDS 2:22, 1991.

Koss MP: Hidden rape: Sexual aggression and victimization in a national sample of students in higher education. *In* Bur-

gess AW (ed): Rape and Sexual Assault II. New York, Garland Publishing, 1988.

Koss MP, Dinero TE, Seibel CA, Cox SL: Stranger and acquaintance rape: Are there differences in the victim's experience? Psychol Women Q 12:1, 1988.

Koss MP, Gidycz CA, Wisniewski N: The scope of rape: Incidence and prevalence of sexual aggression and victimization in a national sample of higher education students. J Consult Clin Psychol 55:162, 1987.

Koss MP, Heslet L: Somatic consequences of violence against women. Arch Fam Med 1:53, 1992.

Koss MP, Koss PG, Woodruff WJ: Deleterious effects of criminal victimization on women's health and medical utilization. Arch Intern Med 151:342, 1991.

Koss MP, Woodruff WJ, Koss PG: Relation of criminal victimization to health perceptions among women medical patients. J Consult Clin Psychol 58:147, 1990.

Lottes IL: Sexual socialization and attitudes toward rape. *In* Burgess AW (ed): Rape and Sexual Assault II. New York, Garland Publishing, 1988.

Resnick HS, Kilpatrick DG, Best CL, Kramer TL: Vulnerability-stress factors in development of posttraumatic stress disorder. J Nerv Ment Dis 180:424, 1992.

Russell DEH: Rape in Marriage. New York, MacMillan, 1982.

Winfield I, George LK, Swartz M, Blazer DG: Sexual assault and psychiatric disorders among a community sample of women. Am J Psychiatry 147:335, 1990.

A Footnote about Violence Prevention

SANDRA K. BURGE

What can we do to prevent domestic violence? Family physicians are in the best possible position to implement strategies that can prevent violence: Victims are more likely to seek help from a physi-

cian than legal or mental health professionals; victims have higher medical utilization than nonvictims; and family physicians see patients at all stages of the family life cycle, enabling them to intervene with intergenerational and cyclical patterns of violence. Prevention can be conceptualized in three ways: Primary prevention guides patients to avoid the problem altogether; secondary prevention identifies a problem in early stages, and prevents damage; and tertiary prevention identifies a problem in later stages, treats the current damage, and seeks to prevent further damage. Family physicians can use all three levels of prevention when working with violent or potentially violent families.

PRIMARY PREVENTION

Good parent education may prevent violence before it happens. Teach parents what to expect from their children at every level of development, reviewing cognitive as well as physical and motor expectations. Offer them nonviolent options for disciplining their children. Allow them to ventilate about the frustrations of parenting, and to discuss the impact of parenthood on their intimate relationship. If partner/spousal conflict becomes serious, remind them that they are the models for their children's future relationships, and guide them to appropriate therapy. Avoiding violence in this generation should also influence relationships in the next generation.

SECONDARY PREVENTION

Especially with young men and women, ask about the quality of their relationships. If they describe "fights" or "problems with temper," ask them about hitting or hurting each other, and ask about their parents' relationships. People in early stages of relationships may not identify violent behaviors as an ongoing problem—men who hurt are very remorseful, women who are hurt are convinced that these events are rare, and both believe it will never happen again. Express concern about physical fights. Describe negative consequences for couples where deliberate harm is inflicted: injuries, divorce, emotional distress in their children, and adult children who become batterers or victims. Even if they do not believe that their conflicts are serious, if hitting has occurred, gently encourage them to seek counseling for a relationship "tuneup" that will help them learn to relate to each other in the best possible ways.

TERTIARY PREVENTION

This is what many physicians (and other professionals in the legal and mental health systems) do now—identify a chronic, cycling, dangerous pattern of behaviors. At this stage, for example, when a battered wife is living in a continual state of fear, it is difficult to save the marriage, and the "treatment of choice" for many professionals is to get the woman out of the marriage before further harm is done. When speaking to the victim, acknowledge the stress she endures in her daily life. Label the violence as a problem, and inform her that there are options she can consider. In a collaborative fashion, list those options with her input—they can include staying, leaving, and getting help for the batterer. Assess current levels of danger, and ask her to devise an escape plan in the event that the batterer becomes dangerous again. Follow up frequently in order to assess ongoing levels of danger, and to provide her a place of safety, support, and empathy.

CHAPTER 7

CARE OF THE ELDERLY

MEL P. DALY and GEORGE A. TALER

DEMOGRAPHICS

There are approximately 35 million people over the age of 65, representing about 13 per cent of the United States population. This number is expected to increase such that, by the year 2030, it is projected that there will be 66 million people over 65 years of age, representing 22 per cent of the population. While it appears that absolute life span cannot be extended, average life expectancy continues to increase, and, for someone currently 65 years of age, is 15 years for a man and 19 years for a woman. The goal of health care delivery initiatives for older Americans therefore must be to delay the onset of disease and disability. As more people are living longer, many accumulate disease and disability. Evidence suggests that interventions directed at preventing the major causes of death and disability can delay their onset and not only reduce early mortality but compress morbidity until late in life (Fries, 1980). Those over 85 represent the fastest growing segment of the population and so will have a significant impact on health care policy decisions in the near future.

Most older persons live in the community, over two thirds living with a family member and one out of three living alone. The majority (66 per cent) of older people have children who live within 30 minutes (travel time), and 60 per cent of community-dwelling elderly people visit at least weekly with their children. Almost 80 per cent of older men are married, but older women are five times more likely to be widowed and are three times more likely to be living alone. About 5 per cent of those over the age of 65 live in nursing homes; however, among those over the age of 85, approximately one in four persons lives in an institutional setting.

Older individuals account for one third of all hospital stays and almost half of all hospital days. An older person is more likely to stay in the hospital longer and visit his or her doctor more frequently. The average health care expenditure for older individuals is approximately four times that spent on younger persons, with hospital costs accounting for the major portion of this expense.

CHANGES WITH AGE

Normal aging is a heterogeneous process characterized by an inevitable erosion in function at a cellular, tissue, and organ level, with wide variation between individuals. The common denominator among all elderly would appear to be an age-related decline in physiologic reserve, resulting in a reduced ability to respond to pathophysiologic stressors. Because of this, even normal older persons have less efficient responses to changes in temperature (either hyper- or hypothermia) and plasma or extracellular fluid volume, and are at more risk for such conditions as orthostatic hypotension and hypertension because of altered autonomic nervous system responses (Kenney, 1989). Frequently, older persons do not manifest the same levels of febrile responses to infection as younger patients. There is a higher prevalence of infection and autoimmune conditions in older people as a result of age-related changes in cell-mediated immunity, which may result in anergy. Thymic involution appears to occur with advanced years, perhaps accounting for the high incidence of impaired immune response in the elderly. While basal hematopoiesis remains unchanged with age (Lipschitz and Udapa, 1986), the ability to mount a rapid hematopoietic response to blood loss or hypoxia is reduced.

There is extreme individual variation in how tissues and organs age, even in the absence of pathology. Many of the "changes" reported in epidemiologic studies of normal elderly individuals reflect environmental and genetic effects, and potentially can be reversed by modifications in behaviors or preventive practices. For example, it has been reported that total body fat composition doubles between the ages of 25 and 75. However, this change does not occur in less developed societies, suggesting that factors other than aging (i.e., diet and physical activities) may be responsible. Also, there is evidence that much of the age-associated decline in lean body mass and bone density can be reversed by regular exercise (Pollock et al., 1987). Truly "age-related" changes are not amenable to intervention; these include declines in skin melanocyte number and function, with resulting greying of hair, and in the collagen content of skin and sub-

TABLE 7–1. STRUCTURAL/FUNCTIONAL AGE-RELATED CHANGES*

1. Cellular Level: Various morphologic changes in nucleus and cytoplasmic organelles; decreased cell number generally throughout tissues; deposition of lipofuscin pigment in both mitotic and postmitotic cells; decreased cell functions, including oxidative phosphorylation, DNA and RNA synthesis and protein synthesis, and decreased adrenergic responsiveness; changes in response to stress and functional effectiveness of enzyme systems.

2. Connective Tissue: Collagen—increased strength, stability, and increase in number of cross-links, resulting in greater stiffness; decreased tissue elasticity in skin, major blood vessels, heart, lungs, and ligaments.

3. Body Composition: Weight generally declines after age 50 in males while remaining relatively constant in females; decrease in lean body weight caused primarily by shrinkage of muscle mass reflected in decreased creatinine production (25% in males and 15% in females); organ size declines (muscles, liver, brain, kidneys) with some exceptions (prostate, lungs, heart, and (?) GI tract).

4. Cardiovascular: Cardiac output falls 1% per year after age 30; impaired heart rate increases to stress; stroke volume decreases 0.7% per year in resting state; heart rate declines; prolonged mechanical refractory period; ECG has small increases in PR, QRS, and QT intervals with decreased amplitude and left-shift of QRS; progressive elastocalcinosis of media of elastic arteries and elastic lamina of muscular arteries resulting in decreased distensibility and increased systolic blood pressure; decreased blood flow to various organs—less to kidney than heart or brain.

5. Excretory: Total nephron count decreases by 30 to 40% between ages 25 and 85; kidney weight decreases 30%; GFR decreases 46% and RPF 53% between ages 20 and 90; filtration fraction increases; a parallel reduction in renal tubular cell mass causes a 43% decrease in max. tubular resorption for glucose; decreased concentrating ability and a slower and prolonged response to acid and base loads; serum creatinine does not reflect creatinine clearance because of decreased production owing to smaller muscle mass; compensatory hypertrophy capabilities are decreased to a max. of 30% vs. 50% in a young kidney.

6. Respiratory: Increased A-P diameter, kyphosis, decreased strength of expiratory muscles = decreased compliance of chest wall; decreased number of alveoli owing to destruction of septa with dilatation of resp. bronchioles and alveolar ducts; increased rigidity of lungs and decreased compliance promotes airway collapse; increased RV, FRC with unchanged TLC; VC decreased 26 and 22 cc per year in males and females, respectively; increased AaO_2 difference (10 to 15%) due to V/Q abnormality with airway collapse in dependent but still perfused lung regions; no change in $PaCO_2$; all timed ventilatory functions decrease, probably owing to decreased elastic recoil and early airway collapse with increased resistance to expiration; increased risk of pulmonary infection owing to decreased projective force of cough and mucociliary clearance rate, increased frequency of aspiration, and gram-colonization rate of oropharynx.

7. Gastrointestinal:
   Dentition: Wearing of enamel and dentin on chewing surfaces; fibrosis and decreased Ca^{++} of pulp space; root resorption and root dentin sclerosis; apical migration of supporting structures; all result in increased chance of loss of teeth—50% are without by age 65.
   Esophagus: Decreased peristaltic response; increased nonperistaltic generalized contractions (corkscrew esophagus on barium swallow); delayed transit time; decreased LES relaxation following swallowing—achalasia; increased incidence of H.H; increase in columnar epithelium in lower esophagus.
   Stomach: Decreased secretion of acid to 20% of volumes in youth; increased intestinal metaplasia and polyposis; increased incidence of atrophic gastritis (Scandinavian study—40% after age 65), but this is probably a genetically determined age-related pathologic process.
   Sm. Intestine: Decreased Peyer's patches and lymphoid tissue; with exception of decreased absorption of Ca^{++} (active transport), which may be affected by endocrine function, and possibly Fe^{++}, which is related to gastric acidity, no significant changes in absorptive function have been noted.
   Colon: Thickened muscularis mucosa; increased incidence of diverticulosis, over 50% by age 80; decreased intestinal motility (increased hypotonia and decreased peristalsis), resulting in increased storage and dehydration of stool, leading to constipation; increased incidence of fecal incontinence owing to decreased external sphincter tone—assoc. (±) with neurologic disease and responds to feedback training.
   Liver: Weight decreased by 20% by age 50; albumin is decreased and globulin is increased with no change in total protein; remainder of common LFTs are normal (bil, SGPT, SGOT, and alk. phos.); there is slow metabolism of several drugs owing to decreased efficiency of enzyme systems.
   Gallbladder: Increased incidence of stones to 40% by age 80, possibly owing to decreasing cholesterol stabilization mechanisms.
   Pancreas: No change in organ weight but possibly decreased functional tissue: trypsin decreased but bicarbonate, lipase, and amylase (with stimulation) are all normal; insulin—see Endocrine.

8. Endocrine:
   Pituitary: ACTH response to stress is possibly decreased; ADH response to hyperosmolarity is increased, resulting in an increased incidence of SIADH.
   Thyroid: T_4 and TSH are normal while T_3 is decreased 25 to 40% after age 60, ^{131}I uptake rate is decreased, as is T_4 metabolism by the liver; response to stress is normal, therefore reduced turnover rates reflect decreased BMR and peripheral need owing to decreased lean body weight.
   Parathyroid: Reports are equivocal as to PTH levels.
   Pancreas: Decreased number and function of insulin-secreting cells; a greater proportion of insulin secreted is in inactive precursor proinsulin form; progressive peripheral insulin resistance owing to relative increase in body fat in relation to decrease in LBW—as stable number of fat cells increase in size, there is a decrease in insulin receptor effectiveness; all this results in an increased glucose response to an oral GTT but a normal fasting glucose.
   Adrenals: Glucocorticoid levels retain normal diurnal rhythms with decreased secretion and excretion rates—i.e., a slower turnover; response to stress is normal to decreased; there are decreased levels of adrenal androgens (50%); estrogens are all adrenal in origin after menopause and are 5 to 10% of normal in females and unchanged in males; testosterone metabolism and production rates both decrease while binding globulin increases—these changes result in decreased free testosterone.

Table continued on following page

TABLE 7–1.   STRUCTURAL/FUNCTIONAL AGE-RELATED CHANGES* *(Continued)*

9. Hematopoietic and Immune: Red cell line is normal, including a normal hematocrit; Fe^{++} absorption is reduced, as are serum Fe^{++} and TIBC slightly; platelets are normal; fibrinogen levels are increased, and consequently the ESR can be increased up to 40 mm per hour; phagocytic function is normal; IgA and IgG are normal while IgM may be decreased; number of B cells is normal but response to antigen challenge of vaccination is reduced, possibly owing to decreased T cell function; there is a reduced ability of T cells to proliferate in response to challenge, possibly owing to changes in cell subpopulations, i.e., an increase in suppressor cells; there is decreased delayed hypersensitivity in elderly; complement levels are normal.

10. Neurologic: Variable degree of neuronal dropout, depending on location and individual differences; decreased interconnections between dendrites with presumed decrease in number of transmitted impulses; lipofuscin pigment accumulation and degeneration of Nissl substance; geometric increase in number of senile plaques, neurofibrillary tangles, and granulovacuolar degeneration; cerebral blood flow declines with age; 15% decrease in nerve conduction velocities with a decrease in motor and sensory latency; increased MAO's and serotonin with possible decreased catechol levels; progressive loss of stage 4 sleep with numerous brief arousals with slight decrease in total sleep, giving the impression of sleeplessness; sedatives decrease the latency to sleep and periods of arousal but only temporarily, with return of usual pattern after a few days; a 7% decline in brain weight by age 80; 20% decrease in blood flow to CNS by age 70.

11. Special Senses:

    Sight: Decreased visual acuity, visual fields, and speed of dark adaptation; increased minimal light threshold reception, and greater loss of VA with dim illumination; increased discoloration and rigidity of lens nucleus, resulting in decreased accommodative ability; pupillary response to light and accommodation decrease so that by age 85 only $\frac{1}{3}$ respond to light and none to accommodation; increased frequency of chronic glaucoma owing to decreased reabsorption of intraocular fluid; increased lens size and abnormalities of shape lead to astigmatism and myopia; increased incidence of cataracts (? pathologic condition).

    Hearing: Tympanic membrane flexibility declines; increased mean pure tone threshold with age for all frequencies, especially for 4000 cps in males after 60; more important is the loss in speech reception and discrimination thresholds.

    Taste: Decrease in number and functional status of taste buds; saliva flow is decreased by $\frac{2}{3}$, leading to dry mouth and decreased taste sense; taste also affected by state of oral hygiene and use of dental prostheses.

    Smell: Decreased to same extent as taste (one study with only 22% normal).

    Touch: Decreased touch acuity; pain sensors appear to be intact.

12. Musculoskeletal:

    Stature: Height progressively decreases primarily owing to shortening of the vertebral column from narrowing of the intervertebral disks and a decrease in vertebral height; there is kyphosis as well; long bones are relatively preserved in length; total height loss is 2 inches between ages 20 and 70.

    Bones: Bone loss is universal beginning after age 40, accelerated in females after menopause and totaling 25% in females and 12% in males; those with the smallest bone mass at maturity are affected most; etiology is still unclear; there is continued appositional bone growth on outside surfaces, resulting in wider hollowed out bones; there is loss of trabeculae along with apatite and protein matrix; increased risk of fracture is present and incidence of vertebral collapse and femur fractures is significantly increased; edentulous state leads to progressive mandibular resorption.

    Joints: Dehydration of intervertebral disks and joint cartilage with wear and tear atrophy (fibrillar degeneration); exposure of subchondral bone leads to ebumation and spur formation at sites of trauma; changes affect weight-bearing joints most but also the glenoid and others; pain is a concomitant symptom.

    Muscles: Decreased number of cells; increased fat content in muscle bundles; decreased numbers of capillaries and neurons per motor unit; increased lipofuscin pigment deposition; decreased myosis-ATPase activity; progressive loss of muscular strength and mechanical efficiency.

From Thompson MP, Tollison JW: Caring for the elderly. *In* Rakel RE (ed): Textbook of Family Practice, 4th edition. Philadelphia, WB Saunders Company, 1990, pp 144–145, with permission.

cutaneous tissue, with thinning of skin and wrinkling. Other tissue and organ changes that occur most consistently with aging are listed in Table 7–1. When disease is superimposed on the normal changes of aging, homeostasis is more easily disrupted, causing greater declines in function and a slower return to premorbid levels of ability.

APPROACH TO THE PATIENT

The variability among older persons that results from age-related physiologic changes, the frequent presence of multiple, concurrent pathology, and the heterogeneous presentations of illness make it difficult for the clinician to develop a uniform approach to elderly patients. Many elderly persons minimize their symptoms and infrequently seek medical assistance. Ageist beliefs are pervasive among the elderly (and their families), with many believing that illness and disability are natural consequences of the aging process. Some believe that little benefit can be gained from seeing a physician and fear seeking medical evaluation, should significant pathology be uncovered.

Illness may present in nonspecific ways as anorexia, self-neglect, malaise, altered mental status, or incontinence (Beers and Besdine, 1987). These symptoms may be manifestations of pathology ranging from infection to myocardial or cerebrovascular disease to depression. For many older persons, the first indication of disease is a decline in previous levels of function, either physically, mentally, socially, or emotionally. Thus, a comprehensive approach is indicated to assess each of these domains, especially for the "frail," multiply impaired older person.

The office should be quiet and warm; chairs and

examination tables should be comfortable and yet high and wide enough for patients with arthritis and muscular weakness. Walkers, wheelchairs, voice amplification, communication aids, and other assistive devices should be available. Additional time should be allowed to address issues such as changes in functional, cognitive, sensory, and emotional performance (Rubenstein et al.,

TABLE 7–2. MINI-MENTAL STATE EXAMINATION (MMSE)

Add points for each correct response.

	Score	Points
Orientation		
1. What is the: Year?	_____	1
Season?	_____	1
Date?	_____	1
Day?	_____	1
Month?	_____	1
2. Where are we? State?	_____	1
County?	_____	1
Town or city?	_____	1
Hospital?	_____	1
Floor?	_____	1
Registration		
3. Name three objects, taking one second to say each. Then ask the patient to repeat all three after you have said them.	_____	3
Give one point for each correct answer. Repeat the answers until patient learns all three.		
Attention and calculation		
4. Serial sevens. Give one point for each correct answer. Stop after five answers. Alternate: Spell WORLD backwards.	_____	5
Recall		
5. Ask for names of three objects learned in question 3. Give one point for each correct answer.	_____	3
Language		
6. Point to a pencil and a watch. Have the patient name them as you point.	_____	2
7. Have the patient repeat "No ifs, ands, or buts."	_____	1
8. Have the patient follow a three-stage command: "Take a paper in your right hand. Fold the paper in half. Put the paper on the floor."	_____	3
9. Have the patient read and obey the following: "CLOSE YOUR EYES." (Write it in large letters.)	_____	1
10. Have the patient write a sentence of his or her choice. (The sentence should contain a subject and an object and should make sense. (Ignore spelling errors when scoring.)	_____	1
11. Have the patient copy the design. (Give one point if all sides and angles are preserved and if the intersecting sides form a quadrangle.)	_____	1
	_____ =	1 Total 30

In validation studies using a cut-off score of 23 or below, the MMSE has a sensitivity of 87%, a specificity of 82%, a false positive ratio of 39.4%, and a false negative ratio of 4.7%. These ratios refer to the MMSE's capacity to accurately distinguish patients with clinically diagnosed dementia or delirium from patients without these syndromes.

SOURCE: Courtesy of Marshall Folstein, MD. Reprinted with permission.

For additional information on administration and scoring refer to the following references:
1. Anthony JC, LeResche L, Niaz U, et al. Limits of "Mini-Mental State" as a screening test for dementia and delirium among hospital patients. *Psych Med.* 1982;12:397–408.
2. Folstein MF, Anthony JC, et al. Meaning of cognitive impairment in the elderly. *J Am Geriatr Soc.* 1985;33(4):228–235.
3. Folstein MF, Folstein S, McHugh PR. Mini-Mental State: a practical method for grading the cognitive state of patients for the clinician. *J Psych Res.* 1975;12:189–198.
4. Spenser MP, Folstein MF. The Mini-Mental State Examination. In: Keller PA, Ritt LG. *Innovations in Clinical Practice: A Source Book.* 1985;4:305–310.

From Beck JC (ed): Appendix A. *In* Geriatrics Review Syllabus: A Core Curriculum in Geriatric Medicine. American Geriatrics Society 1991-1992 Program. New York, American Geriatrics Society, 1991-1992, p 489, with permission.

1989). At times, it may be necessary to enlist the help of a caregiver to clarify details. Questions should be asked about common symptoms often not volunteered, such as incontinence, falls, difficulty with ambulation, forgetfulness, and depression. A thorough list of prescription and nonprescription medications also should be obtained. More formal testing of higher intellectual function may be indicated, especially if the patient has difficulty recalling details or chronology. Other important areas to address in the history include appetite, weight and nutrition, sleep, driving ability, sexual function, and preferences about end-of-life decision making.

The physical examination should pay particular attention to height, weight, and posture. Orthostatic pulse and blood pressure measurements are important because of the high prevalence of high blood pressure and orthostatic hypotension. A sensory evaluation should include an assessment of vision and hearing. Teeth, gums, dentures, and the oral mucosa should be inspected carefully. Cardiac murmurs are common and should be assessed for pathologic significance and hemodynamic compromise. The presence of peripheral pulses and vascular bruits should be noted. Although frequently omitted, all older persons should have a rectal examination because findings such as prostatic hypertrophy or nodules, carcinomas, and hemorrhoids are common. Many older women have not had adequate screening, pelvic examination, and Pap smears. A comprehensive neurologic examination may reveal abnormalities in motor, sensory, or cerebellar function, and a mental status examination should be included as a screen for dementia and delirium. The evaluation should be complemented further by standardized performance-based evaluations and screening questionnaires. A number of instruments have been validated to assess the domains of function frequently found to be abnormal and that are often amenable to interventions. The most commonly used tests include the Mini-Mental State Examination (Folstein et al., 1975), the Geriatric Depression Scale (Yesavage et al., 1983), the Katz Activities of Daily Living (Katz et al., 1963) and the Instrumental Activities of Daily Living (Lawton and Brody, 1969), Scales, the Physical Performance Test (Reuben and Siu, 1990), and the "Get-up-and-go test" to assess gait and mobility (Tinetti, 1986) (see Tables 7–2 through 7–6). Ideally, this type of comprehensive evaluation should be done by a trained interdisciplinary team of professionals.

TABLE 7–3. GERIATRIC DEPRESSION SCALE (SHORT FORM)

Choose the best answer for how you felt over the past week.

1. Are you basically satisfied with your life?	yes/no
2. Have you dropped many of your activities and interests?	yes/no
3. Do you feel that your life is empty?	yes/no
4. Do you often get bored?	yes/no
5. Are you in good spirits most of the time?	yes/no
6. Are you afraid that something bad is going to happen to you?	yes/no
7. Do you feel happy most of the time?	yes/no
8. Do you often feel helpless?	yes/no
9. Do you prefer to stay at home, rather than going out and doing newCyto ?	yes/no
10. Do you feel you have more problems with memory than most?	yes/no
11. Do you think it is wonderful to be alive now?	yes/no
12. Do you feel pretty worthless the way you are now?	yes/no
13. Do you feel full of energy?	yes/no
14. Do you feel that your situation is hopeless?	yes/no
15. Do you think that most people are better off than you are?	yes/no

This is the scoring for the scale. One point for each of these answers. Cut-off: normal (0–5), above 5 suggests depression.

1. no	6. yes	11. no
2. yes	7. no	12. yes
3. yes	8. yes	13. no
4. yes	9. yes	14. yes
5. no	10. yes	15. yes

SOURCE: Courtesy of Jerome A. Yesavage, MD. Reprinted with permission.

For additional information on administration and scoring refer to the following references:
1. Sheikh JI, Yesavage JA. Geriatric Depression Scale: recent evidence and development of a shorter version. *Clin Gerontol.* 1986;5:165–172.
2. Yesavage JA, Brink TL, Rose TL, et al. Development and validation of a geriatric depression rating scale: a preliminary report. *J. Psych Res.* 1983; 17:27.

From Beck JC (ed): Appendix A. *In* Geriatrics Review Syllabus: A Core Curriculum in Geriatric Medicine. American Geriatrics Society 1991-1992 Program. New York, American Geriatrics Society, 1991-1992, p 488, with permission.

TABLE 7–4. ACTIVITIES OF DAILY LIVING (ADL) SCALE

Evaluation Form

Name _____   Day of evaluation _____

For each area of functioning listed below, check description that applies. (The word "assistance" means supervision, direction, or personal assistance.)

Bathing—either sponge bath, tub bath, or shower

☐	☐	☐
Receives no assistance (gets in and out of tub by self, if tub is usual means of bathing)	Receives assistance in bathing only one part of the body (such as back or a leg)	Receives assistance in bathing more than one part of the body (or not bathed)

Dressing—gets clothes from closets and drawers, including underclothes, outer garments, and using fasteners (including braces, if worn)

☐	☐	☐
Gets clothes and gets completely dressed without assistance	Gets clothes and gets dressed without assistance, except for assistance in tying shoes	Receives assistance in getting clothes or in getting dressed, or stays partly or completely undressed

Toileting—going to the "toilet room" for bowel and urine elimination; cleaning self after elimination and arranging clothes

☐	☐	☐
Goes to "toilet room," cleans self, and arranges clothes without assistance (may use object for support, such as cane, walker, or wheelchair, and may manage night bedpan or commode, emptying same in morning)	Receives assistance in going to "toilet room" or in cleansing self or in arranging clothes after elimination or in use of night bedpan or commode	Doesn't go to room termed "toilet" for the elimination process

Transfer

☐	☐	☐
Moves in and out of bed as well as in and out of chair without assistance (may be using object for support, such as cane or walker)	Moves in and out of bed or chair with assistance	Doesn't get out of bed

Continence

☐	☐	☐
Controls urination and bowel movement completely by self	Has occasional "accidents"	Supervision helps keep urine or bowel control; catheter is used or person is incontinent

Feeding

☐	☐	☐
Feeds self without assistance	Feeds self except for getting assistance in cutting meat or buttering bread	Receives assistance in feeding or is fed partly or completely by using tubes or intravenous fluids

SOURCE: Courtesy of Sidney Katz, MD. Reprinted with permission.

For additional information on administration and scoring refer to the following references:
1. Katz S. Assessing self-maintenance: activities of daily living, mobility, and instrumental activities of daily living. *J Am Geriatr Soc.* 1983;31:721–727.
2. Katz S, Akpom CA. A measure of primary sociobiologic functions. *Int J Health Services.* 1976;6:493–508.
3. Katz S, Downs TD, Cash HR, et al. Progress in development of the index of ADL. *J Gerontol.* 1970;10(1):20–30.

From Beck JC (ed): Appendix A. *In* Geriatrics Review Syllabus: A Core Curriculum in Geriatric Medicine. American Geriatrics Society 1991-1992 Program. New York, American Geriatrics Society, 1991-1992, p 469, with permission.

TABLE 7–5. INSTRUMENTAL ACTIVITIES OF DAILY LIVING (IADL) SCALE

Self-Rated Version Extracted from the Multilevel Assessment Instrument (MAI)

1. Can you use the telephone:
   without help,   3
   with some help, or   2
   are you completely unable to use the telephone?   1

2. Can you get to places out of walking distance:
   without help,   3
   with some help, or   2
   are you completely unable to travel unless special arrangements are made?   1

3. Can you go shopping for groceries:
   without help,   3
   with some help, or   2
   are you completely unable to do any shopping?   1

4. Can you prepare your own meals:
   without help,   3
   with some help, or   2
   are you completely unable to prepare any meals?   1

5. Can you do your own housework:
   without help,   3
   with some help, or   2
   are you completely unable to do any housework?   1

6. Can you do your own handyman work:
   without help,   3
   with some help, or   2
   are you completely unable to do any handyman work?   1

7. Can you do your own laundry:
   without help,   3
   with some help, or   2
   are you completely unable to do any laundry at all?   1

8a. Do you take medicines or use any medications?
   (If yes, answer Question 8b) Yes   1
   (If no, answer Question 8c) No   2

8b. Do you take your own medicine
   without help (in the right doses at the right time),   3
   with some help (take medicine if someone prepares it for you and/or reminds you to take it), or   2
   (are you/would you be) completely unable to take your own medicine?   1

8c. If you had to take medicine, can you do it
   without help (in the right doses at the right time),   3
   with some help (take medicine if someone prepares it for you and/or reminds you to take it), or   2
   (are you/would you be) completely unable to take your own medicine?   1

9. Can you manage your own money:
   without help,   3
   with some help, or   2
   are you completely unable to handle money?   1

SOURCE: Lawton MP, Brody EM. Assessment of older people: self-maintaining and instrumental activities of daily living. *Gerontologist.* 1969;9:179–185. Reprinted with permission.

For additional information on administration and scoring refer to the following references:
1. Lawton MP. Scales to measure competence in everyday activities. *Psychopharm Bull.* 1988;24(4):609–614.
2. Lawton MP, Moss M, Fulcomer M, et al. A research and service-oriented Multilevel Assessment Instrument. *J Gerontol.* 1982; 37:91–99.

From Beck JC (ed): Appendix A. In Geriatrics Review Syllabus: A Core Curriculum in Geriatric Medicine. American Geriatrics Society 1991-1992 Program. New York, American Geriatrics Society, 1991-1992, p 471, with permission.

TEAM APPROACH TO CARE

Health care teams are an integral component of geriatric practice. Teams are established more easily in hospital settings, drawing together representatives from various disciplines (see Geriatric Evaluation and Management Units). In ambulatory care, similar resources can be brought together through affiliations with a home care program, because the majority of patients who require this intensive level of professional services are also likely to be eligible for outpatient skilled nursing or physical therapy services. For less severely compromised patients, a core team comprised of a phy-

TABLE 7–6. PHYSICAL PERFORMANCE TEST

Administer the Physical Performance Test (PPT) as outlined below. Subjects are told to perform each task at their usual speed and given up to two chances to complete each item. Assistive devices are permitted for tasks 6 through 8.

1. Ask the subject, when given the command "go," to write the sentence "whales live in the blue ocean." Time from the word "go" until the pen is lifted from the page at the end of the sentence. All words must be included and legible. Period need not be included for task to be considered complete.

2. Five kidney beans are placed in a bowl, 5 inches from the edge of the desk in front of the patient. An empty coffee can is placed on the table at the patient's nondominant side. A teaspoon is placed in the patient's dominant hand. Ask the subject, on the command "go," to pick up the beans, one at a time, and place each in the coffee can. Time from the command "go" until the last bean is heard hitting the bottom of the can.

3. Place a *Physician's Desk Reference* or other heavy book on a table in front of the patient. Ask the patient, when given the command "go," to place the book on a shelf above shoulder level. Time from the command "go" to the time the book is resting on the shelf.

4. If the subject has a jacket or cardigan sweater, ask him or her to remove it. If not, give the subject a lab coat. Ask the subject, on the command "go," to put the coat on completely such that it is straight on his or her shoulders and then remove the garment completely. Time from the command "go" until the garment has been completely removed.

5. Place a penny approximately 1 foot from the patient's foot on the dominant side. Ask the patient, on the command "go," to pick up the penny from the floor and stand up. Time from the command "go" until the subject is standing erect with penny in hand.

6. With subject in a corridor or in an open room, ask the subject to turn 360 degrees. Evaluate using scale on PPT scoring sheet.

7. Bring subject to start on 50-foot walk test course (25 feet out and 25 feet back) and ask the subject, on the command "go," to walk to 25-foot mark and back. Time from the command "go" until the starting line is crossed on the way back.

8. Bring subject to foot of stairs (9 to 12 steps) and ask subject, on the command "go," to begin climbing stairs until he or she feels tired and wishes to stop. Before beginning this task, alert the subject to possibility of developing chest pain or shortness of breath and inform the subject to tell you if any of these symptoms occur. Escort the subject up the stairs. Time from the command "go" until the subject's first foot reaches the top of the first flight of stairs. Record the number of flights (maximum is four) climbed (up and down is one flight).

SOURCE: Reuben DB, Siu AL. An objective measure of physical function of elderly outpatients. *J Am Geriatr Soc.* 1990;38: 1105–1112. Reprinted with permission.

From Beck JC (ed): Appendix A. *In* Geriatrics Review Syllabus: A Core Curriculum in Geriatric Medicine. American Geriatrics Society 1991-1992 Program. New York, American Geriatrics Society, 1991-1992, p 477, with permission.

sician, nurse, and social worker can be coordinated by using office staff and an informal relationship with a social worker from the community.

Regardless of how the team is established, team dynamics are an important consideration in maintaining interdisciplinary working relationships. Each member must learn about the professional services provided by the others, both to appreciate the full extent of resources available and to maintain professional boundaries. Case management responsibilities generally are assumed by the professional whose services are most critical to the patient's needs. A roster of patients that includes their current status, ongoing interventions, and treatment goals helps to assure that continuity of care and communications among the team members is maintained. Team dynamics need constant monitoring and frequent adjustment in roles and methods of interaction to optimize cohesiveness.

HEALTH CARE SETTINGS FOR THE ELDERLY

Comprehensive Geriatric Assessment Programs

Comprehensive geriatric assessment (CGA) is becoming recognized as an important component of health care for frail elderly persons and their caregivers. Programs are offered in either inpatient units or outpatient clinics and are designed to provide interdisciplinary care to address the medical, social, and psychological problems that affect older people and their caregivers. While it might be argued that many elderly people could benefit from CGA, most are healthy. Therefore, targeting programs for the most appropriate patient is a central element of effective CGA. Those most likely to benefit are on the verge of institutionalization, are in lower socioeconomic groups, have had inadequate medical care, and have poor social support networks. The most "at risk" elderly constitute about 10 per cent of hospitalized elderly patients and a small portion (perhaps up to 5 per cent) of community-dwelling elderly (Fretwell, 1988).

Descriptive studies and controlled clinical trials on the effects of interdisciplinary outpatient geriatric assessment programs consistently show improved outcomes. Data would suggest that patients evaluated in these programs are placed more appropriately (Williams et al., 1973), frequently have new medical diagnoses found (Brocklehurst et al., 1978), have significant adjustments made to their medication regimen, and have longer duration and maintenance of independence when compared to controls (Tulloch and Moore 1979). Furthermore, patients randomized to receive routine care are more likely to be rehospitalized and have longer lengths of stay (Williams et al., 1987). However, studies have not yielded convincing evidence to suggest an effect on survival or use of home or nursing home services. A recent meta-analysis of controlled trials of CGA suggested that programs linking assessment to long-term management are most effective in improving survival and function (Stuck et al., 1993).

Few studies of CGA programs have included any data on assessment of caregivers. As the population ages, family care of older persons will increase. Those who require help look first to their spouse and then to daughters or daughters-in-law for assistance. About one in five persons over the age of 45 provides help to an elderly relative; about 40 per cent of caregivers are adult children, and another 35 per cent are spouses (Stone et al., 1987). Caregivers usually fulfill this role with little help from others even though they may be elderly and have their own health, financial, and social problems. Prospective studies of outpatients evaluated by a CGA program suggest that the primary caregivers' burden in providing care was an independent predictor of the use of home services and nursing home placement (Brown et al., 1990). Other consequences of caregiver stress and burden may be neglect or, in extreme cases, elder abuse (O'Malley et al., 1983).

Geriatric Evaluation and Management Units

Geriatric patients often present with multiple, concurrent, and interactive medical, social, and psychiatric problems that are difficult to manage under pressures to reduce both hospital lengths of stay and inpatient expenditures. To address these issues more effectively, several centers have established designated areas within the hospital in which CGA accompanies the diagnosis and management of the presenting illness. As in outpatient CGA programs, these geriatric evaluation and management units (GEMUs) must include strict criteria for admission. The target population are patients from the community who are at risk of institutionalization, but who have potential for adequate community supports on discharge. Patients with a poor prognosis and those who are otherwise healthy are not likely to derive sufficient benefits to justify this intense commitment of resources.

A critical feature of a successful GEMU is primary management of the medical, pharmacologic, and social interventions. This includes a meticulous assessment of the patient's diagnoses, pharmacologic regimen, functional dependencies, and social support systems. Medications are chosen to not only lessen the symptomatic burden of illness, but also to minimize the pharmacologic load, enhance compliance, and reduce side effects. Functional dependencies are addressed through physical and occupational therapies, assessment of vision and hearing, management of incontinence, and the prescription of supporting appliances and devices to foster independence and reduce caregiver burden. Social supports are explored to link patients with community resources and to maximize the benefits of entitlement programs. The likelihood of the patient returning to the community is improved without significantly extending the hospital length of stay when these issues are addressed early in the hospital course (Evans and Hendricks, 1993). Provisions should be made for continued ambulatory care services following discharge. This type of continuity of care assures that the home-based services are in concert with the medical care plan suggested by the GEMU team.

The success of GEMUs was demonstrated conclusively in a recent meta-analysis of controlled trials (Stuck et al., 1993). Patients admitted to GEMUs had a 35 per cent reduction in mortality at 6 months and a 23 per cent reduction at 12 months when compared to patients having routine care on a general medical floor. The odds of living at home at 6 months were nearly doubled, and the benefit persisted for at least 12 months following discharge. Furthermore, the rates of readmission also were reduced significantly. Beneficial effects on both physical and cognitive functions were found at 6 and 12 months (Evans and Hendricks, 1993). Data would suggest that GEMUs have positive effects on caregivers' feelings of emotional well-being and self-reported health at 3 months after hospital discharge (Silliman et al., 1990).

The practical issues to consider in establishing a GEMU are organizing the interdisciplinary team and assuring funding for the program (Lavizzo-Mourey et al., 1993). There may be a lack of availability of certain key members of the team in some communities. Team meetings are expensive in personnel time and are not a reimbursable service. Follow-up consultations may not be reimbursable unless the geriatrician is the primary care provider; also, the expanded role of social services may not be remunerated.

Inpatient Consultation Services

An alternative to the GEMU is to make the interdisciplinary geriatric evaluation team available on a consultative basis. Referral may be requested by a primary health care professional or by establishing set criteria (e.g., age greater than 70, first-time nursing home referral) or as part of an assessment for home care. Common requests for consultation are: general medical management of a patient not responding to initial therapy, discharge planning, evaluation and management of dementia, assessment of rehabilitation potential, and "failure to thrive" (Winograd and Stearns, 1990). The initial screening for appropriateness often is provided by either a social worker or a nurse, with other members of the team seeing the patient individually and coordinating their suggestions through a team meeting. The recommendations of each discipline are reflected in the final verbal and written report.

There is controversy over the effectiveness of inpatient consultation services (Stuck et al., 1993). Benefits include an increased awareness of new diagnoses, adjustments in the medication regimen, and more appropriate referrals to ancillary services such as physical and occupational therapy. Geriatric consultation services are most effective when there is widespread appreciation of the benefits to be derived from consultation, and agreement between the consultation team and the primary care physician. Under these circumstances, improved survival, decreased medication loads, and reduced hospital recidivism can be realized (Hogan and Fox, 1990).

Geriatric Rehabilitation Services

Rehabilitation provides assessment and intervention for functionally impaired older persons with a goal of preserving or restoring function, or accommodating to disability. Almost all elderly patients can benefit from rehabilitation, especially after a medical event that results in loss of function. Rehabilitation parallels the principles of geriatric care by incorporating physical, emotional, and social parameters into the treatment process. Care optimally is provided by an interdisciplinary team consisting of a physician, nurse, social worker, physical therapist, occupational therapist, speech therapist, recreational therapist, and psychologist/psychiatrist.

The current climate of health care delivery has changed with regard to rehabilitation for the elderly. Settings for rehabilitation include dedicated rehabilitation units, skilled nursing facilities, the home, and outpatient facilities. Standards are being developed by the Commission on Accreditation of Rehabilitation Facilities for subacute rehabilitation. These standards are likely to be especially relevant for the elderly person because there is no consensus on the definitions and goals of geriatric rehabilitation, or on the appropriate mix of services needed to achieve these goals (Brummel-Smith, 1993).

Rehabilitation of older persons should begin in the acute care hospital or immediately after an acute medical insult. Because immobility or bed rest results in rapid declines in function, it is important to stabilize the primary condition and prevent secondary complications. These include malnutrition, urinary incontinence, pressure ulcers, contractures, and confusion, all of which commonly occur in elderly hospitalized patients (Inouye et al., 1993).

Rehabilitation of Specific Disorders

STROKE.   Two thirds of completed strokes occur in those over the age of 65, and the functional consequences are often serious. Rehabilitation produces its best results when started within 48 hours of the event, once medical stability has been achieved. The early phase of rehabilitation focuses on preventing complications such as pressure ulcers and deep venous thrombosis by frequently turning patients and by employing range-of-motion exercises for the involved limbs. Close attention to nutrition, bowel and bladder function, and skin integrity is also important in the early stages of recovery. The long-term goals are to compensate for physical losses and to minimize social and economic losses by restoring or maximizing function. The determinants of functional prognosis are the degree of early recovery, the patient's functional status before the stroke, the presence of supportive caregivers and environment, the patient's ability to learn, and the patient's motivation. Poor prognostic indicators include: coma at presentation, incontinence 2 weeks after the stroke, poor cognitive function, severe hemiparesis or hemiplegia after 1 month, previous stroke, visuospatial deficits, neglect or denial of the involved side, significant cardiovascular disease, large or deep lesions on computerized tomography scans, and multiple neurologic deficits (Dombovy et al., 1986). Patients with hemorrhages, if they survive the initial insult, tend to do better in rehabilitation than those with fixed infarcts.

A typical patient with a new stroke presents with flaccid paralysis of the affected limbs. Characteristically, there is gradual progression from flaccidity to spasticity to normal muscle tone, while motor paralysis resolves through muscle synergy patterns to voluntary segmental movements. Typically, proximal function returns prior to distal function. Recovery may halt at any phase, and functional recovery must be reassessed carefully on a regular basis. Most recovery occurs within the first month; however, motor gains can be seen for up to 6 months. Sensory, swallowing, and speech improvements may be seen for up to a year.

There is still controversy as to whether rehabilitation augments recovery beyond that which can be expected to occur spontaneously. Recent randomized studies suggest that inpatient rehabilitation may result in improved functional outcomes, although these gains did not always persist at 12 months (Sivenius and Kaveli, 1985; Smith et al., 1986). Others have reported benefits of stroke rehabilitation programs that include improved gait (Lehmann et al., 1975), more appropriate use of resources (Young and Forster, 1992), and improvements in poststroke mood disorders (Lipsey et al., 1986). It is estimated that, with the help of rehabilitation, 90 per cent of patients can be taught to get out of bed, 60 per cent can become self-sufficient, and 30 per cent of those in the employable age group can return to work (Lehmann et al., 1975).

Rehabilitation is less successful in elderly patients with severe underlying cardiac or pulmonary disease. Emotional lability and depression are common, occurring in up to 50 per cent of patients; however, if recognized, these symptoms can be treated successfully with antidepressants (Robinson et al., 1984). Anther common problem that limits function in patients who have had strokes is dysphagia. Speech–language pathologists or occupational therapists can design programs to treat patients with pharyngeal dysphagia (Miller et al., 1993). Patients with flaccid paralysis of their upper extremities are at risk for developing subluxation of the shoulder and reflex sympathetic dystrophy. Range-of-motion exercises, proper positioning, and splinting may alleviate symptoms of pain and swelling. Short courses of oral steroids and superficial heat or cold prior to passive stretching of the affected extremity also may be helpful.

AMPUTATIONS. The rehabilitation of an elderly amputee is limited only by the degree of cardiovascular disease, compromised blood supply to the "good limb," psychological adjustment to the loss of limb, motivation, and other medical complications in the early postoperative period (Clark et al., 1983; Wolf et al., 1990a,b). The energy necessary to ambulate increases dramatically, with prostheses, with a 30 per cent increase for a unilateral below-knee amputation, 40 to 50 per cent for bilateral below-knee amputations, and 80 per cent for an above-knee amputation (Fisher and Gullickson, 1978). Rehabilitation can be enhanced by preoperative counseling, strength and balance training, pain control, and early postoperative mobilization to prevent contractures and pressure ulcers. Usually, patients can be measured for a temporary prosthesis 4 to 8 weeks after surgery and a permanent prosthesis 8 to 12 weeks after surgery. Weight bearing on a temporary prosthesis is practiced first using parallel bars, and then with the aid of a walker. Patients with unilateral below-knee amputations usually have excellent outcomes (two thirds become ambulatory); however, above-knee amputees (20 per cent become ambulatory) and those with bilateral amputations often do not progress toward ambulation. Recent advances in design and material have resulted in prosthetic limbs that are more comfortable, cosmetic, and functional.

HIP FRACTURES/TOTAL HIP REPLACEMENT. Inpatient orthopedic geriatric rehabilitation unit stays usually are indicated for elderly patients who have had hip surgery if there are other complicating medical problems that limit a patient's ability to regain functional independence, concomitant upper extremity arthritis, weakness, or poor endurance secondary to underlying cardiopulmonary disease. Most patients return to their homes having made significant gains in function (Applegate et al., 1983; Daly et al., 1992) and, of those alive 2 years later, most have sustained these gains and continue to live in their own homes. Studies of the effectiveness of these units also report shorter length of stay in hospitals, less institutionalization,

reduced complication rates, and improved medical care as new medical diagnoses are uncovered and treated before discharge (Sainesbury et al., 1986; Zuckerman et al., 1992). Factors that influence outcomes of rehabilitation include the patient's weight-bearing status (which depends on the type and severity of the fracture and surgical procedure), premorbid level of function, and cognitive status and the presence of comorbid medical illnesses.

DECONDITIONING. Functional declines resulting from bed rest or enforced immobility occur rapidly. Muscle strength and mass decline by 1 to 2 per cent per day of bed rest; similarly, there may be declines in balance, reaction time, and cardiovascular responsiveness. The changes that occur in organ physiology as a result of imposed inactivity depend on the person's prior fitness and level of activity (Hoenig and Rubenstein, 1991). Orthostatic hypotension may result from deconditioning and can lead to complaints of dizziness and falls; patients tend to fatigue more easily and perceive any activity as being more strenuous.

It would appear that much of the functional loss resulting from deconditioning is preventable. Patients should be encouraged to do isotonic and isometric exercises while in bed; range-of-motion exercises should be ordered for patients unable to sit in a chair. A tilt-table may be necessary to regain autonomic responsiveness in patients with orthostatic hypotension. The early focus of rehabilitation is to restore endurance by using graduated resistive exercises prior to embarking on attempts to restore ambulation (Vorhers and Riley, 1993). Even very elderly persons, including those with chronic diseases and resultant deconditioning, can participate in exercise programs and will show improvements in cardiovascular function, fitness, strength, and flexibility (Fiatarone et al., 1990; Morey et al., 1991).

Assistive Devices

For patients with residual deficits in functional abilities, assistive devices can allow them to complete these activities more efficiently. Canes may be useful for patients with minimal gait impairment to provide weight-bearing relief. A cane is of the proper length when the elbow is flexed about 30 degrees with the cane tip 6 inches lateral to the forefoot on the uninvolved side and in contact with the ground at the same time as the affected foot. Quadripod canes are more appropriate for patients recovering from stroke who have both motor and proprioceptive impairments. Walkers are helpful for patients with instability because of general weakness or bilateral deficits, and can displace up to 50 per cent of body weight. For patients who do not have enough upper extremity strength to advance a standard walker, rolling or wheeled walkers may provide the necessary stability, and help the patient maintain propulsion. Modified platform walkers can be used for patients with severely impaired upper extremity strength, such as those with rheumatoid arthritis.

When walkers are not feasible, most older, cognitively intact patients can be trained to use wheelchairs, which can be modified to account for upper extremity strength and dexterity, endurance, balance, weight, and skin condition. Homes may have to be modified for wheelchair accessibility; doorways must be at least 3 feet wide and bathrooms at least 5 to 6 feet wide to permit turning the chair.

Orthotics may be prescribed to help stabilize functional deficits in the musculoskeletal system and may be helpful in the relief of pain by relatively immobilizing and reducing weight on an affected limb or the spine. Commonly used orthotics include ankle–foot orthoses, which are used to preserve joint alignment and to limit weight bearing and are indicated for limb weakness secondary to cerebrovascular accidents or peripheral neuropathies; and knee–ankle–foot orthoses, which provide additional structural support around the knee. Spinal orthotics may help stabilize and reduce pain in patients with vertebral compression fractures or degenerative disc disease. Upper extremity orthotics, such as a "cock-up" splint, frequently are used to reduce compression symptoms in patients with rheumatoid arthritis or carpal tunnel syndrome.

Assistive devices are not limited to mobility aids. Adaptive equipment has been developed to assist with dressing, eating, personal hygiene, and household chores. A long-handled shoe horn is a simple device that may help a patient who has difficulty with flexion of the trunk or lower extremity. Bathroom modifications such as a raised toilet seat, grab bar, or shower chair may help with safe toileting and bathing. A rocker knife, with its sharp curved blade, may help a hemiplegic patient cut food with only one hand.

Home Care Services

Long-term care in the home is the fastest growing sector of health services delivery in the United States (Kavesh, 1986). This growth has been stimulated by the boom in the population over 80 years of age, changes in the hospital environment, and fiscal consequences of institutionalization. Advances in technology and a loosening of restrictions on location of service have allowed the home care industry to respond to the needs of frail, homebound elderly patients. Furthermore, efforts to reduce the costs of care to the chronically ill have led practitioners to explore increasingly more complex services in the home. A recent survey of primary care physicians showed that 53 to 82 per cent make house calls (Siwek, 1985), and on average 5 to 10 per cent of patients in primary care practice receive services in their home under the direction of a physician.

Physician groups that offer home care services generally are perceived in their community as caring and compassionate, thus enhancing the attractiveness of the practice in a competitive market. On the practical side, the kinds of patients appropriate for house calls often are managed more efficiently at home. When seen in the office, multiply impaired patients require additional staff time to assist with dressing, mobility, or continence, and it often takes more physician time to review a complex medical treatment plan (especially if the patient is not accompanied by the primary caregiver). Home care patients also can increase a physician's hospital practice. Homebound patients experience 0.5 admissions per patient per year, a much higher rate than for ambulatory patients, or even those in nursing homes. In addition, familiarity with the potentials of in-home services facilitates discharge planning.

House calls also add an important dimension to care by providing information about the patient's circumstances. A study by Ramsdell et al. (1989) showed that two new problems per patient were found among patients who were evaluated in the office and then subsequently evaluated at home. Twenty-three per cent of these new problems had a potential for significant morbidity or mortality, and they resulted in one to eight new recommendations. Issues that often are overlooked in the office include: safety, barriers to compliance, hygiene, and medications obtained either over the counter, from other family or friends, or from other physicians.

The home setting also has a significant impact on the way historical and physical examination data are collected and how diagnostic tests and therapeutic interventions are considered. Comprehensive medical assessments can be done using equipment that can be carried in a compact "house call bag" capable of carrying 10 to 15 pounds (see Table 7–7). The added costs and inconvenience of diagnostic testing and consultation promote a stepwise clinical algorithmic strategy that may be more appropriate. Finally, negotiating with patients on their own "turf" reinforces the importance of patient autonomy and decision making.

Developing an Office-Based House Call Program

The most effective way to provide care for patients in their homes is to define the geographic catchment area in which home visits can be made efficiently and safely, and to determine the size of the home care practice (American Medical Association Department of Geriatric Health, 1992). Generally, five to seven patients can be seen in a half day, and more when multiple visits can be clustered. The size of the home care practice depends on the number of available sessions per quarter. There are no restrictions on remuneration for the number of visits as long as there is justification in

TABLE 7–7. HOUSE CALL BAG

Equipment

Blood pressure cuffs with interchangeable bulb and gauge (regular, obese, pediatric)
Gloves with lubricant and hemocculture slides
Otoscope/ophthalmoscope kit
Glucometer
Peak flow meter
Digital thermometer
Goniometer
Tape measure
Hammer and tuning fork
Bandage scissors
Toenail clippers
Portable bathroom scale
Optional: Sterile scissors, forceps, and disposable scalpel
          Sterile 4 × 4 gauze and tape
          Hand-held electrocardiogram

Stationery

Prescription blanks
Appointment cards
Progress note paper, history forms, drug flow sheets, etc.
Advance directive forms
Release of information forms
Informed consent forms for tetanus, pneumovax, and influenza vaccinations, and débridement or other procedures
Assessment forms such as Mini-Mental State Examination, elderly abuse checklist, and home safety assessment checklist
Information and referral phone numbers

the progress notes; however, patients who need to be seen by a physician more than once a week should be considered for hospitalization or hospice services. Patients who need nursing supervision may have home care visits up to twice daily, for a short time.

Patients most appropriate for inclusion are those with mobility impairments or those who are disruptive; others to be considered are those with multiple complex chronic medical and psychiatric problems, especially when taking multiple medications, and those in need of medical attention but who frequently fail to comply with office appointments. For some patients, house calls need to be scheduled only once or for a limited number of visits. For patients not responding to what should be adequate therapy, or whose response is variable, a house call may uncover reasons not apparent in the office, such as nutritional problems or dietary indiscretions, unfilled prescriptions, noncompliance, or the presence of medications from other sources that may be interfering with the expected response. Terminally ill patients who find it difficult to come to the office and who have become housebound are better seen at home to address their physical and emotional needs more effectively. Likewise, recently bereaved individuals often are best seen at home. Finally, a home visit for situations of suspected caregiver burnout or elder abuse will uncover more information than can be obtained in the office.

Coordinating the Office-Based House Call Program

To manage an office-based house call program successfully, one person should be designated as the house call coordinator. Relevant telephone calls should be channeled through the coordinator, including those from patients, nurses, laboratories, other ancillary services, and vendors. Emergency triage may be managed through simple algorithms, saving physician time on the telephone. The coordinator can be trained to document patient-related events and take responsibility for coordinating the logistics of handling routine problems, as well as emergencies.

Financial issues are very important in the success of the program, so careful documentation of medical records, of telephone contacts with patients, family, and home care staff, and of team meetings should be maintained to justify higher reimbursement codes. A medical director contract with a local home care agency can offset any losses that might occur through the house call practice. Such contracts usually require approximately 4 to 8 hr/week for quality assurance chart reviews, in-service training for the agency staff, liaison with other physicians, and policy review and development.

As in other aspects of geriatric care, a multidisciplinary team approach to care is the ideal. The house call team may be comprised of the physician, the house call coordinator, representatives from the home care agency, and other ancillary providers with whom the program has a working arrangement. The house call program should align ideally with one home care agency and have associations with a pharmacist and a durable medical equipment vendor. The home care agency should be willing to assign a limited number of nurses to the patients in the house call practice and to participate in team meetings. The pharmacist can work in consultation with the physician in reviewing drug profiles and alerting the team to new medications and formulations. The house call team meetings are important for communication and for interdisciplinary consultation, and allow for the timely completion of all of the required documentation. Weekly meetings generally last an hour for programs that manage 100 patients.

Nursing Homes

Although only 5 per cent of the population 65 and older reside in nursing homes, approximately 22 per cent of those over the age of 85 are institutionalized (Hing et al., 1990). On a national level, there are nearly 1.7 million beds in over 15,000 homes, with an annual expenditure of more than $53 billion (Iglehart, 1992). On an individual basis, it is predicted that, for those who turned 65 in 1990, 43 per cent will spend some time in a nursing home during their remaining life. However, this risk is age dependent, and increases with advancing years (Kemper and Murtaugh, 1991).

Another factor that has increased the need for nursing home beds has been the influence of the Medicare Prospective Payment System (PPS), which has resulted in a dramatic decline in the length of hospital stays. Because there is less time for convalescence and rehabilitation, nursing home placement often is sought for more complex patients. Consequently, as hospital deaths have declined, the percentage of deaths occurring in nursing homes has increased (Sager et al., 1989).

In the near future, the growing market for long-term care insurance is likely to stimulate demand for nursing home care. Currently, the cost of care is paid largely by the patients themselves (51.2 per cent), followed by Medicaid (41.5 per cent); Medicare pays only 2.1 per cent of the total expenditures for nursing homes (Feather and Karuza, 1988). Medicaid loopholes now used by many families to protect assets eventually will be closed, so that insurance will be the only mechanism by which to preserve one's estate. The realization that institutional care may cost from $30,000 to $60,000/year has prompted older people to protect their assets. The financially based reluctance to access nursing home care will evaporate once it is already paid for.

More than half of all nursing home admissions are "short-stay" patients needing convalescence and rehabilitation (approximately 30 per cent) or terminal care (approximately 40 per cent) (Kane et al., 1989). The rest return to the hospital for continued care (approximately 25 per cent) or are transferred to other facilities. The "long-stay" patients, comprising approximately 40 per cent of admissions, have stays beyond 6 months, and remain in the nursing home for an average of 2.9 years. The "long-stay" patients represent the majority of residents in long-term care at any time; they can be categorized into three groups: those with primarily functional dependency, those with cognitive impairments, or those with both. Up to 94 per cent of patients in long-term care have some degree of mental impairment, mainly as a result of degenerative neurologic diseases, multi-infarct dementia, depression, and delirium (Rovner et al., 1986). Those with predominantly functional dependencies have suffered major illnesses that require an increasingly more sophisticated level of service.

The long-term care industry has responded to the increased complexity of care with an impressive array of service delivery capabilities that rivals that in the acute care setting, such as parenteral therapies for the administration of antibiotics, total parenteral nutrition, and, in some facilities, parenteral morphine for the terminally ill. The complexity and acuity of care has led to the growing use of full-time physicians, with nurse-practitioners and physician assistants, to provide on-site supervision and staff support in many larger facilities.

Decisions to Institutionalize

Nursing home placement depends primarily on the intended outcomes, and on the expected length of stay. Short stays for rehabilitation and convalescence are appropriate following an acute illness or an exacerbation of a chronic illness. Short-term respite also may be indicated when the stresses of caregiving threaten to overburden the family, or sometimes as terminal care when the emotional and physical burdens become overwhelming. These admissions generally are covered by Medicare and private insurance.

Long-term placement may be one of the most momentous decisions for the individual and the family, potentially affecting several generations because of disruption of family integrity and guilt, and because the full cost is borne by the patient. The family physician frequently is involved in the decision-making process and usually can present three options: home care, admission to a life-care community, or nursing home placement.

In assessing patients for the most appropriate placement, levels of functional and physiologic impairments, presence of chronic illnesses, patient preferences, and the availability of support systems must be considered carefully (Table 7–8). Although the primary caregiver usually provides the bulk of personal support, secondary caregivers contribute to the support system; secondary caregivers include home care professional services, health aides and chore workers, home-delivered meal programs, and family, friends, and volunteers. It is important to assess the capabilities of the primary and secondary caregivers in defining what ultimately might be the most appropriate disposition.

Alternatives to home care should be considered in the absence of a caregiving system or with an

---

TABLE 7–8. PROCESS FOR CONSIDERING INSTITUTIONALIZATION

- Review the patient's functional disabilities.
- Review the areas of dependency to uncover impairments that are amenable to correction.
- Assess the patient and the caregiver for their appropriateness for a formal rehabilitative program.
- Ask the nursing staff or family about any evidence of nocturnal disturbances, wandering, or other aberrant behaviors.
- Assess the primary caregiver's willingness and ability to provide supervision or assistance in areas of functional disability and tolerance of behavioral problems.
- Assess the financial impact of institutionalization on the patient and family.
- Determine patient preferences.

inability to fill in the gaps in function for a multiply disabled individual. Other factors to consider are the presence of certain patient behaviors that could undermine even the most devoted caregiver. Nocturnal disturbances of any kind are tolerated poorly. Other aberrant behaviors associated with cognitive impairments, such as wandering or noisiness, or the need for frequent assistance for toileting, often cause caregiver distress and lead to placement.

An alternative to either home care or institutional placement for certain patients is admission to a life-care community. In many ways, this disposition includes aspects of both home care and institutionalization. The environment is designed to match the needs of the individual better, and there is a greater opportunity for social integration. As with institutionalization, there can be a significant depletion of assets; however, these costs are agreed on at admission, and in some life-care communities the entrance fees are returned to the family. Because most life-care communities have a continuum of care and on-site medical supervision, health care needs can be met on a timely basis, and the patient supported in the least restrictive environment.

Medical Aspects of Nursing Home Care

Nursing home medicine is becoming a recognized area of interest among geriatricians and family physicians, and has become a financially viable setting for practice. The average patient has multiple, concurrent, and interactive medical and psychosocial problems that require constant monitoring, therapeutic adjustment, and counseling. Care usually is provided through an interdisciplinary team compromised of physicians and physician extenders (physician assistants and nurse-practitioners), nurse specialists, dietitians, therapists, social workers, and clinical pharmacists. Fortunately, Medicare reimbursement is now equivalent to that for acute care, reflecting the complexity and time required for patient management.

DEHYDRATION. Dehydration is among the most common disorders of nursing home patients, and is the most common fluid and electrolyte problem. It is also one of the major risk factors for urinary tract, respiratory, and skin infections, and hypotension secondary to dehydration is one of the leading causes of depressed mental alertness and falls. Patients who become acutely ill and develop coincident dehydration have an excessive rate of mortality.

The risk factors for dehydration include: four or more chronic conditions, age over 85, female, bed boundness, and taking four or more medications, especially laxatives (Lavizzo-Mourey et al., 1988). The elderly are especially prone to dehydration because of an age-related decline in the concentrating ability of the kidney (Rowe et al., 1976) and in neuroendocrine water homeostatic mechanisms. Furthermore, given free access to water, many elderly individuals will not drink sufficient amounts to maintain fluid homeostasis (Miller et al., 1982). The proportion of body mass attributed to water volume also declines with age, especially among women, therefore increasing their risk of dehydration. Finally, patients with Alzheimer's disease demonstrate a diminished thirst response and subnormal arginine vasopressin response to fluid restriction (Albert et al., 1989).

The clinical signs of dehydration that correlate best with severity include: tongue dryness, longitudinal tongue furrows, dryness of the mucous membranes of the mouth, upper body muscle weakness, confusion, slurred speech, and sunken eyes. Commonly found symptoms and signs among younger patients with dehydration are not helpful in older nursing home patients. These include thirst, dryness of the skin, and changes in skin turgor over the forehead, chest, or forearms; postural pulse and blood pressure changes, and the time-honored attribution of low-grade fever to dehydration, have not been demonstrated under study conditions (Gross et al., 1992).

Once identified, dehydration must be treated aggressively to prevent progression. The volume of water required to re-establish fluid tonicity can be calculated roughly by using the following equation:

$$\text{Water deficit} = [60\% \times \text{current body weight (kg)}] \times \left[\left(\frac{\text{current plasma sodium concentration}}{140}\right) - 1\right]$$

Approximately one half the deficit should be corrected over the first 24 hours, and the remainder over the next 48 to 72 hours. Water may be given orally as a specified nursing order, via feeding tube, intravenously, or by clysis. Preferably, fluids are replaced orally or enterally to avoid accidental overload. After hydration has been re-established, it is important to monitor intake and output to assure that overt and insensible losses are accounted for. In some patients, desired daily fluid intake should be specified as part of the standing orders.

FEVER. Elevation in body temperature is a universally accepted sign of an acute change in clinical status. Fever is suggestive of an infection, but it does not specifically identify a pathogen or location, and can signify a noninfectious process. This is particularly true in the older nursing home patient.

Several factors affect the mechanism of the febrile response in the elderly patient (Norman et al., 1985). Although immunologic signals and neurohumoral mechanisms are not altered over the life span, their impact may be blunted by physiologic changes with advanced age, the patient's activity level, and certain medications. Heat production declines with age and debility as the result of diminished muscle mass relative to body weight that accompanies a sedentary lifestyle. Among older and less active individuals, shivering is less efficient as a source of additional heat production. Medications intended to decrease inflammation, such as nonsteroidal anti-inflammatory drugs (NSAIDs), attenuate the neurohumoral signals and blunt febrile responses.

Fever is defined as a temperature above the normal range of healthy individuals (MacKowiak et al., 1992), but the variable response of older persons makes it difficult to establish a "cutoff" temperature above which a patient is febrile. Older individuals tend to have a lower basal body temperature, and the likelihood of finding a significant infection has been reported to increase with body temperature beginning at 99.5°F (Wasserman et al., 1989). There is evidence, however, that many elderly patients with clinically significant illness remain afebrile or have below-normal temperatures. In older nursing home patients, monitoring changes in temperature from baseline may be a more useful approach. Castle et al. (1991) showed that a change of 2.4°F identified 35 per cent of patients with significant infections, and a change of 1.4°F identified 66 per cent, despite the finding that 47 per cent of their patients had a febrile response of less than 101°F and 11 per cent of less than 99°F. Other findings indirectly corroborate the significance of the fever and help to direct the diagnostic evaluation. Nondifferentiating signs include a transient change in blood pressure, pulse, or respiration; symptoms include altered mental status, diminished appetite, malaise, a recent loss of interest in activities, or a fall.

Noninfectious Causes of Fever. The most common noninfectious cause of fever is mechanical blockage of a hollow viscus causing a local inflammatory response. Atelectasis or mucous plugs in the bronchus result in collapse of small airways, leading to activation of macrophages with release of endogenous pyrogens. Repeated microaspirations in patients with dysphasia or during enteral feeding may produce similar local inflammatory responses and fever. Any process that causes distention of the bowel or bladder (e.g., fecal impaction or blockage of a urinary catheter) can result in fever.

Phlebitis is a frequently overlooked noninfectious cause of fever, with or without thrombosis. An immobile, dehydrated nursing home patient who is placed in a chair for a long period of time is at high risk for clot formation. This initiates a local inflammatory reaction, usually in the calves, lower thighs, or pelvis, that may be associated with fever. Large pulmonary emboli are found in approximately 5 per cent of autopsies of elderly patients. Smaller embolic "showers" may manifest only with transient, recurrent fever, sometimes without evidence of tachypnea and tachycardia.

Infectious Causes of Fever. Infections are prevalent in nursing homes because of the frailty of the population, close contact among patients, and poor quality of infection control procedures. Infections cause 54 per cent of acute medically attended problems and 48 per cent of hospitalizations, and are related to 63 per cent of deaths (Mott and Barker, 1988). Approximately 70 to 80 per cent of all fevers are caused by one of three sources of infection: urinary tract infection, pneumonia or bronchitis, and skin or wound infection. Other less frequent causes are episodic outbreaks of viral upper respiratory infections, influenza, viral gastroenteritis, osteomyelitis, and rare outbreaks of tuberculosis or bacterial diarrheas.

Urinary Tract Infections. The incidence of urinary tract infections is proportional to the degree of immobility and the incidence of genitourinary abnormalities. There is a high prevalence of asymptomatic bacteriuria in nursing home patients (15 to 20 per cent for men, 25 to 50 per cent for women), and patients with urinary catheters have up to a 98 per cent rate of bacteriuria with multiple organisms (Warren et al., 1982). Therefore, the findings of bacteriuria and pyuria on urinalysis, and a urine culture with greater than 10^5 colony-forming units/mL is insufficient evidence to ascribe a fever to a urinary tract infection. The diagnosis depends on the additional evidence of new symptoms, or a concordance between blood and urine cultures. The symptoms of an uncomplicated urinary tract infection, such as dysuria, frequency, urgency, and new or worsening incontinence, are found infrequently among elderly nursing home patients. Urinary tract infection may be suggested by back or flank pain, suprapubic discomfort, headache, anorexia, and malaise. Urine may become malodorous and cloudy, with more sediment. Perineal discomfort more often is associated with chronic prostatitis, probably the leading cause of recurrent urinary tract infections among men.

Midstream, clean-caught urine sampling is the preferred method of obtaining specimens in those able to cooperate. Among incontinent men, cleansing of the glans penis with povidone-iodine solution, applying a clean condom catheter, and collecting the specimen within 30 to 120 minutes can yield adequate samples. Those with indwelling catheters should have the catheter replaced and the specimen drawn from the new catheter, to avoid culturing organisms that have colonized only the tubing. Otherwise, the specimen should be obtained by "in-and-out" catheterization. It may be prudent to treat patients who have been catheterized for specimen procurement with a short course (1 to 3 days) of antibiotics because the procedure itself inoculates the bladder (Ronald et al., 1992).

Findings on urinalysis may be more helpful in excluding the presence of a significant urinary tract infection than in confirming infection. When pyuria is absent, the chance of significant bacteriuria is less than 5 per cent, even if bacteria are noted on microscopy (Boscia et al., 1989). The upper limit of normal is less than 10 white blood cells per high-powered field (HPF) in a resuspended sediment of centrifuged urine (Lipsky et al., 1987). Therefore, a change from a recent urinalysis in the number of white blood cells per HPF from "few" to "many" or "too numerous to count" may be a major confirmatory test for the presence of a urinary tract infection in a febrile patient. Microscopic hematuria has not been evaluated as a sign of infection among nursing home patients. Gross hematuria often is not indicative of a urinary tract infection; rather, it usually represents a structural abnormality in the genitourinary system, such as a stone or neoplasm, or simply catheter-induced trauma (Nicolle et al., 1993).

Among patients with pyuria, only 60 per cent have positive urine cultures. This may be due to noninfectious causes of bladder inflammation, such as stones, foreign body reaction to a catheter, or the presence of yeast or fastidious organisms, such as chlamydia, mycoplasma, or mycobacteria, that do not grow under routine culture techniques. Treatment for these organisms may be necessary in a patient with symptoms suggestive of a urinary source.

The organisms associated with urinary tract infections in the nursing home are more varied than those found among community-dwelling elderly, and more often resistant to antibiotics. Although *Escherichia coli* infections are most common, there is a greater incidence of *Klebsiella Proteus Enterobacter Citrobacter Serratia* and *Pseudomonas* species. Patients with catheters also have a higher incidence of colonization with *Providencia* and *Enterococcus* species. The presence of a Foley catheter assures that antibiotic therapy will only alter, not eradicate, the urinary flora; therefore, if at all possible, the catheter should be removed when treating sepsis of urinary origin (Warren et al., 1982).

Respiratory Tract Infections. Pneumonia is one of the most frequent causes of hospitalization and death among nursing home patients. Predisposing factors for developing pneumonia are chronic obstructive pulmonary disease, tracheostomy, and bedfast status; less common factors are congestive heart failure, stroke, cancer, diabetes, and malnutrition. Mortality rates from pneumococcal pneumonia with bacteremia range from 12 to 40 per cent; mortality increases significantly in patients with comorbid conditions (Barker and Mullooly, 1980). Fever accompanied by cough productive of purulent sputum, dyspnea, tachypnea (with a respiratory rate greater than 25 min), and pleuritic chest pain are suggestive of a lower respiratory tract infection. Nonspecific symptoms may include anorexia, mental confusion, malaise, declines in function, and incontinence.

A distinguishing feature between pneumonia and bronchitis is the presence with the former of a new infiltrate on the chest radiograph (McGeer et al., 1991). Progression of the infiltrate may occur even after treatment has been instituted (Fein et al., 1989). Given the high rate of radiographic abnormalities, it is helpful to compare current radiographs with any available previous studies. Other tests that are usually of value in a younger population are not as reliable among nursing home patients. Only a third of patients have a productive cough, and, among those from whom sputum specimens are obtained, only half meet the quality criteria for valid cultures. Finally, many patients have pharyngeal colonization with gram-negative bacilli, further limiting the predictive value of this test (Lentino and Lucks, 1987).

Streptococcus pneumoniae is the most common organism causing pneumonia in nursing home patients. Gram-negative bacilli also are identified frequently. Although some investigators have reported a predominant number of patients admitted to a hospital for acute care with pneumonia caused by *Klebsiella pneumoniae, Staphylococcus aureus,* and *Haemophilus influenzae,* this may represent the hospitalization of patients who have not responded to empiric therapy that was initiated in the nursing home.

Tuberculosis remains a serious potential problem in nursing homes because of the relatively high prevalence of patients previously exposed who are at risk of recrudescence, the general debility of nursing home patients, and the close living quarters, which foster rapid dissemination. Screening purified protein derivative reactivity may wane with age, yielding a false-negative result unless rechallenged, but the reaction to testing in the face of an acute infection is generally reliable (Stead et al., 1985). The signs and symptoms of an acute infection are similar to those in the younger population, with two exceptions: the presence of previous scarring on chest radiographs may obscure recurrent disease, and there is a greater incidence of extrapulmonary spread. The diagnosis should be considered in any patient with a persistent productive cough who has not responded to appropriate therapy.

Skin Infections. Pressure ulcers may develop in up to 25 per cent of patients in nursing homes, and osteomyelitis is a frequent complication of deeper wounds. Skin infections are more common in patients who are nonambulatory, diabetic, and malnourished. The most likely source of a skin infection is a pressure ulcer; closed skin infections such as cellulitis and abscesses occur occasionally, but frequently in association with pressure ulcers at a distant site. Because all wounds are colonized, reliable diagnostic signs of infection include fever, purulent drainage, and inflammation extending more than 1 cm from the wound edge into the surrounding skin.

Swab wound cultures reflect superficial colonization and are unreliable in identifying etiologic organisms in cellulitis surrounding an open wound or sinus tract. Needle aspiration at the leading edge is rarely helpful and, if positive, underestimates the number of bacterial isolates. Only deep tissue biopsy has been shown to provide reliable specimens for identification of infecting organisms (Rudensky et al., 1992). The most frequently cultured organisms are *Proteus mirabilis, S. aureus,* and anaerobes such as *Bacteroides fragilis,* often as polymicrobial infections. Bacteremia is uncommon, but, when associated with pressure ulcers, it is often polymicrobial and is indicative of a grave prognosis.

Bacteremia. The mortality rate associated with bacteremia is related to the underlying source and the number of chronic conditions (Richardson, 1993). A delay in delivery of appropriate therapy may result in grave consequences; however, because bacteremia may present with nonspecific signs and symptoms in nursing home patients, early recognition and diagnosis is difficult.

Although fever is a sensitive indicator of illness, only that associated with an altered mental status, malaise, lethargy, or coma is suggestive of bacteremia (Fontanarosa et al., 1992). Chills are present in only one third of patients but, when present, double the chance of bacteremia. Initial laboratory studies may be helpful in diagnosing bacteremia. In one study, the presence of a body temperature greater than 99.5°F and a leukocytosis of greater than 14,000 mm^3 conferred a 30 per cent chance of bacteremia. Febrile patients with bandemia greater than 6 per cent had a 60 per cent chance of positive blood cultures, and all patients with an elevated body temperature, leukocytosis, and bandemia were found to be bacteremic (Wasserman et al., 1989).

The diagnosis of bacteremia is dependent on a positive blood culture. Adequate blood (10 mL) must be obtained to assure diagnostic accuracy. Multiple samples should be obtained because the first set of blood cultures reveals an infecting organism in only 80 per cent of cases. In an extensive review of blood cultures (Aronson and Bor, 1987), it was suggested that one culture was rarely, if ever, sufficient, especially if the pretest possibility of bacteremia was low to moderate.

Genitourinary tract infections followed by respiratory tract infections account for one third to one half of all cases of bacteremia. Suspected bacteremias without an identified source should be treated with antibiotics that are effective for organisms likely to cause these infections, including *E. coli, S. pneumoniae, S. aureus,* and *Enterococcus.*

Diarrheal Illnesses. Gastrointestinal illness occurs in both sporadic cases and clustered epidemics. The most important pathogen in sporadic diarrhea is *Clostridium difficile,* which is frequently endemic, and can be epidemic in long-term care facilities (Bentley, 1990). *C. difficile* is responsible for approximately 20 per cent of all diarrheal illnesses, and approximately 20 to 25 per cent of all postantibiotic diarrheas.

Clustered cases of gastroenteritis most often result from seasonal viral illnesses caused by rotavirus and Norwalk agent. Random clusters also may occur as a result of food poisoning associated with *S. aureus, Clostridium perfringens,* and *Salmonella.* Diarrheal illnesses caused by enteric pathogens such as *E. coli, Shigella, Campylobacter,* or *Yersinia,* or parasitic diseases such as *Giardia lamblia,* are rare in the nursing home setting.

The *C. difficile*–associated syndrome is characterized by low-grade fever, abdominal discomfort, and diarrhea for at least 1 day. This presentation is not different from the clinical presentation of viral illnesses, food poisoning, or other noninfectious causes of gastrointestinal disorders, such as fecal impaction, ileus, obstruction, and vascular insufficiency. Thus, all diarrheal illnesses lasting more than 1 day should be investigated fully in addition to ordering assays for *C. difficile* cytotoxin. A stool smear for leukocytes is nonspecific. Routine cultures for enteric pathogens are difficult to justify for sporadic cases of gastroenteritis, given the rare occurrence of these infections (Yablon et al., 1993). Only during an outbreak of diarrheal illness is a more thorough evaluation, including stool testing for enteric pathogens, ova and parasites, and viral cultures, warranted to isolate the offending agent.

Empiric Antibacterial Therapy. The oral route is preferable for the administration of antibiotics and is appropriate for mild to moderate infections. Medications that attain similar blood levels whether given orally or intravenously are especially attractive in the treatment of the common infections in nursing homes. Mild infections can be treated with first-line agents such as ampicillin, cephaloxin, and erythromycin. Amoxicillin–clavulanic acid, ciprofloxacin, and trimethoprim-sulfamethoxazole are commonly used agents for moderately severe infections. Intramuscular therapy should be considered only if the intravenous route is unavailable; if needed, ceftriaxone is a reasonable choice. For more severe infections, in which the patient is clinically unstable or toxic but has requested that hospitalization be withheld, intravenous therapies often are effective. Combination therapies using ampicillin, a cephalosporin, and/or an aminoglycoside usually will provide adequate antimicrobial coverage at a reasonable cost.

Because the spectrum of organisms at different sites and the sensitivities to antimicrobial therapies differ geographically, the choice of empiric therapies should be directed by infection control surveillance studies. These reports can be obtained from the laboratory and document the most prevalent organisms by site, and their sensitivity patterns. In this way, more specific empiric treatments can be initiated. Adjustments in therapy can be made once definitive culture and sensitivity results are available.

BOWEL PROBLEMS. Complaints of constipation are common, and laxatives are among the most frequently prescribed medications for patients in nursing homes (Lamy and Krug, 1978). Normal bowel function ranges from three bowel movements per day to three per week (Connell et al., 1965). Therefore, constipation may be defined as having two or fewer bowel movements per week, straining on more than 25 per cent of occasions, and findings of large amounts of feces in the rectum on either digital examination or abdominal radiography.

Bowel transit times may become prolonged, leading to desiccation of the fecal material, decreased bulk, and, therefore, decreased stimulation of colonic motor activity. With age and immobility, myenteric plexus function becomes attenuated and less responsive to colonic stimulants, leading to segmental motor incoordination and further lengthening bowel transit time (Harari et al., 1993). Laxative abuse serves to exacerbate these changes.

A reduced intake of dietary fiber, dehydration, cognitive impairments, and certain medications play important etiologic roles. Diuretics reduce total body water; anticholinergics and calcium channel blockers may decrease smooth muscle contractility in the gut; NSAIDs and angiotensin-converting enzyme inhibitors may reduce prostaglandin stimulation of smooth muscle; narcotic agents reduce endorphin stimulation of the colon; and aluminum antacids may bind the fecal mass to the exclusion of water. Among nursing home patients, there is a high prevalence of chronic illnesses that may cause constipation. Diabetes mellitus may decrease autonomic tone through localized neurologic damage. Strokes also may cause constipation by weakening the abdominal and pelvic musculature. Parkinson's disease, depression, dementia, hypokalemia, and hypercalcemia all may affect neuromuscular tone and result in constipation.

A rational approach to patients with constipation begins with a history and physical examination. Patients who require therapy are those with two or fewer evacuations per week; those who evacuate more than twice per week and without hard stools should be reassured and instructed to avoid laxatives. Patients with chronic constipation most often are identifiable by the presence of a fecal impaction and retained stool on abdominal radiograph. Truly refractory constipation requires evaluation by colonoscopy or barium enema to rule out megacolon or other colonic pathology.

Nonpharmacologic interventions for the treatment of constipation are preferred. The patient should be assessed for fecal impaction, which may require manual disimpaction using a local anesthetic gel. If retained feces is noted on an abdominal radiograph but the rectal antrum is clear, then an oil retention enema followed by tap water ene-

mas is usually effective. This procedure may need to be repeated for 2 to 4 days until the colon is clear (Wrenn, 1989). Patients should attempt defecation approximately one-half hour after breakfast or dinner to take advantage of the gastrocolic reflex. Dietary fiber should be increased by 1 to 2 gm/week to a total of 6 to 10 grams of fiber per day. Slowly increasing fiber intake may reduce the symptoms of bloating and flatulence that often accompany an abrupt change in stool bulk. Finally, patients should be encouraged to drink a minimum of 2 L of fluids per day.

Two classes of pharmacologic agents are available for the treatment of constipation: stimulant laxatives and bulk-forming agents. Senna acts by altering electrolyte transport in the colon, thereby increasing intraluminal fluids, and by directly simulating intestinal motility. Other stimulant laxatives, such as danthron and cascara, are generally effective in 8 to 12 hours, and so should be administered at bedtime, but may be given up to several times daily for the treatment of retained feces. Some patients require maintenance therapy two to three times per week. Bisacodyl suppositories are used most appropriately in patients with poor rectal tone or a loss of sensation as a result of stroke or spinal cord injury; evacuation can be expected in 30 to 60 minutes with rectal stimulation. Other available agents include phenolphthalein and castor oil; however, electrolyte abnormalities, malabsorption, and cramping are common side effects.

Bulk laxatives absorb water, thereby producing a larger, softer fecal mass, which in turn promotes colonic peristalsis and ease of transit. The most common agents are composed of psyllium powder; however, synthetic compounds such as psyllium polycarbophil and methylcellulose often are better tolerated, cheaper, and available in a tablet form. Adequate dietary fluids are necessary for these agents to be effective, and there is a risk of impaction if fluid intake is inadequate. The other preparations act by creating a hyperosmolar environment within the colon, causing shifts of extravascular fluids into the lumen to mix with the fecal mass, increasing bulk and colonic motility. Among these hyperosmolar bulk-forming agents are magnesium salts, sorbitol, and lactulose. Glycerin suppositories act as both a hyperosmolar laxative and a lubricant. The most potent hyperosmolar agent is polyethylene glycol, which is recommended for bowel preparation prior to colonoscopy or barium enema. One to 2 L/day for 2 to 3 days is usually effective in clearing a high fecal impaction.

Stool softeners such as docusate sodium act as a surfactant, but have no laxative action; their primary purpose is to soften stool to relieve straining among patients with normal bowel function. Stool softeners are usually ineffective as a primary treatment for patients with chronic constipation.

FOLEY CATHETERS. Urinary incontinence is found in 40 per cent of patients on admission to a nursing home (Ouslander et al., 1993), and approximately 25 per cent of patients with incontinence will have a Foley catheter on transfer from the hospital. Incontinence alone is not an indication for prolonged Foley urinary catheterization. Catheters should be maintained in only several well-defined circumstances: chronic outlet obstruction caused by strictures or benign prostatic hypertrophy, a requirement for strict fluid intake and output records, or in patients with other medical problems that would be affected adversely by urinary incontinence, such as those with pelvic girdle pressure ulcers or other disruptions of the skin integrity. All other patients should have Foley catheters removed.

Among patients with indwelling urinary catheters, colonization of the urine reaches a prevalence of 85 to 98 per cent within approximately 2 weeks. Prophylactic treatment of asymptomatic bacteriuria in this group of patients is of no benefit (Warren et al., 1982). Although there is a higher incidence of fevers among patients with catheters (Warren et al., 1987), most episodes are transient and self-limited. Patients who remain febrile, or show evidence of systemic illness, should be evaluated and other causes excluded prior to instituting treatment for urinary tract infection (McGeer et al., 1991). At least two sets of blood cultures should be obtained in addition to urinary cultures before treatment is initiated. The catheter should be replaced and a specimen drawn from a new catheter to avoid culturing organisms that have colonized only the tubing. Organisms seen in Grams staining of the urine help with decisions about empiric therapy. Bacilli should be treated with a third-generation cephalosporin plus an aminoglycoside, while treatment of cocci should include vancomycin because methecine-resistant *S. aureus* is endemic in long-term care institutions. Concordance between urine cultures and blood cultures will direct later decisions about appropriate therapy.

Another common problem among patients with indwelling catheters involves repeated blockage of the catheter, characterized by urine leakage, lower abdominal cramping, and recurrent fevers. Chronic irritation of the bladder and partial outflow obstruction may cause excessive mucus production and other changes that promote the formation of concretions. Using the smallest balloon that will be retained and frequently changing the catheter is usually effective. A review of the chart will reveal the periodicity of the blockages, and catheter changes should be scheduled in anticipation. Antibiotic suppressant therapy is rarely effective, and irrigation, even with continuous flow, is of no benefit. Once the urine has cleared of mucus and concretions, the schedule of changes can be advanced slowly.

Following the removal of an indwelling catheter, patients should be treated with a full course of antibiotics, either empirically or based on urine culture and sensitivity tests acquired within 5 days of catheter removal (Harding et al., 1991).

GASTROSTOMY TUBES/FEEDING TUBES. An alternative means of providing adequate nutrition and hydration for nursing home patients is by enteral feeding tubes. Nasogastric tubes can be inserted easily and are acceptable for short-term use. Weighted, narrow-lumen feeding tubes are tolerated better by most patients and have fewer complications. Complications of nasogastric tube feedings include irritation of the nares, exacerbation of sinusitis or pharyngitis, and the possibility that the tube or its contents may be regurgitated and aspirated. Patients with agitation and confusion may have to be restrained to prevent extubation; however, restraints can aggravate the behavioral disturbance.

The preferred method of providing enteral nutrition is through a gastrostomy tube. For patients who are likely to require nutritional assistance for more than several weeks or who are intolerant of a nasogastric tube, a percutaneous endoscopic gastrostomy can be placed safely with intravenous sedation and local anesthesia. Because the entry port is on the abdomen, there is less tendency for patients to attempt to extubate themselves. Nursing staff can change gastrostomy Foley catheters easily without the need for radiographic confirmation of placement, as is often required for nasogastric tubes.

A disadvantage of gastrostomy feeding is the leakage of gastric contents onto the abdominal wall, causing a chemical burn. This complication can be treated successfully with omeprazole 20 mg/day and protecting the skin with zinc oxide ointment. Occasionally, topical steroid, antifungal, or antistaphylococcal preparations may be needed, either singly or in combination under the zinc oxide barrier. In these cases, increasing or decreasing the catheter size is usually not of benefit. Intestinal blockage may be caused by the Foley catheter balloon being carried by peristalsis to occlude the pylorus or duodenum. This complication can be averted by anchoring the tubing to a split 4 × 4 gauze pad that is then taped to the abdominal wall.

Jejunostomy tubes are indicated only in patients who have a surgically absent stomach. This type of tube offers very little advantage and several major disadvantages: The tube may be replaced only surgically; special elemental diets often are needed because the stomach is bypassed; and there is a greater likelihood of "dumping syndrome" and bowel overgrowth, with malabsorption and diarrhea.

All forms of feeding tubes are associated with an equal likelihood of aspiration of gastric contents (Jarnagin, 1992). Patients at high risk of aspiration should be fed only when the head of the bed is elevated at least 30 degrees. There is no difference in aspiration risk between patients fed by either continuous or bolus feedings.

Evidence supporting the association between liquid feedings and diarrhea is inconsistent. Most patients tolerate the hyperosmolarity of tube feeding formulas, and there is no scientifically based reason to begin feedings with diluted formulas. When diarrhea occurs, it frequently is caused by an overgrowth of *C. difficile* in patients who have been treated with antibiotics. Diarrhea also may occur as a result of a failure of the gastrointestinal tract to break down complex sugars, which then act as a hyperosmolar laxative. Sorbitol is found in relatively high doses in liquid formulations of medications and may cause diarrhea by a similar mechanism.

SPECIAL ASPECTS OF GERIATRIC CARE

Atypical Presentations of Common Illnesses

Because people are living longer, illnesses that previously were described as occurring infrequently in the presenium now are found commonly among the elderly. Most notable among these conditions is Alzheimer's disease, which has been found to one of the major causes of dementia in the elderly. In addition, conditions that were described as occurring most often in younger persons now have been shown to have their greatest incidence in old age (e.g., rheumatoid arthritis and osteomyelitis). The incidence of cancer is also greatest among the elderly. Other diagnoses, such as Hodgkin's disease, Crohn's disease, and asymmetric septal hypertrophy, have a second peak of incidence after 60. In addition, some illnesses will present differently when they occur in an older patient. For example, rheumatoid arthritis is often less destructive to joints and has a different pattern of joint involvement; lupus erythematosus may manifest primarily as serositis with pericardial and pleural effusions, rather than with arthritis as the predominant presenting complaint. Other conditions occur mainly or entirely in older patients. Polymyalgia rheumatica/temporal arteritis, osteoporosis, Paget's disease, macular degeneration, and pseudogout rarely are seen in patients under the age of 60.

A further challenge of geriatric medicine is that certain common conditions may occur but the accepted features of the illness may be lacking or may take a different form, thus obscuring the diagnosis. Among the elderly, pain, fever, thirst, and breathlessness are less reliable and consistent symptoms. Instead, the cardinal signs of illness in the elderly relate predominately to changes in mentation, functional status, and a "failure to thrive."

Infections without Fever

Although most neurohumoral mechanisms remain intact throughout life, the ability to mount a fever may be altered by both age and severe debility (see earlier in this chapter). Several studies have documented the absence of fever among elderly patients with significant infectious diseases. This has been reported for elderly patients with pneumococcal bacteremias (Finkelstein et al., 1983) and bacterial endocarditis (Terpenning et al., 1987), and for nursing home patients with pneumonia, urinary tract infections, and cellulitis (Castle et al., 1991).

The importance of recognizing this altered presentation of serious infectious processes is underscored by the negative correlation between fever and mortality. Among patients with bacteremias, studies have shown that the mortality rate of those whose maximal temperature response was between 95° and 100.8°F was 71 per cent, whereas it was less than 50 per cent in patients whose temperature was greater than 100.9°F (Gleckman and Hibert, 1982).

Pneumonia is the infectious disease most often overlooked because of blunted fever and atypical signs and symptoms. Fever on presentation is absent in 20 to 30 per cent of cases, and cough is absent in up to 50 per cent. Conversely, changes in mental status are the principle symptoms in 40 to 50 per cent of patients (Marrie et al., 1986). Several autopsy studies of patients in long-term care facilities have demonstrated that pneumonia is the most common cause of death and is also most often underdiagnosed premortem (Gloth and Burton, 1990).

Pain

Pain perception and pain reaction threshold are decreased in the older patient. This may be exacerbated by decreased alertness as a side effect of medications, and by dementia (Crook et al., 1984). Silent ischemia increases in prevalence with age, as does myocardial infarction without chest pain (McDonald, 1983). Older patients may sustain osteoporotic fractures of the vertebrae, wrist, and hip that may result in diminished function rather than pain and discomfort. Likewise, distention of abdominal organs as occurs in cholecystitis, volvulus, mesenteric artery thrombosis with infarction, appendicitis, and urinary obstruction may present with surprisingly few localizing symptoms. The older patient often will manifest other significant signs of illness, such as delirium, falls, or other changes in function.

Breathlessness

Changes in mental status may mask the sensation of dyspnea, although tachypnea may be evident. The cause for this lack of awareness in some patients is unknown, but is not necessarily related to changes in cognition or general alertness. This presentation is most evident with acute congestive heart failure, pulmonary emboli, and interstitial lung disease, in which symptoms other than breathlessness (i.e., chest pain, lower extremity swelling, or dizziness) may be the patient's chief complaint.

Diseases Occurring More Commonly in the Elderly

Polymyalgia Rheumatica

Polymyalgia rheumatica (PMR) is a disease of the elderly rarely occurring before the age of 50. The presentation is insidious, and the patient complains of aching and stiffness in the muscles of the shoulder girdle and occasionally of the pelvis. The pathology is related to a transient synovitis of the shoulder, hip (Olhagen, 1986), or peripheral joints. Fever, malaise, and weight loss are associated symptoms. The physical examination reveals tenderness of the shoulder and neck muscles, but there is rarely a significant loss of strength. The diagnosis of PMR is based on a combination of the clinical symptoms, an exclusion of other pathology, and the presence of an elevated erythrocyte sedimentation rate (ESR). The condition is also relatively self-limited, usually lasting for up to 2 years. Significant relief occurs in most cases with treatment with low-dose corticosteroids (15 mg of prednisone per day) or NSAIDs continued for approximately 2 years. Typically, patients with PMR respond symptomatically within a few days of institution of prednisone therapy (Goodwin, 1992). Treatment may be discontinued gradually, with careful monitoring of the ESR and symptoms.

Giant Cell Arteritis

Approximately 20 per cent of patients with PMR will develop temporal arteritis. Temporal arteritis is a vasculitis that can affect any large artery; however, the symptoms usually are confined to branches of the internal carotid artery. The most common presentation is headache occurring in the temporal artery area or occasionally in the frontal, occipital, or parietal areas. Patients usually complain of surface pain made worse by resting on a pillow or by cold exposure, and it is characteristically worse at nighttime. Occasionally, patients may complain of pain with chewing, swallowing, or tongue motion. Transient double vision may occur, but the major visual symptom is unilateral, partial, or complete blindness. Other less common clinical findings include tender scalp nodules, Raynaud's phenomena of the limbs, carotid artery tenderness, taste and smell disturbances, decreased peripheral pulses, and occasionally mononeuropathy affecting the median or peroneal nerve (Calama and Hunder, 1980). Because of the potentially disastrous ocular complications of giant cell arteritis, older patients should be managed aggressively with high-dose prednisone (50 mg/day). If temporal artery biopsy fails to confirm the diagnosis, multiple biopsies or contralateral biopsies may be necessary. The signs and symptoms of temporal arteritis should be used as a guide for tapering the steroid dose, which should be continued at high levels for several months before attempts are made to taper.

Cervical Spondylosis

This term describes degenerative changes that occur in the epiphysial joints and intervertebral disks of the neck with or without neurologic signs. One or more of the cervical nerve roots may be compressed or stretched and myelopathy may result. Patients usually present with neck pain, diminished neck movement, headaches, or neurologic compression symptoms, including radicular pain, sensory disturbances in the arms, and weakness of the arms or legs. Compression of the cervical cord may occur secondary to narrowing of the cervical canal and may present with spastic paraparesis of the lower extremities and a neurogenic bladder. If the lower cervical spine is involved, then upper motor neuron signs may be found in the lower extremities with normal findings in the upper extremities. Sometimes these signs are accompanied by posterior column and sensory deficits in the legs. Radiculopathy may present as a segmental pattern of weakness or sensory loss confined to one or more dermatomes and may be found either unilaterally or bilaterally in the upper extremities. Tendon reflexes usually are depressed in the affected distribution. A herniated cervical disk causes acute, subacute, or chronic pain that radiates into the arm, at times accompanied by muscle spasm and tenderness of the neck, scapula, or trapezius regions.

Degenerative disease of the cervical spine is usually progressive, but in many cases the clinical course is asymptomatic despite anatomic abnormalities. When symptoms occur, however, evaluation is always warranted. Plain radiographs of the cervical spine, myelography, or magnetic resonance imaging helps confirm the diagnosis (Russell, 1990). Operative treatment may be necessary to prevent further progression of symptoms if there are significant neurologic deficits or if root pain is severe, persistent, and unresponsive to conservative measures (White and Paryabi, 1988). Full recovery frequently results after decompressive laminectomy if the condition is recognized early.

Lumbar Stenosis

Lumbar spinal stenosis is typically a disorder of older persons, occurring more frequently in persons with a congenitally narrow spinal canal if they develop superimposed vertebral osteophytes or thickening of the ligamentum flavum. Lumbar spinal stenosis frequently coexists with cervical spondylosis. In general, spinal stenosis is asymptomatic and not associated with neurologic abnormalities. The diagnosis should be considered when patients present with low back pain and symptoms and signs related to nerve root compression. Most commonly affected are the muscles in the L5-S1 distribution. A common complaint is "pseudoclaudication"—slow onset of pain, numbness, or weakness in the buttocks, thighs, or legs that occurs with standing, walking, or back extension and is relieved by sitting or lying. Extension of the lumbar spine as occurs with standing, lying prone, or walking downhill produces bulging of the disk into the canal, reduces the length of the posterior canal, and causes protrusion of the ligamentum flavum into the canal. These symptoms also may be associated with arterial insufficiency. Patients with lumbar or spinal stenosis often will adopt a flexed posture as they walk and support themselves with walkers or grocery carts. Persistent pain and neurologic deficits, however, call for neurosurgical evaluation and consideration for surgery. In carefully selected patients, spinal decompression, laminectomy, and fusion may produce resolution of symptoms.

Paget's Disease

Paget's disease is a disorder of the bone characterized by excessive destruction and repair with associated deformities. The etiology is unknown, although it occurs most commonly in families and has a geographic predilection for the northern United States and northern European countries. The condition is most often asymptomatic and localized to a single bone. The first symptom is usually deep bone pain that is worse at night. Affected bones are soft, larger than normal, and deformed. At the cellular level, an initial destructive phase is followed by a phase of disorganized bone repair (Hamdy, 1990). The rate of bone turnover may be increased enormously in patients with active Paget's disease, occasionally more than 20 times normal.

The signs and symptoms of Paget's disease depend on the bones affected. Patients gradually may become aware of a swelling or deformity of a bone or may develop a disturbance of gait because of inequality of leg lengths. Skull enlargement may occur and headaches may become a prominent feature as a result of distortions of cartilage or the periosteum, or secondary osteoarthritis. Patients occasionally may present with blindness, deafness, or various neuralgias.

The characteristic laboratory findings are a significant elevation of the alkaline phosphatase levels, normal serum calcium and phosphorus, and elevated urinary hydroxyproline levels when the disease is active. Serum calcium levels may become elevated when patients are immobilized. The radiologic findings reflect the underlying pathology. The pelvic bones are involved most often,

followed by the femur, skull, tibia, spine, clavicle, and ribs. In the early phases, lesions may be osteoporotic, destructive, and radiolucent, particularly in the skull. Later, new bone formation is seen as areas of increased density.

COMPLICATIONS. Fractures frequently occur through soft bone with minimal trauma. If immobilization and hypercalcemia occur, then kidney stones may develop. If the vertebral column becomes involved, spinal cord compression may occur. Osteosarcoma may occur in pagetic bone and usually is heralded by increased bone pain and a sudden rise in alkaline phosphatase (Haibach et al., 1985). Rarely, the increased vascularity of pagetic bones may give rise to high-output cardiac failure.

TREATMENT. Most cases of Paget's disease require no treatment. Specific antipagetic treatment is indicated for persistent pain that is resistant to analgesics, neural complications, rapidly progressive deformity, hypercalcemia, hypercalciuria, kidney stones, repeated fractures or nonunion of fractures, and high-output cardiac failure, and in preparation for major orthopedic surgery. Agents are available that may reduce excessive bone resorption. Calcitonin acts by reducing osteoclastic activity and can be given in daily doses of 50 to 100 IU subcutaneously, or three times per week for months to years, and usually results in reductions in levels of alkaline phosphatase and rates of urinary hydroxyproline excretion. Variable decreases in bone pain and improvements in neurologic function have been reported. The effectiveness of calcitonin tends to plateau after a few weeks; however, continued therapy may result in further histologic improvements. Human calcitonin can be given to patients who fail to respond to synthetic calcitonin or who have developed antibodies. It is more expensive and causes nausea and flushing in up to 20 per cent of patients.

Diphosphonates are the most commonly used agent in the treatment of Paget's disease. Their advantages include few side effects, low costs, and long periods of remission. Biochemical abnormalities often return to normal and only gradually return to pretreatment levels on discontinuation. Etidronate disodium (Didronel) in 200 to 400-mg doses may be given daily for 3 to 6 months, with a rest period before another course is given (because mineralization of new bone may be inhibited if used for longer periods). Doses must be reduced for patients with renal insufficiency because these agents are excreted in urine. Short courses, on a cyclical basis, can result in remission of disease activity for months or even years (Audran et al., 1989).

Mesenteric Infarctions

The spectrum of intestinal ischemia ranges from mild chronic symptoms to catastrophic collapse, depending on the degree of involvement and the rapidity of the process. Chronic mesenteric vascular insufficiency produces a syndrome of intestinal "angina" characterized by colicky abdominal pain after meals. The pain may be related to the size of the meal and can lead to reduced food intake and weight loss unless the patient consumes small, frequent meals. The etiology is usually atherosclerosis; however, infarction may occur secondary to intermittent vessel compression or vasospasm. If symptoms are unremitting, surgical revascularization of the bowel is the treatment of choice. Abdominal angiography is necessary to confirm the diagnosis of occlusive mesenteric arterial disease in patients who are considered to be candidates for vascular surgery.

Acute mesenteric vascular insufficiency is a catastrophic abdominal disorder characterized by severe abdominal pain with nausea and bloody diarrhea. Frank shock may occur, and is a grave sign associated with high morbidity and mortality. Characteristic findings include abdominal distention, tenderness, and rigidity, with a marked leukemoid reaction and hemoconcentration. Bowel sounds initially may be loud but eventually disappear. The occlusive pathology is usually thromboembolic, but occasionally may be small vessel vasculitis, acute pancreatitis, or visceral perforation. For older patients who present with acute or subacute abdominal pain, and who have an underlying cardiac arrhythmia, the possibility of a mesenteric embolus should be considered. Other common causes of vascular insufficiency are hypotension resulting from medications, hypovolemia, or sepsis, and congestive heart failure, which leads to hypoxemia in areas supplied by branch vessels.

Treatment consists of immediate restoration of fluid volume and hemodynamic monitoring. Antibiotics usually are prescribed because the syndrome mimics sepsis. A laparotomy should be done as soon as possible and the gangrenous bowel resected; corrective vascular surgery is rarely possible. The mortality rate is high in the acute phases of the illness, and, in situations in which hypotension and shock exist, the prognosis is grave (Kahn and Rubenstein, 1984).

Syncope/Dizziness/Orthostatic Hypotension

Syncope is defined as a loss of consciousness and postural tone that begins abruptly and lasts for a limited period of time (usually less than 5 minutes), with spontaneous recovery (Manolis et al., 1990). "Near-syncope" is a state of transient dizziness that may be caused by any of the conditions that cause syncope. Near-syncope is more common, and many patients with its symptoms report the problem to their doctor. The loss of consciousness implies that the blood supply to both cerebral hemispheres, or the reticular formation of the brain stem, is interrupted for more than 8 to 10 seconds. Syncope occurs in about 2 per cent of those between the ages of 65 and 69 and in 12 per cent of those over the age of 85, and it frequently (30 per cent of cases) is recurrent. A higher mortality risk is associated with syncope when the etiology is cardiovascular, although this probably is more reflective of the underlying disease (Kapoor, 1991).

The elderly are predisposed to syncope and orthostatic hypotension because of age- and disease-related changes in cardiovascular responsiveness during postural change or exercise, and in the presence of hypovolemia and hypotension (Lipsitz, 1989). When diseases such as congestive heart failure, coronary artery disease, atherosclerosis, carotid artery disease, and hypertension coexist, an impairment of cerebral blood flow may result.

The common causes of syncope can be divided into disorders associated with failure of the systemic circulation to perfuse the cerebral vasculature adequately, metabolic disorders, drug toxicities, and intracranial pathology. Autonomic insufficiency is suggested by symptoms of orthostatic dizziness, visual difficulties, urinary incontinence, inability to sweat, constipation, chronic fatigue, and impotence (Palolisso et al., 1989). Neurologic disorders associated with autonomic dysfunction include Parkinson's disease, the Shy-Drager syndrome, brain stem disorders, and cerebral infarcts. Peripheral neurologic disorders (secondary to diabetes mellitus, vitamin deficiencies, and alcohol-related disorders) also may cause autonomic dysfunction. Another common cause is the loss of sympathetic tone following immobilization or bed rest, resulting in venous pooling in the lower extremities. Postmicturition and defecation syncope has been described; postprandial hypotension also may result in syncopal episodes in patients with impaired cardiovascular reflexes (Lipsitz, 1989). Cardiovascular disorders that reduce cardiac output predispose to syncopal episodes; these include both brady- and tachyarrhythmias and mechanical outflow obstruction secondary to valvular aortic stenosis or asymmetric septal hypertrophy. Patients with diastolic ventricular dysfunction are particularly prone to syncopal episodes with new-onset atrial fibrillation.

Among the elderly, autonomic impairment as a result of medication effects is not unusual; tricyclic antidepressants, levodopa, nitroglycerin preparations, and neuroleptics are likely offenders. Hypoglycemia, hypoxemia, and electrolyte derangements also should be considered in the differential diagnosis. Only rarely are intracranial conditions such as neoplasms or hematomas implicated as the etiology of syncope.

An accurate history of the episode should be obtained to rule out the conditions listed in Table 7–9. A cardiovascular and neurologic examination is indicated, including orthostatic vital signs. However, orthostatic hypotension, defined as a decline in systolic blood pressure of 20 mm Hg or greater or a decline of 10 mm Hg or greater in diastolic blood pressure, occurs in up to 20 per cent of older

TABLE 7–9. ETIOLOGIC FACTORS IN SYNCOPE

Hypotension
  Vasomotor instability
    Orthostatic hypotension
    Carotid sinus syndrome
    Precipitation of syncope by micturition, defecation,
      coughing, and swallowing
    Postprandial syncope
    Vasovagal syncope
  Volume depletion
  Drugs

Abnormal blood composition
  Acute hypoxemia
  Hypoglycemia

Cardiovascular disease
  Anatomic
    Aortic stenosis
    Mitral prolapse and regurgitation
    Hypertrophic cardiomyopathy
    Myxoma
  Myocardial
    Ischemia and infarct
    Cardiomyopathy
  Electrical
    Tachyarrhythmia
    Bradyarrhythmia
    Heart block
    Sick-sinus syndrome
  Vascular
    Pulmonary embolism

Cerebral disorders
  Vascular insufficiency
  Seizures

From Ryan SM, Lipsitz LA: Syncope in: Common diseases, disorders, and health concerns. Cardiovascular diseases. *In* Beck JC (ed): Geriatric Review Syllabus: A Core Curriculum in Geriatric Medicine. American Geriatrics Society 1991-1992 Program. New York, American Geriatrics Society, 1991-1992, p 273, with permission. Adapted from Lipsitz LA: Syncope in the elderly. Ann Intern Med 99:95, 1983.

persons (Mader, 1989). Syncope should not be attributed to orthostasis if the symptoms are not reproduced in the presence of significant postural blood pressure changes. Laboratory tests should include a complete blood count, electrolyte measures, and serum glucose level. An electrocardiogram (ECG) should be obtained, and a 24-hour ambulatory ECG monitor is highly recommended as part of the evaluation (Kapoor, 1991). A tilt test may be helpful in determining if the cause is a vasovagal reaction (Grubb et al., 1991). Echocardiography and electrophysiologic studies may be helpful. In approximately one third of patients no clear cause for syncope can be determined after thorough investigation.

The management should be directed at treating reversible causes. Orthostatic hypotension initially should be treated with nonpharmacologic interventions, such as discontinuing any potentially causative medications, wearing elastic stockings, maintaining a high-salt diet, and elevating the head of the bed to decrease nocturnal diuresis and volume depletion. If pharmacologic interventions are indicated, then fludrocortisone or phenylpro-

panolamine may be considered. Clonidine has been helpful in patients with reduced central catecholamines, by increasing venoconstriction and venous return to the heart.

Drugs in the Elderly

Americans over 65 spend approximately $3 billion/year for prescription and nonprescription drugs, representing 20 to 25 per cent of the total national expenditure. Up to 90 per cent of elderly patients take at least one medication on an occasional basis, and more than 50 per cent take medications regularly. In long-term care institutions, 80 to 98 per cent of patients take at least one drug on a regular basis, with an average of three to seven prescriptions per patient (Nolan and O'Malley, 1988).

The physiologic changes associated with aging and many of the common illnesses that afflict the elderly have extensive pharmacologic consequences (O'Malley et al., 1983). These changes may have profound effects on the way that drugs are processed (pharmacokinetics) and their effects (pharmacodynamics).

Absorption

Although enteric absorption of drugs is unaffected in normal aging, several common pathologic changes may interfere with the absorption of some medications. Gastric acidity often declines and as a result alters the solubility of the drug vehicle, thus delaying its release. Other prescription and nonprescription medications may interfere with absorption by changing the pH or by binding to the medication. Impaired gastric motility may delay the passage of medications into the small intestine, or prolonged transit times may delay passage into the large intestine, where the drug is metabolized before being absorbed. Conversely, dumping syndromes with diarrhea may not allow sufficient time for medications to enter the circulation.

The absorption of medications through the skin is also subject to changes associated with age. The stratum corneum becomes thickened, and there is less subcutaneous blood flow because of age-related declines in the number and density of dermal capillaries. Dosages and timing of medications may have to be adjusted in consideration of these changes.

Volume of Distribution

Changes in body composition associated with age include an increase in the fat volume and a decrease in water volume per weight, which may have significant effects on the pharmacokinetics of medications. Although such changes usually occurring slowly, there may be periods of more rapid changes. For example, illness or retirement may lead to a more sedentary lifestyle, with resultant loss of muscle mass and consequent decrease in water volume; changes in nutrition as a result of dental problems, or changes in socioeconomic level, also may result a higher fat volume.

Drugs distributed in the water volume may achieve higher concentrations at the same dosage as this volume decreases with age. This may lead to exaggerated therapeutic effects, side effects, or toxicity. Minor changes in the metabolic or elimination pathways can have marked effects on the serum level of these medications. Therefore, adjustments often are required in both the prescribed dose and the frequency of administration in times of clinical instability.

The extent of protein binding also affects drug levels within the water volume of distribution. Drugs that are poorly protein bound, such as most antibiotics, can be titrated by balancing administration and elimination. Medications that are highly protein bound, such as warfarin and hydantoin, initially will be distributed among the protein-binding sites, and, when these become saturated, equilibrium will be established between bound and free drug. Only that portion that is free is pharmacologically active and subject to metabolism and elimination. Subsequent doses add to the free component and, unless eliminated, may cause side effects or toxicity. Therefore, for highly protein-bound medications, greater doses may be needed until saturation of protein-binding sites is completed; with chronic dosing, smaller amounts of this drug may be required.

An increase in fat mass affects the pharmacokinetics of medications that are distributed in fatty tissues. Only that portion of the drug that remains in the serum is active; that which enters the fat creates an increasingly large storage reservoir. Serum levels therefore are determined both by intake and by slow release of drugs from the fat mass. In time, these two sources of drug availability may create very high serum levels, and the effects of the medication may persist long after administration has been discontinued. Among the more common examples are long-acting benzodiazepines and high-potency major tranquilizers.

Elimination

Medications are eliminated either by metabolism or by excretion. The liver is the major site of metabolism and deactivation, while the kidney is the organ through which medications, or their byproducts, are eliminated. Both hepatic and renal function are affected by age, and result in significant changes in pharmacokinetics.

HEPATIC METABOLISM. Phase I drug metabolism involves oxidation and reduction reactions through the cytochrome P-450 system in the endoplasmic reticulum. Phase II hepatic enzyme activity involves the addition of a water-soluble group (e.g., acetylation). While the liver decreases in size

with age, with parallel losses of oxidative/reductive capacity, this is usually only a minor factor in altered hepatic drug metabolism; the elimination of drugs that undergo phase II metabolism is not altered by age. A final consideration is that oxidation and reduction reactions often lead to active metabolites. In some cases, these reactions are necessary for activation of a medication; for example, diazepam is metabolized to oxazepam, one of the principle active constituents, which changes the drug from a lipophilic to a more water-soluble form. Phase II metabolism usually results in inactive metabolites that are highly water soluble and enhances renal excretion (e.g., oxazepam conjugates with glucuronide).

Concurrent pathology and medications also affect liver metabolism. Only phase I metabolism depends on hepatic blood flow, and it is highly sensitive to decreases in cardiac output, which may result in an accumulation of medications. A number of medications influence cytochrome P-450 activity. Phenobarbital and chloral hydrate may increase enzyme activity, while cimetidine and alcohol may decrease it.

RECEPTOR SENSITIVITY. Most medications act as agonists or antagonists on cell membrane hormone and neurotransmitter receptors that have significant effects on the pharmacokinetics of many drugs. These receptors often are affected by age and disease, usually decreasing in number. For example, β-receptor agonist activity has been shown to become attenuated with age, resulting in lower heart rate responses to adrenergic agents. Cholinergic receptors also decrease in concentration throughout the body with advancing years, and, therefore, medications with anticholinergic activity are likely to have enhanced effectiveness and frequently result in side effects and toxicities such as delirium, constipation, and urinary retention. Dopamine receptors decline in number and activity with age, and may predispose patients given dopamine antagonists to parkinsonian side effects.

RENAL ELIMINATION. Creatinine clearance declines with age at the rate of approximately 1 mL/min/year between the ages of 30 and 80 (Rowe et al., 1976). These changes are masked somewhat as a result of the decline in muscle mass with age and a sedentary lifestyle. As muscle mass declines, less creatinine is produced, approximately matching the decline in creatinine clearance. Therefore, serum creatinine remains stable over the decades among healthy individuals. In addition, urine concentrating ability and the ability to retain sodium decline with age. Adequate hydration compensates for the decrement in renal concentrating ability. However, renal function also can be compromised further by chronic disease and by medications. As renal reserves are lost, the ability of the kidney to excrete drugs becomes compromised. Therefore, adjustment of dosing amounts and frequencies must be made for drugs excreted by the kidney or for medications that are nephrotoxic.

Principles of Geriatric Prescribing

1. *Use nonpharmacologic interventions if at all possible.* Potential side effects of medications occur more commonly in the elderly and may exacerbate the patient's condition.

2. *Choose medications based on their characteristic patterns of absorption, receptor action, and elimination.* The patient's concurrent illnesses, other medications, and personal habits also should be considered when choosing the most appropriate drug.

3. *Start low and go slowly.* Lower doses often achieve a therapeutic effect; however, medications that are highly protein bound may have a delayed effect. Fat-soluble compounds may require considerable time before steady state is reached.

4. *Titrate to established treatment goals.* It is important to establish treatment end points and to titrate the medications based on clinical indications of effectiveness, rather than a predetermined dosage range.

5. *Keep it simple.* Compliance decreases proportionally to the number of medications and the number of times per day that dosing is required. Reassess the regimen to ensure that each medication has a specific purpose and is still required. Cluster medications, and strive for no more than two medication administration times per day. Discuss the implications of price versus convenience.

6. *Iatrogenesis is a common causes of illness.* If a patient presents with a new symptom, the drug regimen should be reviewed and the medications that might be responsible eliminated, rather than adding new drugs to relieve the symptoms.

7. *Review the regimen on a regular basis, or when adding a new drug, and eliminate any medications that are ineffective or no longer needed.*

Surgical Care of the Elderly

The overall risk of adverse outcomes for older patients undergoing major surgery has diminished in recent years (Djokovic and Hedley-White, 1979). Although excess mortality occurs, much of this can be attributed to the high incidence of concurrent medical problems and the greater likelihood for older persons to be admitted nonelectively and to require operations for emergency or semiemergent reasons. Especially in these situations, the multiple coexisting medical problems may contribute to a lack of physiologic reserve to withstand the stresses of anesthesia and surgery. Most of the perioperative mortality results from coexistent or new-onset cardiac disease, while much of the morbidity is attributed to respiratory complications, including pneumonia, ventilator dependency, pulmonary embolism, and atelectasis. The elderly are more likely to develop postoperative confusion, pressure ulcers, deep venous thromboses, protein–calorie undernutrition, dehydration, and major declines in levels of function.

Risk Factor Identification and Perioperative Management

The care of the elderly surgical patient requires that all medical conditions that may result in adverse outcomes be managed optimally and to ameliorate the associated risk. The risk factors for adverse cardiac outcomes are listed in Table 7–10. Most important among these are the presence of an S_3 gallop or jugular venous distention and a history of having had a recent myocardial infarction. The extent of myocardial damage and the amount of cardiac functional reserve are predictive of cardiac complications. Unstable angina is an important risk factor, and should be investigated and treated prior to elective surgery (Detsky et al., 1986). Cardiac reserve should be assessed in patients undergoing major surgery, especially if their activity has been limited because of significant peripheral vascular disease, arthritis, or other physical impairments. Dipyridamole thallium testing and ambulatory ECG monitoring are useful tests of cardiac reserve and ischemia, and good predictors of cardiac outcome in these patients (Boucher et al., 1985). Other risk factors include hemody-

TABLE 7–10. COMPUTATION OF THE CARDIAC RISK INDEX

Item	Points
History	
Age > 70	5
Myocardial infarction within 6 months	10
Physical examination	
S_3 or jugular venous distension	11
Important valvular aortic stenosis	3
Electrocardiogram	
Rhythm other than sinus or the presence of atrial premature contractions on the preoperative ECG	7
More than 5 PVCs/min at any time prior to surgery	7
Medical status	
Poor general medical status	3
PO_2 < 60 or PCO_2 > 50	
K < 3.0 or HCO_3 < 20 mEq/L	
BUN > 50 or creatinine > 3 mg/dl	
Abnormal SGOT	
Chronic liver disease	
Bedridden due to noncardiac cause	
Operation	
Intraperitoneal, intrathoracic, aortic surgery	3
Emergency surgery	4
Total points	53

From Goldman L, Calvera DL, Nussbaum SR, et al: Multifactorial index of cardiac risk in noncardiac surgical procedures. N Engl J Med 297:845, 1977, with permission.

namically significant aortic stenosis, the type and urgency of the procedure, and the severity of underlying systemic illness. Factors that have not been found to increase the risk of cardiac complications include: mild stable angina, controlled hypertension (diastolic blood pressure less than 100 mm Hg and systolic blood pressure less than 200 mm Hg), hypercholesterolemia, compensated congestive heart failure, the presence of a pacemaker, previous coronary artery bypass surgery, and diabetes mellitus (Weitz and Goldman, 1987).

Patients with active symptomatic cardiac disease should be evaluated by a cardiologist for monitoring by Swan-Ganz catheterization. Murmurs suggestive of hemodynamically significant aortic stenosis or other valvular pathology should be evaluated by echocardiography. Further treatment, such as coronary artery bypass grafting, percutaneous transluminal angioplasty, or valve replacement surgery, may be indicated prior to noncardiac surgery. Antiarrhythmic medications should be continued up to and including the day of surgery. Prophylaxis against bacterial endocarditis is indicated for patients with prosthetic heart valves, congenital malformations, systemic–pulmonary shunts, rheumatic heart disease, a history of subacute bacterial endocarditis, and possibly mitral valve prolapse (Weitz, 1990). It is important that the ventricular rate is controlled in patients with atrial fibrillation because new-onset or rapid atrial fibrillation can result in cardiac decompensation. Cardiac ischemia can be managed perioperatively using nitroglycerin, β-blockers, and calcium channel blockers.

OTHER RISK FACTORS. Older patients are at risk for pulmonary morbidity because age-related declines in partial pressure of oxygen, elastic recoil, and lung compliance are compromised further by the effects of anesthesia and surgery. Other risk factors include obesity, malnutrition, kyphoscoliosis, muscular weakness, a history of cigarette smoking, and an upper abdominal or thoracic operation (Tisi, 1987). For patients who have a history of cigarette smoking or chronic lung disease, the degree of pulmonary compromise should be assessed by arterial blood gases and spirometry. All patients should be advised to discontinue cigarette smoking at least 4 to 6 weeks before surgery. Optimal bronchodilation should be achieved preoperatively, and patients should be taught how to use an incentive spirometer.

Patients with renal disease have a greater incidence of perioperative electrolyte abnormalities, sepsis, and death. Patients having major surgery, particularly major vascular procedures, are at risk for developing postoperative acute tubular necrosis. Preoperative hydration and invasive hemodynamic monitoring may help reduce the incidence of these complications (Beck, 1990).

Anemia is common in hospitalized elderly patients; however, patients who have compensated to their chronic anemias tolerate surgery well. Older patients undergoing major surgery in which large blood loses are anticipated probably should be transfused preoperatively to a hemoglobin level of 10 gm/dL. The older surgical patient is at increased risk for deep venous thrombosis. This is especially true for persons undergoing orthopedic, cancer, major gastrointestinal, or urogenital procedures. The incidence of postoperative deep venous thrombosis can be reduced by prophylactic anticoagulation with coumadin, subcutaneous heparin, or low-molecular-weight heparin (National Institutes of Health Consensus Development Conference, 1986).

Diabetes is the most common endocrinologic disorder encountered by physicians caring for elderly patients perioperatively. Surgical stress usually results in hyperglycemia, which increases the likelihood of sepsis, impaired wound healing, electrolyte abnormalities, and diabetic ketoacidosis. The goal of management is to maintain serum glucose levels in the range of 200 to 250 mg/dL. One half to two thirds of the patient's intermediate-acting insulin can be given on the morning of surgery, and fingerstick glucose levels should be obtained frequently during the procedure. Elevated levels of blood glucose can be treated with regular insulin. For brittle diabetics, an insulin infusion started a few hours before surgery may result in better blood glucose control (Reynolds, 1985).

Postoperative Care

To reduce the incidence of mortality and morbidity, attention must be given to increasing activity soon after surgery. All patients should be turned regularly and encouraged to sit in a chair within the first 24 hours. Activity levels should be increased daily to prevent pressure ulcers, deep venous thrombosis, and deconditioning as a result of immobility. It is estimated that 1 day of postoperative bed rest results in levels of functional decline similar to those of a year of sedentary lifestyle (Harper and Lyles, 1988). Early ambulation and aggressive physical and occupational therapy may be preventative.

The onset of postoperative medical complications may be heralded by a change in mentation, or by delirium in up to 15 per cent of patients. Potentially important precipitating factors include medications, infections, metabolic disturbances, myocardial infarction, hypovolemia, fecal impaction, and urinary retention. New-onset confusion may be the initial manifestation of a medical emergency and should be investigated promptly. If no reversible medical cause is found, then frequent attempts should be made to reorient the patient to his or her environment. Family members, sitters, and nursing staff should assist in this task. As a last resort, judicious use of major tranquilizers may be successful in calming these behaviors.

Surgical procedures may transform mild levels

of protein–calorie undernutrition into severe states of malnutrition. Patients should be fed high-protein supplements in the operative period and nutritional parameters should be monitored closely. This may require intravenous or enteral hydration and nutritional support until adequate oral intake is achieved.

Conditions Related to Nutritional Disorders

Pressure Ulcers

The management of pressure ulcers has become an issue of growing concern for health care facilities. The prevalence of pressure ulcers is 3 to 11 per cent in acute care hospitals and nursing homes, significantly affecting length of stay, resource utilization, and mortality. Over 50 per cent of patients with pressure ulcers are over the age of 70 (Allman, 1989). Although most pressure ulcers (57 to 66 per cent) are acquired in the acute care setting, the majority of these patients are transferred to long-term care facilities, such that approximately 20 per cent of nursing home admissions arrive with pressure ulcers (Smith et al., 1991).

Pressure ulcers are caused by a combination of forces: pressure and either shear or torsion. Pressure is distributed in an expanding cone of tissue involvement with the apex at the skin and the base toward the bone; the amount of pressure determines the depth, and the time over which the pressure is applied determines the extent of tissue injury. Generally, low pressures may be tolerated for several hours without tissue injury, so that turning patients every 2 hours usually can prevent skin breakdown. With the addition of shear or torsion forces, injury may occur across tissue planes. This either compromises or disrupts vascular supply, leading to ischemia or hemorrhage. When the associated pressure is small, damage occurs in the skin, resulting in an intradermal ecchymosis (stage I) or superficial breakdown into the dermis (stage II). With increasing pressure, there may be involvement of subcutaneous tissues and fat (stage III) or underlying muscle and bone (stage IV). With deeper ulcers, tissue damage may occur principally below the skin, leading to a subcutaneous abscess of necrotic tissue or hematoma. Eventually, these may come to the surface and manifest as a pressure ulcer (stage III or IV).

Risk factors for the development of pressure ulcers include recent weight loss, impaired mobility, and neurologic deficit involving either the brain or spinal cord. Superficial pressure ulcers also are associated with urinary and fecal incontinence. Pressure ulcers that extend into the subcutaneous tissues, including fat, muscle, and bone, often are associated with profound hypoalbuminemia.

The treatment of pressure ulcers is predicated on five basic steps. The first is to promote an environment conducive to wound healing. This requires that devitalized tissue be removed by aggressive surgical débridement. Once the inflammation has subsided, then wound healing may be enhanced by maintaining a moist environment under occlusive dressings with normal saline–moistened gauze packing. Recurrent injury must be prevented by the appropriate application of mattress covers or specialty beds, and avoidance of shear and torsion when moving the patient in bed. Healing can be achieved best by careful attention to adequate nutrition with high-protein supplements, either orally or by enteral routes. Although patients with pressure ulcers are usually sedentary, pressure ulcers are major systemic stressors, and the diet should be adjusted to account for the high metabolic demands of healing. Finally, it is important to stabilize concurrent illnesses such as cardiac and pulmonary disease to assure adequate tissue perfusion, and optimize diabetic control and renal function to avoid toxicity of the immune system.

Surgical closure of a pressure ulcer may be considered when the nutritional status has been re-established and the wounds have stabilized fully so that no remaining necrotic tissue is evident. The success of myocutaneous flap surgery is only 40 to 60 per cent, and many patients will suffer recurrent ulcers within the next 2 years despite initial success (Disa et al., 1992). Conservative management and healing by secondary intention can be equally efficacious, and, therefore, careful consideration of treatment goals must be made for each patient.

Anemia

Anemia exists when the quantity of circulating erythrocytes falls below normal. There is some controversy as to whether older patients have an age-related decline in red cell parameters, while others would suggest that, although anemia is prevalent, it should never be regarded as a normal concomitant of aging (Garry et al., 1983). In selected populations, screened for education and socioeconomic class, few normal elderly people will have a decline in hemoglobin values, even into the eighth decade (Zauber and Zauber, 1987). However, studies reporting normal values for large-scale elderly populations may be confounded by the effects of chronic asymptomatic and subclinical conditions that affect hematologic parameters. The evaluation for cause of anemias is productive only when hemoglobin levels are 12 gm/dL or less in men and 11.5 gm/dL or less in women over the age of 65. In contrast, a high prevalence of anemia has been reported in hospitalized elderly, males, blacks, those in lower socioeconomic groups, and those who are chronically institutionalized. Furthermore, there is a greater likelihood of anemia among patients with poor nutritional status, those with concomitant diseases, and those who have had a gastrectomy.

Bone marrow cellularity declines with age, with bone marrow cells being replaced by fat and fibrous tissue. However, the numbers of the most primitive red cell precursors do not decline and no basal changes of hematopoiesis have been noted in normal elderly people (Lipschitz and Udapa, 1986). In general, the bone marrow responds more slowly to stress caused by bleeding, drugs, or infections, but it is not certain whether this is a consequence of aging or a result of chronic inflammation or low-grade nutritional deficiencies. Red cell survival, iron turnover, and red cell mass remain normal.

The most common types of anemia are the *hypoproliferative anemias*, in which red cell production is reduced. This group includes both iron-deficiency anemia and the anemias of chronic disorders resulting from inflammation and protein–calorie undernutrition. Iron-deficiency anemia almost always results from blood loss in the gastrointestinal tract secondary to peptic ulcer disease, gastrointestinal carcinoma, dysplasia of the gastrointestinal tract, diverticular disease, or gastritis caused by NSAIDs. It is rare for iron-deficiency anemia to occur as a result of nutritional deficiency because iron is ubiquitous in food. Iron absorption is unchanged in the elderly, and iron stores increase with age. Minimal normal daily losses of iron occur. Iron absorption is enhanced by vitamin C and in situations of iron deficiency. Iron is absorbed more efficiently from organic sources such as meat and eggs.

In iron-deficiency anemia, serum iron is usually very low while iron-binding capacity is significantly elevated. A serum ferritin level of 50 μg/L or less, or a serum ferritin level of less than 75 μg/L combined with a transferrin saturation of less than 8 per cent, is virtually diagnostic of iron-deficiency anemia (Guyatt et al., 1990). Treatment with oral iron preparations should result in a hematologic response within 3 weeks, and should be continued for 6 months to replenish stores.

The anemia of chronic diseases is characterized by a mild to moderate anemia that is usually normochromic and normocytic. Common causes include chronic infections (endocarditis, polynephritis, tuberculosis), pressure ulcers, neoplasia (lymphoma, leukemia, myeloma, etc.), collagen vascular disease, endocrine disorders (hypothyroidism), and chronic renal insufficiency. The pathophysiology appears to be a defect in the ability of the reticuloendothelial system to mobilize iron. As a result, serum ferritin levels usually are elevated and iron-binding capacity decreased. In general, hemolytic anemias are uncommon; however, autoimmune hemolytic anemia occurring secondary to medications or in association with myeloproliferative disorders can be seen. Because the anemia associated with chronic diseases is associated with large amounts of storage iron, oral iron treatment is not indicated.

Ineffective erythropoiesis almost always results from *vitamin B_{12} or folic acid deficiency*. The cardinal features of these anemias are an abnormality of nuclear maturation resulting in large red blood cells (mean corpuscular volume > 110 fL), hypersegmented granulocytes, and, because of ineffective erythropoiesis, indirect hyperbilirubinemia. Older patients may have low serum levels of vitamin B_{12} but no evidence of any hematologic abnormality because of coexisting iron deficiency, concomitant folic acid deficiency, thalassemia, or an expression of the deficiency only in the central nervous system. Normal levels of folic acid may be able to substitute for vitamin B_{12} at the bone marrow level but not in the central nervous system; hence, neuropathy and myelopathy may occur prior to hematologic abnormalities (Fine and Soria, 1991).

Approximately 25 per cent of patients over the age of 65 with vitamin B_{12} deficiency have normal absorption of vitamin B_{12} but are unable to extract the vitamin from food because of gastric hypochlorhydria (Camel, 1990). It takes approximately 5 to 6 years for stores of vitamin B_{12} to deplete in patients with pernicious anemia. On a dietary basis alone, it is estimated that it would take 10 to 20 years to deplete body stores. Therefore, it is uncommon for normal elderly persons to become vitamin B_{12} deficient.

Pernicious anemia occurs at increased prevalence with advanced years. It is an autoimmune systemic disorder characterized by megaloblastic hematopoiesis and neuropathy. Pathologically, gastric parietal cell atrophy occurs and intrinsic factor is no longer secreted. Rarely, vitamin B_{12} deficiency occurs because of diseases of the terminal ileum, but this can be distinguished by a Schilling test.

Treatment for vitamin B_{12} deficiency consists of weekly or biweekly injections of 100 μg intramuscularly until stores are replenished, after which lifelong monthly injections are required. Within hours of vitamin B_{12} therapy, the bone marrow becomes normoblastic, and reticulocytosis is seen within a week. The anemia usually corrects within a month, and macrocytosis within a few months.

Folic acid deficiency is second only to iron deficiency as the cause of nutritional anemias worldwide. Folic acid is found predominantly in fresh green vegetables, nuts, yeast, and liver. Alcoholics are particularly vulnerable because of impaired absorption and dietary indiscretions. Folic acid requirements are increased during periods of hemolysis or excessive loss, and metabolism may be impaired by certain medications, such as methotrexate and Dilantin. The diagnosis is made by measuring serum or red cell folic acid levels. Treatment with oral folate supplements, 1 mg/day, is uniformly effective.

The *thalassemias and sideroblastic anemias* are disorders of hemoglobin synthesis associated with ineffective erythropoiesis resulting in production of small red blood cells. These disorders are the most common causes of microcytosis not caused by iron-deficiency anemia. Although usually idiopathic, they may occur secondary to excess alcohol intake, certain medications (antituberculous drugs, phenacetin), or chronic diseases (multiple myeloma, cancer, and rheumatoid arthritis). The definitive diagnosis is made by demonstrating iron granules in the bone marrow. The peripheral smear may be dimorphic, with small red blood cells and cells of normal or increased size, often containing iron granules seen as basophilic stippling.

Some sideroblastic anemias respond to a trial of oral pyridoxine (200 mg three times per day). Because this type of anemia is an "iron-loading anemia" and can lead to hemochromatosis, transfusion should be avoided if possible. Sideroblastic anemias also are associated with certain neoplastic conditions, including gastrointestinal tumors, renal cell carcinoma, and lymphoma, or may represent a preleukemic state.

Finally, *anemias from protein undernutrition* are described with increased frequency in the elderly. These anemias are usually normocytic, and serum iron and ferritin levels are usually normal. Low concentrations of serum transferrin are found (Lipschitz and Mitchell, 1982). This may represent a response to a reduced metabolic rate or reduced oxygen consumption, and the anemia usually responds with correction of the nutritional deficiency.

Non–Insulin-Dependent Diabetes Mellitus

Approximately 12 to 15 million persons in the United States have diabetes mellitus; 40 per cent are over the age of 65. The prevalence of diabetes in individuals over the age of 65 is estimated to be 10 per cent, and in those over 85 it is approximately 25 per cent (Kovar et al., 1987). Diabetes ranks as the seventh leading cause of death; complications of the disease resulting in mortality increase with age. Approximately 10 per cent of diabetics develop end-stage renal disease, accounting for 25 per cent of all new dialysis patients (American Diabetes Association, 1986).

With normal aging, there is a slight increase of fasting blood sugar believed to be due to changes in body composition, diet, physical activity, and insulin sensitivity (Helmrich et al., 1991). It is postulated that changes in insulin receptor sensitivity occur at the postreceptor level, leading to a reduced insulin-mediated uptake of glucose in peripheral tissues. These factors are exaggerated in some patients, resulting in type II, or non–insulin-dependent, diabetes mellitus. At-risk groups include those with a family history of diabetes, obesity, and a history of gestational diabetes.

The diagnosis of diabetes mellitus is made when a fasting blood sugar level of over 140 mg/dL is found on two separate occasions, when postprandial or random levels of over 200 mg/dL are found, or with elevated glycosylated hemoglobin levels. Elderly patients infrequently present with symptoms of polyuria, polydypsia, and glycosuria, which may not appear until the serum blood glucose levels are extremely elevated as the result of an age- and disease-associated increase in the renal threshold for glucose. For the same reason, urine monitoring for glucose control and urine screening for diabetes are ineffective.

The degree of blood glucose control that should be achieved is somewhat controversial. Recent studies of aggressive insulin replacement therapy to control blood glucose levels strictly in young insulin-dependent diabetics showed promising results (Keller et al., 1993) by reducing the risk for end-organ complications such as retinopathy, nephropathy, and neuropathy. Elderly patients have greatly accelerated microvascular disease and suffer significant morbidity from neurovascular disease (Naliboff and Rosenthal, 1989). As yet, it is unclear if tight "glycemic" control in elderly patients with non–insulin-dependent diabetes mellitus can delay or prevent the onset of complications. Depending on the patient's age and prognosis, the risks of hypoglycemia may not warrant the potential long-term benefits. Once diabetic nephropathy has progressed to the stage of hypertension, proteinuria, or renal insufficiency, glycemic control does not influence the course (Feldt-Rasmussen et al., 1986).

Biannual eye examinations by an ophthalmologist may help detect cataracts and diabetic retinopathy in earlier stages. Diabetic nephropathy usually is heralded by macroalbuminuria, proteinuria, and glycosuria, which should prompt more aggressive control. Diabetics should be instructed in appropriate care of their feet because ischemia with gangrene secondary to occlusive microvascular disease and atherosclerosis of large and medium-size arteries is 20 times more common in these individuals than in matched controls. Peripheral neuropathy further may place a person at increased risk of ischemic foot ulcers, infections, gangrene, and trauma. Diabetic autonomic neuropathy manifests by postural hypotension, resting tachycardia, diarrhea, constipation, an inability to empty the bladder, and impotence. Diarrhea secondary to autonomic diabetic neuropathy may respond to broad-spectrum antibiotics or to clonidine, gastric atony may be treated with metoclopramide, and bethanecol occasionally improves bladder emptying. Pain associated with diabetic neuropathy may be treated with amitriptyline in doses of 50 to 75 mg at nighttime. Compression stockings may be helpful in patients with orthostatic hypotension.

A reasonable goal for elderly diabetics is to keep random serum blood sugar levels below 200 mg/dL and fasting levels below 150 mg/dL. Initially, treatment should consist of dietary modification, instructing older patients to lose weight and to maximize their caloric intake from complex carbohydrates, which are also high in fiber. Prescribed exercise has been shown to improve glucose utilization and insulin sensitivity (Goldberg and Coon, 1987). Walking for 20 to 30 minutes three times a week may improve glucose tolerance significantly. Blood glucose control can be monitored by home fingerstick glucose measurements or by regular glycosylated hemoglobin measurements. If diet and exercise fail, then oral hypoglycemic agents should be prescribed. Second-generation agents such as glyburide and glipizide are more effective in the elderly, but more expensive. Persistent elevation of blood glucose levels over 300 mg/dL is indication for insulin treatment.

Obesity

It is estimated that one in five adults in the United States is obese, defined as 20 per cent or more above ideal body weight. Strong positive associations between relative weight and heart disease have been demonstrated in longitudinal prospective studies by the American Cancer Society and the Framingham Heart Study, with a doubling of risk among the obese as compared to subjects at desirable weights (National Institutes of Health Consensus Development Conference, 1985). It is also suggested that the distribution of fat is important in assessing the risk for myocardial infarction. Those with fat deposition primarily in the abdomen are at much higher risk than those with deposition in the hips and thighs (Manson et al., 1990). An association has been established between obesity and hypercholesterolemia, diabetes, hypertension, and certain cancers (colon, rectum, prostate, gallbladder, breast, cervix, endometrium, ovary) (National Institutes of Health Consensus Development Conference, 1985).

Total body fat and the proportion of the body's fat composition approximately doubles between the ages of 25 and 75. Some of the decrease in lean body mass can be prevented or reversed by regular exercise programs. The effectiveness of weight reduction is uncertain because, in most studies, subjects have been unable to sustain weight loss (Stunkard, 1987). The estimated reduction in risk for myocardial infarction associated with maintaining an ideal body weight is approximately 40 to 50 per cent. Treatment programs must be multifaceted, including instruction and monitoring of diet and activity, with ongoing psychological support.

Failure to Thrive

Failure to thrive is defined as unintentional weight loss with metabolic abnormalities that may include anemia, lymphocytopenia, hypoalbuminemia, hypocholesterolemia, and glucose intolerance (Berkman et al., 1989). Unexplained weight loss and failure to thrive may progress to such an extent that irreversible loss of muscle mass, physi-

cal weakness, and impaired immunity result in an inevitable decline toward death (Isaacs et al., 1971).

The causes of weight loss remain unexplained in the elderly. The spectrum ranges from medical conditions, such as cancer, endocrine disorders, chronic infections, or inflammation, to psychological disorders, which may manifest first as anorexia with weight loss. The latter often are overlooked, and clinicians should consider the diagnosis of depression and dementia if an older person progressively loses weight. Because of the high incidence of multiple sensory deficits and functional decline, lack of access to food or an inability to prepare or cook food also may result in significant weight loss. Osteoarthritis, rheumatoid arthritis, deafness, blindness, and Parkinson's disease may limit an older person's ability to open containers and cook food. It is estimated that it takes approximately 45 minutes for a caregiver or nursing assistant to feed a person who is unable to manipulate feeding utensils. Conflicting caregiver demands, caregiver burden, or staffing shortages may limit the availability or desire of someone to assist with meals. An important but overlooked reason why older persons fail to thrive is the neglect and isolation that often accompany poverty.

The assessment of unexplained weight loss in an older person requires a careful evaluation of the patient's medical condition, psychological state, and social circumstances. The extent and severity of the condition can be measured by the degree of documented weight loss and laboratory tests for anemia, hypoalbuminemia, hypocholesterolemia, lymphocytopenia, and thyroid hormone levels. An accurate dietary history should be obtained and medications reviewed, because certain medications, such as major tranquilizers, digitalis, and iron preparations, may alter taste and reduce appetite. Treatment should be directed at any reversible causes. Goals should be set for weight gain and nutritional parameters monitored during supervised feedings. There is evidence that megestrol acetate may be effective in increasing weight in certain patients with cancer and acquired immunodeficiency syndrome. The outcome of use of this agent or any other appetite stimulants in the elderly is unknown (Silverstone and Goodall, 1986). Decisions about enteral tube feeding are difficult, especially if patients are unable to participate in the decision-making process or have not documented their preferences previously.

Osteoporosis

Osteoporosis is a metabolic bone disorder characterized by a reduction in density of normally mineralized bone, in the absence of other recognizable causes of bone loss, resulting in an increased susceptibility to fracture (Consensus Development Conference, 1991). While most bone loss occurs in the immediate postmenopausal period, the impact of osteoporosis occurs much later. Approximately 1.5 million osteoporosis-related fractures occur annually, with 70 per cent of all fractures in people over the age of 50 attributable to this disorder. Almost one third of women over the age of 60 will sustain a spinal compression fracture, and nearly 20 per cent of women will suffer a fractured hip. The cost of osteoporosis-related fractures is estimated to be $7 billion/year. The mortality from hip fractures at 1 year is approximately 20 per cent, and 50 per cent of people who fracture their hip require assistance in functional activities 1 year after the fracture (Melton et al., 1989).

Accelerated losses of calcium of from 0.5 to 1 per cent of bone mass per year occur immediately postmenopausally, primarily as a result of postmenopausal estrogen deficiency. Older persons also develop a relative malabsorption of calcium because of reduced gastrointestinal responsiveness to 1,25-dihydroxy–vitamin D_3 (Amaud, 1990). Increased serum levels of parathyroid hormone and reduced exercise in elderly women are also contributing factors. The most rapid rate of bone loss occurs from trabecular bone, with later losses from cortical bone. Trabecular bone is found mainly in the vertebral bodies, with loss leading to osteoporotic fractures of the vertebrae. Cortical bone loss occurs at a slower rate, so hip and other long bone fractures occur much later.

Although primarily age related, osteoporosis may occur secondary to other conditions, including endocrine disorders (diabetes, thyroid disease, hyperparathyroidism), malignant conditions (multiple myeloma), and immobility following a stroke or other neurologic injury (Lukert and Raisz, 1990). Medications such as corticosteroids and alcohol can cause a secondary loss in bone density.

Prior to a fracture, osteoporosis is mostly asymptomatic. The initial presentation of osteoporosis may be backache as a result of spontaneous fracture or collapse of vertebral bodies, or when a fracture of a long bone occurs. Serum calcium phosphorus and alkaline phosphatase levels are normal; however, urinary hydroxyproline levels may be elevated. Imaging studies such as dual x-ray absorptiometry may be useful in making the diagnosis and may help physicians with decisions about perimenopausal estrogen replacement (Consensus Development Conference, 1993; "DATTA," 1992). In the future, biochemical markers of bone turnover may become available to help clinicians more accurately screen for osteoporosis and make rational decisions about therapy.

The treatment for established osteoporosis is experimental, and no treatment restores bone strength once it has been lost. Calcitonin has been approved by the Food and Drug Administration for the treatment of established osteoporosis; however, while treatment with calcitonin increases vertebral bone density, it has not been shown to reduce the incidence of bone fractures (Christiansen, 1991). Cyclical intermittent sodium etidronate, 400 mg/day for 14 days followed by 76 drug-free days, reportedly has increased vertebral bone density by 5 to 6 per cent and reduced vertebral fractures in a placebo-controlled clinical trial, and with few adverse effects (Watts et al., 1990). There is evidence that estrogen replacement therapy, when instituted in the immediate perimenopausal period, significantly reduces the rate of bone loss and the rate of osteoporotic fractures. Furthermore, prospective clinical trials have shown that estrogen replacement therapy significantly reduces mortality from coronary artery disease (Stampfer et al., 1991), as well as the incidence of flushing and vaginal atrophy. All women should be encouraged to increase their intake of calcium to about 1500 mg/day to prevent loss of skeletal bone (Christiansen, 1991), and most authorities would recommend a daily intake of vitamin D of 600 to 800 IU because requirements are increased in the postmenopausal period. Estrogen replacement therapy is associated with a three- to fivefold increased risk of endometrial cancer, although the disease is uncommon in elderly women. The increased risk of endometrial cancer may be avoided by adding a progesterone for 10 days of each cycle (Barrett-Conner and Bush, 1991). Recent evidence suggests that a combination of estrogen and a low dose progestational agent taken continuously (every day) has a favorable impact on lipoprotein profiles, and early reports suggest significant reductions in the incidence of myocardial infarction. A frequently used combination is 0.625 mg conjugated estrogen and 2.5 to 5.0 mg of medroxyprogesterone acetate (Wolfe and Huff, 1989). There is no consensus as to the point at which hormonal therapy can be terminated electively. A decision to use estrogen replacement therapy should be based on the relative risk of osteoporosis and the desires and preferences of the individual patient.

Sexuality

A recent national survey reported that over 50 per cent of adults over the age of 60 years, and 24 per cent of those over the age of 75, reported having sexual relations at least once within the preceding month. Approximately 75 per cent of married men and 60 per cent of married women report that they are sexually active (Toradello and Boscia, 1985). Although sexual activity decreases with age, there is usually no physiologic reason for this. It frequently simply represents lack of a partner, or a partner's poor health.

Female Sexuality

Older women may report decreased libido, infrequent orgasm, dyspareunia, and vaginal dryness primarily as a result of estrogen deficiency (Osborn et al., 1988). Most problems that affect sexuality are due to reduced secretions and decreased lubrication, absence of a partner, dissatisfaction with marriage, coexisting depression, poor health of the partner, and chronic illnesses. Certain medications (antihypertensives, Dilantin, phenothiazines, tegretol, and others) have been associated with diminished vaginal lubrication and loss of libido. It is postulated that thyroid disease and urinary incontinence may have adverse sexual effects (Greendale, 1993-1994). Cerebrovascular accidents have been associated with decreases in sexual satisfaction in elderly women. Treatment of sexual dysfunction in elderly women must be directed at the underlying cause. Estrogen replacement therapy can be helpful in some patients. Physicians may need to refer their patients to therapists who specialize in treating sexual disorders.

Male Sexuality

Alterations occur in normal sexual responses in elderly men. Erections take longer to achieve, pre-ejaculatory secretions often are decreased, the plateau phase may be prolonged, orgasm is often abbreviated with a decrease in ejaculatory force, and there is a prolonged refractory period (Morley et al., 1990). However, other factors, such as partner availability and health and the patient's own health, also may affect sexual function.

Multiple factors may contribute to erectile dysfunction, with vascular disorders being the most common. Atherosclerosis, diabetes, hypertension, and hyperlipidemia may interfere critically with penile blood flow. Central nervous disorders (e.g., stroke, multiple sclerosis, spinal cord disease), peripheral neuropathies, and autonomic neuropathies may interfere with sympathetic nervous activity and result in impotence. A number of medications have been implicated in causing erectile dysfunction (Table 7–11).

Occasionally, elderly patients may complain of absence of ejaculation, which may be caused by retrograde ejaculation into the bladder. This most frequently occurs after surgery on the bladder neck for prostate disease or secondary to diabetes mellitus. Certain medications also are associated with failure to emit semen; these include serotonin uptake inhibitors and monoamine oxidase inhibitors. Hypogonadism occurs more often with advancing years. Most hypogonadol males have normal luteinizing hormone levels, indicating hypogonadotrophic hypogonadism (Korenman et al., 1990). Other endocrine disorders, such as hypo- and hyperthyroidism, also have been associated with absence of ejaculation.

EVALUATION AND TREATMENT. The history and examination should focus on identifying physical and psychological conditions likely to cause erectile dysfunction. A genital examination should include an inspection of the penis, testes, and pros-

TABLE 7–11. DRUGS THAT HAVE BEEN ASSOCIATED WITH IMPOTENCE (BY CLASSIFICATION)

Diuretics

Antihypertensive drugs

Miscellaneous cardiovascular drugs (eg, clofibrate, gemfibrozil, digoxin)

Anxiolytics (eg, phenothiazines, butyrophenones)

Antidepressants

H_2-receptor antagonists

Hormonal agents (eg, estrogens, progestogens, corticosteroids, gonadotrophin-releasing hormone [GnRH] agonists and antagonists)

Cytotoxic agents

Anticonvulsant agents

Miscellaneous drugs (eg, metoclopramide, baclofen, carbonic anhydrase inhibitors, nonsteroidal anti-inflammatory drugs, tobacco, alcohol, opiates)

SOURCE: Modified from Morley JE, Kaiser FE. Impotence in elderly men. *Drugs & Aging.* 1992;2(4):332. Reprinted with permission.

From Kaiser FE: Sexuality. *In* Reuben DB, Yoshikawa TT, Besdine RW (eds): Geriatrics Review Syllabus Supplement: A Core Curriculum in Geriatric Medicine. American Geriatrics Society 1993-1994 Program. New York, American Geriatrics Society, 1993-1994, p 155S, with permission.

tate. Signs and symptoms of hypogonadism, including gynecomastia and loss of pubic hair, should be sought. A peripheral vascular and neurologic examination also should be done. Nocturnal penile tumescence studies may be helpful in distinguishing psychogenic from organic erectile dysfunction. Screening laboratory tests for diabetes, thyroid disorders, and hypogonadism (testosterone, luteinizing hormone levels, and prolactin levels) should be ordered.

The treatment depends on the underlying cause. Antihypertensive medication regimens or other drug regimens may have to be modified. Counseling or referral to a sex therapist is indicated if a psychological reason for erectile dysfunction is found. For patients with hypogonadism, testosterone may be useful. Patients with peripheral vascular disease may respond to a trial of pentoxifylline. If these measures fail, then a referral to a urologist is indicated for consideration of treatment with either a vacuum tumescence device or injections of papaverine with phentolamine or alprostadil (Sue and Tanagho, 1987). A penile prosthesis may be considered in men who do not respond to these measures. Inflatable penile prostheses with implanted reservoirs also may achieve the desired results.

Genitourinary Disorders

Urinary Incontinence

Urinary incontinence affects approximately one third of women over the age of 60 years. The prevalence is twice as high in women as in men. The medical, psychological, and economic burden of this disorder is great (Urinary Incontinence in Adults Guideline Panel, 1992). Incontinence is not a normal consequence of aging; however, changes in the lower genitourinary tract predispose patients to developing incontinence. These include a decrease in bladder capacity, an inability to postpone voiding, more frequent uninhibited bladder contractions, and increased postvoid residual volumes. Urinary incontinence often results when a superimposed pathologic, physiologic, or pharmacologic insult occurs. Common causes of transient urinary incontinence include an acute medical illness (delirium, congestive heart failure, depression [Resnick and Yalla, 1985]), restricted mobility and access to bathroom facilities, medications (sedatives, hypnotics, alcohol, diuretics, anticholinergics, psychotropics, and α-adrenergic blockers), atrophic vaginitis and urethritis, and stool impaction.

Causes of established incontinence can be divided into two underlying processes: (1) disorders of storage of urine secondary to bladder muscle (detrusor) overactivity or outflow tract incompetence; and (2) disorders of bladder emptying because of detrusor muscle underactivity or outlet obstruction. Detrusor overactivity accounts for approximately two thirds of all cases. Local pathologies (cystitis, a bladder tumor, or a kidney stone) may cause irritation of the bladder and uninhibited detrusor contractions. Alzheimer's disease, cerebrovascular events, and other central nervous pathologies also may cause detrusor muscle overactivity by failing to inhibit bladder contractions. Patients with detrusor overactivity have frequent urges to urinate both during the day and at night. Occasionally, patients with detrusor muscle overactivity also have an impaired bladder contractility (Resnick and Yalla, 1987). In these instances, patients pass small amounts of urine and have postvoid residual volumes in excess of 100 mL. Sphincter incompetence is the second most important cause of urinary incontinence in older women and most commonly occurs secondary to pelvic floor muscle laxity (Blaivus and Olsson, 1988). When abdominal pressure increases, pelvic supports are insufficient to preserve continence. Cystoceles and urethroceles may be found on clinical examination. Patients typically leak urine during the day, often with coughing, straining, or even standing.

Detrusor underactivity is an infrequent cause of urinary incontinence in the elderly, and usually results from damage to the nerve supply to the bladder secondary to diabetic autonomic neuropathy and, more rarely, in patients with tertiary syphilis, pernicious anemia, or autonomic neuropathy secondary to Parkinson's disease. An early spinal cord lesion also can cause this type of incontinence. Large postvoid residual volumes are found, and symptoms of leakage of small amounts of urine

occur frequently during the day or night. Outlet obstruction is a common cause of urinary incontinence in older men, and frequently results from benign prostatic hyperplasia, prostate cancer, or urethral strictures. Anatomic abnormalities other than urethral strictures are rare in elderly women.

The evaluation requires a voiding history, which should quantify continent and incontinent periods during the day and at night. The physical examination should focus on a lower genitourinary system and include a rectal examination. In women, a pelvic examination should be done looking for atrophic vaginitis and pelvic muscle laxity. A neurologic examination always is indicated. A postvoid residual volume measurement should be obtained in all patients; volumes of over 200 mL are abnormal. Laboratory studies should include a urinalysis and a measure of serum electrolytes. If the cause of a patient's incontinence cannot be determined after the clinical evaluation, urodynamic evaluation is the next step (Ouslander et al., 1988). This frequently includes cystometry, urethral profilometry, uroflometry, and occasionally electromyography.

The treatment for established urinary incontinence must be individualized (Table 7–12). For patients with detrusor overactivity, bladder retraining is frequently helpful (Hadley, 1986). Patients are toileted at regular intervals and the frequency of toileting is increased based on when incontinent episodes occur. Drugs may be helpful; however, in general, they do not abolish uninhibited contractions. Calcium channel blockers, smooth muscle relaxers, and anticholinergic agents may be helpful. For refractory cases, pads or special absorbent undergarments may be indicated.

Stress incontinence in older women may be treated successfully with pelvic muscle exercises and/or biofeedback. If these measures fail, then a trial of α-adrenergic agonists may be beneficial. As a final resort, surgery may be indicated. Outflow tract obstruction frequently requires either urethral dilation or prostatic surgery in men. Some recent studies have shown that α-adrenergic antagonists reduce incontinence episodes and improve urinary flow rates. In cases of detrusor underactivity, the goal of therapy is to reduce residual volume and prevent urosepsis. Patients should be instructed in techniques of double voiding, and medications such as bethanecol, alone or in combination with an α-blocker, may help decrease postvoid residuals. Ultimately, intermittent catheterization or an indwelling bladder catheter may be necessary.

Prostate Disease

Benign prostatic hypertrophy is a disease of the elderly, with 90 per cent of men having significant benign prostatic hypertrophy by the age of 80. Symptoms of hesitancy, straining, decreased caliber of the urine stream, dribbling, and a sensation

TABLE 7–12.   TREATMENT OF ESTABLISHED URINARY INCONTINENCE*

Condition	Clinical Type of Incontinence	Treatment†‡
Detrusor overactivity with normal contractility	Urge	1. Bladder retraining or prompted voiding regimens 2. ± Bladder relaxant medication (anticholinergic, smooth-muscle relaxant, calcium channel blocker), if needed and not contraindicated 3. Indwelling catheterization alone is often unhelpful because detrusor spasms often increase, leading to leakage around the catheter 4. In selected cases, induce urinary retention pharmacologically and add intermittent or indwelling catheterization
Detrusor hyperactivity with impaired contractility	Urge§	1. If bladder empties adequately with straining, use behavioral methods (as above) ± low doses of bladder relaxant medication (especially feasible in presence of coexisting sphincter incompetence) 2. If residual urine is high (eg, >150 mL), use augmented voiding techniques‖ or intermittent catheterization (± bladder relaxant medication). If neither is feasible, undergarment or indwelling catheter may be used. UTI prophylaxis can be used for recurrent symptomatic UTIs if catheter is not indwelling
Stress incontinence	Stress	1. Conservative methods (weight loss if the patient is obese; treatment of cough or atrophic vaginitis; rarely, use of pessary/tampon) 2. Pelvic muscle exercises ± biofeedback/weighted intravaginal cones (a set of identically sized but progressively heavier weights) 3. Imipramine (or doxepin) or α-adrenegic agonists, if they are not contraindicated 4. Surgery
Urethral obstruction	Urge¶/Overflow	1. Conservative methods (including adjustment of fluid intake, bladder retraining/prompted voiding ± bladder relaxants) if hydronephrosis, elevated residual urine, recurrent symptomatic UTI, and gross hematuria have been excluded 2. Bladder suppressants if there is coexisting DO, PVR volume is small, and surgery is not desired or feasible 3. In men, α-adrenergic antagonists, antiandrogens, or LHRH analogues if they are not contraindicated and the patient either prefers them or is not a candidate for surgery 4. Surgery
Underactive detrusor	Overflow	1. If duration is unknown, decompress for several weeks and perform a voiding trial 2. If this fails, or retention is chronic, try augmented voiding techniques ± α-adrenergic antagonists, if any voiding is possible; bethanechol is rarely useful 3. If this fails, use intermittent or indwelling catheterization

* DHIC, detrusor hyperactivity with impaired contractility; UTI, urinary tract infection; DO, detrusor overactivity with normal contractility; PVR, postvoiding residual; LHRH, luteinizing hormone-releasing hormone.
† In all patients, adequate toilet access should be ensured, contributing conditions (eg, atrophic vaginitis, heart failure) treated, fluid management optimized, and unnecessary medications stopped.
‡ ± = with or without.
§ But DHIC may also mimic stress or overflow incontinence.
‖ These techniques include Credé's method, Valsalva's maneuver, and double voiding.
¶ This condition can also cause postvoid dribbling alone, which is treated conservatively (eg, by sitting to void and allowing more time, by double voiding, and by gently milking the penile urethra after voiding).
From Resnick NM: Incontinence. *In* Reuben DB, Yoshikawa TT, Besdine RW (eds): A Core Curriculum in Geriatric Medicine. American Geriatrics Society 1991–1992 Program. New York, American Geriatrics Society, 1991–1992, p 151, with permission.

of incomplete bladder emptying start to occur in the fifth to sixth decade. Nocturia, frequency, and urge incontinence are common symptoms. Infection may occur as a result of stasis and urinary retention (O'Brien, 1991). Rectal examination does not identify prostatic hypertrophy reliably because obstruction often is confined to the periurethral prostate. Ultrasound, cystourethroscopy, and urodynamic flow rate studies may be useful adjunctive tests. When obstructive symptoms exist, surgery is the treatment of choice. More recently, medical therapy for benign prostatic disease has been advocated, and some success has been reported with use of α-adrenergic blocking agents such as prozasin (Lepor, 1990). Antiadrenergic agents (flutamide) can reduce prostate size; however, use of these

agents results in impotence. Finasteride, which is an enzyme that inhibits conversion of testosterone to the active form, recently has been shown to be effective in improving urinary flow rates, with benefits seen after a year of therapy (McConnell, 1990).

Prostate Cancer

Cancer of the prostate is rare before the age of 60 and is the most common cancer among men over the age of 65, with both rising incidences and mortality. Autopsy data show a 70 per cent incidence of prostate cancer in men over the age of 80 (Carter et al., 1990). Survival with prostate cancer is related to the stage of the disease. Stage A prostate disease usually is unsuspected on a digital rectal examination but is discovered at the time of prostatectomy or biopsy. Stage B disease is characterized by the presence of a prostate nodule but may involve more than one lobe. Stage C disease involves local extension outside of the capsule or to the seminal vesicles. Stage D represents distant metastases.

The diagnosis of prostate cancer frequently is made only when patients have advanced (stage C or D) disease. More than 50 per cent of nodules found on rectal exam prove to be cancerous. Routine ultrasound of the prostate is not indicated for screening because of its cost and low specificity. Prostatic acid phosphatase lacks enough specificity for the disease to make it a useful screening test. Prostate-specific antigen (PSA) levels are elevated moderately in patients with prostatic cancer, benign prostatic hypertrophy, and prostatitis, which may confound diagnosis in early cancer. The rate of increase in PSA from year to year may be a sensitive and specific marker for early prostate cancer (Carter et al., 1992).

The treatment for late stage A disease or stage B prostate cancer is either surgery or radiation therapy, each of which yields comparable results (Moon, 1992). Radiation treatment currently is recommended for stage C cancers. Surgery and hormonal therapy are experimental treatment modalities for stage C cancer. For symptomatic metastatic prostate cancer, antiandrogen interventions, which may include castration, medications, or a combined approach, are the mainstays of treatment. Although hormonal treatment for late-stage disease may do little to alter disease, a marked improvement in bone pain and quality of life is noted in many patients. For pain unresponsive to hormonal treatment, external radiation, sodium etidronate, or steroids may be effective.

Mental Status Changes

Changes in mental status in the elderly usually are manifested in three ways, frequently in combination: delirium, depression, and dementia. Delirium is often the first indicator of an underlying dementia, and dementia is the leading risk factor for the onset of delirium. Depression often accompanies dementia and, when severe, may make dementia appear to be worse.

Delirium

Delirium is a transient organic mental syndrome of acute onset, characterized by global impairment of cognitive functions, a reduced level of consciousness, attentional abnormalities, increased or decreased psychomotor activity, and a disordered sleep–wake cycle (Lipowski, 1990) (Table 7–13). Symptoms usually develop over hours to days, fluctuate over the course of the day, and often be-

TABLE 7–13. A PRACTICAL SUMMARY OF THE DIAGNOSTIC CRITERIA FOR DELIRIUM (AFTER DSM-III R*)

Reduced ability to maintain and shift attention to external stimuli

Disorganized thinking: rambling, irrelevant, or incoherent speech

At least two of the following:
1. Reduced level of consciousness
2. Perceptual disturbances: misinterpretations, illusions, or hallucinations
3. Disturbances of sleep-wakefulness: insomnia or daytime sleeping
4. Increased or decreased psychomotor activity
5. Disorientation to person, place, or time
6. Memory impairment

Abrupt onset of symptoms (hours or days), with daily fluctuation
1. Evidence from history, physical examination, or laboratory tests of specific organic etiological factors
2. Exclusion of nonorganic mental disorders when no etiologic organic factor can be identified

*Diagnostic and Statistical Manual of Mental Disorders. 3rd edition (revised). Washington, D.C.: American Psychiatric Association, 1987: 103, with permission.

come worse at night. Nocturnal restlessness may be a prodrome to full-blown symptoms associated with serious, impending pathology. Delirium may be a sign of a potentially life-threatening condition and should be treated as a medical emergency.

Delirium most often is found in elderly patients admitted to the hospital but often is overlooked or misdiagnosed as depression or dementia, and can have significant consequences. The incidence is estimated to range from 25 to 60 per cent. Patients who develop delirium while hospitalized have an increased morbidity and mortality, require closer nursing surveillance, have longer hospitalizations, and have a higher rate of nursing home placement on discharge (Inouye et al., 1990).

The causes of delirium in the elderly are most commonly infections, metabolic disturbances, and toxic reactions to medications; less common etiologies include cerebrovascular accidents, mass lesions in the brain, seizures, and vitamin deficiency states (Francis, 1992). Infectious causes of delirium include urinary tract infections, pneumonia, bacteremias, and less often meningitis. Symptoms are mediated through several common pathways. The cholinergic neurotransmitter system may be affected by a variety of medications, including antidepressants, antihypertensives, antiarrhythmics, major tranquilizers, and preoperative anticholinergic medications. Hypoxia and hypoglycemia also may decrease acetylcholine synthesis significantly. Mediators of the inflammatory state, such as interleukins and lymphokines, can provoke the electroencephalographic (EEG) changes associated with delirium and produce similar clinical symptoms. Endorphins also may be implicated, and may account for the delirium associated with the use of narcotic analgesics. Other neurotransmitter systems have been implicated and probably mediate the delirium associated with the use of sedative hypnotics, histamine$_2$ receptor blockers, and antiparkinsonian medications.

The recognition of delirium may be difficult because of its insidious nature and the fact that symptoms may be worse in the evening. Patients at risk include those with an underlying dementia or other neurologic disease, advanced age, and depression, and those admitted with metabolic abnormalities such as azotemia and abnormal sodium levels. Cognitive testing using the Mini-Mental State Examination (see Table 7–2) or clock drawing test on the initial encounter helps to establish a baseline; this is especially important for patients admitted to the hospital or nursing home. Clues to the diagnosis may be obtained from family reports or review of nursing notes for disorientation, inappropriate behavior, and delusions or hallucinations. When delirium is suspected, further history should include questions that pertain to inattention, acute onset and fluctuating course, disorganized thinking, and altered level of consciousness (Inouye et al., 1990).

The physical examination should include a neurologic evaluation for new onset of lateralizing signs and symptoms. Auscultation of the heart and lungs may reveal the presence of pneumonia, arrhythmia, or congestive heart failure. Examination of the abdomen sometimes uncovers evidence of an unsuspected acute abdomen or a distended bladder; rectal examination always should be done to exclude a fecal impaction. Vital signs may be abnormal, and findings of hypotension, fever, or hypothermia should be noted.

Laboratory assessment should begin with simple diagnostic studies (blood count, electrolytes, and urinalysis) to exclude infectious causes and frequently implicated metabolic and fluid and electrolyte disturbances. Blood cultures and a chest radiograph should be ordered if infectious etiologies are suspected. Serum calcium and magnesium levels and assays of serum levels of any potentially etiologic medication should be obtained. Arterial blood gases and lumbar puncture are only rarely helpful in the diagnostic evaluation. Less than 10 per cent of cases of delirium result from acute central nervous system disease, so unless there are neurologic signs and symptoms or a history of trauma, neuroimaging studies are rarely helpful. For patients who present with an insidious onset of confusion over days to weeks, thyroid function tests, vitamin B$_{12}$ and folic acid levels, and heavy metal and drug screens for the presence of unknown medications either accidentally or intentionally ingested may be useful in determining the cause.

The initial management should involve an evaluation and correction of underlying pathophysiol-

ogy. Nonpharmacologic treatment measures are usually sufficient until the underlying condition is controlled. Delirious patients should be placed in quiet surroundings with soft music and lighting, especially in the evenings and at night. Corrective eyeglasses and hearing aids should be made available, if indicated. Physical restraints frequently make delirious patients more agitated, so if at all possible they should not be used. Family members or "sitters" may help to assure and reorient acutely confused patients.

If these measures fail, pharmacologic interventions may be required. Haloperidol in doses of 0.5 mg may be initiated, then doubled at 30-minute intervals until effective. Maintenance dosing at one half the loading dose then should be instituted and tapered as the delirium clears. Other alternatives for the treatment of delirious behaviors include benzodiazepines (e.g., lorazepam, 0.5 to 1 mg intravenously). Narcotics may be useful in controlling agitation in patients with severe pain.

Depression

Depressive symptoms are a major public health problem, affecting nearly one in seven community-residing people 65 years of age and greater. The prevalence of major depression is in the range of 3 per cent in the community, 5 per cent in primary care settings, and up to 15 to 25 per cent nursing homes. Suicide rates are highest among the very old, especially elderly white males. Despite the prevalence, only about one in ten patients with moderately severe to severe depression receives psychiatric treatment. This may be because depression frequently presents in an insidious manner in older persons. Affective changes such as sadness, hopelessness, and a sense of worthlessness often are not as striking in the elderly patient. Ageist beliefs (among patients, physicians, and family) that these symptoms may be "normal" in older persons may contribute to nondiagnosis. Comorbid medical conditions, loss of social integration through separation from the family or the death of friends, financial constraints, loneliness, and diminished vocational opportunities all may be seen as legitimate reasons for the depression. Somatic symptoms may be the primary manifestation of depression. Constipation, musculoskeletal aches and pains, sleeplessness, diminished appetite, weight loss, and anergia often are attributed to age and illness. Finally, somatic symptoms may offer a mechanism for avoiding the stigma of psychiatric disease and masking the underlying depression.

The diagnosis of depression can be made by recognizing the psychiatric and somatic constellation of symptoms and signs (Table 7–14). Screening instruments such as the Geriatric Depression Scale (see Table 7–3) have been validated among older persons. Elderly persons who present for medical evaluation should be asked about symptoms of

TABLE 7–14. A PRACTICAL SUMMARY OF THE DIAGNOSTIC CRITERIA FOR DEPRESSION (AFTER DSM-III R*)

A two-week period of changed mood (sadness, loss of interest or pleasure) not due to physical illness, confusion, or delusions-hallucinations, with at least five of the following:
1. Depressed mood predominantly most of the time
2. Markedly diminished interest or pleasure
3. Significant changes in appetite or weight.
4. Insomnia or hypersomnia.
5. Agitated or retarded activity
6. Fatigue or energy loss.
7. Worthlessness or inappropriate guilt
8. Inability to think, concentrate, or decide
9. Recurrent thoughts of death or suicide

No organic factor is known to have caused or sustains the disturbance, nor is the disturbance a normal bereavement on the death of a loved one.
No delusions or hallucinations have been present for two weeks without accompanying mood symptoms.
Not superimposed on schizophrenia, schizophreniform disorder, or other psychotic disorder

*Diagnostic and Statistical Manual of Mental Disorders. 3rd edition (revised). Washington, D.C.: American Psychiatric Association, 1987: 222, with permission.

depression and be evaluated using a validated geriatric depression scale. Other diagnostic tests, such as the dexamethasone suppression test and urinary metabolites of norepinephrine, are not as accurate because of the frequent presence of concurrent illnesses and other physiologic changes.

The treatment of major depression in the elderly should include consideration of both counseling and pharmacologic interventions. Treatment plans must be individualized and monitored carefully.

A trial of Ritalin, 10 mg daily for 5 to 10 days, may be useful in hospitalized patients, because responders are more likely to benefit from tricyclic antidepressants (TCAs). Nortriptyline is a good choice for the treatment of depression because it has few cardiac side effects, rarely causes orthostatic hypotension, and has a well-defined therapeutic window, which helps to ensure appropriate dosing but it still has more anticholinergia than trazdone or the SSRIs. Other TCAs (amitriptyline, imipramine, desipramine) may be equally effective but frequently are associated with cardiac, sedative, and anticholinergic side effects in the elderly. For patients with cardiac conduction disturbances or intolerance of anticholinergic side effects, other drugs may be considered. Serotonergic agents such as trazodone and sertraline are especially useful in older patients with sleep disturbances and have few sides effects. Fluoxetine may be useful in older patients with symptoms of anergia. Unlike TCAs, fluoxetine, if effective, usually will result in symptomatic relief of depression within a week of institution of therapy. Anorexia and agitation are common side effects and may preclude its use in some elderly patients. Monoamine

oxidase inhibitors also are tolerated well in older patients and should be considered if other agents are not effective. Psychiatric consultation should be obtained if it is thought that these agents should be used. For severe depression or refractory cases, electroconvulsive therapy (ECT) is an important option to consider. In well-selected patients, ECT has been shown to have a more rapid rate of therapeutic onset, fewer side effects, and a higher rate of success than pharmacologic treatments. Complaints of retrograde amnesia, although commonly reported, diminish in time.

Maintenance therapy should be continued following resolution of the acute symptoms of a major depression. Between 40 and 60 per cent of patients will respond well to therapy within 2 to 4 weeks of achieving adequate drug levels, and medications should be maintained for at least 6 months before considering decreasing the dose or withdrawing therapy. Many older individuals require maintenance therapies, often at subtherapeutic drug levels, to prevent the return of depressive symptoms. In patients who relapse, treatment may have to be continued indefinitely.

Dementia

The prevalence of dementia in patients 65 to 74 years of age is approximately 1 to 2 per cent; however, this may increase to 20 per cent for those patients over 85, and approaches 50 per cent among centenarians (Katzman, 1986). Dementia is defined as a syndrome with global impairment of higher cognitive function, most predominately memory, abstract thinking, language and arithmetic skills, orientation and visiospatial abilities. This results in deteriorations of occupational and social functioning, and often affects personal hygiene and attention to nutrition and dressing. There may be accompanying personality changes, and changes in mood expressed as either depression or hypomania with disinhibition (Table 7–15). The symptoms are usually insidious in onset and slowly progressive over time. Although dementia may be accompanied by other illnesses, in the majority of cases patients maintain surprisingly good health.

Alzheimer's disease is the leading cause of insidious-onset dementia and accounts for 40 to 90 per cent of cases, depending on population and settings. Multi-infarct dementia accounts for up to 40 per cent of cases, especially among blacks, who have a high prevalence of hypertension and diabetes. Among the other causes are Parkinson's disease and related syndromes; alcohol and other drug abuse; traumatic, metabolic, or neoplastic injury to the brain; normal-pressure hydrocephalus (NPH); hormonal disorders such as hyper- or hypothyroidism; vitamin B_{12} deficiency and other nutritional disorders; infectious processes (including human immunodeficiency virus, [HIV], neuro

TABLE 7–15. A PRACTICAL SUMMARY OF THE DIAGNOSTIC CRITERIA FOR DEMENTIA (AFTER DSM-III R*)

Impaired short- and long-term memory

At least one of the following:
1. Impaired abstract thinking: difficulty defining words and concepts or finding similarities or differences
2. Impaired judgment: inability to plan or to deal with important issues
3. Disturbances of higher cortical functioning: aphasia, agnosia, apraxia.
4. Personality change

Work and social problems related to criteria above

Not present solely during periods of delirium

Either one of the following:
1. Evidence from history, physical examination, or laboratory tests of specific organic etiological factors
2. Exclusion of nonorganic mental disorders when no etiologic organic factor can be identified, e.g., depression as cause of cognitive problems

*Diagnostic and Statistical Manual of Mental Disorders. 3rd edition (revised). Washington, D.C.: American Psychiatric Association, 1987: 107, with permission.

syphilis, and Creutzfeldt-Jakob disease); neurotoxins, such as heavy metals; and paraneoplastic syndromes.

CLINICAL EVALUATION. There is currently no specific test available to diagnose Alzheimer's disease, but the sensitivity and specificity of the clinical evaluation are approximately 85 to 90 per cent (Larson et al., 1992). The diagnostic evaluation of a patient with suspected Alzheimer's disease consists of a detailed history, complete physical examination, and laboratory testing to exclude reversible causes of dementia. Historical features that suggest Alzheimer's disease are a slow, insidious course with indistinct onset and a progression over months to years; the initial symptoms generally are memory loss, impaired judgment, and disturbed social functioning. Occasionally, the onset may appear to be abrupt, precipitated by surgery, transfer to a new setting or hospitalization, or a seemingly trivial incident, such as a traffic violation or death of a pet. A careful history usually will reveal that function previously was maintained by strict adherence to a routine that had been upset, which resulted in a catastrophic reaction to the event.

Other causes of dementia are associated with distinctive historical features. Symptoms suggestive of multi-infarct dementia may include a stair-step decline in function, generally over the course of 12 to 18 months, that may resemble a progressive, waxing and waning course. There is often a history of hypertension, arteriosclerotic cardiovascular disease, or previous stroke. Degenerative neurologic diseases, such as parkinsonism and Huntington's chorea or lacunar infarctions, fre-

quently cause cognitive declines, and are suggested by progressive bradykinesia with tremor or chorea, flattening of affect, depression, and loss of spontaneity in both activities and conversation. This latter syndrome may be referred to as "subcortical" dementia.

The physical examination should exclude delirium and other reversible medical causes. The presence of lateralizing neurologic signs and symptoms is suggestive of multi-infarct dementia, and a confirmatory computerized tomography (CT) or magnetic resonance imaging (MRI) scan may be useful. Primitive reflexes (palmomental, Hoffman, snout, grasp, etc.) may emerge in patients with progressive cerebral degeneration. The Babinski reflex is usually normal but, if asymmetric, suggests the presence of cerebrovascular disease. Gait and balance testing are important and may suggest the diagnosis of NPH or other focal central nervous system pathology. A number of well-validated, reliable screening tests are available to assist in the clinical evaluation of elderly patients with suspected dementia in the primary care setting. Among these screening instruments, the Mini-Mental State Examination is a frequently used, brief, and accurate evaluative tool easily administered in primary care settings (Folstein et al., 1975) (see Table 7–2). The clock drawing test requires the patient to reproduce the face of a clock with a specific time, and standardized criteria are available to grade performance. The Set Test requires the patient to enumerate five items from five categories suggested by the interviewer; for example, cities, flowers, animals, colors, fruit, or articles of clothing. Patients without cognitive impairment usually will recall more than 22 of 25 items depending on the patient's educational level and the complexity of the sets. More formal neuropsychological testing is indicated in patients suspected of having dementia and in patients in whom the diagnosis is suggested by history but not readily apparent on examination or screening tests.

In up to 10 per cent of patients with cognitive impairment, a reversible or treatable cause is found. Thus, all patients should be evaluated by laboratory testing and other studies that may be indicated depending on the presentation. Laboratory tests that may rule out reversible causes of dementia include those listed in Table 7–16. In general, patients should have laboratory tests that include a complete blood count, general blood chemistry screen, thyroid function tests, folic acid levels, rapid plasma reagin test, and urinalysis. Other tests should be ordered if indicated. Although neurosyphilis is a potential cause of dementia, its incidence is increasingly rare, especially in patients with low rapid plasma reagin, serologic test for syphilis, or Venereal Disease Research Laboratory test titers. Neuroimaging with CT or MRI scans is most helpful in patients with lateralizing neurologic signs, or patients with a

TABLE 7–16. LABORATORY TESTS USED TO EVALUATE COGNITIVE IMPAIRMENT*

CBC
ESR
VDRL
Chemistry panel
T_4
B_{12}
Folate
Urinalysis
ECG
Chest x-ray
CT scan (in selected patients)
MRI scan (in selected patients)
EEG (in selected patients)
LP (in selected patients)

*Abnormal results from any of these tests suggest need for more extensive evaluation.

From Ramsdell JW, Rothrock JF, Ward HW, et al: Evaluation of cognitive impairment in the elderly. J Gen Intern Med 5:55, 1990, with permission.

classic history suggestive of NPH, in which early dementia is preceded by a gait disturbance and incontinence. The value of CT scans in unselected patients is questionable, although most experts recommend that patients with cognitive abnormalities have at least one study in the course of their evaluation. EEG testing is most helpful in patients with evidence suggestive of either a delirium or severe depression. Nonconvulsive seizure disorders may provoke a waxing and waning course over weeks or months; patients with a normal EEG should be evaluated more thoroughly for the possibility of depression or other psychiatric disorders. Lumbar puncture rarely adds to the diagnosis unless a delirium is suspected. In elderly patients who received blood transfusions during the early 1980s, HIV screening also should be considered.

The comprehensive evaluation of dementia also should include a systematic assessment of any potentially reversible factors, such as hearing loss or impairments of visual acuity, that may exacerbate the decline in mental functioning. Thyroid disease, depression, chronic renal failure, subacute infections such as chronic urinary tract infections, and compromised cardiac or pulmonary function may cause declines in higher cognitive function in patients with dementia. If identified, confusion or change in mentation in older patients always should be evaluated carefully and followed over time, because these patients are more likely to show evidence of dementia later in their course.

TREATMENT OF BEHAVIORAL ASPECTS OF DEMENTIA. Behavioral problems associated with dementia are very common and distressing for patients and families. Most disturbing are nighttime disruption, nonspecific agitation and restlessness, wandering, hallucinations, and suspiciousness or paranoia. Less common symptoms include physical or verbal aggression, repetitive quests for attention, hiding and hoarding things, sexual disinhibition, and widely fluctuating mood.

Nocturnal disturbances, restlessness, and agitation may respond to decreasing environmental stimulation by providing soft music, low lighting, and the presence of familiar objects in the evening. For those who are consistently up at night, when others are sleeping, it is usually helpful to increase their daytime physical activity and curtail daytime napping. Medications should be used only as a last resort. Low doses of a sedating major tranquilizer, such as thioridazine (10 to 25 mg), may be helpful. For patients unresponsive to major tranquilizers, short-acting benzodiazepines such as lorazepam (0.5 to 2 mg) or oxazepam (10 to 45 mg) may be given at night. Major and minor tranquilizers rarely work in combination, and only one or the other should be used. Alternatively, a sedative antidepressant, such as trazodone, may be helpful in low doses. Diphenhydramine, chloral hydrate, and alcohol cause sedation initially; however, they rapidly lose their effectiveness, and so are not recommended for the older patient. This approach will be successful in 50 to 75 per cent of patients; for the remainder, psychiatric consultation is helpful for counseling the patient and the family, and for assistance in selecting and managing alternative psychotropic agents.

Patients with hallucinations, delusions or illusions, paranoia, or paraphrenia respond best to low doses of major tranquilizers such as haloperidol. Total daily dosing should be no greater than 4 mg, and should be decreased as behavioral control is achieved. All major tranquilizers are of equal efficacy in comparable doses; the selection is based primarily on the agent's side effect profile. Therefore, if the desired primary effect is not achieved with one agent, another class of medication should be tried. For those in whom aggression is the predominant symptom and who have not responded to major tranquilizers, carbamazepine or valproic acid may be considered as second-line agents; for patients capable of tolerating β-blockers, high-dose propranolol also has been shown to be effective (Warshaw, 1990).

Wandering is a common and serious problem and occurs in one third to two thirds of patients with moderate dementia. Medications usually are ineffective and are more likely to provoke falls and injuries than to control the behavior. Simple environmental measures are recommended, such as using childproof doorknobs or installing new locks or placing them in unusual locations, such as at the bottom of the door. Similarly, windows should be secured. As a safeguard for patients who occasionally escape from the home, an identifying bracelet may be obtained through the Alzheimer's Association. Nighttime wandering is prevented best by encouraging sleep, but safety is paramount. It is important to provide nightlights and remove such hazards as electrical cords and loose rugs. Restraints such as Posey vests or seatbelts usually provoke agitation and are not recommended.

Catastrophic reactions and emotional lability may be very disconcerting to the family. Catastrophic reactions are dramatic and violent outbursts of anger, emotional collapse, or even physically striking out when faced with a frustrating task or situation. It may be possible to prevent catastrophic reactions by treating restlessness and agitation. Other methods include providing structured and repetitive activities, and simplifying tasks into discrete slow steps. Emotional lability over seemingly minor events often will respond to therapeutic doses of nortriptyline or sertraline; lithium carbonate also may prove helpful as adjunctive therapy.

As the behavioral problems respond to these pharmacologic measures, doses should be decreased or eliminated. Because of past abuses of psychotropic medications in nursing homes, the Omnibus Budget Reconciliation Act health Standards have mandated that these medications be evaluated frequently and attempts to wean patients be documented as part of the medical care plan in the institutional setting (Health Care Financing Administration. Federal Register, February 2, 1989, p. 5366). Withdrawal should be planned over the course of several weeks to avoid delirium. As a general guideline, doses should be decreased by half at 2 to 4-week intervals until lowered to one quarter to one eighth the original dose, then discontinued. If the aberrant behavior recurs during the course of withdrawal, returning to the previous dosing level usually will suffice.

Sleep Disorders

Epidemiologic studies show that 30 to 50 per cent of older persons complain about difficulty getting to sleep or staying asleep, and about 20 to 50 per cent use hypnotic drugs (National Institutes of Health Consensus Development Conference, 1991). In 1985, more than 20 million prescriptions were written for sedative hypnotic benzodiazepines, a 40 per cent increase from the late 1970s. These medications were prescribed nearly twice as often for patients over the age of 65 as among those between the ages of 40 and 59. Furthermore, sleep-related problems are poorly tolerated by caregivers and are reported as a major reason for institutionalizing care recipients. In institutions, over 90 per cent of patients receive prescription for hypnotic medications in any given year (Dement et al., 1982).

Older persons frequently complain of difficulty falling asleep and often report "light" or fragmented sleep with early morning awakening. These concerns are not without basis. According to sleep studies of normal older adults, there is great individual variation in sleep patterns but, in general, total sleep time is reduced. Sleep onset is slightly delayed, and sleep is generally lighter and disrupted by frequent awakenings. Rapid eye movement sleep usually is preserved until advanced age, but significantly less time is spent in the deeper restorative stages of non–rapid eye movement sleep (Miles and Dement, 1980). As a result, the elderly person often compensates by spending longer periods of time in bed, or by daytime napping.

The elderly have a higher prevalence of chronic medical illnesses, which also may interfere with normal sleep because of shortness of breath, urinary frequency, or other symptoms. Dementia and depression are prevalent among the elderly and can result in changes in normal sleep patterns. Some commonly prescribed medications also may affect sleep architecture. Nightmares have been associated with the use of quinidine, steroids, and some β-blockers. Sleep disruptions also have been reported among patients taking aminophylline, phenytoin, L-dopa, and nasal decongestants (Guillemicault and Silvestri, 1982).

With advancing years, there is a higher incidence of sleep-related respiratory disorders that may cause episodic oxygen desaturations and nocturnal miniarousals (Ancoli-Israel et al., 1985). Nocturnal myoclonus, a condition characterized by stereotypic kicking movements of the legs during sleep, is also more common among the elderly. The elderly are more prone to desynchronization of their circadian rhythm, resulting in advancements or delays in sleep–wake cycles. Multiple sensory loss, social isolation, and institutionalization may exacerbate this problem further.

In evaluating sleep complaints, it may be helpful to have the patient complete a 2-week sleep–wake diary and confirm diary entries with a partner or caregiver. Patients frequently over- or underestimate the duration and quality of their sleep. A referral to a sleep center is indicated if the cause of a persistent sleep disorder is unclear from the history, examination, and review of the sleep diary. Other indications for this type of referral are: (1) suspicion of a significant sleep-related respiratory disorder, (2) confirmation or diagnosis of sleep-related myoclonus, (3) evaluation of possible narcolepsy or cataplexy, and (4) persistent insomnia.

Sleep apnea is potentially the most serious sleep disorder and is associated with significant morbidity and mortality (Bliwise et al., 1988). This condition is defined as a cessation of respiratory air flow lasting 10 seconds or longer, resulting in multiple episodes of hypoxemia, sleep arousals, and excessive somnolence during the day. Central or obstructive sleep apnea may occur separately or coexist. Most apneic episodes are asymptomatic; however, in patients with daytime sleepiness, snoring, insomnia, unexplained right-sided heart failure, arrhythmias, hypertension, or bradycardia, sleep apnea should be considered. These conditions are found more commonly in older obese men, and in patients with hypothyroidism.

TREATMENT. A comprehensive evaluation first must rule out significant cardiopulmonary pathology. It is important to educate older persons that changes in sleep occur "normally" with advancing years; this reassurance may be all that is required. Nearly all patients benefit from improved "sleep hygiene" (Prinz et al., 1990). The bedroom should be made comfortable and noise reduced to a minimum. Caffeine, nicotine, or alcohol consumption should be discouraged before sleep. Daytime activity and exercise should be encouraged, and bedtime limited to 7 to 8 hours per night. For institutionalized elderly patients, a routine for daytime activity scheduling should be established, including regular meals, exercise, and the avoidance of nighttime drug administration.

Older patients are at increased risk for drug tolerance, drug dependence, and drug interactions when sleep medications are prescribed, and there is little evidence to support long-term or repeat prescription of hypnotics. This is especially true for long-acting benzodiazepines such as flurazepam and diazepam, which may worsen sleep apnea syndrome and sleep complaints caused by depression. Regular use is associated with adverse daytime effects such as daytime sleepiness, risk of injurious falls, and impaired psychomotor function mimicking a dementia (Freedman et al., 1984). Low doses of short-acting benzodiazepines may be beneficial in treating transient insomnia that does not respond to modification of sleep habits. The lowest effective dose of a short-acting compound such as temazepam or oxazepam may be used for short-term therapy. Older persons with chronic insomnia may benefit from treatment with low doses of sedating antidepressants such as trazodone or doxepin.

For moderate to severe sleep apnea syndrome, a decision for therapeutic intervention should be made only after an evaluation at a sleep center. This condition responds somewhat to weight loss and positional changes at nighttime. In some cases, nasal continuous positive airway pressure, surgical widening of the upper airway, and use of nonsedating TCAs have been successful in improving sleep architecture.

Parkinsonism

Parkinson's syndrome describes a combination of symptoms resulting from any process that disrupts the basal ganglia, such as idiopathic degenerative disorders, small-vessel cerebrovascular disease, or drug side effects. The classic findings include resting tremor, rigidity on passive motion of the extremities, slowing of voluntary movements, and abnormalities of posture and gait. Parkinson's disease, an idiopathic degeneration of neurons of the substantia nigra, is the most common cause of this syndrome, typically beginning between the ages of 45 and 65. The prevalence of Parkinson's disease in persons over the age of 50 is 1 per cent, and it occurs slightly more commonly in men (Martilla, 1989).

A number of other conditions must be considered in the differential diagnosis, especially if the presentation is atypical. A rapid onset of symptoms, marked asymmetry, or prominent neurologic findings may suggest Wilson's disease, Huntington's disease, Alzheimer's disease, progressive supranuclear palsy, hydrocephalus, NPH, and occasionally subdural hematomas and multiple cerebral infarctions. Rarely, metabolic disorders such as hepatic, pulmonary, or renal insufficiency may produce encephalopathies that may resemble Parkinson's syndrome. Drug-induced parkinsonism may occur in persons taking neuroleptic antipsychotic medications, usually within 1 to 4 weeks of initiating or increasing the dose. Metoclopramide and reserpine are also potential inducers of parkinsonism.

Parkinson's disease usually presents insidiously, and the patient may be unaware of its onset. The clinical findings may present in any combination. The tremor is characteristically slow and most prominent in the hands as a pill-rolling action, and disappears with intentional movement. The tremor also may present in the arms (with forearm supination and pronation), neck, and tongue, and occasionally as titubation. It usually is accentuated when the patient becomes excited or moves the opposite limb. The rigidity typically is described as cogwheel in quality. The most disabling feature of Parkinson's disease, however, is the bradykinesia, which manifests as slowing of voluntary movement and a reduction in automatic movements, such as swinging of the arms while walking. The facial muscles also may be involved, reducing facial expressiveness and causing muffled speech and infrequent blinking.

Patients adopt a stooped, flexed posture of the head, trunk, arms, and legs; have difficulty initiating gait; may be unable or slow to rise from a chair; and have poor control of balance and, although they may be aware of this, are unable to make corrective movements to prevent falls. At times, patients may freeze suddenly while attempting to walk or make a turn. Other findings include seborrhea and excessive perspiration, constipation, dysphagia, sialorrhea, urinary hesitancy or retention, and hypophonia (Gotham et al., 1986). Most patients with Parkinson's disease develop a depressive illness, and up to 30 per cent develop a dementia that is similar to Alzheimer's disease. The course is variable, but is usually progressive over a period of 5 to 15 years. Prior to the introduction of pharmacologic therapy, the average survival after diagnosis was 9 years.

Treatment

Therapy must be individualized, and careful adjustments must be made to the medical regimen in response to the benefits and side effects of treatment. For most persons, a trial of anticholinergic medications should be initiated once the symptoms begin to interfere with activities of daily living; however, when prompt control of symptoms is essential, initial therapy with L-dopa is appropriate (Koller and Hubble, 1990). The response to treatment is highly individual, but most patients demonstrate a significant improvement in rigidity, bradykinesia, and tremor. L-Dopa is a precursor of dopamine and is usually administered in combination with carbidopa, which inhibits the peripheral conversion of L-dopa to dopamine, thus allowing L-dopa to penetrate the blood–brain barrier for uptake in the central nervous system. The starting dose of the combination regimen is 10 mg of carbidopa and 100 mg of L-dopa three to five times a day, and the dose is increased every 3 days until the patient's symptoms improve or side effects occur. The increased dose should be given at the times of day when the patient reports that symptoms are worse. The total dosage should not exceed 25 mg of carbidopa and 250 mg of L-dopa five times a day. Once an optimal daily dose is found, long-acting preparations may be used to decrease the dosing frequency.

Side effects are common, mostly gastrointestinal problems, orthostatic hypotension, and occasionally cardiac arrhythmias. Dyskinesias occurs in 40 to 90 per cent of treated patients and may worsen with time, but often respond to reduction of total L-dopa dosage (Nutt, 1990). Occasionally, patients develop confusion, bizarre dreams, hallucinations, delirium, and paranoid ideation, which resolve with a reduced L-dopa dose given at more frequent intervals. Disruptive behavior can be treated with thioridazine (Mellaril) or diphenhydramine hydrochloride (Benadryl) while awaiting resolution of the symptoms. With longer durations of therapy, either the response to L-dopa may wear off or patients may develop an "on/off effect" with sudden freezing or bradykinesia. More frequent dosing or increased dosages may alleviate these symptoms in some patients. A new controlled-release preparation of carbidopa-levodopa (Sinemet CR) may be helpful in these situations because this preparation provides more stable plasma concentrations. This formulation also appears to improve sleep patterns in many patients with Parkinson's disease (Ahlshog et al., 1988). However, these phenomena may be unresponsive to treatment and may represent progression of the disease.

Selegiline is a monoamine oxidase B inhibitor that can be given concomitantly with carbidopa-levodopa. This medication has been shown to retard the progression of Parkinson's disease at doses of 10 mg/day when used early in the course of illness (Tetrud and Langston, 1989), and may allow for lower doses of L-dopa. Although few side effects occur when selegilene is used alone, side effects of nausea, dyskinesia, hallucinations, and confusion can occur when used with carbidopa-levodopa. In patients with bradykinesia and rigidity, amantadine may be a useful adjunct to L-dopa therapy. Confusion, agitation, and nightmares are frequent side effects that limit its widespread use. Bromocriptine is a dopamine agonist and may be useful when response to L-dopa diminishes. Frequent side effects, including gastrointestinal symptoms, hypotension, and confusion, have been reported. The anticholinergic medications benztropine and trihexyphenidyl may be helpful if tremors are the predominant symptom. In the elderly, however, side effects are common with these drugs, particularly in patients with prostatic hypertrophy, glaucoma, and constipation, and they may exacerbate dementia. Antidepressant medications are usually helpful in patients with clinical depression secondary to Parkinson's disease. Surgical treatment with stereotactic thalotomy and tissue transplantation is currently experimental and reserved for younger patients who have predominantly unilateral tremor and rigidity. However, thalotomy has little effect in alleviating the bradykinesia and postural instability that are so disabling (Goetz et al., 1989).

Physical therapy and speech therapy help many patients. The quality of life can be improved by providing simple aids to daily living, including rails and grab bars about the home, special table cutlery, nonslip mats, and devices to amplify the voice. Fear of falling is a common symptom experienced by many Parkinson's patients. It may be useful to instruct patients to walk with their hands clasped behind their back, or to use a walker for greater stability.

HEALTH PROMOTION/DISEASE PREVENTION

Value of Prevention

It is evident that some of the most effective interventions available to clinicians for reducing the incidence and severity of the leading causes of disease and disability are those that address personal health practices. This requires empowering patients to take a more active role in identifying risk factors and encouraging them to take steps toward modifying these risks (Kligman et al., 1990).

The goals of preventive strategies change somewhat with advancing years. Whereas disease-specific mortality and morbidity may be important for younger persons, these goals lose some focus with advancing years. The elderly, in general, are more interested in preventing decline in their quality of life and in preserving independence, vitality, and function. The focus of preventive geriatrics should be highly individualized programs taking into consideration the older person's preferences, functional status, comorbidity, affordability, and practicality (U.S. Preventive Services Task Force, 1989a).

Primary Prevention

Primary preventive interventions are designed to reduce the risk of disease onset and pertain mainly to personal behaviors and health practices.

Immunizations (Fedson, 1992; Woolf et al., 1990a).

PNEUMONIA. Pneumococcal disease accounts for approximately 40,000 deaths per year in the United States and is the most common cause of pneumonia in the elderly. Hospitalization rates for pneumococcal pneumonia and bacteremia account for approximately 100,000 admissions per year, especially for patients with chronic cardiopulmonary disease, stroke, diabetes, and cancer. Eighty-five per cent of the excess mortality occurs in the elderly. The new 23-valent pneumococcal vaccine is protective against 80 to 90 per cent of known strains of *S. pneumoniae* causing bacteremic pneumococcal disease. There are minimal side effects associated with the vaccine, usually limited to low-grade fever, myalgias, arrhythmia, and pain for 1 to 2 days. The pneumococcal vaccine is recommended for all elderly persons, particularly those with chronic medical conditions, and should be given to persons with surgical or functional asplenia.

INFLUENZA. There have been 10 influenza epidemics since 1957, each accounting for 40,000 excess deaths. Approximately 10,000 deaths per year result from influenza infections, with 80 to 90 per cent of the excess mortality in those over the age of 65. Influenza vaccines are composed of inactivated preparations containing each of the most recently circulating influenza A and B viruses. Excluding patients who are immunocompromised, the elderly appear to mount a protective antibody response to the vaccine. The only contraindications are an adverse reaction to a previous dose or a history of anaphylactic hypersensitivity to eggs. The immune response is delayed for 3 to 4 weeks, and there is a rapid decline of antibody titers; therefore, vaccinations should be given before the start of the flu season. Health care workers and other persons who can transmit influenza to the high-risk elderly person also should be vaccinated. Antiviral chemoprophylaxis with amantadine may be offered to persons in whom a less than adequate response to the vaccine might be expected, or in high-risk patients who have not yet received the vaccine.

TETANUS. While tetanus is now an uncommon condition, 60 per cent of cases occur in persons over the age of 65. The case fatality rate is four times greater in those over the age of 60. All adults should receive a booster at least once every 10 years, and a complete series of combined tetanus–diphtheria toxoids should be given to patients who have not received a primary series. Patients with pressure ulcers are particularly susceptible because the devitalized tissue provides an optimal medium for anaerobic growth.

Nutrition

The major diseases in which dietary excesses and imbalances are implicated rank among the leading causes of death and illness in the elderly (Manson et al., 1992). These include coronary artery disease, hypertension, cancer (colon, breast, and prostate), cerebrovascular disease, diabetes, osteoporosis, constipation/diverticular disease, and dental disease. Therefore, regular counseling should be offered regarding a patient's dietary intake of calories, fluid, cholesterol, fiber, sodium, and minerals. Patients should be encouraged to maintain a desirable weight. Specific instructions about diet should include recommendations for fat intake of less than 30 per cent of the total calories ingested, and for consumption of less than 300 mg of cholesterol per day. Saturated fat consumption should be less than 10 per cent of all calories, and patients should be encouraged to eat fish and poultry. Specific instructions should be given about increasing lean meat, low-fat dairy products, whole grain products in cereals, vegetables and fruit, and foods low in sodium. Women, especially, should be counseled about the need to maintain an adequate calcium intake.

Alcohol

Although the exact prevalence of alcohol use is unknown in the elderly, it is estimated that up to 10 per cent of those over the age of 65 have a drinking problem. Twenty per cent of nursing home residents have a history of alcohol dependency, and it is estimated that at least 20 per cent of all elderly medical and psychiatric patients are alcohol dependent (Dufour et al., 1992). Clinicians should ask routinely about alcohol use, and all patients should be informed of the health and injury risks from abuse. Of particular concern among the elderly is the high prevalence of alcohol-related dementia, nonintentional injury, and gastrointestinal bleeding. The use of the CAGE screening instrument is equally effective among older patients (see Chapter 57).

Physical Activity

Less than 10 per cent of elderly persons engage in routine physical activity, and most live sedentary lifestyles. A sedentary lifestyle should be considered a modifiable risk factor for coronary artery disease, hypertension, non–insulin-dependent diabetes mellitus, and osteoporosis. Regular physical activity has been associated with reductions in all-cause mortality in both men and women, and over 40 observational epidemiologic studies have demonstrated the beneficial relationship between exercise and coronary artery disease, with 30 of the 40 showing a protective effect (Manson et al., 1992). Regular exercise can slow the rate of decline in maximum oxygen consumption that occurs with aging and result in improvements in resting heart rate, mean arterial blood pressure, lipoprotein profile (increasing high-density lipoprotein, decreasing triglyceride levels), and general psychological well-being. There is also increasing evidence that regular physical activity is associated with maintaining higher levels of functional capability.

The role of exercise in the prevention of osteoporosis is less clear. Bone mass in weight-bearing areas may be increased by regular exercise (Sinaki et al., 1989), or even by low-level increases in activity, especially in high-risk groups. Patients should be encouraged to exercise regularly, and each exercise program should include warm-up, exercise, and cool-down phases lasting approximately 30 minutes in total. Patients should be encouraged to exercise to 60 per cent of maximal heart rate three times a week for approximately 30 minutes. Eventually, it may be possible to advance to vigorous aerobic exercise at 70 per cent of estimated maximum heart rate (220 − age in years = maximum heart rate).

Cigarette Smoking

It is estimated that 20 per cent of persons between the ages of 65 and 74 are current cigarette smokers. The prevalence of smoking among men over the age of 65 has shown a recent decline; however, among older women, there has been a slight increase. The cumulative risk for cigarette-related diseases increases with the number of years and number of cigarettes smoked on average per day (Centers for Disease Control, 1989), and, therefore, the elderly suffer in proportion to their exposure. It is estimated that smoking accounts for one in six deaths in the United States. Death rates from coronary heart disease, cerebrovascular disease, cancer, and respiratory disease are all higher among smokers.

Much of this mortality can be reduced by smoking cessation at any age (U.S. Department of Health and Human Services, 1990). For coronary artery disease, there is an initial rapid decline in risk within 1 to 2 years after smoking cessation, followed by a long period of gradual decline. The risk within 5 years of quitting for both men and women is approximately the same as for those who never smoked. However, the risk reduction benefit for cancer and for chronic obstructive lung disease mortality declines to that of nonsmokers only after 10 to 15 years of abstinence in men and 5 to 10 years in women. There is less convincing evidence that smoking cessation may help slow osteoporosis and reduce the risk of hip fractures, and that former smokers have higher levels of physical function

and better quality of life than continuing smokers (LaCroix and Omenn, 1992).

Approximately 38 million of the 53 million adult smokers can be reached by clinicians, and evidence suggests that counseling can be effective in changing behaviors. Effectiveness depends on many variables, including the number of interventions, the type of face-to-face advice given, patient motivation, the level of nicotine dependence, and the confidence the patient has in the benefits of discontinuing. A history of tobacco use should be obtained on all patients and smoking cessation counseling immediately instituted. Support visits, follow-up telephone calls, and self-help materials may be helpful. Patients also may benefit from community counseling and support programs and a trial of nicotine gum or patches.

Unintentional Injuries

For those over the age of 65, unintentional injuries are the sixth leading cause of death. Motor vehicle accidents are the major category of fatal injuries in adults up to 75 years of age; thereafter, injuries resulting from falls are the leading precipitant of accidental deaths (Williams and Carsten, 1989). Older drivers should be encouraged to take refresher courses and improve their knowledge and driving skills; motor vehicle crash rates adjusted for actual miles driven are higher among the elderly than any other age group except for those under 25 years. Older persons should be made aware of the changes of aging and superimposed pathology, and their potential effects on driving. Dementia and cerebrovascular disease are associated with high risks of unsafe driving, and doctors should ensure that patients and families are informed of the implications of their conditions for driving (Herman and Robertson, 1993-1994). It may be necessary for physicians to report unsafe elderly drivers to the Motor Vehicle Administration. All older persons should be encouraged to wear safety belts because there is good evidence, at least among younger individuals, that injurious accidents and death are decreased in motorists wearing safety belts.

Approximately one in three community-dwelling elderly persons falls in any given year, with 50 per cent sustaining repeated falls. Approximately 5 per cent of all falls result in a fracture of either the wrist or the hip. A further 5 per cent result in serious soft tissue injury, causing a period of bed confinement; these injuries include hematomas, hemarthroses, sprains, and dislocations. Most falls take place in the older person's home as a result of routine activities. Tripping over doorsills, scatter rugs, electric cords, and other obstacles in the home is the most common etiologic factor. Climbing and particularly descending stairs account for approximately one fourth of all falls that occur at home. A significant portion of elderly persons who fall develop a fear of falling, which may limit their willingness to ambulate.

The etiology of falls is multifactorial (Tinetti et al., 1988). Epidemiologic studies show that community-dwelling fallers are more likely to have cognitive impairment, lower extremity disability, foot problems, balance and gait abnormalities, a history of previous falls, or Parkinson's disease, or currently are taking diuretics, antihypertensives, sedatives, tranquilizers, or hypnotic medications (Heidrick et al., 1991). A number of age-related changes place an older person at increased risk of falling, including a reduction in gait velocity, step length, and step height. Subtle changes in balance, such as increased anteroposterior sway and slower righting reflexes, also may contribute to this risk. Superimposed sensory impairments, such as vestibular disorders, proprioceptive changes resulting from pathology in the joints, peripheral neuropathy, and cervical spondylosis, further increase the risk (Nevitt et al., 1989). Other pathologic conditions include musculoskeletal (osteo- and rheumatoid arthritis) and neurologic (cerebrovascular disease, Parkinson's disease, cerebellar disorders, lumbar stenosis) diseases, postural hypotension, and foot disorders. Other risk factors that should be included in a comprehensive history and physical examination are visual and hearing impairments. Medications that may be associated with an increased risk of falling also should be reassessed, and discontinued if possible.

To prevent falls, a home assessment and an environmental safety checklist may help in recognizing potentially correctable fall hazards. It is important that patients and families are instructed about adequate lighting and accessible switches. All floor obstacles should be removed and carpet edges tacked down. Patients should be instructed to buy nonskid shoes with low heels and reminded not to walk in stocking feet or in loose slippers. Stair steps should be in good repair, and step height, if possible, should be 6 inches or less. It may be necessary to install grab bars, nonskid or rubber mats, shower chairs, or raised toilet seats in the bathroom.

Burns are another common cause of accidental injury and death. The housing in which many older Americans live is less than adequate. Over 45 per cent of homes owned by older Americans were built prior to 1950, and about one third were built prior to 1940. Many of these homes do not have smoke detectors installed or have water heaters with high temperature settings. Because the elderly are at increased risk for deaths and morbidity secondary to burns, all homes should have smoke detectors installed, and hot water heaters should be set at 120°F.

Oral Health

While over 50 per cent of persons currently older than 65 years of age are edentulous, tomorrow's older adults will be keeping their teeth longer, probably because of improved dietary habits, visiting their dentist more regularly, and better preventive dentistry (Niessen and Douglass, 1992). This increase in tooth retention will increase the need for restorative dentistry, and for the treatment of caries and gingival and periodontal disease. Older adults are also at increased risk of oral soft tissue pathology, with approximately 30,000 new oral cancers reported annually in the United States. In general, physicians should counsel their patients regarding dental health and encourage regular dental care. Daily brushing with a fluoride-containing toothpaste and cleaning with dental floss should be recommended. Annual visits for prophylactic dental care and screening evaluations by dentists should be encouraged strongly.

Aspirin Prophylaxis

Daily aspirin for prophylaxis can lower the risk of myocardial infarctions significantly in persons at increased risk for atherosclerosis (Peto et al., 1988); (Steering Committee of the Physicians' Health Study Research Group, 1988). These risk factors include: hypertension, male gender, obesity, family history, diabetes mellitus, cigarette smoking, and high-density lipoprotein (HDL) cholesterol less than 35 mg/dL or low-density lipoprotein (LDL) cholesterol greater than 100 mg/dL. A prospective study of 87,000 U.S. nurses suggested that aspirin is also effective in preventing initial myocardial infarction in women (Manson et al., 1991). Side effects include gastrointestinal discomfort and mild bleeding, but occasional serious bleeding and peptic ulcer disease may limit the widespread use of aspirin. The U.S. Preventive Services Task Force (1989b) recommends that consideration be given to low-dose aspirin therapy, 325 mg every other day, for persons at increased risk for myocardial infarction.

Estrogen

The risk of coronary artery disease increases after menopause for elderly women; however, a large number of observational studies have demonstrated a reduced incidence in postmenopausal women taking estrogen replacement therapy. The attributable benefit is estimated to be in the range of 40 to 45 per cent (Manson et al., 1992) and is achieved by increasing HDL and decreasing LDL cholesterol concentrations. These relative benefits must be weighed against the increased risk of endometrial cancer, gallbladder disease, and perhaps breast cancer. As yet, there is insufficient evidence to suggest that estrogen works as well in elderly women as in those who are peri- or immediately postmenopausal, or is beneficial in secondary prevention of heart disease. It would appear that a combined estrogen and progesterone regimen, which reduces the risk of endometrial cancer, does not have the same magnitude of benefit as estrogen alone on HDL levels. However, combined regimens seem to reduce total and LDL cholesterol levels. Given the clear benefit for the symptoms of menopause and preventing osteoporosis, the decision to use estrogen replacement therapy as a tool for primary prevention of coronary artery disease deserves consideration, but must be made on an individual basis.

Secondary Prevention

Secondary prevention refers to strategies aimed at identifying and improving outcomes of persons with preclinical or asymptomatic disease. Early detection through screening is the most common method of secondary prevention (Woolf et al., 1990b).

Heart Disease

Because coronary artery disease accounts for approximately one in three deaths, with an estimated annual cost of $80 billion/year, any intervention that might improve survival would affect thousands of lives (Manson et al., 1992). The primary modifiable risk factors for coronary heart disease include hypertension, hypercholesteremia, cigarette smoking, obesity, and physical inactivity. Advanced age, male sex, and family history of coronary artery disease are nonmodifiable risk factors.

Hypertension

Over 60 million Americans are hypertensive, and approximately 50 per cent of all elderly persons have either systolic or combined systolic–diastolic hypertension (Applegate, 1990). Epidemiologic studies suggest that the average systolic blood pressure increases with advancing years, while diastolic blood pressure rises until about age 60 and then levels off. Although both systolic and diastolic hypertension independently predict future vascular events—in particular cerebrovascular disease, cardiovascular disease, and mortality from all vascular causes (MacMahon et al., 1990)—most of the increase in the prevalence of disease attributed to hypertension is accounted for by isolated systolic hypertension. The risk for morbidity and mortality is at least additive as other risk factors are present.

There is strong evidence from prospective epidemiologic studies that treatment of both systolic and diastolic hypertension is beneficial in the primary prevention of cerebrovascular disease and myocardial infarction (National Heart, Lung and Blood Institute, 1993). This is especially true for patients with severe diastolic hypertension (blood pressure > 115 mm Hg). Only a few studies have evaluated the effects of treating hypertension in the elderly. The European Working Party on Hypertension in the Elderly (EWPHE), demonstrated that cardiovascular mortality rate was reduced sig-

nificantly for older persons with diastolic hypertension treated for 8 years. The morbidity resulting from cerebrovascular disease also was reduced by approximately 50 per cent. Treatment did not have a significant impact on patients with entry-level diastolic blood pressure in the range of 90 to 95 mm Hg (Amery et al., 1985). The Systolic Hypertension in the Elderly Program (SHEP) reported that pharmacologic treatment of isolated systolic hypertension over 5 years resulted in a 35 per cent reduction in cerebrovascular events and a 31 per cent reduction in cardiovascular events (SHEP Cooperative Research Group, 1991). In both trials, diuretic treatment was the first-line therapy of choice. Concerns have been raised about the potential for adverse effects on serum lipids, blood glucose, electrolytes, and serum uric acid in elderly patients taking diuretics. Data from these trials and others would suggest, however, that there is scant evidence that adverse effects occur to a serious degree. Patients who develop significant and persistent alterations of lipid or glucose levels should be prescribed other medications.

Treatment is confounded by the possibility that too great a lowering of diastolic blood pressure may result in reduced coronary artery blood flow, especially during diastole (Applegate, 1990). Mortality from myocardial infarction increases as diastolic blood pressure levels are reduced below 85 mm Hg, especially in patients with symptomatic ischemic heart disease. It is important, therefore, to caution about overly vigorous treatment of hypertension. Conservative targets for systolic blood pressure therapy are no lower than 135 to 140 mm Hg, and for diastolic blood pressure no lower than 85 mm Hg. Both systolic and diastolic hypertension should be treated with medications if the average blood pressure is greater than 160 mm Hg systolic, or greater than 100 mm Hg diastolic, in at least two positions (preferably sitting and standing) on at least two visits. Nonpharmacologic interventions such as exercise and diet should first be tried. In general, diuretics are a good choice for treatment of hypertension in older persons, with second-line agents added as needed. Because the EWPHE did not show a benefit for persons treated for diastolic blood pressures between 90 and 95 mm Hg, these patients probably can be observed safely over time (Amery et al., 1985).

Hypercholesteremia

Total cholesterol and LDL cholesterol levels increase with age until they reach a plateau, for men in their 50s and women in their 60s, after which a decline usually is seen. A positive relationship has been demonstrated between serum cholesterol levels and the risk of coronary artery disease. This holds for all levels of cholesterol, with little evidence of a threshold effect (Expert Panel, 1988). Reducing total blood cholesterol and, in particular, LDL cholesterol decreases the risk of subsequent heart disease. Recently, the National Cholesterol Education Program (1993) has suggested that LDL cholesterol levels of 160 mg are acceptable for those without cardiac risk factors, but a level of 130 mg/dL or less is recommended for those with established coronary heart disease, male sex, and low HDL cholesterol levels. Specific recommendations about prevention and treatment of hypercholesteremia in the elderly are missing, but extrapolation of data from trials showing a reduction in coronary heart disease risk in middle-aged patients seems reasonable.

The decision to screen for and treat hypercholesteremia in the elderly requires judgment and a careful weighing of the risk/benefit ratio. Elevated levels of LDL represent a greater risk for persons in middle age than in their 80s (Hazzard, 1990); however, there is no reason to believe that treatment should be any less effective in the elderly. In contrast, there is no evidence that such interventions are beneficial, and the cost of both screening and medications is prohibitive (Garber et al., 1991). A rational approach should consider age, concomitant risk factors, functional status, predicted longevity, and patient preferences.

Cancer

Cancer is the second leading cause of death in the elderly, with over 50 per cent of all malignancies occurring in those over 65 years of age. To screen for cancer effectively, the disease should be epidemiologically significant, the diagnostic tests must have a high sensitivity and specificity in the preclinical stage and be acceptable to the patient, and early treatment should both be available and lead to better results than treatment started after symptoms arise. Few studies of the efficacy of cancer screening programs have included the elderly. Patient preferences and the likely risk/benefit ratio of detection and treatment should be carefully weighed when considering cancer screening strategies in the elderly.

Colorectal Cancer

Colorectal cancer is the second most common cancer in the United States, with 70 per cent of cases occurring in persons over the age of 65 years. The incidence of colorectal cancer becomes significant after the age of 50, and doubles every decade until the age of 80. The long-term survival of patients with early-stage disease is over 90 per cent, whereas those with disseminated disease at the time of diagnosis have a very poor prognosis. Risk factors include a family history of colon cancer, a history of familial polyposis coli, ulcerative colitis, adenomatous polyps, previous colorectal cancer, or a history of endometrial, ovarian, or breast cancer. Available screening tests include stool testing for occult blood, sigmoidoscopy, and colonoscopy.

Among patients ages 50 to 80 years, annual screening with fecal occult blood testing can reduce the 13-year cumulative mortality by up to one third (Mandel et al., 1993); however, the positive predictive value of this is less than 10 per cent. Sigmoidoscopy is a sensitive method for early detection of cancer and has been shown by case control studies to reduce mortality from cancer of the rectum and distal colon (Selby et al., 1992). Given these recent studies, it would seem prudent, for patients who are willing to undergo periodic screening, that annual fecal occult blood testing should be recommended, with the awareness that the subsequent diagnostic evaluation of positive test results is relatively costly and uncomfortable, and has a low positive predictive value for detecting cancer.

Breast Cancer

More than one half of breast cancers occur in women over the age of 60, with the mortality increasing in this age group in recent years. The age-adjusted mortality from breast cancer has not declined because, until recently, most women have not participated in cancer screening programs. Risk factors for breast cancer include North American or Northern European descent, a family history of premenopausal breast cancer, previous breast cancer, or a history of benign breast disease. Mortality from breast cancer can be reduced by as much as 50 per cent in asymptomatic women who participate in screening programs (Shapiro et al., 1988). It is estimated that the benefits may extend into the 80s for healthy women (Mandelblatt et al., 1992). Most older women, especially less educated minority women, do not obtain regular screening by physician breast exams or mammograms; the most common reason reported is that their physician had not recommended it. All women over the age of 50 should have an annual clinical breast exam by a physician and should have mammograms on an annual or biannual basis at least until the age of 75 (Woolf et al., 1990b). Some authors recommend that screening beyond the age of 75 years should be continued as long as the patient's predicted life expectancy exceeds 5 years (Oddone et al., 1992).

Cervical Cancer

The incidence of invasive cervical cancer has declined in the United States in the last 50 years; however, 15,000 new cases and approximately 7000 deaths occur from this disease annually. Over 50 per cent of deaths occur in women over the age of 65. Up to 40 per cent of black women and 20 per cent of white women have never had a Pap smear (Mandelblatt et al., 1986), especially lower income, poorly educated, and elderly women. The specificity of Pap testing is difficult to determine because women with normal Pap smears are not subjected to a definitive diagnostic test such as biopsy, and the sensitivity and specificity of Pap smears may be lower in older women because of atrophic changes. Nevertheless, there is indirect evidence that regular Pap smear screening reduces the incidence of cervical cancer and cancer-related deaths (Mandelblatt and Fahs, 1988). It therefore would seem prudent that elderly women should have a Pap smear at least once. Older women do not appear to benefit from repeated screening if at least two consecutive smears have been normal, so it is reasonable to discontinue screening at the age of 65 if the woman has had previously documented normal examinations.

Prostate Cancer

Prostate cancer is the second most common malignancy in older men, and the third most common cause of death. There are 122,000 new cases diagnosed per year, with about 32,000 deaths annually (Oddone et al., 1992). The majority of cases are found among patients over age 65, with a greater incidence occurring in blacks and those with a family history of prostate cancer. It appears that early-stage diagnosis is associated with improved survival. The natural history of prostate cancer is unpredictable, and the apparent survival rate of early disease may reflect simply length and lead time biases. The value of screening for prostate cancer is controversial (Catalona et al., 1991). The sensitivity of digital rectal examination is low. Transrectal ultrasound and PSA levels have received much attention recently; however, both tests have low sensitivities and high false-positive rates. No study has proven that PSA is effective as a screening tool, although the specificity of the test increases with serum levels. A prospective, randomized, controlled clinical trial is in progress to determine the effects of screening for prostate cancer on mortality.

Other Cancers

There is no evidence to suggest that screening asymptomatic individuals for lung cancer, pancreatic cancer, ovarian cancer, or oral cancer is justifiable. Patients at high risk, such as those with familial or previous history of skin cancer or an occupational/recreational exposure to sun, probably should have a complete skin examination on an annual or biannual basis. Patients with a history of excessive alcohol consumption or tobacco use have a higher risk of oral cancer, and, although screening may not be effective in the elderly, it is probably worthwhile to examine the oral mucosa regularly in high-risk patients.

Other Screenings/Secondary Prevention Interventions

Hearing Impairment

Almost 20 million Americans suffer from some degree of hearing loss. Older persons develop an age-associated bilateral sensorineural high-frequency hearing loss so that, by the age of 80, almost 50 per cent have self-reported hearing difficulties. However, the individual often is unaware of the hearing deficits early in the course, and less than 10 per cent of hearing-impaired persons over the age of 65 use a hearing aid. Hearing loss is associated with lower levels of self-reported functional abilities, spending more time in bed, and having more physician visits annually (Lichtenstein, 1990). Because of the high prevalence of hearing impairment among the elderly, physicians should screen periodically for hearing loss by audioscopic examination and simple audiometry. Hearing aids substantially improve communication, mood, and cognitive function, and are generally acceptable.

Visual Impairment

About one in seven persons over the age of 65 has some form of visual impairment, and up to 10 per cent are blind in both eyes. Visual disorders that occur more commonly in older persons include glaucoma, macular degeneration, and cataracts (Lichtenstein, 1990). Many older adults are unaware of changes in visual acuity, and up to one quarter may be using incorrect prescriptions. Visually impaired elderly persons have lower feelings of self-esteem, decreased levels of physical activity, and more impairments in function. Most traffic violations that occur among the elderly involve difficulty with traffic signals, turning, and yielding right of way, which are all vision-dependent functions. Data from the Framingham Eye Study suggest that visual loss is associated with an increased risk of falling and fractures. Because of this significant burden of disease, physicians should check visual acuity in asymptomatic older persons regularly. There is insufficient evidence to recommend routine tonometry, especially if done by primary care physicians (U.S. Preventive Services Task Force, 1989c); therefore, patients should be screened by an ophthalmologist or an optometrist.

END-OF-LIFE ISSUES

Advance Directives

Patient autonomy is one of the guiding ethical principles of modern medicine, and is encountered daily in negotiations with patients about diagnostic tests to which they are willing to submit and medications they are willing to take, and through the process of informed consent, which is intended to assure that the patient is aware of the risks and benefits of potentially harmful interventions. These expressions of autonomy are based on a patient's ability to understand and to make reason judgments as a partner in their health care. There may come a time when the patient is incapable of decision making, and, under these circumstances, there are two ways in which the patient's autonomy may be expressed: a living will and a durable power of attorney for health care.

Living Will

Every state has provisions for an advance directive whereby an individual may express his or her wishes about certain types of medical interventions at the end of life. There are several universal elements that define a living will. The individual must have become incompetent, and the provisions come into force only when the patient is declared terminally ill, and when, to a reasonable degree of medical certainty, no further interventions will alter the patient's course. The interventions to be withheld or withdrawn may be enumerated or broadly conveyed; the form depends as much on drafting limitations imposed by state law as those imposed by patient preference.

Although living wills are helpful in certain situations, there are important limitations. First, living wills are nonbinding, and therefore hospitals and physicians are not obligated to conform with all of the requests. Should a family member disagree, or if no one corroborates the intentions expressed through the living will, health care providers may need to seek a court-appointed guardian. Furthermore, living wills are usually applicable only in the event of terminal illness. Degenerative diseases that are associated with mental incapacity, such as Alzheimer's disease, multi-infarct dementia, and Parkinson's disease, are slowly progressive and may not be applicable under a strict interpretation of terminal illness. Therefore, the living will may be of no solace to those afflicted with a lingering illness.

Durable Power of Attorney for Health Care

In order to obviate the problems of the living will, most states have enacted legislation through which individuals can identify an agent to act on their behalf, should they become mentally incapacitated. The decisions of the designated agent are binding to nearly the same extent as if they were made by the patient. These decisions may include such matters as choosing or dismissing health care providers, signing informed consent documents, and other administrative tasks such as admission and discharge from hospitals and nursing homes and access to the medical record. These advance directive documents most often are accompanied by a durable power of attorney over finance, thus providing the financial means to implement health care decisions. Decision-making powers are not restricted to the circumstances of terminal illness. This flexibility allows appropriate decision making, in concert with the patient's wishes, in the event of a lingering illness. These powers are balanced by important safeguards wherein an agent who either contravenes specific statements in the durable power of attorney for health care document or appears to be acting in a potentially abusive or exploitative fashion can be taken to court for judicial review. The court has the power to appoint a guardian to supersede the agent, if needed.

Documentation of Advance Directives

Both forms of advance directives can be executed without incurring the expense of legal counsel. Standard forms are available through Choice in Dying, New York (200 Varick Street, New York, NY 10014; 1-800-989-9455). A review of advance directive documents should be a part of the annual health examination of older adults, and at other times when a reconsideration of general health care interventions seems warranted (e.g., after recovery from a major illness or other major life change). Most patients welcome the opportunity to discuss their wishes and concerns openly with their physician. Patients who wish to avoid the subject are still usually willing to identify their preferred surrogate decision maker. Documentation of this discussion may hold as much credence as the formal document, and is admissible evidence in the event of a guardianship hearing.

Terminal Care

Not all patients who die are terminally ill. For example, many patients die suddenly and unexpectedly, and some patients succumb to acute life-threatening illnesses despite aggressive medical management that saves the majority of those afflicted. The designation of terminal illness connotes an expectation of death within a foreseeable future from an illness that is generally not amenable to medical intervention. Definitions also may include considerations of functional incapacity and unremitting symptoms attributed to the progression of the illness. It is important for physicians to recognize when the conditions of terminal illness have been met so that the medical care plan can be reconsidered appropriately.

There are several salient features of terminal care that should be reviewed as part of the reassessment of the medical care plan. Symptom control—especially relief of pain and other symptoms, such as breathlessness, nausea, itching, and diarrhea, that may be equally discomforting—is of paramount importance and should be addressed appropriately. In the presence of a terminal illness, long-term side effects of medications, such as drug addiction to opiates or parkinsonism secondary to major tranquilizers, no longer hold the same relevance. Should oral or topical analgesics no longer prove effective or acceptable, parenteral therapies, preferably with patient control, should be initiated.

Terminal care also demands a fine balance between aggressive medical interventions and withholding certain therapies. Radiation treatments for pain control or dyspnea, surgical débridement of pressure ulcers for hygienic purposes, and antibiotics for transient infections are usually appropriate. In contrast, hypertension control and maintenance of chemical homeostasis for glucose, electrolytes, renal function, and hematocrit become less important considerations, because these are often asymptomatic. The provision or withholding of a feeding tube should be discussed and the decision documented long before the issue arises.

Cardiopulmonary resuscitation also should be discussed openly. Resuscitative efforts may be appropriate if death is precipitated by a medical intervention, such as surgery, yet be withheld if death ensues from natural causes. Physicians have no obligation to provide futile treatment, even when requested to do so, but the intention to withhold resuscitation should be made known to the patient and the family. Reluctance to accept this decision may be assuaged by a second opinion or review by an ethics committee.

For patients at home or in nursing homes, the decision of whether to seek hospitalization should be considered. Certain interventions that might be needed for symptom control may be available only in the acute care setting. For some families, the prospect of impending death may be frightening and so family members may avoid the patient, with resulting neglect. Some patients may wish to unburden their family as their needs increase; for others, dying at home or in familiar surroundings is the only acceptable alternative.

Social and psychological support are of equal importance to the control of symptoms. If the patient is in a hospital or nursing home, visiting privileges by family and friends should be liberalized and provisions made to allow a family vigil as death becomes imminent. Psychological counseling for both the patient and the family can prove invaluable. Anxiolytics and antidepressants should be made freely available as needed. Involvement of the clergy may be important for certain individuals and their family, and should be encouraged. Finally, it is important that the patient not perceive that the physician has abandoned him or her. Frequent visits are necessary to assure that the medical regimen is effective and that all aspects of comfort care are provided. In settings other than a hospice, constant vigilance is necessary to assure that covering physicians do not initiate unwanted therapies. If possible, a bereavement visit following the death of a patient may help the family to come to closure in their grief.

REFERENCES

Ahlshog JE, Meunter CD, McManus PG, et al: Controlled-release Sinemet (CR-4): A double blind crossover study in patients with fluctuating Parkinson's disease. Mayo Clin Proc 63:876, 1988.

Albert SG, Nakra BR, Grossberg GT, Caminal ER: Vasopressin response to dehydration in Alzheimer's disease. J Am Geriatr Soc 37:843, 1989.

Allman RM: Pressure ulcers among the elderly. N Engl J Med 320:850, 1989.

Amaud CD: Role of dietary calcium in osteoporosis. Adv Intern Med 35:93, 1990.

American Diabetes Association: Diabetes facts and figures. Alexandria, VA: American Diabetes Association, 1986.

American Medical Association Department of Geriatric Health: Guidelines for the medical management of the home care patient. Chicago, American Medical Association, 1992.

Amery A, Birkenhager W, Brixko P: Mortality and morbidity results in the European Working Party on High Blood Pressure in the Elderly trial. Lancet 2:1349, 1985.

Ancoli-Israel S, Kripke DF, Mason W, et al: Sleep apnea and periodic movements in an aging sample. J Gerontol 40:419, 1985.

Applegate WB: High blood pressure treatment in the elderly. Clin Geriatr Med 8:103, 1990.

Applegate WB, Akins D, Zwaag RV, et al: A geriatric rehabilitation and assessment unit in the community hospital. J Am Geriatr Soc 31:206, 1983.

Applegate WB, Miller ST, Graney MJ, et al: A randomized, controlled trial of a geriatric assessment unit in a community rehabilitation hospital. N Engl J Med 322:1572, 1990.

Aronson MD, Bor DH: Blood cultures. Ann Intern Med 106:246, 1987.

Audran M, Clochon P, Etghen D, et al: Treatment of Paget's disease of bone with (4-chlorophenyl)thiomethylene bisphosphonate. Clin Rheumatol 8:71, 1989.

Barker WH, Mullooly JP: Impact of epidemic Type A influenza in a defined adult population. Am J Epidemiol 112:798, 1980.

Barrett-Conner E, Bush TL: Estrogen and coronary heart disease in women. JAMA 265:1861, 1991.

Beck LH: Perioperative renal, fluid, and electrolyte management. Clin Geriatr Med 6:557, 1990.

Beers M, Besdine RW: Medical assessment of the elderly patient. Clin Geriatr Med 3:17, 1987.

Bentley DW: Clostridium difficile associated disease in long-term care facilities. Infect Control Hosp Epidemiol 11:434, 1990.

Berkman B, Foster LWS, Campion E: Failure to thrive: Paradigm for the frail elder. Gerontologist 29:654, 1989.

Blaivus JG, Olsson CA: Stress incontinence: Classification and surgical approach. J Urol 139:727, 1988.

Bliwise DL, Bliwise NG, Pastinen M, et al: Sleep apnea and mortality in an aged cohort. Am J Publ Health 78:544, 1988.

Boscia JA, Abrutyn E, Levison ME, et al: Pyuria and asymptomatic bacteriuria in elderly ambulatory women. Ann Intern Med 110:404, 1989.

Boucher CA, Brewster DC, Darling RC, et al: Determination of cardiac risk by dipyridamole-thallium imaging before peripheral vascular surgery. N Engl J Med 312:389, 1985.

Brocklehurst JC, Carty MH, Leeming JT: Medical screening of old people accepted for residential care. Lancet 2:141, 1978.

Brown LJ, Potter JF, Foster BG: Caregiver burden should be evaluated during geriatric assessment. J Am Geriatr Soc 38:455, 1990.

Brummel-Smith K (ed): Geriatric rehabilitation. Clin Geriatr Med 9:xiii-895, 1993.

Calama KT, Hunder GG: Clinical manifestations of giant cell arteritis. Clin Rheum Dis 6:389, 1980.

Camel R: Subtle and atypical cobalamin deficiency. Am J Hematol 34:108, 1990.

Carter BS, Carter B, Isaacs JT: Epidemiologic evidence regarding predisposing factors to prostate cancer. Prostate 16:187, 1990.

Carter HB, Pearson JD, Melter EJ, et al: Longitudinal evaluation of prostate specific antigen levels in men with and without prostatic disease. JAMA 267:2215, 1992.

Castle SC, Norman DC, Yeh M, et al: Fever response in elderly nursing home residents: Are the older truly colder? J Am Geriatr Soc 39:853, 1991.

Catalona WJ, Smith DS, Ratliff TL, et al. Measurement of prostate specific-antigen in serum as a screening test for prostate cancer. N Engl J Med 324:1156, 1991.

Center for Disease Control: Tobacco use by adults—United States. MMWR 38:685, 1989.

Christiansen C (ed): Proceedings of a Symposium Consensus Development Conference on Osteoporosis. Am J Med 91(suppl 5B):1S, 1991.

Clark GS, Blue B, Bearer JB: Rehabilitation of the elderly amputee. J Am Geriatr Soc 31:439, 1983.

Connell AM, Hilton C, Ervine G, et al: Variation of bowel habit in two population samples. BMJ 2:1095, 1965.

Consensus Development Conference: Prophylaxis and treatment of osteoporosis. Am J Med 90:107, 1991.

Consensus Development Conference: Diagnosis, prophylaxis, and treatment of osteoporosis. Am J Med 94:646, 1993.

Crook J, Rideout E, Browne G: The prevalence of pain complaints in a general population. Pain 18:299, 1984.

Daly MP, Adelman AM, Resnick BM: The Supportive Care Unit—inpatient geriatric rehabilitation: Preliminary data. MD Med J 41:515, 1992.

DATTA: Diagnostic and therapeutic technology assessment: Measurement of bone density with dual x-ray absorptiometry (DEXA). JAMA 267:286, 1992.

Dement WC, Miles LE, Carskordon MA: "White paper" on sleep and aging. J Am Geriatr Soc 30:25, 1982.

Detsky AB, Abrams HB, McLaughlin JR, et al: Predicting cardiac complications in patients undergoing non-cardiac surgery. J Intern Med 1:211, 1986.

Disa JJ, Carlton JM, Goldberg NH: Efficacy of operative cure in pressure sore patients. Plast Reconstr Surg 89:272, 1992.

Djokovic JL, Hedley-White J: Predictions of outcome of surgery and anesthesia in patients over 80. JAMA 242:2301, 1979.

Dombovy M, Sandok B, Basford J: Rehabilitation for stroke: A review. Stroke 17:363, 1986.

Dufour MC, Archer L, Gordis E: Alcohol and the elderly. Clin Geriatr Med 8:127, 1992.

Evans RL, Hendricks RD: Evaluating hospital discharge planning: A randomized clinical trial. Med Care 31:358, 1993.

Expert Panel: Report of the National Cholesterol Education Panel on detection, evaluation, and treatment of high blood cholesterol in adults. Arch Intern Med 148:36, 1988.

Feather J, Karuza J: The funding of nursing home care. *In* Katz PR, Calkins E (eds): Principles and Practice of Nursing home Care. New York, Springer, 1988, pp 15–22.

Fedson DS: Clinical practice and public policy for influenza and pneumococcal vaccination of the elderly. Clin Geriatr Med 8:201, 1992.

Fein AM, Fein-Silber SH, Neiderman MS, et al: What to do when your patient's pneumonia fails to resolve. J Respir Dis 10:83, 1989.

Feldt-Rasmussen B, Mathusen ER, Deckert T: Effect of two years of strict metabolic control on the progression of incipient nephropathy in insulin-dependent diabetics. Lancet 2:1300, 1986.

Fiatarone MA, Marks EC, Ryan ND, et al: High intensity strength training in nonagenarians: Effects on skeletal muscle. JAMA 263:3029, 1990.

Fine EJ, Soria ED: Myths about vitamin B12 deficiency. South Med J 84:1475, 1991.

Finkelstein M, Petkun WM, Freedman ML, et al: Pneumococcal bacteremia in adults: Age dependent differences in presentation and in outcome. J Am Geriatr Soc 31:19, 1983.

Fisher VS, Gullickson G: Energy cost of amputation in health and disability: A literature review. Arch Phys Med Rehabil 59:124, 1978.

Folstein MF, Folstein SE, McHugh PR: "Mini-Mental State": A practical method for grading the cognitive status of patients for the clinician. J Psychiatr Res 12:189, 1975.

Fontanarosa PB, Kaeberlein FJ, Gerson LW, Tomson RB: Difficulty in predicting bacteremia in elderly emergency room patients. Ann Emerg Med 21:842, 1992.

Francis J. Delirium in older patients. J Am Geriatr Soc 40:829, 1992.

Freedman DX, Braun J, Derryberry JS: Drugs and insomnia: NIH Consensus Development Conference. NIH Consensus Dev Conf 4:1, 1984.

Fretwell M: The Consensus Conference on Comprehensive Geriatric Assessment. J Am Geriatr Soc 36:377, 1988.

Fries JF: Aging, natural death, and the compression of morbidity. N Engl J Med 303:130, 1980.

Garber AM, Littenberg B, Sox HC, et al: Costs and health consequences of cholesterol screening for asymptomatic older Americans. Arch Intern Med 151:1089, 1991.

Garry PJ, Goodwin JS, Hunt WC: Iron status and anemia in the elderly: New findings and a review of previous studies. J Am Geriatr Soc 31:389, 1983.

Gleckman R, Hibert D: Afebrile bacteremia: A phenomenon in geriatric patients. JAMA 248:1478, 1982.

Gloth FM, Burton JR: Autopsies and death certificates in the chronic care setting. J Am Geriatr Soc 38:151, 1990.

Goetz CG, Olanow CW, Koller WC: Multicenter study of autologous adrenal medullary transplantation to the corpus striatum in patients with advanced Parkinson's disease. N Engl J Med 320:337, 1989.

Goldberg AP, Coon PJ: Non-insulin dependent diabetes mellitus in the elderly. Endocrinol Metab Clin North Am 16:843, 1987.

Goodwin JS: Progress in gerontology: polymyalgia rheumatica and temporal arteritis. J Am Geriatr Soc 40:515, 1992.

Gotham AM, Brown RG, Marsden CD: Depression in Parkinson's disease: A quantitative and qualitative analysis. J Neurol Neurosurg Psychiatry 49:381, 1986.

Gross CR, Lindquist RD, Woolley AC, et al: Clinical indicators of dehydration severity in elderly patients. J Emerg Med 10:267, 1992.

Grubb BP, Temsey-Amios P, Hahn H, Elliot L: Utility of the upright tile-table testing in the evaluation and management of syncope of unknown origin. Am J Med 90:6, 1991.

Guillemicault C, Silvestri R: Aging, drugs, and sleep. Neurobiol Aging 3:379, 1982.

Guyatt GH, Patterson C, Ali M, et al: Diagnosis of iron deficiency in the elderly. Am J Med 88:205, 1990.

Hadley EC: Bladder training and related therapies for urinary incontinence in elderly people. JAMA 256:372, 1986.

Haibach H, Farrell L, Dittruch FJ: Neoplasms arising in Paget's disease of bone: A study of 82 cases. Am J Clin Pathol 83:594, 1985.

Hamdy RC: Paget's disease of bone. Hosp Pract 30:33, 1990.

Harari D, Gurwitz JH, Minaker KL: Constipation in the elderly. J Am Geriatr Soc 41:1130, 1993.

Harding GKM, Nicolle LE, Ronald AR, et al: How long should catheter-acquired urinary tract infections in women be treated? Ann Intern Med 114:713, 1991.

Harper CM, Lyles YM: Physiology and complications of bedrest. J Am Geriatr Soc 36:1047, 1988.

Hazzard WR: Dyslipoproteinemia in the elderly: Should it be treated? Clin Geriatr Med 8:89, 1990.

Heidrick FE, Stergachis A, Gross KM: Diuretic drug use and the risk of hip fracture. Ann Intern Med 45:1, 1991.

Helmrich SP, Rageand DR, Leung RW, Paffenbarger RS: Physical activity and reduced occurrence of non-insulin dependent diabetes mellitus. N Engl J Med 325:147, 1991.

Herman CJ, Robertson JM: Issues in preventive geriatrics. *In* Ruben BB, Yoshokawa TT, Bestine RW (eds): Geriatric Review Syllabus Supplement. American Geriatrics Society 1993–1994 Program. New York, American Geriatrics Society, 1993–1994, pp 335–385.

Hing E, Sekscenski E, Strahn G: The National Nursing Home Survey 1985: Summary for the United States. Vital Health Stat [13], no. 97, 1990.

Hoenig HM, Rubenstein LZ: Hospital associated deconditioning and dysfunction. J Am Geriatr Soc 39:220, 1991.

Hogan DB, Fox RA: A prospective controlled trial of a geriatric consultation team in an acute-care hospital. Age Aging 19:107, 1990.

Iglehart JK: The American health care system: Introduction. N Engl J Med 326:962, 1992.

Inouye SK, van Dyck CH, Alessi CA, et al: Clarifying confusion: The confusion assessment method. A new method for detection of delirium. Ann Intern Med 113:941, 1990.

Inouye SK, Acampora D, Miller RL, et al: The Yale Geriatric Care Program: A model of care to prevent functional decline in hospitalized elderly patients. J Am Geriatr Soc 41:1345, 1993.

Isaacs B, Gum J, McKechan A, et al: The concept of pre-death. Lancet 1:1115, 1971.

Jarnagin WR, Duh Q, Mulvihill SJ, et al: The efficacy and limitation of percutaneous endoscopic gastrostomy. Arch Surg 127:261, 1992.

Kahn AH, Rubenstein PC: Ischemic bowel disease: Diagnosis and prognosis. Geriatrics 39(11):63, 1984.

Kaiser FE: Sexuality. *In* Reuben DB, Yoshvkawa TT, Besdine RW (eds): Geriatric Review Syllabus: A Core Curriculum in Geriatric Medicine, Supplement. American Geriatrics Society 1993–1994 Program. New York, American Geriatrics Society, 1993–1994, pp 153s–156s.

Kane RL, Ouslander JG, Abrass IB: Essentials of Clinical Geriatrics 2nd ed. New York, McGraw-Hill, 1988.

Kapoor WN: Diagnostic evaluation of syncope. Am J Med 90:91, 1991.

Katz S, Ford AB, Moskowitz RW, et al: Studies of illness in the aged. The index of ADL: A standardized measure of biological and psychosocial function. JAMA 185:914, 1963.

Katzman R: Alzheimer's disease. N Engl J Med 314:964, 1986.

Kavesh WN: Home care: Process, outcome, cost. Annu Rev Geront Geriatr 6:135, 1986.

Keller RJ, Eisenbarth GS, Jackson RA: Insulin prophylaxis in individuals at high risk of Type I diabetes. N Engl J Med 341:927, 1993.

Kemper P, Murtaugh CM: Life time use of nursing home care. N Engl J Med 324:595, 1991.

Kenney RA (ed): Physiology of Aging: A Synopsis, 2nd edition. Chicago, Year Book Medical Publishers, 1989.

Kligman EW, Kamerow DB, Artz LM: Year 2000 health objectives for the family physician. Am Fam Physician 42:851, 1990.

Koller WC, Hubble JP: Levadopa therapy in Parkinson's disease. Neurology 40(suppl 3):40, 1990.

Korenman SG, Morley JE, Mooradian AD, et al: Secondary hypogonadism in older men: Its relationship to impotence. J Clin Endocrinol Metab 71:963, 1990.

Kovar MG, Harris MI, Hadden WC: The scope of diabetes mellitus in the United States population. Am J Publ Health 77:1549, 1987.

LaCroix AZ, Omenn GS: Older adults and smoking. Clin Geriatr Med 8:69, 1992.

Lamy PP, Krug BH: Review of laxative utilization in a skilled nursing facility. J Am Geriatr Soc 26(12):544, 1978.

Larson EB, Kukull WA, Katzman RL: Cognitive impairment: Dementia and Alzheimer's disease. Annu Rev Public Health 13:431, 1992.

Lavizzo-Mourey RJ, Hillman AL, Diserens D, Schwartz JS: Hospitals' motivations in establishing or closing geriatric evaluation management units: Diffusion of a new patient-care technology in a changing health care environment. J Gerontol 48:M78, 1993.

Lavizzo-Mourey R, Johnson J, Stolley P: Risk factors for dehydration among elderly nursing home residents. J Am Geriatr Soc 36:213, 1988.

Lawton MP, Brody EM: Assessment of older people: Self-maintaining and instrumental activities of daily living. Gerontologist 9:179, 1969.

Lehmann JF, DeLater BJ, Fowler RF, et al: Stroke: Does rehabilitation affect outcome? Arch Phys Med Rehab 56:375, 1975.

Lentino JR, Lucks DA: Non-value sputum culture in the management of lower respiratory tract infections. J Clin Microbiol 25:758, 1987.

Lepor H: Role of alpha-adrenergic blockers in the treatment of benign prostatic hyperplasia. Prostate Suppl 3:75, 1990.

Lichtenstein MJ: Hearing and visual impairments. Clin Geriatr Med 8:173, 1990.

Lipowski ZJ: Delirium: Acute Confusional States. London, Oxford University Press, 1990.

Lipschitz DA, Mitchell CO: The correctability of the nutrition immune and hematopoietic manifestations of protein calorie malnutrition in the elderly. J Am Coll Nutr 1:17, 1982.

Lipschitz DA, Udapa KB: Age and the hematopoietic system. J Am Geriatr Soc 34:448, 1986.

Lipsey JR, Spencer WC, Robins PV, Robinson RG: Phenomenological comparison of post-stroke depression and functional depression. Am J Psych 143:527, 1986

Lipsitz LA: Orthostatic hypotension in the elderly. N Engl J Med 321:952, 1989.

Lipsky BA, Ireton RC, Fihn SD, et al: Diagnosis of bacteriuria in men: Specimen collection and culture interpretation. J Infect Dis 155:847, 1987.

Lukert BP, Raisz LG: Glucocorticoid-induced osteoporosis: Pathogenesis and management. Ann Intern Med 112:352, 1990.

MacKowiak PA, Wasserman SS, Levine MM: A critical appraisal of 98.6°F, the upper limit of the normal body temperature, and other legacies of Carl Reinhold August Wunderlich. JAMA 268:1578, 1992.

MacMahon S, Peto R, Cutler J, et al: Blood pressure, stroke, and coronary heart disease: Part 1, Prolonged differences in blood pressure: Prospective observational studies erected for the regression delusional bias. Lancet 335:765, 1990.

Mader SL: Aging and postural hypotension: An update. J Am Geriatr Soc 37:129, 1989.

Mandel JS, Bond JH, Church TR, et al: Reducing mortality from colorectal cancer by screening for fecal occult blood. N Engl J Med 328:1365, 1993.

Mandelblatt JS, Fahs MC: The cost-effectiveness of cervical cancer screening for low income elderly women. JAMA 259:2409, 1988.

Mandelblatt J, Gopal I, Wistreich I: Gynecological care of elderly women: Another look at Papanicolaou smear testing. JAMA 256:367, 1986.

Mandelblatt JS, Wheat ME, Monare M, et al: Breast cancer screening for elderly women with and without comorbid conditions: A decision analysis model. Ann Intern Med 116:722, 1992.

Manolis AS, Lunzer M, Salem D, Estes NAM: Syncope: Current diagnostic evaluation and management. Ann Intern Med 112:850, 1990.

Manson JE, Colditz GA, Stampfer MJ, et al: A prospective study of obesity and risk of coronary heart disease in women. N Engl J Med 323:882, 1990.

Manson JE, Stumpfer MJ, Colditz GA, et al: A prospective study of aspirin use and primary prevention of cardiovascular disease in women. JAMA 266:521, 1991.

Manson JE, Tosteson H, Satterfield S, et al: The primary prevention of myocardial infarction. N Engl J Med 326:1406, 1992.

Marrie TJ, Durant H, Kwan C: Nursing home-acquired pneumonia: A case-control study. J Am Geriatr Soc 34:697, 1986.

Martilla RJ: Epidemiology of Parkinson's disease. *In* Koeller WC (ed): Handbook of Parkinson's Disease. New York, Marcel Decker, 1989, pp 35–50.

McConnell JD: Androgen ablation and blockage in the treatment of benign prostatic hyperplasia. Urol Clin North Am 17:661, 1990.

McDonald JB: Coronary care in the elderly. Age Aging 12:17, 1983.

McGeer A, Campbell B, Emori TG, et al: Definition of infection for surveillance in long-term care facilities. Am J Infect Cont 19:1, 1991.

Melton LJ, Kan SH, Frye MA, et al: Epidemiology of vetebral fractures in women. Am J Epidemiol 129:1000, 1989.

Miles LE, Dement WC: Sleep and aging. Sleep 3:119, 1980.

Miller PD, Krebs RA, Neal BJ, McIntyre DO: Hypodipsia in geriatric patients. Am J Med 73:354, 1982.

Miller RM, Groher ME, Yorkston KM, Rees TS: Speech, language, swallowing, and auditory rehabilitation. *In* DeLisa JA (ed): Rehabilitation Medicine: Principles & Practice, 2nd edition. Philadelphia, JB Lippincott, 1993, pp 213–217.

Moon TD. Prostate cancer. J Am Geriatr Soc 40:622, 1992.

Morey MC, Cowper PA, Feussner JR, et al: Two-year trends in physical performance following supervised exercise among community-dwelling older veterans. J Am Geriatr Soc 39:549, 1991.

Morley JE, Kaiser JE, Johnson LE: Male sexual function. *In* Cassel CK, et al (eds): Geriatric Medicine, 2nd edition. New York, Springer-Verlag, 1990, pp 256–270.

Mott PD, Barker WH: Hospital and medical care use by nursing home patients: The effect of patient care plans. J Am Geriatr Soc 36:47, 1988.

Naliboff BD, Rosenthal M: Effect of age on complications in adult onset diabetes. J Am Geriatr Soc 37:838, 1989.

National Cholesterol Education Program Expert Panel on Detection, Evaluation, and Treatment of High Blood Cholesterol in Adults (Adult Treatment Panel II): Summary of the Second Report. JAMA 23:3015, 1993.

National Heart, Lung and Blood Institute: National High Blood Pressure Education: Fifth Report of the Joint National Committee on Detection, Evaluation and Treatment of high blood pressure. NIH publication no. 93-1088. Washington, DC, National Institutes of Health, 1993.

National Institutes of Health Consensus Development Conference: Health implications of obesity. Ann Intern Med 103:977, 1985.

National Institutes of Health Consensus Development Conference: Prevention of venous thrombosis and pulmonary embolism. JAMA 256:744, 1986.

National Institutes of Health Consensus Development Conference: The treatment of sleep disorders of older people. Sleep 14:169, 1991.

Nevitt MS, Cummings SR, Kidd S, et al: Risk factors for recurrent non-syncopal falls: A prospective study. JAMA 261:2663, 1989.

Nicolle LE, Orr P, Duckworth H, et al: Gross hematuria in residents of long-term care facilities. Am J Med 94:611, 1993.

Niessen LC, Douglass CW: Preventive actions for enhancing oral health. Clin Geriatr Med 8:201, 1992.

Nolan L, O'Malley K: Prescribing for the elderly: Part II, Prescribing patterns: Differences due to age. J Am Geriatr Soc 36:245, 1988.

Norman DC, Grahn D, Yoshikawa TT: Fever and aging. J Am Geriatr Soc 33:859, 1985.

Nutt J: Levadopa-induced dyskinesia: Review, observations, and speculations. Neurology 40:340, 1990.

O'Brien WM: Benign prostatic hypertrophy. Am Fam Physician 44:162, 1991.

Oddone EZ, Feussner JR, Cohen HJ: Can screening older patients for cancer save lives? Clin Geriatr Med 8:51, 1992.

Olhagen B: Polymyalgia rheumatica. Clin Rheum Dis 12:33, 1986.

O'Malley TA, Everitt DE, O'Malley HC, et al: Identifying and preventing family mediated abuse and neglect of elderly persons. Ann Intern Med 98:998, 1983.

Osborn M, Hawton K, Gath D: Sexual dysfunction among middle-aged women in the community. BMJ 296:959, 1988.

Ouslander JG, Leach G, Abelson S, et al: Simple versus multichannel cystometry in the evaluation of bladder function in an incontinent geriatric population. J Urol 40:1482, 1988.

Ouslander JG, Palmer MH, Rovner BW, German PS: Urinary incontinence in nursing homes: Incidence, remission and associated factors. J Am Geriatr Soc 41:1083, 1993.

Palolisso G, Cennamo G, Marfella R, et al: Exaggerated orthostatic hypotension as first sign of diabetic autonomic neuropathy in the elderly. Arch Gerontol Geriat 9:107, 1989.

Peto R, Gray R, Collins R, et al: Randomized trial of prophylactic daily aspirin in British male doctors. BMJ 296:313, 1988.

Pollock ML, Foster C, Knapp D, et al: Effect of age and training on aerobic capacity and body composition of master athletes. J Appl Physiol 62:725, 1987.

Prinz PN, Vitiello MV, Raskind MA: Geriatrics: Sleep disorders and aging. N Engl J Med 323:520, 1990.

Ramsdell JW, Swart JA, Jackson JE, Renvall M: The yield of a home visit in the assessment of geriatric patients. J Am Geriatr Soc 37:17, 1989.

Resnick NM, Yalla SV: Management of urinary incontinence in the elderly. N Engl J Med 313:800, 1985.

Resnick NM, Yalla SV: Detrusor hyperactivity with impaired contractile function: An unrecognized common cause of incontinence in elderly patients. JAMA 257:3076, 1987.

Reuben DB, Siu AL: An objective measurement of physical function of elderly outpatients: The Physical Performance Test. J Am Geriatr Soc 38:1105, 1990.

Reynolds C: Management of the diabetic surgical patient: A systemic but flexible plan is the key. Postgrad Med 77:265, 1985.

Richardson JP: Bacteremia in the elderly. J Gen Intern Med 8:89, 1993.

Robinson RG, Kubos KL, Starr LB, et al: Mood disorders in stroke patients: The importance of location of the lesion. Brain 107:81, 1984.

Ronald AR, Nicolle LE, Harding GKM: Standards of therapy for urinary tract infections in adults. Infection 20(suppl 3):S164, 1992.

Rovner DW, Kafonek S, Phillips L, et al: Prevalence of mental illness in a community nursing home. Am J Psychiatry 143:1446, 1986.

Rowe JW, Andres R, Tobin JD, et al: The effects of age on creatinine clearance in man: A cross-section and longitudinal study. J Gerontol 3:155, 1976.

Rowe JW, Shock NW, DeFronzo RA: The influence of age on the renal response to water deprivation in man. Nephron 17:270, 1976.

Rubenstein LV, Calkins DR, Greenfield S, et al: Health status assessment for elderly patients: Report of the Society of General Internal Medicine Task Force on Health Assessment. J Am Geriatr Soc 37:562, 1989.

Rudensky B, Lipschitz M, Isaacsohn M, Sonnenblick M: Infected pressure sores: Comparison of methods for bacterial identification. South Med J 85:901, 1992.

Russell EJ: Cervical disk disease. Radiology 177:313, 1990.

Sager MA, Easterling DV, Kindig DA, Anderson OW: Changes in the location of death after passage of Medicare's Prospective Payment System. N Engl J Med 320:433, 1989.

Sainesbury R, Gillespie WJ, Armour PC, Newman EF: An orthopedic geriatric rehabilitation unit: The first 2 years experience. N Z Med J 99:583, 1986.

Selby JV, Friedman GD, Quesenberry CP, Weiss NS: A case control study of screening sigmoidoscopy and mortality from colorectal cancer. N Engl J Med 326:653, 1992.

Shapiro S, Venet W, Strax P, et al (eds): Periodic Screening for Breast Cancer. Baltimore, Johns Hopkins Press, 1988.

SHEP Cooperative Research Group: Prevention of stroke by antihypertensive drug treatment in older persons with isolated systolic hypertension: Final results of the Systolic Hypertension in the Elderly Program (SHEP). JAMA 265:3255, 1991.

Silliman RA, McGarvey ST, Ramond PM, Fretwell MD: The Senior Care Study: Does inpatient interdisciplinary assessment help the family caregivers of acutely ill older patients? J Am Geriatr Soc 38:461, 1990.

Silverstone T, Goodall E: Serotinergic mechanisms in human feedings: The pharmacological evidence. Appetite 7(suppl):85, 1986.

Sinaki M, Wahner HW, Offord KP, et al: Efficacy of non-loading exercises in prevention of vertebral bone loss in post-menopausal women: A controlled trial. Mayo Clin Proc 64:762, 1989.

Sivenius J, Kaveli P: The significance of intensity of rehabilitation of stroke: A controlled trial. Stroke 16:928, 1985.

Siwek J: House calls: Current status and rationale. J Am Fam Physician 31:169, 1985.

Smith DM, Winsemius DK, Besdine RW: Pressure ulcers in the elderly: Can this outcome be improved? J Gen Intern Med 6:81, 1991.

Smith DS, Goldenberg E, Ashbum A, et al: Remedial therapy after stroke: A randomized controlled trial. Br Med J 282:517, 1986.

Stampfer MJ, Colditz GA, Willet WC, et al: Postmenopausal estrogen use and cardiovascular disease: Ten-year follow-up from the Nurses' Health Study. N Engl J Med 325:756, 1991.

Stead WW, Lofgren JP, Warren E, et al: Tuberculosis as an endemic and nosiocomial infection among the elderly in nursing homes. N Engl J Med 312:1483, 1985.

Steering Committee of the Physicians' Health Study Research Group: Preliminary report: Findings of the aspirin component of the ongoing physicians' health study. N Engl J Med 318:262, 1988.

Stone R, Cafferata GL, Saryl K: Caregivers of the frail elderly: A national profile. Gerontologist 27:616, 1987.

Stuck AE, Siu AL, Wieland GD, et al: Comprehensive geriatric assessment: A meta-analysis of controlled trials. Lancet 342:1032, 1993.

Stunkard AJ: Conservative treatments for obesity. Am J Clin Nutr 45:1142, 1987.

Sue TF, Tanagho EA: Physiology of erection and pharmacological management of impotence. J Urol 137:820, 1987.

Terpenning MS, Buggy BP, Kauffman CA: Infective endocarditis: Clinical features in young and elderly patients. Am J Med 83:626, 1987.

Tetrud JL, Langston JW: The effect of deprenyl (selegiline) on the natural history of Parkinson's disease. Science 245:519, 1989.

Tinetti ME: Performance oriented assessment of mobility problems in elderly patients. J Am Geriatr Soc 34:119, 1986.

Tinetti ME, Speechley M, Ginter SF: Risk factors for falls among elderly persons living in the community. N Engl J Med 319:1701, 1988.

Tisi GM: Preoperative identification and evaluation of a patient with lung disease. Med Clin North Am 71:399, 1987.

Toradello O, Boscia FM: Sexuality in aging: A study of a group of 300 elderly men and women. J Endocrinol Invest 8(suppl):123, 1985.

Tulloch AH, Moore V: A randomized controlled trial of geriatric screening and surveillance of general practice. J R Coll Gen Pract 29:732, 1979.

U.S. Department of Health and Human Services: The Health Benefits of Smoking Cessation: A Report of the Surgeon General. DHHS publication no. CDC90-8416. Washington, DC: U.S. Department of Health and Human Services, 1990.

U.S. Preventive Services Task Force: Guide to Clinical Preventive Services: An Assessment of 169 Interventions. Baltimore, Williams & Wilkins, 1989a.

U.S. Preventive Services Task Force: Screening for Glaucoma. *In* Guide to Clinical Preventive Services: An Assessment of the Effectiveness of 169 Interventions. Baltimore, Williams & Wilkins, 1989b, pp 187–192.

U.S. Preventive Services Task Force: Screening for Glaucoma: *In* Guide to Clinical Preventive Services: An Assessment of the Effectiveness of 169 Interventions. Baltimore, Williams & Wilkins, 1989c.

Urinary Incontinence in Adults Guideline Panel: Urinary Incontinence in Adults: Quick Reference Guide for Clinicians (AHCPR publication no. 92-0038). Rockville, MD, Agency for Health Care Policy and Research, 1992.

Vorhers D, Riley BE: Deconditioning. Clin Geriatr Med 9:745, 1993.

Warren JW, Damron D, Tenney JH, et al: Fever, bacteremia, and death as complications of bacteriuria in women with long-term urethral catheters. J Infect Dis 155:1151, 1987.

Warren JW, Muncie HL, Bergquist EJ, Hoopes JM: Sequelae and management of urinary infection in the patient requiring chronic catheterization. J Urol 125:1, 1982.

Warshaw GA: New perspectives in the management of Alzheimer's disease. Am Fam Physician 42(suppl 5):41S, 1990.

Wasserman M, Levinstein M, Keller E, et al: Utility of fever, white blood cells, and differential count in predicting bacterial infection in the elderly. J Am Geriatr Soc 37:537, 1989.

Watts NB, Harris ST, Genant HK, et al: Intermittent cyclical etidronate treatment of postmenopausal osteoporosis. N Engl J Med 323:73, 1990.

Weitz HH: Non-cardiac surgery in the elderly patient with cardiovascular disease. Clin Geriatr Med 6:511, 1990.

Weitz HH, Goldman L: Non-cardiac surgery in the patient with heart disease. Med Clin North Am 71:413, 1987.

White AA, Paryabi MM: Biomechanical considerations in the surgical management of cervical spondylitic myelopathy. Spine 13:856, 1988.

Williams AF, Carsten O: Driver age and crash involvement. Am J Publ Health 79:326, 1989.

Williams TF, Hill, JG, Fairbank, ME, et al: Appropriate placement of the chronically ill and aged: A successful approach by evaluation. J Am Med Assoc 226:1332, 1973.

Williams ME, Williams TF, Zimmer JG: How does the team approach to outpatient geriatric evaluation compare with traditional care: A report of a randomized controlled trial. J Am Geriatr Soc 35:1071, 1987.

Winograd CH, Stearns C: Inpatient geriatric consultation, challenges and benefits. J Am Geriatr Soc 38:926, 1990.

Wolf E, Lilling M, Ferber I, Marcus J: Prosthetic rehabilitation of elderly bilateral amputees. Int J Rehabil Res 12:271, 1989.

Wolfe BM, Huff MW. Effects of combined estrogen and progestin administration of plasma lipoprotein metabolism in postmenopausal women. J Clin Invest 83:40, 1989.

Woolf SH, Kamerow KB, Lawrence RS, et al: The periodic health examination of older adults: The recommendations of the U.S. Preventive Services Task Force. Part I, Counseling, immunizations and chemoprophylaxis. J Am Geriatr Soc 38:817, 1990a.

Woolf SH, Kamerow KB, Lawrence RS, et al: The periodic health examination of older adults: The recommendations of the U.S. Preventive Services Task Force. Part II, Screening tests. J Am Geriatr Soc 38:933, 1990b.

Wrenn K: Fecal impaction. N Engl J Med 321:658, 1989.

Yablon SA, Krotenberg R, Fruhmann K: Clostridium difficile related disease: Evaluation and prevalence among inpatients with diarrhea in two free-standing rehabilitation hospitals. Arch Phys Med Rehabil 74:9, 1993.

Yesavage JA, Brink TL, Rose TL, et al: Development and validation of a geriatric depression screening scale: A preliminary report. J Psychiatr Res 17:37, 1983.

Young JB, Forster A: The Bradford community stroke trial results at six months. Br Med J 304:1085, 1992.

Zauber NP, Zauber AG: Hematologic data of healthy very old people. JAMA 257:2181, 1987.

Zuckerman JD, Sakales SR, Sabian DR, Frankle VH: Hip fractures in geriatric patients: Results of an interdisciplinary hospital care program. Clin Orthop Rel Res 274:213, 1992.

CHAPTER 8
CARE OF THE DYING PATIENT

ROBERT E. RAKEL and PORTER STOREY

Medical education and our professional attitude regarding patient care is oriented primarily toward sustaining life and curing disease. This is reasonable, because it was only a short time ago that the major causes of death were the infectious diseases, and they usually attacked young people who died before experiencing the joys of life. With the advent of antibiotics, it was possible to triumph over these diseases and prevent untimely death. Patients had a high probability of complete recovery. It is no surprise, then, that the profession placed an emphasis on preserving life at all costs and became preoccupied with the advancing technology that made such triumphs possible. Today, people no longer die of acute illness but instead of chronic disease for which there is no cure. This calls for medicine to focus on improving the quality rather than the quantity of life and to recognize that the relief of suffering is superior to attempts to cure when there is limited likelihood of success. Patients with chronic diseases and those who are terminally ill will benefit most from good supportive therapy.

In previous centuries, it was assumed that one's whole life should be so lived that one would be able to "die well," but contemporary American culture has refused to accept death as a normal occurrence. Children and young adults have been conditioned to consider death from the viewpoint of the observer or disinterested third party. An individual's attitude toward his or her own death depends to a large extent on experiences of dealing with the deaths of relatives or friends. Rather than being a time of despair, sickness may be used as an opportunity for reflection. For some patients, it may be the first time they have faced their own mortality. However, too often what naturally would be a very personal encounter has been depersonalized by removal of the dying patient to an institutional setting.

Too often, care of a terminally ill patient centers primarily on the disease, and the patient as a whole person is neglected. The value of treatment must be interpreted on the basis of its net value to the individual. When additional treatments no longer provide benefits, the patient then needs concerned care from someone who provides personalized care with attention to the patient's emotional as well as physical comfort. The dying person often is isolated physically and emotionally from familiar surroundings and placed in a social setting that gives very low priority to an individual's personality, fears, and past experiences. Informed physicians, family, and friends can do much to help the terminal patient die with integrity and with dignity. However, if dying is really to be accepted as a normal component of the life cycle, then reintegration of the dying patient into the routine course of living is necessary.

The concept of quality care does not always demand that death be regarded as an enemy to be fought with every weapon at a physician's disposal. An obsession with quantity of life can adversely affect its quality . . . there are times when graceful death with dignity is preferable to lingering torment. (LORAN Commission, 1989, p. 27)

THE PHYSICIAN'S ATTITUDE

In some ways terminal illness is more taxing on the physician than sudden and unexpected death. It is not surprising for an empathic family physician who has enjoyed a long and close relationship with a patient to be uncomfortable in dealing with the patient's impending death. Physicians are most uncomfortable when they feel helpless. Unfortunately, this leads to withdrawal from the patient who is terminally ill because the physician inappropriately feels helpless and impotent, when in fact a great deal of comfort and help can be provided. While expressing concern and compassion for a terminal patient, the family physician still must maintain composure and objectivity to remain effective. Osler (1904) referred to this as "calm equanimity" and added, "Our equanimity is chiefly exercised in enabling us to bear with composure the misfortunes of our neighbors" (p. 8). Medicine long has emphasized the need for physicians to remain objective and deal with problems factually; if a physician is unable to do so effectively, attempts to hide emotion may lead the physician to adopt a facade that appears unsympathetic and insensitive to the patient's needs. A son reported that "with the worsening of my father's condition, the physician stopped being friendly and warm; his visits became rare and brief; his manner became quite detached, almost angry" (Seravalli, 1988, p. 1729). Such a physician fears rejection and alienation.

Physicians sometimes lose enthusiasm for care once an illness has been recognized as incurable and inevitably fatal. If this occurs, interaction with the patient diminishes at the very time emotional support is needed most and the patient's fear of abandonment is greatest. Time–motion studies indicate that nurses and other ward personnel also spend less time with the terminally ill patient when giving baths and providing routine care. During the terminal stages of a fatal illness, it is vital to the dying patient that the family physician maintain a warm and caring relationship and, through the strength of the doctor–patient bond, provide support for the patient.

The physician who is uncomfortable discussing impending death can discourage conversation in many subtle ways. Hospital rounds are made rapidly, perhaps in a superficial, lighthearted manner, never pausing long enough to give the patient an opportunity to express fears and concerns. Comments such as "Everything will be all right" effectively close lines of communication with an intelligent patient who is fully aware of the seriousness of the situation. When the physician tells a patient, "Don't worry," the patient interprets this as, "Don't bother me." Patients are unlikely to initiate discussions regarding their fears of death or feelings of helplessness under such circumstances and will remain silent or avoid these issues unless they feel the physician is willing to listen and is interested in them. The physician easily can squelch such conversation; but a slight indication of willingness to discuss the problems disturbing the patient often results in frank conversations, which relieve much of the patient's anxiety and bring into the open concerns that can be shared with no one other than the physician.

The "Right Time" To Die

Simpson (1976) described the "how dare you die on me" syndrome, in which the patient has the effrontery to die before medical and nursing staff have used all the treatments in their repertoire. The patient is supposed to die "at the right time"—neither before all potential effective therapies have been tried nor too long after all palliative procedures have been utilized. Health professionals often have a need to feel that everything possible was done for the patient prior to death. These attitudes have developed because the health care process too often focuses more on the health professionals' expectations than on the patients' needs.

We might consider what we have done to the patient who dies in the isolation of a laminar flow room, without having been able to touch another person's hand during his last few weeks of life. Such treatment is a false-positive, a treatment inappropriate to the real needs of the patient. (Saunders, 1976, p. 227)

However, it is impossible for physicians to provide adequate support during this difficult time unless they have come to grips with their own mortality. Studies by the Group for the Advancement of Psychiatry have revealed that physicians are afraid of death in greater proportion than controls of patients (Aring, 1971). What better defense against death than to make one's full-time vocation fighting it? Confronting and accepting one's mortality is good mental health practice for anyone, but it is professionally necessary for all who deal regularly with death: physicians, clergy, counselors, police, nurses, firefighters, funeral directors, ambulance drivers, and so on.

COMMUNICATION

When to Tell the Patient

The issue today is not so much whether or not to tell patients they have a terminal illness but how to share this information with them—because most patients know the nature of their disease process to some degree. Because family physicians know their patients well, they should be able to gauge patients' desire to be told and their capacity to withstand the shock of disclosure.

A frank discussion of death or of how long the patient is expected to live may not be necessary or even indicated. A good understanding between doctor and patient may make open disclosure unnecessary. The physician's role may be primarily one of supporting patients during the progressive terminal course of their illness. Such a situation should not be used by the physician who is uncomfortable with the subject as an excuse to avoid discussing the issue, however. The family physician's primary responsibility is to take the time to evaluate the situation, make sure the patient's true desires have been assessed correctly, and provide whatever support is needed, based on the patient's concepts and needs rather than those of the physician.

The physician who can deal with death honestly is able to focus more attention on the patient and can determine the patient's level of awareness by listening and observing nonverbal cues. Clues to the patient's wish to discuss his or her condition may be nothing more than a deep sigh, a tear, or a shaky voice. The physician must be alert during busy hospital rounds for these or similar signs. The physician can pause to sit and encourage conversation if time permits, or return later when more time is available. Whenever possible, however, the response should be at that moment, because the patient is more likely to communicate freely in a spontaneous situation. A physician who is uncomfortable in this situation may be found insulating himself or herself from the issue during hospital rounds by checking every inch of the intravenous tubing for air bubbles or otherwise directing his or her attention away from the patient, effectively ignoring overt as well as subtle clues to the patient's needs.

When the patient is ready to discuss his or her impending death, physician and patient are probably past the most difficult stage and the physician needs merely to listen, accept the patient's feelings, and respond to questions honestly. Most patients will raise questions that indicate how much they wish to know, provided the physician gives them the opportunity. The most supportive and facilitative act the physician can provide is to sit and ask the patient "Do you have any questions?" When asked in a sincere manner, patients who are ready to talk about their death will take advantage of the opportunity, but they may be reluctant under other, more hurried circumstances.

Patients also usually will indicate when they would like to discuss their prognosis, and will let the physician know when they would like to avoid the subject altogether and focus on more pleasant topics. Even patients who have reached a full level of acceptance of their terminal process cannot remain constantly focused on that subject and must divert their attention to more satisfying issues from time to time. Physicians should honor and respond to this need, just as they would respond to a desire to discuss pain or other problems.

What physicians say to dying patients is not nearly as important as their willingness to listen. One of the most comforting steps physicians can take in caring for the dying is to allow them to talk about their fears, frustrations, hopes, needs, and desires. *Talking about problems can be very therapeutic.* Patients who are permitted to examine and discuss their feelings about death and dying are grateful for the opportunity and usually become less anxious, experience less pain, and accept their situation more easily. If they are denied this opportunity, especially when the terminal process is obvious, they may be convinced that the time remaining is too terrible to be discussed, and their anxiety will be significantly increased. Often the terminally ill are more fearful of the manner in which death will occur (e.g., painful, alone and abandoned, weak and helpless) than they are of death itself.

Do all patients wish to be told of their fatal illness, however? Surveys indicate that 80 to 90 per cent of patients say they wish to be told, whereas many physicians prefer not to tell a patient that he or she is dying. A study by Ward (1974) revealed that family physicians are more likely to discuss a fatal diagnosis with women than with men (22 versus 7.5 per cent) and more often with patients in the upper social class than the lower social class (24 versus 5 per cent for men and 30 versus 26 per cent for women). Many physicians who state they theoretically believe in telling the patient of the terminal nature of his or her illness employ evasion in their actual practice as often as most other physicians. Because of this reluctance, which may be based on discomfort with the issue emanating from intensive conditioning to preserve health and maintain life, future medical students must be trained more adequately in assisting patients with the process of living just prior to death.

Most physicians will tell a patient that he or she has terminal cancer if the patient asks a direct question, but otherwise will evade the issue and discuss it openly only with the family. There are many occasions when this is the most appropriate course of action; not infrequently, patients are encountered who clearly indicate they cannot and do not wish to face the fact that they have an incurable disease. It is essential, however, that the physician evaluate the true nature of the patient's desire in the matter and neither avoid the issue when the patient wishes to discuss it nor force a discussion on an unwilling individual. "When the task of telling a patient about an onerous diagnosis is too easy, the doctor has become callous. When it is too difficult, he needs to examine his own guilt or anxiety." (Weisman and Brettell, 1978, p. 251).

Patients should be given adequate time to absorb the knowledge of the terminal nature of their illness and the opportunity to react appropriately before death intervenes. This is not possible if the physician procrastinates or rationalizes that it is better not to inform the patient. The process should not be allowed to advance to so final a stage that there is inadequate time remaining for the individual to react appropriately and put his or her affairs in order.

There is no need to answer questions the patient has not yet asked. One way to approach the subject is to ask patients what they think the problem is, or how sick they think they really are. The response may be straightforward ("I think I have cancer"), or the patient may indicate a wish to avoid the issue by saying, "I hope it's nothing serious." The patient's condition can be revealed gradually or in stages, such as telling him or her following surgery that there is a suspicion of cancer but that further information will have to wait for the pathology report. The physician should observe the patient's response to this initial hint and, based on that reaction, choose a method for presenting subsequent information. Tumulty (1973) supported the concept of gradualism in informing a patient and the family of the terminal nature of the illness:

The total truth is revealed in small doses as the illness unfolds, affording the family the opportunity to get its feet under itself before another blow falls. . . . The patient and the family need to be eased into the truth . . . not slugged with it. (pp. 180–181)

Such a gradual disclosure is likely to lead to acceptance, whereas a harsh, sudden, or abrupt disclosure is likely to result in denial or severe depression. If the patient appears reluctant to accept the information, do not push the issue; merely make sure that openings for discussion are made available periodically and further information provided when the patient is ready.

When sharing information regarding a fatal diagnosis with a patient, eye contact, touch, and personal closeness are important. If possible, sit with the patient and hold his or her hand or touch the forearm. Such gestures convey a sense of support, closeness, and compassion, reinforcing verbal assurance that he or she will not be abandoned during the difficult time remaining. Sitting with the patient on the bed or at the bedside rather than standing puts the physician on the same level and conveys in a clear, nonverbal manner a willingness to talk and listen. A study was done in which physicians visited with hospitalized patients for exactly 3 minutes. Half of the visits they sat down and the other half they remained standing, a little removed from the bed. "Every one of the patients [with whom] the physician had sat down thought the physician had stayed at least 10 minutes. None of the ones [with whom] the physician remained standing estimated that it was as long" (Kubler-Ross, 1975, p. 20).

Prognosticating

One of the most difficult tasks in medicine is predicting how long someone with a terminal illness will live. People enjoy repeating stories of patients who survived long after the date their doctor predicted. In most cases, however, physicians tend to be overly optimistic, and short estimates are more accurate than longer ones (Evans and McCarthy, 1985). Attempts have been made to develop indexes (e.g., the Karnofsky Index) that assist the physician in making objective estimates that correlate with actual survival. However, no accurate method is currently available, largely because of the multiple variables that influence when a patient dies. A good policy is to provide a conservative estimate. It is better to have the patient and family proud that they "beat the odds" or exceeded the physician's prediction than to have the patient die earlier than anticipated.

Conspiracy of Silence

Honesty with the terminal patient will provide the greatest benefits. However, the physician frequently is torn between patient and family, with the patient saying, "Don't tell my wife because she can't handle it," while the wife is saying, "Don't tell my husband because he can't handle it." Al-

though the wishes and desires of the family must be considered when deciding how to care for a dying patient, the physician's primary obligation is to the patient. The method of management must be based on the physician's knowledge of the patient and insight into his or her desires, feelings, and approach to life. Despite all efforts at deception, the patient knows or will soon learn about his or her condition anyway.

By cooperating with the family in a conspiracy of silence, information that really belongs to the patient is withheld. Only if the physician believes the patient is not yet ready to cope with the information or sincerely wishes not to be told should the information be withheld. This is more often the exception than the rule, however. One patient said, "I knew it was cancer from the moment they started lying to me" (Lamerton, 1976, p. 28). Simpson (1976) described a 63-year-old woman whose family insisted she knew nothing of her inoperable gastric carcinoma. When visited by the physician, "She gave a dry chuckle: 'Only a little ulcer . . . and my relatives down from Wales to see me for the first time in 15 years, and the priest here at 6 in the morning?'" (p. 193). Obviously the patient knew the seriousness of her condition, and the mutual deception was nothing more than a charade. When such a game continues, terminally ill patients become more and more isolated because they are unable to communicate honestly and openly with those closest to them about their concerns and fears. The elaborate schemes some families and physicians develop to "protect" the patient lead to a great deal of tension within the family, as everyone attempts to perpetuate the lie while continuing to interact with the patient.

Similarly, failure to provide the information to the patient's family can lead to a decrease in the quality of their relationship in the time remaining, because tensions and fears felt by the patient are not understood by those close to him or her. Dunphy (1976) described an incident in which a patient with terminal cancer asked that his wife not be told. He then quickly planned a world cruise, which they had wanted to take for some time. The wife, unaware of the reason for the hasty departure, was unhappy and complaining throughout the trip, while the husband saw himself as a silent martyr, trying to provide a final measure of happiness for his wife. Only after returning home and reminiscing on this miserable cruise did he tell his wife the truth and the reason for the precipitous departure. Had she been told earlier, each one of their final days together could have been a pleasant and memorable experience.

DENIAL

Most patients tend to deny the reality of their situation after being made aware of the terminal nature of their illness. Denial is one way of coping with or protecting oneself against overwhelming anxiety, which otherwise could be incapacitating. This reaction is more marked in the patient who is told abruptly without being adequately prepared beforehand. Although denial is noted primarily when the patient first learns of his or her impending death, it can appear in different degrees at different times. Even patients who have reached the level of acceptance of the terminal nature of their illness will need to employ denial periodically to avoid feelings of hopelessness. The mental burden of impending death is too heavy to carry all the time, and periodic relief is necessary in order to carry on customary activities and enjoy the limited time left. As Aring (1971) noted, La Rochefoucauld said: "Neither the sun nor death can be looked at steadily."

A patient who avoids asking about his or her illness or prognosis when the physician offers every opportunity for him or her to do so normally is experiencing denial. Excessive denial usually means that the patient subconsciously knows the truth but wishes to avoid facing it consciously. Even when repeatedly given the accurate diagnosis, some patients deny ever having been told. This denial provides constant emotional protection until the patient is ready to face the truth.

WATCH WITH ME

The greatest fear of the dying patient is that of suffering alone and being deserted. There is less fear of a painful death than of the loneliness and alienation that may accompany it. A patient particularly dreads being abandoned by the physician in the face of death, and may need increasing levels of professional support as the illness progresses. This is particularly true if family and friends are not able to cope with the deteriorating condition and begin to avoid contact, thus contributing further to the patient's feelings of loneliness and abandonment. If the patient feels he or she has no one with whom to discuss his or her condition or to relate in an open and honest fashion, despair is likely to ensue. The patient's fear of the unknown is easier to cope with if his or her apprehension can be shared with a caring physician who provides comfort, support, encouragement, and even a modicum of hope.

Each new problem of the dying patient should be viewed as a nuisance requiring relief or removal and approached with the vigor that one would devote to an acute, short-term illness. Whenever a fresh complaint arises, the patient should be reexamined and attempts made to relieve the symptom so the patient will not feel unworthy of further attention. If everyday nuisances can be controlled or lessened, the patient will feel there is sincere concern for making his or her remaining life pleas-

ant. The physician should give attention to details such as improving the taste of food by fixing or replacing dentures or stimulating the patient's appetite, eliminating foul odors, or suggesting occupational therapy in an attempt to avoid boredom. The physician should take advantage of every opportunity to touch and examine the patient rather than standing apart. Gentle palpation of areas of pain or merely taking a pulse can convey a sense of concern and warmth and provide comfort for an apprehensive and lonely patient. The physician and other health professionals can provide a great deal of support merely through conversation. The tendency to withdraw and reduce conversation contributes to the patient's sense of loneliness. Silence is an enemy of the dying and serves to widen their separation from society. Conversation is a social bond that affirms life and reduces anxiety by providing a means of catharsis. Saunders (1976) summed up the needs of a dying patient with the words of one patient: "Watch with me," asking that he not be abandoned in his final days. The readiness to listen and personal, caring contact are comforts that cannot be matched by our modern wonder drugs and procedures.

When dying patients notice that people are avoiding them, they may interpret it as rejection because they have failed to get better or see it as the loss of love from family and friends. The last-mentioned situation is particularly traumatic, because it tends to negate relationships the patient has cherished throughout life. The pleasures and joys of a rewarding life can suddenly appear to lose their value as the dying patient reflects over past events if he or she is ignored or avoided during these final days. The dying patient's contentment is dependent on maintaining warm relationships with loved ones as well as continuing other satisfying interpersonal relationships—such as with the physician. If physicians and others withdraw from interaction with the terminally ill patient, much of the motivation for living disappears and is replaced by despair or terminal depression. The following plea to fellow health professionals is from a young student nurse who was terminally ill (Kubler-Ross, 1975):

I know you feel insecure, don't know what to say, don't know what to do. But please believe me, if you care, you can't go wrong. Just admit that you care. . . . All I want to know is that there will be someone to hold my hand when I need it. I am afraid. Death may get to be a routine to you, but it is new to me. You may not see me as unique! . . . If only we could be honest, both admit of our fears, touch one another. If you really care, would you lose so much of your valuable professionalism if you even cried with me? Just person to person? Then, it might not be so hard to die—in a hospital—with friends close by. (p. 26)

PATIENT CONTROL

Terminally ill patients have a need to believe that they are still in control of their affairs as far as possible, even though they have lost control of their bodies. They should be given the freedom to make choices and assume responsibility over as many aspects of their existence as possible. For many individuals, this is an essential part of living, and its loss may destroy their motivation to live. A terminally ill patient should be helped to focus on and cope with the realities of daily living, because these problems remain very real and can serve as a diversion from constant preoccupation with the prospect of death. When patients have understanding and insight into the treatment and feels they still have some control over the decision-making process regarding their lives, they are more likely to cooperate with prescribed treatment regimens. It is often fear of the unknown that makes a patient suspicious and resistant to therapy. The patient also should be given the opportunity to settle his or her affairs. Concentration on preparing his or her financial business and putting the house in order is a pragmatic approach to active participation in the decision-making process. Some patients may have a burning desire to complete a cherished project, reconcile an estranged relationship, or visit particular places before they die. Positive motivation can be maintained by assisting them to focus on and deal with these issues.

A sense of control is more possible for the patient if pain is controlled and he or she is made comfortable. Sleep should not be forced with medication, because some patients resist going to sleep, fearing they may never awaken, while others frequently have terrifying dreams.

THE IMPORTANCE OF HOPE

Hope is one of the essential ingredients of human existence, without which life is dark and cold and frustrating. It maintains strength and gives substance to courage. In the presence of hope, suffering of all sorts still has some positive qualities. In its absence, suffering is a completely negative experience. (Tumulty, 1973, p. 171)

Twycross (1986) defined hope as having "an expectation greater than zero of achieving a desired goal." The physician should not raise false hopes or be overly aggressive in treating a terminal illness to help the patient maintain hope. However, advanced cancer patients can maintain a positive outlook on life. The physician can help direct a patient toward an achievable goal such as pain relief, support for the family from a hospice service, or making a trip to visit relatives.

Hope increases when honest information is provided, and it is reduced when information is withheld.

Even when death is near, the patient can hope for a measure of happiness during the amount of time he or she has remaining. The physician can support the patient's hope for a good quality of life

in the remaining time, for spiritual healing, and for a final phase of life that has integrity and dignity.

PROLONGING LIVING OR PROLONGING DYING?

It has been a long time since pneumonia was accepted as "the old man's friend." As one organic system after another slowed to a halt, the aged person was released from nausea, pain, delirium, and the degradation of lingering deterioration by finally developing pneumonia and dying. The family doctor merely showed concern and support; before antibiotics there was not much to do but stand by and "let nature take its course." With improved medical care, it is possible that a person whose dying process might have taken only a few days in previous years now can have the unrewarding dying experience dragged out for months (Veatch, 1972). Modern technology makes it possible to carry the benefits of improved medical care to unrealistic extremes; one person was kept alive in a vegetative state for over 37 years (LORAN Commission, 1989).

Protraction of the dying process is a modern epidemic. Some physicians seem to forget that their primary responsibility is to relieve suffering, not to prolong it. Greater clinical skill often is required to provide daily supportive care than to cure acute illness. Tenderness and caring must be included in the protocols of the terminally ill so that the ravaged patient is allowed to die peacefully, without tubing and respirators. Patients should "be allowed to experience those waning moments unencumbered by high-tech devices that serve only to impede their capacity for human interaction. Here it is the patient's comfort, not the caregiver's need "to do something", that should prevail" (LORAN Commission, 1989, p. 29).

Sometimes therapeutic restraint is necessary to permit a patient to die with dignity. When a cure is no longer possible, care should focus on the comfort of patient and family. At St. Christopher's Hospice in London, medical equipment is shunned and feeding is provided by human hands instead of nasogastric or intravenous tubes: "even if the patient does not get enough physical nourishment, he or she gets what is more important—the personal nourishment of someone who cares enough to sit by the bed several hours each day" (Nelson and Rohricht, 1984, p. 174).

MANAGEMENT OF SYMPTOMS

A great deal can be done to help a patient whose disease is incurable. The family physician can help alleviate the fear, symptoms, and family stress that so often make this a distressing time. Care of the dying patient can be one of the most rewarding aspects of the family physician's practice. Yet, too often, the physician's discomfort with this stage of life contributes to the isolation and discouragement of the terminally ill patient. Unwarranted fears of respiratory depression, addiction, or tolerance prevent the prescribing of adequate amounts of analgesics. The resulting uncontrolled pain makes those final weeks a nightmare for all. Families may disintegrate as a result of the sleepless nights, fears, and guilt that come from trying to cope with uncontrolled symptoms. Who needs a physician more than this family?

Good control of pain, nausea, and dyspnea can enable patients to die in the place of their choosing with comfort and dignity. Families can cope with their responsibilities and carry good memories of their loved one's final weeks. Physicians can feel gratified at the excellent relief from distress they can provide in this trying time.

The keys to symptom control, as in all areas of medicine, are a careful history and physical examination to determine the various causes of discomfort and a broad knowledge of the therapeutic agents available.

Pain Control

Chronic pain is influenced by memories of past pain and by the anticipation of pain yet to come. The fear of worsening pain may color the present perception of discomfort. Frustration and anxiety may accentuate the pain. All of these factors can lower the patient's pain threshold so that even minor disturbances take on immense proportions (Twycross, 1993).

Failure to treat the whole person often results in inadequate pain control for patients with terminal cancer. Fatigue, insomnia, anxiety, boredom, and anger all contribute to a lower threshold of pain. Rest, sleep, diversion, and companionship all help to increase the patient's tolerance for pain.

Analgesics should be given in adequate amounts to provide comfort. The approach to analgesic medication in which doses are given as needed should be abandoned in the treatment of dying patients, because it contributes to a lower pain threshold and a need for increasing doses of medication to relieve the pain. When medication is given regularly in adequate doses, the anxiety and fear that accentuate pain are avoided and lower doses of the drug are effective, because the patient no longer fears recurrence or "breakthrough."

High doses of narcotics may be necessary to obtain initial pain control in a patient with severe pain. Dependence is rarely a problem in patients who receive appropriate narcotic doses for chronic severe cancer pain. When medication is given *prior* to the recurrence of pain, craving for medication does not occur. There should be no more than

a 20 per cent reduction in dosage in any 2-day periods otherwise, withdrawal symptoms may occur.

Opioids

A symptom-oriented history and careful examination may reveal a number of different sources of pain. Oral candidiasis, decubitus ulcers, constipation, and infected wounds all have specific remedies. Most patients with pain from cancer (and many patients with pain from non-neoplastic illnesses) will require an opioid analgesic. Opioids are often the safest analgesics available, usually causing only temporary sedation and increased need for laxatives.

Concerns about addiction, respiratory depression, and tolerance usually are unwarranted in these patients (Twycross, 1993). If the dose is titrated carefully, the patient's pain (or dyspnea) usually can be controlled completely and the patient still can be alert and mentally clear on even hundreds of milligrams of oral morphine given every 4 hours (Bruera, 1990).

A number of effective oral narcotic preparations are available (Tables 8–1 and 8–2). If hydrocodone, 5 to 10 mg every 4 hours, is not adequate, oxycodone, 5 to 10 mg every 4 hours, should be used. Oral morphine beginning with 10 to 15 mg every 4 hours is usually the next step, but hydromorphone is a good alternative. The morphine dose should be titrated upward until analgesia lasts the full 4 hours, even if a dose of 300 mg every 4 hours is required.

The particular drug used is less important than the method of administration. In order to *prevent* pain and end the cycle of uncontrolled pain followed by oversedation, an oral narcotic should be administered on a regular schedule around the

TABLE 8–1. SELECTED ORAL NARCOTICS

Narcotic and Dose	Oral Morphine Equivalent (mg)
Codeine 30 mg + acetaminophen 300 mg (Tylenol No. 3)	1–2
Hydrocodone 5 mg + homatropine 1.5 mg (Hycodan)	1–2
Hydrocodone 5 mg + acetaminophen 500 mg (Vicodin)	1–2
Oxycodone 5 mg + aspirin 325 mg (Percodan)	5
Oxycodone 5 mg + acetaminophen 325 mg (Percocet)	5
Oxycodone 5 mg/5 mL (Roxicodone)	5/5 mL
Hydromorphone 2 mg (Dilaudid)	10
Fentanyl patches 50 μg/hr (Duragesic)	15 q 4 hr
Morphine	
Tablets (Lilly, Roxane, Purdue-Frederick)	10, 15, or 30
Syrup (Roxane, Purdue-Frederick)	10 or 20/5 mL
Solution (Roxane, Purdue-Frederick)	20/mL
Slow release (MS Contin 30 mg, Oramorph SR)	10 q 4 hr × 3

TABLE 8–2. DOSING DATA FOR OPIOID ANALGESICS

Drug	Approximate Equianalgesic Oral Dose*	Approximate Equianalgesic Parenteral Dose*	Recommended Starting Dose† (Adults > 50 kg Body Weight)		Recommended Starting Dose† (Children and Adults < 50 kg Body Weight)‡	
			Oral	Parenteral	Oral	Parenteral
Opioid Agonist						
Morphine§	30 mg q 3–4 hr (around-the-clock dosing)	10 mg q 3–4 hr	30 mg q 3–4 hr	10 mg q 3–4 hr	0.3 mg/kg q 3–4 hr	0.1 mg/kg q 3–4 hr
	60 mg q 3–4 hr (single dose or intermittent dosing)					
Codeine‖	130 mg q 3–4 hr	75 mg q 3–4 hr	60 mg q 3–4 hr	60 mg q 2 hr (intramuscular/ subcutaneous)	1 mg/kg 3–4 hr¶	Not recommended
Hydromorphone§ (Dilaudid)	7.5 mg q 3–4 hr	1.5 mg q 3–4 hr	6 mg q 3–4 hr	1.5 mg q 3–4 hr	0.06 mg/kg q 3–4 hr¶	0.015 mg/kg q 3–4 hr
Hydrocodone (in Lorcet, Lortab, Vicodin, others)	Equivalence data not substantiated	Not available	10 mg q 3–4 hr	Not available	0.2 mg/kg q 3–4 hr¶	Not available
Levorphanol (Levo-Dromoran)	4 mg q 6–8 hr	2 mg q 6–8 hr	4 mg q 6–8 hr	2 mg q 6–8 hr	0.04 mg/kg q 6–8 hr	0.02 mg/kg q 6–8 hr
Meperidine (Demerol)	300 mg q 2–3 hr	100 mg q 3 hr	Not recommended	100 mg q 3 hr	Not recommended	0.75 mg/kg q 2–3 hr
Methadone (Dolophine, others)	20 mg q 6–8 hr	10 mg q 6–8 hr	20 mg q 6–8 hr	10 mg q 6–8 hr	0.2 mg/kg q 6–8 hr	0.1 mg/kg q 6–8 hr
Oxycodone (Roxicodone, also in Percocet, Percodan, Tylox, others)	30 mg q 3–4 hr	Not available	10 mg q 3–4 hr	Not available	0.2 mg/kg q 3–4 hr¶	Not available
Oxymorphone§ (Numorphan)	Not available	1 mg q 3–4 hr	Not available	1 mg q 3–4 hr	Not recommended	Not recommended
Opioid Agonist–Antagonist and Partial Agonist						
Buprenorphine (Buprenex)	Not available	0.3–0.4 mg q 6–8 hr	Not available	0.4 mg q 6–8 hr	Not available	0.004 mg/kg q 6–8 hr
Butorphanol (Stadol)	Not available	2 mg q 3–4 hr	Not available	2 mg q 3–4 hr	Not available	Not recommended
Nalbuphine (Nubain)	Not available	10 mg q 3–4 hr	Not available	10 mg q 3–4 hr	Not available	0.1 mg/kg q 3–4 hr
Pentazocine (Talwin, others)	150 mg q 3–4 hr	60 mg q 3–4 hr	50 mg q 4–6 hr	Not recommended	Not recommended	Not recommended

* Note: Published tables vary in the suggested doses that are equianalgesic to morphine. Clinical response is the criterion that must be applied for each patient; titration to clinical response is necessary. Because there is not complete cross tolerance among these drugs, it is usually necessary to use a lower than equianalgesic dose when changing drugs and to retitrate to response.

† Caution: Recommended doses do not apply to patients with renal or hepatic insufficiency or other conditions affecting drug metabolism and kinetics.

‡ Caution: Doses listed for patients with body weight less than 50 kg cannot be used as initial starting doses in babies less than 6 months of age. Consult the *Clinical Practice Guideline for Acute Pain Management: Operative or Medical Procedures and Trauma* section on management of pain in neonates for recommendations.

§ For morphine, hydromorphone, and oxymorphone, rectal administration is an alternate route for patients unable to take oral medications, but equianalgesic doses may differ from oral and parenteral doses because of pharmacokinetic differences.

‖ Caution: Codeine doses above 65 mg often are not appropriate due to diminishing incremental analgesia with increasing doses but continually increasing constipation and other side effects.

¶ Caution: Doses of aspirin and acetaminophen in combination opioid/NSAID preparations must also be adjusted to the patient's body weight.

From Agency for Health Care Policy and Research: Acute Pain Management in Adults: Operative Procedures (Quick Reference Guide for Clinicians) (AHCPR publication no. 92-0019). Rockville, MD, Agency for Health Care Policy and Research, 1992.

clock. "Booster" doses equal to about half of the regular 4-hour dose can be used as needed for breakthrough pain. Long-acting drugs such as methadone (half-life 48 to 72 hours) can be prescribed every 6 to 8 hours, but are unsuitable for "booster" doses. They will accumulate over several days and are difficult to titrate, especially in patients who have fluctuating levels of pain or deteriorating renal or hepatic function. Slow-release morphine preparations such as MS Contin or Oramorph SR can provide excellent analgesia for 8 to 12 hours but are expensive and unsuitable for "booster" doses. These tablets may be given rectally when the patient cannot swallow (Wilkinson et al., 1992). Small, soluble tablets or concentrated solutions of morphine or hydromorphone can be given sublingually when the patient is too weak to swallow, and can be used for both 4-hour and booster doses. Transdermal fentanyl patches (Duragesic) are now available in 25-, 50-, 75-, and 100-μg/hr strengths. Because they are very expensive and deliver a wide variation of plasma levels (25-μg patch = 4 to 11 mg of oral morphine every 4 hours), they should be reserved for patients who cannot utilize the oral or subcutaneous routes. There is no need to use injections when an adequate dose by mouth will work as well. Table 8–3 provides a checklist of items to remember when prescribing an opioid.

Two opioid agents that also are available orally are not recommended for cancer pain. Meperidine (Demerol) has a very low oral potency, a short duration of action, and a toxic metabolite that can cause tremors or even seizures (Kaiko et al., 1983). Pentazocine (Talwin, Talacen) is an agonist–antagonist agent that is no more potent than aspirin with codeine and has a high incidence of psychotomimetic effects (hallucinations, confusion) in cancer patients.

TABLE 8–3. PHYSICIAN'S CHECKLIST WHEN PRESCRIBING OPIOIDS

1. Has an appropriate starting dose been determined?
2. Is a co-analgesic needed?
3. Is an antiemetic needed?
4. Has a laxative been prescribed?
5. Is the drug regimen written out in sufficient detail?
6. Has the patient been warned about possible side effects that might occur initially?
7. Do the patient and family know what to do if the pain remains uncontrolled?
8. Have arrangements been made for follow-up after 1, 3, and 7 days—either by the physician or by a trained hospice nurse?
9. Does the patient know what to do if he or she needs help or advice before the next follow-up visit?
10. Is the patient confident that the pain will improve considerably, probably within a few days, certainly within 1 or 2 weeks?

Modified from Twycross RG: Symptoms Control in Far Advanced Cancer: Pain Relief, 2nd edition. London, Pitman, 1993, with permission.

Co-Analgesics

Co-analgesics are drugs that potentiate the analgesic effects of opioids for particular types of pain (Table 8–4). Nonsteroidal anti-inflammatory drugs (NSAIDs) are quite helpful in the alleviation of pain from lesions in bones or skeletal muscles. The nonacetylated salicylates (e.g., salsalate [Disalcid], choline magnesium trisalicylate [Trilisate]) are less toxic to the gastric mucosa and do not inhibit platelet function (Zucker and Rothwell, 1978) but are less potent analgesics. The newer nonsalicylate NSAIDs are more potent, more convenient, more expensive, and less toxic than aspirin. Although no single agent has been shown to be consistently more efficacious, particular patients do seem to favor one drug over another. If swallowing large tablets becomes a problem, piroxicam (Feldene) capsules, naproxen (Naprosyn) suspension, or indomethacin (Indocin) rectal suppositories may be used.

For the burning, stabbing, or shooting pain caused by nerve damage, a tricyclic antidepressant or an anticonvulsant may be a useful addition. Amitriptyline, in doses smaller than those used to treat depression (10 to 50 mg at bedtime), is often effective. If swallowing problems arise, doxepin (Sinequan) solution should be used. The addition of carbamazepine (200 mg three times daily) or valproate (Depakene, 250 mg three times per day) should be considered if the tricyclic agent alone is not adequate. Both doxepin and carbamazepine can be administered rectally in gelatin capsules (Storey and Trumble, 1992). A short course of steroids also has been helpful in treating difficult, narcotic-resistant pain.

Visceral or Bladder Spasms

These spasms are best treated with an anticholinergic agent such as dicyclomine (Bentyl) or oxybutynin (Ditropan). If only small doses are needed, Transderm Scōp patches may be useful. For more severe cases, the addition of 0.8 to 2.0 mg of scopolamine to a 24-hour subcutaneous infusion of narcotic should be used (Storey et al., 1990).

Anxiety

If anxiety is severe enough to require drug therapy and pain remains a problem, hydroxyzine (Atarax or Vistaril), 10 to 50 mg every 4 to 8 hours, should be considered. This drug also has been shown to potentiate morphine in large doses. If a parenteral agent is needed, methotrimeprazine (Levoprome) can be used. This is the only phenothiazine with analgesic activity, and it is a potent sedative and antiemetic as well. An intramuscular injection of 20 to 30 mg usually will calm a crisis,

TABLE 8–4. CO-ANALGESICS

Pain Source	Pain Character	Drug Class	Examples	Comments
Bone or soft tissue	Tenderness over bone or joint	NSAIDs	Ibuprofen, 400 mg q 4 hr	Inexpensive; *large* pills
	Pain on movement		Sulindac (Clinoril), 200 mg q 12 hr	Well tolerated; preferred in renal impairment
			Naproxen (Naprosyn susp., 125 mg/5 mL), 15 mL q 8 hr	Liquid preparation
			Indomethacin (Indocin 50 mg caps. *or* supp.), q 8 hr	Suppository; more gastritis?
			Piroxicam (Feldene 20 mg caps.), 1 q day	Easiest to swallow; more gastritis?
			Choline magnesium trisalicylate (Trilisate susp., 500 mg/5 mL), 15 mL q 12 hr	No platelet dysfunction; less problem with gastritis; less effective
Nerve damage or dysesthesia	Burning or shooting pain radiating from plexis or spinal root	Tricyclic antidepressant	Amitriptyline (Elavil), 10–50 mg q hs	Best studied; sedating; start with low dose
			alone or with Doxepin (Sinequan), 10–50 mg q hs	10 mg/mL susp. available
			or Trazodone (Desyrel), 25–150 mg q hs	Less anticholinergic effect; 1/3rd as potent as amitriptyline
		Anticonvulsant	Carbamazepine (Tegretol), 200 mg q 6–12 hr	Absorbed from rectum, unlike phenytoin
Smooth muscle spasms	Colic—cramping, abdominal pain, bladder spasms	Anticholinergic	Scopolamine (Transderm-Scōp), 1–2 patches q 3 day	Also may be mixed with narcotic in S.Q. infusion, 0.8–2.0 mg/day
			Dicyclomine (Bentyl), 10 mg q 4–8 hr	Capsules
			Oxybutynin (Ditropan), 5–10 mg q 8 hr	Tablets
Anxiety	Generalized restlessness and discomfort	Antihistamine	Hydroxyzine (Atarax or Vistaril), 10–50 mg q 4 hr	P.O. or by S.Q. infusion
		Phenothiazine	Methotrimeprazine (Levoprome), 50–300 mg/day	I.M. or S.Q. infusion only

and 50 to 300 mg/day can be used by subcutaneous infusion (Storey et al., 1990). Orthostatic hypotension and irritation at the injection site are possible side effects (Oliver, 1985).

Dyspnea

Like pain, dyspnea can have a multitude of causes. When anemia, bronchospasm, and heart failure have been excluded or treated, the focus should be on symptom control. Oxygen can be helpful but is much less effective than narcotics for controlling this distressing symptom. When the dose of narcotic is titrated carefully to control the pain and the narcotic is administered on a regular schedule with "booster doses" available, the patient can get excellent relief without significant respiratory depression (Bruera et al., 1990). Careful consideration should be given to the use of antibiotics for pneumonia in the terminally ill patient. Because dyspnea can be controlled well without antibiotics, the physician must decide whether the antibiotics will improve the quality of life or just prolong the dying.

Constipation

When mobility and oral intake decrease and narcotic analgesics are required, virtually every patient will require regular doses of laxatives to avoid distressing constipation. The laxative should be given once or twice *every* day and the amount increased until an effective dose is found. Bulk laxatives are tolerated poorly and rarely are adequate for these patients. If docusate (Colace), 100 to 200 mg twice daily, is not effective, add senna (Senokot) or bisacodyl (Dulcolax), 1 to 4 tablets twice daily. Sorbitol 70% should be added in doses of 15 to 45 mL two or three times per day if the tablets are inadequate or cause excessive cramping. If a patient has gone several days without a bowel movement or is having small, frequent, liquid stools, an impaction may require manual removal. Bisacodyl suppositories or enemas may be needed occasionally until an effective oral regimen is found.

Nausea and Vomiting

In patients with nausea and vomiting, first look for a reversible cause such as constipation or gastritis from NSAIDs. If increased intracranial pressure is the cause, then the patient may require steroids. Overfeeding may be the problem if a nasogastric or gastrostomy tube is in place. Metoclopramide (Reglan) is the agent of choice when an enormous liver limits gastric emptying. Many patients whose nausea and vomiting have not responded to pro-

chlorperazine (Compazine) or promethazine (Phenergan) will be relieved by haloperidol (Haldol), 0.5 to 2 mg every 8 hours.

Like persistent pain, persistent nausea should be treated with regularly scheduled doses. Combinations of antiemetics that have different modes of action may be needed. A combination of haloperidol with metoclopramide or cyclizine (Marezine) may be effective. When oral antiemetics cannot be tolerated, rectal suppositories can be tried but rarely provide adequate control for persistent nausea and vomiting. Continuous subcutaneous infusions of metoclopromide, haloperidol, or methotrimeprazine (Levoprome) are more effective (Baines, 1988). Even vomiting associated with complete bowel obstruction can be controlled *without* a nasogastric tube or gastrostomy with a continuous subcutaneous infusion of narcotics, antiemetics, and anticholinergic agents (Baines et al., 1985).

Hiccup

Persistent hiccuping can be caused by any lesion affecting the phrenic nerve and by gastric distention or systemic problems, such as uremia. Treatment can consist of chlorpromazine (Thorazine), 25 to 50 mg orally every 4 to 6 hours; metoclopromide (Reglan), 10 to 20 mg orally every 6 to 8 hours; or haloperidol (Haldol), 1 to 2 mg orally every 4 to 6 hours.

Subcutaneous Infusions

When oral narcotics or antiemetics cannot be tolerated because of nausea, vomiting, stupor, or extreme weakness, parenteral medications may be needed. Frequent intramuscular injections or frequently restarting intravenous infusions can be painful and difficult to manage at home. Up to 50 mL of medication per day can be infused through a small-gauge butterfly needle under the skin of the upper chest, arms, abdomen, or thighs using a miniature pump (Fig. 8–1). Morphine and hydromorphone (Dilaudid) have been shown to be safe and effective when administered by this route (Bruera et al., 1988). Metoclopramide (Reglan), 60 to 90 mg/day, methotrimeprazine (Levoprome), 50 to 300 mg/day, and scopolamine, 0.4 to 2.0 mg/day, can be combined with a narcotic for control of nausea, colic, and secretions. Haloperidol also can be combined with the narcotic and infused by this route, but a white crystalline precipitate of pure haloperidol sometimes forms in the syringe at higher (>1.5 mg/mL) concentrations (Storey et al., 1990). This infusion usually is started in the hospital or hospice inpatient unit to ensure proper dose selection. The family can be taught to maintain the

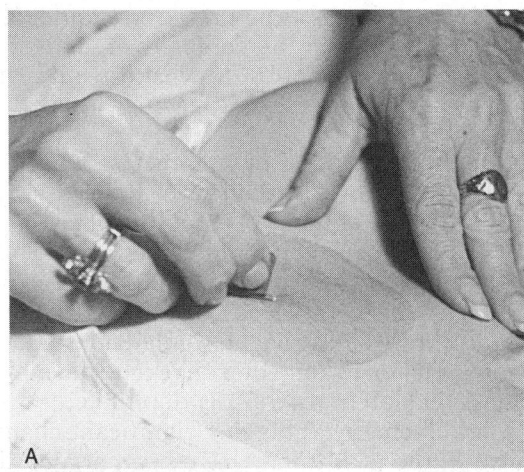

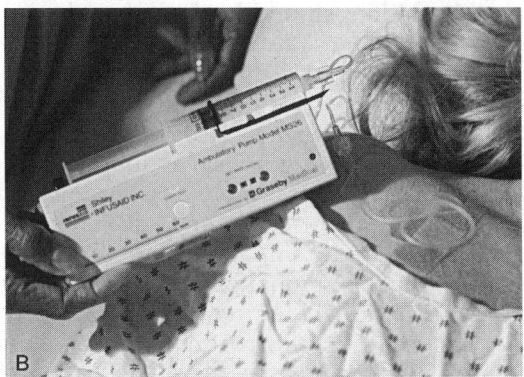

FIGURE 8–1. *A*, Application of subcutaneous infusion. *B*, Syringe driver in place for subcutaneous infusion. (Photos by Mildred Duelburg.)

infusion and give "booster" doses as needed either with the pump or sublingually.

NUTRITION

Although uncontrolled pain is the principal complaint of many patients, their family's principal concern is often how little they are eating. The causes of cancer cachexia are still unknown. Because patients seem to stop eating, lose weight, and eventually die, the natural assumption has been made that, even if we cannot effectively treat the cancer, we can at least treat malnutrition and thereby delay death.

The problem is that more harm than good can come from aggressive dietary therapy. Families sometimes are referred to aggressive dietitians who emphasize the need for multiple cans of supplement each day so strongly that the family feels responsible if the patient loses weight and dies. Unfortunately, the patient's final weeks become a struggle with the family over how much they have eaten. One patient said, "Tell her to stop pushing that spoon into my face, I don't want any more!" This can be carried to extremes, such as inserting

nasogastric tubes in patients who "do not cooperate." Their hands are even tied to bed rails if the tube is tugged on. A study of tube feedings in elderly patients revealed that, within 2 weeks, 67 per cent of patients with nasogastric tubes had attempted self-extubation and 43 per cent had aspiration pneumonia! Gastric or jejunal tubes had a lower self-extubation rate (44 per cent), but 56 per cent of the patients had aspiration pneumonia, 31 per cent had a leak or infection at the insertion site, and 50 per cent had a clogged or kinked tube (Ciocon et al., 1988). Large volumes of supplemental feeding can cause painful gastric distention, nausea, diarrhea, and copious pulmonary secretions.

There is no evidence that forced feeding really prolongs life. Careful metabolic studies on force-fed cancer patients at the National Institutes of Health showed irreversibly increased metabolic rates from force feeding. It was speculated that tumor growth was accelerated (Terepka and Waterhouse, 1956). Animal experiments have shown that growth rates of a variety of different cancers are nutrient dependent—the growth rate slows down with fasting or protein-free diets and speeds up with total parenteral nutrition (Buzby et al., 1980; Stragand et al., 1979). Several trials have been conducted in which patients receiving total parenteral nutrition plus chemotherapy were compared to those receiving chemotherapy alone. The group receiving total parenteral nutrition died faster. This was especially true for patients with adenocarcinoma of the lung (Jordan et al., 1981), colorectal cancer (Nixon et al., 1981), and small-cell lung cancer (Shike et al., 1984). When Klein and associates (1986) pooled the data from papers written on total parenteral nutrition and cancer through 1985, they found that infections were more common in patients receiving total parenteral nutrition, and that these patients were less responsive to chemotherapy and had shortened survival times. After reviewing all of the clinical trials of parenteral nutrition in patients receiving cancer chemotherapy, the American College of Physicians (1989) concluded:

The evidence suggests that parenteral nutritional support was associated with net harm, and no conditions could be defined in which such treatment appeared to be of benefit. Thus, the routine use of parenteral nutrition for patients undergoing chemotherapy should be strongly discouraged. (p. 735)

What should be done to relieve the anorexia of advanced cancer? Table 8–5 lists a number of treatable causes of anorexia. Uncontrolled pain blunts anyone's appetite and can be alleviated. Low-level nausea, oral candidiasis, and constipation certainly can interfere with eating and all are treated easily. Families can be taught how to relieve xerostomia (dry mouth) with a small syringe filled with water or juice and how to prepare soft foods. Corticoste-

TABLE 8–5. MANAGEMENT OF ANOREXIA

Treat "anorexia"
  Aches and pains
  Nausea
  Oral candidiasis
  Reactive depression
  Evacuation problems (constipation)
  Xerostomia (dry mouth)
  Iatrogenic problems (from chemotherapy or radiation
    therapy)
  Acid problems (gastric, ulcers)
Teach the family to prepare soft, easy-to-swallow foods
Consider steroids
Avoid nasogastric or gastrostomy tubes or hyperalimentation
Allay guilt

roids have been beneficial to some. The most important service the family physician can provide is to allay guilt. An appropriate statement would be: "I do *not* feel that how much time your husband has or how comfortable he is depends on how much he eats."

WHERE TO DIE

Death with dignity is easiest to accomplish when the patient dies amid the surroundings that gave meaning to his or her life and in the company of those whose companionship provided most of the rewards of living. Physicians too often deny this, however, in the medically conditioned struggle to prolong life. Medical technology has advanced to the point that too few patients are permitted to die at home, even though improved diagnostic techniques identify the irreversible nature of a terminal process at an earlier stage. A sorry commentary, reflecting the abuse of technology, is the case of a man who had built his house with his own hands and wanted to die there but was prevented from doing so while physicians exhausted their therapeutic armamentarium in an attempt to prolong his life a few days or weeks. The family physician must remain in charge as the patient's advocate when the consultants want to continue aggressive therapy, yet all the patient wants to do is go to sleep. The family physician must have the courage to discontinue aggressive therapy when the evidence points to its futility.

Charles Lindbergh is an excellent example of an individual who insisted on designing his final days in a manner that would preserve dignity and allow him to die as comfortably as possible. When dying of lymphoma, he refused to remain in a medical center on the East Coast and returned to his home in Hawaii, where he made final arrangements regarding his estate and discussed with friends and family the details of his memorial service and bur-

ial site. His death was as he preferred—quiet, dignified, private, and in the company of family and friends—a striking contrast to what it would have been had he not insisted on leaving the medical center.

Although 80 per cent of Americans still die in hospitals, polls show that most of them say they would rather die at home. Jacqueline Onassis is a recent example of a prominent person whose wish to die at home was respected. Similarly, Richard Nixon's wishes were respected when his physicians and family knew that he wanted no extraordinary means taken to keep him alive if he developed an illness that left him seriously debilitated, particularly intellectually. This is a significant change, because in the past it may have been argued that a former president should have all the advantages of modern medicine. Physicians now are recognizing that death is not a disease, but what occurs when the disease has won the battle. The most important actor on this stage is the patient, not the physician who is trying to "save" him or her.

Some patients do not want to be a burden to their family and pride themselves on being able to afford hospitalization or nursing home care. For some of these patients, the gradual withdrawal from family may be an emotional "letting go" that is necessary for all concerned in their particular family and circumstances. In other cases, there may be a spouse of a perfectly good marriage who is simply not equipped either physically or psychologically to deal with the loved one dying right there in the house over a 2-month period. What is important is a network of support for all concerned. However, there should not be an arbitrary judgment as to what is best for all people. The family physician will be sensitive to the style of living and the style of dying that seems most appropriate in a given case once the options have been explained to the family.

HOSPICE CARE

"Hospice" originally meant a way station for pilgrims and travelers—where they could be replenished, refreshed, and cared for. The Irish Sisters of Charity viewed death as one stage of a journey. They opened hospices for dying patients in Dublin in 1879 and in London in 1905. These were places where dying people could be cared for when such care could not be managed at home.

Cicely Saunders was trained as a nurse and social worker in London in the 1940s. She cared for a dying cancer patient who made a £500 donation to "be a window" in the special home for the dying they both knew was needed. Ms. Saunders went to medical school and then worked in St. Joseph's

Hospice in London from 1958 to 1965. She discovered the effectiveness of interdisciplinary team support, scheduled doses of oral opioid, and other methods to relieve the symptoms and stresses of her patients and their families. She opened St. Christopher's Hospice in south London in 1967 and the modern hospice movement was born.

The hospice concept can benefit patients and families wherever death takes place. A hospice program consists of palliative and supportive services that provide physical, psychological, social, and spiritual care for dying persons and their families. Services are provided by a medically supervised interdisciplinary team of professionals and volunteers and are available both in the home and in an inpatient setting. Home care is provided as necessary—on a part-time, intermittent, regularly scheduled, or around-the-clock on-call basis. The hospice concept is directed toward providing

support and care for persons in the last phases of incurable diseases so that they might live as fully and as comfortably as possible . . . [and] that, through appropriate care [and] the promotion of a caring community sensitive to their needs, patients and families may be free to attain a degree of mental and spiritual preparation for death that is satisfactory to them. (National Hospice Organization, 1979, p. 3)

Admission to a hospice program requires that a person have an inevitably fatal illness with a prognosis of weeks or months, that a request be made for the services, and that the attending physician consent to and cooperate with the hospice care. Table 8–6 lists the standards of a hospice program as developed by the National Hospice Organization.

The interdisciplinary hospice team consists of a patient care coordinator, a nurse, a physician, a counselor, a volunteer coordinator, and spiritual support. Medical services are on call 24 hours a day, 7 days a week. Continuity of care by the same group of team members provides a familiarity that is comforting to the patient. Volunteers are an integral part of the program and provide many helpful services.

Support for the Family

Hospice care is not focused only on the patient; the unit of care is the patient and family. The physical, psychological, and interpersonal needs of both the patient and the family are addressed. Following a patient's death, family members may experience increased morbidity and mortality, emphasizing the need for greater family support from the physician. Unfortunately, most physicians do not routinely contact the family following a patient's death, so this need often goes unrecognized.

TABLE 8–6. PRINCIPLES OF HOSPICE CARE

- Hospice offers palliative care, to all terminally ill people and their families regardless of age, gender, nationality, race, creed, sexual orientation, disability, diagnosis, availability of a primary caregiver, or ability to pay.

- The unit of care in hospice is the patient/family.

- A highly qualified, specially trained team of hospice professionals and volunteers work together to meet the physiological, psychological, social, spiritual, and economic needs of patient/families facing terminal illness and bereavement.

- The hospice interdisciplinary team collaborates continuously with the patient's attending physician to develop and maintain a patient-directed, individualized plan of care.

- Hospice offers a safe, coordinated program of palliative and supportive care, in a variety of appropriate settings, from the time of admission through bereavement, with the focus on keeping terminally ill patients in their own homes as long as possible.

- Hospice care is available 24 hours a day, seven days a week, and services continue without interruption if the patient care setting changes.

- Hospice is accountable for the appropriate allocation and utilization of its resources in order to provide optimal care consistent with patient/family needs.

- Hospice maintains a comprehensive and accurate record of services provided in all care settings for each patient/family.

- Hospice has an organized governing body that has complete and ultimate responsibility for the organization.

- The hospice governing body entrusts the hospice administrator with overall management responsibility for operating the hospice including planning, organizing, staffing, and evaluating the organization and its' services.

- Hospice is committed to continuous assessment and improvement of the quality and efficiency of its services.

From Standards of a Hospice Program of Care. Arlington, VA, National Hospice Organization, 1993, with permission.

The hospice team provides follow-up bereavement care to the family up to 1 year after the patient's death. Family members who experience grief following the death of a loved one are more vulnerable to physical and other emotional disturbances than at any other time in their lives. They need help dealing with the grief, guilt, and symptoms associated with this emotional turmoil. The bereavement services of a hospice team can minimize these problems and can help family members cope with the pain of memories that arise from time to time, especially at holidays, birthdays, and other stressful occasions.

One man who was dying of cancer kept it a secret from family and friends in order to spare them having to suffer with him. After his death some admired his ability to suffer in silence, but many were angry and hurt, interpreting his actions to mean that he did not feel they were strong enough to suffer with him. The survivors not only were angry because he did not appear to need them, but also were hurt because he did not even say goodbye ("New Age Hospice Horizons," 1989).

The most remarkable contribution of the hospice movement is not that it provides a special and compassionate setting in which terminally ill persons can die without heroic measures being applied to them, but that the family becomes involved and comfortable in caring for the ill member. With the rapid increase of scientific and technologic competence in the field of medicine, families feel increasingly incompetent and impotent to deal with dying. The hospice movement has reversed that trend and helps family members to work with community support services to provide home care for many of these patients. When symptoms cannot be controlled at home, the hospice inpatient unit can provide medical and nursing expertise in a "home-like" setting.

Selecting a Hospice

Most cities now have more than one hospice. Some organizations consist of good-hearted volunteers with little or no medical expertise. Others have free-standing inpatient units and their own medical staffs. The following questions will help in the selection of a hospice:

1. Is the hospice certified by Medicare and state licensing agencies?

2. Does the hospice employ its own staff to provide home and inpatient care? (A hospice is more than a billing agreement.)

3. Does the hospice employ a physician who will be able to help with particularly difficult problems?

SOCIAL SUPPORT AND RESOURCES IN THE COMMUNITY

In addition to the extended family, there are many other resources that the family physician can use in the care of the dying patient such as the visiting or public health nurse. Most county social service departments have some form of homemaker service. Social workers from both public and private agencies can assist the patient and family in dealing with negative feelings, hostile relationships, economic planning, and financial assistance programs. The social worker is often the key to obtaining tangible assistance such as wheelchairs, walkers, and hospital beds and adapting the home for the handicapped.

For the sensorily deprived, there are talking books, tape cassettes, and other aids from the local public library and the library of the State Commission for the Blind. The chronically and terminally ill child of school age can have a teacher for the homebound to keep up with his or her peers, making every day count in as positive a manner as possible. The patient avoids the burden of feeling rejected because of having the stigma of dying. In-home assistance also increases the number of natural interpersonal relationships, avoiding further isolation of a person who already is limited in locomotion and outreach.

Some persons have built close relationships through membership in churches or synagogues, service clubs, choirs, prayer groups, athletic teams, professional associations, hobby clubs, and so on. If these friends and associates do not show up, it may be, as Orville Kelly found before he organized Make Today Count, that they are embarrassed and insecure in the face of this impending death of a friend, or that they hesitate to intrude. This malady need not go untreated. The family physician does not have time to be a social coordinator, but a brief call to a minister, social worker, or family member usually can start the wheels of social interaction moving again. The physician is simply the catalyst.

Every religion pays special attention to the dying person. Support comes from the priest, minister, or rabbi, who can help the patient work through basic issues of the meaning of life. The question of "why?" and the confusion of guilt that plagues some patients may benefit most from a religious counselor. Even if a particular unresolved issue that now surfaces is in no way related scientifically or medically to the illness, it is still a great relief to get it resolved, whether through confession, sacramental absolution, restitution, or reconciliation with a significant other. This can be fully as important as medication in the care of the whole person. Bereavement on the part of family members or friends also is eased when things are "made right."

The priest, minister, or rabbi not only serves as a symbol of a community of faith that cares about the sick and dying, but also represents a belief system that nurtures hope and trust.

The task of the minister (or priest or rabbi) is both to sustain and nurture hope through the dying process, and to help the person who is dying surrender the unrealistic forms of hope in favor of more appropriate forms as death draws near. (Paterson, 1981, p. 227)

LEGAL AND MORAL ISSUES

Euthanasia or Assisted Suicide

Virtually all dying patients think about suicide and many ask their physician to help them. The greatest difficulties in the care of the dying sometimes are seen in patients who linger much longer than expected—so-called postmature deaths. How should the caring physician respond to such situations?

In any areas in which medicine intersects moral codes, there are bound to be diverse opinions and heated debate. The distinction between "active" and "passive" euthanasia should be kept in mind. "Active" euthanasia involves the purposeful administration of drugs to end life. It is common practice in Holland but unlawful in the United States. "Passive" euthanasia involves the withholding of drugs and permitting the disease to run its course. "Assisted suicide" involves the prescribing of large quantities of drugs for the purpose of empowering a patient to take his or her own life.

Most physicians are uncomfortable managing the suffering of a dying patient. It has been proposed that the physician's wish to be released from such a painful clinical relationship may be a factor influencing the patient's suicidal decision. A patient's suicide has a profound effect on the patient's physician, especially younger physicians. "By some measures, the distress equals in intensity, if not duration, that caused by the death of a parent. Patients' suicides engender anger, guilt, and loss of self-esteem on the part of treating physicians" (Miles, 1994, p. 1787). The emotional strain on Dutch physicians who had assisted suicide left them "disinclined to repeat the act" (Diekstra, 1993).

The principal reason for most patients wanting to end their lives is the high degree of suffering—usually because of uncontrolled pain or intolerable debilitation. However, much can be done to relieve pain, and support systems can be devised to provide the necessary care for an incapacitated patient. One experience of being thanked for *not* agreeing to assist in suicide by a patient whose pain was previously intolerable but is now well controlled makes any physician hesitate before agreeing to participate in assisted suicide. Permanent solutions to temporary problems should be avoided.

The notion that any treatable complication of a terminal illness *must* be treated because it *can* be treated is also wrong. Most patients do not want to die, but they are just as concerned about the *quality* of their time remaining as they are about the *quantity*. The physician may rescue an advanced cancer patient from one potentially lethal complication, only to find that another, which may cause much worse suffering, will end the person's life. Hippocrates' admonition *primum non nocere* (first do not harm) also may apply to treatments that under other circumstances may be helpful.

Living Will

All 50 states now have laws recognizing living wills or similar advance directives. Almost 90 per cent of Americans say they would not want extraordinary steps taken to prolong their lives if they were dying, but only 20 per cent have put that wish in writing in the form of a living will. The version of the living will shown in Figure 8–2 has several advantages over others. While it makes very clear the person's wishes, it is also fair to the physician and hospital administration. Instead of locking things arbitrarily in place, it leaves two witnesses as guardians of the individual's wishes and inten-

---

I wish to live a full and long life, but not at all costs. If my death is near and cannot be avoided, and if I have lost the ability to interact with others and have no reasonable chance of regaining this ability, or if my suffering is intense and irreversible, I do not want to have my life prolonged. I would then ask not to be subjected to surgery or resuscitation. Nor would I then wish to have life support from mechanical ventilators, intensive care services, or other life prolonging procedures. I would wish, rather, to have care which gives comfort and support, which facilitates my interaction with others to the extent that this is possible, and which brings peace.

In order to carry out these instructions and to interpret them, I authorize _____ to accept, plan, and refuse treatment on my behalf in cooperation with attending physicians and health personnel. This person knows how I value the experience of living, and how I would weigh incompetence, suffering, and dying. Should it be impossible to reach this person, I authorize _____ to make such choices for me. I have discussed my desires concerning terminal care with them, and I trust their judgment on my behalf.

In addition, I have discussed with them the following specific instructions regarding my care:

Date _____ Signed _____

Witnessed by _____ and by _____

FIGURE 8–2. Example of a living will.

tions with discretion to use their judgment in the specific circumstances. This statement presumes good will on all sides and should be helpful to all concerned. A statement that simply says "no reasonable expectation of my recovery from physical or mental disability" seems too vague and broad. It is also difficult to define so general a term as "artificial means," which is included in other living wills.

Legislation: "Natural Death" Laws

Beginning in 1976 with the California Natural Death Act, legislation has been enacted or proposed in many states to provide a more structured and legally binding provision for what the living will accomplishes on an individual basis. The California law not only mandates that the wishes of the signer of such a document must be granted but also holds the physician immune from prosecution for malpractice for fulfilling the stipulation of the document. The law varies somewhat from state to state, and each physician should become acquainted with the local legislation.

Recent federal legislation now requires that Directives to Physicians and Durable Power of Attorney documents be offered to every patient on admission to a hospital or hospice program. Because family physicians know the patient within the familial context and the community ethos, and provide greater continuity of care than large tertiary care centers, there should be less of a need to rely on legislation to protect the patient's rights or to guarantee voluntary informed consent. Over a period of time, the family physician can build the kind of relationship of trust wherein a consensus is naturally understood. When such a covenant exists, an adversarial relationship usually does not arise. Although public policy statements and guidelines have their place, they are no substitute for the trust and mutual respect that should characterize the doctor–patient relationship.

"Do Not Resuscitate" Orders

Cardiac arrest often occurs in persons who need not die because the incident is a temporary crisis and is reversible, sometimes even by the intervention of a lay person trained in cardiopulmonary resuscitation. At the other end of the spectrum, it is technically possible, with heart–lung machinery and a pacemaker, to keep a heart stimulated or keep the blood circulating in a body to which, according to consensus, consciousness will never return. Neither of these extremes presents a major problem in medical ethics. Decision making is more difficult in the gray area between these two extremes. There are complex moral and legal is-

sues involved in decisions not to treat or not to resuscitate, or in so-called no code orders.

The physician should be acquainted with any policy statement or guidelines that have been developed by the hospital. In or out of the hospital, persons with unexpected arrest should be resuscitated because it is an emergency and there is no time to assess the cause or attendant circumstances. It is not wise to allow age, mental retardation, or other "quality of life" issues to enter at this time. In the case of a patient with no response on an electroencephalogram, the physician should be alert to the possibility that drug overdose, hypothermia, or barbiturate therapy may be responsible. It is entirely within the physician's prerogative to determine the care that is medically appropriate for a patient. An attending physician may determine that a patient is irreversibly terminally ill and that no course of therapy offers any reasonable expectation of remission or cure of the terminal condition. Once this determination has been made, then the decision not to resuscitate may be appropriate. The essence of terminal illness is the expectation that death is imminent "within a short time." Because it is not possible to predict the time of death precisely, the decision is based on medical judgment. Consultation with a medical colleague should be sought if there is any doubt about the status of the patient. This also may provide reassurance for the family in certain instances.

The patient himself or herself may request that no cardiopulmonary resuscitation be initiated in case of an arrest, raising the issue of "voluntary informed consent" and the patient's rights. The physician needs to assess the mental status of the patient to ascertain that there are no extenuating circumstances, such as disorientation resulting from chemotherapy, metabolic abnormalities, or psychosocial factors. (One patient developed a sudden loss of interest in living when served with divorce papers while receiving treatment in the hospital.)

One way to avoid confusion or misinterpretation is to talk frankly with the terminally ill patient some time prior to the end stage of an illness. The following is an example of a frank but sympathetic approach.

As you know, we have used medicine A, which gave you some relief for a time; then we changed to treatment B, which has not helped you as much as we had hoped it would. We have no cure for this illness, but will continue to do what we can to keep you going and as comfortable as possible for as long as you have yet to live. Do you have any questions about what I have said so far?

Now I want to explain what else we could do for you. Your heart is very weak and may fail to work. I recall you said you hoped that your son could come to visit you and that he is seeking an emergency furlough from his Army duty overseas. You also mentioned that you are so tired of this illness and pain that you are ready to die. If your heart should stop working, we could try to start it again and keep it going with a special treatment. What do you think of this?

The above conversation takes into account the illness, past treatment, future prospects, and interpersonal relationships. It acknowledges individual values and gives the patient a chance to participate in the decision-making process. Meanwhile, the physician does not lose professional standing or authority or the opportunity to provide scientific and medical expertise as the patient's valued consultant and guide.

It is not pleasant to talk about dying. If one perseveres and overrides the initial reticence, however, the rewards of this kind of interaction are great. Many physicians report that their most meaningful relationships with patients have been precisely those that involved deep and personal sharing about the meaning of life, which was allowed to surface by facing death together. There are issues to be considered other than pleasure and the avoidance of pain. Being truly human means being open to all the meanings of existence.

REFERENCES

American College of Physicians: Position Paper: Parenteral nutrition in patients receiving cancer chemotherapy. Ann Intern Med 110:734, 1989.

Aring CD: The Understanding Physician. Detroit, Wayne State University Press, 1971.

Baines M: Nausea and vomiting in the patient with advanced cancer. J Pain Symptom Manage 3:81, 1988.

Baines M, Oliver DJ, Carter RL: Medical management of intestinal obstruction in patients with advanced malignant disease. Lancet 2:990, 1985.

Bruera E, Brenneis C, Michaud M, et al: Use of subcutaneous route for administration of narcotics in patients with cancer pain. Cancer 62:407, 1988.

Bruera E, Macmillan K, Pither J, MacDonald RN: Effects of morphine on the dyspnea of terminal cancer patients. J Pain Symptom Manage 5:341, 1990.

Buzby GP, Mullen JL, Stein TP, et al: Host-tumor interaction and nutrient supply. Cancer 45:2940, 1980.

Ciocon JO, Silverstone FA, Grouer M, et al: Tube feedings in elderly patients. Arch Intern Med 148:429, 1988.

Diekstra RFW: Assisted-suicide and euthenasia: Experience from the Netherlands. Ann Med 25:5, 1993.

Dunphy JE: On caring for the patient with cancer. N Engl J Med 295:313, 1976.

Evans C, McCarthy M: Prognostic uncertainty in terminal care: Can the Karnofsky Index help? Lancet 1:1204, 1985.

Jordan WM, Valdivreso M, Frankmann C, et al: Treatment of advanced adenocarcinoma of the lungs with ftoratur, doxurubicin, cyclophosphamide and cisplatin (FACP) and intensive IV hyperalimentation. Cancer Treat Rep 65:197, 1981.

Kaiko RF, Foley KM, Gravinsky PLJ, et al: Central nervous system excitatory effects of meperidine in cancer patients. Ann Neurol 13:180, 1983.

Klein S, Simes J, Blackburn, GL: Total parenteral nutrition and cancer clinical trials. Cancer 58:1378, 1986.

Kubler-Ross E: Death: The Final Stage of Growth. Englewood Cliffs, NJ, Prentice-Hall, 1975.

Lamerton R: Care of the Dying. Westport, CT, Technomic Publishing Company, 1976.

LORAN Commission: A Report to the Community. Brookline, MA, Harvard Community Health Plan, 1989.

Miles SH: Physicians and their patient's suicides. JAMA 271:1786, 1994.

National Hospice Organization: Standards of a Hospice Program of Care. Arlington, VA, 1993.

Nelson JB, Rohricht JS: Human Medicine: Ethical Perspectives on Today's Medical Issues. Minneapolis, Augsburg Publishing House, 1984.

New Age Hospice Horizons. Houston, TX, New Age Hospice, 1989.

Nixon DW, Moffit S, Lawson DH, et al: Total parenteral nutrition as an adjunct to chemotherapy of metastatic colorectal cancer. Cancer Treat Rep 65(suppl 5):121, 1981.

Office of Cancer Communication: Coping with Cancer; a Resource for the Health Professional. (NIH publication no. 80–2080). Bethesda, MD, National Cancer Institute, 1980.

Oliver DJ: The use of methotrimepraizine in terminal care. Br J Clin Pract 39:339, 1985.

Osler W: Aequanimitas. Philadelphia, P. Blakiston's Son and Company, 1904.

Paterson G: Death, dying, and the elderly. *In* Clements WM (ed): Ministry with the Aging. New York, Harper & Row, 1981, pp 227–228.

Saunders C: Living with dying. Man Med 1:227, 1976.

Seravalli EP: The dying patient, the physician and the fear of death. N Engl J Med 319:1728, 1988.

Shike M, Russell D McR, Detsky AS, et al: Changes in body composition in patients with small-cell lung cancer—the effects of TPN as an adjunct to chemotherapy. Ann Intern Med 101:303, 1984.

Simpson MA: Planning for terminal care. Lancet 2:192, 1976.

Spilling R (ed): Terminal Care at Home. Oxford, England, Oxford University Press, 1986.

Storey P, Hill HH, St. Louis RH, Tarver EE: Subcutaneous infusions for control of cancer symptoms. J Pain Symptom Manage 5:33, 1990.

Storey P, Trumble M: Rectal doxepin and carbamazepine therapy in patients with cancer. N Engl J Med 327:1318, 1992.

Stragand JJ, Braunschweiger PG, Pollice AA, et al: Cell kinetic alterations in marine mammary tumors following fasting and refeeding. Eur J Cancer 15:218, 1979.

Terepka AR, Waterhouse C: Metabolic observations during forced feedings of patients with cancer. Am J Med 20:225, 1956.

Tumulty PA: The Effective Clinician. Philadelphia, WB Saunders Company, 1973.

Twycross RG: Hospice care. *In:* Spilling R (ed): Terminal Care at Home. Oxford, England Oxford University Press, 1986, p 105.

Twycross RC: Principles and practice of pain relief in terminal cancer. *In* Corr CA (ed): Hospice Care—Principles and Practice. New York, Springer Publishing, 1983, pp 55–72.

Twycross RG: Symptoms Control in Far Advanced Cancer: Pain Relief, 2nd edition. London, Pitman, 1993.

Veatch RM: Choosing not to prolong dying. Med Dimensions (December): 8 ff, 1972.

Volkan V: Typical findings in pathological grief. Psychiatr Q 44:231, 1970.

Ward A: Telling the patient. J R Coll Gen Pract 24:465, 1974.

Weisman A, Brettell HR: The pre-terminal and terminal patient. *In* Rakel RE, Conn H (eds): Family Practice, 2nd edition. Philadelphia, WB Saunders Company, 1978, pp 249–257.

Wilkinson TJ, Robinson BA, Begg EJ, et al: Pharmacokinetics and efficacy of rectal versus oral sustained-release morphine in cancer patients. Cancer Chemother Pharmacol 31:251, 1992.

Zucker MB, Rothwell KG: Differential influences of salicylate compounds on platelet aggregation and serotonin release. Curr Ther Res 23:194, 1978.

SUGGESTED READINGS _____

Angell M: The quality of mercy. N Engl J Med 306:98, 1982.

Davidson GW: Living With Dying. Minneapolis, Augsburg Publishing House, 1975.

Driscoll CE: Pain management. Prim Care 14:337, 1987a.

Driscoll CE: Symptom control in terminal illness. Prim Care 14:353, 1987b.

Graham J: In the Company of Others. New York, Harcourt Brace Jovanovich, 1982.

Hively J (ed): Hospice of Marin Information Handbook, 2nd edition. San Rafael, CA, Hospice of Marin, 1981.

Kelly OE, Murray WC: Make Today Count. New York, Delacorte Press, 1975.

Kubler-Ross E: On Death and Dying. New York, Macmillan, 1969.

Kushner HS: When Bad Things Happen to Good People. New York, Schocken Books, 1981.

Lindemann E: Symptomatology and management of acute grief. Am J Psychiatry 101:141, 1944.

Lipman AG: Drug therapy in cancer pain. Cancer Nurs 3:39, 1980.

Nelson JB: Human Medicine: Ethical Perspectives on New Medical Issues. Minneapolis, Augsburg Publishing House, 1973.

Pearson L (ed): Death and Dying. Cleveland, The Press of Case Western Reserve University, 1969.

Shimm DS, Logue GL, Maltie AA, et al: Medical management of chronic cancer pain. JAMA 241:2408, 1979.

Simpson MA: The Facts of Death. Englewood Cliffs, NJ, Prentice-Hall, 1979.

Snow LW: A Death with Dignity: When the Chinese Came. New York, Random House, 1974.

Stedeford A: Couples facing death. II. Unsatisfactory communication. BMJ 238:1098, 1981.

Switzer DK: The Dynamics of Death. New York, Abingdon Press, 1970.

Tolle SW, Elliot DL, Hickam DH: Physician attitudes and practices at the time of patient death. Arch Intern Med 144:2389, 1984.

White RB, Gathman LT: The syndrome of ordinary grief. Am Fam Physician 8:96, 1973.

Wong CB, Swazey JP (eds): Dilemmas of Dying: Policies and Procedures for Decisions Not to Treat. Boston, GK Hall & Company, 1981.

CHAPTER 9

ETHICS IN FAMILY PRACTICE

WARREN L. HOLLEMAN and BARUCH A. BRODY

Economic, social, legal, and political factors have combined in recent years to effect major changes in medical practice and health care policy. Concern for patient rights and patient autonomy, as well as the demands of third-party payers, have transformed the practice of medicine. The ethical issues discussed in this chapter have taken on new dimensions as a result of this transformation.

MEDICINE AS A RELATIONSHIP AND AS A PROFESSION

At its most fundamental level, the practice of medicine should not be regarded as a science, an art, or a business, even though each of these elements is essential. The practice of medicine—particularly primary care medicine—is rooted, instead, in a relationship between the patient as person and the physician as professional (Jonsen et al., 1986; Siegler, 1985; Smith and Churchill, 1986). Two problems currently threaten the quality of that relationship: a misunderstanding of patient autonomy and inappropriate third-party intervention.

When physicians respect the autonomy of their patients so that patients take control of their health care, the physician is in danger of becoming a hired hand of the patient and the physician–patient relationship is in danger of degenerating into a purely commercial relationship. Patients "own" their bodies but they should not "own" their physicians. Physicians have an obligation to practice within professional standards of care as well as a right to refrain from doing anything that would violate their own moral and religious convictions (Christie and Hoffmaster, 1986). Physicians must respect the autonomy of their patients, but they also must avoid the temptation to shirk their own professional and moral responsibilities and must nurture a cooperative relationship with the patient. This is no easy task, but it is through cooperation that the physician and the patient can best work together toward a common goal—to maintain the health of the patient.

The physician–patient relationship also suffers when outside parties interfere inappropriately. When third-party payers set the standard of care, the physician is in danger of becoming a hired hand of the third party. The physician must balance competing loyalties between patients and third parties as well as between professional standards and personal beliefs. In this era of third-party payers, the physician–patient relationship can no longer be exclusive, but it must remain primary. In the remainder of this section, we examine two areas in which these problems are particularly prominent: work-related visits and benefits-related visits.

Work- and School-Related Evaluations

Preplacement examinations, work release evaluations, school absence excuses, and athletic physicals comprise a major component of many primary care practices. Inappropriate third-party interventions in this area challenge the primacy of the physician–patient relationship and the integrity of the medical profession. The following guidelines have been suggested (Holleman and Holleman, 1988; Kelman, 1985; Rosenstock and Hagopian, 1987) and should help alleviate some of the problems most commonly associated with these evaluations.

The purpose of the preplacement examination is to determine a person's fitness for work, to protect workers from illnesses and injuries, to protect employers from the costs of preventable job-related illnesses and injuries, and to collect baseline data for the future treatment of such illnesses and injuries. To enable the physician to make such an evaluation, the employer must provide the physician with a detailed job description, including physical requirements, psychological strains, and exposures to toxins. The physician then should tell the employer whether the prospective employee can perform the job without posing a risk to self or others. As discussed below, the physician should not release any medical records to the employer but should keep them on file as baseline data. At the beginning of the evaluation, the physician should advise the patient of the investigative nature of the visit. The physician must warn the prospective employee regarding health risks of the particular occupation (e.g., toxins affecting pregnancies, stresses affecting hypertensive patients) and must tell him or her of any problems detected in the course of the evaluation, regardless of their effect on job performance.

Work release evaluations, school release evaluations, and athletic physicals should be performed in accordance with the same guidelines as preplacement physicals, but they do present some additional problems of their own. Most work and school release evaluations involve short-term absences for minor problems for which there are few, if any, objective findings. Often, workers and students present after their illness or injury has resolved. These absences often reflect personal, family, or job-related problems that are not strictly medical in nature. Investigating such problems for employers and school administrators damages the physician–patient relationship and discredits medicine as a healing profession. Patients will have difficulty trusting a physician who investigates on one occasion but offers therapy on another. We recommend that physicians encourage employers and school administrators to develop nonmedical strategies for policing casual absenteeism. Physicians who do perform these evaluations should minimize the harm to the physician–patient relationship and to the integrity of the profession by evaluating only in the context of treatment and by refusing to release confidential medical information to employers and school administrators.

Many patients present to family practice physicians seeking to be certified as eligible for worker's compensation, long-term disability, group or individual medical insurance, Medicare, Medicaid, and veteran's benefits. Many others already have been certified and are seeking proper care under the terms of these programs. Physicians must be familiar with the details of the various programs so as to enable their patients to benefit appropriately from them. Physicians also must be aware of the potential abuses of such programs so as to help protect those who legitimately qualify from being harmed by those who do not. For example, if a patient presents with an on-the-job injury but also requests treatment for some other problem, the physician should file separate bills so that the worker's compensation fund only pays for job-related illnesses and injuries. Physicians who detect intentional abuse should attempt to identify the reasons for the abuse, particularly in the case of habitual, long-term abusers (Alexander, 1980; Whiting, 1977). Long-term abuse of benefits programs can be prevented only if family practice physicians insist that patients receive continuing comprehensive care from one physician or from a small team of physicians who know the patient well.

SPECIAL PROBLEMS IN FAMILY PRACTICE SETTINGS

Having introduced the concept of medicine as a relationship and as a profession and having seen what this concept means in many primary care contexts, we turn in the next sections to problem areas that challenge our understanding of the physician–patient relation and of the professional character of medicine.

Confidentiality

The principle of confidentiality is one of the most widely accepted and historically influential principles governing the patient–physician relationship in western cultures. The Hippocratic oath mandates that the physician not divulge "whatsoever I shall see or hear in the course of my profession as well as outside my profession in my intercourse with men, if it be what should not be published abroad." The 1980 Principles of Medical Ethics of the American Medical Association mandate that the physician "shall safeguard patient confidences within the constraints of the law."

Confidentiality is important as a way of encouraging patients to be frank in their communications with physicians, as a way of physicians keeping an implicit promise to patients that their confidence will be respected, and as a way of emphasizing the patient's right to privacy. In all of these ways, preserving confidentiality strengthens the relationship between an autonomous patient and a professional physician.

As the delivery of health care has changed from the model of a single physician caring for individual patients to the model of a team of health care workers in an institutional setting providing care to a wide variety of patients, the mandate of confidentiality has changed. The emphasis has switched from physicians keeping secrets to information about patients being divulged only to those members of the health care team and those institutional employees who have a need for the information, either to provide appropriate care or to meet appropriate institutional needs (e.g., monitoring of quality of care or organizing reimbursement). The underlying theme remains that information should not be provided to anyone else without the patient's consent.

This last point deserves special emphasis because it structures the decision as to when it is appropriate to provide information about the patient to insurance companies and to employers. Providing such information is perfectly appropriate if the patient consents; otherwise, it is not. For this reason, patients commonly are asked to authorize the release of information to particular individuals; the principle of confidentiality is not breached if information is provided pursuant to such a release (Bruce, 1984). However, the scope of information supplied and the persons to whom it is supplied are determined by the patient's instructions. Thus, if a patient requests a statement certifying that he or she is fit to return to work, it is not appropriate for the physician to provide to the employer a full account of the patient's illness and treatment; all that should be provided is the requested statement about the patient's fitness to return to work.

There are circumstances in which our society has judged that the need for information outweighs the principle of confidentiality; these are the circumstances in which the physician is required by law to disclose otherwise confidential information regardless of the wishes of the patient. The exact circumstances vary from jurisdiction to jurisdiction and are determined by state statutes and court decisions. Common circumstances include certain types of judicial proceedings, suspected abuse of dependent individuals such as children and the frail elderly, venereal and communicable diseases, and gunshot wounds (Bruce, 1984). In recent years, following the *Tarasoff* decision in California (*Tarasoff v. Regents of California*, 1974), the concept has emerged that physicians are obligated to warn and/or to take measures to protect third parties threatened by the behavior of their patients, even if doing so involves a breach of confidentiality. The scope of that principle is far from clear (Mills et al., 1987); one obvious controversial example is whether physicians should warn the spouses or regular sexual partners of patients who test positive for human immunodeficiency virus about the threat this illness poses to them (Dickens, 1988).

The principle of confidentiality extends to not providing information to family members of competent adult patients unless the patients want the information to be shared. Often, it will be clear that the patient has no concern about the sharing of information with his or her family. In cases of doubt, the patient should be consulted, especially if the information is of a sensitive nature or if there is evidence of family discord. An appropriate practice on admitting a patient to a hospital is to ask the patient to identify a particular family member, if any, to whom information should be provided for distribution to the family if the patient is not capable of fulfilling that role (e.g., in the immediate postsurgical period).

Certain cases are particularly troublesome. Among the most troublesome are those involving teenage patients. Information about pediatric patients is, of course, provided directly to the parents of the patients and not to the patients themselves; information about adult patients is, of course, provided directly to the patient and not the patient's parents. What about teenage patients seeking abortions, contraceptive advice, or treatment for venereal diseases, substance abuse, or psychiatric problems? Unless confidentiality can be guaranteed, such patients may not seek out the care they need. If confidentiality is protected, such patients may not get the parental counseling and support from which they also could benefit. Considerable confusion exists about the morally appropriate and legally mandated approach to confidentiality of information involving adolescent patients (Holder, 1985; Morrissey et al., 1986). Equally troubling are cases involving elderly patients who are less than fully competent but far from totally demented. Families of such patients often ask physicians to provide them with information about the patient's condition, information that they may not want to share with the patient. Such a request may be perfectly appropriate for the clearly incompetent demented patient, whereas it is obviously inappropriate for normal geriatric patients. How to handle cases that fall between these two extremes is unclear.

Informed Consent

The principle of informed consent is a much more recently articulated principle than the principle of confidentiality; the actual phrase "informed consent" first appeared in 1957 in the court case *Salgo v. Leland Stanford Jr. University Board of Trustees*. However, it has come to be accepted as a fundamental principle governing the relation between patients and physicians.

The principle's basic mandate is that a physician must obtain the free and informed consent of a patient, if the patient is competent to give that consent, or of the patient's surrogate if the patient is not competent, before medical treatment is provided. Two exceptions normally are recognized. The first (the emergency exception) is invoked when emergency treatment is necessary to protect the patient's life or health and consent cannot be obtained in a timely fashion. The second (the therapeutic privilege) is invoked when there is strong reason to believe that the very attempt to obtain consent will be harmful to the patient because of the psychological impact of the information conveyed (Rozovsky, 1984).

Several complementary accounts of the significance of the principle of informed consent are available. One stresses the clinical benefits (in terms of building trust and obtaining compliance) from a therapeutic regimen begun as a result of a joint patient–physician decision rather than as a result of a unilateral physician decision. The other stresses the patient's right to control what happens to his or her body; the resulting obligation of the physician to obtain informed consent is the way in which the physician respects that right.

The standard practice in many institutions is to obtain written documentation of informed consent primarily (if not exclusively) in cases of invasive procedures. This practice should not be understood to mean that the principle of informed consent does not apply to other medical interventions; it applies to all of them. Signed consent forms are merely written evidence of the informed consent already obtained, and the practice reflects the prudent desire to obtain written documentation in cases in which potential liability is highest. Informed consent, as opposed to the written documentation of that consent, should be obtained in all cases, both as a way of obtaining clinical benefits and as a way of respecting patient's rights.

There has been considerable disagreement about the amount and type of information that must be supplied to the patient. Obviously, only a portion of the relevant information known by the physician can be conveyed to the patient. Moreover, any attempt to provide too much information may result in the physician overwhelming and confusing the patient. Some selection of information is required, and the disagreement centers around which principle of selection to adopt.

Two different proposals have been adopted by America's courts (Rozovsky, 1984). The first is the *professional practice standard,* which maintains that a consent is informed if the patient has been provided the information that reasonable medical practitioners would normally provide under similar circumstances. The second is the *reasonable person standard,* which maintains that a consent is informed if the patient has been provided the information that a reasonable person would need to have in order to make a decision about whether to undergo the therapy in question. The information to be provided would presumably fall under the categories shown in Table 9–1.

Most commentators have argued for the second standard, because it best corresponds to the goals of informed consent, but a majority of courts have adopted the usually less demanding professional practice standard (Rozovsky, 1984). Clinicians are, we believe, best advised to adopt the usually more stringent reasonable person standard, because it provides all the clinical and moral benefits of obtaining informed consent while firmly ensuring that the legal requirement of informed consent is satisfied. Clinicians also must be careful to provide that information using terminology that patients are likely to understand.

A very difficult problem arises when one is dealing with patients whose competency is impaired. Informed consent is obtained from the patient when the patient is clearly competent and from the

patient's surrogate (a legally appointed guardian, if available, or the closest family member) if the patient is clearly incompetent. What, however, should one do when the patient's mental capacities are clearly impaired but present to some degree? This problem is alleviated partially when one remembers that the assessment of the patient's competency is not an assessment of the patient's total ability to manage all of his or her affairs; it is just the assessment of whether at this moment the patient can: (1) receive the information relevant to giving or refusing informed consent for this particular treatment; (2) remember that information; (3) appropriately assess and use that information to make a decision; and (4) make a decision (Brody, 1988). Although no formal test exists to ensure that the patient has the capacity to perform items 1 through 4 in the list, a careful discussion with the patient usually will enable the physician to ascertain whether these criteria are satisfied. If doubt remains, one should obtain consent from both the patient and the surrogate.

A second difficulty involves teenage patients. Informed consent is obtained from parents before one treats children, but from patients once they become adults. How should physicians treat teenage patients? Most states have passed special laws allowing physicians to treat them after obtaining only their consent when: (1) the treatment is for venereal disease, pregnancy or contraception, or drug-related problems; (2) they are living away from their parents and are responsible for their own affairs; or (3) they are married. Other cases (particularly abortion) are more problematic (Holder, 1985; Morrissey et al., 1986).

The Noncompliant Patient

Implicit in the principle of informed consent—the principle that medical treatment can be provided only after the patient has freely and knowingly consented to it—is the concept that a patient may choose not to comply with the physician's recommendations and that the choice not to comply must be respected. This concept easily can be misunderstood, however, leading to a quick and facile acceptance of a patient's noncompliance before its meaning is properly understood.

Several studies of noncompliance (Applebaum and Roth, 1983; Connelly and Campbell, 1987) have indicated that the majority of cases of noncompliance involve failures of communication, lack of trust as a result of previous bad experiences with the physician in question or others, and psychological and psychopathologic factors. Only a minority of cases involve a true value difference between the physician and the patient. This finding has profound implications for the clinical management of noncompliance. Physicians confronting noncompliant patients need to assess the

TABLE 9–1.   ELEMENTS OF INFORMED CONSENT UNDER REASONABLE PERSON STANDARD

Nature of the patient's condition (e.g., hypertension)
Description of the treatment proposed (e.g., particular medication)
Benefits of proposed treatment (e.g., control of hypertension and resulting lowering of risk of disease)
Risks of proposed treatment (e.g., side effects for that medication)
Alternatives (e.g., other medications, diet and exercise, no intervention)
Costs of proposed treatment

TABLE 9–2. EVALUATION OF NONCOMPLIANCE

Cause	Clinical Response
Problem in communication	Patient should be reinformed about the need for treatment
Failure of trust	Address question of mistrust; involve other physicians who may be trusted
Psychological factors	Treat anxiety, depression, and so on
Value conflict	Respect patient wishes

noncompliance, evaluate its cause, and react appropriately. Table 9–2 indicates how such a noncompliance assessment would proceed. In short, morality does not call on the physician to accept at face value every episode of noncompliance on the part of the patient. Doing so may in fact constitute a form of disrespect for the patient. What morality does call for is a full evaluation of the cause of the noncompliance, appropriate responses where possible to eliminate the cause, and respect for the patient's noncompliance only when it is an informed and competent refusal that is based on a difference between the patient's and the physician's values.

Even in those cases in which noncompliance represents an informed and competent refusal of the physician's recommendations because the patient's values differ, there may well exist alternative second-best forms of treatment that could be mutually acceptable. Consider a patient who refuses to stay in a hospital for a full evaluation because the patient is concerned about the need to be home to handle personal problems. Such a patient should be scheduled for an outpatient evaluation, even if it is not as satisfactory as a full evaluation in the hospital. (More examples of such compromises are provided later.) Respecting patient values in cases of noncompliance is not a matter of letting the patient win a power struggle; it is, more often, finding a mutually acceptable (even though not necessarily optimal) course of action. A failure to seek out such alternatives often may represent a lack of respect for the patient.

A form of noncompliance that deserves special attention is the patient who doesn't fill the prescription the doctor writes. This is sometimes the result of the patient's financial condition. The optimal medication from the physician's perspective may cost too much from the patient's perspective. Particularly when dealing with patients who have high medication bills because they need so many drugs or with patients who have very limited means, physicians should raise the question of cost frankly and explore less expensive but satisfactory (even if not optimal) medications.

A similar problem often arises when one considers the question of side effects of various drugs.

Different patients with different values and different tolerances may find certain side effects unacceptable. The physician certainly should not assume that a pattern of side effects that are acceptable to the physician will be acceptable to the patient. An important recent study (Croog et al., 1988) has stressed the significance of these matters in connection with the choice of antihypertensive agents, considering the implications of different agents for sexual dysfunction. Taking the patient's values into account in deciding which antihypertensive medication to order is a far clearer example of respecting the patient's values than simply accepting a patient's noncompliance with a prescription for a particular antihypertensive medication. This point can, of course, be generalized to other cases.

SPECIAL PROBLEMS IN TERTIARY CARE SETTINGS

Quality of care can be improved by careful attention to the components examined thus far: the physician–patient relation, medicine as a profession, confidentiality, informed consent, and the promotion of patient compliance. When the focus shifts from primary care provided by the family physician to care provided by subspecialists in tertiary care settings, new problems arise and old problems become even more complicated. The next two sections examine ways of resolving some of these problems.

Referrals

Decisions regarding referrals often are accompanied by great confusion. Referrals to subspecialists practicing in tertiary care institutions can provoke anxiety on the part of patients. The referring physician risks losing a patient and a substantial amount of money and is subject to embarrassment if a mistake is discovered. Referrals sometimes degenerate into power struggles between subspecialists and generalists. Because family practice is a community-based discipline, there is much debate and little consensus as to the family practice physician's role in the tertiary care setting (Christie and Hoffmaster, 1986). The following guidelines about appropriate referrals and about continuity through referrals are intended to help clarify these responsibilities and thus ease the tension and improve the quality of care.

Decisions to refer should be based on a realistic assessment of the potentialities and limitations of family practice as a discipline, of oneself as a physician, and of the facilities available in one's geographic region. Unfortunately, a number of other factors (financial and institutional as well as medical) often cloud the decision-making process and disrupt relations between primary and tertiary care physicians (Weiss, 1985, 1986).

Many subspecialists in oversubscribed areas have taken it on themselves to enter family practice as a means of bolstering their incomes, despite their inadequate training in this area (Aiken et al., 1979; Gillette, 1979; Sigel and Sigel, 1980). Conversely, family practice physicians sometimes feel pressured to go beyond their areas of expertise for financial and professional reasons: They fear losing the patient and the income and fear that their seeking consultation might reinforce the misconception that family practice physicians are inferior (Perkoff, 1986; Sussman et al., 1982; Weary, 1984).

Knowing when to refer requires courage and humility. Courage is the ability to act competently and wisely without being swayed by irrational fears. Some family practice physicians, motivated by unrealistic fears of mistakes and exposure, refer too early. Humility, on the other hand, is the willingness to recognize one's *actual* limitations and to act accordingly. Some family practice physicians, unaware of their limitations, refer too late. A proper combination of courage and humility, along with good working relationships with subspecialists, can prevent most of the problems involved in referring too early or too late.

Even if the family practice physician does decide to refer the patient, he or she remains the patient's primary physician (Christie and Hoffmaster, 1986). Equipped with a strong knowledge of general medicine, of the patient's medical history, and of the patient's personal traits, and committed to treating the disease in the context of the person and the person in the context of the family, the family practice physician is ideally suited to manage the patient throughout the referral.

When initiating a referral, the family practice physician's responsibilities are to educate the patient as to the reasons for referral, to recommend a subspecialist or treatment center best suited to the patient's medical and personal needs, to prepare the patient for what lies ahead, and to provide the specialist with data relevant to the patient's illness. Even after the referral, the family practice physician remains responsible for the quality of the patient's care. This may require translating medical jargon to patients or patient preferences to subspecialists and hospital staff, coordinating the activities of the various consultants, mediating disputes between consultants, ensuring that confidentiality is maintained by the health care team, and counseling patients and their families. The referral process is not complete until the subspecialist and the family practice physician have discussed all findings, treatments, results, and recommendations and the patient has discussed these with the family practice physician (Christie and Hoffmaster, 1986; McPhee et al., 1984; Rakel and Williamson, 1984).

Sometimes, subspecialists disagree as to how to manage a particular disorder. Consider the different way that surgeons and cardiologists may treat carotid artery disease. Or consider the range of approaches, within particular subspecialties, in treating certain disorders: differences among gynecologists regarding indications for a hysterectomy, and differences among neonatologists in managing severely handicapped infants. This makes the referring physician's task a difficult and delicate one. The referring physician must be aware of the differences between subspecialties and between particular physicians within a subspecialty. The referring physician must know the patient and the patient's family well enough to recommend the appropriate subspecialist. In many cases, the principle of informed consent will mandate that the referring physician educate the patient and the family as to the strengths and weaknesses of the available options. Family practice physicians should help their patients find a subspecialist who will be appropriate to both their medical needs and their personal preferences (Froom et al., 1984).

Financial Gatekeeping

The soaring costs of health care have led corporations and government agencies to develop prospective payment systems and capitation plans, with family practice physicians often serving as gatekeepers of the health care network. It is hoped that this will save money and streamline the referral process. However, it might drive a bureaucratic wedge into the physician–patient relationship, allow money to compete with quality in determining the standard of care, and inhibit the physician's freedom to practice an individualized style of medicine.

Prospective reimbursement systems (such as the Medicare Diagnosis-Related Group system) save money by limiting the reimbursement available to physicians, thereby encouraging them to do less (Eastaugh, 1987). Designers of such systems have the legitimate right to require physicians to avoid wasteful procedures and referrals; this prevents unnecessary expenditures and ensures a more just distribution of health care expenditures. Such limitations do not, however, preclude the physician's responsibility to offer the patient the best possible care within the limitations set by those policies. When particular patients require care in excess of the normal level of reimbursement, the family practice physician confronts a major ethical dilemma.

Considerable controversy exists as to whether physicians should do everything that they believe may benefit each patient without regard to costs or other societal considerations (Levinsky, 1984) or whether physicians must not be allowed to ignore the bottom line (Aaron and Schwartz, 1984). Traditionalists tend to ignore the fact that financial considerations always have limited the quality of care available to the poor. The question we are now confronting is whether these considerations may legitimately limit the quality of care available to everyone.

In caring for individual patients, physicians should distinguish between providing what the patient wants and what the patient needs. The controversy concerns whether all procedures and services likely to benefit the patient—as evidenced by outcome data—should be made available to the patient. When patients request unnecessary or marginally beneficial procedures and services, however, physicians must refuse.

It is often recommended (Fried, 1975) that, if societal costs necessitate that care be withdrawn from or limited for certain patients, these decisions must be made not at the bedside but at the policy level, prior to and apart from particular situations and applications. Such difficult policy decisions should not be made by physicians alone but should be negotiated at the policy level by the three major competing parties in the health care delivery system: institutional representatives, whose concern it is that the bills be paid; physicians, whose interest is professional integrity and personal income; and patients, who want the best care and the maximum choice at the lowest price (Pellegrino and Thomasma, 1981). It is an open question whether these recommendations are reasonable, realistic, and appropriate (BA Brody, 1988).

THE PHYSICIAN AS HUMAN BEING

The medical profession has, in the past few decades, achieved truly impressive gains in the battle against sickness, suffering, and death. Diseases that killed their victims just a generation ago are now manageable, curable, or even preventable. Yet physicians seem remarkably inept at maintaining their own health and well-being; they suffer high rates of alcoholism, substance abuse, divorce, burnout, and suicide (Hilfiker, 1985; Jonsen, 1983). Why can't the healers heal themselves, and what can they do to get on the road to recovery? To deal with these problems, we recommend that physicians learn to distinguish between competence and perfectionism, dedication and workaholism, and compassion and sentimentalism.

In medical school and residency, young doctors often learn to put their careers ahead of self and family (Gerber, 1983). This dedication is, in some ways, good. Young physicians want to do everything they can to help their patients. But this is often coupled with an unrealistic perception of their capabilities and those of their profession. They allow their egos to become too closely identified with their successes and failures. They become obsessed with insecurity (they are not good enough) and guilt (they do not work hard enough).

They worry that they might have missed a diagnosis and fear that their patients will die or suffer unnecessarily. Physicians are not supposed to make mistakes, but they do. Their profession requires staying on top of an ever-expanding field of knowledge, adeptness at a wide range of techniques and skills, making the right decision when fatigued or hassled or angry, picking up on subtle clues or poorly articulated symptoms, and juggling a plethora of human needs at once. Mistakes are inevitable, but talking about them is taboo. The only place mistakes are openly discussed, it seems, is the courtroom (Hilfiker, 1985). To be more effective clinicians, physicians must learn to acknowledge their capacity to err and must learn to discuss errors in a constructive manner. Physicians who do not admit their mistakes are doomed to repeat them. Physicians who discuss their mistakes can learn from them and experience healing in the process.

The physician who takes the time to care for personal and family needs is a more effective clinician because he or she is better able to cope with the stresses and strains of a demanding profession. Also, in the case of family practice physicians whose patients know them well, the physician will become a role model for personal health and fitness.

Another area in which physicians must learn to accept their humanity, and the humanity of their patients, is in the area of emotions. Clinicians must help patients recognize, express, and interpret their emotions. Clinicians must become aware of their own emotions, recognize their clinical value, and learn how to express and interpret them. The physician who ignores the emotions dehumanizes the physician–patient relationship. The family practice physician who improperly expresses, utilizes, or interprets emotional factors deprofessionalizes that relationship (Frankel, 1986; Katz, 1963; Zinn, 1988). Traditionally, physicians have been trained to maintain objectivity, affective neutrality, and clinical detachment. To be scientific, however, does not preclude recognizing the legitimacy of emotions or the necessity of empathy as a legitimate clinical and moral response to suffering. Sometimes a patient's feelings offer a clue to his or her symptoms. Sometimes a physician's feelings in response to a patient offer a clue to the patient's problem (Zinn, 1988). Suffering patients need a physician who will suffer alongside them and who will help them to express and interpret their feelings (Reich, 1989). When their patients suffer, physicians suffer too. The physician who suffers alongside a suffering patient or family allows the opportunity for healing of self as well as of the patient or family. Many of the physician's feelings, however, cannot be appropriately expressed in the clinical encounter. To maintain personal well-being, therefore, the physician must find appropriate outlets for expression and interpretation.

THE SPECIAL CASE OF EUTHANASIA AND ASSISTED SUICIDE

No discussion of the ethics of family practice would be complete without examining euthanasia and assisted suicide, issues that have provoked considerable public debate and challenged long-standing notions of the physician–patient relationship and the nature of the medical profession. In the coming years, patients may turn increasingly to their family practice physicians for assistance in dying, and thus it is important for family practice physicians to be prepared to respond appropriately.

Some surveys indicate that most Americans favor legalization of some methods of ending the life of a seriously ill or impaired person. In November, 1993, 1254 adult Americans were asked: "Do you think that the law should allow doctors to comply with the wishes of a dying patient in severe distress who asks to have his or her life ended, or not?" Seventy-three per cent responded "Yes." Public support of assisted death has increased steadily over the past decade. In 1982, 53 per cent responded affirmatively to the same question, and in 1987, 62 per cent (Taylor, 1993).

Many fear that aggressive measures to keep them alive, administered against their will, might inflict more suffering and indignity than they wish to bear. Others worry that the pain and debilitation of the illness itself might become unbearable, and want the assurance that escape through euthanasia or assisted suicide is available. These are legitimate concerns: A recent study suggested that terminally ill patients frequently are overtreated against their will, and that physicians continue to undertreat pain despite advances in pain and symptom management (Solomon et al., 1993). Another study has shown that most terminal geriatric patients prefer palliative care but that these "patients . . . exert strikingly little influence in the making of the treatment decision" and frequently are misinformed regarding the terminal nature of their condition (Prigerson, 1992). A major factor, according to the study, is physicians' own discomfort with death. Physicians practicing in teaching hospitals were found to be particularly uncomfortable with death, less likely to disclose a terminal diagnosis, and more likely to provide curative treatment in the last months of life (Prigerson, 1992).

Some physicians have urged colleagues to take a more active role in helping patients who request assistance in dying (H Brody, 1992a; Kevorkian, 1991; Quill, 1991). They regard such action as an acknowledgment of medical hubris and an expression of medical compassion and willingness to support the autonomous wishes of patients. The American Medical Association (AMA), however, and a number of prominent physicians and ethicists have opposed efforts to legalize euthanasia and physician-assisted suicide (Council on Ethical and Judicial Affairs of the AMA, 1988; Gaylin et al., 1988; Office of the General Council of the AMA, 1989; Reichel and Dyck, 1989). Physician participation in euthanasia and assisted suicide would, in their view, violate the Hippocratic Oath and confuse patients, erode trust, and tarnish medicine's image as a healing profession.

The most widely publicized model of physician-endorsed euthanasia is found in the Netherlands, where the government does not prosecute physicians who abide by an agreed-on standard of care (de Wachter, 1992). The criteria for euthanasia are that the patient's suffering must be intolerable despite aggressive relief efforts; there must be a low probability of improvement; the patient must be rational and fully informed; the patient's requests for euthanasia must be voluntary and repeated consistently over a reasonable period of time; and two physicians must accede to the request.

Some patient advocacy organizations, most notably the Hemlock Society and Choice in Dying (formerly Society for the Right to Die), urge the adoption of similar standards in the United States, with the government protecting physicians from criminal and civil litigation. These parties believe that aggressive attempts to prolong the lives of terminally ill persons are unnatural and torturous, and that euthanasia or assisted suicide are sometimes the most humane alternatives. Others, including many of the pro-life organizations, hold that the taking of a human life is what is unnatural and immoral, and that patients and physicians should always, in the words of the Hebrew scriptures, "choose life." They also express a practical concern that acceptance of this practice will lead to a slippery slope involving involuntary as well as voluntary euthanasia and euthanasia for patients who are not terminally ill or not experiencing unbearable suffering. They point to an apparent erosion of standards in the Netherlands, where, for example, 1000 incompetent patients are euthanized per year (ten Have and Welie, 1992). (Supporters respond that the percentage of life-terminating acts performed without the explicit request of the patient is relatively small, this percentage is stable or shrinking rather than growing, and that most of these cases represent patients who requested euthanasia prior to becoming incompetent [Pijnenborg et al., 1993; van Delden et al., 1993].)

Physician-assisted suicide, as opposed to euthanasia, has been proposed as a way to minimize the role of the physician in the action causing the death of the patient, while enabling the physician to provide expertise and, in some cases, the equipment necessary to make the death as painless as possible. The patient feels a greater sense of control, and the image of the medical profession is not tainted by a stigma of murder attached to the event. However, suicide also can carry a stigma. Moreover, many have suggested that the ethical distinction between euthanasia and assisted suicide may be more cosmetic than substantial, analogous to the now-obsolete distinction between withholding and withdrawing of treatment. Regardless of the methods, the motives and outcome are the same. Preoccupation with taints and stigmas reflects more concern for image than integrity, and also may indicate a lack of courage rather than a commitment to principle.

Another concern is that, in this era of cost containment, dying patients will feel unduly pressured to choose suicide rather than spend society's, and perhaps their family's, limited resources. This raises the question of whether such decisions ever can be truly autonomous and voluntary.

Hospice physicians, who have pioneered in the development of pain and symptom management for terminally ill persons (Ogle et al., 1992; Saunders, 1967), offer help to get beyond the impasse of those physicians who feel torn between wanting to relieve the suffering of the dying but not wanting to serve, directly or indirectly, as the cause of their patient's death. Hospice medicine has shown that the pain of dying persons usually can be palliated by aggressive pharmacologic treatment as well as by attention to "total pain," which includes all the physical, emotional, social, spiritual, and financial sources of the patient's suffering. The existence of this expertise, and the relative ease with which a family physician can master it, implies an obligation to utilize these methods and, when necessary, to seek consultation from palliative care specialists.

An ethical dilemma persists, however, in the occasional case of a patient whose pain or suffering remains unbearable despite the best care available and who requests assistance in dying (H Brody, 1992). Patients with severe physical disabilities, such as those with amyotrophic lateral sclerosis, advanced Parkinson's disease, or quadriplegia, also might request assistance in dying. Hospice care offers much less for these patients, and they may turn to their family practice physician for help. Many family physicians would like to assist such patients but fear legal repercussions. What should those physicians do?

It is disingenuous to deny assistance on the basis of pragmatic considerations, such as slippery slopes, outbreaks of mercy killings, and mistrust of white coats. Withholding and withdrawing treatment also could create slippery slopes and also have been opposed on the basis of inflated fears, but these concerns are now considered insufficient to justify a prohibition against these practices. Most Americans know the difference between the euthanasia-as-murder and the type of assisted dying currently being discussed, limited to patients suffering unbearably despite aggressive efforts to relieve physical and psychological pain, who request assistance voluntarily, and who receive voluntary, compassionate, competent assistance by their physicians. A review process should, of course, be established to assure that these criteria are met (H Brody, 1992).

From an ethical perspective, the essential issue is whether the longstanding prohibition against killing, which many regard as absolute, should outweigh all other considerations, such as the patient's autonomy or the degree of pain and suffering. Or, does the situation of unbearable and suffering pose a special situation that our society ought to regard as an exception to the general prohibition of killing, through granting certain types of patients the right to waive their right not to be killed? These two horns of the dilemma embody the crux of the issue, and all other concerns should be regarded as peripheral.

At the present time, assistance in dying is illegal in the United States and much of the world. Whether the legislatures and the courts should stand in the way of physicians who, with compassion and competence, are willing to assist this small category of patients is an issue that our society is in the process of resolving. The ethical obligation for family practice physicians remains to help patients live and die with as much dignity, control, and comfort as possible in light of whatever decision society makes.

CONCLUSION

The ethical questions faced by physicians have been transformed, in ways we have indicated, by changing economic, social, legal, and political factors. In the end, however, the ethics of medicine remains committed to a view of the patient–physician relationship as a relationship between two autonomous human beings—a patient who is suffering and seeks help, and a physician who maintains his or her humanity as well as his or her professionalism.

REFERENCES

Aaron H, Schwartz W: The Painful Prescription: Rationing Hospital Care. Washington, DC, Brookings Institute, 1984.

Aiken LH, Lewis CE, Craig J, et al: The contributions of specialists to the delivery of primary care: A new perspective. N Engl J Med 300:1363, 1979.

Alexander E Jr: A "truth in mending" act [commentary]. JAMA 243:1239, 1980.

Applebaum P, Roth L: Patients who refuse treatment in medical hospitals. JAMA 250:1296, 1983.

Brody BA: Life and Death Decision Making. New York, Oxford University Press, 1988.

Brody H: Assisted death—a compassionate response to a medical failure. N Engl J Med 327:1384, 1992a.

Bruce JA: Privacy and Confidentiality of Health Care Information. Chicago, American Hospital Association, 1984.

Christie RJ, Hoffmaster CB: Ethical Issues in Family Medicine. New York, Oxford University Press, 1986.

Connelly J, Campbell C: Patients who refuse treatment in medical offices. Arch Intern Med 147:1829, 1987.

Council on Ethical and Judicial Affairs of the American Medical Association: Euthanasia. Chicago, American Medical Association, 1988.

Croog S, Levine S, Sudilovsky A, et al: Sexual symptoms in hypertensive patients. Arch Intern Med 148:788, 1988.

de Wachter MAM: Euthanasia in the Netherlands. Hastings Cent Rep 22:23, 1992.

Dickens BM: Legal limits of AIDS confidentiality. JAMA 259:3449, 1988.

Eastaugh SR: Financing Health Care: Economic Efficiency and Equity. Dover, MA, Auburn House Publishing Company, 1987.

Frankel BL: Affective neutrality [A Piece of My Mind]. JAMA 256:515, 1986.

Fried C: Rights and health care—beyond equity and efficiency. N Engl J Med 293:241, 1975.

Froom J, Feinbloom RI, Rosen MG: Risks of referral. J Fam Pract 18:623, 1984.

Gaylin W, Kass LR, Pellegrino ED, Siegler M: "Doctors must not kill." JAMA 259:2139, 1988.

Gerber LA: Married to Their Careers: Career and Family Dilemmas in Doctors' Lives. New York, Tavistock Publications, 1983.

Gillette RD: The delivery of "primary care" by specialists. N Engl J Med 301:893, 1979.

Hilfiker D: A Physician Looks at His Work. New York, Pantheon Books, 1985.

Holder A: Legal Issues in Pediatrics and Adolescent Medicine. New Haven, CT, Yale University Press, 1985.

Holleman WL, Holleman MC: School and work release evaluations. JAMA 260:3629, 1988.

Jonsen AR: Watching the doctor. N Engl J Med 308:1531, 1983.

Jonsen AR, Siegler M, Winslade WJ: Clinical Ethics: A Practical Approach to Ethical Decisions in Clinical Medicine, 2nd edition. New York, Macmillan, 1986.

Katz RL: Empathy: Its Nature and Uses. London, The Free Press of Glencoe, Collier-Macmillan Limited, 1963.

Kelman GR: The pre-employment medical examination. Lancet 2:1231, 1985.

Kevorkian J: Prescription—Medicine: The Goodness of Planned Death. Buffalo, NY, Prometheus Books, 1991.

Levinsky NG: The doctor's master. N Engl J Med 311:1573, 1984.

McPhee SJ, Lo B, Saika GY, Meltzer R: How good is communication between primary care physicians and sub-specialty consultants? (Special Report). Arch Intern Med 144:1265, 1984.

Mills M, Sullivan G, Eth S: Protecting third parties: A decade after Tarasoff. Am J Psychiatry 144:68, 1987.

Morrissey J, Hofmann A, Thrope J: Consent and Confidentiality in the Health Care of Children and Adolescents. New York, Free Press, 1986.

Office of the General Council of the American Medical Association: Assisted suicide. JAMA 262:1844, 1989.

Ogle KS, Warren D, Plumb JD: Pain management in advanced cancer. Primary Care 19:793, 1992.

Pellegrino EG, Thomasma DC: A Philosophical Basis of Medical Practice: Toward a Philosophy and Ethic of the Healing Professions. New York, Oxford University Press, 1981.

Perkoff GT: Ethical aspects of the physician surplus: Implications for family practice. J Fam Pract 22:455, 1986.

Pijnenborg L, van der Maas PJ, van Delden JJM, Looman CWN: Life-terminating acts without explicit request of patient. Lancet 341:1196, 1993.

Prigerson HG: Socialization to dying: Social determinants of death acknowledgment and treatment among terminally ill geriatric patients. J Health Soc Behav 33:378, 1992.

Quill TE: Death and dignity: A case of individualized decision making. N Engl J Med 324:691, 1991.

Rakel RE, Williamson PS: Use of consultants. In Rakel RE (ed): Textbook of Family Practice, 3rd edition. Philadelphia, WB Saunders Company, 1984, pp 190–197.

Reich WT: Speaking of suffering: A moral account of compassion. Soundings 72:83, 1989.

Reichel W, Dyck AJ: Euthanasia: A contemporary moral quandary. Lancet 2:1321, 1989.

Rosenstock L, Hagopian A: Ethical dilemmas in providing health care to workers. Ann Intern Med 107:575, 1987.

Rozovsky F: Consent to Treatment: A Practical Guide. Boston, Little, Brown, 1984.

Saunders CM: The Management of Terminal Illness. London, Hospital Medicine, 1967.

Siegler M: The progression of medicine: From physician paternalism to patient autonomy to bureaucratic parsimony. Arch Intern Med 145:713, 1985.

Sigel L, Sigel B: The role of subspecialists in primary medical care. Perspect Biol Med 24:122, 1980.

Smith HL, Churchill LR: Professional Ethics and Primary Care Medicine: Beyond Dilemmas and Decorum. Durham, NC, Duke University Press, 1986.

Soloman MZ, O'Donnell LO, Jennings B, et al: Decisions near the end of life: Professional views on life-sustaining treatments. Am J Public Health 83:14, 1993.

Sussman EJ, Tsiaras WG, Soper KA: Diagnosis of diabetic eye disease. JAMA 247:3231, 1982.

Tarasoff v Regents of California, 118 Cal Rptr 1974, 129.

Taylor H: Majority support for euthanasia and Dr. Kevorkian increases. The Harris Poll #63, 1993.

ten Have HAMJ, Welie JVM: Euthanasia: Normal medical practice? Hastings Cent Rep 22:34, 1992.

van Delden JJM, Pijnenborg L, van der Mass PJ: The Remmelink study: Two years later. Hastings Cent Rep 23:24, 1993.

Wanzer SH, Federman DD, Adelstein SJ, et al: The physician's responsibility toward hopelessly ill patients: A second look. N Engl J Med 320:844, 1989.

Weary PE: Behold, the gatekeeper cometh [commentary]. Int J Dermatol 23:33, 1984.

Weiss BD: Family practice in hospitals [commentary]. JAMA 253:549, 1985.

Weiss BD: The effect of malpractice insurance costs on family physicians' hospital practices. J Fam Pract 23:55, 1986.

Whiting RK: The anxious manipulator and disability [letter]. J Occup Med 19:655, 1977.

Zinn WM: Doctors have feelings too. JAMA 259:3296, 1988.

Part II

COMMUNITY MEDICINE

CHAPTER 10

PERIODIC HEALTH EXAMINATION

JOHN W. FEIGHTNER, RENALDO N. BATTISTA,
and JENNIFER LYNN DINGLE

The idea of integrating prevention in clinical care is not new; it can be traced back to Hippocrates, who wrote: "Whoever wishes to investigate medicine properly should consider the mode in which the inhabitants live ... Whether they are fond of drinking and eating to excess ... Or are fond of exercise and labour" (1985, p. 190). However, the popularity of this idea has waxed and waned over the centuries, reflecting an underlying tension between prevention and cure, health and disease (Battista, 1993).

The medical community's interest in prevention has grown during the past 20 years. Surveys show that an increasing amount of office time now is allocated to preventive services in family medicine, general internal medicine, and other primary care practices (Battista, 1983; Lurie et al., 1987; McPhee et al., 1986; Mendenhall, 1981; Romm et al., 1981). In Canada and the United States, task forces have been convened to consider what preventive health care services practitioners should provide (Canadian Task Force on the Periodic Health Exam, 1979; U. S. Preventive Services Task Force, 1989). An expanding awareness of preventive health care by third-party payers can be expected as the demand for coverage mounts (Battista and Fletcher, 1988).

The approach proposed for the periodic health examination is based on a set of age- and sex-related health protection packages and aims at creating a lifetime health care plan. This strategy results from shortcomings discovered in the conventional annual checkup. The scope and the frequency of examinations included in the conventional checkup are challenged on grounds that they bear little relation to the needs of different age and sex groups. Moreover, most of the tests and procedures included in routine examinations have not been demonstrated to be efficacious or effective, and the optimal frequency of their administration has not been ascertained. The health protection package approach addresses these two main criticisms by being targeted specifically to age and sex groups and by being restricted to procedures about which

we have some evidence of efficacy and effectiveness.

THEORETICAL FOUNDATION OF THE PERIODIC HEALTH EXAMINATION

Definition of Terms

Periodic Health Examination. The periodic health examination is composed of a group of tasks designed either to determine the risk of subsequent disease or to identify disease in its early, symptomless state. Other interventions, such as injections for immunization and counseling for the prevention of disease or the maintenance of health, also are covered by the definition.

Health Protection Package. Health protection packages are sets of procedures that are particularly applicable to the periodic health examination at certain ages and in certain "at-risk" groups.

Preventive Intervention. There are basically two types of preventive intervention: primary and secondary. The aim of *primary prevention* is to prevent the occurrence of disease by modifying exposure to ill health behaviors or risk factors; the aim of *secondary prevention* is to identify a disease at such an early stage that application of a subsequent intervention could affect the ultimate outcome positively. Although secondary prevention and *early detection* often are used interchangeably, a secondary preventive intervention subsumes the application of an early detection procedure followed by the appropriate primary preventive or curative intervention. Detection of disease or even risk factors for a disease in patients who consult physicians for unrelated symptoms is also referred to as *case finding*. *Screening* is the application of procedures to populations or subpopulations in order to classify them into two groups: one with a high probability of being affected by fatal or disabling condition, and the other with a low probability of incurring the same conditions. Those with a high probability then are referred to a physician for further diagnosis or consultation. Poor compliance with the second step will compromise the effectiveness of screening.

Efficacy. Efficacy is the attribute of an intervention or maneuver that results in more good than harm to those who accept and comply with the intervention and subsequent treatment.

Effectiveness. Effectiveness is the attribute of an intervention or maneuver that results in more good than harm to those to whom it is offered.

Efficiency. Efficiency is the attribute of an effective intervention that optimizes the use of limited resources.

Scientific Principles of Evaluation of Preventive Services

The efficacy and effectiveness of preventive interventions are ascertained best through the same approaches used to evaluate any therapeutic intervention. The randomized controlled trial remains the preferred strategy of evaluation whenever feasible. Other approaches are the cohort study, the case–control study, quasi-experimental designs such as time series, and descriptive studies or case reports. Measuring health outcomes is a difficult and common problem whatever design is chosen. Ideally, an intervention should be evaluated in terms of such outcomes as mortality, morbidity, or the resulting quality of life.

Clarifying the casual pathway of a preventive maneuver is important. It identifies the type of evidence that must be examined for complete evaluation of effectiveness (Battista and Fletcher, 1988). Figure 10–1 illustrates the causal pathway model for primary preventive measure such as counseling (Canadian Task Force on the Periodic Health Examination, 1989a). The causal pathway for screening tests for preclinical disease clarifies the need to evaluate two causal links to infer effectiveness: the ability of the early detection procedure to identify the target condition and the ability of a treatment intervention to achieve a favorable outcome (Fig. 10–2).

An early detection procedure can be a history item, a physical examination, or a laboratory test;

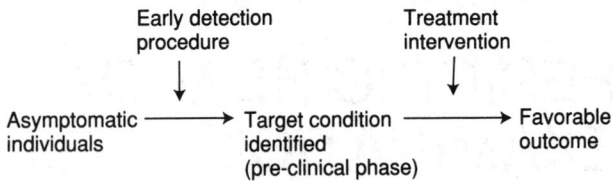

FIGURE 10–2. Causal pathway for secondary preventive interventions. (From Battista RN, Fletcher SW: Making recommendations on preventive practices: Methodological issues. *In* Battista RN, Lawrence RS [eds]: Implementing Preventive Services, a supplement to Am J Prev Med 4(4): 53, 1988, New York, Oxford University Press, with permission.)

ideally it should be accurate, safe, simple, inexpensive, acceptable to both patients and clinicians, and positive (or neutral) in its psychological labeling effects. The performance characteristics of early detection procedures can be determined. *Sensitivity* is defined as the proportion of diseased individuals correctly identified by the procedure; *specificity* is the proportion of healthy individuals correctly classified as disease free by the technique. The positive and negative predictive values of each test also should be ascertained, if at all possible, because they are of utmost importance to the clinician. The *positive predictive value* is that proportion of individuals having a positive test who actually are affected by the disease in question, whereas the *negative predictive value* of a test is the proportion of subjects with a negative test who are free of the disease. When the prevalence of a particular disease is low, the positive predictive value of relevant detection tests will be low, even when they have high sensitivity and high specificity, whereas the negative predictive values will be high. When asymptomatic subjects are being examined, high performance on all of these test properties is crucial to early detection. The principles involved are discussed at length in the epidemiologic literature Fletcher et al., 1988; McNeil et al., 1975; Sackett et al., 1985; Vecchio, 1966).

Several methodologic snares can jeopardize the evaluation of secondary preventive interventions, particularly in the domain of chronic diseases. The advantage sought by early detection is improvement of life expectancy and quality of life, but commonly used indices, such as the 5-year survival from time of diagnosis, can be very deceptive in this context. Early detection does not, in itself, ensure any deferral of the time of death; it may only lengthen the illness by making people aware of their disease sooner. Proper evaluation of secondary preventive strategies always should correct for this potential "lead-time" bias. Detection procedures probably identify slowly evolving conditions more easily than rapidly progressing ones. The more likely identification of conditions with longer natural histories and better prognoses may make a preventive procedure appear to have a better per-

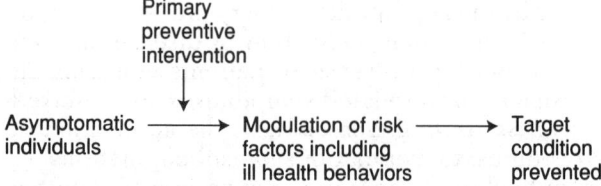

FIGURE 10–1. Causal pathway for primary preventive interventions. (From Battista RN, Fletcher SW: Making recommendations on preventive practices: Methodological issues. *In* Battista RN, Lawrence RS [eds]: Implementing Preventive Services, a supplement to Am J Prev Med 4(4): 60, 1988, New York, Oxford University Press, with permission.)

formance than it actually has (length bias) (Cole and Morrison, 1980; Sackett et al., 1985).

When the efficacy and effectiveness of preventive interventions have been ascertained, their cost–benefit and/or cost-effectiveness ratios should be assessed because the increasing scarcity of resources for health care makes societal choices necessary. Decision makers then can recommend choices from among those with comparable effectiveness but different degrees of efficacy (Russell, 1986; Weinstein and Stason, 1977). Sound practice recommendations also should take into account issues of safety, availability, and acceptability of effective or efficacious interventions.

Formulation Process of Practice Recommendations

The Canadian Task Force on the Periodic Health Examination developed a clinical–epidemiologic approach in making recommendations for the periodic health examination (Woolf et al., 1990). This process subsequently was adopted and amended by the U.S. Preventive Services Task Force at its initiation in 1984. The task force uses a simple method for grading the evidence pertaining to the effectiveness of interventions, based on the methodologic strengths of the designs and approaches used. The highest level of evidence would be associated with randomized controlled trials, while the opinions of experts would be considered as the lowest level (Table 10–1). Task force members prepare background papers using this methodology and present their results to the other members at working meetings of the task force; three to four such meetings are held each year. Through several iterations spread over 1 to 2 years, the task force reaches consensus on recommendations that are graded for inclusion or exclusion as follows (Battista, 1993):

TABLE 10–1. RULES OF EVIDENCE

I: Evidence obtained from at least one properly randomized controlled trial.

II-1:   Evidence obtained from well-designed controlled trials without randomization.

II-2:   Evidence obtained from well-designed cohort or case-control analytic studies, preferably from more than one center or research group.

II-3:   Evidence obtained from comparisons between times or places with or without the intervention. Dramatic results in uncontrolled experiments (such as the results of treatment with penicillin in the 1940s) could also be included in this category.

III: Opinions of respected authorities, based on clinical experience, descriptive studies, or reports of expert committees.

From Wolf SH, Battista RN, Anderson GM, et al: Assessing the clinical effectiveness of preventing manuevers. J Clin Epidemol 43:891, 1990. Adapted from the Canadian Task Force on the Periodic Health Examination: The periodic health examination 1: Introduction. Can Med Assoc J 141:205, 1989, with permission.

A: good evidence for inclusion
B: fair evidence for inclusion
C: evidence for inclusion or exclusion poor, therefore delineating a set of research priorities
D: fair evidence for exclusion
E: good evidence for exclusion

Graded recommendations explicitly acknowledge the different degrees of current scientific certainty about different preventive services. Grades help clinicians attach priorities to preventive activities in their practices. Graded recommendations also may help point the way for reimbursement agencies when considering which procedures to reimburse. Finally, by making explicit the areas where evidence is weak, problems are highlighted for future research agendas.

PRACTICE OF THE PERIODIC HEALTH EXAMINATION

Recommendations and Health Protection Packages

One should reiterate that primary and secondary preventive measures are performed (or their need identified) when a patient comes in to see the physician for intercurrent illness or problems. These are patient-initiated encounters. The patient is given an explanation of the purpose of the procedures and counseling. Over time, it is hoped that a family physician's practice would become "educated" to this lifetime strategy of prevention.

Tables 10–2 through 10–6 provide guidelines for preventive interventions that should be included in the periodic health examination of different patient groups; they summarize the findings of the Canadian Task Force on the Periodic Health Examination and the U.S. Preventive Services Task Force. Importantly, Table 10–7 lists those clinical conditions for which controversy remains regarding inclusion in a periodic health examination. Finally, Table 10–8 identifies conditions for which evidence supports their *exclusion* from a periodic health examination. For each age group, the tables indicate whether or not a given preventive intervention should be directed at high-risk persons and, when possible, its frequency. The references given are for the respective task force publications, which, in turn, contain all the key references used in making the final recommendations and assigning the grades. Conditions currently under an updating review by the Canadian Task Force so indicated. Both task forces will be publishing fully updated recommendations in the near future.

In the following section, we offer three examples of case finding and the practice of the periodic health examination. There are several common themes of preventive practice that pervade all three examples:

TABLE 10–2. PERIODIC HEALTH EXAMINATION PREVENTIVE INTERVENTIONS—*PRENATAL*

Target Condition	Clinical Procedure	Canadian Task Force (CTF)	U.S. Preventive Services Task Force (USPSTF)
Asymptomatic General Population			
Hypertension	Systolic and diastolic blood pressure measurement	At every visit (A).* (CTF, 1984).	At the first prenatal visit and periodically throughout the pregnancy (USPSTF, 1989).
Bacteriuria	Urine culture	Once in each trimester and 6 weeks postpartum (B) (CTF, 1979).†	Urine culture is recommended for detecting asymptomatic bacteriuria (USPSTF).
Blood group incompatibility	Blood typing, Rh antibody test	Screen at first prenatal visit (A) (CTF, 1979).†	Screen at first prenatal visit and at 28 weeks if Rh negative. Unsensitized Rh-negative women should receive Rh(D) immune globulin at 28–29 weeks' gestation and within 72 hours after delivery, as well as after induced abortion, amniocentesis, or transplacental hemorrhage >30 mL (USPSTF, unpublished).
Gonorrhea	Cultures of cervical and urethral smears	Screen at first prenatal visit and in last trimester if woman is at high risk (A) (CTF, 1979).†	At first prenatal visit. An additional test later in pregnancy is recommended for those at increased risk of acquiring gonorrhea (USPSTF, 1989).
Chlamydial genital infection	Cultures of cervical and urethral smears	Screening and treatment may be beneficial in preventing infection in the newborn, but efficacy is not yet proven (B) (CTF, 1984).†	**High-risk women only:** Persons who attend clinics for sexually transmitted diseases (STDs), adolescents, and family planning; those age <20 years; and those with multiple sexual partners, a sexual partner with multiple sexual contacts, or a recent partner who tested positive for chlamydia should be tested for chlamydia at the first prenatal visit (B) (USPSTF, 1989).
Syphilis	Venereal Disease Research Laboratory (VDRL) or rapid plasma reagin (RPR) blood test	Screen at first visit and repeat during last trimester for high-risk women (CTF, 1979).	At first prenatal visit and at delivery. An additional test at 28 weeks' gestation or later is recommended for high-risk patients. (USPSTF, 1989).†
Hepatitis B	Hepatitis B surface antigen (HBsAg)	No recommendation.†	At first prenatal visit. May be repeated in the third trimester if mother engages in high-risk behavior or is exposed to hepatitis B virus; infants born to HBsAg-positive mothers should receive hepatitis B immune globulin and vaccination (USPSTF, 1989).
Rubella, congenital rubella syndrome	Serologic testing for rubella antibodies	No recommendation (see vaccination of infants and adolescents, Tables 10–3 and 10–4).†	At the first clinical encounter with all pregnant and nonpregnant women of childbearing age lacking evidence of immunity. Susceptible pregnant women should not be vaccinated until immediately after delivery. Vaccination without screening also may be offered (USPSTF, unpublished).
Perinatal morbidity and mortality	Ultrasound	Single ultrasound in the second trimester. Benefit mainly through increased detection and abortion of fetuses with malformations (B) (CTF, 1992b).†	Recommended only for women at high risk of delivering a growth-retarded infant (USPSTF, 1989).

Table continued on opposite page

TABLE 10–2. *(Continued)*

Target Condition	Clinical Procedure	Canadian Task Force (CTF)	U.S. Preventive Services Task Force (USPSTF)
Breast-feeding	Counseling	Provide appropriate information about all infant feeding methods. Breast-feeding is recommended (B) (CTF, 1984).†	No recommendation.
Low birth weight, postnatal asphyxia	Counseling, nutritional history, weighing	Promote intrauterine growth through smoking cessation, adequate rest, and good nutrition (B) (CTF, 1979).†	Provide counseling regarding smoking, alcohol, and other drug abuse and nutrition (USPSTF, 1989).
Alcohol consumption/fetal alcohol syndrome	Counseling	Inform of consequences of alcohol consumption and advise to reduce consumption (B) (CTF, 1979).†	Provide information in the first trimester about the harmful effects of alcohol and other drugs on the fetus. Advise to drink moderately, if at all (USPSTF, 1989).
Anemia	Hemoglobin analysis	No recommendation.	All pregnant women at their first prenatal visit (USPSTF, 1989).
Neural tube defect (NTD)	Periconceptual folic acid supplementation	**Low-risk women:** Advise women in reproductive years (except epileptic women) to increase their consumption of folic acid to 0.4 mg/day. Supplementation may be most appropriate route (A) (CTF, 1994b). **High-risk women:** Supplementation with 4 mg folic acid daily during the 3 months before and the 3 months after conception (A) (CTF, 1994b).	No recommendation.
	Counseling, maternal serum alpha-fetoprotein (MSAFP) measurement at 16–18 weeks; elevated levels followed by ultrasonography and amniocentesis if necessary	Quality-controlled screening programs and the offer of abortion for affected pregnancies. There is some risk of terminating unaffected pregnancies, and women should be informed of all the alternatives (B) (CTF, 1994b).	MSAFP should be measured on all pregnant women during weeks 16–18 in locations that have adequate counseling and follow-up services (USPSTF, 1989).

High-Risk Asymptomatic Populations

Target Condition	Clinical Procedure	Canadian Task Force (CTF)	U.S. Preventive Services Task Force (USPSTF)
Down syndrome (DS)	Counseling, MSAFP screening, amniocentesis	**High-risk women only:** Those at high risk include (1) one parent known carrier of faulty chromosome, (2) previous child with DS, (3) familial history of DS, (4) maternal age >35 years. Following a screening protocol, including the offer of abortion, is recommended (B) (CTF, 1979).†	Amniocentesis for karyotyping should be offered to pregnant women age 35 years and older. MSAFP should be measured on all pregnant women during weeks 16–18 in locations that have adequate counseling and follow-up services (USPSTF, 1989).

Table continued on following page

TABLE 10–2. (*Continued*)

Target Condition	Clinical Procedure	Canadian Task Force (CTF)	U.S. Preventive Services Task Force (USPSTF)
Toxoplasmosis	Counseling, serologic testing for *Toxoplasma gondii*	**High-risk women only:** Women with cat at home or who eat raw meat are at high risk. Nonimmune (seronegative) high-risk women should be tested each trimester and counseled to avoid cat litter and raw meat (A) (CTF, 1979).	No recommendation.
Neonatal herpes simplex	Clinical exam, cesarean section	Transmission of herpes simplex to the newborn can be prevented among women with clinical evidence of genital herpes simplex at delivery (d) (CTF, 1989).	Routine screening is not recommended (D). May ask pregnant women at the first prenatal visit whether they or their sexual contacts have had genital herpetic lesions. Women with first-episode genital lesions should be cultured (USPSTF, unpublished, 1993).
Hemoglobinopathies	Hemoglobin electrophoresis	**High risk only:** It is recommended that people of Asian, African, and Mediterranean ancestry who are of parenting age be tested for thalassemia (B) (CTF, 1979).	**High risk only:** Hemoglobin electrophoresis should be performed at the first prenatal visit of all pregnant black women. Carriers should be urged to have the father tested and should receive information on the availability of prenatal diagnosis if the father is positive (USPSTF, 1989).
Human immunodeficiency virus (HIV)/ acquired immunodeficiency syndrome	Voluntary screening with enzyme-linked immunosorbent assay and confirmatory test	Screening should be considered in large cities, where the rate is highest, or in individuals at high risk (C) (CTF, 1992c).	Testing should be offered to pregnant women (or women contemplating pregnancy) who are at increased risk for HIV infection at the first prenatal visit and in the third trimester (USPSTF, 1989).

* Recommendation grade: A, good evidence for inclusion; B, fair evidence for inclusion; C, evidence for inclusion or exclusion poor, therefore delineating a set of research priorities; D, fair evidence for exclusion.
† Currently under review.

1. Prevention was done in the course of management of intercurrent health problems frequently handled by the family physician.

2. Guidelines such as those shown in the tables in this chapter or adaptations of such guidelines created by physicians for their own patient population should be subjected to clinical judgment, based on knowledge of the patient.

3. The presence of a high-risk situation (e.g., a man occupationally exposed to loud noise or a woman with heavy ultraviolet light exposure) should influence the preventive schedule adopted.

4. Although most of these activities can be done in the context of patient-triggered encounters, exceptions must be recognized. For instance, a recall system for patients who would benefit from mammography on an annual basis would be essential to ensure adequate patient adherence to the preventive schedule.

5. Much of what can and should be done in preventive medicine is appropriately undertaken by allied health professionals working with the family physician, especially if the physician works in settings with a team approach.

Physicians involved in lifetime health maintenance should adopt or design flow sheets compatible with their own practices and charting systems. Such flow sheets make it very easy to check the "health protection status" of patients when they come in for any problem.

Clinical Examples

Case 1

A 42-year-old man, who has been known to the physician for 12 years but has not been seen for 3 years, comes in to have pain at the bottom of his spine checked. He has had it for 5 days following a fall on the ice. A physical examination by the physician reveals a possible fracture of the tip of the coccyx with very localized tenderness. Appropriate advice is given for this problem as well as reassurance. While the patient is in the physician's office, his blood pressure is measured (it is within normal

TABLE 10–3.—PERIODIC HEALTH EXAMINATION PREVENTIVE INTERVENTIONS—*NEONATES AND INFANTS* (0–18 MONTHS)

Target Condition	Clinical Procedure	Canadian Task Force (CTF)	U.S. Preventive Services Task Force (USPSTF)
I. Preventive Interventions at Birth			
Asymptomatic General Population			
Ophthalmia neonatorum	Silver nitrate or antibiotic eye drops	Prophylactic agents have comparable efficacy. Immediate as opposed to delayed silver nitrate prophylaxis does not significantly affect parent–infant bonding (A)* (CTF, 1992d).	Erythromycin 0.5% or tetracycline 1% ophthalmic ointment should be applied to eyes of all newborns as soon as possible after birth and no later than 1 hr of age. Silver nitrate is chemically irritating, frequently causes chemical conjunctivitis, and has limited efficacy in preventing chlamydial ophthalmia neonatorum (USPSTF, 1989).
Congenital syphilis	Venereal Disease Research Laboratory test (VDRL) of cord blood	When indicated, weekly quantitative reagin tests recommended during the first month (B) (CTF, 1979).	No recommendation (see Table 10–2).
Neonatal hypothyroidism	T_4 testing from heel prick	Routine screening programs effective (A) (CTF, 1990a).	Screening all neonates between days 3 and 6 after birth (USPSTF, 1989).
Hemorrhagic disease of the newborn	Intramuscular vitamin K	For primary prevention, inject 1 mg at birth (B) (CTF, 1979).	No recommendation.
High-Risk Populations			
Hemoglobin disorders	Hemoglobin electrophoresis of cord or heel prick blood specimen	No recommendation (see Table 10–2).	**High-risk infants only:** Screen those of Caribbean, Latin American, Asian, Mediterranean, and African descent. Where prevalence of sickle cell disease or thalassemia is high, routine screening may be more efficient than selective screening (USPSTF, 1989).
II. Preventive Interventions for Neonates			
Asymptomatic General Population			
Congenital hip dislocation	Ortolani's maneuver, hip flexion–abduction	Perform in first week of life. Outcome is better with early rather than with late detection and treatment (A) (CTF, 1990d).	No recommendation.
Intraventricular septal defect	Clinical examination, history taking	Perform at discharge from nursery and at 6 weeks. Accurate diagnosis important in view of documented labeling effects (B) (CTF, 1979).	No recommendation.
Phenylketonuria (PKU)	Guthrie test, fluorometric test	Screening should be done routinely on newborns (B) (CTF, 1979).†	Screen newborns prior to discharge from nursery. Infants tested before 24 hr of age should receive a repeat screen before the third week of life (USPSTF, 1989).†
High-Risk Populations			
Human immunodeficiency virus (HIV)/acquired immunodeficiency syndrome	Viral DNA polymerase chain reaction, virus isolation	**High risk only:** Infants of HIV-positive women should be screened for vertical transmission (B) (CTF, 1992c).	No specific recommendation but implied as follow-up to seropositive results in mother.

Table continued on following page

TABLE 10-3.   *(Continued)*

Target Condition	Clinical Procedure	Canadian Task Force (CTF)	U.S. Preventive Services Task Force (USPSTF)
III. Preventive Interventions for Infants *Asymptomatic General Population*			
Hearing impairment	History and physical examination	Screening is recommended because outcome is better with early rather than late detection and treatment (A) (CTF, 1990d).	**High risk only:** Screen those with a family history of childhood hearing impairment, congenital perinatal infection with herpes, syphilis, rubella, cytomegalovirus, or toxoplasmosis, malformations involving head or neck, birth weight below 1500 grams, bacterial meningitis, hyperbilirubinemia requiring exchange transfusion, or severe perinatal asphyxia. High-risk children not tested at birth should be screened before age 3 (USPSTF, 1989).
Physical growth disorders	Serial height and weight measurements	At each well baby visit, investigate infants under the 3rd or above the 97th percentile (B) (CTF, 1979).	Measure regularly and plot on a growth chart throughout infancy and childhood (USPSTF, 1989).
Strabismus, amblyopia	Eye inspection, cover–uncover test, stereotesting	Screening should be performed because outcome is better with early rather than late treatment of amblyopia (A) (CTF, 1990d).	Clinicians should be alert for signs of ocular misalignment when examining all infants and children (see Table 10–4) (USPSTF, 1989).
Preventable infectious disease	Diphtheria–pertussis–tetanus, (DPT), polio, measles–mumps–rubella, (MMR) and Haemophilis influenzae tybe b vaccination	Vaccination schedules vary. Caution is advised in infants allergic to egg protein (A) (CTF, 1990d).†	Childhood immunization should include DTP vaccine along with trivalent oral polio vaccine at ages 2, 4, 6 (DTP only), and 15 months (and age 4–6 years). MMR vaccine should be administered at 15 months and 4–6 years and *Haemophilus influenzae* type b conjugate vaccine should be given at 2, 4, 6, and 15 months or 2, 4, and 12 months of age. In areas with recurrent measles transmission, monovalent measles vaccine should be administered at 9 months of age (USPSTF, 1989).†
Nighttime crying	Counseling, anticipatory guidance	Families complying with appropriate counseling have fewer problems with nighttime crying than those not counseled (A) (CTF, 1990d).	No recommendation.
Motor vehicle accident (MVA) injury	Counseling	Occupant protection systems (seat belts and child safety seats) reduce risk of MVA injury by 40–50%. Urge parents to refrain from driving while under the influence of alcohol and other drugs (B). Physicians can influence at least a short-term improvement in use (CTF, in press).	USPSTF (1989) and CTF positions are in agreement.

Table continued on opposite page

TABLE 10–3. (*Continued*)

Target Condition	Clinical Procedure	Canadian Task Force (CTF)	U.S. Preventive Services Task Force (USPSTF)
Accidental injury in the home	Counseling	Reduce hot water to <54.4°C (130°F); safety-proof cupboards, electrical outlets, and drawers with poisonous substances or sharp objects; put gates over stairs (A) (CTF, 1990d).	It may be clinically prudent for clinicians to recommend specific injury control measures for those at risk. Homeowners should be advised to install and periodically test smoke detectors, hot water heaters should be set at 120°F, and firearms should be kept unloaded in a locked, child-resistant compartment. Those with children in the home should be advised to keep a 1-oz bottle of syrup of ipecac, to display the telephone number of the local poison control center, and to place all medications, toxic substances, and matches in child-resistant containers. Collapsible gates or other barriers should be placed at stairway entrances, a 4-foot latch gate installed around swimming pools, and window guards installed in high-rise buildings to prevent falls (USPSTF, 1989).
Anemia	Hemoglobin/hemotocrit, nutritional counseling	In all but severe cases, there is poor evidence regarding the value of treating iron-deficiency anemia, although treatment does raise hemoglobin levels. High-risk groups include: premature babies, babies born of multiple pregnancy or to an iron-deficient woman, and those in low socioeconomic circumstances (C) (CTF, 1979).†	Screen all infants once. Parents should be encouraged to include iron-enriched foods in the diet of infants and young children (USPSTF, 1989).
Smoking	Counseling	No recommendation.	Parents with young children should receive information on the potential harmful effects of secondhand smoke on child health (USPSTF, 1989).
Dental caries	Nutritional counseling	Daily fluoride supplements where water fluoride levels are suboptimal, if dosage carefully followed (A)/(C) (CTF, in press).	Limit sweets (A) and avoid bedtime baby bottle containing cariogenic liquid (B). Children under age 2 years should be treated with fluoride drops if the water concentration is less than 0.3 ppm; recommended dose is 0.25 mg/day. While examining the mouth, clinicians should be alert for obvious signs of oral disease (USPSTF, 1989).
High-Risk Populations Lead poisoning	Erythrocyte protoporphyrin measurement	No recommendation.	No recommendation.

Table continued on following page

TABLE 10–3. *(Continued)*

Target Condition	Clinical Procedure	Canadian Task Force (CTF)	U.S. Preventive Services Task Force (USPSTF)
Cystic fibrosis (CF)	Sweat test, DNA analysis	Screen with sweat test at 4–6 weeks for diagnosis of CF in siblings of children with CF (B). DNA analysis for siblings of children with CF is effective in identifying carrier status (B) (CTF, 1991d).	No recommendation.
Child maltreatment	Home visits	Families of low socioeconomic status, single parents, or teenaged parents. Home visitation by specially trained nurses during the perinatal period through infancy decreased the number of reports of abuse and neglect, emergency department visits, accidents, and hospital admissions (A) (MacMillan et al., 1993).	Clinicians examining children should be alert to the physical findings of child abuse. Guidelines are available to help clinicians interview children who are potential victims of sexual abuse (USPSTF, 1989).

* Recommendation grade: A, good evidence for inclusion; B, fair evidence for inclusion; C, evidence for inclusion or exclusion poor, therefore delineating a set of research priorities.

† Currently under review.

limits) and clinical assessment of hearing is done, because this man is a foreman in a lumber processing mill; the physician stresses the value of wearing ear protection to prevent hearing loss. Alcohol does not appear to be a problem, and the physician reinforces with satisfaction the patient's continuing 6-year abstinence from smoking. The physician notes that, 5 years ago, the patient's cholesterol was within normal limits; another nonfasting total cholesterol measure is ordered. The patient has been a strong advocate of mandatory seat belts for a long time and has been to the dentist within 12 months. His family situation seems to be healthy.

Case 2

A 65-year-old woman consults her physician about headaches she has had for 4 months. This results in three visits in which a careful investigation of the problem is carried out. On the third visit the physician devotes most of the visit to health protection activities. The decision to defer prevention to the third visit was made because the patient was known to adhere strongly to recommendations of physicians. Otherwise, the package would have been administered earlier in the process. The patient's blood pressure is checked. The skin is examined carefully because this patient spends 7 or 8 months of the year in the hot sun of Alabama; she is encouraged to use sun screens routinely. A physical examination of the breasts is done and arrangements are made for a mammography study. She is urged strongly to return for a further physical examination and mammography in approximately 1 year. The practice nurse has a recall card system for that purpose. The patient gives a history of being under dental care every 8 weeks because of bridge work. A tetanus booster is given in accordance with her mid-decade examination. A Papanicolaou smear is performed because the last one had been performed when she was age 62. The importance of wearing seat belts is reinforced by the physician, because she is resistant to this practice.

Case 3

A 16-year-old girl comes to the physician on referral by a friend to receive a certificate of health as a requirement for attending a basketball camp. Her history reveals that she has not been immunized against rubella, and because she has not seen a physician for several years, she did not receive her mid-decade tetanus–diphtheria booster when she was 15 years old; appropriate vaccinations are given. She is slightly underweight for her height but, on inquiry into her eating habits and dieting practices, the physician is assured that her diet is adequate. She wears orthodontic braces and has received regular dental care; the physician suggests that she consult her dentist regarding dental sealants, and that she wear teeth guards while playing basketball. She is commended for not smoking and given advice about seat belt use. She denies being sexually active; the physician urges her to seek contraceptive advice when she is ready to be sexually involved.

Facilitating the Implementation of Preventive Services in Primary Care

The implementation of new evidence and guidelines into clinical practice has received increasing attention in recent years. Through evaluative studies, usually in the continuing medical education, context, we continue to learn more about what

TABLE 10–4. PERIODIC HEALTH EXAMINATION PREVENTIVE INTERVENTIONS—*CHILDREN AND ADOLESCENTS* (AGES 1½–19 YEARS)*

Target Condition	Clinical Procedure	Canadian Task Force (CTF)	U.S. Preventive Services Task Force (USPSTF)
Asymptomatic General Population			
Physical growth disorders	Serial height and weight measurement	Further investigation is recommended in children under the 3rd or above the 97th percentile (B)† (CTF, 1979).	Measure regularly and plot on a growth chart. Those individuals who are 20% or more above desirable weight should receive appropriate nutritional and exercise counseling (USPSTF, 1989).
Hypertension	Blood pressure measurement	Measure at every visit of all adult patients (> age 16) (A) (CTF, 1979).	Measure regularly in all persons age 3 and above (USPSTF, 1989).
Refractive defects, strabismus, amblyopia	Visual acuity testing, stereotesting, cover–uncover test	Routine screening in preschool years decreases the prevalence of uncorrected disorders (B) (CTF, 1989c).	Testing for amblyopia and strabismus is recommended for all children once before entering school, preferably at age 3 or 4. Routine screening for refractive errors is not recommended for schoolchildren, but clinicians should be alert for signs of ocular misalignment. Vision screening of asymptomatic adolescents is not recommended (USPSTF, 1989).
Rubella, diptheria, and tetanus	Vaccination history	Ensure that prepubertal girls are vaccinated for rubella. Ensure that diphtheria and tetanus booster are given 10 years after full immunization (B) (CTF, 1979).	Serologic testing for rubella antibodies should be performed at the first clinical encounter with women of childbearing age lacking evidence of immunity. Susceptible nonpregnant women who agree not to become pregnant for 3 months should be immunized with RA27/3 live attenuated vaccine. Measles–mumps–rubella vaccine should be administered to all nonpregnant persons born after 1956 who lack evidence of immunity to measles. Tetanus–diphtheria booster should be administered at age 14–16 years and every 10 years thereafter (USPSTF, 1989).
Human immunodeficiency virus (HIV)/acquired immunodeficiency syndrome	Counseling, history, voluntary HIV screening	Obtaining a history of sexual practices and of injection drug use has limited sensitivity but may be offered for patient education; counseling reduces but does not eliminate high-risk activities in high-risk populations (C). Offer screening tests routinely to high-risk patients only (A) (CTF, 1992c).	Clinicians should take a complete sexual and drug use history on all adolescent and adult patients. Sexually active patients should be advised that abstaining from sex or maintaining a mutually faithful monogamous sexual relationship with a partner known to be uninfected are the most effective strategies to prevent infection. Patients also should receive counseling about the indications and proper methods for using condoms and spermicides. Intravenous drug users should be encouraged to enroll in a drug treatment program and warned against sharing or using unsterilized drug equipment.

Table continued on following page

TABLE 10–4. *(Continued)*

Target Condition	Clinical Procedure	Canadian Task Force (CTF)	U.S. Preventive Services Task Force (USPSTF)
			High-risk only: Screening for infection with HIV should be offered periodically to persons seeking treatment for sexually transmitted diseases, intravenous drug users, homosexual and bisexual men, and others at increased risk of infection. Testing should not be performed in the absence of informed consent and adequate pretest and post-test counseling (USPSTF, 1989).‡
Unwanted teenage pregnancy	Contraceptive counseling, sexual practices, history	Identify sexually active adolescents; inform them of contraceptive methods and prescribe if necessary (B) (CTF, 1988).‡	Clinicians should obtain a complete sexual history from all adolescent and adult patients. Those who are sexually active but do not want to have a child should receive detailed counseling on methods to prevent unintended pregnancy. Sexually active patients also should receive information on measures to prevent sexually transmitted diseases (USPSTF, 1989).
Malnutrition	Counseling, history	Adolescent girls are at high risk for malnutrition. Enquire into eating habits and possible deficiencies (iron, folic acid, calcium) (B) (CTF, 1979).	Adolescent girls should receive counseling on calcium and iron intake; parents should be counseled about the nutritional requirements of infancy and childhood (USPSTF, 1989).
Dental disease	Dental history and counseling	Water fluoridation to prevent caries (A). Fluoride supplementation for children in areas without water fluoridation if dosage schedule carefully followed (A). Fluoride dentifrice daily (A) with supervision of young children to avoid excessive swallowing. Flossing is ineffective in preventing gingivitis in children but is recommended to establish the habit (C). (CTF, in press).	All patients should be encouraged to visit a dental care provider on a regular basis (C). Primary care clinicians should counsel patients regarding daily tooth brushing and dental flossing (C), the appropriate use of fluoride for caries prevention (A), and avoiding sugary foods (A). Children living in communities with inadequate water fluoridation should receive appropriate dietary fluoride supplements (A). While examining the mouth, clinicians should be alert for obvious signs of oral disease (dental decay, malalignment, premature loss of teeth, mouth breathing) (USPSTF, 1989).
Smoking	Counseling, history	Inform about the risks of smoking and available smoking cessation strategies; schedule follow-up visits to reinforce advice (A) (CTF, 1986).	Tobacco cessation counseling should be offered on a regular basis to all patients who smoke cigarettes, pipes, or cigars and to those who use smokeless tobacco. The prescription of nicotine gum may be an appropriate adjunct for some patients. Adolescents who do not currently use tobacco products should be advised not to start. Parents with young children should receive information on the harmful effects of secondhand smoke. (USPSTF, 1989).

Table continued on opposite page

TABLE 10–4. *(Continued)*

Target Condition	Clinical Procedure	Canadian Task Force (CTF)	U.S. Preventive Services Task Force (USPSTF)
Motor vehicle accidents	Counseling	Physician can influence a significant short-term improvement in the use of seat belts (B). Children should not be permitted to ride in the cargo area of station wagons, vans, or pickup trucks (CTF, unpublished).	Clinicians regularly should urge their patients to use safety belts whenever driving or riding in an automobile. Child safety seats or seat belts should be worn in accordance with the child's size. Children should not be permitted to ride in the cargo area of station wagons, vans, or pickup trucks. Those who operate or ride on motorcycles or bicycles should be counseled to wear safety helmets and the latter counseled regarding avoiding riding in motor vehicle traffic. All patients should be counseled regarding the dangers of operating a motor vehicle while under the influence of alcohol or other drugs, as well as on the risks of riding in a vehicle operated by someone who is under the influence of these substances. Adolescents should be encouraged to discuss with their families transportation alternatives for social activities where alcohol and other drugs are used (USPSTF, 1989).
Household and recreational injury	Counseling	Advise individuals who ride bicycles on roadways to wear helmets (B). Advise parents to never leave young child alone in bathtub (B), regarding burns and scalds (smoking, smoke detectors, nonflammable sleepwear, water temperature) (B), and on prevention of poisoning (B). Counsel adolescents against engaging in water recreational activity while under the influence of alcohol (B) (CTF, unpublished).	Clinicians should urge adolescents and adults who use alcohol or other drugs to avoid engaging in potentially dangerous activities (operating vehicle, swimming, handling firearms, smoking in bed) while intoxicated. It may be clinically prudent to provide counseling on other measures to reduce the risk of unintentional injuries from falls, drowning, fires or burns, poisoning, and firearms (USPSTF, 1989).
Violent injuries	Counseling, referral	No recommendation	Clinicians should ask adolescents and young adults (especially males ages 15–24 years) to discuss previous violent behavior, current alcohol and drug use, and the availability of firearms. Patients with evidence of violent behavior should be counseled regarding nonviolent alternatives to conflict resolution and about the risks of violent injury associated with easy access to firearms and intoxication with alcohol or other drugs (USPSTF, 1989).

Table continued on following page

TABLE 10–4. *(Continued)*

Target Condition	Clinical Procedure	Canadian Task Force (CTF)	U.S. Preventive Services Task Force (USPSTF)
High-Risk Populations Suicide	Evaluation of suicide risk	**High risk:** Evidence of psychiatric disorder (especially psychosis, depression, or substance abuse), recent suicide attempt, or death of family member through suicide. Effectiveness of evaluation by primary caregivers has not been evaluated but is recommended for people at high risk because of burden of suffering (C) (CTF, 1990b).	**High risk:** recent divorce, separation, unemployment, depression, alcohol or other drug abuse, serious medical illnesses, living alone, recent bereavement. Clinicians should assess the emotional well-being of patients at risk; patients with evidence of suicidal ideation should be questioned regarding the extent of preparatory actions and/or referred for psychiatric counseling.

*See Table 10–5 for the following conditions that also apply to high-risk children and adolescents: skin cancer, tuberculosis, influenza, meningococcal meningitis, hemoglobinopathies, hearing impairment, diabetes mellitus, chlamydial genital infection, gonorrhea, syphilis, hepatitis B, lung cancer, pneumococcal pneumonia, and testicular cancer. Some interventions described in Table 10–3 for infants also carry forward into this age group (i.e., child maltreatment, hearing impairment, and lead poisoning).

†Recommendation grade: A, good evidence for inclusion; B, fair evidence for inclusion; C, evidence for inclusion or exclusion poor, therefore delineating a set of research priorities.

‡Currently under review.

works and what does not. Davis et al. (1992) provided an important update of their earlier review regarding effective strategies related to physician behavior change. They drew on categories developed by Green et al. (1988) to group the interventions into predisposing strategies, predisposing plus enabling strategies, predisposing plus reinforcing strategies, and multiple-component interventions.

Guidelines alone are not effective in changing behavior. The current use of reminders and feedback in conjunction with guidelines would appear to be effective in improving the performance of physicians, particularly in the area of prevention. The use of opinion leaders to convey new information and attention to the modification of office systems are also important.

Cognitive Factors in Implementation

Although the proliferation of preventive services guidelines witnessed over the last several years can be helpful, conflicting guidelines can be confusing to the practicing physician. Basing guidelines on a standardized review and evaluation of evidence, an approach used by the Canadian Task Force on the Periodic Health Examination and the U.S. Preventive Services Task Force is an approach being adopted more frequently by bodies issuing guidelines. However, guidelines built on consensus more than evidence continue to be generated and have the potential to create confusion.

It is now well recognized that knowledge alone is insufficient to ensure the implementation of effective preventive services (Lomas and Haynes, 1988). However, awareness and knowledge of effective guidelines can be seen as a predisposing

factor that must be linked to other strategies to ensure successful implementation.

Sociodemographic Characteristics of Implementation

Despite major differences between the Canadian and the American health care systems, the level of integration of preventive services into primary care seems to be comparable in these two countries (Bass and Elford, 1988; Lewis, 1988).

Certain demographic variables appear to be associated with increased provision of preventive services. Younger physicians are more likely than older physicians to comply with preventive service recommendations. Moreover, women physicians have been found to be more likely to include preventive services overall in their practice (Battista et al., 1986), and it would appear that women physicians are more likely to offer preventive services to women than are male physicians (Lurie et al., 1993). Although there is limited evidence that differences in practice patterns result from differences in past medical training, evidence from a recent Canadian study supports the hypothesis that graduates of family medicine residency training are more likely to include preventive services in their clinical practice (Borgiel et al., 1989).

Organizational Factors in Implementation

OPERATIONAL TOOLS. In the review by Davis et al. (1992), reminder systems, particularly computer-based systems, were effective in facilitating the implementation of preventive services. Feedback in the clinical setting—for example, as the result of practice audit—is also an effective strategy. Evidence exists to support the benefit of trans-

TABLE 10–5. PERIODIC HEALTH EXAMINATION PREVENTIVE INTERVENTIONS—*ALL ADULTS*
(AGES 20–64 YEARS)

Target Condition	Clinical Procedure	Canadian Task Force (CTF)	U.S. Preventive Services Task Force (USPSTF)
Asymptomatic General Population			
Hypertension	Blood pressure measurement	Measure at every visit (A)* (CTF, 1984).	Persons thought to be normotensive should receive blood pressure measurements at least once every 2 years if their last diastolic and systolic pressures were below 85 and 140 mm Hg, respectively, and annually if the last diastolic blood pressure was 85–89 mm Hg (USPSTF, 1989).
Breast cancer	Clinical breast examination, mammography	Perform clinical exam and mammography annually for women age >50 years; consider for women age 35+ with a positive family history (A) (CTF, 1986).†	All women over age 40 should receive an annual clinical breast examination. Mammography every 1–2 years is recommended for women ages 50–75. For women with a family history of premenopausally diagnosed breast cancer in first-degree relatives, it may be prudent to begin regular screening at age 35 (USPSTF, 1989).
Cervical cancer	Papanicolaou smear	Annual screening is recommended following initiation of sexual activity or age 18; after two normal smears, screen every 3 years to age 69 (B). Consider increasing frequency for women with risk factors: age of first sexual intercourse <18 years, many sexual partners or consort with many partners, smoking, or low socioeconomic status. (CTF, unpublished, 1992).	Regular testing is recommended for all women who are or have been sexually active, beginning with the onset of sexual activity or age 18 and repeated every 1–3 years at the physician's discretion, depending on risk factors. They may be discontinued at age 65 if previous smears have been consistently normal (USPSTF, 1989).
Hypercholesterolemia	Nonfasting plasma cholesterol analysis, dietary advice	In the primary prevention of coronary artery disease (CAD), treatment is efficacious in reducing incidence of CAD (B) but the effectiveness of screening has not been evaluated; consider screening for men ages 30–59 (C). Perform every 5 years. Repeat at 1–8 weeks if total cholesterol level >6.2 mmol/L. Prescribe low-fat diet if mean total cholesterol level is 6.20–6.85 mmol/L or low-density lipoprotein C (LDL-C) level is 4.15-4.90 mmol/L. Prescribe stepped low-fat diet if mean total cholesterol level >6.85 mmol/L or LDL-C level >4.90 mmol/L; if goal is not achieved within 6 months (mean total cholesterol level >6.85 mmol/L or LDL-C >4.50 mmol/L), add drug therapy. There is fair evidence to provide general dietary advice to men ages 30–69. Decreased intake of total fat, saturated fat, and cholesterol is associated with decreased incidence of CAD (B). For all others, the value of such advice has not been demonstrated (C) (CTF, 1993).	Periodic measurement of total serum cholesterol (nonfasting) is most important for middle-aged men, and it may also be clinically prudent in young men, women, and the elderly; an interval of every 5 years (and more frequently with history of elevated cholesterol) based on expert opinion. Abnormal results should be confirmed with second test. All adults with total blood cholesterol >6.2 mmol/L or those with borderline levels (5.15–6.15 mmol/L) and CAD or two or more cardiac risk factors (male gender, family history of premature CAD in first-degree relative, smoking, hypertension, high-density lipoprotein C <0.90 mmol/L, diabetes mellitus, previous stroke or peripheral vascular disease, severe obesity) should receive counseling on the results, intensive dietary counseling, and follow-up evaluation. Drug therapy should be considered in middle-aged men in whom blood cholesterol remains significantly elevated (>6.85 mmol/L or >6.2 mmol/L in persons with CAD or at least two risk factors) after a 6-month trial of dietary intervention (USPSTF, 1989).

Table continued on following page

TABLE 10–5. *(Continued)*

Target Condition	Clinical Procedure	Canadian Task Force (CTF)	U.S. Preventive Services Task Force (USPSTF)
Osteoporotic fractures	Estrogen/hormone replacement therapy (ERT/ HRT), calcium supplementation, exercise	There is good evidence that ERT slows the rate of bone loss and fair evidence that it decreases the incidence of fractures. Calcium intake and exercise may prevent bone loss. Weigh possible risk of cardiovascular disease, stroke, and fracture versus endometrial and breast cancer; decisions regarding ERT should be made on an individual basis (C) (CTF, 1988).†	ERT should be considered for asymptomatic women who are at increased risk for osteoporosis, who lack known contraindications, and who have received adequate counseling about potential benefits and risks. Women should receive counseling on methods to ensure adequate calcium intake and weight-bearing exercise. (USPSTF, 1989).†
Tetanus	Tetanus booster	Booster recommended once every 10 years (A) (CTF, 1979).	All adults should receive tetanus–diphtheria toxoid boosters at least once every 10 years (USPSTF, 1989).
Household, recreational injuries	Counseling	Advise individuals who ride bicycles on roadways to wear helmets (B). Counsel on household safety (smoke detectors, etc.) (B) (CTF, unpublished, 1992).	Patients who use alcohol or other drugs should be warned against engaging in potentially dangerous activities while intoxicated. It may be clinically prudent to provide counseling on other measures to reduce the risk of unintentional household or environmental injuries from falls, drownings, fires or burns, poisoning, and firearms (USPSTF, 1989).
Motor vehicle accident injury	Counseling	Physician can improve short-term use of seat belts (B) (CTF, unpublished).	Clinicians regularly should urge their patients to use safety belts whenever driving or riding in an automobile. Those who operate or ride on motorcycles or bicycles should be counseled to wear safety helmets. All patients should be counseled regarding the dangers of operating a motor vehicle while under the influence of alcohol or other drugs, as well as on the risks of riding in a vehicle operated by someone who is under the influence of these substances. Counseling is most important for those at increased risk of motor vehicle injury, such as young adults, persons who use alcohol or other drugs, and patients with medical conditions that may impair motor vehicle safety (USPSTF, 1989).
Problem drinking	Case finding and counseling	Active case finding to identify problem drinking, counseling to reduce alcohol consumption, and periodic monitoring of progress. Recommend men drink no more than 3–5 drinks per day and women, 2–3 (B) (CTF, 1989b).	All adults should be asked to describe their use of alcohol and other drugs. Persons in whom alcohol or other drug abuse or dependence is confirmed should receive appropriate counseling, treatment, and referral. All persons who use alcohol should be encouraged to limit their consumption, and all persons who use alcohol or other intoxicating drugs should be counseled about the health risks and dangers of operating a motor vehicle or performing other potentially dangerous activities while intoxicated (USPSTF, 1989).

Table continued on opposite page

TABLE 10–5. *(Continued)*

Target Condition	Clinical Procedure	Canadian Task Force (CTF)	U.S. Preventive Services Task Force (USPSTF)
Physical inactivity	Exercise counseling	No recommendations.	Clinicians should counsel all patients to engage in a program of regular physical activity, tailored to their health status and personal lifestyle (USPSTF, 1989).
Malnutrition	Nutrition counseling	No recommendation (except for hypercholesterolemia; see above).†	Clinicians should provide periodic counseling regarding dietary intake of calories, fat (especially limiting saturated fat; total fat should be <30% of total calories), cholesterol, complex carbohydrates (starches), fiber, and sodium. Specifically, patients should receive diet and exercise prescription designed to achieve and maintain a desirable weight by keeping caloric intake balanced with energy expenditures (USPSTF, 1989).
Dental caries, periodontal disease, malocclusion	Dental history, fluoridation, oral hygiene, dental services, counseling	Fluoride dentifrice should be used daily (A). Toothbrushing (B) and flossing (A) are recommended for primary prevention of gingivitis. There is fair evidence to recommend professional scaling based on the clinical signs of periodontal disease and oral hygiene performance of the individual (B), and fair evidence to avoid smoking (B) to prevent periodontal disease. **High risk only:** Professionally applied topical fluorides and self-applied fluoride mouth rinses are recommended for those with very active decay (A). Anticalculus dentifrice is recommended for high calculus formers. (B) Scaling and chlorhexidine rinse are recommended for individuals with periodontitis or periodontal surgery (A) (Ismail et al., 1993).	All patients should be encouraged to visit a dental care provider on a regular basis (C). Primary care clinicians should counsel patients regarding daily tooth brushing and dental flossing (C), the appropriate use of fluoride for caries prevention (A), and avoiding sugary foods (A). While examining the mouth, clinicians should be alert for obvious signs of oral disease. (USPSTF, 1989).
Smoking	Counseling and follow-up	Inform about the risks of smoking and available smoking cessation strategies; schedule follow-up visits to reinforce advice. Prescribe nicotine gum or patch only as an adjunct (A) (CTF, 1986).	Tobacco cessation counseling should be offered on a regular basis to all patients who smoke cigarettes, pipes, or cigars and to those who use smokeless tobacco. The prescription of nicotine gum may be an appropriate adjunct for some patients. Young adults who do not currently use tobacco products should be advised not to start. (USPSTF, 1989).
High-Risk Populations Skin cancer	Skin examination, counseling	Those with heavy exposure to ultraviolet light or in contact with polycyclic aromatic hydrocarbons; first-degree relatives of patients with dysplastic nevi. Counsel to reduce exposure to ultraviolet light (B) (CTF, 1984).†	**High-risk persons only:** Clinicians should advise patients at increased risk of skin cancer to protect their skin from solar rays (C) (USPSTF, unpublished, 1993).

Table continued on following page

TABLE 10–5. *(Continued)*

Target Condition	Clinical Procedure	Canadian Task Force (CTF)	U.S. Preventive Services Task Force (USPSTF)
Tuberculosis (TB)	Mantoux skin test, bacille Calmette-Guérin immunization and isoniazid chemoprophylaxis	Those living in contact with a person with TB, occupationally exposed to TB, or in communities or groups in which the infection rate is high. For those who react negatively to tuberculin, vaccine is effective; for those who react positively, chemoprophylaxis prevents progression of the disease (A) (CTF, 1979).†	**High risk only:** Household members of persons with TB and others at risk for close contact with TB (staff of TB clinics, shelters for the homeless, nursing homes, substance abuse facilities, dialysis units, correctional institutions); recent immigrants or refugees from countries in which TB is common; migrant workers; residents of nursing homes, correctional institutes, and homeless shelters; persons with certain underlying medical disorders (eg., human immunodeficiency virus [HIV] infection). Screening recommended for all persons at increased risk. Persons with positive skin test should receive a chest radiograph and clinical evaluation and isoniazid prophylaxis if there is no active infection (USPSTF, 1989).
Influenza	Most recent influenza vaccine, amantadine prophylaxis	Annual vaccination of selected populations: institutionalized, chronic heart and pulmonary disease, diabetics, and immunocompromised (B). Amantadine chemoprophylaxis around index case (A). (CTF, in press).	**High-risk persons only:** Individuals suffering from chronic cardiopulmonary disorders, metabolic diseases (including diabetes mellitus), hemoglobinopathies, immunosuppression, or renal dysfunction. Health care workers and residents of long-term care facilities also should be vaccinated. For those at high risk for influenza A or in whom vaccination is contraindicated, amantadine prophylaxis should be used (USPSTF, 1989).
Meningococcal meningitis	Rifamprin chemoprophylaxis	No recommendation.	**High risk:** Indicated for household or day care nonpregnant contacts of persons with meningococcal infection, as well as those with direct exposure to oral secretions (e.g., kissing) (USPSTF, 1989).
Hemoglobinopathies	Hemoglobin electrophoresis	It is recommended that people of Asian, African, and Mediterranean ancestry who are or parenting age be tested for thalassemia (B) (CTF, 1979).	**High risk:** those of Caribbean, Latin American, Asian, Mediterranean, and African descent. Discuss testing with adolescents and young adults at risk for sickle cell trait, thalassemia, and other hemoglobinopathies (USPSTF, 1989).
Hearing impairment	History and physical examination, referral for audiometry	Promote use of ear protection in those with occupational or leisure-time exposure to loud noise (A). For patients with a positive family history and a history of ear problems, early detection and correction of impairment is recommended (B). (CTF, 1984).	**High risk only:** Those exposed to excessive noise in occupational or recreational settings. Frequently left to clinical discretion. (USPSTF, 1989).

Table continued on opposite page

TABLE 10–5. *(Continued)*

Target Condition	Clinical Procedure	Canadian Task Force (CTF)	U.S. Preventive Services Task Force (USPSTF)
Colorectal cancer	Colonoscopy, sigmoidoscopy, hemoccult	Cancer family syndrome—risk of adenocarcinoma approaches 50%; offer colonoscopy because it is a superior test for detecting right-sided cancer (B) (Solomon et al., 1994).	Under review.
Diabetes mellitus	Fasting and oral glucose tolerance test	Positive family history, circulatory dysfunction and frank vascular impairments, obstetric history of birth weight over 4 kg, stillbirth, recurrent abortion or fetal abnormalities. Secondary prevention (B) (CTF, 1979).†	Periodic fasting plasma glucose measurements may be appropriate in persons at **high risk** for diabetes, such as the markedly obese, persons with a family history of diabetes, or women with a history of gestational diabetes. Routine screening in asymptomatic nonpregnant adults is not recommended. (USPSTF, 1989).
Chlamydial genital infection	Culture of cervical or urethral swab or micromethod	Sexual partners of patients with nongonococcal urethritis, those with multiple sexual partners (B) (CTF, 1984).†	Routine testing is recommended for asymptomatic persons who attend clinics for sexually transmitted diseases (STDs), adolescents, or family planning; those age <20 years; and those with multiple sexual partners, or a sexual partner with multiple sexual contacts. (USPSTF, 1989).
Gonorrhea	Culture of cervical or urethral swab	Persons with multiple sexual partners, in active military service, at work camps, or in prisons; homosexuals (A) (CTF, 1979).†	**High risk:** prostitutes, persons with multiple sexual partners or a sexual partner with multiple sexual contacts, sexual contacts of persons with culture-proven gonorrhea, and persons with a history of repeated episodes of gonorrhea. (USPSTF, 1989).
Syphilis	Venereal Disease Research Laboratory (VDRL) or rapid plasma reagrin (RPR) blood tests	Homosexuals, those with multiple sexual partners, in active military service, at work camps, or in prisons. (A) (CTF, 1979).	Routine serologic testing recommended for persons at **increased risk,** such as prostitutes, persons who engage in sex with multiple partners in areas in which syphilis is prevalent, and sexual contacts of persons with active syphilis. (USPSTF, 1989).
Hepatitis B	Hepatitis B vaccination	Dialysis patients, patients receiving multiple blood products, health care personnel exposed to blood or blood products, patients entering institutions for mentally retarded, drug addicts, homosexuals, those in contact with patients or carriers. Vaccinate for primary prevention (A) (CTF, 1984).†	Vaccine should be offered to homosexually active men, intravenous drug users, recipients of certain blood products, and persons in health-related jobs with frequent exposure to blood or blood products (A) (USPSTF, 1989).†
HIV/acquired immunodeficiency syndrome	Counseling, history, voluntary HIV screening	Offer screening to homosexual and bisexual men, prostitutes, injection drug users, people with STDs, sexual contacts of HIV-positive people, and those from countries with a high prevalence rate of HIV infection (A) (CTF, 1992c).	Screening for infection with HIV should be offered periodically to persons seeking treatment for STDs, intravenous drug users, homosexual and bisexual men, and others at increased risk of infection. Testing should not be performed in the absence of informed consent and adequate pretest and post-test counseling. Intravenous drug users should be encouraged to enroll in a drug treatment program and warned against sharing drug equipment or using unsterilized needles and syringes.

Table continued on following page

TABLE 10–5. *(Continued)*

Target Condition	Clinical Procedure	Canadian Task Force (CTF)	U.S. Preventive Services Task Force (USPSTF)
Suicide	Evaluation of suicide risk	Evidence of psychiatric disorder (especially psychosis, depression, or substance abuse), recent suicide attempt, or death of family member through suicide. Effectiveness of evaluation by primary caregivers has not been evaluated but is recommended for people at high risk because of burden of suffering (C) (CTF, 1990b).	**High risk:** recent divorce, separation, unemployment, depression, alcohol or other drug abuse, serious medical illnesses, living alone, recent bereavement. Clinicians should assess the emotional well-being of patients at risk; patients with evidence of suicidal ideation should be questioned regarding the extent of preparatory actions and/or referred for psychiatric counseling.
Lung cancer	Nutritional counseling	Although smoking cessation is much more desirable, smokers who are unable to quit should be advised to follow a diet high in leafy green vegetables and fruit (fair evidence diet beneficial; effectiveness of physician advice unknown) (B/C) (CTF, 1990c).	No recommendation.
Pneumococcal pneumonia	Vaccination	Vaccine only recommended for patients with sickle-cell disease, those having undergone splenectomy, and immunocompetent patients ≥55 years in institutions (A) (CTF, 1991b).	Pneumococcal vaccination should be provided at least once to all persons age ≥65 years and to those with medical conditions that increase the risk of pneumococcal infection (chronic cardiac or pulmonary disease, sickle-cell disease, nephrotic syndrome, Hodgkin's disease, asplenia, diabetes mellitus, alcoholism, cirrhosis, multiple myeloma, renal disease, and conditions associated with immunosuppression). Patients living in special environments or social settings with an identified increased risk of pneumococcal disease also should be vaccinated (B) (USPSTF, 1989).
Peripheral artery disease	Physical exam	No recommendation.	Routine screening is not recommended.
Testicular cancer	Physical exam	Little evidence regarding effectiveness of prevention but the incidence of the disease is higher in individuals who have cryptorchidism, are infertile with atrophic testes, or are of ambiguous sex (C) (CFT, 1984).	Periodic screening for testicular cancer is recommended for men with a history of cryptorchidism, orchiopexy, or testicular atrophy. Clinicians should advise adolescents and young adult males to seek prompt medical attention for testicular symptoms such as pain, swelling, or heaviness. (USPSTF, 1989).

*Recommendation grade: A, good evidence for inclusion; B, fair evidence for inclusion; C, evidence for inclusion or exclusion is poor, therefore delineating a set of research priorities.
†Currently under review.

lating practice recommendations into practical instruments such as flow sheets or health charts to be used by the clinician in the practice setting (Cohen et al., 1982; Knight et al., 1987). Finally, patient education strategies have been demonstrated to be useful in the implementation and provision of preventive services (McPhee et al., 1991).

OFFICE SYSTEM CHANGE.   Increasingly, investigators have recognized the importance of viewing the primary care physician's office from a systems perspective and have identified the need to inter-

vene with strategies that facilitate changes in the system. Studies evaluating such interventions to enhance the implementation of preventive services in the cancer field have demonstrated the power of this approach (Carney et al., 1992; Dietrich et al., 1992).

Additional Factors

A number of other factors have been suggested as influencing implementation of preventive services. However, the evidence is less clear cut. For

TABLE 10–6.   PERIODIC HEALTH EXAMINATION PREVENTIVE INTERVENTIONS—*ELDERLY*
(>65 years of age)*

Target Condition	Clinical Procedure	Canadian Task Force (CTF)	U.S. Preventive Services Task Force (USPSTF)
Asymptomatic General Population			
Hearing impairment	History, referral for auditory testing	Identify those with a history of occupational or leisure-time exposure to loud noise, or who present with loud speech, or tinnitus, or need to have words repeated (B)† (CTF, 1984).	Elderly patients should be evaluated regarding their hearing, counseled regarding the availability and use of hearing aids, and referred appropriately for any abnormalities. (USPSTF, 1989).
Refractive defects	Snellen sight card	The Snellen sight card reliably detects reduced visual acuity (B) (CTF, in press).	Vision screening may be appropriate in the elderly but there is insufficient evidence to recommend an optimal interval (USPSTF, 1989).
Functional incapacity with aging	Physical appraisal, detailed clinical inquiry	Detect impairment in sensory function, psychological function, locomotion, and activities of daily living. This preferably is done in the home setting (B) (CTF, 1979).	Clinician periodically should inquire into the functional status of elderly patients at home and at work, and should remain alert to changes in performance with age (USPSTF, 1989).
Influenza	Influenza vaccination, outreach	Annual vaccination reduces incidence and severity of the disease (B) and outreach increases vaccination rate (A) (CTF, in press).	Influenza vaccine should be administered annually to all persons age 65 and older (A) (USPSTF, 1989).
Household and recreational injuries	Counseling, assessment, referral	Multidisciplinary postfall assessment reduces future falls and injury (A) (CTF, unpublished).	Elderly patients or those responsible for elderly persons should be advised to inspect the home for adequate lighting, to remove or repair floor structures that predispose to tripping, and to install handrails and traction strips in stairways and bathtubs. Clinicians periodically should test visual acuity, counsel patients with medical conditions affecting mobility, and monitor the use of drugs associated with falls. Older patients who lack medical contraindications should be counseled to engage in exercise programs to maintain and improve mobility and flexibility (USPSTF, 1989).
High-Risk Populations			
Diabetic retinopathy (DR)	Funduscopy, retinal photography	Diabetics of at least 5 years' duration should be screened annually. Photocoagulation in proliferative DR preserves vision (B) (CTF, in press).	No recommendation.
Malnutrition	Nutritional history, height and weight measurement	Elderly persons living alone should be assessed (B). Home visits may be useful. (CTF, 1979).‡	No specific recommendation.

* To be performed in addition to procedures recommended in the adult health examination.
† Recommendation grade: A, good evidence for inclusion; B, fair evidence for inclusion.
‡ Currently under review.

example, although some evidence exists to support the increased implementation of preventive services in a community health center as compared to fee-for-service practices (Battista and Spitzer, 1983), the evidence is less clear cut in health maintenance organizations in the United States (Wilner, 1986) and in similar practice settings in Canada (Lomas and Abelson, 1990). Likewise, the evidence regarding reimbursement for services continues to be associated with some controversy (Logsdon and Rosen, 1984; Manning et al., 1984; Pineault, 1976).

Time can be limiting factor in the integration of preventive services into primary care. Preventive services compete with curative services, and a limited number of preventive activities can be offered

**TABLE 10–7. PERIODIC HEALTH EXAMINATION PREVENTIVE INTERVENTIONS THAT REMAIN
CONTROVERSIAL AS TO INCLUSION OR EXCLUSION**

Target Condition	Clinical Procedure	Nature of Controversy
Anemia	Routine iron supplementation in pregnancy	Although it is clear from observational data that pregnant women with anemia (hemoglobin <10 gm/dL) are at increased risk of preterm birth, low birth weight, and other adverse outcomes, it is unclear from such evidence whether anemia is responsible for these outcomes or whether they can be prevented through iron supplementation. It is unclear whether iron supplementation during pregnancy can reduce the incidence of iron deficiency in children, a condition that has been associated with delayed psychomotor development. Although iron supplementation can improve hematologic indices, controlled clinical trials have failed to demonstrate that iron supplementation or changes in hematologic indices actually improve clinical outcomes for the mother or newborn.
Gestational diabetes	Fasting, random blood glucose, oral glucose challenge test (GCT), or search for risk factors and test for glucosuria	The effectiveness of screening has not been evaluated properly in the general population, but screening with GCT may result in a decreased incidence of macrosomia and birth trauma. However, important questions persist regarding the benefits of treatment.
Intrapartum asphyxia	Electronic fetal monitoring (EFM) during labor	There is poor evidence for either inclusion or exclusion of EFM as opposed to active clinical monitoring even for high-risk women. Neonatal morbidity and mortality rates have not been shown definitively to be reduced, and an increase in the rate of cesarean section has been associated with EFM use.
Scoliosis	Physical examination, Adams forward bending test	Screening has a high rate of overreferral, and there is a lack of sound evidence about the efficacy of treatment, even when scoliosis is detected at an earlier and less severe stage.
Bacteriuria	Urine testing	Screening detects some cases, but yield is low and reinfection often follows treatment. It may be clinically prudent to screen diabetics and preschool children based on prevalence and seriousness of complications.
Colorectal cancer*	Fecal occult blood screening in adults over age 40	There is evidence that annual rehydrated hemoccult fecal occult blood screening has a small but significant cancer specific mortality benefit after more than 10 years of screening. However, the high false positivity (9.8%) combined with the poor sensitivity of annual (49%) and biannual (38%) screening make this a poor method for detecting colorectal cancer.
Prostate cancer	Digital rectal examination, PSA prostate-specific antigen	The prevalence of prostate cancer increases with age but may not always be life threatening. Evidence on the benefits of treatment is inconclusive. Prostate-specific antigen testing does not have sufficient evidence to support its effectiveness.
Breast cancer	Teaching breast self-examination	There is insufficient evidence that breast self-examination reduces mortality. Breast self-examination may produce anxiety or cause the performance of unnecessary diagnostic procedures in young women, in whom the incidence of breast cancer is very low.
Oral cancer	Oral cavity exam	Secondary prevention by regular oral examinations to ensure early detection is possible but the effects on the outcome are unknown. Effectiveness of treatment depends on the site of the lesion. It may be clinically prudent in persons at increased risk (smoking or alcohol history or those with suspicious lesions).
Low back injury	Back conditioning exercise	There is no consistent association between common activities (even repetitive lifting, cross-country skiing, and prolonged driving, which probably increase risk) and injury. Screening by history, physical examination, or diagnostic imaging has not been proved to be sensitive or specific. The benefits of exercise are inconclusive and there is insufficient evidence to recommend a single, universally correct lifting technique.
Cervical carotid bruits, stroke	Neck auscultation	The efficacy of early detection and treatment for preventing stroke in asymptomatic patients is not established. The U.S. Preventive Services Task Force suggests screening of persons at high risk for cerebrovascular or cardiovascular disease or with neurologic symptoms (transient ischemic attacks) or history of cerebrovascular disease. The recommendation may change as new evidence emerges regarding the effectiveness of treatment.

Table continued on opposite page

TABLE 10–7. *(Continued)*

Target Condition	Clinical Procedure	Nature of Controversy
Age-related macular degeneration (ARMD), glaucoma*	Funduscopy	Detection of ARMD can be performed reliably by those trained in funduscopy, but sensitivity for its detection by primary care physicians is unknown. Photocoagulation preserves vision in ARMD with neovascularization. Schiøtz tonometry has poor sensitivity and specificity in detecting glaucoma.
Low-dose aspirin prophylaxis	Cardiovascular disease	No clear evidence that routine use in asymptomatic men will reduce the rate of death from all causes, cardiovascular disease, or myocardial infarction (MI); a reduced rate of nonfatal MI needs to be balanced against potential adverse effects (hemorrhage and disabling stroke).
Abdominal aortic aneurysm	Physical examination, ultrasonography	Screening in primary care has not been evaluated in terms of detection rate or impact on death. Death rate is considerably lower for elective resection than for emergency resection of ruptured aneurysm.
Cognitive impairment*	Mental status questionnaire for patients over 6 years	Short Portable Mental Status questionnaire and Mini-Mental State Examination fulfill acceptable methodologic criteria and are practical, but treatment has not been shown to be beneficial. High costs of investigation and labeling are potentially harmful but have not been studied systematically.

* Considered controversial solely by the Canadian Task Force (CTF). 1979, 1984, 1986, 1989d, 1991a, 1991c, 1991e, 1991f, Solomon et al., 1994.

TABLE 10–8.   PERIODIC HEALTH EXAMINATION PREVENTIVE INTERVENTIONS THAT SHOULD *NOT* BE PERFORMED IN ASYMPTOMATIC PERSONS

Target Condition	Clinical Procedure	Canadian Task Force (CTF)	U.S. Preventive Services Task Force (USPSTF)
Preterm birth	Home uterine activity monitoring (HUAM)	No recommendation.	There are no controlled trials of HUAM in pregnancies with no risk factors for preterm labor. Given lack of evidence of benefit, HUAM is not recommended in the management of normal pregnancies (USPSTF, 1993).
Child maltreatment	Screening to identify people at risk of maltreating children	Screening procedures (checklists, self-administered questionnaires, standardized interviews, or clinical judgment) have high false-positive rates, resulting in a high risk of mislabeling people as potential child abusers (D)* (MacMillan et al., 1993).	Routine screening interviews or examinations for evidence of violent injuries are not recommended. Clinicians examining children should be alert to the physical findings of child abuse (USPSTF, 1989).
Developmental delay	Preschool developmental screening with Denver Developmental test	Improved school performance through early intervention has not been demonstrated and parental anxiety is increased (D) (CTF, 1989c).	No recommendation.
Childhood obesity	Very-low-calorie diet	Weight loss on very-low-calorie diets for preadolescent obese children is poorly maintained (D) (CTF, 1994a).	Children are not specifically evaluated, but those individuals who are 20% or more above desirable weight should receive appropriate nutritional and exercise counseling (USPSTF, 1989).
Depression	Depression screening with the General Health Questionnaire or the Zung Self-Rating Depression Scale	Although physicians should maintain a high index of suspicion, routine testing for depression by questionnaire did not improve detection rate or management (D) (CTF, 1990b).†	Routine screening is not recommended. Clinicians should maintain a high index of suspicion for depressive symptoms in adolescents and young adults, persons with a family or personal history of depression, those with chronic illnesses, and those who have experienced a recent loss. Those with sleep disorders or multiple unexplained somatic complaints also should be considered (USPSTF, 1989).

Table continued on following page

TABLE 10–8.   *(Continued)*

Target Condition	Clinical Procedure	Canadian Task Force (CTF)	U.S. Preventive Services Task Force (USPSTF)
Urinary tract infection	Urinalysis	Screening detects some cases, but yield is low. Reinfection often follows treatment (D) (CTF, 1979).†	Screening is not recommended but the strength of recommendation depends on prevalence and evaluation of treatment. High prevalence/treatment not fully evaluated in: Wolmen age ≥60 years (C) Diabetic women (C) High prevalence/treatment not efficacious—don't screen: Women age <60 years (E) Men age ≥60 years (D) Institutionalized elderly (D) Low prevalence—don't screen men age <60 years (E). (USPSTF, 1989).
Hyperthyroidism	Thyroid function tests, thyroid-stimulating hormone level, T₄	The procedure is not sensitive enough to detect subclinical states. Effectiveness of treatment of presymptomatic disease is unknown and symptoms manifest rapidly (D) (CTF, 1990a).	Screening for thyroid disorders is not recommended for asymptomatic adults and children. (USPSTF, 1989).†
Osteoporosis	Bone densitometry	Clinical procedure is expensive. Bone mass is not a sufficiently accurate predictor of fracture (D) (CTF, 1988).†	Routine screening for decreased bone mineral content is not recommended. In perimenopausal women who are at increased risk and for whom estrogen therapy otherwise would not be recommended, measurement may help the patient and clinician determine whether such therapy is appropriate (USPSTF, 1989).†
Lung cancer	Chest radiographic studies, sputum cytology	No clinical procedure has been validated for early detection. Fair evidence that neither procedure significantly changes the mortality rate (D) (CTF, 1990c).	Screening is not recommended (USPSTF, 1989).
Endometrial cancer	Endometrial biopsy; cytologic examination of endometrium	Early detection procedures for benign hyperplasia are unreliable. The effectiveness of screening is unknown. There are no controlled studies on the effectiveness of early treatment (D) (CTF, 1988).	No recommendation.
Bladder cancer	Cytologic examination of the urine, urinalysis (hematuria dipstick)	There is no evidence that early detection improves the prognosis (D) (CTF, 1979).†	Dipstick urinalysis may be clinically prudent in individuals over age 60 (C) but is not recommended for younger individuals (D) (USPSTF, 1989).

* Recommendation grade: C, evidence for inclusion or exclusion poor, therefore delineating a set of research priorities; D, fair evidence for exclusion; E, good evidence for exclusion.
† Currently under review.

during an encounter. For counseling, there is often a limit to the number of topics that can be discussed in one visit.

From a broader perspective, there has been growing interest in the potential impact of opinion leaders and "academic detailing" on the implementation of preventive services in the primary care setting. Many of the general principles have been evaluated in the realm of the implementation of evidence and guidelines in the therapeutic field (Avorn and Soumerai, 1983; Lomas et al., 1989) and have existed in the pharmaceutical industry for decades. The evaluation of such strategies to enhance the implementation of preventive services in primary care is ongoing.

Hence, implementing preventive services into primary care is a complex exercise. Successful implementation of preventive services should result from a balanced and artful orchestration of several factors. The importance of such factors will vary according to the specific condition being considered (Battista et al., 1986).

CONCLUSION

Current recommendations must evolve continually because new evidence on the effectiveness of primary and secondary preventive measures emerges constantly. Moreover, changing social and economic circumstances in Canada and in the United States may require reconsideration of the recommendations and of the strategy that has been advocated in this chapter.

Moreover, physicians are in the midst of a Copernican revolution; in effect, the center of the health care galaxy is progressively shifting from the physician to the patient. Physicians increasingly will need to share responsibility for decision making with other health professionals and with patients.

Our current state of knowledge makes it impossible to make absolute recommendations about most disorders. For certain important preventive interventions, the evidence is either controversial or incomplete (Table 10–7), and bodies such as the Canadian and U.S. Task Forces cannot make recommendations on the basis that a particular preventive measure might be beneficial. For stronger recommendations, more definitive evidence is required to strengthen the scientific basis of preventive practice in family medicine.

In *The Logic of Medicine*, Murphy (1979) offered a pertinent admonishment:

If we can never know the answer, let us be honest and admit that we cannot. If we cannot produce proof, let us withhold the final stamp of intellectual approval until we do. It is better to be an agnostic forever than to worship false gods. (p. 166)

The authors of this chapter have adopted a similar stand. But what of the harried clinician who must act now and cannot wait for the conclusive evidence to be gathered and disseminated?

Thoughtful clinicians act daily on the basis of incomplete evidence, executing those clinical maneuvers that they think are in their patients' best interests. So it is, too, with the preventive interventions discussed in this chapter. Those that have been found, on rigorous validation, to do more good than harm are recommended unequivocally. The rest are presented with open and candid uncertainty as to their value. The worst disservice to the harried clinician would be to fail to distinguish between unquestionably beneficial detection maneuvers and those of dubious value, and to withhold the evidence associated with each preventive act that a family physician contemplates as he or she cares for patients and seeks to protect their health.

Clinical practice guidelines in preventive care can be a powerful instrument for enhancing preventive services. As a crucial link between health science and clinical practice, guidelines should not replace clinical judgment but support it, and make clinical practice an even more dynamic exercise. Successful implementation of preventive services should result from a balanced and artful orchestration of the factors discussed here.

REFERENCES

Avorn J, Soumerai SB: Improving drug therapy decisions through educational outreach: A randomized trial of academically based "detailing". N Engl J Med 308:1457, 1983.

Bass MJ, Elford RW: Preventive practice patterns of Canadian primary care physicians. Am J Prev Med 4(suppl):17, 1988.

Battista RN: Adult cancer prevention in primary care patterns of practice in Quebec. Am J Public Health 73:1036, 1983.

Battista RN: Practice guidelines for preventive care: The Canadian experience. Br J Gen Pract 43:301, 1993.

Battista RN, Fletcher SW: Making recommendations on preventive practice: Methodological issues. *In* Battista RN, Lawrence RS (eds): Implementing Preventive Services. New York, Oxford University Press, 1988, pp 53–67.

Battista RN, Spitzer WO: Adult cancer prevention in primary care: Contrasts among primary care practice settings in Quebec. Am J Public Health 73:1040, 1983.

Battista RN, Williams JI, MacFarlane LA: Determinants of primary medical practice in adult cancer prevention. Med Care 24:216, 1986.

Borgiel AEM, Williams JI, Bass MJ, et al: Quality of care in family practice: Does residency training make a difference? Can Med Assoc J 140:1035, 1989.

Canadian Task Force on the Periodic Health Examination: The periodic health examination. Can Med Assoc J 121:1196, 1979.

Canadian Task Force on the Periodic Health Examination: The periodic health examination 2:1984 update. Can Med Assoc J 130:1278, 1984.

Canadian Task Force on the Periodic Health Examination: The periodic health examination 2:1985 update. Can Med Assoc J 135:724, 1986.

Canadian Task Force on the Periodic Health Examination: The periodic health examination 2:1987 update. Can Med Assoc J 138:618, 1988.

Canadian Task Force on the Periodic Health Examination: The periodic health examination 1: Introduction. Can Med Assoc J 141:205, 1989a.

Canadian Task Force on the Periodic Health Examination: The periodic health examination 2:1989 update. Can Med Assoc J 141:209, 1989b.

Canadian Task Force on the Periodic Health Examination: The periodic health examination 3:1989 update. Can Med Assoc J 141:1136, 1989c.

Canadian Task Force on the Periodic Health Examination: Periodic health examination, 1989 update: 4. Intrapartum electronic fetal monitoring and prevention of neonatal herpes simplex. Can Med Assoc J 141:1233, 1989d.

Canadian Task Force on the Periodic Health Examination: Periodic health examination, 1990 update: 1. Early detection of hyperthyroidism and hypothyroidism in adults and screening of newborns for congenital hypothyroidism. Can Med Assoc J 142:955, 1990a.

Canadian Task Force on the Periodic Health Examination: Periodic health examination, 1990 update: 2. Early detection of depression and prevention of suicide. Can Med Assoc J 142:1233, 1990b.

Canadian Task Force on the Periodic Health Examination: Periodic health examination, 1990 update: 3. Interventions to prevent lung cancer other than smoking cessation. Can Med Assoc J 143:269, 1990c.

Canadian Task Force on the Periodic Health Examination: Periodic health examination, 1990 update: 4. Well-baby care in the first 2 years of life. Can Med Assoc J 143:867, 1990d.

Canadian Task Force on the Periodic Health Examination: Periodic health examination, 1991 update: 1. Screening for cognitive impairment in the elderly. Can Med Assoc J 144:425, 1991a.

Canadian Task Force on the Periodic Health Examination: Periodic health examination, 1991 update: 2. Administration of pneumococcal vaccine. Can Med Assoc J 144:665, 1991b.

Canadian Task Force on the Periodic Health Examination: Periodic health examination, 1991 update: 3. Secondary prevention of prostate cancer. Can Med Assoc J 145:413, 1991c.

Canadian Task Force on the Periodic Health Examination: Periodic health examination, 1991 update: 4. Screening for cystic fibrosis. Can Med Assoc J 145:629, 1991d.

Canadian Task Force on the Periodic Health Examination: Periodic health examination, 1991 update: 5. Screening for abdominal aortic aneurysm. Can Med Assoc J 145:783, 1991e.

Canadian Task Force on the Periodic Health Examination: Periodic health examination, 1991 update: 6. Acetylsalicylic acid and the primary prevention of cardiovascular disease. Can Med Assoc J 145:1091, 1991f.

Canadian Task Force on the Periodic Health Examination: Periodic health examination, 1992 update: 1. Screening for gestational diabetes. Can Med Assoc J 147:435, 1992a.

Canadian Task Force on the Periodic Health Examination: Periodic health examination, 1992 update: 2. Routine prenatal ultrasound screening. Can Med Assoc J 147:627, 1992b.

Canadian Task Force on the Periodic Health Examination: Periodic health examination, 1992 update: 3. HIV antibody screening. Can Med Assoc J 147:867, 1992c.

Canadian Task Force on the Periodic Health Examination: Periodic health examination, 1992 update: 4. Prophylaxis for gonococcal and chlamydial ophthalmia neonatorum. Can Med Assoc J 147:1449, 1992d.

Canadian Task Force on the Periodic Health Examination: Periodic health examination, 1993 update: 2. Lowering the blood total cholesterol level to prevent coronary heart disease. Can Med Assoc J 148:521, 1993.

Canadian Task Force on the Periodic Health Examination: Periodic health examination, 1994 update: 1. Obesity in childhood. Can Med Assoc J 150:871, 1994a.

Canadian Task Force on the Periodic Health Examination: Periodic health examination, 1994 update: 3. Primary and secondary prevention of neural tube defects. Can Med Assoc J 151:159, 1994b.

Carney PA, Dietrich AJ, Kellar A, et al: Tools, teamwork, and tenacity: An office system for cancer prevention. J Fam Pract 35:388, 1992.

Cohen DI, Littenberg B, Wetzel C, Neuhauser D: Improving physician compliance with preventive medicine guidelines. Med Care 20:1040, 1982.

Cole P, Morrison AS: Basic issues in population screening for cancer. J Natl Cancer Inst 64:1263, 1980.

Davis DA, Thomson MA, Oxman A, et al: Evidence for the effectiveness of CME: A review of 50 randomized controlled trial. JAMA 268:1111, 1992.

Dietrich AJ, O'Connor GT, Keller A, et al: Cancer: Improvising early detection and prevention: A community practice randomized trial. BMJ 301:687, 1992.

Fletcher RH, Fletcher SW, Wagner E: Clinical Epidemiology—The Essentials. Baltimore, Williams & Wilkins, 1988, pp 41–58.

Green LW, Eriksen MP, Schor EL: Preventive practices by physicians: Behavioral determinants and potential interventions. Am J Prev Med 4(suppl):101, 1988.

Hippocrates: On air, waters, and places (The genuine works of Hippocrates, Vol. 1). London, The Sydenham Society, 1985, p 190.

Ismail AI, Lewis DW with the Canadian Task Force on the Periodic Health Examination: Periodic health examination, 1993 update: 3. Periodontal disease: classification, diagnosis, risk factors and prevention. Can Med Assoc J 149:1409, 1993.

Knight BP, O'Malley MS, Fletcher SW: Physician acceptance of a computerized health maintenance promoting program. Am J Prev Med 3:19, 1987.

Lewis CE: Disease prevention and health promotion practices of primary care physicians in the United States. Am J Prev Med 4(suppl):9, 1988.

Logsdon DN, Rosen MA: The cost of preventive health services in primary medical care and implications for health insurance coverage. J Ambul Care Manag 7:46, 1984.

Lomas J, Abelson J: Do health service organizations and community health centres have higher disease prevention and health promotion levels than fee for service practices? Can Med Assoc J 142:575, 1990.

Lomas J, Anderson GM, Domnick-Pierre K, et al: Do practice guidelines guide practice? The effect of a consensus statement on the practice of physicians. N Engl J Med 321:1306, 1989.

Lomas J, Haynes RB: A taxonomy and critical review of tested strategies for the application of clinical practice recommendations: From "official" to "individual" clinical policy. Am J Prev Med 4(suppl):77, 1988.

Lurie N, Manning WG, Peterson C, et al: Preventive care: Do we practice what we preach? Am J Public Health 77:801, 1987.

Lurie N, Slater J, McGovern P, et al: Preventive care for women: Does the sex of the physician matter? N Engl J Med 329:478, 1993.

McMillan HC, MacMillan JH, Offord DR with the Canadian Task Force on the Periodic Health Examination:Periodic health examination, 1993 update: 1. Primary prevention of child maltreatment. Can Med Assoc J 148:151, 1993.

Manning WG, Leibowitz A, Goldberg GA, et al: A controlled trial of the effect of a prepaid group practice on use of services. N Engl J Med 310:1505, 1984.

McNeil BJ, Keeler E, Adelstein SJ: Primer on certain elements of medical decision-making. N Engl J Med 193:212, 1975.

McPhee SJ, Bird JA, Fordham P, et al: Promoting cancer prevention activities by primary care physicians—results of a randomized, controlled trial. JAMA 266:538, 1991.

McPhee SJ, Richard RJ, Solkowitz SN: Performance of cancer screening in a university general internal medicine practice: Comparison with the 1980 American Cancer Society guidelines. J Gen Intern Med 1:275, 1986.

Mendenhall RC: Medical practice in the United States: A special report of the Robert Wood Johnson Foundation. Princeton, NJ, Robert Wood Johnson Foundation, 1981.

Murphy E: The Logic of Medicine. Baltimore, The John Hopkins University Press, 1979.

Pineault R: The effect of prepaid group practice on physicians' utilization behavior. Med Care 14:121, 1976.

Romm FJ, Fletcher SW, Hulka BS: The periodic health examination: Comparison of recommendations and internists' performance. South Med J 74:265, 1981.

Russell LB: Is Prevention Better Than Cure? Washington, DC, The Brookings Institution, 1986.

Sackett DL, Haynes RB, Tugwell P: Clinical Epidemiology: A Basic Science for Clinical Medicine. Boston, Little, Brown, 1985, pp 59–155.

Solomon MJ, McLeod RS with the Canadian Task Force on the Periodic Health Examination: Periodic health examination, 1994 update: 2. Screening strategies for colorectal cancer. Can Med Assoc J 150:1961, 1994.

U.S. Preventive Services Task Force: Guide to Clinical Preventive Services: An Assessment of the Effectiveness of 169 Interventions. Baltimore, Williams & Wilkins, 1989.

U.S. Preventive Services Task Force: Home uterine activity monitoring for preterm labour: Review article. JAMA. 270:369, 1993.

Vecchio TJ: Predictive value of a diagnostic test in unselected populations. N Engl J Med 174:1171, 1966.

Weinstein MC, Stason WB: Foundations of cost effectiveness analysis for health and medical practice. N Engl J Med 296:716, 1977.

Wilner S: Health promotion and disease prevention in HMO's. Health Aff 5(1):122, 1986.

Woolf SH, Battista RN, Anderson GM, Logan AG, Wang E, and the Canadian Task Force on the Periodic Health Examination: Assessing the clinical effectiveness of preventive maneuvers: Analytic principles and systematic methods in reviewing evidence and developing clinical practice recommendations. J Clin Epidemiol 43:891, 1990.

CHAPTER 11

PREVENTIVE HEALTH CARE

R. MICHAEL MORSE and WARREN A. HEFFRON

ROLE OF THE FAMILY PHYSICIAN

The family physician has a unique opportunity to be an effective force in disease prevention and health promotion, and can screen effectively for a broad range of risk factors for preventable diseases and encourage healthy lifestyle behaviors. Many preventive activities are most beneficial when applied to an entire family unit. These family-wide activities can serve as the foundation for more age-specific individual recommendations and interventions. The family physician is the specialist to whom patients and other specialists look for provision of this broad range of health promotion and disease prevention activities.

Preventive activities traditionally are classified by the phase of disease process in which intervention occurs: tertiary (disease diagnosed and symptoms present), secondary (disease present and diagnosable but no symptoms present), and primary (no diagnosable disease, no symptoms present, but risk factors evident). Because the bulk of medical education relates to the patient who is already ill, physicians often tend to provide evaluation and treatment in reaction to patient symptoms rather than attempting to anticipate problems and prevent them.

EVALUATING PREVENTIVE ACTIVITIES

Not all diseases lend themselves well to the shift from effective intervention at the tertiary level to intervention at the secondary or primary level. Several parameters are used to determine the validity of such a shift for each disease and to determine the population group to whom the intervention should be applied. The general criteria are:

1. Is the disease worth screening for? Does it have a significant impact on the quality or quantity of life; is it of sufficient prevalence in the population to justify screening?

2. Is sufficient information available to identify accurately, using risk factors and screening tests, the individual or groups likely to develop the disease? Or, by using diagnostic tests, is it possible to identify those likely to have the disease already at a presymptomatic stage?

3. Are the tests that are used to accomplish the screening or early detection acceptable to the patient and physician in terms of accuracy, morbidity, and cost?

4. If it is possible to predict the disease or diagnose it prior to the onset of symptoms, is there a known intervention that will alter the course of the disease significantly?

5. Is the intervention or treatment acceptable in terms of proven effectiveness, risk, morbidity, cost, and patient acceptability?

A number of measures are used to help answer these questions.

Incidence. This is the rate of onset of a disease in a population and is expressed as the number of persons developing the disease per a given number of persons (typically 100,000) per year. Incidence expresses the risk of developing the disease in a given population. Even if the incidence is very low, the benefits of screening may be high enough in identifiable high-risk subgroups (specific age groups, certain nationalities, a specific sex) to qualify for prevention.

Mortality. The death rate of a disease is expressed as the number of persons dying from the disease per population at risk (usually 100,000) per year. Because a disease may not be fatal but may still be preventable, mortality statistics alone cannot set priorities for prevention but are generally more available and accurate. Incidence statistically represents the onset of a disease; mortality represents the end point of fatal illnesses. Table 11–1 shows a typical mortality table.

Prevalence. Prevalence is the proportion of individuals with a trait or disease in the population at a given time. This is a critical value for determining the predictive value of screening procedures.

Sensitivity. Sensitivity is the value derived by applying a test to a group of individuals *known to have a trait or a disease* and is expressed as a percentage of positive tests in that tested group. Thus, sensitivity tells one about a test in a known population but does not itself interpret the likelihood of disease for a test in an individual for whom the presence of disease in unknown. The value tells nothing about the results when applied to an undifferentiated population.

TABLE 11–1. U.S. MORTALITY DATA 1991

Rank Order*	Causes of Death (Ninth Revision, International Classification of Diseases, 1975)	Rate†	Per Cent of Total Deaths	Per Cent Change from 1979 to 1991	Ratio of: Male to Female	Ratio of: Black to White
...	All causes	860.3	100.0	−11.0	1.73	1.60
1	Diseases of heart	285.9	33.2	−25.7	1.89	1.47
2	Malignant neoplasms, including neoplasms of lymphatic and hematopoietic tissues	204.1	23.7	2.8	1.47	1.37
3	Cerebrovascular diseases	56.9	6.6	−35.6	1.19	1.89
4	Chronic obstructive pulmonary diseases and allied conditions	35.9	4.2	37.7	1.74	0.83
5	Accidents and adverse effects	35.4	4.1	−27.7	2.63	1.28
	Motor vehicle accidents	17.3	2.0	−26.7	2.39	0.98
	All other accidents and adverse effects	18.2	2.1	−29.1	2.94	1.69
6	Pneumonia and influenza	30.9	3.6	19.6	1.65	1.46
7	Diabetes mellitus	19.4	2.3	20.4	1.14	2.42
8	Suicide	12.2	1.4	−2.6	4.37	0.57
9	Human immunodeficiency virus infection	11.7	1.4	—	7.44	3.42
10	Homicide and legal intervention	10.5	1.2	6.9	3.84	6.76
11	Chronic liver disease and cirrhosis	10.1	1.2	−30.8	2.25	1.58
12	Nephritis, nephrotic syndrome, and nephrosis	8.5	1.0	—	1.54	2.78
13	Septicemia	7.8	.9	78.3	1.31	2.71
14	Atherosclerosis	6.9	.8	−54.4	1.36	1.12
15	Certain conditions originating in the perinatal period‡	6.7	.8	−39.5	1.27	3.13
...	All other causes	117.4	13.7			

* Rank based on number of deaths.
† Inasmuch as deaths from this cause occur mainly among infants, per cent changes are based on infant mortality rates instead of age-adjusted rates.
‡ Deaths per 100,000 population per year.
From Monthly Vital Statistics Report, Centers for Disease Control and Prevention/National Center for Health Statistics, United States Department of Health and Human Services, 42(2S):1, 1994.

Specificity. Specificity is the complement of sensitivity and is derived by applying a test to a population *known not to have a trait or disease*. It is expressed as a percentage of the disease-free group with a negative test.

Positive Predictive Value. Positive predictive value tells one about the test when applied to a mixed population of individuals both with and without the disease. It is expressed as a percentage of all the positive tests that will be true positives. Thus, it expresses the likelihood of a disease truly being present in an individual when a test is positive. This value is more useful when interpreting a positive test performed on a particular individual.

Negative Predictive Value. This is the converse of the positive predictive value and is expressed as the percentage of negative tests in a mixed population that will be true negatives. Thus, it expresses the likelihood of a negative test representing the absence of a disease.

The sensitivity and specificity are constants that are always true of a certain test when it is performed properly, regardless of the population tested. However, the positive predictive value and the negative predictive value *are dependent on the prevalence of disease* in the population tested. The relationship between calculations of sensitivity, specificity, positive predictive value, and negative predictive value can be shown in a four-square table (Table 11–2).

Table 11–3 demonstrates the interdependence of sensitivity, specificity, prevalence, and positive

TABLE 11–2. THE FOUR-SQUARE TABLE

	Positive tests	Negative tests	
Prevalence = Population with disease = TP + FN	True positive (TP)	False negative (FN)	Sensitivity = $\dfrac{TP}{TP + FN} \times 100$
Population without disease = FP + TN	False positive (FP)	True negative (TN)	Specificity = $\dfrac{TN}{FP + TN} \times 100$
	Positive predictive value (PPV) = $\dfrac{TP}{TP + FP}$	Negative predictive value (NPV) = $\dfrac{TN}{TN + FN}$	

TABLE 11–3. EFFECT OF PREVALENCE ON PREDICTIVE VALUE

	Positive Predictive Value		
Preva-lence	Sens = 90%, Spec = 90%	Sens = 95%, Spec = 95%	Sens = 99%, Spec = 99%
0.1%	0.9%	1.9%	9%
1%	8.3%	16.1%	50%
2%	15.5%	27.9%	66.9%
5%	32.1%	50%	83.9%
50%	90%	95%	99%

predictive value. The prevalence in the population can be seen to have a dramatic effect on the predictive value of a test at various sensitivities and specificities.

Risk Factors

A risk factor is a value or condition that, if present, significantly alters the likelihood of a disease occurring when compared with the likelihood for the population. A risk factor does not necessarily imply a cause-and-effect relationship between the factor and the disease. It may be simply a statistical association. To substantiate such a cause-and-effect relationship, a study must modify a single risk factor and show, as a result, a statistically significant change in the incidence, morbidity, or mortality of the disease being studied. The proportion of risk for a particular disease that thus can be "attributed" to a specific factor is known as the *attributable risk*.

When a multiple risk factors are present, their cumulative effect is most often additive but in some cases may be multiplicative. Likewise, modification of risk factors usually reduces risk in a subtractive manner.

Interventions

When testing the effectiveness of an intervention, the type of study and how well it is designed will determine the believability of the results. Both the Canadian Task Force on the Periodic Health Examination and the U.S. Preventive Services Task Force have embraced a common method of rating the effectiveness of interventions and recommendations for their inclusion in screening (Table 11–4). These ratings are assigned after a thorough review of all the evidence available. They provide specialty groups and individual physicians with critical information to help make judgments concerning the value of various preventive activities.

PREVENTION APPLIED TO SPECIFIC DISEASES

Atherosclerotic Diseases

Coronary Heart Disease

INCIDENCE. An adult male in the United States has a 1 in 5 chance of having a myocardial infarction by 60 years of age, which is twice the incidence in females. However, myocardial infarction is still the number one killer of both men and women. The yearly incidence of myocardial infarction is 1.5 million. Men between the ages of 35 and 84 have myocardial infarction or sudden death as their *initial* onset of symptoms 67 per cent of the time. This is the presenting event for a lesser percentage (43 per cent) of women.

PREVALENCE. By 20 to 24 years of age, about 44 per cent of white men, 34 per cent of black men, 11 per cent of white women, and 43 per cent of black women will have raised lesions in their coronary arteries. The estimated prevalence of coronary heart disease in the U.S. population in 1990 was 2.6 per cent (6.23 million cases).

Because the positive predictive value of screening procedures rises significantly when a group with a high prevalence is screened, it is of importance to know the prevalence in population subgroups. Autopsy studies show a prevalence range from 1.9 per cent in 30- to 39-year-old men to 12.3 per cent for men 60 to 69 years of age. Preva-

TABLE 11–4. U.S. PREVENTIVE SERVICES TASK FORCE CLASSIFICATION CODES

Effectiveness of Intervention	Classification of Recommendations
I: Evidence obtained from at least one properly randomized trial	A: There is good evidence to support the recommendation that the condition be specifically considered in a periodic health examination
II-1: Evidence from well-designed controlled trials without randomization	B: There is fair evidence for inclusion
II-2: Evidence obtained from well-designed cohort or case-control analytic studies, preferably from more than one center or research group	C: There is poor evidence for inclusion
II-3: Evidence obtained from multiple time series studies with or without the intervention	D: There is fair evidence to support the recommendation that the condition be excluded from consideration in a periodic health examination
III: Opinions of respected authorities based on clinical experience, descriptive studies, or reports of expert committees	E: There is good evidence to exclude the condition from consideration in a periodic health examination

lence among women in the same age groups ranged from 0.3 per cent to 7.5 per cent, respectively.

COST AND IMPACT ON SOCIETY. It is estimated that the cost of all cardiovascular disease to our society in 1990 was $117 billion, including direct and indirect costs.

MORBIDITY AND MORTALITY. In 1990, coronary heart disease was responsible for 489,340 deaths in the United States, which is 22.6 per cent of all deaths for the year. The case fatality rate for myocardial infarction is 1 in 3. Three hundred thousand of the 500,000 deaths each year occur prior to reaching the hospital (American Heart Association, 1992).

IMPORTANT FACTS RELEVANT TO PREVENTION.

1. Risk factor reduction will lessen the incidence of coronary heart disease, especially when concentrated on reduction of blood lipid levels, hypertension control, and cessation of cigarette smoking. Other important risk factors to consider for modification include sedentary lifestyle, obesity, and control of diabetes mellitus.

2. Changing the American diet to a low-saturated-fat, low-cholesterol diet will reduce the levels of serum cholesterol.

3. No population in the world has been found with a combination of high total serum cholesterol levels and low rates of coronary heart disease.

4. A 4.8-year study of male physicians ages 40 to 84 has shown that aspirin, in dosages of 325 mg every other day, can reduce the incidence of myocardial infarction by nearly half. Total vascular-related deaths were reduced by 23 per cent. This study may have significant relevance to much broader groups (Steering Committee of the Physicians' Health Study Research Group, 1988).

SCREENING TEST RECOMMENDATIONS. For the general population:

1. Measure total and high-density lipoprotein cholesterol between 20 and 30 years of age and at least every 5 years thereafter.

2. Measure blood pressure each office visit.

3. Update family and smoking history in previous nonsmokers every 5 years.

4. Measure fasting blood sugar every 5 years.

5. Monitor exercise levels at least every 5 years for every patient.

6. Evaluate for obesity yearly.

7. Monitor stress levels yearly.

PREVENTIVE ACTIVITIES RECOMMENDATIONS. All risk factors should be modified whenever possible. *Cholesterol Control.*

1. As outlined in Chapter 42, physicians should prescribe a healthy diet to decrease the risk of heart disease for all patients. It is particularly important that children learn healthy eating habits early in life. The primary dietary goal is maintaining total fat at less than 30 per cent of calories, with specific emphasis on minimizing saturated fat intake. Most authorities believe that increasing the proportion of monounsaturated fats (olive oil, canola oil) in the total dietary fat allowance should be recommended to patients. This is based on epidemiologic studies and on the observation that these oils reduce low-density lipoprotein cholesterol at least as much as the polyunsaturated fatty acids when substituted in the diet for saturated fats. Furthermore, they do not lower high-density lipoprotein levels, as do the polyunsaturated fats. Epidemiologic data show a significant protective effect against coronary heart disease in populations consuming three or more servings of fish weekly. Also, a diet high in soluble fiber (oat bran products, legumes, and fruits) has been shown to reduce serum cholesterol. Antioxidants, particularly vitamin E, have been associated with reduced coronary heart disease.

2. All patients should be evaluated for risk status. The presence of other risk factors (Table 11–5) is used to determine the low-density lipoprotein intervention levels. Table 11–6 shows the recommendations for intervention with diet and medications.

3. Other methods of altering risk secondary to hypercholesterolemia include weight control, exercise (to increase high-density lipoproteins), and drug therapy.

TABLE 11–5. RISK STATUS BASED ON PRESENCE OF CHD RISK FACTORS OTHER THAN LOW-DENSITY LIPOPROTEIN CHOLESTEROL*

Positive Risk Factors
Age
    Male ≥45
    Females ≥55 or premature menopause without estrogen replacement therapy
Family history of premature CHD (definite myocardial infarction or sudden death before 55 y of age in father or other male first-degree relative, or before 65 y of age in mother or other female first-degree relative)
Current cigarette smoking
Hypertension (blood pressure ≥140/90 mm Hg,† or taking antihypertensive medication)
Low HDL cholesterol (<35 mg/dL† [0.9 mmol/L])

Negative Risk Factors‡
High HDL cholesterol (≥60 mg/dL [1.6 mmol/L])

* High risk, defined as net of two or more coronary heart disease (CHD) risk factors, leads to more vigorous intervention. Age (defined differently for men and women) is treated as a risk factor because rates of CHD are higher in the elderly than in the young, and in men than in women of the same age. Obesity is not listed as a risk factor because it operates through other risk factors that are included (hypertension, hyperlipidemia, decreased high-density lipoprotein [HDL] cholesterol, and diabetes mellitus), but it should be considered a target for intervention. Physical inactivity is similarly not listed as a risk factor, but it too should be considered a target for intervention, and physical activity is recommended as desirable for everyone. High risk due to personal history of coronary or peripheral atherosclerosis is assumed.

† Confirmed by measurements on several occasions.

‡ If the HDL cholesterol level is ≥60 mg/dL (1.6 mmol/L), subtract one risk factor (because high HDL cholesterol levels decrease CHD risk).

From Expert Panel on Detection, Evaluation, and Treatment of High Blood Cholesterol in Adults: Summary of the second report of the National Cholesterol Education Program (NCEP) (Adult Treatment Panel II). JAMA 269:3015, 1993.

TABLE 11–6. TREATMENT DECISIONS BASED ON LDL CHOLESTEROL LEVEL*

	Initiation Level	
Patient Category	Dietary Therapy	Drug Treatment
Without CHD and with fewer than two risk factors	≥160 mg/dL (4.1 mmol/L)	≥190 mg/dL (4.9 mmol/L)
Without CHD and with two or more risk factors	≥130 mg/dL (3.4 mmol/L)	≥160 mg/dL (4.1 mmol/L)
With CHD	>100 mg/dL (2.6 mmol/L)	≥130 mg/dL (3.4 mmol/L)

* LDL, low-density lipoprotein; CHD, coronary heart disease.
From Expert Panel on Detection, Evaluation, and Treatment of High Blood Cholesterol in Adults: Summary of the second report of the National Cholesterol Education Program (NCEP) (Adult Treatment Panel II). JAMA 269:3015, 1993.

Control of Hypertension. Aggressive treatment of all patients with a systolic pressure greater than 140 mm Hg or a diastolic pressure greater than 90 mm Hg is essential. Risk is proportional to blood pressure even at diastolic levels between 80 and 90 mm Hg.

Prior to institution of drug therapy for hypertension, nonpharmacologic methods should be considered. These include salt restriction, weight reduction, reduction or elimination of alcohol intake, biofeedback, and regular aerobic exercise.

Smoking Cessation. Control of smoking may be the most correctable risk factor for coronary heart disease. There is increasing evidence that passive smoking also has significant impact on health. Each physician should have a plan for assisting patients in smoking cessation that includes the following elements:

1. Patient recognition of smoking as a health problem.
2. A firm stance by the physician against smoking.
3. Encouraging the patient to make the decision to stop.
4. Setting a target date for starting the program.
5. Multiple methodologies available depending on patient needs and preferences: tapering, "cold turkey," substitution (e.g., nicotine gum or patch), counseling, hypnosis, support groups, buddy systems, and acupuncture.
6. Structured long-term follow-up with maximal support and encouragement from physician and office staff.

Aspirin Prophylaxis. Low-dose aspirin therapy should be considered for men and women age 40 and over who are at increased risk for myocardial infarction and lack contraindications for the drug.

Other Preventive Activities. It is recommended that physicians assist all patients to avoid risk factor development through encouragement of healthy lifestyles. Education to prevent smoking, promotion of physical activity, promotion of stress reduction, maintenance of ideal body weight, and provision of periodic preventive health care should be made available to patients.

RELATED ISSUES. The mortality from coronary heart disease in this country has decreased 32.6 per cent between 1980 and 1990, continuing a trend from 1964. It is estimated that 60 per cent of this reduction is due to lifestyle changes, especially diet modification and smoking cessation. This encouraging information alone provides physicians sufficient reason to pursue further aggressive risk factor prevention and modification on a population-wide basis.

The issue of the effect of personality characteristics on the risk of coronary heart disease is poorly understood. Although traditionally the type A personality (highly stressed, constantly pushed for time, highly competitive, often intolerant of others) has been implicated as a risk factor, recent studies raise doubts about this concept while supporting the hypothesis that suppressed anger may play a significant role.

Treadmill exercise stress testing has been advocated as both a screening test and a diagnostic test. Because of a generally low sensitivity and a prohibitively high false-positive rate, this test has not found a clear indication as a screening test.

IMPACT ON THE FAMILY UNIT. The lifestyles that are important for prevention of coronary heart disease cannot be implemented easily by an individual without due consideration of the person's family and environment. The chances of the patient quitting smoking are dimmed considerably when there are other smokers in the home. Dietary changes, especially, cannot be implemented effectively for only one individual in a family unit. Major changes in knowledge, attitudes, and habits of the entire family often are required so that the desirable foods can be purchased, properly prepared, and consumed with an agreed-on common goal of improved health. Anything less can lead to resentment, confusion, and outright rebellion.

When a family member needs dietary therapy, a family meeting at the beginning will enhance the chances of long-term success. This meeting can be used to educate the family about risk and diet, enlist all family members' cooperation and support, and make plans for flexibility to meet everyone's needs. Fortunately, the diets recommended by the American Heart Association are nutritionally well balanced and can be recommended to all individuals, regardless of risk status.

Very helpful guidelines and educational materials are available from the American Heart Association through local and state chapters (see References). Several excellent cookbooks are also widely available (Brody, 1985; Conner and Conner, 1986; Eshleman, 1984).

Cerebrovascular Disease

INCIDENCE. The incidence of stroke is 500,000 per year The yearly incidence increases with age with 356,000 of the 500,000 strokes per year occurring in those over age 65.

PREVALENCE. There are over 3 million stroke victims still alive, for a population prevalence for completed stroke of 1250 in 100,000 persons. This does not include the additional millions of individuals with significant atherosclerotic cerebrovascular disease who are at high risk of stroke.

COST AND IMPACT ON SOCIETY. The cost of stroke is estimated at $18 billion annually, including direct and indirect costs (American Heart Association, 1992).

MORBIDITY AND MORTALITY. Stroke is the fourth leading cause of death in the United States after coronary heart disease, cancer, and injury. The mortality rate is 28.4 in 100,000 persons per year, resulting in a total of 145,340 deaths in 1990.

In addition to its high mortality rate, stroke carries a very high morbidity. It is the leading cause of serious disability in the United States. The morbidity rate also rises dramatically with age.

IMPORTANT FACTS RELEVANT TO PREVENTION. The major risk factor for stroke is hypertension. The other major risk factors for coronary heart disease are less predictive for stroke risk. The known presence of heart disease carries a high risk. Diabetes mellitus, even when mild, imparts a significantly increased risk that rises dramatically if both hypertension and diabetes are present.

Transient ischemic attacks confer a high risk of subsequent stroke. One out of five stroke victims has had one of four major symptoms suggestive of a transient ischemic attack in the previous year: (1) temporary loss of vision (especially in one eye), (2) unilateral numbness, (3) aphasia, and (4) focal weakness.

Patients with carotid bruits have been reported to have a 2 per cent incidence of stroke per year. These patients are also at significantly increased risk for myocardial infarction. Although most experts recommend prophylactic aspirin therapy, the current data are not sufficient to show that treatment with aspirin, anticoagulants, or surgery will reduce the risk of stroke effectively in patients with asymptomatic carotid bruits. Such studies are in progress and will provide further guidance in the future.

Other risk factors for stroke include family history of stroke, cigarette smoking, oral contraceptive use, hyperlipidemia, and elevated hematocrit.

SCREENING TEST RECOMMENDATIONS. Elevated blood pressure, systolic *or* diastolic, is the single greatest risk factor for stroke and should be evaluated at each office visit. Other risk factors for atherosclerosis should be sought as previously recommended under coronary heart disease. The patient should be checked for the presence of carotid bruits every 5 years after age 40.

PREVENTIVE ACTIVITIES RECOMMENDATIONS. Prevention of stroke is aimed primarily at prevention of sustained, even mild hypertension. Promotion of the healthy lifestyle habits discussed for coronary heart disease is likely, although unproven, to be of benefit. Smokers, in particular, should be advised strongly to stop. Secondary prevention of completed stroke in patients with transient ischemic attacks may include aspirin prophylaxis, anticoagulation, or carotid endarterectomy, depending on the clinical circumstances.

DISCUSSION. The most important reason to listen for carotid bruits is to document the existence of significant atherosclerosis and therefore to alert the physician of the need to modify risk factors more aggressively. There is a risk, however, of initiating a process leading to unnecessary angiography and endarterectomy, which carry a substantial risk in themselves.

IMPACT ON FAMILY UNIT. The common results of stroke—physical disability, intellectual disability, and depression—often cause a loss of independence. The family or friends are suddenly forced to help make parental-type decisions. Active participation in the rehabilitation and care of a stroke victim can create enormous stress, both financially and emotionally, on the family unit. Placement of the patient in a nursing home, however rational, will require a resolution of guilt within the family. The family physician plays a critical central role in the coordination of rehabilitation with the family and in helping the family to resolve conflicting feelings.

Substance Abuse: Alcoholism and Other Drug Dependency

INCIDENCE. Difficulties in clearly identifying the point in time when an individual becomes an alcoholic make incidence rates very difficult to reliably determine. A rough estimate of incidence is 310 in 100,000 persons per year, which is derived by using prevalence rates and the average of 12 to 15 years of untreated alcoholism from onset to death.

PREVALENCE. Alcoholism affects at least 18 million Americans, for a prevalence of 7500 in 100,000 persons, or 7.5 per cent of the entire population. The number of adolescent weekly drinkers dropped from 54.7 million to 41.7 million from 1988 to 1990. In an ambulatory medical setting, the prevalence of alcoholism is at least 10 per cent (Whitfield et al., 1986). The rate for dependency on other drugs is about 2 per cent (2000 in 100,000 persons). The rates of drug use and abuse in adolescents and young adults are particularly striking. The average age of first use of alcohol and marijuana is 13 years. Recent surveys show some encouraging trends. The number of adolescents using cocaine dropped by 49 per cent from 1988 to 1990 (to 2.1 per cent). The use of marijuana dropped by 50 per cent during the 1980s to 13.9 per cent. Unfortunately, crack use has not declined; the highest use is among young people 18 to 25 years old, males, blacks, the unemployed, and those living in large metropolitan areas.

COST AND IMPACT ON SOCIETY. The estimated cost of alcohol abuse in the United States in 1988 was $85.8 billion: $72.3 billion from lost employment, reduced productivity, and other indirect costs, and $13.5 billion in health care costs (American Medical Association, 1993). The total societal cost for drug abuse is estimated at more than $58 billion.

MORBIDITY AND MORTALITY. Patients with alcoholism have an overall risk of mortality 2.5 times that of the normal population. Over 7 per cent of all deaths in any given year are alcohol related.

The morbidity for chemical dependency (alcohol and drug abuse) is substantial, ranging from the extremely high association with crime to the increased incidence of cirrhosis, psychosis, depression, cardiomyopathy, peptic ulcer disease, overdose, cancer of directly exposed organs (lips, mouth, pharynx, esophagus, stomach, and liver), pancreatitis, suicide, various infections (hepatitis, human immunodeficiency virus, endocarditis, and pneumonia), fetal alcohol syndrome, and accidents of all types.

IMPORTANT FACTS RELEVANT TO PREVENTION. The most useful definition of chemical dependency is: The continued habitual use of a substance by a person despite recurring serious adverse effects on the person's life.

Measures to increase enforcement of drinking and driving laws, to increase prices for alcoholic beverages, and to increase the minimum drinking age have been shown either to reduce consumption or to reduce frequency of the legal consequences of drinking. Whether education will, in fact, reduce the rate of alcoholism is not known. Strong cultural biases (e.g., Orthodox Judaism) against drunkenness have a strong effect on the reduction of the prevalence of dependency.

Children of alcoholics are at a three times greater risk of becoming alcoholics, whether or not they are raised by their biologic parents.

While spontaneous recovery of alcoholism is reported in 4 to 26 per cent of patients, treatment can result in a 70 per cent recovery rate. It is unrealistic, dangerous, and delusional for an alcoholic to ever attempt controlled drinking.

SCREENING TEST RECOMMENDATIONS. All patients over 12 years of age should be screened regularly for alcohol and substance abuse. A yearly frequency of screenings will deliver a strong educational message to the patient.

Probably the screening question with the greatest positive predictive value is: "Have you ever had a health, legal, or personal problem as a result of drinking alcohol?" This should be followed by: "When was your last drink?" (The answer is positive if the last drink occurred within 24 hours.) In a high-risk population with a prevalence of 20 per cent (e.g., the average inpatient population), an affirmative answer to *either* of these two questions has a diagnostic accuracy as follows: sensitivity of 91.5 per cent, specificity of 89.7 per cent, positive predictive value of 69.4 per cent, and negative predictive value of 97.6 per cent (Cyr and Wartman, 1988). Two positive answers on the CAGE questions are also highly suggestive, with a 66 per cent positive predictive value (Bush et al., 1987). The Michigan Alcoholism Screening Test (MAST) also can be helpful in the diagnostic evaluation (Selzer, 1971). See Chapter 57 for a discussion of screening.

The presence or absence of alcoholism in first-degree relatives should be a part of the family history. All patients, including children, should be asked yearly if there are any problems within the family that involve alcohol.

PREVENTIVE ACTIVITIES RECOMMENDATIONS. Literature concerning the warning signs of alcoholism and sources of help should be freely available in every medical office. If the subject of chemical dependency is dealt with openly, there is an increased likelihood that the affected individual will seek help through the family physician.

Patients with a family history of alcoholism should be counseled concerning their high-risk status and encouraged to become members of Alanon or the Children of Alcoholics Foundation.

RELATED ISSUES. The same questions used for alcohol may be equally applicable to drug abuse. In addition, certain cues found in alcoholics and other drug-dependent patients will help lead to the correct diagnosis: problems with children, separation, divorce, job changes, depression, anxiety, hypertension, macrocytosis of red blood cells, low resistance to infections, recurrent accidents, any trouble with legal authorities (including driving while intoxicated), upper gastrointestinal complaints, and abnormal liver enzymes.

IMPACT OF THE FAMILY UNIT. The family is at the epicenter of the alcoholic or other drug dependent earthquake. As the rumblings of the disease progress, so does pathology within the family. Most prominent is the role of "co-dependent" or "enabler," the person who assumes the abnegated responsibilities of the alcoholic or drug abuser, covers for him or her, and makes possible the alcoholic's continued drinking or the drug abusers continued use. This person is often the major focus of the alcoholic's hostility. Treatment should include healing of the entire family.

Cancer

General Cancer Information

INCIDENCE. The estimated number of new cancer cases for 1993 (excluding carcinoma in situ and nonmelanotic skin cancers) is 1,170,000, or 488 in 100,000 persons. The six cancers with the highest incidence (excluding skin cancers) are cancers of the lung, the colon–rectum, the breast, the prostate, the urinary tract, and the uterus. Carcinoma in situ and nonmelanotic skin cancers will account for an additional 700,000 cases. Thirty per cent of all Americans (85 million) eventually will develop cancer (American Cancer Society, 1933).

Prevalence. There are over 8 million people alive today with a history of cancer, of whom 5 million have been classified as cured. No data are available to indicate how many Americans have undiagnosed cancer at this time.

Cost and Impact on Society. The overall yearly cost of cancer to society is estimated at $104 billion. The total cost of medical care for cancer is over $35 billion per year.

Morbidity and Mortality. Cancer mortality (22 per cent of all deaths) is second only to cardiovascular disease mortality in the United States. The estimated mortality for 1993 is 526,000, or 219 in 100,000 persons. The six leading causes of cancer death are cancers of the lung, colon–rectum, breast, prostate, pancreas, and urinary system.

From 1930 to 1989, the age-adjusted mortality rate for cancer in the United States rose from 143 to 171 in 100,000 persons. This rise primarily has been due to the increments in mortality from cancer of the lung.

Important Facts Relevant to Prevention. Thirty-five per cent of all cancer deaths are thought to be related to diet (including obesity) (Doll and Peto, 1981). Obese individuals have increased risk of colon, breast, and uterine cancers. High-fat diets have been associated with prostate, breast, and colon cancer. Foods rich in the antioxidant vitamins A (dark green and deep yellow vegetables and fruits) and C (citrus fruits, strawberries, and sweet peppers) and cruciferous vegetables (cabbage, broccoli, brussel sprouts, and cauliflower) all are believed to have protective effects for various cancers. Salt-cured, smoked, and nitrite-cured foods increase the risk of upper gastrointestinal cancers.

Smoking accounts for 160,000 cancer deaths (13.7 per cent), primarily from cancer of the lung, the urinary bladder, the mouth, the throat, and the larynx, whereas alcohol is responsible for approximately 17,000 (1.5 per cent). Occupational exposures are thought to be responsible for 5 per cent of cancer mortality.

Therefore, diet, smoking, alcohol, and occupational exposures may account for over 55 per cent of all cancer mortality. These are potentially preventable causes and are amenable to intervention by the family physician.

Early diagnosis and treatment (secondary prevention) is also of great benefit. The American Cancer Society estimates that 100,000 of the

526,000 yearly deaths (19 per cent) could be prevented by screening and early intervention.

Impact on the Family Unit. For many of the cancers, a positive family history is a significant risk factor that requires the physician to emphasize prevention and early detection for these families. Members of families caring for cancer patients may experience hypochondriasis, depression, phobic disorders, generalized anxiety, and anger and hostility. These may be precipitated when issues of illness and death are dealt with in the family.

Because of the great importance of lifestyle in the prevention of cancer, family health habits are the major source of potential successful cancer prevention. When one considers the fact that cancer will strike three out of four families, the value of generally applied preventive health measures within every family practice becomes evident.

Colorectal Cancer

Incidence. Colorectal cancer has the second highest incidence of all cancers. The American Cancer Society estimated 149,000 new cases in 1994, for an incidence of 62 in 100,000 persons. The incidence of colorectal cancer begins to rise after age 40, roughly doubling each decade. Ninety per cent of cases occur in the population over 50.

Prevalence. The exact prevalence in the population is not known. Most screening trials find one to two cancers and 80 polyps in 1000 screened patients.

Morbidity and Mortality. Mortality from diagnosed colorectal cancer has fallen 29 per cent for women to 16.4 per 100,000, and 6 per cent for men to 23.6 per 100,000, over the past 30 years. Current mortality was approximately 57,000 in 1993. The survival rate varies dramatically with the stage of the cancer, as shown in Table 11–7.

Important Facts Relevant to Prevention. Colorectal cancer appears to arise almost exclusively from benign adenomatous polyps over a period of 5 to 10 years. However, only 20 to 30 per cent of polyps are adenomas, and only 5 to 10 per cent of adenomatous polyps become malignant (Riegelman and Povar, 1988). The initial appearance of adenomas occurs primarily between 40 and 45 years of age, with a significant increase in colorectal cancer every 5 to 10 years later.

The likelihood of malignancy in a polyp increases with size—from 1 to 2 per cent in those

TABLE 11–7. FIVE-YEAR SURVIVAL RATE FOR COLORECTAL CANCER

	Colon	Rectum
Localized	92%	85%
Regional spread	61%	51%
Distant spread	<7%	<7%

From American Cancer Society: Cancer Facts and Figures—1994. Atlanta, American Cancer Society, 1994, with permission.

TABLE 11–8. RISK FACTORS FOR COLORECTAL CANCER

Age >50
History of adenomas
Personal or family history of colorectal cancer or polyps
Ulcerative colitis
Crohn's disease affecting the colon
Personal or family history of genital or breast cancer in females

less than 1.0 cm to 60 per cent in those larger than 4 cm (Bader, 1986).

Although there has been a progressive change toward polyps occurring higher in the large bowel, over 60 per cent are still within reach of the 60-cm flexible sigmoidoscope.

High-fat diets have been strongly associated with the incidence of colorectal cancer. Lack of fiber also has been implicated. Risk factors for colorectal cancer are found in Table 11–8. Other risk factors that are less well established are cutaneous papillomas, a history of cholecystectomy, extensive work-related handling of synthetic fibers, and a history of ureterosigmoidostomy. Recent evidence shows that regular aspirin use may be protective.

SCREENING TEST RECOMMENDATIONS

1. Rectal examination and a six-slide fecal occult blood test yearly on all patients over 40 years of age.
2. Flexible sigmoidoscopy every 5 years on all adults starting after age 50.

The use of both fecal occult blood testing and flexible sigmoidoscopy has been controversial. The U.S. Preventive Services Task Force recommended neither, but the authors believe that data published since then tend to support these tests more strongly (Mandel et al., 1993; Selby et al., 1992, 1993).

PREVENTIVE ACTIVITIES RECOMMENDATIONS. Risk factor analysis should be performed by the time the patient is 40 years of age. Preventive activities include surveillance, noted earlier, for presymptomatic carcinomas and lesions with malignant potential (adenomas). All patients, regardless of age, should be encouraged to eat a high-fiber, low-fat diet.

RELATED ISSUES. Theoretically, the ideal screening method with the highest sensitivity and specificity for high-risk persons is periodic colonoscopy. This method is not practical, cost-effective, or acceptable for the general population. Knowing the 5- to 10-year natural history of progression from adenoma to cancer, one reasonably could begin screening procedures at least this long prior to the age of 50, when the most dramatic increase in actual cancer incidence occurs. Every 5 years is favored for the general population. More frequent testing of those believed to have significant risk factors is justified. It may be possible to define a very low-risk population in which flexible sigmoidoscopy is no longer beneficial by using the risk criteria and perhaps a given number of negative examinations.

IMPACT ON THE FAMILY UNIT. Because family history is a major risk factor, information obtained by the family physician should be used for family education concerning prevention.

Breast Cancer

INCIDENCE. Breast cancer is the most common cancer among women. The 1993 breast cancer incidence was 107 in 100,000 women, and has increased only slightly since 1987. In 1993, there were an estimated 182,000 new cases of breast cancer. In American women, the annual incidence of breast cancer increases rapidly with age, from 20 in 100,000 women at age 30 to 180 in 100,000 women at age 50. The lifetime incidence of breast cancer for women is 1 in 9 and appears to be slowly increasing. Twenty-eight per cent of all new female cancers are breast cancers, compared with 16 per cent for colorectal cancer, the next most common malignancy in women.

MORBIDITY AND MORTALITY. Despite an increasing incidence, the mortality rates for breast cancer from 1974 to 1993 have been stable as a result of earlier diagnosis. In 1993, breast cancer deaths in women were 46,000. This accounts for 18 per cent of all female cancer deaths, which is now second to the 22 per cent of female cancer deaths caused by lung cancer. The 5-year survival rate for localized breast cancer is 93 per cent compared with 78 per cent in the 1940s. In situ breast cancer has a cure rate approaching 100 per cent. The survival rate at 5 years is 71 per cent for breast cancers with regional spread and 18 per cent for cases with distant metastases.

IMPORTANT FACTS RELEVANT TO PREVENTION. The major accepted risk factors are listed in Table 11–9. In addition, there have been suggested associations between breast cancer and certain diets (high fat, low fiber) and a stronger relation with moderate alcohol consumption. Despite evaluation of risk factors, 75 per cent of women with breast cancer will have no risk factor other than their age. The risk rises progressively with age. A woman 65 to 69 years old has over 200 times the risk of a woman 20 to 24 years old and over four times the risk of a woman 35 to 39 years old.

Breast self-examination alone has a sensitivity of 26 per cent compared with 45 per cent for clinical breast examination, 71 per cent for mammography, and 75 per cent for a combination of mammography and clinical breast examination (U.S. Preventive Services Task Force, 1989). The specificity of mammography is 94 to 99 per cent. Of significance, however, is the fact that in the Breast Cancer Detection Demonstration Project, 690 of the total 2675 breast cancers diagnosed were found by breast self-examination between screening visits.

TABLE 11–9.　RISK FACTORS FOR BREAST CANCER

Factor	Relative Risk
* Atypical hyperplasia and family history	11
* Family history of premenopausal bilateral breast cancer	9
* Family history of premenopausal breast cancer	1.5
Family history of postmenopausal breast cancer	1.5
Family history of bilateral breast cancer	5
* History of previous personal breast cancer	5
Fibrocystic disease, proliferative type on biopsy	1.5–4
* Lobular carcinoma in situ	7.2
* Intraductal carcinoma in situ (risk > lobular carcinoma in situ)	N/A
* Atypical lobular or ductal hyperplasia on biopsy	N/A
First pregnancy after age 35	2–3
Nulliparous	3
Early menarche or late menopause	1.3–2.0
Increasing age	(see text)

Factors with Unclear Status
Geographic location (North America and Northern Europe)
Alcohol intake
High-fat, low-fiber diet
Obesity
History of ovarian, endometrial, salivary cancers

* Factors for which there is a consensus to place a patient in a high-risk group needing special attention.
Adapted from Love SM, Gelman RS, Silen W: Fibrocystic disease of the breast—a non-disease? N Engl J Med 312:146, 1985, with permission.

Nevertheless, a definitive study showing a lowered mortality rate for those performing breast self-examination has not been done.

Clinical breast examination is believed to be useful. Studies have shown that up to 16 per cent of cancers may be missed if no breast examination is included in screening. Half of these are minimal cancers and, therefore, highly curable (Potchen and Sierra, 1987).

A number of factors have been shown not to alter the risk of breast cancer significantly. These include breast trauma, fibroadenomas, fibrocystic breast disease of the nonproliferative type, caffeine consumption, mastodynia with negative mammographic and clinical examination, breast-feeding, and use of birth control pills or postmenopausal estrogen therapy.

SCREENING TEST RECOMMENDATIONS. Table 11–10 outlines the official guidelines of the U.S. Preventive Services Task Force (USPSTF) and the American Cancer Society. These recommendations range from conservative to aggressive. Each physician must decide the appropriate level of preventive care to implement in practice. The USPSTF guidelines represent the minimum level of preventive health care expected of primary care physicians.

PREVENTIVE ACTIVITIES RECOMMENDATIONS. Very little has been proven concerning the primary prevention of breast cancer. The role of a high-fat, low-fiber diet remains controversial. Patients should be advised of the concern raised as a result of the association of moderate alcohol ingestion with breast cancer. Because these dietary recommendations can be made on other grounds and are considered to be of general benefit, physicians may wish to make these recommendations before a direct cause-and-effect relationship is firmly established.

Although of unproven benefit, breast self-examination is a logical, low-risk, no-cost activity. It should be taught to each female at the time of her first gynecologic examination and reviewed at each subsequent examination. Every female should have an initial documented evaluation of risk factors for breast cancer at or before age 30. A program for prospective screening should be determined at that time.

Secondary prevention is the goal of current major screening recommendations and is focused

TABLE 11–10.　OFFICIAL RECOMMENDATIONS FOR BREAST CANCER SCREENING

Age	Test*	American Cancer Society: Frequency	U.S. Preventive Services Task Force		
			Frequency	Category of Evidence†	Recommendations†
20–34	BSE	Monthly			
	CBE	q 3 years			
35–39	BSE	Monthly			
	CBE	q 3 years			
40–49	BSE	Monthly		III	C
	CBE	Yearly	Yearly	III	C
	Mamm	q 1–2 years			
50–59	BSE	Monthly		III	C
	CBE	Yearly	Yearly	I	A
	Mamm	Yearly	Yearly	I	A
60+	BSE	Monthly		III	C
	CBE	Yearly	Yearly	II-2	B
	Mamm	Yearly	Yearly	II-2	B

* BSE, breast self-examination; CBE, clinical breast examination; Mamm, mammography.
† See Table 11–4 for explanation.

on the early detection of disease prior to symptoms. All lesions of the breast should be investigated promptly. Any mass found on clinical examination or on mammography should be evaluated by needle aspiration, needle biopsy, or open excisional biopsy, depending on the clinical circumstances. A negative mammogram or a negative clinical examination alone is never fully adequate to rule out cancer.

RELATED ISSUES. Environmental factors deserve more attention. The Japanese have a very low incidence of breast cancer. However, subsequent generations of Japanese immigrants to the United States have increasing incidence rates, eventually equaling the high levels in the United States.

Screening mammography in the 40- to 50-year-old group remains controversial. Most large-scale prospective studies have failed to show a statistically significant reduction in breast mortality for women screened with mammography between 40 and 50 years of age. There may be good reason to do this in high-risk individuals, with some experts recommending yearly mammography starting at age 35. Some physicians will offer screening mammography every 1 to 2 years to all women in this age group. At the other end of the age spectrum, the USPSTF recommends that physicians consider discontinuing mammograms at age 75 for women at low risk.

The positive predictive value of abnormal results (positive clinical breast examination or positive mammography interpretation) of the Breast Cancer Detection Demonstration Project screening program is very low (approximately 15.5 per cent), primarily because of a sensitivity of 87 per cent (Reigelman and Povar, 1988). However, the specificity is very high. Therefore, using the screening program, 87 per cent of women with carcinoma of the breast will be found, but a large number of women will be falsely positive and need to be evaluated with further diagnostic work-up, such as a needle aspiration, needle biopsy, or open biopsy.

The costs of mammographic screening remain a major concern. The 10-year cost of annual screening of only 25 per cent of all women in the 40- to 50-year age range would be $402 million, with a total of 373 lives saved by the year 2000 (Eddy, 1988). Even limiting mammography to those over 50 years of age would result in a yearly cost of $3.3 billion at an average of $100 per examination. This is by far the most expensive preventive health care activity recommended.

The smaller the tumor when discovered, the better the prognosis. A review of several studies shows that nonpalpable mammographically detected cancers have a 13 to 20 per cent incidence of metastatic spread, whereas those found by palpation have positive nodes 40 to 55 per cent of the time (McLellan, 1988). It has been calculated that

the average time between the ability of mammography to first detect the breast cancer and the ability of the physician to palpate the mass is 2 years, which may be of some value in estimating the optimal interval for mammography.

IMPACT ON THE FAMILY UNIT. The fear of breast cancer can produce a great deal of anxiety and may be substantially heightened by a strong family history. As with other diseases with a strong familial predisposition, the elements of guilt and resentment can have profound effects on family functioning.

Once breast cancer is diagnosed, a major issue is the patient's and the husband's perceived loss of feminine identity. This can be allayed in part by a knowledgeable physician willing to discuss these concerns openly and inform the patient and husband of the variety of improved treatment alternatives now available. These include consideration of limited surgical procedures, radiation, and prosthesis implantation.

Once cancer has been diagnosed and a treatment plan decided on, the family physician can play a critical role in preventing subsequent family dysfunction. The patient will need help in dealing with anger, helplessness, fear of recurrence, and the ill effects of treatment. The emotional life and dynamics of the family will be changed forever. The family unit will require guidance and understanding.

Lung Cancer

INCIDENCE. In the United States, lung cancer now has the second highest cancer incidence for men (behind prostate) and the third highest in women (behind breast and colorectal). In 1993, the estimated number of new cases was 170,000—100,000 men and 70,000 women.

MORBIDITY AND MORTALITY. Lung cancer is the leading cause of cancer mortality for both men and women. The estimated number of deaths in 1993 was 149,000. By comparing the similarity of the incidence with the mortality statistics, the grim nature of the prognosis is apparent, reflected in a 13 per cent 5-year survival.

IMPORTANT FACTS RELEVANT TO PREVENTION. Except for the small minority of cases secondary to industrial exposure, the only known way to prevent lung cancer is to not smoke. Eighty-three per cent of all lung cancers are directly attributable to smoking. Adequate intake of vitamin A has been associated with a reduced risk in smokers.

SCREENING TEST RECOMMENDATIONS. Although chest radiographic studies or sputum cytology may detect lung cancer at a presymptomatic stage, there is no study that shows a resultant improvement in the prognosis.

PREVENTIVE ACTIVITIES RECOMMENDATIONS. Patients at all ages should receive a strong health message from their physician concerning smoking: "It's addicting. Don't start. If you have started, stop." All preventive health checks should include an inquiry concerning smoking.

RELATED ISSUES. It is ironic that lung cancer has the highest mortality rate of all cancers and yet is one of the most preventable. Physicians can continue to have a major impact on the risk of this disease through community and patient intervention and education. Excellent support materials are available from the American Academy of Family Physicians, the American Cancer Society, and the American Heart Association. Physician recommendation is a strong contributor to patients' decisions to stop smoking.

IMPACT ON THE FAMILY UNIT. A single smoker in a family can be a source of secondary smoke exposure for the rest of the family. This has been shown to increase the risk of lung cancer, heart disease, and upper respiratory infections in family members. Children from households with smokers have a higher school absentee rate. Couples who smoke create a special problem for the physician who wishes to help. It is difficult to persuade one smoker to quit while the other continues, and it is equally problematic to bring two smokers to the point of wishing to stop at the same time. The withdrawal period is one of great stress and requires family education and support.

Carcinoma of the Cervix

INCIDENCE. The incidence of invasive cervical carcinoma is declining. There were approximately 13,500 new cases of invasive cervical cancer in 1993. The incidence rises steadily through age 50 and then remains steady. Worldwide, cervical carcinoma is the most common malignancy in women, whereas in the United States it ranks seventh.

MORBIDITY AND MORTALITY. The mortality rate for invasive carcinoma of the cervix is 4400 persons per year. The preinvasive cancer lesion of cervical intraepithelial neoplasia (CIN III or carcinoma in situ) has a 100 per cent cure rate with proper treatment, whereas stage I disease has an 89 per cent 5-year survival and stage III has a 30 per cent 5-year survival. Overall, the 5-year survival rate is 66 per cent. The Papanicolaou (Pap) smear screening programs detect disease at earlier stages when cure rates are higher and are have been primarily responsible for the dramatic reduction in mortality.

IMPORTANT FACTS RELEVANT TO PREVENTION. Squamous cell carcinoma of the cervix occurs almost exclusively in women who have had coitus. Although the mean time for progression from mild dysplasia (CIN I) to severe dysplasia or carcinoma in situ (CIN III) is 5.8 years and the mean time for further progression to invasive carcinoma is an additional 10 years (Richart et al., 1981), the rate of progression for any one individual is unpredictable. Carcinoma in situ may regress spontaneously in 30 to 50 per cent of cases. At least 30 per cent of patients with CIN III will have pro-

gression to invasive carcinoma (Hudson et al., 1988).

Major risk factors are early age for first intercourse, multiple sexual partners, herpes simplex virus infection, smoking, and history of condylomata (human papillomavirus) infection. Early sexual intercourse has an especially dramatic association with risk. Females who have had coitus less than 1 year after menarche are 26 times as likely to eventually develop cervical carcinoma as the general population.

Fifteen to 20 per cent of American women do not undergo regular Pap tests, and they account for the majority of cases of carcinoma of the cervix. Most studies show the Pap test is demonstrated to be 55 to 80 per cent sensitive (Richart et al., 1981). Specificity is reported at 91 to 99 per cent.

SCREENING TEST RECOMMENDATIONS. All women should begin having Pap smears when sexual activity begins, but no later than age 18. The American Cancer Society recommends that each woman should have at least three negative annual Pap smears, at which time frequency may be reduced to every 3 years at the discretion of the physician. Many physicians continue to advocate yearly screening. As yet, there appears to be no justification for screening high-risk groups more frequently. However, the 33 per cent incidence of CIN in patients with human papillomavirus infections may represent a high-risk subgroup requiring more frequent monitoring.

PREVENTIVE ACTIVITIES RECOMMENDATIONS. Teenagers and young women should be counseled concerning the marked risk they assume for sexually transmitted diseases and their consequences should they choose to have early sexual relations, particularly with multiple partners. Risk status should be re-evaluated at each preventive health visit, especially in groups who may have an increased likelihood of multiple sexual partners. Women should be advised of their risk status, with emphasis on the importance of regular re-evaluation. Although barrier contraception has only theoretical benefit, it also can be recommended strongly to help prevent sexually transmitted diseases.

RELATED ISSUES. There are other good reasons to see many women more often than every 3 years, such as monitoring use of birth control pills, breast cancer screening, dietary advice, contraceptive counseling, and prepregnancy counseling. It may be only a minority of women who will need to visit their physician less often than once yearly. Women have been educated for many years that the yearly Pap test is essential but *not* that there are other important issues to be dealt with during these visits.

IMPACT ON THE FAMILY UNIT. Invasive cervical cancer occurring during the childbearing years usually will be treated surgically, ending chances of future pregnancy. This will have a profound effect on a single female's approach to possible marriage and on a married couple's plans and relationship. The family physician's role only begins with referral for appropriate treatment. Preventive counseling is necessary in these situations. Women past the childbearing years still may suffer a loss of identity, similar to but not as intense as that of the breast cancer victim.

Skin Cancer

INCIDENCE. There were 600,000 cases of skin cancer in 1993, of which 32,000 were malignant melanoma. This is over three times the incidence of cancer in any other organ system, and incidence continues to rise dramatically.

MORBIDITY AND MORTALITY. Of the 8800 skin cancer deaths each year, 6800 are from malignant melanoma.

IMPORTANT FACTS RELEVANT TO PREVENTION. The major risk factor for all skin cancer is exposure to ultraviolet light. Those who have had severe exposures as children and those with fair complexions are at particular risk. Occupational exposures to coal tar, pitch, arsenic, radium, and creosote all increase risk. A prior history of local treatment with ionizing radiation increases chances of localized skin cancers 25 to 30 years later.

SCREENING TEST RECOMMENDATIONS. During regular preventive health examinations, the skin should be examined thoroughly for suspicious lesions. All lesions suspicious for malignancy should be prophylactically excised and submitted for pathologic interpretation.

PREVENTIVE ACTIVITIES RECOMMENDATIONS. For primary prevention, all patients at risk should be counseled in measures for avoidance of ultraviolet light (sun or artificial tanning), protection with higher number sunscreens (level 15 or greater), and use of protective clothing. Secondary prevention includes regular self-examination, especially for patients with already existing pigmented nevi.

The physician also should be alert to actinic keratoses and treat generalized lesions with 5-fluorouracil topical application and localized lesions with cryocautery.

Endometrial Cancer

INCIDENCE. In 1993 there were 13 cases of endometrial cancer in 100,000 persons (31,000 cases per year).

MORTALITY. The 1993 mortality was 2.4 deaths in 100,000 persons (5700 cases per year).

IMPORTANT FACTS RELEVANT TO PREVENTION. Endometrial cancer occurs primarily in postmenopausal women. The major etiologic factor appears to be the presence of unopposed estrogen, whether physiologic or iatrogenic. The most important early warning sign is abnormal vaginal bleeding. Risk factors are early menarche, late menopause, prolonged treatment with estrogen

alone, history of infertility, age, chronic anovulation, and tamoxifen therapy.

SCREENING TEST RECOMMENDATIONS. Abnormal endometrial cells occasionally are found on Pap smear, but this is not an adequate screen. Any endometrial cells found on a postmenopausal Pap smear should be considered abnormal. All postmenopausal females with bleeding of any amount must have endometrial sampling performed.

PREVENTIVE ACTIVITIES RECOMMENDATIONS. Risk factors should be established at menopause and modified when possible. All females with an intact uterus treated with estrogen replacement therapy also should be cycled with a progestational agent.

Cancer of the Prostate

INCIDENCE. The 1993 incidence of prostate cancer was 165,000 cases; it is now the most common cancer in men. After age 80, the incidence is as high as 1 in 10. Black Americans have the highest incidence in the world.

PREVALENCE. The prevalence of microscopic prostate cancer on autopsy increases with age.

MORTALITY AND MORBIDITY. Prostate cancer resulted in 35,000 deaths in 1993. Despite increasingly aggressive therapy, there has been no improvement in the age-adjusted death rate since 1949.

IMPORTANT FACTS RELEVANT TO PREVENTION. Only 1 in 380 men with histologic evidence of prostate cancer will die from the disease. Although a prostate-specific antigen (PSA) blood test and transrectal ultrasound have been shown to detect prostate cancers otherwise not palpable on rectal exam, no study has shown a reduction in mortality from screening with these procedures. Rectal exam alone has a sensitivity of 70 per cent and a specificity of 80 per cent.

SCREENING TEST RECOMMENDATIONS. No recommendations for screening tests for prostate cancer can be made at this time.

Other Preventable Diseases

Osteoporosis

INCIDENCE. The incidence of fractures secondary to osteoporosis is over 1.5 million per year. By extreme old age, 1 in every 3 women and 1 in every 6 men will have had a hip fracture, and 1 in 3 women over 65 will have vertebral fractures (Riggs and Melton, 1986). Female lifetime incidence of hip fractures is 15 per cent (USPSTF, 1989).

PREVALENCE. It is estimated that 15 to 20 million Americans have osteoporosis and are therefore at markedly increased risk for fractures.

COST AND IMPACT ON SOCIETY. The direct and indirect costs of caring for patients suffering fractures secondary to osteoporosis are $10 billion each year (USPSTF, 1989) and are expected to more than double in the next 30 years unless a comprehensive prevention program is initiated for our aging population (Cummings et al., 1990).

MORBIDITY AND MORTALITY. There is a 15 to 20 per cent reduction in expected survival in the year following a hip fracture. In addition, 50 per cent of hip fractures lead to significant disability (USPSTF, 1989).

IMPORTANT FACTS RELEVANT TO PREVENTION. Bone mass peaks in human beings shortly after the end of linear skeletal growth. There is a strong genetic influence on peak bone mass (Stevenson, 1990). Caucasian women have significantly lower peaks than men or darker skinned women. After age 30, women have a 0.3 to 0.5 per cent loss of bone mass yearly that abruptly increases to 2 to 3 per cent per year at menopause and then, over the next 10 years, gradually returns to premenopausal rates. The rates of loss of trabecular bone and cortical bone (the hip contains both) are somewhat different. Trabecular bone (vertebra, distal radius) loss occurs earlier and in greater proportion during the menopausal years than cortical bone (long bones) loss (Riggs and Melton, 1986). Men follow a similar sequence but without the accelerated phase. Total loss of bone mass in men is about two thirds that in women.

Prior to achieving peak bone mass, inadequate calcium intake (under 100 mg) may affect the peak bone mass adversely and later will affect the rate of loss. In postmenopausal women not receiving estrogen replacement therapy (ERT), increasing this amount to 1.5 grams still will not maintain zero calcium balance and appears to have no additional positive effect on bone density. Most data suggest that maintaining adequate calcium is helpful in reducing the rate of postmenopausal bone loss (Dawson-Hughes et al., 1990). There is an 80 per cent prevalence of inadequate calcium intake among women.

ERT is the most effective method of preventing the accelerated phase of bone mass loss after menopause. Discontinuation of estrogen therapy results in a prompt return of accelerated bone loss. Other methods of maximizing peak mass and slowing bone mass loss include regular weight-bearing exercise. There is a positive effect on the density in the femoral neck (Stevenson, 1990), and one study also has shown an increase in lumbar bone density with exercise (Dalsky et al., 1988).

There are many primary risk factors for osteoporosis, and multiple additional medical conditions also may place an individual at higher risk (Table 11–11). Contributing factors may be overlooked easily when other medical problems that may increase the risk of osteoporosis consume the focus of attention. A good example is the elderly white woman in otherwise good health who develops polymyalgia rheumatica. The diagnosis and treatment with corticosteroids become the major focus.

TABLE 11–11. RISK FACTORS FOR OSTEOPOROSIS

Positive family history
Advancing age
Female sex
Caucasian or Asian race
Early menopause (including surgically induced)
Underweight
Cigarette smoking
History of dietary calcium deficiency
Hypogonadism (men)
Sedentary lifestyle
Alcohol consumption
Subtotal gastrectomy
Hyperthyroidism
Hemiplegia
Chronic obstructive pulmonary disease
Glucorticoid therapy
Anticonvulsant therapy

It is easy to forget that such a person, 2 years later, may be free of symptoms of polymyalgia rheumatica but be debilitated by vertebral fractures.

SCREENING TEST RECOMMENDATIONS. No screening test can be recommended. Specifically, densitometry has no place in routine preventive health care at this time. It may be helpful in establishing a baseline at menopause for high-risk individuals.

PREVENTIVE ACTIVITIES RECOMMENDATIONS. All patients, especially women, should be educated regarding the recommended intake of at least 800 to 1000 mg of dietary calcium; adolescents may need 1200 mg and postmenopausal woman may need 1500 mg. Major nutritional sources of calcium are listed in Table 11–12. Recommendations for use of dairy products include the advice to use low-fat alternatives wherever possible as part of the overall prudent diet. Women of any age unable to meet minimal calcium needs through diet should be advised to use supplemental calcium.

The elderly often have decreased ability to absorb vitamin D and therefore also should be advised to also take 800 U of vitamin D daily. Risk status should be determined for all women, preferably at menarche, and should be re-evaluated at

TABLE 11–12. NUTRITIONAL SOURCES OF CALCIUM

Food	Serving Size	Calcium (mg)
Milk	1 cup	300
Cheese (low fat)	1 oz	185
Yogurt (nonfat)	1 cup	450
Yogurt (whole milk)	1 cup	275
Cottage cheese (1% milk)	½ cup	70
Dark green leafy vegetables	½ cup	150–180
Other vegetables	½ cup	30–100
Fruits	Average serving	<25

the time of routine preventive health visits. Additional counseling concerning osteoporosis prevention should be given to those at higher risk.

Every woman should be evaluated thoroughly at menopause for risk factors and possible ERT. In general, most white women with any other risk factors are candidates unless there are specific contraindications.

All patients should be counseled to maintain regular aerobic weight-bearing activity as part of the overall program for general preventive health care. Although 50 to 60 minutes of exercise performed three times weekly has been shown to increase bone mass, the minimum levels necessary have not been determined (Dalsky et al., 1988). For patients with established osteoporosis, the major treatments to retard further progression include antiresorptive therapy with estrogen, calcitonin, or disodium etidronate. Anabolic steroids, parathyroid hormone, and fluoride also may be indicated in selected cases (Riggs and Melton, 1992).

RELATED ISSUES. When prescribing ERT, a daily dosage equivalent to 0.625 mg of conjugated estrogen has been documented to be effective; 0.3 mg may be equally effective. In women with an intact uterus, it is desirable to add progesterone for at least the last 10 days of each estrogen cycle, followed by 5 to 7 days without either hormone. Progesterone reduces or eliminates the increased risk of endometrial cancer associated with unopposed estrogen therapy. Although ERT appears to affect the lipid profile favorably, the effects of progesterone may negate this partially, and therefore progesterone should be used in the lowest effective dose—the equivalent of 5 mg of medroxyprogesterone acetate.

IMPACT ON THE FAMILY UNIT. Family eating patterns will primarily determine the peak bone mass achieved. Therefore, counseling of women in the childbearing years should include recommendations for the entire family.

Elderly patients who are already at high risk create a dilemma for the family physician. There is little that is of proven value in replacing bone mass that is already lost. Exercise may place the severely osteoporotic patient at some increased risk for fractures. The resulting sudden loss of independence in an elderly family member suffering from a serious fracture has a great impact on the family in emotional, organizational, and financial terms. The major decisions that must be made as a result of the condition often reverse the parent–child roles.

Intimate knowledge of the elderly patient, his or her functional capacities, and the living situation places the family physician in a pivotal role in the prevention of fractures.

Sexually Transmitted Diseases

INCIDENCE. The peak incidence of sexually transmitted disease is in teenagers and young adults; teenagers alone account for 2.5 million cases. The reported incidence of gonorrhea is 2 million cases per year (833 in 100,000 persons), with marked clustering in metropolitan areas. Estimated yearly incidence figures for chlamydia infection are an astounding 3 to 4 million cases. Each year, 120,000 infants are infected with chlamydia at birth. There are an estimated 270,000 new cases of herpes genitalis and 35,000 cases of syphilis each year (USPSTF, 1989). The incidence of congenital syphilis is rising and is currently 10.5 cases in 100,000 live births (USPSTF, 1989).

PREVALENCE. Because of the long duration of infection, the two most prevalent sexually transmitted diseases are herpes simplex virus and human papillomavirus. The cumulative prevalence of herpes simplex genitalis virus alone is 20 million cases at this time. Because of the asymptomatic nature of many chlamydial infections, it is estimated that the prevalence in the general population is 5 per cent.

COST AND IMPACT ON SOCIETY. The yearly economic cost of genital herpes is $500 million and of chlamydia is $1 million (USPSTF, 1989).

MORBIDITY AND MORTALITY. Over 200,000 women per year, one fifth of those with pelvic inflammatory disease, become infertile, and 50 per cent of all ectopic pregnancies are a result of pelvic inflammatory disease. Twenty per cent of women with one episode of pelvic inflammatory disease will develop chronic pain.

IMPORTANT FACTS RELEVANT TO PREVENTION. All of the sexually transmitted diseases have a high asymptomatic carrier rate, making prevention of transmission very difficult. Therefore, the single major risk factor is multiple sexual partners. Only abstinence, monogamy, or condoms will affect the risk dramatically.

SCREENING TEST RECOMMENDATIONS. No screening tests are recommended for the general population. A screening gonorrhea culture test and a direct fluorescent antibody test or enzyme-linked immunosorbent assay for chlamydia should be performed in patients from high-risk groups at the time of routine pelvic examination. Persons with multiple sexual partners should be examined yearly. Screening during pregnancy is particularly important because of the potential for congenital defects and transmission to the fetus. Routine screening for syphilis should be performed in high-risk groups.

PREVENTIVE ACTIVITIES RECOMMENDATIONS. Education should begin before or at the beginning of sexual activity. All sexually active patients should be encouraged to seek medical evaluation for even apparently minor genital tract symptoms. Barrier contraception can reduce transmission significantly in those engaging in high-risk sexual activities.

RELATED ISSUES. Physicians must maintain a high index of suspicion for all sexually transmitted diseases because there is a very high percentage of asymptomatic and minimally symptomatic patients. In high-risk populations, presumptive treatment for chlamydial infection, even with minimal signs or symptoms, is recommended by many experts. Treatment recommendations for gonorrhea now include coverage for chlamydia as well.

IMPACT ON THE FAMILY UNIT. The incrimination that can result when a husband or wife is diagnosed with a sexually transmitted disease may lead to major family disruption. The physician will play the key role in interpreting the meaning of such an episode and bringing the couple to a mutual understanding. It is therefore critical that the physician know the natural course of the disease. For instance, 30 per cent of women with gonorrhea may be asymptomatic carriers (in some populations, men also may be almost this high), 70 per cent of patients with genital herpes have no symptoms, and 70 per cent of female lower genital tract infections with chlamydia are asymptomatic (Office of Disease Prevention and Health Promotion, 1988).

Human Immunodeficiency Virus Infection

INCIDENCE. The incidence of acquired immunodeficiency syndrome (AIDS) secondary to human immunodeficiency virus (HIV) infection was estimated at 17.1 in 100,000 persons in 1991. Fifty-two per cent of cases are attributable to transmission among homosexual/bisexual men (while the case load increased to 25 per cent among women and men who were injecting drug users in 1991). Numbers of cases also are increasing among minority populations as compared to whites in the United States. Within 10 years of HIV infection, about 50 per cent of persons will develop AIDS.

PREVALENCE. The Centers for Disease Control estimates that HIV has infected 1.5 million Americans. The prevalence of AIDS was estimated at 2.4 in 100,000 persons, with 289,000 cases and 182,275 deaths by 1993. The number of cases increased by 10 per cent from 1990 to 1991. Six thousand births a year are to HIV-infected mothers ("Update," 1992).

COST AND IMPACT ON SOCIETY. The Centers for Disease Control estimates total yearly direct and indirect costs of $13 billion.

MORBIDITY AND MORTALITY. The case fatality rate is over 75 per cent for persons diagnosed with AIDS after 2 years.

IMPORTANT FACTS RELEVANT TO PREVENTION. The groups with the highest prevalence are homosexual males, intravenous drug users, individuals with multiple sexual partners, patients with multiple blood transfusions after 1977 and prior to blood screening in 1985, hemophiliacs, and babies born to infected mothers.

SCREENING TEST RECOMMENDATIONS. All patients should be screened for risk status. The frequency of screening will vary depending on the particular patient population. Patients in high-risk groups should be encouraged strongly to be screened for antibodies to HIV. One major reason for screening is to identify those individuals who already are infected so that intervention may be instituted to halt the further spread of the virus.

PREVENTIVE ACTIVITIES RECOMMENDATIONS. Education of patients to modify high-risk behaviors is the first priority for the family physician. At this time, the only real chance for meaningful intervention is to prevent exposure to individuals infected with HIV. Children and teenagers, in particular, must be helped to understand the reality of the risks of sexual contact (especially when condoms are not used) and intravenous drug use (especially using shared needles or syringes).

Women at high risk in the childbearing years should be considered for yearly HIV antibody screening. Any of these women found to be positive for HIV should be counseled strongly against conception.

Within the office, the physician has a responsibility to employees and other patients to implement recommended measures to ensure protection from inadvertent transmission. The Occupational Safety and Health Administration now requires annual courses for health care workers.

Physician education of patients to modify lifestyle practices can be crucial in preventing the spread of AIDS. However, prevention of secondary infections in the AIDS patient can be beneficial in management. Care in preparation of foods can decrease contact with bacterial and parasitic pathogens, avoidance of handling cat litter can help prevent toxoplasmosis, and avoidance of travel to areas endemic for coccidioidomycosis and histoplasmosis can be of value.

Special attention should be given to immunization of patients with HIV infection (Jewell and Hecht, 1993). *Pneumococcus, Haemophilus influenzae,* and hepatitis B vaccines are especially important. Although HIV-infected patients produce lower antibody responses to these three diseases, most will produce protective antibodies if they are not already debilitated. When administering *H. influenzae* type b vaccine, the conjugated vaccine (which is T-cell dependent) appears to be more effective in early HIV infection, whereas the unconjugated vaccine is more effective in persons with AIDS. Vaccination of adults for diphtheria, tetanus, mumps, rubella, polio, and measles also is recommended. Because the response rates decline with more advanced disease, it is advisable to update all vaccinations early in the course of the illness. Attenuated vaccines may be safer when available.

RELATED ISSUES. In addition to individual action, there is a need for immediate, aggressive public health measures. Major preventive recommendations include:

1. Institution of a confidential system whereby an exposed partner would be notified.

2. Notification of all persons having received blood transfusions between 1977 and 1985 that they should be tested.

3. Prevention and treatment of intravenous drug abuse as a top national priority.

4. Aggressive pursuit of drug and alcohol abuse prevention (considered a factor for potential exposure to HIV), especially through education of the nation's young people.

5. Continual monitoring of blood supplies for safety.

6. Prevention of spread within health care facilities.

Secondary prevention will become increasingly important if methods to stop or retard disease progression in its presymptomatic stages become accessible and affordable.

Prevention of opportunistic infections can be facilitated by chemoprophylaxis. For prevention of *Pneumocystis carinii* infection, trimethoprim-sulfamethoxazole is the first line of defense and aerosolized pentamidine or dapsone are the second. Prophylaxis is indicated if the CD4 counts fall below 200/mL, for oral thrush, or for unexplained fevers of more than 2 weeks' duration. Prophylaxis also should be considered for toxoplasmosis and *Mycoplasma avium* complex infection.

Smoking cessation is also important because of its association with a more rapid decline in CD4 counts as well as a greater incidence of opportunistic infections. Continued substance abuse is also a risk factor for more rapid progression of disease.

Prevention of psychological complications may be facilitated by anticipatory counseling and frequent screening for anxiety, depression, social stresses, and suicidal ideation. Physician use of medications and counseling or referral to support groups can be preventive.

A careful sexual history from all patients may identify individuals with high-risk behaviors and permit education for safer sexual practices, such as monogamy, condom and spermicide use, and the special risks associated with anal intercourse. All patients should be offered HIV testing when they are diagnosed with any other sexually transmitted disease.

IMPACT ON THE FAMILY UNIT. A special tragedy is the 65 per cent possibility that HIV will be transmitted from a mother to her unborn baby. Many of these infected babies are now left abandoned in the hospital. Special care needs to be given to uninfected partners of patients.

Other Infectious Diseases and Immunizations

INCIDENCE. There are a number of infectious diseases that can be prevented almost completely by immunization. Many of these diseases have been public health scourges in the past and the sources of great epidemics and even pandemics.

These diseases include measles, mumps, rubella, hepatitis B, pneumococcal disease, influenza, pertussis, diphtheria, tetanus, poliomyelitis, and *h. influenzae* B diseases. The development of immunizations has cut incidence of these infections a hundredfold or even a thousandfold in some cases.

Another group of preventable infectious diseases are those usually encountered by international travelers. The most common are malaria and travelers' diarrhea. The physician should provide information about mosquito avoidance, prophylactic medication, and food and water consumption.

PREVENTIVE ACTIVITIES RECOMMENDATIONS

1. Each physician's office should be equipped to give needed immunizations when the screen reveals a need, or be prepared to refer to a facility that does. A sample schedule of recommended immunizations is found in Table 11–13.

2. All physicians should participate in community health education programs promoting public understanding of the need for appropriate immunizations.

DISCUSSION. Of all the activities carried out by physicians, the prevention of infectious diseases by immunization is the least expensive, takes the least effort, and is the most efficient. The control of the major infectious diseases has been a marked success for preventive medicine in the 20th century.

Yet, despite the proven efficacy, there are major gaps in the full implementation of immunization. Measles has had a dramatic resurgence as a result of lax immunization practices. There are also major deficiencies in the levels of immunization for pneumococcal disease and influenza.

Health care workers in particular have an obligation to assure that they personally have been adequately immunized for hepatitis B.

IMPACT ON THE FAMILY UNIT. A particular challenge for the family physician is the family that refuses to immunize its children for religious reasons or out of neglect. Other parents fear the potential side effects of vaccines (especially pertussis) and will rationalize that, because most other children are immunized, the chances of their child contracting the infection are near zero. Each physician should be aware of the relevant state laws and should have a strategy for dealing with these problems.

Moderate cost and occasional mild side effects such as fever, localized pain, or adenitis may cause some negative impact on the family. Although a rare disastrous complication may occur, such as poliomyelitis in an unimmunized family member, these are so unusual that they are far outweighed by the benefits to the general population. The ultimate impact of a proper immunization program is healthier and more productive families with fewer congenital anomalies, fewer lost children, fewer

TABLE 11–13.   IMMUNIZATIONS: INDICATIONS AND SCHEDULES

Immunization	0–15 Years of Age	16–64 Years	65 or Older
DPT	2, 4, 6, 15 months and 4–6 years		
dT	15 years		Every 10 years
OPV	2, 4, 6,* 15 months and 4–6 years		
Measles	15 months and 4–6 years	College entrance†	
Mumps	15 months		
Rubella	15 months		
Haemophilus B‡	2, 4, 12 months		
Influenza	Yearly, if high risk	Yearly, if high risk	Yearly or at age 65
Pneumococcus		Once only when becomes high risk	
Hepatitis B	Birth, 2 months, 6–18 months	Series of 3, when becomes high risk any age, if not previously immunized	

* Optional, except in endemic areas.
† If no previous booster. Other target groups, if no previous booster, are those leaving for foreign travel and health care workers.
‡ Conjugate vaccine: schedule and number of injections may vary with vaccines from different manufacturers.
From Morse RM, Heffron WA: Disease Prevention. *In* Rakel RE (ed): Essentials of Family Medicine. Philadelphia, WB Saunders Company, 1993, p 135, with permission.

paralyzed children and adults, and longer life spans for the elderly.

Accidents

INCIDENCE. The estimated number of yearly accidents is over 60 million, reflecting a rate of nonfatal injury of 26,400 in 100,000 persons. The highest rate is found in the 18- to 24-year age group.

COST AND IMPACT ON SOCIETY. Estimated direct and indirect costs of injury in 1984 were nearly $97 million.

MORBIDITY AND MORTALITY. Accidents are the fourth leading cause of death in the United States, and the leading cause in persons under age 45. The total is 95,000 deaths per year. Almost half were secondary to automobile accidents. A distant second cause is falls, but these accidents are remarkable in that over 70 per cent of them occur in individuals over age 65. The third most frequent cause of accidental death is drowning, which kills 7000 people each year.

IMPORTANT FACTS RELEVANT TO PREVENTION. Homes are the most common site of overall injuries, whereas the automobile is the most common site for fatal injury. Only 46 per cent of people use seat belts. It is estimated that over half of all fatal automobile accidents and adult drownings involve alcoholic beverages.

SCREENING TEST RECOMMENDATIONS. Screening for alcohol abuse is of top priority. Not only is it the major cause of traffic fatalities, it is also a major factor in all other types of traumatic accidents. Patients should be asked at the time of routine preventive health checks whether or not they regularly use seat belts.

PREVENTIVE ACTIVITIES RECOMMENDATIONS. The guidelines for prevention listed under the sections for alcohol abuse and osteoporosis should be followed. Parents should be encouraged to ensure that all children are taught to swim. Homes should be safety proofed, especially when small children

and the elderly live within the home. Use of seat belts and child restraint devices should be encouraged strongly. Firearms should be locked up carefully in the home. For the elderly, strategies for falls and fire protection in the home are particularly important.

IMPACT ON THE FAMILY UNIT. In addition to the immediate trauma suffered, nonfatal accidents have a direct impact on the individual and the family. An issue that must be confronted is the injured person's and the other family members' own mortality. Although some families will come closer at these times, others may distance themselves from the patient as a defense mechanism.

Fatal accidents present a special problem. The loss is unexpected, and often occurs in those who are otherwise young and healthy. For the family, the process of grieving may become particularly difficult or pathologic.

Glaucoma

PREVALENCE. The prevalence of glaucoma is less than 1 per cent in those under 70 years of age and almost 4 per cent in those over 75. Glaucoma affects 2 million Americans.

IMPORTANT FACTS RELEVANT TO PREVENTION. The ultimate result of untreated glaucoma is blindness. The most common type, primary open-angle glaucoma, is asymptomatic until severe, when irreversible damage often has occurred.

The three major criteria for diagnosis are elevated intraocular pressure, visual field defects, and optic disk pallor, widening, and cupping. In glaucoma, the cup-to-disk ratio is greater than 0.5, and the disk may be elliptical. The funduscopic changes on direct ophthalmoscopy are seen best with a red filter.

Up to 15 per cent of glaucoma patients can have normal intraocular pressure, whereas over 70 per cent of patients with elevated pressures (21 to 35 mm Hg) will not develop glaucoma. Both of these groups represent exceptions to the usual descriptions of pathogenesis.

The risk factors for glaucoma are family history (15 to 20 times the risk), black race (four times the risk), diabetes mellitus, and age.

SCREENING TEST RECOMMENDATIONS. The value of any screening tests for glaucoma is controversial. The use of the Schiøtz tonometer of special concern because of its very low sensitivity and specificity. The risk of relying on pressure measurements for screening is when a "normal" pressure measurement is used to reassure patients that they will not develop glaucoma. If the family physician elects to use this method, patients should be screened starting at age 40 and every 5 years thereafter until age 60, at which time the screening interval should be reduced to every 2 to 3 years. Funduscopic evaluation by a well-trained physician at the time of tonometry may increase the sensitivity of screening. The USPSTF does not recommend routine tonometry by family physicians, but they state that it may be clinically prudent to refer high-risk patients to eye specialists for periodic testing.

Diabetes Mellitus

Diabetes mellitus does not meet the criteria for mass screening, despite its high prevalence, high morbidity and mortality, long presymptomatic stage, and ease of diagnosis. Early diagnosis and treatment has not been shown to alter the prognosis. Nevertheless, screening has been advocated in the recommendations for coronary heart disease because the presence of diabetes is a major risk factor in that evaluation. The only exception in which screening for diabetes provides clear direct benefit is during pregnancy.

OTHER PREVENTION STRATEGIES

Benefits to health may be significant when physicians consider prevention of additional less common entities. The USPSTF has recommended a number of additional screening and counseling prevention strategies in its Guide to Clinical Preventive Services (see References).

LIFESTYLES FOR HEALTH

When one reviews the most common causes of mortality, illness, and disability, there is a strikingly common theme in their etiology and prevention: An individual's lifestyle is the major modifiable determinant of health.

Proper diet is of paramount importance to prevent the nation's number one killer, coronary heart disease, and it is estimated that 35 per cent of cancers, the nation's number two killer, are secondary to diet (Doll and Peto, 1981). Fortunately, the specific dietary components that are recommended for prevention of each individual disease are also beneficial in general. Therefore, it is possible to make broad prudent dietary recommendations as a base on which all physicians and patients can build, including (1) total calories needed to achieve and maintain ideal body weight; (2) fat intake of less than 30 per cent of calories; (3) saturated fat intake of less than 10 per cent of total calories; (4) cholesterol intake of less than 300 mg/day; (5) carbohydrate intake of 50 to 60 per cent of total calories, emphasizing the need for complex carbohydrates; (6) maximal fiber intake in the diet, with emphasis on the need for soluble fiber sources; (7) minimum calcium intake of 800 to 1000 mg daily; (8) sodium chloride intake of less than 3 grams of sodium (7.5 grams of salt); and (9) assurance of adequate amounts of vitamins, minerals, and antioxidants by including a wide variety of fruits and vegetables in the daily intake.

The importance of stress reduction and exercise in preventing disease is a subject of great interest. There is general agreement that they are of real importance. Even moderate amounts of exercise

TABLE 11–14.   RELATIONSHIP BETWEEN COMMON PREVENTABLE DISEASES AND THE MOST COMMON RISK FACTORS

Risk Factor	Diet	Hyper-lipidemia	Obesity	Hyper-tension	Smoking	Alcohol	Sedentary Life Style	Heredity	Stress and Depression
Coronary heart disease	■	■	■	■	■		■	■	■
Stroke	■	■		■	■		■	■	■
Chemical dependence						■		■	■
Osteoporosis	■				■	■	■	■	
Accident/suicide					■	■		■	■
Sexually transmitted diseases and human immunodeficiency virus infection						■			
Lung cancer	■				■			■	
Breast cancer	■		■			■		■	
Colon cancer	■						■	■	
Cervical cancer					■				
Endometrial cancer			■						

have been demonstrated to reduce all causes of mortality dramatically.

Another common theme is the critical importance of avoiding toxins, especially the addictive substances nicotine and alcohol. Smoking accounts for 30 per cent of all cancer deaths and is a major factor in coronary heart disease. It is directly responsible for 390,000 deaths each year. It is estimated that each pack of cigarettes sold results in a cost of $2.17 in medical care and lost productivity. The pervasive social and health effects of alcohol on individuals and society have been outlined.

Table 11–14 shows selected major diseases and the most common risk factors.

DEVELOPING A PREVENTIVE HEALTH CARE FLOW SHEET

A simple and flexible flow sheet is essential for the continuity and comprehensiveness of preventive health care. This form can be used effectively as a tool for educating patients concerning their

TABLE 11–15. PREVENTIVE HEALTH CARE AND RISK ANALYSIS FLOW CHART (UNIVERSITY OF VIRGINIA)

Patient Name: _____ Patient Number: _____ Chart Number: _____

AGE→	50	51	52	53	54	55	56	57	58	59
Lifestyle Risk Assessment	■	■	■	■	■	■	■	■	■	■
Cholesterol, HDL	■					■				
Stool Guaiac X3, Rectal	■	■	■	■	■	■	■	■	■	■
Flexible Sigmoidoscopy	■					■				
Td	■									
Breast Exam	■	■	■	■	■	■	■	■	■	■
Mammogram	■	■	■	■	■	■	■	■	■	■
Pap	■	▪ ▪	▪ ▪	■	▪ ▪	▪ ▪	■	▪ ▪	▪ ▪	■
Glaucoma Vision Screen	▪ ▪					▪ ▪				

Flow Chart Key: ■ = Routine accepted procedure; ▪ ▪ = Optional or controversial procedure.
Flow Chart Instructions: Enter month/year test completed, D/E if done elsewhere, N/A if not applicable; add bars as needed.

Risk Analysis Instructions: Circle items that are patient risk factors. For resolved risk factors, add OK and month/year. Check items that are not risk factors. Unmarked items are assumed not to have been determined yet.

Coronary Heart Disease
High LDL
Low HDL
+Family Hx
Male
Tobacco
Hypertension
LVH
Diabetes mellitus
Sedentary
Obesity
Stress?
BCP > 35 y/o

Colorectal Cancer
+Family Hx
High fat diet
Hx polyps

Lung Cancer
Tobacco use

Suicide
Previous attempt
+Family Hx
Depression

Alcohol Abuse
Felt like Cutting down
Annoyed by criticism
Guilty about drinking
Eye opener
+Family Hx
Previous problems

Glaucoma
+Family Hx
Diabetes mellitus
Black

Sexually Transmitted Disease
Blood transfusions (1978–85)
Multiple sexual partners
Bisexual/homosexual
Nonbarrier contraception
Presence of or exposure to STD
Hx of IV drug use

Breast Cancer
+Family Hx
Nulliparous
Primigravida >35 y/o
High-risk biopsy

Cervical Cancer
Hx condylomata
Hx herpes
Multiple sexual partners
Early first intercourse
Prior dysplasia

Osteoporosis
<1 gm Ca/day
Sedentary
+Family Hx
Thin
White/Oriental
Tobacco

Accident/Injury
Seat belts/airbags
Drink and drive
Speeding
Cycle, no helmet
No smoke detector
Lives in high crime area

Physician Notes: (place the note number next to the appropriate referenced item in the chart)
1.
2.
3.

preventive health care needs. Patients at high risk for certain illnesses may need to have increased frequency of screening tests or special tests added. Also, recommendations for preventive activities will change as new information becomes available. An inflexible form will be of little use after 5 to 10 years.

An *informative* flow sheet will alert the physician to risk factors that have not been identified and procedures that have not been accomplished. Missing pieces of information should be obvious on even a cursory review of the form.

A deterrent to the use of any form or flow sheet is a need to duplicate information that is available elsewhere in the record. Therefore, the more data that are *unique* to the form, the more likely it is to be used.

Tables 11–15 and 11–16 show examples of flow sheets that the family physician may wish to modify for a particular practice.

GETTING STARTED

A comprehensive preventive health program is difficult to implement all at once in a busy physician's office. It often requires adopting a new perspective for the physician and the staff, a support set of educational materials and referral sources, and equipment. Adding new elements one at a time will obviate much of the potential threat posed by such a major undertaking. The office may decide to emphasize mammography, lipid screening, Pap tests, or colorectal cancer screening at the beginning. Necessary staff and physician education, selection of appropriate educational materials, purchase of equipment, and implementation of the program then can take place in a longitudinal fashion at a comfortable pace. Once this is done to everyone's satisfaction, additional screening and preventive modules can be added, once again one at a time.

The important thing is to begin.

TABLE 11–16. HEALTH SCREENING FLOW SHEET (DEPARTMENT OF FAMILY MEDICINE, (UNIVERSITY OF NEW MEXICO)

Categories	Age Date	36	37	38	39	40	41	42	43	44	45	46	47	48	49	50
History and Physical Examination																
Blood pressure measured every year																
Dental examination every year																
Teach breast self-examination																
Menopause symptoms (present?)																
Contraceptive needs reviewed every year																
Laboratory Tests																
Baseline mammogram (under age 50)																
Cholesterol and high-density lipoprotein (baseline)																
Papanicolaou's smear (every 2 years—American Cancer Society; every 5 years—Canada)																
Immunization																
Td (every 10 years)																
Counsel/Patient Education (Annually)																
Cigarette smoking																
Alcohol use																
Occupational hazards																
Skin cancer protection																
Seat belt use																
Exercise																
Life stages Career/achievement Family social stability																
Calcium supplementation																

From Morse RM, Heffron WA: Disease Prevention. *In* Rakel RE [ed]: Essentials of Family Medicine. Philadelphia, WB Saunders Company, 1993, p 139, with permission.

REFERENCES

American Cancer Society: Cancer Facts and Figures—1994. Atlanta, American Cancer Society, 1994.

American Heart Association: An Eating Plan for Healthy Americans. Dallas, American Heart Association, 1985.

American Heart Association: Dietary Treatment of Hypercholesterolemia—A Manual for Patients. Dallas, American Heart Association, 1988.

American Heart Association: 1993 Heart and Stroke Facts Statistics. Dallas, American Heart Association, 1992.

American Medical Association: Factors Contributing to the Health Care Cost Problem. Chicago, American Medical Association, 1993.

Bader JP: Screening of colorectal cancer. Dig Dis Sci 31(suppl): 9, 1986.

Brody J: Good Food Book. New York, WW Norton, 1985.

Bush B, Shaw S, Cleary P, et al: Screening for alcohol abuse using the CAGE questionnaire. Am J Med 82:231, 1987.

Conner WE, Conner SL: The New American Diet. New York, Simon & Schuster, 1986.

Cummings SR, Rubin SM, Black D: The future of hip fractures in the United States: Numbers, costs, and potential effects of postmenopausal estrogen. Clin Orthop 252:163, 1990.

Cyr MG, Wartman SA: The effectiveness of routine screening questions in the detection of alcoholism. JAMA 259:51, 1988.

Dalsky GP, Stocke KS, Ehsani AA, et al: Weight-bearing exercise training and lumbar bone mineral content in post-menopausal women. Ann Intern Med 108:824, 1988.

Dawson-Hughes B, Dallel GE, Krall EA, et al: A controlled trial effect of calcium supplementation on bone density in postmenopausal women. N Engl J Med 323:878, 1990.

Doll R, Peto R: The Causes of Cancer: Quantitative Estimates of Avoidable Risks of Cancer in the United States Today. New York, Oxford University Press, 1981.

Eddy DM: The value of mammography screening in women under age 50 years. JAMA 259:1512, 1988.

Eshleman R: The American Heart Association Cookbook. New York, David McKay Company, 1984.

Hudson TW, Reinhart MA, Rose SD, et al: Clinical Preventive Medicine: Health Promotion and Disease Prevention. Boston, Little, Brown, 1988.

Jewell JF, Hecht FM: Preventive health care for adults with HIV infection. JAMA 269:1144, 1993.

Mandel JS, Bond JH, Church TR, et al: Reducing mortality from colorectal cancer by screening for fecal occult blood. N Engl J Med 328:1365, 1993.

McLellan GL: Screening and early diagnosis of breast cancer. J Fam Pract 26:561, 1988.

Office of Disease Prevention and Health Promotion, United States Public Health Service: Disease Prevention/Health Promotion: The Facts. Palo Alto, CA, Bull Publishing Company, 1988.

Potchen EJ, Sierra AE: The detection and cure of breast cancer. Obstet Gynecol Clin North Am 14:667, 1987.

Richart RM, Barron BA: Screening strategies for cervical cancer and cervical intraepithelial neoplasia. Cancer 47:1176, 1981.

Riegelman RK, Povar GJ: Putting Prevention in Practice. Boston, Little, Brown, 1988.

Riggs BL, Melton LJ: Involutional osteoporosis. N Engl J Med 314:1676, 1986.

Riggs BL, Melton LJ: The prevention and treatment of osteoporosis. N Engl J Med 327:620, 1992.

Selby JV, Friedman GD, Quesenberry CP, Weiss NS: A case-control study of screening sigmoidoscopy from colorectal cancer. N Engl J Med 326:653, 1992.

Selby JV, Friedman GD, Quesenberry CP, Weiss NS: Effect of fecal occult blood testing on mortality from colorectal cancer. Ann Intern Med 118:1, 1993.

Selzer ML: The Michigan Alcoholism Screening Test: The quest for a new diagnostic instrument. Am J Psychiatry 127:1653, 1971.

Steering Committee of the Physicians' Health Study Research Group: Preliminary report: Findings from the aspirin component of the ongoing Physicians' Health Study. N Engl J Med 318:4, 1988.

Stevenson JC: Pathogenesis, prevention, and treatment of osteoporosis. Obstet Gynecol 75:365, 1990.

Update: Acquired immunodeficiency syndrome—United States, 1991. MMWR 42(26):463, 1992.

U.S. Preventive Services Task Force: Guide to Clinical Preventive Services. Baltimore, Williams & Wilkins, 1989.

Whitfield CL, Davis JE, Barker LR: Alcoholism. *In* Barker LR, Burton JR, Zieve PD (eds): Principles of Ambulatory Medicine. Baltimore, Williams & Wilkins, 1986, p 248.

CHAPTER 12

USE OF CONSULTANTS

ROBERT E. RAKEL

All physicians, regardless of their specialty, turn to another physician at some time for advice. This process necessarily became formalized as physicians focused their training and limited their practice to a particular segment of medicine. The first specialty board, the American Board of Ophthalmology, was formed in 1917, and, by 1989, there were 23 specialty boards and 51 subspecialty boards. The American Board of Family Practice was established in 1969 as the 20th primary specialty.

It is a common misconception of medical students that subspecialists know more than generalists. The fact is that the amount of information required to practice each of the 74 specialties and subspecialties is defined clearly and is equivalent. What varies is the degree of breadth and depth in each. In addition to being trained in a wide variety of clinical areas, family physicians also are trained to coordinate the care of seriously ill individuals who require a variety of consultants, orchestrating the skills of each to achieve optimum patient care and satisfaction (see Chapter 1).

Every patient should have a primary care physician who not only sees him for first-contact care, but who actively participates in his secondary and tertiary care by arranging and coordinating his consultant needs, by providing continuity, and by taking the patient back. (Stephens, 1982, p. 33).

The appropriate use of the consultation process is an art that contributes to improved patient care when utilized properly by family physicians. Although there is a definite distinction between consultation and referral, the terms often are used interchangeably. Consultation is by definition the practice of one physician asking another for an opinion or assistance, whereas referral is the transfer of responsibility to another physician for the care of a specific problem. Referral usually involves one physician requesting the services of another for a particular purpose and for a limited time, such as referral to a surgeon for a cholecystectomy or to a cardiologist for coronary angiography. In contrast, consultation is the process whereby one physician requests the opinion of a colleague regarding the diagnosis or management of a patient's problem. Regardless of this distinction, the physician initiating either process is spoken of as

the referring physician, and the physician who is consulted or to whom the patient is referred is called the consultant.

In a study of patterns of consultation and referral, Geyman and associates (1976) found that 97 per cent of the exchanges between family physicians and other specialists were referrals and only 3 per cent were consultations. Fry (1971) noted with regret that consultation is no longer a deliberation between colleagues about diagnosis or proper treatment: "We have come to view our specialist colleagues more as expert 'technicians' than as consultants" (p. 148). Although the system in the United Kingdom has been described as the specialist controlling the hospital and the general practitioner controlling the patient, this separation avoids much of the rivalry over patient care that occurs in the United States. Horder (1977) believes that "patients look to all of us for the same two things, technical competence and personal care. I believe that, at present, we have more cause to be concerned about the supply of personal care than technical competence" (p. 396).

Many consultations are discretionary; they can be divided into urgent or mandatory, in which case the patient is likely to suffer harm if not referred, and elective (the patient is unlikely to suffer harm if not referred). Although only 3 to 4 per cent of patients seen by family physicians are referred, this percentage may be reduced if the consultation requires review by colleagues. In a prospective review of nonurgent consultation requests, Chao et al. (1993) used a committee of two faculty and two residents to review 930 nonurgent consultation requests during a 3-month period. Alternative management was recommended in 28 per cent of cases, resulting in a decline of nonurgent consultations from 4.3 to 3.2 per cent. There were 71 urgent referrals that bypassed the committee and 166 nonurgent referrals that were reviewed. In a similar but retrospective study, Lawler and associates (1990) found that half of all referrals were elective; the specialties receiving the highest proportion of urgent or mandatory referrals were ophthalmology and cardiology.

Family physicians see problems at their early, undifferentiated stage, when it is most difficult to make an accurate diagnosis. The ability to make a diagnosis at this stage comes from experience and depends on a high index of suspicion when key elements of a serious problem are present or suspected. The family physician's ability to make a diagnosis at this early stage is based on prior knowledge of the patient, previous care-seeking behavior of the patient (stoic or frequent complainer), the social situation, and risks based on family history and personal habits. Lawler et al. (1990) evaluated elective versus mandatory referrals in a rural family practice clinic. They found that half of all family practice referrals could be considered elective, and that a large number of referrals were made to assist in making or confirming the diagnosis when the disease was ill defined.

It has been assumed that physicians request a consultation when they are uncertain of the diagnosis or less competent in a particular clinical area. Calman et al. (1992) found just the opposite, that the greater a physician's knowledge in a clinical area, the more he or she consults with specialists in that field. The consultation rate was highest when the referring physician was certain of the diagnosis. They propose that those not referring may have missed the diagnosis and not realized a referral was necessary.

WHEN TO REFER

Dixon (1976) listed five reasons for referral: (1) diagnosis, (2) management, (3) diagnosis and management, (4) patient request, and (5) reinforcement or confirmation of a diagnosis or plan of management. Factors that influence a physician's decision to obtain a consultation or refer include: potential cost to the patient, convenience to the patient, patient request for or expectation of referral, physician loss of income or self-esteem (admitting failure), quality of available consultants, and physician satisfaction with previous referrals.

It is wise to ask for a consultation whenever the patient or family expresses doubt or shows lack of confidence in the diagnosis or management. It is sometimes wise to obtain a second opinion for patients who have a life-threatening illness or a disease with a poor prognosis.

Consultation also should be considered when the family physician is dissatisfied with the patient's progress or is unsure of the diagnosis. Sometimes an agency or special unit has a capability of providing better service, such as in drug detoxification. One rarely gets in trouble asking for help with a difficult problem, but every experienced physician can remember at least one case in which a consultation should have been obtained. A consultation should be initiated promptly any time the patient or family requests or hints that they would like to have one. The physician must be alert to subtle clues of doubt indicating the desire for another opinion. If these clues are recognized and acted on, confidence in the family physician increases. If not recognized, patient dissatisfaction leading to malpractice litigation may result. When doubt is recognized, the patient or family member should be encouraged to discuss this openly; consultation is then often unnecessary.

An early consultation is much less likely to damage patient confidence than a delayed one. The confident and secure physician who considers patient welfare to be of the utmost importance is not threatened and freely utilizes consultants at the appropriate, sometimes early, stage of a problem, before it has progressed to serious proportions that are more difficult to manage.

The patient's family is more apt to display doubt regarding the management of a case than is the patient. The physician who communicates easily with members of the family and is aware of their feelings will detect this insecurity earlier than the physician who is familiar only with the patient. The patient is less likely than other family members to express doubt regarding a diagnosis or method of management for fear of offending the physician. Whenever doubt is noted among the family members, the physician should suggest that the opinion of another physician be obtained.

RESPONSIBILITIES OF THE REFERRING PHYSICIAN

The consultation process involves approximately 12 decision points, beginning with the family physician's decision to refer and concluding with the family physician's providing feedback to the consultant regarding the eventual outcome (see Table 12–1).

TABLE 12–1. THE CONSULTATION PROCESS

1. The decision is made to refer.
2. Consideration is given to the patient's medical, emotional, cultural, and socioeconomic background.
3. Selection of the appropriate discipline (specialty field).
4. Selection of the appropriate physician in that field.
5. Preparation of both the patient and family for the consultation.
6. Preparation of the consultant.
7. The consultant provides feedback to the patient and family.
8. The consultant provides feedback to the family physician.
9. The family physician evaluates appropriateness of the consultant's recommendations.
10. The family physician facilitates the patient and the family's acceptance of recommendations.
11. The family physician acts on the recommendations or selects another consultant in same or different field.
12. The family physician provides feedback to the consultant regarding eventual outcome.

Modified from Barnett BL Jr, Collins JJ Jr: A new look at the consultation continuum. J Fam Pract 5:665, 1977. Reprinted by permission of Appleton & Lange, Inc.

Selection of the Consultant

The referring physician is responsible for the selection of the proper consultant for a particular patient. The family physician, whose comprehensive training involves a broad range of disciplines, has the insight needed to select the appropriate consultant for a specific problem. Care must be taken to select a consultant who has knowledge and skills appropriate to the patient's need, a personality compatible with that of the patient, availability, competency maintained by frequent use of the required skills, and the ability to work well with the referring physician. Compatibility of personalities is an especially important factor to be considered, if at all possible, when selecting a consultant. A surgeon who alienates the patient, no matter how skilled, will be less effective than one who establishes good rapport and has the patient's confidence and cooperation.

Referrals to a psychiatrist sometimes pose special problems and can be among the most difficult, because the family physician must avoid having the patient interpret the referral as rejection. Some patients resist such a referral, and the family physician also may feel uncomfortable making the suggestion. However, the patient frequently welcomes psychiatric help and may be relieved by the recommendation. In a review of psychiatric problems encountered in hospitalized patients (Steinberg et al., 1980), 50 per cent of the patients for whom psychiatric consultation would have been helpful did not receive it because of physician resistance or failure to recognize the psychiatric problem. In those patients who later received psychiatric care, most of them accepted it well.

Patients are likely to benefit more from a psychiatric referral if they enter into the consultation with a positive frame of mind. Once the need for a psychiatric referral has been determined, the patient should be told the reason in an honest, straightforward manner. Questions about psychosocial problems should be incorporated into the history from the beginning of an illness, because they are a part of every problem, rather than being avoided until organic possibilities have been exhausted, resulting in the interpretation by the patient that "the problem is all in my head."

Psychiatric referrals are also a problem because the referring physician is less likely to receive a letter or report from a psychiatrist than from other consultants. This can be interpreted as the psychiatrist hiding behind patient confidentiality, a suspicion that would appear to be confirmed if no report is received.

A perceptive family physician—through knowledge of the patient's personality, lifestyle, and previous reaction to similar situations—can best select the consultant and clinical setting to which the patient will respond positively. Occasionally, it is necessary for the family physician to emphasize the consultant's excellent technical skills and forewarn the patient of possible personality differences or other idiosyncrasies. Patient and family confidence can play a major role in the effectiveness of that consultant. This confidence will be enhanced if the referring physician shows respect for the consultant's skills and makes the recommendation with enthusiasm.

Adequate Transfer of Information

The referring physician must be sure that the referral contract is understood clearly by the consultant. If the referring physician wants help with a diagnosis but does not say so, the consultant may assume that the request is for help with management, leading to dissatisfaction and unwarranted charges of "patient stealing." The referring physician should state the reason for the consultation request and the action desired so that the consultant knows clearly whether the request is for an opinion only or also involves management.

The most common breakdowns of communication between referring and consulting physicians are the consultation request and the consultant's report. The referring physician must evaluate the problem adequately and transmit all necessary information to the consultant. Complete and accurate background information should avoid unnecessary duplication of diagnostic tests. Adequate transfer of information does not consist of a few notes scribbled on a prescription blank, nor is it proper to provide the consultant only with sketchy details by telephone.

The process of information transfer varies with the nature of the problem. Some are straightforward, as, for example a 67-year-old patient with a intertrochanteric fracture. If there are no medical problems and the patient is a good surgical risk, the transfer report can be brief. Other problems may require a complete summary of the office record, as in the referral of a 9-year-old patient for recurring fever that lasts approximately 1 week every month despite negative laboratory studies.

An outpatient referral is facilitated by using a standard form such as that shown in Figure 12–1. It should be in the mail within 24 hours or, better still, carried by the patient to the consultant, accompanied by a copy of the problem list and other pertinent items from the data base, including recent progress notes, laboratory reports, and x-ray films. The problem-oriented medical record is ideally suited to this, because it summarizes all major disorders affecting the individual and alerts the consultant to other past and potentially significant complications that should be considered in the management of the patient's current situation. An extensive referral note is not needed when adequate information is provided by the medical record.

BAYLOR FAMILY PRACTICE CENTER
5510 Greenbriar
Houston, Texas 77005
(713) 798-7700

DATE: _____

TO: _____

FROM: _____

PLEASE SEE: _____

REGARDING: _____

_____

_____

_____

_____
BAYLOR FAMILY PRACTICE DOCTOR'S SIGNATURE

INITIAL RESULTS OF CONSULTATION: _____

_____

_____

_____

_____

_____
CONSULTANT'S SIGNATURE

PLEASE SEND A NARRATIVE WITH FINAL REPORT.

FIGURE 12–1. Standard physician referral form. (Used with permission from Baylor College of Medicine, Department of Family Medicine, Houston, TX.)

Family physicians often complain that they do not receive reports from consultants, and consultants often complain that they do not receive adequate information from the referring physician. The two are probably related, with the quality of the consultant's report depending on the adequacy of information supplied by the referring physician. Patient satisfaction with the consultant also may depend on the quality of this communication between physicians. Williams and Peet (1994) found that both the referring and consulting physicians prefer an initial verbal communication that is followed by a written report. They confirm the need for referring physicians to improve the quality of information provided consultants. The fax is facilitating this process. The referring physician can send records to the consultant and receive a report almost immediately if the system is used properly.

Patient Preparation and Compliance

Ten to 20 per cent of all patients never keep the appointment with the consultant. Patient compliance may be improved if the patient feels more involved in the referral process. First, the referring physician should inform the patient adequately regarding the need for referral and ensure his or her understanding and cooperation. (The consent is particularly important if the patient is hospitalized, because almost half of the complaints to medical society grievance committees stem from patients receiving bills for hospital consultations that they had not authorized.) The informed patient understands what will occur and that the family physician will remain in charge or will resume responsibility at the conclusion of the referral. This understanding is important if the patient is to avoid feeling rejected or "sent away."

It is also likely that compliance will be increased if the patient is given some choice of consultants and control over the time of appointment. When the family physician recommends a consultation, the patient should be asked if a specific consultant is preferred. If not, then three qualified individuals should be suggested, with the positive features of each being identified. If the patient does not indicate a preference, then the family physician should make the final decision. Hines and Curry (1978) encourage the patient to review the referral form and accompanying materials when carrying them to the consultant. They believe this increases patient insight and cooperation, reducing "no shows" in the consultant's office.

Details about the appointment with the consultant may be difficult for the patient to remember, so providing a written note containing the consultant's name, address, and telephone number is helpful. It also may help to include directions to the consultant's office and to discuss with the patient what to expect during the visit, especially the amount of time it will take.

Contrary to previous belief, Lloyd and associates (1993) found that patient compliance with referrals was not related to the nature, severity, or duration of the problem or to the patient's perception of the need for referral. They did find, however, that patients were less likely to follow through with the referral if they had been unable to discuss their problem adequately with their family physician, emphasizing the need to address all of the patient's worries and concerns thoroughly before referring them to another physician.

Evaluation of Information

It is the family physician's responsibility to continue to interact with the physician to whom the patient is referred and to lend assistance in the management of the case to the degree that is necessary for the best care of the patient. Even referrals that are for specific surgical procedures require that the family physician remain involved to manage concomitant medical problems, especially if they require cooperation from other family members. Carson (1982) found that only 7.8 per cent of referrals were for the purpose of establishing a diagnosis. As in other studies, most referrals were

for specific procedures, in this study to orthopedists, obstetricians, general surgeons, and dermatologists. Even when the consultation involves surgical or other technical skills, the family physician is responsible for ensuring that other aspects of the patient's medical background are not ignored and that the family is kept adequately informed.

Newly discovered information must be coordinated with that already recorded. When information is received from the consultant, the family physician must evaluate it within the context of the individual patient and the patient's family situation, work environment, expectations, and ability to comply. The family physician also should guide the consultant in the amount of information that should be given the patient and family, being aware of how much information the family can tolerate and how it should be provided in order to enlist maximum support. Continued involvement of the family physician improves compliance with the treatment program and facilitates long-term rehabilitation.

Feedback to Consultants

It may be of value to keep a log of all referrals. Such a log, containing the patient's name, name of consultant, and date of referral, then could be checked when the report is returned to ensure that the patient actually sees the consultant and that a report is obtained. It also would help identify consultants who do not return information on patients. The log could be reviewed weekly and the consultant or patient contacted if no information is received after a specified time.

Family physicians should give feedback to the consultant regarding the outcome of an unusual case, and not leave the consultant wondering whether the diagnosis was correct or the treatment successful. This is an especially appropriate courtesy if the consultant was prompt in reporting and in returning the patient. If the consultant has not provided information of value in managing the patient, then a second consultation should be considered seriously. Clarfield (1980) found that referring physicians believed that one third of the time (31 per cent of consultations) they had learned nothing of value from the referral. It is also important to let the consultant know if the consultation was inadequate. Experienced family physicians can help young consultants improve their "art of consultation" and should accept this as a responsibility, because consultants rarely are taught this skill during residency training. Bates (1979) believes that "nothing better expresses the ideal fraternity of medicine than an older family doctor helping a young specialist with professional relationships" (p. 177).

Suspecting that faulty consultation practices may be learned during residency training, McPhee and colleagues (1984) studied the communication between 27 general internists at a university medical center and their subspecialty colleagues who practiced in the same building in San Francisco. Even in this close academic setting, where the referral rate was 9.4 per cent, the referring physician did not receive a report 45 per cent of the time. The poorest responding consultants were ophthalmology (no response 69 per cent of the time), obstetrics and gynecology (61 per cent), orthopedics (57 per cent), and dermatology (52 per cent). A response was most likely to be received if the referring physician personally contacted the consultant and if the patient had a return appointment.

RESPONSIBILITIES OF THE CONSULTANT

The consultant is expected to provide a prompt and concise report to the referring physician. The specific questions posed on the consultation request should be addressed and action limited to the amount of involvement requested. When the consultation involves a hospitalized patient, the consultant should see the patient promptly, should provide an opinion and give therapeutic suggestions in a concise note on the consultation sheet, and, in general, should not write orders unless requested to do so by the referring physician.

The consultant has a responsibility to the patient and the referring physician to avoid unnecessary expense through duplication of studies recently obtained by the primary physician, unless there is good reason to doubt the results or there is sufficient need to repeat the test. Of course, the referring physician must have included the actual radiographs and adequate laboratory data as part of the referral document if such duplication is to be avoided. Adequate communication via the consultation request is essential, so that the consultant is made aware of the tests that already have been performed, the methods used, and the results obtained. The consultant's obligation is to build on this information, repeating procedures only when necessary to verify an abnormality or evaluate a change.

When a patient is referred for care, the consultant should remain in contact with the referring physician throughout the period of care and return the patient with a full written report when the problem is resolved or when no further involvement by the consultant is warranted.

A consultant should not refer patients to other consultants without the knowledge and consent of the primary physician, who should be coordinating or at least closely involved with this process. When the consultant is trying to decide whether the referring physician is capable of resuming care of the patient, the wisest course may be simply to ask rather than run the risk of underestimating or over-

estimating the family physician's level of competency or desire to resume care at that point.

The most common reason for discontinuing referrals to a particular consultant is failure to receive adequate reports or failure of the consultant to return the patient for continuing care. The latter occurs most frequently when physicians who also function as primary physicians are used as consultants. The patient may "stay on" for continuing care if the consultant does not encourage his or her return to the referring physician. Even though a specific request was made for follow-up information, Cummins and associates (1980) received a report from the consultant only 62 per cent of the time. Seventy-eight per cent of consultants who were in private practice responded, but only 59 per cent of those in university clinics did so. It was disappointing to note that the follow-up information was not better for patients who required continuing care by the family physician than for those with self-limiting problems. Even though one university stressed to its staff the importance of providing such follow-up information, the faculty did so only 75 per cent of the time. It is distressing for the family physician who is responsible for continuing care of the patient to have the patient return after being hospitalized at a university center with no information having been sent regarding the treatment given or plans for follow-up. It is even more embarrassing to learn from a family member that a patient who recently was referred to a nearby medical center has died.

Curry and associates (1980) found that enclosing a return mailer with the consultation request (including a stamped, self-addressed envelope and a form specifically requesting feedback from the consultant) increased the percentage of consultant feedback from 39 per cent to 60 per cent and also increased the speed of the reply. These rates were significantly higher if the lack of reply from Veterans Administration Hospitals was excluded. Even with the higher response rate, it is unfortunate that 40 per cent of the referrals resulted in no report to the referring physician. Another method that may improve the response rate is to use a two-part pressure-sensitive form, the top half of which includes the referring physician's information. The bottom half then is available for the consultant's report (Fig. 12–1).

Providing appropriate feedback to both patient and referring physician is a talent possessed by too few referral centers. The Mayo Clinic has an excellent reputation for providing good feedback to the referring physician. The Clinic also has a talent for maintaining or bolstering patients' respect for their family physician. Bates (1979) noted that

the top notch consultant will render a report that informs without patronizing, educates without lecturing, directs without ordering and—sometimes most difficult of all—solves the problem without making the referring physician appear to be stupid. The real stars in this play are the consultants who discuss the differential diagnosis in such a way that they make a good case for the referring physician's previous diagnosis even when it was wrong (p. 178).

Although most consultation requests instruct the consultant to proceed with diagnosis and treatment of a problem, this should not be assumed unless specifically indicated. Tumulty (1973) outlined the basic code of ethics for a consultant as follows:

After completing his examination, the consultant should simply state to the patient and to his family that he will thoroughly discuss the problem with the responsible physician . . . Under no circumstances at this time should a consultant give to a patient or his family any information of a specific nature relating to diagnosis, treatment, or prognosis unless he is directly requested to do so by the primary physician (pp. 45–46).

The consultant's opinion should be weighed by the referring physician and the appropriate action taken, depending on the conclusions reached. The family physician already may have considered many of the recommendations the consultant makes but discarded them based on factors that may be unknown to the consultant.

Shortell and Anderson (1971) described the rewards for both referring physician and consultant when their exchange is effective. For the referring physician, it is a positive and rewarding experience, knowing the patient has received proper treatment. It will be a negative experience if the patient does not return or is disappointed with the consultant. The consultant will be flattered at being chosen as an expert and will enjoy receiving a well-prepared, cooperative patient. This could change to a negative feeling if the consultant receives an unpleasant, problem patient because the family physician does not want to be "bothered" any longer (i.e., the "dumping syndrome"), or if the consultant is called on to treat patients without having been provided adequate background information.

REFERRAL RATES

Rates of referral by family physicians in the United States and Canada average 3.5 per cent, with a range of 1.0 to 5.4 per cent, as shown in Table 12–2. Referral rates are greater for women than men and are highest in 15- to 44-year-old individuals (Mayer, 1982). The National Ambulatory Medical Care Survey (unpublished data, National Center for Health Statistics, 1985) noted a 4.2 per cent consultation rate in general and family practice. Lawler found a referral rate of only 1.31 per cent among second- and third-year family practice residents. Second-year residents had lower referral rates than third-year residents, supposedly because of differences in case mix and a lack of referral experience by second-year residents (Lawler, 1987).

The largest study of outpatient consultation rates by family physicians has been conducted by Crump and Massengill (1988) at the University of Alabama in Huntsville. This was a 9-year study involving 177,838 patient visits to 143 residents and 18 faculty members. The overall consultation rate was 1.4 per cent: little year-to-year variation was noted (range 1.1 to 1.6 per cent). Most of the referrals were to specialists in otolaryngology and orthopedics, followed by obstetrics and gynecology, general surgery, neurology, and urology.

In pediatrics and internal medicine, the two other primary care specialties, referral rates are somewhat higher. Internal medicine has a referral rate of 2.2 to 18.2 per cent, and pediatrics a range of 1.0 to 9.5 per cent (Penchansky, 1970); however, the referral process in these specialties has not been studied in as much detail. It appears that this difference in rates can be explained by the less comprehensive nature of internists' and pediatricians' practices and their need for assistance in fields peripheral to areas of major emphasis in training. As noted in Table 12–3, most referrals are to a surgical specialty for a diagnostic procedure or specific therapy.

Ruane (1979) reviewed 108 consecutive referrals in a family practice and found a 1.5 per cent referral rate. He noted that, "The well trained family physician provides definitive care for the vast majority (in this study 98.5 percent) of patient encounters, contrary to the cherished beliefs of many medical school faculty" (p. 1040). Twenty per cent of the referrals were for the specific treatment of clearcut problems (usually surgery). Sixty-four per cent were for diagnostic tests not available to the primary care physician, such as allergy testing or arthrography. One family physician in his third year of practice found that less than one half of 1 per cent of patients were referred to a tertiary care center, and these referrals were usually for the management of uncommon problems such as leukemia, sepsis, bone tumor, or cardiac bypass rather than for diagnosis (Schmidt, 1977). Dixon (1976) studied a small rural community in Ontario (referral rate of 3.3 per cent) and found that referrals were primarily to specialists in general surgery, orthopedics, and obstetrics for specific surgical procedures such as appendectomy, cholecystectomy, and cesarean section.

Consultations in a rural practice have been documented according to the International Classification of Health Problems in Primary Care (Glenn et al., 1983). By far the most frequent problems requiring consultation involved the nervous system and sense organs. More than 86 per cent of these problems were referred to specialists in neurology, ophthalmology, or otolaryngology. The second most common problems that needed referral were those associated with the genitourinary system, requiring consultation from a urologist or gynecologist. Data of this type may assist residency

TABLE 12–2. RATES OF REFERRAL BY FAMILY PHYSICIANS FOR THE UNITED STATES, CANADA, AND EUROPE

Investigators	Location	Number of Patients	Referral Rate (%)
United States			
Calman et al. (1992)	New York	35,218	2.5
Chao et al. (1993)	Ohio	37,174	2.5 urgent,
			3.2 nonurgent
Crump and Massengill (1988)	Alabama	177,838	1.4
Dolezal et al. (1980)	South Dakota	15,609	1.0
Geyman et al. (1976)	California	6,409	1.6
Glenn et al. (1983)	Missouri	30,131	1.7
Hansen et al. (1982)	North Carolina	6,579	2.1
Mayer (1982)	Minnesota	12,228	3.9
Metcalfe and Sischy (1973)	New York	4,604	2.2
Moscovice et al. (1979)	Washington	6,586	2.4
Ruane (1979)	Vermont	7,220	1.5
Schmidt (1977)	Massachusetts	5,814	3.0
White (1984)	Illinois	3,975	3.0
			Average: 2.3
Canada			
Brock (1977)	Ontario (London)	8,616	5.4
Dixon (1976)	Ontario (Rainy River)	6,584	3.3
Hines and Curry (1978)	Ontario (Toronto)	35,351	5.3
			Average: 4.6
Europe*			
	United Kingdom	11,827	4.7
	Belgium	1,190	3.8
	Denmark	1,532	6.4
	France	396	2.4
	German Democratic Republic	688	4.1
	Federal Republic of Germany	2,077	5.5
	Hungary	2,196	3.5
	Republic of Ireland	528	4.2
	Italy	6,146	6.6
	Netherlands	1,566	4.4
	Norway	913	8.1
	Portugal	3,243	5.6
	Spain	6,943	5.5
	Switzerland	1,096	3.8
	Yugoslavia	3,384	6.4
			Average 5.0

* All data from "European study of referrals" (1992).

TABLE 12–3. SPECIALTIES MOST FREQUENTLY CONSULTED BY FAMILY PHYSICIANS IN THE UNITED STATES*

General surgery
Orthopedics
Obstetrics/gynecology
Otolaryngology
Ophthalmology
Urology
Neurology
Dermatology
Cardiology
Psychiatry

* In decreasing order of frequency. Compiled from 12 studies: Calman et al. (1992), Chao et al. (1993), Crump and Massengill (1988), Dolezal et al. (1980), Geyman et al. (1976), Glenn et al. (1983), Hansen et al. (1982), Mayer (1982), Metcalfe and Sischy (1973), Moscovice et al. (1979), Ruane (1979), and White (1984).

directors in emphasizing those areas during graduate training, although most referrals will continue to be for specific subspecialty procedures.

When referral rates for fee-for-service patients were compared with those for members of a health maintenance organization (HMO) in Minnesota (Mayer, 1982), the fee-for-service patients had a lower referral rate (3.19 per cent) than the HMO patients (4.46 per cent). Although the percentages of referral differed, the rank order of specialties to which patients were referred was remarkably similar and matched the referral specialties most commonly noted in other studies (see Table 12–3).

Referral rates in Europe are similar to those in North America. A study was conducted among 15 European countries to define and compare national referral patterns. Over 1500 general practitioners documented 44,134 referrals. The United Kingdom had the largest data set, with 407 participating physicians referring 4.7 per cent of their patients to, in order of frequency, general surgery, gynecology, orthopedics, otolaryngology, obstetrics, and ophthalmology specialists. The study also looked at the percentage of referrals in each country that were thought to be influenced (requested) by the patient, and the delay between specialist appointment and the first communication received by the referring physician. Reports were received within 2 weeks of the specialist appointment in 78 per cent of the referrals ("European study of referrals," 1992).

What is not clear is whether a low rate of referral indicates that the physician is competent and requires assistance infrequently or that the physician is incompetent and does not recognize problems that require referral. Other factors may play a role as well; the practice may consist mostly of healthy young adults, or consultants may not be available and referral may be difficult.

PHYSICIAN SELF-REFERRAL

Physicians have come under considerable criticism when suspected of referring patients to colleagues or laboratories in which they have an interest or from which they derive some financial benefit as a result of the referral. The most common types of self-referral are those to laboratories or medical equipment suppliers in which the physician has a significant investment. Professional "kickbacks," in which the physician is paid for referring a patient, long have been unethical. Receiving or paying a kickback for referring a Medicare patient is now a felony in the United States. Although few physicians would refer a patient to a poor-quality physician or laboratory purely because of a financial kickback, it is also clear that "anyone's judgement can be subtly influenced by financial interests" (Stark, 1989, p. 146). Any time a physician referral is thought to be in the physician's best interest rather than the patient's, the profession of medicine is at risk of losing its valued place in society. Physicians must avoid any referral that involves personal gain because this practice runs the risk of influencing decisions and affecting patient care.

THE TEACHER–PUPIL RELATIONSHIP

The consultation process works best when two physicians work together as colleagues to solve a difficult patient problem. The process is usually a learning opportunity for the referring physician, so it is easy for the consultant to assume the role of teacher and the referring physician the role of pupil. However, the process is not a superior–inferior or teacher–pupil relationship but rather two skilled physicians working together. The consult-

ant has the responsibility to confirm the findings of the referring physician if no new information is detected. The consultant should not enter into a series of exotic tests merely because it is thought to be "expected" or because of fear that his or her prestige as a consultant will be jeopardized. The family physician may have requested another opinion primarily to confirm the diagnosis, perhaps wishing to obtain reassurance before telling the patient he or she has a permanent and incurable disease state.

If the referring physician places the consultant in the role of "teacher," the consultant may feel obliged to make comments or recommendations that may not be necessary. The "pupil" likewise feels obliged to follow these recommendations. If the consultant's report is superficial, the referring physician is obliged to take only those actions that he or she feels are in the best interest of the patient. The family physician should accept full responsibility for interpreting and using the opinions of the consultant, in a manner similar to the evaluation of laboratory test results. The referring physician is as free to ignore the consultant's advice as to solicit it in the first place.

Balint (1964) believes that this teacher–pupil relationship interferes with patient care if the family physician is dissatisfied with the consultant's report but follows the advice solely out of respect for the consultant as the "expert." The consultant may have formed an opinion based on insufficient information or without total knowledge of the patient's emotional and medical background; or it may have been generated, or even manufactured, as a result of having little additional information to offer. A good consultant will admit when he or she has nothing further that needs to be done and will not pursue unnecessary additional testing.

The consultation process is more successful when there is a personal interchange between two physicians rather than when communication is solely by letter. When the referring physician responds only to recommendations made in a report, without the opportunity to discuss them with the consultant, inappropriate assumptions may be made. The more personal the interchange that occurs between the two physicians, the more effective will be the consultation.

COLLUSION OF ANONYMITY

A "collusion of anonymity" exists when neither the referring physician nor the consultant accepts responsibility for the patient (Balint, 1964). Inappropriate decisions regarding patient care can be made when neither physician accepts full responsibility. The problem is amplified when the family physician turns to a variety of consultants for advice, yielding to each, with no one person accepting ongoing responsibility for the patient. The consultation process is not a ritual of "passing the buck" but an integral part of the family physician's continuing responsibility for patient care. If the consultant does not provide meaningful or useful information, then additional consultations must be obtained until the problem is resolved satisfactorily. The term "primary physician" implies primary responsibility for the patient, not just physician of first contact.

THE FAMILY PHYSICIAN AS A CONSULTANT

It is unfortunate that too much responsibility for primary care is burdening many subspecialists. Cardiologists who treat acne and general surgeons who remove ingrown toenails are wasting years of specialized training. Referrals to family physicians frequently are made by physicians in the surgical disciplines for the care of families when psychosocial problems are prominent, for geriatric care, for the long-term management of a chronic illness, and for medical emergencies. Pediatricians frequently refer teenagers or young adults who have outgrown their practice.

In a survey of family physicians from five midwestern states, Amundson and Vogt (1989) found that 35 per cent of the respondents received consultations and referrals from other generalist specialists and 28 per cent received them from subspecialists. The most common reason for the referral was that the patient did not have a family physician, but the second most common reason, when the referring physician was another generalist, was for a procedure such as flexible sigmoidoscopy or vasectomy. One of the most common reasons for referral overall was for the family physician to serve as a coordinator of care (i.e., "captain of the ship").

The family physician can be a valuable consultant when comprehensive and continuing health care is in the patient's best interest or there is a need for a physician skilled in coordinating the care of multiple specialists.

REFERENCES

Amundson LH, Vogt HB: The consultant family physician. J Am Board Fam Pract 2:34, 1989.

Balint M: The Doctor, His Patient, and the Illness. London, Sir Isaac Pitman and Sons, 1964.

Bates RC: The two sides of very successful consultation. Med Econ 56(26):172, 1979.

Brock C: Consultation and referral patterns of family physicians. J Fam Pract 4:1129, 1977.

Calman NS, Hyman RB, Licht W: Variability in consultation rates and practitioner level of diagnostic certainty. J Fam Pract 35:31, 1992.

Carson ME: The referral process. Med J Aust 1:180, 1982.

Chao J, Galazka S, Stange K, Fedirko T: A prospective review system of nonurgent consultation requests in a family medicine residency practice. Fam Med 25:570, 1993.

Clarfield AM: A study of all referrals from a family practice unit. Can Fam Physician 26:527, 1980.

Crump WJ, Massengill P: Outpatient consultations from a family practice residency program: Nine year's experience. J Am Board Fam Pract 1:164, 1988.

Cummins RO, Smith RW, Inui TS: Communication failure in primary care: Failure of consultants to provide follow-up information. JAMA 243:1650, 1980.

Curry RW Jr, Crandall LA, Coggins WF: The referral process: A study of one method for improving communication between rural practitioners and consultants. J Fam Pract 10:287, 1980.

Dixon AS: Survey of a rural practice: Rainy River, 1975. Can Fam Physician 22:693, 1976.

Dolezal JM, Amundson LH, Sinning NJ, et al: PriCare and ambulatory referrals. Cont Educ Fam Physician 12:84, 1980.

European study of referrals from primary to secondary care: Report to the Concerted Action Committee of Health Services Research for the European Community (Fleming DM, project leader). Occasional paper 56. London, Royal College of General Practitioners, 1992.

Fry J: Hospital referrals: Must they go up? Changing patterns over 20 years. Lancet 2:148, 1971.

Geyman JP, Brown RC, Rivers K: Referrals in family practice: A comparative study by geographic region and practice setting. J Fam Pract 3:163, 1976.

Glenn JK, Hofmeister RW, Neikirk H, Wright H: Continuity of care in the referral process: An analysis of family physicians' expectations of consultants. J Fam Pract 16:329, 1983.

Hansen JP, Brown SE, Sullivan RJ Jr, Muhlbaier LH: Factors related to an effective referral and consultation process. J Fam Pract 4:651, 1982.

Hines RM, Curry OJ: The consultation process and physician satisfaction: Review of referral patterns in three urban family practice units. Can Med Assoc J 118:1065, 1978.

Horder JP: Physicians and family doctors: A new relationship. J R Coll Gen Pract 27:391, 1977.

Lawler FH: Referral rates of senior family practice residents in an ambulatory care clinic. J Med Educ 62:177, 1987.

Lawler FH, Purvis JR, Glenn JK, et al: Physician referrals from a rural family practice residency clinic: A pilot study. Fam Pract Res J 10:19, 1990.

Lloyd M, Bradford C, Webb S: Non-attendance at outpatient clinics: Is it related to the referral process? Fam Pract 10:111, 1993.

Ludke RL: An examination of the factors that influence patient referral decisions. Med Care 20:782, 1982.

Mayer TR: Family practice referral patterns in a health maintenance organization. J Fam Pract 14:315, 1982.

McPhee SJ, Lo B, Saika GY, Meltzer R: How good is communication between primary care physicians and subspecialty consultants? Arch Intern Med 144:1265, 1984.

Metcalfe DH, Sischy D: Patterns of referral from family practice. N Y State J Med 73:1690, 1973.

Moscovice I, Schwartz CW, Shortell SM: Referral patterns of family physicians in an underserved rural area. J Fam Pract 9:677, 1979.

Nyma KC: Referral patterns in general practice. Aust Fam Physician 2:173, 1973.

Penchansky R, Fox D: Frequency of referral and patient characteristics in group practice. Med Care 8:368, 1970.

Ruane TJ: Consultation and referral in a Vermont family practice: A study of utilization, specialty distribution, and outcome. J Fam Pract 8:1037, 1979.

Saunders RC: Consultation-referral among physicians: Practice and process. J Fam Pract 6:123, 1978.

Schmidt DD: Referral patterns in an individual family practice. J Fam Pract 5:401, 1977.

Shortell SM, Anderson OW: The physician referral process: A theoretical perspective. Health Serv Res 6:39, 1971.

Stark EH: Ethics in patient referrals. Acad Med 64:146, 1989.

Steinberg H, Torem M, Saravey SM: An analysis of physician resistance to psychiatric consultations. Arch Gen Psychiatry 37:1007, 1980.

Stephens GG: The Intellectual Basis of Family Practice. Tucson, AZ, Winter Publishing Company, 1982.

Tumulty PA: The Effective Clinician. Philadelphia, WB Saunders Company, 1973.

White FZ: Referral patterns among family practitioners. Illinois Med J 166(1):31, 1984.

Williams PT, Peet G: Differences in the value of clinical information: Referring physicians versus consulting specialists. J Am Board Fam Pract 7:292, 1994.

CHAPTER 13
COMMUNITY-ORIENTED PRIMARY CARE

PAUL A. NUTTING and LARRY A. GREEN

An unprecedented growth in knowledge and technology dating from the mid-1940s has engulfed the medical profession, producing many miracles of modern medicine but also leading to an unfortunate overemphasis on the biotechnology of health care. By the mid-1960s, this technological revolution had nearly eliminated the practice of primary care, but, fortunately, the pendulum has begun to reverse its swing, aided by the timely development and growth of family medicine. Over its nearly 20 years, family medicine has been uniquely committed to providing primary care to individuals and family units. Compared with other disciplines, family medicine makes no claim to subspecialty care, but rather devotes its energies to practicing, teaching, and developing the knowledge base of primary care, an all-encompassing field that takes patients and their problems as its focus of attention. With the growing strength of family medicine and the sustained momentum for health care reform, primary care slowly is becoming once again the foundation of the U.S. health care system.

As primary care has begun to gain prominence, renewed interest also is being given to community-oriented primary care (COPC). Once considered to be the domain of publicly funded health programs treating underserved populations, the principles of COPC now are being embraced by private practices and other health care delivery organizations as well. *Community-oriented primary care is a modification of the traditional model of primary care in which a primary care practice or program systematically identifies and addresses the health problems of a defined population.* This is accomplished by combining primary care skills and the principles of epidemiology. Although not the prevailing form of primary care in this country, the challenges of COPC increasingly are attracting the interest and attention of primary care physicians, educators, researchers, and health policy experts.

COPC has become part of the vocabulary of primary care only recently, but the underlying concepts have been expressed by primary care advocates in the United States for some time (Geiger, 1967; Haggerty et al., 1975; Sheps, 1978; White et al., 1961). These and other proponents of primary care have stressed the need to harness and direct the technical capability of our health care system toward addressing the health and health care needs of defined populations. Each has argued for a central strategy that marries epidemiology and primary medical care. Sidney Kark first introduced the term "community-oriented primary care" to the primary care literature in describing his work first in South Africa and more recently in Israel (Kark, 1981). He defined COPC as "a strategy whereby elements of primary health care and of community medicine are systematically developed and brought together in a coordinated practice" (p. 12). Donald Madison, writing in a U.S. context, characterized a community-responsive practice as "one which assumes a larger than ordinary share of responsibility for safeguarding the health of a community, and which follows through on this responsibility by taking action beyond the traditional mode of treating the complaints and problems of patients as they approach the practice one-by-one" (Madison and Shenkin, 1978, p. 23). In describing the future of COPC in the United States, Fitzhugh Mullan characterized COPC as "the reunion of the traditions of public health and personal clinical health services" (1982, p. 1077).

The principles of COPC have a long-standing tradition, having provided the philosophical foundation for publically funded health programs for many years (Yach and Tollman, 1993). As one example, community health centers strive to address the health problems of local communities in underserved areas and target primary care services toward medically needy populations. On another front, the Indian Health Service has delivered health care services to American Indians and Alaskan natives since 1955. Over a 40-year period, a comprehensive, integrated primary care program has been developed that operates within and is tailored to the health needs of particular Indian communities. Community involvement has been an integral philosophical underpinning of both the community health centers and the Indian Health Service.

More recently, the mainstream of primary care

has begun to adopt elements of COPC as well. A study from the Institute of Medicine described the implementation of COPC principles in different U.S. primary care settings. The study concluded that although not a prevalent form of primary care practice, the COPC approach offers great promise as a form of primary care that is responsive to the health care needs of defined populations, ranging from geopolitical communities to the enrolled populations of prepaid health plans (Institute of Medicine, 1984a). Seven case studies demonstrated the feasibility of COPC in vastly different health care environments, illustrating the spectrum of COPC expression in settings typical of today's U.S. health care system (Institute of Medicine, 1984b). This is particularly the case with prepaid group practices and other organized systems for health care delivery. With a contractual obligation to a fixed enrollment, health maintenance organizations (HMOs) have economic incentives to respond effectively to the health needs of their enrolled communities.

In recent years, family physicians have begun to shift the focus of medicine from care of unusual problems to the care of common maladies, from the care of specific organ systems to the care of the entire individual, from care limited by artificial boundaries between specialty to problems as they present in the community. This broadened focus offers a rich substrate for the principles of COPC to take root and grow. Although family medicine has no monopoly on COPC, it represents the most promising opportunities for growth because its broad mandate permits a physician to be attentive to the full breadth of the community's problems, such as unplanned pregnancy, child abuse, hypercholesterolemia, somatization, inadequate immunization, and substance abuse. In sum, family medicine offers the best hope for incorporating the central principles of COPC into the mainstream of primary care, and COPC offers a context for the family physician to expand beyond the focus of the examining room to consider systematically the larger population from which patients emerge occasionally for care (Nutting and Garr, 1989).

COMPONENTS OF COPC

The basic elements of COPC are simple: (1) a primary care practice or program, (2) a defined population that the practice wishes to serve, and (3) a process by which the major health problems of the target population are addressed. Given the dramatic variations in the organization and financing of primary care, it is not surprising that the basic elements have been adapted widely to the practice environments of different communities, as demonstrated by the case studies in the Institute of Medicine (1984b) report on COPC. A model of COPC has been proposed that accommodates different expressions of COPC while providing enough

structure to support research, education, and practice (Nutting, 1986). Its components are described in the next sections.

Primary Care Practice or Program

The face of primary care in the United States continues to evolve with rising expectations for primary care. Practices that differ in their organizational structure and methods of financing nonetheless will find that the COPC model is flexible enough to accommodate a vast range of organizational characteristics. The only requirement is that the practice meet the basic characteristics of primary care, namely, that it *offers an array of personal health services that are accessible and acceptable to the patient, comprehensive in scope, and coordinated and continuous over time, and for which the physician is accountable for the quality and potential effects of services.* The primary care component of the model speaks to the services a practice provides, but not to the composition or organization of the physicians, nor the manner by which the costs are reimbursed (directly or indirectly by the patient, patient groups, or third parties).

Community or Target Population

There is a myth that there is an ideal definition of a community. In reality, the target population changes continually and usually requires explicit definition before a particular program can be mounted or a problem assessed. For example, a practice might define its population as all patients seen in the past 2 years. Even this simple population will change as each day removes some patients and adds others. Accepting ongoing changes in this population, such a definition might be relevant to an immunization campaign. By comparison, however, a program to detect early developmental delays would need to focus on a subset of the population. The critical concept is not to define "the" population, but to define a relevant population and accept responsibility at some level for offering a mix of health services that are relevant to its needs and demands.

In some settings, the COPC practice will address "true" communities, those sharing common social, cultural, economic, and political systems. In other cases, the community may consist of less clearly defined, and perhaps less organized, groups such as individuals enrolled in a health plan, occupational or workplace populations, or school populations. Where the community is difficult to define, the practice may choose to limit its focus to its active patient population or, more broadly, to its practice population, the latter consisting of all members of households of active patients.

Involving the community or members of the target population in the COPC process is an important feature of COPC, and one to be encouraged where possible. However, the manner and extent to which it is feasible for the community participants to collaborate in the COPC process will vary widely across different settings, whether they be small fee-for-service practices in rural areas, large urban HMOs, or publicly funded community health centers. Although a fee-for-service suburban practice might appear to be the least conducive to community participation, at least one excellent example has been described (Seifert, 1990).

The range of variation for community participation can be thought of in terms of (1) the organization and mechanisms of input, (2) the level of involvement, and (3) the focus of attention. Of these, the focus of attention is perhaps the most critical. Just as physicians have a tendency to focus their attention on their most active patients (the numerator of the practice), the community participants also often develop a "numerator bias." For example, the consumer boards of federally funded community health centers frequently focus on administrative issues surrounding the daily operation of the health facility. When attention is broadened to the "denominator" population, community involvement can add a distinctly new, and vitally important, dimension to the identification of community health problems. For example, group consensus techniques can enhance the involvement of consumers and physicians in setting priorities among competing health needs and in allocating constrained resources among competing health programs (Horowitz and Gallagher, 1990). The critical role for the patient and community participants is to develop a "denominator bias" and to represent the interests of the entire target population while participating in the functions of the COPC process.

The COPC Process

The third component of the model is the process by which the major health problems of the community are identified and systematically addressed. This process can be described as a set of activities that fall into four functional categories, and each can be accomplished through a variety of strategies (Nutting, 1990a).

Defining and Characterizing the Community

The tradition of primary care has stressed the importance of understanding the community from which individual patients present for care. The COPC model extends this notion to the denominator group, recommending that the health status of the population be analyzed with the same rigor that the physician uses when approaching the individual patient. The physician needs to know who are the individuals who comprise the denominator population, where they live, how their behavior influences their health, where and when they seek care for ailments, and how they perceive and finance their care.

Many family physicians, through years of practice and observation, will have developed a basic knowledge of their community, based on subjective analysis of information gained from patients and the fact of living and often raising a family in the community. In the absence of a systematic approach to collecting and analyzing data on the community, however, family physicians erroneously may generalize patterns of health and health behavior from their most familiar patients (the numerator) to the target community (the denominator). Most physicians can recall from their training examples of this error made by specialists who assume the importance of some obscure disease that appears commonly in their specialty practice.

In many instances, valuable information on the community can be derived from secondary data obtained from the local health department. Census data and vital statistics also can be useful in the early development of an information base on the community, and clearly are most relevant when drawn from a population that corresponds closely to the target population of the practice.

Identifying the Community Health Problems

The second step follows logically from the first and includes the activities necessary to identify the major health problems of the community, characterize their determinants and correlates, and set priorities among them. Initially, it may be appropriate to identify important problems based on the physician's practice impressions and the perceptions of community members. The use of group process techniques can improve the rigor of these activities (Horowitz and Gallagher, 1990). In addition, information often can be obtained at reasonable expense through secondary data sources (vital statistics, epidemiologic studies).

Community surveys can be helpful and potentially yield important information, but they are expensive and time consuming, and too often the momentum for COPC dissipates during the long process of designing, conducting, and analyzing survey information. It is important to realize that, in the nearly 60 examples of community problems addressed by 26 programs and practices surveyed during the Institute of Medicine (1984a) study, not a single health problem was discovered from primary data collection that was not suspected previously by either the physicians or the community (Nutting et al., 1985).

This is not to suggest that primary data collection may not be important in the COPC process. New data often are needed to clarify the extent and severity of the problem and to develop an intervention that will be successful within that particular population. At the same time, however, when primary data collection is not feasible, practice impressions and secondary data can help delineate health problems that warrant the practice's attention.

Most practices that undertake this process will find a number of important health problems, and some attention will be required to set priorities among them. For the family physician this may require deciding between such disparate problems as teen pregnancy, breast cancer screening, or *Haemophilus influenzae* type B immunization in children.

Modifying Practice Patterns

Once a priority health problem has been identified, the COPC practice should develop an intervention strategy to address the problem better. In practice, these strategies generally fall into two categories. First, the physician can initiate an emphasis program entirely within the practice by modifying practice patterns. In this case, the emphasis program will consist largely of varying the mix and array of services provided, targeting services toward high-risk individuals, and/or changing patterns of accessibility to services. Second, the physician can develop or collaborate in an emphasis program beyond the scope of the practice. In this case the physician may retain the traditional role of the physician or may assume the role of an active citizen. The active COPC physician will be involved simultaneously in emphasis programs that mix both categories.

Most interventions are not intended to blanket all members of the community, nor are they intended to be limited to those individuals who present for or request certain services. Often those individuals who might benefit most from the emphasis program are not active users of the health care system at all. In this case, efforts to target high-risk individuals and mount aggressive outreach activities may be necessary to achieve the desired effect. Even simple interventions may have a dramatic impact when successfully targeted at specific individuals at increased risk (Nutting et al., 1975).

Monitoring Impact of Program Modifications

Of the four COPC functions, this is the one that is most often neglected. Although it is tempting to move to the next health problem, some level of effort should be devoted to assessing the impact of practice modifications. In addition to identifying refinements that may increase the impact of emphasis programs, monitoring practice activities permits elimination of those activities that already may have served their purpose with little or no continuing benefit, thus freeing up energies and resources for program activities with potentially higher impact.

In reality, all programs are evaluated at a subjective level. Practitioners and patients alike form opinions of new programs, and both are often vocal in their views. Where more formal evaluation and primary data collection are needed, the evaluation plan should be simple enough to be implemented realistically, but rigorous enough to provide information that is locally useful in determining the future of the intervention effort under study. The first and most important step in accomplishing this is to state as precisely as possible the evaluation question to be addressed and to frame it in the context of the entire denominator population. Too often emphasis programs are designed to address an important problem within the target population, but evaluation efforts focus only on those individuals who emerge from the community as active users of the practice. Evaluations that are "numerator based" can lead to erroneous judgments of program benefit (Nutting, 1990b).

The simultaneous re-emergence in the 1980s of interest in COPC and practice-based research is probably not accidental (Green and Lutz, 1990; Iverson et al., 1988). Both represent corrective actions to balance the extraordinary success of the modern health science center with its unforeseen adverse consequences. These centers have emphasized the unusual phenomena in medicine, which White et al. (1961) characterized as the smallest box in the ecology of medical care, leaving in relative neglect the common concerns of free-living people in local communities. In response, family practice leaders are recognizing the urgent need to apply with greater vigor the methods of science to phenomena occurring at the primary care level. Of course, all practice-based research is not COPC and the major thrust of COPC is not research; however, they are syntonic in their intent and process, and they both seek to overcome similar selection and observer biases by concentrating attention on a defined population. Because of this common interest, progress in practice-based research is likely to fuel COPC, and the COPC process will, in turn, stimulate critical inquiry into important and neglected problems.

OBSTACLES TO IMPLEMENTING COPC

The development of a COPC practice or program will encounter several difficult problems (Madison, 1983; Rogers, 1982) that will vary with the practice setting. First, for many practices the community may be extremely complex and difficult to define, particularly in urban areas, where the community can be subdivided into neighborhoods, each with a unique ethnic and social structure. Many communities, especially suburban communities, are served by a multitude of practices and health programs, making it difficult for physicians to distinguish their own community from those of other practices. Indeed, many families and individuals do not look to a single practice or program for all of their health care services, instead using multiple physicians.

Most physicians have a limited set of resources at their disposal that can be directed to the COPC activities. It is uncommon to find a primary care practice that has an abundance of financial reserves, staff commitment, or time and energy to be devoted to activities beyond direct patient care. Most practices have only a basic data system, in many cases limited to the hard copy of the medical record. Although many practices are moving into data automation, most computer systems in primary care are devoted to billing and other practice management tasks. Even those practices with well-developed patient care information systems often find that data are limited to their active patients and do not serve well in identifying and characterizing the health problems of the larger target population.

Primary care physicians generally lack specific skills, knowledge, and experience in the principles, strategies, and methods of COPC. This lack is reminiscent of the predicament of medical graduates of two decades ago. On entering a primary care practice, physicians found that they lacked many of the skills necessary to provide care for those common problems that were prevalent in their patient population but rare in the teaching curriculum of the tertiary care centers where they trained. The current dilemma is an extension of the old problem: Although specialty programs are now providing improved training in the care of primary care problems, they are deficient in training physicians to define and respond to health problems within their target population or community. Much has been accomplished through academic departments of community medicine, but regrettable gaps remain between the training for primary care, community medicine, and public health.

There is a relative lack of analytic tools and techniques that are feasible for COPC activities in most primary care settings. Although methods have been well developed in the parent disciplines of demography, epidemiology, anthropology, health services and evaluation research, and biostatistics, they have not been distilled and fitted to the unique needs of the busy primary care setting. To be useful and to support the practice of COPC, tools and techniques must strike a careful balance between the ease and simplicity with which they can be used and the rigor required to alter the health care program confidently. To use a clinical analogy, working diagnoses are made with an information base that could be challenged if submitted for publication in a leading medical journal. Nonetheless, they are quite adequate in the primary care setting, where care is continuous and vigilant enough to detect early changes in health status.

Finally, the most vexing problem facing COPC, and indeed facing all of primary care, is that the current mechanisms of reimbursement do not support, much less encourage, the additional activities of COPC. Many new practice forms are developing in an attempt to gain an edge in the increasingly competitive medical care marketplace; unfortunately, few provide incentives for the additional activities of COPC. Even HMOs do not provide a clear incentive to act prospectively to improve the health of a population that is free to disenroll before the impact of an emphasis program may be realized.

COPC FOR FAMILY PRACTICE

The first obstacle described above can be overcome by virtually any family physician who wishes to define and address a target population consisting of all members of the households of active patients (Nutting and Garr, 1989; Nutting et al., 1991). In caring for patients of all ages, family physicians have a unique opportunity to apply the principles of COPC to a "practice population" that consists of active patients, inactive patients, and household members who have not been patients. Although not a community in a sociopolitical sense, such a practice population represents an excellent opportunity for family physicians to expand their scope of clinical concern beyond the stream of patients that encounter the practice.

An example of how this might be accomplished in a large practice has been described (Nutting et al., 1991). In this practice, registration of each new patient included collecting name, date of birth, and gender *of each member of the household* and entry of these data into the billing system. Data from the billing system could be downloaded subsequently for analysis on a personal computer. Although this practice is not common to all family physician's offices, it is not difficult to accomplish.

With data on all members of the practice population, distinctions can be made among active patients, inactive patients, and nonpatients. In the example, active patients were defined as those making contact with the practice within the previous 24 calendar months. This defined the practice population, which included 1147 members of 559 households, made up of 615 (54%) active patients, 366 (32%) inactive patients, and 166 (14%) nonpatients.

Comparison of the age and gender distributions of the active, inactive, and nonpatients (Fig. 13–1) suggests a preponderance of females of childbearing age and children among the active patient population. Young adult males are common in the inactive patients but dominate the nonpatient population. There also appears to be a relative excess of adolescents among the inactive patients.

The distribution of the practice population by composition of the household is shown in Table 13–1. The most common *household* consists of a single adult under age 50 (42.9%), but most of the *people* in the practice population live in house-

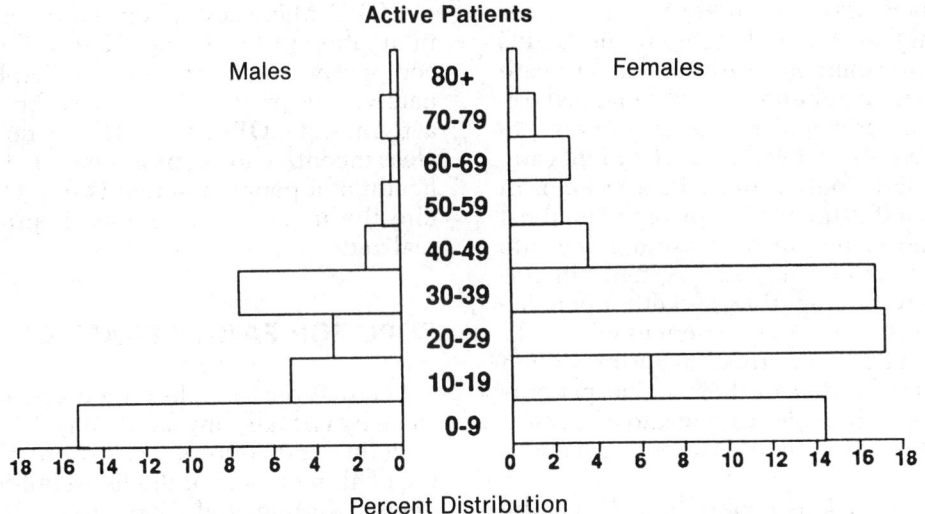

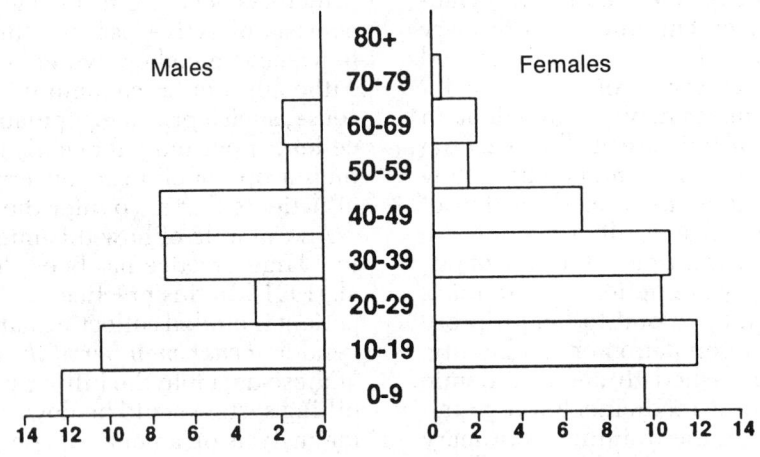

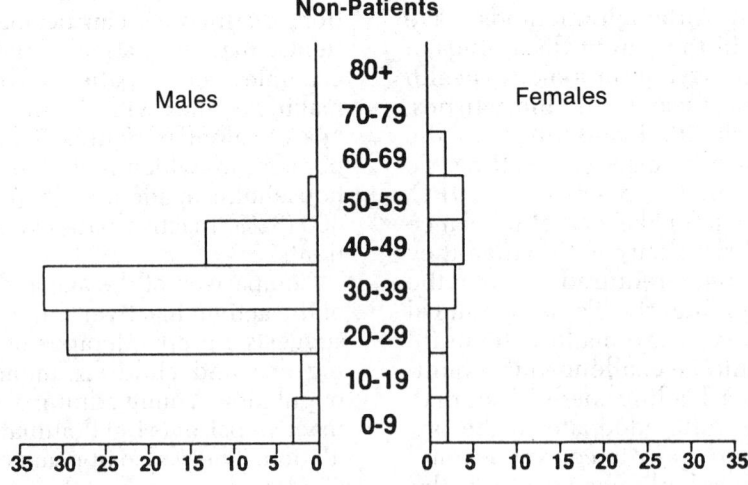

FIGURE 13–1. Age/gender distribution of active, inactive, and nonpatients. (From Nutting PA, Nagle J, Dudley T: Epidemiology and practice management: An example of community-oriented primary care. Fam Med 23: 218, 1991.)

TABLE 13–1. DISTRIBUTION OF PRACTICE POPULATION BY COMPOSITION OF HOUSEHOLD

	Number of Households		Number of Children		Total Number of Individuals	
	N	(%)	N	(%)	N	(%)
Two adults with children	110	(19.6)	265	(58.2)	485	(42.3)
Single adult with children	92	(16.5)	190	(41.8)	282	(24.6)
Two adults with no children						
Over 50 years	17	(3.0)	–	–	34	(3.0)
Under 50 years	6	(1.1)	–	–	12	(1.0)
Single adult with no children						
Over 50 years	94	(16.8)	–	–	94	(8.2)
Under 50 years	240	(42.9)	–	–	240	(20.9)
Totals	559	(99.9)	455	(100)	1147	(100)

holds consisting of two adults with children (42.3%) or a single adult with children (24.6%). This was surprising to all physicians in the practice, who thought that they rarely saw anything resembling a nuclear family.

Prior to planning outreach activities beyond the active patients, two characteristics of the practice population were investigated. *First,* the physicians in the practice were concerned that reaching out to nonactive patients might appear to be aggressive marketing and attempting to "steal" patients from other practices in the area. A survey of active patients provided an estimate of to whom each individual in each household (that is, each individual in the practice population) looked for primary medical care. The results suggest that all the active and inactive patients and over 85% of the nonpatients identified the practice as their primary source of medical care. Although based on a nonrandom sample, these results provided sufficient reassurance that reaching out to this group of nonpatients should not be construed as marketing the patients of other practices in the vicinity. *Second,* the practice managers were concerned that the physicians not reach out to a population that would further increase the already strained financial liability of the practice. Data collected in the survey also suggest that the active patients and nonpatients did not differ markedly by method of payment for services.

Identifying a practice population of all members of the household of active patients of the practice created a potential target population, including substantial numbers of inactive patients and nonpatients. Descriptive analysis suggested that there were a substantial number of individuals not currently active in the practice who were neither patients identified with other practices nor patients differing substantially in their coverage. This practice proceeded to identify a number of health care problems in the practice population that would be amenable to correction by modifying practice patterns and behaviors (Nutting et al., 1991). Knowing the names and addresses of all members of the

practice population, combined with regular contact with at least one member of the household, suggested a number of innovative strategies for efficient outreach.

Creating and describing a practice population provides an opportunity for any family physician to look beyond the stream of patients passing through the examining room one at a time, and to begin applying the principles of COPC to the practice population. Doing so invites physicians to examine their practice population with the kind of awe and wonder that characterizes the best traditions of family practice.

THE ROAD TO SUCCESS: TAKING AN INCREMENTAL APPROACH TO COPC

Clearly, there are significant impediments to implementing a COPC practice, yet it is quite possible to integrate the COPC principles into the practice of primary care in an incremental fashion. To many physicians, the decision to develop a COPC practice is seen as one requiring momentous and largely irreversible changes in the practice or program. Because the COPC literature in the last several years has described relatively well-developed forms of COPC, many physicians perceive a gulf between their current practices and the COPC practice model, which has, in turn, discouraged many potential COPC physicians from taking the first steps. In reality, the transition to a COPC practice involves the addition of only two elements to a primary care practice—a definition of the target population and the development of activities that systematically address the health problems of that population. Both of these additional elements can be approached incrementally and at a pace appropriate to any setting.

Start with a Definable Target Population

Many physicians may find it difficult to address the health problems of their total community. The characteristics of the community may appear overwhelmingly complex, with a bewildering mix of ethnic groups and political factions. In addition, the presence of other primary care programs may complicate efforts to distinguish one practice population from another, and call into question the appropriateness of the physician's assuming responsibility for patients presumably cared for through another practice or program. In such cases, the COPC process might be started by targeting a community consisting of the active patients of the practice, or a "practice community" consisting of the active patients and all members of their households. Similarly, other target populations may be addressed, such as populations defined by location (e.g., school or workplace), by health problem (e.g., hypertension, homeless), by age group (e.g., elderly, infancy), or by risk group (e.g., teenage pregnancy). COPC is an iterative process, and the practice starting with a "bite-sized" subset of the community can expand its scope later.

Start with Simple Tools

Similarly, the process adopted for addressing the community's health problems can vary widely. Each of the four functions can be approached with differing levels of rigor at differing costs and with differing requirements for physician time and energy. At the most basic level, the physician can rely on subjective information gleaned from the practice impressions of professional colleagues and the wealth of information that can be mined from the opinions and experience of individuals from the community. Subjective information of this sort can be obtained at little expense, and the combined wisdom of the health professional and consumers offers a richness of information not often possible with quantitative data alone. Moreover, through collaboration, professional and consumers can approach cooperatively the difficult task of setting priorities among competing health problems.

The use of secondary (or existing) data offers another inexpensive alternative for initiating the COPC functions. Most communities have a wealth of data available, ranging from census data to vital statistics. The appropriateness of secondary data will, of course, vary across settings and largely will be a function of the "fit" between the target population of the practice and the population for which the data were collected. Increasingly, basic socioeconomic data are becoming available by zip code, enabling many practices with a billing system to estimate some population parameters for their active patients.

Starting with simple tools and a definable target population offers the practice ways of moving toward a more mature COPC model, as shown in

LEVELS OF THE TARGET POPULATION

	ACTIVE PATIENTS	PRACTICE COMMUNITY	TOTAL COMMUNITY
STAGE 1: use of subjective information			Teen-age pregnancy
STAGE 2: use of secondary data.		Hypertension	
STAGE 3: use of newly collected and analyzed data	Dysuria in working women		

FIGURE 13–2. An iterative approach to COPC. A practice may address different target populations and do so with methods of differing levels of quantitative rigor.

Figure 13–2. On one dimension, the increasing rigor of the processes of COPC can be described in terms of the scope of input information used. At Stage 1, the practice may be characterizing the community and identifying health problems using the subjective impressions of the physicians and/or patients. At Stage 2, secondary data may be used, while at Stage 3, new data are collected and analyzed to describe the community and its health problems. Along the other dimension, a COPC practice can define its denominator population at three levels. The first is the population of active patients, defined as all individuals who have contacted the practice within the previous 2 years. The next level is the practice community, which includes all members of the household to which active patients belong. Finally, there is the larger population encompassing, for example, school populations, the enrolled members of a health plan, participants in a workplace health program, and/or a geographic community.

Viewed in this context, physicians may locate their current pattern of practice and identify feasible steps toward a more rigorous practice of COPC. Many practices may be operating simultaneously in more than one cell of the matrix. For example, a practice that has a strong quality assurance activity may be engaged in activities at Stage 3 in examining the quality of care provided for dysuria among the working women in the practice. At the same time, the physicians may be concerned about members of the practice community with undiagnosed or untreated hypertension, based on prevalence figures extrapolated from secondary data (Stage 2). Finally, the practice may be collaborating with other community programs to address the problem of unwanted teenage pregnancy based on subjective information within the larger community (Stage 1). If the practice is involved in an HMO or has a contract with a major employer in the community for occupational health services, other denominator populations may be addressed at differing stages of implementation of the COPC process.

While the matrix scheme of Figure 13–2 implies a value associated with higher levels of rigor, COPC activities on either dimension appropriately vary with the issues and should adapt to local resources and requirements. In some settings, the philosophy of the physicians or the needs of the area may argue for defining the denominator population as a social, cultural, or geographic community, whereas other practices or programs may find it more appropriate to address a practice community. Along the other dimension, Stage 3 may represent a high level of development for a given function, but attaining the ideal in a practical world may not always be worth the marginal cost. For example, some programs may be able to extract more information about their community from the diligent use of secondary data than from the use of a sophisticated, but undoubtedly more expensive, data system.

GETTING STARTED

Preparatory Inventory

For physicians interested in incorporating some of the principles of COPC into their practice, a preparatory inventory may be made by reflecting seriously on five questions.

How Committed Am I to Trying COPC?

One's own personal commitment is critical and should be judged objectively and without bias. Initiating a COPC practice requires a great deal of time and personal commitment and requires individual leadership from at least one physician in the practice.

Do I Have Professional Colleagues Who Are Equally Committed?

The commitment of the other professional staff is important. At least one other fellow traveler committed to the principles of COPC can make the journey through largely uncharted terrain less hazardous and more stimulating. Importantly, the division of labor that colleagues within the practice or in other community programs permit may allow more time for alternative pursuits.

Is My Practice or Program on Reasonably Stable Ground, in Terms of Both Financial and Professional Growth?

The costs of initiating COPC activities are largely unknown, and such activities may not generate additional income. The practice that is struggling financially or that is in a period of rapid transition in terms of personnel, physical facilities, or definition of goals may have a full agenda without taking on the challenges of COPC. In contrast, physicians who have established their practice and are looking for further challenge in their professional life may find that moving toward a COPC model is less expensive (and professionally more rewarding) than embarking, for example, on an expensive hobby.

Is There Sufficient Interest and Commitment among the Community or Target Population That I Would Address?

Important allies in the COPC process, often not relied on heavily enough in the early phases of COPC, are the patients and community participants. What constitutes the community and whom the key participants are must be defined early in the process, and will vary greatly among practices. The commitment of the target population and its major participants can be an extremely important resource to recognize and incorporate at the time of the initial decision to implement COPC.

Do I Have Access to a Reasonable Amount of Data on the Target Population?

Depending on how the target community is defined, there may or may not be a great deal of data available, a difference that can be critical in the early stages of defining and characterizing the community and identifying its major health problems. For practices that plan to start with the active patient population, it is helpful (but certainly not necessary) to have an operational data system within the practice. For those planning to address a geographic community, a few hours spent with an epidemiologist at the local health department can provide an important reconnaissance of the available data and a reasonable assessment of the additional effort that will be required in the early COPC activities.

Suggestions for Program Development

If the initial inventory of resources affirms moving toward the COPC model, the following suggestions may be useful.

1. *Define your community in a manageable way.* Starting with the active patients of your practice or with the households of your active patients may be a more than adequate initial challenge. An expansion of the definition of the community will be relatively easy downstream.

2. *Develop allies for the COPC effort, within your practice or program, within the community you plan to address, and wherever possible among other practices and/or community programs.* Developing allies means gaining partners, an important asset even at the price of possible modification

in initial goals or timetables. Remember, however, that the practice of COPC is a continuing journey. Partners are important and usually well worth the inconvenience of altering the initial travel plan.

3. *Take your time and don't rush—maintain modest and achievable expectations.* Although difficult to appreciate at the beginning, many of the early successes will appear small but will be viewed later as the most critical in the history of your efforts. Plan them carefully and enjoy accomplishing them well. Subsequent progress (and success) will build on these initial efforts.

4. *Plan for initial success.* Nothing reinforces commitment and generates new allies like an initial success. Taking on the most critical (and often the most vexing) health problem of the community at the outset is risky. A good strategy is to direct initial efforts at a visible problem for which there is considerable enthusiasm, but particularly one for which a positive impact is achievable in a relatively short period of time and will be apparent when achieved. Attempting to reduce cardiac mortality, for example, through a community-based blood pressure control program is a frequently selected COPC emphasis program. It also may be an unsatisfactory problem *for the initial* effort, however, because success, even if achieved, will occur far in the future and may be modest relative to the community's total cardiac mortality. Long before the data show that the initial efforts had an important impact, you and your allies may have moved on.

5. *Maintain a healthy perspective.* You are among the first to discover and explore the territory of COPC. There is not a great deal known of how to accomplish COPC in your setting. You will rapidly become an expert. Document your experiences and share them with others, because you are helping to develop the field.

CONCLUSIONS

Community-oriented primary care remains an unrealized innovation in the delivery of primary care services. It has the potential to improve the quality of care and the health status of a defined population. For the practitioner so inclined, COPC offers the rewards of expanding one's health care activities beyond the confines of the examining room. Yet, there remains a general malaise among physicians and a remarkable lack of recognition by key decision makers concerning the great potential of COPC. There are few organizational supports for a practice inclined to pursue a better understanding of a community and its problems, and appropriate investigative tools applicable to practice settings are sometimes lacking. Other than the fees for services that may be incidentally billable as part of customary care, there are virtually no financial incentives for physicians to adopt COPC. However, reform of health care delivery systems, medical education, and clinical research may offer, in various settings, unprecedented opportunities to practice and understand community-oriented primary care. If so, the principles of COPC and the capacities of practice-based research are available, and further progress is critical and indicated. Advancements depend in part on physicians being able to recognize the inadequacy of the biomedical model alone and to accept the challenge to enrich it with the methods and fruits of COPC and practice-based research. If these opportunities are ignored, the interface between people and their personal physicians indeed will remain ill-defined and poorly understood, and many important concerns of our communities will remain neglected. If realized, patients in their communities should get the care they need rather than what we simply have to offer, and the care they get should be more demonstrably effective, and ultimately more personally satisfying.

REFERENCES

Geiger HJ: The neighborhood health center. Arch Environ Health 14:912, 1967.

Green LA, Lutz LJ: Notions about networks: Primary care practices in pursuit of improved primary care. *In* Mayfield J, Grady ML (eds): Primary Care Research: An Agenda for the 90s. Rockville, MD, Agency for Health Care Policy and Research, 1990, pp 125–132.

Haggerty RJ, Roghmann KJ, Pless IB: Child Health and the Community. New York, John Wiley & Sons, 1975.

Horowitz C, Gallagher KM: Group process techniques for COPC practice. *In* Nutting PA (ed): Community-Oriented Primary Care: From Principle to Practice. Albuquerque, University of New Mexico Press, 1990, pp 174–178.

Institute of Medicine: Community-Oriented Primary Care: A Practical Assessment, Vol. I: The Committee Report. Washington, DC, National Academy Press, 1984a.

Institute of Medicine: Community-Oriented Primary Care: A Practical Assessment, Vol. II: The Case Studies. Washington, DC, National Academy Press, 1984b.

Iverson DC, Calonge BN, Miller RS, et al: The development and management of a primary care research network, 1978–87. Fam Med 20:177, 1988.

Kark SL: Community-Oriented Primary Health Care. New York, Appleton-Century-Crofts, 1981.

Madison DL: The case for community-oriented primary care. JAMA 249:1279, 1983.

Madison DL, Shenkin BN: Leadership for Community-Responsive Practice. Chapel Hill, NC, The Rural Practice Project, 1978.

Mullan F: Community-oriented primary care: An agenda for the '80s. N Engl J Med 307:1076, 1982.

Nutting PA: Community-oriented primary care: An integrated model for practice, research, and education. Am J Prev Med 2:140, 1986.

Nutting PA (ed): Community-Oriented Primary Care: From Principle to Practice. Albuquerque, University of New Mexico Press, 1990a.

Nutting PA: The evaluation function in COPC: Quality assurance for the community. *In* Nutting PA (ed): Community-Oriented Primary Care: From Principle to Practice. Albuquerque, University of New Mexico Press, 1990b, pp 344–351.

Nutting PA, Garr DR: Community-Oriented Primary Care (Monograph 124). Kansas City, MO, American Academy of Family Physicians, 1989.

Nutting PA, Nagle J, Dudley T: Epidemiology and practice management: An example of community-oriented primary care. Fam Med 23:218, 1991.

Nutting PA, Strotz C, Shorr GI: Reduction of gastroenteritis morbidity in high risk infants. Pediatrics 55:354, 1975.

Nutting PA, Wood M, Conner EM: Community-oriented primary care in the United States. JAMA 253:1763, 1985.

Rogers DE: Community-oriented primary care. JAMA 248:1622, 1982.

Seifert MH: An incremental patient participation model. In Nutting PA (ed): Community-Oriented Primary Care: From Principle to Practice. Albuquerque, University of New Mexico Press, 1990, pp 379–383.

Sheps CG: Primary care—the problem and the prospect. Ann NY Acad Sci 310:265, 1978.

White KL, Williams TF, Greenburg BG: The ecology of medical care. N Engl J Med 265:885, 1961.

Yach D, Tollman SM: Public health initiatives in South Africa in the 1940s and 1950s: Lessons for a post-apartheid era. Am J Public Health 83:1043, 1993.

CHAPTER 14

ASSESSMENT OF FUNCTIONAL HEALTH STATUS

PATRICK J. O'CONNOR and SYDNEY H. CROOG

The maintenance and improvement of patients' functional status is often one of the fundamental goals of the family physician (Parkerson et al., 1993). In order to do this effectively, the physician must have a practical and accurate method of screening and assessing function. At present, many methods of screening and assessing patients' functional status are available, including the physician's traditional approach of questions and observations as well as standardized scales and measures that have been developed recently.

In primary care office practice, however, the presence of functional impairment in many patients, as well as marked time constraints, creates a persisting clinical dilemma. How can the busy physician accurately detect significant functional impairment in a routine office visit that necessarily may be very brief?

The need for functional assessment has stimulated the recent development of a number of innovative methods of screening and assessing functional status in the office. The explosion of information on functional status presents clinicians with many new options (Lohr, 1989, 1992; McDowell and Newell, 1987; Stewart and Ware, 1992). However, given this array of options, how effective are the various methods? Can they be used on large numbers of patients daily in office practice without disrupting patient flow? Should they be applied to all patients or only to those at greatest risk of functional impairment? Finally, what advantages, if any, do these newer techniques have over traditional clinical methods of screening and assessing functional impairment?

DEFINITION AND CLINICAL SIGNIFICANCE OF FUNCTIONAL STATUS

The definition of functional status is a matter of some controversy. This derives in part from semantic confusion in the use of certain terms (World Health Organization, 1980) and in part from differences in the theoretical concepts of functional status (Wright and Feinstein, 1992).

Functional status, as considered in this chapter, includes those dimensions of health that extend beyond but are related to the purely biologic dimension. Considering functional status as a multidimensional construct, there is general agreement that physical, emotional, cognitive, and social function are critical components. Physical function is a measure of the ability to perform certain activities, such as bathing, toileting, cooking, eating, walking, climbing stairs, dressing, and peeling an apple. Emotional status may include measures of depression, anxiety, self-esteem, and coping. Cognitive function includes measures of orientation, memory, language, reasoning, judgment, attention span, and alertness. Social function includes measures of the intactness and extent of a person's interpersonal contacts, social resources, and performance of usual role activities (Levine and Croog, 1984; Ware, 1987) and sexual function (Croog et al., 1988). Other dimensions sometimes included in functional status are feelings of well-being and satisfaction and inventories of symptoms or assessment of pain (Nelson et al., 1990).

Functional status is related to but not necessarily dependent on physiologic homeostasis. For example, two persons with diabetes of similar type and duration and with similar treatment, control, and complications may have quite different configurations of functional status. One person may have made appropriate family and lifestyle adjustments and maintained work and social involvements. The other may have greater difficulty adjusting to the disease, and may have stopped working and reduced social involvements. A thorough grasp of the patient's physiologic state does not necessarily provide accurate knowledge of functional status.

Historically, clinical assessment of those dimensions of health referred to as functional status has always been an important part of primary care (Starfield, 1992), and many clinicians use questions to probe these dimensions. Yet in office practice, time pressures often limit the depth of exploration of physical, emotional, cognitive, and social functions. Organic problems (such as elevated blood pressure or serum glucose) demand time and attention, and the average time spent by family physicians in an office visit with most patients is less than 15 minutes, even for patients with complex medical problems (Radecki et al., 1988).

Much acute illness indeed can be dealt with purely in terms of the biomedical model; that is, no extended inquiry into functional status is required. However, for the chronically ill, the elderly, the caretakers of these patients, and some other special groups of patients, *screening* for functional deficits or change in functional status may be critical in providing good care. When functional impairments are identified by screening, *comprehensive functional assessment* followed by specific treatment or *intervention strategies* is warranted.

A SYSTEMATIC APPROACH TO SCREENING AND ASSESSMENT OF FUNCTIONAL STATUS

In office practice, traditional clinical techniques of questioning and observation may not be effective in evaluating the nature and severity of functional impairment (Calkins et al., 1991). Evidence suggests that in office practice a substantial proportion of functional impairment may elude detection. For example, Nelson and associates (1987), using a sophisticated method of assessing functional status in a network of primary care practices, found that 32 per cent of patients reported moderate or major limitation of physical function, 45 per cent of patients reported moderate or major limitation of emotional function, and 34 per cent of patients reported moderate or major limitation of social function. However, only about half of these functional limitations were recognized by the patients' regular physicians. The implications of these discrepancies of functional outcomes, patient satisfaction, and doctor–patient relationships clearly merit consideration.

In a sense, functional impairment is a problem or "disease" in its own right. Hence, standard criteria for screening, diagnosis, and treatment have been developed for functional impairment just as they have for other diseases (Maeland et al., 1992; Parkerson et al., 1992; Stewart et al., 1989). However, because data suggest that existing informal methods of screening and diagnosis of functional impairment are not always sufficiently effective in office practice, we advocate use of a three-step formal approach, leading from screening to assessment to treatment:

1. *Office-based screening* of selected high-risk groups of patients can be incorporated using brief, standardized, self-administered instruments. (These data can be viewed, perhaps, as analogous to an additional vital sign.)

2. *Comprehensive functional assessment* (CFA) can be used for those individuals who are identified by screening to have a significant functional impairment (American College of Physicians, 1988). The physician can construct a "functional problem list" based on the CFA and include it along with the usual medical problem list of the problem-oriented medical record.

3. An *effective treatment or intervention strategy,* guided by the functional problem list, can be used to stabilize or improve the functional status of the patient.

Systematic screening methods can provide an effective, brief way of identifying functional impairment in office practice. At present, many useful CFA methods are available for physical, emotional, cognitive, and social functional assessment (Duke University Center for the Study of Aging and Human Development, 1978; Granger et al., 1987; Kane and Kane, 1981). Functional problems, once identified, also may merit more in-depth assessment. Detailed evaluation of the patient and the construction of a functional problem list thus can provide a rational basis for treatment or intervention strategies. When employing these or other methods, the physician carrying out CFA of a particular patient should focus first on those functional dimensions that are most important to the patient.

CFA often can be done by the physician alone, but it sometimes may require a multidisciplinary team. Moreover, although many intervention strategies cannot be carried out solely by the physician, the physician is often in the best position to screen for functional problems, initiate CFA, and coordinate referral to other services.

Given the current state of the art, it is often difficult to demonstrate specifically that detection of more subtle functional impairments leads to better health outcomes. However, a considerable body of data suggests that certain interventions, when applied appropriately and early, may lead to better functional outcomes. Such interventions include changing pharmacotherapy to reduce functional impairment (Croog et al., 1988), emotional support by physicians and other health professionals (Novak, 1987), disease-specific patient and caregiver support groups, and caregiver education groups. They also may include physical therapy or job retraining (Granger et al., 1987), family therapy or individual counseling, respite care, hospice care, visiting nurse support, special transportation services, or systematic intervention based on CFA (Cohen et al., 1992; Epstein et al., 1990; LV Rubenstein et al., 1985, 1989; LZ Rubenstein, 1987).

Thus, efficient screening, comprehensive assessment, and effective treatment and intervention strategies can improve functional status. In particular, screening for functional status seems justified in certain high-risk groups (Feinstein, 1992; Greenfield and Nelson, 1992; Jenkins, 1992; Wasson et al., 1992).

WORKING WITH GROUPS AT HIGHEST RISK OF FUNCTIONAL IMPAIRMENT

Several groups of patients are at high risk for impaired physical, emotional, cognitive, or social function. These include the elderly, the chronically ill, the caregivers of the elderly and the chronically ill, and patients being treated with pharmacologic agents that may impair function.

The Chronically Ill

Estimates are that 30 to 50 million people in the United States suffer some dysfunction related to chronic disease or the sequelae of injuries. About 15 million people have dysfunction that is severe enough to cause limitation in their work or school performance or their ability to run a household. The rates of functional impairment are highest in the elderly; 12 per cent of the population over age 65 accounts for about 33 per cent of disabilities (Dawson et al., 1987). However, about two thirds of those with limitations are found in younger age groups, particularly among the chronically ill and survivors of serious injuries.

Data from many sources confirm high rates of functional impairment in the primary care setting. A survey of 11,186 patients of 526 physicians in three regions of the United States found that 45 per cent reported limited physical function, 28 per cent had limited role function, 9 per cent had limited social function, 31 per cent had limited metal function, 52 per cent had low health perceptions, and 29 per cent reported moderate or greater pain (Stewart et al., 1989). Each of these levels of impairment was much greater than those reported in a general population survey of 2008 patients using the same questions. Such data confirm very high levels of functional impairment in many dimensions among patients seeking primary medical care.

Screening of chronically ill patients, particularly patients who have more than one disease, is important because of the functional impact of the diseases (which may act synergistically) and the sometimes veiled functional impacts of therapy (Croog et al., 1988). CFA then can be brought to bear on these multiple identified problems.

The impact of chronic diseases on physical function has been well described (Stewart et al., 1989), and evaluation of physical function in patients with a wide range of chronic diseases (Bergner et al., 1992) has proved to be of great clinical utility. Functional measures that tap emotional, cognitive, and social dimensions in patients with chronic diseases have been developed for research purposes, but are not yet well adapted for use in office practice (Wells et al., 1989).

The Elderly

Among the elderly, in particular, functional status is commonly impaired. As many as 50 per cent of elderly living at home may have some physical disability that interferes with performing activities of daily living, and nearly 80 per cent of those 65 years old suffer from at least one chronic illness (Rowe and Besdine, 1988).

Systematic screening of functional status in the elderly can be applied usefully in the office as (1) an aid in diagnosis, (2) a way to anticipate needed social interventions, and (3) a guide in developing plans for treatment and approaching possible institutionalization of an elderly person. Functional status provides an empirical yardstick against which to measure risks and benefits of alternative therapeutic strategies. An additional advantage of systematic and periodic functional assessment of the elderly is that the process may facilitate communication among various specialists or disciplines involved in care of the elderly.

An axiom of geriatric medicine is that reliable and objective screening of functional status should be done at regular intervals, and that this screening should be supplemented by CFA whenever problems are detected. Dimensions of function that may require particular attention include vision, hearing, physical, emotional, cognitive, and social function as well as general well-being. Such screening and assessment are needed not only because they help to determine the best supportive strategies to compensate for loss of function over time but also because subtle deterioration in function (e.g., mobility, mental status, continence, or intake) may herald the onset of serious new disease or worsening of chronic disease (Applegate et al., 1990).

However, realistic and accurate screening for functional impairment in the elderly may be difficult (Bowman et al., 1990; Siu et al., 1993). Visual and auditory deficits or impaired cognitive status may make data from examinations, interviews, or questionnaires unattainable or inaccurate (Myers et al., 1993). Hence, it may be necessary to question caregivers and family members in order to obtain a clinically useful picture of a patient's functional status.

Caregivers of the Chronically Ill and Elderly

Another group at high risk of functional impairment is composed of the caregivers, spouses, or family members of elderly or chronically ill patients. Although the phenomenon was not systematically examined until recently, there is now an expanding literature on the stress and health risks to people in caregiver roles (Andolsek et al., 1988). The expression "hidden patient" has been used to describe their situation. These persons are *themselves* often at high risk for impairment of emotional status (depression, anxiety, and exhaustion) and of social function (sleep deprivation, missed work, inability to leave the home, and so on) (Zarit et al., 1985). Although some physicians question whether searching for such problem situations is their proper role or prerogative, others strongly argue that this is a vitally important role for which the family physician in particular is ideally suited.

Making a home visit or getting the "hidden patient" to accompany the identified patient on office visits can provide valuable information about caregiver function and coping as well as give additional information about the identified patient. Information provided by relatives, neighbors, or clergy also may be useful. Such data can lead to more informed management of both the patient and the caregiver in the context of the family system; they can help avoid disasters such as undetected depression or suicide of a caregiver (Cohen and Eisdorfer, 1988) and premature or delayed institutionalization of the identified patient.

Other Groups at High Risk of Functional Impairment

Patients with acute conditions who are being treated with drugs that might impair walking, memory, sleep, vision, sexual function, continence, or appetite form another group at high risk of functional impairment. Even a short course of medication for an acute problem can cause significant emotional or social dysfunction, occasional physical injury, or serious adverse drug effects. For example, among patients being treated with psychotropic medications, there is an increased risk of functional impairment ranging from drowsiness to falls with associated hip fractures. Thus, continuing evaluation of changes in functional status of patients being treated for acute illness may provide data that help the clinician choose treatments that are both biologically and functionally optimal.

OVERVIEW OF AVAILABLE INSTRUMENTS TO SCREEN FOR FUNCTIONAL STATUS IN THE OFFICE SETTING

Pioneer multidisciplinary research teams have developed a number of comprehensive instruments to assess functional health status for research purposes. Three of the most comprehensive are the Sickness Impact Profile (Bergner et al., 1981), the Rand Adult Health Status Measures (Brook et al., 1979), and the Older Americans Resource Survey (Duke University Center for the Study of Aging and Human Development, 1978). Because of their length, these instruments are not

appropriate for routine screening in the office setting, but they have been used in CFA protocols. Many of the short, practical office methods of assessing functional status discussed in the following sections were derived from these longer instruments or standardized against them.

A number of *disease-specific* multidimensional measures of functional status are available. These include instruments designed for musculoskeletal conditions, cardiac disease, pulmonary disease, cancer, and other conditions. In the last 5 years, hundreds of publications and dozens of new disease-specific measures have become available, but most are designed for research rather than for screening in a busy office practice (Guyatt et al., 1991; Patrick and Deyo, 1989). Furthermore, several comparative studies have shown that, in the office, setting global measures of functional status are often as good as, or even superior to, disease-specific measures as a general screening tool for functional impairment (Ganiats et al., 1992; Parkerson et al., 1993). Therefore, we will focus on the practical office use of global measures of functional status rather than disease-specific measures.

Some argue that observational methods of assessing functional status, especially physical function, are superior to patient self-report in response to questions. A number of creative observational techniques to assess function have been developed. However, a number of well-designed studies have shown that self-reported functional status is nearly as sensitive as observed function in office screening for functional impairment, and is less disruptive of patient flow. In contrast, observational measures of functional status may be more useful in inpatient or intensive care settings (Knaus et al., 1991). We will focus on self-reported measures rather than observational ones.

Several relatively short, global, multidimensional functional scales are useful to the busy office-based practitioner who wants to assess functional status in a quantitative and objective fashion (Katz et al., 1992). Most of the instruments discussed here can be self-administered or administered by office personnel. Most were developed and tested for use in primary care settings. All have been shown to be useful in assessing functional status at one point in time, and some are useful in assessing changes over time.

The Duke Health Profile

The Duke Health Profile (DUKE) is a 17-item instrument derived from a longer instrument developed by a team of family physicians, internists, and health service researchers for use in primary care (Parkerson et al., 1981, 1990). The DUKE is easy to understand and can be self-administered by the patient in 2 to 4 minutes. It assesses six health measures (physical, mental, social, general,

DUKE HEALTH PROFILE (The DUKE)

Copyright ● 1989 by the Department of Community and Family Medicine,
Duke University Medical Center, Durham, N.C., U.S.A.

INSTRUCTIONS:

Here are a number of questions about your health and feelings. Please read each question carefully and check (√) your best answer. You should answer the questions in your own way. There are no right or wrong answers. (Please ignore the small scoring numbers next to each blank.)

	Yes, describes me exactly	Somewhat describes me	No, doesn't describe me at all
1. I like who I am	12	11	10
2. I am not an easy person to get along with	20	21	22
3. I am basically a healthy person	32	31	30
4. I give up too easily	40	41	42
5. I have difficulty concentrating	50	51	52
6. I am happy with my family relationships	62	61	60
7. I am comfortable being around people	72	71	70

TODAY would you have any physical trouble or difficulty:

	None	Some	A Lot
8. Walking up a flight of stairs	82	81	80
9. Running the length of a football field	92	91	90

DURING THE PAST WEEK: How much trouble have you had with:

	None	Some	A Lot
10. Sleeping	102	101	100
11. Hurting or aching in any part of your body ..	112	111	110
12. Getting tired easily	122	121	120
13. Feeling depressed or sad	132	131	130
14. Nervousness	142	141	140

DURING THE PAST WEEK: How often did you:

	None	Some	A Lot
15. Socialize with other people (talk or visit with friends or relatives)	150	151	152
16. Take part in social, religious, or recreation activities (meetings, church, movies, sports, parties)	160	161	162

DURING THE PAST WEEK: How often did you:

	None	1-4 Days	5-7 Days
17. Stay in your home, a nursing home, or hospital because of sickness, injury, or other health problem	172	171	170

FIGURE 14–1. Duke Health Profile. (From Parkerson GR, Broadhead WE, Tse C-KJ: Comparison of the Duke Health Profile and the MOS Short-Form in healthy young adults. Med Care 29:679, 1991, with permission.)

perceived health, and self-esteem) along with four measures of dysfunction (anxiety, depression, pain, and disability). The complete DUKE is shown in Figure 14–1.

The DUKE is designed specifically for use in busy clinical practices (Parkerson et al., 1990). The questions have good face validity and are easy to understand and score. However, the reliability of the scales is not as good as it would be if more questions were asked (Parkerson et al., 1991), and the ability of the DUKE to detect change in function over time has not yet been assessed fully. The DUKE provides a quick, practical way to identify areas of concern, allowing the clinician to delve further into problems as he or she sees fit (Fig. 14–1).

The brevity of the DUKE is its strength. The creators of this profile argue persuasively that standard reliability tests, such as Cronbach's alpha (Cronbach, 1951), require a certain amount of redundancy in item selection. When instruments are developed, such redundancy in item focus adds reliability but makes the instrument less useful in practice settings (Parkerson et al., 1993). It is important for clinicians who may be considering the use of an instrument in practice to look at the questions, consider why the instrument is to be used, and consider the inevitable trade-offs between psychometric properties and practicality. If the clinician wishes to screen for functional problems in high-risk patients, a short but less psychometrically sophisticated instrument such as the DUKE may well prove useful. However, much more work is needed to establish the usefulness of the DUKE in a wider variety of practice settings.

The Dartmouth Cooperative Charts

Nelson and coworkers (1987, 1990) have developed a system of assessing functional status using nine pictorial charts. Patients view each chart and then select one of five choices reflecting varying levels of function. The charts cover physical condition, emotional condition, daily work, social activities, pain, change in conditions, overall condition, social support, and quality of life. A sample chart is shown in Figure 14–2.

The charts have been tested on over 2000 patients in four clinical settings. They can be self-administered or staff-administered in only 2 minutes at the time usual vital signs are taken. They are acceptable to patients, office staff, and physicians (Fig. 14–2). The test–retest reliability of the charts ranged from .73 to .98 in older patients and low-income patients. The sensitivity of the charts to change over time has not been reported in detail but is likely to be suboptimal; internal consistency reliability measures are not applicable because each dimension is scored by only one response (one chart). Validity was assessed by comparing pa-

DAILY ACTIVITIES

During the past 4 weeks . . .
   How much difficulty have you had doing your usual activities or task, both inside and outside the house because of your physical and emotional health ?

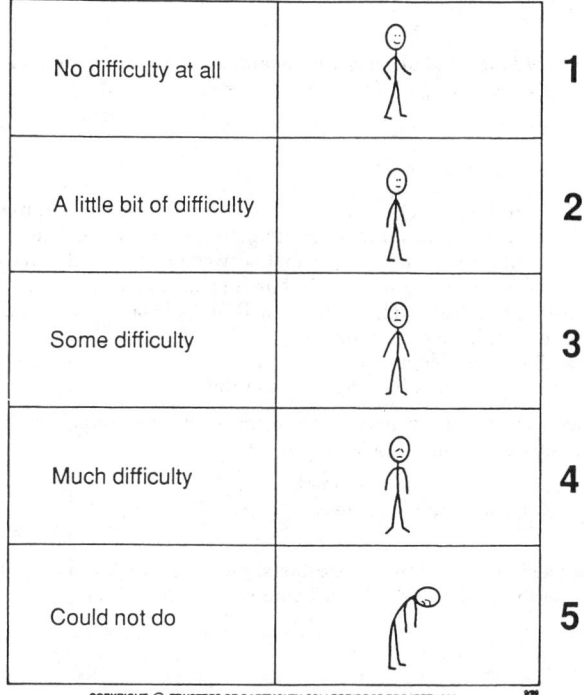

COPYRIGHT © TRUSTEES OF DARTMOUTH COLLEGE/COOP PROJECT 1989
SUPPORT PROVIDED BY THE HENRY J. KAISER FAMILY FOUNDATION

FIGURE 14–2.   One sample chart of the nine that comprise the Dartmouth Cooperative Charts. (From Nelson E, Wasson J, Kirk J, et al: Assessment of function in routine clinical practice: Description of the COOP chart method and preliminary findings. J Chron Dis 40:55S, 1987, with permission. Copyright Trustees of Dartmouth College.)

tient's Dartmouth Cooperative Chart responses with scores on longer, standard measures, and was good (Nelson et al., 1990). Convergent validity ranged from .40 to .74 and averaged .64. Discriminant validity was good except for some collinearity between physical and role function scores ($r = .50$). The authors believe that the charts have good face validity and improve physician–patient communication (Nelson et al., 1987). Use of the charts led to discovery of new information in 25 per cent of cases, and to changes in management for 40 per cent of those. More work is needed to refine the Dartmouth Cooperative Charts and to assess further their utility in office practice.

The charts have been compared directly to the Rand 36-item health survey (SF-36) in one study (McHorney et al., 1992) involving 638 well adults, 168 adults with chronic medical illnesses, and 163 adults with known psychiatric conditions. In general, the psychometric properties of instruments is markedly improved as the number of items per

TABLE 14–1. SAMPLE QUESTIONS FROM THE RAND SHORT-FORM HEALTH SURVEY: MEDICAL OUTCOMES STUDY (SF-20)

In general, would you say your health is:
1 ☐ Excellent
2 ☐ Very good
3 ☐ Good
4 ☐ Fair
5 ☐ Poor

How much bodily pain have you had during the past 4 weeks?
1 ☐ None
2 ☐ Very mild
3 ☐ Mild
4 ☐ Moderate
5 ☐ Severe

For how long (if at all) has your health limited you in each of the following activities? (Check One Box on Each Line)

	Limited for more than 3 months 1	Limited for 3 months or less 2	Not limited at all 3
a. The kinds or amounts of vigorous activities you can do, like lifting heavy objects, running, or participating in strenuous sports	☐	☐	☐
b. The kinds or amounts of moderate activities you can do, like moving a table, carrying groceries, or bowling	☐	☐	☐
c. Walking uphill or climbing a few flights of stairs	☐	☐	☐
d. Bending, lifting, or stooping	☐	☐	☐
e. Walking one block	☐	☐	☐
f. Eating, dressing, bathing, or using the toilet	☐	☐	☐

Does your health keep you from working at a job, doing work around the house, or going to school?

1 ☐ Yes, for more than 3 months
2 ☐ Yes, for 3 months or less
3 ☐ No

Have you been unable to do certain kinds or amounts of work, housework, or schoolwork because of your health?

1 ☐ Yes, for more than 3 months
2 ☐ Yes, for 3 months or less
3 ☐ No

For each of the following questions, please check the box for the one answer that comes closest to the way you have been feeling during the past month. (Check One Box on Each Line)

	All of the Time 1	Most of the Time 2	A Good Bit of the Time 3	Some of the Time 4	A Little of the Time 5	None of the Time 6
How much of the time, during the past month, has your health limited your social activities (like visiting with friends or close relatives)?	☐	☐	☐	☐	☐	☐
How much of the time, during the past month, have you been a very nervous person?	☐	☐	☐	☐	☐	☐
During the past month, how much of the time have you felt calm and peaceful?	☐	☐	☐	☐	☐	☐
How much of the time, during the past month, have you felt down-hearted and blue?	☐	☐	☐	☐	☐	☐
During the past month, how much of the time have you been a happy person?	☐	☐	☐	☐	☐	☐
How often, during the past month, have you felt so down in the dumps that nothing could cheer you up?	☐	☐	☐	☐	☐	☐

Please check the box that best describes whether each of the following statements is true or false for you.
(Check One Box on Each Line)

	Definitely True 1	Mostly True 2	Not Sure 3	Mostly False 4	Definitely False 5
a. I am somewhat ill	☐	☐	☐	☐	☐
b. I am as healthy as anybody I know	☐	☐	☐	☐	☐
c. My health is excellent	☐	☐	☐	☐	☐
d. I have been feeling bad lately	☐	☐	☐	☐	☐

From Stewart AL, Hays RD, Ware JE Jr: The Medical Outcome Study (MOS) Short-Form General Health Survey: Reliability and validity in a patient population. Med Care 26:724, 1988, with permission. Copyright Rand Corporation.

scale increases. However, the charts performed relatively well, especially with emotional function, suggesting that they are useful as a screening tool for functional impairment.

The authors of the charts have developed other sets of charts for pregnant women, adolescents, alcoholism, violence, diabetes, and asthma. Most of these versions are still being pilot tested, but some may soon be available. The cartoon approach may be especially advantageous in certain groups of patients, such as those with low literacy.

The Rand 20-Item and 36-Item Health Surveys

The Rand 20-item Health Survey, popularly known as the SF-20, has not been developed further since the late 1980s and has been supplanted by the SF-36, a longer version that is now the most widely used and best studied global functional health status measure (McHorney et al., 1992; Ware, 1993; Ware et al., 1992). The SF-36, like the SF-20 before it, measures functional status in six dimensions: physical functioning, role functioning, social functioning, mental health, health perceptions, and pain. Both these instruments were derived from the much longer Adult Health Status Measures developed by the Rand Institute in the late 1970s as part of the Health Insurance Study (Brook et al., 1979).

The item pool from which the SF-20 and SF-36 were derived was tested by phone interviews with a national sample of 2008 adults and also with 11,186 patients of 526 health care providers in three communities (Stewart et al., 1989). Correlation among health measures, comparison of patient and general population samples, and correlations between health measures and sociodemographic traits all suggested adequate to good scale validity. Although the SF-36 replaces the SF-20, and was lengthened to improve its psychometric properties, the SF-20 may be superior for use in office practice as a screening tool for functional status. For research purposes, the improved psychometric properties of the SF-36 may justify its longer administration time and item redundancy. Neither one of these instruments has been evaluated carefully for its ability to measure change over time (Hays et al., 1993; Stewart et al., 1992). Selected questions from the SF-20 are shown in Table 14–1.

Functional Status Index

The Functional Status Index was developed by MacKenzie and associates (1986) at Cornell University Medical Center. This simple index is designed to be sensitive to change in maximal function over time in individual patients. It starts with a "baseline component"; changes from baseline are

detected using a "transition component." The index has three dimensions: physical, mental, and emotional.

Maximal functional status is scored as better than, the same as, or worse than baseline. Validity was measured against Sickness Impact Profile scores, and the Functional Status Index scores were well correlated with Sickness Impact Profile scores over time for the physical dimension. The validity of the emotional and mental dimensions has not been reported.

The Functional Status Index is limited by the fact that only *directionality* of change in maximal function is indicated; the magnitude of the change cannot be measured. There are only three dimensions in the Functional Status Index; thus it lacks the breadth of other scales such as the SF-36 or the DUKE. Nevertheless, the method is innovative and deserves further development, because the office-based practitioner is often interested in changes in functional status over time.

Activities of Daily Living and Instrumental Activities of Daily Living

The Activities of Daily Living (ADL) index was one of the earliest and remains one of the most widely used methods of assessing certain elements of functional status (Katz et al., 1963). Respondents are scored on a 3-point scale for their need for assistance in using the toilet, bathing, dressing, eating, and getting in and out of bed or chairs.

The Instrumental Activities of Daily Living (IADL) index subsequently was proposed as a measure of more subtle impairment in functional status, and includes measures of a person's ability to prepare meals, shop for groceries, do routine household chores, manage money, do laundry, take medications, get to places out of walking distance, and use the telephone. The IADL in particular has been endorsed enthusiastically as a practical and useful set of questions that clinicians can use in office practice to detect unsuspected functional impairments (Kane and Kane, 1981, pp. 55–67; Myers, 1992). Because these measures do not fall into neat conceptual catagories, their psychometric properties are difficult to quantify. However, the practical nature of the questions has appeal to many clinicians, and they may be useful in various clinical scenarios.

SUMMARY

Of the multidimensional global functional health status instruments reviewed here, the SF-20, the DUKE, and the Dartmouth Cooperative Charts are potentially useful as screening tools in office practice to identify patients who may have unsuspected functional impairments. Among patients at high risk for functional impairment, or among patients with known functional problems, the use of these instruments may lead to early identification and intervention to stabilize or improve function. As these instruments are refined and others are developed, specific recommendations may change.

A major need is development of a practical instrument that can detect changes in an individual patient's functional status over time. Practical office tools such as flow sheets and problem lists that assist clinicians in monitoring functional status over time also need further development.

As experience with practical and systematic methods of screening, assessing, and treating functional impairment accumulates, more sophisticated evaluations of the effectiveness of office screening for functional impairment as a means of improving the health status of patients will become available.

REFERENCES

American College of Physicians, Health and Public Policy Committee: Comprehensive functional assessment for elderly patients. Ann Intern Med 109:70, 1988.

Andolsek KM, Clapp-Channing NE, Gehlbach SH, et al: Caregivers and elderly relatives: The prevalence of caregiving in a family practice. Arch Intern Med 148:2177, 1988.

Applegate WB, Blass JP, Williams TF: Instruments for the functional assessment of older patients. N Engl J Med 322:1207, 1990.

Bergner M, Barry JJ, Bowman MA, et al: Where do we go from here? Opportunities for applying health status assessment measures in clinical settings. Med Care 30(suppl 5):MS219, 1992.

Bergner M, Bobbitt RA, Carter WB, Gilson BS: The Sickness Impact Profile: Development and final revision of a health status measure. Med Care 19:787, 1981.

Bowman MA, Sharp PC, Herndow A, Dignan M: Methods for determining patient improvement following visits to family physicians. Fam Med 22:275, 1990.

Brook RH, Ware JE Jr, Davies-Avery A, et al: Overview of adult health status measures fielded in Rand's Health Insurance Study. Med Care 17(suppl 7):1, 1979.

Calkins DR, Rubenstein LV, Cleary PD, et al: Failure of physicians to recognize functional disability in ambulatory patients. Ann Intern Med 114:451, 1991.

Cohen D, Eisdorfer C: Depression in family members caring for a relative with Alzheimer's disease. J Am Geriatr Soc 36:885, 1988.

Cohen HJ, Saltz CC, Samsa G, et al: Predictors of two-year post-hospitalization mortality among elderly veterans in a study evaluating geriatric consultation teams. J Am Geriatr Soc 40:1231, 1992.

Cronbach LJ: Coefficient alpha and the internal structure of tests. Psychometrics 16:297, 1951.

Croog SH, Levine S, Sudliovsky A, et al: Sexual symptoms in hypertensive patients: A clinical trial of antihypertensive agents. Arch Intern Med 148:788, 1988.

Dawson D, Hendershot G, Fulton J: Aging in the eighties: Functional limitations of individuals age 65 years and over. Advance Data from Vital and Health Statistics of the National Center for Health Statistics 133:1, 1987.

Duke University Center for the Study of Aging and Human Development: Multidimensional Functional Assessment: The OARS Methodology. Durham, NC, Duke University Press, 1978.

Epstein AM, Hall JA, Fretwell M, et al: Consultative geriatric assessment for ambulatory patients: A randomized trial in a health maintenance organization. JAMA 263:538, 1990.

Feinstein AR: Benefits and obstacles for development of health status assessment measures in clinical settings. Med Care 30(suppl 5):MS42, 1992.

Ganiats TG, Palinkas LA, Kaplan RM: Comparison of Quality of Well-Being Scale and Functional Status Index in patients with atrial fibrillation. Med Care 30:958, 1992.

Granger CU, Seltzer GB, Fishbein CF: Primary Care of the Functionally Disabled: Assessment and Management. Philadelphia, JB Lippincott, 1987.

Greenfield S, Nelson EC: Recent developments and future issues in the use of health status assessment measures in clinical settings. Med Care 30(suppl 5):23, 1992.

Guyatt G, Feeny D, Patrick D: Issues in quality-of-life measurement in clinical trials. Controlled Clin Trials 12:81s, 1991.

Hays RD, Sherbourne CD, Mazel RM: The Rand 36-item health survey 1.0. Health Econ 2:217, 1993.

Jenkins CD: Assessment of outcomes of health intervention. Soc Sci Med 35:367, 1992.

Kane RA, Kane RL: Assessing the Elderly: A Practical Guide to Measurement. Lexington, MA, Lexington Books, 1981.

Katz JM, Larson MG, Phillips CB, et al: Comparative measurement sensitivity of short and longer health status instruments. Med Care 30:917, 1992.

Katz S, Ford AB, Moskowitz RW, et al: Studies of illness in the aged. The index of ADL: A standardized measure of biological and psychosocial function. JAMA 185:94, 1963.

Knaus SA, Wagner DP, Draper EA, et al: The APACHE III prognastic system: Risk prediction of hospital mortality for critically ill patients. Chest 100:1619, 1991.

Levine S, Croog SH: What constitutes quality of life? A conceptualization of the dimensions of life quality in healthy populations and patients with cardiovascular disease. In Wegner NK, et al (eds): Assessment of Quality of Life in Clinical Trials of Cardiovascular Therapies. New York, Le Jacq, 1984, pp 46–59.

Lohr KN (ed): Advances in health status assessment (conference proceedings). Med Care 27(suppl 3):S1, 1989.

Lohr KN (ed): Advances in health status assessment: Fostering the application of health status measures in clinical setting (proceedings of a conference). Med Care 30(suppl 5):MS1, 1992.

MacKenzie CR, Charlson ME, DiGiola D, et al: A patient specific measure of change in maximal function. Arch Intern Med 146:1325, 1986.

Maeland JG, Laerum E: Measuring quality of life in general practice. Scand J Primary Health Care 10:1, 1992.

McDowell L, Newell C: Measuring Health: A Guide to Rating Scales and Questionnaires. New York, Oxford University Press, 1987.

McHorney CA, Ware JE, Rogers W, et al: The validity and relative precision of MOS short- and long-form health status scales and Dartmouth COOP Charts. Med Care 30(suppl):MS253, 1992.

Myers AM: The clinical Swiss army knife: Empirical evidence on the validity of IADL functional status measures. Med Care 30(suppl):MS96, 1992.

Myers AM, Holliday PJ, Harvey KA, Hutchinson KS: Functional performance measures: Are they superior to self-assessments? J Gerontol Med Sci 48:M196, 1993.

Nelson EC, Landgraf JM, Hays RD, et al: The functional status of patients: How can it be measured in physicians' offices? Med Care 28:1111, 1990.

Nelson E, Wasson J, Kirk J, et al: Assessment of function in routine clinical practice: Description of the COOP chart method and preliminary findings. J Chron Dis 40:55S, 1987.

Novak DH: Therapeutic aspects of the clinical encounter. J Gen Intern Med 2:346, 1987.

Parkerson GR, Broadhead WE, Tse C-KJ: The Duke Health Profile, a 17-item measure of health and dysfunction. Med Care 28:1056, 1990.

Parkerson GR, Broadhead WE, Tse C-KJ: Comparison of the Duke Health Profile and the MOS Short-Form in healthy young adults. Med Care 29:679, 1991.

Parkerson GR, Broadhead WE, Tse C-KJ: Quality of life and functional health of primary care patients. J Clin Epidemiol 45:1303, 1992.

Parkerson GR, Connis RT, Broadhead WE, et al: Disease-specific versus generic measurement of health-related quality of life in insulin-dependent diabetic patients. Med Care 31:629, 1993.

Parkerson GR, Gehlbach SJ, Wagner EH, et al: The Duke-UNC Health Profile: An adult health status instrument for primary care. Med Care 19:806, 1981.

Patrick DL, Deyo RA: Generic and disease-specific measures in assessing health status and quality of life. Med Care 27(suppl 3):S217, 1989.

Radecki SE, Kane RL, Solomon DH, et al: Do physicians spend less time with older patients? J Am Geriatr Soc 36:713, 1988.

Rowe JW, Besdine RW (eds): Geriatric Medicine, 2nd edition. Boston, Little, Brown, 1988.

Rubenstein LV, Calkins DR, Fink A, et al: Topics in primary care medicine: How to help your patients function better. West J Med 143:114, 1985.

Rubenstein LV, Calkins DR, Young RT, et al: Improving patient function: A randomized trial of functional disability screening. Ann Intern Med 111:836, 1989.

Rubenstein LZ: Geriatric assessment: An overview of its impacts. Clin Geriatr Med 3:1, 1987.

Siu AL, Hays RD, Ouslander JG, et al: Measuring functioning and health in the very old. J Gerontol Med Sci 48:M10, 1993.

Starfield B: Primary Care: Concept, Evaluation, and Policy. New York, Oxford University Press, 1992.

Stewart AL, Greenfield S, Hays RD, et al: Functional status and well-being of patients with chronic conditions. JAMA 262:907, 1989.

Stewart AL, Ware JE (eds): Measuring Functioning and Well-Being: The Medical Outcomes Study Approach. Durham, NC, Duke University Press, 1992.

Ware JE: SF-36 Health Survey: Manual and Interpretation Guide. Boston, Nimrod Press, 1993.

Ware JE Jr: Standards for validating health measures: Definition and content. J Chron Dis 40:473, 1987.

Ware JE, Sherbourne CD, Davies AR: Developing and testing the MOS 20-item short-form health survey: A general population application. *In* Stewart AL, Ware JE (eds): Measuring Functioning and Well-Being: The Medical Outcomes Study Approach. Durham, NC, Duke University Press, 1992, pp 277–290.

Wasson J, Keller A, Rubenstein L, et al: Benefits and obstacles of health status assessment in ambulatory settings: The clinician's point of view. Med Care 30(suppl):MS42, 1992.

Wells KB, Hays RD, Burnam A, et al: Detection of depressive disorder for patients receiving prepaid or fee-for-service care: Results from the Medical Outcomes Study. JAMA 262:3298, 1989.

World Health Organization: International Classification of Impairments, Disabilities and Handicaps. Geneva, World Health Organization, 1980.

Wright JG, Feinstein AR: A comparative contrast of clinimetric and psychometric methods for constructing indexes and rating scales. J Clin Epidemiol 45:1201, 1992.

Zarit SH, Orr NK, Zarit JM: The Hidden Victims of Alzheimer's Disease: Families under Stress. New York, New York University Press, 1985.

Part III

COMMUNICATION IN FAMILY MEDICINE

CHAPTER 15

ESTABLISHING RAPPORT

ROBERT E. RAKEL

Compassion, interest, and thoroughness are essential components of successful patient care. These features traditionally have been embodied in the term "bedside manner," which also connotes qualities of concern, kindness, friendliness, wit, and cheerfulness, all of which result in an atmosphere of trust and confidence between physician and patient. The physician with the best bedside manner actually may be the one who makes no special effort to communicate these feelings but simply acts in a concerned, natural, and comfortable manner.

The health care relationship involves trust and a certain degree of control over another person, so the provider must be skilled and effective in the requisite technical services. Charm, a warm bedside manner, or a pleasant personality, in the absence of skill, sound judgment, and knowledge, is hollow. Conversely, competence of the highest level, in the absence of rapport, results in less than optimal clinical outcome. Patients and staff may tolerate a boorish, tactless, and insensitive physician of exceptional ability, but such relationships usually are characterized by friction, anxiety, anger and, sooner or later, disloyalty.

Oliver Wendell Holmes said that the physician, in order to be effective, should "speak softly, be well-dressed, have quiet ways and have eyes that do not wander" (1883, p. 388). Lack of eye contact may be interpreted as a lack of concern. A good first impression is certainly a great help in establishing rapport. You do not get a second chance to create a first impression. The physician should approach the patient in an assured, confident (but not cocky or arrogant) manner, and present a personal appearance that is acceptable to the patient. Empathetic frankness and honesty are also important factors in instilling confidence and trust.

Personal appearance is a significant part of nonverbal communication. Patients consider house staff who wear white coats with conventional street clothes as more competent than those who wear scrub suits. Negative attitudes toward physicians are associated with casual clothing (such as blue jeans, athletic shoes, and clogs), with overly feminine items such as prominent ruffles and dangling earrings, and with temporarily fashionable items (such as long hair on men, male earrings, and pat-

terned hose on women) (Gjerdingen et al., 1987). If white coats are worn, the patient sees only the collar, tie, and shoes, so it is important to keep these neat.

A genuine smile can be helpful in quickly establishing a friendly atmosphere and developing a warm interpersonal relationship. A grin can be the physician's most effective weapon for breaking down resistance or apprehension in patients, especially children or young adults. A number of studies have shown that patients are more positively disposed to physicians who smile. The smile must be genuine, however. Patients can spot a phony smile a mile away.

Posture is also important in conveying an image of confidence and competence. Standing erect, moving briskly with head up and stomach in, is better than slouching. Energetic people seldom slump; they sit upright and appear alert. A listless or lethargic appearance can be interpreted as lack of concern.

Before entering the examining room or hospital room to see a patient, review the chart briefly and become familiar with the patient's name and its proper pronunciation. If the pronunciation is either unusual or difficult, place phonetic markings on the chart as a reminder for future use. Repeat the patient's name when first given it to confirm the pronunciation, then use the name twice in the first minute to help it register. Review the chart also for particular aspects of the previous visit that should be remembered and commented on, such as the illness treated at that time, family conditions, or other problems. Patients will believe that the well-informed physician is truly interested in them. Additional courtesy, such as opening the door and assisting patients with their coats (especially an elderly patient) shows a consideration that aids in establishing and maintaining rapport.

RESPECT

The greatest deterrent to establishing patient rapport is an attitude of indifference or lack of interest by the physician. Patients should believe that their comments are being listened to, carefully considered, and taken seriously. They must believe that the physician values their comments and opinions before trusting him or her with information of a more personal nature. As long as the physician's attitude toward the patient embodies respect, concern, and kindness and a sincere effort is made to understand the patient's difficulties, the patient will overlook or forgive a myriad of other problems.

Oliver Wendell Holmes advised patients to:

Choose a man who is personally agreeable, for a daily visit from a intelligent, amiable, pleasant, sympathetic person will cost you no more than one from a sloven or a boor, and his presence will do more for you than any prescription the other will order. (1883, p. 391)

Ideally, there will be a bond of mutual respect between physician and patient. A physician can show respect for patients, and accept their respect, only insofar as respect is an integral part of his or her personality. There must be a concept of self-respect before one can respect others.

It may be that it is a lack of security rather than an excess of it that leads physicians to appear aloof and unconcerned. Too often physicians think that a god-like image of omnipotence is necessary for the maintenance of patient respect and confidence. It is usually a lack of self-confidence that causes physicians to retreat behind this protective image, which in turn limits their ability to help. Secure physicians are more free to establish close personal relationships with patients without fearing their position will be threatened. A physician with a positive self-image is also willing to recognize and admit the limits of personal competence and feels comfortable seeking help from a colleague when such consultation is of value to the patient's care.

The bond of mutual respect is enhanced if the physician makes positive statements about other people. Patients find it difficult to respect a physician who is regularly detractive, making negative statements about other people or other physicians. Any comments that can be interpreted as "building yourself up by tearing someone else down" merely accomplish the reverse.

The effectiveness of physicians depends on the degree of their insight into the limitations of their personalities and the psychological defenses that distort their perceptions of patients. Physicians must recognize those situations or patients that make them unreasonably angry or provoked (e.g., a whining, complaining individual who shows no interest in being rehabilitated, preferring a role of social dependency). Obviously, the physician's emotions, if they go unrecognized, can serve as a barrier to the development of mutual respect. If the physician is aware of negative feelings toward a patient, an effort can be made to avoid showing signs of irritation or anger. It has been said that clenching of the physician's fist is a clinical sign of the hysterical patient. The physician should attempt to remain objective and analyze the situation for its diagnostic value.

Patients with trivial complaints or somatic manifestations of emotional disease sometimes are given less attention than those with clear-cut organic abnormalities. The frequency with which a physician complains about the triviality and inappropriateness of patients' problems has been found to be related to the volume of patients seen and the degree to which the physician feels overburdened. The more patients that physicians see and the more overloaded their practices, the more likely they are to describe patient complaints as trivial, inappropriate, or bothersome. Physicians who either have more time or take more time per patient and investigate the patient's complaints more thoroughly frequently uncover significant factors and have less tendency to view the complaints as trivial. Respect for patients involves taking their fears and apprehensions seriously and withholding value judgments. Patients who frequently seek help for nonspecific somatic and functional complaints may be depressed (Widmer, 1980).

PATIENT SATISFACTION

Clearly, there is a close relationship between rapport and patient satisfaction, and this entire chapter deals with the many facets of that relationship. It is important that the physician make an effort to understand what patients are going through—not only their pain and discomfort but the effect these have on their lives—and communicate this understanding to them.

Most studied indicate that patient satisfaction depends on information, and the degree to which the patient understands the illness. Joos and associates (1993) found that patients whose desires for information and attention to emotional and family problems went unmet were significantly less satisfied with their physicians than those whose desires were met. They found that even patients with chronic diseases who had lived with the problem for years had questions they wanted answered. Their satisfaction was related more strongly to the desire for information and affective support than to whether or not the physician conducted examinations and tests. It is also clear that the greater the patients' satisfaction, the more likely they are to comply with treatment recommendations.

Factors that interfere with patient satisfaction, in addition to poor communication, are a perception of physician insensitivity and office foul-ups such as appointment delays, billing mistakes, and frustration with the telephone system.

COMMUNICATION AND RAPPORT

Even the most knowledgeable and skilled physician will have limited effectiveness if unable to develop rapport with patients. Unfortunately, rapport is one of those intangibles that is more than the sum of its parts. Rapport is not analyzed easily within any one body of knowledge, yet it is fair to say that the basis of rapport is the development of communication skills that instill in patients a sense of confidence and trust by conveying sincerity and an interest in their care and well-being. The patient's satisfaction and compliance with the physician's instructions (both measures of rapport, so to speak) depend on the ability of the physician to communicate understanding, compassion, and genuine interest in the patient and to display a thorough approach to solving the patient's problems. Patient satisfaction also is related to the physician's talent for educating patients regarding the disease process and for motivating them to participate in their treatment.

The majority of complaints against physicians—and those that all too frequently lead to legal action—are simply the result of a lack of communication between doctor and patient. The potential for a serious problem always exists when a patient is inadequately informed regarding a diagnostic procedure, treatment, prognosis, or anticipated cost. The misunderstandings that result cause a great deal of unnecessary expense and grief for both parties.

Similarly, the worries that result from distorted information can jeopardize the doctor-patient relationship severely. When a patient is discussed on hospital rounds or with a colleague in the office, take care that the discussion is not within the patient's hearing distance or within that of other patients. Another patient, overhearing the conversation, may believe that the comments apply to him or her, or may know the patient involved and relay the information in a distorted manner. Fragments of such conversations, overheard by the patient or others, are too easily taken out of context and can become the focus of fearful fantasies that only serve to increase uneasiness and apprehension.

Failure of communication between physician and patient also can affect the outcome of treatment, often as seriously as can an error in treatment. More complaints against physicians result from a breakdown of the caring aspect of the doctor–patient relationship than from the technical quality of treatment.

Unfortunately, there are no criteria for the establishment of rapport, as there are criteria for the diagnosis of this or that disease. Each physician must develop his or her own unique style. However, communications theory identifies most of the major elements of rapport, and a brief acquaintance with relevant portions of that theory may be helpful.

First, communication suggests an exchange of information between persons over some type of channel. Establishing an open channel is the first element of the communication process and influences all that follows. In the clinical setting, the channel is the face-to-face conversation of patient and clinician in the interview or examination; the telephone is an important secondary channel.

Establishing communication means that the patient can gain access to the clinician—on the phone or by an early appointment—without having to run an obstacle course created by an overly protective staff. Delay in returning a phone call may result in a patient remaining home all day waiting; if the call is not returned at all, the negative effect on rapport is great.

Unwillingness to make communication convenient for the patient usually results in a spiral of increasingly frequent attempts to reach the physician and mounting frustration for everyone. In contrast, physicians who give a high priority to communicating discover that most patients are considerate and even protective of the physician's time. At the beginning of a practice, a certain amount of testing is done by patients to determine how accessible a physician is; those who pass the test find that they are rarely inconvenienced by unnecessary calls or visits.

In any face-to-face encounter, communication is both intended and unintended, and the distinction is important. *Intended* messages are verbal statements that transmit fact and nonverbal messages that the sender hopes will elicit predictable responses from the receiver. One patient, for example, may enact by a sophisticated blend of verbal and nonverbal communications the role of "strong, brave, unafraid, and willing to face reality." Another patient (or, indeed, the same patient in another setting) may communicate verbally and nonverbally a message of "weak, helpless, needing support and sympathy." Such a performance is not the result of a well-thought-out, conscious decision; it results mostly from learned processes that are unconscious but accessible to scientific analysis.

Unintended communication refers to messages that are given off by individuals beyond their awareness. However, subtle clues are perceptible to the astute observer. The patient who wishes to create an impression of bravery, for example, may contradict the intended message by a slight hand tremor, a barely noticeable weakness of the voice, or beads of perspiration on the forehead. In clinical practice, the recognition of the patient's true thoughts and feelings is a central skill in establishing and maintaining rapport (see Micro-Expressions and Nose Rub).

Verbal Communication

Much of the communication process in the clinical interview centers on verbal interchange. Symptoms, past medical history, family medical history, and psychosocial data are transmitted primarily by verbal means (see Chapter 18). Some aspects of verbal communication play an important role in establishing and maintaining rapport. Slips of the tongue or major areas of omission (e.g., a married person who never mentions a spouse) may signify problem areas that, when explored, help establish the interviewer as a perceptive person who understands what lies beneath the surface. The interviewer constantly must consider: Why is the patient telling me that? Even simple, casual remarks may be the patient's way of sending up a trial balloon about issues of great concern—for example, the man who says, "Oh, by the way, a friend of mine has been having some chest pain when he walks a lot—do you think that sounds serious?" may be actually talking about a concern of his own that he is unable to face directly. Or, a child may be brought to the office with a trivial problem in order that the mother might have a chance to discuss with the physician something that is troubling her; the child is a calling card, signaling the need to open the communication channel. The physician who is sensitive to these subtle clues and encourages the patient to discuss what is actually troublesome will find that the rapport thus established allows future interviews to be much more open and direct.

Physicians in practice who have established rapport during an ongoing relationship with patients communicate more easily than do physicians seeing a patient for the first time in an emergency department. Studies by Korsch and Negrete (1972) showed that doctors in an emergency room did more talking than the patients, although their perception was just the opposite. This was attributed to interaction with unfamiliar patients by house staff in a setting in which the stress level is high and the orientation therapeutic. Yet Arntson and Philipsborn (1982) found that physicians in private practice for 26 years, who knew their patients and saw them in a low-stress situation for diagnosis or health maintenance, also talked more than the patients (twice as long). One difference in the two settings, however, was that in the private office there was a strong reciprocal affective relationship between doctor and patient. If either made an affective statement, the other would respond similarly, whereas in the emergency room, mothers expressed twice as many affective statements as did the physicians.

Vocabulary

The use of appropriate vocabulary assists in establishing rapport by ensuring easy and accurate communication. Phrasing questions in simple language appropriate to the patient's level of understanding and avoidance of medical jargon help establish a sense of working together. The patient's cultural background and educational level should be considered, and the physician should avoid using slang (or a contrived accent), because the pa-

tient will detect the artificiality and consider this patronizing. However, a language style easily can be assumed that is different from the physician's normal speech yet natural and comfortable for both physician and patient.

Medical terminology should be avoided unless it is familiar to the patient. More than once a lumbar puncture has been interpreted by the patient to mean an operation to drain the lungs. No longer does the physician gain a therapeutic advantage by writing prescriptions in Latin or impressing the patient with medical words. Today's patients prefer to be enlightened and demand maximum insight into their care. It is best to start all explanations at a basic level and proceed only as rapidly as patient understanding permits.

Physicians also should be sure of what patients mean to convey by their word selection and make certain they are operating at a common level of understanding. When the patient says he or she "drinks a little," inquire further to find out what is meant by a little; or if he or she "spits up blood," determine whether it is truly spitting or vomiting. A major barrier to accurate interpersonal communication is the tendency of people to react to a statement from their own points of view, rather than attempting to interpret it from the speaker's vantage point. If a question exists regarding the clarity of the interpretation, it is best to repeat it to the speaker's satisfaction. Contract negotiators have found that, when parties in a dispute realize that they are being understood and each party sees how the situation appears to the other, there is less need to exaggerate and act defensively.

Korsch and Negrete (1972) found that some of the longest interviews between physician and patient were due to failures in communication; the doctor and patient had to spend considerable time trying to get on the same wavelength. An analysis of the conversations revealed that less than 5 per cent of the physician's conversation was personal or friendly in nature and that, although most of the physicians believed that they had been friendly, fewer than half of the patients had this impression. The following partial transcript of an interview from Korsch and Negrete (1972) is a vivid illustration of failure to communicate because of inappropriate vocabulary and lack of attention to patient understanding:

Father: How does his heart sound?
Doctor: Sounds pretty good. He's got a little murmur there. I'm not sure what it is. It's . . . it uh . . . could just be a little hole in his heart.
Mother: Is that very dangerous when you have a hole in your heart?
Doctor: No, because I think it's the upper chamber, and if it's the upper chamber then it means nothing.
Mother: Oh.
Doctor: Otherwise they just grow up and they repair them.

Mother:	What would cause the hole in his heart?
Doctor:	H'm?
Mother:	What was it that caused the hole in his heart?
Doctor:	It's 'cause . . . uh . . . ust developmental, when their uh . . .
Mother:	M-h'm.
Doctor:	There's a little membrane that comes down, and if it's the upper chamber, there's a membrane that comes down, one from each direction. And sometimes they don't quite meet, and so there's either a hole at the top or a hole at the bottom and then . . . it's really uh . . . uh . . . almost never causes any trouble.
Mother:	Oh.
Doctor:	It's uh . . . one thing that they never get SBE from . . . it's the only heart lesion in which they don't.
Mother:	Uh-huh.
Doctor:	And uh . . . they grow up to be normal.
Mother:	Oh, good.
Doctor:	And uh . . . if anything happens they can always catheterize them and make sure that's what it is, or do heart surgery.
Mother:	Yeah.
Doctor:	Really no problem with it. They almost never get into trouble so . . .
Mother:	Do you think he might have developed the murmur being that my husband and I both have a murmur?
Doctor:	No.
Mother:	No. Oh, it's not hereditary, then?
Doctor:	No.
Mother:	Oh, I see. [Someone whistling in the room]
Doctor:	It is true that certain people . . . tendency to rheumatic fever, for instance.
Mother:	H'mm.
Doctor:	There is a tendency for the abnormal antigen-antibody reaction to be inherited, and therefore they can sometimes be more susceptible.
Mother:	Oh, I see. That wouldn't mean anything if uh . . . I would . . . I'm Rh negative and he's positive. It wouldn't mean anything in that line, would it?
Doctor:	Uh-huh.
Mother:	No? Okay.
Doctor:	No. The only thing you have to worry about is other babies.
Mother:	M'h'm.
Doctor:	Watch you Coombs' and things.
Mother:	Watch my what?
Doctor:	Watch your Coombs' and things.
Mother:	Oh, yeah.
Doctor:	Your titres, Coombs' titres. (p. 68)

Nonverbal Communication

Verbal communication occupies so much of daily social interaction that nonverbal communication often is ignored. However, much that is said is unspoken. Communications specialists have demonstrated convincingly the major importance nonverbal messages have in validating or contradicting verbal messages, and their enormous influence as communication symbols in their own right.

Communication between two people is usually one-third nonverbal. What is said verbally often is emphasized nonverbally, and personal attitudes and emotions usually are communicated at the nonverbal level. Nonverbal communicative signals are under less censorship from conscious control than are verbal messages, so they are likely to be more genuine.

Charles Darwin held that there is a unique pattern of nonverbal actions for each emotion. In *Expressions of the Emotions in Man and Animals* (1872), Darwin suggested that emotional expressions are evolutionary remnants of previous adaptive behavior that persist even though currently useless. Snarling as a sign of aggression is one example. While more recent knowledge indicates that emotional expression is learned as well as genetically mediated, Darwin's idea of a unique pattern of actions has been shown for depression and anxiety and is likely in the future to be demonstrated for other emotional states as well.

The elements of nonverbal communication have been classified in the following categories (Knapp, 1978): *Body language* or *kinesics* (including gestures and facial expressions), *physical characteristics* (such as age, skin coloration, evidence of health), *touching, paralanguage* (tone of voice, rate of speech, and so on), *proxemics* (spatial factors), *artifacts* (clothing and accessories), and *environmental factors* (furniture, decor, and so on). All of these aspects of nonverbal communication have relevance for the physician–patient encounter.

Paralanguage

Paralanguage is the voice effect that accompanies or modifies talking and often communicates meaning. It includes velocity of speech (fast, slow, hesitant), tone and volume of voice, sighs and grunts, pauses, and inflections. Urgency, sincerity, confidence, hesitation, thoughtfulness, gaiety, sadness, and apprehension all are conveyed by qualities of voice. McCaskey (1979) believes that the literal interpretation (definition) of words accounts for only 10 per cent of communication between two people, while facial expression and tone of voice account for up to 90 per cent of the communication.

Certainly there is a real difference between verbal and vocal information. The verbal message refers to the words literally transmitted. The vocal message includes the emotional quality, the tone of voice, and the frequency and length of pauses—information that is lost when the words are written. Tone of voice, for example, actually can reverse the meaning of words. Sarcasm is a common example of a contradiction between vocal and verbal messages. Comparative studies have shown that, when the vocal and verbal messages transmit contradictory information, the vocal is more accurate.

Physicians should be alert to subtle changes of tone, such as when patients ask whether everything will be all right. Are they asking for reassurance, showing fear, or doubting the diagnosis? Rather than concentrating exclusively on *what* patients are saying, the astute physician will concentrate on *how* they are saying it.

Touch

A close personal interest in the patient can be communicated by the appropriate use of touch. The most socially acceptable method in this country is a handshake, enabling the physician to establish early contact with the patient. The handshake, properly used, can convey to the patient sincerity and interest as well as security and poise. It is an inoffensive intrusion into the other person's area of privacy and can be extended under certain circumstances to include the application of the left hand to the upper or lower arm. This technique is often used by politicians to emphasize sincerity and concern.

The handshake as a traditional greeting of friendship began by the raising of exposed hands by two approaching individuals to give evidence that they held no weapons. This proceeded to the grasping of hands, or in the Roman society, the forearms. In the United States, a firm handshake is most acceptable. Usually, the limp or "wet dishrag" handshake indicates lack of interest or insincerity, especially if it is rapidly withdrawn. A moist palm is a sign of nervousness or apprehension, and the "halfway there," fingers-only handshake indicates reluctance or indecision. However, the handshake continues to be modified culturally, and one should be extremely wary of misinterpreting another person's handshake without understanding his or her cultural background.

In China, the Confucian code of etiquette dictated that there should never be a touching of persons, and even today Chinese officials may appear reluctant to grasp an extended hand (a Chinese formerly shook his own hand) (Butterfield, 1982). Some young people in the United States have modified the traditional palm-to-palm handshake to a grasping of the thumb and thenar eminence and continue to develop new variations reminiscent of the secret handshakes of fraternal groups.

Touching can be an effective method for communicating concern or compassion and can break down some of the defensive barriers to communication. Caution should be exercised, however, not to use it excessively or earlier than is socially permissible. If used without adequate preparation, touch can be interpreted as an invasion of privacy and a forward and inconsiderate act. Touch by a physician can be viewed as aggressive behavior if it is used before rapport is established. During the physical examination, it is best to talk before touching by explaining to the patient what will be done next. Studies of primates have shown that touching gestures usually are considered nonaggressive and calming in nature. When used properly by the physician, touch can be facilitative and welcome.

The tremendous symbolic value of touch as a healing power was demonstrated during the Middle Ages when people sought relief from scrofula (tuberculous lymphadenitis) through the king's touch, or royal touch, in spite of the notoriously low cure rates. This power has been transferred to physicians, and patients often feel better after a routine physical examination. Friedman (1979) stated that 85 per cent of patients leaving a physician's office feel better even if they have not received medication or treatment, and 50 per cent of patients in the waiting room feel better in anticipation of the help they will receive.

Touch, or laying on of the hands, may indeed promote healing, especially if it is imbued by the patient with a special symbolic value. Franz Mesmer (1734–1815) was among the first to emphasize the medical importance of "laying on of the hands." Mesmer, however, believed that there was a magnetic power in his hands, which he called animal magnetism and which he applied to ailing individuals. His theory was unscientific, and although he became famous for successfully treating a number of hysterical patients, he finally was discredited by a committee that included Benjamin Franklin and Antoine Lavoisier. They found his treatments to be without magnetism and essentially useless. They did agree, however, that he had helped many people and had brought about many cures. They attributed these cures to as yet unknown factors rather than to the animal magnetism he claimed. Incidentally, mesmerism was the forerunner of hypnosis (initially called artificial somnambulism), which was developed by Puysegur, a disciple of Mesmer.

The magic of touch can be good medicine, especially when combined with concern, support, and reassurance. Stroking, a special kind of touching, describes a physical or symbolic recognition of a person's finer attributes. A stroke may be a kind word, a warm gesture, or a simple touch of the hand. Infants deprived of touch and stroking suffer mental and physical deterioration. Adults also require stroking to maintain a healthy emotional state. Stroking occurs whenever an interchange between two people leaves one or both with a good, or fulfilled, feeling.

Kinesics (Body Language)

The astute physician will cultivate observational skills that enable the detection of hidden or subtle clues to diagnosis contained in the patient's nonverbal behavior. Kinesics is the study of nonverbal gestures, or body movements, and their meaning as a form of communication. It is essential to remember, however, that specific gestures and their interpretation are of importance only when judged in the context of the circumstances surrounding them. Body language alone does not reveal the entire behavioral image any more than does verbal language alone. Just as one word does not make a sentence or even have much meaning without the sentence, a single gesture has clinical relevance only as part of a sequence of actions. Although individual signs have significance, they are not reliable when they stand alone; they are meaningful only when considered in the context of a person's total behavioral pattern.

When there is congruence between the verbal and nonverbal message—that is, when the gesture conveys the same message as the spoken word—communication and its meaning are almost sure to be in agreement. When one indicates something different from the other, however, the nonverbal message usually will be the more accurate.

Attempts by the patient to mask feelings can be detected readily by observing body behavior. True feelings are more likely to leak through conscious efforts to conceal one's feelings. Likewise, a physician's attempt at deception will be detected by patients and can destroy confidence and damage rapport. Positive verbal communication, such as "You're looking better today," when accompanied by negative nonverbal cues, will be interpreted by the patients as insincere. For example, a patient who is not told the true nature of a terminal illness usually knows it anyway and may distrust family, friends, and physician if they persist in the charade.

Reassuring a patient that "nothing is wrong," rather than putting the patient at ease because the physician found nothing abnormal, instead may be interpreted as "the doctor is unable to make me better." Premature reassurance may be interpreted as rejection. If reassurance is used, it must be genuine and and realistic and given only after a thorough evaluation of the problem (Lau, 1989).

Alan Alda, in a medical school commencement address, challenged new physicians to be able to read a patient's involuntary muscles as well as their radiographic studies. He asked, "Can you see the fear and uncertainty in my face? If I tell you where it hurts, can you hear in my voice where I ache? I show you my body, but I bring you my person. Will you tell me what you are doing and in words I can understand? Will you tell me when you don't know what to do?" (*Time*, May 28, 1979, p. 68). The physician will see the fear and uncertainty in the patient's face only if he or she is looking at the patient rather than the medical record. Alda's statement reflects the concern and compassion that patients desire. By using appropriate body language, the physician can convey this attention and concern in the most effective manner possible.

BODY POSITION. The body position when sitting can show varying degrees of tension or relaxation. The tense person sits erect with a fairly rigid posture. One who is moderately relaxed has a forward lean of approximately 20 degrees and a side lean of up to 10 degrees. A very relaxed position (usually too relaxed for physicians interacting with patients) is a backward lean (recline) of 20 degrees and a sideways lean of over 10 degrees.

Higher patient satisfaction is associated with a physician's forward body lean and rotation of the torso toward the patient. Larsen and Smith (1981) found that "the patient also responds more favorably to the physician who relaxes his chin in his hands and gazes directly at the patient, rather than a physician who elevates his chin (unsupported) as if to imply a more superior status." Physicians whose communication styles have been considered patient oriented have been noted to change body position more frequently than physicians whose conversations were physician centered.

An attempt should be made, whenever possible, to sit rather than stand when interviewing a patient. Rapport is improved if the physician does not intimidate the patient by placing them in a submissive position. Patients feel more comfortable, and less helpless, speaking in a sitting position rather than prone. Sitting on the patient's bed has been frowned on, but for some patients it is an effective means of establishing closeness and conveying warmth in a relaxed yet attentive manner.

MIRRORING. When good rapport exists between two people, each will mirror the other's movements. Some people consciously try to establish rapport with another by mirroring that person's movements. Some people consciously try to establish rapport with another by mirroring that person's body posture (Fig. 15–1). Disruptions in this mirroring may signal that one member disagrees with what the other has said or feels betrayed or insulted but cannot express this verbally. If the physician notices this sudden disruption of mirroring activity by the patient, more attention should be focused on the comment that led to the change of position. Renegotiation or further explanation may be indicated.

HEAD POSITION. Typically, the head is held forward in anger and back in defiance, anxiety, or fear. It is down or bowed in sadness, submissiveness, shame, or guilt. The head tilted to one side indicates interest and attention (Fig. 15–2); when circumstances are appropriate, this can be a flirtation. The erect head indicates self-confidence and maturity.

When listening to a patient, the physician should show interest and concern by an attentive position—best illustrated by sitting forward in the chair with an interested, attentive facial expression and the head slightly tilted. Darwin was one of the first to note that animals assume a head tilt when listening intently.

FACE. Darwin (1872) proposed that cultures throughout the world express similar emotions or states of mind with remarkably uniform body movements. His information was gathered from missionary friends working with aborigines, persons under hypnosis, infants, and the insane. He also studied the blind and deaf, who, without bene-

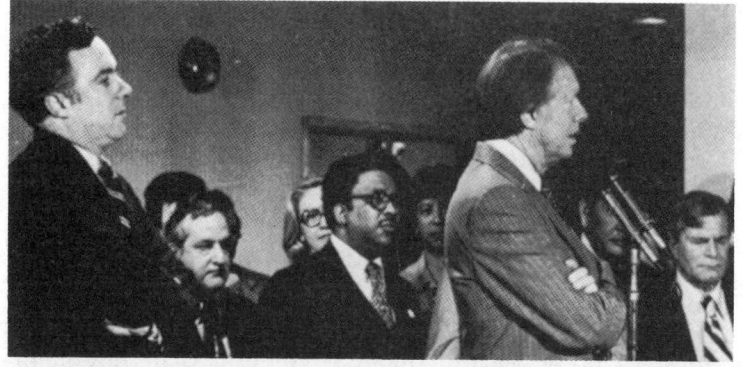

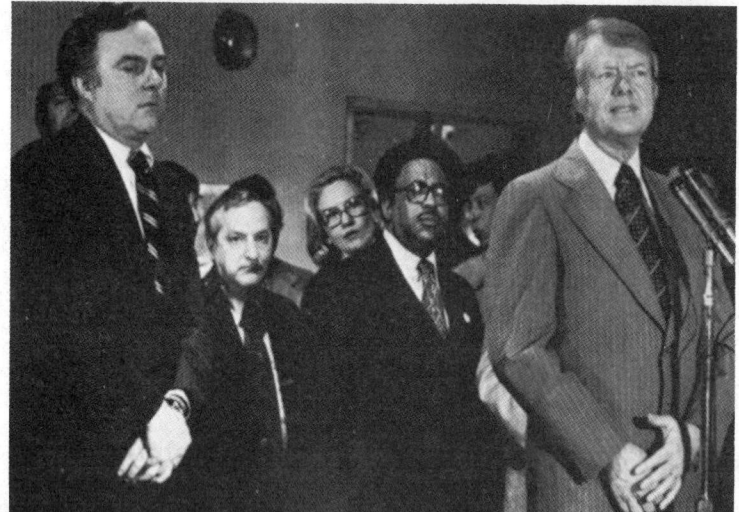

FIGURE 15–1. Joseph Califano (left), Secretary of Health, Education and Welfare, mirrors his boss, President Jimmy Carter, through his posture and gestures. (*In* Key MR [ed]: The Relationship of Verbal and Nonverbal Communication. New York, Mouton Publishers, 1980, p. v, with permission.)

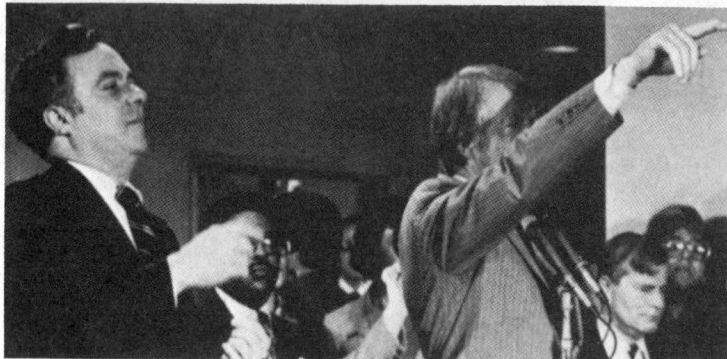

fit of learning from others, were noted to raise eyebrows when surprised and shrug their shoulders to indicate helplessness.

Darwin held that the facial expression of emotion, when undisguised, is independent of culture and is identical throughout the world. Thus, the facial expressions of joy, sadness, and anger are the same in the Australian aborigine, the American farmer, and the Norwegian fisherman. Various cultures, however, do disguise the facial expression in different ways. In the American culture, the mouth most commonly is used to disguise feelings. A person in a social gathering may be smiling, although inwardly sad or angry. The eyebrows, eyes, and forehead are least affected by these cultural dis-

guises and are the most consistently dependable indicators of emotion. As Shakespeare wrote, "I saw his heart in his face" (*The Winter's Tale*, Act I, Scene II).

Ekman and Friesen (1975) found that the facial expressions of fear, disgust, happiness, and anger were the same in countries with widely disparate language and culture. They also found that these expressions involve both sides of the face, but contempt involves only one side, such as tightening one corner of the mouth. Videotapes of college students in the United States and Japan, taken without their knowledge while they were watching a stress-inducing film, showed identical facial expressions of disgust. When they discussed the

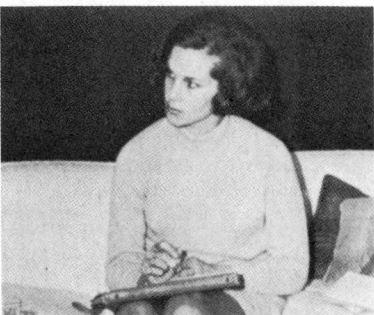

FIGURE 15–2. This woman signals attentiveness and serious-ness by holding very still, cocking her head, and looking in-tently at the speaker. (From Scheflen AE: Body Language and the Social Order—Communication as Behavioral Control. En-glewood Cliffs, NJ, Prentice-Hall, 1972, with permission.)

film with other people, however, the Japanese masked their facial expressions of unpleasant feel-ings much more than did the Americans.

Ekman and Friesen used composite facial photo-graphs to show how each part of the face contrib-utes to the expressions of emotion, especially sur-prise, fear, disgust, anger, happiness, and sadness (see Fig. 15–3). In our culture, when people wish to disguise their true feelings and convey an impression that is more socially acceptable, they do so by smiling. This may be especially true in patients who are sad or depressed. Figure 15–4 is a composite showing sadness in the eyes, brow, and forehead being masked by a smile.

MICRO-EXPRESSIONS. Ekman and Friesen (1975) also described micro-expressions, a valuable indi-cation of masking or deception. "Micro-expres-

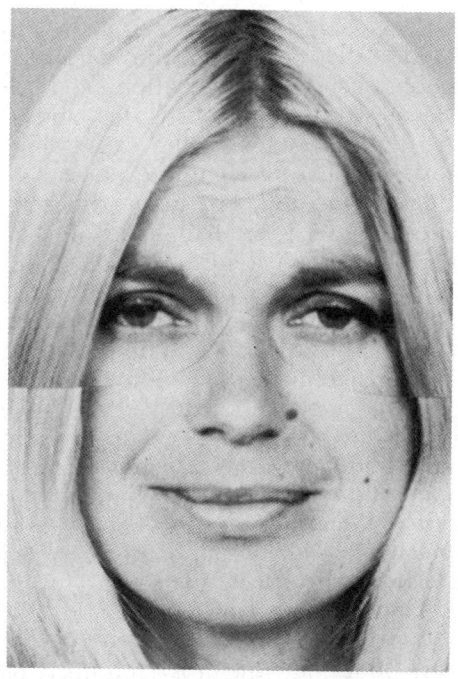

FIGURE 15–4. Masking of sadness by smiling (see eyes and forehead). (From Ekman P, Friesen WV: Unmasking the Face: A Guide to Recognizing Emotions from Facial Clues. Engle-wood Cliffs, NJ, Prentice-Hall, 1975, with permission.)

sions are caused by the face's all too rapid effi-ciency in registering inner feelings" (Morris, 1977, p. 110). Most facial expressions last more than 1 second, but micro-expressions last only one fifth to one twenty-fifth of a second. This is approxi-mately the time it takes to blink an eye, and micro-

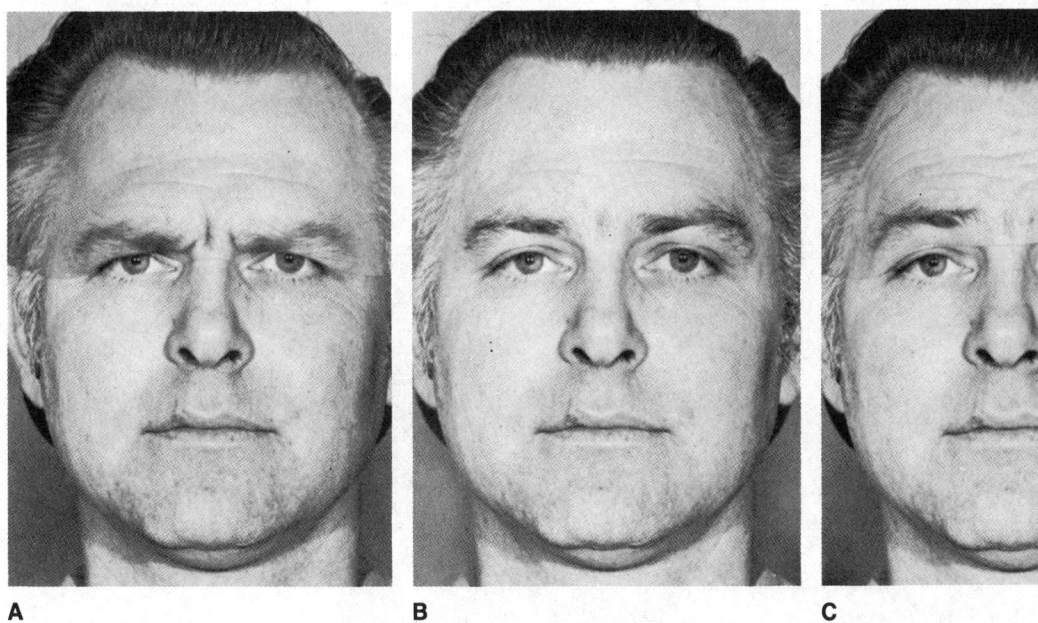

A   B   C

FIGURE 15–3. This man shows the anger brow with the rest of the face uninvolved *(A)*; a neutral face *(B)*; and, for comparison, the fear brow with the rest of the face uninvolved *(C)*. (From Ekman P, Friesen WV: Unmasking the Face: A Guide to Recognizing Emotions from Facial Clues. Englewood Cliffs, NJ, Prentice-Hall, 1975, with permission.)

expressions easily can be missed if the physician is not carefully observing the patient. Micro-expressions occur when the patient begins to show a true facial expression, senses this, and immediately neutralizes or masks the expression. Some micro-expressions are complete enough to show the true emotion felt, but many times they are squelched to such extent that the physician has only a clue that the patient is managing his or her facial expression.

EYES. The eyes are probably the principal organs of expression. They are so important to a person's appearance that, when anonymity is desired, only the eyes need to be covered. The eyebrows have been shown to have 40 different positions of expression and the eyelids 23. Consider the magnitude of possible combinations when all facial elements are involved as indicators of expression. The message conveyed by each position can be further modified by the length of a glance and its intensity.

The eyes can give more information for some emotions than others. Knapp (1978) found that the eyes were better than the brow, forehead, or lower face for the accurate portrayal of fear but were less accurate for anger and disgust. Even the lower eyelid alone can convey considerable information. In Figure 15–5, it is apparent that *B* depicts more sadness than *A*, but the pictures differ only in one respect—the lower eyelid.

It long has been known that *pupils* dilate when the person sees something pleasant and contract when something unpleasant is viewed. This involuntary signal can be a valuable indication of what is really going on. Oriental jade dealers wore dark glasses so that no one could see their pupils dilate when they discovered an especially valuable piece of jade. Likewise, a magician doing card tricks can tell when a preselected card is seen by a subject because of the sudden pupil enlargement. In one experiment (Hess, 1975), the pupils of males dilated when the men were shown photographs of nude females and constricted for nude males. Homosexuals demonstrated the opposite. Baby pictures produced pupil dilation in both single and married women and in married men with children. The pictures produced pupil constriction in single men and married but childless men. Dilated pupils also can indicate that listeners are interested, while constricted pupils suggest that they do not like what is being said (as well as viewed).

Sincerity is expressed with the eyes. The best method for conveying sincerity is frequent eye contact, a technique most appropriately used when listening to the other person. One trait of good listeners is that they constantly look at the speaker. A listener who does not maintain eye contact, but continues to look down or away from the speaker, may be shy, depressed, or indicating rejection of either the speaker or the comments being made. One patient recently said, "I had one student doctor who looked at his toes instead of me. If he ever opens a practice, I don't believe I would trust him." Conversely, speakers frequently may break eye contact when talking and are permitted a distant stare when formulating ideas and selecting phrases. However, they still should try to make frequent, although less prolonged and intense, eye contact.

A special kind of human-to-human awareness is conveyed by eye contact. Prolonged eye contact, or staring, can be offensive. Monkeys can be provoked to combat by a person staring at them be-

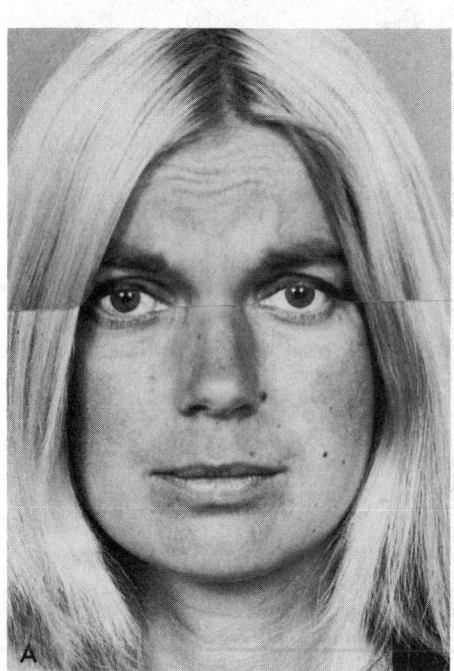 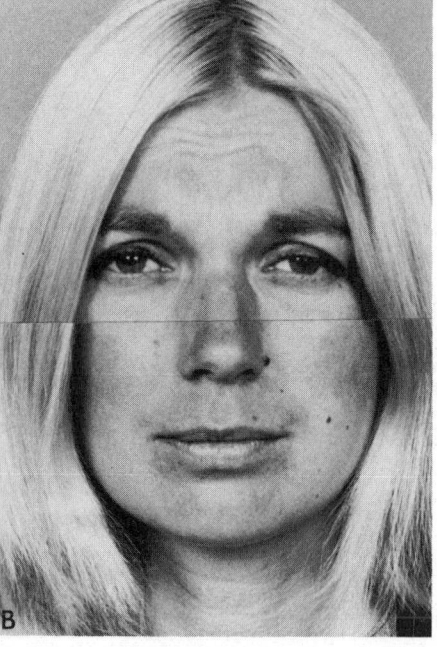

FIGURE 15–5. Sadness shown in the eyes and forehead (the mouth is neutral). The importance of the eyelids can be seen because *B* is obviously sadder than *A* but differs only in that a sad lower eyelid has been substituted for a neutral lower eyelid. (From Ekman P, Friesen WV: Unmasking the Face: A Guide to Recognizing Emotions from Facial Clues. Englewood Cliffs, NJ, Prentice-Hall, 1975, with permission.)

cause of the threat of aggression that this represents. Under other circumstances, however, staring can be flirtatious, emphasizing that the meaning of eye behavior depends on other factors in the situation.

The acceptability of eye contact varies significantly among different cultures. In the United States, focusing one's eyes on the speaker indicates respect and attention regardless of the age of the individuals involved. However, Mexican-Americans and blacks tend not to maintain as much eye contact while listening as do other Americans and may look away from the speaker more often. This is not a sign of disrespect or inattention. In Latin American countries, a younger person may be thought disrespectful if his or her eyes meet those of the adult who is speaking. A physician could be considered seductive in that culture if he or she maintained steady eye contact while talking to a patient. In the United States, it is impolite to maintain eye contact with a stranger for more than 3 seconds, but Europeans believe that longer periods of eye contact are perfectly normal. Obviously, then, the physician needs to consider the patient's cultural background when interpreting the meaning of eye contact behavior. Looking away from the speaker from time to time may be a sign of respect and sensitivity rather than the opposite. At the same time, the physician's failure to look a patient in the eye can be dehumanizing and cause the patient to feel more like an object than a person. Patients are most comfortable when the physician looks at them approximately 50 per cent of the time and are uncomfortable when eye contact is avoided.

The frequency of eye contact also can provide clues to whether the patient is anxious or depressed. Waxer (1977) demonstrated that both the presence of anxiety and its intensity could be determined on the basis of nonverbal cues alone. Prominent cues involved the hands, mouth, and torso. Anxious patients generated more stroking of themselves, such as hand on hand or hand on face, and had more twitches and tremors. They smiled less, and their torsos were stiff and rigid as though they were afraid to move. They also had a more rapid respiratory rate. The eyes of anxious patients blinked frequently or darted back and forth. They looked at the interviewer as frequently as low-anxiety patients but maintained eye contact for less time on each gaze. (Similarly, the patient may interpret the physician's lack of eye contact as indicative of anxiety or discomfort, even rejection.)

Depressed patients also maintain eye contact only one fourth as long as nondepressed patients. Downward contraction of the mouth and a downward angling of the head are also cues to depression. As with the anxious patient, there is no difference in frequency of eye contact in the depressed patient; the difference is only in the duration of contact.

Patients with abdominal pain that is due to organic disease are more likely to keep their eyes open during palpation of the abdomen than those with nonspecific pain (Gray et al., 1988). This may be because the patient with genuine abdominal tenderness apprehensively watches the doctor's hand as it approaches the tender area.

HANDS. The hands will be droopy and flaccid with sadness, fidgety or grasping in anxiety, and clenched in anger. When a speaker joins his or her hands, with fingers extended and fingertips touching, it is called steepling and indicates confidence and assurance in the comments being made (Fig. 15–6).

Palms usually are held in the palm-in position. Turning the palms outward can be a subtle courting behavior (usually used by women), but more likely indicates a warm and friendly greeting (Davis, 1975).

The hands of an anxious patient can be noted to shake when holding a pen or cigarette, to twitch, or to be braced unnaturally. The white-knuckle pose of tightly locked fingers can be an effort to mask the jitters.

Hands also can be a subtle indicator of the urge to interrupt. Be alert for this sign in a patient so that important information will not be suppressed, and the patient can be given every opportunity to supply valuable information. Indications of this urge to interrupt are a slight raising of the hand or perhaps the index finger only, pulling at the ear lobe, or raising the index finger to the lips. The latter also may indicate an attempt to suppress a comment and should alert the physician to inquire further and elicit the hidden information. A patient listening in "The Thinker" position, with the index finger across the lips or extended along the cheek, or one sitting with elbows on the table and hands clenched in front of the mouth, although listening intently, may not be buying what the physi-

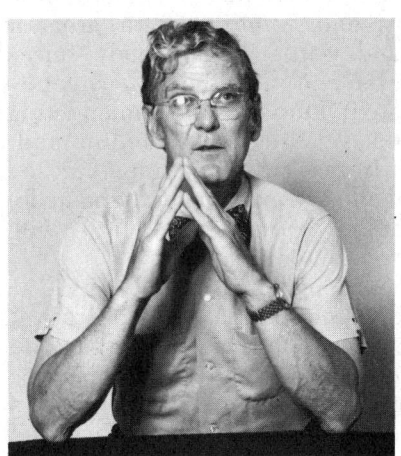

FIGURE 15–6. Steepling.

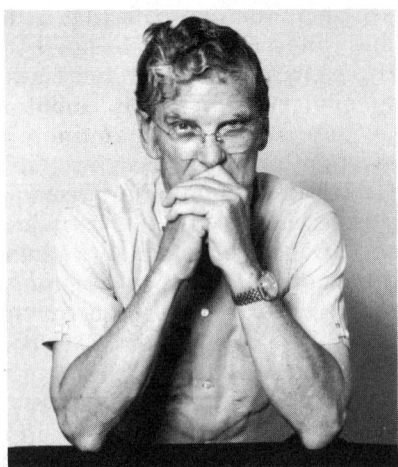

FIGURE 15–7. The defensive or "doubting Thomas" position.

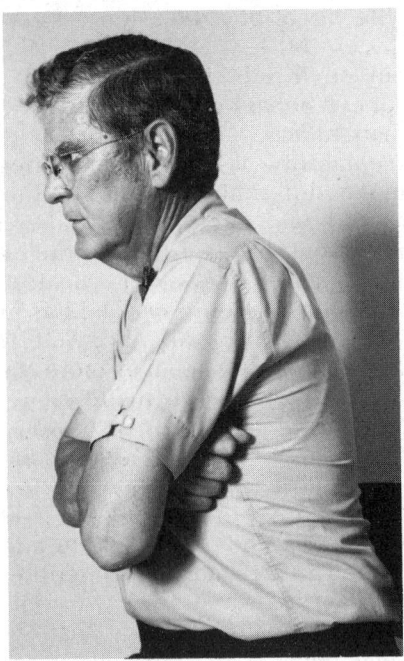

FIGURE 15–8. The resistant position, suggesting suppressed anger.

cian is saying (Fig. 15–7). Take additional time to amplify the issue or explain the diagnosis or treatment regimen further.

ARMS. Although folded arms are found in all cultures, this is considered a discovered action rather than an inborn trait, because it is a natural position of comfort that is as easily discovered by the African tribesman as the New York banker. It is the subtle ways in which the arms are held that can give clues to underlying emotions. Crossed arms can be a defensive posture, indicating disagreement with another's view, or it can be a sign of insecurity. It can also be nothing more than a position of comfort and should, as with all other signs, be considered in the context of the individual's total behavior.

Note the manner in which the arms are crossed. Are they relaxed in the normal position of comfort, or are they in a hugging posture, reflecting insecurity or sadness and indicating a need for reassurance? Anger can be seen in clenched fists that are held tightly against the body in a holding-back manner, preventing them from hitting (Fig. 15–8). If the patient has assumed a position of resistance or defensiveness, sitting with arms and legs crossed and perhaps with body turned away, search for the reason for this defensiveness and try to eliminate it. Perhaps a recommendation that the patient stop smoking is threatening and difficult to accept. In that case, it is important to make an additional effort to explain the rationale for the recommendation; do not hurry over it with a brief comment or admonition.

LEGS. Although crossing the legs is a common position of comfort, it can also indicate a shutting out of, or protection against, the outside world. If crossed legs in a patient confirm the total kinesic picture of resistance, including crossed arms and other signals discussed earlier (Fig. 15–9), make every effort to identify the reason for the resistance and correct it before proceeding further. Diagnos-

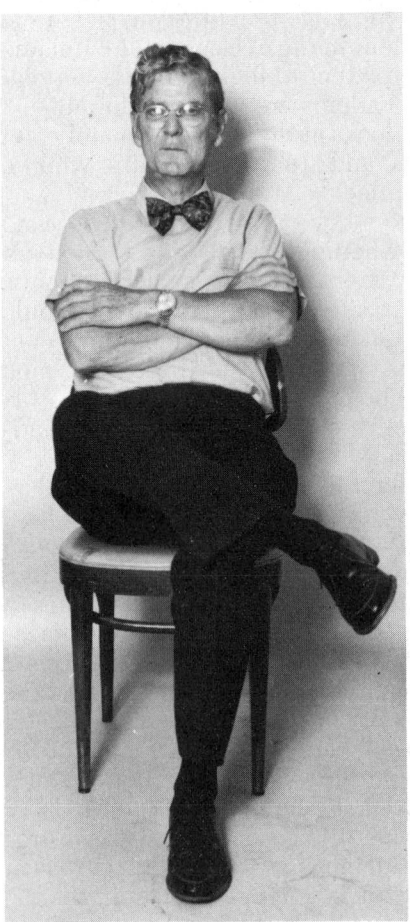

FIGURE 15–9. The defensive position.

tic information obtained from a resistant patient is likely to be incomplete, and instructions are unlikely to be followed.

Note also the position of the feet and their movement. Just as anxiety is associated with fidgety hand movements, so it is with the fidgety, constantly moving foot. An anxious or scared person may sit forward in the chair with feet placed in the ready-to-run position, one foot in front of the other. The angry person is more likely to place the feet widely apart in a position of stability, while the feet of a sad person tend to move in a slow, circular pattern.

PREENING GESTURES. Preening gestures, such as the male pulling up socks, adjusting a tie, or combing hair and the female adjusting clothing or using a mirror to review makeup, may not necessarily be seductive in nature but can be an attempt to establish rapport and good interpersonal relations. If the preening is intended to be flirtatious, however, the woman may cross her legs, place a hand on her hip, caress her leg, or stroke the arm or thigh in some fashion. The flirtatious male usually will utilize gaze holding and head tilt to accentuate normal preening gestures. The physician should remain alert to the accentuation of normal preening gestures into courtship actions in order to identify the seductive patient and deal with the issue early, before unknowingly encouraging the patient to proceed further along this course.

RESPIRATORY AVOIDANCE RESPONSE. The respiratory avoidance response involves a frequent clearing of the throat when no phlegm or mucus is present. All animals exhibit a respiratory avoidance response as a means of clearing something unpleasant or undesirable from the respiratory tract. This action also can be a nonverbal indication of disgust or rejection. When physicians find themselves doing this, they should observe the accompanying circumstances and note whether posterior pharyngeal mucus is truly present.

NOSE RUB. Another component of the respiratory avoidance response is the nose rub (Fig. 15–10). This involves a light or subtle rub of the nose with the index finger and signals rejection of a statement being made either by the subject or by another individual. The nose rub to relieve an itch is usually vigorous and involves a repeated series of rubs, whereas that of the respiratory avoidance response is soft and consists of one or two light strokes, often involving nothing more than a light flick of the nose. Morris (1977) described the nose flick as "a reflection of the fact that a split is being forced between inner thoughts and outward action" (p. 111). It can be associated with lying or with the struggle to appear calm while suppressing anger or discomfort.

This sign can be quite useful in patient interviewing. For example, the physician may ask a patient, "How are things at home?" The patient may answer, "Fine," then clear his or her throat and

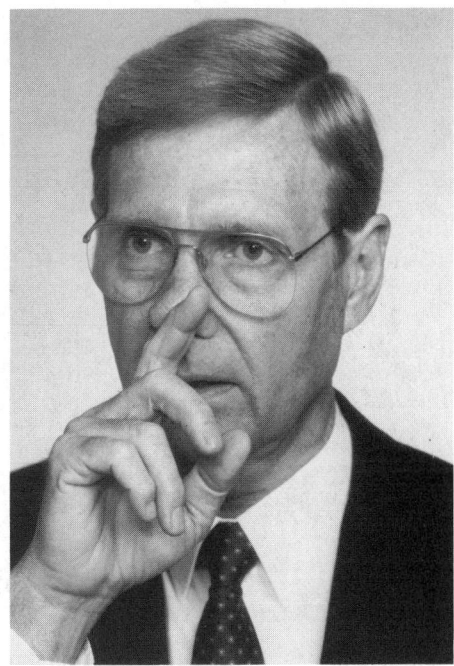

FIGURE 15–10. The nose rub, a variation of the respiratory avoidance response.

lightly rub the nose with the index finger. He or she is actually saying, "I don't like what you are asking me," or "I feel uncomfortable with my answer; things really aren't going very well at home." If there is a cause to pursue the issue further, a simple comment such as "Really?" or "You mean not even an occasional argument?" may lead to a flood of information masked by the previous response.

VERBAL–NONVERBAL MISMATCH. Another example that what a patient is saying may be in conflict with what is being felt is a "verbal–nonverbal mismatch," for example, when the patient answers "fine" to "how are things between you and your husband" while looking sad and avoiding eye contact (Quill, 1989). If the patient answered negatively to the question "Have you ever had a venereal disease" and at the same time exhibited a nose rub, this topic should be followed up with a similar inquiry later, perhaps while doing the physical examination, when the patient may feel more comfortable after better rapport has been established.

Other clues that the patient may not be telling the truth or that there are repressed feelings are asymmetrical facial expressions and a prolonged smile or expression of amazement. Almost all authentic facial expressions fade after 4 or 5 seconds (Ekman, 1985).

Proxemics (Spatial Factors)

Proxemics is the study of how people unconsciously structure the space around them. This structuring varies with every culture. North Ameri-

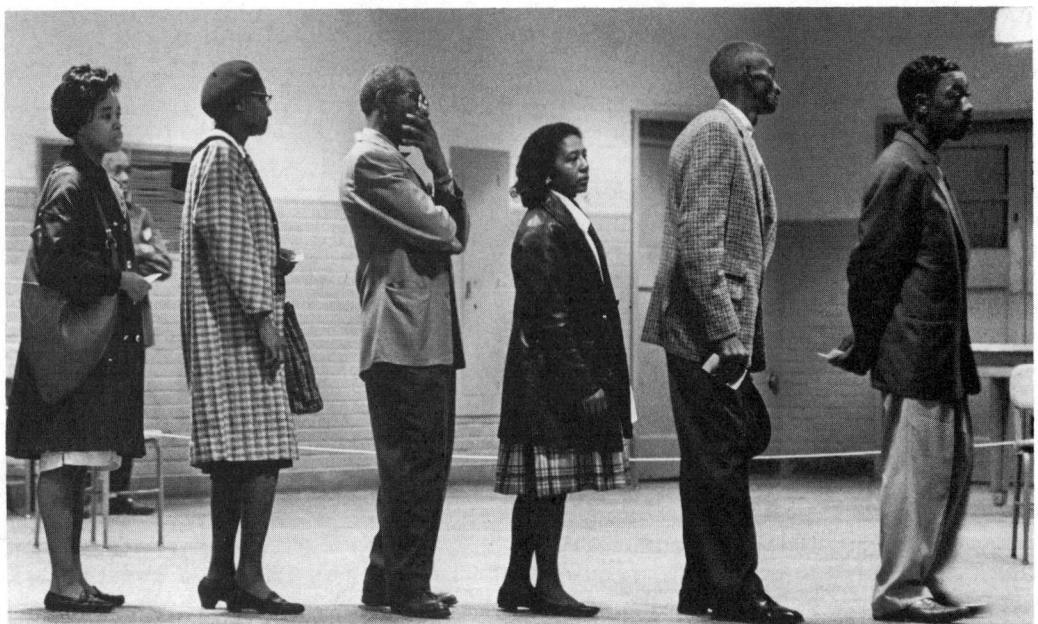

FIGURE 15–11.   The "body bubble" surrounding strangers in a queue. (Reproduced by permission of Magnum Photos, Inc., New York.)

cans, for example, maintain a protective "body bubble" of space about 2 feet in diameter (close enough to touch) around them when they interact with strangers or casual acquaintances. Violators of that space are considered intruders and cause the person to become defensive (see Fig. 15–11). In the Middle East, no such bubble exists, and it is proper to invade this area. In fact, not to do so may be interpreted as unfriendly and standoffish. Arabs prefer to stand close enough to touch and smell the other person. Americans, however, if forced to stand close together, as on a crowded subway, will use their eyes (distant gaze) to maintain a more proper distance. An arm's length is a good measure of the appropriate personal distance for most people. A wife can stand inside her husband's bubble, but she will be unhappy if another woman invades this sphere of privacy (and vice versa).

Robert Frost said that "good fences make good neighbors." In suburbs and small towns, people are more likely to talk to each other while in their backyards if a fence indicates the boundary than if there is a communal yard (McCaskey, 1979). Marking the boundary helps maintain territoriality and actually brings the neighbors closer together than when there is no fence.

Intimate space has been classified as that ranging from close physical contact to 18 inches, *personal* space from 18 inches to 4 feet, *social* space from 4 feet to 12 feet, and *public* space 12 feet and beyond. Placing a desk between two people shifts personal space to social space. The office desk also can be a barrier to communication when it is placed between the physician and patient, thereby emphasizing the illusion of the physician's impor-

tance and power. There may be occasions when this is desired, but it usually is not necessary in a family physician's office. Office furniture should be arranged so that a minimum number of obstacles lie between physician and patient. The patient also should be made to feel as comfortable as possible, with a minimum of bright lights, smoke, and other irritating stimuli present in the room.

Hidden (or Masked) Communication

Although the average person has a symptom about every 6 days, he or she visits a physician only once every 4 months. Some people will visit a physician much more frequently than others for the same symptom. The group that visits more frequently tends to have a higher level of anxiety, fear, grief, or frustration. It is the physician's responsibility to search for, identify, and treat organic disease if it is present, yet in about half of the cases none will be found. Of course, it is equally important to identify the reason for these visits—the basis for the heightened concern or increased anxiety. A person may see a minor symptom as a potential catastrophe if he or she thinks it may be a sign of cancer similar to that causing a parent's death. Is the patient really there "just for a blood pressure check" or because of concern over the condition of his or her coronary arteries since a friend recently had an acute myocardial infarction? If the physician deals only with the symptoms, the real concerns may go undetected, and the result will be a dissatisfied and noncompliant patient.

Barsky (1981) cautioned that "patients who express dissatisfaction with their medical care should be questioned about this, as they may be dissatisfied because their real motivation in seeking care has not been illuminated" (p. 492). He also advised the physician to investigate the patient's current life stresses when visits are made if there is no change in clinical status.

Patient Expectations

Patients may come to a physician because of what they imagine is causing their symptoms rather than because of the symptoms themselves. Identifying what patients hope can be done for them—that is, focusing on their expectations for the visit—often will reveal hidden reasons for the visit. The physician should be sure to address the patient's expectations and make certain that the interpretation is correct. Rapport and satisfaction will be enhanced if the physician identifies and satisfies the patient's expectations for the visit. Dissatisfaction results when these expectations go unmet.

Hand-on-the-Doorknob Syndrome

The patient's parting phrase is sometimes a clue to the primary reason for the visit, or it may reflect another issue of great concern that is emotionally threatening and could not be voiced until adequate courage was summoned at the moment of departure. It sometimes finally surfaces as a last, desperate attempt to communicate—because, with hand on door, escape is readily accessible if the physician's reaction is unfavorable. Reasons for this hidden communication by the patient are important and must be recognized and dealt with. Because of fear of rejection or humiliation, the patient may test the physician with minor complaints before mentioning the real reason for the visit (Quill, 1989). The physician must be alert to any unusual behavior during an interview, such as slips of the tongue, unexpected responses, and overly enthusiastic denials. Further search should be made for the underlying reason for the visit when a patient presents with a trivial complaint that appears inappropriate at that time. It is a good practice to ask the patient routinely at the end of a visit "Is there anything we have not covered or anything else you would like to ask me?"

Patients with a fear of cancer, for instance, often are unable to voice their concern to the physician. Instead, they present with somatic complaints or contrived reasons that necessitate a complete examination. They are hopeful that the examination will allay their fears without it being necessary to express them openly. For example, a female patient presenting for a complete physical examination actually may be concerned over the possibility of a carcinoma of the breast, which her elder sister may have had at the same age or for which a friend recently had surgery. Such situations emphasize the need for a complete family history and a discussion of any patient concerns, in an effort to allow these feelings to surface. Attention then should be paid to alleviating the anxiety. Apprehension regarding cancer is widespread, and often the only cure for this fear is a therapeutic conversation with the physician. It is very likely that most patients harbor some fear of cancer, and, therefore, following a complete history and physical examination, specific mention should be made that no signs of cancer can be detected at this time. If this precaution is not taken, a patient with a hidden anxiety or fear of cancer may remain suspicious that a cancer could be present, because there was no apparent attempt to look specifically for it.

The "Oh, by the way" is a variation of the hand-on-the-doorknob syndrome. White and associates (1994) found that 21 per cent of patients in their study raised new problems at the end of the visit. Only one fourth of the physicians asked the patients at the end of the visit if they had any more questions.

Listening Well

A good family physician must be a good listener. Of all the communication skills essential to rapport, the ability to listen well is probably the most important. All the information in the world about body language, vocal messages, and nonverbal cues is of limited value unless it helps the family physician be a better listener.

The appearance of readiness to listen is aided by bending forward and maintaining eye contact. The physician can discourage a patient from talking simply by looking away or writing in the medical record. Well-chosen questions can be rendered useless by inappropriate nonverbal behavior.

Physicians should listen to patients in an alert and uncritical manner. They should appear relaxed yet attentive. They should be nonjudgmental, so as not to inhibit the patient's expression and willingness to relate problems of a sensitive nature.

Analyses of doctor–patient interviews reveal that, on the average, the doctor rather than the patient does most of the talking, although the physicians, when questioned, usually imagine the reverse. In general, the less the physician says during an interview, the more the patient will say.

Silence

Silence can be as effective a means of eliciting further information as direct questions. The timing is important, however, and silence should be used as a technique only when the physician is relatively certain that there is more information to follow the last statement. A shift of position, or a nod and a smile, properly timed and coupled with silence, can be more effective than an encouraging comment. Nonverbal encouragement to continue is less distracting and may be more facilitative than the verbal form.

Attorneys use silence in the courtroom to get witnesses to say more than they had intended. They wait silently as if the witness has not given a complete answer, and usually do get additional information. Silence can be effective as long as the patient feels more inclined to fill the void than the physician. This is of value, however, only when there is more information to be obtained. It is said that Charles DeGaulle thought that silence was the ultimate power tool, and in his speeches he would gain control by looking at the audience, never breaking eye contact, and saying nothing.

Interruption

The patient may be following a line of thought and may be about to open up more but must stop and refocus if the physician "captures" the patient's attention with a question. The physician should interrupt a patient's statement only if it is necessary to change the conversation to a new topic, clarify an issue, elicit information not produced spontaneously, offer reassurance, or reduce patient anxiety.

Physicians usually use closed-ended questions to interrupt the patient and thereby inappropriately control the interview. Beckman and Frankel (1984) found that 69 per cent of patients (52 of 74) had only 18 seconds to complete their initial complaint before being interrupted by their physician. This usually occurred after the patient stated only a single concern and it effectively halted the further flow of information from the patient. This prematurely terminates opportunities for patients to present their primary concerns. Only 1 of the 52 patients subsequently returned to and completed their opening statement. In these recorded office interviews, only 23 per cent of the patients were permitted to complete their list of problems uninterrupted, and, when they were, the complete statements usually took less than 60 seconds and none required more than 2.5 minutes. Male physicians tend to interrupt more often than female physicians, and black female patients are interrupted much more frequently than white males (West, 1984).

Interviewing Effectively

The skilled family physician can spend 10 minutes with a patient and the patient feels it was 20. This is far better than the physician who spends 20 minutes but leaves patients feeling that the physician was in a hurry and they were encroaching on the physician's precious time every minute of the visit.

Overly brief or abrupt conversations in the office or at the bedside can damage rapport severely. Physicians signal how much time they plan to spend by a variety of nonverbal cues, and patients rarely have the courage to counter this by asking for more time. The physician who hurriedly asks "How are you?" while flipping through a chart with only a quick glance at the patient destroys communication. Even the busiest physicians can accomplish wonders in a very few minutes by indicating that their full attention is on the patient: Everyone remembers an outstanding physician who, for whatever time was available, would, by a relaxed posture and attentive manner, truly communicate with the patient.

The interesting and revealing study by Korsch and Negrete (1972), involving analysis of taped doctor–patient encounters in a pediatric clinic, revealed that many of the mothers were dissatisfied because the physician paid too little attention to their concern and apprehension about their child. Their attitude had little relationship to the amount of attention that the physician actually paid to the infant, which was usually very adequate.

Even in an established family practice where essentially none of the patients was dissatisfied with the physician, 54 per cent of the patients either forgot to mention something of concern or misunderstood facts about diagnosis or treatment (Snyder et al., 1976). Twenty-nine of the 84 patients forgot to tell the physician something that was bothering them. This illustrates the wisdom of concluding every interview with the statement "Is there anything else bothering you that we haven't discussed?" Snyder et al. suggested that "the physician will be well advised to consciously underestimate his ability to communicate" (p. 276). Rather than assume that patients have understood the instructions, ask them to repeat the instructions as they understood them. Patients with chronic illnesses, and those visiting the physician for the first time, are most likely to misunderstand treatment instructions. When seeing a patient with a chronic illness, assess the patient's understanding of instructions given at a previous visit by asking, "What medications are you taking?" or "How are you taking your medication?" A patient seen for the first time can be asked, "How have you been treating this problem?"

When meeting a new patient, the method used to address the patient during the introduction can help establish rapport by conveying an atmosphere of mutual respect. Use the patient's name during the introduction, during the interview, and on leaving. An appropriate introduction would be, "Good morning, Mrs. Brown, I'm Dr. ___" or "Good morning, Mrs. Brown. I'm ___ ___, a second-year medical student, and I'll be taking your medical history and examining you today." It is also better to show concern for the patient with an opening statement like "How can I help you?" rather than "What brings you here today?"

Rapport can be influenced positively or negatively by how the physician addresses the patient.

Although the majority of patients prefer to be addressed by their first name, some may be irritated by this if sufficient familiarity has not been established. A good policy is to ask the patient what they prefer to be called (e.g., by a nickname) and note this in the chart, or wait until adequate familiarity has been established. Bergman et al. (1988) found that 96 per cent of patients preferred to be addressed by their first name, and 40 per cent preferred to address the physician by first name, although only 14 per cent actually did so.

Facilitating Techniques

In addition to the nonverbal facilitating techniques of silence and body positioning mentioned previously, patients can be encouraged to talk further with simple comments such as, "And then?" or by repeating a portion of the statement just made. For example:

Patient: I have been very nervous lately.
Doctor: Nervous?

Humor

Humor can be helpful in establishing rapport, but it is also a two-edged sword and can cut the other way if used inappropriately. It can be used to "break the ice" and is most useful if it communicates the feeling that "we are all in this together." A clever airplane pilot can diffuse a tense situation or lighten the mood of delayed passengers through the appropriate use of humor. More research is needed on the value of humor in medicine so that we will know when and how to use it effectively. Norman Cousins, former editor of the *Saturday Review*, obtained relief from the pain of ankylosing spondylitis by watching comedy videotapes like "The Three Stooges" and "Abbott and Costello."

Confrontation

Confrontation, wisely used, can help establish communication and rapport. Statements such as "you look unhappy" or "you appear very anxious" are based on the physician's observation of the patient. If the physician has been unable to establish rapport, it may help to approach the issue openly and frankly: "We don't seem to be communicating very well. Can you tell me what is wrong?" This is also a useful maneuver when a previously good relationship suddenly turns sour.

Summarization (or Paraphrasing)

Summarization is a brief restatement of what the patient has said and gives both the interviewer and patient a chance to correct errors or misunderstanding. It demonstrates the physician's interest in the patient's history and his or her effort to collect the facts accurately. A summary gives the patient an opportunity to add more details but also lets him or her know you were listening. The physician can restate what the patient has said and em-

phasize the important points to assure clear understanding. Summarization assures that both parties are using the same definitions and minimizes inappropriate assumptions. "Let me see if I have understood you correctly" or "Am I understanding this correctly?" are good ways to introduce a paraphrase.

Summarizing is also a subtle way of focusing on the important facts in the history without asking closed-ended questions that may inhibit the patient. A summary also can be used to change the subject when the physician wants to move on to another topic.

Concluding a History

In an effort to avoid leaving gaps in the history or allowing patient concerns to go unattended, it is wise to conclude every complete history with the statement "Is there anything else you would like to mention?" or "Is there anything that we have not discussed?" This excellent practice is of little value, however, if at the same time the physician puts away pen and pad, closes the chart, and starts edging toward the door.

Open-Ended Questions

Probably the single most valuable rapport-promoting element of verbal communication is the use of open-ended questions at the onset of an interview. "Tell me more about it" is both an interview technique and a state of mind. The physician who understands that no checklist of "yes/no" questions can possibly portray the patient as a unique human being will create an atmosphere of sensitivity and interest that contributes greatly to the early establishment of rapport. Once the broad outlines of the patient's unique situation are indicated, detailed questioning moves along quickly.

Specific questions beget specific answers and rarely anything more. However, the physician may wish to use this technique on occasion, as when dealing with the verbose, rambling patient who refuses to stick to the point or when specific information is needed. When more general or hidden data are sought, however, the physician must choose questions and gestures that offer the maximal potential for obtaining information. In order to be effective, open-ended questioning requires that the physician appear relaxed and ready to listen regardless of the amount of pressure from waiting patients. Once it becomes apparent that more time is necessary than is available, a new appointment should be made so that adequate time is assured.

Signals That Discourage Communication

While appearing to respond affirmatively and facilitate the conversation, people in fact can turn off the speaker if they frequently comment "yes" in a manner that conveys disinterest or impatience. Everyone has experienced the person who says "yes" before the sentence is finished or the point made. Patients can be subdued and reduced to silence in a similar manner—intentionally or unintentionally.

Confidentiality

Confidentiality is a cardinal principle of professionalism. Effective communication requires that the patient feel secure in the knowledge that all information will be kept strictly confidential. It is the ethical responsibility of each physician to maintain this bond of confidentiality. The family physician must appreciate this intimate and confidential bond and avoid any threat to its dissolution. Hippocrates said, "And whatever I shall see or hear in the course of my profession, as well as outside my profession in my intercourse with men, if it be what should not be published abroad, I will never divulge, holding such things to be holy secrets."

Assurance that all information and actions will be kept confidential is especially important when dealing with adolescents. They may not be aware of this basic ethical principle in the medical profession or realize that it applies to them. They may be reluctant to share information and trust completely for fear that parents or peers may find out.

Complex problems of confidentiality can arise for the physician who cares for several members of the same family. Family members often can provide important information that supplements what the clinician learns directly from the patient. Unfortunately, information sometimes may be offered only on the promise that it will not be disclosed to the patient. Remembering who said what and about whom and what information is privileged and what is not quickly can result in an impossible situation for the family physician. Secrets rarely can be kept for long; the patient sooner or later learns what has been confided, thus straining the bonds of trust. In general, it is best not to be a party to secrets but rather to find a way to discuss sensitive material. Not infrequently, the very issues about which secrecy is requested are central to the patient's problem. If rapport is to be maintained, the physician must diplomatically explore the possibility of dealing with such problems in a constructive fashion as soon as the patient's situation permits.

Rapport with Families

No patient exists in a social vacuum. Visible or invisible, family and friends provide a social environment that exerts an important influence on the clinical course of disease. The family usually has a stronger emotional influence on the patient than does the physician, so effective communication with the patient's family is an important element in successful patient care. Their positive support is necessary if the physician's plan of management

is to be carried out. Family support of the physician's treatment regimen can help ensure that a patient remains on a prescribed diet, takes medication as instructed, rests appropriately, or maintains a proper exercise program. An unsupportive family attitude could negate or severely jeopardize previous gains in treatment.

Family, friends, and colleagues can be valuable sources of important information regarding the patient's illness beyond that given by the patient, including facts that were forgotten, repressed, or even unknown to the patient. Communication should be established through the most responsible family member (other than the patient). However, it is important that such discussion be known to patients and a summary of the discussion shared with them by the physician to avoid a misunderstanding or conflict of ideas when patient and family interact. If the patient and the family have different sets of information, they may become suspicious of future communications with the physician. Any frustration on the patient's part resulting from inadequate communication will be magnified considerably by family members. Any defect in family communication can create difficulties directly related to the number of interested individuals within the family, often causing a small problem to reach enormous proportions.

Communication with concerned family and friends need not be time consuming. If a serious or prolonged illness is involved, a family conference can outline what can be expected and what will be done. It is usually possible to identify one family member as the communication channel to whom future reports will be given, thus avoiding frequent and repetitious calls. Many clinicians find that optimal control and satisfaction is achieved by initiating the calls themselves on a regular schedule.

Lack of understanding the family's concerns and inadequate communication with family members is a major factor leading to malpractice suits. Beckman et al. (1994) found that devaluing the patient or family views and failing to understand their concerns was a major reason mentioned by plaintiffs. The most common complaint was the feeling of being deserted by the physician and feeling alone when the physician would not return calls or return to the bedside as promised, especially after an adverse event.

Rapport with Children

Working with children is one of the delights of practice. Children have a quality of freshness and directness that adults often lack. There are no secret formulas for interacting with the young, although there are cautions to be observed. Most procedures are not uncomfortable if one exercises patience, but forced gaiety and false promises that "it won't hurt" immediately are perceived as dishonest, and, once trust is destroyed, it may never be regained by any physician. It is usually possible to find ways to elicit the cooperation of the apprehensive child. A separate pediatric examination room, with appropriate decor, is reassuring. White coats need not be worn if the child has unpleasant associations with such uniforms. Examining the ear of the mother or an older sibling, for example, before examining the child often allays anxiety. Let the child handle the stethoscope or otoscope. Simple rewards also can make the physician's office a place of interest for the child. Accompanying other members of the family on visits to the physician helps the child gain familiarity with the office and staff. The physician who spends a few extra minutes with children and family early in the professional relationship will reap enormous dividends in years to come.

Rapport with the Elderly

The older patient is becoming an increasingly large part of the typical family practice. Treating the senior citizen can be rewarding if viewed with a positive attitude. The basis of such a perspective is a sound knowledge of geriatric medicine, which offers creative approaches for dealing with problems once viewed as frustrating or hopeless.

Elderly patients may feel that their lives are empty or meaningless and may seek satisfaction in memories of past accomplishments; usually they are appreciative of any attention paid to these meaningful segments of their lives. Whenever possible, preserve their sense of dignity and foster their feeling of continuing usefulness. Loneliness, depression, and increased dependency, where they exist, must be addressed in any treatment plan. The effort to see beyond the patient's immediate problem to the strengths and accomplishments of the older individual can lay the foundation for a positive relationship based on mutual respect. A house call can establish rapport as nothing else can; the physician gains an important perspective on the patient as a person.

A few geriatric patients can be difficult to deal with on a creative basis; the vast majority, however, will enrich a practice by bringing to it all the wisdom, insight, and maturity that comes with having successfully lived through the difficulties and gratifications that are an inevitable part of our era.

CARE WITH CARING

"One of the essential qualities of the clinician is interest in humanity, for the secret of the care of the patient is in caring for the patient." This statement by Francis Peabody (1930, p. 57) could well serve as the maxim for establishing patient rapport. While continuing to emphasize the curing aspects of medicine, family medicine places increased emphasis on its caring aspects. Caring is the opposite of apathy and implies the application of human tenderness and compassion to the curing of individuals. It involves respect for the individual as a human being and enables the physician to motivate patients to participate in their care. Physicians must convince patients that they care and are sincerely interested in providing help.

Allen Gregg has said that more mistakes in medicine are made by those who do not care than by those who do not know. The caring implies an empathetic relationship between physician and patient. Empathy is the capacity of physicians to understand what the patient is experiencing, and is best accomplished if physicians place themselves in the role of patients in an effort to understand their feelings. The capacity to understand another person's feelings is the foundation of the physician–patient relationship. This does not imply a sharing of feelings with the patient (sympathy), because the physician then would become emotionally affected. It is best that the physician avoid becoming emotionally involved in order to maintain professional equanimity and objectivity when caring for the patient.

Chekov, a physician himself, believed that medical students should spend half of their time learning what it feels like to be ill. Although this may be an extreme method for developing empathy, it is important that the student, before becoming immersed in the technical and cognitive aspects of medicine, be able to identify with the patient's feelings, fears, apprehensions, and expectations so that the knowledge acquired during medical school can be applied meaningfully in the context of these needs. Exposing students to patients in the first year of medical school, before they have been preoccupied with the diagnosis and treatment of disease, offers them an opportunity, under the watchful gaze of an instructor, to focus on the process of communication. Barriers to effective communication then can be identified. For example, a student may have difficulty permitting a patient with terminal cancer to talk about impending death. More than one student has been known to convey discomfort nonverbally by conducting the interview standing at the foot of the hospital bed, adjacent to the door, ready to escape.

Although the physician may be able to cure a disease only occasionally, he or she always can console the patient. An unknown French author has admonished the medical profession "to cure sometimes, to relieve often, to comfort always." The family physician provides personalized patient care and attempts to minimize the often frightening and dehumanizing experience to which patients are subjected in our highly structured modern medical system. The physician must strive constantly to preserve personal dignity for the patient, especially when his or her identity is threatened by a strange and somewhat frightening hospital environment. Care *for* a patient is more personal than the care *of* a patient.

Most patients have some degree of stress related to their presenting complaint, so it is important that we convey a sense of caring when attempting to resolve their problem. Fuller (1993) stated

On a daily basis I assess the disease process and adjust the medical management as needed, but my joy comes from listening carefully, helping people to identify their stressors, providing my best advice when I think it is appropriate, but always offering my caring and understanding ... I am both rewarded and fascinated to observe that people feel better just by recognizing that I care (p. 1033).

One of his patients said it best: *"No one cares how much you know, until they know how much you care."*

REFERENCES

Arntson PH, Philipsborn HG: Pediatrician-parent communication in a continuity-of-care setting. Clin Pediatr 21:302, 1982.

Barsky AJ: Hidden reasons some patients visit doctors. Ann Intern Med 94:492, 1981.

Beckman HB, Frankel RM: The effect of physician behavior on the collection of data. Ann Intern Med 101:692, 1984.

Beckman HB, Markakis KM, Suchman AL, Frankel RM: The doctor-patient relationship and malpractice: Lessons from plaintiff depositions. Arch Intern Med 154:1365, 1994.

Bergman JJ, Eggertsen SC, Phillips WR, et al: How patients and physicians address each other in the office. J Fam Pract 27:399, 1988.

Butterfield F: China: Alive in the Bitter Sea. New York, Times Books, 1982.

Darwin C: Expressions of the Emotions in Man and Animals. London, John Murray, 1872.

Davis F: Inside Intuition. New York, New American Library, 1975.

Ekman P: Telling Lies. New York, WW Norton, 1985.

Ekman P, Friesen WV: Unmasking the Face: A Guide to Recognizing Emotions from Facial Clues. Englewood Cliffs, NJ, Prentice-Hall, 1975.

Friedman HS: Nonverbal communication between patients and medical practitioners. J Soc Issues 35:82, 1979.

Fuller LE: Primary caring. JAMA 270:1033, 1993.

Gjerdingen DK, Simpson DE, Titus SL: Patients' and physicians' attitudes regarding the physicians' professional appearance. Arch Intern Med 147:1209, 1987.

Gray DW, Dixon JM, Collin J: The closed eye sign: An aid to diagnosing non-specific abdominal pain. BMJ 297:837, 1988.

Hess ET: The Telltale Eye. New York, Van Nostrand Reinhold, 1975.

Holmes OW: Medical Essays: 1842–1882. Boston, Houghton Mifflin, 1883.

Joos SK, Hickam DH, Borders LM: Patients' desires and satisfaction in general medicine clinics. Public Health Rep 108: 751, 1993.

Key MR (ed): The Relationship of Verbal and Nonverbal Communication. New York, Mouton Publishers, 1980.

Knapp ML: Nonverbal Communication in Human Interaction, 2nd edition. New York, Holt, Reinhart & Winston, 1978.

Korsch BM, Negrete V: Doctor-patient communication. Sci Am 227:66, 1972.

Larsen KM, Smith CK: Assessment of nonverbal communication in patient-physician interview. J Fam Pract 12:481, 1981.

Lau BWK: Reassurance does not always help. Can Fam Physician 35:1161, 1989.

McCaskey MB: The hidden messages managers send. Harv Bus Rev Nov-Dec: 135, 1979.

Morris D: Manwatching: A Field Guide to Human Behavior. New York, Harry N. Abrams, 1977.

Peabody FW: Doctor and Patient. New York, Macmillan, 1930.

Quill TE: Recognizing and adjusting to barriers in doctor-patient communication. Ann Intern Med 111:51, 1989.

Scheflen AE: Body Language and the Social Order—Communication as Behavioral Control. Englewood Cliffs, NJ, Prentice-Hall, 1972.

Snyder D, Lynch JJ, Gruss L: Doctor-patient communication in a private family practice. J Fam Pract 3:271, 1976.

Waxer PH: Nonverbal cues for anxiety: An examination of emotional leakage. J Abnorm Psychol 86:306, 1977.

West C: Routine Complications: Troubles with Talk between Doctors and Patients. Bloomington, Indiana University Press, 1984.

White J, Levinson W, Roter D: "Oh, by the way": The closing moments of the medical visit. J Gen Intern Med 9:24, 1994.

Widmer RB, Cadoret RJ, North CS: Depression in family practice: Some effects on spouses and children. J Fam Pract 10: 45, 1980.

SUGGESTED READINGS

Levinson D: A Guide to the Clinical Interview. Philadelphia, WB Saunders Company, 1987.

Nierenberg GI, Calero HH: How to Read a Person Like a Book. New York, Hawthorn Books, 1917.

Peck SR: Atlas of Facial Expression. New York, Oxford University Press, 1987.

Polhemus T (ed): The Body Reader: Social Aspects of the Human Body. New York, Pantheon Books, 1978.

CHAPTER **16**

PATIENT COMPLIANCE

C. EDWARD EVANS and R. BRIAN HAYNES

[The physician] should keep aware of the fact that patients often lie when they state that they have taken certain medicines.

Hippocrates

The recognition of poor compliance in ancient times belies the fact that over 90 per cent of the literature on compliance has been published since the early 1970s. Thus, although physicians have dispensed medicines and potions through the centuries in vast quantities, it is only in recent years that there has been systematic examination of whether patients actually take the treatment.

This interest in patient compliance seems to parallel the introduction of more and more efficacious medications. Whether this is fortuitous or not, it was perhaps to the patient's benefit in the past that little attention was paid to compliance, because poor compliance probably saved the patient's life on many occasions. Some treatments, especially the massive purges and bleeding of the 18th century and arsenic and hydrochloric acid of this century, certainly had lethal rather than therapeutic potential. Such lessons of the past should not be forgotten in considering compliance today, because we still prescribe many treatments of dubious value. Nevertheless, our armamentarium of useful treatments is now sizable and expanding rapidly; low patient compliance stands squarely in the way of achieving the full benefit of modern therapy.

The extent of poor compliance is distressing. Fifty per cent is a representative compliance figure for many classes of long-term therapy. Only about two thirds of those who continue under care take enough of their prescribed medication to achieve adequate blood pressure control (Haynes et al., 1979). If we look at compliance with diets and lifestyle changes, such as stopping smoking, the figures are even more dismal (Best and Block, 1979). For example, when asked to give up smoking, only about 4 per cent of patients will be able to do so and remain successful for a year.

Added to this, physicians—even family physicians—are not good at estimating compliance levels in patients (Gilbert et al., 1980). Physicians have a strong tendency to overestimate the compliance of their own patients and usually are unable to predict which patients will comply with treatment.

Fortunately, the story does not end here. There are practical methods of detecting poor compliance and strategies for improving it, as we shall see as this chapter unfolds.

DEFINITIONS

The trend in medicine, and particularly in family medicine, is away from the authoritarian caregiver toward a more democratic role that involves the patient in decisions. Thus, the use of the word "compliance" has raised objections from many physicians because it implies obedience to a superior will or intellect and anything but an adult-to-adult relationship between physician and patient. Unfortunately, no better term has surfaced. "Adherence" and "defaulting" are probably the most common alternatives, but they still carry many negative connotations. Although we recognize the problems and sympathize with the views of those who oppose the term, we will use *compliance* throughout this chapter because it is widely used and generally accepted.

Compliance has been defined as the extent to which a person's behavior (in terms of keeping appointments, taking medications, and executing lifestyle changes) coincides with medical advice (Sackett, 1976). Poor compliance is more difficult to define. What percentage of prescribed medication can a patient forget or omit before being classed as a poor complier? How are patients who take too much medication classified? These are questions without simple, straightforward answers. One way of looking at the problem is to use patient outcomes as a guide. For instance, in hypertension studies, patients taking 80 per cent or more of prescribed medication were considered compliant because this amount of medication is required to produce systematic blood pressure reduction (Sackett et al., 1975). It makes sense that efforts directed at poor compliers should be concentrated on those not achieving therapeutic goals. This obviously makes for more efficient use of resources. However, this pragmatic approach is not entirely satisfactory in that some patients who respond to treatment may be doing so because of overprescribing rather than good compliance. In the event that these patients are hospitalized or placed

269

in some other situation in which compliance may be near to 100 per cent, they may well run into serious effects of overdose.

FACTORS INFLUENCING COMPLIANCE

Many approaches, ranging from complex psychological theories to simplistic or intuitive ideas, have been taken to explain compliance behavior. None is entirely satisfactory, and many are lamentably wrong (Leventhal and Cameron, 1987).

In looking at the many factors involved, there is a natural tendency for the physician to believe that poor compliance is the patient's fault. In the final analysis this may be true. After all, it is the patient who must swallow the pill, but there are many other factors leading up to the final act of pill taking that need to be considered. For instance, what about the disease or condition being treated: Is it symptomatic or asymptomatic? Life-threatening or purely a nuisance? What about the treatment itself: Is it unpleasant to take, inconvenient, or expensive? Does it work? Is the environment in which the treatment is prescribed conducive to regular follow-up? Does the physician inspire confidence in the treatment? Do his or her attitudes interfere with compliance? All these factors could have important effects on compliance behavior, but, as we shall see, only some of them do.

The Patient

The sociodemographic characteristics or attitudes of the patient have received a great deal of attention, and such attributes as age, sex, marital status, education, intelligence, and economic status bear no consistent relationship to compliance. Two exceptions are the very young and very old, whose compliance characteristics tend to conform to those of their caregivers. Economic status can affect access to medical care, but, once a patient is in care, it does not consistently affect compliance.

Perhaps the most widely held theory of compliance behavior, probably because of its intuitive appeal, is that of the communications approach (Leventhal et al., 1984). In this model, it is proposed that patients generally do not know enough about their illness or treatment and that it is this ignorance that leads to poor compliance. It follows that adequate instruction or message generation and reception, comprehension, and retention of the message should result in improved compliance. Although it appears that this is true for short-term treatments (less than 2 weeks in duration), knowledge bears little relationship to compliance with chronic disease regimens (Haynes, 1979).

Another popular theory looks at patient motivation and beliefs. The Health Belief Model (Becker, 1976) argues that the likelihood of an individual undertaking a recommended health action is dependent on his or her perception of the level of personal susceptibility to the particular illness or condition; the degree of severity of the consequences of contracting the condition; the potential benefits or efficacy of the treatment in preventing or reducing susceptibility and/or severity; and the physical, psychological, financial, and other barriers or costs involved in initiating or continuing the treatment. The model also requires a stimulus or cue to action to trigger the appropriate behavior (compliance); this cue can be either internal (e.g., a symptom) or external (e.g., screening campaign or physician's advice). This model has been shown to have predictive value for some preventive and short-term therapeutic health actions, such as immunizations and medical regimens for acute disease, but the extent of its predictive value is modest at best (Janz and Becker, 1984).

Other models have been studied, including the behavioral learning model, which is based on cognitive and social learning theory, and the self-regulating model. As yet, no model has been developed that adequately explains a person's compliance behavior or gives a clear rationale for modifying it (Haynes et al., 1982).

The Disease

In general, disease factors are relatively unimportant as determinants of compliance. There are, however, a few exceptions to this generalization. Psychiatric patients with schizophrenia, paranoid features, and personality disorders are less compliant than other psychiatric patients—a fact that probably reduces the compliance of psychiatric patients as a whole below that of patients with nonpsychiatric disorders.

Surprisingly, no relationship has been demonstrated between the severity of symptoms and compliance, but the more symptoms a patient reports, the lower his or her compliance is likely to be. In contrast, increasing disability produced by a disease appears to be associated with better compliance. Whether this is a result of increased severity of disease or simply the result of the *increased supervision* that often accompanies increased disability has not been examined directly.

Chronic diseases requiring long-term treatment have been shown clearly to result in increasingly poor compliance. This fact is of great clinical importance in such potentially serious diseases as tuberculosis and hypertension and is more likely to be a function of the duration of the *treatment* regimen than the duration of the *disease* itself.

The Regimen

On the whole, the greater the behavioral demands of a treatment, the poorer the compliance.

This means that regimens requiring changes in lifestyle, such as dieting, exercising, and stopping bad habits, result in much poorer compliance than simply taking pills, because of the substantially greater behavioral changes demanded.

Nevertheless, it is quite clear that the greater the number of drugs or treatments prescribed for a patient, the greater the probability of poor compliance. This includes both errors of omission and commission. Although the frequency of pill taking is not so important, it also has an effect in that patients are less likely to comply with a regimen requiring four or more doses a day than with one requiring one or two daily doses.

Although alternative oral medications for the same condition do not appear to result in substantial differences in compliance, there does appear to be a difference between different treatments for different problems. This ranges from 17 per cent compliance with antacids to 89 per cent compliance with cardiac drugs (Closson and Kikugawa, 1975).

One form of alternative treatment that has been shown to have a beneficial effect is the injection of long-acting parenteral preparations. Examples of this are the use of benzathine penicillin for acute streptococcal pharyngitis and rheumatic fever prophylaxis and long-acting phenothiazines for schizophrenia, both of which have been shown to be both acceptable to patients and more successful than oral preparations. This also has been demonstrated with twice-weekly injections of streptomycin for tuberculosis. The fact that diabetics comply so poorly with self-injected insulin suggests that the success of long-acting preparations is less likely to be due to their parenteral nature than to result from the medical supervision necessary to administer them.

Another disappointment for intuitive reasoning is the fact that there is very little evidence that side effects of treatment are a major cause of poor compliance. Studies have shown that there is no difference in the reported frequency of side effects between compliers and noncompliers (Latiolais and Berry, 1969; Willcox et al., 1965). In studies in which patients were asked for reasons for their noncompliance, only 5 to 10 per cent implicated side effects (Glick, 1965; Rickels et al., 1964).

The cost of treatment is an important barrier to compliance for many people, although the total effect of cost is not obvious, as might first appear. For instance, one study showed that hospital admissions *increased* among psychiatric outpatients given drugs at nominal cost compared to a group paying regular prices (Cody and Robinson, 1977).

The Physician

The physician is obviously in a key position to influence compliance. After all, it is the physician who initiates the treatment in the majority of cases. For example, if the frequency of dose affects compliance, then, by the very act of prescribing a four-times-a-day regimen, the physician potentially is reducing compliance below the level achievable with a prescription requiring a single daily dose.

More complex than the mechanics of prescribing, however, is the interaction between physician and patient. Patients are more likely to comply with treatment if their expectations are met by the visit and if they are well satisfied with their care (Francis et al., 1969; Kincey et al., 1975). The concept of a personal physician or the feeling of knowing a physician well also has been associated with increased compliance (Ettlinger and Freeman, 1981). The problem is that dissecting the physician–patient relationship and measuring factors resulting in increased satisfaction are not easy. This is demonstrated in one study in which some patients felt they knew their physician *well* after only one visit, while others felt they still did not know their physicians after as many as *14* visits (Ettlinger and Freeman, 1981).

It is conceivable that a long-term relationship between physician and patient might even result in decreased knowledge by the physician of the patient's level of compliance. A long-time patient may not want to hurt his or her physician by admitting to poor compliance. Certainly, there is evidence that physicians are no better at estimating compliance in patients they have known for more than 5 years compared to those they have known for shorter periods; they do abysmally with both groups (Gilbert et al., 1980).

DETECTION OF POOR COMPLIANCE

Clinical Judgment

Most of us would like to believe that a good physician can detect poor compliance in his or her patients; surely, this goes along with increasing clinical experience. Unfortunately, studies have shown that this is not the case: Using clinical judgment has been shown to be no better than flipping a coin as a detection method. The first studies demonstrating this were carried out in specialty settings and with physicians who did not have an ongoing relationship with patients. Unfortunately, the hope that family physicians, with their ongoing relationships with their patients, might be in a better position to make predictions also has been dispelled. Family physicians were not only unable to detect poor compliers among their patients, but the length of time they had known their patients had no effect on their ability to predict.

The emphasis of the unreliability of clinical judgment is important in that it serves to direct us to a more systematic approach toward detection of poor compliance.

Monitoring Attendance

As referred to previously, over 50 per cent of hypertensives stop visiting their physicians within a year of starting treatment, and patients who do not show up for follow-up appointments are unlikely to be in a position to be good compliers with treatment. What is not so obvious, however, is that many physicians are unable to detect this type of noncompliance because their appointment systems are inadequate or because the patients do not take the step of making an appointment in the first place.

It follows, then, that an important method of detecting poor compliance is to watch the appointment book and day sheet. Although there is no guarantee that patients who keep appointments will comply with treatment, there is no doubt that those who do not appear for follow-up will not be in a position to comply with treatment. The importance of monitoring attendance cannot be overstressed: Dropping out of care is one of the most frequent and most severe forms of noncompliance.

Response to Treatment

Provided that the treatment prescribed is known to be efficacious, failure of a patient to respond to treatment can be used as a readily available indicator of compliance levels. However, this method of assessing compliance is not infallible. For example, patients who appear to respond to treatment may do so because they were misdiagnosed and do not have the condition of interest or because their physicians' overprescribing is compensating for their poor compliance. Nevertheless, from the compliance perspective at least, there is little need to be concerned about patients who have reached the therapeutic goal. In contrast, patients not showing a response to treatment will include patients who genuinely do not respond to therapy or who have been prescribed inadequate amounts and also will include a high proportion of poor compliers or noncompliers. Further detection methods are desirable to identify the latter positively.

Asking the Patient

Although it is not always reliable, asking the patient directly about compliance can be a very valuable and practical way of determining the pattern of medication consumption (Table 16–1). When asked directly, about half of noncompliant patients will admit to missing at least some medication (Haynes et al., 1980). One can be assured that it is highly improbable that a *compliant* patient will admit to poor compliance, so patients admitting to missing medication have a very high likelihood of being poor compliers. The converse is not true,

TABLE 16–1.   A SIMPLE METHOD TO DETECT NONCOMPLIANCE

Asking the Patient

The easiest way to detect medication noncompliance is to ask the patient.

About 50% of noncompliant patients will admit to missing at least some medication.

If a patient admits to noncompliance, you can believe him or her.

Patients admitting to poor compliance are most responsive to attempts to improve compliance.

How to Ask

Use a "matter-of-fact," nonjudgmental, nonthreatening manner.

Use an introduction that allows a patient to "save face": "Most people find it difficult to remember to take medicines. About how many pills have *you* missed in the past week?"

however, because, even under optimal interview conditions, about half of noncompliant patients will deny the fact. Patients who admit to missing medication generally overestimate the amount of medication they do take. In one study, the average overestimate was 17 per cent (Haynes et al., 1980).

It must be emphasized that the method of questioning is of paramount importance. Asking in a threatening or belligerent manner will result in reflex denial. Approaching the patient with a face-saving, nonthreatening, nonjudgmental question will yield a higher proportion of accurate responses. One way of doing this is to use an approach such as the following: "Most people find it difficult to remember to take medicines. About how many pills have *you* missed in the past week?" Because of patients' tendency to overestimate compliance, it is important to take into account that admission of any noncompliance implies a compliance rate of less than 80 per cent or as low as 40 per cent on average.

The methods of detecting low compliance described so far can be applied easily in any treatment setting and, if applied with care, will detect the majority of poor compliers (Stephenson et al., 1993). The following methods may be of help in detecting some of the remainder.

Counting Pills

As a method of proving a quantitative estimate of compliance over a period of time, pill counts can be relatively reliable so long as they are carried out in the patient's home with strict attention to bookkeeping (Haynes et al., 1980). Unless the count can be carried out in such a manner that the patient is unaware of what is going on, it becomes a one-time-only procedure. It follows that, although pill counts are very important research tools, they are not very practical for most clinical situations. It can be reasoned that using pill counts in the office or clinic will result in a bias in the direction of overestimating compliance in that patients will consciously or unconsciously only bring *some* of their unused pills with them, giving the appearance that they have taken more of the medication than is actually the case. Studies using microprocessor-equipped medication containers have shown that some patients actually dump medication in the days prior to a physician visit. In one study, 14 per cent of patients actuated their aerosol inhalers more than 100 times in a 3-hour interval (Mallion et al., 1992, Rand et al., 1992). It is virtually impossible for the bias to go in the opposite direction unless the patient is receiving the same prescriptions from two or more physicians at the same time.

In general, pill counts give higher estimates of compliance than quantitative drug assays and lower (but more accurate) estimates than patient self-reports.

Drug Levels

A laboratory test to detect the presence or absence of good compliance is an unrealistic dream. However, for some drugs, especially those with long serum half-lives resulting in relatively steady serum levels, the measurement of serum levels can be an extremely useful indication of compliance. The best examples of this are digoxin and phenytoin, for which plasma levels have been used successfully to both monitor compliance and improve it through feedback to the patient. Other drugs commonly measured in this way are phenobarbitone and other anticonvulsants, theophylline, tricyclic antidepressants, lithium, and a variety of cardiac drugs. The caution is, however, that there is a great deal of individual variation in drug absorption, metabolism, and excretion. In addition, serum levels of drugs with short half-lives only indicate how recently a dose was taken and give no information on long-term compliance.

Drug levels in urine also have been used as compliance indicators. For instance, the presence or absence of penicillin can be detected easily using inhibition of growth of the microorganism *Sarcina lutea* (Cummins et al., 1991). Although these methods and others involving inactive markers such as riboflavin, carbon-14, and nonpharmacologic traces of digoxin (Mäenpää et al., 1992) have been used in research, they are not practical methods for the clinician. What is more, single qualitative assessments of urine samples have been shown to be inferior measures of compliance to simply asking the patient (Haynes et al., 1980).

PREVENTION AND TREATMENT OF POOR COMPLIANCE

Misconceptions

Before discussing prevention and treatment, it is worthwhile to re-examine some popular misconceptions about compliance.

The first misconception is that a good clinician can identify poor compliers. In fact, clinical judgment has a poor record of detecting compliance levels. *There is no stereotypical poor complier.* This is very important, because restricting prevention and treatment strategies to patients thought to be potentially poor compliers must result in neglect of a large number of patients who need attention as well as unnecessary attention to some patients who do not require it.

Another popular and important misconception is that all that stops patients from being near-perfect compliers is their ignorance of either the condition being treated or the treatment being used. Although there is some evidence that written instructions help improve compliance for short-term regimens, even "mastery learning", in which patients were given detailed step-by-step instruction on hypertension, had no beneficial effect on long-term compliance (Sackett et al., 1975). The belief that it is possible to scare a patient into complying with treatment also has been dispelled (Leventhal et al., 1967).

Although these popular beliefs have been discredited, Logan (1978), in a survey of primary care physicians, has shown that the methods they employed to improve compliance were predominantly those that have been found lacking. What is more, methods that *have* been shown to be effective were not generally applied. Furthermore, changing the long-term behavior of physicians to manage compliance successfully cannot be done by simply informing or instructing them about efficacious interventions (Evans et al., 1984; Haynes et al., 1984).

Figure 16–1 provides a framework for thinking about strategies for helping patients to comply. Success for long-term treatments generally re-

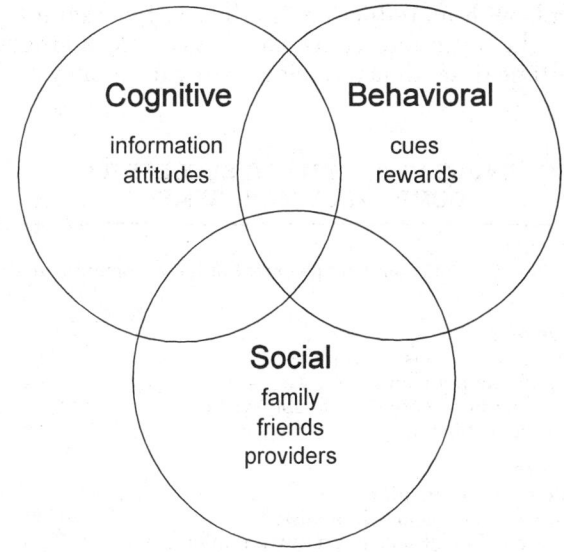

FIGURE 16–1. Factors influencing compliance. (From Evans CE, Haynes RB: Patient Compliance. *In* Rakel RE [ed]: Essentials of Family Medicine. Philadelphia, WB Saunders, 1993, p 115, with permission.)

quires adopting tactics from at least two of the areas in the figure. Thus, while addressing cognitive factors (providing the patient with clear information about the reason for and administration of the treatment) is usually sufficient for a course of treatment that lasts 1 to 2 weeks, for longer treatments instruction must be supplemented by periodic reminders (cues) and reinforcement (rewards), and the patient's family may have to be recruited to help out. Methods of detecting poor compliance were discussed earlier in the chapter; the details of the various prevention and treatment approaches follow.

Prevention

The main thrust in the prevention of poor compliance is to remove barriers to compliance. Preventing patients from dropping out from care is of primary importance. Longer waiting times are associated with higher "no-show" rates (Rockart and Hoffman, 1969), so that one aim is to keep patient waiting time to a minimum. Individual appointments at mutually convenient times help to achieve this goal. A system for follow-up, ensuring that patients leave the office with a *specific time* for a future appointment rather than with instructions to call for an appointment in, for example, 3 months, makes detection of those who do drop out much easier (Table 16–2).

Simplifying the treatment regimen will remove another barrier to compliance. An essential element of this approach is to *eliminate unnecessary medications*. In addition, medications should be prescribed that need to be taken as few times daily as possible. The frequency of dosing with many drugs can be reduced below usually prescribed levels with no reduction in efficacy. For example, tricyclic antidepressants can be given as a single bedtime dose, thus reducing dosing frequency and

---

TABLE 16–2. KEYS TO SUCCESSFUL COMPLIANCE MANAGEMENT

Detection
Monitor attendance and achievement of the therapeutic goal
Ask the patient

Prevention
Make appointments convenient
Simplify the regimen
Give clear instructions, preferably written
Make the patient an active participant

Treatment
Follow up nonattenders
Increase attention and supervision
Use cueing, feedback, and positive reinforcement
Titrate frequency of visits to compliance need
Involve spouse or other partner
Maintain compliance interventions as long as compliance is desirable

---

timing side effects so that they occur mainly during sleep. A final strategy is to prescribe the least amount of medication necessary to achieve the therapeutic goal.

It has been shown that patients who feel that they are actively involved in their own care are better compliers than those who do not (Schulman, 1979). Studies also have shown that negotiating care with the patient, rather than simply dictating or prescribing it, results in better compliance (Eisenthal et al., 1979; Kelly and Scott, 1990; Tracy, 1977). Encouraging patients to take greater responsibility for their care by asking more questions of their physicians results in improved attendance (Roter, 1977). It follows that encouraging patients to participate in and take more responsibility for their own care is another strategy for preventing poor compliance, and it not only makes scientific sense but follows contemporary trends in physician–patient relationships.

Treatment

Dropping out of care constitutes a *compliance crisis*. Mail, telephone, or physician reminders, orienting patients to the clinic, or contracting with patients can reduce broken appointments (Macharia et al., 1992). If the patient does fail to attend, there must be prompt action by the receptionist or office nurse to reschedule him or her (Takala et al., 1979). A simple method of identifying those patients for whom compliance is important (e.g., the use of chart stickers or special symbols on the day sheet) may make the receptionist's task simpler. Personal contact of persistent nonattenders by the physician himself or herself or the use of outreach services such as public health nurses are other ways of "treating" nonattendance.

Low compliance is a chronic condition without a "one-shot" cure, so treatment of poor compliance must continue as long as the regimen of prescribed treatment. To make matters worse, none of the following has improved compliance when tested alone: special learning packages (Sackett et al., 1975) and pamphlets (Swain and Steckel, 1981); special unit dose reminder pill packaging (Becker et al., 1986); counseling about medication and compliance by a health educator (Levine et al., 1979) or by nurses (Shepard et al., 1979); visits to patients' homes (Johnson et al., 1978); provision of care at the worksite (Sackett et al., 1975); self-monitoring of blood pressure (Johnson et al., 1978; Shepard et al., 1979); tangible rewards (Shepard et al., 1979); and group discussions (Shepard et al., 1979). Although these tactics have not worked alone, many have been part of more complex interventions that have been successful; whether they are essential parts of these complex interventions or just along for the ride is difficult to say.

Most successful compliance interventions have

two features in common: (1) increased supervision of, or attention to, the patient; and (2) intentional reinforcement, reward, or encouragement of compliance (Haynes et al., 1987).

A variety of inducements to comply have been used, including feedback of blood pressure response to hypertensive patients either by the provider (McKenney et al., 1973; Takala et al., 1979) or by the patient taking his or her own blood pressure (Haynes et al., 1976; Nessman et al., 1980); small tangible rewards for improved compliance and/or therapeutic response (Haynes et al., 1976; Shepard et al., 1979; Swain and Steckel, 1981); medication tailored to daily schedules to decrease forgetting and inconvenience (Haynes et al., 1976; Logan et al., 1979); encouragement of family support (Levine et al., 1979); stimulation of self-help through group support and discussion (Levine et al., 1979; Nessman et al., 1980); negotiation of a brief written contract with the patient to improve health behavior (Swain and Steckel, 1981); and calling back patients who miss appointments (Bass et al., 1986; Peterson et al., 1984; Takala et al., 1979).

Many individuals other than physicians have taken an effective part in this process. Nurses, pharmacists, health educators, psychologists, and even individuals with no formal health training have played a key role in successful interventions.

In summary, the treatment of poor compliance involves many approaches. For short-term treatments, simple, clear instructions are sufficient. For longer term treatments, there must be follow-up of nonattenders by telephone or mailed reminders. In addition, the practitioner must increase attention to and supervision of poor compliers and provide rewards or positive reinforcement for good compliance that could include, among other simple maneuvers, simple praise and extending the time between appointments for those responding to treatment. Inui et al. (1976) have shown that most of these maneuvers can be incorporated with success into regular practice by simple focusing on compliance for a few moments during each encounter with the patient, emphasizing the importance of following the regimen, and tailoring medication to daily routines. This can be accomplished without necessarily prolonging the visit. Most importantly, it is clear that all compliance interventions applied to noncompliers must be maintained as long as treatment is prescribed.

ETHICAL ISSUES

"Am I my brother's keeper?" (Genesis 4:9). This question highlights the dilemma in which most physicians find themselves when they are pressed to extend their compliance-improving strategies beyond a simple office visit. As with most questions of ethics, there is no easy answer.

The decision to apply tactics deliberately designed to change the compliance behavior of patients should meet several ethical standards, which apply to all therapeutic interventions (Levine, 1980). First, the diagnosis must be correct. Second, the therapy to be complied with must be of established efficacy. Third, neither the illness nor the proposed treatment should be trivial. Fourth, the patient must be an informed and willing partner in any attempt to alter his or her compliance. Finally, the method employed to improve compliance also must be of demonstrated effectiveness.

Having applied these standards and embarked on a course of treatment, it makes no sense, ethically or otherwise, for the physician to abandon a patient at the first sign of poor compliance. Most physicians consider it *unethical* to withhold efficacious treatment from a patient with a serious physical disease. Why then should it be *ethical* to consider withholding treatment when the condition is *noncompliance?*

FUTURE TRENDS

The advent of the personal computer has resulted in increasing use of microcomputers and microcomputer networks in physicians' offices. Although initial applications have been for business and office management purposes, the computerization of health records affords a potential for monitoring patient compliance and assisting in the management of poor compliers (Haynes and Walker, 1987).

Computerized appointment systems make it possible to provide patients with appointment times for long periods ahead and easily can be modified to flag nonattenders and produce automatic reminders. The ability to record age, sex, and diagnoses makes it possible to design a system that can improve *provider* compliance with screening and preventive maneuvers (Bypass et al., 1988; Hogg, 1990). Medication systems that store prescribing information can form the basis of a system that monitors whether patients are at least requesting prescription refills on time (Steiner et al., 1988). The potential is great, but it will require both effort and expense by physicians to make it work.

What of other advancements? The technology that brought us the efficacious treatments also is helping with compliance—drugs with long half-lives, long-acting parenteral preparations, and conjunctival inserts. As more drugs become available for continuous transdermal absorption, it may be that the administration of medication by transdermal patches will result in better compliance than drugs given by the oral route (Burris et al., 1991). Although the use of microprocessor-equipped pill boxes as a monitoring or surveillance tool raises ethical problems, the use of the same technology as a patient reminder could prove worthwhile (McKenney et al., 1992).

CONCLUSION

In dealing with compliance, we have concentrated consciously on compliance with medication, emphasizing long-term medications. This is not because we believe that compliance with short-term medications is inconsequential or that there is no problem of compliance with lifestyle or other behavioral changes. On the contrary, both of these areas are very important and, in fact, the exploration of noncompliance with lifestyle changes is a field of study in its own right.

It is our hope that we have raised the level of compliance consciousness in the reader. Being aware of the problem and the difficulties in detecting it are essential before any treatment can be carried out.

The approaches to treatment we suggest are practical and well within the reach of practicing physicians. At last, after centuries of ineffectual ministrations, we have treatments that actually work; it behooves us as providers of those treatments to give them every opportunity to be effective.

The past one or two decades have brought the therapist together with the patient, his or her family, and other members of the health care team in jointly working toward the full effectiveness of potent treatments. The rewards of this alliance are great—reduction of morbidity, disability, and preventable deaths. The family physician is in an ideal position to share in these rewards.

REFERENCES

Bass MJ, McWhinney IR, Donner A: Do family physicians need medical assistants to detect and manage hypertension? Can Med Assoc J 134:1247, 1986.

Becker LA, Glanz K, Sobel E, et al: A randomized trial of special packaging of antihypertensive medications. J Fam Pract 22:357, 1986.

Becker MH: Sociobehavioral determinants of compliance. *In* Sackett DL, Haynes RB (eds): Compliance with Therapeutic Regimens. Baltimore, Johns Hopkins University Press, 1976, pp 40–49.

Best JA, Block M: Compliance in the control of cigarette smoking. *In* Haynes RB, Taylor DW, Sackett DL (eds): Compliance in Health Care. Baltimore, John Hopkins University Press, 1979, pp 202–222.

Burris JF, Vasilios P, Wallin JD, et al: Therapeutic adherence in the elderly: Transdermal clonidine compared to oral verapamil for hypertension. Am J Med 91(1A):22S, 1991.

Bypass P, Hanlon PW, Hanlon LCS, et al: Microcomputer management of a vaccine trial. Comput Biol Med 18:179, 1988.

Closson R, Kikugawa C: Non-compliance varies with drug class. Hospitals 49:89, 1975.

Cody J, Robinson A: The effect of low-cost maintenance medication on the rehospitalization of schizophrenic outpatients. Am J Psychiatry 134:73, 1977.

Cummins D, Heusschkel R, Davies SC: Penicillin prophylaxis in children with sickle cell disease in Brent. BMJ 302:989, 1991.

Eisenthal S, Emery R, Lazare A, et al: "Adherence" and the negotiated approach to patienthood. Arch Gen Psychiatry 36:393, 1979.

Ettlinger PRA, Freeman GK: General practice compliance study: Is it worth being a personal doctor? BMJ 282:1192, 1981.

Evans CE, Haynes RB, Birkett NJ, et al: Does a mailed continuing education program improve physician performance? Results of a randomized trial in antihypertensive care. JAMA 255:501, 1984.

Francis V, Korsch BM, Morris MJ: Gaps in doctor-patient communication. N Engl J Med 280:535, 1969.

Gilbert JR, Evans CE, Haynes RB, et al: Predicting compliance with a regimen of digoxin therapy in a family practice. Can Med Assoc J 123:119, 1980.

Glick BS: Dropout in an outpatient, double-blind drug study. Psychosomatics 6:44, 1965.

Haynes RB: Determinants of compliance: The disease and the mechanics of treatment. *In* Haynes RB, Taylor DW, Sackett DL (eds): Compliance in Health Care. Baltimore, Johns Hopkins University Press, 1979, pp 49–62.

Haynes RB, Davis DA, McKibbon A, et al: A critical appraisal of the efficacy of continuing medical education. JAMA 251:61, 1984.

Haynes RB, Mattson ME, Chobanian AV, et al: Management of patient compliance in the treatment of hypertension. Hypertension 4:415, 1982.

Haynes RB, Sackett DL, Gibson ES, et al: Improvement of medication compliance in uncontrolled hypertension. Lancet 1:1265, 1976.

Haynes RB, Sackett DL, Taylor DW: Practical management of low compliance with antihypertensive therapy: A guide for the busy practitioner. Clin Invest Med 1:175, 1979.

Haynes RB, Taylor DW, Sackett DL, et al: Can simple clinical measurements detect patient noncompliance? Hypertension 2:757, 1980.

Haynes RB, Walker CJ: Computer-aided quality assurance: A critical appraisal. Arch Intern Med 147:1297, 1987.

Haynes RB, Wang E, Gomes MD: A critical review of interventions to improve compliance with prescribed medications. Patient Educ Counseling 10:155, 1987.

Hogg W: The role of computers in preventive medicine in a rural family practice. Can Med Assoc J 143:33, 1990.

Inui T, Yourtee E, Williamson J: Improved outcomes in hypertension after physician tutorials. Ann Intern Med 84:646, 1976.

Janz N, Becker M: The health belief model: A decade later. Health Educ Q 11:1, 1984.

Johnson AL, Taylor DW, Sackett DL, et al: Self-recording of blood pressure in the management of hypertension. Can Med Assoc J 119:1034, 1978.

Kelly GR, Scott JE: Medication compliance and health education among outpatients with chronic mental disorders. Med Care 28:1181, 1990.

Kincey J, Bradshaw P, Ley P: Patients' satisfaction and reported acceptance of advice in general practice. J R Coll Gen Pract 25:558, 1975.

Latiolais CJ, Berry CC: Misuse of prescription medication by outpatients. Drug Intell Clin Pharmacy 3:270, 1969.

Leventhal H, Cameron L: Behavioral theories and the problem of compliance. Patient Educ Counseling 10:117, 1987.

Leventhal H, Watts J, Pagano F: Effects of fear and instructions on how to cope with danger. J Pers Soc Psychol 6:313, 1967.

Leventhal H, Zimmerman R, Gutman M: Compliance: A self-regulation perspective. *In* Gentry D (ed): Handbook of Behavioral Medicine. New York, Pergamon Press, 1984, pp 369–434.

Levine DM, Green LW, Deeds SG, et al: Health education for hypertensive patients. JAMA 241:1700, 1979.

Levine RJ: Ethical considerations in the development and application of compliance strategies for the treatment of hypertension. *In* Haynes RB, Matteson ME, Engebretson TO Jr (eds): Patient Compliance to Prescribed Antihypertensive Regimens, (NIH Publication no. 81-2102). Washington, DC, U.S. Department of Health and Human Services, 1980, pp 229–246.

Logan AS: Investigation of Toronto General Practitioners' Treatment of Patients with Hypertension. Toronto, Canadian Facts, 1978.

Logan AS, Milne BJ, Achber C, et al: Worksite treatment of hypertension by specially trained nurses: A controlled trial. Lancet 2:1175, 1979.

Macharia WM, Leon G, Rowe BH, et al: An overview of interventions to improve compliance with appointment keeping for medical services. JAMA 267:1813, 1992.

Mäenpää H, Manninen V, Heinonen OP: Compliance with medication in the Helsinki Heart Study. Eur J Clin Pharmacol 42:15, 1992.

Mallion JM, Meilhac B, Tremel F, et al: Use of a microprocessor-equipped tablet box in monitoring compliance with antihypertensive treatment. J Cardiovasc Pharmacol 19(suppl 2):S41, 1992.

McKenney JM, Munroe WP, Wright JT Jr: Impact of an electronic medication compliance aid on long-term blood pressure control. J Clin Pharmacol 32:277, 1992.

McKenney JM, Slining JM, Henderson HR, et al: The effect of clinical pharmacy services on patients with essential hypertension. Circulation 48:1104, 1973.

Nessman DG, Carnahan JE, Nugent CA: Improving compliance: Patient-operated hypertension groups. Arch Intern Med 140:1427, 1980.

Peterson GM, McLean S, Millingen KS: A randomized trial of strategies to improve patient compliance with anticonvulsant therapy. Epilepsia 25:412, 1984.

Rand CS, Wise RA, Nides M, et al: Metered-dose inhaler adherence in a clinical trial. Am Rev Respir Dis 146:1376, 1992.

Rickels K, Boren R, Stuart HM: Controlled psychopharmacological research in general practice. J New Drugs 4:138, 1964.

Rockart JF, Hoffman PB: Physician and patient behavior under different scheduling systems in a hospital outpatient department. Med Care 7:463, 1969.

Roter D: Patient participation in the patient-provider interaction: The effects of patient question asking on the quality of interaction, satisfaction and compliance. Health Educ Monogr 5:281, 1977.

Sackett DL: Introduction. *In* Sackett DL, Haynes RB (eds): Compliance with Therapeutic Regimens. Baltimore, Johns Hopkins University Press, 1976, p 1.

Sackett DL, Haynes RB, Gibson ES, et al: Randomized clinical trial of strategies for improving medication compliance in primary hypertension. Lancet 1:1205, 1975.

Schulman B: Active patient orientation and outcomes in hypertensive treatment. Med Care 17:267, 1979.

Shepard DS, Foster SB, Stason WB, et al: Cost-effectiveness of interventions to improve compliance with antihypertensive therapy. Prev Med 8:229, 1979.

Steiner JF, Koepsall TD, Fihn SD, et al: A general method of compliance assessment using centralized pharmacy records: Description and validation. Med Care 26:814, 1988.

Stephenson BJ, Rowe BH, Haynes RB, et al: Is this patient taking the treatment as prescribed? JAMA 269:2779, 1993.

Swain MA, Steckel SB: Influencing adherence among hypertensives. Res Nurs Health 4:213, 1981.

Takala J, Niemela N, Rosti J, Sivers K: Improving compliance with therapeutic regimens in hypertensive patients in a community health center. Circulation 59:540, 1979.

Tracy J: Impact of intake procedures upon client attrition in a community mental health centre. J Consult Clin Psychol 45:192, 1977.

Willcox DR, Gillan R, Hare EH: Do psychiatric out-patients take their drugs? BMJ 2:790, 1965.

CHAPTER 17

PATIENT EDUCATION

ROBERT B. KELLY and DONNA R. FALVO

There has been literally an explosion of attention given to the area of patient education in the last 20 years. Education has been suggested as a way to increase adherance, to improve satisfaction, to lower cost, to reduce morbidity and mortality, to enhance quality of life, and to empower patients or increase their autonomy. There was relatively little research in the field at first, but this area has developed considerably. Although the impact of patient education varies by the type of educational intervention and by the target outcome or the target population studied, careful reviewers have concluded that substantial benefits have been demonstrated from a wide range of strategies (Mullen et al., 1985). The more that interventions adhere to sound educational principles, the better they work (Simons-Morton et al., 1992).

Within the discipline of family medicine, patient education has found a home. The American Academy of Family Physicians (AAFP) has a standing Health Education Committee. The first general objective in the AAFP's mission statement is to "encourage health promotion, disease prevention and patient education, and to assume a leadership role in improving the health of the American public" (AAFP, 1993a, p. 1). The Society of Teachers of Family Medicine (STFM) has had a Working Group on Patient Education since the late 1970s (STFM, 1979). A series of annual Patient Education Conferences began in 1978, now jointly sponsored by the AAFP and STFM, drawing currently more than 300 family physicians, nurses, and other health educators. The AAFP has developed guidelines for residency curricula in the area; includes written patient education materials in its journal, *American Family Physician;* and in 1992 began to produce a series of patient education brochures for physician offices. Other professional societies have adopted policy statements that strongly support patient education. These include the American Medical Association, the American Nurses' Association, the American Hospital Association, and the American Society of Hospital Pharmacists.

We have summarized an optimistic appraisal of the effectiveness of patient education and its acceptance by professional organizations. However, its potential impact currently is limited by lack of coordination of services, by inadequate training of physicians and nurses, and by poor reimbursement for educational services that are not paired with other forms of service delivery. There is also a legitimate question of whether education has been designed to fulfill the needs of health care providers rather than to empower the patient (Webber, 1990). The AAFP sees these barriers as "challenges which are being overcome or which require attention" (AAFP, 1993b, p. 2). We assume that the future face of health care will be oriented toward improved outcomes at lower cost. We believe that patient education certainly will have a place in such a framework, but only when education as a preventive or therapeutic intervention can stand up to careful scrutiny, judged in the same manner as any other aspect of care.

DEFINITIONS

A confusing array of terms relating to education can be found in the literature. Although they often have been used interchangeably, there has been increasing divergence of meaning as concepts have evolved. The term *patient education* dates to the early 1950s, when Veterans Administration hospitals began education programs as part of an effort toward total patient care (Falvo, 1985). Other terms, such as *health education, health promotion,* and *health* or *patient instruction, teaching,* or *information,* also have been used.

For the purposes of our discussion, we define *patient education* as a process of teaching and learning that takes place in the context of the relationships between health care providers and patients. The STFM similarly has defined it as "the process of influencing patient behavior, producing changes in knowledge, attitudes, and skills required to maintain or improve health" (STFM, 1979, p. 3). We define the related concept of *health education* as a process of teaching and learning outside of a provider–patient relationship. It typically encompasses topics such as growth and development, physical or psychological processes of health and illness, or lifestyle behaviors. Health or human biology and physiology classes offered by schools are examples of health education. Health education also "includes the physician's role in

**TABLE 17–1. TOPIC AREAS OF COUNSELING
SERVICES RECOMMENDED BY THE USPSTF***

Tobacco use
Exercise
Nutrition
Motor vehicle injury
Household and environmental injury
Human immunodeficiency virus and other sexually transmitted
  diseases
Unintended pregnancy
Dental care

---

* U.S. Preventive Service Task Force

---

influencing the health status of the public through involvement with community groups and the media" (AAFP, 1993b, p. 2). When the major goal of education is to encourage healthier lifestyle behaviors in order to prevent illness and disability, this can be called *health promotion*. Health promotion is therefore a subset of patient education, health education, and disease prevention. In addition to screening interventions and immunizations, *preventive services* include "counseling," an example of health promotion as patient education (U.S. Preventive Services Task Force, 1989). Areas of patient education that are also recommended as preventive services by the U.S. Preventive Services Task Force (USPSTF) are summarized in Table 17–1.

RATIONALE

Incorporating patient education into practice meets current agendas of the public, health providers, expert panels, and policy makers. It is clear that the public wants to be better informed about every aspect of their health care. This state of affairs is a natural outgrowth of the consumer rights and feminist movements of the last 30 years. Examples of this trend include the National Consumer Health Information and Health Promotion Act of 1976 and the 1975 *Patient's Bill of Rights* of the American Hospital Association. People basically want more ability and autonomy in decision making about their health, and are more satisfied with their medical care when they perceive that their need for information has been met. Knowledge and skills gained through education are empowering, leading to improved self-image, and ultimately to better health outcomes. This societal change also accounts for the development and refinement of concerns about informed consent, living wills, advance directives, and health care proxies.

Apart from patients' expectations and satisfaction, there are a number of compelling reasons for physicians and other health providers to educate patients. The most important of these are better adherence and improved quality of care. It is clear that compliance with providers' instructions and prescriptions is enhanced by education (Shumaker

et al., 1990). For such adherence to prescribed treatment, education is necessary not only for the nuts and bolts of how to do it and for how often and how long to do it, but also for why to do it. To the extent that compliance with treatment improves outcomes and education improves compliance, education leads to improved health outcomes and reduced morbidity. For physicians and other providers, the direct benefits of health promotion efforts are more nebulous, because the health impacts of successful intervention are avoidance of future health problems. Ideally, providers internalize a system of values that are self-reinforcing when they promote health. Attempts to instill such a value system should be incorporated into medical student, nursing, and resident education. One also can find many examples of managed care organizations that provide for health promotion as part of a quality-of-care standard. This regulatory approach is likely to become even more common.

Additional benefits to the physician include practice marketing through enhanced patient satisfaction. There is also evidence that education reduces unnecessary office visits and phone contacts, which have become increasingly important as managed and capitated medical care have become more commonplace. Legal issues also must be considered. The current legal standard of informed consent holds the physician accountable for injuries resulting from undisclosed risks. Enhanced patient satisfaction that results from education, together with more realistic expectations, can contribute greatly to prevention of malpractice actions. The process of patient education, together with its documentation, thus also serves as a method for reducing liability risk.

From the perspective of expert panels and policy makers, it is clear that the U.S. health care system is in the midst of profound change. The lion's share of this change has been prompted by problems of access to care and the high cost of care. At the same time, there are significant changes occurring based on a paradigm shift from curative care to preventive care. This paradigm shift was heralded and encouraged by the USPSTF in 1989 in their first report. By curative care, we mean the paradigm of interaction in which people present to health professionals with a perceived illness, seeking cure of that illness. The USPSTF pointed out that existing data "suggest that among the most effective interventions available to clinicians for reducing the incidence and severity of the leading causes of disease and disability in the United States are those that address the personal health practices of patients" (1989, p. xxii). This implies movement of health care providers and patients toward a nontraditional relationship, in which encouragement of healthy lifestyles by providers and acceptance of responsibility for health behaviors by patients become the cornerstones of a new preventive care paradigm. Education of patients will be critical to the implementation of this paradigm. Prevention must become the agenda of both patients and health care providers; education gradually can make this a reality. In addition, patients will need to aquire knowledge and skills relating to specific areas such as nutrition and accident prevention.

It has been argued by many policy makers that an emphasis on prevention will both improve health and reduce costs. Although health improvement is likely, cost reduction is more questionable and will have to stand the test of experience. Current examples of potential cost savings include reduced utilization of services, reduced length of hospital stay, and decreased use of emergency services for conditions such as asthma and diabetes. Our belief is that we will, at a minimum, achieve higher health quality for each dollar spent when those dollars include spending for patient education.

APPROPRIATENESS

When is patient education appropriate? The easiest answer is that it is always appropriate. It is hard to imagine a medical interaction in which education of the patient or his or her family cannot make a contribution. Obviously, in the case of infants, the education will be directed to a parent or guardian, and in the case of children to both the child and parent(s). In the case of a comatose patient, the education will be directed to a family member. However, there are circumstances in which one must be sensitive to the ability of patients and families to benefit from the education. For example, people who have just been told of a major diagnosis, such as cancer, may not be able to deal with or remember further information given at that time, even if they request it. In these instances, it will be important to schedule additional contacts to continue the process.

It is possible to view patient education as a separate part of the process of care, distinct from history taking, examination, and therapy. Any recent medical school or residency graduate is familiar with the SOAP note format (Subjective data, Objective data, Assessment, and Plan) for documenting a medical encounter. In this rubric, the physician can "add education to the plan," using a SOAPE note. The benefit of this approach is that it serves as a reminder to educate patients and as an organized way to document the education. The SOAPE note is a particularly useful construct to incorporate into student and resident teaching.

The reality, however, is that education is a critical thread throughout the fabric of high-quality primary care. There is no excellent family physician who is not also an excellent teacher. When observing such a physician, it is typically evident that education is incorporated continuously during the interaction with the patient, not segregated as a separate step. When taking a history, one can assess attitudes, knowledge, and skills. When performing an examination, one can instruct about the purpose of the examination and the meaning of findings. When discussing a diagnosis, one can share its meaning and the process of decision making in approachable terminology. When suggesting therapy, one can assess understanding, willingness, and barriers to implementation.

OPPORTUNITIES

Whereas *patient education* may in large part occur in the context of individual provider–patient interactions, there are many additional opportunities to get involved in *health education*. Health education is a regular part of curricula in schools, may be found in workplace programs in many communities, and is featured routinely in the mass media. Family physicians who have become involved in health education benefit from the knowledge that their health messages are reaching a wider audience with greater potential impact, from the related networking in their community, and from enhanced reputations leading to practice growth. Involvement can begin with something small and manageable. Physicians can offer to come for question-and-answer sessions during health classes, offer to be a consultant to the school board regarding health curricula, or become a team physician for junior high or high school teams. Other possibilities include being available to give health talks for community organizations, sponsoring a community health fair, or advising local employers and their employees on avoiding workplace injuries. Media involvement can come from volunteering to comment on current issues in health for local radio and television stations or from writing a regular health column for the local newspaper.

Within their own practices, many family physicians wonder how to find the time to include all of the education they would like to provide. There are a variety of creative solutions to this problem. One is to expand services to include group classes for common topics such as smoking cessation, perinatal care, and healthy diet. Another is to make patient education the responsibility of the entire practice, involving office nurses, medical assistants, and receptionists as a team. Larger practices may have access to dietitians or pharmacists as well. Even small practices sometimes can share the help of "circuit riders" who divide their time among practices. Motivation and creativity are the keys to success.

It is also important not to overlook existing resources in the community. These include national and local disease-specific support organizations such as the American Diabetes Association, American Heart Association, American Cancer Society, American Lung Association, Weight Watchers, and Alcoholics Anonymous. Educational resources in the form of groups or short courses also may be sponsored by local libraries, YMCA chapters, churches, or other community organizations. Becoming familiar with these resources allows the physician to anticipate what patients can expect, and to utilize the resources appropriately.

PRINCIPLES OF PATIENT EDUCATION

We already have noted the existence of a growing movement to encourage patients to take responsibility for their health behaviors. There is a corresponding need for a fundamental shift in the attitudes of health care professionals. One arguably might propose that physicians, in particular, became rather parentalistic during the explosion of medical knowledge, technology, and new pharmaceuticals in the latter half of this century. The fantasy of patients accepting the advice of all-knowing physicians in an unquestioning and docile manner is a thing of the past. We should strive toward a doctor–patient partnership, in which patients see physicians (and the physicians see themselves) as "health consultants." The role of health consultant has education at its core.

In such a role, it is only natural to wonder how to educate most effectively. Fortunately, much is known about this question, derived from research into child and adult learning, as well as specific research in the field of patient education. This research has demonstrated consistently that benefits are greatest when interventions follow sound educational principles. As summarized in a recent review, these principles are *feedback, reinforcement, individualization, facilitation, relevance,* and use of *multiple educational channels* (Simons-Morton et al., 1992). Feedback simply means that the patient is informed about progress toward goals and objectives. Reinforcement refers to encouragement or rewards for progress. Individualization takes into account the needs, desires, and characteristics of the patient and demands that specific

TABLE 17–2.   USPSTF RECOMMENDATIONS FOR PATIENT EDUCATION AND COUNSELING*

Develop a therapeutic alliance
Counsel all patients
Ensure that patients understand the relationship between behavior and health
Work with patients to assess barriers to behavior change
Gain commitment from patients to change
Involve patients in selecting risk factors to change
Use a combination of strategies
Design a behavior modification plan
Monitor progress through follow-up contact
Involve office staff

* U.S. Preventive Service Task Force

goals and objectives be negotiated for each patient. Facilitation refers to materials, cues, or skill training that assist the patient in making changes. Relevance to the learner means that the content is appropriate for an individual patient's circumstances. Multiple channels implies combined learning strategies as well as a team approach to education. These principles have been incorporated into the USPSTF's (1989) recommendations for patient education and counseling, shown in Table 17–2.

A MODEL OF HEALTH BEHAVIOR

Sometimes the goal of patient education is to influence patients' knowledge about their health and health care. However, more often the purpose of patient education efforts is not simply to inform, but rather to change behavior. Typically, the goal is to improve adherence to therapeutic regimens, encourage new lifestyles, or help the patient adopt other behaviors that prevent disease and disability.

A great deal of research has been devoted to the understanding of health behavior; much of this work is directly applicable to an expanded definition of patient education. The bulk of the important findings have been published in the sociologic, anthropologic, and public health literature. Unfortunately, these papers are not routinely accessed by primary care physicians, who have the greatest opportunity to make practical application of their results. We will present briefly two of the most well-studied theoretical models, and combine them into a working model of health behavior that has clear implications for the practice of patient education.

The *health belief model* (HBM) has received more study than any other (Shumaker et al., 1990). Basically, this model assumes that much of health behavior can be explained by four factors: *perceived susceptibility*, meaning essentially how vulnerable or susceptible an individual feels to a given condition or problem in the future; *perceived severity* of the condition or problem, should it occur; *perceived benefits* of taking a particular health action; and *perceived barriers* or *obstacles* to taking the action. In contrast to what has been shown for illness behaviors, the role of perceived severity is less important for preventive health behaviors, probably because of the remoteness of the preventable outcome. Some investigators have added to the HBM various social support factors that incorporate the individual's context of family or others' support. Many researchers have added the factor of *motivation* to the HBM, meaning generally a predisposing health attitude, or an intention to take health-related actions. However, with or without these additions, the HBM has been shown repeatedly to explain a variety of health behaviors, including both illness behavior and prevention behavior.

A more recently developed but increasingly popular theoretical construct, first described by Bandura, has been termed *social learning theory* (SLT) (Shumaker et al., 1990). This theory postulates that health behavior is determined by expectancies and incentives. Expectancies include primarily *outcome expectations* and *efficacy expectations*. Outcome expectations are the beliefs about whether or not a given behavior will lead to given outcomes (e.g., Will I prevent lung cancer from developing if I stop smoking?). Efficacy expectations, or *self-efficacy*, consists of beliefs about how capable one is of performing a specific behavior that leads to the outcome in question (e.g., Will I be able to stop smoking?). *Incentives* refers to the value that the person attributes to the outcome. SLT incentives and outcome expectations are closely to related to perceived benefits, risks, and severity in the HBM framework. Self-efficacy is a more unique concept. In the HBM it probably would be related most closely to the concept of perceived obstacles, but it incorporates additional nuances not included in the HBM. A growing body of research has demonstrated clearly the important impact of self-efficacy on behavior. There also has been at least one attempt to justify an integration of the HBM and self-efficacy into a new model.

There are examples of studies of health promotion that have investigated the contributions of health beliefs, social support, motivation, and self-efficacy in the prediction of behavior change (Kelly, 1988; Kelly et al., 1991). In these studies,

motivation for change (but not beliefs or efficacy) was found to be clearly associated with behavioral responses to health promotion interventions. Second, health beliefs and self-efficacy predicted motivation for change in most lifestyle areas. Perceived support was not found to be important in predicting motivation, but did have associations with self-efficacy for some lifestyle areas, as did beliefs. These findings strongly suggest that motivation, or a state of interest in making a change, is an extremely important intervening step in the adoption of new behavior. Other studies have supported the key role of motivation. It is clear that even brief but direct and confidently worded messages from their physician can have significant impacts on patients' attempts to change behavior, and on the proportion who do adopt new behaviors. This finding probably is related to changes that occur in motivated patients, for whom the physician's message serves as the cue they need to take action.

In light of this and other empirical data, we propose an integration of the HBM and SLT into a practical understanding of health behavior change, incorporating motivation as a critical intermediate step on the way to new behavior. Figure 17–1 shows a diagram of this integrated model. The size and direction of the arrows are drawn roughly in proportion to the strength of associations. The model implies that a motivated patient who has the necessary knowledge to act, and some kind of

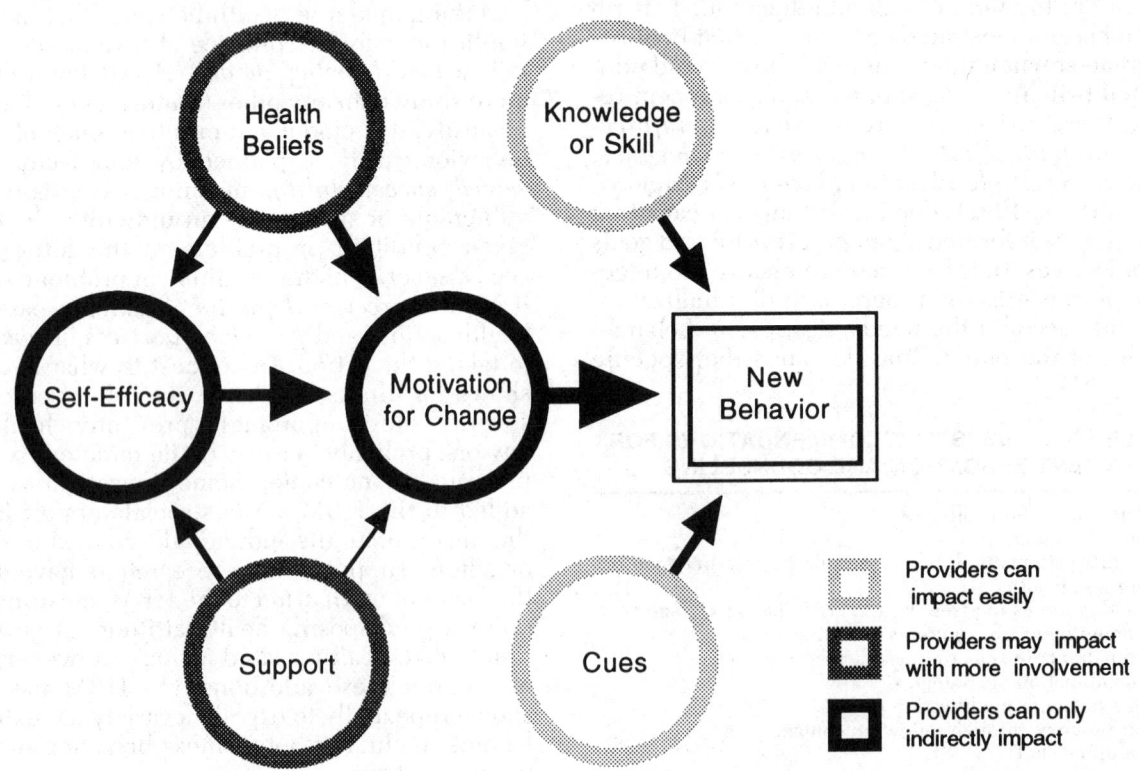

FIGURE 17–1. Integrated model of health behavior.

internal or external cue to action, will take a health action. Motivation, in turn, is determined primarily by self-efficacy and health beliefs, with social support playing a more minor role. The model also incorporates the relationship of health beliefs and social support to self-efficacy. When the former change, self-efficacy can be expected to change as well. Although not all-inclusive, this model incorporates two important theoretical frameworks in the context of empirical data. We believe that it is a useful framework to look critically at patient education in practice.

We are not alone in proposing a model that incorporates motivation or related concepts as a central construct. Prochaska and DiClemente's (1983) transtheoretical model has a similar theoretical underpinning, although it defines five stages through which patients progress during periods of lifestyle changes.

IMPLICATIONS OF THE MODEL

Busy family physicians and other health care providers know that a typical office visit does not accommodate lengthy discussions with patients to examine comprehensively their beliefs, expectations, or social support. The "good news" of the model relates to the critical importance of motivation. Fortunately, motivation can be assessed easily with simple questions such as: "What do you want to work on?" or "Are you interested in making a change?" Given typical constraints of time and resources in a primary care practice, it often may make sense to focus the majority of patient education efforts on motivated patients. Giving such patients the proper cue or knowledge to make a beneficial change is generally easy to accomplish. For simple behaviors (such as stretching before exercise), simple recommendations or an instructional pamphlet may be all that is needed to accompany the physician's strong statement of support for the new behavior. For other more complicated behaviors (such as dietary changes), one or more additional scheduled visits with the physician, a dietitian, or other provider may be needed to set goals, convey knowledge or skills, and reinforce behavior change.

The "bad news" of the model is that it probably does not make much sense to spend time giving cues and knowledge per se to unmotivated patients. Instead, if the behavior is an important one, the goal of the health care provider would be to increase the patient's motivation for change. The model implies that this can be accomplished by changes in health beliefs, social support, or self-efficacy, which could in turn impact on motivation. Short of giving up, the constraints of clinical practice dictate repeated brief attempts to assess and address these areas over a number of visits, with the hoped-for result of changes in the patient's be-

liefs, social support, or efficacy expectations over time.

A simple structural diagram can be used to summarize these implications (Fig. 17–2). First, education is a dynamic process, most akin to a cycle of assessment, planning, instructing, and evaluation. A number of factors must be assessed. These include the patient's current medical condition, risk for future health problems, and motivation to address any identified needs or behaviors. Ideally, this assessment should be a collaborative process between physician and patient, so that both become invested in its outcome.

For motivated patients, it makes sense to proceed with cues, instruction, and skill training as appropriate. It is always important to establish the patient's existing understanding before launching into a plan for education. For some behaviors, it is also important to involve family members or other social influences. A good example of this is dietary change in a male patient whose wife does all of the shopping and cooking for the family. In order to "close the loop," a final step is an evaluation of the outcome of the education, returning to the first step of identification of a problem or need.

The assessment process will have determined the necessary content, and also should indicate the patient's preferences for learning. Given motivation to learn a skill or change a behavior, the next step is to plan the delivery or process of education. Planning will include a joint decision on the use of various modalities based on preferences and resources, but also a decision about who will be involved. In many cases, the physician will involve other providers or agencies, particularly for complex problems. Once the education has been provided, a key step that unfortunately often is overlooked is to evaluate the behavior, skill, or knowledge that was targeted. This evaluation logically leads to another cycle of assessment, planning, and providing further education as needed.

This may sound quite complex and involved to busy practitioners. There certainly are conditions, such as diabetes, that do require extensive educational assessment, planning, performance, and evaluation. However, in most circumstances these principles are much less daunting to apply. The initial assessment of needs, expectations, and beliefs begins the moment the physician and patient interact. The first few moments of the interaction tell the patient what he or she can expect from the doctor and in turn tell the physician what the patient expects from the visit. A simple question such as "Tell me how I might help you today" communicates to the patient an interest and concern in what they have to say. Patients' responses to such questions also provide insight into their perspective of the visit and provide information or cues that may be explored in further depth. In addition, patients' responses provide information about their perceptions of their condition and about their

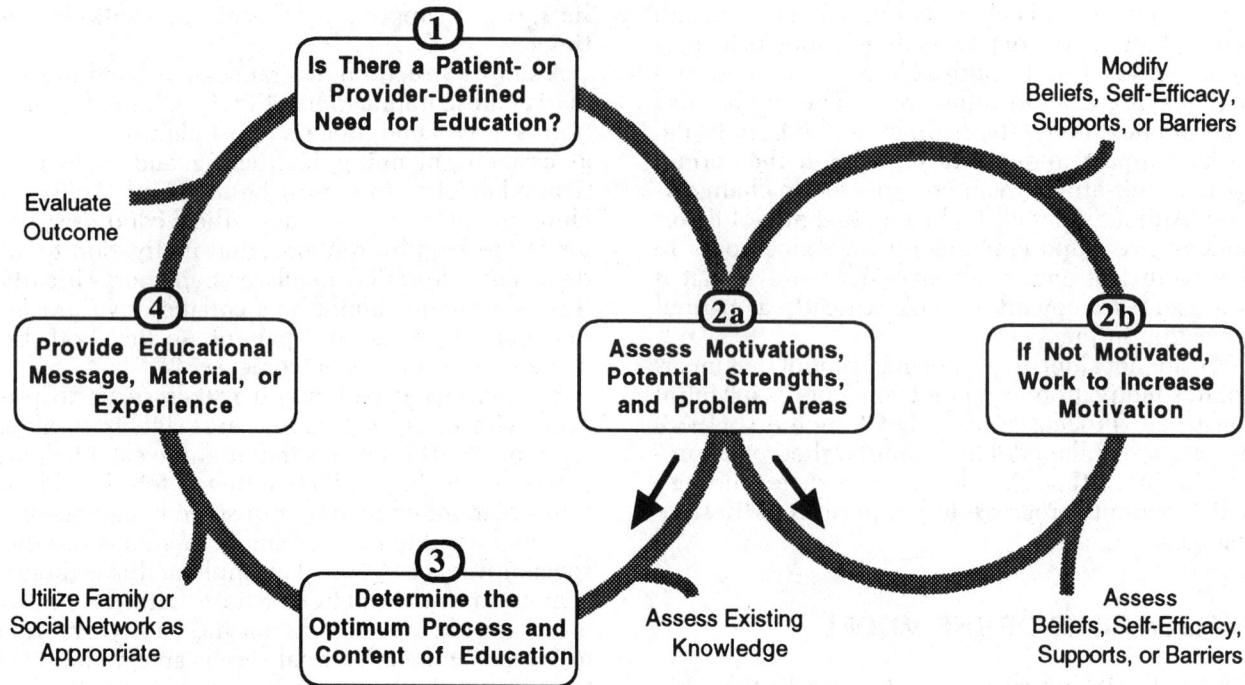

FIGURE 17–2.   Practice implications of the integrated model of health behavior.

expectations for the visit. For example, a patient might say "I'm here again with a cough. I know it comes from smoking, but I just can't seem to quit." This statement has embedded suggestions about the patient's health beliefs and self-efficacy for smoking cessation. Further exploration would help assess motivation for change, and give other clues regarding beliefs, barriers, supports, and other factors that may need to be addressed in any attempt to help this patient change his or her behavior.

The trick is not to think that all of this must be accomplished in one 15-minute office visit. In fact, conducting effective patient education is not so much a matter of time as it is a matter of efficiency. Collecting data necessary for rational patient education planning is possible in a relatively small amount of time, if it is integrated properly into the medical interview. To accomplish this goal, the health provider must become skilled in recognizing how various components of the normal health provider–patient interaction contribute to the patient teaching process. Assessment, planning, implementation, and evaluation can be woven into the fabric of routine care. In many instances, much important assessment information is already known to the family physician, and can be utilized without further time spent in data gathering.

When patients are unmotivated, the physician should decide whether or not to try to increase motivation through an assessment and modification of beliefs, self-efficacy, and supports or barriers. At a minimum, an "open door" policy should be adopted. The physician must convey the message

that he or she is willing and ready to help the patient make changes when the patient becomes motivated to make them. Motivation to change should be assessed on a regular basis as the patient is cared for over time.

If one takes up the challenge of the unmotivated patient, how should beliefs, support, or self-efficacy be assessed and addressed in the context of routine office visits? First, from the patient's verbal and nonverbal communication, the health provider can learn what is important from the patient's standpoint. For example, one may ask: What is the problem as the patient sees it? What are the patient's expectations and goals? What factors are available, both internal and external, that will facilitate or hinder resolution of the problem as the patient sees it? During the interaction, the patient's current perceptions about his or her condition or level of risk can be explored. Sometimes a health belief is just the result of misinformation. A question as simple as "Could you tell me briefly what you already know about . . ." helps the health provider determine the patient's beliefs and existing understanding. It is also important to assess the patient's perceptions about the treatment or new behavior the health provider would like to prescribe. Patients' potentials for following this recommendation are affected by the degree to which they believe the treatment will lead to the outcome desired, the degree to which they believe the benefit to outweigh any inconvenience or discomfort, and the degree to which they perceive that the results of not following treatment recommendations are worse than the results of following recommendations. By clarifying these issues, the health provider has the opportunity to correct misunderstandings, give new information, and potentially change the perceptions or beliefs over time.

Also important to identify are potential supports or barriers the patient perceives as enhancing or hindering his or her ability to follow the health provider's recommendations. By attention to these issues, patients can be helped to find ways in which they can utilize the supports to enhance their ability to follow the treatment regimen, or to overcome or modify the barriers they perceive. Family or cultural concerns may play a role in facilitating or resisting behavior change as well, and are part of this area of assessment. Other social realities also may come into play. These might include the patient's residential location, living arrangements, employment situation, income, and working hours. Only by identifying factors that potentially could hinder the patient from carrying out the recommendations can the health provider work with the patient to devise a plan that is better suited to the patient's individual situation.

Just as beliefs, supports, and barriers can be explored over time with patients, one also can determine how successful patients think they would be in accomplishing the desired behavior change, or their self-efficacy expectations for that behavior. Low self-efficacy is likely to contribute to low motivation for change. When this seems to stem from misinformation, health beliefs, or low support, it may be possible to address self-efficacy through these factors. In other cases, anecdotes about others' successes or direct exposure to successful role models may be more fruitful. In most patients, when a behavior can be broken down into manageable smaller steps, the mastery of each step can be used to enhance self-efficacy for later steps. Physician–patient contracting for mutually agreeable goals that the patient believes he or she can accomplish is another example of an approach that incorporates self-efficacy.

Because many patients are not motivated, and because the health rewards of behavior change are often not immediate, physicians also must take steps to avoid burnout. The first step toward avoiding frustration is to focus first on motivated patients. This group will respond to brief, time-efficient messages and interventions that are well within the reach of busy practitioners. Tangible rewards and personal satisfaction gained from these efforts can "charge the batteries" for attempts to expand activities to unmotivated patients. For unmotivated patients, a long-term view is often helpful. The goal is to change motivation in small increments over time, and to be ready to detect a change in motivation that will allow for meaningful change in behavior. It also can be the case that events will take place that cause a dramatic shift in motivation, usually as a result of a change in perceived risk.

The classic example is personal illness or illness in a friend or family member that is due to lifestyle behaviors. Women who are pregnant are much more likely to stop smoking, because of their new concern for risk to their baby. Those who have a myocardial infarction (or whose coworker of the same age suffers a myocardial infarction) often change diet and physical activities in ways that never interested them before. These events are opportunities to explore and to capitalize on when it seems that health beliefs have changed. In the meantime, the best strategy is to be nonjudgmental, to feel rewarded for small changes that patients make, to provide further encouragement to them, and to accept that some people will not change despite one's best efforts. For example, if the annual smoking quit rate in a practice increases to 10 per cent from a baseline of 5 per cent of smokers per year, the physician should not despair about the other 90 per cent, but instead should congratulate himself or herself on doubling the rate of smoking cessation, and leave the door open to the other 90 per cent.

OTHER PRACTICAL ISSUES

Assessing Knowledge

A common mistake that is made in patient education is to forge ahead with the educational message or content without first assessing existing knowledge. For example, not all diabetics in poor control need further instruction in dietary management. The pertinent issue might be signs and symptoms of hyperglycemia and hypoglycemia, skill training in use of home blood glucose testing equipment, or planning for extra insulin dosing based on the results of home testing. Physicians also must be careful to define needed knowledge in a functional, outcome-driven sense. A dietitian or physician may need to be able to calculate the percentage of calories derived from fat in a food. In contrast, it may be both more important and more realistic for many patients to learn what foods tend to be high in saturated fat, and to make changes in the way they prepare meals to avoid excess fat.

For some disease entities, there are published knowledge scales that have been used in research, but few of these are practical for routine practice. Fortunately, a number of simple questions are almost always useful to assess knowledge, and have added benefit in enriching the physician's understanding of health beliefs and other important issues. These questions are:

What have you been told the problem is?
What does that mean to you?
How did you get this problem?
What are you doing now to treat the problem?
How do you believe this treatment is supposed to help?

Are you satisfied with the results of this treatment? What questions do you have about the problem or its treatment?

Answers to these and similar questions will bring out misconceptions and gaps in knowledge about causation, physiology, and therapeutics. These areas then can be prioritized jointly by physician and patient to construct an agenda for education, and can be revisited following the delivery of the education.

Literacy

Most physicians and other health providers depend on printed material to augment verbal or other instruction. Reading comprehension is therefore the most important aspect of literacy that relates to patient education. Studies consistently have found large discrepancies between the reading comprehension of average patients and the ability levels needed to read patient education materials. For example, one study of public clinic patients determined an average reading comprehension level of 6th grade, while a variety of patient education materials used in the setting required a comprehension level of 11th to 14th grade (Davis et al., 1990). Even when asked about it, illiterate patients generally do not admit to their deficiency voluntarily (Doak et al., 1985). National surveys have estimated a prevalence of functional illiteracy of 13 to 55 per cent (Davis et al., 1990). Physicians often have used educational grade level attainment as a surrogate for reading comprehension, but this may overestimate reading comprehension by an average of three or four grade levels.

It is therefore likely that patients known to have low literacy are only the tip of the iceberg in an average practice. Further research is needed to develop rapidly administered screening tests for literacy. Physicians practicing in public clinics should be especially concerned about the problem. In these settings, it may be justified to use existing longer instruments to screen for deficient reading comprehension. One example of such a measure is the Peabody Individual Achievement Test (Dunn and Markwardt, 1970). This includes a reading recognition section that takes 5 to 10 minutes to complete and a reading comprehension subtest that takes 5 to 40 minutes to complete (Davis et al., 1990). Although the recognition subtest is not as accurate as the comprehension subtest, it may be a more practical screen for those with constraints of staff time.

PLANNING FOR PATIENT EDUCATION IN YOUR PRACTICE

Careful planning is the major factor in the success of any patient education efforts in a practice,

whether or not the physician actually delivers the education. In a typical practice, physicians recruit and hire staff, set policies for how patients will be treated, make decisions about the physical layout of the office, and plan for the equipping and furnishing of a waiting area, exam rooms, and other spaces. All of these involvements have an impact on patient education.

Who Will Be Involved

Formal studies and anecdotal reports consistently have indicated that involvement of all of the office staff in patient education makes the total impact all the more powerful, and saves physician time. The physician always will need to be involved in defining the educational goals, delivering brief messages about the importance of goals, prescribing an educational process, and following up regularly to assess progress. Depending on the physician's interest and the nature of the problem, the education can be given by the physician himself or herself or delgated to others. There are many examples of office nurses and other staff taking on the role of education in particular areas such as smoking cessation and proper nutrition. Reception staff can suggest printed materials or other available modalities to patients while they wait, or can be involved in giving patients printed materials "prescribed" by the physician. Group classes can be offered in the evening, organized around common topics within the practice. If these are run in conjunction with existing evening clinic hours, group classes can become a very time-efficient method of delivering education to selected patients. In larger practices, interested staff can form a "patient education committee" that sets priority areas for the practice, evaluates or develops printed materials and other resources, and uses a quality improvement process to foster higher quality patient education.

Available community resources should not be overlooked. This includes professionals such as dietitians or diabetes educators who may be hired on a full-time or part-time basis by a larger practice, or who can split their time as a "circuit rider," spending a few hours a week at a number of practices. Many communities have existing programs for smoking cessation, weight loss, stress reduction, or exercise. Some of these may be commercial ventures; others may operate on a cost recovery basis or may be free of charge, sponsored by a school system, library, or community center. Physicians can spend some of their time or their staff's time to become familiar with the programs, their costs, and their schedules. It is best to recommend the ones that seem most suited for individual patients and follow up the outcome to determine whether the program merits continued referrals. In some cases, a physician's involvement as a medical consultant can lead to an improved program.

It is easy to focus on individual patients, without considering that almost all patients have a family context. Presence or absence of family support and related issues can be critical to the success of patient education, arguing for family involvement in the process. It is important to recognize that families can aid or hinder achievement of educational goals. Everything that has been said already about motivation, health beliefs, and self-efficacy also can be applied to family members or even the family unit as a whole. For example, it is rather self-evident that whether or not a spouse smokes will be an important factor in a smoking patient's efforts to quit. Similarly, if a patient needs to learn about dietary change to lower cholesterol and his or her spouse does all the food preparation for the household, the instruction will not be likely to affect the target behavior without involvement of that spouse. Simple questions often provide very useful information. One can ask the patient: "Who have you talked to about your symptoms (problem)?" "What did they say?" "Who do you generally turn to for help?" One can ask family members: "What do you believe is causing the symptoms (problem)?" "What are your major concerns?" "What can be done to help?" (Falvo and Bosshart, 1990). In some circumstances, simply gaining an understanding of family issues and concerns may be all that is required to modify the educational approach effectively. In other cases, it will be critical to bring family members into the educational process or even make them the targets of the education. This is obviously true for young children, but is also indicated for family members or other caregivers, of elderly patients with poor recent memory.

Using Verbal Instruction

The most common form of patient education lies in talking to patients within the context of routine doctor–patient contacts dealing with medical problems and health maintenance issues. This interaction serves as the foundation for further education that may be provided in the form of printed materials, video materials, classes, or other instructional modalities. Information must be given in a relevant and comprehensive way, embedded in appropriate goals and realistic expectations that are shared between provider and patient.

An atmosphere of acceptance, but not necessarily approval, is the first prerequisite to effective communication. This implies that the physician maintain a nonjudgmental stance when inquiring about the patient's experiences, beliefs, and behaviors. Physicians must demonstrate that they understand the patient's perspective, even if they do not agree with it. These crucial steps lead to a teaming with the patient toward achievement of common goals. Without the establishment of such an accepting atmosphere, patients will be reluctant to share feelings and other information about themselves.

Effective messages are based in an understanding of the patient's circumstances, including existing motivation for change, knowledge and skills, and beliefs, as already discussed. Understanding anxieties and fears is also important. Research has shown that mild to moderate fear can be motivating, whereas extreme fear tends to lead to denial, and is therefore counterproductive. For this reason, one must be careful in making frightening statements, or giving "fear messages," such as: "If you don't stop smoking, you'll be dead in a year."

Medical jargon also should be avoided. Physicians often do not realize just how much of their vocabulary is actually highly technical and outside of the average patient's understanding. As an example, few patients know that they even have a spleen or a thymus gland, much less where they are in the body or what they do. Adults have very poor functional understanding of medical terms. Nearly 50 per cent define "hypertension" as meaning nervous or easily upset. To 25 per cent, "orally" means how often one takes medicine (Gibbs et al., 1987). One approach to helping patients decode the jargon is to embed synonyms in the information provided. For example, say: "There is an atherosclerotic lesion *or blockage* in one of the coronary arteries, *the vessels that carry blood to the heart muscle itself.*" Whenever possible, avoid medical terms altogether.

Specificity and clarity are equally important principles. It is best not to use language such as: "Cut down on the fat you eat," or "Exercise more," or "Avoid heavy lifting", or even "Take your medicine three times a day." In the case of exercise, for example, one can indicate the type of exercise, how often to do it, how long to do it, how intensely to do it (e.g., by using a target pulse), how to warm up and cool down before and after, and any warning symptoms to watch out for. This level of specificity will go a long way toward ensuring that motivated patients will have the information they need to change their behavior in an effective manner.

A final tip for effective verbal instruction is to check continually patients' understanding of what they have been told. At a minimum, patients should be encouraged to ask questions and seek clarification. It is an even better strategy to ask patients to summarize their understanding of the information they have been given. Questions are most effectively stated in a fashion that accepts blame for any misunderstandings and is therefore not condescending: "Just so I can be sure that I've been clear about the information I've given you, would you repeat back to me in your own words what you are to do?" (Falvo and Bosshart, 1990).

Using Printed Materials

Printed materials are the next most commonly used patient education modality after verbal instruction. Unfortunately, they often are used alone or without sufficient preceding verbal instruction, as a surrogate for provider–patient interaction. In this sense printed materials are overused. Volumes of research have shown that they are not effective when used this way (Simons-Morton et al., 1992). However, in another sense they are not used enough. Studies have shown that printed materials are desired by patients and lead to improved outcomes when given to supplement other instruction.

Printed materials can be classified into two principle types that we will call *prescriptive* and *nonprescriptive*. Although there is some overlap between the genres, prescriptive materials are, by definition, usually given by the provider to the patient with a specific goal in mind. Their use often is triggered by the onset or recurrence of a medical problem. For example, if the patient has strained his or her lower back muscles, a brochure might be given that explains back mechanics, avoidance measures to prevent reinjury, and a physical program to improve flexibility and strength during and after healing. This material would serve to supplement the physician's instructions about the care of this injury. In contrast, nonprescriptive materials are put out for patients to take freely or read as desired, usually in a waiting room or exam room area. They are more general and topic oriented, and serve more a function of health education than patient education. Examples would include a brochure that describes the four basic food groups, a pamphlet about warming up before exercise, or a description of common sexually transmitted diseases. Such nonprescriptive materials serve more to inform than to change behavior, but may lead to patient questions and resulting expanded opportunities for patient education during the office visit.

Physicians or practice-based patient education committees have options of using existing materials or developing their own for any topics deemed to be important. It is important to recognize that physicians are responsible for the accuracy of any materials they distribute. Hundreds of materials are available free of charge or at low cost. Sources of free materials are primarily pharmaceutical companies and national voluntary associations such as the American Cancer Society. Other national organizations, such as the American Heart Association, and medical specialty societies, such as the AAFP and the American Academy of Pediatrics, offer materials at low cost, usually in the range of $.10 to $.20 per copy. In most cases, single copies for review can be ordered so that physicians can decide on the appropriateness of the material for their practice.

Several issues are important to consider before using existing materials. First, is the content appropriate? Materials provided by pharmaceutical companies may advertise a product or present information in a biased way. Voluntary organizations' guidelines may not agree with the physician's own judgments about proper screening and treatment. Second, is the material clearly presented, with a reading comprehension level appropriate for the patients served by the practice? In some cases, materials are developed with a target reading level in mind. An example is the series of "Health Notes from Your Family Doctor" that have been produced by the AAFP, which are designed to be at about an 8th grade comprehension level, and rarely exceed this guideline. Unfortunately, the majority of materials that are widely available have not been produced with lower literacy patients in mind, and are typically written at a 12th grade or higher comprehension level. A third type of concern is logistical: Will additional copies of the material continue to be available for replenishing supplies, or might the material go out of print? This is particularly a concern for pharmaceutical company–funded productions. Finally, is the format of the material suitable for storage and display in whatever system is used in the practice?

Writing One's Own

It is likely for a variety of reasons that the practice will want to develop some of its own printed materials. This has the advantage of control over content and format, but also carries with it the responsibility for accuracy and the not insignificant work of developing a good product. We suggest that practices begin with a planning process that identifies the most important needs, based on the common educational issues that the practice deals with, and the existing materials and their quality and usefulness for these issues. Because accuracy is a critical issue, the physician should broaden the knowledge base with a recent literature search before starting to write. This is most important if a physician is writing about a topic for nonprescriptive material to use in the waiting room. However, it remains a useful process for prescriptive materials, even if the goal is simply to put down in writing the physician's usual advice for a problem, to save time and amplify what messages are delivered in the exam room.

A common pitfall is to try to include too much information in the material. When writing, the physician should restrict the content to three or four salient teaching points; avoid jargon, extensive use of statistics, and fear messages; be clear with advice and specific with instructions; and use short words and short sentences to improve readers' comprehension. A number of computer programs, such as Grammatik and PC-Style, are available to test a material for reading level using established formulas that rely on items such as sentence length and numbers of polysyllabic words. Programs even can point out the words or areas of the text that could be simplified for improved comprehension. Ideally, material should be tested on colleagues and on a few patients before final reproduction in quantity. Such a review process can be invaluable.

Simple line drawings with a few labels are usually more effective than complex illustrations, and have the added benefit of reproducing better on the office copy machine. Subheads help readers find information, and sparing use of bold and italic type help to emphasize terms when needed. Writers should use the active tense, avoid negatives, and not use absolutes such as "never," "must," and "always." Expert writers recommend use of the first person in phrasing questions and the use of the second person in answering them: "How often and how long should *I* exercise?" "For best results, *you* should exercise for at least 30 minutes, at least three times each week." When laying out material, the writer should leave plenty of white space on the page, avoid long strings of capital letters, use a type face with serifs (the small tails at the edges of letters, as in this text), use a 10- or 12-point type size (slightly larger than the size of this text), and use a two- or even a three-column format if possible. Modern word processors and page layout software have brought a great deal of sophistication to what can be accomplished with the personal computer that many physicians and practices already own. Even two-color materials are not difficult to develop with a little help from a local printer or by getting a second color toner cartridge for the copy machine.

Other Materials and Modalities

It is generally helpful to supplement printed materials with models, anatomic charts, and other visual aids that can be used during the process of instruction. Such helps can be invaluable in trying to explain what a 3-ounce serving of meat looks like, how to check the fit of a vaginal diaphragm, or how a herniated lumbar disk presses on nerves in the back. Models and charts can be purchased from supply houses or sometimes are offered at no charge by pharmaceutical companies that market a related product.

Alternative modalities include audiotape, videotape, and computer-assisted instruction. Audiotape instruction has been available for quite some time, and requires only a small investment in equipment. It is best used in combination with printed material, with the possible exception of audiotapes used for relaxation training and stress reduction. Use of videotape instruction is expanding, although still not commonplace. It has been shown to be quite good at increasing short-term knowledge and in role modeling, although it offers no advantages in the areas of long-term retention of information or adherence (Gagliano, 1988). Videotapes may be very useful for illiterate patients and also may lend themselves to replacing the waiting room television programs with educational messages. They have the disadvantage of relatively great expense (typically $100 to $200 per topic from commercial sources).

Computer-assisted instruction is an emerging technology that offers great promise (Hannah et al., 1989). A computer in theory can customize its interaction with a patient based on an assessment of existing knowledge, patient and physician preferences, and the patient's retention of information already provided. Computers can be anonymous, nonjudgmental, and infinitely patient—all desirable traits in an educator. Well-written software can individualize the process of instruction to a given patient's needs quite cleverly. Currently available systems using videodisk or CD-ROM technology can store and retrieve text, graphics, and short video segments. As processors and storage devices continue to become faster and less costly and more software and packaged products become available, we expect this modality to become much more important.

Office Systems and Design

One of the ways to be most effective in patient education is to view the practice setting in its totality as an educational experience for patients. From this perspective, health providers can examine critically each physical area and each staff person for their potential to contribute to patient education. For example, the waiting area need not be just an attractive area with comfortable chairs and a magazine rack or a television. Physicians can make available a rack of nonprescriptive educational brochures, decorate the walls with posters that reinforce simple educational messages, and even play educational videotapes or use computer-assisted instruction. Exam rooms also can have posters and racks of printed materials, particularly materials that patients might be embarrassed to pick up while others are watching. Some practices use monthly or quarterly health "themes" and rotate posters and materials that relate to the theme. Practices that use audiotapes or videotapes may find it effective to create a patient education room, or (if space is lacking) create a mobile cart with the necessary audiovisual equipment.

Most practices will need to establish some mechanism for storing, retrieving, indexing, and ordering of printed materials. There is not a single best way to do this. Physical systems range from racks to filing cabinets to shelves to computer-based programs that print materials on demand. Functionally, the important aspects of any system are that providers (1) know what types of material are available, (2) agree with their content, (3) know how to find desired materials, (4) periodically review existing materials for applicability and accuracy, and (5) order or produce more as stocks run low. It is often practical to delegate responsibility for many of these tasks to office personnel. Office staff also may be quite eager to participate in a patient education committee that identifies priority areas and reviews printed and other materials before they are added to the practice's resources.

FUTURE DIRECTIONS

For many years, professionals have been concerned about inadequate reimbursement for patient education. It has been practiced "on faith" in many cases, as an adjunct to reimbursed services. As the health care needs of a larger proportion of patients become covered by capitated payment for total health services, patient education may truly come into own. However, in this environment, the rationale for including patient education in the mix of services will have to be either higher quality outcomes of care, lower cost of care, or both. This leads to a clear research mandate for investigations of the effects of patient education on outcomes and cost. Those of us who believe that patient education makes a difference should take a leadership role in the planning and execution of such research.

The potential usefulness of computers in health education and patient education is largely untapped at this time. Information networks such as the global InterNet are growing at an extremely rapid pace. More and more information is available at lower cost, and public-access computing at little or no cost is available in many areas. It is not clear how this emerging technology will be used, but it has the potential to be the next generation of public library. When this information base becomes combined with "artificial intelligence" capabilities and advanced computer-assisted instruction methods, there is little theoretical limit to what might be accomplished. While we wait for these advances to reach their full potential, computers can be used now to share information among providers, to store and retrieve materials, and to prepare copy for printed material.

REFERENCES

American Academy of Family Physicians: 1993-1994 Compendium of AAFP Positions on Selected Health Issues. Kansas City, MO, American Academy of Family Physicians, 1993a.

American Academy of Family Physicians: Patient education: A leadership role for family physicians and the AAFP. Kansas City, MO, American Academy of Family Physicians Committee on Health Education, 1993b.

Davis TC, Crouch MA, Wills G, et al: The gap between patient reading comprehension and the readability of patient education materials. J Fam Pract 31:533, 1990.

Doak CC, Doak LG, Root JH: Teaching Patients with Low Literacy Skills. Philadelphia, JB Lippincott, 1985.

Dunn LM, Markwardt FC: Peabody Individual Achievement Test. Circle Pines, MN, American Guidance Service, 1970.

Falvo DR: Effective Patient Education—A Guide to Increased Compliance. Rockville, MD, Aspen Publishers, 1985, p 244.

Falvo DR, Bosshart DA: Patient education. *In* Rakel RE, (ed): Textbook of Family Practice, 4th edition. Philadelphia, WB Saunders Company, 1990, pp 380–389.

Gagliano ME: A literature review on the efficacy of video in patient education. J Med Educ 63:785, 1988.

Gibbs RD, Gibbs PH, Henrich J: Patient understanding of commonly used medical vocabulary. J Fam Pract 25:176, 1987.

Hannah KJ, Conley-Price P, Fenty D, et al: Computer applications for staff development and patient education. Methods Inf Med 28:261, 1989.

Kelly RB: Controlled trial of a time-efficient method of health promotion. Am J Prev Med 4:200, 1987.

Kelly RB, Zyzanski SJ, Alemagno SA: Prediction of motivation and behavior change following health promotion: Role of health beliefs, social support, and self-efficacy. Soc Sci Med 32:311, 1991.

Mullen PD, Green LW, Persinger GS: Clinical trials of patient education for chronic conditions: A comparative meta-analysis of intervention types. Prev Med 14:753, 1985.

Prochaska IO, DiClemente CC: Stages and processes of self-change of smoking: Toward an integrative model of change. J Consult Clin Psychol 51:390, 1983.

Shumaker SA, Schron EB, Ockene JK (eds): The Handbook of Health Behavior Change. New York, Springer, 1990.

Simons-Morton DG, Mullen PD, Mains DA, et al: Characteristics of controlled studies of patient education and counseling for preventive health behaviors. Patient Educ Couns 19:175, 1992.

Society of Teachers of Family Medicine: Patient Education: A Handbook for Teachers. Report of the National Task Force on Training Family Physicians in Patient Education. Kansas City, MO, Society of Teachers of Family Medicine, 1979.

U.S. Preventive Services Task Force: Guide to Clinical Preventive Services—An Assessment of the Effectiveness of 169 Interventions. Baltimore, Williams & Wilkins, 1989, p 419.

Webber GC: Patient education: A review of the issues. Med Care 28:1089, 1990.

CHAPTER 18

INTERVIEWING TECHNIQUES

F. MARIAN BISHOP and ROBERT E. FROELICH

COMMUNICATION AND INTERVIEWING

There is a barrage of mass communication on the lives of most individuals in today's environment that has both a direct and an indirect effect on the physician–patient interaction and the interviewing process. The public has come to expect instant information exchange and 30-second sound bites that provide few details or backup data.

The commercialization of mass communication has led to a depersonalization of human relations and to a glorification of cliches and slogans. The standardized response begins more and more to substitute for deeply felt, personalized expression ... the human ear has adapted itself to sort *and disregard* a considerable number of verbal messages that emerge from radio loudspeakers and the television sets, just as it formerly accommodated itself to the task of absorbing what was being said. (Ruesch and Kees, 1970, pp. 3–7)

These observations suggest that interviewers have been unconsciously trained by mass communication media to not hear and have the task of retraining themselves to hear what is being said by patients. Interviewers have the problem of being sure that they fill in the missing details and required data base accurately, which requires utilizing a multiplicity of skills that are neither utilized nor required in the daily barrage of mass communication.

Time after time, interviewers listen to a word a patient says and jump to the conclusion that they understand what the patient meant by the word. A common misconception of all interviewers is the belief that the patient is using a word to mean what the interviewer believes it to mean. To illustrate this point, let us consider the professor who writes, rewrites, and reviews a test question on a topic that he and his students have been discussing for several weeks. They have been using a set of words common to the field of study. What happens when the professor puts the question on a test? Undoubtedly, some students will misinterpret the question and answer a meaning of the question that the professor had no intention of asking.

Greater opportunity for confusion is present if the question was not previously written, was not reviewed for possible misinterpretations, and is only presented in the oral form. This is the precise situation of an interview. Taken one step further, let us say that the question can be answered with a "yes" or "no." How much misinformation can be developed by such a question and answer?

Semantics is the basic study of all verbal communication (Hayakawa, 1964). A basic semantic concept is that a word is to what it represents as a map is to a territory. No map *is* the territory. No two maps of the same territory are the same. Each map is a unique abstraction of that territory, and the same applies to words and what they represent. As an illustration, consider a sensation that a patient notes and refers to as pain. The sensation the patient experiences is the territory. The patient's description of the pain is his or her map of the territory. The words paint the verbal picture of the sensation. It is only through clarification of the patient's use of the words that an interviewer can get a relatively accurate idea of what the territory is.

Most diagnoses can be made if one is able to get an accurate description of the patient's internal sensation or territory. Consider the situation in which ten neurons from deep pain fibers are firing into the spinal cord dorsal root. One person may refer to this sensation as very painful while a second person may refer to it as an ache. The territory is the same but each person uses a different map to represent the territory.

Every communication has two components. One component is the cognitive, dictionary definition of the words that make up the communication—the description of the territory. The second component is the affective or emotional tone of the communication. It is important to hear both components and to have the ability to respond to either component. For example, when people are angry, the dictionary definitions of their words may convey very little of the intended message. To react only to the words may be to miss the message completely.

The nonverbal accompaniment to the words (the context, the voice quality and emphasis, the facial expression, the body posture, the setting, the attire, the patient's age and culture) help the interviewer fill in the unexpressed. However, the only way to be sure that this understanding is accurate is for the interviewer to check it with the patient. The use of summary statements and asking, "What I hear you saying is. . . . Am I correct?" is an effective technique to be sure that the patient is being heard correctly. This kind of interviewer intervention reassures patients that the interviewer is focused on them, which they will appreciate.

The communication process is understood further when we realize that "if words are to be used significantly, they must still evoke pictorial images in the mind of a reader or listener" and "that only through the use of words that evoke exact and striking images can an emotional response be produced in the reader" (Ruesch and Kees, 1970, pp. 3–7). The reverse of this statement is that no communication occurs when the listener has no experience or image to connect to the words being spoken. "We do not first experience or understand some reality and then find words to name that understanding. We understand in and through the languages available to us" (Tracy, 1987, p. 48).

If we understand that we see out of our eyes and hear out of our ears (i.e., we do not see or hear that which we are not trained or set to see or hear), we begin to focus our attention in interviewing on seeing and listening, rather than asking. To be open to hear whatever is said and to see whatever happens is a most difficult task. Once we begin to see and hear what is not familiar, then the next task begins—that of giving meaning to these observations. It is only through time spent with patients that we finally understand their communication and what meaning to apply to it.

PURPOSE OF THE INTERVIEW

The interview has several purposes. The one most often identified is that of gathering data from the patient that will lead to an understanding of the disease process and the underlying physiologic status. Equally important is the purpose of establishing a relationship and a treatment contract between the patient and the physician and the physician's staff. This relationship and the associated treatment contract is an essential common element of all successful patient care.

Prior to establishing a successful contract with a patient, another purpose of the interview takes place. The assessment of the patient's attitudes, beliefs, understandings, and biases as they relate to his or her illness, the role of medications, and the patient role is necessary for successful treatment. In the extreme situation, a patient may understand the role of patient as a passive recipient of care, while the physician may expect the patient to take active care of himself or herself. If this difference in expectations is not understood, the chance of successful treatment is endangered.

The final purpose of the interview is to meet the needs of the patient and the needs of the physician. In most patient visits, when the physician and patient are from the same cultural background, their expectations are harmonious and synchronized to the point that their individual needs never enter conscious awareness. Only when the expectations are not harmonious, when there are friction, discomfort, and noncompliance, do the needs and expectations of the patient and physician come into awareness and become an issue for discussion, working through, and resolution.

EMPOWERING THE PATIENT

There is a considerable body of research that suggests that more patient involvement in the interview process results in greater patient satisfaction (Brody et al., 1989). Many times patients feel angry because they feel powerless to affect their own medical care process. They feel hesitant or embarrassed to ask questions. This disempowerment of the patient is a critical barrier in the physician–patient encounter. Also, it is clear from research such as that of Greenfield and colleagues (1985) that greater involvement of patients in their own medical care management and treatment leads to better health.

Although patients generally wish to be involved in decisions about their medical care and physicians do not wish to exclude them, there seems to be a mismatch between expectation and perception.

Patients say their physicians don't listen to them, explain things clearly, or want to be bothered with questions. Meanwhile, physicians say that they wish their patients would have more realistic expectations and take a more active role in the management of their own care. The picture is that the medical encounter is like two ships passing in the night. (Feffer, 1992, pp. 8–10)

Awareness of the slippage between expectation and perception is important. It can be useful for both the physician and the patient to outline clearly their mutual expectations at the beginning of the interview and review their perception of success before concluding the encounter. Physicians should take the lead in this process. "Physicians, with their training historically focused on taking charge and making decisions, have greater than average needs to unlearn habitual disempowering practices" (Feffer, 1992, pp. 8–10).

Physician need to help patients overcome the barriers of being active participants and see that their needs are met. One way to encourage greater patient involvement is to be sure the patient feels secure enough to ask questions and be an active participant. In addition, asking patients for their opinions and responding to what they say is empowering in and of itself. There is no substitute for routinely eliciting feedback from patients regarding both medical and interpersonal issues.

There are several indicators that patients feel disempowered and there are problems in communication. These include patient unresponsiveness, patient statements that are unclear to the physician in content or relationship to the topic being discussed, and direct disagreement between the patient and the physician.

A patient becomes empowered by being given responsibility for sharing his or her medical history. This is accomplished through facilitations, reflections, and empathic responses, rather than by asking direct questions. Critical listening is not a passive process. It is accomplished by the physician listening and responding to what patients say. If the interview narrative concerns the disease rather than the patient and the encounter turns into 20 questions aimed at discovering a disease, the patient is neither empowered nor a full participant in the doctor–patient relationship.

A cookbook approach to interviewing overlooks the unique features of the patient, the current situation and problem, and the physician's own personality and interpersonal style. Thus, interviewing is more an art than a science. Nevertheless, there are some useful techniques and approaches that can be utilized. The authors of this chapter, along with others such as Sanson-Fisher et al. (1991), contend it is not necessary to interview patients by trial and error. Some of these techniques and approaches are discussed in the following sections.

ORGANIZING THE MEDICAL INTERVIEW

A good interview should result in an accurate and comprehensive story of the patient's situation. This story is sometimes referred to as the medical history. A commonplace phrase is, "taking a medical history."

But medical histories, like written histories of nations or institutions, are not taken but made . . . made from oral accounts of the patient's present and past illnesses by the patient, family, and friends, as well as the oral and written statements of colleagues, records of previous hospitalizations, and so on. Selection, interpretation, and ordering of information pervade the process of writing the case history. The point of all of this is that medical histories are created, not found. (Donnelly, 1988, p. 6)

A broad point of view suggests that the interchange between physician and patient is a problem-solving process made up of seven or eight steps depending on the definition of each step. From this perspective, the medical interview can be organized as follows.

Step 1: Purpose and Willingness to Consider Problems

By seeing the physician, the patient expresses a willingness to talk about an acute or chronic problem, illness, or discomfort with the physician. Occasionally, the patient comes for other reasons, such as to get out of work or obtain disability. The session can be frustrating if its purpose is not clear to both the patient and the physician.

By seeing the patient, the physician expresses a willingness to consider and deal with the patient's problems. Some physicians have other reasons, such as earning a living or fulfilling an educational requirement. If one of these other reasons prevails, the session may be very frustrating to the patient.

Step 2: Greeting and Sizing Up

In the first 20 seconds, visual input dominates the awareness of the two participants. For the patient, the warmth or coldness of the room's decor, the light level, and the privacy or lack of it are important first impressions. Next, the posture, dress, attitude, physical distance, sex, age, and body build of the physician are noted. The physician's voice pitch, volume, and expression are judged by the patient and fitted into prejudices built up by past experiences. What the physician actually says is then judged in this context. Thus, who says it, how it is said, and when it is said play as big a role as what is said.

Similarly, the physician judges the patient's body build, posture, sex, age, dress, and gestures. Quickly, the physician imagines the patient is sick, a complainer, an alcoholic, and so on and guesses the economic resources and type of work the patient does. Based on past experiences, the physician also stereotypes the patient before a word is spoken. With a new patient, it is probably best for the physician to be quiet for 5 seconds to allow this "sizing up" process to take place.

Step 3: The Problem or Chief Complaint

Opening the medical interview varies with the setting and style of the physician. Generally, a nurse, clerk, or secretary obtains descriptive data about a patient, such as name, address, age, other family members, medical insurance, and telephone number, before the interview. Some physicians prefer to acquire this information themselves as a way to open an interview on a nonthreatening topic. By gathering this information firsthand, the physician also can observe and obtain information concerning the patient's memory, orientation, and problem relationships.

Once the descriptive data are obtained, the next step is to ask what led the patient to make an appointment. Usually the record will indicate a reason for the visit. It is best to remember that a patient needs an admission ticket to see a physician. An admission ticket is a socially and medically acceptable excuse for the visit, but it may be just that—an excuse. To find the real reason, it is helpful to ask for the chief complaint, using a facilitation or an open-ended question, not a specific question. For example, asking "What is the situation that brings you here today?" is more useful than saying, "The nurse says you have an earache. What seems to be the trouble?"

Once the chief complaint is identified and clarified, the patient and physician need to agree that both are willing to share information, to explore the complaint, and to do what is necessary to understand, diagnose, or treat it. Ideally, the contract also defines the type of relationship they will have; that is, they are going to relate as a superior and an inferior, as two equals, as a teacher and a student, or as two advocates with veto power over the other's decision.

Most often, the contract is understood by behavior and willingness to respond to each other. However, when there is hesitancy to respond, when the patient asks questions of the physician, or when either person is uncomfortable, it is important to define a contract verbally and see if the other will agree. (e.g., "You seem a bit hesitant to answer my questions. Are you willing to share information with me about this problem?"). Such a question will bring out what each expects and is willing to do. If the answer is "No," the next question might be, "What are you willing to do?"

The type of relationship usually is established by the style and personality of the physician, but the physician can learn to adapt and modify the approach to meet the needs of each patient best. Sometimes the type of relationship contract is established and agreed to nonverbally through posture, tone of voice, relative physical positions, and the medical problem.

Step 4: Data Gathering

Once the chief complaint is understood and clarified, data concerning the present illness are encouraged and elicited from the patient. The interview process for a simple acute problem generally is limited to several specific questions, such as "Where did the fall occur?" or "How did the cut happen?" The interview process for a complex or chronic condition usually follows an overall guideline of obtaining specific details of the present symptoms, related diet, exercise, medications, work and home environments, social stresses, financial stresses, and emotional and behavioral reactions to the symptoms, and what the patient does to alleviate them.

The successful, efficient process for a medical interview has been described as: open the topic with open-ended questions followed by facilitations, reflections, empathic replies, and silences to learn as much as the patient is able to tell without physician suggestion and interference (Enelow

and Swisher, 1986). Once patients have said as much as they can, they are facilitated further by laundry list questions, direct questions, yes–no questions, and summary statements of clarification. The topic is closed and a bridging comment is made to move to the next topic. This process is repeated many times during a medical interview in dealing with each topic.

Once the present condition is defined, the onset of the problem should be dealt with. The physician needs a detailed description of the symptoms, how they were precipitated, how they progressed, and any data associated with each period of symptoms up to the present time. Table 18–1 sets out the types of physician interventions most suited for each phase of medical interview topic exploration.

The most common mistake in medical interviewing is for the physician to deal with the onset of the illness before knowing enough about the patient's present state to have a good idea of the organ of involvement. Without this understanding, the physician does not know where to focus attention in obtaining details of the progression of the present illness. If it is not known whether the pain described in the chest is cardiac, esophageal, or chest wall, it is not known on which organ to focus the review of the history of the present illness.

Relevant data from the past medical, social, work, and family histories are obtained using the

---

TABLE 18–1.   PHYSICIAN INTERVENTIONS FOR PHASES OF THE MEDICAL INTERVIEW

I. Opening a Topic
Facilitation
Open-ended question
Bridging phrase

II. Assisting the Patient's Narrative
Support and reassurance
Empathy
Confrontation
Reflection
Interpretation
Silence
Modified laundry-list

III. Focusing Upon a Topic
Confrontation
Reflection
Probing
Interpretation
Summation

IV. Obtaining Specific Information
Direct question
Yes-no question
Probing
Problem question
Laundry-list

V. Closing Topic or Interview
Summation
Prescription for action

From Froelich RE, Bishop FM: Clinical Interviewing Skills: A Programmed Manual, 3rd edition. St. Louis, CV Mosby, 1977, with permission.

same techniques and process of opening the topic, assisting the narrative, closing the topic, and bridging a new topic (Table 18–1).

Step 5: Analysis and Definition of the Problem

Once the data are obtained, they must be analyzed to give meaning to the symptoms, history, and associated data. This analysis defines the patient's discomforts as a physiologic or disease process. Thus, a tentative diagnosis is formed. Although dependent on the interview, the diagnostic process is related to training, information, and ability to synthesize numerous types of data.

Step 6: Treatment Alternatives and Decisions

After the physiologic process is defined, diagnostic or treatment alternatives are considered. In the ideal problem-solving process, the patient has enough understanding to suggest some of the diagnostic or treatment alternatives. The physician presents suggestions and alternatives along with their probable outcomes, cost, and side effects. Ideally, this decision is a joint decision between the physician and the patient.

Step 7: Action and Evaluation

The diagnostic or treatment alternative is instituted and the results are evaluated by both the physician and the patient. If the decision involves a treatment and it solves the problem, this episode of health care for this patient is concluded with questions and suggestions of how to avoid similar illnesses in the future. If the decision is a diagnostic activity or an unsuccessful treatment, the physician and patient return to Step 3 or Step 4 with the new data.

Although primarily written as a textbook for medical students, Coulehan and Block's (1987) text presents materials that are relevant to specific patient encounters with numerous examples of doctor–patient interactions.

PITFALLS IN INTERVIEWING

The effectiveness of an interviewer to conduct a good medical interview and to create and make a medical history is dependent in part on the ability to avoid some of the following common pitfalls. These pitfalls can, at times, become an unconscious detriment to both the experienced and the novice interviewer. With practice and conscious effort, they can be avoided; with attention and vigi-

lance, they can be utilized appropriately rather than routinely.

Direct Questions

The temptation to resort to direct questions is probably the major pitfall for the inexperienced interviewer and the interviewer who lets skills languish. An interview made up of direct questions gathers little information per unit time, because most of the time is spent by the interviewer framing and asking questions, each of which elicits a specific bit of information.

The direct question approach does not permit patients to give information they have experienced, and the interviewers may never obtain the piece of information the patients wanted to give—that is, unless interviewers just happened to ask the one specific question that taps the information.

"Why" Questions

A second pitfall is asking "why" questions: "Why did you take that medicine?" "Why did you leave work?" "Why did you get a divorce?" The problem with these questions is that they call on patients to account for their behavior and encourage defensive attitudes. "Why" questions of a patient imply that the patient did something wrong. Because much of the patient's behavior may be derived from the unconscious or be related to reasons that are not socially acceptable, patients may be antagonized by the implication in the question that they did something wrong. Patients may feel that such a question finds fault with them and thus may become irritated or annoyed. It is difficult to ask a "why" question and avoid the overtones of accusation. In addition, "why" questions come from a whining transactional position on the part of the interviewer. The whining position may be described as a position of helplessness, pleading, or angry frustration.

The above questions could be rephrased as: "Tell me about taking that medicine." "You needed to leave work?" "Are you willing to tell me about the divorce?"

Suggestive Questions

A third pitfall is a question that has within it the answer. This is called a suggestive question. An example is, "When you discussed your problem, your breathing was a little rapid. Were you a little nervous at the time?" What choice does the patient have in responding to such a question? Obviously, much misinformation can be obtained by using suggestive questions. This is especially true when the patient feels put down or inferior to the physician and feels a need to be compliant.

"Yes" and "No" Questions

With many patients there is a danger in using questions requiring yes and no answers. The patient's answer may be more dependent on the immediate milieu than on the facts. When a question is answered with a "Yes," it is not clear what the "Yes" means. Is it given to please, to give the interviewer what the patient thinks he or she wants to hear, to avoid discussing an area that the patient wants to avoid, or is it a factual response? Similarly, when the question can be answered with a "No," the patient may wish to disagree, wish to please, wish to avoid discussing a topic, or wish to give a factual response. Much inaccurate information can be obtained by using this type of question. Even an experienced interviewer can get misinformation from any patient by asking a question that can be answered most appropriately by a "Yes" or "No."

Unsignaled Topic Changes

When the physician asks the patient for information and there is a longer than usual pause before answering, the topic has probably been changed without signaling this intention to the patient. This interviewing pitfall slows the interviewing process and, because the topic change is unsignaled, gives the patient the impression the interviewer has no clear plan of action. When it is time to change a topic, it is best to use a bridging phrase such as, "Let's shift to talking about . . . ," to guide the patient in the direction the interview is to go.

Lack of Eye Contact

A pitfall that sometimes is forgotten is that lack of eye contact through concentration on a note pad, a chart, or a referral note will affect greatly the information obtained from a patient. In addition to giving the message that the paper is more important than the patient, the interviewer misses out on all of the gestures, facial expressions, and shifts in position that add so much to the meaning of what is said. At times, when listening to only the words, the interviewer even misses the intonation of the voice, the guttural emphasis, the slight laugh, or the held-back cry.

Lack of Feedback to Patients

Giving no feedback to the patient is an interviewing pitfall that will interfere with the doctor–patient relationship. Giving no feedback is im-

possible if both the doctor and the patient are in the same room in view of each other and able to hear each other. As one patient said to her physician, "I knew how you felt about that by your raised eyebrows." The physician, however, had been unaware of any eyebrow movement. Whatever we do either is interpreted by the patient as encouraging or discouraging his or her current responses. With practice and videotape review of interviews, an interviewer can gain increasing conscious control of the nonverbal feedback given to patients.

PROBLEM PATIENTS

The effectiveness of an interview in large part is dependent on the number and variety of interviewing techniques the physician can utilize to meet the variety of situations that arise in an interview. For example, the same techniques will not work with the overtalkative and the reticent, the sad and the angry, or the frightened and the stoic patient.

Some of the interviewing literature focuses on problem patients. Although this focus has led to some meaningful understandings, the broader view of the problem patient being a part of an interview system has led to additional insights with a focus on the physician as well as the patient. A problem patient to one physician may be an ideal patient to the next physician. This section will focus on both the patient and the physician, using a personalized approach to attitudes and feelings of the physician in the discussion.

Defensive Patient

Patients are usually defensive because of an expected negative outcome if they were to talk freely about the topic at hand. For instance, the patient may expect anger, rejection, blame, or ridicule, and there is fear or anxiety about the expected outcome. Several techniques may be used to deal with defensiveness and the obstacle it poses to evaluation and diagnosis.

One technique is to ask, "What might happen if you were to talk about . . . ?" The patient's answer is pursued until the physician understands the fear. In rare instances, the physician may agree that the expected outcome is a probable outcome (e.g., information used in a pending lawsuit) and that the patient should not discuss the topic. More likely, once the outcome is discussed, it becomes evident to the patient that nothing bad will happen if the topic is discussed. As the topic is dealt with, the defensiveness begins to melt away.

A second technique is to ask, "What is the worst possible thing or catastrophe that could happen if you talked about . . . ?" Again, the physician may agree that the catastrophe might occur or, as is more usually the case, the patient will realize the unlikeliness of the catastrophic action actually taking place.

A third technique, especially if the patient is teasing or appears to be suggesting there is important information and then withholds the information, is to agree not to discuss the topic and go on to another one. If this is a "tease," the topic will be brought up later in the session or in the next session if it is of great importance to the patient. By not responding, the physician reinforces a straightforward, open discussion rather than a continuation of teasing innuendos.

A fourth technique is to comment on the defensiveness, such as: "You seem very reluctant to discuss this topic," followed initially by silence on the physician's part. If the patient does not respond, the physician may proceed with, "Is there anything that will make it easier for you to discuss this topic?" or "Are there any questions you want to ask before proceeding?" or "Can you identify your concerns in talking about this topic?" Finally, the physician might ask, "Is there some problem about your trusting me with the information about this topic?" or "Is there something that concerns you about my reaction to or feelings toward you if we discuss this topic?"

Should any of the latter questions be asked, the physician needs to be prepared to discuss the patient's replies honestly, directly, objectively, and without personal distance in the sense that the patient is reacting to the person in the physician role. The patient may be reacting to his or her fantasy of the physician-person (transference), putting expectations on the physician. These expectations need to be checked for accuracy before proceeding. The first time the relationship between the physician and the patient is the focus, it may be helpful to record the session on tape and review the session with a peer or supervisor who can provide some objective observations on the doctor–patient relationship. When dealing with defensiveness, it is a transference problem rather than a reality problem most of the time.

Fearful Patient

One can produce anxiety in one's self with a scary thought and restricted breathing. By doing the opposite—relaxing the breathing and avoiding the fear-producing thoughts—anxiety can be controlled.

A decision needs to be made as to whether the patient's fear is related to a real threat, sometimes referred to as reality fear, or to an imagined threat, referred to as neurotic fear. Fear associated with a real threat is considered healthy. Relaxation techniques, focusing the person's attention away from the threat, and caring support are useful ways to comfort these patients. It is important to let patients experience their real fear and help them through it.

The neurotic fear of an imagined threat should be handled through exploration of the threat and the probability that it would actually occur, along with the consequences if it did occur. Again, what is the catastrophic fear and how realistic or likely is it to happen? The question, "So what if it does happen?" may help. This process confronts the unreality of the fear and imagined threat.

The next step is to encourage the patient to agree to breathe slowly and deeply and to stop the scary thoughts. The patient should focus on some pleasant thoughts instead. This uses a positive approach, rather than a negative approach.

Angry Patient

Several issues are raised when dealing with an angry patient:

1. What is the direction and quality of the anger?

2. Can the physician accept or allow the patient to be angry?

3. Is the patient's anger affecting the medical problem?

4. How is the patient justifying the anger?

5. Is the anger caused by frustration or is it a cover-up for sadness?

In the normal, healthy person, anger is the natural result of frustration. To overcome the frustration in a socially acceptable manner, the anger takes the form of aggression. Once the anger changes to hostility, it becomes destructive rather than constructive and is considered maladaptive.

Physicians vary widely in their ability to recognize anger and tolerate it in a patient. One physician may enjoy the spunk of the angry patient while another fears, withdraws from, or denies a patient's anger. The issue is, how can the physician be comfortable with an angry patient? Is the physician willing to learn how to be comfortable with an angry patient? Some physicians answer this question with, "Yes, if I am sure the patient is in control and will not hurt me." This is a diagnostic decision that needs to be addressed.

Whether or not a person is angry at a given moment is under his or her own control. A person who chooses not to be angry cannot be made angry. Invitations to be angry may be ignored or viewed as just idiosyncrasies. Also, attention can be focused on what might motivate others to send out such behavioral signals or invitations. Any of these techniques will effectively help a person avoid becoming angry in response to another's hostile behavior.

Understanding anger as a feeling under the control of the individual suggests a way to manage it. An additional factor to consider is how the person uses anger in the interpersonal process. Anger is frequently used as blackmail (i.e., "If you do . . . , I will be angry and when I get angry you better watch out."). Anger is also frequently used as an attempt to control the behavior of others. Thus, the treatment of anger is to acknowledge it and then ignore it with such a statement as, "You sure are angry. If you want to be angry it's OK with me." And, if it fits, add "I really think it is kind of stupid to stay angry in this situation."

These statements acknowledge the anger, accept the patient being angry, and allow the physician avoid being a part of the game with subsequent payoff. The physician might follow these statements with, "If you want to look at how you make yourself so angry, I am willing to look at it with you," or "I will be happy to refer you to someone who will help you find a way to be more comfortable rather than angry."

Manipulative or Demanding Patient

A manipulative patient is skilled in getting something wanted from other people by using a variety of artful maneuvers, such as threats to produce a fit of temper, attempts at suicide that are aimed at influencing others, and behavior that otherwise plays on the guilt of others, such as seduction.

The issue is "Can I accept the patient being manipulative?" or "Can I outmanipulate the patient for his or her own good?" The issue of manipulation becomes potentially pathologic when the patient becomes dishonest or deceives the physician as a way to obtain more drugs, hospital admission, unwarranted surgery, or some special treatment. At this level of manipulation, consultation with a psychiatrist or someone who knows how to manage such patients may be needed. Most manipulative patients can be managed by the family physician by the use of a very specific contract regarding the issues of discomfort, such as demands to be seen after hours or unnecessary night calls.

Changing Reactions to Problem Patients

The key to changing behavior is answered by the question, "How?" When the process, mechanism, or procedure for the behavior—in this case, interview style—is understood, it is possible to change some part or all of the process, mechanism, or procedure in order to initiate a new behavior.

For example, if a physician becomes angry with a patient and wishes to change this feeling, the question should be asked, "How did I make myself angry?" or "How did I interpret the patient's statements or behavior to make myself angry?" or "What meaning did I assign to the patient's behavior?" Once these "how" and "what" questions are answered, the physician can ask, "Is there another

way to interpret the patient's behavior?" or "Would I still be angry if I interpreted the behavior another way and gave it a different meaning?"

The conclusive step to institute change is to decide to interpret the behavior in another way and decide to feel something other than anger the next time the physician is faced with the patient's behavior. This process involves asking:

1. How do the physician's behaviors or feelings come about?
2. What meaning is assigned to the patient's behavior?
3. How can the perception of the behavior be interpreted differently?

The process also involves deciding on an alternate way to interpret the behavior to initiate change. In learning medical interviewing, this process of change is key to improving medical interviewing skills.

ALTERNATIVES TO THE FACE-TO-FACE INTERVIEW

The Questionnaire

The questionnaire completed by a patient (either on paper or from the interviewer's memory) is quite different from an interview. They differ in two major ways. First, the questionnaire lacks the human qualities of a human interaction—a constantly renegotiated give and take. It lacks all of the nonverbal aspects of meaningful communication. Second, the questionnaire lacks the ability to make meaning out of the patient's responses. Without meaning, the physician has limited or no use of the information. To illustrate, the datum that a patient was married at age 15 is of little use in and of itself. However, knowing the circumstances surrounding the decision to marry at age 15 may have profound meaning in understanding the patient's reactions to a present illness. The raw datum, "married age 15," is made meaningful and useful in the present context by elaboration in the interview.

Although a written questionnaire given to a patient may result in information, there is no human relationship established between a patient and a questionnaire. Because the relationship is important to the treatment of the patient and the patient's cooperation, the human interview is an essential element of the patient's visit.

The Computerized History

By not being able to make meaning out of the patient's words, computerized histories have the semantic problem of not being able to explain further to the patient just what is meant by the question being asked, and the reverse problem of not being able to ask the patient just what he or she meant by what was said. A study of computerized histories found that only "68% [of patients] could express all or most of their complaints, but some of their physical complaints could not be entered (at all)," and only "52% of the women" and "74% of the male patients found the range of answers from which to choose sufficient" (Quaak et al., 1986, pp. 551–564). As the authors of this chapter found as early as 1968, the computer is unable to understand a patient's communication because communicating includes verbal and nonverbal messages. The meaning of the words is shaded by the nonverbal as well as linguistic aspects of the message, and the computer is unable to pick up this meaning. Remember the problem of direct questions noted earlier in the chapter. Computer-generated questions, by necessity, must be direct questions because the computer is unable to interpret dialogue as a response.

The major activity of the interviewer is to make meaning out of the words chosen by the patient. Only after the meaning is confirmed by the interviewer can the physiologic processes be understood. "It is crucial not to put man-machine interaction and human dialogue on the same footing. A computer is quite unable to understand anything, but it can help health professionals in gathering medical history data" (Houziaux, 1986, pp. 129–143).

ORGANIZATIONS INVOLVED IN ENHANCING INTERVIEWING SKILLS

Family practice organizations have been involved in emphasizing and teaching interviewing techniques from the beginning of the specialty. Since the late 1960s, the Behavioral Sciences Task Force of the Society of Teachers of Family Medicine (STFM) has presented numerous workshops on skills development in teaching medical interviewing. However, this has not been the only focus of this task force; other STFM committees and task forces touch on curriculum development and faculty development in interviewing techniques and the doctor–patient relationship.

The Society of General Internal Medicine also was interested in medical interviewing and, in 1978, appointed a Task Force on Medical Interview and Related Skills, which interested a number of individuals from other disciplines, including family practice. In 1989, the task force changed its name to the Task Force on the Doctor and Patient in anticipation of forming a separate academy and to reflect a broader range of interests.

In January 1993, invitations were issued to all interested persons representing a large variety of disciplines to join the new organization, called the American Academy on the Physician and Patient. One of the reasons stated for the new academy was that

it was clear that this work equally concerned each primary care discipline—medicine, pediatrics, and family practice. In order for pediatricians and family practitioners to feel a partnership in our efforts, they needed to be on equal footing. This was the principal reason to separate from the Society of General Internal Medicine. (Lipkin, 1993, pp. 1–2)

The mission of the academy is "to continually improve the quality of the doctor-patient relationship, and to promote the integration of biological and psychosocial approaches within clinical practice, teaching, and research." The first objective is "to develop and teach skills in the medical interview and clinical reasoning that integrate biological, psychological and social domains."

Practitioners with a special interest in medical interviewing may wish to access the academy videotapes. Rather than being didactically oriented, these resources include a variety of provocative trigger tapes and scenarios. Most of the offerings include some teaching materials, strategies, and references. Some of the tapes address more targeted topics such as alcoholism, cancer, acquired immunodeficiency syndrome, and bilingual medical interviewing.

REFERENCES

Brody DS, Miller SM, Leman CE, et al: Patient perception of involvement in medical care: Relationship to illness, attitudes, and outcomes. J Gen Intern Med 4:506, 1989.

Coulehan, JL, Block, MR: Medical Interview: A Primer for Students of the Art. Philadelphia, FA Davis, 1987.

Donnelly WJ: Righting the medical record: Transforming the chronicle into story. JAMA 260:6, 1988.

Enelow AJ, Swisher SN: Interviewing and Patient Care. New York, Oxford University Press, 1986.

Feffer D: The patient's turn. Medical Encounter—American Academy on Physician and Patient 9(1):8, 1992.

Greenfield S, Kaplan S, Ware JE: Expanding patient's involvement in care: Effects on patient outcomes. Ann Intern Med 102:520, 1985.

Hayakawa SI: Language in Thought and Action. New York, Harcourt, Brace & World, 1964.

Houziaux MO: Historical and methodological aspects of computer-assisted medical history-taking. Med Inf 11(2):129, 1986.

Lipkin M: The formation of AAPP. Medical Encounter—American Academy on Physician and Patient 10(suppl):1, 1993.

Quaak MJ, Westerman RF, Schouten JA, et al: Appraisal of computerized medical histories: comparisons between computerized and conventional records. Comput Biomed Res 19:551, 1986.

Ruesch J, Kees W: Nonverbal Communication. Berkeley, University of California Press, 1970, pp 3–7.

Sanson-Fisher RW, Redman S, Walsh R, et al: Training medical practitioners in information transfer skills: The new challenge. Med Educ 25:322, 1991.

Tracy D: Plurality and Ambiguity: Hermeneutics, Religion, Hope. New York, Harper & Row, 1987.

Part IV

PRACTICE OF FAMILY MEDICINE

CHAPTER 19

CLINICAL PROBLEM SOLVING IN FAMILY PRACTICE

I. R. McWHINNEY

Although the general principles of problem solving are the same in all branches of medicine, each discipline has its way of applying them. The differences between disciplines are due to differences in the problems they encounter and to differences in their roles within the health care system. The problem-solving strategies of family physicians have evolved in response to a number of special features of family practice:

1. The pattern of illness in family practice approximates the pattern of illness in the community. This means that there is a high incidence of acute, short-term illness, much of it transient and self-limiting; a high prevalence of chronic illness; and a high prevalence of behavioral problems. Contrary to the conventional view, patients do not present with either physical or behavioral problems. They come with problems that are often a complex mixture of physical, psychological, and social elements.

The incidence and prevalence of disease in family practice have, as we will see, an important effect on the predictive value of symptoms and tests. To deal successfully with this pattern of problems, the family physician's problem-solving strategies must be especially adapted for two purposes. First, they must be capable of separating, in the early stages of illness, the serious and life-threatening diseases from the transient and minor. Because the serious diseases come in the midst of the more common minor and transient illnesses and because the symptoms are often very similar, this is no easy task. Second, these strategies must be capable of teasing out the physical, social, and psychological elements of the patient's problem.

2. When the patient first sees the family physician for a new episode of illness, the illness is likely to be both undifferentiated and unorganized. The meaning of these concepts is discussed below.

3. Because the family physician is available for all types of problems, no prior assumptions can be made about the type of problems likely to be encountered. Problem-solving methods therefore must be adaptable enough to deal with any health-related problem. Because the family physician's commitment to patients is unconditional, he or she cannot make the categorization "my problem/not my problem" that is made by organ and system specialists.

4. In family practice, disease often is seen early, before the full clinical picture has developed. Information on which to base a precise diagnosis—the kind of information discussed in textbooks—is often not available to the family physician when the patient is first seen. Decisions must be made with fewer cues than are available in the later stages of disease. They also must be made with different cues. Symptoms change as an illness advances. The symptoms and tests that have diagnostic value in the early stages may be quite different from those that have diagnostic value in the later stages.

5. The family physician's relationship with patients is continuous and transcends individual episodes of illness. This has two important consequences. Because the relationship is open ended, the physician need be in no hurry to solve all the patient's problems in one or two visits. Observation over time can be used as a method for testing hypotheses, assessing probabilities, and attempting to understand the context of problems.

6. Because family physicians are directly available to their patients, their workload can be predicted and planned only to a limited extent. This means that decisions often must be made under pressure of time. To be effective decision makers under these conditions, family physicians must be particularly skilled in ascertaining at an early stage what is the patient's main problem. They must develop the skills of formulating a strategy for dealing with the problems in the time available, focusing on the decisions that must be made immediately, selecting the most efficient strategy for arriving at these decisions, and devising a plan for the longer term assessment and management of the problem. Finally, the physician must put other problems in a priority order and devise a similar plan for their longer term assessment and management.

CENTRAL CONCEPTS IN FAMILY MEDICINE

Undifferentiated Illness

By undifferentiated illness we mean an illness that has not previously been assessed, categorized, and named by a physician. In the process of diagnosis, the physician takes raw data presented by the patient, adds the data acquired by his or her own search, and tries to fit the illness into a disease category within his or her own frame of reference. In this way, many of the patients presenting to family physicians have their "raw" illnesses differentiated into well-known disease categories.

However, many patients have illnesses that defy this kind of differentiation. There are at least four reasons why this may be so. First, an illness may be transient and self-limiting, creating a functional disturbance that clears completely, leaving no evidence on which a diagnosis can be based. These illnesses are usually short lived, but not invariably so. Sometimes, a patient may suffer for months from an illness that eventually clears without ever having been diagnosed.

Second, there are, at the edge of every disease category, borderline and intermediate conditions that are difficult or impossible to classify. Our disease categories are not as sharply outlined as we sometimes think. Because family physicians see all variants of disease, they are especially liable to encounter milder variants and borderline conditions that may never reach the system specialist.

Third, an illness may remain undifferentiated for many years before its true nature unfolds in time. For example, it may be years before an attack of transient blurring of vision is followed by other evidence of multiple sclerosis.

Fourth, an illness may be so closely interwoven with the personality and personal life of the patient—so individual—that it defies classification. Patients with chronic pain are often examples of this type of illness.

The family physician's assessment of an illness therefore may, have a number of outcomes. Some illnesses will be diagnosed in the conventional manner in a comparatively short period of time; some eventually will be diagnosed after a longer period of observation; some will come and go without ever being diagnosed; and some will never be diagnosed because they defy classification. Whatever type he or she is dealing with, the family physician must have a strategy that is appropriate for the problem. Harm may be done if the wrong strategy is used. For example, the use of the conventional diagnostic strategy in a patient with an ill-defined pain syndrome may result in a spurious "diagnosis," overinvestigation, overmedication, and iatrogenic disease. Using data from the National Ambulatory Care Survey, Carmichael (1980) has calculated that only in half the ambulatory encounters with the family physician does the patient have an illness with objective evidence of physical pathology. Of these, the majority are in the effective domain, and many of the remainder are visits for preventive or administrative purposes. Carmichael argued that, for self-limiting and behavioral problems and for preventive services (between them accounting for 80 per cent of all encounters), the crucial factor is the relationship between patient and physician rather than the action of the physician.

Unorganized Illness

The concept of the organization of illness is an important one for family medicine. When patients first tell a physician about their problems and symptoms, they usually do so with little insight into the nature or cause of those problems. A patient who has had malaise, anorexia, and discolored urine for 5 days and a 3-month history of fatigue, depression, and headaches does not know that in the physician's mind these add up to two clusters of symptoms, one suggesting hepatitis and the other depression. When these problems are presented for the first time, they usually will not come out in an orderly sequence that reflects a clear concept of their nature and cause. The patient may, of course, have his or her own ideas about the significance of the symptoms, but these often will be very different from the assessment made by the physician. The way symptoms are presented also will be influenced strongly by the patient's fears and anxieties and by his or her ability to describe these sensations.

Once the patient has been through the process of assessment by a physician, all this changes. He or she learns that the malaise, anorexia, and discolored urine are not isolated phenomena, but a cluster of symptoms associated with hepatitis. He or she learns that the tiredness is related to depression, that the headaches are tension headaches, and that these are quite separate problems from the hepatitis. If we now imagine that the hepatitis becomes worse and the patient is referred to a specialist, it is not difficult to see that the history given to the specialist will be quite different from the one given to the family physician. It will be "organized" around the concepts of infectious hepatitis and depression.

Five facts contribute to the lack of organization in the data presented to the family physician:

1. Patients often present more than one problem at the same visit.

2. The problems often are not presented in order of priority. The most serious problem may be left until last or not even mentioned at all.

3. The most sensitive problems may be expressed in indirect or metaphoric language.

4. The problem is not necessarily the same as the disease.

5. Much of the information presented by the patient is "noise" (i.e., it is not useful in solving the patient's presenting problems). At this stage, the patient usually has little insight into the significance of the data he or she is presenting. Even "noise," however, may be useful to the physician as background information.

Diagnosis

Although there is no agreed-on definition of the terms "diagnosis" and "making a diagnosis," in modern usage they usually refer to the process of classifying a patient's illness into one of the recognized disease categories. This has not always been so. In other periods of history, diagnosis meant diagnosis of a patient rather than diagnosis of a disease. Nevertheless, I think it is better to adhere to modern usage and define diagnosis (the process) as "the assignment of a patient's illness to a category that links the symptoms with a pathologic process, a known outcome, and—whenever possible—a cause."

Successful classification of the illness has four very important results. First, by knowing the natural history of the disease category, clinicians can predict the outcome of the illness if it remains untreated. Second, they can make inferences about the cause or causes of the illness. Third, they can make inferences about the patient that go beyond the evidence of their senses. Fourth, they can, by using the common taxonomic language of medicine, communicate their findings to other clinicians. For example, if a patient with fatigue, pallor, and loss of weight is classified as having "pernicious anemia," the clinician can infer that the patient, if deficient in intrinsic factor, will die if untreated and will respond rapidly to injection of vitamin B_{12}.

It is clear that classification is a very powerful tool. The successful application of technology to medicine depends on it, because unless we can predict the outcome of untreated illness, we cannot know whether or not our interventions are effective. It helps us organize our thoughts about the phenomena of illness. It also, as we shall see, helps us organize our thoughts about human behavior. While recognizing the central role of classification, however, we must not lose sight of its limitations. Classification is a generalizing process that tacitly ignores individual differences. It works by reducing the complex phenomena of illness or behavior to relatively simple categories. Neither illness nor behavior, however, is as simple as this. No two patients are the same. In making clinical decisions, therefore, the clinician must go through two processes at the same time: one a generalizing and the other an individualizing process. As we shall see

when we discuss management decisions, this can lead to different management decisions for patients with the same "diagnosis" or disease label. The distinction between illness and disease—discussed below—provides us with a useful conceptual framework for thinking about these complex phenomena.

Diagnosing (classifying and naming) the patient's illness is a crucial part of the problem-solving process, but it is by no means the whole of it. At the same time, the clinician must assess the personal and environmental context of the illness. This will involve the individual description of a unique person as well as other types of classification. The clinician also must make complex management decisions in which risk/benefit, prognostic, and ethical calculations play a part.

The family physician learns, to the extent few other physicians do, the limitations of the conventional classification system. It is estimated that in only 50 per cent of patients seen by family physicians is it possible to make a diagnosis in the sense I have defined it. The reasons for this already have been given. Of course, patients who cannot be diagnosed always can be given labels such as "low back syndrome" or "pleurodynia," but this is not diagnosis as defined above, and labels of this type have little predictive value. Even when a diagnosis is made, the family physician also knows that he or she may not have solved the problem, because the problem may be different from the diagnosis.

Howie (1973) has provided evidence that, with some types of illness, family physicians base their management decisions on the presence or absence of certain clinical features rather than on the diagnostic label applied. In a large study done in 62 general practices, 1000 patients with respiratory illness were reported. Cough and chest signs were present in 163, and of these 152 (93 per cent) received an antibiotic. The presence of cough and chest signs therefore had a predictive value for antibiotic treatment of 0.93. Twelve different diagnostic labels were applied to the 163 patients. Five of the labels had a predictive value of only 0.45. It appears, therefore, that family physicians, when dealing with certain kinds of illness, make management decisions based on their clinical findings and then apply a diagnostic label after the decision is made.

Illness and Disease

The conceptual distinction between illness and disease is a useful one for the family physician (Kleinman et al., 1978). An illness may be described as all the sensations of a patient and all the ramifications of the disorder. It includes symptoms, feelings, discomforts, disabilities, defenses and supports, attitudes toward the condition and the physician, and the effect of the disorder on personal relationships and work. A disease is a theoretical construct that a physician uses to explain something about the patient's illness. Given a certain constellation of findings, we say that a patient has a disease called pernicious anemia. The category "pernicious anemia" is a useful conceptual tool that enables us to make certain inferences and predictions about the patient.

As I have defined them, disease and illness belong to two different universes of discourse: one to the world of theory and the other to the world of experience. The patient experiences the illness; the physician diagnoses the disease (i.e., puts the illness into his or her own explanatory frame of reference). It is important to note that the patient may have his or her own explanatory frame of reference, which may be derived from his or her culture, religion, social class, or personal experience (Kleinman et al., 1978).

UNDERSTANDING PATIENTS' BEHAVIOR

From all that has been said so far, it will be clear that an understanding of patients' behavior is crucial to the accurate identification of undifferentiated clinical problems. For any patient visit, the physician should be able to answer the following questions:

1. Why did the patient come?
2. Why did the patient come at this particular time?
3. What does the patient mean by these complaints? What type of language is the patient using?
4. What is the patient's own perception of the problem(s)?
5. What is the chief problem?
6. What is the context of the problem(s)? How does it relate to the patient's life situation and stage of development?

The process of finding answers to these questions often goes on in parallel with the process of clinical diagnosis. The steps in the first process are essentially the same as those in the second: The physician responds to certain cues, formulates a hypothesis about the patient's behavior, and then conducts a search to verify the hypothesis. The difference between the two processes is that, in clinical diagnosis, we have as a guide a precise and universally recognized classification of disease. For patient behavior, we have no universally agreed on schema.

In the course of problem solving, the family physician makes use of categories that are different from the recognized taxa of disease. In the early part of the process, for example, he or she may have to place the illness into one of two broad categories: A/B and A/Not A. Examples are given in Figure

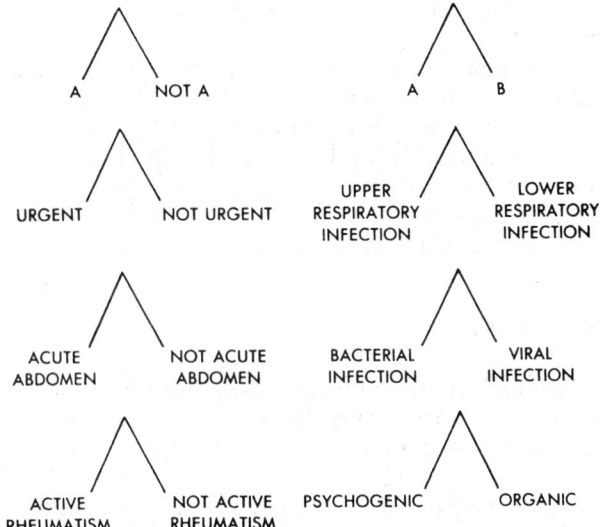

FIGURE 19–1. Examples of broad categories of illness used in family practice. (From McWhinney IR: An Introduction to Family Medicine. New York, Oxford University Press, 1981, p 89, with permission.)

19–1. Several points should be borne in mind about this binary categorization:

1. Although many patients can be categorized usefully in this way, the physician always must remember that patients' problems may fall in both categories, such as psychogenic and organic, or upper and lower respiratory infection.
2. This broad categorization is used early in the problem-solving process. Obviously, if a patient falls into some of the categories, the process will continue toward a much more precise clinical diagnosis.
3. In contrast, if the illness is categorized as "not an acute abdomen" or "virus infection (not serious)," the clinician may discontinue the search and observe the patient, because he or she expects the illness to be minor and self-limiting. In these cases, the clinician can achieve his or her objective by defining what the patient does not have—the so-called eliminative diagnosis of Crombie (1963).
4. If the illness is categorized as "psychogenic," this may be the end of the classification process. The physician then may proceed to explore the individual aspects of the illness.
5. The tests that are useful for separating illness into these broad categories are different from those that are useful for attaining a precise clinical diagnosis. The erythrocyte sedimentation rate (ESR), for example, is a very useful test for discriminating between categories such as psychogenic/organic and active rheumatism/no active rheumatism; it is much less useful for distinguishing among the subcategories of rheumatic disease.

One of the reasons that family practice is so confusing to new students and residents is that the descriptions of disease they see in standard medical textbooks are based on observations made in the advanced stages of disease. The family physician works at the other end of the time scale, where the pattern is very different and much less complete. The first stage of the problem-solving process, in this situation, is to identify cues to the patient's illness.

THE PROBLEM-SOLVING PROCESS

Figure 19–2 shows a model of the process of clinical problem solving that applies to all fields of medicine (McWhinney, 1989). The model is based on the work of Elstein et al. (1978). When presented with a problem, the clinician responds to cues by forming one or more hypotheses about what is wrong with the patient. He or she then embarks on a search (the history, examination, and investigation) to test the hypothesis. In the course of the search, he or she looks for positive (confirming) and negative (nonconfirming) evidence. If the evidence does not confirm the hypothesis, the hypothesis is revised and the search begins again. As indicated by the feedback loop in Figure 19–2, the process is a cyclical one, with the clinician constantly revising, testing, and further revising the hypothesis until he or she has refined it to the point at which it seems justifiable to make management decisions. Even after this point, the clinician still must be prepared to revise the hypothesis if the progress of the patient is not as predicted.

CUES

A cue is an item of information. When a patient presents his or her problems, the family physician is confronted by a mass of data of varying value, from the highly significant to "noise." Out of this mass of data, he or she responds to cues that have meaning because they give him or her an idea about what is wrong with the patient.

Cues can be classified in a number of ways:

1. *Single or multiple.* Sometimes cues are single; more usually they form a cluster, so that the physician responds to a pattern.

2. *Symptom cues, sign cues, behavioral cues, contextual cues.* Symptom and sign cues need no explanation. Behavioral cues are those the physician receives from the patient's behavior or from his or her own subjective sensations. "I feel I could cry" is a cue to the patient's emotional state. "This patient makes me feel depressed" may be a cue to the patient's mood. Contextual cues are those that come from some incongruity the physician senses in the whole pattern of the consultation. For example: "Why did the patient not mention her husband?"

3. *Certain and probabilistic cues.* A certain cue enables the physician to say with certainly what is wrong with the patient. This is what we usually mean by spot diagnosis. Certain cues are unfortunately rare in family practice, as they are in most fields of medicine. Most cues are probabilistic; that is, they may indicate a number of different diseases with varying probabilities, and the physician can only formulate hypotheses about what is wrong with the patient. The hypotheses then must be tested by a search for further information.

Of all the cues presented to family physicians, symptoms are the most important. In the early stages of illness, and in the varieties of illness seen by the family physician, signs are less frequently available. The family physician is especially concerned with two aspects of a symptom. One is its capacity to bring the patient to see him or her (i.e., its significance for the patient). This has been called by Feinstein (1967) the "iatrophic stimulus." For example, hemoptysis has a greater value as an iatrophic stimulus than cough. The other is the sensitivity, specificity, and predictive value of

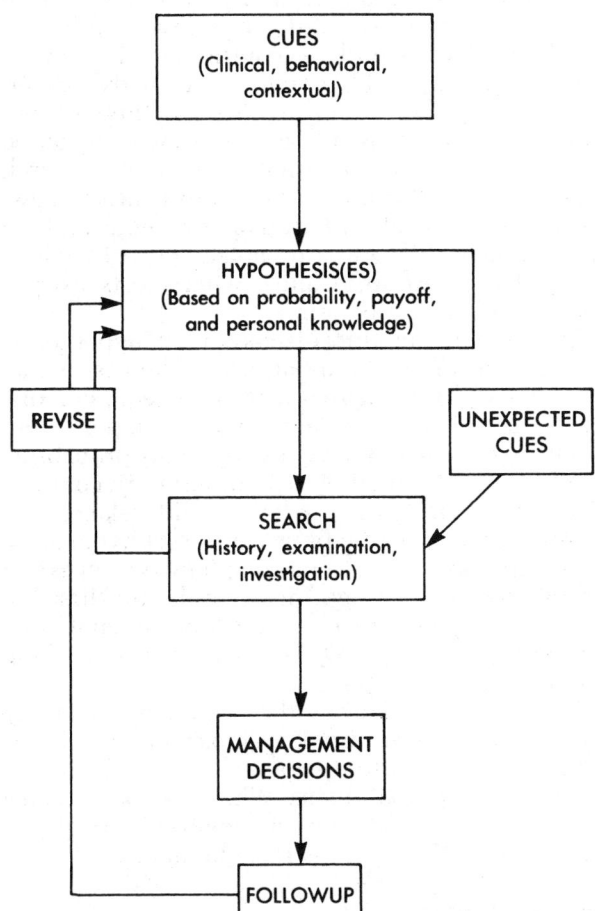

FIGURE 19–2. Model of the diagnostic process. (From McWhinney IR: An Introduction to Family Medicine. New York, Oxford University Press, 1981, p 83, with permission.)

the symptom in the early stages of illness. These terms will be defined later when we discuss the search. All of them are measures of how effective a symptom or test is in identifying a disease and in discriminating between it and other disease or a state of health.

To learn family medicine, one must learn the value of symptoms in the early stage of illness. Naturally, cues to the early detection of serious and life-threatening illness are of special importance for the family physician. Even though the physician may see only one every 10 years, he or she still must know how to separate the patient with subarachnoid hemorrhage from the thousands presenting with headache. The physician does this by the recognition of key cues, described by Williams (1977) as "red flags," that alert him or her to danger.

HYPOTHESIS

Investigators of the clinical process have found consistently that clinicians form their first hypothesis very soon after the patient has presented his or her first problem. Hypothesis formation is a mark of the clinician's creativity. We do not know how clinical hypotheses are generated, any more than we know how they are generated in scientific discovery. They are certainly not the result of linear logic: They seem to spring into consciousness as we respond to cues. Experience is certainly a factor: The incoming information is matched with other information stored in our mind's filing system. Generally speaking, the greater the clinician's experience in his or her field, the more powerful will be his or her hypotheses. Generation of a hypothesis does depend, however, on what use the physician has made of his or her experience. There is a well known comparison between a physician with 20 years' experience and one who has 1 year of experience 20 times.

The clinician usually has between two and five hypotheses at any one time: To handle more than six is difficult for the human mind. As old hypotheses are discarded and new ones called up, the clinician can consider many more in the course of his or her investigation.

The hypotheses are placed in ranking order, based on two main criteria: probability and payoff. Payoff is an indication of the consequences of diagnosing or not diagnosing a disease. The more serious a disease and the more amenable to treatment, the greater the positive payoff of making the diagnosis and the greater the negative payoff of missing it. If a disease has a high payoff, it may be ranked high on the clinician's list, even though it has a low probability. In a child with abdominal pain, for example, acute appendicitis may be ranked high—even though of low probability—because of the high positive value of an early diagnosis.

If considerations of payoff do not arise, the hypotheses are ranked in order of probability. Note that this is not the prior probability (the prevalence of the disease in the practice population) but *the conditional probability* (the probability of the disease, given the patient's symptoms). A synonym for conditional probability is predictive value: the predictive value of symptom X for disease A.

Predictive value varies with prevalence. Because of differences in disease prevalence, there may be a big difference between the predictive values of the *same symptom* in family and specialty practice. For example, in a patient with fatigue but with no other presenting data, my first-ranking hypothesis usually would be depression. For a hematologist, the first-ranking hypothesis might be anemia. Each would be correct in its own context, given the differences in predictive value of the symptom fatigue. Similarly, my first-ranking hypothesis in a patient with a headache might be different from that of a neurologist.

How much does the ranking order matter? It matters because the order of hypothesis determines the search strategy. If depression is my first-ranking hypothesis, I would begin by seeking evidence of depression. If my hypothesis is supported, I would test it further by ruling out other causes of fatigue—usually by a few simple and economical tests and by continuing observation over time. If my first hypothesis is a blood disorder, I would begin by seeking evidence of this and consider depression only if the findings were negative or did not explain the fatigue. Again, each search strategy would be appropriate in its context. However, a search strategy based on erroneous ranking (assuming payoff factors are not operative) can lead to waste of resources and—where tests carry a risk—harm to the patient.

Before leaving this discussion of hypotheses, two fallacies must be mentioned. The first is that the family physician always thinks of common diseases first. This is not always so: It depends entirely on the cues. If the cues are highly probabilistic, such as fatigue, this will hold true. In contrast, if the cue indicates a rare disease with relative certainty, this will be the physician's first hypothesis. If a hypertensive patient complains of attacks of sweating and flushing, for example, the first hypothesis may be pheochromocytoma, even though the physician may only see one case in a whole lifetime.

The second fallacy is that diagnosis in family practice is different from diagnosis in other fields of medicine because it is probabilistic. All clinical diagnosis is probabilistic. Where family practice differs is in the relatively low levels of probability at which many decisions must be made.

THE SEARCH

The purpose of the search is twofold: to test and validate the physician's hypothesis(es), and to bring to light new and unexpected cues. These purposes are fulfilled respectively by the directed and the routine search.

The Directed Search

Because the purpose of the directed search is to test the physician's initial hypothesis, it follows that the search strategy will vary with the hypothesis. In selecting a search strategy, the family physician must make two kinds of choices: which tests to use and what the extent of the search should be.

The word "tests" embraces history questions, items of physical examination, and laboratory and imaging investigations. Tests are selected according to two kinds of criteria: (1) the capacity of the test to change the prior or pretest probability that the patient has or does not have the disease in question, and (2) the risks and benefits of doing the test. The measures used to determine the usefulness of a test are its sensitivity, specificity and predictive value.

One way of understanding these indices is by means of a 2 × 2 table, illustrated in Table 19–1. Patients with the disease (infectious mononucleosis) are in the two left-hand boxes, those without the disease in the two right-hand boxes. Patients testing positive (with the Monospot test) are in the upper two boxes, those testing negative in the lower two boxes. The boxes are identified, starting from the upper left, as *a*, *b*, *c*, and *d*. Box *a* contains those patients who have the disease and who test positive (true positives). Box *b* contains those without the disease who test positive (false positives). Box *d* contains those without the disease who test negative (true negatives). Box *c* contains those with the disease who test negative (false negatives).

With the help of the table, we now can look at the meaning of the three indices.

Sensitivity

Sensitivity is the proportion of patients with the disease who have a positive test result, which has been called (Galen and Gambino, 1975) "positivity in disease." In the table, boxes $a + c$ give us those patients with the disease and box *a* gives us those with the disease who test positive. Sensitivity expressed as a percentage is therefore:

$$\frac{a}{a + c} \times 100$$

Another way of putting this would be:

$$\frac{\text{True positives (TP)}}{\text{True positives (TP)} + \text{False negatives (FN)}} \times 100$$

In Table 19–1, the boxes have been completed for the Monospot test in infectious mononucleosis. The sensitivity of the test is:

$$\frac{17}{17 + 3} \times 100 = 85\%$$

Some aspects of sensitivity are especially important for family physicians. A highly sensitive test is very good for ruling out hypotheses. If we have a test that is 100 per cent sensitive, and the patient tests negative, we can say with confidence that the patient does not have the disease. Because the test is 100 per cent sensitive, we know that there are no false negatives. A positive test, however, is not so helpful, because we do not know whether it is a true or false positive. If a test is 100 per cent sensitive, it certainly will not be 100 per cent specific, and there will be some false positives. Let us consider some examples.

In a study of headache in family practice (unpublished data), we found that tenderness on pressure over the sinuses was 100 per cent sensitive for sinusitis: Absence of tenderness ruled out sinusitis. Presence of tenderness, however, was of little value because so many patients without sinusitis tested positive. In headache patients over the age of 50, an ESR rate of greater than 50 mm/hr was 100 per cent sensitive for cranial arteritis. This is very tentative because the disease is rare and there was only one case among the 272 patients in the study. There was also only one false positive, a patient who turned out to have pernicious anemia. Our study supported a clinical impression that the ESR is very useful for ruling out cranial arteritis.

Sensitivity varies with the stage of the disease. Failure to understand this can lead to difficulties for the newcomer to family medicine.

A second-year resident saw a 12-year-old boy in the office during his morning session. The boy had com-

TABLE 19–1. SENSITIVITY, SPECIFICITY, AND PREDICTIVE VALUE OF THE MONOSPOT TEST FOR INFECTIOUS MONONUCLEOSIS IN PATIENTS WITH SORE THROATS*

		Infectious Mononucleosis		
		Present	Absent	
Monospot Test	Positive	17 *a*	*b* 69	
	Negative	*c* 3	*d* 911	
		20	980	

$$\text{Sensitivity} = \frac{a}{a + c} \times 100 = \frac{17}{20} \times 100 = 85\%$$

$$\text{Specificity} = \frac{d}{b + d} \times 100 = \frac{911}{69 + 911} \times 100 = 93\%$$

Positive Predictive Value

$$= \frac{a}{a + b} \times 100 = \frac{17}{17 + 69} \times 100 = 19\%$$

* Prevalence of infectious mononucleosis in patients with sore throats = 20/1000.

plained of continuous central abdominal pain for several hours. On examination, there was no abdominal tenderness and the temperature was normal. Because there was some frequency of micturition, the resident diagnosed a urinary infection. That same evening, the mother called the doctor on duty because the pain was worse and the boy was vomiting. Examination of the abdomen showed tenderness and muscular rigidity in all areas. A perforated appendix was diagnosed and the boy made a full recovery after emergency surgery.

The pitfall here was that the abdominal tenderness and pyrexia, although sensitive signs in the later stages of appendicitis, are not 100 per cent sensitive in the early stages. The family physician therefore cannot rely on these for ruling out appendicitis. In this case, the history of continuous abdominal pain should have been sufficient to require re-examination of the patient within 4 hours. An additional error was to make urinary infection a top-ranking hypothesis, because it is uncommon in boys of this age and not usually associated with continuous abdominal pain.

There are many examples of this variation of sensitivity with evolution of a disease: the chest radiograph in pneumonia, lung cancer, and pulmonary embolus; the electrocardiogram in myocardial infarction; and splenic enlargement in infectious mononucleosis, to mention some of them. Few are well documented: Textbooks are not written about the early stages of illness.

Specificity

Specificity is the proportion of patients without the disease who have a negative test result. This is sometimes referred to as "negativity in health" (Galen and Gambino, 1975), but note that absence of the disease in question is not synonymous with health. The patient may have some other disease. In Table 19–1, boxes *b* and *d* give us those patients without the disease, and box *d* gives us those without the disease who test negative. Specificity, expressed as a percentage, is therefore:

$$\frac{d}{b + d} \times 100$$

Another way of putting this would be:

$$\frac{\text{True negatives (TN)}}{\text{True negatives (TN) + False positives (FP)}} \times 100$$

In Table 19–1, the specificity of the Monospot test is:

$$\frac{911}{69 + 911} \times 100 = 93\%$$

A highly specific test is very good for ruling in hypotheses. If a test is 100 per cent specific and the patient tests positive, we can say with certainly that the patient has the disease. Because the test is 100 per cent specific, we know that there are no false positives. The test is diagnostic. A negative test, however, is less helpful, because we do not know whether it is a true or false negative. If a test is 100 per cent specific, it almost certainly will not be 100 per cent sensitive.

Predictive Value

As we have seen, sensitivity tells us nothing about the false positives and specificity tells us nothing about the false negatives. Yet it is very important for us to know about them. The trouble with false positives and false negatives is that both carry penalties for the patient. A false positive can be hazardous in two ways: by imposing a disease label on a healthy person and by exposing him or her to risky investigations and therapies. A false negative carries a penalty because it "misses" the diagnosis in a sick patient. Thus, we need a measure that tells us about the false positives and negatives. The predictive value does this.

The positive predictive value (PPV) is the proportion of positive results that are true positives:

$$\text{PPV} = \frac{\text{TP}}{\text{TP} + \text{FP}} \times 100$$

The negative predictive value (NPV) is the proportion of negative test results that are true negatives:

$$\text{NPV} = \frac{\text{TN}}{\text{TN} + \text{FN}} \times 100$$

The denominator in each case is the number of positive or negative test results, rather that the number of patients with or without the disease. In Table 19–1, the positive predictive value is:

$$\frac{a}{a + b}$$

and the negative predictive value is:

$$\frac{d}{c + d}$$

Synonyms for positive predictive value are the conditional probability of a positive test result and the post-test probability of disease following a positive result. Synonyms for negative predictive value are the conditional probability of a negative test result, and the post-test probability of no disease following a negative result.

In Table 19–1, the positive predictive value of the Monospot test is:

$$\frac{17}{17 + 69} \times 100 = 19.7\%$$

and the negative predictive value is:

$$\frac{911}{3 + 911} \times 100 = 99\%$$

The predictive value is a key index, because it tells us the power of a test to change the probability that the patient has the disease in question. There is, however, something very important to bear in mind. We have already mentioned it: The predictive value varies with the prevalence of the disease. Let us see how this works in the case of the Monospot test. In Table 19–1, the prevalence of

TABLE 19–2. SENSITIVITY, SPECIFICITY, AND PREDICTIVE VALUE OF THE MONOSPOT TEST FOR INFECTIOUS MONONUCLEOSIS IN PATIENTS WITH SORE THROAT*

		Infectious Mononucleosis	
		Present	Absent
Monospot Test	Positive	86 _a_	_b_ 63
	Negative	_c_ 14	_d_ 837
		100	900

$$\text{Sensitivity} = \frac{a}{a+c} \times 100 = \frac{86}{86+14} \times 100 = 86\%$$

$$\text{Specificity} = \frac{d}{b+d} \times 100 = \frac{837}{63+837} \times 100 = 93\%$$

Predictive Value Positive
$$= \frac{a}{a+b} \times 100 = \frac{86}{86+63} \times 100 = 58\%$$

* Prevalence of infectious mononucleosis in patients with sore throats = 100/1000.

mononucleosis in patients with sore throat is 2 per cent; in Table 19–2, the prevalence is 10 per cent. This could be the difference between a family practice and a student health service practice. The effect of this is to increase the positive predictive value to 58 per cent, while the sensitivity and specificity remain virtually the same. The reason is that, as the prevalence increases, the proportion of people with the disease increases and the number of false positives decreases. The variation of predictive value with prevalence can mean that a test that is indicated in a specialty clinic may be contraindicated in family practice.

Having said that predictive value varies with prevalence, we must go on to say that there is one exception. If the sensitivity of a test is 100 per cent, the predictive value of a negative test does not vary with prevalence. There are no false negatives and the negative predictive value is also 100 per cent. Conversely, if the specificity of a test is 100 per cent, the predictive value of a positive test does not vary with prevalence. There are no false positives and the positive predictive value is also 100 per cent. Unfortunately, there are not many tests that reach 100 per cent either for sensitivity or for specificity. Those that we have, we treasure for their capacity to rule out or to rule in a diagnosis.

For the more common tests with sensitivity and specificity of between 80 and 95 per cent, the variation with prevalence is important. Table 19–3 shows how predictive value changes with prevalence for a test that has 95 per cent sensitivity and specificity. Note that a test has a greater power to change the pretest or prior probability in the mid-

dle ranges of prevalence (40 to 80 per cent). When we get to prevalence rates of 90 per cent and 10 per cent, the change in pretest probability is less than 10 per cent. Whether or not this makes the test justifiable depends on the payoff of the diagnosis and the risk of the test. A disease may be so devastating if undiagnosed, and so amenable to treatment, that we do the test even though the disease has a very low level of prevalence. The test for phenylketonuria is an example of this.

A reminder is in order here. Remember that our definition of test includes elements of the history, examination, and investigation. The experienced clinician selects his or her questions and items of physical examination for their capacity to change the prior probability. Even before the clinician starts, the patient's presenting symptoms have changed the prior probability in some way. Despite the panoply of investigations available to us, the history and physical examination—in family practice, especially the history—are still the most effective ways of increasing the probability.

Decision Analysis and Likelihood Ratios

Before leaving the question of how to select tests, mention must be made of two other tools for helping us to make choices: likelihood ratios and decision analysis. As a tool for helping us with decisions about individual patients, *decision analysis* has little application in family practice. It comes in useful mainly in developing optimal strategies for complex clinical conditions. Sackett et al. (1985) defined decision analysis as "a method of describing complex clinical problems in an explicit fashion, identifying the available courses of action (both diagnosis and management), assessing the probability and value (or utility) of all possible outcomes, and then making a simple calculation to select the optimal course of action" (p. 126). For a description of how decision analysis works, the reader is referred to Sackett et al. (1985).

Likelihood ratios are another way of expressing how good a test is for increasing the probability of a diagnosis. The calculation of the ratio uses indices with which we are already familiar: sensitivity and specificity. The likelihood ratio for a positive result is the odds that a test will be positive in a patient with the disease, in contrast to a patient without the disease. The likelihood ratio for a negative result is the odds that a test will be negative in a patient with the disease, contrasted with a patient without the disease.

The first figure in the positive likelihood ratio (positivity in disease) is the sensitivity of the test. The second figure (positivity in nondisease) is 100 minus the specificity (expressed as a percentage). For example, the likelihood ratio of a positive Monospot test in infectious mononucleosis (from Table 19–1) is:

TABLE 19–3.   EFFECT OF PREVALENCE ON THE PREDICTIVE VALUE OF AN EXCELLENT SIGN, SYMPTOM, OR LABORATORY TEST*

	99%	95%	90%	80%	70%	60%	50%	40%	30%	20%	10%	5%	1%	0.5%	0.1%
Prevalence (pretest likelihood or prior probability of disease)	99%	95%	90%	80%	70%	60%	50%	40%	30%	20%	10%	5%	1%	0.5%	0.1%
Predictive value of a positive test (posterior probability of disease following a positive test result)	99.5%	99.7%	99.4%	99%	98%	97%	95%	93%	89%	83%	68%	50%	16%	9%	2%
Predictive value of a negative test Posterior probability *no* disease following a negative test result	15%	50%	68%	83%	89%	93%	95%	97%	98%	99%	99.4%	99.7%	99.9%	99.97%	99.99%
Posterior probability *of* disease following a negative test result	84%	50%	32%	17%	11%	7%	5%	3%	2%	1%	0.5%	0.3%	0.1%	0.03%	0.01%

* Both sensitivity and specificity equal 95% in every case.
From Sackett DL, Hayes RB, Guyatt GH, et al: Clinical Epidemiology: A Basic Science for Clinical Medicine. Boston, Little, Brown, p 80, 1985, with permission.

$$\frac{\dfrac{a}{a+c} \times 100}{100 - \left(\dfrac{d}{b+d} \times 100\right)} = \frac{90}{5} = \frac{18}{1}$$

Thus, the odds of a patient with a positive test result having the disease are 18 to 1.

By multiplying the ratio with the pretest odds, we can arrive at the post-test odds for the diagnosis. The predictive value told us how our diagnostic test had altered the probability or likelihood of the patient having the disease; likelihood ratio tells us how our test has changed the odds on the patient having the disease. If we prefer to think in probabilities, odds can be converted to probabilities and vice versa. To convert odds to probability, we divide it by itself plus one. The post-test odds on infectious mononucleosis become a post-test probability of:

$$\frac{18}{18+1} = 0.947, \text{ or } 94.73\%$$

To convert probabilities to odds, we divide the probability by its complement (1 minus itself). The post-test probability of 94.7% becomes a post-test odds of:

$$\frac{0.9473}{1 - 0.9473} = \frac{0.9473}{0.0527} = 18$$

In this example we have treated the test as if the result will be either positive or negative, rather than a continuous variable. It is also possible to express likelihood ratios for different levels of a test result that varies over a range. For serum uric acid level, for example, we can express the likelihood ratio for gout at 7.0, 8.0, and 9.0 mg/100 mL.

Because likelihood ratios are calculated from the sensitivity and specificity data, they do not vary with the prevalence of the disease. Like sensitivity and specificity, however, they do vary with the stage of the disease.

As time goes on, information about the likelihood ratios and predictive values of tests probably will become increasingly available. As family physicians, we should not only get to know these indices for the symptoms, signs, and tests we use ourselves, but also become accustomed to asking our consultants for the likelihood ratios or predictive values of tests they recommend to us. As our patients become more informed, we may also find that they begin to ask these questions themselves.

In testing a hypothesis, the clinician seeks both positive and negative evidence: He or she seeks not only to support the hypothesis but also to refute it, to rule it in and to rule it out. Suppose that the first two hypotheses in a patient with weight loss are thyrotoxicosis and diabetes. Suppose that the search has yielded evidence in support of thyrotoxicosis. The clinician then will proceed with tests such as urinalysis and blood sugar measurement, which should be negative if the first hypothesis is correct (unless both conditions are present). Studies of problem solving have shown that clinicians, like problem solvers in other fields, show a marked preference for positive over negative evidence. They would much rather try to support their hypothesis than refute it. As Elstein et al. (1978) have observed, this is an experimental confirmation of an observation made centuries ago by Francis Bacon: "It is the peculiar and perpetual error of the human intellect to be more moved and excited by affirmatives than by negatives."

The Last Part of the Directed Search

The testing of hypotheses raises the difficult question of when the directed search should be ended. When have we collected enough evidence? What is the appropriate level of probability? This brings us face to face with the problem of uncertainty, and with the potential conflict between precision on the one hand and the patient's well-being on the other. Uncertainty is inherent in medicine. The data we collect are of uncertain value; the observations we make and the tests we perform are subject to error; our diagnoses are probabilistic; and both the outcome of the patient's illness and the results of treatment are to varying degrees unknown. The main purpose of our search is to reduce uncertainty. The problem comes when we must balance the pursuit of greater precision against the risk of further testing. In modern times, precision in medicine has been the overriding value. It is of course a great good and worthy objective, but greater precision does not necessarily reduce uncertainty. The quest for precision can become mindless, as in the inexorable search for a diagnosis in a patient who is already recovering from an illness. The quest for precision can become a false trail when the true need is to gain a better understanding of the patient.

Until recently, an excessive pursuit of precision did not carry many risks. Now the technology of investigation has advanced so rapidly as to create many hazards, not to speak of enormous expense. Not the least of the hazards is finding a spurious abnormality, with all the attendant risks of inappropriate treatment.

The Routine Search

The routine search comprises the routine systems inquiry and physical examination. The chief aims of the routine part of the search are to prompt alternative hypotheses by bringing to light cues that have not emerged in the directed part of the search, to collect baseline and background data on the patient, and to screen for symptomless conditions such as hypertension.

The routine search is sometimes referred to as a "complete history and physical." This is a misnomer, because even the routine search is a selection from a much larger number of possible tests. As in the directed search, the tests are selected for their usefulness in achieving the objective. Internists probably would include ophthalmoscopy in their routine, but not laryngoscopy—for the very good reason that ophthalmoscopy is more useful in generating new cues in patients seen in internists. For similar reasons, otolaryngologists probably would make the opposite choice.

For three reasons, the family physician tends to make different use of routine searches than do some other clinicians. First, because the patient is usually well known to the physician, he or she may have all the baseline data needed. Second, in minor and transient disorders, little in the way of a routine search is required. Third, because the family physician deals with such a wide range of clinical problems, from minor to life threatening, no single routine is appropriate for every patient. He or she therefore develops different routines for different problems: one for sore throat, one for fatigue, one for dyspepsia, and so on.

The End Point in Family Practice

Traditionally, the end point of the search has been a diagnosis. In family practice, however, this is not always realistic. For reasons already discussed, many of the illnesses seen in family practice do not have a diagnosis in the strict sense of the term. The illness may be at too early a stage for definitive diagnosis; it may be clear spontaneously before diagnosis is possible; or it may be so interwoven with the personal life of the patient as to defy categorization.

In all patients, however, decisions must be made, even if no diagnosis is made. It is more helpful, therefore, to describe the end point in terms of a management decision. The end point of the search on any particular occasion is the point at which enough information is available for an informed decision to be made without avoidable risk to the patient.

It is important to understand that the end points are often different in family practice than in referral specialties. A consultant seeing a referred patient probably will feel the need to make a definitive diagnosis before referring the patient back to the patient's own physician. A family physician is not under the same constraint. The continuing relationship with patients means that all problems do not have to be solved right away. Because the relationship itself has no formal end point, the search can be discontinued and resumed according to need. In this sense, there is no final end point, because the family physician always should be ready to revise his or her hypothesis if new evidence becomes available.

The family physician, because of his or her role, makes two types of decisions that do not arise as often in other branches of medicine:

1. *The decision to wait.* In making this decision, the physician is using the evolution of the illness over time as a test of his or her hypothesis. It is obviously inherent in this decision that no extra risk should be incurred by waiting. The use of time to validate hypotheses in this way can make many investigations redundant. One example of this decision is the eliminative diagnosis referred to earlier, in which the physician decides that the illness is transient and minor, then waits for this hypothesis to be verified.

2. *The decision to refer.* The end point of a search may be the decision to consult with or refer to another physician. This decision may have to be made before arriving at a definitive diagnosis—for example, with a severely ill baby or a patient with an acute abdomen. It is clear that the objective of the family physician in these cases is different from that of the specialist. The family physician has fulfilled his or her obligation if he or she has decided to refer the patient in time for the patient to receive effective treatment. The physician has failed this obligation if he or she has worsened the outcome of the illness by delaying referral in an effort to provide a more definitive diagnosis.

MANAGEMENT DECISIONS

Diagnosis, as defined above, is a categorizing process. Its end point is a probabilistic statement about what is wrong with the patient. A decision, in comparison, cannot be probabilistic. A clinician cannot "probably" prescribe an antibiotic, or "probably" refer a patient. Management decisions must be either/or. When the clinician arrives at such a decision, he or she takes the probabilistic statement and integrates it with a large number of other variables, many of them unique to the patient. Whereas diagnosis is a reductive, generalizing process, decision making is a synthesizing, individualizing process.

Among the variables the clinician must take into account are: the patient's wishes; the diagnosis of the patient's main problem; other problems the patient may have; the prognosis; the personality and life situation of the patient; the risks and benefits of the decision alternatives; the family's wishes; and ethical issues. First on this list are the patient's wishes, because if we have a true regard for his or her automony, it is the patient who makes the decision, on the advice of his or her physician, after being informed as fully as possible about the alternatives.

The complexity of problems, the frequent difficulty in achieving diagnostic precision, and the close personal knowledge of patients combine to make management both the most challenging and the most rewarding part of family practice. Stephens (1975) has called it "the quintessential skill of clinical practice and the ground of what family physicians know that is unique" (p. 423). Management is probably more individualized in family practice than in any other field of medicine. Obviously, the more precisely defined the problem, the less scope for variation in management. If a patient has pernicious anemia, the treatment in all cases is vitamin B_{12}. Even in this case, however, there may be individual aspects of management that, if neglected, may lead to failure of treatment. For example, how likely is the patient to comply? What is to be done to ensure that he or she is fol-

lowed up? Few problems in family practice are as easy to define as pernicious anemia.

Extraneous Factors in Clinical Decision Making

In this chapter, emphasis has been placed on the logic of decision making. The process has been presented as a rational one, with a logic arising out of the clinical situation itself. It is important to recognize, however, that factors outside the clinical situation may have a powerful influence on the process. Some of these are:

1. *Institutional factors.* In deciding on a search strategy, a physician may be heavily influenced by the rules of the institution. Such rules, applied regardless of individual situations, lie behind some of the overinvestigation that is done in teaching hospitals. The rules are no less powerful for being unwritten.

2. *Patient's expectations.* As a result of reading medical articles in the press, or of hearsay, or of a belief that they are exercising their rights as consumers, patients may make demands for tests that the physician may find very difficult to resist, even though there is no logical justification for them.

3. *Fear of litigation.* The prevalence of malpractice suits has had a powerful influence on the search strategies of physicians, the effect being to encourage overinvestigation.

4. *Physician factors.* Another influence on the diagnostic process is the physician's own personality, feelings, and experience. Physicians who feel insecure or who cannot tolerate uncertainty tend to carry out more tests than those who feel secure and tolerate uncertainty well. A physician's strategy may be influenced by feelings of anxiety about a particular patient or type of problem. A physician who believes he or she has made past errors with a patient, or with a particular problem, for example, may tend to be overly meticulous in investigations or especially liable to refer the patient to a specialist.

IDENTIFICATION OF ERRORS IN PROBLEM SOLVING

It is important for both teacher and learner to be able to identify where in the process an error has occurred. Problem-solving errors in family practice can be classified according to the level at which they occur: cues, hypotheses, search, or management decisions. Some common examples are given below.

Cue Blindness

This describes the situation when the clinician fails to respond to cues presented by the patient.

The problem may be inexperience, as when the clinician does not recognize the information as a cue, or the cue may, for some reason, be "blocked out." This is especially common with late cues. One example from my own experience is of a patient who for some time had had a fever of unknown origin, with a high ESR. Exhaustive investigation had failed to provide a diagnosis. After a time, the patient began to complain of headaches, a cue missed until a consultant recognized it as a predictor of cranial arteritis, a diagnosis that proved to be correct.

Another reason for missed cues is the "mental set" of the clinician. The following story was told by a resident about a clinician with whom he was working. The patient suffered from anterior chest pain, and the clinician was taking a history with a diagnosis of ischemic heart disease in mind. Suddenly the patient interjected "and I feel like crying all the time." The clinician failed to respond to this cue and continued to ask questions about the patient's pain. The eventual diagnosis was depression. In this case, the clinician had a "set" on a certain line of inquiry, which blinded him to the most valuable cue of them all.

Premature Convergence on a Hypothesis

In the early stage of hypothesis formation, it is important for the clinician's thinking to be lateral and divergent, considering many possible explanations for the patient's symptoms. One common error at this level is premature convergence on a hypothesis of virus infection in a patient with a mild febrile illness. This leads to failure to test such alternative hypothesis as urinary tract infection.

Errors in the Search

Two opposite errors are common in the search strategy. The first is *redundancy*. In this case, investigations are continued far beyond the point necessary for making an informed decision. Over-investigation is perhaps the most common error in medicine today, although it is more typical of the teaching hospital than of family practice. Sometimes it is due to the inexorable search for a diagnosis in a patient who is already recovering from an illness. Another example of this error, often found early in family medicine residency, is the use of investigations when clinical observation would provide a better search strategy. For many illnesses encountered in family practice, such as herpes zoster and measles, clinical observation is the only way of making the diagnosis.

A second common error is *inadequate testing*. Sometimes very simple procedures will increase the validity of a diagnosis without additional risk or expense: an ESR in a patient with fatigue and depression, a rectal examination in a patient with abdominal pain, or a urinalysis in a patient with fever. Yet these opportunities for validation often are not taken if the clinician believes that there is good positive evidence for his or her hypothesis. This is an example of the well-known preference of all problem solvers for positive rather than negative evidence.

Management Errors

A common fault in management is failure to consider some of the important variables that should enter into the decision, such as the risks of treatment or the ethical issues. The fault often can be identified by asking two questions: (1) What were the decision alternatives? and (2) What is the evidence for and against each alternative? It is by reflecting on their decisions and the ensuing consequences that clinicians can continue to improve their skills.

CONCLUSION

The methods used by family physicians do not "come naturally"; they must be learned. Nowadays students can be introduced to them as undergraduates and can learn them formally during vocational training. In former days, young physicians were plunged into family practice after a hospital-based education and experienced the confusion described by Sir James Mackenzie (Mair, 1973):

> I had not long been in the practice when I discovered how defective was my knowledge. I left college under the impression that every patient's condition could be diagnosed. For a long time I strove to make a diagnosis and assiduously studied my lectures and textbooks, without avail. . . . For some years I thought this inability to diagnose my patient's complaints was due to personal defects, but gradually, through consultations and other ways, I came to recognize that the kind of information I wanted did not exist. . . . (p. 47)

It has been assumed erroneously that clinical methods learned in a hospital, on selected patients with advanced disease, will be transferable to the problems encountered in family practice. All evidence from experimental psychology is that such a transfer does not take place. The learning process must take place in an environment similar to the future environment of practice. Practitioners in former days did learn eventually, but they did so by the slow and painful process of trial and error.

The description of the methods used by family physicians has been a liberating influence in family medicine. For years it was assumed—even by family physicians themselves—that their methods were a debased form of the purer and more thorough methods used in other fields of medicine. Now we know that those of family medicine are admirably suited to the problems encountered in family practice.

The analysis of clinical decision making therefore has been an important process for family medicine. We cannot teach or learn clinical family practice until we can anatomize the clinical process, give the reasons for our decisions, and identify and correct the errors. A physician who can examine his or her own decisions in this way will continue to grow in clinical wisdom throughout his or her career.

To achieve maximum benefit from this learning process, we obviously must review each case after we know its outcome. Because, in family practice, the interval between the onset of an illness and the outcome may be several years, a good records system is a necessity. Not only should individual patients' records be kept accurately, but there also should be a diagnostic index by which the physician can review his or her experience of all patients within a single diagnostic rubric.

REFERENCES

Bursztajn H, Feinbloom RI, Hamm RM, et al: Medical Choices, Medical Chances: How Patients, Families, and Physicians Can Cope with Uncertainty. New York, Delacorte Press, 1981.

Carmichael LP: The relational model: A paradigm of family medicine. J Fl Med Assoc 67:860, 1980.

Crombie DL: Diagnostic methods. Practitioner 191:539, 1963.

Elstein AS, Shulman LS, Sprafka SA: Medical Problem-Solving: An Analysis of Clinical Reasoning. Cambridge, MA, Harvard University Press, 1978.

Feinstein A: Clinical Judgment. Baltimore, Williams & Wilkins, 1967.

Galen RS, Gambino SR: Beyond Normality: The Predictive Value and Efficiency of Medical Diagnosis. New York, John Wiley & Sons, 1975.

Howie JGR: A new look at respiratory illness in general practice: A reclassification of respiratory illness based on antibiotic prescribing. J R Coll Gen Pract 23:895, 1973.

Kleinman A, Einberg L, Good B: Culture, illness and care: Clinical lessons from anthropologic and cross-culture research. Ann Intern Med 88:251, 1978.

Mair A: Sir James Mackenzie, M.D., General Practitioner, 1853–1925. Edinburgh, Churchill Livingstone, 1973.

McWhinney IR: A Textbook of Family Medicine. New York, Oxford University Press, 1989.

Sackett DL, Hayes RB, Tugwell P: Clinical Epidemiology: A Basic Science for Clinical Medicine. Boston, Little, Brown, 1985.

Stephens GC: The intellectual basis of family practice. J Fam Pract 2:423, 1975.

Williams T: A strategy for defining the clinical content of family medicine. J Fam Pract 4:497, 1977.

CHAPTER 20

INFECTIOUS DISEASES

MICHAEL F. PARRY, HAROLD C. NEU, and JOSEPH V. CONNELLY

ANTIMICROBIAL THERAPY

Successful treatment of an infectious disease requires early diagnosis and prompt administration of appropriate antimicrobial agents. Above and beyond this, however, the outcome of the illness depends to a considerable extent on the nature of the infecting agent, its virulence, its portal of entry, the natural history of the untreated infection, and the integrity of the host's defense mechanisms. Conditions present in the host, such as malnutrition, immunodeficiency, or undrained abscesses, are more important determinants of outcome than selection of a specific drug for treatment. Nevertheless, in patients with comparably severe underlying disease, the selection of an appropriate antibiotic clearly enhances outcome.

Antibiotic Susceptibility Testing

Tests of antimicrobial susceptibility provide useful information both to maximize the effectiveness of treatment and to minimize toxicity by enabling the physician to select the most appropriate drug, dose, and route of administration. Susceptibility testing is indicated for all organisms that contribute to an infectious process when the susceptibilities cannot be predicted uniformly on the basis of species identification. Such organisms traditionally have included members of the Enterobacteriaceae (gram-negative enteric bacilli), staphylococci, and nonfermentative gram-negative bacilli, such as *Pseudomonas*. More recently, the emergence of penicillin-resistant strains of *Streptococcus pneumoniae* (pneumococcus) and ampicillin/vancomycin-resistant enterococci calls for wider use of such testing.

Techniques for determining antibiotic susceptibility fall into two broad categories: dilution tests and diffusion tests. *Diffusion susceptibility testing* (the Kirby-Bauer method) has been widely available since the mid-1960s. The principle of the method is that a drug, contained in filter paper disks and applied to an agar surface, will diffuse into the surrounding medium and generate a gradient of concentrations from the disk's edge. Zones of inhibition occur where antibiotic concentrations are just sufficient to inhibit bacterial growth on the agar surface. The diameter of the zone produced varies inversely with the concentration of the drug needed to inhibit growth. Results thus are reported as susceptible, moderately susceptible, or resistant in relationship to antimicrobial drug concentrations that are easily achievable in blood or urine with standard doses of a given agent.

In contrast to the disk diffusion method, which is qualitative and reflects bacterial inhibition rather than killing, *broth dilution methods* are quantitative and can be used to determine killing as well as inhibition. Tubes or wells of broth containing an antibiotic are inoculated with a suspension of bacteria and examined for growth, or turbidity, after incubation. Failure of growth to occur indicates effective inhibition, and the lowest concentration of drug inhibiting bacterial growth is called the *minimum inhibitory concentration* (MIC). Bacterial killing can be assessed by subculturing samples from the tubes or wells without apparent growth to see if viable organisms remain. The lowest concentration of drug at which killing is achieved is called the *minimum bactericidal concentration* or (MBC). Results reported as MIC or MBC values can be related directly to achievable blood, urine, or tissue concentrations of an antimicrobial agent. Dosage features of most antimicrobial agents are listed in Table 20–1.

It is important for the microbiology laboratory to test bacterial susceptibility to antimicrobial agents known to be representative of other compounds in their class. For example, routine susceptibility testing of *Staphylococcus aureus* includes only one penicillinase-resistant penicillin derivative, such as oxacillin. The class representative, oxacillin, indicates susceptibility to nafcillin and methicillin and the oral agents cloxacillin and dicloxacillin as well.

Antibiotic Selection

Organism-specific therapy is the ultimate goal of antimicrobial selection. The use of several, or broader spectrum, agents will be less cost-effec-

TABLE 20–1. ANTIMICROBIAL DRUG THERAPY*

| Drug | Dosage | | | | | Modification in Renal Failure: Creatinine Clearance (mL/min) | | |
| | Children | | | Adults | | | | |
	Newborn	Oral	Parenteral	Oral	Parenteral	30–60	10–30	<10
Acyclovir† (Zovirax)	30 mg/kg/day q 8 hr	NA‡	30 mg/kg/day q 8 hr	1000 mg/day q 4 hr	15–30 mg/kg/day q 8 hr	5 mg/kg q 12 hr	5 mg/kg q 24 hr	2.5 mg/kg q 24 hr
Amantadine (Symmetrel)	NA	6.6 mg/kg/day q 24 hr	—	200 mg q 24 hr	—	100 mg q 24 hr	100 mg q 48 hr	200 mg q 7 days
Amikacin§ (Amikin)	15 mg/kg/day q 12 hr	—	15 mg/kg/day q 8–12 hr	—	15 mg/kg/day q 8–12 hr	5 mg/kg q 12–18 hr	2.5 mg/kg q 12–18 hr	2.5 mg/kg q 24–36 hr
Amoxicillin (Amoxil, others)	NA	20–40 mg/kg/day q 8 hr	—	750–1500 mg/day q 8 hr	—	NC‖	q 12 hr	q 24 hr
Amoxicillin plus clavulanic acid (Augmentin)	NA	20–40 mg/kg/day q 8 hr	—	750–1500 mg/day q 8 hr	—	NC	q 12 hr	q 24 hr
Amphotericin B (Fungizone)	0.25–1.0 mg/kg/day q 24–48 hr	—	0.25–1.0 mg/kg/day q 24–48 hr	—	0.25–1.0 mg/kg/day q 24–48 hr	NC	NC	NC
Ampicillin	75–200 mg/kg/day q 6–8 hr	50–100 mg/kg/day q 6 hr	100–200 mg/kg/day q 4–6 hr	1–4 gm/day q 6 hr	2–12 gm/day q 4–6 hr	NC	q 8 hr	q 12 hr
Ampicillin plus sulbactam (Unasyn)	NA	—	100–200 mg/kg/day q 6 hr	—	3–12 gm/day q 6 hr	NC	q 8 hr	q 12 hr
Azithromycin (Zithromax)	NA	NA	—	500 mg × 1, then 250 mg q 24 hr × 4	—	NC	NC	NC
Aztreonam (Azactam)	90–120 mg/kg/day q 6–8 hr	—	90–120 mg/kg/day q 6 hr	—	2–8 gm/day q 6 hr	NC	q 8 hr	q 12 hr
Carbenicillin (Geocillin, Pyopen, others)	200–400 mg/kg/day q 6–8 hr	50–65 mg/kg/day q 6 hr	200–600 mg/kg/day q 4–6 hr	1.5–3 gm (4–8 tablets)/day q 6 hr	30–40 gm/day q 4–6 hr	q 6 hr	2–4 gm q 8 hr	2 gm q 12 hr
Cefaclor (Ceclor)	NA	20–40 mg/kg/day q 6 hr	—	1–2 gm/day q 6 hr	—	NC	NC	NC
Cefadroxil (Duricef)	NA	30 mg/kg/day q 12 hr	—	1–2 gm/day q 12 hr	—	NC	q 12–24 hr	q 24–36 hr
Cefamandole (Mandol)	NA	—	50–150 mg/kg/day q 6 hr	—	2–12 gm/day q 6 hr	NC	q 8 hr	q 12 hr
Cefazolin (Ancef, Kefzol)	40–60 mg/kg/day q 8 hr	—	25–100 mg/kg/day q 8 hr	—	1–6 gm/day q 8 hr	NC	q 12–24 hr	q 24–36 hr

Drug								
Cefixime (Suprax)	NA	8 mg/kg/day q 24 hr	—	200–800 mg/day q 24 hr	—	NC	NC	200 mg q 24 hr
Cefmetazole (Zefazone)	NA	—	NA	—	4–8 gm/day q 6–12 hr	q 12 hr	q 24 hr	q 48 hr
Cefonicid (Monocid)	NA	—	NA	—	1–2 gm/day q 12–24 hr	NC	q 24 hr	q 48 hr
Cefoperazone (Cefobid)	50–100 mg/kg/day q 12 hr	—	50–200 mg/kg/day q 12 hr	—	2–12 gm/day q 12 hr	NC	NC	NC
Cefotaxime (Claforan)	100–150 mg/kg/day q 8–12 hr	—	100–200 mg/kg/day q 8 hr	—	2–12 gm/day q 6–8 hr	NC	NC	q 8 hr
Cefotetan (Cefotan)	NA	—	40–80 mg/kg/day q 12 hr	—	2–6 gm/day q 12 hr	NC	q 24 hr	q 48 hr
Cefoxitin (Mefoxin)	40–120 mg/kg/day q 6–8 hr	—	80–160 mg/kg/day q 4–6 hr	—	2–12 gm/day q 4–6 hr	q 8 hr	q 12 hr	q 24 hr
Cefpodoxime (Vantin)	NA	8–10 mg/kg/day q 12 hr	—	200–800 mg/day q 12 hr	—	NC	q 24 hr	q 48 hr
Cefprozil (Cefzil)	NA	30 mg/kg/day q 12 hr	—	500–1000 mg/day q 12 hr	—	NC	NC	q 24 hr
Ceftazidime (Fortaz, Tazicef, Tazidime)	100–150 mg/kg/day q 8–12 hr	—	50–150 mg/kg/day q 8 hr	—	2–6 gm/day q 8 hr	q 12 hr	q 18 hr	q 36 hr
Ceftizoxime (Cefizox)	NA	—	150–200 mg/kg/day q 6–8 hr	—	2–12 gm/day q 8–12 hr	q 12–24 hr	q 24–36 hr	q 48–72 hr
Ceftriaxone (Rocephin)	50–75 mg/kg/day q 12–24 hr	—	50–100 mg/kg/day q 24 hr	—	0.25–4 gm/day q 24 hr	NC	NC	NC
Cefuroxime (Zinacef, Ceftin)	20–50 mg/kg/day q 12 hr	30 mg/kg/day q 12 hr	50–100 mg/kg/day q 8 hr	250–1000 mg/day q 12 hr	2.25–4.5 gm/day q 8 hr	NC	q 12 hr	q 24 hr
Cephalexin (Keflex, others)	NA	25–50 mg/kg/day q 6 hr	25–50 mg/kg/day q 6 hr	1–4 gm/day q 6 hr	—	NC	q 12 hr	q 24 hr
Cephalothin (Keflin, others)	40–60 mg/kg/day q 8 hr	—	80–160 mg/kg/day q 4–6 hr	—	2–12 gm/day q 4–6 hr	NC	q 8 hr	q 12 hr
Cephradine (Velosef, others)	NA	25–50 mg/kg/day q 6–8 hr	50–100 mg/kg/day q 6–8 hr	1–4 gm/day q 6 hr	2–12 gm/day q 6 hr	q 8 hr	q 12 hr	q 24 hr
Chloramphenicol (Chloromycetin)	NA	50–100 mg/kg/day q 6 hr	50–100 mg/kg/day q 6 hr	1–4 gm/day q 6 hr	1–4 gm/day q 6 hr	NC	NC	NC
Ciprofloxacin (Cipro)	NA	NA	NA	500–1500 mg/day q 12 hr	800 mg/day q 12 hr	NC	NC	q 24 hr

Table continued on following page

TABLE 20–1. *(Continued)*

| Drug | Dosage | | | | | Modification in Renal Failure: Creatinine Clearance (mL/min) | | |
| | Newborn | Children | | Adults | | 30–60 | 10–30 | <10 |
		Oral	Parenteral	Oral	Parenteral			
Clarithromycin (Biaxin)	NA	15 mg/kg/day q 12 hr	—	500–1000 mg/day q 12 hr	—	NC	NC	NC
Clindamycin (Cleocin, others)	20–40 mg/kg/day q 6 hr	10–30 mg/kg/day q 6–8 hr	25–40 mg/kg/day q 6–8 hr	450–1200 mg/day q 8 hr	900–2700 mg/day q 8 hr	NC	NC	NC
Cloxacillin (Tegopen, others)	NA	50–100 mg/kg/day q 6 hr	—	2–4 gm/day q 6 hr	—	NC	NC	NC
Dicloxacillin (Dynapen, others)	NA	12.5–50 mg/kg/day q 6 hr	—	1–4 gm/day q 6 hr	—	NC	NC	NC
Didanosine (Videx)	NA	200 mg/m²/day q 12 hr	—	250–600 mg/day q 12 hr	—	NC	NA	NA
Doxycycline (Vibramycin, others)	NA	NA	NA	100–200 mg/day q 12–24 hr	100–200 mg/day q 12–24 hr	NC	NC	NC
Enoxacin (Penetrex)	NA	NA	—	400–800 mg/day q 12 hr	—	NC	q 24 hr	q 24 hr
Erythromycin (Erythrocin, EES, E-mycin, others)	20–40 mg/kg/day q 6–8 hr	30–50 mg/kg/day q 6–8 hr	20–50 mg/kg/day q 6–8 hr	1–2 gm/day q 6–8 hr	1–4 gm/day q 6–8 hr	NC	NC	NC
Ethambutol (Myambutol)	NA	15 mg/kg/day q 24 hr	—	15–25 mg/kg/day q 24 hr	—	NC	10 mg/kg/day q 24 hr	5 mg/kg/day q 24 hr
Fluconazole† (Diflucan)	NA	3–6 mg/kg/day q 24 hr	3–6 mg/kg/day q 24 hr	50–400 mg/day q 24 hr	100–400 mg/day q 24 hr	NC	50–200 mg/day q 24 hr	50–100 mg/day q 24 hr
Flucytosine§ (Ancobon)	80–160 mg/kg/day q 6 hr	50–150 mg/kg/day q 6 hr	—	50–150 mg/kg/day q 6 hr	—	q 12 hr	q 24 hr	q 48 hr
Foscarnet† (Foscavir)	NA	—	NA	—	180 mg/kg/day q 8 hr (induction)	q 24 hr	Avoid	Avoid
Ganciclovir† (Cytovene)	NA	—	10 mg/kg/day q 12 hr (induction)	—	10 mg/kg/day q 12 hr (induction)	NC	q 24 hr	q 48 hr
Gentamicin§ (Garamycin, others)	7.5 mg/kg/day q 8–12 hr	—	5–7.5 mg/kg/day q 8 hr	—	3–5 mg/kg/day q 8 or q 24 hr	1.5 mg/kg q 12–16 hr	0.75 mg/kg q 12–16 hr	0.75 mg/kg q 24–36 hr

Imipenem plus cilastatin (Primaxin)	NA	—	50–100 mg/kg/day q 6 hr	—	1–4 gm/day q 6 hr	NC	q 8–12 hr	q 18–24 hr
Isoniazid	10–20 mg/kg/day q 24 hr	10–20 mg/kg/day q 24 hr	10–20 mg/kg/day q 24 hr	300 mg/day q 24 hr	300 mg/day q 24 hr	NC	NC	100–200 mg/day q 24 hr
Kanamycin§ (Kantrex)	20–30 mg/kg/day q 8 hr	15–30 mg/kg/day q 8 hr	15–30 mg/kg/day q 8–12 hr	—	15 mg/kg/day q 8–12 hr	5 mg/kg q 18 hr	2.5 mg/kg q 18–24 hr	2.5 mg/kg q 24–48 hr
Ketoconazole (Nizoral)	NA	5–10 mg/kg/day q 12–24 hr	5–10 mg/kg/day q 12–24 hr	200–400 mg/day q 24 hr	—	NC	NC	NC
Lomefloxacin (Maxequin)	NA	NA	NA	400 mg q 24 hr	—	NC	200 mg q 24 hr	200 mg q 24 hr
Loracarbef (Lorabid)	NA	NA	30 mg/kg/day q 12 hr	400–800 mg/day q 12 hr	—	q 24 hr	q 48 hr	q 72 hr
Methicillin (Staphcillin, others)	50–200 mg/kg/day q 8 hr	50–200 mg/kg/day q 6 hr	100–400 mg/kg/day q 4–6 hr	—	4–12 gm/day q 4–6 hr	NC	q 6 hr	q 8 hr
Metronidazole	30–50 mg/kg/day q 6–12 hr	30–50 mg/kg/day q 6–12 hr	30–50 mg/kg/day q 6–12 hr	1–3 gm/day q 6–12 hr	1–3 gm/day q 6–12 hr	NC	NC	q 12 hr
Mezlocillin (Mezlin)	200–300 mg/kg/day q 6–8 hr	200–300 mg/kg/day q 6–12 hr	200–300 mg/kg/day q 4–6 hr	—	6–24 gm/day q 4–6 hr	NC	q 6 hr	q 8 hr
Minocycline (Minocin)	NA	NA	NA	100–200 mg/day q 12–24 hr	100–200 mg/day q 12–24 hr	NC	NC	NC
Nafcillin (Unipen, Nafcil, others)	50–100 mg/kg/day q 8 hr	50–100 mg/kg/day q 6 hr	100–200 mg/kg/day q 4–6 hr	1–4 gm/day q 6 hr	2–12 gm/day q 4–6 hr	NC	NC	NC
Netilmicin§ (Netromycin)	4–6.5 mg/kg/day q 12 hr	5–8 mg/kg/day q 8–12 hr	5–8 mg/kg/day q 8–12 hr	—	3–6 mg/kg/day q 8–12 hr	1.7 mg/kg q 12–18 hr	0.8 mg/kg q 12–18 hr	0.8 mg/kg q 24–36 hr
Nitrofurantoin (Macrodantin, others)	NA	5–7 mg/kg/day q 6 hr	5–7 mg/kg/day q 6 hr	200–400 mg/day q 6 hr	—	NC	Avoid	Avoid
Norfloxacin (Noroxin)	NA	NA	NA	800 mg/day q 12 hr	—	NC	q 12–24 hr	q 24 hr
Ofloxacin (Floxin)	NA	NA	NA	400–800 mg/day q 12 hr	400–800 mg/day q 12 hr	NC	q 24 hr	q 48 hr
Oxacillin (Prostaphlin, others)	75–100 mg/kg/day q 8 hr	100–200 mg/kg/day q 4–6 hr	100–200 mg/kg/day q 4–6 hr	2–4 gm/day q 6 hr	2–12 gm/day q 4–6 hr	NC	NC	q 6 hr
Penicillin G	100,000–200,000 units/kg/day q 6 hr	100,000–400,000 units/kg/day q 4 hr	100,000–400,000 units/kg/day q 4 hr	—	2–24 million units/day q 4 hr	q 6 hr	q 8 hr	q 12 hr

Table continued on following page

TABLE 20-1. *(Continued)*

| Drug | Dosage | | | | | Modification in Renal Failure: Creatinine Clearance (mL/min) | | |
| | Children | | | Adults | | | | |
	Newborn	Oral	Parenteral	Oral	Parenteral	30-60	10-30	<10
Penicillin V	NA	25-50 mg/kg/day q 6 hr	—	2-4 gm/day q 6 hr	—	NC	q 8 hr	q 12 hr
Pentamidine† (Pentam 300)	NA	—	4 mg/kg q 24 hr	—	4 mg/kg q 24 hr	NC	NC	NC
Piperacillin (Pipracil)	200 mg/kg/day q 12 hr	—	200-300 mg/kg/day q 4-6 hr	—	6-24 gm/day q 4-6 hr	NC	q 8 hr	q 12 hr
Piperacillin plus tazobactam (Zosyn)	NA	—	NA	—	12 gm/day as piperacillin q 6 hr	NC	q 8 hr	q 12 hr
Pyrazinamide	NA	15-30 mg/kg/day q 12 hr	—	25 mg/kg/day q 6-8 hr	—	q 8 hr	Avoid	Avoid
Rifampin† (Rifadin, Rimactane)	10 mg/kg/day q 24 hr	10-20 mg/kg/day q 24 hr	10-20 mg/kg/day q 24 hr	600 mg/d q 24 hr	600 mg/d q 24 hr	NC	NC	NC
Rimantidine (Flumadine)	NA	5.0 mg/kg/day q 24 hr	—	200 mg/day q 12-24 hr	—	NC	NC	q 24 hr
Streptomycin§	NA	—	20-30 mg/kg/day q 12-24 hr	—	15 mg/kg/day q 12-24 hr	q 24 hr	q 48 hr	q 72 hr
Sulfonamides (Gantrisin, Gantanol)	NA	150 mg/kg/day q 6 hr	—	2-4 mg/day q 6 hr	—	q 8 hr	q 12 hr	q 24 hr
Tetracycline HCl	NA	NA	NA	1-2 gm/day q 6 hr	Use doxycycline or minocycline	NC	Avoid	Avoid

Drug							
Ticarcillin (Ticar)	200–300 mg/kg/day q 8 hr	200–300 mg/kg/day q 4–6 hr	—	200–300 mg/kg/day q 4–6 hr	q 6 hr	q 8 hr	q 12 hr
Ticarcillin plus clavulanic acid (Timentin)	200–300 mg/kg/day as ticarcillin q 8 hr	200–300 mg/kg/day as ticarcillin q 4–6 hr	—	12.4 gm/day q 6 hr	NC	q 8 hr	q 12 hr
Tobramycin§ (Nebcin)	7.5 mg/kg/day q 8 hr	6–7.5 mg/kg/day q 8 hr	—	3–5 mg/kg/day q 8 hr	1.5 mg/kg q 12–18 hr	0.75 mg/kg q 12–18 hr	0.75 mg/kg q 24–36 hr
Trimethoprim (Proloprim, Trimpex)	NA	—	200 mg/day q 12–24 hr	—	NC	100 mg/day q 12–24 hr	Avoid
Trimethoprim plus sulfamethoxazole† (Bactrim, Septra)	NA	5–20 mg/kg/day q 6–12 hr	320–1600 mg/day q 12 hr	5–20 mg/kg/day q 6–12 hr	NC	4–10 mg/kg/day q 12 hr	3–8 mg/kg/day q 24 hr
Vancomycin§ (Vancocin, others)	30 mg/kg/day q 8 hr	30–40 mg/kg/day q 12 hr	500 mg/day q 6 hr	2.0 gm/day q 12 hr	1.0 gm q 24–36 hr	1.0 gm q 48–72 hr	1.0 gm q 5–7 days
Zalcitabine (Hivid)	NA	—	1.125–2.25 mg/day q 8 hr	—	NC	q 12 hr	q 24 hr
Zidovudine (Retrovir)	NA	6–12 mg/kg/day q 4 hr	600 mg/day q 8 hr	—	NC	NC	q 12–24 hr

* Antimicrobial drug therapy is expressed as total daily dose, followed by usual dosing intervals. Antimicrobial agents are alphabetized generically. Newborn doses are calculated for normal-weight, term babies between 7 and 30 days of age; note that premature infants, low-birth-weight infants, or newborns less than 7 days old may have different kinetics and should be dosed according to more detailed guidelines (e.g., Johnson KB [ed]: The Harriet Lane Handbook. St. Louis, CV Mosby, 1993).
† Doses may differ when drug is used for prophylaxis instead of treatment, or maintenance instead of induction.
‡ NA, not advised because of toxicity, insufficient data, or lack of indication.
§ Antimicrobial levels should be measured for optimal safety and efficacy, especially when renal function is impaired.
‖ NC, no change in dose.

tive, may increase the risk of toxicity, and actually may increase the incidence of superinfection.

The choice between bactericidal and bacteriostatic antibiotics has plagued clinicians for years. Despite theoretical advantages (with certain exceptions, such as infective endocarditis, meningitis, and infections in the neutropenic patient), bactericidal drugs have not proved clinically superior to bacteriostatic compounds. In the aforementioned exceptions, bactericidal drugs (such as penicillins or cephalosporins) are necessary because of impaired host defenses or sites of infection that are inaccessible to normal host defenses. A two-drug regimen is sometimes necessary in order to assure bactericidal activity. Enterococci are not killed by penicillin alone, and enterococcal endocarditis requires treatment with a combination of a penicillin plus an aminoglycoside antibiotic. Two-drug therapy also may be indicated in situations in which either drug is only marginally effective against the offending pathogen but the two drugs together may be manyfold more active than either drug alone (i.e., they may be synergistic); or in mixed infections in which more than one antimicrobial agent is necessary to provide coverage of multiple pathogens.

Ultimately, the choice of antimicrobial agent is based on past clinical experience as well as on the results of antimicrobial susceptibility testing. Some drugs, such as penicillin or cephalosporin derivatives, can be given in extremely high doses with little toxicity; this is not true of others, such as aminoglycoside antibiotics. Additional concerns may include degree of protein binding, lipid solubility, routes of excretion and metabolism, and available modes of administration. Failure to cure typhoidal *Salmonella* infections with aminoglycoside antibiotics despite in vitro susceptibilities emphasizes the difficulties encountered in interpreting laboratory data without a clinical correlation. The preferred drugs for treatment of specific microorganisms are listed in Table 20–2.

Antimicrobial Prophylaxis

Controlled clinical trials have demonstrated clearly the value of prophylactic antibiotics in reducing the incidence of postoperative infection in certain situations. Unfortunately, much prophylaxis is administered inappropriately, resulting in excessive costs and the risks of superinfection and drug toxicity.

Perioperative infections usually arise from contamination of the wound or operative site by microorganisms from contiguous skin or mucosal surfaces transected during surgery. Less commonly, exogenous sources, such as unsterile equipment or airborne bacteria, are to blame. Factors influencing the development of wound infection include local conditions, such as the number of bacteria inocu-

lated into the wound, the adequacy of local defense mechanisms, and the condition of the tissue with respect to necrosis, debris, or ischemia; and systemic factors, such as obesity, old age, malnutrition, prolonged preoperative hospitalization, or lengthy operative procedures.

The principle of antimicrobial prophylaxis is that antibiotics administered at the time of, or immediately before, inoculation of bacteria into the wound will prevent infection. Administration of antimicrobial prophylaxis after inoculation is ineffective. Accordingly, administration of prophylactic antibiotics is best achieved by a single preoperative dose. Maintenance of intraoperative antibiotic levels may require redosing during prolonged surgical procedures, but the value of continuing antibiotics after surgery has not been demonstrated convincingly. If antibiotics are continued, their administration should be limited to 24 hours postoperatively.

The indications for perioperative prophylaxis are listed in Table 20–3. Prophylaxis is indicated in certain situations only for high-risk patients. For example, prophylaxis is not indicated for most gastroduodenal surgery unless bleeding, obstruction, or achlorhydria (e.g., chronic antacid or histamine$_2$ [H$_2$] antagonist therapy) is a factor. Patients at high risk for infection after biliary surgery include those individuals over 70 years of age, patients with obstructive jaundice or previous biliary tract surgery, patients with common duct stones, and patients operated on for or during acute cholecystitis. The indications for prophylactic antibiotics in cesarean section include patients in labor, patients with ruptured membranes, and those who have had internal fetal monitoring during labor prior to cesarean section. Patients receiving antibiotics while undergoing surgery for traumatic wounds or a ruptured viscus are considered to be receiving treatment rather than prophylaxis. Accordingly, therapy usually is continued for some time after surgery.

Patients with valvular heart disease, who may be predisposed to bacterial endocarditis after bacteremia associated with manipulation of infected or potentially infected tissues, should receive prophylaxis directed against organisms that produce endocarditis. This requires a regimen different from the standard surgical prophylactic program listed in Table 20–3, and is discussed in the section on cardiovascular infections.

Classes of Antimicrobial Agents

Aminoglycoside Antibiotics

Aminoglycoside antibiotics are complex amino sugars produced by a variety of fungi. They are active against most aerobic gram-negative bacilli and some staphylococci. Gentamicin, the most commonly used derivative, is active against nearly all strains of *Escherichia coli, Klebsiella,* and *Pro-*

TABLE 20–2.　ANTIMICROBIAL AGENTS OF CHOICE FOR TREATMENT OF SPECIFIC MICROORGANISMS

Infecting Organism	Morphology*	Drug of First Choice†	Alternate Choices†
Bacilli			
Achromobacter‡	GNB	Imipenem	TMP/SMX, APP, ceftazidime, AG
Acinetobacter anitratus‡	GNB	APP + AG	Imipenem, fluoroquinolone, ceftazidime
Actinomyces	GPB	Penicillin	Clindamycin, tetracycline
Aeromonas‡	GNB	Fluoroquinolone	AG, TGC, TMP/SMX
Bacteroides fragilis‡	GNB	Metronidazole	Clindamycin, BLI, cefoxitin, cefotetan, imipenem
Bacteroides species‡	GNB	Clindamycin or metronidazole	Penicillin, APP, BLI, cefoxitin, cefotetan, imipenem
Bordetella	GNCB	Erythromycin	Ampicillin, tetracycline, TMP/SMX
Borrelia burgdorferi	GNS	Doxycycline	Amoxicillin, azithromycin, ceftriaxone, cefotaxime
Borrelia recurrentis	GNS	Tetracycline	Erythromycin, chloramphenicol
Brucella	GNB	Tetracycline + gentamicin	TMP/SMX or fluoroquinolone or tetracycline + rifampin
Camplyobacter jejuni	GNB	Fluoroquinolone	Erythromycin, gentamicin
Capnocytophaga	GNB	Penicillin	Erythromycin, cephalosporin, clindamycin
Chlamydia pneumoniae	NA	Tetracycline	Erythromycin, ofloxacin
Chlamydia psittaci	NA	Tetracycline	Chloramphenicol, erythromycin
Chlamydia trachomatis	NA	Tetracycline	Erythromycin, sulfonamide, azithromycin
Citrobacter diversus‡	GNB	TGC	AG, BLI, fluoroquinolone, TMP/SMX, aztreonam
Citrobacter freundii‡	GNB	Imipenem or fluoroquinolone	AG, TGC, TMP/SMX, aztreonam, APP
Clostridium difficile	GPB	Metronidazole	Vancomycin (P.O.), bacitracin (P.O.)
Clostridium species	GPB	Penicillin	Metronidazole, clindamycin, cephalosporin
Corynebacterium diphtheriae (illness)	GPB	Erythromycin + antitoxin	Penicillin G + antitoxin
Corynebacterium diphtheriae (carrier)	GPB	Erythromycin	Clindamycin
Corynebacterium jeikeium	GPB	Vancomycin	
Coxiella burnetti	NA	Doxycycline	Erythromycin
Cytomegalovirus	V	Ganciclovir	Foscarnet
Eikenella corrodens‡	GNB	Penicillin	BLI, erythromycin, cefoxitin, TGC, imipenem
Enterobacter‡	GNB	AG or APP or imipenem	TGC, aztreonam, fluoroquinolone, TMP/SMX
Enterococcus	GPC	Ampicillin ± AG	Vancomycin ± AG, fluoroquinolone (urine)
Escherichia coli‡	GNB	Cephalosporin	Ampicillin, BLI, TGC, fluoroquinolone, TMP/SMX, AG
Erysipelothrix rhusiopathiae	GPB	Ampicillin	Tetracycline
Eubacterium	GPB	Penicillin	Clindamycin, tetracycline
Flavobacterium‡	GPB	Vancomycin	Imipenem, fluoroquinolone, TMP/SMX, rifampin
Francisella tularensis	GNCB	AG ± tetracycline	Tetracycline, chloramphenicol
Fusobacterium	GNB	Penicillin	Clindamycin, metronidazole, imipenem, cefoxitin
Gardnerella vaginalis	GVB	Metronidazole	Clindamycin
Haemophilus influenzae, type b‡	GNCB	TGC	Ampicillin, TMP/SMX, BLI, fluoroquinolone
Haemophilus influenzae, other‡	GNCB	Amoxicillin or BLI	Fluoroquinolone, TMP/SMX, SGC, macrolide
Haemophilus ducreyi	GNCB	Ceftriaxone or fluoroquinolone	TMP/SMX, erythromycin, BLI
Herpes simplex (ocular)	V	Trifluridine	Vidarabine, IUDR
Herpes simplex (other)	V	Acyclovir	Foscarnet
Human immunodeficiency virus	V	Zidovudine	Didanosine, zalcitabine
Influenza A	V	Amantidine or rimantadine	
Klebsiella‡	GNB	TGC or fluoroquinolone	AG, TMP/SMX, aztreonam, BLI, imipenem
Legionella	GNB	Erythromycin ± rifampin	Fluoroquinolone, TMP/SMX
Leptospira	GNS	Cefotaxime or ceftriaxone	Penicillin, tetracycline
Listeria monocytogenes	GPB	Ampicillin ± gentamicin	TMP/SMX
Moraxella catarrhalis‡	GNDC	TGC or BLI	TMP/SMX, fluoroquinolone, macrolide, SGC
Morganella morganii‡	GNB	TGC	AG, APP, imipenem, fluoroquinolone, TMP/SMX

Table continued on following page

TABLE 20–2. *(Continued)*

Infecting Organism	Morphology*	Drug of First Choice†	Alternate Choices†
Mycobacterium avium complex‡	AFB	Macrolide + rifampin + ethambutol + fluoroquinolone	+ Clofazimine, + amikacin
Mycobacterium fortuitum complex‡	AFB	Macrolide + amikacin	+ Imipenem, +doxycycline, + fluoroquinolone
Mycobacterium leprae	AFB	Dapsone + rifampin	+ Clofazimine
Mycobacterium marinum‡	AFB	Rifampin + ethambutol	Minocycline, macrolide
Mycobacterium tuberculosis‡	AFB	Isoniazid + rifampin + pyrazinamide ± ethambutol	+ Streptomycin, + fluoroquinolone
Mycoplasma pneumoniae	NA	Erythromycin	Tetracycline
Neisseria gonorrhoeae‡	GNDC	Ceftriaxone or cefixime	Fluoroquinolone, BLI, ampicillin, spectinomycin
Neisseria meningitidis (illness)	GNDC	Penicillin	TGC, chloramphenicol
Neisseria meningitidis (carrier)	GNDC	Rifampin	Minocycline
Nocardia	GPB	Sulfonamide	TMP/SMX, minocycline, imipenem, amikacin
Pasteurella multocida	GNCB	Penicillin or ampicillin	Tetracycline, TMP/SMX, fluoroquinolone, TGC
Peptostreptococcus	GPC	Penicillin	Clindamycin, vancomycin, cephalosporin
Propionibacterium acnes	GPB	Tetracycline	Clindamycin (topical), erythromycin
Proteus mirabilis‡	GNB	Ampicillin	AG, TGC, aztreonam, TMP/SMX, fluoroquinolone
Proteus vulgaris‡	GNB	TGC or aztreonam	Imipenem, AG, APP, fluoroquinolone, TMP/SMX
Providencia‡	GNB	TGC or fluoroquinolone	Imipenem, AG, aztreonam, TMP/SMX
Pseudomonas aeruginosa‡ (systemic or neutropenic)	GNB	Tobramycin + APP or ceftazidime	Ciprofloxacin, imipenem, aztreonam
Pseudomonas aeruginosa‡ (other)	GNB	Ciprofloxacin or ceftazidime	APP, AG, aztreonam, imipenem, other quinolone
Pseudomonas cepacia‡	GNB	TMP/SMX	
Rhodococcus equi‡	GPC	Vancomycin	Erythromycin, TMP/SMX
Rickettsia species	NA	Tetracycline	Chloramphenicol
Rochalimaea henselae	GNB	Erythromycin or doxycycline	Fluoroquinolone
Salmonella typhi‡	GNB	TMP/SMX or fluoroquinolone	Ceftriaxone, chloramphenicol, amoxicillin
Salmonella species‡ (systemic)	GNB	Ceftriaxone or fluoroquinolone	TMP/SMX, ampicillin
Serratia‡	GNB	TGC	AG, fluoroquinolone, imipenem, TMP/SMX
Shigella‡	GNB	Fluoroquinolone	TMP/SMX
Staphylococcus aureus‡ (methicillin sensitive)	GPC	PRP	Cephalosporin, vancomycin, clindamycin, BLI, TMP/SMX, imipenem
Staphylococcus aureus‡ (methicillan resistant)	GPC	Vancomycin	TMP/SMX + rifampin ± mupirocin (topical)
Staphylococcus, coagulase-negative‡	GPC	Vancomycin	PRP, cephalosporin, TMP/SMX

Organism	Morphology	Drug of choice	Alternatives
Streptobacillus moniliformis	GPB	Penicillin	Tetracycline
Streptococcus agalactiae (group B)	GPC	Ampicillin ± AG	Cephalosporin, vancomycin, erythromycin
Streptococcus pneumoniae‡	GPC	Penicillin	Cephalosporin, erythromycin, vancomycin
Streptococcus pyogenes (group A)	GPC	Penicillin	Erythromycin, clindamycin, cephalosporin
Streptococcus, viridans group	GPC	Penicillin	Cephalosporin, vancomycin
Treponema pallidum	GNS	Penicillin	Erythromycin, tetracycline
Ureaplasma	NA	Tetracycline	Erythromycin
Varicella-zoster	V	Acyclovir	Foscarnet
Vibrio cholerae	GNB	Tetracycline	TMP/SMX, fluoroquinolone
Vibrio parahaemolyticus	GNB	Fluoroquinolone	Tetracycline, ampicillin
Vibrio vulnificus‡	GNB	Tetracycline	Ampicillin, fluoroquinolone, chloramphenicol
Xanthomonas maltophilia‡	GNB	TMP/SMX	Ciprofloxacin, ticarcillin/clavulanate
Yersinia enterocolitica‡	GNB	TGC	Cefoxitin, TMP/SMX, fluoroquinolone
Yersinia pestis	GNB	Streptomycin	Tetracycline, chloramphenicol
Fungi			
Aspergillus species		Amphotericin	Itraconazole
Blastomyces dermatitidis		Itraconazole	Ketoconazole, amphotericin
Candida species, systemic		Amphotericin ± flucytosine	Fluconazole
Candida species, urinary		Fluconazole	Amphotericin, flucytosine
Candida species, chronic mucocutaneous		Ketoconazole	Fluconazole, amphotericin
Candida species, cutaneous		Clotrimazole (topical)	Fluconazole, ketoconazole, other topicals
Coccidioides immitis		Fluconazole or ketoconazole	Itraconazole, amphotericin
Cryptococcus neoformans		Amphotericin or fluconazole	± Flucytosine
Chromomycosis		Fluconazole or itraconazole	Amphotericin, flucytosine
Dermatophytes		Ketoconazole (systemic), clotrimazole (topical)	Griseofulvin, itraconazole; Miconazole, econazole, tioconazole, tolnaftate; Ketoconazole
Histoplasma capsulatum		Itraconazole or amphotericin	
Phycomycosis (zygomycosis)		Amphotericin	
Sporothrix schenckii		Itraconazole	SSKI (lymphocutaneous), amphotericin

* Morphology: AFB, acid-fast bacillus; GNB, gram-negative bacillus; GNCB, gram-negative coccobacillus; GNDC, gram-negative diplococci; GNS, gram-negative spirillary or spirochetal organism; GPB, gram positive bacillus; GPC, gram-positive cocci; NA, not applicable; V, virus.

† Antimicrobial agents: APP, antipseudomonal penicillin (ticarcillin, mezlocillin, piperacillin); AG, aminoglycoside (gentamicin, tobramycin, amikacin, netilmicin); BLI, β-lactam plus β-lactamase inhibitor (ampicillin + sulbactam, amoxicillin + clavulanate, ticarcillin + clavulanate, piperacillin + tazobactam); IUDR, idoxuridine; Macrolide, new macrolide (azithromycin or clarithromycin); PRP, penicillinase-resistant penicillin (oxacillin, cloxacillin, dicloxacillin, methicillin, nafcillin); SGC, second-generation cephalosporin, oral (cefuroxime, cefpodoxime, loracarbef, cefaclor, cefprozil); SSKI, saturated solution of potassium iodide; TGC, third-generation cephalosporin (cefotaxime, ceftriaxone, ceftizoxime, cefoperazone, cefixime, ceftazidime); TMP/SMX, trimethoprim + sulfamethoxazole.

‡ Susceptibilities vary; alter therapy according to antimicrobial susceptibility test results.

TABLE 20–3.   PREVENTION OF WOUND INFECTION AND SEPSIS IN SURGICAL PATIENTS

Nature of Surgery	Most Common Pathogens	Recommended Drugs	Preoperative I.V. Dose*
Cardiovascular Prosthetic valve insertion Open heart surgery Pacemaker insertion	Staphylococci, diphtheroids	Cefzolin or vancomycin	1 gram
Arterial Reconstructive Aortic surgery, groin incision Prosthetic vascular material Leg amputation for ischemia	Staphylococci, enterococci, enteric gram-negative	Cefazolin or vancomycin	1 gram
Noncardiac Thoracic With bronchial transection	Staphylococci, streptococci, *Haemophilus*	Cefazolin or cefuroxime	1–1.5 gram
Neurosurgery Craniotomy or spinal surgery	Staphylococci	Cefazolin or vancomycin	1 gram
Orthopedic Total joint replacement Internal fixation of fracture	Staphylococci	Cefazolin or vancomycin	1 gram
Head and Neck With mucosal incision	Staphylococci, streptococci, oral anaerobes	Cefazolin or clindamycin	1 gram 600 mg
Gastroduodenal High-risk surgery (obstructed, achlorhydric, bleeding)	Streptococci, oral anaerobes, enteric gram-negatives	Cefazolin or cefotetan	1 gram
Biliary Tract High-risk surgery (acute cholecystitis, obstruction, elderly)	Enteric gram-negative bacilli	Cefazolin or cefotetan	1 gram
Colorectal	Enteric gram-negative bacilli, anaerobes, streptococci	Oral neomycin + erythromycin + mechanical prep with cefoxitin or cefotetan	1 gram
Gynecologic Vaginal or abdominal hysterectomy, high-risk cesarean section	Enteric gram-negative bacilli, anaerobes, streptococci	Cefazolin (after cord clamping for C-section)	1 gram

* If surgery is prolonged, additional doses of antimicrobial agent should be given every 4 to 6 hours during surgery. For a discussion of the value of continuing antibiotics postoperatively, see text.

teus as well as *Pseudomonas* and other nonfermentative gram-negative bacilli. Streptococci and anaerobes, however, are intrinsically resistant to aminoglycoside antibiotics.

Aminoglycosides work by binding to ribosomes. Such binding is usually irreversible, and, therefore, these drugs are bactericidal. Resistance to aminoglycoside antibiotics is mediated either by a decrease in permeability to the compound (streptococci and anaerobes) or by enzymatic inactivation (which may be plasmid mediated and, therefore, transferable from one organism to another). Amikacin is less susceptible to such inactivation and, therefore, may be of value when gentamicin- and tobramycin-resistant strains are frequent.

Aminoglycoside antibiotics are not absorbed after oral administration. After parenteral administration, they are not metabolized and are excreted by glomerular filtration. Impairment of renal function profoundly affects the excretion of these compounds, and dosage modification is necessary (Table 20–1). In order to assure adequate blood and tissue levels and to avoid toxicity, measurement of blood concentrations is recommended in patients receiving aminoglycoside antibiotics for systemic infections. Gentamicin or tobramycin peak blood concentrations should be maintained between 4 and 8 μg/mL, and trough levels between 1 and 2 μg/mL, for patients with normal renal function receiving every-8-hours dosing. Recent data suggest that once-daily administration using a 4- to 5-mg/kg dose of gentamicin or tobramycin results in equivalent or less toxicity and similar clinical success as a result of the prolonged postantibiotic effect. The tissue penetration of aminoglycoside antibiotics is poor, and cerebrospinal fluid (CSF) concentrations are generally subtherapeutic even in the presence of inflammation.

Toxicity is the major drawback to the use of aminoglycoside antibiotics. Ototoxicity, both auditory and vestibular, neuromuscular blockade, and nephrotoxicity are the major problems. Ototoxicity is seen most frequently in patients with underlying renal disease and pre-existing auditory disease, and its occurrence is related to the total dose received, duration of therapy, and treatment with other ototoxic drugs, particularly prior aminoglycoside antibiotics or loop diuretics. Neuromuscular blockade occasionally is seen after surgical procedures, where prolonged muscular weakness after anesthesia is the presentation. Occasionally, acute neurologic deterioration is seen in patients with other neuromuscular disorders, such as myasthenia gravis.

Nephrotoxicity is the most frequently encountered adverse reaction to aminoglycoside antibiotics. It usually is seen after prolonged administration (over 2 weeks) to elderly patients with preexisting renal or liver disease. Typically, it presents as nonoliguric renal failure, with variable urinary microscopic findings and gradually rising blood urea nitrogen (BUN) and creatinine levels. Azotemia is usually reversible if the drug is stopped early and if other complicating factors, such as septic shock, are absent.

Aminoglycoside antibiotics are of value because of their broad aerobic gram-negative spectrum and low cost (gentamicin). Their clinical use is primarily for the empiric treatment of gram-negative bacillary infections; for the treatment of difficult infections caused by gram-negative aerobic bacilli, in combination with a β-lactam antibiotic; and, with ampicillin or penicillin, for the treatment of serious enterococcal infections.

Cephalosporins

Cephalosporins are β-lactam antibiotics, active by virtue of their interference with the synthesis of bacterial cell wall components, and are bactericidal for most susceptible microorganisms. The multitude of cephalosporin derivatives has been popularly divided into first-, second-, and third-generation derivatives based on the timing of their development and their spectrum of activity.

Cefazolin is the workhorse parental first-generation derivative and has a spectrum of activity similar to cephapirin, cephradine, and cephalothin. It is active against most gram-positive cocci, with the exception of enterococci; most gram-positive anaerobes; many strains of *E. coli*, *Klebsiella*, and *Proteus mirabilis*; and some gram-negative anaerobes but not *Bacteroides fragilis*. Cephalexin, cefadroxil, and cephadine are available orally and possess similar spectra.

Cefuroxime and cefamandole are second-generation cephalosporin derivatives, possessing the same basic spectrum as cefazolin but also active against *Moraxella*, *Haemophilus*, and some other gram-negative bacilli. Cefoxitin and cefotetan, properly called cephamycins because of their resistance to gram-negative β-lactamases, are active against *B. fragilis* and many strains of enteric gram-negative bacilli that are resistant to first-generation cephalosporins. However, they possess weaker activity than other second-generation derivatives against gram-positive bacteria and *Haemophilus*.

A plethora of oral second-generation cephalosporins have become available in recent years, with a spectrum of activity close to that of cefuroxime. These expensive compounds have found a niche for the treatment of upper and lower respiratory infections for which simpler and cheaper compounds may be excluded because of allergy, resistance, or clinical failure. They include oral cefuroxime, cefaclor, cefpodoxime, cefprozil, loracarbef, and cefixime. Cefixime has no useful antistaphylococcal activity.

Further development in this class has created so-called third-generation derivatives, such as cefotaxime, ceftizoxime, ceftriaxone, cefoperazone, and ceftazidime. These drugs are significantly more active against members of the Enterobacteriaceae and certain streptococci. Cefoperazone and ceftazidime also have activity against many strains of *Pseudomonas aeruginosa*. In addition, they are all very active against *Neisseria*, *Moraxella*, and *Haemophilus* species, including ampicillin-resistant strains, but have weaker activity against staphylococci than the earlier cephalosporins. None of these derivatives has activity against enterococci, and their anaerobic coverage is variable.

Cephalosporin pharmacokinetics vary from one derivative to another (Table 20–1). Most are excreted renally, some have considerable biliary excretion, and others are metabolized (particularly cephalothin and cefotaxime). The third-generation derivatives penetrate the blood–CSF barrier and achieve CSF concentrations effective for the treatment of most gram-positive and gram-negative bacillary meningitis. First- and second-generation derivatives do not enter the CSF reliably and should not be used for the treatment of meningitis.

Cephalosporins retain, along with penicillins, relative freedom from major toxicity. Hypersensitivity reactions, local reactions to infusion or injection, and rare instances of leukopenia, thrombocytopenia, or hemolytic anemia are seen. Cefamandole, cefotetan, and cefoperazone possess a unique side chain that has weak anti–vitamin K activity. Patients on a vitamin K–deficient diet (such as postoperative or malnourished patients) may experience unexpected rises in prothrombin time and bleeding correctable by administration of vitamin K. These agents also can provoke an Antabuse-like reaction.

The cephalosporins are of clinical value for a wide variety of infections because they lack major toxicity, are bactericidal, and have a broad spectrum of activity. They are useful for prophylaxis, are of value in complicated and mixed infections, and are used effectively as substitutes for penicillin in some patients allergic to penicillin (see later in this chapter). Third-generation cephalosporins are the drugs of choice for resistant *Haemophilus* and gram-negative bacillary meningitis, and ceftazidime for *P. aeruginosa* and *Acinetobacter* species.

Chloramphenicol

Chloramphenicol is an antibiotic isolated from *Streptomyces*. It inhibits protein synthesis at a ribosomal level and is either bactericidal or bacteriostatic depending on the particular isolate involved. Chloramphenicol has a broad spectrum of activity. It is active against most gram-positive cocci, including *S. pneumoniae*. Its activity against aerobic gram-negative bacteria is also broad and includes *Haemophilus* species, most *E. coli*, *Enterobacter*, *Klebsiella*, *Proteus*, *Serratia*, and *Salmonella*. It is not active against *Pseudomonas*. Chloramphenicol is active against the majority of anaerobes, including *B. fragilis*.

Chloramphenicol is well absorbed and highly lipid soluble, accounting for its ability to cross the blood–brain barrier, thereby achieving CSF concentrations adequate to treat some forms of meningitis.

Although an extremely active compound, chloramphenicol is potentially toxic. Bone marrow depression is the major adverse reaction. This may be a dose-related, reversible phenomenon. A more severe, aplastic anemia is seen as an idiosyncratic reaction, independent of dose, and occurs with a frequency of approximately 1 in 50,000. It seems impossible to predict who will develop marrow aplasia as a result of chloramphenicol administration. At least triweekly blood counts are indicated in all patients receiving chloramphenicol, with termination of therapy if the white blood cell counts fall to less than 4000/mm^3 or platelet counts to less than 120,000/mm^3. Other side effects of chloramphenicol include optic neuritis after prolonged oral administration, and, rarely, hypersensitivity reactions. Chloramphenicol inhibits the activity of microsomal liver enzymes, thereby interfering with the metabolism of many other drugs.

With the development of safer and more potent antimicrobial agents, chloramphenicol has been relegated to a role of largely historical interest. However, it remains useful for the treatment of systemic *Salmonella* infections and rickettsial infections. Because of its central nervous system penetration, it may be a useful alternative to penicillin G or cephalosporins for the treatment of gram-positive meningitis, brain abscesses, and *Haemophilus influenzae* infections of the central nervous system.

The Lincinoids

Lincomycin and clindamycin are antibiotics similar in activity to erythromycin. They act by competitively binding to ribosomes, thereby inhibiting protein synthesis. They appear to occupy the same binding sites as erythromycin, so that concomitant administration of both drugs results in antagonism. The spectrum of activity of clindamycin includes most gram-positive bacteria, with the exception of enterococci, and most anaerobes, including *B. fragilis*. Clindamycin is much more potent in the latter regard and lincomycin is no longer used. However, many institutions report that up to 10 per cent of *B. fragilis* isolates are now also resistant to clindamycin. Neither drug is active against aerobic gram-negative bacilli. Clindamycin also has useful activity against certain protozoa, such as *Babesia* (in combination with quinine) and *Toxoplasma*.

Clindamycin is well absorbed after oral administration. It is distributed throughout the body but does not reach adequate levels in CSF. Clindamycin is excreted primarily through the liver, and the normal half-life is not altered appreciably in patients with renal impairment. Only small amounts are excreted in the urine.

The major toxicity of clindamycin is gastrointestinal. Diarrhea occurs in 10 per cent of patients. Pseudomembranous colitis, resulting from overgrowth of *Clostridium difficile*, occurs in perhaps 1 per cent of patients. It occurs as frequently with parenteral therapy as with oral, is not related to duration of therapy, and may be exacerbated or precipitated by coadministration of antiperistaltic drugs, such as diphenoxylate (Lomotil). Hypersensitivity reactions occur occasionally. Hepatotoxicity is seen rarely.

Clindamycin is valuable for the treatment of staphylococcal and streptococcal infections, particularly in bone and soft tissue. Clindamycin is also useful for the treatment of anaerobic infections, particularly those caused by *B. fragilis*. Because it is ineffective against aerobic gram-negative bacilli, clindamycin usually must be used in combination with other drugs for the treatment of infradiaphragmatic infections. As an alternate to penicillin G, it is excellent for the treatment of anaerobic and mixed aerobic and anaerobic pleuropulmonary infections.

Macrolide Antibiotics

Erythromycin is a broad-spectrum macrocyclic antibiotic. It is active against many staphylococci and most streptococci, excluding enterococci. In addition, it is active against many gram-positive bacilli, including anaerobes, *Listeria*, and *Corynebacterium*. Gram-negative organisms are infrequently sensitive, although some strains of *Haemophilus* and *Moraxella* may be inhibited effectively. *Treponema pallidum*, *Mycoplasma*, *Chlamydia*, and some *Rickettsia* are susceptible to erythromycin. It is the agent of choice for the treatment of *Legionella* infections. Erythromycin acts by binding competitively to ribosomal proteins, thereby inhibiting protein synthesis.

Erythromycin is absorbed erratically after oral administration. A variety of oral forms are available, and it has not been established that any of the various erythromycin salts, esters, or base preparations has a clinical advantage over any other in the treatment of infections caused by susceptible microorganisms. Erythromycin distributes well to most body tissues except CSF. It is excreted primarily in the bile and penetrates prostatic fluid, but urinary levels are marginal.

Two new macrolides, clarithromycin and azithromycin, recently have been approved for use. They possess a spectrum of activity similar to erythromycin and clinical outcomes appear equivalent. However, they are two- to fourfold more potent against *Moraxella* and *Haemophilus* and possess activity against some atypical mycobacteria. These expensive compounds are well absorbed, distribute widely throughout the body, achieve exceedingly high intracellular concentrations, and have prolonged half-lives allowing twice-daily (clarithromycin) or once-daily (azithromycin) dosing. Indeed, azithromycin is not eliminated from the body for over 5 days.

Macrolides are relatively safe compounds. Nausea, vomiting, and abdominal cramps are fairly frequently complaints with erythromycin but uncommon with clarithromycin and azithromycin. Cholestatic hepatitis may follow use of estolate. Hypersensitivity reactions are unusual. Phlebitis after intravenous administration is common. Transient sensorineural hearing loss has appeared as a rare complication of high-dose intravenous therapy.

Clinical uses of macrolide antibiotics include treatment of gram-positive infections, particularly in penicillin-allergic patients; treatment of *Legionella*, *Chlamydia*, and *Mycoplasma* infections; alternatives to penicillin for the treatment of uncomplicated syphilis in penicillin-allergic patients; and as valuable agents for the treatment of *Corynebacterium diphtheriae* infections.

Metronidazole

Metronidazole is an imidazole derivative with unique activity against certain protozoa (*Trichomonas*, *Entamoeba*, and *Giardia*) and anaerobic bacteria, including *B. fragilis*. It has no activity against aerobic microorganisms and in the treatment of mixed infections must be used with an antibiotic effective against aerobes. Metronidazole interferes with DNA synthesis and is bactericidal against susceptible microorganisms.

Metronidazole is well absorbed after oral administration. It penetrates all body tissues well and reaches a particularly high concentration in the brain and CSF. Most of the drug is metabolized in the liver and excreted in the urine as inactive metabolites. Moderate to severe liver disease will prolong the half-life from 8 to 18 hours and requires dose adjustment.

Metronidazole is well tolerated but can cause gastrointestinal upset and, rarely, leukopenia, peripheral neuropathy, and seizures. Although extensive studies have not shown an increase in bacterial mutation or carcinogenicity in humans, it should not be used in pregnant women. Metroni-

dazole interferes with ethanol metabolism, producing an Antabuse-like reaction, and also may inhibit the metabolism of warfarin and phenytoin.

Metronidazole is of great clinical use for the treatment of protozoal infections, particularly trichomoniasis, amebiasis, and giardiasis. It is not a very effective intraluminal amebicide and, therefore, must be followed by an effective intraluminal drug, such as diiodohydroxyquin (Diodoquin). Metronidazole is very valuable for the treatment of anaerobic infections but, when mixed infection is present, it must be combined with an antibiotic effective against aerobic bacteria. Metronidazole is the agent of choice for the treatment of anaerobic infections of the central nervous system (such as brain abscesses) and for the treatment of pseudomembranous colitis.

Penicillin Derivatives

Penicillin and its many derivatives remain safe, effective, and potent despite the appearance of β-lactam–destroying enzymes in many genera of gram-positive and gram-negative bacteria. Derived from the *Penicillium* group of fungi, penicillins are bactericidal inhibitors of cell wall synthesis.

Penicillin G is becoming less active against gram-positive bacteria. Ninety per cent of staphylococci are resistant. Penicillins are not bactericidal for enterococci, and certain strains of *S. pneumoniae* have become relatively (MIC values of 0.1 to 1.0 μg/mL) or totally (MIC values >1.0 μg/mL) resistant to penicillin G as a result of altered penicillin-binding proteins within the cell membrane. The frequency of such strains varies from 3 to 22 per cent of isolates, depending on geographic region. Although many of these pneumococcal strains can be killed by high doses of penicillin G, increasing numbers of isolates are totally resistant to penicillin. Penicillin is active against *Listeria*, *Treponema*, and *Borrelia* (including *B. burgdorferi*). Ampicillin and amoxicillin have an antimicrobial spectrum similar to penicillin G but are more active against gram-negative bacilli and are effective for the treatment of many infections caused by non-β-lactamase–producing *Haemophilus*, *E. coli*, *P. mirabilis*, and *Salmonella* species.

Methicillin, nafcillin, and oxacillin are resistant to the hydrolytic action of gram-positive β-lactamases. Accordingly, these derivatives have become the drugs of choice for treating infections caused by staphylococci. They are less active than penicillin G against other gram-positive organisms and have inadequate activity against anaerobes and gram-negative microorganisms.

Mezlocillin, ticarcillin, and piperacillin are the antipseudomonal penicillins in common use. They have a basic spectrum of activity similar to ampicillin but, in addition, are effective against many strains of *Enterobacter*, *Serratia*, *Acinetobacter*, *Morganella*, and *Pseudomonas*. Mezlocillin and piperacillin also are active against 60 to 80 per cent of community-acquired *Klebsiella* species and have better enterococcal activity than other members of this group. Piperacillin has greater in vitro potency against *P. aeruginosa*, although it has not been shown convincingly superior to other derivatives for the treatment of clinical infections caused by *Pseudomonas*.

In order to expand the spectrum and retain the usefulness of some penicillin derivatives threatened by the increased prevalence of β-lactamase production in both gram-positive and gram-negative bacteria, the β-lactamase inhibitors clavulanic acid, sulbactam, and tazobactam have been developed. These compounds effectively block the activity of staphylococcal β-lactamases and many gram-negative β-lactamases, allowing the parent penicillinase-susceptible derivative to regain activity against previously resistant bacteria. Thus, Augmentin (amoxicillin–clavulanate), Unasyn (ampicillin–sulbactam), Timentin (ticarcillin–clavulanate), and Zosyn (piperacillin–tazobactam) (Table 20–1) are active against β-lactamase–producing staphylococci, *Haemophilus*, *Moraxella*, *Neisseria gonorrhoeae*, *Bacteroides*, *E. coli*, and *Klebsiella*. Microorganisms producing primarily cephalosporinases of the type 1 variety are not susceptible to this inhibitory function, and these combinations offer no advantage over amoxicillin, ampicillin, ticarcillin, or piperacillin alone. Such microorganisms include *Enterobacter*, *Serratia*, *Morganella*, and *Pseudomonas*. Owing to the clinical distribution of β-lactamases, the β-lactamase–blocking compounds provide broad-spectrum, polymicrobial coverage in skin and soft tissue infections, intra-abdominal and pelvic infections, and upper and lower respiratory infections.

Penicillin derivates are excreted primarily in urine, although the antistaphylococcal penicillins and mezlocillin and piperacillin are metabolized in the liver and excreted in the bile. Penicillin G is not acid stable and, therefore, penicillin V is preferred for oral administration. Amoxicillin is absorbed better orally and reaches twice the blood level of ampicillin or penicillin V at equivalent doses. The tissue penetration of these compounds is good, but CSF levels are low in the absence of inflammation. The concentrations of amoxicillin in sinus and middle ear fluids are greater than those achieved by ampicillin, making it preferable for the treatment of otitis media and sinusitis.

Penicillin derivatives are free from major toxicity. Anaphylaxis is the most serious adverse reaction, occurring in approximately 0.05 per cent of penicillin-treated patients. Other hypersensitivity reactions include eosinophilia, interstitial nephritis, maculopapular skin eruptions, and serum sickness. High doses of penicillin derivatives, particularly in the presence of renal failure, can produce myoclonus and seizures. Inadvertent intravenous injection of procaine penicillin produces acute pro-caine toxicity with fever, tachycardia, anxiety, and hallucinations.

When ticarcillin and carbenicillin are administered in large doses, inhibition of platelet aggregation may occur, and clinical bleeding is observed in from 1 to 5 per cent of patients treated with these compounds. Hypokalemia also is seen as a result of the effect of the nonreabsorbable anion and resultant hyperkaluria. The amount of sodium in ticarcillin and carbenicillin is approximately 5 mEq/gm and may be sufficient to exacerbate congestive heart failure. Rarely, leukopenia, hemolytic anemia, and thrombocytopenia are seen as a result of the administration of penicillins.

Patients reporting allergy to penicillin often lack true hypersensitivity. Some reactions to ampicillin and methicillin are not immunologically mediated and do not recur on re-exposure. Such reactions occur commonly (50 to 90 per cent of cases) in patients with infectious mononucleosis treated with ampicillin or amoxicillin. Late hyersensitivity reactions (i.e., occurring several days or weeks after starting penicillin) are immunoglobulin (Ig) G mediated and are not usually dangerous. Penicillin may be continued if necessary, with symptomatic treatment of the rash and pruritus. In this setting, however, the occurrence of clinically significant serum sickness, interstitial nephritis, or exfoliation should prompt withdrawal of the drug. Immediate hypersensitivity reactions, mediated by IgE, are rare and represent true hypersensitivity. Such reactions usually can be detected by skin testing with penicilloyl-polylysine (commercially available as Prepen) and a dilute mixture of degraded penicillin G, known as the minor determinant mixture. A positive reaction to these tests has a high predictive value for immediate hypersensitivity and contraindicates the use of penicillin. If absolutely necessary, desensitization may be undertaken by a trained allergist or infectious disease specialist.

The incidence of cross-allergenicity with cephalosporin derivatives is debated frequently but is probably less than 10 per cent. However, patients with true anaphylaxis to penicillin G should not be given cephalosporin antibiotics without extreme caution. Patients with late reactions to penicillin derivatives usually can be given cephalosporin derivatives without incident, and the cephalosporins play a valuable role in this regard.

Monobactams

Aztreonam is the first of a group of monocyclic β-lactam antibiotics, also known as the monobactams. These antibiotics are potent, bactericidal drugs active against most aerobic gram-negative bacilli, including aminoglycoside-resistant strains, and *P. aeruginosa*. Aztreonam is also active against *Neisseria* species and *Haemophilus*, including β-lactamase–producing strains. It has no activity against gram-positive bacteria or anaerobes.

Aztreonam is not orally bioavailable. Intravenous or intramuscular administration produces effective blood and tissue concentrations for 4 to 6 hours in patients with normal renal function. There is insignificant metabolism, and the drug is excreted almost entirely in the urine, requiring dosage adjustment in renal failure (Table 20–1).

Because of its unique spectrum, aztreonam has proven a useful, albeit costly, replacement for aminoglycoside antibiotics in many clinical situations. It has proven effective for the treatment of urinary tract infections, lower respiratory tract infections, skin and soft tissue, and bone and joint infections as a single agent. In polymicrobial infections or where gram-positive or anaerobic bacteria are suspected, a second agent to cover these additional pathogens must be used in addition.

The adverse effects associated with the use of aztreonam are similar to those seen with other β-lactams. Aztreonam is not nephrotoxic or ototoxic, and, because of its lack of anaerobic activity, diarrhea is uncommon. A major advantage of aztreonam is its lack of immunologic cross-reactivity with penicillin and cephalosporin derivatives. It has been used without incident to treat infections in patients with positive penicillin skin tests and a documented history of anaphylactic reaction to penicillin.

Carbapenems

Imipenem is a carbapenem, a semisynthetic β-lactam with an unusually broad spectrum of activity. It is active against most gram-negative bacilli, including *P. aeruginosa*, most gram-positive bacteria, except for methicillin-resistant staphylococci and some enterococci, and all anaerobic bacteria, including *B. fragilis*. Cross-resistance with other β-lactams is infrequent, so it is useful for the treatment of infections caused by multi–drug-resistant flora.

No oral formulation of imipenem is available. When administered intravenously, it undergoes rapid inactivation by renal peptidases. This inactivation is blocked effectively by combining imipenem with cilastatin, an enzyme inhibitor, to provide a clinically useful combination known commercially as Primaxin. The pharmocokinetics of this combination are similar to those of other β-lactams, achieving good concentrations in most body fluids except the central nervous system. Renal dysfunction requires dosage adjustment (Table 20–1).

Imipenem is useful for a wide variety of bacterial infections, particularly polymicrobial infections in which aerobes and anaerobes are present. Intraabdominal and soft tissue infections are examples. Because of its broad spectrum, imipenem has an important role in treating drug-resistant nosocomial infections. For this reason, together with its cost, many experts reserve Primaxin for use in exceptional clinical situations.

Primaxin, like other β-lactams, is usually well tolerated. Cross-allergenicity with penicillins does occur. Administration of large doses in renal failure may produce seizures, so close monitoring of renal function and appropriate dose adjustment (Table 20–1) are necessary. The maximum daily dose of Primaxin should not exceed 4 grams.

Quinolones

The newly introduced fluorinated quinolones are synthetic antimicrobial agents. They are bactericidal compounds, inhibiting DNA gyrase, an enzyme crucial to bacterial cell function and replication. Fluoroquinolones are highly active in vitro against enteric gram-negative bacilli such as *E. coli* and *Klebsiella* and also against nonfermenters such as *Pseudomonas* and *Aeromonas*. They possess some activity against staphylococci, including methicillin-resistant strains, although resistance resulting from overuse has emerged in many institutions. Activity against enterococci and other streptococci is somewhat less, and their therapeutic value in infections caused by these microorganisms is not well established. The anaerobic activity of most quinolones is weak and probably not clinically valuable. Fluoroquinolones are also active against *Legionella, Mycoplasma, Haemophilus,* and *Neisseria* species. They possess variable activity against *Chlamydia, Ureaplasma,* and *Mycobacterium.*

Resistance to fluoroquinolone antibiotics was rare prior to their introduction in 1987. However, excessive and frequently inappropriate use in both health care institutions and the community has led to a dramatic increase in resistance among staphylococci, especially methicillin-resistant strains, *Pseudomonas*, and enterococci. Cross-resistance occurs within the fluoroquinolone class but does not generally cross to other classes of antimicrobial agents. The fluoroquinolones, therefore, are frequently useful for the treatment of infections caused by multi–drug-resistant gram-negative bacilli.

Fluoroquinolones are absorbed readily after oral administration. Their relatively small molecular weight and low degree of protein binding result in excellent tissue penetration. Particularly high concentrations are achieved within phagocytic cells and in prostatic tissue, bronchial epithelium, bile, urine, and stool. The serum half-lives of these antimicrobial agents are long, permitting dosing intervals of 8 to 12 hours or more. Although metabolized to varying degrees in the liver, urinary concentrations of active drug are high at all levels of renal function, far in excess of those needed to inhibit most urinary pathogens.

Norfloxacin, ciprofloxacin, ofloxacin, enoxacin, and lomefloxacin are the fluoroquinolone derivatives currently available. All compounds are effective orally for the treatment of uncomplicated and complicated urinary tract infections, and uncomplicated gonorrhea, and are drugs of choice for prostatitis and urinary tract infections caused by *P. aeruginosa*. These drugs are also agents of choice for the treatment of infectious diarrhea because they inhibit essentially all enteric pathogens except *C. difficile*. Ciprofloxacin and ofloxacin also have been shown to be effective in skin, soft tissue, bone and joint, and lower respiratory infections caused by susceptible pathogens, particularly gram-negative bacilli. In these roles as oral agents, quinolones may shorten the course of, or replace entirely, intravenous antimicrobial therapy of certain infections.

Fluoroquinolones are well tolerated. The most frequent adverse reactions are gastrointestinal—chiefly nausea, occurring in 8 to 10 per cent of patients. Vomiting and diarrhea occur less frequently. Some patients experience central nervous system effects, such as headache, dizziness, restlessness, or tremor. These reactions are seen most frequently in elderly patients. Other adverse reactions, such as drug fever, rash, and pruritus, occur in 1 to 2 per cent of patients. Photosensitivity reactions and interstitial nephritis have been reported. Because of fetal and juvenile cartilage toxicity in some animal models, administration of these agents to pregnant or lactating women is contraindicated and no pediatric indication currently exists.

A significant drug interaction between some fluoroquinolones and xanthine derivatives results in increased serum concentrations of theophylline and caffeine during therapy. Divalent cations, including antacids and calcium, iron, and zinc compounds, prevent absorption of the fluoroquinolones by chelation. Concomitant administration of H_2 antagonists, however, does not alter antimicrobial serum concentrations significantly.

Sulfonamides and Trimethoprim

The sulfonamides, first synthesized for clinical use in 1935, initiated a new era in the chemotherapy of infectious diseases. They are bacteriostatic compounds and act by inhibiting dihydrofolate synthetase activity, because they are structural analogues for its substrate, *para*-aminobenzoic acid. In combination with trimethoprim, which inhibits the next step in purine synthesis, dihydrofolate reductase, they are frequently synergistic.

Sulfonamides are active against a wide variety of gram-positive bacteria, except enterococci, and gram-negative organisms. Most members of the Enterobacteriaceae are susceptible. In addition, *Chlamydia*, *Nocardia*, and *Toxoplasma* are inhibited. Trimethoprim has a similar range of activity against aerobic gram-positive and gram-negative bacteria. Because of their sequential activity in blocking bacterial purine synthesis, sulfamethoxazole and trimethoprim (Bactrim, Septra) are synergistically active against the vast majority of susceptible microorganisms, particularly *H. influenzae*, staphylococci, members of Enterobacteriaceae,

and protozoa such as *Pneumocystis* and *Isospora*. *Pseudomonas aeruginosa*, enterococci and anaerobes are not inhibited effectively, but an emerging pathogen of nosocomial importance, *Xanthomonas maltophilia*, is usually susceptible.

Both sulfonamides and trimethoprim are well absorbed after oral administration and penetrate well to all body tissues, including the central nervous system. Trimethoprim penetrates prostatic tissue particularly well and, either alone or in combination with sulfamethoxazole, is useful for the treatment of bacterial prostatitis. Both drugs are excreted predominantly in the urine, reaching levels higher than those found in serum.

Adverse reactions resulting from sulfonamides and trimethoprim are primarily those of hypersensitivity: a variety of cutaneous eruptions and serum sickness. Erythema multiforme or the Stevens-Johnson syndrome is the most severe form of hypersensitivity and can be seen with either drug. It is particularly severe with long-acting sulfonamides. Therefore, short-acting sulfonamides (sulfisoxazole or sulfamethoxazole) are the derivatives of choice for the treatment of most infections. Drug fever, nausea, vomiting, diarrhea, pulmonary reactions, and hypersensitivity meningitis are seen on rare occasions. Agranulocytosis resulting from sulfonamide derivatives has been described, and megaloblastic anemia resulting from inhibition of human dihydrofolate reductase occasionally is seen in patients receiving trimethoprim chronically or in large doses. Such patients usually are malnourished or receiving other antifolates for the treatment of malignancy. Administration of folinic acid (Leukovorin) will reverse the folic acid deficiency induced by these agents.

The clinical utility of sulfonamides and/or trimethoprim primarily has been for treatment of urinary tract infections. However, in combination, these drugs are particularly effective for the treatment of upper and lower respiratory tract infections caused by *Pneumococcus*, *Moraxella*, or *Haemophilus* species, including sinusitis, otitis media, and bronchitis. The combination is also effective for the treatment of *Nocardia* infections, infections caused by *Pneumocystis carinii*, *Chlamydia trachomatis* infections, and toxoplasmosis. Because of bacterial resistance, the sulfonamides are no longer drugs of choice for the treatment or prophylaxis of meningococcal infections. Trimethoprim plus sulfamethoxazole is a popular choice for the treatment of enteric infections, particularly those caused by *Salmonella* or *Shigella*, but not *Campylobacter*.

Tetracyclines

The tetracyclines are complex compounds with a broad range of activity. They are primarily bacteriostatic and act by inhibiting protein synthesis at a ribosomal level. Tetracyclines are active against many gram-positive bacteria, including *S. aureus*, and gram-negative bacteria, including most members of the Enterobacteriaceae, except *Proteus* species. Many other gram-negative bacteria are also susceptible, including *Haemophilus* species, *Neisseria* species, *Borrelia,* and some nonfermentative bacteria (but not *P. aeruginosa*) at achievable serum levels. The tetracyclines also are active against a wide variety of other microorganisms, including *Rickettsia, Chlamydia, Mycoplasma,* and some *Plasmodium* species. Minocycline has improved activity against staphylococci, including methicillin-resistant strains, and some atypical mycobacteria.

Tetracyclines are absorbed well orally, except in the presence of food or divalent cations, such as antacids or ferrous compounds. Minocycline and doxycycline, however, are less affected by such agents and essentially are absorbed completely, even in the presence of food. Doxycycline and minocycyline are excreted primarily by the liver and not in the urine. All other tetracyclines are excreted to a large extent in urine and are effective for the treatment of some urinary tract infections. Tetracycline and minocycline are more lipid soluble, an important property in determining their tissue penetration.

The side effects of tetracycline are primarily gastrointestinal, with nausea, vomiting, and diarrhea common. Hypersensitivity reactions are uncommon. Photosensitivity, however, is particularly troublesome. Tooth discoloration contraindicates the use of tetracycline in pregnancy and under the age of 10 years. Hepatotoxicity may be seen with intravenous tetracycline, particularly during pregnancy or in renal failure. Doxycycline and minocycline are the parenteral tetracyclines of choice, because they are excreted by extrarenal means and have not been associated with hepatotoxicity. Minocycline is unique in the frequent production of reversible vestibular toxicity.

Tetracyclines have a broad clinical role. They are useful for the treatment of a variety of respiratory tract infections, particularly exacerbations of chronic bronchitis. They are effective for the treatment of mycoplasm and staphylococcal infections, uncomplicated urinary tract infections, prostatitis, and infections caused by *Rickettsia.* Tetracyclines are effective drugs for the treatment of chlamydial infections, particularly nongonococcal urethritis, and mucopurulent cervicitis. They are drugs of choice for treatment of early Lyme disease.

Vancomycin

Vancomycin is a glycopeptide antibiotic isolated from *Nocardia* species. Its use has had a resurgence as a result of the increased prevalence of methicillin-resistant staphylococci, multi–drug-resistant enterococci, and the emergence of *C. difficile.* Its mode of action is the bactericidal inhibition of cell wall synthesis. It is active against most aerobic and anaerobic gram-positive bacteria, including staphylococcal species, *Corynebacteria,* enterococci, and *Clostridia.* It is not active against gram-negative bacteria. Some enterococci recently have become resistant.

Vancomycin is not absorbed after oral administration, and parenteral administration is not effective for the treatment of *C. difficile* colitis. The drug is not metabolized but is excreted by the kidneys in unchanged form. Vancomycin diffuses well into most body compartments except CSF. Because of its total dependence on the kidney for excretion, major adjustments in dose are necessary in the presence of renal insufficiency (Table 20–1).

Deafness is the most serious adverse effect of vancomycin administration. It is more common in the elderly and in those with renal insufficiency and is related to excessively high serum levels. Blood levels of vancomycin should be monitored during therapy and peak levels maintained at less than 40 μg/mL. Occasionally, hypersensitivity reactions are seen, and thrombophlebitis is frequently troublesome. Too-rapid infusion produces facial and upper body flushing and pruritus ("red man syndrome"). This is not an allergic reaction and should be managed by slowing infusion rates.

Vancomycin is a valuable but expensive drug for the treatment of staphylococcal infections, particularly those resulting from methicillin-resistant staphylococci or serious staphylococcal infections in penicillin-allergic patients. It is also very useful for the treatment of enterococcal infections as an alternative to penicillin. Metronidazole has replaced vancomycin as the drug of choice for the treatment of pseudomembranous colitis (caused by *C. difficile*) because of the increasing prevalence of vancomycin-resistant strains of *Enterococcus faecium.*

BONE AND JOINT INFECTIONS

Infectious Arthritis

Infectious arthritis may be of hematogenous origin, may be due to direct percutaneous inoculation of a joint, or may be secondary to a contiguous focus of infection in adjacent soft tissues or bone. In children below 1 year of age, septic arthritis usually is associated with adjacent osteomyelitis, because capillaries perforate the epiphyseal growth plate, allowing infection to spread from bone to joint. Over the age of 1 year, infection is likely to be localized to the joint without concomitant osteomyelitis. Distant infection, trauma, and pre-existing osteoarthritis or rheumatoid arthritis are common predisposing risks for the development of septic arthritis. Arthritis may be seen in certain systemic infections, such as meningococcemia, as a result of immune complex disease rather than joint infection. The arthritis that follows *Salmonella, Shigella,* or *Yersinia* intestinal infection is immunologically similar, and occurs most often in persons with histocompatibility antigen (HLA) B27.

The frequency with which certain microorganisms cause arthritis is dependent on the patient's age (Table 20–4). In the newborn, group B streptococci and staphylococci are most common, although some gram-negative bacilli, such as *E. coli*, may cause septic arthritis as a consequence of bacteremia. The most common organisms in children between the ages of 2 months and 2 years are *H. influenzae* and streptococcal species, although the prevalence of *H. influenzae* septic arthritis is strikingly decreased in recent years as a result of the efficacy of the *Haemophilus* vaccine. After 2 years of age, *S. aureus* causes most bacterial arthritis. In adults ages 15 to 50, *N. gonorrhoeae*, must be considered. Lyme disease is a common cause of large-joint monarticular arthritis at all ages in southern Connecticut, southeastern New York, and the north central states. Gram-negative bacilli are implicated uncommonly as a cause of infectious arthritis in all age groups. Most afflicted patients have underlying disease or longstanding arthritis in the affected joint. Intravenous drug users are prone to develop *Pseudomonas* septic arthritis, particularly in sternoclavicular and sacroiliac joints. *Salmonella* arthritis occurs in individuals with hemolytic disorders, such as sickle cell disease. Anaerobes, although uncommonly reported, appear to be important causes of septic arthritis in the elderly. Mycobacteria characteristically produce an indolent monoarticular arthritis of the knees. Such infections also may involve tendon sheaths. *Sporothrix schenkii* is the most common fungus isolated from the infected joints, particularly the knee and wrist. Monarticular arthritis also occurs with other fungi, such as *Coccidioides immitis*. Viral infections commonly manifesting arthritis include rubella (and rubella vaccine), parvovirus, mumps, Epstein-Barr virus (EBV), and hepatitis B virus.

Individuals with septic arthritis present with fever, pain, limitation of motion, swelling, and redness of the joint. Small children may have only limited movement of the joint and appear to have pa-

TABLE 20–4. MICROBIOLOGIC ETIOLOGY OF SUPPURATIVE ARTHRITIS BY AGE (EXCLUDING LYME DISEASE)

Organism	Per Cent Etiology by Age (years)			
	<2	2–14	15–40	>40
Staphylococcus aureus	40	60	40	70
Haemophilus influenzae	30	10	<1	<1
Streptococci	20	20	15	15
Neisseria gonorrhoeae	<1	5	40	<1
Gram-negative bacilli	5	5	5	10
Anaerobes	<1	<1	<1	5

TABLE 20–5. FREQUENCY OF JOINT INVOLVEMENT IN SUPPURATIVE ARTHRITIS

Joint	Children (%)	Adults (%)
Knee	40	50
Hip	20	25
Ankle	15	7
Elbow	15	10
Wrist	5	7
Shoulder	5	15
Interphalangeal, metacarpal	1	1
Sternoclavicular	<1	10
Sacroiliac	<1	2

ralysis. In the majority of cases, an effusion will be demonstrable, although the hip may be difficult to evaluate. The knee is the most commonly affected joint in both children and adults (Table 20–5).

Laboratory findings in septic arthritis are nonspecific. The sedimentation rate and white blood cell count are usually elevated. Anemia may be present but is more likely related to the underlying disease. Examination of the joint aspirate reveals purulent fluid with a leukocyte count over 50,000/mm^3. Joint fluid protein is elevated, and the glucose level usually will be less than 40 mg/dL, although in children it may be normal. Gram-stained smears of joint fluid will show the organism in most cases of staphylococcal arthritis but in less than 30 per cent of cases of arthritis caused by other bacteria. Cultures should be performed using special media for fastidious organisms, such as *Haemophilus* and *Neisseria*, and blood cultures are indicated because they will be positive in many patients. Latex agglutination is a useful supplementary tool to identify bacterial antigen in joint fluid. Radiographic studies are not helpful unless concomitant osteomyelitis exists. Lyme and viral serologies should be performed when epidemiologically and clinically indicated.

Although all individuals who present with acute monarticular arthritis should be evaluated for a bacterial etiology, other diseases may mimic septic arthritis. Rheumatoid arthritis, juvenile rheumatoid arthritis, osteoarthritis, gout, pseudogout, acute flares of systemic lupus erythematosus, hemarthroses, and viral arthritis may produce similar findings. A high polymorphonuclear leukocyte count in synovial fluid is seen in many of these diseases, particularly gout and pseudogout. Joint fluid must be examined for crystals as well as culturing and Gram's staining.

After proper joint fluid examination and culture, therapy is initiated based on the results of the Gram's stain and the anticipated pathogens. To avoid joint destruction, empiric therapy should be begun immediately without waiting for culture confirmation and subsequently should be tailored to the isolated microorganism. Infectious arthritis generally is treated for 3 to 4 weeks, usually with parenteral antibiotics, although recent studies indicate that oral therapy in children may be effective after 1 week of parenteral therapy, and, in adults with gram-negative bacillary arthritis, oral fluoroquinolone therapy is effective. Antibiotics penetrate joint fluid well, and intra-articular administration is of no additional value. Infected joint fluid should be removed as it accumulates to prevent leukocyte enzyme destruction of articular cartilage. Closed-needle aspiration is the preferred mode of drainage and appears to result in greater recovery of joint function than open drainage. The exception to this is septic hip infection, in which the mechanical difficulties of closed-needle aspiration make open drainage preferred, or in small children, in whom repeated aspirations may be more traumatic than open drainage.

Lyme Disease

Lyme disease is a multisystem disorder with prominent rheumatologic and cutaneous manifestions. Originally recognized in 1975 as a cluster of pediatric arthritis in Old Lyme, Connecticut, it has become clear in the last decade that Lyme disease is a common illness with protean manifestations affecting adults as well as children throughout the world. It is a spirochetal infection caused by *B. burgdorferi*, and is transmitted by ticks of the *Ixodes* genus (the deer tick).

Early Lyme disease is manifest by rash (erythema chronicum migrans [ECM]; see Figure 20-1, p. 367) and a "flu-like" syndrome with headache, body aches, malaise, fatigue, and a low-grade fever. Many patients do not recall a tick bite because the deer tick is so small. With a median incubation period of 7 days (range 5 to 21 days), a small, red macule or papule appears, expanding with a flat or raised red border to a diameter of up to 20 or more cm. The center may become pale, vesicular, or hemorrhagic. Subsequent to the initial lesion, approximately 30 per cent of patients develop smaller, secondary annular lesions, but in total only 60 to 70 per cent of infected patients develop a rash. The appearance of ECM is almost pathognomonic for Lyme disease, but atypical forms occur and may be mistaken for cellulitis, traumatic lesions, or allergic rashes.

Subsequent to the initial infection, and a variable latent period of well-being, neurologic manifestations may appear. These may take the form of aseptic meningitis, neuritis with cranial nerve palsies such as Bell's palsy, and motor or sensory peripheral neuropathies. Up to two thirds of patients exhibit subtle signs of encephalitis, such as memory loss, emotional lability, irritability, fatigue, depression, and headache. Cardiac abnormalities may be manifested by rhythm disturbances, atrioventricular block, myocarditis, or pericarditis.

Late Lyme disease usually is manifested by arthritis. This occurs weeks, months, or even years after the initial infection and presents as a monarticular or oligoarticular arthritis affecting primarily large joints. Arthritis may migrate, may fluctuate in intensity, and, in children, may be accompanied by significant fever. In untreated patients, the arthritis may become chronic, resulting in erosive joint damage and disability. Late neurologic manifestations, although described frequently, are rare and include radiculopathy, demyelinating-like syndromes, dementia, and polyneuropathy.

The diagnosis of Lyme disease depends on a high index of clinical suspicion, particularly for the multisystem manifestations of the disease. Serologic testing is readily available, but tests are frequently negative in early disease. False-positive tests may occur in patients with hypergammaglobulinemia, other spirochetal diseases, autoimmune disease, endocarditis, and infectious mononucleosis. Isolation of the spirochete from tissue or body fluids is difficult and impractical in most cases.

The treatment of Lyme disease depends on its stage. In early disease associated with ECM and constitutional symptoms, tetracycline, doxycycline, or amoxicillin administered for 14 days is generally curative. Oral cefuroxime, cefixime, or azithromycin also may be effective. Lower cure rates are seen with erythromycin. Patients with more advanced disease or established arthritis may require longer courses of oral antibiotics (doxycycline or amoxicillin for 4 to 6 weeks). If central nervous system involvement or carditis is present, parenteral therapy with ceftriaxone, cefotaxime, or penicillin G administered for 2 to 4 weeks is preferred.

With early and aggressive treatment, the prognosis in early Lyme disease is excellent. The response rates in later stages are lower, in part because of lingering fatigue and arthralgia that commonly occur after an adequate course of antibiotic therapy. Adjunctive therapy with nonsteroidal anti-inflammatory agents and antidepressants, psychological support, and infectious disease consultation may be helpful. Adrenocortical steroid therapy is not advised, and extended course(s) of intravenous antibiotics (over 4 weeks) are rarely if ever indicated.

Osteomyelitis

Osteomyelitis can be divided into categories by pathogenesis. Hematogenous osteomyelitis is blood borne from a distant source; contiguous osteomyelitis develops from an adjacent soft tissue infection; and osteomyelitis may be associated with vascular insufficiency.

Hematogenous Osteomyelitis

Acute hematogenous osteomyelitis occurs primarily in children. Seventy per cent of such cases occur before the age of 10 years. The favorite anatomic site for hematogenous osteomyelitis in children is rapidly growing long bones, most frequently the distal epiphyses of the lower extremities. Bacteria are seeded into the dilated capillary loops of the metaphysis, where sluggish and turbulent blood flow allows bacterial growth. The infective process may cross the epiphyseal plate in infants, resulting in joint space infection. Many studies report notable but physically minor trauma immediately prior to the onset of symptoms.

Infecting microorganisms, as in septic arthritis, depend on the age of the patient (Table 20–6). In infantile osteomyelitis, *H. influenzae*, group B streptococci, and staphylococci are important pathogens. In childhood hematogenous osteomyelitis, *S. aureus* is overwhelmingly predominant. In adults, hematogenous osteomyelitis is associated with severe debility or parenteral narcotic abuse. *Staphylococcus aureus* remains the most common isolate, but gram-negative organisms, particularly *Pseudomonas*, are found with increased frequency, especially in vertebral osteomyelitis associated with drug abuse.

The presenting signs and symptoms of hematogenous osteomyelitis vary from minimal to pronounced depending on the site of the involvement, age of the patient, and severity of illness. In the newborn and infant, physical findings are few. Clinical illness ranges from benign, with minimal symptoms, to a fulminant disease with symptoms resulting from bacteremia rather than from osteomyelitis itself. Physical examination may show edema and tenderness over the entire extremity, making localization difficult. Less severely involved infants will guard the affected limb, especially if septic arthritis is present as well. A high index of suspicion must be maintained in the infant who refuses to use a limb or who has tenderness and swelling of the limb.

Despite difficulties in interpretation because of new bone formation in infants, radiographic studies frequently show soft tissue swelling, foci of necrosis, and rarefaction in the metaphysis adjoining the epiphyseal plates. Radiographic changes occur earlier in infants than in older children and may appear within 7 to 10 days of onset.

Most hematogenous osteomyelitis in older children occurs in boys between the ages of 1 and 14. Forty per cent have a history of preceeding minor trauma. The distal femur, proximal and distal tibia and fibula, foot, and proximal humerus are involved in 80 per cent. History and physical findings in this age group lend themselves to earlier diagnosis, although many cases remain unsuspected and result in avoidable disability. Most patients have fever and chills. Limping, regional bone pain, localized swelling, warmth, erythema, and guarding of the affected limb are found in most patients. Pain may be severe enough to cause pseudoparalysis of the affected member. Specific physical localization can be difficult before the process involves a subperiosteal area, allowing discrete pain.

Hematogenous osteomyelitis in adults frequently involves the spine. The vertebral body is the prime focus, with the lumbar area most frequently involved. Patients usually present with nondescript complaints of fever, chills, and backache. Paravertebral spasm may be present. Paraspinal abscesses frequently occur and may result in serious neurologic deficits that require emergent myelography and decompression. Laboratory findings are limited, but the white blood cell count and sedimentation rate usually are elevated. Radiographic studies, bone scan, and computerized tomography (CT) usually are needed to confirm the diagnosis.

The diagnosis in all ages is facilitated by the use of bone scanning. Technetium-labeled phosphate compounds accumulate in areas of rapid bone turnover and may define an area of involvement within 48 hours of the onset of symptoms. However, a negative bone scan does not rule out osteomyelitis and a positive bone scan is not pathognomonic for infection. Bone lysis on plain films appears at 10 to

TABLE 20–6. ETIOLOGIC AGENTS OF ACUTE HEMATOGENOUS OSTEOMYELITIS BY PATIENT AGE

Organism	Per Cent Etiology by Age (years)					
	<2	2–5	6–10	11–15	Adult	Average
Staphylococcus aureus	33	60	76	73	62	61
Coagulase-negative staphylococci	14	<1	<1	8	2	5
Streptococci	16	11	5	8	5	9
Streptococcus pneumoniae	5	<1	<1	<1	2	1.5
Haemophilus influenzae	11	2	<1	<1	<1	2.5
Pseudomonas aeruginosa	<1	2	2	4	3	2.5
Enterobacteriaceae	3	3	2	<1	9	3.5
Salmonella	<1	3	<1	<1	2	1
Mixed	9	4	<1	<1	2	3
Unknown	18	19	15	7	15	15

21 days, although radiographic changes may never develop if antibiotics are administered early. Ultrasound examination, magnetic resonance imaging (MRI), and CT scanning are useful adjuncts to evaluate for subperiosteal collections or concomitant soft tissue foci. The latter two also may reveal bone destruction earlier than plain films.

The prognosis of hematogenous osteomyelitis is good if the diagnosis is made early. Disability is usually related to delayed diagnosis. This is particularly true in infants, whose epiphyseal growth plate may be disturbed as a result of the infection. In adults, the frequent presence of underlying debilitating disease makes overall outcome worse.

Contiguous and Traumatic Osteomyelitis

Contiguous osteomyelitis usually affects patients over 50 years of age who have an adjacent soft tissue infection or an infected wound extending directly to bone. Surgical procedures most often implicated are open reduction of fractures, insertion of prosthetic devices, and spinal surgery. Soft tissue infections causing contiguous osteomyelitis include lung abscesses spreading to ribs or spine, infected teeth resulting in mandibular infections, sinus or ear infections leading to involvement of the skull and mastoid, and traumatic infections, including puncture wounds.

Staphylococcus is the primary pathogen in most cases, but gram-negative bacteria and anaerobes also are isolated with regularity (Table 20–7). The bacteriology is reflective of the particular contiguous focus; for example, osteomyelitis of the mandible is caused by mouth flora such as streptococci and anaerobes, and gram-negative microorganisms and staphylococci are implicated in infections involving the feet.

Physical examination is the key to diagnosing contiguous osteomyelitis. Pain, swelling, and erythema developing in the postoperative period or after initial control of a soft tissue infection should arouse the suspicion of osteomyelitis. A radiographic study is the cornerstone of diagnosis, with rarefaction, periosteal reaction, and necrosis of bone. Radionuclide scans are difficult to interpret

because postoperative changes, healing fractures, or contiguous soft tissue inflammation may give misleading results. If the diagnosis is delayed, continued pain and swelling with development of sinus tracts and persistent drainage are the usual complaints. Fever is not commonly present. At this stage, the diagnosis is obvious.

Traumatic osteomyelitis most commonly follows compound fractures, surgical procedures, and puncture wounds in which the underlying bone is traumatized. Men ages 15 to 30 constitute the majority of patients. Bacteria involved are primarily skin flora, such as staphylococci and occasionally gram-negative environmental organisms. Osteomyelitis of the foot following puncture wounds, particularly in children, requires special consideration because *P. aeruginosa* is a common isolate as a result of its propensity for growing in the soles of sneakers.

Osteomyelitis Resulting from Vascular Insufficiency

Patients with osteomyelitis associated with vascular insufficiency present special problems. Most are elderly, with severe underlying atherosclerotic vascular disease, smoking history, and/or diabetes mellitus. There is frequently a history of neuropathy, minor trauma, abrasions, and blisters with recurrent foot ulceration and chronic drainage. Patients have few systemic symptoms; fever and septicemia are uncommon. Multiple phalanges and metatarsals ultimately are affected. Radiographic studies reveal demineralized bone, new bone formation, sequestra, and soft tissue swelling. An unsuspected foreign body, such as a pin or needle, may be evident.

The bacteriology of such cases is frequently polymicrobial, with staphylococci, streptococci, gram-negative bacilli, and anaerobes involved. Sinus tract and wound cultures in patients with underlying osteomyelitis are not helpful, because they often are colonized by irrelevant microorganisms. Cultures must be obtained by biopsy or percutaneous needle aspirate directly from the involved bone.

Treatment

Surgical therapy is usually required to establish a microbiologic diagnosis, to drain collections of pus, and to remove dead bone and other foreign material. Failure of response to appropriate antibiotic therapy, continued pain, swelling, fever, and a persistently elevated sedimentation rate may be clues to the need for further surgery. In vertebral osteomyelitis, neurologic compromise requires immediate surgical intervention to relieve cord compression. Surgery should be used to drain an infected hip joint when it complicates osteomyelitis, but closed-needle aspiration is usually adequate to drain septic arthritis in other joints when it accompanies osteomyelitis.

TABLE 20–7. MICROORGANISMS RECOVERED FROM OSTEOMYELITIS CAUSED BY A CONTIGUOUS FOCUS OF INFECTION

Microorganism	Average Per Cent Recovered
Staphylococcus aureus	49
Coagulase-negative staphylococci	2
Streptococci	9
Anaerobes	15
Pseudomonas	7
Other aerobic gram-negative bacilli	16
Other	8
Mixed	8
Unknown	12

Prolonged antibiotic therapy is a cornerstone of therapy. In acute hematogenous osteomyelitis, antibiotics are frequently effective alone if given before extensive bone damage has occurred. In contrast, in chronic osteomyelitis or osteomyelitis associated with a foreign body, antibiotics alone are of little value unless all dead bone and foreign bodies are removed. Antibiotic therapy is selected based on the pathogens isolated from bone culture and generally is administered parenterally in high doses for 4 to 6 weeks. Oral antibiotic therapy for acute hematogenous osteomyelitis in children and with fluoroquinolones for gram-negative osteomyelitis in adults has been of value, although such patients require careful follow-up, good compliance, and the documentation of adequate serum bactericidal activity. Empiric therapy frequently is needed, however, because cultures are commonly not available or are negative as a result of prior administration of outpatient antibiotics.

CARDIOVASCULAR INFECTIONS

Infective Endocarditis

Endocarditis is an infection of the heart valves or endocardium. It may present as an acute, fulminant illness with rapid valve destruction and severe systemic toxicity. More frequently, however, it presents as an indolent illness with weeks or months of predominantly constitutional symptoms, and, in this form, is known as subacute endocarditis. Although an appreciation of the tempo of illness is helpful in understanding its pathogenesis and the organisms involved, there is great variation from case to case.

Infective endocarditis is not uncommon, accounting for 1 to 2 in 1000 hospital admissions. In recent years, rheumatic heart disease has become a less important predisposition to endocarditis than intravenous drug use, prosthetic heart valves, or atherosclerotic valvular disease. With increasing longevity and cardiovascular surgery, the relative shift in predisposing conditions probably will continue. There also has been an increase in aortic valve involvement, although mitral valve infections remain the most common.

Pathogenesis

The pathogenesis of endocarditis as it occurs on a previously damaged valve is well understood. The pre-existing valve lesion creates turbulent flow, which produces endothelial damage and the formation of sterile platelet–fibrin thrombi. Bacteremia with an organism that has the ability to adhere to endothelium or platelet–fibrin thrombi may result in infection. Because phagocytosis does not occur on valve leaflets, bacteria multiply within the thrombus to form a vegetation.

Understanding the pathogenesis of endocarditis explains a number of clinical observations. Patients with chronic congestive heart failure, atrial septal defects, chronic atrial fibrillation, or purely stenotic valvular lesions generally have low pressure gradients and, therefore, less turbulent flow. These lesions are all low risk for infective endocarditis. In contrast, insufficient valvular lesions associated with a high pressure gradient and markedly turbulent flow are at greater risk. Patients with mitral valve prolapse are at higher risk if a regurgitant murmur is audible than if only a click is present. The predominant right heart involvement in intravenous drug abusers suggests that tricuspid valve damage may occur as a result of injected particulate material.

As the infection progresses, it may extend into supporting valve structures, leading to further damage and compromised valve function. Vegetations may embolize, resulting in vascular occlusion. Suppurative metastatic lesions may follow these embolic phenomena, particularly if gram-negative bacilli or staphylococci are the etiologic agents. Infections with more indolent organisms, such as viridans streptococci (*Streptococcus mutans, Streptococcus sanguis*, etc.), are associated not with suppuration but with immunologic events (see later in this chapter).

The sources of the infecting bacteria in endocarditis are usually mucosal surfaces with transient bacteremia precipitated by local trauma. Bacterial seeding from the gums, sinuses, genitourinary tract, or gastrointestinal tract may precipitate endocarditis. Intravenous drug use or indwelling intravenous catheters also may produce bacteremia and endocarditis.

Clinical Presentation

The clinical presentations of endocarditis vary widely. Indolent onset, with low-grade fever, constitutional and musculoskeletal symptoms, weight loss, malaise, easy fatigability, and anorexia, is common in patients with subacute infection. In contrast, patients with acute endocarditis present with systemic toxicity, shaking chills, and high fever of short duration. Many patients will have suppurative or embolic extracardiac manifestations, such as a focal central nervous system deficit, pleuritis, meningitis, flank pain and pyuria, or cough and hemoptysis.

Up to 10 per cent of patients have no audible murmur. This is particularly true for individuals with endocarditis involving only the tricuspid valve. Petechiae may be visible in the nail beds, conjunctivae, and mucous membranes. They are due to small vessel infarction or emboli and, when seen in the retina, are particularly striking. Retinal infarcts, referred to as Roth spots, appear as oval hemorrhages with pale centers. They are not pathognomonic for endocarditis but can be seen in other vascular diseases, such as systemic lupus erythematosus. Janeway lesions are large, nontender macules occurring on the palms or soles and probably represent embolic phenomena. Osler's nodes are tender subcutaneous erythematous nodules in the pulp of the fingers or toes. They may represent either antigen–antibody complex vasculitis with infarct or embolic phenomena. Similarly to Roth spots, they are not pathognomonic for endocarditis. Clubbing and splenomegaly rarely are seen nowadays.

Laboratory Findings

Anemia is the most common hematologic abnormality in endocarditis. It is normochromic and normocytic and is usually due to marrow suppression associated with infection. Hemolysis is unusual in endocarditis involving natural heart valves but frequently is seen in prosthetic valvular endocarditis. The white blood cell count is elevated in acute infections but may be normal in subacute infections. The erythrocyte sedimentation rate is elevated in almost all patients. The rheumatoid factor may be positive, particularly in patients with longstanding disease. This is a nonspecific finding and is due to elevated IgM anti-IgG. Serum complement levels usually are elevated as acute-phase reactants but may be depressed if antigen–antibody complex disease is present. Cryoglobulins are positive in many patients and represent circulating immune complexes. Other nonspecific immunologic events may be seen, including a false-positive Veneral Disease Research Laboratories (VDRL) test and antinuclear antibody test. The urinalysis frequently shows proteinuria and microscopic hematuria. Microscopic hematuria may be due to immune-complex glomerulonephritis and may be associated with red blood cell casts.

Blood cultures are positive in greater than 90 per cent of patients with endocarditis. Numerous studies have shown that three blood cultures will yield the causative organism in over 95 per cent of culture-positive cases. The bacteremia of endocarditis is continual; therefore, random cultures are most appropriate, the diagnosis being dependent on the volume of blood drawn rather than the number of cultures performed. In suspected endocarditis, therefore, three samples should be obtained prior to initiation of therapy. Each sample should be taken by separate venipuncture.

Despite improved techniques and special media, 10 per cent of cases of bacterial endocarditis will be culture negative. High levels of antibacterial antibody, poor viability of the microorganism, cell wall–deficient or particularly fastidious microorganisms, and prior antibiotic therapy all cause culture-negative endocarditis. If clinical evidence is particularly strong, empiric therapy may be indicated.

Endocarditis represents a sustained bacteremia and should be so documented. A single blood culture positive for viridans streptococci or coagulase-negative staphylococci could represent transient bacteremia from the mouth, intestine, or skin rather than endocarditis.

Microbiology

Streptococci and staphylococci account for 80 per cent of all endocarditis on natural heart valves (Table 20–8). Although the viridans group streptococci of presumably oral origin still account for the majority of cases, recent dental work can be implicated in only 30 per cent of cases. Group D streptococci have become increasingly important in recent years as a result of the increased frequency of elderly patients with underlying genitourinary or gastrointestinal disease. *S. bovis*, a nonenterococcal group D streptococcus, is associated with occult colonic neoplasia in over 50 per cent of cases. Staphylococci also are found with increased frequency as a result of the prevalence of intravenous drug use and prosthetic heart valves. Gram-negative endocarditis remains uncommon but is a particular problem for patients with prosthetic heart valves and intravenous drug users. The reason for the preponderance of streptococci in infective endocarditis is their ability to adhere to valve tissue. Gram-negative bacilli adhere poorly, which explains the paucity of cases of gram-negative endocarditis despite the fact that these organisms commonly cause bacteremia.

Fungal endocarditis occurs only in specific settings. Open heart surgery patients, patients receiving prolonged intravenous therapy (particularly total parenteral nutrition), and intravenous drug abusers are prone to fungal endocarditis. *Candida* species are isolated most commonly, although *Aspergillus* may cause infection as well. Fungal endocarditis in drug addicts usually is related to prolonged intravenous therapy for a preceding bacterial infection. The diagnosis of fungal endocarditis is difficult because blood cultures may be negative. However, bulky vegetations frequently produce major organ emboli, the pathology of which may make a diagnosis.

Prosthetic valve endocarditis may be divided temporally into two groups: early infection, occurring less than 60 days postoperatively, and late infection, occurring more than 60 days postoperatively (Table 20–8). Early prosthetic valve infections are due to organisms acquired perioperatively, including fungi, staphylococcal species, diphtheroids, and gram-negative bacilli. These microorganisms may be acquired intraoperatively or in the perioperative period as a result of intubation and prolonged use of indwelling intravenous and bladder catheters. Late infections resemble natural valve infections in their microbiology (Table 20–8).

Differential Diagnosis

A variety of conditions mimic infective endocarditis. The prolonged fever and constitutional symptoms typical of subacute endocarditis may be

TABLE 20–8. MICROBIOLOGY OF HEART VALVE INFECTIONS

	Per Cent of Isolates			
Microorganism	Natural Valve	Intravenous Drug User	Early Prosthetic Valve	Late Prosthetic Valve
Viridans streptococci	35	5	5	30
Enterococci	10	6	3	10
Streptococcus bovis	15	2	2	10
Staphylococcus aureus	15	60	10	10
Coagulase-negative staphylococcus	5	2	35	20
Gram-negative bacilli	5	10	15	5
Fungi	3	10	15	5
Others*	12	5	15	10

* Includes diphtheroids, other streptococci, *Haemophilus*, and related organisms.

due to such conditions as neoplasia, tuberculosis, viral infection, or collagen vascular disease. Prolonged fever in the patient with rheumatic heart disease may be rheumatic fever itself. Fever after open heart surgery may have many causes other than an infected prosthesis, including pneumonia, postpericardiotomy syndrome, urinary tract infection, or thrombophlebitis. Acute endocarditis, which frequently presents with extracardiac manifestations, may be mistaken for a primary pulmonary infection, meningitis, cerebrovascular accident, or pyelonephritis. Attention to the cardiovascular examination and clinical setting together with appropriate cultures of blood and other body fluids should help in the diagnosis, as long as the possibility of endocarditis is at least considered.

Treatment

The treatment of infective endocarditis is with microbicidal antibiotics. Because neutrophils are not involved in the resolution of endocarditis, antibiotics alone are the mainstay of therapy. Treatment must be prolonged to kill those microorganisms resting deep within the vegetation. Acute endocarditis should be treated as soon as blood cultures are obtained, without waiting for culture results, in order to minimize valve destruction and spread of infection to the supporting valve structures. In subacute illness, treatment usually can be delayed for 1 to 2 days until blood cultures are known to be positive. Effective programs for the treatment of endocarditis are outlined in Table 20–9.

Most viridans streptococci and *S. bovis* remain exquisitely sensitive to penicillin G. However, up to 20 per cent of such strains may be tolerant or only intermediately sensitive to penicillin, requiring individualization of therapy based on MIC and MBC values of the bacterial isolate. Short-course (2 weeks of penicillin plus aminoglycoside) therapy is established only for uncomplicated endocarditis caused by penicillin-susceptible strains in young patients. Enterococci are not killed by penicillin or ampicillin alone and require, in addition, a synergistic aminoglycoside antibiotic, such as gentamicin. Duration of symptoms, valvular calcification, the recent emergence of multi–drug-resistant strains, and other factors impact on the selection and duration of therapy, and infectious disease consultation should be sought.

The role of testing for serum bactericidal activity is controversial. Tests are difficult to perform and poorly predictive. They are probably of value only in selected cases caused by unusual microorganisms.

Staphylococci should be considered penicillin resistant until susceptibility tests prove otherwise. Left-sided staphylococcal endocarditis must be treated for 6 weeks for optimal results. The addition of an aminoglycoside antibiotic for synergy has not been shown to enhance cure rates in the treatment of staphylococcal endocarditis. Gram-negative and fungal endocarditis present extremely difficult problems. Surgery is almost always necessary for cure and should be performed early to avoid irreversible damage to the valve and supporting structures.

The management of prosthetic valve infections is difficult. Early prosthetic valve infection occurring within 60 days of surgery almost always requires valve replacement in addition to antibiotic therapy. However, late prosthetic valve infections, particularly when these infections are due to penicillin-sensitive streptococci, frequently respond to medical therapy alone. The need for surgery is dictated by the response to medical therapy.

Ancillary therapy should include cardiovascular support as necessary. Corticosteroid therapy is of no value. Anticoagulants should be used as needed for thromboembolic events and are not specifically contraindicated.

Surgical removal of infected valves plays an increasingly important role in the treatment of endocarditis. Indications for surgery include persistent infection despite appropriate antibiotic therapy (e.g., for fungal or gram-negative endocarditis), intractable or progressive congestive heart failure unresponsive to standard carditonic regimens, and major organ emboli. Patients with bulky vegeta-

TABLE 20–9. TREATMENT OF ENDOCARDITIS

Microorganism	Preferred Regimen	Penicillin-Allergic Regimen
Streptococcus viridans group	Penicillin G 12–18 million units/day for 3–4 weeks *or* Penicillin G 12–18 million units/day plus gentamicin 4–5 mg/kg/day for 2 weeks	Cefazolin 6 gm/day or vancomycin 2 gm/day
Streptococcus bovis	Same as *S. viridans*	Same as *S. viridans*
Enterococcus	Penicillin G 18–24 million units/day plus gentamicin 4–5 mg/kg/day for 4–6 weeks	Vancomycin 2 gm/day plus gentamicin 4–5 mg/kg/day for 4–6 weeks
Staphylococcus		
Non–penicillinase producing	Penicillin G 18–24 million units/day for 4–6 weeks	Cefazolin 6 gm/day or vancomycin 2 gm/day for 4–6 weeks
Penicillinase producing	Oxacillin 12 gm/day or nafcillin 12 gm/day for 4–6 weeks	Cefazolin 6 gm/day or vancomycin 2 gm/day for 4–6 weeks
Pneumococcus or β-hemolytic streptococcus	Penicillin G 18–24 million units/day for 4–6 weeks	Cefazolin 6 gm/day or vancomycin 2 gm/day for 4–6 weeks
Haemophilus species, *Actinobacillus*, or *Cardiobacterium*	A third-generation cephalosporin for 4–6 weeks	Ampicillin 12 gm/day plus gentamicin 5 mg/kg/day for 4–6 weeks
Gram-negative bacillus	A β-lactam antibiotic plus an aminoglycoside antibiotic according to susceptibility tests for 4–6 weeks; surgery probably also required	
Fungus	Amphotericin B plus early surgery; 5-flucytosine, fluconazole, or ketoconazole may be useful adjuncts	

tions seen on echocardiogram, particularly if they involve the aortic valve, may be candidates for early surgery in the absence of these indications. Early valve replacement is not associated with an increased risk of infection as long as effective antimicrobial agents are being administered at the time of surgery.

Even after effective therapy is instituted, the patient may remain febrile for some time. Prolonged or recurrent fever should prompt re-evaluation for a febrile drug reaction, thrombophlebitis, embolization, myocardial abscess, or superinfection. Embolic phenomena may occur late, despite adequate therapy, and are not an indication of failure to achieve adequate killing with the antimicrobial regimen.

Prevention

Bacteremia is the prerequisite for endocarditis. When bacteremia is anticipated, prophylactic antibiotics should be administered to prevent endocarditis in patients with pre-existing valvular lesions. Prophylaxis must be administered so that *peak blood levels* are achieved at the time of anticipated bacteremia. This concept differs from that of surgical wound prophylaxis, in which *peak tissue levels* are required at the time of surgery. Antibiotics are selected to kill the microorganisms most likely to produce bacteremia from a given source. In the mouth, this is α-hemolytic streptococcoci, and, in the gastrointestinal and genitourinary tract, it is enterococci. Prophylactic antibiotics should be administered immediately prior to the procedure and may be repeated once 6 to 8 hours later (Table 20–10). Cephalosporins should not be used. Administration of antibiotics for several days prior to the procedure promotes the emergence of resistant microorganisms and decreases the effectiveness of prophylaxis.

Pericarditis and Myocarditis

Pericarditis is an inflammation of the visceral and parietal pericardium. A variety of agents are associated with infectious pericarditis; most are viral or bacterial (Table 20–11). Fever, chest pain, and fatigue may be the presenting problem. The chest pain is usually retrosternal, with radiation to the neck and arms. It may be increased by inspiration or motion and is frequently lessened by sitting or leaning forward. In chronic pericarditis and rare cases of acute pericarditis, however, pain may not be present, and the manifestations may be only those of increasing congestive heart failure resulting from constriction or tamponade.

The diagnosis of pericarditis is based on clinical suspicion, electrocardiographic abnormalities suggesting pericarditis, echocardiography, and a chest radiograph showing cardiac enlargement. It should be noted that, in constrictive pericarditis, cardiac enlargement may not be marked.

Coxsackie B virus infections are the best documented causes of viral pericarditis. Coxsackieviruses are ubiquitous, and infections caused by these agents are prevalent in the summer and early fall. Children and young adults are affected most commonly and frequently have a history of cough and

TABLE 20–10. PROPHYLAXIS OF ENDOCARDITIS IN PATIENTS WITH VALVULAR HEART DISEASE*

For Dental and Upper Respiratory Tract Procedures

Parenteral (High-Risk Patients)	
Ampicillin	2 grams I.V. or I.M. 30 minutes before procedure; then ampicillin 1 gram I.V. or I.M., or amoxicillin 1.5 grams P.O., 6 hours later
or	
Vancomycin	1 gram over 1 hour immediately before procedure; no follow-up dose necessary
with or without	
Gentamicin	1.5 mg/kg I.M. or I.V. 30 minutes before procedure; may repeat 8 hours later
Oral (Low-Risk Patients)	
Amoxicillin	3 grams P.O. 1 hour before procedure; then 1.5 grams P.O. 6 hours later
or	
Erythromycin	1 gram P.O. 1–2 hours before procedure; then 500 mg 6 hours later
or	
Clindamycin	300 mg P.O. 1 hour before procedure; then 150 mg 6 hours later

For Gastrointestinal and Genitourinary Procedures

Parenteral (High-Risk Patients)	
Ampicillin	2 grams I.M. or I.V. 30 minutes before procedure; then ampicillin 1 gram I.M. or I.V., or amoxicillin 1.5 grams P.O., 6 hours later
plus	
Gentamicin	1.5 mg/kg I.M. or I.V. 30 minutes before procedure; may repeat 8 hours later
or	
Vancomycin	1 gram I.V. over 1 hour immediately before procedure; no follow-up dose necessary
plus	
Gentamicin	1.5 mg/kg I.M. or I.V. 30 minutes before procedure; may repeat 8 hours later
Alternate Oral Regimen (Low-Risk Patients)	
Amoxicillin	3 grams P.O. 1 hour before procedure; then 1.5 grams P.O. 6 hours later

* Parenteral regimens are recommended for high-risk patients, including those with prosthetic heart valves, with prior episodes of endocarditis, or with surgically constructed systemic–pulmonary shunts.

coryza 10 to 14 days prior to the onset of pericarditis. Diagnosis is made by virus isolation, but, because of the late onset of pericarditis, the virus may not be recovered. Serodiagnosis is usually difficult because of multiple antigenically different serotypes of coxsackievirus.

Purulent pericarditis is a medical and surgical emergency. It may be due to bacteremic seeding of the pericardium or contiguous spread from a pulmonary or mediastinal focus. *Staphylococcus aureus, H. influenzae,* and pneumococci account for the majority of cases.

The differential diagnosis of infectious pericarditis should include noninfectious etiologies such as systemic lupus erythematosus, congestive heart failure, uremia, radiation pericarditis, trauma, myocardial infarction, pulmonary emboli, nephrosis, neoplasia, or acute rheumatic fever. Myxedema, rheumatoid arthritis, serum sickness, and other connective tissue diseases also should be considered.

Agents responsible for *myocarditis* are usually those responsible for pericarditis (Table 20–12). Both myocarditis and pericarditis may occur in the

TABLE 20–11. CAUSES OF INFECTIOUS PERICARDITIS

Viral	Bacterial
Adenovirus	*Borrelia burgdorferi*
Coxsackie A, B	*Francisella*
Cytomegalovirus	Gonococcus
Echo virus	*Haemophilus*
Epstein-Barr virus	*Legionella*
Influenza	Meningococcus
Mumps	*Mycobacterium tuberculosis*
Varicella	Pneumococcus
	Staphylococcus
Fungal	Streptococcus
Aspergillus	
Blastomyces	**Protozoal**
Coccidioides	*Entamoeba*
Cryptococcus	*Toxoplasma*
Histoplasma	*Trypanosoma*

TABLE 20–12. INFECTIOUS CAUSES OF MYOCARDITIS

Viral	Bacterial
Adenovirus	*Borrelia burgdorferi*
Arbovirus	*Chlamydia psittaci*
Coxsackie A, B	*Corynebacterium diphtheriae*
Cytomegalovirus	*Leptospira*
Echo virus	Meningococcus
Epstein-Barr virus	*Mycobacterium tuberculosis*
Hepatitis B	*Treponema pallidum*
Herpes simplex	
Human immunodeficiency virus	**Parasitic**
	Toxoplasma
Influenza	Trichinosis
Lymphocytic choriomeningitis	*Trypanosoma*
Measles	
Mumps	**Fungal**
Poliovirus	*Aspergillus*
Rabies	*Coccidioides*
Rubella	*Histoplasma*
Varicella	

same patient, and the differential diagnosis is similar. Most cardiomyopathies in adults are idiopathic, but some may originate from a primary infectious process.

Management of pericarditis or myocarditis should be directed at treatment for the causative agent (if applicable) and maintenance of a stable cardiovascular system by bed rest and administration of anti-inflammatory and cardiotonic drugs. The role of steroids remains controversial, particularly in individuals for whom infection can be documented. Pericardiotomy may be indicated if effusions prove persistent. No specific drug therapy is available for most viral causes of pericarditis or myocarditis.

CENTRAL NERVOUS SYSTEM INFECTIONS

Bacterial Meningitis

Pathophysiology

Despite advances in the prevention and treatment of many infectious diseases, meningitis remains a profoundly serious infection. Death and serious disability from bacterial meningitis are decreased only by early recognition and the immediate institution of appropriate therapy.

Microorganisms reach the central nervous system by one of two routes: direct extension from an extracerebral source or hematogenous spread from a remote focus of infection. Remote foci are often the lung, bowel, skin, and heart. Local foci of infection include the paranasal sinuses, ears, and other facial areas. Most meningitis is hematogenous in origin. Organisms reaching the spinal fluid spread rapidly throughout the subarachnoid space. The brain itself is remarkably resistant to bacterial infection, although cortical vasculitis with small-vessel thromboses may produce focal signs.

The cellular response to infection in the subarachnoid space is polymorphonuclear if bacterial, and mononuclear if fungal, tuberculous, or viral. The cellular response and attendant cytokine release may damage surrounding tissues and produce disturbances in CSF production and flow, resulting in hydrocephalus. In small children, inflammation in the subdural space may produce subdural effusions. Cerebral edema secondary to cortical vasculitis may produce herniation and brain stem compression.

Normal spinal fluid glucose concentration is greater than 40 per cent of simultaneous blood glucose concentration, although at values over 250 mg/dL this relationship may no longer hold. The decrease in CSF glucose concentration seen in meningitis is a result of both a decrease in active transport of glucose into the CSF and the interaction of bacteria and leukocytes, resulting in glucose consumption because of phagocytosis. In viral meningitis, the mononuclear cell response does not usually result in a fall in CSF glucose concentrations. CSF protein levels in meningitis are increased primarily as a result of the entry of plasma proteins from alteration in the permeability of the blood–brain–CSF barrier. Cellular response is dictated by the infecting organism (Table 20–13).

Neonatal Meningitis

Neonatal meningitis occurs in 1 to 2 in 1000 births. Risk factors include maternal infection, prematurity, small size, complicated delivery, and prolonged (over 24 hours) rupture of membranes. The organisms responsible for neonatal meningitis are usually those acquired from the maternal vaginal flora. Occasionally, they may be acquired from the nursery environment during prolonged hospital stay.

Group B streptococci account for 30 to 40 per cent of cases of neonatal meningitis. Fifty per cent of babies born to mothers colonized with group B streptococci will be themselves colonized, and 1 in 100 colonized babies will become ill. *Escherichia coli* are the next most common cause, and 80 per cent of the responsible *E. coli* strains have K1 capsular polysaccharide, compared to less than 15 per cent of *E. coli* strains isolated from septicemic adults. Organisms such as *Klebsiella*, *Proteus*, *Enterobacter*, and *Citrobacter* may be acquired at birth, as are most *E. coli*, but they are more likely due to colonization within the nursery or neonatal intensive care unit. Such organisms may be multi–drug-resistant and present major treatment problems.

The clinical presentation of neonatal meningitis is subtle. Irritability, lethargy, changes in feeding habits, respiratory distress, or periodic apnea may be the only manifestations. Neck stiffness rarely is seen. Bulging fontanelles and seizures are late phenomena and, if present, are associated with high mortality.

The laboratory features of neonatal sepsis and meningitis are few. The peripheral white blood cell count is rarely helpful. Lumbar puncture is usually diagnostic; however, results must be interpreted in light of the fact that normal neonatal CSF contains up to 30 white blood cells and has a protein content of up to 120 mg/dL. Gram's stain and cultures should be performed promptly, and ancillary tests, such as bacterial antigen detection in CSF, may be useful. Blood cultures are frequently positive.

The empiric treatment of neonatal meningitis consists of a combination of ampicillin plus a third-generation cephalosporin, such as cefotaxime, to cover the likely gram-positive and gram-negative microorganisms. Treatment should be continued for a minimum of 3 weeks. Despite effective therapy, however, the mortality in both group B streptococcal and *E. coli* meningitis occurring in the first week of life is close to 50 per cent. Fifty per

TABLE 20–13.   CEREBROSPINAL FLUID PROFILES IN MENINGITIS

	Bacterial	Viral	Fungal/Tuberculosis
Pressure	Increased	Normal or slightly increased	Increased
Protein	>300 mg/dL	50–150 mg/dL	>300 mg/dL
Glucose	<40 mg/dL	Normal	<40 mg/dL
Cells	>500/mm^3	<500/mm^3	20–400/mm^3
	>90% neutrophils	>50% mononuclear	>50% mononuclear

cent of the survivors will have major neurologic residuals, such as mental retardation, seizure disorders, and learning disability.

Childhood Meningitis

Bacterial meningitis in children ages 2 months to 10 years is due to *H. influenzae, Neisseria meningitidis,* or *S. pneumoniae.* All these organisms possess a polysaccharide capsule that contributes to their pathogenicity. Asymptomatic nasopharyngeal carrier rates range from 5 to 50 per cent depending on the time of year and age of the patient. Protective maternal antibody falls between 3 and 6 months of age and corresponds to the increasing incidence of meningitis. Bacterial meningitis peaks in incidence from December to April and parallels the prevalence of pharyngeal colonization with each organism. The factors that cause a colonized individual to develop meningitis are unknown, although antecedent viral infection is probably important.

Prior to the widespread use of *H. influenzae* type b vaccine, *H. influenzae* was the main cause of meningitis in children ages 3 months to 3 years of age in the United States. Because of successful vaccination, however, the incidence of meningitis resulting from this pathogen has fallen by 80 per cent in the past 5 years. *Neisseria meningitidis* peaks in incidence at age 1 to 4 years and again at 15 to 30 years. Capsular types B, C, and Y have been the most common cause of meningitis in recent years. As with immunity to *Haemophilus,* immunity to *Neisseria* species is stimulated by exposure to other, cross-reacting, microorganisms. Although development of antibody protects against bacteremia and meningitis, it does not prevent nasopharyngeal colonization with either *Haemophilus* species or *N. meningitidis.* Such colonized, but immune, individuals remain a reservoir for these organisms within the family and population at large.

Pneumococcal meningitis may develop as a primary bacteremic illness or as a complication of pneumonia, otitis, mastoiditis, or sinusitis. Hypogammaglobulinemia, the absence of the spleen, or concomitant sickle cell disease also predisposes to pneumococcal bacteremia and meningitis. The large number of pneumococcal serotypes (84) means that infection with one type does not confer protection against future infections with another type. The incidence of pneumococcal meningitis

peaks later in life than that for *Haemophilus* or *Neisseria* infection and is the most common cause of meningitis over age 10.

The clinical manifestations of meningitis in the older infant and child are more dramatic than those of the neonate. Fever, headache, confusion, lethargy, vomiting, or convulsions may be the presenting signs. Physical examination may reveal altered consciousness and a stiff neck. The presence of a petechial or purpuric rash should suggest *Neisseria,* although *Haemophilus,* pneumococcus, and *S. aureus* occasionally can produce this rash. Coexistent pneumonitis, sinusitis, or otitis should suggest pneumococcal or *Haemophilus* meningitis.

Adult Meningitis

Bacterial meningitis in adults is overwhelmingly likely to be due to *S. pneumoniae.* In certain settings, however, staphylococci (after trauma or associated with intravenous drug use) or gram-negative bacilli (after neurosurgery or in immunosuppressed individuals) may produce meningitis. *Cryptococcus* and *Listeria* must be considered in the differential diagnosis in patients with depressed cell-mediated immunity, as seen with lymphoma or human immunodeficiency virus (HIV) infection. The presentation of meningitis in older, particularly immunosuppressed, adults may be atypical. Mental confusion, absence of fever, or lack of a stiff neck may make the diagnosis difficult.

Diagnosis and Treatment

The laboratory diagnosis of meningitis is made by examining the CSF (Table 20–13). Normal CSF should contain less than four cells, all lymphocytes. Gram's stain should be performed on the centrifuged sediment and must be interpreted with caution. Detection of bacterial antigen by latex agglutination may provide some help in assisting with rapid diagnosis.

Purulent CSF, associated with hypoglycorrhachia, is characteristic of untreated bacterial meningitis but also may be seen with parameningeal infections or meningeal carcinomatosis. Conversely, partially treated bacterial meningitis may have a lymphocytic predominance (Table 20–14).

The prognosis in meningitis is dependent on the speed with which appropriate therapy is initiated. If the clinical setting and examination of the spinal fluid give a clue to the specific organism, treatment based on past experience and known susceptibility

TABLE 20–14. CEREBROSPINAL FLUID PROFILES

Purulent Profile (Polymorphonuclear Leukocytes)

Bacterial meningitis
Early viral meningitis
Embolic cerebral infarction in endocarditis
Parameningeal infections (brain abscess, subdural empyema, venous sinus thrombophlebitis)
Chemical meningitis

Lymphocytic Low-Glucose Profile

Tuberculous meningitis
Fungal meningitis
Partially treated bacterial meningitis
Certain bacterial meningitides (spirochetal, *Listeria*, Lyme disease)
Certain viral meningitides (mumps, lymphocytic choriomeningitis, herpes simplex, varicella-zoster)
Sarcoidosis
Carcinomatous meningitis

Lymphocytic Normal-Glucose Profile

Viral meningitis or encephalitis
Postinfectious or postvaccinal encephalomyelitis
Parameningeal infection (brain abscess, subdural empyema, epidural abscess, venous sinus thrombophlebitis)
Early fungal meningitis
Early tuberculous meningitis
Parasitic infection (e.g., toxoplasmosis)

---

patterns can be initiated promptly. If the diagnosis is unknown, empiric therapy must be begun.

In neonates, treatment must cover *E. coli* and group B streptococci. Experience suggests that a third-generation cephalosporin with concomitant ampicillin is most appropriate. In young children, the organisms of concern are *Haemophilus*, meningococcus, and pneumococcus, and, because many (15 to 30 per cent) strains of *Haemophilus* are ampicillin resistant, initial therapy should be with cefotaxime or ceftriaxone. Rifampin should be administered at the end of treatment for *H. influenzae* meningitis (see Prophylaxis). In older adolescents and adults, pneumococcus or meningococcus are the most likely microorganisms, and empiric treatment with penicillin G is usually adequate. The presence of immunosuppression, intravenous drug abuse, or recent neurosurgery should raise consideration of more unusual microorganisms, and therapy should be selected on the basis of likely pathogens. Most meningitis should be treated parenterally for a minimum of 10 days; gram-negative meningitis requires a minimum of 3 weeks. Intrathecal or intraventricular antibiotics are not indicated except for fungal or multi–drug-resistant gram-negative bacillary meningitis.

Animal model data and now recent pediatric studies have shown that corticosteroid administration will modulate the inflammatory response and decrease morbidity in childhood meningitis. Dexamethasone, 0.6 mg/kg/day in two or four divided doses for 4 days, starting 15 to 20 minutes *before* antibiotics, has been shown to decrease sensorineural hearing loss and also may lessen mortality. The role of steroid therapy in adult meningitis is unclear, but it should not be used in aseptic meningitis.

Prophylaxis

The occurrence of meningococcal disease requires contact prophylaxis. Furthermore, both group A and group C meningococcal vaccines are available and very effective in epidemic settings. Family members and nursery school and intimate contacts of cases of meningococcal disease should be treated prophylactically with rifampin 10 mg/kg (maximum 600 mg) every 12 hours for four doses. Casual contact and contacts in the hospital setting (unless mouth-to-mouth resuscitation or laboratory accidents have occurred) do not require prophylaxis. Family contacts, and perhaps close and nursery school contacts of patients with invasive *Haemophilus* infections (such as meningitis), also warrant rifampin prophylaxis, 20 mg/kg/day (maximum 600 mg) for 4 days. A single dose of ciprofloxacin, 500 mg, can be used in rifampin-allergic adult patients.

Aseptic Meningitis

Viral infections of the central nervous system occur at all ages and most commonly are seen in the summer and early fall. Aseptic meningitis is usually an illness of abrupt onset and short duration. Fever, headache, nausea and vomiting, and neck stiffness are the cardinal manifestations. Children show irritability with drowsiness or lethargy. Multiple attacks of aseptic meningitis, although uncommon, do occur. A variety of agents are implicated (Table 20–15). It is important to remember

TABLE 20–15. CAUSATIVE AGENTS OF ASEPTIC MENINGITIS AND ENCEPHALITIS

Adenovirus
Arthropod-borne (arbovirus) viruses
  California encephalitis
  Eastern equine encephalitis
  Western equine encephalitis
  St. Louis encephalitis
Borrelia (Lyme disease)
Brucella
Colorado tick fever
Cytomegalovirus
Epstein-Barr virus
Enterovirus
  Echovirus
  Coxsackieviruses A and B
  Poliovirus
Herpes simplex virus
Human immunodeficiency virus
Leptospira
Lymphocytic choriomeningitis
Mumps
Mycoplasma pneumoniae
Rickettsia rickettsii (Rocky Mountain spotted fever)
Treponema pallidum (syphilis)
Varicella-zoster virus

that Lyme disease and syphilis are causes of "aseptic" meningitis.

Laboratory abnormalities include a relatively normal peripheral white blood cell count and a CSF pleocytosis that is predominantly mononuclear (Table 20–13). However, polymorphonuclear leukocytes may predominate in the first several hours of a viral infection, and repeat lumbar puncture in 12 hours may be necessary to clarify the etiology. In some cases of mumps, lymphocytic choriomeningitis, and herpes infection, hypoglycorrhachia may occur (Table 20–14).

The differential diagnosis of "aseptic meningitis" includes tuberculous meningitis, fungal meningitis, brain abscess or other parameningeal infection, endocarditis, and hypersensitivity meningoencephalitis (Table 20–14). Occasionally, neoplastic involvement of the meninges can mimic aseptic meningitis.

Agents causing aseptic meningitis also may produce encephalitis (Table 20–15). The distinction between aseptic meningitis, meningoencephalitis, and encephalitis is primarily clinical. Coxsackieviruses and echoviruses usually produce aseptic meningitis rather than encephalitis. Arboviruses produce primarily encephalitis. Herpes simplex virus type 1 produces characteristic frontotemporal encephalitis. The prognosis is poor, and treatment with parenteral acyclovir is effective only when started early. In contrast, herpes simplex virus type 2 produces primarily aseptic meningitis. The resurgence of sylvatic rabies in the Northeast and its potential for transmission to humans should be remembered.

The management of aseptic meningitis and encephalitis, with the exception of *Herpesvirus* or bacterial etiologies (Table 20–15), is purely supportive. The outcome of viral meningitis and encephalitis is extremely variable. Mortality in herpes simplex encephalitis is high, but the morbidity in mumps meningitis is extremely low. In general, the very young and the very old have a greater morbidity.

Parameningeal Infections

Subdural empyema and brain abscess are parameningeal collections that manifest themselves primarily as central nervous system mass lesions. Infection may occur by direct extension from a contiguous focus, such as sinusitis or otitis; septic thrombosis of a penetrating venous system from an underlying focus of infection; or hematogenous seeding from a distant focus, such as a pulmonary infection, endocarditis, or skin infection.

The organisms implicated in infection depend on the source. If the source is sinusitis or otitis, streptococci (including *S. pneumoniae*), anaerobes, and *S. aureus* predominate. After intracranial surgery or head trauma, staphylococcal species and gram-negative bacilli are the likely organisms. Hematogenous seeding implicates *S. aureus*, streptococci, anaerobes, and the Enterobacteriaceae. Most cryptogenic brain abscesses of unknown primary origin are due to streptococcal species and anaerobes. Mixed infections are common, and Gram-stained smears of abscess material always should be made, because 20 per cent of cultures fail to grow any organism. In immunocompromised or HIV-infected patients, toxoplasmosis, *Nocardia*, or fungal abscesses must be considered.

Subdural empyema presents with abrupt onset of fever and headache. Altered consciousness and seizures may be present. Signs of meningeal irritation frequently are found. In contrast, parenchymal brain abscesses present insidiously, with drowsiness, confusion, vomiting, seizures, and focal neurologic signs. Fever is uncommonly prominent in brain abscesses, with 50 per cent of patients having fever less than 100.5° F. Because of the absence of fever, the diagnosis of brain abscess is frequently overlooked, with early diagnoses primarily those of a neoplastic lesion or psychiatric disturbance.

Laboratory data are not particularly helpful in the diagnosis of parameningeal infections. The peripheral white blood cell count and sedimentation rate may be normal or elevated. CSF reveals moderately elevated protein and a mild pleocytosis of mixed cell type. Caution must be exercised in performing a lumbar puncture, because pressure changes may precipitate herniation. CT scan and MRI are helpful in localizing the infectious process.

The management of subdural empyema and brain abscess is twofold. Antibiotic therapy should be directed against the likely microorganisms, with surgical intervention timed appropriately. Early surgical drainage is the keystone of therapy for subdural empyema, and antibiotics should be continued a minimum of 3 weeks after surgery. The timing of surgical intervention for brain abscesses is more controversial. Experts favor either complete excision of the abscess cavity and abscess wall or stereotactic needle aspiration. Toxoplasmosis and small bacterial abscesses may resolve with medical therapy alone. Signs of increased intracranial pressure are an indication for early surgical intervention, but it may be desirable to delay surgery until there is evidence of abscess encapsulation. Antibiotics should be initiated as soon as a diagnosis is considered and should be continued for at least 3 weeks postoperatively. Because anaerobes are involved so commonly in brain abscesses, metronidazole is favored as part of the initial regimen. Ampicillin, oxacillin, or third-generation cephalosporins are also valuable and should be used in addition to metronidazole, pending the results of microbiologic studies. The role of steroids is controversial, and their use should be minimized because they may interfere with adequate encapsulation and resolution of the infection.

FEVER

Fever is the most celebrated manifestation of infectious disease and the foremost patient complaint. Studies performed in the 1800s showed that fever could be produced by the injection of microbial free extracts of human cells, and Beeson demonstrated in 1948 that fever associated with infection was due primarily to a substance isolated from human phagocytic cells. This mediator, initially named "endogenous pyrogen" and later known as lymphocyte-activating factor or leukocytic pyrogen, is now known as interleukin-1.

Pathogenesis of Fever

A variety of experimental and clinical data clearly define the role of interleukin-1 in the production of fever. It is a heat-labile protein, synthesized and released by monocytes and tissue macrophages. Interleukin-1 production can be evoked by a variety of both microbial and nonmicrobial stimuli. The systemic effects of this mediator include fever resulting from the action of interleukin-1 on the thermal regulatory center in the brain, an increase in the number of neutrophils as a result of a direct action on the bone marrow, and modulation of a variety of subcellular acute-phase responses. The fact that fever is a regular occurrence in patients with agranulocytosis, certain blood dyscrasias, viral infections, and granulomatous infections supports the role of monocytes and tissue macrophages as the most prominent inflammatory cells responsible for releasing pyrogen.

The regulation of body temperature is performed mostly by the autonomic nervous system, which adjusts blood flow to body surfaces, thereby regulating the amount of heat lost or gained by vasodilation or vasoconstriction. Normally, humans generate body heat from the metabolism of dietary fats, proteins, and carbohydrates. At rest, the viscera supply 60 per cent of body heat; during exercise up to 90 per cent of body heat may be generated by muscular activity. Shivering produces a fourfold increase in heat production. Heat loss from the body occurs primarily through radiation or evaporation, as in sweating.

The hypothalamus normally maintains body temperature at 98.6° F, or 37° C. The equilibrium between heat production and heat loss in healthy people is regulated tightly, with a normal diurnal variation producing peak temperatures in late afternoon and early evening. Fever, resulting from the effect of interleukin-1 on the hypothalamus, raises the body's temperature to a new "set point" around which the new temperature is regulated. When interleukin-1 is withdrawn, the set point is lowered, the body sweats, the skin vasodilates, and the temperature falls.

Although fever physiologically follows the effect of interleukin-1 on the hypothalamus, there are situations in which normal mechanisms do not function. In thyrotoxicosis, metabolic activity and heat production exceed the body's ability to dissipate heat by vasodilation and sweating, resulting in fever. In heat stroke, environmental temperature overwhelms the body's ability to dissipate heat and the regulatory function of the hypothalamus is impaired, resulting in high fever without effective vasodilation or sweating. Finally, central nervous system lesions resulting from tumors or vascular disease may produce fever as a result of direct malfunction of the hypothalamic regulatory centers. Patients with "central fever" usually manifest wide swings of temperature without a diurnal pattern.

Fever is not usually harmful to the host, with some exceptions. Sustained core temperatures over 105° F (40.5° C) may produce cerebral damage. Intracranial pressure rises with increases in body temperatures in patients with central nervous system mass lesions. Fever may exacerbate the increased intracranial pressure. The metabolic demands of fever may be detrimental to patients with acute myocardial infarction, and febrile seizures are seen in young children. In these situations, fever may need to be treated specifically. In other circumstances, administration of antipyretic drugs frequently does more to confuse than to help the clinical situation.

Fever of Unknown Origin

Fever of unknown origin (FUO) has been defined as an illness of at least 3 weeks' duration with a temperature exceeding 101° F, or 38.3° C, on several occasions and with no established diagnosis after 1 week of evaluation in the hospital. This definition, proposed in 1960, may not be applicable today because patients are evaluated more extensively and promptly by better laboratory screening and more sophisticated radiologic procedures. Nevertheless, it serves as a useful way to categorize febrile illnesses of long duration. It should be noted that febrile illnesses of short duration are most often due to infection, whereas prolonged fevers are frequently noninfectious.

Diagnostic categories of FUO vary in frequency according to age and population group. Approximately 40 per cent of FUOs are due to infectious diseases, 20 per cent are due to neoplasia, 15 per cent are due to collagen vascular diseases, and 15 per cent are due to miscellaneous causes. Approximately 10 per cent of FUOs remain undiagnosed. In pediatric populations, infection represents a greater percentage and neoplasia a smaller percentage of the total cases when compared with adults. Prolonged fever in patients with underlying HIV infection is discussed separately (Chapter 21).

Infection is the most common single cause of

TABLE 20–16. DIAGNOSTIC CATEGORIES OF FEVER OF UNDETERMINED ORIGIN

I. Infection
   A. Systemic infection
      1. Tuberculosis
      2. Infective endocarditis
      3. Miscellaneous infections: cytomegalovirus, Epstein-Barr virus, human immunodeficiency virus, disseminated mycoses, malaria, babesiosis, brucellosis
   B. Localized infection
      1. Hepatic infection (liver abscess, cholangitis)
      2. Other visceral infections (pancreatic abscess, tubo-ovarian abscess, psoas abscess)
      3. Urinary tract infections (pyelonephritis, renal carbuncle, perinephric abscess, prostatic abscess)
II. Neoplasms
III. Collagen vascular disorders
IV. Miscellaneous causes
   A. Inflammatory bowel disease
   B. Pulmonary emboli
   C. Granulomatous disorders
   D. Drug fever
   E. Factitous fever
   F. Hepatic cirrhosis with active hepatocellular necrosis
   G. Miscellaneous rare causes (familial Mediterranean fever, Whipple's disease)
V. Undiagnosed

prolonged fever (Table 20–16). *Tuberculosis* remains a major cause of FUO. Many such patients are elderly, and have a negative chest radiograph and a negative purified protein derivative test. A single organ, such as the endometrium or kidney, may be involved. Biopsy and/or culture of blood, bone marrow, and liver are helpful diagnostically, as are a history of HIV infection, foreign birth, family history of tuberculosis, and prior episode of prolonged pulmonary infection.

Infective endocarditis is a frequent cause of FUO. In recent studies, patients are more likely to be elderly, may or may not have a heart murmur, and usually do not have the classic manifestations of embolic phenomena, splinter hemorrhages, or splenomegaly. Multiple blood cultures, echocardiograms, and repeated careful physical examinations are most helpful in diagnosis.

Viral infections, especially those resulting from HIV, cytomegalovirus, or EBV, are common causes of prolonged fever. In the pediatric age group, viral infections are the single most common cause of FUO.

Visceral abscesses may present as a FUO. Perirectal abscesses are commonly a focus of infection in the neutropenic patient, and subphrenic or pelvic abscesses are common causes in the postoperative patient. Liver abscesses should be considered, especially in travelers (amebic) or in individuals with biliary disease. Perinephric abscesses occur in patients with a history of urinary tract infection, especially in young women, or in patients with obstructive uropathy or calculous disease. Prostatic abscesses should be considered in older men with

underlying prostatic disease. Abscesses presenting as a FUO may be manifest not by localized pain, tenderness, or mass, but as fever alone in the appropriate historical setting.

Fever may be due to *neoplasia* without infection. Such is commonly the case with reticuloendothelial neoplasms. In lymphoma, fever is often remittent, irregular, or spiking and accompanied by night sweats. Fever responds to appropriate chemotherapy, and its reappearance may suggest recurrent disease. When fever in acute leukemia is present on admission or at discovery of disease, it is usually associated with a readily diagnosable localized infection or is due to the leukemia itself. Fever also may be associated with nonreticuloendothelial tumors; renal cell tumors and hepatoma are particularly noteworthy. Atrial myxoma may present with fever, anemia, and a heart murmur and must be differentiated from infective endocarditis. Fever frequently accompanies the liver metastases of any primary neoplasm.

Collagen vascular diseases may present with prolonged fever. Juvenile rheumatoid arthritis is one of the two most common causes of FUO in children, the other being viral infection. In adults, rheumatoid arthritis frequently presents with fever, and temporal arteritis or polymyalgia rheumatica may present with prolonged fever in the older adult. Systemic lupus erythematosus may be manifest by fever and should be suspected when rash, leukopenia, and serositis are also present. Most of these collagen vascular diseases have prominent constitutional and musculoskeletal symptoms and markedly elevated sedimentation rates, suggesting their diagnosis.

Drug fever is particularly common, not only as a cause of FUO but also as a cause of short-term fever. Other manifestations of hypersensitivity, such as rash and eosinophilia, may or may not be present. Fever may be due to an allergic or direct effect of the drug. Phenothiazines, for example, impair temperature regulation through their effects on the autonomic nervous system. Drugs most commonly associated with fever are antiarrhythmic drugs such as procainamide and quinidine; anticonvulsants, particularly phenytoin; antimicrobial agents, especially penicillins, cephalosporins, isoniazid, and sulfonamides; the antihypertensives hydralazine and α-methyldopa; and bleomycin, iodides, and cimetidine. Fever is usually low grade but may be spiking, and usually is associated with a normal white blood cell count.

Fevers frequently are associated with a variety of *granulomatous disorders,* such as sarcoidosis, Wegener's granulomatosis, granulomatous hepatitis, and infectious diseases such as fungal disease or tuberculosis. The diagnosis may be difficult, and tissue diagnosis is frequently necessary.

Inflammatory bowel disease always should be considered in the differential diagnosis of a FUO. There may be few bowel symptoms, and thus the

TABLE 20–17. EVALUATION OF FACTITIOUS (FALSIFIED) FEVER

Clinical Clues
Pulse–temperature dissociation
High temperature (>106°F)
Lack of diurnal variation
Absence of sweating or shivering
Well looking, no weight loss
Normal laboratory data

Diagnostic Clues
Oral–rectal temperature discrepancy
No fever when under direct observation, as when taken electronically
Temperature of freshly voided urine

diagnosis may be elusive. Joint symptoms may predominate, particularly in Crohn's disease or Whipple's disease.

Pulmonary emboli, especially small and multiple, frequently are overlooked as the cause of prolonged fever. Such patients may have a normal chest radiograph and no evidence of thrombophlebitis. Predisposing factors include recent surgery, venous disease, prolonged inactivity, and prostatic or pelvic inflammatory disease.

Factitious fever (Table 20–17) always should be considered, particularly in young, usually female, often paramedical personnel who have prolonged fever without evidence of weight loss and a relatively good appearance. It should be remembered, however, that factitious fever may appear on a background of organic disease, so that such patients already may have a distracting, alternative diagnosis. Factitious fever may be falsified, through manipulating the thermometer, or may be created through self-injection of foreign material. Clues to the diagnosis of falsified fever are listed in Table 20–17. Factitious fever traditionally has been the diagnosis of 1 to 2 per cent of all patients with FUO.

In the evaluation of a patient with FUO, a thorough history and physical examination are of utmost importance. Detailed recent and remote travel, drug use, animal and sexual exposure, and occupational histories are mandatory. Important symptoms to elicit are subtle gastrointestinal or genitourinary symptoms, myalgias, arthralgias, or rash. Repeated physical exams must be performed to detect the presence of adenopathy, splenomegaly, abdominal tenderness, abnormalities of joints or skin, heart murmurs, and fleeting findings on funduscopic exam. The lack of an adequate history and physical examination is responsible for the fact that 50 per cent of prolonged fevers are undiagnosed. Other omissions, such as failure to perform an indicated laboratory test or ignoring an abnormal test, account for another 20 per cent of misdiagnosis.

If the diagnosis of prolonged fever is not established after a thorough history and repeated physi-

cal examinations, standard laboratory and radiographic tests, including abdominal and pelvic CT scans, and a tissue biopsy may be necessary to provide the diagnosis. Blind biopsies are not usually helpful; they should be guided by abnormal laboratory tests, symptoms, or physical findings. Liver biopsy and bone marrow biopsy are useful in certain settings. Infectious disease consultation should be sought before blind therapeutic trials of antibiotics are begun.

Finally, it is important to realize that patients presenting with prolonged fever usually have common illnesses with atypical presentations rather than exotic diseases. In all cases, it behooves the clinician to pursue the diagnosis, because most patients with prolonged fever recover only after a specific diagnosis is made and therapy tailored to that diagnosis is administered.

GASTROINTESTINAL INFECTIONS

Diarrheal disease is a topic of passing interest to many physicians. Indeed, in industrial nations, it is considered more a nuisance than a serious illness. However, in the United States, diarrheal diseases are among the five leading causes of death in small children, and, in underdeveloped countries, diarrheal disease results in more infant deaths than any other cause.

Although systemic conditions such as age and nutritional status are important protective factors, the gastrointestinal tract itself plays the most important role in protection from exogenous infection (Table 20–18). *Gastric acid* destroys most ingested bacteria. Gastrectomy or administration of antacids or histamine antagonists will increase susceptibility to infection with ingested microorganisms. The *indigenous intestinal flora*, from stomach to colon, maintain ecologic stability of the gastrointestinal tract and interfere with the establishment of residence by invading microorganisms. This seems to be accomplished by competition for essential nutrients, by the production of toxic metabolites such as short-chain fatty acids, and by competition for epithelial cell–binding sites, by which disease is mediated. Bile acids, deconjugated by enteric bacteria, are inhibitory to other microorganisms and probably play a significant role in the maintenance of normal intestinal flora. *Bowel motility* is an important element of protection because it moves

TABLE 20–18. HOST DEFENSES AGAINST GASTROINTESTINAL INFECTION

Gastric acid
Indigenous flora
Bowel motility
Secretory immunoglobulin
Digestive proteases

bacteria along the intestinal tract, inhibiting attachment to and penetration of the gastrointestinal epithelium. Interference with bowel motility by administration of antiperistaltic drugs can worsen the course of an established enteritis significantly. *Local immunity* with production of secretory IgA is important for protection against invading microorganisms. Secretory IgA prevents attachment of the organisms to the epithelial cell surface and aids in their immobilization within the intestinal mucus. The secretion of *digestive proteases* or enzymes into the lumen of the intestine destroys toxins elaborated by pathogenic organisms.

Diarrheal Disease

Pathogenesis

Acute diarrheal disease may be caused by a variety of bacteria, parasites, and viruses singly or in combination. Each agent has distinct epidemiologic and clinical features that aid in diagnosis. Diarrhea may occur in epidemics, as in food-borne outbreaks, or as a sporadic illness without a clearcut vehicle. Almost all diarrheal disease is due to fecal–oral transmission, directly or indirectly.

Common etiologic agents of diarrheal disease are listed in Table 20–19. However, it is important to note that, in up to 50 per cent of diarrheal outbreaks, no pathogen is isolated. Whether these are chemical, viral, or due to other unidentifiable or unrecognizable pathogens is not clear. The type and severity of diarrheal illness will be determined by the age and underlying disease of the patient, the geographic location and time of year, the patient's dietary and personal hygiene habits, and the economic development and industrialization of the patient's country of origin.

There are a number of properties of microorganisms that enable them to cause diarrheal illness. Many microorganisms elaborate toxins that produce disease. Preformed toxins (Table 20–20) are frequently neurotoxins and produce their effects through activity on the central nervous system. Enterotoxins stimulate secretion of electrolytes and/or fluids by the intestinal mucosa. There is no inflammation associated with enterotoxin production. In contrast, some enteric pathogens produce cytopathic toxins that cause mucosal destruction and inflammatory colitis. Some organisms invade the epithelium, and cause tissue destruction locally (e.g., *Shigella*), while others invade without much inflammatory response (e.g., *Salmonella*). An important virulence factor is the ability of the microorganism to adhere to the intestinal mucosa, even for those agents that produce disease by toxin elaboration (e.g., *Vibrio cholerae*).

Approach to Diarrheal Disease

An adequate history is the best approach to the differential diagnosis of diarrheal illness. The patient's age and the severity, type, and duration of illness are all important. The presence or absence of fever, severe abdominal pain, and hematochezia suggest different pathogens than those for profuse, watery diarrhea without pain, blood, or fever (Table 20–20). A detailed history of prior antibiotic use, travel, contact with illness, and diet (Table 20–19) is necessary. Physical examination should be done promptly to determine the degree of fluid loss, particularly in children.

Stool must be examined to provide objective evidence of illness. Whether it is watery, mucoid, or bloody provides specific information as to etiology. Microscopic examination will show fecal leukocytes in invasive disease (Table 20–20). Cultures should be obtained promptly. This is particularly true if *Shigella* is suspected, because this organism will not survive even short periods of storage. It is essential to notify the laboratory if certain organisms are suspected, because *Vibrio*, *E. coli* 0157, and *Yersinia* require selective culture techniques.

Diarrhea in the Infant

Diarrhea in newborn infants usually occurs in epidemic situations and is frequently due to rotaviruses or toxin-producing strains of *E. coli*. Occasionally, *Shigella*, *Salmonella*, *Campylobacter*, and other viral enteritides occur in infants, particularly during institutional outbreaks. The index cases in such outbreaks may acquire the infection at birth through contact with infected maternal fecal or perineal flora. Because the majority of diarrheal disease in infants is not invasive, septic com-

TABLE 20–19.   COMMON ETIOLOGIC AGENTS OF DIARRHEAL DISEASE

Microorganism	Vehicle
Bacillus cereus	Foods (cereal products, fried rice)
Campylobacter	Foods (poultry), animals
Clostridium difficile	Person-to-person, environmental
Clostridium perfringens	Foods (prepared meat dishes)
Cryptosporidium	Water, animals
Entamoeba histolytica	Water, person to person, institutions
E. coli, enterotoxigenic	Food, water, travel
E. coli, enterohemorrhagic	Food (undercooked hamburger)
Giardia	Water, person to person
Norwalk virus	Foods (salads, shellfish), water
Rotavirus	Person to person, institutions
Salmonella	Foods (eggs, poultry), animals, birds
Shigella	Person to person, prepared foods, institutions
Staphylococcus aureus	Foods (prepared dishes)
Vibrio cholera	Water, shellfish
Vibrio parahaemoliticus	Shellfish
Yersinia	Water, unpasteurized milk, person to person

TABLE 20–20. TYPES OF ENTERIC DISEASE

Mechanism	Preformed toxin Noninflammatory	Enterotoxin Noninflammatory	Invasion/cytotoxin Inflammatory	Invasion Penetrating
Location of effect	Central nervous system	Small bowel, proximal	Colon	Small bowel, distal
Microorganisms	*Staphylococcus aureus, Bacillus cereus*	*Vibrio cholerae, E. coli, Salmonella* spp., *Vibrio paraphaemolyticus, Clostridium perfringens, Bacillus cereus, Shigella dysenteriae, Campylobacter*	*Shigella, E. coli, Campylobacter, Clostridium difficile, Salmonella* spp., *Entamoeba histolytica*	*Salmonella typhi, Salmonella paratyphi, Yersinia,* Viral (proximal)
Illness	Vomiting, watery diarrhea	Watery diarrhea	Fever, dysentery, diarrhea	Fever, diarrhea
Stools	No leukocytes	No leukocytes	Fecal polymorphonuclear leukocytes	Fecal monocytes and polymorphonuclear leukocytes

plications are unusual and dehydration is the major clinical problem. The use of antimicrobial agents or antimotility and antisecretory drugs is rarely necessary or successful.

Treatment of diarrhea in infants and young children is primarily with fluid and electrolyte replacement. Oral rehydration therapy is satisfactory unless dehydration is severe. Recommended solutions are highly effective, inexpensive, and readily available. The oral rehydration solution recommended by the World Health Organization contains 3.5 grams NaCl, 1.5 grams KCl, 2.5 grams $NaHCO_3$, and 20 grams glucose per liter. The active intestinal transport of glucose promotes coupled absorption of sodium and water, thereby accelerating the replenishment of fluid and electrolytes. Oral rehydration should begin at 15 to 25 ml/kg/h for 4 hours for mild to moderate dehydration, and be followed by maintenance fluids equivalent to measured stool, urine, and insensible losses. Oral intake of food, including breast milk, should continue if clinically possible.

Diarrhea in Children

Children ages 6 months to 5 years represent the bulk of patients with infectious diarrhea. Organisms of particular importance in this age group include rotavirus, *Salmonella*, and *Shigella*.

Rotaviruses are the main cause of winter gastroenteritis in children in temperate climates. After an incubation period of 48 hours, vomiting and diarrhea begin suddenly and may last from 2 to 14 days. Fever is unusual. Stools are watery, with mucus, but do not contain blood or leukocytes. Treatment is supportive, using the oral rehydration therapy described for infant diarrhea. Milk products should be avoided because of the appearance of a temporary lactase deficiency in viral gastroenteritis.

Shigellosis occurs predominantly in the same age group, particularly in a family milieu or institutional setting. The incubation period is 2 to 4 days, followed by fever, diarrhea, and dysentery (bloody stools of small volume). Vomiting may occur in younger children, and respiratory symptoms are

also frequent at this age. Meningismus may be present. The abdominal findings in shigellosis are typical of invasive disease. Tenderness, hyperactive bowel sounds, and even rebound tenderness occasionally are seen. Sigmoidoscopy shows intense hyperemia with mucus, pus, and multiple ulcerations. Microscopic examination of the stool reveals large numbers of polymorphonuclear leukocytes.

Individuals with shigellosis should be treated according to the severity of their illness. The drug of choice at present is trimethoprim–sulfamethoxazole for children or a fluoroquinolone for adults. In recent years, however, antibiotic-resistant *Shigella* species have become common. Treatment of shigellosis substantially shortens the period of diarrhea and fever compared with placebo treatment. Antiperistaltic drugs such as diphenoxylate, loperamide, or opiates are contraindicated in invasive diarrheal diseases.

The prevalence of *Salmonella* gastroenteritis peaks in children between the ages of 6 months and 2 years. House pets, from dogs to turtles, and food products, particularly poultry and egg products, are the major reservoirs. Person-to-person transmission is also implicated. Seventy per cent of *Salmonella* infections manifest themselves as diarrheal disease. The incubation period is 8 to 48 hours, and symptoms include abdominal cramps, vomiting, and fever. Stools are foul smelling and bile colored. Bacteremia is more common in children less than 1 year of age, and respiratory symptoms and meningismus also occur in this age group. Physical examination shows mild abdominal tenderness and hyperactive bowel sounds. Examination of the stool may reveal a few white cells, and occasionally blood will be found.

Salmonella enteritis is self-limited except when bacteremia occurs. In children below 3 years of age, blood cultures always should be obtained. Treatment is indicated if bacteremia is present, the host is compromised, or the illness is prolonged. Oral antibiotics may prolong the carrier state and increase the risk of person-to-person transmission because of prolonged fecal carriage. The drugs of choice for treatment of *Salmonella* infections in children include trimethoprim–sulfamethoxazole, ampicillin, and amoxicillin. Oral cephalosporins are less effective but parenteral third-generation cephalosporins have been used successfully.

When bacteremia occurs with *Salmonella* in this age group, a typhoidal illness is not usually seen. However, salmonella may seed discrete organs, such as bone, spleen, or liver, particularly in children with hematologic disorders. This may result in focal *Salmonella* infections requiring specific medical and/or surgical therapy, or may result in a chronic carrier state.

Yersinia enterocolitica is an organism responsible for a variety of clinical syndromes. In children less than 5 years old, fever and gastroenteritis may occur. In older children and adolescents, abdominal pain is the most prominent feature and is due to suppurative mesenteric lymphadenitis. This may mimic appendicitis and has prompted appendectomy on many an occasion. A self-limited diarrheal illness also may be seen.

Diarrheal Disease in Older Children and Adults

Viral diarrhea occurs regularly in adolescents and adults. Epidemics occur in late fall and early winter. The clinical features include various combinations of diarrhea, nausea, vomiting, low-grade fever, abdominal cramps, headache, and malaise lasting 24 to 48 hours. The agents most frequently implicated are Norwalk-like agents, and the treatment is symptomatic. Stool examination shows no leukocytes, thereby ruling out invasive bacterial infection. A diagnosis of Norwalk-like illness can be suspected on clinical and epidemiologic grounds in the absence of other documented pathogens. Microbiologic confirmation is currently difficult because of the limited availability of immunodiagnostic testing.

Shigellosis and salmonellosis also occur in adults, particularly those having traveled to foreign countries. The clinical manifestations are similar to those in children, and most cases are self-limited, but protracted or severe illness should be treated with a fluoroquinolone antimicrobial. *Salmonella* bacteremia in older adults has an unfortunate predilection for vascular endothelium, with the development of mycotic aneurysms.

Salmonella typhi infections in adults may present clinically as typhoid fever. The incubation period varies from 8 to 14 days. Onset of illness is gradual, with headache, anorexia, lethargy, and malaise. Nonproductive cough is common, but only 20 per cent of patients have diarrhea. Constipation is a more frequent complaint. Fever fluctuates between 102° and 105° F for 2 to 3 weeks in untreated patients. Physical findings are variable, but the pulse may be slow, there may be scattered rhonchi, and splenomegaly frequently is present. Laboratory data show leukopenia and sometimes thrombocytopenia. *Salmonella typhi* can be isolated from the stool at any time in the illness and from the blood in 90 per cent of patients during the first week. *Salmonella* agglutinins are helpful but not definitive, and a diagnosis must be based on culture. Although a number of antimicrobial agents are effective in vitro against *S. typhi* infections, chloramphenicol, ampicillin (and amoxicillin), trimethoprim–sulfamethoxazole, and the quinolones are clinically useful. An individual who continues to excrete *S. typhi* in the stool may respond to prolonged fluoroquinolone therapy or require cholecystectomy.

Campylobacter jejuni is a short, curved, gram-negative bacillus and a major cause of bacterial diarrhea in humans. Commonly acquired from sick pets, unpasteurized milk, or ill-prepared poultry products, it produces an acute illness with frequently bloody diarrhea, fever, and tenesmus. Abdominal pain may be severe. Symptoms last from 2 to 7 days, but may be more protracted. Sigmoidoscopy appearance may be indistinguishable from that of ulcerative colitis. The treatment of choice is a fluoroquinolone antibiotic or erythromycin by mouth. Occasionally, septicemia is present and requires parenteral therapy with a third-generation cephalosporin, imipenem, or a quinolone.

Vibrio species are halophilic, gram-negative rods found in marine water and shellfish throughout the world. *Vibrio parahaemolyticus* is the most common species seen in the United States, where it produces outbreaks of illness in the summer. *Vibrio parahaemolyticus* may produce a toxigenic illness similar to that produced by *E. coli* or an invasive illness similar to shigellosis. In contrast, *V. cholerae* produces only a toxigenic diarrhea. Cholera is rare in the United States, although the organism is endemic in the Gulf Coast and may be found in crustaceans and shellfish harvested from this area. Epidemic cholera exists in South America, particularly, Peru, Bolivia, and Chile, and should be anticipated in travelers returning from this area.

Traveler's diarrhea is an illness acquired by travelers to tropical or semitropical countries. *Enterotoxigenic E. coli* is the most frequent pathogen, although viruses, *Shigella*, *Salmonella*, *Entamoeba*, and *Giardia* all are seen in this setting (Table 20–21). Toxigenic *E. coli* produces watery diarrhea of sudden onset, with abdominal cramps but no fever and no tenesmus. Stools are watery and free of blood and fecal leukocytes. Treatment is symptomatic. Prophylactic Pepto-Bismol has been found to be useful, but prophylactic antibiotics may predispose to infection with drug-resistant organisms and are not routinely recommended. Empiric treatment with trimethoprim–sulfamethoxazole or a quinolone will shorten the course of severe illness.

Enterohemorrhagic E. coli produces epidemic and sporadic diarrhea in children and adults.

TABLE 20–21. ENTERIC PATHOGENS AND TRAVELERS' DIARRHEA

Etiologic Agents	Frequency of Association with Travelers' Diarrhea
Enterotoxigenic *E. coli*	30–60
Shigella	5–10
Campylobacter jejuni	5–15
Salmonella strains	3–5
Aeromonas hydrophila	1–5
Rotavirus	1–5
Norwalk agent	1–5
Cryptosporidium	5–15
Giardia	1–3
Multiple agents	5–15
Unknown	15–25

These strains, most often serotype O157:H7, produce a verotoxin that mediates the clinical syndrome of abdominal cramps and grossly bloody diarrhea. Most patients are afebrile. Undercooked hamburger is the vehicle most often implicated. Complications include the hemolytic-uremic syndrome and there is a high mortality in elderly patients.

Antibiotic-associated diarrhea is common. Most cases are self-limited and not associated with significant colitis. True pseudomembranous colitis is rare. It has been associated most commonly with clindamycin administration (perhaps 1 per cent of those receiving clindamycin develop this condition), although it is now seen with a variety of β-lactam antibiotics, tetracyclines, and sulfonamides. Pseudomembranous colitis is due to overgrowth of antibiotic-resistant *C. difficile*, which produces a cytopathic toxin. The clinical findings are those of diarrhea, fever, abdominal pain, distention, and systemic toxicity. Stools are usually watery and mucoid, and may contain blood and fecal leukocytes. The treatment of choice is oral metronidazole, 500 mg three times a day.

Intra-Abdominal Infections

Intraperitoneal infections may be generalized or localized depending on the host response and pathogenesis. Because intraperitoneal recesses all interconnect, infection in one area may spread to another during the course of any intra-abdominal infection.

Primary peritonitis occurs without a definite cause. It is seen at all ages, particularly in children with nephrotic syndrome and in adults with alcoholic cirrhosis. About 10 per cent of patients with alcoholic cirrhosis and ascites will develop primary peritonitis, although the diagnosis may be difficult because of subtle physical signs.

The most common agents in children are *S. pneumoniae* and group A streptococci. In adults, *E. coli* is most common, followed by *S. pneumoniae*,

Bacteroides, and other bowel flora. Streptococcal infection is usually considered to be hematogenous, while infection caused by bowel flora suggests an intestinal transmural route. Clinical manifestations include fever, distention, and abdominal tenderness. Rigidity and/or paralytic ileus may be present. Children show more signs of inflammation than the adult cirrhotic. Ascitic fluid protein content is of little help in the diagnosis, but the peritoneal white blood cell count is usually over 300/mm^3.

Secondary peritonitis usually occurs as a result of injury to the gastrointestinal tract, such as perforated ulcer, ischemic bowel, or diverticulitis, or as a result of the spread from infection originating in an intra-abdominal or juxtaperitoneal organ such as the uterus, fallopian tube, or appendix. Most cases of secondary peritonitis are caused by microorganisms from a ruptured viscus. The stomach, duodendum, and upper small bowel contain mouth flora such as S. viridans group streptococci, staphylococci, and oral anaerobes (Table 20–22). Some individuals, particularly those with gastric outlet obstruction, achlorhydria, bleeding, or prolonged administration of antacids or H$_2$ blockers, also may be colonized with colonic flora such as *E. coli*, *Klebsiella*, enterococci, and *B. fragilis*. The flora of the colon are primarily anaerobic (Table 20–22).

Intraperitoneal abscesses frequently follow peritonitis, particularly in cases of appendicitis or diverticulitis, or after bowel surgery. Characteristically, as with peritonitis, infections are polymicrobial, with anaerobes predominating, particularly *B. fragilis* and anaerobic streptococci. The appearance of fever and chills 5 to 7 days after bowel surgery should suggest a localized area of peritonitis or abscess resulting from an anastomotic leak.

The clinical diagnosis of peritonitis is usually not difficult except in the compromised host, in whom physical findings may be blunted. There is usually leukocytosis, and there may be evidence of hemoconcentration resulting from pooling of fluid in the intestine or abdomen. Radiographs re-

TABLE 20–22. FLORA OF THE INTESTINAL TRACT

Aerobes	Anaerobes
Mouth, Esophagus, and Proximal Small Bowel	
Streptococci	*Bacteroides oralis*
Staphylococci	*Bacteroides melaninogenicus*
Neisseria	*Fusobacterium*
Haemophilus	*Peptococcus*
Lactobacilli	*Peptostreptococcus*
Colon and Distal Small Bowel	
E. coli	*Bacteroides fragilis*
Klebsiella	*Clostridium* species
Proteus	*Peptostreptococcus*
Enterobacter	*Peptococcus*
Enterococci	*Eubacterium*
	Bifidobacterium

veal distention of the bowel, and, if a viscus has ruptured, free air may be seen below the diaphragms. Needle aspiration of the abdomen may yield cloudy fluid, with leukocytes and bacteria on smear.

The diagnosis of intra-abdominal abscess may be more difficult. This is particularly true in the postsurgical patient, in whom physical findings are obscured by recent surgery. Gallium scan is of limited value because of postsurgical inflammation. The use of ultrasound, radionuclide, and CT scanning or MRI may be necessary in combination to determine the presence or absence of an abscess.

The treatment of intraperitoneal infection secondary to bowel flora requires aggressive surgical correction of the primary lesion, drainage of sequestered collections of pus, and administration of appropriate antimicrobial agents. Because most such infections are polymicrobial, broad-spectrum therapy is indicated to cover aerobic and anaerobic gram-positive and gram-negative microorganisms if and until definite cultures are available. Many fastidious anaerobes may not be recovered, and empiric therapy for anaerobes often must be continued even in the face of negative cultures. Gram-stained smears of peritoneal exudate will assist in determining the likely pathogens.

Equally effective antimicrobial regimens include clindamycin or metronidazole plus an aminoglycoside, fluoroquinolone, extended-spectrum penicillin or cephalosporin; cefoxitin or cefotetan; ticarcillin plus clavulanic acid; piperacillin plus tozobactam; or ampicillin plus sulbactam or imipenem. The selection is made by personal preference, severity of illness, relative risks of drug toxicity, the results of Gram-stained smears and cultures, and cost. Duration of therapy varies with clinical circumstances but is generally continued until the white blood cell count is normal and the patient has been afebrile for 3 to 5 days.

INFECTION IN THE COMPROMISED HOST

Individuals with altered host defenses comprise a significant proportion of the hospital population and are increasingly being cared for by primary care practitioners. Patients may be compromised in a variety of ways and are susceptible to different pathogens according to the type of immunosuppression (Tables 20–23 and 20–24). Bacteria, fungi, viruses, or parasites may be responsible for disease, depending on the particular defect in host defense (Table 20–24). For example, the use of indwelling percutaneous catheters provides a means by which bacteria or fungi may circumvent normal skin barriers and enter the vascular system. Such intravascular devices are responsible for the fact that gram-positive skin flora have emerged as the most common cause of bacteremia in the neutro-

TABLE 20–23. HOST DEFENSE SYSTEMS

1. Anatomic barriers and secretions (integument, mucosal surfaces)
2. Normal bacterial flora
3. Phagocytes (granulocytes, monocytes, macrophages)
4. Reticuloendothelial system (spleen, liver, tissue macrophages)
5. Complement system
6. Cell-mediated immunity (T lymphocyte, macrophage)
7. Humoral immunity (B lymphocyte, plasma cell, immunoglobulin)

penic host. The HIV-infected patient has depressed cellular immunity, resulting in an increased risk of infection with fungi, protozoa, and intracellular bacteria such as *Salmonella* and mycobacteria. Many diseases, such as hematologic malignancies treated with steroids and chemotherapy, compromise multiple defense systems and therefore render the patient susceptible to a wide variety of pathogens.

Mechanisms of Immune Defense

Phagocytes and immunoglobulin are important for protection against bacterial infection. In neutropenic patients, the majority of infections are caused by bacteria, particularly staphylococci and gram-negative bacilli. Humoral immunity is important for protection against encapsulated microorganisms such as *S. pneumoniae* and *H. influenzae*. In the absence of pre-existing antibody, the spleen has a special role in clearing the blood stream of such organisms. Overwhelming sepsis caused by these organisms may occur in asplenic individuals, particularly children. T lymphocytes are important in a permissive role for the development of humoral immunity by facilitating B-cell differentiation to antibody-producing plasma cells. Defects in cell-mediated immunity therefore also may predispose to bacterial infection such as pneumococcal sepsis, as seen, for example, in HIV infection. The intimate relationship between B cells, T cells, and macrophages makes isolated deficiencies uncommon.

Protection of the host from invasive fungal infections involves multiple systems. Fungi such as *Candida*, *Aspergillus*, and *Mucor* generally produce systemic infection only in those individuals with absent normal flora, damaged cutaneous defenses, defective humoral and cell-mediated immunity, and abnormal leukocyte function. Serious infections caused by *Candida*, for example, are seen in patients receiving antibiotics, thereby suppressing normal flora; individuals with surgical or ulcerative disruption of the gastrointestinal mucosa, allowing *Candida* to enter the blood stream; and patients receiving corticosteroid therapy, whose cell-mediated immunity and neutrophil

TABLE 20–24. COMMON PATHOGENS ASSOCIATED WITH SPECIFIC IMMUNOLOGIC DEFECTS

Depression of:	Pathogens
Humoral immune response (globulins, B lymphocyte)	*Pneumococcus, Haemophilus*, gram-negative bacilli
Cellular immune response (macrophage, T lymphocyte)	Mycobacteria, *Candida, Cryptococcus, Listeria, Legionella, Salmonella, Nocardia*, herpes, *Toxoplasma*, cytomegalovirus
Neutrophil	Staphylococci, gram-negative bacilli, *Candida, Aspergillus*
Reticuloendothelial system (e.g., splenectomy)	*Pneumococcus, Haemophilus*, gram-negative bacilli

function are compromised. In individuals with depressed immunity resulting from HIV infection, neoplasia, and/or cancer chemotherapy, *Aspergillus, Cryptococcus, Histoplasma*, and *Coccidioides* may produce disease. The diagnosis of such infections requires a high index of suspicion, appropriate cultures (which frequently require tissue biopsy), and attempts at serologic diagnosis.

Viral infections occur primarily in individuals with depressed cell-mediated immunity. Infections in this category include herpes viruses (both varicella-zoster and herpes simplex), and cytomegalovirus. The defenses against protozoal and parasitic infections are combined humoral, phagocytic, and cell mediated. Cell-mediated immunity appears to play the most important role in the control of infection by most of these pathogens, particularly *P. carinii, Toxoplasma gondii*, and *Strongyloides stercoralis*. However, because most disease is associated with multiple immune defects, the differential diagnosis is wide and should not be limited by such categorization.

Treatment

It is clear that, in patients with neoplastic disease, infection is still the leading cause of death, and the risk of bacterial infection is proportional to the degree of neutropenia in such patients (Table 20–25). The treatment of infection in the compromised host requires a precise diagnosis because of the wide variety of microorganisms that may be implicated. An understanding of the type of immune defect in the individual will help to suggest particular pathogens.

In severe neutropenia, systemic bacterial infection must be suspected and empiric therapy begun at the onset of fever. Failure to do so may result

TABLE 20–25. RISK OF INFECTION IN NEUTROPENIA ASSOCIATED WITH MALIGNANCY

Neutrophil Count	Number of Episodes of Infection per 1000 Days
>1000/mm^3	5
500–1000/mm^3	10
100–500/mm^3	20
<100/mm^3	45

in death from overwhelming infection. The initial regimen should consist of two antibiotics, an aminoglycoside (either gentamicin, tobramycin, or amikacin), plus a β-lactam (such as ticarcillin, mezlocillin, ceftazidime). A double–β-lactam regimen (e.g., piperacillin plus cefotaxime) also may be used. Monotherapy with a single broad-spectrum antibiotic such as ceftazidime or imipenem recently has become popular but is not to be used without caution. Vancomycin may be a useful adjunct when methicillin-resistant diphtheroids or staphylococci are suspected, as in patients with indwelling central venous catheters. Blood and other accessible body fluids (or tissues) should be obtained for culture prior to initiation of therapy; serologic studies should be performed when indicated for fungi; and a history of exposure to tuberculosis, parasites, or animals should be documented. If feasible, intravenous and bladder catheters should be changed or removed because they may be the source of infection. If the infection is associated with a pulmonary focus, fiberoptic bronchoscopy and lavage, shielded brushing, or biopsy may be necessary to identify the pathogen. Failure to identify an offending pathogen may result in lack of response to therapy and worsening of the patient's condition. If an etiology is not established by routine work-up, physical examination, and repeated radiographs and cultures, additional empiric therapy in the face of continued immunosuppression may be indicated. Failure to respond to a combination of antibiotics in neutropenia may warrant the addition of empiric antifungal therapy. Neutropenic patients who become afebrile on empiric antibiotic therapy, even if a microorganism is not isolated, should be treated for a minimum of 14 days. While neutropenic, they will continue to be at risk of additional serious systemic bacterial or fungal infections. Clinical cure is ultimately dependent on bone marrow recovery.

Prophylactic antimicrobial agents are beneficial in certain situations (e.g., for prevention of *Pneumocystis* pneumonia), but other ancillary measures, such as granulocyte transfusions and protected environments (reverse isolation), are of questionable value. Supplemental immunoglobulin therapy is valuable for patients whose IgG level is less than 300 mg/dL, and careful attention to maintenance of normal skin and mucous membrane integrity is vital. Selected use of granulocyte or granulocyte/macrophage colony-stimulating factors has been shown to decrease the duration of neutropenia and its associated febrile morbidity. Further prevention of infection may be achieved by good nutrition; avoidance of invasive procedures and the indiscriminate use of antibiotics; avoidance of unnecessary hospitalization, when increased colonization with gram-negative, frequently multi–drug-resistant, bacilli may occur; and decreasing or eliminating immunosuppressive therapy as soon as possible.

RESPIRATORY TRACT INFECTION

Respiratory tract infection is one of the most common illnesses seen by the primary care physician. Ten per cent of hospital admissions are for the treatment of serious respiratory tract infections, and such infections are a major cause of mortality, particularly in those with underlying cardiopulmonary disease or alcoholism. Despite the introduction of antimicrobial agents, a large number of patients still die of pneumonia. These patients are usually elderly, with a variety of associated diseases, and present complex diagnostic and therapeutic problems.

Host Defenses Against Respiratory Infection

A variety of protective factors exist that prevent respiratory infections and maintain normal functioning of the bronchopulmonary tree.

The mouth, nasopharynx, and oropharynx are colonized by a variety of normal flora. Large numbers of aerobic gram-positive cocci (particularly viridans streptococci) and gram-negative cocci (*Neisseria* species), as well as anaerobic bacteria (*Fusobacterium*, anaerobic streptococci, and oral *Bacteroides* species), maintain the integrity of a mucosal defense system. Interference with this normal flora, such as by administering antibiotics, can increase susceptibility to colonization with more pathogenic organisms. Seasonal changes in normal flora do occur, with S. *pneumoniae* colonizing 15 to 30 per cent of normal individuals during the winter months. Expectorated sputum samples from such individuals may grow S. *pneumoniae*, reflecting only pharyngeal colonization.

Bronchial mucus secretion and ciliated respiratory epithelium remove most bacteria and fungi. In addition, secretory immunoglobulin (IgA) immobilizes bacteria and prevents their invasion. Absence of IgA and disrupted bronchial mucosa and ciliated epithelium, as is found in chronic obstructive pulmonary disease, cystic fibrosis, or acute influenza, increases the risk of pulmonary infection.

The cough and epiglottic reflexes prevent particulate matter from entering the lower respiratory tract. Impairment of these reflexes occurs in individuals with neurologic disease, alcoholism, or drug overdose and may lead to aspiration pneumonia. The final line of defense is alveolar macrophages, lymphocytes, neutrophils, and circulating immunoglobulin. Pneumonia can develop when there is a breakdown of any of these elements, such as in systemic immunodeficiency, neutropenia, or congestive heart failure with accumulation of alveolar fluid.

Viral infections predispose to bacterial pulmonary infections by damaging the bronchial epithelium, with a resultant decrease in mucociliary clearance and precipitation of infection by small amounts of aspirated oral flora. Small-volume aspiration is a common phenomenon in most individuals, but normal clearance mechanisms usually prevent disease.

Upper Respiratory Tract Infections

Upper respiratory tract infections are a frequent cause of visits to the family physician. Acute *pharyngitis* is usually due to viral upper respiratory tract infections, particularly rhinovirus and coronavirus. Adenovirus, herpes simplex, EBV, and cytomegalovirus also produce pharyngitis, which may be severe. Conjunctivitis accompanies adenoviral pharyngitis, and exudate is common with EBV or herpes simplex virus. Vesicles and shallow ulcers of the palate, gingiva, and lips suggest herpetic pharyngitis. Herpes esophagitis may occur as a result of mucosal inoculation with swallowed virus. This need not suggest underlying HIV infection.

Fifteen to 20 per cent of pharyngitis cases are bacterial, usually due to *Streptococcus pyogenes*. Occasionally, *Corynebacterium* species, particularly *diphtheriae*, gonorrhea, *Myocoplasma*, and *Chlamydia pneumoniae* are involved etiologically. Streptococcal pharyngitis is difficult to distinguish from severe viral pharyngitis. Exudate, tender cervical adenopathy, and high fever may or may not be present. Uvular edema is often pronounced. Infection may be complicated by scarlet fever as a result of the production of erythrogenic toxin, or rheumatic fever in cases of delayed treatment.

The development of rapid antigen detection tests has been a significant advance in the diagnosis and treatment of streptococcal pharyngitis, allowing early diagnosis and specific therapy. In the absence of such testing, empiric therapy may be useful but will overtreat a large number of severe or exudative viral pharyngitides. The presence of concomitant rhinorrhea or cough should suggest a nonbacterial etiology. Recent high-risk sexual exposure should raise suspicions of herpes simplex or gonococcal infection. Treatment of streptococcal pharyngitis is with oral penicillin or amoxicillin, erythromycin, or clindamycin. Clinical failures are frequently due to misdiagnosis of a viral infection, persistent suppurative foci with intratonsillar abscesses, or the presence of coexistent β-lactamase–producing organisms. Alternative measures in such cases include the use of a non–β-lactam compound, Augmentin, or prolonged therapy.

Otitis media is the most frequent diagnosis for illness in the first 3 years of life. By age 3, one third of children have had three or more episodes. Congestion of pharyngeal and eustachian tube mucosa resulting from viral infections produces obstruction complicated by suppuration. *Streptococcus pneumoniae, H. influenzae,* and *Moraxella catarrhalis* are the most frequent bacterial pathogens. Pure viral otitis media may account for 25 to 50 per cent of all cases. Although most cases of otitis media resolve within a few days after initiation of antimicrobial therapy, 50 per cent of children will still have middle ear fluid 1 month after onset.

The preferred antimicrobial agent for treatment of otitis media is amoxicillin. However, β-lactamase production in most *Moraxella* and 10 to 25 per cent of *Haemophilus* species, and the increasing prevalence of penicillin-resistant pneumococci, may require alternate therapy in children who do not respond promptly to treatment. Amoxicillin-clavulanate, trimethoprim–sulfamethoxazole, oral cephalosporins (such as cefixime, cefpodoxime, or cefuroxime) may be necessary. Toxicity with persistent or recurrent fever should prompt consideration of tympanocentesis to dictate better therapy. Nasal and oral decongestants are useful adjuncts. Chronic or recurrent otitis media may require consideration of long-term antimicrobial prophylaxis, administration of pneumococcal in addition to *Haemophilus* vaccine, or myringotomy. Such cases obviously require thoughtful evaluation by the otolaryngologist and infectious disease specialist.

Acute *sinusitis* is diagnosed more commonly in adults. Most cases are due to bacterial complications of viral upper respiratory tract infections or allergic conditions. Occasionally, obstructive processes such as polyps, deviated septa, or foreign bodies may precipitate infection. Sinusitis also may originate from maxillary dental infection or nasal packing for epistaxis.

Most cases of acute sinusitis are due to *S. pneumoniae, H. influenzae,* or *M. catarrhalis.* Less commonly, *S. aureus* or *S. pyogenes* are isolated. In chronic sinusitis, sinusitis of dental origin, or hospital-acquired disease, the flora may be more complex and include anaerobes or gram-negative bacilli. Complications include osteomyelitis or meningitis and brain abscess resulting from retrograde spread of infection through the dural venous sinuses. Diagnosis is facilitated by a thorough history and physical examination, including dental evaluation. Transillumination of maxillary and frontal sinuses may be helpful. Radiographic procedures, particularly CT scanning, may be necessary for confirmation.

Empiric therapy, as in otitis media, will produce a good response in most cases of acute sinusitis. Adjunctive therapy with nasal decongestants is helpful. In refractory cases, irrigation and drainage or surgical decompression may be necessary. Control of allergic rhinitis and corrective surgery for septal abnormalities may prevent recurrence. However, repeated instrumentation for therapeutic irrigation actually may promote mucosal edema and lead to superinfection with gram-negative bacilli, such as *Pseudomonas.*

Lower Respiratory Tract Infections

Infections in the Newborn

Bronchopulmonary infections are an important cause of morbidity in infants. Risk factors include prematurity and prolonged rupture of membranes prior to delivery. Congenital pneumonia, seen within the first few days of life, is acquired either transplacentally or from aspiration of infected amniotic or vaginal fluid. The latter is more common and is usually due to gram-negative bacilli (particularly *E. coli*) or group B streptococci. Occasionally staphylococci, other gram-negative bacilli, or *Chlamydia* may be the cause (Table 20–26).

Hospital-acquired neonatal pneumonia usually occurs between 2 and 14 days after birth. In these instances, pneumonia is usually the result of resuscitation efforts or contamination of infants by bacteria present on the hands of personnel in the nursery. Occasionally it is due to hematogenous spread of organisms from infected sites such as the umbilicus or an intravenous catheter. Staphylococci and gram-negative bacilli are the predominant pathogens.

The presentation of pneumonia in the newborn

TABLE 20–26. TYPES OF PNEUMONITIS ACCORDING TO AGE

Newborns
Escherichia coli, group B streptococci, *Staphylococcus aureus, Chlamydia*

Children Ages 1–8 Years
Viruses, *Streptococcus pneumoniae, Haemophilus influenzae*

Older Children, Young Adults
Mycoplasma pneumoniae, adenovirus, *Streptococcus pneumoniae*

Adults
Streptococcus pneumoniae, Haemophilus influenzae, oral anaerobes, *Staphylococcus aureus, Klebsiella, Legionella pneumophila, Mycoplasma pneumoniae, Chlamydia pneumoniae*

Immunocompromised Patients
All the above microorganisms, plus *Pneumocystis carinii, Nocardia asteroides, Aspergillus, Candida, Cryptococcus,* cytomegalovirus

is one of respiratory distress. The neonate may be cyanotic, may or may not be febrile, and usually has minimal sputum production. Grunting, intercostal retraction, and nasal flaring may be present. Radiographs show patchy infiltrates and are crucial for diagnosis because of the paucity of physical findings.

Chlamydial pneumonitis usually occurs between 3 and 6 weeks after birth. The onset is gradual, with a dry cough. The child is usually afebrile but has tachypnea and rales, and radiographs show hyperinflated lungs with patchy infiltrates. Conjunctivitis may be present, and eosinophilia is frequent. The diagnosis may be established by culture, enzyme immunoassay, or direct fluorescent antibody.

Bacteriologic diagnosis of pneumonitis in the newborn is necessary for specific therapy. Blood cultures and Gram's stains and cultures of tracheal or gastric aspirates are frequently helpful in diagnosis. Initial therapy should be directed at likely pathogens, including group B streptococci and gram-negative bacilli. Ampicillin plus gentamicin is the most commonly used regimen but should be altered according to the results of culture and susceptibility tests. Chlamydial pneumonitis is treated with erythromycin.

Infections in Children Ages 2 Months to 12 Years

Upper and lower respiratory tract infections account for 80 per cent of illnesses experienced by children. Normal children ages 3 to 5 years have six to eight infections per year, ranging from pharyngitis and otitis to pneumonia. Most lower respiratory tract infections in this age group are due to viruses, particularly respiratory syncytial virus (RSV), parainfluenza virus, and adenovirus. Of these, RSV and parainfluenza viruses are responsible for most lower respiratory tract illnesses below the age of 2 years. *Mycoplasma pneumoniae* produces most disease in the preadolescent and adolescent age group. Recurrent infections resulting from *H. influenzae* or pneumococcus, or diffuse lung infiltrates suggesting lymphoid interstitial pneumonia or *Pneumocystis*, should prompt a search for HIV infection (Chapter 21).

Croup occurs primarily in children 3 months to 3 years of age. It usually begins with a mild but distinctive cough that progressively worsens. There is little sputum production, but low-grade fever and associated coryza are present. The disease is primarily subepiglottic, and the epiglottis is not markedly inflamed or edematous. Croup is most often due to parainfluenza virus infection. Treatment is symptomatic, with a stress on humidification. Antibiotics are not indicated because this is a viral infection.

Epiglottitis occurs primarily in children 2 to 7 years of age. The illness is of sudden onset, with sore throat, high fever, hoarseness, dysphagia, drooling, and respiratory distress. Stridor may develop. Cough is not prominent, in contrast to croup. The epiglottis is edematous and cherry red. It should not be examined repeatedly because this may precipitate acute airway obstruction. Lateral soft tissue radiographs of the neck demonstrate an enlarged epiglottis. The etiology is usually *H. influenzae* type b, and cultures of pharynx and blood are frequently positive. The initial treatment of choice is a third-generation cephalosporin or cefuroxime modified when culture and susceptibility results are available.

Bronchiolitis occurs in children 6 months to 2 years of age and is most commonly due to RSV. It begins with a mild cough, coryza, and rhinorrhea, progressing to tachypnea, wheezing, and respiratory distress. Rales and rhonchi may be evident. Radiographs show hyperinflation, peribronchial cuffing, and perihilar infiltrates. The disease may be particularly severe in infants less than 1 year of age and may lead to respiratory failure. Treatment is primarily humidification and bronchodilation. Ribavirin is indicated for treatment of severe cases of RSV, but antibiotics should be reserved for bacterial superinfection.

Pneumonia in children is usually viral. When bacterial, *S. pneumoniae* and *H. influenzae* are the main causes. *Mycoplasma* in the child produces a tracheobronchitis rather than the pneumonia typical of young adulthood. Children with sickle cell disease are predisposed to particularly severe pneumococcal or *Mycoplasma* pneumonia.

Infections in the Adult

Acute bronchitis is an inflammation of the tracheobronchial tree. In patients without underlying lung disease, it is predominantly due to viruses such as influenza, adenovirus, and parainfluenza virus, occasionally *Mycoplasma*, and less frequently bacterial pathogens. The illness usually begins with rhinorrhea, sore throat, and coryza. Cough follows quickly and may persist after many of the upper respiratory symptoms have abated. Sputum production increases with duration of the illness, particularly in those who are smokers.

Physical examination reveals rhonchi and occasional wheezes. Rales and signs of consolidation are not present unless concomitant pneumonia exists. Fever is usually less than 101° F. Chest radiographs reveal no pulmonary infiltrates but may show peribronchial cuffing or hyperinflation. Laboratory studies are usually unremarkable.

Treatment should consist of hydration and possibly expectorants. Bronchodilators may be necessary if wheezing occurs. The role of antibiotics is unclear, but they are not indicated for most patients. If examination of the sputum reveals a predominant pathogen on Gram's stain or culture, antibiotics then may be useful.

Acute bacterial exacerbations of chronic bronchitis in patients with structural disease of the tracheobronchial tree represent a different problem.

Most of these patients have a history of smoking, chronic cough, and sputum production, and may have attendant pulmonary or cardiac insufficiency. These exacerbations frequently are manifested by an increase in sputum production, change in viscosity or color of sputum, and increasing dyspnea and wheezing. Most patients do not have chills, fever, or leukocytosis.

Evaluation of such patients is difficult. The sputum is usually full of leukocytes in the absence of an acute exacerbation. Organisms also may be present in such secretions. Although the exacerbations may be precipitated by a viral infection, a concomitant increase in leukocytosis or bacterial counts in the sputum of such patients suggests a bacterial component. Because *Haemophilus* species and pneumococci are the most commonly isolated organisms, antibiotic administration should be directed at these pathogens and is of value. Perhaps more important is attention to pulmonary toilet, discontinuance of smoking, bronchodilators, and humidification. Cough suppressants, antihistamines, and other drying agents should be avoided. Occasionally, pathogens other than *Haemophilus* species and *S. pneumoniae* may be present and may need alternative therapy, including parenteral antibiotics. Useful empiric agents include amoxicillin, tetracycline, and trimethoprim–sulfamethoxazole. If resistant flora are isolated, more potent oral agents such as cefuroxime, amoxicillin plus clavulanic acid, a fluoroquinolone, or macrolide may be effective.

Prophylactic administration of antibiotics to patients with a history of chronic bronchitis is of value in those individuals with severe underlying lung disease who have a history of repeated decompensation during the winter months. Cyclic antibiotic regimens include any of the previously mentioned three agents.

Pneumonia in the Adult

Identification of the etiologic agent of pneumonia is frequently difficult and requires a thorough history and physical examination and thoughtful interpretation of Gram's stains, cultures, and radiographic studies. Important clues to the diagnosis are patient age (Table 20–26), season, duration of illness, and concomitant clinical features such as alcoholism, loss of consciousness, underlying cardiac disease, travel history, exposure to birds or animals, recent surgical procedure or hospitalization, and concomitant extrapulmonary disease. Physical examination and radiographic findings are rarely specific, although certain suggestive features may emerge (Tables 20–27 and 20–28).

Influenza

Influenza is an illness of short incubation and rapid onset. Cough, malaise, chills, severe headache and retro-orbital pain, coryza, rhinorrhea, and watery eyes are common. Myalgias are marked, particularly in the low back and legs. Fever is prominent and may be as high as 104° F. Cough is usually nonproductive. Influenza occurs in epidemics, an important clue to its diagnosis.

The early phase of the illness is due to a bronchitis and there is decreased mucociliary clearance as a result of the direct effects of viral infection on the respiratory epithelium. These abnormalities predispose to bacterial superinfection. Typically this occurs after 5 to 7 days of illness, at which time the patient has begun to improve, when purulent sputum and return of fever suddenly develop. Physical examination now reveals signs of pneumonia. Organisms most commonly implicated include *S. pneumoniae, H. influenzae,* and *S. aureus.* Occasionally *Klebsiella* or *Moraxella* is a secondary infecting organism. Bacterial superinfection occurs particularly in smokers and in individuals with chronic bronchitis.

Influenza may require 2 to 4 weeks to resolve in the absence of superinfection, and postviral fatigue may be prominent, particularly in the elderly. Although no specific therapy of established infection is available, amantidine or rimantadine may be of value in speeding defervesence and decreasing the degree of peripheral airway resistance.

TABLE 20–27. DIFFERENTIAL CHARACTERISTICS OF BACTERIAL AND VIRAL OR *MYCOPLASMA* PNEUMONIA*

Feature	Bacterial	Mycoplasma/Viral/Chlamydia
Onset	Sudden	Gradual
Shaking chills	Common	Uncommon
Cough	Variable	Prominent
Fever	High	Low grade, <102°F
Tachycardia >120 bpm	Common	Uncommon
Tachypnea >30 breaths/min	Common	Uncommon
Chest pain	Common	Uncommon
Sputum	Purulent	Scant, mucoid
Radiographic consolidation	Frequent	Unusual
Pleural effusion	Occasional—large	Infrequent—small
Leukocytosis	Frequent	Rarely >12,000/mm^3

* None of these characteristics are absolute; they are most useful in the nondebilitated or nonimmunosuppressed host without significant underlying pulmonary disease.

TABLE 20-28.   RADIOGRAPHIC FINDINGS IN PNEUMONIA*

Bacterial Pneumonia

Pneumococcus	Usually RLL or LLL infiltrate or consolidation in healthy adult; bronchopneumonia in alcoholics or debilitated patients
Staphylococcus	Multiple infiltrates, early abscess formation, pneumatoceles
Klebsiella	Upper or RML consolidation, loss of volume, bulging fissure, early abscess formation
Haemophilus	Bronchopneumonia
Pseudomonas	Usually lower lobes, multiple small abscesses, perihilar infiltrates, wedge shaped
Anaerobes	Dependent areas, lower lobes, right greater than left, empyema, abscess
Legionella	Patchy alveolar infiltrates, lobar or segmental

Nonbacterial Pneumonia

Adenovirus	Diffuse interstitial infiltrates
Cytomegalovirus	Diffuse interstitial infiltrates
Influenza	Diffuse interstitial infiltrates
Varicella	Fine, widespread nodular infiltrates, especially lower lobes
Psittacosis	Perihilar infiltrates, often bilateral
Mycoplasma, chlamydia	Scattered patchy infiltrates, small effusions, rare consolidation
Tuberculosis	Child: lower or middle lobe infiltrate, hilar adenopathy; adult: upper lobe, cavitary; HIV: any, frequently atypical

Fungal Pneumonia

Aspergillus	Perihilar, necrotizing, wedge shaped (infarct)
Histoplasmosis	Perihilar and diffuse with adenopathy; calcifications; upper lobe, cavitary
Cryptococcosis	Basilar streaky to dense infiltrate
Coccidioidomycosis	Multiple infiltrates, pleural effusions, thin-walled cavities

Other

Pneumocystis	Perihilar and interstitial infiltrates, "ground glass," bilateral, extensive, more variable in HIV

* LLL, left lower lobe; RLL, right lower lobe; RML, right middle lobe.

Consideration should be given to prophylaxis of influenza by *annual* vaccination (in October or November) of susceptible individuals (Table 20–29). Current vaccines are safe and effective. Two to 3 weeks are required after vaccination for immunity to develop. Amantidine or rimantadine are less satisfactory but also effective methods of prevention of influenza A infection. They must be taken daily (200 mg/day) to be effective. Pneumococcal vaccine also should be administered to high-risk patients, including asplenic patients. One dose of pneumococcal vaccine provides effective immunity for at least 5 years after administration. It does not need to be repeated annually.

Bacterial Pneumonia

Pneumonia caused by *Mycoplasma pneumoniae* or *C. pneumoniae* (TWAR) occurs most frequently, although by no means exclusively, in young adults. The onset is gradual, with a hacking, nonproductive cough. Later, scant, white then purulent, sputum appears as bronchial epithelial cells slough and initiate a polymorphonuclear leukocyte response. At this time differentiation from bacterial disease may be difficult. Systemic symptoms are prominent and include malaise, headache, and fever between 100° and 103° F. Rash, serous otitis, and joint symptoms occasionally may accompany the pulmonary complaints of *Mycoplasma* infection. Pharyngitis is common in *Chlamydia* infections. Additionally helpful diagnostic features include occurrence in the late summer and early fall, associated family cluster of respiratory complaints, or an outbreak in a summer camp or similar institution.

Physical findings may be unremarkable. Auscultation of the chest reveals only scattered rhonchi or fine localized rales in most cases. The radiograph, in contradistinction to the benign physical exam, is often impressive, with fine or patchy lower lobe or perihilar infiltrates. Consolidation may occur, particularly in older patients, and small pleural effusions are not uncommon. Laboratory data reveal white blood cell counts of 10,000 to

TABLE 20-29.   TARGET GROUPS FOR INFLUENZA VACCINE

Groups at greatest risk of influenza-related complications
1. Adults and children with chronic cardiovascular or pulmonary diseases
2. Residents of nursing homes or other chronic care facilities

Groups at modest risk of influenza-related complications
1. Otherwise healthy individuals over 65 years of age
2. Adults and children with diabetes mellitus, renal dysfunction, anemia, immunosuppression or immunodeficiency (including HIV infection)
3. Children (6 months through 18 years of age) receiving long-term aspirin therapy

Groups capable of nosocomial transmission
1. Physicians, nurses, and other medical care personnel having extensive contact with high-risk patients
2. Providers to high-risk patients in the home care setting, including family members

Any individuals who wish to receive vaccine to reduce their chance of acquiring influenza infection

15,000/mm^3 with a polymorphonuclear leukocyte predominance. Cold agglutinin titers may be helpful early in *Mycoplasma* infections but are not specific and are negative in approximately one third of cases. The diagnosis of *Mycoplasma* is confirmed by acute and convalescent complement fixation titers. *Chlamydia pneumoniae* serology, both IgG and IgM, is now performed reliably in many laboratories. Although cultures can be done, they are uncommonly available.

The treatment of choice is erythromycin, tetracycline, or a new macrolide such as clarithromycin or azithromycin. Symptomatic improvement occurs with administration of any of these agents, but cough and malaise may persist. Therapy should continue for 3 weeks. The organism may not be eradicated from the sputum and therefore secondary cases in the family may still occur. Even in the absence of treatment, resolution is spontaneous in the vast majority of patients. Persistent cough with wheezing may follow an episode of *Chlamydia* pneumonia for 3 to 6 months.

Nonbacterial Pneumonia

Other, nonbacterial pneumonias may be seen in both children and adults. *Adenoviral* pneumonia cannot be differentiated clinically or radiographically from *Mycoplasma* pneumonia. *Psittacosis* occurs in individuals exposed to infected birds. Sporadic cases most frequently are associated with parrots or parakeets, although outbreaks occasionally occur in poultry processing plants or from contacts with infected turkeys. The onset is usually abrupt, with prominent dry cough and severe headache. Temperature–pulse dissociation is frequent, and infiltrates may be perihilar or peripheral. The infection responds promptly to administration of tetracycline. Q fever and tularemia pneumonia are extremely rare.

Fungal Pneumonia

Fungal pneumonia should be considered in the differential diagnosis of nonbacterial pneumonia. Travel to the Southwest should suggest coccidioidomycosis. Exposure to bird droppings, chickens, or starlings should suggest histoplasmosis. Cryptococcal pulmonary disease also should be suggested in this setting. All of these illnesses present with moderate fever, flu-like symptoms, and a nonproductive cough. Their presence or absence should be considered by appropriate history. The diagnosis is made serologically and by examination of lung tissue. Cultures are rarely positive in the early stages of such illnesses.

Pneumocystis Pneumonia

Pneumocystis pneumonia must be considered in the young adult with fever and nonproductive cough, especially when a history of sexual promiscuity or intravenous drug abuse is elicited. Chest radiograph findings may be subtle, but dyspnea,

hypoxemia, thrush, and other signs of HIV infection may be present.

Legionella *Pneumonia*

Legionella infection is relatively common, accounting for approximately 2 to 10 per cent of community-acquired pneumonias. *Legionella* also may cause a hospital-acquired pneumonia, particularly in immunosuppressed or transplant patients. *Legionella pneumophila* is a weakly gram-negative–staining bacillus whose source is usually water (e.g., showerheads or faucets) and soil (particularly in areas of excavation). Person-to-person transmission is not important. Disease is most common in the summer and fall.

Fever, myalgias, chills, and a nonproductive cough occur 2 to 10 days after exposure. Abdominal pain, nausea, vomiting, and confusion may be prominent. Most patients are male, elderly, and smokers. Physical examination reveals an acutely ill patient with a temperature of 103° to 105° F. Rales and rhonchi may be present, but signs of consolidation are not found early. Radiographic findings vary from patchy infiltrates to lobar consolidation. Solitary lung abscesses have been reported, and pleural effusions may occur.

Laboratory data reveal a leukocytosis, sometimes exceeding 20,000/mm^3. Other findings are proteinuria, hyponatremia, and hypophosphatemia. Sputum Gram's stains are negative, but fluorescent antibody stains and DNA probes are available to identify the organisms in respiratory secretions. A special medium (charcoal yeast extract agar) is necessary to isolate the organism, with greatest yields obtained from bronchoscopic specimens or transtracheal aspirates. The diagnosis can be confirmed serologically, allowing 3 weeks between acute and convalescent serology and demonstrating a fourfold antibody rise.

Legionella infections carry a high mortality, in part because of delayed diagnosis and because the infection is frequent in elderly and immunosuppressed patients. The diagnosis should be considered in an individual with rapidly progressive pneumonia, with no organisms isolated by standard culture techniques, and who does not respond to usual antibiotic therapy. Mortality in the absence of specific therapy is over 50 per cent. With appropriate antibiotics, this mortality can be reduced to 10 per cent. Erythromycin is the drug of choice, administered at a dose of 3 to 4 gm/day, intravenously initially, for 3 weeks. Rifampin, trimethoprim–sulfamethoxazole, tetracycline, or a fluoroquinolone may be useful alternative agents.

Pneumococcal Pneumonia

Streptococcus pneumoniae (pneumococcus) is the most common cause of pneumonia in the adult, with an incidence of one to two cases per 1000 individuals per year. Pneumococcal pneumonia is also common in small children, especially those with sickle cell disease or immunoglobulin dysfunction. Underlying diseases in the adult, such as chronic lung or cardiac disorders, alcoholism with cirrhosis, diabetes mellitus, and HIV infections, predispose to illness. Pneumococcal pneumonia is most frequent during the winter months.

The classic presentation of pneumococcal pneumonia is a sudden onset of fever, pleuritic chest pain, and cough with purulent or rusty sputum. Antecedent viral upper or lower respiratory tract infection is present in many cases. However, atypical presentations are common, particularly in the elderly and alcoholic populations. In such patients, fever may be low grade, behavior disturbances may seem more significant than respiratory symptoms, and cough may not be prominent. Patients appear acutely ill, frequently with dyspnea and chest splinting. Signs of consolidation are frequently present, a pleural friction rub or signs of pleural fluid may be present, and there may be abdominal pain and ileus.

Laboratory findings include an elevated white blood cell count with a left shift. In the elderly or alcoholic patient, however, the white count may be normal or depressed. Chest radiograph usually shows disease confined to one lobe, frequently a lower lobe, but several lobes may be involved with either consolidation or bronchopneumonia. Chronic changes in the lung architecture in chronic lung disease make both auscultation and radiographic analysis difficult, so the presence of pneumonia may be unclear. Gram's stain of the sputum will show polymorphonuclear leukocytes and "lancet-shaped" gram-positive diplococci. However, up to 40 per cent of patients with bacteremic pneumococcal pneumonia will have negative sputum cultures, so that blood cultures should be obtained in all patients. Because bacteremia is so common and because meningitis or other metastatic foci of infection also may occur, alteration in mental status should be viewed with suspicion and lumbar punctures performed in such cases.

The treatment of uncomplicated pneumococcal pneumonia is with parenteral penicillin G, 6 to 18 million units/day until afebrile. The emergence of penicillin-resistant strains now requires close attention to clinical response and consultation with the microbiology laboratory. A third-generation cephalosporin or vancomycin may be necessary. In the penicillin-allergic patient, erythromycin or a first-generation cephalosporin (e.g., cefazolin) may be used. Attention should be paid to adequate hydration, oxygenation and ventilatory support, postural drainage, and adequate humidification. Pleural effusions, if present, should be aspirated diagnostically and empyemas drained.

Staphylococcal Pneumonia

Staphylococcal pneumonia accounts for less than 5 per cent of adult pneumonia, but carries a high mortality. It is seen particularly in the wake of influenza and as a hospital-acquired infection. In addition, staphylococcal pneumonia is seen as a consequence of bacteremic spread from another focus of infection, particularly endocarditis in the intravenous drug user.

The clinical features of staphylococcal pneumonia are frequently more striking than the radiographic examination. Recurrent chills, high spiking fever, dyspnea, cyanosis, and pleuritic chest pain are common. Sputum is frequently purulent, with blood streaking. Physical findings are variable, but a pleural effusion and pleural friction rub frequently are detected. Leukocytosis is usually marked. Chest radiograph findings include multiple infiltrates with abscess formation, empyema, pyopneumothorax, and pneumatoceles (thin-walled cavities). Sputum examination usually shows many polymorphonuclear leukocytes and gram-positive cocci in clusters. However, in bacteremic staphylococcal pneumonia, the sputum may be normal.

The treatment of staphylococcal pneumonia is with parenteral administration of an antistaphylococcal penicillin, such as oxacillin, in a dose of 8 to 12 gm/day in the adult and 100 to 200 mg/kg/day in the child. Cephalosporins or vancomycin are alternative therapy. Blood cultures always should be performed prior to therapy. Tricuspid valve endocarditis always should be considered in the intravenous drug user. The presence of pleural fluid should prompt evaluation for empyema, with surgical drainage as necessary. Despite effective therapy, the severity of illness and the rapidity of its progression contribute to the still-high mortality of 20 to 30 per cent.

Aerobic Gram-Negative Bacillary Pneumonia

Aerobic gram-negative bacillary pneumonia accounts for less than 20 per cent of community-acquired pneumonia but for 50 per cent or more of hospital-associated cases. Most pneumonia deaths in the hospital setting are due to these organisms. Gram-negative pneumonia is usually acquired by aspiration of endogenous oropharyngeal flora in those individuals colonized with gram-negative bacilli. It is seen less commonly as a complication of contaminated aerosols, particularly in patients on ventilatory support for other pulmonary conditions, or as a complication of bacteremia from an extrapulmonary source. Pharyngeal colonization with gram-negative bacilli varies from less than 10 per cent in the normal host to over 50 per cent in the debilitated, hospitalized, particularly bedridden, individual. Twenty-five per cent of colonized and intubated patients will develop gram-negative pneumonia.

Haemophilus influenzae produces pneumonia in infants and children and in the elderly. As a cause of childhood pneumonia, it frequently is associated with bacteremia. In elderly patients, chronic bronchitis and alcoholism are usual concomitant illnesses. Radiographs show patchy, bilateral infiltrates, and the sputum Gram's stain is usually diagnostic.

Klebsiella pneumonia typically is seen in elderly males with a history of alcoholism or other underlying lung disease. It is also an important cause of pneumonia in nursing homes and in hospitalized patients. The onset is sudden, with severe toxicity. Pleuritic chest pain and hemoptysis are features. Sputum is thick, often bloody.

Pseudomonas pulmonary infections occur as a result of aspiration of pharyngeal flora; from seeding of the lung by bacteremia from distant foci; and from aerosols of contaminated solutions. *Pseudomonas* pneumonia associated with bacteremia occurs in individuals with severely compromised host defenses, such as neoplasia with neutropenia, severe burns, or prolonged confinement in an intensive care unit. The mortality in bacteremic *Pseudomonas* pneumonia is over 75 per cent. This is primarily a reflection of severity of underlying disease in the host rather than an attribute of the microorganism per se.

Therapy of all gram-negative bacillary pneumonias depends on the antimicrobial susceptibility of the involved microorganisms, and single-drug therapy, particularly with newer and more potent agents, will be adequate in many cases. In addition to specific antibiotic therapy, adequate humidification, oxygenation, and ventilation is necessary. Intubation may be appropriate for such patients but provides an added risk of superinfection.

Laboratory Diagnosis of Pneumonia

Sputum examination and culture are essential for appropriate diagnosis of pneumonia. Saliva or nasopharyngeal secretions are of little value in determining the etiology. Whether secretions are obtained by expectoration, endotracheal suction, or bronchoscopy, such material must be confirmed adequate by smear. If there are more than 25 squamous epithelial cells per low-power field of specimen, such material should be considered inadequate for culture because it represents oral flora. Expectorated sputum is adequate for culture if fewer than 5 epithelial cells are present per low-power field and polymorphonuclear leukocytes are seen. The neutropenic patient may have no neutrophils seen on smear but should have no epithelial cells in the specimen. The morphology of a microorganism may enable a presumptive diagnosis from Gram's stain alone, but it is not distinctive in most instances. Transtracheal cultures or bronchoscopic specimens obtained by shielded brush techniques may be cultured anaerobically or for fastidious organisms such as *Legionella.* Anaerobic cultures of expectorated sputum samples are of no value, because they contain oral anaerobic flora.

Differential Diagnosis of Pneumonia

Other conditions may mimic the signs and symptoms of pneumonia. *Pulmonary emboli* should be considered, particularly in individuals with prolonged bed rest, recent immobilization, or abdominal or pelvic surgery. *Atelectasis* in the postoperative patient may present with fever and linear infiltrates. *Mucus plugging* may cause segmental or lobar atelectasis with or without infection. *Pulmonary contusion* secondary to trauma may present as pleuritic chest pain, fever, and tachypnea with infiltrates on chest radiograph. *Congestive heart failure* may be manifested by nonproductive cough and dyspnea. However, fever is unusual, sputum production is minimal, and cardiomegaly is usually present on radiograph.

Anaerobic Lung Disease

Anaerobic lung infection is usually due to aspiration of oral microorganisms, although occasionally metastatic foci from an anaerobic infection distant to the lung may be the cause. Predisposing factors to anaerobic pleuropulmonary infections include those conditions that result in altered consciousness or dysphagia and are primarily structural or functional rather than immunologic. Alcoholism, seizure disorders, narcotic addiction, sedative overdose, esophageal dysfunction resulting from tumor or motility disorder, cerebrovascular accidents, gastrointestinal disease with prolonged vomiting, or neurologic defects frequently are present. Local pulmonary conditions such as infarction, obstruction resulting from carcinoma, bronchiectasis, or foreign bodies are also important risk factors. Anaerobic pulmonary infections are located in dependent segments, particularly the posterior segments of the upper lobes and the superior segments of the lower lobes.

Pleuropulmonary disease resulting from anaerobes may take several forms. Simple pneumonitis, necrotizing pneumonia, lung abscess, or empyema may occur. Necrotizing pneumonia may be rapidly progressive, whereas lung abscesses are usually indolent. The majority of patients with lung abscesses have symptoms for over 7 days; fever, weight loss, and other constitutional symptoms are common. Foul-smelling sputum is a helpful sign but its absence does not rule out an anaerobic pulmonary infection. Furthermore, although aspiration pneumonia is usually due to anaerobes, the edentulous patient, lacking gingivae, which are the source of anaerobes, may have an aerobic pneumonia resulting from aspiration. In hospitalized patients, although anaerobes may be present, colonizing gram-negative aerobes may be important copathogens.

Penicillin G or clindamycin is the antibiotic of choice for anaerobic pleuropulmonary infections. Tetracycline, erythromycin, and cephalosporin de-

TABLE 20–30. GRAM-NEGATIVE BACTEREMIA IN THE UNITED STATES

Microorganism	Per Cent of Cases	Per Cent Mortality
E. coli	35	30
Klebsiella	25	38
Pseudomonas	15	54
Bacteroides	10	30
Proteus	10	33
Enterobacter	5	25
Serratia	4	37

rivatives also may be effective in some patients. Patients with lung abscesses usually have adequate drainage via the bronchial tree by expectoration of sputum. If there is obstruction, however, drainage may need to be established surgically. Anaerobic empyema demands surgical drainage.

SEPSIS AND BACTEREMIA

Epidemiology

In the 1930s and the 1940s, 90 per cent of all bacteremia was due to gram-positive microorganisms; most of these were streptococci and staphylococci. After the introduction of penicillin and streptomycin in the 1940s, the rate of gram-positive sepsis fell markedly relative to gram-negative sepsis. By the 1970s and early 1980s, three fourths of all bacteremia was due to gram-negative bacilli. However, in the past decade, gram-positive organisms have re-emerged as the most prevalent causes of bacteremia as a result of the exponential use of indwelling intravascular devices (chiefly implantable central lines and vascular access ports) and the overuse of extended-spectrum cephalosporins. Between 14 and 16 cases of bacteremia occur for every 1000 hospital admissions. This is triple the rate for 1970 and ten times the rate for 1950. *Escherichia coli* is the single most common gram-negative pathogen, accounting for 30 to 40 per cent of cases, followed by *Klebsiella, Enterobacter,* and *Bacteroides* (Table 20–30). Approximately 10 per cent of patients have polymicrobial bacteremia.

Knowing the source of bacteremia allows one to predict the pathogen (Table 20–31). Genitourinary tract infections cause 40 per cent of all septic epi-

sodes, usually resulting from *E. coli, Proteus,* or *Pseudomonas.* The gastrointestinal tract, respiratory tract, skin, and soft tissues are additional sources in decreasing order of frequency. Soft tissue infections include such sources as decubitus or venous stasis ulcers, subcutaneous abscesses, and cellulitis from intravenous sites (Figure 20–1).

Septic Shock

Not all bacteremia is accompanied by clinical shock. The factors that determine whether shock will occur are not clearly understood, although it is the cell wall lipopolysaccharide, or endotoxin in gram-negative bacilli, that provokes most of the biochemical, functional, and clinical changes that characterize septic shock. Endotoxin directly injures endothelial cells, resulting in prostaglandin synthesis, exposure of vascular collagen, and activation of Hageman factor with subsequent complement, kinin, and clotting factor consumption. Endotoxin also interacts with macrophages to release interleukin-1, which causes fever and leukocytosis, and tumor necrosis factor or cachectin, which further activates prostaglandin and leukotriene systems. The resultant endothelial damage, vascular dilation, increased vascular permeability, and capillary occlusion diminish microcirculation to vital organs, with resultant tissue hypoxia. Peripheral oxygen utilization is decreased, lactic acidosis develops, and, if the process continues, cell death and patient demise will follow.

The clinical manifestations of septicemia may be subtle (Table 20–32). In early septic shock the patient is warm, vasodilated, hypotensive, tachycardic, and tachypneic. The patient may or may not be febrile. As a consequence of tissue hypoxia, the patient may be agitated or confused. The urine output in early septic shock may be good, but the central venous pressure will be low, reflecting a decreased intravascular volume as a result of venous pooling and loss of fluid through damaged vessel walls. As septic shock progresses, vasoconstriction supervenes. The patient becomes cold, mottled, and dusky. Blood pressure remains low, the pulse is weak, and myocardial contractility is now impaired. The patient becomes more acidotic, tachypneic, and confused. Urine output decreases, and a paralytic ileus may be prominent. Diffuse rales

TABLE 20–31. SOURCE OF BACTEREMIA AND PATHOGENS TO BE SUSPECTED

Source	Per Cent of Cases	Most Common Pathogens
Genitourinary	40	E. coli, Proteus mirabilis, Pseudomonas, Candida
Gastrointestinal	25	E. coli, Klebsiella, Bacteroides, Streptococcus, Candida
Respiratory	20	Pneumococcus, Staphylococcus, Enterobacter, Pseudomonas
Skin and soft tissue	15	Streptococcus, Staphylococcus, Bacteroides, Enterobacter, E. coli, Pseudomonas

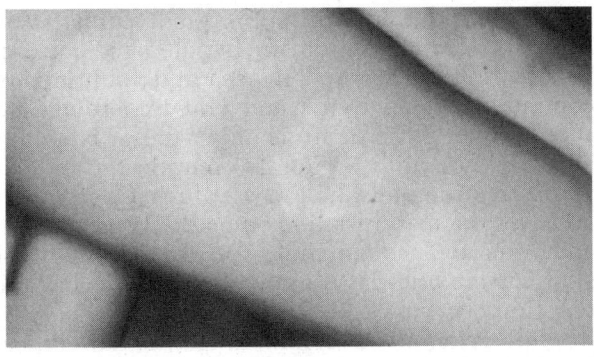
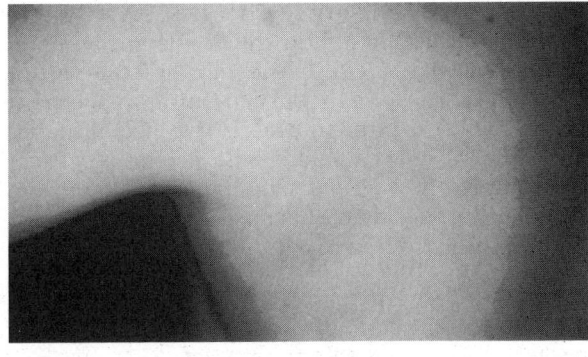

A **B**

FIGURE 20–1. Erythema chronicum migrans of the forearm of a four-year-old child *(A)* and the shoulder of a 25-year-old man *(B)*. Note the central vesiculation.

are audible throughout the lungs and reflect a combination of cardiac and noncardiac pulmonary edema resulting from vascular damage.

The laboratory findings in septic shock are numerous. The most reproducible hematologic abnormality is thrombocytopenia resulting from disseminated intravascular coagulation. Elevated prothrombin time and thrombin time and increased fibrin split products are observed. Although the biochemical parameters of disseminated intravascular coagulation are reversed with heparin, the use of heparin does not decrease the mortality or morbidity of septic shock. Other hematologic abnormalities in sepsis include an early rise in hematocrit resulting from hemoconcentration, and a later fall resulting from hemolysis in conjunction with disseminated intravascular coagulation. The white blood cell count initially falls as a result of margination of cells and perhaps as a direct effect of endotoxin on the release of neutrophils from the bone marrow. Subsequently, the white count should rise in a response appropriate to the severity of infection.

The hemodynamics of septic shock change with time. Early on, the total peripheral resistance is low and the cardiac output is normal or high. Central venous and pulmonary artery pressures are low as a result of venous pooling and vasodilation. As septic shock progresses, total peripheral resistance rises and cardiac output falls. The central venous and pulmonary artery pressures may remain low if fluid losses are not replaced.

TABLE 20–32. VARIED CLINICAL MANIFESTATIONS OF SEPSIS

Chills, fever, hypotension
Hyperpnea, tachypnea, respiratory alkalosis
Unexplained confusion, agitation
Oliguria or anuria
Thrombocytopenia
Tachycardia
Paralytic ileus
Metabolic acidosis

The pulmonary findings in septic shock are those of noncardiac pulmonary edema, or adult respiratory distress syndrome, as a result of vascular damage with leakage of intravascular fluid into interstitial spaces. Intravascular aggregates of platelets, neutrophils, and fibrin are observed microscopically. Arterial blood gases initially show a respiratory alkalosis, with decreased pCO_2 and decreased pO_2 resulting from ventilation–perfusion abnormalities and interstitial edema. Subsequently, metabolic acidosis appears as a result of accumulation of lactic acid.

Renal function in septic shock remains normal early. Renal blood flow and urine flow decrease later. Oliguric renal failure in septic shock has an extremely poor prognosis, with a mortality greater than 50 per cent in most series.

Treatment

The treatment of septic shock is logical if one understands its pathophysiology. Treatment is twofold: (1) restoration of the microcirculation, and (2) elimination of the microorganism. Attempts to modify the effects of endotoxin and other biochemical mediators of septic shock through the use of immune modulators or antiendotoxin antibodies are subjects of active study but have not yet proven clinically valuable.

Intravenous fluids are important early in treatment. They should be administered aggressively while monitoring central venous or pulmonary artery pressure and urine output. Intravascular volume measurements are particularly important in late septic shock, when myocardial depression and/or renal failure may have developed. The fluid deficit may be several liters prior to adequate repletion of intravascular volume. Isotonic saline is the preferred solution. Supplemental colloid in the form of albumin, fresh frozen plasma, or whole blood also may be of value.

Partial correction of metabolic acidosis should be attempted. Overcorrection may lead to cerebral vasoconstriction, hypokalemia, and a leftward shift in the oxyhemoglobin dissociation curve, with decreased oxygen delivery to vital tissues. The role of corticosteroids in septic shock is controversial. Recent evidence suggests they are of little value.

Vasopressors are secondary to fluid replacement in importance. Administration in the face of inadequate intravascular volume will exacerbate vasoconstriction and worsen tissue hypoxia. Dopamine is the preferred agent because it produces less renal vasoconstriction than other compounds when used in the correct dosage.

Antibiotics should be selected based on the spectrum of activity necessary to cover most anticipated pathogens (Table 20–31). They are always given intravenously to assure total and adequate absorption. A two-drug or even three-drug regimen may be necessary to assure adequate coverage of potential gram-negative and gram-positive pathogens based on their anticipated susceptibility patterns (Table 20–2). One also must look for a correctable lesion, such as an abscess, an obstructing ureteral stone, or an infected intravenous site, that can be eliminated.

The prognosis is primarily dependent on the severity of the host's underlying disease. Patients with rapidly fatal underlying disease (such as acute leukemia or acute renal failure) have a mortality of up to 80 per cent, compared with patients with nonfatal underlying disease (such as trauma or surgery), among whom the mortality is 20 per cent. Mortality increases with age, a gastrointestinal or respiratory tract source versus a genitourinary tract source, and acquisition of infection in the hospital rather than the community. Finally, prognosis is also dependent on early recognition of infection, vigorous treatment of shock, and prompt administration of an appropriate antimicrobial agent.

Toxic Shock Syndrome

Several toxin-mediated syndromes appear clinically similar to septic shock. Staphylococcal toxic shock syndrome is the most well described, although recent reports indicate that some strains of S. *pyogenes* can produce a similar clinical illness. Originally described in 1978, staphylococcal toxic shock syndrome received more widespread publicity in 1980 when its association with tampon use became evident. Despite changes in tampon use and structure, several hundred cases of toxic shock syndrome occur annually, now predominantly nonmenstrual. Such patients are likely to be colonized or infected with toxin-producing strains of S. *aureus* in the upper respiratory tract, or to have soft tissue foci such as postoperative wound infections. Nonmenstrual cases are divided equally between men and women.

The clinical manifestations of toxic shock syndrome vary from fulminant shock with multiple organ failure to milder cases manifested primarily by fever and rash. Temperature of over 102° F, dif-fuse erythroderma with subsequent palmar desquamation, and symptomatic hypotension occur in most patients. Diarrhea, nausea and vomiting are common. Conjunctivitis and oral hyperemia are seen in over three quarters of patients. Myalgia is also common and frequently complicated by elevated creatine phosphokinase values. Central nervous system manifestations include disorientation and lethargy, but generally no focal findings or signs of meningitis. Abnormal renal and hepatic function occur in over 50 per cent of patients and thrombocytopenia is common. Additional clinical findings of importance include headache, edema of the hands and feet, abdominal pain, and patchy hair or nail loss subsequent to recovery.

The treatment of toxic shock syndrome is primarily hemodynamic support, removal of any sequestered focus of staphylococci (such as tampon removal or abscess drainage), and the administration of an effective antistaphylococcal antibiotic. Aggressive treatment usually leads to full recovery. The risk of recurrence in menstrually associated toxic shock syndrome varies from 20 to 40 per cent and should interdict future tampon use. The role of adrenocortical steroids in the treatment of this disease has not been well studied.

The differential diagnosis of toxic shock syndrome should include other hypotensive illnesses, such as septicemic or hemorrhagic shock, and illnesses associated with similar cutaneous manifestations, such as leptospirosis, scarlet fever, Kawasaki disease, and drug eruptions. Appropriate cultures, serologic testing, history and physical exam, and appreciation of the spectrum of illness of toxic shock syndrome should allow differentiation among these various illnesses.

SEXUALLY TRANSMITTED DISEASES

Although syphilis and gonorrhea are considered the prototypic venereal diseases, it is clear that a host of viral, bacterial, and protozoal pathogens may be transmitted by sexual activity. This is particularly true for anal sex. Furthermore, the incidence of most sexually transmitted diseases (STDs) is increasing annually despite educational programs stemming from the acquired immunodeficiency syndrome (AIDS) epidemic. Pathogens with documented sexual transmission are listed in Table 20–33. It is useful to approach the differential diagnosis of STDs by the manifestations of infection (Table 20–34), whether they be exudative or ulcerative.

Gonorrhea

Although second in frequency to nongonococcal urethritis in men, gonorrhea remains a major public health problem with serious systemic conse-

TABLE 20–33. SEXUALLY TRANSMITTED DISEASES

Agent	Disease
Bacteria	
Neisseria gonorrhoeae	Gonorrhea
Treponema pallidum	Syphilis
Haemophilus ducreyi	Chancroid
Calymmatobacterium granulomatis	Granuloma inguinale
Gardnerella (prev. *Corynebacterium* or *Haemophilus*) *vaginalis*	"Nonspecific" vaginitis
Shigella, Salmonella	Gastroenteritis
Campylobacter species	Gastroenteritis, proctitis
Mycobacterium tuberculosis	Genital tuberculosis
Chlamydia/Ureaplasma	
C. *trachomatis* (serotypes L_1–L_3)	Lymphogranuloma venereum
C. *trachomatis* (serotypes D–K)	Nongonococcal urethritis, cervicitis, proctitis
U. (prev. *Mycoplasma*) *urealyticum*	Nongonococcal urethritis
Viruses	
Herpes simplex virus	Herpes genitalis, proctitis
Papillomavirus	Genital warts
Poxvirus (?)	Molluscum contagiosum
Cytomegalovirus (CMV)	CMV mononucleosis, disseminated CMV
Hepatitis B virus	Hepatitis B (serum hepatitis)
Human immunodeficiency virus	AIDS
Fungi	
Candida species	Vaginitis; balanitis
Parasites	
Trichomonas vaginalis	Trichomonas vaginitis, urethritis
Giardia lamblia	Giardiasis
Entamoeba histolytica	Amebiasis
Enterobius vermicularis	Vaginitis (pinworm)
Phthirus pubis	Pediculosis pubis
Sarcoptes scabei	Scabies

quences, particularly in women. Almost half-a-million cases are reported annually. Seventy per cent of infected women are asymptomatic and represent the reservoir for the heterosexual population. About 10 per cent of heterosexual men are also asymptomatic, as are homosexual men who engage in anal intercourse. The disease transmits almost entirely by sexual means, because the gonococcus is unable to survive even short periods outside the human body. Uninfected women exposed to infected men during sexual intercourse will become infected 50 to 70 per cent of the time. In contrast, only 20 to 30 per cent of men exposed to infected women will become infected. Gonorrhea is an illness that fails to confer immunity; therefore, reinfection is the rule.

Local symptoms in men occur after an incubation period of 3 to 7 days. Typically, urethritis manifests as burning on urination and a spontaneous, purulent penile discharge. Individuals engaging in anal intercourse may develop proctitis, although the majority of rectally infected individuals are asymptomatic. Proctitis is manifested by tenesmus and pain or burning on defecation. Anoscopy reveals punctate ulcerations and intraluminal pus. Most anal symptoms in individuals engaging in rectal intercourse are due to local trauma or fissures rather than proctitis. Pharyngitis may occur in individuals engaging in oral–genital sex, although many of these individuals also will be asymptomatic. There are no characteristic clinical manifestations of gonococcal pharyngitis, and the appearance of the throat is variable. Conjunctivitis may occur as a result of direct inoculation of gonococcus into the conjunctivae. Rapid progression and corneal ulceration ensue if treatment is not prompt. Failure of treatment in men may result in spread of infection to the posterior urethra, prostate, seminal vesicles, and epididymis. Untreated urethritis may result in urethral stricture and the later sequela of obstructive uropathy.

Localized cervical and vaginal colonization is

TABLE 20–34. MANIFESTATIONS OF SEXUALLY TRANSMISSIBLE DISEASE

Diseases Manifested by Discharges
Gonorrhea
Nongonococcal urethritis

Diseases Manifested by Ulcers
Syphilis
Herpes simplex
Chancroid
Granuloma inguinale

Diseases Manifested by Nodules
Molluscum contagiosum
Genital warts
Secondary syphilis (condylomata lata)

the rule in infected women. Neither vaginitis nor urethritis occurs. Spread to the uterine cavity and fallopian tubes may follow, particularly at the time of menstruation, and result in acute salpingitis and pelvic peritonitis. The exact role of the gonococcus in the production of pelvic inflammatory disease, however, is unclear. Anaerobes and enteric gram-negative bacilli may be more important and lead to superinfection, abscess formation, tubal stricture, and sterility. Gonococci rarely are recovered from such infections.

Gonococci may disseminate in both men and women. Systemic gonococcal infection, however, rarely is seen in men owing to the local symptoms that prompt early treatment, in contrast to the asymptomatic nature of infection in women. Gono-coccemia may manifest as the gonococcal arthritis-dermatitis syndrome. Bacteremia with fever, chills, and characteristic hemorrhagic, vesicopustular skin lesions occurs (Figure 20–2). Tenosynovitis, particularly of the small joints of the hands and feet, is seen frequently. Skin lesions are painful and may evolve into a necrotic eschar. Blood cultures are usually positive and joint fluid aspirates are negative in this syndrome, but organisms may be recovered from the skin lesions. Occasionally, monarticular arthritis is the presenting manifestation of disseminated gonococcal infection, and the skin lesions, bacteremia, and tenosynovitis are not present. In these cases, gonococci usually can be recovered from the joint fluid but not the blood.

Disseminated gonococcal infection may produce endocarditis, although this is very uncommon. Peri-hepatic involvement may occur by direct spread from infected fallopian tubes. Right upper quad-rant pain and tenderness are the manifestations, making the disorder difficult to distinguish from acute cholecystitis. Blood cultures are usually neg-ative, but fine, "banjo-string" adhesions may be seen on peritoneoscopy. This presentation fre-quently is referred to as the Fitz-Hugh–Curtis syn-drome, and should be considered in the differen-tial diagnosis of right upper quadrant pain and fever in sexually active women.

Gonococcal ophthalmia, as it may occur in the adult, also may occur in the newborn who acquires the microorganism from contact with infected vagi-nal secretions. The disease is prevented by pro-phylactic administration of erythromycin or silver nitrate eye drops. Genital gonococcal infections in children usually are due to sexual abuse by an in-fected adult, usually a relative.

Gram's stain of urethral exudate is an accepted technique for diagnosis of gonorrhea in men. In women, however, only a minority of cases can be diagnosed correctly because of confusing normal flora. Cultures should be taken from the cervix, rec-tum (not contaminated with feces), and pharynx of women suspected of having gonorrhea. Culture of urethral exudate in men is adequate to confirm the diagnosis, except in homosexual men, from whom oral and anal cultures also should be obtained. In disseminated infection, samples of cul-de-sac fluid and joint fluid and aspirates of skin lesions should be obtained and inoculated onto chocolate agar. Cultures taken from the areas with normal flora (pharynx, rectum, or female genital tract) should be inoculated onto selective media to inhibit growth of competing normal bacterial flora. Cul-tures should be inoculated promptly and placed in a high–carbon dioxide atmosphere. Refrigeration of specimens will kill the gonococcus.

In recent years, *N. gonorrhoeae* has become more resistant to penicillin. Even relatively sensi-tive strains require high doses of penicillin for cure. However, strains of gonococci that dissemi-nate tend to remain more penicillin sensitive than those causing purely local disease. In the last 10 years, many strains of *N. gonorrhoeae* have become totally resistant to penicillin by production of a β-lactamase (penicillinase). These penicillinase-pro-ducing *N. gonorrhoeae* (PPNG) strains comprise 5 to 20 per cent of isolates nationwide. For this rea-son, penicillin G can no longer be considered the drug of choice for the treatment of infections result-ing from *N. gonorrhoeae*.

Treatment regimens are outlined in Table 20–35. Men and women *exposed* to gonorrhea should be examined, cultured, and treated at once with any of the primary treatment regimens. Ceftri-axone or cefixime is preferred, particularly in indi-viduals with anorectal or pharyngeal infection.

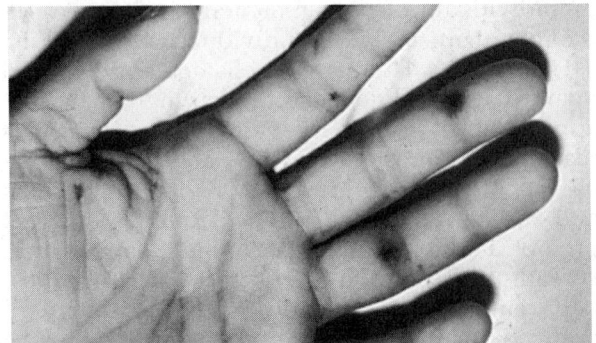
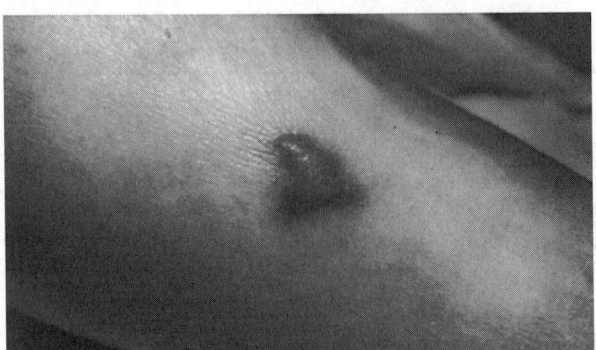

FIGURE 20–2.   Hemorrhagic vesicopustules on the hand *(A)* and hemorrhagic bullae on the ankle *(B)* in a case of gonococcal bacteremia.

TABLE 20–35. RECOMMENDED TREATMENT SCHEDULES FOR GONORRHEA AND PELVIC INFLAMMATORY DISEASE

Condition	Drug of Choice	Dosage	Alternative
Gonorrhea			
Uncomplicated urethritis, cervicitis, rectal, or pharyngeal infection	Ceftriaxone	125 mg I.M. once	Cefixime, 400 mg P.O. once, or ciprofloxacin, 500 mg P.O. once, or ofloxacin, 400 mg P.O. once, plus treatment for coexistant chlamydia
Conjunctivitis	Ceftriaxone	1 gm I.M. once plus saline solution lavage	
Disseminated infection	Ceftriaxone	1 gm I.M. or I.V. daily for 7–10 days; oral follow-up as listed	Cefotaxime or ceftizoxime, 1 gm I.V. q 8 hr until improved, then P.O. cefixime, 400 mg q 12 hr, or ciprofloxacin, 500 mg P.O. q 12 hr to complete 7 days of therapy
Meningitis	Ceftriaxone	1–2 gm daily for 10–14 days	
Endocarditis	Ceftriaxone	1–2 gm daily for 4 weeks	
Ophthalmia neonatorum	Ceftriaxone	25–50 mg/kg I.V. or I.M., single dose	
Disseminated infection in infants and children	Ceftriaxone	50 mg/kg/day I.V. or I.M. for 7–14 days	
Chlamydia Trachomatis			
Urethritis or cervicitis	Doxycycline	100 mg P.O. q 12 hr for 7 days	Ofloxacin, 300 mg P.O. q 12 hr for 7 days, or erythromycin base, 500 mg P.O. q 6 hr for 7 days, or sulfisoxazole, 500 mg q 6 hr for 10 days
	or azithromycin	1 gm P.O. once	
Ophthalmia neonatorum	Erythromycin	50 mg/kg P.O. divided q 6 hr for 10–14 days	
Pneumonia in infants	Erythromycin	50 mg/kg P.O. divided q 6 hr for 10–14 days	
Infections in infants and children <8 years of age	Erythromycin	50 mg/kg P.O. divided q 6 hr for 10–14 days	
Pelvic Inflammatory Disease			
Inpatients	Cefoxitin	2 gm I.V. q 6 hr	Clindamycin, 900 mg I.V. q 8 hr, plus gentamicin, 1.5 mg/kg q 8 hr, to improvement, then oral regimen for chlamydia to complete 14 days
	or cefotetan	2 g I.V. q 12 hr	
	plus doxycycline	100 gm I.V. q 12 hr, then oral follow-up to complete 14 days	
Outpatients	Ceftriaxone	250 mg I.M. once	Ofloxacin, 400 mg P.O. q 12 hr, plus clindamycin, 450 mg P.O., or metronidazole, 500 mg q 12 hr P.O., for 14 days
	plus doxycycline	100 mg P.O. q 12 hr for 14 days	
Epididymitis	Ceftriaxone	250 mg I.M. once	
	plus doxycycline	100 mg P.O. q 12 hr for 10 days	

Modified from Centers for Disease Control: 1993 sexually transmitted diseases treatment guidelines. MMWR 42:RR-14, 1993.

Pharyngeal infections are difficult to treat, and high failure rates are reported with both oral amoxicillin and intramuscular spectinomycin. Gonococcal regimens should be followed by azithromycin or doxycycline to eliminate potentially coexistent *Chlamydia* or *Ureaplasma* infection. Follow-up cultures should be obtained 3 to 7 days after completion of treatment for all cases of uncomplicated gonorrhea. Long-acting forms of penicillin G (i.e., benzathine penicillin) are effective for the treatment of syphilis but have no role in the treatment of gonorrhea. Oral penicillin V is similarly ineffective. Patients with incubating syphilis are likely to be cured by all treatment regimens for uncomplicated gonorrhea except for spectinomycin, and serologic tests for syphilis should be done for all patients with suspected STD.

In treating pelvic inflammatory disease, early hospitalization and intravenous therapy should be considered to prevent tubal scarring and infertility. An intrauterine device, if present, should be removed. For disseminated gonococcal infection, hospitalization is indicated for those who may be unreliable or who have uncertain diagnoses. Open drainage of infected joints other than the hip is not indicated. Follow-up examination and cultures should be performed in all instances.

Chlamydia Infections

With the advent of reliable culture techniques, enzyme immunoassay, and monoclonal antibody methods, the spectrum of disease produced by

Chlamydia has broadened. Several serovars of *C. trachomatis*, designated A through L, have been described and are responsible for a multitude of clinical conditions, including trachoma, nongono-coccal urethritis (NGU), mucopurulent cervicitis, inclusion conjunctivitis, proctitis, epididymitis, prostatitis, salpingitis, endometritis, perihepatitis, neonatal conjunctivitis and pneumonitis, and lymphogranuloma venereum.

NGU is probably more prevalent than gonorrhea. However, it is not a reportable disease so the exact incidence is unknown; estimates range from 3 to 5 million new cases annually. *Chlamydia trachomatis* is isolated from 50 per cent of NGU cases, although many men with *Chlamydia* urethritis are asymptomatic. Symptoms, when present, are those of dysuria and discharge. The urethral exudate is usually scant and mucoid, in contrast to the spontaneous and purulent discharge of gonorrhea. Epididymitis and possibly prostatitis may follow untreated infection. Concurrent conjunctivitis resulting from self-inoculation is not uncommon.

Chlamydial infections in women produce a mucopurulent cervicitis and acute dysuria ("the urethral syndrome"). Dysuria resulting from *Chlamydia* causes pyuria without bacteriuria. Mucopurulent cervicitis is diagnosed by the presence of mucopurulent endocervical secretions seen on swab and confirmed on Gram's stain, together with cervical erythema and friability. As a consequence of ascending infection, *Chlamydia* is thought to cause up to 50 per cent of the 1 million annual cases of pelvic inflammatory disease in the United States. In this role, it is implicated as a cause of infertility, premature delivery, and postpartum and neonatal infections.

The diagnosis of chlamydial infection must be made primarily on clinical grounds because laboratory methods are imperfect. Cell culture, although most sensitive, is not widely available. Direct fluorescent antibody testing is useful but of low sensitivity, particularly in screening low-risk populations. Enzyme immunoassay is more sensitive but less specific; false-positive tests occur in women with heavy bacterial growth. Serologic testing is rarely useful.

Drugs of choice for the treatment of *C. trachomatis* infections are tetracycline or macrolide antibiotics. Sulfamides are also useful. Azithromycin in a single 1-gram oral dose is equivalent to 1 week of doxycycline, 200 mg daily, for uncomplicated infections or documented exposure. Longer courses of therapy should be given for complicated infections such as epididymitis or salpingitis.

Syphilis

Syphilis remains a widespread disease. Reported cases of both primary and secondary syphilis have shown no decrease in recent years. In 1992, 30,000 cases were reported to public health authorities, an increase of over 20 per cent since 1980. Most cases are reported from large urban areas.

Primary syphilis occurs 10 to 90 days after sexual contact. The typical chancre is single, indurated, and nonpainful. Regional lymphadenopathy is usually present. Although most occur in the genital area, lesions may occur on the lip, tongue, breast, and elsewhere. Dark-field examination is positive, but serologic tests do not become reactive until the chancre begins to heal. The fluorescent treponemal antibody absorption (FTA-ABS) test becomes positive earliest but, by the fourth week, both the VDRL and FTA-ABS tests are usually reactive.

Secondary syphilis develops 2 to 6 weeks after the primary infection. It is manifested by a flu-like illness with headache, malaise, generalized lymphadenopathy, arthralgia, and rash. Cutaneous lesions are bilateral, involve the palms and soles, and are nonpruritic; they may be pustular, anular, or follicular. Mucous membranes are involved, with a thin gray exudate (mucus patches) or broad-based wart-like lesion (condyloma lata). Such lesions are teeming with spirochetes and highly contagious. Nephritis, meningitis, uveitis, and hepatitis also may occur at this stage. Lesions resolve spontaneously in 2 to 5 weeks, although relapses may occur within the first 2 years. Serology is always positive in secondary syphilis, with the VDRL frequently in high titer.

Late syphilis may be symptomatic or asymptomatic. In asymptomatic late syphilis, there are no signs or symptoms of infection. Diagnosis is made by routine serology. Symptomatic late syphilis may present with skin lesions, usually gummas, which are painless, ulcerating lesions particularly of the face and palate. Skeletal lesions, either Charcot joints or osteomyelitis, may occur. Cardiovascular syphilis, involving the aortic ring with the development of aortic regurgitation, is well appreciated.

Central nervous system involvement in late syphilis may be meningeal (most commonly seen in secondary or early late syphilis), parenchymatous (as tabes dorsalis or general paresis), or asymptomatic. Meningeal involvement is associated with a positive serology in both the blood and CSF and is reversible with treatment. Late asymptomatic parenchymatous syphilis frequently is associated with a negative serum VDRL, and a high index of suspicion therefore must be maintained to make the diagnosis. The spinal fluid VDRL frequently will be positive. Response to treatment is variable in late central nervous system infections.

The diagnosis of syphilis in the primary stage is made by dark-field examination. In subsequent stages, the diagnosis is made on clinical grounds and by serology. Two basic tests are available: (1) nonspecific antibody tests directed against cross-reacting lipid antigens of *Treponema*; and (2) specific antitreponemal antibody tests. The VDRL (or

TABLE 20–36. RESULTS OF COMMONLY USED SEROLOGIC TESTS FOR SYPHILIS

Test	Frequency of Positivity by Stage (%)		
	Primary	Secondary	Late
VDRL	70	99	70
ART or RPR	80	99	70
FTA-ABS	85	100	98

its simplified counterparts, the automated reagin test [ART] and rapid plasma reagin [RPR]) is the standard flocculation test for nontreponemal antibody. It is used as a screening test in most laboratories. The FTA-ABS test is the specific antitreponemal antibody test most frequently used (Table 20–36).

The FTA-ABS test is positive in 85 per cent of late primary syphilis and in 99 per cent of other forms. The FTA-ABS may be positive in early syphilis when the VDRL is still negative, and in late syphilis the VDRL may become negative while the FTA-ABS will remain positive. The VDRL titer is most useful in following response to treatment, but patients with longstanding positive serologies may remain positive even in the face of adequate treatment (i.e., they are "serofast"). As with all serologic reactions, the VDRL is subject to false-positive results (Table 20–37). Although false-positive reactions of the FTA-ABS do occur, they are rare, are associated with abnormal globulins, and frequently can be distinguished techni-

TABLE 20–37. CONDITIONS REPORTED TO CAUSE FALSE-POSITIVE VDRL

Addison's disease	Malaria
Atopic dermatitis	Measles
Brucellosis	Mumps
Chancroid	Multiple myeloma
Cirrhosis	Myocardial infarction
Coccidioidomycosis	Narcotic addiction
Cryoglobulinemia	Pellagra
Dermatomyositis	Pemphigus
Diabetes mellitus	Pernicious anemia
Diphtheria	Pneumonia
Epstein-Barr virus infection	Pregnancy
Glomerulonephritis (acute)	Polyarteritis nodosa
Hashimoto's thyroiditis	Rat-bite fever
Hemolytic anemia	Relapsing fever
Hepatitis	Rheumatic fever
Histoplasmosis	Sarcoidosis
Human immunodeficiency virus infection	Scleroderma
Idiopathic thrombocytopenic purpura	Subacute bacterial endocarditis
Infectious mononucleosis	Systemic lupus erythematosus
Influenza	Trypanosomiasis
Leprosy	Tuberculosis
Leptospirosis	Typhus
Lymphocytic leukemia	Vaccinia
Lymphogranuloma venereum	Varicella
Lymphosarcoma	Vincent's angina

cally from true positives. A positive VDRL, ART, or RPR in the face of a negative FTA-ABS test is due to disease other than syphilis and is referred to as a biologic false positive.

Penicillin is the preferential agent for the treatment of syphilis (Table 20–38). The VDRL usually will become negative 6 to 12 months after effective treatment of primary syphilis and 1 to 2 years after treatment of secondary syphilis but may remain positive for life after treatment of late syphilis. Because penetration of the central nervous system by benzathine penicillin is essentially nil, intravenous aqueous penicillin G is preferred for the treatment of active neurosyphilis.

Approximately 50 per cent of patients with secondary syphilis will develop fever, malaise, myalgia, and a flare of cutaneous lesions after penicillin treatment. This is referred to as a Jarisch-Herxheimer reaction and is due to systemic release of treponemal antigens. Very early treatment of primary or incubating syphilis, before the development of a significant antibody response, may create a negative serology in an individual who has no protective antibody.

Herpes Simplex Infections

It is estimated that genital herpes occurs with an annual incidence of 1 million primary cases and 20 million recurrences. Most infections are caused by herpes simplex virus type 2, although herpes simplex virus type 1 has become increasingly common, accounting for 10 to 15 per cent of all genital cases.

The manifestations of illness are multiple vesicular lesions that develop on the external or internal genitalia with an incubation period of approximately 1 week. Vesicles in moist areas ulcerate and become exquisitely painful. First infections are usually more severe and may be accompanied by considerable fever and autonomic neuropathy with urinary retention. Dysuria, pain, and paresthesias are the local manifestations in women, whereas in men the lesions are less prone to ulcerate and are less painful. Active genital herpes in the parturient woman is an indication for cesarean section, because the morbidity and mortality of disseminated herpes infection in the neonate is extremely high.

The diagnosis of herpes simplex is made by observing the characteristically multiple vesicles or ulcers and by examining Giemsa-stained scrapings or Papanicolaou (Pap) smears made from the base of the lesions. Intranuclear inclusions or multinucleated giant cells can be seen. Viral cultures are useful to confirm the diagnosis.

Acyclovir is the only effective therapy for herpes simplex virus infections currently available. It is most efficacious by the parenteral route for primary infections, and for prevention of frequent recurrences. It is of questionable value for treatment of

TABLE 20–38. RECOMMENDED TREATMENT SCHEDULES FOR SYPHILIS

Stage	Preferred Treatment	Alternative Treatment
Early syphilis (primary, secondary latent less than 1 year's duration)	Benzathine penicillin G, 2.4 million units I.M. once	Tetracycline hydrochloride, 0.5 gm P.O. 4 times a day for 15 days *or* Erythromycin, 0.5 gm P.O. 4 times a day for 15 days
Late syphilis (more than 1 year's duration, cardiovascular)	Benzathine penicillin G, 2.4 million units I.M. weekly for 3 doses	Tetracycline hydrochloride, 0.5 gm 4 times a day orally for 30 days *or* Erythromycin, 0.5 gm 4 times a day P.O. for 30 days
Neurosyphilis	Aqueous penicillin G, 12–24 million units/day I.V. divided every 4 hours for 10 days	Tetracycline hydrochloride, 0.5 gm 4 times a day P.O. for 30 days *or* Erythromycin, 0.5 gm 4 times a day P.O. for 30 days
Congenital syphilis	Aqueous penicillin G, 25,000 units/kg I.M. or I.V. twice a day for 10 days *or* Procaine penicillin G, 50,000 units/kg I.M. daily for 10 days	

symptomatic recurrences but does decrease viral shedding, perhaps important for minimizing transmission. Current treatment recommendations are listed in Table 20–39.

Papillomavirus Infections

Genital human papillomavirus (HPV) infections are increasing in frequency and are now the most common viral STD, twice as common as genital *Herpesvirus* infections. With recognition that most genital HPV infections are subclinical, their epidemiologic and clinical significance has been redefined.

Long considered a nuisance STD, it is now clear that certain DNA types of HPV possess tissue specificity and potential oncogenicity. HPV types 6 and 11 are most prevalent in exophytic genital warts and HPV types 16 and 18 are most commonly associated with cervical neoplasia. Indeed, the prevalence of HPV type 16 or 18 in cervical dysplasia (cervical intraepithelial neoplasia [CIN] I) is 70 per cent, and in carcinoma in situ (CIN III), it is 85 per cent. The prevalence of HPV DNA in sexually active women is high even without clinical disease; 5 to 15 per cent of cytologically (Pap smear) normal women possess HPV DNA in cervical cells.

The spectrum of clinical illness produced by HPV ranges from asymptomatic infection to exuberantly hypertrophic warts. Condylomata acuminata are usually flesh colored but may be hyperpigmented, with plaques, papules, and pointed (acuminate) projections. Flatter, sessile lesions also may occur and are overlooked easily. Warts occur predominantly on the vulva and cervix in females and on the penile shaft in males. Anal and oral warts are seen in relationship to specific sexual practices. HPV infections of the cervix and vagina

TABLE 20–39. TREATMENT RECOMMENDATIONS FOR GENITAL HERPES SIMPLEX VIRUS (HSV) INFECTIONS

Infection Type	Treatment
Immunocompetent Host First episodes	Acyclovir, 200 mg P.O. five times/day for 10 days *or* Acyclovir, 5 mg/kg body weight I.V. q 8 hr for 5–7 days (for severe local or systemic symptoms, neurologic complications, or dissemination)
Symptomatic recurrences of genital HSV infection	Acyclovir, 200 mg P.O. 5 times/day for 5 days, if associated with significant symptoms (of uncertain benefit)
Suppression of recurrent genital HSV infection	Acyclovir, 400 mg P.O. two to three times daily for up to 12 months, intended for patients with frequent (more than six times per year) symptomatic recurrences
Immunosuppressed Host First episodes or symptomatic recurrences	Acyclovir, 400 mg P.O. five times/day for 7–10 days *or* Acyclovir, 10 mg/kg body weight I.V. q 8 hr for 7 days
Suppression of reactivation of HSV infection during periods of immunosuppression	Acyclovir, 2.5–5 mg/kg body weight I.V. q 8 hr for high-risk periods; high-dose oral may be adequate
Genital HSV Infection during Pregnancy	Acyclovir not indicated

Modified from Webb DH, Fife KH: Genital herpes simplex virus infections. Infect Dis Clin North Am 1:113, 1987, with permission.

are usually subclinical. Their presence is suspected by colposcopic application of 3 to 5 per cent acetic acid, resulting in the appearance of white lesions, or by cytology. Serologic studies and direct antibody staining of infected tissues are insensitive and of limited availability.

All modes of treatment suffer from a high relapse rate after apparently successful therapy. Podophyllin, a resin extract of the May apple, has been used most widely but is followed by a relapse rate of 60 to 70 per cent. Cryotherapy is more successful but usually requires several treatments for cure. Surgery or laser ablation are useful adjuncts but recurrence rates are also high, particularly for laser therapy. The roles of 5-fluorouracil and intralesional interferon compared to or combined with standard therapy are not clear.

Chancroid

Chancroid is a localized, ulcerative lesion of the genitalia of increasing frequency. The ulcers are usually multiple, painful, and soft, with associated adenopathy. Mucous membranes are not affected, and the disease is caused by a fastidious gram-negative rod, *Haemophilus ducreyi*. The organism is rarely grown or cultured but can be suspected on Gram's stain. The treatment of choice is ceftriaxone or a fluoroquinolone. The major differential diagnosis is syphilis, which, in contrast, to chancroid, is usually painless and associated with a positive dark-field examination.

Lymphogranuloma Venereum

Lymphogranuloma venereum is an uncommon form of chronic lymphadenitis caused by *C. trachomatis*. Lymphadenopathy, fever, chills, arthralgias, and headaches are prominent. Obliterative lymphadenitis of the penis or vulva and rectal strictures develop. The diagnosis is made serologically and clinically, and the treatment of choice is tetracycline, 2 gm/day for 2 weeks.

Molluscum Contagiosum

Molluscum contagiosum is a viral illness presenting with grouped, umbilicated papules on genital skin. Occasionally, these lesions may appear on the limbs, face, or trunk and are spread by contact, with an incubation period of 6 to 8 weeks. The lesions are painless and asymptomatic. The diagnosis is made clinically and established by crushing a lesion and examining the contents for intracytoplasmic inclusions. Treatment is by desiccation or cryosurgery, although lesions usually regress spontaneously over several weeks to months.

Vaginitis

Vulvovaginitis in women may be due to a variety of organisms. *Candida albicans*, *Trichomonas vaginalis*, and *Gardnerella vaginalis* are most common. Clinical distinction among these various etiologies may be difficult, and smears and cultures are helpful in making a definitive diagnosis. Mixed infections are frequent. Although the type of discharge varies from one individual to another, *Trichomonas* generally causes a profuse, frothy, malodorous discharge, and *Candida* causes a scant, thick, and cheesy white exudate.

Smears of vaginal exudate will show yeast and pseudohyphae in vaginal candidiasis and clue cells (vaginal epithelial cells coated with masses of gram-variable coccobacilli) in *Gardnerella* infection (also known as nonspecific vaginitis or bacterial vaginosis). Cultures are necessary to rule out *N. gonorrhoeae*. The treatment of *Trichomonas* and *Gardnerella* vaginitis is with metronidazole. Treatment of *Candida* is accomplished best with intravaginal antifungals, ketoconozole or fluconazole. Oral treatment with fluconazole is preferred for refractory cases.

SKIN AND SOFT TISSUE INFECTIONS

Skin and soft tissue infections are an important cause of visits to the family physician. They can be classified best by their clinical appearance and can be grouped together as *pyodermas*, a term signifying bacterial infections of the skin and sometimes underlying subcutaneous tissues.

Impetigo is a disease of the superficial layers of skin. It may be vesicular, erosive, or pustular, then crusted. Many are mixed infections, although *S. pyogenes* (group A) is implicated in most cases. *Staphylococcus aureus* is involved in 20 to 40 per cent of cases, and the presence of bullae should suggest infection resulting from *S. aureus*. Impetiginous lesions occasionally may be confused with herpes simplex, particularly because they occur around the lips and chin. Most impetigo occurs in children and is probably precipitated by a skin abrasion or insect bite. A nonsuppurative complication of concern is acute poststreptococcal glomerulonephritis. Strains of group A streptococci causing skin infections are different serologic types from those causing pharyngeal infection, and they do not, in general, cause acute rheumatic fever.

Furunculosis is usually due to *S. aureus*. Infections may vary from a small pimple to a deep, multipocketed carbuncle extending into the subcutaneous fat. Furuncles and carbuncles occur at areas of perspiration and friction, such as the neck, axillae, thighs, and buttocks. The lesions are more common in individuals with diabetes or obesity, in those receiving corticosteroids, and in individuals with defects of phagocytic cell function. Whereas furuncles are well localized and may drain spontaneously, carbuncles are more indurated and may spread in deep tissue planes. Bacteremia may accompany the latter.

Erysipelas is a superficial infection of the skin with extensive lymphatic involvement, usually resulting from group A streptococci. It occurs more often in infants, children, and the elderly. There is frequently an antecedent upper respiratory tract infection, and the lesion tends to recur in the same site. The lesion is expanding, red, and edematous with a sharply raised border. Leukocytosis is common and patients are frequently toxic. Bacteremia, however, is uncommon. Streptococci may be cultured from the advancing edge of the lesion.

Cellulitis is a spreading infection of deep skin layers usually caused by *S. aureus* or group A streptococcus. There is frequently a history of trauma with a puncture wound or laceration. The patient complains of local tenderness, erythema, and pain. Fever, chills, and malaise are frequent. Ascending lymphangitis or regional adenopathy also may be present. Occasionally, septic thrombophlebitis may occur.

Under certain circumstances, organisms other than staphylococci and streptococci may cause cellulitis. *Erysipelothrix* causes cellulitis after handling contaminated fish or meat products. Gram-negative bacteria such as *E. coli* or *Proteus* may be involved after abdominal or perineal surgery or, together with anaerobes, in cellulitis associated with foot ulcers. *Aeromonas hydrophila* is an important cause of cellulitis after injuries in fresh water. Injuries associated with salt water activity may result in cellulitis caused by *Vibrio* species. Cellulitis associated with cat or dog bites, particularly if ascending lymphangitis is present, is likely to be due to *Pasteurella multocida*. Cellulitis from human bites involves anaerobic bacteria such as *Fusobacterium* as well as staphylococci or streptococci. Culture and Gram's stain of the lesions, particularly if there is a history of trauma, will help to elucidate the pathogen(s) and allow appropriate and specific therapy.

Certain skin lesions are accompanied by extensive necrosis, marked systemic toxicity, and rapid progression. The classification of these necrotizing infections is sometimes difficult because of the multiple organisms involved and their varied clinical presentation. Necrotizing infections frequently follow contaminated wounds or abdominal or perineal surgery. Predisposing factors in addition to surgery include diabetes, devitalized tissue, and blunt trauma with hematoma infection. Multiple organisms frequently are involved, and utmost attempts should be made to define the infecting pathogens by biopsy or tissue aspiration, Gram's stains, and blood cultures. The presence of gas within the wound does not necessarily imply *Clostridia*. The majority of gas-forming infections are nonclostridial, caused by a mixed flora of anaerobes, microaerophilic streptococci, and enteric gram-negative bacilli.

The treatment of skin and subcutaneous infections is dictated by their depth and severity. Superficial infections, such as impetigo and erysipelas, usually respond to conservative therapy with penicillin. In the penicillin-allergic patient, erythromycin, clindamycin, or a first-generation cephalosporin is usually effective.

Surgical drainage alone is frequently adequate for the treatment of furuncles and carbuncles. If antibiotics are necessary, an oral penicillinase-resistant penicillin, such as cloxacillin, is the drug of choice, because staphylococci are the most common pathogens.

The treatment of cellulitis depends on the pathogen. Because a variety of microorganisms may be present, a thorough history and Gram's stain of wound exudate will be valuable in selecting appropriate initial therapy. All such lesions should be cultured aerobically and anaerobically. Empiric antimicrobial therapy should be directed at staphylococci and streptococci if no other pathogens are suspected. In bite wounds, infection with mouth anaerobes must be considered, and all bite victims should receive prophylactic antibiotics.

Diabetic foot infections are a common outpatient problem. Tissue ischemia, recurrent trauma resulting from neuropathy, poorly fitting shoes, tinea pedis, and neglect lead to ulcerations, necrotizing soft tissue infection, osteomyelitis, and gangrene. Such patients require a multidisciplinary approach to care, including orthotics and podiatric care, diabetes control, revascularization, and appropriate antibiotic treatment. Patient education for optimal self-care is paramount (Table 20–40).

TABLE 20–40. PRINCIPLES OF DIABETIC FOOT CARE

Do not use tobacco in any form
Keep warm at all times
Wear wide-toed shoes that have good arch support and warm cotton socks
Do not use garters that encircle the leg
Do not sit with knees crossed
Do not apply any heat or medicine on your feet unless instructed
Wash your feet every day; dry thoroughly, especially between the toes
Apply lanolin or oil if your feet are dry and scaly
Apply powder if your feet are moist
Examine your feet closely every day
Keep toenails trimmed correctly; use a podiatrist if necessary
Consult your physician promptly when you notice redness, blistering, pain, swelling, or any break in the skin
Seek medical help for athlete's foot
Do not swim in cold water or in the ocean
Avoid sunburn
Walk slower but walk often
Avoid pressure points; use cotton wicks between toes if necessary
Maintain good diabetic control

The treatment of necrotizing skin and subcutaneous infections is also dependent on definition of pathogens. Surgical débridement is essential. Necrotic tissue must be excised, abscesses drained, and fasciotomies performed to decompress and drain swollen fascial compartments if infection extends beneath the subcutaneous tissue. Antibiotic therapy should be directed at multiple pathogens, with initial therapy determined by Gram's stain of wound exudate. Blood cultures should be obtained, because bacteremia is present in many patients with necrotizing infections. It is essential to remember that all necrotic tissue must be removed. Attempts to save nonviable tissue invariably end in disaster.

TUBERCULOSIS

The incidence of tuberculosis had declined in recent decades as a result of improvements in socioeconomic conditions and nutrition. Mortality also declined with the introduction of effective chemotherapy. In 1985, however, the downward trend in annual incidence observed since 1930 began to reverse itself. Over 30,000 new cases are anticipated in 1994, particularly in residents of urban areas, HIV-infected persons, immigrants, and nonwhites. Furthermore, multi–drug-resistant strains have emerged in alarming numbers in AIDS patients, resulting in epidemics in prisons, hospitals, and AIDS care facilities.

Pathophysiology of Tuberculosis

Most human tuberculosis is due to *Mycobacterium tuberculosis*. Infection is acquired through inhalation of aerosolized droplets of sputum known as droplet nuclei, which, when inhaled, pass through terminal airways and are deposited in the alveolae. Fomites (inanimate objects) generally do not transmit tuberculosis. Following deposition in alveolae, the bacteria multiply without extensive tissue reaction, spreading through regional lymphatics to the hilar lymph nodes and then the blood stream. During this asymptomatic blood stream dissemination, mycobacteria are seeded to all parts of the body. Tuberculin-delayed hypersensitivity, representing the establishment of cell-mediated immunity, develops between 2 and 10 weeks after acquisition of infection.

As the primary focus resolves, infected lymph nodes may calcify, yielding a Ghon complex. Subsequent, postprimary, disease is the form of tuberculosis most commonly recognized. It represents reactivation of dormant foci inoculated at the time of primary bacteremia. Reactivation usually occurs months to years after the primary infection and usually is precipitated by depression in cell-mediated immunity resulting from intercurrent disease or administration of immunosuppressive drugs.

Clinical Manifestations of Pulmonary Tuberculosis

Primary pulmonary tuberculosis is usually a disease of children and young adults, in whom it is manifest as a flu-like illness. A brassy cough with scant sputum production, myalgias, low-grade fever, and malaise may last only a few days. Auscultation is usually unremarkable and chest radiographic studies may show a small, lower lung field infiltrate with hilar adenopathy. Acid-fast bacilli usually are not demonstrable on smears at this time, although the tuberculin skin test will be positive at the time of clinical illness.

Postprimary pulmonary tuberculosis is usually an upper lobe disease and represents reactivation of dormant foci. However, atypical radiographic findings, particularly in AIDS patients (Table 20–41), may include lower lobe infection, multiple lobe involvement, or primarily pleural disease. The onset is usually insidious, with constitutional symptoms predominating. Anorexia, weight loss, fatigue, fever, chills, and night sweats are common. Occasionally, patients do not realize they are ill, and the disease is incidentally discovered on a chest radiographic study. When cough and sputum production develop, they frequently are not severe at onset. Hemoptysis may occur if ulceration of a bronchial wall or blood vessel occurs. Pleuritic pain may be present if the pleura is involved in the inflammatory response. The differences in presentation of tuberculosis in HIV-infected compared to non–HIV-infected persons is summarized in Table 20–41.

Physical examination in postprimary disease is

TABLE 20–41. PULMONARY TUBERCULOSIS: DIFFERING MANIFESTATIONS IN HIV-INFECTED AND NON–HIV-INFECTED INDIVIDUALS

	HIV (−) (%)	HIV (+) (%)
Tuberculosis		
Pulmonary	85–100	30–70
Extrapulmonary	15	15–70
Lymphatic	5	30–50
Meningitis	2	10
Positive PPD (>10 mm)	85–95	30–80
Sputum acid-fast bacilli smear positive	50–80	30–80
Blood culture positive	<10	25–40
Chest radiograph		
Hilar adenopathy	5	30–40
Pleural effusion	20–25	25–30
Upper lobe infiltrate	70–90	20–30
Miliary pattern	<2	10–15
Cavitation	10–35	0–40
Normal	0–5	10–15

often of little value unless there is a large cavity or extensive pneumonitis. Laboratory data are also of little assistance, although there may be anemia, elevated sedimentation rate, and mild leukocytosis. Acid-fast bacilli smears should be positive. Invasive techniques may be necessary to demonstrate the organism if expectorated sputum is scant or if smears are negative.

The Tuberculin Skin Test

The tuberculin skin test contains an extract prepared from culture filtrates of tubercle bacilli. It is called purified protein derivative (PPD) and is administered intradermally to evaluate delayed hypersensitivity. Intermediate PPD (the usual skin test preparation, representing 5 tine units) is injected as 0.1 mL of solution, and the injection site is evaluated at 48 to 72 hours for induration. New guidelines have been created for PPD interpretation because the test possesses differential sensitivity in different populations (Table 20–42).

Approximately 10 per cent of normal individuals with culture- and biopsy-proven tuberculosis are skin test negative. A negative skin test, therefore, does not conclusively eliminate the diagnosis. A borderline reaction may represent prior tuberculosis exposure with no recent antigenic stimulus or atypical mycobacterial infection. In the former instance, a second intermediate PPD, performed 1 week after the initial test, will be positive in those individuals with true *M. tuberculosis* exposure.

Interpretation of tuberculin reactions in individuals who have received bacille Calmette-Guérin (BCG) vaccine is often difficult. These patients usually have positive tests for 5 to 10 years after immunization. However, positive tests more than 10 years after immunization should suggest new infection with *M. tuberculosis*. Falsely negative tuberculin tests may be seen with old PPD preparations; intercurrent viral illness, vaccination, or other intracellular infection; inadequate application of the test material; overwhelming illness; concomitant administration of adrenal corticosteroids or immunosuppressive drugs; or diseases such as malnutrition, HIV infection, or neoplasia.

Extrapulmonary Tuberculosis

Although pulmonary tuberculosis accounts for most mycobacterial infection, extrapulmonary forms of the disease, particularly common in HIV-infected individuals, present both diagnostic and therapeutic problems. Extrapulmonary tuberculosis represents reactivation of dormant foci seeded at the time of primary bacteremia.

Genital tuberculosis in men is usually secondary to renal involvement with foci in the kidney, seminal vesicles, prostate, or epididymis. Genital lesions presenting with swelling and tenderness may suggest neoplasm or bacterial infection. In women, genital tuberculosis also results from reactivation and involves the fallopian tubes most commonly. Symptoms are nonspecific, and the diagnosis frequently is made during evaluation for sterility. The majority of patients with genitourinary tuberculosis are of foreign birth and nonwhite. Fifty per cent have normal chest radiographic studies, and the diagnosis is made by biopsy of involved tissue or by urine cultures for evaluation of culture-negative pyuria. Urine cultures must be processed immediately, because storage of urine will result in death of mycobacteria.

Lymph node tuberculosis is the most common form of extrapulmonary disease, resulting from reactivation of organisms hematogenously disseminated at the time of the primary pulmonary infection. The usual presentation is a painless swelling of the anterior cervical lymph nodes. Posterior cervical, mediastinal, and supraclavicular lymph nodes are involved less frequently. Fever, weight loss, and pain are usually not present. Laboratory evaluation is normal and biopsy is needed for diagnosis.

Tuberculous peritonitis is a disease of insidious onset, uncommon in the United States, with a predilection for women of foreign birth. The hallmarks are abdominal pain, fever, and exudative ascites. Organisms seed the peritoneal cavity from hematogenous spread during primary tuberculosis or from contiguous spread from infected peritoneal lymph nodes, fallopian tubes, or intestinal foci. Ascites is prominent on physical examination and an abdominal mass may be palpated as a result of adhesions of bowel, omentum, and mesentery. Laboratory values reveal anemia, a normal white blood cell count, and elevated sedimentation rate. As in genitourinary tuberculosis, the chest radiograph is

TABLE 20–42.   INTERPRETIVE CRITERIA FOR TUBERCULIN (PPD) SKIN TEST POSITIVITY

Induration at 48 Hours	Patient Risk Factor for Positivity
≥5 mm	Recent close contact with active tuberculosis case
	Abnormal chest radiograph suggesting old tuberculosis
	HIV infection
≥10 mm	Diabetes mellitus, gastrectomy, silicosis
	Injection drug use without HIV infection
	Immunodeficiency caused by non-HIV conditions
	Prolonged steroid therapy or cancer chemotherapy
	Birth in high-prevalence country
	Correctional institution or nursing home resident
	Hospital and microbiology laboratory employee
	Medically underserved, low-income population
≥15 mm	All others

normal in 50 per cent of patients. The diagnosis is dependent on culture and histologic examination of the peritoneum. Ascitic fluid smears and cultures are usually negative.

Tuberculous pericarditis may develop from reactivation of dormant foci or from contiguous spread from infected mediastinal lymph nodes. The peak incidence is in the fourth to fifth decades of life, and the presenting symptoms are cough, dyspnea, fever, and chest pain. Cardiomegaly is present in 95 per cent, but pulmonary infiltrates or evidence of active pulmonary tuberculosis is present in less than one half. A positive tuberculin skin test is present in 85 per cent, and the diagnosis is made by culture of pericardial tissue obtained at surgery.

Skeletal and joint tuberculosis is uncommon. In the United States, it is primarily a disease of older adults, intravenous drug users, or HIV-infected patients. Organisms reach the bones during the hematogenous phase of primary tuberculosis. The spine is involved most frequently, followed by the hip and knee. Immunosuppressed patients may have numerous sites of involvement, with rib involvement predominating. Tuberculous arthritis is monarticular, characteristically involving the weight-bearing joints. Diagnosis can be established only by biopsy.

Tuberculous meningitis is a disease of older adults and young children. Headache, weight loss, night sweats, and other vague symptoms are the presenting complaints. Classic signs of meningitis may or may not be present. The CSF profile is mononuclear and low in glucose.

Miliary tuberculosis results from massive hematogenous dissemination of tubercle bacilli from an established, reactivated focus. Numerous lesions of the same age and size occur in many organs of the body. Characteristically, the large numbers of granulomata seen in the lungs on chest radiographs are likened to millet seeds. It is a disease of HIV-infected or elderly, frequently malnourished, individuals. The presenting manifestations are vague, and the diagnosis is difficult. Weakness, anorexia, weight loss, and fever are present in over 50 per cent of patients. The tuberculin skin test is positive in less than half the patients. Radiographic studies may not show miliary lesions at the outset, and sputum analysis is not helpful because cavitary disease with endobronchial microorganisms is not present. Diagnosis must be made by lung biopsy, bone marrow biopsy, liver biopsy, or blood culture.

Diseases Caused by Other Mycobacteria

It long has been known that acid-fast microorganisms other than *M. tuberculosis* can cause clinical disease. The current classification of mycobacteria

TABLE 20–43. CLASSIFICATION OF ATYPICAL MYCOBACTERIA AND THE DISEASES THEY MAY CAUSE

Organisms	Disease
I. Slow-growing potential pathogens	
A. *M. avium* complex	Lymphadenitis, pulmonary, disseminated
B. *M. scrofulaceum*	Lymphadenitis
C. *M. kansasii*	Pulmonary and disseminated
D. *M. ulcerans*	Cutaneous and soft tissue
E. *M. marinum*	Cutaneous and soft tissue
F. *M. xenopi*	Pulmonary
G. *M. szulgai*	Very rare
H. *M. simiae*	Very rare
II. Rapid-growing potential pathogens	
A. *M. fortuitum* complex	Soft tissue, bone, pulmonary

and the diseases they may cause are listed in Table 20–43.

Mycobacterium avium complex (MAC) is now the most frequently isolated mycobacterium. Because of its environmental prevalence (soil and water), it is a frequent contaminant in culture processing and it is commonly a cause of disseminated infection in AIDS patients. Twenty to 30 per cent of AIDS patients with CD4 counts less than 100/mm^3 have disseminated MAC infection, which is multi–drug resistant and requires innovative, complex chemotherapeutic regimens for suppression. Cure is rarely achieved. MAC also can cause pulmonary infections in nonimmunosuppressed patients, particularly those with structural lung disease, lung cancer, or pneumoconiosis.

Mycobacterium kansasii causes pulmonary disease identical to that of *M. tuberculosis* and frequently responds well to chemotherapy. *Mycobacterium scrofulaceum* produces cervical adenitis, primarily in children under 2 years of age, and is treated by excision of the involved lymph nodes. Lymphadenitis in adults is usually due to *M. tuberculosis*. *Mycobacterium marinum* is a cause of granulomatous skin lesions, nodular lymphangitis, and soft tissue infection after trauma sustained in fresh or salt water, particularly while handling fish, and usually responds well to antimicrobial therapy.

Chemotherapy of Tuberculosis

The goal of chemotherapy in tuberculosis is to administer enough agents to prevent the emergence of resistant microorganisms and to administer them for an adequate period of time to prevent relapse. Because of the emergence of multi–drug-resistant strains, a supervised three-drug regimen is advised for the initial treatment of most minimal

TABLE 20–44. CRITERIA FOR ISONIAZID PROPHYLAXIS

1. Recent (<2 years) converters of any age
2. Tuberculin (intermediate PPD) reactors below age 35
3. Household contacts of infectious cases, particularly if children less than 4 years of age
4. Immunosuppressed patients with a positive intermediate PPD if never previously treated
5. Any-age patient with a positive intermediate PPD and old granulomatous disease on chest radiograph (not a Ghon complex) who has never been treated

to moderate active pulmonary disease caused by *M. tuberculosis.* Isoniazid, rifampin, and pyrazinamide are the drugs of choice. Recent data suggest that a four-drug regimen using isoniazid, rifampin, pyrazinamide, and either ethambutol or an aminoglycoside (streptomycin or amikacin) is indicated if there is any likelihood of drug resistance. If susceptibility testing reveals no resistance, the regimens can be simplified. A 6-month regimen is adequate for most minimal disease in non–HIV-infected patients, 9 to 12 months is required in more extensive disease, and possibly indefinite therapy is necessary in AIDS patients. Surgery is rarely necessary except in far-advanced, cavitary disease. Attention also must be given to nutrition, psychological, and sociological problems that co-exist. Every attempt must be made to assure that the medications are taken for the prescribed amount of time, and intermittent supervised therapy may be useful. Extrapulmonary tuberculosis is treated in the same fashion as pulmonary tuberculosis, except for meningitis or miliary disease, which may require more aggressive therapy.

The family and contacts of active cases must be evaluated, skin tested, and/or radiographed. Certain contacts will benefit from prophylactic treatment with isoniazid. The conversion from a negative to a positive skin test carries a high risk of developing active tuberculosis within 2 years. The benefits of prophylaxis must be weighed against the risk of isoniazid toxicity (i.e., hepatitis), which is seen in approximately 1 per cent of all patients but is lowest in individuals under 35 years of age. Administration of isoniazid seems to decrease the risk of reactivation, although its actual effect on dormant bacilli is not known. Based on these principles, isoniazid prophylaxis is recommended for those individuals listed in Table 20–44. In these patients, the risk of developing active disease is high, and isoniazid is administered to eradicate the small numbers of actively growing bacilli living in sequestered foci. Isoniazid is administered in a dose of 300 mg/day for 6 months in these situations, but for 1 year in HIV-infected individuals.

URINARY TRACT INFECTIONS

Urinary tract infections are second in frequency only to respiratory tract infections as a clinical problem encountered by the practicing physician. Our understanding of the etiology, pathogenesis, and natural history of urinary tract infections has improved in recent years, and a more rational approach to therapy has been developed both for the management of acute infections and for the prevention of recurrent infections.

Terminology

Traditionally, urinary tract infections are designated as pyelonephritis or cystitis based on purely clinical criteria without objective evidence to indicate whether the infection is confined to the kidney or urinary bladder. However, in order to utilize the best therapeutic regimen, it is essential to understand where the infection is localized.

Cystitis describes a clinical symptom complex of dysuria, frequency, urgency, and suprapubic tenderness. This symptom complex may be caused by urethritis, bacterial infection of the bladder, local infection caused by herpes simplex, or other inflammatory conditions. *Acute pyelonephritis* describes a syndrome of flank pain, costovertebral angle tenderness, and fever, with or without the symptoms of cystitis or urethritis. The clinical manifestations of pyelonephritis, however, can be mimicked by renal infarction, renal calculi, or ureteral obstruction without infection and sometimes are seen with purely bladder bacteriuria.

Repeated episodes of urinary tract infection may be *relapses* or *reinfections.* Relapse indicates recurrence of infection with the same microorganism. Reinfection means that bacteriuria is due to a microorganism different from the preceding one. Relapse suggests either inadequate therapy as a result of an inappropriate drug or duration of therapy, or a focus of infection not adequately treated by antimicrobial therapy alone, such as a calculus, stricture, diverticulum, or other obstructive uropathy. Reinfection implies predisposition to infection from an exogenous source without structural disease. Patients with *asymptomatic bacteriuria* have significant numbers of organisms in the urine without symptoms. *Symptomatic bacteriuria,* or the *urethral syndrome,* refers to the presence of lower tract symptoms without organisms being cultured from the urine. *Chronic pyelonephritis* does not necessarily mean infection; it is a pathologic diagnosis. It is most often due to vascular disease, analgesic abuse, or uric acid nephropathy. It may or may not be complicated by infection.

Pathogenesis of Urinary Tract Infection

Ascending infection is the major route of entry for microorganisms into the urinary tract. Hematogenous seeding of the urinary tract is a rare event, except with bacteremia resulting from *S. aureus*.

The bladder itself is normally sterile. It is removed from contact with bacteria by the urethra. The distal urethra has a normal bacterial flora composed of diphtheroids, lactobacilli, streptococci, and coagulase-negative staphylococci. In women, gram-negative bacteria from the colon colonize the anterior vagina, the vulva, and subsequently the distal urethra. Microorganisms then migrate into the bladder, sometimes with the help of mechanical massage, as occurs in sexual intercourse. Failure to remove all of the bacteria with urination, particularly if there is residual urine in the bladder, allows multiplication of microorganisms within the bladder and subsequent infection. The short urethra of women, its closeness to the perirectal area, and the nature of sexual intercourse make colonization of the female lower urinary tract easy.

Both bacterial and host factors are important in the pathogenesis of urinary tract infection. Although there are many different strains of *E. coli*, only a small proportion of these strains cause infection. The presence of surface proteins or adhesins on the surface of such bacteria allows them to attach to vaginal, vulvar, and uroepithelial cells. Adherence occurs by attachment of these bacterial surface proteins to epithelial cell surface glycolipid receptors (also known as glycocalyx). Adhesive capacity is associated with the severity of infection and the propensity of a given strain of *E. coli* to cause pyelonephritis rather than cystitis or asymptomatic bacteriuria.

Host factors also contribute to the pathogenesis of, or protection from, urinary tract infection. It has been shown that *E. coli* organisms adhere more avidly to the uroepithelial cells of women who develop recurrent infection than to the cells of women who do not. Thus, a combination of bacteria with surface proteins of high affinity for certain types of epithelial cell surface receptors and the presence of such receptive cells in a specific individual will predispose to urinary tract infection.

Protective elements that inhibit growth of bacteria in the urine include a high urea concentration, high osmolality, and low pH. The bladder mucosa itself has antibacterial activity, which, combined with the removal of bacteria by urination, acts as a major protective factor. The low pH of vaginal secretions and the presence of cervicovaginal antibody in some women also protects against perineal colonization by fecal bacteria and decreases the risk of infection.

Structural abnormalities in the urinary tract interfere with these protective functions. Most important is obstruction of flow resulting from such conditions as urethral strictures, calculi, retroperitoneal fibrosis, uterine enlargement, tumors, prostatic hypertrophy, and neurologic disease. Furthermore, intraluminal lesions, such as calculi or diverticuli, may provide a residual focus in which

bacteria may survive, sequestered from the effects of antimicrobial therapy.

Vesicoureteral reflux resulting from congenital abnormalities or bladder distention provides an easy route for bacteria to reach the kidney. Incomplete emptying of the bladder, whether due to obstruction or neurologic disease, promotes urinary stasis, allowing growth of microorganisms. Patients with obstruction or stasis often have bacteria introduced by cystoscopy or bladder catheterization, thereby producing an infection that is difficult to eradicate.

Bacteria Involved

Escherichia coli is by far the most common pathogen. In female outpatients, more than 85 per cent of infections are due to *E. coli*, whether first-time infections or recurrences. The remaining 15 per cent of infections are due to *P. mirabilis*, *Klebsiella* species, and *Staphylococcus* species. It is exceedingly rare for an outpatient to develop infection caused by *Pseudomonas*, *Serratia*, or *Enterobacter*. These organisms cause infection primarily in hospitalized patients after instrumentation of the urinary tract. Occasionally, however, these organisms may occur without instrumentation in the bedridden patient who is ill and incontinent and has received antibiotics that alter the bowel and perineal flora. Nonetheless, even as a cause of nosocomial (hospital-acquired) infection, *E. coli* is more frequent than *Klebsiella*, *Proteus*, or *Pseudomonas*.

It has become apparent in recent years that coagulase-negative staphylococci may produce symptomatic urinary tract infections. *Staphylococcus saprophyticus* is the chief culprit and can be differentiated from *Staphylococcus epidermidis* by its resistance to novobiocin. It causes bladder infections, primarily in young women, with a seasonal preponderance in the summer months. *Staphylococcus aureus* present in a urine culture should prompt a search for distant foci of infection with secondary bacteremic seeding of the urinary tract. *Chlamydia* are also an important cause of lower urinary tract symptoms in young women whose urine is culture negative and who have primarily urethritis. *Proteus mirabilis* is seen most frequently in patients with urinary tract calculi, and its presence should be suspected in this setting. The production of a urease by *P. mirabilis* results in an abnormally high urine pH, which is a clue to its presence.

Epidemiology of Urinary Tract Infection

Although the prevalence of bacteriuria increases with age, urinary tract infections occur at all ages

TABLE 20–45. PREVALENCE OF BACTERIURIA

Age Group	Women (%)	Men (%)
Newborn	<0.5	0.5–1
Preschool	3–5	<0.5
School	1–5	<0.5
Adults 15–50 years old		<0.5
Sexually active	4–8	
Nuns	0.5–2	
Adults over 60 years old	10–20	2–10

(Table 20–45). In the neonate, the frequency of bacteriuria is approximately 1 per cent. The majority of such children are male, and the bacteriuria is usually associated with congenital abnormalities of the urinary tract. During the preschool and school years, urinary tract infection is more common in girls than boys. Large surveys have found from 1 to 5 per cent prevalence of bacteriuria in female schoolchildren (see Table 20–45). Infection in either boys or girls in the preschool age frequently is associated with structural lesions or vesicoureteral reflux and may be responsible for significant renal damage in this situation.

From ages 5 to 15, between 5 and 6 per cent of girls will have at least one episode of bacteriuria. Each year approximately 25 per cent of those who are bacteriuric will spontaneously cure, or be treated and cured, but a similar proportion will become bacteriuric. It is clear from long-term studies that bacteriuria in young girls defines a person who is at greater risk of developing symptomatic urinary tract infections later in life, but it is not clear that, in the absence of obstruction or major degrees of vesicoureteral reflux, there is any risk of permanent, clinically significant renal damage.

In adults, the frequency of bacteriuria increases with sexual activity. Between 4 and 8 per cent of sexually active young women have bacteriuria, a percentage that increases with increasing age, debility, and bed rest. At least 30 per cent of women will have a urinary tract infection at some time in their life, whether symptomatic or asymptomatic.

During pregnancy, there is a much higher frequency of symptomatic upper tract infection as a result of a number of physiologic changes that occur during the last trimester. Ureteral compression and hydronephrosis resulting from uterine enlargement and decreased ureteral peristalis occur. In addition to the risk of renal infection, there is an increased risk of prematurity, perinatal death, stillbirth, and intrauterine growth retardation in pregnant bacteriuric women. Routine screening of all pregnant women for bacteriuria is justified, because treatment can reduce the risk of pyelonephritis and perinatal complications.

Bacteriuria is rarely seen in men between the ages of 1 and 50 in the absence of instrumentation. However, about 3 to 4 per cent of men over 70 years of age have bacteriuria, and 10 per cent of hospitalized elderly males are bacteriuric. This increase is due to the presence of prostatic disease.

Clinical Presentations

The manifestations of urinary tract infection vary with age. Neonates and children younger than 2 years of age do not complain of dysuria but present with fever, failure to thrive, and vomiting. Dysuria and abdominal or back pain are complaints of children over 3 years of age. In adults, the symptoms of lower tract infection are frequent urination of small amounts, urgency, dysuria, and suprapubic pain. Upper tract infection (acute pyelonephritis) usually presents with fever and chills, flank pain, and nausea. Frequency, urgency, and dysuria of lower tract origin may or may not be present.

Acute dysuria in young women does not always signify bacterial cystitis (Table 20–46). Indeed, 10 per cent of such women have symptoms resulting from local disease, such as vaginitis or herpes simplex infection. An additional 40 per cent have either bladder bacteriuria with numbers smaller than the benchmark 10^5 organisms/mL, or they have isolated urethritis, usually caused by *Chlamydia*. Appropriate clinical and microbiologic evaluation can distinguish between these etiologies.

Not every patient with a urinary tract infection will have classic symptoms. Many will be asymptomatic, and many symptomatic patients present in atypical fashion. An individual may feel tired. A child who is toilet trained may wet her bed. A man may have low back pain. The illness may present as a fever of unknown origin. Pain may be referred to the right lower quadrant or anterior abdomen rather than the flank. Paralytic ileus may be the most prominent finding. A diagnosis of urinary tract infection obviously should be considered in all these situations.

Diagnosis

A diagnosis of urinary tract infection is made by examining the urine. A clean, voided, midstream urine specimen is the method of choice because it has no morbidity. Attention should be paid to the technique of collection, because poor technique may lead to misdiagnosis.

Microscopic examination of the urine is performed after centrifugation. The presence of 5 to 10 leukocytes per high-power field represents 50 to 100 cells/mm^3, and white blood cell casts indicate renal parenchymal injury. Pyuria (over 10 leukocytes per high-power field), however, is an unreliable prediction of infection (i.e., bacteriuria) because both false-positive (30 per cent) and false-negative (30 per cent) results are frequent.

Hematuria and proteinuria may occur in urinary

TABLE 20–46. DISTRIBUTION OF DIAGNOSIS IN 200 OTHERWISE HEALTHY ADULT WOMEN PRESENTING WITH URINARY FREQUENCY AND DYSURIA

Local Disease	Cystitis	Pyelonephritis	"Urethritis"
Herpes simplex infection Vaginitis of various cause	$>10^5$ bacteria/mL of urine Lower tract infection	$>10^5$ bacteria/mL of urine Upper tract infection	$<10^5$ bacteria/mL of urine (bladder infection) *Chlamydia* urethritis
10%	40%	10%	40%

Modified after Stamm WE, Wagner KF, Amsel R, et al: Causes of the acute urethral syndrome in women. N Engl J Med 303:409, 1980, with permission. Copyright 1980, Massachusetts Medical Society.

tract infections. Most patients, however, excrete only small amounts of protein (less than 1 gm/24 hr) unless concomitant glomerular disease is present.

The most useful rapid test for presumptive diagnosis of a urinary tract infection is the presence of bacteria on a smear of unspun urine. A drop of fresh urine is placed on a glass slide and allowed to dry, and then treated with Gram's stain. More than one organism visible per oil field indicates over 10^5 organisms/mL of urine. It is absolutely essential that the urine be processed immediately, because the number of bacteria changes with time. The visibility of bacteria on spun urine specimens is inappropriate for quantitation.

The use of commercial dipsticks for urinalysis may be very helpful. Leukocyte esterase and nitrite detection strongly correlate with significant pyuria and bacteriuria, although false-negative nitrite tests occur in the face of inadequate dietary nitrate and with some particular microorganisms (e.g., *Candida*).

Urine culture is performed by collecting a midstream specimen of urine in order to wash out urethral bacteria and obtain a normally sterile bladder specimen. Numerous studies have established that greater than 10^5 bacteria/mL of urine is indicative of infection. However, 10^2 to 10^5 bacteria occasionally may be significant, because other factors, such as degree of hydration, prior antibiotic administration, and methods of collection, also influence the number of bacteria present.

Urine samples should be obtained in a sterile container and promptly processed. A dipslide method has become popular in which an agar slant is inoculated immediately with a thin film of freshly voided urine. This latter method avoids changes in bacterial counts associated with transportation or storage. Urine that cannot be inoculated immediately should be refrigerated until processing. For male patients in whom prostatitis is suspected, a divided urine specimen is necessary. The first voided 10 mL represents urethral flora. A midstream collection is then obtained, representing bladder flora. Prostatic massage is performed, and the following 10 mL of urine collected represents prostatic flora. Infection can be localized easily by comparing quantitative cultures of the aforementioned specimens.

In children with urinary tract infections, particu-

larly neonates, suprapubic aspiration of the bladder is a simple and useful method. Even small numbers of bacteria (e.g., 10^2 to 10^4) are indicative of infection if obtained by suprapubic aspiration.

Urethral catheterization should be avoided. One should realize that this carries a risk of introducing infection. The risk of infection following single catheterization depends on the patient population, with a low of 1 per cent in a healthy, young, female outpatient to a high of 30 per cent in an elderly, bedridden woman.

Treatment

The goals for treatment of urinary tract infection are (1) resolution of the acute infection and (2) prevention of irreversible renal damage.

Patients with asymptomatic bacteriuria in the absence of pregnancy, obstruction, or gross vesicoureteral reflux, although at increased risk of symptomatic urinary tract infections, do not appear to suffer any adverse long-term consequences of their bacteriuria. Patients with asymptomatic bacteriuria who clearly need treatment include pregnant women, men, children with vesicoureteral reflux, individuals with obstructive uropathy, and diabetics. Elderly nursing home patients with asymptomatic bacteriuria also may benefit from treatment to reduce morbidity.

Acute symptomatic infections in outpatients without underlying urologic pathology are usually caused by *E. coli* sensitive to all antibiotics. This is particularly true for young women. Each episode therefore should be treated with the least expensive, most readily available agent, such as trimethoprim–sulfamethoxazole. For difficult infections, including failure of primary therapy, relapse, or infection caused by resistant microorganisms, a fluoroquinolone may be indicated. In those individuals with recurrent symptomatic episodes, long-term prophylaxis is useful. Such prophylaxis will decrease the risk of recurrent symptomatic episodes as long as it is continued. However, after terminating prophylaxis, bacteriuria will return. A variety of prophylactic regimens have been found to be effective and are listed in Table 20–47.

The duration of treatment needed to cure a urinary tract infection depends on the site of infec-

TABLE 20–47. EFFECTS OF LOW-DOSE PROPHYLACTIC ANTIBIOTIC REGIMENS ON FREQUENCY OF RECURRENT SYMPTOMATIC BACTERIURIA

Regimen	Episodes/Patient/Year
None	2.8–4.2
Sulfamethoxazole, 500 mg qod	2.0–2.5
Sulfamethoxazole–trimethoprim, 1 tablet qd–qod	<0.2
Nitrofurantoin, 100 mg qd	<0.2
Trimethoprim, 100 mg qd	<0.2

tion. Acute dysuria in young women is usually of bladder or urethral origin and likely will respond to a 3-day course of treatment. Single-dose therapy should not be used. Three-day short course regimens have a low rate of adverse reactions and a cure rate equal to that achieved with longer courses of treatment. Such programs include trimethoprim–sulfamethoxazole, 1 double-strength tablet every 12 hours; sulfisoxazole, 500 mg every 6 hours; and ciprofloxacin, 250 mg every 12 hours.

Complicated urinary tract infections (see Table 20–48) require longer courses of treatment and the presumption of upper tract infection (pyelonephritis). Antimicrobal therapy for acute pyelonephritis is best selected from drug susceptibility testing results and continued for 14 days. Parenteral therapy is needed for septicemia, extreme illness, dehydration, or concomitant paralytic ileus. Courses of treatment longer than 14 days may be required for relapse of pyelonephritis or persistent prostatic foci of infection.

The role of ancillary measures is unclear. Although adequate hydration is important, the role of forced diuresis is unknown. Indeed, increasing urine output decreases the urinary concentration of antimicrobial agent and so actually may be counterproductive. Attention should be paid to good voiding habits, with avoidance of prolonged voluntary deferral of micturition, voiding after intercourse if sexual habits seem to promote recurrent infections, and maintenance of adequate hydration. Perineal cleansing after defecation should be

TABLE 20–48. RISK FACTORS FOR COMPLICATED URINARY TRACT INFECTIONS

Male sex
Age <12, >65 years
Hospital-acquired infection
Known urologic abnormality or stone
Indwelling catheter
Recent instrumentation
Diabetes mellitus
Prior relapse after treatment
History of recent pyelonephritis
Symptoms for <7 days pretreatment
Persistent symptoms (>4 days) during therapy
Pregnancy

established as a front-to-back maneuver to minimize fecal contamination of the periurethral area. Attention to such detail has been shown to be of some value in preventing recurrent infections.

Finally, the management of patients with infected urine and an indwelling bladder catheter must be discussed. Treatment of asymptomatic bacteriuria in such patients is not indicated because it will select out resistant microorganisms as long as the catheter remains in place. Removal of the catheter usually will not result in spontaneous elimination of bacteriuria, but specific therapy then can be administered. Treatment of bacteriuria in patients with indwelling catheters should be reserved for symptomatic episodes. Avoidance of catheterization is the best method of preventing catheter-associated infections.

VIRAL INFECTIONS

Viruses are obligate intracellular parasites. They are transmitted by close contact between an infected host (human or otherwise) and an immunologically naive recipient. Failure to respond to antimicrobial agents and difficulties in cultivation make the diagnosis of most viral infections a presumptive one based on the presenting epidemiologic and clinical features. Table 20–49 summarizes the modes of transmission, means of prevention, and treatment of common viral infections.

Adenovirus

Adenoviruses are important causes of febrile and respiratory diseases. These infections occur most often in children, students, and military recruits. Many infections are asymptomatic. Virus can be isolated from a high percentage of tonsillar and adenoid (hence its name) tissue. Viral shedding from the gastrointestinal tract can last for years. Adenovirus infections can present with a wide variety of clinical features. Patients typically develop an acute febrile illness associated with cough, sore throat, rhinorrhea, headache, and mild chills. Pneumonia develops as a complication in about 10 per cent of cases. Pharyngoconjunctival fever is a highly contagious adenoviral illness characterized by unilateral conjunctivitis, preauricular adenopathy, and pharyngitis. Enteric adenoviral infections are common. Other possible manifestations of adenoviral infections include epidemic keratoconjunctivitis, hemorrhagic cystitis, a pertussis-like syndrome, bronchiolitis, and necrotizing pneumonitis. Neonatal infections are rare but very serious. There are no specific treatments or prophylactic measures against adenovirus.

TABLE 20–49.　DISEASES CAUSED BY VIRUSES—THEIR MODES OF TRANSMISSION, PREVENTION, AND TREATMENT

Disease State	Virus	Transmission	Prevention*	Treatment†
Bronchiolitis	Adenovirus	Respiratory	None	None
	Parainfluenza	Respiratory	None	None
	Respiratory syncytial virus (RSV)	Hands, respiratory	Hand washing	Ribavirin
Bronchitis	Adenovirus	Respiratory	Vaccination (military use only)	None
	Influenza	Respiratory	Vaccination, amantidine, rimantidine	Amantidine, rimantidine
	Parainfluenza	Respiratory	None	None
	RSV	Hands, respiratory	Hand washing	Ribavirin
Conjunctivitis/ keratitis	Adenovirus		Hand washing	None
	Coxsackievirus A		Hand washing	None
	Enterovirus 70		Hand washing	None
	Herpes simplex virus		Hand washing	Trifluridine, vidarabine
Croup	Parainfluenza	Respiratory	None	None
Febrile exanthem	Coxsackievirus	Fecal–oral, respiratory	Hand washing	None
	Echovirus	Fecal–oral, respiratory	Hand washing	None
	Measles	Respiratory	Vaccination	None
	Parvovirus B19	Respiratory	None	None
	Roseola	Respiratory	None	None
	Rubella	Respiratory	Vaccination	None
Gastroenteritis	Adenovirus	Hands, respiratory	Hand washing	None
	Coronavirus	Hands, respiratory	Hand washing	None
	Norwalk virus	Fecal–oral, respiratory	Hand washing	None
	Rotavirus	Fecal–oral	Hand washing	None
Hemorrhagic fever	Dengue	Mosquito	Repellant	None
	Hantavirus	Rodent	None	None
	Yellow fever	Mosquito	Repellant, vaccination	None
Hepatitis	Cytomegalovirus	Respiratory, blood	None	Ganciclovir, foscarnet
	Epstein-Barr	Respiratory, blood	None	None
	Hepatitis A	Fecal–oral	Passive antibody (ISG)	None
	Hepatitis B	Blood, secretions	Passive antibody (HBIG), vaccination	Interferon α
	Hepatitis C	Blood	? Passive antibody (ISG)	Interferon α
	Yellow fever	Mosquito	Repellant, vaccination	None
Lymphadenopathy	Cytomegalovirus	Respiratory, blood	None	Ganciclovir, foscarnet
	Epstein-Barr	Respiratory, blood	None	None
	HIV	Blood, sexual	Blood precautions, condoms	Zidovudine, ddC, ddI, d4T
Meningitis/ encephalitis	Arboviruses	Mosquito	Repellant, vaccination	None
	Coxsackievirus	Fecal–oral, respiratory	Hand washing	None
	Echovirus	Fecal–oral, respiratory	Hand washing	None
	Herpes simplex virus	Respiratory, contact	None	Acyclovir
	HIV	Blood, sexual	Blood precautions, condoms	Zidovudine, ddI, ddC, d4T
	Mumps	Respiratory	Vaccination	None
	Rabies	Bite or saliva contact	Passive antibody (RIG), vaccination	None
Paralytic illness	Coxsackievirus	Fecal–oral, respiratory	Hand washing	None
	Echovirus	Fecal–oral, respiratory	Hand washing	None
	Poliovirus	Fecal–oral	Vaccination	None
Parotitis	Coxsackievirus	Fecal–oral, respiratory	Hand washing	None
	Mumps	Respiratory	Vaccination	None
Pharyngitis	Adenovirus	Respiratory	Vaccination (military only)	None
	Coxsackievirus	Fecal–oral, respiratory	Hand washing	None
	Cytomegalovirus	Respiratory, blood	None	Ganciclovir, foscarnet
	Echovirus	Fecal–oral, respiratory	Hand washing	None
	Epstein-Barr	Respiratory, blood	None	None

Table continued on following page

TABLE 20–49.   *(Continued)*

Disease State	Virus	Transmission	Prevention*	Treatment†
Pharyngitis, vesicular	Coxsackievirus A	Fecal–oral, respiratory	Hand washing	None
	Herpes simplex virus	Respiratory, contact	None	Acyclovir
Pneumonia/ pneumonitis	Adenovirus	Respiratory	Vaccination (military only)	None
	Cytomegalovirus	Respiratory, blood	None	Ganciclovir, foscarnet, IVIG
	Hantavirus	Rodent	None	? Ribavirin
	Influenza	Respiratory	Vaccination, amantidine, rimantidine	Amantidine, rimantidine
	RSV	Hands, respiratory	Hand washing	Ribavirin
Upper respiratory infection	Adenovirus	Respiratory	Vaccination (military only)	None
	Coronavirus	Hands, respiratory	None	None
	Influenza	Respiratory	Vaccination, amantidine, rimantidine	Amantidine, rimantidine
	Parainfluenza	Respiratory	None	None
	RSV	Hands, respiratory	Hand washing	Ribavirin
	Rhinovirus	Hands, respiratory	None	None
Vesicular exanthem	Coxsackievirus	Fecal–oral, respiratory	Hand washing	None
	Echovirus	Fecal–oral, respiratory	Hand washing	None
	Herpes simplex virus	Respiratory, contact	None	Acyclovir
	Varicella-zoster	Respiratory, contact	None	Acyclovir, foscarnet

* Diseases spread by respiratory routes or direct contact may be prevented in some cases by isolation of infected patients.
† Supportive treatment (e.g., intravenous fluids, oxygen) may be indicated but is not listed as specific antiviral therapy.

Arbovirus

Arthropod-borne viruses (arboviruses) cause several important diseases. Eastern and western equine encephalitis, St. Louis encephalitis, and California (Lacrosse) encephalitis are all caused by arboviruses. Regional outbreaks of these infections occur periodically during summer months. Dengue virus is endemic to many tropical areas, including the Caribbean and Central and South America. Dengue fever is characterized by high fever, severe headache, retrobulbar pain, myalgias, extremity pain, and a characteristic facial flushing. Travelers to endemic areas are at risk of acquiring this disease. Yellow fever and Rift Valley fever are important causes of morbidity and mortality in endemic areas. Treatment of these arbovirus infections, like the others, is supportive only. No specific treatments are yet available. There is now a vaccine effective against Japanese encephalitis virus, a severe encephalitis that occurs in south and eastern Asia.

Coronavirus

Coronaviruses are among the most common agents to cause the common cold in adults and children. Symptoms are clinically indistinguishable from colds caused by rhinovirus. They occasionally cause lower respiratory disease and also may be an important cause of viral gastroenteritis in children.

Because of antigenic diversity and frequent reinfection, it is unlikely a vaccine will be developed to prevent coronavirus infections.

Cytomegalovirus

By late adulthood, most people have been infected by cytomegalovirus (CMV). The virus is transmitted perinatally from mother to child, through contact with infected body fluids, and through sexual contact. It rarely causes disease in the immunocompetent patient but exhibits protean manifestations in immunosuppressed patients. Most infections in newborns are asymptomatic. Five to ten per cent of infected newborns develop a disease characterized by jaundice, hepatosplenomegaly, microcephaly, petechial rash, pneumonitis, or chorioretinitis. Sensorineural hearing loss occurs in 20 per cent of these infants. CMV most commonly presents as mononucleosis in immunocompetent adults. Retinitis, interstitial pneumonia, esophagitis, and colitis frequently are seen in immunosuppressed adults. Less commonly seen are meningoencephalitis, hepatitis, and adrenal gland involvement. Treatment of CMV infections is problematic. Ganciclovir and foscarnet have been used with some success in retinitis and gastrointestinal disease. They are less effective in pneumonitis.

Enteroviruses

Nonpolio enteroviruses that cause illness include many serotypes of echovirus, coxsackievirus, and enterovirus. These are extremely common infections. All children are likely to experience at least one infection each summer and fall, although 50 to 80 per cent of these are asymptomatic. There is a large spectrum of diseases caused by these viruses that in most cases are clinically indistinguishable. A nonspecific febrile illness ("summer grippe") lasting 3 to 4 days and characterized by the abrupt onset of fever and malaise is probably the most common manifestation of enteroviral infections. Exanthems and enanthems of many varieties are seen with these infections. Most of these are not distinctive enough on clinical grounds to differentiate the etiologic agent. The exceptions are hand-foot-and-mouth disease and herpangina, which are caused predominantly by group A coxsackieviruses. Aseptic meningitis is caused by an enterovirus in most cases. Epidemic pleurodynia—a disease of muscle, not pleura—is characterized by the abrupt onset of fever and spasmodic pain of the rib cage or abdomen. The illness usually is caused by group B coxsackieviruses and lasts 4 to 6 days. Acute hemorrhagic conjunctivitis is a highly contagious illness caused by enterovirus 70. It is characterized by eye pain, swelling of the eyelids, and subconjunctival hemorrhages. Recovery is usually complete by 10 days. Myocarditis, paralysis, pericarditis, orchitis, gastroenteritis, and myositis sometimes are caused by enteroviruses.

Epstein-Barr Virus

As with other members of the *Herpesvirus* family (e.g., CMV, herpes simplex, varicella-zoster), almost all people become infected with EBV by adulthood. Approximately 50 per cent of the population seroconverts by age 5. The virus appears to be of low contagiousness and probably is spread by intimate contact. Many infections are subclinical, and virus shedding persists for up to 18 months after infection. The most common manifestation of primary EBV infection is infectious mononucleosis. The classic presentation of this disease is the triad of pharyngitis, lymphadenopathy, and fever. Other common features are malaise, headache, anorexia, myalgias, hepatosplenomegaly, ampicillin-associated rash, and a palatal enanthem. The infection tends to be more severe in older patients. Almost all patients recover uneventfully in 1 to 3 weeks, although malaise and fatigue can persist considerably longer. Potential complications include laryngotonsillar obstruction, splenic rupture, encephalitis, granulocytopenia, and thrombocytopenia. Treatment is supportive except in patients with impending airway obstruction, severe thrombocytopenia, or hemolytic anemia. A short course of corticosteroids is beneficial in these circumstances. Burkitt's lymphoma in Africa, nasopharyngeal carcinoma, and primary central nervous system lymphoma in AIDS patients probably are caused by EBV infection.

Hantavirus

The hantavirus, carried by rodents in various regions of the world, is responsible for two known conditions with relatively high mortality rates. Korean hemorrhagic fever, first reported during the Korean War in the early 1950s, is characterized by fever, headache, hemorrhages, shock, and renal failure. In 1993, cases began to be reported in the Southwest of a syndrome characterized by fever, myalgias, headache, acute respiratory distress, and a high mortality rate. Both of these syndromes are acquired through contact with infected animals. No vector or human-to-human transmission seems to take place. Ribavirin has been used with some success in cases of severe Korean hemorrhagic fever. Experience with the American hantavirus infection and ribavirin is limited so far.

Herpes Simplex Virus

Herpes simplex virus (HSV) infections are among the most common infections of human beings. HSV-1 most frequently affects the lips, oral mucosa, eye, and finger. HSV-2 has a predilection for the genital, anal, and perianal areas and neonates. However, either type can be found in any site. Primary infections of both types are frequently asymptomatic. Symptomatic primary HSV-1 infections usually are manifested as gingivostomatitis, pharyngitis, or ocular infection in a child. Primary HSV-2 infections typically present as tender vesicular genital, anal, or perianal lesions in adolescents or young adults. HSV infections tend to recur at variable rates in different people. Severity tends to wane with recurrences. As in primary infections, recurrences can be asymptomatic and the infection is easily transmitted during these times. HSV-1 occasionally causes encephalitis and HSV-2 aseptic meningitis. HSV infections are much more severe in the immunocompromised patient. Acyclovir is used in the treatment and prophylaxis of HSV infections. Acyclovir given early in the course of primary mucocutaneous HSV infection substantially reduces the severity and duration of disease.

Influenza Virus

Influenza virus has been responsible for epidemics of respiratory disease for at least the past 400 years. Pandemics of influenza occur periodically and are responsible for enormous morbidity and mortality. The most well-known pandemic, in 1918–1919, was associated with over 21 million deaths worldwide. Outbreaks of differing severity occur each winter in temperate climates. The disease is characterized by the sudden onset of fever, cough, headache, myalgias, and prostration. It typically lasts 3 to 5 days. The most serious complication is either a primary viral or secondary bacterial pneumonia. Less common complications include Reye's syndrome, myocarditis, pericarditis, and myositis. Amantadine and rimantidine are effective in reducing the duration of influenza symptoms if taken early in the course of the disease. They are also effective prophylactic agents against influenza A in those people who cannot be or have not been vaccinated. The most effective prophylactic agent is the inactivated virus vaccine. This vaccine is recommended annually for high-risk individuals, including those over 65; people with any underlying pulmonary, cardiac, or chronic metabolic disease; health care providers; residents of nursing homes; and children on chronic aspirin therapy.

Measles Virus

A resurgence of measles was noted between 1989 and 1992. Unimmunized immigrants, inadequate rates of vaccination in preschool children, and vaccine failure in high school and college students were responsible. Measles is an extremely contagious disease spread by airborne droplets. Classically, it is characterized by a prodrome of fever, anorexia, malaise, conjunctivitis, cough, and coryza lasting several days. This is followed by the development of Koplik's spots, bluish gray specks on a red base on the buccal mucosa. The typical macular confluent rash beginning on the face and then migrating down the body follows. The most common complications are pneumonia and encephalitis. The disease tends to be much more severe in the immunocompromised patient. Treatment is supportive. Current recommendations for prophylaxis are that each child be given two doses of live measles vaccine, one at 15 months of age and another at entry into elementary or middle school. Young adults born after 1957 should have documentation of administration of one dose of live measles vaccine after their first birthday. Entrants to colleges, universities, and other institutions of learning, and employees of health care facilities should have documentation of two doses.

Mumps Virus

Cases of mumps declined by 98 per cent from 1967 to 1985 as a result of the widespread use of an effective live virus vaccine. There has been a slight increase subsequent to this secondary to lower vaccination rates. Transmission is through direct contact, droplets, or fomites. Subclinical infection occurs in 30 per cent of cases. In the remainder, the classic manifestation is nonsuppurative swelling and tenderness of the parotid glands. Extrasalivary gland involvement is more common in the postpubertal patient. Meningitis, orchitis, and pancreatitis are the most important extrasalivary manifestations. Treatment is supportive. Prevention is through the administration of live attenuated virus vaccine. Two doses are now recommended, one after 12 months of age and the other at entry into elementary or middle school.

Norwalk Virus

Epidemic viral gastroenteritis most often is associated with the Norwalk virus. It predominantly affects older children and adults. It rarely is serious enough to warrant hospitalization. Transmission is fecal–oral. It can be associated with the ingestion of contaminated food or water. After an incubation period of 12 to 48 hours, the infected person experiences nausea and abdominal cramping. Vomiting and diarrhea usually occur together, although either may be present alone. Symptoms usually resolve within 48 to 72 hours. Treatment is supportive. An effective vaccine will be difficult to develop because immunity is short lived.

Papillomavirus

HPV infections produce epithelial tumors of the skin and mucous membranes. The virus is widespread through the population. Common, plantar, and flat warts are prevalent in children. Condyloma acuminata, or anogenital warts, is a STD whose incidence is rapidly increasing. HPV infection has been found in numerous sites, including conjunctiva, nasal cavity, sinuses, oral cavity, tracheobronchial mucosa, esophagus, larynx, urethra, anogenital tract, and skin. Evidence is suggestive that HPV infection leads to the development of squamous epithelial precancerous lesions and carcinomas in some of these sites. Transmission is through close contact. Treatment consists of physical or chemical destruction of visible lesions. Prevention is through avoidance of contact with infectious lesions.

Parainfluenza Virus

Parainfluenza virus infections are an important cause of respiratory infections in young children. They are the most common known agents causing croup. They rank second only to RSV as a cause of lower respiratory disease in infants. Transmission is person to person by contact or aerosolized droplets. Clinical features are primarily respiratory. They can range in severity from a mild cold to severe croup or bronchiolitis requiring hospitalization. Asymptomatic infections appear to be common. Primary infections, although generally more severe than reinfections, rarely are serious. There is no specific treatment for parainfluenza infections. Development of an effective vaccine is problematic because of the frequency of reinfection with this virus.

Parvovirus B19

Human parvovirus B19 causes erythema infectiosum ("fifth disease"), transient aplastic crisis in patients with hemolytic anemias (sickle cell, thalassemia, etc.), and chronic anemia in immunodeficiency states (e.g., HIV infection). It also has been associated with acute arthropathy and fetal illness (hydrops fetalis, spontaneous abortion). Infection occurs throughout the year, and periodic community epidemics can occur. Seroprevalence ranges from 1 to 15 per cent in young children to 50 to 60 per cent in adults. Transmission is through respiratory droplets. Erythema infectiosum is the most commonly recognized manifestation of parvovirus B19 illness. Its hallmark is a rash that erupts on the face ("slapped cheek" appearance) following a mild prodromal illness. A rash of variable appearance sometimes occurs on other parts of the body. The facial rash may reappear for weeks after the initial illness. Treatment of most B19 infections is not necessary because of the mild self-limited nature of the illnesses. Immune globulin has been shown to be effective in some patients with B19-caused anemia and red cell aplasia.

Poxvirus

Poxvirus infections in humans include smallpox (now eradicated), orf, paravaccinia, and molluscum contagiosum. Humans are only incidental hosts for orf and paravaccinia. Molluscum contagiosum is a human virus whose incidence has been increasing. It is seen most commonly in the 15 to 24-year age group but also is seen in children. Transmission is through skin-to-skin contact. It is characterized by multiple, painless, umbilicated, pearly white papules 3 to 5 mm in diameter. A more widespread, treatment-resistant form of the infection occurs in the immunocompromised patient. Although lesions frequently resolve spontaneously, treatment may involve currettage, liquid nitrogen, or chemical eradication.

Rabies Virus

The rabies virus occurs in animals throughout the continental United States and on most continents of the world. In the United States, wild animals (skunks, raccoons, woodchucks, bats, foxes) most commonly are infected, whereas in other parts of the world the domestic dog is the major source of infection. The disease is transmitted primarily when the saliva of an infected animal is inoculated into a host by biting. The incubation period is usually 20 to 90 days. A prodrome of nonspecific symptoms such as malaise, headache, fever, and anorexia lasts for 2 to 10 days. Coma followed by death occurs after a 2- to 7-day period of neurologic symptoms that include paresthesias, paralysis, delirium, hyperactivity, and the pathognomonic hydrophobia and aerophobia. Once symptoms develop, rabies has the highest case fatality rate of any known human infection. No specific treatment is available. Rabies can be prevented by appropriate postexposure treatment with rabies immune globulin and rabies vaccine.

Respiratory Syncytial Virus

RSV is the most common cause of lower respiratory tract illness in young children. It is responsible for 40 to 50 per cent of hospitalizations for bronchiolitis and 25 per cent of hospitalizations for pediatric pneumonia in the United States. Primary infection usually occurs within the first 2 years of age. Reinfection is common. Primary infection typically begins with coryza, congestion, and low-grade fever that progresses to cough, wheezing, and dyspnea. Otitis media is common. The peak frequency of infections is in the 3- to 6-month age range. Peak hospitalization rates occur in 1- to 3-month-olds. Adult infections present as upper respiratory infections. Transmission occurs through hand–nose, hand–eye, and fomite contact. Infections are most common in the winter and spring. Treatment is primarily supportive, with oxygen and hydration. The data on bronchodilator efficacy are conflicting. Specific therapy with aerosolized ribavirin is indicated for seriously ill high-risk children.

Rhinovirus

The rhinovirus causes approximately 50 per cent of common colds. Adults and children experience one to two infections per year, of which approximately three fourths are symptomatic. Peak incidence is in the fall and spring. Transmission is person to person, with autoinoculation through hand–eye or hand–nose contact. Complications of rhinovirus colds include sinusitis, otitis media, bronchitis, and asthma exacerbation. Treatment is supportive. Immunity is type specific, but because there are over 100 different serotypes of rhinovirus, this immunity is of little clinical significance and the development of an effective vaccine is unlikely soon.

Rotavirus

Rotaviruses are the most frequent cause of diarrhea in young children in developed countries. They predominantly affect children 3 to 24 months of age, although older children and adults can develop minor disease. The severity of illness ranges from completely asymptomatic to severe, dehydrating illness. Death from rotaviral infections is rare in developed countries; however, it is a major cause of childhood mortality in developing countries. Peak seasonal incidence is in the late fall in the Southwest. It then spreads northeastward, peaking in eastern Canada in the spring. After an incubation period of 1 to 3 days, the affected child develops vomiting and fever followed by diarrhea and dehydration. Typically the illness lasts 5 to 7 days. Treatment is supportive. Considerable effort is being expended to develop an effective vaccine. It is likely these efforts will be successful.

Rubella Virus

Rubella infections are generally benign and self-limited, but intrapartum infection can be associated with disastrous effects in the fetus. Although the incidence has declined enormously since the introduction of rubella vaccine, limited outbreaks continue to occur. Postnatally, the infection presents as a nonspecific illness consisting of adenopathy (posterior auricular, posterior cervical, and suboccipital) and a maculopapular rash spreading from the face downward. Congenital rubella syndrome is associated with protean manifestations, including those that are temporary (low birth weight, thrombocytopenia, hepatosplenomegaly), permanent (deafness, cataracts, patent ductus), and developmental (mental retardation, behavior disorders, seizures). No treatment is needed in postnatal rubella because the symptoms are so mild. Prevention is through two doses of live attenuated virus, one given after 12 months of age and the second before entry into elementary or middle school.

Varicella-Zoster Virus

Varicella-zoster virus (VZV), a member of the *Herpesvirus* group, causes varicella (chickenpox) and herpes zoster (shingles). Varicella is the presentation of the primary illness. It is a highly contagious disease primarily of young children. Ninety per cent of cases are in children under 9 years of age. Infections are most common in the winter and spring. Transmission is through close contact with an infected person. The illness is characterized by the development of successive crops of vesicles on an erythematous base. Most cases resolve in 7 to 10 days. Complications are more common in adolescents and adults and may include pneumonia and encephalitis. Morbidity and mortality are significantly higher in the immunocompromised patient. Herpes zoster is the clinical manifestation of VZV reactivation. It is most common in elderly patients but may occur at any age. It is characterized by a painful vesicular eruption of one to three dermatomes. Susceptible individuals can contract chicken pox if exposed to a person with zoster. The most common complication of zoster is postherpetic neuralgia. Treatment of normal hosts with VZV infections is with high-dose acyclovir begun as early as possible in the course of the illness. Immunocompromised hosts require intravenous treatment.

SUGGESTED READINGS

General

Benenson AS (ed): Control of Communicable Diseases in Man, 15th edition. Washington, DC, American Public Health Association, 1990.

Bennett JV, Brachman PS (eds): Hospital Infections, 3rd edition. Boston, Little, Brown, 1992.

Hoeprich PD (ed): Infectious Diseases, 4th edition. Philadelphia, Harper & Row, 1989.

Krugman S, Katz SL (eds): Infectious Diseases of Children, 9th edition. St. Louis, CV Mosby, 1992.

Mandell GL, Douglas RG Jr, Bennett JE (eds): Principles and Practice of Infectious Diseases, 3rd edition. New York, John Wiley & Sons, 1990.

Remington JS, Klein JO (eds): Infectious Diseases of the Fetus and Newborn Infant, 3rd edition. Philadelphia, WB Saunders Company, 1990.

Warren KS, Mahmoud AAF (eds): Geographic Medicine for the Practitioner, 2nd edition. New York, Springer-Verlag, 1985.

Antibiotics

Kucers A, Bennett NM: The Use of Antibiotics, 4th edition. Philadelphia, JB Lippincott, 1987.

Lambert HP, O'Grady F: Antibiotic and Chemotherapy, 6th edition. New York, Churchill Livingstone, 1992.

Neu HC (ed): Update on antibiotics I and II. Med Clin North Am 71:1051, 1987; 72:555, 1988.

Nichols RL (ed): Current approaches to antibiotic prophylaxis in surgery. Infect Dis Clin Pract 2:149, 1993.

Paluzzi RG: Antimicrobial prophylaxis for surgery. Med Clin North Am 77:427, 1993.

The Medical Letter Handbook of Antimicrobial Therapy. New Rochelle, NY, The Medical Letter, 1992.

Bone and Joint Infection

Buchstein SR, Gardner P: Lyme disease. Infect Dis Clin North Am 5:103, 1991.

Emslie KR, Nade S: Pathogenesis and treatment of acute hematogenous osteomyelitis. Rev Infect Dis 8:841, 1986.

Esterhai JL Jr, Gelb I: Adult septic arthritis. Orthop Clin North Am 22:503, 1991.

Mackowiak PA, Jones SR, Smith JW: Diagnostic value of sinus-tract cultures in chronic osteomyelitis. JAMA 239:2772, 1978.

Malane MS, Grant-Kels JM, Feder HM Jr, et al: Diagnosis of Lyme disease based on dermatologic manifestations. Ann Intern Med 114:490, 1991.

Shaw BA, Kasser JR: Acute septic arthritis in infancy and childhood. Clin Orthop 257:212, 1990.

Spach DH, Liles WC, Campbell GL, et al: Tick-borne diseases in the United States. N Engl J Med 329:936, 1993.

Stechenberg BW: Lyme disease: The latest great imitator. Pediatr Infect Dis J 7:402, 1988.

Steere AC, Schoen RT, Taylor E: The clinical evolution of Lyme arthritis. Ann Intern Med 107:725, 1987.

Waldvogel FA, Vasey H: Osteomyelitis: The past decade. N Engl J Med 303:360, 1980.

Cardiovascular Infections

Karchmer AW, Dismukes WE, Buckley MJ, et al: Late prosthetic valvular endocarditis. Am J Med 64:199, 1978.

Pesanti EL, Smith IM: Infective endocarditis with negative blood cultures: An analysis of 52 cases. Am J Med 66:43, 1979.

Venezio FR, Westenfelder GO, Cook FV, et al: Infective endocarditis in a community hospital. Arch Intern Med 142:789, 1982.

Watanakunakorn C, Burkert T: Infective endocarditis at a large community teaching hospital. Medicine (Baltimore) 72:90, 1993.

Wilson WR, Geraci JE: Treatment of streptococcal infective endocarditis. Am J Med 78(suppl 6B):128, 1985.

Central Nervous System Infections

Geiseler PJ, Nelson KE, Levin S, et al: Community-acquired purulent meningitis: A review of 1316 cases during the antibiotic era, 1954–1976. Rev Infect Dis 2:725, 1980.

Luby JP: Infections of the central nervous system. Am J Med Sci 304:379, 1992.

Odio CM, Faingezicht I, Paris M, et al: The beneficial effects of early dexamethasone administration in infants and children with bacterial meningitis. N Engl J Med 324:1525, 1991.

Sande MA: Antibiotic therapy of bacterial meningitis: Lessons we've learned. Am J Med 71:507, 1981.

Fever

Baraff LJ, Bass JW, Fleisher GR, et al: Practice guideline for the management of infants and children 0 to 36 months of age with fever without source. Pediatrics 92:1, 1993.

Dinarello CA, Cannon JG, Wolff SM: New concepts on the pathogenesis of fever. Rev Infect Dis 10:168, 1988.

Esposito AL, Gleckman RA: A diagnostic approach to the adult with fever of unknown origin. Arch Intern Med 139:575, 1979.

Mackowiak PA, LeMaistre CF: Drug fever: A critical appraisal of conventional concepts. Ann Intern Med 106:728, 1987.

McNeil BJ, Sanders R, Anderson PO, et al: A prospective study of computed tomography, ultrasound and gallium imaging in patients with fever. Radiology 139:647, 1981.

Petersdorf RG, Beeson PB: Fever of unexplained origin: Report of 100 cases. Medicine 40:1, 1961.

Gastrointestinal Infection

Bartlett JG, Chang TW, Gurwith M, et al: Antibiotic associated pseudomembranous colitis due to toxin-producing *Clostridia*. N Engl J Med 298:531, 1978.

Blacklow NR, Greenberg HB: Viral gastroenteritis. N Engl J Med 325:252, 1991.

Cantey JR: Infectious diarrhea: Pathogenesis and risk factors. Am J Med 78:65, 1985.

Cheney CP, Wong RK: Acute infectious diarrhea. Med Clin North Am 77:1169, 1993.

Ericsson CD, DuPont HL: Traveler's diarrhea: Recent developments. Infect Dis Clin North Am 2:66, 1985.

Gorbach SL: Intraabdominal infections. Clin Infect Dis 17:961, 1993.

Guerrant RL, Shields DS, Thorsan SM, et al: Evaluation and diagnosis of acute infectious diarrhea. Am J Med 78(suppl 6B):91, 1985.

Infection in the Compromised Host

Bodey GP: Antimicrobial prophylaxis for infection in neutropenic patients. Curr Clin Top Infect Dis 9:1, 1988.

Glenn J, Cotton D, Wesley R, et al: Anorectal infections in patients with malignant diseases. Rev Infect Dis 10:42, 1988.

Pizzo PA: Management of fever in patients with cancer and treatment induced neutropenia. N Engl J Med 328:1323, 1993.

Sickles EA, Greene WH, Wiernik PH: Clinical presentations of infection in granulocytopenic patients. Arch Intern Med 135:715, 1975.

Young LS: Nosocomial infections in the immunocompromised adult. Am J Med 70:398, 1981.

Respiratory Tract Infections

Ching WT, Meyer RD: Legionella infections. Infect Dis Clin North Am 1:595, 1987.

England AC, Fraser DW, Plikaytis BD, et al: Sporadic legionellosis in the United States: The first thousand cases. Ann Intern Med 94:164, 1981.

Finland M: Pneumonia and pneumococcal infections with special reference to pneumococcal pneumonia. Am Rev Respir Dis 120:481, 1979.

McGowan JE: Respiratory tract infections due to *Branhamella catarrhalis* and *Neisseria* species. Curr Clin Top Infect Dis 8:181, 1987.

Murphy TF, Henderson FW, Clyde WA Jr, et al: Pneumonia: An eleven-year study in a pediatric practice. Am J Epidemiol 113:12, 1981.

Wallace RT (ed): Lower respiratory tract infections. Infect Dis Clin North Am 5:3, 1991.

Sepsis and Bacteremia

Bone RC: The pathogenesis of sepsis. Ann Intern Med 115:457, 1991.

Freedman, RM, Ingram DL, Gross I, et al: A half-century of neonatal sepsis at Yale. Am J Dis Child 135:140, 1981.

Kreger BE, Craven DE, McCabe WR: Gram-negative bacteremia. IV. Reevaluation of clinical features and treatment in 612 patients. Am J Med 68:344, 1980.

Parrillo JE, Parker MM, Natanson C, et al: Septic shock in humans: Advances in the understanding of pathogensis, cardiovascular dysfunction, and therapy. Ann Intern Med 113:227, 1990.

Todd JK: Staphylococcal toxin syndromes. Annu Rev Med 36:337, 1985.

Sexually Transmitted Diseases

Centers for Disease Control and Prevention: 1993 Sexually transmitted diseases treatment guidelines. MMWR 42(no. RR-14), 1993.

Handsfield HH (ed): Sexually transmitted diseases. Infect Dis Clin North Am 1:1, 1987.

Mertz GJ, Jones CC, Mills J, et al: Long-term acyclovir suppression of frequently recurring genital herpes simplex virus infection. JAMA 260:201, 1988.

Quinn TC, Corey L, Chaffee RG, et al: The etiology of anorectal infections in homosexual men. Am J Med 71:395, 1981.

Skin and Soft Tissue Infections

Cruse PJE, Foord R: The epidemiology of wound infection: A 10-year prospective study of 62,939 wounds. Surg Clin North Am 60:27, 1980.

Fleisher G, Ludwig S, Campos J: Cellulitis: Bacterial etiology, clinical features and laboratory findings. J Pediatr 97:591, 1980.

McDonough JJ, Stern PJ, Alexander JW: Management of animal and human bites and resulting human infections. Curr Clin Top Infect Dis 8:11, 1987.

Meislin HW, Lerner SA, Graves MH, et al: Cutaneous abscesses: Anaerobic and aerobic bacteriology and outpatient management. Ann Intern Med 87:145, 1977.

Tuberculosis

American Thoracic Society/Centers for Disease Control: Treatment of tuberculosis and tuberculous infection in adults and children. Am Rev Respir Dis 134:355, 1986.

Huebner RE, Schein MF, Bass JB Jr: The tuberculin skin test. Clin Infect Dis 17:968, 1993.

Iseman MD: Treatment of multidrug-resistant tuberculosis. N Engl J Med 329:784, 1993.

Snider DE, Rieder HL, Combs D, et al: Tuberculosis in children. Pediatr Infect Dis 7:271, 1988.

Woods GL, Washington JA: Mycobacteria other than *Mycobacterium tuberculosis*: Review of microbiologic and clinical aspects. Rev Infect Dis 9:275, 1987.

Urinary Tract Infection

Andriole VT: Urinary tract infections. Infect Dis Clin North Am 1:713, 1987.

Gillenwater JY, Harrison RB, Kunin CM: Natural history of bacteriuria in schoolgirls. N Engl J Med 301:396, 1979.

Kunin CM: Detection, Prevention and Management of Urinary Tract Infections, 4th edition. Philadelphia, Lea & Febiger, 1987.

Stamm WE: Diagnosis of *Chlamydia trachomatis* genitourinary infections. Ann Intern Med 108:710, 1988.

Stamm WE, Hooten TM: Management of urinary tract infections in adults. N Engl J Med 329:1328, 1993.

Viral Infection

Bale JF: Viral encephalitis. Med Clin North Am 77:25, 1993.

Fishbein DB, Robinson LE: Rabies. N Engl J Med 329:1632, 1993.

Mertz GJ: Genital herpes simplex virus infections. Med Clin North Am 74:1443, 1990.

Whitley RJ: Therapeutic approaches to varicella-zoster virus infections. J Infect Dis 166(suppl 1):s51, 1992.

CHAPTER 21

CARE OF THE ADULT HIV-1–INFECTED PATIENT

SUSAN M. MILLER

The first cases of the acquired immunodeficiency syndrome (AIDS) were reported in June 1981. The human immunodeficiency virus (HIV) has since become a focus of medical, legal, political, sociological, and public health concerns and remains one of the most controversial and frightening pandemics in modern medicine. This epidemic has precipitated a discussion of many disparate attitudes concerning public health, individual rights, research, therapeutic alternatives, infectious diseases, and health care reimbursement.

Early in the epidemic, the etiologic agent of AIDS was identified as HIV, a retrovirus of the lentivirus subfamily (Barre-Sinoussi et al., 1983; Gallo et al., 1984). Retroviruses have an unusual replicative enzyme known as reverse transcriptase (RNA-directed DNA polymerase) that is not found in normal eukaryotic cells. The enzyme allows the virus to copy its viral RNA into DNA precursors. This proviral DNA then is incorporated permanently into host cell chromosomes, thereby protecting the HIV's DNA from host cell defenses and ensuring its survival by transmission through host genes.

AIDS itself is a constellation of illnesses that result from the progressive impairment and destruction of immune function secondary to HIV infection. The loss of vitality in immune function makes the host organism vulnerable to malignancies and infections it normally would resist. The immunodeficiency of AIDS is similar to that seen in patients with chemotherapy-induced immunosuppression or in organ transplant recipients; that is, the opportunistic infections occur in the context of the immunodeficiency. Patients do not die from HIV infection per se, but rather from the opportunistic infections that result from the acquired impairment in immune function. The purpose of this chapter is to help physicians (1) recognize physical findings associated with immunodeficiency, (2) interpret HIV serologic test results, (3) initiate outpatient primary care management, (4) discern common opportunistic infections, (5) summarize guidelines for treatment, (6) address common complications of therapy, and (7) preview new drugs and treatment strategies.

EPIDEMIOLOGY

HIV infection has variable epidemiologic characteristics depending on which region of the world is examined. For example, in Africa entire populations are disappearing because the heterosexual epidemic is further complicated by malnutrition, malaria, tuberculosis, indigenous diarrhea, and poverty. In Cuba, HIV infection in part was introduced by soldiers returning from Angola, where they had acquired infection through heterosexual transmission. In the United States, the epidemic has predominant features of both sexual behavior (homosexual and heterosexual) and substance abuse. In 1992, HIV infection was the leading cause of death among men 25 to 44 years of age; among women, it was the fourth leading cause of death in the same age group ("MMWR Update," 1993).

The changing demographics of HIV infection within the United States show increasing rates of HIV infection in adolescents and women. Nineteen ninety-three marked the first year that heterosexual transmission was the risk factor in greater than 50 per cent of women with AIDS (eclipsing intravenous drug use).

HIV transmission is as simple and complex as individual behaviors. Behaviors that may increase the likelihood of HIV transmission include anal intercourse, concomitant sexually transmitted diseases, multiple sexual partners, lack of circumcision, cervical ectopy, menstruation, advanced HIV disease, viral virulence, and baseline host immune status. Behaviors that decrease the risk of infection with HIV include abstinence, decreasing the number of sexual partners, and condoms. Management and modification of behavior often is complicated by poverty, discrimination, group alienation, and misinformation (Merson, 1993; Sande and Volberding, 1992).

Epidemics occurring in tandem with HIV include the resurgence of *Mycobacterium tuberculosis*, intravenous drug use, and sexually transmitted diseases.

ETIOLOGY AND PATHOGENESIS

The initial step in the immunopathogenesis of AIDS is host infection by HIV. This infection is characterized by a chronic, progressive, and usually fatal clinical course. The biologic features of HIV and the host immune response(s) that trigger functional and qualitative immune suppression and lead to advanced HIV disease progression still remain an enigma, and are the subjects of intensive research (Pantaleo et al., 1993; Weiss, 1993).

Although HIV preferentially infects monocytes, macrophages, and helper T lymphocytes, it may affect other host cells, including bone marrow precursors, Langerhans' cells, glial cells, the central nervous system, and lymph node reservoirs (DeVita et al., 1992; Sande and Volberding, 1992).

There are two overlapping arms of the immune response: humoral and cellular. The humoral (antibody) response consists of B lymphocytes. The cellular arm is composed of all subsets of T lymphocytes, monocytes, and macrophages.

The subpopulation of T lymphocytes known as helper T cells are the primary regulators of the immune response and proliferate in response to antigenic stimulation. Furthermore, HIV-infected helper T cells are susceptible to cytopathic effects and resultant cellular abnormalities and depletion. Additional mechanisms of immune dysregulation associated with HIV infection may include a series of immunologic and nonimmunologic mechanisms: syncytia formation, HIV-specific cytotoxic T lymphocytes, autoimmune mechanisms, anergy, superantigen formation, and apoptosis (Pantaleo et al., 1993).

Monocytes and macrophages are essential in activating the immune response and may be necessary for the further development of antibody responses, in addition to their traditional role of scavengers. Infected macrophages have the ability to cross the blood–brain barrier, and may be a mechanism for central nervous system penetrations by HIV. The generalized lymphadenopathy seen throughout the course of HIV may reflect seeding and sequestration of HIV within lymph nodes. This reservoir of continued HIV replication may be a vital component of disease progression/reactivation in spite of the early neutralizing antibody responses by the host organism (Pantaleo et al., 1993).

To conceptualize the clinical picture of this disease, an understanding of the (theorized) replicative process of HIV is essential. HIV preferentially (although not exclusively) infects cells with a specific protein receptor known as the CD4 molecule. Attachment of HIV-1 requires successful interaction between the CD4 expressed on the surface of the target cell and the viral envelope glycoprotein, gp120. Once HIV has entered the cell cytoplasm by endocytosis, it is rapidly uncoated, and a single strand of complementary DNA is generated from the HIV RNA genome via the HIV reverse transcriptase enzyme. A second strand of DNA then is synthesized, and now a double-stranded copy of the original viral RNA is available for incorporation into the host genome. This viral DNA is translocated into the nucleus and inserted into host cell chromosomes by a virally encoded integrase enzyme. Any unintegrated HIV DNA remains in the cell cytoplasm and may have a role in the cytopathicity associated with HIV. HIV progeny released from cells then may elicit an antibody response or infect other susceptible cells (DeVita et al., 1992; Pantaleo et al., 1993).

The HIV reverse transcriptase enzyme does not have the ability to correct for spontaneous mutations that occur during the transcription process. These mutations lead to increased diversity of HIV, and results in different strains existing within the same host. These viral strains may have different genotypic and phenotypic traits and are capable of being transmitted to other individuals.

After HIV infection is established, it persists throughout the lifetime of the infected person, avoiding microbiologic clearance by the host immune response. After repetitive and sequential replication of HIV, a subsequent depletion of T4 lymphocytes occurs that results in a disarray of cell-mediated and humoral immune responses. This depletion of T4 lymphocytes is a variably paced process without spontaneous reversal that parallels the prolonged clinical course between the appearance of antibodies to HIV (seroconversion) and the subsequent appearance of an AIDS-defining illness. The longer an individual is infected with HIV, the greater the risk of disease progression. However, not all CD4 loss appears to be the result of direct killing by HIV. The gp120 envelope protein of HIV has a strong affinity for the CD4 receptor. An infected cell then may bind with the CD4 receptor of uninfected cells, forming syncytia and indirectly resulting in CD4 cell depletion. If the rate of CD4 cell regeneration is less than the rate of depletion, the host will experience CD4 cell decline, with a resultant loss in immune stability. Another indirect mechanism may be apoptosis, or "programmed" cell death. A virologically asymptomatic carrier state has not been identified (DeVita et al., 1992; Pantaleo et al., 1993; Phair, 1994; Weiss, 1993).

The Centers for Disease Control (CDC) has established a classification system for HIV infection based on the natural history of this illness. The categories in this definition have been standardized to gather epidemiologic data and to simplify the clinical description in local and national reporting (see Table 21–1) (CDC, 1985, 1987c, 1992b).

Occupational Infection

HIV is not easily transmissible. Its communicability is related to an individual's high-risk behav-

TABLE 21–1. REVISED HIV-1 CLASSIFICATION SYSTEM FOR ADOLESCENTS AND ADULTS

CATEGORY A: Consists of one or more of the conditions listed below in an adolescent or adult (>13 years) with documented HIV infection. Conditions listed in categories B and C must not have occurred.

- Asymptomatic HIV infection
- Persistent generalized lymphadenopathy
- Acute (primary) HIV infection with accompanying illness or history of acute HIV infection

CATEGORY B: Consists of symptomatic conditions in an HIV-infected adolescent or adult that are not included among conditions listed in Category C and that meet at least one of the following criteria:

a) the conditions are attributed to HIV infection or are indicative of a defect in cell-mediated immunity; or
b) the conditions are considered by physicians to have a clinical course or to require management that is complicated by HIV infection.

EXAMPLES of conditions in clinical Category B include, BUT ARE NOT LIMITED TO:

- Bacillary angiomatosis
- Candidiasis, oropharyngeal (thrush)
- Candidiasis, vulvovaginal; persistent, frequent, or poorly responsive to therapy
- Cervical dysplasia (moderate or severe/cervical carcinoma in situ)
- Constitutional symptoms, such as fever (38.5°C) or diarrhea lasting >1 month
- Hairy leukoplakia, oral
- Herpes zoster (shingles), involving at least two distinct episodes or more than one dermatome
- Idiopathic thrombocytopenic purpura
- Listeriosis
- Pelvic inflammatory disease, particularly if complicated by tubo-ovarian abscess
- Peripheral neuropathy

For classification purposes, Category B conditions take precedence over those in Category A.

CATEGORY C: Includes the clinical conditions listed in the AIDS surveillance case definition. For classification purposes, once a Category C condition has occurred, the person will remain in Category C.

- CD4+ lymphocyte count <200 cells/mm^3
- Candidiasis of bronchi, trachea, or lungs
- Candidiasis, esophageal
- Cervical cancer, invasive*
- Coccidioidomycosis, disseminated or extrapulmonary
- Cryptococcosis, extrapulmonary
- Cryptosporidiosis, chronic intestinal (>1 month's duration)
- Cytomegalovirus disease (other than liver, spleen, or nodes)
- Cytomegalovirus retinitis (with loss of vision)
- Encephalopathy, HIV-related
- Herpes simplex: chronic ulcer(s) (>1 month's duration); or bronchitis, pneumonitis, or esophagitis
- Histoplasmosis, disseminated or extrapulmonary
- Isosporiasis, chronic intestinal (>1 month's duration)
- Kaposi's sarcoma
- Lymphoma, Burkitt's
- Lymphoma, immunoblastic
- Lymphoma, primary, of brain
- *Mycobacterium avium* complex or *M. kansasii,* disseminated or extrapulmonary
- *Mycobacterium tuberculosis,* any site (pulmonary* or extrapulmonary)
- *Mycobacterium,* other species or unidentified species, disseminated or extrapulmonary)
- *Pneumocystis carinii* pneumonia
- Pneumonia, recurrent*
- Progressive multifocal leukoencephalopathy
- *Salmonella* septicemia, recurrent
- Toxoplasmosis of brain
- Wasting syndrome due to HIV

* Added in the 1993 expansion of the AIDS surveillance case definition.
From Centers for Disease Control: 1993 revised classification system for HIV infection and expanded surveillance case definition for AIDS among adolescents and adults. MMWR 41(RR-7):3–4, 15, 1992.

ior. These behaviors include sexual intercourse (i.e., homosexual, bisexual, or heterosexual), parenteral exposure (i.e., intravenous drug use, blood, blood products, or organ transplantation), and vertical transmission (i.e., transplacental, postpartum, perinatal). Human breast milk, oral sex, shared razors, dental procedures, and contaminated open wounds have been implicated as a mechanism of infection in rare instances.

The occupational rate of nosocomial HIV transmission following parenteral exposure is approximately 0.32 per cent (six infections in more than 2008 needle sticks involving HIV-infected blood) (Sande and Volberding, 1992). The National Institutes of Health has studied more than 2100 skin exposures with zero seroconversions (D.M. Bell, personal communication, 1993). In contrast, the risk of needle-stick or cutaneous hepatitis B virus infection is approximately 25 per cent under similar circumstances of exposure. The risk from mucous membrane contact or inoculation of nonintact skin is too low for quantification despite the fact that at least 1000 exposures of this type have been assessed. All clinical HIV exposures are not comparable. Factors that may increase the risk stratification of occupational infection include intramuscular penetrations, injections of blood, or large-bore hollow needles. The portal of entry for mucocutaneous cases may be related to the volume of blood and duration of contact. Other factors for transmission may include stage of illness in the source patient, source patient viremia, and the immune status of the recipient health care worker (Sande and Volberding, 1992). The minimal infective dose of HIV is not known. Safer discarding of needles and proactive universal implementation of universal precautions decreases the likelihood of exposure. The use of safety devices is being explored.

The implementation of universal precautions has decreased the occupational risk of transmission of not only HIV, but also hepatitis B virus (CDC, 1987b, 1988, 1989, 1991b). Additional reasonable precautions include avoidance of needlesticks and use of disposable gloves if there is a chance of exposure to infected substances. If a surface has been contaminated with HIV, ordinary household bleach will rapidly destroy the virus. HIV is not transmitted by hepatitis B vaccine, RhoGAM, heat-treated factor VIII, or immunoglobulin preparations. Furthermore, insect vectors, casual contact (e.g., environmental surfaces, skin, sweat, tears, changing diapers), and social contact (e.g., hugging, sneezing, coughing, shaking hands) have not been implicated as routes of transmission (Sande and Volberding, 1992).

AMBULATORY MANAGEMENT

The clinician and patient first must consider the potential for a positive diagnosis prior to treatment for HIV. A routine sexual behavior and substance abuse discussion, in addition to a blood transfusion/organ transplant history, should be part of any foundation of a physician–patient relationship. The interview must include not only current but also past behaviors, including adolescent or single-time experimentation. Acknowledgment of a patient's behavior does not mandate that the physician accepts the behavior. However, if the physician uses nonjudgmental language, the patient is more likely to reveal accurate information, thereby allowing the physician to assess whether the high-risk behavior is ongoing or relapsing.

The history taking can provide a forum for educational interventions and facilitate behavior modification. An open discussion about the impact of HIV on individual health also can be a mechanism to educate patients and their families about behavior prevention. In addition, individualized physician education may provide a mechanism to assist indirectly in decreasing the transmission of HIV. Finally, patients may be unaware that their behavior and that of their sexual partners is considered high risk, especially if they are misinformed and believe that only certain groups of individuals are at risk of HIV exposure.

The first step in the management of HIV-infected individuals involves primary care physicians educating themselves and their staff regarding the CDC's recommendations about universal precautions (CDC, 1987b, 1988, 1989, 1991b) and tuberculosis (CDC, 1989, 1990a, 1991a). The concept of universal precautions stresses that all patients should be assumed to be infectious for HIV and other blood-borne pathogens. Universal precautions should be followed when health care workers are exposed to blood, amniotic fluid, pericardial fluid, peritoneal pleural fluid, synovial fluid, cerebrospinal fluid, semen, vaginal secretions, or any body fluid visibly contaminated with blood. Adherence to these guidelines minimizes occupational risk for hepatitis B and C virus, *M. tuberculosis*, and HIV for health care providers. Other infectious diseases for which one's medical occupation may be a risk factor for the nonimmune adult are rubella, measles, mumps, varicella, and influenza.

In addition to coping with the fears of contagion and occupational risk, primary care physicians need to develop an understanding of their patients' sexual behaviors and assess their own attitudes about injection drug use. Physicians also will need to be comfortable with hospice, home, or terminal care.

Diagnosis

Identification of individuals with past (e.g., blood transfusion), current (e.g., intravenous drug use), and potential (e.g., adolescent) high-risk status is imperative. After the history is obtained, a possible sequence of HIV testing may include enzyme-linked immunosorbent assay (ELISA) serologic testing, and then, if positive, independent confirmation with a Western blot test (Table 21–2). An informed consent must be obtained prior to testing. Serologic testing may be obtained at anonymous testing centers or in collaboration with community health departments or family planning agencies. Positive test results must be given face to face in order that appropriate post-test counseling can be provided. Essential components of a

**TABLE 21–2. ADULT HIV SEROLOGIC
TESTING—UNITED STATES RECOMMENDATIONS**

Pretest and Post-Test Counseling

Pretest and post-test counseling must address the following issues: determination of individual potential risk status (past, current, future); implications of positive, negative, and indeterminate test results; pregnancy and contraception issues; behavior modification to reduce risk; low-risk sexual activities; and referral to appropriate agencies for follow-up.

Note: Pretest and post-test counseling provides an opportunity to tailor risk reduction education. Health care providers may wish to consider the use of an informed consent form. Finally, a sample that is repetitively positive must be confirmed by an independent antibody assay.

Anonymous or Confidential Testing

A system must be implemented that has the ability to protect the anonymity and confidentiality of test specimens and results.

Note: If testing is performed in a private office, the physician may wish to use numerically coded samples. If this is not feasible, use of alternative testing sites may be advisable.

Voluntary versus Mandatory Testing

Although voluntary testing is preferable, in certain situations mandatory testing is performed.

Mandatory testing: Testing of blood, plasma, sperm, and organ donation. Mandatory testing also occurs within the military, and in specific legal interactions.

Interpretation of Results (Postexposure)

A negative enzyme-linked immunosorbent assay screen and absence of antibody bands on the Western blot test at 0, 3, 6, 9, and 12 months after a one-time exposure provides evidence that no immune response to HIV has occurred. Indeterminate test results must be followed closely.

Polymerase chain reaction (PCR) testing may have a role in confirming HIV serostatus if an indeterminate test result occurs. PCR may delineate an individual who is seroconverting from one who is falsely positive.

Clinical follow-up of patients with indeterminant test results requires observation and repeat testing.

From Centers for Disease Control: Public Health Service Guidelines for counseling and antibody testing to prevent HIV infection and AIDS. MMWR 36:509, 1987.

post-test counseling session include the following (CDC, 1987a):

The meaning of the test result

The possible need for additional testing, including sexual contacts

Appropriate measures to prevent or decrease the risk of HIV transmission

Appropriate medical and mental health care support services

The benefits of partner notification and a mechanism for referral

The complexity of post-test counseling strictly warrants *against* giving HIV test results over the telephone. For example, the physician may not be giving the test results to the person tested. It is often helpful to explain that the test only reveals antibodies against HIV, and is not diagnostic of AIDS. HIV is a chronic infection and is not immediately fatal. Seroreversion has not been documented conclusively. The increased prevalence of factitious HIV infection belies the need for accurate serological documentation.

Immunodiagnostic Tests

Numerous immunodiagnostic tests to ascertain HIV infection have been developed for laboratory and clinical use. All are designed to detect directly or indirectly infection with HIV, not AIDS per se. For example, viral presence can be detected by viral co-cultures, polymerase chain reaction (amplification of nucleic acid sequences), radio immunoprecipitation assay, or indirect immunofluorescence assay techniques. These methods are not practical in the ambulatory environment secondary to the time, expense, and expertise required for their performance.

ANTIGEN TESTING.   p24 antigen testing, a test measuring the amount of free viral protein (p24), is widely available. p24 Antigenemia is most prevalent during initial seroconversion and during later stages of active disease. A decrease in p24 antigen levels may be a mechanism to gauge a patient's response to antiretroviral therapy. An increase in levels may be an indirect measure of failure of antiretroviral therapy or disease progression.

ANTIBODY TESTING.   The most commonly utilized HIV-specific detection techniques are the ELISA and Western immunoblotting antibody tests. ELISA is used in blood screening because it is inexpensive and simple to perform. The Western blot test is technically more difficult to perform and interpret, and is used as an independent confirmation technique of a positive ELISA test. Neither test requires the use of live virus and is safer than those techniques requiring viral culture.

INTERPRETATION OF TEST RESULTS.   Antibody and antigen tests identify individuals with prior HIV infection, but do not measure host immunity. Furthermore, they cannot reveal the precise moment of initial infection or the patient's remaining life expectancy. Neither the ELISA nor the Western blot test is 100 per cent sensitive or specific. They are limited by a "reliance" on host antibody production and the absence of host cross-reacting antibodies. The median time period for host production of detectable antibodies is 2.1 months, and 95 per cent of individuals will develop antibody within 5.8 months of initial infection (Sande and Volberding, 1992). Hence, an individual will have a "false-negative" test during the "window period" between infection and antibody production. Being exposed to HIV does not mandate subsequent infection with HIV. This can be confusing because people do not realize high risk is not an absolute risk. Current testing techniques only ascertain HIV infection. A list of possible associative causes for false-positive and false-negative HIV antibody tests and recommendations for testing are listed in Table 21–3.

TABLE 21–3. POTENTIAL SOURCES OF FALSE-POSITIVE OR FALSE-NEGATIVE ANTIBODY TESTS

False Positive	False Negative
Populations with low seroprevalence	Prior to host antibody response (i.e., "window period")
Passive transfer of antibody in immunoglobulin preparations	Late infection, resulting from deterioration of host antibody response
Cross-reactive antibodies secondary to multiple blood transfusions, multiparity, serum proteins (cryoglobulins, rheumatoid factor), other retroviruses, or human leukocyte antigens (HLA class I, HLA class II)	Laboratory error*
Transplacental transfer of maternal antibody	
Flu vaccine (transiently)	
Laboratory error*	

* Laboratory error may include misinterpretation of weakly positive bands, or the incorrect application of interpretive criteria.

Baseline Evaluation of the HIV-Infected Patient

Usually patients are significantly distressed after receiving positive serologic results. A pro-actively scheduled medical follow-up provides a mechanism to provide ongoing counseling and support. Early diagnosis of HIV infection provides an opportunity for early intervention and monitoring of the disease process.

Medical History

Interpersed in the history and physical exam (Table 21–4) are questions that might suggest immunodeficiency that previously had not been diagnosed or labeled as HIV infection. Also, questions about transmission that the general public would not necessarily attribute to themselves as a risk behavior are included. For example, adolescents may have intercourse in the context of alcohol (thus impairing judgement), and not consider the resulting sexual behavior as a risk. Anyone treated for a sexually transmitted disease must be educated that the same behavior that exposed them to that disease also can expose them to HIV. Birth control pills do not prevent the transmission of HIV infection, so teenagers trying to prevent pregnancy need additional counseling on the prevention of sexually transmitted diseases.

Education to modify behavior is difficult at best. Because the behavior that transmits HIV is a high risk but not an absolute risk, individuals who have in the past participated in high-risk behaviors but are not (yet) infected may feel a certain invulnerability to HIV.

The following information for clinical classification or delineation of potential co-factors of disease progression may be helpful: recent herpes zoster infection, aseptic meningitis, Bell's palsy, sexually transmitted disease history (syphilis, gonorrhea, herpes simplex, chlamydia, nongonococcal urethritis, pelvic inflammatory disease), health of significant others, weight loss, prior or recent tuberculosis treatment or testing, prior hepatitis A, B, or C infection, possession of household pets, foreign travel, drug allergies, sexual partner history, use of alcohol, and illicit or prescription drug use.

The use of needles is not limited to hypodermic syringes. Tattooing devices may transmit HIV and hepatitis B virus. In shooting galleries, individuals may share needles or buy "clean works," but the intensity of injection drug use and associated sexual behaviors is increased. Any alcohol or illicit or prescription drug use impairs judgment. The presence of a sexually transmitted disease correlates with HIV and may act as a co-factor for transmission. Incarceration may lead to sexual behaviors (voluntary or assault) that are not admitted to on release. Even if both individuals in a sexual encounter are HIV positive, HIV genotypes may vary; hence the use of condoms is essential. Anonymous sexual behavior and use of prostitutes (foreign or United States) contribute to the hierarchy of high-risk behaviors.

Physical Findings

The physical exam often provides the first clue that a person is immunosuppressed, and therefore signals the need to obtain a risk history and serologic testing. The following physical abnormalities may be associated with HIV infection: oral candidiasis, recurrent tinea infections, recurrent vaginal candidiasis, seborrheic dermatitis, molluscum contagiosum, Reiter's syndrome, oral hairy leukoplakia, extrainguinal lymphadenopathy, peripheral neuropathy, cognitive changes, parotid gland enlargement, and chronic sinusitis. A subset of these symptoms is highly predictive of the development of AIDS (oral candidiasis, hairy leukoplakia, generalized wasting, and multidermatomal zoster). Accurate staging of disease alerts the clinician to potential complications of HIV infection and guides the choice of therapeutic options. Sande and Volbeding (1992) provide an excellent review of clinical symptoms and physical findings. Staging of HIV infection may be simplified by the use of the CDC classification schema for HIV infection (Table 21–1).

The entire clinical spectrum of HIV disease in women is not fully known at this time. Women are far more likely to develop invasive candidal infections rather than disseminated Kaposi's sarcoma. Women frequently develop recurrent bacterial pneumonias, pelvic inflammatory disease, and cervical dysplasis. Dysfunctional uterine bleeding may make it more difficult for a woman to maintain iron reserves. Breast milk is capable of transmitting HIV. Artificial insemination does not prevent the

TABLE 21–4. ESSENTIAL COMPONENTS OF HISTORY AND PHYSICAL EXAM (BRIEF)

Current and Past Transmission Risk

High-Risk Behavior History
Number of sexual partners
Types of sexual behavior(s)
Patient or partner treated for a venereal disease (e.g., syphilis, gonorrhea, herpes simplex, chlamydia, nongonococcal urethritis, pelvic inflammatory disease, chancroid); site of sexually transmitted disease
Patient or sexual partner(s) ever in jail or prison
Use of dirty needles (e.g., shooting galleries, shared needles or works, tatoo, steroid injections)
Alcohol, illicit or prescription drug use (e.g., crack)
Risk of domestic violence; history of domestic or sexual violence
Prostitution history (as a source of sexual gratification, as a source of financial support, or to buy drugs)
Safer sex practices; use of condoms
HIV history of sexual partners; zidovudine (or other anti-retroviral) history of sexual partners
Needlestick; blood-borne pathogen exposure
Mycobacterium tuberculosis, multi–drug-resistant tuberculosis exposure

Medication History
Allergic reactions to antibiotics (especially sulfa)
Previous antiretroviral therapy
Participation in research protocols
Use of alternative therapies

Surgical History
Past surgical treatment
Blood or blood products (1978–1985)
Self or partner skin graft/organ transplant/artificial insemination (1978–1985)
Bilateral tubal ligation, colposcopy, hysterectomy
History of lymph node biopsy
Gender surgery

Medical History
Review of systems
?Symptoms of advanced HIV disease (weight loss, night sweats, fever, chills, diarrhea, alteration in mental status, arthralgias, myalgias, neuropathy, cough, shortness of breath, change in visual acuity, vaginal discharge, etc.)
Hepatitis A, B, C
Pregnancy, last menstrual period, contraception methods
Abnormal Pap smear, mammography, estrogen replacement therapy, dysfunctional uterine bleeding
Psychiatric history and previous therapy
Tuberculin skin test in last year; treatment for tuberculosis
Herpes zoster

Bell's palsy
Household pets
Foreign travel
Vaccination history
Chronic medical conditions (hypertension, heart disease, diabetes, etc.)
Rubella titer

Physician Examination
Vital signs, weight changes
Generalized lymphadenopathy (biopsy if asymmetric)
Recurrent or persistent skin rashes (e.g., psoriasis, folliculitis, cat scratch disease, seborrheic dermatitis)
Chronic nail infections
Track marks, tattooing, carbon tattooing
Cardiac murmur (esp. if intravenous drug user)
Nail pigmentation secondary to zidovudine
Abdominal scars (?splenectomy)
Oral candidiasis
Recurrent vulvovaginal candidiasis
Oral hairy leukoplakia
Periodontal disease
Parotid enlargement
Stomatitis
Kaposi's sarcoma
Herpes zoster
Any sexually transmitted disease and location (e.g., rectal herpes, trichomonas)
Breast masses or gynecomastia (e.g., marijuana, ketoconazole)
Cervical carcinoma in situ
Hepatomegaly, splenomegaly
Recurrent oral, anal, vaginal, genital condyloma or ulcerations
Cotton wool spots
Sinusitis
Myositis
Mental status exam (e.g., dementia)
Neurologic exam (e.g., neuropathy, alterations in gait)

Social History
Sexual orientation
Presence/absence of infected offspring, sexual partners
Source of HIV infection
?Survived other HIV-infected partners
?Caregiver
Living arrangements
Financial arrangements
Incarceration history
Power of attorney
Living will
Need for case management referral

transmission of HIV for discordant couples wishing to conceive. Vasectomy is also not protective. Furthermore, the optimal management of breast cancer in an HIV-infected woman is completely unknown. The use of zidovudine during pregnancy apparently reduces the vertical transmission of HIV (MMWR, 1994).

Baseline Laboratory Analysis

Suggested baseline laboratory studies include: complete blood count (to rule out HIV-associated anemia, thrombocytopenia, and granulocytopenia); absolute CD4 lymphocyte count (to assess degree of relative immunosuppression); chemistry profile (e.g., an elevated lactate dehydrogenase level may be associated with *Pneumocystis carinii* pneumonia [PCP] or crack use); rapid plasma reagin (RPR)/microhemagglutinin *Treponema pallidum* tests; hepatitis profile (rule out chronic active hepatitis); urine toxicology screen; sputum for acid-fast bacilli testing; Papanicolaou (Pap) smear; urine pregnancy test; and toxoplasmosis immunoglobulin G antibody titer.

The CD4 lymphocyte count (i.e., T4 counts, helper count) forms the basis for current antiretroviral and opportunistic infection prophylaxis therapy guidelines (CDC, 1992a, 1992c, Sande et al., 1993). It has been used as a surrogate marker for disease progression, and, in conjunction with clinical findings, has had a prominent role in monitoring disease progression.

Aggressive management of syphilis, including lumbar puncture to rule out neurosyphilis (if the RPR > 1:32) is essential. Aggressive assessment to rule out *M. tuberculosis* (MTB) infection is mandatory. A baseline application of five tuberculin units of purified protein derivative (PPD) and a screening chest radiograph are suggested to screen for occult tuberculosis. Greater than 5 mm induration requires prophylaxis with isoniazid. In the context of HIV infection, a negative PPD test is not sufficient to rule out MTB infection. All HIV-infected patients must be assessed routinely for MTB, and all MTB patients must be assessed routinely for HIV infection. Annual chest radiographs and induced sputum for acid-fast bacilli testing are recommended. Research studies are ongoing to determine if routine isoniazid prophylaxis is warranted for patients with CD4 lymphocyte counts of less than 200 cells/mm^3 or for any HIV-infected patient with MTB exposure (CDC, 1990a, 1990b, 1991a). Awareness of local patterns of tuberculosis drug resistance are essential. Patients with active tuberculosis require directly observed therapy. The management of multi–drug-resistant tuberculosis (MDRTB) is beyond the scope of this chapter.

Active chemical dependency (illicit and prescription and alcohol) complicates the management of HIV infection. Antiretroviral compliance may be nonexistent or complicated by azidothymidine (AZT) having a street value based on the folklore that taking AZT before shooting up or having sex is "protective." Shooting galleries increase the risk of transmission not only of HIV but also of tuberculosis (including MDRTB) and sexually transmitted diseases (Cherubin and Sapira, 1993). Chemical dependency increases the risk of prostitution (male and female). Long-term cocaine use is associated with increasing risk of intravenous drug use. If his or her sexual partners are using intravenous drugs, an indvidual's risk of intravenous drug use and HIV exposure also increases. Early results from needle exchange programs suggest a decrease in the transmission of hepatitis B (Friedman et al., 1993). Awareness of and close collaboration with drug treatment facilities is also essential.

There are increasing numbers of HIV-infected women in whom the HIV diagnosis is made during pregnancy or in the later stages of HIV disease. If an HIV diagnosis is made following childbirth, this may be the woman's initial notification. She then must deal with her child's infection, her own infection, plus the source of her infection. A woman may seek testing because her partner is sick and she desires a mechanism to get him tested. Frequently the diagnosis in women is made at a later stage than in men because HIV is not in the routine differential diagnosis for many clinicians (e.g., an older woman with altered mental status whose husband had a blood transfusion during previous bypass surgery).

Laboratory Abnormalities

Interpretation of nonspecific symptoms or physical findings in HIV infection is often difficult. After completion of an HIV-oriented review of the patient's symptoms, the following laboratory studies *may* have diagnostic utility based on individual symptomatology. Patients with central nervous system complaints may require a cryptococcal antigen test, toxoplasmosis titer, lumbar puncture, computerized tomography scan, or magnetic resonance imaging studies. Patients with prior serologic evidence of toxoplasmosis are at increased risk for reactiviation of disease. If a patient complains of shortness of breath or a chronic nonproductive cough, measurement of arterial blood gases, gallium scanning, or bronchoscopy may clarify the clinical diagnosis. An elevated lactate dehydrogenase may suggest PCP, *Mycobacterium avium-intracellulare* lymphoma, or crack use. Female patients need relatively frequent Pap smears to screen for cervical dysplasia, human papillomavirus and cervical carcinoma. Cervical, vulvar, and vaginal dysplasia requires aggressive diagnosis, including colposcopy and biopsy. Standard antibiotic regimens for the treatment of pelvic inflammatory disease should be effective in HIV-infected women, who are at increased risk for genital tract disease. An endometrial biopsy with suction curettage may serve as a complement to therapy to identify microbiologic pathogens. Menstrual irregularities require appropriate management. Women may require serum pregnancy tests before the initiation of many therapies (Minkoff and DeHovitz, 1991).

HIV-infected obstetric patients should be referred to an HIV subspecialist who is experienced in antiretroviral therapy during pregnancy. Furthermore, research protocols are ongoing to decrease the chance of HIV transmission to the infant. Pregnancy can provide an opportunity for a women to withdraw from illegal drugs. In contrast, HIV seropositivity may limit access to voluntary termination of pregnancy.

The epidemiologic role of menstruation in the transmission of HIV is not fully known. Patients are advised to avoid intercourse during menses. Genital ulcer disease caused by herpes simplex, chancroid, syphilis, and HIV itself may further the transmission of HIV. Depending on the stage of immunosuppression, women with extensive genital ulcer disease may require intravenous therapy for chronic herpes infections.

Acute or chronic gastrointestinal symptoms commonly have a treatable etiology. Hence, stool or colonoscopy studies for *Amoeba, Mycobacterium, Shigella, Salmonella, Isospora, Cryptosporidum, Microsporidia, Histoplasma,* or *Clostridium dificile* toxin may be warranted. Finally, suspicious skin lesions or lymph nodes should be biopsied.

Tests that are not routinely helpful include cytomegalovirus titers, Epstein-Barr virus titers, and *P. carinii* antigen and antibody tests.

Prognostic Markers

In patients with advanced immune dysfunction, study results that may indicate a short-term risk of developing AIDS are rapidly falling CD4 lymphocyte counts, newly elevated p24 antigen levels, a decrease in antibody levels to p24 antigens, or loss of lymphadenopathy (Sande et al., 1992).

Immunization

The patient's vaccination status should be determined. Adult recommendations for symptomatic and asymptomatic individuals are listed in Table 21–5. Also, childhood infections and immunizations should be reviewed. For example, if the person is exposed to children, chicken pox becomes a risk and varicella immune globulin may be considered. Patient not vaccinated as children should receive inactivated, not oral, polio vaccine. Prior bacille Calmette-Guérin vaccination is not a contraindication to use of a PPD test, nor is it an adequate explanation for a positive PPD test. Review of immunization history is important prior to foreign travel (CDC, 1992d; Jewett and Hecht, 1993).

TREATMENT

Antiretroviral Therapy

None of the HIV treatment regimens currently available are curative, nor is viricidal therapy or vaccine prophylaxis anticipated in the near future. The scientific obstacles to vaccine development include transmission of HIV as a free or cell-bound virus, genetic diversity of isolates, lack of completely neutralizing antibody responses, reservoirs of HIV infection, and potential enhancing antibody responses (DeVita et al., 1992; Pantaleo et al., 1993).

Zidovudine (AZT, Retrovir) was the first nucleoside analogue approved for the palliative treatment of HIV infection (Fischl et al., 1987). Along with didanosine (ddI, Videx) and zalcitabine (ddC, HIVID), stavudine (d4T, Zerit), zidovudine specifically inhibits the HIV reverse transcriptase enzyme by chain-terminating the synthesis of proviral DNA. All three approved agents lead to transient decreases in p24 antigen levels, temporary elevation of CD4 lymphocyte counts, and delayed onset of opportunistic infections. A beneficial effect on long-term survival has not been demonstrated by currently available studies.

Recommendations regarding the appropriate use of antiretroviral therapy are in a state of flux since the Concorde data were presented in Berlin (and represent differing philosophies for the management of a chronic viral infection). The currently approved agents have limited antiviral efficacy and limited duration of effect. None of the currently approved agents are able to eradicate the viral infection or sustain host immunologic improvement. Progressive HIV disease appears at sometime during antiretroviral therapy. Prospective studies are underway to compare sequential, simultaneous, and combination therapy with nucleoside reverse transcriptase inhibitors. Research is also underway to examine the role of non-nucleoside reverse transcriptase inhibitors, but the findings are too preliminary to offer clinical recommendations. Sande et al. (1993) offer a useful, preliminary framework for individualizing therapy using representative clinical scenarios stratified on whether the patient is experiencing symptomatic or asymptomatic HIV infection (Table 21–6).

Clinical decision making is determined by prior antiretroviral therapy, intolerance to specific antiviral agents, symptomatic stage of HIV infection, and patient preference. In general, in patients with no prior antiretroviral therapy, zidovudine monotherapy, 200 mg three times daily, is offered to patients with CD4 lymphocyte counts of less than 500 cells/mm^3 (Fischl et al., 1987, 1990; Sande et

TABLE 21–5. IMMUNIZATION OF ADULTS INFECTED WITH HIV—UNITED STATES RECOMMENDATIONS

Vaccine	Administration Recommendation*
Pneumovax†	Yes
Influenza	Yes
Hepatitis B‡	Yes
Tetanus toxoid	Yes
Yellow fever	No
Oral poliovirus§	No
Cholera	N/E
Typhoid	N/E
Rabies‖	Yes
Tuberculosis (bacille Calmette-Guérin)	No
HbCV	¶
Rubeola	#

* Yes, safe to administer; No, do not administer; N/E, not efficacious. *Note:* Vaccination of an HIV-infected individual may not provoke protective or measurable antibody titers.

† Especially in splenectomized patients; may not induce an immune response in symptomatic persons.

‡ In high-risk individuals, it may be prudent to check serology first; this is especially important for individuals who continue to practice high-risk behavior, and for health care workers.

§ Oral attenuated poliovirus vaccine should not be administered to an immunosuppressed individual if not vaccinated as a child; consider inactivated polio vaccine.

‖ Use of this vaccine must be in a context of administration: pre-exposure in an asymptomatic individual for whom job exposure is likely may be warranted; postexposure vaccination is recommended.

¶ *Haemophilus* b conjugate vaccine; although current recommendations are only for pediatric patients, future recommendations may include use for adult and elderly patient populations.

Administration of single antigen vaccine to HIV-infected adults is controversial. The safest course is to update immune status of noninfected family members. Pre-exposure: individuals born before 1957 are considered "immune" regardless of their clinical history. Postexposure: gammaglobulin 0.5 mL/kg (maximum dose 15 mL) within 6 days of exposure.

TABLE 21–6.   ANTIRETROVIRAL THERAPY FOR HIV-INFECTED ADULTS*

Clinical Status	CD4+ Range, Cell Count × 10^9/L	Recommendation
No Previous Antiretroviral Therapy		
Asymptomatic	>0.50	No therapy
Asymptomatic	0.20–0.50	Zidovudine or no therapy
Symptomatic	0.20–0.50	Zidovudine
Asymptomatic	<0.20	Zidovudine
Symptomatic	<0.20	Zidovudine
Previous Antiretroviral Therapy		
Stable	≥0.30	Continue zidovudine
Stable	<0.30	Continue zidovudine or change to didanosine
Progressing	0.05–0.50	Change to didanosine or zalcitabine
Progressing	<0.05	Change to didanosine or zalcitabine
Intolerant to Zidovudine		
Stable or progressing	<0.50	Change to didanosine or zalcitabine

* Recommendations from the 1993 National Institute of Allergy and Infectious Diseases State-of-the-Art Conference. The role of stavudine remains in transition.
From Sande MA, Carpenter CC, Cobbs CG, et al: Antiretroviral therapy for adult HIV-infected patients. JAMA 270:2583, 1993, with permission. Copyright 1993, American Medical Association.

al., 1993). Of the available antiretroviral agents, zidovudine probably has the superior therapeutic profile for initial therapy. If the CD4 lymphocyte count is less than 200 cells/mn^3, then antiretroviral therapy is more strongly recommended (whether the patient is experiencing symptomatic or asymptomatic disease) and prophylaxis against PCP is started. For patients with CD4 counts of greater than 500 cells/mn^3 who are asymptomatic, no antiretroviral therapy is recommended at this time (Sande et al., 1993).

In patients with prior zidovudine antiretroviral therapy, who are stable, and who have CD4 counts greater than 300 cells/mm^3, continued therapy with zidovudine is recommended. For patients who have disease progression with zidovudine, or intolerance to this drug, a change to either didanosine, 125 to 200 mg twice daily, or zalcitabine, 0.75 mg three times daily, is recommended. Included in this group are patients with CD4 counts of less than 500 cells/mm^3 who have disease progression. In contrast, when patients have a CD4 cell count of less than 50 cells/mm^3, the clinician and patient may wish to defer antiretroviral therapy if significant toxicity is occurring without apparent clinical benefit (Sande et al., 1993).

Monitoring of CD4 lymphocytes is frequently used as a surrogate marker for clinical decision making and to determine a relative level of immune function. In any therapeutic decision, it is the overall trend of immune deterioration that is important, rather than a single CD4 cell level. Note that if a CD4 sample is stored overnight prior to processing, a spuriously low value may be obtained.

Future studies may provide recommendations regarding combination therapy, or guidelines in the management of HIV resistance. In general, if resistance emerges, changing to or adding a second reverse transcriptase inhibitor is reasonable (Collier et al., 1992; Fischl et al., 1993). However, combination therapy may not delay the emergence of resistant strains of HIV (Richman, 1994).

Opportunistic Infections

The inherent difficulties in treating HIV-infected patients are related to the increased severity of opportunistic infections, increased frequency of adverse reactions to standard doses of medications (e.g., sulfa compounds), multiplicity of infections, likelihood of recurrent infections, and diminished host immune function. Because of the high relapse rate after successful treatment of opportunistic infections, prophylactic therapy has become standard.

Because there is a lack of successful treatment for certain opportunistic bacterial (MTB), fungal, and protozoal (i.e., microsporidiosis) infections, there is a continued need for either research medications or research applications of previously approved medications. A summary of treatment guidelines for the most common opportunistic infections is listed in Table 21–7 (DeVita et al., 1992; "Drugs for AIDS," 1993; Miller, 1990; Sande and Volberding, 1992; Sanford et al., 1993).

Pneumocystis carinii *Pneumonia*

Primary and secondary PCP prophylaxis has improved survival rates in HIV-infected patients. The drug of choice for prophylaxis and treatment of acute PCP is trimethoprim-sulfamethoxazole (TMP-SMX) (CDC, 1992c). Advantages of this medication include ease of administration and oral or intravenous dosage formulations. For patients who are unable to take the medication secondary to allergic reactions, desensitization protocols are available. Patients who must discontinue TMP-SMX during acute therapy secondary to side effects may be able to tolerate a lower dose on subsequent rechallenge. Intravenous pentamidine has far more side effects than TMP-SMX and has a delayed onset of action until adequate pulmonary tissue levels are reached. For PCP prophylaxis, the current aerosolization formulation has a significant failure rate on an annual basis, and is not used for the treatment of acute PCP. Dapsone in combination with trimethoprim is an additional oral regimen that has efficacy in the treatment of mild to moderate PCP. Patients who are intolerant of TMP-SMX frequently are able to tolerate this drug combination.

TABLE 21–7.   SUGGESTED REGIMENS FOR PRIMARY AND PROPHYLACTIC TREATMENT OF COMMON OPPORTUNISTIC INFECTIONS IN AIDS

Standard Adult Therapy (Daily Dose)	Alternative Therapy	Prophylactic or Maintenance Therapy
Protozoa		
Pneumocystis carinii pneumonia*		
Trimethoprim-sulfamethoxazole (15–20 mg/kg/day P.O. or I.V. divided q 6 hr)†	Pentamidine isethionate (3–4 mg/kg/day I.V.)	Trimethoprim-sulfamethoxazole DS (qd or 3 times/week)‡
Trimethoprim (15 mg/kg/day) + dapsone (100 mg P.O./day) divided q 6 hr × 21 days	*or* Clindamycin (900 mg P.O./I.V. q 6–8 hr)	Dapsone (25–100 mg P.O./day or 100 mg (2 times/week)
Note: if po$_2$ < 70 mm Hg, add Prednisone (40 mg P.O. b.i.d. × 5 days, then 40 mg qd × 5 days, then 20 mg qd × 11 days)	*plus* Primaquine (30 mg P.O. qd × 21 days) *or* Atovaquone (750 mg P.O. t.i.d. × 21 days)§	Pentamidine isethionate (aerosolized) (300 mg q 28 days)‡ Sulfadoxine and pyrimethamine (Fansidar)
	Trimetrexate‖ (45 mg/m^2 I.V. qd) *plus* Leucovorin (20 mg/m^2 q 6 hr)	
Toxoplasma gondii encephalitis¶		
Pyrimethamine (100 mg b.i.d. × 1 day [loading dose], then 50–75 mg P.O. qd)	Clindamycin (450 mg P.O. t.i.d. [or 600 mg I.V. q 6 hr]) may be substituted for sulfadiazine	Suppressive therapy required: Pyrimethamine (50 mg qd) *plus*
plus Leucovorin (folinic acid) (10 mg P.O. qd) *plus*	Atovaquone (750 mg P.O. t.i.d.) ?Azithromycin ?Clarithromycin	Leucovorin (folinic acid) (10 mg qd) *plus* Sulfadiazine (2 gm P.O. qd)
Sulfadiazine 4–6 grams in divided doses		
May need Decadron if edema or mass effect and/or Dilantin (if seizures)		**Primary prophylactic treatment has not been established**
Cryptosporidium colitis		
Paromomycin (500–750 mg P.O. t.i.d.)	?Azithromycin (Supportive care: fluids, analgesics, antispasmodics, opiate-derived antidiarrheals) ?Octreotide ?Hyperalimentation, Vivonex	Maintenance therapy required
Bacteria		
Mycobacterium tuberculosis, #,**		*Maintenance therapy:*
If MTB pansensitive, for initial therapy Isoniazid (300 mg P.O./day) *plus*	Streptomycin (15 mg/kg I.M./day) MDRTB is beyond the scope of this chapter.	If MTB isolate is pansensitive, ethambutol and pyrazinamide may be discontinued after 2 months of negative cultures. Isoniazid and rifampin then are continued for at least 9–12 months.
Rifampin (600 mg P.O./day) *plus* Pyrazinamide (15–30 mg/kg P.O./day) *plus*		*Prophylaxis:* Isoniazid (300 mg P.O. qd) *plus*
Ethambutol (15–25 mg/kg/day) *plus* Pyridoxine (50 mg P.O. qd)		Pyridoxine (50 mg P.O. qd) *or* Rifampin (600 mg P.O. qd)
Mycobacterium tuberculosis‡,**		*Maintenance therapy:* If MTB isolate is pan sensitive, ethambutol and pyrazinamide may be discontinued after 2 months of negative cultures. Isoniazid and rifampin then are continued for at least 9–12 months.
If MTB pansensitive for initial therapy Isoniazid (300 mg P.O./day) *plus*	Beyond the scope of this chapter	Prophylaxis: Isoniazid (300 mg P.O. qd) *plus*
Rifampin (600 mg P.O./day) *plus* Pyrazinamide (15–30 mg/kg/P.O./day) *plus*		Pyridoxine (50 mg P.O. qd) *or* Rifampin (600 mg P.O. qd)
Ethambutol (15–25 mg/kg/day) *plus* Pyridoxine (50 mg P.O. qd) or streptomycin (15 mg 1 kg 1 M/day)		

Table continued on following page

TABLE 21–7.   *(Continued)*

Standard Adult Therapy (Daily Dose)	Alternative Therapy	Prophylactic or Maintenance Therapy

Mycobacterium avium-intracellulare infection
    Clarithromycin (500–1000 mg P.O. b.i.d.)
        or
    Azithromycin (500–100 mg P.O. qod)
        plus
    Ethambutol (15 mg/kg P.O. qd)
        plus
    Clofazimine (100 mg P.O. qd)
	Amikacin (7.5 mg/kg I.V. qd)††
	Ciprofloxacin (750 mg P.O. b.i.d.)††
	?Rifabutin
		Maintenance therapy required:
		    Clarithromycin (500 mg P.O. b.i.d.)
		        plus
		    Clofazimine (100 mg P.O. qd)
		
		Primary prophylaxis:
		    Rifabutin (300 mg/day)
		    ?Clarithromycin

Treponema syphilis
    Primary, secondary, latent
 	
    Benzathine penicillin (2.4 million U I.M.)
        or
    Doxycycline (100 mg P.O. b.i.d. × 14 days)
        or
    Erythromycin (500 mg P.O. q.i.d. × 14 days)
    Late latent
    Benzathine penicillin (2.4 million U I.M. weekly × 3)
        or
    Doxycycline (100 mg P.O. b.i.d. × 28 days)
    Neurosyphilis
    Aqueous penicillin G (12 million U /day I.V. × 10 days)
        or
    Procaine penicillin (2.4 million U I.M. daily × 10 days)
        plus
    Probenecid (500 mg P.O. b.i.d. × 10 days)
	Amoxicillin (2 gm P.O. t.i.d. × 14 days)
	        plus
	Probenecid (500 mg P.O. t.i.d. × 14 days)
	        or
	Doxycycline (200 mg P.O. b.i.d. × 21 days)
	        or
	Ceftriaxone (1 gm I.M. daily × 5–14 days)
	        or
	Benzathine penicillin (2.4 million U I.M. weekly × 3 doses)
	        plus
	Doxycycline (200 mg P.O. b.i.d. × 21 days)
	
	?Ceftriaxone (2 gm I.V./day × 14 days)
		No maintenance therapy required

Fungi and Yeasts
Candida stomatitis‖‖
    Clotrimazole (10 mg 3–5 times/day)
    Nystatin (3 × 10⁶ units, 3–5 times/day)
    Ketoconazole (200–400 mg P.O. qd)§
	Fluconazole (50–100 mg/day)
	Amphotericin B (0.3–0.5 mg/kg/day)
	?Itraconazole
		Maintenance therapy required

Candida vaginitis
    Clotrimazole cream (1%) (qd × 7)
    Miconazole suppository (100 mg qid × 7 days)
	Ketoconazole (200 mg P.O. qd or b.i.d.)
	Fluconazole (100–200 mg P.O. qd)
	Amphotericin B (0.3–0.5 mg/kg/day)
		Maintenance therapy may be required

Candida esophagitis
 	
    Ketoconazole (400–600 mg P.O. qd)
    Fluconazole (200–400 mg P.O. qd)
Cryptococcosis
	Amphotericin B (0.3–0.5 mg/kg I.V. qd)	Maintenance therapy required:
		    Ketoconazole (200 mg P.O. qd)
		    Fluconazole (50 or 100 mg P.O. qd)

    Amphotericin B (0.5–0.8 mg/kg/day to 1 gm)
Histoplasmosis
	Fluconazole (400 mg P.O. qd) (if normal mental status)
	Itraconazole (200 mg P.O. b.i.d.)
		Maintenance therapy:
		    Fluconazole (200 mg P.O. qd)
		        or
		    Amphotericin B (0.5–1.0 mg/kg/week)

    Amphotericin B (0.5–1.0 mg/kg/day I.V. for 4–8 weeks)
	Itraconazole (200 mg P.O. b.i.d.) (after 500 mg amphotericin B)	Maintenance therapy:
		    Amphotericin B (1 mg/kg/week)
		        or
		    Itraconazole (200 mg b.i.d.)

Coccidioidomycosis Amphotericin B (0.6 mg/kg/day) (may need intrathecal dosing)	Fluconazole (400–800 mg P.O. qd) ?Itraconazole (200 mg P.O. b.i.d.)	

Table continued on opposite page

TABLE 21–7. *(Continued)*

Standard Adult Therapy (Daily Dose)	Alternative Therapy	Prophylactic or Maintenance Therapy
Viruses		
Cytomegalovirus retinitis	None	Ganciclovir (5 mg/kg I.V./day) (lifelong)
Ganciclovir (15 mg/kg I.V. b.i.d. × 14–21 days) (may require colony-stimulating factor therapy for neutropenia)	?Combination therapy of gangiclovir and foscarnet	Foscarnet (90 mg/kg I.V. qd) (lifelong)
		?Oral ganciclovir
Foscarnet (60 mg/kg (I.V. q 8 hr × 14–21 days)§§		

* Empiric therapy is a temporary measure until a diagnostic procedure can be performed. Simultaneous use of two treatment regimens does not increase survival. Alternatives for failed initial therapy may involve changing from one conventional regimen to another and repeating the bronchoscopy to rule out a second opportunistic infection. The clinician may wish to monitor serum sulfamethoxazole levels.

† Dosage based on trimethoprim component.

‡ When CD4 lymphocyte count is less than 200 cells/mm^3.

§ *Must* be taken with fatty food to increase absorption. Current formulation has poor bioavailability. Can only be used in mild to moderate disease.

‖ For moderate to severe disease in patients who fail or are intolerant of trimethoprim–sulfamethoxazole or pentamidine therapy. *MUST* be given with leucovorin.

¶ Folic acid prevents action of pyrimethamine. Folinic acid decreases toxicity of pyrimethamine.

Isolation of organism + sensitivity patterns are essential. Directly observed therapy is preferred. Patient isolation may be required.

** HIV-seropositive patients with positive skin tests need at least 12 months of isoniazid/pyridoxine for prophylaxis. An absence of skin test reactivity, however, is not exclusionary. Report cases to health department. Therapeutic failures occur when isoniazid and rifampin are coadministered with ketoconazole because of drug interactions. Rifampin may increase methadone maintenance requirements. Adjuvant steroids for PCP may need re-evaluation in areas of increased MTB/MDRTB.

†† In combination with macrolide antibiotics.

‡‡ Better absorption if ingested with acidic fluid (e.g., orange juice or Coca-Cola). Avoid taking with antacids.

§§ Hydrate with 1000 mL normal saline during induction. All dosages must be adjusted for renal function.

‖ ‖ Candida strains resistant to azoles are increasing in frequency, especially in patients with advanced HIV disease.

Data from "Drugs for AIDS" (1993), Miller (1990), Sanford et al. (1993), Gallant (1994), and Lane (1994).

In addition, suppressive toxoplasmosis therapy with pyrimethamine + sulfadiazine or pyrimethamine + clindamycin offers protection for PCP.

Atovaquone has not been approved for prophylaxis of PCP. The medication is undergoing formulation changes in order to improve its bioavailability and absorption. For patients with severe hypoxemia associated with PCP, adjuvant steroids have decreased the occurrence of respiratory failure. Side effects of steroid use may include dissemination of mycobacterial illness, reactivation of herpes infection, and thrush. Clinicians practicing in areas of high MTB/MDRTB incidence may wish to use caution in the concomitant use of prednisone. Intravenous alternatives for the treatment of PCP include TMP-SMX, pentamidine or trimetrexate (plus leucovorin).

Toxoplasmosis

Toxoplasma gondii is a major opportunistic infection in patients with AIDS and may result from reactivation of latent disease or acute infection. It frequently affects the central nervous system. Geographic origin, residence, and dietary habits of patients may reflect the relative risk of acquiring toxoplasmosis, especially in Hispanic patients. Empiric diagnosis and therapy based on serology and magnetic resonance imaging/computerized tomography findings frequently is initiated in order to avoid stereotactic brain biopsies in the early management of this illness. The administration of anticonvulsant agents to prevent seizures may be reasonable. Lifelong suppressive therapy is required because current therapeutic agents are not effective against cyst forms.

Mycobacterium tuberculosis

A resurgence of tuberculosis has been seen for the last 6 years, especially in metropolitan areas heavily affected by the HIV epidemic. Outbreaks of tuberculosis have occurred in health care, community, and incarceration centers. These outbreaks also have included MDRTB. Because of these drug-resistant MTB outbreaks, the initial management of tuberculosis is now a four-drug regimen in areas without a high prevalence of MDRTB. It is mandatory that antimicrobial sensitivities be obtained on all initial isolates. Because of a rising incidence of drug resistance, most experts recommend that patients with tuberculosis receive their medications under directly observed therapy.

In HIV-infected patients, a tuberculin reaction of 5 mm or greater induration requires at least 1 year of isoniazid (or rifampin) prophylaxis regardless of age. HIV-infected patients with anergy, high risk of exposure, or known MTB exposure also should be considered for isoniazid prophylaxis (CDC, 1990a, 1990b). The CDC has ongoing studies to delineate further recommendations for this guideline. If patients have an exposure to known MDRTB, additional prophylactic agents may include concomitant pyrazinamide, ethambutol, or a quinolone. The use of aerosolized pentamidine prophylaxis or rifabutin *M. avium-intracellulare* prophylaxis should be avoided at centers with high MTB prevalence.

Cytomegalovirus

Cytomegalovirus (CMV) retinitis occurs in 25 per cent of patients with HIV infection, usually when their CD4 lymphocyte counts are less than 50 cells/mm^3. Current treatment for invasive disease requires induction and maintenance therapy with intravenous medications and the placement of permanent long-line catheters. Despite maintenance therapy, CMV progression may occur because neither ganciclovir nor foscarnet are viricidal. The emergence of resistant strains of CMV has been observed. No oral or prophylactic medication exists at the present time, although research protocols examining the role of oral ganciclovir are in progress. CMV encephalitis, colitis, esophagitis, and pneumonia may respond to antiviral therapy with ganciclovir or foscarnet. Other anti-CMV agents are under active development including oral ganciclovir and HPMPC.

Syphilis

A co-epidemic of syphilis parallels the HIV epidemic. The incidence of neonatal syphilis is resurging. In HIV-infected patients, syphilis may have an atypical presentation, an accelerated course to tertiary states, failure of repetitive standard therapy, and significant neurologic symptomology. Positive RPRs require aggressive assessment and management, including lumbar puncture. Suspicious lesions need biopsy, especially if serologic tests for syphilis are negative. Patients with positive RPRs need HIV serologic testing. Treatment alternatives are summarized in Table 21–7.

Prophylactic Polypharmacy and Drug Interactions

The use of prophylaxis creates a problem of polypharmacy, with its attendant risk of drug toxicities (Table 21–8) and interactions. Some of the potential pharmacokinetic difficulties experienced by HIV-infected patients include hypoalbuminemia, impaired gastrointestinal absorption (secondary to HIV enteropathy and malabsorption), and decreased gastrointestinal transit time (diarrhea). The multiplicity of medications leads to unknown drug interactions and drug toxicities, especially in the context of other approved medications (such as histamine$_2$ blockers and antihypertensives). Clinicians must be aware of the potential for additive toxicities (i.e., bone marrow suppression, or combination of agents that are neurotoxic). The effects of chronic versus intermittent antibiotic use on immune function are unknown. The long-term effects of medications are becoming important because HIV-infected patients are living longer; for example, does prolonged immunosuppression lead to the appearance of new malignancies, or are they a result of early antiretroviral intervention?

Research interventions, antiviral therapy, and opportunistic infection prophylaxis usually are guided by the patient's CD4 lymphocyte count or clinical classification status. However, the use of primary prophylaxis is changing clinical presentations of infections (i.e., PCP presenting as extrapulmonic pneumocystosis secondary to aerosolized pentamidine). The long-term use of chronic antibiotic, antiviral, and antifungal agents is now resulting in the emergence of resistant organisms (i.e., zidovudine-resistant HIV, azole-resistant *Candida*, ganciclovir and foscarnet-resistant CMV). The safety of these agents during pregnancy is now being scrutinized more closely as more HIV-infected women are remaining pregnant. Guidelines for prophylaxis have been summarized by Gallant et al., 1994.

Finally, the clinician must become aware of the potential for drug interactions. Examples of some of the more common potential drug interactions include:

1　Zidovudine + ganciclovir: synergistic bone marrow suppression
2　Didanosine or zalcitabine + vincristine: neuropathy
3　Rifampin + methadone: increased methadone requirements
4　Rifabutin + zidovudine: decreased zidovudine levels
5　Histamine$_2$ blockers + ketoconazole: decreased ketoconazole absorption
6　Didanosine + ethambutol or pyrazinamide: hyperuricemia
7　Rifampin + ketoconazole or fluconazole: increased azole requirements

Psychological Issues

Many psychological issues confront patients with HIV infection. Although referral for counseling may be necessary in some situations, the family practice physician may alleviate a majority of these concerns by addressing these issues within the framework of longitudinal care. The following organization of psychosocial issues may enable physicians and their support staff to provide assistance to patients and families. Awareness of community programs, hotlines, education programs, drug treatment facilities, anonymous testing programs, community-based research, indigent care facilities, community health departments, churches, hospices, outreach programs, and home health care options may facilitate continuity of care for HIV-infected patients and their families.

Issues Directly Related to the Patient

Numerous psychological issues interface with the medical complications of HIV infection. On initial discovery of seropositivity, the patient may

TABLE 21–8. MAJOR TOXICITIES ASSOCIATED WITH TREATMENT MODALITIES

Therapeutic Agent	Toxicity
Acyclovir	High doses may be associated with thrombocytopenia, renal insufficiency, nervous system depression, seizures, encephalopathy, phlebitis, hives
Amikacin	Ototoxicity, nephrotoxicity
Amphotericin B	Renal failure, hypokalemia, thrombophlebitis, marrow suppression, headache, hypomagnesemia, hypotension, delirium, rigors
Ampicillin	Anaphylaxis, rash, marrow suppression, epigastric distress, pseudomembrane colitis
Atovaquone	Rash, nausea, diarrhea, increased liver enzymes; poor absorption can lead to treatment failure
Ciprofloxacin	Nausea, vomiting, abdominal pain, pruritus, central nervous system effects, arthralgias, rash, papilledema
Clindamycin	Pseudomembranous colitis, rash, increased hepatic enzymes
Clofazimine	Abdominal pain, blue discoloration of skin, gastrointestinal obstruction, splenic infarction, bowel obstruction, ichthyosis
Chloramphenicol	Pseudomembranous colitis, anaphylaxis, rash, polyarthritis, anemia
Dapsone	Hemolytic anemia, rash, renal, i.e., toxicity (albuminuria, nephrotic syndrome) increased methemoglobin (if glucose-6-phosphate dehydrogenase deficiency, peripheral neuropathy, nephrotic syndrome), insomnia
Didanosine (ddI)*	Pancreatitis, peripheral neuropathy, diarrhea (related to buffer), hypertension (related to buffer), cardiomyopathy, increased amylase, increased triglycerides, leucopenia, anemia, thrombocytopenia, hyperuricemia; drug interactions with dapsone, ketoconazole, tetracyclines, quinolones
Erythropoietin	Hypertension, seizures, thrombosis
Ethambutol	Optic neuritis, anaphylaxis, epigastric distress, peripheral neuritis, skin rash
Ethionamide	Epigastric distress, peripheral neuritis, optic neuritis, jaundice
Fluconazole	Elevated hepatic enzymes, seizures, nausea, prolonged prothrombin time with coumadin, low phosphate, hypokalemia, anaphylaxis, thrombocytopenia
Foscarnet	Anemia, liver enzyme elevation, decreased calcium levels, renal failure, seizures, ulcers; dosage based on creatinine clearance, not serum creatinine
Ganciclovir	Dose adjustment necessary for renal insufficiency; neutropenia, rash, thrombocytopenia, confusion, epigastric distress, fever, neuropathy, central nervous system symptoms
Isoniazid	Hepatitis (risk increased with alcohol), peripheral neuropathy, nausea, epigastric distress, diarrhea, allergic reactions, hyperglycemia, central nervous system changes
Itraconazole	Nausea, epigastric pain, headache, rash, hypokalemia, edema, adrenal insufficiency, rhabdomyolysis
Ketoconazole	Adrenal suppression, hepatotoxicity, anaphylaxis, menstrual changes
Neupogen	Bone pain, fever, myalgias, arthralgias, fluid accumulation (pleural, pericardial), increased lactate dehydrogenase, ? antibody formation
Nystatin	Diarrhea, nausea, vomiting
Pentamidine isethionate (intravenous)	Renal, pancreatic, and hepatic toxicities; bone marrow insufficiency; hypotension; hypoglycemia; hyperglycemia, cardiac arrhythmias
Pentamidine isethionate (aerosolized)	Bronchospasm, cough, metal taste in mouth, increased triglycerides, pneumothorax
Pyrazinamide	Hepatotoxicity, epigastric distress, rash, arthralgias, hyperuricemia
Pyrimethamine	Thrombocytopenia, neutropenia, folic acid deficiency, gastrointestinal intolerance, central nervous system changes
Rifabutin	Neutropenia, rash, gastrointestinal distress, thrombocytopenia, hepatitis, arthralgias, changed color of body fluids, uveitis
Rifampin	Hepatic dysfunction, epigastric distress, headache, thrombocytopenia (especially when combined with ethambutol), hypersensitivity, reddish or orange discoloration of urine and body secretions
Stavudine (d4T)	Peripheral neuropathy, leucopenia, increased liver function abnormality, ataxia
Streptomycin	Ototoxicity, nephrotoxicity
Sulfadiazine	Thrombocytopenia, neutropenia, rash, acute renal failure
Sulfadoxine and pyrimethamine (Fansidar)	Stevens-Johnson syndrome, bone marrow suppression

Table continued on following page

TABLE 21–8. *(Continued)*

Therapeutic Agent	Toxicity
Trimethoprim-sulfamethoxazole	Drug fever, nausea, rash, neutropenia, thrombocytopenia, hepatitis
Trimetrexate	Neutropenia, thrombocytopenia, increased transminases, rash, mucositis, fever, increased serum creatinine
Zalcitabine (ddC)*	Peripheral neuropathy, apthous ulcers, esophageal ulcers, pancreatitis, nausea/vomiting, pruritus, headaches, arthralgias, myalgias, thrombocytopenia, leukopenia
Zidovudine (AZT)*	Anemia, macrocytic anemia, granulocytopenia, nausea, headaches, abdominal pain, myalgias, myopathy, fatigue, cardiomyopathy, nail pigmentation, seizure, hypomania

* In vitro resistance to zidovudine, didanosine, and zalcitabine is being reported. Transmission of zidovudine-resistant HIV isolates also has been reported.

experience a spectrum of responses ranging from fear, denial, and anxiety to anger, guilt, depression, and suicidal ideation. Unless these emotional responses are acknowledged, they have the potential to undermine patient care by confounding the presentation of clinical illness.

Significant unmet needs may overshadow medical treatment and include housing assistance, medications, transportation, substance abuse services, food, and direct emergency assistance. Patients who are incarcerated face additional barriers to care whether within the judicial system or in public facilities. Working with local social service agencies may provide a mechanism to facilitate allocation of these resources.

Women frequently have difficulty arranging child care or day care services. Addressing who will have guardianship over their children is becoming a more frequently raised concern. The clinician may wish to assess whether exposure to violence is a risk factor.

Family Issues

As in other chronic diseases, the family may not have the capacity to offer unconditional support. Oftentimes, these families have been unaware of the individual's risk behavior and may, once informed, exhibit anger, blame, hostility, or abandonment. Frequently they need reassurance concerning their own safety and perceived risk of infection. Educating patients and their families about universal precautions is required. In addition, peer or societal alienation may further stigmatize and isolate the family. The physician can serve a valuable role in addressing these concerns.

Many patients are also caregivers for other HIV-infected patients. Having a sense of this, in addition to a historical sense of how many people an individual patient has *survived,* may provide a depth of insight for the physician caring for these individuals. In contrast, an uninfected individual may feel a sense of guilt or isolation for *not* being infected and may relapse into high-risk behaviors.

Legal Issues

The debate concerning legal issues is exacerbated by rapidly changing public policy. Legal guidelines governing informed consent in serologic testing and disability definitions remain in transition. For example, controversy exists over testing programs for infants, and the use of this information as a surrogate for maternal seropositivity. Access to various forms of insurance and loss of insurance is being deliberated via the judicial system.

Controversies surrounding mandatory testing, quarantine, confidentiality, and duties to warn close contacts and family members further compromise the public health response to this epidemic. The judicial system is in the process of clarifying these dilemmas. Frequently, in the preterminal stages of HIV infection, neurologic impairment or dementia occurs. Prior to this complication, the patient must obtain a will and durable power of attorney. Documentation of advance directives for resuscitation can assist the physician in abiding with the patient's wishes.

Sexuality

Women are being exposed to sexual intercourse at earlier ages. Children do not have the ability to insist that their sexual partners use a condom. Teenage girls may have rectal intercourse in order to protect their "virginity." Ten- and 11-year-old girls may be viewed as desirable sexual partners under the assumption that their virginity decreases the risk of their being seropositive. Very frequently, however, their heterosexual partners have frequently participated in high-risk behaviors.

In examining young adult behaviors, we are seeing increased rates of crack use, male sex with men, sex with high-risk heterosexual partners, multiple sexual partners, intravenous drug use, and sex trading. Adolescents and young adults are more likely to be infected through their sexual behaviors. Drug addiction itself is a surrogate for high-risk sexual behaviors, leading to increased rates of sexually transmitted diseases and HIV. Sexual behavior is complicated by young adults' experimentation and their sense of invulnerability. Young adults and children also may be victims of child abuse or incest and not have any control over what happens to their bodies. Furthermore, sexual intercourse may be the only mechanism for an individual to achieve monetary survival. Prostitutes may not routinely use condoms, particularly if their clients pay more for them "not to."

Even if both partners are HIV positive, safer sex measures still need to be utilized to decrease the risk of transmitting sexually transmitted diseases, virulent HIV, AZT-resistant HIV, hepatitis, and CMV, and the risk of pregnancy.

Adjuvants to Care

Patient education that focuses on holistic care may diminish the desperation and hopelessness observed in many patients. For this educational process to be credible, it should address alcohol and drug abuse, the existence of alternative treatment regimens, and special needs of minority populations. However, patients need to understand that quack regimens are ubiquitous and potentially harmful. In addition, individual and family therapy, assessment of spiritual needs, and nutritional counseling will facilitate management of this disease.

Palliation

The role of palliation for primary care providers is determined by the clinical stage of HIV infection. A patient with a relatively intact immune system will require treatment interventions that stabilize and maintain health. Those patients with acute infectious emergencies require aggressive medical management. Eventually, however, some patients in the terminal stage of their illness will decline further treatment. In this scenario, pain control and palliation supersede other concerns.

Future Directions

At this point in time, no single medication is able to eradicate HIV. The benefits of zidovudine, didanosine, zalcitabine and stavudine are modest and quickly fade, probably secondary to HIV's ability to form resistant mutations. Multidrug combination therapy studies examining agents that inhibit different steps in the viral life cycle (e.g., protease inhibitors, anti–reverse transcriptase enzymes, ribozymes) are emerging. It is hoped that the use of combination therapy either simultaneously or sequentially will overcome or avoid resistance. Combination therapy also may provide a mechanism to reduce drug-related toxicity.

3TC, FTC, nevirapine, TIBO, and tat inhibitor drugs have resulted in the rapid emergence of HIV resistance, and clinical studies for these is drugs are stalled. Convergent therapy has been discarded.

The main strategies for managing HIV are to determine mechanisms to prevent HIV from proliferating within an infected person. The argument is that a decreased viral load may delay damage inflicted by the virus. The ability to cure AIDS will not occur until there is a mechanism to eliminate the latently infected cells. Although significant information exists about the HIV life cycle, much less is understood about how HIV and the host immune system interact and the mechanisms of pathogenesis. New studies about the role and regulation of host cytokines may clarify this issue. Further studies of the importance of syncytia-inducing HIV in disease pathogenesis are also underway (Johnston and Hoth, 1993). Until a clearer understanding about the immune response to HIV, and the nuances of pathogenicity, is achieved, a vaccine to prevent HIV infection or delay progression of disease will not be available (Hoth, 1994).

Finally, as patients are living longer with immunosuppression, new illnesses are being diagnosed with increased frequency: microsporidiosis, AZT/didanosine/zalcitabine-resistant viral strains, increasing progressive multifocal leukoencephalopathy, increasing lymphoma, adrenal insufficiency, endocarditis, cardiomyopathy, Sjögren's (autoimmune) disease, *Mycobacterium kansasii* infection, *Nocardia asteroides*, infection, azole-resistant *Candida* infections, *Rhodococcus equi* infection, *Bartonella henselae* infection, and CMV resistance to ganciclovir and foscarnet. This expanding spectrum of illness will provide many challenges to the clinicians caring for the HIV-infected patient.

_____ REFERENCES

Barre-Sinoussi F, Chermann JC, Rey F, et al: Isolation of a T-lymphotropic retrovirus from a patient at risk from acquired immunodeficiency syndrome (AIDS). Science 220:868, 1983.

Centers for Disease Control: Public Health Service guidelines for counseling and antibody testing to prevent HIV infection and AIDS. MMWR 36:509, 1987.

Centers for Disease Control: Guidelines for prevention of transmission of human immunodeficiency virus and hepatitis B virus to health-care and public-safety workers. MMWR 38(S-6):1, 1989.

Centers for Disease Control: Guidelines for the performance of CD4 + T-cell determinations in persons with human immunodeficiency virus infection. MMWR 41(RR-8):1, 1992a.

Centers for Disease Control: 1993 Revised classification system for HIV infection and expanded surveillance case definition for AIDS among adolescents and adults. MMWR 41(RR-7):1, 1992b.

Centers for Disease Control: Public health service guidelines for counseling and antibody testing to prevent HIV infection and AIDS. MMWR 36:509, 1987a.

Centers for Disease Control: Purified protein derivative (PPD)-tuberculin anergy and HIV infection: Guidelines for anergy testing and management of anergic persons at risk of tuberculosis. MMWR 40(RR-5):27, 1991a.

Centers for Disease Control: Recommendations for preventing transmission of human immunodeficiency virus and hepatitis B virus to patients during exposure-prone invasive procedures. MMWR 40(RR-8):1, 1991b.

Centers for Disease Control: Recommendations for prevention of HIV transmission in health-care settings. MMWR 36:1S, 1987b.

Centers for Disease Control: Recommendations for prophylaxis against *Pneumocystis carinii* pneumonia for adults and adolescents infected with human immunodeficiency virus. MMWR 41(RR-4):1, 1992c.

Centers for Disease Control: Recommendations of the Advisory Committee on Immunization Practices (ACIP): Use of vaccines and immune globulins in persons with altered immunocompetence. MMWR 42(RR-4):1, 1992d.

Centers for Disease Control: Revision of the CDC surveillance case definition of acquired immune deficiency syndrome. MMWR 35(suppl):1S, 1987c.

Centers for Disease Control: Revision of the CDC surveillance case definition of acquired immunodeficiency syndrome for national reporting—United States. MMWR 34:373, 1985.

Centers for Disease Control: Screening for tuberculosis and tuberculosis infection in high-risk populations. MMWR 39(RR-8):1, 1990a.

Centers for Disease Control: The use of preventive therapy for tuberculous infection in the United States. MMWR 39(RR-8):9, 1990b.

Centers for Disease Control: Update: Universal precautions for prevention of transmission of human immunodeficiency virus, hepatitis B virus, and other bloodborne pathogens in health-care settings. MMWR 37:377, 1988.

Cherubin CE, Sapira JD: The medical complications of drug addiction and the medical assessment of the intravenous drug user: 25 years later. Ann Intern Med 119:1017, 1993.

Collier AC, Coombs RW, Fischl MA, et al: Combination therapy with zidovudine and didanosine in patients with advanced human immunodeficiency virus infection: A phase I/II study. Ann Intern Med 116:13, 1992.

DeVita VT, Hellman S, Rosenberg SA: AIDS: Etiology, Diagnosis, Treatment, and Prevention, 3rd edition. Philadelphia, JB Lippincott, 1992.

Drugs for AIDS and associated infections. Med Let 35:79, 1993.

Fischl MA, Olson RM, Follanshe SE, et al: Zalcitabine compared with zidovudine in patients with advanced HIV-1 infection who received previous zidovudine therapy. Ann Intern Med 118:762, 1993.

Fischl MA, Parker CB, Pettinelli C, et al: A randomized controlled trial of a reduced daily dose of zidovudine in patients with the acquired immunodeficiency syndrome. N Engl J Med 323:1009, 1990.

Fischl MA, Richman, DD, Grieco MH, et al: The efficacy of azidothymidine (AZT) in the treatment of patients with AIDS and AIDS-related complex: A double-blind, placebo-controlled trial. N Engl J Med 317:192, 1987.

Friedman SR, Des Jarlais DC, Wenston J, et al: Stable racial/ethnic differences in HIV seroprevalence among IDUS. In: Abstracts of the First National Conference on Human Retroviruses. Washington, DC, American Society for Microbiology, Abstr #285, 1993.

Gallant JE, Moore RD, Chaisson RE: Prophylaxis for opportunistic infections in patients with HIV infection. Ann Intern Med 120:932, 1994.

Gallo RC, Salahuddin SZ, Popovic M, et al: Frequent detection and isolation of cytopathic retroviruses (HTLV-III) from patients with AIDS and at risk for AIDS. Science 224:500, 1984.

Hoth DF, Bologres DP, Corey L, et al: HIV vaccine development: A progress report. Ann Intern Med 121:603, 1994.

Jewett JR, Hecht FM: Preventive health care for adults with HIV infection. JAMA 269:1144, 1993.

Johnston MI, Hoth DF: Present status and future prospects for HIV therapies. Science 260:1286, 1993.

Lane HC, Laughon BE, Falloon J, et al: Recent advances in the management of AIDS-related opportunistic infections. Ann Intern Med 120:945, 1994.

Merson MH: Slowing the spread of HIV: Agenda for the 1990s. Science 260:1266, 1993.

Miller SM: Treatment of opportunistic infections associated with acquired immune deficiency syndrome. Primary Care 17:543, 1990.

Minkoff HL, DeHovitz JA: Care of women infected with the human immunodeficiency virus. JAMA 266:2253, 1991.

MMWR Update: Mortality Attributable to HIV infection among persons aged 25–44 years—United States, 1991 and 1992. MMWR 52:869, 1993.

MMWR Recommendations of the U.S. Public Health Service task force on the use of zidovudine to reduce perinatal transmission of human immunodeficiency virus. MMWR 43:1, 1994.

Pantaleo G, Graziosi C, Fauci AS: The immunopathogenesis of human immunodeficiency virus infection. N Engl J Med 328:327, 1993.

Phair JP: Keynote address: Variations in the natural history of HIV infection. AIDS Research and Human Retroviruses 10:883, 1994.

Richman DD: Resistance drug failure, and disease progression. AIDS Research and Human Retroviruses 10:901, 1994.

Sande MA, Carpenter CCJ, Cobbs CG, et al: Antiretroviral therapy for adult HIV-infected patients. JAMA 270:2583, 1993.

Sande MA, Volberding PA: The Medical Management of AIDS, 3rd edition. Philadelphia, WB Saunders Company, 1992.

Sanford JP, Sande MA, Gilbert DN, et al: Guide to HIV/AIDS Therapy. Dallas, Antimicrobial Therapy, Inc., 1993.

Weiss RA: How does HIV cause AIDS? Science 260:1273, 1993.

CHAPTER 22

PULMONARY MEDICINE

JOHN G. PRICHARD and LAWRENCE M. TIERNEY, Jr.

Most respiratory illnesses encountered in family medicine practice are benign and self-limited. It is the great challenge of a generalist's practice to distinguish those milder afflictions from serious diseases that often present in an undifferentiated form. As in all areas of practice, it is the ability to note unique susceptibilities of one's patients and to find in the multitude of historical points, physical findings, and laboratory data those often small pieces of information that set apart one disease process from another that is important.

The diagnosis and management of respiratory illnesses require knowledge of the epidemiology of diseases of the chest, an understanding of the natural history of individual disorders, and an ability to enable patients to note deviations from expected clinical courses of self-limiting diseases. For example, the knowledge that influenza activity is beginning within the community often allows one to make a presumptive diagnosis given the proper clinical setting. Because complications of this disease are few, patients or their families must, under the direction and guidance of the physician, observe the course of the illness and report findings or symptoms that may forewarn of complications. It is frequently the persistence of a particular symptom with the passage of time that becomes the only reasonable way to distinguish it as having a possibly serious underlying cause.

The prevention of respiratory disease is an especially important responsibility of the family physician. The prevention of pertussis and diphtheria, now taken to be routine, presently may be extended to include the prevention of influenza, tuberculosis, pneumococcal pneumonia, and infections caused by *Haemophilus influenzae* and *Pneumocystis carinii*. Nearly all cases of lung cancer and the majority of cases of chronic obstructive pulmonary disease (COPD) could be eliminated by smoking prevention. Efforts in this regard, as in environmental air pollution, are a form of preventive medicine that must be pursued on an individual basis with our patients and in the community as both social and political problems.

To review in detail even the most common of respiratory illnesses seen in the family physician's office would be a formidable undertaking. We therefore have limited the text to areas of pulmonary medicine in which diagnosis or management recently has changed or is controversial. We also have elected to include entities that, although perhaps uncommon, represent diagnostic dilemmas or are not discussed in other readily available sources.

RADIOLOGY

Because most of the chest is hidden, even to those most accomplished in auscultation, radiographic studies are a crucial part of our diagnostic armamentarium. The radiologist's ability to provide a reasonable differential diagnosis based on the pattern of radiographic abnormalities is greatly hampered by the absence of historical information.

Under ideal circumstances, a radiographic study is ordered to solve a clinical difficulty. The radiologist then reviews the film and notes a particular pattern from which a differential diagnosis may be generated. That list is further refined, ideally in consultation with the family physician, by distinguished features in the history and physical examination. Supplemental radiographic studies then may be chosen and, depending on the results of those studies, further diagnostic interventions or treatment undertaken.

Chest radiographs ordered in asymptomatic people are not helpful as part of routine screening for the early diagnosis of lung cancer in patients who smoke or as a means of screening for tuberculosis. Additionally, routine chest films do not influence the overall management of patients with chronic lung diseases such as asthma or chronic bronchitis–emphysema, unless there is clinical evidence indicating worsening.

However, the chest radiograph can be of immense value in attempting to sort out the cause of persistent cough, determine the origin of fever in a young child or elderly person, or distinguish between acute bronchitis and pneumonia. If chest radiographs are ordered, the aim should be toward resolving a particular clinical problem or in investigating clinically unapproachable or silent areas in a complex patient.

TESTS OF RESPIRATORY FUNCTION

Spirometric units that measure the forced expiratory volume in 1 second (FEV_1) and the forced vital capacity (FVC) are satisfactory for office testing of respiratory function. Reliable and inexpensive spirometers are now readily available. For children or young adults, hand-held peak flow meters can be used easily and give reproducible results. Standard reference tables for normal values (as functions of age, height, and sex) are available from instrument manufacturers or may be found in standard texts of respiratory disease.

Oximetry is becoming widely used in hospital emergency rooms and outpatient respiratory therapy departments. Pulse oximetry is a useful and noninvasive method of determining the per cent oxygen saturation. Its greatest use is in evaluating patients with acute respiratory illness, such as pneumonia, in whom the need for supplemental oxygen must be assessed. It is also useful for patients with chronic respiratory disease in whom there has been a worsening of symptoms. Oximetry results may, at times, be helpful in deciding on the need for hospital admission or supplemental home oxygen therapy for patients with obstructive lung disease or to document desaturation for insurance or disability purposes.

Arterial blood gases are invaluable for the evaluation of patients with pulmonary disease. Blood gases allow a determination as to the presence or absence of hypoxemia, the adequacy of ventilation, and the degree of metabolic compensation for respiratory dysfunction. Although expensive and uncomfortable for patients compared with oximetry, arterial blood gases provide more information and are very precise.

Determination of the *partial pressures* of oxygen (Po_2) and carbon dioxide (Pco_2) is especially useful in the initial evaluation of patients with chronic obstructive or restrictive lung disease, both to assess the severity of disease and as a baseline to which one later can refer during periods of clinical deterioration or improvement.

PERSISTENT COUGH WITHOUT APPARENT CAUSE

Persistent cough is a common complaint in ambulatory practice. Nonproductive but persistent cough in children most frequently is due to allergy or recurrent viral infections. In both children and adults, a persistent cough may follow a lower respiratory tract viral infection. In this circumstance, the cough most often is due to otherwise clinically silent reactive airways. The symptoms frequently can be managed with a combination of bronchodilator and a cough suppressant, such as dextromethorphan or codeine. Should a postviral cough persist, despite these interventions, some clinicians advise a brief course of an inhaled corticosteroid.

Environmental changes may bring about a persistent cough; chemical pollutants, such as smoke from a wood-burning stove or fireplace, tobacco smoke, or industrial exposures, may produce cough that remits only with a change in climate or location of work. An atmosphere of very low humidity, whether occurring naturally at higher altitudes or as a consequence of home heating, may produce tracheobronchial irritation and subsequent cough. In younger children, a bronchial foreign body, or a foreign body lodged deep within the ear canal, may produce a persistent cough.

An evening cough is particularly associated with reactive airways, especially in children. Similarly, an evening cough may be associated with postnasal discharge resulting from respiratory allergy. In these instances, an empiric trial of a bronchodilator or antihistamine may bring relief.

Disease of the pulmonary interstitium, congestive heart failure, and pulmonary neoplasms may produce chronic cough. The chest radiograph is crucial diagnostically and should be employed early in evaluating persistent cough, particularly if initial empiric therapy fails.

Endobronchial disease (tuberculosis, tumors) may cause persistent nonproductive cough without abnormalities on chest radiograph. Hence, a rare patient with persistent cough eventually may require bronchoscopy for diagnosis. Bronchoscopy should be advised early if there are worrisome symptoms, such as hemoptysis, fever, or weight loss, associated with persistent cough.

Angiotensin-converting enzyme inhibitors (enalapril, captopril) may produce cough in certain susceptible individuals; however, the underlying mechanism is not presently understood.

Finally, a persistent cough may represent a tic or habit cough. Psychogenic coughs are related to anxiety, and questioning may reveal, particularly in the adolescent, signs of adjustment difficulty in several areas. Clues to the nature of the cough may include its disappearance during sleep or its resolution during weekends or school holidays.

In most instances, a chronic cough will respond to empiric therapy with antihistamines and/or bronchodilators or resolve spontaneously without treatment. Otherwise, a chest radiograph, and occasionally bronchoscopy, will provide answers to its cause. In rare circumstances, despite one's best efforts at history taking and various diagnostic maneuvers, the cause of cough remains obscure. In this instance, it is best to start the diagnostic process over again with particular attention to recognizable exacerbating factors, recent environmental changes, and a survey of all medications consumed. A ear–nose–throat examination and repeat radiographic examination of the chest may prove helpful. Pulmonary function tests may demonstrate abnormalities of diffusing capacity (interstitial lung disease), or spirometry may reveal reversible bronchospasm that then may justify an intensive course of bronchodilator therapy.

PLEURAL EFFUSION

Diagnostic approaches to pleural effusion have not changed substantially over the last several years. The history, physical examination, chest radiograph, and laboratory analysis of pleural fluid yield a definitive or presumptive diagnosis in over 90 per cent of cases. Pleural effusions are expected in many clinical settings and often may be followed until the underlying condition is controlled and resolution occurs.

Pathophysiologic mechanisms in pleural fluid accumulation are generally well understood. In the individual patient, however, they are often multiple. These mechanisms, with a single example of each, are presented in Table 22–1.

Physical findings in cases of pleural effusion are well known and are not recounted here. Signs are not likely to be elicited unless the effusion is greater than 300 mL. Patients with pleural effusion are seen in consultation most commonly because of the underlying disorder associated with, or directly producing, the effusion. Symptoms and signs associated with the present illness guide the immediacy with which the effusion must be evaluated and determine approaches to diagnosis. Depending on its cause, pleuritic pain may be present, and moderate effusions (800 to 1000 mL) may be associated with breathlessness.

In defining the cause of an effusion, attention should be directed to associated complaints of the patient. Pleuritic pain, fever, and the production of purulent sputum would make a diagnosis of par-apneumonic effusion likely. Worsening dyspnea on exertion, paroxysmal nocturnal dyspnea, and clinical signs of heart failure will implicate increased hydrostatic pressure. Weight loss and a recent or remote history of breast malignancy would suggest a malignant effusion.

Pleural fluid first accumulates in the most dependent regions of the thorax, recesses that lie posteriorly. With increasing amounts, the lateral recesses, and eventually the anterior recess, will be occupied as well. Occasionally, pleural fluid accumulates between the lung and the hemidiaphragm rather than the posterior or lateral sulcus. Subpulmonary collections may be quite large. Once suspected, lateral decubitus radiographs confirm the suspicion of fluid.

Occasionally, pleural collections may become encapsulated between fissures and form a tumor-like, rounded density. In the majority of cases, such pseudotumors occur at the horizontal fissure and vanish with control of the underlying cause, congestive heart failure in most cases. In addition to defining the amount of pleural fluid and its precise location, associated parenchymal infiltrates, or congestive heart failure, radiograhic studies also may provide clues to the presence of subdiaphragmatic pathology. Bilateral decubitus views sometimes will allow imaging of the entire ipsilateral lung.

Analysis of Pleural Fluid

In most instances, analysis of pleural fluid obtained by thoracentesis will define the cause of the collection. Because there are many biochemical, cytologic, and microbiologic tests obtainable on pleural fluid, test selection must evolve from the clinical setting. Table 22–2 briefly lists various test and their significance. In some instances, the clinical circumstances point so strongly toward a particular etiology that ordering specific tests with the initial thoracentesis is justified.

When the clinical picture is less obvious, the most useful tests are those that allow one to distinguish between exudative and transudative effusions. This is done best by obtaining total protein and lactate dehydrogenase (LDH) levels simultaneously on the pleural fluid and serum. Table 22–3 shows the values for these findings that will allow a confident separation into the two types of effusions.

Transudative effusions occur in conditions in which intravascular oncotic pressures are diminished (nephrotic syndrome, advanced liver disease) or in circumstances of elevated venous pressures (congestive heart failure, constrictive pericarditis). Transudative effusions are more frequently bilateral and, in the majority of cases, can be observed confidently while managing the underlying cause. In contradistinction, exudative ef-

TABLE 22–1. MECHANISMS UNDERLYING PLEURAL FLUID COLLECTIONS

Mechanism	Example	Type of Effusion
Increase in hydrostatic pressure	Congestive heart failure	Transudate
Decrease in oncotic pressure	Nephrotic syndrome (hypoalbuminemia)	Transudate
Increase in negative intrapleural pressure	Atelectasis	Transudate
Increased capillary permeability	Infection	Exudate
Decreased lymphatic drainage	Obstruction of lymphatics as result of malignancy	Exudate
Increased transport of fluid across diaphragm	Pancreatitis	Exudate

TABLE 22–2. LABORATORY FINDINGS ON PLEURAL FLUID AND THEIR SIGNIFICANCE

Test	Significance and Special Instruction
Total protein	Obtain serum protein determination. An exudative effusion is defined by a pleural fluid protein divided by serum protein equaling 0.5 or more.
Lactate dehydrogenase	Obtain serum LDH level. An exudate is indicated if pleural fluid LDH divided by serum LDH = 0.6 or greater, or LDH is more than two thirds above upper limit of normal for serum.
Differential count	
Red cells	Collect in tube with anticoagulant. Frankly bloody effusions suggest malignancy, lung infarct, or trauma.
White cells	Total count of 10,000 is common in many causes of exudative effusions. Very large numbers seen with empyema.
Lymphocytes	If lymphocytes predominate (≥50%), malignancy or tuberculosis is most likely. Pleural biopsy and/or cytologic studies should follow.
Mesothelial cells	Presence of mesothelial cells common; absence is of more importance. Tuberculosis very unlikely if large numbers are present and *is* likely in lymphocyte-predominant exudates with few or no mesothelial cells.
Plasma cells	Seen in association with many causes of exudative effusions, including trauma. Very large numbers may suggest myeloma.
Eosinophils	Associated with pulmonary embolus, malignancy, hemothorax, resolving parapneumonic effusion, viral pleuritis, tuberculosis, and coccidioidomycosis.
Glucose	Useful if effusion is thought to be associated with rheumatoid disease (in which case the value is usually 30 mg/dL or less) and in parapneumonic effusions.
Amylase	Elevated in pancreatic disease, esophageal rupture, and, occasionally, nonpancreatic malignancies.
pH	Draw into heparinized blood gas syringe. Obtain only when pneumonia is present. A value of 7.10 or less is indication for chest tube, but only if effusion is due to bacterial infection.
Gram's stain	If positive, very useful in parapneumonic effusion. Will help guide antimicrobial therapy.
Acid-fast stain	Almost *never* positive even in proven cases. Histology and culture of pleural biopsy preferred. If pleural fluid is cultured for acid-fast bacilli, send *large* volume (300 mL).
Cytology	Add heparin to collection tube or place directly in fixative such as 60 per cent ethanol. Volume needed will depend on method cytologist uses.
Cell block	Often very helpful addition to cytology. Larger volumes required—discuss with pathologist before thoracentesis is performed.
Cultures	Preferable to collect in syringe; exclude remaining air. Take to laboratory with covered new needle. Be selective in ordering fungal and acid-fast bacilli cultures.

fusions almost invariably are caused by one of the serious illnesses listed in Table 22–4.

The pH of pleural fluid should be obtained in cases in which an effusion complicating bacterial pneumonia is the principal diagnostic consideration. There is general agreement that a pleural fluid pH of 7.10 or less indicates need for tube thoracostomy. Draining the pleural space obviates the development of empyema thoracis or loculation of parapneumonic fluid. The pH of pleural fluid in circumstances other than underlying bacterial pneumonia has no prognostic or diagnostic significance.

Cytologic analysis of pleural fluid has become the cornerstone of diagnosis in malignant effu-

sions. Combining the examination of Papanicolaou-stained smears and sections prepared from paraffin-imbedded cell buttons yields a diagnosis in more than 90 per cent of cases. False-positive results occasionally are reported, usually as a result of misinterpretation of reactive mesothelial cells as malignant. If initial studies are negative or inconclusive, and malignant effusion remains the principal clinical diagnosis, repeated cytologic studies are warranted.

Pleural Biopsy

Needle biopsy of the pleura finds its greatest use in circumstances in which a pleural effusion is exudative, lymphocyte predominant, and relatively lacking in mesothelial cells. These findings are characteristic, but not diagnostic, of pleural tuberculosis. If pleural biopsy specimens are examined histologically and cultured, this more than doubles the diagnostic yield of tuberculosis over culturing pleural fluid only. By combining all three methods, a definitive diagnosis of tuberculosis can be achieved in roughly 80 per cent of cases. Pleural

TABLE 22–3. ANALYSIS OF PLEURAL FLUID: EXUDATIVE VERSUS TRANSUDATIVE EFFUSION

Laboratory Test	Transudate	Exudate
Pleural fluid protein divided by serum protein	<0.5	>0.5
Pleural fluid LDH divided by serum LDH	<0.6	>0.6

TABLE 22–4. CAUSES OF EXUDATIVE PLEURAL EFFUSIONS

Malignancy
Infections
   Bacterial parapneumonic effusion
   Viral
   Tuberculosis
   Fungal (rare)
   Parasitic (rare)
Serositis
   Rheumatic pleuritis
   Lupus erythematosus
   Drug hypersensitivity
Pulmonary infarction
Trauma
Subdiaphragmatic disorders
   Pancreatitis
   Peritoneal carcinomatosis
   Peritonitis
   Subphrenic abscess
   Subphrenic trauma (e.g., spleen hematoma)
   Hepatic abscesses
Miscellaneous disorders
   Uremia
   Sarcoidosis (rare)
   Meigs' syndrome
   Post–radiation therapy
   Chronic atelectasis
   Abnormalities of lymphatic drainage
   Benign effusion with asbestos

biopsy also improves diagnostic accuracy in cases of malignant effusion. Because pleural biopsy is not without risk and is frequently uncomfortable, it is probably best reserved for cases of suspected tuberculosis or suspected malignant effusions when initial cytologic studies are inconclusive.

Etiologies of Pleural Effusion

Pleural effusion resulting from *malignancy* is most often a consequence of primary tumors having their origin in the lung. Breast malignancy and tumors arising from the lymphoreticular system are the second and third most common causes, respectively. Adenocarcinoma of unknown primary site produces malignant effusions at a rate comparable to that for tumors arising in the lymphatic system (12 per cent). Primary tumors of the genitourinary or gastrointestinal tract involve the pleura less often.

Pleural effusions associated with malignancies other than breast tumors or lymphoma signify advanced disease and a poor prognosis. If the tumor is responsive to chemotherapy, the collection may resolve and not recur. Frequently, management will require removal of the collection by tube thoracostomy followed by pleurodesis. Tube drainage can be accomplished with relative comfort if a small-bore chest tube is placed under adequate systemic and local analgesia. When drainage is minimal (less than 50 mL/24 h), pleurodesis may

be undertaken. This most often is accomplished by instillation of doxycycline or bleomycin. Some patients tolerate this procedure well while others find it very painful. Thus, every effort should be made to ensure adequate intrapleural analgesia.

Recent studies have shown that a dose of 250 mg of lidocaine in a 1% or 0.5% solution will achieve good pleural anesthesia without toxic serum levels. Ensuring contact of the lidocaine solution with all pleural surfaces is essential before instilling the pleurodesis solution. Local pleural anesthesia should be augmented by systemic analgesia with opiates. Pleurolysis can be expected in the majority of patients. On the rare occasions when this method fails, repeated application of doxycycline may be effective. Talc also has been used successfully to effect pleurodesis, being insufflated into the pleural space via a thoracoscope.

Tuberculous effusions may be seen in the absence of underlying parenchymal disease. These effusions occur as a consequence of rupture of a caseous focus subjacent to the pleura. A low-grade fever is frequently present and, unless the collection represents an empyema, the skin test is almost invariably positive. The collection is exudative, and usually, although not exclusively, lymphocytes predominate. Treatment is identical to that used for pulmonary tuberculosis.

Effusion commonly occurs coincident with *pneumonia*. Initially, the fluid is thin, with a relatively low number of inflammatory cells. With prompt antibiotic therapy, such effusions are arrested and resorb without further difficulty. Effusions associated with more virulent organisms, or in cases in which treatment is delayed, become more heavily laden with inflammatory cells and fibrin. These effusions may form loculated collections in dependent, posterior regions of the chest.

If loculations are small, unassociated with persistent fever, and painless, they likely will cause no great difficulty and resorb with time. Conversely, large collections and persistent fever are indications for drainage. The location of loculated collections is defined easily by ultrasound. Percutaneous drainage often brings dramatic resolution of fever and radiographic abnormalities.

Empyema, or the appearance of grossly purulent material and viable organisms in the pleural space, may occur following a parapneumonic effusion or rupture of a tuberculous or bacterial abscess into the pleural space. Aerobic organisms are the cause in 40 per cent of cases, and streptococcal species are isolated most frequently. Mixed anaerobes are found exclusively in 30 per cent of cases, with *Bacteroides* species being the predominant organism.

When a parapneumonic effusion is noted, early thoracentesis may have valuable diagnostic as well as therapeutic implications. A Gram's stain may detect organisms and direct specific antibiotic therapy. In a nonloculated effusion, pleural pH, glu-

Weight loss of 4.5 kg or more
Fever
Large effusion
Reactive tuberculin test
>95% lymphocytes in pleural fluid

cose, and LDH determinations will help indicate the need for tube thoracostomy.

A minority of patients with pleural effusion will remain undiagnosed following initial endeavors at defining its etiology. Recent studies have suggested certain criteria that, if present, strongly predict an underlying malignant or other treatable cause. Those patients with small exudative effusions (800 mL or less), and who are not associated with the criteria set forth in Table 22–5, may be followed expectantly. Should the clinical circumstances change, then further diagnostic efforts are warranted.

The use of fiberoptic bronchoscopy in the evaluation of pleural effusion of unknown cause provides a very low diagnostic yield. Thoracoscopy may allow direct visualization of the pleura, thereby permitting directed biopsies in cases in which diagnosis has not been determined by usual methods.

PULMONARY EMBOLISM

Pulmonary embolism remains a daunting illness of high morbidity and mortality for all physicians. Autopsy studies have revealed that as many as 20 per cent of all deaths are at least associated with this finding; estimates of incidence indicate that over 600,000 cases occur yearly in the United States, with perhaps a third of these resulting in the death of the patient. What makes pulmonary embolization challenging for the physician is the difficulty in establishing the diagnosis, as well as the risks of therapy. Many episodes take place in already terminally ill patients in whom this problem is agonal; however, a majority are observed in patients who have a temporary predisposing factor and in whom recovery from the embolism is associated with good health subsequent to it.

Pulmonary embolism may be defined as the transfer of thrombus or other material from the systemic venous circulation, through the right side of the heart, and into the pulmonary vasculature. The majority of such thrombi originate in the veins of the lower extremities, above the popliteal. In some instances, embolization may occur from the pelvic veins, periprostatic plexus, subclavian veins, and even from the right atrium or ventricle; in the latter instances, there is often clinical information pres-

ent leading the clinician to suspect these sources. There are several types of patients in whom pulmonary embolization from veins of the pelvis and the legs is more likely to occur. Patients with deep venous thrombophlebitis are a common example, and, likewise, patients with any kind of major pelvic trauma, either spontaneous or surgical, fall into this group. Chronic venous insufficiency (postphlebitic syndrome) also may give rise to pulmonary embolization, and prolonged immobility for any reason is associated with both venous thrombosis and pulmonary embolization.

Patients with congestive heart failure, and its associated stagnation of the venous circulation, are more apt to suffer pulmonary embolization, and symptoms may be very difficult to separate from those of the primary cardiac condition. Systemic hypercoagulability—as observed in patients with malignancy, those with various congenital defects (such as antithrombin III deficiency), and, in particular, in women receiving oral contraceptive pills—also is associated with both deep venous thrombosis and pulmonary embolization. Indeed, the past history of the patient presenting with suspected pulmonary embolization is an important determinant of the utility of diagnostic studies, as will be described below.

Diagnosis

It long has been noted that the major difficulty in the diagnosis of pulmonary embolization results from the nonspecificity of the symptoms and signs associated with it. Indeed, the most common symptom is dyspnea, which itself has countless other causes. Chest pain, often pleuritic in quality, is frequent but not constant; the same is true of cough and, less commonly, hemoptysis, the latter when pulmonary infarction has taken place. The onset of the above symptoms is typically crisp, but recurrent episodes may result in the patient's perception that the onset of these complaints was gradual. There is little correlation between the severity of symptoms and the size of the embolus; in the rare patient in whom syncope is caused by pulmonary embolization, it is more likely to be massive.

Physical examination may be no more rewarding. Most commonly found are tachycardia and tachypnea, both of which have numerous other causes. Fever, most often low grade but occasionally more than 39°C, is observed in less than half of patients. Occasionally, adventitious sounds or pleural friction rub may be appreciated; more often, they are absent. Evidence of right ventricular overload, such as a palpable systolic parasternal lift and an increased intensity of the second heart sound, is seldom present but highly suggestive of the diagnosis when it is. Also helpful on physical examination is a search for a potential source, such as thrombophlebitis; however, physical signs for that condition are themselves undependable, with numerous false positives and negatives being encountered. The clinician occasionally measures the diameter of the lower extremities to determine if venous obstruction might be present; however, in most people, the left leg is slightly larger than the right as a result of the normal passage of the left common iliac vein under the aorta. In short, the symptoms and signs of pulmonary embolization are seldom discriminant diagnostically.

As might be anticipated, the differential diagnosis of suspected pulmonary embolization is broad. Pneumonia, especially with pleural involvement, is a typical mimic; the *Pneumococcus* variant is particularly apt to do this. Other infections causing pleuritic chest pain and dyspnea include epidemic pleurodynia. Episodic shortness of breath also may be caused by left ventricular dysfunction resulting from primary heart disease; when chest pain is not pleuritic, then myocardial infarction may be suspected. It has been stated that pulmonary embolization also may result in bronchospasm, thus producing confusion between it and asthma and/or COPD; this probably occurs rarely. The differential diagnosis may be summed by saying that nearly any cardiac or pulmonary disease, of any etiology, may be confused with pulmonary embolization; perhaps more importantly, pulmonary embolization may coexist with these conditions, further adding to the diagnostician's dilemma.

A wide variety of diagnostic imaging studies are available to investigate potential pulmonary embolism and its sources. Prior to undertaking any investigation, however, the physician should decide if the patient is a candidate for treatment, which consists for the most part of systemic anticoagulation. Commonly performed blood studies are usually not helpful; there may be mild leukocytosis and, very rarely, a slight elevation in serum bilirubin and LDH levels if pulmonary infarction has taken place. Arterial blood gases typically show slight hypoxemia and, with it, some hypocarbia, resulting in an increased A-a gradient. The electrocardiogram most often shows sinus tachycardia; evidence of right ventricular conduction disturbance, although helpful diagnostically, is usually absent. The plain chest radiograph may be completely normal; the most common abnormality is simple plate-like atelectasis and an elevation of one hemidiaphragm. Less frequent are reduced blood flow into the embolized lung and a prominent pulmonary artery on the affected side. Pleural effusions occasionally are observed. A wedge-shaped peripheral infiltrate in the lung parenchyma that is pleural based and pointing toward the ipsilateral hilum (Hampton's hump), although helpful when present, is most often absent.

The radionuclide ventilation–perfusion lung scan is the most useful imaging study. This is an extremely sensitive test, and a perfectly normal perfusion scan excludes any consideration of pulmonary embolism. However, abnormalities may be caused by numerous cardiopulmonary processes, including COPD and congestive heart failure. For this reason, a ventilation scan of the lung is compared with perfusion abnormalities. This study has its highest predictive value when there is a large (lobar) perfusion defect associated with normal ventilation; 90 per cent of such patients have pulmonary embolism at arteriography. Many variations of this pattern are seen however. Segmental or subsegmental unmatched perfusion defects make pulmonary embolism less likely; if the defects are matched by reduced ventilation, it is less likely still, with subsegmental matched defects representing a likelihood in the range of 10 per cent for pulmonary embolization. It is in this instance that consideration of the clinical likelihood of embolization guides the clinician. For example, the complete absence of any predisposing factors toward embolism may lead the physician to discontinue investigation after a low-probability scan; other studies may be considered if one or more risk factors have been documented.

The gold standard for the diagnosis of pulmonary embolism is a pulmonary arteriogram. This is appreciably more invasive and expensive than the ventilation–perfusion scan, exposes the patient to radiation and intravenous contrast agents, and carries with it the risk of potential cardiovascular abnormalities associated with the passage of the catheter through the right ventricle. A pulmonary angiogram never needs to be performed if a perfusion lung scan has been normal; when abnormal, the scan may direct the radiologist to the affected parts of the lung, thus minimizing the exposure to contrast. The presence of pulmonary hypertension constitutes a relative contraindication to this study. Precise guidelines on when to perform pulmonary angiography are difficult to enumerate, and it is often left to the clinician to weigh the risk of empiric anticoagulation for 3 to 6 months against the risk of the procedure. In most instances, it is performed in patients who constitute moderate anticoagulation risks. When anticoagulation is absolutely contraindicated, this study may be performed if the physician considers the patient a candidate for vena caval interruption (see Treatment of Pulmonary Embolism). Although there is considerable interest in such techniques as magnetic resonance imaging to visualize major proximal pulmonary emboli, these investigations are not applied widely for the diagnosis of pulmonary embolism at this time.

An alternative, and sometime supplemental, approach to the diagnosis of pulmonary embolism involves identifying a potential source. Because over 90 per cent of these emboli originate from the deep venous system of the pelvis and lower extremities, diagnostic techniques aimed at studying these vessels can be used with much efficacy to stratify the risk for embolism in a given patient. For example, the combination of a low- or moderate-probability ventilation–perfusion scan in a patient possessing one or more risk factors for pulmonary embolism and a positive study indicating deep venous thrombosis may be sufficient reason to anticoagulate the patient, obviating the need for pulmonary angiography.

The procedure that is most sensitive and specific for evaluating deep venous thrombosis in the legs is contrast venography. At the same time, this study is expensive. It is at times difficult to perform, requires an experienced radiologist to interpret, and exposes the patient to both contrast and radiation. Two types of less invasive studies are in widespread use: Doppler ultrasonography and impedance plethysmography. Both studies are painless and may be performed repetitively and on an outpatient basis. The sensitivity of both of these studies approaches 90 per cent for the presence of impaired flow of blood in the deep femoral systems. Of the two, Doppler is more sensitive in the calf veins, although these are rarely the source of a pulmonary embolism .Some clincans prefer the use of both studies, believing that the sensitivity and specificity are increased. Doppler ultrasonography has the added advantage of being able to diagnose valvular incompetence in the venous system, but at the same time the interpretation of any Doppler study is operator dependent, thus requiring experience. Increasingly, advances are being made in noninvasive visualization of vascular structures, and it can be expected that duplex ultrasonography, which combines imaging plus the use of ultrasonography, will provide additional diagnostic information.

In short, many patients with pulmonary embolism may be diagnosed exclusively on noninvasive grounds. The most important aspect of the process is the pretest assessment by the clinician of the probability of the clinical event, plus a risk–benefit analysis of treatment in a given patient. Thus, in some patients, the clinician may choose not to perform even a simple lung scan if the patient is not a candidate for any therapy; in others, any combination of the above-described studies may be employed. Above all, it is important to consider each patient individually, rather than obtaining all possible studies on any patient with suspected pulmonary embolism.

Treatment

The treatment of pulmonary embolism is systemic anticoagulation, although it still remains an area of some debate. Indeed, there exist very few studies, likely for ethical reasons, comparing the natural history of untreated pulmonary embolism with that of anticoagulated patients. Nevertheless, anticoagulation is widely accepted as a standard of care in the medical community. In nearly all patients, the initial therapy of pulmonary embolism is intravenous heparin, administered in a dose aimed at maintaining the patient's partial thromboplastin time (PTT) between 1.5 and 2 times the patient's baseline level. For patients with baselines higher than a laboratory's control values, the PTT should be assumed to be in the middle of the laboratory range; when a patient's PTT is below the control range, then the clinician should aim for a therapeutic value of at least twice that baseline. Doses necessary to achieve this level of anticoagulation vary from patient to patient and may vary within the same patient during an episode of treatment. Clinically, patients appear more resistant to the anticoagulant effects of heparin in the early days after pulmonary embolization, so that the clinician should be wary of an increasing PTT on a stable dose of heparin.

A standard maintenance dose of heparin is generally in the range of 1000 units/hr, after a loading dose of 10,000 units; most clinicians prefer to administer it by constant infusion. Although the proper duration of intravenous heparin remains uncertain, most physicians settle on a 7- to 10-day course, followed by 3 to 6 months of additional anticoagulation. This may be accomplished by intermittent subcutaneous heparin in doses adequate to prolong the PTT to 1.5 times control halfway between doses, or warfarin in doses capable of prolonging the patient's prothrombin time to 1.5 times control. It appears that little additional value, but a considerably increased bleeding tendency, is observed if the prothrombin time is between 1.5 and 2 times control, so that a range between 1.3 and 1.5 is ideal. When warfarin is used for subsequent anticoagulation, it generally is instituted a few days before the intended discontinuation of heparin; this drug is contraindicated in pregnancy because of its toxicity to the fetus and because of teratogenicity, so that subcutaneous heparin is administered in this instance. Although 3 to 6 months of anticoagulation is frequently the rule in these patients, assuming there are no contraindications, this is by no means proved. A shorter duration may be chosen for a person with risk factors that may be transient; in some instances, prolonged or even permanent anticoagulation might be chosen for other patients. This latter group might include those with permanent immobilization, previous episodes of pulmonary thromboembolic disease, or rare inherited clotting tendencies, such as antithrombin III deficiency.

The occasional patient with pulmonary embolization may be a candidate for thrombolytic therapy, with either streptokinase or urokinase. Although no survival advantage has been shown for these therapies, it is agreed that there is more rapid resolution of symptoms and signs, especially of large and potentially life-threatening emboli. Thus, this type of treatment is best reserved for patients who are judged to have massive embolization by imaging studies or those who showed unstable cardiovascular systems (i.e., hypotension requiring pressors). It can be anticipated that there may be a role for tissue plasminogen activator in the future in this condition, but, at the moment, it is largely an experimental agent for this indication.

Finally, vena caval interruption may be performed in certain circumstances. In patients with proved pulmonary embolization with absolute contraindications to anticoagulation, this is a valuable therapy; additionally, in those in whom documented recurrence of embolization occurs despite at least 24 to 48 hours of adequate anticoagulation, this may be offered. The mode of interruption in most widespread application is the Greenfield filter, which may be inserted through a neck vein, advancing through the superior vena cava to the inferior vena cava, and positioned just below the renal veins. The filter remains in place permanently and, in experienced hands, is relatively easy to insert. However, complications reported have included tearing of the vena cava or embolization of the filter itself, so it is important that it be reserved for the precise indications noted.

Prevention

Considerable attention has been paid in recent years to the prevention of pulmonary embolization, and there is general agreement on the classes of patients to whom this should be offered. Prevention may be carried out by several therapies: low-dose subcutaneous heparin, full heparin anticoagulation, and external pneumatic compression of the lower extremities. Elastic stockings and early ambulation after a surgical procedure are less useful. The highest risk for pulmonary embolization exists in patients with femoral fractures or those having orthopedic operations on the pelvis or legs. The risk is lower, but still increased, for gynecologic, abdominal, or urologic surgery. Less well studied, but assumed to be a higher risk, are medical patients who will be at prolonged bed rest. There are a variety of other conditions, including neoplasms and acquired anticoagulation (which paradoxically produces an *increased* clotting tendency, such as the lupus anticoagulant), that usually do not receive prophylaxis therapy. The following constitute prophylactic recommendations.

For patients undergoing orthopedic procedures on the hip or femur, heparin should be given in doses sufficient to anticoagulate in the same way as described previously for acute pulmonary embolization. Pneumatic compression is also helpful; low-dose subcutaneous heparin is ineffective in this group. For a patient undergoing gynecologic, abdominal, or urologic surgery, low-dose heparin (5000 units every 12 hours) affords protection. It has been suggested that pneumatic compression may be substituted for low-dose heparin in these

patients, and it may prove to be equally efficacious. Although there is less information to justify it, the same low-dose heparin therapy often is administered to patients with medical conditions at bed rest, particularly those with acute myocardial infarction but also those with chronic congestive heart failure or septicemia. Concerning neurosurgical procedures, any anticoagulation, including low-dose heparin, is contraindicated; here external pneumatic compression is the therapy of choice.

The contraindications to full-dose anticoagulation, which would interdict either heparin or warfarin, include recent trauma, bacterial endocarditis, advanced diabetic retinopathy, recent or contemplated neurosurgery, and recent gastrointestinal bleeding (10 to 14 days).

Low-Molecular-Weight Heparin

The introduction of low-molecular-weight heparin has added new considerations to the analysis of treatment strategies in pulmonary thromboembolic disease. Low-molecular-weight heparin does not prolong the PTT, and appears to be associated with appreciably fewer bleeding complications when compared with standard formulations of the drug. Studies indicate its efficacy to be similar to that of conventional heparin for treatment of deep venous thrombosis and for prevention of postoperative thromboembolic disease. Although its use in established pulmonary embolization has been investigated less thoroughly, there is little reason to suspect it would not be equally efficacious. Low-molecular-weight heparin is currently considerably more expensive than the standard-weight drug; the cost differential is offset by the lack of necessity for clotting studies to monitor therapy. It may well be that low-molecular-weight heparin will become the drug of choice in many of the clinical situations noted above.

DISORDERS OF THE PROXIMAL AIRWAYS

Most of the disorders of the proximal airways encountered in ambulatory practice affect children. The proximal airways and larynx of the child have a small surface area with an extensive submucosal vasculature. Infection or inflammation of these structures results in edema with consequent narrowing of the lumina. The most common disorders affecting the proximal airways in childhood and adolescence include epiglottitis (see Chapter 23) laryngotracheitis, bacterial tracheitis, and laryngotracheobronchitis. Although these diseases have factors in common and may overlap in terms of severity, a diagnosis usually can be made on the basis of history, physical findings, and the results of therapeutic interventions.

Laryngotracheitis (spasmatic croup) is encountered most commonly in the fall and winter months and usually affects children between 1 and 4 years of age. The onset of the illness is usually sudden, predominantly nocturnal, and characterized by a barking cough. There is a paucity of prodromal or concurrent symptoms of upper respiratory tract infection, and fever is usually absent. The disorder is considered to be caused by a viral infection or allergy causing subglottic edema. Exposure to humidified air, cold or warm, often brings relief of cough and stridor promptly. Hence, children brought to the hospital for evaluation may be rendered nearly free of symptoms simply by exposure to the evening or night air.

Viral laryngotracheitis must be distinguished from a bronchial foreign body, angioneurotic edema, and extrinsic or intrinsic laryngeal or tracheal masses. The onset of the illness and surrounding circumstances usually can lead to the exclusion of these disorders. Treatment includes the provision of humidified air, whether at home or in the hospital. Corticosteroids have shown benefit in decreasing the duration of symptoms. Laryngotracheitis is distinguished from epiglottitis by the latter's association with a somewhat less precipitous onset, fever, and a toxic appearance.

In *laryngotracheobronchitis*, cough becomes associated with symptoms and signs of a viral upper respiratory tract infection. Cough progresses in severity and becomes associated with stridor, bronchospasm, and fever. Signs and symptoms frequently worsen in the evening hours. Although the illness is encountered more frequently in winter, it may be seen during any season, and most commonly between the age of 3 months and 3 years. The syndrome may accompany outbreaks of influenza virus, respiratory syncytial virus, and other viral respiratory pathogens.

Physical examination reveals a febrile child with a croup-like cough. Respiratory distress may be manifested by retractions, and stridor may be present to a minor or marked degree. There are usually signs indicating upper respiratory tract inflammation, including rhinorrhea. Audible wheezing is usually present, and a chest radiograph may show narrowing of the tracheal shadow. Differential diagnosis includes epiglottitis, inhaled foreign body, and spasmodic croup.

Therapy consists of humidified air and oxygen therapy. Racemic epinephrine, given by aerosol, is indicated in other than mild cases and may bring rapid, albeit transient, relief. Repeated aerosol treatments may be warranted, but refractiveness to this modality may occur. Although benefit is not proven, some clinicians occasionally employ corticosteroids because some children seem to respond to them. In the minority of cases, airway narrowing progresses and respiratory distress worsens. Naso-

tracheal intubation may be required, and the tube may need to be left in place for several days.

Occasionally, children thought to have laryngotracheobronchitis are found, at the time of intubation, to have purulent secretions in the airway. Bacterial cultures may grow *Staphylococcus aureus*. *Bacterial tracheitis* may occur as a primary event but generally is thought to occur following viral injury to the proximal airway. Treatment usually involves placing a nasotracheal tube, providing supplemental oxygen, humidification of inspired air, and administration of a β-lactamase–resistant penicillin or a cephalosporin.

ACUTE BRONCHITIS

Acute bronchitis is the illness diagnosed fifth most commonly by family physicians. This condition accounts for an enormous amount of time missed from work and school. During particular seasonal outbreaks, especially of influenza, acute bronchitis can account for more than half of telephone consultations and one third of office visits.

Viruses cause the vast majority of episodes of acute bronchitis, with influenza A and B and respiratory syncytial virus being associated with distinct seasonal outbreaks. Adenoviruses, rhinoviruses, coxsackievirus, and parainfluenza viruses also cause episodes of acute tracheobronchitis. In young adults, *Mycoplasma pneumoniae* and a particular strain of *Chlamydia psittaci* have been documented to cause a small proportion of cases of acute bronchitis.

With the exception of *Bordetella pertussis*, the etiologic agent of whooping cough, bacterial agents are more difficult to incriminate as definite causes of bronchitis. Most of the organisms thus far incriminated (*H. influenzae*, *Streptococcus pneumoniae*, and *Moraxella [Branhamella] catarrhalis*) are part of normal flora of the upper respiratory tract. The isolation of these organisms in cases of acute bronchitis therefore is expected. However, their presence in increased numbers in persons with chronic disease of smaller airways and their common association with pneumonia lend credence to their presumed role as causative agents of acute bronchitis.

The diagnosis of acute bronchitis usually rests on clinical grounds. Patients complain of acute, usually productive cough and, occasionally, minimal hemoptysis, frequently in association with mild to moderate fever, chills (without true rigors), myalgias, and fatigue. In many cases, pharyngitis and/or rhinitis either precede or accompany the lower respiratory tract symptoms. Persons who smoke develop acute bronchitis more frequently, with more severe and persistent symptoms.

On examination of the chest, signs of consolidation are absent. Fine crackles, representing secretions in the airways, may be demonstrated, and wheezing may be evident or discovered on auscultation during forced expiration. In the elderly febrile patient, and occasionally in febrile infants and children with signs and symptoms of bronchitis, a chest radiograph is warranted to differentiate acute bronchitis from pneumonia. In most patients, neither radiographic studies nor additional laboratory tests, such as leukocyte counts, are of value.

Treatment of acute bronchitis remains largely symptomatic. For those in whom cough is severe and wheezing can be demonstrated, temporary use of inhaled bronchodilators may be of benefit. If the cough is associated with substernal pain and lack of sleep, a cough suppressant, such as dextromethorphan or codeine, may bring improvement. For patients with rhinitis, the addition of an antihistamine may be helpful. Acetaminophen or other nonsteroidal anti-inflammatory agents may help control fever and myalgias.

Antibiotics frequently are prescribed for acute bronchitis, although their benefit remains unproven. Although bronchitis may be a harbinger of pneumonia, this is an infrequent complication and antibiotic therapy has not been shown to decrease the frequency with which it evolves.

The use of antibiotic therapy in acute bronchitis, although often demanded by patients, is both elective and empiric. The choice of antibiotic in acute bronchitis is also problematic. Clinical syndromes overlap sufficiently that one cannot distinguish easily between potential causative agents, and no laboratory tests can differentiate reliably among the various pathogens. Although serologic tests and viral cultures are available, these are not practical in the ambulatory setting.

Erythromycin frequently is prescribed; however, there is an increasing rate of resistance to this agent among strains of *H. influenzae* and a high rate of discontinuance because of gastric intolerance, even with enteric-coated formulations. Erythromycin and tetracycline have been shown to decrease the duration of illnesses caused by *Mycoplasma*; however, there is no reliable constellation of symptoms or signs that favor *Mycoplasma* over other agents as the cause of bronchitis.

If antibiotic therapy is elected, a Gram's stain of sputum may be helpful in guiding selection of an antimicrobial. If *S. pneumoniae* or Haemophilus is recognized, then trimethoprim-sulfamethoxazole or amoxicillin-clavulinate represent rational choices. If the patient is between 5 and 40 years of age, has purulent sputum without a predominant organism on Gram's stain, or lives in a relatively closed environment in which *Mycoplasma* illness has been documented in others, erythromycin then may be prescribed.

During outbreaks of influenza A activity, patients with compatible symptoms may reasonably be treated with amantadine. To be effective, it must be instituted within the first 72 hours of illness.

BRONCHIOLITIS

Acute bronchiolitis is a febrile disease of infancy and early childhood caused by infection of the respiratory epithelium of smaller airways. Peribronchial edema and inflammatory cell infiltration occur, becoming associated with obstruction of small airways from cellular debris and mucus plugs.

The disease is encountered most commonly in children from 2 to 12 months of age. During epidemics of bronchiolitis, which occur predominantly between January and May, more than 80 per cent of cases are due to respiratory syncytial virus. During nonepidemic outbreaks, respiratory syncytial virus is found in slightly over 50 per cent of cases, with parainfluenza viruses, adenoviruses, influenza viruses, rhinoviruses, and *Mycoplasma* being associated with the remainder of cases. Concomitant infection with either another virus or a bacteria occurs in roughly 5 per cent of cases.

Following an incubation period of 5 to 7 days, the child develops fever, often associated with signs of upper respiratory tract infection, and copious production of tenacious nasal secretions. Progressive cough and dyspnea then ensue during the first 5 days of illness. Irritability and respiratory distress usually bring the child to medical attention.

On examination, the most striking findings are rhinorrhea, respiratory distress, and wheezing. The chest radiograph may show marked hyperinflation with depression of both diaphragms, thereby explaining the frequent ability to palpate both spleen and liver on physical examination. Peribronchial and interstitial infiltrates may be noted in multiple lobes, in addition to atelectasis.

The differential diagnosis includes gastric aspiration, inhaled foreign body, and asthma associated with viral infection. Pneumonia often is considered because of the high frequency of abnormal chest radiographs associated with respiratory syncytial virus infection. The white blood cell count may be elevated, and in some children a left shift is seen. An initial episode of asthma precipitated by a viral infection may not be distinguishable from bronchiolitis on clinical grounds. Definitive etiologic diagnosis is possible using viral cultures or immunofluorescence assays on nasopharyngeal secretions; however, these studies rarely are ordered outside of research or teaching institutions.

The treatment of bronchiolitis is aimed at the management of respiratory distress. Supplemental oxygen is provided and antibiotics sometimes are prescribed because of the uncertainty concerning bacterial pneumonia. Although children less than 2 years old are relatively unresponsive to inhaled β-agonist therapy, this often is provided along with intravenous theophylline to seriously ill children. The mortality rate in large series varies from 0.5 to 5 per cent, with death more likely in children with pre-existing lung disease (i.e., bronchopulmonary dysplasia) or heart disease.

It long has been recognized that children with severe bronchiolitis, once recovered, may have persistent chest symptoms several years hence. Recurrent lower respiratory tract infections with evidence of airway obstruction may occur and mandate readmission. Because of these findings, an etiologic role of respiratory syncytial virus in the pathogenesis of asthma has been postulated. Current evidence does not support an association of recurrent chest symptoms following bronchiolitis with a family history of asthma or evidence of atopy. The extent to which antiviral therapy is effective in treating bronchiolitis or in preventing its sequelae is presently unknown. For children who experience wheezing following bronchiolitis, most episodes can be shown to be precipitated by a recurrent viral illness. Additionally, most of these children have come from homes where parents smoke.

PNEUMONIA

The term "pneumonia" encompasses an extraordinary range of severity of illness and of causative agents. Although here we are concerned mainly with infectious causes of pneumonia, the same symptoms and signs can be caused by a host of noninfectious illnesses, including inhaled chemicals, hypersensitivity disorders, and other noninfectious inflammatory disorders such as sarcoidosis. Certainly, most cases of pneumonia are transient, self-resolving infections that go unrecognized or respond to empiric therapy on an outpatient basis. In the majority of instances, even among hospitalized patients, no etiologic agent is defined. Approximately 1 million cases occur annually, and pneumonia results in about 3 per cent of hospitalizations.

Given the variety of organisms capable of causing pneumonia, and the overlapping clinical and radiographic findings caused by them, a clinical diagnosis based solely on possible etiologic agents will be unrewarding. For example, S. pneumoniae, the most common cause of community-acquired pneumonia in hospitalized patients, may produce a relatively mild illness with inflammation limited to a single lobe. This same organism also may cause an overwhelming illness with panlobar involvement, bacteremia, and multiple distant sites of infection.

Radiographic patterns are extremely helpful in the diagnosis of pneumonia. Although certain patterns may be characteristic of a particular pathogen, none are pathognomonic. Similarly, laboratory studies, such as the white blood cell count or degree of left shift, offer only general guidance. Most laboratory tests are nonspecific and a good deal of variation is to be expected.

Hence, whereas knowledge of the usual pattern of illness caused by distinct pathogens is essential in the evaluation of an individual patient with pneumonia, an epidemiologic approach is more useful. Factors that bear on unique susceptibilities and influence the presentation or likely course are found in the patient's history; age, race, occupation, local endemicity, and associated illnesses such as diabetes, human immunodeficiency virus (HIV) infection, or a recent episode of influenza each may help to incriminate a particular pathogen.

Subjective data will lead one to suspect an *acute* or *chronic* pneumonia—a distinction that carries great etiologic significance. Whether the disease was *acquired in the hospital or in the community* raises suspicion for certain pathogens and the likelihood that the organism will be resistant to antibiotics.

Combining epidemiologic, historical, and clinical information with specific patterns found on the chest radiograph is enormously helpful. Whether the lung involvement is localized or diffuse, is associated with effusion, is predominantly cavitary, or demonstrates involvement far out of proportion to the degree of illness influences one's further diagnostic attempts. A recent history of altered consciousness (e.g., seizure) and the finding of pulmonary infiltrates in dependent segments leads one to the consideration of *aspiration pneumonia* and immediately influences choice of antibiotic therapy.

The diagnosis of pneumonia is, in most instances, made clinically on the basis of lower respiratory tract signs. No single clinical sign or symptom predicts accurately the presence of infiltrates on the chest radiograph. However, abnormal auscultatory findings on chest examination in patients with acute respiratory tract symptoms are most predictive of an abnormal chest radiograph.

The extent to which efforts should be directed toward etiologic diagnosis before beginning therapy will be influenced both by the severity of illness and the relative likelihood of complications. The etiologic diagnosis of pneumonia must take into account historical and clinical data in addition to patterns obtained from the chest radiograph. These guide the evaluation, while definitive diagnosis is based on sputum Gram's stain and cultures, blood cultures, serologic assays, and, at times, lung biopsy. Tests such as the total leukocyte count are nonspecific and provide little insight as to potential pathogens. A Gram's stain and culture of adequate sputum specimens are most useful; if adequate specimens cannot be produced spontaneously, they often can be obtained by saline aerosol induction. If positive, blood cultures provide highly specific information and should be considered, particularly for patients who are to receive parenteral therapy for pneumonia on an outpatient basis.

Again, most cases of pneumonia are self-limiting, and in many patients, empiric therapy is entirely warranted. Further attempts at diagnosis may be reasonable only if empiric therapy is failing or the diagnosis can be obtained by relatively simple and inexpensive diagnostic tests. Urgent and invasive diagnostic methods may be necessary, however, either because of the severity of illness or the setting in which it is evolving.

The choice of laboratory tests and the sequence in which they are employed will depend on whether one considers the pneumonia to represent typical bacterial pneumonia or an atypical process more likely to be caused by mycobacteria, viruses, fungi, mycoplasma, or parasitic disease. Table 22–6 lists some features helpful in distinguishing atypical from typical pneumonia in older children or adult patients.

Despite efforts to identify clinical and laboratory factors that might aid in differentiating bacterial pneumonia from viral pneumonia in children, the positive predictive value of any single finding or group of combined laboratory and clinical findings is poor. Judgment as to the severity of illness within the context of the patient and his or her community consistently has been found to be of greater importance than any single laboratory determination, or group of laboratory findings, in deciding proper disposition of the patient.

Factors that favor a bacterial rather than viral cause of pneumonia include the following: age greater than 6 months, fever greater than or equal to 103° F, and total band count greater than 500. Certain radiographic features also may be helpful. If a single lobe is involved with a definite infiltrate or if multiple lobes are involved by well-defined infiltrates, this favors a bacterial cause as well. Conversely, interstitial or peribronchial infiltrates that involve multiple sites associated with segmental atelectasis favor a viral etiology.

Whether one evaluates a child with a lower respiratory tract infection by a formal scoring system or a more global clinical evaluation based on clinical experience and judgment is less important than recognizing that viral or bacterial causes of lower respiratory tract infections are not mutually exclusive. Indeed, most bacterial infections of the lower respiratory tract probably arise as a consequence of disordered local defense mechanisms induced by a viral infection.

The most immediate difficulty in managing patients with pneumonia is the decision whether to admit the patient to the hospital or begin therapy on an ambulatory basis. Obviously, patients who lcak the ability to care for themselves or who do not have capable family members to look after them may require admission. Those who appear toxic, display an increased work of breathing, or are compromised by alcoholism or other illnesses that may place them at risk similarly should be hospitalized. In uncertain cases, oximetry or arterial blood gases may be reassuring or indicate the need for supplemental oxygen therapy in the hospital. Reasonable and insightful patients who have concerned family members to supervise their course often can be managed satisfactorily as outpatients.

Because most cases of community-acquired pneumonia are likely to be due to either *S. pneumoniae* or *H. influenzae*, oral agents chosen for treatment should cover these bacteria. β-Lactamase–producing strains of *H. influenzae* are isolated increasingly; thus amoxicillin–clavulinic acid represents a reasonable first choice for oral therapy. Trimethoprim-sulfamethoxazole and erythromycin-sulfisoxazole represent satisfactory alternatives.

The course of *Mycoplasma* pneumonia can be shorted by treatment with erythromycin. Tetracycline is an alternative agent, except in children. The newer macrolides (clarithromycin, azithromycin) also share in vitro anti-*Mycoplasma* activity. Unfortunately, the diagnosis is difficult; there are no reliable clinical or radiologic findings, either in children or adults, that can distinguish *Mycoplasma* from other causes of atypical pneumonia, especially early in its course (Table 22–7). A cold agglutinin titer of 1:32 or greater is supportive of the diagnosis but is nonspecific. Complement fixation titers may not increase to a diagnostic level until the second or third week of illness. Culture of sputum for *Mycoplasma* is difficult and is not helpful in deciding on initial antibiotic therapy. Hence, erythromycin may be reasonable empiric therapy in young patients with an atypical pneumonia syndrome and a compatible chest radiograph, and whose sputum shows leukocytes but no evident pathogens on Gram's stain.

In the management of adults with community-acquired pneumonia, there may be instances when oral antibiotic therapy is not deemed adequate. Yet, for a variety of reasons, hospitalization may not be desirable, or the patient may refuse admis-

TABLE 22–6. FEATURES DIFFERENTIATING TYPICAL AND ATYPICAL PNEUMONIA

Feature	Typical	Atypical
Prodromal illness	+ +	+ + +
Sudden onset (or sudden worsening of prodrome)	+ + +	+
Rigors	+ + + +	+ +
Chest pain	+ + + +	+ +
Fever (>102°F)	+ + + +	+ +
Purulent sputum	+ + + +	+ +
White cell count with left shift	+ + + +	+ +
Dyspnea	+ + +	+ +
Degrees of illness	+ + +	+ +
Radiographic study worse than anticipated	+ + + +	+ + + +
Lobar distribution of infiltrate	+ + + +	+
Pleural effusion	+ + + +	+

+ + + + = common; + = rare.

TABLE 22–7. SIGNS AND SYMPTOMS ASSOCIATED WITH *MYCOPLASMA PNEUMONIAE* PNEUMONIA

Symptom or Finding	Expected Occurrence (%)
Cough	90
Fever	80
Sore throat	50
Injected pharynx	45
Nausea, vomiting	40
Headache	30
Chills	30
Otitis, myringitis	30
Chest pain	25
Muscle aches	25
Lung consolidation	25
Dyspnea	25
Adenopathy (cervical)	25

Adapted from Mansel JU, Rosenow EC, Smith TF, et al: *Mycoplasma pneumoniae* pneumonia. Chest 95:639, 1989.

sion. In these circumstances, parenteral therapy may be initiated using a long–half-life cephalosporin administered once every 24 hours by the intramuscular route or via an indwelling heparin lock. Parenteral therapy may be discontinued and replaced with oral therapy as soon as the patient's clinical course indicates that the pneumonic process is resolving.

TUBERCULOSIS

Tuberculosis is a chronic, relapsing, systemic illness that is transmitted almost exclusively via the respiratory route. Similar to other chronic granulomatous diseases of the lung, such as histoplamosis or coccidioidomycosis, a primary infection is followed by healing in the majority of cases; only 15 per cent of infected individuals develop an illness that at some time will be diagnosed as tuberculosis.

In most of the world, infection is acquired during childhood, although a new infection may occur at any age. Symptoms following initial infection are usually mild and, unless suspicion is aroused because of additional epidemiologic or skin test data, often do not lead to further investigation. Cough may or may not be present and constitutional symptoms are highly variable, being seen less frequently in the very young or elderly.

Concomitant with the development of pneumonia, there is subclinical dissemination of *M. tuberculosis* to virtually all organs. Within 6 weeks following infection, delayed hypersensitivity develops with arrest of bacterial replication. From time to time, however, factors that enforce local control at such infected sites may falter. Mycobacterial replication may resume and a variety of syndromes then may occur, depending on the location of bacterial regrowth. Reactivation of tuberculosis usually occurs in the lung, resulting in so-called reactivation-type tuberculosis. Infiltrates most commonly are seen in the upper lobes, often with cavities. Formation of the latter requires some degree of hypersensitivity. In some patients, cavitation does not occur, and the infiltrates may take on the appearance of pneumonia of any cause or may appear as nodules simulating neoplasm.

As evidenced by the foregoing, the diagnosis of tuberculosis often is made by inference, taking the history, epidemiologic clues, and clinical and radiographic information into account. In children, the finding of a reactive tuberculin skin test in association with an abnormal chest radiograph is usually grounds for a full course of antituberculosis chemotherapy. If warranted (uncertain diagnosis, suspicion of resistant organisms), three successive early morning gastric aspirates may be obtained or fiberoptic bronchoscopy performed. In those able to cooperate, the induction of sputum samples using hypertonic saline is superior to spontaneously produced sputum in terms of recovery of organisms.

Biopsy of affected organs (pleura, lymph nodes, or bone) may be required to obtain a histologic diagnosis and for cultures. At times, despite one's best efforts, treatment must proceed on an empiric basis. This is nearly always the case in smear-negative pulmonary tuberculosis, because cultures often take as long as 6 weeks before a definitive identification is possible. Recent advances using fluorescent microscopy and newer methods of culture, however, have improved greatly the rapidity with which definitive diagnosis can be made.

The treatment of pulmonary and extrapulmonary tuberculosis affecting both children and adults has become more complicated over the past several years because of the emergence of multi–drug-resistant organisms in several metropolitan areas of the country. It has been said that there exists only one opportunity to treat tuberculosis properly. Several principles guide the treatment of tuberculosis. Indeed, adherence to such guidelines will help to limit treatment failures and subsequent emergence of resistant strains of tuberculosis:

1. Used isoniazid monotherapy only for prevention—this presupposes exclusion of active disease.
2. Start therapy *after* collection of relevant clinical samples.
3. Initiate treatment with at least three drugs (usually isoniazid, rifampin, and pyrazinamide).
4. Never add a single drug to a failing regimen.

Such principles apply to adults as well as children who are infected with tuberculosis. For patients in whom there is a likelihood of nonadherence to the prescribed regimen, local public health personnel may be able to assist with treatment by providing an opportunity to observe the administration of oral antituberculosis medication directly.

During pregnancy, isoniazid and rifampin may

be used without concern for teratogenicity and, if drug resistance is suspected, ethambutol should be added.

With the use of multiple drugs, the duration of therapy for tuberculosis has shortened. Regimens lasting 6 to 9 months are now standard, although therapy may be extended for a variety of reasons, including treatment of drug-resistant organisms or the presence of immunodeficiency from a variety of causes. In the latter instances, the precise duration of therapy is uncertain but may extend from 12 months to 2 years in some cases.

The prevention of tuberculosis is accomplished not only by the treatment of contagious patients but by the identification of infected, asymptomatic individuals as well. The tuberculin skin test may identify individuals who have been infected with tuberculosis, but it cannot distinguish between those with active versus inactive disease. Current recommendations for otherwise well individuals suggest screening with intradermal or multipuncture skin tests at 1 year of age, again at the time of entry to preschool or kindergarten, and at some point during adolescence. Tuberculin skin testing also should be considered for all new immigrants and young people planning to study or travel extensively in areas where tuberculosis is endemic.

As a result of screening either in the office or by school health services, the physician may be confronted with the patient who is well but has a reactive tuberculin skin test. Figure 22–1 suggests a management scheme for asymptomatic adults. Although 10 mm of induration at 48 to 72 hours usually is taken to represent a prior tuberculosis infection, it may be appropriate to lower this threshold to 5 mm. For example, a 5-mm area of induration in a 6-month-old child known to have been exposed to a family member with active pulmonary tuberculosis might well be considered to indicate infection. It is especially the case in a young adult or child that a reactive tuberculin skin test indicates the presence of an infectious individual in the young person's environment. Hence, the reactive tuberculin test represents a sentinel event that should prompt investigation of the child's siblings, parents, or other persons with whom significant contact has been made.

The decision to use preventive therapy, usually isoniazid, presumes that active disease has been reasonably eliminated and compliance with either a year-long or 6-month regimen can be anticipated. Isoniazid usually is tolerated very well, although parents occasionally complain that a child may seem somewhat hyperactive. This usually can be resolved satisfactorily by providing the drug in the evening hours.

Although drug-induced hepatitis represents a rare complication of isoniazid therapy, it is an age-related phenomenon usually occurring in older individuals. Periodic determination of hepatic transaminases in an otherwise well individual generally is not warranted.

CHRONIC DISORDERS OF THE AIRWAYS

Three disorders commonly are recognized under the term "chronic obstructive pulmonary disease": chronic bronchitis, asthma, and emphysema. Although often thought of as mutually exclusive and distinct clinical entities, they share either common precipitants, pathophysiology, or response to therapeutic intervention. Obstruction to airflow can be demonstrated in each, as can anatomic abnormalities such as bronchial muscle hypertrophy, glandular hypertrophy, and varying degrees of airway narrowing. Therapeutic interventions, specifically cessation of smoking and the use of various bronchodilating drugs, may have a salutary effect.

Although asthma typically is regarded as paroxysmal episodes of reversible bronchospasm, in some patients the obstruction to airflow eventually becomes less reversible, resembling that in patients with chronic bronchitis.

In some individuals who smoke, an increase in

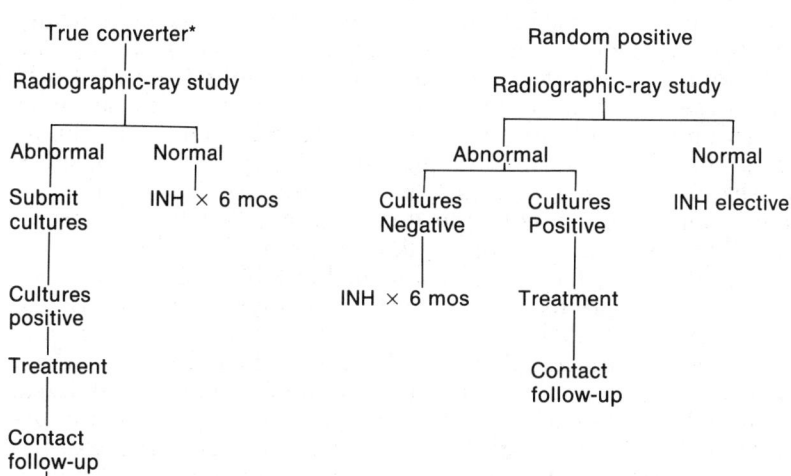

FIGURE 22–1. Management of adult tuberculin-positive patients. *Documented change from negative skin test to positive within 2 years. INH, isoniazid.

elastase and various mediators of the inflammatory response can be demonstrated within alveoli. The result is the destruction of very small distal airways and a concomitant increase in the size of alveolar spaces. Although rare patients may be demonstrated to have relatively pure emphysema (e.g., α_1-antitrypsin deficiency), most can be demonstrated to have bronchorrhea and reversible limitations of airflow.

The terms "blue bloater" and "pink puffer" occasionally are used to distinguish between, respectively, individuals with chronic bronchitis and emphysema. However, anatomic studies have shown more similarities than differences between these two clinically identifiable groups. It appears that the clinical abnormalities in these patients can be attributed to differing central responses to hypoxemia, rather than fundamental differences in type or severity of pulmonary disease.

Asthma

Asthma is defined by several criteria and must be differentiated from other causes of paroxysmal dyspnea. In childhood, asthma must be distinguished from acute bronchiolitis, lower respiratory tract infections, cystic fibrosis, congestive heart failure, recurrent pulmonary aspiration, and retained bronchial foreign body. Asthma attacks are characteristically paroxysmal and may bear temporal relationships to environmental or emotional stimuli or become manifest only with upper or lower respiratory tract infections. There may be a seasonal incidence, with return of normal respiratory function during intervening periods. A family history of asthma or a personal history of eczema or other atopic phenomena may support a diagnosis of asthma.

Physical examination may show wheezing during all phases or only part of the respiratory cycle that usually clears promptly with institution of treatment and remains clear during asymptomatic intervals. The chest radiograph is characteristically normal during asymptomatic periods. Eosinophils may or may not be found in sputum and sometimes are increased on the differential white cell count.

Since 1979, there has been a consistent increase in the reported number of deaths resulting from asthma, only in part explained by a change in disease classification and reporting. Increases in asthma mortality have been reported from other countries as well and have been most striking within the 5- to 34-year age group. The rising mortality in metropolitan areas may be related in part to increasing air pollution; however, as indicated by asthma death rates in Montana (third highest rate in United States), other factors are also important. A lack of definite seasonal variation in mortality argues against viral infections or environmental allergens playing a significant role.

Studies from New Zealand, where the highest increase in death rate thus far has been reported, showed that more than 50 per cent of those who died were *in extremis* at the time of presentation to the hospital. As testimony to their circumstances, no deaths occurred in those surviving more than 30 minutes after reaching the emergency room.

In childhood cases that have been reviewed intensively, certain high-risk factors have emerged: discontinuity of medical supervision, nearly exclusive reliance on emergency rooms for asthma care, and frequent admissions for status asthmaticus. Recent hospitalization, tapering of relatively high steroid doses, and minority racial status also are associated with the higher likelihood of sudden death resulting from asthma. Dysfunctional family circumstances or an expressed wish to die has been documented in a number of adolescent asthma deaths. Overreliance on the use of inhaled β-mimetic agents and a tendency to delay seeking emergency care appear to contribute to a large proportion of deaths resulting from asthma.

Most asthma attacks are terminated readily. This usual experience may lull patients, their families, and even their caregivers into a false sense of security. In contrast, unpredictable attacks of breathlessness, especially in children, may cause great anxiety. Thus, in the care of asthmatic patients and their families, the physician must walk the narrow path of providing confidence and competency to the patient and family, while acknowledging concern and the importance of seeking care urgently either with severe attacks or when usual home treatment is failing.

Asthma is a heterogeneous disorder, both in severity and in natural history, that is multifactorial in its causation and persistence. Traditionally, asthma has been divided into intrinsic and extrinsic forms, a distinction that may have some clinical merit but appears to be becoming less significant in terms of distinguishing underlying mechanisms. Individuals with paroxysmal episodes of wheezing related to hypersensitivity to environmental agents have been considered to have *extrinsic asthma*. These patients have tended to have a family history of asthma, cutaneous manifestations of allergy, and elevated levels of immunoglobulin (Ig) E. Patients with *intrinsic asthma* tend to be somewhat older and more frequently have abnormal radiographic studies that demonstrate hyperinflation and fibrosis. Paroxysms of wheezing are associated more often with purulent sputum, and the illness assumes a course akin to chronic bronchitis.

The relationship of heritable factors that may predispose to reactive airways, early experience with lower respiratory tract viral infections, and the acquisition of hypersensitivity in the development of asthmatic syndromes remain unknown. Recent data indicate a very strong association between asthma prevalence and increasing age-specific IgE levels. However, among unselected individuals with very high IgE levels, only a minority suffer from asthma. Clearly, then, there are other factors that predispose to the onset of asthma and perpetuate its occurrence. As many as one third of asthma attacks in childhood and adulthood can be shown to be associated with lower respiratory tract viral infections, especially those caused by respiratory syncytial virus. The majority of children recovering from respiratory syncytial virus infections will experience lower respiratory tract symptoms over the succeeding several years.

The therapy of asthma involves use of pharmacologic and nonpharmacologic therapy that is based on an understanding of precipitating factors and the severity and constancy of symptoms. There is considerable individual variation in the degree to which pharmacologic therapy is tolerated and effective. Therefore, therapy proceeds in a stepped manner, using objective methods (e.g., FEV_1 peak flow rates) to monitor benefits while noting drug-associated toxicity.

For patients with asthma who smoke, persistent efforts toward achieving complete smoking cessation should be undertaken. Specific precipitating events, drugs, or environmental circumstances should be alleviated when possible. Intensive efforts toward home dust control by the use of air purifiers are expensive and disruptive and are of unproven benefit. The value of dietary restrictions, allergy testing, and immunotherapy remains controversial. The latter are time consuming and expensive. Their use might be considered in circumstances in which there is evidence of other immune-mediated disorders, such as atopy or allergic rhinitis, and pharmacotherapy has not satisfactorily controlled wheezing. Indeed, referral to a pediatrician or pulmonary physician experienced in the treatment of asthma should precede referral for immunotherapy.

Asthma represents a variety of syndromes, the course of which will change from time to time as a result of a host of factors; the therapy one employs must change accordingly. An indicator of the successful management of asthma is not simply the absence of bronchospasm, but also minimizing disruption of school performance or other aspects of daily living brought about by therapy. Over the past few years, the inflammatory component of asthma has become the main target of pharmacotherapy. Hence, there has been a shift away from using inhaled β-agonists as first-line therapy for moderate to severe disease, and in their place employing inhaled corticosteroids, cromolyn sodium, or nedocromil sodium. Anti-inflammatory therapy is supplemented by inhaled β-agonist therapy when necessary. Inhaled bronchodilator therapy may be considered first-line treatment for those children or adults with infrequent bouts of wheezing. Typically, this would include circumstances wherein the patient experiences bronchospasm in association with viral respiratory tract infections but is otherwise free of symptoms. Primary therapy for children or adults with moderate to severe asthma should focus on the use of inhaled corticosteroids. Trials of inhaled corticosteroids or cromolyn may be unsuccessful unless the goals and expectations for such therapy are clearly understood by the patient or the child's family. Relief of bronchospasm over the short term is not to be expected. Indeed, abrupt discontinuance of inhaled β-agonists and attempted replacement with cromolyn or corticosteroids likely will end in therapeutic failure. If exercise, exposure to cold air, or unavoidable exposure to allergens predictably induces bronchospasm, cromolyn may be used on a prophylactic basis.

With more severe bouts of asthma, such as may accompany acute viral illness, the early use of parenteral or oral corticosteroids will decrease the need for inhaled bronchodilators and may obviate the need for emergency room visits or hospitalization. Long-term use of oral corticosteroids should be avoided, especially in children. However, prolonged use of inhaled corticosteroids has been shown to be safe and efficacious and may replace the need for oral corticoids in the majority of patients.

Short–half-life theophylline preparations may be useful for patients who develop bronchospasm only at night. The use of theophylline in the control of asthma has declined because of the efficacy of steroids, cromolyn, and selective β-agonists. Importantly, the toxicity and behavioral problems associated with theophylline also have become more widely appreciated. This is especially true in the older adult, in whom seizures, cardiac dysrhythmias, severe nausea and vomiting, hypoglycemia, and the like complicating theophylline use are not rare events. Such difficulties with theophylline can be ascribed to its narrow therapeutic index and, particularly, its extensive and complicated interactions with an ever-expanding number of other therapeutic agents.

Chronic Bronchitis–Emphysema

Patients with persistent airway obstruction, chronic production of sputum, and usually a long history of cigarette use commonly are considered to have chronic bronchitis–emphysema. Postmortem studies have shown both airspace destruction and airways disease, thereby justifying inclusion of both disorders under COPD. Studies concerning the natural history of chronic airway obstruction have demonstrated a dismal prognosis. Ten-year survival data varied little between those nonatopic smokers with chronic sputum production and those with a more pure form of emphysema who also were smokers. These findings were in sharp distinction to nonsmoking asthmatics, whose 10-year survival was excellent.

Despite the fact that COPD is not a reversible

disease process, both the duration and quality of life can be improved on with careful management. The single most important factor slowing the inevitable decline in FEV_1 is complete cessation of smoking. Although numerous clinical trials using varied modalities for smoking cessation have been conducted, it appears that consistent advice from a concerned physician to both the patient and his or her family is as effective as any other type of intervention. However, some patients appear to respond to adjunctive measures, such as smoking cessation classes or pharmacologic interventions.

Similar to asthma therapy, the approach to pharmacologic treatment of (COPD) has taken on new directions. Whereas theophylline represented the cornerstone of long-term therapy of chronic bronchitis–emphysema in years past, inhaled bronchodilator therapy has emerged as first-line pharmacologic treatment presently. The anticholinergic drug ipratropium bromide probably represents the initial drug of choice for inhalational bronchodilator therapy. Its duration of action and efficacy is superior to that of β-agonists. However, selective β-agonists are effective and are at least additive in terms of bronchodilating effect when used in conjunction with ipratropium bromide.

Corticosteroids, whether used orally or inhaled, are controversial in terms of the benefit they provide in management of COPD. As with many therapeutic modalities, benefit easily may be seen in some individuals while having no measurable effect in most. Hence, in patients receiving optimal bronchodilator therapy and who remain symptomatic, a trial (monitored by serial measurements of FEV_1) of corticosteroids may prove to be of benefit. If a trial of corticosteroids is deemed to be beneficial, then inhaled corticosteroids may completely and safely replace the use of systemic corticoids even over the long term.

The precise role of bacteria in acute worsening of chronic bronchitis–emphysema remains unknown. *Moraxella catarrhalis*, *S. pneumoniae*, and *H. influenzae* are the most common organisms isolated from the airways of symptomatic, or asymptomatic, patients with COPD. Not only is the role of these organisms unclear in terms of their contribution to the inevitable decline in pulmonary function in COPD patients, but the extent to which they may play a role in exacerbations is similarly uncertain. Antibiotics effective against the above-mentioned organisms have been shown in some studies to be of benefit in shortening hospital stays, whereas in other similarly designed studies no such efficacy could be demonstrated. Despite the lack of clarity concerning this issue, many clinicians use antibiotics during periods of exacerbation of symptoms whether the patient is ambulatory or hospitalized.

The development of acute lower respiratory tract infection in the setting of moderate to severe COPD carries a very serious prognosis. Providing yearly influenza vaccine and immunizing with polyvalent pneumococcal vaccine may reduce the incidence or severity of this complication.

Rehabilitation of the patient with severe COPD is an important aspect of overall management; benefit may be noted by both objective and subjective determinants, such as improved exercise tolerance and self-esteem and lessening of depression. Pulmonary rehabilitation programs may be prescribed through nonprofit community organizations or hospitals that sponsor such programs.

Patients with chronic bronchitis–emphysema have a sustained increased work of breathing. It is particularly the pink puffer who frequently is noted to be thin and undernourished. It long has been considered that this may contribute to poor respiratory muscle function; indeed, recent weight loss is a poor prognostic sign. In undernourished patients with severe airflow obstruction, supplementing the diet improves respiratory muscle power, breathlessness scores, and a sense of well-being.

The natural history of chronic bronchitis–emphysema is one of an inexorable decline in FEV_1. In some individuals, the work of breathing is not maintained, resulting in hypercarbia and sustained hypoxemia. These patients often are overweight, edematous, and cyanotic and have elevated hematocrits (blue bloaters). Right heart failure, which produces edema, hepatomegaly, and jugular venous distention, is a direct consequence of pulmonary hypertension induced by chronic hypoxemia.

Long-term oxygen therapy, when used at least 15 to 18 hours a day, has been shown clearly to improve both the quality of life and its duration. In addition to long-term bronchodilator therapy, cessation of smoking, and control of purulent secretions, long-term home oxygen therapy should be prescribed for those patients with sustained arterial Po_2 below 55 mm Hg. If cor pulmonale is evident, and can be attributed to sustained hypoxemia, home oxygen therapy should be prescribed even if daytime arterial blood gas determinations show a Po_2 greater than 55 mm Hg. The reason for the latter is that some patients desaturate during sleep for sufficiently long periods to produce pulmonary hypertension. Despite the long-term benefits of oxygen therapy, it is expensive and cumbersome. Newer methods of oxygen delivery, however, can improve patient mobility and efficiency of oxygen use at reasonable cost.

BRONCHIECTASIS

Bronchiectasis occurs as a consequence of weakness of the bronchial wall brought about by inflammation. Persistent inflammation and obstruction contribute to atelectasis, retained secretions, and repeated episodes of focal pneumonia. Subsequent healing and fibrosis place traction on bronchial walls, resulting in further dilation. External compression of the bronchi, usually as a consequence of adjacent nodal inflammation, also may cause obstruction. The disorder is decreasing in prevalence as a result of more effective treatment of pneumonias and the less frequent occurrence of tuberculosis.

Bronchiectasis may be diffuse or focal. Diffuse bronchiectasis may occur consequent to massive gastric aspiration, chemical injury, severe episodes of tuberculosis, staphylococcal pneumonia, fungal pneumonias, or allergic bronchopulmonary aspergillosis. Focal disease may be due to retention of an aspirated foreign body, obstruction by endobronchial tumors, localized pneumonia, or recurrent pulmonary aspiration of gastric contents.

Chronic productive cough associated with intermittent, minor hemoptysis is now the most frequent presentation. Recurrent bouts of fever with purulent secretions may occur and, with progressive disease, dyspnea, weight loss, and fatigue may supervene.

Physical findings will vary depending on the stage of disease; however, wheezing, coarse rales, and clubbing may be noted. Laboratory studies may reveal leukocytosis if an intercurrent pneumonia is present. A mild anemia, hyperglobulinemia, or an elevated erythrocyte sedimentation rate may be present. A chest radiograph may show evidence of localized or diffuse disease. The diagnosis may be confirmed by computerized tomography (CT) scan of the chest, which can demonstrate segments of lung involvement.

Bronchoscopy is usually of limited value unless there is focal bronchiectasis, and a tumor or retained foreign body is to be excluded. Pulmonary function tests will vary with the extent of disease but usually show a combined obstructive and restrictive defect.

In younger patients, bronchiectasis commonly is seen as a manifestation of an underlying systemic disorder rather than a consequence of prolonged or recurrent bouts of pneumonia. Impaired immune function (hypogammaglobulinemia), dysfunction of mucociliary transport (cystic fibrosis, Kartagener's syndrome), or reactive airways disease (asthma–bronchopulmonary aspergillosis) may be associated with diffuse bronchiectasis.

An approach to the patient with bronchiectasis should include securing anatomic proof of diagnosis by the least invasive method and ceasing cigarette use. A historical review, searching for precipitating events (recurrent pneumonias, tuberculosis) or conditions known to predispose to bronchiectasis, should be undertaken.

Long-term treatment is aimed at management of the underlying disorder, prescribing antibiotics to control infections, and effecting drainage of secretions. One should immunize patients against influenza and pneumococcal pneumonia and promptly treat bacterial infections when they occur. Revers-

ing bronchospasm will be important in certain patients, as will maintaining an adequate level of nutrition. In patients with localized disease who experience repeated hemoptysis or pneumonia, surgical treatment should be considered.

CYSTIC FIBROSIS

During the past two decades, the median survival of patients with cystic fibrosis (CF) has increased dramatically. Most affected children will now live to nearly 30. Such progress is owed chiefly to the establishment of subspecialty centers. Improved management of nutrition and pulmonary infections largely accounts for the enhanced quality and duration of life. The family physician has an important role in the diagnosis of CF and the treatment of non-CF illnesses, and a shared responsibility in the management of its complications.

CF is an autosomal recessive disorder, occurring once in 2000 live births, and may be suspected by a variety of signs or symptoms (Table 22–8). Assays to detect most carriers of cystic fibrosis are available and should be offered to those with a family history of the disorder. The pathophysiology of cystic fibrosis is expressed at the level of the epithelial cells of small airways. Defects of chloride secretion and sodium reabsorption result in mucus of abnormally high viscosity.

Although most cases are diagnosed before age 3, depending on the severity of disease, it may not be considered until adolescence or, in rare circumstances, adulthood. Once the diagnosis is considered, the patient should be referred to a CF center for definitive diagnosis.

Patients with CF, and their families, face enor-

TABLE 22–8. PRESENTING SIGNS AND SYMPTOMS OF CYSTIC FIBROSIS

Age	Signs and Symptoms
Infancy	Meconium ileus Rectal prolapse Failure to thrive Recurrent pneumonia Diarrhea Persistent cough Hyponatremia Heat prostration
Childhood	Intussusception Constipation Abnormal stools Bowel obstruction
Adolescence	Sputum cultures positive for *Pseudomonas* Short stature Delayed sexual development
Adulthood	Infertility Steatorrhea–malnutrition Bronchiectasis

mous burdens. Daily management of the disorder itself, an almost constant fear of loss of life, delayed maturation, hampered development of physical and social skills, isolation, poor self-esteem, and unpredictable crisis brought about by pulmonary infections are issues that the family physician must be prepared to help manage.

Particularly early on in the course of the illness, parents will be especially perceptive of any area of disagreement, no matter how trivial, between their personal physician and the CF center's staff. Opinions regarding the care of patients with CF differ even among those well experienced in its management. Hence, issues such as timing of immunizations, use of antibiotics during minor respiratory tract infections, nutrition, participation in school exercise programs, and genetic counseling of siblings or parents should be agreed on mutually by the primary care physician and the subspecialist. Indeed, the successful long-term management of these children, and even their eventual loss, is eased tremendously by the experience and compassion of their team of physicians.

INTERSTITIAL LUNG DISEASES

The interstitium of the lung may be defined as that part of the alveolar wall that separates the capillary endothelial cells from alveolar epithelial cells. In excess of 125 different diseases have been considered to be interstitial when they involve the lung, although it to be recognized that many involve other tissues and organ systems. As regards chronic diffuse diseases of the lung, then, they may be principally interstitial; mainly alveolar filling; or, more often, a combination of both. Thus, the term "interstitial lung diseases" can be confusing to the clinician but perhaps less so if it is remembered that these processes are uncommonly restricted specifically to that part of the pulmonary anatomy.

The so-called interstitial diseases, irrespective of their cause, tend to show either inflammation or fibrosis pathologically and often both; when inflammation dominates, the process is frequently termed "alveolitis." Any number of different cells of inflammation may be observed, including mononuclear cells, lymphocytes, polymorphonuclear neutrophils, and eosinophils, with the prevalence of one or another determined by the cause of the disease. In addition, an important feature of some interstitial lung diseases is the presence of granulomas; sarcoidosis (see later) is an example. However, most interstitial lung diseases may not be separated from each other based solely on histopathologic examination. Thus, only in certain circumstances is it necessary to obtain biopsy material in the assessment of interstitial lung disease. The pathogenesis of all these conditions may be summed up by considering that an abnormal inflammatory response exists in the pulmonary interstitium; that it may be initiated by numerous processes—some known but others idiopathic; that varying types of histology may be observed in the acute phase (but with the two broad groups being lymphocytic/granulomatous and neutrophilic); and that all ultimately may result in pulmonary fibrosis.

As might be anticipated by this localization of the pathology within the lung, interstitial lung diseases share many functional abnormalities. Lungs affected with these conditions show consistently decreased compliance; the lungs are stiff and require greater pressures to achieve any volume of expansion, resulting in an increased work of breathing. At the same time, the higher pressures required for expansion secondarily result in a lower lung volume and lower total lung capacity. Damage to the exchange surface between the circulation and the inspired air results in impairment of diffusion capacity, because of a reduced total area for effective gas exchange. Together, these result in a typical pattern seen in interstitial lung diseases of hypoxia with slight reduction in Po_2. Although diffusion is impaired as noted previously, the hypoxia more likely results from impairment of the matching of ventilation and perfusion than it does from abnormal diffusion, as had been believed previously. The hypoxia and hypocarbia tend to be progressive, and when oxygen saturation of hemoglobin is consistently below 90 per cent, which occurs at a Po_2 of approximately 50 to 55 mm Hg, then consequent pulmonary hypertension may be expected. This in turn exacerbates the process by inflicting additional trauma on the pulmonary microvasculature.

Diagnosis

Many observers prefer to differentiate interstitial lung diseases into those of known and unknown causes (Table 22–9), and it is clearly in the patient's best interest for a meticulous search to be carried out for any potentially reversible cause. The general history obtained from the patient with suspected interstitial lung disease therefore is directed in a fashion aimed at identifying such causes. The specific pulmonary symptoms, however, are remarkably similar irrespective of cause: The typical patient notes the insidious onset of dyspnea, usually exertional; the breathlessness is not episodic; and orthopnea is not a feature. Depending on the rate of progression, the patient may be dyspneic at rest when first observed, but the considerable majority of patients have a more indolent onset of this complaint. The other common symptom is cough. This is typically dry and nonproductive. Hemoptysis is seldom present unless extensive fibrosis has occurred. On physical examination, the patient usually appears comfortable, although very slight tachypnea may be observed if

TABLE 22–9. CAUSES OF INTERSTITIAL PULMONARY DISEASE

Known Cause	Unknown Cause
Inorganic dusts	Idiopathic pulmonary
Silica	fibrosis
Silicates (including	Sarcoidosis
asbestos)	Eosinophilic granuloma
Beryllium	Rheumatic disease
Hard metal dusts	associated
Organic dusts	Goodpasture's syndrome
(hypersensitivity	Idiopathic pulmonary
pneumonitis)	hemosiderosis
Gases, fumes, vapors	Wegener's
Chlorine	granulomatosis
Sulfur dioxide	Angioimmunoblastic
Mercury	lymphadenopathy
Drugs	Ankylosing spondylitis
Antineoplastic agents	Amyloidosis
Antibiotics	Pulmonary
Sulfonamides	lymphangiomyomatosis
Nitrofurantoin	Whipple's disease
Drugs inducing lupus	Alveolar proteinosis
erythematosus	Inflammatory bowel
Sulfonylureas	disease associated
Gold	
Phenytoin	
Amiodarone	
Poisons	
Paraquat	
Radiation	
Infections	
Disseminated mycobacterial	
or fungal infections	
Viral pneumonia	
Pneumocystis carinii	
pneumonia	
Residue of active infection	
of any type	
Pulmonary edema	
Lymphangitic carcinoma	

the respiratory rate is counted over a minute. The only finding on auscultation is inspiratory crackles, most often appreciated at both bases. Some clinicians believe the dry rales to be characteristic of an interstitial process.

In clinical practice, the combination of a complaint of dyspnea and/or cough with or without the presence of crackles on physical examination is sufficient reason to obtain a radiograph of the chest. It is at this point that the interstitial nature of the process is appreciated, and further historical inquiries typically are made. Likewise, additional abnormalities on the chest film, when present, allow the clinician to narrow the differential diagnosis considerably.

As concerns additional history, there are several fruitful areas of inquiry. For example, the presence of symptoms suggesting a systemic autoimmune disease, such as dermatomyositis or lupus erythematosus, would lead the clinician to recognize that this would be interstitial lung disease complicating those disorders. Many drugs have been reported to cause interstitial pneumonitis; the most typical

encountered in family practice would likely be nitrofurantoin, although numerous antineoplastic agents, gold, and even radiation itself can produce the same process. An occupational history is quite important in the patient with an interstitial abnormality on chest radiograph. Exposure to metals (such as beryllium, silica, coal, and asbestos) or organic matter (such as sugar cane, hay, sawdust, and many others) may cause this. Similarly, the presence of additional systemic symptoms, such as fever, may lead the clinician to consider more seriously an infectious etiology. Tuberculosis, fungal diseases (such as histoplasmosis and coccidioidomycosis), many viral infections, and atypical pneumonitides (such as Q fever) may result in an interstitial process.

Given implications for therapy, it is of special importance to consider infection (Table 22–10) in all such cases. Of particular interest in the patient's history is the presence or absence of risk factors for acquired immunodeficiency syndrome (AIDS); additional inquiries could concern the presence or absence of pets, especially birds. A previous history of malignancy might alert the physician to the presence of lymphangitic carcinoma presenting as an interstitial radiologic pattern. Other aspects of the physical examination, once the clinician is aware of the presence of interstitial radiographic diseases, become important. Lymphadenopathy, synovitis, hepatomegaly, a palpable spleen, and evidence of cardiomegaly all can help the clinician assign priorities to various etiologies in order to tailor the subsequent investigation.

Additional evaluation of the chest film itself also provides additional clues. Of prime importance is the initial distinction between a mostly interstitial abnormality and one that is caused primarily by an alveolar filling process. Although most of the latter are associated with more acute illnesses, such as bacterial pneumonia or pulmonary edema, there are several chronic abnormalities of alveolar filling that clinically resemble the interstitial lung diseases. These include alveolar proteinosis, Goodpasture's syndrome, and eosinophilic pneumonia; all are quite rare. Roentgenographically, an alveolar abnormality results in the loss of the distinction of adjacent parenchymal vessels and of the boundaries of neighboring structures such as the heart

TABLE 22–10. INFECTIOUS CAUSES OF INTERSTITIAL LUNG DISEASES

Bacterial chlamydial: tuberculosis, atypical mycobacteriosis, actinomycosis, *Nocardia* infection, psittacosis, leptospirosis, Whipple's disease, Lyme disease, legionnaires' disease (occasionally), mycoplasma (occasionally) infections
Viral: acute HIV, Epstein-Barr virus, cytomegalovirus, herpes simplex virus infections
Parasitic: *Pneumocystis carinii*, *Echinococcus* infections
Fungal: sporotrichosis, histoplasmosis, coccidioidomycosis
Rickettsial: Q fever

border or diaphragm. The infiltrate of interstitial diseases, by contrast, appears in the early phase as linear, or sometimes nodular, with many patients showing elements of both. With chronicity of disease, scarring and retraction may result in an appearance referred to as honey-combing, which is the development of small cystic spaces throughout the lungs. Prominent pulmonary arteries also are noted in this late stage of interstitial lung disease.

Associated abnormalities may be quite helpful in diagnosis. If there is concomitant pleural thickening or effusion, then considerations such as the interstitial diseases associated with autoimmune processes, asbestosis, lymphangitic carcinomatosis, and nitrofurantoin lung are more likely. Associated hilar and/or mediastinal lymphadenopathy favor sarcoidosis, lymphoma with lymphangitic involvement, primary or metastatic lung carcinoma, or pneumoconiosis, particularly berylliosis. If pneumothorax is present, then eosinophilic granuloma is worthy of consideration; the latter also is associated with lytic bone lesions that can be appreciated in ribs. Interstitial disease that is most prominent in the upper lung fields suggests end-stage sarcoidosis; infections such as tuberculosis; and pneumoconiosis, particularly silicosis. When cardiomegaly is present with an interstitial lower lobe infiltrate, the clinician should keep congestive heart failure in mind; in this case, the infiltrates are linear and subpleural, the so-called Kerley's B lines. Finally, approximately 10 per cent of patients who ultimately develop radiographically abnormal interstitial lung disease may be symptomatic with a normal chest film at the time of first presentation; this can be observed in small recurrent pulmonary embolization and *Pneumocystis* pneumonia.

In short, the combination of numerous details of history, physical examination, and thorough inspection of the chest radiograph allows the physician a reasonable opportunity to establish the diagnosis and, more importantly, to select subsequent studies of higher predictive value. Any subsequent investigation of interstitial lung diseases is tempered by the fact that, in more than two thirds of cases, no identifiable cause will be found. Similarly, although many conditions have been reported to be associated with an interstitial abnormality by radiograph, in many of these conditions, this pattern is an atypical or unusual manifestation. Thus, a panel of studies obtained on a routine basis is to be avoided. For example, culture of the expectorated sputum for typical bacterial pathogens, as well as for fungus and tuberculosis, is seldom likely to be helpful. Hematologic studies are usually within normal limits; the occasional patient with longstanding hypoxia may show erythrocytosis, but the white cell count is usually within normal limits. Chemistries are revealing only when certain conditions are under active consideration; for instance, the elevated alkaline phospha-

tase and hypercalcemia of sarcoidosis may be illuminating, as is the elevated LDH of *Pneumocystis* pneumonia, but these studies are only supportive of a hypothesis and not diagnostic. As implied earlier, examination of expectorated sputum is in general not helpful. In many centers, however, the diagnosis of *Pneumocystis* pneumonia may be made after sputum induction by ultrasonic nebulization; in this instance, the patient may be spared more invasive studies.

Invasive Diagnostic Procedures

The principal conundrum in the approach to interstitial lung diseases relates to the appropriateness of bronchoscopy, bronchoalveolar lavage, and open lung biopsy in patients with this problem. Thus, a preprocedure assessment of the likelihood of finding a treatable lesion, and consideration of whether the patient is a candidate for such treatment, is prudent. Occasionally, invasive diagnostic studies are employed to establish a diagnosis related to occupational exposure for purposes of compensation; asbestosis is an example.

Of these studies, an *open lung biopsy* is the most sensitive and specific. It is excellent in identifying infectious or neoplastic causes of interstitial lung disease, demonstrates granulomas when they are present, and is also accurate for many other parenchymal processes. A biopsy also allows the clinician the opportunity to determine how much a radiographic process is contributed to by active inflammation, and how much by fibrosis, even if the specific etiology of the process cannot be determined. Open lung biopsy, however, requires general anesthesia and thus carries a small but finite risk of significant morbidity or even mortality; similarly, recuperation requires a chest thoracostomy tube. Furthermore, the majority of open lung biopsies will not yield a specific cause of the problem.

In the last few years, open lung biopsy has been replaced by a less invasive approach, *thorascopic biopsy*. This procedure, similar conceptually to other fiberoptic endoscopic diagnostic studies, is far less morbid and requires much less recovery time. It can be performed with negligible mortality, unlike an open lung biopsy; furthermore, it appears as though its sensitivity and specificity, although not studied prospectively as yet, may be similar to those of open procedures. Thorascopic biopsy is becoming increasingly available throughout the country.

A less invasive diagnostic approach than either of these is a *transbronchial lung biopsy*. Although highly sensitive for sarcoidosis and *Pneumocystis* pneumonia, this is less likely to reveal definitive information about other parenchymal processes. Complications of transbronchial biopsy include hemoptysis, pneumothorax (in about 5 per cent of cases), and the worsening of hypoxia. Pulmonary hypertension and coagulation disorders constitute contraindications.

Another study performed in increasing numbers of centers is *bronchoalveolar lavage*. In this procedure, irrigation of the distal airways is carried out by bronchoscopy, and an analysis of the fluid for the type of cells present is carried out. Predominance of lymphocytes suggests a granulomatous process such as sarcoidosis; increased numbers of neutrophils are observed in idiopathic pulmonary fibrosis. It is safe to say, however, that this procedure is not in widespread use and remains more of a research tool than a clinically useful investigation.

In short, a lung biopsy, whether open or thorascopic, is more sensitive and specific but more invasive. Transbronchial biopsy is diagnostic in certain conditions but is less useful in many diffuse pulmonary processes in which involvement of the lung is patchy.

Etiology

Because certain causes of interstitial pulmonary diseases are of particular interest, they will be discussed individually, starting with several conditions of identified cause. *Silicosis* results from the inhalation of silicon dioxide and occurs in sand blasters and quarry workers. The development of pulmonary disease requires many years of exposure, and the highest doses occur with occupations such as sand blasting. Early in the disease, there are small nodular densities distributed interstitially in the lungs; these nodules become larger over time and are particularly marked in patients who have rheumatoid arthritis (Caplan's syndrome). Silicosis is more prominent in the upper lobes, and it often is associated with dense calcification of regional hilar nodes. Patients with silicosis also have a very much higher risk for the development of tuberculosis. The diagnosis generally can be made from the history along with a plain chest film; more invasive investigation is seldom necessary.

Although its major effects are pulmonary, *sarcoidosis* is a systemic disease of unknown cause. It most commonly affects blacks and is more frequent among women than men; it is a young person's disease. Because of its systemic nature, the clinical manifestations are protean. Pulmonary sarcoidosis may present with bilateral hilar adenopathy alone (stage I), hilar adenopathy plus parenchymal interstitial disease (II), or parenchymal disease by itself (III). It is likely that the disorder progresses through all three stages, but the occasional patient may not come to medical attention until it is rather advanced, at which time it is also more difficult to diagnose. Unusual pulmonary manifestations include nodules, with or without cavitation, and, rarely, pleural effusions. Extrapulmonary manifestations and indications for steroid therapy include hypercalcemia, caused by granulomatous elabora-

tion of a vitamin D–like substance; granulomatous hepatitis; arthritis; iritis; carditis (characterized typically by conduction disturbance abnormalities); and nodular skin lesions. All or none of these may be present in patients with pulmonary involvement. Most observers would favor establishing a histologic diagnosis, even with a high pretest probability, and sarcoidosis is a condition in which transbronchial biopsy demonstrative of noncaseating granulomas has high sensitivity. Generally, the combination of this pathology in the proper clinical situation allows the clinician to establish the diagnosis. Approximately three quarters of patients with sarcoidosis have skin test anergy, a sometimes useful feature helping to separate this process from similar conditions.

Asbestosis is another common interstitial lung disease. Asbestos also is capable of causing mesotheliomas of pleura and peritoneum and is synergistic with cigarette smoke in inducing bronchogenic neoplasm. Patients who have exposure to asbestos include shipyard and construction workers and those who have worked extensively with brake linings. Inadvertent exposure still may occur in the remodeling of buildings where asbestos had been used during construction. The chest radiograph in asbestosis shows prominent bibasilar nodular streaking. Typically, associated pleural disease is present, including calcification of the diaphragmatic pleura and irregular thickening of the pleura elsewhere in the lung. Asbestosis also may be associated with a benign exudative pleural effusion, with or without interstitial lung disease. In general, the diagnosis of asbestosis may be made by the clinical history in concert with the chest film, although the occasional patient may require histologic confirmation; asbestos fibers may be identified readily in histologic specimens, but this requires electron microscopic analysis.

Hypersensitivity pneumonitis is perhaps an unfortunate term, but this condition is one in which immunologic attack on inhaled particles occurs in the interstitium of the lung. The inhaled antigens in hypersensitivity pneumonitis are invariably organic, being derived from nonpathogenic microorganisms or plant or animal proteins. The list of such antigens is now a long one, although the prototype disease of this category is *farmer's lung*, in which the microorganisms in damp hay are inhaled and produce immunologic pulmonary injury. Clinically, the dyspnea in hypersensitivity pneumonitis is typically episodic, occurring shortly after exposure. In some cases, however, inhalation and symptoms may not be related temporally. In these cases, it may be difficult to appreciate the relationship between the exposure and the illness, and thus a higher index of suspicion is required on the part of the physician. Hypersensitivity pneumonitis is thus an example of the importance of a detailed occupational history in all patients presenting with interstitial abnormality by chest radiograph. Histopathologically, one observes prominent lymphocytic infiltration in the interstitium as well as occasional poorly formed granulomas, which thus may be distinguished from those seen in sarcoidosis. This correlates with the belief that the pathogenesis of this condition is related to a cell-mediated immune response to the antigen. Although it might be anticipated that corticosteroids would be of some value in this condition, the most obvious therapeutic intervention is the alteration or discontinuation of the patients' exposure to the responsible antigen.

Interstitial lung disease induced by radiation is seen in up to 10 per cent of patients who receive therapeutic radiation for lymphomas and carcinomas involving thoracic structures. Symptoms may begin as early as 1 month after the completion of treatment, in which case symptoms are more acute, although the indolent onset of dyspnea may reflect a more fibrotic process and may not present until a year after the radiation. In the early phase, patients may be febrile in addition to experiencing pulmonary symptoms. Radiation pneumonitis characteristically is not confined to an anatomic segment of lung but rather involves the part that receives the radiation. Perhaps the biggest dilemma facing the clinician in this situation is whether the pulmonary infiltrate is due to radiation, to concomitantly administered chemotherapy, to recurrence of the tumor itself, or to superimposed infection. Steroids may be effective for early occurring disease but are less valuable if fibrosis is present.

Although there are many identifiable causative agents of interstitial lung diseases, and many other diseases with which interstitial lung disease is associated, the majority of interstitial lung disease cases encountered by the clinician are of unknown cause and generally are termed *idiopathic pulmonary fibrosis*. The diagnosis of this process is one of exclusion. Patients who present with idiopathic pulmonary fibrosis are usually in the fifth to seventh decades of life, with an equal incidence in both sexes. In addition to the symptoms of dyspnea and cough, the occasional patient will have fever and arthralgias; on exam, clubbing of the fingers may be present in addition to basilar crackles. It is believed by many that idiopathic pulmonary fibrosis is a process that undergoes an evolution from desquamative interstitial pneumonitis, in which inflammatory cells in the interstitium and the alveolar spaces are observed, to a picture of usual interstitial pneumonitis, in which the most notable pathologic abnormality is fibrosis. Other investigators believe these are two separate processes. In any event, theories advanced to account for either possibility invariably conclude that some unknown antigen initiates the disease, and that antigen–antibody complexes are important in its pathogenesis. This view also would hold that these complexes stimulate the activation of macrophages, which in turn release chemotactic factors for neutrophils and perhaps other mediators of inflammation. Although neutrophils are not prominent histopathologically, they are more numerous on bronchoalveolar lavage than in other forms of interstitial lung disease. Many patients with idiopathic pulmonary fibrosis have nonspecifically positive studies for antinuclear antibodies and rheumatoid factors. These test abnormalities occur in the absence of other more specific clinical evidence for autoimmune diseases; at the same time, several primary immunologic diseases may in fact be associated with interstitial pulmonary disease. A biopsy of the lung in idiopathic pulmonary fibrosis will show several of the nonspecific findings that have been referred to. Such a study is more important for excluding other etiologies. If granulomas are present, idiopathic pulmonary fibrosis is excluded. The prognosis for this problem is better for patients whose initial biopsy specimens reveal more active inflammation than fibrosis, and many clinicians believe that this group responds more favorably to treatment with immunosuppressive agents, particularly corticosteroids.

Treatment

The treatment of interstitial lung diseases, then, depends entirely on the cause. In those instances in which a specific infectious cause can be demonstrated, the outlook is excellent. Similarly, in those cases in which an inhalant or drug is responsible, therapy consists of withdrawing the offending agent. In the majority of cases, however, the clinician is left without an identifiable etiology and must decide whether to institute steroids empirically or to proceed to lung biopsy first. Because response to this type of treatment is inconsistent, and in view of the long-term toxicity of steroids, empiric treatment is unwise for most patients. Similarly, there is little correlation between the radiographic appearance and the histologic presence or absence of fibrosis. For all these reasons, there are few instances in which histologic confirmation is not obtained. Occasionally, very rapid progressive interstitial pulmonary fibrosis, or other immunologically mediated lung disease, may progress rapidly enough to render the patient a poor candidate for either open lung biopsy or bronchoscopy. In these few patients, a course of steroids may be attempted, but it is often necessary to treat simultaneously for infectious diseases. Otherwise, the treatment is entirely supportive, with supplemental oxygen of value in patients who are symptomatic at rest or whose ambient Po_2 concentrations are consistently less than 55 mm Hg.

PNEUMOTHORAX

In ambulatory practice, pneumothorax is seen most often as a spontaneous and idiopathic event.

Occasionally, patients with emphysema will develop pneumothorax, often associated with acute bronchitis. Deceleration injuries, thought to be minor at the time of their occurrence, may be followed shortly by dyspnea and/or chest pain and a pneumothorax subsequently is recognized on a chest film, even in the absence of rib fractures.

Patients with expanding pneumothoraces, or those with limited respiratory reserve, may require immediate tube thoracostomy. In contrast, there are instances when a pneumothorax may be managed expectantly. Individuals who have excellent respiratory reserve and are minimally symptomatic and generally responsible may be observed by frequent radiographs until it is quite clear that the pneumothorax is stable. Depending on its size, a pneumothorax may resolve over days to weeks.

For cases of spontaneous pneumothorax in which tube thoracostomy is not indicated immediately, a series of radiographic studies, following hours on the initial one, would seem prudent to ensure the stability of the pneumothorax before discharging the patient for expectant management. Occasionally, one may wish to attempt aspirating free air from within the pleural space using a small-bore catheter and syringe with stopcock. When successful, this technique is less painful and costly than tube thoracostomy and hospitalization. Whether one elects catheter aspiration or expectant management will depend entirely on the degree to which the patient is symptomatic and can gain immediate care should the need occur.

An increasingly common cause of pneumothorax is *P. carinii* pneumonia associated with AIDs. Particularly in patients who have received inhaled pentamidine for prophylaxis against this infection, small upper lobe bullae or cysts develop, and pneumothorax develops when one ruptures. In the occasional patient with severe infection treated with mechanical ventilation, positive pressure increases this risk. Pneumothorax associated with *Pneumocystis* infection is particularly difficult to treat, in part because of the often poor nutritional status of the patient and difficulty in healing the tear in the cyst. This has led to the use of the Heimlich valve, which can be placed for chronic pneumothorax. This results in loss of negative interpleural pressure, but effectively acts as a check valve to prevent the development of tension. It may be used for long-term treatment of pneumothorax and results in considerably reduced hospital stays.

For relatively small pneumothoraces, the availability of small-bore thoracostomy tubes with attached Heimlich valves may allow ambulatory management. For patients with recurrent episodes of pneumothorax, the current availability of thoracoscopy allows direct visualization and stapling of blebs usually located on the anterior surface of the upper lobe. Heretofore, definitive treatment for recurrent pneumothorax usually required a formal thoracotomy.

SOLITARY PULMONARY NODULE

A commonly encountered problem in primary care practice is the asymptomatic pulmonary nodule. The clinician typically encounters this problem on a chest radiograph obtained as a matter of routine or for some other indication, such as a pre-employment examination. The approach to the asymptomatic pulmonary coin lesion is aimed at stratifying the risk of cancer and removing the lesion in those patients in whom carcinoma cannot be excluded safely by clinical evaluation.

Factors favoring malignancy in an asymptomatic person include age over 35, absence of calcification, size greater than 4 cm, history of smoking, and chest film showing recent growth. Such lesions are likely benign if they have shown no growth in the previous 2 years, if the lesion has sharp margins, if it occurs in a young patient, and if it has a high density on CT scan. Solid calcification and stability in size over 5 years indicate near-certain benignity.

Other factors important in stratifying risk include residence of the patient, because some areas of the country are endemic for histoplasmosis and coccidioidomycosis; this is particularly helpful in the young patient who is not a smoker. Other aspects of the history, physical examination, or skin tests are seldom valuable. In young men, particular attention should be paid to examination of the testicles because of the implications for treatment in the presence of a gonadal tumor. Coexistence of rheumatoid arthritis is important, especially in the presence of peripheral rheumatoid nodules, because they may also occur within the lung parenchyma.

Diagnostic investigation of the solitary pulmonary nodule need not be extensive. Unless the history and physical examination, and inexpensive tests such as blood count, urinalysis, and basic study of serum chemistries, are abnormal, the coin lesion is very unlikely to represent metastasis from an extrapulmonary primary tumor. For this reason, extensive imaging studies of the gastrointestinal or genitourinary systems rarely are indicated.

Probably the most important, and most commonly overlooked, aspect of the investigation of the asymptomatic pulmonary nodule is a vigorous attempt to recover previous chest radiographs. Often the entire question can be rendered moot by finding the presence of a similar abnormality on studies performed years earlier.

If chest CT does not exclude a benign disorder, then transthoracic needle aspiration may preclude the need for thoracotomy and achieve a diagnosis in 80 per cent or more of cases. This is particularly true of the nodule that is greater than 2 cm in diameter. If the needle aspiration is nondiagnostic, thoracotomy still may be necessary. Bronchoscopy may be helpful for lesions closer to the hilus, the yield being greater for nodules 3 cm or larger in size. Should the nodule be small and within 1 to 2 cm of the plural surface, thorascopic excisional biopsy should be considered as a possible alternative to transthoracic needle biopsy or thoracotomy in occasional high-risk patients.

Occasionally, observation of a solitary nodule may be indicated. Factors that influence this approach include the patient's age and overall condition, associated illnesses, and surgical risk. Current recommendations regarding radiographic surveillance are a chest radiograph every 3 months for 1 year followed by repeat films every 6 months during the second year. Growth of the nodule during this interval ordinarily would indicate a need for biopsy.

LUNG CANCER

Carcinoma of the lung remains the leading cause of death from malignancy in the United States in both sexes. Approximately 150,000 new cases are diagnosed yearly, of which about two thirds are in men. The incidence in both sexes has been rising dramatically, more so than in any other malignant neoplasm. Despite advances in diagnostic technology and in therapy for many diseases, there had been little change in the outlook for patients with lung cancer, 90 per cent of whom will die of their disease. Thus, this constitutes a major health risk, especially in light of the fact that as many as 80 or 90 per cent of these tumors can be prevented.

Causes for bronchogenic carcinoma are several, with cigarette smoking topping the list; nine cases in ten are linked directly to their use. Other exposures producing malignant deterioration of bronchial epithelium include asbestos, radiation (uranium), and chemicals such as nickel and chromic acid. Furthermore, the occasional tumor arises in an area of the lung scarred from previous injury. As regards the association with smoking, the risk relates to total exposure as measured by the number of years a person has smoked, the total number of cigarettes smoked, the age at initiation of the habit, whether or not the person inhales, and the concentration of carcinogen in the smoke. After discontinuation, the risk decreases slowly and, after 10 to 15 years, reaches the level observed in individuals who have never smoked. The role of passive smoking is controversial. Although passive smoke may contain even higher levels of carcinogen, there has not been a consistent positive association between passive smoking and new cases of lung cancer, although many epidemiologists believe it exists. Special mention of the risk of asbestos is merited. Those nonsmokers exposed to it have a severalfold increase in the incidence of bronchogenic carcinoma, which rises to nearly 100

times control in individuals exposed to the substance who also smoke.

There are four commonly encountered histologic types of carcinoma of the lung: adenocarcinoma, squamous cell carcinoma, large-cell carcinoma, and small-cell carcinoma. Adenocarcinoma and squamous cell each represent approximately one third of the total, with small-cell accounting for another one fifth or so. The remainder are large-cell, with an additional 1 per cent (approximately) caused by other types, such as bronchoalveolar carcinoma. Oncologists prefer to evaluate therapeutic options and prognosis based on a staging system, described later, for all cancers save small-cell. This system utilizes size of primary tumor, regional nodal involvement, and presence or absence of metastatic disease to stage cancers.

There are a number of clinical manifestations encountered in these patients. Tumors arising within the lung parenchyma produce symptoms through involvement of a bronchus, distant metastasis, or extension into mediastinal or chest wall structures. Less than 10 per cent of patients are totally asymptomatic at the time of diagnosis; in these, a chest radiograph has been obtained for other purposes and the abnormality is an incidental finding. A subset of this group includes patients with asymptomatic coin lesions (see Solitary Pulmonary Nodule). Common symptoms caused by the primary tumor include a persistent cough, with or without hemoptysis. Many patients have dull and poorly characterized chest pain. Nonspecific complaints include weight loss, fatigue, and malaise. The occasional patient will come to attention because of the symptoms of pneumonia caused by the tumor obstruction of a bronchus. If the primary tumor is located in the apex of the lung, symptoms caused by invasion of the brachial plexus, such as pain in the arm, may be reported. Centrally located primaries also can compress the great veins, resulting in superior vena cava syndrome. In both the syndrome and apical tumors, relatively small, and thus potentially treatable, lesions may be responsible for prominent symptoms.

In fewer patients, medical attention is sought because of symptoms produced by metastasis. Many lung cancers spread to the central nervous system, and a seizure or stroke may be the first sign of this problem; similarly, bone pain or abdominal discomfort caused by hepatomegaly may bring the patient to a physician. Other manifestations caused by intrathoracic invasiveness of the tumor include hoarseness, caused by compromise of the left recurrent laryngeal nerve, and facial or conjunctival suffusion on the basis of superior vena cava syndrome. Less commonly, a paraneoplastic syndrome is the presenting problem; the polyuria and constipation of hypercalcemia or the abnormal mental status or seizure caused by the hyponatremia of the syndrome of inappropriate antidiuretic hormone are examples.

Diagnosis

The physical examination may be entirely within normal limits in patients with lung cancer, but most have one or another abnormality helpful in diagnosis. There may be temporal wasting resulting from weight loss, and evidence for COPD, with hyperexpanded lung fields and reduced breath sounds. Rales in the chest are almost never heard in patients with obstructed bronchi; their presence favors an infectious cause of a pulmonary process. Helpful when present are localized wheezes on auscultation and/or evidence for atelectasis or pleural effusion (reduced breath sounds, diminished percussion note). Finger clubbing is a common skeletal sign of bronchogenic carcinoma; interestingly, this seldom is observed in small-cell cancer and tends to be confined to the other three histologic types. Physical examination also may reveal neck vein distention, conjunctival suffusion, and prominent chest wall venous collaterals indicative of superior vena cava compromises; or Horner's syndrome may be associated with apical tumor. Finally, there may be evidence on exam of metastasis in the form of focal neurologic signs, bony tenderness, or hepatomegaly.

The study leading to the diagnosis of lung cancer is in nearly all instances the plain chest radiograph. Although it has had some advocates in the past, routine chest radiographs, even in patients at higher risk (e.g., cigarette smoker over the age of 40), do not result in a survival advantage related to early diagnosis. An asymptomatic patient with a small peripheral nodule that turns out to be malignant is in a better prognostic group, but the incidence of this type of presentation is not sufficiently great to justify the chest radiograph as a screening procedure. The radiographic changes of primary lung cancer are diverse. A hilar prominence or mass is characteristic of squamous cell and small-cell carcinoma; a peripheral nodule is more likely to be adenocarcinoma. Any cell type may result in atelectasis of a lobe by occlusion of the bronchus; cavitation is observed most often in squamous cells. Large-cell carcinoma often begins as a peripheral nodule but grows rapidly and is often a large mass by the time of presentation; like small-cell carcinoma, it spreads early to hilar and mediastinal lymph nodes. Any of the cell types may compromise a bronchus sufficiently to result in pneumonia, which may obscure the primary lesion. A large pleural effusion may be the only visible abnormality on plain chest film in patients presenting with lung cancer. Blood studies are performed frequently in these patients, but few are genuinely helpful. Many patients have a mild anemia, and some have pseudonormal abnormalities resulting from pre-existing erythrocytosis from chronic hypoxia associated with COPD. Occasionally, the first clue to a lung primary may be the hyponatremia or hypercalcemia caused by ectopic hormone production by the tumor.

Histologic Diagnosis

Once lung cancer is suspected, the histologic diagnosis may be made in a number of ways. The least invasive test available is expectorated sputum cytology. Maximum yield is reached by obtaining three first-morning specimens. Although this should be an ideal study to perform on an outpatient, most institutions report a higher yield from inpatients. This is likely due to more prompt processing of specimens once obtained. Sputum cytology has an excellent yield in proximal tumors but is rarely if ever positive in peripheral coin lesions. Like the routine chest radiograph, obtaining random sputum cytologies in an asymptomatic patient at high risk confers no survival advantage from early diagnosis. In theory, because small-cell carcinoma of the lung is almost invariably metastatic by the time of diagnosis, a positive expectorated sputum cytology for this cell type could save more invasive diagnostic procedures, such as bronchoscopy, for such patients. In practice, however, most patients with an unexplained pulmonary process in which lung carcinoma is in the differential diagnosis will undergo bronchoscopy. Thus, in practice, the role of sputum cytology is chiefly in stable, ambulatory patients.

Definitive histologic diagnosis is frequently made by the bronchoscopic approach. Squamous cell carcinoma often may be visualized in this fashion as an exophytic mass, and brush biopsy for cytologic study is obtained directly. In small-cell carcinoma, subepithelial invasion is common and the bronchus may appear to be compressed extrinsically. For more peripheral lesions, a fine-needle aspiration of the lung may be performed, which in experienced hands has a high yield. The complications of bronchoscopy are few, the main one being bleeding from a tumor or postprocedural bronchospasm; needle aspirations, however, frequently result in pneumothorax. Furthermore, with fine-needle aspiration, a negative result does not in all cases assure the clinician that the lesion is benign and, thus, may not ultimately change the clinical approach. In patients who are not surgical candidates, a diagnosis obtained in this way may guide subsequent nonsurgical therapies; likewise, the occasional patient who is resistant to undergoing surgery may find histologic proof of malignancy persuasive.

Staging and Localizing Metastases

Once a histologic diagnosis is secure, the tumor is staged to guide therapy and assess prognosis. Because of the aforementioned propensity of small-cell carcinoma to be metastatic at the time of diagnosis, a staging system is most pertinent for non–small-cell tumors. In widespread usage is the TNM method, in which the primary neoplasm (T), nodal involvement (N), and metastasis (M) are assessed separately, with resultant grouping into three stages. In general, the TNM system reflects increasingly more extensive disease as the number rises. For instance, T1 disease is a tumor of less than 3 cm in size, surrounded by lung or pleura, with no evidence of invasion proximal to a lobar bronchus; N1 disease defines ipsilateral hilar nodal involvement. Depending on the outcome of these assessments, the patient is typed in stages I through IV, in which I indicates local, operable disease and IV distant metastasis and thus inoperable disease, with II and III intermediate groups in which therapy is more unsettled.

The principal areas of concern in this staging process, for the most part, are intrathoracic structures in the hilum and mediastinum. Thoracic CT scans now are obtained nearly invariably, even if the plain chest film does not indicate hilar or mediastinal involvement. CT scan with contrast allows distinction of tumor masses and involved lymph nodes from vasculature and gives the clinician more information on which to base decisions concerning further invasive procedures. When hilar or mediastinal nodes are abnormal but still of the size at which infectious or inflammatory etiologies could be present (1.5 cm or less), mediatinoscopy or limited surgical exploration through a small parasternal incision may be performed. Occasionally, this may be scheduled as a preliminary to more definitive surgery, and, if the results indicate operability, an immediate thoracotomy may be performed, with the intent of curative resection.

Obviously, the presence of any distant metastases in non–small-cell, or any small-cell, lung cancer renders the patient inoperable. As a result, many patients are subjected to extensive diagnostic investigations of distant sites searching for a metastasis. The most common sites for metastasis of lung cancer are brain and bone. For obscure reasons, up to 30 per cent of all lung cancers also metastasize to the adrenal glands. There is no general agreement about the applicability of diagnostic studies in these patients. In general, any test, such as a CT scan of the brain, is more apt to be positive if symptoms or signs suggest a focal lesion to begin with. Similarly, a bone scan is more likely to show involvement if the patient has symptoms referable to the skeleton. Thus, many clinicians would obtain a brain CT scan, bone scan, or abdominal CT scan only if symptoms, signs, or initial blood studies indicate a higher likelihood of metastasis; others believe these studies should be performed on all patients, because of the occasional asymptomatic individual with subsequently proven metastasis. The disadvantage of imaging studies in patients with lower pretest probabilities of metastasis is that the incidence of a false-positive test increases. For example, CT scanning of the normal population demonstrates adrenal abnormalities in approximately 5 per cent; this is particularly troublesome in that the adrenals are (in most centers) now routinely visualized as part of the thoracic CT scan performed in nearly all patients with lung cancer. Thus, the issue of assessment for distant metastasis is not settled, but suffice to say that it is of crucial importance to establish its presence in the staging process, in view of the considerable effect it has on subsequent management.

With respect to small-cell carcinoma, the TNM staging does not correlate as well with prognosis. Most observers prefer to view small-cell carcinoma, once diagnosed, in one of two ways: clinically limited disease, in which there is no gross tumor in the contralateral lung or in distant sites, or extensive disease, when there is considerable tumor obvious even on the initial chest radiograph or in which distant metastasis is clinically obvious.

In sum, the diagnostic assessment of carcinoma of the lung is of considerable importance in planning therapy. In certain clinical situations, the assessment may consist simply of history and physical examination, chest film, and positive expectorated sputum cytologies; in others, more extensive and invasive diagnostic studies are indicated.

Differential Diagnosis

The differential diagnosis of lung cancer includes several considerations. Most important to exclude are infectious processes mimicking a tumor. Cavitary lung abscess or tuberculosis may look quite similar to bronchogenic carcinoma; it should be noted that in the *edentulous* person, bacterial lung abscess is a rare event, and a cavity almost always indicates tumor. Pulmonary embolism sometimes may resemble lung cancer, especially when chest pain and hemoptysis are prominent. The occasional patient with autoimmune diseases, such as rheumatoid arthritis with pleural effusion, may be thought to have a bronchogenic neoplasm. In patients with trauma, a bloody pleural effusion may resemble one that is malignant. Perhaps of most concern is the assumption that any persistent cough reflects either a smoker's cough or bronchitis, delaying the proper assessment for a potential malignancy. Other conditions similar to primary bronchogenic carcinoma include other tumors metastatic to lung or lymphoma originating in the hilar or mediastinal nodes; in these patients, diagnostic assessment and treatment are altered considerably. Sarcoidosis, particularly when hilar adenopathy is prominent, also may be confused with malignancy. Any pulmonary process in smoking patients over 40 years of age always should be regarded as potentially reflecting lung cancer.

Treatment

The ideal treatment of bronchogenic carcinoma is surgical, and although only a small percentage of patients are cured of this disease, the appreciable majority of those that are owe this cure to surgical resection of the tumor. Given the patient population at risk, many patients with lung cancer have coincident coronary artery disease and obstructive lung disease; in addition, some are quite elderly.

Thus, it can be argued reasonably that an assessment of suitability for operative approach should precede any extensive diagnostic and staging work-up. In patients with COPD, a FEV_1 of 2 liters or more indicates that a pneumonectomy would be tolerated; if this figure is less than 1 liter, surgical treatment is relatively contraindicated. In those patients whose FEV_1 is between 1 and 2 liters, a ventilation–perfusion scan may be helpful in predicting how much function will remain after resection of a lung. An FEV_1 of 750 mL or more is ordinarily compatible with tolerable function, so that a calculation using the percentage of contribution to the total FEV_1 of the segment in question may be made and subtracted from the overall FEV_1 to determine acceptability. This method of estimating postoperative pulmonary status is more reliable for pneumonectomy than for resection of smaller amounts of lung. Some clinicians merely prefer to walk with patients up two or more flights of stairs and observe whether or not the individual is still able to carry on a normal conversation; if so, these clinicians believe that the risk for pneumonectomy is acceptable. In addition to limited pulmonary reserve, patients with obstructive lung disease are more likely to experience postoperative complications, such as infection, atelectasis, or bronchopleural fistula, further compounding the difficulty of making this decision. As concerns the coexistence of coronary artery disease, although this increases the risk for surgery and for additional postoperative complications, it does not pose an absolute contraindication to operation.

The surgical outcome in non–small-cell cancer, not surprisingly, is closely related to the TNM stage, and thus to the extent of disease. In addition to the contraindications noted previously, a malignant pleural effusion, primary tumor within 2 cm of the hilum, or tumor directly invading the chest wall, diaphragm, mediastinum, or pericardium constitutes a contraindication to surgery. Exceptions to this rule are peripheral tumors involving the chest wall without pleural effusion and those that arise in the apex. Controversy remains about the surgical management of cases with ipsilateral mediastinal node positivity, in whom many clinicians favor surgical removal of the primary, with mediastinal lymph node dissection, followed by postoperative radiotherapy. Others consider these patients to be inoperable. For patients with stages I and II disease, who undergo thoracotomy and in whom no additional positive lymph nodes are found, the 5-year survival is between 40 and 80 per cent. In the occasional stage III patient who is offered operative therapy, this figure slips to 20 to 40 per cent.

The nonoperative treatment of patients with non–small-cell cancer is disappointing. A number of regimens of combination chemotherapy have been tried, although benefits have been modest. Radiotherapy is applied more often in a palliative fashion and may be effective in selected patients in whom hemoptysis or bronchial obstruction poses clinical difficulties. Similarly, it may provide temporary remission in patients with superior vena cava syndrome, and it is the modality of choice for epidural metastases with threatened compromise of spinal cord function. Radiation also is used as an initial therapy in cancer rising in the superior sulcus, which is followed by surgical removal; despite the local invasivity, the prognosis with this treatment is quite good.

The management of small-cell cancer differs appreciably from the above, with the exception of the radiation therapy applied to symptomatic bony, nervous system, or mediastinal lesions. In small-cell carcinoma, systemic combination chemotherapy is the principal treatment. With modern regimens, many including drugs such as cisplatin and doxorubicin, 15 to 20 per cent of patients who have disease clinically localized to one hemithorax will enjoy a survival in excess of 2 years. A higher percentage than this obtains symptomatic relief, because of the relative sensitivity of this tumor; however, recurrence tends to be the rule. The role of radiation therapy in patients with clinically localized disease is under active investigation. Empiric radiation therapy of the brain reduces the incidence of clinically evident cerebral metastasis in patients who have obtained remission of disease elsewhere through chemotherapy. Very occasionally, subsequent surgical removal of a primary tumor is carried out if a mass has shrunk appreciably, but has not entirely disappeared, by chemotherapy. Similarly, in the very unusual patient with small-cell cancer presenting as an asymptomatic coin lesion, primary surgical resection may be attempted. Those patients with small-cell carcinoma who have extensive disease at the time of presentation have a very bleak outlook. Here, nearly all treatment is palliative, and less than 5 per cent survive for more than 2 years.

In sum, carcinoma of the lung remains a daunting clinical problem. Its natural history and prognosis are quite dependent on cell type, but the overall survival still is in the range of 10 to 15 per cent for 5 years. Patients with squamous cell carcinoma do well if hilar nodes are histologically negative; many dying of the disease do so with tumors still confined to the chest, where they tend to be locally invasive. Individuals with small-cell carcinoma, although having a poor overall prognosis because of the propensity for the disease to metastasize widely early in the course, may do well if they are free of disease 2 years after the institution of therapies; in them, treatment is, with few exceptions, nonsurgical. Adenocarcinoma of the lung remains unpredictable; although numerous surgical cures have been reported, absence of disease in the lymph nodes is not as good a predictor of subsequent recurrence elsewhere in the body as it is in squamous cell carcinoma. Large-cell carcinoma also is a rapid-growing neoplasm, and although surgical therapy remains the treatment of first choice, the outcome is seldom a good one.

SUGGESTED READINGS

Radiology

Oboler SY, LaForce FM: The periodic physical examination in asymptomatic adults. Ann Intern Med 110:214, 1989.

Owens MW, Kinasewitz GT, Lambert RS, et al: Influence of spirometry and chest radiograph on the management of pulmonary outpatients. Arch Intern Med 147:1966, 1987.

Spillane RM, Shepard JO, Deluca SA: High Resolution CT of the lungs. Am Fam Physician 48:493, 1993.

Persistent Cough

Pratter MR, Bartter T, Akers S, DuBois J: An algorithmic approach to chronic cough. Ann Intern Med 119:977, 1993.

Pleural Effusion

Feinsilver SH, Barrows AA, Buaman SS: Fiberoptic bronchoscopy and pleural effusion of unknown origin. Chest 90:516, 1986.

Himelman RB, Callen PW: The prognostic value of loculations in parapneumonic pleural effusions. Chest 90:852, 1986.

Irani R, Underwood RD, Johnson EH: Malignant pleural effusion: Clinical pathophysiologic study. Arch Intern Med 147:1133, 1987.

Leslie WK, Kinasewitz GT: Clinical characteristics of the patient with nonspecific pleuritis. Chest 94:603, 1988.

Light RW, Girard WM, Jenkinson SG: Parapneumonic effusions. Am J Med 69:507, 1980.

Prakash UBS, Reiman HM: Comparison of needle biopsy with cytologic analysis for the evaluation of pleural effusion: Analysis of 414 cases. Mayo Clin Proc 60:158, 1985.

Sahn S: Management of complicated paraneumonic effusions. Am Rev Respir Dis 148:813, 1993.

Sherman S, Ravikrishnan KP, Patel AS: Optimum anesthesia with intrapleural lidocaine during chemical pleurodesis with tetracycline. Chest 93:153, 1988.

Sieskin A, Hirasuna J: Evaluation of pleural effusion. Med Rounds 1:54, 1988.

Varkey B, Rose HD, Kutty CP: Empyema thoracis during a ten-year period. Arch Intern Med 141:1771, 1981.

Pulmonary Embolism

Clagett GP, Anderson FA Jr, Levine MN, et al: Prevention of venous thromboembolism. Chest 102(suppl 4):391, 1992.

Hyers TM, Hull RD, Weg JG: Antithrombotic therapy for venous thromboembolic disease. Chest 102(suppl 4):408, 1992.

Triplett DA: Low-molecular-weight heparins: Is smaller better? Arch Intern Med 153:1525, 1993.

Pneumonia

American Thoracic Society: Guidelines for the initial management of adults with community-acquired pneumonia: Diagnosis, assessment of severity, and initial antimicrobial therapy. Am Rev Respir Dis 148:1418, 1993.

Farr BM, Sloman AJ, Fisch MJ: Predicting death in patients hospitalized for community-acquired pneumonia. Ann Intern Med 115:428, 1991.

Gardner P, Schaffner W: Immunization of adults. N Engl J Med 328:1252, 1993.

Grossman LK, Caplan SE: Clinical, laboratory and radiological information in the diagnosis of pneumonia in children. Ann Emerg Med 17:43, 1988.

Mansel JU, Rosenow EC, Smith TF, Martin JW: *Mycoplasma pneumoniae* pneumonia. Chest 95:639, 1989.

Ostergaard L, Anderson PL: Etiology of community-acquired pneumonia. Chest 104:1400, 1993.

Tuberculosis

Iseman MD: Treatment of multi-drug-resistant tuberculosis. N Engl J Med 329:784, 1993.

Prichard JG: Pulmonary tuberculosis. Med Rounds 1:107, 1988.

Stead WW, To T, Harrison RW, Abraham JH: Benefit-risk considerations in preventive treatment for tuberculosis in elderly persons. Ann Intern Med 107:843, 1987.

Chronic Disorders of the Airways

Burrows B, Martinez FD, Halonen M, et al: Association of asthma with serum IgE levels and skin-test reactivity to allergens. N Engl J Med 324:271, 1989.

Ferguson GT, Cherniack RM: Management of chronic obstructive pulmonary disease. Am Rev Respir Dis 146:1067, 1992.

International Consensus Report on Diagnosis and Management of Asthma (Publication no. NIH 92-3091). Bethesda, MD, U.S. Department of Health and Human Services, 1992.

Li JTC, Reed CE: Proper use of aerosol corticosteroids to control asthma. Mayo Clin Proc 64:205, 1989.

McFadden ER, Gilbert IA: Asthma. N Engl J Med 327:1928, 1992.

Petty TL: Home oxygen therapy. Mayo Clin Proc 62:841, 1987.

Rodnick JE, Gude JK: The use of antibiotics in acute bronchitis and acute exacerbations of chronic bronchitis. West J Med 149:347, 1988.

Bronchiectasis

Barker, AF, Bardana EJ: Bronchiectasis: Update of an orphan disease. Am Rev Respir Dis 137:969, 1988.

Cystic Fibrosis

Stern RC: The primary care physician and the patient with cystic fibrosis. J Pediatr 114:31, 1989.

Interstitial Lung Disease

DePaso WJ, Winterbauer RH: Interstitial lung disease. DM 37:61, 1991.

Tierney LM Jr: Idiopathic pulmonary fibrosis. Semin Respir Med 12:229, 1991.

Pneumothorax

Light RW: Management of spontaneous pneumothorax. Am Rev Respir Dis 148:245, 1993.

Solitary Pulmonary Nodule

Midthun DE, Swensen SJ, Jett JR: Approach to the solitary pulmonary nodule. Mayo Clin Proc 68:378, 1993.

Lung Cancer

Jett JR: Current treatment of unresectable lung cancer. Mayo Clin Proc 68:603, 1993.

Patel AM, Dunn WF, Trastek VF: Staging systems of lung cancer. Mayo Clin Proc 68:475, 1993.

Patel AM, Peters SG: Clinical manifestations of lung cancer. Mayo Clin Proc 68:273, 1993.

General Review

Weinberger SE: Recent advances in pulmonary medicine. N Engl J Med 328:1389, 1993a.

Weinberger SE: Recent advances in pulmonary medicine. N Engl J Med 328:1462, 1993b.

CHAPTER 23

OTOLARYNGOLOGY

BYRON J. BAILEY, CHESTER L. STRUNK,
and CHARLES W. SMITH, Jr.

EMERGENCIES

Croup

Croup is a syndrome characterized by inspiratory stridor, most often caused by parainfluenza virus. It is most likely to occur in children under the age of two, in late fall or early winter epidemics (Strome et al., 1985). The trachea is inflamed below the glottis, usually sparing the lungs, the distal bronchi, and the supraglottic regions.

Children with croup usually develop fever, a barking cough, inspiratory stridor, and hoarseness over a 24-hour period. Physical findings include inspiratory (and occasionally expiratory) stridor and tachypnea. The diagnosis is made clinically, but a lateral neck radiograph may help to differentiate croup from supraglottitis or foreign body aspiration. Blood gases always should be obtained if signs of respiratory distress are present.

The most important treatment decision is whether to hospitalize the child. Generally, a child with a respiratory rate under 40 breaths/min can be managed as an outpatient if the parents are reliable and if the child is able to maintain hydration. Relief may be obtained by using a hot shower to generate humidification. A cool-mist ultrasonic humidifier also should be run constantly for several days until symptoms abate.

Patients who are hospitalized should receive intravenous fluid replacement and humidified air. Racemic epinephrine, 0.25 to 0.5 mL mixed with 2 mL normal saline by nebulization, may be repeated every 30 to 60 minutes as needed to relieve respiratory distress. The use of steroids in controversial because the data are conflicting as to their effectiveness. If used, the recommended drug and dosage is dexamethasone, 0.5 to 1 mg/kg intravenously or intramuscularly as a single treatment. If the above treatment fails to result in improvement, intubation or tracheotomy is required.

The decision whether to intubate or perform a tracheotomy is always difficult. Intubation is less invasive but may be complicated by the age of the child and the degree of subglottic edema. Nasotracheal intubation is preferred, with emergency tracheotomy capability immediately available if the attempt is unsuccessful.

Supraglottitis

Supraglottitis (epiglottitis) is an acute infection of the larynx above the vocal cords, usually caused by bacteria. The majority of cases occur in children under the age of 6, and are almost always the result of *Haemophilus influenzae* infections. In adults, however, β-hemolytic streptococcus, *Pneumococcus*, or *Staphylococcus aureus* also may be be causative (Dayal, 1981).

The illness is characterized by the abrupt onset of high fever (>102° F) and a severe, often progressive course. Severe throat pain is present, which makes it difficult for the patient to swallow secretions. Respiratory difficulty is an ominous sign, and may begin to occur a short time after the onset of symptoms. The rapidity of progression of symptoms is dependent on the age of the child and the virulence of the organism involved. The diagnosis should be suspected strongly whenever fever, dysphagia, and respiratory difficulty are seen simultaneously.

On physical examination, the patient appears acutely ill, and may have difficulty swallowing secretions. Nuchal rigidity occasionally may be seen, raising the possibility of meningitis. Tachypnea and use of accessory muscles of respiration may be seen. Severe cases also may be accompanied by cyanosis.

The presumptive diagnosis should be made from the history and general appearance of the patient, and should be confirmed at the time the airway is secured. Once an airway is in place, laryngeal secretions should be obtained for culture. Blood cultures and serologic antigen studies also should be performed.

Because supraglottitis is a life-threatening condition, these patients are admitted to the hospital and usually referred to an otolaryngologist for management. Antibiotics are given to ensure coverage against the relatively common occurrence of ampicillin-resistant *H. influenzae*. Acceptable initial choices include sulbactam-ampicillin (Unasyn), cefuroxime (Zinacef), ceftriaxone (Rocephin), or chloramphenicol. Therapy should be continued for at least 7 days. In addition to antibiotics, humidified air—usually with low-flow oxygen—should be administered. The period of extubation requires an environment that allows very close observation by nursing staff. The prognosis for recovery is excellent. Virtually all deaths occur because of respiratory embarrassment from inadequate airway management.

Peritonsillar Abscess

Abscesses in the peritonsillar space are most commonly a complication of acute tonsillopharyngitis and, thus, are almost always due to infection with group A β-hemolytic streptococci. Symptoms of acute pharyngitis progress to severe unilateral throat pain and difficulty swallowing. Severe pain may limit oral intake and cause drooling from pooled saliva and muffled speech, sometimes referred to as a "hot potato" voice.

Examination usually reveals a patient with fever, mild dehydration, increased oral secretions, and difficulty opening the mouth (trismus). The involved tonsil is swollen and displaced toward the midline and downward. It may be difficult to determine whether swelling is due to an abscess or cellulitis. Palpation of a fluctuant area with a gloved finger is useful to confirm an abscess. Other diagnostic possibilities include infectious mononucleosis, other parapharyngeal space infections, and tonsillar or pharyngeal tumors. Diagnostic tests should include a throat culture or a latex slide test for streptococcus, culture of any aspirated material, a complete blood count, and a Monospot test.

All children should be admitted to the hospital. Adults who have significant dehydration, or who cannot cooperate with outpatient drainage procedures, also must be admitted. Others may be managed as outpatients with either needle aspiration or outpatient incision and drainage. For example, after inducing topical anesthesia with benzocaine or lidocaine, an 18-gauge spinal needle is inserted into the area of fluctuance and the fluid aspirated. The patient then should be placed on oral penicillin, 500 mg four times a day for 10 to 14 days or until the episode resolves. If symptoms recur, the patient should be hospitalized for incision and drainage and treated with intravenous antibiotics. Tonsillectomy is recommended following resolution because of the tendency for recurrence.

Foreign Body Aspiration

Foreign body aspiration is seen most commonly in small children, but may occur at any age. Objects may become lodged in the pharynx, larynx, trachea or bronchi. Symptoms depend on the site of the foreign body. *Pharyngeal* locations primarily produce discomfort, whereas *laryngeal* foreign bodies cause total or near-total occlusion. *Tracheobronchial* occlusions cause coughing and intermittent or constant stridor, wheezing, and/or cyanosis. More distal foreign bodies initially may go unnoticed but subsequently will result in wheezing, respiratory distress, and/or pneumonia.

Physical findings are variable and also depend on location and severity of respiratory obstruction. Any combination of tachypnea, cyanosis, stridor and wheezing may be found. Obstruction of the right mainstem bronchus causes decreased breath sounds and reduced chest expansion. A one-way ball valve effect may occur, resulting in hyperexpansion and hyperresonance to percussion.

The chest radiograph may show signs of local, lobar, or whole-lung atelectasis and, if the object is radiopaque, it also may be seen. If sufficient time has elapsed (usually 24 hours or more), pneumonic infiltrates may be present. Anteroposterior and lateral views of the neck also should be obtained. If the diagnosis is still in doubt, fluoroscopy often allows the site of obstruction to be localized.

Management involves maintenance of the airway and removal of the foreign body. Pharyngeal objects usually can be removed with a mirror and forceps. Laryngoscopy or endoscopy under anesthesia is required for removal at the level of the larynx and beyond. Removal usually is followed by immediate relief of symptoms, unless infection is present.

Head and Neck Trauma and Respiratory Embarrassment

Trauma to the head and neck region may cause respiratory difficulty in a number of ways, including dislodged dentures, aspiration of blood and mucus, tongue trauma, or laceration of the airway. Patients presenting with facial trauma and respiratory distress must be immediately assessed, suctioned, and given an oral or nasopharyngeal airway. If the patient is still in distress, an emergency tracheotomy or cricothyrotomy should be performed. Once the airway is stabilized, attention can be directed to other traumatized areas.

Laryngeal trauma will result in local pain and dysphonia. Laryngoscopy should be performed to confirm the diagnosis and assess the damage. A tracheostomy should be performed if the airway is unstable. *Tracheal trauma* or *separation* may result in similar signs and symptoms, including subcutaneous emphysema. In addition to respiratory endoscopy, the *esophagus* also should be assessed for concomitant injury. A tracheotomy should be placed as far from the injury as possible, and the tracheal separation repaired surgically.

Epistaxis

Epistaxis most commonly originates from the rich capillary network in the anterior septum known as Kiesselbach's plexus. In hypertensive and elderly patients, it may occur posteriorly in areas of the nose that are very difficult to visualize. The most common causes of nosebleed are drying of the nasal mucosa and trauma from picking the nose (Kirchner, 1982).

If manual pressure, applied to the nasal septum with the head upright for 10 full minutes, does not stop the bleeding, careful examination and identification of the point of bleeding is required. Proper equipment and lighting is an absolute must, and should include a *nasal speculum, bayonet forceps,* and *suction capability* (Johnson and Rood, 1981). The physician first must determine whether the bleeding is anterior or posterior. If the bleeding site is not readily apparent, nasal vasoconstriction is accomplished with cotton balls impregnated with 5% cocaine solution or a mixture of 4% lidocaine and 1/100,000 epinephrine. After several minutes, the bleeding should be slowed so that identification of the bleeding point is possible. *Cautery* with 25% trichloroacetic acid or silver nitrate is usually effective in controlling bleeding. Care should be taken to dry the nasal mucosa prior to cauterization. A silver nitrate stick should be applied to the bleeding site for about 20 seconds (Johnson and Rood, 1981). Following cauterization, patients should be advised not to blow the nose, to open the mouth when sneezing, to avoid aspirin, to use a cool-mist humidifier, and to apply antibiotic ointment or Vaseline to the nose several times per day.

If cautery is unsuccessful and the bleeding is anterior, half-inch iodoform gauze should be impregnated with Vaseline or antibiotic ointment and inserted into the nose in layers with bayonet forceps. As much packing as possible without deforming the septum should be used, and should be left in place for 2 to 5 days. Patients who have nasal packing in place generally should be treated with antibiotics because of the high likelihood of sinusitis. Pain medication is often necessary. Patients should be cautioned that nasal obstruction often persists for several days after the packing has been removed. An alternative to the use of gauze packing is the use of an *epistaxis balloon* inserted into the nose and filled with air or saline.

If the bleeding is posterior, packing must be performed differently. A *posterior pack* is fashioned using two or three 4-inch gauze pads with three silk sutures tied around the middle. A soft rubber catheter is introduced into the nose, grasped by a hemostat, and pulled from the nasopharynx through the mouth. Two of the sutures are tied to the end of the catheter, which is then pulled back through the nose, bringing the posterior pack into the nasopharynx. It is usually necessary to guide the pack into the nasopharynx with a finger. The third suture is left trailing from the mouth. A firm anterior pack is then placed, followed by a rolled gauze pad across the nose, secured by the two sutures hanging from the nose, which also secures the posterior pack firmly in place. Epistaxis catheters or Foley catheters also may be used to control bleeding from a posterior site; however, excessive pressure on the nasal ala or columella will cause tissue necrosis.

If bleeding cannot be controlled by any of the above methods, or if it is recurrent, a referral for arterial ligation must be considered.

THE EAR

Otalgia

Otalgia (ear pain, earache) is a symptom and not a diagnosis. Otalgia can be either primary or secondary. Primary otalgia arises from pathologic conditions of the ear itself. Secondary otalgia is from periauricular sites or referred from a distant origin. More than 50 per cent of otalgia originates from a source other than the ear. The intensity of the otalgia is not necessarily proportional in seriousness to the disease causing it; mild otalgia or vague pain may result from laryngeal or esophageal carcinoma, whereas dental caries may cause severe pain.

The cause of pain originating from the external ear and canal will be obvious from inspection in most instances (i.e., a furuncle of the external canal or an otitis externa). Exceptions include an early neoplasm of the external canal or the neuralgia of herpes zoster oticus. Otalgia of middle ear origin should be readily apparent. Tic-like pain may originate from the geniculate complex of the seventh nerve or the tympanic branch of the ninth nerve. The most common periauricular causes of otalgia include parotitis, lymphadenitis, and temporomandibular joint dysfunction. Periauricular lymphadenitis may arise from lesions in the scalp.

Temporomandibular joint dysfunction is a common cause of otalgia and is often a result of faulty dental occlusion or excessive jaw movement (Guralnick et al., 1978; Talaat et al., 1986).

Lesions in the area of the palatine, pharyngeal, and lingual tonsils, as well as adjacent tongue, may cause ear pain via the glossopharyngeal nerve. Squamous cell carcinomas of the base of the tongue may present with referred otalgia and require palpation and biopsy for diagnosis. Laryngeal, hypopharyngeal, esophageal, and lung lesions may cause secondary otalgia from branches of the vagus nerve.

If the cause of otalgia is not readily apparent from a routine otorhinolaryngologic examination, then office laryngoscopy followed by a chest radiograph and barium swallow may be required (Paparella and Shumrick, 1980).

Otorrhea

Drainage from the ear is a common otologic complaint. It is important to document the nature of the otorrhea, as well as related symptoms and events, such as trauma. The most common cause of otorrhea is *cerumen,* which may range from pale yellow to dark brown and from liquid to solid. Profuse bleeding from the ear is rare except in severe trauma or in patients with clotting disorders. Middle ear and mastoid infections, acute perforations, tumors, and external otitis may be associated with mild bleeding. Serous drainage may occur with bleb rupture from bullous myringitis, otitis externa, or external canal dermatitis. Purulent otorrhea indicates infection. The color may range from yellow to green. A malodorous discharge is associated with tissue necrosis and is usually found in infected cholesteatoma. A mucoid discharge without odor is an indication of middle ear mucosal disease and/or eustachian tube dysfunction, often of a temporary nature.

Spontaneous cerebrospinal fluid otorrhea is rare. It may accompany a temporal bone fracture or may be secondary to a tumor or surgery. The fluid is clear and the diagnosis may be confirmed by analysis for sugar, protein, sodium, and cells. Cerebrospinal fluid also will produce a halo sign when a drop is placed on filter paper. The halo sign is a ring of clear fluid surrounding a circle of blood-stained moisture produced by the greater diffusion of spinal fluid than blood.

Otoscopy

The most convenient method to illuminate the external canal and tympanic membrane is the diagnostic otoscope (Fig. 23–1). It includes a halogen light source, an air-sealed head, and rubber tubing for pneumatic otoscopy. An open operating head should be available for removal of cerumen. When performing otoscopy, the physician should remember that the bony canal is very tender when manipulated. Prior to any instrumentation of the ear canal, the patient should be warned to prevent a sudden head movement. Infants should be examined while in the parent's arms. A bottle or pacifier may help to distract the infant. Young children often will respond positively to games such as watching the "Tinkerbell" otoscope light, blowing out the light, and looking for "bunnies in the ears." Every effort should be made to avoid the injected eardrum of a crying child.

To visualize the tympanic membrane, the pinna must be pulled posteriorly and superiorly. The entire annulus should be seen, including the pars flaccida. The largest speculum possible should be used in order to obtain a tight seal for pneumatic otoscopy. A handheld bulb or tubing in the mouth is used for changing pressure in the external canal.

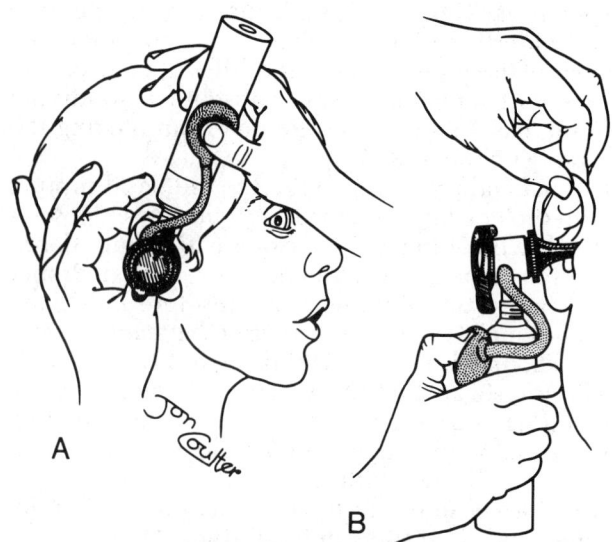

FIGURE 23–1. Methods of positioning otoscope to enhance visualization and to minimize the chance that head movement will result in trauma to the ear canal. Both of the otoscopist's hands can be used (*A*), or, when the child is cooperative, a finger touching the child's cheek is sufficient (*B*). (From Bluestone CD, Klein JO. Methods of examination: clinical examination. *In* Bluestone CD, Stool SE [eds]: Pediatric Otolaryngology. Philadelphia, WB Saunders Company, 1990, p 111, with permission.)

The normal tympanic membrane and middle ear will allow the eardrum to move crisply in both directions. A weak tympanic membrane or one affected by negative middle ear pressure will move out with negative pressure, then passively return without the need of positive pressure. The malleus should be examined for fixation or diminished mobility. With a retracted tympanic membrane, the short process of the malleus is very prominent while the manubrium becomes more horizontal and foreshortened. The tympanic membrane in serous otitis changes from a shiny gray to amber, sometimes with air bubbles. Pus produces a white color to the tympanic membrane and causes it to bulge and lose landmarks. Blood causes the tympanic membrane to appear blue. Dense white plaques represent tympanosclerosis and indicate healed otitis media. In many normal ears, the incus can be seen shining through the posterosuperior quadrant of the drumhead (Strome et al., 1985).

Hearing Evaluation

Office hearing evaluation consists of tuning fork tests and clinical speech testing. *Tuning fork tests* will help detect abnormal hearing, and will differentiate conductive loss from sensorineural loss. These tests provide a gross estimate of hearing but are not as accurate as an audiogram. Tuning fork tests are not usually successful in children less than 4 years of age.

Clinical speech testing may be performed in patients over 5 years of age. The whispered voice test is performed by using bisyllabic words of equal stress, such as *baseball, airplane, cowboy, railroad, eardrum, ice cream,* and *hot dog.* The opposite ear is masked by using a Bárány's box or a partially occluded suction tubing. The hand should be held in such a way as to prevent the patient from lip reading. The results of the test should be expressed as normal hearing or as mild-moderate or severe hearing loss. This type of testing is much more accurate than the use of a watch tick. For children, calibrated noise makers are available that give some frequency information. Again, one must be careful to shield the noisemaker from the visual field of the child to eliminate visual cues.

Another indirect measure of hearing in a young child is an assessment of his or her speech. If by 18 months of age a child has not said at least one word that is intelligible to an outsider, then he or she is at risk for hearing loss. By age 2 years, a child should be able to put two words together and be understood. By age 3 years, the child should be able to put three-word sentences together.

Audiometric Diagnosis

A hearing evaluation should be an extension of a physical examination and can range in complexity from a simple office evaluation to sophisticated audiometry.

Tuning fork tests using a 512-Hz tuning fork always should be performed and can define normal from abnormal hearing, conductive loss versus sensorineural loss, and the frequency range of the loss. These tests provide a gross estimate and are not a substitute for an audiogram.

The *Rinne test* is performed by first placing a tuning fork on the mastoid tip (Fig. 23–2A) and then aligning the prongs next to the meatus and parallel to the ear canal (Fig. 23–2B). The patient is asked which position sounds louder. If the air-conducted sound is louder than the bone-con-

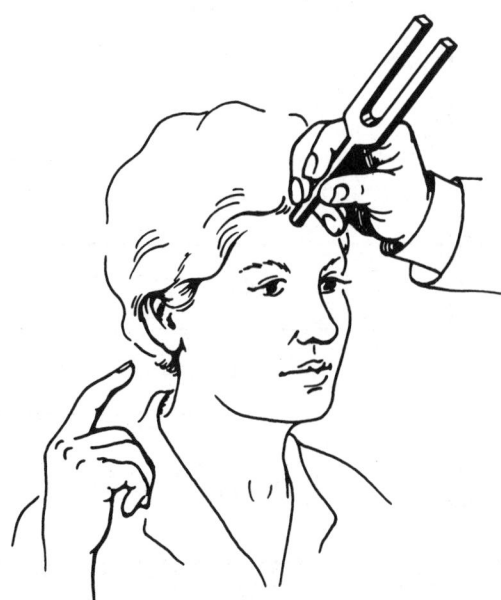

FIGURE 23–3. The Weber test. (From Meyerhoff WL, Roland PS: Physical examination of the ear. *In* Paparella MM, Shumrick DA [eds]: Otolaryngology, Vol. II. Philadelphia, WB Saunders Company, 1991, p 909, with permission.)

ducted sound, then either the hearing is normal or there is a sensorineural loss. If the bone-conducted sound is louder than the air-conducted sound, then there is a conductive loss in that ear.

The *Weber test* (Fig. 23–3) evaluates symmetry of hearing by placing the 512-Hz tuning fork on the forehead or over the central incisors. The patient reports whether the sound is heard loudest in the middle or whether it lateralizes to one ear or the other. If the tone is loudest in the middle, then either the hearing is normal or the hearing loss is symmetrical. Lateralization indicates a conductive hearing loss in that ear or a significant sensorineural loss in the opposite ear.

Basic audiometry involves pure-tone testing and

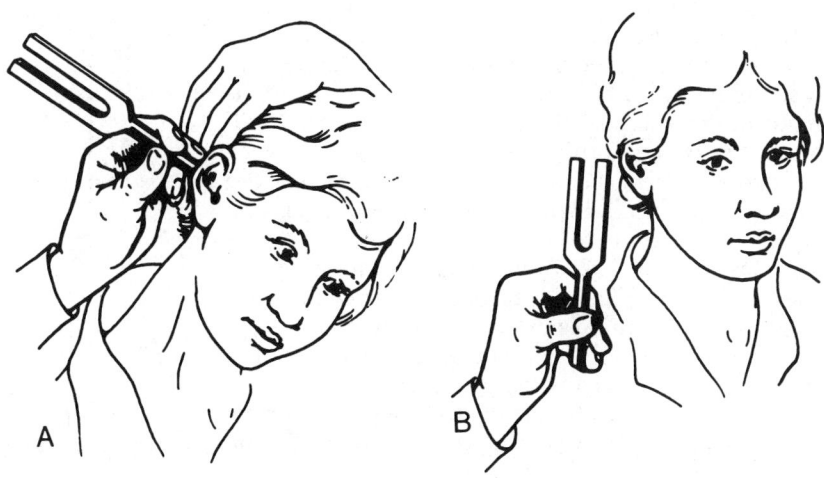

FIGURE 23–2. The Rinne test. (From Meyerhoff WL, Roland PS: Physical examination of the ear. *In* Paparella MM, Shumrick DA [eds]: Otolaryngology, Vol. II. Philadelphia, WB Saunders Company, 1991, p 909, with permission.)

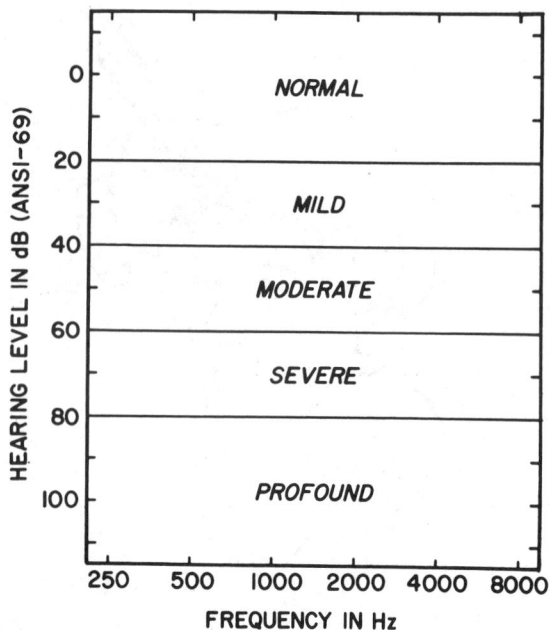

FIGURE 23–4. An audiogram form. The frequency scale ranges from 250 to 8000 Hz. The intensity scale ranges from −10 to 110 dB. The five general categories used to classify a patient's hearing loss according to degree of impairment are illustrated. (From Yellin MW: Hearing measurement in children. *In* Paparella MM, Shumrick DA [eds]: Otolaryngology, Vol. II. Philadelphia, WB Saunders Company, 1991, p 962, with permission.)

speech reception threshold (SRT) testing. In *pure-tone testing*, a single-frequency tone is presented via headphones. The intensity is varied until the tester determines the lowest intensity that is audible. This is repeated in each ear at various frequencies. The test is then repeated using a bone-conduction vibrator placed over the mastoid. Air conduction is equal to bone conduction in sensorineural losses and in normal hearing. In conductive hearing loss, bone-conduction scores are better than air-conduction scores. The results are expressed as decibels of hearing loss, with a range of 0 to 100 dB (Fig. 23–4).

The *SRT* is determined by presenting a list of bisyllabic words at a frequency of 1000 Hz. The intensity of the words is varied until a level is reached at which the patient can repeat half of the test items. The SRT for each ear should approximate the average of the pure tones at 500, 1000, and 2000 Hz (± 5 dB) in each ear.

Speech discrimination tests are used to test the clarity of articulated speech. A list of monosyllabic words are given at 40 dB above the SRT. The results are reported as a percentage of the words on the list that are repeated correctly. Normal discrimination scores are 90 per cent or above.

There are *special audiometric tests* to determine if a hearing loss is caused by a cochlear or retrocochlear lesion (eighth nerve to auditory cortex). Other than auditory brain stem response, tone

decay and reflex decay tests are the most commonly used basic audiometric tests for a retrocochlear lesion.

Impedance Audiometry

There are three important components of impedance audiometry: tympanometry, physical volume test, and acoustic reflex threshold.

Tympanometry is an objective measure of the compliance of the tympanic membrane as a function of mechanically varied air pressures in the external auditory canal. Tympanic membrane mobility reflects pathology of the middle ear space. With eustachian tube obstruction, there is absorption of the static air in the middle ear space by blood vessels. This creates negative air pressure in the middle ear space followed by a transudation of fluid and retraction of the tympanic membrane. This negative middle ear pressure can be identified by tympanometry.

There are five different curves produced by tympanometry (Fig. 23–5). The *type A curve* is found in patients with normal middle ear function. The curve shows normal middle ear pressures at the point of maximal compliance. The *type A_S curve* is found in patients with normal middle ear function. The curve shows normal middle ear pressures at the point of maximal compliance. The *type A_S curve* is characterized by normal middle ear pressure and limited compliance relative to the mobility of the normal tympanic membrane. The "S" denotes stiffness, which is seen in otosclerosis, scarred tympanic membranes, and some cases of tympanosclerosis. The *type A_D curve* shows large

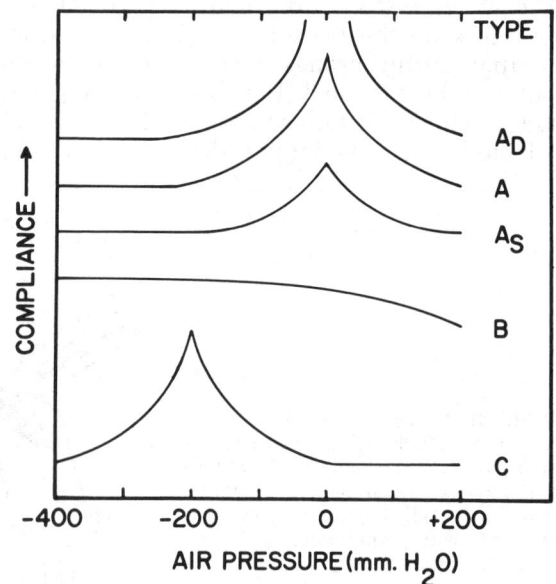

FIGURE 23–5. The three basic tympanometric shapes (see text for description). (From Yellin MW: Hearing measurement in children. *In* Paparella MM, Shumrick DA [eds]: Otolaryngology, Vol. II. Philadelphia, WB Saunders Company, 1991, p 957, with permission.)

changes in compliance with relatively small changes in air pressure. The "D" indicates disarticulation, as seen in discontinuity of the ossicular chain or in large monomeric tympanic membranes.

The *type B curve* demonstrates little or no compliance with changes in air pressure in the middle ear. This type of curve is seen in instances of middle ear fluid, adhesive otitis media, and perforations of the tympanic membrane, or with a patent ventilating tube in the eardrum. Finally, the *type C curve* indicates negative middle ear pressure of -200 mm H_2O. This may or may not indicate the presence of middle ear fluid.

The *physical volume test* will help clarify the etiology responsible for type B tympanograms. A type B tympanogram with volumes larger than 2.0 mL in children is usually indicative of a perforation or patent ventilation tube. Type B tympanograms with normal volume measurement are indicative of a nonmobile intact tympanic membrane.

The *acoustic reflex threshold* is a measurement of the level at which the stapedial muscle contracts. The normal-hearing individual will produce an acoustic reflex with pure tone signals between 70 and 100 dB hearing threshold level. Because the acoustic reflex is mediated by loudness, it is a sensitive indicator of cochlear pathology. The acoustic reflex test also can be used to confirm the presence of a conductive hearing loss. Another application of the acoustic reflex test is the detection of retrocochlear pathology.

Auditory Brain Stem Response Audiometry

Auditory brain stem response (ABR) audiometry is an objective auditory test that does not require a subjective response from the patient. The aim of ABR audiometry is to record the potentials that arise in the auditory system as a result of sound stimulation. This test can be used to assess or approximate the threshold of hearing in the higher frequencies. ABR is also useful in detecting retrocochlear lesions, such as an acoustic neuroma. The patient with multiple sclerosis and hearing loss also may demonstrate an abnormal ABR.

Sensorineural Hearing Loss in Children

Sensorineural hearing loss in childhood may go undetected for years, particularly if it is restricted to the high frequencies. This can result in speech and language difficulties that can have a profound effect on intellectual development. It is important to detect these losses at an early age so that corrective measures can be undertaken.

Hearing actually begins in utero. It has been shown clinically that a 3-month-old infant responds preferentially to a tape recording of his or her mother's voice. The first word is spoken at about 1 year, with two-word sentences by age 2 years. By age 4, the basic steps to normal language acquisition have been completed.

It is important to determine the cause of a hearing loss in children. This begins with a detailed interview with the parents covering the gestational, perinatal, postnatal, and family histories. The gestational history should seek to uncover maternal infection, trauma, immunologic disorder, nutritional disturbance, or endocrine imbalance. Maternal infections that can affect the fetus include rubella, cytomegalovirus, toxoplasmosis, influenza, syphilis, and herpes simplex types 1 and 2. Maternal trauma may take the form of a disturbance in the placenta or umbilical cord, irradiation, drug ingestion, maternal alcoholism, and associated nutritional disturbances.

Endocrine disturbances of the mother, such as thyrotoxicosis, diabetes, and psuedohypoparathyroidism, also may predispose the fetus to aural damage.

Perinatal events that lead to hypoxia and hearing loss include placenta previa, abruptio placentae, prolonged difficult labor, nuchal or prolapsed cord, and prematurity. Neonatal jaundice and an unconjugated bilirubin level of greater than 25 mg/dL may lead to hearing loss. The use of aminoglycosides to treat septicemia or meningitis in patients with an immature renal system also may cause a hearing loss.

The postnatal history must include careful questioning of the parents with regard to the response of the infant to sound and the onset of vocalization. Postnatal viral infections that cause hearing loss include adenovirus, chickenpox, Epstein-Barr virus, herpes zoster oticus, influenza, measles, mumps, encephalitis, and viral hepatitis. Of these, *mumps* is the leading cause of acquired unilateral sensorineural hearing loss in children. Bacterial meningitis may cause either a unilateral or bilateral sensorineural hearing loss.

The family history is very important because congenital deafness is inherited in 50 per cent of cases. Up to 80 per cent of these cases are inherited in an autosomal recessive fashion, and the remaining 20 per cent as an autosomal dominant disorder. The majority of these are single-gene mendelian inheritance and not part of a recognizable syndrome associated with malformations of other organs or body systems. Autosomal dominant hearing loss is usually mild, flat, and progressive when compared to autosomal recessive losses. Only 1 to 3 per cent of genetic deafness is caused by X-linked inheritance.

The physical examination should include a thorough inspection of the pinna. The tympanic membranes should be examined with the pneumatic otoscope or the microscope. An effort should be made to uncover a recognized syndrome by using an organ system approach. A search for craniofacial, dental, cardiac, and renal abnormalities should be undertaken. In addition, endocrine dysfunction, neurologic disease, dermal abnormalities, and skeletal dysplasia may be found. Finally, a consideration of metabolic storage disease and chromosome abnormalities completes the evaluation.

A hearing evaluation using ABR should be obtained in all high-risk newborn infants.

Medication Ototoxicity

Ototoxic drugs in clinical practice include aminoglycosides, furosemide and ethacrynic acid, salicylates, *cis*-platinum, and erythromycin.

The *aminoglycoside antibiotics* destroy the hair cells and stria vascularis of the inner ear, resulting in irreversible hearing loss. The degree of ototoxicity is increased by noise exposure and use with other ototoxic drugs. Streptomycin, gentamycin, and tobramycin are primarily vestibulotoxic. Nethecillin is a new synthetic aminoglycoside that is apparently less ototoxic than any of the presently available aminoglycosides. The effect of most aminoglycosides is insidious. Hearing loss may not become apparent until weeks or months after therapy has been discontinued. Early effects can be detected by high-frequency audiometry and electronystagmography. Because aminoglycosides are excreted by the kidney, renal impairment renders a patient much more susceptible to these ototoxic drugs. Aminoglycosides can cross the placental barrier, resulting in hearing loss in unborn children. Monitoring peak and trough blood levels when administering these medications is helpful in preventing toxicity.

Quinine can be the cause of temporary or permanent sensorineural hearing loss. Elderly patients taking quinine for leg cramps may develop tinnitus and hearing loss from this medication. The ingestion of therapeutic doses of quinine by the pregnant woman may cause severe bilateral sensorineural hearing loss in the fetus.

Salicylates cause reversible hearing loss and tinnitus. The salicylates block an enzyme system within the inner ear, resulting in the uncoupling of oxidative phosphorylation within the cochlea. Normal hearing returns 24 to 72 hours after discontinuation. Ingestion of 6 to 8 gm/day are required to reach toxicity. Hearing loss occurs whenever salicylate serum levels reach 20 mg/dL or above.

Cis-platinum has both auditory and vestibular toxicity. The hearing loss is usually bilateral and appears first at high frequencies (6000 and 8000 Hz). The hearing loss may be asymmetric and may not appear until several days after treatment.

Patients at high risk for ototoxicity from *erythromycin* include individuals with hepatic or renal failure or those with legionnaires' disease. The daily dose of erythromycin should not exceed 1.5 grams if the serum creatinine concentration is above 1.8 mg/dL. The otoneurologic changes observed with erythromycin administration are reversible following cessation of therapy (Meyerhoff, 1984).

Dizziness Evaluation

The office evaluation of the patient who has a chief complaint of dizziness begins with a detailed history. The history can be divided conveniently into five parts. First is the differentiation of true vertigo from lightheadedness or disequilibrium. True vertigo has a rotational component, which can be in the form of objects spinning or turning around the individual, or severe spinning or turning feeling from inside. This is to be differentiated from the lightheadedness, giddiness, or "swimming-type" sensation in the head. True vertigo most often is associated with a disorder of the vestibular system. Rarely is loss of consciousness associated with a vestibular disorder. Inquiries regarding the association of the vertigo with nausea or vomiting are important to ascertain the severity of the vertigo.

The second part involves associated phenomena, precipitating factors, the periodicity of the attacks, and their frequency. Inquiries regarding allergies, head injuries, position change, hyperventilation, fatigue, neck injury, and history of seizures are important events that may be associated with dizziness.

The next part is specific for symptoms of ear disease. Questions about hearing, tinnitus, fullness or stuffiness in the ears, otalgia, or discharge from the ears should be asked. The fourth part attempts to rule out associated brain stem phenomena such as double vision; numbness of the arms, face, or legs; weakness of the arms or legs; difficulty with speech; confusion; or loss of consciousness. The final part involves questions about high blood pressure, diabetes, or previous ear surgery.

After a thorough history, the physical examination should begin with the vital signs, including blood pressure in the supine, sitting, and standing positions. The pulse should be taken carefully to evaluate arrhythmias. A thorough ear, nose, and throat evaluation is next. Tuning fork evaluation, including the Weber and Rinne tests, also should be performed. The eyes should be examined carefully for nystagmus and the fundi examined carefully for papilledema. A neuro-otologic evaluation should include a careful examination of the cranial nerves, followed by cerebellar testing. Rhomberg testing should be performed as well as tandem walk, heel walk, and toe walk. If there is a positional component to the dizziness, then a test involving rapid position changes should be performed to look for nystagmus and evidence of benign paroxysmal positional vertigo. Further tests usually should include an audiogram. If there is a vertiginous component to the dizziness, then an electronystagmogram should also be considered. Additional tests will be directed by the history and physical but may include magnetic resonance imaging, computerized tomography, and various blood tests such as fluorescent treponemal antibody absorption and erythrocyte sedimentation rate.

Electronystagmography

Electronystagmography is an objective study of the vestibular system, based on the principle that the eye is a dipole with a positive charge at the cornea and a negative charge at the retina. Electrodes are placed about the eye to detect any movement of the eye such as might occur with nystagmus. This nystagmus may either be spontaneous or induced by position change or caloric stimulus. By comparing one ear with the other, a relative *e* hypofunction can be identified. Other tests within the electronystagmographic battery include positional testing, optokinetic testing, pendulum tracing, and spontaneous nystagmus.

The electronystagmograph will not provide a diagnosis for vertigo but will help localize the lesion if it is in the vestibular system.

Ménière's Disease

Ménière's disease is a term for the coexistence of recurrent vertigo, tinnitus, and hearing loss. Although the cause is uncertain, symptoms are produced by distention and pressure buildup in the vestibular and cochlear apparatus of the inner ear. The disease most commonly occurs in women around the age of 50, and often progresses from isolated vertigo to include tinnitus and hearing loss. Although the vertigo tends to lessen over time, the hearing loss tends to worsen because of gradual destruction of the vestibular and cochlear receptor sites.

The episodes of vertigo occur suddenly and without warning and often are accompanied by nausea and vomiting. Dizziness may last from a few minutes up to several hours, but patients often report feeling unsteady for several days. Although most patients have disease on one side only, about one third of cases eventually will become bilateral. Examination between attacks is normal except for hearing loss, if present. During attacks, nystagmus away from the involved ear may be seen.

No effective cure for Ménière's disease exists. Management of acute attacks of vertigo include bed rest and antivertiginous medication. Severe attacks may require hospitalization for parenteral fluids and medication. Long-term management strategies to reduce frequency of attacks include cessation of smoking, decreased caffeine consumption, and a low-salt diet. Several surgical approaches have been used to treat intractable cases. About 10 per cent of patients eventually require surgery, primarily because of frequent uncontrolled attacks of vertigo. A decompressive shunt procedure performed on the endolymphatic sac will resolve the vertigo in two thirds of patients while retaining reasonable hearing. A vestibular nerve section will resolve the vertigo in 95 per cent of patients but will not improve the hearing loss.

No current operation consistently will improve the hearing loss. Confirmation of the effectiveness of these procedures is still in progress.

Vestibular Neuronitis

Vestibular neuronitis primarily affects adults, causing the abrupt onset of severe vertigo, nausea, and vomiting without hearing loss. Although proof is lacking, it is thought to be caused by a viral infection of the labyrinth and is self-limited, usually lasting a few days. Like most patients with acute vertigo, a change of head position markedly exacerbates symptoms. Patients may experience residual vertigo for several weeks.

Examination usually reveals only horizontal nystagmus. Caloric testing shows depression of the vestibular response. Treatment should include antihistamines, bed rest, and hydration. Progressive positional exercises should be performed once the acute vertigo is gone. The Cawthorne-Cooksey exercises are designed to retrain the eye and body musculature to use vision and proprioceptive signals to compensate for the lost vestibular signals (Table 23–1).

Benign Paroxysmal Positional Vertigo

Benign paroxysmal positional vertigo is the most common cause of vertigo in the elderly, and is thought to be the result of stimulation of the labyrinthine mechanism from displacement of some of

---

TABLE 23–1. CAWTHORNE-COOKSEY EXERCISES FOR PATIENT WITH VERTIGO

May Be Done in Bed, during Acute Phase
Eye movements, first slow, then fast
  Up and down
  Side to side
  Focus on a finger from 10 to 30 cm from face
Head movements, first slow, then fast, then with eyes closed
  Forward and backward
  Side to side

Should Be Done while Sitting
Head movements as above
Shoulder shrugging and circling
Bending forward to pick up objects from the ground

Should Be Done while Standing
Eye and head movements, shoulder shrugging, and circling as above
Go from sitting to standing position with eyes open, then closed
Throw small balls from hand to hand above eye level
Throw ball from hand to hand under knee
Change from sitting to standing position, turning around in between

Done while Moving About
Circling around center person, who throws large ball to and fro
Walking across room with eyes open, then closed
Walk up and down slope with eyes open, then closed
Walk up and down steps with eyes open, then closed
Perform a game involving stooping and stretching and aiming, such as skittles, bowling, or basketball

Adapted from Baloh RW: The dizzy patient: Symptomatic treatment of vertigo. Postgrad Med 73:317, 1983, with permission.

the otoconia that rest atop of hair cells in that organ (Slater, 1988). Vertigo may be severe initially, but gradually improves over several weeks to months. Examination reveals nystagmus in the affected head position that is characterized by a 2- to 20-second latent period and that fatigues after 20 to 30 seconds. Because the nystagmus may be subtle and brief, it may not be detectable with the naked eye. The use of Frenzel glasses can help the physician make the diagnosis of this form of nystagmus. Many believe that the condition will resolve more quickly if the patient will continually stimulate the vertigo by putting the head into the precipitating position. Patients should be instructed not to avoid the offending head position. Positional exercises are also helpful, presumably by helping the patient adapt to the asymmetrical input from the two labyrinths.

Labyrinthitis

Labyrinthitis is the *most frequent complication of otitis media*, resulting from extension of infection within the temporal bone. There are three types of labyrinthitis: perilabyrinthitis, serous labyrinthitis, and suppurative labyrinthitis, in order of descending severity. *Perilabyrinthitis* or labyrinthine fistula, which may be produced surgically, occurs secondary to bone erosion by cholesteatoma, or develops after a Valsalva maneuver or explosion. The patient complains of dizziness and/or hearing loss, particularly if he or she presses against the tragus, manipulates the auricle, or quickly turns the head. A Valsalva-type maneuver may reproduce the dizziness, and a loud noise also may cause vertigo momentarily. A positive fistula test is present in two thirds of the cases with a labyrinthine fistula. The positive fistula test consists of nystagmus and vertigo and is produced when positive and negative pressure is applied to the soft tissue covering the fistula. A strong positive fistula test is always an indication for surgical examination of the labyrinth. When erosion is associated with chronic otitis media, then a radical or modified-radical mastoidectomy is performed.

Serous labyrinthitis is due to diffuse intralabyrinthine inflammation without pus formation and is not followed by permanent loss of auditory and vestibular function. Serous labyrinthitis may be secondary to acute or chronic otitis media with or without cholesteatoma formation. Serous labyrinthitis in acute otitis media is treated with intravenous antibiotics and a myringotomy for drainage. Serous labyrinthitis secondary to chronic otitis media usually requires surgical intervention for drainage of the suppurative process or removal of the cholesteatoma matrix.

Suppurative labyrinthitis is a diffuse intralabyrinthine infection with pus formation and is associated with permanent loss of auditory and vestibular function. Suppurative labyrinthitis may be secondary to direct extension of the purulent process in the middle ear or may result from the spread of meningeal inflammation into the labyrinth through the internal auditory canal or, less frequently, the cochlear aqueduct. Clinical symptoms include nausea and vomiting, intense vertigo, tinnitus, hearing loss, and nystagmus. Treatment consists of intense antibiotic treatment and surgical drainage of the labyrinth.

Herpes Zoster Oticus

Herpes zoster oticus (*Ramsay Hunt syndrome*) is characterized by cutaneous eruptions about the auricle and external ear canal, facial nerve paralysis or palsy, vertigo, and hearing loss. There may be a prodromal period of general malaise and neuralgia prior to the onset of cutaneous eruption. The facial paralysis, hearing loss, and vertigo may occur alone or in various combinations after the onset of pain. The management consists of topical or systemic antibiotic therapy for control of any secondary bacterial infection. Systemic analgesics also may be necessary for pain control. The role of corticosteroids in the management of herpes zoster oticus has not been well established. Acyclovir may be helpful in decreasing the healing time and lessening the pain associated with these lesions. The facial paralysis of herpes zoster oticus is generally more severe than that seen in Bell's palsy and may be persistent. Sensorineural hearing loss also may persist following the resolution of the infection.

Otitis Externa

Otitis externa (*swimmer's ear*) commonly occurs during the summer months. Moisture from frequent swimming, in combination with high temperatures, creates optimum conditions for growth of bacteria in the external canal. Another common cause of recurrent otitis externa is excessive cleaning of the protective cerumen in the canal (Bell, 1985). The bacteria most commonly responsible for otitis are *Pseudomonas*, *Proteus*, and, occasionally, staphylococcus and streptococcus. The patient first experiences itching, which usually progresses to ear pain, occasionally becoming quite severe. In addition, the patient often complains of a plugged sensation, which also may be quite bothersome.

The most common physical finding is pain on traction of the external ear. The canal is erythematous and edematous, and may contain whitish exudate and desquamated debris. Treatment should begin with gentle cleansing and suction of the ear canal. In cooperative patients, this often can be accomplished with the use of a small tuft of cotton on a wire applicator. Instillation of antibiotic-steroid drops (e.g., polymyxin B–neomycin-hydrocortisone) four to five times a day usually results in healing within a few days. Marcy (1985) noted that 2% to 5% acetic acid ear drops are also effective in eliminating the infectious agent. If severe swelling is present, a cotton wick should be inserted, so that the drops can penetrate the canal. The wick then may be removed by the patient in 1 or 2 days. If cellulitis is present in the periauricular area, an oral antibiotic such as cephelexin should be prescribed.

An unusual form of external otitis is referred to as *necrotizing* (or malignant) *external otitis.* This entity most often is seen in diabetic patients, and is due to *Pseudomonas* or *Proteus* infection. It usually involves not only the canal but surrounding subcutaneous tissues and, often, bone. Pain is usually more severe, and examination may reveal granulation tissue on the floor of the ear canal at the bone–cartilage junction. A diabetic or immunosuppressed individual with swimmer's ear deserves careful consideration to exclude this entity. Management requires long-term parenteral antibiotics and judicious débridement in an inpatient setting.

Otomycosis

Individuals especially susceptable to otomycotic external infections include hearing aid users, the immunocompromised, or those who have undergone open-cavity mastoidectomies. The organisms are usually saprophytes rather than pathogens and occur superimposed on underlying bacterial infection of the external or middle ear. Fungal infections occur more frequently in tropical or subtropical climates, and are associated with intense heat and humidity. Among the more commonly seen fungi are *Aspergillus, Mucor,* yeast-like fungi, dermatophytes, and actinomyces. Itching is the initial and most prominent symptom, followed by a sense of fullness, hearing loss, and pain. The ear canals of such patients are mildly erythematous and may have a moist accumulation of debris. The primary management of saprophytic fungal infections is complete cleansing and débridement of the ear canal. This usually is performed under microscopic control with suction and/or irrigation and instruments. The canal is then wiped with *m*-cresyl acetate or 1% thyanol and 70% alcohol. After cleansing, the insufflation of 5% iodochlorhydroxyquin in boric acid powder is effective in preventing recurrence. This may have to be repeated at weekly intervals for 1 or 2 weeks.

Furuncles of the External Auditory Canal

Furuncles are staphylococcal infections of the pilosebaceous units of the outer third of the external auditory canal. They present as localized swellings that may become fluctuant and extremely tender. Early lesions are treated with local heat and antistaphylococcal antibiotics. Fluctuant lesions should be drained. Narcotics may be necessary for the first 24 to 48 hours for pain control.

External Auditory Canal Foreign Body

Impacted cerumen is one of the most common ear complaints in family practice. Prevention always should be stressed by discouraging the use of cotton-tipped applicators. Even for patients who produce large amounts of cerumen, avoiding insertion of objects smaller than the little finger usually will result in flaking and natural extrusion. Once impaction has occurred, cerumen may be removed by an ear curette or by irrigation. Irrigation should not be used if there is a history of a draining ear or a perforation of the tympanic membrane. Use of body-temperature water (37° C) will help prevent the occurrence of vertigo (Black, 1986). A large amount of dry cerumen may need to be softened with Ceruminex or a similar preparation. Patients with very hard, dry wax may require the use of drops for several days prior to irrigation. A combination of curetting and irrigation also may be employed in difficult cases. If minor trauma results, antibiotic–steroid ear drops should be used for 24 to 48 hours.

Bullous Myringitis

Bullous myringitis most commonly is associated with a viral or *Mycoplasma* upper respiratory infection. Symptoms usually are limited to mild to moderate ear pain or a sensation of ear fullness. Examination reveals blebs on the surface of the tympanic membrane that are thin walled and contain fluid. The pain usually subsides in 1 or 2 days. If it is difficult to determine whether an associated otitis media is present, antibiotics should be prescribed, followed by re-examination in 48 to 72 hours.

Otitis Media

Acute Otitis Media

Acute otitis media is second only to viral upper respiratory infections in prevalence during childhood. Over two thirds of all children will experience at least one episode of otitis media during the first 3 years of life. At least 10 per cent of these will have persistent effusions lasting 3 months or more. Most cases occur during the winter and early spring months, and are associated with respiratory syncytial virus, influenza virus, and adenovirus infections (Henderson et al., 1982). The most common causative organism, accounting for about one third of cases, is the pneumococcus (*Streptococcus pneumoniae*), followed by *H. influenzae* and *Mora-*

xella (*Branhemella*) *catarrhalis* (about 20 per cent each). Streptococci, staphylococci, and viruses are responsible for the remainder. Bodor (1982) reported that, when otitis media is accompanied by purulent conjunctivitis, 73 per cent of patients had *H. influenzae* infections.

Symptoms of acute otitis media consist of ear pain, mild to moderate fever, and unilateral hearing loss. Diagnosis depends on careful examination of the tympanic membrane. Erythema, bulging of the membrane with distortion of landmarks, and discoloration from middle ear fluid are diagnostic of acute otitis. Patients who are acutely ill, newborns, and those who have not responded satisfactorily to antibiotic treatment should be considered for tympanocentesis and culture of middle ear fluid.

Because the organism is not usually known, antibiotic choice is empiric. The initial drug of choice is amoxicillin, 50 to 100 mg/kg/day. If the patient does not respond to this antibiotic, alternatives include erythromycin, 50 mg/kg/day, combined with sulfamethoxazole, 150 mg/kg/day, in four divided doses; trimethoprim-sulfamethoxazole, 8 and 40 mg/kg/day in two divided doses; cefaclor, 40 mg/kg/day; or amoxicillin–K clavulanate, 40 mg/kg/day in three divided doses. Follow-up examination should be performed 2 to 3 weeks later. Those patients who have failed to respond to antibiotic therapy after two adequate regimens may have underlying pathology, such as persistent eustachian tube obstruction or cholesteatoma. These patients cannot be managed adequately by medical therapy alone and should be referred for evaluation by an otolaryngologist.

In patients who have early recurrences of otitis, Carlin et al. (1987) noted that they were more likely to be harboring a different organism than the one that caused the initial infection. Persistence of middle ear fluid is common, but gradual progress toward resolution should be expected. In patients with middle ear effusion, decongestants or another course of antibiotic therapy may be tried. Cantekin et al. (1983) showed in a double-blind, randomized trial that use of decongestants resulted in no better results than giving a placebo. Most clinicians prefer a conservative, noninterventional approach unless the patient continues to have significant symptoms. The decision to place ventilation tubes or to perform tonsillectomy and/or adenoidectomy is very subjective and difficult to make. If significant hearing loss or speech delay is present following recurrent otitis media, or if resolution of effusion is delayed longer than 12 weeks, consideration should be given to performing a ventilating procedure (Ghory, 1982).

Chronic Otitis Media

Chronic otitis media describes a process whereby irreversible changes have occurred in the tympanic membrane, middle ear, or mastoid.

Treatment of this disease may vary from the correction of a small central perforation to the removal of an extensive cholesteatoma and drainage of a posterior fossa abscess. (Chronic otitis media can be active, with continuous suppuration, or inactive, representing the sequela of previous infections.)

The etiology of chronic otitis media is usually eustachian tube dysfunction or trauma and involves a defect in the structure of the tympanic membrane. The eustachian tube dysfunction may be a result of a cleft palate, obstructing adenoids, tumor, chronic sinusitis, allergic rhinitis, hypothyroidism, smoking, or collagen diseases.

Chronic otitis media can be divided further into tubotympanic disease and attic–antrum disease. *Tubotympanic disease* may be either a permanent perforation or a persistent tubotympanic mucosal infection. In a persistent perforation, there is a hole in the pars tensa whose margin is completely covered with a healed epithelium. The ear is usually dry, although it may discharge intermittently secondary to water passing through the external meatus or from spread up the eustachian tube from nose blowing or sneezing. When the middle ear is infected, the mucosa is red and edematous and the discharge is mucopurulent and odorless. Hearing loss depends on the size and location of the perforation. The hearing may be normal in a small anterior perforation. Large posterior perforations cause a greater degree of hearing loss. A hearing loss of greater than 30 dB usually indicates ossicular involvement.

The patient should be instructed to avoid getting water in the ear by plugging with a molded wax plug or with a tightly fitted petrolatum cotton plug. Any pathology of the nose, paranasal sinuses, or nasopharynx should be treated. The discharging ear should be cultured and cleaned, preferably with a microscope and suction or alternatively with the operating head of an otoscope and a cotton-tipped applicator. Appropriate antibiotic drops and/or powder then may be used in the ear.

Small, predominantly dry, central perforations that do not interfere with hearing may never need to be closed surgically. However, if the patient wishes to be active in water sports, then repair is preferable. The small to medium size perforation sometimes will close with a paper-patch procedure performed in the office. The ear should be free of infection for a few months prior to any procedure. Closure of a perforation will prevent the recurrent infections that cause mucosal changes of the windows and ossicles that may "stiffen" them or lead to disruption of the ossicular chain.

The chronically draining ear without cholesteatoma presents with an odorless, mucopurulent discharge through a near-total defect in the tympanic membrane. The exposed ossicles are buried in a thick, exuberant, red mucosa. Polyps may be present and should not be removed except under microscopic control. Any pathology of the nose, paranasal sinuses, or nasopharynx must be corrected. These patients typically do not have otalgia, fever, or vertigo.

Cultures of the discharge should be obtained and appropriate antimicrobial drops and daily middle ear suctioning begun. Alternatively, the patient can be hospitalized and administered a parenteral β-lactam antipseudomonal drug. The patient who does not respond to this regimen or develops an intratemporal suppurative complication requires surgery on the middle ear and mastoid.

Complications of Otitis Media

Suppurative intracranial complications of otitis media have decreased with the advent of antimicrobial agents. The complications that do occur are associated more often with chronic suppurative otitis media and mastoiditis, with or without cholesteatoma. The middle ear and mastoid air cell system is adjacent to many important structures, including the sigmoid sinus, the posterior fossa dura, and the middle fossa dura. Suppuration in the middle ear and mastoid may spread to these structures, resulting in the following intracranial complications: meningitis, extradural abscess, subdural empyema, focal encephalitis, brain abscess, lateral sinus thrombophlebitis, and otitic hydrocephalus (Fig. 23–6). The patient who has acute or chronic otitis media and develops one or more of the following signs or symptoms—especially while receiving medical therapy—should be suspected of having a suppurative intracranial

complication: *persistent headache, lethargy, malaise, irritability, severe otalgia, onset of fever, nausea,* and *vomiting.* The following would be signs and symptoms demanding an intensive search for an intracranial complication: stiff neck, focal seizures, ataxia, blurred vision, papilledema, diplopia, hemiplegia, aphasia, dysdiadochokinesia, intention tremor, dysmetria, and hemianopsia. Fever is common with acute otitis media, but persistent or recurrent fever, particularly after appropriate antimicrobial therapy, may be a sign of spread of infection.

Meningitis is the *most common* intracranial suppurative complication of acute and chronic otitis media. The most common cause of meningitis is an upper respiratory infection with a simultaneous middle ear infection. When meningitis is suspected, tympanocentesis and a myringotomy should be performed for identification of the causative organism and establishment of drainage.

Extradural abscess develops from either cholesteatoma or infection, causing destruction of bone adjacent to the dura. This results in granulation tissue and purulent material collecting between the lateral aspect of the dura and the adjacent temporal bone. Symptoms can include severe earache, low-grade fever, and headache in the temporal region with deep, local, throbbing pain. Otorrhea may accompany the extradural abscess and is characteristically profuse, creamy, and pulsatile. Computerized tomography may reveal a sizeable extradural abscess. Treatment consists of appropriate

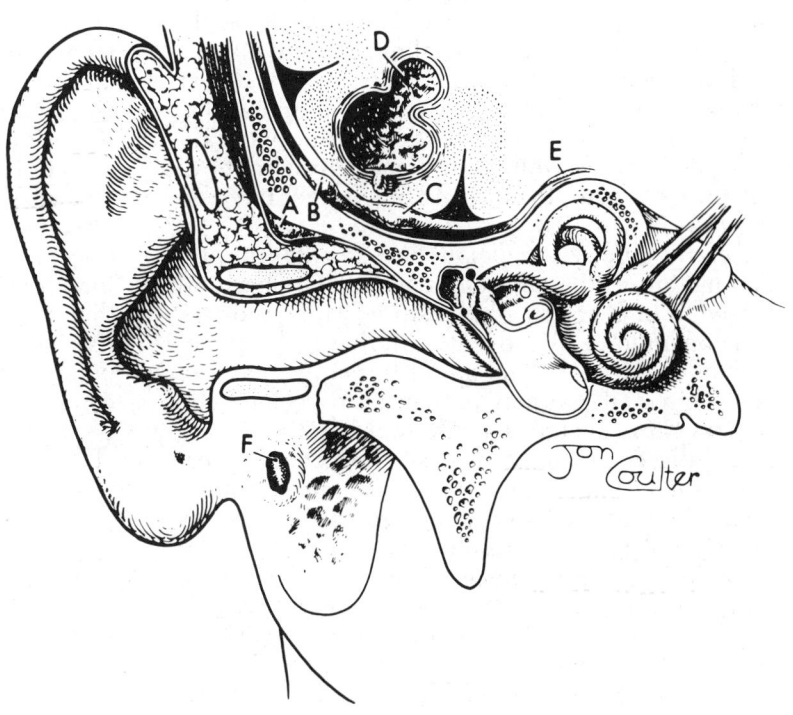

FIGURE 23–6. Suppurative complications of otitis media and mastoiditis. *A,* Subperiosteal abscess; *B,* extradural abscess; *C,* subdural empyema; *D,* brain abscesses; *E,* meningitis; *F,* lateral sinus thrombosis. (From Bluestone CD, Klein JO: Intracranial suppurative complications of otitis media and mastoiditis. *In* Bluestone CD, Stool SE [eds]: Pediatric Otolaryngology. Philadelphia, WB Saunders Company, 1990, p 537, with permission.)

antimicrobial therapy and surgical drainage, including a mastoidectomy.

Subdural empyema is a collection of purulent material between the dura externally and the subarachnoid membrane internally. This can occur by direct extension or, more rarely, by thrombophlebitis through venous channels. Patients with empyema are very toxic and febrile, and have severe headache in the temporoparietal region. Central nervous system findings may include seizures, hemiplegia, dysmetria, belligerent behavior, somnolence, stupor, deviation of the eye, dysphagia, sensory deficits, stiff neck, and a positive Kernig's sign. Hemiplegia and recurrent seizures in a patient with suppurative middle ear and mastoid disease are indicative of a subdural empyema. A subdural empyema may be confirmed with computerized tomography. Treatment includes intensive intravenous antimicrobial therapy and neurosurgical drainage.

Otogenic abscess of the brain may follow from acute or chronic middle ear and mastoid infection, or follow the development of an adjacent infection such as lateral sinus thrombophlebitis, petrositis, or meningitis. Temporal lobe abscesses are more common than cerebellar abscesses. Signs of invasion of the central nervous system occur about a month after an episode of acute otitis media or an acute exacerbation of chronic otitis media. Systemic signs include fever and chills. Signs of generalized central nervous system infection may occur and include severe headache, vomiting, drowsiness, seizures, irritability, personality changes, altered levels of consciousness, anorexia, weight loss, and meningismus. In addition, there may be specific signs of temporal or cerebellar involvement, such as vertigo, focal seizures, visual field defects, and nystagmus. Temporal lobe abscesses may be completely silent. Terminal signs include coma, papilledema, or cardiovascular changes. Treatment consists of antimicrobial agents and drainage or resection of the brain abscess or both, as well as surgical débridement of the primary focus, the mastoid or adjacent infected tissues.

Lateral sinus thrombophlebitis results from inflammation in the adjacent mastoid. The mastoid infection in contact with the sinus walls produces inflammation of the adventitia followed by penetration of the vein. The mural thrombus may become infected and may propagate to occlude the lumen. Clinical signs include high, spiking fevers and chills, and signs of increased intracranial pressure, including altered states of consciousness, headache, papilledema, and seizures. Bacteremia is frequent and may result in spread of infected thrombi, causing pneumonia and empyema; bone and joint infection; and, less commonly, thyroiditis, endocarditis, and abscess of the kidney. Computerized tomography is an invaluable aid in making the diagnosis and should precede a lumbar puncture. Management includes appropriate use of antimicrobial agents. The sinus should be uncovered and any perisinus abscess drained. The lateral sinus should be opened and the thrombus removed. On rare occasions the internal jugular vein may have to be ligated.

Chronic Otitis Media with Effusion

Chronic otitis media with effusion develops secondary to eustachian tube obstruction, barotrauma, or radiotherapy. The fluid may be either serous or mucoid. Clinical experience and experimental evidence suggest that a continuum of serous to mucoid fluid is seen. The pathogenesis of serous effusions involves negative pressure within the middle ear, which occurs as the result of mucosal absorption of middle ear gas, which causes transudation of fluid fro the blood vessels of the mucoperiosteum. *Serous otitis media* is the most common cause of hearing loss in children. More than 30 per cent of all children have had three or more episodes of otitis by their second birthday. If the effusion persists, secondary infection can develop, which results in proliferation and activation of secretory cells in the middle ear.

As the fluid thickens, it then is known as a mucoid effusion. The patient with *chronic otitis media with effusion* will present with a hearing loss and a fullness or pressure in the involved ear. Infants and toddlers with the disorder may present with pulling at the ears, nocturnal awakening, and general fussiness.

Physical exam reveals retracted eardrums and fluid with or without bubbles. With serous fluid the tympanic membrane is amber, while mucoid effusion presents a dull-appearing drum but with distinct margins. Pneumatic otoscopy reveals little or no movement. Tuning fork tests and audiometry show a conductive hearing loss that rarely exceeds 40 dB. Management involves the removal or elimination of any precipitating factors, including sinusitis, allergic rhinitis, and obstructing or chronically infected adenoid tissue.

Eighty per cent of patients with otitis media with effusion will be effusion free within 2 months of an episode of acute otitis media or upper respiratory infection. If the effusion is still present at 2 months, then a 2-week trial of an antimicrobial agent effective against β-lactamase–producing bacteria might be of benefit prior to consideration for surgery. Decongestants and antihistamines have not proven to be effective management for effusions (Cantekin et al., 1983); however, they may be helpful in patients with documented nasal allergy. The insertion of pressure-equalizing tubes is indicated if an effusion persists for 3 months or longer (Fig. 23–7). Approximately 80 per cent of patients with pressure-equalizing tubes respond after one insertion and require no further therapy.

The child with a persistent conductive hearing loss secondary to otitis media with effusion is at

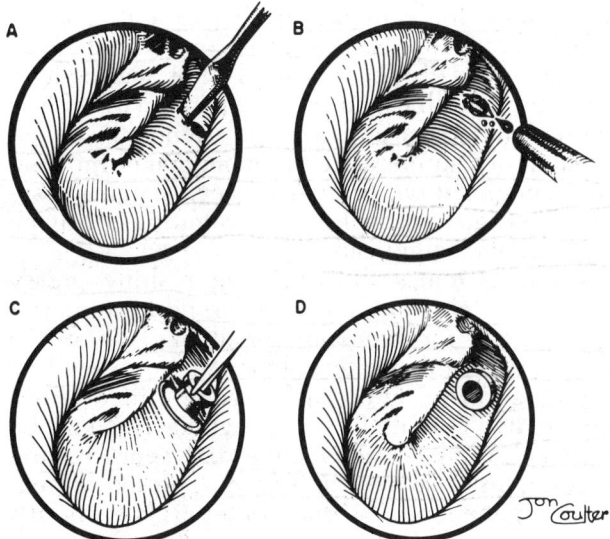

FIGURE 23–7. Method of insertion of a tympanostomy tube. *A,* Radial incision in the tympanic membrane. *B,* Middle ear effusion aspirated. *C,* Short, biflanged tympanostomy tube (Armstrong type) inserted using alligator forceps. *D,* Tube position in anterosuperior portion of tympanic membrane. (From Bluestone CD, Klein JO: Otitis media, atelectasis, and eustachian tube dysfunction. *In* Bluestone CD, Klein JO [eds]: Pediatric Otolaryngology. Philadelphia, WB Saunders Company, 1990, p 320, with permission.)

risk for cognitive and language delay. The nasopharynx of adults with a unilateral effusion should be examined carefully for a nasopharyngeal carcinoma (Bluestone and Klein, 1988).

Tympanic Membrane Perforations

Tympanic membrane perforations may be secondary to infection or trauma or may be iatrogenically produced by a ventilating tube. Perforation resulting from acute otitis media is pinpoint in size and occurs in the pars tensa region. These perforations heal within 24 hours and are of no clinical significance. They are often so small that tympanometry is required to detect their presence. A rare acute otitis media may produce a larger perforation. Traumatic perforations produce a perforation of the pars tensa. These are often quite large and are accompanied by pain, bleeding, a hollow feeling in the ear, and hearing loss. These patients require careful examination and audiometric evaluation to rule out an ossicular chain discontinuity or sensorineural hearing loss. Associated vertigo must be investigated to rule out a problem at the oval or round windows.

Uncomplicated pars tensa perforations are treated expectantly. If a perforation does not heal spontaneously in 3 months, then it may require surgical closure. Antibiotic drops are indicated only if there has been contamination by water or debris.

Systemic antibiotics are not necessary, but pain medication may be required for the first few days. The patient should be cautioned to avoid water contamination of the middle ear by using cotton impregnated with Vaseline for plugging of the ear. An audiogram should be obtained at the end of treatment to document the return of hearing.

Perforations also may occur secondary to placement of ventilating tubes for middle ear effusions and/or infections. These perforations occur when large-diameter or "long-term" tubes are used. They occur more commonly in patients who have had a tube in place for 2 years or longer. These can be repaired when the underlying eustachian tube dysfunction has resolved.

Acute Mastoiditis

Acute mastoiditis consists of three stages. The first stage involves signs and symptoms consistent with acute otitis media. There is pain, fever, and hearing loss. Radiographs of the mastoid air cell system show clouding. If resolution does not occur at this stage, then it may progress to the second stage, *acute mastoiditis with periosteitis.* At this stage, the infection has spread to the periosteum, covering the mastoid process. Patients with acute mastoiditis with periosteitis have fever, otalgia and postauricular erythema, tenderness, and slight swelling. The pinna may be displaced inferiorly and anteriorly, with loss of the postauricular crease. Radiographs again will show clouding of the mastoid air cell system. These patients should be hospitalized and have a tympanocentesis followed by a myringotomy for drainage and perhaps insertion of a tympanostomy tube. They are placed on appropriate antimicrobial therapy and observed for the first 24 to 48 hours. Most will improve, but if they do not, a complete simple mastoidectomy is performed.

The most advanced stage of acute mastoiditis is *acute mastoid osteitis.* These patients present with swelling, redness, and tenderness to touch over the mastoid bone. The pinna is displaced outward and downward, and swelling or sagging of the posterosuperior canal wall is present. Purulent discharge may issue through a tympanic membrane perforation. An occasional patient with acute mastoid osteitis may present with a normal-appearing middle ear and tympanic membrane. In these patients, the middle ear involvement drains through the eustachian tube. Computerized tomography will show the haziness and distortion of the mastoid air cell system. There is loss of the sharpness of the shadows of the cellular walls as a result of demineralization, atrophy, and ischemia of the bony septa. When this occurs, the process is known as *coalescent mastoiditis.* Management of acute coalescent mastoiditis involves a complete simple cortical mastoidectomy with an accompanying myringotomy and drainage of the middle ear air cell system. Intravenous antibiotic therapy also is administered.

Congenital and Acquired Cholesteatoma

Keratinizing stratified squamous epithelium within the middle ear or other pneumatized portions of the temporal bone is called *keratoma* or *cholesteatoma*. Cholesteatomas may be either congenital or acquired. A *congenital cholesteatoma* represents a congenital cyst of epithelial tissue and appears as a white, cyst-like structure within the middle ear or temporal bone.

The most common cholesteatoma is the *acquired type*, which is secondary to middle ear disease. Seventy-five per cent of acquired cholesteatomas are located in the attic or posterosuperior quadrant. The pathogenesis involves a functional obstruction of the eustachian tube resulting from constriction rather than dilation of the tube during swallowing. This results in impaired ventilation of the middle ear–mastoid air cell system, which in turns causes fluctuating or sustained high-negative middle ear pressure. The tympanic membrane becomes flaccid and eventually collapses onto the ossicles and medial wall of the middle ear. The most flaccid parts are the posterosuperior and pars flaccida areas. A retraction pocket develops that may become adherent to the ossicles or surrounding structures or both. Cholesteatoma formation then can occur, as demonstrated in Figure 23–8.

The signs and symptoms of cholesteatoma may be completely absent for many years. Recurrent or continuous foul-smelling discharge and progressive hearing loss are the usual presenting signs. Children usually do not complain of hearing loss, tinnitus, or fullness in the ear, particularly if it is unilateral. Otalgia and fever may signify the development of a suppurative intratemporal or intracranial complication. Similarly, facial paralysis, severe vertigo, headache, and vomiting signify a suppurative complication.

Cholesteatomas appear as white, shiny, greasy flakes of debris in the attic or posterosuperior quadrant of the tympanic membrane. They also may be accompanied by polyps and a foul-smelling discharge. The audiogram usually will reveal a conductive hearing loss, although hearing may be normal. A mixed conductive and sensorineural hearing loss also may be present. The sensorineural component may be due to a serous labyrinthitis or a fistula.

Cholesteatomas are managed surgically. It is beyond the scope of this writing to describe the various surgical approaches used in the management of cholesteatoma. The goals of surgery, from most important to least important, are as follows: (1) removal of disease to give a dry, safe ear; (2) preservation of hearing; and (3) improvement of hearing. One or more operations may be required to achieve these results (Bluestone and Klein, 1988).

Otosclerosis

Otosclerosis is an inherited autosomal dominant trait with poor penetrance. It is much more common in Caucasians, less common in blacks, and rare in orientals. About 10 per cent of Caucasians develop otosclerosis and 1 per cent become symptomatic. Women present clinically with otosclerosis twice as often as men. Most of the patients present between the ages of 11 and 30 years. Eighty per cent eventually become bilateral. Pregnancy seems to accelerate the process.

Patients with otosclerosis present with hearing loss. A positive family history is elicited in 50 to 70 per cent of the cases. The otoscopic examination is usually unremarkable. Tuning fork tests usually confirm the diagnosis. A conductive or mixed hearing loss is detected. The conductive component will vary between 10 and 50 dB, depending on the degree of fixation. If there is cochlear involvement, the hearing loss either will be flat or sloping down across all frequencies, or have a "cookie-bite" configuration.

There are generally four management options to consider in otosclerosis. Observation may be chosen, particularly if the hearing loss is mild. The option of the use of a hearing aid to improve the hearing always should be discussed with the patient. Sodium fluoride has been recommended as a medication that might halt or retard the progression of otosclerosis. Surgery is the final option. The

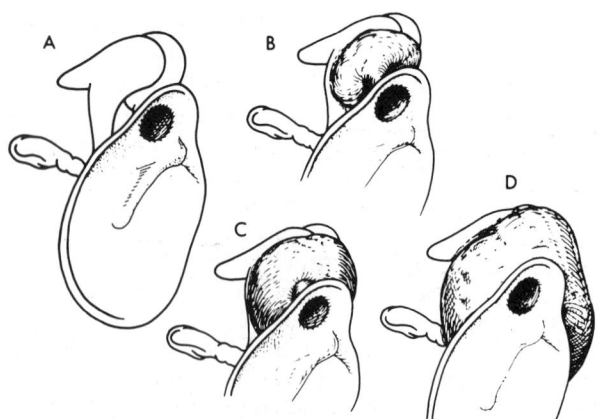

FIGURE 23–8. Evolution of acquired attic cholesteatoma. *A,* Attic retraction pocket that appears on otoscopic examination to be a "perforation." *B,* A narrow neck sac developing. *C,* Enlargement of the sac with erosion of the ossicles. *D,* A large cholesteatoma sac, a portion of which can be seen through the eardrum. (From Bluestone CD, Klein JO: Intratemporal complications and sequelae of otitis media. *In* Bluestone CD, Stool SE [eds]: Pediatric Otolaryngology. Philadelphia, WB Saunders Company, 1990, p 487, with permission.)

aim of surgical management is to restore a mobile mechanism for transmitting sound vibrations to the inner ear. Stapedectomy or stapedotomy surgery is highly successful in the properly prepared and selected patient.

Tumors of the Ear

Benign Tumors

Benign tumors of the ear include osteomas, exostosis, Winkler's disease, keratosis obterans, and glomus jugulare tumors. *Osteomas* consist of cancellous bone that arises as a pedunculated tumor from either the tympanosquamous suture or the tyampanomastoid suture. Symptoms include hearing loss and discomfort. Surgical treatment is necessary only when symptomatic. *Exostoses* are dense compact bone, and are the most common tumors of the external auditory canal. They become symptomatic when they cause an accumulation of debris in the canal, resulting in infection or obstruction. The one causative factor is believed to be prolonged swimming in cold salt water. *Winkler's disease* consists of a benign nodular painful growth on the helical rim, occurring mostly in men. The nodule is tender, preventing some patients from sleeping on that side. Treatment consists of cortisone injections. Surgical excision may be required if cortisone does not relieve the pain.

Keratosis obterans is a rare collection or accumulation of large plugs of desquamating squamous epithelium deep within the external auditory canal. This process may cause an erosion of the bony portion of the external auditory canal. It is associated with chronic pulmonary disease, sinusitis, and bronchiectasis. Pain is the presenting complaint. The etiology is unknown but the plugs are thought to represent faulty migration of squamous epithelium. Treatment consists of periodic débridement of the desquamated squamous epithelium.

Glomus jugulare tumors, also called nonchromaffin perigangliomas, arise from glomus bodies located in the adventitia of the dome of the jugular bulb, or along branches of the tympanic plexus. These tumors grow slowly but are destructive by invasion of surrounding structures. They are sometimes multicentric in origin; up to 10 per cent have a definite association with carotid body tumors. The tumor presents typically as a pulsating tinnitus, followed by hearing loss and, finally, invasion of the tympanic membrane. An isolated facial paralysis may develop, followed by multiple cranial nerve involvement, including nerves IX, X, XI, and XII. Examination in the early stages may reveal a reddish swelling behind the tympanic membrane, which pulsates. Radiologic techniques employed for diagnosis include high-resolution computerized tomography scanning, arteriography, and jugular venography. Unless there are contraindications, glomus tumors should be removed surgically. If there are contraindications to surgery, then radiotherapy may arrest tumor growth.

Acoustic Neuroma

Acoustic neuroma (schwannoma) accounts for approximately 8 *per cent* of all brain tumors and 80 *per cent* of all posterior fossa tumors. Patients with acoustic neuromas typically present with a gradual, progressive, unilateral sensorineural hearing loss with poor speech discrimination. At first patients may notice only the accompanying unilateral tinnitus and not the hearing loss. Therefore, any unexplained unilateral, progressive hearing loss and/or tinnitus should raise suspicion of an acoustic neuroma.

Approximately 10 per cent of patients with acoustic neuroma will present with a sudden unilateral sensorineural hearing loss. Any patient who presents with an unexplained unilateral sensorineural hearing loss of 1 month or greater in duration should undergo contrast-enhanced computerized tomography, or a magnetic resonance imaging study. Approximately *10 per cent* of acoustic neuroma patients will present with episodic vertigo. More commonly, the vestibular presentation is one of unsteadiness rather than true vertigo. The majority of acoustic neuromas arise from the vestibular division of the eighth cranial nerve. The tumors damage vestibular function slowly enough for compensation of the resulting asymmetry to occur. Acoustic neuromas usually are removed surgically, although poor surgical candidates with small tumors may undergo gamma knife radiation therapy. Schwannomas also may arise from other sites, as indicated in the magnetic resonance imaging scan in Figure 23–9.

Malignant Neoplasms

Eighty-five per cent of ear malignancies involve the auricle, while 10 per cent involve the external auditory canal and only 5 per cent involve the middle ear and mastoid. Otorrhea and pain are the earliest symptoms. The pain is often intense and out of proportion to the pathologic and clinical findings. Bleeding, a sense of fullness in the ear, and a conductive hearing loss also may be present. Late findings include perceptive deafness (15 per cent), vertigo (13 per cent), and facial nerve paralysis (13 to 35 per cent).

Squamous cell carcinoma makes up two thirds of the malignancies of the external ear, while basal cell carcinoma make up the remaining one third. In general, surgical resection provides a better prognosis than radiotherapy. The most common tumor of the middle ear is squamous cell carcinoma. Computerized tomography is useful in delineating the extent of bone destruction in carcinoma of the ear. Early attempts at treatment of cancer of the temporal bone consisted of radical mastoidectomy followed by radiotherapy, and re-

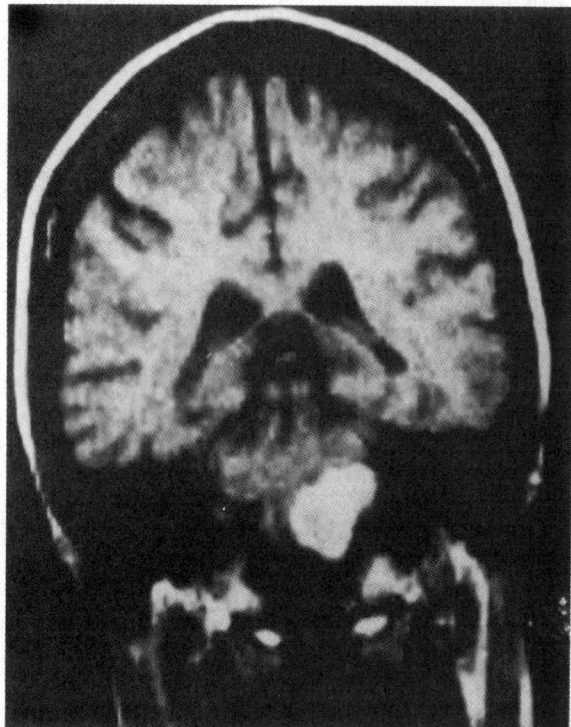
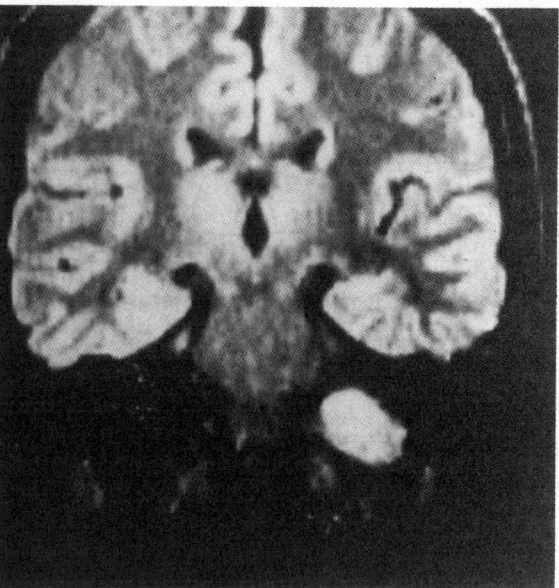

FIGURE 23–9. Schwannomas of jugular foramen demonstrated by magnetic resonance imaging. *A,* Hemorrhagic schwannoma of left cranial nerve XI is seen as high-intensity mass in region of jugular foramen. *B,* High-intensity mass within jugular foramen represents schwannoma of cranial nerve XII. Both views are in coronal projection, with imaging performed on 0.35-Tesla Diasonics unit. (From Cummings CW, Harker, LA, et al. (eds): Otolaryngology—Head and Neck Surgery, Vol. 4. St Louis, CV Mosby, 1986, p 2858, with permission. Courtesy of William P. Dillon, M.D., San Francisco.)

sulted in a 5-year cure rate of less than 25 per cent. Recent development of temporal bone resection techniques have increased the 5-year cure rate to 44 per cent.

Traumatic Injuries of the Ear

Auricle Trauma

Auricle trauma can be divided into lacerations, hematoma, burns, and frostbite. *Lacerations* can range from simple lacerations to complete avulsion and often are associated with multiple trauma. The ear should be cleaned carefully of all foreign debris. Cartilage should not be sutured except to reform the contour of the ear. Perichondrium should be closed using fine absorbable suture. The skin should be approximated using interrupted 6-0 monofilament nylon, and a sterile mastoid dressing should be applied. An avulsed auricle should be repaired in the operating room. The auricle can be preserved in sterile iced saline.

Hematomas are usually secondary to blunt trauma that produces a collection of blood between the perichondrium and the cartilage that presents as a smooth blue mass. Prompt drainage is required to prevent aseptic necrosis of the underlying cartilage. If hematomas or seromas are seen early be-

fore clot formation, they may be aspirated with an 18-gauge needle and a pressure dressing applied. If they recur or cannot be aspirated, they should be opened, drained, and compressed. The dressing rolls should be left undisturbed for 1 week and the patient placed on an antistaphylococcal antibiotic.

Acute management of the *burned auricle* involves gentle local cleansing, topical antibiotic application, and the avoidance of any pressure on the ear. Late complications include perichondritis and chondritis, which require intravenous antibiotics and drainage if fluctuance develops.

Frostbite of the auricle occurs particularly when the temperature falls below 10° C, which blocks the sensory nerve input, depriving the patient of the warning of impending danger. The ear becomes white and shiny, with bulla formation. Rapid rewarming is necessary with compresses at a temperature of 38° to 42° C. The ear then is treated as for a burn by applying antibiotic cream to any breaks in the skin and avoidance of any pressure. No débridement should be performed until lack of viability is determined with certainty.

Barotrauma

Barotrauma results from a change in atmospheric pressure while the eustachian tube is occluded. Barotrauma is increasing in frequency because of increased air travel and scuba diving.

The eustachian tube functions as a one-way valve. Air can leave the middle ear passively, but an active process is required for air to enter the middle ear. Airplane ascent produces a decrease in pressure, leading to an increased volume of air. Descent leads to an increase in ambient pressure, which collapses the cartilagenous portion of the eustachian tube.

Factors that favor the development of barotitis include swelling of the nasopharyngeal end of the eustachian tube secondary to an upper respiratory infection or allergy, ignorance of the need to equalize pressure, rapid rate of descent, and sleeping during descent.

With moderate barotrauma, there is vascular engorgement and mild hemorrhage in the tympanic membrane. With more severe barotrauma, hemotympanum or perforation of the tympanic membrane may result. Symptoms vary with the severity of the barotrauma, and may include severe pain, decreased hearing, a sense of fullness, low-pitched tinnitus, and, occasionally, vertigo.

The condition may be treated by performing a Valsalva maneuver when a sensation of fullness is first noted. Topical and systemic decongestants may be helpful. For hemotympanum, a myringotomy is performed only if the individual is a pilot and must immediately return to flying. Perforations are repaired only if not healed within 3 months.

Recurrent barotitis should be treated by eliminating any underlying pathology in the nose or sinuses, such as severe septal deviation, hypertrophic lymphoid tissue, allergic rhinitis, and chronic sinusitis. Insertion of ventilation tubes may be necessary for barotitis secondary to flying.

Temporal Bone Fractures and Labyrinthine Concussion

Temporal bone fractures are described as being either longitudinal, transverse, or mixed. *Longitudinal fractures* constitute 80 per cent of temporal bone fractures and result from direct lateral blunt trauma to the skull in the parietal region of the head. The fracture extends from the squamous portion of the temporal bone along the roof of the external auditory canal. These fractures often disrupt the tympanic membrane, resulting in bleeding from the ear. There may be a conductive hearing loss secondary to disruption of the middle ear ossicles. Spinal fluid leaks are rare in longitudinal fractures. Vestibular and cochlear function usually are preserved, although a mild high-frequency sensorineural hearing loss sometimes is seen secondary to the concussive effect. Facial paralysis is rare and, if present, often is delayed in onset, being secondary to trauma and edema instead of interruption of the nerve.

Transverse fractures account for approximately 20 per cent of temporal bone fractures and usually are caused by a severe blow to the occipital portion of the skull. They occur in severely injured patients and result in a profound sensorineural hearing loss and total loss of vestibular function. Facial paralysis may be present in up to 50 per cent of cases and usually is caused by interruption of the facial nerve. Transverse fractures result in a hemotympanum rather than exterior bleeding. Cerebrospinal fluid leaks frequently are seen in transverse fractures and are detected when clear fluid drains from the eustachian tube into the nasopharynx. Labyrinthine concussion is secondary to head injury. The patient complains of mild unsteadiness or lightheadedness, particular with change of head position. Audiometric testing reveals a high-frequency hearing loss. The electronystagmogram may show spontaneous or positional nystagmus. Occasionally, the caloric response is hypoactive.

Hearing Loss

Hearing Loss from Acoustic Energy

Hearing loss from acoustic energy is the most commonly acquired and preventable cause of sensorineural hearing loss. The hearing loss may be secondary to extremely high levels of acoustic energy (e.g., an explosion or chronic noise exposure in excess of 80 dB). At least 10 million people in industry suffer from noise-induced hearing loss (NIHL). Noise may be recreational, military, environmental, or social in origin and may produce either temporary or permanent hearing loss. Temporary threshold shifts last less than 16 hours and have their greatest effect at 4000 Hz. With continued exposure, the audiogram at 4000 Hz becomes deeper and wider until high-frequency perception is completely gone; then low frequencies are affected increasingly. A 16-hour interval is required between last noise exposure and the measurement of hearing. For compensation purposes, at least 1 month should lapse between last exposure and final assessment (Clark and Bohne, 1984).

There is no age or sex difference in susceptibility to NIHL. When noise is combined with ototoxic drugs, there is more organic damage than either would produce alone. There is no evidence that a person with pre-existing sensorineural hearing loss is more susceptible to NIHL. There is a large amount of individual variation in susceptibility to NIHL.

Other factors that must be considered before attributing a sensorineural hearing loss to noise include presbycusis, ototoxic chemicals and drugs, familial hearing loss, trauma, and chronic otitis media (Rose, 1981).

There is no treatment that will reverse a *permanent* threshold shift. Hearing aid amplification and lip-reading are of benefit. Prevention is the key to reducing the incidence of NIHL. Reduction at the source of the noise would be best but is also the most difficult to achieve. The best ear protection is a combination of earplugs and fluid-sealed muffs. Cotton is not effective as an earplug. A hearing conservation program should be instituted if difficulty in hearing occurs while in noise, if tinnitus develops after working in noise, or if there is a temporary loss of hearing perceived by the worker.

Sudden Sensorineural Hearing Loss

One definition of sudden sensorineural hearing loss is a loss that is greater than 30 dB in three contiguous frequencies that occurs in less than 3 days. In the majority of cases, the hearing loss occurs suddenly and the cause is not clinically apparent. Approximately half of the patients have some associated imbalance or vertigo. The reported incidence of 1 in 10,000 persons per year is probably lower than the true incidence, because many people recover before seeking medical attention. Prognosis for recovery is poor in those with vertigo, profound hearing loss, or age greater than 40 years.

The most common cause of idiopathic sensorineural hearing loss is viral cochleitis. Multiple viruses, including mumps, influenza B, rubeola, and cytomegalovirus, have been found to be responsible for idiopathic sensorineural hearing loss. Partial or complete occlusion of the cochlear vasculature may occur in Waldenström's macroglobulinemia, polycythemia vera, and sickle cell anemia, or following cardiopulmonary bypass surgery and can result in sudden hearing loss. Cochlear membrane breaks are also potential causes of sudden hearing loss. Round or oval window fistulas may occur following abrupt compression or decompression of the ears, head injuries, heavy lifting, or straining. Physical findings include fluctuating hearing and/or tinnitus, which may improve overnight and worsen during the day.

The initial work-up should include a history, otologic and neurologic examination, audiologic testing, and laboratory studies (see Table 23–2 for suggested tests). If hearing loss does not return in 1 month or is progressive, then computerized tomography with contrast or magnetic resonance imaging is obtained.

Patients with moderate hearing loss of presumed viral etiology who have no vestibular symptoms may respond to steroid therapy. Carbogen (5% CO_2 and 95% O_2) has been found to improve perilymphatic oxygen levels. There is evidence to suggest that this may help improve hearing in the speech frequencies.

Finally, patients who have a definite history of antecedent barotrauma should have an immediate middle ear exploration to repair a fistula. Patients with an uncertain diagnosis of a fistula should be placed at bed rest with head elevation.

Presbycusis

Prebycusis is defined as the effect of aging on the auditory system, characteristically resulting in a bilateral symmetrical neurosensory hearing loss

---

TABLE 23–2. ASSESSMENT OF PATIENTS WITH SUDDEN HEARING LOSS

Initial Assessment (within 2 Weeks of Hearing Loss)
History and otoneurologic examination
Laboratory data
  Complete blood count
  Complete erythrocyte sedimentation rate
  Glucose
  Glucose tolerance test or hemoglobin A_{1c} (optional)
  Fluorescent treponemal antibody absorption test
  Cholesterol level
  Triglyceride level
  Acute and convalescent sera for viral antibody titers (optional)
Audiologic evaluation
  Air and bone conduction
  Speech audiometry
  Alternate binaural loudness balance
  Auditory brain stem response
  Upright and recumbent audiograms (for suspected fistulas only)
Hallpike's caloric test with electronystagmography (ENG); positional tests, fistula test, or EMG with impedance testing (for suspected fistulas only)

Further Evaluation if Hearing Loss Does Not Return in 1 Month, or if Hearing Loss Progresses
Radiographic views of internal auditory meatus
Computerized tomography scan, with contrast

---

in the frequencies above 2000 Hz, although other patterns occur. At first, conversation is not impaired because the frequencies involved are typically above those of speech, which is 500 to 2000 Hz. As the higher speech frequencies become involved, the patient typically complains of the inability to understand speech. This lack of understanding is the result of a decreased ability to discriminate consonants, particularly those spoken by women and children. When speech discrimination begins to fail, conversation becomes more and more difficult, particularly in a group setting. The ability to ignore competing speech also becomes impaired, and maintaining communication becomes increasingly difficult, which often results in isolation of the individual.

Approximately *one-third* of the population over age 65 has a significant hearing impairment. It is difficult to ascertain what portion of hearing impairment is caused by aging of the auditory system and what is caused by other traumatic or metabolic factors. Efforts have been made to identify histologic and audiologic correlates. Schuknecht (1964) divided presbycusis into four types: sensory presbycusis, neural presbycusis, strial presbycusis, and cochlear presbycusis. Whatever type of presbycusis is present, the individual can be helped with a properly fitted hearing aid. There are also many less expensive *assistive listening devices* available on the market that may be helpful in certain listening situations. There is current research involving an implantable hearing device that would drive the ossicular chain by electromagnetic means. This may become available in the near future to improve sensorineural hearing loss from many causes.

Facial Nerve Paralysis

Although trauma or surgery can result in facial nerve paralysis, the cause is usually never determined, and the condition is referred to as Bell's palsy. Current theories favor a viral etiology (Olsen, 1984). It is relatively common, affecting about 1 in 60 or 70 persons. Paralysis occurs abruptly and is complete within 48 hours of onset. About 80 per cent of the patients will recover complete function within a few weeks or months, but recurrences are seen in about 10 per cent.

Examination reveals partial or complete paralysis in all branches of the seventh nerve. A complete neurologic examination should be performed. Electroneurography performed within the first 2 weeks may help to determine prognosis. Evidence of denervation on electroneurography indicates that a much longer recovery period is expected. Treatment should include protection and splinting of the eye, massaging facial muscles, and corticosteroids.

Corticosteroids (e.g., prednisone, 60 to 80 mg daily) given during the first 5 days and tapered over the next 5 days may help to shorten and lessen the paralysis. If the patient does not seek treatment before 48 hours, the use of prednisone is probably not worthwhile. If complete facial paralysis lasts longer than 2 weeks, electroneurography provides some degree of prognostic information. Surgical decompression of the facial nerve has been performed in patients with severe denervation, but with inconsistent and controversial results.

THE NOSE AND SINUSES

Choanal Atresia

Choanal atresia is a unilateral or bilateral obstruction of the posterior choanae (openings from posterior nose to nasopharynx). The condition occurs in 1 in 5000 to 8000 births, and the obstructing tissue may be membranous only (10 per cent) but is usually osseous (90 per cent). It usually occurs in females and is usually unilateral. The nasal cavities form as the nasal placodes invaginate posteriorly until they encounter the nasobuccal membrane, which usually attenuates and ruptures around the sixth week of gestation. Theories that explain choanal atresia include persistence of the buccopharyngeal membrane, persistence of the nasobuccal membrane, or misdirection of mesodermal elements in the choanal region.

Because neonates are obligate nasal breathers, acute respiratory distress usually occurs with bilateral atresia, and it may be life-threatening. Adaptation to oral breathing may take several weeks. Unilateral atresia can be overlooked until it is diagnosed later in life on the basis of persistent unilateral nasal discharge. There are often associated anomalies, including the CHARGE syndrome (*c*oloboma, cardiac [*h*eart] anomalies, choanal *a*tresia, *r*etarded growth, and *g*enital and *e*ar abnormalities).

Diagnosis requires a high index of suspicion. A wisp of cotton or a cold mirror will demonstrate lack of air flow through the nose. A no. 6 French catheter will not pass beyond 3 to 4 cm from the nostril, and radiopaque dye will reveal the nature of the obstruction. Treatment usually requires emergency airway management, and a small oral airway is effective for a short time. As soon as the infant can tolerate general anesthesia safely, a transnasal, transseptal, or transpalatal approach is employed by the surgeon to open up the choanal region.

Allergic Rhinitis

Allergic rhinitis is encountered commonly in family practice and usually begins in patients younger than 20 years of age (Busse, 1983). It may occur seasonally from pollen allergies, or perenially as a result of allergy to house dust, animal dander, or food. Patients usually present with itching of the nose and eyes, sneezing, nasal obstruction, watery nasal discharge, and increased lacrimation.

Examination reveals narrowing of the nasal airway with a pale, purplish hue to the mucosa and a clear, watery discharge. Nasal polyps also may be noted. Diagnosis is usually evident from a careful history of the relationship of symptoms to allergen exposure. A nasal smear for eosinophils may help in differentiating this condition from nonallergic nasal problems. Other helpful diagnostic procedures may include skin tests and radioallergosorbent tests.

Treatment requires a multifactorial approach, including elimination of exposure, desensitization therapy, antihistamines, and nasal instillation of corticosteroids. Recently a nasal preparation of cromolyn has become available that may help to prevent symptoms when used prior to exposure. In severe cases, and for episodes that are limited to short periods in the year, a short course of systemic corticosteroids may be very helpful. Topical steroid sprays such as beclomethasone and flunisolide are also helpful for patients whose symptoms have not responded to antihistamines. Concomitant bacterial infection, especially sinusitis, is common.

Nasal Polyposis

Nasal obstruction, partial or complete, may be caused by nasal polyps. These polyps are soft, smooth, translucent, lobulated tissue masses that arise from nasal or sinus mucosa. They consist of edematous mucosa and submucosa and may be unilateral or bilateral, single or multiple. They are the most commonly seen intranasal masses, occurring with equal frequency in both sexes and at any age.

Nasal polyps usually occur in association with other specific clinical entities, such as allergic disorders, cystic fibrosis, aspirin-induced asthma, chronic sinus infection, and the recently described syndrome of recurrent respiratory disease, azoospermia, and nasal polyposis. There is a particularly high correlation between polyps and allergic rhinitis, with about half of these patients developing significant nasal polyposis. Also, over half of the patients with aspirin intolerance and asthma are noted to have nasal polyposis.

Diagnosis is made on the basis of the history and physical examination. Polyps differ from most other nasal masses by their pale, wet appearance and because they are mobile, insensitive to pain, and do not bleed. Sinus radiographs are indicated to assess the degree of associated sinus disease so that an effective management plan can be undertaken. A sweat test should be performed in any child with polyposis in order to rule out cystic fibrosis. The differential diagnosis includes encephalocele, inverting papilloma, carcinoma, olfactory neuroblastoma, and angiofibroma.

The first approach in therapy should be medical, using antibiotics, antihistamines, steroids, and/or allergic hyposensitization as appropriate. Surgical management is used secondarily and may include polypectomy, ethmoidectomy, and possibly other sinus surgical techniques.

Vasomotor Rhinitis

Vasomotor rhinitis is a misnomer because it does not result in inflammation. It is due to dilation of the nasal vessels and consequent nasal discharge. The condition appears to be more common in patients who are suffering from chronic anxiety states. Many of these patients may simply be intolerant of the normal production of nasal mucus (500 to 700 mL/day). The condition occurs more commonly in adolescents and young adults, and is more common in women. Patients primarily complain of nasal obstruction and clear nasal discharge. Examination often reveals mild swelling of the nasal mucosa. Systemic decongestants and antihistamines are the primary treatment of this condition. Patients must be educated about the deleterious effects of long-term use of topical decongestants. Patients complaining of chronic, intractable symptoms may be considered candidates for submucous resection or cryosurgery of the nasal turbinates.

Rhinitis Medicamentosa

Rhinitis medicamentosa is not an inflammatory condition, but rather a chronic, reactive vasodilation caused by excessive use of topical nasal vasoconstrictors. After several days of use of topical vasoconstrictors, a rebound phenomenon occurs that consists of rhinorrhea, edema, and loss of ciliary function. A vicious cycle develops that leads to increasingly frequent use of the offending medication. Patients soon come to feel dependent on the use of the nasal drops or sprays, and typically have a great deal of trouble discontinuing their use. The patient's only recourse is to suffer nasal obstruction for about 2 to 3 weeks, after which the normal tone returns to the nasal vasculature. Systemic decongestants, nasal instillation of normal saline, and aerosolized nasal corticosteroids may help to relieve symptoms during this period of withdrawal from the medication.

Viral Rhinitis

Colds are humans' most common infection, occurring at least once or twice a year in adults and five to eight times per year in children. Although they are little more than a nuisance in the adult, they are often accompanied by sinusitis and middle ear infections in children. The main culprit is one of many strains of rhinovirus. Other agents that may cause a similar condition include *Mycoplasma, Neisseria, H. influenzae,* and *S. aureus.* Peak occurrences of viral rhinitis occur in September, January, and April.

Low-grade fever is followed rapidly by irritability, sneezing, and nasal discharge. Nasal secretions become progressively thicker, often purulent. Myalgias, headache, and a nonproductive cough are also common.

Treatment recommendations include acetominophen, fluids, rest, and decongestants. Aspirin should not be given to children because of the increased risk of Reye's syndrome in cases of influenza or varicella infections. Instillation of nasal decongestants is useful for infants who have trouble eating and breathing because of nasal obstruction. Saline or 0.125% to 0.25% phenylephrine may be used. Symptoms rarely last for more than a week.

Sinusitis

Acute Sinusitis

Acute sinusitis may involve any or all of the paranasal sinuses, which include the frontal, maxillary, sphenoid, and ethmoids. Acute sinusitis, as contrasted with subacute and chronic infections, is defined as lasting from 1 day to 3 weeks. It most commonly follows nasal obstruction from viral rhinitis.

Mucosal swelling causes blockage of the ostia, resulting in obstruction and subsequent progression of the infection. Other predisposing causes include allergic rhinitis, deviated nasal septum, foreign body, and frequent swimming. Systemic predisposing factors include diabetes, malnutrition, and blood dyscrasias (Kern, 1988). The most common organisms are streptococci, pneumococci, *H. influenzae*, and staphylococci. Sinusitis occasionally may be caused by gram-negative and anaerobic organisms, fungi, and mycobacteria.

The early symptoms of sinusitis are those of viral rhinitis, followed by a feeling of fullness over one side of the face or a dull, localized headache. Frontal involvement is often associated with a generalized headache and may progress rapidly. Maxillary sinusitis often causes radiation of pain to the teeth. Ethmoid sinusitis results in pain over the bridge of the nose and behind the eye. Sphenoid involvement also causes retro-orbital pain and may cause an occipital headache. On examination, patients also may have evidence of periostitis leading to swelling and erythema over the involved sinus. The nasal mucosa is often erythematous and edematous, and purulent nasal drainage is often present. Tenderness to palpation may be present over the frontal or maxillary sinus (Bailey, 1973).

Sinus radiographs are helpful in confirming questionable cases and may show mucosal thickening or air–fluid levels. If symptoms are limited to the maxillary sinus, a simple Waters view usually will suffice. Cultures may be taken from the posterior nasopharynx, but their usefulness is debated.

Treatment is directed at the infection itself, and to decongesting the nasal mucosa to allow drainage of the involved sinus. Either amoxicillin or erythromycin will be effective against the majority of organisms causing sinusitis (Table 23–3). Amoxicillin with clavulinate (Augmentin) is an appropriate selection for the 15 to 20 per cent of patients

TABLE 23–3. CAUSATIVE ORGANISMS IN ACUTE SINUSITIS

Agent	Incidence (Per Cent of Cases)
Bacteria	30
Streptococcus pneumoniae	30
Haemophilus influenzae	20
Anaerobic bacteria	10
Staphylococcus aureus	4
Streptococcus pyogenes	2
Moraxella (Branhamella) catarrhalis	2
Aerobic gram-negative bacteria	9
Viruses	
Rhinovirus	15
Influenza	5
Parainfluenza	3
Adenovirus	<1

Adapted from Kern EB: Suppurative (bacterial) sinusitis. Postgrad Med 81:194, 1987, with permission.

whose infection is caused by β-lactamase–producing strains of *H. influenzae* and *M. catarrhalis*. Other antibiotics that have been advised include cefuroxime axetil (Ceftin), cefaclor (Ceclor), or cefixime (Suprax). It is recommended that antibiotic therapy be continued for 2 to 3 weeks. A topical nasal decongestant spray should be used three times a day for a maximum of 5 days. Systemic decongestants also may be used.

Ethmoid Sinusitis

The ethmoid sinus complex is the primary key to the health of the nose and the other pairs of sinuses. Ethmoid sinus development begins with the appearance of small slits along the lateral wall of the nose during the fifth month of fetal development. At birth, the maxillary and ethmoid sinuses are the only sinus cavities, and during childhood these two groups are responsible for most of the complications of sinusitis occurring in children. Each ethmoid sinus complex consists of 4 to 17 cells, with the anterior group draining into the recess just beneath the middle turbinate and the posterior group beneath the superior turbinate.

Clinical manifestations of ethmoid sinusitis include upper facial pain, discharge, visual dysfunction, headaches, fever, and chronic cough. Because only a thin bony wall separates the ethmoid complex from the eye and the brain, complications of ethmoiditis may threaten both of these regions.

In addition to the history and physical examination, radiographic studies are essential for adequate assessment of the ethmoid sinuses. The computerized tomography scan has become the gold standard for precise evaluation.

Medical management includes antibiotics, antihistamines, decongestants, topical steroids, and allergic hyposensitization as appropriate for each individual patient. Chronic sinus infection is more likely to be secondary to agents such as *S. aureus* or anaerobes such as *Bacteroides fragilis*. Therapy often includes an antibiotic such as amoxicillin with clavulinate (Augmentin) plus a second antibiotic such as metronidazole (Flagyl) or clindamycin (Cleocin). It is important to remember that, in the immunocompromised patient, one should always suspect the possibility of *Pseudomonas* infection. Persistent chronic sinus infections should be referred for further evaluation and management by an otolaryngologist. The goal is to relieve sinus obstruction and re-establish drainage and aeration of these cells. Usually, this can be accomplished with medical management, but, when this fails, surgical intervention is indicated to avoid complications.

Chronic Nasal/Sinus Infection

Chronic or recurrent infection involving the nose and paranasal sinuses (Fig. 23–10) is a common and often frustrating challenge for primary care physicians and otolaryngologists. Most instances of *chronic rhinosinusitis* are the result of pathologic conditions in the nasal airway, and

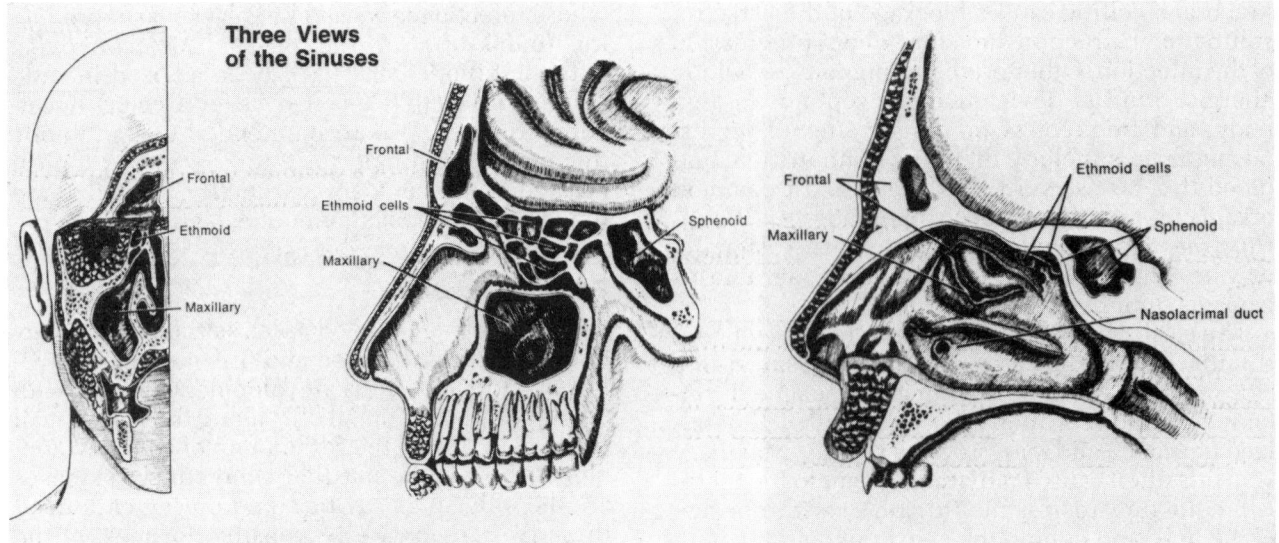

FIGURE 23–10.   Three views of the paranasal sinuses.

many of these patients cannot be controlled by medical management alone. With time, chronic infection results in disruption of normal airflow patterns (obstructed nasal breathing) and nasal ciliary clearance of mucus (anterior and posterior nasal discharge). When this occurs, more serious and even life-threatening complications become likely.

In some patients there are correctable predisposing causes for the development of chronicity. These include such factors as environmental smoke, dust, fumes, and pollen—all of which must be assessed and limited or controlled. Trauma to the nose or abnormal growth/development may result in internal deformity of the nasal septum, a problem reviewed later in this chapter.

Endoscopic nasal and sinus diagnosis and surgery provide an important advance in this field. The ability to identify precisely the source and nature of the pathology is now linked with new techniques that permit removal of abnormal tissue and preservation of areas that can regain their normal function. Procedures now are performed on an outpatient basis that are safer and more effective than prior operations that required several days of hospitalization.

Acute and Chronic Frontal Sinusitis

The frontal sinus begins to develop between the first and second years after birth and reaches its full size at about age 20. This sinus drains into the middle meatus under the middle turbinate.

Acute frontal sinusitis may develop secondary to various conditions that interfere with adequate sinus aeration and drainage. Typical predisposing problems are allergic rhinitis, polys, septal deviation, tumors, or nasal infection. Common symptoms are headaches that are worse in the morning, mucopurulent discharge, and fever. Examination often reveals edema and tenderness over the sinus. Radiographic studies may show an air–fluid level or complete opacification of the sinuses. Complications include osteomyelitis, Pott's puffy tumor of the forehead, orbital cellulitis, and intracranial infection.

Treatment of acute frontal sinusitis is directed at re-establishing sinus drainage using topical and systemic decongestants along with antibiotic therapy. Heat, humidified air, and rest are often helpful adjunctive measures. When medical management fails, the frontal sinus may require a drainage procedure (trephination).

Chronic frontal sinusitis may result from inadequately treated acute frontal sinusitis and is a surgical problem. The common symptoms are nasal discharge and frontal headaches. Radiographs show thickened mucosa and/or bony sclerosis. The surgical procedure used is osteoplastic fat obliteration.

Nasal Tumors

Tumors of the nasal passage and sinuses, other than polyps, are uncommon but of considerable importance because of their location and their tendency to impair nasal function. They usually become symptomatic by causing obstruction, pressure, or bleeding. Radiographic studies are useful in determining tumor extension to adjacent sites, and biopsy is required to define the precise nature of the growth.

Tumor-Like Lesions

Tumor-like lesions of the nose and paranasal sinuses include *giant cell reparative granulomas*, which are thought to be an aberrant form of local reparative reaction in response to an inflammatory process. These may occur in any of the sinuses, but they are found most commonly in the maxillary or ethmoid region, and they are seen more frequently in young patients.

Ossifying fibroma is a cellular fibroma that produces calcified intercellular material. Seen most often in children as a painless cheek mass, it can expand and obliterate the maxillary sinus. Excision usually results in cure. A similar disorder, *fibrous dysplasia*, differs in that it arises from the proliferation of fibro-osseous tissue inside the affected facial bones and is not a true neoplasm. The more common monostatic form usually involves the frontal or sphenoid bones, causing a single, unilateral facial swelling. The polyostotic form affects females more frequently and may be associated with skin lesions and sexual precocity, in which case it is termed Albright's syndrome.

Benign Neoplasms

Nasal *papilloma* is the most common example of benign neoplasm. Exophytic papillomata are very firm and usually are cured by simple excision. *Inverting papilloma* is a softer, verrucous lesion that usually arises from the lateral nasal wall. These neoplasms grow slowly and invade the underlying bone. They tend to recur following excision, and 4 to 15 per cent eventually are found to be malignant.

Osteoma is a benign neoplasm that grows slowly and is often asymptomatic. These tumors arise more frequently in pubertal males, and they usually involve the frontal sinus, with the ethmoid region being the next most common site. Surgical excision is necessary if the osteoma grows sufficiently large to obstruct the sinus ostium.

Malignant Neoplasms

Malignant neoplasms are relatively rare, accounting for about 3 per cent of all upper aerodigestive tract cancer. Known etiologic factors are nickel, wood dust, and Thorotrast. Most patients are past age 50, most of these tumors arise in the maxillary sinus, and over half of the tumors are advanced (T3 or T4) when the diagnosis is made. *Squamous cell carcinoma* is the most common histologic type, and combined surgery and radiation therapy are employed in managing these patients. Cure rates of about 30 per cent are reported.

Adenocarcinoma is found predominately in the ethmoid sinuses. The patients are slightly younger, the tumors somewhat more slow growing, and the prognosis slightly better than for squamous cell carcinoma. *Lymphoma* may arise in extranodal form in the nose or paranasal sinuses. Subclasses of nasal lymphoma include reticulosarcoma, lymphosarcoma, and plasmacytoma. Most of these tumors arise in the maxillary antrum and they present at a younger age than most carcinomas. Unlike lymphoma elsewhere, dissemination of sinus tumors is not common, and the prognosis is better than for other lymphomas and carcinomas.

Melanoma is rare and is found in older patients, with the mean age being about 75. These tumors tend to arise high in the nasal cavity and to invade the ethmoid sinuses. In contradistinction to skin melanoma, these malignancies do not appear to arise in pre-existing lesions and many of them may remain localized for a prolonged period. However, they carry a very poor prognosis, with a 5-year survival rate of about 5 per cent.

Esthesioneuroblastoma is a rare tumor arising in the roof of the nose. Most of the patients are young adults, and the common symptoms are obstruction and loss of sense of smell. These tumors tend to spread submucosally, making it difficult to assess accurately the extent of the disease. Metastasis occurs in about 20 per cent of patients, and aggressive surgical excision is combined with radiation therapy in most instances. Cure rates are approximately 50 per cent with aggressive treatment.

Nasal Trauma

The nose is the most frequently injured structure in the head and neck region. The bony skeleton of the external nose is formed by the paired nasal bones that join in the midline and are supported by the nasal process of the frontal bone and the frontal process of each maxilla. The middle third of the nasal skeleton is composed of the upper lateral cartilages, while the lower lateral cartilages support the lower third. Internal nasal structures of importance are the quadrangular cartilage and the bony vomer on which it rests.

Nasal Bone Fractures

In adults, the nasal bones remain attached to each other when fractured, while they frequently separate in children. Therefore, unilateral depressed nasal bone fractures are much less common in adults than in children. Inside the nose, displacement of the quadrangular cartilage from the vomer or angulation of the quadrangular cartilage is a common occurrence in response to a strong blow from anteriorly. Hematoma formation is common at these various fracture sites, making these areas susceptible to infection after a few days. In most cases, fibroblasts are activated but quickly are replaced by osteoblasts, which begin to lay down callus, leading to overall thickening of the bone and rapid healing that is quite advanced within 10 days.

Diagnosis of fracture is made on the basis of visually apparent deformity or the palpation of loose or displaced fragments. Prior studies have shown that less than half of these patients have had an intranasal examination, an essential component of a thorough work-up and an important step in planning the proper treatment. Radiographic studies usually are not helpful and may be confusing.

In the absence of a significant septal fracture, reduction of displaced nasal bones can be accom-

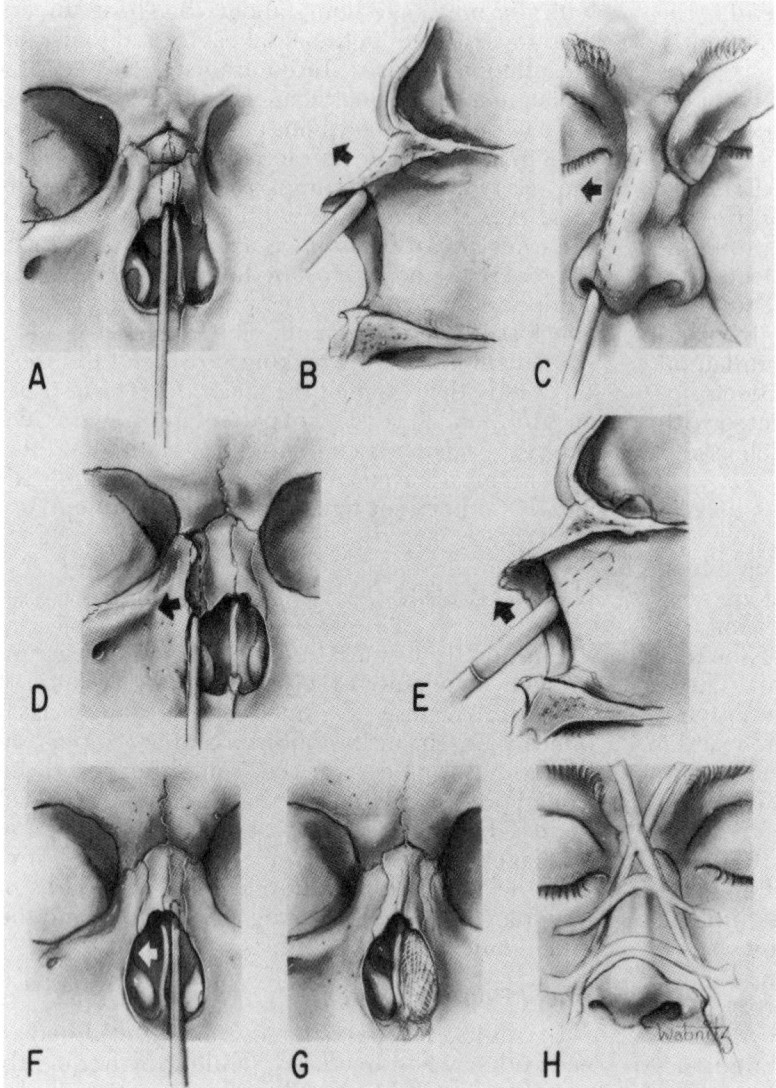

FIGURE 23–11. Reduction of nasal bone fractures. *A*, Elevator inserted into right nares. *B*, Narrow edge is placed high in nasal pyramid. *C*, With counterpressure on the laterally displaced left nasal bone, the elevator is moved outward, forward, and laterally. *D*, The elevator is inserted into the right nares. *E*, The elevator is thrust outward and laterally. *F*, Reduction of the nasal septum with medial pressure. *G*, Nasal packing with ½-inch gauze strip. *H*, Foam rubber-covered aluminum splint or dental molding compound is used for severe comminution. (From Loré JM Jr [ed]: An Atlas of Head and Neck Surgery, Vol. 1. Philadelphia, WB Saunders Company, 1973, p 415, with permission.)

plished using regional anesthesia (Bailey, 1982). Reduction is best performed between 3 and 7 days after injury. Intranasal packing is required for 7 to 10 days and an external splint is useful to maintain the reduction (Fig. 23–11).

Fracture of the Nasal Septum

If there is a concomitant fracture of the nasal septum with the external pyramid, alignment of the septum must be accomplished and maintained to prevent a later shift of the external nose by the internal structures. In the case of an isolated fracture–dislocation of the quadrangular cartilage, reduction is necessary to prevent the late complication of nasal airway obstruction. Open reduction, sometimes requiring general anesthesia, may be needed to avoid the 40 per cent failure rate reported with closed reduction techniques.

In the instance of delayed treatment for septal deviation, the goals of surgery are twofold: to correct any dorsal deviation that gives the impression of a crooked nose and to restore a patent nasal airway on each side. Osteotomy or refracturing of misaligned nasal bones may be necessary, often combined with straightening and repositioning the nasal cartilages that shape the contours of the lower two thirds of the external nose.

Nasal and septal surgery in the child raises concern over the possible disruption of nasal and facial growth centers. Experience has shown that severe nasal trauma also may displace and disrupt nasal structures and redirect the lines of growth, resulting in deformity. Therefore, most surgeons have concluded that there is less potential for harm in operating carefully on selected patients than in delaying correction of traumatic deformities until these young patients become adults.

Frontoethmoid Complex Fractures

Severe traumatic injury may result from high-energy impact at the junction of the nose and forehead. Anatomically, this nasal complex region is not a single unit but a combination of adjacent structures that are relatively fragile. When fractured, the upper portion of the nasal skeleton can be driven inward and superiorly toward the anterior cranial fossa. This may result in heavy bleeding from tearing of the anterior ethmoid arteries, disruption of the medial palpebral ligaments of the eyelids, injury to the lacrimal system, and/or cerebrospinal fluid leak. The trochlea can be avulsed, causing diplopia (double vision).

On clinical examination, the cardinal sign of this injury is a broad, flat, depressed, and unstable nasal dorsum. There is usually a laceration over the nasal bridge and considerable edema of the adjacent soft tissue. There may be epistaxis and nasal obstruction as well.

Ophthalmologic assessment is a mandatory step for any patient with an injury in this area, to detect any associated eye injuries. Radiographic studies are necessary to define the exact status of the facial bones and skull base.

Definitive repair of ethmoid complex fractures must be accomplished quickly, before fragments become fixed and healed in poor position. Open reduction techniques with wiring of fractures, repair of the palpebral ligaments, and reconstruction of the other soft tissue elements is required to prevent serious late complications.

Traumatic Cerebrospinal Fluid Leak

Cerebrospinal fluid otorrhea occurs in about 6 per cent of basilar skull surgery. Fortunately, 90 per cent of these leaks close spontaneously, but persistent cerebrospinal fluid otorrhea is not uncommon following longitudinal fractures of the temporal bone. The diagnosis is made on the basis of chemical testing of the fluid, which reveals a glucose content that is two thirds of the blood glucose level. The most accurate test involves identifying two electrophoretic bands of transferrin.

Cerebrospinal fluid rhinorrhea may follow closed head injury or mid-facial fractures. About 80 per cent of these leaks will be evident within 48 hours. A high index of suspicion is important because 20 per cent of the patients found to have a leak within 1 week of the injury will develop meningitis.

Treatment of cerebrospinal fluid leak usually is carried out by otolaryngologists and neurosurgeons. Antibiotic coverage usually is employed initially, and surgical repair is indicated for those patients whose leaks do not cease spontaneously in a timely manner.

Turbinate Dysfunction

The nasal turbinates are three shelf-like projections from the lateral wall of the nose. Their mucous membrane covering is lined with pseudostratified, columnar ciliated epithelium. The turbinates warm and moisten the inspired air, and they participate in the movement of the blanket of mucus that acts as a filter by catching and holding 95 per cent of the particles in the inspired air. By this function, they play a vital role in the body's overall defense against infection.

The turbinates become involved in many disease processes, such as *acute rhinitis* (common cold), *allergic rhinitis*, *vasomotor rhinitis* (autonomic imbalance), and *rhinitis medicamentosa* (abuse of nose drops).

Chronic hypertrophic rhinitis is the end stage of the above types of rhinitis, and it is characterized by enlarged, meaty, obstructive turbinates. The diagnosis is confirmed by spraying the nose with a topical sympathomimetic solution (ephedrine) and observing the lack of a decongesting effect. Surgical management is the only effective treatment for this problem.

ORAL CAVITY–PHARYNX

Acute Pharyngitis and Tonsillitis

Acute pharyngitis is one of the most common reasons patients visit a family physician. The two most common causes are viral and streptococcal. Recently the role of other agents such as *Chlamydia* and *Mycoplasma* has been debated. McMillan and colleagues (1986) reported that 40 per cent of 320 patients with sore throat had positive strep cultures compared to 11.9 per cent of controls. Sixteen per cent had positive viral cultures compared to 2.9 per cent of controls. While 15.8 per cent were positive for *Mycoplasma*, 17.6 per cent of controls also had positive cultures. This study supports the common belief that β-hemolytic streptococci represent the majority of cases of significant bacterial pharyngitis (Mandel, 1985).

Patients with streptococcal pharyngitis present with sore throat, fever, and odynophagia. Myalgias, arthralgias, abdominal pain, headache, and vomiting also may occur. When cough and rhinorrhea are present, a viral etiology is much more likely. Physical exam reveals pharyngeal erythema, often with a patchy, purulent tonsillar exudate. Petechiae in the soft palate and tender anterior cervical lymph nodes are often present.

Diagnosis is made by either a throat culture or a latex fixation test for streptococcal antigen (rapid strep test). Evidence suggests that this technique is as sensitive and specific as the throat culture and therefore is likely to replace that procedure in the near future (Fischer and Mentrup, 1986). Rapid identification allows early treatment of streptococcal pharyngitis, which can reduce the duration of symptoms to less than 24 hours (Bass, 1986). De-Neef (1986) noted that use of the rapid test minimizes costs and time away from work. When the rapid test is negative, a culture generally should be performed to clarify the diagnosis, because false-negative rates have been reported to range between 5 and 10 per cent.

Treatment consists of increased fluids, acetaminophen, warm saline gargles, and antibiotics. Penicillin is the drug of choice. If oral medication is preferred, penicillin V, 250 mg four times a day for 10 days, should be given to adults and about 50,000 units/kg/day should be given in four divided doses to children. Alternatively, intramuscular benzathine penicillin may be given according to the following guidelines: 600,000 units for children under 6; 900,000 units for children between 6 and 9 years of age; and 1.2 million units for anyone over 9 years of age. Erythromycin is the drug of choice for patients who are allergic to penicillin.

Stomatitis and Oral Manifestations of Systemic Disease

Many oral problems are localized and not associated with systemic diseases (e.g., gingivitis, glossitis). In other instances, disease processes involving the rest of the body affect the mouth. It may be difficult to differentiate between these two categories and to decide which consultant to involve.

Infection of the oral cavity may be of bacterial etiology. *Streptococcal gingivostomatitis* is an example and is caused by *Streptococcus viridans* or β-hemolytic streptococcus. It differs from other forms of gingivitis in that it does not result in loss of gingival tissue. *Tuberculosis* may present in the oral cavity on rare occasions, with a predilection for the dorsum of the tongue. In other instances, the palate or the gingiva will be primary sites.

Viral stomatitis may take several forms, including *herpes zoster*, *herpes labialis* (herpes simplex virus), *herpangina* (Coxsackie virus), or a *viral wart*.

Acute necrotizing gingivitis (trench mouth) is a fusospirochetal infection that causes a grayish yellow pseudomembrane that bleeds easily, fetid breath, fever, and cervical lymphadenopathy. It causes necrosis of the interdental papillae and recession of the gingival margin. *Oral syphilis* is rare, but may present in tertiary syphilis as a palatal perforation or a tongue mass.

Mycotic stomatitis is a category that includes acute and chronic conditions. *Acute pseudomembranous candidiasis* (thrush) is caused by *Candida albicans* and is seen most often in infants and debilitated, diabetic, or immunocompromised patients. It may occur as a side effect of the administration of antibiotics, corticosteroids, or cytotoxic drugs. *Chronic hyperplastic candidiasis* presents as an isolated white patch resembling oral leukoplakia. Both of these infections respond to antifungal agents such as nystatin or miconazole.

Actinomycosis (lumpy jaw) is a chronic infectious–granulomatous disease usually caused by *Actinomyces israelii* and characterized by tissue invasion and spread with the formation of multiple sinus tracts. It presents as a bluish swelling of the tongue or gum or as a palpable neck mass. It is quite responsive to treatment with penicillin or sulfas.

Several categories of systemic disease may cause lesions in the oral cavity. These categories include endocrine, nutritional, and metabolic system diseases as well as hematopoietic system and nervous system disorders. *Diabetes mellitus* may cause tongue dryness in addition to gingival bleeding, hypertrophy, and purple discoloration. *Addison's disease* often results in changes of oral mucosal pigmentation (white or very dark-appearing areas). *Acromegaly* is associated with mandibular hyperplasia and marked enlargement of the tongue (macroglossia). *Ascorbic acid deficiency* (scurvy) causes the gingival tissue to become quite swollen and to bleed easily. *Severe protein depletion* (kwashiorkor) results in an acute necrotizing gingivitis, candidiasis, atrophy of the tongue papillae, and cracking of the skin at the angles of the mouth. Waldenström's *macroglobulinemia* may present with mucosal purpura and bleeding gums. *Amyloidosis* is associated with tongue enlargement.

Other systemic diseases causing oral cavity abnormalities are summarized in Table 23–4.

Juvenile Nasopharyngeal Angiofibroma

Juvenile nasopharyngeal angiofibroma is a highly vascular, locally aggressive tumor that is found almost exclusively in adolescent males. Grossly, the tumor is a reddish purple, lobulated, sessile mass arising in the roof of the nasopharynx. As it enlarges, it causes progressive nasal obstruction and spontaneous epistaxis. Hearing loss, sinusitis, cranial nerve deficits, and even facial swelling may be noted as the tumor expansion continues. Radiographs reveal anterior bowing of the posterior wall of the maxillary sinus, posterior bowing of the anterior wall of the pterygopalatine fissure, and a characteristic tumor blush on angiography. Biopsy is quite hazardous because of the potential for very heavy bleeding. The differential diagnosis includes a nasopharyngeal polyp, lymphoepithelioma, craniopharyngioma, chordoma, and dermoid cyst. Treatment is surgical excision, sometimes preceded by hormone therapy or embolization as steps to reduce the operative blood loss. Radiotherapy is reserved for those tumors that are unresectable because of expansion intracranially.

Oral Cavity Malignancy

Squamous cell carcinoma of the *tongue* and *floor of the mouth* are the most common oral cavity

TABLE 23–4. DISEASES THAT CAUSE ABNORMALITIES OF THE ORAL CAVITY

Hematopoietic System

Iron-deficiency anemia	Loss of lingual papillae, pale or fiery red tongue
Sideropenic dysphagia (Plummer-Vinson syndrome)	Angular cheilosis, thin vermilla, atrophy of lingual papillae, esophageal webs
Pernicious anemia	Oral cavity paresthesias, taste disturbances, xerostomia (dry mouth), lobulated tongue, loss of papillae
Thrombocytopenia	Bleeding, ecchymoses, purpura, and petechiae
Malignant neutropenia (may be drug induced)	Infective ulcerations, fever, sore throat, sweating, headache, and prostration
Chronic idiopathic neutropenia	Subacute gingivitis, loosening of teeth, recurrent aphthous ulcers

Nervous System

Melkersson-Rosenthal syndrome	Unilateral facial paralysis, facial swelling, fissured tongue

Musculoskeletal System

Dermatomyositis	Gingival edema
Scleroderma	Fibrotic, rigid lips; pale oral mucosa; immobility of tongue
Sjögren's syndrome (sicca syndrome)	Xerostomia, enlarged salivary glands, keratoconjunctivitis
Mikulicz's disease	Enlarged salivary glands

Skin

Pemphigus vulgaris	Large bullae in oral cavity
Erythema multiforme (Stevens-Johnson syndrome)	Stomatitis, skin bullae
Discoid lupus erythematosus	Erythematous lesions, followed by scaling, then atrophic lesions
Psoriasis vulgaris	Geographic tongue
Reticular lichen planus	Delicate white–gray buccal lesions

malignancies. These tumors comprise 7 per cent of all cancers in the United States and 45 per cent of all cancers in Bombay, India. Alcohol and tobacco are the most important etiologic factors and act synergistically to induce the development of oral squamous cell carcinoma. These growths usually are preceded by an area of superficial leukoplakia (white patch) that is easily detected during a thorough examination. Bimanual palpation of the tongue and floor of the mouth should be routine during the examination of all patients older than 40. Diagnosis is confirmed by biopsy, and treatment planning must include assessment of the adjacent mandible and the cervical lymph nodes. Small, superficial cancers in this area can be managed by wide local excision. Larger tumors usually require combined surgery and radiation therapy.

Carcinoma of the palate is usually of the squamous cell type and usually arises near the posterior, free edge of the soft palate. The lesions are ulcerative and cause pain, odynophagia, and a sensation of a mass in the palate. Trismus is a late sign and indicates a poor prognosis. Surgery is utilized for early lesions and is combined with radiotherapy for advanced tumors. After resection, the anatomic and functional palatal defect is rehabilitated by a prosthesis. Prognosis depends on the stage of the malignancy and ranges from 65 to 95 per cent for T1 lesions to 30 per cent for T3 lesions.

Minor salivary gland cancer commonly occurs on the palate and presents as an asymptomatic, mucosa-covered mass. These tumors grow slowly and are not considered to be radiotherapy curable. Surgical resection is the therapeutic mainstay.

Buccal (cheek) carcinoma usually occurs in older (60s to 70s) patients with a history of smoking or chewing tobacco. These tumors may be either the superficial verrucous form or deeply invasive. About a third of the patients present with disease limited to the cheek, but, unfortunately, patients frequently ignore early symptoms beyond the point of curability. Small tumors may be cured using either surgery or radiotherapy.

Malignant melanoma of the oral cavity arises most often on the palate. Grossly, the lesions appear brownish gray with a smooth, lacy pattern, giving a benign appearance. Some authorities recommend biopsy of all pigmented oral cavity lesions arising in Caucasian patients. Treatment is surgical, and the 5-year survival rates are very low (10 to 15 per cent).

Swallowing Disorders (Dysphagia)

Dysphagia is a very common complaint, especially among the older patient population. Advances in the field of endoscopy and radiology have increased our understanding of the act of swallowing and our ability to assess individual patients. The most common disorders causing disturbances of swallowing include achalasia, diffuse spasm, esophagitis, diverticulae, and tumors.

Achalasia is a disorder of esophageal motility involving the body of the esophagus and the lower esophageal sphincter. It is characterized by a decreased number of ganglion cells in Auerbach's myenteric plexus. This defect causes diminished or absent peristalsis and failure of the lower esophageal sphincter to relax. As the disease progresses, the esophagus becomes increasingly dilated until an entire meal may be lodged in its lumen. The onset of achalasia is usually insidious, and the most common sensation is that of food "sticking" in the lower esophagus. Pain is infrequent and regurgitation is common. Treatment consists of dilation of milder cases and an esophagomyotomy for more intractable cases.

Diffuse spasm of the esophagus is characterized

by failure of the muscular contractions to follow the usual progressive peristaltic pattern in the distal half. The normal pattern is replaced by a series of repetitive contractions. The etiology is unclear, but is thought to be a disturbance of vagal tone. Histologically, there is an extreme degree of muscular hypertrophy. Diagnosis is based largely on radiologic studies that document the functional disturbance. Patients complain of dysphagia and substernal pain that may radiate to the jaw or arms, in some cases mimicking angina. Treatment is similar to that for achalasia.

Esophagitis may be caused by chemical agents (alcohol, spices, tobacco), physical trauma (thermal, foreign body), infection (bacterial, viral, *Candida*, parasites), or radiation. Systemic disease may be a factor in some patients (blood dyscrasias, scleroderma, pemphigus, or immunosuppression). Therapy depends on the predisposing factors.

Diverticulae are pouches that form as the result of increased luminal pressure (pulsion diverticulum) or external pulling forces on the esophageal wall (traction diverticulum). *Zenker's diverticulum* is a pharyngoesophageal pouch that usually is seen in elderly males. These pouches cause regurgitation of food, foul odor, dysphagia, and aspiration. The treatment is surgical excision.

Benign esophageal tumors are uncommon and usually present after the fourth decade. They usually give no symptoms when they are small, so consequently they are usually quite large when diagnosed. *Leiomyoma* is the most common of the benign tumors, with cysts, papillomas, polyps, and hemangiomas being quite rare. Endoscopic excision is usually possible for these benign tumors.

Malignant esophageal tumors usually occur in male patients in the 50 to 70-year age group. Squamous cell carcinoma is the most common malignancy, and symptoms include dysphagia (solids initially, then liquids), weight loss, hoarseness (recurrent laryngeal nerve involvement), cough, and pneumonia. Radiographic studies and esophagoscopy are employed for diagnosis. Radiation therapy or surgery may be utilized for treatment, but cure rates are only 10 to 15 per cent.

THE LARYNX

Fiberoptic and Mirror Laryngoscopy

Mirror laryngoscopy can be accomplished in most patients unless they have a very sensitive gag reflex. Better visibility is gained by using the largest mirror that can be tolerated by the patient (Johnson, 1984). Spraying the throat with *benzocaine* prior to examination may help, but if the exam is still difficult, 2 to 5 mg of intravenous *diazepam* will facilitate matters. The patient should be seated upright, leaning forward slightly. The mirror should be warmed slightly to prevent fog-

ging. The tongue should be grasped with a gauze pad and the mirror introduced until it just touches the soft palate. The patient may be asked to "pant like a dog" to suppress the gag reflex, and to say "eee" to approximate the cords and facilitate visualization of the anterior larynx. If only the base of the tongue is visible, it is probably because the patient is not leaning far enough forward.

Both rigid and flexible *fiberoptic laryngoscopes* are available for office use. The flexible instrument is inserted through the nose while the rigid scope is inserted through the mouth. The flexible scope is a small version of the flexible fiberoptic sigmoidoscope and is being used increasingly by primary care physicians as a diagnostic instrument. An additional benefit of the fiberoptic scope is the ability to photograph lesions for documentation or future consultation purposes (Dewitt, 1988).

Laryngitis

Acute laryngitis in children usually manifests as croup and was discussed earlier in this chapter. Acute laryngitis in the adult is usually viral in etiology and is a mild, self-limited illness. Patients develop hoarseness and cough and often become gradually unable to talk above a whisper. Fluids, humidification, and voice rest should be advised until symptoms have resolved.

Chronic laryngitis is primarily a problem of adults who use their voice for extended speaking or singing. An acute inflammation is often aggravated by an inadequate period of rest. Chronic bronchitis, excessive alcohol ingestion, and cigarette smoking are also frequent contributing factors. Examination usually reveals edema and, occasionally, thickening or nodularity of the cords. Therapy must focus on removal of all irritating factors and resting the voice, to which the patient is often resistant. A beclamethasone inhaler may help to decrease the inflammation.

Airway Obstruction in the Neonate

Airway obstruction in neonates is characterized by stridor, a rasping, rattling, or musical sound that coincides with the respiratory effort. *Inspiratory stridor* suggests a high obstruction (tongue, pharynx, supraglottis), while *expiratory stridor* indicates obstruction of the intrathoracic trachea or bronchi. The most likely causes for neonatal stridor are laryngomalacia, subglottic stenosis, vocal cord paralysis, and vascular ring anomalies.

The nature of the stridor differs with each of the above-mentioned disorders, and careful analysis of the stridor may be pathognomonic. *Laryngomalacia* is characterized by a soft, floppy laryngeal skeleton and immaturity of neuromuscular function. Airway intervention is not usually necessary, and the problem resolves by 12 to 18 months of age. Laryngomalacia causes a coarse inspiratory stridor, but the vocalizing sounds of the infant are normal. Because of the redundant nature of the arytenoid and aryepiglottic mucosa, the neonate's cry may have a harsh component that is relieved in a prone position. A neonate with *subglottic stenosis* will have normal-sounding but weak vocalizations obscured by stridor. The cry may be weakened by poor air exchange. The subglottic stenosis usually appears to be concentric, and the point of greatest obstruction is about 2 to 3 mm below the true cords.

Vocal cord paralysis represents about 10 per cent of all congenital laryngeal abnormalities, with unilateral paralysis being more common than bilateral. Tracheotomy is often required in the case of bilateral paralysis. Unilateral vocal cord paralysis usually results in a breathy cry only, but if stridor is present it is usually louder when awake and may be positional. The infant may sleep quietly when lying on the side of the paralysis and become stridorous when placed on the other side.

Laryngeal webs may cause changes ranging from mild hoarseness to aphonia and from mild stridor and cough to gross obstruction with severe distress. The severity of the stridor and the obstruction are proportional to the degree of webbing anteriorly. About three fourths of the webs are glottic, with the remainder divided equally between supraglottic and subglottic webs.

Gradual onset and progression of stridor suggests the possibility of an enlarging mass, such as a *subglottic hemangioma*. Feeding difficulties that cause aspiration or cyanosis suggest that the sphincteric mechanism of the laryngeal muscles is deficient (neurologic sensory or motor deficit). Subglottic hemangiomas usually become symptomatic within the first 6 months of life. They occur more commonly in female infants and more often on the left side. About half of these neonates will have skin hemangiomas. Laser excision currently is recommended as the treatment of choice.

Unsuspected *foreign bodies* may be another possibility for these problems in neonates and infants. Radiographic studies and endoscopy are often essential steps in pinpointing the exact cause for stridor in this age group.

Among slightly older infants and children, acquired processes become more important as causes for airway obstruction. Prominent among these airway disorders are *viral laryngotracheobronchitis*, *bacterial tracheitis* (usually *S. aureus*), *spasmodic croup*, and *epiglottitis*.

Laryngeal Trauma

The cartilaginous skeleton of the larynx is suspended from the hyoid bone and generally serves to support and protect the airway. The thyroid cartilage is composed of two halves that join in the midline in a keel-like configuration to form the prominence, or Adam's apple. The cricoid cartilage is shaped like a signet ring and completely encircles the subglottic lumen, the smallest area of the upper airway.

Laryngeal trauma can be categorized according to the mechanism of tissue injury as blunt trauma, penetrating injuries, thermal burns, and radiation injury. Each of these groups poses special problems in diagnosis and management.

Blunt external trauma is the most common form of laryngeal trauma, and it may result in cartilage fractures. Oftentimes with a motor vehicle accident, the neck is extended and the laryngeal region impacts the dashboard or steering wheel, driving it posteriorly and compressing it against the cervical spine. These patients may fracture the thyroid or cricoid cartilages and lacerate the soft tissue inside the cartilages. Common symptoms are voice changes (hoarseness, aphonia), dysphagia, stridor, pain, local tenderness, subcutaneous emphysema (air in the neck tissues), and hemoptysis. Radiographic studies are essential to rule out cervical spine fracture, and a computerized tomography scan is best for assessing the degree of laryngeal injury. After the airway is secured, laryngoscopy may be required to clarify the need for surgical repair. In general, surgical exploration is necessary if there is evidence of airway obstruction, subcutaneous emphysema, vocal cord paralysis, mucosal laceration, arytenoid displacement, or cartilage fracture.

Penetrating trauma usually results from a stab or gunshot wound. The signs and symptoms are similar to those of blunt external trauma, with the difference being the presence of an obvious neck wound on physical examination. All penetrating laryngeal injuries require operative exploration and repair, along with antibiotic coverage and tetanus prophylaxis.

Thermal laryngeal injuries usually are caused by the aspiration of hot/caustic liquids or by inhalation. These injuries produce an intense inflammatory response in the larynx, often compromising the airway. Intubation is generally required for airway maintenance for the initial postinjury period. Thermal injuries may produce severe pulmonary damage as well. Baseline arterial blood gases, antibiotics, fluid replacement, aminophylline, steroids, and ventilatory support are components of the complex therapeutic regimen that is required in these circumstances.

Radiation injury is an uncommon complication of radiation therapy but, when encountered, requires immediate recognition and treatment. Chondritis and cartilage necrosis have the potential to cripple the larynx or even require its removal. Antibiotics, steroids, and tracheotomy are used to manage this problem.

Laryngeal Papillomatosis

Juvenile laryngeal papillomatosis is the most common benign neoplasm of the larynx in children. It is caused by the human papillomaviruses, a group of related DNA viruses that also cause cutaneous and genital warts. The lesions are red, sessile lesions of the glottis primarily, but often involve the palate, tonsil, pharynx, and nose. The two clinical forms are juvenile onset and adult onset. The juvenile-onset type almost always presents by age 4 and usually is associated with a history of maternal genital warts. The lesions are almost always multiple, aggressive, and recurrent. The adult-onset type presents in two patterns: as multiple lesions in young adults or as single warts in older adults.

Laryngeal papillomas almost always cause major voice changes and hoarseness. They may become obstructive and at times also will cause problems with aspiration. Laryngoscopy and laser excision is the customary treatment. Interferon has been shown to produce remission and regression of the process, but the effect is temporary, and progression resumes when the interferon is discontinued.

Laryngeal Malignancy

Laryngeal carcinoma (almost exclusively squamous cell carcinoma) affects over 10,000 new persons in the United States each year. Cigarette smoking and alcohol consumption are the major etiologic factors. Most laryngeal tumors originate on the true vocal cords (glottic), with nearly all of the remainder involving the false cords and epiglottis (supraglottic) or the piriform sinuses and vallecula (marginal). The symptoms, signs, treatment, and prognosis differ for each of these sites.

Glottic carcinoma causes hoarseness as an early sign resulting from the interference with vocal fold movement and glottic closure. Indirect laryngoscopy reveals an irregular, red or white growth (Fig. 23–12). Direct laryngoscopy provides an opportunity for biopsy confirmation of the diagnosis and for planning the most appropriate therapy. Early lesions of the true cords can be managed by endoscopic excision, intermediate lesions by partial laryngectomy (Fig. 23–13), and advanced lesions by total laryngectomy and/or radiotherapy. Cure rates range from over 90 per cent for T1 glottic carcinoma to about 50 per cent for T4 lesions.

Supraglottic and marginal zone laryngeal cancer usually presents with a sensation of a lump in the throat, dysphagia, or an asymptomatic neck node mass. The supraglottic lymphatics are much more plentiful, and early spread to cervical lymph nodes is much more common than with glottic carcinoma. Early tumors can be treated by supraglottic partial laryngectomy, while more advanced lesions require total laryngectomy and/or radio-

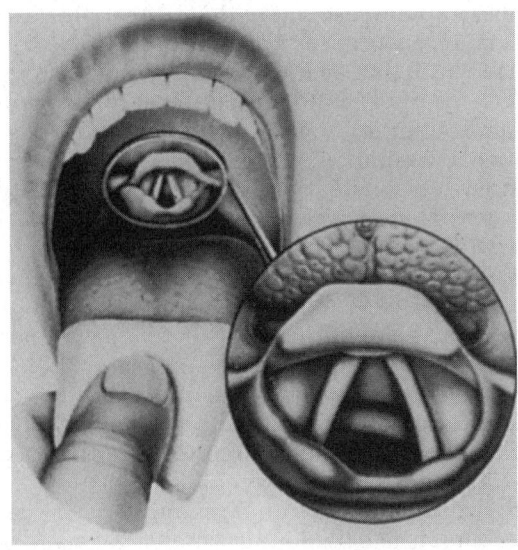

FIGURE 23–12. The hypopharynx should be examined, at least by indirect and preferably also by direct, laryngoscopy because of the high frequency of involvement of these sites by primary squamous cell carcinoma. (From Clark W: Diagnosis: Evaluation of neck masses. Hosp Med 19:64, 1983, with permission.)

therapy. Cure rates for supraglottic cancer range from 85 per cent for T1 lesions to about 40 per cent for T4 tumors.

The bottom line for primary physicians is the maintenance of a high index of suspicion for laryngeal cancer in patients past 40. The history of smoking should be a red flag in the case of older patients with any voice change, dysphagia, sore throat, or neck mass. Persistence of symptoms beyond 2 weeks shifts the burden of proof to the primary physician to rule out the diagnosis of malignancy.

Subglottic (Laryngotracheal) Stenosis

The cross-sectional area of the airway is proportional to the fourth power of the radius of the lumen, so that small changes produced by edema or scarring (particularly in the infant larynx) are greatly magnified. For example, 1 mm of edema in the normal neonatal subglottic larynx reduces the airway by 32 per cent. The subglottic region is particularly prone to damage from an endotracheal tube because the cricoid cartilage is the only rigid structure completely encircling the airway and the submucosa is particularly susceptible to an edematous inflammatory reaction.

Acquired laryngotracheal stenosis has increased in incidence over the past two decades following the widespread use of prolonged intubation of neonates, especially those with prematurity and even smaller larynges. Use of a ventilator adds a piston-like action to the injury caused by an endotracheal

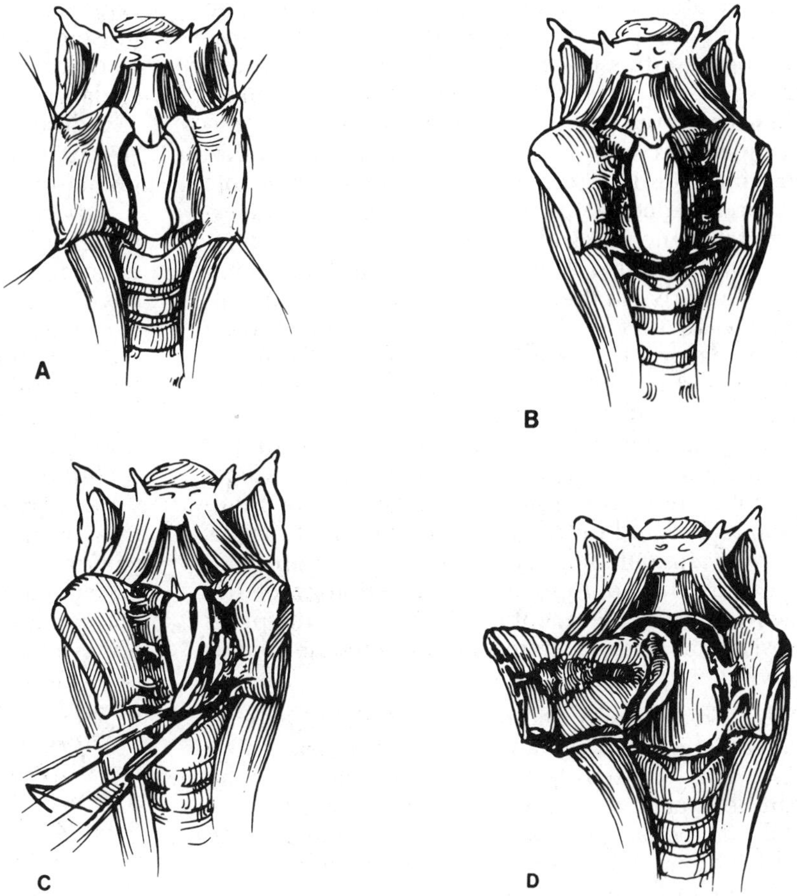

FIGURE 23–13. Management of anterior commissure carcinoma. *A*, Creation of a central cartilage segment. *B*, Elevation of the internal thyroid perichondrium on both sides. *C*, Laryngeal entry away from the tumor as first step in resection. *D*, Primary tumor resected with adequate margins as exposure is gained. (From Bailey BJ, Stiernberg CM: Extended partial laryngeal surgery. *In* Jacobs C [ed]: Cancers of the Head and Neck. Boston, Martinus Nijhoff Publishers, 1987, p 36, with permission.)

tube. Birth weight, tube size, duration of intubation, multiple intubations, and infection are key factors in producing subglottic stenosis. Congenital stenosis also has been a major factor in some reported series.

The usual clinical picture involves an infant who cannot be extubated after prolonged intubation. Other etiologic factors are predominate in older age groups, with external trauma, burns, and granulomatous disease leading the list of causes. Stridor is a common sign, often being biphasic and somewhat subtle at rest but obvious with crying or exertion. Radiographic studies are helpful in localizing and evaluating the extent of the stenosis. The final step in assessment is endoscopic inspection of the subglottic region to establish the exact nature and configuration of the stenosis.

Treatment methods include dilation and the injection of steroids to decrease obstructive scar formation. Serial laser excision of cicatrix is useful in some instances. Severe stenosis requires open surgical resection of scar and reconstruction of the subglottic region. For neonates, the anterior cricoid splitting procedure has proven to be useful as an early measure for the infant who fails extubation. By releasing the constraint of the cricoid ring, the subglottic dimensions can be increased to accommodate the endotracheal tube without producing scar tissue. Fortunately, the prognosis for successful management of this problem is quite high, with less than 10 per cent of infants being left with a permanent tracheotomy.

Chronic Aspiration

Chronic aspiration results from processes that disrupt the normal act of swallowing so as to permit saliva or ingested food to enter the laryngotracheobronchial airway. The first phase of swallowing is voluntary and consists of using the tongue to push a food bolus into the oropharynx while contracting the palate to seal off the nasopharynx. All subsequent phases are involuntary, beginning with the movement of the food bolus down the pharynx by the contraction of the pharyngeal constrictors. Then the cricopharyngeus muscle relaxes, allowing the bolus to flow into the proximal esophagus. The larynx is simultaneously elevated up to lie under the posteriorly displaced tongue base. The true and false cords move to the midline to close and protect the airway. The pathologic processes that may interfere with normal swallowing include *neurologic*, *neoplastic*, and *traumatic* disorders.

Evaluation of the patient with chronic aspiration begins with a careful history designed to narrow the possibilities to one of the three major groups above. Then a complete head and neck examination is performed with particular attention to evaluating cranial nerve and laryngeal function. Radiographic studies (especially a cinefluoroscopic exam) and endoscopic examination may be necessary to define precisely the nature of the problem.

Many of these patients are elderly and weak, and the major risk to their survival is *aspiration pneumonia*. In this group, the use of small feeding tubes, raising the head of the bed at a 45-degree angle, and changing their habits to reduce bolus size can be effective therapy.

Surgical therapy must be considered if the patient cannot be managed successfully by medical means. This could be manifested by signs of pneumonia, or could develop as a requirement for improved alimentation. The type of procedure chosen must be appropriate for the etiology of the aspiration, the therapeutic objective, and the prognosis for recovery. Surgical options include the following:

1. Tracheotomy and use of an inflated balloon cuff around the tracheotomy tube to prevent aspiration. This is a short-term solution for patients who can be expected regain normal swallowing.

2. Hypopharyngostomy/esophagostomy, in which a surgical opening is made for temporary or permanent feeding purposes.

3. Teflon injection into a paralyzed vocal cord, which will expand the cord medially to close any opening that permits aspiration.

4. Surgical thyroplasty procedures that medialize the vocal cord, which will provide protection from aspiration and better postoperative voice quality.

5. Cricopharyngeal myotomy, a cutting of the muscle fibers in those patients who are aspirating because of a holdup of the bolus caused by cricopharyngeus spasm or paralysis.

6. Laryngeal closure procedures plus tracheotomy, which seals off the larynx surgically to prevent aspiration.

The key to successful management of these patients lies in precise assessment of the cause and thoughtful consideration of the patient's prognosis. A plan must be chosen that is safe and effective, but potentially reversible in the event of recovery of function.

Vocal Cord Paralysis

The larynx is a complex neuromuscular organ with several key functions: phonation, respiration, and protection of the lungs, to name a few. Vocal cord movement is controlled by the coordination action of the vagus nerve through the superior laryngeal nerve, which supplies the cricothyroid muscle (tenses the cords), and the recurrent laryngeal nerve, which innervates the remaining intrinsic laryngeal muscles. Only one pair of muscles act to pull the vocal cords apart for breathing, whereas several muscle pairs bring them to the midline for phonation and airway protection.

Superior laryngeal nerve paralysis may be rather subtle, because there are remaining muscles to compensate for the motor function loss. It produces a paralysis of one or both cricothyroid muscles, which results in bowing of the true vocal cord on phonation. Inability to tense the cord causes a loss of ability to sing or speak in the higher pitch range. There may be mild problems with aspiration, but these are usually transient.

Unilateral recurrent laryngeal nerve paralysis usually produces an immobile vocal cord situated in a position just off the midline. The voice becomes hoarse and breathy, and the patients have a weakened cough and may aspirate. In many cases there is a gradual compensation process, with the opposite cord taking up much of the slack. If compensation is incomplete, Teflon injection of the paralyzed cord is indicated.

Bilateral recurrent laryngeal nerve paralysis usually presents as airway obstruction with stridor. The voice is usually strong because the cords are paralyzed near the midline of the airway. Tracheotomy is necessary if the airway obstruction is severe.

In general, vocal cord paralysis is classified as being either central or peripheral in origin. *Central paralysis* is caused by diabetic neuropathy, aortic aneurysm, inflammatory disease (viral, influenza, tuberculosis), bronchogenic carcinoma, esophageal cancer, thyroid tumors, mediastinal or neck metastic cancer, surgical trauma (thyroidectomy), basal skull fracture, chest surgery, or penetrating neck trauma. Therefore, the work-up must include a comprehensive history and physical exam, with particular attention to neurologic problems. Chest, skull base, esophageal, and neck radiographs may be necessary. Lab studies include complete blood count, Venereal Disease Research Laboratory tests, fasting blood sugar, viral antibody titers, rheumatoid factor, and a heavy metal screen.

Management options include watchful waiting, tracheotomy, neck exploration for trauma, Teflon injection, and arytenoidectomy. Neuromuscular pedicle reinnervation techniques show promise for restoring laryngeal function in many patients, but these procedures are still in the process of clinical refinement and are not accepted universally.

THE NECK

Deep Neck Infections

The deep cervical fascia completely envelopes the neck, extending from the nuchal line of the

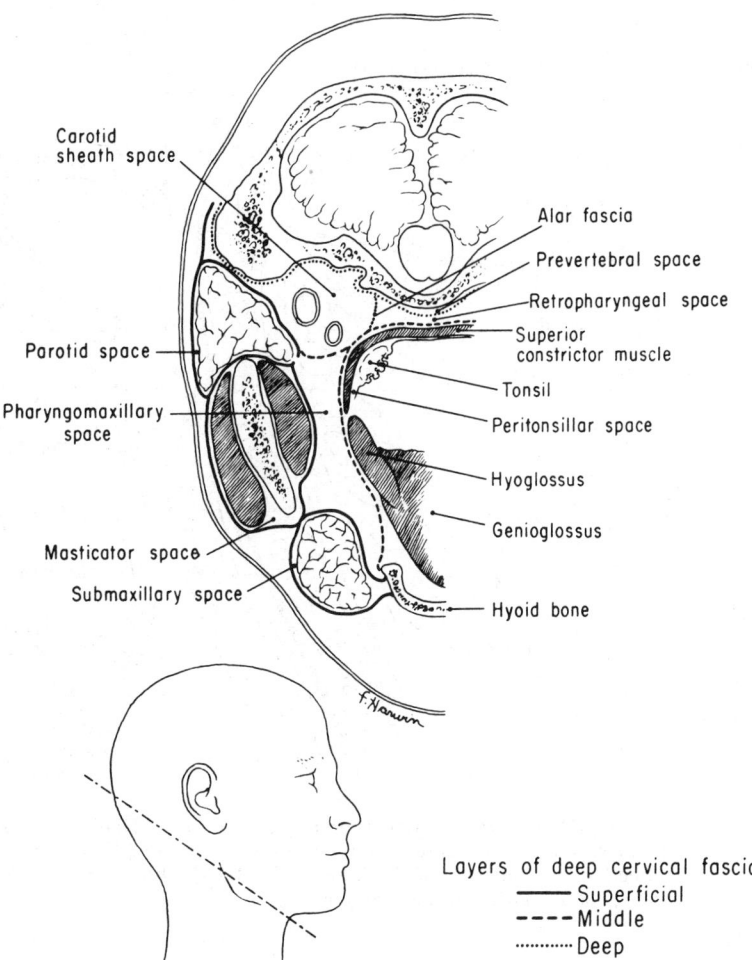

FIGURE 23–14. Cross section of neck at level of the oropharynx. Potential spaces bounded by deep cervical fascia are depicted. (From Everts EC, Echevarria J: Diseases of the pharynx and deep neck infections. *In* Paparella MM, Shumrick DA [eds]: Otolaryngology, Vol. III. Philadelphia, WB Saunders Company, 1980, p 2313, with permission.)

skull and the cervical spine and wrapping around to attach to the hyoid bone and the clavicle (Figs. 23–14 and 23–15). In the preantibiotic era, nearly all deep neck infections originated in the pharynx and tonsils, but now dental, otologic, nasal, and salivary gland origins are quite common. Most deep neck infections are caused by *Streptococcus* species, but *S. aureus* and anaerobes are also significant pathogens. There are five major distinct types of deep neck infection: pharyngomaxillary, retropharyngeal, submandibular, parotid, and masticator space infections.

Pharyngomaxillary space infections arise in the space bounded by the hyoid bone, the temporal bone, the lateral pharyngeal wall, and the mandible. The most common sources are infections of the pharynx and tonsils. Initial manifestations include fever, sore throat, and pain on swallowing (odynophagia). Trismus and medial displacement of the tonsil soon follow. Treatment for this abscess is intravenous antibiotics and drainage through an incision below the angle of the mandible.

Retropharyngeal space infection occurs in the region deep to the posterior pharyngeal wall. Sites of origin include the nose, sinuses, and adenoids/

nasopharynx. These abscesses usually are seen in children younger than 4 years, and, when seen in adults, the physician should consider tuberculosis. Early signs and symptoms include refusal of food followed by fever and respiratory obstruction. Later signs are neck extension and tilting of the head toward the side of less involvement. The infection may spread into the mediastinum. Intravenous antibiotics, incision and drainage, and (occasionally) a tracheotomy are the main therapeutic steps.

Submandibular space infections involve the anatomic space bounded by the floor of the mouth and the deep cervical fascia between the mandible and the hyoid bone. Most follow dental infections or a tooth extraction. There may be skin redness and fluctuance or mouth and tongue swelling. The tongue may be sufficiently displaced posteriorly to require a tracheotomy for airway obstruction. Intravenous antibiotics and incision and drainage are mainstays of therapy.

Parotid space infections usually follow acute parotitis, often in postoperative, dehydrated, or debilitated patients. There is pain, swelling, and warmth over the parotid gland. *Staphylococcus au-*

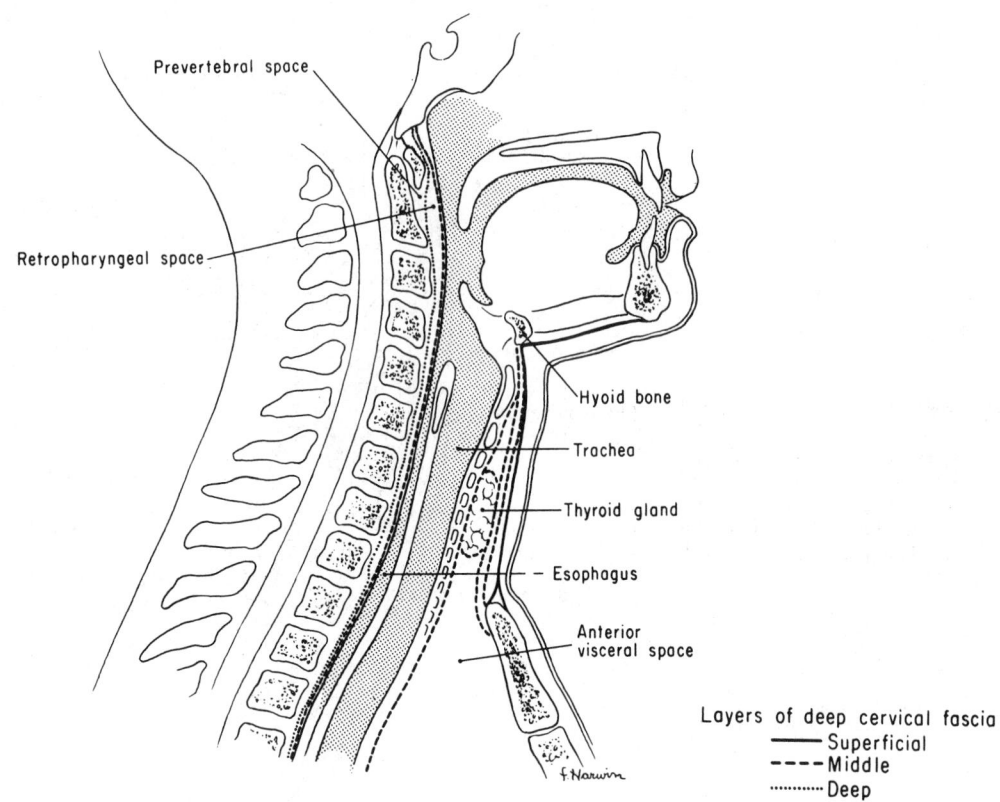

FIGURE 23–15. Midsagittal section diagram of neck. Deep neck space infections can progress inferiorly into mediastinum or down spinal column. (From Everts EC, Echevarria J: Diseases of the pharynx and deep neck infections. *In* Paparella MM, Shumrick DA [eds]: Otolaryngology, Vol. III. Philadelphia, WB Saunders Company, 1980, p 2312, with permission.)

reus is a common pathogen, and successful treatment may require intravenous antibiotics, hydration, sialogogues, low-dose radiotherapy, and incision and drainage.

Masticator space infections involve the region just anterior to the pharyngomaxillary space and often result from infection around an impacted third molar. There is trismus and swelling over the angle of the mandible. Intravenous antibiotics and incision and drainage are therapeutic.

Congenital Neck Cysts and Sinuses

The branchial apparatus is a system of segmental arches separated by external grooves and internal pouches that develop during the fourth week of intrauterine life. Grossly, this apparatus resembles a system of gill slits, and in some children disorders of development result in the appearance of cysts, draining sinuses, or lymphatic vascular tumors. The most common of these are branchial cleft cysts, thyroglossal duct cysts, and lymphangiomas (Fig. 23–16).

Branchial cleft cyst usually appears as a smooth, round, nontender mass along the anterior border of the sternocleidomastoid muscle, and deep to that muscle. These cysts usually do not become appar-

ent until the second decade of life, when the slow accumulation of fluid or the onset of infection involving the cyst calls attention to its presence. These cysts generally are lined by stratified squamous epithelium with hair follicles plus sweat and sebaceous glands. Cysts are more common than fistulas or sinus tracts. The exact location of the cyst and its associated tract varies depending on which branchial cleft is the origin. Diagnosis is based on the history of a progressively enlarging neck mass that is not consistent with cervical lymphadenopathy and is located in an appropriate site. Treatment is by surgical excision of the cyst and its tract, and recurrence postoperatively is quite uncommon.

Thyroglossal duct cyst originates during the descent of the mesodermal tissues in the region of the ventral (thyroid) diverticulum to its final developmental status as the thyroid gland. Along the way, this tissue passes through the hyoid bone region, and occasionally duct tissue remnants are left along the route and form midline cysts. These cysts usually are located immediately inferior to the hyoid bone, but they may be located anywhere from the submental region to the suprasternal notch. The cysts are lined by squamous, ciliated, or transitional epithelium and are surrounded by a fibrous tissue capsule. The cyst fluid is mucinous and often contains cholesterol crystals. About half

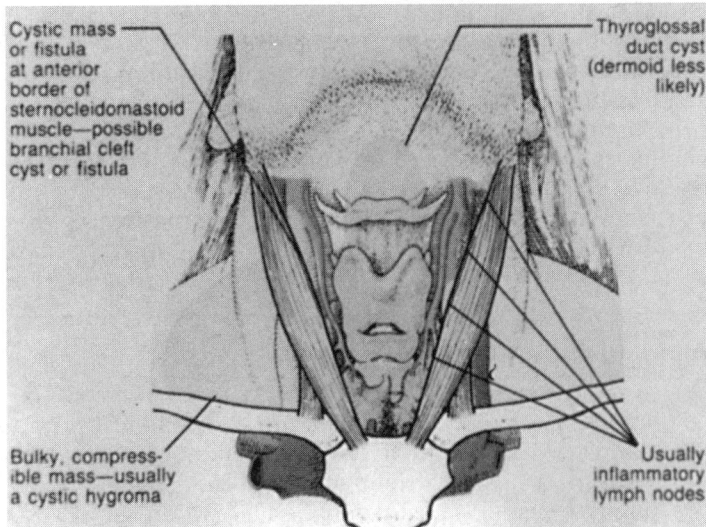

FIGURE 23–16. Common neck masses in children.

of these cysts become apparent prior to the age of 10 years as a painless, midline neck mass. Protrusion of the tongue usually will cause the mass to move superiorly. Treatment consists of complete excision of the cyst and its tract in patients with infection or cosmetically unacceptable appearance. The procedure includes removal of the central portion of the hyoid bone plus a deep cone of midline tongue tissue. These steps have reduced the incidence of cyst recurrence greatly (from nearly 50 per cent in earlier years to less than 5 per cent).

The third most common congenital neck mass is *cystic hygroma* (often used synonymously with *lymphangioma*). This tumor is composed of lymphatic elements that are arranged like a cluster of grapes to form a soft, usually compressible mass that can be located at any level between the maxilla and the axilla. Typically, the mass is situated in the lower half of the neck and is noted during the neonatal period. Another pattern of presentation is that of a smaller mass located in the upper neck or lower portion of the face that becomes apparent after the age of 3 to 4 years.

Diagnosis is made on the basis of painless, progressive enlargement in size plus the typical physical findings. Treatment is surgical excision, with great care taken to avoid injury to important head and neck structures.

Salivary Gland Disease in Children

With the exception of mumps, salivary gland disorders are more common in adults than in children. Most pediatric salivary gland problems are characterized by painful swelling or a gradually enlarging mass. The parotid gland and the submandibular gland are both surrounded by capsules that tend to constrain any swelling or infection that arises within the gland. Each gland is composed of a set of lobulated glandular units that drain through a branching series of ducts into one main excretory duct. This arrangement predisposes the gland to recurrent infection if there is blockage of a major duct by inflammation or a stone. The sole function of the salivary glands is the production of saliva for hydration, lubrication, and digestion. Glandular secretion results from both sympathetic and parasympathetic stimulation.

The most common cause of parotid gland swelling in children is *acute viral parotitis*, or mumps, which is a febrile illness that causes painful parotid enlargement. Physical exam shows a red punctum (opening of duct inside cheek) with clear saliva. The disease is usually caused by mumps virus, but it may be caused by echovirus or coxsackievirus A. There is an 18- to 21-day incubation period after exposure. Often, all four salivary glands are involved, and important complications include encephalitis, orchitis, pancreatitis, and deafness (usually unilateral).

Lymphoma, sarcoidosis, and *granulomatous diseases* (tuberculosis, atypical mycobacteria, actinomycosis, or cat-scratch disease) are related pathologic changes involving adjacent lymph nodes, and any of these conditions may mimic salivary gland disease. There are also several endocrine and metabolic diseases (such as *Sjögren's syndrome, cystic fibrosis,* and *allergic disorders*) that may be difficult to differentiate from salivary gland disease.

Several noninfectious, primary, non-neoplastic diseases may cause swelling of the salivary gland in children. *Sialectasis* is a condition in which congenital, saccular degeneration of the smallest set of ducts causes stasis of the saliva and recurrent parotitis. The exacerbations are usually unilateral, last about a week, recur in 3 or 4 months, and generally are considered to be self-limiting. Diagnosis is by sialography, a radiographic dye study. *Sialolithiasis,* an inflammatory disease caused by an obstructing stone in the main duct, is more common in the submandibular salivary glands than in the parotid. Search for and removal of the offending stone is the management strategy.

Hemangioma and *lymphangioma* are the most common neoplasms of the salivary glands in children. *Benign mixed tumor* (pleomorphic adenoma) is essentially the only benign, solid, neoplastic mass in children.

Salivary Gland Disease in Adults

Sjögren's syndrome is characterized by a triad of xerostomia, keratoconjunctivitis, and a connective tissue disorder (usually rheumatoid arthritis). The presumptive diagnosis is made when two of these three features are present. On physical exam there is a dry mouth (xerostomia) secondary to a decrease in salivary flow. The parotid glands are enlarged bilaterally with a diffuse, firm, irregular contour. Fever and glandular tenderness are common. Patients complain of dryness of the eyes with a burning sensation and photosensitivity. On inspection, there is often a superficial ocular keratitis. Dryness and scaling of the skin are common. Diagnosis is confirmed by increased gammaglobulins, rheumatoid factor, and antinuclear antibodies. Biopsy of the lip will show histopathologic changes similar to those of the salivary glands (acinar atrophy, lymphocytic sialoadenitis, and ductal hyperplasia). Early treatment with corticosteroids is recommended.

Benign salivary gland neoplasms are characterized by the appearance of a slowly enlarging, painless mass in most instances. *Mixed tumor (pleomorphic adenoma)* is the most common. Salivary gland tumor represents about 65 per cent of all parotid tumors and 50 per cent of all submandibular gland neoplasms. Mixed tumors are more common in female patients and usually present during the fifth decade of life. They almost always are limited to the superficial lobe in the parotid, and superficial parotid lobectomy is nearly always curative.

Warthin's tumor represents about 5 per cent of all parotid tumors and is the second most common parotid neoplasm. It most frequently arises in older males and is felt as a rubbery, smooth mass in the tail of the gland (posteriorly and inferiorly). Surgical excision is curative in almost all instances.

Other important benign tumors are *oncocytoma, monomorphic adenoma,* and *sebaceous lymphadenoma.*

The most common malignancy of the parotid gland is *mucoepidermoid carcinoma,* a tumor that most often presents in middle-aged women. Surgical excision carries a 90 per cent 5-year survival for low-grade tumors and a 40 to 50 per cent 5-year survival for high-grade malignancy.

Adenoid cystic carcinoma is the most common malignant tumor of the submandibular and minor salivary glands. Sex distribution is about equal, and the patients are usually in their 40s. Treatment is surgical excision, but postoperative radiation therapy is employed frequently because of the high percentage of late tumor recurrence. About 40 per cent of these patients develop distant metastases (usually lungs): the 5-year survival is 65 per cent but the 20-year survival is only about 15 per cent.

Other significant malignant neoplasms include *acinous cell carcinoma, malignant mixed tumor* (or carcinoma ex pleomorphic adenoma), *squamous cell carcinoma, adenocarcinoma, undifferentiated carcinoma,* and *lymphoma.*

Salivary Gland Trauma

Salivary gland injuries are serious and frequently associated with long-term morbidity. Unfortunately, they often are overlooked or underestimated in patients who have suffered multiple trauma. These injuries are classified as *acute* (blunt, lacerating, penetrating, avulsion, or blast) or *chronic* (irritation from dentures, foreign bodies, stones, or irradiation). The origin of the injury may be primarily external, intraoral, or both. Careful history and thorough physical exam are necessary to clarify the exact injury to adjacent soft tissue, muscle, nerve, vascular tissues, and facial skeleton. A laceration of the salivary gland or main duct usually results in the presence of saliva in the wound. Ductal injuries should be repaired if at all possible prior to any efforts to repair concomitant facial lacerations (Bailey, 1993).

Facial nerve injuries are also of great importance, and careful assessment of facial muscle function is a high priority, with attention to the forehead, eyes, nose, and mouth. The patient should be asked to smile, show the teeth, pucker the lips, close eyes tightly, and wrinkle the forehead. All details should be recorded as soon as possible to avoid confusion concerning neurologic deficits that might occur at a somewhat later date after the injury (and therefore carry a different significance).

Penetrating wounds of the lower face carry a high potential for injury to the parotid or submandibular glands. Knife or shotgun wounds and human or animal bites place the area of wounding at risk for serious infection. In addition to the management of the initial injury, the job is not complete until tetanus prophylaxis (and rabies investigation in appropriate circumstances) has been considered.

The major point to be emphasized in assessing and treating lacerations around the parotid is that early recognition and repair of major salivary ducts or primary branches of the facial nerve is the key to a successful outcome (Fig. 23–17). This requires the use of microsurgical techniques, and referral injury is indicated by hemoptysis, hoarseness, crepitus, or sucking wounds. Pharyngeal–esophageal injury is suggested by dysphagia, crepitus, tachycardia, and fever. The findings with vascular injury are an expanding hematoma, central nervous system deficit, pulse deficit, thrills, bruits, shock, or persistent bleeding. Particular importance should be attached to hoarseness, cranial nerve deficit, or hemiplegia.

In addition to the careful history and physical exam, direct laryngoscopy may be necessary to rule out lacerations of the larynx or pharynx and injury of the recurrent laryngeal nerves.

Radiographic assessment of the pharynx or esophagus is accomplished by swallowing contrast material (thin barium still is used most commonly). Angiography is valuable for diagnosis and may be useful in treatment when embolizing techniques are needed. Even though nearly all (92 per cent) of the carotid arteriograms will be negative in these patients, this study is indicated in all patients with central neurologic findings (if their clinical status permits it) because of the importance of a positive finding.

In earlier years (prior to World War II), almost all patients were managed by careful observation and surgical intervention only if the patients' condition worsened. During World War II, a policy of mandatory neck exploration decreased the mortality from these wounds but carried a 60 per cent rate of negative explorations. Today the policy of selective exploration is employed based on the presence of any of the following:

1. Unstable vital signs.
2. Evidence of airway injury (hemoptysis, hoarseness, crepitus, or subcutaneous emphysema).
3. Evidence of pharyngeal–esophageal penetration (dysphagia, crepitus, positive contrast swallowing study).
4. Signs of vascular disruption (expanding hematoma, bruit, thrill, positive angiogram).
5. Neurologic deficit (cranial nerve deficit, hemiplegia, etc.).

Basically, surgical exploration is performed as a means of determining precisely the nature of the injury and of repairing nerves, vessels, and soft tissue of the airway and pharyngoesophageal passages. Maintaining a high degree of suspicion and pursuing the diagnostic steps promptly are the key elements of managing these patients appropriately.

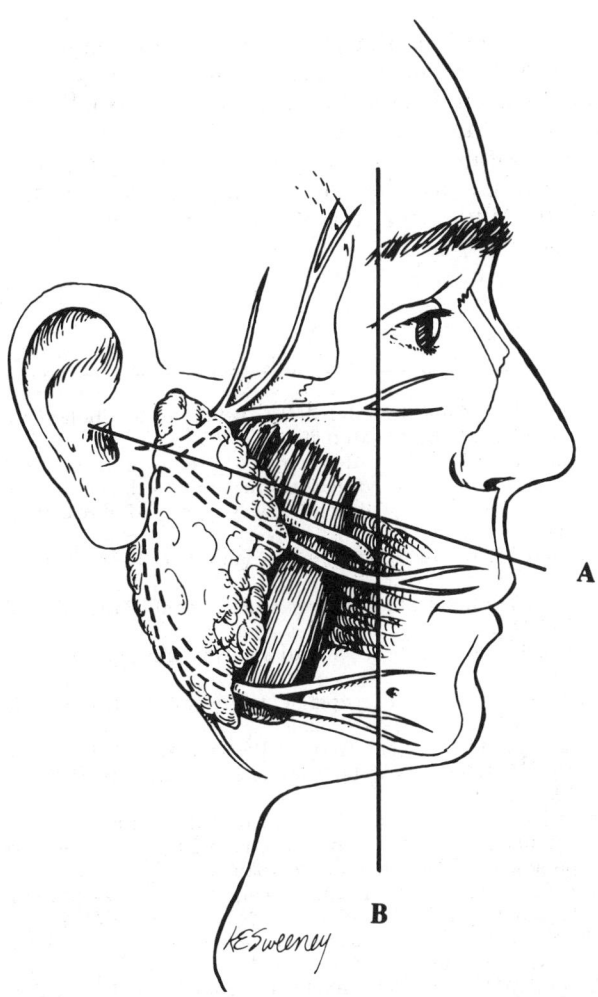

FIGURE 23–17. Treatment and repair of parotid lacerations. Line A, marking position of parotid duct, extends from tragus to middle of upper lip. Salivary duct occupies central third of this line. Buccal branch of facial nerve runs parallel to line A near duct. Line B runs from lateral canthus vertically to mental foramen. Fibers of the facial nerve anterior to line B need not be repaired and recover function if soft tissues are approximated accurately in layers. (From Cummings CW, Schuller DE, et al (eds): Otolaryngology—Head and Neck Surgery, Vol. 2. St. Louis, Mosby-Year Book, 1993, p 1022, with permission.)

to an otolaryngologist/head and neck surgeon is appropriate.

Penetrating Neck Injuries

Stab and gunshot wounds are the main causes of *penetrating neck injuries.* Emergency management of these patients focuses on protecting or restoring the airway, control of bleeding, and prevention or treatment of hypovolemic shock during the initial minutes of stabilization and evaluation.

Attention then is focused on assessment of the exact nature of the deeper injuries, with particular attention to systems that may be disrupted. Airway

Thyroid Nodules

Thyroid nodules most often are due to single or multiple colloid goiter. Other causes include thyroglossal duct cysts, toxic nodular goiter, adenomas, and thyroid carcinoma. Benign tumors must be differentiated from thyroid malignancies. Palpation of a thyroid nodule should be followed by fine-needle aspiration or open biopsy to determine the histology of the lesion.

Thyroid Carcinoma

Thyroid carcinoma arises from either epithelial or medullary tissue. Epithelial carcinomas are of three types: papillary, follicular, and anaplastic. The great majority of lesions are papillary; both follicular and anaplastic lesions are unusual. Anaplastic lesions are seen most commonly in elderly patients and have a very poor prognosis. Most other thyroid malignancies are treated surgically and have a relatively favorable prognosis.

REFERENCES

Bailey BJ: Management of maxillofacial trauma. Res Staff Physician December:57:23, 1982.

Bailey BJ: Management of sinus infections. Am Fam Physician 7(6):100, 1973.

Bailey BJ: Trauma. In Cummings CW, Frederickson JM, et al (eds): Otolaryngology–Head and Neck Surgery, Vol. 2. St. Louis, CV Mosby, 1993, pp 1018–1028.

Bass JW: Treatment of streptococcal pharyngitis revisited. JAMA 256:740, 1986.

Bell DN: Otitis externa: A common, often self-inflicted condition. Postgrad Med 78:101, 1985.

Black B: Cleaning the ear. Aust Fam Physician 15:1354, 1986.

Bluestone C, Klein J: Otitis Media in Infants and Children. Philadelphia, WB Saunders Company, 1988, pp 217–229.

Bodor FF: Conjunctivitis-otitis syndrome. Pediatrics 69:695, 1982.

Busse WW: Chronic rhinitis: A systematic approach to diagnosis and treatment. Postgrad Med 73:325, 1983.

Cantekin EI, Mandel EM, Bluestone CD, et al: Lack of efficacy of a decongestant-antihistamine combination for otitis media with effusion in children. N Engl J Med 308:298, 1983.

Carlin SA, Marchant CD, Shurin PA, et al: Early recurrences of otitis media: Reinfection or relapse? J Pediatr 110:20, 1987.

Clark WW, Bohne BA: The effects of noise on hearing and the ear. Med Times December:17fm, 1984.

Dayal VS: Clinical Otolaryngology. Philadelphia, JB Lippincott, 1981, p 213.

DeNeef P: Comparison of tests for streptococcal pharyngitis. J Fam Pract 23:551, 1986.

DeWitt DE: Fiberoptic rhinolaryngoscopy in primary care. Postgrad Med 84:125, 1988.

Fischer PM, Mentrup PL: Comparison of throat culture and latex agglutination test for streptococcal pharyngitis. J Fam Pract 22:245, 1986.

Ghory JE: OME: Leading cause of preventable hearing loss. J Respir Dis 3:127, 1982.

Guralnick W, Kaban LB, Merrill RG: Temporomandibular-joint afflictions. N Engl J Med 299:123, 1978.

Henderson FW, Collier AM, Sanyal MA, et al: A longitudinal study of respiratory viruses and bacteria in the etiology of acute otitis media with effusion. N Engl J Med 306:1277, 1982.

Johnson JT: Indirect laryngoscopy. Fam Pract Recert 6(9):23, 1984.

Johnson JT, Rood SR: Epistaxis management. Postgrad Med 70:231, 1981.

Kern EB: Suppurative (bacterial) sinusitis. Postgrad Med 81:194, 1988.

Kirchner JA: Current concepts in otolaryngology: Epistaxis. N Engl J Med 307:1126, 1982.

Mandel JH: Pharyngeal infections. Postgrad Med 77:187, 1985.

Marcy SM: Infections of the external ear. Pediatr Infect Dis 4:192, 1985.

McMillan JA, Sandstrom C, Weiner LB, et al: Viral and bacterial organisms associated with acute pharyngitis in a school-aged population. J Pediatr 109:747, 1986.

Meyerhoff WL: Diagnosis and Management of Hearing Loss. Philadelphia, WB Saunders Company. 1984, pp 74–75.

Olsen KD: Facial nerve paralysis: General evaluation, Bell's palsy. Postgrad Med 75:219, 1984.

Paparella MM, Shumrick DA: Otolaryngology, Vol. II: The Ear. Philadelphia, WB Saunders Company, 1980, pp 1354–1357.

Rose DE: Noise and hearing loss. Postgrad Med 70:119, 1981.

Schuknecht HF: Further observations on presbycusis. Arch Otolaryngol 80:369, 1964.

Slater R: Vertigo: How serious are recurrent and single attacks? Postgrad Med 84:58, 1988.

Strome M, Kelly JH, Fried MP, et al: Manual of Otolaryngology: Diagnosis and Therapy. Boston, Little, Brown, 1985, pp 4–7.

Talaat AM, El-Dibany MM, El-Garf A: Physical therapy in the management of myofacial pain dysfunction syndrome. Ann Otol Rhinol 95:225, 1986.

CHAPTER 24

ALLERGY

PAUL P. VanARSDEL, Jr. and GREG L. LEDGERWOOD

DEFINITION AND CLASSIFICATION

Originally, immunology meant the study of immunity: the resistance to microbial infection acquired as a result of natural or deliberate exposure. Such immunity can be mediated either by circulating antibody, by cells (T lymphocytes), or by both. In any event, the reaction is with the organism or antigenic substance involved. This is called *specific immunity*. The scope of immunology expanded in the last century when scientists began to inject foreign proteins into animals and humans to produce active or passive immunity. Unanticipated adverse reactions occurred. Portier and Richet described anaphylaxis in 1902 in dogs. With Schick, von Pirquet described serum sickness in 1905 and coined the word *allergy* in 1906.

Today, the word *anaphylaxis* generally is used as it was originally, to designate an acquired adverse reactivity to a foreign substance, manifested by the rapid onset of generalized symptoms that may be fatal. It also may be applied to any reaction caused by antigen-induced mediator release, even a positive immediate-type skin test (see later). *Allergy*, in contrast, has acquired a broader connotation. Any injurious reaction caused by acquired sensitivity (appearance of specific blood antibody or T cell) is an allergic reaction. Some prefer the word *hypersensitivity*, feeling that the meaning of the term *allergy* has degenerated through inappropriate usage. *Atopy* was coined in the early 1920s to designate a subset of allergic patients who had acquired sensitivity to environmental substances (pollens, mold spores, house dust, animal danders, foods, and so on) that were innocuous for most people. This type of sensitivity is familial and is manifested most often by asthma, allergic rhinitis, and infantile eczema, affecting from 15 to 20 per cent of the population. The mode of genetic transmission is complex (Marsh and Bias, 1988).

What has happened to the word *immunology* since the 19th century? It is now used for all conditions ("immunologic diseases") in which antibodies/T cells are helpful, harmful, or deficient. The first category, representing the original basis for immunology, is a component of preventive medicine and is covered in that chapter.

Coombs and Gell (1975) enhanced our under-standing of harmful allergic reactions by developing a well-known classification that has come into general medical use (Table 24-1). The most frequent problems faced by the clinical allergist are in Type I reactions (immediate hypersensitivity). When exposed to antigens ("allergens") by inhalation, ingestion, or injection, allergic patients develop vascular dilation, edema, glandular hypersecretion, and smooth muscle spasm; symptoms may be local (asthma, hay fever) or systemic (urticaria, anaphylactic shock). These symptoms are produced by the reaction of allergens with specific antibodies of the immunoglobulin (Ig) E class that are bound to receptors on tissue mast cells and blood basophils, resulting in a release of chemical mediators. Some are pre-formed (histamine, chemotactic factors) while others (leukotrienes, platelet-activating factor) are newly generated from membrane lipids and are extremely potent. Platelet activating factor (PAF) may be 1000 times as potent as histamine and is produced by human mast cells as well as neutrophils, monocytes, and platelets (Serafin and Austen, 1987).

Type II reactions are primarily hematologic and are usually complement dependent; allergic drug reactions may or may not be. Penicillin can induce hemolytic anemia in patients who develop antibodies to red cell–bound penicillin determinants without complement activation. In contrast, methyldopa can result in a complement-dependent autoimmune reaction through the production of antibodies with Rh specificity (VanArsdel, 1988).

Type III reactions produce various antigen–antibody complex diseases. Systemic lupus erythematosus is the prime example. Although most type III reactions are autoimmune, some, such as bacterial endocarditis, involve microbial antigens. With most of the nonhuman (xenogeneic) therapeutic antitoxic sera having been supplanted by those of human origin, most serum sickness now occurs in transplant patients receiving antithymocyte globulin.

Finally, type IV reactions are dependent on the acquisition of specific sensitivity by the T (i.e., thymus-derived) lymphocytes. Such cell-mediated sensitivity is an exaggeration of the normal host protective responses to foreign substances. It can result in contact dermatitis when low-molecular-

TABLE 24–1. THE COOMBS AND GELL CLASSIFICATION OF ALLERGIC REACTIONS

Type	Antigen	Antibody	Mechanism	Clinical Problems
I	Free, soluble	IgE-bound to mast cells, basophils	Release or synthesis of several potent chemical mediators	Anaphylaxis, allergic rhinitis
II	Cellular, or bound to cells	Circulating IgG, IgM, complement activation	Complement-induced tissue injury	Transfusion reactions, autoimmune anemia
III	Bound to antibody in blood as complex lattice	Circulating IgG, IgM, complement activation	Complement-induced tissue injury	Serum sickness, systemic lupus erythematosus
IV	Any, except polysaccharides	None	Sensitive T lymphocytes release mediators ("lymphokines")	Contact dermatitis, tissue graft reactions

Adapted from Coombs RRA, Gell PGH: Classification of allergic reactions responsible for clinical hypersensitivity and disease. *In* Gell PGH, Coombs RRA (eds): Clinical Aspects of Immunology, 3rd edition. Oxford, England, Blackwell Scientific Publications, 1975, pp 761–781.

weight chemicals in contact with the skin conjugate with skin proteins to become active sensitizers, and is also responsible in part for tissue graft rejection.

GENERAL EVALUATION OF THE PATIENT

The *history* is usually the most important component in the evaluation of a patient suspected of having an allergic problem. When interviewing a new patient, the physician should take pains to identify any previous allergic problems in the patient and also allergy in close family members. This is particularly helpful in providing support for the diagnosis of an atopic disease. A careful search of environmental factors should be undertaken. Variation in symptoms with the seasons and with changes in location should be recorded carefully. The patient should be questioned in detail regarding the home environment: location, type of heating, type and quality of construction, insulation, humidity, nature of furnishings, draperies and bedding, pets and their habits, method of house cleaning, cigarette smoking, and so on. The work environment must be examined for air pollution, other exposure to chemical irritants or sensitizers, physical demands, and job stresses. Sometimes the patient's clothing habits must be recorded, and a dietary history should not be overlooked—especially in children. Finally, previous and present use of drugs should be noted, including laxatives, antacids, and other over-the-counter remedies that the patient may not recognize as drugs.

Most allergic problems involve the skin or respiratory tract, and these should receive the most attention on the *physical examination*. The location of skin lesions as well as their description should be recorded, and urticarial lesions, if present, should be outlined in ink to aid in determining if they are evanescent or persistent. The nose is often overlooked or is given only a cursory examination. The color and degree of swelling of its mucous membrane, the amount and consistency of secre-

tions, and the presence or absence of polyps (not to be confused with turbinates!) should be noted. The lungs, if free of rales, should be examined during forced expiration, which may bring out asthmatic wheezing.

The atopic child may have dark circles under the eyes ("allergic shiners") and a transverse crease above the tip of the nose from frequent nose rubbing. Of particular importance in children is the observation of the tympanic membrane and its motility using a tympanometer and/or the pneumatic otoscope (see below). Sinusitis can be present at the initial evaluation. Mucopurulent discharge from the nares or seen in the posterior pharynx raises the possibility of the same. Occult sinusitis can be identified further either with a plain radiograph using a Waters view or, in more complex cases, a limited coronal computerized tomography (CT) scan of the sinus cavities.

A few general *laboratory* procedures may be helpful, such as the nasal or sputum smear, which should be examined for eosinophils. Eosinophils are best visualized with an eosin–methylene blue stain (Hansel's). Blood eosinophilia is helpful if present, but its absence does not exclude allergic disease. The measurement of total serum IgE is of limited value and rarely worth the expense.

For further evaluation of obstructive airways disease, several recording spirometers that are simple, durable, and accurate are available. We use the Vitalograph spirometer extensively for the purposes of (1) confirming or ruling out airway disease, (2) establishing the degree of response to an inhaled bronchodilator, and (3) monitoring the progress of the patient. Several inexpensive peak flow meters are also available for monitoring patients' progress.

Provocation testing involves the measurement of ventilatory function before or after some stimulus. It can be used by most physicians as an aid in diagnosing exercise bronchospasm. However, the methacholine provocation test, which is useful in doubtful situations to confirm or exclude the diagnosis of asthma in general, is time consuming and rather risky, so is best left to experienced laboratories.

Skin testing should be selective and based on clues provided by the history whenever possible. In adults testing is limited to pollens, house dust (dust mite), feathers, animal danders, and mold spores. If the history is suggestive, skin tests to some foods also may be done. Food testing is more useful in young children. The *prick test* is performed by placing a drop of 1:10 or 1:20 allergen extract on the skin and then "tenting" up the skin under the drop with the tip of a lancet or small needle until the tip pops free. The excess allergen is blotted off and the site is inspected for the development of a wheal-and-erythema reaction 15 minutes later. The prick test is sufficiently sensitive to identify practically all pollen or food allergies. However, the intradermal test may be needed to identify dust mite, dander, or mold allergens. This is performed by injecting just enough of a dilute, sterile solution (prepared by the manufacturer specifically for intradermal testing) to produce a 1- to 2-mm bleb. The positive result again is a whealing reaction that should have a diameter of at least 5 mm but preferably 10 mm greater than that of the control.

Specific IgE antibodies to a variety of antigens can be measured using the radioallergosorbent test (RAST), but this test is expensive and provides no more information than skin testing. The physician who is not equipped to do skin testing may get helpful information by sending a patient's serum to a laboratory that does the RAST, but results are not always reliable.

Some other procedures purported to identify allergy, particularly food allergy, have received considerable attention recently in the lay press. These are cytotoxic testing, subcutaneous or sublingual provocation testing, and neutralization testing. None of these has been established as reliable in properly controlled trials (VanArsdel and Larson, 1989).

THE ROLE OF THE FAMILY PHYSICIAN IN ALLERGY DIAGNOSIS AND MANAGEMENT

Never in the recent history of medicine has a field such as allergy, with its basis in immunology, expanded so much in scientific development and in treatment options as in the last two decades. Unfortunately, the field of allergy also has been subject to a comparable expansion in questionable practices, including the inappropriate or controversial use of new technology. The family physician is deluged with new information on a daily basis. With this new information, the family physician's role in diagnosing and treating allergic conditions has expanded greatly. Reference laboratories have provided "kits" for allergy testing, and "in-house" evaluation studies utilizing RAST methods are all too commonplace. It therefore becomes important for the family physician to understand the limitations of the testing when applied to the allergic patient. Foremost in importance should be the careful history and physical examination and the use of appropriate medications prior to even considering diagnostic testing such as RAST or skin testing. Even in qualified hands, these tests alone are not diagnostic because they are subject to interpretation of the person performing the test, and can lead the most well-meaning physician astray. The family physician can manage a great deal of the allergic problems presented to him or her, but, when conservative methods fail to control symptoms, one must consider referral to an appropriate allergy specialist.

ALLERGIC RHINITIS

Allergic rhinitis is a symptom complex caused by airborne antigens. It occurs as *seasonal rhinitis* (hay fever) when pollens are in high concentration in the air. It may be intermittent or continuous without seasonal variation, and then is termed *perennial allergic rhinitis*. Occurring often in families with an allergic history and estimated to occur in 8 to 10 per cent of the population under 20 years of age, seasonal allergic rhinitis was found to occur twice as commonly as perennial allergic rhinitis (Broder et al., 1974).

Manifestations

In *seasonal allergic rhinitis*, exposure is followed by complaints of paroxysmal sneezing, a watery nasal discharge with congestion, and nasal itching. Conjunctival and pharyngeal itching is often present. Less specific symptoms are postnasal drainage with a sense of fullness or aching in the frontal areas.

In children, nasal irritation may result in nose picking and recurrent epistaxis. Parents may complain of restless sleeping, snoring, or nighttime coughing associated with postnasal mucus drainage and mild hoarseness. As a result of a lack of smell, appetite may be decreased. An allergic "salute" may be present as seen by the upward thrust of the palm against the nares to relieve itching and to open the nasal airways. A gaping expression from mouth breathing is common, as are "allergic shiners" (described previously). Denne's line (a wrinkle beneath the lower lid) is described as being associated with allergic rhinitis and atopic dermatitis. Speech may have a nasal quality. The nasal mucosa is typically moist, with enlarged pale turbinates and serous discharge.

In *perennial allergic rhinitis*, nasal congestion, itching, obstruction, and the need to sniff constantly may be associated with a loss of sense of taste or smell and a feeling of being "stuffed up," with decreased hearing and a popping sensation in the ears. A lower sneezing threshold often occurs with altered autonomic reflexes in perennial allergic rhinitis such that paroxysms of sneezing and rhinorrhea may result from changes in ambient temperature, head movement, odors, perfume, tobacco smoke, irritants, alcohol, and exposure to small quantities of antigen. Exercise reverses nasal congestion temporarily, from minutes to hours.

The turbinates are usually swollen and edematous, and may be mistaken for nasal polyps, which are pearl-gray gelatinous masses unusual in uncomplicated allergic rhinitis. Below the turbinates, the floor of the nostril is often prominent as a result of mucosal edema. In one third to one half of children with allergic rhinitis, eustachian tube obstruction may be present, with resultant serous otitis. Otoscopy may reveal a retracted or bulging tympanic membrane, impaired mobility, or a fluid level. In patients with intact tympanic membranes, tympanometry to measure middle ear pressures provides an indirect measure of eustachian tube function (Bluestone and Cantekin, 1981). The edematous nasal mucosa may obstruct sinus ostia, resulting in congestion or sinusitis with pressure symptoms or headache, particularly notable when bending down.

Diagnosis

A seasonal history or, even better, an association with an inhaled allergen, is helpful. It is often difficult to associate specific allergens with perennial rhinitis. Occasionally, a change in environment, such as a vacation, may point to the existence of environmental allergens. For confirmation of an allergic state, a smear of nasal secretions is made easily by having the patient blow the nose directly onto a sheet of plastic, with transfer of secretions to a glass slide, which is then stained with Hansel's stain. An eosinophil count greater than 10 per cent of the total white cells indicates a probable allergic cause, while 80 to 90 per cent eosinophils are diagnostic of an allergic state. A peripheral eosinophil count, when elevated, is helpful; however, this is of limited use because marked allergic symptoms can occur in the absence of blood eosinophilia.

Treatment of Allergic Rhinitis

Nonspecific

Removal of exposure to known allergens is of prime importance, because this will eliminate symptoms. When exposure is unavoidable, *environmental control* should reduce symptoms and prevent exacerbations. General measures such as the use of an air conditioner or electronic filters can reduce the number of particulate allergens.

The use of a mask over the nose and mouth with replaceable microfoam filters significantly reduces the effects of a temporary exposure to inhaled allergens.

It is the patient or the family who must assume responsibility for environmental control, so it is helpful to provide an understanding of allergens. Commonly inhaled allergens include pollens, which are widely recognized as producing symptoms of seasonal allergic rhinitis, conjunctivitis, and asthma. Allergenic pollens may derive from tree, grass, and weed sources. Pollens from flowering plants are insect borne and are not generally important allergens. In general, there is a direct relationship between pollen exposure and allergic symptoms. However, the intensity of reaction to pollen exposure is increased by recent exposure to other allergens, which appear to "prime" the nasal mucosa. Hence, the best indication of intensity is the symptom, not the pollen count. Pollen prevalence commonly is determined by the use of "gravity" slides, which sample pollen fallout without regard to environmental wind direction, speed, and turbulence, so that reports of pollen prevalence in daily news media often do not reflect the true concentration in the air or individual exposure. Inhaled fungal allergens in fungus-sensitive subjects may produce seasonal symptoms during situations that promote fungal growth, such as humid and rainy weather and exposure to hay, mulches, commercial peat moss, compost piles, and leaf litter. Indoors, areas of spore formation can be identified at sites of water condensation, such as shower curtains, window moldings, and damp basements. In addition, it may be important to recognize that "cool-mist" vaporizers can be contaminated and serve as sources of fungal contamination.

A prime role for the patient and family is in the environmental control of house dust, which, although a heterogeneous mixture of bacteria, fibrous matter of plant and animal origin, human epidermis, food remnants, fungi, insect debris, and animal danders, contains one major source of antigen, the dust mite. Mites are ubiquitous in households and are most prevalent in bedding, mattresses, carpeting, and upholstered furniture, particularly where warmth and humidity are high (Platts-Mills and Chapman, 1987). Animal allergens are derived from dried saliva on the shed fur of cats, rodent urine, and epidermal material from farm animals. The allergic respiratory reactions produced by animal allergens are species specific. Finished furs and wood are not allergenic. Feathers are often nonallergenic when fresh and produce allergic symptoms only after degradation. A careful history to identify environmental allergens is an important element in advising avoidance and treatment. When explanations for allergic exacerbations are provided by the physician to the patient, frustration can be decreased.

Control of Symptoms

Antihistamines are effective for symptomatic control of allergic rhinitis, whether seasonal or perennial. For optimal results, they should be used before exposure to the know allergen. Complete control may not be achieved with many patients who use antihistamines only sporadically. During the implicated season, an around-the-clock administration provides maximal symptomatic relief. To improve compliance and to encourage continued use, one should explain that mild drowsiness and other side effects may subside after a few days of continual antihistamine therapy. If more significant side effects occur, such as somnolence, excitation, nervousness, palpitations, and dryness of the mouth, the dose might be reduced or the patient switched to one of the new nonsedating antihistamines. The newer nonsedating antihistamines (terfenadine, astemizole, loratidine) generally provide excellent control of symptoms for patients greater than 12 years of age. Care must be taken to instruct patients using terfenadine and astemizole to avoid concomitant use of these agents with erythromycin or antifungal drugs such as ketoconazole (possible cardiac arrhythmias). If allergic rhinitis is associated with asthma, antihistamines should be used with care during acute attacks of asthma because they occasionally worsen the inspissation of bronchial secretions.

In general, antihistamines are less effective alone than when used in combination with α-adrenergic decongestant drugs in controlling nasal obstruction, which may be the main problem in chronic perennial allergic rhinitis. α-Adrenergic drugs are effective not only in combination with antihistamines but also topically. Topical vasoconstrictors (sprays and drops) are best restricted to temporary use (e.g., when taking an airplane trip or during a severe temporary flare-up of symptoms). For more sustained control of chronic nasal obstruction unresponsive to oral antihistamines–decongestants, the topical glucocorticoids beclomethasone and flunisolide are effective, and they produce no adrenal suppression when properly used. Their therapeutic effects are not immediate. This should be explained to the patient in order to ensure cooperation and continuation of treatment. One to 3 weeks may be required for some patients to achieve maximum benefit. If no improvement is evident by 3 to 4 weeks, the glucocorticoid should be discontinued. When symptoms are severe and nonresponsive to trials of therapy as outlined previously, oral glucocorticoid therapy can be used as a last resort and only for limited duration, as for the remainder of a pollen season. The rationale for glucocorticoid therapy for allergic rhinitis is that the condition, although IgE antibody mediated, has a dual component: the immediate phase of edema and hypersecretion and a late inflammatory phase (Bascom et al., 1988). This dual reaction occurs in asthma as well (see later in this chapter).

Specific Therapy

On identification by skin tests of sensitivity to an unavoidable inhalant allergen, immunotherapy may be indicated in the treatment of allergic rhinitis. Its efficacy has been shown to be 80 per cent for pollen symptom control and 60 per cent for molds and house dust symptom control. It is therefore more effective in seasonal allergic rhinitis than perennial allergic rhinitis. In the consideration of the use of immunotherapy, the ease of control of other therapy should be weighed in respect to the frequency and severity of symptoms.

NASAL POLYPS

Perennial allergic rhinitis may be associated with nasal polyps, but usually only when complicated by sinus infection. In the adult, the presence of polyps may be associated with a sensitivity to aspirin manifested by aggravation of rhinitis, asthma, and even shock. Nasal polyps often develop in the absence of, or only coincidentally with, allergy. They arise from infected ethmoid or maxillary sinuses and are easily visible in the nasal cavity. They can cause obstruction and aggravate the pre-existing sinus disease. The size of nasal polyps may be reduced by treating briefly with systemic glucocorticoids or by using topical glucocorticoids two or three times daily for 3 or 4 weeks and then once daily for a longer period. If sinus infection or the underlying allergic factors are not controlled appropriately, polypectomy may be necessary. Unfortunately, this procedure, without sinus surgery, often is not curative, and polyps tend to recur.

SINUSITIS

Chronic allergic rhinitis predisposes to sinus disease, although, as implied previously, sinus disease can develop in the absence of allergy. Acute sinusitis is characterized by a persistent rhinorrhea, postnasal drip, purulent drip, purulent discharge after an upper respiratory tract infection, and a dull throbbing pain over the affected sinus, with fever. In younger children the ethmoid sinuses commonly are involved, while in older children and adults the maxillary and frontal sinuses are infected most frequently. Such acute sinusitis usually is caused by bacterial infection and associated with pain and pressure over sinuses, headaches, and fever. When complicating allergic rhinitis, sinus disease may be associated with a sore throat, middle ear disease, and characteristically a persistent cough, especially at night. Periorbital edema, facial pallor, and circles under the eyes may be striking. The nasal mucosa is covered with purulent discharge, and a coexisting serous otitis may be present.

With persistent postnasal discharge, bacterial seeding from infected sinuses may result in recurrent bronchitis. Examination of the chest may reveal some wheezing resulting from a reflex bronchospasm. In the presence of acute bacterial sinusitis, the nasal smear will show a large number of neutrophils rather than the eosinophils of preexisting allergic disease. Transillumination of the sinuses, although helpful, is not always reliable. Sinus radiographs may reveal opacification, an air–fluid level, or marked membrane thickening. However, even in the presence of severe allergic mucosal edema with or without secretions, radiologic changes may be minimal. Occasionally, a limited coronal CT of the sinus cavities is very helpful in situations in which a definitive diagnosis is mandated either by worsening of symptoms or asthma refractory to standard therapy, or in which surgery has been contemplated previously. Chronic antihistamine therapy and topical glucocorticoids may be helpful in preventing recurrent episodes of sinusitis in patients with chronic allergic rhinitis.

EOSINOPHILIC NONALLERGIC RHINITIS

Some patients with perennial rhinitis are not atopic by history or skin testing. Chronic nasal obstruction is the predominating symptom, and the condition may be associated with sinus disease and nasal polyps. Although there is no evidence of allergy by skin testing, numerous eosinophils are present, and the diagnosis is made readily by examining the nasal secretions for eosinophils (Mullarkey, 1988). The condition is also called nonallergic rhinitis with eosinophilia (NARES). Topical glucocorticoid therapy is much more effective than antihistamines or decongestants. As with asthmatics, the patients with associated sinus disease and nasal polyps are at risk for adverse reactions to aspirin and nonsteroidal anti-inflammatory agents.

VASOMOTOR RHINITIS

A substantial number of patients have chronic rhinitis with rhinorrhea, postnasal drainage, and chronic or intermittent nasal obstruction. Symptoms are aggravated by many factors of a physical or irritating character, such as cold air, odors, and smoke. Skin tests are negative, and there are no eosinophils in the tissues or secretions. No drug therapy is particularly satisfactory, although some patients benefit from antihistamine–decongestant combinations, and occasionally topical glucocorticoids. The regular use of buffered saline lavage may be the most satisfactory treatment.

ALLERGY IN THE EYE

Conjunctivitis is the usual ocular reaction to airborne allergens. Itching is the first symptom and may be associated with lacrimation. Dilation of the conjunctival blood vessels produces a "red" eye. Transudation of fluid through vessel walls results in edema of the conjunctiva, while exuded cells with increased glandular mucus secretion result in ocular "discharge." In most atopic patients, conjunctivitis and allergic rhinitis occur together, but some may be bothered only by the eye symptoms. In contrast to other forms of conjunctivitis, the secretions contain eosinophils.

Vernal conjunctivitis is so called because of its occurrence in spring and summer months. It is characterized by a bilateral recurrent inflammation of the conjunctiva. Vernal conjunctivitis commonly occurs between the ages of 5 and 20 years. It often spontaneously resolves in 5 to 10 years. More than 50 per cent of children with vernal conjunctivitis also have an atopic disorder such as allergic rhinitis, eczema, or asthma. Acute itching, tearing, and photophobia occur with excess mucus production. Frequently a sense of a foreign body in the eye is present. The topical conjunctival appearance as described establishes the diagnosis, which is confirmed by cytologic smears showing numerous eosinophils. In the tarsal (palpebral) form, there are flat-topped cobblestone papillae; in the limbal form, gelatinous hypertrophy may be present, with limbal papillary hypertrophy frequently associated with white dots (Trantas' spots). Despite the seasonal nature and the predilection for atopic patients, no allergens have been identified as causal or aggravating factors.

The usual therapy of atopic conjunctivitis is an oral antihistamine and a topical decongestant. Cromolyn (4% ophthalmic solution) is also effective, particularly in preventing the development of anticipated symptoms. Both ketorolac and lodoxamide ophthalmic solution also have been shown to be effective. However, regular daily use is necessary to obtain maximum positive results. Contact lenses should not be worn. In severe cases, and in vernal conjunctivitis, a soluble steroid such as a fluorometholone ophthalmic solution is effective. The dose should be titrated to the minimum required to control symptoms. Use should be intermittent, because glucocorticoids can lead to the development of cataracts, can potentiate secondary bacterial infection or a herpes simplex keratitis, and can increase intraocular pressure.

The eyelids rather than the conjunctiva are likely to be involved in angioedema or urticaria. Contact (type IV) allergy may be caused by various chemicals that may be conveyed by the fingers to the eyelids. Obviously, however, contact allergy to ophthalmic solutions will involve the conjunctiva as well as the eyelids.

ASTHMA

Asthma is a reversible obstructive disorder of the tracheobronchial tree characterized by paroxysmal episodes of respiratory distress often interspersed with periods of apparent well-being. However, asthma is also an inflammatory process involving mucosal edema, mucus production, and increased vascular permeability. It can begin at any age, but most often appears in childhood. It commonly has a familial predisposition; the majority of childhood-onset cases begin between 3 and 6 years of age, and the onset often is associated with a respiratory infection. When onset is early, prognosis is excellent and most patients improve at puberty. Until puberty, asthma is twice as common among men as women. This distribution reverses between puberty and early adulthood, so that, among adults with asthma, women are affected more frequently than men. In many children who have outgrown asthma in puberty, there may be a recurrence of asthmatic symptoms later in life. When asthma appears in the adult, remission is less common than in children.

Asthma can be separated conveniently by etiologic factors into two main groups, as seen in Table 24–2. In *intrinsic asthma* (most commonly seen in adults), symptoms are provoked and worsened by infection, exertion, emotion, and nonspecific environmental factors and are not related to allergen exposure. The majority of *extrinsic* asthma patients are atopic, with symptoms related to environmental allergens. The remaining nonatopic patients have extrinsic asthma related to occupational factors.

The *Guidelines for the Diagnosis and Management of Asthma* published in August of 1991 under sponsorship of the National Institutes of Health (Expert Panel Report, 1991), followed by the *International Consensus Report on Diagnosis and Treatment of Asthma* in March 1992 under the same sponsorship, have set the standard for diagnosis and treatment of this disease (Table 24–3).

Pathophysiology

The characteristic physiologic change in asthma is airway obstruction caused by bronchial smooth muscle spasm, mucous plugging, edema, and inflammation of the bronchial wall. As a result of such airway narrowing, inspiration and expiration are impeded. Obstruction to air flow results in air trapping and hyperinflation of lungs. Smooth muscle spasm can occur in the large, medium, or small airways. This airway hyperreactivity is associated with, and probably aggravated by injury to and loss of, the epithelial cell lining. Biochemical mediators so far identified in these events include histamine, a variety of enzymes, and chemotactic factors (important in the late phase), as well as newly generated mediators of the arachidonic acid pathway—prostaglandins, leukotrienes, and PAFs (Creticos, 1992). When large airways are involved (50 per cent of asthmatic patients), wheezing predominates. When small airways are involved, the predominant symptoms are dyspnea and cough rather than wheezing.

With air flow obstruction during an asthmatic attack, there is an increase in residual volume and a decrease in vital capacity proportionate to the degree of severity. With uneven airway obstruction in various parts of the lung, air flow is not uniform, while blood perfusion of the lungs continues through the poorly ventilated segments. The result is arterial hypoxemia as seen in a reduced PaO_2. In subclinical asthma, the PaO_2 may be the only abnormality. In mild to moderate asthma, ventilation rate is increased and $PaCO_2$ is reduced while the pH remains normal, expressing compensated respiratory alkalosis. In more severe attacks, with impending respiratory failure, there is alveolar hy-

TABLE 24–2. CLINICAL FEATURES OF EXTRINSIC AND INTRINSIC ASTHMA

	Extrinsic Asthma		Intrinsic Asthma (Idiopathic)
	Atopic	Nonatopic	
Age of onset	Usually childhood	Adult	Usually after age 25
Symptoms	Variable with environment and season	Usually occupation related	Unpredictable fluctuations, often chronic
Associated conditions	Allergic rhinitis, atopic dermatitis	None	Bronchitis, sinusitis, nasal polyps
Family history of atopic disease	Strong	Minor	Asthma only (?)
Skin tests (wheal-erythema)	Several positive, related to history	Negative, or one reaction only	Usually negative
Total IgE	High	Usually normal	Normal
Eosinophilia	High during allergen exposure	Sometimes high during allergen exposure	High
Prognosis	Good, especially with allergen avoidance	Good, especially with allergen avoidance	Fair, remissions uncommon

TABLE 24–3. CLASSIFICATION OF ASTHMA SEVERITY*

Asthma Severity	Clinical Features before Treatment	Lung Function†	Regular Medication Usually Required to Maintain Control
Mild	• Intermittent, brief symptoms <1–2 times a week • Nocturnal asthma symptoms <2 times a month • Asymptomatic between exacerbations	• PEF >80% predicted at baseline • PEF variability <20% • PEF normal after bronchodilator	• Intermittent inhaled short acting beta$_2$-agonist (taken as needed) only
Moderate	• Exacerbations >1–2 times a week • Nocturnal asthma symptoms >2 times a month • Symptoms requiring inhaled beta$_2$-agonist almost daily	• PEF 60–80% predicted at baseline • PEF variability 20–30% • PEF normal after bronchodilator	• Daily inhaled anti-inflammatory agent • Possibly a daily long-acting bronchodilator, especially for nocturnal symptoms
Severe	• Frequent exacerbations • Continuous symptoms • Frequent nocturnal asthma symptoms • Physical activities limited by asthma • Hospitalization for asthma in previous year‡ • Previous life-threatening exacerbation‡	• PEF <60% predicted at baseline • PEF variability >30% • PEF below normal despite optimal therapy	• Daily inhaled anti-inflammatory agent at high doses • Daily long-acting bronchodilator, especially for nocturnal symptoms • Frequent use of systemic corticosteroids

Notes:

The characteristics noted in this table are general, and the characteristics may overlap because asthma is highly variable. Furthermore, an individual's classification may change over time.

One or more features may be present to be assigned a grade of severity.

An individual should usually be assigned to the most severe grade in which any feature occurs.

Once the minimum medication required to maintain control of asthma has been identified, then this medication requirement reflects the overall severity of the condition.

† PEF, peak expiratory flow.

‡ The potential severity—related to a patient's past history (for example, a previous life-threatening exacerbation or a hospitalization for asthma in the previous year) as well as present status—should be considered at all times.

From International Consensus Report on Diagnosis and Management of Asthma (publication no. [NIH] 92-3091). Bethesda, MD, U.S. Department of Health and Human Services, 1992, p 4.

poventilation with a rise in PaCO_2 and a fall in pH, resulting in respiratory acidosis. Pulmonary artery pressure increases as a result of air trapping and hyperinflation. In acute and rapidly reversible attacks, bronchospasm is the most significant abnormality; in chronic asthma and more prolonged irreversible acute attacks, dysfunction is due to mucus plugging, edema, and inflammation of the bronchial wall.

It is becoming clear that asthma has both immediate (bronchospastic) and late-phase (inflammatory) components in the response to inhaled allergens and certain other provoking agents (Cockcroft, 1988). The occurrence of this dual asthmatic response has important therapeutic implications.

Approach to the Patient

The history often provides a diagnosis. Asthma should be suspected in any person with unexplained episodes of dyspnea, cough, repeated chest colds, or bronchitis, particularly in children. Even cough by itself may be a symptom of asthma. In evaluation of the acute attack, severity is related to frequency, duration, intensity, and response to previous medication with side effects, as well as symptom-free intervals. When symptoms are chronic and/or continuous, the condition may be confused with irreversible chronic obstructive pulmonary disease. A family history may be positive for asthma or atopy, and a search for provocative environmental factors, including occupational exposure, smoking, stress, infection, exercise, and medication (aspirin, propranolol), may yield important information.

Signs

In the symptom-free, uncomplicated asthmatic individual, there are no specific findings. However, examination of the upper respiratory tract may reveal signs of allergic rhinitis and/or the presence of nasal polyps. In children, a comparison of the growth grid is important because growth retardation may be caused by chronic hypoxemia or previous medication with glucocorticoids, or both. Recording the blood pressure is of importance because steroids, adrenergic agents, and theophylline may elevate blood pressure.

During an asthmatic episode, the patient presents with difficulty in respiration with an increased respiratory rate, using accessory muscles with suprasternal retraction, pursed lip expiration, and flaring of the nostrils. Cyanosis may be present. Expiration is prolonged, with intercostal retraction. There may be evidence of hyperinflation, with an increased anteroposterior diameter, hyperresonance, and reduced diaphragmatic excursion. On auscultation, an unevenness of ventilation may be present, with high-pitched inspiratory and expiratory dry rales. Rhonchi are accentuated during forced expiration. In children, compression of the chest during expiration may produce latent wheezes. It may be difficult to persuade older children and adolescents to exhale forcefully to induce latent wheezes, because the patient has learned that this might induce coughing and increase bronchial constriction. In patients with marked hyperinflation in whom there is little air exchange, wheezing may be absent. Cardiac dullness may be decreased and the liver edge may be palpable because of a lowered diaphragm from pulmonary hyperexpansion.

Assessment

To supplement the history and physical examination, the response to a bronchial dilator may be used to establish the presence of reversible obstructive lung disease. To do this, the ventilatory function is measured, using a forced expiration volume in one second (FEV_1), before and after the patient inhales an aerosol of a bronchodilator drug. If there is no change, the patient may be retested after a subcutaneous injection of 1:1000 epinephrine. Examination of sputum is simple, and can be done quickly. A predominance of lymphocytes suggest viral respiratory infection, while a predominance of neutrophils and ingested bacteria is indicative of secondary infection. Sputum analysis in an acute attack in the absence of infection usually shows some ciliated columnar epithelial cells, eosinophilia greater than 20 per cent, and varying amounts of neutrophils. With bronchial or bronchopulmonary infection, neutrophils predominate, with lower ranges of eosinophils (5 to 20 per cent). Worsening of asthma symptoms usually is accompanied by an increase in total blood eosinophil count. Depression of the blood eosinophil count and sputum eosinophilia is seen with glucocorticoid therapy, and this response occasionally is used to assess the adequacy of the dosage.

The complete blood count is often normal. Moderate leukocytosis does not necessarily indicate infection. Inflammation and stress of the disease, fear or crying in a young individual, and epinephrine administration all can elevate the white count. While blood eosinophilia is common in asthma, it may be suppressed by stress, epinephrine, or steroid therapy at the time the patient is being assessed.

A chest radiograph is not often helpful in the evaluation of noncomplicated asthma, because it is usually normal. However, it provides a baseline for future comparison. In adults, chest radiographs may not be necessary with each episode in patients with predictable recurrent attacks. However, in young children first presenting with asthma, it is important to differentiate asthma from bronchiolitis in infancy. A chest radiograph is also useful in ruling out a congenital anomaly and the presence of a foreign body. If the asthmatic attack is sufficiently severe as to necessitate hospitalization, an admitting chest radiograph is advisable to rule out infiltrates, atelectasis, and free air in the chest, mediastinum, or soft tissues. A majority of asthmatics will show hyperinflation with increased bronchial markings and flattening of the diaphragm during an acute episode.

The total serum IgE is not particularly useful information for the management of asthma. It is normal in intrinsic asthma but not always elevated in extrinsic asthma. Its main significance is as an aid in diagnosing bronchopulmonary aspergillosis, which commonly has markedly elevated serum IgE levels.

Skin tests are selected according to the information obtained from the history. Obvious limitations are present, because some ubiquitous allergens may not be identified by history alone. The value of skin testing is greatest in the extrinsic asthmatic patient when respirable allergens are suspected from the history to be clinically significant causative agents. When all tests are negative, skin testing helps to establish the diagnosis of intrinsic asthma.

Pulmonary Function Tests

Pulmonary function tests provide information important in assessing airway function in the long-term evaluation of bronchial asthma. In the use of office spirometry, it is important to determine the "normal" pulmonary function value for each individual, because predicted limits are derived from a normal reference population and the individual's asymptomatic normal value may not be in conformance with that population. In general, determination of pulmonary function in children less than 5 to 6 years of age is not practical, because cooperation may not be optimal.

The clinical picture of obstructive airways disease is characterized by a slow loss of ability to expel air from the lung. The decreased maximum expiratory flow rate can be measured by spirometry in the office setting. In the use of spirometry the patient is first instructed thoroughly in the performance of the test. Conditions during testing should be consistent. Test results are valid only if the patient developed a maximal expiratory effort following full inspiration. The technician operating the pulmonary function equipment should first demonstrate how to perform the test. Reliable spirometric tests depend on individual motivation in addition to proper technique. When the patient has pain or a coughing spasm, maximal expiratory effort is not achieved. Premature termination of expiration or a Valsalva maneuver during the expiration produces errors. In general, no more than three consecutive spirometry tests are advisable for measuring pulmonary functions at any given time, because additional effort by an asthmatic can induce bronchospasm with progressive decrease in the flow rate.

Because an important use of pulmonary function tests is to determine the degree of reversibility of airways obstruction, bronchodilating medication should be discontinued at least 6 hours before this test. A baseline pulmonary function is obtained first and then the test is repeated 15 minutes after inhaling a bronchodilating drug. In normal subjects, no change is observed in pulmonary function after the inhalation of a bronchodilator. In patients with reversible obstructive airways disease and a low baseline flow rate, significant improvement should occur (more than 15 to 20 per cent in the FEV_1, or peak flow rate). If no change occurs after inhalation of the bronchodilator, the patient may have irreversible airway disease (chronic bronchitis and emphysema) or the airway obstruction may be primarily due to inflammation and respond only to glucocorticoid therapy.

In patients who do not have abnormal pulmonary function when examined but complain of symptoms occurring at other times that suggest asthma, a bronchial challenge with histamine or methacholine (Mecholyl) may be useful. Although bronchial challenge can be used to demonstrate that the bronchi are or are not hyperactive, and this can rule out the diagnosis of asthma, such testing when positive is potentially dangerous and should be done only by experienced, properly equipped personnel. It can be particularly useful in consideration of occupational asthma. The bronchoprovocation test using inhaled allergen is rarely necessary. It may produce an immediate fall in lung function but also may produce a 6- or 8-hour–delayed response. Again it should be undertaken only by experts in a controlled setting.

Differential Diagnosis

In children, it is important to differentiate asthma from bronchiolitis in infancy, bronchitis, croup, epiglottitis, and aspiration of foreign body. An inspiratory stridor differentiates hypertrophic tonsils, laryngeal disease, subglottic stenosis, or a foreign body from asthma. Among the chronic conditions, childhood cystic fibrosis is distinguished by malabsorption and failure to thrive and a sweat chloride concentration greater than 60 mEq/L. In young adults, hyperventilation generally is associated with anxiety and nonpulmonary symptoms, and relaxation with reassurance often differentiates it from asthma. Rebreathing from a bag is helpful, although this is not advisable during an acute attack or when hypoxemia is suspected. In the older patient, pulmonary embolism may be differentiated by a history of predisposing factors (thrombophlebitis, cardiac failure, oral contraceptives, prolonged bed rest, or malignancy). Cardiac asthma may be associated with a history of cardiac disease, moist rales in the chest, and a third heart sound, which distinguishes it from asthma. Cardiac asthma usually presents as such in a patient with underlying obstructive lung disease who develops heart failure.

Management

The aim of management is to keep the patient as symptom free as possible with minimal medication. It is essential that the patient understand the disease and its precipitating and aggravating factors and recognize its early manifestations, so that an acute episode can be treated early in order to forestall hospitalization. Recognition of the emotional impact of asthma from a personal, family, and work standpoint can facilitate an acceptance of the limitations of the disease without overreaction and frustration. In schoolchildren, problems can be reduced by providing guidelines to parents and teachers in relation to appropriate activity. Asthmatic patients can be taught to practice relaxed breathing in association with medication or autohypnosis to decrease the anxiety and to prevent the panic that often is associated with the onset of acute symptoms. Breathing instructions include conscious slow exhalation through pursed lips while allowing abdominal muscles to relax and at the same time monitoring diaphragmatic movement with a hand placed on the upper abdomen. In children, if major allergens identified cannot be eliminated or avoided, immunotherapy can be useful. Compliance in drug therapy is particularly important.

The concept of preventive therapy is the rule. This encompasses the use of specific pharmacologic agents capable not only of ablating the immediate phase of the asthmatic reaction but also of suppressing the ensuing late-phase inflammatory component (discussed later). For a patient with mild paroxysmal asthma, albuterol or metaproterenol (β-adrenergics) delivered via a metered-dose inhaler attached to a "spacer" device generally provide excellent relief for 6 to 8 hours. Longer acting inhaled sympathomimetic aerosols will soon be available in the United States, and their availability may improve our treatment of asthma considerably (Bone, 1993). The oral form of these drugs does not seem to offer much more therapeutic benefit, and they have more side effects than the same drug given by inhalation. Theophylline, once considered the "foundation medication" in the treatment of asthma, has fallen out of favor as our understanding of the pathophysiology of asthma has evolved. However, it still has a beneficial effect given at bedtime, in a sustained-release form, for those patients with nocturnal symptoms.

When the patient with an acute attack of asthma does not respond to the measures outlined above, management should proceed in a controlled setting such as an emergency room of a hospital. Blood gases are obtained to assess the severity of the attack. Oxygen saturation should be monitored continuously. The patient is treated first with a nebulized β-adrenergic bronchodilator. In younger adults and in the absence of cardiac disease, this treatment can be supplemented with subcutaneous epinephrine or terbutaline if necessary. The nebulizer treatment can be repeated every 15 minutes for three doses and the subcutaneous drug once in 20 to 30 minutes. Improvement in bronchospasm is usually rapid. If response is sustained, the patient can be discharged on inhaled β-adrenergic therapy with consideration given to a "tapering" course of glucocorticoids (prednisone). Appropriate follow-up is important. If the PaO_2 is below 60 mm Hg, supplemental humidified oxygen is administered at 2 to 4 L/min and blood gases should be re-evaluated to maintain the PaO_2 level above 65 mg Hg. Intravenous fluids then should be given. Aminophylline may be added intravenously, although there is now mounting evidence that it offers no additional benefit over adequate adrenergic therapy in emergency room management. The usual loading dose of aminophylline is 6 mg/kg over 20 to 30 minutes, with a lower dose if oral theophylline has been taken recently. Infusion of aminophylline in a maintenance dose of 0.5 mg/kg/hr is continued, with monitoring of serum theophylline levels. In patients who have needed glucocorticoid therapy in the past or are on a maintenance regimen of glucocorticoid, an intravenous infusion of methylprednisolone, 125 mg, is advisable. When sufficiently improved, the patient can be sent home with instructions to take oral steroid and bronchodilator drugs regularly for several days with appropriate follow-up. If the patient is not responsive to therapy as outlined, hospitalization for status asthmaticus is required for more intense management. A typical asthma therapy flow chart for emergency room use is depicted in Figure 24–1.

Status Asthmaticus

A patient is considered to have status asthmaticus when severe asthma is unresponsive to the usual emergency methods of treatment and ventilatory failure is imminent. Status asthmaticus has a 1 to 3 per cent mortality risk and is a medical emergency requiring prompt hospital management. While there may be no obvious precipitating factors, status asthmaticus may be triggered by inhaled allergens or irritants, a viral respiratory infection, an emotional crisis, or medication (especially steroid) withdrawal. Some patients may have a premonitory pattern with increasing disability

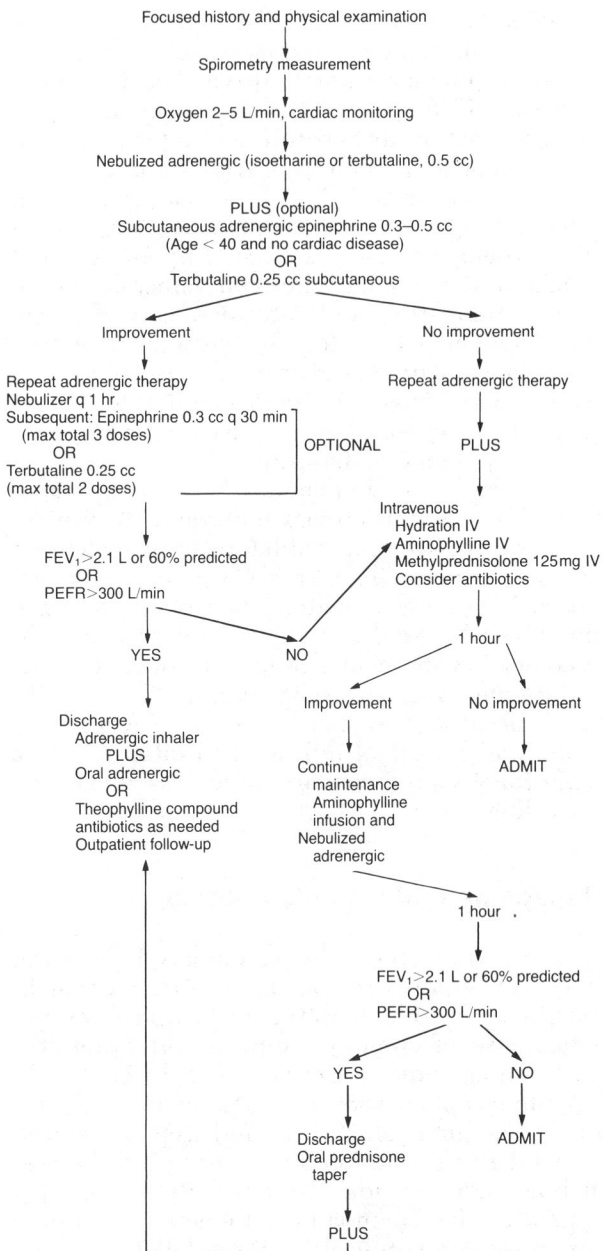

FIGURE 24–1. Flow chart for management of acute asthma. (From Eisenberg MS, Compass MK: Flow management of acute asthma. *In* Eisenberg MS, Copass, MK [eds]: Emergency Medical Therapy, 3rd edition. Philadelphia, WB Saunders Company, 1988, p 454, with permission.)

and wheezing associated with scantier, more tenacious sputum, and a decreased efficacy of maintenance therapy. The patient is usually anxious, irritable, and tachypneic, with tachycardia and impaired speech caused by labored breathing.

Status asthmaticus must be treated aggressively. The following changes provide an indication of severity. A paradoxical pulse correlates with an FEV_1 of less than 20 per cent of the predicted value. An arterial blood PCO_2 of 45 mm Hg or more and a PO_2 of 60 mm Hg or less indicates the patient has developed alveolar hypoventilation as a result of either fatigue of the respiratory muscle or a depression of respiratory-centered drive. This is an ominous sign. If the patient is able to cooperate, pulmonary function tests before and after treatment with a bronchodilator also provide information on severity, because an FEV_1 of less than 10 per cent of the predicted value, nonresponsive to bronchodilator therapy in the presence of hypoxemia and metabolic acidosis, indicates ventilatory failure requiring intubation and intensive care therapy. Other obvious parameters for hospitalization and intensive care are disturbance of consciousness; a "silent chest," in which air movement is too inadequate to generate a wheeze; and obvious pneumothorax or pneumomediastinum.

In general, sedation should be avoided, especially if the Paco$_2$ is normal or elevated, to prevent depression of a central ventilatory drive, which can augment hypoventilation and cause respiratory acidosis. If necessary, hydroxyzine or benzodiazepine may be used cautiously for severe anxiety or to counteract the central effects of drug therapy. Barbiturates and phenothiazines are contraindicated, because they can depress the respiratory center and bronchial reflexes and often add to a confusional state secondary to decreased cerebral blood flow.

Management of Chronic Asthma

Asthma is chronic if the patient has daily symptoms and requires regular medication to remain symptom free. Pharmacotherapy emphasizes the regular use of cromolyn, topical corticosteroids, ipratropium, and/or nedocromil (Table 24–4).

Acute symptoms can be treated as needed with a β-adrenergic agonist delivered from a metered dose inhaler or via "updraft" using a nebulizer such as a Pulmonaide. Regular daily use of a β$_2$-agonist as the "foundation" therapy for chronic asthma is contraindicated. Recent data (Li and Reed, 1993) has suggested that these agents *might* be responsible for the increase in asthma morbidity and mortality. Several mechanisms have been proposed, including the exposure of a greater portion of the tracheobronchial tree to allergens by diminishing bronchospasm while enhancing long-term inflammatory damage produced by this exposure.

Cromolyn sodium can be used in the patient with extrinsic asthma either to prevent allergen-induced attacks or after steroids have produced maximal improvement and are being tapered. Cromolyn sodium is considered the drug of choice for children under the age of 10. It may be used either with a metered-dose inhaler (two inhalations, four times a day, used with a spacer) or delivered via a "nebulizer," sometimes combined with a "unit dose" β-adrenergic. If effective, treatment can be

continued, with regular attempts to lower the dosage by dropping one dose every 1 to 2 weeks. Cromolyn sodium should be discontinued in an acute asthmatic attack. Patient compliance is frequently a problem. In the chronic patient, older than 10 years of age, and who is threatened with steroid dependency, topical glucocorticoids (beclomethasone, flunisolide, and triamcinolone acetate) should be initiated. Up to 4 weeks of use may be necessary before maximum improvement is seen. In some cases, higher doses than recommended (200 mg four times/day) will offer additional benefit; however, this must be monitored carefully. Such inhalations can be given in conjunction with oral glucocorticoids to reduce the systemic dosage (Konig, 1988). If these inhalations themselves cause bronchospasm, pretreatment with a metaproterenol or albuterol inhalation can facilitate peripheral penetration. With time, the β$_2$-agonists usually can be discontinued. Rinsing of the throat and mouth after inhalations of glucocorticoids can decrease risks of oropharyngeal candidiasis. Nedocromil, also an anti-inflammatory agent, seemingly works in a fashion similar to that of Cromolyn: inhibition of mediator release from a variety of inflammatory cell types. It, too, can be used for initial treatment (two puffs, four times/day with a spacer). If continuous oral glucocorticoid therapy is necessary, giving the drug on alternate days will minimize side effects; however, asthma often appears on the off day. In the patient with chronic asthma who has thick tenacious sputum, maintenance of a high fluid intake is important.

In the long-term management of chronic asthma with frequent flare-ups related to a hyperreactive airway, the value of long-term use of cromolyn, nedocromil, and glucocorticoid therapy is now well established. All three drugs inhibit the late, or inflammatory, phase of asthma, whereas β-adrenergic bronchodilators and theophylline do not. Cromolyn and nedocromil may have some advantage over inhaled glucocorticoids because of their lack of systemic side effects, but glucocorticoids are effective in a higher proportion of patients. Combining one or more of these agents with glucocorticoids in the more severe asthmatic patient is effective, the therapeutic goal being control of symptoms with the least amount of medication (Expert Panel Report, 1991).

Some other drugs are used under special or investigative circumstances for treatment of patients with severe, chronic, steroid-dependent asthma. These include troleandomycin (with methylprednisolone), methotrexate, and gold salts. Their use is beyond the scope of this chapter.

One other drug should be mentioned. Ipratropium bromide is an anticholinergic bronchodilator available in this country in a metered-dose inhaler. Its main usefulness is in treatment of patients with bronchospasm associated with chronic bronchitis and emphysema (Gross, 1988). Its effect in asth-

TABLE 24–4. MANAGEMENT OF CHRONIC ASTHMA*

Step-up: Progression to the next higher step is indicated when control cannot be achieved at the current step and there is assurance that medication is used correctly. If PEFR $\leq$ 60% predicted or personal best, consider a burst of oral corticosteroids and then proceed.

Step-down: Reduction in therapy is considered when the outcome for therapy has been achieved and sustained for several weeks or even months at the current step. Reduction in therapy is also needed to identify the minimum therapy required to maintain control.

Outcome: Control of Asthma
- Minimal (ideally no) chronic symptoms, including nocturnal symptoms
- Minimal (infrequent) episodes
- No emergency visits
- Minimal need for p.r.n. beta$_2$-agonist
- No limitations on activities, including exercise
- PEF circadian variation <20%
- (Near) normal PEF
- Minimal (or no) adverse effects from medicine

Outcome: Best Possible Results
- Least symptoms
- Least need for p.r.n. beta$_2$-agonist
- Least limitation of activity
- Least PEFR circadian variation
- Best PEFR
- Least adverse effects from medicine

Therapy†
- Short-acting inhaled beta$_2$-agonist p.r.n. not more than 3 times a week
- Short-acting inhaled beta$_2$-agonist or cromolyn before exercise or exposure to antigen

Therapy†
- Inhaled anti-inflammatory daily
  - Initially: Inhaled corticosteroid 200–500 μg or cromolyn or nedocromil (Children begin with a trial of cromolyn)
  - If necessary: inhaled corticosteroid 400–750 μg (Alternatively, particularly for nocturnal symptoms, proceed to Step 3 with additional long-acting bronchodilator) and
- Short-acting inhaled beta$_2$-agonist p.r.n., not to exceed 3–4 times a day

Therapy†
- Inhaled corticosteroids 800–1000 μg daily (>1000 μg under specialist's supervision) and
- Sustained-release theophyline, oral beta$_2$-agonist, or long-acting inhaled beta$_2$-agonist, especially for nocturnal symptoms; may consider inhaled anticholinergics and
- Short-acting inhaled beta$_2$-agonist p.r.n., not to exceed 3–4 times a day

Therapy†
- Inhaled corticosteroid 800–1000 μg daily (>1000 μg under specialist's supervision) and
- Sustained-release theophyline and/or oral beta$_2$-agonist, or long-acting inhaled beta$_2$-agonist, especially for nocturnal symptoms with or without
- Short-acting inhaled beta$_2$-agonist once a day; may consider inhaled anticholinergic and
- Oral corticosteroids (alternate-day or single daily dose) and
- Short-acting inhaled beta$_2$-agonist p.r.n., up to 3–4 times a day

Step-Down
- Once control is reached at any step, and sustained, a step-down—reduction in therapy—may be carefully considered and is needed to identify the minimum therapy required to maintain control.
- Advise patients of signs of worsening asthma and actions to control it.

Clinical Features Pretreatment*‡
- Intermittent, brief symptoms <1–2 times a week
- Nocturnal asthma symptoms <1–2 times a month
- Asymptomatic between exacerbations
- PEFR or FEV:
  - >80% predicted
  - variability <20%

Clinical Features Pretreatment*‡
- Exacerbations >1–2 times a week
- Exacerbations may affect activity and sleep
- Nocturnal asthma symptoms >2 times a month
- Chronic symptoms requiring short-acting beta$_2$-agonist almost daily
- PEFR or FEV:
  - 60–80% predicted
  - variability 20–30%

Clinical Features Pretreatment*‡
- Frequent exacerbations
- Continuous symptoms
- Frequent nocturnal asthma symptoms
- Physical activities limited by asthma
- PEFR or FEV:
  - <60% predicted
  - variability >30%

| STEP 1: MILD | STEP 2: MODERATE | STEP 3: MODERATE | STEP 4: SEVERE |

---

* PEFR, peak expiratory flow rate; PEF, peak expiratory flow.

† All therapy must include patient education about prevention (including environmental control where appropriate) as well as control of symptoms.

‡ One or more features may be present to be assigned a grade of severity; an individual should usually be assigned to the most severe grade in which any feature occurs.

From International Consensus Report on Diagnosis and Management of Asthma (publication no. [NIH] 92-3091). Bethesda, MD, U.S. Department of Health and Human Services, 1992, p 34.

matic patients is variable; generally it is less effective than an adrenergic agent, and it has no effect on the late-phase asthmatic reaction. In some settings, atropine (1 mg/mL) can be added to β-adrenergics to be delivered via nebulization. Whether this offers any benefit in an acute setting is debated.

Monitoring peak flow rates in children and adults alike has offered an additional tool in recognizing changes in pulmonary performance that often precede an acute asthma attack. Inexpensive, these peak flow meters allow the patient and physician to assess pulmonary stability continuously and alert both to the potential need for re-evaluation.

Exercised-Induced Asthma

Asthma following exercise is common in children and young adults. It is usually brief and indistinguishable from asthma resulting from other causes. Some patients have asthma only after exercise. Patients may complain of mild chest tightness, irritation, and cough, or they may wheeze overtly and become severely short of breath and disabled when severe hypoxia is present.

The most reliable method for evaluation of exercise-induced asthma is an exercise challenge, which can be performed easily in an office setting. Pulmonary functions using a peak flow meter or spirometer usually are measured before exercise. The pulmonary response is assessed after 5 to 8 minutes of a slow run. If a treadmill is available, it, too, can be utilized. A decrease of 10 per cent in the peak expiratory flow rate or 12 to 15 per cent in the FEV_1 is considered abnormal. A change of 30 to 45 per cent is considered a moderately severe response, and a change greater than 45 per cent a severe response. Epinephrine and oxygen should be on hand for rare emergencies during exercise testing.

In general, exercise-induced asthma is not a contraindication to activity. Particularly in children, in whom physical activity is a major part of normal development, counseling can provide a choice for an appropriate activity that is least likely to induce asthma. Swimming, baseball, gymnastics, and golf are usually well tolerated. In general, some individuals may need to have restrictions from time to time, particularly on cold days or when environmental pollution or the pollen load is heavy. Such restrictions, when adequately understood, usually are accepted.

Premedication can prevent asthmatic attacks by the inhalation of cromolyn or an adrenergic drug immediately before exercise. When theophylline is used 1½ to 2 hours before exercise, a therapeutic drug level is achieved for full effectiveness at the time of exercise. For international athletic competition, the use of adrenergic bronchodilators is not allowed.

Occupational Asthma

Occupational asthma is due to an agent or agents encountered at work. It is often aggravated by nonspecific stimuli such as cold air, exercise, smoking, and respiratory infections. Symptoms such as acute bronchospasm or cough may not appear until several hours after the workers has left the place of work, so that the diagnosis may be difficult. Cough may be superimposed on chronic obstructive pulmonary disease, with airways obstruction unresponsive to bronchodilators in the work place but responsive when tested outside of the work place. Recurrent "chest colds" may be present, with improvement away from work and recrudescence 1 to 2 weeks after returning to work. The deleterious effect of the work environment is determined by measuring the peak expiratory flow rate at regular intervals for 2 weeks at work and 1 week at home, differentiating between work exposure values and non–work exposure values. Table 24–5 lists common causal agents.

TABLE 24–5. CAUSAL AGENTS OF OCCUPATIONAL ASTHMA

Agents	Workers at Risk
Flour, grain dust, mites	Bakers, millers, dock workers, farmers, silo workers
Cotton, flax, sisal, hemp	Textile workers
Wood dusts (western red cedar, redwood, mahogany, other hardwoods)	Sawmill workers, carpenters, builders
Cork dust (suberosis)	Cork makers, lumbermen
Epoxy resins (phthalic anhydride, triethylene tetramine)	Plastics, adhesives, synthetic rubber makers
Metals (nickel, cobalt, platinum, chromates)	Metal and chromium platers, metal refiners, grinders, jewelers
Enzymes (*Bacillus subtilis*)	Detergent industry workers
Coffee bean dust	Coffee workers
Polyvinyl chloride (PVC)	Meat wrappers
Ammonia, chlorine, sulfur dioxide, hydrochloric acid	Chemical, petroleum, paper mill workers
Henna extracts, persulfates	Hairdressers
Organic phosphorus	Farmers
Soldering fluxes, rosin (colophony)	Electrical solderers, hot-melt gluers, chemists, feather pluckers
Formaldehyde, formalin, toluene diisocyanate (TDI)	Plastic molders, medical technicians
Penicillin, sulfonamides, piperazine, cimetidine, propranolol	Pharmaceutical workers
Animal dander, rat urine protein	Laboratory technicians, veterinarians, farmers

Allergic Bronchopulmonary Aspergillosis

Allergic bronchopulmonary aspergillosis is an immediate hypersensitivity and immune complex disease caused by *Aspergillus fumigatus*. It is associated with a history of asthma in atopic adult patients. It presents with episodes of wheezing, fever, cough productive of brownish plugs, and dyspnea. Leukocytosis and eosinophilia occur in both blood and sputum. Microscopy of the sputum often yields the fungus. Culture, when repeatedly positive, suggests the diagnosis. Transient or fixed pulmonary infiltrates are seen radiologically. Bronchoscopy or tomograms often reveal proximal bronchiectasis. On prick or intradermal testing with *Aspergillus* antigens, skin reactivity is positive in 15 minutes and 8 hours. Precipitating antibodies to *Aspergillus* and elevated serum IgE confirm the diagnosis.

During acute episodes, a bronchodilator (and antibiotics if bacterial infection is present) is helpful in controlling symptoms, but oral prednisone, 25 to 50 mg/day, is the treatment of choice. After 2 weeks, this can be tapered to an alternate-day regimen and stopped after 3 months. Repeat courses of steroids may be necessary. When untreated, destruction of lung tissue progresses to recurrent irreversible bronchiectasis and pulmonary fibrosis, with eventual respiratory failure (Patterson et al., 1986).

Drug Treatment and Pregnancy

During pregnancy, the increase in chorionic gonadotropin and plasma cortisol and a slight increase in cyclic AMP combine to reduce the effects of histamine release. In addition, serum IgE levels tend to decrease in pregnancy. Asthma improves in approximately one third of pregnant asthmatic patients, slightly more than one third remain the same, and less than one third worsen. In women with mild asthma prior to pregnancy, there is likely to be little change or some improvement during pregnancy. In women with severe asthma, there is a tendency to worsen during pregnancy. If asthma worsens during the initial pregnancy, it is likely to worsen during subsequent pregnancies, and this may reflect a general worsening of asthma with time.

Treatment in the first trimester should be limited to essential medications to prevent maternal hypoxemia. Uncontrolled asthma leading to hypoxemia is a greater risk to the fetus than any of the usual drugs. Conventional therapy with theophylline is not associated with teratogenic effects, and cromolyn sodium can be used for prevention of attacks. Glucocorticoids should be used only when absolutely necessary to control asthma adequately. If steroids have been used during pregnancy, sup-

plemental steroids at delivery may be necessary. An acceptable schedule is cortisone acetate 100 mg intravenously or intramuscularly every 8 hours through labor and delivery. Newborns of mothers treated with high-dose glucocorticoid therapy should be observed for adrenal insufficiency.

Decongestants have not been established as safe during pregnancy. If used, they should be used sparingly and given topically if possible. Pseudoephedrine may be the safest oral decongestant. Judicious use of some antihistamines, such as diphenhydramine (Benadryl), tripelennamine (Pyribenzamine), and chlorpheniramine (Chlor-Trimeton), is considered acceptable during pregnancy, but all should be used sparingly, especially during the first trimester (Weber and Nelson, 1986).

Breast Feeding

Less than 1 per cent of oral theophylline appears in the breast milk. At therapeutic blood levels in the mother, the infant would receive only about 2 mg/kg/24 hr. Occasionally, infant hyperirritability has been attributed to maternal theophylline therapy. No known adverse effects have been related to β_2-adrenergic bronchodilators in the breast milk. While secreted in trace amounts in breast milk, antihistamines are without adverse effect to the infant other than sleepiness. Secretion of glucocorticoids in breast milk is less than 1 per cent of the administered dose and never approaches the normal amount produced by the fetus. There is no contraindication to immunotherapy of the nursing mother. Antigens used may be secreted in trace amounts; however, absorption by the infant is considered to be clinically unimportant. Severe antigen-induced systemic reactions during immunotherapy have produced lower abdominal cramping and uterine bleeding. Although no adverse fetal effects have been reported, immunotherapy should not be started during pregnancy, and the dose of each ongoing immunotherapy injection should be kept constant or decreased during the pregnancy (Weber and Nelson, 1986).

HYPERSENSITIVITY PNEUMONITIS

Hypersensitivity pneumonitis is an infiltrative lung disease caused by inhaled antigen, and may be manifest as a combination of type III (immune complex) and type IV (delayed or cellular hypersensitivity) immunologic reactions. Individual susceptibility varies. Clinical manifestations include fever, chills, malaise, and cough, rather than bronchospasm and wheezing, developing 4 to 6 hours after exposure to the antigen. Pulmonary function tests reveal restrictive rather than obstructive lung disease, and the chest radiograph will show signs of alveolitis. Examples of commonly seen conditions produced by the antigens are mushroom worker's disease, farmer's lung, maple bark stripper's disease, cheese worker's lung, and pigeon breeder's disease. A high index of suspicion often leads to the diagnosis. Environmental caution and the use of glucocorticoids are the mainstays of management.

ATOPIC DERMATITIS

Atopic dermatitis is a chronic, or relapsing, highly pruritic skin eruption that usually develops in patients with a personal or family history of respiratory atopic problems. Onset is after the age of 5 in only about 10 per cent of cases. In contrast with other forms of infantile eczema, atopic dermatitis rarely appears before the infant is 2 months old.

The pathogenesis of atopic dermatitis is complex and only partially understood. The pathophysiologic response of the skin is abnormal. There is an increased tendency to diaphoresis, yet sebum production is low and generalized dryness is often a problem. The response of the cutaneous vasculature is diagnostic. Stroking the skin produces vasoconstriction rather than vasodilation (white dermographism) and injection of methacholine produces the gradual appearance of vasoconstriction (the "delayed blanch" phenomenon) rather than erythema-and-wheal formation. Usually there is no flare response to histamine either. In addition, there is some experimental evidence, mostly indirect, that skin responds abnormally to adrenergic stimuli (Hanifin, 1982).

The central problem is itch. The above-described abnormalities are contributory to, or at least associated with, a low itch threshold. Any stimuli, including allergens, irritants, emotional stress, and the irritation produced by scratching, can aggravate itching. Once the skin is inflamed, it is entirely possible that the itch–scratch cycle can lead to a chronic problem in the absence of any other aggravating factors. Allergens are not of primary importance in the pathogenesis of atopic dermatitis, because as many as 20 per cent of patients have low serum levels of IgE and few if any positive allergen skin test reactions. However, allergens, especially foods, can induce or aggravate symptoms such as pruritus, erythema and edema, as determined by double-blind oral challenge studies (Sampson, 1986).

The clinical features vary with age. In infants, the lesions often appear on the face first and may extend to the scalp, trunk, and extensor aspects of the extremities. Vesiculation, oozing, and crusting are prominent, and secondary infection is common. In older children, the lesions tend to localize in flexural sites—antecubital and popliteal fossae and the neck in particular. Vesiculation is less prominent; the lesions are papular and with time become lichenified. Generalized dryness of the skin is a common problem. If remission does not occur and the inflammation is not adequately controlled, the lesions become progressively lichenified—especially in the flexural area—and scattered excoriated, crusted papules commonly occur on the face, forearms, hands, and even wrists. The lesions of about 80 per cent of children under 2 years of age with atopic dermatitis will clear up gradually as they get older, but the remainder will have a chronic relapsing problem indefinitely, often into adult life. The clinical appearance is similar in adults.

Resistance to infection is impaired in some patients in proportion to the severity of the disease. The more severe cases of atopic dermatitis may be associated with host-defense deficiencies, but how these relate to the pathogenesis is uncertain. There is no doubt that many patients with atopic dermatitis have impaired T-cell function and relative cutaneous anergy, and thus are at considerable risk for development of disseminated viral or fungal infection. An impaired T-cell suppressor function may be one of the reasons for elevated IgE production. During severe atopic dermatitis, neutrophil and monocyte chemotaxis is also impaired. Generalized vaccinia, sometimes fatal, was a serious risk when smallpox vaccination was in common use. Generalized herpetic infection is still a threat, and the susceptibility to other viruses (e.g., warts and molluscum contagiosum) is substantial. Excoriations, vesiculation, and probably the chemotactic defects mentioned previously render patients vulnerable to superficial staphylococcal or streptococcal infections.

Acute lesions, especially in infants, contain vesicles, and in chronic lesions hyperkeratosis is prominent and there is an increased number of mast cells in the tissue. The histopathologic appearance of atopic dermatitis is inflammatory, with mononuclear cells and occasional plasma cells. Only a small proportion of infiltrating cells are eosinophils or basophils.

The laboratory is of limited value in making the diagnosis of atopic dermatitis. An increased blood eosinophil count and/or serum IgE level may be helpful, for example, in excluding the diagnosis of seborrheic dermatitis in an infant, but the diagnosis can usually be made on clinical grounds. One would expect skin tests for IgE-mediated sensitivity to be positive to several inhaled and ingested allergens in these patients, and such information may be helpful in confirming the atopic state but not in establishing the cause.

Treatment is directed at relieving pruritus, controlling infection, and promoting healing. The patient or parent must understand that typical therapy is of primary importance in management. Acute, vesicular, exudative, crusting dermatitis is treated with cool dressings of Burow's solution several times daily. An oral antihistamine such as diphenhydramine (Benadryl) or hydroxyzine (Atarax) aids in relieving pruritus. Terfenadine, astemizole, or loratadine also can be used in patients older than 12. Scratching may be minimized by trimming fingernails and/or having the patient wear cotton gloves at night. A short course of systemic glucocorticoid therapy may be necessary. Appropriate antibacterial therapy may hasten recovery.

Except during the acute exudative phase, the foundation of topical therapy consists of an emollient for dry skin and a glucocorticoid for inflammation. There are many emollient creams, lotions, and ointments available, and the patient should be advised to obtain small supplies of several to find out which is most effective. Preparations containing 10 per cent urea may be particularly effective in treatment of dry skin. A fluorinated steroid cream or ointment (whichever of the many on the market is chosen) should be used in the lowest effective concentration available to minimize both side effects and cost. Because of the risk of skin atrophy and telangiectasis as local side effects of the fluorinated steroids, they should not be used on the face; hydrocortisone or a similar nonfluorinated steroid cream should be used instead. Conventional bathing, which promotes dry skin, should be avoided. Instead, the patient should use a nonlipid cleansing solution such as Cetaphil. Regular use of hydroxyzine as an oral antipruritic drug is often helpful; antihistamines should never be applied topically.

Most patients with atopic dermatitis will be sensitive to some allergens as determined by skin tests. As an adjunct to topical therapy, an empirical trial of environmental control (minimizing contact with dust, feathers, animals, and irritant substances such as wool garments) may be worthwhile. Also, a trial elimination of foods, such as wheat, eggs, nuts, and legumes, may be helpful—especially in youngsters below age 2. Skin testing for food and inhalant allergens might add some information if the empiric trials are inconclusive, but positive tests should be interpreted conservatively and in a way consistent with the history and, perhaps, food challenge testing (Sampson, 1986).

URTICARIA AND ANGIOEDEMA

The pruritic evanescent, edematous, erythematous, and circumscribed lesions (or hives) of urticaria are familiar to physician and layman alike. They can vary widely in size, from pinhead-sized papules to the size of a rather large pancake. Angioedema may occur alone, but often occurs with urticaria. It is deeper, more diffuse, and likely to develop in thin, distensible, subcutaneous tissue such as lips, eyelids, genitalia, and mucous membranes.

The appearance of the lesions suggests that the pathogenesis of urticaria involves a type I hypersensitivity mechanism: the IgE antibody–antigen triggering of the release of histamine and other vasoactive mediators from mast cells. This is often the case in acute urticaria, but, in many cases of acute, and most cases of chronic, urticaria, the trigger responsible for mediator release is unknown. The histologic appearance of urticaria is usually simple. Edema fluid separates collagen fibers and bundles, particularly in the reticular dermis. There are a few inflammatory cells, and those that exist are perivascular. In a few cases, the biopsy shows vasculitis in addition to edema.

About 20 per cent of the population has experienced acute urticaria at least once. However, at any given time, the prevalence is little more than 1 in 1000. Of these, about two third have chronic urticaria. Whether the problem is acute or chronic, each urticarial wheal develops and then fades away over a space of a few hours. Persisting lesions should raise the question of vasculitis.

Urticaria is a disease of diversity, and its complex classification is outlined in Table 24–6. Allergic urticaria is usually acute and mediated by IgE antibody. By far the most common cases are reactions to drugs, stinging insect venoms, and allergenic extracts used in immunotherapy. In older children and adults, the skin and gastrointestinal tract are fairly effective barriers to allergens. Only the atopic person who is extremely sensitive is likely to react to an ingested food or to contact of an allergen with the unbroken skin. Urticaria caused by an inhaled allergen is extremely rare.

Certain drugs can cause release of histamine directly; allergy is not involved. Radiographic contrast media, polymyxins, tubocurarine, and opiates can produce such toxic-idiosyncratic reactions. Contact urticaria can be a toxic effect of dimethylsulfoxide and formaldehyde. Shellfish and certain fruits, when eaten in large amounts, can product "urticaria of gluttony." Coffee, alcoholic beverages, and aspirin may aggravate urticaria on a nonallergic basis.

The physical urticarias include three fairly common ones that can be mediated by IgE antibodies. It is thought that the antibodies are directed at some dermal proteins that are altered by the physical trauma and thus appear to be "foreign." Cholinergic urticaria is also fairly common. It is a unique generalized eruption consisting of highly pruritic small wheals that often are surrounded by a large flare. The eruption can be provoked by emotional stress, heat, or exercise. Indeed, an exercise test is the most reliable way to confirm the diagnosis.

All the familial conditions are rare. *Hereditary angioedema* will be discussed here because it may be life-threatening and can be treated very effectively. It is characterized by the acute development of an indurated, edematous, subcutaneous swelling occurring spontaneously or following trauma or infection. The reaction is not pruritic. It may be preceded by evanescent reticulate erythema but is never associated with urticaria. It may

TABLE 24–6. CLASSIFICATION OF URTICARIA AND ANGIOEDEMA

Allergic
Drugs
Foods, food additives
Contact allergens
Inhaled allergens
Venoms and other injectables

Toxic
Histamine-releasing drugs and chemicals
Foods

Intrinsic Host Abnormalities
Increased stores of mediator
Urticaria pigmentosa
Systemic mastocytosis

Physical sensitivity, nonfamilial
Cholinergic
Cold: Sporadic (IgE)
Secondary
Light: 6 types (IgE)
Dermographism (IgE)
Pressure
Aquagenic
Decompression

Genetic (all autosomal dominant)
Familial cold
Localized heat
Vibratory
Urticaria with deafness, limb pain, and amyloidosis
Erythropoietic protoporphyria
Hereditary angioedema

Underlying Disease
Infection
Viral: Hepatitis B, infectious mononucleosis, rubella, coxsackievirus
Fungal: *Candida albicans*
Parasitic

Other
Malignancy, especially lymphomas
Systemic lupus erythematosus
Vasculitis
Polycythemia vera
Porphyria
Sjögren's syndrome

Contributing Factors
Alcohol ingestion
Coffee and other stimulants
Exercise
Fever
Emotional stress, depression
Hyperthyroidism
Pregnancy

Unknown
Idiopathic mast cell lability (?)

occur in any cutaneous or mucous membrane location, including the bowel. Crampy gastrointestinal symptoms, sometimes mimicking bowel obstruction, occur at one time or another in almost everyone with the disease. Although it is hereditary, the family history may be negative, and the first symptoms do not necessarily appear during childhood.

The inherited defect in hereditary angioedema is a lack or dysfunction of a serum inhibitor of the activated first component of complement (C1 esterase). When complement is activated, the reaction accelerates without restraint in the absence of this inhibitor and leads to generation of potent vasoactive kinins. The diagnosis can be made by an assay for inhibitor function and/or by measuring C4 (the fourth component of complement), which is almost always low, even between attacks. Treatment is specific and highly effective. The impeded androgens stanozolol and danazol prevent attacks by improving synthesis of the functional inhibitor (Sheffer et al., 1987).

Acute urticaria is a fairly common event during viral infections. It may be the first sign of hepatitis B infection; the surface antigen has been identified in the dermis of some patients. However, infection as a cause of chronic urticaria is decidedly unusual. Although some have claimed that many cases are caused by sensitivity to a low-grade *Candida* infection, that has not been our experience. Also, a search for a parasitic disease is rarely productive.

Urticaria may be the first sign of some other underlying disease, such as lymphomas and systemic lupus erythematosus. Invariably, other manifestations of these diseases soon will appear. Cutaneous vasculitis, diagnosed by the presence of persistent lesions and a positive biopsy, should produce other lesions, such as palpable purpura, in due time, but sometimes urticaria remains the only visible manifestation. It is not known if the prognosis for this type of urticaria differs from that for chronic urticaria.

Among the contributing factors, emotional stress is often discussed. In fact, it is not often a recognizable problem except in patients with cholinergic urticaria.

No cause can be identified in about 75 per cent of patients with chronic urticaria (Monroe, 1981). Once established, it may continue as an annoying but benign disease for several years.

In evaluating the patient with acute urticaria and angioedema, one should expect the cause to be fairly obvious from the history alone in many patients. If a viral infection is responsible, time alone will provide the answer. (Incidentally, the first signs of infection may precede the appearance of urticaria by several days. *If an antibiotic is given before urticaria appears, the eruption may be falsely attributed to drug allergy.*) Occasionally, skin testing is helpful to differentiate food allergy from overindulgence. Perhaps half the cases of acute urticaria will not have an identifiable cause.

The patient with chronic urticaria should be questioned carefully about the chronic use of drugs and remedies and foods containing dyes, preservatives, and other additives. Skin testing for type I allergy is rarely helpful. Underlying disease should be excluded by means of a thorough physical examination and routine screening laboratory tests. However, such screening tests and the more specialized serum complement tests so rarely detect an underlying disease that their cost-effectiveness is questionable (Jacobson et al., 1980).

Treatment of acute urticaria, whether the cause is identified or not, consists of hydroxyzine or diphenhydramine, to relieve itching. Being nonsedating, terfenadine may be more acceptable for some patients but is likely to be less effective than the other agents. If the reaction is severe, especially if angioedema threatens the airway, then subcutaneous and topical epinephrine also should be given (see Systemic Allergy). Hydroxyzine and the new agents (terfenadine, etc.) are effective drugs for treatment of most patients with chronic or recurrent urticaria. Cyproheptadine may be more effective in some patients, particularly those with cold urticaria. Doxepin may be effective in some others. Patients who are not well controlled by one of these drugs sometimes have been helped by the addition of a histamine₂ antihistamine (cimetidine) or the β-adrenergic drug terbutaline; in our experience, however, the results have been disappointing. Patients should be counseled to try to avoid aggravating factors such as coffee, aspirin, and stress, and should be reassured about the benign nature of chronic urticaria, which often remits spontaneously.

ALLERGIC CONTACT DERMATITIS

This is a pruritic eruption that progresses from erythema and induration to a vesiculobullous state if contact with the offending substance continues. It is produced by substances that are not primary skin irritants or are irritating to the skin only in unusually high concentrations. As with any allergic state, contact dermatitis develops only after prior exposure of from a few days to several years. This acquired sensitivity is of the delayed or T-lymphocyte–mediated type. Most sensitizers are low-molecular-weight chemicals and are not capable of eliciting reactions directly. Instead, it is thought that they conjugate to some dermal protein and function as allergic *haptens* rendered active by the carrier protein. Certain dendritic cells in the epidermis, called Langerhans cells, have been recognized as probably responsible for the hapten processing that leads to sensitization (Thiers, 1982). The microscopic appearance consists of intracellular edema, round cell infiltration, and epidermal vesiculation.

Clinically, the erythematous, vesicular lesion proceeds to a weeping and crusting stage and may become secondarily infected. Occasionally the reaction develops slowly, with induration fissuring, lichenification, and pigmentation rather than vesiculation (Fisher, 1986). The location of the lesion, as much as its appearance, may suggest the diagnosis. Forearms, ears, eyelids, lips, groin, and dorsa of the feet frequently are involved. The eyelids are particularly sensitive and may react to a substance rubbed on them by fingers that do not react.

A few substances will sensitize almost everyone. These include the *Rhus* oleoresins (poison ivy, oak, and sumac) and a few chemicals, one of which, dinitrochlorobenzene (DNCB), is used to induce sensitivity as a test for cell-mediated immune competence. Other common sensitizers affecting 1 to 10 per cent of the population are dyes, especially paraphenylenediamine, chromates used as tanning agents, rubber compounds, nickel found in costume jewelry and in garment fastenings, and mercury. Among drugs, the more common are ethylenediamine, a stabilizer in some creams that cross-reacts with aminophylline, the preservatives thimerosal and parabens, bacitracin, benzocaine, formaldehyde (also a primary irritant), idoxyuridine, neomycin, sunscreen lotions, and therapeutic dyes.

Other substances produce photoreactivity. Some have this property as an inherent toxicity and thus will affect susceptible people on the first application. These include psoralens, eosin, and other dyes used in cosmetics and coal tar derivatives and residues. Others must be applied for a while before an allergic, cell-mediated reaction develops on exposure to sunlight. The more common are the halogenated salicylanilides (found in some deodorant soaps) and stilbenes (textile whitening). No topical medicine now available in the United States is known to induce photoallergy.

The treatment of contact dermatitis is similar to that for atopic dermatitis, except that one can use systemic glucocorticoids with less concern for side effects because it should be a self-limited condition. If the reaction is detected early enough, recognizing and removing the offending contactant may be all that is necessary. If doubt exists about the cause, then patch tests can be done with the suspected substances.

The patch test is carried out by placing each substance in question in contact with a small (5- to 6-mm) area of the skin and keeping it in place with hypoallergenic tape. It may be practical to use a small amount of the actual substance, but in some situations one must obtain specially prepared solutions made up in subirritating concentrations. A detailed listing of chemicals and other substances suitable for patch testing and the appropriate dilutions and diluents can be found in Fisher (1986). The patches are left on for 48 hours or longer, and the patient is warned to remove the patch and wash off any site that begins to itch or burn before then. A positive test at 48 hours is a reproduction in miniature of the original lesion: erythema, induration, and vesiculation. Occasionally a borderline reaction evolves into a definite positive reaction over the next day or two. The risks of patch testing consist of ulceration at the site of an intense reaction and a flaring of the original skin lesions.

SYSTEMIC ALLERGY

Anaphylaxis is any clinical reaction caused by the potent vasoactive mediators that are released explosively after allergen triggering of IgE antibody–sensitized mast cells (type I reaction). *Systemic* or generalized anaphylaxis is a potential life-threatening reaction to injected or ingested allergens. It can be caused by insect venoms, allergenic extracts used for immunotherapy, drugs (especially injected enzymes or horse antisera, and oral or injected penicillin), and certain foods (shellfish, nuts, legumes, egg, and rarely others). Some other agents can produce a similar clinical reaction in the absence of allergic sensitivity because they cause the release of histamine from mast cells directly. The most important are the radiographic contrast media, which also generate vasoactive kinins. Such reactions are referred to as *anaphylactoid* rather than *anaphylactic*, because of the lack of evidence for allergy. In recent years, an increasing number of anaphylactoid reactions have been reported that are exercise induced (Sheffer et al., 1985), and even more that have no identifiable cause (Boxer et al., 1987).

Any substance that can produce urticaria can produce systemic reactions if the dose, rate of administration, or reactivity of the recipient is great enough. Fortunately, most are not sufficiently potent to do this when given or taken in the customary way. Massive and explosive mediator release affects not only the skin but also the respiratory tract, the gastrointestinal tract, and the circulation. Angioedema may so obstruct the upper airway that the patient is asphyxiated. This is the major recognizable cause of death found at autopsy (James and Austen, 1964). Anaphylactic *shock* is the result primarily of a drop in plasma volume caused by a loss of vascular integrity. If the reaction is sufficiently severe and not treated, cardiogenic shock may develop.

The symptoms of systemic anaphylaxis are, in the usual order of progression, a feeling of apprehension, tingling of the extremities, a flushing sensation, itching, palpitations, urticaria, angioedema, nausea, abdominal discomfort, cough, difficulty in breathing, vomiting, diarrhea, intestinal and uterine cramping, incontinence, convulsions, coma, and death. On examination, the typical patient has a generalized flush, with some urticarial wheals beginning to develop. The pulse is rapid, and the blood pressure is initially normal. Later, with sustained hypotension and compensatory peripheral vasoconstriction, the patient may appear pale.

The risk of anaphylaxis can be reduced by taking certain precautions. A careful history of previous adverse drug reactions is important. As many as 25 per cent of anaphylactic deaths from penicillin occurred in patients who were not asked about previous reactions, according to a World Health Organization report. Skin testing to detect IgE-mediated sensitivity is advisable before giving anyone xenogenic serum, parenteral enzymes, or polypeptide hormones, and also should be performed before administering penicillin to a person with a history suggestive of a previous reaction or a chick embryo vaccine to a person with a history of egg sensitivity. The patient with a history of reaction to radiographic contrast media can be premedicated if another procedure is needed, or the newer nonionic, low osmolar agents can be considered. The person who has had a systemic reaction to an insect sting should obtain an emergency kit that contains a prefilled syringe of epinephrine, and be trained in its injection. Immunotherapy to the appropriate venom, starting with the injection of a fraction of a microgram and gradually increasing the dose to 100 μg, is highly effective in preventing reactions to subsequent stings (Valentine and Lichtenstein, 1987). Patients at risk for adverse drug reactions should wear a warning identification bracelet such as those provided by Medic-Alert.

The treatment of anaphylaxis is summarized in Table 24–7. Note that epinephrine is central to all aspects. If a reaction is developing from an injection or sting in an extremity, it often can be aborted by the prompt application of a tourniquet above the site of the injection and administration of 0.3 mL of 1:1000 epinephrine (0.01 mg/kg in children) in a different extremity. The site of injection also can be infiltrated with about 0.2 mL of epinephrine in the same dilution to retard absorption. An intravenous line should be inserted and a glucose–saline solution administered. If the blood pressure begins to fall, the fluid should be run in rapidly. Several liters sometimes must be given to maintain or restore the blood pressure. The patient should be monitored to detect saline overload. Use of a colloid solution is rarely necessary, nor is a vasopressor drug. Epinephrine injection can be re-

TABLE 24–7. ANAPHYLAXIS TREATMENT

Isolate antigen
  Tourniquet
  Epinephrine

Maintain or restore plasma volume
  Epinephrine (I.V. rapidly if blood pressure falls)
  I.V. fluids

Maintain airway, give oxygen
  Upper: add topical epinephrine I.V. antihistamine
  Lower: add theophylline

Restore cardiac output
  Epinephrine
  Theophylline
  Isoproterenol
  Dopamine

peated as early as 15 minutes after the initial dose. If the patient is in shock, it should be given slowly intravenously, 0.25 to 0.5 mg in a 1:100,000 solution at 5 to 10 µg/min. If there is any hint of respiratory embarrassment, the patient should be given oxygen. Oropharyngeal angioedema can be treated topically with an aerosol of epinephrine. Diphenhydramine, 50 to 100 mg (adult dose) intravenously, also may be helpful. If upper airway obstruction is imminent, insertion of an airway (difficult!) or a tracheostomy may be necessary. If there is any sign of bronchospasm, intravenous aminophylline, 6 mg/kg, should be given. Very rarely, one may need to give a direct β-adrenergic stimulant such as isoproterenol, which has an advantage over dopamine or dobutamine because it is also a bronchodilator. Glucocorticoid therapy provides no benefit over the critical first few minutes. When all other appropriate therapy has been given, it is prudent to give a glucocorticoid over the next 24 hours to suppress any late-phase reaction (usually urticaria but may be generalized) that may develop.

DRUG ALLERGY

Most adverse drug reactions result from excessive intake (toxicity) or unusual susceptibility to the toxic effects. Some patients are unusually susceptible because of underlying disease and some are unusually susceptible for unknown reasons. Their reactions are called *intolerance* if the adverse event is an expected pharmacologic effect of the drug and *idiosyncrasy* if it is substantially different.

Allergic drug reactions usually can be differentiated from the others by means of the features listed in Table 24–8. One feature of special importance is that the risk of reacting exists far below

TABLE 24–8. FEATURES OF ALLERGIC DRUG REACTIONS

1. Prior exposure (usually for treatment) occurs without adverse effects.
2. The reactions usually appear only after several days of treatment after first exposure to the drug.
3. The risk of reaction still exists at doses far below the therapeutic range.
4. Clinical manifestations do not resemble the general pharmacologic effects of the drug and cannot be predicted from animal testing.
5. The reactions occur in a small proportion of the population.
6. The reactions usually are restricted to a limited number of syndromes generally accepted as allergic in nature.
7. In a few instances antibodies or T lymphocytes have been identified that react specifically with the drug or a metabolite.
8. The same reactions can be reproduced on administering a small amount of the suspected drug or drugs of similar chemical structure.

the therapeutic range. If one can establish that the reaction to a drug is toxic-idiosyncratic, then treatment with a modest reduction in dose may be successful. This stratagem is unlikely to be successful, and may be dangerous, if the reaction is allergic.

Testing for drug allergy is reliable only in special circumstances. These have been alluded to earlier. Skin testing for immediate sensitivity does identify allergy to a high-molecular-weight protein or polypeptide substances. However, most drugs have a low molecular weight, usually less than 1000, and thus can only sensitize by forming a firm covalent bond with a large carrier protein. This cannot happen directly; it occurs only after the drug has been modified in the body to a chemically reactive intermediate. The intermediates of penicillin are the only ones to have been definitely identified so far. One has been conjugated with polylysine to form penicilloyl polylysine (PPL). It is available commercially for skin testing as Pre-Pen. Unfortunately, PPL skin testing usually fails to identify those few patients at risk for systemic anaphylaxis. They have positive skin reactions to what are called the minor determinants, but the minor determinant mixture for skin testing is not yet on the market. Until it is, penicillin allergy can be excluded most of the time, when the need for treatment with one of the penicillins is especially pressing, by testing with PPL and a solution of 1000 units/mL penicillin G (prick test first, followed by intradermal testing if necessary). If the skin tests are negative, treatment can be cautiously started, using a small test dose first.

Except for some technically difficult tests that can be used to confirm hematologic drug reactions, in vitro tests that have been proposed for the diagnosis of drug allergy are unreliable. These include RAST (with the single except of PPL), lymphocyte stimulation, basophil or mast cell histamine release, and leukocyte cytotoxicity. This is not surprising, because the appropriate conjugates capable of producing specific immunologic reactions have not been identified, except for penicillin (VanArsdel, 1982).

The most reliable test is to readminister the drug to see if the clinical reaction can be reproduced. As mentioned earlier, this is the purpose of the patch test. Otherwise, the risk of doing so is usually unacceptable unless treatment is essential and no alternative drug is available.

Other types of clinical reactions than those discussed above are reviewed in detail elsewhere (VanArsdel, 1988), so they will be mentioned only briefly here. *Serum sickness* probably depends on both type I and type III (immune complex) mechanisms. Fever, adenopathy, and arthralgias occur with a urticarial rash when the reaction is due to foreign serum. A reaction similar to serum sickness may occur during or after treatment with a penicillin (or homologue), sulfonamide, or hydralazine, but is distinctly uncommon.

"Rashes" are the erythematous maculopapular or morbilliform eruptions that are sometimes only minimally pruritic. Close to half of the drug reactions presumed to be allergic fall into this category. The most common substances involved are the semisynthetic penicillins, sulfonamides (especially trimethoprim-sulfamethoxazole), blood products, dipyrone, cephalosporins, allopurinol, and acetylcysteine (Bigby et al., 1986).

Fixed eruptions are pigmented macules that sometimes are eczematous. They can be produced by metronidazole, penicillins, sulfonamides, some analgesics and sedates, gold salts, and even phenolphthalein. Reproducing the reaction by giving the drug again confirms the diagnosis.

Vasculitis most characteristically appears as an erythematous eruption that may become tender, purpuric, and palpable. Sometimes other organ systems besides the skin are affected. Allopurinol, cimetidine, furosemide, hydantoins, penicillins, and sulfonamides are commonly used drugs that can product vasculitis. However, only about 10 per cent of reported cases of vasculitis seem to be drug induced, so any association may be coincidental.

Fever alone may be produced by allopurinol, cephalosporins, penicillins, barbiturates, methyldopa, phenytoin, procainamide, and quinidine. It is not usually associated with any constitutional symptoms, so the patient may not be aware of it. The diagnosis is supported if treatment with the suspected drug is stopped and the temperature drops to normal within 48 hours (except for phenytoin, where this drop may take several days). The diagnosis is confirmed, if necessary, by readministering a small dose of the drug; this is reasonably safe.

Pulmonary reactions are bronchospastic or infiltrative. *Asthma* is very rare except in association with systemic anaphylaxis. *Interstitial pneumonitis* develops with cough, dyspnea, fever, and malaise and is produced most often by gold salts, nitrofurantoin, and thiazide diuretics. *Eosinophilic pneumonitis* is less symptomatic but is associated with blood eosinophilia. It can be produced by gold salts, penicillin, and sulfonamides.

Hepatic reactions can be primarily cholestatic and relatively benign or primarily hepatocellular and potentially fatal. The former can be caused by erythromycins (particularly the estolate form), phenothiazines, imipramine, nalidixic acid, and nitrofurantoin. The latter can be produced by allopurinol, hydantoins, isoniazid, methyldopa, monoamine oxidase inhibitors, rifampin, sulfonamides, and valproic acid.

Interstitial nephritis is the usual allergic renal reaction, and the best known responsible drug is methicillin. However, other penicillins, cephalosporins, and sulfonamides have been implicated, as well as cimetidine, diuretics, nonsteroidal antirheumatic drugs, and allopurinol.

Systemic lupus erythematosus is a self-limited reaction similar to the natural disease (but lacking the cerebral, cutaneous, and renal changes) and is associated with the appearance of circulating antinuclear antibodies. It often develops during treatment with hydralazine or procainamide and less frequently with chlorpromazine, isoniazid, penicillamine, and phenytoin treatment.

Hematologic reactions include blood *eosinophilia* alone (antimicrobials, digitalis glycosides, allopurinol, penicillamine, and phenothiazines); *hemolytic anemia* (high-dose penicillin, chlorpromazine, isoniazid, quinidine, rifampin, and sulfonamides); *thrombocytopenia* caused by immune destruction (quinine, quinidine, cephalosporins, gold salts, hydantoins, antituberculous drugs, analgesics, sulfonamides, and thiazide diuretics); and *granulocytopenia* caused by immune destruction (chlorpromazine, gold salts, phenylbutazone, procainamide, quinidine, and sulfonamides).

Toxic epidermal necrolysis is a rare but potentially fatal reaction that may be related to drugs such as allopurinol, penicillins, phenytoin, sulfonamides, and sulindac. Reactions that are occasionally drug induced but more commonly are related to infection or unknown causes include *exfoliative dermatitis* and *erythema multiforme*. There is no good evidence that *erythema nodosum* or *Henoch-Schönlein purpura* are drug induced.

Pseudoallergic drug reactions are reactions caused by the pharmacologic or toxic action of certain drugs. Reactions caused by histamine-releasing drugs were mentioned earlier. Rhinitis is a well-recognized side effect of reserpine, but also can be found during treatment with other antihypertensive drugs. Asthma is a recognized side effect of treatment with β-blocking drugs, even timolol eye drops.

The prevention and treatment of allergic drug reactions is reviewed elsewhere (VanArsdel, 1988). Briefly, if a reaction occurs, the suspected drug or drugs should be stopped immediately. Symptoms should be treated with antipruritic and analgesic drugs as needed. If these are inadequate, a glucocorticoid drug should be given in ample doses.

FOOD ALLERGY

There are few topics so subject to confusion, misinterpretation, argument, and outright exploitation as that of food allergy. The word *allergy* itself is used so indiscriminately by laymen and professionals alike when food is involved that substitute words such as *sensitivity* and *hypersensitivity* have been proposed as being more precise. However, allergy, as it was originally intended, and as it has been used in this chapter, refers only to conditions produced by antibody-mediated or lymphocyte-mediated tissue injury following contact with a specific allergen.

Allergy mediated by IgE antifood antibodies usually develops in infancy as the diet is liberalized. There is some evidence also that some foods eaten by the mother appear in milk and can sensitize the nursing infant. As expected, the individual with a strong family history of atopy is likely to acquire sensitivity to some foods, but which ones are determined largely by chance and by the age at which the food is introduced. The infant's incomplete digestion, high mucosal permeability, and perhaps weak immunologic defense (by secretory IgA) favor both sensitization and the production of symptoms after sensitization has been established. As the young child grows older, food-induced symptoms become less significant, probably because of maturation of the digestive action of the gastrointestinal tract. However, the IgE antibodies may persist for many years. Skin tests to the originally allergenic foods may remain positive long after those foods have ceased to cause symptoms.

The evidence that immunologic mechanisms other than IgE play a role is much less impressive. Several gastrointestinal diseases have been associated with IgG antibodies in the serum, especially to milk, but these antibodies are probably secondary to the diseases rather than causative. Celiac sprue, caused by sensitivity to wheat gluten, is one example of food sensitivity that is probably due to an IgG antigluten antibody. Delayed or cell-mediated sensitivity may be involved in some adverse food reactions, but because these reactions are not associated with positive delayed skin tests, supporting evidence is entirely circumstantial.

Some of the atopic diseases associated with food allergy were discussed earlier. Atopic dermatitis can be aggravated by food allergens, and asthma and allergic rhinitis can be provoked by them as well. Gastrointestinal symptoms—nausea, vomiting, abdominal cramps, and diarrhea—may occur alone, but more often they accompany respiratory and cutaneous symptoms in the atopic patient with or without atopic dermatitis.

The above manifestations of food allergy are most common in early childhood, but the highly allergic person may continue to have trouble into adult life. Indeed, such a person, if highly sensitive to some food, runs a risk of systemic anaphylaxis from that food that does not seem to diminish with time.

The importance of gastrointestinal digestion in preventing symptoms from food allergens is best brought out by the many examples of patients who react on contact or inhalation to a particular food that gives a positive skin test but they have no trouble eating it. "Baker's asthma" caused by inhaled wheat flour is the best known example.

Another interesting, although rare, disease that can occur in adults as well as children is eosinophilic gastroenteritis, a chronic, symptomatic disease associated with anemia and protein-losing enteropathy. It is made worse by the ingestion of food allergens but, unfortunately, usually persists to a certain degree even if no recognizable allergens are eaten.

Other symptoms that occasionally are provoked by food allergens are headache, irritability, malaise, myalgias, or arthralgias. Usually, each accompanies one or more of the major symptoms rather than being the only symptom of food allergy.

The most common food allergens are milk, egg, nuts and legumes, shellfish, other fish, wheat, chocolate, and pork, but any food is potentially allergenic.

Food *intolerance* is a condition in which the adverse reaction is based on a nonallergic mechanism or in which the mechanism is unknown. Thus, cow's milk intolerance, responsible for gastrointestinal symptoms, may be due to an intestinal deficiency in disaccharidase, but milk also can produce gastrointestinal, and even respiratory, symptoms in a few patients for no identifiable reason (Lessof et al., 1980). It even has been found responsible for intestinal blood loss in infants sufficient to cause significant anemia. The mechanism responsible for intolerance to some food additives or coloring agents is also unknown, but is probably pharmacologic rather than immunologic. Asthma related to food ingestion actually may be produced by the yellow food dye tartrazine.

Food allergy or intolerance has been blamed for certain other conditions. The so-called allergic tension–fatigue syndrome is an example. Enuresis is another, and the "total allergy syndrome" (multiple symptoms attributed to allergy to practically everything) is a third that has received a good deal of recent attention by the press. Much publicity also has been given to the claim that abnormal hyperactivity in children is often due to food additives. All these alleged associations are controversial, because they have not yet been supported by well-controlled clinical trials.

The diagnosis of food allergy depends to a great extent on the history. Symptoms should be recorded in terms of both time and severity in relationship with the types and amount of food ingested. This may be done best by asking the patient to keep a food-symptom diary over a 2-week period, being careful to note all ingredients of any given item. Any suspicious foods then are eliminated from the diet for 2 weeks. If improvement occurs, they are added back to the diet one at a time until symptoms reappear or get worse. If several items are suspected, one should look for an allergenic common ingredient, such as soybean. If no improvement occurs, or the history is not helpful, an empiric elimination diet can be used to restrict the patient to one food in each category (grain, vegetable, fruit, meat), switching to a different food after a week. If the elimination diet is successful, then the one-by-one reintroduction of additional foods proceeds as before until symptoms are provoked (Dong, 1984).

If the empiric diet adjustment is not successful, then testing for IgE food antibodies should be done. The prick test, using a 1:10 or 1:20 weight/volume glycerinated extract, correlates well with true clinical food allergy, as proven by double-blind, placebo-controlled oral challenge experiments (Bock, 1980). Intradermal testing can result in positive skin tests at levels of sensitivity insufficient to be responsible for the symptoms of most patients. The serologic test (RAST) offers no advantage over skin testing unless dermatitis is so extensive that the skin cannot be used. No other tests are advisable. Serum precipitating antibodies to milk or wheat, for example, do not indicate allergy. Other tests, such as cutaneous or sublingual provocation, the pulse and leukopenic test, and the leukocytotoxic serum test, have not been validated by acceptable scientific means.

The obvious treatment for food allergy or intolerance is to avoid the offending food. However, when allergy to many foods is suspected, one may need to establish which are clinically important by placebo-controlled blind challenges. These may become necessary if the alternative is a nutritionally deficient diet. Drug treatment of the cutaneous or respiratory symptoms of food allergy has been covered in earlier sections. The original hope that oral cromolyn sodium would not only control gastrointestinal symptoms but block food allergen absorption has not been realized, and immunotherapy to food allergens is risky and probably ineffective.

The greatest stumbling block that family physicians face in discussing food allergy is understanding what is and what is not food allergy. Unfortunately, the lay press along with popular "talk shows" have invited misunderstanding among patients. It becomes important for the family physician to become familiar with these misconceptions so that a sound and medically helpful evaluation can be done. The foregoing discussion is an attempt to clarify what, at this time, is medically known and understood.

REFERENCES

Bascom R, Pipkorn U, Lichtenstein LM, Naclerio RM: The influx of inflammatory cells into nasal washings during the late response to antigen challenge: Effect of systemic steroid pretreatment. Am Rev Respir Dis 138:406, 1988.

Bigby M, Jick S, Jick H, Arndt K: Drug-induced cutaneous reactions: A report from the Boston Collaborative Drug Surveillance Program on 15,438 consecutive inpatients, 1975 to 1982. JAMA 256:3358, 1986.

Bluestone RD, Cantekin EI: Panel of experience with testing eustachian tube function. Ann Otol Rhinol Laryngol 90:552, 1981.

Bock SA: Food sensitivity: A critical review and practical approach. Am J Dis Child 134:973, 1980.

Bone RC: Inhaled β-agonists: A critical analysis. J Respir Dis 14:979, 1993.

Boxer M, Greenberger PA, Patterson R: Clinical summary and course of idiopathic anaphylaxis in 73 patients. Arch Intern Med 147:269, 1987.

Broder I, Higgins MW, Mathews HP, Keller JB: Epidemiology of asthma and allergic rhinitis in a total community, Tecumseh, Michigan. J Allergy Clin Immunol 54:100, 1974.

Cockcroft DW: Airway hyperresponsiveness and late asthmatic responses. Chest 94:178, 1988.

Coombs RRA, Gell PGH: Classification of allergic reactions responsible for clinical hypersensitivity and disease. In Gell PGH, Coombs RRA (eds): Clinical Aspects of Immunology, 3rd edition. Oxford, England, Blackwell Scientific Publications, 1975, pp 761–781.

Creticos PS: Drug therapy of asthma. In Smith EM, Reynard A (eds): Textbook of Pharmacology. Philadelphia, WB Saunders Company, 1992, pp 1051–1066.

Dong FM: All About Food Allergy. Philadelphia, George F. Stickley Company, 1984.

Expert Panel Report: Guidelines for the Diagnosis and Management of Asthma. Resources (publication no. [NIH] 91-3042). Bethesda, MD, U.S. Department of Health and Human Resources, 1991.

Fisher AA: Contact Dermatitis, 3rd edition. Philadelphia, Lea & Febiger, 1986.

Gross NJ: Ipratropium bromide. N Engl J Med 319:486, 1988.

Hanifin JM: Atopic dermatitis. J Am Acad Dermatol 6:1, 1982.

International Consensus Report on Diagnosis and Management of Asthma. (publication no. [NIH] 92-3091). Bethesda, MD, U.S. Department of Health and Human Services 1992.

Jacobson KW, Branch LB, Nelson HS: Laboratory tests in chronic urticaria. JAMA 243:1644, 1980.

James LP Jr, Austen KF: Fatal systemic anaphylaxis in man. N Engl J Med 270:597, 1964.

Konig P: Inhaled corticosteroids—their present and future role in the management of asthma. J Allergy Clin Immunol 82:297, 1988.

Lessof MH, Wraith DG, Merrett TG, et al: Food allergy and intolerance in 100 patients—local and systemic effects. Q J Med 49:259, 1980.

Li JTC, Reed CE: Inhaled β-agonists: Weighing risks and benefits. J Respir Dis 14:991, 1993.

Marsh DG, Bias WB: The genetics of atopic allergy. In Samter DW, Talmage DW, Frank MM, et al (eds): Immunological Diseases, 4th edition. Boston, Little, Brown, 1988, p 1027.

Monroe EW: Urticaria. Int J Dermatol 20:32, 1981.

Mullarkey MF: Eosinophilic nonallergic rhinitis. J Allergy Clin Immunol 82:941, 1988.

Patterson R, Greenberger PA, Halwig JM, et al: Allergic bronchopulmonary aspergillosis: Natural history and classification of early disease by serologic and roentgenographic studies. Arch Intern Med 146:916, 1986.

Platts-Mills TAE, Chapman MD: Dust mites: Immunology, allergic disease, and environmental control. J Allergy Clin Immunol 80:755, 1987.

Sampson HA: Food hypersensitivity as a pathogenic factor in atopic dermatitis. NER Allergy Proc 7:511, 1986.

Serafin WE, Austen KF: Mediators of immediate hypersensitivity reactions. N Engl J Med 317:30, 1987.

Sheffer AL, Fearon DT, Austen KF: Hereditary angioedema: A decade of management with stanozolol. J Allergy Clin Immunol 80:855, 1987.

Sheffer AL, Tong AKF, Murphy GF, et al: Exercise induced

anaphylaxis: A serious form of physical allergy associated with mast cell degranulation. J Allergy Clin Immunol 75: 479, 1985.

Thiers BH: The Langerhans cell. J Am Acad Dermatol 6:519, 1982.

Valentine MD, Lichtenstein LM: Anaphylaxis and stinging insect hypersensitivity. JAMA 258:2881, 1987.

VanArsdel PP Jr: Diagnosing drug allergy. JAMA 247:2576, 1982.

VanArsdel PP Jr: Drug hypersensitivity. *In* Bierman CW, Pearlman DS (eds): Allergic Diseases from Infancy to Adulthood, 2nd edition. Philadelphia, WB Saunders Company, 1988, p 684.

VanArsdel PP Jr, Larson EB: Diagnostic tests for patients with suspected allergic disease: Utility and limitations. Ann Intern Med 110:304, 1989.

Weber RW, Nelson HS: Immunologic and atopic aspects of pregnancy and lactation. Ann Allergy 57:159, 1986.

CHAPTER 25

PARASITOLOGY AND TRAVEL MEDICINE

Parasitology

CYNTHIA L. CHAPPELL

Parasites are organisms that live on or in another species at the expense or disadvantage of their host. There are more parasitic species in the world than there are free-living species, even when one excludes viruses, bacteria, and fungi. Humans are host to 100 species of ecto- and endoparasites. *Endoparasites* live within the host's body and can be divided into protozoan species and helminths or parasitic worms. *Ectoparasites*, such as mites, lice, or ticks, live on or in the skin of the host. Parasites by definition damage their hosts, but in many cases, especially in light infections, the degree of injury may be imperceptible. Indeed, many individuals unknowingly harbor one or a few parasites without any evidence of symptoms. In contrast, heavy infections typically are associated with symptomatic illness and in some cases can be very severe and, in selected individuals, even life-threatening. Thus, asymptomatic, as well as symptomatic, parasitic diseases should be treated because they may be a source of infection for others.

There is a common perception by the public that parasitic diseases are only found in developing countries or in the lower socioeconomic classes. Both, of course, are untrue. Many parasitic species are endemic in the United States and may, in fact, be more widespread than once thought. Current estimates indicate that 55 million Americans harbor some parasite. Also, large numbers of people, including military personnel, business persons, and vacationers travelling to other countries around the world, often are exposed to parasites that are not endemic to or commonly found in our own country. In addition, individuals immigrating to the United States from many areas around the globe sometimes bring with them parasitic infections that are not easily recognized by U.S. physicians and may, in some cases, be directly infectious to others. Thus, family physicians may be faced with an increasing number of diseases that in the past were considered exotic for the United States.

It is impossible to cover the full range of parasitic diseases in one chapter, even those that cause the highest morbidity and mortality worldwide. Instead the text will focus on those infections that physicians are most likely to encounter in practice, with a brief mention of some of the more unusual endemic species. For a complete, in-depth description of the full gamut of parasitic infections, a definitive text (Strickland, 1991; Sun, 1988; Warren and Mahmoud, 1990) is most helpful; other sources of basic information include papers by Kappas et al. (1991) and Moore et al. (1993) (see also "Drugs for parasitic infections," 1993).

GASTROINTESTINAL PROTOZOAN PARASITES

Gastrointestinal protozoan infections have decreased greatly over the decades with the advent of water treatment and sanitation. However, waterborne outbreaks of parasitic diseases, such as giardiasis and cryptosporidiosis, still occur when water treatment plants are inadequately maintained or are overwhelmed by area flooding. Small outbreaks may be more common than realized because recent serologic surveys suggest that a high proportion of the population has evidence of past exposure to these organisms. In addition to water, protozoan cysts can be transmitted through food, through exposure to infected domestic animals, and by person-to-person contact. The latter is especially important in institutions, such as day care centers and nursing homes, and in any situation that brings individuals in constant close contact with one another.

Although several species of protozoans can be found in stool, only four are considered truly patho-

TABLE 25–1. PROTOZOAN SPECIES INHABITING THE GASTROINTESTINAL TRACT OF HUMANS*

Amoebae	Flagellates
Entamoeba histolytica	***Giardia lamblia***
Entamoeba coli	*Chilomastix mesnili*
Entamoeba hartmanni	*Retortamonas intestinalis*
Endolimax nana	*Enteromonas hominis*
Iodamoeba butschlii	*Pentatrichomonas hominis*
Dientamoeba fragilis	Coccidians
Ciliates	***Cryptosporidium parvum***
Balantidium coli	***Isospora belli***
	Enterocytozoon bieneusi
	Cyclospora cayetanensis

* Recognized pathogens appear in bold type.

genic in immunocompetent hosts (Table 25–1), *Entamoeba histolytica, Balantidium coli, Giardia lamblia,* and *Cryptosporidium parvum.* Another three species—*Isospora belli, Enterocytozoon* species (microsporidia), and a newly described species, *Cyclospora cayetanensis*—are disease-producing organisms in immunosuppressed individuals. On rare occasions other protozoan species, such as *Dientamoeba fragilis* and *Entamoeba coli,* are associated with symptoms. In these cases no other pathogens are found, and the protozoan species is typically present in high numbers. Many physicians often will treat these patients empirically, usually resulting in clinical improvement. However, it should be noted that these species are not proven pathogens and stools still may contain low numbers of these organisms after treatment.

Giardiasis

Life Cycle

Giardiasis is an infection of the upper bowel caused by *G. lamblia.* The trophozoite, which adheres to the intestinal mucosa, is 10 to 20 μ in length and shaped like a teardrop. The infectious cyst (8 × 12 μ) has two to four nuclei located at one end with characteristic axostyles visible as a linear structure down the center of the cyst. When cysts are ingested with water or food or by person-to-person transmission, the trophozoites passing through the stomach are exposed to digestive enzymes and low pH, which stimulate them to emerge in the duodenum. After excystment, they divide asexually and adhere to the microvillar surface, where they tend to concentrate in the crypts. It is presumed that they live on the mucosal secretions. As the trophozoites move down the colon, they undergo a process of encystment and cyst maturation. The rate at which encystment and subsequent excretion occurs varies widely from day to day.

Epidemiology

Giardia is found worldwide and is a common contaminant of surface waters. *Giardia duodenalis* infects many different mammalian species and cannot be distinguished morphologically from *G. lamblia.* However, the ability of *G. duodenalis* to infect humans is still unknown. *Giardia* cysts remain viable for approximately 5 weeks in cold water and are resistant to the usual concentrations of chlorine. The great majority of cysts are removed from the drinking water supply by filtration; however, low numbers still may be found in tap water. Cysts are killed by temperatures above 50° C; thus, campers and hikers should be cautioned to boil water from rivers and streams before drinking. With the advent of day care centers, *Giardia* has become a more commonly diagnosed infection. Longitudinal studies have found that 33 to 37 per cent of children were infected at some time during the 12 to 15 months of study (Ish-Horowicz et al., 1989; Rauch et al., 1990), and that 22 per cent of the infected children were symptomatic. Furthermore, 37 per cent of the symptomatic children had two or more episodes during the study period. Although the majority of infections are asymptomatic, parents and other close contacts may contract the infection and exhibit symptoms. As expected, the risk of disease in caregivers is associated with the person who has the greatest exposure (i.e., the diaper-changer). Young animals, such as kittens and puppies, also become infected with *Giardia*; however, the risk of human infection from such sources remains unknown.

Pathogenesis and Symptoms

Giardia trophozoites "graze" along the intestinal surface epithelium, congregate in the crypts, and occasionally infect the bile duct epithelium. Mild disease is associated with some reduction in absorption and minor histologic abnormalities. The trophozoites do not invade the mucosal tissues actively, but in severe disease can be associated with microvillar blunting and a submucosal infiltration of lymphocytes and polymorphonuclear leukocytes. It is unclear whether the microvilli are damaged by the parasite or the host immune response. Malabsorption of fat, D-xylose, and vitamin B_{12}, as well as lactose intolerance, are well documented. Specific pathogenic mechanisms are not well understood, but may involve a combination of host immunity and parasite adherence factor(s) and strain differences. Mucosal immunoglobulin (Ig) A has been implicated as a factor in the susceptibility to symptomatic infection and the course of disease. Serum IgA was decreased in children with persistent infection compared to those with acute, nonpersistent infection (Vinayak et al., 1989). Furthermore, breast-fed babies appear to be protected from initial, but not chronic, infection (Morrow et al., 1992).

The classical presentation of acute giardiasis includes two or more of the following symptoms with explosive, watery diarrhea: foul-smelling stools, upper abdominal cramping or discomfort, bloating and flatulence, excessive tiredness, and nausea (Lewis and Freedman, 1992; Hopkins and Juranek, 1991). The incubation period averages 7 to 9 days, and the illness persists in most individuals for approximately 2 weeks. However, in one epidemiologic study, 30 per cent of individuals were symptomatic for 4 or more weeks (Birkhead and Vogt, 1989). Chronic infection is now recognized in infants (Ish-Horowicz et al., 1989; Varga and Delage, 1990), in whom prolonged cyst excretion generally is associated with asymptomatic infection. However, chronic symptomatic infection also occurs, although the incidence has not been established. In both children and adults, symptoms do not always follow the classical pattern, but may present as intermittent mild diarrhea; abdominal discomfort and bloating, especially after meals; or lactose intolerance. Preliminary evidence suggests that a high percentage of individuals with chronic gastrointestinal complaints and unrevealing gastrointestinal work-up are infected with *Giardia* (Chappell and Matson, 1992; Gunasekaran and Hassall, 1992; Leonhardt et al., 1992). It is important to consider giardiasis early in the evaluation of such patients in order to avoid unnecessary, costly procedures.

Diagnosis and Treatment

The standard in diagnostic procedures long has been the microscopic evaluation of stained fecal specimens. This technique, however, is affected adversely by the extreme day-to-day variation in cyst excretion and often requires multiple stool specimens to evaluate the patient effectively. The advent of new, immunologically based assays has dramatically improved the diagnostic capability with a single stool specimen (Addiss et al., 1991; Chappell and Matson, 1992; Isaac-Renton, 1991). The tests, which are produced in an enzyme-linked immunosorbent assay (ELISA) or immunofluorescent, assay (IFA) format, are available from several manufacturers and rely on antibody binding to cysts (IFA) or on antibody capture of parasite products (ELISA). These testing procedures undoubtedly will improve the diagnosis of both acute and chronic infections.

The mainstay of therapy (Table 25–2) is metronidazole in adults and furazolidone in children. Both

drugs are associated with side effects in a some patients, the most common of which are nausea and/or vomiting and abdominal pain. Metronidazole is mutagenic and should be avoided during pregnancy, particularly in the first trimester. Paromomycin, an nonabsorbed aminoglycoside, may be substituted.

Cryptosporidiosis

Cryptosporidiosis is caused by the coccidian parasite *C. parvum*. Prior to the acquired immunodeficiency syndrome (AIDS) epidemic, this organism generally was thought to be nonpathogenic in humans. However, the role of *Cryptosporidium* as an opportunistic infection in immunocompromised individuals and its role in community outbreaks has established its place in the list of pathogenic protozoa.

Life Cycle

The infectious stage of *Cryptosporidium* is the oocyst, a round to oval-shaped organism that is approximately 3 to 5 μ in diameter (Fig. 25–1). When oocysts are ingested, the low pH of the stomach and exposure to digestive enzymes contribute to the weakening of the protective cell wall and subsequent excystation of the organism. Two to four cylindrical sporozoites emerge in the upper bowel and rapidly interact with the enterocyte surface. The mechanism of attachment has not been elucidated; however, it is clear that sporozoites have a limited existence free in the gut lumen. Once the sporozoite interacts with the cell membrane, it gains entry into the cell and inhabits a parasitophorous vacuole just under the enterocyte membrane. Thus, the organisms is intracellular but extracytoplasmic. Within the parasitophorous vacuole, the sporozoite undergoes developmental stages to produce type 1 and type 2 meronts. Type 1 meronts escape from the cell and are responsible for spread of the infection to neighboring cells. Type 2 meronts further mature into gametocytes, fuse, and form oocysts. Some of the oocysts also can be responsible for autoinfection, while thick-walled oocysts are excreted into the environment and pass the infection on to others.

Epidemiology

Oocysts typically are transmitted via contaminated water or contact with an infected animal or person (Janoff et al., 1990). They are commonly present in surface water and can survive in adverse environments for long periods of time. Oocysts must be removed from water by filtration because they are resistant to the usual concentrations of chlorine. Although few *Cryptosporidium* are usually present in treated water, suboptimal flocculation or filtration in times of water stress (flooding, etc.) may lead to community outbreaks in which a

TABLE 25–2. TREATMENT OF GIARDIASIS

	Treatment	
	Metronidazole	Furazolidone
Adult dose*	200–250 mg 3 times daily for 14 days	100 mg 4 times daily for 7–10 days
Pediatric dose	15 mg/kg/day in 3 divided doses for 7 days	8 mg/kg/day in 4 divided doses for 7–10 days

* For pregnant women, use paromomycin, 25 to 30 mg/kg/day in three doses for 7 days.

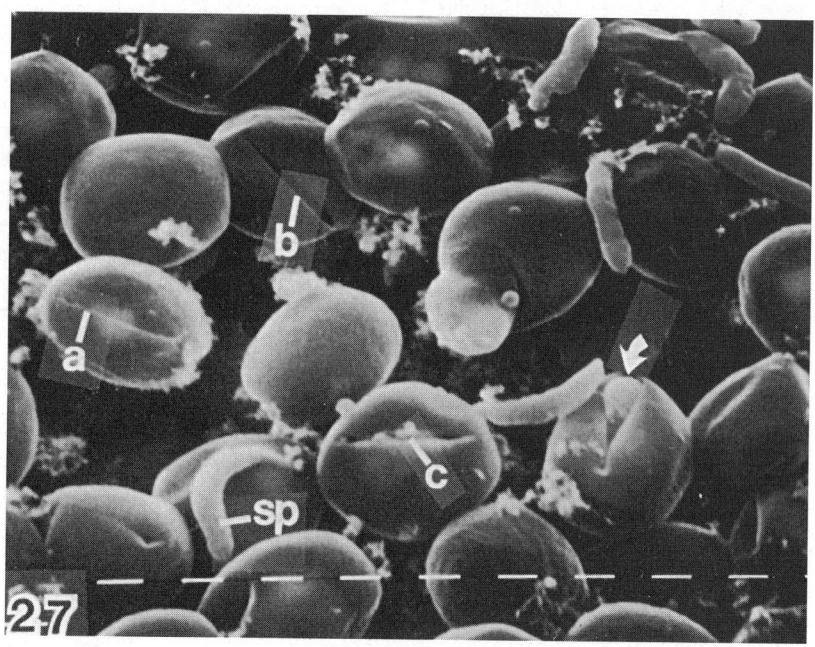

FIGURE 25–1. Scanning electron micrograph of oocysts of a human isolate of *C. parvum*. Oocysts were cleaned and concentrated from the feces of an experimentally infected calf, preincubated in H_2O at 37° C for 2 hours, and then incubated in 0.25% trypsin plus 0.75% sodium taurocholate (w/v) in phosphate-buffered saline (pH 7.4) for 40 minutes at 37° C. Parasites then were deposited on Nucleopore filters, fixed with 3% (w/v) glutaraldehyde in phosphate buffer (pH 7.4), and processed for scanning electron microscopy. The oocyst wall suture begins to dissolve, forming an indention (a). Further dissolution results in the formation of a cleft (b), which widens (c). Sporozoites (sp) escape through the widened cleft (arrow). Lines at the bottom of the micrograph each represent 1.0 μm. (From Walzer PD, Genta RM [eds]: Parasitic Infections in the Compromised Host. New York, Marcel Dekker, 1989, p. 295, with permission.)

large portion (60 per cent or more) of the population report gastrointestinal symptoms (Edwards, 1993; Hayes et al., 1989). Young animals also can be a source of human disease. Calves are especially susceptible to *Cryptosporidium* and excrete oocysts in high numbers. Animal handlers, veterinarians, and dairy farmers often are exposed to oocysts and may become ill. Young children are also especially susceptible to infection. Day care centers have rates of infection that range from approximately 2 per cent during asymptomatic periods to 50 to 60 per cent in times of "in-house" diarrheal outbreaks. Serologic surveys in the United States reveal *Cryptosporidium* antibodies in approximately 32 per cent (Ungar et al., 1989) of immunocompetent individuals, depending on the specific population tested. It is believed that infection typically stimulates a serologic response persisting 12 months or more, but it is not known if the presence of serum antibodies has a protective effect on subsequent exposures.

Pathogenesis and Symptoms

The most heavily infected region of the gastrointestinal tract is the jejunum, although virtually any portion of the gut may be involved in AIDS patients. Little is known about pathogenic mechanisms in this disease. The requirements for parasite adherence, invasion, growth, and development have not been described. Based on the impressive amount of diarrhea seen in some patients, investigators have surmised that a cholera-like toxin may be elaborated by the parasite; however, no direct evidence yet exists to support the notion. In the immunocompetent host, the infection may result in varied reactions. While some individuals are asymptomatic, others have mild to severe symptoms including profuse, watery diarrhea, abdominal cramps, nausea and vomiting, and a low-grade fever (Fayer and Ungar, 1986; Jokipii and Jokipii, 1986). Symptoms generally appear after a 5 to 7 day incubation period and persist for approximately 2 to 4 weeks. Oocysts can be found in the stool for 1 to 2 weeks after symptoms have abated. Chronic carriage has not been a generally recognized phenomenon, but recent studies in children suggest that *Cryptosporidium* may be the cause of chronic diarrhea in some infants and young children (Phillips et al., 1992).

In contrast to the normal host, the immunosuppressed individual is at risk for developing a chronic, progressive, and potentially life-threatening disease (Current et al., 1983). *Cryptosporidium* is a prominent organism in AIDS patients with diarrhea. Some investigators have found that about 20 per cent of AIDS patients are infected (Madi et al., 1991), and others suggest that more than 50 per cent will become infected at some point during their illness. In these individuals, the usual profuse diarrhea is even more dramatic, with fluid losses of 3 to 6 liters/day. In extreme cases, fluid replacement is unable to keep pace with loss, resulting in dehydration and death. The severity of disease is correlated with the CD4+ lymphocyte count. Chronic and progressive disease tends to develop in patients with a CD4+ count less than 200/mm[3] (Flanigan et al., 1992). Histologic analyses of intestinal biopsies from *Cryptosporidium*-infected AIDS patients often show normal villous architecture and no or only moderate inflammation. Villous blunting, crypt hyperplasia, and a mononuclear and lymphocytic inflammatory infil-

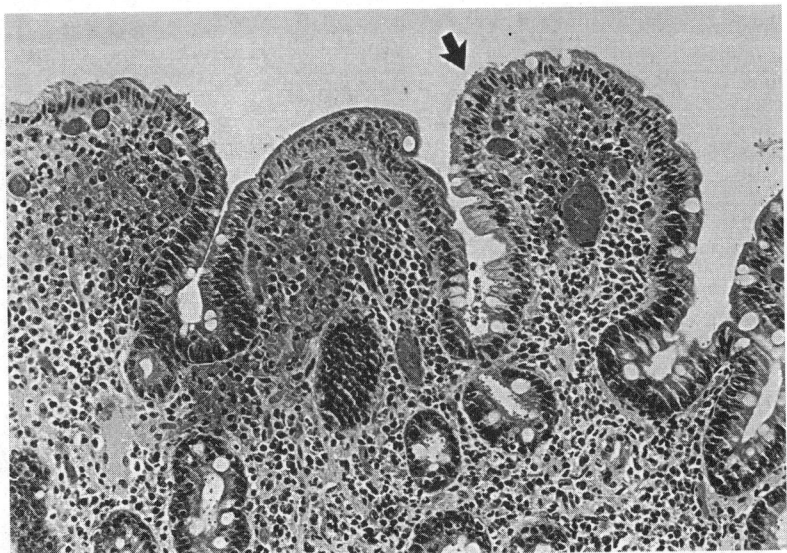

FIGURE 25–2. Photomicrograph of a duodenal mucosal biopsy specimen from a patient with moderately heavy *Cryptosporidium* infection and partial villous atrophy. Grossly broadened and shortened villi are seen. There is a dense *Cryptosporidium* lining in some areas (arrow) and in virtually all crypts; in contrast, only sparse organisms are seen in other parts of the mucosa. The inflammatory infiltrate is predominantly mononuclear, and numerous lymphocytes, but no neutrophils, infiltrate the surface epithelium (H&E; original magnification × 200). (From Genta RM, Chappell CL, White AC, et al: Duodenal morphology and intensity of infection in AIDS-related intestinal cryptosporidiosis. Gastroenterology 108:1769, 1993, with permission.)

trate (Fig. 25–2) are associated with heavier *Cryptosporidium* infections (Genta et al., 1993). Abnormal absorption is also a prominent finding. Extraintestinal disease involving the biliary tract and gallbladder (Teixidor et al., 1991) or respiratory tract (Moore and Frenkel, 1991) also may occur in profoundly suppressed patients.

Diagnosis and Treatment

New laboratory techniques have made *Cryptosporidium* diagnosis easier and more reliable than earlier acid-fast staining methods. An immunofluorescent method using a monoclonal antibody to an oocyst cell wall antigen recently has become available (Arrowood and Sterling, 1989). This method, which assays fresh or preserved fecal samples, has improved sensitivity over staining techniques (Garcia et al., 1992) but does require a fluorescence microscope. ELISA-based antigen capture methodologies are just becoming available and are undergoing clinical testing in several laboratories. To date, the sensitivity of ELISA-based assays appears to be similar to that of the IFA. Both of these diagnostic approaches should improve the detection of *Cryptosporidium* in instances in which there is a low level of infection.

Over 60 antimicrobial agents have been tested for anti-*Cryptosporidium* activity without success. Anecdotal evidence has suggested that drugs such as spiramycin (Moskovitz et al., 1988) and octreotide (Romeu et al., 1991) may improve symptoms in some patients, but no randomized, controlled studies have been done. Paromomycin is another compound that has been used in AIDS-associated cryptosporidiosis with some success (Armitage et al., 1992; Fichtenbaum et al., 1993). The search for efficacious compounds continues. An immunologic approach to treatment, involving the use of hyperimmune colostrum, has produced promising results in a few patients (Connolly et al., 1988; Ungar et al., 1990), but randomized, controlled trials of this therapy will be necessary to establish its efficacy.

Coccidiosis

Other coccidian infections also are associated with enteropathy in AIDS patients. These include *Isospora belli*, the microsporidia *Enterocytozoon bieneusi* and *Septata intestinalis* (Cali et al., 1993; Molina et al., 1993), and a newly described organism, *Cyclospora cayetanensis* (Ortega et al., 1993). All of these organisms cause protracted diarrhea in immunocompromised patients. In several studies of AIDS diarrhea, microsporidia or *Isospora* have been the only identifiable agent in 33 per cent and 2 to 10 per cent of such patients, respectively. The prevalence of *Cyclospora* infection is not yet known. These infections are clinically indistinguishable, and physicians must rely on staining of fecal specimens and/or electron microscopy of biopsy material for their identification.

Detection of *Isospora* and the microsporidial species is especially important because potentially effective treatments may be initiated. In *I. belli* infection, the drug of choice is trimethoprim-sulfamethoxazole (TMP-SMX), 160 mg TMP plus 800 mg SMX four times a day for 10 days, then twice a day for 3 weeks; however, in the event of sulfonamide sensitivity, pyrimethamine, 50 to 75 mg daily, has been effective. Anecdotal experience suggests that *C. cayentanensis* also can be treated successfully with co-trimoxazole, 160 mg TMP plus 800 mg SMX twice a day (Madico et al., 1993). The microsporidia, *S. intestinalis* and *E. bieneusi*, may be treated with albendazole, 400 mg twice a day, although *E. bieneusi* may respond more favorably to mebendazole or octreotide (Cello et al., 1991). Albendazole for the treatment of *E. bieneusi* infections in AIDS patients may be obtained for compassionate use through an Investigational New Drug (IND) protocol from the FDA.

HELMINTHIC INFECTIONS

Parasitic worms are responsible for major worldwide morbidity and mortality. Several helminthic infections are endemic to the United States and others commonly are brought to the United States by immigrants and travellers from endemic regions. Some of these species, such as *Taenia solium* (cysticercosis) are directly infectious to others and pose a significant public health problem in border towns and areas visited by migrant workers. Zoonotic infections also can occur when children or adults are exposed to the infective stages of pet parasites. Cutaneous larva migrans can be contracted when *Toxocara* larvae penetrate the skin of humans and migrate under the dermis. *Dipylidium caninum*, the dog tapeworm, can infect children who accidentally ingest infected fleas after petting a dog or playing on an infested carpet. Patients with these or one of the many helminths prevalent in other countries may at some time present to the family physician. It is important to consider travel history and the possibility of helminthic infection in the work-up. Space limitations require that only the most common species are discussed herein; however, a basic medical parasitology text is an essential resource for every practice.

Taeniasis and Cysticercosis (Pork Tapeworm)

The taeniid species, *Taenia saginata* (beef tapeworm) and *Taenia solium* (pork tapeworm), are both parasites of the human gastrointestinal tract. It is the adult stage of these parasites that is found attached to the intestinal mucosa. *T. solium*, however, is also the causative agent of a second disease entity, cysticercosis, that is the manifestation of the larva stage infection. Because humans can be both the definitive and intermediate host, *T. solium* has a much greater impact on the population than does *T. saginata*. In addition to the enormous impact of the human disease, *T. solium* infection in pigs results in major economic losses in countries already stressed by a variety of other social and economic problems. It is estimated that 50 million cases of neurocysticercosis exist worldwide with 50,000 deaths annually (CDC, 1992). Since Mexico, Central and South America are areas of high endemicity for *T. solium*, travellers, immigrants from those areas or persons in close contact with infected individuals may contract cysticercosis. New trade agreements with Mexico and a relaxation of border regulations are expected to increase the number of cases seen in the United States.

Life Cycle

The *T. solium* life cycle involves an intermediate host (pig) and a definitive host (human) (Figure 25–3). Individuals become infected when the larval cysts, cysticerci, are ingested with the flesh of undercooked pork. These small cysticerci (5 to 20 mm dia) consist of a fluid-filled bladder and an invaginated scolex, the tapeworm "head". Once the cysticerci pass through the stomach, the bladder is disrupted, and the scolex evaginates and attaches to the intestinal wall. The segmented adult matures within about 2 months, can attain a length of 2 to 7 meters, and can survive for up to 25 years. The intestinal infection with the adult worm is called taeniasis. The 700 to 1000 segments or proglottids comprising the adult worm each contain both testes and uterus. The more mature proglottids, containing approximately 50,000 eggs, are found at the distal end of the tapeworm, where one or more (sometimes 2 to 3 are attached in a chain) may break off and be passed with the stool. It is the proglottids (1.2 × 0.6 cm) which will be seen by the infected person since the ova (31 to 43 microns in dia; Figure 25–4) are microscopic. Proglottids may move slowly in an undulating fashion for several minutes after being passed.

In areas where sanitation is lax, human feces may be deposited in open privies or may contaminate the soil where pigs forage. When pigs ingest the ova, they hatch in the small intestine and actively burrow through the intestinal wall. This migratory stage, called the oncosphere, may localize to many tissues including the musculature. The invasive larval infection is termed cysticercosis. Likewise, cysticercosis in humans occurs when *T. solium* ova are accidentally ingested. The ensuing process of ova hatching and migration is much the same as in the pig. Cysts in humans may also be found in

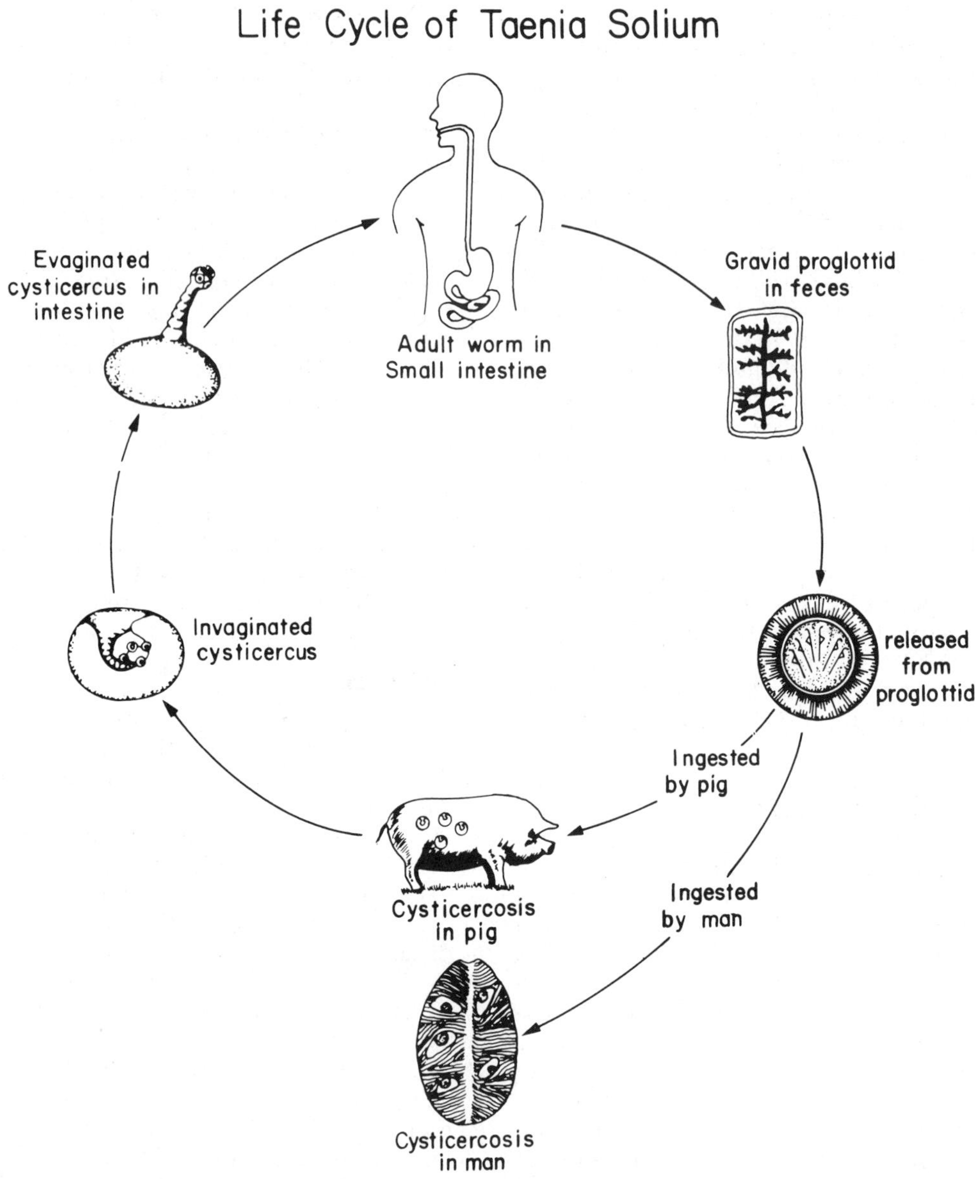

Life Cycle of Taenia Solium

FIGURE 25–3. Taenia solium life cycle. (From Sun T: Color Atlas and Textbook of Diagnostic Parasitology. New York, Igaku-Shoin Medical Publishers, 1988 p. 263, with permission.)

many tissues, including musculature, ocular tissues, and in the brain. Neurocysticercosis is caused by one or many cysts localizing to the brain parenchyma or, in some cases, the ventricles.

Epidemiology

T. solium is endemic in many areas of the world, such as Southeast Asia, India, Africa (central and southern), Mexico, Central and South America (Schantz, 1989). The 5 million cases of *T. solium* infections worldwide almost surely represents an underestimate since no sensitive method of establishing intestinal infection exists. New serodiagnostic assays for invasive disease indicate that in China, India, Peru, Rwanda, and Mexico cysticercosis has been found in 11 to 44 per cent of

patients with neurological complaints, which also suggests that this infection is more widespread than previously appreciated. Indeed, direct observation at autopsy from hospital patients in Mexico have found that 3.8 per cent of individuals had neurocysticercosis (Del Brutto and Sotelo, 1988). Moreover, in Mexico cysticercosis accounts for more cases of adult onset of seizures than all other causes (Medina, 1990). The number of cysticercosis cases have increased in the United States along with increased immigration. In a recent study in Houston, of 112 cases of cysticercosis, 82 (73 per cent) occurred in Hispanics (Shandera et al., 1994, This paper is also an excellent and current review of all aspects of neurocysticercosis).

Studies have shown that approximately 20 to 25

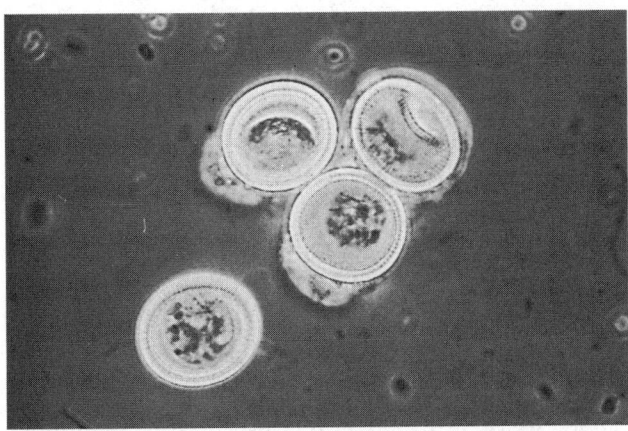

FIGURE 25–4. Four eggs of *Taenia* species examined by phase-contrast microscopy. Hooklets can be seen in the embryo. (×160). (From Sun T: Color Atlas and Textbook of Diagnostic Parasitology. New York, Igaku-Shoin Medical Publishers, 1988, p. 269, with permission.)

per cent of individuals with cysticercosis also harbor the adult tapeworm, suggesting an autoinfection via direct fecal-oral contamination. In other cases, however, the lack of a concurrent intestinal infection suggests that ova were transmitted through contact with a person harboring the adult parasite. Since these worms can survive for up to 25 years, a person with taeniasis can potentially be the focus of one or more cases of cysticercosis. For example, several cases of cysticercosis in a New York Jewish community were traced to a domestic employee (Schantz et al., 1992), and other cases have been reported in persons who have never left the United States (Sorvillo et al., 1992). Further, studies in Mexico and Central America support the notion of transmission via close contact with infected individuals, such as household members (Lara-Aguilera et al., 1992; Diaz-Camacho et al., 1990; Kaminsky, 1991).

Pathogenesis and Symptoms

Taeniasis typically involves only one tapeworm and is usually asymptomatic. There may be some irritation at the attachment site and occasionally some mild symptoms, including indigestion, diarrhea or constipation. If eosinophilia is present, it is usually less than 15 per cent. On rare occasions, tissue necrosis and even perforation may occur when the local blood supply becomes compromised.

Cysticercosis is caused from the migration of oncospheres to various body tissues and their subsequent development into cysticerci. These cysts can localize to all areas of the body, including the musculature, spinal cord, eyes, peritoneal cavity, lungs, intestinal submucosa, thyroid glands, spinal cord and brain (Figure 25–5). Symptoms vary

widely depending upon the tissue affected, as well as the size and number of cysts. Viable cysts are space-occupying lesions that appear to cause little overt damage to surrounding tissues beyond a mechanical compression. Some mild fibrosis is typically seen, but there is essentially no cellular response. The immune response only becomes apparent when the cysts die and begin to leak antigens. At that time there is a brisk inflammatory response characterized by the influx of neutrophils, lymphocytes, plasma cells, histiocytes and some eosinophils. The size of the cyst can vary, but tends to be around 1 cm in diameter in tissues, such as the muscle. Cysts may enlarge, however, in more open areas, such as the peritoneal cavity and in the ventricles of the brain. Cysts in the muscles, including the myocardium, and the subcutaneous tissues are usually asymptomatic. Calcified cysts in these locations may be found incidentally on x-rays.

Ocular cysticercosis is found in about 20 per cent of neurocysticercosis patients. The cysts are usually localized in the vitreous humor and in subretinal tissues, but may also be found in the orbit, conjunctiva or anterior chamber. Visual problems are related to obstruction or scarring.

Neurocysticercosis is the most important pathological condition of *T. solium* infection. Cysts can be present for years without causing significant problems. One to hundreds of cysts have been found in the human brain; however, the more usual number is about 10 or fewer cysts. Studies of soldiers revealed that the incubation period could be 1 to 30 years with an average of 4.5 years. Children, however, may have a shorter course. As in other tissues, dying cysts elicit an inflammatory response that is thought to be an important part of the symptomatology. This was confirmed when corticosteroid treatment was found to lessen the symptoms. The most common complaints are adult onset sei-

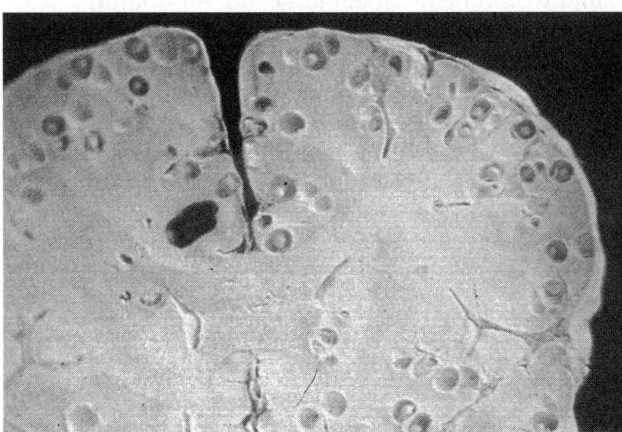

FIGURE 25–5. A case of cerebral cysticercosis shows numerous cysticerci on the cut surface of the brain. Notice that most bladder worms have a protoscolex. (From Sun T: Color Atlas and Textbook of Diagnostic Parasitology. New York, Igaku-Shoin Medical Publishers, 1988, p. 270, with permission.)

zures (79.5 per cent) and headache (40.2 per cent) (Shandera et al., 1994). Other symptoms may vary widely depending on the particular location of the lesion(s) and the state of the cyst. In a multiple cyst infection, there is an asynchrony in the development. Cysts may be different sizes and may have different survival times. Thus, in a patient some cysts may be viable while others are dying and, yet others, may be dead and calcified. Refecting this disparity, seizures may be focal or generalized, sporadic or progress to status epilepticus. The onset may be insidious or sudden. Occasionally, especially in intense infections, mental disturbances may also be noted.

Increased intracranial pressure can be caused by a mechanical occlusion of the ventricular circulation. The condition often persents with hydrocephalus and is characterized by a steady progression to vomiting, pain and visual abnormalities. Cysticerci found within the ventricle can become enlarged and are associated with a racemose form of the disease. In this instance, the larvae develop abnormally, dividing to form a cluster-like collection of cysts. The percentage of cases with ventricular disease varies widely (0.7 to 40 per cent) from study to study (Sotelo et al., 1985a; Grisolia and Wiederholt, 1982; Loo and Braude, 1982). Such conditions are very serious and usually require surgical intervention and shunting.

Diagnosis

Diagnosis of taeniasis is problematic since ova from *T. solium* and *T. saginata* are indistinguishable. In cases where the tapeworm is recovered, the species can be identified through the number of uterine branches in the proglottid or the morphological features of the scolex. Fecal smears for ova identification may often be negative since the proglottids do not immediately disintegrate and release eggs into the stool. Sensitive and specific immunologically-based tests for *T. solium* antigens in stool would be of great benefit for epidemiological studies and for identification of active infections posing the added risk of cysticercosis.

Radiologic methods, including computerized tomography (CT) scans and magnetic resonance imaging (MRI), are the standards in the diagnosis of cysticercosis (Chang et al., 1991; Rodriquez-Carbajal et al., 1987; Zee et al., 1988). Enhancement with contrast medium is necessary to visualize inflammation surrounding recently non-viable or dying cysts. CT is somewhat better at detecting cortical calcifications, while MRI appears to be more reliable for parenchymal, intraventricular and leptomeningeal forms (Shandera et al., 1994). These techniques can often visualize the scolices within the cysts and, in the case of a single cyst, can provide an important clue in differentiating cysticercosis from other pathological processes. These imaging techniques are also useful for following the response to therapy (Jena et al., 1992).

Detection of *T. solium* antibodies is at present a useful confirmatory, rather than diagnostic, test. Although advances have been made in the test's specificity (Tsang et al., 1989), its sensitivity was 94 per cent and 64 per cent in cases of multiple cysts and single cysts, respectively (Wilson et al., 1991). However, the improved specificity has yielded positivity in both serum and CSF, thus making testing possible without requiring a spinal tap. This test is being employed by the CDC and may be obtained upon request. CSF analysis is not particularly helpful in diagnosis since normal values have been reported for 37 per cent of confirmed cases and abnormalities, when they were seen, were minimal and nonspecific (Shandera, 1994).

Treatment

Treatment of cysticercosis is controversial, and outcomes may not differ significantly from the natural course of the disease. Even though no placebo-controlled trials have been done, praziquantel is widely used since patients with non-inflammatory cystic lesions showed a decreased number of cysts (Sotelo et al., 1984; Sotelo et al., 1988) and improvement in seizures (Del Brutto et al., 1992; Robles et al., 1987; Sotelo et al., 1985b). Although corticosteroids have been used concurrently with praziquantel by some in the past, a recent review suggests that in the absence of increased intracranial pressure its use is not warranted (McGowan et al., 1992). Further, in their series of 112 patients with cysticercosis, Shandera et al. (1994) observed a poorer outcome when corticosteroids were combined with praziquantel treatment. Albendazole has been compared with praziquantel in the treatment of parenchymal disease (Escobedo et al., 1987; Takayanagui and Jardim, 1992), where it was found to be equally effective. Dosages for both drugs are shown in Table 25–3.

Hydrocephalus and increased intracranial pressure can result from obstruction by cysts and/or associated inflammation. In such cases, surgical intervention is warranted. Patients receiving shunts, however, must often undergo revision (Colli et al., 1986; Rueda-Franco, 1987). In one study praziquantel therapy was associated with a need for fewer shunt revisions (Shandera et al., 1994); however, further study is needed to firmly establish the role of praziquantel in extraparenchymal disease.

Enterobiasis (Pinworms)

Enterobiasis is the most common and, perhaps, one of the more ancient parasitic infections in the United States (Fig. 25–6). The parasite, along with other nematode and protozoan species, has been detected in 2000-year old human feces (Faulkner, et al., 1989). Almost all individuals acquire pinworms at one time or another during their lifetimes, usually as children. Recent studies, how-

TABLE 25–3.   TREATMENT OF HELMINTHIC INFECTIONS

Helminth species	Pyrantel pamoate	Mebendazole	Levamisole
Enterobius vermicularis	Single dose: 11 mg/kg P.O. (max. 1 g); Repeat after 2 weeks	100 mg P.O.	150 mg (adults); 3–5 mg/kg (children)
Ascaris lumbricoides	Single dose: 11 mg/kg P.O. (max. 1 g); Repeat after 2 weeks		
Taenia solium	Praziquantel Single dose: 5–10 mg/kg	Albendazole	
Taeniasis	50 mg/kg/day in 3 doses × 15 day	15 mg/kg/day in 3 doses × 28 day	
Cysticercosis			

ever, suggest that the infection may be declining in the United States (Vermund and MacLeod, 1988). Early infections do not prevent reinfection during childhood (Gilman et al., 1991) or later; however, the susceptibility to symptomatic infection decreases with age. This ubiquitous parasite, *Enterobius vermicularis*, is an unassuming passenger that causes perianal irritation in its host but rarely is responsible for any serious tissue damage.

Life Cycle

The *Enterobius* life cycle is relatively simple compared to that of many other parasitic nematodes. Humans are virtually the only known host and no intermediate host species is required, which also means that autoinfection occurs. Infection is initiated when a parasite egg is ingested.

The larvae hatch in the jejunum and develop as they move through the ileum. The time to maturation to the adult stage can vary between 1 and 3 months, with an average of approximately 7 weeks. The adult female worm measures 0.5 mm in width and 5 to 11 mm in length and inhabits the appendix, cecum, and colon. Males are smaller, measuring 0.1 to 0.2 mm in diameter and 2 to 5 mm in length. Each female produces approximately 10,000 eggs, which are shed after the worm migrates out of the body onto the perianal region. The female then dies and rapidly disintegrates. The eggs (approximately 28 × 57 μ) are oval shaped with a slight flattening on one side. The larva, which is visible through the transparent shell, quickly develops and is infectious within about 4 to 6 hours.

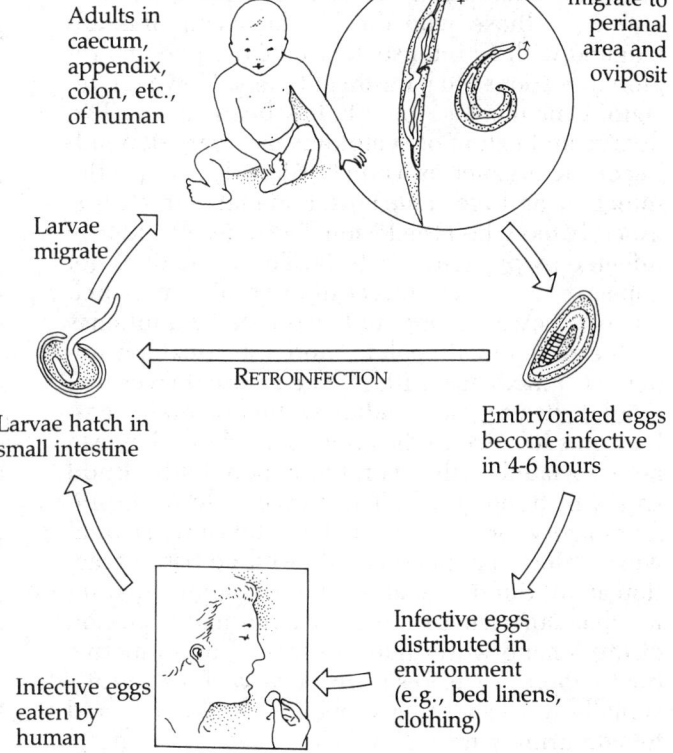

FIGURE 25–6. *Enterobius* life cycle. (From Bogitsh BJ, Cheng TC: Human Parasitology. Philadelphia, WB Saunders Company, 1990, p. 330, with permission.)

Gravid females migrate to perianal area and oviposit

Adults in caecum, appendix, colon, etc., of human

Larvae migrate

RETROINFECTION

Larvae hatch in small intestine

Embryonated eggs become infective in 4-6 hours

Infective eggs distributed in environment (e.g., bed linens, clothing)

Infective eggs eaten by human

Epidemiology

Enterobius infections are spread most easily when population density is high and environmental conditions are conducive to egg survival. Thus, classrooms, day care centers, and other groups of children provide excellent opportunities for parasite spread. Pinworms are transmitted most efficiently by hand-to-mouth contact, a common occurrence when children contaminate their fingers by scratching the anal region and subsequently handle toys, books, or other objects. Transmission also can occur when bedclothes or linens are handled. Eggs are dispersed into the environment by shaking bed linens and can be found in the dust throughout the house. The larva within the eggshell can survive in the environment for about 2 weeks, depending on the temperature and humidity of the surroundings, but generally lose their infectivity within 1 to 2 days after oviposition. Eggs can be inhaled with dust particles or can infect others indirectly when dust settles on objects, food, and the like. Thus, once introduced into the household, *Enterobius* becomes firmly established in the family by continuous passage among the members. The latest Centers for Disease Control results (1987 data) gathered from state diagnostic laboratories show that 11.4 per cent of tape tests for suspected pinworm cases were positive; most (61.6 per cent) of these cases were reported from the Southern Atlantic states (Kappus et al., 1991).

Pathology and Symptoms

As in many parasitic infections, the majority of individuals (about 75 per cent) are asymptomatic. However, those who do develop symptoms are plagued with an intense itching of the perianal region in response to parasite antigens. However, no significant increase in IgE has been noted. The degree and extent of symptoms may vary depending on factors such as worm burden, duration of the infection, and age of the host. Perianal dermatitis is exacerbated when the lesions become secondarily infected by pyogenic bacteria. The worm does not appear to cause any direct injury to the intestinal mucosa; however, one study has noted granulomas of the abdominal, pelvic, and intestinal peritoneum (Sinniah et al., 1991). The granuloma formed around disintegrating adult worms or their eggs. Parasites localize in the appendix, where they can be associated with a chronic appendicitis (Budd and Armstrong, 1987). Their exact role in the inflammatory process is unclear, because several worm-infested appendices showed no tissue reaction at all (Sinniah et al., 1991). Extraintestinal infections can occur as a result of abnormal migration of the female worm into the female reproductive tract, where it can result in vulvovaginitis. Occasionally worms also have been found in male and female urinary tracts.

Diagnosis and Treatment

The "Scotch tape test" remains the standard in diagnosis. This is a simple procedure that can be carried out at home. The components of the test are a piece of clear tape and a microscope slide. After the child has gone to sleep, the gravid females migrate to the perianal region to deposit eggs. Thus, the nighttime or early morning hours are best for egg collection. A piece of tape is placed on the perianal skin and gently peeled away. The tape is then adhered to a microscope slide and delivered to the physician for examination. The characteristically shaped eggs can be seen easily under the microscope, and a diagnosis can be confirmed. One test will detect more than 50 per cent of infections. Additional tests increase the number of cases detected, but negative results are valid only after seven tests performed every second day (Pawlowski, 1990). Fecal samples are not generally useful, because the eggs are not dispersed until the female migrates out of the body.

Pyrantel pamoate and mebendazole are effective agents for killing adult worms. The exact dosages can be found in Table 25–3. These agents, however, are ineffective against newly hatched larvae, and retreatment in 2 weeks often is required to eradicate the parasite. For individuals, such as schoolchildren, under constant exposure to infection, treatment may be given every 3 to 4 months to prevent heavy infection. In a household in which more than one family member is suspected of having pinworm infection, all members should be treated twice.

Ascariasis

According to World Health Organization estimates, ascariasis is the most common parasitic disease in the world, infecting an estimated 900 million people, or approximately 25 per cent of the human population. *Ascaris lumbricoides*, the roundworm, is the largest human nematode, with the female measuring 22 to 35 cm in length and 3 to 6 mm in diameter. The male roundworm is slightly smaller, with a diameter of 2 to 4 mm and a length ranging from 15 to 31 cm. The male easily can be distinguished by its coiled tail and copulatory spicules (Fig. 25–7A). Ascariasis is worldwide in its distribution and is endemic to the U.S. southern and Gulf Coast states.

Life Cycle

Infection in humans is initiated with the ingestion of *A. lumbricoides* ova. The microscopic ova ($40 \times 60\ \mu$) are produced in quantity and excreted with the feces. Mature female worms typically release approximately 200,000 eggs every day for their 12 to 18-month life span. When ova are ingested, they hatch in the upper intestine, penetrate

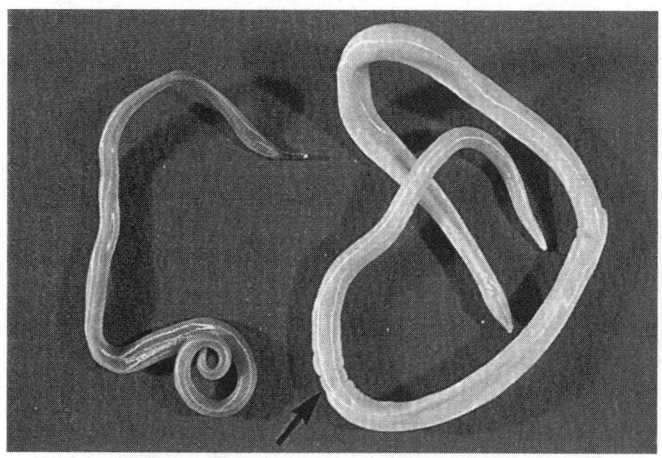
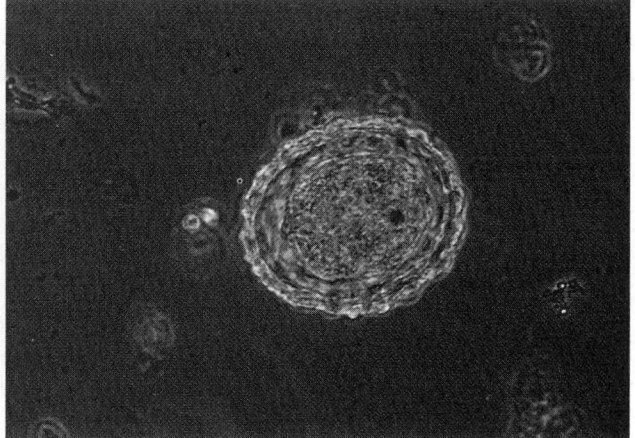

A   **FIGURE 25–7.** *A*, A pair of female and male worms of *A. lumbricoides.* Note the vulvar waist (arrow) of the   **B**
female worm and the coiled end of the male worm. *B*, A fertilized egg of *A. lumbricoides* has a translucent
shell and an albuminous outer coat and contains a large, unsegmented ovum. (Unstained, ×160.) (From Sun
T: Color Atlas and Textbook of Diagnostic Parasitology. New York, Igaku-Shoin Medical Publishers, 1988, p
179, with permission.)

the gut mucosa, and migrate through the portal system to the liver and eventually to the lung, where they arrive 5 to 6 days after exposure. After 7 to 8 more days, the immature worms penetrate the alveoli and move to the bronchi and trachea, aided by coughing spasms in the host. Once in the trachea, the worms are swallowed and eventually inhabit the jejunum, where they reach their full maturity and begin to produce ova within approximately 2 to 2.5 months after infection. The excreted ova each contain a single larva that must progress through developmental stages before becoming an infective larva. This process takes place in the soil. Under optimal environmental conditions, ova can become infectious in 10 to 14 days and can remain viable for up to 6 years.

Epidemiology

Because infection is through contact with contaminated soil, prevalence is directly related to population density, sanitary conditions, and environmental factors. Maximum infection rates typically are found in children from approximately 4 to 14 years old. Some studies show a declining infection rate with age; however, reinfection in endemic environments is common. In developing countries, the prevalence of *A. lumbricoides* may reach 90 per cent or more, but varies widely with socioeconomic conditions. Infection rates of approximately 45 per cent are reported in the rural areas of Central and South America, Africa, and China. In the United States, ascariasis can be found in immigrants and in individuals living in endemic regions. The overall U.S. infection rate is estimated to be low; however, no recent population-based surveys have been done. From stool samples submitted to state laboratories in 1987, 1735 infections were identified in 44 states (Kappus et al., 1991).

Pathogenesis and Symptoms

Pathologic changes in the host are related to the migration of the parasite through tissues and the intensity of infection. *Ascaris* produces potent allergens, which during lung migration may elicit a hypersensitivity response characterized by pulmonary infiltration and asthmatic attacks. Other symptoms may include urticaria, low-grade fever, cough, dyspnea, substernal discomfort and occasionally a bloody sputum. In contrast, typical intestinal infections of 10 to 20 worms often produce little to no symptomatology. When they do occur, symptoms may include one or more of the following: abdominal discomfort, nausea, vomiting, anorexia, and diarrhea or constipation. There is a compelling body of evidence that supports the notion that roundworms (usually heavy infections) contribute to malnutrition in children with low caloric intake. Each worm competes with the host for 22.7 mg of total nitrogen and 2.8 grams of carbohydrate each day. *Ascaris* infection in well-nourished children, however, is not associated with any significant dietary deficiency.

Adult roundworms do not invade the intestinal mucosa unless they are disturbed by high fevers, certain drugs, or other irritants. In such an event, the parasites can migrate out of the gastrointestinal tract through the mouth or anus or into the biliary ducts and liver, or on occasion will perforate the intestine, causing a peritonitis and/or abscess. Another serious complication of ascariasis is bowel obstruction, which occurs in heavy infections when worms aggregate, usually in the ileum. Treatment can sometimes be helpful in clearing the obstruction, but, for those who do not improve rapidly, surgical intervention is necessary. Presurgical treatment has the added benefit of preventing migration of remaining worms through sutured areas (Weirsma and Hadley, 1988).

Diagnosis and Treatment

The large number of roundworm eggs that are produced each day help to ensure the survival of the parasite through the spread of infection, but also afford the relative ease of diagnosis. A single worm will produce enough eggs to be detected in a smear of a single fecal specimen. *Ascaris* ova may be identified by their characteristic morphology (Fig. 25–7*B*) in smears from fresh or preserved fecal specimens with or without the aid of stains. Roundworms occasionally are an incidental finding on radiographs of barium studies. The worms ingest the contrast medium and are revealed distinctly within the intestinal lumen. Nevertheless, barium studies are not the method of choice for diagnosis of ascariasis. Serologic diagnosis has not proven effective because the complex nature of the antigen preparation leads to a lack of specificity. An increase in total IgE and eosinophilia may be detected in the migratory phase of the infection, but decline rapidly after the worms reach the intestine.

Treatment for pulmonary ascariasis is not available, but symptoms may be eased with the use of corticosteroids. In contrast, the treatment for intestinal *Ascaris* infection is straightforward and effective. Pyrantel pamoate, mebendazole, and levamisole commonly are used as single agents and have cure rates of 80 per cent or better (Asaolu et al., 1991; Tankhiwale et al., 1989) (Table 25–3). The drugs are efficacious for the adult worm in the dosages shown, but have no effect on larvae in the migratory phase of infection or encased in the egg (Massara et al., 1991).

ECTOPARASITES

Lice

Lice inhabiting clothing (body lice; *Pediculus humanus humanus*) (Fig. 25–8) or hair on the head

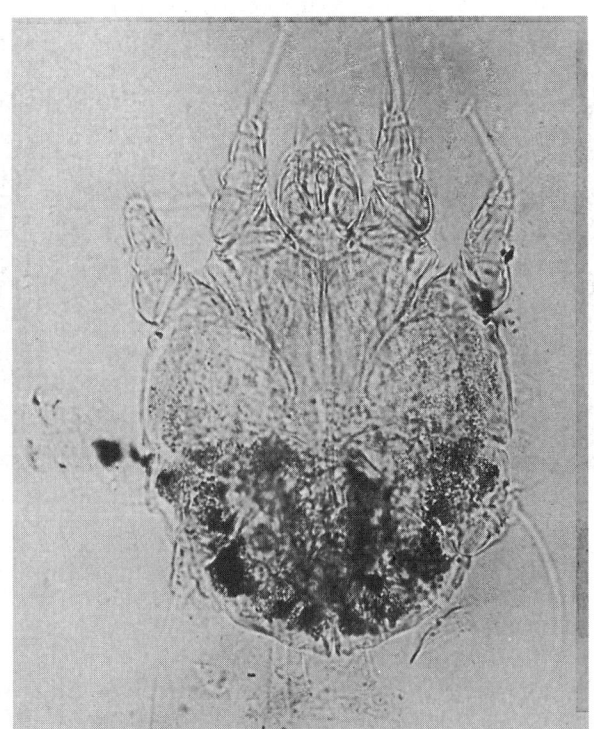

FIGURE 25–9. Adult mite, *Sarcoptes scabiei hominis.* (From Strickland: Hunter's Tropical Medicine, 7th edition. Philadelphia, WB Saunders Company, 1991, with permission.)

(*Pediculus humanus capitis*) or in the pubic area (*Phthirus pubis*) are contracted easily through direct contact with infected individuals or their clothing, or objects such as combs or brushes that they have used. The infestation is associated with population density and lack of adequate sanitary conditions. However, the insects may be passed in virtually any place where people gather, such as schoolrooms. The adult louse deposits eggs (nits) on the hair shaft (head lice) or on clothing (body lice). Eggs hatch to produce larval stages that undergo a series of moults to become adult lice. Continuous infestation with lice can persist indefinitely.

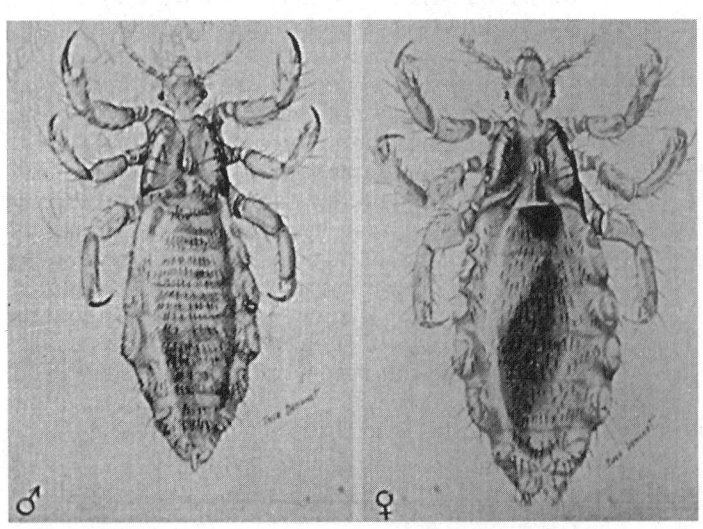

FIGURE 25–8. *Pediculus humanus humanus* male and female. (Courtesy of the National Institutes of Health, U.S. Public Health Service.)

Lice bite host skin in order to access blood, their main source of nourishment. Thus, infected individuals experience cutaneous lesions, papules, and intense pruritis. Also, lesions can become infected with bacteria secondarily from scratching. In times of stress to a population, such as in war, lice are an effective vector for the spread of epidemic typhus or louse-borne relapsing fever.

Adult lice sometimes can be seen in fine-toothed combs, or the nits can be detected by examination of the hair shaft. The infestation responds well to therapy with shampoos or ointments containing 1% permethrin or 1% lindane. Infested areas, such as bedding and clothing, can be treated with 1% malathion or fumigated with ethylformate.

Mites

The most common mite infesting humans is the itch mite or scabies (*Sarcoptes scabiei*). Scabies is characterized by small skin vesicles formed when the mites burrow into the skin. Mites live off the blood of their hosts and burrow into the skin to lay their eggs. Invasion of the dermis results in intense itching. The adults may invade virtually any part of the body, but particularly are found in crevices between the fingers or toes, on wrists and elbows, between the penis and scrotum, and on the buttocks, backs of knees, or under the breasts. The mite is best detected by placing a drop of mineral oil on an early papule or burrow and scraping the area with a sterile scalpel. The material then can be examined under the microscope. The adult mites (Fig. 25–9) are approximately 215 to 390 μ in size, and the eggs are $170 \times 92\,\mu$. Occasionally, yellow-brown fecal particles ($15 \times 30\,\mu$) also can be visualized. Specific identification of the mite species is often difficult because of the many morphologic stages of the life cycle. Topical preparations containing 5% permethrin, 1% lindane, or 10% crotamiton are effective treatment, but one to three applications may be required. The lotion or ointment should be applied to clean, dry skin.

Other mite species infesting animals, such as pets or birds, or grain mites occasionally can cause discomfort in sensitive individuals. These mites do not burrow into skin for nourishment, but can elicit hypersensitivity reactions from the deposition of their products on the skin. Treatment of such infestations requires ridding of the mites from the environment rather than topical treatment for the individual.

REFERENCES

Addiss DG, Mathews HM, Stewart JM, et al: Evaluation of a commercially available enzyme-linked immunosorbent assay for *Giardia lamblia* in stool. J Clin Microbiol 29:1137, 1991.

Armitage K, Flanigan T, Carey J, et al: Treatment of cryptosporidiosis with paromomycin: A report of five cases. Arch Intern Med 152:2497, 1992.

Arrowood MJ, Sterling CR: Comparison of conventional staining methods and monoclonal antibody-based methods for *Cryptosporidium* oocyst detection. J Clin Microbiol 27:1490, 1989.

Asaolu SO, Holland CV, Crompton DW: Community control of *Ascaris lumbricoides* in rural Oyo State, Nigeria: Mass, targeted and selective treatment with levamisole. Parasitology 103:291, 1991.

Birkhead G, Vogt RL: Epidemiologic surveillance for endemic *Giardia lamblia* infection in Vermont: The roles of waterborne and person-to-person transmission. Am J Epidemiol 129:762, 1989.

Budd JS, Armstrong C: Role of *Enterobius vermicularis* in the aetiology of appendicitis. Br J Surg 74:748, 1987.

Cali A, Kotler DP, Orenstein JM: *Septata intestinalis* N.G., N. Sp., an intestinal microsporidian associated with chronic diarrhea and dissemination in AIDS patients. J Eukaryot Microbiol 40:101, 1993.

Cello JP, Grendell JH, Basuk P, et al: Effect of octreotide on refractory AIDS-associated diarrhea: A prospective, multicenter clinical trial. Ann Intern Med 115:705, 1991.

Centers for Disease Control and Prevention (CDC): Neurocysticercosis. Update: International Task Force for Disease Eradication. MMWR 41:697, 1993.

Chang KH, Seung YC, Hesselink J: Parasitic disease of the central nervous system. Neuroimaging Clin North Am 1:159, 1991.

Chappell CL, Matson CM: *Giardia* antigen detection in patients with chronic gastrointestinal disturbances. J Fam Pract 35:49, 1992.

Colli BO, Martelli N, Assitari JA, et al: Results of surgical treatment of neurocysticercosis in 69 cases. J. Neurosurgery 65:309, 1986.

Connolly GM, Dryden MS, Shanson DC, Gazzard BG: Cryptosporidial diarrhea in AIDS and its treatment. Gut 29:593, 1988.

Current WL, Reese NC, Ernst JVD, et al: Human cryptosporidiosis in immunocompetent and immunodeficient persons: Studies of an outbreak and experimental transmission. N Engl J Med 308:1252, 1983.

Del Brutto OH, Santibanez R, Noboa CA, et al: Epilepsy due to neurocysticercosis: Analysis of 203 patients. Neurology 42:389, 1992.

Del Brutto OH, Sotelo J: Neurocysticercosis: An update. Rev Infect. Dis. 10:1075, 1988.

Diaz-Camacho S, Candil-Ruiz A, Uribe-Beltran M, et al: Serology as an indicator of *Taenia solium* tapeworm infections in a rural community in Mexico. Trans Roy Soc Trop Med Hyg 84:563, 1990.

Drugs for parasitic infections. Med Lett Drugs Ther 35:111, 1993.

Edwards DD: Troubled waters in Milwaukee. ASM News 59:342, 1993.

Escobedo P., Penagos P., Rodriquez J, et al: Albendazole therapy for neurocysticercosis. Arch Intern Med 147:738, 1987.

Faulkner CT, Patton S, Johnson SS: Prehistoric parasitism in Tennessee: Evidence from the analysis of desiccated fecal material collected from Big Bone Cave, Van Buren County, Tennessee. J Parasitol 75:461, 1989.

Fayer R, Ungar BLP: Cryptosporidium spp. and cryptosporidiosis. Microbiol Rev 50:458, 1986.

Fichtenbaum CJ, Ritchie DJ, Powderly WG: Use of paromomycin for treatment of cryptosporidiosis in patients with AIDS. Clin Infect Dis 16:298, 1993.

Flanigan T, Whalen C, Turner J, et al: *Cryptosporidium* infection and CD4 counts. Ann Intern Med 116:840, 1992.

Garcia LS, Shum AC, Bruckner DA: Evaluation of a new monoclonal antibody combination reagent for direct fluorescence detection of *Giardia* cysts and *Cryptosporidium* oocysts in human fecal specimens. J Clin Microbiol 30:3255, 1992.

Genta RM, Chappell CL, White AC, et al: Duodenal morphology and intensity of infection in AIDS-related intestinal cryptosporidiosis. Gastroenterology 108:1769, 1993.

Gilman RH, Marquis GS, Miranda E: Prevalence and symptoms of *Enterobius vermicularis* infections in a Peruvian shanty town. Trans R Soc Trop Med Hyg 85:761, 1991.

Grisolia JS, Wiederholt WC: CNS cysticercosis. Arch Neurol 39:540, 1982.

Gunasekaran TS, Hassall E: Giardiasis mimicking inflammatory bowel disease. J Pediatr 120:424, 1992.

Hayes EB, Matte TD, O'Brien TGR, et al: Large community outbreak of cryptosporidiosis due to contamination of a filtered public water supply. N Engl J Med 320:1372, 1989.

Hopkins RS, Juranek DD: Acute giardiasis: An improved clinical case definition for epidemiological studies. Am J Epidemiol 133:402, 1991.

Isaac-Renton JL: Immunological methods of diagnosis in giardiasis: An overview. Ann Clin Lab Sci 21:116, 1991.

Ish-Horowicz M, Korman SH, Shapiro M, et al: Asymptomatic giardiasis in children. Pediatr Infect Dis J 8:773, 1989.

Janoff EN, Mead PS, Mead JF, et al: Endemic *Cryptosporidium* and *Giardia lamblia* infections in a Thai orphanage. Am J Trop Med Hyg 43:248, 1990.

Jena A, Sanchetee PC, Tripathi R., et al: MR observations on the effects of praziquantel in neurocysticercosis. Magn Reson Imaging 10:77, 1992.

Jokipii L, Jokipii AMM: Timing of symptoms and oocyst excretion in human cryptosporidiosis. N Engl J Med 315:1643, 1986.

Kaminsky RG de: Taeniasis-cysticercosis in Honduras. Trans Roy Soc Trop Med Hyg 85:531, 1991.

Kappus KK, Juranek DD, Roberts JM: Results of testing for intestinal parasites by state diagnostic laboratories, United States, 1987. MMWR 40(SS-4):25, 1991.

Lara-Aguilera R, Mendoza-Cruz JF, Martinez-Toledo, JL, et al: Taenia solium taeniasis and neurocysticercosis in a Mexican rural family. Am J Trop Med Hyg 46:85, 1992.

Leonhardt U, Ebert R, Bommer W, Schauer A: Diagnostic and therapeutic problems in lamblia infections. Dtsch Med Wochenschr 117:96, 1992.

Lewis DJ, Freedman AR: *Giardia lamblia* as an intestinal pathogen. Dig Dis 10:102, 1992.

Loo L, Braude AL: Cerebral cysticercosis in San Diego. Medicine 61:341, 1982.

Madi K, Trajman A, daSilva CF, et al: Jejunal biopsy in HIV-infected patients. J Acquir Immune Defic Syndr 4:930, 1991.

Madico G, Gilman RH, Miranda E, et al: Treatment of *Cyclospora* infections with cotrimoxazole (letter). Lancet 342:122, 1993.

Massara CL, Costa HM, DeSouza DW, et al. Viability of *Ascaris Lumbricoides* eggs eliminated after anti-helminthic therapy. Mem Inst Oswaldo Cruz 86:233, 1991.

McGowan JE Jr, Chesney PJ, Crossley KB: Guidelines for the use of systematic glucocorticosteroids in the management of selected infections. Working Group on Steroid Use, Antimicrobial Agents Committee, Infectious Disease Society of America. J Infect Dis 165:1, 1992.

Medina MT, Rosas E, Rubio-Donnadieu F, et al: Neurocysticercosis as the main cause of late-onset epilepsy in Mexico. Arch Intern Med 150:325, 1990.

Molina JM, Sarfati C, Beauvais B, et al: Intestinal microsporidiosis in human immunodeficiency virus-infected patients with chronic unexplained diarrhea: Prevalence and clinical and biologic features. J Infect Dis 167:217, 1993.

Moore AC, Herwaldt BL, Craun GF, et al: Surveillance for water-borne disease outbreaks—United States, 1991–1992. MMWR 42(SS-5):1, 1993.

Moore JA, Frenkel JK: Respiratory and enteric cryptosporidiosis in humans. Arch Pathol Lab Med 115:1160, 1991.

Morrow AL, Reves RR, West MS, et al: Protection against infection with *Giardia lamblia* by breast-feeding in a cohort of Mexican infants. J Pediatr 121:363, 1992.

Moskovitz BL, Stanton TL, Kusmierek JJ: Spiramycin therapy for cryptosporidial diarrhoea in immunocompromised patients. J Antimicrob Chemother 22:189, 1988.

Ortega YR, Sterling CR, Gilman RH, et al: *Cyclospora* species—a new protozoan pathogen of humans. N Engl J Med 328:1308, 1993.

Pawlowsk ZS: Enterobiasis. In Warren KS, Mahmoud AAF (eds): Tropical and Geographical Medicine, 2nd edition. New York, McGraw-Hill, 1990, pp 404–407.

Phillips AD, Thomas AG, Walker-Smith JA: *Cryptosporidium*, chronic diarrhoea and the proximal small intestinal mucosa. Gut 33:1057, 1992.

Rauch AM, Van R, Bartlett AV, Pickering LK: Longitudinal study of *Giardia lamblia* infection in a day care center population. Pediatr Infect Dis J 9:186, 1990.

Robles C, Sedano AM, Vargas-Tenori N: Longterm results of praziquantel therapy in neurocysticercosis. J Neurosurg 66:359, 1987.

Rodriquez-Cabajal J, Boleaga-Duran B, Dorfsman J: The role of computed tomography (CT) in the diagnosis of neurocysticercosis. Childs Nerv Syst 3(4):199, 1987.

Romeu J, Miro JM, Sirera G, et al: Efficacy of octreotide in the management of chronic diarrhoea in AIDS. AIDS 5:1495, 1991.

Rueda-Franco F: Surgical considerations in neurocysticercosis. Child's Nerv Syst 3:212, 1987.

Schantz PM: Surveillance and control programs for cestode diseases. In Miller MJ, Lover EJ (eds.): Parasitic Diseases: Treatment and Control. Ch. 35. Boca Raton: CRC Press, 1989.

Schantz PM, Moore AC, Munoz JL, et al: Neurocysticercosis in an othodox Jewish community in New York City. N Engl J Med 327:692, 1992.

Shandera WX, White AC Jr, Chen JC, et al: Neurocysticercosis in Houston, Texas. A report of 112 cases. Medicine (Baltimore) 73(1):37, 1994.

Sinniah B, Leopairut J, Neafie RC, et al: Enterobiasis: A histopathological study of 259 patients. Ann Trop Med Parasitol 85:625, 1991.

Sorvillo FJ, Waterman SH, Richards FO, et al: Cysticercosis surveillance: Locally acquired and travel-related infections and detection of intestinal tapeworm carriers in Los Angeles County. Am J Trop Med Hyg 47:365, 1992.

Sotelo J, Escobedo F, Penagos P: Albendazole vs praziquantel for therapy for neurocysticercosis: A controlled trial. Arch Neurol 45:532, 1988.

Sotelo J, Escobedo F, Rodriguez-Carbajal J, et al: Therapy of parenchymal brain cysticercosis with praziquantel. N Engl J Med 310:1001, 1984.

Sotelo J, Guerrero V, and Rubio F: Neurocysticercosis: A new classification based on active and inactive forms. Arch Intern Med 145:442, 1985a.

Sotelo J, Torres B, Rubio-Donnadieu F, et al: Praziquantel in the treatment of neurocysticercosis: Longterm follow-up. Neurology 35:752, 1985b.

Strickland GT (ed): Hunter's Tropical Medicine, 7th ed. Philadelphia, WB Saunders Company, 1991.

Sun T: Color Atlas and Textbook of Diagnostic Parasitology. New York, Igaku-Shoin Medical Publishers, 1988.

Takayanagui OM, and Jardim E: Therapy for neurocysticercosis: Comparison between albendazole and praziquantel. Arch Neurol 49:290, 1992.

Tankhiwale SR, Kukade AL, Sarmah HC, et al: Single dose therapy of ascariasis—a randomized comparison of mebendazole and pyrantel. J Commun Dis 21:71, 1989.

Teixidor HS, Godwin TA, Ramirez EA: Cryptosporidiosis of the biliary tract in AIDS. Radiology 180:51, 1991.

Tsang VC, Brand JA, and Boyer AE: An enzyme-linked immunoelectric-transfer blot assay and glycoprotein antigens for diagnosing human cysticercosis (*Taenia solium*). J Infect Dis 159:50, 1989.

Ungar BL, Mulligan M, Nutman TB: Serological evidence of *Cryptosporidium* infection in US volunteers before and during Peace Corps service in Africa. Arch Intern Med 149:894, 1989.

Ungar BL, Ward DJ, Fayer R, Quinn CA: Cessation of *Cryptosporidium*-associated diarrhea in an acquired immunodeficiency syndrome patient after treatment with hyperimmune bovine colostrum. Gastroenterology 98:486, 1990.

Varga L, Delage G: *Giardia lamblia* infestation at child day care centers: Nutritional impact in infested children. Arch Fr Pediatr 47:5, 1990.

Vermund SH, MacLeod S: Is pinworm a vanishing infection? Laboratory surveillance in a New York City medical center from 1971 to 1986. Am J Dis Child 142:566, 1988.

Vinayak VK, Kumkum, Khanna R: Serum antibodies to giardial surface antigens: Lower titres in persistent than in non-persistent giardiasis. J Med Microbiol 30:207, 1989.

Warren KS, Mahmoud AAF (eds): Tropical and Geographical Medicine, 2nd ed. New York, McGraw-Hill, 1990.

Weirsma R, Hadley GP: Small bowel volvulus complicating intestinal ascariasis in children. Br J Surg 75:86, 1988.

Wilson M, Bryan RT, Fried JA, et al: Clinical evaluation of the cysticercosis enzyme-linked immunoelectrotransfer blot in patients with neurocysticercosis. J Infect Dis 164:1007, 1991.

Zee CS, Segali HD, Boswell W, et al: MR imaging of neurocysticercosis. J. Comput Assist Tomogr 12:927, 1988.

Emporiatrics (Travel Medicine)

JANE E. CORBOY

THE FAMILY PHYSICIAN'S ROLE IN TRAVEL MEDICINE

Family physicians frequently provide advice for their patients embarking on foreign travel. Inquiries range from requests for antibiotics to information on flying with small children. Many travel agents offer travelers' advice that is quite practical and generally accurate, but when a patient asks a physician for guidance, he or she wants solid medical information. The functions family physicians most frequently perform for travelers are:

1. Risk assessment and counseling for risk reduction

2. Provision of appropriate preventive and therapeutic measures

3. Diagnosis and treatment of complications of travel

Physician easily may carry out these three activities in the setting of a formal pretravel visit and a post-trip visit scheduled if needed.

THE PRETRAVEL VISIT

The goals of the pretravel visit are (1) to assess relative risks of acquiring disease, (2) to provide risk reduction counseling, and (3) to provide appropriate prophylactic medication or immunizations.

The physician should assess the traveler's relative risk in light of the specifics of the trip planned. The determinants of relative risk are factors related to the trip itself, such as the location, length of stay, means of travel, and activities planned, and factors related to the traveler's underlying diseases or conditions. For example, a person traveling by bus to a remote area of an underdeveloped country and working for several weeks in a relief project clearly has a greater risk for infectious diseases, malaria, and exposure to local hazards than a person flying to a resort area for a weekend on the beach. The information can be obtained using a checklist-type questionnaire (Fig. 25–10).

After learning the traveler's plans, the physician should plan to provide information on immunizations, malaria prophylaxis, traveler's diarrhea, avoidance of other complications of travel, and resources available to the traveler during the trip.

Need for Immunizations

Because many vaccine-preventable diseases, including measles, polio, tetanus, diphtheria, and pertussis, are endemic in developing countries worldwide, it is especially important that travelers' routine immunizations are current. Infants and children may have their immunization schedules accelerated, especially for polio and measles (Anderson, 1992). Oral polio vaccine may be given at 4- to 6-week intervals beginning in the newborn period in order for the child to have three doses prior to departure. If an infant is traveling to an underdeveloped country, the physician may administer single-antigen measles vaccine as early as 6 months of age, followed by measles–mumps–rubella (MMR) vaccine at 15 months and a second MMR vaccine at elementary or high school entry.

Travel medicine

TRIP PLANNING QUESTIONNAIRE
Travelers, please answer the questions on this sheet
as best you can. It will help us to help you.

Today's date: _____ Name: _____ Sex: M ____ F ____ Age: _____

Allergies to drugs or vaccines: _____

Current medical conditions: _____

Current medications/hormones: _____

Female patients: Are you pregnant or   Referred by: _____
planning pregnancy? Yes _____ No _____

Itinerary (List countries and dates in order of travel):

      City, country _____ Dates _____

                      _____ _____

                      _____ _____

Purpose of travel (check one):

      Business _____ Foreign study _____ Volunteer agency _____

      Missionary _____ Vacation _____ Field work _____

      Diving _____ Teaching _____ Climbing _____

                                                    Other _____

Type of travel (check choices):

      Independent travel: Fixed itinerary_____ Flexible itinerary _____

      Guided or escorted tour _____

Accommodations (check choices):

      Hotel _____ Rented foreign home _____ Camp _____ Youth hostel _____

      Safari _____ Resort _____ Private home _____ Other _____

Home departure date _____ Home return date _____

Total length of trip: wk _____ mo _____ yr _____

Goals of your visit(s) to this office: _____
_____

Do you need a pretravel physical exam and forms to be filled out? Yes ____ No ____
(You may need a special appointment for this).

_____

This section to be filled out by nurse or doctor

Information sheets given to patient.

_____Vaccine information	_____Proguanil HCl (Paludrine)	_____Diarrhea	_____Low lactose diet
_____High altitude	_____Malaria	_____Jet lag diet	_____Travelers' medical kit
_____Schistosomiasis	_____Hepatitis	_____Japanese encephalitis	_____Malaria/pregnancy
_____Food/water precautions	_____Rabies	_____Chagas' disease	_____Insect repellents

Adapted with permission from the University of Washington Travel Medicine Service, Seattle, Wash.

FIGURE 25–10. Travel planning questionnaire. (From Dupont HL, Jong EC, Zanick DC: When a patient
wants travel advice. Patient Care, July:55, 1991, with permission.) *Illustration continued on following page.*

TRIP PLANNING QUESTIONNAIRE *(Continued)*
(To be filled out by MD or RN)

Today's date: _____ BP: _____ Temp.: _____ Pulse: _____

Immunizations	Date of last shot	This trip	Clinical dates (Initial after giving)		
Diphtheria-tetanus toxoids and pertussis vaccine adsorbed (children 2 mo–7 yr)	_____	Y/N	_____	_____	_____
Tetanus-diphtheria toxoids adsorbed (adults and children older than 7 yr)	_____	Y/N	_____	_____	_____
Poliovirus vaccine live oral trivalent (Orimune)	_____	Y/N	_____	_____	_____
Poliovirus vaccine, inactivated (IPOL, Poliovax)	_____	Y/N	_____	_____	_____
Measles-mumps-rubella virus vaccine live (M-M-R II)	_____	Y/N	_____	_____	_____
Yellow fever virus vaccine, live, attenuated (YF-Vax)	_____	Y/N	_____	_____	_____
Cholera vaccine	_____	Y/N	_____	_____	_____
Typhoid fever vaccine live oral Ty21A (Vivotif Berna)	_____	Y/N	_____	_____	_____
Typhoid fever vaccine, inactivated	_____	Y/N	_____	_____	_____
Meningococcal polysaccharide vaccine groups A, C, Y, and W-135 (Menomune-A/C/Y/W-135)*	_____	Y/N	_____	_____	_____
Rabies vaccine, human diploid cell (Imovax Rabies, Imovax Rabies I.D.)	_____	Y/N	_____	_____	_____
Rabies vaccine, adsorbed	_____	Y/N	_____	_____	_____
Influenza virus vaccine (Flu-Imune, Fluogen, Fluzone, etc.)	_____	Y/N	_____	_____	_____
Immune globulin intramuscular (Gamastan, Gammar)†	_____	Y/N	_____	_____	_____
Hepatitis B vaccine (Engerix-B, Recombivax HB)	_____	Y/N	_____	_____	_____
Plague vaccine	_____	Y/N	_____	_____	_____
Pneumococcal vaccine, polyvalent (Pneumovax 23, Pnu-Imune 23)	_____	Y/N	_____	_____	_____
Haemophilus b conjugate vaccine (HibTITER, PedvaxHIB, PROHIBIT) (children 2 mo-5 yr)	_____	Y/N	_____	_____	_____

Prescriptions given

Malaria prophylaxis
_____ Chloroquine phosphate (Aralen Phosphate)
_____ Doxycycline hyclate (Doryx, Vibramycin, Vibra-Tabs, etc.) (chloroquine-resistant *Plasmodium falciparum* malaria)
_____ Mefloquine HCl (Lariam) (chloroquine-resistant and/or sulfadoxine/pyrimethamine-resistant *P. falciparum* malaria)

Malaria treatment
_____ Sulfadoxine/pyrimethamine (Fansidar) (chloroquine-resistant strains of *P. falciparum* malaria)

Traveler's diarrhea
_____ Diphenoxylate HCl/atropine sulfate (Lomotil) tablets or liquid
_____ Loperamide HCl (Imodium) 2-mg capsules
_____ Trimethoprim/sulfamethoxazole (Bactrim DS, Cotrim DS, Septra DS, etc.) double-strength tablets
_____ Doxycycline hyolate (Doryx, Vibramycin, Vibra-Tabs, etc.) 100-mg capsules or tablets (or tetracycline)
_____ Ciprofloxacin HCl (Cipro) 500-mg tablets

Other treatment
_____ Triazolam (Halcion) 0.25-mg tablets (nonbarbiturate hypnotic)
_____ Acetazolamide (Diamox) 250-mg tablets (prevention/treatment of acute mountain sickness)

Notes: _____

_____

RN: _____ MD: _____

* Booster dose recommended for children first vaccinated when less than 4 yr who remain at high risk. † For prophylaxis against hepatitis A.

FIGURE 25–10. *Continued*

Adolescents and adults may need boosters for tetanus (as diphtheria and tetanus toxoids) and measles (as MMR) if these are not current.

Travelers may need other vaccines when required by countries for entry or because of unavoidable risks to the traveler (Cohen-Abbo and Edwards, 1992). Some of the more commonly requested vaccines are yellow fever, typhoid, cholera, immune globulin, and hepatitis B. Only state-designated centers may administer *yellow fever vaccine* because of its perishable nature. Many countries in or neighboring endemic areas require a validated International Certificate of Vaccination for entry. Endemic areas include sub-Saharan Africa and tropical South America. Physicians should contact the local public health agency for information about their community's sites authorized to administer and certify yellow fever vaccinations. *Typhoid fever vaccine* is available in oral or parenteral form. It is not an entry requirement for any country and is indicated only if ingestion of contaminated food or water is unavoidable. *Cholera vaccine* is a parenteral vaccine required by some Asian countries. It is not proven to be effective, however, and a single dose of 0.2 mL for children and 0.5 mL for adults, rather than the two-dose series, will satisfy most local requirements. *Immune serum globulin* may be effective for preventing hepatitis A in travelers to high-prevalence areas. A single intramuscular dose of 0.02 mL/kg gives 3 months' protection; travelers staying longer than 3 months should receive 0.06 mL/kg intramuscularly every 6 months. *Hepatitis B* is endemic in Southeast Asia, the South Pacific islands, the Amazon Basin, sub-Saharan Africa, Haiti, and the Dominican Republic. Although the vaccine is not required for entry into any country, physicians should give the three-dose series to health care and laboratory workers, or to anyone who will have close contact with a high-prevalence population, including children.

Other available vaccines, depending on the traveler's destination and itinerary, include meningococcus, rabies, plague, and Japanese and tick-borne encephalitis.

Malaria Prophylaxis

The first step in counseling for malaria prevention is stratification of the traveler's risk of acquiring the disease. As noted earlier, the risk varies with the geographic area visited and the activities planned. The *Plasmodium* species causing malaria are endemic to tropical and semitropical areas. Travelers acquire the infection through bites from infected *Anopheles* mosquitoes. Therefore, the cornerstone of prevention is avoidance of mosquitoes through knowledge of their nocturnal feeding habits and the use of physical barriers and chemical repellents. Travelers should restrict outdoor activities to the daytime, wear clothing that covers as much of the skin as possible, and use mosquito screens and chemical repellents in their living quarters. Repellents containing Deet (*N,N*-diethyl-*m*-toluamide) are most effective, but can cause neurotoxic reactions if used in excess. Repellents should be applied only to intact, exposed skin, and rinsed off after returning indoors. Permethrin may be applied to clothing and pyrethrum sprays may be used to reduce the flying insect population in sleeping areas. These measures reduce travelers' risk of malaria, but physicians also should recommend a chemoprophylaxis program for travelers to malarious areas (Centers for Disease Control, 1990). The regimens shown in Table 25–4 are the most commonly recommended. Usually the traveler starts the drug 1 to 2 weeks before arrival in

TABLE 25–4. DRUGS FOR MALARIA PREVENTION

Drug	Regimen
For Prophylaxis	
Chloroquine phosphate (Aralen), 300 mg	5 mg/kg base, up to 300 mg base P.O. weekly
Hydroxychloroquine (Plaquenil), 310 mg	5 mg/kg base, up to 310 mg base P.O. weekly
Mefloquine (Lariam), 250 mg	<15 kg: not recommended 15–19 kg: ¼ tablet/week 20–30 kg: ½ tablet/week 31–45 kg: ¾ tablet/week >45 kg: 1 tablet/week
Doxycycline (Vibramycin), 100 mg tablets or capsules	Over 8 years of age, 2 mg/kg up to 100 mg orally per DAY beginning 1–2 DAYS before entry into malarious area
Primaquine	0.3 mg/kg base up to 15 mg base P.O., daily for last 14 days of travel to areas with high level of *P. ovale* and *P. vivax.*
For Presumptive Treatment Only	
Pyrimethamine-sulfadoxine (Fansidar), to be taken *once* for symptoms of malaria	5–10 kg: ½ tablet 11–20 kg: 1 tablet 21–30 kg: 1½ tablets 31–45 kg: 2 tablets >45 kg: 3 tablets

the malarious areas and continues for the duration of the trip and for 1 month after departure. Chloroquine resistance is increasingly prevalent in most areas, except the Middle East, western Central America, Haiti, and the Dominican Republic. Chloroquine is recommended for these areas, while mefloquine or doxycycline are the drugs of choice for chloroquine-resistant areas. If a person cannot take either of these drugs (e.g., children weighing under 15 kg), the physician should provide chloroquine and instruct the patient to take a "treatment dose" of pyrimethamine-sulfadoxine if a febrile illness develops, and to seek medical care as soon as possible. Travelers spending longer than 1 month in malarious areas should prevent "relapsing malaria" (hepatic *P. vivax* or *P. ovale* sequestration) with primaquine taken the last 14 days of their prophylactic regimen. Pregnant women may take chloroquine, but other drugs are not safe. Because malaria is more severe in pregnancy and there is increased risk of stillbirth and prematurity, women should avoid elective travel to chloroquine-resistant areas during pregnancy.

Traveler's Diarrhea Counseling

Traveler's diarrhea is a common problem among international travelers, most commonly among those traveling from developed into developing countries. The disease, usually associated with cramps and watery diarrhea, may result from a variety of bacteria, viruses, and parasites. The most commonly isolated bacterial pathogens are *Escherichia coli* (enterotoxigenic, enteropathogenic, enteroinvasive, and enteroadherent strains), *Salmonella*, *Shigella*, and *Campylobacter*. Common viral pathogens include rotaviruses and Norwalk-like viruses, while common parasitic causes include *Giardia lamblia* and *Entamoeba histolytica*. Risk factors for infection, as with malaria, include travel to countries or parts of countries with poor sanitation, failure to carry out behavior modifications, and the presence of underlying disease or immune compromise. Stratification of countries' risk is shown in Table 25–5. The key behavioral measures are those that minimize exposure to enteric pathogens. These include avoidance of "high-risk" foods and beverages, frequent hand washing, and brushing teeth with boiled, purified or carbonated water. Table 25–6 lists safe and unsafe foods and beverages.

Despite these measures, many travelers become ill with diarrhea, and many request a prophylactic antibiotic to take during their trip. There are three general approaches to reducing the morbidity of traveler's diarrhea: (1) bismuth subsalicylate, (2) prophylactic antibiotics, and (3) early symptomatic and antibiotic therapy after the development of symptoms. A number of clinical trials have analyzed the cost–benefit balance of the three ap-

TABLE 25–5. RISK FOR TRAVELER'S DIARRHEA BY COUNTRY

High Risk (40%)
Mexico and Latin America
Africa
Middle East
Southeast Asia

Intermediate Risk (10–15%)
Caribbean Islands
Northern Mediterranean
Unified Commonwealth (former Soviet Union)
China

Low Risk (2–5%)
Canada and the United States
Northwestern Europe
Australia and New Zealand
South Africa
Japan

TABLE 25–6. SAFE FOODS AND BEVERAGES FOR PREVENTION OF TRAVELER'S DIARRHEA

Safe Foods
Well-cooked meats and fish that are steaming hot when served
Fruits that the traveler peels
Foods with high acid or sugar content
Dry foods like breads and crackers
Canned fruits and vegetables

Safe Beverages
Carbonated, bottled water
Water that has been boiled or purified
Full-strength canned fruit juices
Hot coffee or tea
Wine and beer

Tap water and ice made from tap water are *not* safe.

proaches, especially since the introduction of the quinolone antibiotics. Because of medication side effects, and risks that include the development of resistant organisms, and because of the efficacy of early treatment if needed, prophylactic therapy should be limited to debilitated patients or those taking a short trip with a "critical mission" when even 24 hours of morbidity would be unacceptable. The physician may provide travelers with appropriate instructions on early assessment and therapy (DuPont et al., 1986). The patient should measure his or her temperature with the first watery stool. If the temperature is less than 100° F, and there is no blood in the stool, the patient may start loperamide and antibiotics; antibiotics alone should be started if the temperature is over 100° F or there is blood present. Table 25–7 lists the prophylactic and therapeutic regimens that may be prescribed.

Other Illnesses or Complications of Travel

In addition to infectious agents, travelers are exposed to unfamiliar surroundings and the illnesses

TABLE 25–7. CHEMOPROPHYLAXIS AND THERAPY OF TRAVELER'S DIARRHEA

Prevention Only
Bismuth subsalicylate (Pepto-Bismol) 2 tablets four times daily during travel and for 2 days after leaving area

Prophylactic and Therapeutic Antibiotics

Location	Drug	Prophylactic Dosage	Therapeutic Dosage
Non-Caribbean Mexico	Trimethoprim-sulfamethoxazole DS	1 tablet/day	1 tablet b.i.d.
Caribbean Mexico,	Norfloxacin (Noroxin)	400 mg/day	400 mg b.i.d.
Latin America,	Ciprofloxacin (Cipro)	500 mg/day	500 mg b.i.d.
Africa, Asia	Ofloxacin (Floxin)	200 mg/day	200 mg b.i.d.

or complications that may follow. The physician may be able to prevent these complications by offering anticipatory guidance about environmental, behavioral, and medical risks to the traveler. Common environmental risks include heat, cold, sun exposure, and high altitude. Travelers frequently want advice on avoiding jet lag, which may be ameliorated by a special 3-day diet with alternating feasts and fasts that may help reset the biologic clock (Hill and Pearson, 1988). It is also important to counsel about the risk of sexually transmitted diseases, including human immunodeficiency virus and hepatitis B. Finally, patients with pre-existing medical conditions should carry all medications and prescriptions with them, including prescriptions for corrective lenses. The stress of travel or an unusual diet or activity may cause exacerbation of some conditions, such as seizure disorders, asthma, diabetes, or heart disease, so patients should have explicit sick day rules and extra medications as needed.

Resources Available to the Traveler during the Trip

Despite excellent advice and careful adherence to risk-reducing behavior, some travelers will become ill during their trip. There are two major sources for obtaining care overseas (Table 25–8). The International Association for Medical Assistance to Travelers (IAMAT) is a nonprofit organization that maintains a worldwide directory of English-speaking physicians who have agreed to provide medical care to international travelers at reasonable rates. The nearest American consulate or embassy can recommend additional resources in case of an emergency, so the traveler should know how to contact the embassy at all times during the trip.

At the conclusion of the pretravel visit, the physician should provide the traveler with guidelines for the need for a post-travel visit. The three major reasons for requesting a post-travel visit are (1) the patient is symptomatic (fever, diarrhea) on return; (2) the patient has had a health problem abroad; and (3) the patient is returning from a lengthy stay in a high-risk area.

RESOURCES AVAILABLE TO THE PHYSICIAN FOR ADVISING INTERNATIONAL TRAVELERS

Although much of the information about maintaining wellness during travel is simply sound health advice, there is an ever-changing, ever-increasing volume of information related to travelers' health. Family physicians may access this information in a variety of ways (Table 25–8). Someone who sees a large number of international travelers may wish to subscribe to one of the computer-based services that has weekly or monthly updates on vaccine requirements, distribution of chloroquine resistance, and even current political conditions that affect travelers, and can print an individualized report for the traveler at the time of the

TABLE 25–8. RESOURCES FOR PHYSICIANS

Overseas Medical Assistance Service
  International Association for Medical Assistance to Travelers (IAMAT)
  417 Center Street
  Lewiston, NY 14092

Publications
Health Information for International Travel ("Yellow Book") (HHS publication No. 90-8280)
Summary of Health Information for International Travel ("Blue Sheet")
  Centers for Disease Control and Prevention (CDC)
  (404) 332-4559
Travel Medicine Advisor, a loose-leaf notebook with bimonthly updates and patient education handouts that may be reprinted
  American Health Consultants, Inc.
  Box 740056
  Atlanta, GA 30374
  (800) 688-2421

Recorded Information
CDC FAX Information Service: (404) 332-4565
CDC hotline: (404) 332-4559

Subscription Services
Immunization Alert, a computer-based information system, updated weekly or monthly with IBM-compatible or Macintosh diskettes
  93 Timber Drive
  Storrs, CT 06268
  (203) 487-0611

pretravel visit. A physician who receives only rare requests for advice may be well served by having the Centers for Disease Control and Prevention (CDC) publication, *Health Informational for International Travel* (the "Yellow Book"), one copy of which is free to physicians on request. Another readily accessible source of travel information is the CDC's hot line or FAX Information Service. Table 25–8 gives the address or telephone numbers for these and other resources.

REFERENCES

Anderson EL: Preparation for travel. Semin Pediatr Infect Dis 1:3, 1992.

Centers for Disease Control: Recommendations for the prevention of malaria among travelers. MMWR 39(RR-3):1, 1990.

Cohen-Abbo A, Edwards KM: Vaccines for foreign travel. Semin Pediatr Infect Dis 1:6, 1992.

DuPont HL, Ericsson CD, Johnson PC, et al: Antimicrobial agents in the prevention of travelers' diarrhea. Rev Infect Dis 8(suppl 2):S167, 1986.

Hill DR, Pearson RD: Health advice for international travel. Ann Intern Med 108:839, 1988.

CHAPTER 26

OBSTETRICS

KENNETH L. NOLLER and RANDY WERTHEIMER

The discipline of family medicine is well suited to the provision of family-centered obstetric care. Family physicians have the opportunity to know the medical and psychosocial dynamics of the family prior to the pregnancy, to support the family through the pregnancy, to manage the acute challenge of labor and delivery, to care for the expanded family in transition, and to help them adjust to their new and changing roles.

The longitudinal experience of knowing patients before they are pregnant, being the provider of the news that they are pregnant, dealing with the patient's fears and hopes about the process, following the changes in the patient's state at different stages of the pregnancy, observing changing family dynamics with the expectation of the new baby, being present during the labor process, mediating that process to both mother and father and extended family, participating with the family in the delivery, assuring the family of normalcy or explaining the event of any abnormality in either mother or baby or the process itself, and of course following mother, baby and family back into the home setting—this by nature longitudinal practice is at the center of the experience of family practice. (Candib, 1976, p 393)

Although the medical advances in obstetrics, including fetal monitoring, epidural anesthesia, neonatal intensive care units, and the specialties of perinatology and neonatology, have strengthened our abilities to care for the pregnant woman and her newborn, the modernization and new technology have significant limitations. For example, the cesarean section rate in our country has risen at an alarming rate; many of the now routine interventions are without proven benefit to low-risk women; and strict adherence to a "maximum" strategy, routinely intervening in anticipation of potential complications, often without measuring the effect of this approach on the majority of low-risk women (Rosenblatt, 1988), clearly has led to unnecessary obstetric procedures and the distancing of the woman from the process of her pregnancy, labor, and delivery. Furthermore, we have been unable to reduce the rate of low-birth-weight births since 1980. Our infant mortality rates are high for our minority populations, and there are significant differences in perinatal morbidity and mortality among different ethnic groups.

Family physicians have much to offer in this context. Our focus on prevention and our ability to provide continuing care can have an important role in reversing these trends. We practice mainly in the community rather than the hospital, and can bring our community, family-centered approach to our pregnant and laboring women. We use our skills to provide intergenerational care in the context of the family, and apply a humanistic approach to the natural process of birth while using the newer interventions when appropriate.

PREPARATION FOR PREGNANCY—PRECONCEPTION CARE

In 1989, the U.S. Public Health Service Expert Panel on the Content of Prenatal Care, a multidisciplinary group with representation from the Academies of Family Practice and Pediatrics, the American College of Obstetricians and Gynecologists, and the American College of Nurse-Midwives, recommended we initiate the practice of preconception care ("Caring for Our Future," 1989). During this time, risk assessment, health promotion, and medical and psychosocial intervention should be addressed by the physician (Table 26–1). This planned preconception visit should take place within the year prior to pregnancy, and may make unnecessary many tasks usually accomplished at the first prenatal visit. The greatest sensitivity to the environment for the developing fetus occurs during the 17 to 56 days after conception, yet many studies show that as many as one quarter of pregnant women fail to initiate care until after the first trimester, and many experience limited care throughout their pregnancy. Because healthy women are more likely to have healthier babies, the time to treat illnesses or change unhealthy behavior is prior to pregnancy, when the developing fetus is not at risk. As primary care physicians, we should approach all women during their reproductive years with these goals in mind. In addition, preconception care should involve the male partner whenever possible. Potential fathers also may need risk assessment, health promotion, and psychosocial intervention. The Expert Panel further recommended that the concept of preconception

TABLE 26–1. EXPERT PANEL PRECONCEPTION CARE RECOMMENDATIONS

Risk Assessment for All

Medical history
  Sociodemographic data
  Menstrual
  Past obstetric
  Contraceptive*
  Sexual*
  Medical/surgical
  Infection
  Family and genetic
  Nutrition
Psychosocial history
  Smoking
  Drugs
  Alcohol
  Stress
  Mental status*
  Exposure to teratogens
  Social support
  Physical abuse
  Pregnancy readiness
  Housing, finances, etc.
  Extremes of physical work, exercise, and other activity
Physical examination
  General physical examination*
  Blood pressure/pulse
  Height/weight profile
  Pelvic examination/pelvimetry
  Breast examination*

Laboratory Tests

Recommended for all
  Hemoglobin/hematocrit
  Rh factor
  Rubella titer
  Urine (protein, sugar)
  Papanicolaou smear*
  Gonococcal culture
  Syphilis test
  Hepatitis B
Offer to all
  Human immunodeficiency virus
  Toxic drug screen
Offer to some or all†
  Cytomegalovirus
  Herpes simplex
  Toxoplasmosis
  Varicella
Recommended for some
  Tuberculosis screen
  Chlamydia culture or rapid screen
  Hemoglobinopathies
  Tay-Sachs screen
  Parental karyotype

Health Promotion Counseling and Information

Nutrition‡
Avoidance of smoking
Avoidance of alcohol
Avoidance of illicit drugs
Avoidance of teratogens
Safer sex*
Need for early entry into prenatal care*
Preparation for screening and diagnostic tests

---

  * Accepted by Panel but not specifically reviewed.
  † Panel could not agree.
  ‡ Unable to reach agreement whether for all or for those at risk.
  From Rosen M, Merkatz I, Hill J: Caring for our future: A report by the Expert Panel on the Content of Prenatal Care. Obstet Gynecol 77: 784, 1991, with permission.

care "be introduced as part of prenatal care with accompanying reimbursement and coverage included in all health insurance plans" ("Caring for Our Future," 1989, p. 26).

Medical Risk Assessment

A detailed medical and psychosocial history is the cornerstone of risk assessment. Medical assessment should include menstrual, past obstetric, contraceptive, sexual, medical or surgical illness, and family and genetic histories, as well as medications, both prescription and over the counter. Environmental or chemical exposures in the workplace must be reviewed.

Contraceptive Practices

In the preconception period, the return of menses and pregnancy may be delayed slightly after oral contraceptive use, although the fertility rate is within the normal range by 1 year. Post-pill amenorrhea of greater than 6 months' duration occurs in less than 1 per cent of women. Studies have not confirmed fetal anomalies following any type of contraceptive use during the first trimester of pregnancy.

Medical Illnesses

DIABETES. The preconception control of hyperglycemia is related to lower rates of spontaneous abortions as well as a reduction in congenital malformations, macrosomia, and stillbirth. One recent study comparing glucose control prior to conception to diabetic control beginning at 8 weeks' gestation found that the preconception group had a significantly lower frequency of congenital malformations (Fuhrmann et al., 1983). Certainly in women with risk factors such as a prior large baby or a prior unexplained stillbirth, or in women with a positive family history, preconception diabetic screening should be considered.

OTHER MEDICAL CONDITIONS. Cervical dysplasia is easily detected and treated prior to pregnancy. Similarly, other relatively common medical conditions such as asthma, seizure disorders, and hypertension are best recognized and treated with possible pregnancy in mind. The choice of medications, particularly in illnesses such as seizure disorders, can be modified because of potential teratogenic effects.

Infections

Common sexually transmitted diseases such as chlamydia and gonorrhea are best detected prior to pregnancy.

HUMAN IMMUNODEFICIENCY VIRUS. Of particular importance is the woman's knowledge of her human immunodeficiency virus (HIV) status. HIV-positive women must be advised of the increased morbidity for both themselves and their potential offspring. Studies suggest that the risk of acquired immunodeficiency syndrome (AIDS) or AIDS-related complex is higher in infants born to mothers who have AIDS symptoms during pregnancy, as well as in women who continue to engage in high-risk behaviors such as intravenous drug use. About 30 per cent of HIV-positive pregnant women will transmit the disease to the infant. It appears that the virus is transmitted both in utero and during the birth process.

HEPATITIS B. All women should be screened for hepatitis B in the preconception period. This is particularly important for those with a history of illicit drug use, acute episodes of other sexually transmitted diseases, multiple sexual partners, employment in a health care or public safety field, or household contact with a hepatitis B virus carrier. Because primary vaccination consists of three vaccine doses over a 6-month period, and immunity usually is not obtained until the completion of the series, this problem should be addressed prior to pregnancy. Prevention can protect the mother and fetus from acute and chronic hepatitis, cirrhosis, and primary hepatocellular carcinoma.

TOXOPLASMOSIS. The pathogen *Toxoplasma gondii* is spread by the ingestion of oocytes found in raw meat or in the feces of infected cats. An acute infection often will cause vague, nonspecific symptoms, including fever, fatigue, and lymphadenopathy. Eight per cent of children born to mothers who acquire a primary infection are severely affected, with complications including mental retardation, chorioretinitis, and sensorineural hearing loss (Wilson and Remington 1980). Serologic testing during pregnancy is often not helpful because of the difficulty in establishing the existence of a primary infection. If the preconception titer were known, an immune woman would not be at risk, and a nonimmune woman would be counseled to avoid close contact with cats or cat litter (Jack and Culpepper, 1991). However, the cost of generalized screening would be significant, and it is not presently recommended for all women during the preconception visit.

RUBELLA. A rubella titer should be drawn routinely in all women of childbearing age at the preconception visit because rubella infection in pregnancy can result in spontaneous abortion, stillbirth, or a baby with congenital rubella syndrome. Prospective studies have shown that the risk of fetal anomalies was 25 per cent when the mother contracted rubella in the first trimester, compared to less than 1 per cent with infection in the second trimester. A history of rubella is not adequate to predict prior immunity. Only persons with detectable antibodies are considered immune. However, a woman with no history of disease or vaccination can be vaccinated without prior serologic testing. The woman then should be advised to allow 3 months to pass prior to becoming pregnant. However, the actual observed risk of vaccination in early pregnancy causing congenital malformations is no greater than the risk of malformations occurring by chance ("Rubella and Pregnancy," 1992).

VARICELLA (CHICKEN POX). Most women in the United States are immune to chickenpox before they become pregnant. However, some small percentage of women have not been exposed to the disease. It is helpful if women are asked in the preconception period if they already have had the disease. If not, a varicella titer should be obtained, and most women will be found to be immune even if they do not remember having the disease. If the woman is found to be nonimmune to varicella, consideration should be given to providing the vaccine prior to conception. If the woman chooses not to receive the vaccine, she should be counseled to avoid contact with young children who have been exposed to chickenpox. At the present time, varicella vaccine is not to be used during pregnancy. Should an infection occur early in the first trimester, some authors report an increase in spontaneous abortion. Late first trimester, second trimester, and early third trimester infections are relatively innocuous for both mother and fetus. However, maternal infection occurring 7 to 14 days prior to delivery may cause life-threatening neonatal infections.

Genetic Diseases

Genetic risk assessment also should be performed prior to conception, because nearly 3 per cent of births are associated with major congenital anomalies. Specific risk is associated with advanced maternal age (>35), a family history of genetic disease, or a previously affected child. Common disorders for which genetic screening may be recommended include Tay-Sachs disease in Ashkenazi Jews, β-thalassemia in Greeks and Italians, α-thalassemia in Southeast Asians and Filipinos, sickle cell anemia in blacks, and cystic fibrosis in whites with a family history. However, the list of genetic diseases that are detectable by prenatal testing grows almost daily. Thus, any history with a genetic component deserves investigation.

Nutrition

In recent years we have come to realize the profound effect a woman's nutritional status can have on the outcome of her pregnancy. Both ends of the weight spectrum (i.e., severe underweight or significant obesity) can cause difficulties during pregnancy. Underweight women who gain weight poorly during their pregnancy have a higher incidence of low-birth-weight infants and of neonatal and fetal demises. Similarly, obese women are more likely to present with gestational diabetes, hypertension, and macrosomic infants, and are at risk for dysfunctional labors. The prepregnant body mass index governs the total weight gain recommended in pregnancy (ACOG Technical Bulletin no. 179, 1993).

Some women may have diets that are deficient in folic acid. These women's fetuses are at greater risks for neural tube defects. All women with a history of a neural tube defect in a previous pregnancy should begin folic acid, 4 mg daily, at least 1 month prior to conception and should continue this through the first 3 months of pregnancy. Furthermore, in 1993 the Centers for Disease Control and Prevention (CDC) recommended that all women of childbearing age who are capable of becoming pregnant should consume 0.4 mg of folic acid a day for the purpose of reducing the risk of spina bifida or other neural tube defects (Morbidity and Mortality Weekly Report, 1993). Currently there are about 2500 births per year in the United States compromised by neural tube defects. It is estimated that the preconception ingestion of folic acid would reduce the risk of this anomaly by 50 per cent (Oakley, 1993).

Psychosocial Risk Assessment

We know that pregnancy imparts great psychosocial stress on the family unit. It is helpful to evaluate the adequacy of income and housing for the soon-to-be-pregnant woman. The level of education, and in some cases the marital status, can help define the risk profile. It is helpful to know the woman's support system to understand who potentially will support her through this period of transition. We should evaluate her stress level, her exposure to and risk of physical abuse, any underlying psychiatric conditions, and eating disorders. Also, we should assess the environment for potential teratogen exposures both at home and at work. Alcohol and smoking have significant effects on the developing fetus, and ideally are best addressed prior to pregnancy. We must use this information to effect behavior change whenever possible, and to make referrals to appropriate community agencies when necessary.

PRENATAL CARE

The First Prenatal Visit

The first pregnancy visit is simplified vastly if preconception care has occurred or if the patient is well known and has had regular visits to the family physician. Ideally this first visit should occur between 6 and 8 weeks of gestation. Table 26–2 documents what should occur at the first visit, as suggested by the U.S. Public Health Service Expert Panel on Prenatal Care. If a preconception visit has not occurred, then several tests will be needed in addition to those listed in Table 26–2. These additional tests can be found in Table 26–1. In addition, the medical and psychosocial history must be reviewed.

TABLE 26–2. EXPERT PANEL RECOMMENDATIONS FOR FIRST PREGNANCY VISIT

Risk Assessment for All
Medical history
  Medical/surgical update
  Nutrition update
  Current pregnancy to date*
Psychosocial history
  Smoking
  Alcohol
  Drugs
  Social support
  Extremes of physical work, exercise, and other activity
  Stress
Physical examination
  Blood pressure*
  Weight
  Breast examination*
  Pelvic examination for uterine size, dating, abnormalities*

Laboratory Tests
Recommended for all
  Hemoglobin/hematocrit
  Urine culture
Recommended for some
  Rh screen
  Syphilis test
  Blood glucose level
  Gonococcal culture

Health Promotion Activities and Information for All
Avoidance of teratogens
Safer sex*
Physical and emotional changes in pregnancy*
Sexuality*
Self-help strategies for discomforts (for some)
Fetal growth and development
Classes on nutrition, physical changes, exercise, psychological adaptation
Nutritional counseling (some or all)
Preparation for screening and diagnostic tests
Content and timing of visits*
Need to report danger signs*

---

* Accepted by panel but not specifically reviewed.
From Rosen M, Merkatz I, Hill J: Caring for our future: A report by the Expert Panel on the Content of Prenatal Care. Obstet Gynecol 77: 785, 1991, with permission.

A woman may perceive early signs of pregnancy within a few days of the first missed menstrual period. Usually the earliest signs are breast tenderness, fatigue, and some abnormal reaction to food. Although these three signs may not always be present or always be recognized by the woman, they are common and suggestive of intrauterine pregnancy. These symptoms are often reliable indicators, even in women who have irregular menses and who frequently skip menstrual periods.

The date of the last menstrual period should be determined. If not known exactly, the date should be estimated. Very often dates such as birthdays, national holidays, and school vacations can help pinpoint the dates. Information about the normal menstrual cycle should be obtained. The usual method of determining an estimated date of confinement (EDC) in the United States is to employ

Nägele's rule. By this convention, the EDC is determined by subtracting 3 months and adding 7 days to the date of onset of the last menstrual period. However, extra days should be added for menstrual cycles longer than 28 days or subtracted for cycles less than 28 days. Also, any history of an unusually light or heavy period just before pregnancy should be noted.

Rapid, inexpensive, and reliable urine pregnancy tests are now readily available both from medical laboratories and over the counter in most pharmacies. Each test has a slightly different sensitivity, but most should be positive 14 days after the first missed menstrual period. Over-the-counter home pregnancy tests are reliable but not infallible; occasionally false-positive results occur. If a precise and accurate pregnancy test is needed, the amount of human chorionic gonadotropin (hCG) present in the serum may be determined. Quantitative determination of hCG should be used when it is important to know the actual level—for example, in cases of hydatidiform mole or ectopic pregnancy.

Psychosocial History

The psychosocial history should include a review of smoking, alcohol, and drug use. Smoking contributes to low birth weight, placenta previa, congenital anomalies, and spontaneous abortion. Somewhere between 20 and 35 per cent of women smoke during their pregnancy. With physician support and smoking cessation programs, studies show that 12 to 25 per cent of pregnant women will stop smoking. Women who had no interest in stopping prior to pregnancy suddenly may show interest in quitting. The physician should explore this potential change in attitude.

Caffeine intake, both before and during pregnancy, may be associated with a slight increase in risk of fetal loss, according to a recent study (Infante-Rivard et al., 1993). Furthermore, the risk appears to be a linear connection increasing with each 100 mg of caffeine ingested daily during pregnancy. (One cup of caffeinated coffee equals 100 mg of caffeine.)

Alcohol intake must be discussed specifically. Fetal alcohol syndrome (FAS) includes intrauterine growth retardation, mental retardation, maxillary hypoplasia, flat philtrum, thin upper lip, and reduction in the width of the palpebral fissures. A dose–response relationship and a period of greatest sensitivity have not been established definitively. Binge drinking early in pregnancy may be associated with neural tube defects, perhaps mediated through poor nutritional intake. Decreased brain growth and differentiation results from high alcohol consumption in the second and third trimesters. Chronic consumption of 6 ounces a day places the fetus at high risk. It is unlikely that the child of a woman who drinks less than 2 ounces per day would have the full syndrome, but infants of these mothers still may be at risk for physical or behavioral impairment. The incidence of FAS in the general population is now 3 to 5 per 1000 live births (Brent and Beckman, 1992).

Cocaine is a commonly used recreational drug associated with spontaneous abortion, congenital anomalies, fetal growth retardation, premature delivery, and placental anomalies. Cocaine use correlates significantly with heavy smoking, excessive alcohol use, and the use of other illicit drugs.

Heroin use in pregnancy is associated with many of the same poor outcomes of pregnancy noted for cocaine use. Because sudden heroin withdrawal may cause fetal death, methadone maintenance—ideally in the setting of a community drug program—should be considered. The neonate born to an addicted woman must receive maintenance narcotics and only slowly be weaned to avoid catastrophic withdrawal symptoms that can cause neonatal death.

Identification of social risk factors or poverty is important and may merit intervention. For example, the food supplementation program for Women, Infants and Children, Aid to Families with Dependent Children, and other local community support programs can help dramatically. In the case of adolescent pregnancy, it is important for the physician to help the patient explore means to continue her education during pregnancy. All patients should be questioned about abuse, either physical or verbal, regardless of socioeconomic or ethnic background. All positive answers are treated as important information that places the patient at high risk. Many physicians do not have the time to address adequately all social problems of their pregnancy patients. In such cases, the practicing physician can establish a close relationship with a social worker, nurse, or other health care provider who can respond appropriately to the nutritional, psychological, environmental, and habit problems of the pregnant patient together with the physician. The team approach maximizes what can be accomplished for the disadvantaged patient.

Physical Exam

The initial physical examination should include measurement of blood pressure and weight, breast exam, and pelvic exam for uterine sizing and abnormalities. The external genitalia, vagina, and cervix should be inspected carefully for abnormalities that may lead to difficulties in pregnancy, labor, or delivery.

An examiner may have difficulty determining the presence of pregnancy in the first 6 to 8 weeks of gestation. Although the uterus is usually palpably enlarged and soft within 6 weeks from the last menstrual period, the exact size often is not easy to determine. This is particularly true in obese women and in women who have had several children. Chadwick's sign, a purplish discoloration of the uterine cervix resulting from the increased blood supply, is often present by 6 weeks from the last menstrual period. Between 8 and 12 weeks, the examiner should be able to estimate the size of the uterus to within 2 weeks of gestational age. Any discrepancy between the size of the uterus and the last menstrual period should be noted, and may be an indication for further clarification, including ultrasound.

The examiner should perform clinical pelvimetry. The diagonal conjugate is the most significant pelvis measurement. In order to obtain this measurement correctly, the fingers of the examining hand must reach the promontory of the sacrum. At this point, the hand is elevated to the inferior aspect of the symphysis, and the distance between the tip of the middle finger and the symphysis is noted. Once the diagonal conjugate is determined, the examining finger should trace the concavity of the sacrum and the pelvic side walls. The fingers then sweep between the ischial spines, and the distance between is them noted. An inadequate pelvis for vaginal delivery could be suspected if the diagonal conjugate is less than 12 cm, the sacrum has an unusual shape, the pelvic side walls are straight, or the distance between the ischial spines is less than 10 cm.

Laboratory Studies

A Papanicolaou smear should be obtained for every patient at her first prenatal visit unless a negative exam has been obtained within the last 6 months. A hematocrit and a urine culture should be obtained for all patients as well. Anemia is defined as a hemoglobin of less than 11.0 gm/dL in the first and third trimester and less than 10.5 gm/dL in the second trimester, or, equivalently, a hematocrit of 33 and 32 per cent, respectively. The most common cause of anemia in pregnancy is iron deficiency.

It has become a common practice in many areas of the United States routinely to obtain an endocervical smear for *Neisseria gonorrhoeae* and *Chlamydia trachomatis* at the initial evaluation, as well as a serologic test for syphilis. In some practices, however, these infections are sufficiently rare to make this unnecessary. It is estimated that 5 to 7 per cent of women are culture positive for *Chlamydia*. Among poor and minority populations, the rate rises to higher than 20 per cent. The CDC has recommended that pregnant women who satisfy at least one of the following criteria have at least one prenatal culture: younger than 20, unmarried, history of other sexually transmitted diseases, multiple sexual partners, or a partner with multiple sexual partners. *Chlamydia* is often asymptomatic in the woman and may not be evident during an exam. The newborn acquires *C. trachomatis* through contact with infected genital secretions at birth. Inclusion conjunctivitis develops in 18 to 50 per cent of infants born to mothers with chlamydial infections, and chlamydial pneumonia develops in 11 to 20 per cent.

Syphilis has not been a major health problem during pregnancy in our country for many years. However, in some communities this infection has been on the rise again. Among mothers who have the disease and remain untreated, 25 per cent of fetuses will die in utero and 25 per cent will die shortly after birth, and 40 per cent of survivors will develop syphilis after the third week of life. The manifestations of congenital syphilis include skin lesions, periostitis and osteochondritis of long bones, hepatosplenomegaly, facial and dental defects, eighth nerve deafness, and neurosyphilis.

Gonococcal infections are very common. Both females and males may be asymptomatic. Neonatal gonorrhea is acquired in utero or during delivery. In utero infections result in chorioamnionitis and neonatal sepsis. Infections acquired during delivery cause conjunctivitis, otitis externa, and vulvovaginitis.

Health Promotion

Anticipatory guidance during the first visit should include avoidance of teratogens, nutritional counseling, preparation and screening for diagnostic tests, timing of visits, and danger signs that need to be reported. Exercise should be encouraged. Even the trained athlete can continue vigorous physical training during pregnancy, but all should avoid raising their core temperature or exercising to the point of extreme breathlessness or dehydration.

Safe sex should be advocated by the physician, because limitations for the pregnant woman only center on comfort and position. Many patients will be hesitant to ask about sex, and the physician should raise the topic for discussion. Patients should be reminded about the importance of seat belts when traveling in an automobile. The lap belt should be strapped below and the shoulder belt above the gravid uterus. Patients should be told to call their physician immediately if severe pelvic pain or vaginal bleeding occurs.

The nutritional demands on the patient will vary according to her pregravid weight. The prepregnant body mass index (the weight divided by the height) governs the recommended total weight gain and the weight gain per month to achieve it. There is a positive linear relationship between maternal weight gain and newborn weight, and a positive linear relationship between maternal prepregnant weight and newborn weight.

The basal metabolic rate increases by about 50 kcal/day through the early part of the third trimester and then increases to approximately 150 kcal/day for the remainder of the pregnancy. The calorie content of the diet required to supply daily energy needs and to achieve appropriate weight gain is estimated by multiplying the patient's optimal body weight, in kilograms, by 35 kcal and adding 300 kcal to the total.

For women of normal weight during pregnancy, the optimal weight gain is between 13.6 and 16.8 kg (30 to 37 pounds). Underweight teenagers should gain near the upper end of the range. Studies show that, in severely underweight women, the perinatal mortality risk is lowest when their weight gain is greater than 16.8 kg (37 pounds). Babies born to underweight women who gain little during pregnancy have a higher rate of fetal and neonatal death, intrauterine growth retardation, and low birth weight. At the other extreme, perinatal morbidity begins to increase when obese women gain more than 6.8 kg (15 pounds) and fetal death increases significantly after an 11.4-kg (25-pound) weight gain in this population (ACOG Technical Bulletin no. 179, 1993). Extreme obesity increases the risk of gestational diabetes, hypertension, macrosomia, dysfunctional prolonged labor, and shoulder dystocia. In an obese woman, a weight gain of 15 pounds or less is recommended. Weight loss is never appropriate in pregnancy. If a minimal weight gain is desired, an 1800-calorie diet should be recommended.

Women should be encouraged to eat a balanced, nutritious diet, including whole-grain cereals and breads, vegetables and fruit, protein-rich foods, and dairy products. A healthy diet is achievable from many cultural perspectives, and the starting point has to be with foods that are familiar and enjoyed by the patient. Vitamin and mineral supplementation is not indicated in women who eat well-balanced diets, except for iron and folic acid.

Folic acid, 0.4 mg daily, if not already started in the preconception period, should be begun at the first prenatal visit and continued through the first 3 months of pregnancy in an attempt to reduce the risk of neural tube defect. Because neural tube closure is completed by 4 to 6 weeks following conception, beginning folic acid after that time may not be of value.

The net additional requirement for iron in pregnancy is about 1 gram. It is not necessary to begin iron supplementation at the first prenatal visit. Rather, for most women it should be started in the second trimester and continued throughout pregnancy, at a dose of 30 mg of elemental iron per day. This is available as ferrous sulfate or as ferrous gluconate. Some of the constipating effects of iron appear to be minimized in the ferrous gluconate preparation. Maximum absorption occurs when iron tablets are taken between meals with water. For maintenance therapy, there is no advantage to taking additional iron and the gastrointestinal side effects can be problematic. Calcium supplementation is recommended only in women who cannot eat dairy products. The recommended daily allowance of calcium for the pregnant woman is the same as that for the nonpregnant woman, 1200 mg/day.

Follow-up Visits

Traditionally, women have been seen at least monthly throughout pregnancy, and somewhat more frequently in the third trimester, with weekly visits recommended after 36 weeks' gestation. The U.S. Public Health Service Expert Panel has suggested a more patient-centered scheduling of visits, with varying frequencies for low-risk women and more frequent visits for those with medical or psychosocial risk factors (Table 26-3). They recommend a follow-up visit at 12 weeks for all nulliparous women, and electively for multigravidas, to review laboratory results and to reinforce health promotion activities.

A 16-week visit is advised for all pregnant

TABLE 26-3. EXPERT PANEL RECOMMENDATIONS FOR VISITS THROUGHOUT PREGNANCY

Activity	Week/Trimester
Check for Any Exposure to Infection*	
Physical examination	
Blood pressure	24†
Weight	Each visit
Fundal height/growth	16†
Fetal lie/presentation/ engagement/fetal heart rate*	24†
Cervical examination	41†
Laboratory Tests	
Hemoglobin/hematocrit	24–28
Rh‡	26–28
Diabetic screen	26–28
Repeat syphilis‡	Third trimester
Repeat gonococcal and human immunodeficiency virus‡	36
Serum α-fetoprotein	14–16
Ultrasound*‡	When indicated
Health Promotion Activities	
Teratogen avoidance	Each visit
Safer sex*	Each trimester
Maternal seatbelt use	Each trimester
Smoking cessation‡	Each visit
Work/nutrition counseling‡	Each visit
Signs of preterm labor	Second/third trimester
Physical/emotional changes*	First/third trimester
Sexuality counseling*	Last half of pregnancy
Fetal growth/development	Each visit
Self-help for discomforts‡	Each visit
General health habits	Each visit
Breast feeding	26†
Infant car seat safety	Each visit
Childbirth/parenting classes	32
Family roles adjustment	38
Information about laboratory tests*	Before testing
Birth plan*	Third trimester
Labor (when to call/where to go)*	Third trimester

* Accepted by panel but not specifically reviewed.
† That week and each week thereafter.
‡ For some.
From Rosen M, Merkatz I, Hill J: Caring for our future: A report by the Expert Panel on the Content of Prenatal Care. Obstet Gynecol 77: 785, 1991, with permission.

women to offer α-fetoprotein (AFP) screening. AFP screening should be considered on all women at 16 to 18 weeks' gestation, as a screening test for neural tube defects and Down syndrome. Ninety per cent of neural tube defects occur in the absence of positive history, with an overall incidence of 1 to 2 in 1000 births in the United States. Maternal AFP serum levels will be elevated in 80 to 90 per cent of women whose fetuses have open neural tube defects, as well as in women with multiple gestations and in cases of other rare fetal anomalies, including omphalocele, congenital nephrosis, and fetal bowel obstruction. The levels will not be elevated in cases of closed neural tube defects, including hydrocephalus. A positive screening test is an AFP level greater than 2.5 times the median value for normal controls at the corresponding gestational age. Eighty per cent of cases of Down syndrome occur in women under 35 years of age, and approximately 20 to 25 per cent of Down syndrome cases in this population will be identified through AFP screening. A low AFP level in combination with the maternal age helps predict the risk.

The Expert Panel does not recommend a routine visit at 20 weeks, unless the patient is at high risk for either medical or social reasons. Blood pressure measurement should be made at the preconception and first pregnancy visits and, if elevated, closely followed over the first half of the pregnancy; if normal, the measurement does not need to be repeated until the 24-week visit. Similarly, the panel recommends dropping the urine dip as a routine screen after the first two prenatal visits. Albuminuria is a rare development without other coexisting signs of pregnancy-induced hypertension or preeclampsia (Rosen et al., 1991). Risk assessment and health promotion should be ongoing at each visit, and will dictate the future appointment schedule.

The Expert Panel concluded that, in the absence of risk, 10 visits for nulliparous women and 8 visits for parous women would be adequate. Blood pressure, weight gain, fundal height, fetal position, and heart rate should be documented at all visits in the second half of the pregnancy. McDonald's measurements of the uterine fundus are useful. These are obtained by measuring the distance from the top of the symphysis pubis to the top of the uterine fundus. Between 20 and 30 weeks of gestation, the height of the uterine fundus in centimeters should be approximately equal to the number of weeks of gestation, assuming the woman is not obese (Fig. 26–1) Any significant difference between the number of weeks of gestation and the uterine size should alert the physician to the possibility of multiple gestation if larger than expected, or growth retardation if smaller than expected. Either condition then can be defined more specifically by use of ultrasound.

A repeat hematocrit should be done routinely at 24 to 28 weeks, as should a diabetes screening test. The latter is performed by giving the patient a 50-

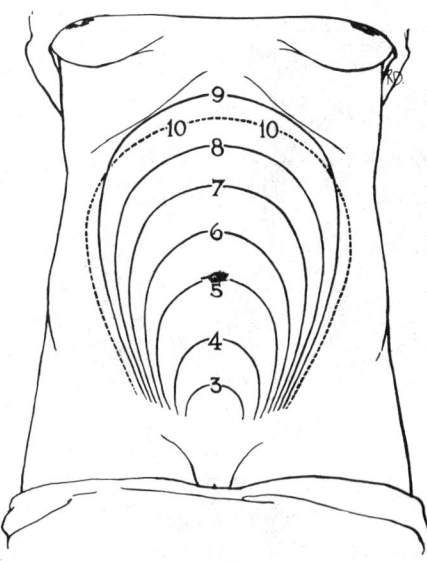

FIGURE 26–1. Relative height of the fundus at the various human months of pregnancy. (From Hellman LM, Pritchard JA: Williams Obstetrics, 14th edition. New York, Appleton-Century-Crofts, 1971, p 280, with permission.)

gram glucose load and drawing a blood sample 60 minutes later. Values of 135 mg/dL or higher require a 3-hour glucose tolerance test (Table 26–4). The patient is instructed to eat a high-carbohydrate diet for a few days prior to the 3-hour glucose tolerance test.

Beginning at about 30 weeks, the uterus should be examined at each visit using Leopold's maneuvers (Fig. 26–2; Table 26–5). The physician should discuss the signs of the onset of labor and the appropriate actions to take, as well as the importance of rupture of membranes and the necessity for evaluation of the patient if rupture of membranes is thought to occur. Breast-feeding should be encouraged. Childbirth/parenting classes should begin by 32 weeks. Physical and emotional changes that occur in pregnancy should be reviewed. Fatigue will become more pronounced in the third trimester. Many relationships become more stressed at this time as a fatigued, and sometimes more emotionally vulnerable, woman attempts to maintain her routine schedule. A sensitive physician who raises these issues can be an enormous support to the pregnant woman.

TABLE 26–4. GLUCOSE SCREENING AT 28 WEEKS' GESTATION

Test	Upper Limit of Normal (mg/dL)
50-gm glucose tolerance	135
3-hr GTT*	Fasting: 105
	1 hour: 190
	2 hour: 105
	3 hour: 145

* Glucose tolerance test.

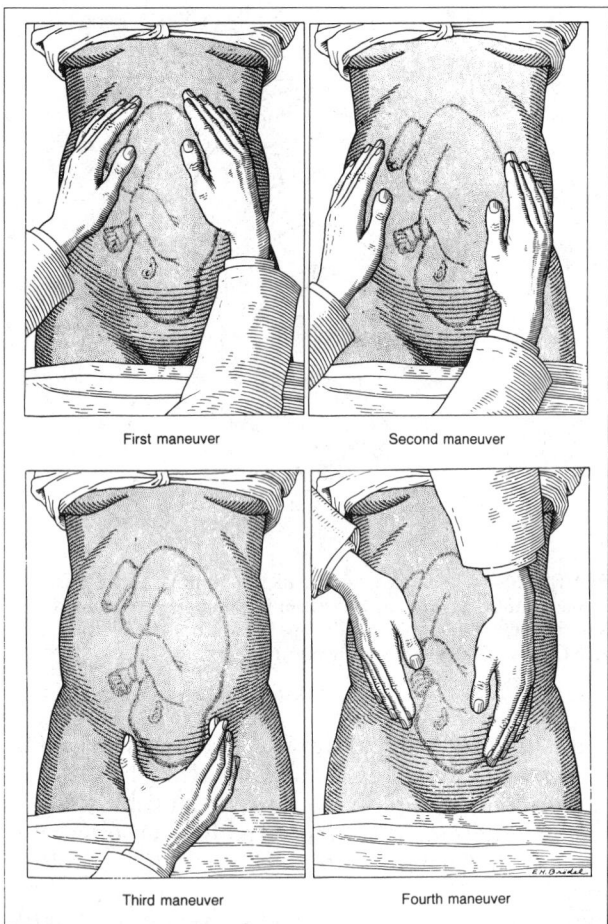

First maneuver

Second maneuver

Third maneuver

Fourth maneuver

FIGURE 26–2. Palpation in left occiput anterior position. (From Cunningham FG, MacDonald PC, Gant NF [eds]: Williams Obstetrics, 18th edition. East Norwalk, CT, Appleton & Lange, 1989, p 183, with permission.)

Syphilis and gonorrhea testing should be repeated in high-risk women during the latter half of the third trimester. Weekly visits begin at 37 weeks. Blood pressure, weight, and fetal height and position should be evaluated at each visit. Breech presentation at 37 weeks should prompt consideration of an attempt at external version. Unless there is concern about early cervical dilation, the cervix need not be checked until 41 weeks, according to the consensus of the Expert Panel.

TABLE 26–5. LEOPOLD'S MANEUVERS

Maneuver	Action	Question
First	Examine the fundus	What fetal part is in the fundus?
Second	Palpate the lateral abdomen	Where is the fetal back?
Third	Palpate the suprapubic area	Is the presenting part engaged?
Fourth (vertex only)	Find the cephalic prominence	Is the head flexed?

Postmaturity is defined as a gestation that goes beyond 42 weeks. Antenatal testing should begin at that point. Most experts now believe that the single most important requirement for fetal well-being is the quantity of amniotic fluid. The total amniotic fluid index, the cumulative measurement of fluid pockets from all four quadrants, should measure 5 cm. Otherwise, the woman may be at risk for oligohydramnios.

The other standard accepted method of post-dates monitoring involves a biweekly nonstress tests (see Fetal Testing in Patients with Toxemia or PIH, later in this chapter). In most hospitals, this nonstress test can be done as part of the biophysical profile.

ACCIDENTS OF EARLY PREGNANCY

Spontaneous Abortion

Despite the best efforts of physicians and the hopes of parents, approximately one in six clinical pregnancies in the United States ends in spontaneous abortion (Barnes et al., 1980). When sensitive tests for pregnancy have been used for research purposes, it has been shown that up to one half of all human gestations end in abortion. These early losses result from many causes, but major chromosomal defects and poor implantation—causes not amenable to medical intervention—are believed to be the most frequent. Other causes, such as smoking, alcohol use, environmental toxins, drug exposure, and poor nutrition, can be reduced by medical intervention and counseling.

The term "spontaneous abortion" refers to the spontaneous passage of the products of conception. Such passage may be either complete or incomplete. If the products of conception are passed intact, if bleeding ceases promptly after such passage, and if the cervical canal and uterine size rapidly return to normal, the abortion is considered to be complete and manipulation of the uterus is not advised. To avoid continued bleeding, it has been common practice in the United States to use ergot derivatives such as methylergonovine, 0.2 mg four times a day for 2 to 3 days, unless a medical history of hypertension or asthma is present.

A woman often passes only part of the products of conception, and then the term "incomplete spontaneous abortion" is appropriate. Incomplete abortion is more likely if the pregnancy is of greater than 12 weeks' gestation or if infection has occurred. In these women, the endocervical canal usually remains dilated, fetal membranes or placental tissue may be seen in the canal, bleeding continues unabated, and the uterine size remains enlarged. Medications alone rarely cause complete uterine emptying. Therefore, it has been our practice to perform uterine evacuation when fragments of fetal tissue remain within the uterus. Evacuation of the uterus may be accomplished easily and safely by vacuum curettage if it is of less than 12 weeks' size. If the equipment for this procedure is not available, then curettage using sharp curettes may be accomplished. Dense uterine synechiae causing amenorrhea (Asherman's syndrome) and other complications of dilation and curettage occur more commonly after sharp curettage than after vacuum curettage. Oxytocin or ergot derivatives may be given to cause uterine contraction and to decrease the chances of perforation. Any uterus that is larger than 12 weeks' size presents a particular problem and is at high risk for perforation or rupture at evacuation.

Threatened Abortion

The term "threatened abortion" is defined as bleeding occurring during the first 4 months of pregnancy. Although nearly 50 per cent of all women who are pregnant will bleed some time during the pregnancy, bleeding is a sign that is suggestive of a high risk of fetal death. Although it is never easy to predict the outcome of threatened abortion, in general the amount of bleeding and the presence or absence of severe uterine cramping can be predictive signs. Thus, heavy bleeding and severe cramping are usually prodromal symptoms of impending spontaneous abortion.

In past years, women who have experienced a threatened abortion often were placed at bed rest or given medications to prevent spontaneous abortion. We now know that, once bleeding has started, the use of medication and bed rest are of no benefit. Although a woman probably should be counseled against vigorous exercise or strenuous physical activity, data suggest that bed rest is not helpful.

Ultrasonography may be useful in cases of threatened abortion to determine whether a viable pregnancy is present, and to help distinguish it from ectopic pregnancy. The presence of a normal-appearing gestational sac with a fetal pole is an encouraging sign; if a fetal heart rate is identified, spontaneous abortion rarely occurs. However, if the uterus is empty or if an empty sac or an abnormal sac is identified, the chance of a normal pregnancy is minimal.

Ectopic Pregnancy

Although the term "ectopic pregnancy" refers to a pregnancy that implants anywhere except the endometrial cavity, it is used almost synonymously with tubal pregnancy. Intra-abdominal and ovarian pregnancies do occur, but they are extremely rare.

An extrauterine pregnancy in the fallopian tube occurs in approximately 1 of every 70 pregnancies, and its incidence is increasing at an alarming rate

(Lawson et al., 1989). Therefore, any physician who cares for pregnant women sees this complication with some frequency. The major contributing factor to this disease is the pre-existence of tubal scarring as a result of pelvic inflammatory disease or tubal surgery. Another common factor is previous ectopic pregnancy, because women who have experienced this complication previously have a 5 to 20 per cent chance of it occurring in subsequent pregnancies.

In the past, the diagnosis of ectopic pregnancy was made almost exclusively on the basis of physical findings and history. A woman who presented in an emergency setting with a history of delayed or missed menses and was experiencing unilateral vaginal pain and bleeding was considered to have an ectopic pregnancy until proven otherwise. Most of these women were taken to the operating room immediately, with the result that many unnecessary laparotomies were performed. Fortunately, it is now possible to utilize several newer diagnostic techniques that aid in the diagnosis or exclusion of ectopic pregnancy. In addition, it is now often possible to follow a woman as an outpatient until exact determination of her pregnancy status has been accomplished, rather than requiring immediate surgery.

Vaginal probe ultrasonography can be particularly helpful if it identifies either an intrauterine pregnancy or an adnexal mass that is diagnostic of implantation. Unfortunately, many ultrasound scans are nondiagnostic or equivocal. In these cases, the use of quantitative β-hCG determinations may be helpful. In general, a woman with a normal intrauterine pregnancy, during the first several weeks of gestation, will exhibit a twofold increase in the level of β-hCG approximately every 48 hours. Although normal pregnancies may vary considerably from this "48-hour doubling" norm, absence of such increase is worrisome.

A patient who is evaluated in an emergency facility, is stable, has no evidence of adnexal mass by examination or ultrasound, has no intraperitoneal free fluid detected by ultrasound, is not bleeding heavily, and is reliable may be followed as an outpatient if properly instructed. The patient must be told to return immediately if her symptoms increase. Repeat evaluation also is indicated if the β-hCG level does not rise in a predictable fashion.

If the strongly likelihood of an ectopic gestation is present, laparoscopy is the next step. In virtually every case, an ectopic pregnancy can be differentiated easily and correctly from a ruptured corpus luteum cyst or pelvic inflammatory disease. Additionally, in recent years almost all ectopic pregnancies—ruptured or not—can be managed with operative laparoscopic techniques rather than open laparotomy. The reduced morbidity from this technique is remarkable. Many patients with ectopic pregnancies leave the hospital in less than 24 hours and are back at work within a few days.

If rupture is present, partial salpingectomy occasionally may be necessary, and this usually can be accomplished with operative laparoscopic techniques. If the ectopic gestation is intact, linear salpingostomy and removal of the products of conception is the procedure of choice.

Recently, some ectopic pregnancies have been treated medically utilizing methotrexate. This method of management appears to be safe and effective for early gestational ages. However, the limits of its usefulness have not yet been established clearly (Stovall et al., 1989).

OBSTETRIC ULTRASOUND

The use of B-scan ultrasonography of the uterus has become almost routine during the care of pregnant patients in the United States, despite documentation of little if any benefit in low-risk pregnancies (Ewigman et al., 1993). "Routine" scans commonly are done at 14 to 16 weeks' gestation. At this point in pregnancy, it is possible to (1) date the pregnancy with accuracy, (2) detect multiple gestation, (3) detect complete placenta previa, and (4) detect most major fetal structural abnormalities. However, routine use of ultrasonography also can lead to misinformation. For example, ultrasound examination at 14 to 16 weeks' gestation often will show a low-lying placenta, which may increase both the patient's and the physician's anxiety yet never result in a clinical abnormality. As the uterus grows, most "low-lying placentas" become fundal. Likewise, examinations performed later than 20 weeks' gestation are not very useful for pregnancy dating.

Ultrasonography remains a very useful technique in high-risk pregnancy. All women with a history of a suboptimal pregnancy outcome should be considered for early ultrasonography, and repeat examinations as indicated. In addition, women who develop complications of the current pregnancy (e.g., vaginal bleeding, pre-eclampsia, suspected decreased or increased fetal growth, diabetes) should have ultrasound examination. Ultrasonography is also necessary prior to amniocentesis for placental, umbilical cord, and fetal localization and needle direction; prior to external version; and on rare occasions for evaluation of fetal position. Ultrasonography is not recommended for determination of fetal sex unless it is important because of a sex-linked inherited disorder.

AMNIOCENTESIS

There are numerous indications for amniocentesis. Although the technique was developed largely for determining the severity of fetal Rh disease, this is now a rare indication. Years of experience and refinement of the technique have now made it a procedure with very low morbidity.

Perhaps the most common indication for early prenatal amniocentesis is concern regarding the possibility of a fetal chromosomal abnormality. It now has become common practice throughout many areas of the United States to offer amniocentesis to all pregnant women age 35 or greater. The age is now somewhat arbitrary, but was originally chosen because 35 years is approximately the age at which the total risk of detectable chromosomal abnormalities becomes more common than 1 in every 200 pregnancies—the original morbidity rate of amniocentesis. Although Down's syndrome is the most commonly detected chromosomal abnormality in women beyond age 35, many trisomies occur more frequently with increasing maternal (and in some cases paternal) age. Women with a history of previously delivering a child with a detectable chromosomal abnormality also should be offered amniocentesis.

There is an ever-increasing number of metabolic/genetic abnormalities that can be detected by amniocentesis. For example, it is possible to detect the presence of cystic fibrosis, Tay-Sachs disease, and many other inherited disorders.

With the widespread use of maternal serum AFP (MSAFP) testing for the detection of neural tube defects, amniocentesis has become a common adjunct when either high or low levels of MSAFP are detected. Although it has been known for some time that high levels are associated with an open neural tube defect, it is only more recently that Downs' syndrome has been linked to a very low level of MSAFP. Some laboratories now offer routine evaluation of the maternal serum level of other factors, which may increase the sensitivity and specificity of the AFP test for the detection of both Downs' syndrome and open neural tube defects. However, not all authorities and not all laboratories support the use of these additional techniques at this time.

Amniocentesis also often is used for the determination of fetal lung maturity. A sample of amniotic fluid (in a nondiabetic patient) can be examined for the presence of sphingomyelin and lecithin. If the lecithin/sphingomyelin (L/S) ratio is greater than 2.0 to 1 (some laboratory techniques require a level of 3.0 to 1), there is great likelihood that the fetal lungs are mature enough to support independent respiration. The addition of testing for the presence of phosphatidylglycerol to the determination of the L/S ratio further assures fetal lung maturity. When phosphatidylglycerol is present in the face of a mature L/S ratio, the chance of respiratory distress syndrome is extremely small. Determination of fetal lung maturity is particularly important when elective delivery is planned. Unfortunately, inappropriate induction of labor and repeat cesarean section remain common causes for respiratory distress syndrome in the

United States. Determination of fetal lung maturity also is important in certain abnormal conditions (e.g., placenta previa). In such cases, it is often advantageous to perform cesarean section as soon as lung maturity has been established because significant bleeding that can jeopardize maternal and fetal health may occur at any time.

Amniocentesis also is performed in some cases of premature onset of labor when there is a concern that the initiation of labor is the result of chorioamnionitis. Failure to detect bacteria or white blood cells in the amniotic fluid is good evidence that chorioamnionitis has not occurred.

Amniocentesis always should be performed with the aid of ultrasound guidance. With the addition of ultrasonography, the risk of fetal damage has been reduced markedly. Once a pocket of fluid has been identified, if possible well away from the placenta, the abdomen is prepped with an antiseptic solution and a small-bore spinal needle is inserted into the amniotic cavity under ultrasound guidance. Sufficient fluid is withdrawn for the performance of all necessary tests (usually 10 to 25 mL) and the needle is removed. If the fetal heart rate tracing remains normal, the patient may resume normal activities immediately.

MEDICAL DISEASES IN PREGNANCY

Many medical diseases commonly occur in pregnancy. Only those that result in permanent infertility or that so debilitate the woman that she is unable to achieve pregnancy are not seen. Currently, many chronic, disabling diseases are seen associated with pregnancy, whereas in previous years life expectancy with such diseases did not extend into the reproductive years, or the woman was so debilitated that pregnancy virtually never occurred.

The ability to care properly for a pregnant woman with a medical disease requires a different approach during gestation than when she is not pregnant. In the nonpregnant woman, treatment is directed entirely toward her care. If the same woman is pregnant, however, treatment of her condition must be tempered by the presence of the pregnancy/fetus. For many medical diseases, it is important to recognize two separate viewpoints: what is the effect of pregnancy on this disease, and what is the effect of this disease and its treatment on the pregnancy?

Such thinking is quite different from that usually employed in medicine. For example, insulin-dependent diabetes mellitus is a common, well-understood disease. Women with this disease lead relatively normal lives for decades. Yet pregnancy causes profound changes. In pregnancy, diabetes is much harder to control, and insulin requirements increase markedly (effect of pregnancy on disease). In addition, without extremely tight control of blood sugar levels, the disease results in a marked increase in congenital anomalies, macrosomia, and stillbirth (effect of disease on pregnancy).

In this section of this chapter, selected medical diseases will be discussed within this framework. It is important to realize, however, that most medical diseases, whether they be inherited or acquired, infectious or metabolic, system specific or generalized, must be managed differently in the pregnant woman.

Integumentary System

Many women report profound changes in their skin during pregnancy. Unfortunately, the changes are unpredictable. The marked increase in the circulating levels of all steroid compounds (and the addition of several steroids that are not found in the nonpregnant state) lead to some changes. More women report "dry" skin in pregnancy than those who note an increase in oiliness. Thus, some women have a marked improvement of several common skin diseases, including acne (? due to increased estrogen). However, other women experience a marked flare of acne (? due to increased levels of androgenic substances). Those dermatologic diseases that are improved by the use of corticosteroids may improve somewhat during pregnancy.

Most women will notice some increased skin pigmentation during their first pregnancy. The areola of the nipples often darkens considerably and the abdominal linea alba becomes the "linea nigra." In addition, facial pigmentation (chloasma) may be noted on the forehead and cheeks. Fortunately, chloasma often rapidly disappears following delivery.

Many pregnant women will notice an increase in body hair during pregnancy. Typically this is very thin and soft and usually disappears shortly after delivery. The increase in hair may be most noticeable in the cheeks, neck, breasts, abdomen, and pubic region. Hair may be affected in another way, also. Because there is a dramatic sudden change in the hormonal milieu at the time of delivery, the body's hair follicles may be somewhat synchronized by this event. This may result in the loss of large amounts of hair from the scalp some weeks following delivery. It is important to reassure the patient that such loss is not permanent, but rather a normal response to a hormonal change.

Herpes gestationis is a poorly understood disease of later pregnancy and the puerperium that results in severe pruritis and widespread ulceration of the skin. This disease is *not* due to the herpes virus. In many cases, the lesions become worse throughout pregnancy and ultimately may result in total incapacitation. Systemic corticosteroids may relieve the itching and decrease the occurrence of new lesions. In some cases, the disease is severe enough that termination of the pregnancy is considered. The disease is limited to pregnancy.

Pruritis gravidarum (also known by many other names) will be discussed with gastrointestinal disease.

Cardiovascular System

Mitral Valve Disorders

With the near disappearance of rheumatic heart disease in the United States, many fewer cases of organic heart disease are seen now than previously. In fact, mitral valve stenosis, the most frequent condition resulting from rheumatic heart disease, used to comprise nearly 90 per cent of all organic heart disease in pregnancy. This lesion now accounts for less than 50 per cent. Nonetheless, it is still the most frequently seen cardiac lesion in young pregnant women (Noller and Hill, 1991).

Mitral valve stenosis in young women presents a particular problem. In general, the cardiac muscle is still normal and the only lesion is the diseased mitral valve. Usually, there is good cardiac reserve. Although many sophisticated tests are available, the New York Heart Association Functional Classification of Cardiac Disease has remained a very useful, quick screen for the severity of cardiac disease (Table 26–6). However, patients still need appropriate cardiovascular testing to determine cardiac indices with some certainty.

Generally, patients with functional cardiac class I disease should be managed with little interference except for adequate rest and monitoring of the hemoglobin. Class II cardiac patients also generally do well, although they should avoid strenuous exercise. Functional class III and IV patients are at extremely high risk for fetal and maternal death. These patients are all in cardiac failure, and consultation with a high-risk perinatal center is strongly recommended.

The most important consideration is that *cardiac disease should be diagnosed and treated before the onset of pregnancy*. The demands made on the heart by a normal pregnancy may cause heart failure in a person who has no particular difficulty except with extreme exercise (cardiac class II). Patients with mitral valve stenosis may die if they suddenly have atrial fibrillation during pregnancy (Etheridge and Peperell, 1977). Because of the necessity of pumping large amounts of blood through a diseased valve, atrial fibrillation may prevent adequate pumping, or severe fatal pulmonary edema may occur.

The peripheral vascular system also presents particular problems in pregnancy, with the most frequent problem being varicose veins and their complications. Patients with varices or a family history of varices should be encouraged to wear good-quality support panty hose throughout pregnancy. Patients should be instructed to wear these hose at all times when upright. Calf-length and thigh-high hose should be discouraged because the tight tops tend to cause distal edema. Frequent rest in the left lateral recumbent position may help drain the legs and prevent edema and venous stasis. All patients should be instructed in the signs of acute thrombophlebitis and should be advised to report any leg pain, red or warm areas, or obviously discolored areas over varices. Patients with varices also should be cautioned against riding in cars or airplanes for long periods without frequent breaks.

Mitral valve prolapse is a very common condition in young women. There continues to be controversy regarding the need for prophylaxis against bacterial endocarditis. If prophylaxis is to be used, great care must be taken to ensure that the antibiotic agents are safe for both the mother and the fetus.

Chronic Hypertension

Chronic hypertension accompanies many pregnancies. Pregnancy may make the disease worse, and the disease may affect the fetus directly. In general, pregnancy is a physiologic state characterized by vascular relaxation. Therefore, some women with relatively mild hypertension may notice a beneficial effect during the early and middle portions of pregnancy. However, as pregnancy continues, blood pressure typically returns to prepregnant levels and pregnancy-induced hypertension (PIH) and frank toxemia of pregnancy are found to develop in women with chronic hypertension at a rate greater than that in nonhypertensive women (see Complications of Pregnancy, later in this chapter). Frequent blood pressure determinations—always obtained in the left lateral recumbent position—should be made. Any increase in blood pressure is an ominous maternal and fetal sign.

Treatment of high blood pressure in pregnancy must be tempered by the presence of the fetus. That is, only those drugs that are safe for use in pregnancy (i.e., have no adverse effects on the fetus) should be utilized. Fortunately, many of the

---

TABLE 26–6. NEW YORK HEART ASSOCIATION FUNCTIONAL CLASSIFICATION

Class	Criteria
I	No limitation of physical activity
II	No symptoms at rest
	Minor limitation of physical activity (fatigue, palpitations, minor dyspnea)
III	No symptoms at rest
	Marked limitation of physical activity due to symptoms of cardiac disease
IV	Symptoms at rest
	Discomfort increased with any physical activity

common antihypertensive agents are safe for use in pregnancy. Diuretics are not recommended for initiation during pregnancy; however, if a woman is already on a thiazide-type diuretic, it may be continued. Hydralazine and Aldomet classically have been used in pregnancy with excellent results. More recently, nifedipine has been used with great success. In general, calcium channel blockers and cyanide-containing agents should be avoided.

Gastrointestinal System

Although minor aversion to food is common during the early weeks of pregnancy, this is rarely of consequence. However, in a small percentage of pregnant patients, a severe form of pregnancy-related gastrointestinal disease occurs called *hyperemesis gravidarum*. It is characterized by loss of body weight, acidosis, and electrolyte imbalance. Prompt hospitalization and treatment with intravenous fluid is necessary for the safety of both the patient and the fetus. The patient should receive support from the physician and nursing staff, and should be restarted gradually on a full diet. Most patients can be treated and, within a few days, leave the hospital and suffer no recurrence. No organic basis has been found for this disease. Support is probably the most important feature of treatment. Antiemetics often are utilized despite a lack of evidence that they contribute to treatment. None of these has been approved by the Food and Drug Administration as safe and effective during pregnancy. Psychiatric consultation is advised if there are recurrent episodes or if the initial event is serious and prolonged.

Pre-existing *peptic ulcer disease* generally becomes less symptomatic in pregnancy because there is a decrease in the hydrochloric acid secretion of the stomach. In fact, if peptic ulcer disease is diagnosed first in pregnancy, the diagnosis is usually incorrect. In pre-existing disease, nonconstipating antacids may be used if symptoms do not abate with pregnancy.

The diagnosis of *cholecystitis* may be masked in pregnancy. It is often confused with the far more common symptoms of reflux esophagitis and even hyperemesis gravidarum. Fortunately, it is now possible to image the gallbladder without the use of ionizing radiation. If diagnosed, cholecystitis should be treated with a low-fat diet as in the nonpregnant state. Prompt attention to the diagnosis is important because reflux pancreatitis may be particularly difficult to manage in pregnancy. Cholecystectomy, either open or laparoscopic, may be performed in pregnancy (Hill et al., 1975).

Pancreatitis may occur in pregnancy and may be a life-threatening event if it is of the hemorrhagic type. Although this occurs predominantly in alcholic women, pregnancy-induced stasis of the biliary system occasionally may result in pancreatic enzyme reflux, causing a chemical pancreatitis that may be severe.

Regional enteritis may be severe in pregnancy. It is important that adequate maternal nutrition be established and maintained throughout pregnancy when this disease is present (Hanan and Kirsner, 1985). If the woman has severe disease and is in very poor nutritional balance, she probably will not become pregnant. However, if she does, vigorous attempts to maintain adequate nutrition are essential.

Chronic ulcerative colitis also may present problems in pregnancy, but these are rarely as significant as regional enteritis. The patient should be followed with nutritional support and the fetus monitored carefully for evidence of growth retardation (Webb and Sedlack, 1974).

Hepatitis will be covered in Infectious Diseases, later in this chapter.

After hepatitis, the most common cause for *jaundice in pregnancy* is a disease that is identified by many names: the most accepted term at the present time is "cholestatic jaundice of pregnancy" or "cholestasis of pregnancy." This disease presents as pruritus in late pregnancy. Mild jaundice is often present. This is an idiopathic disease usually occurring during the last 10 weeks of pregnancy. In the past, it was believed that the disease, although annoying, did not cause significant fetal or maternal problems. However, it is now recognized that up to 30 per cent of women with this disease have premature labor. The fetus is also at risk for asphyxia in late pregnancy and during labor, and must be monitored closely. Therefore, all patients with cholestatic jaundice are, by definition, high risk and require close follow-up (Noller, 1981; Reid et al., 1976).

Urinary System

The kidneys experience a markedly increased work load during pregnancy. Renal blood flow dramatically increases, as does creatinine clearance. Indeed, a creatinine clearance of 100 liters/24 hours in late pregnancy is significantly decreased and is a sign of renal compromise. A serum creatinine of greater than 0.8 mg/dL is suggestive of renal insufficiency in a normally hydrated pregnant woman.

Because of the increased renal tubular workload, it is sometimes impossible for complete reabsorption of nonelectrolyte solutes to occur. Therefore, some signs, such as glycosuria, may be normal in a pregnant woman. However, normal kidneys may be expected to maintain electrolyte balance in the pregnant patient with normal fluid and electrolyte intake.

Two to 8 per cent of women, whether pregnant or not, will have asymptomatic bacteriuria. One to

2 per cent of pregnant women will develop pyelonephritis, a higher percentage than among non-pregnant women, because changes in pregnancy cause stasis and dilation of the upper urinary tract. The common pathologic organisms are usually aerobic gram-negative rods (*Escherichia coli, Klebsiella,* and *Proteus* species) as well as gram-positive cocci such as *Streptococcus faecalis.* Group B streptococci and *Pseudomonas* are less frequent causes of infection in pregnancy.

All patients should be screened at the first prenatal visit with a urine culture. Women with *asymptomatic bacteriuria* should be treated. Most organisms are susceptible to ampicillin, nitrofurantoin, or one of the cephalosporins. Sulfonamide may be used in the second trimester. Treatment should last for 10 to 14 days, and a follow-up culture should be obtained within the next month. In women with recurrent bacteriuria or cystitis, suppressive low-dose therapy is indicated. Such patients should be checked monthly throughout the pregnancy to assure that there is no worsening of the infection.

Obstetric patients with *pyelonephritis* require admission to the hospital and treatment with intravenous antibiotics pending culture results. Antibiotics of choice include a cephalosporin, ampicillin, or gentamicin combined with a penicillin. Once they are asymptomatic, patients may be switched to oral antibiotics for a 10-day course of therapy. As many as one third of women in this group will have a recurrent urinary tract infection. Therefore, suppressive therapy with monthly cultures is indicated in the pregnant woman with a history of pyelonephritis.

As pregnancy progresses and the uterus enlarges, the ureters may become obstructed or nearly obstructed at the area of the pelvic rim. Severe flank and pelvic pain may result from this "kinking" of the ureters. The patient who arrives at the emergency ward complaining of severe pain in this area—very similar to the renal colic caused by renal stones—may require hospitalization and extensive evaluation. Whereas passage of stones usually results in rather rapid resolution of symptoms, renal colic caused by *ureteral obstruction* at the pelvic rim in late pregnancy may continue for long periods of time. Although ultrasonography occasionally may be helpful in the detection of a renal stone, if present, it is often necessary to perform a "one-shot" intravenous pyelogram to make the diagnosis. Narcotic pain medications usually are necessary to relieve the pain. If no improvement is noted in 1 to 2 days, and the diagnosis has been established firmly, ureteral stenting usually results in prompt resolution of the pain. Pregnant patients with stents in place should receive chronic infection prophylaxis with medications such as nitrofurantoin.

Hematologic System

Iron-deficiency anemia is the most common disorder of the hematologic system seen in pregnancy in the United States. Women who are iron deficient and become pregnant, or women who have borderline iron stores at conception (history of menorrhagia) may exhibit signs of iron deficiency later in pregnancy. Because, in pregnancy, the plasma volume expands more than the red cell mass, there is a physiologic decrease in the hematocrit/hemoglobin concentration of the blood as usually measured. The diagnosis of iron-deficiency anemia should not be made in a woman with a hematocrit greater than 33 per cent or a hemoglobin greater than 11 gm/dL.

The fetus requires a relatively large amount of iron for growth and red blood cell production. Thus, it is advised that all pregnant women receive iron supplementation throughout pregnancy. In most cases this can be administered as part of a prenatal multivitamin. However, for those women with unusually low iron stores or who have known iron-deficiency anemia, additional supplementation is necessary. This can be treated with 60 to 120 mg of elemental iron a day. Additional copper (2 mg) and zinc (15 mg) are needed if more than 60 mg of elemental iron is prescribed daily, because the excess iron can interfere with the absorption of these ions. Maintenance therapy can be resumed when the hematocrit returns to normal.

Folic acid deficiency rarely was observed in the United States and, with now near-universal supplementation of a minimum of 400 μg of folic acid daily, it will become even rarer. However, macrocytic anemia occurring after the 30th week of pregnancy could represent folic acid deficiency.

Sickle cell disease (hemoglobin type S/S) is a devastating disease. Although most individuals with this disease will have been diagnosed prior to pregnancy, in the case of unusually young teenage girls, the first crisis occasionally occurs during pregnancy. Extreme pain, often localized in the bony skeleton, is a common presenting symptom. (See Chapter 45 for more information concerning sickle cell diseases.)

Thrombocytopenia

There are several diseases that cause thrombocytopenia in the pregnant woman. Immune thrombocytopenic purpura and systemic lupus erythematosis are more common in women than in men. The HELLP syndrome (see Toxemia of Pregnancy, later in this chapter) and thrombotic thrombocytopenic purpura are relatively pregnancy specific. Certain drugs also may cause a decrease in platelets. In some ways, immune thrombocytopenic purpura diagnosed and treated prior to pregnancy may be more problematic than that which is diagnosed during pregnancy. Often a woman who has been diagnosed previously has undergone splenectomy and has no particular platelet problem. It must not be forgotten, however, that she may continue to carry one or more antiplatelet antibodies/factors that are transferred to the fetus. Therefore, the fetus may be born with relatively few platelets and may experience significant bleeding problems. Women diagnosed during pregnancy usually are placed on corticosteroids and often have a prompt response. The maternal response does not guarantee the fetal condition, however, and the fetus may have a very low platelet level when born.

It is unclear whether fetal scalp sampling in labor to determine the fetal platelet level is necessary. Nonetheless, it is commonly practiced. Specifically, when a woman begins labor and the fetal scalp is accessible, a small incision is made in the scalp in routine fashion as is done for scalp pH determination. The sample is then sent for platelet determination. If the fetal platelets are found to be less than $50,000/mm^3$, cesarean section is recommended by some authors in an attempt to decrease the likelihood of intracerebral bleed. However, it is not universally accepted that vaginal delivery poses more of a threat to the fetus from intracerebral bleeding than does cesarean section delivery. Thus, some authors now recommend no fetal scalp sampling if the maternal platelets are within normal range.

Maternal–Fetal Blood Incompatibilities

Although the CDE (Rhesus) blood group is the best known, several of the major and minor blood groups may be the cause of significant risk of fetal anemia and hydrops fetalis. Every woman should have a screen for irregular blood group antibodies at her first prenatal visit. If evidence of a dangerous incompatibility is found, the patient must be monitored by serum antibody titers and amniotic fluid.

RH DISEASE. Rh incompatibility between mother and fetus is largely a problem of the past. The pregnant woman's blood group and Rh factor should be determined at the first visit. All Rh-negative women should be counseled by their physicians about the process by which Rh sensitization occurs. Prophylaxis with 300 mg of Rh immune globulin (RhIG) is performed routinely at 28 weeks' gestation, after any manipulation (amniocentesis, version), and after a significant bleeding episode. At birth, the Rh factor of the infant should be determined, and if it is positive, the mother should be treated with another dose of RhIG.

If traumatic delivery has taken place (all operative deliveries, cesarean section, mid-forceps deliveries, and manual removal of the placenta), the Kleihauer test for fetal red cells in the maternal serum should be performed. This test is routinely available from most laboratories and can determine accurately the volume of fetal blood that has transferred into the mother's circulation. Despite years of use, the amount of fetal blood that can be neu-

tralized by one 300-μg vial of RhIG is still debated. Some authorities believe that only 15 mL of fetal blood can be neutralized by one vial of RhIG, while others believe it is 30 mL. It is always better to use too much RhIG rather than too little in the nonallergic woman.

The D^u test is performed routinely in most laboratories but can only detect fetal–maternal bleeding in excess of 25 mL. Therefore, the test is not sensitive enough to identify bleeding of 15 to 25 mL. Two vials of RhIG are indicated for bleeding in this range.

There are some women who have been Rh sensitized in earlier pregnancies or who become sensitized through therapeutic abortion, spontaneous abortion, inadvertent transfusion with inappropriate blood, or spontaneously during an apparently normal gestation. When sensitization occurs, it is a very high-risk situation for the fetus, and consultation with a maternal–fetal medicine specialist is recommended. Frequent amniocenteses and fetal transfusion with red blood cells may be necessary.

Neurologic System

Seizure Disorders

Women who are receiving treatment for the various seizure disorders require special attention during pregnancy. Seizure activity may be slightly increased and harder to control, perhaps because of increased renal clearance of anticonvulsant drugs. In addition, several commonly used medications are associated with a significant increase in birth defects. Valproic acid is associated with a 1 to 2 per cent risk of a neural tube defect. Both Dilantin and phenobarbital have been implicated as possible causes of congenital abnormalities. Some authors have suggested this is a result of medication-induced folic acid deficiency, and may be avoided by treating all pregnant women with seizures with 4 mg of folic acid a day. Even without maternal therapy, neonates born to women with seizures have an increased risk of congenital malformation (Bjerkadel, 1982).

Medications for which there are established serum levels for the prevention of seizures should be monitored closely during pregnancy to assure that adequate levels are maintained to avoid a recurrence of convulsions.

Carpal Tunnel Syndrome

Many pregnant women experience symptoms of carpal tunnel syndrome during the last few weeks of pregnancy. In some women this may become profound, with marked loss of sensation and dysesthesias throughout the palm and fingers. Fortunately, these symptoms usually abate rather quickly following delivery. During pregnancy, symptoms may be decreased by avoidance of activity that tends to worsen these symptoms, namely repetitive wrist and hand motions. Orthopedic splints often are helpful in extreme cases.

Respiratory System

Many women experience the "breathlessness of pregnancy" during the third trimester. This symptom appears to be largely due to pressure from the enlarging uterus on the diaphragm. In most cases, reassurance alone is sufficient treatment. Breathlessness must be distinguished from dyspnea, and if there is a suspicion that the patient is experiencing any degree of breathing difficulty, careful percussion and auscultation of the lungs as well as measurement of the tidal volume and blood gases may be indicated. The incidence of pulmonary embolism is slightly increased in pregnancy.

Asthma is a common disease in young women. During pregnancy, some one third of women with this disease will be found to improve markedly. Unfortunately, the majority of women with asthma experience no change in their symptoms and a few are somewhat worse. The drugs most commonly used for the treatment of asthma—β-blockers and prednisone—may be utilized during pregnancy. However, as for all drugs, patients should be advised to use minimum effective dosages.

Endocrine System

Diabetes Mellitus

Shortly after the introduction of insulin, the first successful pregnancy and delivery occurred in a woman affected with this condition. Yet it very quickly became apparent that the control of diabetes in pregnancy demanded unusual care by both the patient and the physician. Whole clinics became devoted solely to the treatment of pregnant women with insulin-dependent diabetes.

The interactions between pregnancy and diabetes are dramatic. Whereas diabetic women often maintain stable insulin dosages for years, pregnant women require frequent, even daily, changes; pregnant women were among the first to be noted to require multiple insulin dosages per day. Also, diabetic women often follow urine sugars alone, whereas pregnant women require frequent blood glucose determinations by their physicians. However, even with this close monitoring, pregnant women still experienced many unfavorable pregnancy outcomes: increased congenital malformations, increased stillbirths, and increased macrosomia. Only recently has it been learned that improvement in all three of these abnormalities is possible with extremely strict control of plasma glucose beginning *before conception* (Reece et al.,

1988). Only those diabetic women who are very well controlled from the outset and who maintain this control throughout pregnancy can expect to achieve the same good pregnancy outcome results as nondiabetic women.

Before it was recognized that strict control of blood sugar was necessary, various attempts were made to improve fetal/neonatal survival in diabetic women. The use of estriol determinations and early cesarean delivery are but two of many. It is now recognized that the patient who carefully guards against elevated glucose levels may be allowed to experience spontaneous labor at term. Nevertheless, it is suggested that the pregnant diabetic have ultrasonography for determination of fetal weight during the last month of pregnancy to assure that macrosomia has not occurred. Attempted vaginal delivery of a macrosomic infant (greater than 4000 grams) carries an unusually high risk of complication, most commonly shoulder dystocia and nerve injury.

All authorities on pregnancy and diabetes agree that increased fetal surveillance is necessary. However, the age of gestation at which to start fetal testing, and the type and frequency of testing, is hotly debated. Nonstress tests may be done twice weekly; contraction stress tests or biophysical profiles may be done once weekly. Testing probably should start around the 32nd week of gestation.

Ketoacidosis in a pregnant woman may result rapidly in fetal death. This condition, which is also life threatening to the pregnant woman, must be managed aggressively utilizing an intravenous insulin drip. The sooner the patient can be returned to normal glucose levels, the less danger to the fetus. Except in very rare conditions, the use of infusions of bicarbonate are not indicated and may be harmful.

Gestational Diabetes

It is now recommended that all pregnant women undergo screening for gestational diabetes (see Prenatal Care). Typically this is done by administering a 50-gram glucose load in a nonfasting woman between 26 and 28 weeks' gestation (see Table 26–4). If the blood glucose is greater than 135 mg/dL 1 hour following ingestion of the glucose load, the patient should undergo a 3-hour glucose tolerance test. If the results are abnormal, the patient should be seen immediately, counseled, and placed on a strict American Diabetes Association–recommended diet. She should be monitored closely and, if glucose control is not achieved within 2 weeks, she should be placed on insulin. Women who have experienced gestational diabetes previously or who have a strong family history should be tested earlier.

Fetal macrosomia is the most common complication of gestational diabetes. Because most fetal weight increase occurs following the 28th week, it is not important to perform ultrasonography for fetal size before this time. However, in the woman newly diagnosed with gestational diabetes, it is important to follow fetal growth carefully after the 28th week.

Infectious Diseases

Virtually any infection that occurs in a nonpregnant woman may occur in pregnancy. For years it has been suggested that pregnant women are unusually susceptible to many infections because of the "immunocompromised" state induced by pregnancy. It now appears that pregnancy may not alter the immune status of the pregnant woman significantly. It is not possible in this chapter to present both sides of this issue. However, it is important to recognize that infections can and do occur in pregnant women, and that prompt diagnosis and treatment are essential. In addition, the treatment (and on occasion the diagnostic methodology) must be altered in the pregnant woman.

Respiratory Infections

Upper respiratory tract infections are particularly troublesome to pregnant women. Estrogen induces hyperemia of all mucous membranes. Thus, the sinuses and nasal passages of pregnant women may be occluded partially solely because of the presence of excess estrogen, even without viral infection. "Rhinitis of pregnancy" is a noninfectious physiologic state that is particularly bothersome to many pregnant women. Use of decongestants and antihistamines should not be encouraged unless the patient finds it impossible to continue her normal activities.

Upper respiratory tract viral infections (the common cold) may cause more symptoms than in the nonpregnant woman, but have no more consequences. Pneumonitis may occur in pregnant women. *Mycoplasma* infections are perhaps the most common and may be treated with erythromycin as in the nonpregnant state. Pneumococcal and streptococcal pneumonias remain potentially life threatening in both pregnant and nonpregnant women. Prompt treatment with appropriate antibiotics is essential.

Hepatitis

Hepatitis is a common disease in the United States. All types are seen in pregnancy, but hepatitis B is the most problematic. Nutritional support is the most important element in the treatment of all types of hepatitis in pregnancy. Both the fetus and the mother usually will survive without sequelae if nutritional support is adequate (Noller, 1981). Acute fulminant hepatitis B is the only exception to this rule. This disease cannot be distinguished easily from the fatty necrosis of the liver that occurs infrequently in late pregnancy.

If a woman develops hepatitis B in pregnancy

TABLE 26–7. HEPATITIS B STATUS OF NEONATE

Time of Maternal Infection	Neonatal Status
Early pregnancy	Often no active disease; infant may be chronic carrier
Late pregnancy	Usually active disease; carrier status common
Positive "e" antigen	Usually active disease; carrier status common

or is a chronic carrier, the fetus is at risk for either active disease or carrier status (Table 26–7). At birth, the neonate should receive hepatitis B hyperimmune globulin and the first dose of hepatitis vaccine. Although this may seem not to be indicated in the infant who has active disease, there is some evidence that such treatment might shorten the disease course and prevent carrier status.

In cases of hepatitis B, it is extremely important to take precautions against the spread of the virus to medical and nursing personnel via the blood and amniotic fluid at delivery. This is especially important in dealing with certain high-risk patients, such as intravenous drug users.

On rare occasions, women with severe chronic active hepatitis will achieve pregnancy. If portal hypertension is present, it likely will become more severe during pregnancy. Severe bleeding from esophageal varices is common, and pregnancy termination may be necessary.

Hepatitis C (non-A, non-B) also occurs in pregnancy. There is no evidence that the disease is more severe in pregnant women than in nonpregnant women.

Sexually Transmitted Diseases

Sexually transmitted diseases (STDs) comprise a long list of diseases. While syphilis and gonorrhea are the only "classic" disease entities, herpes, human papilloma virus, trichomonas, HIV, hepatitis, yeast infections, and several other diseases commonly are transmitted by sexual activity. Some of these diseases have important implications during pregnancy, which are discussed below.

SYPHILIS. The only acceptable treatment of syphilis in pregnancy is penicillin. Although erythromycin will treat syphilis in the pregnant woman, it often does not eradicate the disease in the fetus. No other drug is known to have good activity against this organism. Thus, penicillin is required, even in penicillin-allergic women. In this case the patient must be desensitized to penicillin rapidly and treated (Centers for Disease Control and Prevention 1993).

GONORRHEA. Gonorrhea infections are relatively common in the United States. Treatment with ceftriaxone remains the standard and can be used in pregnancy. If the patient is cephalosporin allergic, erythromycin may be used. Pelvic inflammatory disease is rarely, if ever, observed in a known pregnant woman.

CHLAMYDIA. Infections with *C. trachomatis* are common in women less than 35 years of age. Many authors now recommend routine screening for this organism in all pregnant women, although the cost-effectiveness of this screening procedure has not been well established. If the test for *Chlamydia* is positive, it is recommended that the woman receive oral erythromycin, either as erythromycin base, 500 mg, or as erythromycin ethylsuccinate, 800 mg four times a day for 7 days. Erythromycin estolate should not be used during pregnancy because of hepatotoxicity. Sexual partners must be treated as well. In women sensitive to high-dose erythromycin, the dose can be halved and the duration of therapy doubled. Sulfonamide can be used with caution in penicillin-allergic women, with the knowledge of the potential development of neonatal hyperbilirubinemia. Safer but less effective regimens exist, including amoxicillin, 500 mg three times a day for 7 days, and clindamycin, 450 mg four times a day for 7 days.

HERPES SIMPLEX VIRUS. Genital infection with herpes simplex virus (usually type II, although type I may be involved) has important implications in pregnancy. Patients who experience primary infection early in pregnancy may undergo spontaneous abortion. Primary infection later in pregnancy is not associated with increased pregnancy loss or malformation.

Exposure of the fetus to active herpes simplex virus at the time of delivery may result in neonatal infection. Such infection may be mild, resulting in only a few skin lesions, or may be systemic, with severe neurologic sequelae and/or death. Full-term healthy infants are less likely to develop systemic infection than premature or compromised infants.

A woman who has a known history of genital herpes simplex virus should have thorough inspection of the vulva and the remainder of the lower genital tract at the time of the initiation of labor. If active lesions are found, the patient should undergo cesarean section. However, if the woman has no active lesions and has experienced none in the previous few days, vaginal delivery may be accomplished and cesarean section reserved for obstetric indications only.

β-HEMOLYTIC STREPTOCOCCUS. β-Hemolytic streptococcus infection of the cervix and lower genital tract is present in 10 to 15 per cent of all pregnant women. Infants who develop β-hemolytic streptococcus infections soon after birth may develop a life-threatening condition. Thus, it has been proposed by some authors that all pregnant women be screened for the presence of this organism. Unfortunately such screening—and treatment of women who are positive—does not ensure that neonates will not develop β-hemolytic streptococcus infections.

Carriers of β-hemolytic streptococcus are very difficult to clear permanently of such colonization. In studies of women who have been treated, repeat cultures several weeks later almost always show recurrence of the infection. Thus, most authorities do not recommend routine culture of pregnant women for β-hemolytic streptococcus.

However, there are two suggestions that currently are being followed by many labor and delivery units. First, all women with a premature onset of labor are cultured routinely for β-hemolytic streptococcus and penicillin therapy is begun at the time of admission to the hospital. The penicillin is continued until the streptococcus culture is returned as negative. If the culture is positive, the patient is treated for a full 5 days. If a woman has ruptured membranes for more than 18 hours, penicillin prophylaxis is begun. Neonatal β-hemolytic streptococcus infections occur most frequently in women who have experienced ruptured membranes for more than 18 hours.

TRICHOMONIASIS. *Trichomonas vaginalis* may present a treatment dilemma for the pregnant woman. Metronidazole, the only effective treatment, is not recommended in the first trimester, although in fact no adverse fetal outcomes are documented from the use of this drug. The CDC alternatively recommends clotrimazole 100 mg intravaginally for 7 days (Centers for Disease Control and Prevention, 1993). Symptoms may lessen, although the cure rate is low. Metronidazole may be used in very symptomatic women after 14 weeks' gestation.

YEAST INFECTIONS. Yeast infections are common in pregnancy, and the intense itching can be quite uncomfortable. There are no contraindications to the use of clotrimazole or miconazole.

EFFECTS ON RUPTURE OF MEMBRANES AND ONSET OF LABOR. Certain STD organisms have been associated with premature rupture of the membranes and/or premature onset of labor. These include gonorrhea, *Chlamydia*, *Mycoplasma*, and bacterial vaginosis. Although many of the studies that implicate these organisms are technically flawed, overall it is assumed that the patient with any of these infections carries a slightly increased risk of premature delivery.

COMPLICATIONS OF PREGNANCY

Premature Rupture of Membranes

Premature rupture of membranes, defined as rupture of membranes 2 hours or longer prior to the onset of labor, occurs in 5 to 10 per cent of all pregnancies. Over 60 per cent of cases occur in term patients. The family physician must have a clear, rational plan to handle this common event. All patients should be directed to come to the hospital for evaluation and documentation of membrane rupture. Although many patients do not contact their physician until hours after the event, management requires that the physician document membrane rupture and assess cervical dilation. The history is accurate in 90 per cent of cases. However, some patients who think they have ruptured their membranes in fact may not have, and may be confusing vaginal secretions or urine with ruptured membranes. No large studies have evaluated outpatient management of this condition.

On admission to the hospital, a sterile speculum examination first must be done. Often one can confirm pooling of fluid in the posterior fornix. Nitrazine paper frequently is used; however, false-positive results are very common with contamination by blood, urine, and infected vaginal secretions. The test is reliable only if negative. The diagnosis is confirmed by analyzing a drop of fluid under a microscope at medium/high power. Fern-like leaf patterns will appear as the fluid dries (Fig. 26–3). Samples should not be obtained from the internal cervical os, because secretions from this area can appear fern-pattern positive even with intact membranes.

The next crucial step is to assess the ripeness of the cervix. Although visual inspection may not be able to distinguish subtle differences in ripeness, it should allow one to distinguish a very unfavorable cervix from a more favorable one. The Bishop method for scoring of the cervix is described in Table 26–8. One should make every attempt to evaluate the cervix by visual inspection only, because manual exam increases the likelihood of infection.

A fetal heart tracing should be obtained to be certain that there is no fetal compromise. Lower genital tract cultures should be done, screening for group B streptococcus. A baseline white blood cell count should be drawn. Patients who have medical indications for induction, such as hypertension or insulin-dependent diabetes, should be induced immediately. However, if all is otherwise normal, the physician has two options: (1) to manage the patient conservatively and expectantly, or (2) to induce labor (Fig. 26–4). It is expected that at least 75 to 85 per cent of women managed expectantly will go into labor within 24 hours, and the vast majority of the remainder within 48 hours. If the cervix is not ripe, the physician can appropriately wait for the patient to go into spontaneous labor, monitoring her in the hospital with daily white blood cell counts and monitoring for maternal fever and fetal heart rate every 4 hours. Only if the woman develops signs of infection would induction then occur. There does not appear to be any advantage to inducing a woman at the 24-hour point, according to the most recent review of clinical investigations (Duff, 1991). Patients who were

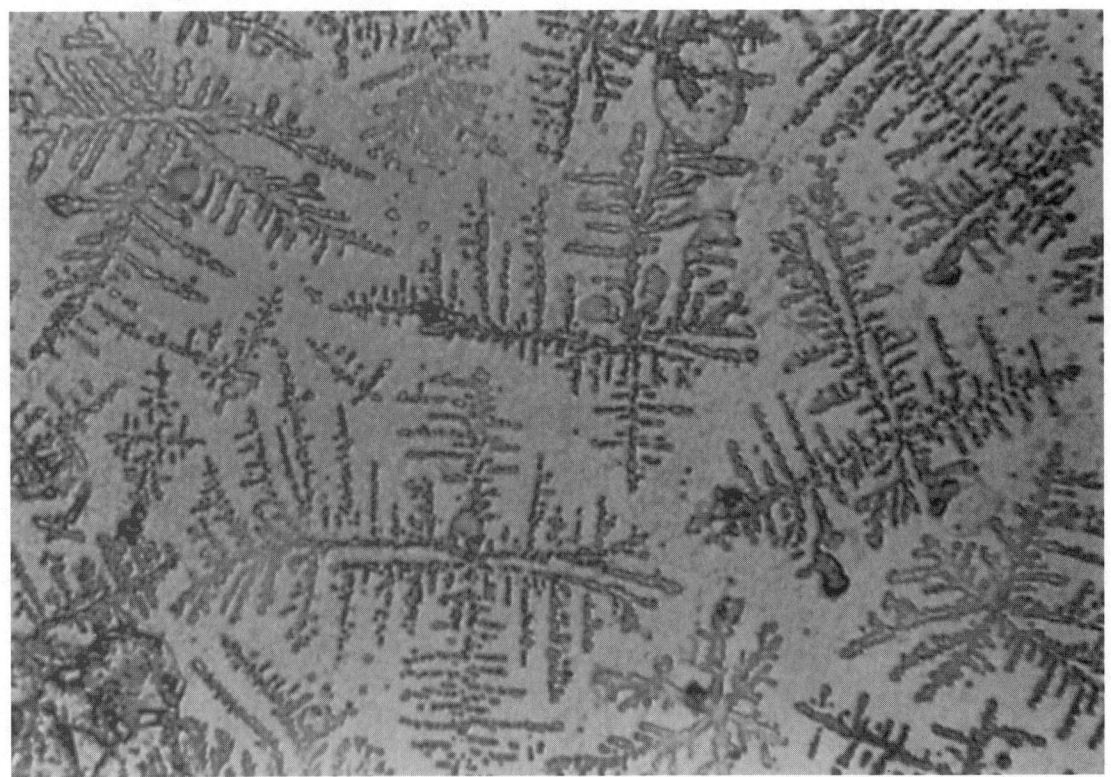

FIGURE 26–3. Photomicrograph of amniotic fluid ferning. (×45) (From Greenwald JL: Premature rupture of the membranes: Diagnosis and management strategies. Am Fam Physician 48:297, 1993, with permission.)

TABLE 26–8. THE BISHOP SCORE*

Dilation	0 cm	1 to 2 cm	3 to 4 cm	5 to 6 cm
Score:	0	1	2	3
Effacement	0 to 30%	40 to 50%	60 to 70%	80%
Score:	0	1	2	3
Station	−3	−2	−1 to 0	+1 to +2
Score:	0	1	2	3
Consistency	Firm	Medium	Soft	
Score:	0	1	2	
Position of cervical os	Posterior	Middle	Anterior	
Score:	0	1	2	

* The score prior to the onset of labor is generally 11 or less. A score of 9 or greater is highly favorable for induction.
From Greenwald JL: Premature rupture of the membranes: Diagnostic and management strategies. Am Fam Physician 48:298, 1993, with permission.

induced at this late point had a higher incidence of maternal and fetal complications. A second alternative in the group of women with unfavorable Bishop scores is to begin induction immediately, anticipate a long latent phase of labor, and minimize vaginal exams. Both the expectant and the aggressive management styles have had favorable outcomes.

In the patient with ruptured membranes and a ripe cervix, early induction of labor is recommended if the patient does not start into labor within a few hours. "In such patients, there is little to be gained by an extended period of observation, and an increased duration of the latent period correlates with an increased risk of maternal and neonatal infection" (Duff, 1991, p. 728).

Premature rupture of membranes in a preterm pregnancy, defined as less than 37 weeks' gestation, will be handled differently. Digital exam should never be performed in that case, and further antepartum testing must be done to assess the maturity of the infant (Lewis et al., 1992).

Toxemia of Pregnancy (Pre-eclampsia, Eclampsia, Pregnancy-Induced Hypertension)

Despite centuries of study, toxemia of pregnancy is still not fully understood. This disease (characterized by maternal hypertension, proteinuria, rapid weight gain, and edema) may remain mild

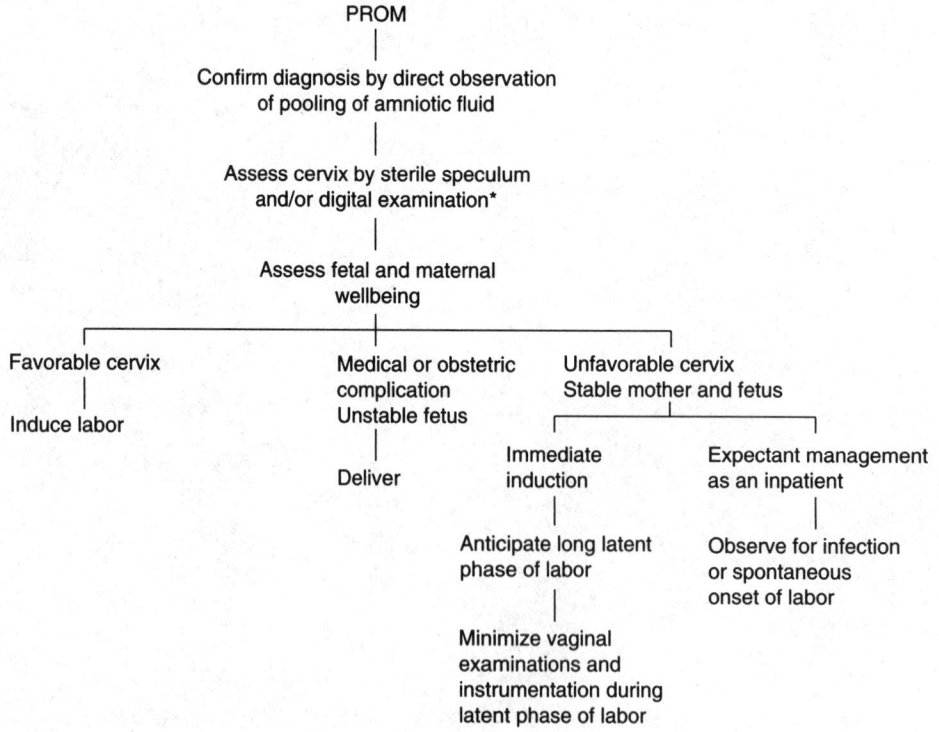

FIGURE 26–4. Algorithm for management of a term patient with premature rupture of membranes (PROM). *Do not perform digital exam on a patient with PROM prior to 37 weeks' gestation.

or may develop fully to include maternal seizure activity, fetal demise, and maternal death. The disease process includes an abnormal maternal response to angiotensin, constriction of the arteriolar and arterial bed, and malperfusion of the placenta. Maternal hypertension is thought to result from the body's attempt to overcome the arterial constriction, rather than being a cause of the disease. Recently the disease has been considered to result from the maternal immune system's recognition of the fetal antigens as alien. The disease occurs most commonly in women who are pregnant for the first time or who have experienced the disease previously. The disease is also more common in multiparous women who have a new sexual partner. Despite some evidence to suggest that the use of low-dose aspirin may reduce the occurrence of toxemia in low-risk women, the risk of aspirin-induced abruptio placentae outweighs the small reduction in pre-eclampsia (Sibai et al., 1993).

Toxemia may occur at any time in pregnancy, although it is most common after 28 weeks of gestation. Toxemia occurring before this time is most often due to gestational trophoblastic disease or multiple gestation. Early disease is particularly ominous because the pregnant woman often has no symptoms in the early phases of the disease.

The presence of an elevated blood pressure at the time of a routine prenatal visit or the detection of protein in a voided urine specimen represent the two most common ways in which the disease is diagnosed. Detection of an elevation of blood pressure of more than 30 mm Hg systolic or 15 mm Hg diastolic above the initial baseline on two occasions more than 6 hours apart, along with the detection of more than 300 mg of protein in a 24-hour urine sample, confirms the diagnosis. Although rapid weight gain and edema classically have been part of the diagnosis of toxemia, they are now known to be only secondary factors and do not, by themselves, support the diagnosis.

Patients suspected of having toxemia should be placed at restricted activities. It has been shown that women with early stages of the disease who are placed at bed rest and who receive no other medical intervention often have no exacerbation of the disease and, on occasion, have remission. At the present time, bed rest, preferably in the left lateral recumbent position, is the only treatment for this disease other than delivery of the fetus.

Women with toxemia must be followed closely. If the disease progresses, this must be done in the hospital with blood pressure monitoring, collection of 24-hour urines, and close observation. Additionally, the disease affects the fetus as well as the mother and therefore frequent fetal testing is important. Nonstress testing and biophysical profiles are the most commonly used methods of ascertaining fetal well-being (see Fetal Testing in Patients with Toxemia and PIH).

If, despite rest, the mother continues to deterio-

rate, delivery must be accomplished. Blood pressure readings in the dangerous range (systolic near 200 with diastolic above 100) or urine protein in excess of 3 grams in 24 hours suggest a condition serious enough to warrant delivery, despite gestational age. Indeed, in most cases the fetus is so affected that premature delivery is preferable to the fetus remaining in the uterus. If the decision is made to effect delivery, vaginal delivery should be attempted first unless the fetus shows signs of severe stress.

In past years, salt and/or water restriction as well as the use of diuretics was recommended. It is now known that toxemia causes intravascular hypovolemia, and water and salt restriction, as well as the use of diuretics, only exacerbates the disease.

HELLP Syndrome

In some cases, toxemia of pregnancy progresses rapidly and the HELLP syndrome develops. This acronym was developed after observation of the signs of *h*emolysis, *e*levated *l*iver enzymes, and *l*ow *p*latelets. Patients with the HELLP syndrome have anemia, markedly abnormal liver enzymes, and rapidly falling platelets. In addition, they usually (although not always) exhibit severe hypertension and profound proteinuria. Right upper quadrant pain may be present and represents stretching of Glisson's liver capsule from hepatic edema. Hyperreflexia is almost always present, with clonus detected in many patients. Seizure activity may occur if the patient is not treated promptly. In normal pregnancy, platelets are elevated; in the HELLP syndrome, they are often under 100,000/mm^3 and may rapidly fall to less than 50,000/mm^3.

The only treatment for the HELLP syndrome is prompt delivery. In addition, the patient routinely should receive magnesium sulfate ($MgSO_4$) therapy to prevent seizure activity. $MgSO_4$ usually is given as a 4-gram intravenous loading dose over a period of 20 to 60 minutes followed by approximately 2 gm/hr intravenously through a metered intravenous infusion mechanism. $MgSO_4$ may cause cardiac asystole and respiratory failure unless administered with great care. It should never be administered by any method other than intravenous infusion through a metered pump. The use of direct drip $MgSO_4$ or intramuscular injection is no longer recommended. Urinary output must be watched carefully because magnesium toxicity may occur as a result of reduced urinary output in severe cases of toxemia. Monitoring of magnesium levels is suggested because this can help avoid Mg^{++} toxicity.

$MgSO_4$ does little to control hypertension and, if the hypertension is severe, rapid-acting antihypertensives such as hydralazine should be used. Ten milligrams of hydralazine may be given by slow intravenous push, if needed. The blood pressure must be watched very closely because prolonged hypotension occasionally is observed after the use of this drug. The maximal effect will be seen within 20 minutes. Follow-up dosages must be given with care because of a potential additive effect. Nifedipine has been used recently in cases of extreme hypertension.

In the past, when a pregnant woman with severe toxemia was admitted to the hospital, standard practice was to spend 24 hours "stabilizing" the patient before delivery was attempted if the HELLP syndrome was present. This management is not acively debated since delay may follow for progression of the disease process. After control of the reflexes and blood pressure has been established with MgSO₄ and antihypertensive agents (usually in less than 2 hours), in most cases of severe disease, delivery should be considered, regardless of gestational age.

Disseminated Intravascular Coagulation

Many women with severe toxemia have disseminated intravascular coagulation (DIC). The platelet concentration and a coagulation profile should be obtained at admission for all women with this disease. If DIC is profound, only delivery will correct the condition. Although there is no longer any indication for the use of fibrinogen, large amounts of platelet concentrate and fresh frozen plasma should be available for use at the time of delivery, if necessary.

Postdelivery Treatment

Following delivery, the patient usually will return rapidly to normal. However, seizure activity may occur up to several days following delivery, although the first 24 hours are the most worrisome. Intravenous MgSO₄ therapy usually is continued for 24 to 48 hours following delivery, depending on the severity of the disease process.

Hypertension Conditions

TOXEMIA AND CHRONIC HYPERTENSION. For reasons unknown, chronic hypertension results in the development of superimposed toxemia with greater frequency than in the nonhypertensive woman. Assuming that hypertension is controlled with appropriate medications, toxemia is treated as described earlier.

PREGNANCY-INDUCED HYPERTENSION/TRANSIENT HYPERTENSION. Some pregnant women develop PIH without signs or symptoms of toxemia. This disease is usually self-limited and the patient rapidly returns to a normotensive state following delivery. If the hypertension is in a dangerous range, she should be treated with antihypertensive medications. Women who fail to return to normotensive levels 6 weeks following delivery should be investigated thoroughly for other causes of hypertension, such as renal artery stenosis.

Fetal Testing in Patients with Toxemia and PIH

A useful aid for monitoring the fetus is the *nonstress test* (see Fig. 26–5). For nonstress testing, the patient is placed in a reclining position and the fetus is monitored for 20 minutes. The fetal heart rate pattern is observed after spontaneous fetal movement, and accelerations of the fetal heart rate of 15 beats or greater for more than 15 seconds should occur after movement on at least two occasions during the 20-minute test period. If no accelerations occur within that time period, the test is continued for at least 40 minutes, during which time the clinician may attempt to stimulate the fetus with abdominal palpation. If the fetus does not respond to nonstress testing, the test is considered nonreactive and is suggestive of fetal sleep or fetal compromise. Nonreactive tests should be repeated in 8 hours and, if still nonreactive, they should be followed by a biophysical profile.

The *biophysical profile* is a more sophisticated version of nonstress testing. Nonstress testing is performed in the usual fashion. Ultrasonography then is done to assess fetal breathing, tone, and motion, and the amniotic fluid volume is estimated. Scores of 0, 1, or 2 are given to each of these five variables (nonstress test, fluid volume, fetal tone, fetal breathing, and fetal motion) and a total of 10 indicates adequate placental perfusion. The biophysical profile has largely supplemented contraction stress testing, in which low levels of oxytocin are used to cause at least three contractions in 10 minutes.

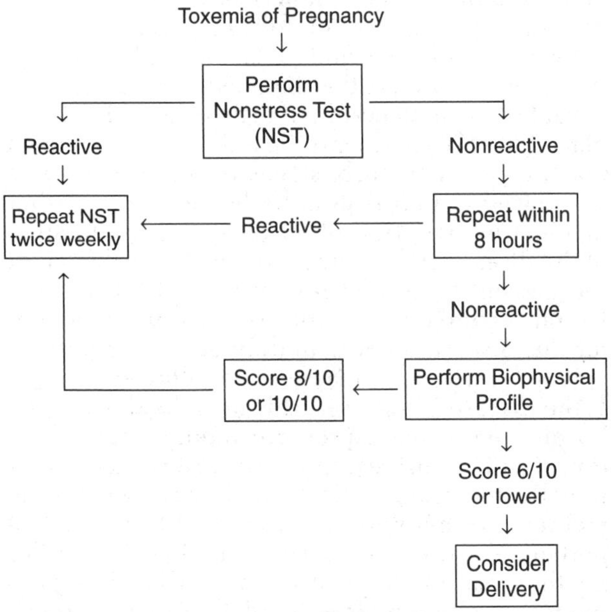

FIGURE 26–5. Fetal testing in mothers with toxemia of pregnancy.

Third-Trimester Bleeding

This is a common complication of pregnancy and is usually the result of either placenta previa or abruptio placentae. *Placenta previa* is a life-threatening situation for both mother and fetus. Electronic maternal and fetal monitoring should be instituted on admission. When ultrasound examination has been performed during prenatal care, the diagnosis of placenta previa can be excluded if a woman has vaginal bleeding when she enters the labor and delivery suite. If the placenta is not low lying, vaginal examination may be undertaken. However, if ultrasonography has not been performed, vaginal examination should be deferred because a finger can be placed inadvertently through the placenta and can cause severe hemorrhage, with possible fetal and maternal death. Total placenta previa requires cesarean section.

Abruptio placentae is similarly a life-threatening event for both mother and fetus. Depending on the portion of the placenta that has been torn from the uterine wall, the fetus may be little affected or may be dead. The area of placental separation occasionally may be identified using ultrasonography in the labor and delivery suite. Usually, the main symptom is pain and the signs are uterine tetany and vaginal bleeding. Large retroplacental hematomas may occur with sequestration of blood, depletion of the coagulation factors, and rapid onset of disseminated intravascular coagulation. Consideration should be given to immediate delivery, with blood products immediately available.

Vaginal delivery may be accomplished, but cesarean section often is needed. The fetus should be monitored continuously electronically with a scalp electrode because it may show signs of impending death during attempts at vaginal delivery. When treating a patient who has abruptio placentae, an efficient and accurate hematologic laboratory should be available. Blood should be drawn for prothrombin time, fibrinogen levels, and a complete blood count. The treatment of choice is delivery. If loss of blood has been significant, whole blood, packed red blood cells, fresh frozen plasma, and platelet concentrate can be used to restore the depleted blood and coagulation factors. Fibrinogen should not be administered because of the high risk of hepatitis.

Placental abruption is seen with increased frequency in women who use cocaine. Women who present with an abruption should be considered for drug screening.

Multiple Gestation

Twins occur spontaneously in approximately 1 in every 80 pregnancies in the United States. Triplets occur in approximately 1 in 6500 to 8000 pregnancies. Because of the widespread use of advanced reproductive technologies, multiple pregnancies are now much more common in the United States. These are significant complications of pregnancy and experience is required to deal with them properly. It used to be a commonly accepted fact that women with multiple gestation went into labor very early, with prematurity being the most common complication of twin birth. However, multiple gestation usually is identified early in pregnancy by means of ultrasonography, and, if the patient is placed at bed rest, she often will carry to term.

Cesarean section for twin deliveries is recommended unless both twins are in the vertex position, there are definitely two separate sacs, both twins are the same size (±300 grams), and electronic fetal monitoring is available. Electronic fetal monitoring of the second twin should be performed during and after delivery of the first twin.

Premature Labor

Prematurity is the most frequent cause of neonatal death in the United States. Certain women are at high risk for premature labor and deliveries (Table 26–9). Proper risk assessment at the time of the initial obstetric visit may identify many of these associated problems, if present.

If premature labor occurs, it should be documented. The diagnosis should not be made unless there is progressive cervical dilation. If the gestation is of less than 36 weeks, consideration should be given to attempting to stop labor using β-sympathomimetic agents or $MgSO_4$. Currently, ritodrine

---

TABLE 26–9. FACTORS ASSOCIATED WITH INCREASED RISK OF PREMATURE DELIVERY

Medical
Primigravidity
History of previous premature delivery
In utero diethylstilbestrol exposure
Maternal hypertension
Multiple gestation
Previous cervical manipulation (dilation, conization)
Sexually transmitted diseases
Pyelonephritis

Social
Age < 18 or > 35
Low level of education
Nonmarried status
Poor or absent prenatal care
Low income
Abusive relationship

Behavioral
Smoking
Alcohol abuse
Illicit drug use

TABLE 26–10.   RITODRINE PROTOCOL

Patient placed in left lateral position
Obtain baseline K^+, glucose
Record: Maternal vital signs
     Blood pressure and pulse—baseline, then every 10
       min until stabilized, then every 60 min
     Input and output
Fetal heart rate
    Continuous electronic fetal monitoring
Start intravenous infusion with 5% dextrose in lactated Ringer's
    solution
Administer ritodrine
    Infusion pump mandatory
    Piggyback to intravenous infusion
    Solution: 15 mg ritodrine in 500 mL 5% dextrose (300 μg/
      mL)
    Infusion rate (per minute): Increase until contractions cease
      Initial: 0.3 mL (100 μg)
      10 min: 0.5 mL (150 μg)
      20 min: 0.7 mL (200 μg)
      30 min: 0.9 mL (250 μg)
      40 min: 1.0 mL (300 μg)
      50 min: 1.2 mL (350 μg)
    Do not exceed 350 μg/min
Maintain maternal: Pulse < 130/min
                  Systolic blood pressure > 90 mm Hg
Obtain K^+, glucose in 4 hr
Continue infusion for 12 hr after contractions cease
Maintenance schedule (after 12 hr without contractions)
    10 mg ritodrine orally
    Discontinue intravenous infusion 30 min later
    10 mg ritodrine orally every 2 hr for 24 hr
    20 mg ritodrine orally every 4 to 6 hr until delivery

is approved for this use. Table 26–10 shows one method of administration of this medication. Terbutaline is equally effective but requires a different regimen and is not marketed for this indication. $MgSO_4$ has become popular and, if used, must be given intravenously with all precautions as listed in the section on HELLP Syndrome.

Intrauterine Growth Retardation

The astute physician can detect evidence of poor growth of the fetus in utero. In these situations, ultrasound should be obtained to document fetal size. A weight below the 10th percentile of expected weights for the population suggests intrauterine growth retardation. The estimate of weight requires measurement of the biparietal diameter, head and abdominal circumference, and femur length at a minimum. The measurements must be obtained in exactly the correct plane to be meaningful. Only a trained ultrasonographer can assess intrauterine fetal weight accurately. However, with experience, the estimate is accurate to within a few grams.

If the fetus is not growing as expected, the cause may be intrinsic maternal or fetal disease or other extenuating circumstances such as smoking, alcoholism, malnutrition, or infection. In all cases, the fetus is considered at high risk and must be monitored closely for evidence of maladaptation to stress. Nonstress testing is indicated.

Fetal Demise

Although fetal demise before viability (spontaneous abortion) is very common, losses in the late second and third trimesters are relatively rare. Appropriate management of coexistent medical diseases has decreased fetal death resulting from these complications greatly. Therefore, as part of the risk assessment at the first and subsequent prenatal visits, preexisting medical illnesses should be reviewed carefully to determine increased fetal risk.

A profound change has occurred in the frequency of intrapartum deaths during the past few years. Intrapartum deaths should rarely, if ever, occur except in some cases of congenital anomalies that are incompatible with life. Electronic fetal monitoring has shown that deaths during labor and delivery do not occur suddenly. The fetus will exhibit evidence of its compromised state for many hours (even days) before death. In all cases of high-risk pregnancy, electronic fetal monitoring during labor is required.

LABOR AND DELIVERY

Uterine contractions and a changing cervix commonly are used as indicators of the onset of labor. The starting dilation and effacement of the cervix will vary, because many multiparous women will be a few centimeters dilated during the third trimester. It is not uncommon for women, particularly multiparous women, to experience Braxton-Hicks contractions prior to the onset of actual labor. These contractions are characterized by having no observable effect on the cervix. In general, the contractions of true labor are characterized by (1) regular occurrence, (2) gradual shortening intervals between them, and (3) an increasing discomfort located usually in the back and abdomen. Generally the contractions of "false" labor differ in that (1) they occur at irregular intervals, (2) the intervals remain long, and (3) the intensity of the discomfort remains the same and is usually located in the lower abdomen.

Classically, labor has been divided into three stages: the first stage starts with the onset of labor and lasts until the cervix has become completely dilated. The second stage of labor extends from the time of complete cervical dilation until the delivery of the infant. The third stage is the time from the delivery of the infant to the delivery of the placenta.

First- and Second-Stage Labor

The early or latent phase of labor is quite variable in duration and usually lasts until about 4 cm in dilation. Simultaneous effacement of the cervix occurs in this phase as well. In the primigravid patient, the latent phase may be long and is best tolerated in the familiar atmosphere of the patient's home rather than in the hospital. Most nulliparas have latent phases less than 20 hours in duration. Most multiparas rarely exceed a latent phase of 14 hours.

Prolongation of the latent phase is a common problem that the family physician may face. If sedation or anesthesia is given too early, it can cause this labor dysfunction. For some, the prolonged latent phase may be accompanied by an inability to sleep, and the woman may become exhausted even before the active phase of labor has begun. In this instance, rest is beneficial. The use of morphine sulfate, 15 mg given subcutaneously, often diminishes contractions and allows the patient to sleep. Most patients treated this way will progress to the active phase within 6 to 10 hours. For women who are experiencing early labor at home, signs and symptoms that should alert the patient to go to the hospital immediately are significant bleeding or an unusual degree of pain. Also, if a patient believes

there has been rupture of membranes, she should be checked at the hospital in a timely fashion.

The active phase of labor is more rapid, although there remains considerable physiologic variability. The average cervical change is 1.2 cm/hr in the primiparous and 1.5 cm/hr in the multiparous woman. The Friedman curve (Fig. 26–6) describes the average labor. However, strict adherence to these parameters need not occur, and the woman may still experience a normal labor. Several disorders of protracted active phase length and protracted fetal descent may occur. Reasons for these are varied, including malposition (such as persistent occiput posterior), excess sedation, anesthesia, and cephalopelvic disproportion. True arrest of labor is defined as no cervical change in 2 hours during the active phase.

In the first stage of labor, women should have their blood pressure, the fetal heart rate, and the frequency and duration of contractions measured and recorded every 15 to 30 minutes. The fetal heart rate should be auscultated after a contraction at least every 30 minutes during the first stage. This can be accomplished easily with a fetoscope, with Doppler ultrasound, or electronically (see Fetal Monitoring). Continuous fetal monitoring is less optimal because it forces the woman to be in a supine position and limits her freedom of move-

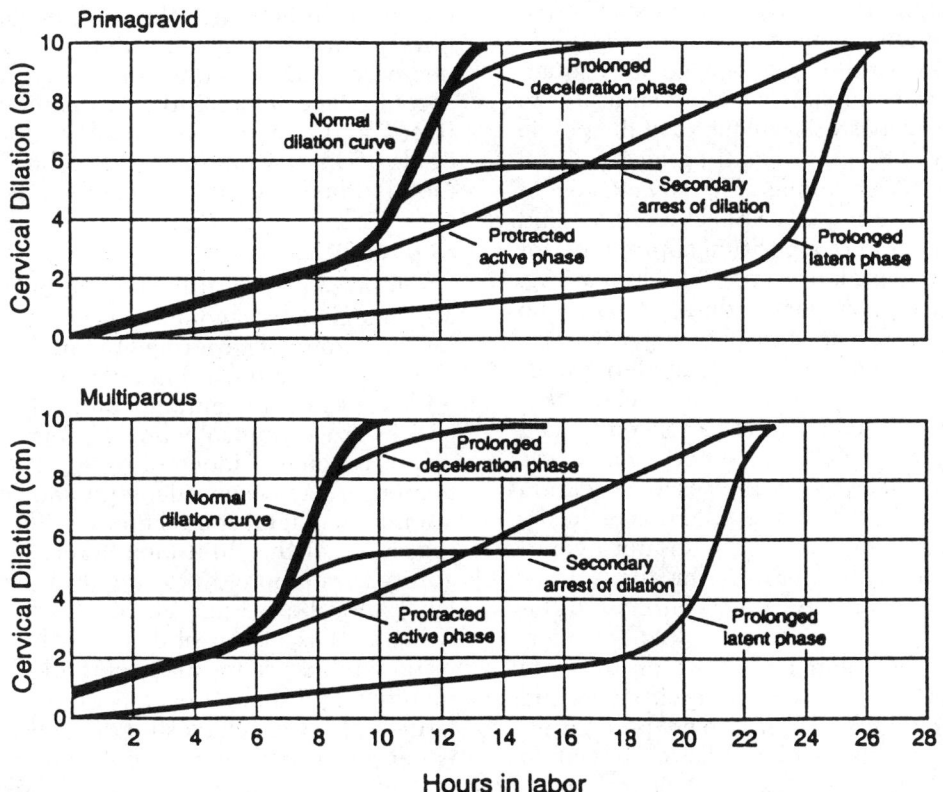

FIGURE 26–6. Composite curves of abnormal labor progress. (From Scherger J, Levitt C, Acheson L: Teaching family-centered perinatal care in family medicine, Part 2. Fam Med 24:369, 1992, with permission.)

ment. Furthermore, there have been no proven benefits to the use of continuous electronic fetal monitoring in the low-risk patient, and it has been associated with increased medical intervention, including cesarean section. Specific indications for the use of electronic fetal monitoring include oxytocin induction or augmentation of labor, abnormal fetal heart rate by auscultation, multiple gestation, hypertension or pre-eclampsia, dysfunctional labor, meconium staining, diabetes, or prematurity.

Support of the Laboring Woman

Oral fluids should be given to women in labor unless there is a demonstrated need for intravenous fluids, such as vomiting or dehydration. Support and observation are key to managing a normal labor. A woman should be free to choose a variety of positions while laboring, and to ambulate if she so desires. Without interference, most women will change positions frequently in labor. Some studies support the claim that women who are upright during labor report less pain. Certainly in the vertical position there is greater pressure on the cervix, which may account for the more rapid labors in women who are not routinely placed in the dorsal position. A fatigued woman may rest on her side.

In the second stage of labor, women should be encouraged to use their instincts about pushing, and often will do more effective pushing when they are sitting, squatting, or kneeling. The lithotomy position is the least physiologic for effective pushing. An upright semisitting position actually may work to shorten the second stage. The squatting position has been shown radiographically to enhance the anteroposterior diameter of the pelvic outlet by 0.5 to 2.0 cm. Semisitting also may be useful because it combines the advantages of squatting, with its efficient expulsive efforts, and the increased comfort of a position appropriate for women not used to prolonged periods of squatting.

The role of a support person during labor, who is present continually, appears to have positive effects on birth outcome. Studies in a modern inner-city U.S. hospital and in Guatemala revealed that the presence of a "duola", an experienced female labor support person who need not be a nurse, was associated with a decrease in the cesarean section rate, a lessening of the use of epidural anesthesia, a decreased use of pitocin, and a shorter overall duration of labor. The reasons for these findings—the mechanisms by which support influences labor and delivery—are not totally understood. While duolas and male partners provide similar roles for laboring women, their styles and means of offering support appear to be quite different. Duolas physically touch the laboring women more than four times as frequently as do male partners. In addition, male partners tend to spend less time with the laboring woman.

Labor support is centuries old, but its advantages have now been validated in three controlled studied and its positive benefits should not be overlooked in the trend towards more and increasingly complex technology. For those who provide care for mothers during labor, the challenge is to turn to obstetric technology only when necessary, relying instead on the practice of continuous labor support to help the birth process follow its natural normal course. (Kennell et al., 1991, p. 2201)

Pain Control

Not all women will want to tolerate the pain of labor by natural means. However, all nonpharmacologic methods should be employed, including continuous support, position change, rest, physical contact, breathing techniques, a warm shower, or use of locally applied heat. A prepared patient will be better able to tolerate the pain. Prenatal courses and physician-initiated conversations about the pain of labor and the side effects of analgesia should occur prior to the onset of labor. The physician must know what the patient wants and be comfortable with her changing her mind based on the course of labor. A short-acting narcotic may be quite effective in helping the woman through an intensely painful period without altering the course of labor.

Epidural anesthesia is the method of choice in many large perinatal centers (see Obstetric Anesthesia and Analgesia, later in this chapter). Documented side effects from this medication include prolongation of the first stage of labor, decreased uterine contractions, relaxation of the pelvic diaphragm predisposing to minor malpresentations, decreased maternal urge and ability to push in the second stage, increased instrumental vaginal delivery, and increased cesarean section rate (Thorp et al., 1990). Its routine use in labor is not recommended because of these common complications.

Amniotomy

Amniotomy, or artificial rupture of membranes, appears in many randomized trials to shorten labor by 1 to 2 hours if performed before 6 cm of dilation. Certainly the issue of infection is more paramount with ruptured membranes and repeated cervical checks in a woman who is progressing slowly. There is some evidence to suggest increased formation of caput succedaneum and increased disalignment of fetal cranial bones without the buffering effect of the fluid membranes. However, the ability of amniotomy to speed up a slow-moving labor may be a huge advantage to the laboring woman. It is also useful to check for meconium or to gain access for placement of electronic fetal monitoring if there are signs of fetal distress. One large-scale study suggested that, when amniotomy is not performed, 66 per cent of women will have unruptured membranes at the end of the first stage of labor and 12 per cent would remain unruptured at delivery.

Amnioinfusion

Increased, prolonged, and severe variable decelerations sometimes are noted following rupture of membranes or in fetuses with oligohydramnios. It is believed that these variable decelerations are often the result of cord compression during contractions. Recently, the technique of amnioinfusion has been developed to "refloat" the cord. In some cases the procedure results in rapid cessation of the variable decelerations and allows for vaginal delivery when cesarean section otherwise would have been necessary.

In order to perform amnioinfusion, an intrauterine pressure catheter with an infusion port should be utilized. It is important for the fetal head to be applied well to the cervix because the infused fluid will merely leak out if the fetal vertex does not tamponade the cervix. A bolus of 500 mL of sterile, room-temperature normal saline is infused into the uterus over 15 to 30 minutes and the fetal heart pattern observed. If the severe variable decelerations are helped or disappear, the infusion may continue at a rate that continues to show resolution of decelerations, usually 20 to 100 mL/hr. Ultrasonography is useful to prevent overdistention of the uterus.

Third-Stage Labor: Delivery of Infant and Placenta

Ideally, low-risk women should be able to labor and deliver in the same physical space. All delivery rooms must be equipped properly to manage the neonate during the first few minutes of life. The room should be large enough to include an area where the neonate can be examined. All delivery rooms must have facilities available for infant suction and intubation. Additionally, a radiant warmer should be available or the ambient temperature in the delivery room maintained at 80° F (26.7° C).

The delivery of the infant should occur in whatever position the woman finds most comfortable, so long as the physician still has access to the head as the baby emerges. The four basic positions commonly used are lithotomy, lateral, semisitting or squatting, and dorsal (modified lithotomy). The lithotomy position provides easier access to the perineum, allows easier monitoring of the fetal heart, and allows for a more comfortable position for the person delivering the baby. The lateral Simms position (Figs. 26–7 through 26–10), with the patient lying on her left side, the dependent leg flexed, and the superior leg elevated with pushing, is more physiologic. The perineum is also in full view and easily accessible.

As the infant's head begins to distend the perineum, the patient experiences intense pain and often burning from the stretching of the perineum. In a primiparous woman, this aspect of labor may take 20 to 30 minutes. Often a warm cloth applied to the perineum between contractions is soothing.

Some physicians use lubricating oils to massage the distending perineum. The efficacy of these maneuvers has not been studied well. Patience and support are key issues if one wishes to avoid an episiotomy. An episiotomy should not be performed routinely, unless it is obvious that a perineal laceration will occur. In those instances, a clean surgical incision is preferable to a jagged tear. There is no evidence to support the concept that episiotomy before distention will result in a more stable perineum in later years or that episiotomy prevents third- and fourth-degree perineal lacerations.

The infant's head should not be allowed to "pop" over the perineal body. The head is best delivered slowly and in a controlled fashion. Sometimes it is beneficial to have the woman push between contractions. Immediately on delivery of the head, the physician should run a hand over the fetal head to the area of the neck and shoulders to determine whether the umbilical cord is around the neck. If it is, it usually can be slipped easily over the head. If this cannot be accomplished, the cord should be double-clamped, cut, and unwrapped from the fetal head. The oral pharynx should be suctioned with a bulb syringe with the physician's finger placed in the baby's mouth. If there is meconium, DeLee suction through both the oral pharynx and the nasopharynx is done with the head on the perineum. The goal is to avoid aspiration of amniotic fluid. The physician need not rush to deliver the shoulders unless there are signs of fetal distress. If necessary, the shoulders should be rotated gently to the anteroposterior or oblique position and with very gentle traction on the head. After delivering the first shoulder, the posterior shoulder usually delivers easily.

On completion of the delivery, the infant's head should remain dependent to allow for drainage and further suctioning. The baby should be placed on the mother's chest immediately unless further resuscitation is needed. The cord should be clamped electively and cut at a comfortable moment for the bonding mother. There appears to be no advantage to early or delayed cutting of the cord; however, the cord should not be "stripped" of blood because transfusion of the infant may occur. The father or other support person may be asked to cut the cord once double-clamping is accomplished.

If amniotic fluid is contaminated with meconium, the delivery must proceed slightly differently. Immediately on delivery of the infant, the head should be kept down, the cord clamped, and the infant placed immediately in the warmer. The infant should be intubated and suctioned. If meconium is at or below the cords, intubation is performed repeatedly until suctioning returns only clear fluid. Once the laryngoscope has been placed, if no meconium is seen in the pharynx, the procedure can be terminated.

Infant assessment should be accomplished at 1 and 5 minutes, and an Apgar score assigned. The

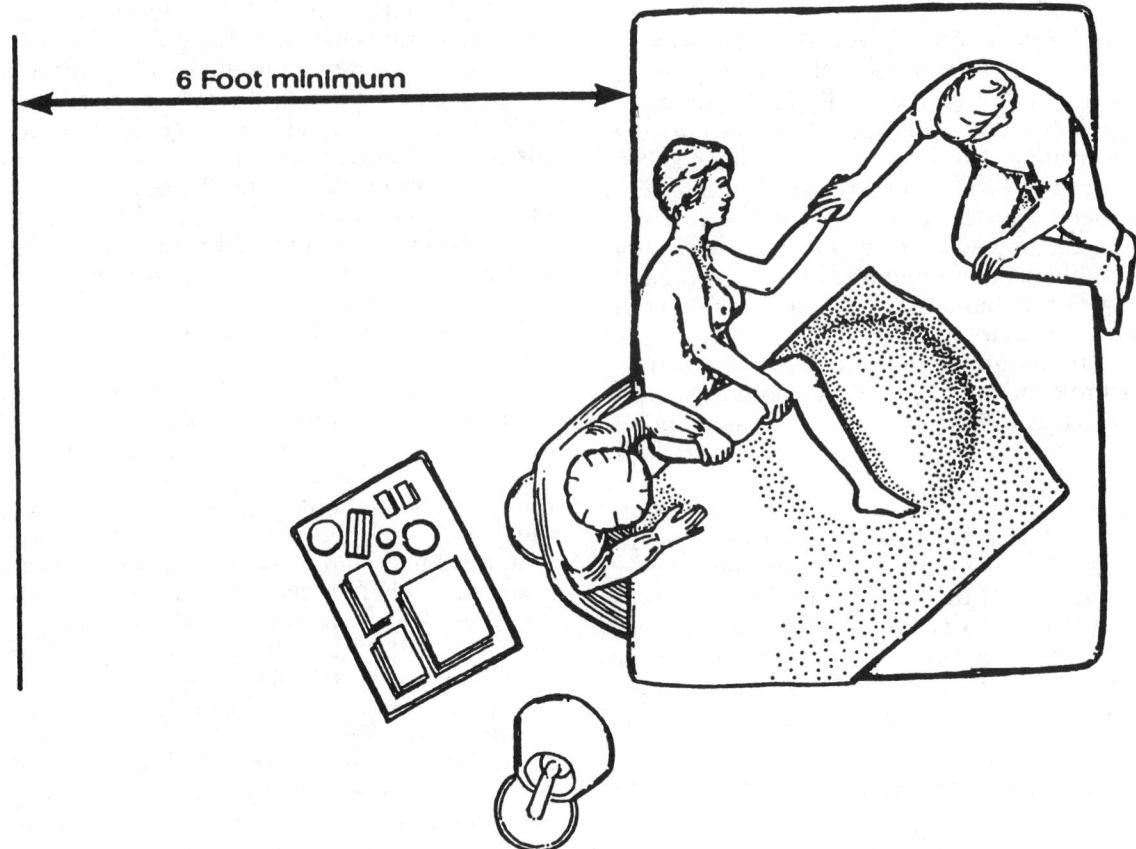

FIGURE 26–7. Positioning of equipment and patient prior to lateral Sims' delivery. (From Kirkwood C, Clark L: Lateral Sims' deliveries: A new application for an old technique. J Fam Pract 17:703, 1983. Reprinted by permission of Appleton & Lange.)

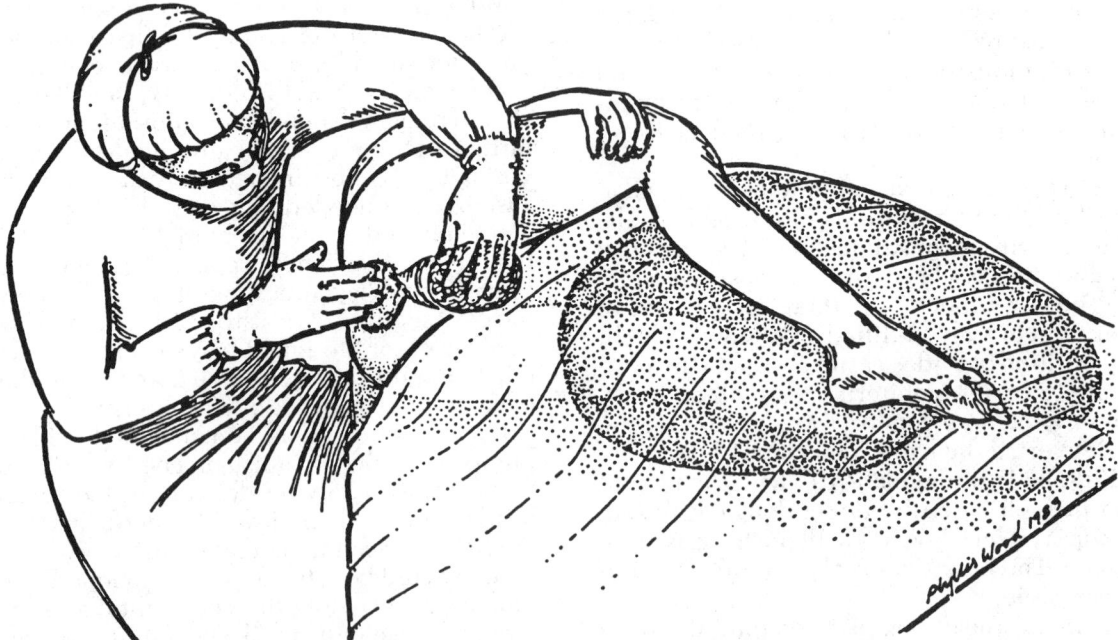

FIGURE 26–8. Management of crowning. Obstetrician sits with left side at patient's sacrum, using the left hand to control the disease of the fetal head, leaving the right hand free for assisting the delivery of the chin and suctioning. (From Kirkwood C, Clark L: Lateral Sims' deliveries: A new application for an old technique. J Fam Pract 17:704, 1983. Reprinted with permission of Appleton & Lange.)

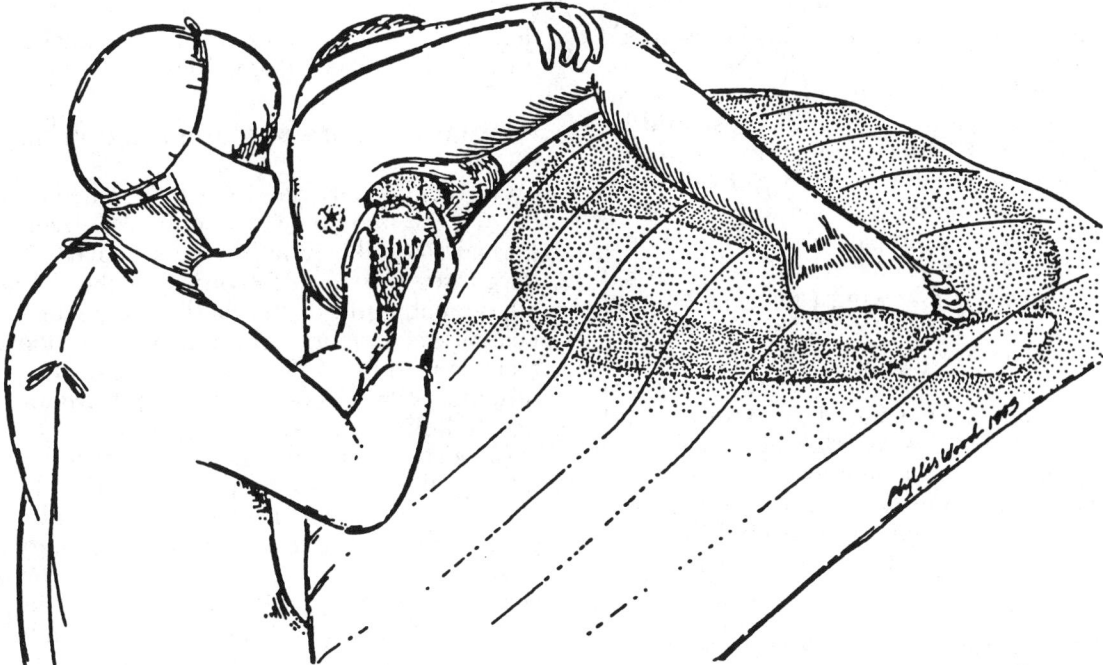

FIGURE 26–9.   Delivery of the shoulders and aftercoming parts. The physician has turned 180 degrees and faces the perineum. (From Kirkwood C, Clark L: Lateral Sims' deliveries: A new application for an old technique. J Fam Pract 17:704, 1983. Reprinted with permission of Appleton & Lange.)

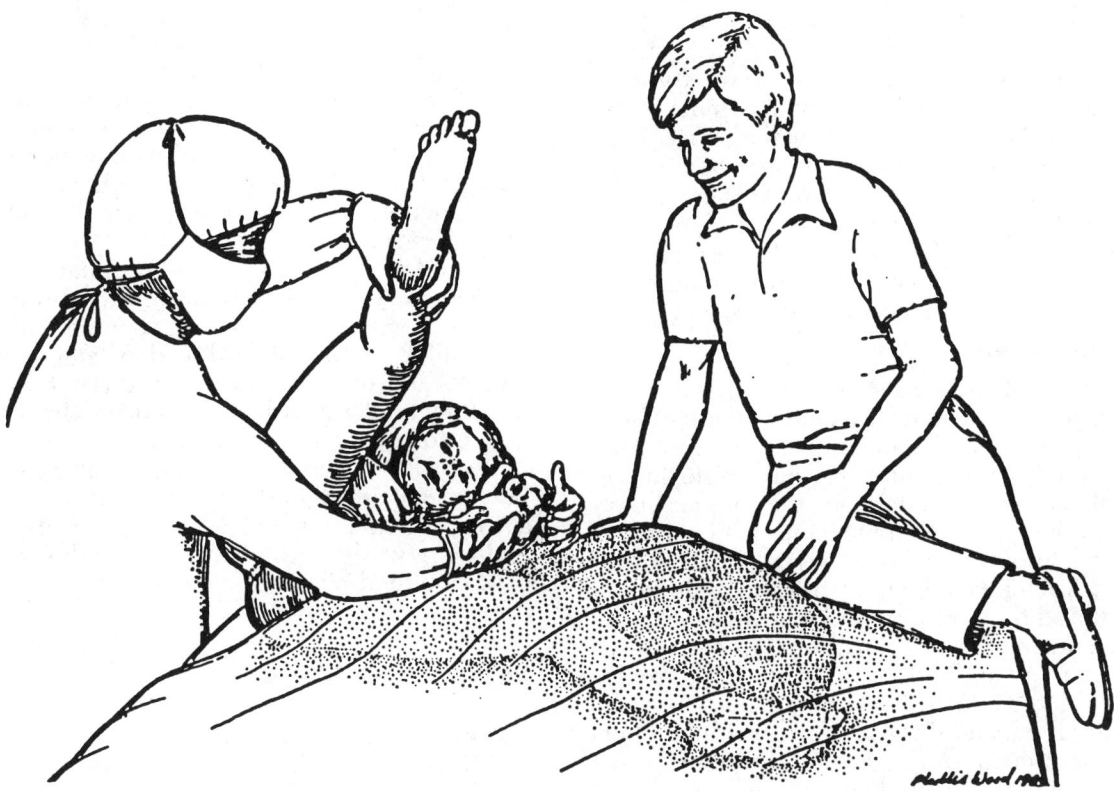

FIGURE 26–10.   Delivery completed. The baby may be placed directly on the mother's chest before the cord is cut by handing it between the mother's legs. (From Kirkwood C, Clark L: Lateral Sims' deliveries: A new application for an old technique. J Fam Pract 17:705, 1983. Reprinted with permission of Appleton & Lange.)

delivering physician should not assign the Apgar score. The infant should remain in the mother's arms if possible.

The third stage of labor usually can be accomplished easily. A sample of cord blood should be obtained and sent for blood type of the newborn. A cord pH may be helpful if there was fetal stress. This stage of labor routinely can last up to 30 minutes, and patience on the part of the physician is required. Gentle traction on the cord may facilitate separation, and often, following a gush of bleeding, the placenta may be removed easily from the uterus and vagina. Strong traction should never be placed on the cord because the cord could rupture or, more ominously, inversion of the uterus could occur. If, after 30 minutes, the placenta has not separated, manual removal should be considered. After either spontaneous or manual removal of the placenta, the organ should be inspected carefully to ensure that removal is complete.

Vacuum Extraction

The vacuum extractor may be used to aid in the delivery of an infant if maternal exhaustion or anesthesia has resulted in the patient's inability to complete the delivery spontaneously. Several different devices are currently available. All utilize a soft suction cup; a metal or nonmalleable hard rubber cup should not be used. Careful placement is of prime importance. The cup should never be placed over the anterior fontanelle. In most cases application should be restricted to (1) a fetus at at least +2 station, (2) fetal vertex in an anterior position, and (3) estimated fetal weight less than 4000 grams.

The vacuum extractor has become popular in the United States primarily because of the widely held belief that it is safer than forceps. However, it is not clear, when cases are matched for fetal size, station, and position, that this is true. Indeed, fetal damage can occur from misuse of the vacuum extractor. Cephalohematoma and scalp laceration are but two of the observed complications.

Forceps Delivery

Forceps also may be used as an aid in delivery of the fetus in a patient who is exhausted or in whom anesthesia prevents spontaneous delivery. Although forceps procedures are quite safe in the hands of experienced operators, they are also dangerous in the hands of an inexperienced operator. In general, forceps use should be restricted to those physicians who have been instructed in the technique during their training and who have been supervised during their use on numerous occasions.

If forceps are applied to a fetus at +2 or greater station with the fetal head aligned in an anteroposterior direction, and if the forceps are applied correctly, the procedure is safe and efficacious. Forceps should never be applied if there is any doubt concerning the position of the fetal head. Likewise, forceps delivery should not be attempted if there is any question of fetal macrosomia, because

shoulder dystocia may occur. Forceps delivery may be life saving in cases of acute fetal compromise in the second stage of labor.

Postpartum Care of Mother and Infant

Oxytocic agents need not be used routinely in the nursing mother with a normal delivery and a normal-size baby. A multiparous woman with more than three previous deliveries, or the delivery of a large baby, places the mother at greater risk for postpartum hemorrhage, and the addition of pitocin is warranted. Ten or 20 units can be given intramuscularly or added to the intravenous solution to help the contracting uterus.

Inspection of the vagina and cervix follows. Optimally all 360 degrees of the cervix should be visualized. The anterior lip may need to be grasped gently with a ring forceps to coax the cervix into view. If lacerations are present, they should be sewn immediately with sutures placed in a running lock fashion. Generally it is a difficult procedure to perform without assistance.

After inspection, the cervix is pushed high using sponges and the upper vault is inspected for tears. The lateral fornical area and periurethral and perineal areas are inspected carefully. Periurethral abrasions are common and need not be repaired unless heavy bleeding occurs.

Mother and baby should be watched carefully over the next several hours, preferably together. The fundus must be checked regularly. If the fundus is rising in the abdomen, this is a reliable indication of relaxation and accumulation of blood clots. The uterus then must be massaged vigorously and frequently and all clots expelled. The patient can be taught to help with the massage. The blood pressure must be watched closely during recovery.

The infant is given vitamin K intramuscularly in the delivery room. Erythromycin ointment is placed in each eye to prevent conjunctivitis. Both these interventions should be done at the bonding mother and child's convenience. It is not necessary that they be done within moments of the delivery.

The length of a normal postpartum stay is now 24 hours. The woman should be encouraged to ambulate soon after her delivery and to begin normal activities in the hospital. Classes on newborn care, including washing the baby, care of the umbilical cord, and feeding of the baby, should occur in this time frame.

FETAL MONITORING

Although only occasionally indicated (see Labor and Delivery), when the decision has been made to employ electronic fetal monitoring, the procedure should be discussed with the patient. If the patient is aware of the way in which the sensors pick up the fetal heart rate and contractions, she often can

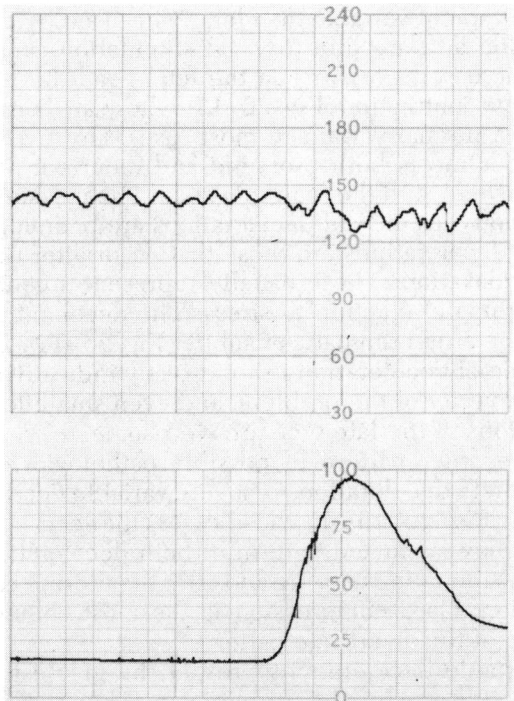

FIGURE 26–11. Normal fetal heart rate with normal beat-to-beat variability and a normal baseline (top line). The bottom line shows a normal uterine contraction. (From Hill LM: Diagnosis and management of fetal distress. Mayo Clin Proc 54:784, 1979, with permission.)

help in the maintenance of a quality signal. For those patients in whom it is sufficient to know the pattern of the fetal heart rate and only the occurrence of uterine contractions, external electronic fetal monitoring is sufficient. However, external monitoring gives no information concerning the strength of contractions. This can be obtained only by means of an intrauterine pressure monitor. It has been our experience that, when electronic fetal monitoring is employed, external monitoring usually is sufficient. However, if worrisome patterns become evident, if it is essential to know the intrauterine pressure, or if there is great difficulty in establishing an adequate external signal, internal electronic fetal monitoring is employed.

A number of factors of the fetal heart beat are followed: the rate, the variability of the rate, and changes in the rate in relation to uterine contractions (Hill, 1979). In general, the fetal heart rate during active labor should be between 110 and 150 beats/min. In a normal, uncompromised fetus, this rate will vary. In fact, lack of beat-to-beat variability of 10 to 15/min is suggestive of fetal compromise. However, many drugs—such as medications commonly used for analgesia—and fetal sleep may cause a temporary flattening of the normal variability. In the case of medication, this appears to be a direct effect of the maternal medication on the fetus through transplacental passage of the drug(s). Figure 26–11 demonstrates normal fetal heart rate variability, and Figure 26–12 shows an example of decreased variability.

FIGURE 26–12. Decreased variability and normal baseline. This may be due to distress, medications, or fetal sleep. (From Hill LM: Diagnosis and management of fetal distress. Mayo Clin Proc 54:784, 1979, with permission.)

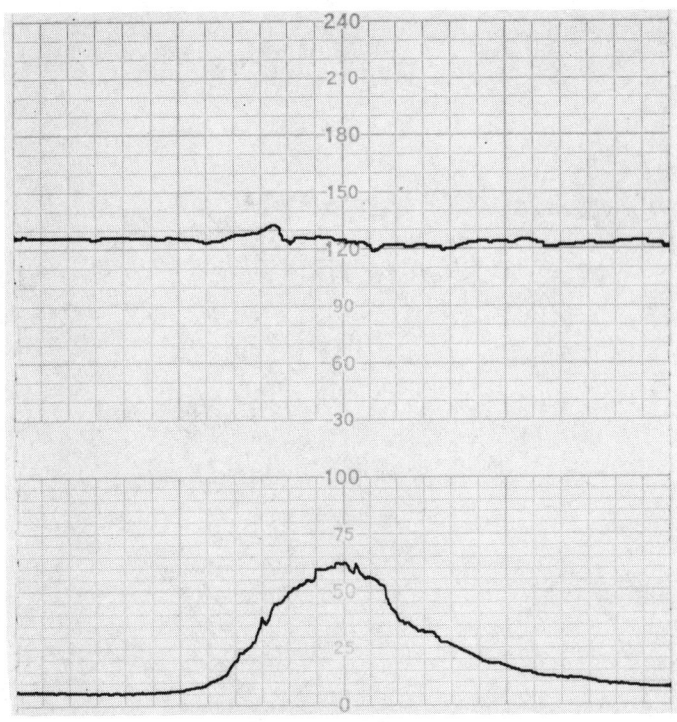

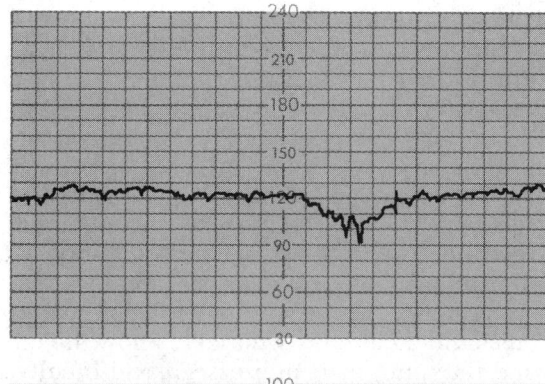

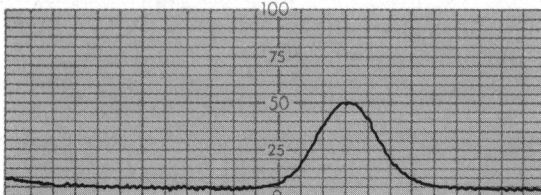

FIGURE 26–13. Normal baseline and variable deceleration with decreased variability. (From Hill LM: Diagnosis and management of fetal distress. Mayo Clin Proc 54:784, 1979, with permission.)

The pattern of the fetal heart rate during and after uterine contractions gives the observer considerable information concerning the status of the fetus. Two patterns are considered normal. In many pregnancies, the fetal heart rate varies little during and just after uterine contractions. In others, a deceleration of the rate is noted that is coincident with the onset of the contraction and ceases at the time of relaxation of the uterus. These dips

are a type of variable deceleration caused by contraction and are due to vagal stimulation caused by increased pressure on the fetal head during a uterine contraction (Fig. 26–13). These are considered a normal variant in most cases. However, if the decline is both profound and recurrent, it is worrisome, and the scalp pH should be measured.

Two types of fetal decelerations are pathologic. Late decelerations are those that occur after uterine relaxation. These usually represent a central (neurologic) reaction to stress. The decelerations may be either dramatic or subtle (Fig. 26–14). The degree of deceleration is not directly indicative of the severity of the problem, and even small decelerations of the late type are worrisome.

The other pattern of possible pathologic fetal heart rate decelerations is severe variable deceleration (Fig. 26–15). In these cases, the fetal heart rate shows a mixed pattern of both decelerations and accelerations during and after the uterine contraction. Cord compression is the most common cause of this heart rate pattern.

Variable decelerations present the greatest interpretive problem for the clinician. When variable decelerations are present, fetal scalp pH can be a most useful adjunctive means of determining the true status of the fetus. The use of this test involves obtaining a small sample of blood from the fetal scalp in a heparinized capillary tube and determining the pH using a pH meter adapted for microvolumes. The technique of obtaining the sample is relatively simple. A scalp pH of between 7.25 and 7.45 is a reliable indication of fetal well-being. The clinician can be reassured that the variable dece-

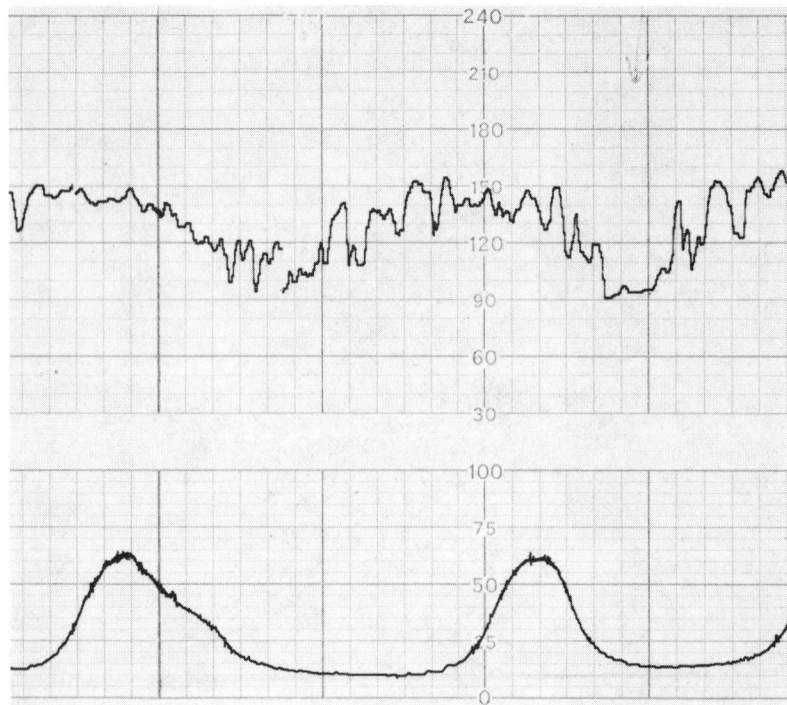

FIGURE 26–14. Internal monitor tracing showing persistent, severe late decelerations. (From Hill LM: Diagnosis and management of fetal distress. Mayo Clin Proc 54:784, 1979, with permission.)

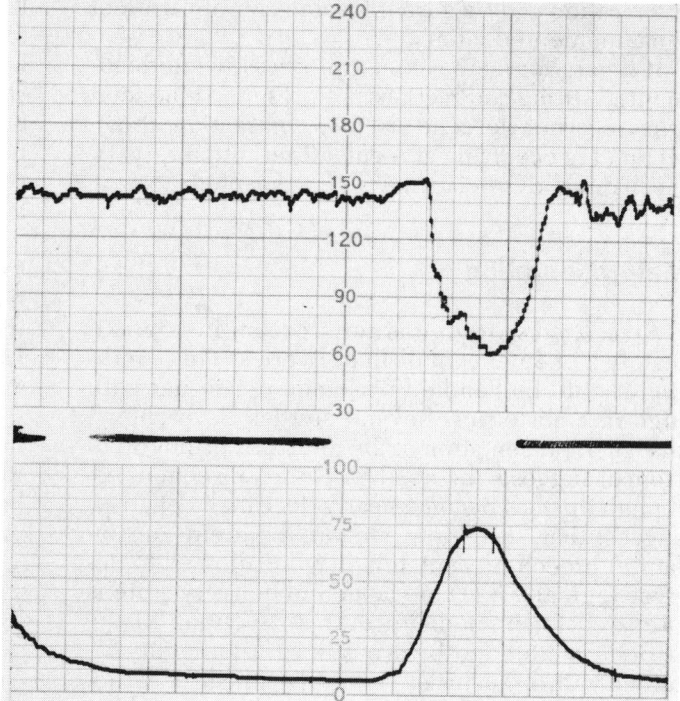

FIGURE 26–15. Decreased variability, normal baseline, and variable deceleration. Note the slight acceleration at the start of the contraction. (From Hill LM: Diagnosis and management of fetal distress. Mayo Clin Proc 54:784, 1979, with permission.)

lerations that are seen *at that time* have not caused fetal compromise. However, if the pattern continues, repeated scalp samples are advised.

If the scalp pH is 7.25 or less, another sample should be obtained to guard against laboratory error. If the second sample is also low or borderline, steps must be taken to either correct the acidosis or deliver the fetus. At times, the use of oxygen by mask and changing the position of the woman resolves both the deceleration pattern and the acidosis. Once an abnormal pH sample is obtained, a repeat sample is indicated within a few minutes. In fact, it is always advisable to take a repeat sample if the pH is indicative of abnormality.

The status of the fetus cannot be determined on the basis of an isolated observation of a deceleration or of a single scalp sample alone. Interpretation of the findings must be individualized based on the risk status, the progress of labor, the use of analgesic drugs, and other known extrinsic factors. The decision to intervene should be made only after these factors have been considered carefully.

Electronic fetal monitoring should not be utilized unless the personnel observing the patterns are thoroughly familiar with their interpretation. Without these interpretive skills, a large number of inappropriate cesarean sections and difficult deliveries will occur. Companies that market the technical equipment for electronic fetal monitoring often provide detailed educational services for the paramedical and medical personnel who use the equipment.

COMPLICATIONS OF LABOR AND DELIVERY

Prolonged or Arrested Labor

When labor is not progressing as expected, very frequently the cause is uterine inertia. Even an experienced examiner may have difficulty in being certain that contractions are of sufficient length and duration to effect a normal labor. Whenever labor is prolonged, an intrauterine pressure monitor should be placed. If the intrauterine pressure is not at least 50 mm Hg, the contractions will not have the desired effect. In this case, oxytocin given intravenously may help to augment labor.

In labor, oxytocin should be given only through an infusion pump. Many accidents occur when oxytocin is given intravenously without such a device. Initially, the oxytocin infusion should be prepared at a concentration of 10 units in 1 liter of solution and started at an infusion rate of approximately 1 milliunit/min. The patient is observed very carefully, and the rate of infusion is increased 1 to 2 milliunits/min every 15 to 20 minutes until effective contractions occur. It is rarely necessary to go above 30 milliunits/min to effect adequate contractions. In fact, if adequate contractions are not achieved at this infusion rate, other causes for the uterine inertia should be considered. If it appears that oxytocin at this infusion rate will be needed over a long time, the concentration should be increased to 20 or even 30 units/liter in order that smaller volumes of fluid will be given. Water intoxication can be a troublesome complication of long-augmented labors.

It is rare for a labor to not progress when documented strong contractions are present. If the fetal part does not descend despite contraction above 50 mm Hg occurring at regular 3-minute intervals, mechanical dystocia should be suspected.

Malpresentation

Breech presentation at term occurs in approximately 2 or 3 per cent of all deliveries. This condition should be handled by someone familiar with high-risk obstetrics. Several studies have shown that such presentation of the fetus in a primigravid woman suggests the need for cesarean section. Although this has become nearly doctrinal, data now suggest that, in some primigravid patients, an infant in breech presentation may be allowed to deliver vaginally if (1) the labor and delivery suite is prepared for immediate cesarean section, (2) the patient is attended by a physician thoroughly familiar with breech delivery, (3) clinical or radiographic pelvimetry has shown an adequate pelvis, (4) the fetal head is flexed, (5) the fetus is estimated to weigh at least 2500 grams and less than 4000 grams, and (6) neonatal care is immediately available (Collea, 1980; Collea et al., 1978).

However, breech presentation during labor is becoming a rare event. External fetal version at 37 weeks' gestation has become the norm when breech presentation is present in late pregnancy. Version can be accomplished safely in a delivery suite that is equipped with ultrasonography, electronic fetal monitoring, and facilities for the performance of immediate cesarean section if necessary. After a period of 15 to 20 minutes of external fetal monitoring to assess fetal stability, low doses of intravenous tocolytic agents are administered to completely relax the uterus. External version then often can be accomplished with ease. This usually requires two individuals to manipulate the fetus. Following version, the position of the fetus should be documented by ultrasonography, the tocolytic infusion stopped, and reassessment of fetal well-being using electronic fetal monitoring reinstituted. If the fetus shows signs of stress, the tocolytic agent should be started again and the fetus returned to breech presentation. This problem occurs rarely. If fetal heart rate deceleration persists, immediate cesarean section is indicated. Although this procedure is quite safe, it should be undertaken only by someone thoroughly familiar with the procedure and its risks.

The most frequent malpresentation is *transverse or posterior arrest of the fetal head* in the mid-pelvic region. A transverse position of the fetal head is normal as the infant is transversing the mid-pelvis, and should be considered abnormal only if it persists after complete dilation and descent of the head below the spines. In many patients, a transverse or posterior position may be corrected by manual rotation. If the woman is multiparous, she then may be allowed to push and usually will deliver rapidly. If she is primiparous, it is often necessary to hold the infant's head in the anterior position for some time while the patient continues to push the infant to the pelvic floor.

If the fetus is in good condition (as determined by electronic fetal monitoring), transverse positions may be watched without intervention. Continued pushing may effect rotation and delivery. Infants in the posterior position usually will persist and may deliver spontaneously.

Mid-forceps rotations were performed commonly in the past to correct transverse and posterior fetal positions. It is now clear that harm can be done through the inappropriate use of these instruments.

Cephalopelvic Disproportion

In this condition, the relationship between the size of the maternal pelvis and the infant's head size is the important factor. A large infant may pass easily through a very large pelvis, but a small pelvis can cause difficulties with the progression of labor of a normal fetal head. If cephalopelvic disproportion is present, as demonstrated by lack of fetal descent despite documented adequate contractions, a cesarean section should be performed.

Toxemia

Although discussed in some detail earlier in this chapter, it is well to reconsider the possibility of toxemia occurring for the first time during and immediately after parturition. Severe pre-eclampsia is an indication for delivery. If the labor is progressing well, hyperreflexia should be controlled with the use of $MgSO_4$ and severe hypertension should be controlled with the use of hydralazine or other appropriate antihypertensive drugs.

Fetal Stress

The use of the electronic fetal monitor and fetal scalp pH to evaluate fetal stress has been discussed. The delivering physician should consider the status of the fetus throughout labor and during delivery. It is unfortunate that many physicians who monitor women during labor remove the monitor when the patient is taken to the delivery room. Particularly in primigravid women, this period may exceed 1 hour, and fetal stress may occur without being detected.

Intrapartum and Postpartum Hemorrhage

Intrapartum hemorrhage is usually due to abruptio placentae. Should this occur, the status of the fetus must be monitored and the woman must be delivered as soon as possible.

Postpartum hemorrhage can be a life-threatening complication of delivery. When it occurs on the delivery table, it usually responds to vigorous uterine massage and the intravenous use of oxytocic agents. It is perhaps even more dangerous when it occurs after the woman has left the delivery room. In many hospitals, close observation of a normal patient does not occur. A woman may collect several units of blood in the uterus and vagina without feeling uncomfortable. Consequently, the fundus should be checked frequently.

If postpartum hemorrhage occurs during the first 4 to 6 hours, the most common cause is uterine relaxation. This condition should respond quickly to massage and oxytocic agents. If it does not, the possibility should be considered that a portion of the placenta has remained inside the uterus or that a previously unrecognized vaginal or cervical tear is present. The patient should be returned to the operating room and should be re-examined. Postpartum curettage should be avoided if possible because it can cause uterine perforation and scarring.

Uterine rupture is a rare cause of postpartum hemorrhage. Such rupture should be considered if a forceps delivery has been performed or if the woman has had a previous cesarean section.

Late postpartum hemorrhage also may occur. If it has been more than 24 hours since delivery, the most common cause is infection, and endometritis should be suspected. A retained placenta is second in frequency, and, in this situation, curettage should be considered.

SURGICAL OBSTETRICS

Episiotomy

Episiotomy is performed commonly during vaginal delivery; it should not be performed routinely but should be reserved for specific indications (Belizan, 1993). If it is clear that a sizeable tear will occur unless episiotomy is performed, a surgical incision seems preferable. However, the indications and consequences have not been studied in great detail (Sultan et al., 1993).

Episiotomy repair has been standardized throughout most of the United States (Fig. 26–16). Absorbable suture material should be used. Repair begins at the apex of the vaginal portion of the incision. The suture should be placed approximately 1 cm above the apex and tied. The vagina then is closed using a running-lock suture. Tension should be maintained on the suture throughout this portion of the repair or bleeding from the epithelial edge may occur. The operator always should be careful to avoid placing a suture in the rectum.

The only landmark in the vagina is the hymenal ring. Once the vaginal repair has reached the hymenal ring, the suture should be either tied off or held out of the way while any necessary deep perineal sutures are placed. These may be either simple or figure-of-8 sutures and should accomplish hemostasis and provide good perineal support. Care must be taken so that the rectal mucosa is not perforated. It is important to be certain that the rectal sphincter is intact. If it is not, it may be repaired by placing several figure-of-8 sutures in the fascial sheath surrounding the muscle.

After placement of the deep interrupted sutures, the same suture that was used for the vagina usually is extended down the perineal defect in the subcutaneous tissue until it reaches the bottommost point of the incision. The suture then is turned around and brought up subcuticularly. The suture is tied at the hymenal ring.

Cesarean Section

Cesarean section is a straightforward surgical procedure in the hands of an experienced, trained operator. It requires close cooperation with the anesthesiology and nursing staffs. The procedure should never be attempted in a setting where there is not adequate anesthesia coverage, a well-stocked blood bank, adequate neonatal care, and a physician experienced in performing the procedure. Anyone who performs this procedure should be prepared to perform a cesarean hysterectomy should the need arise. Although this step is rarely needed, occasionally it may be necessary. Usually, the patient cannot be moved.

Anesthesia must be individualized (Bonica, 1969). In the past, most cesarean sections have been performed with the patient under general anesthesia. This is safe for the fetus only if very low concentrations of inhalation and intravenous agents are used for a short time; all anesthetic agents rapidly cross the placenta and affect the fetus directly. Within minutes, the fetus can be anesthetized and will be at extreme risk for fetal distress and asphyxia. General anesthesia is now rarely used for cesarean section in the United States.

Spinal and epidural anesthesia techniques are the most common methods employed and are much safer for the fetus. However, hypotension must be avoided carefully, mostly by the use of intravenous fluids. Hypotension may be life threatening for the fetus.

Whenever possible, the cesarean section should be of the low cervical transverse type. In this procedure, the abdomen is opened through a Pfannenstiel incision. A bladder flap then is taken down

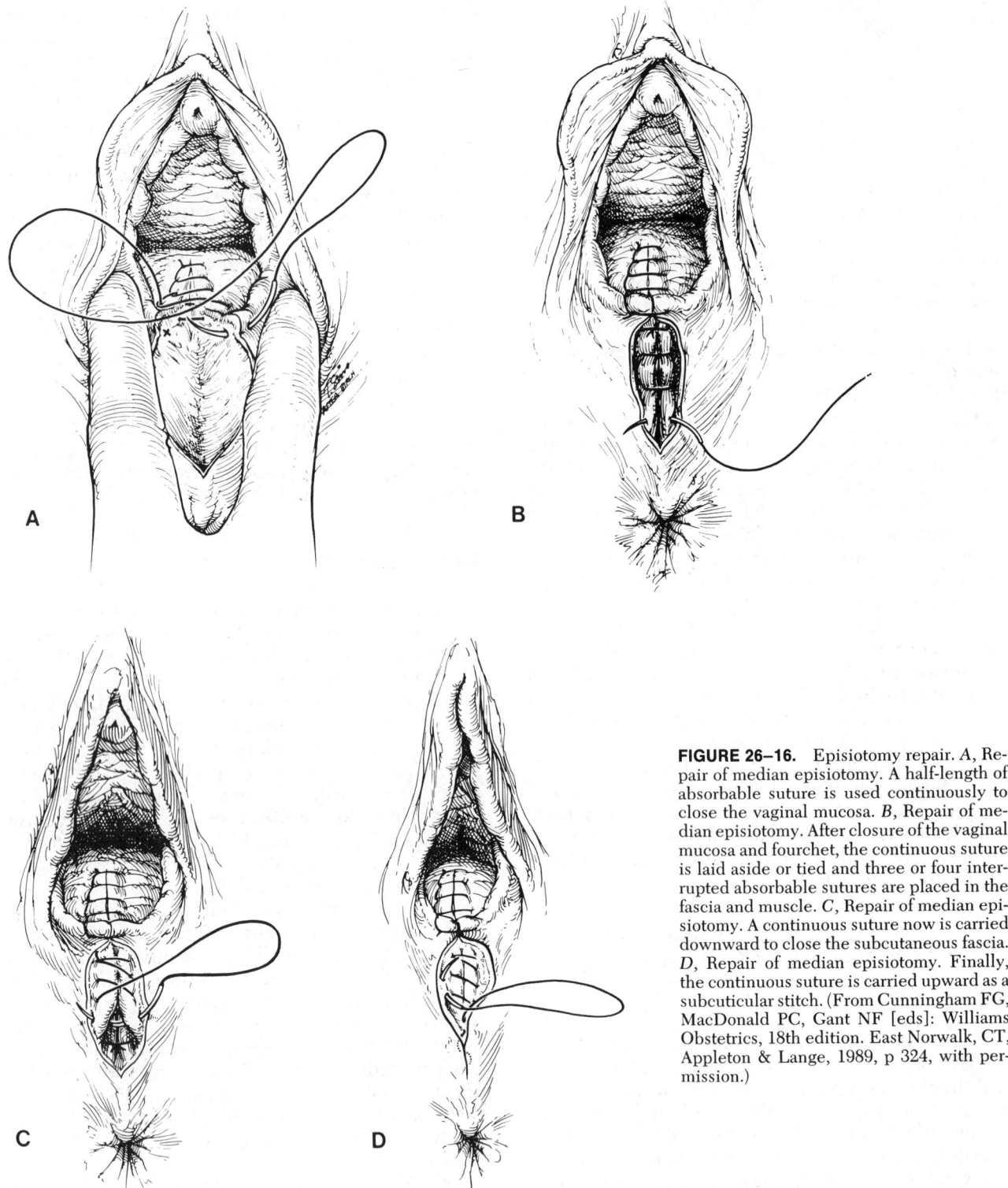

FIGURE 26–16. Episiotomy repair. *A*, Repair of median episiotomy. A half-length of absorbable suture is used continuously to close the vaginal mucosa. *B*, Repair of median episiotomy. After closure of the vaginal mucosa and fourchet, the continuous suture is laid aside or tied and three or four interrupted absorbable sutures are placed in the fascia and muscle. *C*, Repair of median episiotomy. A continuous suture now is carried downward to close the subcutaneous fascia. *D*, Repair of median episiotomy. Finally, the continuous suture is carried upward as a subcuticular stitch. (From Cunningham FG, MacDonald PC, Gant NF [eds]: Williams Obstetrics, 18th edition. East Norwalk, CT, Appleton & Lange, 1989, p 324, with permission.)

from the lower uterine segment, and the uterus is opened transversely. Care must be taken that the incision does not extend into the area of the vessels of the broad ligament. In some cases—for example, when placenta previa has caused tremendous dilation of the vessels of the lower uterine segment—a low vertical incision is preferable.

Uterine Rupture

Spontaneous uterine rupture occurs very rarely. Most ruptures are the result of either overstimulation of the uterus from oxytocic agents or labor after classical cesarean section.

Time is essential in uterine rupture. The patient

must undergo laparotomy as soon as possible. The fetus usually dies unless the rupture occurs in a hospital where cesarean section is available within a very few minutes. At the time of rupture, the patient often will relate a "tearing" feeling.

Uterine rupture may be repaired occasionally, but cesarean hysterectomy may need to be performed. This procedure requires the utmost care to prevent damage to the ureters or bladder, or both.

Vaginal Birth after Cesarean Section

During the last several years, it has been demonstrated repeatedly that vaginal birth after cesarean section (VBAC) may occur safely if the operation was performed transversely in the lower uterine segment. Both the American College of Obstetricians and Gynecologists and the National Institutes of Health Consensus Conference Committee have stressed the need to employ VBAC in an attempt to lower the escalating rate of cesarean section in the United States. Whereas VBAC was performed in past years with great trepidation, it has been shown that VBAC is less likely to cause maternal complications than repeat cesarean section.

VBAC is indicated except in extremely unusual circumstances. Only in the most unusual cases of pelvic deformity, gross fetal macrosomia, or classical uterine incision would VBAC be contraindicated. The labor and delivery suite attempting VBAC must, however, be prepared to perform emergency cesarean section on short notice. The anesthesia and operating teams must be present in the hospital. Adequate supplies of replacement fluids and blood must be available.

Inverted Uterus

Spontaneous inversion of the uterus almost never occurs. In virtually all cases, inversion occurs as a complication of vigorous traction on the umbilical cord. Interestingly, severe maternal hypotension usually immediately follows uterine inversion.

The condition is corrected by immediately replacing the uterus, if possible. If the cervix has clamped down around the uterine fundus, inhalation agents can be used to relax the uterus, after which it may be replaced. In this case, uterine packing should be performed to maintain the uterus in place. Generally, these packs may be removed after 24 hours. Severe hemorrhage also may accompany this complication.

OBSTETRIC ANESTHESIA AND ANALGESIA

Analgesia

Narcotic medications have been used extensively for relief of pain in labor. Although these are effective for pain relief, they cross to the placenta and can depress the fetus or newborn. If needed for pain relief, these drugs should be given in only small doses and should be administered intravenously. Because many of these drugs and their metabolic products build up in the fetus, doses should not be repeated more than one or two times.

The timing of the peak action of the narcotic agent should be calculated so that is does not occur at the expected time of delivery. For example, meperidine has its peak action after an intravenous dose in about 30 minutes. If delivery occurs at this time, neonatal depression may be observed.

General Anesthesia

There is no place for the use of general anesthesia in routine deliveries. It should be reserved only for cesarean section when conduction anesthesia is not possible.

Regional Anesthesia

Pudendal

A frequent form of anesthesia given to women in labor in the United States is the pudendal block. This block is accomplished by injection of approximately 10 mL of a 1% solution of an anesthetic agent such as lidocaine just medial and inferior to the ischial spine on each side of the pelvis. When properly performed, this will provide good anesthetic effect in the posterior vulva, the lower third of the vagina, and the area around the anus. This method allows for ease in delivery and episiotomy repair (Fig. 26–17).

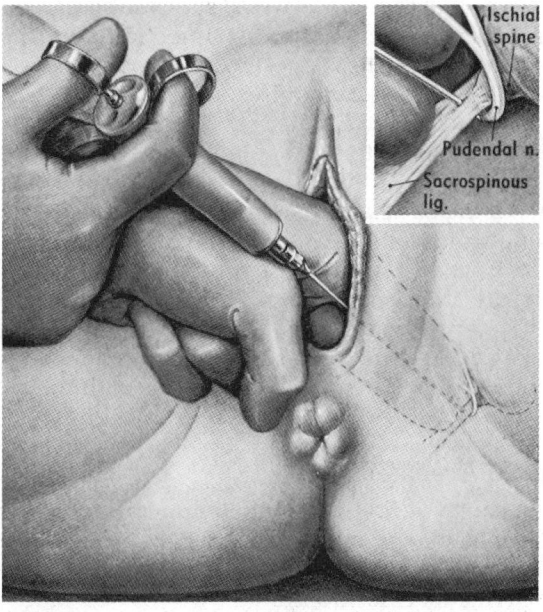

FIGURE 26–17. Technique of pudendal block. (From Bonica JJ: Principles and Practice of Obstetric Analgesia & Anesthesia, Vol. 1. Philadelphia, FA Davis, 1967, p 493, with permission.)

Even in the hands of an experienced operator, the block is not always effective. It is common practice to repeat the injection at least once. However, anesthetic agents can reach maximal doses with repeated attempts at pudendal block. If the block cannot be accomplished on a single reinjection, the use of local anesthesia should be considered.

Local

The use of local anesthesia for the repair of episiotomy has become more frequent during the past few years. Many women who wish a "natural" delivery prefer not to have a pudendal block. This is an adequate type of anesthesia for repair of episiotomy.

Paracervical Block

The use of paracervical block during labor has decreased throughout the United States. Paracervical block frequently causes prolonged fetal bradycardia. Although this generally does not result in serious fetal consequences, the bradycardia produced is of sufficient concern that this form of anesthesia should be avoided or used with great caution. Electronic fetal monitoring always should be used when paracervical block is administered.

Epidural Block

Lumbar epidural block has become a very common anesthetic technique in the United States. Correct utilization of this technique allows for adequate anesthesia during labor and delivery (Clark, 1981). A correctly placed epidural catheter can alleviate the pain from cervical dilation in labor without affecting uterine contractions. When the patient is ready for delivery, she can be placed in an upright position, another injection given, and satisfactory perineal anesthesia accomplished.

This technique requires considerable experience for its safe use. One of the possible major complications is maternal hypotension with resultant fetal bradycardia and distress. This is almost never seen if the patient has been pretreated with an adequate fluid volume and is monitored closely. Maternal blood pressure should be measured frequently after institution of lumbar epidural block. If hypotension begins to develop, this usually can be corrected quickly by increasing the rate of intravenous fluid infusion. The lumbar epidural block also is ideal for cesarean section.

Spinal Anesthesia

Because of the frequent complication of severe spinal headache, spinal anesthesia has become less commonly used than in the past. Additionally, the women must be monitored very closely and the blood pressure taken almost continuously once the agent has been placed in the subarachnoid space. This technique allows for good perineal relaxation but often completely blocks the patient's ability to push adequately.

The technique sometimes is used for cesarean section, but severe spinal headache also may follow in this situation unless very small-bore needles are used. For this reason, lumbar epidural anesthesia is superior.

PUERPERIUM

The postpartum exam is usually performed about 6 weeks after the delivery of the infant. The new mother already should have been seen with her newborn prior to that visit. The newborns should be checked within the first 2 weeks following delivery to monitor weight gain, evaluate for feeding problems or jaundice, and ascertain how the family is coping with the new infant.

By 6 weeks, the family has begun its adjustment to the new infant. Postpartum bleeding and discharge should have ceased by this point. Usually the vaginal and perineal epithelial and deep structures have healed sufficiently within 3 or 4 weeks after delivery. The uterus is back to normal size and the cervix closed. If the mother is breast-feeding, breast engorgement and nipple soreness will have resolved.

The physical exam of the mother should include blood pressure check, breast exam, and pelvic exam, including Pap smear. A hematocrit should be drawn. The mother should be instructed to remain on iron and folic acid supplementation if she is nursing.

Discussion about contraception should have commenced prior to the woman leaving the hospital, because for many women pelvic healing will be sufficient to resume sexual activity within 3 or 4 weeks of delivery. Diaphragms may be fitted with ease at the 6-week examination. Oral contraceptives may be started at any time, but there is more chance of difficulties with regulation and irregular bleeding if they are started before the first menstrual period. Although it has been recommended that women who breast-feed not use oral contraceptives, statements by the American Academy of Pediatrics indicate that the use of low-dosage oral contraceptives in mothers who breast-feed does not create significant risk to the infant, although there is some evidence that lactation may be affected adversely (Committee on Drugs, 1981). The steroid hormones are excreted in small amounts in the breast milk and do reach the infant. Intrauterine devices or provera injections are other viable options.

The family physician should ask about family adjustment. Is the mother getting enough help? Is she feeling sleep deprived? How are siblings adjusting to the new baby? What is happening in the relationship between the mother and her significant other? Women and their partners should be told about increased vaginal dryness and decrease in libido associated with nursing. The family physician needs to explore how the family is coping with transition and evaluate the need for support services.

REFERENCES

ACOG Technical Bulletin no. 179. Nutrition during Pregnancy. Washington DC, American College of Obstetricians and Gynecologists, 1993.

Barnes AB, Colton T, Gundersen J, et al: Fertility and outcome of pregnancy in women exposed in utero to diethylstilbestrol. N Engl J Med 302:609, 1980.

Belizan J: Routine vs selective episiotomy: A randomized controlled trial. Lancet 342:1517, 1993.

Bjerkadel T: Outcome of pregnancy in women with epilepsy, Norway, 1966–1978: Congenital malformations. In Janz D, Dam M, Richens A (eds): Epilepsy, Pregnancy, and the Child. New York, Raven Press, 1982, p 289.

Bonica JJ: Principles and Practice of Obstetric Analgesia & Anesthesia, Vol. II. Philadelphia, FA Davis Company, 1969.

Brent R, Beckman D: Prescribed drugs, therapeutic agents, and fetal teratogenesis. In Reece E, Hobbins J, Mahoney M, Petrie R (eds): Medicine of the Fetus and Mother. Philadelphia, JB Lippincott, 1992, pp 300–316.

Candib L: Obstetrics in family practice: A personal and political perspective. J Fam Pract 3:391, 1976.

Caring for our future: The content of prenatal care. Washington DC, U.S. Public Health Service, 1989, p 51.

Centers for Disease Control and Prevention: 1993 Sexually Transmitted Disease Treatment Guidelines. Washington, DC, U.S. Department of Health and Human Services, 1993.

Clark RB: Conduction anesthesia. Clin Obstet Gynecol 24:601, 1981.

Collea JV: Current management of breech presentation. Clin Obstet Gynecol 23:525, 1980.

Collea JV, Rabin SC, Weghorst GR, et al: The randomized management of term frank breech presentation: Vaginal delivery vs. cesarean section. Am J Obstet Gynecol 131:186, 1978.

Committee on Drugs, American Academy of Pediatrics: Breast feeding and contraception. Pediatrics 68:138, 1981.

Duff P: Management of premature rupture of membranes in term patients. Clin Obstet Gynecol 34:723, 1991.

Etheridge MJ, Peperell RJ: Heart disease and pregnancy at the Royal Women's Hospital. Med J Aust 2:277, 1977.

Ewigman BG, Crane JP, Frigoletto FD, et al: Effect of prenatal ultrasound screening on perinatal outcome. N Engl J Med 329:821, 1993.

Friedman E: Disordered labor: Objective evaluation and management. J Fam Pract 2:167, 1975.

Fuhrmann K, Reiher H, Semmier K, et al: Prevention of congenital malformations in infants of insulin dependent diabetic mothers. Diabetes Care 6:219, 1983.

Hanan IM, Kirsner JR: Inflammatory bowel disease in the pregnant woman. Clin Perinatal 12:669, 1985.

Hill LM: Diagnosis and management of fetal distress. Mayo Clin Proc 54:784, 1979.

Hill LM, Johnson CE, Lee RA: Cholecystectomy in pregnancy. Obstet Gynecol 46:291, 1975.

Infante-Rivard C, Fernandez A, Gauthier R, et al: Fetal loss associated with caffeine intake before and during pregnancy. JAMA 270:2940, 1993.

Jack B, Culpepper L: Preconception care—risk reduction and health promotion in preparation for pregnancy. JAMA 264:1147, 1990.

Kennell J, Klaus M, Robertson S, et al: Continuous emotional support during labor in a US hospital. JAMA 265:2197, 1991.

Lawson HW, Atrash HK, Saftlas AF, Finch EL: Ectopic pregnancy in the United States, 1970–1986. MMWR 38:1, 1989.

Lewis DF, Major CA, Towers CV, et al: Effects of digital vaginal examinations on latency period in preterm premature rupture of membranes. Obstet Gynecol 80:630, 1992.

Morbidity and Mortality Weekly Report: Recommendations for use of folic acid to reduce number of spina bifida cases and other neural tube defects. JAMA 269:1233, 1993.

Noller KL: Liver disease in pregnancy. In Iffy L, Kaminetzky H (eds): Principles and Practice of Obstetrics and Perinatology, Vol II. New York, John Wiley & Sons, 1981, pp 1328–1330.

Noller KL, Hill LM: Cardiac disease associated with pregnancy and its management. In Guiliani ER, Fuster V, Gersh BJ, et al. (eds): Cardiology: Fundamentals and Practice, 2nd edition. St. Louis, Mosby–Year Book Publishers, 1991, pp 1207–2122.

Oakley G: Folic acid-preventable spina bifida and anencephaly. JAMA 269:1292, 1993.

Reece EA, Gabrielli J, Abdalla M: The prevention of diabetes-associated birth defects. Semin Perinatol 12(4):292, 1988.

Reid R, Ivey KJ, Rencoret RH, et al: Fetal complications of obstetric cholestasis. BMJ 1:870, 1976.

Rooks J, Weatherby N, Ernst E, et al: Outcomes of care in birth centers. N Engl J Med 321:1804, 1989.

Rosenblatt R: The future of obstetrics in family practice: Time for a new direction. J Fam Pract 26:127, 1988.

Rubella and Pregnancy (ACOG Technical Bulletin no. 171). Washington, DC, American College of Obstetricians and Gynecologists, 1992.

Sibai BM, Caritis SN, Thom E, et al: Prevention of preeclampsia with low-dose aspirin in healthy, nulliparous pregnant women. N Engl J Med 329:1213, 1993.

Stovall TG, Ling FW, Buster JE: Outpatient chemotherapy of unruptured ectopic pregnancy. Fertil Steril 51:435, 1989.

Sultan AH, Kamm MA, Hudson CN, et al: Anal-sphincter disruption during vaginal delivery. N Engl J Med 329:1905, 1993.

Thorp J, McNitt J, Leppert P: Effects of epidural analgesia: Some questions and answers. Birth 17:3, 1990.

Webb MJ, Sedlack RE: Ulcerative colitis in pregnancy. Med Clin North Am 58:823, 1974.

Wilson CB, Remington JS: What can be done to prevent congenital toxoplasmosis. Am J Obstet Gynecol 138:357, 1980.

SUGGESTED READINGS

ACOG Technical Bulletin no. 154. Alpha-Fetoprotein. Washington DC, American College of Obstetricians and Gynecologists, 1991.

Antepartum Fetal Surveillance (ACOG Technical Bulletin no. 107). Washington, DC, American College of Obstetricians and Gynecologists, 1987.

Antimicrobial Therapy for Obstetric Patients (ACOG Technical Bulletin no. 117). Washington, DC, American College of Obstetricians and Gynecologists, 1988.

Carroll J: *Chlamydia trachomatis* during pregnancy. Can Fam Physician 39:97, 1993.

Chasnoff I, Burns W, Schnoll S, Burns K: Cocaine use in pregnancy. N Engl J Med 313:666, 1985.

Chavez G, Mulinare J, Cordero J: Maternal cocaine use during early pregnancy as a risk factor for congenital urogenital anomalies. JAMA 262:795, 1986.

Dunne K: Characteristics associated with perineal condition in an alternative birth center. J Nurse Midwifery 29:29, 1984.

Fraser W, Marcoux S, Moutquin J, Christen A, Canadian Amniotomy Study Group: Effect of early amniotomy on the risk of dystocia in nulliparous women. N Engl J Med 328:1145, 1993.

Freeman R: Intrapartum fetal monitoring—a disappointing story. N Engl J Med 322:624, 1990.

Gjerdingen D, Fontaine P: Preconception health care: A critical task for family physicians. JABFP 4:237, 1991.

Greenwald JL: Premature rupture of the membranes: Diagnostic and management strategies. Am Fam Physician 48:293, 1993.

Guideline for Hepatitis B Virus Screening and Vaccination during Pregnancy (ACOG Committee Opinion no. 111). Washington, DC, American College of Obstetricians and Gynecologists, 1992.

Jack B, Culpepper L: Preconception care. J Fam Pract 32:306, 1991.

Larimore W: Family practice obstetrics in America: A future or a funeral??? Keynote Address, AAFP/STFM National Conference on Obstetrics for the Family Physician: Family Centered Perinatal Care, City, May 14, 1993.

Larimore W: Family-centered birthing: A niche for family physicians. Am Fam Physician 47:1365, 1993.

Management of Diabetes Mellitus in Pregnancy (ACOG Technical Bulletin no. 92). New York, American College of Obstetricians and Gynecologists, 1986.

Olson R, Olson C, Cox N: Maternal birthing positions and perineal injury. J Fam Pract 30:553, 1990.

Premature Rupture of Membranes (ACOG Technical Bulletin no. 115). Washington, DC, American College of Obstetricians and Gynecologists, 1988.

Prentice A, Lind T: Fetal heart rate monitoring during labour—too frequent intervention, too little benefit. Lancet II:1375, 1987.

Reynolds J, Rudkin P: Changes in the management of labour: 1. Length and management of the second stage. Can Med Assoc J 136:1041, 1987.

Rosen M, Merkatz I, Hill J: Caring for our future: A report by the Expert Panel on the Content of Prenatal Care. Obstet Gynecol 77:782, 1991.

Rosenberg I: Folic acid and neural-tube defects—time for action: N Engl J Med 327:1875, 1992.

Scherger J, Levitt C, Acheson L, et al: Teaching family-centered perinatal care in family medicine, Part 1. Fam Med 24:238, 1992a.

Scherger J, Levitt C, Acheson L: Teaching family-centered perinatal care in family medicine, Part 2. Fam Med 24:368, 1992b.

Smith M, Ruffin M, Green L: The rational management of labor. Am Fam Physician 47:1471, 1993.

Viscomi C, Eisenach J: Patient-controlled epidural analgesia during labor. Obstet Gynecol 77:348, 1991.

Warren K, Bast R: Alcohol-related birth defects: An update. Public Health Rep 103:638, 1988.

Werler M, Shapiro S, Mitchell A: Periconceptional folic acid exposure and risk of occurrent neural tube defects. JAMA 269:1257, 1993.

CHAPTER 27
CARE OF THE NEWBORN

ROBERT HUNT SPRINKLE

The well-trained family physician, among all potential caregivers, is best prepared to reduce perinatal risk by integrating the care of the sexually active adolescent, the expectant and newly delivered mother, and the newborn baby. When the same physician oversees pregnancy, labor, delivery, and newborn care, highly coherent perinatal management should result. When several physicians are involved, integrated management is less automatic but still must be sought, because it is the only acceptable standard of perinatal care.

MANAGING THE NEWBORN IMMEDIATELY AFTER DELIVERY

Assisting Physiologic Adaptation

During fetal life, when circulation to the pulmonary bed is low, fluid produced in the lungs mostly flows out through the tracheobronchial tree to mix with fluid in the amniotic sac. During vaginal delivery but not during cesarean delivery, some residual pulmonary fluid is "squeezed out" through the nose and mouth. When the umbilical cord is clamped, cutting off the low-pressure placental circulatory bed, fetal cardiovascular systemic pressures rise abruptly, and complex events, many of them prostaglandin mediated, take place. The lungs begin to fill with air when high negative pulmonary air pressure is generated by respiratory effort or, in the compromised infant, when high positive pulmonary air pressure is generated by resuscitative effort. Negative-pressure alveolar aeration contributes to a lowering of pulmonary vascular pressure. As the pulmonary vascular bed becomes more fully perfused, more residual lung fluid is resorbed into the circulation. Increasing pulmonary vascular return to the left atrium raises left atrial pressure, and this pressure rise effectively closes the foramen ovale. Progressive narrowing of the ductus arteriosus over the next several days then completes the functional separation of the higher pressure systemic arterial circulation from the lower pressure systemic venous and pulmonary circulations (Reller et al., 1988).

There are many potential impediments to normal transition from intrauterine to extrauterine life.

Pulmonary surfactant deficiency or surfactant immaturity, corresponding roughly to a ratio of lecithin (phosphatidylcholine) to sphingomyelin of less than 2.0, may not allow adequate alveolar inflation. Pulmonary hypoplasia, associated with diaphragmatic herniation or caused by low fetal urinary output or chronic amniotic fluid leakage through the mechanism of oligohydramnios, may make adequate gas exchange anatomically impossible. Cardiovascular malformations, the effects of cardiovascular-active drugs, and acquired problems, such as pulmonary infections or aspiration syndromes, also may prevent or impede successful adaptation.

Cold stress to the wet newborn is the most common and the most easily avoided transitional problem. To reduce cold stress, ambient temperature, if adjustable, should be brought to between 75° and 80° F (24° and 27° C). In well-equipped delivery environments, a radiant warmer, preferably self-regulating, should be brought to equilibrium, and warm sterile towels should be opened on the warmer. Other common impediments to adaptation often can be removed by easy interventions using simple instruments. Oxygen masks, a resuscitation bag and pressure manometer, oxygen flow, suction and suction catheters, laryngoscope blades and lights, a bulb syringe, a DeLee catheter and trap, and several sizes of endotracheal tubes routinely should be located, positively identified, and functionally confirmed.

Initial Inspection and Maneuvers

Blood and other fluids with which staff may come in contact in the delivery room may contain infectious agents; practices lessening, if not eliminating, skin and mucous membrane contact with these substances must prevail.

The rough amount, color, gross contents, and odor of the amniotic fluid should be assessed during the delivery process. In selected cases, a sample of fluid should be dispatched for microscopic examination and culture or for lecithin/sphingomyelin determination.

First the oropharynx and then the nose should be suctioned on the perineum during or immediately after vaginal delivery or on the abdomen immediately after cesarean delivery. If thick meconium is present, routine oropharyngeal and nasal suctioning may be bypassed in favor of immediate laryngoscopic examination, ideally performed before the initial breath. If thick meconium is found, first the trachea and then the hypopharynx, oropharynx, and nose should be suctioned with a DeLee catheter or, preferably, through an endotracheal tube hooked up to a suction device. If standard suctioning is performed first in these high-risk babies, gagging, gasping, and deep inspiration of meconium may be stimulated. Aggressive suctioning of lightly stained infants is not advisable, however, and has been shown to cause more problems than it prevents (Linder et al., 1988; Sepkowitz, 1987).

Neonatal blood volume is increased by stripping or "milking" the umbilical cord prior to clamping, holding the infant in a dependent position before clamping, or delaying clamping beyond the time needed to clear the infant's nasal and oropharyngeal secretions. These maneuvers are not ordinarily necessary and are not routinely advisable; they may increase iron stores at the price of hypervolemia or exaggerated neonatal jaundice. Cord blood samples for laboratory studies should be collected from the placental end of the cord.

The infant's umbilical cord stump should be clamped no closer than 2 cm from the abdominal wall to facilitate umbilical vessel catheterization, should it become necessary. The infant should be placed under a radiant warmer. A Trendelenburg position favors the suctioning of secretions and, if necessary, laryngoscopy and intubation. The infant should be dried in a soft, prewarmed towel. This maneuver decreases evaporative heat loss and stimulates mildly depressed infants.

Sometimes, an otherwise normal infant will exhibit marked acrocyanosis immediately after delivery. Although central hypoxemia is seldom responsible, an oxygen stream commonly is directed at the baby's nose. This brief therapeutic maneuver may be harmless, but "wall oxygen" is typically pure oxygen, and even transient hyperoxemia may cause spasm of the retinal vasculature in the occasional infant. Blowing cold oxygen, air, or mist in the face also may stimulate a generalized vagal response.

At 1 minute and again at 5 minutes, the infant is given an Apgar score (Apgar, 1953). Criteria for Apgar scoring are presented in Table 27–1. A 1-minute Apgar score greater than 9 is rare as a result of physiologic acrocyanosis. Infants scoring 3 or less at 1 minute probably will need extended resuscitative efforts; those scoring from 4 to 6 may do well after vigorous stimulation or brief respiratory support; those scoring 7 and above likely will do well with no special treatment or with light or even incidental stimulation. Infants whose scores at 5 minutes have not risen to 7 or above and infants whose scores actually have fallen may be quite ill.

The placenta should be inspected for size and quality; infarcts, calcifications, and other defects; gross clotting; membrane cloudiness suggesting infection; umbilical cord length and number of vessels; and evidence of a pseudovascular umbilical structure suggesting a patent urachus or a freshly severed loop of bowel. The placenta should be preserved until the infant is discharged.

The initial physical examination includes birth weight and body measurements as well as the Apgar scores that predict clinical course. This provides a better opportunity to estimate gestational age than does an examination performed after an interval as short as 6 to 12 hours, because of rapid epidermal drying, although some neurologic aspects of the estimation actually may become clearer with time in the temporarily depressed infant. Patency of the nares may be demonstrated by passage of a no. 8 French catheter bilaterally, although this procedure need not be routine. Anal patency and the passage of meconium and urine should be noted, as should obvious birth trauma.

Prophylactic Measures

Effective postexposure prophylaxis against *Neisseria gonorrhoeae* conjunctivitis can be achieved by the application of 1% silver nitrate, 0.5% erythromycin, or 1% tetracycline to the conjunctivae soon after delivery. Silver nitrate may be a superior prophylactic for penicillinase-producing *N. go-*

TABLE 27–1. CRITERIA FOR APGAR SCORING

Sign	Score		
	0	1	2
Heart rate	Absent	Below 100 beats/min	100 beats/min or above
Respiratory effort	Absent	Hypoventilation or weak cry	Good effort or strong cry
Muscle tone	Absent	Some flexion or motion	Good flexion or active motion
Reflex irritability (to foot slap or nasal catheter)	Absent	Grimace only	Vigorous response, cry, sneeze, cough
Color	Blue all over or pale	Pink body and blue extremities	Pink all over

Adapted from Apgar V: A proposal for a new method of evaluation of the newborn infant. Curr Res Anesth Analg 32:260, 1953.

norrhoeae, and tetracycline and erythromycin arguably may be superior for *Chlamydia trachomatis.* Yet, clearly, none of these agents is effective enough to allow the neglect of prepartum maternal surveillence (Hammerschlag et al., 1989); some even question their superiority to no prophylaxis as antichlamydials (Chen, 1992). Silver nitrate works by stimulating an inflammatory response in the conjunctivae; a mild chemical conjunctivitis often results. Herpes simplex virus (HSV), another cause of ophthalmia neonatorum, is discussed in Chapter 47.

Until the infant's gut is colonized by autochthonous flora, vitamin K cannot be produced and inactive forms of coagulation factors II, VII, IX, and X cannot be activated. Unless vitamin K is administered soon after birth, the infant will pass through several days unprotected from hemorrhagic disease of the newborn. Both intramuscular and oral forms of vitamin K are effective prophylactically, but the intramuscular form is better studied, and a needle mark in a standard site can serve as reassurance that vitamin K has in fact been given.

All newborns should be immunized actively against hepatitis B virus (HBV) (Halsey, 1993); this recommendation is especially important in areas of HBV endemicity (Moyes et al., 1987). Newborns known to be at risk for the vertical acquisition of HBV need both active and passive immunization in the delivery room.

Parental Contact and Participation

Unless the new mother is unconscious or unless, as a relinquishing mother, she has explicitly requested not to see her baby, the newborn should never leave the delivery room without being seen by and, if possible, touched by its mother. The same rule must apply to the father when present. No exception need be made even for severely ill infants. More happily, the vigorous newborn, dried and swaddled head to toe or dried and naked if ambient temperature permits, should be handed to a fully conscious mother and offered a first feeding while being cuddled against the breast (Righard and Alade, 1990).

COMPLETE HISTORY AND PHYSICAL EXAMINATION

The newborn's complete history is the full family history, the mother's past obstetric and recent preconception and periconception history, and the entire prenatal history, including any record of extrauterine or intrauterine fetal monitoring and the details of delivery and early neonatal life. These topics, excepting the last, have been covered in Chapter 26. In practice, the newborn history usu-

ally can be written in a few short paragraphs and presented verbally in less than a minute.

The physician must record a full physical examination of the newborn within 24 hours of delivery. In babies not obviously the product of term gestations, a formal estimation of gestational age should be performed within 6 to 12 hours of delivery. Abnormalities are found through routine examination in about 9 per cent of newborns; minor findings often are missed or are found only prior to discharge on a "second look" (Moss et al., 1991). The examiner must be attentive not only to significant pathology but also to trivial abnormalities and physiologic curiosities, because these lesser findings can cause needless parental anxiety if left undiscussed.

General Inspection

Size and Color

Even in the full-term baby, size may not be normal. A small or skinny baby may be the product of a poorly nourished, chronically diseased, or drug-abusing mother; or may have been maintained by an insufficient placenta; or may have been infected in utero; or may be expressing a chromosomal or metabolic abnormality. A post-term baby may appear long and thin, may have a "little old man" face, and may show dry, peeling skin and long fingernails and toenails, often stained green with meconium. Unusually large, fat babies may be the infants of diabetic mothers.

The normal newborn almost always will have a pink tongue. Unwrapped in a warm examination room and lying on a blanket, the infant may appear pink all over or may appear pink centrally while displaying bluish extremities. Acrocyanosis is common in the newborn period, especially under cold conditions, and is usually, although not always, physiologic. Acrocyanosis occurs when the concentration of reduced (unsaturated) hemoglobin reaches about 5 gm/dL in capillary blood. Slow flow through the periphery will produce this condition, but slow flow through the periphery can be caused not only by cold stress but also by shock, heart failure, or vascular obstruction. Central cyanosis suggests the presence of about 3 gm/dL of reduced hemoglobin in *arterial* blood. Central cyanosis persisting 20 minutes or so beyond delivery in a noncrying infant is not physiologic. Central cyanosis clearing only with crying—a paradoxical sign—suggests choanal atresia. Persistent central cyanosis implies an excess of reduced hemoglobin and can be caused by polycythemia, right-to-left shunting, heart failure with or without right-to-left shunting, pulmonary disease, central nervous system disease affecting respiratory drive, shock of any cause, or, rarely, methemoglobinemia. It should be noted that sick babies who happen to have relatively high concentrations of fetal hemoglobin may not display central cyanosis until their oxygen tensions reach dangerously low levels, so the absence of central cyanosis should not by itself deflect an investigation of oxygen delivery (Fanaroff and Martin, 1991).

Pale babies may be anemic. Plethoric babies, cyanotic or not, may be polycythemic. Icterus appearing on the first day of life suggests a hemolytic process, hepatitis, or hepatobiliary malformation.

Activity

The normal full-term newborn exhibits several patterns of activity, ranging from quiet sleep to crying. During the first day of extrauterine life, many babies are more alert than they will be later on in the first week, but some sleep almost constantly and show little interest in feeding. The term baby should exhibit flexor tone even during sleep and especially when agitated; babies born from abnormal presentations may not exhibit the usual flexor positions in all extremities; and babies of different races may vary markedly in tone. Jittery babies are usually normal (Parker et al., 1990), although their glucose, calcium, and magnesium levels often are checked, and they are sometimes held over for electroencephalography. Beyond the usual range of jitteriness is the baby withdrawing from a maternal drug of abuse. Inspection of the drug-withdrawing baby also may suggest other signs of autonomic dysfunction. Seizure activity in newborns is much different from seizure activity in older children and adults. Paroxysmal, repetitive activity of almost any sort can indicate abnormal discharge from the central nervous system. Hypoventilation and absence of limb motor function suggest spinal cord trauma (MacKinnon et al., 1993).

Respirations and Phonations

Respirations should be quiet and unlabored, the chest and abdomen moving together. Normal respiratory rate varies from about 30 to 60 breaths/min. Respiratory pattern also varies widely, with sporadic breath-to-breath intervals as long as 15 seconds, causing occasional false alarms. Nonstridorous, unlabored respirations and a lusty cry are strong evidence against airway obstruction, such as choanal atresia or laryngomalacia, and against significant pulmonary disease. Persistently weak or unusual cry suggests a broad range of pathologies. Tachypnea, retractions, nasal flaring, grunting, and, ultimately, cyanosis are the hallmarks of respiratory distress, although normal newborns in early transition to extrauterine life and hypothermic, hypoglycemic, anemic, or polycythemic newborns can show some or all of these signs as well.

Pulsations and Contours

Some congenital cardiovascular problems may be suggested by abnormally placed or abnormally timed superficial chest pulsations, pulsations sometimes better seen than felt. Unusually obvious peripheral arterial pulsations may be noticed in a baby whose ductus arteriosus remains patent; pulsations of the posterior tibial artery are often observable in this circumstance.

The abdomen may be rounded, flat, or scaphoid (meaning boatlike). Babies yet to pass their meconium may be a bit distended, as may those who have swallowed large amounts of air during crying or during bag-and-mask ventilatory stimulation. The abdomen may be enlarged by an intra-abdominal solid mass; by a viscus distended with air, urine, or fluid; or by free intraperitoneal fluid. A scaphoid abdomen implies a deficiency of intra-abdominal contents, as in diaphragmatic herniation. If diaphragmatic herniation is suspected in a baby needing ventilatory resuscitation, intubation is required immediately because bag-and-mask ventilation may distend the intrathoracic gut with air, further compromising pulmonary function. Abdominal musculature may be incompletely approximated, as in diastasis recti or umbilical herniation.

Asymmetry of the head, neck, or extremities may suggest intrauterine molding, abnormal intrauterine lie, abnormal underlying structure, or birth trauma, such as brachial plexus injury or facial palsy. Symmetrical deformity of the feet or hips also may be due to molding or to abnormal intrauterine lie, respectively. Persistent tilting of the head to one side suggests fibrosed hemorrhage into the sternocleidomastoid muscle. The dorsa of the hands and feet or the skin over the pubis may be mildly edematous; marked edema of the dorsa of the feet in a phenotypic female should suggest Turner's syndrome.

Vital Signs

Temperature

Normal newborn core temperature ranges from 36° to 37.5° C (96.8° to 99.6° F). In well babies, core (i.e., rectal) temperature readings often are not taken. Axillary temperature readings are popular, although unreliable; aural infrared thermometry is also unreliable in newborns (Yetman et al., 1993). Skin temperature readings are useful only in special care settings.

The newborn baby can compensate for evaporative, radiant, convective, and conductive heat loss over a narrower temperature range than adults. The newborn also makes relatively more use of nonshivering thermogenesis, accomplished predominantly by the catabolism of brown fat.

The thermal shock of delivery is a challenge to the baby's compensatory mechanisms, especially following cesarean delivery (Christensson et al., 1993). If left undried and unwrapped in a room made thermally comfortable for laboring adults, the newborn's core temperature can drop by 2° to 3° C. Cold stress can occur even if only the scalp is improperly dried and covered. Cold stress can present as an illness, such as respiratory distress or hypoglycemia, and it can make the course of any illness more difficult. Placing an infant in an incubator is not a guarantee that thermal neutrality will be achieved or maintained; improperly serviced or poorly designed incubators, many of obsolete, single-walled construction, are still in common use.

Hyperthermia is less frequently a problem and is more likely to be caused by high room temperature, equipment malfunction, or overwrapping than by infection, metabolic derangement, or brain injury. An environmentally overheated baby is vasodilated, and the extremities may not be much cooler than the trunk. A septic baby is likely to be vasoconstricted peripherally, at least at some stage in the course of the infection, and his or her extremities may be noticeably cooler than the trunk (Klaus and Fanaroff, 1993).

Pulse Rate

Pulse rate is rapid in the first few minutes after birth, normally topping 180 beats/min. In the delivery room, the pulse is felt most conveniently at the umbilicus, but peripheral pulses also should be easy to feel because persistent flow through the ductus arteriosus produces a wide pulse pressure. By 20 minutes, heart rate is usually around 140 beats/min. Mean peaks are lower for preterm infants. At no time in the delivery room should heart rate fall below 100 beats/min. Heart rate is quite variable in the newborn period and can be expected to rise and fall quickly within broad limits with stimulation, irritation, or agitation and as a function of state of arousal. Most neonatal tachycardias and bradycardias are physiologic or procedure-related and are self-limited; others are caused by drugs or various pathologic conditions (Fanaroff and Martin, 1991).

Respiratory Rate

Respiratory rate and pattern have been described earlier.

Blood Pressure

Blood pressure should be measured in every newborn. The auscultatory or Doppler methods usually are employed; palpation readings are less reproducible and can approximate only the mean arterial pressure. Normal systolic pressure for term infants born by vaginal delivery is about 65 to 70 mm Hg; for term infants delivered by cesarean section it is about 60 mm Hg. Pressures for premature babies are somewhat lower. Aortic pressures obtained after catheterization of the umbilical artery (Fig. 27–1) have been used to establish reference values (Versmold et al., 1981). Because cuff pressures commonly are measured only in the arm in apparently normal babies and are not measured routinely in both arms and in one leg, it is unlikely

that readings placed on the nursery day sheet will identify nonhypertensive babies with coarcted aortas.

Measurements

Weight

Birth weight should be measured in metric units. Babies who weigh up to 1500 grams at delivery are very-low-birth-weight babies, those who weigh from 1501 to 2500 grams at delivery are low-birth-weight babies, and those who weigh from 2501 to 4000 grams are babies of normal birth weight. A baby of any birth weight up to 4000 grams may be described as "appropriate for gestational age" (AGA), "small for gestational age" (SGA), or "large for gestational age" (LGA), according to reference values (Fig. 27–2). Babies who weigh 4001 grams or more are LGA and "macrosomic." AGA, SGA, and LGA determinations depend on sure knowledge of date of conception or on the result of an estimation of gestational age by Dubowitz or Ballard criteria, as described later in this chapter.

Most babies lose weight over the first 3 days of extrauterine life, an interval during which even vigorous babies may not feed avidly and mothers may find their milk has not yet "come in." In an otherwise well baby, this early weight loss, assuming it does not exceed about 7 per cent of birth weight, should be considered physiologic. Most of this weight loss is due to negative water balance, although brown fat also is expended. Head circumference, if studied carefully, can be shown to decrease during this period. Some small full-term AGA babies may fall below 2501 grams during the first few days; these babies do not "become" SGA.

Length

Length usually is measured incorrectly in the healthy, full-term baby because of hip and knee flexion, while usually being measured more accurately in the premature, sick, or floppy baby. Babies with good tone are best placed supine on a paper sheet; a vertically held pen can be used to mark the paper at the level of the baby's vertex; the hips and knees then can be straightened gently and another pen mark made at the level of the heel surfaces; the distance between the two marks can be measured in the baby's absence.

Head Circumference

The head is measured at its greatest circumference, the fronto-occipital circumference.

Skin

Signs of Trauma and Stress

Babies normally suck on their fingers, hands, and forearms in utero, sometimes vigorously

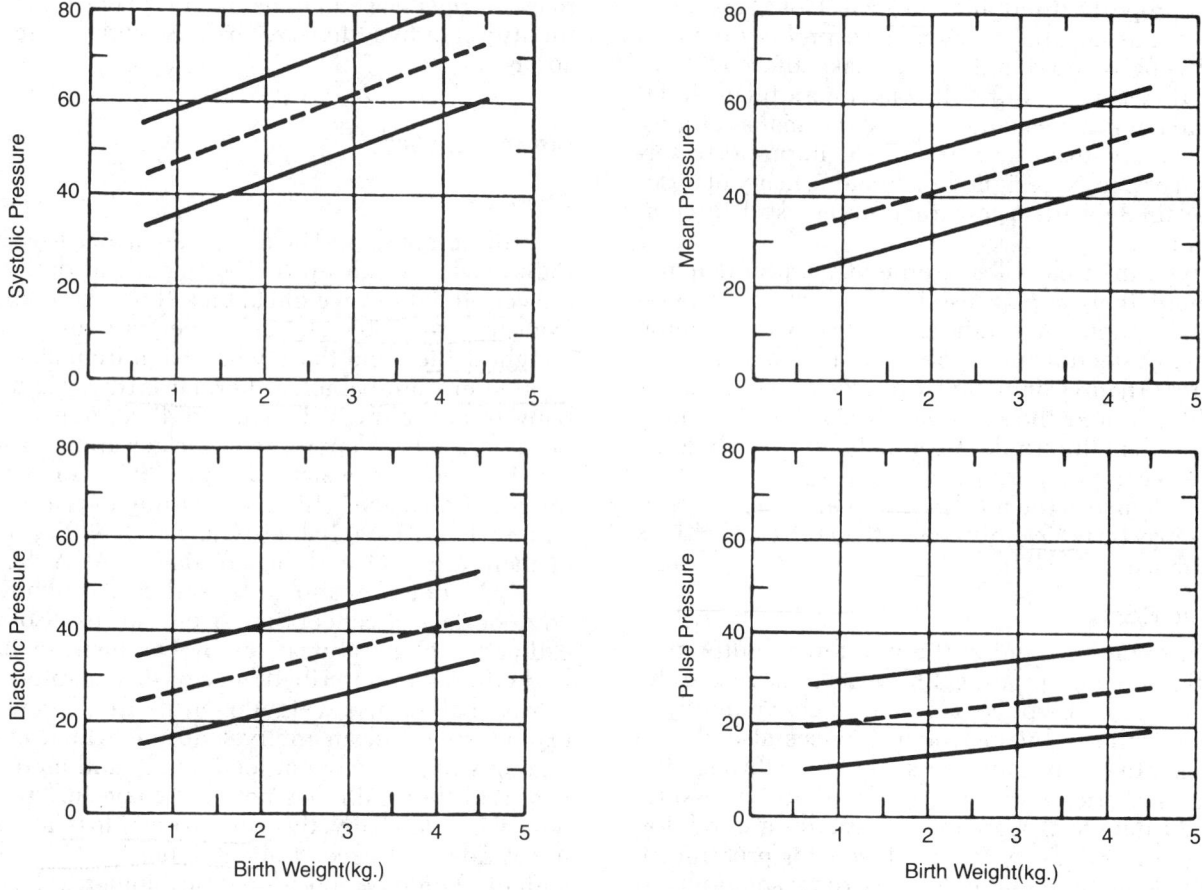

FIGURE 27–1.   Arterial blood pressure values in newborns. Aortic pressures obtained by catheterization of the umbilical artery in stable infants of various weights within 12 hours of birth. (From Versmold HT, Kitterman JA, Phibbs RH, et al: Aortic blood pressure during the first 12 hours of life in infants with birth weight 610 to 4220 grams. Pediatrics 67:607, 1981, with permission.)

enough to cause sucking blisters. Many are monitored invasively during labor and show electrode screw marks on the skin of the presenting part, usually but not always the vertex. Forceps marks often are seen on the face, external ear, and scalp, and vacuum extractor marks on the presenting part. Scalpel wounds sometimes are seen after cesarean deliveries. Ecchymoses are common on the scalp, face, neck, and extremities, especially in premature babies and after difficult or precipitous deliveries. Localized showers of petechiae suggest increased venous pressure, as may be found above a tight nuchal cord or in the presenting part. Inguinal petechiae are also common. Fixed petechial rashes must be distinguished from those that progress after delivery, because the latter suggest serious, evolving medical problems, such as sepsis, and not birth trauma. Nodular areas of subcutaneous fat necrosis occasionally are seen as early as the second day but more often are noticed after a week or so; they are most common at sites of trauma in large, difficult-to-deliver babies. A needle mark should be identified at the site of vitamin K administra-

tion. Meconium passed in utero may stain the skin and nails green.

Signs Correlated with Gestational Age

The skin of preterm babies is thin, smooth, and shiny; in particularly immature babies, the skin is translucent and almost gelatinous and is easily traumatized. The back, head, and even the face may be covered by a light growth of short, fine hairs called the lanugo.

The skin of freshly delivered full-term babies is pink, soft, and well supported by subcutaneous fat but still easily wrinkled, and it is covered with a waxy, yellowish–whitish paste of dead cells and sebum called the vernix caseosa, or, literally, the "cheesy varnish."

Post-term babies lose subcutaneous fat and vernix caseosa before birth and present as long, thin babies with loose, dry, already desquamating skin.

In full-term babies, desquamation typically begins after a physiologic reddening of the skin that starts within several hours of delivery and lasts several hours more. Livedo reticularis, a bluish mot-

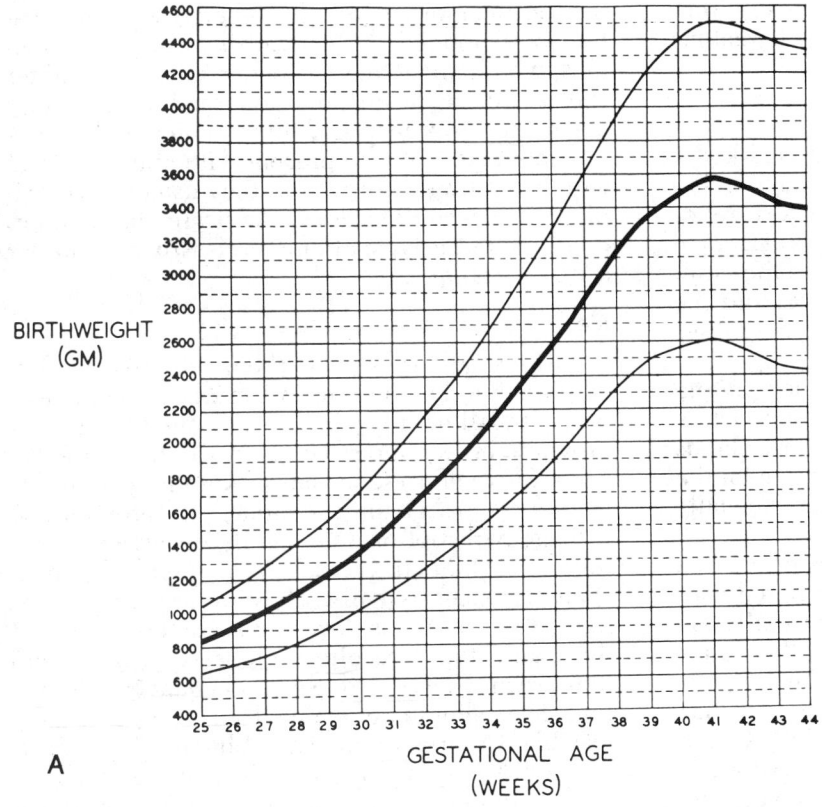

A

GESTATIONAL AGE
(WEEKS)

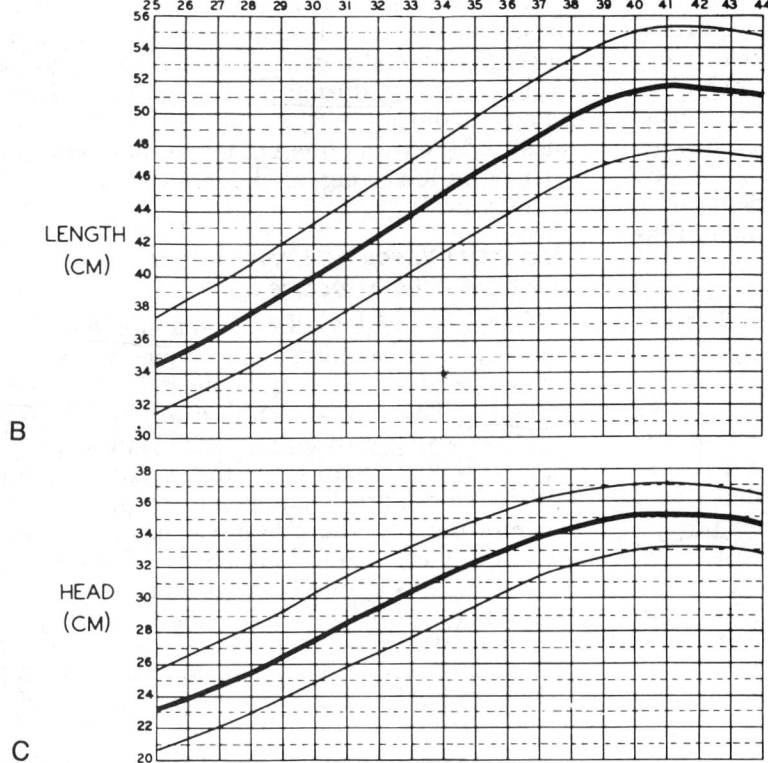

B

C

FIGURE 27–2. Intrauterine growth charts for live-born Caucasian infants at sea level: birth weight *(A)*, length *(B)*, and head circumference *(C)* (smoothed curves ± 2 standard deviations). (From Usher R, McLean F: Intrauterine growth of live-born Caucasian infants at sea level: Standards obtained from measurements in 7 dimensions of infants born between 25 and 44 weeks of gestation. J Pediatr 74:901, 1969, with permission.)

tling of the skin most prominent in a cool environment, also may follow this brief erythematous phase.

Appendages, Cysts, and Inclusions

Hair distribution and hair quality vary markedly in normal full-term newborns. Hypertrichosis, hypotrichosis, and abnormal appearance, texture, or morphology can be clues to the diagnosis of a range of congenital problems. Abnormalities in the other obvious skin appendages, the fingernails and the toenails, similarly can suggest specific diagnoses (Fanaroff and Martin, 1991).

Sweating is unusual during the first day, but facial sweating commonly is seen in warm or active babies by about the third day. Sebaceous glands are active in utero and continue to be active for the first few months or even the first few years; usually they then become dormant until puberty.

Tiny, firm, noninflammatory, yellowish–whitish keratogenous cysts very often are distributed over the forehead, nose, and cheeks. They usually are gone within the first month. Because they once brought to mind millet seeds scattered just below the surface of the skin, they were named "milia" (plural form of *milium*, Latin for millet). Other, quite different lesions carry the name "miliaria," from *febris miliarius*, meaning "miliary fever," because some of these lesions were thought to be inflammatory forms of milia. They are not. Miliaria crystallina, miliaria pustularis, and miliaria rubra are all disorders of sweat retention, the first characterized by delicate clear vesicles, the second by delicate cloudy vesicles, and the third by crops of small reddish papules. This third version is often identified as a heat rash. Miliaria occurs in skin folds and over the face and scalp, particularly in warm, humid conditions. It is less common in the neonatal period than later on.

Squamous cell inclusions can be found in several areas, including the prepuce, where they can be confused with pustules.

Pigmentary Lesions

Babies are born with a full complement of melanocytes, regardless of race, but they are lighter skinned than they will be in later childhood and adulthood. Bluish macular patches called *Mongolian spots* are common findings in most racial groups—oriental, black, American Indian, and Hispanic—and also sometimes are found in Caucasian babies. They routinely are seen in the lumbosacral area and usually disappear within a few years; Mongolian spots occurring elsewhere more likely may persist.

Café au lait spots, named for the color of coffee with cream, may be light to dark brown, depending on racial pigmentation. They are almost always inconsequential; small solitary spots are seen in as many as one fifth of normal newborns. Less dismissable are spots over 1.5 cm in length, spots numbering more than six, or otherwise unremarkable spots noticed in the company of axillary freckles, which are actually tiny versions of the larger spots. Any of these three abnormal settings suggests neurofibromatosis. Some babies with tuberous sclerosis likewise present with abnormal café au lait spotting patterns, but they usually also display white macules shaped classically like slender, nondigitated leaves, often more easily seen under a Wood's lamp.

Nevi

Various nevi are seen in the newborn. Congenital pigmented nevi occur in 1 to 2 per cent of newborns. Small nevi can be distinguished from other brown spots by their texture or by their uneven color. Some of these lesions may undergo transformation to malignant melanomas in later life, so management options should be discussed sometime in childhood. Giant hairy nevi must be managed more aggressively. They are much more disfiguring, sometimes covering substantial areas of the trunk; they are often intensely pruritic; and they are much more prone to malignant transformation. They should be removed as soon as surgically feasible. Compound nevi and blue nevi also occur and are less ominous, but still may be managed best by surgical removal. Epidermal nevi are hamartomas made up of epidermis and epidermal appendages. They present as verrucous nevi of warty appearance or as sebaceous nevi of waxy appearance. Epidermal nevi may degenerate into basal cell carcinomas during puberty and so should be removed during early adolescence. Many if not most babies with large epidermal nevi will prove to have serious congenital defects on thorough examination.

Abnormal Vascular, Lymphatic, or Erythropoietic Structures

Vascular macules called "salmon patches"—irregular, flat, blanching spots on the forehead, glabella, eyelids, or nape of the neck—are extremely common. They are transient capillary hemangiomas and usually disappear well within the first year, although marks on the neck, sometimes called "stork bites," may persist longer.

Unfortunately, the evocative term *nevus flammeus* or "flame nevus" has come to have two distinct uses. It is applied to transient capillary hemangiomas of the forehead, glabella, and eyelids, and it is also used as a synonym for "port-wine stain," a permanent lesion that may exist independently or may appear as part of an encephalofacial angiomatosis (i.e., Sturge-Weber syndrome) or as part of several other congenital syndromes (Fanaroff and Martin, 1991).

Cutaneous hemangiomas are capillary, cavernous, or mixed—the first kind constructed of dilated vessels superficially situated, the second containing blood-filled cavities deeper in the skin, and the third showing both features histologically and grossly. Most of the cutaneous hemangiomas diagnosed are superficial, looking like single ripe strawberries stuck to the skin, often on the face and more often in girls than in boys. Many others are subcutaneous, looking mushy, lumpy, and bluish red. Some are mixed, and some others are too deep to be detected except by palpation. Only about a quarter of the superficial lesions are apparent at birth (Tan and Gilchrest, 1988). A lumbar cutaneous hemangioma may indicate the otherwise entirely occult tethering of the spinal cord; magnetic resonance imaging should be considered (Albright et al., 1989).

Cutaneous lymphangiomas, like cutaneous hemangiomas, can be superficial or cavernous. Most need not be treated in the newborn period but eventually may require surgery, which is often unsuccessful. Cystic hygromas are large lymphangiomas, usually in the neck. They often compress the airway acutely and, for many reasons, are extremely difficult to manage.

Purplish subcutaneous nodules may represent intradermal erythropoiesis associated with intrauterine infection, particularly congenital rubella, or may indicate congenital metastatic neuroblastoma. A baby so affected often is referred to as a "blueberry muffin baby."

Macules, Papules, Pustules, and Vesicles

Erythema toxicum neonatorum is, despite its name, a benign condition. It is observed almost exclusively in full-term babies, coming on in the first several days in one third to two thirds of a nursery's population and lasting from a few hours to a few weeks. Erythema toxicum is characterized by irregular erythematous macules and yellowish papules and pustules, the latter packed with eosinophils. Any part of the skin surface, usually excepting the palms and soles, can be involved, and the general appearance is well described as "flea-bitten." Flare reactions to touch sometimes are observed, and dermatographia sometimes can be elicited, suggesting an increased level of histamine in the skin of affected babies. Similar rashes in adults might be expected to stimulate complaints of pruritus, but there is no evidence that newborns are distressed by this eruption.

Transient neonatal pustular melanosis is an idiopathic vesiculopustular condition of intrauterine onset in which primary vesiculopustules form and resolve quickly, leaving behind postinflammatory hyperpigmented macules, briefly surrounded by the scaly remnants of the original lesions. The vesiculopustules may form on any skin surface, including palms, soles, and scalp, but often congregate on the forehead, under the chin, and on the lower back. They remain intact no more than a few days, but the macules they leave behind fade over several months; therefore, macules usually predominate, even at birth. The primary lesions can be distinguished from common bacterial pustules by noting that they contain no conventionally stainable organisms. They may be distinguished from the pustules of erythema toxicum by noting the neutrophilic staining of their polymorphonuclear leukocytes; unlike the pustules of erythema toxicum, they contain few if any eosinophils. If first noticed in its postvesiculopustular stage, this condition may cause some confusion, because its freckles occasionally may be misidentified as petechiae. Careful search for and characterization of a remaining vesiculopustule should help diagnose late-recognized cases.

Papules, pustules, and vesicles may be seen in miliaria, as discussed earlier. The skin lesions of HSV infection can be confused with benign conditions (see Infectious Problems, later in this chapter).

Dimples, Pits, and Sinuses

Lumbosacral dimples and pits are common and normal. However, lumbosacral sinuses, which may look like dimples or pits, suggest serious underlying abnormalities. Similarly, when found in the lumbosacral area or along the dorsal midline, skin tags, hairy patches other than hairy nevi, and discolorations other than Mongolian spots should prompt consideration of occult craniospinal defects.

Other Findings

Many other abnormalities of the skin occur as isolated minor abnormalities, as parts of recognizable patterns of malformation, or as distinct entities, sometimes tragically impressive (see Chapter 40). Reference to specialized texts is encouraged.

Head

Shape and Sutures

Babies delivered vaginally from a vertex presentation have characteristically long, pointed heads. Different molding patterns correspond to different presentations; molding is unlikely if cesarean delivery has been accomplished before pelvic head engagement.

The sagittal, coronal, lambdoid, and frontal sutures should be palpated. The anterior and posterior fontanelles should be located and measured. The posterior fontanelle frequently is not palpable in term babies. Wide sutures and large fontanelles may be associated with prematurity, increased intracranial pressure or other serious intracranial pathology, or congenital hypothyroidism; as isolated findings, however, they may be normal. Fused sutures are not normal.

Fractures

Skull fractures are infrequent because the cranial plates are relatively unmineralized in early life and because their joining by fibrous sutures allows overriding. All fractures are more common after difficult deliveries. Small, linear fractures predominate. Depressed fractures, which are easy to see and feel, usually are associated with forceps application. Basilar fractures are more difficult to diagnose. They often present as shock because of severe intracranial bleeding.

Craniotabes

Craniotabes is a physical sign elicited by indenting a resilient cranial plate. Craniotabes is most often physiologic and needs no work-up, especially when found only at a plate's periphery. However, craniotabes can be a pathologic sign pointing to congenital syphilis (to which association it owes its name), osteogenesis imperfecta, or, in the older infant, rickets.

Caput Succedaneum

In vertex deliveries or cesarean deliveries achieved after engagement of the head, scalp edema may form a caput succedaneum, a boggy swelling often crossing suture lines and resolving spontaneously over a few days.

Cephalohematoma

Rupture of small, low-pressure subperiosteal vessels may produce a slowly enlarging cephalohematoma, a fluctuant outpouching of nondiscolored scalp confined within boundaries corresponding to suture lines. Cephalohematomas most often are found over the parietal bones but may appear over the occipital bone or even the frontal bones; they are typically single, but need not be. Boundaries may be surprisingly distinct and, later on, may even be ridge-like. Some physicians are made uneasy by their inability to palpate for a depressed skull fracture through a cephalohematoma, and about 1 in 20 cephalohematomas does indeed overlie a skull fracture, but these are almost always linear fractures needing no special treatment. More serious cranial and intracranial injuries may coexist with cephalohematomas, but, in otherwise normal babies, routine radiographic examination is hard to justify. However, some authorities do advocate follow-up radiographs at 4 to 6 weeks to look for evidence of leptomeningeal cyst formation (Fanaroff and Martin, 1991). Resorption of old blood may accentuate or prolong neonatal jaundice, and slowly resolving cephalohematomas may become infected. Infection is especially correlated with attempts at aspiration or surgical drainage, so these procedures should be reserved for strong diagnostic and therapeutic indications, respectively. Cephalohematomas resolve over 2 weeks to 3 months, often leaving newly formed bone at the margins of the elevated periosteum.

Face

In normal vertex deliveries, and especially when it has been the presenting part, the face can be bruised and abraded. It may display a petechial rash, reflecting functional obstruction to venous return from the skin and head during the second stage of labor, particularly if the umbilical cord has been wrapped tightly around the neck. Facial bones occasionally may have been fractured, and the cartilaginous nasal septum may have been dislocated, causing noisy respirations and even respiratory distress. Facial nerve palsies, best observed with crying, can follow either spontaneous or forceps-assisted deliveries but also can be atraumatic signs of Möbius's syndrome.

Many congenital disorders are first recognized by facial examination. The range and subtlety of facial signs defy summary, but a "normal facies" can be distinguished from an "abnormal facies" by any systematic observer.

Ears

The external ears are apt to be traumatized during forceps application or traction. Hematomas must be evacuated to prevent "cauliflower" deformities of the cartilage.

The helix of the ear normally joins the scalp at a point on a horizontal line drawn from the lateral angle of the eye. Low position and posterior rotation of the ears may result jointly from premature arrest of tissue migration in embryonic life. Low-set, posteriorly rotated ears are often also small or malformed or "simplified."

Preauricular tags or pits can be associated with other specific abnormalities, but they are usually isolated findings in otherwise normal babies. Some preauricular pits can be the ostia of sinus tracts liable to become infected chronically in later life.

Abnormalities of the external ear should raise suspicions about ear canal patency and middle ear and inner ear function, and, sometimes, renal function.

The tympanic membrane often is obscured by vernix and debris and usually is not worth examining in otherwise normal newborns. If examination is indicated, some peculiarities should be kept in mind. The pinna should be retracted inferiorly and posteriorly to straighten the ear canal, not superiorly and posteriorly as in older children. The tympanic membrane is whitish gray, not pearly gray; it is normally opaque, not translucent; and it is normally highly vascular—which is to say that it looks edematous and injected by the standards of later childhood. Pneumo-otoscopy, which allows the examiner of older children to "palpate" the tympanic membrane visually, is less helpful in the newborn because the more pliable canal walls expand and collapse with induced oscillations of air pressure, dampening the effect on the membrane and even obscuring it physically.

Hearing testing is possible in the newborn both by direct, nontechnical, behavioral means and by various technologically sophisticated means. Newborns who have been sick, especially those exposed to ototoxic or neurotoxic infectious agents or drugs, should be evaluated formally for hearing loss before or shortly after going home, as should babies with family histories of sensorineural hearing loss.

Eyes

Comprehensive Versus Noncomprehensive Examination

In babies in whom nonocular congenital abnormalities already have been noticed or in whom intrauterine infection has been suspected or birth-related ocular trauma discovered, examination of the eyes should be comprehensive. Otherwise, noncomprehensive examination is reasonable and can be performed with just a few routines and maneuvers. Gross appearance, ocular size, position, symmetry, and extraocular details, such as palpebral fissure angle, should be noted. Behavioral reaction to light or visual stimulus and pupillary reaction to light should be elicited. Anisocoria up to 1.0 mm is not unusual in newborns, and pupillary response is quite inconsistent before 32 weeks' gestational age (Isenberg et al., 1989). Gross functional integrity of the extraocular muscles may be confirmed by simple observation or by passive motion of the head. Congenital strabismus and nonphysiologic nystagmus are important findings. Conjunctival inflammation (common after prophylaxis for ophthalmia neonatorum) and conjunctival hemorrhage (common after vaginal delivery) should be recorded. Corneal size and clarity and defects of iris circularity or coloration should be noted. The pupil should be black on direct illumination and red when examined through an ophthalmoscope. The retina need not be examined in detail in the apparently normal baby.

Cornea, Lens, Vitreous, and Fundus

Normal corneas may be a bit cloudy for the first few days, more so in premature infants. Persistent cloudiness or marked cloudiness associated with an enlarged cornea should bring congenital glaucoma forcefully to mind. Suspect eyes must be examined by an ophthalmologist as soon as possible.

A cataract may be idiopathic; may be a sign of a genetic or inborn metabolic disease, intrauterine infection, or other congenital syndrome; or may be the result of trauma. Early evaluation is the key to preservation of sight. A cataract always should raise the possibility of congenital rubella or congenital cytomegalovirus infection.

Ectopia lentis, or dislocation of the lens, is often a sign of a recognizable syndrome or a sign of trauma.

Retinoblastoma, the most common malignant neonatal eye tumor, is well known as a cause of leukokoria and secondary glaucoma, but it often presents less strikingly. The opportunity to detect a premetastatic retinoblastoma should be a chief inducement to routine ophthalmoscopic examination.

Leukokoria, or white pupil, is easily noted in an alert newborn and always indicates an abnormality of the lens, vitreous, or fundus, fundus being the joint term for retina and choroid. However, the abnormalities to which diagnosis of leukokoria is such an obvious clue often do not in fact produce a grossly white pupil. Therefore, a quick ophthalmoscopic examination must be performed on every newborn. Primary description of an abnormal finding should note the level at which it comes into ophthalmoscopic focus: cornea, iris, lens, vitreous, or fundus (see Chapter 47).

Sclera

The sclera is normally bluish white to white in full-term newborns. The underdeveloped sclera of premature babies is more noticeably blue, as is the collagen-deficient sclera found in osteogenesis imperfecta, Marfan's syndrome, Ehlers-Danlos syndrome, and Crouzon's syndrome. Various scleral pigmentary abnormalities may occur as isolated defects.

Iris

Aniridia, or absence of the iris, unilateral or bilateral, may be associated with significant visual problems. It also may be associated with Wilms' tumor and, therefore, should prompt vigorous investigation.

Iris coloboma, an eccentric iris defect usually found in the inferonasal quadrant, is the most common congenital eye defect; it may or may not be associated with other eye defects or somatic syndromes.

Lid

Lid coloboma is a notchlike or larger defect of the eyelid. Some lid colobomas preclude full coverage of the cornea and must be repaired surgically.

Lid masses easily should be classifiable as hemangiomas, lymphangiomas, neurofibromas, or dermoid cysts, and they should be managed accordingly. Dermoid cysts are benign lesions found at the closure sites of embryonic clefts, typically in the lateral eyebrow or upper lid but sometimes occultly within the orbit itself. External dermoid cysts are firm, pea-like masses attached to the underlying periosteum but unattached to the overlying skin. Because dermoid cysts may connect to the cranial, orbital, or sinus cavities, some authorities urge radiographic studies of the involved area. However, most experienced clinicians regard dermoid cysts of the brow or eyelid as incidental findings of little consequence.

Lid droop, or ptosis, if unilateral, suggests Horner's syndrome. In post-traumatic Horner's syndrome, iris pigmentation, to whatever extent it may be established at birth, should match bilaterally. If Horner's syndrome has developed in utero, as it might in the case of a congenital mediastinal neuroblastoma, for instance, ipsilateral iris pigmentation may not be occurring normally, and heterochromia may be apparent. Heterochromia also may be found in aganglionic megacolon (Hirschsprung's disease). Bilateral ptosis is more suggestive of a neonatal myasthenia gravis syndrome or abnormal innervation of both levator palpebrae superioris muscles.

Nose

The newborn should be considered an obligate nose breather, although this nasal obligation is not absolute. Traumatic dislocations of the nasal septum sometimes can cause respiratory distress and can be reduced by lifting the nares with cotton swabs bilaterally or simply by grasping and lifting the nose with the fingers. Choanal atresia should be suspected in the otherwise normal but persistently stridorous or tachypneic infant and in the infant whose central cyanosis improves, rather than worsens, with crying. Nasal patency can be demonstrated indirectly in various ways—listening in a quiet room or fogging a cool mirror—and directly by passage of a no. 8 French catheter into the nasopharynx. Dogged pursuit of subtle findings may result in an iatrogenic obstruction caused by traumatic mucosal swelling. True congenital nasal stenosis usually can be managed nonsurgically with temporary nasopharyngeal intubation (Leiberman et al., 1992).

Rhinorrhea is unusual early in the newborn period, and its differential diagnosis is not what it will be later on in life. Cerebrospinal fluid rhinorrhea can be a sign of basilar skull fracture. Syphilitic rhinitis, called "snuffles," can be present shortly after birth in transplacentally infected babies, although it more commonly presents after a few days to a few weeks or months; snuffling discharge should be considered potentially infective. Excoriating discharge from a saddle-shaped nose is a classic image that always should prompt consideration of congenital syphilis.

Bleeding from the newborn nose is almost always secondary to traumatic suctioning, sometimes performed reflexively by nursery staff in babies who sneeze, as babies do physiologically. Absent any sign of mucosal trauma, investigation should include confirmation of vitamin K administration and, perhaps, a platelet count.

The nose is deformed in many congenital syndromes.

Jaw, Lip, Palate, Mouth, Tongue, and Oropharynx

Intrauterine molding of the jaw is common, a shoulder-shaped concavity being the usual sign. Affected babies may rest their heads toward the molded side preferentially.

Micrognathia, or very small jaw, is found in many syndromes. The Pierre Robin malformation complex is composed of micrognathia, glossoptosis, and a high-arched palate or U-shaped cleft palate. These babies may have serious difficulty breathing and nursing.

Cleft deformities range from isolated lip pitting and lip notching to isolated cleft of the upper lip or the palate to bilateral clefts of the upper lip extending through to the nose and combined with cleft palate. Bifid uvula suggests a submucous cleft of the hard palate. A gloved finger should be placed in the mouth in all babies to feel for a submucous cleft, whether or not the uvula is bifid.

Several intraoral lesions are fairly common. Natal teeth, usually lower central incisors, can interfere with nursing and can be aspirated when shed. They also can be signs of broader congenital problems (Leung, 1986). Ranulas are bluish sublingual salivary retention cysts that may need to be aspirated if they interfere with nursing. Lymphangiomas of the alveolar ridges, except for their location, look much the same; they usually regress. Bohn's nodules are nonmidline cysts of the hard palate or cysts of the alveolar ridges. Epstein's pearls, epithelial rests in the midline of the hard palate, are routine findings.

Macroglossia is seen in congenital hypothyroidism and various congenital syndromes, including mucopolysaccharidoses and Beckwith's syndrome. The frenulum normally attaches nearly at the tip of the tongue; parents may need reassurance that the tongue does not have to be "untied" by frenulectomy.

Excessive oropharyngeal secretions may suggest a high gastrointestinal blockage, such as esophageal atresia.

Neck

Clavicular fractures (Joseph and Rosenfeld, 1990) are commonly of the greenstick variety, in which case they may be overlooked pending callus formation, but they also may be complete, in which case deformity and discoloration may be obvious and crepitus elicitable. The Moro reflex may be asymmetrical in the presence of clavicular fracture. Another important sign of neck trauma is seen not in the neck but in the arm: brachial plexus injury.

There are three patterns of brachial plexus injury. Only one, the Duchenne-Erb palsy of the upper arm, is common; it is caused by injury to cervical roots five and six. Babies with brachial plexus injuries sometimes also have sustained ipsilateral phrenic nerve injuries. Radiographic examination is recommended.

A firm, fusiform fibrous mass is sometimes found in the belly of one sternocleidomastoid muscle at birth or several weeks thereafter. Such masses traditionally have been assumed to be organizing or fibrosed traumatic hematomas, but this view no longer seems fully satisfactory. At any rate, this mass is associated with torticollis (Latin for "twisted neck"), whose common cosmetic result is wryneck and whose more extreme consequence is distortion of the face and skull. Early institution of physical therapy is advisable and can prove an adequate remedy, but parents also should be introduced to the idea that surgical resection may be needed within the first year.

Branchial cleft cysts also present in the area of the sternocleidomastoids. Cystic hygromas are large lymphangiomas arising in the anterior triangle of the neck. They can compress the airway acutely and often require complicated surgical and medical interventions during prolonged hospitalizations. Thyroglossal duct cysts present in the midline, as do congenital goiters.

The involution of ectatic lymphatic vessels results in webbing of the neck, a sign of several congenital syndromes, including Turner's, Noonan's, Klippel-Feil, and trisomies 18 and 21.

Nipples and Breasts

Supernumerary nipples occur in 2 to 3 per cent of newborns. They are found along the milk line from above the true breast toward the inguinal canal. They usually do not overlie breast tissue. Extra nipples are associated with renal anomalies; however, the association is a weak one in otherwise normal babies and in babies with recognizable malformations not independently associated with renal lesions (Hersh et al., 1987; Kenney et al., 1987).

Breast tissue may be present and may even excrete small amounts of milk ("witch's milk") if squeezed. Neonatal breast hypertrophy is a normal response to maternal hormone secretion; it may persist for weeks to months. If squeezed frequently, functioning neonatal breasts may more easily become infected and abscessed and, if abscessed, scarred. Parents should know that ignoring this oddity will hasten its resolution (Madlon-Kay, 1986).

Chest

Inspection of the chest has been discussed earlier.

Palpation of the chest is performed as it would be in an adult patient except that the hand must be applied to several areas of interest at once. Abnormal cardiac pulsations, including thrills, should be noted.

Percussion is useful only for the assessment of gross pathology, such as pneumothorax, effusion, or diaphragmatic hernia; newborn heart borders cannot be located easily by percussion.

Auscultation of the chest demonstrates shallow respirations punctuated by deep, noisy sighs and preponderantly tubular breath sounds transmitted through a thin chest wall. Localizing findings to a particular lobe is difficult. During transition from intrauterine to extrauterine life, retained lung fluid and still-unopened alveoli are associated with fine crepitant rales and some rhonchi, and flow through the ductus arteriosus may produce a characteristic murmur. The heart sounds should be identified and an attempt made to note splitting of the second sound; normal splitting is a good indicator of normal pulmonary circulation.

See also Respiratory Problems, later in this chapter.

Cardiovascular System

See Chapter 35; see also Chest earlier and Arterial Pulses and Cardiovascular Problems later in this chapter.

Abdomen

A warm-handed examiner can assess a sleeping or sucking newborn's abdomen quickly. Placing the nondominant hand behind the baby's flank allows bimanual examination. Alternatively, the hips can be flexed by lifting the ankles, and it is sometimes helpful to flex the spine by lifting the baby's neck and shoulders with the nonexamining hand. In an agitated baby, the examiner will have to divide the palpation between periods of inspiration when tension of the abdominal musculature relaxes momentarily; to take best advantage of these intervals, the hand simply should rest in the area of interest until a deep breath softens the belly.

Normal findings may include a smooth, soft liver edge several centimeters below the right costal margin; rarely, a spleen tip just within the left costal margin; vaguely palpable kidneys within the retroperitoneal wall; and a small bladder above the symphysis. Pathologic abdominal masses are mostly of renal and adrenal origin: horseshoe kidney, pelvic kidney, polycystic kidney, multicystic kidney, duplicated kidney, postobstructive hydronephrotic kidney, Wilms' tumor, neuroblastoma, and adrenal hemorrhage. Other lesions, such as choledochal cyst, also are found.

A stomach bubble may be felt, as may air-filled

loops of bowel. Peristalsis may be observed, especially shortly after birth and in babies with thin abdominal walls. When air in a viscus causes concern, well-organized bowel sounds can be reassuring; re-examination in an hour or two often will demonstrate a change in pattern. The rectum must be inspected for patency and the day sheet checked to confirm passage of meconium; virtually all normal full-term babies will have passed a meconium stool by the end of their first 24 hours, while premature babies may take much longer (Verma and Dhanireddy, 1993). A gloved, short-nailed fifth finger can examine a well-lubricated rectum safely up to several centimeters if necessary and may stimulate passage of a meconium plug. The stools of low-birth-weight babies and babies identified as ill often will be tested routinely for the presence of occult blood; occult hematochezia is surprisingly common in these babies and is usually not a sign of necrotizing enterocolitis (Abramo et al., 1988).

Emesis and excessive salivation may indicate gastrointestinal obstruction, especially in the setting of gestational polyhydramnios. To confirm esophageal patency, a feeding tube can be passed into the stomach and its presence confirmed by auscultation of injected air and by cross-table lateral radiography. (These maneuvers can confirm esophageal patency but cannot by themselves confirm tracheoesophageal integrity.) If an unexpectedly large amount of stomach fluid is found—over 30 mL in a full-term baby—an upper gastrointestinal obstruction is likely, whether functional, as with an ileus, or mechanical. The source of bloody stomach fluid—swallowed maternal blood or gastrointestinal bleeding—can be differentiated by an Apt test.

Umbilicus

The clamped cord once again should be inspected to confirm the presence of two arteries and one vein. Finding a single umbilical artery should prompt further investigation, particularly renal ultrasonography; in about one half of these babies, at least one additional congenital malformation can be identified (Leung and Robson, 1989). Rarely, a patent urachus or a severed loop of herniated bowel can be present in the umbilical stump; cord clamping makes discharge from these structures unlikely and careful inspection more critical. Mild erythema of the periumbilical skin is physiologic; frank erythema, classically in a triangular area above the umbilicus, purulent discharge, and putrid odor are signs of omphalitis. Necrotizing funisitis, an inflammation in the umbilical cord matrix, recently has been re-recognized as a specific indicator of congenital syphilis; the "barber pole" cord, its classic presentation, should prompt immediate precautions (Fojaco et al., 1989). Umbilical

herniation of various degree is common and is occasionally part of a recognizable syndrome. More striking errors in abdominal wall development require emergent fluid resuscitation, sterile regimen, and urgent surgical consultation; these include gastroschisis, a failure of closure on the right side of the umbilicus; omphalocele, a herniation of peritoneum-covered intra-abdominal contents, frequently malformed; and exstrophy of the bladder. Diastasis recti, manifested during crying by a midline abdominal outpouching, is normal and is not a mild form of failure of abdominal wall closure.

Genitalia, Perineum, and Inguinal Regions

Almost all babies urinate within the first 24 hours. A dry diaper should prompt a look at the nursery day sheet; if urination has not been recorded, the examiner should repeat the abdominal examination to check bladder and kidney size.

On removing the baby's diaper, the examiner may notice a reddish stain at the point of urination. This is usually just a "red brick dust" stain caused by uric acid crystals; a Hematest or guaiac test should be negative. Later on, vicarious menstruation may stain the diaper in girls. Like red brick dust staining, vicarious menstruation is physiologic.

The inguinal regions and the scrotum or labia majora should be checked for masses and indirect hernias. Inguinal hernias are more common in premature babies.

In males, inguinal herniation may be associated with cryptorchidism or with a hydrocele. Descended testicles may retract into the inguinal canal when cold or when examined. They usually can be coaxed back into the scrotum for examination. True bilateral cryptorchidism immediately raises doubts as to genotypic sex. Fluctuant, translucent scrotal masses are hydroceles, often bilateral. Most congenital hydroceles, as opposed to hydroceles of later onset, resolve spontaneously and do not indicate a coexistent inguinal hernia. Nontransilluminating scrotal masses may represent tumors or testicular torsion. Hypospadias comes in three degrees: first, urethral opening low on the ventral glans; second, urethral opening on the ventral penile shaft; third, urethral opening on the perineum at the base of the shaft. Epispadias exists when the urethra opens onto the dorsal surface of the shaft; epispadias is rare in otherwise normal babies. Circumcision should not be performed if the urethral meatus is not in the normal position because prepuce skin will be needed for surgical repair.

In females, the ovary may herniate into the labia majora, where there is some risk of its infarction. In the testicular feminization syndrome, an inguinal mass in a phenotypic female may in fact be a testicle. A vaginal tag may protrude from between the labia majora in normal females. A mucoid vaginal secretion is normal. Apparently, all otherwise normally formed females have hymens (Jenny et al., 1987; Mor and Merlob, 1988). Hydrometrocolpos presents as a white mass protruding from between the labia majora; spontaneous rupture or surgical incision releases the retained fluid. Ambiguous genitalia must be described carefully and formal sex-determination procedures undertaken as soon as possible.

Arterial Pulses

Meticulous palpation of the femoral triangles almost always locates femoral arterial pulses. Frustrated examiners sometimes find it reassuring to check arterial pulses in the lower legs before resuming their search. Once located, the femoral arteries must be palpated in simultaneous comparison to the brachial arteries, because "congenital" coarctation of the aorta may not yet be expressed fully (Ward et al., 1990). A baby's first complete physical examination should occur within 24 hours of birth; during this period, the ductus arteriosus still may be patent. A baby who ultimately will be recognized as having coarctation of the aorta in fact may have palpable femoral pulses on first examination either because blood still flows freely through the patent ductus or because the old distal opening of the now-closed ductus still distorts the aortic lumen just enough to allow blood temporarily to squirt around the impending coarctation (Thoele et al., 1987). Femoral arterial pulses may seem decreased only when compared with the brachial arterial pulse. Babies whose coarctations are proximal to the ductus may have full femoral arterial flow thanks to persistent ductal patency, but these babies should be recognizable on the basis of other findings.

Skeleton and Extremities

The examiner should assure himself or herself that the baby can move all extremities actively. Gross deformities and the effects of molding should be noted. Fixed joint deformities should be differentiated from passively reducible deformities.

Fracture of the clavicle, described earlier, is common; so is fracture of the humerus. Supernumerary digits, usually on the hands and more common in blacks than in whites, may or may not contain bone. If they do contain bone, their management requires orthopedic consultation; if not, they can be tied off with a ligature and left to necrose and shed. Constriction bands arising from a ruptured amnion may compromise an extremity; occasionally, an amniotic band still may be found at a constriction site.

Examination of skeleton and extremities probably could be carried out adequately by inspection alone were it not for the hips. Examination of the hip joints requires that the examiner perform Ortolani's reduction maneuver and Barlow's dislocation maneuver (Fig. 27–3). Very frequently, hip "clicks" stimulate requests for radiographic and orthopedic consultations. As in adults, clicks are caused by the movement of articular and periarticular parts, but the "clunks" attending subluxation and rearticulation are felt easily and often even grossly visible. Dislocatable hips often are missed on first examination; a predischarge re-examination of the hips should be routine (Jones, 1989; Moss et al., 1991), but positive examinations should not be repeated excessively because damage to the articular cartilage can result. Hip real-time ultrasonography of all "high-risk" babies—those with family histories of congenital displasia of the hip, birth histories of breech presentation or oligohydramnios, or observed postural abnormalities—has been described as potentially cost-effective (Walter et al., 1992). Management options vary (Burger et al., 1990) (see Chapter 38).

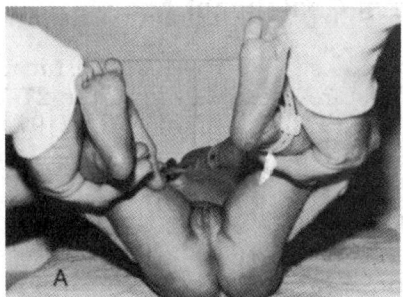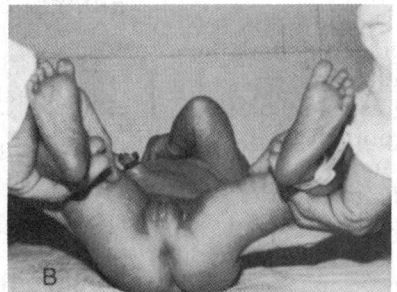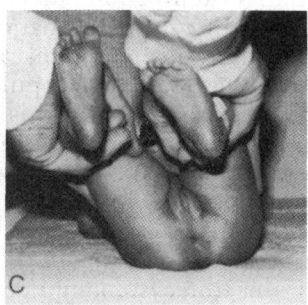

FIGURE 27–3. Screening examination for congenital dislocation of the hip. *A,* Initial position. *B,* Ortolani's reduction maneuver. *C,* Barlow's dislocation maneuver. (Adapted from Asher MA: Screening for congenital dislocation of the hip, scoliosis, and other abnormalities affecting the musculoskeletal system. Pediatr Clin North Am 33:1335, 1986.)

TABLE 27–2. FUNCTION AND TESTING OF THE CRANIAL NERVES

Cranial Nerve	Name	Function and Testing
I	Olfactory	Smell—not tested. May use peppermint to stimulate sucking or an arousal–withdrawal response.
II	Optic	Vision—tested by blink response to light and by visual fixation with eyes following brightly colored object or examiner's face.
III IV VI	Oculomotor Trochlear Abducens	Control pupillary response to light (III) and extraocular muscle movements (III, IV, and VI). Latter may be tested by observing spontaneous eye movements or movements elicited by turning head from side to side (doll's eye maneuver).
V	Trigeminal	Sensory component displayed by rooting reflex and eye blink reflex. Strength of masseter and pterygoid muscles is assessed best by evaluation of suck and biting (motor V).
VII	Facial	Evaluated by carefully noting presence of nasolabial folds and position and movement of corners of mouth. Facial expressions are under control of VII.
VIII	Auditory	Vestibular component tested by rotating infant clockwise or counterclockwise and simultaneously noting that eyes turn in direction of rotation. Auditory component may be demonstrated by startle response to loud sound or simply speaking into one ear and noting infant's head turn toward voice.
IX	Glossopharyngeal	Tongue movement and taste—tested by gagging infant with tongue blade and noting normal midline positioning of uvula.
X	Vagus	Evaluated by noting normal cry and autonomic visceral functions.
XI	Accessory	Controls sternocleidomastoid muscle. Can be tested by observing the head move from side to side.
XII	Hypoglossal	Controls tongue movement. Tested by simply observing tongue thrusting and tongue movements when inspecting oropharynx.

From Coen RW, Koffler H: Primary Care of the Newborn. Boston, Little, Brown, 1987, p. 45; adapted from Volpe JJ: Neurology of the Newborn, Philadelphia, WB Saunders Company, 1981, with permission.

Neurologic System

As stressed earlier, sophisticated, systematic inspection satisfies most requirements of the neurologic examination.

Function and testing of the cranial nerves are summarized in Table 27–2.

Deep tendon reflexes should be elicited at the biceps, knee, and ankle. Ankle clonus should be unsustained, although it sometimes may be surprisingly prolonged in clearly normal babies. Stroking the side of the mouth should stimulate a turning of the head toward the stimulus. Suck should be strong in alert babies.

The Moro and startle reflexes are elicited by physical shocks and sudden changes in support, such as first lifting slightly and then dropping one end of the examining table; the baby reaches out the arms and hands and then grasps in a manner recalling a lower primate offspring trying to regain a grip on its running mother's underbelly.

Placing a finger on the palm should elicit the palmar grasp reflex; the trunk and sometimes the head of a normal baby can be pulled off the examining table on the strength of this grasp. The plantar grasp reflex is more difficult to appreciate.

On picking up the baby, tone and head control should be noted. Holding the infant up under the chest and belly, the examiner should run a finger along either side of the back; the baby should squirm, the trunk becoming concave on the side of the stimulus.

The Babinski reflex, important in assessing upper motor neuron damage in older children and adults, is not reliable in newborns.

Seizure activity in newborns is more often tonic or clonic than tonic–clonic and is often subtle. Typical newborn seizures include abnormal movements or changes in tone in the trunk or extremities and rhythmic or tonic activity of the muscles innervated by the cranial nerves. The range of presentations includes—but is certainly not limited to—posturing, sucking or chewing, tonic deviation of the eyes or batting of the eyelids, bicycling movements of the legs, rhythmic twitching, and even apnea.

Depressed infants may have been devastated neurologically during the birth process, or they may be showing the effects of maternal analgesia or anesthesia. Other seemingly depressed babies actually may be hypotonic, suffering from a myasthenic syndrome or a motor neuron disease. Highly agitated infants may be withdrawing from intrauterine habituation to a psychoactive drug.

Estimation of Gestational Age

Dubowitz et al.'s (1970) criteria for estimation of gestational age are presented in Table 27–3 and Figures 27–4 and 27–5. Ballard et al.'s (1979) simplified criteria are presented in Figure 27–6.

ROUTINES FOR THE FIRST FEW DAYS

Observation, Stabilization, and Screening

The baby's physiologic transition period extends for many hours or even several days; it is made

**TABLE 27–3. DUBOWITZ CRITERIA FOR ESTIMATION OF GESTATIONAL AGE:
EXTERNAL PHYSICAL FINDINGS**

External Sign	Score*				
	0	1	2	3	4
Edema	Obvious edema of hands and feet; pitting over tibia	No obvious edema of hands and feet; pitting over tibia	No edema		
Skin texture	Very thin, gelatinous	Thin and smooth	Smooth; medium thickness; rash or superficial peeling	Slight thickening; superficial cracking and peeling, especially of hands and feet	Thick and parchment-like; superficial or deep cracking
Skin color	Dark red	Uniformly pink	Pale pink; variable over body	Pale; only pink over ears, lips, palms, or soles	
Skin opacity (trunk)	Numerous veins and venules clearly seen, especially over abdomen	Veins and tributaries seen	A few large vessels clearly seen over abdomen	A few large vessels seen indistinctly over abdomen	No blood vessels seen
Lanugo (over back)	No lanugo	Abundant; long and thick over whole back	Hair thinning, especially over lower back	Small amount of lanugo and bald areas	At least half of back devoid of lanugo
Plantar creases	No skin creases	Faint red marks over anterior half of sole	Definite red marks over > anterior half; indentations over < anterior third	Indentations over > anterior third	Definite deep indentations over > anterior third
Nipple formation	Nipple barely visible, no areola	Nipple well defined; areola smooth and flat, diameter < 0.75 cm	Areola stippled, edge not raised, diameter < 0.75 cm	Areola stippled, edge raised, diameter > 0.75 cm	
Breast size	No breast tissue palpable	Breast tissue on one or both sides, < 0.5 cm diameter	Breast tissue on both sides, one or both 0.5–1.0 cm	Breast tissue on both sides, one or both > 1 cm	
Ear form	Pinna flat and shapeless, little or no incurving of edge	Incurving of part of edge of pinna	Partial incurving of whole of upper pinna	Well-defined incurving of whole of upper pinna	
Ear firmness	Pinna soft, easily folded, no recoil	Pinna soft, easily folded, slow recoil	Cartilage to edge of pinna but soft in places, ready recoil	Pinna firm, cartilage to edge, instant recoil	
Genitals: Male	Neither testis in scrotum	At least one testis high in scrotum	At least one testis right down		
Genitals: Female (with hips half abducted)	Labia majora widely separated, labia minora protruding	Labia majora almost cover labia minora	Labia majora completely cover labia minora		

* For scoring, see legend of Figure 27–5.
From Dubowitz LM, Dubowitz V, Goldberg C: Clinical assessment of gestational age in the newborn infant. J Pediatr 77:1, 1970; adapted from Farr V, Kerridge DF, Mitchell RG: The definition of some external characteristics used in the assessment of gestational age of the newborn infant. Develop Med Child Neurol 8:507, 1966, with permission.

smoother by the maintenance of a neutral thermal environment. During the early transition period, vital signs should be checked hourly until stable. Ophthalmia neonatorum prophylaxis and vitamin K should be administered. Several routine laboratory studies—blood glucose, hematocrit, and thyroid-stimulating hormone—should be performed on a lateral heel stick capillary blood sample. Phe-

nylalanine level, also performed on a heel stick sample, must follow the digestion of a milk feeding and therefore would be meaningless if collected immediately after delivery. Other studies already should have been run on cord blood dispatched from the delivery room: blood type and Coombs' test, a syphilis test, hemoglobin electrophoresis, and, at the physician's discretion, immunoglobulin

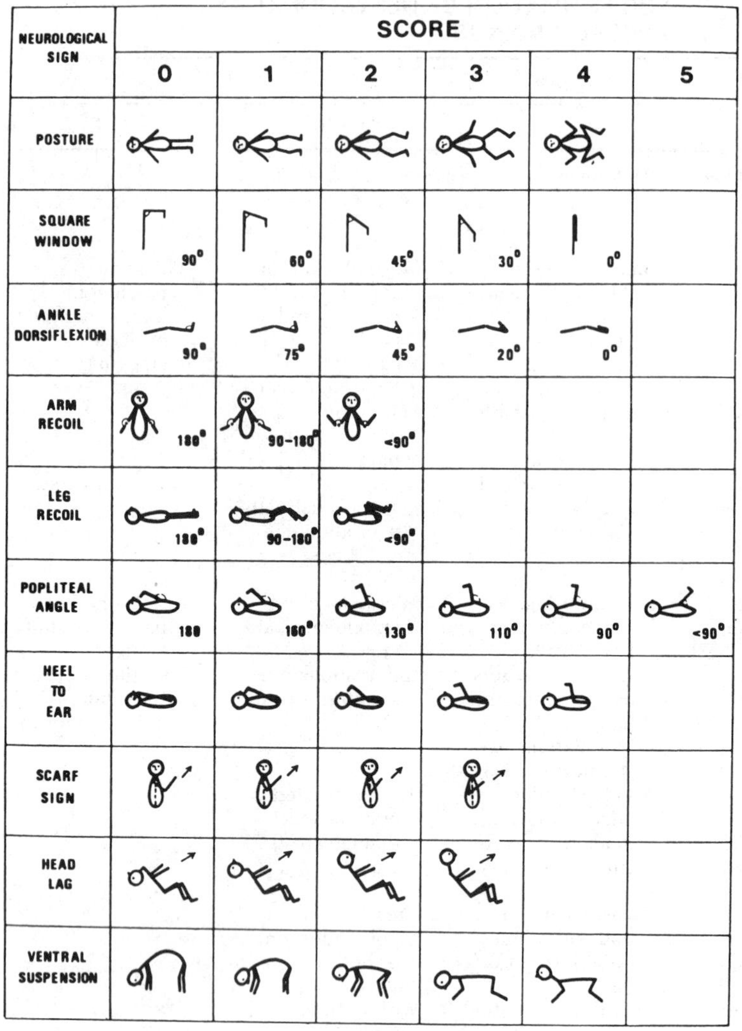

NEUROLOGICAL SIGN	SCORE					
	0	1	2	3	4	5
POSTURE						
SQUARE WINDOW	90°	60°	45°	30°	0°	
ANKLE DORSIFLEXION	90°	75°	45°	20°	0°	
ARM RECOIL	180°	90–180°	<90°			
LEG RECOIL	180°	90–180°	<90°			
POPLITEAL ANGLE	180	160°	130°	110°	90°	<90°
HEEL TO EAR						
SCARF SIGN						
HEAD LAG						
VENTRAL SUSPENSION						

FIGURE 27–4. Dubowitz criteria for estimation of gestational age: neurological and neuromuscular findings. (Adapted from Dubowitz LM, Dubowitz V, Goldberg C: Clinical assessment of gestational age in the newborn infant. J Pediatr 77:1, 1970; and Amiel-Tison C: Neurological evaluation of the maturity of newborn infants. Arch Dis Child 43:89, 1968.)

(Ig) M level. Further discussion of these and additional tests routinely or frequently run on presumably normal newborns will appear later in this chapter under Postnatal Screening. Routine body surface cultures yield no useful information (Evans et al., 1988).

Bathing

Preservation of the vernix caseosa makes good sense; it protects the skin from drying and is somewhat bacteriocidal. However, its virtues are lost on most families, who usually think it unclean and unsightly, especially when mixed with maternal blood. So, after stabilization in a neutral thermal environment, the baby may be bathed with warm, freshly drawn, standing water. Bathing in running water is unwise, because it encourages observant mothers to adopt the practice at home, where inattention to changing water temperature may result in burns, some severe. Soap (Morelli and Weston, 1987) is not necessary, except to suppress a documented nursery epidemic, such as bullous dermatitis or periumbilical cellulitis. Immersion above the umbilicus should be avoided until the umbilical stump has sloughed and the umbilicus has become covered in granulation tissue.

Umbilical Cord Care

The umbilical cord stump may become colonized with pathogenic bacteria—typically streptococci, *Staphlococcus aureus,* and coliforms—and may provide access for such organisms to the umbilicus itself, to the umbilical vein, to the anterior abdominal wall, and to the systemic circulation. It is advisable, therefore, to encourage drying and to apply to the stump an antiseptic agent, such as triple dye, despite its limited effectiveness (Rosenfeld et al., 1990), or alcohol or an antibiotic ointment.

First Feeding

An "artificial" first feeding is a modern nursery tradition difficult to displace. Two justifications

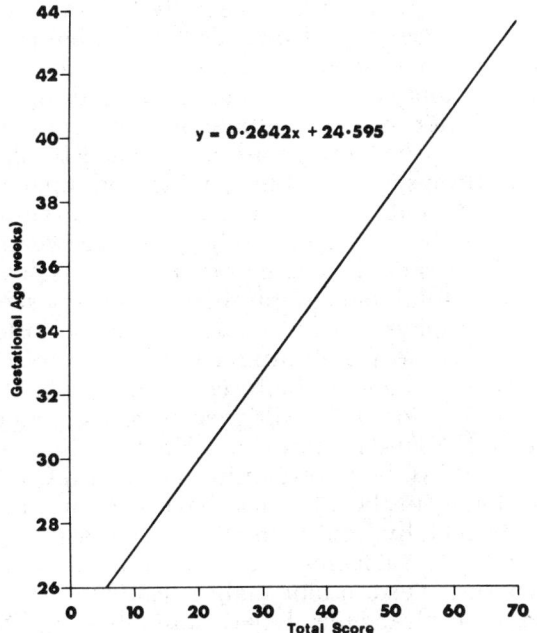

FIGURE 27–5. Gestational age scoring graph for Dubowitz criteria for estimation of gestational age. Scoring: A maximum-score case would be arrived at by adding the Table 27–3 score (e.g., 2 + 4 + 3 + 4 + 4 + 4 + 3 + 3 + 3 + 3 + 2 = 35) and the Figure 27–4 score (e.g., 4 + 4 + 4 + 2 + 2 + 5 + 4 + 3 + 3 + 4 = 35). The total score of 70, found on the graph presented here, corresponds to a gestational age of 43 to 44 weeks. (From Dubowitz ML, Dubowitz V, Goldberg C: Clinical assessment of gestational age in the newborn infant. J Pediatr 77:1, 1970, with permission.)

commonly are heard: some babies at risk for mild hypoglycemia may benefit from an "early" feeding of dextrose 5% in water, and some babies with upper gastrointestinal obstruction and some with tracheoesophageal fistula may come safely to medical attention by vomiting or coughing after a sterile water feeding. Still, the optimal first feeding is human colostrum sucked immediately after delivery. The often negligible volume of this first feeding need not prompt supplementation. Normal, term babies are born fully hydrated; they come with a several days' supply of "excess" water already on board. It is this "excess" whose expenditure is primarily responsible for physiologic postnatal weight loss. If bottle feeding is the maternal choice, a standard formula can be offered.

Postnatal Screening

Blood Glucose Level

At birth, blood glucose is about two thirds the mother's level. Within an hour or two, blood glucose falls to a level no lower than 35 to 40 mg/dL and then rises to a 6-hour value between 45 and 60 mg/dL. Levels in premature babies are a little lower, in part because glycogen stores are relatively deficient. Newborns normally consume glucose at about twice the adult rate; if they are physically stressed or if they are the hyperinsulinemic products of diabetic gestations, their glucose demand may exceed the supply deliverable by glyco-

PHYSICAL MATURITY

	0	1	2	3	4	5
Skin	gelatinous red, transparent	smooth pink, visible veins	superficial peeling &/or rash few veins	cracking pale area rare veins	parchment deep cracking no vessels	leathery cracked wrinkled
Lanugo	none	abundant	thinning	bald areas	mostly bald	
Plantar Creases	no crease	faint red marks	anterior transverse crease only	creases ant. 2/3	creases cover entire sole	
Breast	barely percept.	flat areola no bud	stippled areola 1–2 mm bud	raised areola 3–4 mm bud	full areola 5–10 mm bud	
Ear	pinna flat, stays folded	sl. curved pinna; soft with slow recoil	well-curv. pinna; soft but ready recoil	formed & firm with instant recoil	thick cartilage ear stiff	
Genitals ♂	scrotum empty no rugae		testes descending, few rugae	testes down good rugae	testes pendulous deep rugae	
Genitals ♀	prominent clitoris & labia minora		majora & minora equally prominent	majora large minora small	clitoris & minora completely covered	

MATURITY RATING

Score	Wks
5	26
10	28
15	30
20	32
25	34
30	36
35	38
40	40
45	42
50	44

Neuromuscular Maturity

	0	1	2	3	4	5
Posture						
Square Window (wrist)	90°	60°	45°	30°	0°	
Arm Recoil	180°		100°–180°	90°–100°	<90°	
Popliteal Angle	180°	160°	130°	110°	90°	<90°
Scarf Sign						
Heel to Ear						

FIGURE 27–6. Ballard's simplified criteria for estimation of gestational age. The sum of scores on all items of physical and neuromuscular maturity provides a maturity in weeks (see Maturity Rating). (Modified from Ballard JL, Novak KK, Driver M: A simplified score for assessment of fetal maturation of newly born infants. J Pediatr 95:769, 1979.)

genolysis and gluconeogenesis combined. Blood glucose below 40 mg/dL requires a diagnostic explanation. Hypoglycemic babies may be jittery and may even experience seizure, or they may be depressed. Most cases of transient neonatal hypoglycemia can be anticipated on the basis of prematurity or perinatal stress; early nutritive feeding or an intravenous dextrose infusion may prevent symptoms. To prevent scarring of the heel pad, capillary blood samples should be drawn from the side of the heel. The heel should be warm, because cold-induced vascular stasis produces a localized relative hypoglycemia. Samples should be analyzed immediately with fresh materials, or they should be placed on ice, because blood glucose levels fall at room temperature.

Hematocrit

Peripheral vascular stasis increases the hematocrit of capillary blood obtained by lateral heel stick, more so if the leg and foot are squeezed during sampling. Hematocrits spun from freely flowing heel stick blood are preferable but still give higher values than those spun from either peripheral venous or arterial blood. Average full-term day 1 hematocrit is 53 per cent; by day 2, the average hematocrit peaks at about 58 per cent. Normal hematocrit values range from about 45 to 60 per cent (hemoglobin from about 15 to 20 gm/dL). Hematocrit over 70 per cent defines polycythemia and implies hyperviscosity. Obviously, high capillary values must be checked with peripheral venous or arterial samples. Polycythemic babies are usually plethoric and may be lethargic. Immediate concerns are thrombosis and sludging, particularly in the brain. A partial exchange transfusion, not simple phlebotomy, may be indicated, although it has proved difficult to define babies whose ongoing risk from polycythemia exceeds their risk from therapy (Baba et al., 1992; Oh, 1986).

Differential Leukocyte Count

Neither total nor differential leukocyte counts should be considered routine postnatal screening tests. However, babies coming to special attention because of perinatal history or physical examination should have these tests performed. An increased ratio of immature to total neutrophils may suggest acute systemic infection (Manroe et al., 1979).

Blood Type and Coombs' Test

Maternal–infant ABO incompatibility or a positive direct Coombs' test should prompt serial hematocrits and indirect serum bilirubin levels. Severe ABO isoimmunization or Rh isoimmunization of any degree demands intermediate to intensive care.

Syphilis Test

A positive serologic test for syphilis in an asymptomatic newborn may reflect antireponemal IgG antibody acquired transplacentally from a treated or untreated mother. However, this benign possibility cannot be confirmed on serologic grounds alone without observation of a fall in antitreponemal IgG titer over several months. Consequently, any positive maternal, cord, or neonatal serology almost always requires full syphilis work-up in the nursery (Chhabra et al., 1993). Physical examination must be repeated carefully (while wearing gloves). Darkfield examination of nasal discharge may be helpful; radiography of the long bones may show metaphyseal demineralization or periosteal bone formation. Cerebrospinal fluid (CSF) must be examined and a CSF fluorescent treponemal antibody absorption (FTA-ABS) test performed. A positive CSF FTA-ABS test is not proof of congenital neurosyphilis, however; antitreponemal IgG antibody found in the CSF may have been acquired transplacentally. IgM antibody, in contrast to IgG antibody, does not cross the blood–brain barrier in newborns. Western blot analysis can demonstrate specific antitreponemal IgM antibodies in CSF, confirming a diagnosis of congenital neurosyphilis (Sanchez, 1989). Even when active congenital syphilis cannot be demonstrated definitively, antibiotic treatment of suspect cases is almost always advisable, and, in the context of parental unreliability, it is mandatory (Zenker and Berman, 1991). Some women infected late in pregnancy will deliver infants without serologic or clinical signs of syphilis in the nursery. A serologic test for syphilis has been advocated in the routine evaluation of febrile infants in areas of high prevalence (Dorfman and Glaser, 1990) (see Chapter 20).

Hemoglobin Electrophoresis

Detection of sickle cell disease in the newborn period is very helpful (Vichinsky et al., 1988), because it allows early parental counseling and education and early initiation of daily oral penicillin prophylaxis against overwhelming sepsis. Several other hemoglobinopathies also may be detected by this test (see Chapter 45).

Thyroxine or Thyroid-Stimulating Hormone Screening Test

In most North American jurisdictions, thyroxine (T_4) is the only thyroid screening test performed if it is normal; if it is low, a thyroid-stimulating hormone (TSH) screen also is run. Unfortunately, some babies with T_4 in the normal range will have an elevated TSH. In Japan and in most of Europe, the testing order is reversed. Neither policy is perfect; testing TSH first will not uncover babies with some of the more unusual congenital thyroid problems. Further problems result when early discharge or out-of-hospital delivery necessitates testing before 3 days of age, because TSH may be physiologically elevated during the first 2 days after delivery. Abnormal screening results should prompt immediate full maternal and infant evaluations and testing of both T_4 and TSH in a serum sample drawn from the baby's venous blood, not from another heel stick. Treatment for congenital hypothyroidism is with *l*-thyroxine 10 to 15 μg/kg/day, the goal being maintenance of T_4 levels in the upper half of the normal range throughout the first year of life (American Academy of Pediatrics and American Thyroid Association, 1987).

Nearly universal thyroid screening has been a great advance in developed countries, but it still misses from 6 to 12 per cent of congenitally hypothyroid babies and falsely implicates others. Congenital hypothyroidism still must be suspected on clinical grounds in babies who have large open fontanelles or umbilical hernias or who are hypothermic, hypotonic, macroglossic, excessively mottled, coarsely featured, somnolent, slow to feed, or persistently jaundiced, whether or not their thyroid glands are enlarged and whether or not their screening tests are normal.

Phenylalanine Level

In classic phenylketonuria (PKU), phenylalanine hydroxylase activity is greatly decreased or absent, so dietary phenylalanine accumulates, and tyrosine, which is made from phenylalanine, is depressed. Affected babies are asymptomatic in the newborn period, but, if they have begun feeding, the blood phenylalanine level will be elevated, making them identifiable and making phenylalanine-related organ damage, particularly brain damage, largely preventable by dietary restriction.

Galactosemia Testing

In babies with a deficiency of galactokinase, galactose accumulates in the lenses, causing cataracts. The urine of affected babies who are ingesting galactose or lactose (whose hydrolysis yields glucose and galactose) will contain a non–glucose-reducing substance, specifically, galactose. Dietary restriction therapy is easy and effective if instituted early enough. Babies with a deficiency of galactokinase do not have classic galactosemia.

In babies with deficient activity of galactose-1-phosphate uridyltransferase, dietary galactose accumulates in and damages the liver and kidneys and eventually the brain and the lenses. The urine contains non–glucose-reducing substances, specifically, galactose and galactose 1-phosphate. Affected babies appear normal at birth but become fulminantly ill within a few days and usually are assumed to be septic; occasionally, galactosemic babies are indeed septic as well as galactosemic. Other do not become critically ill but simply fail to thrive in the first year. Babies with a deficiency of galactose-1-phosphate uridyltransferase do have classic galactosemia. Non–glucose-reducing substances in the urine can be demonstrated by the combination of a negative Clinistix or Tes-Tape with a positive Clinitest.

Immunoglobulin M Level

Cord blood IgM below 20 mg/dL is normal. Elevated values suggest fetal response to intrauterine infection.

Other Postnatal Screening Tests

Other congenital problems for which screening tests have been mandated or have been under trial evaluation in United States jurisdictions have included adenosine deaminase deficiency, adrenal hyperplasia (Caravella et al., 1987), biotinidase deficiency, cystic fibrosis (Gregg et al., 1993; Hammond et al., 1991), hearing loss, histidinemia, homocystinuria, hyperleucinemia, lead exposure, and maple syrup urine disease. Individual family histories may prompt tests not employed for general newborn population screening.

Circumcision

Circumcision should *never* be performed if there is any doubt whatsoever about the anatomic normality of the penis. Circumcision prevents phimosis, paraphimosis, and balanoposthitis, and it decreases the incidence of cancer of the penis and, possibly, in ultimate sexual partners, cancer of the uterine cervix (American Academy of Pediatrics, 1989). More immediately, circumcision decreases the already small chance of urinary tract infection in the young male infant (Ginsburg and McCraken, 1982; Wiswell and Roscelli, 1986; Wiswell et al., 1988). That said, the "need" to excise normal tissue strikes a Darwinian dissonance in many ears (Winberg et al., 1989), and potential benefits must be weighed against known risks (Brown and Brown, 1987; Fergusson et al., 1988; Herzog and Alvarez, 1986; Poland, 1990; Schoen, 1990; Wallerstein, 1980; Wiswell and Geschke, 1989). Freehand circumcision is learned easily but often is abandoned in favor of the Gomco or Plastibell techniques (Figs. 27–7 and 27–8).

Circumcision is painful (Anand and Hickey, 1987); local anesthetic infiltration is a compassionate option (Toffler et al., 1990).

Once the genital area is prepped and draped, a straight hemostat is inserted into the preputial orifice and the ring is dilated gently. A blunt flexible probe is inserted between the glans and the inner epithelium of the prepuce. The external urethral meatus *must* be identified clearly. Usually, to free the glans from adherent tissue, a straight hemostat is clamped in the midline for about a minute; a dorsal slit then is made in the crushed area. This incision is extended to within 0.5 cm of the coronal sulcus. The foreskin is pulled back and blunt dissection continued until the entire glans is free of adherent tissue. The circumcision then may be completed using either a Gomco clamp or a Plastibell.

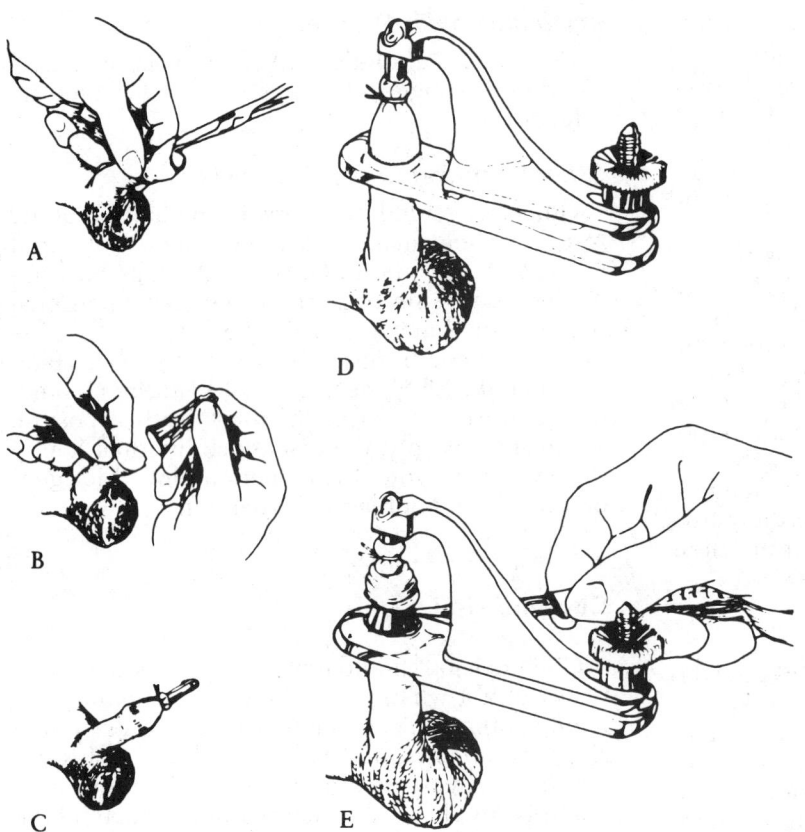

FIGURE 27–7. Gomco device and circumcision technique. (From Coen RW, Koffler H: Primary Care of the Newborn. Boston, Little, Brown, 1987, p 232; as adapted from Wallerstein, E: Circumcision: An American Health Fallacy. New York, Springer, 1980, with permission.)

If a Gomco clamp is used, it should be tightened for a minimum of 5 minutes before incising the foreskin. Once the clamp is removed, the penis should be wrapped with a petroleum-jelly–coated gauze pad to keep it from sticking to the diaper.

If a Plastibell is used, it should be tightened in place securely for about 5 minutes before the redundant foreskin is incised. The Plastibell handle is separated from the cap, leaving the base of the foreskin fastened tightly. The opening in the cap permits urine to pass. About 5 to 10 days later, the cap and remaining foreskin fall off together.

Following the circumcision, the parents must be instructed to watch for problems in urination, bleeding, and signs of infection. Perineal hygiene should be stressed.

STANDARD CARE THROUGH THE FIRST MONTH OF LIFE

Many recommendations for standard newborn care are implicit or explicit in previous sections, especially in Routines for the First Few Days.

Safety

In developed countries, the baby's trip home and all subsequent motorized trips should be taken in a well-designed and properly used infant car seat (Bull et al., 1988a, 1988b). Car seat teaching can be managed conveniently postpartum by videotape, and car seat office education can be accomplished cheaply and effectively (Hletko et al., 1987). Besides vehicular trauma, major safety risks during the first month of life include airway obstruction caused by defective multipiece pacifiers, airway compression caused by necklaces and pacifier strings, suffocation caused by improper bedding or by face-down positioning for sleep (Kemp and Thach, 1991; Ponsonby et al., 1993), thermal burns during bathing, pet and rat bites, hyperthermia from overwrapping in warm weather (Cheng and Partridge, 1993), and abusive reactions to crying. Infant resuscitation teaching by videotape may be feasible (Kaiserman et al., 1989).

Care of the Perineum, Umbilical Stump, and Penis

Diapering and its complications are discussed in Chapter 40. Umbilical stump management was discussed earlier in Routines for the First Few Days. The uncircumcised penis should be cleaned carefully at each diaper change. The foreskin should not be retracted fully during the newborn period. Until healed, the circumcised penis should be wrapped in a petroleum-jelly–coated gauze pad changed with each diapering (or at least daily).

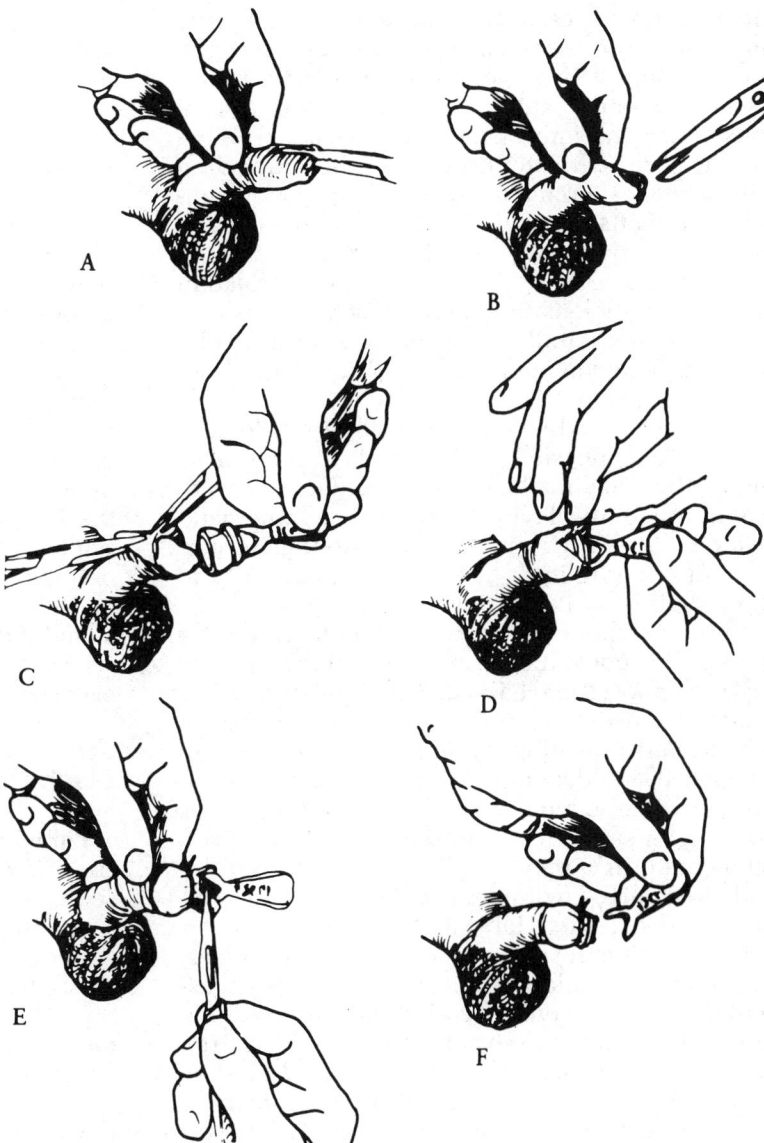

FIGURE 27–8. Plastibell circumcision technique. (From Coen RW, Koffler H: Primary Care of the Newborn. Boston, Little, Brown, 1987, p 233; as adapted from Wallerstein, E: Circumcision: An American Health Fallacy. New York, Springer, 1980, with permission.)

Feeding Advice

Expectant mothers should be encouraged strongly to plan on nursing their babies. Exceptions to this rule are rare: mothers who may, in their breast milk, pass on the human immunodeficiency virus (HIV) (Van de Perre et al., 1991), the human T-cell leukemia/lymphoma virus, type I (HTLV-I) (Tsuji et al., 1990), and, perhaps, cytomegalovirus (CMV) (Oxtoby, 1988); mothers who have active pulmonary tuberculosis; mothers needing certain prescription drugs; mothers addicted to certain substances; and mothers who, for whatever private reasons, clearly do not want to nurse. Even mothers from demographic groups with low breast-feeding rates can be influenced favorably by professional advice (Joffe and Radius, 1987; Kurinij et al., 1988; Winikoff et al., 1987); inclusion of a breast pump in hospital discharge packs also helps (Dungy et al., 1992). Although they may not nurse for long, ambivalent breast-feeders still can impart to their babies the immunologic advantages of colostrum and, apparently, the less well characterized advantages of transitional and mature milk.

Normal newborns, who are usually alert or easily arousable for an hour or so after birth, should be offered the breast as soon as possible. Suckling stimulates maternal secretion of oxytocin from the posterior pituitary and prolactin from the anterior pituitary. In the mother, oxytocin stimulates contraction of the myometrium, helping to prevent uterine hemorrhage, and stimulates contraction of the mammary myoepithelial cells, propelling milk toward and through the nipple. Prolactin stimulates milk production primarily.

The keys to successful lactation are the mother's confidence and the baby's sucking reflex. It is almost always the case that confident mothers have no serious problems nourishing alert, hungry, healthy babies. However, maternal anxiety inhibits oxytocin-stimulated myoepithelial contraction, thus giving the impression that milk is not being produced in adequate quantity, further degrading self-assurance. Premature babies, babies with neurologic deficits or cardiovascular or pulmonary disease, or sleepy babies not being fed "on demand" may not suck actively enough to maintain prolactin at levels sufficient to stimulate lactation. Breast pumping, breast milk storage or banking, and tube feedings may be indicated (Helsing and King, 1982).

"Demand" feeding matches milk supply to milk requirement physiologically, and it minimizes fussing by allowing the baby's circadian rhythm to mature smoothly. Trying to "normalize" a demand schedule too early is unwise, because it gives parents an opportunity to fail and an opportunity to think their baby is refusing to cooperate.

In the newborn period, energy requirement for growth is about 120 kcal/kg/day. Many competently composed and packaged nonhuman milk formulas are available, most providing about 0.6 to 0.7 kcal/mL; leading formulas are detailed in Chapter 28. In developed countries, these formulas can be used safely as primary feedings or as convenient supplements to breast milk. In developing countries, they usually are transported dry and then mixed with local water, which is frequently not sterile (Habicht et al., 1988).

Iron supplementation of breast milk is not necessary until some months beyond the newborn period as a result of enhanced iron absorption. Vitamin supplementation sometimes is provided. Iron supplementation of artificial formulas is desirable. Many infants fed cow's milk lose iron in nutritionally important amounts through occult gastrointestinal bleeding (Ziegler et al., 1990). The common suspicion that iron supplementation causes "colic" is unfounded (Nelson et al., 1988).

Neither human milk nor cow's milk contains a significant amount of fluoride, and an infant's intake of fluoridated tap water is hard to predict. Accordingly, fluoride intake often must be supplemented; 2 weeks of age is the recommended starting time and 0.25 mg/day the recommended intake. However, oversupplementation—even just twice the recommended daily intake—can discolor tooth enamel, so supplementation should be prescribed only for those babies unlikely to receive 0.25 mg/day from diet and tap water (Herrmann and Roberts, 1987).

Colic connotes excessive, "unjustified" crying in otherwise healthy infants within the first 12 weeks. The term is antiquated and a misnomer; there is no colic in colic. Although a consensus on pathophysiology and behavioral dynamics is yet to form (McKenzie, 1991; Moore et al., 1988; Schmitt, 1986; Taubman, 1988; Woolridge and Fisher, 1988; Zuckerman et al., 1990), pharmacologic therapies for colic remain sharply inconsistent with most leading theories.

Postpartum Depression

At some point before baby and parents go home, specific mention should be made of postpartum depression, a common phenomenon of largely somatic origin. The emerging neuroendocrine model of postpartum depression can be described in simple terms and should be stressed; older behavioral models are poorly supported scientifically, and their emphasis is ill-advised psychologically. Parents should know in advance that postpartum depression, in its myriad forms, may subtract from the happiness of early motherhood but does not imply maternal incapacity or unconscious rejection of infant or consort. Postpartum depression should not be feared, but it is unpleasant and even occasionally dangerous, and the physician should describe its symptoms and ask to be informed of their occurrence (see Chapter 52).

Discharge and the First Return Visit

Babies need not be born in hospitals, and, absent specific contraindications, those who are may be sent home "early" at little disadvantage, other than a somewhat higher chance of readmission during the newborn period (Conrad et al., 1989). Just prior to discharge is a good time to discuss parental expectations, which sometimes need tactful amendment (Delight et al., 1991), as well as common problems (e.g., postpartum depression and "colic"), and the mother's plans, if any, to return to work outside the home. Parental smoking once again should be discouraged vigorously, especially in the abstinent mother looking forward to a resumption of her tobacco use (Greenberg et al., 1989). A short check-in at 2 weeks is advisable, especially for inexperienced parents. Nursery problems may need follow-up, and PKU and galactosemia screens may need repetition if hospital discharge preceded full feedings. In developing countries, bacillus Calmette-Guérin inoculation (Sirinavin et al., 1991) and rotavirus vaccination may be performed.

Fever in the First Month of Life

In-hospital parental teaching often will have included safe use of a thermometer, but temperature determination and interpretation in the baby's first month of life are so tricky that physicians should discourage parents from using thermometer readings when making care-seeking decisions. Most temperature elevations in the newborn period do not imply true emergencies, and rapidly progressive diseases, such as infection caused by the group B β-hemolytic streptococcus, enteric bacteria, or *Streptococcus pneumoniae,* may present with elevated, depressed, or normal core temperature.

A well-wrapped baby normal on physical examination except for a mildly elevated core temperature should be re-examined after lying unwrapped on a blanket in a comfortably warm examining room. If, after an interval of 20 to 30 minutes, temperature normalizes, the parents may be reassured. They should be advised not to overwrap their baby and should be asked to report on their baby's condition after 6 to 12 hours. With this sole exception—environmental fever—prudent practice would dictate further diagnostic procedures, such as total and differential leukocyte counts, and, most important, re-examination in several hours—in other words, at the return of laboratory values—either in an outpatient or an inpatient setting. Many physicians also would culture blood, examine and culture urine and CSF (Bonadio et al., 1992), and perform a chest radiograph. Some physicians would, in addition, hospitalize all febrile babies under 1 month old and administer systemic antibiotics pending the maturation of cultures. All in all, meticulous physical examination and early repeat evaluation are the best guides to management.

No baby in the first month of life should have a fever evaluated over the telephone. No baby in the first month of life should have a fever treated with antipyretics. A baby in the first month of life whose fever needs symptomatic control is clearly sick enough to be hospitalized for definitive diagnosis and well-chosen therapy.

MAKING SENSE OF SHOCK, DISTRESS, AND DEPRESSION

Timing

A baby depressed immediately after birth is likely to have been distressed in utero, injured in labor or delivery, or overwhelmed by the metabolic demands of the birth process. Explanations include placental insufficiency, placental hemorrhage or fetomaternal transfusion, hypoxic or traumatic encephalopathy, anesthetic or narcotic depression, acute ascending infection, lethal chromosomal defect, or secondary apnea from another cause. Many such babies, once removed from difficult intrauterine conditions, will improve, either spontaneously or with stimulation or, in the case of opioid depression, with naloxone. Others will respond only slowly or not at all to full ventilatory support and pharmacologic intervention.

A baby vigorous at birth but distressed shortly thereafter may be suffering the effects of prematurity generally, pulmonary immaturity specifically, a pulmonary malformation, a pulmonary aspiration syndrome, excess residual lung fluid, or a cardiovascular malformation or malfunction of little consequence under the conditions of fetal circulation but of much greater consequence in extrauterine life.

A baby apparently normal at birth but in trouble some hours or even a day or so later may be "running low" on a vital substance, such as glucose, calcium, magnesium, blood, or a dependency-producing drug; may be showing signs of infection; or may be evolving another type of pathology, such as cerebral edema from otherwise unsuspected head trauma or hypoxia.

A sick baby, particularly a premature baby, having unexpected problems after steady progress may be declaring a systemic infection; a gastrointestinal catastrophe (classically, necrotizing enterocolitis); a cerebral problem, such as a seizure; or a neurodevelopmental problem, such as an apneic spell.

A baby apparently normal at discharge from the nursery but now sick later in the first month of life may be demonstrating a problem previously overlooked, such as a congenital heart lesion, pulmonary malformation, or central nervous system defect, or may be presenting with a disease, usually infectious, that was acquired before, during, just after, or long after delivery. Late-onset group B β-hemolytic streptococcal sepsis, listeriosis, chlamydial infection, and HSV infection, although acquired antepartum or intrapartum, may present after a considerable interval (as may other infections not so likely to cause shock, distress, or depression).

Clinical Setting

Many problems predisposing to shock, distress, or depression can be anticipated antepartum: prematurity, postmaturity, intrauterine growth retardation from whatever cause (such as pregnancy-induced hypertension), multiple gestation, sonographically resolvable malformations, erythroblastosis fetalis, diabetic gestation, certain congenital and perinatally acquired infections, drug effect, and drug dependency. Other predispositions to shock, distress, or depression should come quickly to mind once delivery has been accomplished: hyaline membrane disease in the premature baby; meconium aspiration syndrome in the meconium-stained baby; intracranial hemorrhage in the traumatized baby; hypoglycemia in the premature, stressed, or macrosomic baby; and addisonian crisis in the masculinized phenotypic female. Even after discharge, clinical setting can be a clue to diagnosis; pyloric stenosis (Breaux et al., 1988) in the thin but hungry firstborn male is a classic example.

Predominant Finding

Shock may be differentiated on clinical grounds into hypovolemic, cardiogenic, or septic varieties. Hypovolemic and cardiogenic shock are common final expressions of the full range of lethal pathologies; babies who are septic or who have sustained a critical cerebral insult may present in cardiovascular collapse.

Distress in the newborn is typically respiratory. The term "respiratory distress" connotes difficult air movement and suggests labored or stridorous breathing. The term "respiratory distress syndrome" (RDS) indicates hyaline membrane disease specifically and implies expiratory grunting, a classic RDS sign found also in pneumothorax, hypothermia, and polycythemia. Babies who are tachypneic are often in respiratory distress, although their distress may be only the transient tachypnea that marks the incomplete resorption of residual lung fluid. However, tachypnea also may be seen in babies whose distress is not at all respiratory but, rather, metabolic, as in respiratory compensation of a metabolic acidosis, or neurologic, as in central hyperventilation.

Depression is a nonspecific sign and is best evaluated empirically. Babies who are stimulated easily physically or with a few positive-pressure breaths may be perfectly normal. Those responding to naloxone may need no special care beyond the first few hours. Those whose depression is not easily reversed or whose depression deepens probably are damaged significantly or seriously ill.

Other predominant signs, such as cyanosis, have been discussed in previous sections.

Response to Early Diagnostic and Therapeutic Interventions

Diagnostic procedures and therapeutic trials must be undertaken systematically. Their goals are the reliable narrowing of differential diagnoses. Their triple risks are the suggestion of unwarranted conclusions, the exacerbation of existing pathology, and the creation of iatrogenic damage.

RESUSCITATION OF THE NEWBORN

Attitude

The amazing costs and the tragic outcomes of many newborn hospitalizations have affected attitudes toward newborn resuscitation (Berseth et al., 1986). Intensive efforts applied to the newborn are sometimes *mis*applied, but resuscitation saves many babies—even some "stillborns"—who eventually prove undamaged or only mildly damaged (Grogaard et al., 1990; Jain et al., 1991). An intraresuscitative re-evaluation may demonstrate the futility of full or continued efforts, particularly in very-low-birth-weight babies already receiving intensive support, but resuscitation should not be withheld entirely without compellingly humane cause. In the United States, the "Baby Doe" problem has complicated these decisions, although largely through misapprehension of the relevant rulings, regulations, and statutes (Edens et al., 1990; Todres et al., 1988; Walters, 1988).

In the developed world, professionals skilled in newborn resuscitation should—*and can* (Bailey and Kattwinkel, 1990)—attend or be immediately available to every delivery, *even in small community hospitals.*

Adapting Adult Resuscitative Methods to Newborns

Physicians accustomed to the resuscitation of adults must adapt their critical-care practices thoughtfully to the resuscitation of newborns, in which population respiratory insufficiency predominates. Resuscitative habits acquired during the revival of asystolic, fibrillating, failing, or ischemic adult hearts will not save many babies. Primary cardiac arrest does occur in newborns, but it is distinctly rare. Acute cardiogenic pulmonary edema and acute pulmonary embolization are likewise much less common (although the latter may be under-recognized in instrumented babies).

Response to volume expansion is not the same in newborns as in adults. Newborn stroke volume is practically fixed; therefore, cardiac output is rate-dependent and is not increased substantially by preload augmentation. Rapid volume expansion may cause the ductus arteriosus to dilate, producing a seemingly paradoxical hypotension. Rapid volume expansion, as might occur with sodium bicarbonate therapy for presumed metabolic acidosis, may cause periventricular or intraventricular hemorrhage, especially in premature babies. Nonmeticulous adult fluid practices are unacceptable in newborn resuscitation.

In adult resuscitations, hyperoxemia is a welcome sign that vigorous efforts, including the liberal use of supplemental oxygen, have been successful. In newborns, particularly prematures, supplemental oxygen must be administered more carefully, because even brief periods of hyperoxemia may increase the risk of blindness from retrolental fibroplasia (the retinopathy of prematurity) (Flynn et al., 1992), and hyperoxia of uncertain duration predisposes to bronchopulmonary dysplasia. That said, failure to administer sufficient supplemental oxygen in a resuscitation may result in brain damage or death.

Compared with adult resuscitation, acute vascular access is much more easily obtained in freshly delivered newborns with patent umbilical veins, but much more tediously secured if peripheral veins must be used or if central venous catheters must be placed at nonumbilical sites. Arterial blood gas sampling is harder, and acceptable sites are somewhat different: umbilical, radial, temporal, and posterior tibial arteries, but not brachial or femoral arteries. Smaller samples of both venous and arterial blood can be used for testing, and reported potassium values are much more likely to be spuriously high, reflecting erythrocyte lysis.

Finally, pharmacokinetics are hard to predict in individual babies (Morselli, 1989).

Carrying an age-appropriate "code card" can be reassuring (American Academy of Pediatrics, 1988; Rockney, 1988).

Step-By-Step Resuscitation Immediately after Delivery

Step 1: Consider meconium aspiration as a risk in the baby needing resuscitation.

If thick meconium is evident, suction the trachea, hypopharynx, oropharynx, and mouth and then the nares and nasopharynx, preferably before stimulating a respiratory gasp and *always* before initiating positive-pressure ventilation. Asphyxia tolerance is greater in the newborn than in the older child or the adult, and extending asphyxia just long enough to prevent or lessen the severity of meconium aspiration is a good trade-off. If breathing has begun, suctioning still should be tried, because meconium may persist in accessible locations for 20 minutes or more. If a meconium-stained baby suddenly deteriorates, consider the possibility of a pulmonary air leak; percuss, auscultate, and transilluminate the chest for evidence of pneumothorax or pneumomediastinum.

Meconium is found in amniotic fluid in about 10 per cent of births; its "terminal" passage is usually not a respiratory risk. Overly aggressive suctioning itself can cause trouble, and meconium-stained babies born apneic obviously have other serious problems as well. The risk of meconium aspiration should be assessed quickly, and retrieval maneuvers either should be skipped or should be performed efficiently.

Step 2: Check for spontaneous movement and try to elicit spontaneous respirations.

The baby born totally limp, cyanotic, unresponsive, and bradycardic, although "stillborn" in the true sense of the word, sometimes can be resuscitated with reasonable results. If spontaneous respiratory movement can be elicited by sensory stimulation, the baby is exhibiting primary apnea and might begin gasping if left alone; if spontaneous respiratory movement cannot be elicited by sensory stimulation, the baby is exhibiting secondary apnea and probably would not gasp again without resuscitation. The majority of babies needing re-

suscitation are born in primary apnea. Although every depressed newborn deserves a resuscitative trial, those born in secondary apnea are less likely to respond and are less likely to recover without major sequelae. Quick, initial differentiation of primary from secondary apnea can help the resuscitating physician decide how long these efforts should persist.

Step 3: Dry the skin and hair.

Cold stress is a frequently unremembered impediment to successful resuscitation. If the baby is lying on a blanket, drying can be incorporated into step 2 as the stimulatory maneuver used in the attempt to elicit spontaneous respirations. If not, a warm dry towel should be requested as step 4 is begun.

Step 4: Commence bag-and-mask ventilation.

The pharynx should be cleared of any obstruction and a birth-weight–appropriate mask fitted snuggly over the baby's nose and mouth, the baby held slightly head down, and the head itself held in the "sniffing" position. Initial pressures of 20 to 30 cm H_2O or higher may be needed. Compensatory hyperventilation—about 50 breaths/min—is the best way to deal with metabolic acidosis during newborn resuscitation. However, rapid pH change, even rapid pH "improvement," is dangerous; steady, gradual raising of the pH should be the goal of compensatory hyperventilation.

Do not commence bag-and-mask ventilation if a scaphoid abdomen suggests diaphragmatic herniation, because air under pressure will enter the stomach and thence, perhaps, the intrathoracic gut, making the ventilation of presumably hypoplastic lungs even more difficult. If diaphragmatic herniation is suspected, proceed directly to tracheal intubation.

Depending on their configuration, self-inflating bags may not be able to deliver oxygen at high concentrations or any gas at high pressures. Anesthesia bags do not have the limitations of self-inflating bags, but their safe use requires prior familiarity and they *must* be used with pressure manometers. Pure oxygen is still the gas available in most delivery rooms; monitored retreat from 100 per cent supplemental oxygen is advisable to lessen the risks of retrolental fibroplasia and bronchopulmonary dysplasia.

Step 5: Commence external cardiac massage if the heart rate does not rise rapidly to above 80 beats/min despite adequate ventilatory support.

A second operator is necessary if cardiac massage is required. Both thumbs should be placed over the midsternum and the other fingers placed under the spine; the two-handed, thumbs-on-the-sternum technique has been shown superior to the one-handed technique (David, 1988). Smooth compressions of 1 to 1.5 cm should be made 100 to 120 times per minute. It is wise to coordinate ventilations and chest compressions to lessen the detrimental venous-return effect of positive-pressure ventilation and to lessen the risk of pneumothorax and pneumomediastinum; in practice, good coordination is hard to achieve. Heart rate is monitored most easily at the umbilicus, and less easily at the femoral arteries.

Step 6: Intubate the trachea if bag-and-mask ventilation seems inadequate.

A size 1 Miller laryngoscope blade—the term-infant-sized blade—can be used on babies of all sizes. Endotracheal tubes in 2.5, 3.0, 3.5, and 4.0-mm sizes should be available, as should a bendable metal obturator or stylette with which to stiffen the endotracheal tube for better control. An obturator can be dangerous; its tip must never extend beyond the end of the endotracheal tube; an obturated endotracheal tube must never be forced against tissue. Obturators often are used because endotracheal tubes, kept at the ready under radiant warmers, have become flaccid by the time they are needed. Keeping endotracheal tubes cool makes obturator use less of an issue. Sticking endotracheal tubes in a cup of sterile ice is very helpful, although a bit unorthodox.

As shown in Figure 27–9, take the laryngoscope in the left hand. Open the baby's mouth with the right hand. Slip the laryngoscope blade into the right side of the mouth and displace the tongue gently to the left. If it is comfortable to do so, place the fourth and fifth digits of the laryngoscope hand under the baby's chin or, in smaller babies, under the neck, and lift slightly. Visualize the epiglottis. Advance the blade tip into the vallecula (the "little valley" just anterior to the epiglottis itself); alternatively, "pick up" the epiglottis with the blade tip. Either way, lift straight up gently on the laryngoscope handle. Suctioning may be needed, and, sometimes, the light pressure of an assistant's finger on the trachea may be helpful.

The larynx must be visualized! Accept no substitutes! If the larynx cannot be identified positively, give up and return to bag-and-mask ventilation immediately. Try again after about 30 seconds. The endotracheal tube must be seen passing through the larynx and into the trachea. If the tube is not seen actually passing through the larynx, esophageal intubation must be assumed. Listening for ventilation sounds over the chest is a good habit but is not a definitive way to confirm endotracheal intubation in the newborn.

The endotracheal tube used should be the largest one that will allow an audible air leak at ventilatory pressures around 30 to 40 cm H_2O. Some tubes are tapered at the optimal laryngeal level; nontapered tubes, which generally are preferred, often are marked with a black circle—the "vocal cord line"—at this same level, the object being tube tip placement above the carina, not in the right mainstem bronchus. After securing the tube to the face with tape, compare breath sounds in the right lateral lung field to breath sounds in the left lateral lung field. If only the right lung is being ventilated, withdraw the tube a little, listen again, and retape. Eventually, safe tube position should be confirmed by portable anteroposterior chest radiography. Nasotracheal intubation, a procedure requiring the use of McGill forceps, may be preferred primarily in some babies with micrognathia or may be preferred generally to enhance tube stability.

Step 7: Insert an orogastric feeding tube to decompress the stomach.

Gastric distention can interfere with diaphragmatic excursion, and gastric contents easily can be aspirated, whether or not an endotracheal tube (always uncuffed in newborns) has been placed. Gastric content is relatively greater in babies born by cesarean section. Proper placement of an orogastric tube incidentally confirms esophageal patency.

Step 8: Assess volume status and replete absolute or functional deficiencies.

Blood pressure is often difficult to measure during resuscitation. It is frequently very low, and even when it is not low, auscultating Korotkoff sounds can be challenging, even when using a Doppler device. Hypotensive babies have weak peripheral pulses, but newborns with substantial right-to-left shunting have large pulse pressures, and so may have pulses that are relatively easy to feel.

Respiratory support, with or without short-term external cardiac massage, should bring the heart rate to above 100 beats/min in most newborns. When it does not, absolute or functional volume depletion should be considered. Using sterile technique, place a radiopaque plastic catheter into the umbilical vein, no more than 5 cm plus the umbilical stump length to avoid physical, osmotic, or pharmacologic trauma to the liver. Dispatch blood for a spun hematocrit, but remember that acute blood loss may not yet be reflected in the hematocrit. Consider inoculating a blood culture.

If acute blood loss is suspected (as it might be from inspection of the placenta), if fetomaternal transfusion is suspected (as it might be after cesarean delivery because of cord clamping above the level of the placenta), or if massive hemolysis is suspected (as it should be in babies born to Rh-negative mothers), a transfusion of fresh whole blood, a plasma expander, Ringer's lactate, or normal saline should be considered. Low-antibody-titer, O-negative, fresh whole blood crossmatched against maternal blood is the volume expander of choice in this setting, but it is available only as a result of forethought. Blood can be drawn from the placental umbilical vein or from a vein on the pla-

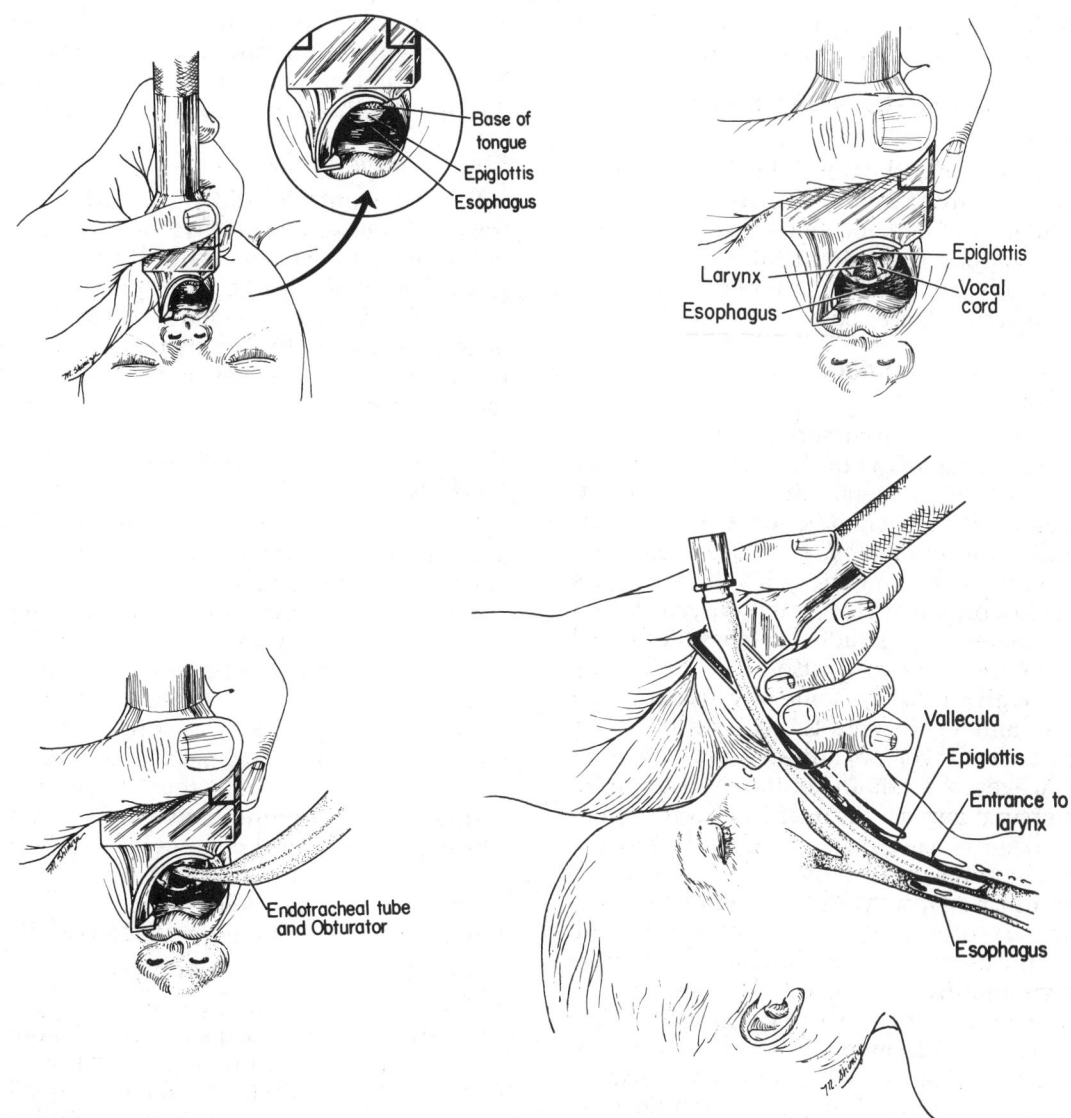

FIGURE 27–9. Direct laryngoscopy and intubation of the neonate. (From Fisher DE, Paton JB: Resuscitation of the newborn. *In* Klaus MH, Fanaroff AA [eds]: Care of the High-Risk Neonate, 4th edition. Philadelphia, WB Saunders Company, 1993, p 47, with permission.)

cental surface. Placental blood is the baby's own blood and, barring ongoing immune-mediated hemolysis, is theoretically ideal. However, bacterial contamination and microembolization are risks; careful asepsis, use of a heparin-washed syringe, and interposition of a blood filter between syringe and catheter can reduce these risks. Whichever fluid is used, 10 mL/kg can be administered once or, as indicated, more than once.

Septic or otherwise acidotic babies also may have a functional volume deficit needing repletion. If they are not judged also to be anemic, a plasma expander or a saline solution should be administered instead of blood. Sodium bicarbonate may be a good choice here, because its administration combines a volume effect and a hydrogen ion buffering effect (see step 11). Volume expansion

has been overstressed and overpracticed in the past. The first candidate for blame in continuing vascular collapse should be the quality of ventilatory support.

Step 9: Consider administering naloxone.

If the mother of a depressed newborn has received a narcotic within about 4 hours of delivery or if she might have self-administered a narcotic before coming under professional care, consider giving naloxone as Narcan, 0.01 to 0.02 mg/mL, 1 mL to premature babies and 2 mL to full-term babies intravenously or endotracheally, or, if perfusion is adequate, subcutaneously or intramuscularly. The dose may have to be repeated several times at 5- to 20-minute intervals. Initiating full-blown withdrawal in a severely drug-addicted newborn may not simplify management.

Step 10: Assess acid–base and arterial blood gas status.

To monitor ongoing therapy, a heparinized arterial sample—ideally, a sample from the right radial artery—should be sent for acid–base and blood gas determination. If frequent arterial sampling seems necessary, an umbilical artery catheter later should be inserted under controlled conditions.

Step 11: Consider pharmacologic intervention.

Naloxone has been discussed in step 9.

Sodium bicarbonate can be used to treat primary metabolic acidosis or metabolic acidosis complicating prolonged resuscitation. However, in this second and more common case, its use is often inappropriate, because ventilatory insufficiency is a feature of most prolonged resuscitations, and ventilatory insufficiency precludes the hoped-for pH rise. Sodium bicarbonate 1 mEq/mL, 1 to 2 mEq/kg should be given slowly; some physicians prefer to dilute sodium bicarbonate 1:1 with sterile water. Readministration every 5 minutes may be indicated. However, overadministration of sodium bicarbonate is dangerous; iatrogenic hyperosmolarity and alkalosis can damage or kill. Further treatment should be guided by arterial (or venous) pH determinations if available. Acidosis itself sometimes can elevate the blood pressure; alkali therapy in these cases may simultaneously correct the acidosis and drop the blood pressure.

Epinephrine 1:10,000, 0.01 to 0.03 mg/kg, 0.1 to 0.3 mL/kg can be delivered endotracheally (mixed with 1 to 2 mL of normal saline to aid dispersal in the pulmonary tree) or through an umbilical venous catheter. It can be given in response to asystole or heart rate persistently below 80 beats/min despite adequate ventilatory support, pure oxygen delivery, and external cardiac massage. Epinephrine may be readministered every 5 minutes if needed. No longer is atropine or calcium recommended for use in newborn resuscitation (Peckham et al., 1986). Calcium chloride often has been used in desperation. Calcium chloride (or epinephrine) can be given directly into the heart in moribund babies, but this practice is almost never successful. Laceration of vital structures is routine and salvage of more than the heart extremely rare.

Pharmacologic interventions of many types are mainstays of modern newborn intensive care but are not often important in initial resuscitation. Ventilatory and circulatory support in a neutral thermal environment are surely the essential elements in most successful "saves."

Step 12: Arrange further management.

Transfer to the in-house nursery or special care unit should be accomplished or transport to a regional referral center should be arranged. If the mother is conscious and if she alone or she and the baby's father are still in the delivery room, move the infant within arm's length on the way out.

Step 13: Talk to the family.

Report events candidly and ask for whatever treatment consent seems warranted; excessive detail is neither necessary ethically or legally nor desirable psychologically at this juncture (Broyles et al., 1992). If transfer to another institution seems necessary, assure the family that continuity of care need not suffer, either immediately or over a longer term.

Step 14: Write temporary monitoring and fluid orders.

Until disposition is fully determined, vital sign and monitoring orders should be individualized to address anticipated risks.

Fully normal newborns can manage nicely with no fluid intake for well over a day; they do not need vascular access routes; they are not sick; and they have not just been resuscitated. However, babies who have just been severely stressed or who are otherwise sick have particular needs, and fluid orders written for them must be individualized. Using "normal requirements" only as a guide, the physician often must compose fluids from scratch, ordering each constituent separately. Newborn maintenance requirements are based on the following standards (Levin and Morriss, 1990):

Water, 100 mL/kg every 24 hours
Sodium (Na^+), 4 mEq/kg every 24 hours
Potassium (K^+), 2 mEq/kg every 24 hours
Chloride (Cl^-), 4 mEq/kg every 24 hours
Calcium (Ca^{2+}), 50 to 200 mg/kg every 24 hours
Magnesium (Mg^{2+}), 0.4 to 0.8 mEq/kg every 24 hours
Phosphate (PO_4^-), 15 to 50 mg/kg every 24 hours
Glucose, 100 to 200 mg/kg every 24 hours.

During the first day of life, water and glucose requirements likely would be met by a solution of dextrose 10% in water pumped at 4 mL/kg/hr. However, resuscitated babies should be fluid restricted to no more than two thirds the water rate for at least the first postresuscitation day. Whether their base rate is full or restricted, babies under radiant warmers should be given 20 per cent more water and babies under bilirubin lights 10 per cent more water. Furthermore, babies whose rectal temperature varies above or below 37.8° C should have their water rates compensated up or down 12 per cent per degree centigrade.

Blood glucose screening may prompt an adjustment in dextrose administration. Calcium, as calcium gluconate, may or may not be required; until recently, calcium gluconate supplementation was provided compulsively to many babies who did not need it. When urine finally is produced, isostheuria suggests that renal "work" has been minimized by the administration of well-ordered fluids. Sodium, potassium, and chloride may be added on the second day of life if urination has begun. Regular serum sodium, potassium, and chloride measurements should guide further adjustments.

PROBLEMS IN NEWBORN CARE

Respiratory Problems

Respiratory Distress Syndrome

Respiratory distress syndrome—or hyaline membrane disease—is caused by surfactant deficiency or surfactant immaturity, perhaps exacerbated by pulmonary hypoperfusion (Klaus and Fanaroff, 1993). The classic histologic finding is a hyaline-staining pseudomembrane lining an uninflated alveolus. RDS affects about 10 per cent of all premature babies and some full-term babies as well. It is the greatest single cause of nursery mortality in developed countries. RDS presents with difficulty initiating respirations, expiratory grunting or whining, sternal and intercostal retractions, nasal flaring, tachypnea or bradypnea, and, often, cyanosis. Chest radiography shows lung fields with a "ground glass" appearance and air bronchograms (Fig. 27–10). Supplemental oxygen is sufficient for mildly affected babies, and continuous positive airway pressure (CPAP) for some others, but many require mechanical ventilation (Carlo and Martin, 1986). Mild water and electrolyte restriction is helpful early in treatment. Frequent arterial blood gas determinations or indirect continuous hemoglobin oxygen saturation monitoring by pulse oximetry (Bowes et al., 1989) is indispensable. Arterial blood gas determinations provide more information, and pulse oximetry may not be reliable in the least stable patients. However, if samples are obtained by needle sticks, damage to arteries, nerves, or tendons may be sustained; vascular puncture itself has been shown to change P_{aCO_2} and P_{aO_2} in patients not being ventilated mechanically (Kim et al., 1991); and, if samples are obtained through indwelling lines, arterial embolization (or sepsis) may occur.

Recovery occurs when endogenous surfactant production reaches adequate levels and classically is presaged by a spontaneous diuresis. Recovery is impeded by a host of common complicating problems, and slow pulmonary progress makes almost inevitable residual damage to lungs and, often, to other organs as well.

Many therapeutic innovations, intensive nutritional support chief among them, have improved salvage rates and quality. Others have been less successful. Novel ventilatory modes, such as high-frequency oscillatory ventilation, may or may not have a role (HIFI Study Group, 1989, 1990a, 1990b). Therapeutic use of artificial and nonhuman

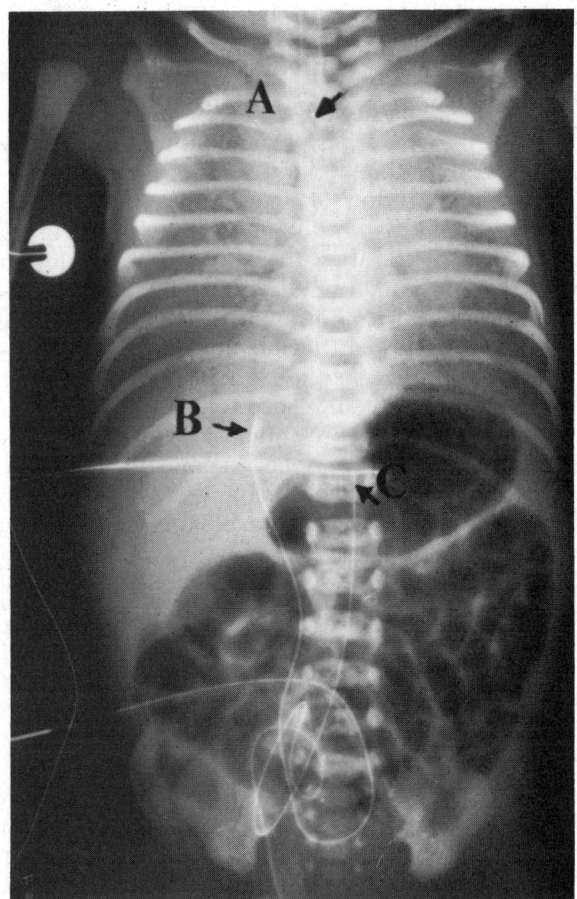

FIGURE 27–10. Anteroposterior roentgenogram of infant with hyaline membrane disease. Note granular lungs, air bronchogram, and air-filled esophagus. A, endotracheal tube; B, umbilical venous catheter at the junction of the umbilical vein, ductus venosus, and portal vein. (From Kliegman RM, Behrman RE. The fetus and the neonatal infant/diseases of the newborn infant: premature and full-term. *In* Behrman RE, Vaughan VC [eds]: Textbook of Pediatrics, 13th edition. Philadelphia, WB Saunders Company, 1992, p 465. Courtesy of Walter E. Berdon, Babies Hospital, New York, with permission.)

animal surfactants has been disappointing, although synthetic human surfactant, produced in large amounts by recombinant DNA techniques, can be highly effective both prophylactically and therapeutically (Bose et al., 1990; Corbet et al., 1991; Davis et al., 1988; Long et al., 1991). Some severely affected babies can be saved by the ventilatory rest achieved with venoarterial extracorporeal membrane oxygenation (ECMO), but at significant risk to all organs other than the lungs, because thrombosis and thromboembolization are routine (Vogler et al., 1988), and at special risk to the brain, because ligation of the right internal carotid artery is necessary (Frattallone et al., 1988; Schumacher et al., 1988), at least temporarily (Crombleholme et al., 1990; Taylor, 1992). Although most venoarterial ECMO survivors seem to develop normally by 12 months of age (Glass et al., 1989), venovenous ECMO, which is simpler and safer, largely may replace venoarterial bypass (Cornish et al., 1993).

Transient Tachypnea of the Newborn

The baby with transient tachypnea of the newborn (TTN) is typically otherwise normal and classically is the product of a cesarean delivery. Tachypnea without distress other than a little grunting, and usually without cyanosis, is observed; normal or mildly abnormal breath sounds are heard. Chest radiography shows central perihilar streaking and, often, a generous cardiac shadow.

Lack of a "vaginal squeeze" during cesarean delivery and incomplete resorption of fetal lung fluid are the reasons usually offered to explain TTN. Perihilar streaking may correspond to decreased pulmonary compliance. Tachypnea is presumably the most efficient way for these babies to minimize pulmonary work.

Special observation is needed, but either no treatment or just supplemental oxygen under 40 per cent is required. Sometimes CPAP is indicated. Tachypnea persisting beyond 24 hours is not usually considered transient.

Meconium Aspiration

Meconium aspiration syndrome is caused by the presence of ball-valve collections of meconium in distal airways. Ventilation is made difficult primarily by airway obstruction and secondarily by air trapping and air leaking. Severely affected babies suffer multiple pneumothoraces and pneumomediastinum. Multiple complications make many of these babies unsalvageable. ECMO, despite its problems, has proved useful in otherwise hopeless cases.

Pneumothorax and Pneumomediastinum

Pneumothorax or pneumomediastinum may be the first sign of the meconium aspiration syndrome. Spontaneous pneumothorax, if asymptomatic, requires no therapy. If it is associated with clinical signs of tension or other signs of respiratory distress, then evacuation is necessary. Chest radiography is needed, but sometimes action must be taken on clinical findings alone. A butterfly needle and catheter are used. The distal hub of the catheter is placed in a basin of sterile water, and the needle is introduced into the pneumothoracic region by "walking over" the appropriate rib, as if a pleural effusion were being tapped. Air under pressure will bubble into the basin. Alternatively, the hub can be connected to a two-way stopcock and the stopcock connected to a syringe containing a small amount of sterile water. The syringe can be used to evacuate several volumes of air. If air reaccumulates, chest tube placement becomes necessary. Breathing supplemental oxygen hastens absorption of pleural air (Klaus and Fanaroff, 1990).

Pneumonia

Perinatally acquired pneumonias, particularly group B β-hemolytic streptococcal pneumonia, may closely resemble hyaline membrane disease (see Infectious Problems later in this chapter and Chapter 20).

Cardiovascular Problems

Disorders of Transition

Although fetal circulation may have been perfectly normal, the ductus arteriosus may close slowly, may close incompletely, may close and reopen during illness or during intravascular volume repletion or overexpansion, or may remain widely open for no apparent reason. Sick newborns with a patent ductus arteriosus (PDA) may develop congestive heart failure and may need pharmacologic PDA closure or surgical PDA ligation. Often, a mechanically ventilated baby failing to progress has an otherwise unsuspected PDA, after whose closure ventilatory support requirements start to decrease.

Persistent pulmonary hypertension of the newborn (or "persistence of fetal circulation") may present idiopathically or in association with other serious illnesses. Affected babies are mostly full term. Pulmonary vascular resistance does not decline from, or it returns to, fetal levels, making adequate gas exchange impossible. Extremely intensive medical treatment is necessary in all cases; some babies survive (Levin and Morriss, 1990).

Cyanotic Congenital Heart Lesions

Central cyanosis should be evaluated as follows:

1. Physical examination should be performed with particular attention to breath sounds, arterial pulses, precordial configuration, precordial palpation and auscultation, and liver size.
2. A drop of blood should be smeared on a glass slide and exposed to 100 per cent oxygen. Color change to red excludes methemoglobinemia.
3. Hemoglobin and hematocrit should be measured, because polycythemia can cause both central cyanosis and congestive heart failure.
4. Arterial blood gas tensions and pH should be determined in room air (or at current supplemental oxygen settings) and then repeated in 100 per cent oxygen. In patients with cyanotic congenital heart disease, P_aO_2 might rise by 10 to 15 mm Hg but no higher. A rise of more than 25 mm Hg suggests pulmonary disease.
5. A chest radiograph should be inspected for
   a. Primary pulmonary disease.
   b. Heart size.
   c. Heart shape.
   d. Pulmonary vascular markings, which should be classed as showing

i. normal pulmonary blood flow.
ii. increased pulmonary blood flow.
iii. decreased pulmonary blood flow.

6. An electrocardiogram should be inspected for dysrhythmia and, with the help of a pediatric cardiologist, for other gross findings as well. Electrocardiograms performed or interpreted according to adult standards are useless except as rhythm strips.

7. An echocardiogram should be arranged at the earliest opportunity if it can be performed by an operator experienced with babies. Otherwise, echocardiography should be delayed pending transport to a regional center.

8. In babies with cyanotic congenital heart disease, cardiac catheterization (or, in special circumstances, a less invasive procedure) should be performed as soon as possible to define anatomy and guide therapy.

Cyanotic congenital heart lesions with diminished pulmonary blood flow include tetralogy of Fallot, pulmonary atresia with ventriculoseptal defect (pseudotruncus), pulmonary atresia without ventriculoseptal defect, critical pulmonary valvular stenosis, tricuspid atresia, Ebstein's anomaly of the tricuspid valve, and various other complex lesions.

Cyanotic congenital heart lesions with increased pulmonary blood flow include complete transposition of the great vessels, total anomalous pulmonary venous return, hypoplastic left heart syndrome, and persistent common truncus arteriosus (Levin and Morriss, 1990).

Noncyanotic Congenital Heart Lesions

Noncyanotic congenital heart lesions include transposition of the great vessels with ventricular septal defect, aortic coarctation syndrome, and PDA with pulmonary artery hypertension (see Chapter 35).

Dysrhythmias

Bradycardia can be seen in certain neurologic and metabolic disorders. Congenital heart block usually is seen in babies born to mothers with systemic lupus erythematosus; pacing is required. Paroxysmal atrial tachycardia (PAT), sometimes associated with Wolff-Parkinson-White syndrome, may convert to normal sinus rhythm with vagal stimulation, such as rectal examination or elicitation of the diving reflex (not recommended for the inexperienced). PAT requires digitalization and, often, cardioversion. Dysrhythmias should be treated in consultation with a pediatric cardiologist.

Peripheral Pulmonic Stenosis

Peripheral pulmonic stenosis (PPS) is characterized by a soft systolic murmur heard best over the peripheral lung fields, usually in an otherwise normal, often small, newborn. The PPS murmur is assumed to be due to turbulent flow in multiple branches of the pulmonary artery and evidently is associated with closure of the ductus arteriosus (Maroto et al., 1991). It is usually transient. Without other evidence of right-heart pressure elevation, it can be followed as a benign finding. PPS is discussed much more commonly in practice than in print.

Infectious Problems

After enjoying certain gestational protections (e.g., placental and membranous barriers) and despite many perinatal advantages (e.g., placental passage of maternal IgG, intrapartum and puerperal acquisition of normal skin and alimentary flora, vernix caseosa, "high" levels of circulating granulocytes, umbilical stump granulation tissue, colostrum), the newborn, by adult standards, is less than fully competent immunologically (Quie, 1990).

Various problems in newborns may be caused by maternal infection with—or maternal carriage of—certain microorganisms:

Those known to be teratogenic: *Toxoplasma gondii*, rubella virus, CMV, HSV, *Treponema pallidum*, and HIV (known jointly as "TORCH-SH").

Those known to be acquired by otherwise normal babies either in utero or at delivery: *Chlamydia trachomatis*, pathogenic coliforms, CMV, HBV, HSV, HIV, *Listeria monocytogenes*, *Mycobacterium tuberculosis*, N. *Gonnorrhoeae*, rubella virus, the group B β-hemolytic streptococcus, *T. gondii*, and *T. pallidum*.

Those known to be or suspected of being passed in breast milk: CMV, HIV, and HTLV-I.

Outside developed countries, additional infectious disease risks obtain.

Chorioamnionitis is a common cause of premature labor (Hillier et al., 1988) and neonatal infection. Babies born to mothers in whom chorioamnionitis has been suspected must be examined and observed carefully; total and differential leukocyte counts, blood cultures, and, often, lumbar punctures should be performed. Urine cultures, which must be obtained by suprapubic tap, are neither useful nor desirable in the early newborn period (DiGeronimo, 1992). Empiric administration of systemic antibiotics should be considered but should not be automatic.

Early-onset sepsis from perinatal acquisition of maternal organisms presents within 5 days of birth. Late-onset sepsis presents after 5 days and is likely to coexist with localized infection, such as meningitis. Organisms likely to cause early-onset sepsis include the group B β-hemolytic streptococcus (Payne et al., 1988), maternal gut bacteria, and *L.*

monocytogenes. Organisms likely to cause late-onset sepsis include, in addition to the early-onset pathogens, *Haemophilus influenzae* and *S. pneumoniae.* Ampicillin and an aminoglycoside have long been first-choice antibiotics for both early-onset and late-onset sepsis, although newer agents, particularly cephalosporins, have come increasingly into use to cover strains less sensitive to older agents and to cover the wider variety of late-onset pathogens.

HIV infection is hard to diagnose in the newborn, because transplacental acquisition of anti-HIV IgG is more common than pre- or perinatal acquisition of HIV itself and because serial HIV cultures may be negative for many months in infected infants. Although also sometimes falsely negative, antiviral IgA Western blot and dot blot assays using recombinant HIV-1 proteins are often truly positive in cord blood (Martin et al., 1991). Polymerase chain reaction (PCR) can be employed to find otherwise-occult HIV proviral DNA in peripheral blood mononuclear cells; unfortunately, PCR is occasionally falsely positive in this setting. Recommendations continue to evolve quickly, and the evaluation and management of potentially HIV-infected newborns has improved greatly over the past decade (Prober and Gershon, 1991).

Babies born vaginally to mothers suffering a primary genital herpetic eruption are at high risk for serious herpetic infection. Babies born vaginally to mothers suffering a recurrent eruption are at lower risk (Brown et al., 1987). However, neonatal herpetic infection also occurs in the offspring of unsuspected, asymptomatic HSV shedders (Prober et al., 1988). Babies delivered by cesarean section to avoid vaginal herpetic contact are not protected absolutely; rarely, ascending infection will prove to have occurred already. Any herpetiform skin lesion must be examined by Tzank preparation and viral culture, and every newborn with even one herpetic lesion must be treated expectantly for herpes encephalitis. The drug of choice is acyclovir.

The full range of intrauterine and newborn infections is extremely wide, in terms of both site and organism. Prophylactic, diagnostic, and therapeutic protocols depend on gestational and neonatal age, clinical presentation, instrumentation, and local flora and sensitivities. Some chronic infections, such as toxoplasmosis (Hohlfeld et al., 1989) and syphilis, are treatable both gestationally and postnatally. The vertical transmission of others, such as CMV, HSV, and HTLV-I, may be avoided knowingly; that of HBV, although perhaps unavoidable, still may be interdicted through passive and active immunization; and that of varicella-zoster virus, when manifested as maternal peripartum chickenpox (Miller et al., 1989), may be interdicted or modified through passive immunization. Current recommendations should be followed in every case (Nelson, 1993) (see previous sections and Chapter 20).

Neurologic Problems

Hypoxic encephalopathy (Brann, 1986), periventricular and intraventricular hemorrhage (Allan and Volpe, 1986), and seizure disorders (Painter et al., 1986) require specialized evaluation and management. *Neonatal seizures* always must be explained as soon as possible but need not always be suppressed immediately. Traumatic, metabolic, toxic, infectious, and postasphyxial explanations should be considered quickly but as thoroughly as possible. When a correctable cause is discovered, such as hypoglycemia, seizure therapy can be definitive, not suppressive. However, when neonatal seizures must be suppressed, first therapy should be phenobarbital, 10 to 20 mg/kg given intravenously over 5 to 10 minutes. If seizures persist or recur, an additional 10 mg/kg may be given an hour later and, if suppression is still inadequate, once more an hour after that. If phenobarbital maintenance seems necessary, 4 to 5 mg/kg per day may be given, intravenously or orally, divided into two doses. Phenytoin and other drugs sometimes must be added, but their use is more complicated. Prognosis for newborns with seizures is a function of ultimate diagnosis but is often optimistic (see Chapter 48).

Drug exposure syndromes (e.g., sedation in the babies of drug-treated epileptic mothers) and *drug withdrawal syndromes* (i.e., cases of jitteriness, irritability, hypertonicity, convulsions, hyperventilation, vomiting, diarrhea, and sweating) may occur in babies born to mothers taking various substances: narcotics (including methadone), benzodiazepines, phenobarbital, alcohol, pentazocine, cocaine, and others. Onset of withdrawal symptoms is typically shortly after birth but in some cases of methadone exposure may be days or weeks later. Babies of marijuana-using mothers may have short, dysphonic cries (Lester and Dreher, 1989).

Maternal history should be reviewed confidentially. Birth following placental abruption may suggest immediately antecedent maternal cocaine (or "crack" cocaine) use. Samples of blood and urine from mother and baby should be screened for narcotics and other toxic substances. Meconium, a drug "sink," may be a superior substance for testing, particularly for cocaine (Ostrea et al., 1989, 1993). Supportive care may have to be supplemented with phenobarbital or opiates and other depressants. Babies born to intravenous drug abusers or to women whose sexual partners inject drugs should be evaluated for HBV and HIV exposure. Mothers being maintained on methadone should not breast-feed their babies (Graef et al., 1988).

Cerebral palsy is a nonprogressive motor disorder with origins in pre- or perinatal life. It often can be anticipated. A low 5-minute Apgar score, seizure activity, and certain other neonatal signs, taken together, are significantly predictive (Ellenberg and Nelson, 1988). However, events occurring *before* labor and delivery are particularly important, relatively underappreciated (Ellis et al., 1988; Naeye et al., 1989; Torfs et al., 1990), and hard to affect positively (Cummins et al., 1993). Cerebral palsy can occur in infants and children with completely normal newborn histories (Nelson and Ellenberg, 1987). Many embryopathies involving the central nervous system are recognized consequences of intrauterine infection or drug exposure. In developed countries, the fetal alcohol syndrome, often overlooked (Little et al., 1990), is the most common preventable cause of mental retardation.

Metabolic Problems

Diabetic progeny require special evaluation and management. Residual hyperinsulinemia makes severe hypoglycemia a constant danger. Compulsive monitoring is required: blood glucose determinations at hours 0, 1, 2, 3, 6, 12, 24, and 48; and serum calcium determinations at hours 6, 12, 24, and 48. Dextrose supplementation is required by the oral, the orogastric, or, usually, the intravenous route. Sometimes, while intravenous access first is being secured or after it inadvertently has been lost, glucagon 300 μg/kg (maximum dose 1.0 mg) can be given subcutaneously. Chronic hyperglycemia has many adverse effects, direct and indirect, and diabetic progeny have increased rates of specific congenital anomalies (Becerra et al., 1990), perinatal asphyxia and trauma, RDS, polycythemia, hyperbilirubinemia, neurobehavioral deficits (Rizzo et al., 1990), and other problems.

Congenital adrenal hyperplasia (CAH) is the outcome of various autosomally recessive defects in the enzymes needed to synthesize cortisol. Because pituitary feedback stimulation of the adrenal produces excess androgens, CAH often presents in the newborn period as virilization in the phenotypic female; in many phenotypic males, the correct diagnosis is not made during life. In its common, salt-wasting form, CAH is caused by a deficiency of the enzyme 21-hydroxylase. The affected baby is deficient in both hydrocortisone and aldosterone, and the renal distal tubular activity of whatever aldosterone is produced may be inhibited by 17-hydroxyprogesterone and progesterone. Presentation in addisonian crisis is therefore common. Emergent goals are the intravenous repletion of volume deficiency, initiation of glucocorticoid and mineralocorticoid maintenance therapy, and suppression of adrenocorticotropic hormone release. The most immediate needs are met by dextrose 5% in normal saline, 20 mL/kg intravenously over 20 minutes, then hydrocortisone hemisuccinate (Solu-Cortef), 25 mg by intravenous push, and then deoxycorticosterone acetate (DOCA), 1 mg in-

tramuscularly. Early consultation with a pediatric endocrinologist is essential.

Unexplained poor feeding, lethargy, irritability, convulsions, hypertonia, hypotonia, hyperventilation, or coma can be seen in babies whose blood ammonia is elevated. Many hyperammonemic babies lack specific urea cycle enzymes.

See also Postnatal Screening.

Gastrointestinal Problems

Many gastrointestinal problems have been described earlier. Management often must include pediatric subspecialists and pediatric surgeons (see chapter 43).

A meconium plug may obstruct the rectum or the distal colon (and even the entire colon and terminal ileum). A contrast enema may prove both diagnostic and therapeutic. Most babies with meconium plugs are otherwise normal, but a few ultimately will prove to have Hirschsprung's disease (congenital aganglionic megacolon). Some babies with meconium plugs really have the meconium ileus of cystic fibrosis.

Necrotizing enterocolitis (NEC) classically is seen in improving premature babies and often presents after the institution or advancement of enteral feedings. However, larger babies also can develop NEC, usually in combination with another illness. An insult to the bowel wall, perhaps an ischemic insult, may compromise a section of mucosa physically or immunologically, allowing bacterial entry. Vomiting or failure to digest an orogastric tube feeding is often the first sign, soon followed by abdominal distention, ileus, gastrointestinal bleeding, sepsis, gut perforation, peritonitis, abdominal wall inflammation, and death. Serial radiograms first may show a fixed loop of bowel, then air in the bowel wall (pneumatosis intestinalis), then air in the portal system and the liver. Initial stabilization involves gut rest, volume repletion, and antibiotics. Intensive medical support, including total parenteral nutrition, always is needed, and surgical intervention often is required on short notice. Consultation with a neonatologist is essential; transport to a level III facility is usually necessary.

Neonatal hepatitis and biliary atresia usually present several weeks after birth as jaundice and hepatomegaly; their long-term management is complex.

Hematologic Problems

See also previous sections and Chapter 45.

Erythroblastosis Fetalis

Erythroblastosis fetalis is caused by fetomaternal rhesus (Rh) incompatibility or ABO blood group incompatibility. Obstetric management has been discussed in Chapter 26.

Some Rh-positive babies born to Rh-negative mothers are affected only mildly, but severely affected babies are profoundly anemic, icteric, hydropic, and unstable. Rh-negative blood typed and crossmatched against maternal blood should be available in the delivery room and should be administered in a single-volume exchange transfusion as soon as an umbilical venous catheter can be placed. Subsequently, multiple double-volume exchange transfusions must be performed to prevent kernicterus, a clinical syndrome in which bilirubin crosses the blood–brain barrier. Intrauterine death or hydrops at birth is rare in cases of ABO incompatibility, but hyperbilirubinemia is sometimes severe. Anti-A sensitization is more common and less dangerous than anti-B sensitization.

Rare blood group incompatibilities also sometimes can cause severe hemolytic disease. When rapidly deepening jaundice is caused by an ongoing hemolytic process, phototherapy cannot be considered an appropriate defense against kernicterus. Physical removal of sensitized erythrocytes, free hemoglobin, and hemoglobin's catabolites, including bilirubin, is necessary.

Bleeding

The differential diagnosis of bleeding in the newborn can be simplified on clinical grounds. The most frequent causes of bleeding in "sick" newborns are disseminated intravascular coagulation, consumptive thrombocytopenia, and liver failure. The most frequent causes of bleeding in "well" newborns are immune thrombocytopenia, vitamin K deficiency, hemophilia (80 per cent A, 20 per cent B), and anatomic vascular disruption (such as in an ulcer or hemangioma). Work-up should include careful maternal and family histories, a careful physical examination of the baby, and, to begin with, a platelet count, prothrombin time, and partial thromboplastin time performed on the baby. Maternal laboratory work-up should be individualized (Buchanan, 1986).

Physiologic Jaundice

All bilirubin derives from heme. In the newborn, bilirubin can be (1) *overproduced* in cases of acute or chronic hemolysis, resorption of extravasated blood, and polycythemia; (2) *undersecreted* in metabolic or endocrine disorders or in biliary obstructive disorders; (3) *underexcreted* in cases of intestinal defect or obstruction, in which situations the enterohepatic circulation of bilirubin, in large part a holdover from fetal life, may be accentuated, compounding the problem; and (4) *overproduced*, undersecreted, and underexcreted *simultaneously* in sick babies.

When, after the first day of extrauterine life, the hepatic conjugation of bilirubin is still too slow to prevent the accumulation of albumin-bound, lipid-soluble, unconjugated bilirubin in the serum, physiologic jaundice is described. When the serum level of unconjugated bilirubin threatens to exceed the bilirubin-binding capacity of albumin, exaggerated physiologic jaundice is described. When the serum level of unconjugated bilirubin does in fact exceed the bilirubin-binding capacity of albumin, kernicterus becomes a risk. In kernicterus, free lipid-soluble unconjugated bilirubin stains the basal ganglia and brainstem nuclei, and possible consequences range from a transient subclinical encephalopathy to neurologic devastation.

Jaundice occurs physiologically in half of all full-term babies and in more than half of all premature babies. It peaks and recedes within a week. Jaundice presenting during the first postpartum day is not physiologic. Unconjugated bilirubin levels exceeding 15 mg/dL in full-term babies and 10 mg/dL in premature babies usually are considered exaggerated and often prompt the institution of phototherapy. Kernicterus more often occurs occultly in premature than in full-term babies; autopsy evidence shows it to occur at lower serum levels in premature—or, at least, in sick premature—babies, even occurring at levels below 10 mg/dL. Exogenous factors, such as the now-abandoned use of benzyl alcohol as a preservative in intravenous flush solutions, may have contributed to this association (Jardine and Rogers, 1989). Although the handicap risk—the cerebral palsy risk—is demonstrably a function of maximum serum total bilirubin (van de Bor et al., 1989), rules defining threshold levels for clinical response in full-term, premature, and sick babies are inherently arbitrary and often informal.

When exaggeration of physiologic jaundice occurs, history and physical examination must be reviewed; clinical correlates are numerous (Johnson et al., 1989), although otherwise unsuspected sepsis is probably not one of them (Maisels and Kring, 1992). Samples must be collected for hematocrit, reticulocyte count, blood smear, and total and direct serum bilirubin concentration. Results of the direct Coombs' test and both the mother's and the baby's blood type and Rh factor must be retrieved and evaluated.

If exaggerated physiologic jaundice is diagnosed, several options may be considered:

1. The baby can be observed further. Intervention in the past often has been needlessly aggressive, particularly for full-term babies. Transcutaneous bilirubin monitoring can be useful in this setting.

2. Feedings can be supplemented. Breast-fed babies may not yet be receiving enough milk to stimulate gut motility sufficiently to blunt the effectiveness of the enterohepatic circulation of bilirubin.

3. Breast-feeding can be interrupted for a day

or so. Breast-feeding contributes to physiologic jaundice in some babies, evidently by enhancing the intestinal absorption of bilirubin in enterohepatic circulation (Alonso et al., 1991).

4. Phototherapy can be initiated. Light in the 425- to 475-nm range transforms unconjugated bilirubin into photoisomers that are more water soluble than the native species. These photoisomers still must pass through the liver, but they need not be conjugated by glucuronyl transferase to be secreted into the bile. Babies under "bililights" need a 10 per cent increment in their fluid maintenance; if they become temporarily lactose intolerant, as many do, they may need to be compensated for ongoing volume losses. Diarrhea under the lights is inconvenient, because diapers, which greatly decrease skin exposure to light, cannot be worn. Eyes must be covered, and the eye cover must not be allowed to work its way off the eyes or down over the nose. Some babies become "bronzed" during phototherapy, with unknown consequences.

5. Rarely, conservative steps cannot obviate the need for one or more double-volume exchange transfusions. Otherwise healthy term babies probably do not need exchange transfusions until their unconjugated bilirubin levels exceed 20 mg/dL; some physicians temporize until levels reach 25 mg/dL or even more (Newman and Maisels, 1992). Exchange transfusions are not risk-free procedures.

6. In future, it may become common practice to slow bilirubin production by inhibiting heme oxygenase with tin-protoporphyrin, even in some cases of autoimmunization (Kappas et al., 1988).

COMMUNITY CARE OF THE NICU GRADUATE

Family physicians increasingly are called on to care for neonatal intensive care unit (NICU) graduates, many of them former premature babies, some of them handicapped, some of them multiply transfused (Donowitz et al., 1989), and many of them at increased risk of one sort or another (Trachtenberg and Miller, 1986). Failure to thrive is comparatively common, even when correction is made for gestational age. Bronchopulmonary dysplasia often follows prolonged oxygen therapy or mechanical ventilation (Bancalari and Gerhardt, 1986). Babies with bronchopulmonary dysplasia often do poorly when infected with respiratory syncytial virus (Groothuis et al., 1988) and other common pathogens; pertussis infection in these babies is extremely dangerous. Postintubation airway scarring and tracheomalacia may complicate otherwise minor respiratory infections (Sotomayor et al., 1986). Weak suck, poorly coordinated swallowing, and gastroesophageal reflux (Giuffre et al., 1987) may impede growth and increase the risk of pulmonary aspiration. Intestinal scarring can make common diarrheal illnesses difficult to manage. Sudden infant death syndrome is a well-known risk, as is child abuse, which seems easier to predict than to prevent (Brayden et al., 1993). Nevertheless, most NICU graduates survive, and most survivors ultimately thrive.

REFERENCES

Abramo TJ, Evans JS, Kokomoor FW, et al: Occult blood in stools and necrotizing enterocolitis: Is there a relationship? Am J Dis Child 142:451, 1988.

Albright AL, Gartner JC, Weiner ES: Lumbar cutaneous hemangiomas as indicators of tethered spinal cords. Pediatrics 83:977, 1989.

Allan WC, Volpe JJ: Periventricular-intraventricular hemorrhage. Pediatr Clin North Am 33:47, 1986.

Alonso EM, Whitington PF, Whirington SH, et al: Enterohepatic circulation of nonconjugated bilirubin in rats fed with human milk. J Pediatr 118:425, 1991.

American Academy of Pediatrics: Emergency drug doses for infants and children. Pediatrics 81:462, 1988.

American Academy of Pediatrics: Report of the Task Force on Circumcision. Pediatrics 84:388, 1989. [See erratum in Pediatrics 84:761, 1989.]

American Academy of Pediatrics and American College of Obstetricians and Gynecologists: Guidelines for Perinatal Care. Washington, DC, American College of Obstetricians and Gynecologists, 1988.

American Academy of Pediatrics and American Thyroid Association: Newborn screening for congenital hypothyroidism: Recommended guidelines. Pediatrics 80:745, 1987.

Amiel-Tison C: Neurological evaluation of the maturity of newborn infants. Arch Dis Child 43:89, 1968.

Anand KJS, Hickey PR: Pain and its effects in the human neonate and fetus. N Engl J Med 317:1321, 1987.

Apgar V: A proposal for a new method of evaluation of the newborn infant. Curr Res Anesth Analg 32:260, 1953.

Asher MA: Screening for congenital dislocation of the hip, scoliosis, and other abnormalities affecting the musculoskeletal system. Pediatr Clin North Am 33:1335, 1986.

Athreya BH, Silverman BK: Pediatric Physical Diagnosis. Norwalk, CT, Appleton-Century-Crofts, 1985.

Bada HS, Korones SB, Pourcyrous M, et al: Asymptomatic syndrome of polycythemic hyperviscosity: Effect of partial plasma exchange transfusion. J Pediatr 120(4, pt 1):579, 1992.

Bailey C, Kattwinkel J: Establishing a neonatal resuscitation team in community hospitals. J Perinatol 10:294, 1990.

Ballard JL, Novak KK, Driver M: A simplified score for assessment of fetal maturation of newly born infants. J Pediatr 95: 769, 1979.

Bancalari E, Gerhardt T: Bronchopulmonary dysplasia. Pediatr Clin North Am 33:1, 1986.

Becerra JE, Khoury MJ, Cordero JF, et al: Diabetes mellitus during pregnancy and the risks for specific birth defects: A population-based case-control study. Pediatrics 85:1, 1990.

Berseth CL, Kenny JD, Durand R: Longitudinal development in pediatric residents of attitudes toward neonatal resuscitation. Am J Dis Child 140:766, 1986.

Bonadio WA, Stanco L, Bruce R, et al: Reference values of normal cerebrospinal fluid composition in infants ages 0 to 8 weeks. Pediatr Infect Dis J 11:589, 1992.

Bose C, Corbet A, Bose G, et al: Improved outcome at 28 days of age for very low birth weight infants treated with a single dose of a synthetic surfactant. J Pediatr 117:947, 1990.

Bowes WA 3d, Corke BC, Hulka J: Pulse oximetry: A review of the theory, accuracy, and clinical applications. Obstet Gynecol 74(3, pt 2):541, 1989.

Brann AW: Hypoxic ischemic encephalopathy. Pediatr Clin North Am 33:451, 1986.

Brayden RM, Altemeier WA, Dietrich MS, et al: A prospective study of secondary prevention of child maltreatment. J Pediatr 122:511, 1993.

Breaux CW, Georgeson KE, Roya SA, et al: Changing patterns in the diagnosis of hypertrophic pyloric stenosis. Pediatrics 81:213, 1988.

Brown MS, Brown CA: Circumcision decision: Prominence of social concerns. Pediatrics 80:215, 1987.

Brown ZA, Vontver LA, Benedetti J, et al: Effects of infants of a first episode of genital herpes during pregnancy. N Engl J Med 317:1246, 1987.

Broyles S, Sharp C, Tyson J, Sadler J: How should parents be informed about major procedures? An exploratory trial in the neonatal period. Early Hum Dev 31:67, 1992.

Buchanan GR: Coagulation disorders in the neonate. Pediatr Clin North Am 33:203, 1986.

Bull MJ, Weber K, Stroup KB: Automotive restraint systems for premature infants. J Pediatr 112:385, 1988a.

Bull MJ, Stroup KB, Gerhart S: Misuse of car safety seats. Pediatrics 81:98, 1988b.

Burger BJ, Burger JD, Bos CF, et al: Neonatal screening and staggered early treatment for congenital dislocation or dysplasia of the hip. Lancet 336:1549, 1990.

Caravella SJ, Clark DA, Dweek HS: Health codes for newborn care. Pediatrics 80:1, 1987.

Carlo WA, Martin RJ: Principles of neonatal assisted ventilation. Pediatr Clin North Am 33:221, 1986.

Chen JY: Prophylaxis of ophthalmia neonatorum: Comparison of silver nitrate, tetracycline, erythromycin and no prophylaxis. Pediatr Infect Dis J 11:1026, 1992.

Cheng TL, Partridge JC: Effect of bundling and high environmental temperature on neonatal body temperature. Pediatrics 92:238, 1993.

Chhabra RS, Brion LP, Castro M, et al: Comparison of maternal sera, cord blood, and neonatal sera for detecting presumptive congenital syphilis: Relationship with maternal treatment. Pediatrics 91:88, 1993.

Christensson K, Siles C, Cabrera T, et al: Lower body temperatures in infants delivered by caesarean section than in vaginally delivered infants. Acta Paediatr 82:128, 1993.

Coen RW, Koffler H: Primary Care of the Newborn. Boston, Little, Brown, 1987.

Conrad PD, Wilkening RB, Rosenberg AA: Safety of newborn discharge in less than 36 hours in an indigent population. Am J Dis Child 143:98, 1989.

Corbet A, Bucciarelli R, Goldman S, et al: Decreased mortality rate among small premature infants treated at birth with a single dose of synthetic surfactant: A multicenter controlled trial (American Exosurf Pediatric Study Group 1). J Pediatr 118:277, 1991.

Cornish JD, Heiss KF, Clark RH, et al: Efficacy of venovenous extracorporeal membrane oxygenation for neonates with respiratory and circulatory compromise. J Pediatr 122:105, 1993.

Crombleholme TM, Adzick NS, deLorimier AA, et al: Carotid artery reconstruction following extracorporeal membrane oxygenation. Am J Dis Child 144:872, 1990.

Cummins SK, Nelson KB, Grether JK, et al: Cerebral palsy in four northern California counties, births 1983 through 1985. J Pediatr 123:230, 1993.

David R: Closed chest cardiac massage in the newborn infant. Pediatrics 81:552, 1988.

Davis JM, Veness-Meehan K, Notter RH, et al: Changes in pulmonary mechanics after the administration of surfactant to infants with respiratory distress syndrome. N Engl J Med 319:476, 1988.

Delight E, Goodall J, Jones PW: What do parents expect antenatally and do babies teach them? Arch Dis Child 66:1309, 1991.

DiGeronimo RJ: Lack of efficacy of the urine culture as part of the initial workup of suspected neonatal sepsis. Pediatr Infect Dis J 11:764, 1992.

Donowitz LG, Turner RB, Searcy MA, et al: The high rate of blood donor exposure for critically ill neonates. Infect Control Hosp Epidemiol 10:509, 1989.

Dorfman DH, Glaser JH: Congenital syphilis presenting in infants after the newborn period. N Engl J Med 323:1299, 1990.

Dubowitz LM, Dubowitz V, Goldberg C: Clinical assessment of gestational age in the newborn infant. J Pediatr 77:1, 1970.

Dungy CI, Christensen-Szalanski J, Losch M, et al: Effect of discharge samples on duration of breast-feeding. Pediatrics 90(2, pt 1):233, 1992.

Edens MJ, Eyler FD, Wagner JT, Eitzman DV: Neonatal ethics: Development of a consultative group. Pediatrics 86:944, 1990.

Ellenberg JH, Nelson KB: Cluster of perinatal events identifying infants at high risk for death or disability. J Pediatr 113:546, 1988.

Ellis WG, Goetzman BW, Lindenberg JA: Neuropathologic documentation of prenatal brain damage. Am J Dis Child 142:858, 1988.

Evans ME, Schaffner W, Federspiel CF, et al: Sensitivity, specificity, and predictive value of body surface cultures in a neonatal intensive care unit. JAMA 259:249, 1988.

Fanaroff AA, Martin RJ (eds): Neonatal-Perinatal Medicine: Diseases of the Fetus and Infant, 5th edition. St. Louis, CV Mosby, 1991.

Fergusson DM, Lawton JM, Shannon FT: Neonatal circumcision and penile problems: An 8-year longitudinal study. Pediatrics 81:537, 1988.

Flynn JT, Bancalari, E, Snyder ES, et al: A cohort study of transcutaneous oxygen tension and the incidence and severity of retinopathy of prematurity. N Engl J Med 326:1050, 1992.

Fojaco RM, Hensley GT, Moskowitz L: Congenital syphilis and necrotizing funisitis. JAMA 261:1788, 1989.

Frattallone JM, Fuhrman BP, Kochanek PM, et al: Management of pulmonary barotrauma by extracorporeal membrane oxygenation, apnea, and lung rest. J Pediatr 112:787, 1988.

Ginsburg CM, McCracken GH: Urinary tract infections in young infants. Pediatrics 69:409, 1982.

Giuffre RM, Rubins S, Mitchell I: Antireflux surgery in infants with bronchopulmonary dysplasia. Am J Dis Child 141:648, 1987.

Glass P, Miller M, Short B: Morbidity for survivors of extracorporeal membrane oxygenation: Neurodevelopmental outcome at 1 year of age. Pediatrics 83:72, 1989.

Graef JW, (ed); Alleyne CM et al (editorial board): Manual of Pediatric Therapeutics, 4th edition. Boston, Little, Brown, 1988.

Greenberg RA, Bauman KE, Glover LH, et al: Ecology of passive smoking by young infants. J Pediatr 114:774, 1989.

Gregg RG, Wilfond BS, Farrell PM, et al: Application of DNA analysis in a population-screening program for neonatal diagnosis of cystic fibrosis (CF): Comparison of screening protocols. Am J Hum Genet 52:616, 1993.

Grogaard JB, Lindstrom DP, Parker RA, et al: Increased survival rate in very low birth weight infants (1500 grams or less): No association with increased incidence of handicaps. J Pediatr 117(1, pt 1):139, 1990.

Groothuis JR, Gutierrez KM, Lauer BA: Respiratory syncytial virus infection in children with bronchopulmonary dysplasia. Pediatrics 82:199, 1988.

Habicht J-P, DaVanzo J, Butz WP: Mother's milk and sewage: Their interactive effects on infant mortality. Pediatrics 81:456, 1988.

Halsey NA: Discussion of Immunization Practices Advisory Committee/American Academy of Pediatrics recommendations for universal infant hepatitis B vaccination. Pediatr Infect Dis J 12:446, 1993.

Hammerschlag MR, Cummings J, Butz WP, et al: Efficacy of neonatal ocular prophylaxis for the prevention of chlamydial and gonococcal conjunctivitis. N Engl J Med 320:769, 1989.

Hammond KB, Abman SH, Sokol RJ, et al: Efficacy of statewide neonatal screening for cystic fibrosis by assay of trypsinogen concentrations. N Engl J Med 325:769, 1991.

Helsing E, King FS: Breast-feeding in Practice: A Manual for Health Workers. Oxford, England, Oxford University Press, 1982.

Hensinger RN: Congenital dislocation of the hip. Ciba Found Symp 31:5, 1979.

Herrmann HJ, Roberts MW: Preventive dental care: The role of the pediatrician. Pediatrics 80:107, 1987.

Hersh JH, Bloom AS, Cromer AD, et al: Does a supernumerary nipple/renal field defect exist? Am J Dis Child 141:989, 1987.

Herzog LW, Alvarez SR: The frequency of foreskin problems in uncircumcised children. Am J Dis Child 140:254, 1986.

HIFI Study Group: High-frequency oscillatory ventilation compared with conventional mechanical ventilation in the treatment of respiratory failure in preterm infants. N Engl J Med 320:88, 1989.

HIFI Study Group: High-frequency oscillatory ventilation compared with conventionalintermittent mechanical ventilation in the treatment of respiratory failure in preterm infants. Neurodevelopmental status at 16 to 24 months of postterm age. J Pediatr 117:939, 1990a.

HIFI Study Group: High-frequency oscillatory ventilation compared with conventional mechanical ventilation in the treatment of respiratory failure in preterm infants: Assessment of pulmonary function at 9 months of corrected age. J Pediatr 116:933, 1990b.

Hillier SL, Martius J, Krohn M, et al: A case-control study of chorioamnionic infection and histologic chorioamnionitis in prematurity. N Engl J Med 319:972, 1988.

Hletko PJ, Robin SS, Hletko JD, et al: Infant safety seat use: Reaching the hard to reach. Am J Dis Child 141:1301, 1987.

Hohlfeld P, Daffos F, Thulliez P, et al: Fetal toxoplasmosis: Outcome of pregnancy and infant follow-up after in utero treatment. J Pediatr 115(5, pt 1):765, 1989.

Isenberg SJ, Dang Y, Jotterand V: The pupils of term and preterm infants. Am J Ophthalmol 108:75, 1989.

Jain L, Ferre C, Vidyasagar D, et al: Cardiopulmonary resuscitation of apparently stillborn infants: Survival and long-term outcome. J Pediatr 118:778, 1991.

Jardine DS, Rogers K: Relationship of benzyl alcohol to kernicterus, intraventricular hemorrhage, and mortality in preterm infants. Pediatrics 83:153, 1989.

Jenny C, Kuhns ML, Arakawa F: Hymens in newborn female infants. Pediatrics 80:399, 1987.

Joffe A, Radius SM: Breast versus bottle: Correlates of adolescent mothers' infant-feeding practices. Pediatrics 79:689, 1987.

Johnson CA, Liese BS, Hassanein RE: Factors predictive of heightened third-day bilirubin levels: A multiple stepwise regression analysis. Fam Med 21:283, 1989.

Jones DA: Importance of the clicking hip in screening for congenital dislocation of the hip. Lancet 1:599, 1989.

Joseph PR, Rosenfeld W: Clavicular fractures in neonates. Am J Dis Child 144:165, 1990.

Kaiserman K, Martin GI, Sindel BC, et al: The effectiveness of a cardiopulmonary resuscitation program for mothers of newborn infants. J Perinatol 9:49, 1989.

Kappas A, Drummond GS, Manola T, et al: Sn-protoporphyrin use in the management of hyperbilirubinemia in term newborns with direct Coombs-positive ABO incompatibility. Pediatrics 81:485, 1988.

Kemp JS, Thach BT: Sudden death in infants sleeping on polystyrene-filled cushions. N Engl J Med 324:1858, 1991.

Kenney RD, Flippo JL, Black EB: Supernumerary nipples and renal anomalies in neonates. Am J Dis Child 141:987, 1987.

Kim EH, Cohen RS, Ramachandran P: Effect of vascular puncture on blood gases in the newborn. Pediatr Pulmonol 10:287, 1991.

Klaus MH, Fanaroff AA (eds): Care of the High-Risk Neonate, 4th edition. Philadelphia, WB Saunders Company, 1993.

Kurinij N, Shiono PH, Rhoads GG: Breast-feeding incidence and duration in black and white women. Pediatrics 81:365, 1988.

Leiberman A, Carmi R, Bar-Ziv Y, Karplus M: Congenital nasal stenosis in newborn infants. J Pediatr 120:124, 1992.

Lester BM, Dreher M: Effects of marijuana use during pregnancy on newborn cry. Child Dev 60:765, 1989.

Leung AKC: Natal teeth. Am J Dis Child 140:249, 1986.

Leung AKC, Robson WLM: Single umbilical artery: A report of 159 cases. Am J Dis Child 143:108, 1989.

Levin DL, Morriss FC (eds): Essentials of Pediatric Intensive Care, 2nd edition. St. Louis, Quality Medical Publishing, 1990.

Linder N, Arand JU, Tsur M, et al: Need for endotracheal intubation and suction in meconium-stained neonates. J Pediatr 112:613, 1988.

Little BB, Snell LM, Rosenfeld, et al: Failure to recognize fetal alcohol syndrome in newborn infants. Am J Dis Child 144:1142, 1990.

Long W, Thompson T, Sundell H, et al: Effects of two rescue doses of a synthetic surfactant on mortality rate and survival without bronchopulmonary dysplasia in 700- to 1350-gram infants with respiratory distress syndrome (the American Exosurf Neonatal Study Group I). J Pediatr 118(4, pt 1):595, 1991.

MacKinnon JA, Perlman M, Kirpalani H, et al: Spinal cord injury at birth: Diagnostic and prognostic data in twenty-two patients. J Pediatr 122:431, 1993.

Madlon-Kay DJ: "Witch's milk": Galactorrhea in the newborn. Am J Dis Child 141:252, 1986.

Maisels MJ, Kring E: Risk of sepsis in newborns with severe hyperbilirubinemia. Pediatrics 90:741, 1992.

Manroe BL, Weinberg AG, Rosenfeld CR, et al: The neonatal blood count in health and disease. I. Reference values for neutrophilic cells. J Pediatr 95:89, 1979.

Maroto E, Fouron JC, Ak'e E, et al: Closure of the ductus arteriosus: Determinant factor in the appearance of transient peripheral pulmonary stenosis of the neonate. J Pediatr 119:955, 1991.

Martin NL, Levy JA, Legg H, et al: Detection of infection with human immunodeficiency virus (HIV) type 1 in infants by an anti-HIV immunoglobulin A assay using recombinant proteins. J Pediatr 118:354, 1991.

McKenzie S: Troublesome crying in infants: Effect of advice to reduce stimulation. Arch Dis Child 66:1416, 1991.

Miller E, Cradock-Watson JE, Ridehalgh MK: Outcome in newborn babies given anti-varicella-zoster immunoglobulin after perinatal maternal infection with varicella-zoster virus. Lancet 2:371, 1989.

Moore DJ, Robb TA, Davidson GP: Breath hydrogen response to milk containing lactose in colicky and noncolicky infants. J Pediatr 113:979, 1988.

Mor N, Merlob P: Congenital absence of hymen only a rumor? Pediatrics 82:679, 1988.

Morelli JG, Weston WL: Soaps and shampoos in pediatric practice. Pediatrics 80:634, 1987.

Morselli PL: Clinical pharmacology of the perinatal period and early infancy. Clin Pharmacokinet 17(suppl 1):13, 1989.

Moss GD, Cartlidge PH, Speidel BD, et al: Routine examination in the neonatal period. BMJ 302:878, 1991.

Moyes CD, Milne A, Dimitrakakis M, et al: Very-low-dose hepatitis B vaccine in newborn infants: An economic option for control in endemic areas. Lancet 1:29, 1987.

Naeye RL, Peters EC, Bartholomew M, et al: Origins of cerebral palsy. Am J Dis Child 143:1154, 1989.

Nelson JD: 1993–1994 Pocketbook of Pediatric Antimicrobial Therapy, 10th edition. Baltimore, Williams & Wilkins, 1993.

Nelson KB, Ellenberg JH: The asymptomatic newborn and risk of cerebral palsy. Am J Dis Child 141:1333, 1987.

Nelson SE, Ziegler EE, Copeland AM, et al: Lack of adverse reactions to iron-fortified formula. Pediatrics 81:360, 1988.

Newman TB, Maisels MJ: Evaluation and treatment of jaundice

in the term newborn: A kinder, gentler approach. Pediatrics 89(5, pt 1):809, 1992.

Oh W: Neonatal polycythemia and hyperviscosity. Pediatr Clin North Am 33:523, 1986.

Ostrea EM, Brady MJ, Parks PM, et al: Drug screening in infants of drug-dependent mothers: An alternative to urine testing. J Pediatr 115:474, 1989.

Ostrea EM Jr, Romero A, Yee H: Adaptation of the meconium drug test for mass screening. J Pediatr 122:152, 1993.

Oxtoby MJ: Human immunodeficiency virus and other viruses in human milk: Placing the issues in broader perspective. Pediatr Infect Dis J 7:825, 1988.

Painter MJ, Bergman I, Crumrine P: Neonatal seizures. Pediatr Clin North Am 33:91, 1986.

Parker S, Zuckerman B, Bauchner H, et al: Jitteriness in full-term neonates: Prevalence and correlates. Pediatrics 85:17, 1990.

Payne NR, Burke BA, Day DL, et al: Correlation of clinical and pathologic findings in early onset neonatal group B streptococcal infection with disease severity and prediction of outcome. Pediatr Infect Dis J 7:836, 1988.

Poland RL: The question of routine neonatal circumcision. N Engl J Med 322:1312, 1990.

Ponsonby A-L, Dwyer T, Gibbons LE, et al: Factors potentiating the risk of sudden infant death syndrome associated with the prone position. N Engl J Med 329:377, 1993.

Prober CG, Gershon AA: Medical management of newborns and infants born to human immunodeficiency virus-seropositive mothers. Pediatr Infect Dis J 10:684, 1991.

Prober CG, Hensleigh PA, Boucher FD, et al: Use of routine viral cultures at delivery to identify neonates exposed to herpes simplex virus. N Engl J Med 318:887, 1988.

Quie PG: Antimicrobial defenses in the neonate. Semin Perinatol 14(4, suppl 1):2, 1990.

Reller MD, Ziegler ML, Rice MJ, et al: Duration of ductal shunting in healthy preterm infants: An echocardiographic color flow Doppler study. J Pediatr 112:441, 1988.

Righard L, Alade MO: Effect of delivery room routines on success of first breast-feed. Lancet 336:1105, 1990.

Rizzo T, Freinkel N, Metzger BE, et al: Correlations between antepartum maternal metabolism and newborn behavior. Am J Obstet Gynecol 163(5, pt 1):1458, 1990.

Rockney RM: Pediatric code cards. Am J Dis Child 142:73, 1988.

Rosenfeld CR, Laptook AR, Jeffery J: Limited effectiveness of triple dye in preventing colonization with methicillin-resistant *Staphylococcus aureus* in a special care nursery. Pediatr Infect Dis J 9:290, 1990.

Sanchez P: Nelson JD, McCracken GH (eds). Congenital Neurosyphilis. Pediatr Infect Dis J Newsletter 15:1, 1989, in Pediatr Infect Dis J 8(1), 1989.

Schmitt BD: The prevention of sleep problems and colic. Pediatr Clin North Am 33:763, 1986.

Schoen EJ: The status of circumcision of newborns. N Engl J Med 322:1308, 1990.

Schumacher RE, Barks JD, Johnston MU, et al: Right-sided brain lesions in infants following extracorporeal membrane oxygenation. Pediatrics 82:155, 1988.

Sepkowitz S: Influence of the legal imperative and medical guidelines on the incidence and management of the meconium-stained newborn. Am J Dis Child 141:1124, 1987.

Sirinavin S, Chotpitayasunondh T, Suwanjutha S, et al: Protective efficacy of neonatal bacillus Calmette-Guérin vaccination against tuberculosis. Pediatr Infect Dis J 10:359, 1991.

Sotomayor JL, Godinez RI, Borden S, et al: Large-airway collapse due to acquired tracheobronchomalacia in infancy. Am J Dis Child 140:367, 1986.

Standards and guidelines for cardiopulmonary resuscitation (CPR) and emergency cardiac care (ECC): Part VI: Neonatal advanced life support. JAMA 255:2969, 1986.

Tan OT, Gilchrest BA: Laser therapy for selected cutaneous vascular lesions in the pediatric population: A review. Pediatrics 82:652, 1988.

Taubman B: Parental counselling compared with elimination of cow's milk or soy milk protein for the treatment of infant colic syndrome: A randomized trial. Pediatrics 81:756, 1988.

Taylor BJ: Evaluation of the reconstructed carotid artery following extracorporeal membrane oxygenation. Pediatrics 90:568, 1992.

Thoele DG, Muster AJ, Paul MH: Recognition of coarctation of the aorta: A continuing challenge for the primary care physician. Am J Dis Child 141:1201, 1987.

Todres ID, Guillemin J, Grodin MA, et al: Life-saving therapy for newborns: A questionnaire survey in the state of Massachusetts. Pediatrics 81:643, 1988.

Toffler WL, Sinclair AE, White KA: Dorsal penile nerve block during newborn circumcision: Underutilization of a proven technique? J Am Board Fam Pract 3:171, 1990.

Torfs CP, van den Berg, Oechsli FW, et al: Prenatal and perinatal factors in the etiology of cerebral palsy. J Pediatr 116:615, 1990.

Trachtenberg DE, Miller TC: Office care of the premature infant. Am Fam Physician 33:119, 1986.

Tsuji Y, Doi H, Yamabe T, et al: Prevention of mother-to-child transmission of human T-lymphotropic virus type-I. Pediatrics 86:11, 1990.

Usher R, McLean F: Intrauterine growth of live-born Caucasian infants at sea level: Standards obtained from measurements in 7 dimensions of infants born between 25 and 44 weeks of gestation. J Pediatr 74:901, 1969.

van de Bor M, Ens-Dokkum M, Schreuder AM, et al: Hyperbilirubinemia in preterm infants and neurodevelopmental outcome at 2 years of age: Results of a national collaborative survey. Pediatrics 83:915, 1989.

Van de Perre P, Simonon A, Msellati P, et al: Postnatal transmission of human immunodeficiency virus type 1 from mother to infant: A prospective cohort study in Kigali, Rwanda. N Engl J Med 325:593, 1991.

Verma A, Dhanireddy R: Time of first stool in extremely low birth weight (< or = 1000 grams) infants. J Pediatr 122:626, 1993.

Versmold HT, Kitterman JA, Phibbs RH, et al: Aortic blood pressure during the first 12 hours of life in infants with birth weight 610 to 4,220 grams. Pediatrics 67:607, 1981.

Vichinsky E, Hurst D, Earles A, et al: Newborn screening for sickle cell disease: Effect on mortality. Pediatrics 81:749, 1988.

Volpe JJ: Neurology of the Newborn. Philadelphia, WB Saunders Company, 1981.

Wallerstein E: Circumcision: An American Health Fallacy. New York, Springer, 1980.

Walter RS, Donaldson JS, Davis CL, et al: Ultrasound screening of high-risk infants: A method to increase early detection of congenital dysplasia of the hip. Am J Dis Child 146:230, 1992.

Walters JW: Approaches to ethical decision making in the neonatal intensive care unit. Am J Dis Child 142:825, 1988.

Ward KE, Pryor RW, Matson JR, et al: Delayed detection of coarctation in infancy: Implications for timing of newborn follow-up. Pediatrics 86:972, 1990.

Winberg J, Bollgren I, Gothefors L, et al: The prepuce: A mistake of nature? Lancet 1:598, 1989.

Winikoff B, Myers D, Laukaran VH, et al: Overcoming obstacles to breast-feeding in a large municipal hospital: Applications of lessons learned. Pediatrics 80:423, 1987.

Wiswell TE, Geschke DW: Risks from circumcision during the first month of life compared with those for uncircumcised boys. Pediatrics 83:1011, 1989.

Wiswell TE, Roscelli JD: Corroborative evidence for the decreased incidence of urinary tract infections in circumcised male infants. Pediatrics 78:96, 1986.

Wiswell TE, Miller GM, Gelston HM Jr, et al: Effect of circumcision status on periurethral flora during the first year of life. J Pediatr 113:442, 1988.

Woolridge MW, Fisher C: Colic, "overfeeding," and symptoms of lactose malabsorption in the breast-fed baby: A possible artifact of feed management? Lancet 2:382, 1988.

Yetman RJ, Coody DX, West MS, et al: Comparison of temperature measurements by an aural infrared thermometer with measurements by traditional rectal and axillary techniques. J Pediatr 122(5, pt 1):769, 1993.

Zenker PN, Berman SM: Congenital syphilis: Trends and recommendations for evaluation and management. Pediatr Infect Dis J 10:516, 1991.

Ziegler EE, Fomon SJ, Nelson SE, et al: Cow milk feeding in infancy: Further observations on blood loss from the gastrointestinal tract. J Pediatr 116:11, 1990.

Zuckerman B, Bauchner H, Parker S, et al: Maternal depressive symptoms during pregnancy, and newborn irritability. J Dev Behav Pediatr 11:190, 1990.

SUGGESTED READINGS

Farr V, Kerridge DF, Mitchell RG: The definition of some external characteristics used in the assessment of gestational age of the newborn infant. Dev Med Child Neurol 8:507, 1966.

Vogler C, Sotelo-Avila C, Lagunoff, et al: Aluminum-containing emboli in infants treated with extracorporeal membrane oxygenation. N Engl J Med 319:75, 1988.

CHAPTER 28

GROWTH AND DEVELOPMENT

SANFORD R. KIMMEL and LORRAINE FAY

Growth is a dynamic process in which increasing cell size and number in various tissues results in a physical increase in the size of the body as a whole. Simultaneously, development occurs as tissues differentiate in form and mature in function, reflecting the individual's genetic heritage and environmental interaction. Nutritional, family, emotional, sociocultural, and community, as well as physical, factors play a role in shaping the child's psychologic and physiologic development (Vaughan and Litt, 1992). The child emotionally responds to a particular stimulus in an apparently innate and characteristic style that reflects his or her temperament (Sahler and McAnarney, 1981).

Knowledge of normal as well as abnormal patterns of growth and development enables the physician to assist the child in maximizing his or her fullest potential. Growth in height and weight are sensitive reflections of a child's general health (Green, 1986). Deviations from normal may reflect the presence of physical illness or a disturbance in the child's environment. Consequently, such deviations warrant an evaluation of those factors influencing growth and development (Table 28–1).

MEASURING PHYSICAL PARAMETERS OF GROWTH

Weight, length, and head circumference are the most useful routine measurements in infants. The weight should be determined on a balance beam scale and recorded at each visit. Infants under 24 months should be weighed nude, while older children may wear light clothing but not shoes.

Total body length in children up to age 2 is obtained most accurately by placing them in the recumbent position and measuring from crown to heel. This procedure is facilitated in infants by the use of a measuring board (Tanner, 1986). Older children should have their shoeless standing height determined with heels, buttocks, scapulae, and occiput touching a vertical wall to which a fixed ruler has been attached. The child should look straight ahead while a right triangular board is placed firmly against the top of the head. The examiner then reads and records the height (Silverstein and Rosenbloom, 1988). The usual mea-

suring rod attached to a weight scale is not precise (Green, 1986).

Head circumference reflects the growth of the cranium and its contents. It should be determined and recorded at all routine physical examinations during the first 2 years of life (American Academy of Pediatrics [AAP] Committee on Psychosocial Aspects of Child and Family Health, 1988). This also may be done as part of the initial exam at any age. A nonstretchable measuring tape (usually paper or flexible plastic) is used to obtain the greatest circumference encompassing the occipital, parietal, and frontal prominences. A small head circumference, or microcephaly, may be familial, may be due to craniosynostosis, congenital viral infections, fetal drug syndromes, underlying structural abnormalities, or may be secondary to trauma, infections, or dysmorphic syndromes. A large head circumference, or macrocephaly, most frequently is caused by hydrocephalus but may be familial, due to intracranial bleeding or masses, due to thickening of the skull, or associated with fragile X syndrome and other conditions (Green, 1986).

Proper Use and Interpretation of Growth Charts

The growth charts shown in Figure 28–1 are those constructed by the National Center for Health Statistics (NCHS) from a survey of generally well-nourished children representing a cross section of ethnic and economic groups in the United States (Vaughan and Litt, 1992). These graphs provide a normal range of weight and length or height for a given chronologic age. Recumbent length is recorded on the chart for children from birth to 36 months old, while standing height is recorded on the chart for children from 2 to 18 years old. Premature infants should have their chronologic age adjusted according to their degree of prematurity up to age 2 years because most catch-up growth is complete by this time. Alternatively, an infant growth record beginning several months prior to term may be utilized for premature infants under 1 year of age (Fig. 28–2). Although a height or weight above the 95th percentile or below the 5th percentile should alert the physician

TABLE 28-1. FACTORS INFLUENCING PHYSICAL GROWTH

Genetic
1. Parental height
   a. Familial (tall or short) stature
   b. Constitutional growth delay
2. Chromosomal abnormalities
   a. Down syndrome
   b. Turner syndrome
   c. Other syndromes or disorders
3. Race

Environmental
1. Intrauterine
   a. Maternal size
   b. Maternal nutrition
   c. Maternal smoking and drug use
   d. Congenital infection
   e. Placental function
2. Postnatal
   a. Nutrition
   b. Socioeconomic status
   c. Cultural or home environment

Endocrinologic
1. Thyroid hormone
2. Cortisol
3. Androgens
4. Estrogens
5. Growth hormone–somatomedin axis
6. Diabetes mellitus (poorly controlled)

Chronic or Recurrent Systemic Illness
1. Congenital heart disease
2. Central nervous system disease
3. Pulmonary disease
   a. Asthma
   b. Cystic fibrosis
4. Gastrointestinal disease
   a. Inflammatory bowel disease
   b. Malabsorption syndromes
5. Renal disease
   a. Chronic renal insufficiency
   b. Renal tubular acidosis
   c. Bartter's syndrome
   d. Nephrogenic diabetes insipidus

Metabolic Disease or Status
1. Chronic acidosis
2. Storage diseases

Chronic Mediations
1. Exogenous steroids

Adapted from Lipsky MS, Horner JM: The child with short stature. Am Fam Physician 37:233, 1988, with permission.

to a possible problem, the child may represent the outer fringe of the normal range.

Linear growth in infants has been shown to occur in incremental bursts rather than continuously (Lampl et al., 1992). A growth curve constructed by a series of heights and weights taken over a period of time allows the physician to compare the child's current growth with his or her previous pattern. A child whose growth curve parallels the normal curve regardless of his or her absolute percentile has a normal rate of growth for that particular child. In comparison, a child whose height or weight crosses multiple percentile lines or whose

linear growth rate drops below 4 cm/year requires further evaluation for nutritional, psychosocial, or organic problems that could impede or accelerate growth (Lipsky and Horner, 1988). Children who are large at birth but destined to be small and children who are small at birth but destined to be large usually will reach their genetic isobar on the growth chart by age 2 (Silverstein and Rosenbloom, 1988).

Rules of Thumb

Although careful measuring and plotting of growth parameters is the most accurate method by which to follow a child's physical growth, rules of thumb (Keefer, 1988) are helpful to the physician in remembering and forming an overall impression of the child's progress (Table 28–2). The growth velocity, or rate of gain in height or weight, actually decreases from the time of birth until the onset of the pubertal growth spurt (Fig. 28–3).

Familial Short Stature and Constitutional Growth Delay

Each child has a different rate of maturation, or what Boas termed "tempo of growth" (Tanner, 1986). Consequently, if a child's growth falls outside the range of normal, it may be useful to obtain bone age films, usually of the hand and wrist. By comparing the development of the ossification centers and epiphyseal–diaphyseal unions to known standards, it is possible to estimate skeletal maturity (Green, 1986). Some causes of retarded or accelerated bone age are listed in Table 28–3.

Calculation of midparental height also is useful

TABLE 28-2. RULES OF THUMB: GROWTH GUIDELINES FOR CHILDREN

Age	Length or Height	Weight
Newborn	50 cm (20 in) average	3.4 kg (7.5 lbs) average
Newborn– 3 months		1 kg/month (0.5–1 oz/day)
4–5 months		Doubles birth weight
6 months		0.5 kg/month
12 months	Increases by 50%	Triples birth weight
12–24 months		0.25 kg/month
>2 years	>5 cm (2 in)/year until adolescent growth spurt	2.3 kg (5 lb)/year until adolescent growth spurt
4 years	Doubles (40 in approximately)	40 lbs approximately

Adapted from Keefer CH: Normal growth and development: An overview. *In* Dershewitz RA (ed): Ambulatory Pediatric Care. Philadelphia, JB Lippincott, 1988, p 24, with permission.

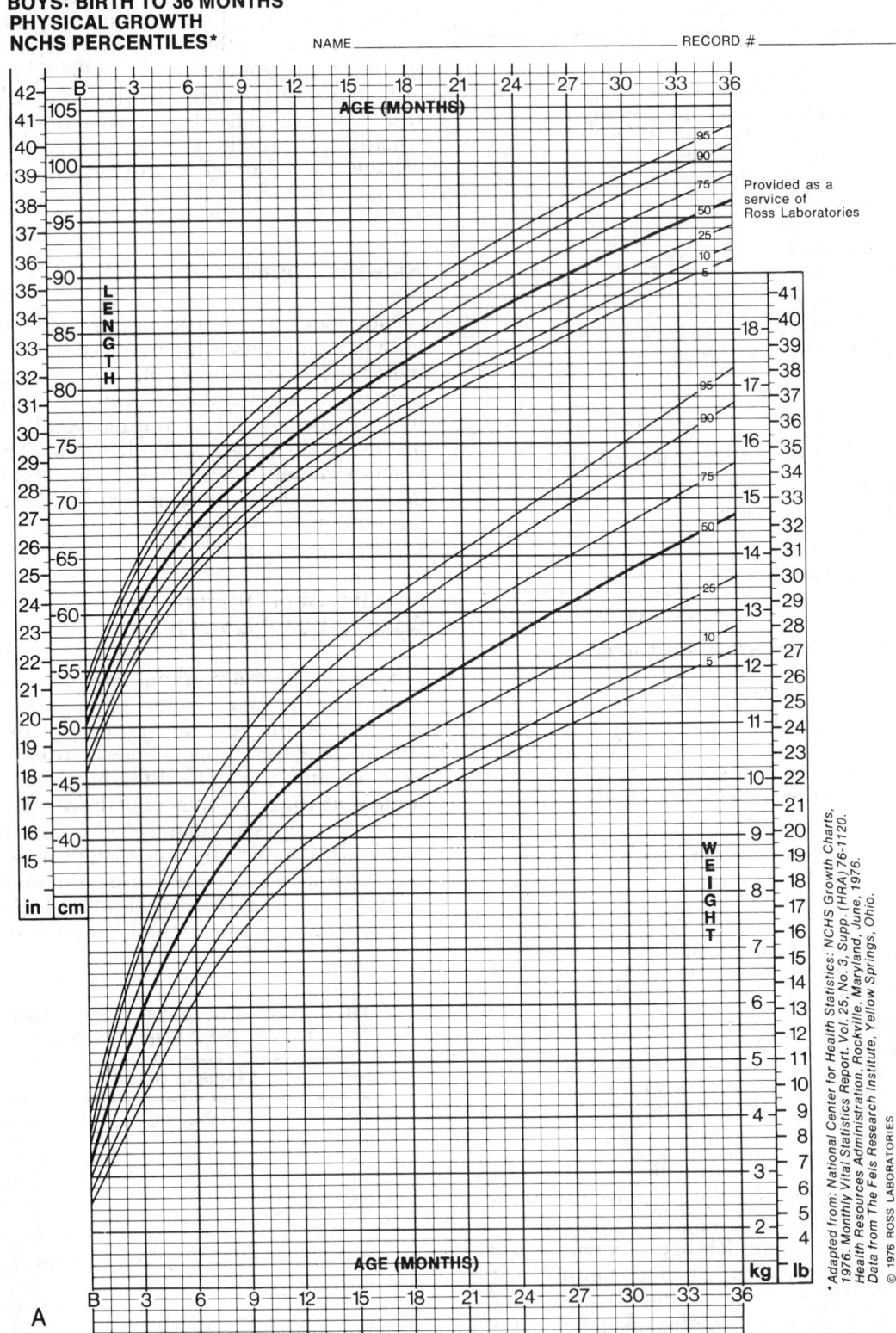

BOYS: BIRTH TO 36 MONTHS
PHYSICAL GROWTH
NCHS PERCENTILES*

NAME_____ RECORD #_____

Provided as a
service of
Ross Laboratories

* Adapted from: National Center for Health Statistics: NCHS Growth Charts, 1976. Monthly Vital Statistics Report. Vol. 25, No. 3, Supp. (HRA) 76-1120. Health Resources Administration. Rockville, Maryland, June, 1976. Data from The Fels Research Institute, Yellow Springs, Ohio.

© 1976 ROSS LABORATORIES

FIGURE 28–1. These growth charts for boys (*A, B*) and girls (*C, D*) plot length *A, C*) or height (*B, D*) for age on their upper curves and weight for age on their lower curves. (Percentiles are constructed from NCHS data and used with permission of Ross Products Division, Abbott Laboratories, Columbus, OH, copyright 1982.) *Illustration continued on opposite page*

**BOYS: 2 TO 18 YEARS
PHYSICAL GROWTH
NCHS PERCENTILES***

NAME_____   RECORD #_____

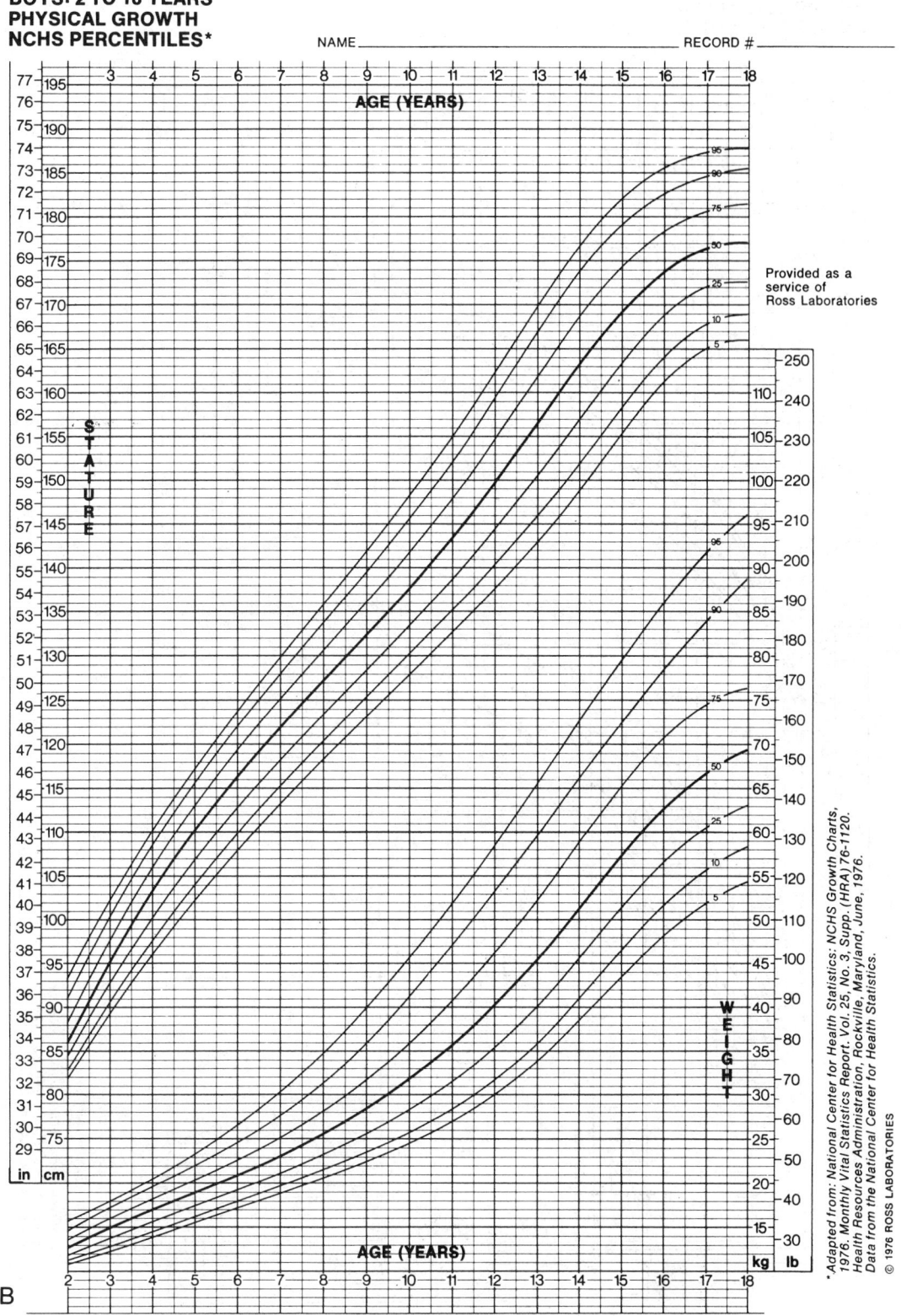

Provided as a
service of
Ross Laboratories

Adapted from: National Center for Health Statistics: NCHS Growth Charts, 1976. Monthly Vital Statistics Report. Vol. 25, No. 3, Supp. (HRA) 76-1120. Health Resources Administration, Rockville, Maryland, June, 1976. Data from the National Center for Health Statistics.

© 1976 ROSS LABORATORIES

FIGURE 28–1. *Continued.   Illustration continued on following page*

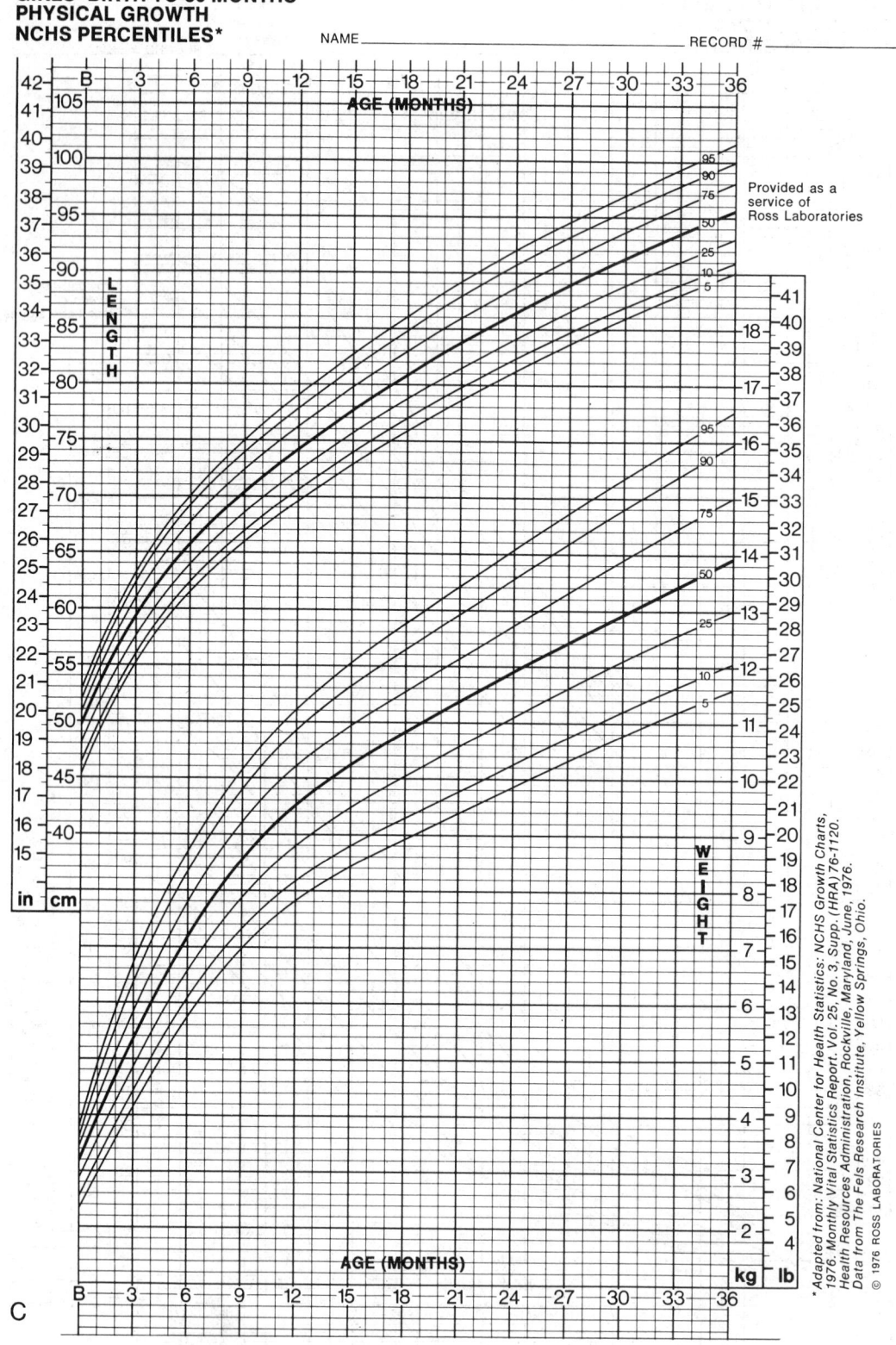

GIRLS: BIRTH TO 36 MONTHS
PHYSICAL GROWTH
NCHS PERCENTILES*

NAME_____ RECORD #_____

FIGURE 28–1. *Continued.   Illustration continued on following page*

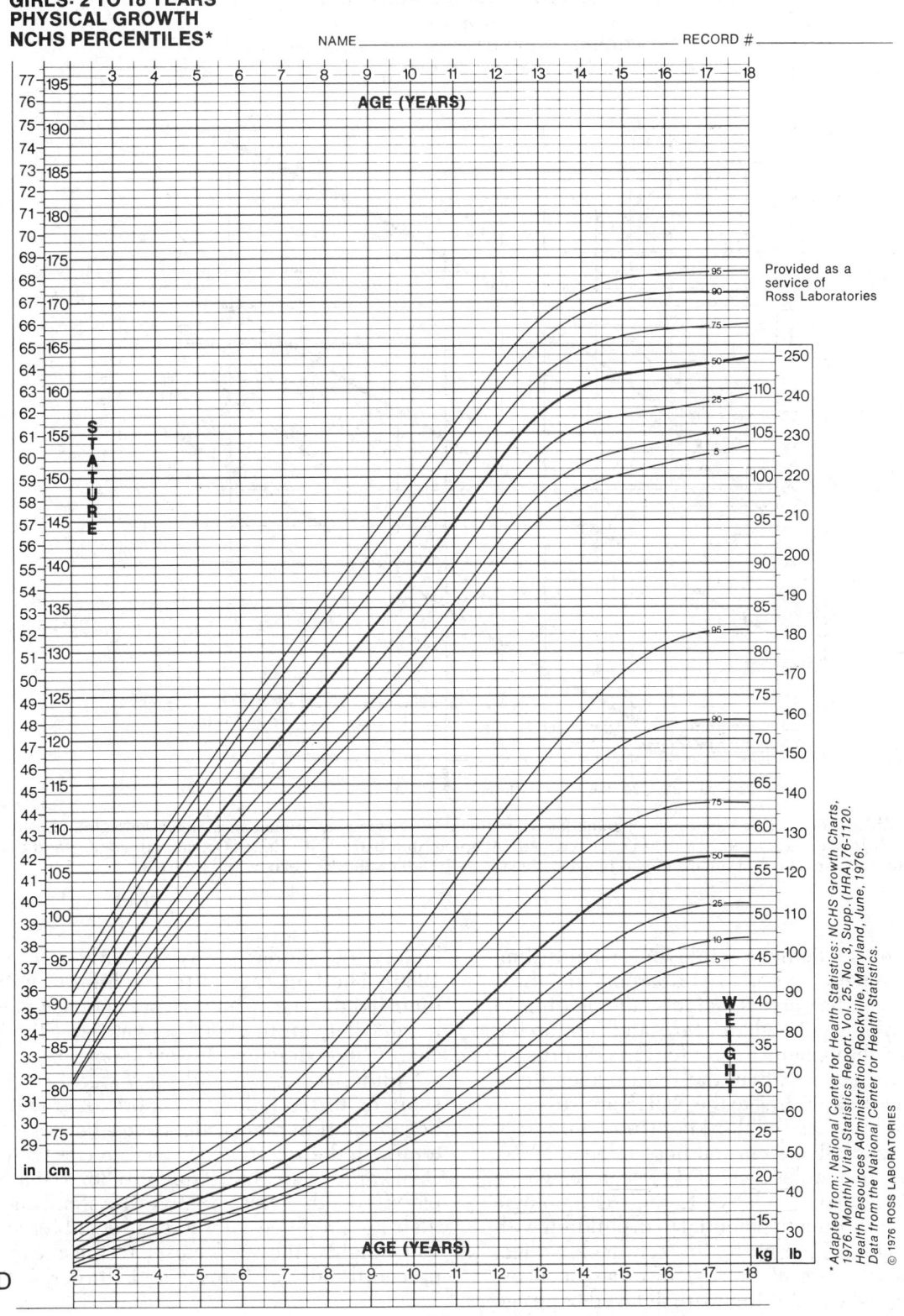

GIRLS: 2 TO 18 YEARS
PHYSICAL GROWTH
NCHS PERCENTILES*

FIGURE 28–1. *Continued.*

* Adapted from: National Center for Health Statistics: NCHS Growth Charts, 1976. Monthly Vital Statistics Report. Vol. 25, No. 3, Supp. (HRA) 76-1120. Health Resources Administration, Rockville, Maryland, June, 1976. Data from the National Center for Health Statistics.
© 1976 ROSS LABORATORIES

GROWTH RECORD FOR INFANTS
in relation to
GESTATIONAL AGE AND FETAL AND INFANT NORMS
(combined sexes)

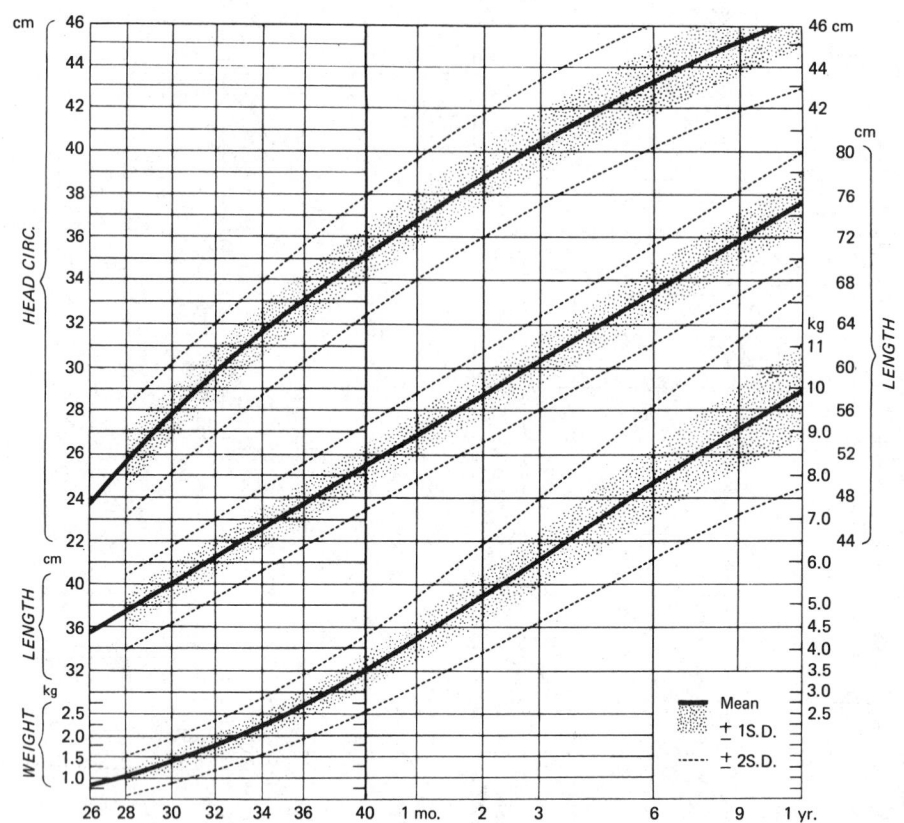

FIGURE 28–2. This infant growth graph for white infants of varying gestational ages plots growth from birth until 1 year of age after "term" has been reached. (Adapted from Babson SG, Benda GI: Growth graphs for the clinical assessment of infants of varying gestational age. J Pediatr 89:815, 1976, with permission.)

in determining whether a child is or is not fulfilling his or her genetic potential. Midparental height is the average of the parents' heights, after adding 13 cm to the mother's height for boys and subtracting 13 cm from the father's height for girls. Short stature is defined as less than the third percentile of normal for age according to the NCHS growth chart or a height less than the third percentile for midparental height (Silverstein and Rosenbloom, 1988).

Children and adolescents of short stature, whose bone age is delayed relative to their chronologic age, have more growth potential than children with a skeletal age appropriate for their chronologic age. If an organic cause of short stature has been excluded, then these children with delayed bone age are likely to have *constitutional growth delay*. The majority of these children are boys who were of normal length and weight at birth. Their growth rate shifts downward during the first 2 years of life and stabilizes at 4 to 5 cm/year until the onset of their pubertal growth spurt, which often occurs later than their peers. Frequently, there is a family history of similar delayed maturation (Green, 1986). The bone age of these children will equal their height age, which is the age at which their height plots on the 50th percentile of the growth chart (Silverstein and Rosenbloom, 1988).

Children with *familial short stature* tend to be short at birth, follow the normal growth curve below the fifth percentile, have a bone age consistent with their chronologic age, and reach puberty at an appropriate time (Green, 1986). Usually, their parents or other close relatives are short, and, when their height percentiles are corrected for midparental heights, they fall closer to the mean height percentile for age (Lipsky and Horner, 1988).

Pubertal Growth and Development

All children grow at a different tempo, with some maturing earlier than others and some later. This difference is most apparent during puberty. As a result, the usual NCHS growth charts are least able

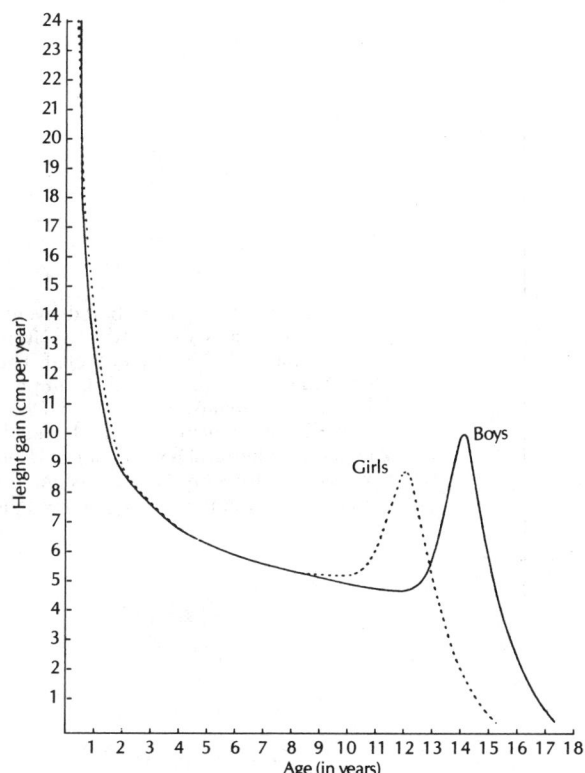

FIGURE 28–3. Average linear growth velocity curves for boys and girls from infancy through the pubertal growth spurt. Note the rapid deceleration of linear growth in infancy, its relative stability throughout childhood, and its rapid acceleration at puberty. Also note that the pubertal growth spurt in boys is later and greater than that in girls. As a result, the average adult stature of men is greater than that of women. (From Lipsky MS, Horner JM: The child with short stature. Am Fam Physician 37:232, 1988, with permission.)

to account for variations in normality during this time. Tanner and Davies (1985) have taken the NCHS data and constructed height and weight velocity curves for American boys and girls that account for the early and later maturers. These charts also allow for notation of the various stages of puberty that have been described by Tanner (1986) (Table 28–4).

The onset of puberty generally occurs at age 9

TABLE 28–3. CONDITIONS AFFECTING BONE AGE

Some Causes of Retarded Bone Age
1. Hypopituitarism
2. Hypothyroidism
3. Malnutrition
4. Constitutional dwarfism
5. Chronic disease
6. Severe illness
7. Male hypogonadism
8. Delayed adolescence

Some Causes of Accelerated Bone Age
1. Sexual precocity
2. Obesity

in American girls, with the peak height velocity occurring at age 11.5 years (range 9.7 to 13.5 years for early to late maturers), while American boys have onset of puberty at age 11 and peak height velocity at 13.5 years (range 11.7 to 15.3 years) (Tanner and Davies, 1985). Because boys have 2 additional years of prepubertal growth and a peak height velocity greater than girls, their ultimate height is usually taller. Head, hands, and feet are first to reach their adult size, followed by leg length, trunk length (which accounts for much of the spurt), and body breadth. Pubertal boys develop greater shoulder breadth than pubertal girls, who develop wider hips. Adolescents can be reassured that their bodies eventually will become more proportionate with their hands and feet. Boys ultimately gain greater muscle size and strength than girls while losing limb fat. This is due to their increased secretion of testosterone, which also increases red cell mass and hemoglobin (Tanner, 1986).

The adolescent growth spurt in skeletal and body dimensions is associated closely with the development of the reproductive system. Although the onset and rate of maturation varies according to the individual, the sequence is usually the same within sexes (Figs. 28–4 and 28–5).

The first sign of puberty in boys is an increase in growth of the testes and scrotum, with reddening and wrinkling of the scrotal skin. Pubic hair appears within 6 months, followed by phallic enlargement in 12 to 18 months and peak height velocity 2 to 2.5 years after testicular enlargement (Copeland, 1986). Axillary hair usually appears 2 years after the beginning of pubic hair growth (stage 4 pubic hair), but there is considerable variability. Some boys may have enlargement of the breasts midway through adolescence. Following the attainment of peak height velocity, boys develop mature spermatozoa, full facial hair, and voice change. However, breaking of the voice is a late and often gradual process.

In girls, the breast bud is the first sign of puberty, and the pubertal growth spurt typically occurs concurrently, peaking at stage 3 breast and pubic hair. The uterus and vagina develop simultaneously with the breast, but menarche usually does not occur until stage 4 breast and pubic hair. Although the peak height velocity has been passed, girls may grow an average of 6 cm more after menarche. Early cycles may be irregular and anovulatory, but early sterility should never be presupposed (Tanner, 1986).

NUTRITION: FROM INFANCY THROUGH ADOLESCENCE

Proper physical growth and appropriate cognitive development are clearly dependent on adequate nutrition. Infants with iron-deficiency ane-

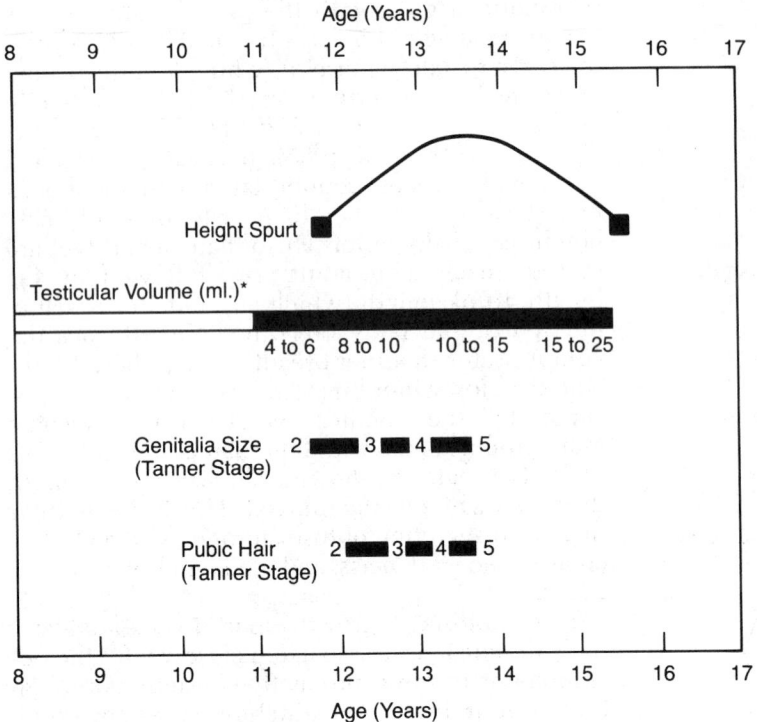

FIGURE 28–4. Sequence of pubertal events in average American males. (Adapted from Brookman RR, Rauh JL, Morrison JA, et al: The Princeton Maturation Study, 1976, unpublished data for adolescents in Cincinnati, Ohio. *In* Copeland KC, Brookman RR, Rauh JL [eds]: Assessment of Pubertal Development. Used with permission of Ross Products Division, Abbott Laboratories, Columbus, OH, copyright 1986, p 4.)

*Testicular volume less than ml. using orchidometer (Prader Beads) represents prepubertal stage.

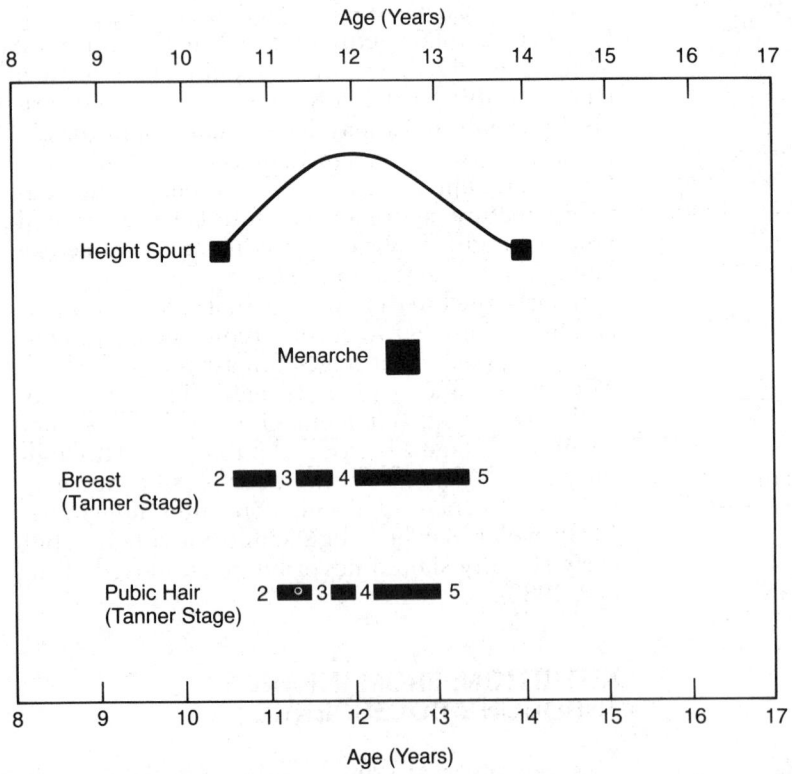

FIGURE 28–5. Sequence of pubertal events in average American females. (Adapted from Brookman RR, Rauh JL, Morrison JA, et al: The Princeton Maturation Study, 1976, unpublished data for adolescents in Cincinnati, Ohio. *In* Copeland KC, Brookman RR, Rauh JL [eds]: Assessment of Pubertal Development. Used with permission of Ross Products Division, Abbott Laboratories, Columbus, OH, copyright 1986, p 4.)

TABLE 28–4. SEXUAL MATURITY STAGES IN BOYS AND GIRLS

Stage	Male Genitalia	Pubic Hair	Breasts
1	Preadolescent—testes, scrotum, and penis are of childhood size	None; may be vellus hair, as over abdomen	Preadolescent, elevation of papilla only
2	Slight enlargement of scrotum with reddening of skin; little or no enlargement of penis	Sparse growth of long, slightly pigmented, downy hair, straight or slightly curled, primarily at base of penis or along labia	Breast bud stage; breast and papilla form a small mound; areolar diameter enlarges
3	Further enlargement at scrotum; penis enlarges, mainly in length	Hair considerably darker, coarser, and more curled; spreads sparsely over junction of pubes	Further enlargement of breasts and areola with no separation of their contours
4	Further enlargement and darkening of scrotum; penis enlarges, especially in breadth; glans develops	Adult-type hair that does not extend onto thighs, covering a smaller area than in adult	Areola and papilla project to form a secondary mound above the contour of the breast; stage 4 development of the areolar mound does not occur in 10% of girls and is slight in 20%; when present, it may persist well into adulthood
5	Adult in size and shape	Adult in quantity and type with extension onto thighs but not up linea alba	Mature female; papilla projects and areola recesses to general contour of breast
6		Spreads up linea alba (80% of men, 10% of women)	

Data from Tanner JM: Normal growth and techniques of growth assessment. Clin Endocrinol Metab 15:436, 1986, with permission.

mia have been found to have lower scores on the Bayley mental development index. Adolescents with iron deficiency may have poor exercise tolerance and impaired short-term memory (Oski, 1993). Mealtime also represents a time for social interaction within the family unit, whether this be the bonding of mother and child during breast-feeding or discussion of the day's events during dinnertime.

Malnutrition is still a problem in the United States, but inappropriate nutrition, especially calorie/nutrient imbalance, is even more commonplace. Frequent consumption of fast foods often adds an excessive amount of calories to the diet in the form of fat. Information from population surveys, such as the National Health and Nutrition Examination Surveys (NHANES 1 and 2), documents a greatly increasing prevalence of obesity in the pediatric age group. This is associated with a greater risk of elevated systolic and diastolic blood pressure in obese children and adolescents (Gortmaker et al., 1987). Adolescent obesity is associated with an increased death rate from coronary artery disease and colorectal cancer in men later in life (Must et al., 1992). Sociocultural factors, such as increased television viewing among young people, may lead to decreased activity, excessive snacking on high-calorie junk foods, and subsequent obesity (Dietz and Gortmaker, 1985). In contrast, dieting in pursuit of the media's representation of the ideal woman may lead to eating disorders, such as bulimia and/or anorexia.

Infants and Toddlers

Infants require 80 to 120 kcal/kg/day to meet basal metabolic requirements and the energy demands of growth and activity during the first year of life. This decreases by about 10 kcal/kg/day for each subsequent 3-year period. Increased physical activity or stress imposed by disease processes, such as fever, increase the body's basal energy requirements. For example, fever may increase basal caloric needs by 10 per cent for each degree centigrade, while peak physical activity may double or triple the body's usual requirement of 15 to 25 kcal/kg/day. Human milk, most formulas, and a well-balanced diet usually have approximately 10 per cent of calories derived from protein, 50 per cent from carbohydrate, and 40 per cent from fat (Barness, 1992). A comparison of some common milks and formulas is shown in Table 28–5.

The ideal food for full-term infants during the first 12 months of life is human milk. Oliver Wendell Holmes once noted, "A pair of substantial mammary glands has the advantage over the two hemispheres of the most learned professor's brain in the art of compounding a nutritious fluid for infants" (Cone, 1979, p. 138). Human milk is fresh, readily available at the proper temperature, and generally free of contaminating bacteria. It contains secretory immunoglobulin IgA antibodies, macrophages, and lactoferrin, a whey protein that binds iron and inhibits the growth of *Escherichia coli* in the intestine (Barness, 1992). The protein in human milk consists predominantly of whey

TABLE 28–5. COMPARISON OF COMMON MILKS AND INFANT FORMULAS

Milk/Formula	Kcal/oz	Protein (gm/dL)	CHO* (gm/dL)	CHO Type	Fat (gm/dL)	Fe (mg/L)	Comments
Human milk	22	1.1	7.2	Lactose	3.6	.5	Small flocculent curd: iron easily absorbed. Low vitamin D (22 IU/L) indicates need for supplement or sunlight.
Pasteurized cow's milk	20	3.3	4.8	Lactose	3.7	.45	Tough curd. Do not use before age 12 months.
Evaporated milk	22	3.8	5.4	Lactose	4.0	1	Softer, smaller curd; less allergenic than whole cow's milk. Universal availability. Supplement with Fe and vitamin C.
Prepared formula–cow's milk based	20	1.4–1.6	6.9–7.4	Lactose	3.4–3.8	1.1–1.5 10.0–12.7†	Iron-fortified formula preferred. Need for fluoride supplement if using ready-to-feed formula.
Prepared formulas–soy based	20	1.8–2.1	6.7–6.9	Sucrose, corn syrup, polycose, tapioca	3.6–3.8	12.0–12.7	25–40% cross reactivity with cow's milk protein.

* CHO, carbohydrates.
† Iron-fortified formula.
Adapted and compiled from Barness L: Formula feeding. *In* Berhman, RE, Kliegman RM, Nelson WE, Vaughan VC (eds): Nelson Textbook of Pediatrics, 14th edition. Philadelphia, WB Saunders Company, 1992, p 122; *and* American Academy of Pediatrics Committee on Nutrition (Barness LA, ed): Pediatric Nutrition Handbook, 3rd edition. Elk Grove Village, IL, American Academy of Pediatrics, 1993, pp 354, 362–364, 369–370, with permission.

proteins and is of higher quality than cow's milk because it contains higher amounts of essential and sulfur-containing amino acids (Benkov and Le-Leiko, 1987).

The lower protein content of human milk produces a lower renal solute load and a fluid requirement of 130 to 190 mL/kg/day for infants under 6 months of age (Barness, 1992). Commercial cow's milk and soy-based formulas must contain higher levels of protein to compensate for their lower quality (Table 28–5). However, they are quite acceptable for the mother who is unable to nurse her infant or for the parents who wish to bottle-feed their child. Soy formula should be used in infants with lactase deficiency or galactosemia and may be tried in infants intolerant to milk (AAP Committee on Nutrition, 1993). Because cow's milk and soy protein are potentially antigenic in some infants, it is advisable to use a protein hydrolysate formula in cases of true milk allergy or malabsorption (Benkov and LeLeiko, 1987). These are usually lactose free and may contain medium-chain triglycerides to improve fat absorption (AAP Committee on Nutrition, 1993).

Human breast milk or iron-fortified infant formula is now recommended for the first 12 months of life. Whole cow's milk is not suitable for infants because of excessive sodium, potassium, and protein intake, accompanied by low intakes of iron, linoleic acid, and vitamin E (AAP Committee on Nutrition, 1993). Significant intestinal blood loss may occur in infants under 12 months of age receiving whole cow's milk. Very low-fat milks are calorically inadequate and lack the polyunsaturated fats and cholesterol required for the developing nervous system. Breast-fed infants seldom develop iron-deficiency anemia before 4 to 6 months of age because the iron present in breast milk is well absorbed. Iron-fortified infant cereal is a good source of the 1 mg/kg/day of elemental iron required by full-term infants. Breast-fed preterm infants should be supplemented with 2 to 3 mg/kg/day of elemental iron to a maximum of 15 mg/day until solid foods are begun (AAP Committee on Nutrition, 1993). Parents should be warned that iron is toxic in excessive amounts and appropriate precautions should be taken. Breast-fed infants and infants fed commercial ready-to-feed formula, who do not receive additional fluoridated water, may be given 0.25 mg/day of supplemental fluoride. The breast-fed infant who is darkly pigmented or receiving little exposure to sunlight also may benefit from an additional 400 units of vitamin D daily because only small amounts of vitamin D are present in human milk (AAP Committee on Nutrition, 1993).

Solid foods generally are introduced between 4 and 6 months of age, when the extrusion reflex of early infancy has disappeared and the ability to swallow nonliquid foods has become established. Single-grain infant cereals, such as rice, are usually well tolerated and can provide a source of fortified iron. The order of introduction of other solid foods is generally not critical, but the child should be tried on each new single-ingredient food for a week prior to introducing mixtures of foods. Homemade infant foods should not have salt or sugar added to suit adult tastes. Honey is associated with infant botulism and should not be given to infants less than 1 year old. Foods such as hot dogs, nuts, grapes, or rounded candies should not be offered to infants or toddlers because they pose the risks of choking, aspiration, and even death (AAP Committee on Nutrition, 1993).

The toddler's food intake may be quite variable from day to day or even meal to meal. An increasing variety in taste, color, consistency, and temperature will help to maintain an adequate nutritional intake (AAP Committee on Nutrition, 1993). The basic food groups constitute a pyramid, with grains such as breads, cereals, rice, and pasta at the base supplying the most servings per day; then fruits and vegetables; then dairy products, meat, fish, poultry, eggs, and legumes; and with fats, oils, and sweets used sparingly at the top ("The Food Guide Pyramid," 1992). This is shown in Figure 28–6.

Parents should be counseled that toddlers are often picky eaters but generally grow well despite this. Parents need to guide children in their selection of food but should not turn mealtime into a battleground. Forcing the child to be a clean-plater does not benefit disadvantaged children elsewhere and may serve to promote obesity in later life. Snacking or eating while watching television should be discouraged while physical activity should be encouraged (AAP Committee on Nutrition, 1993).

Healthy children eating from the basic food groups usually do not require a multivitamin supplement. Children who eat only vegetables but no dairy products, meat, or eggs require supplemental vitamin B_{12}. A dietitian also should be consulted because children following such a strict vegetarian

diet may be lacking other nutrients. Children with malabsorption or hemolytic anemia may require additional folic acid (AAP Committee on Nutrition, 1993). Parents who insist on utilizing a vitamin supplement without any obvious deficiency on the part of the child should be counseled to use a preparation that does not exceed the recommended daily allowances (RDAs) of the National Research Council of the National Academy of Sciences. Vitamins A and D, in particular, can produce toxicity if given in excessive dosages.

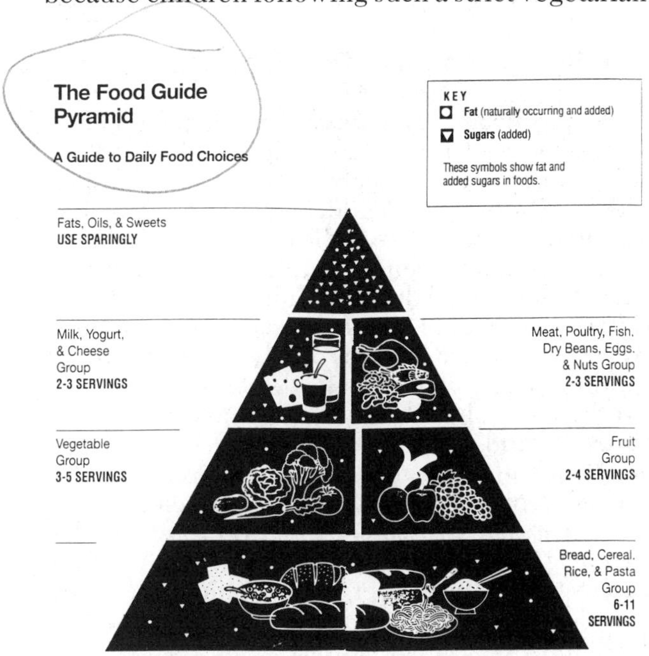

Adolescent Nutrition

Although the common picture of a hungry teenage boy is one with his head immersed in a refrigerator or wolfing down a burger, adolescent boys have the same risk of developing iron-deficiency anemia as adolescent girls. This is due to their greater increase in lean body mass and blood volume. Teenage boys and girls often replace milk and juice with soft drinks, coffee, tea, and alcoholic beverages, thereby lowering their intake of calcium as well as vitamins A and C. Because girls frequently are dieting to limit body weight, their overall food intake is diminished in comparison to that of boys, who eat relatively greater amounts of food (AAP Committee on Nutrition, 1993).

Energy requirements vary greatly in adolescents depending on their activity and stage of adolescence. The athletic teenager at the peak of his or her growth spurt may require an additional 600 to 1200 kcal/day in comparison to the sedentary teenager. This will add 22 to 45 grams of protein to meet the need for building muscle mass and blood volume during training (AAP Committee on Nutrition, 1993).

Special considerations include the pregnant teenage girl, the teenager following a vegetarian diet, or the teenager with hyperlipidemia. In addition to the deficiencies in calcium, iron, and vitamin A common to adolescent diets, deficiencies of folate or zinc may occur, having a deleterious effect on the outcome of the pregnancy or maternal growth. The U.S. Department of Health and Human Services now recommends that all women of childbearing potential take 0.4 mg of folic acid per day to decrease the risk of giving birth to children with neural tube defects (Centers for Disease Control and Prevention, 1992). The prenatal diet should be tailored to allow for a total weight gain of 12 to 15 kg or an additional 300 kcal/day. The teenager following a strict vegetarian diet is also at risk for deficiencies of vitamins D and B_{12}, riboflavin, calcium, iron, zinc, and possibly other trace elements (AAP Committee on Nutrition, 1993).

Universal screening for hypercholesterolemia in children is not currently recommended. A serum lipid profile should be obtained in children who have a family history of premature (55 years of age

The Food Guide Pyramid

A Guide to Daily Food Choices

KEY
☐ **Fat** (naturally occurring and added)
◤ **Sugars** (added)

These symbols show fat and added sugars in foods.

Fats, Oils, & Sweets
USE SPARINGLY

Milk, Yogurt, & Cheese Group
2-3 SERVINGS

Meat, Poultry, Fish, Dry Beans, Eggs, & Nuts Group
2-3 SERVINGS

Vegetable Group
3-5 SERVINGS

Fruit Group
2-4 SERVINGS

Bread, Cereal, Rice, & Pasta Group
6-11 SERVINGS

FIGURE 28–6. The Food Guide Pyramid emphasizes foods from a variety of groups. Each provides different nutrients to complete a healthy diet. Preschool children require the lower number of servings with the equivalent of 2 cups of milk/day. Older children and teenage girls require an intermediate number of servings. Teenage boys require the maximum number of servings from each group. (From The Food Guide Pyramid. Washington, DC, U.S. Department of Agriculture, 1992, pp 2–3.)

or younger) coronary heart disease or peripheral vascular or cerebrovascular disease in parents or grandparents. This should include total and high-density lipoprotein cholesterol as well as fasting triglycerides to enable the calculation of low-density lipoprotein cholesterol. Children whose parent(s) have a blood cholesterol level of 240 mg/dL or higher should be screened with a total blood cholesterol determination. A blood cholesterol level of 170 to 199 mg/dL indicates that the measure should be repeated and the two values averaged. If retesting confirms that level or the initial blood cholesterol is 200 mg/dL or greater, then a lipoprotein analysis also should be done (National Cholesterol Education Program [NCEP] Expert Panel, 1992). It is recommended that all healthy children over the age of 2 years follow a diet in which a wide variety of foods provide adequate caloric intake to achieve proper growth and development as well as desirable weight. Total fat and saturated fat intake should be no more than 30 per cent and 10 per cent, respectively, of total calories, while dietary cholesterol should be less than 300 mg/day. Other risk factors for coronary heart disease, such as cigarette smoking, hypertension, obesity, and diabetes mellitus, should be identified and treated, and regular aerobic activity should be encouraged (NCEP Expert Panel, 1992).

PSYCHOSOCIAL DEVELOPMENT

One of the rewards of caring for children in medical practice is in experiencing the developmental progress of cognitive, motor, social, and language skills as these children grow. Individually, children develop at their own rate, with a great deal of variability occurring in the normal range.

Children acquire developmental tasks in a predictable sequence. For example, children typically do not learn to walk until they have mastered crawling and then standing. Although the majority of children are able to crawl by 9 months of age and walk by 14.5 months, even severely delayed children will follow the sequence of crawl, stand, and walk (Milani-Comparetti and Gidoni, 1967). This information is important when providing anticipatory guidance to parents about their child's development, or when prescribing intervention therapy for developmentally delayed youngsters; intervention strategies must work with a child to attain the next step in the sequence at his or her present developmental level, regardless of the chronologic age of the child.

This predictable sequence is dictated not only by learning on the part of the child, but by maturation of the central nervous system (CNS) as well (Springate, 1981). Prior to a critical stage in the maturation of the CNS, certain skills may not be learned regardless of the intellectual potential of the individual. For instance, because CNS control

to the external anal sphincter is incomplete before 18 to 24 months of age, it is impossible to truly toilet train even the most precocious toddler before this age.

Development commonly is categorized into the following domains: cognitive function, language development, fine motor, gross motor, and personal social development. Developmental disabilities may occur in one or any combination of the above domains, which may help the practitioner in arriving at a diagnosis. For example, a child with mental retardation is likely to have cognitive and language delays. Conversely, a child with cerebral palsy may have normal or near-normal cognitive development with significant delays in gross and fine motor function.

An outline of salient features of development based on age is presented in Table 28–6. This is intended as a guide to normal development to be considered along with historical information, physical findings, and developmental screening results when evaluating child development.

The relative roles of heredity and environment in predicting developmental potential have been debated widely. Most researchers in child development believe that developmental outcomes are a product of intrinsic child factors, including genetic potential and temperament, and extrinsic environmental factors, such as intrauterine, infectious, traumatic, chemical, and sociocultural factors (Vaughan, 1992).

Identifying Abnormal Development

The physician caring for the growing child must be well versed in normal child development in order to provide anticipatory guidance to families and to ensure that a child is meeting his or her potential. Studies have indicated that early intervention programs benefit children with, or at risk for, developmental delays (Bennett and Guralnick, 1991), regardless of whether the cause of their delays is intrinsic or extrinsic. Early identification of children with developmental delays also may benefit the family by allaying anxiety about the undiagnosed child who seems "different." Such families frequently engage in "doctor shopping," to the detriment of continuity of care for the child.

The passage of PL 99-457, the Education of the Handicapped Act Amendments, in 1986, ensured improvements in delivery of educational services to children from birth to age 5 with, or at risk for, developmental abnormalities (Blackman et al., 1992). The role of the physician was expanded by mandating physician input in diagnosing conditions that would allow a child access to early intervention services.

Developmental Surveillance

The concept of "developmental surveillance" was introduced recently as a means for health care

TABLE 28–6. DEVELOPMENTAL MILESTONES IN YOUNG CHILDREN

Age	Gross Motor	Fine Motor	Reflex Motor	Social/Adaptive/ Cognitive	Language
Neonate	Flexed attitude, turns head side to side in prone without lifting, head sags if unsupported, body sags on ventral suspension		Moro symmetrical, grasp reflex, stepping reflex, suck reflex, placing reflex	Fixates on face or light, moves in cadence with sound	Alerts to voice
1 mo	Extends legs more, holds chin up briefly in prone, head lag persists		Persistence of neonatal reflexes; tonic neck posture	Watches person, visually tracks to midline, begins to smile, body moves in cadence with voice	Throaty noises, range of cries to signal hunger, pain, etc.
2 mos	Raises head from prone, sustains head in plane with body or ventral suspension, head lag on pull to sit		Stepping reflex fades	Smiles on social contact, attracts to voice	Coos
4 mos	Head up to vertical axis in prone, bears weight on arms, extends legs, symmetric posture with hands in midline in supine, no head lag on pull to sit, pushes with feet in standing, holds head erect in sitting	Grasps and attains object, brings to mouth	Grasp, Moro, tonic neck fade; downward parachute present	Laughs out loud, voices displeasure if contact broken, excites at sight of food, regards a small pellet	Vowel sounds, visually searches for speaker
6 mos	Sits alone with rounded back, rolls over, pivots, creeps	Rakes at pellet, transfers, turns body to reach	Sideways parachute present	Prefers mother, responds to emotion, imitates banging, visually follows dropped object	Polysyllabic babble, blows bubble ("raspberry"), laughs
9 mos	Sits with erect back, crawls, walks holding both hands, pulls to stand, can get to sitting	Pokes with forefinger, uses assisted pincer grasp	Forward (7 mo) and backward parachute present, plantar grasp fades	Plays "peek-a-boo," "pat-a-cake"; waves bye-bye; finds an object after watching it hidden; may cry at sight of unfamiliar person	Responds to some verbal commands: "no"; imitates some sounds; uses "mama," "dada" nonspecifically
12 mos	Cruises holding on, stands alone, may take several steps, walks holding hand	Neat pincer grasp, releases on request; puts 2 cubes in cup, pellet in bottle		Plays ball, adjusts posture when dressing, drinks from a cup, imitates activity (talks on toy phone)	1–2 true words, symbolic gestures (i.e. shakes head "no"), points to indicate wants
15 mos	Walks alone, crawls up stairs, walks backward, rises after stooping	Dumps pellet from bottle or draws line with crayon when demonstrated, scribbles spontaneously, stacks 2 cubes		Feeds self with utensils, performs simple household tasks (pick up toys), hugs parent	Points to body parts, jargons, follows 1-step command without gestures
18 mos	Runs stiffly, sits on small chair, walks up stairs with hand holding rail	Tower of 4 cubes, dumps pellet on request, imitates line with crayon		Feeds self with utensils; kisses parent with pucker; explores drawers, wastebaskets; removes garment; seeks help when in trouble	10 words, says "no," names pictures, points to 1 body part
24 mos	Runs well; walks up and down stairs, one at a time; jumps in place, climbs on furniture; kicks ball	Tower of 7 cubes, "train" of 4 cubes; imitates vertical and circular crayon stroke, imitates folding paper		Listens to story with pictures, helps to undress, dresses with help, parallel play, uses spoon well	30–50 words; 2- or 3-word sentences; uses pronouns, sometimes incorrectly; relates recent experience; speech 50% intelligible

Table continued on following page

TABLE 28–6. *(Continued)*

Age	Gross Motor	Fine Motor	Reflex Motor	Social/Adaptive/ Cognitive	Language
36 mos	Alternates feet climbing stairs, stands on one foot briefly, broad jumps with both feet, pedals tricycle, throws ball overhand	Tower of 10 cubes, imitates "bridge" of 3 cubes, imitates cross, copies circle, attempts to draw person		Knows age and sex, counts 3 objects, repeats 3 serial numbers, understands turn-taking, washes and dries hands, helps with dressing (dons shirts, shoes, unbuttons)	States full name; uses complete sentences; speech 75% intelligible to stranger; uses plurals, past tense, pronouns correctly
48 mos	Hops on one foot, throws ball overhand, balances on each foot 2–3 sec	Uses scissors to cut out pictures; copies cross, square; draws man with head and 2–4 body parts (pairs count as 1 part); tells a story		Counts 4 objects correctly, group play with role playing, toilets independently, dresses with little supervision	
60 mos	Skips, balances on each foot 4–5 sec	Copies triangle, 8–10-part person		Counts 10 objects, prints first name, domestic role playing, asks meaning of words, dresses and undresses independently	Uses complete sentences, names 4 colors, repeats 10-syllable sentence, follows 3-stage command

Compiled from Vaughn VC, Litt IF: Growth and development. *In* Behrman RE, Kliegman RM, Nelson WE, Vaughn VC (eds): Nelson Textbook of Pediatrics, 14th edition. Philadelphia, WB Saunders Company, 1992, pp 41–42, with permission.

providers to monitor child development (Dworkin, 1993). There are four key components to developmental surveillance: (1) eliciting and attending to parental concerns, (2) longitudinal tracking of children's developmental progress, (3) seeking input from other professionals involved with the child (i.e., preschool teachers), and (4) interpretation of all findings within the context of the child's well-being.

There is no one "ideal" way to conduct developmental surveillance in the physician's office. Many physicians rely on informal questioning of parents regarding developmental milestones, and informal observation of the child's abilities. Although quick and inexpensive, this method is not standardized and is likely to miss many children with significant delays. Although parental suspicion of language delay correlates well with actual delay, parental recall of other milestones is less reliable and is likely to result in under-reporting of significant developmental lags (Levy and Hyman, 1993). In addition, physicians, regardless of their years in practice, also have been found to be inaccurate in their predictions about developmental status when specific screening criteria are not used consistently (Bierman et al., 1984).

Routine, periodic screening of all children, utilizing one of several available developmental screening tools, is a strategy believed by many to optimize the physician's ability to detect early developmental delay. One advantage of such a strategy is that significant and potentially treatable developmental delay is less likely to be missed. Disadvantages include relatively low cost-effec-

tiveness, given that most of the screened population will be normal; and the substantial time involved in screening, generally 20 to 30 minutes. Because of variable sensitivity, mild but significant delays may be missed, and the family and physician may be assured falsely that all is well when, indeed, the child could benefit from intervention. There is also a fairly low specificity for many of these instruments, prompting over-referral of normally developing children. Many screening instruments are available; however, longitudinal outcome studies of children screened by these instruments are lacking. Table 28–7 presents a partial listing of some available instruments considered to be appropriate for use in a physician's office. A more cost-effective, practical method of screening for developmental delay in a busy office setting is by utilizing a tiered approach to developmental surveillance, as illustrated in Figure 28–7.

Utilizing this approach, children with medical conditions known to be associated with delays in language, motor, and/or personal social development should forego screening and be referred at once for early intervention services. Table 28–8 presents a partial listing of some such conditions. Children with conditions that place them at high physical or environmental risk for developmental delays, such as those in Table 28–8, need close surveillance. These children are managed best with periodic (every 6 to 12 months) formal developmental surveillance utilizing an instrument such as the Denver II as an adjunct to careful history and physical examination (Frankenburg, 1994). Although the Denver II has many more language

TABLE 28–7.   DEVELOPMENTAL SCREENING INSTRUMENTS

Screening Test	Source	Description
Denver	Denver Developmental Materials P.O. Box 6169 Denver, CO 80200	Screens personal–social, fine motor, language, gross motor, Ages 0–6 Takes 20–30 min Use as a surveillance rather than a screening tool
Minnesota Infant Development Inventory (MIDI)	Behavior Science Systems, Inc. Box 580274 Minneapolis, MN 55458	Screens gross motor, fine motor, language, comprehensive social Ages 0–15 months Parent report; takes 10 min
Minnesota Early Child Development Inventory (ECDI)	Behavior Science Systems, Inc. Box 580274 Minneapolis, MN 55458	Screens self-help, fine motor, expressive language, comprehensive, memory, and letters; includes adjustment and symptom scales Ages 1–3 years Parent report; takes 10 min
Minnesota Preschool Inventory	Behavior Science Systems, Inc. Box 580274 Minneapolis, MN 55458	Same scales as ECDI, determines child's school readiness Ages 3–6 years Parent report; takes 10 min
Early Language Milestones (ELM)	J. Coplan PRO-Ed. Inc. Austin, Texas 78758	Screens auditory expressive, auditory receptive, and visual skills Age 0–3 years Takes 15–20 min
Clinical Linguistic Auditory Milestones Scale (CLAMS)	Kennedy Krieger Institute Dept. of Developmental Pediatrics Baltimore, MD 21205	Assesses receptive, expressive language by observation and parent interview Ages 1–36 months

items than its predecessor (Frankenburg et al., 1992), the addition of a specific language screen, such as the Early Language Milestones or Clinical Linguistic Auditory Milestones Scale, may enhance detection of language delays. Children at low risk may be screened periodically at recommended intervals by parental questionnaires, history, and physician observation. The Minnesota inventories, consisting of the Minnesota Infant Development Inventory, Minnesota Early Child Development Inventory, and Minnesota Preschool Inventory, are useful and brief tools for screening

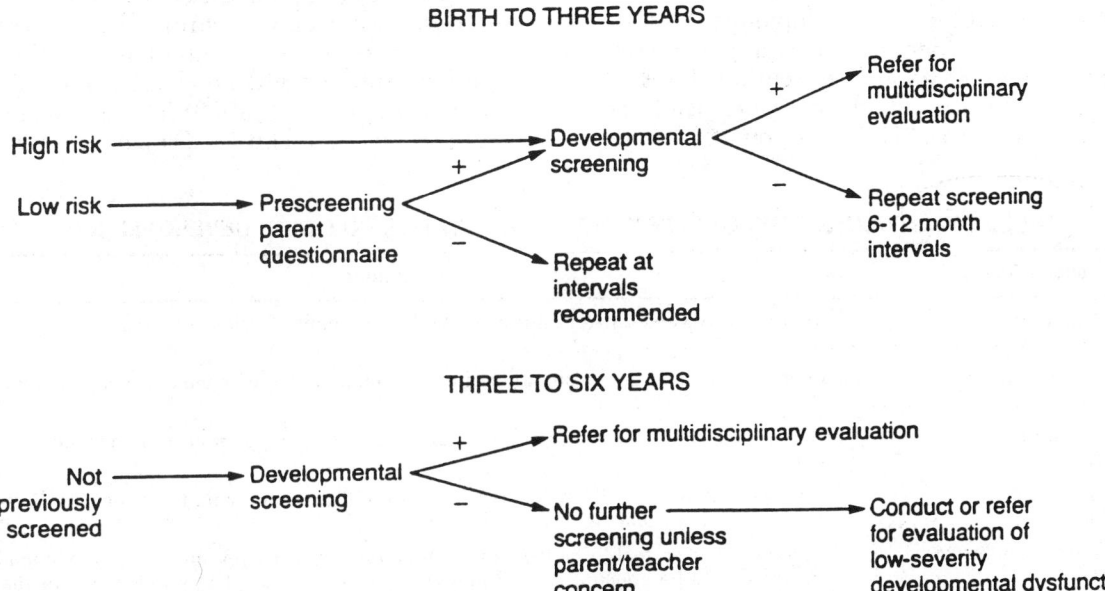

FIGURE 28–7.   Developmental surveillance flowsheet. (From Blackman JA: Developmental screening: Infants, toddlers, and preschoolers. *In* Levine MD, Carey WB, Crocker AC [eds]: Developmental-Behavioral Pediatrics. Philadelphia, WB Saunders Company, 1992, p 622, with permission.)

TABLE 28–8. DEVELOPMENTAL IMPAIRMENT SURVEILLANCE

Conditions Associated with Developmental Impairment (Refer for Early Intervention)
Hearing impairment
Visual impairment
Down syndrome
Other chromosomal anomalies
Myelomeningocele
Severe limb anomalies
Cleft palate

Conditions Associated with High Risk of Developmental Impairment (Require Regular Developmental Screening)
Extreme prematurity
Neonatal seizures
5-minute Apgar score <3
Hydrocephalus
Meningitis/encephalitis
Congenital infections
Maternal substance abuse
Intrauterine growth retardation
Parent with mental illness
Lead toxicity
Chronic illness
Child abuse
Head injury

low-risk children. Longer parent questionnaires taking 20 minutes to complete (the Minnesota Child Development Inventory and Minnesota Pre-Kindergarten Inventory) are also available from the same company for more comprehensive developmental surveillance (Kenny and Culbertson, 1993). If these measures arouse concern about potential delay, then formal screening should be performed. If the index of suspicion is high, prompt referral to a developmental center or early intervention program for further evaluation is warranted.

Regardless of the approach adopted by the physician to monitor children's development, it is critical always to consider seriously any concerns raised by the parents about their child's development. Such concerns should never be dismissed with comments such as "He'll outgrow it." If care-

ful developmental assessment of the child finds development to be progressing normally, this may be shared with the family, along with anticipatory guidance about upcoming developmental milestones to be expected. The parent should always be invited to return if these milestones are not forthcoming as expected, or if additional concerns arise. Discussion of age-appropriate play activities to stimulate development are always welcomed by parents, and convey to them that the physician is interested in discussing developmental issues.

Personality Development

Behavior, or how an individual interacts with his or her environment, is influenced in part by neuro-developmental status. As a consequence, children at different developmental ages are expected to behave in different ways. Certain vexing childhood behaviors, such as attachment to a blanket in an 18-month-old, negative behavior marked by temper tantrums at age 2, and fear of the dark at age 3, are all normal expressions of a child's struggling to achieve age-appropriate developmental tasks.

One of the most widely referenced theories of personality development is Erikson's psychosocial stages theory (Table 28–9). At each of eight stages through life, individuals are confronted with a crisis requiring integration of personal needs with sociocultural demands. Successful integration of needs and development indicates normal adaptation. Familiarity with these stages allows the practitioner to counsel families about the emotional needs of children at different ages and explain the appropriateness of these challenging behaviors.

Temperament is an additional factor to be considered in understanding child behavior. Temperament is believed to be an inborn trait, influencing how infants interact with and learn from their environment (Thomas et al., 1968). Three basic temperament profiles based on nine separate infant char-

TABLE 28–9. USING ERIKSON'S PSYCHOSOCIAL STAGES TO GUIDE DEVELOPMENT

Psychosocial Stage	Guidance
Basic Trust and Mistrust (0–2 years; infancy)	Parent can provide consistent nurturing to development of attitude of trust.
Autonomy vs. Shame and Doubt (2–4 years)	Parent should allow safe exploration of environment and encourage decision making.
Initiative vs. Guilt (5–7 years)	Limits on child should be for child's, family's, and society's protection, and not random or condemning.
Industry vs. Inferiority (8–12 years)	Caregiver must work with the school to assure child is achieving to his or her abilities and feeling sense of competence versus inferiority.
Identity vs. Role Confusion (13–17 years)	Selection of career goal; establishment of relationship with opposite sex; independence from family should be encouraged by caregiver. Failures to adapt in previous stages make this stage more difficult.
Intimacy vs. Isolation (18–22 years)	Need to make personal/occupational commitments.

TABLE 28–10. TEMPERAMENT: CHARACTERISTICS AND PROFILES

Temperament Characteristics

Activity	Frequency and speed of involvement
Rhythmicity	Regularity of physiologic functions such as hunger, sleep, elimination
Approach/Withdrawal	Immediate reaction of child to new stimuli
Adaptability	Degree of ease or difficulty with which child adjusts to new stimuli
Intensity	Energy level of responses, without regard to positive or negative quality of the response
Mood	Predominance of pleasant and friendly versus unfriendly behavior during waking
Attention span/ persistence	Length of time the child will engage in a single activity with or without interruption
Distractibility	Degree of ease with which extraneous stimuli interfere with child's task performance
Sensory threshold	Amount of external stimulation required to evoke a response

Temperament Profiles

Easy (40%)	Regularity of biological functions, positive approach responses to new stimuli, high adaptability to change, mild to moderately intense mood that is predominantly positive.
Difficult (10%)	Irregularity of biological functions, negative withdrawal responses to new stimuli, non- or slow adaptability to change, intense expressions of mood that are predominantly negative.
Slow to warm up (15%)	Negative responses of mild intensity to new stimuli, with slow adaptability with repeated contact. Mild intensity of reactions.

Adapted from Chess S, Thomas A: Dynamics of individual behavior development. *In* Levine MD, Carey WB, Crocker AC (eds): Developmental-Behavioral Pediatrics. Philadelphia, WB Saunders Company, 1992, p 86, with permission.

acteristics are outlined in Table 28–10. These are broad generalizations, and not all infants will fit easily into one of these three categories. One application of this information in a physician's practice may be to counsel families about the inborn nature of temperament characteristics. Each family's personal value system influences their reaction to a child of a particular temperament. For instance, in a highly competitive, athletically oriented family, high-energy, high-intensity characteristics may be viewed more positively than in a family in which studiousness is valued. Qualities such as introversion–extraversion often are based on character-

istics of temperament and are not modified readily by the environment. In the family in which "goodness of fit" between individual members' temperaments does not exist, knowledge of the inborn nature of temperament can help the family accept the child's unique characteristics. Anticipatory guidance then may focus on achieving a better "mesh" between family and child.

IMMUNIZATIONS

Indications and Contraindications

Routine immunizations are essential for the control and prevention of previously common childhood infectious diseases. Although approximately 95 per cent of school-age children in the United States are immunized, the measles epidemic of 1989–1991 primarily was caused by failure to vaccinate young children at the recommended age. Reasons for this include missed opportunities to vaccinate, deficient health care delivery in the public sector, inadequate access to medical care, and lack of public awareness (Peter, 1992). Recommended standards for increasing access and improving administration of pediatric immunizations have been developed subsequently (Ad Hoc Working Group for the Development of Standards, 1993).

Parents or guardians should be questioned about possible contraindications, precautions, and any prior adverse events in response to vaccine administration as listed in Table 28–11. They should be informed about the potential benefits as well as the risks of the vaccine and the risks of the natural disease should the immunization not be given. Federal regulations now require health care providers administering measles, mumps, rubella, polio, diphtheria, tetanus, and pertussis vaccines to provide and review vaccine information statements (VIS's) detailing these potential risks and benefits with the parents or guardians (Federal Register, 1994). Copies of VIS's may be obtained from the Centers for Disease Control and Prevention, the American Academy of Pediatrics, the American Academy of Physicians, or state health departments.

Prior to vaccine administration, inquiry regarding the child's current state of health as well as that of other family members should be made. An immunosuppressed member of the household may contraindicate the administration of certain live virus vaccines, such as oral polio vaccine (OPV). Minor febrile illnesses are not contraindications to vaccine administration. Absolute contraindications to immunizations are "concurrent moderate or severe illness, a previous anaphylactic reaction to the specific vaccine, and a severe hypersensitivity reaction to a vaccine constituent such as egg protein

TABLE 28–11. GUIDE TO CONTRAINDICATIONS AND PRECAUTIONS TO IMMUNIZATIONS*

True Contraindications and Precautions	Not True (Vaccines May Be Given)
General for All Vaccines (DTP/DTaP, OPV, IPV, MMR, Hib, HBV)†	
Anaphylactic reaction to a vaccine contraindicates further doses of that vaccine.	Mild to moderate local reaction (soreness, redness, swelling) following a dose of an injectable antigen
Anaphylactic reaction to a vaccine constituent contraindicates the use of vaccines containing that substance.	Mild acute illness with or without low-grade fever
Moderate or severe illnesses with or without a fever	Current antimicrobial therapy
	Convalescent phase of illnesses
	Prematurity (same dosage and indications as for normal, full-term infants)
	Recent exposure to an infectious disease
	History of penicillin or other nonspecific allergies or fact that relatives have such allergies
DTP/DTaP	
Encephalopathy within 7 d of administration of dose of DTP	Temperature of <40.5° C (105° F) following a previous dose of DTP
Precaution: Fever of ≥40.5° C (105° F) within 48 h after vaccination with a dose of DTP‡	Family history of convulsions§
Precaution: Collapse or shocklike state (hypotonic–hyporesponsive episode) within 48 h of receiving a prior dose of DTP‡	Family history of an adverse event following DTP administration
Precaution: Seizures within 3 d of receiving a prior dose of DTP‡ (see footnote § regarding management of children with a personal history of seizures at any time)	Family history of sudden infant death syndrome
Precaution: Persistent, inconsolable crying lasting ≥3 h, within 48 h of receiving a dose of DTP‡	
OPV‖	
Infection with HIV or a household contact with HIV	Breast-feeding
Known altered immunodeficiency (hematologic and solid tumors; congenital immunodeficiency; and long-term immunosuppressive therapy)	Current antimicrobial therapy
Immunodeficient household contact	Diarrhea
Precaution: Pregnancy‡	
IPV	
Anaphylactic reactions to neomycin or streptomycin	None identified
Precaution: Pregnancy‡	
MMR‖	
Anaphylactic reactions to egg infection and to neomycin¶	Tuberculosis or positive for purified protein derivative (PPD) of tuberculin
Pregnancy	Simultaneous tuberculosis skin testing#
Known altered immunodeficiency (hematologic and solid tumors, congenital immunodeficiency, and long-term immunosuppressive therapy)	Breast-feeding
	Pregnancy of mother of recipient
Precaution: Recent (within 3 mo) immunoglobulin administration‡	Immunodeficient family member or household contact
	Infection with HIV
	Nonanaphylactic reactions to eggs or neomycin
Hib	
None identified	None identified
HBV	
None identified	Pregnancy

* This information is based on the recommendations of the Advisory Committee on Immunization Practices (ACIP) and those of the Committee on Infectious Diseases (Red Book Committee) of the American Academy of Pediatrics (AAP). Sometimes these recommendations vary from those contained in the manufacturers' package inserts. For more detailed information, providers should consult the published recommendations of the ACIP, the AAP, the American Academy of Family Physicians, and the manufacturers' package inserts.

† DTP indicates diphtheria and tetanus toxoids and pertussis vaccine; DTaP, diphtheria, tetanus, and acellular pertussis vaccine; OPV, oral poliovirus vaccine; IPV, inactivated poliomyelitis vaccine; MMR, measles, mumps, rubella vaccine; Hib, *Haemophilus influenzae* b vaccine; HBV, hepatitis B vaccine; and HIV, human immunodeficiency virus.

‡ Although not a contraindication, this should be carefully reviewed. The benefits and risks of administering a specific vaccine to an individual under the circumstances should be considered. If the risks are believed to outweigh the benefits, the immunization should be withheld; if the benefits are believed to outweigh the risks (for example, during an outbreak or foreign travel), the immunization should be given. Whether and when to administer DTP to children with proven or suspected underlying neurologic disorders should be decided on an individual basis. It is prudent on theoretical grounds to avoid vaccinating pregnant women. However, if immediate protection against poliomyelitis is needed, OPV, not IPV, is recommended.

§ Acetaminophen given prior to administering DTP and thereafter every 4 h for 24 h should be considered for children with a personal or family history of convulsions in siblings or parents.

‖ There is a theoretical risk that the administration of multiple live virus vaccines (OPV and MMR) within 30 d of one another if not given on the same day will result in a suboptimal immune response. There are no data to substantiate this.

¶ Persons with a history of anaphylactic reactions following egg ingestion should be vaccinated only with extreme caution. Protocols have been developed for vaccinating such persons and should be consulted (*J Pediatr.* 1983;102:196–199, and *J Pediatr.* 1988;113:504–506).

Measles vaccination may temporarily suppress tuberculin reactivity. If testing cannot be done the day of MMR vaccination, the test should be postponed for 4 to 6 wk.

From Ad Hoc Working Group for the Development of Standards for Pediatric Immunization Practices: Standards for pediatric immunization practices. JAMA 269:1817, 1993.

or antibiotic" (Peter, 1992). Specific contraindications and precautions are listed in Table 28–11.

Vaccine Administration

Most immunizations must be given by deep intramuscular or subcutaneous injection. Intramuscular injections should be given in the anterolateral thigh or the deltoid muscle of the upper arm. The sciatic nerve potentially may be injured by deep intragluteal injections. Theoretical concerns exist that immune responses may be impaired to two live viral vaccines given within 30 days of each other. Live viral vaccines must be given simultaneously or at least 1 month apart. OPV must be dosed at least 6 weeks apart. If gamma globulin is given, then further vaccine administration should be delayed for 3 months to allow optimal antibody production (AAP Committee on Infectious Diseases, 1991). Acetaminophen administered at the time of immunization in a dose of 10 to 15 mg/kg and continued every 4 hours for up to 24 hours may moderate the fever, pain, and fussiness of diphtheria–tetanus–pertussis (DTP) vaccination (Lewis et al., 1988).

Schedule of Immunizations

The recommended schedule for active immunization is given in Table 28–12. A lapse in the immunization schedule does not require starting over the entire series. Doses of DTP or any vaccine should not be divided or reduced because this can result in an inadequate response. Premature infants should receive the same dose at the same chronologic age as full-term infants (AAP Committee on Infectious Diseases, 1991).

Measles, Mumps, and Rubella Vaccine

The measles–mumps–rubella (MMR) vaccine should be given to children who are 15 months of age. Children who live in a high-risk area having a large unvaccinated population or a recent outbreak of measles should be vaccinated at 12 months of age. A second MMR is recommended or required by law in many areas prior to entrance to elementary (age 4 to 6 years) or junior high (age 11 to 12 years) school because outbreaks of measles still occur on college, high school, and junior high school campuses. Children may be immunized with MMR even if there is a pregnant or immunosuppressed family member because the vaccine viruses are not transmitted (AAP Committee on Infectious Diseases, 1989).

Haemophilus influenzae *Type b* Conjugate Vaccines

Several *Haemophilus influenzae* type b conjugate vaccines (HbCVs) have been licensed for use in infants beginning at age 2 months. HbOC (Hibtiter), PRP-OMP (Pedvax HIB), and PRP-T (Ac-

tHIB) are conjugated to different carrier proteins, while HbOC-DTP (Tetramune) combines HbOC with whole-cell DTP. The schedule of administration varies according to the type of vaccine, as shown in Table 28–12. Children age 15 to 60 months of age need only one dose of any conjugate vaccine. Children age 5 years or older generally are not given HbCV unless they have a chronic illness associated with an increased risk of *H. influenzae* type b disease. Sickle cell anemia, asplenia, human immunodeficiency virus (HIV) infection, and chemotherapy for malignancies are indications for administration of HbCV. The combination HbOC-DTP should not be used in infants in whom pertussis vaccination is contraindicated or in persons 7 years of age or older (AAP Committee on Infectious Diseases, 1993).

Acellular Pertussis Vaccines

Two acellular pertussis vaccines combined with diphtheria and tetanus toxoids (Acel-Imune and Tripedia), currently are licensed in the United States for use as the fourth and fifth booster doses of DTP in children 15 months of age or older (Kimmel, 1993). These vaccines are immunogenic and produce fewer adverse reactions than whole-cell pertussis vaccines. Because they are less likely to produce moderate to high fever than the whole-cell DTP vaccine, they are particularly recommended for children who have had previous seizures or have a history of seizures in the immediate family (Immunization Practices Advisory Committee, 1992).

Hepatitis B Vaccines

Approximately 200,000 to 300,000 new hepatitis B infections occurred annually from 1980 to 1991 despite attempts to vaccinate selectively persons with identified risk factors. Universal immunization with hepatitis B vaccine is now recommended for all infants beginning at birth or in the first 2 months of life. The dose varies according to the type of vaccine used and follows the schedule in Table 28–12. The infant born to a mother positive for hepatitis B surface antigen should receive an initial dose of 5 μg Recombivax HB or 10 μg Engerix-B and 0.5 mL of hepatitis B immune globulin (HBIG) intramuscularly at separate sites within 12 hours of birth. Repeat vaccine doses should be given at ages 1 and 6 months. Adolescents who have multiple sex partners, use injectable drugs, or engage in other high-risk behaviors also should receive hepatitis B vaccine. Children who are institutionalized, on hemodialysis, receive clotting-factor concentrates, or have household contacts infected with hepatitis B also should be considered candidates for immunization with hepatitis B vaccine (Immunization Practices Advisory Committee, 1991).

"Catching Up" with Immunizations

Although all 50 states in the United States mandate immunization of children prior to school

TABLE 28–12. RECOMMENDED CHILDHOOD IMMUNIZATION SCHEDULE UNITED STATES – JANUARY, 1995

Age ▶ Vaccine ▼	Birth	2 mos	4 mos	6 mos	12‖ mos	15 mos	18 mos	4–6 yrs	11–12 yrs	14–16 yrs
Hepatitis B°	HB-1	HB-2		HB-3						
Diphtheria, Tetanus, Pertussis†		DTP	DTP	DTP	DTP or DTaP at 15+m			DTP or DTaP	Td	
H. influenzae type b‡		Hib	Hib	Hib	Hib					
Polio		OPV	OPV	OPV				OPV		
Measles, Mumps, Rubella§					MMR			MMR or MMR		

Approved by the Advisory Committee on Immunization Practices (ACIP), American Academy of Pediatrics (AAP), and American Academy of Family Physicians (AAFP)

° Infants born to HBsAg-negative mothers should receive the second dose of Hepatitis B vaccine between 1 and 4 months of age, provided at least one month has elapsed since receipt of the first dose. The third dose is recommended between 6 and 18 months of age.

Infants born to HBsAg-positive mothers should receive immunoprophylaxis for Hepatitis B with 0.5 ml Hepatitis B Immune Globulin (HBIG) within 12 hours of birth, and 0.5 ml of either Merck Sharpe & Dohme vaccine (Recombivax HB) or of SmithKline Beecham vaccine (Engerix-B) at a separate site. In these infants, the second dose of vaccine is recommended at 1 month of age and the third dose at 6 months of age. All pregnant women should be screened for HBsAg in an early prenatal visit.

† The fourth dose of DTP may be administered as early as 12 months of age, provided at least 6 months have elapsed since DTP3. Combined DTP-Hib products may be used when these two vaccines are to be administered simultaneously. DTaP (diphtheria and tetanus toxoids and acellular pertussis vaccine) is licensed for use for the 4th and/or 5th dose of DTP vaccine in children 15 months of age or older and may be preferred for these doses in children in this age group.

‡ Three *H. influenzae* type b conjugate vaccines are available for use in infants: HbOC [HibTITER] (Lederle Praxis); PRP-T [ActHIB; OmniHIB] (Pasteur Merieux, distributed by SmithKline Beecham; Connaught); and PRP-OMP [PedvaxHIB] (Merck Sharp & Dohme). Children who have received PRP-OMP at 2 and 4 months of age do not require a dose at 6 months of age. After the primary infant Hib conjugate vaccine series is completed, any licensed Hib conjugate vaccine may be used as a booster dose at age 12–15 months.

§ The second dose of MMR vaccine should be administered EITHER at 4–6 years of age OR at 11–12 years of age.

‖ Vaccines recommended in the second year of life (12–15 months of age) may be given at either one or two visits.

NOTE: This schedule is provided by the American Academy of Family Physicians only as an assistance for physicians making clinical decisions regarding the care of their patients. As such, they cannot substitute for the individual judgment brought to each clinical situation by the patient's family physician. As with all clinical reference resources, they reflect the best understanding of the science of medicine at the time of publication, but they should be used with the clear understanding that continued research may result in new knowledge and recommendations.

From Recommended Childhood Immunization Schedule, United States–January 1995, American Family Physician 50(8):1826, 1994, with permission.

entry, physicians still encounter young children who are not immunized. For unimmunized children between the ages of 15 months and 6 years of age, a tuberculosis skin test, DTP or DTaP, OPV, MMR, and HbCV may be given simultaneously at separate sites. A second DTP and OPV are given 2 months later. A third DTP can be given 2 months later if needed to complete the primary series. Booster doses of DTP and OPV can be given 6 to 12 months after completion of the primary series and again between ages 4 and 6 years prior to school entry. In some areas, the booster MMR also may be required prior to entry to elementary school. Children 7 years old or older are given the adult tetanus–diphtheria toxoid formulation (Td) in place of DTP and do not require HbCV.

Special Clinical Situations

Bacille Calmette-Guérin (BCG) and live viral vaccines such as OPV are usually contraindicated in the patient who is immunocompromised or infected with HIV and in their household contacts.

TABLE 28–13. REPORTABLE EVENTS FOLLOWING VACCINATION

Vaccine/Toxoid	Event		Interval from Vaccination
DTP, P, DTP/Polio Combined	A.	Anaphylaxis or anaphylactic shock	24 hours
	B.	Encephalopathy (or encephalitis)*	7 days
	C.	Shock-collapse or hypotonic-hyporesponsive collapse†	7 days
	D.	Residual seizure disorder*	(See Aids to Interpretation†)
	E.	Any acute complication or sequela (including death) of above events	No limit
	F.	Events in vaccinees described in manufacturer's package insert as contraindications to additional doses of vaccine† (such as convulsions)	(See package insert)
Measles, Mumps, and Rubella; DT, Td, Tetanus Toxoid	A.	Anaphylaxis or anaphylactic shock	24 hours
	B.	Encephalopathy (or encephalitis)*	15 days for measles, mumps, and rubella vaccines; 7 days for DT, Td, and T toxoids
	C.	Residual seizure disorder*	(See Aids to Interpretation†)
	D.	Any acute complication or sequela (including death) of above events	No limit
	E.	Events in vaccinees described in manufacturer's package insert as contraindications to additional doses of vaccine†	(See package insert)
Oral Polio Vaccine	A.	Paralytic poliomyelitis	
		—in a non-immunodeficient recipient	30 days
		—in an immunodeficient recipient	6 months
		—in a vaccine-associated community case	No limit
	B.	Any acute complication or sequela (including death) of above events	No limit
	C.	Events in vaccinees described in manufacturer's package insert as contraindications to additional doses of vaccine†	(See package insert)
Inactivated Polio Vaccine	A.	Anaphylaxis or anaphylactic shock	24 hours
	B.	Any acute complication or sequela (including death) of above event	No limit
	C.	Events in vaccinees described in manufacturer's package insert as contraindications to additional doses of vaccine†	(See package insert)

* **Aids to Interpretation:**

Shock–collapse or hypotonic–hyporesponsive collapse may be evidenced by signs or symptoms such as decrease in or loss of muscle tone, paralysis (partial or complete), hemiplegia, hemiparesis, loss of color or turning pale white or blue, unresponsiveness to environmental stimuli, depression of or loss of consciousness, prolonged sleeping with difficulty arousing, or cardiovascular or respiratory arrest.

Residual seizure disorder may be considered to have occurred if no other seizure or convulsion unaccompanied by fever or accompanied by a fever of less than 102° F occurred before the first seizure or convulsion after the administration of the vaccine involved.

AND, if in the case of measles-, mumps-, or rubella-containing vaccines, the first seizure or convulsion occurred within 15 days after vaccination OR in the case of any other vaccine, the first seizure or convulsion occurred within 3 days after vaccination.

AND, if two or more seizures or convulsions unaccompanied by fever or accompanied by a fever of less than 102° F occurred within 1 year after vaccination.

The terms seizure and convulsion include grand mal, petit mal, absence, myoclonic, tonic–clonic and focal motor seizures and signs. Encephalopathy means any significant acquired abnormality of, injury to, or impairment of function of the brain. Among the frequent manifestations of encephalopathy are focal and diffuse neurologic signs, increased intracranial pressure, or changes lasting at least 6 hours in level of consciousness, with or without convulsions. The neurologic signs and symptoms of encephalopathy may be temporary with complete recovery, or they may result in various degrees of permanent impairment. Signs and symptoms such as high-pitched and unusual screaming, persistent inconsolable crying, and bulging fontanel are compatible with an encephalopathy, but in and of themselves are not conclusive evidence of encephalopathy. Encephalopathy usually can be documented by slow wave activity on an electroencephalogram.

† The health-care provider must refer to the CONTRAINDICATION section of the manufacturer's package insert for each vaccine.

From National Childhood Vaccine Injury Act: Requirements for permanent vaccination records and for reporting of selected events after vaccination. MMWR 37:198, 1988.

Enhanced-potency inactivated polio vaccine (e-IPV) should be given to these children (AAP Committee on Infectious Diseases, 1991). Measles can cause severe disease, including fatalities, in symptomatic HIV-infected patients. MMR should be administered to all HIV-infected children at age 15 months or earlier if there is a measles outbreak. If exposed to measles, symptomatic HIV-infected children should receive immune globulin at 0.5 mL/kg to a maximum dose of 15 mL regardless of vaccination status. Exposed asymptomatic HIV-infected children should receive 0.25 mL/kg of immune globulin (AAP Committee on Infectious Disease, 1991).

Yearly immunization with split-virus influenza vaccine is recommended for children 6 months to 12 years with chronic pulmonary, cardiac, renal, or metabolic diseases, those receiving immunosuppressive or long-term aspirin therapy, and those who have sickle cell disease. The 23-valent pneumococcal vaccine is recommended for children 2 years and older who have increased risk of serious systemic infections as a result of sickle cell disease, functional or anatomic asplenia, nephrotic syndrome, or HIV infection or who are preparing to undergo chemo- or radiation therapy (AAP Committee on Infectious Disease, 1991).

Future Vaccines

A live, attenuated varicella vaccine currently is licensed in Japan and some European countries.

It is immunogenic and well tolerated in normal children, with 5 to 10 per cent experiencing mild fever, rash, or local reactions. The vaccine is less immunogenic in leukemic children, who have more reactions and require two doses of the vaccine, as do adults (Phillips, 1993). Further combinations of vaccines also may be expected in the future.

The National Childhood Vaccine Injury Act

The National Childhood Vaccine Injury Act was passed to provide compensation for children inadvertently injured by any of the routinely recommended childhood vaccines and to provide liability protection for manufacturers and health care providers who administer the vaccines. The intent of the law is to ensure a stable supply of vaccine and allow routine immunizations to continue. The physician or other health care provider must maintain permanent documentation of the date, vaccine type, manufacturer, lot number, and name, address, and title of the person administering the vaccine. A list of reportable but not necessarily compensible events is given in Table 28–13. Significant adverse events should be reported to the Vaccine Adverse Event Reporting System (VAERS) at 1-800-822-7967.

REFERENCES

Ad Hoc Working Group for the Development of Standards for Pediatric Immunization Practices: Standards for pediatric immunization practices. JAMA 269:1817, 1993.

American Academy of Pediatrics Committee on Infectious Diseases: *Haemophilus influenzae* type b conjugate vaccines: Recommendations for immunization with recently and previously licensed vaccines. AAP News June:17, 1993.

American Academy of Pediatrics Committee on Infectious Diseases: Measles: Reassessment of current immunization policy. Pediatrics 84:1110, 1989.

American Academy of Pediatrics Committee on Infectious Diseases: Report of the Committee on Infectious Diseases (the Red Book), 22nd edition. Elk Gove Village, IL, American Academy of Pediatrics, 1991, pp 9–32, 46–51, 124–125, 274–281, 308–323, 376–378, 383–389, 465–470.

American Academy of Pediatrics Committee on Nutrition (Barness LA, ed): Pediatric Nutrition Handbook, 3rd edition. Elk Grove Village, IL, American Academy of Pediatrics, 1993, pp 1–63, 133–143, 227–236, 252–262, 354–359, 362–364, 369–370.

American Academy of Pediatrics Committee on Psychosocial Aspects of Child and Family Health: Guidelines for Health Supervision II, 1985–1988. Elk Grove Village, IL, American Academy of Pediatrics, 1988, p 59.

Barness LA: Nutrition and nutritional disorders. In Behrman RE, Kliegman RM, Nelson WE, Vaughan VC (eds). Nelson Textbook of Pediatrics, 14th edition. Philadelphia, WB Saunders Company, 1992, pp 105–130.

Benkov KJ, LeLeiko NS: A rational approach to infant formulas. Pediatr Ann 16:225, 1987.

Bennett FC, Guralnick MJ: Effectiveness of developmental intervention in the first five years of life. Pediatr Clin North Am 38:1513, 1991.

Bierman JM, Connor A, Vaage M, et al: Pediatricians' assessment of the intelligence of two-year-olds and their mental test scores. Pediatrics 34:680, 1984.

Blackman JA, Healy A, Ruppert ES: Participation by pediatricians in early intervention: Impetus from Public Law 99-457. Pediatrics 89:98, 1992.

Centers for Disease Control and Prevention: Recommendations for the use of folic acid to reduce the number of cases of spina bifida and other neural tube defects. MMWR 41(RR-14):1, 1992.

Cone TE: History of American Pediatrics. Boston, Little, Brown, 1979, p 138.

Copeland KC: Variations in normal sexual development. Pediatr Rev 8:47, 1986.

Dietz WH, Gortmaker SL: Do we fatten our children at the television set? Obesity and television viewing in children and adolescents. Pediatrics 75:807, 1985.

Dworkin PH: Ready to learn: A mandate for pediatrics. J Dev Behav Pediatr 14:192, 1993.

Federal Register, New vaccine information materials notice 59 [59 FR 31888]: 31889, 1994.

Frankenburg WK. Preventing developmental delays: Is developmental screening sufficient? Pediatrics 93:586, 1994.

Frankenburg WK, Dodds J, Archer P, Shapiro H, Bresnick B.

The Denver II: a major revision and restandardization of the Denver Developmental Screening Test. Pediatrics 89: 91, 1992.

Gortmaker SL, Dietz WH, Sobol AM, Wehler CA: Increasing pediatric obesity in the United States. Am J Dis Child 141: 535, 1987.

Green M (ed): Pediatric Diagnosis, 4th edition. Philadelphia, WB Saunders Company, 1986, pp 278–285.

Immunization Practices Advisory Committee: Hepatitis B virus: A comprehensive strategy for eliminating transmission in the United States through universal childhood vaccination. MMWR 40(RR-13):1, 1991.

Immunization Practices Advisory Committee: Pertussis vaccination: Acellular pertussis vaccine for reinforcing and booster use—supplementary ACIP statement. MMWR 41(RR-1):1, 1992.

Keefer CH: Normal growth and development: An overview. *In* Dershewitz RA (ed): Ambulatory Pediatric Care. Philadelphia, JB Lippincott, 1988, pp 23–27.

Kenny TJ, Culbertson JL: Developmental screening for preschoolers. *In* Culbertson JL, Wills DW (eds): Testing Young Children. Austin, TX, PRO-ED, 1993, pp 73–100.

Kimmel SR: Answers to questions about the acellular pertussis vaccine. Am Fam Physician 47:1825, 1993.

Lampl M, Veldhuis JD, Johnson ML: Saltation and stasis: A model of human growth. Science 258:801, 1992.

Levy SE, Hyman SL: Pediatric assessment of the child with developmental delay. Pediatr Clin N Am 40:465, 1993.

Lewis K, Cherry JD, Sachs MH, et al: The effect of prophylactic acetaminophen administration on reactions to DTP vaccination. Am J Dis Child 142:62, 1988.

Lipsky MS, Horner JM: The child with short stature. Am Fam Physician 37:230, 1988.

Milani-Comparetti A, Gidoni EA: Routine developmental examination in normal and retarded children. Dev Med Child Neurol 9:63, 1967.

Must A, Jacques PF, Dallal GE, et al: Long-term morbidity and mortality of overweight adolescents. N Engl J Med 327: 1350, 1992.

National Cholesterol Education Program Expert Panel on Blood Cholesterol Levels in Children and Adolescents: Highlights of the report of the Expert Panel on Blood Cholesterol Levels in Children and Adolescents. Pediatrics 89: 495, 1992.

Oski FA: Iron deficiency in infancy and childhood. N Engl J Med 329:190, 1993.

Peter G: Childhood immunizations. N Engl J Med 327:1794, 1992.

Phillips CF: Vaccine update, 1993. Contemp Pediatr February: 75, 1993.

Sahler OJ, McAnarney ER: The Child from Three to Eighteen. St. Louis, CV Mosby, 1981, pp 3–20.

Silverstein JH, Rosenbloom AL: Evaluating growth failure: Diagnostic tools. Fam Pract Recert 10:43, 1988.

Springate JE: The neuroanatomic basis of early motor development: A review. Dev Behav Pediatr 2(4):146, 1981.

Tanner JM: Normal growth and techniques of growth assessment. Clin Endocrinol Metab 15:411, 1986.

Tanner JM, Davies PSW: Clinical longitudinal standards for height and height velocity for North American children. J Pediatr 107:317, 1985.

The Food Guide Pyramid. Washington, DC, U.S. Department of Agriculture, 1992, pp 1–29.

Thomas A, Chess S, Birch HG: Temperament and Behavior Disorder in Children. New York, New York University Press, 1968.

Vaughan VC: Assessment of growth and development during infancy and early childhood. Pediatr Rev 13(3):88, 1992.

Vaughan VC, Litt IF: Growth and development. *In* Behrman RE, Kliegman RM, Nelson WE, Vaughan VC (eds): Nelson Textbook of Pediatrics, 14th edition. Philadelphia, WB Saunders Company, 1992, pp 13–43.

CHAPTER 29

CHILDHOOD AND ADOLESCENCE

CHRISTOPHER V. CHAMBERS

One of the special joys of a family physician derives from providing care to children and adolescents within the context of their families. The family doctor functions not only as the health care provider and advocate for the child, but also as the physician for the entire family, thereby bringing a more global perspective to both the issues of normal development and the disruptive effects of illness. Children and adolescents represent a significant portion of a family physician's practice. Between 20 and 35 per cent of patient care activities of the average family physician are devoted to the care of children and adolescents less than 21 years of age.

Pediatricians and other specialists also provide medical care for children and adolescents. According to one source, pediatricians provide most of the care given to infants and preschool children but, after age 4, the health care of children is distributed nearly equally between pediatricians and family physicians. After age 10, family physicians and general practitioners provide the great majority of care (Starfield et al., 1983).

The range of health care provided for children and adolescents by family physicians has been studied and is similar to that documented by primary care pediatricians. Table 29–1 presents data for the 25 most common diagnoses of children and adolescents (less than 18 years of age) seen in family practice, representing 77.5 per cent of all diagnoses made on these patients in 1 year (Poole et al., 1982). As evidenced from this table, family physicians provide a wide range of services, including health supervision and the diagnosis and management of acute and chronic medical problems, as well as the evaluation and management of emotional disease. The social problems of the 1980s and 1990s, related to drug use and the human immunodeficiency virus (HIV) epidemic among other factors, have challenged primary care physicians further. The family physician therefore must possess broad-based clinical skills in order to be able to address the diversity of problems. The physician's practice also must make certain accommodations to meet the varied needs of different populations appropriately. The overall objective in providing medical care for children and adolescents should be to help them achieve their full potential in growth and development.

ROUTINE HEALTH CARE OF CHILDREN

Utilization

The majority of health care for infants and toddlers is well-baby and well-child care, organized around recommended immunization schedules. Children under 2 make an average of four to five visits per year to physicians. For most children over the age of 2, the basic immunization schedules are nearly completed and most of the medical care provided to these children is related to the evaluation and management of acute or chronic medical problems. In general, this is a healthy group. Children between the ages of 2 and 14 make an average of less than two visits per year to physicians (National Center for Health Statistics, 1978).

Nevertheless, there is much to be accomplished in the routine health supervision visit for children. In addition to obtaining an interval history, the child's growth and development are assessed by recording the height and weight and systematically reviewing developmental and behavioral milestones. The child is examined and appropriate sensory screening is done and recorded. Simple laboratory tests also have been recommended to screen for clinically unrecognized diseases, although the appropriate frequency for screening remains elusive. At all visits, there is the opportunity to provide anticipatory guidance regarding future development and possible protection against illness.

There are no compelling guidelines regarding the frequency of routine visits for children over 2 years of age (Strain, 1984). Annual visits prior to each school year have been recommended, but visits may be most appropriate around the approach or arrival of other milestones. For older children in particular, the onset of puberty or menarche may be a good time for a visit to a trusted family physician. Although the "best" interval has not been determined, regular visits are recommended because

TABLE 29–1. MOST COMMON DIAGNOSES IN CHILDREN (<18 YEARS OLD) SEEN IN FAMILY PRACTICE

Diagnoses	Percent of All Pediatric Diagnoses	Percent of All Pediatric Patients
1. Well-child care	25.2	53.8
2. Upper respiratory tract infection	12.0	31.2
3. Acute otitis media	7.6	14.2
4. Prenatal care	4.3	3.5
5. Pharyngitis/tonsillitis	3.5	9.0
6. Laceration	2.7	6.5
7. Sprains/strains	2.0	4.8
8. Chronic or serous otitis media	1.9	4.8
9. Bronchitis/bronchiolitis	1.8	4.8
10. Viral syndrome	1.4	4.6
11. Hayfever	1.3	2.5
12. Fracture	1.3	2.2
13. Bruise/contusion	1.2	4.0
14. Administrative*	1.2	3.6
15. Conjunctivitis	1.2	3.7
16. Infectious diarrhea	1.1	3.2
17. Abdominal pain (unknown etiology)	1.1	2.9
18. Warts	1.0	2.1
19. Cystitis	1.0	2.5
20. Asthma	0.9	1.7
21. Pneumonia	0.8	1.7
22. Eczema	0.7	2.0
23. Psychophysiologic gastrointestinal symptoms	0.7	1.8
24. Acne	0.6	1.6
25. Fever without an identified source	0.6	2.0
TOTAL	77.5	

* Administrative services for which the patient was billed, including filling out forms, writing letters, and making referrals.

From Poole SR, Morrison JD, Marshall J, et al: Pediatric health care in family practice. J Fam Pract 15:945, 1982. Reprinted by permission of Appleton & Lange.

they establish a relationship of trust for the discussion of future problems as well as allowing the physician to assess a child's growth and development over time.

Conduct of the Routine Visit

Preschool and school-age children generally are brought to the office by one or both of their parents. The parents should be given the opportunity to define the agenda. A simple question such as "What had you hoped we would accomplish in today's visit?" may help to elicit any underlying concerns that the parent may have about the child's growth and development.

Although the parents provide the reason for the visit and most of the history, older children should be given the chance to tell the physician why they have come to the office. With even young children,

however, important nonverbal communication takes place during the first few minutes of the office visit. Preschool children keep a wary eye on the physician and make value judgments based on their perceptions of their parents' reactions to the physician. Because of this, it is a good idea to start off visits with small children by engaging in relaxed conversation with the parents and tentative playful interaction with the child in the parent's lap. Most of the physical exam of the 2- and 3-year-old child can be performed while the child is held by the parent. By alternating parts of the physical exam with playful conversation and gestures, a skillful clinician can examine even an ill 2- or 3-year-old without increasing the child's anxiety.

Older children are generally more comfortable in the physician's office, particularly if they have developed a sense of trust for the doctor. School-age children usually enjoy telling the physician why they have come, and, conversely, it is a good idea for the physician to explain what is going to happen during each part of the visit. The physician's relationship with the adult members of the family, as well as the child's level of cooperation and maturity, help to determine the best approach. Again, patience and flexibility are essential in evaluating children of various ages.

A brief mention should be made regarding physician availability for problems other than those addressed at regularly scheduled appointments. One of the most important factors in a parent's decision in choosing a physician for a child is the availability of the doctor. As previously mentioned, the great majority of visits for the preschool child, and only a slightly lesser number for the school-age child, are for acute problems. The family physician taking care of children must have some available time in the practice schedule for seeing children on short notice. Availability by phone in off hours or during the day is also an issue. Although children over 2 are less likely to have urgent problems than infants and toddlers, there are still a great many questions that arise during the night. Many physicians have found it worthwhile to have a designated phone hour each morning before office hours begin to allow parents the chance to ask questions about less urgent problems or to discuss having their child seen that day for an unscheduled appointment.

Growth and Development Measurements

During health supervision visits for children, growth and development are assessed routinely. Measurements are recorded and compared with published standards. The sequence of growth in children is usually uncomplicated and orderly. The challenge for the physician is to determine whether any deviation from this orderly sequence is a variation of normal or an indication of an underlying problem. Any major variation from accepted standards becomes a red flag for the physician. The physician then must decide between "watchful waiting"—that is, a passive monitoring of indices of improvement or worsening—or diagnostic evaluation (i.e., looking for a specific diagnosis and a course of intervention). Often, the choice is a combination of the two.

Height and Weight

The height and weight of children should be recorded at least yearly after the age of 2. Routine head circumference measurements are no longer necessary unless there is specific clinical concern. The height and weight measurements also should be plotted on the standard growth curves and reviewed with parents. As an example, most parents find that visualizing the tracking of height over time helps them understand how their child can be shorter than other children of the same age and still be growing normally.

Deviations from normal merit brief mention here. On the one hand, growth curves can be used to identify the obese child in whom a more structured evaluation of diet should follow. Recent studies linking childhood obesity with risk factors for heart disease in adults suggest that there may be value in early identification and interventions for these children. On the other hand, a very thin child may be found to have a calorie-poor diet. Appropriate dietary changes should be suggested for this child as well. Failure to grow or gain weight also can be a consequence of any of a number of physical and psychological problems. There is no universally accepted definition for "failure to thrive," but various authors have suggested that children with weight below the third percentile for age or children whose weights are significantly "crossing percentiles" should be considered to be failing to thrive (Berwick, 1980). When organic disease is not readily apparent by clinical examination, failure to thrive is an uncommon diagnosis in children over 2. In most instances, deviations from the accepted growth standards are the result of individual, familial, or ethnic variations from published charts. Clinical judgment dictates whether an aggressive medical evaluation or watchful waiting is appropriate.

Developmental Screening

After the age of about 12 months, height and weight do not change as dramatically from visit to visit, and the parents' attention should be refocused on the developmental growth of their child. A standardized developmental screening test, such as the Denver Developmental Screening Test (see Chapter 28), should be administered routinely and the results recorded at each well-child visit. Preschool children with repeatedly abnormal findings in fine or gross motor function, language develop-

ment, or interpersonal/social skills require referral for further evaluation.

By law, school-age children must receive any developmental assessments deemed necessary by the school district to make an appropriate educational plan. In many instances this evaluation does not involve the child's family physician, but for others (e.g., those requiring medications, such as the attention-deficit/hyperactivity disorder), the physician must maintain two-way communication with the school's developmental psychologist and the child's teacher to optimize therapy.

Nutrition Screening

Appetite normally decreases in the second year of life coincident with the previously mentioned slowing of the growth rate. From ages 2 through 5, there is a great variability in caloric intake from meal to meal (Birch et al., 1991). Parents should be forewarned about these changes to prevent mealtime from being a period of conflict.

For children between the ages of 1 and 10, attention to the four basic food groups is generally sufficient to meet the daily requirements for all nutrients. Children usually prefer finger foods and single food items to combination foods. In addition, frequent meals and snacks are often necessary because of a child's limited gastric capacity.

Some specific principles are important for review. Fats are necessary for small children because of their caloric density and essential role in neurologic development. Parents should be advised to use whole milk in the diet until age 2. The fat content of a small child's diet should comprise 35 per cent of the total caloric intake. Calcium is necessary for bone and tooth development and primarily is provided through dairy products. Children who are lactose intolerant or vegetarians need appropriate intervention. Fluoride prevents dental caries, but excessive intake may mottle teeth. The need for supplementation is dependent on the child's water supply. If the water is not fluoridated, daily supplementation with sodium fluoride is recommended (0.25 mg/day for children under 2, 0.50 mg/day for children 2 to 3 and 1.0 mg/day for children over 3).

Blood Pressure Monitoring

Although clinical hypertension is far less prevalent in children than in adults, there is increasing concern about the relationship between elevated blood pressure in youths and the development of essential hypertension and cardiovascular disease in adulthood. Consequently, recommendations for the regular monitoring of blood pressure have been established and standards for comparison are now available (Task Force on Blood Pressure Control, 1987).

It is accepted generally that routine monitoring of blood pressure as a part of continuing medical care should begin at age 3. For the normotensive child, annual measurements at the time of well-child visits are appropriate. Blood pressure measurements also should be made in the child over 3 at the time of presentation for acute illnesses such as poststreptococcal glomerulonephritis, where increased blood pressure may complicate the primary illness.

Because of the rapid changes in growth during childhood, several different pediatric cuffs should be available. The appropriate-size cuff should be long enough to encircle the circumference of the arm completely and wide enough to cover approximately three fourths of the upper arm between the shoulder and the olecranon. The bell of the stethoscope should fit comfortably in the antecubital fossa without being placed under the lower margin of the cuff. For less cooperative children, the systolic pressure alone can be determined by deflating the cuff while palpating for the return of the brachial or radial pulse.

The blood pressure in children is measured best when environmental stress and anxiety about the measurement have been reduced. Blood pressure in children is more labile than in adults and can be affected greatly by endogenous catecholamines. As a result, acute illness or even anxiety can lead to transient elevations of the blood pressure.

The blood pressure measurement should be recorded in the patient's chart and compared with standard nomograms (Fig. 29–1). These nomograms were compiled using cumulative data from several studies. Black, Mexican-American, and white children were represented in the studies sampled, and there were no differences in the blood pressure readings among these groups. The curves therefore appear to be applicable to all races.

In conjunction with the recommendations from the Task Force on Blood Pressure Control in Children published in 1987, normal blood pressure is defined as systolic and diastolic blood pressures less than the 90th percentile for age and sex. High-normal blood pressure is defined as systolic and/or diastolic blood pressure between the 90th and 95th percentiles for age and sex. High blood pressure or hypertension is defined as average systolic and/or diastolic blood pressure equal to or greater than the 95th percentile for age and sex on at least three occasions. There are remarkable differences between children and adults with respect to the readings that determine high blood pressure and, consequently, comparisons to published standards must be done. For example, a systolic pressure of 111 mm Hg is in the 90th percentile for a 6-year-old boy.

The significance of high blood pressure in children is often unclear. For young children, there is a poor correlation between high blood pressure measurements and the development of essential hypertension as an adult (Shear et al., 1986). It is not until the onset of puberty that elevated blood pressure predicts well the development of essential hypertension. There are no clear data regarding the number of children with high blood pres-

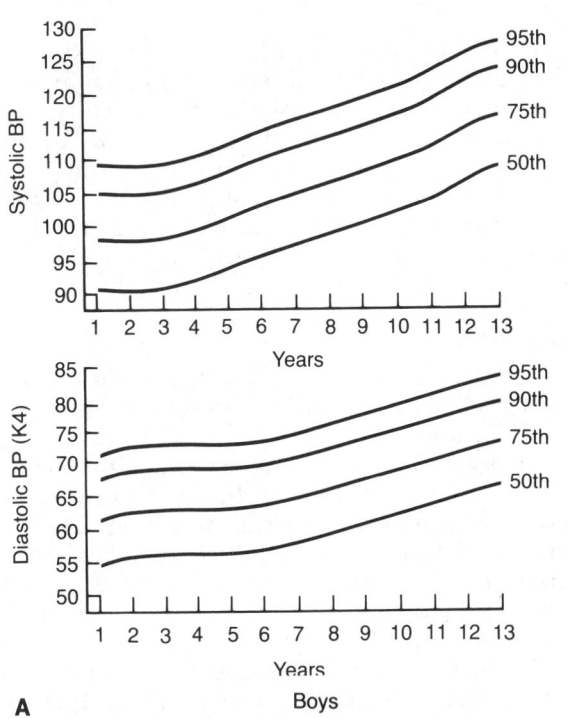

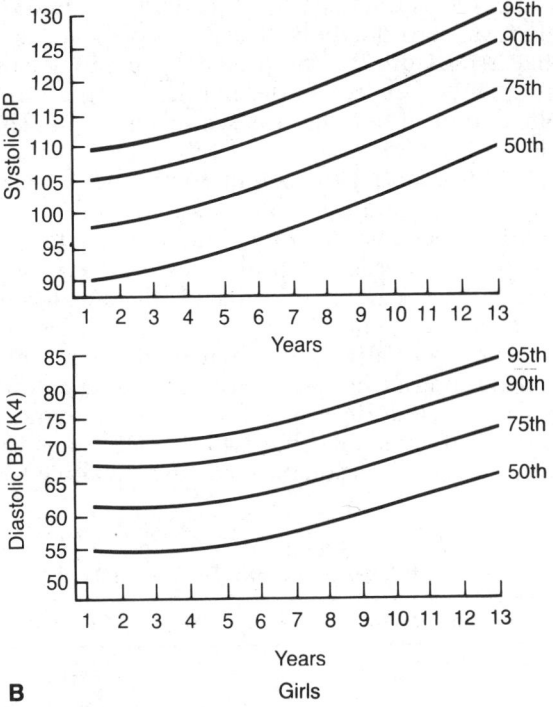

A   Boys   **B**   Girls

FIGURE 29–1. Age-specific percentiles of blood pressure measurements in boys (*A*) and girls (*B*) 1 to 13 years of age; Korotkoff Phase IV (K4) used for diastolic blood pressure. (From Task Force on Blood Pressure Control in Children, National Heart, Lung and Blood Institute: Report of the Second Task Force on Blood Pressure Control in Children—1987. Pediatrics 79:1, 1987, with permission.)

sure in whom an underlying cause will be found. Previous studies that found secondary hypertension in 80 per cent or more of young children were studies of referral populations to specialty care. Good data regarding primary care populations are not available. However, it is still true that the younger the patient and the more severe the hypertension, the more likely one is to find an underlying cause of the elevated blood pressure.

The medical evaluation of high blood pressure in children must be individualized for each patient and must take into account the age, race, sex, family history, and level of the blood pressure. Repeated blood pressure measurements are necessary to demonstrate that the elevation is sustained, but the extent of the medical evaluation and the urgency to initiate therapy will depend on the severity of the elevation.

Sensory Screening

Evaluation of Hearing

Much of the early evaluation of hearing in infants and toddlers is based on subjective reports by the parents regarding the child's response to environmental sounds. However, the development of abnormal speech in the young child may make more formal evaluation appropriate. The human ear normally detects sounds in the range of 20 to 20,000 Hz but is most sensitive in the range of 1000 to 6000 Hz, the normal speech frequency. In this range, the normal ear has threshold for sound levels near zero decibels. The level of hearing loss that is measured is the threshold level measured in decibels relative to the normal hearing threshold. A typical hearing loss scale is given in Table 29–2.

Children under the age of 3 in whom a hearing loss is suspected probably should be referred to a hearing specialist for formal audiometry to quantify the hearing loss. Children over 3 years of age generally can be screened with the headphones used in routine office audiometry. An office audiometer is a relatively inexpensive item and minimal training is necessary for screening children. No clear guidelines regarding the frequency of testing are available, but two annual exams prior to school seem reasonable. Testing usually is done

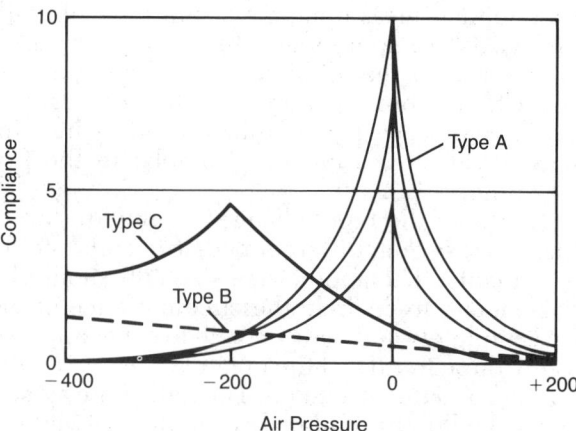

FIGURE 29–2. Common types of tympanograms.

at four different frequencies (500, 1000, 1500, and 2000 Hz) for three different sound levels (25, 40, and 60 dB) to quantify the extent of hearing loss, if any. The results of the audiometric evaluation can be recorded on a simple graph.

Children suspected of having middle ear disease also may be candidates for office tympanometry. This technique quantitates the change in tympanic membrane mobility or compliance as air pressure in the external ear canal is varied. The tympanic membrane is most compliant when the pressures on either side of it are equal. The test is performed by placing a three-channel probe into the ear canal to create a seal. A graph called a tympanogram is produced (Fig. 29–2).

In the normal or type A tympanogram, the point of peak tympanic membrane compliance is at the point where the air pressure in the ear canal varies from atmospheric pressure by less than 100 mm H_2O. Abnormal tympanograms that are flat (type B) or in which the peak compliance occurs when the air pressure within the ear canal is reduced (type C) may occur in the presence of a middle ear effusion or with other middle ear pathology.

Evaluation of Vision

Again, the evaluation of vision in children under 3 years of age generally is based on subjective reports by the parent. More formal testing should begin routinely at age 3. Visual acuity normally may be in the 20/30 to 20/40 range at age 3 or 4 but should improve to 20/20 by the age of 6 or 7. Squinting during testing, which creates a pinhole aperture effect, suggests the presence of an uncorrected refractive error. The family physician also may note strabismus, a misalignment of the eyes, during testing. Strabismus may be intermittent and benign but, if it persists, can result in decreased visual acuity (i.e., amblyopia). Referral to an ophthalmologist is appropriate.

Allen Cards, which have pictures of easily recognized items such as a telephone and a tree, can be

TABLE 29–2. HEARING LOSS SCALE

Hearing Impairment	Hearing Threshold (dB)
None	10–25
Mild	26–40
Moderate	41–55
Moderate to severe	56–70
Severe	71–90
Profound	>91

used to test the visual acuity of children around 3 and 4 years of age. Once a child can read letters or numbers, acuity can be determined easily with the Snellen Chart. Interest and cooperation are obviously necessary to obtain optimal visual acuity. A difference between the right and left eye of more than one line on the chart is significant and should lead to further evaluation.

Routine screening probably should be performed annually for the preschool child and for school-age children through the second or third grade. Testing again should be recommended around the onset of puberty because of the increased likelihood of uncovering myopia around this age of development.

Dental Screening

Primary dentition is usually complete by the age of 2 years. The permanent teeth generally being erupting around the age of 6 to 7 years and are complete through the second molars by the age of 12 or 13. Children should be encouraged to brush their own teeth from the age of 2 to 3 years, but parents should assist in the brushing. Most children lack the manual dexterity to brush satisfactorily until 6 years of age. Flossing is also difficult for children, and parents should take responsibility for flossing if tight contact between adjacent teeth is present. Routine dental appointments should begin at age 2 to 3 and are still recommended twice yearly by pediatric dentists.

Screening Healthy Children for Disease

Only a limited number of screening tests and procedures are recommended in the evaluation of the healthy child. The general purpose of a screening test is to identify normal individuals who have a disease or who are at high risk of getting that disease. This contrasts with a diagnostic test, which is used to confirm a clinical suspicion. A given test therefore is classified as screening or diagnostic depending on the purpose and clinical setting.

Iron-Deficiency Anemia

The hemoglobin and hematocrit vary normally with age and, after the onset of puberty, are different for males and females. As seen in Table 29–3, the mean corpuscular volume (MCV) also increases with age. Although recent studies have documented a decline in the prevalence of anemia over the past decade (Yip et al., 1987), concerns regarding behavioral and developmental disturbances associated with iron deficiency and the availability of simple, inexpensive tests to identify this condition suggest that screening some populations is still appropriate (Stockman, 1987). Iron-deficiency anemia is particularly prevalent in children with poor nutritional habits.

Several different tests can be used to screen for iron deficiency. The complete blood count or hematocrit, which can be performed in the office, detect iron deficiency at a late stage, well after iron stores are exhausted. The serum ferritin is a sensitive and specific test in children but is more expensive than these other tests. Routine screening for iron deficiency is recommended for children between 8 and 10 months of age, when changes in the diet may result in the depletion of iron stores. Additional or annual testing should be performed on children at high risk as determined by nutritional assessment.

Children with laboratory studies suggestive of an iron-deficiency anemia reasonably can be given a trial of iron therapy. If the anemia is microcytic and not responsive to iron therapy, it probably represents a thalassemia syndrome, particularly if the family is of Mediterranean, Asian or black heritage. In the healthy child, no further evaluation is generally necessary.

TABLE 29–3.　VALUES (MEAN AND LOWER LIMITS OF NORMAL) FOR HEMOGLOBIN, HEMATOCRIT, AND MCV

Age (years)	Hemoglobin (g/dL)		Hematocrit (%)		MCV (μm^3)	
	Mean	Lower Limit	Mean	Lower Limit	Mean	Lower Limit
0.5–1.9	12.5	11.0	37	33	77	70
2–4	12.5	11.0	38	34	79	73
5–7	13.0	11.5	39	35	81	75
8–11	13.5	12.0	40	36	83	76
12–14						
Female	13.5	12.0	41	36	85	78
Male	14.0	12.5	43	37	84	77
15–17						
Female	14.0	12.0	41	36	87	79
Male	15.0	13.0	46	38	86	78

Adapted from Oski FA, Nathan DG (eds): Hematology of Infancy and Childhood. Philadelphia, WB Saunders Company, 1987, with permission.

Lead Poisoning

There is increasing recognition that blood lead levels once thought to be safe are in fact associated with cognitive deficits, behavior disorders, and slowed growth (Centers for Disease Control, 1991). For this reason, the definition of the blood level at which lead poisoning occurs was revised downward to 10 μg/dL in 1991 by the Centers for Disease Control and Prevention (CDC). In response to this new definition, the U.S. Public Health Service issued a strategic plan to reduce or eliminate childhood lead poisoning ("Strategic Plan to Eliminate," 1992). According to this plan, the identification and treatment of children with toxic lead levels is still recommended, but of greater importance is the identification of the lead source and the prevention of subsequent exposure for that child and other children.

Family physicians and pediatricians will play an important role in this program of screening and primary prevention (Committee on Environmental Health, 1993). Physicians first should provide instruction in general measures to prevent exposures. Second, any history of possible lead exposure should be assessed at routine well-child visits between the ages of 6 months and 6 years using a number of specific questions (Table 29–4).

Children with identified risks should have a venous blood lead level measurement. The CDC also recommends routine testing of children at about 9 to 12 months of age and again at about 24 months of age. A finger-stick sample may be used for screening but has a high false-positive rate from contamination by environmental lead. Confirmatory tests should be performed (Table 29–5).

Elevated lead levels should be reported to the local public health or housing authorities so that environmental investigation and cleanup can begin. Chelation therapy is recommended for children with very elevated levels.

TABLE 29–4. ASSESSING THE RISK OF HIGH-DOSE EXPOSURE TO LEAD: SAMPLE QUESTIONNAIRE

Does your child—
1. Live in or regularly visit a house with peeling or chipping paint built before 1960? This could include a day-care center, preschool, the home of a babysitter or a relative, etc.
2. Live in or regularly visit a house built before 1960 with recent, ongoing, or planned renovation or remodeling?
3. Have a brother or sister, housemate, or playmate being followed up or treated for lead poisoning (i.e., blood lead level ≥15 mg/dL)?
4. Live with an adult whose job or hobby involves exposure to lead?
5. Live near an active lead smelter, battery recycling plant, or other industry likely to release lead?

From the Centers for Disease Control: Preventing Lead Poisoning in Young Children. Atlanta, GA, U.S. Department of Health and Human Services, 1991.

TABLE 29–5. SUGGESTED TIMETABLE FOR CONFIRMING CAPILLARY BLOOD LEAD RESULTS WITH A VENOUS BLOOD LEAD MEASUREMENT

Blood Lead Level (μg/dL)	Time within Which Blood Lead Level Should Be Obtained
<10	Not applicable
10–14	Not applicable
15–19	Within 1 month
20–44	Within 1 week
45–69	Within 48 hr
≥70	Immediately

From the Centers for Disease Control: Preventing Lead Poisoning in Young Children. Atlanta, GA, U.S. Department of Health and Human Services, 1991.

Routine Urinalysis

The Guidelines for Health Supervision of Children and Youth (Strain, 1984) recommend a screening urinalysis at age 6 months and again in the preschool years. The rationale behind this recommendation is that abnormal findings might point to clinically undetected reflux-induced nephropathy or other renal disease secondary to congenital anatomic anomalies. Unfortunately, high false-positive rates for hematuria and proteinuria make the costs of screening all children prohibitive. Similarly, although cases of unrecognized infection have been identified in large trials (Kunin et al., 1962), cost-effectiveness analyses have concluded that the screening urinalysis for asymptomatic bacteriuria should be eliminated from the periodic health maintenance visit in children (Kemper and Avner, 1992).

Urinalysis testing is necessary when specific urinary symptoms are present or in the evaluation of a patient with nonspecific clinical indications, including fever or failure to thrive, for example. In these children with a higher probability of having urinary tract disease, the use of the urinalysis or other tests is more for diagnostic than screening purposes.

Cholesterol Screening

Cholesterol screening in childhood remains controversial. Unresolved issues include the question of which children with elevated cholesterol levels are at increased risk for cardiovascular disease, the questionable effectiveness of an intervention, and the cost of implementing a universally applied program. Nonetheless, reference values for lipids in children are available (Table 29–6).

Lipid screening should be recommended for children with a family history of hypercholesterolemia or premature heart disease. A low-cholesterol, low-saturated-fat diet (e.g., the American Heart Association's Step One Diet) should be recommended for all children over 2 years of age (American Heart Association, 1988). Children at high risk (i.e., those with cholesterol levels above

TABLE 29–6. LIPID REFERENCE VALUES (mg/dL) FOR CHILDREN AGES 3 TO 19

Lipid*	Percentile			
	50	75	90	95
Cholesterol	155	175	190	200
LDL-C	95	110	125	135
HDL-C	52	60	68	73
Triglycerides	60	80	100	115

* LDC-C, low-density lipoprotein cholesterol; HDL-C, high-density lipoprotein cholesterol.

Adapted from Lipid Research Clinics Population Studies Data Book, Vol. I: The Prevalence Study (U.S. Department of Health and Human Services Report no. [NIH] 80-1527). Bethesda, MD, National Institutes of Health, 1980.

the 95th percentile) should be targeted for more specialized management.

Tuberculosis Screening

Routine screening for tuberculosis had been recommended widely in the past, in part as a result of the high effectiveness of antituberculous therapy in children. Recent changes in the epidemiology of tuberculosis and the emergence of multiple–drug-resistant strains have increased the public's awareness of this problem. However, mass screening of children is not justified given the low prevalence of positive skin reactors in most communities and the high likelihood of false-positive results caused by previous exposure to atypical mycobacteria in the reactors. One study suggests that tuberculosis screening is not cost-effective unless the prevalence of skin reactors is greater than 1 per cent (North, 1974). In most areas of the United States, the prevalence of infection in children is between 0.1 and 0.5 per cent. Therefore, a knowledge of local public health statistics is needed before making a practice-wide strategy.

The most important criterion in defining the individual child at high risk is a clinical history of previous exposure to tuberculosis. There is also a higher prevalence of reactivity among children from Central American and Southeast Asia. In these children, "screening" for tuberculosis should be done using 5 tuberculin units (5 TU) of purified protein derivative (PPD), with interpretation at 48 to 72 hours. Induration of 15 mm or more is generally diagnostic of infection. Among low-risk groups, an area of induration of 5 to 14 mm usually suggests exposure to atypical mycobacteria. This intermediate response may be consistent with infection by *Mycobacterium tuberculosis* in high-risk populations. Less than 5 mm of induration is a negative test. Tine (multipuncture) testing is not standardized and yields high numbers of false-positive and false-negative results. Although it is an easier test to perform, it should be avoided. Repeat screening generally is not indicated in low-risk populations unless there is evidence of new

exposure to tuberculosis but is recommended annually for high-risk groups.

Anticipatory Guidance

Disease Prevention

In addition to monitoring growth and development, a portion of the routine visit for the preschool and school-age child should be used to provide education about disease prevention.

Accident Prevention

One half of all deaths in childhood are attributable to accidents. There are more than 19 million medical visits by children for accidents and injury care each year, and 100,000 permanent disabilities result from accidents annually. The type of accidents that result in fatalities are most commonly motor vehicle accidents, followed by drowning, fires and burns, and aspirations and asphyxiations. Different-age children are more susceptible to each of these types of accidents, and the physician can take the opportunity at the routine screening visit to discuss measures that might help prevent future disability (Alpert and Guyer, 1985).

AUTOMOTIVE SAFETY. All states currently have laws requiring that infants and small children sit in appropriate safety seats while in a moving automobile. It is important for the physician to review with the parents the appropriate seat for their child. Children who are 17 to 20 pounds can go from an infant carrier to a toddler's seat. Once the child is 40 to 44 pounds, he or she should use a booster seat or the seat belt. However, the shoulder harness is not appropriate until the child is at least 4.5 feet tall. Under no circumstances should a child be carried in a parent's lap while in a moving automobile.

One half of all traffic-related deaths in children are pedestrian deaths. Consequently, children above the age of 2 should be taught about street safety and the dangers of following thrown balls out into the street.

DROWNING. Drowning is the second leading cause of death among children age 5 to 14. Most drownings take place in pools and in bathtubs. Therefore, younger children should be supervised at all times around the tub, and older children should be encouraged to develop their skills in swimming.

FIRES AND BURNS. Parents should be instructed to equip their house with fire detectors and to regularly run through simulated fire drills. To prevent burns, hot water heaters should be set at 125° F or less. Other burns occur near the stove, and parents should remember to turn pot handles away from the front of the stove so that toddlers and preschool children cannot overturn the pots and pans. Cigarette smoking is a common cause of house fires and

TABLE 29–7.   IMMUNIZATION SCHEDULE FOR CHILDREN 7 YEARS OF AGE OR OLDER WHO WERE NOT IMMUNIZED IN INFANCY

Immunization Timing	Td (Adult Dose)	TOPV*	MMR
First visit	Td1	TOPV1	MMR1
2 months after Td1 (minimum interval)	Td2 (4 weeks)	TOPV2 (6 weeks)	MMR2 (1 month)
6–12 months after Td2 (minimum interval)	Td3 (6 months)	TOPV3 (6 weeks)	
10 years after Td3	Td		
Number of doses in basic series	3	3	2

Td = tetanus and diphtheria toxoids; TOPV = trivalent oral poliovirus vaccine; MMR = measles–mumps–rubella vaccine.

* Routine poliovirus immunization is not recommended for adults 18 years of age or older who are residing in the United States. If vaccine is indicated, adults usually should receive enhanced inactivated poliovirus vaccine.

Adapted from Zimmerman RK, Giebink GS: Childhood immunizations: A practical approach for clinicians. Am Fam Physician 45:1759, 1992, with permission.

yet another reason for physicians to recommend smoking cessation.

ASPIRATION.   The foods that children most commonly aspirate are nuts, grapes, raisins, and other small, firm foodstuffs. Obviously, parents should be instructed to avoid these in young children. They also should be instructed in the basics of the Heimlich maneuver and the use of intrascapular blows to the back to dislodge aspirated food.

POISONINGS.   The parents of toddlers and young children should examine their house carefully and safety proof lower cabinets that contain poisonous cleansers and other substances. Houses with small children should have Ipecac and activated charcoal available in the bathroom for use in emergencies and the physician should review their use at the time of routine visits.

Immunizations

Preschool children who have received their previous immunizations require the final diphtheria–pertussis–tetanus and oral polio vaccine boosters to complete the childhood schedules. These are given together between the ages of 4 and 6, prior to entering school or day care. A second measles–mumps–rubella vaccine is also recommended prior to starting kindergarten or first grade. Complete schedules are shown in Table 28–12 of the previous chapter.

Immunization schedules for children who have not received their immunizations on time are listed in Table 29–7.

CHILDHOOD MORBIDITY

Preschool and school-age children make fewer visits than infants and toddlers to physicians for routine preventive health care. The great majority of office visits by children beyond the toddler stage are for the evaluation and treatment of minor, acute medical problems. As seen in Table 29–8, upper and lower respiratory problems account for a significant percentage of the visits to physicians by both preschool and school-age children. A brief discussion of the evaluation and management of some of these common diagnoses follows.

Otitis Media

Acute otitis media, or purulent otitis media, is the most common medical diagnosis made in children (Paradise, 1980). By the age of 3, nearly three fourths of children have had at least one episode

TABLE 29–8.   PERCENT AND CUMULATIVE PERCENT OF VISITS BY CHILDREN FOR MOST FREQUENT DIAGNOSES BY AGE

	Percent of Visits	Cumulative Percent of Visits
Age 2–5 years		
General exam	19.7	19.7
Otitis media	16.9	36.6
Upper respiratory infection	8.7	45.3
Pharyngitis	5.9	51.2
Tonsillitis	3.9	55.1
Bronchitis	3.9	59.0
Streptococcal pharyngitis	2.2	61.2
Asthma	2.2	63.4
Evaluation of suspected problem	2.0	65.4
Other viral illnesses	1.8	67.2
Age 6–10 years		
General exam	15.2	15.2
Otitis media	9.2	24.4
Pharyngitis	8.0	32.4
Upper respiratory infection	6.1	38.5
Asthma	4.6	43.1
Allergic rhinitis	4.3	47.4
Tonsillitis	4.1	51.5
Streptococcal pharyngitis	2.3	53.8
Bronchitis	2.2	56.0
Influenza	2.0	58.0

From National Center for Health Statistics (Cypress BK): Patterns of Ambulatory Care in Pediatrics. The National Ambulatory Medical Care Survey, United States, January 1980–December 1981. Vital Health Stat [13], no. 75, 1983.

of otitis media and almost one third have had three or more episodes.

The pathophysiology of this disease seems to be related to eustachian tube dysfunction. The eustachian tube normally drains and ventilates the middle ear space. In children, the anatomy of the tube is different and the function often is impaired. Viral infections also may affect the function of the eustachian tube apparatus. The role of allergies in predisposing children to middle ear infections is unclear.

Although viral infections are thought to predispose children to middle ear infections, viruses are rarely isolated from middle ear cultures. Bacteria are much more important as pathogens in otitis media. *Streptococcus pneumoniae* is the most important organism in children of all ages. *Haemophilus influenzae* and *Moraxella catarrhalis* are also important pathogens. Other bacteria, including group A streptococci, are isolated less often.

Clinically, children with otitis media usually have ear pain and often fever. Unlike smaller children, children over the age of 2 generally can localize the pain to the affected ear. Malaise, nausea and vomiting, or other less specific symptoms as presenting features are not as common as in younger children.

The diagnosis of otitis media is made by otoscopy. The classic findings include a bulging tympanic membrane with obscured bony landmarks. Diffuse or localized erythema is an inconsistent finding. Pneumatic otoscopy is less difficult than in the younger child and very helpful in the diagnosis. With a good seal, insufflation will reveal decreased or absent mobility of the tympanic membrane.

There are many options for treatment of acute otitis media. The choice of antibiotics is in part dependent on the importance of β-lactamase–producing *H. influenzae* and *M. catarrhalis* in each geographic region. Nevertheless, amoxicillin still has proven to be a reasonable first-line antibiotic. Other first-line choices may include trimethoprim-sulfamethoxazole or erythromycin-sulfazoxazole. Cefaclor and other newer cephalosporins and the combination antibiotic amoxicillin/clavulonate also provide good coverage but are more expensive. Single-dose intramuscular ceftriaxone is effective treatment for otitis media but has not achieved wide acceptance (Green and Rothrock, 1993). In general, otitis media responds within a 2- to 3-day period. If there has been no adequate clinical response, then an empiric switch to a different antibiotic is appropriate.

Residual effusions after treatment of otitis media are common, and up to 70 per cent of children will have an effusion still present at 2 weeks. Therefore, most experts recommend that follow-up examination in the patient with a satisfactory clinical response to antibiotic therapy be delayed until about 2 months after treatment. Any child who still has symptoms should, of course, be seen earlier. A follow-up tympanogram may be helpful to assess successful treatment.

Recurrences of otitis media within 1 month of the initial episode are frequently due to the same organism. Consequently, a change in the choice of antibiotics probably is indicated for early recurrences. Antibiotic prophylaxis should be considered for any child with multiple episodes of otitis media within a 6-month period. Effective antimicrobial choices include twice-daily sulfisoxazole or once-daily amoxicillin or trimethoprim-sulfamethoxazole (not formally approved for this indication). Antihistamines and decongestants have no proven benefit in the treatment of persistent middle ear effusions (Cantekin et al., 1983). The indications and relative benefits of surgical interventions for recurrent otitis media and persistent ear effusions have not been defined clearly.

Viral Upper Respiratory Infection (Including the "Common Cold")

Children of all ages get several colds per year, with a slight increase in the number of infections during the wintertime. Parents can anticipate that their child will get three to eight colds per year. There is some evidence that young children in day care centers will experience more respiratory infections than children who remain at home, although this may be true only for the first year (Wald et al., 1988).

Many viruses cause colds in children. Rhinovirus and coronaviruses are responsible for most of these infections. Other less common causes of colds include parainfluenza, influenza, and respiratory syncytial viruses. Viruses appear to be transmitted by small droplets during close contact. The viruses replicate in the upper respiratory epithelium and result in sloughing of the superficial layer of cells. Symptoms and viral shedding generally last from 3 days to a week or more.

The usual clinical symptoms of a cold include nasal congestion, cough, and variable fevers. The nasal discharge can be thin and clear or mucoid and purulent. Most viral upper respiratory infections are uncomplicated. Suppurative complications, although infrequent, include otitis media, sinusitis, or lower respiratory bacterial infections, including bronchitis and pneumonia.

The nonspecific clinical presentation of a cold may mimic the prodrome of other childhood viral illnesses, including measles or chicken pox. In children with an allergic history, the nasal congestion of an upper respiratory infection should be distinguished from allergic rhinitis.

On physical exam, children with colds are not toxic appearing. The general appearance of a sick child should lead to a careful search for one of the suppurative complications listed above. The non–ill-appearing child should receive a careful head and neck exam as a minimum to rule out early otitis media. For the child with possible allergic rhinitis, a Wright's stain can be done on the nasal discharge. The finding of many eosinophils suggests allergic rhinitis.

Colds resolve spontaneously without specific treatment, and no treatment or symptomatic relief only should be recommended. Antibiotics have no benefit unless bacterial suprainfection has occurred. Acetaminophen is preferred over aspirin because of the association between the use of aspirin during certain viral illnesses and the subsequent development of Reye's syndrome. Decongestants and antihistamines often produce side effects worse than the symptoms for which they are prescribed. Antihistamines may provide some sedation for children in the evening. Older children may be able to use topical decongestants effectively without suffering systemic symptoms.

Pharyngitis and Tonsillitis

Sore throats are one of the most common problems among preschool and school-age children. The peak incidence for sore throats occurs between the ages of 5 and 8 years.

More than 80 per cent of all pharyngitis is caused by viruses. A sore throat is often one of several symptoms associated with a viral upper respiratory infection. Occasionally, the sore throat is the predominant symptom. Adenoviruses may cause an exudative pharyngitis with or without other symptoms of nasal discharge and cough, particularly in younger children. Herpangina, which is caused by coxsackieviruses or Echoviruses, is suggested by vesicles or small ulcers on the tonsillar pillars or soft palate. These may be accompanied by high fever and other symptoms such as headache or malaise. One coxsackievirus, type A16, is the agent responsible for hand-foot-and-mouth disease. The pathognomonic findings include ulcerations of the buccal mucosa in conjunction with papulovesicular lesions on the palms of the hands and the soles of the feet. Infectious mononucleosis also may cause a sore throat and petechial lesions of the soft palate in addition to its characteristic cervical adenopathy. Other viruses may cause pharyngitis but are less common.

Among the bacterial agents that cause pharyngitis, the most important is the group A β-hemolytic streptococcus, which may be responsible for as much as 15 per cent of this disease in children. Streptococcal pharyngitis remains important because untreated cases infrequently may be complicated by the development of acute rheumatic fever. Strep throats are suggested by tonsillar erythema with exudates and an enanthem on the soft palate, and occasionally clinically confirmed by the presence of the erythematous "sandpapery"

rash of scarlet fever. Other bacterial infections causing pharyngitis are uncommon. Diphtheria causes a membranous exudate of the pharynx that is exceptionally rare in the immunized child. Gonorrhea and chlamydia may be found in the sexually abused child and always should lead to a more comprehensive evaluation.

On physical exam, bacterial causes of pharyngitis are less likely if other symptoms of viral upper respiratory infection, such as cough and rhinorrhea, are present. The pharynx should be examined carefully to rule out uvular deviation seen with peritonsillar abscess or clinical signs consistent with epiglottitis.

Most children do not need a culture or quick antigen test for strep throat because of the low likelihood of infection. The strep culture should be used selectively based on clinical symptoms or signs in conjunction with a carefully obtained history of exposure and knowledge of regional epidemiology.

One of the difficult issues is the management of the child carrier of streptococcus. About 50 per cent of children from whom streptococcus is cultured have no serologic evidence of infection and, therefore, treatment is of no proven benefit. However, the problem is that, at the time of evaluation, it is not known whether the patient is infected or merely a carrier with symptoms of pharyngitis. In practice, the symptomatic carrier routinely is treated with antibiotics. The asymptomatic carrier, when discovered by culture, also usually is treated with antibiotic. Because the carrier state is difficult to eradicate and the risk of developing acute rheumatic fever for the carrier is unknown but appears low, experts currently are recommending that reculturing of children after completion of antibiotic therapy and culturing of asymptomatic contacts of children with strep pharyngitis not be done routinely.

The recommended treatment for strep pharyngitis is penicillin orally for 10 days. Erythromycin is an effective, inexpensive alternative for the child allergic to penicillin.

Lower Respiratory Tract Infections

Lower respiratory tract infections are less common than upper respiratory tract infections in children. Several clinical syndromes of lower respiratory tract infections in children are recognized (Table 29–9). Most children with lower respiratory tract infections are not ill enough to require hospitalization. Viruses and *M. pneumoniae* are responsible for most of these infections, and antibiotics therefore are not required (Denny and Clyde, 1986).

Croup

Croup is a relatively common syndrome in children characterized by respiratory obstruction and a

**TABLE 29–9. LOWER RESPIRATORY TRACT
INFECTIONS IN CHILDREN**

Infection	Signs and Symptoms
Croup	Hoarseness, cough, inspiratory stridor with laryngeal obstruction
Tracheobronchitis	Cough and rhonchi; no laryngeal obstruction or wheezing
Bronchiolitis	Expiratory wheezing with or without tachypnea, air trapping and substernal retractions
Pneumonia	Rales or evidence of pulmonary consolidation on physical examination or radiograph

barking cough. Croup generally occurs in children ages 1 to 5, with a peak incidence during the second year of life. The cause of croup is generally viral. The parainfluenza viruses have been implicated in up to 80 per cent of cases. Children with croup generally are afebrile or have low-grade fevers. The symptoms typically begin at night and recur nightly for several days. The symptoms usually can be improved by putting the child in the bathroom with the shower on or exposing him or her to the outside night air.

Tracheobronchitis

Tracheobronchitis is a syndrome involving the lower respiratory tract associated with a productive cough. On physical examination, there is no evidence of lung parenchymal involvement. Tracheobronchitis generally has a viral etiology, and secondary bacterial infection is rare. In a very ill child, a diagnosis of epiglottitis or bacterial tracheitis must be entertained and urgent management, including maintenance of the airway, is essential.

Bronchiolitis

Bronchiolitis is a syndrome that occurs in small children and is unusual after the age of 2. It is generally viral in etiology. Respiratory syncytial viruses have been implicated in a large proportion of cases. Bronchiolitis can be difficult to differentiate from asthma. In borderline cases, it is useful to think of the pathophysiology as reactive airway disease associated with a lower respiratory infection. Recurrence of symptoms in a child with a family history of asthma suggests the possibility of asthma as the true diagnosis. An empiric trial of a bronchodilator is often useful.

Pneumonia

The diagnosis of pneumonia is considered in the child with rales or clinical evidence of pulmonary consolidation. Most pneumonias in children are due to viruses and *Mycoplasma*. Less than one third are bacterial in origin. In general, children with nonbacterial pneumonias have only mild respiratory distress, and a chest radiograph, when obtained, shows hyperinflation, segmental atelectasis, and interstitial infiltrates. The child with bacterial pneumonia may be more ill-appearing and have lobar consolidation. Small children generally cannot produce sputum and, therefore, sputum cultures and Gram's stains are not of benefit. For the older child with presumed bacterial pneumonia, erythromycin may be the appropriate antibiotic because of its effectiveness against *Pneumococcus* and *Mycoplasma* species.

Asthma

Asthma is one of the most common chronic medical conditions in childhood and is the most frequent cause for hospital admission among children. The prevalence of this disease in children is about 5 to 10 per cent. The incidence appears to be increasing among black children and in urban areas (Gergen et al., 1988). Most asthmatics have their first episode before the age of 3, although new cases are diagnosed at all ages and the peak prevalence is among children ages 10 to 12.

Asthma is defined as recurrent episodes of reactive airway disease. Common triggers of smooth muscle spasm in the distal airways include viral infections, environmental allergens, and exercise or cold weather. In some children, emotional factors also may precipitate bronchospasm.

The asthmatic child often presents 1 to 2 days following the onset of an upper respiratory infection. Less commonly, asthma is diagnosed in the child with recurrent cough, which typically is worse at night. Sometimes the diagnosis is suspected in the child with repeated viral infections associated with mild respiratory distress, and confirmed by the empiric response to bronchodilator therapy.

On physical exam, there is a variable degree of respiratory distress and air hunger. Characteristic of the child with asthma is a prolonged expiratory phase. There may be use of accessory respiratory muscles.

The treatment of acute asthma has changed somewhat in the past few years. ("Guidelines for the Diagnosis," 1991). Because of a decrease in side effects, inhalation treatment with β_2-adrenergic agents is preferred to subcutaneous epinephrine. Treatment may be repeated after 20 to 30 minutes for a total of three doses. Children who have not improved after one or two inhalation treatments usually require intravenous theophylline and steroid therapy, as well as hospitalization. If there is improvement, the child can be managed as an outpatient with oral β_2-adrenergic agents. Children over 5 can use metered-dose inhalers effectively but may require a spacer device.

Children with chronically recurrent symptoms of asthma should receive anti-inflammatory medications to treat the underlying pathology of the disease as well as having access to β-agonists for immediate symptom control. The two anti-inflammatory medications recommended for maintenance therapy are cromolyn sodium and inhaled corticosteroids. Cromolyn can be given via inhaler or nebulizer three or four times a day without any anticipated problems. Inhaled steroids are an acceptable first-line therapy as well. Anecdotal reports of growth retardation mandate that inhalation schedules be titrated to the lowest effective dose. The long-acting theophylline preparations often are used for maintenance therapy, although their side effect profile and relatively narrow therapeutic window may make them a better second-line medication. Children under 9 years of age are rapid metabolizers of theophylline and often need 20 to 24 mg/kg/day for maintenance therapy. Older children and adolescents usually are treated with doses of 300 to 400 mg twice daily of a long-acting theophylline. For children on long-term theophylline therapy, a steady-state level should be obtained and children ideally should be kept in the lower end of the therapeutic range of 10 to 20 μg/mL. Several commonly prescribed drugs, including erythromycin, can interfere with the metabolism of theophylline and lead to toxic levels. Children on chronic theophylline therapy with steady-state therapeutic levels probably should receive a reduced dose of their theophylline preparation when concomitant therapy with erythromycin is prescribed. Further adjustments in dosing can be determined by measured drug levels. Oral steroids are not recommended for prolonged use in asthmatics, except as indicated for hospitalized patients or for children with frequent exacerbations of asthma in spite of maximum treatment with other agents.

Atopic Dermatitis

Atopic dermatitis is a chronic condition characterized by dry, eczematous skin in a typical distribution. This condition often is found in association with a personal or family history of other atopic disorders, including allergies and asthma. Atopic dermatitis affects between one and three per cent of children.

Atopic dermatitis generally begins during infancy, but occasionally presents in the older child. By childhood, the rash most commonly involves the flexural surfaces of the antecubital and popliteal fossae, the wrist, and the area around the neck and face. Occasionally, small vesicles and pustules develop on the hands, particularly the interdigital areas. This "dyshidrotic eczema" probably is due to exposure to irritants in the child with atopy.

The most common complication of atopic dermatitis is secondary bacterial infection of affected areas. The infections usually are due to staphylococcus or streptococcus species.

The treatment of atopic dermatitis depends on the degree of inflammation present. Children should be instructed to avoid exacerbating irritants and to avoid frequent hand washing. Harsh, drying soaps should be replaced with mild, moisturizing soaps. Lubricants or moisturizing creams can be used following hand washing. Topical corticosteroid preparations are usually necessary to clear the inflammatory lesions. A general rule is to use the weakest preparation that will work. Fluorinated steroids should be used only for severe lesions and for short periods of time. One useful approach is to apply a small amount of a steroid cream and then cover the area with a lubricating agent. Systemic antibiotics may be necessary to clear up inflammatory lesions that have become infected secondarily.

Gastroenteritis

Gastroenteritis is a common problem in children, with a decreasing incidence after the age of 2. In small children, most infections occur via the fecal–oral route. Not surprisingly, recent data have shown an increased likelihood of gastroenteritis in children attending day care centers (Child Daycare Infectious Disease Study Group, 1984). When looked for, a pathogen can be found in about one half of all cases. About 80 per cent of the pathogens identified are viral (Isaacs et al., 1986). In particular, the rotavirus has been implicated as a major cause of gastroenteritis in children.

Most cases of gastroenteritis in children over 2 are not severe and can be managed without medical intervention, often over the phone. In the otherwise healthy child, putting the bowel at rest with clear liquids for 24 to 48 hours is generally sufficient. Oral rehydration solutions have been used successfully in the United States as well as in Third World nations and can be recommended for moderately dehydrated children. These solutions contain more sodium and less glucose than the oral electrolyte solutions that were previously available. Parents should be advised against feeding the child dairy products because these often exacerbate the symptoms. The diet can be advanced slowly and dairy products added after 3 or 4 days.

Diarrhea and abdominal pain of nonviral etiology generally resolves without antibiotic therapy as well. *Campylobacter* is now the most common bacterial cause of childhood diarrhea. Most episodes are of short duration, although the abdominal pain may be remarkable, and no therapy is indicated. Prolonged episodes with a positive culture should be treated with erythromycin. *Shigella* usually causes mild symptoms, but may be associated with bloody diarrhea. Oral ampicillin or trimethoprim-sulfamethoxazole will shorten the duration of symptoms and lessen the period of infectivity to others. *Salmonella* usually causes relatively mild symptoms, and treatment is not indicated unless the child is at risk for invasive disease. *Giardia* is a protozoan that may cause diarrhea in children and has been found in up to 25 per cent of children in day care centers, most of whom are asymptomatic. Treatment with furazolidone probably is indicated in most cases. Metronidazole has not been approved for use in children under 12.

Urinary Tract Infection

Urinary tract infections (UTIs) are relatively uncommon in children but require aggressive diagnostic and therapeutic management because of their potential to do renal damage. After infancy, girls are much more likely than boys to present with a UTI. Up to 90 per cent of first infections are caused by *Escherichia coli*. Other bacteria that may cause UTIs in children include *Klebsiella*, *Proteus*, *Enterococcus* species, and *Staphylococcus saprophyticus*. The clinical presentation of a UTI in children is dependent on the age of the child. Toddlers often present with nonspecific symptoms, including abdominal discomfort, fever, and a change in their voiding pattern. Preschool children may have discomfort and secondary enuresis in addition to fever and abdominal pain. Older children are more likely to have the "classic" symptoms of a UTI, including frequency, urgency, and dysuria.

Appropriate collection of a urine specimen in a child is difficult. Bagged urine is generally contaminated and can be considered reliable only if the specimen is sterile. Because of perineal contamination, a catheterized specimen may be necessary to confirm ambiguous results. After an appropriate collection, bacteria seen on an unspun specimen suggest infection. The number of white cells seen on a spun specimen is variable, but more than five to ten per high-power field implies inflammation.

A specimen for culture should be refrigerated until plated to prevent bacterial overgrowth. On a noncatheterized specimen, bacterial counts greater than 50,000 are consistent with an infection. On a catheterized specimen, any bacterial growth is significant.

Up to 50 per cent of children under age 4 or 5 will have some vesicoureteral reflux in conjunction with a UTI and fever. Therefore, treatment should be continued for 10 to 14 days. Shorter courses in young children are not warranted. Older children and adolescents have had successful treatment with shorter courses of therapy.

The recommended further evaluation of children with UTIs is contingent on several factors. All males with a first UTI and females with repeat infection or clinical evidence of pyelonephritis or growth retardation should be evaluated further. The test of first choice is a voiding cystourethrogram (VCUG) to look for reflux. The VCUG should be obtained 4 to 6 weeks after treatment of the acute infection because of the high incidence of reflux during a UTI in young children. Prophylactic antibiotics may be necessary to reduce the likelihood of recurrent infection until VCUG can be completed. The renal structure also should be evaluated with intravenous pyelography or ultrasound. The finding of significant reflux or obstructive uropathy should result in referral to a urologist.

ADOLESCENT HEALTH CARE

Family physicians are in a unique position to provide health care to adolescents during the transition from childhood to adulthood. Adolescence often is characterized as a period of chaotic development marked by risk-taking behaviors. Although the reality is usually not so bleak, the developmental changes can be unsettling to even the most healthy-appearing teens. Rapid changes in growth are accompanied by an increasing self-awareness and often self-doubt. In addition, influential forces such as the media and peer pressure conspire against a smooth assimilation of change. Finally, the family often has difficulty in coping with these rapid, uneven changes. With the perspective that adolescence is but one phase in the life cycle and not the culmination of development, and with the understanding of the adolescent's family dynamics, a family doctor has an opportunity to facilitate a teenager's evolution into adulthood that is not available to other specialists.

A common pitfall for physicians is to address adolescents' health needs based solely on their chronologic age. For the most part, our society groups adolescents by age or grade in school, assuming a progressive, linear increase in knowledge, maturity, and socialization skills. Development may be neither orderly nor even, and there may be disparities between physiologic and psychosocial growth in the same individual at a given time. The task of addressing adolescent health care needs requires sensitivity to the stage of development attained by the individual and the skills and emotional resources they have at their disposal. Tailoring health care delivery to find the most developmentally appropriate interventions therefore requires assessments of the stage of maturity in several different areas.

By most criteria, adolescents are a healthy group with low morbidity and mortality. However, adolescents themselves report much greater concerns about their health than might be expected (Levenson et al., 1984). These concerns focus not only on medical problems per se, but also on issues regarding interpersonal relationships, sexuality, substance abuse, and anxiety or nervousness. In other words, adolescents see themselves as needing more comprehensive professional care than that to which they generally have access.

Health Care Utilization Issues

There are many reasons for the apparent underutilization of health care by adolescents (Irwin, 1986). These barriers include the issue of confidentiality and the physician's previous alignment with the patient's family, legal and ethical issues, and economics.

Confidentiality

Family physicians generally have ongoing relationships with the family members of an adolescent patient. Many studies have demonstrated that teenagers will not seek any or all of their health care from a physician if their parents have access to information about the visit (Herold and Goodwin, 1979). Adolescents are particularly reluctant to discuss issues of sexuality or contraception with a physician who has a previous alliance with the family. From the outset, the physician should establish that the doctor–patient relationships assures the patient's right to confidentiality. Occasionally families prefer a two-physician arrangement to avoid conflict of allegiance. However, this represents an option of second choice and is generally unnecessary if the physician defines the ground rules from the start.

Legal and Ethical Issues

The adolescent's right to confidentiality must be balanced against the rights of the parents to supervise the health of their minor child and the physician's desire not to divide the family. Most states have laws that protect both adolescents and physicians regarding the provision of care without parental consent for specific health issues, including the diagnosis and management of pregnancy, the provision of contraception, the diagnosis and management of sexually transmitted diseases, substance use and abuse, and the initial evaluation and treatment of emotional illness. Without assurances of confidentiality, many of these problems would go unevaluated. These laws vary from state to state, and physicians should be familiar with the laws in their own state (Morrisey et al., 1986).

The "mature minor doctrine" states that minor individuals sufficiently mature to understand the benefits and risks of a medical evaluation and treatment are legally able to give valid informed consent (Hofmann, 1980). In most instances, the family physician should gain the consent of the adolescent before sharing the information with the parents. This procedure empowers the adolescent, but also keeps him or her a part of the larger family unit.

Economics

Although adolescents may desire confidentiality regarding their medical care, they often do not have financial resources to pay for their visits. If the physician has a good relationship with the parents, one possible arrangement is for the parents to agree to pay for medical visits that are deemed necessary by the physician. An alternative arrangement is for the teenager to assume part of the cost of each visit. In this era of third-party insurance, there are potential snags in the system to maintaining confidentiality. Bills listing procedures such as a dilation and evacuation, Papanicolou (Pap) smear, or the application of podophylline to venereal warts will be sent to the insured family member, usually a parent. If this arrangement is unsatisfactory, alternative plans must be made in advance.

Conduct of the Visit with an Adolescent

Medical visits for adolescents are frequently more emotionally charged than visits for younger children. In some situations, the adolescent patient is distrustful of the physician, particularly of the potential for an alliance of the physician with the patient's parents. The doctor also must be aware of certain emotions elicited by adolescent patients. Physicians often negatively stereotype adolescents as sexually promiscuous or as substance abusers. Alternatively, physicians may present themselves as more knowledgeable regarding salient adolescent issues than is really the case. These judgmental attitudes increase the adolescent's distrust.

For these reasons, certain guidelines are helpful in the conduct of a medical visit for an adolescent. Most physicians who take care of adolescents see the patient with the parents for part of the visit and then the patient alone. This gives the mother and father an opportunity to discuss their concerns but still empowers the teenager as the patient. It is helpful to explain to the parents that issues discussed with the adolescent in private will be held confidential. Of course, the protection of information discussed does not hold in life-threatening situations, such as for the suicidal adolescent. Most parents are comfortable with this arrangement, particularly when it is laid out at the beginning of the visit. The purpose of this separation is not to divide the family. On the contrary, the family physician often can help the teenager figure out ways to discuss problems with the parents. Developmentally, however, it is often difficult for the teenager to discuss openly issues regarding sexuality and concerns about growth and development, for instance, in front of the parent.

One benefit of this strategy is that the adolescent will begin to accept some of the responsibility for his or her own health care. This transition can be facilitated by initiating this visit format for well-child visits in the preadolescent years. A few minutes of each routine visit can be set aside to allow the older child or preadolescent to discuss any concerns in private. This may foster a trusting relationship for the physician, patient, and family in years to come when developmental issues make confidentiality more important.

Developmental Assessment

Physical Development

Although the changes of puberty tend to follow a predictable sequence, the onset and the rapidity of the changes are extremely variable. Chronologic age therefore correlates poorly with biological maturity. A sexual maturity scale such as the one developed by Tanner can be used to assess the physical developmental stage of a patient. This scale assigns a Tanner stage of 1 (prepubertal) to 5 (adult) to girls based on breasts and pubic hair and to boys based on genitalia and pubic hair (see Table 29–10).

Sexual development in the female generally is heralded by the finding of breast buds, a small amount of tissue beneath the nipple and areola, or thelarche (Fig. 29–3). The growth spurt generally occurs relatively early in puberty in females, around Tanner stage 3. Menarche typically occurs at the end of the growth spurt and signals closure of the epiphyseal growth plates. The mean age of menarche in the United States is 12.8 years, with only minor racial or regional variation.

In males, the first sign of puberty is testicular enlargement, which typically begins between 9.5 and 13.5 years of age. The growth spurt in males occurs late in puberty, around Tanner stage 4. Therefore, males start puberty after females and have their growth spurt later in puberty.

There are many other somatic changes during puberty that are better correlated with sexual maturity than with age (Slap, 1986). Approximately 25 per cent of final adult height is accounted for during pubertal growth. Weight gain also increases appreciably during adolescence, and this change accounts for over 40 per cent of the ideal adult weight in both sexes. However, there are marked differ-

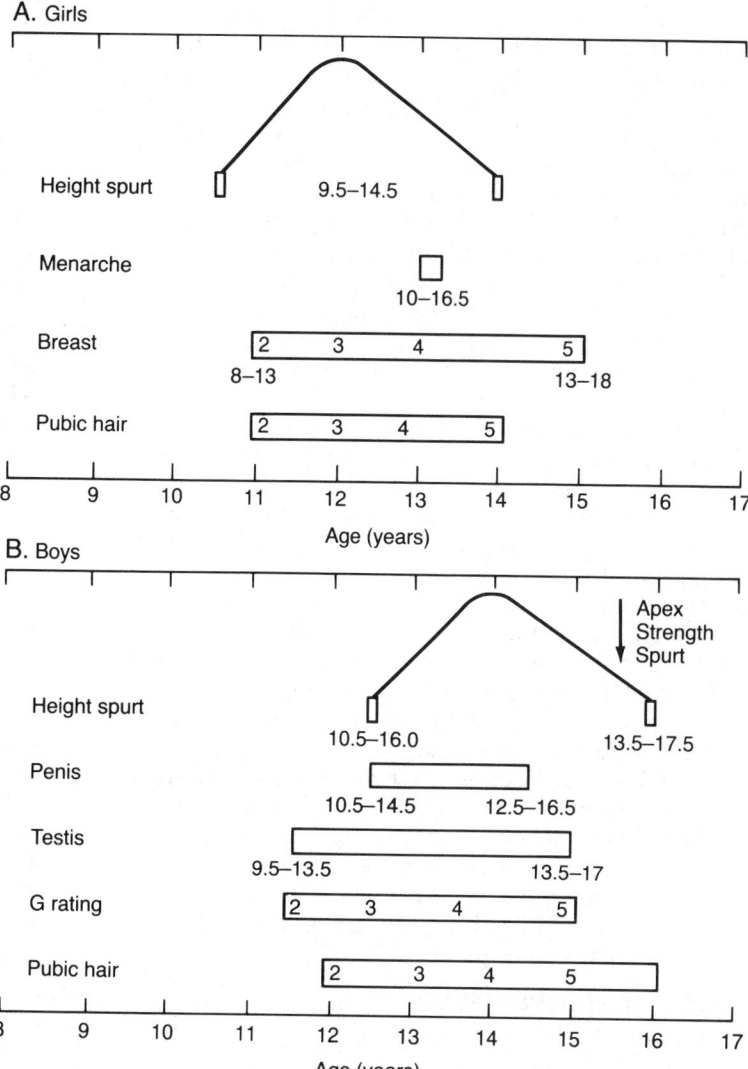

FIGURE 29–3. Sequence of events in puberty for girls *(A)* and boys *(B)*. (From Slap GB: Normal physiological and psychosocial growth in the adolescent. J Adoles Health Care 7:13S, 1986, with permission. Copyright 1986 by the Society for Adolescent Medicine.)

TABLE 29–10.   CLASSIFICATION OF SEXUAL MATURITY STAGES IN GIRLS AND BOYS

Stage	Pubic Hair	Breasts/Genitalia
Girls		
1	Preadolescent	Preadolescent
2	Sparse, lightly pigmented, straight, medial border of labia	Breast bud under areola, areolar diameter increased
3	Darker, beginning to curl, increased amount	Breast and areola enlarged, no contour separation
4	Course, curly, abundant but amount less than in adult	Areola and papilla form secondary mound
5	Adult feminine triangle, spread to medial surface of thighs	Mature, no contour separation, deepening color of areola
Boys		
1	None	Preadolescent: testicles 1–2 cm
2	Scanty, long, slightly pigmented	Testicles >2 cm, scrotum enlarged
3	Darker, starts to curl, small amount	Penis longer; testicles larger
4	Resembles adult type, but less in quantity; course, curly	Widening of glans; scrotum darker
5	Adult distribution, spread to medial surface of thighs	Adult

Adapted from Tanner JM: Growth at Adolescence, 2nd edition. Oxford, England, Blackwell Scientific Publications, 1962, with permission.

ences between males and females in terms of body composition. In girls, the lean body mass decreases from 80 to 75 per cent, whereas in boys it increases from 80 to 90 per cent. Prior to the onset of puberty, males and females are similar in many physiologic measures. As a result of the effects of testosterone, heart weight nearly doubles and vital capacity increases dramatically in boys. Blood volume, red blood cell mass, and hematocrit increase steadily throughout puberty in boys, but remain fairly constant in girls, as shown in Figure 29–4.

Blood pressure measurements also change fairly dramatically with puberty. Systolic blood pressures rise rapidly in boys and reach a plateau in girls (Fig. 29–5). There is a much higher correlation between high blood pressure in adolescents of later maturity stages and adults than in young children. As a result, with each successive sexual maturity stage, a greater proportion of patients with high blood pressure will be found to have essential hypertension.

In addition to providing information regarding physiologic changes, the sexual maturity rating at the time of a visit can be used to help the adolescent with his or her concerns about normal development. For example, late-developing males can be reassured that, because of their early stage of development, they still have several years of growth, including their growth spurt, ahead. As another example, males with gynecomastia can be told that nearly two thirds of boys have gynecomastia at Tanner stage 2, but that more than 95 per cent have resolution by the end of puberty. Adolescents who are most preoccupied with changes in their body and concerned about being examined generally benefit the greatest from information provided by physicians regarding normal developmental processes. Many physicians provide a "running explanation" of their findings during the physical examination of an adolescent.

Psychosocial Development

Although biologic measures are the most obvious signs of puberty, the period of adolescence

is, in fact, a complicated process in which psychosocial growth is intertwined with physical development. Several tasks characterize this biopsychosocial process in adolescents. These "tasks of adolescence" include:

1.   Emancipation from family and formation of self-identity.
2.   Sexual identification and achievement of intimacy.

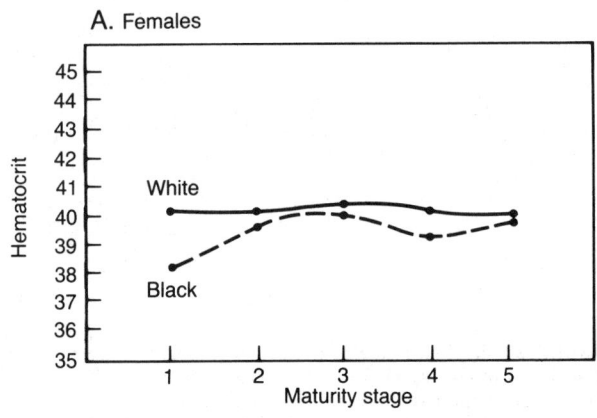

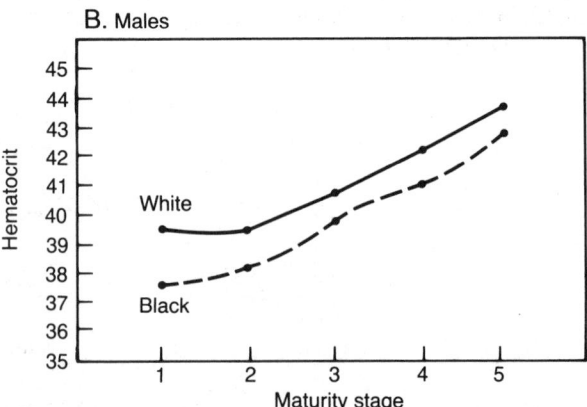

FIGURE 29–4. Hematocrit values for females (*A*) and males (*B*), showing changes during puberty. (From Daniel WA Jr: Adolescents in Health and Disease. Pediatrics 3:388, 1973, with permission.)

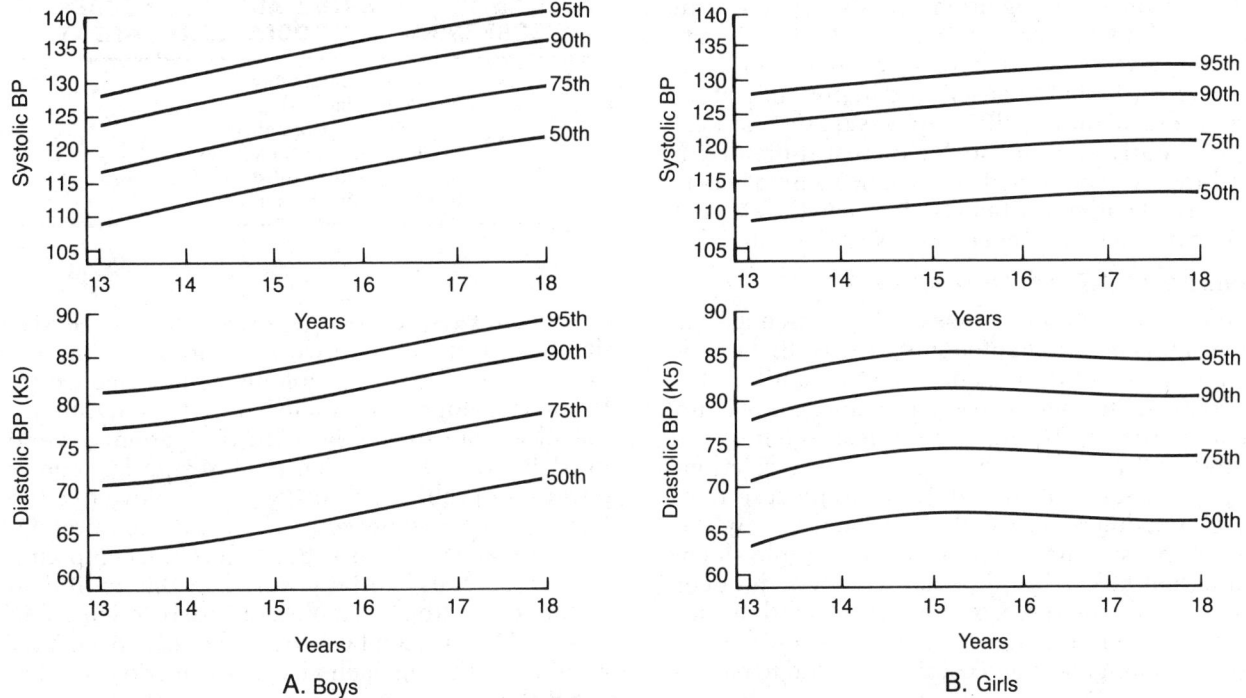

FIGURE 29–5. Age-specific percentiles of blood pressure measurements in boys *(A)* and girls *(B)* 13 to 18 years of age; Korotkoff Phase V (K5) used for diastolic blood pressure. (From Task Force on Blood Pressure Control in Children, National Heart, Lung and Blood Institute: Report of the Second Task Force on Blood Pressure Control in Children—1987. Pediatrics 79:1, 1987, with permission.)

3. Future orientation and career choice.

Although adolescents are not a homogenous group, Table 29–11 can be used to assess normal or abnormal development in adolescent patients.

Cognitive Development

The changes that occur in intellectual development during adolescence are harder to quantify than the sexual maturity ratings. In late childhood and early adolescence, concrete thought processes give way to more abstract thinking. This ability to think abstractly coincides with the introduction of courses in school such as algebra and geometry. Consequently, teenagers who do not move beyond concrete thinking often manifest problems or frustrations with learning around the time of middle school or junior high school. This is an important time for knowledgeable physicians to intervene and help the slow learner find an appropriate educational pace.

TABLE 29–11. PSYCHOSOCIAL DEVELOPMENT OF ADOLESCENTS

Area of Growth	Early Adolescence	Middle Adolescence	Late Adolescence
Family independence	Less interest in parental activities	Peak of parental conflicts	Reacceptance of parental advice and values
Body image	Preoccupation with self and pubertal changes Uncertainty about appearance	General acceptance of body Concern over making body more attractive	Acceptance of pubertal changes
Interpersonal relationships	Intense relationships with same sex	Peak of peer involvement Conformity with peer values Increased sexual activity and experimentation	Peer group less important More time spent in sharing intimate relationships
Self-perception (identity)	Increase cognition ("personal fantasy") Idealistic vocational goals Increased need for privacy Lack of impulse control	Increased scope of feelings Increased intellectual ability Feelings of omnipotence Risk-taking behavior	Practical, realistic vocational goals Refinement of moral, religious, and sexual values Ability to compromise and to set limits

Adapted from Neinstein LS: Adolescent Health Care: A Practical Guide. Baltimore, Urban & Schwartzenberg, 1984, with permission.

The changes in cognition are also apparent in teenagers' future orientation and future events planning. With cognitive maturity comes the ability to set realistic life goals. The importance of future events planning often impacts on the medical system. Early adolescents have great difficulty in handling their own medications, not only because of issues of autonomy but also because they do not anticipate their own needs hours or days ahead.

Interpersonal/Social Development

One of the important "tasks of adolescence" is the establishment of autonomy, that is, the attainment of an identity separate from the family. This process usually begins early in adolescence with the adolescent showing less interest in family activities and perhaps substituting a close relationship with a same-sex friend. In the clinical setting, the early adolescent usually is brought in by the parent and sits there quietly while the physician and parent talk. By middle adolescence, the peer group has assumed greater importance and the adolescent often conforms with peer group values. This often heightens any conflicts related to parental authority. These are the typical angry adolescents that are dragged in to the office by a parent and, unless handled with care, refuse to talk or be examined. By late adolescence, the peer group is less important because the adolescent has established a more stable identity separate from the peer group or the family. With this increased maturity comes an ability to enter an intimate relationship. The relationship with the family is much less conflictual and the late adolescent can assimilate or let go of parental values. These patients often make their own appointments, or if the parent comes with them, they are comfortable letting the parent give his or her view of any problems.

Psychological Development

Coincident with changes in cognitive function, early adolescents commonly have daydreams. The early adolescent often lives a "personal fantasy," and may feel that everyone is watching but that no one can understand his unique problems. This is the time when the adolescent is preoccupied with the physical and the changes of puberty, the "Am I normal?" period. With midadolescence comes a greater acceptance of one's body and, for some, feelings of being indestructible. During this period many adolescents take great risks, often through experimentation with drugs and sexual activity or, alternatively, with motor vehicles. By late adolescence, the body changes have been assimilated into a stable identity, and values from other parts of the adolescent's life help him or her to compromise and set limits in interpersonal settings.

"Screening" the Adolescent Patient

For developmental reasons, adolescents often have difficulty identifying a specific reason for

TABLE 29–12. ESSENTIAL AREAS TO ADDRESS IN "SCREENING" THE ADOLESCENT PATIENT

1. Family interactions.
2. Peer relationships.
3. School performance.
4. Intimacy/sexual activity.
5. Drugs/other substance use.
6. Other risk-taking behaviors.

their visit. Frequently, there is a "hidden agenda" that the physician must work to find. Furthermore, because many of the problems of adolescence relate to developmental issues, it is often helpful for the physician to review with the patient several important areas in which adolescents frequently encounter problems. Most experts believe that the health care of adolescents should be comprehensive and not simply directed at the chief complaint. The "essentials" to be covered in the additional history taken from an adolescent are listed in Table 29–12. This list can be reviewed easily in a matter of minutes during each visit with an adolescent to see if there are any unrecognized problems.

Information about family interactions and peer relationships helps the physician understand how connected or isolated the adolescent feels. By reviewing school performance, the physician can see if the adolescent has the cognitive skills to handle the abstract thinking required in many subjects beyond the sixth grade. If there are problems, the physician can work with the school to find a more appropriate learning plan. Intimate relationships and sexual activity, if any, should be discussed. Adolescents who are not sexually active should have the opportunity to discuss the pressures on them to become sexually active, and supported in their decision to continue their abstinence. Adolescents who are already sexually active should be offered contraception or referred elsewhere where they can receive appropriate counseling and contraception, when indicated. The last menstrual period should be noted for female adolescents who are sexually active. Concern about a possible pregnancy is a common reason for a visit among females. Drug and alcohol use also should be recorded and appropriate intervention planned for adolescents with identified problems. Other risk-taking behavior should be reviewed. This may include skateboard and bicycle use in the younger adolescent, and particularly risky behavior such as drinking and driving in the older adolescent.

Anticipatory Guidance

Adolescents worry about their health more than physicians realize. By self-report, fewer than 10 per cent of adolescents claim never to think about their health, but nearly 40 per cent think about it often and 20 per cent worry about it all the time (Parcel et al., 1977). Through an understanding of normal developmental processes, family physicians may be able to allay some of this anxiety by reassuring the adolescent about normal physical findings at the time of exam and by discussing what changes the adolescent can expect in the months and years ahead. This is particularly true for the early to midadolescent who is so preoccupied with physical changes.

Following the developmental assessment and physical exam, the physician also can provide appropriate information to help limit the teenager's future health risks. Adolescents who have a "steady" boyfriend or girlfriend and are at Tanner stage 4 or 5 are more likely to become sexually active in the near future. It is appropriate to review with the adolescent communication skills between partners regarding intimacy; the risks associated with sexual activity, including pregnancy and sexually transmitted diseases; and the need for contraception. Similarly, adolescents who are engaged in one risk-taking behavior, such as smoking cigarettes, are at greater risk for experimenting with drugs and alcohol, and the assumed risks should be discussed (Irwin and Millstein, 1986). With regard to anticipatory guidance for adolescents, several studies have shown that adolescents prefer a

TABLE 29–13. ANTICIPATORY GUIDANCE REGARDING HEALTH RISK BEHAVIORS

History	Discussion/Evaluation	Intervention
Dating	Adolescent's partner (heterosexual, homosexual) Knowledge of sexual activity and consequences Partner pressure to initiate activity	Delay of premature sexual activity (discussion with partner about sexual activity) Preparation: if sexually active, to prevent adolescent pregnancy (contraception) and sexually transmitted disease (condom use)
Sexual activity Heterosexual Homosexual	Knowledge of risk of pregnancy, sexually transmitted diseases (particularly HIV and AIDS) Knowledge of risk of sexually transmitted diseases	Contraception Sexually transmitted disease prevention Difficulties being gay Specific morbidities
Cigarette smoking	Family history of cigarette smoking Specific medical morbidities of cigarette smoking (cardiovascular, pulmonary) Specific medical morbidities from passive smoking, especially if adolescent is a parent Expense	If not started, encouragement not to start If started, discontinuation
Drug or alcohol use/abuse	Family history of use of specific substances If using, possibility of depression (decreased school grades and concentration difficulties, early morning awakening, uncontrolled anger, crying, and use of drugs as self-medication) Marijuana and cocaine—illegal drugs and legal consequences Medical and psychosocial morbidities Driving vehicles while using substances	If not started, encouragement not to start Discussion of moderate use of alcohol Discussion of drug use and impairment of function—school, work, driving If started, discontinuance individually or through participation in Alcoholics Anonymous or specific drug program Avoidance of driving while under influence of drugs
Serious accidents/injuries	Risk behaviors (driving too fast, use of motorcycles, other dangerous vehicles; use of cigarettes, drugs, alcohol) Possibility of depression Impulsiveness, hyperactivity Number of accidents and exact circumstances of accident Use of seat belts and helmets when driving or riding motorcycles	Discussion of thinking out consequences of behavior before engaging in it Discussion of peer pressure and means of handling other than joining the crowd Discussion of specific intervention if depressed
Violence/homicide	Experience with violence: setting and circumstance Friends injured or killed through violence Carrying guns, knives, other potentially harmful instruments Peer pressures	Protection of adolescent and others by avoiding settings where violent behaviors occur (arguments, gang fights, drug trafficking) and circumstances in which violent behaviors are likely
Suicide	Exact nature of thoughts (general versus specific plan) History of gesture or attempt, or both Family history of depression or suicidal behavior Depression Family knowledge of distress	Discussion with provider, knowing adolescent is distressed Further evaluation, depending on immediacy and risk to adolescent Discussion with family Decision about hospitalization versus ambulatory care

Adapted from Marks A: Well adolescent care. *In* McAnarney ER, Kriepe RE, Orr DP, Comerci GD (eds): Textbook of Adolescent Medicine. Philadelphia, WB Saunders Company, 1992, p 204, with permission.

physician who offers information in a nonjudgmental way. Developmentally, it is difficult for an adolescent to ask the physician to discuss the risks of sexual activity or drug use, but most adolescents want to hear this information from an expert. Recommendations for specific areas of review are provided in Table 29–13.

Morbidity and Mortality in Adolescence

Adolescence was the only age group in the United States that showed an increase in mortality from 1960 through 1981, a period of decreasing mortality for all other age groups. Approximately 75 per cent of the deaths in this group are due to accidents, homicide, and suicide. Accidents alone account for 60 per cent of the mortality during adolescence (Brown, 1979).

Data regarding morbidity during adolescence are harder to come by. The most common reason that adolescents seek medical care is for a comprehensive physical exam, generally for school or camp. Data from the National Center for Health Statistics (1978) suggest that adolescents have many of the same problems as preadolescent patients. However, data from an office specifically directed to adolescent health care show that teenagers have several problems that are unique to their age group (Neinstein, 1984) (see Table 29–14). Some of the specific diagnoses are discussed in the following sections.

Accidents

Accidents account for more than half of the mortality during adolescence. Motor vehicle accidents alone account for 37 per cent of teenage deaths (Brown, 1979). In addition, nonfatal injuries account for the largest number of hospital days among teenagers (National Center for Health Statistics, 1983). National data show that accidents

TABLE 29–14. SPECIFIC PROBLEMS IDENTIFIED DURING VISITS TO A TEEN HEALTH CENTER

Problem Type	Incidence (%)
Gynecologic	18
Dermatologic	15
Adolescent adjustment reaction	14
Headache	10
Obesity	8
Endocrine	7
Gastrointestinal	6
Orthopedic	6
Asthma	4
Seizure disorder	4

Adapted from Neinstein LS: Adolescent Health Care: A Practical Guide. Baltimore, Urban & Schwartzenberg, 1984, with permission.

and poisonings account for about 15 per cent of ambulatory visits to physicians in adolescence.

There is evidence that the frequency of accidents in adolescents may be related to developmental issues (Brown, 1979). Mortality data regarding motor vehicle accidents cite excessive speed as a factor in more than half of accidents among adolescents compared to only 30 per cent of accidents among adults. Alcohol is also a more frequent contributing factor in motor vehicle fatalities among young drivers than it is in other age groups. Risk taking in adolescents serves to fulfill developmental needs related to autonomy and to mastery of new activities. Mastering a skill or activity requires experimentation and often involves testing limits and taking risks. Most teenagers do not have the cognitive ability and life experiences to understand the degree of risk associated with these behaviors. Experts have suggested that interventional strategies should include: (1) providing alternatives to the risk-taking behaviors that are safer and still fulfill the developmental needs, and (2) insulating adolescents from the most negative consequences of risk-taking behaviors (Irwin and Millstein, 1986). An example of this would be to encourage the family of the young driver who is exposed to drinking at high school parties to sign a contract that will guarantee the young person a ride home from a party by an adult if the adolescent has been drinking.

Issues Related to Sexual Activity

Sexual activity among adolescents is common and is occurring at earlier ages than ever before. Nearly 60 per cent of females and 70 per cent of males report having had intercourse by the age of 18 (O'Reilly and Aral, 1985). Between 20 and 30 per cent of 15-year-olds are sexually active. Approximately one fifth of all sexually active females become pregnant each year, and half of these pregnancies occur within the first 6 months of sexual activity. Contraception is used consistently by only a small minority of teenagers. A combination of developmental factors, including misinformation, poor ability to plan for future events, inability to communicate with a partner, and risk-taking behavior, as well as ambivalence in the female about the outcome of pregnancy, conspire against effective contraceptive use.

Provision of Contraception

A thorough developmental assessment is necessary before providing contraception to an adolescent. A discussion of the developmental advantages and disadvantages of some of the contraceptive methods used by adolescents follows (Gruber and Chambers, 1987).

Barrier methods pose no significant medical risk to adolescents and provide protection against acquisition of sexually transmitted diseases, as well as preventing pregnancy. *Condoms,* which do not require a prescription, can be kept readily available by adolescents, who as a rule have intercourse infrequently and sporadically. Additionally, condom use is the only method that allows the male to take primary responsibility for contraception (although sexually active females also should be encouraged to carry condoms). Unfortunately, this method requires consistency of use, and only a small percentage of the males who ever use condoms report consistent use. Furthermore, a stated reliance on condoms may discourage use of more effective methods in some adolescents. The *diaphragm* has perhaps the lowest likelihood of continued use in adolescents for whom it is prescribed. Effective use of the diaphragm requires the female adolescent to have comfort both with touching the genital area during insertion and with communicating with her partner before sexual activity. Clinical experience has shown that this method should be recommended only for relatively sophisticated, mature adolescents in stable relationships who have demonstrated good communication skills.

When the *intrauterine device* (IUD) was first on the market, it seemed like an excellent contraceptive method for adolescents because compliance was not an issue and no communication with the partner was necessary. However, there is an unacceptably high incidence of pelvic inflammatory disease and its sequelae of infertility and ectopic pregnancy related to use of this method, and the IUD cannot be recommended for teenagers.

Oral contraceptives containing 30 to 35 µg of estrogen are the contraceptive method of choice for the sexually active adolescent female. They can be recommended safely for most patients, with only the usual absolute contraindications restricting their use. Several practical issues are important for the physician who provides oral contraceptives to adolescents. Teenage females who by developmental assessment do not have good planning skills will need more frequent follow-up than adult patients for whom oral contraceptives are provided. All adolescents should be given more thorough counseling regarding the possibility of minor side effects such as intramenstrual bleeding or nausea, which may lead to the teenager stopping the pills. Similarly, the patient should be reassured that physiologic changes, including small elevations in blood pressure or rashes, are readily reversible. It is generally a good idea to allow the teenager to discuss any concerns that she has about taking the pill and to address each of the concerns carefully. Many offices benefit by having a nurse or other person designated to handle troubleshooting regarding oral contraceptive use by teenagers.

Two *long-acting hormonal methods* of contraception have become available recently. One of these, marketed as Norplant, requires the insertion under local anesthesia of six small, levonorgestrol-releasing implants, usually in the upper arm. Effective contraception is provided for 5 years. The other, injectable medroxyprogesterone acetate (Depo-Provera), is given intramuscularly in a dose of 150 mg every 3 months. Both of these methods list irregular menstrual bleeding as the most common side effect. No protection against sexually transmitted diseases is provided by either agent, and concomitant use of condoms should be recommended routinely. Although these two long-acting methods of contraception appear to have few medical contraindications, the risks and benefits of prescribing either must be considered carefully from a developmental perspective for each adolescent.

Sexually Transmitted Diseases

Sexually transmitted diseases (STDs) are a common problem among adolescents (Rosenfeld, 1991). About one fifth of all cases of gonorrhea reported in the United States occur in teenagers. Chlamydia, which is not a reportable infection but which causes many of the same clinical syndromes as gonorrhea, is recognized as the most common STD in this age group. The importance of infections caused by the human papillomavirus (HPV) is unclear, but the number of teenagers infected with this agent appears to be increasing. Finally, although acquired immunodeficiency syndrome (AIDS) is uncommon among adolescents, the level of sexual activity in this group and the increasing incidence of other STDs suggest that individuals who develop AIDS in their third decade may have become infected during their teenage years.

There are many factors that may put teenagers at increased risk for acquiring STDs. Like other processes of adolescence, development of sexuality may be marked by experimentation and risk taking. Contraception (and, relevant to STD transmission, barrier methods) is used infrequently. There may be multiple partners. There are biologic factors for this increased risk as well. Both chlamydia and gonorrhea have a predilection for the columnar epithelium on the immature cervix of an adolescent female. Moreover, adolescents have an unchallenged immune system that offers no local protection against STD agents.

Cervicitis in adolescent females is diagnosed by the finding of a mucopurulent cervical discharge and cervical friability. Cultures are positive for chlamydia or gonorrhea in more than 50 per cent of cases; *herpes simplex* is found less commonly. *Chlamydia trachomatis* has a reported prevalence of 8 to 33 per cent among sexually active adolescents, and may be present without obvious clinical signs of cervicitis. Recent decision analysis studies recommend screening all sexually active females for chlamydia if the prevalence of infection is greater than 7 per cent (Phillips et al., 1987).

The major concern regarding unrecognized and

untreated cervical infections is related to the development of upper genital tract infection or pelvic inflammatory disease (PID). There is a 10 to 30 per cent chance of an ascending infection in females with cervical gonorrhea or chlamydia (McGregor, 1985). One fifth of all cases of PID occur in adolescents (Washington et al., 1985). It is estimated that one out of eight sexually active 15-year-olds develops PID yearly. Given the recognized sequelae of PID, including infertility, ectopic pregnancy, and chronic pelvic pain, sexually active adolescent females should be evaluated thoroughly for STDs and treated aggressively with careful follow-up.

Human papillomavirus has been linked with cervical dysplasia. Until recently, HPV infection has been diagnosed by the finding of condylomata acuminata or indirectly on Pap smear. Recent studies have isolated HPV from up to 33 per cent of sexually active adolescents (Rosenfeld et al., 1988). Only a small percentage of these patients had abnormal Pap smears or genital warts. The current management of females with signs of HPV infection includes colposcopy. Pap smears may be indicated more frequently in sexually active adolescents than in adult women.

Male adolescents may present for evaluation of symptoms of urethritis. Nongonococcal (generally chlamydial) urethritis is diagnosed when the Gram's stain of the urethral discharge, if present, shows no intracellular diplococci. Physicians may have some success in recommending the use of condoms for the egocentric male adolescent who has experienced an STD.

HIV/AIDS

Only about 1 per cent of the total cases of AIDS have been diagnosed in adolescents. Nonetheless, HIV transmission may be the highest priority health concern for this age group. The current estimate for the mean latency between exposure to HIV and the clinical diagnosis of AIDS is more than 10 years. Therefore it is safe to assume that many of the people who develop AIDS in their 20s, the second most common decade of life for this diagnosis to be made, contracted the virus during their teenage years.

The modes of transmission for HIV are well known. However, for developmental reasons, adolescents who engage in risk-taking behaviors may not be capable of understanding the potential long-term consequences of their behaviors. National data indicate that, when compared with adults, there are a greater proportion of females (14 versus 7 per cent), minorities (53 versus 38 per cent), and heterosexually acquired cases (47 versus 22 per cent) among adolescents with AIDS. Heterosexual contact was the most frequently cited risk factor among females, accounting for 50 per cent of the cases (Kepke and Hein, 1992).

Prevention and risk reduction remain the mainstays of any program designed to limit the transmission of HIV. All adolescents should receive a risk assessment and those identified as high risk should be targeted for special efforts in risk reduction. General information regarding HIV infection, transmission, and prevention should be provided to all teens.

Acne

Acne, which affects up to 85 per cent of all teenagers, is one of the most common medical problems for this age group. Although acne poses no serious medical risk, the psychological effects of inflammatory lesions can be devastating. Lesions of acne may be as mild as an occasional papule or pustule or as severe as inflammatory, nodulocystic lesions. Areas commonly involved include the face, back, and upper chest.

The etiology of acne is well understood. Androgenic hormones stimulate a proliferation of sebaceous glands. These glands are colonized by skin bacteria, including *Propionibacterium acnes*, which release lipases among other substances. These enzymes act on the sebum to release free fatty acids, which cause inflammation in the dermis and act with other substances to produce abnormal keratinization of the glandular ducts.

Treatment of acne is directed by an understanding of the pathogenesis of this disease. Noninflammatory comedones can be treated with a topical keratolytic agent such as benzoyl peroxide or retinoic acid. When inflammatory lesions are present, antibiotics also are indicated. Most physicians treat acne with a topical antibiotic such as tetracycline, erythromycin, or clindamycin and reserve systemic antibiotics for unresponsive cases. Severe cystic acne, which has the potential for long-term scarring, may require isotretinoin. Substantiated concerns regarding this drug's teratogenicity mitigate against its use in adolescent females. Regular monitoring of laboratory parameters, including liver and lipid profiles, is required when this drug is prescribed. This dangerous drug should be considered only in severe, refractory cases for which careful follow-up is assured.

Special Orthopedic Problems

Scoliosis

Scoliosis, a side-to-side curvature of the spine, is found in 5 to 10 per cent of adolescents. It usually is noted on examination of the back by the finding of asymmetry of the hips, scapulae, or shoulders. Having the patient bend forward at the waist usually accentuates the asymmetry.

Scoliosis may be a result of an underlying problem; however, up to 70 per cent of cases are idiopathic. This is particularly true in girls. Occasionally, the curvature in the spine is compensatory for a leg length discrepancy. This may be detected by differences in the height of the iliac crests. Congenital abnormalities of the spine, including occult spina bifida or hemivertebrae, are responsible for less than 10 per cent of cases. Neuromuscular abnormalities and other problems account for a very small percentage of cases.

The management of scoliosis depends on the degree of curve noted, as well as the sexual maturity rating of the adolescent. Teenagers in early Tanner stages may require close follow-up because scoliosis tends to progress during the growth spurt. Radiographs have been overused in the past and generally are not indicated when the physician is secure with the assessment. Similarly, exercises are of no proven benefit to halt the progression of scoliosis, although lower back exercises may strengthen muscles that easily fatigue. Radiographs are required when more aggressive interventions are being considered. The Cobb angle is determined by the intersecting lines extrapolated from the articular surfaces of the vertebral bodies that define the ends of the scoliotic curve. Adolescents with curvatures of more than 15 degrees who are entering a period of rapid growth probably warrant orthopedic evaluation. Braces often are prescribed for patients with scoliosis of greater than 20 degrees, but surgery usually is reserved for more severe cases.

Osgood-Schlatter Disease

Osgood-Schlatter disease is a painful swelling of the tibial tubercle at the insertion of the infrapatellar tendon. It is a common problem, particularly in males in the early pubertal stages. Traction stress from the patellar tendon may lead to avulsion of small fragments of cartilage or of the ossification center.

This entity tends to occur in active adolescent males around Tanner stage 2 or 3. The pain is aggravated by activity and relieved by rest. On physical exam, there is soft tissue swelling and tenderness over the tibial tubercle. Radiographs are not essential for the diagnosis and are used only to eliminate the possibility of other disease in atypical cases.

Treatment recommendations are made easily, but implementation is often difficult. Restriction of running and jumping activities is usually sufficient to allow improvement. However, most adolescent males are unwilling to completely stop their sports participation and a compromise must be met. Swimming and other sports that do not stress the area involved may be substituted. Ice applied to the area before and after activity and mild anti-inflammatory drugs, such as aspirin, may provide some additional relief. If symptoms are severe or fail to respond to restriction of activity, rare cases may require immobilization.

Substance Use and Abuse

Nationally obtained data substantiate high rates of substance use among both younger and older adolescents (Irwin and Millstein, 1986). In one study, the incidence of cigarette smoking among 12- to 13-year-olds, 14- to 15-year-olds, and 16- to 17-year-olds was 3, 10, and 30 per cent, respectively. The incidence of alcohol use in these same three age groups was 10, 23, and 45 per cent, and that of marijuana use was 2, 8, and 23 per cent. Other cross-sectional studies have confirmed these trends. In a survey of high school seniors in 1984, 93 per cent of the sample reported using alcohol (72 per cent within the past month) and 65 per cent reported using illicit drugs (Johnston et al., 1984).

Certain patterns regarding substance use occur in adolescence. Although many teenagers do not experiment with all of these substances, the use of alcohol or cigarettes is predictive of experimentation with marijuana or other drugs. Another interesting observation from these data is that the period around the seventh and eighth grades appears to be a critical time regarding an adolescent's experimentation with or use of these potentially harmful substances. Physicians taking care of adolescents may be able to identify the teenager at risk for these behaviors and provide counseling and support. The family is often a source of some conflict and must be involved in any ongoing counseling (Muramoto and Leshan, 1993). Adolescents who regularly use illegal substances probably should be referred to a professional trained in adolescent substance abuse. Inpatient treatment is usually necessary when the patient continues to use drugs despite appropriate interventions or exhibits abusive or dangerous behavior.

Psychiatric Disease

Depression/Suicide

Suicide is the third leading cause of death in adolescents (Greydanus, 1986). The number of attempted suicides far exceeds the number of completed suicides, with the ratio reported at between 50:1 and 120:1. Many deaths attributed to accidents also may be completed suicides. In general, female adolescents are more likely to make a suicidal gesture and male adolescents are more likely to complete a suicide attempt. Suicide attempts in adolescents generally occur in the setting of chronic stresses, such as results from a broken family, a learning disability, or the diagnosis of a chronic disease. The acute precipitating event may be the breakup of a relationship or the concern about a pregnancy.

A depressed adolescent may present differently than the typical adult. Whereas the older adolescent may have the classic vegetative signs of depression and report low self-esteem, depression in the younger adolescent may be marked by acting out behavior, excessive anger, a fall off in school performance, or new drug use. For developmental reasons, young adolescents are unable to articulate their troubles.

The physician should evaluate a depressed teenager carefully for the possibility of suicide. Direct questions about suicidal thoughts are appropriate. Similarly, any teenager who has made a suicide attempt or gesture should be handled seriously. Often it is best to hospitalize such a teenager for 24 to 48 hours to "cool off" a volatile situation and to plan an appropriate evaluation and management.

Eating Disorders

Criteria for the diagnosis of anorexia nervosa include a weight loss of more than 15 per cent of original body weight, a disturbance of the body image, onset of the disease at less than 25 years of age, and no other illness that could account for the weight loss. Other commonly associated findings are amenorrhea, a ritualistic exercise history, and excessive preoccupation with food. This illness is far more common in females and occasionally coexists with bulimia. Bulimia is characterized by episodic binge eating followed by self-induced vomiting, use of laxatives, and often abdominal pain.

Patients with eating disorders first present to their family doctor. Although treatment of these illnesses is complicated, a thorough medical evaluation is the appropriate first step. Thereafter, the family physician may seek involvement of a psychiatrist or psychologist with expertise in treatment of eating disorders. Often, the treatment plan is three-pronged and includes medical follow-up and individual as well as family counseling. Anorexia is a serious, potentially fatal diagnosis that requires long-term management.

REFERENCES

Alpert JJ, Guyer B (eds): Injuries and injury prevention. Pediatr Clin North Am 32:5, 1985.

American Heart Association: Dietary Treatment of Hypercholesterolemia: A Manual for Patients. Dallas, American Heart Association, 1988.

Berwick DM: Non-organic failure to thrive. Pediatr Rev 1:265, 1980.

Birch LL, Johnson SL, Andresen G, et al: The variability of young children's energy intake. N Engl J Med 324:232, 1991.

Brown SS: The health needs of adolescents in the U.S. *In* Healthy People: The Surgeon General's Report on Health Promotion and Disease Prevention, Background Papers (Publication no. [PHS] 79-55071A). Washington, DC, U.S. Department of Health, Education and Welfare, 1979, pp 333–364.

Cantekin EI, Mandel EM, Bluestone CD, et al: Lack of efficacy of a decongestant-antihistamine combination for otitis media with effusion ("secretory" otitis media) in children. N Engl J Med 308:297, 1983.

Centers for Disease Control: Preventing Lead Poisoning in Young Children. Atlanta, GA, U.S. Department of Health and Human Services, 1991.

Child Daycare Infectious Disease Study Group, Centers for Disease Control: Special Article: Public health considerations of infectious diseases in child daycare centers. J Pediatr 105:683, 1984.

Committee on Environmental Health: Lead poisoning: From screening to primary prevention. Pediatrics 92:176, 1993.

Denny FW, Clyde WA: Acute lower respiratory tract infections in nonhospitalized children. J Pediatr 108:635, 1986.

Gergen PJ, Mullaly D, Evans R: National survey of prevalence of asthma among children in the United States, 1976 to 1980. Pediatrics 81:1, 1988.

Green SM, Rothrock SG. Single-dose intramuscular ceftriaxone for acute otitis media in children. Pediatrics 91:23, 1993.

Greydanus DE: Depression in adolescence. J Adolesc Health Care 7:109S, 1986.

Gruber E, Chambers CV: Cognitive development and adolescent contraception: Integrating theory and practice. Adolescence XXII:661, 1987.

Guidelines for the Diagnosis and Management of Asthma. (Publication no. 91-3042). Washington, DC, US Department of Health and Human Services, 1991.

Herold ES, Goodwin MS: Why adolescents go to birth-control clinics rather than to their family physicians. Can J Pub Health 70:317, 1979.

Hofmann AD: A rational policy toward consent and confidentiality in adolescent health care. J Adolesc Health Care 1:9, 1980.

Irwin CE: Why adolescent medicine? J Adolesc Health Care 7:2S, 1986.

Irwin CE, Millstein SG: Biopsychosocial correlates of risk-taking behaviors during adolescence. J Adolesc Health Care 7:82S, 1986.

Issacs D, Day D, Crook S: Childhood gastroenteritis: A population study. BMJ 293:545, 1986.

Johnston LD, Bachman JG, O'Malley PM: Use of licit and illicit drugs by America's high school students, 1975–84 (Publication no. 85-1394). Rockville, MD, National Institute of Drug Abuse, 1984.

Kemper KJ, Avner ED: The case against screening urinalyses for asymptomatic bacteriuria in children. Am J Dis Child 146:343, 1992.

Kipke MD, Hein K: Acquired immunodeficiency syndrome and human immunodeficiency virus-related syndromes. *In* McAnarney ER, Kreipe RE, Orr DP, Comerci GD (eds): Textbook of Adolescent Medicine. Philadelphia, WB Saunders Company, 1992, pp 711–719.

Kunin CM, Zacha E, Paquin AJ: Urinary tract infections in schoolchildren. N Engl J Med 266:1287, 1962.

Levenson PM, Morrow JR, Pfefferbaum BJ: Attitudes toward health and illness: A comparison of adolescent, physician, teacher, and school nurse views. J Adolesc Health Care 5:254, 1984.

McGregor JA: Adolescent misadventures with urethritis and cervicitis. J Adolesc Health Care 6:286, 1985.

Morrissey JM, Hofmann AD, Thrope JC: Consent and Confidentiality in the Health Care of Children and Adolescents. New York, Free Press, 1986.

Muramoto ML, Leshan L: Adolescent substance abuse: Recognition and early intervention. Primary Care 20:141, 1993.

National Center for Health Statistics: Utilization of short-stay hospitals by adolescents, United States, 1980: Advance Data Vital Health Stat no. 93:1, 1983.

National Center for Health Statistics (Ezzau TM): Ambulatory Care Utilization Patterns of Children and Young Adults. The National Ambulatory Medical Care Survey, United States,

January–December 1975. Vital Health Stat [13], no. 39, 1978.

Neinstein LS: Adolescent Health Care: A Practical Guide. Baltimore, Urban & Schwartzenberg, 1984.

North AF: Screening in child health care: Where are we now and where are we going? Pediatrics 5:631, 1974.

O'Reilly KR, Aral SO: Adolescence and sexual behavior. J Adolesc Health Care 6:262, 1985.

Paradise JL: Otitis media in infants and children. Pediatrics 65: 917, 1980.

Parcel GS, Nader PR, Meyer MP: Adolescent health concerns, problems and patterns of utilization in a triethnic urban population. Pediatrics 60:157, 1977.

Phillips RS, Aronson MD, Taylor WC, et al: Should tests for *Chlamydia trachomatis* cervical infection be done during routine gynecologic visits? Ann Intern Med 107:188, 1987.

Poole SR, Morrison JD, Marshall J, et al: Pediatric health care in family practice. J Fam Pract 15:945, 1982.

Rosenfeld WD: Sexually transmitted diseases in adolescents. Pediatr Ann 20:303, 1991.

Rosenfeld WD, Vermund SH, Wentz SJ, et al: Positive association of human papillomavirus with adolescent pregnancy. Paper presented at the Society for Adolescent Medicine 15th Annual Research Meeting, New York City, March 24–27, 1988.

Shear CL, Burke GL, Freedman DS, et al: Value of childhood blood pressure measurements and family history in predicting future blood pressure status: Results from 8 years of follow-up in the Bogalusa Heart Study. Pediatrics 77:6, 1986.

Slap GB: Normal physiological and psychosocial growth in the adolescent. J Adolesc Health Care 7:13S, 1986.

Starfield B, Hoekelman RA, McCormick M, et al: Who provides health care to children and adolescents in the United States? Pediatrics 74:991, 1983.

Stockman JA: Iron deficiency anemia: Have we come far enough? [Editorial] JAMA 258:1645, 1987.

Strain JE: AAP Periodicity Guidelines: A framework for educating patients. Pediatrics 74:924, 1984.

Strategic Plan to Eliminate Childhood Lead Poisoning. Washington, DC, U.S. Department of Health and Human Services, 1992.

Task Force on Blood Pressure Control in Children, National Heart, Lung and Blood Institute: Report of the Second Task Force on Blood Pressure Control in Children—1987. Pediatrics 79:1, 1987.

Wald ER, Dashefsky B, Byers C, et al: Frequency and severity of infections in day care. J Pediatr 112:540, 1988.

Washington AE, Sweet RL, Shafer MB: Pelvic inflammatory disease and its sequelae in adolescents. J Adolesc Health Care 6:298, 1985.

Yip R, Binkin NJ, Fleshood L, et al: Declining prevalence of anemia among low-income children in the United States. JAMA 258:1619, 1987.

CHAPTER 30

BEHAVIORAL PROBLEMS IN CHILDREN AND ADOLESCENTS

ALICE ANNE O'DONELL and DOROTHY B. TREVINO

The behavioral and emotional problems of children and adolescents constitute a significant proportion of any family practice. Disorders of this nature are influenced by a wide range of both biologic and environmental factors. All behavior both is influenced by and influences the various contexts in which it occurs, including biology, parent and family interaction patterns, cultural beliefs and norms, and school and community activities. The purpose of this chapter is to present a biopsychosocial approach and philosophy for diagnosis and management. Only the most commonly seen disorders will be addressed here. These will be organized around child and family developmental stages. An emphasis on prevention will be presented for each disorder because this is the economical and parsimonious approach to care. Attention will be given to the individual diagnostic characteristics as well as the family and environmental patterns that influence these. Management will focus on early, brief interventions the physician can make with the patient and family as well as suggestions about referral.

The management of behavioral and emotional problems is most effective when one adopts a health rather than illness philosophy. Not only should emphasis be placed on dysfunctional behaviors and problems present in a patient and his or her environment, but the strengths and abilities of each also should be identified, underscored for the patient, and utilized in management. It is helpful to approach children and parents with the attitude and belief that, regardless of the severity of the problems, each patient is doing the best he or she can given the particular circumstances, experiences, insight, and knowledge (Budman and Gurman, 1988). Such an attitude lends an air of optimism and acceptance that will encourage patient participation as well as reduce negative feelings on the part of the physician. Beginning both the assessment and the management of behavioral problems with an emphasis on strengths rather than deficits further improves the probability of patient compliance.

DISORDERS OCCURRING DURING INFANCY

Individual Developmental Task

The primary developmental task of infancy is the establishment of trust versus mistrust within a context influenced by socioeconomic issues, parenting skills and stressors, and cultural supports and beliefs.

Attachment Difficulties

The attachment theory and research of Bowlby (1982, 1988) and Ainsworth et al. (1978) provide an excellent guideline for assessing very early difficulties and intervening to prevent later ones. This theory, based on animal and cross-cultural early childhood developmental research, describes the biologic function served when infants develop an emotional attachment to caregivers. Infants exhibit attachment behavior (i.e., looking at parent, smiling, clinging, moving body in parent's direction, crying, reaching toward parent, seeking physical proximity, etc.). Sensitive parents and caregivers respond to each of these by giving physical and emotional comfort, food, attention, and security. Four patterns of emotional attachment have been identified in infants and found to be related to later healthy or dysfunctional emotional development (Ainsworth and Eichberg, 1991; Stern, 1985).

The majority of infants, by age 1, can be seen to have what is called a *secure attachment*. In the physician's office, this pattern of attachment might reveal itself when the infant is picked up by a nurse or moved out of the mother's view, or during a procedure that frightens or upsets. In such situations, the secure infant will cry, the mother quickly will respond in a reassuring, soothing way, and the infant quickly will be comforted and quieted by this. This pattern results from fairly consistent, appropriate and immediate response by the parent (or caregiver) to the infant's attachment signals. These secure infants are best prepared for subsequent developmental stages. They have attained the development task of being able to trust those in their environment to get their needs met. Cross-generational data associates this secure attachment interaction pattern with later social competence (Grossmann et al., 1988, Main et al., 1985; Stroufe and Fleeson, 1988).

A minority of infants will reveal an *avoidant pattern* of attachment. In normally distressing situations such as being separated from parents, being in unfamiliar surroundings, or experiencing uncomfortable procedures in the doctor's office, these infants express little or no distress and actually may avoid contact with the parent when he or she reappears. These parents have been found to be actively and repetitively rejecting of the infant's attachment behaviors at home. The parent does not respond consistently to cries, searching eyes, and reaching up, and may even respond with yelling or hitting when the baby cries in protest. The infants may give up and become withdrawn and listless. This detached behavior is believed to be related to early and later childhood depression and inorganic failure to thrive. In the extreme forms of abuse and neglect, avoidant attachment is related directly to depression.

A third pattern of attachment is described as *anxious–resistant*. These infants react with great distress when separated from the parent but are not quickly relieved when the parent returns or attempts to care for them. At home, these caregivers have been found to be very unpredictable in their availability and response to the baby's signals for comfort or care. They also are very intrusive when the baby is exploring its environment. This interactional pattern, if continued, later may be related to oppositional defiant disorders of childhood as well as other disorders.

A fourth type of attachment pattern recently has been identified by Main and Soloman (1986, 1990). The *disoriented–disorganized* pattern is characterized by infant behavior such as staring blankly at an approaching parent, moving toward a parent and suddenly stopping, and looking away blankly with a glazed appearance. These behaviors occur in the absence of any neurologic deficits. They are very brief and may be difficult to notice if one is not looking for them. Parents of these babies have been found to be very preoccupied with losses or past traumas in their own lives. This preoccupation is to such a degree that they are unable to give appropriate and sufficient attention to the child. The parent frequently displays frightened or frightening behavior around the infant. Researchers in child development have begun to link this form of parent–child relating to the development of dissociative disorders (Liotti et al., 1991). Indeed, the blank stares are believed to be brief dissociations (Main and Hesse, 1992). In general, authoritarian and stressful parental environments tend to be associated with aggressive or unstable children (Macoby and Martin, 1983). A reinforcing dynamic between problem behavior in children and unstable ties in the family was found across four generations in a study by Caspi and Elder (1988).

Management

The best opportunity for assessment, early detection, and intervention for possible problems in the infant–parent relationship occurs during prenatal and well-baby visits. Many pediatricians and family physicians now urge both parents to attend some or all of these visits (McDaniel et al., 1990). In a very short time, the physician can detect both the strengths and difficulties of the parents and their environment that may relate directly to future infant, child, and adolescent behavior. Small interventions during this early period may very well avoid or significantly reduce the magnitude of later problems. Before the baby is born, information already should be gathered about significant supports and strengths as well as stressors in such areas as finances, work, marital and family relationships, and cultural values and beliefs. This is an important time to look for abuse or violence in either parents' history because this may (but not necessarily) predispose them to the use of aggressive or abusive parenting styles. As noted earlier, such traumas, if unresolved, also may leave the parent emotionally unavailable to attend appropriately to the baby's needs and signals.

Well-baby visits are the time to be observant of small signs of attachment pattern problems. If a baby exhibits any of the danger behaviors described previously, it is important to begin immediately to look for conditions that may make it difficult to give fairly consistent attention to the baby's needs. Fortunately, studies show that the consequences of adverse early experiences can be ameliorated greatly by later supportive, attentive relationships (Grossman et al., 1988; Main et al., 1985; Rutter, 1988). Intervention may require referral for social services or referral of parents for marital therapy or individual counseling, especially where histories of abuse or violence are uncovered.

When attachment problem behavior is observed by the physician, the following management is suggested as a model for the initial approach to all behavioral problems:

1. Enumerate the various strengths identified, especially those exhibited in the face of stress and adversity.
2. Note nonjudgmentally the behavior of the baby that is of concern. Briefly educate the parent about the behavior most infants would display in that situation.
3. Inquire about feeding, crying, and sleeping behaviors, being careful to listen to the parents' feelings and frustrations. Ask for descriptions of

good times and times when the parents feel it is difficult.

4. Let the parents know they need support and nurturance themselves if they are to be sensitive and consistent with their children. Give a homework assignment requesting the parent to observe what is going on in themselves, their thoughts and feelings, and what is happening in the rest of the family or environment during the infant's problem behavior.

5. Enumerate the specific cues babies give for help and acknowledge that some of these may be irritating. Ask the parent to use their strengths to allow them to be more responsive to the baby's cues for a set number of days or weeks and then return for a follow-up.

These principals and steps are reflected in the following case example.

Dr. Ramirez saw 27-year-old Sarah J. and her 10-month-old infant for a well-baby visit. Dr. Ramirez has been Ms. J's physician for 3 years and knows she is an anxious, single parent who must work full time to make ends meet. He also knows that on occassion she abuses alcohol to relieve her own loneliness and stress. During prenatal visits, he consistently complimented her for diligently keeping appointments, eating well, and abstaining from alcohol during the pregnancy. He referred her to a support group as a better way to deal with her social isolation. In a well-baby visit, he noticed that the infant seemed to cry excessively on examination and did not easily quiet when the mother attempted to comfort her. (He had to invite the mother to reach out to her infant, Annie). As he continued his exam, he told Mrs. J. "You've really been doing a good job keeping Annie physically healthy. I'm impressed given your schedule and the stress in your life. By the way, what are you doing to take care of yourself these days?" After encouraging her to see friends and seek support, he continued with preventive work. "I noticed when Annie was crying, she had a hard time calming down even after you went to her. Do you notice that much?" This was followed with a discussion of the mother's observations, anxieties, and frustrations.

After listening and sympathizing with the stressful situation, Dr. J. initiated a plan. "Let's see if we can give a little attention to this now so it doesn't develop into a problem. You know most infants at this stage can calm down a little faster than Annie. I know you are already really busy and tired, so we want to make this as easy a time for both of you as possible. I am very impressed, given your schedule, with how aware you are of Annie's behavior. (She had listed in detail all of the things that annoyed her about her infant. The physician wisely turned this into a positive). I'd like you to keep that up and, just for the next 2 weeks, when you are at home, become very observant of what is going on when Annie cries and can't be calmed. What are you thinking and feeling? What else was going on in the household or surroundings? Just for these 2 weeks I would like to suggest that, when you are home, you watch Annie even more closely. Whenever you first see her do such things as hold her arms up to you, follow you with her eyes, make noises, or cry, try to respond warmly immediately even if you are feeling irritated or tired. I know this is asking a lot, but it's an experiment for just 2 weeks. Then observe how she does. This parent work is really hard. It's why you need as much help and support as you can get. Let's follow-up on this with a visit in 2 weeks." This physician practiced all of the principals of early detection and positive management.

There also will be times when the situation is so severe that it is clear such treatment will not be enough. When there is enormous stress, abuse, depression, or relationship issues, the same procedure should be followed but a referral for psychotherapy for parent or family should be initiated.

Feeding Problems in Infancy

Problems in feeding vary from parents who are so insensitive to the clues that the infant fails to gain weight adequately to parents are so overbearing and anxious that the infant eats too much. These problems reflect a distortion in the parent–child interaction and can interfere with the child's subsequent psychosocial development.

One of the first skills a new parent learns is the ability to nourish and nurture the infant during the feeding process. Feeding goes well when parents depend primarily on the information coming from the child about timing, amount, preference, pacing, and eating capability (Ainsworth and Bell, 1969). Skillful parents develop a certain amount of flexibility and resourcefulness, such as interpreting the infant's behavior and keeping the infant in an alert, active state while avoiding other interactions that arouse the infant unnecessarily.

Observation by the primary care physician of the caregiver feeding the infant will provide an assessment of attachment. With secure attachment, the mother smiles, looks at and speaks to the infant, and appears to enjoy the interaction. The infant appears to enjoy this interaction by smiling, cuddling, seeking out the nipple, and appearing to be actively engaged in the feeding process.

Feeding concerns expressed by parents during infancy include "Does he have colic?" and "Is she gaining enough weight?" Colicky babies demonstrate more paroxysmal crying than the average baby. Thus they may cry more than 3 hr/day. Colic is more common in first-born infants but appears to be unrelated to gender or feeding method. Colicky babies are observed to be dysthymic infants: Not only do they cry frequently, they often also sleep poorly, fuss or vomit after feeding, release much flatulace, and display a general increased intensity of reaction to all types of stimulus (Salgranati and Dworkin, 1992). Theories of food allergy, difficult temperament, parental anxiety, and neurologic maturation immaturity do not offer an adequate explanation for colic.

A comprehensive history, including drug use, allows the physician to rule out drug withdrawal, developmental disorders, and neuromuscular, or gastrointestinal diseases and to explore feeding, including underfeeding, overfeeding, or maladaptive technique. The physical exam should focus on the determination that the patient is a healthy, vigorous infant with no evidence of congenital abnormalities, child abuse, or intestinal obstruction.

Life events, such as illness in the child or family member or loss of job, can overwhelm the parent's coping responses temporarily. Awareness of illnesses in the family, financial difficulties, and emotional or social problems in the parents (depression, substance abuse, stress-related disorders) should alert the physician that additional support services for the parents may be needed. The goal of intervention is to establish a congenial relationship around feeding that is appropriate for a child's nutritional needs and neuromuscular development (Satter, 1990). Satter reported that training in sensitivity and responsiveness to the child's clues should be the central theme of feeding interventions with parents. Physicians and their staff can assist parents in understanding the child's feeding clues and the individual variations in intake, frequency of feeding, and food selection.

After reassuring the parent of the child's "good health," treatment is focused on assisting the parent to develop specific responses to the crying episodes and a review of feeding techniques that avoid overfeeding and the swallowing of excess air. Some infants appear to be hypersensitive to external stimuli, so efforts should be made to decrease the sensory input by swaddling and limiting the numbers of "handlers" with whom the child may interact. On rare occasions, colic could be secondary to the infant's diet (Lindbergt, 1989). Although the studies have not been validated consistently, many physicians find that a reasonable approach may be to make a formula change for a period of 10 days to 2 weeks. If an improvement has been made, the parent then can return to the original formula after 1 to 2 months.

There is no proven, effective, safe therapy for colic. Simethicone has been found to be of no proven benefit. The anticholinergics, which are intended to relieve smooth muscle spasm, have been associated with drowsiness and apnea in young infants. The physicians' acknowledgment of the frustration and anxiety experienced by the parents and reassurance that they have a healthy infant will assist parents during the 3-month "colic" period.

Sleep

Parental frustration and worry about infant and toddler sleep patterns are very common. An understanding of normal infant sleep patterns can be helpful reassurance. Sleep consists of two states that are distinguished by the presence or absence of rapid eye movements (REMs). Sleep in which these eye movements occur is called REM sleep,

and sleep devoid of eye movements is referred to as non-REM sleep. The non-REM sleep has four stages ranging from drowsiness (stage I) to deep sleep (stage IV). Newborns sleep about 16 hr/day. The newborn goes from alert to REM activity, missing out on non-REM sleep. By 3 months of age, 70 per cent of infants have concentrated their sleep during the night. Sleep studies show infants to awaken intermittently during the night.

The most common sleep problems are seen because of difficulties in settling and remaining asleep. The infant or toddler becomes hyperexcited either by handling, excessive crying, or, in the case of older children, acrimonious arguments. Having a routine bedtime with regular rituals (bath, story telling or reading), showing of affection, and providing a secure environment (such as night light) provides the older child with an opportunity to "wind down" from the day's activities and excitements.

For a comprehensive review of sleep disorders and common problems and their management, including nightmares, night terrors, and sleep walking and talking, the reader is referred to Ferber's book, *Solve Your Child's Sleep Problems* (1985).

DISORDERS IN THE PRESCHOOL AND SCHOOL-AGE CHILD

Individual Developmental Task

During these stages, children are attempting to develop some sense of autonomy rather than doubting themselves, to develop the ability to initiate new activities and not feel excessively guilty, and to develop an eagerness to learn from others, building skills and cooperation. Of course, this occurs in the context of family, culture, schools, and neighborhood.

Adjustment Disorders

A great number of the disturbances in childhood are adjustment reactions to identifiable stressors. Often the parents will identify the stressor but continue to worry about the severe reaction and at this time bring the child to the doctor. Care should be taken to determine whether or not family members are over-reacting to the child, thus setting up the possibility for creating vulnerability. As defined in the DSM-IV (American Psychiatric Association, 1994), to be diagnosed as a disorder, the child's reaction must be seen as being in excess of the normal or expectable reaction to the stressful event. The behavior must cause impairment in school, in relationships, or in usual social functioning. If this is not true, it may be bothersome behavior but is not an adjustment disorder. The reaction to stressors may take many forms, including depressed or anxious mood, a mixture of anxiety and depression, conduct disturbance, and schoolwork problems. In an adjustment reaction to stress, these problem behaviors should abate within 6 months of inception.

The identification of these relatively minor problems early in the child and family development offers an opportunity to intervene in a manner that may be a major mental health promotion venture for the entire family. It is at these early stages that the physician may be able to help the family avoid or alter interaction patterns that reinforce later problems. The approach suggested here not only will help with the adjustment reaction and other behavior problems, but will help any family establish healthy interactions. This can be a preventive measure for all family members.

Management

In addition to the previously discussed step of discussing strengths and education, a homework task may be taught to the family at this time that is based on well-researched communications theory. It is most effective when taught and modeled in the physician's office first. The physician should suggest that the family institute regular family meetings in which they will practice healthy communication patterns that will be helpful throughout life. The meetings should be held as much as possible at the same time each week and for only 30 to 45 minutes to allow for children's attention span. Parents call the meetings, but children may request them if needed. There may be a family issue to discuss or the time may be used simply to check in with each member to hear how their day or week went. Parents are asked to model the communication rules:

1. Everyone gets a chance to talk without interruption and may talk for at least 5 minutes.

2. All others should listen respectfully, as shown through quietly looking at the speaker with an interested expression. Small children should be allowed to listen quietly while moving around a little and playing with a small, quiet toy. Tolerance of younger children's needs and abilities may need to be taught.

3. During discussions, each person is encouraged to label his or her feelings rather than act on them (i.e., to say "I feel angry, hurt, sad, embarrassed, confused," etc. rather than scream, hit, or throw). Tears should be encouraged as acceptable expressions of sadness and hurt rather than withdrawal, depression, or conversion to anger. Adults will be responsible for looking for feelings (e.g., "You are frowning. Do you feel angry?").

4. Some time should always be spent letting each person know how he or she is appreciated or praising him or her for positive actions.

5. When negative feedback is necessary, it should be given by saying, "when you . . . (describe the hurtful behavior, e.g., don't call to tell me you will be late for dinner), I feel . . . (describe the feeling, e.g., hurt, angry, frustrated).

These care communication techniques are useful at all times. No one uses them perfectly and practice is necessary to make them into patterns. Families that work toward these patterns are typically much healthier. This assignment should be described as fun, and family members are encouraged to laugh and catch themselves when they are not perfect.

Encopresis

Encopresis is defined as repeated, involuntary defecation into the clothing. The children are usually more than 4 years of age, and it is more common in boys than girls. Recent studies using manometry and surface electromyography of the external and internal anal sphincters have demonstrated that about 30 to 50 per cent of the children who have difficulty with encopresis have abnormal or prolonged external anal sphincter contraction while straining to defecate (Nolan and Oberklaid, 1993). They proposed the following etiologic factors: anysmus; rectal hypersensitivity; association with oppositional behavior pattern, toilet phobia, or limited attention concentration span; and a high level of motor activity. Nolan and Oberklaid suggested that encopresis is an evacuation release disorder rather than the consequence of constipation. The history should include whether this is primary or secondary; frequency, consistency, and quantity of the soiled stools; the patient's awareness of soiling; and whether spontaneous defecation occurs. The toilet routine and the child's, family's, and school's reaction to the fecal soiling should be explored. The physical exam should rule out a neurologic disorder affecting the lumbosacral spinal cord.

Treatment

Major emphasis should be put on developing a structured toileting program. This can be assisted by using a daily diary. Nolan and Oberklaid (1993) recommended thrice-daily sits on the toilet using predetermined times. The sits should last between 5 and 10 minutes. Laxative use depends on the extent of the fecal retention. Bowel stimulants, such as senna derivatives or bisacodyl, alternating with a lubricant such as mineral oil, may be adequate. For those patients who have substantial fecal impaction, 3-day cycles using enemas plus oral stimulus may be necessary. The duration of the treatment should be until the child has developed either a daily or an every-other-day pattern of self-initiation of defecation in the toilet, as well as the disappearance of fecal soiling. The general management principles proposed in childhood depression also should be followed here.

Attention Deficit Disorder

Parental concerns, clinical observations of a child during an office visit, or observations by other professionals such as teachers, and school nurses alert primary care providers to potential behavioral problems encountered during childhood and adolescence. Of these problems, attention-deficit/hyperactivity disorder (ADHD) is among the most common. The prevalence is estimated at between 3 and 5 per cent in the school-age population. It is six times more frequent in boys than in girls, and may persist into adulthood in 40 to 60 per cent of individuals who were hyperactive as children. Although presently labeled attention-deficit/Hyperactivity disorder, in the past it has been called minimal brain dysfunction, attention deficit disorder, and hyperkinesis. The symptom complex of inattention, impulsivity, and overactivity that is inappropriate for the child's developmental age and interferes with optimal functioning is the hallmark of the clinical syndrome. Table 30–1 outlines the DSM-IV criteria for diagnosis.

Few children present with clear symptoms of ADHD. Most have other problems, including learning disabilities, oppositional defiant behavior, aggressive behavior, mood disorders (particularly depression), anxiety disorders, and, among adolescents and young adults, substance abuse and personality disorders. Numerous psychiatric conditions also can present as attention deficit syndromes (Rostain, 1991).

Information about the parents medical and psychiatric history, including substance abuse, psychosis, depression, anxiety, past developmental or learning disorders, and antisocial behavior, should be explored. Fifteen to 20 per cent of the mothers and 20 to 30 per cent of the fathers of children who have attention deficient disorders also may have had attention deficit disorders themselves. There is, likewise, a very high incidence of alcoholism, (15 to 27 per cent), hysteria affective disorders (10 to 27 per cent), and conduct problems and antisocial behavior (25 to 28 per cent) (Reiff et al., 1993).

The history is the most important tool in diagnosing attention deficit disorders, with an effort being made to identify predisposing factors, associated neurologic and psychotic disorder, early developmental delay, and family strengths and stressors. The physical exam should focus on behavioral observations, abnormal movements, dysmorphic features, abnormal minor physical abnormalities, and disordered or delayed language. A neurologic exam looking for clusters of soft neurologic signs in the area of fine and gross motor movement, motor or focal tics, growth, and stage of sexual development should be done.

A comprehensive history should begin with a detailed description of the parents' concerns and include information regarding the following:

TABLE 30–1. DIAGNOSTIC CRITERIA FOR ATTENTION-DEFICIT/HYPERACTIVITY DISORDER

A. Either (1) or (2):

  (1) Inattention: At least six of the following symptoms of inattention have persisted for at least six months to a degree that is maladaptive and inconsistent with developmental level:

    (a) often fails to give close attention to details or makes careless mistakes in schoolwork, work, or other activities

    (b) often has difficulty sustaining attention in tasks or play activities

    (c) often does not seem to listen to what is being said to him or her

    (d) often does not follow through on instructions and fails to finish schoolwork, chores, or duties in the work place (not due to oppositional behavior or failure to understand instructions)

    (e) often has difficulties organizing tasks and activities

    (f) often avoids or strongly dislikes tasks (such as schoolwork or homework) that require sustained mental effort

    (g) often loses things necessary for tasks or activities (e.g. school assignments, pencils, books, tools, or toys)

    (h) is often easily distracted by extraneous stimuli

    (i) often forgetful in daily activities

  (2) Hyperactivity-impulsivity: At least four of the following symptoms of hyperactivity-impulsivity have persisted for at least six months to a degree that is maladaptive and inconsistent with developmental level:

Hyperactivity

    (a) often fidgets with hands or feet or squirms in seat

    (b) leaves seat in classroom or in other situations in which remaining seated is expected

    (c) often runs about or climbs excessively in situations where it is inappropriate (in adolescents or adults, may be limited to subjective feelings of restlessness)

    (d) often has difficulty playing or engaging in leisure activities quietly

Impulsivity

    (e) often blurts out answers to questions before the question has been completed

    (f) often has difficulty waiting in lines or awaiting turn in games or group situations

B. Onset no later than seven years of age.

C. Symptoms must be present in two or more situations (e.g., at school, work, and at home).

D. The disturbance causes clinically significant stress or impairment in social, academic, or occupational functioning.

E. Does not occur exclusively during the course of a Pervasive Developmental Disorder, Schizophrenia or other Psychotic Disorder, and is not better accounted for by a Mood Disorder, Anxiety Disorder, Dissociative Disorder, or a Personality Disorder.

From American Psychiatric Association: Diagnostic and Statistical Manual of Mental Disorders, 4th edition. Washington, DC, American Psychiatric Press, 1994, with permission.

Pregnancy: general health and prenatal care; infections, alcohol, smoking and drugs; weight gain

Perinatal period: type of delivery, complications, Apgar scores, weight, estimated gestational age, hyperbiliruinemia, problems in the nursery

Developmental milestones

Medical history: trauma, central nervous system infections, seizures, recurrent otitis media, visual disturbances, vaccination reactions, medications, toxic exposures

Speech: delay, articulation, poor comprehension, hearing difficulties

Sleep: history of difficulty falling asleep or waking up, nightmares, night terrors, sleepwalking

Early temperament, personality traits, social abilities, family interactions, discipline

Diet: fads, behavior at meal time, allergies

Drug use and abuse

Social and family history: parents' occupation and education, history of prenatal learning or behavior problems, evidence of ADHD in parents, family history of psychiatric disorders (including substance abuse and antisocial behavior)

School history: type of school, grades, report cards, test performance, teacher reports, classroom behaviors

Miscellaneous: hand preference, drooling, difficulty chewing or swallowing, pica, encopresis, enuresis, tantrums

During the physical exam, the physician should observe the child's ability to cooperate, general mood, spontaneous verbalizations, motor activity, attention span, play, and organization of activities. Height, weight, and head circumference should be determined and growth curves should be completed. Minor congenital anomalies of the limbs and facies (including signs of fetal alcohol syndrome and fragile X syndrome) should be sought. The neurologic examination should include an emphasis on the cranial nerves, especially II (visual acuity, visual fields, fundi); III, IV, and VI (strabismus, nystagmus); and XII (tongue mobility and control). Tone, bulk, and strength of muscles, hand preference, involuntary movements, dysmetria, dysdiadochokinesis, choreiform movements, and balance should be observed. Two-point discrimination, finger naming, and left and right discrimination should be evaluated. Speech, including dysarthria, stuttering, mispronunciation, and aphasia, should be noted. Mental status, including overactivity, distractibility, impulsivity, affect, relatedness, play organization, evidence of autism or thought disorder, fund of information, vocabulary, and general intelligence, should be evaluated.

Rating scales are part of the standard evaluation of children suspected of attention deficit syndrome. They are completed by the parents, the patient, and the teacher. Commonly used scales are the Conners Teacher and Parent Rating Scales, Child Behavior Checklist, ADHD Comprehensive Teacher Rating Scale, and Yale Children's Inventory (Table 30–2).

The psychological evaluation allows the examiner to assess the child's perception of his or her functioning in school, peer relations and family, as well as an assessment of self-worth and feelings about his or her behavior. Not only do these assessments yield information that supports or refutes a diagnosis of attention deficit disorder, but they may identify other disorders such as oppositional defiant disorder, conduct disorder, depression, or anxiety disorders (Reiff et al., 1993).

Many children, by the time they are seen in the

TABLE 30–2. RATING SCALES FOR DIAGNOSIS OF BEHAVIORAL PROBLEMS IN CHILDREN

Scale	Authors	Source
ADHD Comprehensive Teacher Rating Scale	G. J. DuPaul	George G. DuPaul, Ph.D. Department of Psychiatry University of Massachusetts Medical Center 55 Lake Avenue North Worcester, MA 01655
Child Behavior Checklist	T. M. Achenbach and C. S. Edelbrock	Thomas M. Achenbach, Ph.D. Department of Psychiatry University of Vermont Burlington, VT 05401
Conners Teacher Rating Scale; Conners Parent Rating Scale	C. K. Conners	C. Keith Conners, Ph.D. Department of Psychiatry Duke University Medical Center Durham, NC 27710
Yale Children's Inventory	S. Shaywitz, C. Schnell, and B. Shaywitz	Sally Shaywitz, M.D. Yale University School of Medicine Department of Pediatrics 333 Cedar Street New Haven, CT 06510
Children's Depression Inventory	M. Kovacs	Multi-Health Systems, Inc. 908 Niagara Falls Boulevard North Tonawanda, NY 14201-2060
Children's Manifest Anxiety Scale (Revised)	C. R. Reynolds and B. O. Richmond	Western Psychological Services 12031 Wilshire Boulevard Los Angeles, CA 90025-1251

TABLE 30–3.   MEDICATIONS USED IN TREATMENT OF ATTENTION DEFICIT DISORDERS

Drug	Trade Name	How Supplied	Suggested Dosage	Comment
Stimulants				
Methylphenidate	Ritalin	Regular tablets (5, 10, 20 mg) Sustained Release (SR) tablets (20 mg)	0.3–0.6(0.8) mg/kg/dose; titrate dose by 2.5- to 5-mg increments	Take with or shortly before breakfast and lunch. (midafternoon dose if rebound)
Dextroamphetamine	Dexedrine	Regular tablets (5 mg)	0.2–0.4 mg/kg/dose	Alternative if methylphenidate not effective or produces side effects;
		Sustained release ("Spansule") capsules (5, 10, 15 mg)	Start at twice the regular tablet dose (given in AM)	Slightly longer duration of action
Pemoline	Cylert	Regular tablets (18.75, 37.5, 75 mg) Chewable tablets (37.5 mg)	0.5–3.0 mg/kg/day (usually 2.25 mg/kg/day)	Monitor liver functions
Tricyclic Antidepressants				
Imipramine, desipramine, others	Tofranil Norpramin	Tablets (10, 25, 50 mg)	1–4 mg/kg/day (preferably divided b.i.d.; can be given once daily)	Closely monitor cardiac status (EKG)
Clonidine	Catapres	Tablets (0.1, 0.2 mg) Transdermal patch (programmed delivery of 0.1–0.3 mg/day)	4–5 μg/kg/day (usually 0.05 mg q.i.d.)	Do not stop medication abruptly

From Kelly DP, Aylward GP: Attention deficits in school-aged children and adolescents: Current issues and practices. Pediatr Clin North Am 39: 504, 1992, with permission.

primary care physician's office, will already have had some testing performed by the school. The Wechsler scales, including the WISC III, are the most widely administered tests of intellectual ability. Academic achievement tests, such as the Woodcock-Johnson Psychoeducational Battery Test of Achievement, provide the physician with information on intellectual functioning (high or normal IQ or borderline or low IQ) as well as evidence for learning disabilities and speech and language disorders.

It is essential that psychopharmacologic agents are considered as only *one* part of the treatment plan and *only* used after the diagnosis of ADHD has been established firmly. Side effects of the medications must be explained to the child and parents. Close monitoring and periodic reassessment are essential. Trials on and off medication must be observed closely by parents and teachers. Stimulant medications are the most widely used. They have been found to improve the behavioral domains of attention, impulsivity, task, irrelevant activity, aggressiveness, compliance, and noise (Culbert et al., 1994). Methylphenidate, 0.3 to 0.5 mg/kg given at 4-hour intervals two to three times per day, has become the most frequently prescribed medication. Others include dextroamphetamine and pemoline. Successful responses are seen in approximately 70 per cent of the children (Culbert et al., 1994).

Tricyclic antidepressants may be a good choice in children in whom stimulant medication is con-

traindicated or who have comorbid conditions that suggest their use. Imipramine and desipramine are administered in doses of 0.5 to 3 mg/kg/day. An electrocardiogram is recommended before and during treatment because of adverse cardiac effects. Serum blood levels occasionally should be monitored. Clonidine has been found to be effective in treating children and adolescents who have ADHD, Tourette's syndrome, or both. A subset of children who are hyperaroused, aggressive, or both have been found to benefit from clonidine. The dosage is 0.1 to 0.3 mg/day, beginning at 0.05 mg and increasing every 3 days. Blood pressure should be monitored. The associated somnolence of clonidine is usually transient (Culbert et al., 1994). Table 30–3 lists medications and dosages and Figure 30–1 outlines medication management specific to attention deficit disorder presentations.

A home intervention program is essential. Establishment of a daily routine and the use of behavioral management techniques are key to success and long-term outcomes. Acceptable and unacceptable behavior should be defined, consequences for transgressions should be consistent, and implementation should be at the time of occurrence. Predictable routines for waking, eating, play, homework, and sleeping must be established. Behavior therapy techniques that stress positive reinforcement, modeling, and negative consequences for unacceptable behavior are well presented in the books by Goldstein and Goldstein (1990), and Coleman (1993).

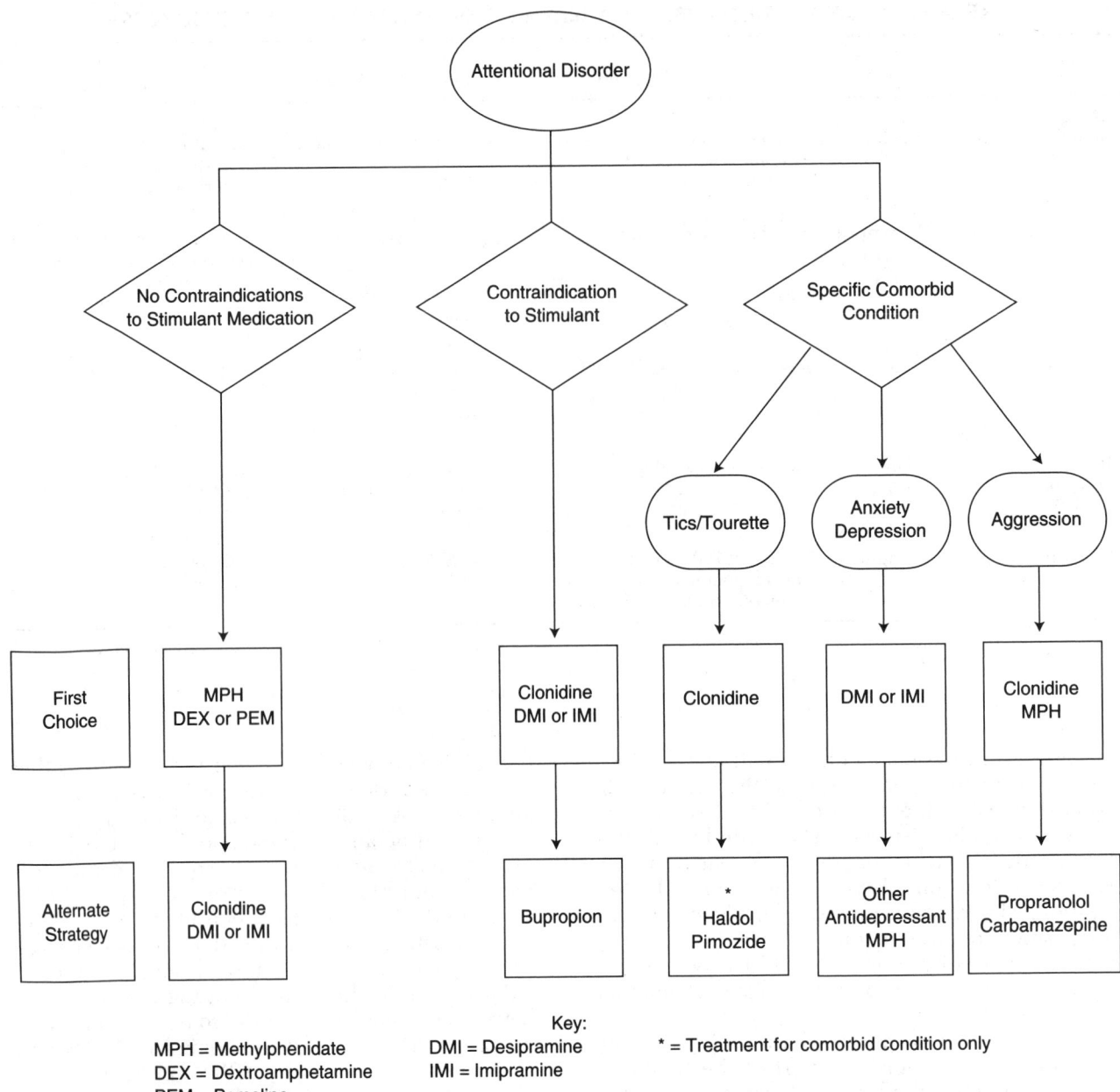

FIGURE 30–1. Medication management specific to attention disorder presentations. (From Culbert TP, Banez G, Reiff MI: Children who have attentional disorders: Interventions. Pediatr Rev 15:10, 1994, with permission.)

The school is key in both diagnosis and management of ADHD. Public Law 94-142, the Education for All Handicapped Children Act of 1975, requires states to "provide free, appropriate, public education" for all handicapped children. Learning disabilities were described as

a disorder in one or more psychological processes involved in understanding or in using language, spoken or written, which may manifest itself in an imperfect ability to listen, think, speak, read, write, spell, or to do mathematical calculations. The first term includes conditions such as perceptual handicaps, brain injury, minimal brain dysfunction, dyslexia, and developmental aphysasia.

Many children with attention deficit disorder suffer from a learning difficulty of sufficient magnitude that school performance is affected negatively. The school, the physician, and the family all should participate in planning the child's individualized education plan (IEP). This will require attention to learning style and the development of educational strategies and social skills training, enhancement of self-esteem, and classroom behavior management.

The physician must provide close follow-up, with review of medication response, parent and child interactions, school progress, and behavior management. Each unit should stress the child's

TABLE 30–4. DIAGNOSTIC CRITERIA FOR OPPOSITIONAL DEFIANT DISORDER

A. A pattern of negativistic, hostile, and defiant behavior lasting at least six months, during which at least four of the following are present:

   (1) often loses temper
   (2) often argues with adults
   (3) often actively defies or refuses to comply with adults' requests or rules
   (4) often deliberately does things that annoy other people
   (5) often blames others for his or her mistakes or misbehavior
   (6) is often touchy or easily annoyed by others
   (7) is often angry and resentful
   (8) is often spiteful or vindictive

B. The disturbance in behavior causes significant impairment in social, academic or occupational functioning.

C. Does not occur exclusively during the course of a Psychotic or Mood Disorder.

D. Does not meet criteria for Conduct Disorder and, if 18 or older, does not meet criteria for Antisocial Personality Disorder.

From American Psychiatric Association: Diagnostic and Statistical Manual of Mental Disorders, 4th edition. Washington, DC, American Psychiatric Press, 1994, with permission.

personal strengths and accomplishment, with the formulation of goals to be accomplished by the next visit.

Oppositional Defiant Disorder and Conduct Disorder

These two conditions are among the most prevalent behavioral disorders in children. Although they seem to be similar in some ways, they differ in important ways (Loeber, 1991). *Oppositional defiant disorder* symptoms include behaviors such as loss of temper, arguments with adults, refusal to comply, blaming others for own behavior, and other somewhat common childhood behaviors (Table 30–4). However, they differ from normal childhood misbehavior and from adjustment reaction disorders. Their rate and intensity of occurrence is atypical. The symptoms may not occur in reaction to an identifiable stressor, and they persist through a later age. Symptoms of oppositional defiant disorder consist of overt, confrontive behavior. In contrast, conduct disorder behavior tends to result in personal harm or property damage rather than verbal confrontation. These behaviors are not overt, but are of a covert, concealing nature, such as theft, truancy, and drug usage. They are more antisocial.

Generally, the symptoms of oppositional defiant disorder appear in earlier childhood before the onset of most conduct disorder symptoms. Very serious conduct disorder behaviors generally do not appear until later adolescence. The early onset of serious conduct disorder symptoms, such as major theft or drug use, is predictive of later persistence

and seriousness. This is not necessarily true for the early onset of oppositional defiant symptoms. The prevalence of oppositional defiant disorder symptoms has been found to decrease with age, whereas the prevalence of conduct disorder symptoms increases with age. Some children with oppositional defiant disorder later develop conduct disorder. It is important to identify these children early.

The DSM-IV diagnosis of *conduct disorders* requires designation by age of onset and by severity (Table 30–5). In child-onset conduct disorder, at

TABLE 30–5. DIAGNOSTIC CRITERIA FOR CONDUCT DISORDER

A. A repetitive and persistent pattern of behavior in which either the basic rights of others or major age-appropriate societal norms or rules are violated, lasting at least six months, during which at least three of the following are present:

   (1) often bullies, threatens, or intimidates others
   (2) often initiates physical flights
   (3) has used a weapon that can cause serious physical harm to others (e.g., a bat, brick, broken bottle, knife, gun)
   (4) has stolen with confrontation with a victim (e.g., mugging, purse snatching, extortion, armed robbery)
   (5) has been physically cruel to people
   (6) has been physically cruel to animals
   (7) has forced someone into sexual activity
   (8) often lies or breaks promises to obtain goods or favors or to avoid obligations (i.e., "cons" others)
   (9) often stays out at night despite parental prohibitions, beginning before 13 years of age
   (10) has stolen items of nontrivial value without confrontation with the victim either within the home or outside the home (e.g., shoplifting, burglary, forgery)
   (11) has deliberately engaged in fire setting with the intention of causing serious damage
   (12) has deliberately destroyed others' property (other than by fire setting)
   (13) has run away from home overnight at least twice while living in parental or parental surrogate home (or once without returning for a lengthy period)
   (14) often truant from school, beginning before 13 years of age (for employed person, absent from work)
   (15) has broken into someone else's house, building, or car

B. If age 18 or older, does not meet criteria for Antisocial Personality Disorder.

Specify type based on age of onset:

Childhood onset type: onset of at least one conduct problem prior to age 10.
Adolescent onset type: no conduct problems prior to age 10.

Specify severity:

Mild: Few if any conduct problems in excess of those required to make the diagnosis, and conduct problems cause only minor harm to others.
Moderate: Number of conduct problems and effect on others intermediate between "mild" and "severe".
Severe: Many conduct problems in excess of those required to make the diagnosis, or conduct problems cause considerable harm to others, e.g., serious physical injury to victims, extensive vandalism or theft.

From American Psychiatric Association: Diagnostic and Statistical Manual of Mental Disorders, 4th edition. Washington, DC, American Psychiatric Press, 1994, with permission.

least one serious behavior (as listed in DSM-IV) had its beginning before the age of 10. The disorder further must be defined as mild, moderate, or severe. Mild conduct disorder is one in which there are few or no conduct behaviors present beyond the number needed for diagnosis. In a moderate condition, the number and severity of negative behaviors are in between mild and severe. Severe conduct disorders involve many negative behaviors of a serious nature.

Management

Conduct disorders in childhood are predictive of more serious later problems. These should be referred for both individual and family therapy as soon as identified because later, more serious conduct behaviors are fairly resistant to therapy. Most children with conduct disorder grow up in very unstable, stressful families. Consequently, the entire family needs to be in family treatment. More than ever, the strengths of family members must be enumerated and utilized. This may seem impossible, but even the most chaotic families have strengths and need to be reminded of them. The angry exasperation of parents may be seen as concern for the child's future, while the child's antisocial behavior may be labeled as a cry for help for the whole family.

It is also very important to attend quickly to childhood oppositional defiant disorders. Those cases of a mild nature may be cared for by the physician, family, and school, while more severe conditions should be referred. Once again, both individual therapy for the child and family therapy are recommended. The individual therapy probably should include behavioral and cognitive techniques as well as an emphasis on establishing a therapeutic relationship that counteracts negative family patterns.

When behavior problems begin to be persistent, parents may request information about discipline. There are a number of parenting programs available in social services and family service agencies to which parents may be referred. Most of these programs include teaching the basic communication techniques described under Adjustment Disorders earlier in this chapter and also teach the use of behavior reinforcement techniques. The basic tenets may be summarized as follows:

1. Avoid power struggles as much as possible; these tend to reinforce negative behaviors.

2. Establish realistic, meaningful consequences for bad behavior and consistently enforce these. However, begin with positive approaches.

3. Establish a point system in which children automatically receive points for tasks accomplished. These points may be turned in for special activities. The family is asked to make a chart of every behavior and task expected of each child. Points are given for timely arrival, appropriate and timely dressing, eating, school attendance and schoolwork, and tasks around the house. A reasonable number of points is required to secure a special activity at the end of the week. Points for daily chores and schoolwork may be required to participate in favorite daily activities, such as television, play with friends, and games. Fairly chaotic families may be unable to follow through with such plans and may need some therapy first to bring order to the household.

Childhood Depression

Mood disorders in children have only been recognized widely for 10 to 20 years. Bipolar disorders are rare in childhood. Major depression is rare up to the age of 3 and remains infrequent before puberty, occurring in less than 3 per cent of these children. However, a 1992 community study found moderate to severe symptoms of depression in 10 to 15 per cent of children in grades 3 to 9 (Weller and Weller, 1991).

The diagnosis of major depression requires the presence of five of the following symptoms during the same 2-week period: depressed mood, markedly diminished interest or pleasure in almost all activities most of the day, significant weight loss or gain, insomnia or hypersomnia, psychomotor agitation or retardation, fatigue or loss of energy daily, feelings of worthlessness or excessive guilt, difficulty thinking or concentrating, and recurrent thoughts of death or suicide. At least one of the symptoms must be either depressed mood or loss of interest/pleasure, and all symptoms must represent a change from prior functioning.

One problem in diagnosing childhood depression is that its symptoms are expressed somewhat differently from those of adult depression (Geller and Carr, 1988). Appetite and weight loss are rare in children, while listlessness, apathy, and inability to enjoy life are much more prominent. Until the age of 5, children do not express guilt or even sadness clearly, but may reveal these indirectly by excessively apologizing for minor infractions. They may complain of headaches and stomachaches, and may be sulky or irritable. By ages 6 to 8, depressed children have few friends, do poorly in school, and may call themselves ugly or stupid. By ages 9 to 12, depressed children daydream often and may have morbid thoughts. They blame themselves for their failures. The depression often seems chronic rather than episodic. The diagnosis of major childhood depression requires ruling out organic causes and other conditions such as adjustment reaction and ADHD.

The causes of childhood depression are uncertain and probably vary (Weller and Weller, 1991). Some childhood depression is certainly genetic. Studies have found that, in 60 per cent of identical twins reared apart, where one child is depressed, the other will be also. Other causes of childhood depression include early attachment problems, abuse, and neglect. Studies indicate high rates of abuse among depressed children. Children who are physically or sexually abused, or are not often spoken to, touched, or hugged or comforted when hurt, become apathetic.

A parent's own depression or preoccupation with unresolved losses or traumas is associated with childhood depression. In a study in which parents were asked to simulate depressed affect for only a few minutes, the infants immediately looked worried, cried, and turned away from their mothers. The babies continued to frown and cry for awhile even after the mothers behaved normally. This is a dramatic argument for assessing and treating the family members of infants and children. Childhood depression is probably a result of a complex combination of biologic vulnerability, problems in upbringing, and social experiences that differ in each case. The course of depression, however, always is impacted by the child's environment.

Management

Once a diagnosis of childhood depression has been made, it is important to begin interventions quickly. Even if the criteria for major depression are not met, milder forms should get early attention. Studies show that 70 per cent of children with mild, chronic depression develop severe depression within 5 years. Antidepressant drugs have not been found to be very effective. Some experts have found that monoamine oxidase inhibitors or selective serotonin reuptake inhibitors, especially Prozac, are more effective. Most do not suggest their use unless the depression has been present for at least 6 months and has not responded to other treatment.

Psychotherapy for children has not been studied as carefully as for adults. Although studies show the vast majority of children are significantly better off after treatment, no one treatment is known to work better than another. Relapse is frequent and, therefore, continued help and follow-up are necessary. Once again, early intervention in as many parts of the child's environment as possible is needed.

Soon after the diagnosis is made, the physician should have a family session including the parents, patient, and siblings. The session will remain fairly brief if it is highly structured. The physician will want to define the purpose of the meetings, educate about depression, inquire about solutions the family has attempted, get them to define their family strengths, describe typical patterns known to reinforce depression and ask the family to spend time specifically counteracting these patterns where they exist in their daily life. The following case example illustrates such a family session.

In the Montgomery family, 6-year-old James finally was brought to the family physician because his parents thought he either had a physical illness or was for some reason trying to irritate the family. The parents described James as being withdrawn for at least 9 months. In the family session, James sat with his head down and physically apart. His parents said they had tried everything to "cheer him up" and now were clearly irritated that he had not responded. Their daughter was a vibrant, active 9-year-old and they often compared the two, pushing James to be more like his sister. After the physician heard their "solutions," she asked each of them to describe what their family strengths were. The described a family that loved one another, was loyal, and worked and played together. Then the physician asked the parents to tell James what his strengths were in great detail. At first, they had difficulty because they were focused on his depressive symptoms. Next the physician described how often, in the case of depression, family, peers, and school personnel begin to push the child to change and perhaps eventually begin to blame, avoid, or reject the depressed person. This is a natural outcome because they do not know the child is not purposefully behaving the way he does, but instead has a condition that is very uncomfortable. Finally, the physician asked the family to each spend time just being empathic with James, encouraging activities, not pushing, and praising every small step. The parents were asked to have a similar discussion with James' teacher and to talk with the Cub Scouts leader to reach out to James.

After several follow-up sessions, if a depressed child is not better, he or she definitely should be referred for additional therapy along with ongoing work with the family and environment. In adults, cognitive therapy, interpersonal therapy, and family therapy have been found helpful with depression. These may be useful for children, but it is essential that the therapy include support, acceptance, and guidance.

DISORDERS IN ADOLESCENTS

Individual Developmental Task

Adolescents must attempt to achieve an identity separate from family.

Adjustment Reactions

As in childhood, adjustment reactions constitute one of the most frequent behavioral conditions in adolescents. The diagnostic features are the same as for childhood and have just as many ways of being expressed. Adolescents experience even more opportunities to be stressed, and those who have shown vulnerabilities earlier may react more strongly to such disappointments as rejections by friends, school problems, and embarrassing events. It is very important to identify the stressful event that has resulted within 3 months in the teen's disturbed reactions. Careful interviewing of the parents and the adolescent separately should make it possible to distinguish adjustment depressions, anxieties, misconduct, and the like from the more severe disorders. The most obvious diagnostic sign is that, before the identifiable stressor, the adolescent did not have the symptoms; also, the symptoms should abate within 6 months after onset.

Management

Often adjustment reactions may be managed with understanding and reassurance to both the patient and family. As with other conditions, it is recommended that a brief family session be held to educate and reassure. Family members may be asked to be extra empathic and understanding of how upsetting the stressful event was to this particular young person. The teenager should be offered a chance to explain, without interruption or negation, exactly how he or she feels about the stressful event that occurred. Often this amount of respectful listening, followed by empathic statements by the family indicating true understanding, will create a significant positive change. At times an adolescent's reaction to a stressor will be severe enough to lead to a major conduct disturbance, such as truancy, vandalism, or fighting. The physician should point out that this behavior is highly unusual for this teenager. The teen's usual positive behavior should be discussed while creating an air of expectation that the latter will resume quickly. If the behavior was serious enough, as in theft or vandalism, the physician should state openly that the parents may want to establish consequences for the behavior. However, it would be helpful if they express empathy for their child's feelings even though they must discipline the actions.

The adolescent must be helped to learn more adaptive ways of dealing with upsets. The family members all may be engaged in a discussion of acceptable means of dealing with whatever strong emotions the adolescent experienced. If the symptomatic behaviors later are repeated and begin to occur more frequently, a more serious diagnosis may need to be entertained. However, it is best to begin with positive expectations rather than utilizing a more negative label prematurely.

Depression

Research (Kashani and Sherman 1989; Weller and Weller, 1991) has found that only 4 to 6 per cent of adolescents have major depression, but another 3 per cent suffer from a milder chronic form. Often depressive symptoms in teenagers are dismissed as adjustment reactions or as typical adolescent turmoil. However, research has shown that normal adolescents do not have times that are so upsetting that they resemble adult depression. Most teenagers get along fairly well with adults and do not feel miserable for extended periods. Adolescent depression, like that in adults (Akiskal and Weller, 1989), is seen in symptoms of loss of appetite, hopelessness, sleep disturbance, and thoughts of suicide. A depressed teenager is at least as likely to commit suicide as a depressed adult. In the past 30 years, the overall rate of suicide in the population has not risen; however, it has risen substantially among teenagers. Suicide attempts may occur after almost any personal conflict or crisis in an already depressed adolescent. Adolescents are impulsive and influenced by the depressive behavior of friends and relatives. Suicide as a possibility is worsened with the use of drugs.

As in childhood depression, little is known about the biologic contributors to adolescent depression. There are many causes of adolescent depression, but some are unique to the developmental stage. Adolescence is a stage in which identity is not yet established, and independence is sought yet dependence remains. There is a heightened sensitivity to embarrassments and rejections, which may play a part in depression. Some adolescents take on a role in the family of caring for depressed or ill parents. Others try unsuccessfully to live up to unrealistic adult expectations. These stressors play a part in the etiology of some teenage depression. Just as in other disorders, adolescent depression must be distinguished from other psychiatric disorders and must be diagnosed and treated in the context of family, peer group, and culture.

Management

As in childhood depression, adolescent depression tends to recur in later stages and to be a precursor to other problems. Some follow-up studies have found that one third of depressed adolescents later became involved with the police. These may be adolescents who always have had both depression and conduct disorder, or it may be that the social costs of depressive symptoms lead to acting out. According to several studies (Dadds et al., 1992), adolescents who have only depression exhibit little or no anger or aggression, nor do their family members. Those who have depression and conduct disorder are quite angry, while little aggression is found in their family. Those who have conduct disorder without depression are very antisocial and come from families with marked patterns of chaos, aggression, and anger.

Once again, a management program that is contextual in nature is extremely important. Depression is affected by the emotions, separations, and depressions of those around the teenager. Depression creates thoughts of self-doubt and deprecation, feelings of hopelessness and meaninglessness, and behaviors of isolation or irritability. These behaviors make others avoid the patient or blame the teen. All of this reinforces depressed symptoms. It is imperative that the physician approach management with the view that no one is trying to make the depression worse. However, everyone, including the teen, his or her family, peers, and school, must work together to make things better. Until a diagnosis is made, it is easy for the teen to be scapegoated because depressed behaviors are indeed not attractive. Perhaps nowhere is the principle of utilizing strengths and positives more important than in work with adolescents. Family, school, and friends may see nothing positive in the teen patient and, by now, the teen may be equally down on others and self. Congratulating each for coming for help (even when the adolescent is there reluctantly) is an important place to begin.

Although diagnostic interviews should be held separately with adolescents and parents, family counseling sessions should be held periodically. The format of labeling strengths, educating the group about depression, and utilizing strengths to interrupt depression-reinforcing interaction patterns is once again the preferred model. Periodic individual and family group follow-up sessions should be held even when the adolescent and/or family is referred for therapy.

Just as in childhood depression, antipressants have not been found to be very effective in adolescents. Prozac has been found to have some effectiveness. However, the use of any drugs should be avoided until symptoms have persisted for at least 6 months and have not responded to other therapy. Once again, research on therapy with adolescents is not as good as with adults. Cognitive, interpersonal, and/or family therapy all may work. Most importantly, some intervention is needed in all parts of the teenager's life—home, peers, and school relationships. Parents and school personnel should be asked to search out and attend to every positive behavior. It will be helpful if all can take the attitude that they know this is very hard for the adolescent and that he or she is not merely being bad. Once again, aggressive intervention at this time may save a teenager from sinking further into dysfunction.

Eating Disorders in Adolescents

Anorexia nervosa is defined by refusal to eat, weight loss or failure to gain weight at 15 per cent below expected body weight, an intense fear of gaining weight or becoming fat, and a misconception of body size. Bulimia is defined by episodes of binge eating and some purging or calorie-consuming activities, such as laxative abuse, vomiting, or vigorous exercise; feeling out of control during binges; and being overconcerned with body shape and weight.

The highest risk group for anorexia nervosa are middle- and upper-class white females, with an incidence range of 1 to 10 per cent. Age at onset for anorexia is 12 to 16 years, and for bulimia, 15 to 20 years. Female anorexics outnumber males by 9 to 1; and in bulimics, females outnumber males 5 to 1 (Harper 1994). Comorbid disorders, such as major depression, sexual abuse, addictive behavior, and anxiety disorder, also can be seen. Patients with anorexia nervosa tend to be less mature than their stated age, both psychologically and physiologically. Our "culture of thinness" is implicated by the patient's obsession with thinness.

Girls may present with amenorrhea as a complaint. The physician often observes the severity of the weight reduction in relation to height. Other physical findings observed are lanugo hair, bradycardia, hypothermia, an orange-like color to the skin (carotenemia), enlarged parotid glands, and lacerations on the soft palate resulting from the induction of vomiting. Abnormal blood work, low blood urea nitrogen and creatines levels, hypocholesterolemia, carotenemia, and potassium deficiencies may be present.

Management

As for other disorders previously discussed in this chapter, management of eating disorders includes an understanding of the emotions of frustration, anger, blame, and guilt in both parents and child. Better nutrition long has been regarded as necessary before meaningful psychological change can occur. Hospitalization often is required for three very different purposes: (1) acute stabilization, when a severely eating-disordered patient develops dehydration or electrolyte imbalance or severe emaciation; (2) treatment of intermediate length to correct dehydration or starvation, to stabilize eating, and to initiate change to being an outpatient; and (3) long-term admission with the more ambitious goal of substantial change in the patient's relationship to food to that of eating for himself or herself (Harper, 1994). Tricyclic antidepressants have been recommended when depression is present, and antianxiolitics have been used when there appears to be a significant mealtime anxiety. A referral to a team of health professionals involved in the care of patients with eating disorders is often necessary.

REFERENCES

Adair H, Bauchner H: Sleep problems in childhood. Curr Probl Pediatr 4:147, 1993.

Ainsworth MDS, Bell SM: Some contemporary patterns of mother infant interaction in the feeding situation. *In* Ambrose A (ed): Stimulation in Early Infancy. New York, Academic Press, 1969, p S182.

Ainsworth MDS, Blehar M, Waters E, Wall S: Patterns of Attachment. Hillsdale, NJ, Lawrence Erlbaum Associates, 1978.

Ainsworth MDS, Eichberg C: Effects on infant-mother attachment of mother's unresolved loss of an attachment figure or other traumatic experiences. *In* Parkes CM, Stevenson-Hinde J, Marris P (eds): Attachment across the Life Cycle. London, Routledge, 1991, pp 33–51.

Akiskal HS, Weller EB: Mood disorders and suicide in children and adolescents. *In* Kaplan HI, Saddock BJ (eds): Comprehensive Textbook of Psychiatry, 5th edition, Vol. 2. Baltimore; Williams & Wilkins, 1989, pp 1981–1994.

Algranati PS, Dworkin PH: Infancy problem behaviors. Pediatr Rev 13:16, 1992.

Ambrosini PJ, Bianchi MD, Rabinovich H, Elia J: Antidepressant treatments in children and adolescents: II. Anxiety, physical, and behavioral disorders. J Am Acad Child Adolesc Psychiatry 32:483, 1993.

American Psychiatric Association: Diagnostic and Statistical Manual of Mental Disorders, 4th edition. Washington, DC, American Psychiatric Press, 1994.

Bowlby J: Attachment and Loss, Vol. 1: Attachment, 2nd edition. London, Hogarth Press, 1982.

Bowlby J: A Secure Base. London, Routledge, 1988.

Brent DA: Depression and suicide in children and adolescents. Pediatr Rev 14:380, 1993.

Budman SH, Gurman AS: Theory and Practice of Brief Therapy. New York, Guilford Press, 1988.

Campbell M, Malone RP: Mental retardation and psychiatric disorders. Hosp Community Psychiatry 42:374, 1991.

Caspi A, Elder GH: Emergent family patterns: The intergenerational construction of problem behavior and relationships. *In* Hinde RA, Stevenson-Hinde J (eds): Relationships within Families: Mutual Friends. Oxford, England, Oxford University Press, 1988, pp 218–240.

Coleman WS: Attention Deficit Disorders, Hyperactivity & Associated Disorders, 6th edition. Madison, WI, Calliope Books, 1993.

Culbert TP, Banez G, Reiff MI: Children who have attentional disorders: Interventions. Pediatr Rev 15:10, 1994.

Dadds MR, Sanders MR, Morrison M, Rebgetz M: Childhood depression and conduct disorder: II. An analysis of family interaction patterns in the home. J Abnorm Psychol 101:505, 1992.

Dahl RE: The pharmacologic treatment of sleep disorders. Pediatr Psychopharmacol 15:161, 1992.

Ferber R: Solve Your Child's Sleep Problems. New York, Simon & Schuster, 1985.

Geller B, Carr LG: Similarities and differences between adult and pediatric major depressive disorders. *In* Georgotas A, Cancro R (eds): Depression and Mania. New York, Elsevier, 1988, pp 565–580.

Goldstein S, Goldstein M: Managing Attention Disorders in Children: A Guide for Practitioners. New York, John Wiley & Sons, 1990.

Grossmann K, Fremmer-Bombik E, Rudolph J, Grossman KE: Maternal attachment representations as related to patterns of infant/mother attachment and maternal care during the first year. *In* Hinde RA, Stevenson-Hinde J (eds): Relationships within Families: Mutual Influences. Oxford, England, Oxford University Press, 1988, pp 241–260.

Harper G: Eating disorders in adolescence. Pediatr Rev 15:72, 1994.

Kashani JH, Sherman DD: Mood disorders in children and adolescents. *In* Tasman A, Halls RE, Frances AJ (eds): Review of Psychiatry, Vol. 8. Washington, DC, American Psychiatric Press, 1989, pp 197–216.

Lindbergt L: Cow's milk, whey, protein, elicit symptoms of infantile colic in colicky formula fed infants: A double line crossover study. Pediatrics 83:262, 1989.

Liotti G, Intreccialagli B, Cecere F: Unresolved mourning in mothers and development of dissociative disorders in children: A case-control study (in Italian). Rev Psichiatr 26:283, 1992.

Loeber R: DSM-IV in progress: Oppositional defiant disorder and conduct disorder. Hosp Community Psychiatry 42:1099, 1991.

Macoby EE, Martin JA: Socialization in the context of the family: Parent child interaction. *In* Mussen PH (ed): Handbook of Child Psychology, Vol. IV. New York, John Wiley & Sons, 1983, pp 88–103.

Main M, Hesse E: Disorganized/disoriented infant behavior in the strange situation, lapses in the monitoring of reasoning and discourse during the parents' adult attachment interviews and dissociative states: In support of Liotti's hypothesis. *In* Ammanuniti M, Stern D (eds): Attachment and Psycho-Analysis. London, Routledge, 1992, pp 86–140.

Main M, Kaplan N, Cassidy J: Security in infancy, childhood and adulthood: A move to the level of representation. Monogr Soc Res Child Dev 209:50, 1985.

Main M, Soloman J: Discovery of a new, insecure-disorganized/disoriented attachment pattern. *In* Brazelton TB, Uogman N (eds): Affective Development in Infancy. Norwood, ST, Ablex, 1986, pp 95–124.

Main M, Soloman J: Procedures in identifying infants as disorganized/disoriented during the Ainsworth Strange Situation. *In* Greenberg MT, Cicchetti D, Cummings EM (eds): Attachment in the Pre-School Years. Chicago, University of Chicago Press, 1990, pp 121–182.

McDaniel S, Campbell TL, Seaburn DB: Family Oriented Primary Care: A Manual for Medical Providers. New York, Springer-Verlag, 1990, pp 105–135.

Mercugliano M: Psychopharmacology in children with developmental disabilities. Pediatr Clin North Am 40:593, 1993.

Nolan T, Oberklaid F: New concepts in the management of encopresis. Pediatr Rev 14:447, 1993.

Popper CW: Psychopharmacologic treatment of anxiety disorders in adolescents and children. J Clin Psychiatry 54:52, 1993.

Reiff MI, Banez GA, Culbert TP: Children who have attention disorders: Diagnosis and evaluation. Pediatr Rev 14:455, 1993.

Rostain AL: Attention deficit disorders in children and adolescents. Pediatr Clin North Am 38:607, 1991.

Rutter M: Functions and consequence of relationship: Some psychopathological considerations. *In* Hinde RA, Stevenson-Hinde J (eds): Relationships within Families: Mutual Influences. Oxford, England, Oxford University Press, pp 332–353.

Ryan ND: The pharmacologic treatment of child and adolescent depression. Pediatr Psychopharmacol 15:29, 1992.

Salgranati P, Dworkin PH: Infancy Problem Behaviors. Pediatr Rev 13:16, 1992.

Satter E: The feeding relationship: Problems and interventions. J Pediatr 117(2, pt 2):S181, 1990.

Schmitt BD: Your Child's Health, 2nd edition. New York, Bantam Books, 1991.

Seagull EA: Childhood depression. Curr Probl Pediatr 20:707, 1990.

Sloman L: Use of medication in pervasive developmental disorders. Psychiatr Clin North Am 14:165, 1991.

Sproufe LA, Fleeson J: The coherence of family relationships. *In* Hinde RA, Stevenson-Hinde J (eds): Relationships within Families: Mutual Influences. Oxford, England, Oxford University Press, 1988, pp 27–47.

Stern D: The Interpersonal World of the Infant. New York, Basic Books, 1985.

Weller EB, Weller RA: Mood disorders in children. *In* Wiener GM (ed): Textbook of Child and Adolescent Psychiatry. Washington, DC, American Psychiatric Press, 1991, pp 240–247.

Wilens TE, Biederman J: The stimulants. Psychiatr Clin North Am 15:191, 1992.

CHAPTER 31

OFFICE SURGERY

CHARLES V. WRIGHT, Jr., and JOSEPH E. RONAGHAN

The scope of office surgery changes steadily. New procedures and refinements of old procedures contribute to this change. Many time-honored office surgical procedures, such as skin surgery, continue largely unchanged. However, cryosurgery and laser procedures on the skin offer enhancements. For the family physician, the office continues as the main site of practice and office procedures continue to expand.

Historically, the emphasis on office surgery has come full circle. Before the advent of anesthesia, most surgery occurred to treat trauma or emergency conditions. The physician's office, the patient's home, tents, and hospitals served equally well as sites for surgery. After the advent of anesthesia, more complicated procedures involving the abdominal, pleural, and cranial cavities required complex equipment and trained personnel. As a result, the site of most surgery shifted to the hospital.

For most of the 20th century, the hospital continued as the primary site for surgery, leaving the office for only "minor" procedures. These minor procedures, usually not requiring general anesthesia, included draining small abscesses, removing skin lesions, and repairing lacerations. During the middle part of this century, emphasis on specialist care ushered in an era of decreasing family physician involvement in hospital-based surgical procedures. Office surgery, however, did not go away, but persevered.

During the last quarter of the 20th century, outpatient surgery units, ambulatory surgery centers, and independent surgical centers claimed the focus of surgical trends. The trend was to perform at such sites those procedures that allowed the patient to go home the same day on an outpatient basis. In these facilities, patients come to the surgical unit the morning of surgery and go home after recovering from the anesthesia. Some physicians developed day surgery units as a part of their office.

Economic conditions, rather than advances in surgery, caused this shift to outpatient surgery. Patients and third-party insurers found hospital-based surgery too expensive. By eliminating the need for overnight care, the outpatient surgical centers decreased the costs of surgical care. Third-party insurers paid the lower total costs at a higher percentage, encouraging further development of more outpatient surgical centers. These centers often left hospitals with a higher percentage of the less profitable trauma and emergency surgeries.

The same economic forces that shifted many major procedures to outpatient-type centers also caused more procedures to be performed in the office. Office surgery is even more important now than earlier in this century.

Office surgery still consists largely of skin surgery, drainage of small abscesses, and laceration repair. The addition of cryosurgery allowed a simple, effective treatment for many skin lesions that previously required excision. Lasers in the family physician's office represent a frontier in office surgery. Although currently not in most office procedure rooms, lasers offer a treatment modality for conditions not currently treated in the office, such as tattoos. Also, lasers offer a new tool for performing some of the established office surgical procedures.

This chapter presents a review of preprocedure patient evaluation, office facilities, principles of wound healing, and traditional office surgery. We also present cryosurgery as an economical modality for office surgery. Finally, we present lasers as an upcoming technique for the office. Even though lasers represent the frontier of office surgery now, we believe all family physicians should become more familiar with lasers as a surgical tool in the office.

EVALUATION OF THE PATIENT

The physician should perform a thorough preoperative evaluation of every surgical patient. For office surgery, questionnaires are helpful in evaluating the patient's history, especially if a complete history and physical was not performed earlier. Patients can complete questionnaires in the office reception area, the examination room, or the procedure room. Physicians need not be present while patients are completing questionnaires. This saves time and allows physicians to perform other duties. Questionnaires should contain questions regarding current symptoms; a history of previous procedures with dates, reasons, and complications; past hospitalization; current medications; a family history with specific questions concerning bleeding disorders and cardiovascular events; and history of any allergic reactions. The physician or nurse should obtain expanded information about any questionable areas in the history before performing the procedure.

Addressing specific areas may enhance the patient's safety during the procedure. Specifically, history of seizures, angina pectoris, and pacemakers needs documentation. Larger doses of anesthetics may induce seizures. Documented therapeutic seizure medication levels lessen patient and physician anxieties about intraoperative seizures. Vasoconstricting agents, such as epinephrine, used in some anesthetic preparations, increase the risk of angina pectoris in patients with coronary artery disease. In patients with angina pectoris, avoidance of drugs containing epinephrine simplifies the task of the procedure. Physicians using electrocautery should exercise caution with patients using a cardiac pacemaker. The demand-type pacemakers present a particular problem because the electrical current may falsely indicate the presence of a heartbeat to the electronic pacemaker. In this situation, the pacemaker does not send the electrical current to induce a cardiac contraction.

A complete examination of the entire skin surface before skin surgery may uncover bacterial, viral, or fungal disease in areas distant from the surgical site. Examination of the skin in its entirety produces a better safeguard against infection than simply questioning the patient about lesions. Observation of adequate precautions prevents infections from being absolute contraindications to skin surgery at a different location.

Surgery planned for the genital area necessitates questioning about herpes simplex. Both physician and patient should be aware that the trauma of a surgical procedure in an area where recurrent herpes simplex occurs may precipitate the herpetic infection. Poor cosmetic effect may occur if herpetic infection develops. Herpes simplex can be problematic not only in the genital area but also in the perioral region, resulting in poor cosmetic results.

Physicians should instruct patients to report any infection or other physical ailment developing between the time of the preoperative visit and the scheduled procedure.

Anticoagulants and aspirin-containing medications may complicate surgical procedures by causing profuse bleeding. Epinephrine used with the local anesthetic infiltration helps prevent bleeding complications in these patients. Performance of many small procedures may be acceptable even with prolonged bleeding times. However, the physician must evaluate carefully the risks of complications from hematoma or bleeding at the surgical site. If aspirin-containing products are necessary

for the management of arthritis or other severe inflammatory problems, these products may be continued in most circumstances. However, most patients should be warned to avoid any aspirin or aspirin-containing products for 7 to 10 days before any surgical procedure. As little as one aspirin tablet will induce the maximum bleeding defect. Acetaminophen or acetaminophen with codeine offers an excellent analgesic alternative to aspirin.

The necessity of blood testing depends on the size and location of the procedure. Small procedures usually require no blood testing at all. If the procedure is extensive or in a particularly vascular area, a complete blood count with differential, prothrombin time, partial thromboplastin time, bleeding time, and platelet count should suffice for patients without a family history of coagulation disorders (Schultz and McKinney, 1985).

There is no need for routine screening for hepatitis B or human immunodeficiency virus (HIV). Physicians performing office surgery who are not currently immunized against hepatitis B should consider immunizing themselves with the hepatitis B vaccine. Physicians should instruct their patients to continue all current medications except aspirin or anticoagulants. Interruption of cardiac medications, antihypertensive medications, and antiarrhythmic medications should not occur. For diabetics taking hypoglycemic agents or insulin, procedures should not be scheduled during the patient's mealtime.

In severe or uncontrolled diabetes, insulin resistance, hyperglycemia, and depressed leukocyte function interfere with collagen synthesis and impair wound healing. The granulocyte influx into the wound slows. Associated with these changes, a depressed protocollagen and collagen synthesis occurs. Reduction of blood glucose levels below 250 mg/dL correlates with improved granulocyte function. The granulocyte dysfunction associated with the insulin resistance of type II (non–insulin-dependent) diabetes improves with administration of either sulfonylurea drugs or extra insulin. Measuring postprandial glucose levels to assure that the blood glucose level does not exceed 250 mg/dL helps assure better wound healing for the diabetic patient (McMurray, 1984).

FACILITIES AND EQUIPMENT

The Procedure Room

Although office surgery can be performed in individual exam rooms using mobile equipment, most offices have designated procedure rooms. Procedure rooms can be as small as 10 × 10 feet, but 12 × 15 or 15 × 15 feet allows more equipment in the operative area and provides a more comfortable setting. Rooms greater than 15 × 15 feet may prove so large that efficiency decreases because of the time required to get items from the far side of the room.

The procedure room should be placed away from the major traffic areas of the office to decrease the noise level and decrease contamination risk. Soft but cheerful colors provide a soothing atmosphere for patients. Adequate cabinet and drawer space for storage of tools, supplies, and medical equipment must be provided.

The examining and operating table, lighting fixtures, and procedure trays constitute the most important equipment in the procedure room. These items vary widely by the number of features and cost. Other equipment may be present depending on the procedures performed and physician desire.

The examining and operating table should have devices for raising, lowering, tilting, and bending at the appropriate spots. This allows the patient to assume the supine, prone, jackknife, and other positions. Many newer electrically operated tables provide comfort by the soft cushions provided and appear warm and attractive, with a variety of colors available. Added features such as arm boards provide additional comfort to patient and physician. The arm board should allow extremity rotation to a position above the patient's head or below the patient's lower abdomen.

Lighting provides an essential aspect of office surgery. The traditional gooseneck lamp provides poor light, obstructs the surgical field, and serves as a source of heat and discomfort for both patient and surgeon. Floor-mounted lamps allow moving the lamp from one side of the procedure table to another or even to another room. However, these lamps sometimes adjust poorly to the angles required for some wounds. Floor-mounted units are less expensive than overhead mounted units. At least one, and preferably two, fixed mounted overhead room lights provide good mobility and high-efficiency lighting for surgical procedures.

An inexpensive substitute for floor-mounted lighting or overhead-mounted lighting, the operating head lamp with plastic headband provides adequate lighting of the surgical field. Such units are mobile, allowing use in other rooms. The headbands adjust to different sizes and provide minimal discomfort to the physician. The operating head lamp also may be used to augment lighting from overhead lighting or floor-mounted lighting. The cost of most head lamp units justifies more than one unit in the physician's office.

A mobile stand to hold surgical trays containing sterile equipment and other items is necessary. Mobile stands, such as the Mayo tray, allow movement of the equipment to a position comfortable for the physician. These stands also keep sterile equipment away from contamination. Most procedure rooms contain only one or two Mayo stands.

The procedure room must contain a sink and surgical soap for the physician's scrub before procedures. The ordinary sink with hand faucets is most common and acceptable. Such units can be installed initially or added later when converting a room to a procedure room. Most office examination rooms already contain a standard sink with hand faucets. Also, the procedure room sink allows for preliminary washing of dirty instruments before sterilization.

There must be provisions for sterilization of instruments and surgical packs. Office autoclaves vary in complexity, size, and expense. Some units sit on the countertop, consuming little space. Other free-standing units rest on the floor, occupying a large area of the room. Sterilizing instruments one at a time rather than as a surgical pack is cumbersome and expensive. We recommend sterilizing instruments in a surgical pack as described later in this chapter. The office autoclave should allow sterilization of the largest surgical pack used in the office.

Additional equipment may prove desirable. Such items include a suction device with tubing, catheters, and tips. Suction devices can be wall mounted or floor mounted. Wall-mounted suction devices are more complex, requiring installation when initially building or remodeling the procedure room. Floor-mounted suction devices with a mobile cart provide a less expensive alternative. The mobile suction units cost much less than the wall-mounted units. We advise that most physicians purchase the mobile units with cart.

Sterilization and Universal Precautions

Hospital or ambulatory surgery unit operating rooms provide large areas for sterile procedures. In contrast, the office procedure room is a clean room rather than a sterile room. Sterile areas in the procedure room are much smaller, usually limited to the small operating field and procedure tray. After every procedure (especially any contaminated procedure), the entire procedure room, furniture, and fixtures should be cleaned. Commercial solutions, available from medical supply dealers, provide ample coverage.

The flooring in the procedure room should be a hard surface such as tile to allow easy movement of equipment around the room. Hard flooring also allows easy cleaning of the inevitable spills and contamination of the floor surface. Avoid using carpet in a procedure room. Carpets do not clean well and serve as a reservoir for bacteria and odors.

Similarly, all wall surfaces must clean easily without ruining the finish. Some paints withstand repeated washing with bacteriostatic or antiseptic solutions; others cannot withstand such use. Consider using a durable, washable wallpaper instead of wall paint. Wallpaper comes in a wide variety of soothing, cheerful colors and textures that make the procedure room more comforting to patients.

TABLE 31–1. RESUSCITATION EQUIPMENT

Defibrillator
Laryngoscope
Endotracheal tubes (3, 5, 7 mm)
Oral airway (small, medium, large)
Suction
Oxygen with tubing, cannula/mask
Disposable bag-valve-mask device

TABLE 31–3. SURGICAL PACK

2 × 2 or 4 × 4 sponges
Towel drapes
4 towel clamps
1 no. 3 scalpel handle
4½-inch needle holder
1 forceps without teeth
2 skin hooks
1 dissecting scissors
1 straight suture scissors
1 Adson forceps
3 curved mosquito hemostats

The ever-present danger of blood-borne pathogens necessitates universal precautions in the procedure room. A supply of sterile and nonsterile gloves should be available to physician and staff. In addition to the traditional face mask, eye protection should be provided for all personnel in the procedure area. Universal precautions also require sharps containers for disposal of needles, intravenous catheters, and scalpel blades. The disposal of body fluids, blood, or any material contaminated with blood or body fluids must comply with all local, state, and federal regulations.

Resuscitation Equipment

Every procedure room should contain resuscitation equipment for patient safety and physician peace of mind. The "crash cart" must contain equipment and drugs to allow for full cardiopulmonary resuscitation (Table 31–1). Although there is some medical–legal responsibility, the major concern should be patient safety. The minimum set of equipment includes defibrillator, bag-valve-mask device, endotracheal tubes, intravenous access materials, oxygen and related tubing, cannulae, masks, and aerosol adapters. Be sure to include equipment for both adult and pediatric resuscitation.

Table 31–2 lists drugs to be included on the crash cart. Every office should establish a routine schedule for inspection and replacement of the drugs on the crash cart to ensure that no out-of-date drugs are present. Physicians or their staff should keep a log of drug expiration dates, dates of inspection, and other documentation that the crash cart is ready for immediate use. Additionally, defi-

brillators should be tested on a routine basis and a log of defibrillator testing should be kept.

Resuscitation kits can be assembled from individual items or purchased as a preassembled package. Individually assembled items are then kept in tool boxes with folding trays and sliding drawers. Commercially available kits, are available and come in suitcase-sized cases with each drug or piece of equipment having its own place in the kit. Regardless of whether the crash cart is assembled individually or purchased as a prepackaged kit, every member of the physician's office working in the procedure room must know the contents and location of every item in the crash cart.

The Surgical Pack

By packaging and sterilizing commonly used instruments, supplies, and equipment together to form a surgical pack, the efficiency of the office procedure increases. The surgical pack forms the basic unit of the procedure equipment. The exact contents of each pack vary widely. Instrument type, size, and number depend largely on the preference of the operator rather than set standards. Table 31–3 lists the components of our most often used surgical pack and Table 31–4 lists items added to the pack after opening. Most physicians develop separate packs for individual procedures such as circumcision, endometrial biopsy and colposcopy, laceration repair, and skin surgery. For example, Table 31–5 lists the items on a simple shave biopsy tray.

At the completion of each procedure, the instruments should be scrubbed with a cleansing solution, dried, and placed back in the surgical tray

TABLE 31–2. RESUSCITATION DRUGS

Aminophylline	Isoproterenol
Amyl nitrite	Furosemide
Aromatic spirits of ammonia	Lidocaine
Atropine sulfate	Narcan
Benadryl injectable	Nifedipine capsule
Bretylium	Nitroglycerin
Calcium chloride	Romazicon
Calcium gluconate	Sodium bicarbonate
Dextrose 5% in water	Solu-Cortef
Dopamine	Solu-Medrol
Epinephrine	Verapamil

TABLE 31–4. ADDITIONS TO SURGICAL PACK

Disposable 5-mL syringe with 18-gauge needle
25- to 30-gauge needle
Disposable drape with adhesive backing
1 no. 15 scalpel blade
Handle for electrocoagulator
Appropriate absorbable suture
Appropriate nonabsorbable suture

TABLE 31–5. SOFT TISSUE BIOPSY TRAY

1 straight hemostat
1 scalpel handle
Punch biopsy, various sizes
1 no. 11 blade
4 × 4 gauze pads

along with new supplies to complete the surgical pack. Then, the surgical packs can be autoclaved and stored. To autoclave the surgical pack, it should be wrapped in suitable cloth material such as surgical towels or autoclave paper and closed and secured with autoclave tape that turns color when sterilization is complete. Using colored autoclave tape permits coding the packs according to type. Handwritten notes on the autoclave tape describe the individual pack and record the date of sterilization. Most autoclaves sterilize using steam under pressure. This type of sterilization may dull sharp edges. Avoiding the dulling of sharp edges requires sterilization with dry heat. Dry heat, however, requires additional equipment and expense.

ANESTHESIA, ANALGESIA, AND SEDATION

The performance of office surgery can be accomplished only with adequate control of pain and anxiety. General anesthesia is usually not available in the office environment. Instead, office surgery requires the use of local, topical, or regional anesthetics with or without sedative or analgesic agents.

Topical Anesthesia

Currently, the best topical anesthetic for use in small areas (less than 5 × 5 cm) is a mixture of lidocaine 2.5% and prilocaine 2.5% in a cream base (EMLA Cream). Apply the EMLA Cream generously to the area and then cover it with nonporous tape for 30 to 40 minutes. This allows adequate anesthesia for small procedures such as skin biopsy, needle aspiration, needle biopsy, and even excision of small cutaneous and subcutaneous lesions. Do not apply EMLA Cream to open wounds or lacerations.

In the past, a topical mixture of tetracaine, adrenaline, and cocaine (TAC) was used as topical anesthesia for the repair of lacerations. Although this combination worked well and avoided injection of local anesthetic, experience soon showed that the intense vasoconstriction caused by the adrenaline and cocaine caused significant wound ischemia, and increasing incidence of ischemic necrosis of wound edges. We recommend avoiding this type of agent.

Local Anesthesia

The majority of office surgical procedures utilize injectable local anesthesia. The most common and effective agent of this type is Lidocaine (xylocaine HCl), which comes in concentrations of 0.5%, 1%, 2%, and 4%, all of which may or may not include epinephrine. Epinephrine has a local vasoconstrictive effect that minimizes bleeding and decreases the rate of uptake and degradation of the anesthetic, prolonging its duration of action. Physicians should avoid using epinephrine in patients with cardiac or hypertensive disorders. NEVER use epinephrine when treating lesions of the fingers, nose, ears, toes, or penis because of vasoconstriction and possible necrosis. The total dose of lidocaine without epinephrine should not exceed 5 mg/kg. If the procedure requires doses exceeding these limits, stage the procedure, allowing 2 or 3 hours for the medication to metabolize between sessions.

Local Infiltration

A 25- or 26-gauge needle is optimal for this procedure. The area should be marked with indelible ink before proceeding. Next, the superficial skin and dermis are infiltrated, raising a wheal, and then the needle is advanced, continuously creating a larger wheal. The infiltration is extended slightly beyond the intended line of incision. After adequate infiltration of the skin, the subcutaneous tissue beneath the lesion is infiltrated. The area is massaged for a short period, and then sensation is checked (Shane, 1983). The addition of 8.4% sodium bicarbonate in a ratio of 1 mL to every 9 mL of lidocaine will markedly decrease or eliminate the burning discomfort during infiltration.

Digital Block

This type of anesthesia is very useful in instances in which local infiltration would be very difficult or very painful because of the lesion's location or extent on the fingers or toes. Epinephrine always should be avoided when performing this type of block. The local anesthetic is injected at the proximal end of the digit, perpendicular to the bone. After injecting approximately 1 mL, the needle is withdrawn slightly and redirected upward and then downward at a 45-degree angle, injecting approximately 0.5 mL above and below the bone. This maneuver is performed on each side of the digit. The injections sites should be massaged for 10 to 15 seconds after injection. Approximately 5 minutes should elapse before checking sensation. Additionally, to produce further anesthesia, the physician may infiltrate local anesthetic circumferentially into the subcutaneous tissue at the digit base (Shane, 1983).

Sedatives and Analgesics

As an adjunct to local or topical anesthesia when the patient has pain or anxiety not controlled by more conservative measures, the physician may elect to use sedative and analgesic medications. Extreme caution must be employed in deciding to use these medications because both types have the potential for significant respiratory depression and adverse reactions.

Sedatives

The benzodiazepines (diazepam, midazolam) typify this category of medications. In addition to excellent sedation, they have the benefit of retrograde amnesia, which enhances the patient's comfort because minimal or no memory of discomfort persists. Use these intravenous medications in very small doses, adjusting the dose for age and medical condition. These drugs can cause respiratory depression in higher doses, so they should be used very cautiously in patients with chronic lung disease. Generally, the dose of diazepam should not exceed 10 mg, and the dose of midazolam should not exceed 5 mg. Should respiratory depression occur, the effects usually can be minimized markedly or reversed by administering flumazenil (Romazicon) promptly. These medications are controlled substances, so they should be maintained in a locked and closely inventoried environment.

Analgesics

The need for significant injectable analgesia in the office surgical environment should be very small. However, certain procedures (reduction of dislocations, repair of a large laceration, endoscopic procedures) may require analgesia in addition to sedation. In this situation, avoid using true narcotics (morphine or meperidine), and, if possible, employ agonist/antagonist drugs (nalbuphine, ketorolac) instead. True narcotics, especially when combined with benzodiazepines, have a much higher incidence of respiratory depression, nausea, and somnolence compared to the agonist/antagonists. When using the narcotic analgesics, nalorphine reverses the effects of these medications. Ketorolac (Toradol) currently does not have indications for intravenous use, so its intramuscular administration should occur at least 30 minutes before the procedure starts. As with benzodiazepines, all injectable analgesics should be maintained in a locked and inventoried environment.

PRINCIPLES OF WOUND CLOSURE

Avoiding tension on the wound edges is one of the keys to good wound closure. Closing a wound too tightly reduces the blood supply to the edges of the wound and inhibits the body's own defenses against infection. Tight sutures, rough handling of the wound, and crushing forces from forceps or retractors contribute to this phenomenon. Direct undermining, detaching the skin from the underlying fascia and advancing the skin, often permits closure of the wound with little tension (Fig. 31–1). In the preoperative evaluation, pinching the skin to see if the skin slides together easily in the area of the planned incision estimates the laxity of the

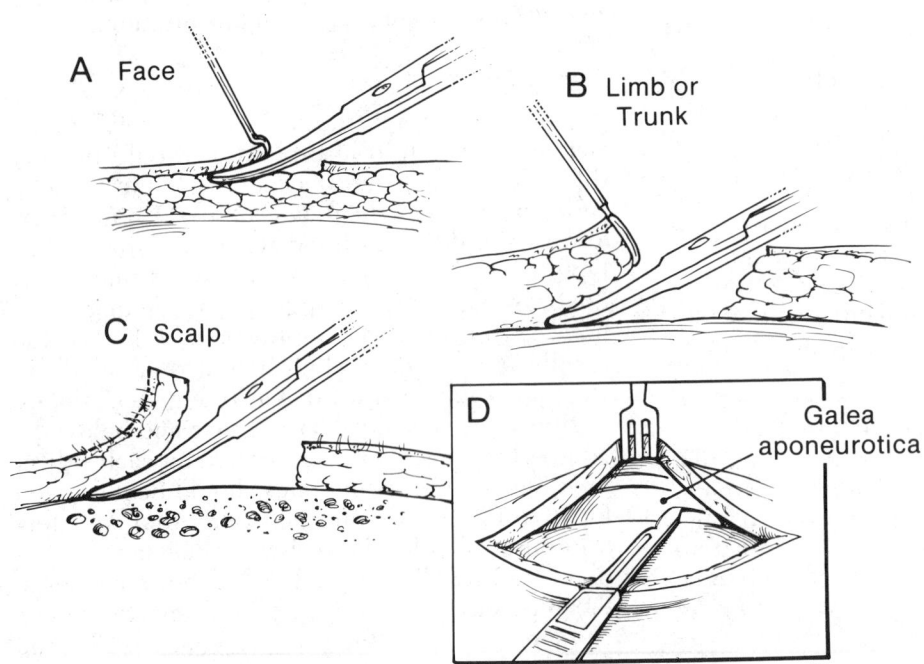

FIGURE 31–1. Undermining tissue adjacent to the incision can relieve tension of wound edges. On the face, tissue is undermined just under the dermal level (A). Undermining below the subcutaneous tissue and above the muscle fascia is appropriate for the limbs and trunk (B).

A Face

B Limb or Trunk

C Scalp

D   Galea aponeurotica

© Baylor College of Medicine 1988

skin. If skin laxity is not sufficient to allow wound closure even with undermining of the edges, consider flaps, V-Y plasty, skin grafting, or other procedures.

Most wound infections occur not from gross contamination but as a result of wound edges drawn together too tightly, reducing blood supply at the edges of the wound and thus inhibiting the body's own defenses against infection. Generally, pressures greater than 30 mm Hg on any wound cause delayed healing as a result of interference with capillary blood flow. Vascularity of the operative area influences wound healing also. Areas of greater vascularity tolerate greater tension on the wound edges. The skin of the face and upper trunk tolerates greater tension than does that of the lower extremities, which have a poorer blood supply. Tissue pressures equal to or greater than mean arterial pressure stop blood circulation in the skin completely, causing skin necrosis. Another important factor, the age of the patient, affects how much tension the skin tolerates. Children's skin tolerates greater wound tension than the skin of geriatric patients.

Accurate approximation of all layers assures optimal wound closure. Good lighting of the wound surface, as well as comfortable positions for both patient and surgeon, plays a paramount role in achieving this goal. The use of small instruments helps avoid excessive injury to cells. Damaged and dead cells provide a culture medium for bacteria.

For most wounds, a simple one-layered closure suffices. In areas of increased skin tension, closure may require several layers. However, a layered closure requires fascia or thick dermis to allow the placement of a deeper layer of sutures. Fat contains very little fibrous tissue and holds sutures for only a few hours. Sutures only draw the wound edges together. In wound healing, it is collagen, not sutures, that provides true permanent wound adhesion. This invalidates the concept of permanent sutures holding tissue together.

The type of suture is less important than the principles of its use. Sutures applied too tightly cut through the skin, enlarge the tunnel, and form a small scar at right angles to the incision. These scars at right angles to the incision are known as "cross hatching" or "railroad tracks." Ideally, a suture should not leave a permanent external mark. If a wound requires leaving sutures in place more than 3 or 4 days, use a buried stitch. External sutures left in place more than 3 to 4 days result in cross hatching around the suture. For wounds about the face, use synthetic material with external interrupted or continuous sutures. Facial wounds with very little tension permit sutures removal in 3 to 4 days and the application of adhesive strips. A buried subcuticular absorbable suture with adhesive strips on the surface provides better cosmetic result for the trunk and extremities, where sutures must be left longer.

Physicians should place sutures at right angles to the skin so that the skin edges evert. Sutures placed too shallow form an inversion of the skin edge. Using interrupted sutures permits better control over the approximation of the wound edges (Fig. 31–2). However, interrupted sutures consume more time, both in placing the suture and removing the suture. In areas of thin skin—for example, on the eyelid or periauricular area, where approximation of the dermis is less important—an external continuous suture provides adequate wound closure. Sutures of synthetic material will evoke less reaction in the skin, making them more useful for external sutures. A continuous stitch allows easier removal. A cut in the center allows a pull on each end to remove the entire stitch. With individual sutures, swelling may bury the knot, which complicates suture removal, especially in children.

A subcuticular suture placed in the dermis under the skin may remain there. Synthetic absorbable sutures rarely cause a long-term problem. Permanent nonabsorbable suture proves less useful because it eventually loses its effectiveness or becomes visible or palpable. Subcuticular sutures stay in place for weeks to months before dissolving and provide good tensile strength. A subcuticular sutures leaves no suture marks, so it proves most useful in the extremities or trunk, where sutures must be left in place for up to 3 weeks. Using subcuticular sutures in children proves advisable because suture removal in pediatric patients can turn out to be a challenging experience.

Staples provide excellent skin approximation and give evidence of low tissue reaction. Staples prove especially useful on the hair-bearing scalp, where suture marks do not form. Use of staples in other areas sometimes causes permanent scars from the puncture wounds. For small wounds, regular sutures usually give better results (Pories and Thomas, 1985).

Wound Healing in Geriatric Patients

The skin of geriatric patients requires special consideration in wound closure. Skin thins as it ages. Changes associated with thinning of the skin include (1) flattening of the dermoepidermal junction, (2) loss of dermal and subcutaneous mass, (3) shortened capillary loops, and (4) a decrease in the number of enzymatically active melanocytes. As a result, open wounds contract more slowly, and incised wounds gain strength more slowly. Cellular proliferation, wound metabolism, and collagen remodeling occur later in older skin than in younger skin (Gilchrest, 1982).

Other conditions found in the elderly may also affect wound healing. Any condition causing poor microvascular circulation, poor tissue oxygenation, or poor nutrition also impairs wound healing in the

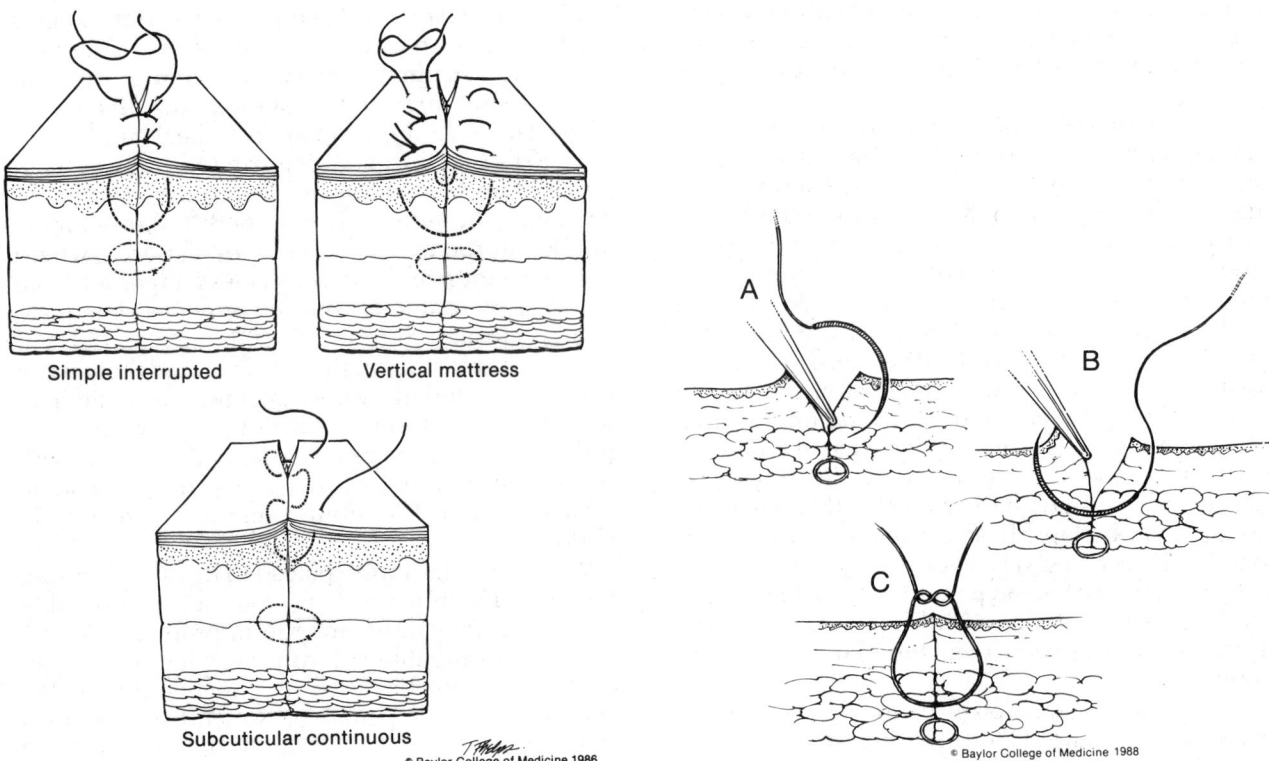

FIGURE 31–2. Skin suture methods. The simple interrupted suture is inserted with the needle entering the skin at an angle of 90 degrees or greater *(A)*. This allows sufficient subcutaneous tissue to be included to encourage eversion of skin edges *(B)*. The needle should exit with the same amount of tissue on each side of the suture *(C)*.

elderly. Hyperglycemia retards wound healing in the same manner as in younger patients (Orgill and Demling, 1988).

Sutures and staples sometime give less than ideal cosmetic results when used on geriatric skin. Both sutures and staples tend to pull through or tear the thin skin, especially if wound edges are under tension. Sutures may cause increased skin damage and necrosis because of decreased circulation in the thin skin. Closure with microporous adhesive strips offers a better alternative to closure with sutures or staples (Goodson and Hunt, 1979). For excision of lesions, simply undermining the skin and closing the wound with microporous adhesive strips suffices to ensure good wound closure and healing. More complicated excisions may require special techniques such as V-Y plasty using microporous adhesive strips. The V-Y plasty serves as a useful technique especially in V-shaped lacerations occurring over the anterior tibia, the dorsum of the hand, and both surfaces of the forearm. Microporous adhesive strips can prove useful in closing more complicated wounds, such as T-shaped wounds. After coapting wound edges with adhesive strips, covering the wounds with a gel paste dressing or a hydrocolloid occlusive dressing (DuoDerm, Convatec, or Teguderm) promotes faster healing and lessens pain.

OFFICE SURGICAL PROCEDURES

The extent and complexity of in-office surgical procedures are primarily a function of the desires and training of the individual practitioner. The following procedures represent the most commonly performed procedures in the office setting. The following brief descriptions present one, but not the only, method of performing the procedure in the office.

Incision and Drainage

The incision and drainage of cutaneous collections of purulent material is an extremely common procedure. Cutaneous abscesses—for example, boils, pilonidal abscesses, and infected sebaceous cysts—are very commonplace, often presenting in an acute stage of inflammation and infection.

Cutaneous abscesses present with redness, swelling, tenderness, and warmth. An area of induration extends well beyond the actual area of purulent material. Fluctuance, or the softening of the central area of skin infection, is the easiest means by which to localize the area requiring drainage. Unless an area of fluctuance is present, drainage should be deferred and the patient placed on appropriate antibiotics and applications of local warm compresses until the infection localizes. The drainage can be performed during a subsequent visit, if needed. Often, this treatment causes the infection to localize and drain spontaneously, thus obviating the need for surgical therapy.

If the collection of pus or fluid requires surgical drainage, the site should be prepared by applying EMLA Cream as an anesthetic. The skin then is painted with povidone-iodine solution. (Local infiltration with xylocaine is uniformly unrewarding because the local pH of the infected tissue causes deactivation of the anesthetic agent.) After the skin is prepped with antibiotic paint, the area is draped with sterile towels, and the area of maximum fluctuance is incised using a no. 11 blade scalpel. Care must be taken to incise completely the skin overlying the area of fluctuance. The incision must not be continued into the indurated, nonfluctuant tissue. Samples for culture and sensitivity tests always should be obtained for any purulent material present. The cavity then is irrigated with a mixture of sterile water and hydrogen peroxide, mixed 50:50. After the cavity appears relatively clean, it is irrigated with 1:2 strength povidone-iodine solution and packed with iodoform gauze. It is NOT necessary to digitally disrupt loculations within the abscess cavity. The area is covered with a gauze dressing and the patient is given a prescription for an appropriate analgesic. The patient is instructed to keep the area dry for 48 hours and remove the dressing with the gauze packing while in the shower. Soap and water usually suffice to keep the wound site clean, and a dry dressing absorbs most drainage that occurs. The patient should return to the office 1 week after the procedure for follow up (Pories and Thomas, 1985; Zacarian, 1985).

Skin Surgery

The skin, being the largest organ of the body, is also the most frequent site of surgical therapy. Both diagnostic (biopsy) and therapeutic (excision) modalities are employed, and most are amenable to the office environment.

Skin Biopsy

The biopsy of skin lesions can be performed in many different fashions, depending on the type and location of the lesion. Raised, small lesions usually warrant shave biopsy. The physician should apply EMLA Cream or inject local anesthetic before prepping the area with povidone-iodine solution. Using a no. 15 blade scalpel, shave off the protruding mass of tissue flush with the skin surface (Fig. 31–3). Direct pressure, electrocautery, silver nitrate, or a combination of these methods usually achieves hemostasis. Typically, shave biopsies do not require a suture. After completion of the procedure, application of an antibiotic ointment and a Band-Aid suffices to allow the patient to go home. Routine cleansing of the site with soap and water can begin the following day. The physician should send the specimen for microscopic analysis, and, if desired, send a small portion for culture, Gram's stain, or other studies.

For lesions too large to allow complete removal in the office, the incisional biopsy technique is utilized. This technique involves routine skin preparation and appropriate local or topical anesthesia, followed by making an elliptical incision beginning on the surface of the lesion, extending across the border of the lesion onto normal skin, and returning to the origin of the incision (Fig. 31–4). The incision must extend through the skin surface and the dermis and terminate at the uppermost level of subcutaneous fat. The specimen should have roughly equal length of pathologic and normal skin. The width of the incision should not be so large as to make closure difficult. Direct pressure controls bleeding in most cases, and coapting the skin edges frequently terminates oozing. Interrupted sutures of 3-0 to 4-0 nylon or polypropylene accomplishes adequate closure. Soap and water

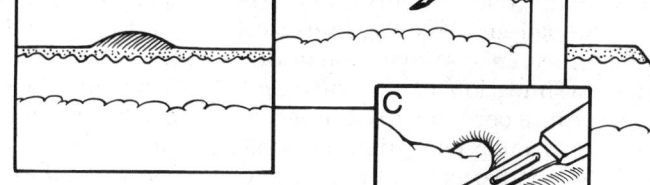

FIGURE 31–3. Technique of shave biopsy (see text for description).

© Baylor College of Medicine 1989

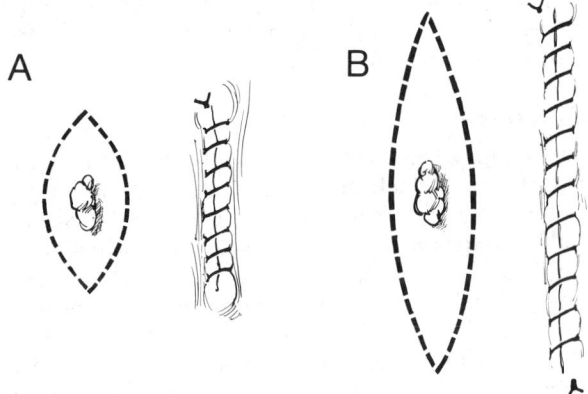

FIGURE 31–4. Excision of a lesion with a short ellipse forms dog ears at the end of the wound (*A*). A length-to-width ratio of 4:1 allows for good approximation of the wound without bunching at the ends (*B*).

usually provides sufficient wound care, and acetaminophen or ibuprofen usually proves adequate for analgesia. Depending on the location of the lesion, a return visit to the office for suture removal should occur in 5 to 10 days. Excisional biopsy is performed in the same manner as incisional biopsy, except that the lesion is small enough to allow an elliptical incision completely around it, thus allowing total removal. The area of excision must include a rim of normal skin measuring approximately 5 mm in width if the lesion is suspicious for malignancy (Pories and Thomas, 1985; Zacarian, 1985).

Lacerations

Lacerations are traumatic incisions of the skin and can vary from simple to complex. *Simple lacerations* are relatively small, clean, straight, and shallow. These lesions are easy to clean, anesthetize, and repair. This type of laceration also has a very low risk of infection. *Complex lacerations* are long and irregular in shape and involve structures below the subcutaneous tissue. These have a much higher risk of infection resulting from outside contamination and possible vascular compromise of the wound edges. The mechanism of injury resulting in a laceration is often emotionally stressful to the patient, especially if a child. The physician may need to spend extra time reassuring the patient and relieving the patient's anxiety. Preservation of function and appearance, prevention of further contamination or infection of the site, and control of bleeding require correct management of a laceration. When repairing a laceration, remember that the goal is to remove contamination and nonviable tissue to allow the simplest repair possible.

REPAIR OF SIMPLE LACERATIONS. Initially, simple lacerations should be irrigated copiously using sterile saline solution. Then, the wound is anesthetized with infiltration of a local anesthetic solution.

After the wound is anesthetized, the laceration and surrounding skin are scrubbed gently with an antibacterial soap such as povidone-iodine or chlorhexidine. The wound is inspected for any loose tissue or debris, which is removed gently with forceps. The wound is painted with a solution of povidone-iodine or chlorhexidine and the area draped with sterile towels. If the skin edges permit easy approximation without significant tension, the wound is closed in a single layer using monofilament 3-0 or 4-0 nonabsorbable suture in either a simple or interrupted mattress fashion. Lesions on the face require closure with monofilament 5-0 or 6-0 nonabsorbable suture in an interrupted simple fashion. Do not use mattress sutures on the face. Lacerations on the extremities or trunk also repair easily using one of the many types of surgical skin staplers now available. After the completion of wound repair, antibiotic ointment and a dry bandage can be applied. Home care of the wound consists of routine bathing; a dry dressing is applied only if clothing irritates the lesion. After removing sutures or staples, tincture of benzoin and adhesive strips are applied over the site to relieve tension on wound edges. Ibuprofen usually provides adequate postrepair analgesia. Occasionally, adequate pain relief may necessitate using acetaminophen with codeine. Note that direct pressure to the wound before closure readily controls most nonpulsatile bleeding from lacerations. Wound repair rarely requires reapproximating the subcutaneous tissue as a separate layer. If significant pulsatile bleeding occurs, direct pressure should be applied to the wound and more expert surgical consultation obtained. The physician should never attempt blindly to clamp a bleeding site in the depth of a wound. Inadvertent nerve, vascular, or tissue damage may occur.

REPAIR OF COMPLEX LACERATIONS. Complex lacerations often extend deep below the subcutaneous tissue and may involve fascia, muscle, nerves, ligaments, and tendons. If a question of nerve or tendon involvement exists, appropriate specialty consultation should be obtained before proceeding with the repair. The general principle in closure of a complex laceration is to convert it to a simple laceration. Initial cleansing, anesthesia, and wound preparation are the same as for a simple laceration. The wound then is closed in layers, starting with the deepest layer. Muscle tissue does not retain suture well, so the fascia over the muscle is usually the deepest layer of the closure. The fascia is coapted using absorbable 2-0 or 3-0 suture, preferably chromic or polyglycolic acid (Vicryl/Dexon). After closure of one layer, the next layer is irrigated with sterile saline. If the subcutaneous layer requires separate closure, a 3-0 or 4-0 absorbable suture is employed. The skin is closed with monofilament nonabsorbable suture or with skin staples. Wound care is the same as for repair of a simple laceration.

SPECIAL SITUATIONS IN LACERATION REPAIR. In cases of extreme patient anxiety or if the patient is an agitated child, lack of patient cooperation may compromise the repair of the laceration. In this instance, the physician should consider using mild sedation before repair. In the adult, a combination of nalbuphine, 1 to 15 mg, and midazolam, 2 to 5 mg, given intravenously can provide excellent sedation, allowing a more controlled approach to repair of the laceration. In children, midazolam, 0.1 to 0.15 mg/kg, combined with fentanyl citrate, 1 to 2 μg/kg, intravenously will give good sedation and amnesia. Physicians should avoid the use of the old "lytic cocktail" (meperidine/promethazine/chlorpromazine) because of the possibility of significant untoward effects (e.g., extrapyramidal symptoms, respiratory arrest, and dyskinesia). The complex laceration may require débridement to allow good approximation and to minimize scarring. Débridement entails removal of devitalized tissue at the wound edges and in deeper layers if necessary. Sometimes ragged or severely contused tissue at the wound edges requires excision to obtain a straight, viable edge to approximate. Wounds with large amounts of avulsed or absent tissue may necessitate referral to other physicians, such as plastic surgeons, more experienced in complicated wound closure. Undermining the wound edges at the time of closure may relieve tension on the skin. Using tissue scissors or a scalpel and incising along the layer separating the dermis from the subcutaneous tissue undermines the wound edges. This maneuver may result in a temporary increase in bleeding. This bleeding usually responds to direct pressure, resulting in skin reapproximation without tension. If the incision requires undermining, the physician must be sure to undermine both sides and each end of the incision.

Surgery of the Nail and Digits

Surgical procedures involving the toenails, fingernails, and digits are a common occurrence in the family physician's practice and involve only a few conditions.

Subungual Hematoma

This condition usually results from a crushing injury involving the compression of the distal phalanx of a digit. A hematoma develops between the nailbed and the nail, causing significant pressure, discomfort, and pain. The diagnosis is made based on history and simple visual inspection of the affected digit. The nailbed has a dark purple to black discoloration. Treatment consists of nailbed decompression and relief of the pressure symptoms. This can be accomplished by any of several simple methods:

1. Drilling a hole in the nail with a special drill device.

2. Melting a hole in the nail with a heated paper clip or hot-loop cautery device.
3. Drilling a hole in the nail with a no. 15 scalpel blade.

The special nail drill instrument is very effective but more expensive than the other methods. Melting a hole in the nail and drilling a hole in the nail are also effective, and certainly less expensive. After hematoma evacuation, relief of pain occurs almost immediately and the nail requires no further treatment.

Fungal Infections (Onychomycosis)

Most fungal infections of the nail do not require surgical therapy. Instead, most onychomycoses respond at least 50 to 60 per cent of the time to oral griseofulvin or ketoconazole therapy when used for 6 to 12 months. Combining topical therapy (Halotex drops, Loprox solution) to oral therapy sometimes hastens improvement. However, should conservative measures fail, removal of the affected nail and its nail matrix may be the only solution. First, a digital block is used to anesthetize the digit, then a rubber band tourniquet is applied just distal to the metacarpophalangeal joint of the digit. The digit is prepped using povidone-iodine solution and the area draped to give a more sterile work field. After verifying anesthesia, a closed hemostat is inserted under the front edge of the nail. A spreading motion of the instrument is used to loosen the nail from the nailbed. The nail then is grasped with the clamp and disrupted from the nail matrix using traction and a side-to-side motion. Direct pressure usually controls minor oozing. If needed, the nail matrix can be ablated using silver nitrate sticks. The tourniquet then is released and direct pressure applied to stop any further oozing. After controlling the oozing, antibiotic ointment is applied, followed by wrapping the area with a piece of petrolatum gauze and applying a tube-gauze dressing. The patient should remove the dressing after 48 hours and begin soaking the foot in clear, warm water three times daily for 15 minutes. For dressings after 48 hours, a small amount of antibiotic ointment should be applied and the area covered with a Band-Aid. If a toenail is involved, closed shoes should be avoided for 7 to 10 days after the procedure. A prescription of a mild analgesic usually suffices for pain control during the first 48 hours following the procedure. The operating physician should re-evaluate the patient in the office in 7 to 10 days. Complete healing usually occurs over 4 to 6 weeks.

Ingrown Toenail

Ingrown toenail is an infection involving the lateral and distal aspect of the nailbed. It usually occurs as a result of trauma or inappropriate trimming of the nail. If seen early, most cases respond to antibiotics, soaks, and local manipulation of the affected side of the toe. The nail must grow beyond the end of the nailbed in order to trim it straight across from side to side. If local measures and antibiotics are ineffective, then the nail requires partial or complete excision. Partial excision is a more complex procedure than complete removal of the nail, and over time usually proves to be an inadequate procedure. Therefore, if a patient has a severe infection or has had multiple, recurring episodes, then complete nail excision offers complete and permanent therapy with a single procedure. The procedure is identical to that described under Fungal Infections, except that the operating physician must remove all granulation tissue and hypertrophic material, either with a curette or by using cautery ablation. Postprocedure care and follow up are identical to that described previously.

Paronychia

Paronychia is an infection (usually staphylococcus) involving the cuticle of the nail. The infection may involve the entire cuticle, but sometimes localizes into an abscess. Treatment of this condition usually is successful using warm soaks and antibiotics, with the lesion either resolving or "pointing" and draining spontaneously. If pain or abscess size are significant, the paronychia may require surgical drainage of the purulent material.

Physicians obtain optimal drainage by establishing digital anesthetic block of the affected digit, followed by povidone-iodine skin preparation. A no. 11 blade scalpel is used to incise and drain the area of fluctuance. The scalpel should parallel the nail at the point of most fluctuance. Providing relief usually does not require an extensive incision, and the release of even a small amount of pus can bring significant relief. The patient should continue soaks and antibiotics after drainage of the abscess. Office follow-up in 7 to 10 days is appropriate (Pories and Thomas, 1985).

Felon

Felon is an infection involving the palmar aspect of the distal phalanx. Frequently, these are very painful as a result of the accumulation of purulent material in a closed space. Treatment consists of institution of oral antibiotics followed by drainage of the pus. Drainage is accomplished by employing a digital anesthetic block and prepping the skin with povidone-iodine. Then an incision is made with a no. 11 blade knife on the side of the inflamed area. The incision should *not* be made on the palmar aspect of the digit pad. Usually, a single incision is adequate. Physicians should avoid the classic "fish mouth" incision extending from side to side across the front of the pad because this causes significant scarring and permanent tactile dysfunction. A small wick of iodoform gauze inserted at the point of drainage and left in place for 24 to 48 hours enhances continued drainage. After removal of the wick, warm soaks are begun to increase local

circulation and aid in healing. A tube gauze dressing applied immediately after drainage usually suffices to control further bleeding or drainage. Follow-up in 7 to 10 days is sufficient (Pories and Thomas, 1985).

Hemorrhoids

Most patients consider hemorrhoids to be a bothersome condition associated with anal irritation and constipation. In actuality, hemorrhoids are normal venous pads or cushions that line the anal canal. These vascular cushions normally assist in defecation, and they work with the neuromuscular reflexes of the anal sphincters. In the process of normal stool elimination, the hemorrhoidal veins swell slightly while guiding the stool out of the rectum and across the anus. With constipation, the straining required to effect elimination causes significant elevation of the venous pressure in the hemorrhoidal veins, causing abnormal distention. Chronic constipation often results in recurrent and permanent distention of the hemorrhoidal veins. This distention can cause secondary symptoms such as bleeding, itching, pain, mucus discharge, prolapse, and thrombosis. The hemorrhoidal veins lying above the pectinate line (mucocutaneous border) in the anal canal are the internal hemorrhoids, and those lying below the pectinate line are the external hemorrhoids.

Internal Hemorrhoids

The most common symptom associated with internal hemorrhoid irritation is painless rectal bleeding. The blood usually occurs on the outside of the stool, but blood may present mixed with the stool or even drip into the commode water. The bleeding is usually bright red and not of significant volume, although the first episode can be very disconcerting to the patient. Occasionally, patients notice blood only on the toilet tissue. If internal hemorrhoids become significantly engorged, a condition called prolapse can occur. In this situation, the mass of dilated hemorrhoidal tissue protrudes across the anal sphincters with defecation. In some cases, manual reduction of the tissue is necessary. Dilated internal hemorrhoids are usually painless because the mucosal tissue above the pectinate line contains minimal innervation.

Treatment of internal hemorrhoid irritation is initially medical. A regimen of psyllium, Proctofoam-HC (for 10 days only), and Tucks pads is effective for over 90 per cent of patients. The patient needs counseling about the benefits of a high-fiber diet and adequate oral fluid intake in order to avoid constipation. The use of Proctofoam-HC is superior to suppositories because the foam has a much more intense local effect, and it will not migrate as do suppositories. (Reverse peristalsis can pull a suppository from the rectum into the duodenum).

The Tucks pads promote better hygiene and add a soothing aspect to the anal area. This "triple combination" can even help resolve some cases of prolapsing hemorrhoids if the patient is compliant. If medical therapy fails, the patient may require surgical relief. Banding is an easily accomplished office procedure if one has the appropriate equipment. The area of interest is visualized via an anoscope, and the hemorrhoid is grasped with the banding instrument. One or two small rubber bands are applied near the base of the hemorrhoid. In a few days, the tissue distal to the rubber bands becomes necrotic and sloughs in the stool. Some small amount of bleeding may occur. This procedure is for internal hemorrhoids only because presence of cutaneous nerve endings on external hemorrhoids make the application of rubber bands extremely painful.

Other methods employed to treat internal hemorrhoid disease include infrared photocoagulation, cryotherapy, and sclerotherapy. Infrared photocoagulation involves the exposure of the hemorrhoid to intense local infrared light that causes the lesion to thrombose and slough. This technique, although effective, results in a foul discharge, tissue slough, and more bleeding than in the banding procedure. The infrared generator and applicator probes are also very expensive. Cryotherapy utilizes liquid nitrogen applied topically to the hemorrhoid by direct application or spray application. The result is similar to that of the infrared therapy. Sclerotherapy involves submucosal injection of a caustic solution to cause inflammation and edema, thus compressing the venous lumen and possibly causing thrombosis. Tissue slough and some increased bleeding also occur with this technique. The operating physician must obtain special training before attempting sclerotherapy because of the expertise required. It bears repeating that, except in special circumstances, medical management of internal hemorrhoid irritation provides better relief.

External Hemorrhoids

The most common complaint associated with external hemorrhoid irritation is pain. The most common presentation of external hemorrhoid irritation is that of thrombosis. The thrombosed external hemorrhoid appears as a firm, purple–red or dark blue, tender nodule lying at the very outer edge of the anus. The patient is usually noticeably uncomfortable. The physician almost inevitably elicits a history of recent or frequent constipation. It also is not unusual that patients with symptomatic external hemorrhoids also will have internal hemorrhoidal dilation. The optimal treatment for a thrombosed external hemorrhoid is again medical. The regimen should be the same as that for internal hemorrhoids with two simple additions. EMLA Cream or benzocaine ointment (Nupercainal) can provide local pain relief. The patient needs to take very warm sitz baths at least four times daily until the pain has resolved. Physicians should avoid the practice of performing incision and drainage or unroofing of a thrombosed external hemorrhoid with removal of the thrombus. The pain relief from such a procedure is minimal, and significant bleeding and infection may occur after the procedure. Many surgeons believe that allowing the thrombus to undergo autolysis while affording pain relief is a better and safer alternative. Once the thrombus has lysed, the edema and induration resolve very rapidly.

Gynecologic Office Surgery

The management of gynecologic surgical problems in the office is an important aspect of office surgery. The procedures presented here are those most frequently encountered in the family physician's office practice.

Bartholin's Gland Cyst or Abscess

This lesion arises as a result of blockage of the duct draining the affected Bartholin's gland. This blockage is usually the result of infection or trauma but also might occur as a postsurgical change. The purpose of therapy is to decompress the engorged gland, control infection, and return the gland to normal function. The use of a Word catheter is the simplest method to employ. With the patient in the dorsal lithotomy position and after application of EMLA Cream, the area of swelling is painted with povidone-iodine solution. The physician makes a stab wound in the cyst or abscess using a no. 11 blade scalpel. Next the fluid and pus that may be present are evacuated and cultured. Then, the Word catheter is inserted and the balloon inflated to a volume of 2 to 3 mL using water or saline. The catheter should remain in place for 3 to 4 weeks to allow a well-epithelialized tract to form and to allow drainage after the catheter removal. The patient should abstain from intercourse until after the catheter removal. Marsupialization of the cyst involves a more complicated procedure in which the top of the cyst cavity is incised and the contents drained. The physician then sutures the edges of the cyst lining to the surrounding normal vaginal mucosa using absorbable suture. This procedure requires significantly more equipment, light, assistants, and anesthesia, and may need to be performed in an outpatient surgery setting rather than the office. Excision of the cyst is even more complex and may require referral to a gynecologist. Before performing any gynecologic procedure, be sure to obtain signed informed consent from the patient.

Cervical Biopsy

Uses of cervical biopsy include investigation of lesions found during routine pelvic exam or investigation of the abnormal Papanicolaou (Pap) smear. Cervical biopsies frequently occur during performance of colposcopy. Obtaining appropriate signed consent is mandatory. This procedure requires no anesthesia. With the patient in the dorsal lithotomy position, the speculum is inserted and the cervix visualized. A Pap smear then is obtained in a routine fashion. After the Pap smear, Lugol's solution is applied to the cervix and any areas that do not stain a dark brown or black are biopsied. Appropriate biopsy forceps are used to obtain specimens from the center of each unstained area, as well as the border area of unstained and stained regions of each suspicious lesion. Biopsies are obtained from the anterior, posterior, and both lateral lips of the cervix. All specimens are placed in separate specimen containers and forwarded for tissue analysis. Usually bleeding responds to direct pressure with a temporary packing, and the patient is allowed to go home with a tampon in place. She should refrain from intercourse for 1 week, and then be followed up in the office.

Endometrial Biopsy or Aspiration

Before proceeding with an endometrial biopsy or aspiration, the operating physician first should determine pregnancy status and document appropriate clinical indications. As with most other office procedures, appropriate informed consent is mandatory. If the patient has not had a Pap smear within the past year, one should be obtained now. The uterine sound is inserted gently through the cervical os to determine the depth and position of the uterine cavity. If the cervical canal is stenotic and requires dilation, a paracervical block is performed first using 1% lidocaine without epinephrine. Proceed gently with cervical dilation. After accomplishing adequate dilation, insert an appropriate aspiration device (Vabra, Karman, Vacutage). Methodically passing the cannula back and forth within the endometrial cavity while slowly advancing the cannula in a rotational manner around the entire cavity usually produces an adequate sample. The patient may experience some cramping or a pressure sensation, but this abates within minutes after cessation of the procedure. Once collected, the specimen is placed in fixative and sent for analysis. After the patient is observed to be sure no excessive bleeding occurs, she can go home with instructions to use ibuprofen or a similar medication for cramps or pain. She should refrain from intercourse for 1 week, then she should be followed up in the office.

Office Procedures on the Female Breast

As an entry point to the health care system, the family physician should take a very active role in screening of female patients for breast disease.

During the screening process, some patients will be found to have glandular pathology of the breast. The more common lesions and their treatment are presented here (Baker and Niederhuber, 1992; Isaacs, 1992).

Lump in the Breast

Patients discover over 50 per cent of abnormal breast lumps. The evaluation of a questionable tumor of the breast should be thorough and precise. History is extremely important in this evaluation process. Age of menarche, number of pregnancies, hormone use, caffeine intake, breast trauma, breast-feeding history, family history of first-degree relatives with breast cancer, smoking history, dietary history, nipple discharge, skin changes, and time of last menstrual period are all important aspects to investigate in determining the patient's risk for breast malignancy. Physical examination of the suspicious area should be thorough and meticulous. Size of the lesion, characteristics of the margins, shape, and mobility of the lesion are all important physical findings. Benign or cystic lesions often appear as round, well-circumscribed, firm, mobile, and sharply bordered. In contrast, malignant lesions usually appear flat or thickened, hard, and irregularly or indistinctly bordered. Benign fibrous lesions present as thick, rubbery, mobile, and irregularly but usually distinctly bordered. Presence or absence of tenderness of the lesion is no indicator of malignant potential. Although 85 per cent of breast lesions are benign, a high index of suspicion for malignancy is necessary, regardless of the age of the patient. All female patients should receive instruction in monthly breast self-exam, which they should perform on the same day of each month, irrespective of their menstrual cycles. The breast consistency should remain essentially unchanged at each exam because the monthly hormonal changes will be the same at the same day each month. The patient must pick a day she can remember easily from month to month and perform her exam on that day.

BREAST CYST. Cystic lesions of the breast are very common and can occur at any age before menopause. The size is completely variable, and tenderness may or may not be present. Cysts sometimes regress during the monthly menstrual cycle and sometimes will spontaneously disappear.

FIBROADENOMA OF THE BREAST. This benign lesion usually occurs during pregnancy or in younger patients. The lesion is firm, rubbery, well circumscribed, mobile, and sometimes large. This type of lesion often will regress after completion of pregnancy, but sometimes it only decreases in size. The lesion is usually nontender and over time will slowly fibrose and sometimes develop small calcifications within it.

BREAST ABSCESS. This lesion usually occurs after trauma to the breast. The lesion sometimes presents as a complication of attempted intravenous drug abuse. Redness, induration, pain, and possible fluctuance are present, and the patient can be toxic. These patients sometimes require hospital admission and intravenous antibiotics. Treatment is the same as for any cutaneous abscess, and the response to therapy is usually prompt.

BREAST CANCER. Unless a patient has advanced local breast cancer, the diagnosis of malignancy on physical examination is very difficult. The classic "orange peel" skin changes signify late and advanced disease. Fortunately, this finding is rare in the routine family physician's practice today. Screening mammography allows early detection of even nonpalpable malignancies. This tool should serve as an adjunct to physical examination. Any patient with a breast tumor associated with ipsilateral axillary lymphadenopathy should be considered to have a malignancy until proven otherwise.

Management of the Breast Lump

The easiest method of evaluation of a breast lesion is via needle aspiration. This simple procedure usually does not require local anesthesia. After povidone-iodine preparation of the skin, the lesion is immobilized between the index and middle fingers of the nondominant hand. Then, a 20-gauge needle attached to a 10-mL syringe is inserted into the lesion. Loss of resistance usually indicates entry into a cyst cavity. When the needle tip lies approximately in the center of the lesion, aspiration is applied. If fluid returns, the lesion obviously is cystic and most often will resolve completely with aspiration. Any fluid obtained is prepared for Pap smear and routine cytology examinations. If no fluid returns on aspiration, several passes should be made into the lesion with suction applied to the syringe. On withdrawing the needle, any cellular material ejected from the needle is prepared for Pap smear evaluation. Fine-needle aspiration is a technique that employs an autoaspiration syringe and supplies very small samples for cytologic evaluation. The method of collection is the same as for routine needle aspiration. Remember that needle aspiration samples of breast lesions can be very difficult to analyze. We recommend using only pathologists with significant experience in this field. When performing any needle aspiration procedure, the physician must be cognizant that the chest wall is close to the breast lesion and that overly vigorous attempts at needle aspiration have resulted in pneumothorax.

Some office surgery texts describe the performance of actual open excisional biopsy in the family physician's office. We believe that, if open biopsy is indicated, the preferred procedure is a tylectomy ("lumpectomy"). If malignancy is discovered, the same surgeon can perform the requisite axillary dissection and assure that the specimen margins are clear of tumor. The performance of open breast biopsy usually necessitates more than local anesthesia. The intravenous sedation required often exceeds office safety standards. Hemostasis is often difficult. Adequate lighting and assistance may be unavailable. We believe that, if open biopsy becomes necessary, the hospital or outpatient surgery center settings and surgical referral presents a better alternative to the office procedure room.

Management of Fibrocystic Breasts

The fibrocystic changes in the female breast are mostly normal and not a disease. Fibrotic changes in the suspensory ligaments of the breast, as well as benign fibrotic changes and cyst formation, occur as a result of hormonal changes and inflammation, lactational changes after and during pregnancy, and sometimes because of exogenous hormone use (i.e., birth control pills). The nodularity of the breast also increases with age because, in the normal aging process, subcutaneous fat replaces normal breast parenchyma. Some authors have postulated that caffeine and other methylxanthine-containing foods, such as chocolate, exacerbate this syndrome of tender, nodular, fibrotic breasts. Smoking also may play an exacerbating role. The management is symptomatic, and utilizes nonsteroidal anti-inflammatory drugs whenever breast tenderness occurs. Patients always should wear a good supportive brassiere, and the use of daily vitamin E (400 I.U.) has been associated with less tenderness and nodularity in some patients. Some patients do not respond to conservative therapy, and further evaluation, such as determining serum prolactin levels, should occur. If levels are elevated, institute a trial of therapy with bromocryptine (Parlodel). In attempts to avoid surgery, testosterone-like drugs (Danazol) also may help, but the side effects usually are not well tolerated. In rare instances, the syndrome is so severe and the breasts so tender and nodular that adequate monthly examination is impossible. In this case, family physicians should obtain plastic surgery consultation for their patient to evaluate them for possible bilateral subcutaneous mastectomy with simultaneous implant reconstruction (Isaacs, 1992; Schwartz et al., 1994).

CRYOSURGERY

Cryosurgery is an extremely useful office procedure. Appropriately selected lesions allow simple and complete treatment without sutures, anesthesia, or significant preparation.

Principles and Equipment

The purpose of cryosurgery is to accomplish local destruction of a skin lesion by applying an intensely cold medium to the lesion, resulting in a partial-thickness thermal injury equivalent to frostbite. The most common freezing medium employed is liquid nitrogen, but devices using nitrous oxide and carbon dioxide are also available.

Liquid nitrogen is cheap, effective, and easy to apply. Keeping the material in a simple thermos-type bottle during use permits application using cotton swabs or ejector-type applicators (Cryac). In the office, storing the liquid nitrogen in a special container designed for liquid nitrogen storage allows periodic dispensing of small amounts for use. Companies supplying liquified gases also can supply the storage containers and maintain the supply for a moderate monthly charge. If nitrous oxide or carbon dioxide is chosen as the freezing agent, these require more expensive applicator units, especially if using gynecologic cryotherapy, because of the need for special applicator tips.

Evaluation of the Lesion

No specimen is obtained for histologic examination, so cryosurgery must be reserved for use in treating obviously benign lesions only. Any lesion suspicious for malignancy should be excised surgically and sent for pathologic analysis. Many common skin lesions, such as skin tags, seborrheic keratosis, actinic keratosis, verruca vulgaris, plantar warts, and benign pigmented nevi, are examples of lesions that are amenable to cryosurgery. Exercise caution when using cryosurgery involving the eyelids, nose, and genitalia.

Techniques

The use of liquid nitrogen applied via a device such as a Cryac applicator is the safest and most effective method. We prefer surgical excision of large lesions (areas greater than 1 cm) because this amount of tissue requires excessive application of agent to freeze the lesion completely. The liquid nitrogen is sprayed onto the lesion in a tangential fashion, aiming away from the physician. Treatment is continued until the lesion and a surrounding 1- to 2-mm area of normal skin become whitened and firm. The patient will experience a slight stinging or burning sensation initially. This is followed by an aching or burning sensation after the lesion rewarms and the whiteness disappears. The uncomfortable sensations continue while the vesicle forms. This discomfort should subside within a few hours after treatment. Using ibuprofen, as needed, provides sufficient analgesia. No skin preparation is required before application of the liquid nitrogen.

Follow-Up

Patients should be advised that the treated lesions will remain slightly red for 24 to 48 hours, during which time blister formation will occur. Patients should protect the blister until it drains spontaneously. If the blister fluid becomes green or turbid before drainage, the patient should contact the physician for evaluation. After the blister ruptures, the area should be allowed to dry normally. Patients should be instructed to leave the skin of the blister intact, keep the area clean with soap and water, and allow an eschar or scab to form normally. As the eschar falls away, so should the treated lesion. The entire sequence, from application of agent to resolution of the eschar, should take 10 to 14 days. Scarring is virtually absent, and smooth, clean skin is the usual result.

Some lesions only partially respond to the cryosurgery. If any or all of the lesion persists after 2 weeks, the patient should return for evaluation and possible re-treatment. If the lesion has not completely resolved after two treatments, surgical excision should be considered.

Summary

We should remember that cryosurgery is for use on lesions confined to the epithelium and dermis only. Subcutaneous lesions (lipoma, sebaceous cyst) are not candidates for this form of therapy. The gynecologic uses of cryosurgery require special applicators and different freezing agents and require more formal training in the use of these devices. If the slightest concern exists about malignancy in a lesion, cryosurgery should be deferred and a standard surgical excision performed to allow tissue analysis.

LASERS IN OFFICE SURGERY

The acronym Laser stands for light amplification by stimulated emission of radiation. The term now refers to the process by which light waves are amplified, and to the device that amplifies the light. The theory of stimulated emission comes from Einstein's work at the turn of the century. However, it was not until 1960 that Theodore Maiman developed the first ruby laser.

Laser light affects tissue through vaporization, photocoagulation, and sonic effects. The first two, vaporization and photocoagulation, refer to the conversion of radiant energy into heat. With vaporization, the conversion of radiant energy to heat occurs rapidly and intensely. The result is tissue temperatures well above the boiling point of water. Vaporization of tissue then occurs, allowing cutting in a finely focused manner similar to that with surgical steel blades. By using different power set-

TABLE 31–6. TYPES OF LASERS

Solid
  Ruby
  Neodymium: yttrium–aluminum–garnet (Nd:YAG)
Gas
  Carbon dioxide (CO_2)
  Argon–krypton
  Helium–neon
Liquid-dye
Semiconductor

tings and a more widely focused beam, tissue vaporization can debulk large amounts of tissue, such as condylomata accuminata. Photocoagulation, in contrast, results in much lower tissue temperatures, coagulating the tissues by the denaturation of protein and similar thermal processes. Photocoagulation produces necrosis of tissue but also produces hemostasis. Photoradiation therapy, a nonthermal event, occurs when a laser interacts with an exogenous or indigenous drug, resulting in a chemical reaction that produces a cytotoxic substance. The sonic effects of lasers produce membrane disruption and cell destruction (Fuller, 1984).

Four components make up a laser unit: (1) the active medium, (2) the excitation mechanism, (3) the feedback mechanism, and (4) the output coupler. The active medium that produces the laser action also gives the name for the device. The active medium can be a solid, a gas, a liquid, or a semiconductor. Table 31–6 shows the classification of the various lasers. The excitation mechanism creates the stimulation in the active medium. The excitation mechanism varies depending on the active medium. The feedback mechanism allows light waves to oscillate back and forth between mirrors. Light waves oscillating back and forth stimulate increasing energy in the active medium. One of the mirrors is partially transmissive and allows light to leave the feedback mechanism through that end. This partially transmissive mirror serves as the output coupler. Light leaving the output coupler then is transmitted to the target, either by mirrors or by fiberoptics. Lenses then can intensify or scatter the light to produce the desired effect (Ratz, 1986).

Lasers are classified by their output power and wavelength. The delivery of laser power varies from continuous levels of power (continuous wave, CW) to a single pulse or series of pulses called pulsed lasers. Most laser oscillators produce a beam too large for most surgical applications. This large beam typically produces insufficient energy intensity to vaporize or coagulate tissue effectively. Lenses placed in the beam of laser light focus the beam to an appropriate stop size. Using lenses provides a beam small enough to limit the size of the surgical incision and increase the effective use of the laser's power. This concentration of power, known as power density (PD), is of principle importance to the surgeon desiring to predict and control the effectiveness of the laser beam. Power density describes the measure of the power contained in a unit beam area, the number of watts per square centimeter (W/cm^2) (Ratz, 1986).

The ability to increase or decrease the PD by altering either the spot size or power carries great importance in laser surgery. Changing spot size or power determines the depth of penetration and the cutting properties of the laser beam. For example, the usual unfocused CO_2 laser without a lens produces a beam of approximately 1 mm in diameter. When set to deliver 10 watts of power (PD = 10 W/cm^2), the PD would be insufficient to vaporize tissue. Using a lens to focus the same 10-W laser beam to a 1.0-mm spot size produces a power density of approximately 1000 W/cm^2, enough to remove tissue rapidly by vaporization. Thus, changing the PD allows changes in the cutting properties of the laser beam (Ratz, 1986).

Safety Measures

Laser safety depends on precise knowledge of laser physics and laser tissue effects. Physicians desiring to use lasers in the office setting must attend a 1- to 2-day course that provides hands-on training before using or purchasing laser equipment. For hospital privileges, physicians must document adequate training. Laser safety depends on operator training and additional precautions not found in other routine office procedures. We describe some precautions for laser surgery here.

Wet cloth towels should be used around any CO_2 laser surgical field. The paper surgical drapes commonly used do not wet and will ignite easily with a stray laser beam. For additional safety, drapes and other flammable materials should be rewetted periodically.

The use of blackened instruments or glass bead–dusted instruments prevents full reflection of the laser beam should an accidental stray beam strike the instruments.

The use of any oil-containing compound should be avoided because these are combustible. Water-soluble solutions should be used on areas the surgeon desires to lase, because water and water-soluble compounds almost entirely absorb laser energy. The physician must ensure that the laser is always on "stand by" or "off" when lasing is not in progress. To prevent accidental discharge, the physician should avoid placing the foot on the foot pedal when not using the laser. Any smoke produced by the laser must be removed from the environment so patients, procedure room personnel, and the operating physician do not inhale the smoke. The smoke is probably mutogenic and/or carcinogenic. Additionally smoke impairs the vision of the operator. Smoke particles heat suction lines and can cause costly repairs. This mandates filters in the suction lines. Additionally, smoke is composed of flammable particles that may reflect the laser beam.

The safety of laser surgical procedures depends on the user's knowledge of the laser's effects on tissue. Using short spurts of energy increases laser safety. The physician should use the highest power and lowest time setting that is comfortable, and avoid continuous lasing by using rest periods. To prevent heat transfer to surrounding tissues, intermittent iced saline irrigation should be used (Mohr et al., 1984).

Basic Surgical Technique

Over the last 10 to 15 years major advances have occurred in cutaneous laser surgery. The majority of the original studies used the argon laser because these devices were more readily available to dermatologic surgeons than the CO_2 laser. Recent literature contains many articles about the use of CO_2 lasers for cutaneous surgery.

The CO_2 laser functions predominantly as a vaporizer, not a coagulator. The CO_2 laser works because water (85 per cent of living tissue) absorbs the energy of the beam. The energy then converts to heat and causes flash boiling of intracellular and extracellular water. Then, denaturation of tissue protein occurs and the cell explodes. Steam and cellular debris rise as a puff of smoke. The amount of destruction varies directly with the product of the duration of exposure and the power in watts. Vessels up to 0.5 mm seal as the tissue vaporizes. Defocusing the beam or decreasing the power permits sealing of vessels up to 2 mm. Both methods decrease power density. The use of lenses can focus a coherent, collimated, monochromatic light beam to a very tiny point, permitting thermally induced tissue destruction to occur with little damage to surrounding normal tissues. Histologically, the laser induces tissue necrosis in an area less than 0.1 mm adjacent to the laser incision. The zone of cellular damage varies from 0.3 mm to 0.5 mm, facilitating reduced scarring during the healing process. Using a defocused beam controls bleeding better than the focused beam. The operator may need to switch to another laser, such as the Nd:YAG or argon laser, to coagulate the bleeding tissue.

Training physicians to use lasers usually requires only 1 to 2 days. Physicians must learn the nuances of each type of laser used. The type of eye protection may vary according to the type of laser used. Training courses vary from 8-hour courses to 2-day comprehensive courses designed to offer training in advanced procedures such as CO_2 laser hemorrhoidectomy. Training in the use of lasers should be accomplished before purchasing of laser devices.

Currently, lasers cost more than most family physicians desire to spend. Although lasers increase the expense of office surgery, the increase in scope of practice may justify the expense. Prices should decrease as more companies enter the office laser surgery market (Mohr et al., 1984).

Refined Laser Techniques

Initially, lasers performed only conventional type procedures. The laser usage was the same as the scalpel blade, dermatologic curette, or electrocautery unit. Using lasers in this method obtained results that were not superior to those of conventional methods. Lasers in office surgery now offer refinements of older techniques and introduce additional techniques for the office surgery practice. These techniques, described by Kirshner (1984), provide useful additions to office surgery. Condylomata accuminata, tatoos, cervical intraepithelial neoplasia, and rhinophyma exemplify some expanded areas of office surgery offered by lasers.

Shave Biopsy

Shave biopsy with CO_2 laser ablation combines an older technique with laser technology. Only obviously benign lesions should be treated in this fashion. In this procedure, the area around the lesion is prepped carefully. The prep solution must be washed carefully from the operative site so there is no residual solution left, because many of the prep solutions contain alcohol that may catch fire when using the laser. The operative area is draped with towels thoroughly soaked in sterile saline to prevent combustion of the drapes by stray laser radiation. After the injection of local anesthetic in a circumferential manner, local anesthetic is injected below the lesion area so the area becomes slightly raised. Using a traditional scalpel blade, a superficial specimen is shaved for pathologic evaluation. Then the base of the shaved area is ablated with the CO_2 laser.

Laser Ablation

For ablation, the laser is used in a focused attitude except if a larger vessel in encountered. In this instance, a defocused laser beam is employed to achieve hemostasis. This method usually provides adequate hemostasis for the usually encountered cutaneous bleeders. Either intermittent or continuous-wave mode is acceptable depending on the choice of the operator. With experience, the physician utilizes the continuous mode more frequently, reducing the overall operative time. The photothermal peel, another technique for superficial lesions, serves as an alternative procedure to using conventional dermabrasion. Areas of superficial scarring, lentigo senilis, or seborrhic keratosis are examples of lesions treated by this technique.

This is another technique in which there must be no question about the benign nature of the lesion.

Laser Dermabrasion

As with all superficial techniques of this nature, such as dermabrasion or skin peel, the most suitable patient possesses lightly pigmented skin, such as those of Celtic origin. These patients with lightly pigmented skin suffer the least amount of pigment irregularity following the procedure. Patients with more deeply pigmented skin typically have less satisfactory results. The physician must proceed with extreme caution in those patients who have thin, atrophic skin. The thermal effects of laser radiation appear to inflict much greater damage on such skin. Using ice to cool the area of the procedure before surgery decreases the thermal effects.

The patient is prepped, draped, and locally anesthetized similarly to the procedure used for shave biopsy. Using a light handpiece, the beam is set in a focused or slightly defocused position. The physician then rapidly moves the laser handpiece back and forth over the affected area with a quick oscillating motion. Between each pass of the instrument over the area, a wet sponge or hydrogen peroxide is used to gently débride the superficial area. The oscillating motion must be very even to obtain a smooth result. The control of treatment depth with this procedure can be very precise. Physicians must practice this procedure technique in a laboratory-type setting until obtaining a secure feeling with the use of the instrument. The wattage setting for this procedure may vary, but in all cases the very low range should be used.

Following surgery, the patient is instructed to use a light application of antibiotic ointment three times daily. After 7 to 10 days, the eschar separates from the skin, leaving a slightly reddened skin surface resembling skin that has undergone a chemical peel.

Treatment of "Red Lesions"

Traditionally, the argon laser has been used extensively to treat "red lesions," a term that loosely groups such entities as port-wine nevi, hemangiomata, and arteriovenous malformations (Dolsky, 1984). CO_2 lasers also treat a number of red lesions (Kirschner, 1984).

To prevent changing the skin color, the physician should avoid povidone-iodine and prep the treatment area with 70% alcohol. Then the area is infiltrated with 1% lidocaine solution and washed with sterile saline to remove any vestige of the alcohol. If the area contains small vessels discernible with either the naked eye or a low-power loupe, treatment is directed to the vessels. If the area contains only vessels not discernible individually, a stippling technique is used in which the laser is applied intermittently to the entire area. The physician omits lasing small segments of cutaneous tissue between the areas irradiated with the laser. For this technique, a 0.2-mm spot size and a lightweight handpiece that directs the beam perpendicular to the surface are used. The duration of each exposure ranges from 1/20th to 1/10th of a second, and wattage settings may vary. Postoperatively, a light application of antibiotic ointment is used (Kirschner, 1984).

Tattoo Removal

Carbon dioxide lasers also can help ablate tattoos. The tattoo itself primarily determines the eventual degree of success in tattoo removal. The more professional the original tattoo, the better the possibility of successful cosmetic obliteration. With amateur tattoos, the depth and concentration of the pigment may be grossly irregular. This makes removal by any method a significantly more complicated prospect. Before beginning the procedure, the patient must be counseled carefully regarding the possibility of successful tattoo removal and alternate methods of treatment reviewed.

Tattoo removals usually require multiple treatment sessions. The number of treatment sessions depends on the size and quality of the tattoo, on the overall condition of the skin, and on individual healing characteristics. The surface to be treated is iced for 5 to 7 minutes before the procedure, allowing the tissues to cool and reducing the degree of thermal effect. The area then is prepped with 70% alcohol and infiltrated with 1% lidocaine with 1:100,000 epinephrine for local anesthesia. As with all other cutaneous laser procedures, sterile saline is used to wash the prep solution from the surface. The area is draped with towels saturated with normal saline solution. The CO_2 laser is used in a perpendicularly to the skin, working intermittently over heavily pigmented areas and sparing normal skin between applications. Laser settings vary from 10 to 14 watts and 1/20th to 1/10th of a second.

Keloid Removal

The CO_2 laser often allows successful removal of keloidal tissue. However, the laser may prove to be the offending instrument in producing some keloid. Thermal effects on the tissue may affect keloid production. A greater tendency toward keloid formation occurs when wattage settings are low and duration of exposure is high.

Use of the Laser as a Cutting Tool

The CO_2 laser used in the focused mode serves as an excellent cutting tool, controlling most small bleeders encountered in cutaneous surgery. Vessels up to 2 mm in diameter usually seal well with the defocused laser beam. This allows using the laser as a scalpel for cutaneous surgery, permitting the surgeon to work in an almost bloodless field using a "no-touch" technique with a high degree of accuracy.

Healing time benefits from manually removing the char in the underlying tissue that develops with laser surgery. Saline flushes or saline-soaked swabs remove the char satisfactorily. If excess char remains, serum accumulates in the area. The excess serum predisposes to development of subsequent problems (Kirschner, 1984).

Gynecologic Surgery

Treating cervical intraepithelial neoplasia (CIN) represents the most frequent reason for using CO_2 laser in gynecology. The treatment of CIN by the CO_2 laser is either by vaporization, excisional biopsy, or a combination of the two. The lesion must occur on the ectocervix without endocervical extension. The operating physician must visualize the entire abnormal transformation zone to exclude the invasive cancer. Patients treated in an ambulatory setting without anesthesia experience minimal cramping and heat discomfort.

For this technique, the laser is attached to the operating microscope. A plastic speculum with an attached smoke-evacuating tube is inserted into the vagina. The cervix is washed with a 3% acetic acid solution to identify all lesions. The transformation zone is outlined with a 3-mm margin. The laser is used in a continuous mode with 20 to 25-W output and less than 1-mm spot size; this attains power densities of approximately 4000 to 5000 W/ cm^2. If using a spot size of 2 mm, the power density ranges are much less. The physician should use the highest power density that can be controlled safely. To prevent furrowing, the beam is moved rapidly in horizontal, vertical, and diagonal directions, vaporizing the transformation zone to a measured depth of 5 to 7 mm. The patient is instructed to expect a watery, reddish discharge for 7 to 10 days and told to put nothing in the vagina for 3 weeks (no douching, no tampons, no coitus). Laser excisional biopsies clarify or confirm discrepancies between colposcopy, Pap smear, and pathology report (Stein, 1984).

REFERENCES

Baker RR, Niederhuber J: The Operative Management of Breast Disease. Philadelphia, WB Saunders Company, 1992.

Dolsky RL: Argon laser skin surgery. Surg Clin North Am 64: 861, 1984.

Fuller TA: The characteristics in operation of surgical lasers. Surg Clin North Am 64:843, 1984.

Gilchrest BA: Age associated changes in the skin. J Am Ger Soc 30:139, 1982.

Goodson WH, Hunt TK: Wound healing and aging. J Invest Dermatol 73:88, 1979.

Isaacs JH: Textbook of Breast Disease. St Louis, Mosby–Year Book, 1992.

Kirschner RA: Cutaneous plastic surgery with the CO_2 laser. Surg Clin North Am 64:871, 1984.

McMurray JF: Wound healing with diabetes mellitus: better glucose control for better wound healing in diabetes. Surg Clin North Am 64:769, 1984.

Mohr RM, McDonnell BC, Unger M, Mauer TP: Safety considerations and safety protocol for laser surgery. Surg Clin North Am 64:851, 1984.

Orgill D, Demling RH: Current concepts and approaches to wound healing. Crit Care Med 16:899, 1988.

Pories WJ, Thomas FT: Office Surgery for Family Physicians. Boston, Butterworth, 1985.

Ratz JL: Lasers in Cutaneous Medicine and Surgery. Chicago, Year Book Medical Publishers, 1986.

Schultz BC, McKinney P: Office Practice of Skin Surgery. Philadelphia, WB Saunders Company, 1985, pp 1–11.

Shane SM: Conscious Sedation for Ambulatory Surgery. Baltimore, University Park Press, 1983.

Schwartz SJ, Shires GT, Spencer FC: Principles of Surgery, 6th edition. New York, McGraw-Hill, 1994.

Stein S: CO_2 laser surgery of the cervix, vagina, and vulva. Surg Clin North Am 64:885, 1984.

Zacarian SA: Cryosurgery for Skin Cancer and Cutaneous Disorders. St. Louis, CV Mosby, 1985.

CHAPTER 32
GYNECOLOGY

KATHLEEN McINTYRE-SELTMAN and
CHRISTINE C. MATSON

APPROACH TO THE PATIENT

The "annual gynecologic examination" provides an opportunity for the family physician to perform a comprehensive health assessment and plan health promotion strategies with the patient. At a minimum, assessment should include current medical problems, risk factor identification and lifestyle issues, need for contraception or estrogen replacement, marital and sexual satisfaction, family function, and work or role satisfaction. Risk issues, including smoking, substance abuse, sexual practices, history of sexual abuse or domestic violence, occupational exposures, exercise, and diet, should be updated regularly.

This survey may reveal specific problems on which the physician will focus, or responses that will allow the physician to recognize special needs. For example, a 25-year-old patient may respond to a routine inquiry about contraceptive practices with "I don't need contraception." The physician who assumes that this response means that the patient is not sexually active or is infertile may miss the fact that her sexual partner is female. Estimates of the percentage of women who have experienced sexual victimization vary widely (Walch and Broadhead, 1992); an intermediate estimate is approximately 27 per cent (Finkelhor et al., 1990). Few will volunteer that information spontaneously in the interview, so sensitivity to the patient's emotional tone when describing family and sexual relationships and specific questions regarding very early, involuntary, or negative sexual experiences are necessary.

Domestic violence affects approximately 10 per cent of women, crossing all age, race, and socioeconomic groups. The physician should be especially sensitive to the possibility of abusive relationships; unwillingness to volunteer this information is characteristic of those who are abused. Bruises or injuries on the face, breasts, thighs, buttocks, or genitals should raise the question of possible abuse. If domestic violence is suspected, whether or not the woman confirms the suspicions, information regarding local safe shelters should be offered. All physicians should be aware of local resources and be able to provide this information at the same visit.

Women of childbearing age comprise the fastest growing cohort of individuals diagnosed with human immunodeficiency virus (HIV). Women are diagnosed later in the course of HIV infection than men, in part because of physicians' low index of suspicion. Risk factors for HIV—intravenous drug abuse or sexual relationship with an intravenous drug abuser, exchanging sex for drugs, multiple sexual partners or partners with multiple partners, a history of sexually transmitted disease, sexual intercourse with bisexual men, or history of transfusions—should be explored, and HIV testing offered liberally. Any woman requesting HIV testing should have her request honored, along with counseling regarding prevention strategies.

Offering anticipatory guidance based on the patient's current individual and family life cycle will include issues such as the following:

Adolescents—developing self-image and self-esteem; increasing independence from family; peer pressure regarding sexual activity; smoking, drugs, and alcohol; establishing intimate relationships; knowledge of sexual risk factors and strategies for decreasing risk; need for contraception; safety.

Young adults—choice of career and goal-setting, methods for dealing with stress, renegotiating relationship with parents, establishing intimate relationships, contraception or conception planning, pregnancy-related issues, establishing a new nuclear family, knowledge of sexual risk factors and strategies for decreasing risk, smoking or substance abuse, safety.

Older adults—work satisfaction, life satisfaction, revising life goals, changing role in family, coping with children and aging parents, plans for maintaining health and function, dealing with physical limitations, dealing with stress, smoking or substance abuse, safety.

Elderly—role transition, life satisfaction, revising life goals, generativity/productivity, changing relationships in family, plans for maintaining health and function, dealing with physical limitations, substance abuse, safety, end-of-life issues.

THE GYNECOLOGIC EXAMINATION

Attention to details of the patient's comfort and sensitivity to her level of anxiety about the pelvic examination are critical in facilitating her relaxation for the procedure. If at all possible, meeting the patient to elicit her history while she is still dressed provides the best beginning for the examination. For women who have been exposed to sexual abuse, a gynecologic examination can trigger feelings of helplessness or panic, even when the antecedent abuse may not be part of conscious awareness. The examiner should be attuned to any signals that the patient has more than expected anxiety regarding the examination, and allow adequate time to explore the patient's feelings and address her concerns. Important details for the patient's privacy and comfort include avoiding unrelated conversations and especially laughter within earshot, an appropriate chaperone, and placing the examination table so that the perineum is not exposed if the door is opened. A warm ambient temperature as well as a warmed and lubricated speculum, a gown that is large enough to provide coverage, and appropriate draping assist with with the patient's relaxation. Raising the table back to approximately 45 degrees allows the patient to meet the examiner's eyes and signal any discomfort or anxiety without tensing her abdominal muscles to lift her head (see Fig. 32–1). The drape should be depressed to allow this eye contact, and a mirror may be provided so that the patient can see any perineal lesions pointed out by the examiner.

In general, it is best to carry on a conversation with the patient about what is being done and the findings as the examination is conducted. After inspection and palpation of the inguinal area and perineum, the warmed speculum, lubricated only with water if a Papanicolaou (Pap) smear is to be performed, is inserted obliquely and rotated to the horizontal to visualize the cervix. The speculum is rotated during its removal to visualize the circumference of the vagina. During the bimanual examination the uterus is palpated by inserting two lubricated gloved digits into the vagina, and gently elevating the cervix so that the size, contour and tenderness of the uterus can be assessed with the other hand on the abdomen. The ovaries are assessed best by using the abdominal hand to sweep the adnexa down to be palpated with the vaginal fingers in each fornix. The examination is completed by palpating the rectovaginal septum and the posterior aspect of the uterus via rectovaginal examination. It is important to describe the results of the examination to the patient without delay, and to reassure when appropriate.

CERVICAL SCREENING

Papanicolaou Smear

Papanicolaou screening has proven effective in reducing deaths from cervical cancer by allowing identification and treatment of premalignant lesions and early malignancies. Deaths have decreased in spite of an increase in the incidence of human papillomavirus (HPV), now well established as a risk factor for cervical cancer (Chow et al., 1986; Chu and White, 1987; Korn and Stern, 1993). The Pap test is an excellent screening test because it is easy to perform, relatively inexpensive, well accepted by patients, and adequately sensitive and has a low false-positive rate in an unselected population; in addition, treatment for early disease is effective. The Pap test is among the most cost-effective screening modalities commonly employed, with its greatest efficiency in younger sexually active women.

Frequency of Screening

The frequency of Pap screening should be chosen according to the patient's risk for cervical cancer. The routine recommendations of the American Cancer Society (Fink, 1988) and the American Col-

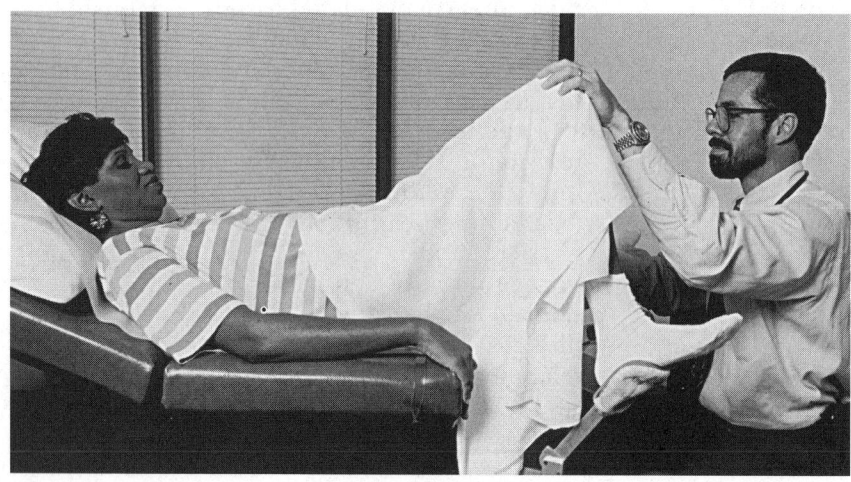

FIGURE 32–1. Proper patient positioning for gynecologic exam allows eye contact between patient and examiner.

TABLE 32–1. RISK FACTORS FOR CERVICAL NEOPLASIA

HPV infection or partner with the infection
Previous abnormal Pap smear
More than two lifetime sexual partners, or partner(s) with more than two partners
Onset of sexual activity before age 20
Smoking
HIV infection or other immunosuppressed states

lege of Obstetrics and Gynecology (1993) address patients at *low risk*—that is, those who are not sexually active or whose sexual relationship is mutually monogamous, and who have no history of an abnormal Pap smear or other identified risk factors for cervical cancer. Even though a woman may have only one sexual partner, her partner having additional partners clearly increases her risk of sexually transmitted disease, including cervical cancer. The American Cancer Society suggests that cervical screening should begin at the age of 18 years, or when sexual activity begins. Testing should be performed annually until three negative tests are obtained; the interval then can be 1 to 3 years, depending on the patient's level of risk and concern, until the age of 36. Between 36 and 60 years of age, annual testing is recommended. After the age of 60, the interval may be increased to 3 years. The U.S. Preventive Services Task Force (1990) suggests that routine screenings may be discontinued in women older than 65 years, but only in women who have had regular screening, including two consecutive normal Pap smears. The American College of Obstetrics and Gynecology (1984) continues to recommend annual cervical screening.

Any of the following risk factors for cervical cancer move a patient from the low risk to a higher risk category, and should suggest greater frequency of Pap testing: history of HPV infection or partner with the infection, history of abnormal Pap smear, more than two lifetime sexual partners, or sexual partner(s) with more than two partners, onset of sexual activity before age 20, smoking, and HIV infection (Table 32–1) (Nelson, 1989; Oriel, 1988; Slattery, 1989). Adenocarcinoma is being diagnosed in an increasing percentage of cervical cancers; neither Pap smears nor colposcopy is an effective screening technique for this cancer type.

Collection Technique

The effectiveness of the cytologic sampling technique introduced by Papanicolaou and Traut in 1943 is based on the fact that almost all cervical cancers originate within a few millimeters of the squamocolumnar junction. Both types of epithelium should be sampled. The presence of endothelial cells on the smear is a marker for an adequate collection (Council on Scientific Affairs, 1989).

The squamocolumnar junction is usually on the ectocervix in younger women, but may be within the endocervix in older women.

For an optimal Pap smear, the patient should be instructed not to douche prior to the examination. A warmed, moistened vaginal speculum without lubricant is inserted, and the cervix is visualized using good lighting. Excess mucus, if present, is removed with a large cotton-tipped applicator. An endocervical brush should be introduced gently into the endocervix and rotated 360 degrees. The brush then is rolled carefully on one half of a glass slide to transfer the fragile epithelial cells. Next, a protruding lip spatula (e.g., an Ayre's spatula) is placed at the os and rotated 360 degrees, then drawn across the other half of the slide. Separate slides may be used for the two samples, but this increases the cytology cost and does not increase sensitivity. The slide then is sprayed immediately with a cytologic fixative. Delay in fixation, excessive numbers of red or white cells, or contamination of the sample by lubricant or vaginal creams can interfere with the interpretation. Use of an endocervical brush followed by an Ayre's spatula significantly increases the sensitivity of the Pap smear for the detection of epithelial abnormalities (Reissman, 1988; Weitzman et al., 1988).

Reporting Systems

The 1988 Bethesda System for Reporting Cervical/Vaginal Cytologic Diagnoses (National Cancer Institute Workshop, 1989) is an attempt to standardize cytologic reporting and reflect current understanding of the pathophysiology of cervical abnormalities. Its format includes a statement of adequacy of the smear, a general category (normal or other), and a description of the smear. In contrast to former systems, only two categories of premalignant lesions are used, reflecting a consensus that the effect of HPV cannot always be distinguished from mild dysplasia (Fig. 32–2; Table 32–2). Low-grade squamous intraepithelial lesions include lesions previously classified as koilocytotic atypia (associated with HPV) and cervical intraepithelial neoplasia (CIN 1). High-grade squamous intraepithelial lesions include lesions formally designated as CIN 2 and CIN 3. Those squamous cells with nondyskaryotic changes that also fall short of koilocytotic atypia are designated as atypical squamous cells of undetermined significance. This designation denotes changes in excess of those usually associated with inflammation or repair. Because of the wide range of changes that can be designated squamous atypia, most pathologists will provide an explanatory note and/or recommendations.

The Papanicolaou system of reporting cervical cytology should no longer be accepted, because its categories do not address elements required for clinical decision making, such as specific characteristics of atypia, or gradations of dysplasia.

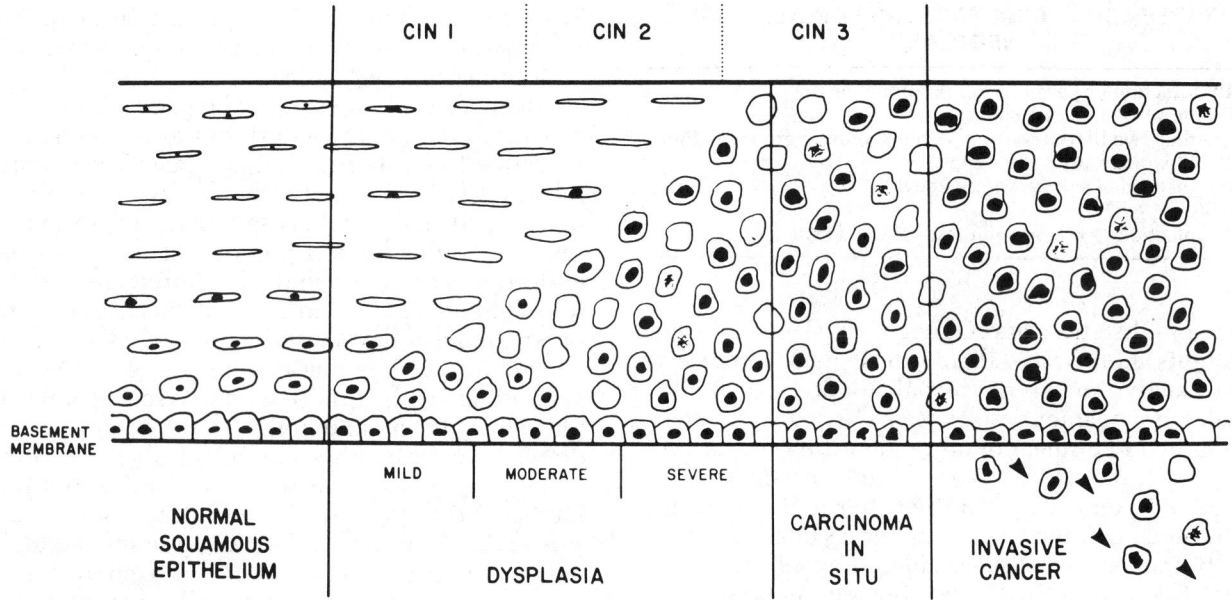

FIGURE 32–2. Diagram of cervical epithelium showing the varying terminology used to characterize progressive degrees of cervical intraepithelial neoplasia (CIN). CIN 1, 2, and 3 are the same as CIN I, II, and III, respectively. (Modified from Richart RM: Cervical intraepithelial neoplasia and the gynecologist. Can J Med Tech 38:177, 1976.)

Assuring Quality in the Interpretation of the Pap Smear

In addition to assuring that the smear has been collected appropriately as described previously, the physician has the responsibility to select a laboratory that maintains a quality assurance program, that provides adequate supervision of cytotechnicians by experienced cytopathologists, and that uses appropriate reporting nomenclature (Council on Scientific Affairs, 1989). It is helpful to compare the rate of reporting of abnormals by different laboratories for the same population.

Patient information always should accompany the cytology request, including age, last menstrual period, use of exogenous hormones, and previous cervical pathology. The cytopathology report frequently will contain a recommendation for specific follow-up of an abnormal smear. This information is most useful if the cytopathologist is aware of pertinent patient data. However, the decision whether to follow or evaluate a patient always should be a clinical judgment based on assessment of the patient's risk, cytologic findings, and availability for further monitoring.

Assuring Evaluation for Abnormal Pap Smears

Each medical office should have a mechanism to assure that evaluation for an abnormal Pap smear

TABLE 32–2. CLASSIFICATION OF CERVICAL SMEARS*

	Papanicolaou System	CIN System	Bethesda System
Class I	Normal smear, no abnormal cells	Normal smear	Normal smear
Class II	Atypical cells below the level of cervical neoplasia	Atypical cells below the level of cervical neoplasia	Inflammatory or reparative atypia
		KCA/HPV effect	Low-grade SIL
Class III	Abnormal cells consistent with dysplasia	KCA/HPV effect Mild dysplasia = CIN1	
		Moderate dysplasia = CIN2	High-grade SIL
Class IV	Abnormal cells consistent with carcinoma in situ	Severe dysplasia and Carcinoma = CIN3	
Class V	Abnormal cells consistent with carcinoma of squamous cell origin; adenocarcinoma	Invasive squamous cell carcinoma	Invasive squamous cell carcinoma

* *Key:* CIN, cervical intraepithelial neoplasia; KCA, koilocytotic atypia; SIL, squamous intraepithelial lesion; HPV, human papillomavirus.

is accomplished. Whether the recommendation to return for a repeat Pap smear or for colposcopic evaluation of a dysplastic lesion is given over the telephone or by mail, a "tickler" file should be used to provide reminders if the patient does not return as recommended.

Other Methods of Cervical Evaluation

Application of *Lugol's solution* to the cervix has been used in the past to identify areas of dysplastic cells that do not take up the stain because they contain less glycogen than normal cells. However, iodine staining is very nonspecific, because normal metaplasia, infection, scar, and atrophy also may be associated with lack of glycogen. Therefore, colposcopy is much more precise in identifying dysplastic epithelium.

The Papanicolaou smear is a screening and not a diagnostic test. Its purpose is to detect lesions that are not visible to the naked eye. Therefore, performing a Pap test to investigate an identified lesion is inappropriate because the rate of false negatives under these circumstances is unacceptably high. An identified lesion of the cervix must be biopsied or at least be evaluated colposcopically to determine need for biopsy. The biopsy instrument should be chosen based on the size and position of the lesion.

Another screening test for cervical cancer is *cervicography*, or photographing the cervix for expert review (Ferris et al., 1993). Although a more expensive technique than the Pap smear, its sensitivity for detection of cervical lesions is increased. However, specificity is only approximately 88 per cent (Szarewski et al., 1991).

COLPOSCOPY

Colposcopy is a technique used for magnified examination of the visible portion of the female genital tract (i.e., the vulva, vagina, and cervix) when the possibility of a lesion has been identified by screening. Its primary benefit is allowing definition of abnormalities detected by the Pap test and in many instances avoiding the morbidity of a cervical conization. The instrument is basically a dissecting microscope with a magnification range from 6 to 20x, fixed on a stand that provides excellent illumination of the area to be studied. A wide variety of instruments are available (Ferris et al., 1991).

The technique of colposcopy involves systematic inspection of the vulva, then visualization of the cervix with a vaginal speculum. After inspection of the cervix and obtaining a Pap smear if indicated, the cervix and the vaginal fornices are cleansed with a 4% acetic acid (vinegar) solution. Application of vinegar produces acetowhitening of some types of abnormal epithelium, including dysplastic epithelium and that infected with HPV (Fig. 32–3). The squamocolumnar junction and transformation zone are examined carefully, and biopsies are taken of any suspicious areas in nonpregnant individuals. For a colposcopic examination to be adequate, all of the squamocolumnar junction must be seen clearly, and any lesions found must be fully visible. Endocervical curettage confirms the presence or absence of dysplasia extending into the cervical canal; its role in routine colposcopic evaluation remains controversial. The endocervical brush has been shown to be similar to endocervical curettage in detecting abnormalities of the canal (Weitzman et al., 1988).

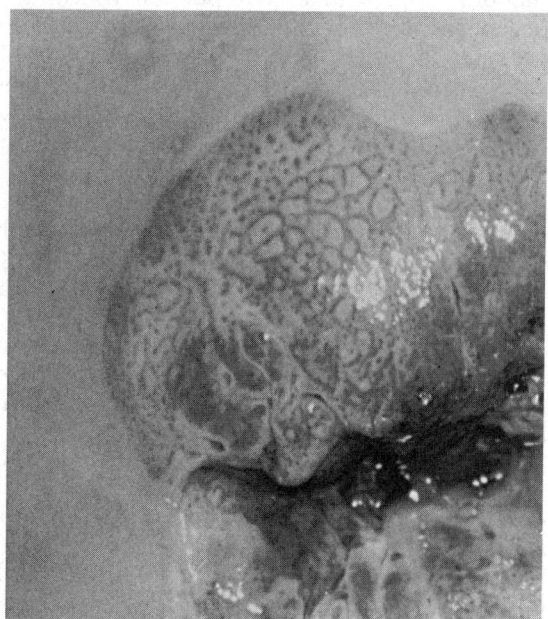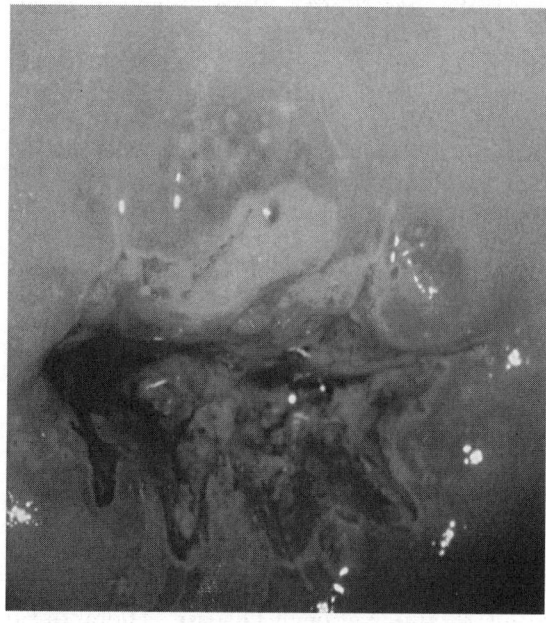

FIGURE 32–3. Colpophotomicrograph of cervix with HPV lesion.

Treatment options for squamous intraepithelial lesions include cryotherapy, laser, loop electrical excision (LEEP), and conization after invasive cancer is ruled out by colposcopy with directed biopsies.

SPECIFIC PROBLEMS

Interpretation of Abnormal Pap Smear Findings

Much of the significance of a Pap smear result depends on the patient's history. Pap testing has a *low* false-positive rate (3 to 15 per cent) but a *high* false-negative rate (10 to 65 per cent), with the highest rate of false negatives associated with repeating the smear after an abnormal result.

The finding of inflammation or reactive atypia on Pap smear usually indicates an infection or the reparative phase of a previous infection or injury. Concomitant dysplasia may be present in 20 to 42 per cent of these patients (Kohan et al., 1985; Lawley et al., 1990; Noumoff, 1987). If a specific etiology can be identified (e.g., *Trichomonas*, bacterial vaginosis, *Chlamydia*), the appropriate treatment should be provided and the Pap smear repeated in 3 months (repeating it sooner can result in falsely positive results). If no specific etiology is found, either following the patient closely or doing colposcopic evaluation is appropriate. Nonspecific treatment (e.g., sulfa cream) is not helpful, and may delay appropriate diagnostic evaluation.

The appropriate evaluation when squamous atypia is identified on Pap smear remains controversial. Studies in referral populations have demonstrated amply that repeatedly atypical Pap smears suggest the presence of dysplasia in up to one third of cases (Reiter, 1986). Slawsen et al. (1994) demonstrated that 55 per cent of patients identified as having squamous atypia from a primary care population had abnormalities on biopsy. Whether an initial atypical smear from a low-risk patient requires colposcopic evaluation depends on an assessment of risk, cost and availability of colposcopic expertise, and the likelihood that the patient can be monitored over time. Repeating the test and finding a negative result is not sufficient evaluation.

Colposcopic evaluation is necessary when "koilocytotic atypia" or "HPV effect," any degree of dysplasia, and, of course, microinvasive or invasive carcinoma is the Pap smear reading. The finding of koilocytosis, characterized primarily by nuclear atypia and perinuclear haloes associated with HPV infection, has become very common. The incidence of HPV infection has increased greatly: initial visits to physicians for genital warts increased more than 800 per cent between 1966 and 1987, according to the National Disease Therapeutic Index.

Endometrial biopsy should be performed when atypical endometrial cells are recognized on a Pap smear, or "out of phase" in the last 2 weeks of the menstrual cycle. Either of these two situations, or histiocytes with evidence of estrogen effect in an estrogen-deficient woman, must prompt endometrial biopsy.

Human Papillomavirus

More than 60 types of HPV are known to infect humans, including more than 10 affecting the lower genital tract. The prevalence of HPV infection in women increases with age through the reproductive years, with peak age of acquisition at ages 20 to 25. The exact prevalence in a given population is difficult to determine, because estimates vary greatly with the diagnostic test used. The presence of HPV effect on Pap smear in an unselected population varies between 2 and 7 per cent, whereas subclinical infection may be detected in 10 to 82 per cent of women by DNA hybridization techniques depending on the population tested (Korn and Stern, 1993). Knowing the type of HPV associated with early dysplastic lesions of the cervix does not allow prediction with certainty of which lesions will progress. Therefore, these more sensitive DNA hybridization or polymerase chain reaction techniques are not currently recommended for routine clinical use.

HPV has been implicated as the sexually transmissible agent primarily responsible for cervical cancer. HPV DNA is detected in more than 90 per cent of cervical cancers, with certain "high-risk" types such as types 16, 18, 31, and 33 disproportionately present. However, HPV infection alone may not be enough to induce neoplasia. It appears that only approximately 10 per cent of women who test positive for HPV DNA go on to develop disease. Co-factors thought to play a role in neoplastic transformation include cigarette smoke metabolites, other infectious agents (herpes simplex virus, cytomegalovirus, and others), dietary deficiencies, immune defects, and hormonal effects.

Transmission of HPV is almost entirely by sexual contact, and efficiency of transmission through one exposure is estimated to be approximately 60 per cent. Incubation is 3 weeks to 8 months, with the average about 3 months. The documentation of HPV DNA on equipment in the medical office (Ferenczy et al., 1989) underscores the need to properly sterilize office instruments in virucidal solutions or through heat sterilization.

When HPV produces disease, it may take the form of overt condylomata, CIN, or subclinical disease detectable with colposcopy. Condylomata should be treated (after significant epithelial atypia is excluded) with local ablative or excisional modalities. Options include bi- or trichloroacetic acid, podophyllin or podophyllotoxin, cautery, cryotherapy, laser, or local excision. Immune modulation with interferon can be helpful in persistent or recurrent disease, especially in immunocompromised patients.

MENSTRUAL ABNORMALITIES

Menstrual Physiology

The menstrual cycle involves a complex interplay among the hypothalamus, pituitary, ovary, and endometrium (see Fig. 32–4). Ovarian follicle development begins a few days prior to the onset of menses. It results from stimulation of granulosa cells by pituitary follicle-stimulating hormone (FSH), controlled in turn by hypothalamic gonadotrophin-releasing hormone (GnRH). As the follicle grows, it secretes increasing amounts of estrogen, resulting in endometrial proliferation. Via a complex feedback process, a mid-cycle surge of luteinizing hormone (LH) is triggered, leading to ovulation. The granulosa and theca cells of the corpus luteum begin to produce progesterone as well as estrogen, causing the endometrium to become secretory. If conception occurs, human chorionic gonadotropin secreted by the embryo maintains the corpus luteum, allowing continued estrogen and progesterone secretion. If conception does not occur, the corpus luteum "self-destructs" after about 10 days. The resulting fall in estrogen and progesterone stimulates GnRH and in turn FSH release, initiating the next follicular cycle. Menstruation also occurs in response to the drop in ovarian steroid levels, with a global sloughing of the functional layer of endometrium associated with release of prostaglandins and other vasoactive substances.

Abnormal Bleeding

The normal menstruation is cyclic (every 23 to 35 days) and self-limited (lasting 3 to 7 days). Average blood loss is approximately 40 mL each cycle. **Menorrhagia** refers to regular menses that are longer and/or heavier than average. Common causes include uterine fibroids, adenomyosis, polyps or coagulation disorders. **Metrorrhagia** refers to bleeding at frequent intervals that may be associated with local vaginal or cervical lesions, uterine polyps, or hormonal dysfunction. **Menometrorrhagia** refers to irregular heavy or prolonged bleeding.

There are many causes of abnormal uterine bleeding (Table 32–3). First, complications of pregnancy must be considered, including threatened abortion, incomplete abortion, ectopic pregnancy, and gestational trophoblastic disease. A sensitive pregnancy test must be done if there is even a remote chance of pregnancy.

Lesions of the vulva, vagina, or cervix that may lead to bleeding include condylomata, malignancies, cervical polyps, and infections such as *Chlamydia* or gonorrhea.

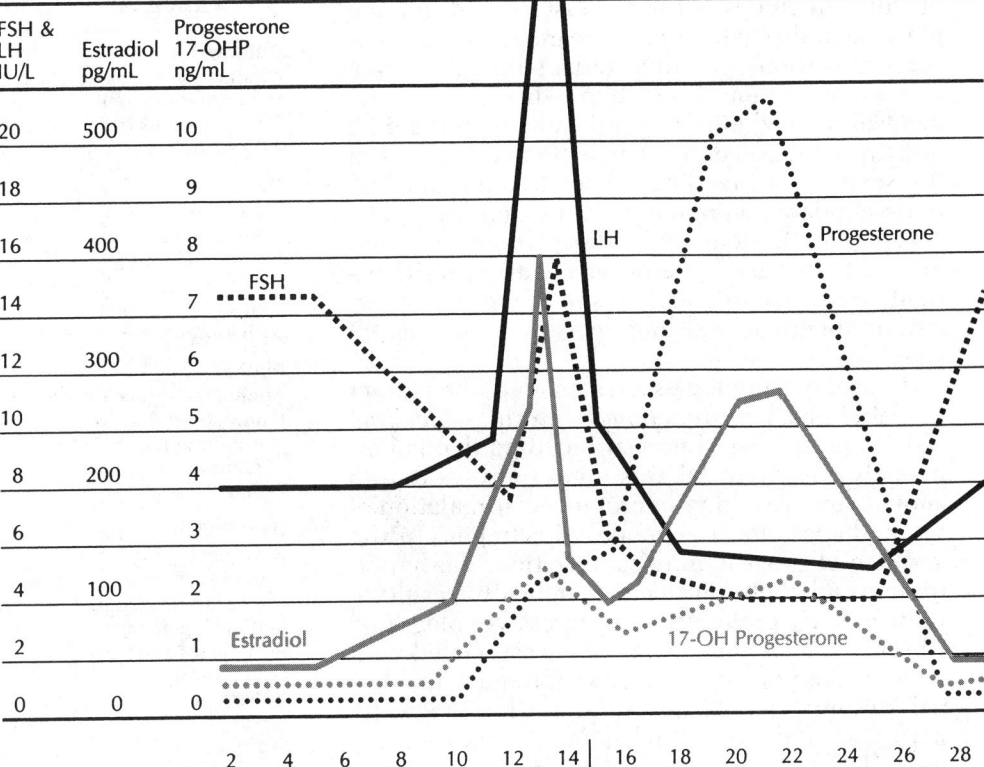

FIGURE 32–4. Hormone levels during menstrual cycle. (From Speroff L: Clinical Gynecologic Endocrinology and Infertility, 5th edition. Baltimore, Williams & Wilkins, 1994, p 191, with permission.)

TABLE 32–3. CAUSES OF ABNORMAL BLEEDING

Pregnancy related	Spontaneous or threatened abortion
	Ectopic pregnancy
	Gestational trophoblastic disease
Hormonally mediated	Dysfunctional uterine bleeding (usually anovulation)
Lower genital tract	Condylomata
	Vulvar, vaginal, cervical cancer
	Cervicitis
	Cervical polyps
	Trauma
Uterus	Fibroids
	Endometrial polyps
	Chronic endometritis
	Cancer or hyperplasia
Ovaries	Neoplasms, benign or malignant
Systemic	Hepatic or renal disease
	Platelet abnormality
	Coagulopathy
	Drug induced (e.g., warfarin, hormones)

Abnormalities of the uterus, such as fibroids, uterine polyps, endometritis, or adenomyosis, are common. Ovarian neoplasms may cause abnormal bleeding whether or not they secrete steroid hormones. Systemic conditions should be considered, including renal, hepatic, or thyroid disease and coagulopathies such as autoimmune thrombocytopenia or drug-induced bleeding diatheses. Oral contraceptive use and intrauterine contraceptive devices also can cause abnormal bleeding.

Evaluation of the patient with abnormal uterine bleeding includes a careful history and general physical and pelvic exam to search for vaginal or cervical lesions, uterine enlargement, ovarian masses, or evidence of systemic diseases. Assessment of hemoglobin, red cell indices, and serum ferritin should be done as an objective measure of the severity of bleeding; platelet count and thyroid-stimulating hormone measurement should be considered. Endometrial biopsy should be performed to rule out hyperplasia or cancer if the patient is at risk, particularly if she is obese, has persistent abnormal bleeding, or is over 40 years of age.

If the above etiologies are excluded, the patient probably has *dysfunctional uterine bleeding* (DUB), defined as abnormal bleeding that is hormonally mediated. DUB is almost always due to anovulation, resulting in prolonged stimulation of the endometrium by unopposed estrogen. In the absence of progesterone stabilization, the hypertrophic endometrium sloughs erratically, resulting in irregular, prolonged, or excessive bleeding. Chronic anovulation commonly is associated with obesity, the polycystic ovary syndrome, and adrenal dysfunction. Anovulation is physiologically normal in the perimenarchal and perimenopausal years. DUB can be controlled medically by administration of a progestin (medroxyprogesterone acetate, 10 mg daily for 10 days) or with oral contraceptives. If the patient desires pregnancy, ovulation should be induced with clomiphene. Antiprostaglandin agents also have been shown to decrease menstrual blood flow, and iron supplementation should be instituted where appropriate.

Endometrial biopsy can be performed in the office, although most women experience moderate uterine cramping during the procedure. After pregnancy is ruled out, and a bimanual exam is done to assess uterine size and position, the cervix is cleansed and stabilized if necessary with a single-tooth tenaculum. Paracervical block with local anesthesia is sometimes helpful. A disposable suction catheter is introduced through the os all the way to the fundus and rotated circumferentially while suction is applied. If a Novak curette is used, it is drawn against each uterine wall from fundus to lower uterine segment. Use of *Laminaria* sometimes may be helpful if the cervix is stenotic and will not admit the curette. The endometrial specimen thus obtained is placed immediately into fixative for histologic evaluation.

Amenorrhea

Amenorrhea, or absence of menses for at least 6 months, may be due to abnormalities of the hypothalamus, pituitary, ovary, or "outflow tract," which includes the uterus, cervix, and vagina (see Table 32–4). Adolescents with primary amenor-

TABLE 32–4. CAUSES OF AMENORRHEA

Outflow Tract
Absence of vagina or uterus, androgen insensitivity
Imperforate hymen, vaginal septum
Cervical stenosis (congenital or acquired)
Asherman's syndrome (endometrial scarring)

Ovary
Premature ovarian failure
  Autoimmune
    Infection (e.g., mumps)
    Toxins
Gonadal dysgenesis
Radiation or chemotherapy

Pituitary
Adenoma—prolactin producing or other
Panhypopituitarism
  Autoimmune
  Trauma
  Radiation

Hypothalamic
Structural
Tumor (e.g., craniopharyngioma)
Increased intracranial pressure
GnRH deficiency
Postencephalitis
Granulomatous disease
Functional
Stress
Weight loss
Anorexia
Exercise
Drugs
Systemic illness

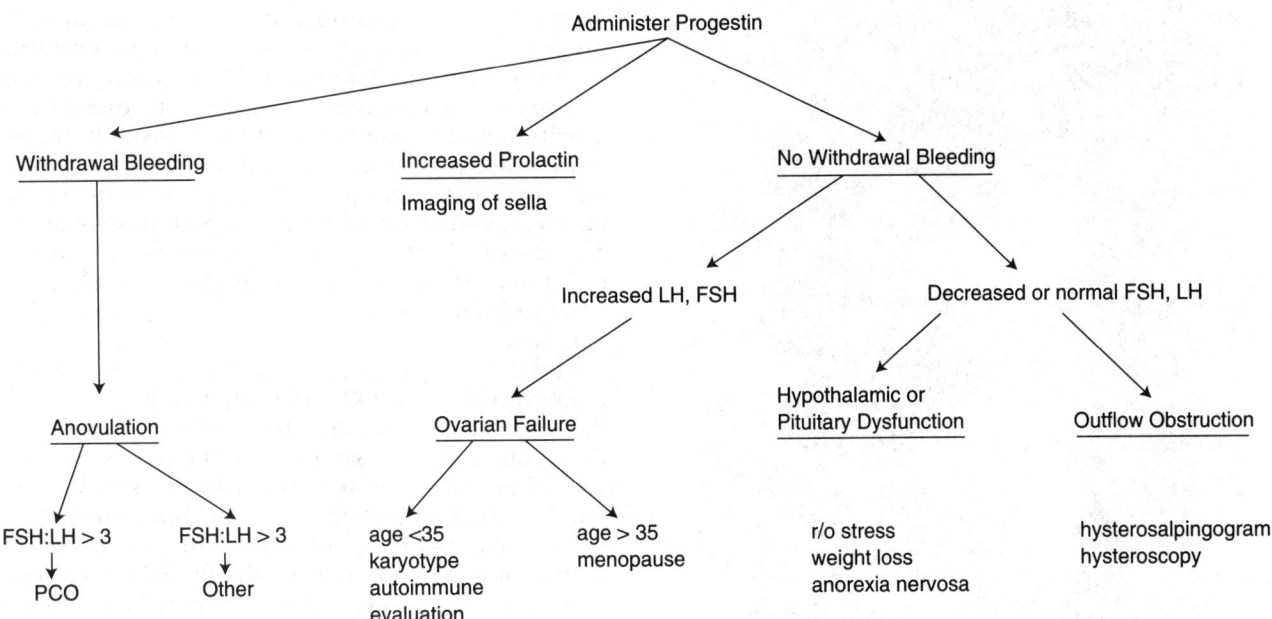

1. Rule out pregnancy
2. Measure LH, FSH, Prolactin

FIGURE 32–5. Evaluation of amenorrhea.

rhea, or absence of menses by age 16, can be divided into those with normal secondary sex characteristics and those with sexual infantilism. In the former group, congenital absence of the uterus, imperforate hymen, and androgen insensitivity should be considered; in the latter group, gonadal dysgenesis, adrenal enzyme deficiencies, and hypothalamic–pituitary disorders are possible etiologies.

Evaluation begins with a careful history and physical exam, including a neurologic exam and assessment of secondary sex characteristics by Tanner staging. If the cause is not evident by examination and a pregnancy test is negative, serum LH, FSH, and prolactin levels should be measured and a progestin challenge administered (10 mg medroxyprogesterone acetate for 10 days, or progesterone in oil, 100 mg intramuscularly) (Fig. 32–5). The presence of withdrawal bleeding means that the endometrium has been primed with estrogen and the patient is anovulatory. The etiology of anovulation should be sought, as outlined in Table 32–4. If bleeding does not occur after the progestin challenge and the LH and FSH are high, the patient has ovarian failure (premature menopause), which may be due to gonadal dysgenesis, autoimmune factors, or ovarian destruction (see Fig. 32–5). If the patient is younger than age 35, further testing should be done to determine the etiology of ovarian failure. If LH and FSH are low, the patient

either has hypothalamic–pituitary failure or an abnormality of the uterus, cervix, or vagina. Rarely, it may be necessary to give estrogen followed by a repeat progestin challenge to assess whether the outflow tract is capable of response to appropriate hormone stimulation.

VAGINAL DISCHARGE

Vaginal Infections

Bacterial Vaginosis

Bacterial vaginosis is the most commonly diagnosed cause of vaginal symptoms (Brown and Kaufmann, 1993). This condition, formerly attributed to infection with an organism known as *Haemophilus vaginalis* or *Gardnerella vaginalis,* is now understood to be an ecologic disturbance of the vaginal flora, characterized by reduced numbers of normally predominant lactobacilli, and increased numbers of anaerobes and gram-negative bacteria, with which *Gardnerella* probably acts synergistically. Women who present with symptoms that are diagnosed as bacterial vaginosis frequently note a white, gray, or green, or brown discharge accompanied by an unpleasant "fishy odor," and sometimes pelvic pain and tenderness. Irritation may be mild or absent. This infection frequently is diagnosed after contact with a new sexual partner or in associ-

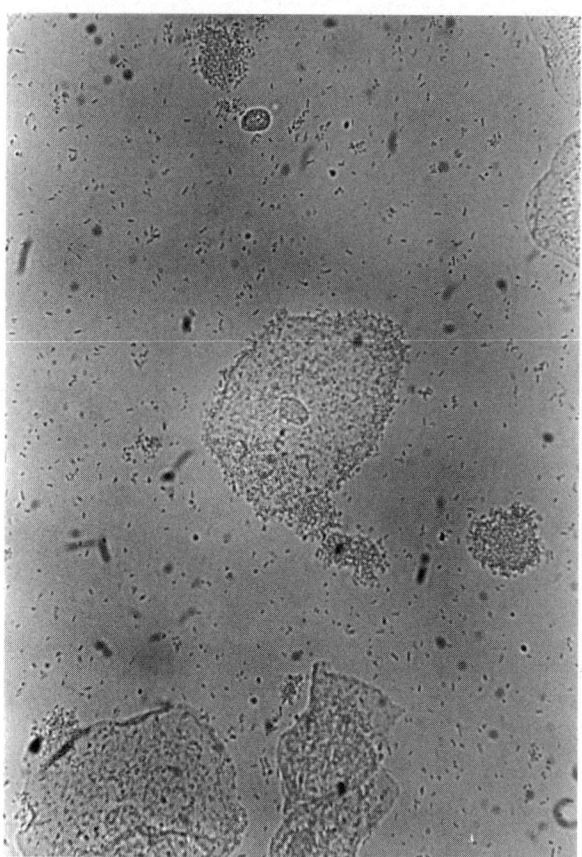

FIGURE 32–6.   Microscopic appearance of "clue cells" (vaginal epithelial cells coated with bacteria) seen in *bacterial vaginosis.*

ation with another sexually transmitted disease. This association makes its diagnosis in a child suggestive of sexual abuse, although it has been described in asymptomatic girls with no history of abuse (Spiegal, 1991) and in virginal females (Eschenbach et al., 1988). Among women with microbiologic findings suggesting bacterial vaginosis, approximately 50 per cent are asymptomatic. These cases of apparent colonization can either spontaneously resolve or become symptomatic, for reasons that are poorly understood (Bump et al., 1984).

Diagnosis of bacterial vaginosis in based on finding at least three of four of the following Amsel criteria (Amsel et al., 1983): pH greater than 4.5; clue cells (see Fig. 32–6); a positive "whiff" test (a fishy odor produced by aromatic amines when potassium hydroxide is added on the wet mount), and a homogeneous white or gray adherent discharge (see Table 32–5). Alternatively, a Gram's stain showing an abundance of flora but an absence of gram-positive rods (lactobacilli) may be used rather than a wet mount.

TREATMENT. When the microbiologic charac-teristics of bacterial vaginosis are documented in the absence of symptoms, no treatment is necessary. Treatment could be considered when a vaginal surgical procedure is planned, because of the association with postoperative infections, and in pregnancy, because of an association with preterm delivery and chorioamnionitis. Whether or not treatment is given, the patient's risk factors for acquisition and transmission of other sexually transmitted diseases should be explored, including sexual and contraceptive practices, number of sexual partners, and other partners her partner may have. The diagnosis of bacterial vaginosis can be an opportunity for primary prevention of currently noncurable infections such as HIV, HPV, and herpes simplex.

The first drug of choice, and the least expensive, is metronidazole, 500 mg orally twice a day for 7 days. The common side effects of gastrointestinal irritation and occasional neurologic symptoms should be discussed with the patient, as well as its emetic effect when taken with alcohol. Alternative treatments include metronidazole gel 0.75%, 5 grams intravaginally twice daily for 5 days, or clindamycin 2% cream, 5 grams intravaginally once daily for 7 days. Effective oral agents include ciprofloxacin, amoxicillin plus clavulanic acid, clindamycin, and cephalexin; previously recommended agents, including ampicillin and triple sulfa cream, are ineffective and should not be used. Chlorhexidine or povidone-iodine suppositories also may be helpful. According to the Food and Drug Administration, use of metronidazole is not recommended during pregnancy, but it frequently is used during the second and third trimester when treatment is required.

Concurrent treatment of the sexual partner remains controversial, with few studies demonstrating improved outcomes (Vejtorp et al., 1988). It is usually recommended only for recurrent or persistent cases. For these cases, re-evaluation may demonstrate the presence of other sexually transmitted diseases that also require treatment.

Candidal Infection

Candida albicans accounts for approximately 85 per cent of candidal vulvovaginitis, although non-candidal species, especially *C. glabrata, C. tropicalis,* and *C. Kruse,* have increased in frequency in the last 20 years. More than 25 per cent of asymptomatic women harbor the organism. Pregnancy, antibiotic use, oral contraceptives, diabetes, and immunosuppression are conditions often associated with candidal infections. Other factors that have been implicated include vaginal pH changes in the week prior to menses; intestinal colonization by *Candida;* sexual transmission, including oral–genital contact; increased dietary intake of carbohydrates or artificial sweeteners; and de-

TABLE 32–5. DIFFERENTIAL DIAGNOSIS AND TREATMENT OF VULVOVAGINITIS

Diagnostic Criterion	Normal	Bacterial Vaginosis	Candida Vulvovaginitis	Trichomonas Vaginitis	Reactive Vaginitis	Atrophic Vaginitis
History	Variable discharge	Malodorous discharge, ± sexual contact, ± after intercourse	Frequently premenstrual; pruritic discharge	Sexual contact; vaginal odor/itching; watery discharge, ± frothy; ± dysuria	Hygiene product use	Burning, dyspareunia
Physical features discharge	Clear mucoid	Homogenous thin, white or gray adherent; ± increased amount	White, curdy; ± thrush patches; ± increased	Greenish yellow; increased; ± frothy, ± friable hyperemic cervix	Vaginal erythema; occasional foreign body	Thinned vaginal mucosa; friable
pH	<4.5	>4.5	4.0–5.0	5.0–6.6	<4.5	<4.5
Laboratory findings	Few WBCs; epithelial cells, lactobacilli predominate	+ "whiff" test (amine odor with KOH); clue cells (see Fig. 32–6); decrease in normal lactobacilli	Mycelia, budding yeast, pseudohyphae on KOH prep	Motile flagellates on saline prep	Increased WBCs	Predominance of peribasal epithelial cells on Pap smear
Culture		Not usually indicated; mix of aerobic and anaerobic bacteria	When necessary, on Sabouraud's agar	When necessary in modified Diamond's media		
Treatment		Metronidazole, 500 mg b.i.d. × 5–7 days *or* 250 mg t.i.d. × 7 days If recurrent, treat sexual partner(s)	Miconazole, clotrimazole; if recurrent: butoconazole, terconazole, sporoconazole or other	Metronidazole, 2 grams in a single dose for patient and partner(s)	Eliminate offending agent; ± corticosteroids	Topical estrogen

creased air circulation because of synthetic clothing. Any condition associated with decreased cell-mediated immunity may predispose to candidal infection; recurrent monilial vulvovaginitis today should raise the question of infection with HIV as well as the possibility of diabetes.

Vulvar pruritus is the most common symptom of candidiasis, occurring in approximately 90 per cent of patients. A white, "cottage cheese" discharge may be present. Vulvar erythema and edema of the labia minora are the most frequently observed signs. Thrush patches sometimes are observed, more commonly in pregnancy. The vaginal pH is usually 4.0 to 4.7. Because these symptoms and signs do not always predict candidal infection (Berg et al., 1984; Reed et al., 1989), laboratory confirmation is desirable, including a wet mount to exclude other etiologies. A postinflammatory or post-treatment sloughing of epithelial cells can produce a discharge that can simulate a monilial discharge and can cause irritation and pruritus as well. The absence of hyphae and spores on the KOH preparation distinguishes this condition from candidal infection. Demonstration of both filaments (pseudohyphae) and spores on potassium hydroxide preparation are necessary to confirm *C. albicans* (Fig. 32–7). Other candidal species may differ in structural components present. Culture on Sabouraud's agar can confirm the diagnosis, although culture rarely is required.

TREATMENT.   The relative safety and efficacy of the imidazole derivatives have resulted in several being approved for over-the-counter use, including clotrimazole (Gyne-Lotrimin, Mycelex) and miconazole (Monistat). Use of these or butoconazole (Femstat) according to recommendations results in cure in about 85 per cent of acute cases. Patients should be aware that these oil-based creams may weaken latex condoms and diaphragms. The best candidates for self-treatment with over-the-counter products are those with previous confirmed *Candida* infections who experience the same symptoms. Those with new or persistent symptoms after treatment should consult a physician. Examination of women who present with persistent symptoms after a trial of an over-the-counter agent is important to distinguish between treatment failure and incorrect diagnosis.

Candidal infections that persist after imidazole treatment are more likely to be a non-*albicans* spe-

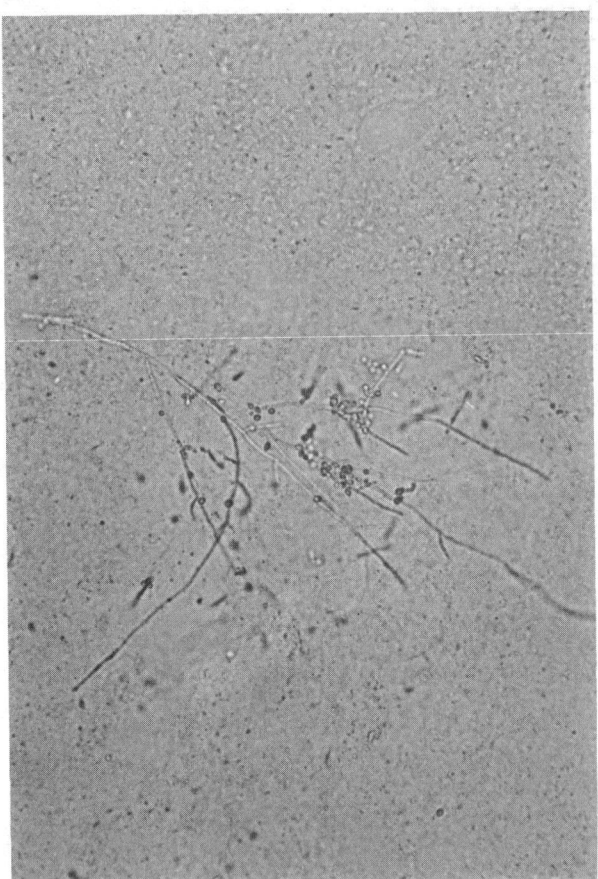

FIGURE 32–7. Yeast and mycelia, seen in potassium hydroxide preparation of candidiasis discharge.

Trichomoniasis

Trichomonas vaginalis, a flagellated anaerobic protozoan, is the causative organism in *Trichomonas* vaginitis. Transmission is usually by sexual contact, although infection through fomites and inadequately chlorinated swimming pools and jacuzzis have been reported. Infection with *Trichomonas* is asymptomatic in approximately 50 per cent of women and 90 per cent of men (Thomason and Gelbart, 1989). Infection in women can be acute or chronic. Chronic infections are characterized by voluminous malodorous, watery discharge but minimal or no inflammatory reaction of the vulvovaginal tissues. In acute infections, irritative manifestations such as pruritus, edema, and erythema are present, as well as profuse discharge. Dysuria and urinary frequency related to urethrocystitis are not uncommon. The most remarkable symptom, the discharge, can be white or colored (greenish, gray, or yellow) and sometimes frothy. The classic "strawberry cervix" is seen in fewer than 10 per cent of cases. The diagnosis of trichomoniasis is confirmed by the finding of an elevated pH (greater than 5), and motile flagellated protozoa on normal saline preparation. Finding more than 10 white blood cells per high-power field is also common (Fig. 32–8). A falsely negative examination can result from using concentrated or cold saline solution, or delayed examination of the slide. *Trichomonas* also can be observed on Pap smear, but this test should not be relied on for detection. Rarely, culture of *Trichomonas* on modified Diamond's media may be required to identify a resistant strain.

TREATMENT. Simultaneous treatment is required for the patient and her sexual partner(s), with instructions to avoid sexual contact until treatment has been complete and symptoms have resolved. A single 2-gram dose of metronidazole or 500 mg every 12 hours for five days are both effective (see Bacterial Vaginosis for discussion of side effects and cautions in pregnancy). Some relief from symptoms can be achieved in pregnancy by using clotrimazole vaginal cream. For persistent or recurrent cases, first verify that no re-exposure occurred before completion of treatment for both partners, and that no additional source of exposure exists. Exclude other sexually transmitted infections. If persistence of the infection after appropriate therapy is confirmed, retreat the patient and her partner(s) using standard doses. Occasionally metronidazole resistance occurs; these individuals, with their partners, can be treated with metronidazole 2 grams orally each day for 3 to 5 days (Centers for Disease Control and Prevention, 1993) or 500 grams orally twice daily for 14 days, along with vaginal povidone-iodine or intravaginal metronidazole gel.

cies (e.g., *C. tropicalis* and *C. glabrata*), which usually respond to the newer triazoles such as terconazole (Terazol), 3- or 7-day vaginal therapy. Systemic absorption occasionally may result in flu-like symptoms. Oral agents such as ketoconazole (200 mg twice daily for 5 to 14 days), fluconazole (100 to 140 mg one time), or itraconazole (200 mg once daily for 3 days) also may be used. Other treatments for chronic or recurrent infection include careful cleansing of the preputial folds; good hygiene, including wearing loose-fitting clothing and avoiding synthetic underwear; continuous vaginal therapy for 3 to 4 weeks; use of intravaginal agents at bedtime for 7 to 10 days before the menstrual period and during any antibiotic use; discontinuing oral contraceptives; and using 600-mg boric acid formulated into suppositories as vaginal suppositories twice daily for 14 days (Jovanovic et al., 1991). Topical imidazole treatment for the foreskin in uncircumcised partners may be helpful. More than three episodes of vulvovaginal candidiases in a year, including self-treated episodes, should prompt evaluation for predisposing conditions such as diabetes and HIV infection.

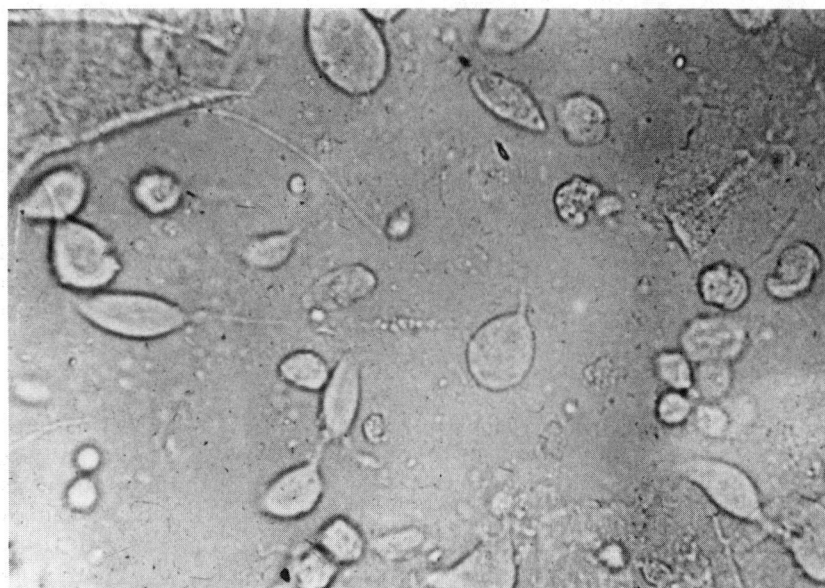

FIGURE 32–8. Flagellated *Trichomonas vaginalis* organisms, seen under high-power magnification. (From Kaufman RH, Freidrich EG Jr, Gardner HL: Benign Diseases of the Vagina and Vulva, 3rd edition. Chicago, Year Book Medical Publishers, 1989, with permission.)

Other Causes of Vaginal Discharge or Irritation

Other infections sometimes can cause vaginal discharge, such as gonorrhea or *Chlamydia* cervicitis, or endometritis. These should be identified by culture or immunodiagnostic testing and treated accordingly. Neoplasms of the lower genital tract may produce discharge. Contact irritation or allergic response to latex or to contraceptive or other vaginal products may cause irritation and discharge; diagnosis is by history. In estrogen-deficient women, the thinned epithelium may result in burning and soreness; topical estrogen is an effective treatment. A physiologic discharge may be mistaken for an abnormal one; exploring the patient's concerns, education, and reassurance are the appropriate interventions. Using a menstrual calendar to follow changes in the character of the discharge through the cycle can be a helpful tool.

ACUTE PELVIC PAIN

Pelvic Inflammatory Disease

Pelvic inflammatory disease (PID) is a common cause of acute pelvic pain, especially in the young patient with multiple sexual partners and inconsistent contraceptive use. The infection usually begins with cervicitis caused by *Chlamydia* or gonorrhea. At the time of menses, the organisms gain access to the upper genital tract and set up an inflammatory process that results in secondary involvement with multiple bacteria, especially coliforms and anaerobes. Clinical sign and symptoms in PID are nonspecific and include lower abdominal pain and tenderness, purulent cervical discharge, cervical motion tenderness, and fever, nausea, and leukocytosis. Women who are not acutely ill can be treated as outpatients with a follow-up pelvic exam in 72 hours to assess response to therapy. Those with peritonitis, vomiting, intrauterine device in place, prior pelvic instrumentation, positive pregnancy test, pelvic mass on exam or ultrasound, or failed outpatient therapy should be hospitalized. Antibiotic regimens are outlined in Table 32–6. Treatment of PID should include a discussion of risk factors and counseling regarding safer sexual practices, as well as a discussion of sequelae of PID, including infertility, ectopic pregnancy, and chronic pelvic pain.

Ectopic Pregnancy

Ectopic pregnancy remains an important cause of pregnancy-related death in this country. Approximately 1 per cent of known pregnancies are ectopic, and the incidence appears to be increasing. Women with a history of PID, endometriosis, or tubal surgery (including tubal ligation) and those using an intrauterine device or progestin-only contraception are at increased risk. Previous ectopic pregnancy is also a risk factor because there is a 15 per cent recurrence rate. Symptoms include pelvic pain that is often unilateral, and amenorrhea asso-

TABLE 32–6.   ANTIBIOTIC REGIMENS FOR PID TREATMENT

Outpatient
- ceftriaxone 250 mg intramuscularly *plus* doxycycline 100 mg orally twice daily for 7 days

Alternatives
- Spectinomycin 2 gm intramuscularly plus oral doxycycline as above
- Ofloxacin 400 mg orally twice daily for 14 days

Inpatient
- Cefoxitin 2 gm intravenously every 6 hours or cefotetan 2 gm intravenously every 12 hr, *plus* doxycycline 100 mg orally or intravenously twice daily
- Clindamycin 900 mg intravenously every 8 hours plus gentamycin 2 mg/kg loading dose followed by 1.5 mg/kg every 8 hr. Follow up with doxycycline orally 100 mg twice daily for 7 days
- Metronidazole 1 gm intravenously every 8 hr plus gentamycin as above, followed by oral doxycycline as above

Note: there is limited evidence to recommend one regimen over another.
Derived from CDC recommendations MMWR 1993;42.

ciated with abnormal spotting or bleeding. Findings on examination include pelvic mass, abdominal and pelvic tenderness, cervical motion tenderness, and evidence of peritoneal irritation. Rupture of an ectopic pregnancy may result in acute, rapidly progressive shock and represents a surgical emergency.

In the past, pregnancy tests were often negative in women with ectopic pregnancy; however, currently available urine pregnancy tests, which can detect levels of human chorionic gonadotrophin (hCG) as low as 50 mIU, are almost always positive. In a patient who is hemodynamically stable, pelvic ultrasound and quantitative measurement of serum hCG are useful diagnostic tests. Ultrasound examination can determine the presence of an intrauterine pregnancy, making concurrent ectopic pregnancy extremely unlikely. In addition, ultrasound findings suggestive of ectopic pregnancy include a complex mass or gestational sac in the adnexa, or significant free fluid in the pelvis. The absence of an intrauterine gestation on ultrasound is highly suggestive of ectopic pregnancy if the hCG is above the level at which an intrauterine pregnancy is large enough to be visualized (2000 mIU/mL for vaginal ultrasound, 6500 mIU/mL for abdominal ultrasound). If the diagnosis remains uncertain and the patient is stable, a repeat hCG level in 48 hours can be helpful, because hCG levels can be expected to double in this time period with a normal pregnancy. An abnormally slow rise in hCG suggests ectopic pregnancy when associated clinical signs and symptoms are present. Because of the risk of rupture, ectopic pregnancy demands a high index of suspicion and early consultation to ensure timely treatment.

Other Causes of Acute Pelvic Pain

Leakage or rupture of an ovarian cyst can cause acute pelvic pain associated with signs of peritoneal irritation. The symptoms are usually self-limited but, if persistent or severe, laparoscopy may be required for diagnosis. Torsion of an ovarian mass or a normal adnexa usually causes acute pain that is crampy at first, then progressively more severe. As the tissue undergoes necrosis, signs of an acute abdomen may appear, with peritoneal irritation, vomiting, fever, leukocytosis, and marked pelvic tenderness. Surgery should be undertaken as soon as possible in an effort to salvage the ovary. Degeneration or infarction of a uterine fibroid, particularly during pregnancy, also may cause severe acute abdominal pain with peritoneal irritation as a result of tissue necrosis. Finally, nongynecologic abdominal emergencies must be considered, including appendicitis, diverticulitis, bowel infarction, nephrolithiasis, cholecystitis, and so on.

CHRONIC PELVIC PAIN

Chronic pelvic pain can be a disabling problem. Many gynecologic and nongynecologic conditions can contribute to chronic pelvic pain, including endometriosis, pelvic adhesions, fibroids, genital prolapse, irritable bowel syndrome, inflammatory bowel disease, intestinal cystitis, and musculoskeletal disorders. Depression or substance abuse may be associated with chronic pelvic pain. Studies have shown that up to 25 per cent of women with chronic pelvic pain have a history of physical or sexual abuse.

The evaluation should begin with a thorough history and physical examination, including a detailed description of the pain, pain in other areas, associated symptoms, past infections or surgeries, social history, and family history. Evaluation of bowel or bladder may be appropriate. While abnormal findings on pelvic exam should prompt further gynecologic evaluation, it is important to recognize that laparoscopy will detect pathology in approximately 50 per cent of women with a normal examination.

A multidisciplinary approach to the evaluation and management of women with chronic pelvic pain is beneficial. In addition to the primary health care provider, gynecologic, urologic, psychological, and/or physical therapy input may be helpful.

PELVIC MASS

The finding of a pelvic mass on exam or imaging procedure is a common clinical dilemma. In formulating a differential diagnosis, it is important to consider first whether the mass might represent a functional ovarian cyst. Normally, the ovum develops in a bed of follicular fluid, which may reach 2.5 cm in diameter just before ovulation. After ovulation, there is some bleeding into the corpus luteum, which may reach up to 4 cm in size. Sometimes, as a result of either inappropriate gonadotrophin stimulation or inappropriate follicular response, these physiologic cysts of the ovary may grow up to 7 cm in size. Such functional cysts are generally minimally symptomatic, unilateral, freely mobile, nontender, and are not associated with other abnormal findings, such as ascites. They generally will resolve by the next menstrual cycle. Many authors believe resolution can be hastened by oral contraceptive suppression. In a woman of reproductive age who is *not* on oral contraceptives, the finding of a mass fitting the above criteria warrants observation for 1 month with or without the administration of oral contraception. If the mass disappears, the patient can be followed safely. If the mass does not disappear, further evaluation should be carried out.

If the mass does not fit the description of a possible functional cyst or if it does not regress after observation, then other diagnostic possibilities should be pursued (Table 32–7). A history of pelvic pain and infertility with an abnormal pelvic exam might suggest endometriosis or chronic PID. Menorrhagia and dysmenorrhea might suggest a fibroid uterus. Vague bloating, dyspepsia, and discomfort should prompt evaluation for ovarian carcinoma. A history of bowel dysfunction would suggest inflammatory bowel disease or colon neoplasms. A detailed gynecologic history, thorough review of systems, and pelvic exam noting the size, consistency, tenderness, and degree of fixation of the mass as well as associated nodularity or ascites will help narrow the diagnostic possibilities. Ultrasound can help to determine whether a mass is cystic or solid, unilocular or complex, and whether ascitic fluid is present. There are, however, both false positives and false negatives associated with ultrasound; therefore, physical examination findings should not be ignored.

Assay of Ca-125, an epithelial ovarian cancer antigen, may be helpful, but it is important to recognize that only 80 per cent of serous carcinomas and 20 per cent of mucinous carcinomas will produce an elevated Ca-125 level; conversely, benign gynecologic disease such as endometriosis may markedly elevate Ca-125 levels. If a diagnosis of ovarian cancer is suspected, referral for surgical exploration should not be delayed on the basis of Ca-125 results.

If these further evaluations suggest a gynecologic cause for the pelvic mass, referral should be arranged to a gynecologist or gynecologic oncolo-

TABLE 32–7. DIFFERENTIAL DIAGNOSIS OF ADNEXAL MASS

Ovarian
Functional cyst
Neoplasm, benign or malignant
Tubo-ovarian abscess
Endometriosis

Tubal
Ectopic pregnancy
Paratubal cyst
Chronic PID/hydrosalpinx

Uterus
Fibroids
Uterine anomaly
Pregnancy

Gastrointestinal
Inflammatory bowel disease
Appendicitis
Carcinoma
Diverticulitis
Stool

Genitourinary
Pelvic kidney
Bladder stone/diverticulum
Full bladder

Retroperitoneum
Lymphadenopathy
Congenital cyst/mass

Abdominal Wall
Hernia
Lipoma/other neoplasm

gist where appropriate. Additional evaluation may be needed if a gastrointestinal or other abdominal source of the mass is suspected.

VULVAR LESIONS

Symptoms of vulvar abnormalities include itching, burning, bleeding, presence of a lump, pain, or dyspareunia. Any skin disorder may present on the vulva. It is important to biopsy vulvar lesions, because gross appearance alone is insufficient to make a diagnosis. Biopsy can be carried out easily in the office after infiltration with local anesthetic, either with a snip or shave biopsy after tenting the lesion with a needle, or with a dermal punch biopsy. Hemostasis can be obtained with silver nitrate, Monsel's solution, or a 3-0 or 4-0 absorbable suture. Magnification may be helpful in targeting the most appropriate biopsy site, by locating areas of atypical epithelium, abnormal vessels, ulceration, or friability that might suggest neoplasm.

Squamous epithelial lesions (formerly known as

vulvar dystrophy) include squamous epithelial hyperplasia and lichen sclerosis. *Squamous epithelial hyperplasia* appears as thickened, leathery, often white lesions, usually on the labia majora. Biopsy is mandatory to rule out atypia. These lesions are best treated with topical steroids and local hygiene measures. A cream compounded of Eurax and a steroid may be needed to control itching. *Lichen sclerosis* appears as thin, crinkled white areas, often in a figure-of-8 distribution extending around the anus. Telangiectasia, subepithelial hemorrhage, and hyperkeratosis are common, and with advanced disease there is may be loss of labial tissue and clitoral phimosis. The diagnosis is made by biopsy. Lichen sclerosis is treated with topical testosterone, 2% in petrolatum once or twice daily, with steroids added if needed to control itching. Treatment response is slow. Once symptoms remit, frequency of administration may be decreased gradually to a maintenance regimen once or twice weekly. Prolonged maintenance therapy often is required.

Vulvar intraepithelial neoplasia (previously termed dysplasia or carcinoma in situ) may be unifocal or multifocal and may appear white, gray, brown, or red. Most commonly the lesions are thickened and raised; there may be surface ulceration. There is an increasing incidence of multifocal vulvar intraepithelial neoplasia in young women, often associated with HPV infection. Multiple biopsies are mandatory to establish the diagnosis and rule out invasion. Several treatment options are available, including wide local excision, laser, electrocautery, and topical 5-fluorouracil. Excision must be performed if there is any question of invasion.

Vulvodynia is a recently described condition in which there is chronic debilitating pain or burning of the labia minora and vestibule, often associated with diffuse or focal erythema. The cause of this condition is unknown. Multiple treatment approaches have been tried, including systemic antifungal agents, topical tissue destruction with acid or laser, topical or intradermal steroids, low-dose tricyclic antidepressants, and surgical resection of the involved tissue. None of these approaches is entirely satisfactory. Many patients will experience remission after 1 to 2 years. Women with vulvodynia require much counseling and support as an integral part of any treatment approach.

MENOPAUSE

The average age of menopause in the United States is 51. The ovaries gradually become less responsive to gonadotrophin stimulation, resulting in low estradiol and high FSH and LH levels. In a woman near 50 years of age, menopause usually can be diagnosed clinically when menstrual irregularity occurs associated with hot flushes and vaginal dryness. In a younger woman, measurement of gonadotrophins may be needed to confirm a clinical suspicion. Women in the United States can be expected to live over one third of their lives after menopause; therefore, the health impact of physiologic changes in this period are important to consider.

Symptoms of menopause include hot flushes, vaginal dryness, and urinary urgency. The hot flush, a sudden perception of increased heat in the upper body and face lasting several minutes, can range in severity from mildly uncomfortable to debilitating. Night hot flushes can lead to sleep disturbance, which can in turn result in irritability, moodiness, inability to concentrate, and lethargy. Untreated, hot flushes generally subside within several years after menopause. Estrogen replacement can prevent or stop hot flushes. Decreased estrogen support of the lower genital tract leads to vaginal dryness and dyspareunia as well as urinary urgency, frequency, and stress incontinence. Estrogen replacement systematically or topically will alleviate these symptoms.

Menopause is associated with an increased risk of cardiovascular disease, possibly related to adverse changes in lipid profile. Menopausal women have an increase in total cholesterol, low-density lipoproteins, and triglycerides and a fall in high-density lipoproteins. Estrogen replacement decreases the risk of myocardial infarction by 50 per cent, appears to slow the development of atherosclerosis assessed by angiography, and decreases the adverse lipid changes associated with menopause.

The rate of bone loss also accelerates at menopause, leading to an increased risk of osteoporosis and associated hip, arm, and vertebral fractures. Estrogen replacement reduces the rate of bone loss as long as it is continued; if estrogen is stopped, bone loss occurs at a rate similar to that in untreated menopause. Although estrogen replacement is clearly effective at preventing bone loss, its ability to increase bone mass once osteoporosis has progressed remains uncertain.

Estrogen replacement therapy has been shown to be effective at preventing symptoms of menopause, decreasing cardiovascular risk, and slowing osteoporosis. There are adverse effects of estrogen therapy as well. Women with an intact uterus who are treated with unopposed estrogen have a six- to eight-times increased risk of developing endometrial carcinoma; however, the addition of progestins decreases this risk to below baseline. Epidemiologic data regarding the influence of estrogen therapy on breast cancer have been conflicting.

Meta-analysis of multiple studies shows no increased risk of breast cancer with estrogen alone or estrogen plus progestin; however, it is possible that an estrogen-dependent breast cancer may grow more rapidly if estrogen replacement is used. Other nonlipid metabolic effects of estrogen replacement are minimal, with no significant change in coagulation factors, glucose metabolism, or blood pressure. In contrast, these factors are altered significantly in oral contraceptive users because of the markedly increased potency of the synthetic ethinyl estradiol found in these agents. Some progestins used for replacement therapy may increase depressive symptoms. Side effects that may be uncomfortable but not health-threatening include breast tenderness, bloating, and breakthrough bleeding.

There are numerous regimens that can be used for estrogen replacement (Table 32–8). The woman with an intact uterus should receive estrogen plus a progestin, either sequentially or continuously. Sequential therapy usually produces regular monthly withdrawal bleeding episodes. Continuous therapy is associated with irregular bleeding for the first several months, but most women become amenorrheic after 6 months. Women who have undergone hysterectomy may be treated with estrogen alone. Routine pretreatment endometrial sampling is not necessary. However, biopsy should be done in women with abnormal bleeding before initiating therapy, and during therapy if unscheduled bleeding occurs on sequential therapy or persists after the first 6 months of continuous therapy. Regular breast examination and mammography are prudent in women receiving estrogen replacement, and patients should be taught and encouraged to perform self–breast examination.

INFERTILITY

Infertility—no pregnancy after 1 year of unprotected intercourse—occurs in approximately 15 to 20 per cent of couples. Possible etiologies include abnormal sperm production or transport, ovulatory dysfunction, tubal blockage, uterine abnormalities, and abnormal semen–cervical mucus interaction. Up to 30 per cent of infertile couples will have more than one abnormality found on evaluation.

A couple should be offered evaluation after 1 year of attempting pregnancy, or sooner if the woman is over 30 or an etiology is obvious (e.g., amenorrhea). Counseling regarding frequency and timing of intercourse is appropriate. A thorough history and physical exam should be performed on both partners, with attention to prior pregnancies, sexually transmitted infections, exposure to toxins, medical and illicit drug use, menstrual and ejaculatory dysfunction, systemic illness, and abnormalities on genital exam. Basic testing of each component is outlined in Table 32–9. The male factor is assessed by semen analysis to evaluate sperm count, abnormal sperm morphology, and leukocytes in the semen. Ovulatory function can be assessed using basal body temperature charting, wherein the basal temperature is recorded for several menstrual cycles. A sustained rise of 0.5° C generally indicates ovulation, which can be documented further with properly timed serum progesterone level and endometrial biopsy. Tubal patency and intrauterine structure can be assessed via hysterosalpingogram, during which radiopaque dye is injected through the cervix under fluoroscopic guidance. Cervical mucus quantity, quality, and sperm interaction are evaluated by microscopic examination of mid-cycle mucus some hours after intercourse.

There are many treatment strategies available for the infertile couple (Table 32–9). If a single cause is identified (e.g., anovulation), specific treatment should be initiated. If treatment is unsuccessful or multiple factors are identified, consultation with a specialist is appropriate. In addition, early consultation with a specialist should be considered strongly in women over age 30, because time becomes critical. Assisted reproduction techniques, such as in vitro fertilization, currently result in a clinical pregnancy rate of 15 to 20 per cent per cycle, with cumulative rates up to 70 per cent.

TABLE 32–8. ESTROGEN REPLACEMENT THERAPY

	Dose Range
Estrogens	
Conjugated estrogen	0.625–1.5 mg q day
Estropipate	0.625–1.5 mg q day
Micronized estradiol	1–2 mg q day
Transdermal estradiol	0.05–0.1 mg twice weekly
Vaginal creams	½–1 applicator twice weekly
Progestins	
Medroxyprogesterone acetate	10 mg × 10 days/month (sequential)
	2.5 mg q day (continuous)
Norethindrone	2.5 mg q day
Regimens	
Sequential	Estrogen days 1–25; progesterone days 14–25 (both off day 26—end of month)
	Estrogen: daily; progesterone days 1–14 (no break in estrogen)
Continuous	Estrogen + progesterone daily
	Estrogen + progesterone 5 days/week, off 2 days

TABLE 32–9. INFERTILITY INVESTIGATION AND INTERVENTIONS

Factor	Incidence	Evaluation	Interventions
Male factor	30–40%	Semen analysis Postcoital test	Intrauterine insemination Varicocele repair Endocrine manipulation Donor insemination
Ovulation	10–15%	Basal body temperature Serum progesterone Timed endometrial biopsy	Ovulation induction Bromocriptine
Tubal/uterine	30–40%	Hysterosalpingogram	Surgical
Cervical	5–10%	Postcoital test	Antibiotics Estrogen/steroids Intrauterine insemination
Rare/unknown	10%		Assisted reproductive techniques

PELVIC RELAXATION

The pelvic organs are supported by ligaments, fascia, and pelvic floor muscles. These support structures can be stretched or damaged by pregnancy and childbirth, obesity, chronic coughing or straining, or pelvic surgery. Mild pelvic relaxation often is exacerbated at menopause, resulting in new onset of symptoms.

Symptoms of genital prolapse correlate poorly with the degree of anatomic relaxation found on examination. Common complaints include sacral backache, pelvic heaviness or a dragging sensation, a sense of "something falling out," and dyspareunia. Symptoms are worse in the evening or after prolonged standing and relieved by supine position. Anterior vaginal wall prolapse (cystocele) may produce urinary urgency, frequency, urinary retention, or urinary incontinence. Posterior vaginal wall relaxation (rectocele) may cause constipation and a need to apply counterpressure with fingers in the vagina in order to pass stool. Complete prolapse of the uterus or vaginal vault may lead to mucosal ulceration, urinary retention, and inability to walk because of the bulky perineal tissue mass.

Genital prolapse usually is diagnosed readily on physical exam. Using the posterior blade of a disarticulated speculum allows individual inspection of the anterior and posterior vaginal walls. It is important to assess the degree of descent at rest and with Valsalva maneuver of each pelvic structure individually, including the uterus, vaginal vault, bladder, and rectum.

Symptoms caused by minor degrees of prolapse often can be improved with Kegel exercises and estrogen replacement therapy where appropriate.

The primary treatment modality for symptomatic prolapse is surgical, with repair of each structure as indicated. In women who are poor surgical risks, vaginal pessaries can be used to support pelvic structures; however, they are associated with discharge and odor that may be troublesome, and they require frequent cleaning. A neglected pessary may cause vaginal ulceration or urinary or bowel obstruction.

The evaluation of *urinary incontinence* deserves special mention. Anatomic stress incontinence occurs when bladder pressure exceeds urethral pressure with coughing or straining; thus, the patient loses urine immediately on coughing with no preceding urge to void. It is usually associated with genital relaxation and it can be suspected on physical examination and by having the patient cough while the bladder is full. Urge incontinence is associated with uninhibited detrusor contractions. The patient may complain of frequency, urgency, nocturia, and loss of urine a few seconds following an urge to void. Overflow incontinence occurs when the bladder is unable to empty because of neurologic dysfunction or obstruction, and varying amounts of urine leak with increased abdominal pressure. Overflow incontinence may be confused with anatomic stress incontinence. Total incontinence (constant urinary leakage) is usually due to a fistula between the ureter, bladder, or urethra and the vagina.

Women with incontinence should undergo careful evaluation, including history and physical exam, catheterization for postresidual and culture, and focused neurologic exam. Cystometric evaluation of bladder and urethral pressures is usually necessary, and cystoscopy may be helpful. Treatment is tailored to the type of incontinence diagnosed and the general medical status of the patient.

REFERENCES

American College of Obstetricians and Gynecologists ACOG Technical Bulletin no. 183. Washington DC, 1993.

Amsel R, Totten PA, Spiegel CA, et al: Nonspecific vaginitis: Diagnostic criteria and microbial and epidemiologic associations. Am J Med 74:14, 1983.

Berg AO, Heidrich FE, Fihn SD, et al: Establishing the cause of genitourinary symptoms in women in a family practice: Comparison of clinical examination and comprehensive microbiology. JAMA 251:520, 1984.

Brown D, Kaufman RH: Vulvovaginitis. *In* Glass RH (ed): Office Gynecology, 4th edition. Baltimore, Williams & Wilkins, 1993, pp 77–85.

Bump RC, Quspan FP, Buesching WJ 3rd, et al: The prevalence, six-month persistence, and predictive values of laboratory indicators of bacterial vaginosis (non-specific vaginitis) in asymptomatic women. Am J Obstet Gynecol 150:917, 1984.

Centers for Disease Control and Prevention: 1993 sexually transmitted diseases treatment guidelines. MMWR 42:RR-14, 1993.

Chow WH, Greenberg RS, Liff JM: Decline in the incidence of carcinoma in situ of the cervix. Am J Public Health 76:1322, 1986.

Chu J, White E: Decreasing incidence of invasive cervical cancer in young women. Am J Obstet Gynecol 157:1105, 1987.

Council on Scientific Affairs: Quality assurance in cervical cytology. JAMA 262:1672, 1989.

Eschenbach DA, Hillier S, Critchlow C, et al: Diagnosis and clinical manifestations of bacterial vaginosis. Am J Obstet Gynecol 148:819, 1988.

Ferenczy A, Bergeron C, Richart RM: Human papillomavirus DNA in fomites on objects used for the management of patients with genital human papillomavirus infections. Obstet Gynecol 74:950, 1989.

Ferris DG, Payne P, Frisch LE, et al: Cervicography: Adjunctive cervical cancer screening by primary care physicians. J Fam Pract 37:158, 1993.

Ferris DG, Willner WH, Ho JJ: Colposcopes, a comprehensive selected critical review. J Fam Pract 33:506, 1991.

Fink D: Change in American Cancer Society Checkup guidelines for detection of cervical cancer. CA 38:127, 1988.

Finklehor D, Hotaling G, Lewis IA, et al: Sexual abuse in a national survey of adult men and women: Prevalence, characteristics, and risk factors. Child Abuse Negl 14:19, 1990.

Jovanovic R, Congema E, Nguyen H: Antifungal agents vs. boric acid for treating chronic mycotic vulvovaginitis. J Reprod Med 35:593, 1991.

Kohan S, Noumoff J, Beckman EM, et al: Colposcopic screening of women with atypical Papanicolaou smears. J Reprod Med 30:383, 1985.

Korn AP, Stern JL: Human papilloma infections of the female genital tract. *In* Glass RH (ed): Office Gynecology, 4th edition. Baltimore, Williams & Wilkins, 1993, pp 55–76.

Lawley TB, Lee RB, Kapela R: The significance of moderate and severe inflammation on class I Papanicolaou smear. Obstet Gynecol 76:997, 1990.

National Cancer Institute Workshop: The 1988 Bethesda System for reporting cervical/vaginal cytological diagnosis. JAMA 262:931, 1989.

Nelson JH Jr, Averette HE, Richart RM: Cervical intraepithelial neoplasia and early invasive cervical carcinoma. CA 39:157, 1989.

Noumoff JS: Atypia in cervical cytology as a risk factor for intraepithelial neoplasia. Am J Obstet Gynecol 156:628, 1987.

Oriel JD: Sex and cervical cancer. Genitourinary Med 64: 81, 1988.

Papanicolaou GN, Traut HF: Diagnosis of uterine cancer by the vaginal smear. New York: Commonwealth Fund, 1943.

Reed BD, Eyler A: Vaginal infections: Diagnosis and management. Am Fam Physician 47:1805, 1993.

Reed BD, Huck W, Zazove P: Differentiation of *Garderella vaginalis*, *Candida albicans*, and *Trichomonas vaginalis* infections of the vagina. J Fam Pract 28:673, 1989.

Reissman SE: Comparison of two Papanicolaou smear techniques in a family practice setting. J Fam Pract 26:525, 1988.

Reiter RC: Management of initial atypical cervical cytology: A randomized, prospective study. Obstet Gynecol 68:237, 1986.

Slattery ML, Overall JC Jr, Abbott TM, et al: Sexual activity, contraception, genital infections, and cervical cancer: support for a sexually transmitted disease hypothesis. Am J Epidemiol 130:248, 1989.

Slawson DC, Bennett JH, Simon LJ, et al: Should all women with cervical atypia be referred for colposcopy: A HARNET* study. J Fam Pract 38:387, 1994.

Spiegal CA: Bacterial vaginosis. Clin Microbiol Rev 4:485, 1991.

Szarewski A, Cuzick J, Edwards R, et al: The use of cervicography in a primary screening service. Br J Obstet Gynaecol 98:313, 1991.

Thomason JL, Gelbart SM: Trichomonas vaginalis. Obstet Gynecol 74(3, Pt 2):536, 1989.

U.S. Preventive Services Task Force. 1990. Guide to clinical preventive services: an assessment of the effectiveness of 169 interventions. Report of the U.S. Preventive Services Task Force. Baltimore. Williams & Wilkins, 1989.

Vejtorp M, Bollerup AC, Vajtorp L, et al: Bacterial vaginosis: A double-blind randomized trial of the effect of treatment of the sexual partner. Br J Obstet Gynaecol 95:920, 1988.

Walch AG, Broadhead WE: Prevalence of lifetime sexual victimization among female patients. J Fam Pract 35:511, 1992.

Weitzman GA, Korhonen MO, Reeves KO, et al: Endocervical brush cytology: An alternative to endocervical curettage? J Reprod Med 33:677, 1988.

SUGGESTED READINGS

Pelvic Inflammatory Disease

Eschenback DA: Epidemiology and diagnosis of acute pelvic inflammatory disease. Obstet Gynecol 55:1425, 1980.

Hager WD, et al: Criteria for diagnosis and grading of salpingitis. Obstet Gynecol 61:113, 1983.

Jacobson LJ: Differential diagnosis of acute pelvic inflammatory disease. Am J Obstet Gynecol 138:1006, 1980.

Infertility

Guzick DDS, et al: Cumulative pregnancy rates for in-vitro fertilization. Fertil Steril 46:663, 1986.

Mishell DR, et al: Infertility, Contraception and Reproductive Endocrinology, 3rd edition. New York, Blackwell Scientific Publications, 1991.

Amenorrhea

Kletzky DA, Davajan V, Nakamura RM, et al: Clinical categorization of patients with secondary amenorrhea using progesterone-induced uterine bleeding and measurement of serum gonadotrophin levels. Am J Obstet Gynecol 121:695, 1975.

Reindollar RH, et al: Adult onset amenorrhea: A study of 262 patients. Am J Obstet Gynecol 155:531, 1986.

Speroff L: Clinical Gynecologic Endocrinology and Infertility, 3rd edition. Baltimore, Williams & Wilkins, 1983.

Tulandi T, Finch RA: Premature ovarian failure. Obstet Gynecol Surv 26:521, 1981.

Abnormal Bleeding

Claessens EA, Cowell CL: Acute adolescent menorrhagia. Am J Obstet Gynecol 139:277, 1981.

Fraser IS, et al: Long term treatment of menorrhagia with mefermanic acid. Obstet Gynecol 61:109, 1983.

Van Eijkeren MA, et al: Menorrhagia—a review. Obstet Gynecol Surv 44:421, 1989.

CHAPTER 33
CONTRACEPTION

JANET P. REALINI

Control of reproductive capacity is extremely important to individuals and families. With available contraceptives, men and women can choose when—and whether—they will have children. They can choose childbearing at a time and under circumstances that are optimal for their physical, emotional, social, and economic well-being. Family physicians are in a unique position to help their patients in this important area with education and counseling about the available methods of contraception.

Current contraceptive technology offers a variety of safe and effective methods from which to choose. No method is perfect; each has its risks, benefits, advantages, and disadvantages. The effectiveness of contraceptive methods is a primary concern of patients and may be described in several ways. Two measures of effectiveness are listed in Table 33–1. Use of a contraceptive is an elective therapy, and the choice of a contraceptive method is a personal and individual one; therefore, the family physician's task is to help patients make an informed choice of a suitable method.

Unfortunately, the existence of contraceptive technologies does not assure that they will be used fully or well. Over half of the pregnancies in the United States are unintended. Adolescents account for over 1 million unintended pregnancies each year. Family physicians have an opportunity and an obligation to help their patients, regardless of age, make responsible, healthy decisions about sexual activity and contraception. Family physicians also can help their communities to deal with these issues.

Prevention and care of sexually transmitted diseases (STDs) are linked closely to contraception. With the growing epidemic of human immunodeficiency virus (HIV) infection, the potential consequences of unprotected sex now include a fatal disease. Unfortunately, there is no method or device that is nearly perfect in preventing both pregnancy and STDs. Family physicians must individualize their contraceptive recommendations based on the risk of STD exposure, as well as on other factors and preferences. For many patients, using more than one method simultaneously may be appropriate.

ORAL CONTRACEPTIVES

Oral contraceptives (OCs) are the most popular form of reversible contraception in the United States: an estimated 16 million American women currently are taking OCs. Since they became available over 30 years ago, OCs have been studied extensively and have undergone an evolution to the current preparations with low doses of both estrogens and progestins. The safety, efficacy, and noncontraceptive benefits of OCs are documented voluminously. Unfortunately, OCs are often misunderstood by the general public. Untrue myths about OCs include that they cause cancer and that they are more dangerous than childbearing. It is thus important that family physicians offer their patients a balanced view of the benefits—as well as the risks—of OCs.

Effectiveness

Theoretically, OCs have a pregnancy rate that is close to zero (see Table 33–1). However, the effectiveness of OCs in actual use is less than perfect and depends a great deal on patient motivation and ability to remember to take the pill.

Oral contraceptives prevent pregnancy primarily by inhibiting ovulation through a negative feedback mechanism on the hypothalamus or anterior pituitary, or both. The midcycle gonadotropin surge is inhibited, and ovulation does not occur. Additional contraceptive mechanisms probably include alterations of cervical mucus, endometrial metabolism, and fallopian tube motility.

Products Available

There are many products commercially available (Table 33–2). Several pills contain only a small dose of progestin; these "mini-pills" will be discussed separately later. Each of the rest of the preparations contains both an estrogen and a progestin.

The two estrogens that have been used in OCs, ethinyl estradiol and mestranol, are synthetic estrogens that are well absorbed orally. For all practi-

TABLE 33–1. PERCENT OF WOMEN WITH ACCIDENTAL PREGNANCY IN THE FIRST YEAR OF USE OF COMMON CONTRACEPTIVE METHODS

Method	Percentage Accidental Pregnancy	
	Typical Use	Perfect Use
Chance	85	85
Spermicides	21	6
Periodic abstinence	20	1–9*
Withdrawal	19	4
Cap (with spermicide)		
Parous	36	26
Nulliparous	18	9
Sponge		
Parous	36	20
Nulliparous	18	9
Diaphragm (with spermicide)	18	6
Condom (without spermicide)		
Male	12	3
Female (Reality)	21	5
Oral contraceptives		
Combined	3	0.1
Progestin only	3	0.5
IUD		
TCu 380A	0.8	0.6
Progesterone T	2.0	1.5
Depo-Provera	0.3	0.3
Norplant	0.09	0.09
Female sterilization	0.4	0.4
Male sterilization	0.15	0.10

* Varies with type of method used. Lowest rates with postovulation method.

From Hatcher RA, Trussell J, Stewart F, et al: Contraceptive Technology. New York, Irvington Publishers, 1994. Adapted with the permission of Contraceptive Technology Communications, Inc.

cal purposes, they are considered to be roughly equipotent. Most of the progestins used in OCs are chemically derived from nortestosterone, and thus have some androgenic effects, in addition to their progestogenic and antiestrogenic effects. Several new progestins with less androgenic effects (desogestrel, norgestimate, and gestodene) are becoming available (Klitsch, 1992).

Predicting the estrogenicity and progestogenicity of OC products is difficult. Many variables are involved, including the types and dosages of the progestins and estrogens; the estrogenic, antiestrogenic, and androgenic effects of the progestins; and the variability of the individuals taking the medication. Moreover, the relative estrogenicity and progestogenicity of various OC combinations have never been studied adequately in humans.

Instructions for Use

Effective patient education is essential to reduce confusion, answer concerns, and prevent unnecessary discontinuation of OCs (Association of Reproductive Health Professionals, 1991). Patients should be encouraged to ask questions and to contact the physician with any concerns.

The first pill of the first pack is started either on the first day of the menstrual period ("day 1 start") or on the first Sunday after the period starts ("Sunday start"). The latter method requires use of a backup contraceptive such as condoms for 7 days after beginning the first pack. Sunday starters should take the first pill on the first day of their period if it falls on a Sunday.

Combined OCs are taken daily for 21 days, followed by a 7-day hiatus, during which withdrawal bleeding of the endometrium occurs. The number of pills that can be missed in one cycle without risking pregnancy is unknown. Patients usually are advised to take the forgotten pill as soon as it is remembered, without postponing the next pill. Two or more missed pills are "made up" by taking two pills a day. It is wise to use a backup method of contraception for 7 days if two or more pills are missed.

There is no evidence of a need to discontinue OCs periodically. The risks associated with OC use do not appear to be related to the length of time a woman is on the pill.

Risks and Side Effects

Serious complications from OC use are rare, and large-scale epidemiologic studies are required to demonstrate their associations with oral contraception. Much of the data we have on side effects is from studies of women taking older preparations containing 50 μg or more of estrogen.

Cardiovascular Risks

Several serious cardiovascular events have been associated with the use of OCs (Stadel, 1981). Venous thromboembolism (i.e., deep vein thrombosis or pulmonary embolism) consistently has been associated with OC use. The relative risk of these venous events is estimated to be 2 to 11 times that of women who do not use OCs, and the risk probably is related to the estrogen component of the pill.

The risk of arterial events associated with OC use—stroke and myocardial infarction—appears to be confined to older women with risk factors, especially cigarette smokers (Royal College of General Practitioners Oral Contraception Study, 1981). The mortality risks of OC use are primarily due to these arterial events, which appear to be related to thrombosis rather than to atherosclerosis. The mortality risk is primarily among women over 35 who smoke cigarettes (Ory, 1983), so OCs are contraindicated for this group of women. Women without cardiovascular risk factors may continue OCs until the time of the menopause, if they so choose.

Reversible hypertension develops in a few patients who are taking OCs. In addition, small elevations in the mean systolic blood pressure levels have been documented in some populations.

TABLE 33–2. AVAILABLE ORAL CONTRACEPTIVE PREPARATIONS

Brand Name	Estrogen (µg)	Progestin (mg)
High-Dose (50-µg) Pills		
Ortho-Novum 1/50, Norinyl 1 + 50, Norethin 1/50, Nelova 1/50, Genora 1/50	Mestranol (50)	Norethindrone (1)
Demulen 1/50	Ethinyl estradiol (50)	Ethynodiol diacetate (1)
Norlestrin 1/50	Ethinyl estradiol (50)	Norethindrone acetate (1)
Norlestrin 2.5/50	Ethinyl estradiol (50)	Norethindrone acetate (2.5)
Ovcon-50	Ethinyl estradiol (50)	Norethindrone (1)
Ovral	Ethinyl estradiol (50)	Norgestrel (0.5)
Low-Dose Monophasics		
Demulen 1/35	Ethinyl estradiol (35)	Ethynodiol diacetate (1)
Ortho-Novum 1/35, Norinyl 1 + 35, Norethin 1/35, Nelova 1/35, Genora 1/35	Ethinyl estradiol (35)	Norethindrone (1)
Modicon, Brevicon, Genora 0.5/35, Nelova 0.5/35	Ethinyl estradiol (35)	Norethindrone (0.5)
Ovcon-35	Ethinyl estradiol (35)	Norethindrone (0.4)
Lo-Ovral	Ethinyl estradiol (30)	Norgestrel (0.3)
Nordette, Levlen	Ethinyl estradiol (30)	Levonorgestrel (0.15)
Loestrin 1.5/30	Ethinyl estradiol (30)	Norethindrone acetate (1.5)
Loestrin 1/20	Ethinyl estradiol (20)	Norethindrone acetate (1)
Ortho-Cept, Desogen	Ethinyl estradiol (30)	Desogestrel (0.15)
Ortho-Cyclen	Ethinyl estradiol (35)	Norgestimate (0.25)
Low-Dose Multiphasics		
Ortho-Novum 10/11	Ethinyl estradiol (35)	Norethindrone (0.5) × 10 days, norethindrone (1.0) × 11 days
Ortho-Novum 7/7/7	Ethinyl estradiol (35)	Norethindrone (0.5) × 7 days, norethindrone (0.75) × 7 days, norethindrone (1.0) × 7 days
Tri-Norinyl	Ethinyl estradiol (35)	Norethindrone (0.5) × 7 days, norethindrone (1.0) × 9 days, norethindrone (0.5) × 5 days
Jenest	Ethinyl estradiol (35)	Norethindrone (0.5) × 7 days, norethindrone (1.0) × 14 days
Triphasil, Tri-Levlen	Ethinyl estradiol (30), ethinyl estradiol (40), ethinyl estradiol (30)	Levonorgestrel (0.05) × 6 days, levonorgestrel (0.075) × 5 days, levonorgestrel (0.125) × 10 days
Ortho Tri Cyclen	Ethinyl estradiol (35)	Norgestimate (0.18) × 7 days, norgestimate (0.215) × 7 days, norgestimate (0.25) × 7 days
Mini-Pills		
Micronor	None	Norethindrone (0.35)
Nor-Q.D.	None	Norethindrone (0.35)
Ovrette	None	Norgestrel (0.075)

OCs and Cancer

Oral contraceptive use appears to reduce the risk of endometrial carcinoma by 50 per cent and that of ovarian cancer by 40 per cent (Cancer and Steroid Hormone Study, 1986). The reduction in these risks is related to the duration of use of OCs and persists for years after OC use is discontinued.

Concern that breast cancer might be caused by exogenous hormones has led to many studies and intense surveillance. Overall, there appears to be no increase in risk of breast cancer with OC use. However, some studies suggest a slightly increased risk of breast cancer diagnosed in younger women (Hawley et al., 1993). Research in this area continues. In the meantime, the U.S. Food and Drug Administration (FDA), along with other regulatory and authoritative bodies, has recommended no change in labeling or prescribing of OCs.

Cancer of the cervix is particularly difficult to study from an epidemiologic standpoint, and its relationship to OC use is not clear. Several studies suggest an increased risk of cervical dysplasia or cervical carcinoma, whereas many do not. Performance of Papanicolaou (Pap) smears at least yearly is recommended for women on OCs so that cervical dysplasia may be detected and treated early.

Rarely, benign hepatic tumors (hepatocellular adenomas)—and perhaps hepatocellular carcinomas—occur in association with long-term OC use. These tumors may present with hypovolemic shock resulting from rupture and intra-abdominal hemorrhage. Liver tumors are so rare that they are not considered a significant risk.

Metabolic Effects

The effect of OCs on serum lipid levels is complex. In general, estrogens tend to have beneficial effects: they decrease low-density lipoprotein

(LDL) cholesterol, which is related directly to coronary risk, and increase high-density lipoprotein (HDL) cholesterol, which is related inversely to coronary risk. Most of the progestins used in OCs tend to do just the opposite: increase LDL cholesterol and decrease HDL cholesterol. When estrogens and progestins are combined in oral contraceptive preparations, their effects on serum lipids are due to both components.

Potentially adverse effects on lipids are minimized by minimizing the progestin dose, such as with multiphasic low-dose preparations. The newer progestins (gestodene, norgestimate, and desogestrel) are expected to have even less adverse effect on lipids. The actual effect of these lipid changes on the coronary risk of young women, however, is unclear. Premenopausal women enjoy relative protection from atherosclerotic coronary disease, and the beneficial effect of estrogen is likely due to other factors in addition to lipoprotein levels (Baird and Glasier, 1993).

OC use does not cause diabetes mellitus per se, although it may uncover diabetes in susceptible women. Even when fasting glucose levels are normal, however, OC use may be associated with glucose intolerance and relative insulin resistance. These effects appear to be due to the progestin component of the pill, and often return to normal after 6 months of use. Low-dose pills and OCs containing the new progestins have minimal effects on glucose metabolism. In women with diabetes mellitus, taking OCs may increase insulin requirements.

OCs and STDs

The risk of *Chlamydia trachomatis* infection of the cervix is higher among women on OCs than in nonusers. This effect may be mediated by the induction of cervical ectropion in women on OCs (Cates and Stone, 1992b). However, the risk of clinical pelvic inflammatory disease (PID) is reduced by half by current use of OCs.

The effects of OC use on the risks of acquiring and transmitting HIV infection are under study. There is some evidence from Africa that OC use may be associated with a greater risk of HIV seroconversion and that OC use may increase the likelihood that a woman with HIV will shed the virus (Cates and Stone, 1992b; Clemetson et al., 1993). Whether OC use increases the risk of HIV infection is not clear; however, it is clear that OC use offers no protection from the deadly virus.

"Minor" Side Effects

Low-dose combination OCs are generally well tolerated. However, some women on OCs experience side effects that are bothersome but not serious. Nausea and "breakthrough" spotting or bleeding are relatively common in the first few months of use and usually subside spontaneously. Patients should be reassured and encouraged to continue taking the pill. Nausea is sometimes helped by taking the pill at bedtime. Spotting may respond to taking the pill at the same time every day.

"Late" breakthrough bleeding (that which occurs after several months on the pill) should prompt evaluation for infections of the genital tract, especially *Chlamydia,* bacterial vaginosis, and trichomoniasis (Association of Reproductive Health Professionals, 1991). When other etiologies are excluded, then the problem can be attributed to the OC formulation. Late breakthrough bleeding sometimes resolves with changing to another low-dose OC preparation. An alternative is to provide small supplemental doses of estrogen (e.g., 20 μg/day of ethinyl estradiol) for one to two pill cycles.

If "amenorrhea"—or lack of withdrawal bleeding—occurs, pregnancy must be excluded. Patients should be reassured that light monthly bleeding is normal on OCs, and that it is not harmful to have no withdrawal bleeding. They should be encouraged to continue the pill and discuss any concerns with the physician. If the lack of withdrawal bleeding persists, it can be managed by switching to a preparation containing 50 μg of estrogen for 1 to 3 months.

Acne is occasionally a side effect, but more frequently acne improves on OCs. Patients with acne usually are advised to avoid pills containing the relatively androgenic progestins norgestrel and levonorgestrel.

Symptoms such as breast tenderness, weight gain, and headache sometimes are experienced by women on the pill. These symptoms may be minimized by prescribing OC preparations with low estrogen dose. Authorities differ on whether women with migraine headaches are candidates for estrogen-containing OCs. However, there is consensus that progressive or severe headaches should prompt discontinuation of OCs.

Other Adverse Effects

An increased risk of symptomatic gallstone disease has been noted in young women in the early years of OC use. OC use appears not to affect the overall risk of gallbladder disease, however. It may be that OC use precipitates the development of symptoms in susceptible women.

Because of experience with high-dose progestins and diethylstilbestrol taken early in pregnancy, there was concern that OCs might cause congenital anomalies. However, careful study has failed to reveal convincing evidence that taking OCs early in pregnancy is teratogenic (Simpson, 1985). Similarly, pregnancies conceived shortly after discontinuing OCs are *not* at increased risk of congenital anomalies.

A short delay in the return of fertility is common after discontinuing OCs, but "postpill amenorrhea" is not considered to be a distinct entity. Women who fail to menstruate within 6 months of discontinuing OCs have diverse underlying problems and should undergo careful evaluation for the cause of the amenorrhea.

Drug interactions may occur in women on OCs (Table 33–3). OC use may affect other drugs taken. Antibiotics and anticonvulsants may reduce OC effectiveness; some cases of accidental pregnancy have been reported. With the exception of rifampin, however, the risk of pregnancy with antibiotic use appears to be elevated only mildly. Many physicians recommend use of a backup method of contraception during short-term antibiotic therapy. Patients on long-term therapy with antibiotics or anticonvulsants should be informed of their slightly higher pregnancy risk with OCs. To reduce this risk, these patients should use higher dose (50 μg estrogen) pills or another method of contraception.

TABLE 33–3. DRUG INTERACTIONS WITH ORAL CONTRACEPTIVES

Drugs Reported To Cause OC Failure
Antibiotics
  Rifampicin (best documented)
  Penicillins, especially ampicillin
  Tetracyclines
  Griseofulvin
  Chloramphenicol
  Erythromycin
  Metronidazole
  Sulfonamides
  Others
Anticonvulsants
  Phenobarbital and other barbiturates
  Phenytoin
  Most others, except valproic acid
Mineral oil (theoretically, in large amounts)
Any drug or condition that decreases intestinal transit time

Drugs Reported To Increase OC Steroid Blood Levels
Acetaminophen
Ascorbic Acid

Drugs Reported To Be Affected by OC Use
Increased Drug Levels or Effects
Antipyrine
Benzodiazepenes (some)
  Alprazolam
  Chlordiazepoxide
  Clorazepate
  Diazepam
  Flurazepam
  Halazepam
  Midazolam
  Prazepam
  Triazolam
Caffeine
Corticosteroids (e.g., prednisolone)
Cyclosporine
Metoprolol (possibly also propranolol, timolol)
Theophylline
Tricyclic antidepressants

Decreased Blood Levels or Effects
Acetaminophen
Benzodiazepenes (some)
  Lorazepam
  Oxazepam
  Temazepam
Morphine
Salicylates, including aspirin
Thyroid hormone

Increased or Decreased Blood Levels or Effects
  Anticoagulants
  Phenytoin

Other Interactions
Troleandomycin (combination may increase risk of cholestasis)

TABLE 33–4. NONCONTRACEPTIVE BENEFITS: CONDITIONS FOR WHICH OC USE OFFERS PROTECTION

Ovarian carcinoma
Endometrial carcinoma
Ectopic pregnancy
Pelvic inflammatory disease
Functional ovarian cysts
Menstrual irregularities
Dysmenorrhea
Iron-deficiency anemia
Benign breast disease
Premenstrual syndrome

Noncontraceptive Benefits

Table 33–4 lists conditions for which OC use confers protection. Ovarian and endometrial carcinoma are reduced by about half among OC users (and former users). Because OCs prevent ovulation, ectopic pregnancy is less likely to occur and primary dysmenorrhea often is relieved.

OC users have a reduced risk of PID when compared to women using no contraception. Ovarian activity is inhibited, and functional ovarian cysts are reduced in frequency, although this beneficial effect appears to be less noticeable with lower dose pills.

Because women on OCs tend to lose less blood each month, iron-deficiency anemia is less common with OC use than among nonusers. Benign breast disease is less common among OC users than among nonusers. Menstrual irregularities are less likely, and some women have relief of premenstrual symptoms on OCs. In addition, some evidence suggests that rheumatoid arthritis, toxic shock syndrome, and uterine fibroids occur less frequently among OC users than among users of other forms of contraception. Ory (1982) estimated that 50,000 hospitalizations are prevented by OC use annually in the United States and that 1 user in 750 is spared a hospitalization.

Contraindications

The contraindications to OC use are listed in Table 33–5. In addition, there are many conditions for which OC use may pose additional risks. In these situations, the patient's lack of other contra-

TABLE 33–5. CONTRAINDICATIONS TO ORAL CONTRACEPTIVES

Contraindications
Thromboembolism
Cerebrovascular disease
Coronary artery disease
Breast cancer, known or suspected
Estrogen-dependent malignancy, known or suspected
Pregnancy, known or suspected
Undiagnosed abnormal vaginal bleeding
Liver neoplasm, benign or malignant
Active liver disease
Cholestatic jaundice of pregnancy, or jaundice with prior use

Other Conditions That May Make OC Use Less Desirable
Hypertension
Diabetes mellitus
Hyperlipidemia
Smoker over 35 years old
Gallbladder disease
Migraine headaches
Seizure disorder
History of serious depression
Chloasma (melasma)
Morbid obesity
Vasomotor rhinitis
Congenital or rheumatic heart disease
Inflammatory bowel disease
Neurofibromatosis
Hereditary hemorrhagic telangectasia
Psoriasis
Systemic lupus erythematosus
Renal disease
Porphyria
Lactation (controversial)
Sickle hemoglobinopathies (controversial)
Elective surgery (controversial)

ceptive options and her risk of pregnancy without OCs may be reasons to consider OCs. The family physician should help her weigh the risks and benefits of OCs as well as those of other contraceptive methods.

Hypertension, diabetes mellitus, and hyperlipidemias are listed in Table 33–5 because they may be worsened by OC use. In addition, these conditions, as well as smoking cigarettes, are risk factors for cardiovascular disease and thus may increase the risks of OC use. Leiomyomata and varicose veins are no longer considered contraindications. Most authors recommend avoiding OCs after acute hepatitis until the liver enzymes have remained normal for several months.

Although they are not mentioned in most lists of contraindications, a number of other conditions may make OCs a less desirable contraceptive choice. Sickling hemoglobinopathies are controversial contraindications. In many parts of the world, OCs are prescribed for women with these conditions without apparent problems. Sickle trait is not a contraindication to OC use. Patients with neurofibromatosis are known to experience worsening of their symptoms at puberty; therefore, the administration of exogenous hormones may pose a risk. Patients with hereditary hemorrhagic telangectasia and psoriasis have been reported to

have exacerbations with OC use. The relationship of the activity of systemic lupus erythematosus to pregnancy and OC use is controversial. Some types of renal disease, especially those that involve hypertension, may contraindicate OC use. Patients with porphyria may have exacerbations of skin lesions or abdominal pain with OC use.

Breast-feeding sometimes has been considered a reason to avoid using combined OCs because of the inhibitory effect of estrogens on breast milk formation. However, in many parts of the world, combined OCs commonly are prescribed for women whose supply of milk is well established, with no discernable adverse effects on infant growth or development. A seizure disorder is unlikely to worsen on OCs, but most anticonvulsants speed the metabolic degradation of steroid contraceptives and may render them less effective. Elective surgery is debated as a contraindication to OC use. Some authors recommend stopping OCs 6 weeks prior to surgery; others believe the risk of pregnancy outweighs the risk of thromboembolism. Morbid obesity predisposes a woman to venous thromboembolism, so it may be viewed as a contraindication to OC use. However, most obese women are able to take OCs without increased risk of serious adverse effects.

Women with a history of serious depression could have a recurrence or worsening of symptoms on OCs. Women with melasma, or chloasma, may have irreversible worsening of skin lesions on OCs. Exogenous hormones and pregnancy have been known to cause vasomotor rhinitis. There have been reports of pulmonary hypertension in congenital or rheumatic heart disease patients who have taken OCs. Because of a possible association of inflammatory bowel diseases with OC use, some authors caution against OC use among women with these disorders.

Choosing a Pill

There is a large selection of effective and well-tolerated OC preparations (Table 33–2). One should start with a "low-dose" pill (i.e., a product containing 30 to 35 μg of estrogen per day). All of these low-dose pills are effective and well tolerated. Lower doses of estrogen (i.e., 20 μg/day) are associated with a slightly higher pregnancy rate, however.

There are theoretical reasons, such as the metabolic effects of OCs, to try to minimize the dose of progestin, as well as that of estrogen. The multiphasic preparations allow a lower total monthly progestin dose. Preparations with the newer progestins (gestodene, norgestimate, and desogestrel) also have theoretical advantages. There are few studies involving direct comparisons of any of the low-dose preparations, and therefore there is little evidence to show that one pill is better than another.

Progestin-Only "Mini-Pills"

Several OCs on the market contain no estrogen, only a small dose of progestin. These mini-pills are not as widely used as are the combined OCs. Their effectiveness is somewhat lower than that of combined OCs (see Table 33–1). Mini-pills prevent pregnancy by affecting cervical mucus viscosity, fallopian tube motility, and endometrial suitability for implantation. Ovulation sometimes is inhibited, but much less consistently than with combined OCs.

Mini-pills are taken every day of the month, with no 7-day hiatus. They require excellent patient compliance to maintain their effectiveness; even one missed pill may result in pregnancy.

The side effects of progestin-only pills are primarily problems with menstrual irregularities. As many as two thirds of users experience menstrual irregularities, especially breakthrough bleeding and amenorrhea.

Mini-pills generally are reserved for selected women whose contraceptive choices are limited. They are used most commonly in lactating women, and do not reduce the milk supply. Because the progestin enters the breast milk in small quantities, there is a theoretical risk of affecting the nursing infant, but most authorities consider this risk to be insignificant.

The systemic effects of the small doses of progestin in mini-pills are presumed to be less significant than those of combined OCs. The actual risks of mini-pills, however, are largely unknown because they have been studied much less than those of combined oral contraceptives.

Mini-pills—and all of the continuous, very-low-dose progestin methods—prevent ectopic pregnancy less well than they do intrauterine pregnancy. Thus, if a pregnancy occurs while the patient is taking mini-pills, it is more likely to be an ectopic one than if she were using no contraception. Most authorities do not consider mini-pills to *cause* ectopic pregnancies, however.

LONG-ACTING HORMONAL METHODS

Long-acting hormonal methods offer highly effective long-term, reversible contraception. Unfortunately, like OCs, they offer no protection against STDs, including HIV infection. Two long-acting hormonal methods are available in the United States, and several others are under development.

Implants

The levonorgestrel implant (Norplant; Wyeth-Ayerst Laboratories) is a system of six flexible Silastic capsules, each containing 36 mg of levonorgestrel, that are inserted under the skin of the inside of the upper arm in a minor surgical procedure. The implant is highly effective (see Table 33–1) from about 24 hours after insertion for up to 5 years. The implant prevents pregnancy by making cervical mucus thicker and smaller in amount and by preventing normal endometrial development, as well as by suppressing ovulation in about half the menstrual cycles.

Side effects resemble those of the mini-pill; irregular bleeding patterns, including spotting, infrequent bleeding, and scanty bleeding, are common. Blood loss is usually less than that of normal menstrual cycles. Women who weigh less are more likely to experience complete amenorrhea. Women who weigh over 150 pounds are more likely to continue to have regular periods, and may have a slightly higher pregnancy rate after several years of use. It is anticipated that the new, softer implant tubing in use in the United States will have lower pregnancy rates, even among heavier women.

Other side effects include headache, nervousness, nausea, dizziness, dermatitis, acne, a change in appetite, breast tenderness, weight gain or loss, hair loss, or an increase in facial or body hair. Adnexal enlargement occasionally occurs, is due to delayed follicular atresia, and generally resolves spontaneously. Insertion site infections are rare, but temporary discomfort and bruising after insertion and removal are common.

Implants prevent ectopic pregnancy less well than they do intrauterine pregnancy. The absolute risk of ectopic pregnancy is lower than that using no contraception, but a higher percentage of pregnancies occurring are ectopic.

The effect of the implants on lipoprotein levels is not yet clear. Some studies suggest beneficial effects, and others suggest detrimental effects. Studies of the implants' effect on clotting factors also vary; the product's labeling reflects a conservative posture, proscribing use in women with active venous thromboembolic disease. Implants may be used by older women and by those who are breast-feeding, waiting 6 weeks after delivery. Women taking anticonvulsant medication probably should consider other methods of contraception; anticonvulsants may render the implants less effective (McCauley and Geller, 1992).

Insertion should be accomplished in the first 5 to 7 days of the menstrual cycle to assure that the patient is not pregnant at the time of insertion. The insertion procedure takes about 10 to 15 minutes and is performed in a sterile fashion under local anesthesia in the office. The implants are generally palpable but not visible. Contraindications to use of the implants are listed in Table 33–6.

Removal of the implants should be performed after 5 years, or whenever the patient requests it. Removal usually takes longer than insertion, and is similar to the insertion procedure. If the patient desires to continue implant use, a replacement set

TABLE 33–6. CONTRAINDICATIONS TO LONG-ACTING HORMONAL CONTRACEPTIVE METHODS

Levonorgestrel Implants
Active thromboembolic disease
Undiagnosed vaginal bleeding
Known or suspected pregnancy
Active liver disease
Benign or malignant liver tumor
Known or suspected breast cancer

Depot Medroxyprogesterone Acetate (DMPA)
Known or suspected pregnancy
Undiagnosed vaginal bleeding
Known or suspected breast cancer
Active thromboembolic disease, or past history of thromboembolic disorder
Cerebrovascular disease
Active liver disease
Known sensitivity to DMPA

of implants may be inserted through the same incision, close to the previous site.

Depot Medroxyprogesterone Acetate

Depot medroxyprogesterone acetate (DMPA) (Depo-Provera; Upjohn) is a highly effective, long-acting injectable contraceptive (see Table 33–1). It is given in a dose of 150 mg intramuscularly in the arm every 12 weeks. The first dose should be administered within 5 days of the onset of the menstrual period, within 5 days of delivery if the patient is not breast-feeding, and at 6 weeks after delivery if she is breast-feeding. Contraindications to DMPA use are listed in Table 33–6.

The progestin dose of DMPA is substantially larger than that of progestin-only mini-pills or levonorgestrel implants. Ovulation is inhibited reliably with regular DMPA use. Like other progestin-only methods, most DMPA users experience bleeding irregularities. However, the rate of amenorrhea rises with continued use, exceeding 50 per cent at 1 year. There is a tendency to gain weight on DMPA. The average weight gain in the first year is about 5 pounds, but is less with each subsequent year. Other adverse reactions reported include headache, depression, nervousness, dizziness, and weakness, as well as other symptoms associated with progestin administration. A disadvantage of DMPA is that it cannot be discontinued rapidly; it may take up to 3 months for associated side effects to dissipate.

The return of fertility after the use of DMPA is delayed for at least 3 months after the last injection, and the median time to conception is 10 months. There is no evidence that DMPA causes permanent infertility.

Concern about cancer risk kept the FDA from approving DMPA for contraceptive use for many years, and several epidemiologic studies have sought to clarify the relationship. Breast cancer risk overall is not significantly elevated with DMPA, although there may be an increased risk of breast cancer in the first few years of use. DMPA reduces the risk of endometrial cancer by about 80 per cent, but does not appear to affect the risk of ovarian cancer. The risk of cervical cancer appears not to be significantly elevated with DMPA use. Further epidemiologic surveillance of DMPA and cancer risks will be important (Klitsch, 1993).

There is also concern that DMPA may reduce bone mineral density and predispose to osteoporotic fractures. In addition, there is evidence that pregnancies in which there is inadvertent fetal exposure to DMPA may result in a higher risk of low birth weight and infant mortality.

INTRAUTERINE DEVICES

Intrauterine devices (IUDs) are used by millions of women throughout the world. IUDs cause endometrial inflammation, which has been theorized to interfere with implantation of the fertilized ovum. However, mounting evidence suggests that IUDs prevent pregnancy by preventing fertilization of the ovum by the spermatozoa.

IUDs are a highly effective form of long-term, reversible contraception that is appropriate for many women. Nevertheless, IUDs tend to be used much less frequently in the United States than in other countries. The lowest expected pregnancy rates of IUDs are somewhat higher than those of OCs (see Table 33–1). However, because little patient compliance is required to use the method properly, the typically observed pregnancy rates with IUDs are comparable to those of OCs. In fact, the observed effectiveness of the TCu-380A (Paragard) is superior to that of OCs in many populations (Treiman and Liskin, 1988).

Two IUDs are commercially available in the United States. The TCu-380A (Paragard; Gyno-Pharma) is a polyethylene T-shaped device with coiled copper wire around the stem and copper sleeves on the two arms. Barium is impregnated in the frame to make it radioopaque. The TCu-380A is approved for 8 years of use. The progesterone T (Progestasert; Alza) is also impregnated with barium, as well as with the natural hormone progesterone, which is released at a rate of 65 μg/day. The progesterone T has a slightly higher pregnancy rate than the TCu-380A, and it must be changed yearly. Several new IUDs are being developed.

Proper insertion of the IUD with sterile technique high in the uterine fundus is essential to ensure optimal contraceptive function. IUDs may be inserted at any time in the cycle, as long as pregnancy is excluded. Some clinicians prefer to insert IUDs during the menses. Some authorities recommend prophylactic antibiotics prior to insertion. Although immediate postpartum IUD insertion is

TABLE 33–7. CONTRAINDICATIONS TO USE OF IUDs

Known or suspected pregnancy
Undiagnosed abnormal genital bleeding
Known or suspected uterine or cervical malignancy, including unresolved abnormal Pap smear
Active genital infection
    PID
    Acute cervicitis
    Vaginitis
    Genital actinomycosis
    Postpartum or postabortal endometritis within the last 3 months
Uterine abnormality resulting in a distorted uterine cavity
High risk of STDs
    Patient or her partner has multiple sexual partners
    History of PID
Decreased resistance to infection (e.g., acquired immunodeficiency syndrome, chronic steroid therapy)
Presence of a previously inserted IUD
For copper-bearing IUDs
    Wilson's disease
    Allergy to copper
History of ectopic pregnancy (controversial)

safe, it is recommended that insertion be delayed until 6 to 8 weeks after delivery because of high expulsion rates after earlier insertions.

Currently available IUDs are very safe. In the first few weeks of use, there is a risk of IUD-associated PID that is related to the insertion process. Older studies of IUDs and PID were flawed by inclusion of patients with Dalkon Shields and by control groups at reduced risk of PID. New studies show that, apart from the first few weeks after insertion, IUDs do not cause PID in women who are at low risk for STDs (Farley et al., 1992). Women with multiple partners, those with a history of STDs, and younger, nulliparous women are at increased risk of PID based on these risk factors; they are thus poor candidates for IUDs. The contraindications to IUD use are listed in Table 33–7.

Bleeding is the most common problem associated with IUD use. A small amount of bleeding often occurs at the time of IUD insertion. Intermenstrual bleeding resulting from the inflammation caused by an IUD may occur at any time but must be differentiated from other causes of bleeding. Menstrual blood loss is typically increased with use of the TCu-380A and reduced with the progesterone T.

There are several other problems that may occur with use of IUDs. Pain and cramping are common with the insertion of an IUD but usually resolve within several days. Dysmenorrhea is sometimes a problem and may prompt the patient to request removal of the device. Expulsion of the device occurs occasionally, usually in the first few months of use. Patients should learn to check for the presence of their IUD string after each menstrual period, and a follow-up visit 3 months after insertion is recommended.

Perforation of the uterus is an uncommon complication (1 to 3 per 1000 insertions). Most perforations occur at the time the IUD is inserted, but may go undetected for some time. Perforating copper-bearing IUDs may cause peritoneal inflammation and adhesions and should be removed. Downward cervical perforations occasionally occur with T-shaped devices. In addition, an IUD may become embedded in the uterine wall without perforating it.

IUDs do not cause ectopic pregnancy. However, they prevent ectopic pregnancy less well than they do intrauterine pregnancy. Thus, a woman who becomes pregnant with an IUD in place has a greater chance that the pregnancy is ectopic than does a non–IUD user.

If a pregnancy occurs with an IUD in place, it is likely to be complicated. More than half will end in spontaneous abortion, and a few of these abortions may be complicated by maternal sepsis and death. If a woman becomes pregnant with an IUD in place and the string is visible, the IUD should be removed as soon as possible. The risk of miscarriage is *less* if the device is removed. If a pregnancy occurs and the string is not visible, ultrasonography should be performed to determine the presence of the IUD. A pregnant woman with an IUD-in-situ that cannot be removed should be counseled about the risk of spontaneous septic midtrimester abortion. If she carries to term, there is an increased risk of chorioamnionitis, premature labor, and stillbirth. IUDs do not cause congenital anomalies, however.

BARRIER METHODS

Barrier methods of contraception are mechanical and chemical devices used at the time of intercourse that prevent spermatozoa from reaching the upper genital tract. Their effectiveness varies considerably depending on the ability and willingness of the couple to use the method correctly with each coitus (see Table 33–1). The failure rates tend to be lower for older and for more highly motivated couples.

The barrier methods offer the advantage of local contact only and freedom from systemic effects. The risks associated with these methods are primarily those of pregnancy, if the method should fail. Notably, these methods provide protection against some forms of STDs.

Diaphragm

The diaphragm is a thin, shallow latex cup with a firm, circular, flexible rim to hold it in place in the vagina. The diaphragm covers the cervix and holds spermicidal cream or jelly at the cervical os. The spermicide placed inside the cup of the diaphragm and along the rim ensures a chemical barrier to sperm. When fitting a diaphragm, one should use the largest size that fits snugly above and behind the symphysis pubis. Sizes range from 55 to 90 mm in diameter, increasing in 5-mm increments. A diaphragm that is too small may not completely cover the cervix or may be dislodged easily during intercourse. A diaphragm that is too large may buckle in the vagina and feel uncomfortable or may lie vertically and ineffectively cover the cervix. When proper fit is obtained, the patient will not feel the presence of the diaphragm. After the fitting, the patient is instructed to insert and remove the device while still in the examination room, so that it is clear she understands these techniques.

The diaphragm is inserted prior to intercourse and left in place for at least 6 hours after coitus. For each additional act of coitus, additional vaginal spermicide is used without removing the diaphragm. Intercourse with the woman on top of the man is sometimes associated with dislodgement of the diaphragm. Some couples incorporate insertion of the diaphragm into their sexual foreplay.

The diaphragm should be removed within 24 hours to avoid any risk of vaginal infection or toxic shock syndrome (TSS). After each use, the diaphragm should be washed with mild soap and water, rinsed, dried, and dusted with cornstarch or unscented talcum powder.

The flexible ring contains one of three types of springs: arcing, coiled, or flat. The arcing spring allows for easier insertion and is the most popular. A plastic introducer is available for flat and coil spring diaphragms.

Diaphragm use is associated with urinary tract infection in some women, and rarely with TSS. Contraindications to diaphragm use include a history of TSS, sensitivity to latex or spermicide, inability of the patient to learn the proper insertion technique, or the presence of anatomic abnormalities such as prolapse, vaginal septum, or recent (within 6 weeks) childbirth.

Cervical Cap

The Pretif Cavity Rim cap is a small, cup-shaped latex rubber device with a firm flexible rim that fits tightly over the cervix. It is held in place by its close fit, producing suction. The use of spermicide inside the cap enhances the seal and ensures a chemical barrier to spermatozoa.

The cap is left in place for up to 48 hours. Compared with the diaphragm, caps allow separation of contraceptive and sexual activity to some extent because coitus can occur multiple times without adding spermicide. Contraindications are the same as for the diaphragm; in addition, a normal Pap smear must be obtained before prescribing a cap.

Cervical cytology should be repeated after 3 months of cap use.

Caps come in several sizes and must be fitted to an individual patient. Special training is required in order to fit caps.

Condoms

Condoms have received increased attention because they reduce the risk of transmission of HIV and other STDs (Cates and Stone, 1992a). Most condoms are made of latex; only 1 per cent are made from sheep intestine—the so-called "natural" condoms. Only the latex condoms have been shown to prevent transmission of HIV effectively. Latex condoms are made in various sizes, shapes, and colors in order to appeal to personal preference. Condoms are available with lubrication, and some are lubricated with spermicide. Condoms with reservoir tips break less readily.

The typically observed contraceptive failure rate of condoms is in the range of 12 per cent in the first year of use. With ideal use, the failure rate may be as low as 2 per cent. To be effective in the prevention of STD transmission, condoms must remain intact and be used consistently and correctly.

The condom is placed on the erect penis prior to any genital contact. The rim of the condom is rolled all the way to the base of the penis. If there is not a reservoir on the tip of the penis, about half an inch of empty condom should be left at the end of the penis to catch the semen. This is accomplished by pinching the end of the condom as it is rolled on. Oil or petroleum-based lubricants should not be used because they may weaken the condom. If lubrication is needed, K-Y jelly, water, saliva, or contraceptive foam or jelly may be used. After coitus, the penis must be withdrawn while still erect, holding the condom at the base of the penis. The condom should be inspected to assure it is intact, and then it is discarded. Condoms should not be reused.

A small number of people are sensitive to the latex material or to the spermicide. The most common complaints of male condom users are of a reduction in sensitivity of the glans and disliking the interruption of foreplay to put on the condom. Use of a condom requires cooperation of the male partner, so it may be impractical for some women who feel they cannot influence their partner.

Vaginal Pouch

A vaginal pouch, or "female condom" (Reality; Wisconsin Pharmacal Company) is now available, and similar devices are under study. The Reality female condom is a loose-fitting polyurethane pouch with two flexible rings. The smaller ring is inserted into the vagina similarly to inserting a diaphragm. The larger ring is worn outside against the vulva and prevents the device from being pushed into the vagina. The penis then penetrates into the vagina inside this lubricated sheath and has no contact with the vagina.

The chief advantage of the female condom is that it is under the woman's control; this may afford some women better protection from pregnancy and STDs. At least one study suggests that female-dependent barrier contraceptives may be associated with better STD protection for women than male condoms (Rosenberg et al., 1992). However, there are fewer data on the Reality pouch than exist for condoms, both in regard to HIV transmission and in regard to pregnancy prevention. The cautious labeling of this over-the-counter device estimates a 26 per cent pregnancy rate at one year, although there are data that suggest lower rates (see Table 33–1). The patient package insert states that, if male condoms are not used, the Reality pouch can help protect the woman and her partner from HIV and other STDs.

Vaginal Spermicides

Vaginal spermicidal preparations include foams, jellies, creams, suppositories, sponges, and films. Each consists of an inert base and a spermicide, either nonoxynol-9 or octoxynol-9. Typical contraceptive failure rates of 15 to 21 per cent are observed when spermicides are used alone (see Table 33–1).

In vitro, spermicides effectively kill many STD organisms, including *Neisseria gonorrheae*, *Trichomonas vaginalis*, herpes simplex virus, *Treponema pallidum*, HIV, and *C. trachomatis*. Clinical studies show that spermicides offer some protection from gonorrhea, chlamydial infection, and PID. Whether spermicides used without mechanical barriers protect against transmission of HIV is not yet known. One study of the sponge found no decrease in seroconversion among high-risk women (Kreiss et al., 1992).

Spermicides have the advantage of being available without a physician's examination or prescription. A contraindication is a sensitivity reaction. Spermicide use has not been shown to cause congenital anomalies.

Foam preparations have the best dispersal in the vagina and thus may cover the cervix best. Creams and jellies primarily are used in conjunction with the diaphragm or cervical cap but can be used alone. These preparations are forced into an applicator tube, which is then placed into the vagina. The plunger is depressed and about a tablespoon of material is deposited.

The vaginal contraceptive sponge (Today; Whitehall Laboratories) contains 1 gram of nonoxynol-9 spermicide. One side has a concave dimple that fits against the cervix, and the other side has a fabric tape to facilitate removal. The sponge is moistened with tap water and inserted into the vagina to fit up against the cervix. It may be left in place up to 24 hours, and is more effective in nulliparous women.

Spermicidal suppositories such as Encare Oval and Semicid have the disadvantage that they require 10 to 30 minutes to dissolve and may not dissolve completely. The packages may be difficult to open and the tablets erroneously used rectally or orally. A contraceptive film, VCF (Apothecus, Inc.), is a wafer-thin, 2×2-inch film that contains 70 mg of nonoxynol-9. It is pushed deeply into the vagina no less that 5 minutes before coitus, and remains effective for about an hour and a half. Its small size is an advantage.

PERIODIC ABSTINENCE

Natural family planning, or rhythm, methods are based on the fact that a woman is fertile for only a few days each cycle, near the time of ovulation. Patients practice abstinence during the fertile period and confine intercourse to the "safe days." Charting materials are available to aid in the record keeping and calculations in each of these techniques. These methods are inexpensive and free of side effects. In addition, this type of contraception is the only method approved by some religions. The method is unsuitable for women with irregular cycles or for couples with a low level of self-discipline.

The calendar method requires keeping a record of at least eight menstrual cycles. The earliest day a woman is likely to be fertile is determined by subtracting 18 from the number of days in the shortest cycle. The latest day of likely fertility is determined by subtracting 11 from the number of days in the longest cycle. Abstinence is then practiced on these "likely" fertile days.

The basal body temperature method for predicting ovulation has a woman measure her temperature each morning before arising. A rise of about $1°$ F occurs following ovulation. Pregnancy may be avoided by avoiding coitus until the temperature rise has been present for 3 days.

The cervical mucus, or Billings, method of natural family planning relies on an awareness of changes in the cervical mucus during the menstrual cycle. The woman checks the character of the mucus daily by inserting a finger into the vagina. Around the time of ovulation, the discharge becomes abundant, thin, slippery, clear, and elastic. Intercourse is avoided until at least 4 days after the "peak" mucus symptom. The sympto-thermal method combines checking the cervical mucus (symptoms) and the basal body temperature to determine the likely time of ovulation.

Effectiveness rates depend on motivation and self-control and are highly variable (see Table

33–1). Typical failure rates for periodic abstinence are about 20 per cent. Rates as low as 2 per cent have been observed only for methods restricting intercourse to the postovulatory portion of the cycle.

STERILIZATION

When a couple has completed its family and desires no further children, sterilization becomes an option. Although progress has been made in techniques to reverse both female sterilization and vasectomy, these operations should be considered permanent. Sterilization is inappropriate for individuals or couples with uncertainty about wanting more children.

Both female tubal sterilization and vasectomy of the male are safe and highly effective methods of contraception. Because of the intraperitoneal location of the female internal genitalia, female sterilization involves slightly higher rates of serious complications than does vasectomy. Proper preoperative evaluation and counseling are essential.

Tubal Sterilization

Obliteration or interruption of the fallopian tubes prevents pregnancy by preventing the ovum from reaching the uterus and the sperm from reaching the ovum. Methods of tubal sterilization include mini-laparotomy with ligation of the tubes (the Pomeroy technique and others), and laparoscopy with banding, clipping, or electrocoagulation of the tubes. Mini-laparotomy can be performed in the immediate postpartum period, or 6 weeks or more after delivery. Laparoscopic procedures are not done until at least 6 weeks after delivery. Both techniques may be done under local anesthesia (American College of Obstetricians and Gynecologists, 1988).

The effectiveness of tubal sterilization is high—but not 100 per cent. A high percentage of pregnancies after tubal occlusion are ectopic when compared with women using no contraception. Operative complications are unusual, and fatalities are rare. It is controversial whether tubal sterilization involves an increased risk for subsequent abnormal bleeding patterns or pelvic pain.

Vasectomy

Interruption of the vas deferens prevents spermatozoa from becoming part of the ejaculate. Vasectomy is a simple and safe office procedure because of the accessibility of the vas in the scrotum. A segment of each vas is excised, and the ends are sealed with ligation, electrocoagulation, or clips.

The "no-scalpel" technique involves less tissue trauma and a lower infection risk, but requires special instruments and training (Stockton et al., 1992).

Contraindications include current infection of the genital tract or scrotal skin, marital or psychologic instability, or the expectation that the procedure will cure a sexual dysfunction. Patients with varicocele, hydrocele, inguinal hernia, filariasis, or previous scrotal surgery may need to be referred to a urologist for the procedure.

Vasectomy failures are uncommon but can occur because of faulty surgical technique, recanalization, or failure of the couple to protect themselves from pregnancy just after the procedure. Azoospermia is not immediate; about 12 ejaculations are required to clear the genital tract of viable sperm. Another form of contraception should be used until the semen analysis demonstrates complete absence of sperm.

Ecchymosis, swelling, and discomfort are common after the procedure and subside within 1 to 2 weeks. Less common complication of the procedure include infection, hematoma, and epididymitis. Serious complications are rare. Although antibodies to sperm often develop, no increased risk of autoimmune disease or heart disease has been observed. Vasectomy has been associated with a slightly increased risk of prostate cancer in some studies, but not in others (Healy, 1993).

OTHER METHODS

Coitus interruptus, or withdrawal, in which the penis is withdrawn from the vagina prior to ejaculation, has a failure rate of approximately 19 per cent in actual use (see Table 33–1). With ideal use, the failure rate is lower. Pregnancy can occur even when the method is used properly because the seminal fluid present prior to ejaculation may contain sperm. This method is inexpensive and always available, but it requires a high degree of self-control and motivation during sexual activity.

Douching is not an effective method of contraception. Sperm penetration of the cervical canal can occur within 15 seconds of ejaculation. If a spermicide has been used, a douche may wash out the spermicide and increase the risk of pregnancy.

Noncoital sex can be an important option for some couples. Some couples use this as an adjunct to periodic abstinence. Care must be taken to avoid semen being spilled near the vagina, or motile sperm may reach the cervix, even without penile penetration.

Abstinence from sexual activity may be a viable option for some individuals. While theoretically effective, typical failure rates of 20 per cent are observed.

Lactation reduces fertility, but not reliably so. To be effective in preventing ovulation, breast-feeding must occur frequently and around the clock, and no other feeding or sucking options should be offered to the infant. Ovulation—and thus pregnancy—may occur even before menstruation is resumed. Other methods should be started by the end of the third postpartum month with full breast-feeding, and by the end of the third postpartum week with partial (or no) breast-feeding.

POSTCOITAL FERTILITY CONTROL

Too often, situations arise in which coitus occurs without protection from pregnancy. Several measures are available that will prevent or interrupt pregnancy after unprotected intercourse. These methods are inappropriate for ongoing contraception.

Emergency contraceptive pills (ECPs), or "morning-after pills," are not approved as such by the FDA, but nevertheless are used by many practitioners for selected patients. The first dose of 100 μg of ethinyl estradiol plus 1.0 mg of norgestrel (i.e., 2 Ovral tablets*) is taken as soon as possible after the exposure—and certainly within 72 hours. The dose is repeated 12 hours later. Nausea is common and may be prevented by use of an antiemetic. The risk of pregnancy after a single midcycle exposure is estimated to be about 14 per cent; use of ECPs reduces the risk to about 2 per cent. Informed consent is essential; a theoretical (but probably not actual) risk of congenital anomalies exists should pregnancy continue.

Mifepristone (RU 486) is more effective and just as safe as the above regimen. High-dose estrogens seldom are used because of their toxicity. Insertion of a copper-bearing IUD within 5 days of unprotected intercourse is also effective.

Several procedures are available to terminate pregnancy once it is established. Early pregnancy termination with the progesterone antagonist mifepristone (RU 486) is used in Europe. This agent interferes with hormonal support of the endometrium and thus of any implanted ovum. When administered with the prostaglandin analogue misoprostol (Cytotec), mifepristone is effective and safe for terminating early pregnancy (Peyron et al., 1993).

The type of abortion procedure and the risks of having a legal abortion are directly related to the duration of the gestation. Abortions up to 12 to 13 weeks from the beginning of the last menstrual period usually are accomplished by cervical dilation followed by suction curettage. The procedure may be performed on an outpatient basis, usually under local anesthesia. After 14 weeks' gestation, the technique of amnioinfusion has been used, but dilation and evacuation, which requires special expertise, appears to be the safer procedure.

Counseling of the patient both before and after a therapeutic abortion is important. A woman with an unplanned pregnancy may have difficulty deciding on a course of action, and misunderstanding about abortion is common. The family physician's task is to apprise her of her options, to assist her in making an informed decision, and to help her deal with the stress of the situation. Future contraception also should be discussed.

CHOOSING A METHOD

In choosing a method of contraception, there are a number of factors to be considered. Patients or couples may have personal preferences, concerns, and previous experiences that influence their options. The importance of high effectiveness is different for different people. Some people have difficulty complying with methods that require daily pill-taking; others may find it difficult to use a method at the time of intercourse. Some couples seek permanent contraception; others need reversible measures. Options may be limited by method contraindications or health risks.

The number of sexual partners that a woman and her partner(s) have influences the choice of a contraceptive method. Persons at high risk of STDs should use condoms to reduce their risk—or refrain from the high-risk behavior. Other methods of contraception can be used at the same time as condoms. Many authors recommend both hormonal contraceptives *and* condoms to women with multiple or high-risk partners if they wish to prevent pregnancy as well as STDs reliably.

Age and parity affect the options. Older parous women are more likely to be good candidates for IUDs; they also tend to use barrier methods more consistently than younger women. Parous women have higher pregnancy rates with the vaginal sponge and cervical cap, however. Older women who smoke should avoid using OCs. However, older women without coronary risk factors may use OCs safely.

The expected frequency of intercourse may also influence the choice of a method. A woman who anticipates intercourse to occur only occasionally may find barrier methods particularly appropriate.

Postpartum patients should have received counseling about contraceptive methods during their prenatal care. In the absence of full breast-feeding, contraceptive measures should be started by the end of the third postpartum week. If OCs are chosen, they commonly are begun 1 to 3 weeks after delivery. There is no theoretical reason why levonorgestrel implants cannot be inserted immediately after delivery, although the product labeling

---

*Other OC preparations also have been used. For Nordette, Levlen, and Lo/Ovral, the dose is four pills. For Triphasil and Tri-Levlen, the dose is four yellow pills. As with Ovral, the dose is repeated 12 hours later.

recommends waiting until 6 weeks after delivery if the patient is breast-feeding. DMPA injections should be started within 5 days of delivery if the patient is not breast-feeding and at 6 weeks after delivery if she is breast-feeding. Barrier methods are options for most postpartum patients. They also may be used until 6 to 8 weeks after delivery, when a diaphragm or cap may be fitted or when an IUD may be inserted, if appropriate. Planning for tubal sterilization should occur during the pregnancy. The procedure may be performed during the first few days after delivery or as an interval procedure at least 6 weeks after delivery.

If a woman breast-feeds her baby, an additional method of contraception should be begun by the end of the third postpartum month to avoid accidental pregnancy. If supplemental bottle feedings are given, contraceptive methods should be begun by the end of the third postpartum week. Breast-feeding women may choose mini-pills, levonorgestrel implants, and DMPA injections. In many countries, combination OCs are used after the milk supply is established. Barrier methods, IUDs, and sterilization also may be considered by breast-feeding women.

Adolescents form a group with special contraceptive needs. Abstinence is not a reliable alternative for many teenagers, and teens often fail to use contraception. Family physicians can play important roles by discussing contraception, STDs, and responsible decision-making with teenagers frankly—and confidentially—*before* their needs become apparent. Hormonal contraception and barrier methods are appropriate choices for teens to consider. The combination of hormonal methods with condom use can help to protect against STDs as well as pregnancy.

Patients and couples should be counseled and educated about the contraceptive options available to them. Family physicians should present the advantages, disadvantages, risks, and benefits of the various methods and assist their patients in making an informed choice of an appropriate method.

REFERENCES

American College of Obstetricians and Gynecologists: Sterilization. ACOG Tech Bulletin 113, 1988.

Association of Reproductive Health Professionals: Maximizing Oral Contraceptive Effectiveness: A Clinician's Handbook. New Jersey: Association of Reproductive Health Professionals, 1991.

Baird DT, Glasier AF: Hormonal contraception. N Engl J Med 328:1543, 1993.

Cancer and Steroid Hormone Study, Centers for Disease Control and the National Institute of Child Health and Human Development: Oral-contraceptive use and the risk of breast cancer. N Engl J Med 315:405, 1986.

Cates W Jr, Stone KM: Family planning, sexually transmitted diseases and contraceptive choice: A literature update—Part I. Fam Plann Perspect 24:75, 1992a.

Cates W Jr, Stone KM: Family planning, sexually transmitted diseases and contraceptive choice: A literature update—Part II. Fam Plann Perspect 24:122, 1992b.

Clemetson DBA, Moss GB, Willerford DM, et al: Detection of HIV DNA in cervical and vaginal secretions: Prevalence and correlates among women in Nairobi, Kenya. JAMA 269:2860, 1993.

Farley TMM, Rosenberg MJ, Rowe PJ, et al: Intrauterine devices and pelvic inflammatory disease: An international perspective. Lancet 339:785, 1992.

Hawley W, Nuovo J, DeNeef CP, Carter P: Do oral contraceptive agents affect the risk of breast cancer? A meta-analysis of the case-control reports. J Am Board Fam Pract 6:123, 1993.

Healy B: From the National Institutes of Health: Does vasectomy cause prostate cancer? JAMA 269:2620, 1993.

Klitsch M: The new pill: Awaiting the next generation of oral contraceptives. Fam Plann Perspect 24:226, 1992.

Klitsch M: Injectable hormones and regulatory controversy: An end to the long-running story? Fam Plann Perspect 25:37, 1993.

Kreiss J, Ngugi E, Holmes K, et al: Efficacy of nonoxynol 9 contraceptive sponge use in preventing heterosexual acquisition of HIV in Nairobi prostitutes. JAMA 268:477, 1992.

McCauley AP, Geller JS: Decisions for Norplant programs. Popul Rep [K], No 4, 1992.

Ory HW: The noncontraceptive health benefits from oral contraceptives. Fam Plann Perspect 14:182, 1982.

Ory HW: Mortality associated with fertility and fertility control. Fam Plann Perspect 15:57, 1983.

Peyron R, Aubeny E, Targosz V, et al: Early termination of pregnancy with mifepristone (RU 486) and the orally active prostaglandin misoprostol. N Engl J Med 328:1509, 1993.

Rosenberg MJ, Davidson AJ, Chen JH, et al: Barrier contraceptives and sexually transmitted diseases in women: A comparison of female-dependent methods and condoms. Am J Public Health 82:669, 1992.

Royal College of General Practitioners Oral Contraception Study: Further analyses of mortality in oral contraceptive users. Lancet 1:541, 1981.

Simpson JL: Do contraceptive methods pose fetal risks? Res Front Fertil Regul 3(6):1, 1985.

Stadel BV: Oral contraceptives and cardiovascular disease. N Engl J Med 301:612, 672, 1981.

Stockton MD, Davis LE, Bolton KM: No-scalpel vasectomy: A technique for family physicians. Am Fam Physician 46:1153, 1992.

Treiman K, Liskin L: IUDs—a new look. Popul Rep [B], no. 5, 1988.

CHAPTER 34

INTERPRETATION OF THE ELECTROCARDIOGRAM

CARLOS VALLBONA

The electrocardiogram (ECG) is a simple test that family physicians can use effectively to analyze the electrical activity of the heart. The analysis can yield important information about cardiac function and may lead to the diagnosis of specific cardiovascular disorders.

STEPS IN THE ANALYSIS OF THE ECG

Analyzing the ECG includes the following steps:

1. Determination of the average heart rate.
2. Analysis of the predominant rhythm and detection of arrhythmias.
3. Computation of the QRS axis in the frontal plane.
4. Analysis of P, QRS, and T waves in the frontal and horizontal planes (if there is a deviation of the ST segment, it should be analyzed also).
5. Measurement of the standard time intervals.
6. Assessment of the extent to which the ECG is normal or abnormal and, in the latter case, diagnosis of the specific abnormalities and their clinical significance.

BASIC CONCEPTS

Electrical Field Generated by the Heart

Electrically, the heart should be considered as a dipole. The transmembrane action potentials (TAPs) generated during the cardiac cycle create an electrical field. Its center is the electrical center of the heart. At various locations in the electrical field it is possible to record whatever changes in potential (electromotive forces [EMFs]) occur during the cardiac cycle. The positive and negative portions of the field are separated by an isoelectric plane (Fig. 34–1).

Electrodes placed below the isoelectric plane will record positive potentials. Electrodes set above the plane will record negative potentials. Electrodes placed at the plane will record zero (isoelectric) potentials. Thus, in the example of

Figure 34–1, an exploring electrode in the right arm will be above the plane and record negative potentials. An electrode in the left foot will be below the plane and record positive potentials. An electrode in the chest at the edge of the plane will record an isoelectric potential.

The electrical field is three-dimensional, but its projection in a frontal plane can be assessed by analyzing the standard limb leads (I, II, III, aVR, aVL, and aVF) and its projection in a horizontal plane by analyzing the precordial or chest leads (V_1 through V_6).

The following basic assumptions are made in the analysis of the frontal and horizontal plane projections: (1) the body is a uniform conductor, (2) the heart is at the center of the body and functions as a dipole, and (3) all electrodes placed on the body surface are equidistant from the electrical center of the heart. Of course, these assumptions are not quite valid because the heart is not at the center of the body, and the electrodes, especially those placed in the precordial area, are not equidistant from the electrical center.

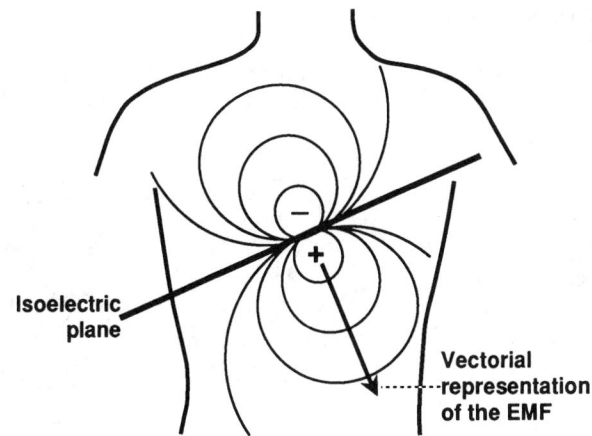

FIGURE 34–1. Electrical field generated by a transmembrane action potential (TAP) of the heart. The TAP can be represented by a vector that indicates its direction and magnitude.

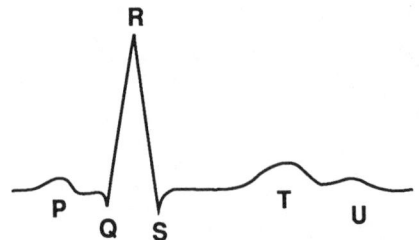

FIGURE 34–2. The normal components of the ECG.

Components of the ECG

The EMFs generated by the heart during systole are recorded as: (1) P wave caused by depolarization of the atria, (2) QRS wave of depolarization of the ventricles, and (3) T wave caused by repolarization of the ventricles (Fig. 34–2). The U wave is an afterwave of repolarization. It always occurs, but in general it has a very small magnitude and can be detected only in those precordial leads where the electrodes are close to the myocardial mass. Certain electrolyte disturbances (e.g., hypokalemia) produce a large U wave in practically all leads.

Measurements of ECG Components

The ECG components may be analyzed as follows:

Pattern analysis: Assessment of the shape and amplitude of the ECG waves in various leads.
Vector analysis: Determination of the vector values (direction in degrees and magnitude in millivolts).
Scalar analysis: Measurement of the duration of various ECG components (in hundredths of a second). Although the measurement of voltages in various leads is a scalar analysis also, it is necessary for the pattern or vector analysis.

The Electrical Axis

It is easy and useful to analyze the QRS complex from the standpoint of the direction of the mean

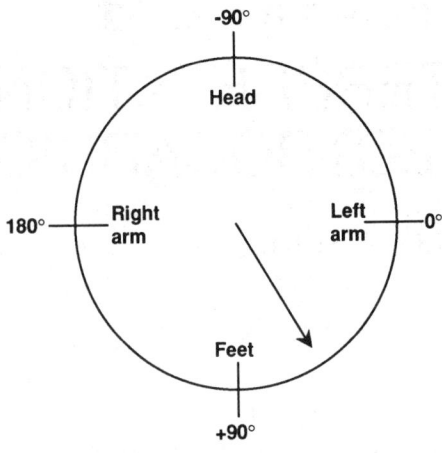

FIGURE 34–3. Reference points for measurements of the direction of the electrical axis of the heart.

of all forces of depolarization in the frontal plane (electrical axis). Figure 34–3 shows the reference points that are used to compute the QRS electrical axis. It is equally feasible to compute the axes of the P and T waves, although this cannot be done as accurately as the computation of QRS axis.

SEQUENCE OF DEPOLARIZATION AND REPOLARIZATION

Atrial Depolarization

During atrial depolarization, there is a slow progression of more or less parallel EMFs from the sinoatrial (SA) to the atrioventricular (AV) node. The resultant P axis has a direction of +45 degrees in the frontal plane and the amplitude is less than or equal to 0.25 mV (Fig. 34–4a). The atrial repolarization seldom is recorded because it takes place at the time of recording of the QRS complex, which is of greater magnitude and therefore cancels out the atrial repolarization forces.

AV Nodal Pause

There is no recorded electrical activity for a period of time (0.06 to 0.10 second) when the impul-

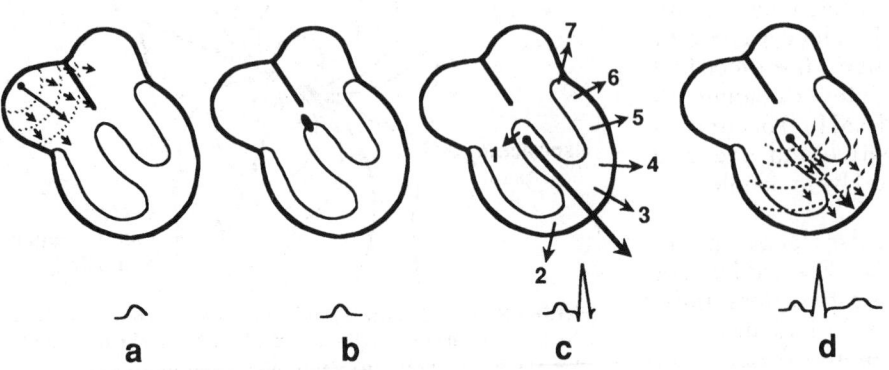

FIGURE 34–4. Sequence of depolarization and repolarization of atria and ventricles.

ses are detained at the AV node before transmission to the bundle of His (Fig. 34–4*b*).

Ventricular Depolarization

During ventricular depolarization, there is a rapid generation of nonparallel EMFs in a sequence that can be described arbitrarily in terms of seven axes distributed as shown in Figure 34–4*c*. The resultant axis of the QRS wave has a direction of +60 degrees in the frontal plane and the amplitude is less than or equal to 1.5 mV.

Ventricular Repolarization

The ventricular repolarization occurs as a slow wave of more or less parallel EMFs that, when summated, can be expressed with an axis almost parallel to that of the QRS wave, with a direction of +60 degrees in the frontal plane and an amplitude of less than or equal to 0.5 mV (Fig. 34–4*d*).

ECG LEAD SYSTEM FOR THE FRONTAL PLANE

Measurement of Potentials at the Body Surface

Traditionally, electrodes are placed on each limb. The potential measured by an electrode on the right arm is expressed as VR, that on the left arm as VL, and that on the left foot as VF. Potentials measured on the right foot are almost identical to those on the left, so the electrode placed on the right foot is for grounding purposes only.

Standard Limb Leads in the Frontal Plane (Einthoven's Triangle)

Einthoven's law states that VR + VL + VF = 0. Lead I = VL − VR when the potential recorded

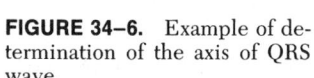

FIGURE 34–5. ECG system for the frontal plane.

by the electrode in the right arm (R) is negative in relation to the left arm (L). Lead II = VF − VR when the electrode in R is negative in relation to the foot electrode (F). Lead III = VF − VL when the electrode in L is negative in relation to F. The standard limb leads I, II, and III constitute Einthoven's triangle (Fig. 34–5*a*). A triaxial system may be constructed by placing the three standard leads at the center of the triangle (Fig. 34–5*b*).

Projection of QRS Axis in Limb Leads

The mean QRS axis projects itself in all the leads. From these projections, it is possible to compute the direction and magnitude of the QRS axis. Similarly, the axes of the P and T waves and even the ST segment may be computed. The Einthoven's triangle method and its equivalent triaxial coordinate system provide a useful but cumbersome model to compute the QRS axis. As an illustration, assume an ECG with the QRS tracings shown in Figure 34–6. The amplitude of the tracings in leads I, II, and III can be projected in each lead. From these projections, it is possible to mea-

FIGURE 34–6. Example of determination of the axis of QRS wave.

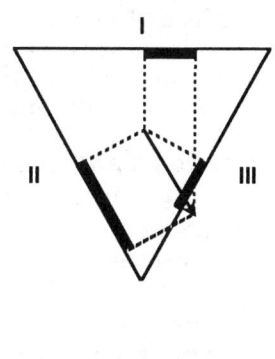

a

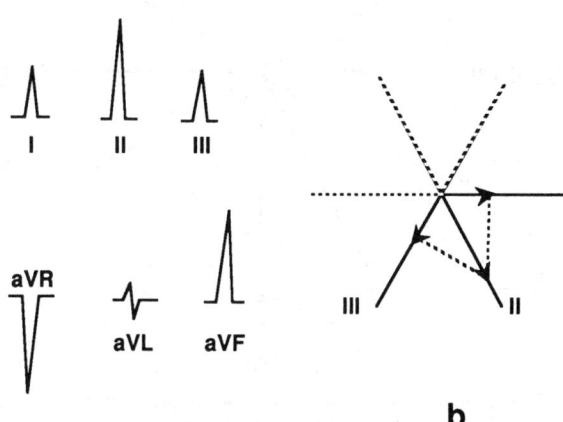

b

sure the mean direction and amplitude of the QRS fairly accurately in the frontal plane (Fig. 34–6*a*).

In addition to leads I, II, and III derived from the Einthoven's triangle, there are leads aVR, aVL, and aVF that, when superimposed with leads I, II, and III, constitute a hexaxial system. Lead aVR records the difference in potential between the electrical center of the heart and a positive electrode in the right arm (R). Similarly, aVL and aVF record the difference in potential between the electrical center and the left arm electrode (L) or the left foot electrode (F), respectively. The amplitudes of the QRS axis can be plotted in each of their respective six leads to obtain the mean direction and amplitude of the QRS axis in the frontal plane. This method offers the advantage of allowing for greater accuracy than the Einthoven's triangle method, but it is still cumbersome (Fig. 34–6*b*).

A simpler approach is to find the lead that has an isoelectric complex. The axis is perpendicular to that lead and falls in the same direction as a lead that would be ideal to measure the direction and amplitude of the QRS axis.

The diagram in Figure 34–7 is very useful in computing the electrical axis and amplitude in the frontal plane. For example, the tracing in Figure 34–6 shows an isoelectric QRS wave in aVL (whose direction is from –30 degrees to +150 degrees). This means that the QRS axis direction is either –120 to +60 degrees. The lead parallel to the axis is II (from –120 to +60 degrees). The QRS complex in lead II is positive, so the axis direction is +60 degrees. The amplitude of the QRS wave in lead II is 14 mm. The standard calibration is 10 mm = 1 mV, so the average amplitude is 1.4 mV.

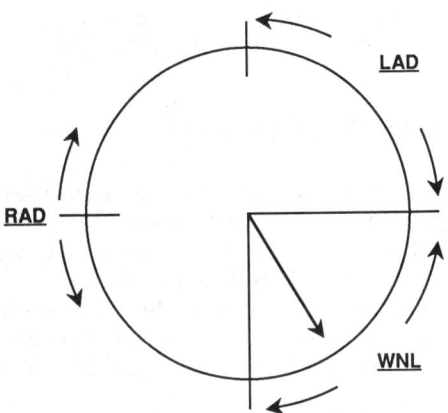

FIGURE 34–8. Normal ranges of values of QRS axis in the frontal plane. WNL, within normal limits.

NORMAL VALUES IN THE FRONTAL PLANE

QRS Axis

Adults

The *direction* of the QRS axis is normally between 0 and +90 degrees, although some textbooks indicate that the normal range is from –20 to +110 degrees. The *magnitude* is less than or equal to 1.5 mV.

If the direction is between 0 and +90 degrees, it is considered within normal limits. If the direction is between +90 and +180 degrees, it is considered to be a right axis deviation (RAD). Extreme RAD occurs if the axis falls between +180 and –90 degrees. If the direction is between 0 and –90 degrees, there is a left axis deviation (LAD) (Fig. 34–8). An undifferentiated axis occurs whenever all leads are nearly isoelectric.

It is clear from this figure that normally the axis of the QRS wave is projected in the positive part of leads I and aVF, whereas a RAD will cause a negative QRS axis in I and a LAD will cause a negative QRS axis in aVF. In the rare cases of extreme RAD, the QRS axis will be negative in both lead I and lead aVF. Thus, a much simplified pattern analysis of the QRS axis can be done by assessing leads I and aVF. The diagrams and QRS patterns in these two leads (Fig. 34–9) show the most common locations of the QRS axis in normal and abnormal conditions.

Newborns and Infants

There is RAD in the QRS axis of newborns and infants because of the relative preponderance of right ventricular forces in the neonatal period.

Elderly

There is a horizontal QRS axis or slight LAD in the elderly because of the preponderance of left

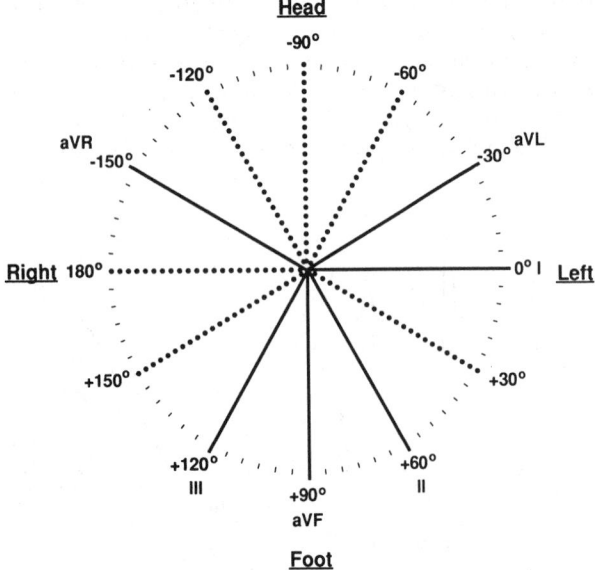

FIGURE 34–7. Diagram for the computation of the electrical axis and amplitudes in the frontal plane.

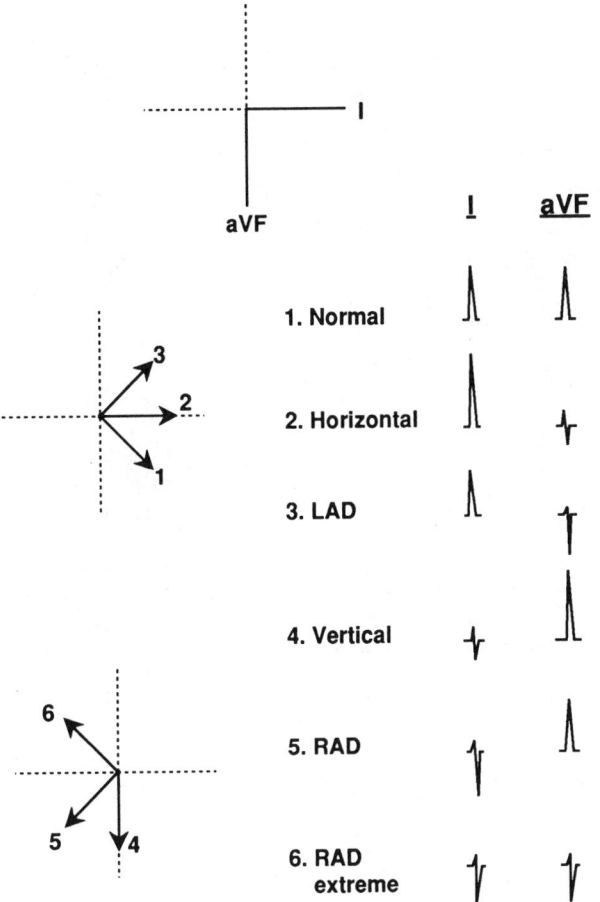

FIGURE 34–9. Pattern analysis of the electrical axis using leads I and aVF as references.

ventricular forces in the majority of persons beyond the sixth decade of life.

P Axis

The P axis has almost the same *direction* as that of the QRS axis, but the range of normal is from +20 to +70 degrees. The magnitude is less than 0.25 mV.

In a pattern analysis, the P axis is considered normal if it is positive in lead II. If the P axis is

negative in aVF, it suggests a marked left atrial enlargement or a nodal rhythm. If the P axis is very small, isoelectric, or negative in lead I, it is likely due to right atrial enlargement.

T Axis

In adults, the *direction* of the T axis is within +60 degrees counterclockwise of the QRS axis or within +45 degrees clockwise of the QRS axis. The magnitude is less than 0.5 mV (Fig. 34–10).

Whenever the angle between the QRS and T axes exceeds 60 degrees counterclockwise or 45 degrees clockwise, the diagnosis of electrical strain is warranted. A T axis of strain points *away* from the ventricle where the strain occurs. Usual causes of strain are hypertrophy, bundle-branch block, ischemia, digitalis, epinephrine effect, metabolic disturbances, and cerebral hemorrhage.

A simple pattern analysis of the T wave can be made by looking at the T wave in the lead of highest QRS positivity. If the T wave is also positive, it is considered normal. The condition referred to as ventricular strain occurs when the T wave is negative in the lead of highest QRS positivity, or when it is positive in the lead of highest QRS negativity.

Examples

Tracings 34–1 through 34–5 show various locations of the QRS axis. Tracing 34–6 shows a left ventricular strain (LVS).

HORIZONTAL OR TRANSVERSE PLANE LEADS

The precordial leads, notwithstanding their staggered placement across the chest, may be considered to lie on a horizontal plane whose center is the electrical center of the heart. Their location on the chest wall is shown in Figure 34–11*a* and their approximate direction in a hexaxial system is shown in Figure 34–11*b*.

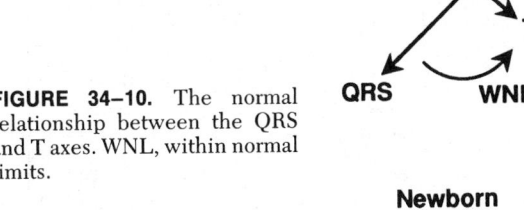

FIGURE 34–10. The normal relationship between the QRS and T axes. WNL, within normal limits.

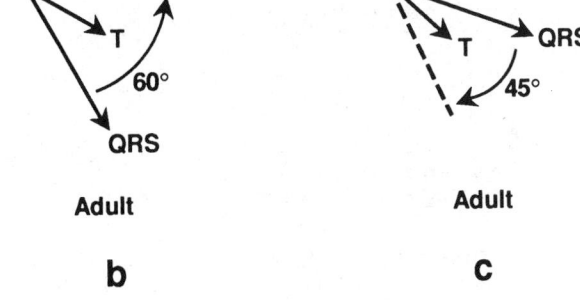

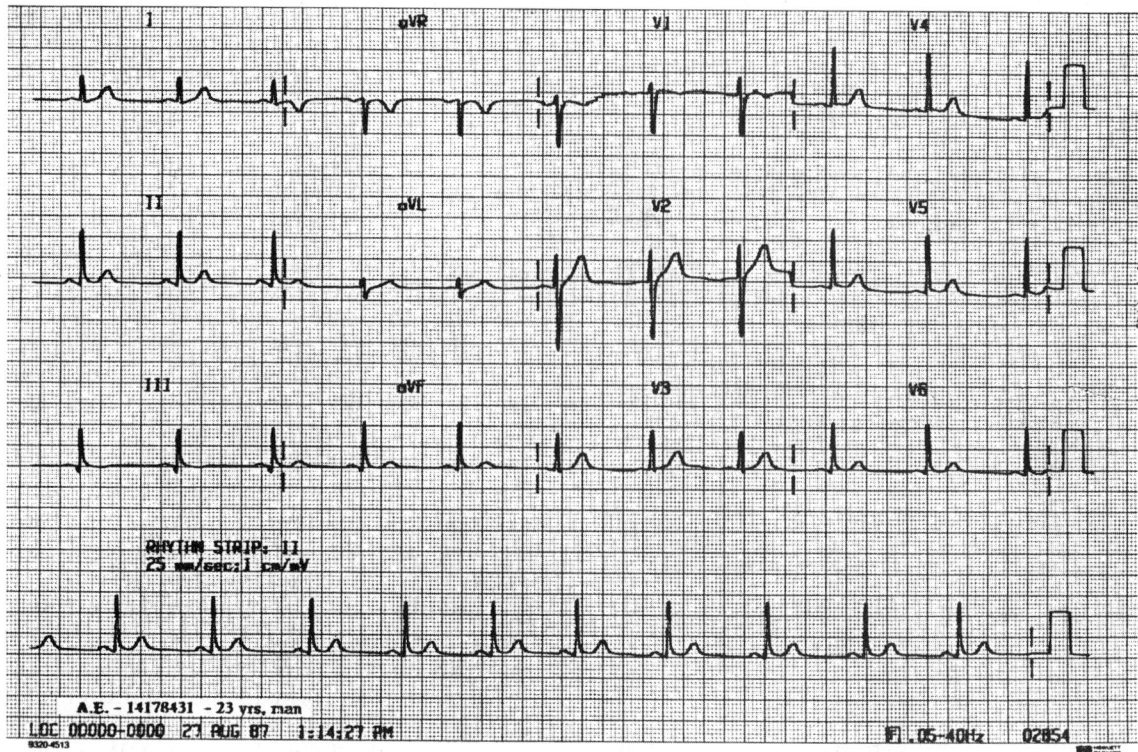

TRACING 34–1.   Example of a normal ECG. Axis of QRS wave, +60 degrees. Axis of T wave, +30 degrees. P, QRS, and T waves are normal in the precordial leads.

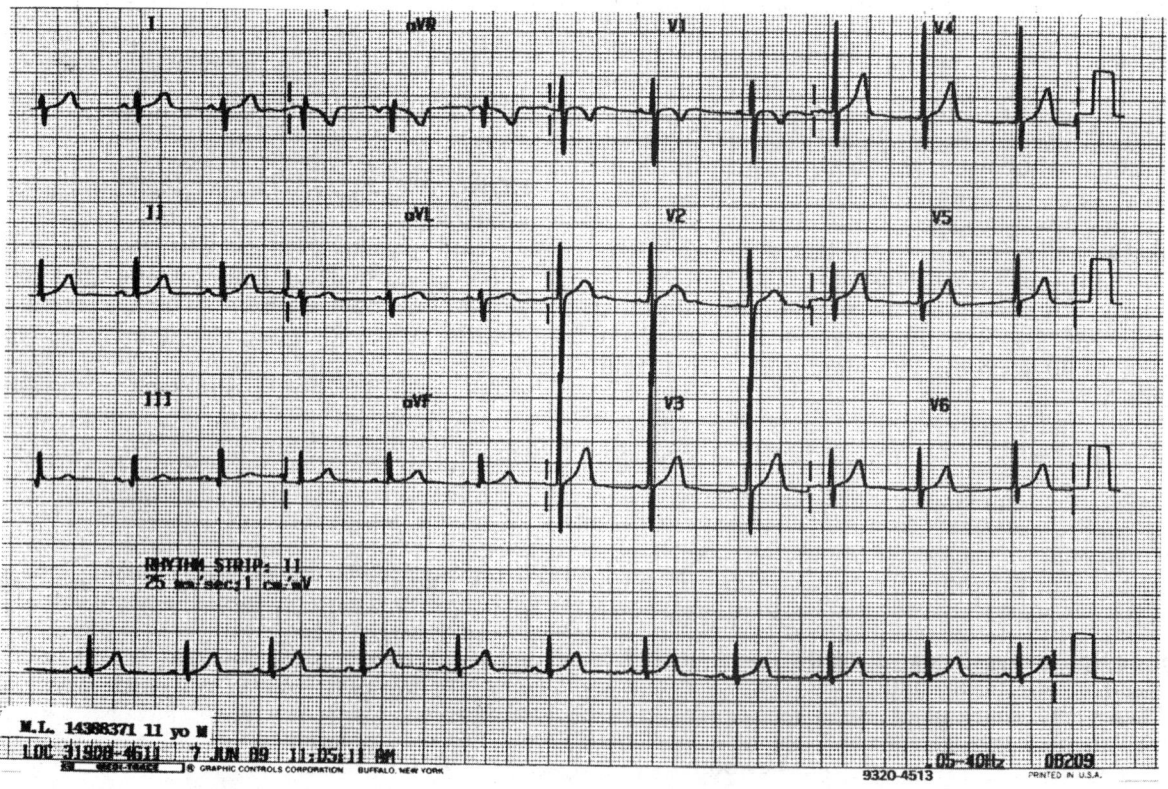

TRACING 34–2.   Example of a normal ECG. Axis of QRS wave, +90 degrees (vertical). Axis of T wave, +40 degrees. P, QRS, and T waves are normal in the precordial leads. A negative T wave in V₁ is normal for children.

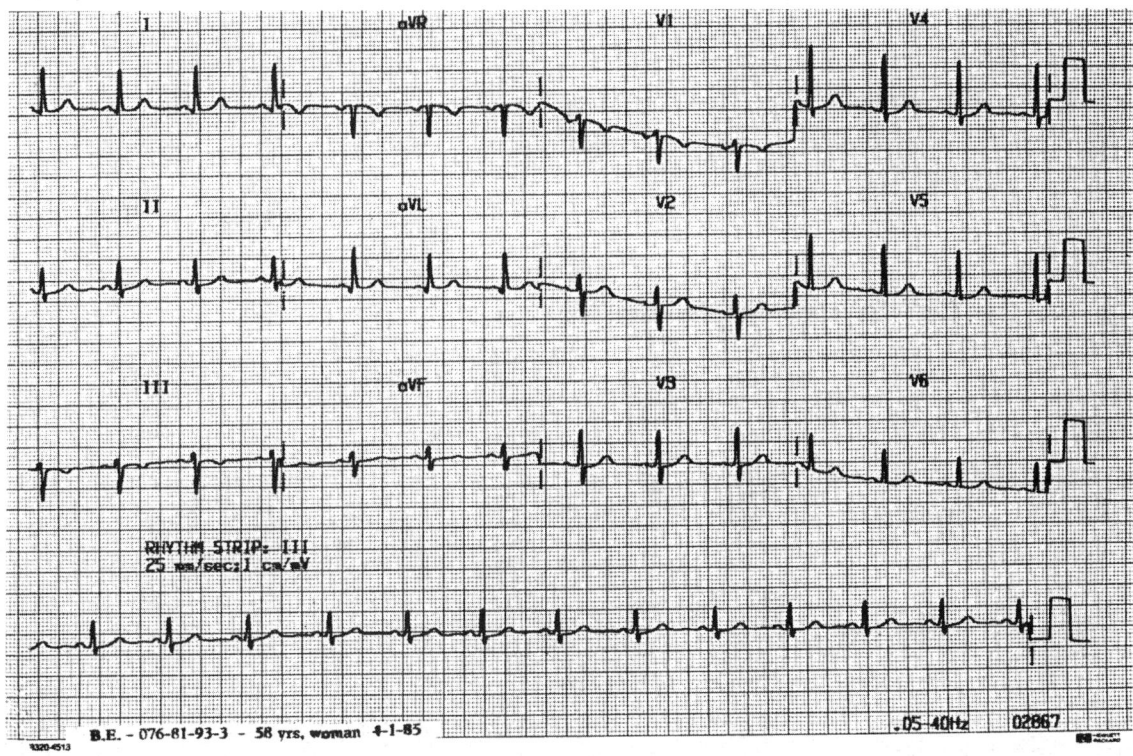

TRACING 34–3.   Example of a normal ECG. Axis of QRS wave, 0 degrees (horizontal). Axis of T wave, +5 degrees. P, QRS, and T waves are normal in the precordial leads.

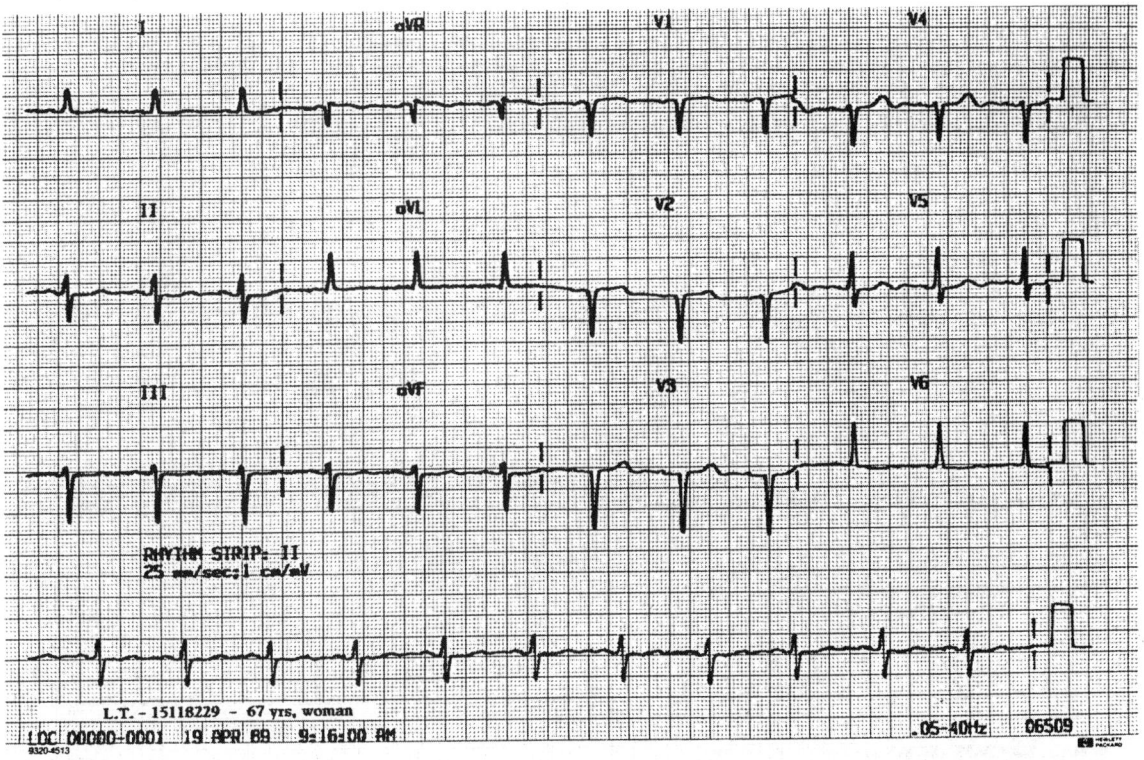

TRACING 34–4.   Example of a left axis deviation. Axis of QRS wave, −40 degrees. Axis of T wave, +60 degrees. Poor R wave progression in the precordial leads caused by an old anterior wall myocardial infarction.

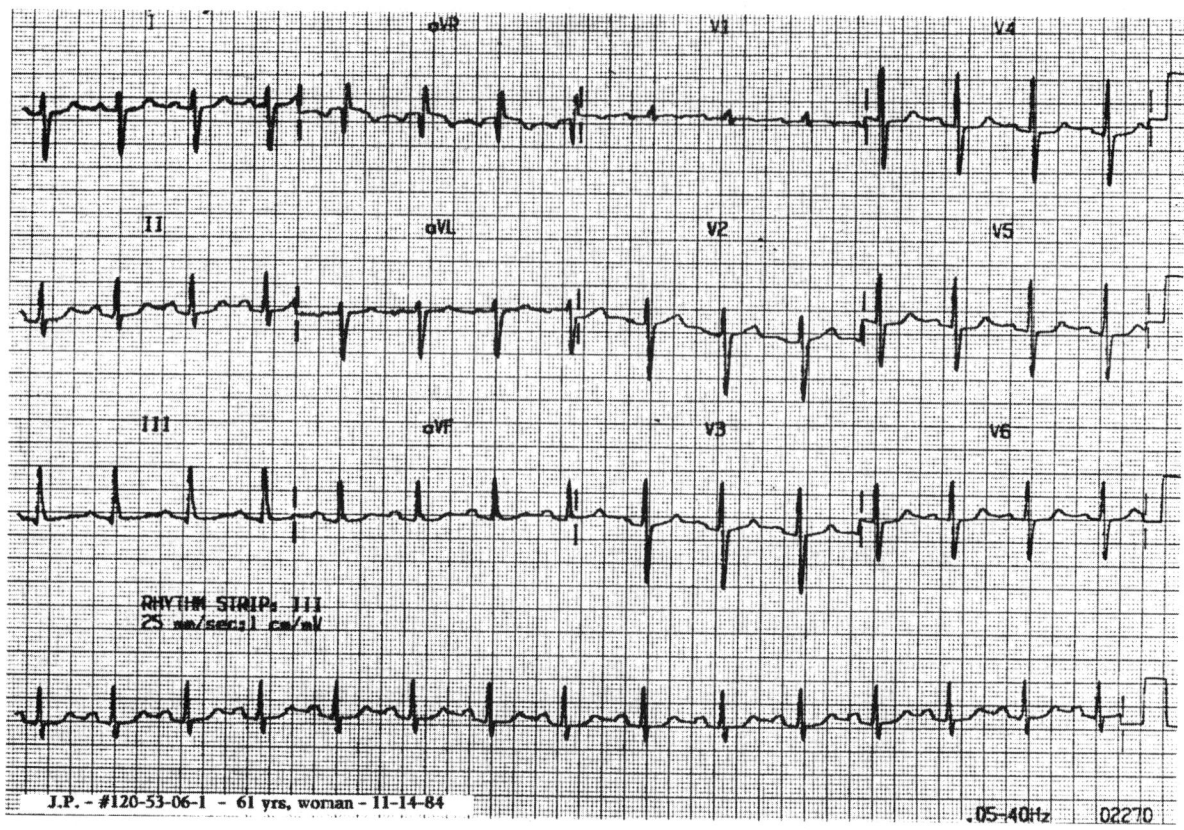

TRACING 34–5.   Example of a right axis deviation. Axis of QRS wave, +125 degrees. Axis of T wave, +30 degrees. The QRS complexes are almost isoelectric in precordial leads V₃ through V₆ because the respective electrodes lie in an isoelectric plane that is perpendicular to the QRS axis.

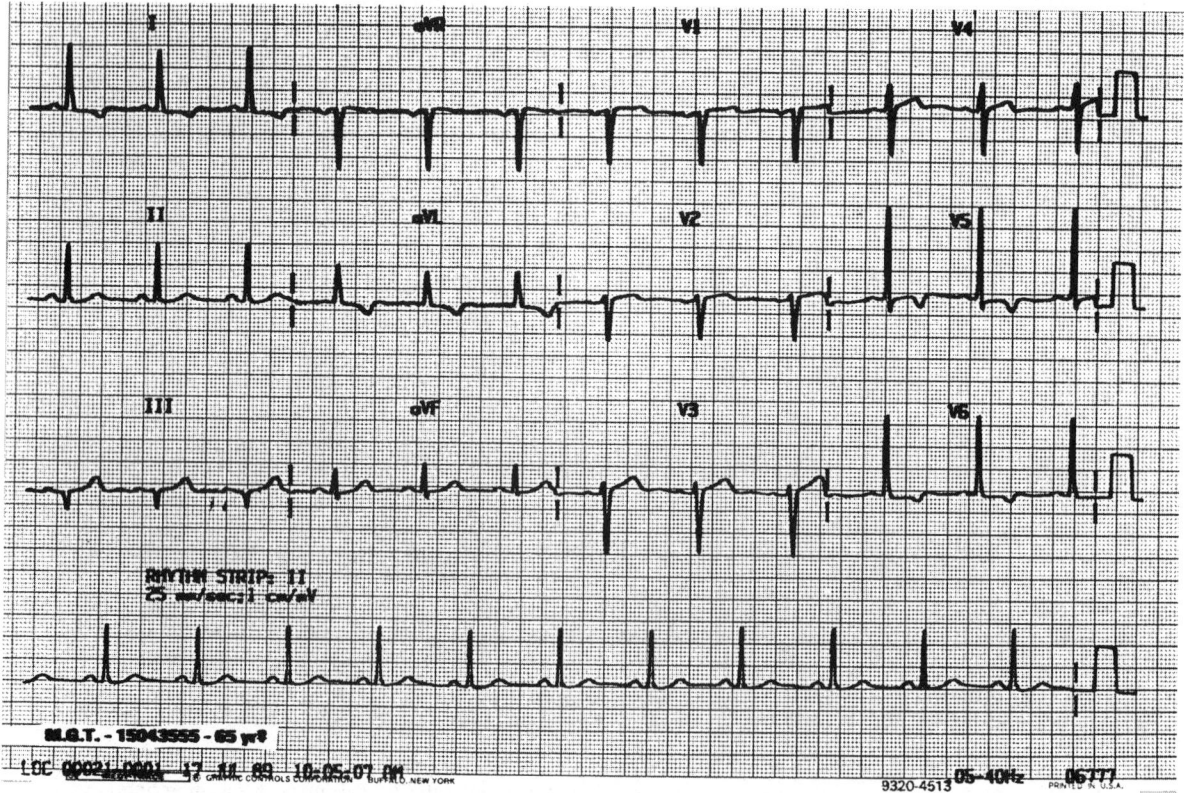

TRACING 34–6.   Example of left ventricular strain. Axis of QRS wave, +15 degrees. Axis of T wave, +120 degrees. There are negative T waves in V₅ and V₆.

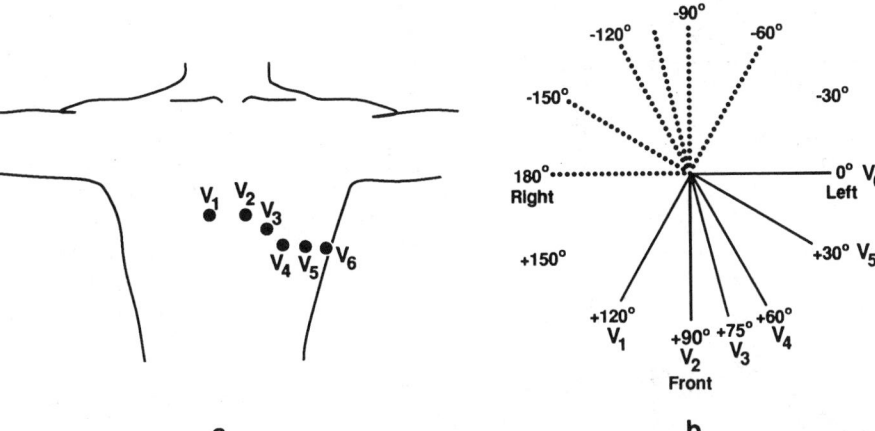

FIGURE 34–11. Placement of electrodes for the chest leads (*a*) and lead system in the horizontal plane (*b*).

a

b

V_1 is placed in the fourth intercostal space at the right sternal border, V_2 at the fourth intercostal space in the left sternal border, V_3 at the fifth intercostal space in the midclavicular line, V_5 at the same plane as V_4 but at the anterior axillary line, and V_6 in the same plane as V_4 at the midaxillary line.

Problems with V Leads

Several problems with the V leads preclude accurate computations of the P, QRS, or T axis in the horizontal plane.

The positive side is toward the front for all leads (except V_6) and toward the left (except V_1 and V_2). However, the horizontal projection of the QRS axis usually is oriented toward the back and to the left, so in general the QRS axis does not lie parallel to any V lead.

The electrical center of the heart is actually displaced to the left and to the front of the center of the transverse plane. This precludes accurate measurements of the amplitude and direction of the QRS axis.

Lung impedance causes decreased amplitudes in V_1, V_2, and V_6, which actually record approximately 60 per cent of the true amplitudes that would be recorded in these leads if there were no lung impedance.

The close proximity of the electrodes to the heart causes the amplitudes on V_3, V_4, and V_5 to be approximately 150 per cent larger than the true am-

plitudes that would be recorded if the electrical center of the heart coincided with the center of the transverse plane. Thus, high voltages of the QRS and T waves and ST segment in these leads may not necessarily indicate the presence of pathology.

The staggered disposition of the electrodes (as shown in Fig. 34–11*a*) precludes computation of the transverse plane axis in the case of a vertical axis in the frontal plane.

Pattern Analysis of Precordial Leads

P Wave

Practically all V leads show a positive P wave (Fig. 34–12).

QRS Wave

There is a gradual increase in voltage of the R wave as it progresses from V_1 to V_5. In a normal R progression, V_2 or V_3 becomes the transitional lead (i.e., the lead that is isoelectric with a RS pattern), V_1 has an rS pattern (i.e., a small R wave and a large S wave), and V_6 has an Rs pattern (i.e., a large R wave and a small S wave) (Fig. 34–12).

T Wave

Practically all V leads show a positive T wave, with the exception of V_1, which may be isoelectric or negative (Fig. 34–12). Negative T waves in V_1 through V_3 indicate strain in the right (anterior) ventricle or in the anterior wall of the left ventricle

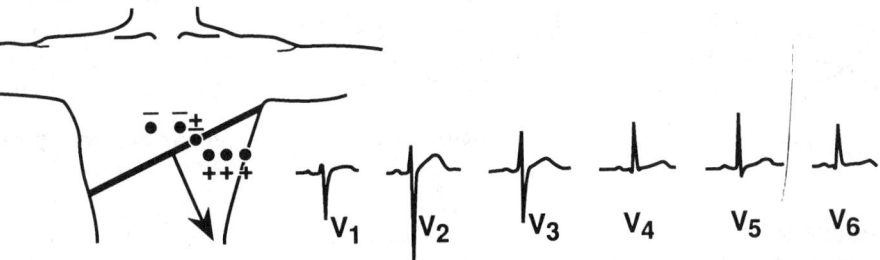

FIGURE 34–12. Normal configuration of P, QRS, and T waves in the precordial leads.

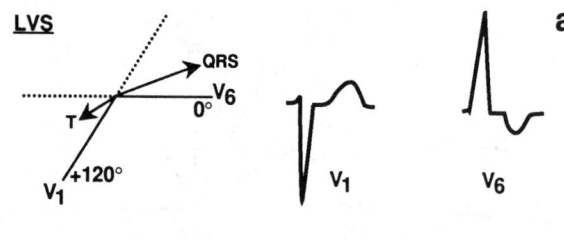

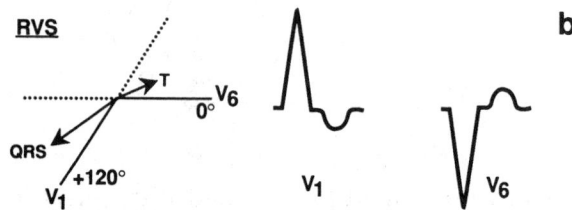

FIGURE 34–13. Abnormal T wave patterns in the precordial leads. LVS, left ventricular strain; RVS, right ventricular strain.

(Fig. 34–13*a*). Negative T waves in V_4 through V_6 indicate strain in the left (posterior) ventricle. This pattern is referred to as "flipped Ts" because normally the T waves are positive in these leads (Fig. 34–13*b*).

LEFT VENTRICULAR HYPERTROPHY

Axis Changes

As a result of the large size of the left (posterior) ventricle in left ventricular hypertrophy (LVH), there is an increased number of EMFs originating from this ventricle. Consequently, most instantaneous EMFs point leftward and backward (Fig. 34–14).

Criteria for Diagnosis of LVH

Frontal Plane

1. LAD or horizontal axis (except when the heart is displaced downward).

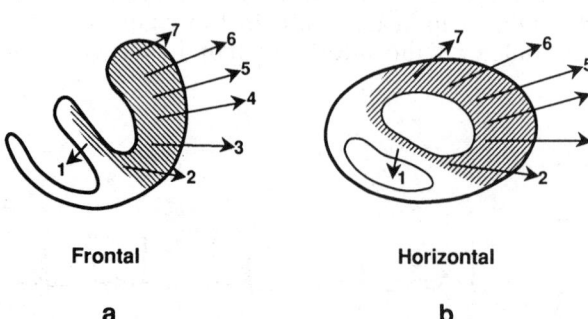

FIGURE 34–14. Genesis and sequence of electromotive forces in left ventricular hypertrophy.

2. Magnitude of QRS wave in the lead of the mean axis greater than 1.5 mV.
3. LVS occurs very often because of a delay in the sequence of repolarization. The changes in the sequence of repolarization account not only for the changes in the T axis but also for the usual presence of ST segment displacement (opposite in direction to QRS axis).
    a. LVH + LVS: systolic overloading (as in aortic stenosis or in hypertension).
    b. LVH without LVS: diastolic overloading (as in aortic insufficiency or ventricular septal defect).
4. Duration of QRS wave greater than 0.08 second but less than 0.12 second.

Horizontal Plane

1. Posterior axis (i.e., transitional lead in V_3 or V_4). The axis may not be posterior when the heart is displaced forward.
2. High magnitude: $S_1 + R_5$ greater than 3.5 mV (index of Sokolow and Lyon). This empirical index states that, when the negative portion of the QRS wave (S_1) in V_1 added to the positive portion of the QRS wave (R) in V_5 exceeds 35 mm (equivalent to 3.5 mV), the diagnosis of LVH should be considered.
3. LVS very often seen (i.e., flipped T waves in V_4, V_5, and V_6).

Example

Tracing 34–7 shows a left ventricular hypertrophy with left ventricular strain.

RIGHT VENTRICULAR HYPERTROPHY

Axis Changes

In Congenital Hypertrophy (Infants and Children)

The ECG changes in right ventricular hypertrophy (RVH) are quite different in infants and adults. In early infancy, the normal heart shows a relative preponderance of the right ventricle, with a greater number of EMFs generated by the right ventricular mass than later on in life. As a result, the majority of QRS instantaneous forces point to the right and to the front. In the frontal plane, there is a right axis deviation. In the horizontal plane, the axis of the QRS wave points to the right and to the front. In cases of congenital RVH, this infantile pattern persists for a long time (Fig. 34–15).

In Acquired Hypertrophy (Older Children and Adults)

In acquired RVH, the sequence of depolarization begins in the right ventricle, with a preponderance of early forces pointing to the front. Subse-

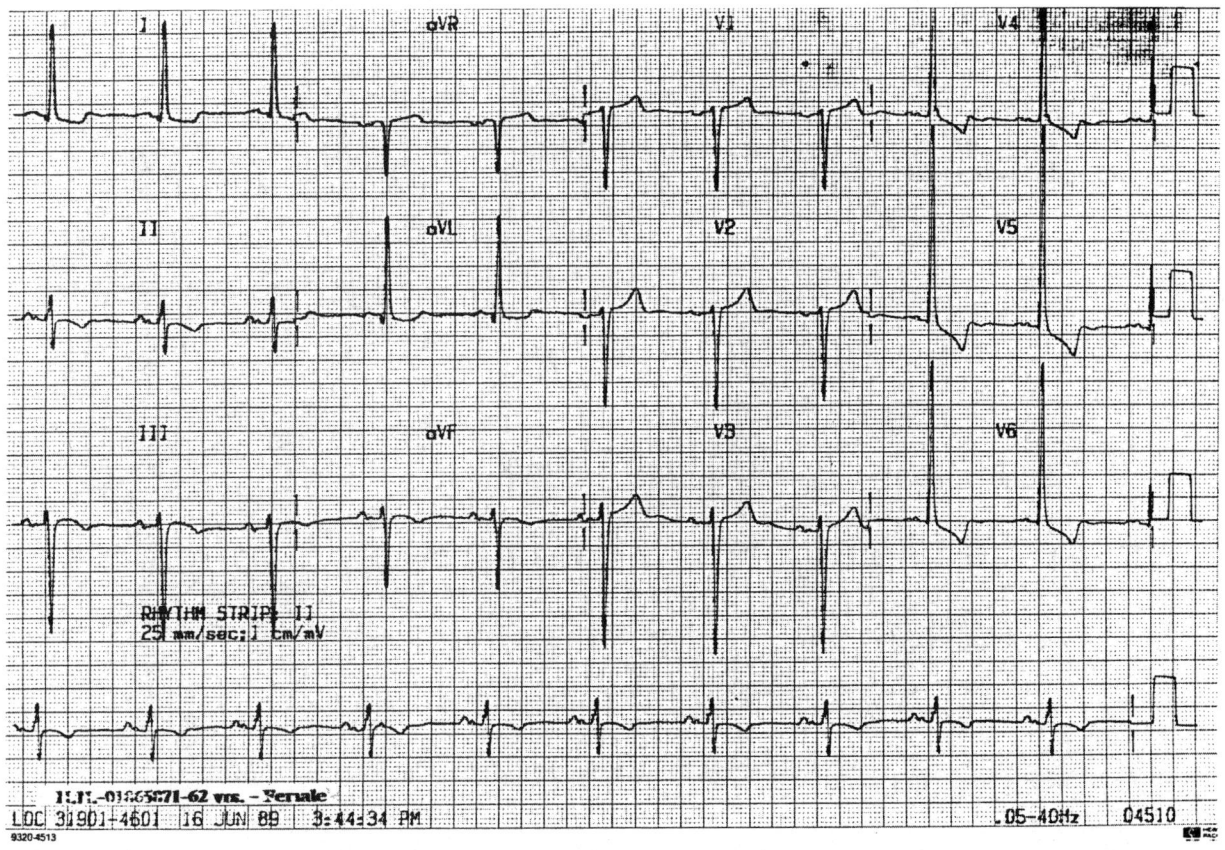

TRACING 34–7. Example of left ventricular hypertrophy with left ventricular strain. Axis of QRS wave, -30 degrees in the frontal plane. Axis of T wave, -120 degrees. The precordial leads show $S_1 + R_5 = 5.5$ mV. Abnormal negative T waves on V_4, V_5, and V_6. Also, P-mitrale.

quently, the forces point to the left because, in spite of the RVH, there is still a relative preponderance of the left ventricle. The terminal forces point to the right and to the front because of the late depolarization of the upper part of an enlarged right ventricle (Fig. 34–16).

Criteria for Diagnosis of RVH

Frontal Plane

1. RAD or vertical axis.
2. Magnitude of QRS wave is normal in the lead parallel to the QRS axis (exceptionally > 1.5 mV).
3. Right ventricular strain (RVS) often seen (especially in infants and/or with systolic overloading).
4. Normal duration of QRS wave.

Horizontal Plane

1. Initial forces very anterior: tall R wave in V_1 ($R_1 > 0.7$ mV) or R_1/S_1 greater than 1, and/or
2. Terminal forces to the right: deep S wave in V_6 ($S_6 > 0.3$ mV) or R_6/S_6 less than 1, or $R_1 + S_5$

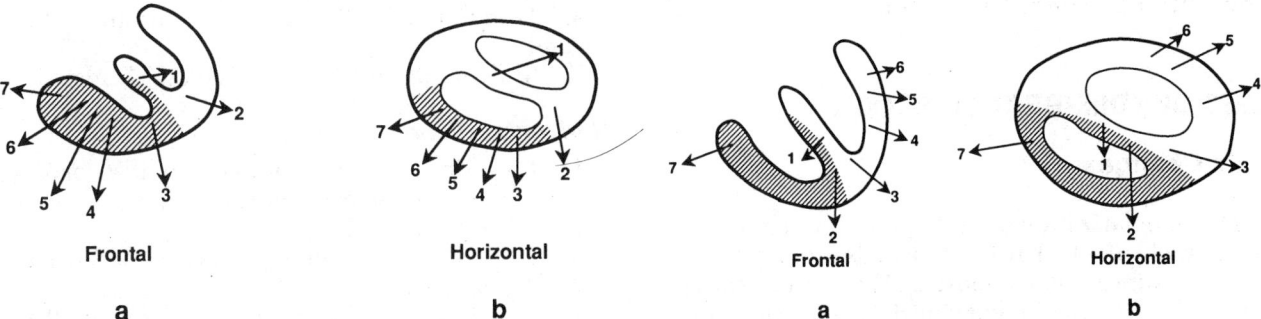

FIGURE 34–15. Genesis and sequence of electromotive forces in congenital right ventricular hypertrophy.

FIGURE 34–16. Genesis and sequence of electromotive forces in acquired right ventricular hypertrophy.

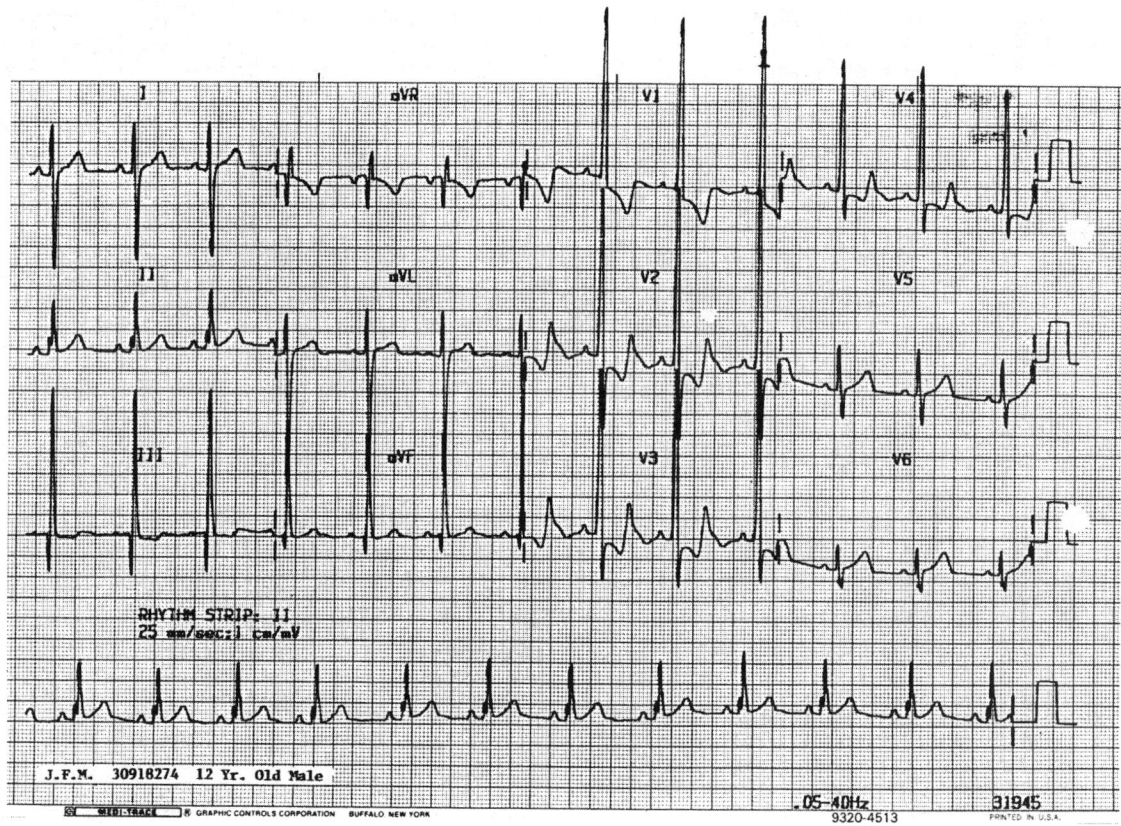

TRACING 34–8. Example of congenital right ventricular hypertrophy with right ventricular strain. Axis of QRS wave in the frontal plane, +120 degrees. Axis of T wave, +30 degrees. High voltage of R wave in V_1, V_2, and V_3. Negative T wave in V_1 and biphasic in V_2 and V_3.

greater than 1.0 mV. These terminal forces also may be displaced to the front (showing a non-slurred R′ in V_1).

3. RVS often found (especially with systolic overloading).

4. Normal duration of QRS wave.

Examples

Tracing 34–8 shows congenital right ventricular hypertrophy with right ventricular strain. Tracing 34–9 shows an acquired right ventricular hypertrophy with right ventricular strain.

LEFT BUNDLE-BRANCH BLOCK

Axis Changes

The depolarization of the septal area in left bundle-branch block (LBBB) proceeds from right to left, but subsequently most EMFs are generated rather slowly from the left ventricle. The right ventricle depolarizes early and rapidly, but the forces generated in the right ventricle are relatively small

and counteracted by the more predominant left ventricular forces (Fig. 34–17).

Criteria for Diagnosis of LBBB

Frontal Plane

1. LAD.

2. Magnitude of QRS wave within normal limits in the lead of mean axis (except where there is LVH also).

3. LVS very often seen (caused by a change in the sequence of repolarization).

4. Duration of QRS wave greater than 0.12 second.

5. Slurring of QRS wave in several leads.

Horizontal Plane

1. Posterior axis (transitional lead at V_3 or V_4).

2. Magnitude within normal limits (except when there is LVH also).

3. LVS very often seen (i.e., flipped T waves in V_4, V_5, and V_6).

4. Duration of QRS wave greater than 0.12 second.

5. Slurring of QRS wave in several leads.

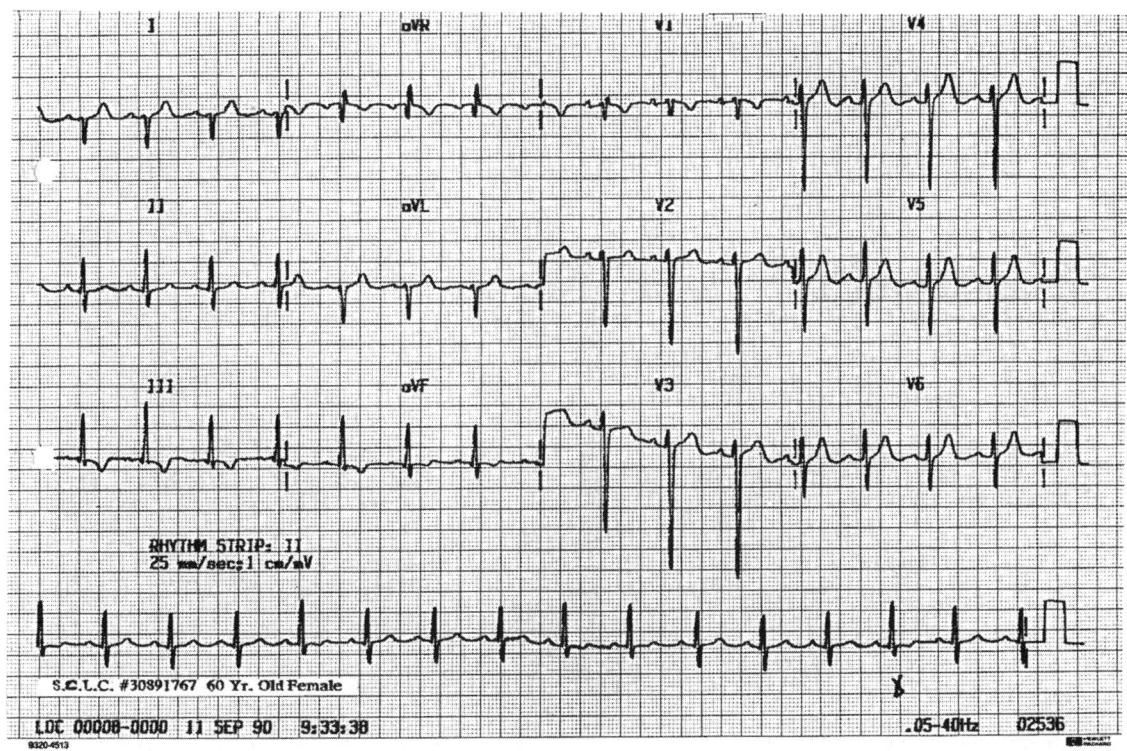

TRACING 34–9. Example of acquired right ventricular hypertrophy with right ventricular strain. Axis of QRS wave, + 120 degrees. Axis of T wave, − 15 degrees. There is a small RR′ pattern in V_1 and a deep S wave in V_6.

Example

Tracing 34–10 shows a left bundle branch block.

RIGHT BUNDLE BRANCH BLOCK

Axis Changes

The sequence of depolarization in right bundle-branch block (RBBB) is similar to that in RVH. However, the anterior displacement of the initial forces is not as marked as in RVH, and the terminal portion of depolarization occurs very slowly (Fig. 34–18).

Criteria for Diagnosis of RBBB

Frontal Plane

1. Normal or near-vertical axis; horizontal axis or LAD if there is also a left anterior hemiblock.
2. Low magnitude of QRS wave in lead parallel to mean axis (usually <1.0 mV).
3. RVS (may not be present).
4. Duration of QRS wave less than 0.12 second.
5. Slurred S wave in lead I.

Horizontal Plane

1. Posterior or undifferentiated axis.
2. Low magnitude of QRS wave.
3. RVS (may not be present).
4. Terminal forces of depolarization to the right (showing a slurred S wave in V_6). These terminal forces also may be displaced to the front (showing an RR′ pattern with a slurred R′ wave in V_1)
5. Slow speed in terminal forces (slurring of S_6 and of R′ waves in V_1 if present).
6. Duration of QRS wave 0.12 second or less.

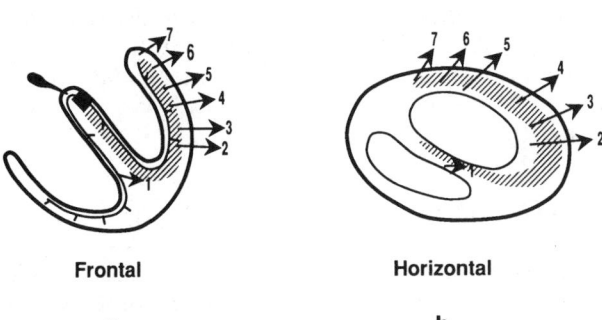

Frontal   **Horizontal**

a   **b**

FIGURE 34–17. Genesis and sequence of electromotive forces in left bundle-branch block.

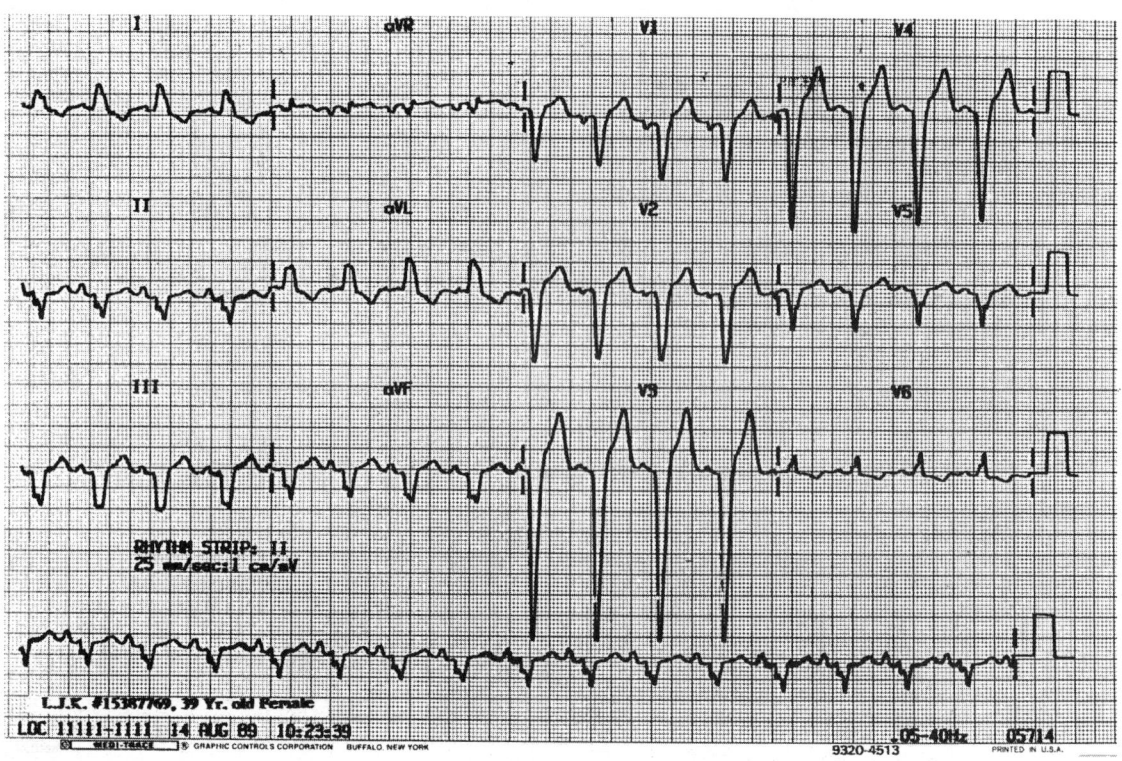

TRACING 34–10. Example of left bundle-branch block. Axis of QRS wave in the frontal plane, −60 degrees. Axis of T wave, +130 degrees (left ventricular strain). Poor R wave progression in the horizontal plane. There are slurred and wide QRS complexes in all leads. ST segment displacement is secondary to the bundle-branch block.

Example

Tracing 34–11 shows a right bundle-branch block.

HEMIBLOCKS

General Concepts

Normally, the conduction of impulses and the generation of QRS EMFs through the bundle of His and its branches occur as shown in Figure

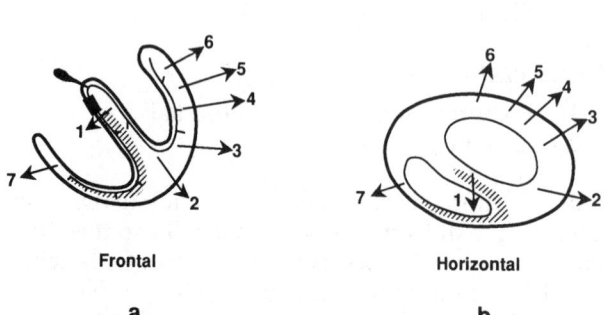

Frontal

a

Horizontal

b

FIGURE 34–18. Genesis and sequence of electromotive forces in right bundle-branch block.

34–19*a*. Conduction disturbances may occur as a result of a lesion in one or several locations of the bundle of His, as shown in the diagram in Figure 34–19*b*.

A conduction defect at 1 produces an atrioventricular block (AVB)

A conduction defect at 2 produces a (RBBB)

A conduction defect at 3 produces a (LBBB)

A conduction defect at 4 produces left anterior or superior hemiblock (LAHB).

A conduction defect at 5 produces a left posterior or inferior hemiblock (LPHB).

Conduction defects at two of the above locations will produce a *bifascicular block*. The most frequent combinations are LAHB + RBBB and LAHB + AVB. Conduction defects at three of the above locations will produce a *trifascicular block*. The most common combination is AVB + LAHB + RBBB.

Axis Changes

The sequence of ventricular depolarization is altered whenever there is a lesion in one of the fascicles of the left bundle, as shown in Figure 34–20. A clinical history usually reveals the existence of coronary artery disease in most cases of hemiblock.

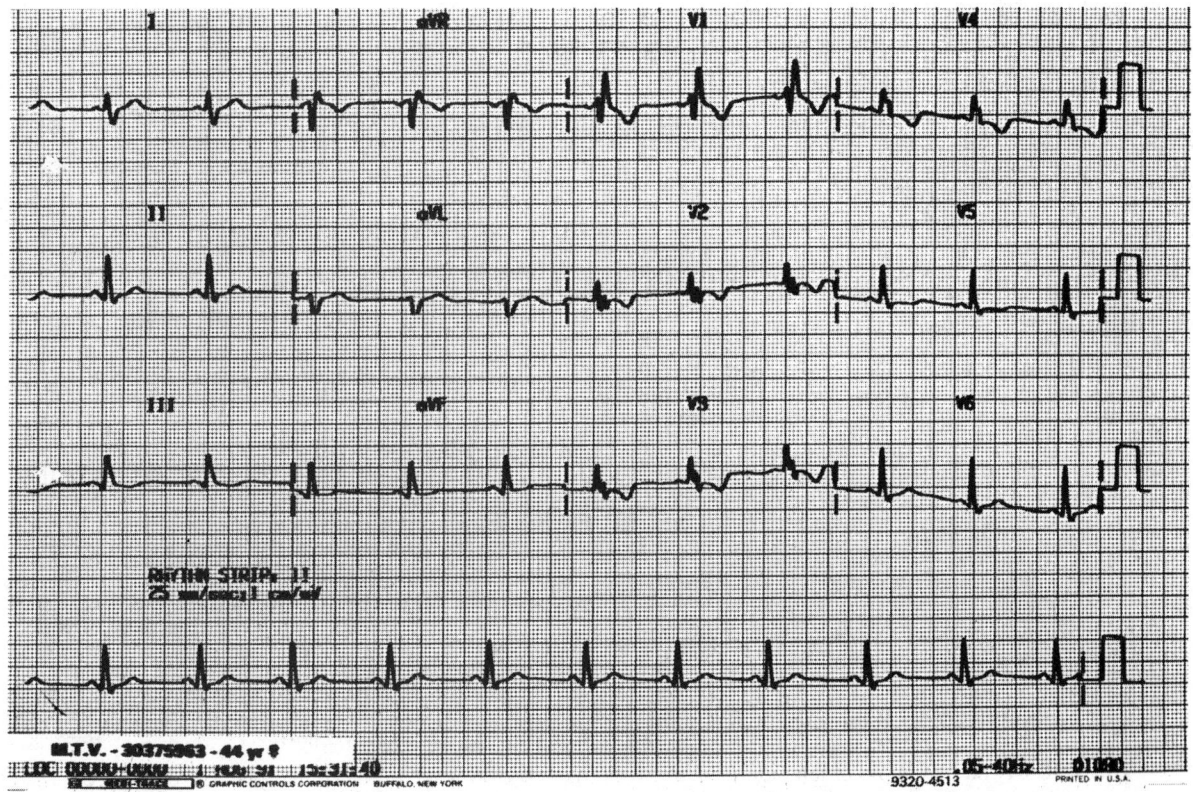

TRACING 34–11. Example of right bundle-branch block. Axis of QRS wave, +90 degrees. Axis of T wave, 0 degrees. Slurred terminal portion of QRS wave in the frontal plane. There is a RR′ pattern in V₁, a notched QRS wave in V₂ through V₄, and slurring of the terminal portion of the QRS wave in V₆.

Criteria for Diagnosis

LAHB or Left Anterior Fascicular Block

FRONTAL PLANE

1. Left axis deviation of at least −30 degrees (not due to other causes) (Figure 34–20a).
2. Low or normal magnitude of QRS wave.
3. Initial forces of depolarization away from the main axis (with Q wave in aVL and occasionally in I).
4. No slurring or only a small notch in one or two leads.

5. QRS wave duration less than 0.12 second.

HORIZONTAL PLANE

1. Usually posterior axis (i.e., transitional lead in V₃ and V₄).

EXAMPLE. Tracing 34–12 shows a left anterior hemiblock.

LPHB or Left Posterior Fascicular Block

This type of hemiblock occurs much less often than the LAHB. As in the case of LAHB, ECG changes resulting from coronary artery disease or

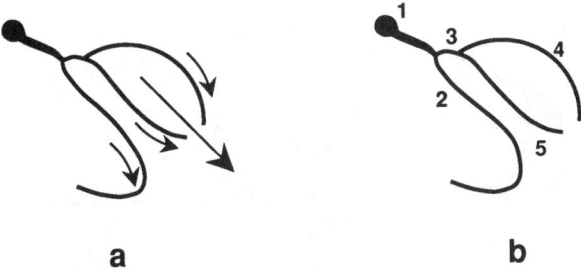

a   **b**

FIGURE 34–19. Normal conduction of electromotive forces in the ventricles and subdivision of the bundle of His: 1, AV junction; 2, right bundle branch; 3, left bundle branch; 4, left anterior fascicle; 5, left posterior fascicle.

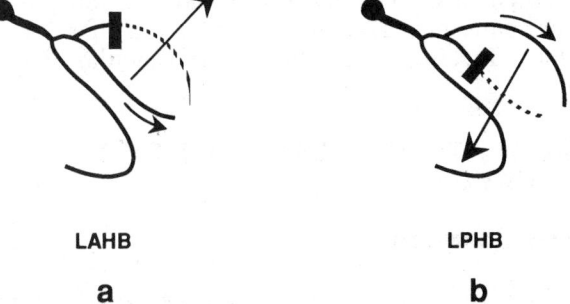

LAHB   **LPHB**

a   **b**

FIGURE 34–20. Axis deviation in hemiblocks. LAHB, left anterior hemiblock; LPHB, left posterior hemiblock.

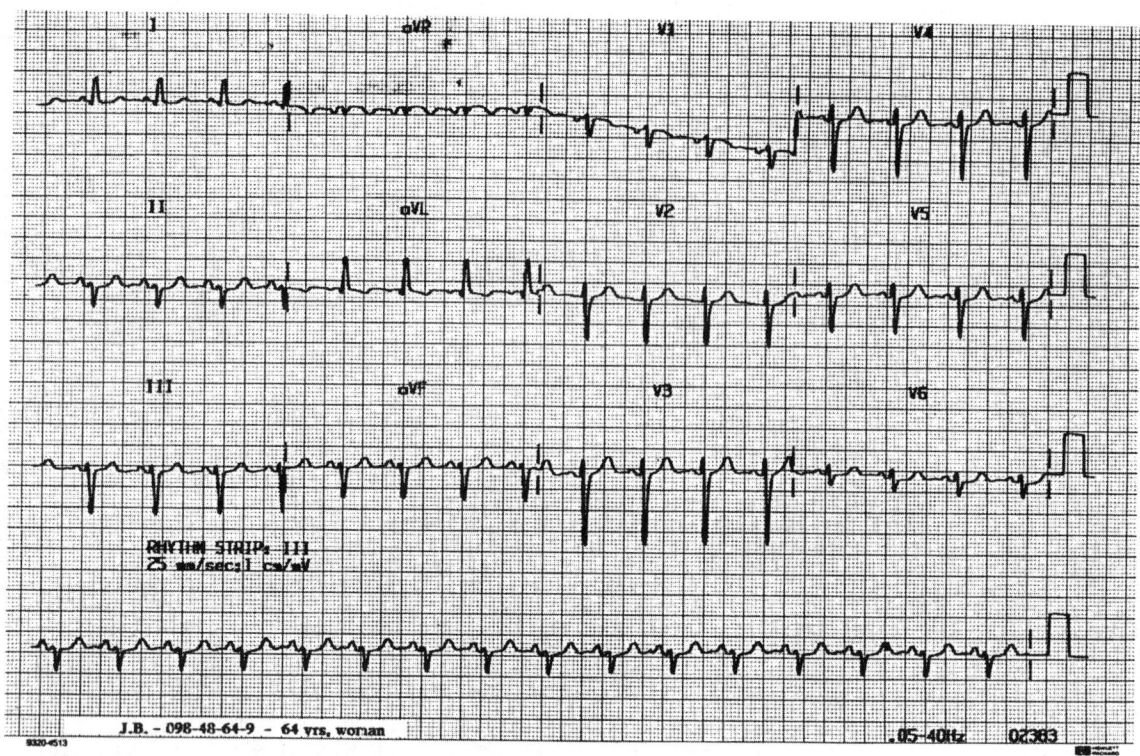

TRACING 34–12.   Example of left anterior hemiblock. Axis of QRS wave in the frontal plane, –50 degrees. Axis of T wave, +75 degrees. The QRS complexes are not as wide as in left bundle-branch block. There is a small Q wave in leads I and aVL.

myocardial infarction may be present in addition to the changes caused by the fascicular block.

FRONTAL PLANE

1.   RAD (otherwise unexplained) (Figure 34–20b). In some cases, there is no RAD but the axis has shifted rightward from its prehemiblock direction.

2.   Low or normal magnitude of QRS wave.

3.   No slurring or a small notch in one or two leads.

4.   QRS wave duration less than 0.12 second.

HORIZONTAL PLANE

1.   An isolated LPHB usually causes a posterior axis (i.e., transitional lead in V_3 and V_4).

EXAMPLES.   Tracing 34–13 shows a left posterior hemiblock. Tracing 34–14 shows a bifascicular block. Tracing 34–15 shows a trifascicular block.

RIGHT ATRIAL ENLARGEMENT OR P-PULMONALE

Axis Changes

As a result of the increased size of the right atrium in right atrial enlargement (RAE), most EMFs originate in that atrium and proceed in a slightly more rightward direction than normal (Fig. 34–21). Most cases of RAE are due to pulmonic valve or pulmonary artery disease, so the term *P-pulmonale* may be used synonymously with right atrial enlargement.

Criteria for Diagnosis of RAE

Frontal Plane

1.   Direction of the P axis is vertical, almost vertical, or deviated to the right (small P wave in I and negative P wave in aVL).

2.   Magnitude of P wave greater than 0.25 mV (peaked P wave in II).

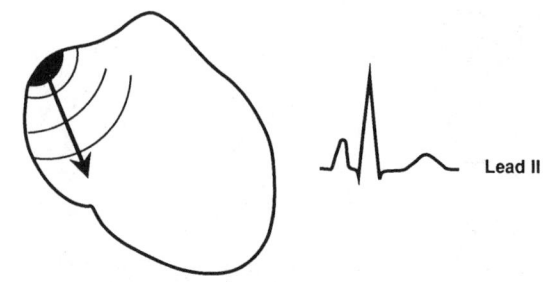

FIGURE 34–21.   Genesis and sequence of electromotive forces in right atrial enlargement.

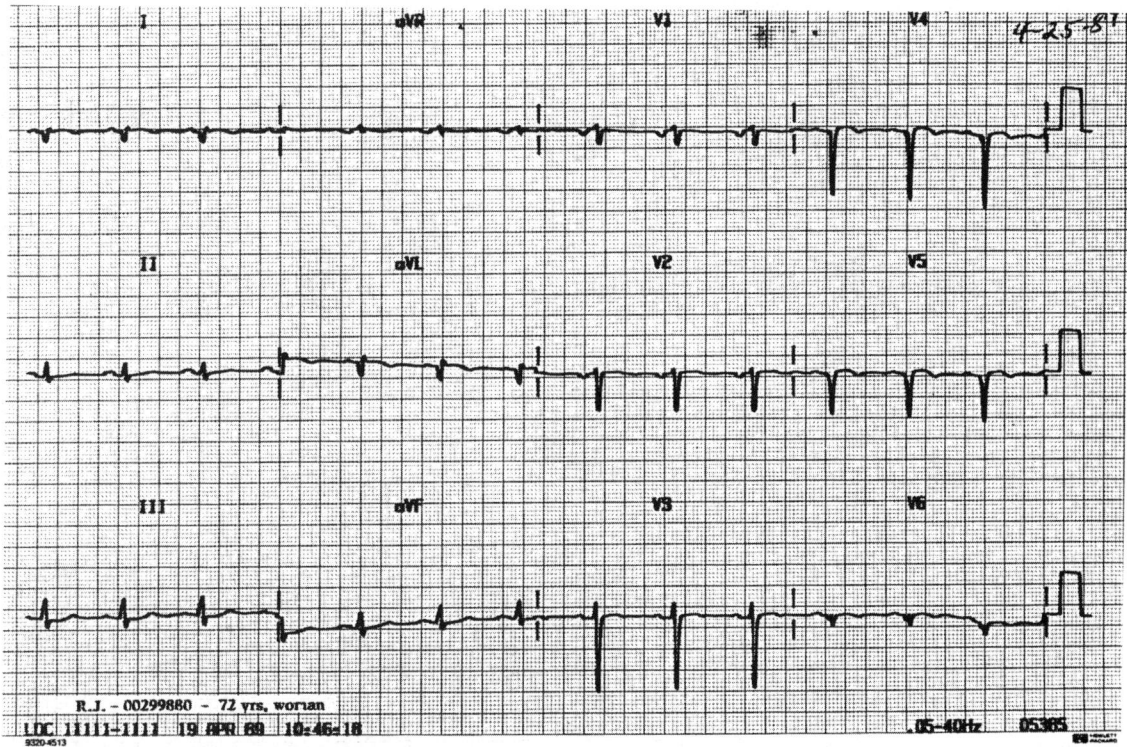

TRACING 34–13. Example of left posterior hemiblock. Axis of QRS wave, +120 degrees. Axis of T wave, +120 degrees. Poor R wave progression in horizontal leads. There is a history of an old myocardial infarction that affected the left posterior fascicle.

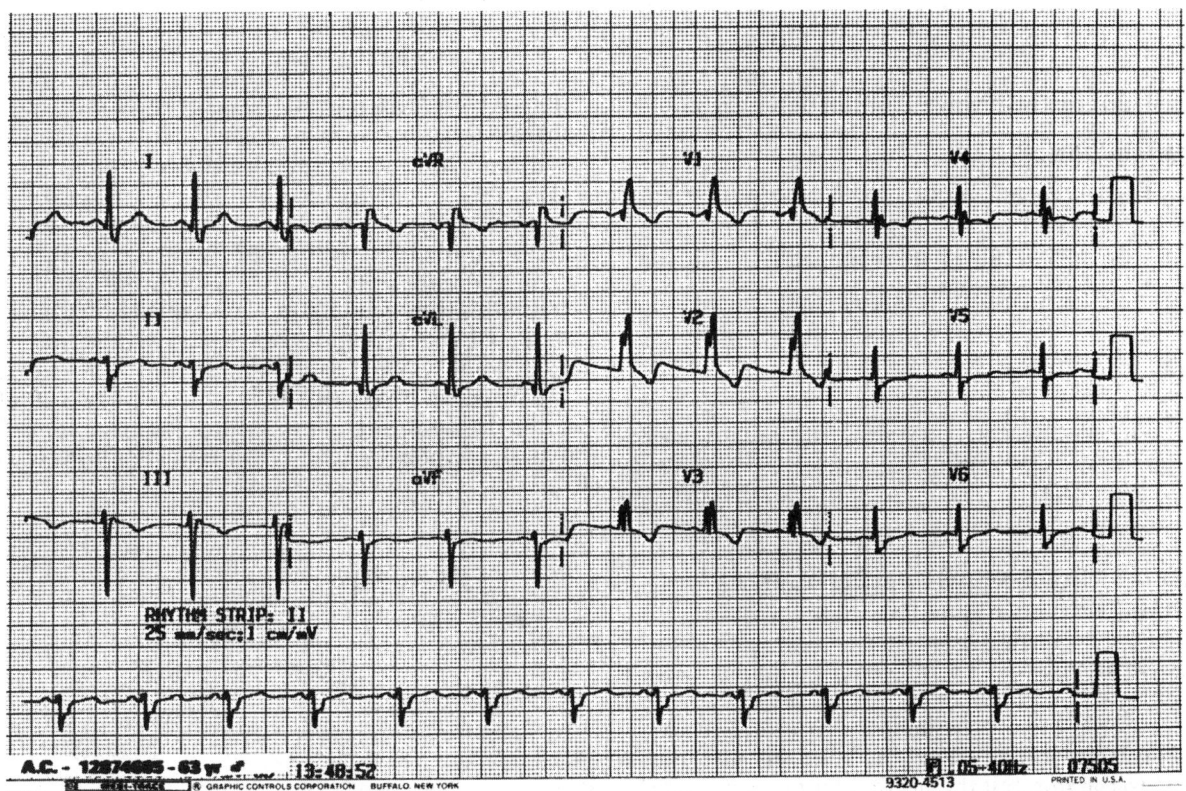

TRACING 34–14. Example of bifascicular block. Axis of QRS wave, −45 degrees. Axis of T wave, 0 degrees. The left axis deviation is suggestive of left anterior hemiblock. The RR' pattern on V_1 through V_3 and the slurring of the terminal portion of the QRS wave in leads I and V_6 indicate a right bundle-branch block.

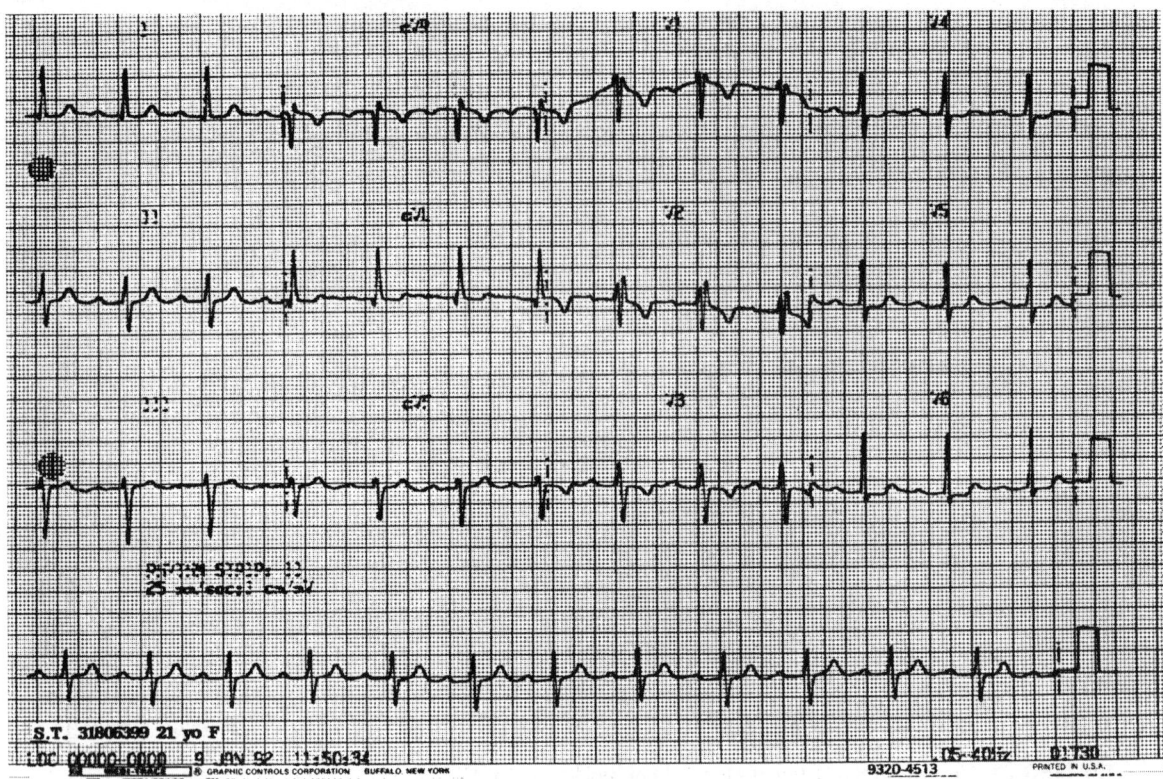

TRACING 34–15. Example of trifascicular block. Axis of QRS wave, −30 degrees. Axis of T wave, +50 degrees. The left axis deviation is indicative of a left anterior hemiblock. The precordial leads show a right bundle-branch block (RR′ pattern in V_1 and V_2). The rhythm strip shows a P-R interval of 0.24 to 0.26 second that indicates a first-degree atrioventricular block.

3. Duration of P wave 0.08 second or less.

Horizontal Plane

1. P axis may be anterior (with a prominent upright P wave in V_1).

Criteria based on the relative duration of P wave/ P-R interval are not reliable.

Example

Tracing 34–16 shows a right atrial enlargement (P-pulmonale) and chronic obstructive pulmonary disease (COPD).

LEFT ATRIAL ENLARGEMENT OR P-MITRALE

Axis Changes

The increased size of the left atrium in left atrial enlargement (LAE) causes a shift of late atrial EMFs to the left, but the normal forces of depolarization of the right atrium occur earlier and in the normal direction. This explains the existence of two P waves. The first is due to depolarization of the right atrium and the second to depolarization of the left atrium. The P wave in several of the standard limb leads shows a double-hump pattern (Fig. 34–22). Most cases of LAE are due to mitral valve disease, so the term *P-mitrale* may be used synonymously with left atrial enlargement.

In patients with diffuse myocardial damage of the left atrium (as in atherosclerotic cardiovascular disease), the depolarization progresses slowly, first to the right atrium and then to the left. As a result, the P wave is broad and small and has a double hump resembling a P-mitrale. The problem here is not hypertrophy but delayed depolarization

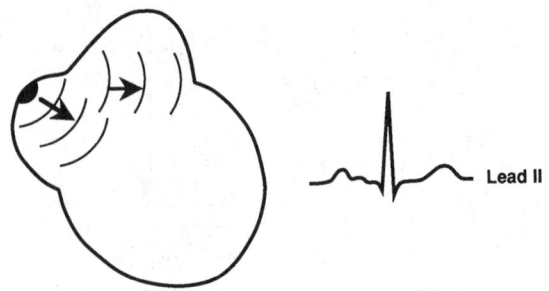

FIGURE 34–22. Genesis and sequence of electromotive forces in left atrial enlargement.

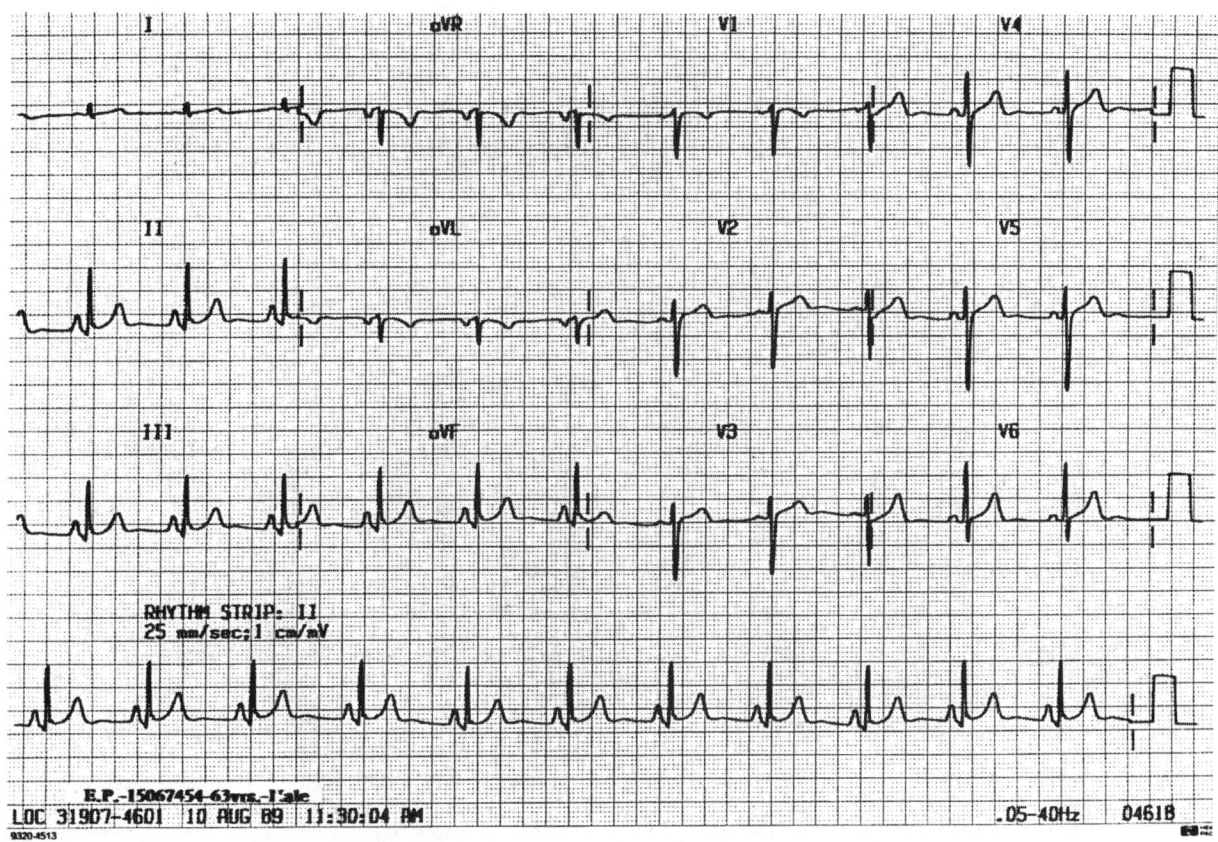

TRACING 34–16.   Example of right atrial enlargement (P-pulmonale) and COPD. Very tall P wave (3.5 mm) on lead II with a vertical axis. Axis of QRS wave, +85 degrees. Axis of T wave, +75 degrees.

through a damaged myocardium, so the preferred term is *left atrial abnormality* (LAA).

Criteria for Diagnosis of LAE or LAA

Frontal Plane

1.   Usually there are two small P axes, the first in the normal direction of about +60 degrees and the second (and often smaller) 30 to 60 degrees to the left of the first. This causes a double-humped P wave in lead II.
2.   Highest amplitude of either one of the two P waves is 2.5 mm (0.25 mV). In cases of LAA, the magnitude is very small.
3.   Duration of P wave usually greater than 0.08 second.

Horizontal Plane

1.   The two P axes (one anterior and quite small, the other posterior and larger) usually produce a biphasic P wave in V_1.

Example

Tracing 34–17 shows a left atrial enlargement (P-mitrale). Tracing 34–7 also shows a P-mitrale.

CHANGES CAUSED BY CHRONIC OBSTRUCTIVE PULMONARY DISEASE

As a result of COPD, there is an increase in the volume of air contained in the lungs. This creates a large area of high electrical impedance that prevents the transmission of the EMFs generated in the heart during depolarization. Although one would expect patients with COPD to have right ventricular and right atrial preponderance (cor pulmonale), the ECG manifestations of such a syndrome may not be evident because of the impedance effect on the transmission of the EMF from an enlarged right ventricle.

ECG Changes Attributable to the Effect of COPD on Cardiac Dynamics

Frontal Plane

1.   RAE (or P-pulmonale).
2.   Vertical axis or RAD.
3.   RVS.

Horizontal Plane

1.   Usually undifferentiated axis.
2.   Late forces of depolarization point to the right (i.e., deep S wave on V_6, not slurred).

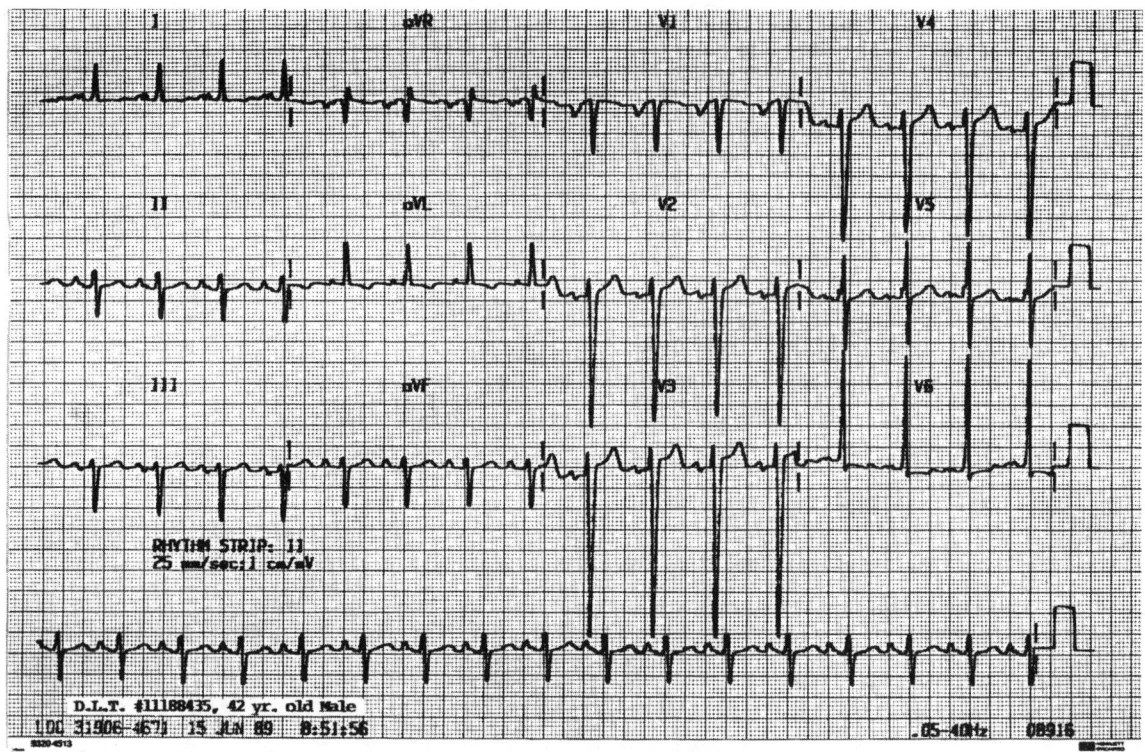

TRACING 34–17. Example of left atrial enlargement (P-mitrale). Axis of QRS wave, −45 degrees. Axis of T wave, +120 degrees. Double-humped P wave in most leads. Negative P wave in V_1. Poor R wave progression in the precordial leads. (See also Tracing 34–7 for an example of P-mitrale.)

Effect on the Transmission of EMFs

As a result of the effect of COPD on electrical impedance, the above changes attributable to the cor pulmonale syndrome may be masked by a distorted transmission of EMFs from the heart to the precordial electrodes. As a result, the following changes are noticeable.

Frontal Plane

1. Overall decrease in the magnitude of QRS wave in the frontal plane.
2. Undifferentiated axis or LAD that mimicks an LAHB.

The presence of P-pulmonale and the clinical history help to establish the diagnosis of COPD.

Horizontal Plane

1. Decrease in the amplitude of QRS wave.
2. Absence of the anteriorly displaced initial forces of depolarization (poor R wave progression).

These criteria mimick an old anterior wall myocardial infarction, but the presence of a P-pulmonale and the clinical history help establish the diagnosis of COPD.

Example

Tracing 34–18 shows chronic obstructive pulmonary disease causing a left axis deviation that mimicks a left anterior hemiblock.

CHANGES CAUSED BY MYOCARDIAL INFARCTION

Axis Changes

The pathologic changes that occur in the myocardium as a result of a myocardial infarction (MI) produce characteristic changes in the QRS and T waves and the ST segment. The following are the important ECG components that help to diagnose MI:

Initial forces of QRS wave (first 0.04 second of the QRS complex). These forces point *away* from the *dead zone* because no EMFs are generated in the dead area. The presence of significant Q waves provides information on the direction of the initial QRS forces.

Axis of ST segment. This axis can be determined in the same way as other axes—that is, by finding a lead with an isoelectric ST segment. This axis points *toward* the area of *injury*.

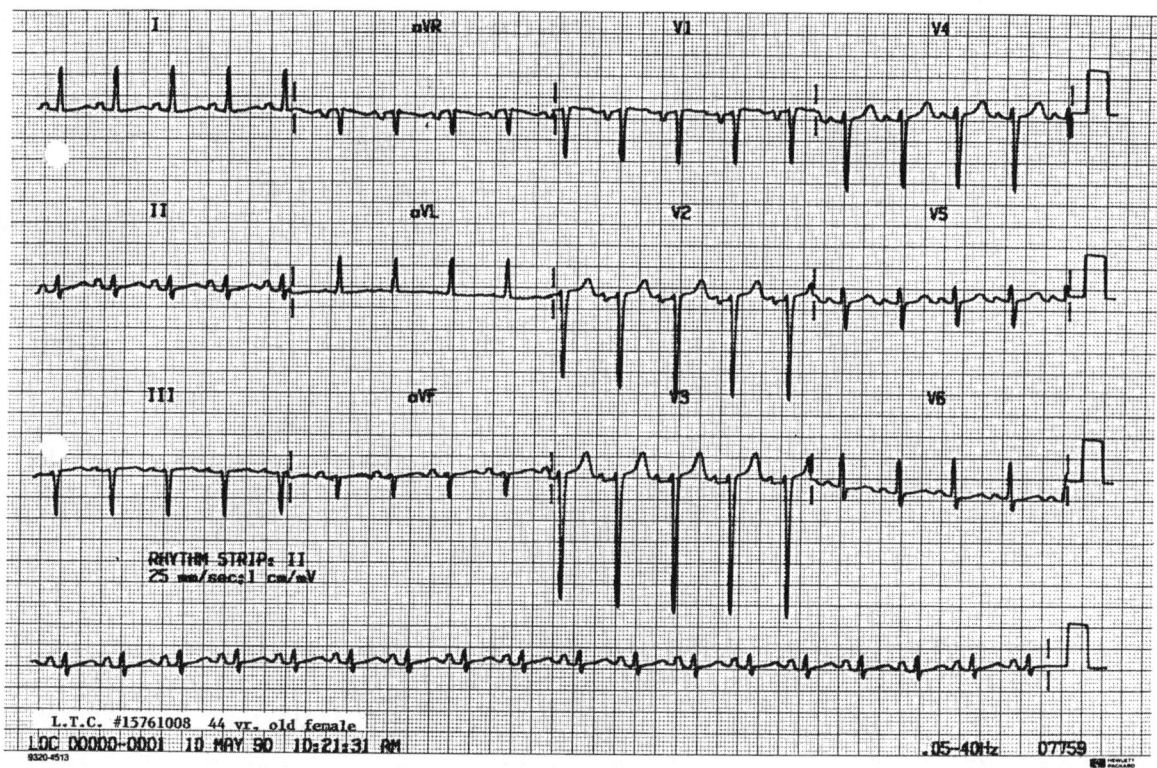

TRACING 34–18. Example of a COPD left axis deviation mimicking a left anterior hemiblock. Axis of QRS wave, −30 degrees. There is P-pulmonale. The poor R wave progression in the precordial leads mimics an old anterior wall myocardial infarction but is due to the impedance produced by the expanded lungs.

Axis of T wave. This axis points *away* from the area of *ischemia* (ECG pattern of strain).

Figure 34–23 shows the effect of the three basic types of pathology on the QRS, ST, and T components of ventricular electrical activity. Clinical information is essential for an accurate diagnosis.

Evolution of the Axis Changes

At each stage in the evolution of an infarction (acute, subacute, and postinfarction or old MI),

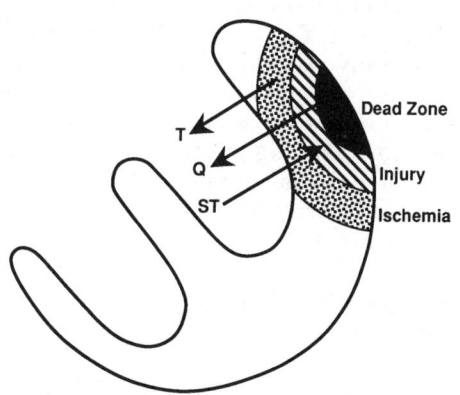

FIGURE 34–23. Relationship between the ECG and pathologic changes in myocardial infarction.

there are prominent ECG changes that are characteristic. Table 34–1 indicates the relative prevalence of changes in each stage.

Criteria for Diagnosis of Stage of MI

Acute Stage (about 1 Week)

1. A prominent ST segment displacement (up or down).
2. Deep and wide Q waves may be present in leads that do not normally have Q waves.

Subacute Stage (1 to 8 Weeks)

1. A prominent negative T wave is present in the leads with a positive QRS wave (strain pattern).
2. Deep and wide Q waves may be present.

TABLE 34–1. EVOLUTION OF ECG CHANGES AT VARIOUS STAGES OF MYOCARDIAL INFARCTION*

Stage of MI	Initial QRS Wave	ST Segment	T Wave
Acute (About 1 week)	±	+ +	±
Subacute (1–8 weeks)	±	±	+ +
Post-MI (>8 weeks)	+ +	−	±

*(−), not present; (±), may be present; (+), apparent; (+ +), very apparent.

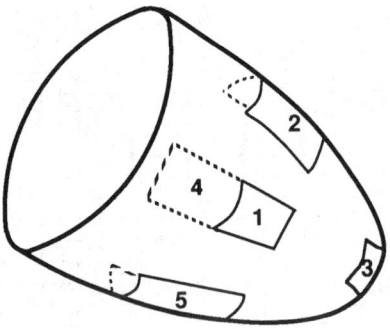

1. **Anterior or Anteroseptal**

2. **Anterolateral or Anterobasal or Superior**

3. **Apical**

4. **Posterior**

5. **Inferior--Diaphragmatic**

FIGURE 34–24. Common locations of myocardial infarction.

Old MI (>8 Weeks)

1. Deep and wide Q waves.
2. Slurring in S waves.

Common Locations of MI

The most common locations of a MI are shown in Figure 34–24. In this figure, the ventricles are drawn like a cone with a single chamber whose anterior wall includes the septum. The free anterior portion of the right ventricular wall is rarely the site of a localized infarction.

Anterior or anteroseptal: caused by an occlusion of the left anterior descending artery.

Anterolateral or anterobasal or superior: caused by an occlusion of the circumflex artery.

Apical: caused by an occlusion of the terminal portion of the left anterior descending artery.

Posterior: caused by an occlusion of the right coronary artery (or one of its branches). May affect the SA and AV nodes and cause dysrhythmia.

Inferior or diaphragmatic: caused by an occlusion of the dominant right coronary artery or dominant left coronary artery. If it results from an occlusion of the right coronary artery, it may affect the SA and AV nodes and cause dysrhythmia.

Criteria for Diagnosis of *Location* of MI

General

1. Significant Q wave of 0.04 second or longer in duration *and* one third the height of QRS wave.

2. Significant ST segment of 2 mm (0.2 mV) or more.

3. Significant T wave: inverted in leads with a positive QRS wave (ventricular strain) and with a deep symmetrical shape of the inversion

Anterior or Anteroseptal

1. ST segment positive in the first or anterior V leads (acute).

2. T wave negative in the first V leads (subacute).

3. QS pattern in V_1 and V_2 (i.e., poor R progression) (old).

Anterolateral or Superior

1. ST segment negative in the inferior lead aVF (acute).

2. T wave positive in III and possibly in aVL (subacute).

3. Q wave in the lateral leads I and aVL (old).

Apical

1. ST segment positive in I (acute).

2. T wave negative in I (subacute).

3. Q wave in I (old).

Posterior

1. ST segment negative in the first or anterior V leads (acute).

2. T wave positive in the first V leads (subacute).

3. R wave prominent in the first or anterior V leads (old).

Inferior or Diaphragmatic

1. ST segment positive in the so-called inferior leads, II, III, and aVF (acute).

2. T wave negative in II, III, and aVF (subacute).

3. Q wave in II, III, and aVF (old).

Examples

Tracing 34–19 shows an acute anterior wall myocardial infarction. Tracing 34–20 shows a subacute anterior wall myocardial infarction. Tracing 34–21 shows an anterolateral myocardial infarction. Tracing 34–22 shows a subacute inferior wall myocardial infarction. Tracing 34–23 shows an old posterior wall myocardial infarction. Tracing 34–24 shows an old inferior wall myocardial infarction.

CAUSES OF ST SEGMENT DISPLACEMENT

In addition to MI, there are other conditions that may produce a measurable ST segment displacement.

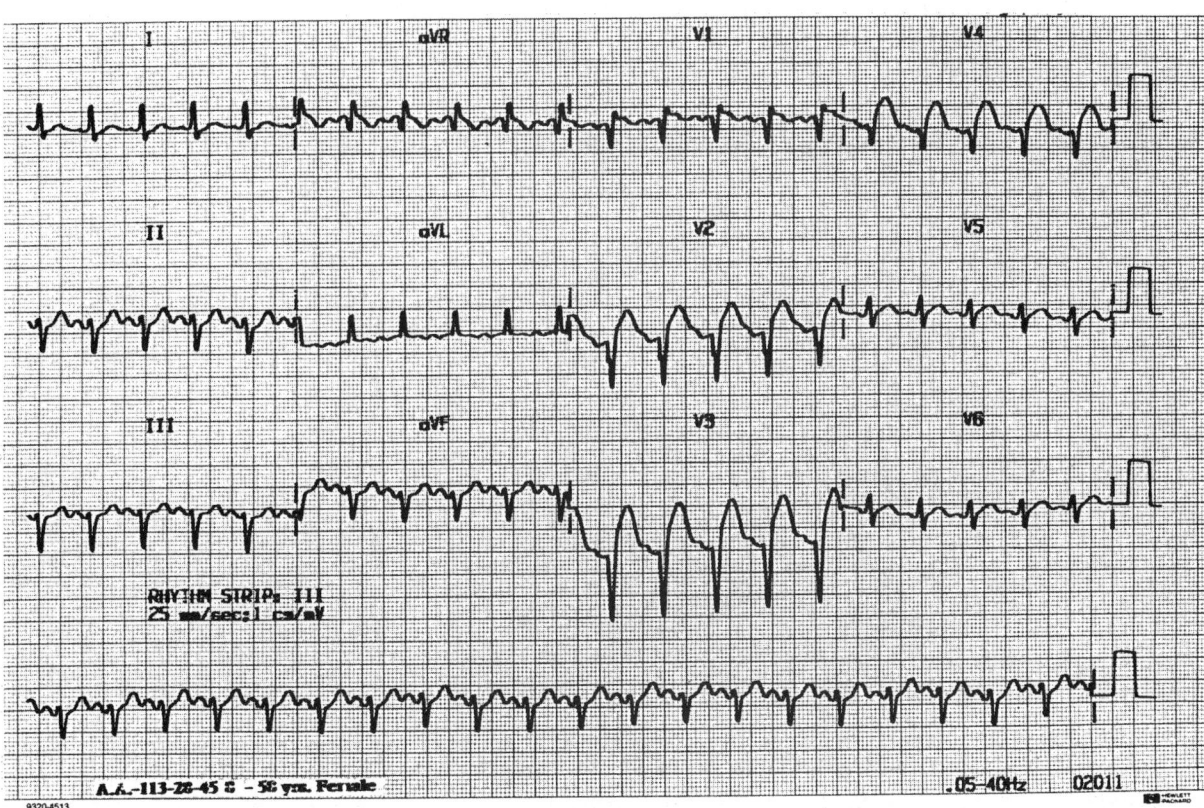

TRACING 34–19. Example of an acute anterior wall myocardial infarction. ST segment elevated in V₁ through V₄. Very poor R wave progression. Tachycardia.

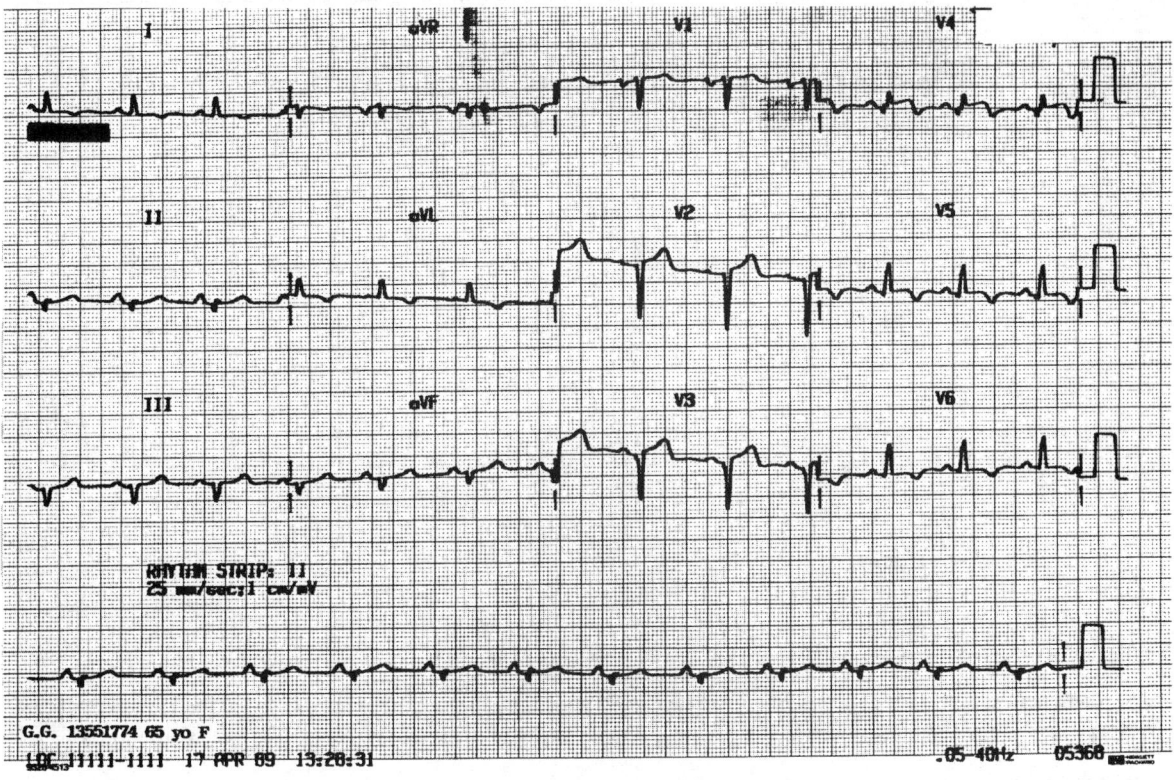

TRACING 34–20. Example of subacute anterior wall myocardial infarction. Negative T waves in lead I and in V₄ through V₆. Poor R wave progression in the precordial leads. Residual ST segment elevation in V₁ through V₄.

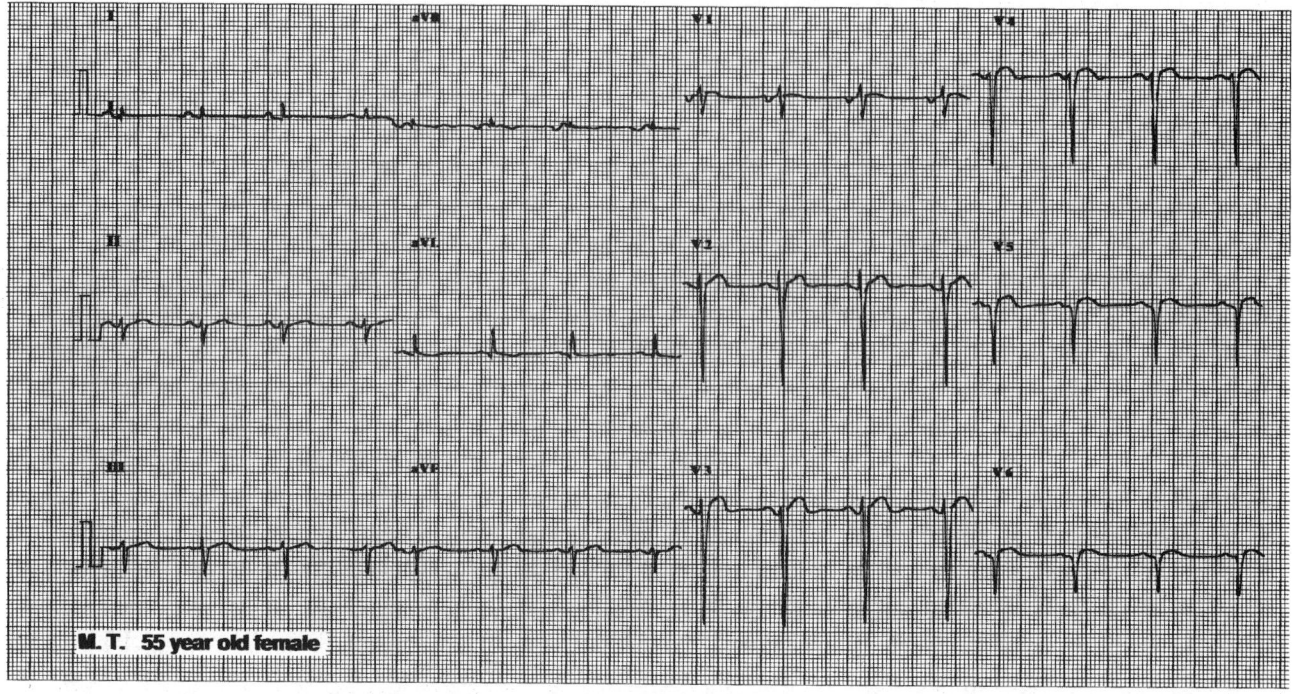

TRACING 34–21. Example of an anterolateral myocardial infarction. Poor R wave progression in the precordial leads. Deep Q waves with a QS pattern in V_5 and V_6. Slight ST segment elevation in precordial leads.

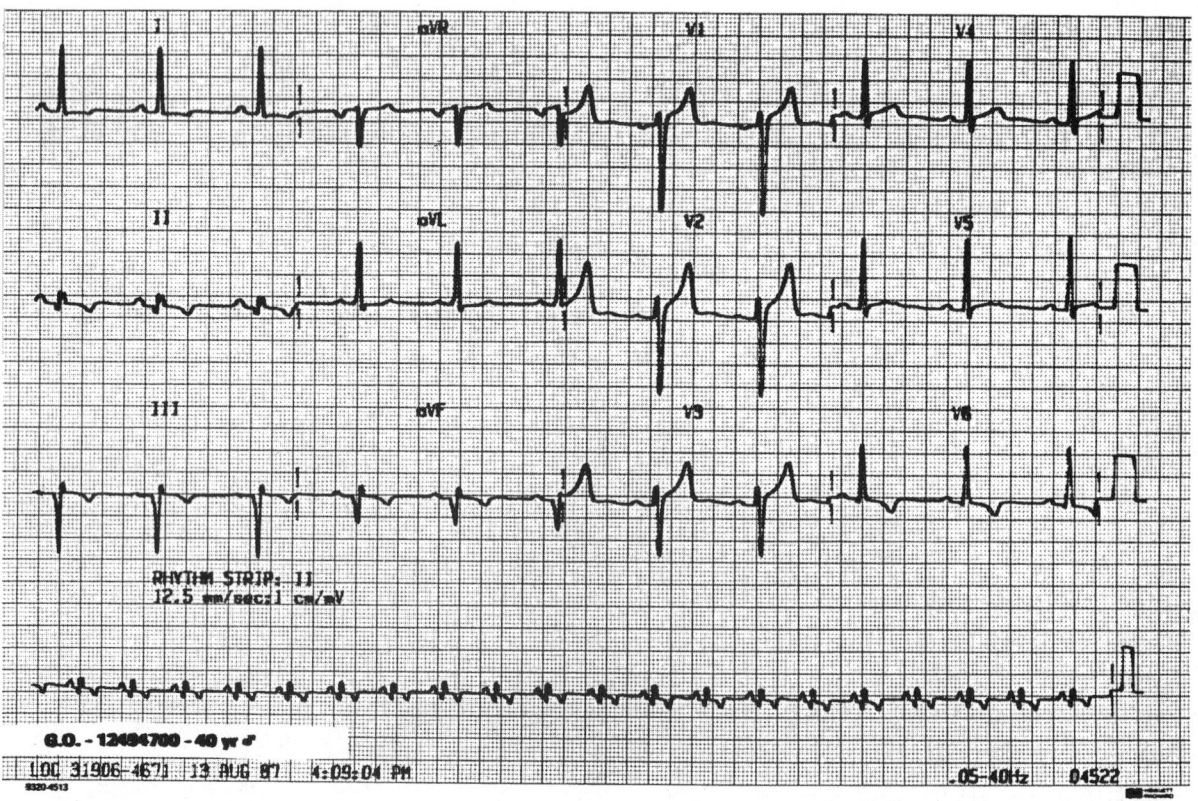

TRACING 34–22. Example of a subacute inferior wall myocardial infarction. Deep Q waves in II, III, and aVF. Negative T waves in II, III, and aVF. T wave in I is slightly negative. Negative T wave in V_6. Despite its appearance, the rhythm strip does not show a tachycardia because it was recorded at 12.5 mm/sec.

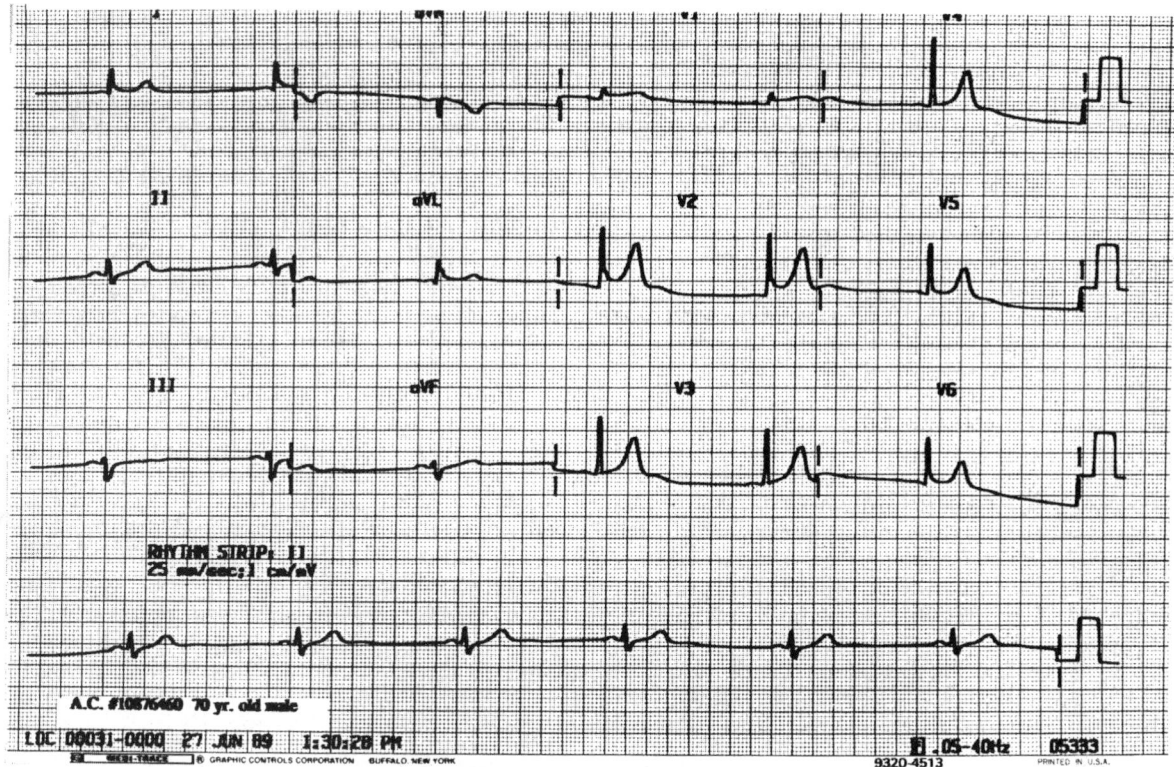

TRACING 34–23. Example of an old posterior wall myocardial infarction. Prominent R waves in all V leads. The slightly elevated ST segment in V₁ through V₄ may be early repolarization (unrelated to myocardial infarction).

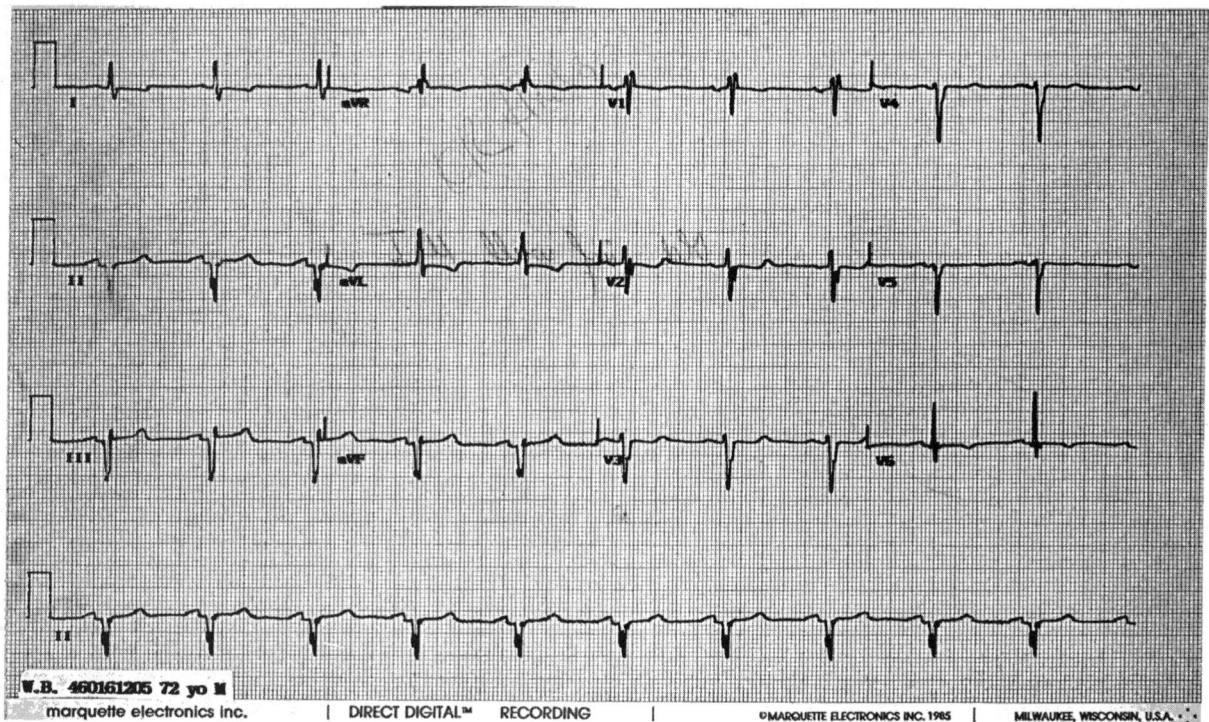

TRACING 34–24. Example of an old inferior wall myocardial infarction. Deep Q waves in II, III, and aVF. There is evidence of a conduction defect (RR′ pattern on V₁ and notched QRS wave in practically all leads), probably resulting from a right bundle-branch block caused by the infarction.

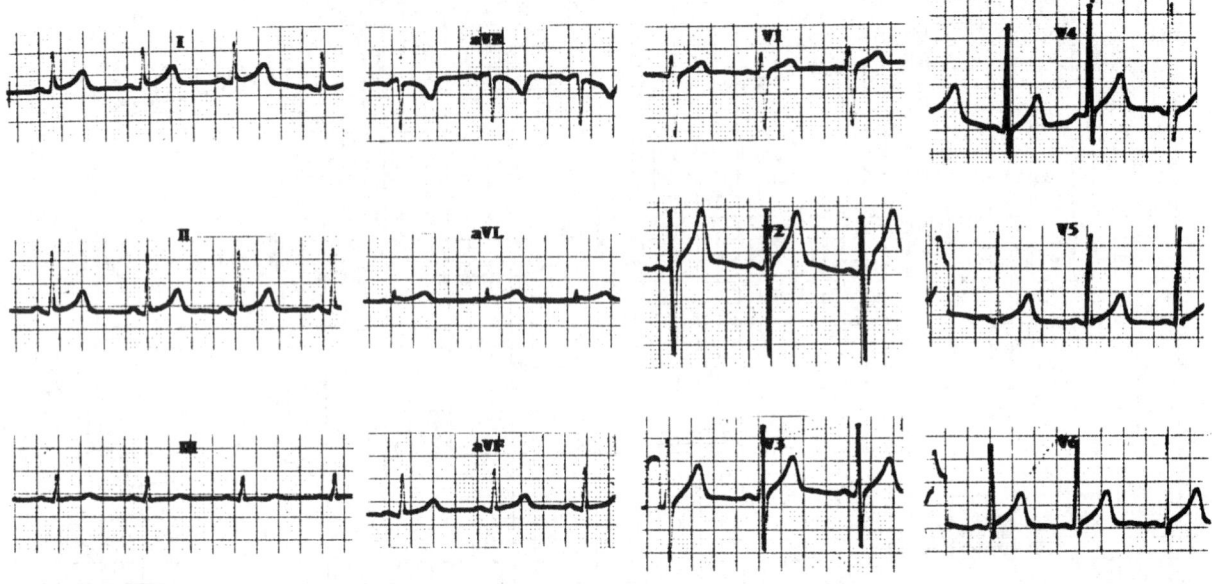

B.C. - 6787983 - 40 yrs. man

TRACING 34–25. Example of acute pericarditis. Small ST segment elevation in all leads except aVR (where ST segment is slightly depressed) and III (where ST segment is isoelectric).

Pericarditis

As a result of the inflammation of the pericardial sac, there is a small current of injury in the subepicardial area that is oriented toward the front. This current causes an ST segment displacement with an axis that points downward and forward (i.e., toward the anterior wall of the ventricles).

Criteria for Diagnosis

1. Displacement of ST segment of 2 mm (0.2 mV) or less.
2. Axis of ST segment almost in the same direction as the QRS axis in the frontal plane (ST segment elevated in leads where QRS wave is positive).
3. Axis of ST segment anterior in the horizontal plane (ST segment elevated in anterior V leads).
4. Patient age often younger than in cases of MI.
5. Evolution:
   a. ST segment displacement disappears within 1 to 2 weeks from onset of illness.
   b. Usually there is no evidence of ischemia (strain).
   c. There is no dead zone (Q waves).

Example

Tracing 34–25 shows an acute pericarditis.

Early Repolarization

In some healthy persons, there may be a difference in the sequence of repolarization between the subepicardial and subendocardial areas. As a result, there is an ST segment displacement that apparently does not have any clinical significance.

Criteria for Diagnosis

1. Small elevation of ST segment of less than 2 mm (0.2 mV)
2. Axis of ST segment in almost the same direction as QRS wave in frontal plane (ST segment elevated in the leads where QRS wave is positive).
3. ST segment elevated in anterior V leads (V_1 and V_2).
4. Most often observed in young persons with a slow heart rate.
5. No clinical manifestations of pericarditis.

Example

Tracing 34–26 shows an early repolarization syndrome.

Prinzmetal Syndrome

This syndrome consists of brief periods of anginal chest pain at rest as a result of spasm of the epicardial coronary arteries. It produces a transient ST elevation that is a manifestation of an injury current in the subepicardial region.

The ST segment changes and pain usually are not detected during exercise. Most of the recorded ST segment changes are obtained with a Holter monitor.

Criteria for Diagnosis

1. Displacement of ST segment of variable magnitude (usually small, but sometimes large).

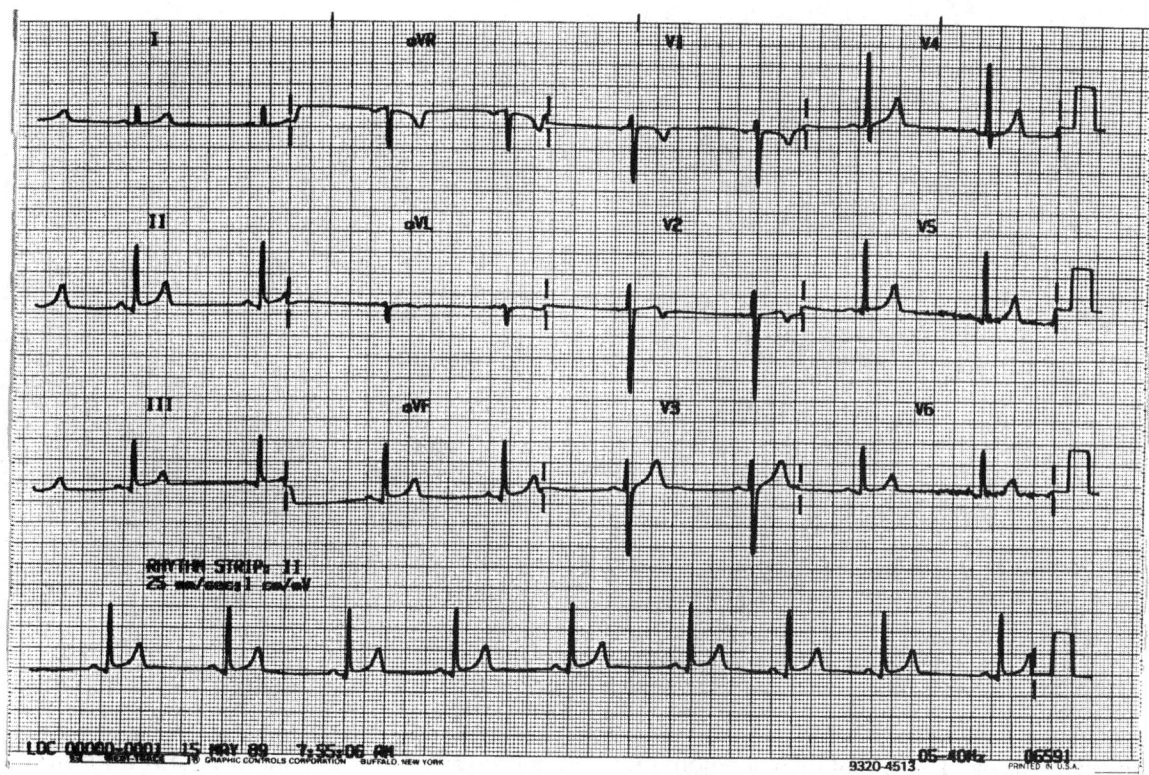

TRACING 34–26. Example of early repolarization syndrome. Notice significant ST segment elevation in all leads that have a positive QRS wave.

2.   Axis of ST segment almost in the same direction of the QRS vector in the frontal plane (ST segment elevated in leads where QRS wave is positive).

3.   Axis of ST segment anterior in the horizontal plane (ST segment elevated in anterior leads).

4.   Usually observed in young or middle-age women.

5.   No clinical manifestations of pericarditis. Brief duration of pain that occurs at rest.

Example

Tracing 34–27 shows a Prinzmetal syndrome.

Ventricular Aneurysm

In cases of a post-MI ventricular aneurysm of the anterior or anteroseptal wall, there is an ST segment displacement that is produced by a difference in the speed of repolarization at the subendocardial and subepicardial areas of the anterior wall. It is not due to an injury potential.

Criteria for Diagnosis

1.   Very small or nonexistent ST segment displacement in the frontal plane.

2.   Axis of ST segment anterior and prominent, 2 mm (0.2 mV) or more in the horizontal plane (ST segment is elevated in anterior leads).

3.   Evidence of dead zone effect in anterior wall (very poor R progression or QS pattern in V_1 through V_4 leads).

4.   History of anterior wall MI.

Example

Tracing 34–28 shows an anterior wall ventricular aneurysm.

Ischemia of Exercise

During exercise, patients with coronary artery disease may develop acute insufficiency of coronary blood flow (ischemia), and this is reflected in a significant ST segment displacement. The mechanism for this displacement may be a difference in the sequence of repolarization between the subendocardial and the subepicardial area. The diagram in Figure 34–25 shows the "ischemic" and "nonis-

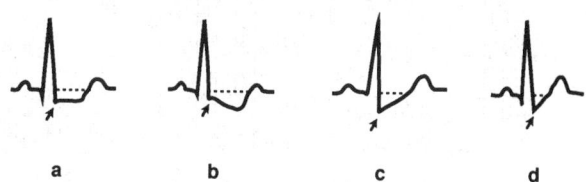

a   b   c   d

FIGURE 34–25. Ischemic and nonischemic changes during exercise.

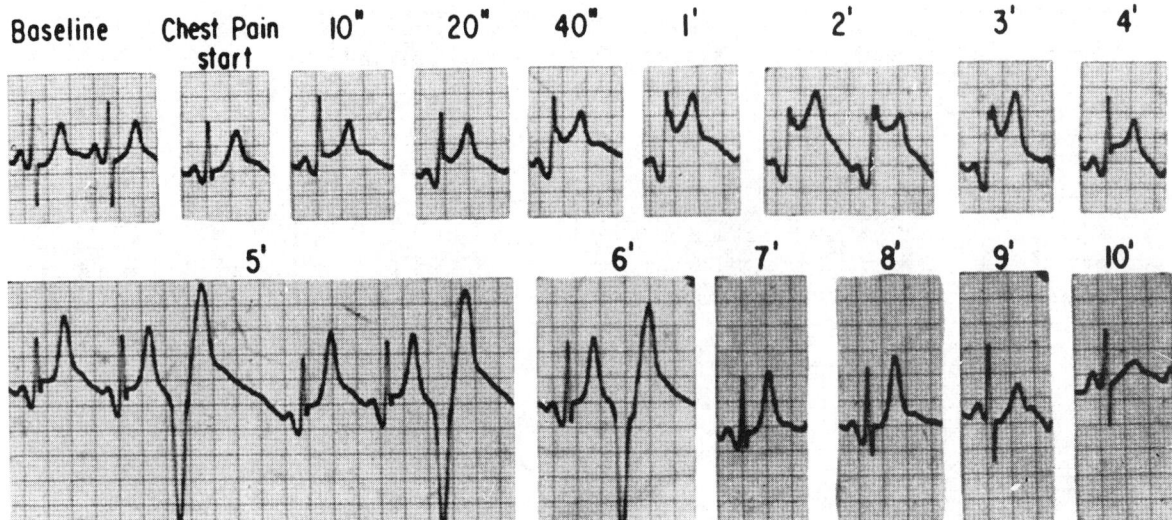

TRACING 34–27. Example of Prinzmetal angina. Sequential tracings of 1 lead of the electrocardiogram on a patient developing Prinzmetal angina. Slight ST elevation occurred when chest pain started and it became more and more pronounced in the subsequent 3 minutes. It gradually subsided after administration of NTG. There was angiographic correlation between the ST elevation and spasm of the coronary artery which re-opened after NTG. (Courtesy of Dr. A. Raizner, Baylor College of Medicine.)

chemic" patterns of ST segment displacement during exercise. Figure 34–25a and b show the ST segment changes suggesting significant ischemia. The ST segment displacement must be of at least 0.08 second duration and is either horizontal or downsloping. Figure 34–25c and d show changes considered to be indicative of nonischemia. The ST segment displacement is of brief duration and upsloping.

The presence of an ST segment ischemic pattern in an ECG obtained at rest suggests the existence of subendocardial ischemia. LVH or LBBB may cause an ST segment displacement not due to ischemia.

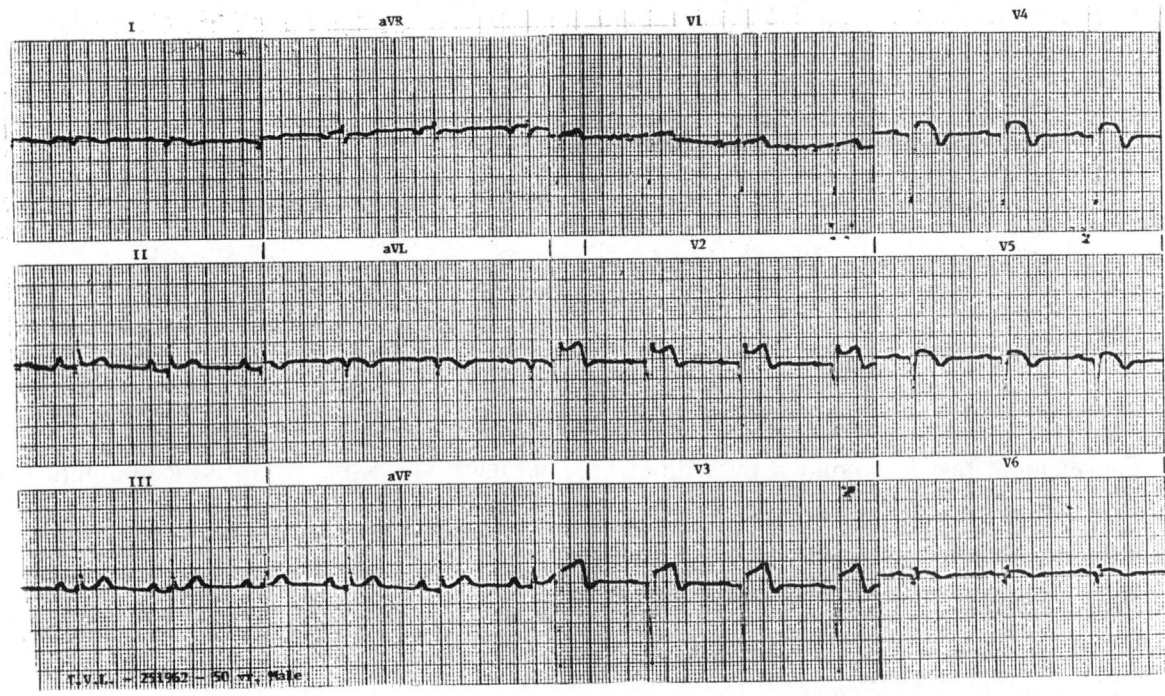

TRACING 34–28. Example of anterior wall ventricular aneurysm. Elevated ST segment in V_1 through V_5. Changes in early depolarization forces (Q waves) in leads II, III, and aVF as well as in precordial leads. History of acute anteroseptal myocardial infarction 5 months earlier. (Courtesy of Dr. H. Starke, Baylor College of Medicine.)

Criteria for Diagnosis

1. Displacement of ST segment of 2 mm (0.2 mV) or more lasting 0.08 second or longer.

2. Axis of ST segment in opposite direction of the QRS axis in the frontal plane (ST segment depressed in the leads where QRS wave is positive).

3. Axis of ST segment in opposite direction of QRS wave in the horizontal plane (ST segment depressed in V_4 through V_6).

Digitalis

Digitalis usually speeds up the repolarization process (short Q-T interval), but the effect is slightly different in the subepicardial and subendocardial areas. The difference accounts for the ST segment displacement.

Criteria for Diagnosis

1. Small ST segment depression, usually 2 mm (0.2 mV) or less, with downsloping and coving in leads with a positive QRS wave.

2. Q-T interval shorter than normal.

3. History of digitalis treatment.

Example

Tracing 34–29 shows a digitalis effect.

Left Ventricular Hypertrophy

The ST segment displacement may be small in the frontal plane but quite prominent in V leads.

It is caused by differences in the repolarization process between the subendocardial and subepicardial areas. The ST segment displacement is in the same direction as the negative T wave.

Example

Tracing 34–7 shows a left ventricular hypertrophy.

Left Bundle-Branch Block

The ST segment displacement is also due to differences in the repolarization process between the subendocardial and subepicardial areas. It has the same direction as the negative T waves.

Example

Tracing 34–10 shows a left bundle-branch block.

DEXTROCARDIA AND REVERSED LEADS

Dextrocardia

In cases of dextrocardia (or situs inversus), the ECG is a mirror image of the normal ECG. Persons with dextrocardia who develop cardiac abnormalities (e.g., ventricular hypertrophy, bundle-branch block) have ECG abnormalities that are also the

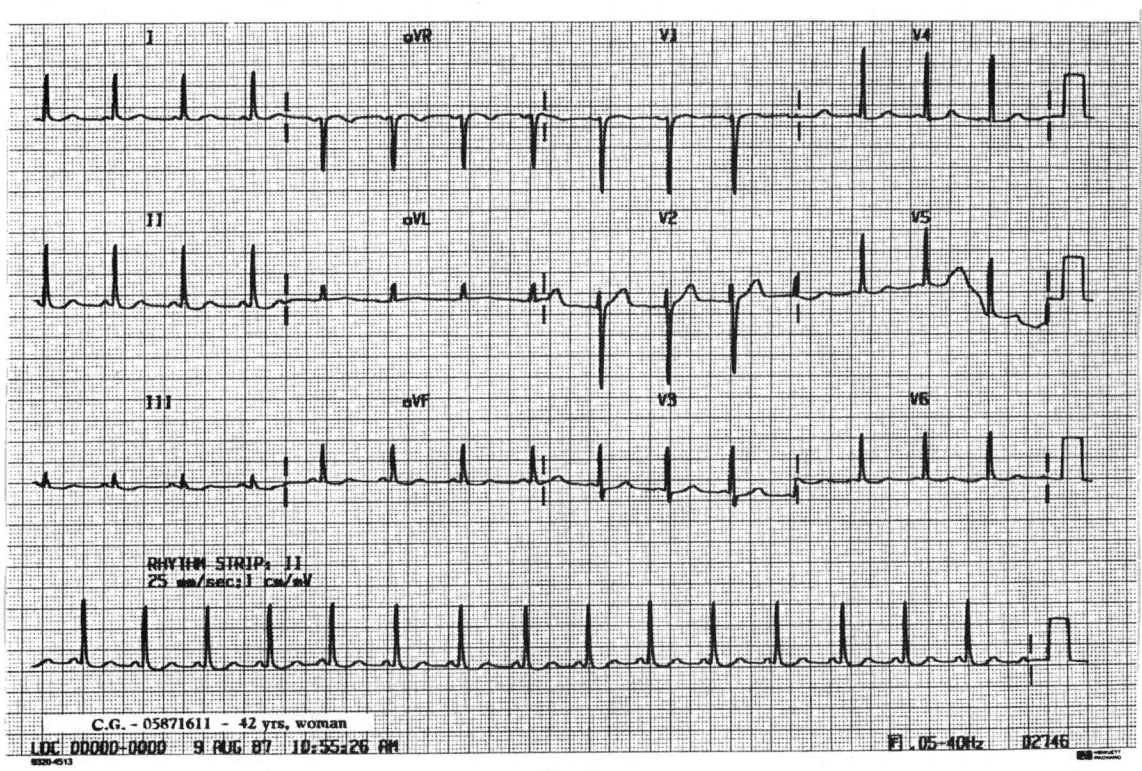

TRACING 34–29. Example of digitalis effect. Small and coved ST segment depression in most leads except aVR.

mirror image of those affecting persons whose heart is in the normal location. The physical examination and chest radiograph reveal placement of the heart in the right hemithorax.

Criteria for Diagnosis

FRONTAL PLANE

1. RAD.
2. Axis of T wave within 60 degrees from QRS wave and usually separated in a clockwise direction (negative T wave in aVL) from the axis of QRS wave.

HORIZONTAL PLANE

1. Axis of QRS wave posterior and to the left (negative QRS wave in V leads).
2. Axis of T wave anterior and to the left (usually negative T wave in V leads).

Example

Tracing 34–30 shows dextrocardia.

Reversed Leads

On occasion, the electrodes for the recording of the standard leads are inadvertently misplaced. If

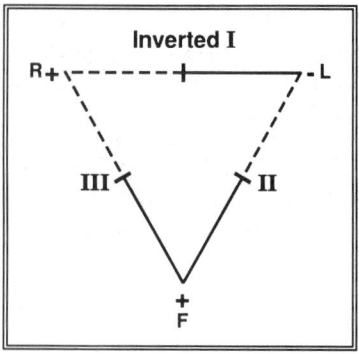

FIGURE 34–26. Changes in the Einthoven triangle produced by reversed placement of the arm electrodes.

the electrode of the left foot is placed on the right, or vice versa, there are no noticeable ECG changes because either electrode is in the lower vertex of the Einthoven triangle. In contrast, if the electrodes of the right and left arm are reversed, then lead I is reversed from its normal disposition, and similar changes occur in leads II and III, aVR, and aVL (Fig. 34–26). Seldom, if ever, there is a simultaneous misplacement of the precordial leads.

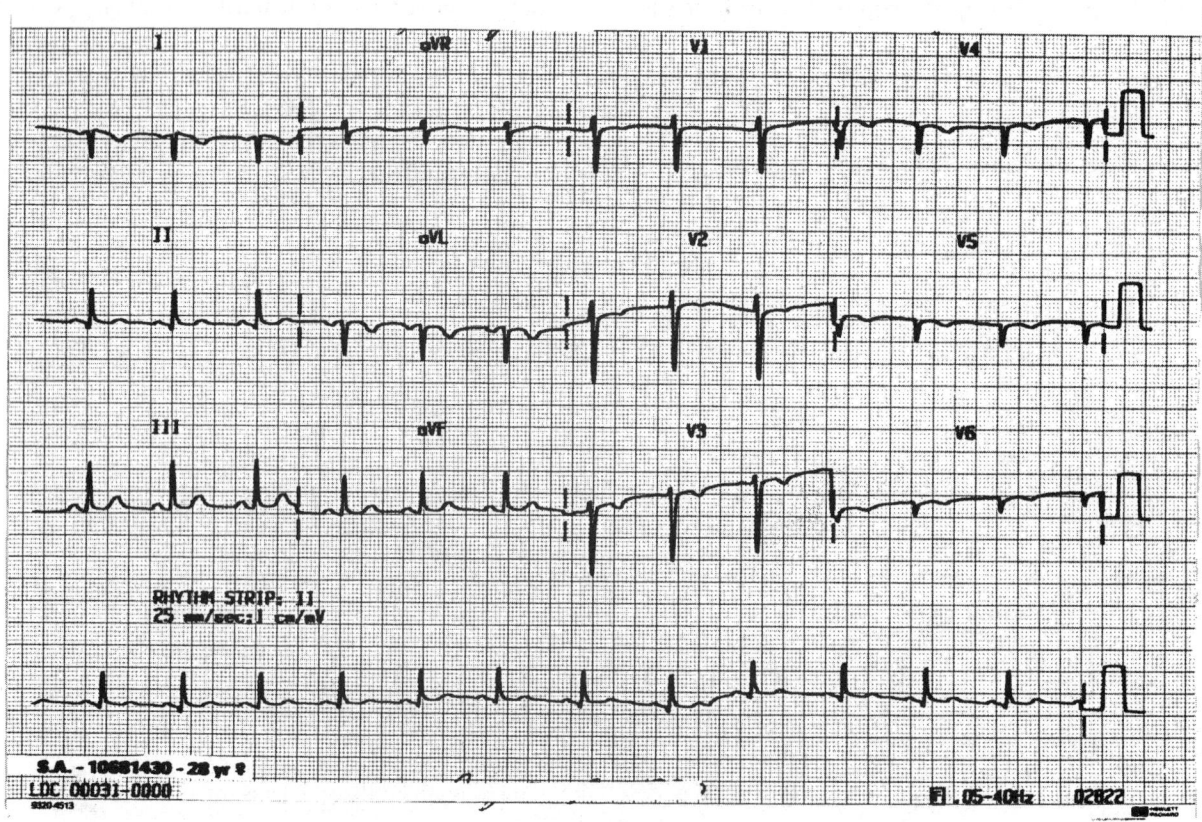

TRACING 34–30. Example of dextrocardia. Negative QRS wave on lead I and negative P, QRS, and T waves on leads I and aVL. Isoelectric aVR. Negative QRS and T waves in all the precordial leads.

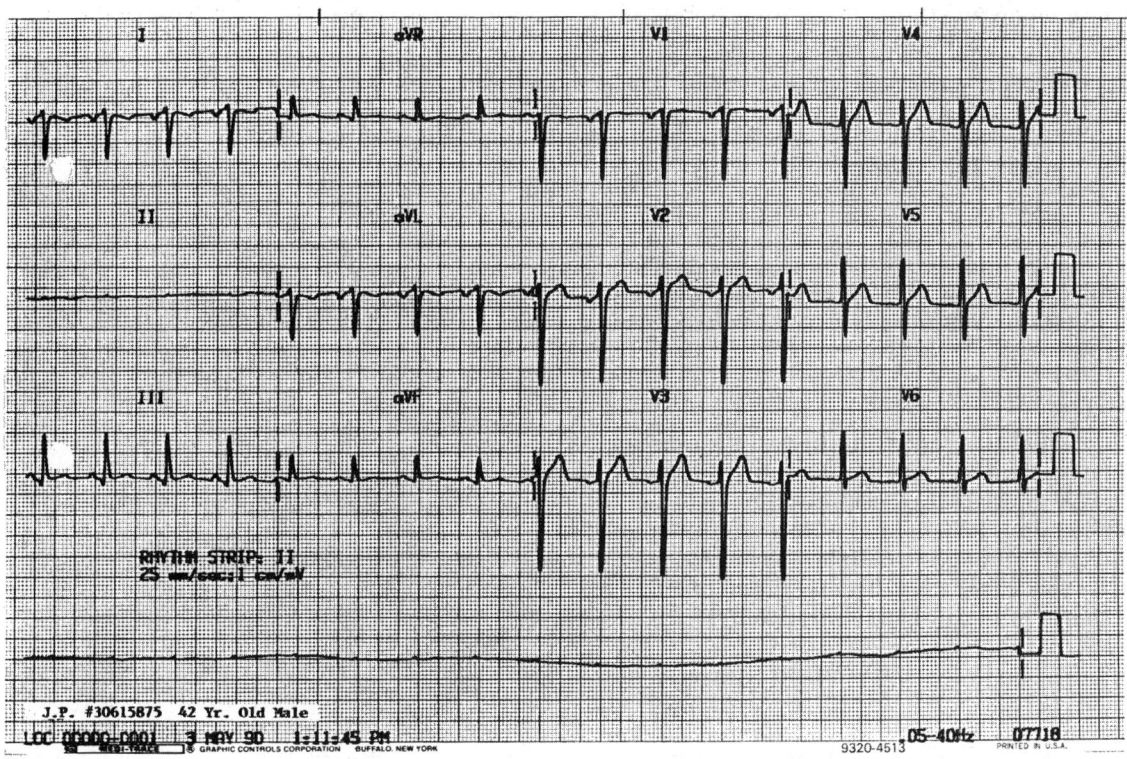

TRACING 34–31. Example of a tracing obtained with reversed leads. Lead I is a mirror image of a normal lead I. Lead II is in reality lead III, and lead III is lead II. Lead aVR is aVL and vice versa. Note that the precordial leads show a normal pattern for the QRS and T waves, although the transitional lead for the QRS wave is V₅ (more to the left than normal).

Thus, the coordinate systems for the frontal and the horizontal planes are not compatible. The physical examination and chest radiograph show the normal location of the heart.

Criteria for Diagnosis

FRONTAL PLANE

1. Right axis deviation in the frontal plane (negative QRS wave in lead I and aVR looks like the normal aVL).

2. Axis of T wave also deviated to the right and usually within 60 degrees from QRS wave.

HORIZONTAL PLANE

1. Axis of QRS wave posterior and to the left in the horizontal plane, thus becoming incompatible with the measurements in the frontal plane (QRS waves in V leads follow the normal pattern).

2. Axis of T wave to the left and to the front in the horizontal plane, thus becoming incompatible with measurements in the frontal plane (T waves in V leads follow the normal pattern).

Example

Tracing 34–31 shows reversed leads.

SCALAR VALUES OF ECG

By scalar values, it is meant the measurements of time intervals between ECG events as well as the measurements of voltages of P, QRS, and T waves in various leads. The time intervals shown in Figure 34–27 may convey very useful information. The usual paper speed is 2.5 cm/sec, so the

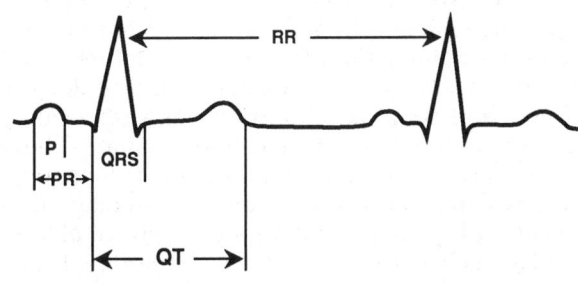

P:	Atrial depolarization time
PR:	Atrial depolarization + AV conduction time
QRS:	Ventricular depolarization time
QT:	Electrical systole time
RR–QT:	Electrical diastole time
RR:	Cardiac cycle time

FIGURE 34–27. The standard time intervals of the ECG in the cardiac cycle.

interval between two thin vertical lines is 0.04 second. The interval between two heavy vertical lines is 0.20 second.

Normal Values for Adults

P Wave

The P wave value is 0.08 second. It is prolonged in P-mitrale and in diffuse atrial damage and shorter in children. It usually is not affected by the heart rate.

P-R Interval

This interval is affected by heart rate and age, so that a sustained increase in rate produces a shorter P-R interval. The upper limit of normal at a rate of 60/min is 0.20 second. Causes of prolonged P-R interval include: (1) first-degree AV block caused by coronary artery disease, rheumatic fever, or diphtheria (infrequent in United States); (2) digitalis; and (3) increased vagal tone. Causes of short P-R interval include: (1) Wolff-Parkinson-White syndrome; (2) other pre-excitation syndromes, especially Lown-Ganong-Levine syndrome; (3) wandering pacemaker; (4) nodal rhythm; and (5) premature atrial beats or contractions.

QRS Interval

This interval is 0.08 second. It is prolonged in bundle-branch block, shorter in children, and usually not affected by the heart rate.

Q-T Interval

This interval also is affected by the heart rate. There are several regression equations to predict the normal value of the Q-T interval for a given heart rate. A commonly used equation is:

$$QT = \sqrt{R - R} - R \pm 0.04 \text{ seconds}$$

At 60 beats/min, the upper limit of normal for the Q-T interval is 0.40 second in men and 0.44 second in women. It is shorter than predicted in hypercalcemia and hyperkalemia and in the early stages of digitalization. It is longer than predicted in hypocalcemia and hypokalemia and under the influence of some psychotropic drugs (especially tricyclic antidepressants and thioridazine). There are two rare congenital syndromes of prolonged Q-T interval that may occur in families and may cause episodes of syncope with a special pattern of ventricular tachycardia (*torsades de pointes*) and sometimes death. The congenital Jervell-Lange-Nielsen syndrome is associated with deafness while the Romano-Ward syndrome is not.

R-R Interval

This interval measures the length of the cardiac cycle and is inversely proportional to the heart rate. If the interval measures one division, or 0.20 sec-

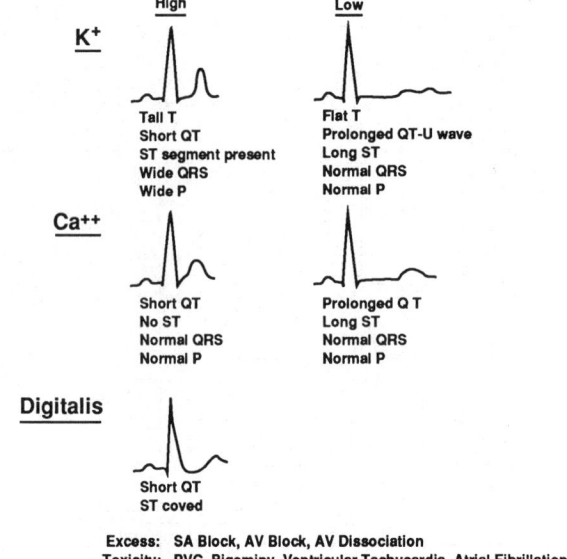

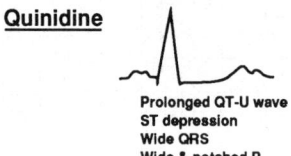

FIGURE 34–28. Typical patterns of ECG changes caused by electrolyte disturbances and drugs. PVC, premature ventricular contraction.

ond, the heart rate is 300 beats/min. If it measures three divisions, or 0.60 second, the rate is 100 beats/min. If it measures six divisions, or 1.20 seconds, the rate is 50 beats/min.

ELECTROLYTE AND DRUG EFFECTS

The typical changes brought about by electrolyte disturbances or by drugs are shown in Figure 34–28.

PRE-EXCITATION SYNDROMES (SHORT P-R INTERVAL)

Wolff-Parkinson-White Syndrome

In Wolff-Parkinson-White (WPW) syndrome, the atrial impulses bypass the AV node and the ventricular excitation occurs via the Kent bundle. The genesis of WPW syndrome and the intervals that should be assessed for its diagnosis are shown in Figure 34–29.

Criteria for Diagnosis

1. Short P-R interval.
2. Normal P wave.

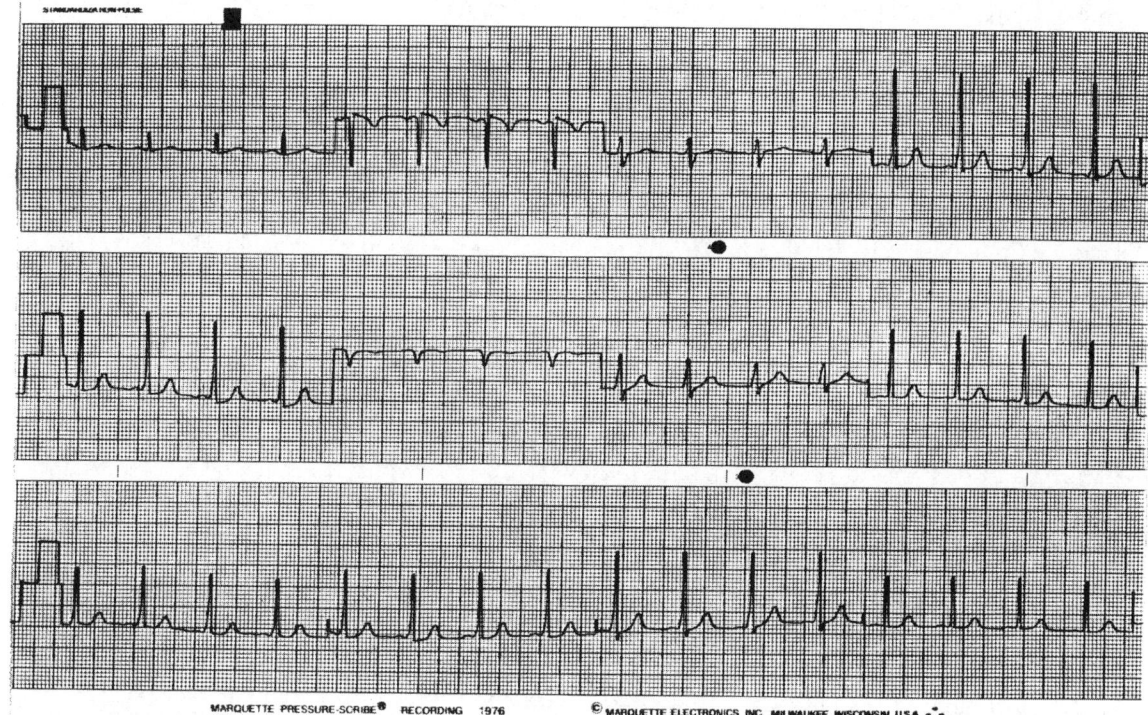

TRACING 34–32. Example of Wolff-Parkinson-White syndrome, type A. The Δ wave is recognized clearly in leads II, III, aVF, and V₁ through V₄.

3. Delta (Δ) wave.
4. Prolonged QRS wave.
5. Prolonged Q-T interval (there may be an inverted T wave).

There are two types of WPW syndrome. In *type A*, the Δ wave is anterior (i.e., there is a slurred R wave in V₁). In *type B*, the Δ wave is posterior (i.e., there is a slurred Q wave in V₁). Patients with WPW syndrome may have episodes of supraventricular tachycardia brought about by fast re-entry of impulses into the atria.

Examples

Tracing 34–32 shows WPW syndrome, type A. Tracing 34–33 shows WPW syndrome, type B.

Lown-Ganong-Levine or Short P-R Interval Syndrome

In Lown-Ganong-Levine (LGL) syndrome, the atrial impulses bypass the AV node and the ventricular excitation occurs via the James bundle. The genesis of LGL syndrome and the intervals that

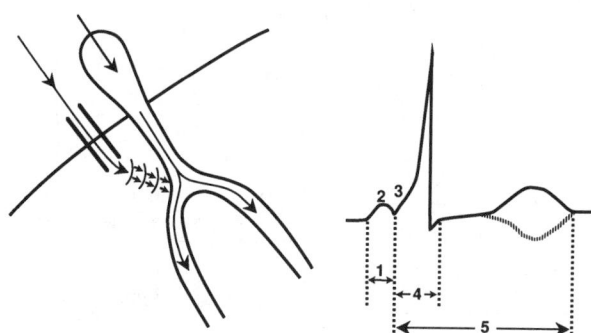

FIGURE 34–29. Transmission of electromotive forces in Wolff-Parkinson-White syndrome: 1, short P-R interval; 2, normal P wave; 3, Δ wave; 4, prolonged QRS wave; 5, prolonged Q-T interval (there may be an inverted T wave).

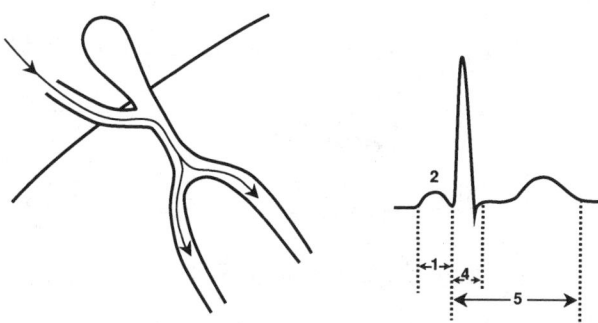

FIGURE 34–30. Transmission of electromotive forces in Lown-Ganong-Levine (short P-R) syndrome: 1, short P-R interval; 2, normal P wave; 3, no Δ wave; 4, normal QRS wave; 5, normal Q-T interval.

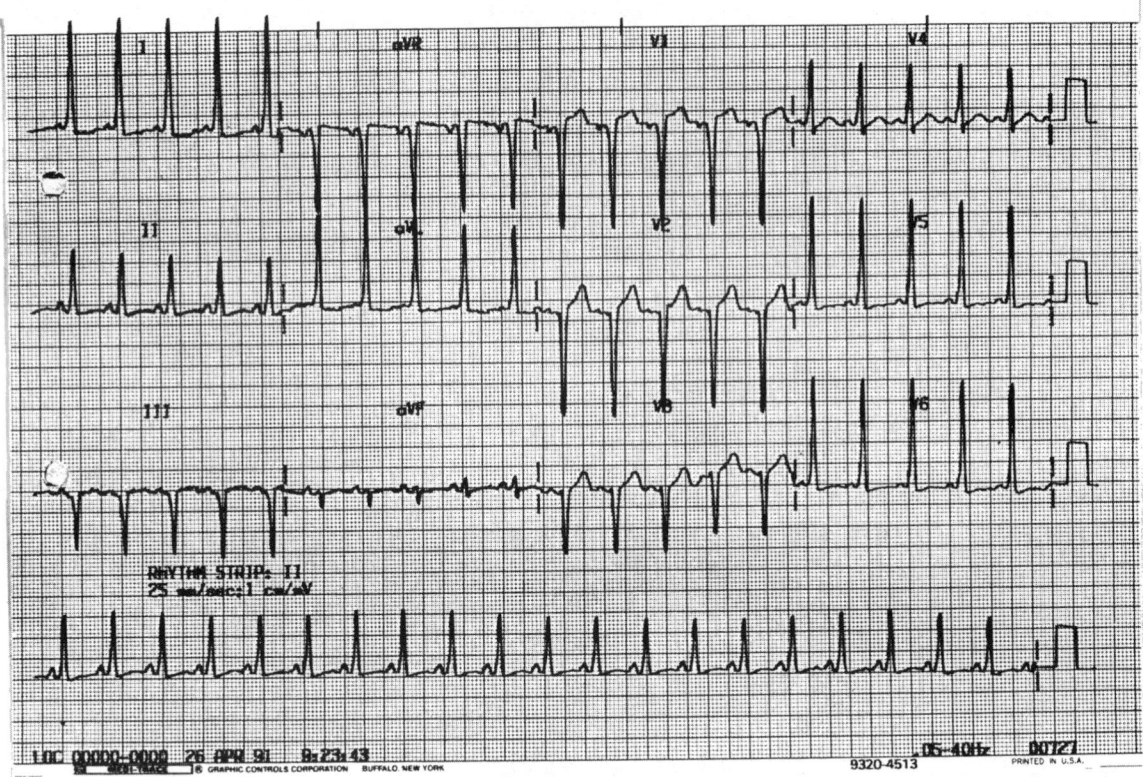

TRACING 34–33. Example of Wolff-Parkinson-White syndrome, type B. The tracing also shows LVH. Note the tachycardia, which may be due to a re-entry phenomenon.

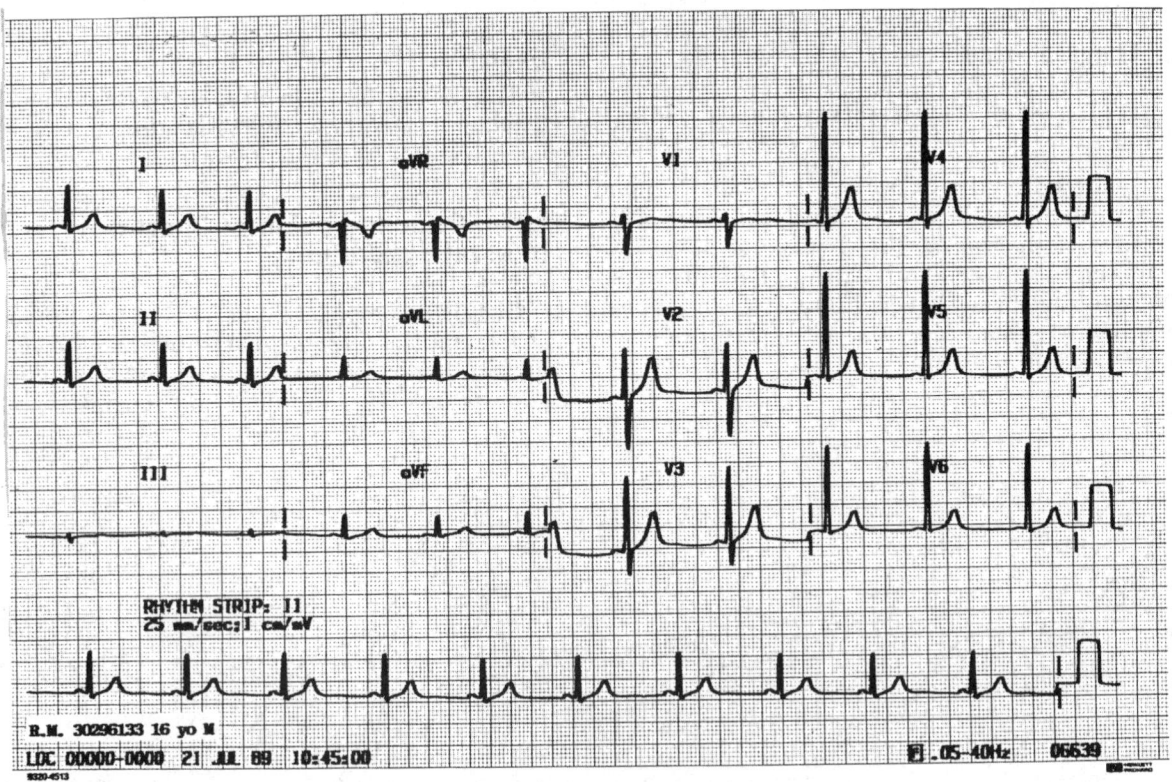

TRACING 34–34. Example of Lown-Ganong-Levine syndrome (short P-R interval syndrome). Note the end of the P wave coinciding with the beginning of the QRS wave. There is no Δ wave.

should be assessed for its diagnosis are shown in Figure 34–30.

The original description of this syndrome indicated the occurrence of episodes of supraventricular tachycardia. Subsequently, the diagnosis of LGL syndrome has been made on the basis of the above criteria regardless of supraventricular tachycardia. The World Health Organization recommends the term *short P-R interval syndrome* rather than LGL syndrome.

Criteria for Diagnosis

1. Short P-R interval.
2. Normal P wave.
3. No Δ wave.
4. Normal QRS wave.
5. Normal Q-T interval.

Example

Tracing 34–34 shows a Lown-Ganong-Levine syndrome.

DISTURBANCES OF THE RHYTHM

Normally, the rhythm of cardiac activity is determined by the regular activation of the SA node, with rapid transmission of impulses to the atria and to the ventricles as described earlier. It is common, however, to detect abnormalities of the rhythm, which are referred to as dysrhythmias or arrhythmias. The section on Diagnosis and Treatment of Arrhythmias in Chapter 35 includes a discussion of the most common patterns of arrhythmia and their pathogenesis and treatment.

SUGGESTED READINGS

Beckwith JR: Grant's Clinical Electrocardiogram: The Spatial Vector Approach. New York, McGraw-Hill, 1970.

Chung EK: Electrocardiography: Practical Applications with Vector Principles. Norwalk, CT, Appleton and Lange, 1985.

Dubin D: Rapid Interpretation of the EKG's, 2nd edition. Tampa, FL, Cover Publishing Co, 1988.

Halhuber MJ, Gunther R, Ciresa M: ECG: An Introductory Course. Berlin, Springer-Verlag, 1979.

Hurst JW, Myerburg RJ: Introduction to Electrocardiography. New York, McGraw-Hill, 1973.

Marriott HJL: ECG. Baltimore, Williams & Wilkins, 1987.

Rosenbaum MB, Erlizari MV, Lazzari JO: The Hemiblocks. Tampa, FL, Tampa Tracings, 1970.

Sandóe E, Sigurd B: Arrhythmia: Diagnosis and Management, A Clinical Electrocardiographic Guide. St. Galen, Verlag für Fachmedien, 1984.

Scheidt S: Basic Electrocardiography. West Caldwell, NJ, Ciba-Geigy, 1986.

CHAPTER **35**

CARDIOVASCULAR DISEASE AND ARRHYTHMIAS

Cardiovascular Disease

STEVEN J. YAKUBOV and EDWARD T. BOPE

PHYSICAL EXAMINATION

Physical Appearance

The cardiovascular physical examination begins with evaluation of the physical appearance. This includes assessing the patient's clinical condition. Many clinical clues can be determined solely by examination of body habitus (long extremities with an arm span exceeding height suggesting Marfan's syndrome; extreme obesity and somnolence suggesting Pickwickian syndrome) or by noticing that the patient is short of breath at rest.

Examination of the head and face can reveal various congenital cardiac diseases associated with structural facial abnormalities. Down syndrome, which is associated with a prominent medial epicanthus and a large protruding tongue, often is accompanied by endocardial cushion defects and ventricular septal defects. Patients with Turner's syndrome characteristically have webbing of the neck and widely set eyes, as well as coarctations of the aorta and bicuspid aortic valves. Patients with Noonan's syndrome also have widely set eyes, webbing of the neck, a small chin, and low-set ears, as well as pulmonic stenosis.

Examination of the eyes may demonstrate exophthalmos, which is characteristic of hyperthyroidism. Arcus senilis is a light-colored ring around the iris associated with hypercholesterolemia in young adults. This finding, however, is normal in the elderly. Xanthalasma, lipid-filled plaques noted around the eyes, are associated with hypercholesterolemia. Blue sclera are associated with a number of connective tissue diseases, such as Marfan's syndrome, Ehlers-Danlos syndrome, and osteogenesis imperfecta. These also are associated with aortic dissection.

Vital Signs

Vital signs are extremely important. The pulse rate is determined best by palpating the radial pulse, noting its strength and regularity. Blood pressure is recorded with an appropriately sized sphygmomanometer. In patients with large or obese arms, the standard blood pressure cuff will overestimate arterial blood pressure; therefore, a leg cuff should be used on the arm. As the cuff is deflated, the first appearance of a clear tapping sound (phase I of Korotkoff sounds) is the systolic pressure. The disappearance of sounds (phase IV of Korotkoff sounds) is the diastolic pressure. An auscultatory gap occurs between phase I and phase II of Korotkoff sounds. This auscultatory gap is caused by a reduced velocity of blood flow to the brachial pulse, and may suggest aortic stenosis.

Phase II of Korotkoff sounds is the period during which the clear tapping sounds of phase I are replaced by soft rumblings. Phase III of Korotkoff sounds occurs as louder murmurs replace the soft rumbling of phase II. If this reappearance of sound is mistakenly interpreted as the systolic blood pressure, underestimation of the true systolic blood pressure occurs.

Blood pressure should be measured in both arms, and it is useful to measure blood pressure in both the supine and standing positions. Normally, there is a small, transient decrease in systolic arterial pressure of 5 to 15 mm Hg and a rise in diastolic pressure when the patient is in a standing position. Systolic blood pressure in the legs may be up to 20 mm Hg higher than in the arms, but diastolic blood pressure in the leg tends to be the same as in the arms.

Pulsus paradoxus is a fall in arterial pressure greater than 10 mm Hg during inspirations. This clinical condition is associated with pericardial tamponade, chronic obstructive pulmonary disease, pleural effusions, and asthma. *Pulsus alternans* is a condition in which every other heart beat has a higher systolic pressure. This is associated with end-stage left ventricular failure.

Jugular Venous Pulse

The internal jugular vein is more visible for examination than the external jugular vein. The venous pulses are best examined with light directed tangentially at the neck with the patient at a 45-degree angle. Normally, the height of the pulse wave is less than 4 cm above the sternal angle. The sternal angle is typically 5 cm above the right atrium; therefore, central venous pressure is normally less than 9 mm Hg. Typically, two waves are determined in the jugular venous pulse. The first is the *a* wave, which reflects atrial contraction and occurs before the carotid pulse. The *x descent* follows the *a* wave and occurs before the second heart sound. The *v* wave follows the second heart sound and is resultant of a rise in right atrial pressure as blood flows into the right atrium while the tricuspid valve is closed. The *v* wave is followed by the *y descent*. The *y* descent occurs as a result of a fall in right atrial pressure as the tricuspid valve opens. As jugular venous pressure rises, the *v* wave becomes higher and the *y* descent more prominent. This rise in jugular venous pressure occurs in right heart failure, pericardial diseases such as constrictive pericarditis and cardiac tamponade, and restrictive cardiomyopathies. This also can be seen in superior vena cava obstruction.

Carotid Pulse

Abnormalities of the carotid pulse occur in a number of disease states. *Pulsus tardus* or delayed systolic upstroke is typical of aortic stenosis. *Pulsus bisferiens* occurs when there are two systolic peaks. It is associated with aortic regurgitation or a combination of aortic stenosis and aortic regurgitation, as well as with hypertrophic obstructive cardiomyopathy.

Examination of the Heart

Typically, the apex demonstrates the point of maximal impulse. It is characteristically in the fifth left intercostal space at the mid-clavicular line. The normal precordial pulse is an outward systolic motion, as the left ventricular strikes the anterior chest wall, followed by retraction as blood is ejected from the left ventricular cavity. Left ventricular hypertrophy exaggerates this outward systolic motion. Aneurysms of the left ventricle produce prominent apical impulses.

Auscultation of the heart is typically the most important examination technique.

Heart Sounds

FIRST HEART SOUND. Classically, the first heart sound has been attributed to the closure of the mitral and tricuspid valves. The first heart sound is typically split, with the first component representing mitral closure and the second component representing tricuspid valve closure. These two components are separated by 0.02 second.

Clinical conditions that increase the intensity of the first heart sound include mitral stenosis, thyrotoxicosis, hypertension, and a short P-R interval. Conditions decreasing the intensity of the first heart sound include a prolonged P-R internal, aortic insufficiency, mitral insufficiency, and cases of mitral stenosis in which the valve is very rigid and calcified. The first heart sound varies in atrial fibrillation and complete heart block.

SECOND HEART SOUND. There are two components of the second heart sound. The first component represents closure of the aortic valve while the second represents closure of the pulmonic valve. The two components usually are fused with expiration and separated by 0.02 to 0.06 second with inspiration.

Wide splitting of the second heart sound with preservation of respiratory variation occurs with complete right bundle-branch block and premature ventricular beats arising from the left ventricle. This condition also can occur in patients with severe mitral regurgitation and pulmonic stenosis. Broad fixed splitting of the second heart sound occurs in atrial septal defect. Paradoxical splitting of the second heart sound occurs with left bundle-branch block and aortic stenosis. Congenital abnormalities of the heart that are associated with no splitting of the second heart sound include tetralogy of Fallot, pulmonary atresia, hypoplastic left heart syndrome, and truncus arteriosus.

In adults, the first component of the second heart sound is greater in intensity than the second component. Systemic hypertension results in a loud first component of the second heart sound. Pulmonary hypertension accelerates or intensifies the second component. The intensity of the second heart sound typically is reduced in patients with chronic obstructive pulmonary disease or pericardial effusion.

THIRD HEART SOUND. The third heart sound is a low-pitched sound occurring approximately 0.15 second after the second heart sound. It is due to rapid expansion and filling of the left or right ventricle in early diastole. The third heart sound may be normal in young patients, but it is termed a "gallop" when it is associated with pathologic conditions. Common clinical conditions causing a third heart sound are congestive heart failure with a dilated left ventricle, mitral insufficiency, anemia, and thyrotoxicosis. Any condition causing volume overload of the left ventricle, such as atrial septal defect, ventricular septal defect, aortic insufficiency, and patent ductus arteriosus, can cause third heart sounds. The third heart sound may be confused with the pericardial knock of constrictive pericarditis. A pericardial knock tends to have a higher frequency and occurs earlier (<0.12 second) after the second heart sound. The third heart sound also can be confused with the opening snap of mitral stenosis. The opening snap is a higher frequency sound that is also earlier (<0.12 second) than the third heart sound.

FOURTH HEART SOUND. The fourth heart sound is a low-frequency vibration that occurs during atrial contraction. This typically is apparent because of noncompliance of the left ventricle, secondary to left ventricular hypertrophy or ischemic heart disease. Any clinical condition causing left ventricular hypertrophy, such as systemic hypertension, aortic stenosis, or hypertrophic obstructive cardiomyopathy, often is associated with fourth heart sounds. This heart sound is determined best using the bell of the stethoscope at the apex.

When heart rates are very rapid, the presence of a third and fourth heart sound in combination, can merge to produce a "summation gallop".

MID-SYSTOLIC CLICKS AND OPENING SNAPS. Mitral valve prolapse is a common clinical condition causing a mid-systolic click and often is associated with a late systolic murmur. Multiple clicks also can occur. The clicks are associated with maximum prolapse of the mitral valve.

The opening snap is a high-frequency sound heard in early diastole with mitral or tricuspid stenosis. Severe mitral stenosis is associated with a very short interval between the second heart sound

and the opening snap. The opening snap is determined best at the mid-left sternal border and the apex when it is due to mitral stenosis.

Heart Murmurs

Murmurs are a vibration secondary to turbulence of blood flow. The intensity of a murmur is graded on a scale of 1 to 6. Grade 1 is the faintest murmur that can be heard with the stethoscope. A grade 3 murmur is extremely loud but with no associated thrill. Grades 4, 5, and 6 are associated with a palpable thrill. A grade 6 murmur is so loud that it can be heard without the use of a stethoscope and is associated with a thrill on palpitation of the heart. The intensity of a murmur is dependent on the volume of blood flowing across the sound-producing area, as well as the blood velocity and the distance from the sound-producing area to the stethoscope. The duration of heart murmurs depends on the duration of the pressure gradient across the sound-producing areas (see Fig. 35–1).

SYSTOLIC MURMURS. Systolic murmurs are either mid-systolic ejection murmurs or pansystolic, regurgitant murmurs. Mid-systolic crescendo–decrescendo ejection murmurs occur as blood is ejected into the aorta or into the pulmonary arteries. These murmurs begin after the first heart sound and end before the second heart sound. Holosystolic regurgitant murmurs occur secondary to the backward flow of blood across the mitral or tricuspid valve. Holosystolic murmurs also can be heard with ventricular septal defects. These murmurs begin with the first heart sound and cease at the second heart sound. The intensity and duration of pansystolic murmurs depend on

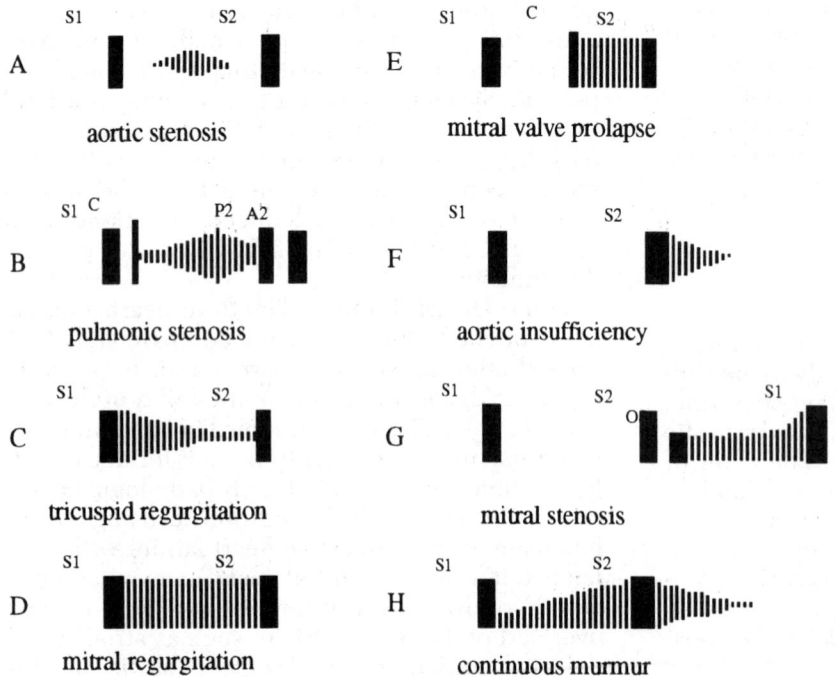

FIGURE 35–1. Diagrammatic representation of common cardiac murmurs.

the duration of the pressure difference across the orifice producing the murmur. These murmurs tend to be of higher frequency compared to systolic ejection murmurs, which are characterized as harsh murmurs. Tricuspid regurgitation producing a holosystolic murmur increases with inspiration.

Systolic ejection murmurs may be functional (not associated with clinical cardiac disease) or may be caused by aortic stenosis, mitral stenosis, hypertrophic obstructive cardiomyopathy, and states of high cardiac output (anemia, fever, exercise, thyrotoxicosis). Functional murmurs are probably aortic in origin and generally peak in early systole. Severe aortic stenosis or pulmonary stenosis produce murmurs that are prolonged and peak in mid to late systole. Longer duration murmurs secondary to aortic stenosis with late peaking tend to be associated with more severe disease.

Late systolic murmurs most commonly are associated with mitral valve prolapse and often are accompanied by a mid-systolic click.

DIASTOLIC MURMURS. Diastolic murmurs are secondary to regurgitation of the aortic or pulmonic valves or to obstruction of flow across the mitral or tricuspid valve.

Regurgitant murmurs across the aortic or pulmonic valve produce murmurs beginning very early in diastole, just after the second heart sound. These murmurs can begin with the second heart sound and are higher in frequency and decrescendo in nature. These murmurs are best heard with the diaphragm of the stethoscope. Aortic insufficiency most commonly is detected while the patient is sitting upright and leaning forward.

It is often difficult to differentiate the murmur caused by pulmonic regurgitation from that of aortic regurgitation. Accentuation of the murmur with deep inspiration favors pulmonic regurgitation. Diastolic murmurs occurring secondary to flow obstruction across the atrial ventricular valves tend to occur in mid-diastole. At this point, ventricular pressure has fallen below atrial pressure and the valve opens. This may be associated with an opening snap when the cause of the murmur is secondary to mitral stenosis (Fig. 35–2). This murmur tends to be low pitched and rumbling. There can be presystolic accentuation of the murmur that is secondary to atrial contraction before the first heart sound. Atrial fibrillation eliminates this presystolic accentuation. The duration of the murmur in mitral stenosis is very important. The longer the duration of the murmur, the more significant the obstruction tends to be. Mitral stenosis murmurs are heard best at the apex with the bell of the stethoscope and the patient in the left lateral decubitus position.

Murmurs secondary to tricuspid stenosis tend to be somewhat higher in frequency than that of mitral stenosis. This murmur typically is augmented with inspiration and is best heard at the left lower sternal border.

CONTINUOUS MURMURS. These murmurs begin in systole and extend into all or part of diastole. There must be a continuous pressure difference between two cardiac chambers for this type of murmur to exist. Typical causes of continuous murmurs include patent ductus arteriosus, rupture of the sinus of Valsalva, or systemic or pulmonic atrioventricular fistulas. Continuous murmurs also can be detected secondary to coarctation of the aorta.

DIAGNOSTIC PHYSIOLOGIC MANEUVERS. Numerous physiologic maneuvers can be employed to discriminate the causes of systolic or diastolic murmurs.

Isometric Exercise. Isometric exercise, such as fist clenching, results in an increased systemic blood pressure and heart rate, as well as an increase in cardiac output. Systolic murmurs secondary to aortic stenosis and hypertrophic cardiomyopathy tend to decrease during isometric exercise. Murmurs secondary to ventricular septal defects and mitral insufficiency tend to increase with this maneuver. Increasing cardiac output accentuates the murmur of mitral stenosis. Increasing systemic blood pressure increases the murmur of aortic insufficiency. The click and murmur of mitral valve prolapse are delayed by isometric exercise.

Postural Positions. Venous return is affected by rapid changes in posture. Arising from the lying position decreases venous return. Murmurs that

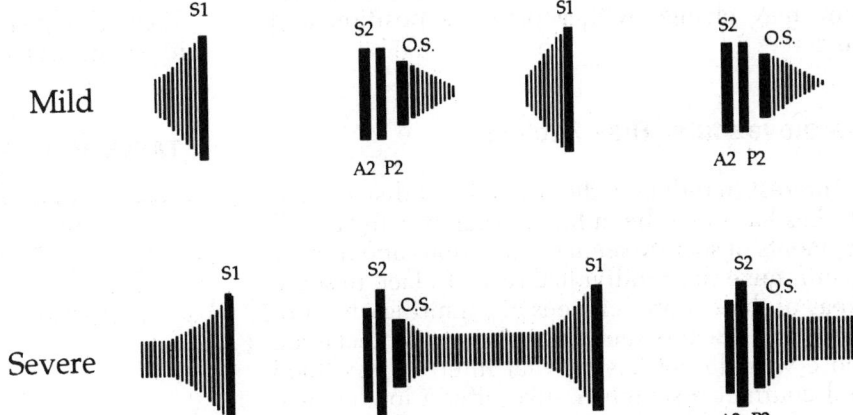

FIGURE 35–2. The murmur of mitral stenosis.

are accentuated by an increase in venous return include mitral and tricuspid regurgitation, functional systolic murmurs, ventricular septal defects, and aortic and pulmonic stenosis. The murmur of hypertrophic obstructive cardiomyopathy is diminished as preload is increased.

Respiration. Deep inspiration results in an enhanced right ventricular filling and decreased left ventricular filling. Generally, murmurs arising from the right side of the heart are enhanced with deep inspiration. Murmurs arising from the left side of the heart typically have very little change with deep inspiration. However, mitral valve prolapse is affected with deep inspiration by causing the click to occur earlier in systole and accentuating the heart murmur.

Valsalva Maneuver. The Valsalva maneuver is a multifaceted physiologic maneuver. It is secondary to forced expiration against a closed glottis. During the first phase of the Valsalva maneuver, intrathoracic pressure rises, with a concomitant increase in left ventricular output and blood pressure. During the second (strain) phase, the venous return is impaired, with reduced right ventricular filling and ultimately a reduction in left ventricular filling. This produces a decrease in left-sided cardiac output. During the second phase, only the murmur of hypertrophic cardiomyopathy is intensified. Any maneuver that reduces left ventricular volume will increase the murmur of hypertrophic obstructive cardiomyopathy. During the third phase of the Valsalva maneuver, which is secondary to release of the respiratory pressure, blood flow to the right side of the heart increases. Therefore, murmurs originating from the right side of the heart return to normal or may be accentuated. Murmurs of the left side of the heart typically recover their intensity later in this phase than those secondary to right-sided causes.

PERICARDIAL FRICTION RUBS. These rubs are described as grating or scratching sounds heard usually at the left sternal border. There may be up to three components to the pericardial friction rub. Often only one or two components can be heard, however, causing confusion with other cardiac murmurs. The murmurs may be inconstant and they may change with a patient's position and posture.

Cardiovascular Risk Factors

Interest in reducing the risk of heart disease and strokes has never been higher than it is today. All segments of society seem to be curious about ways to minimize their individual risks. In fact, in some areas of the country citizens are limiting environmental risk factors such as smoking to protect even those who do not have a vital interest. Fast food and gourmet restaurants alike offer a low cholesterol–low fat list of entrees. So, it is likely that we will see social changes that will benefit the population as a whole.

The great advances in cardiovascular technology often give patients a second chance to consider their lifestyle and decide if changes in their behavior and habits would be appropriate. It is no small job to help patients modify their lifestyle. Greater yield as well as reward could come from early intervention and prevention through education.

Family physicians have an unusual opportunity to implement an education program. We see patients of all ages, so there is the opportunity to teach good health habits at an early age and monitor for compliance and success. Because we care for the entire family, there is the opportunity to recognize familial risk factors and intervene. The ongoing doctor–family relationship allows special insights and possible interventions that other health care providers might not enjoy.

Some risk factors for coronary heart disease cannot be altered. Age and male sex are two known risk factors that cannot be changed. Family history of coronary heart disease is also somewhat fixed. Recent opinion is that family history has at least two effects. The first is the recognition that some of the changeable factors are common to family members. An example might be cigarette smoking, which could be common behavior within a family. Second, it is recognized that some families are more susceptible to the cardiovascular harm created by the behavioral risk factors. Together these reasons put some families at greater risk than others.

Risk Factor Modification

As stated previously, the family physician is extremely well positioned to intervene in risk factor modification. Table 35–1 divides the risk factors between those that are fixed and those that are changeable. While guidelines for children and adolescents seem less well defined, the American Heart Association (AHA) has issued specific screening protocols for adults (Fig. 35–3). Naturally, children should be advised to reduce risks by avoiding inactivity, preventing obesity, and not smoking.

Each changeable risk factor will be discussed with suggestions given for treatment. Enough can-

TABLE 35–1. RISK FACTORS FOR CORONARY HEART DISEASE

Fixed	Changeable
Male Sex	Cigarette smoking
Age	Diabetes mellitus
Family history	Hypertension
	Inactivity
	Lipid abnormalities
	Obesity
	Type A behavior

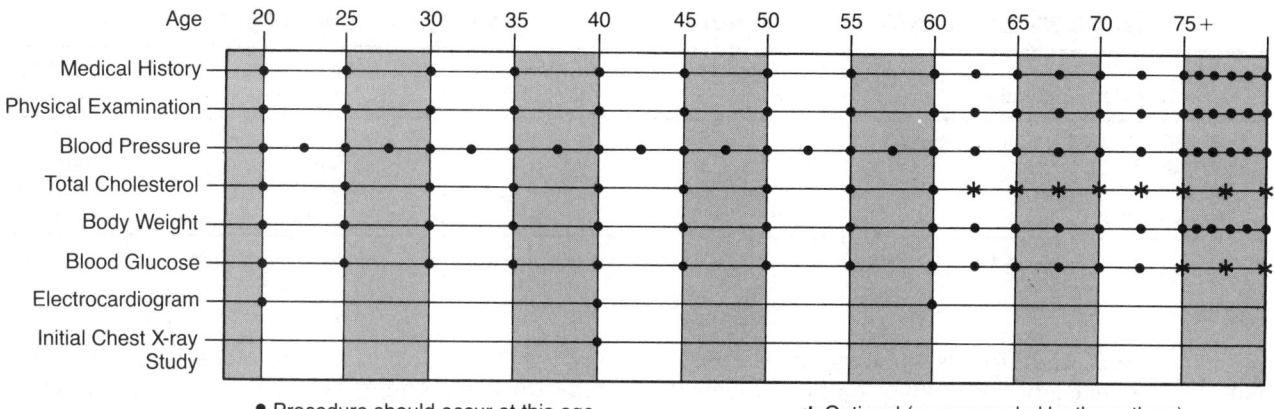

FIGURE 35–3. Periodic health examinations as recommended by the American Heart Association.

not be said for education of patients and the public about the risk factors and the success of modification of those risk factors.

CIGARETTE SMOKING. Since 1964, every report from the Surgeon General has pointed to cigarette smoking as a major contributor to cardiovascular death and a cause of lung cancer. About 350,000 deaths annually are attributed to cigarette smoking. Cigarette smokers have their risk of death and/or myocardial infarction increased by 70 per cent. A variety of mechanisms probably exist for this relationship. Some believe that smoking promotes atherosclerosis. Other contributing factors may be the decrease in high-density lipoprotein (HDL) and increase in plasma fibrinogen in smokers. Each cigarette smoked reduces life by 5.5 minutes as an estimate. Intervention is extremely important. The risk of a coronary event is decreased by 50 per cent 1 year after cessation and approaches the risk of a nonsmoker after a decade (U.S. Department of Health and Human Services, 1983).

DIABETES MELLITUS. Most clinicians recognize a relationship between diabetes and cardiovascular disease. Patients with diabetes often have other coexisting risk factors such as obesity and dyslipidemia. The now-famous Whitehall Study in England studied 18,403 healthy men and found that the risk of coronary heart disease mortality was nearly doubled when impaired glucose tolerance existed (Fuller et al., 1980). Controlling the serum glucose level does reduce the coronary heart disease risk and improve the lipid measures.

LIPID ABNORMALITIES. The most referenced studies regarding the role of lipids in coronary heart disease are the Framingham Heart Study, the Multiple Risk Factor Intervention Trial, Brown and Goldstein's research on low-density lipoprotein (LDL) receptors, the Coronary Primary Prevention Trial (CPPT), and the Helsinki Heart Study. In these studies, the relationship between cholesterol levels and incidence of coronary heart disease was positive. Brown et al. (1981) showed that increased levels of LDL correlated with an

increased risk of coronary heart disease. Others have demonstrated a reduction in risk with the reduction of cholesterol, particularly LDL. Additional studies have shown that, when HDL increased, coronary events decreased. The CPPT followed men for 7 years (Lipids Research Clinics Program, 1984). Those who reduced cholesterol by 25 per cent experienced almost 50 per cent fewer coronary events than a placebo group of men. The CPPT and Framingham studies suggested that a 2 per cent reduction in coronary heart disease risk can be achieved by lowering cholesterol by 1 per cent. Recent analysis says that this ratio may be even more dramatic—in the range of a 3 per cent reduction in risk for each 1 per cent cholesterol decrease. of 1%. It seems worthwhile for every family doctor to screen patients and encourage each one to keep the total cholesterol at or below 200 mg/dL.

Every effort should be made to reach the target of 200 mg/dL by nonpharmacologic methods before considering drug therapy. The chief methods are diet, exercise, and weight loss. The AHA recommends a diet for the general public (Table 35–2). Those with cholesterol above 200 mg/dL should start the step 1 diet and, if control is not achieved, move on to a step 2 diet. Most people can expect a 10 per cent reduction through diet alone. Those with higher cholesterol can achieve even greater than 10 per cent reduction. Exercise, weight loss, cessation of smoking, and the moderate consumption of alcohol all will increase the HDL cholesterol, a desired effect. Of course, consideration should be given to discontinuing lipid-elevating medications. If after 6 months these nonpharmacologic methods have not decreased the cholesterol to 200 mg/dL or less or increased the HDL to above 35 mg/dL, one or more lipid-lowering medications should be considered (Table 35–3). The National Cholesterol Education Program recommends basing treatment decisions on the level of LDL. Those otherwise healthy adults with LDL levels greater than 160 mg/dL would

TABLE 35–2. DIETARY RECOMMENDATIONS OF THE AMERICAN HEART ASSOCIATION

Targeted Population	% of Calories as Fat	% of Calories as Saturated Fat	% of Calories as Carbohydrate	Total Cholesterol/ Day (mg)
Adults with elevated serum cholesterol				
Step 1 diet*	≤30	<10	50–60	<300
Step 2 diet*	≤30	<7	50–60	<200
General public	<30	<10	50–55	≤300

* Same as those recommended by the National Cholesterol Education Program Expert Panel ("Report of the National," 1988).

need treatment. Individuals with established coronary heart disease or with two or more risk factors should be treated to keep LDL below 130 mg/dL.

Obesity. Obesity now has been designated an independent risk factor for coronary heart disease. Whereas for years it was considered a co-factor, a 16-year follow-up of participants in the Framingham Study by Hubert et al. (1983) has shown it to be independent. It is still true that obesity may worsen other risk factors, such as diabetes. At this time it is advisable to avoid weight gain in early and middle adults years.

HYPERTENSION

At least 50 million Americans have elevated blood pressure. These individuals are at increased risk for cerebrovascular disease, cardiovascular disease, renal failure, and cardiomyopathy. The incidence of these diseases increases with higher levels of systolic and diastolic pressure. It is clear that the prevalence of high blood pressure is greater in blacks. The incidence is also higher in less educated populations. These groups deserve special screening emphasis. The Joint National Committee on Detection, Evaluation, and Treatment of High Blood Pressure has benefited the population and physicians as well with education regarding the diagnosis and management of hypertension. Their Fifth Report (1993) is extremely valuable for the clinician.

Numerous studies exist to support the fact that lowering blood pressure will decrease the incidence of stroke and cardiovascular disease. The goal of treatment of hypertension is to prevent end-organ damage and premature death. Proper screening of each patient will identify those at risk and thereby bring more people to treatment.

Diagnosis

Symptoms of high blood pressure are unusual until the disease is far advanced, so most people discover their elevation during a screening or at a routine office visit. Some take note of their family history of hypertension and make themselves available for screening more regularly. The Joint National Committee on Detection, Evaluation, and Treatment of High Blood Pressure has suggested a new classification for hypertension (Table 35–4). This system utilizes stages 1 through 4 rather than descriptive terms such as "mild," which might have lead to complacency in the past. The diagnosis of hypertension is based on the average of two

TABLE 35–3. PHARMACOLOGIC TREATMENT OF LIPID ABNORMALITIES

	Intended Effect					
Agent	Total Cholesterol	HDL	LDL	Triglycerides	Side Effects	Treatment Notes
Bile acid sequestrants, cholestyramine, and colestipol HCL	↓	↑	↓	None or ↑	Constipation, malabsorption of other meds	Take other medications 1 hr before or several hours afterward
Nicotinic acid	↓	↑	↓	↓	Flushing, liver enzyme elevation, gastritis, gout, abnormal glucose tolerance	Check liver enzymes, uric acid and glucose levels
Probucol (Lorelco)	↓	↓	↓	None	Prolong Q-T interval, nausea, diarrhea	Monitor ECG
Gemfibrozil (Lopid)	↓	↑	↓	↓	Gallstones, liver dysfunction, nausea, myositis, abnormal glucose tolerance	Check liver enzymes
HMG-CoA reductase Lovastatin (Mevacor) Prevastatin Sodium (Pravachol)	↓	↑	↓	↓	Liver enzyme elevation, headache, fatigue, gastrointestinal discomfort	Check liver enzymes, examine for lens opacities

TABLE 35-4. CLASSIFICATION OF BLOOD PRESSURE FOR ADULTS AGED 18 YEARS AND OLDER*

Category	Systolic (mm Hg)	Diastolic (mm Hg)
Normal †	<130	<85
High normal	130–139	85–89
Hypertension‡		
Stage 1 (mild)	140–159	90–99
Stage 2 (moderate)	160–179	100–109
Stage 3 (severe)	180–209	110–119
Stage 4 (very severe)	≥210	≥120

* Not taking antihypertensive drugs and not acutely ill. When systolic and diastolic pressures fall into different categories, the higher category should be selected to classify the individual's blood pressure status. For instance, 160/92 mm Hg should be classified as stage 2, and 180/120 mm Hg should be classified as stage 4. Isolated systolic hypertension is defined as a systolic blood pressure of 140 mm Hg or more and a diastolic blood pressure of less than 90 mm Hg and staged appropriately (e.g., 170/85 mm Hg is defined as stage 2 isolated systolic hypertension).

In addition to classifying stages of hypertension on the basis of average blood pressure levels, the clinician should specify presence or absence of target-organ disease and additional risk factors. For example, a patient with diabetes and a blood pressure of 142/94 mm Hg, plus left ventricular hypertrophy, should be classified as having "stage 1 hypertension with target-organ disease (left ventricular hypertrophy) and with another major risk factor (diabetes)." This specificity is important for risk classification and management.

† Optimal blood pressure with respect to cardiovascular risk is less than 120 mm Hg systolic and less than 80 mm Hg diastolic. However, unusually low readings should be evaluated for clinical significance.

‡ Based on the average of two or more readings taken at each of two or more visits after an initial screening.

From the fifth report of the Joint National Committee on Detection, Evaluation and Treatment of High Blood Pressure. Arch Intern Med 153:154, 1993.

TABLE 35-5. RECOMMENDATIONS FOR FOLLOW-UP BASED ON INITIAL SET OF BLOOD PRESSURE MEASUREMENTS FOR ADULTS

Initial Screening Blood Pressure (mm Hg)*		Follow-up Recommended†
Systolic	Diastolic	
<130	<85	Recheck in 2 y
130–139	85–89	Recheck in 1 y‡
140–159	90–99	Confirm within 2 mo
160–179	100–109	Evaluate or refer to source of care within 1 mo
180–209	110–119	Evaluate or refer to source of care within 1 wk
≥210	≥120	Evaluate or refer to source of care immediately

* If the systolic and diastolic categories are different, follow recommendation for the shorter time follow-up (e.g., 160/85 mm Hg should be evaluated or referred to source of care within 1 month).

† The scheduling of follow-up should be modified by reliable information about past blood pressure measurements, other cardiovascular risk factors, or target-organ disease.

‡ Consider providing advice about lifestyle modifications.

From the fifth report of the Joint National Committee on Detection, Evaluation and Treatment of High Blood Pressure. Arch Intern Med 153:154, 1993.

TABLE 35-6. PHYSICAL FINDINGS SUGGESTIVE OF SECONDARY HYPERTENSION

Physical Finding	Suggested Diagnosis
Abdominal masses	Polycystic kidneys
Abdominal bruits	Renal artery stenosis
Lower leg blood pressure with delayed or absent femoral pulse	Coarctation of aorta
Truncal obesity with striae	Cushing's syndrome
Tachycardia, tremor, pallor, orthostatic hypotension, sweating	Pheochromocytoma

or more blood pressure measurements taken at two or more visits after an initial elevation has been measured (Table 35–5). Most clinicians factor in family history, race, age, and obesity in finalizing a diagnosis. Automated ambulatory monitoring is available and is useful when inconsistencies occur, such as elevated pressures in the office only or symptom occurrence outside the office.

The diagnosis of hypertension in children is important for family physicians to understand, although the incidence is very low. Blood pressure should be measured at yearly visits after age 3. Children of hypertensive parents are at higher risk. The report of the Second Task Force on Blood Pressure Control in Children (1987) contains narrative data on 70,000 children of all races and is a good resource for managing children.

After confirming the diagnosis of hypertension, it is necessary to decide if the patient has primary or secondary hypertension. History should rule out medications as the cause. Those known to contribute most commonly are oral contraceptives, thyroid hormone, steroids, and vasopressor drugs. Physical findings often will point to the other causes of secondary hypertension (see Table 35–6). Urinalysis and measurement of levels of serum creatinine, potassium, and aldosterone would help rule out renal parenchymal disease and primary aldosteronism.

The Joint National Committee and many others recommend the initial work-up illustrated in Table 35–7 for patients with hypertension. A good physical with funduscopic exam and special attention to the heart and peripheral pulses is required.

TABLE 35-7. DIAGNOSTIC TESTING FOR NEW HYPERTENSIVES

ECG
Urinalysis
Complete blood count
Glucose level
Potassium level
Calcium level
Creatinine level
Uric acid level
Cholesterol and HDL levels
Triglyceride levels

Management

Having made the diagnosis of hypertension, a management course must be set. If a secondary cause has been identified, a specific treatment is indicated for the disease uncovered. The approach for primary hypertension is less specific and is more often individualized for the patient. An algorithm for treatment has been created and is useful for management (Fig. 35–4).

Lifestyle modification is extremely important but often difficult for the patient. Each visit must stress these factors and check for compliance, especially when the patient is not achieving control.

If an inadequate response is achieved by lifestyle modification, then pharmacologic intervention is needed (Table 35–8). Adequate time should be allowed for patients to adjust to the medications. Rapid changing from one dose or drug to another will only add confusion.

A great deal has been written about individualiz-

ing the pharmacologic choice for the patient. In summary, the idea is to choose the drug with the most efficacy, easiest compliance (cost and frequency), and least side effects. Taylor (1990) has identified four special groups of hypertensive patients who need careful medication selection (Table 35–9).

Hypertensive emergencies may occur requiring the rapid decrease of blood pressure. Three situation calling for immediate action include accelerated or malignant hypertension, progressive target organ symptoms, and severe perioperative hypertension (Table 35–10).

Every effort should be made to educate the patient about hypertension. Each visit should review the medications and modifiable lifestyle choices. Patients should be seen every 3 to 6 months depending on their individual needs and coexisting illnesses. Early detection of changes in blood pressure control can lead to prevention of complications by lifestyle modification or change in medication.

ISCHEMIC CORONARY ARTERY DISEASE

Ischemia is the mismatch of oxygen supply with oxygen demand, with resultant inadequate removal of metabolites. Chest pain is the clinical manifestation of ischemia. Location of the chest pain is helpful in determining whether the cause is ischemic coronary artery disease or other factors causing chest discomfort (see Table 35–11). Angina pectoris typically is described as substernal heaviness or pressure that often radiates to the neck, left shoulder, and subscapular area and often down the left arm. It often is exacerbated by exertion and relieved with rest. It is relieved often with sublingual nitroglycerin. Angina pectoris typically lasts greater than 15 seconds and less than 30 minutes. It is unusual for angina pectoris to be localized at a single point on the chest wall. It is often to helpful to elicit from the patient exacerbating conditions.

Angina pectoris also can be induced by coronary artery spasm (Prinzmetal's angina). Other exacerbating factors of angina pectoris include fever, tachycardia, anemia, and hyperthyroidism. Medications that increase heart rate, such as dobutamine, or increase oxygen consumption, such as dopamine, often can elicit angina. While exertional angina often is relieved within 5 minutes of rest or within 2 minutes of taking sublingual nitroglycerin, angina pectoris caused by other underlying conditions does not respond as well.

Diagnosis

A history of significant risk factors for coronary artery disease also should be taken in determining

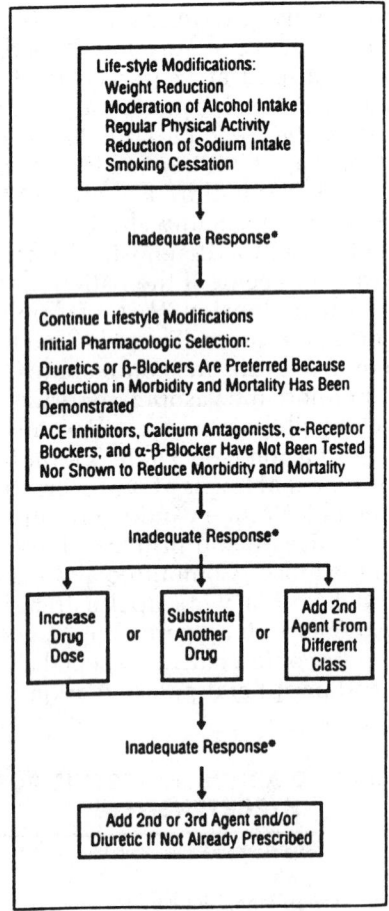

FIGURE 35–4. Treatment algorithm for primary hypertension. Asterisk indicates that response means the patient achieved goal blood pressure or is making considerable progress toward this goal. ACE, angiotensin-converting enzyme. (From the fifth report of the Joint National Committee on Detection, Evaluation and Treatment of High Blood Pressure. Arch Intern Med 153:154, 1993.)

TABLE 35–8. ANTIHYPERTENSIVE AGENTS*

Type of Drug	Usual Dosage Range (Total mg/day)†	Frequency (Times/day)	Mechanisms	Comments
Initial Antihypertensive Agents				
Diuretics				For thiazide and loop diuretics, lower doses and dietary counseling should be used to avoid metabolic changes
Thiazides and related agents			Decreased plasma volume and decreased extracellular fluid volume; decreased cardiac output initially, followed by decreased total peripheral resistance with normalization of cardiac output; long-term effects include slight decrease in extracellular fluid volume	More effective antihypertensive than loop diuretics except in patients with serum creatinine ≥221 μmol/L (2.5 mg/dL)
Bendroflumethiazide	2.5–5	1		
Benzthiazide	12.5–50	1		
Chlorothiazide	125–500	2		
Chlorthalidone	12.5–50	1		Hydrochlorothiazide or chlorthalidone is generally preferred; used in most clinical trials
Cyclothiazide	1.0–2	1		
Hydrochlorothiazide	12.5–50	1		
Hydroflumethiazide	12.5–50	1		
Indapamide	2.5–5	1		
Methyclothiazide	2.5–5	1		
Metolazone	0.5–5	1		
Polythiazide	1.0–4	1		
Quinethazone	25.0–100	1		
Trichlormethiazide	1.0–4	1		
Loop diuretics			See thiazides	Higher doses of loop diuretics may be needed for patients with renal impairment or congestive heart failure
Bumetanide	0.5–5	2		
Ethacrynic acid	25.0–100	2		Ethacrynic acid is only alternative for patients with allergy to thiazide and sulfur-containing diuretics
Furosemide	20.0–320	2		
Potassium sparing			Increased potassium resorption	Weak diuretics
Amiloride	5–10	1 or 2		Used mainly in combination with other diuretics to avoid or reverse hypokalemia from other diuretics
Spironolactone	25–100	2 or 3	Aldosterone antagonist	
Triamterene	50–150	1 or 2		Avoid when serum creatinine ≥221 μmol/L (2.5 mg/dL)
				May cause hyperkalemia, and this may be exaggerated when combined with ACE inhibitors or potassium supplements
Adrenergic Inhibitors				
β Blockers			Decreased cardiac output and increased total peripheral resistance; decreased plasma renin activity; atenolol, betaxolol, bisoprolol, and metoprolol are cardioselective	Selective agents will also inhibit β_2 receptors in higher doses (e.g., all may aggravate asthma)
Atenolol	25–100‡	1		
Betaxolol	5–40	1		
Bisoprolol	5–20	1		
Metoprolol	50–200	1 or 2		
Metoprolol (extended release)	50–200	1		
Nadolol	20–240‡	1		
Propranolol	40–240	2		
Propranolol (long acting)	60–240	1		
Timolol	20–40	2		
β Blockers with ISA			Acebutolol is cardioselective	No clear advantage for agents with ISA except in those with bradycardia who must receive a β blocker; they produce fewer or no metabolic side effects
Acebutolol	200–1200‡	2		
Carteolol	2.5–10‡	1		
Penbutolol	20–80‡	1		
Pindolol	10–60‡	2		
α-β Blocker			Same as β blockers, plus α_1 blockade	Possibly more effective in blacks than other β blockers
Labetalol	200–1200	2		May cause postural effects; titration should be based on standing blood pressure
α_1-Receptor blockers			Block postsynaptic α_1 receptors and cause vasodilation	All may cause postural effects; titration should be based on standing blood pressure
Doxazosin	1.0–16	1		
Prazosin	1.0–20	2 or 3		
Terazosin	1.0–20	1		

Table continued on following page

TABLE 35–8.   ANTIHYPERTENSIVE AGENTS *(Continued)*

Type of Drug	Usual Dosage Range (Total mg/day)†	Frequency (Times/day)	Mechanisms	Comments
ACE inhibitors			Block formation of angiotensin II, promoting vasodilation and decreased aldosterone; also increased bradykinin and vasodilatory prostaglandins	Diuretic doses should be reduced or discontinued before starting ACE inhibitors whenever possible to prevent excessive hypotension
Benazepril	10.0–40‡	1 or 2		
Captopril	12.5–150‡	2		
Cilazapril	2.5–5.0	1 or 2		
Enalapril	2.5–40‡	1 or 2		Reduce dose of those drugs marked with double dagger in patients with serum creatinine ≥221 μmol/L (2.5 mg/dL)
Fosinopril	10.0–40	1 or 2		
Lisinopril	5.0–40‡	1 or 2		
Perindopril	1.0–16‡	1 or 2		
Quinapril	5.0–80‡	1 or 2		May cause hyperkalemia in patients with renal impairment or in those receiving potassium-sparing agents
Ramipril	1.25–20‡	1 or 2		
Spirapril	12.5–50	1 or 2		Can cause acute renal failure in patients with severe bilateral renal artery stenosis or severe stenosis in artery to solitary kidney
Calcium Antagonists			Block inward movement of calcium ion across cell membranes and cause smooth-muscle relaxation	
Diltiazem	90–360	3		These agents also block slow channels in heart and may reduce sinus rate and produce heart block
Diltiazem (sustained release)	120–360	2		
Diltiazem (extended release)	180–360	1		
Verapamil	80–480	2		
Verapamil (long acting)	120–480	1 or 2		
Dihydropyridines				Dihydropyridines are more potent peripheral vasodilators than diltiazem and verapamil and may cause more dizziness, headache, flushing, peripheral edema, and tachycardia
Amlodipine	2.5–10	1		
Felodipine	5–20	1		
Isradipine	2.5–10	2		
Nicardipine	60–120	3		
Nifedipine	30–120	3		
Nifedipine (GITS)	30–90	1		
Supplemental Antihypertensive Agents				
Centrally Acting α₂-Agonists			Stimulate central α₂ receptors that inhibit efferent sympathetic activity	Clonidine patch is replaced once/wk
Clonidine	0.1–1.2	2		
Clonidine (patch)§	0.1–0.3	1 weekly		
Guanabenz	4–64	2		None of these agents should be withdrawn abruptly; avoid in patients who do not adhere to treatment
Guanfacine	1–3	1		
Methyldopa	250–2000	2		
Peripheral-acting Adrenergic Antagonists			Inhibits catecholamine release from neuronal storage sites	May cause serious orthostatic and exercise-induced hypotension
Guanadrel	10–75	2		
Guanethidine	10–100	1		
Rauwolfia alkaloids			Depletion of tissue stores of catecholamines	
Rauwolfia serpentina	50–200	1		
Reserpine	0.05‖–0.25	1		
Direct Vasodilators			Direct smooth-muscle vasodilation (primarily arteriolar)	Hydralazine is subject to phenotypically determined metabolism (acetylation)
Hydralazine	50–300	2–4		
Minoxidil	2.5–80	1 or 2		For both agents, should treat concomitantly with diuretic and β blocker due to fluid retention and reflex tachycardia

* In all patients, lifestyle modifications should also be advised. ACE indicates angiotensin-converting enzyme; ISA, intrinsic sympathomimetic activity; and GITS, gastrointestinal therapeutic system.

† The lower dose indicated is the preferred initial dose, and the higher dose is the maximum daily dose. Most agents require 2 to 4 weeks for complete efficacy, and more frequent dosage adjustments are not advised except for severe hypertension. The dosage range may differ slightly from the recommended dosage in the *Physicians' Desk Reference* or package insert.

‡ Indicates drugs that are excreted by the kidney and require dosage reduction in the presence of renal impairment (serum creatinine ≥221 μmol/ L [≥2.5 mg/dL]).

§ Weekly patch is 1, 2, 3, equivalent to 0.1 to 0.3 mg/d.

‖ A 0.1-mg dose may be given every other day to achieve this dosage.

From the fifth report of the Joint National Committee on Detection, Evaluation and Treatment of High Blood Pressure. Arch Intern Med 153:154, 1993.

TABLE 35–9.   ANTIHYPERTENSIVE DRUG THERAPY IN SPECIAL PATIENT POPULATIONS

Hypertensive Patient Population	Generally Useful Therapy	Potentially Problematic Therapy
Pregnant women	Methyldopa (Aldomet) Hydralazine (Alazine, Apresoline) Beta-blocking agents	Diuretics ACE inhibitors* Calcium antagonists
Blacks	Diuretics Calcium antagonists	Beta-blocking agents ACE inhibitors
Recreational athletes	ACE inhibitors Calcium antagonists Clonidine (Catapres)	Beta-blocking agents Diuretics
Elderly persons	Calcium antagonists ACE inhibitors Diuretics	Beta-blocking agents Alpha-adrenergic antagonists

* ACE = angiotensin-converting enzyme.
From Taylor RB: Patient profiling: Individualization of hypertension therapy. Am Fam Physician 42(suppl):295, 1990, with permission.

TABLE 35–10.   MANAGEMENT OF HYPERTENSIVE CRISIS: EMERGENCIES AND URGENCIES*

Drug	Dose	Onset	Cautions
Parenteral Vasodilators			
Sodium nitroprusside	0.25–10 μg/kg per min as IV infusion; maximal dose for 10 min only	Instantaneous	Nausea, vomiting, muscle twitching; with prolonged use may cause thiocyanate intoxication, methemoglobinemia acidosis, cyanide poisoning; bags, bottles, and delivery sets must be light resistant
Nitroglycerin	5–100 μg as IV infusion	2–5 min	Headache, tachycardia, vomiting, flushing, methemoglobinemia; requires special delivery system due to drug binding to PVC tubing
Diazoxide	50–150 mg as IV bolus, repeated, or 15–30 mg/min by IV infusion	1–2 min	Hypotension, tachycardia, aggravation of angina pectoris, nausea and vomiting, hyperglycemia with repeated injections
Hydralazine	10–20 mg as IV bolus 10–40 mg IM	10 min 20–30 min	Tachycardia, headache, vomiting, aggravation of angina pectoris
Enalaprilat	0.625–1.25 mg every 6 h IV	15–60 min	Renal failure in patients with bilateral renal artery stenosis, hypotension
Parenteral Adrenergic Inhibitors			
Phentolamine	5–15 mg as IV bolus	1–2 min	Tachycardia, orthostatic hypotension
Trimethaphan camsylate	1–4 mg/min as IV infusion	1–5 min	Paresis of bowel and bladder, orthostatic hypotension, blurred vision, dry mouth
Labetalol	20–80 mg as IV bolus every 10 min; 2 mg/min as IV infusion	5–10 min	Bronchoconstriction, heart block, orthostatic hypotension
Methyldopate	250–500 mg as IV infusion every 6 h	30–60 min	Drowsiness
Oral Agents			
Nifedipine (not extended release)	10–20 mg PO, repeat after 30 min	15–30 min	Rapid, uncontrolled reduction in blood pressure may precipitate circulatory collapse in patients with aortic stenosis
Captopril	25 mg PO, repeat as required	15–30 min	Hypotension, renal failure in bilateral renal artery stenosis
Clonidine	0.1–0.2 mg PO, repeated every hour as required to a total dose of 0.6 mg	30–60 min	Hypotension, drowsiness, dry mouth
Labetalol	200–400 mg PO, repeat every 2–3 h	30 min–2 h	Bronchoconstriction, heart block, orthostatic hypotension

* It is sometimes appropriate to administer a diuretic agent with any of these drugs. IV indicates intravenous; IM, intramuscular; PO, orally; and PVC, polyvinyl chloride.
From the fifth report of the Joint National Committee on Detection, Evaluation and Treatment of High Blood Pressure. Arch Intern Med 153:154, 1993.

TABLE 35–11. DIFFERENTIAL DIAGNOSIS OF CHEST PAIN

Aortic dissection	Gastrointestinal (esophageal,
Mitral valve prolapse	peptic ulcer disease,
Psychological	cholecystitis)
Pneumothorax	Coronary artery disease
Pulmonary embolus	Prinzmetal's angina
Pneumothorax	Aortic stenosis
Neuromuscular	Pericarditis
(costochondritis,	
radiculopathy)	

TABLE 35–12. END POINTS OF EXERCISE TREADMILL TESTING

Test completion
Severe chest pain typical of angina pectoris
ST segment depression ≥ 1.5 mm
Ventricular tachycardia
Hypotension during exercise

whether the patient's chest pain is related to coronary artery disease. A family history of heart disease or a history of diabetes mellitus, hyperlipidemia, hypertension, or cigarette smoking are important considerations in evaluation of the patient with chest pain.

Physical examination can give clues to the likelihood of significant coronary artery disease. Decreased peripheral pulses or bruits in the femoral or carotid area increase the suspicion of atherosclerotic disease. The presence of xanthomas suggest hyperlipidemia and may increase the suspicion of coronary artery disease. Unfortunately, there are very few other physical characteristics that can increase suspicion for coronary artery disease. If point tenderness is elicited over the chest wall, it is highly unlikely that the chest pain is secondary to coronary artery disease.

Unfortunately, not all ischemia is clinically apparent. Silent (ischemia without chest discomfort) myocardial ischemia is a well-known clinical condition. Data from the Framingham study suggest that 35 per cent of myocardial infarctions in women and nearly 30 per cent in men are clinically unrecognized. Up to 75 per cent of all episodes of myocardial ischemia detected by Holter monitoring are silent in nature. Given the limitations of history, physical examination, and laboratory testing in patients with angina pectoris, further diagnostic testing is necessary.

Electrocardiogram

An electrocardiogram (ECG) can be especially helpful in the patient with angina pectoris if there are Q waves or T wave inversion present. Occasionally, especially in the presence of chest discomfort, ST segment depression can be noted. A normal ECG does not exclude coronary artery disease.

Exercise Treadmill Testing

The first diagnostic test for angina pectoris following a routine ECG should be exercise treadmill testing. If the patient is unable to walk, pharmacologic means of stress testing are equally applicable. Exercise treadmill tests are interpreted along a continuum. The events constituting a positive ex-

ercise treadmill test are depicted in Table 35–12. Angina pectoris or ST segment changes occurring very early in the exercise treadmill test are of more significance than those occurring after 10 minutes of exercise. An exercise treadmill test is not a perfect test for the diagnosis of coronary artery disease. Depending on the study population involved, the sensitivity and specificity of exercise treadmill testing is approximately 65 per cent. However, completion of the standard Bruce protocol for 12 minutes on the treadmill imparts an excellent cardiovascular risk profile.

Exercise Echocardiography

Echocardiography is an excellent imaging modality used in conjunction with treadmill testing or pharmacologic means of performing stress testing. Echocardiography has been used extensively with dobutamine, dipyridamole, and adenosine. Echocardiography has numerous advantages when used with treadmill testing (see Table 35–13). The sensitivity of exercise echocardiography tends to be slightly less than that of exercise thallium testing; however, the specificity is somewhat higher. The disadvantages of exercise echocardiography are that wall motion abnormalities occur later in the pathogenesis of ischemia than perfusion abnormalities, 5 to 10 per cent of images are inadequate, and greater prognostic information is available with thallium imaging techniques.

Exercise Thallium-201 Testing

Thallium-201 perfusion imaging has been the gold standard adjunctive imaging technique used with exercise treadmill testing. It also has been used extensively with dipyridamole and adenosine for the detection of coronary artery disease. Thallium is dependent on adequate perfusion to areas of myocardium. Those areas that are not receiving adequate blood supply appear as "cold spots." Thallium is injected intravenously at the end of

TABLE 35–13. ADVANTAGES OF EXERCISE ECHOCARDIOGRAPHY

Wall motion assessment
Localization of ischemic zone possible
Assesses valvular function
No radiation to patient
Cost-efficient
Time-efficient

exercise treadmill testing. The patient is encouraged to exercise at least 1 minute longer after thallium has been injected. Approximately 3 hours later, the rest images are obtained. Comparison of resting and exercise images detect areas of significant coronary stenoses. Areas of prior myocardial infarction present fixed defects. Thallium has a sensitivity of approximately 85 per cent and a specificity of 75 per cent in the detection of coronary artery disease.

When compared to exercise echocardiography, thallium testing is more expensive. However, perfusion abnormalities occur prior to wall motion abnormalities. Therefore, the sensitivity of exercise thallium testing is slightly higher, with slightly lower specificities, than exercise echocardiography.

Indications for the use of an adjunctive imaging agent to treadmill testing include patient medications (lanoxin, quinidine), complete left bundle-branch block, right bundle-branch block, left ventricular hypertrophy, and resting electrocardiographic abnormalities. Women tend to have higher false-positive treadmill tests and may require imaging agents. Thallium tends to be a superior agent when detecting myocardial viability following myocardial infarction.

Newer radionuclide imaging agents, such as Zestamibi, may improve the efficiency of radionuclide testing and may improve images. A combination of Zestamibi and thallium may be the most useful technique. The disadvantage of these newer agents is increased cost.

Exercise thallium testing is often useful in patients following percutaneous transluminal coronary angioplasty (PTCA). This is performed for patients with recurrent chest pain after PTCA has been performed or as a routine screening technique in patients with prior PTCA. It is not wise to use thallium within 4 to 6 weeks after PTCA. Persistent thallium defects can be present in these patients, even with an adequate angioplasty result.

Pharmacologic Testing

Pharmacologic stress testing can be performed with adjunctive echocardiography or thallium imaging. The three medications most commonly used are dobutamine, adenosine, and dipyridamole. Dobutamine acts to increase myocardial oxygen consumption, with smaller increases in heart rate and little or no effect on systolic blood pressure. Sometimes vasodilation will predominate, resulting in slightly lower systolic blood pressures. The tachycardic response to dobutamine is much less than that achieved in exercise treadmill testing. The inotropic response to dobutamine is much greater than that of exercise treadmill testing. Dobutamine is infused in incremental doses up to 40 to 50 µg/kg/min. Therefore, the level of ischemia can be determined at any stage of increase of dobutamine infusion. Echocardiographic images are obtained at each stage of increase of dobutamine infusion.

Dipyridamole and adenosine act in similar ways to produce an ischemic response. Both medications induce greater amounts of adenosine to be available at the cellular level. Adenosine is a very potent vasodilator; it induces maximal vasodilation of coronary vasculature. Nondiseased segments of coronary arteries dilate more significantly than those affected by coronary artery disease. This induces a "steal" phenomenon and an ultimate perfusion defect. Vasodilation is a prime mode of action of these medications, so there is less dependence on the typical responses seen on the exercise treadmill testing. Blood pressure tends to fall slightly and heart rate increases only as a reflex mechanism. Inotropic activity is relatively unchanged. Dipyridamole and thallium imaging has been used extensively for screening patients who cannot exercise and are about to undergo peripheral vascular surgery.

Cardiac Catheterization

Cardiac catheterization is considered the gold standard test for patients for coronary artery disease. Cardiac catheterization provides anatomic information regarding severity and location of coronary stenoses. It provides important diagnostic information so that medical therapy, PTCA, or coronary bypass grafting can be recommended. Cardiac catheterization is useful in patients with unstable symptoms and who are not good candidates for treadmill testing. It is also the next step after an abnormal stress thallium or stress echocardiographic study.

Pathogenesis

Atherosclerosis is an accumulation of lipid-laden foam cells, smooth muscle cells, and calcification, often complicated by various amount of thrombus and platelet aggregation. Progressive luminal narrowing leads to decreased perfusion, especially during times of exertion. The ultimate end points are myocardial infarction and death.

Factors that worsen a given coronary artery obstruction include coronary vasospasm and thrombus formation. Coronary vasospasm can be induced by cold temperatures, emotional stress, and cigarette smoking.

Heavily lipid-laden atherosclerotic plaques tend to fracture at higher frequencies. The etiology of plaque fracture is not quite clear, but plaque fractures may be initiated by emotional stress or cigarette smoking. The event of plaque fracturing induces localized thrombus formation. This may result in acute myocardial infarction. It is not necessary to have a severe stenosis for plaque fracturing to occur.

Treatment

The goals of therapy for coronary artery disease are to minimize ischemia. Therefore, myocardial oxygen demand would be minimized and myocardial oxygen supply would be maximized. Other goals are to minimize episodes of ischemia (both silent and nonsilent) and to avoid future cardiac events.

General measures involve dietary modification, cessation of smoking, control of hypertension, weight loss, control of diabetes mellitus, and alterations of lifestyle. A low-cholesterol, low-fat diet is necessary to minimize the risk factor of hypercholesterolemia. Control of hypertension is helpful, especially when left ventricular hypertrophy is present. Left ventricular hypertrophy increases myocardial oxygen demand. Smoking acts to stimulate platelet aggregation. It also stimulates catecholamines, thereby increasing oxygen demand. Cigarette smoke contains carbon dioxide, which increases blood levels of carboxyhemoglobin. This decreases the capacity of blood to deliver oxygen to cardiac cells.

Exercise is encouraged in patients with coronary artery disease; however, overexertion is not recommended. Exercise acts to decrease systemic vascular resistance and improves overall conditioning. Exercise may help to improve the development of collateral circulation of the heart.

β-Blockade Therapy

There are two types of β-adrenergic receptor sites, β_1 and β_2. β_1 Receptors act to increase heart rate and increase contractility. β_2 Receptors cause bronchodilation and dilation of peripheral blood vessels. Therefore, activation of β_1 receptors will result in elevation of the heart rate and inotropic action of the heart, which also results in increased myocardial oxygen demand. Also, blocking β_2 receptors will affect myocardial oxygen supply adversely by causing peripheral vascular constriction and thereby decreasing oxygen delivery to the heart. Therefore, the most potential benefit to the cardiovascular system derived from β blockade would be directed toward only blocking β_1 receptors.

β Blockers have been shown to cause definite decreases in heart rate and contractility. They have been very beneficial in improving coronary blood flow to ischemic regions. These medications are very effective in patients with angina pectoris. There is a significant amount of data to support the use of β blockers in patients with acute myocardial infarction. Large trials have been conducted demonstrating improvement in mortality and morbidity with timolol, metoprolol, and atenolol in acute myocardial infarction.

The ideal β blocker would have specific cardioselectivity, hydrophilic properties (inability to easily penetrate the central nervous system), and a long half-life. The β blockers that demonstrate cardioselectivity include metoprolol, acebutolol, and esmolol. The β blockers with low lipid solubility include nadolol, atenolol, and acebutolol. The β blockers with the longest half-life include nadolol and atenolol.

β blockers have a profound effect on control of heart rate and also can be effective medications for the treatment of hypertension. Goals for the patient with angina pectoris should be to obtain a heart rate between 50 to 60 beats/min and with blunting of heart rate response to approximately 100 beats/min with exercise. Another adequate goal would be for the systolic blood pressure to be adequately maintained below 120 mm Hg with a diastolic blood pressure of nearly 80 mm Hg.

Adverse effects of β blockers are well known (see Table 35–14). Patients with congestive heart failure may tolerate β blockers poorly secondary to the negative inotropy. Some patients experience profound central nervous system side effects, including headaches, depression, and hallucinations. Withdrawal of β blockers should proceed very slowly. Abrupt withdrawal can precipitate severe angina and even myocardial infarction. Some patients tolerate one β blocker better than another. It is not unreasonable to change from one agent to another if the side effects are intolerable.

Calcium Channel Blockers

Calcium channel blocking agents have had an increasing role in the treatment of coronary artery disease. There are numerous calcium antagonists currently approved in the United States. Calcium channel blockers decrease the availability of intracellular calcium. This results in decreased vasoconstriction of pulmonary, coronary, and peripheral vasculature. It also decreases myocardial contractility and can play a role in decreasing atrioventricular (AV) nodal and sinoatrial (SA) nodal conduction times.

Heart rate control by calcium antagonists is important for decreasing myocardial oxygen demand. Of all currently available calcium antagonists, verapamil has the most profound SA nodal and AV nodal effects. Diltiazem also has a significant SA nodal slowing effect; however, this is less common with nifedipine or nicardipine. Verapamil also has the most profound negative inotropic effect of all calcium antagonists. Again, diltiazem has less profound negative action than verapamil but much more so than nifedipine. In some instances, a reflex

TABLE 35–14.   BLOCKADE SIDE EFFECTS

Congestive heart failure	Insomnia
Bradycardia	Bronchoconstriction
Fatigue	Sexual dysfunction
Mental depression	Claudication
Hallucinations	

TABLE 35–15. CALCIUM CHANNEL BLOCKER SIDE EFFECTS

Congestive heart failure	Constipation/diarrhea
Hypotension	Headache
Bradycardia	Peripheral edema
Flushing	

tachycardia and mild increase in contractility can occur with nifedipine. This occurs because the dihydropiridine class of calcium antagonists (to which nifedipine belongs) has more profound effects on systemic vascular tone than the other classes. Decreased peripheral vascular tone enhances coronary blood supply. Therefore, all calcium antagonists, even with slightly different mechanisms of action, have significant antianginal effects.

Depending on the desired heart rate response and negative inotropic response, the correct calcium antagonist can be chosen. There are a variety of adverse effects of calcium antagonists, but not all effects are found with each medication (see Table 35–15). Constipation is much more common with verapamil while peripheral edema is a much more common side effect with using nifedipine. Congestive heart failure, hypotension, bradycardia, flushing, and headache can occur with any of the calcium antagonists. Recently, newer agents of the dihydropiridine class have been released in order to minimize the side effects of existing agents.

Calcium antagonists can be used alone or with nitrates or β-blocking agents. Patients may have a different response to each of these separate drug classifications. Therefore, a particular drug regimen can be tailored to each patient. The patient with peripheral vascular disease in addition to coronary artery disease, may feel better with calcium antagonists rather than β blockers. β blockers in this particular instance may exacerbate the peripheral vascular disease. Patients with prior myocardial infarction may show decreased mortality with the use of β blockers. Again, the calcium antagonists along with β blockers are effective in controlling blood pressure, in addition to their antianginal effects.

Nitrates

Nitrates are well-known standard therapy for patients with coronary artery disease. The administration of nitrates can occur by varying routes, and they have very few side effects. Nitrates can be used easily with other medications for treating angina, with excellent added benefit. Nitrates' action on the coronary blood vessels is not clearly understood; however, they do cause vasodilation and inhibit coronary vasospasm. Nitrates also act to decrease preload by venodilation.

Intravenous nitroglycerin often is used with patients who are admitted to the hospital and fail oral or topical nitroglycerin preparations. Tachyphylaxis to intravenous nitroglycerin can occur after several days of continuous infusion.

Transdermal nitroglycerin can be given in the form of ointment and is easily removed should the patient become hypotensive. However, it is typically an inconvenient way to administer nitroglycerin. Transdermal nitroglycerin patches, in contrast, are a very convenient way of delivering nitroglycerin over a prolonged period of time. Nitroglycerin patches typically were worn for 24 hours in the past; however, because of tachyphylaxis associated with constant nitroglycerin delivery, current recommendations are that nitroglycerin patches be removed prior to the patient going to bed at night. A new patch then can be placed on the patient in the morning. These "nitrate-free" intervals help reduce the phenomenon of tolerance to the medication.

Oral nitrate preparations consist of isosorbide dinitrate and isosorbide mononitrate. Isosorbide mononitrate has a longer duration of action, is well tolerated, and is more convenient. The onset of action is 15 to 30 minutes, and therefore taking an oral medication is not recommended for acute attacks of angina pectoris.

Sublingual nitroglycerin has been the standard form of therapy for patients with acute episodes of angina pectoris. The onset of action is within 3 minutes and the duration of action is maintained for approximately 15 minutes. The dose can be repeated up to three times with 5-minutes intervals for relief of chest discomfort. The side effects of headache, hypotension, and flushing are very common with sublingual nitroglycerin. Nitroglycerin pills are light sensitive and should be replaced every 6 months. Sublingual nitroglycerin spray has a longer shelf life. Sublingual nitroglycerin is also very useful for patients who are about to perform exertional activities that typically bring on angina. Using sublingual nitroglycerin prior to this exertional episode prolongs exercise duration.

Aspirin

Aspirin has become a mainstay in the therapy of patients with coronary artery disease. Aspirin is a very effective antiplatelet agent and has demonstrated benefit in patients with unstable angina. It also decreases the incidence of myocardial infarction, cardiac death, and refractory angina. Patients with known coronary artery disease are recommended to be on aspirin therapy unless there is a significant contraindication. Aspirin is a useful adjunct to patients who also are on other anticoagulants, such as heparin or coumadin. The risk of bleeding is somewhat higher with the use of other anticoagulants; however, the different mechanisms of action convey added benefit. The optimal dose of aspirin is not quite clear. It is still reasonable to treat all patients with chronic stable angina with 325 mg/day unless there are significant aspirin side effects.

ACUTE MYOCARDIAL INFARCTION

Acute myocardial infarction is responsible for nearly 500,000 deaths annually in the United States. Nearly one fourth of all deaths in the United States per year are attributable to acute myocardial events. Most deaths occur within the first hour of myocardial infarction and most are attributable to ventricular arrhythmias, especially ventricular fibrillation. Mortality rates for myocardial infarction were once extremely high. Now, with the advent of thrombolytic therapy, coronary care units, cardiac defibrillators, and other methods of controlling ventricular arrhythmias, the mortality rate has dropped dramatically. In the correct setting, the mortality for myocardial infarction can be as low as 4 per cent. Now the goal for treatment of myocardial infarction is to preserve left ventricular function and decrease mortality. This is achieved with prompt intervention with thrombolytic therapy and/or coronary interventional techniques.

Patients with myocardial infarction typically present with severe substernal chest pain. Up to 30 per cent of patients with acute myocardial infarction have silent events. When chest pain does occur, it is usually intolerable and the patient is often restless. Most commonly, the chest pressure radiates to the neck, the subscapular area, and the left arm. Commonly, patients have had episodes of angina preceding the acute myocardial infarction event. The pain of acute myocardial infarction lasts much longer than that of typical anginal events and is not relieved with rest or nitroglycerin. Acute myocardial infarctions can occur with exertion or they may occur when the patient is at rest.

There tends to be a propensity for myocardial infarction to occur between the hours of 4:00 A.M. and 7:00 A.M. Symptoms of nausea and vomiting often accompany acute inferior myocardial infarction. Anterior myocardial infarctions often are complicated by congestive heart failure and pulmonary edema. Occasionally, cerebral emboli may originate from anterior myocardial infarctions. Although most patients with acute myocardial infarction have tachycardia, occasionally bradycardia may be present, especially with inferior myocardial infarctions.

Physical examination can demonstrate a patient with cool or clammy extremities secondary to low perfusion. Bradycardia or tachycardia may be present. Ventricular arrhythmias are not unusual. Lung examination may reveal the presence of rales at the bases of the lungs if the patient has congestive heart failure. Other signs of congestive heart failure, such as jugular venous distention and peripheral edema, may be present. Occasionally, murmurs may accompany acute myocardial infarction.

Mitral insufficiency murmur may be present if papillary muscle ischemia is involved. The holosystolic murmur of ventricular septal defect may be present as a complication of a septal myocardial infarction. Pericardial friction rubs are not uncommon in the first few days following myocardial infarction.

Differential diagnosis of the patient with severe chest discomfort includes acute myocardial infarction, aortic dissection, pulmonary embolism, and pneumothorax. Occasionally, less severe disorders such as severe gastroesophageal reflux may be present and may mimic the pain of acute myocardial infarction.

Electrocardiographic Diagnosis

The most important diagnostic test for acute myocardial infarction is the ECG. A variety of changes can be found to indicate acute myocardial infarction, but the typical evolutionary changes most commonly found are ST segment elevation and ultimately Q waves in the leads affected by the myocardial infarction. Some patients will present with only ST segment depression or T wave inversion. Up to 20 per cent of patients with acute myocardial infarction have only a history that is consistent with the syndrome and no ECG evidence to back suspicion of acute myocardial infarction.

The first ECG abnormality to occur in acute myocardial infarction is localized hyperacute T waves peaking in leads nearest to the location of the myocardial infarction. Ischemia causes localized release of potassium, causing peaking of the T waves. ST segment elevation then follows and ultimately Q waves develop. It may take several hours or even days for T wave changes to develop. ST segment elevation eventually will return to baseline. Occasionally, ST segments will remain elevated if an aneurysm is formed at the site of the infarction. T wave inversion occurs as the ST segment elevation returns to baseline. Posterior myocardial infarctions present with ST segment depression in leads V_1 and V_2. Right ventricular infarction is seen best with the right-sided ECG, with the most specific lead for right ventricular infarction being V_4R. Patients with severe posterior infarctions or inferior infarctions should have right-sided ECGs performed to document the evidence of right ventricular ischemia or infarction.

Q waves that develop following myocardial infarction may persist or they may be evanescent. The most common location for Q waves to disappear over time are in the inferior leads. T wave inversion in areas affected by myocardial infarction also may persist for years. Resolution of electrocardiographic changes immediately after the initiation of thrombolytic therapy indicates that patency of the vessel likely has been restored.

Non–Q wave myocardial infarction indicates

that myocardial enzymes have risen without the true evolutionary pattern of a Q wave infarction being present. This may involve ST segment elevation or depression or T wave inversion at some point during the patient's anginal chest pain. The essential criterion for documenting non–Q wave myocardial infarction is creatine phosphokinase (CPK) elevation. Some patients with non–Q wave myocardial infarction have no ECG changes at all. Implications of non–Q wave infarctions will be discussed later.

Localization of myocardial infarction can be accomplished according the ECG (Table 35–16). Prediction of the affected artery involved also can be made by ECG findings.

Other events can mimic ECG changes of myocardial infarction. ST segment elevation can occur in coronary vasospasm without truly indicating myocardial injury. Pericarditis also produces ST segment elevation and T wave inversion. The difference between pericarditis and myocardial infarction is that ST segment elevation in pericarditis returns to baseline prior to T wave inversions. In myocardial infarction, T wave inversion occurs as the ST segment elevation is returning to baseline.

Also, P-R segment depression is not seen in acute myocardial infarction. Repolarization variant often can mimic myocardial infarction. In this condition, ST segment elevation may seem to occur because of J point elevation. Digoxin and left ventricular hypertrophy can produce ST segment depression without being indicative of myocardial infarction. It may be more difficult to discern the presence of an acute myocardial infarction in patients with left bundle-branch block and right bundle-branch block. Conduction abnormalities such as hemiblocks may mimic or mask myocardial infarction.

Although Q waves had been thought to indicate transmural infarction, this is not necessarily true. The presence or absence of Q waves on the ECG does not necessarily correlate with pathologic findings of transmural or nontransmural myocardial infarction. Therefore, the terms *Q wave* and *non–Q wave myocardial infarction* should be applied to the ECG and *transmural* and *nontransmural* should be applied to pathologic specimens.

Laboratory Diagnosis

The most useful enzyme determination of myocardial infarction, essential to the diagnosis of acute myocardial infarction, is that of CPK. Serum levels rise in 6 to 8 hours after the onset of infarction and peak within 24 hours. CPK returns to normal within 48 to 72 hours after myocardial infarction. Re-establishing patency of the coronary artery quickly reduces the time of peak elevation of CPK. If successful thrombolysis or successful coronary intervention occurs for acute myocardial infarction, the level of CPK is not as reliable in correlating severity of myocardial injury. The MB isoenzyme of CPK is more specific for myocardial cells. Typically, it does not increase after a skeletal muscle injury. The level of the MB isoenzyme peaks slightly earlier than does total CPK and normalizes within 72 hours of elevation. When the MB isoenzyme is greater than 4 per cent of the total CPK level, the reliability of diagnosing myocardial infarction is greater. If a patient has an MB isoenzyme greater than 15 per cent of total CPK level, even if the total CPK is normal, a diagnosis of myocardial infarction can be made if the total CPK level demonstrates a typical rise and fall. CPK MB isoenzymes can be released with cardiac trauma, defibrillation, and myocarditis.

Lactate dehydrogenase (LDH) often has been used in the past for diagnosis of myocardial infarction. Its peak is within 3 to 5 days following myocardial infarction and elevation may persist up to 10 days. LDH isoenzymes are useful if the CPK is negative and the myocardial infarction is thought to have occurred at least 2 days prior to the time of presentation. Other enzymes for diagnosing myocardial infarction are less helpful.

Imaging Modalities

Echocardiography has played a greater role in helping to determine etiology of chest discomfort. Often, echocardiography can be performed at the time of ongoing ischemia to determine wall motion abnormalities. If regional wall motion abnormality is determined by echocardiography at the time of chest discomfort, a suspicion of significant coro-

TABLE 35–16. ECG LOCALIZATION OF ACUTE MYOCARDIAL INFARCTION

Location	ECG Leads	Infarct Artery
Inferior	II, III, AVF	Right coronary
Posterior	V_1, V_2	Circumflex/posterior descending
Anteroseptal	V_1, V_2	Left anterior descending
Anterior	V_1, V_2, V_3	Left anterior descending
Anterolateral	V_4, V_5, V_6	Left anterior descending/diagonal or circumflex
High lateral	I, AVL	Diagonal
Right ventricular	V_4R	Acute margin of right coronary

nary artery disease is greater. Echocardiography also can be of considerable benefit when diagnosing major complications of acute myocardial infarction, such as ventricular septal defects, cardiac perforation, severe mitral regurgitation with papillary muscle dysfunction, flailed mitral leaflets, and the presence of left ventricular apical thrombus.

Radionuclide studies are of some advantage in the diagnosis of myocardial infarction. Technetium pyrophosphate scanning is helpful in the diagnosis of a remote myocardial infarction. This tracer binds to calcium within an area of damaged myocardium. When scanning is performed between 24 and 72 hours after myocardial infarction, maximal information is obtained. The test has higher sensitivities when performed in patients with transmural infarction.

Pathogenesis

There are different mechanisms of acute myocardial infarction. Most infarctions occur with thrombotic occlusions of a significantly narrowed coronary artery. Plaque disruption at the site of a severely stenotic lesion may lead to localized platelet aggregation and thrombus formation. Approximately 15 per cent of all patients with acute myocardial infarction have demonstrated less than a 50 per cent stenosis at the site responsible for the acute occlusion. Once occlusion has occurred, and if it is prolonged, myocardial injury and ultimately infarction result. Understanding the concepts of plaque fissuring and fracture, platelet aggregation, and thrombus formation help direct therapy toward acute intervention and interruption of the acute myocardial infarction.

Once occlusion occurs, oxygen delivery to the myocardium ceases and ATP becomes depleted, leading to myocardial injury. The wave theory of cellular death indicates that cell death proceeds from the subendocardium to the subepicardium. Necrosis can persist from as little as 2 hours to as long as 8 to 12 hours from the onset of chest discomfort. Much of this depends on the patient's collateral circulation and the effectiveness of each patient's own fibrinolytic system. The size of the myocardial infarction is determined by the area of myocardium supplied by the occluded coronary artery, the amount of collateral blood supply, and whether reperfusion is established. When reperfusion is established, oxygen once again is delivered to the myocardial cells. Some cells will be irreversibly damaged; however, salvage of ischemic but viable myocytes may occur. Reperfusion often is accompanied by resolution of ECG abnormalities and arrhythmias of any type, and resolution of clinical chest pain. Spontaneous thrombolysis can occur in up to one-half of infarct-related arteries that are not treated with thrombolytic therapy. Spontaneous thrombolysis may occur quickly, resulting in a non–Q wave infarction, or it may occur in a delayed fashion, up to 7 days after the time of total occlusion.

Patients without significant stenoses and thrombotic occlusion often are heavy smokers or may have vasculitis (e.g., systemic lupus erythematosus or polyarteritis nodosa). Kawasaki disease can be associated with myocardial infarction and coronary artery aneurysms. Occasionally, embolic phenomena from the aortic valve can result in myocardial infarction. Cocaine use has been associated with intense coronary vasospasm and coronary infarction.

Complications

Hemodynamic complications of myocardial infarction include congestive heart failure and cardiogenic shock. Myocardial infarction causes a decrease in systolic functioning in the area of myocardium affected by the ischemic zone. Often, there is a decrease in diastolic relaxation. Compensatory mechanisms result in hyperdynamic forces in the area not involved by infarction. More than half of patients with acute myocardial infarction have elevated pulmonary capillary wedge pressures. This is a mechanism to maintain cardiac output. Congestive heart failure is diagnosed by the clinical presentation of pulmonary rales, dyspnea, and right-sided heart failure signs. Hypotension is very common. Mortality increases as the signs of congestive heart failure worsen and in the presence of atrial fibrillation.

Cardiogenic shock is secondary to profound left ventricular failure at the time of acute myocardial infarction. This results in inadequate tissue perfusion and significant systemic hypotension. A further increase in vascular resistance causes increased ischemia and worsening ventricular function. Cardiogenic shock can occur at the time of initial presentation or later during the hospital course. Hemodynamic hallmarks of cardiogenic shock include systolic blood pressure of less than 90 mm Hg and a cardiac index of less than 1.8 L/min/m². The pulmonary wedge pressure is greater than 18 mm Hg and there are systemic signs of hypoperfusion.

The goals of treatment for cardiogenic shock and congestive heart failure include maintaining cardiac output and perfusion pressure. Adequate fluid resuscitation is necessary in cases in which pulmonary capillary wedge pressure may be marginally low. Once pulmonary capillary wedge pressure is adequate, vasodilators and inotropic agents are often necessary. Intra-aortic balloon catheterization is necessary in certain instances of severe cardiogenic shock. Right ventricular infarctions often require intensive fluid resuscitation to sustain cardiac output.

Immediate Therapy

When the diagnosis of acute myocardial infarction is made, therapy is directed at restoring patency of the infarct-related vessel as soon as possible. Unless contraindicated, all patients should receive aspirin and β blockers immediately. Intravenous use of metoprolol has been shown to decrease mortality at the time of myocardial infarction. Reinfarction rates are also decreased by the immediate institution of β blockade therapy. Patients with significant left ventricular dysfunction or severe bradycardia are not candidates for immediate β blockade.

Aspirin is given immediately unless an aspirin allergy is present. The ISIS-2 trial showed that aspirin, in conjunction with thrombolytic therapy, had a significant decrease in mortality rates and reinfarction (ISIS-2 Collaborative Group, 1988). Bleeding does not seem to be increased when aspirin is combined with heparin or thrombolytic agents. Aspirin is useful in the secondary prevention of myocardial infarction. Intravenous nitroglycerin is useful in alleviating ischemia at the time of acute myocardial infarction. The venodilation offered by intravenous nitroglycerin is helpful to patients who present with congestive heart failure. There is some evidence that intravenous nitrates decrease mortality in patients with anterior myocardial infarction. This benefit is less clear in those with inferior myocardial infarction.

Patients who present with non–Q wave myocardial infarction and have no evidence of congestive heart failure may benefit from diltiazem therapy. There is no sure indication that calcium channel blockers benefit patients with Q wave myocardial infarctions.

Thrombolytic Therapy

The most effective means for re-establishing patency of occluded coronary arteries remains thrombolytic therapy. Thrombolytic agents that have been used for therapy of acute myocardial infarction include tissue plasminogen activator (tPA), streptokinase, and anisoylated streptokinase. All medications can be given intravenously. The immediate goal is to re-establish vessel patency with the fewest number of complications. Characteristics of thrombolytic agents are outlined in Table 35–17. The highest rates of reperfusion have been established with front-loaded tPA therapy. The

GUSTO trial (Topol, 1993) demonstrated mortality benefit with front-loaded tPA therapy compared to intravenous streptokinase and a combination of streptokinase and tPA. All regimens included the immediate use of heparin therapy, either in intravenous or subcutaneous form. Heparin is helpful in decreasing reocclusion with the use of tPA. The use of heparin with streptokinase is less clear because reocclusion rates are diminished by this longer acting preparation of thrombolytic agent.

Restoration of coronary patency is associated with clinical signs of resolution of chest pain, ECG resolution of ST segment changes, and reperfusion arrhythmias. The reperfusion arrhythmias may take the form of sinus bradycardia, atrial ventricular block, ventricular tachycardia, or even ventricular fibrillation. Accelerated idioventricular rhythm has been thought to be the most common of these perfusion arrhythmias. When all three clinical markers of reperfusion occur, there is a high degree of certainty that the vessel has been opened by thrombolytic agents.

Criteria for thrombolytic agent administration include chest pain lasting greater than 30 minutes and no relief with nitroglycerin, with associated with ST segment elevation in two or more continuous leads. The use of thrombolytic therapy in patients with unstable angina is not clear, although it currently is being studied. Thrombolytic therapy in non–Q wave myocardial infarction has not been shown to have a clear mortality benefit.

The greatest benefit in mortality with thrombolytic therapy occurs in patients with anterior infarction and in those of age greater than 70. However, the risk of thrombolytic therapy also increases as age increases. Inferior myocardial infarctions also benefit from thrombolytic therapy, although the mortality reduction is not as great as that for anterior infarctions. Therefore, all patients with acute myocardial infarctions are considered candidates for thrombolytic therapy regardless of infarct location. Contraindications to thrombolytic therapy are detailed in Table 35–18.

Survival benefit has been maintained in patients with persistent chest pain up to 12 hours after the onset of myocardial infarction. The greatest benefit is achieved within 4 hours of and certainly within 2 hours of the onset of chest discomfort. Although survival benefit is less clear between 6 and 12 hours after onset of symptoms, there is justification

TABLE 35–17. THROMBOLYTIC AGENT CHARACTERISTICS

Agent*	Half-Life (min)	Systemic Lysis	Reperfusion Rate (%)	Antigenicity	Cost
rtPA	5	Mild	75–90	None	3+
Streptokinase	23	Severe	50–60	Yes	+
APSAC	90	Severe	60–70	Yes	3+

* rtPA, reverse tissue plasminogen activator; APSAC, anisoylated plasminogen streptokinase activator complex.

TABLE 35–18. CONTRAINDICATIONS TO THROMBOLYTIC THERAPY

Absolute	History of cerebrovascular bleeding or tumor
	Active peptic ulcer disease
	Recent major trauma or surgery
	Severe uncontrollable hypertension
Relative	Age greater than 75
	Prolonged cardiopulmonary resuscitation
	History of hematologic abnormality
	History of gastrointestinal bleeding

for thrombolytic therapy in patients in this subgroup who continue to have chest pain.

Bleeding complications are the major drawback to thrombolytic therapy. Central nervous system hemorrhagic events are the most serious complication of thrombolytic therapy. Not all cerebrovascular events are hemorrhagic, and such events may not be related to the thrombolytic agent given. Central nervous system events occur in approximately 1.5 per cent of patients given thrombolytic therapy. Transfusion is necessary in nearly 10 to 20 per cent of patients receiving thrombolytic therapy. In patients who undergo PTCA very close to the time of thrombolytic therapy, the need for transfusion is slightly higher. Risk factors for cerebrovascular bleeding events include advanced age, hypertension, and previous cerebrovascular disease.

Thrombolytic therapy reduces mortality from myocardial infarction by approximately 50 per cent. It is greater in those who received earlier therapy and in whom there is anterior infarction. The survival benefit maintained after discharge is roughly correlated with maintaining infarct artery patency.

The major effect of thrombolytic therapy is preservation of left ventricular mass. The most powerful long-term predictor of survival following myocardial infarction is left ventricular ejection fraction. Whether reperfusion occurs by mechanical means, thrombolytic therapy, or spontaneously, preservation of left ventricular wall motion is necessary. The phenomenon of "stunning" may occur up to 10 days following myocardial infarction. Return to normal wall motion may occur in these patients, with beneficial effects on long-term survival benefit.

Reocclusion and reinfarction have been minimized with the use of intravenous heparin therapy following tPA therapy. Judicious use of stress testing and coronary angiography, with or without balloon angioplasty, also has improved long-term results following the initial myocardial event.

Angioplasty

An alternative therapy to thrombolytics for acute myocardial infarction is the use of balloon angioplasty. There are different strategies of balloon angioplasty following acute myocardial infarction.

Immediate revascularization by balloon angioplasty can be performed in place of thrombolytic therapy. Direct angioplasty, in comparison to thrombolytic therapy, demonstrates enhanced immediate patency rate. There may be an slightly enhanced decrease in mortality with immediately angioplasty. There has been greater improvement in ventricular function and less residual stenosis compared with intracoronary streptokinase use. However, the rate of reocclusion with emergent angioplasty is significantly higher than that with elective angioplasty. Bleeding risks with balloon angioplasty and thrombolysis are very similar.

Another approach may be to use balloon angioplasty as a *salvage* technique following unsuccessful thrombolysis. The TAMI trials demonstrated a 14 per cent mortality rate in those patients who needed salvage angioplasty following unsuccessful thrombolysis (Topol et al., 1992). This group also demonstrated a 29 per cent reocclusion rate with no significant impact on left ventricular ejection fraction. The poorer survival in the group needing salvage angioplasty may reflect a greater clot burden.

Routine catheterization and angioplasty immediately after thrombolytic therapy for all patients is currently not favored. The TAMI I trial found that there was no significant benefit to immediate cardiac catheterization after thrombolytics are infused (Califf et al., 1991; Topol et al., 1987). There has been recent evidence that patients can be stratified according to stress testing after successful thrombolytic therapy. When stress testing is abnormal, diagnostic coronary angiography can be performed.

Indications for Cardiac Catheterization

The typical length of in-hospital stay following acute myocardial infarction is 5 to 7 days. Early discharge may be possible following successful thrombolysis followed by stress testing or PTCA. Postinfarction care can be broken down into three categories: medical therapy, identifications of high-risk subgroups, and dysrhythmia evaluation.

The mainstay of medical therapy remains aspirin, which has been noted to have significant benefit in prevention of second infarction. Diltiazem appears useful early in the course of uncomplicated non–Q wave infarction. β Blocker therapy is useful in Q wave infarction.

Identification of high-risk subgroups is important. Cardiac catheterization is indicated for patients with Q wave infarction with congestive heart failure or postinfarction angina. Indications for cardiac catheterization following non–Q wave infarction include congestive heart failure, postinfarct angina, persistent ECG abnormalities (ST segment changes, T wave inversion), or failure of resolution of anterior ECG changes. The long-term mortality of non–Q wave infarction is not different than that of Q wave infarctions because of higher recurrence rates.

All postinfarction patients who do not need cardiac catheterization should undergo stress testing (submaximal or maximal exercise, or pharmacologic testing) prior to discharge. Additional imaging modalities (e.g., echocardiography or thallium) may be helpful to identify "salvageable" myocardium and to quantify myocardial damage. The best predictor of long-term survival is left ventricular ejection fraction. In most instances, abnormal stress tests are followed up with cardiac catheterization. Patients who are able to complete stress testing successfully at 4 to 6 weeks are recommended to return to work.

Ventricular arrhythmias are the major cause of sudden death in the postinfarction patient. Complex ventricular ectopy is an independent predictor of poor prognosis after infarction. Most episodes of sudden death occur within the first 7 months after infarction. A signal-averaged electrocardiogram (SAECG) can predict arrhythmic events in the first year after myocardial infarction. Patients with abnormal SAECGs have a five-fold higher incidence of ventricular tachycardia or sudden cardiac death than those with normal SAECGs. Using a combination of Holter monitoring, SAECG, and assessment of left ventricular ejection fraction, it is possible to identify those patients at high risk for arrhythmic events. Electrophysiologic testing is useful when these noninvasive tests identify high-risk patients.

Postinfarction Myocardial Care

Risk factor modification and rehabilitation is essential for patients following myocardial infarction. Cessation of smoking, modification of dietary fat, and regular exercise are recommended. Control of diabetes and hypertension are essential. Education of the postinfarct patient is very important for long-term benefit.

MYOCARDIAL AND PERICARDIAL DISEASES

Myocarditis and pericarditis are inflammatory processes affecting the cardiac muscle or the pericardial sac surrounding the heart. There are numerous causes of these entities, including drugs, infectious agents, tumor, and radiation.

Myocarditis

Myocarditis has varying clinical manifestations, ranging from an asymptomatic state to severe congestive heart failure. Symptoms of chest pain, fatigue, and dyspnea can be present. Poorer myocardial function correlates with elevation of heart rate. Myocarditis can be associated with abnormal atrial and ventricular rhythms. ECG abnormalities include diffuse, nonspecific findings and low voltage and other conduction disturbances. Echocardiography often reveals reduced left ventricular wall motion and occasional left ventricular dilation. Detection of regional wall motion abnormalities by echocardiography is not common.

Therapy for myocarditis is primarily supportive. Prognosis after an episode of myocarditis is unpredictable. Congestive heart failure as the result of myocarditis is treated in the usual manner with the exception of the use of digitalis, which often exacerbates arrhythmias associated with myocarditis. The use of steroids is controversial.

There are numerous causes of myocarditis (see Table 35–19). The most common form in South America is caused by the protozoan *Trypanosoma cruzi*. The protozoan is transmitted to humans through an insect bite. It elicits an autoimmune reaction that is ultimately responsible for the myocarditis. This cause of myocarditis is very unusual in the United States.

Diphtheria was once a more common cause of myocarditis. Approximately 25 per cent of all cases of diphtheria resulted in myocardial involvement. In some cases, sudden death occurred. Treatment of diphtheria includes administration of antitoxin and penicillin G. Trichinosis, caused by the larva *Trichinella spiralis*, and Lyme disease, caused by the spirochete *Borrelia burgdorferi*, are also causes of myocarditis. Again, the incidence of myocarditis secondary to these two agents is relatively rare.

The incidence of cardiac involvement secondary to the acquired immunodeficiency syndrome (AIDS) is nearly 50 per cent. Mortality secondary to cardiac complications in patients with AIDS is nearly 18 per cent, usually secondary to ventricular arrhythmia. Cardiac manifestations of AIDS include myocarditis, pericarditis, and cardiac tumor infiltration. The etiology of the myocarditis is not

TABLE 35–19. ETIOLOGIES OF MYOCARDITIS

Viral	Coxsackie virus (esp. group B), echovirus, poliovirus, Epstein-Barr virus, poliovirus, retrovirus, influenza
Bacterial	Diphtheria, tuberculosis, salmonella, streptococcus, bucellosis
Spirochetes	Syphilis, leptospirosis, Lyme disease
Rickettsia	Typhus, Rocky Mountain spotted fever, Q fever
Chlamydia	Psittacosis
Fungal	Candidiasis, aspergillosis, histoplasmosis, blastomycosis
Metazoal	Schistosomiasis, trichinosis, ascariasis
Chemicals or toxins	Antineoplastic agents, lead, arsenic, pheochromocytoma, lithium
Physical agents	Radiation, hypothermia

clear. AIDS predisposes to other viral infiltrations of the myocardium, as well as bacterial and non-bacterial endocarditis. Malignant lymphomas have been associated with cardiac involvement in these patients also. Treatment is directed against the offending agent. Pentamidine, which often is used for prophylaxis of *Pneumocystis carinii* pneumonia, can precipitate ventricular tachycardia in patients with myocardial disease secondary to AIDS.

Viral myocarditis is the most common etiology of myocarditis in the United States. The most common viruses involved are coxsackie A and B and the echo virus. Many cases of idiopathic dilated cardiomyopathy are thought to be secondary to late sequelae from previous viral infections of the myocardium. It is very difficult to prove this theory. Endomyocardial biopsy in order to obtain tissue for viral cultures is not a well-established procedure because the results are not known to change therapy or prognosis. Supportive therapy is indicated for viral myocarditis. Rest is certainly indicated. The use of corticosteroid therapy is unclear. Afterload reduction with the use of angiotensin-converting enzyme (ACE) inhibitors is probably the most beneficial medication. Most patients do recover from viral myocarditis, although the recovery period can last from months to years. Rarely is myocarditis fatal.

Cardiomyopathies

Cardiomyopathy is a condition of abnormal cardiac muscle function secondary to various etiologies. Cardiomyopathy is classified as either dilated, hypertrophic, or restrictive.

Dilated Cardiomyopathy

Dilated cardiomyopathy is associated with left ventricular dilation with abnormal systolic and diastolic dysfunction. The most common form of dilated cardiomyopathy is idiopathic (Table 35–20). Typically, all four chambers of the heart are dilated. Symptoms consist of exertional fatigue and dyspnea progressing to resting dyspnea. Right heart failure symptoms also can occur, as well as peripheral embolic events originating from the heart.

Physical examination can demonstrate typical signs of right heart failure, including rales, jugular venous distention, hepatomegaly, and ascites. Auscultation can demonstrate the presence of a third

TABLE 35–20. ETIOLOGIES OF DILATED CARDIOMYOPATHY

Idiopathic	Glycogen storage disease
Myocarditis	Toxins, antineoplastic agents
Alcoholism	Peripartum status
Connective tissue disease	Neuromuscular disease

and fourth heart sound. There may be associated mitral regurgitation secondary to annular dilation. The ECG demonstrates a wide variety of abnormalities, including atrial and ventricular arrhythmias and nonspecific diffuse ECG changes.

Echocardiography is the best diagnostic tool. It is able to determine chamber sizes and valvular function. It is also useful to rule out thrombus in the left ventricle and quantitate left ventricular ejection fraction. Cardiac catheterization is useful for determining right heart pressures, as well as left ventricular end-diastolic pressure. Coronary angiography is useful to rule out coronary artery disease as the etiology for the dilated cardiomyopathy.

Therapy for dilated cardiomyopathy is mainly supportive. Fluid restriction, afterload reduction, and diuretic therapy are useful initially. In severe cases, intravenous inotropic agents may be necessary to improve left ventricular function. Digitalis may be helpful in improving cardiac muscle function; however, proarrhythmic effects must be monitored closely. ACE inhibitors are probably the most effective agents for long-term benefits in patients with dilated cardiomyopathy. ACE inhibitors have been shown definitely to decrease mortality in symptomatic patients with poor ejection fractions. Although ACE inhibitors decrease hospitalizations in patients who are asymptomatic with poor left ventricular function, the mortality benefit is less clear.

The effects of calcium channel blockers and β blockers are not certain. Calcium antagonists and β blockade therapy may be necessary in patients with concomitant coronary disease. However, there is no well-proven benefit to either of these agents in decrease of mortality for dilated cardiomyopathy alone.

Cardiac transplantation can be considered for improved survival. The 1-year survival rate for cardiac transplantation is greater than 80 per cent with current immunosuppressive agents.

Predictions of poor prognosis following the diagnosis of dilated cardiomyopathy include age greater than 50, cardiac index of less than 3 L/min/m^2, a cardiothoracic ratio greater than 0.55, and very poor left ventricular function. Commonly, the cause of death is ventricular arrhythmias; however, the roles of electrophysiologic testing or implantation of cardiac defibrillators are not clear. Anticoagulation therapy is necessary for patients with dilated cardiomyopathy, especially in the face of thrombus detected on echocardiography.

Hypertrophic Cardiomyopathy

Hypertrophic cardiomyopathy (HCM) is usually asymmetric, involving the septum more so than the posterior free wall. This condition previously was referred to as idiopathic hypertrophic subaortic stenosis (IHSS). The prominent characteristic of HCM is abnormal left ventricular relaxation. As ventricular thickness increases, the left ventricle becomes more noncompliant. Therefore, diastolic filling is impaired while systolic function remains intact. During systole, the anterior mitral leaflet moves forward and produces an outflow obstruction with the thickened interventricular septum. The obstruction worsens with volume-depleted states and with low systolic blood pressures. HCM is more common in males than in females and blacks than in whites.

Symptoms of HCM include syncope, exertional dyspnea, and occasionally angina. Angina may occur even in the absence of significant coronary artery disease as a result of the thickened left ventricle. Syncope is multifactorial. It can be secondary to cerebral microemboli originating from the mitral valve, decreased left ventricular outflow in volume-depleted states, or ventricular arrhythmias. The incidence of stroke in HCM is nearly 3 per cent. Patients with HCM tend to present clinically before the age of 30.

Physical examination characteristics of HCM include pulsus bisferiens, wherein the carotid pulse rises rapidly with a double peak. Auscultation often reveals a fourth heart sound and a harsh crescendo–decrescendo murmur heard best at the lower sternal border during systole. The murmur increases with Valsalva maneuver and decreases with hand grip. An accompanying mitral regurgitation murmur often occurs. The diagnosis of HCM is made best with echocardiography. The left ventricular walls are hypertrophied, with disproportionate thickness of the left ventricular septum. Systolic anterior motion of the mitral valve often is seen. There is a large intracavitary gradient within the left ventricle detected on Doppler echocardiography.

Electrophysiologic testing and/or Holter monitoring have been recommended for patients with HCM. High-grade ventricular arrhythmias have been associated with this condition. Atrial fibrillation is not uncommon with long-standing diastolic dysfunction.

Therapy for HCM is aimed at improving left ventricular compliance. β Blockers and calcium channel blockers have been shown to reduce left ventricular outflow gradient and improve diastolic relaxation. These medications reduce myocardial oxygen demand also. Surgical myomectomy of the left ventricular septum has been recommended in refractory cases. This has been shown to alleviate the intraventricular gradient; however, its effect on long-term mortality is less clear.

Pregnant women with HCM still may give birth by vaginal delivery unless there is a history of syncope or documentation of a severe outflow tract gradient. If anesthesia is necessary, epidural and spinal anesthesia should be avoided. General anesthesia with intravenous propranolol or verapamil provides a safer setting in this instance.

For patients with atrial fibrillation and obstruc-tive cardiomyopathy, anticoagulation is necessary to decrease the risk of systemic embolization. All patients should receive antibiotic prophylaxis before dental procedures. All patients are instructed to avoid strenuous physical activity because of the risk of sudden death. The incidence and occurrence of sudden death are unpredictable. Sudden death tends to occur more commonly in patients who are very young at the time of initial diagnosis, those with a family history of hypertrophic cardiomyopathy and/or sudden death, and those patients with a history of syncope. Unfortunately, sudden death may develop in any patients regardless of medical or surgical therapy.

Restrictive Cardiomyopathy

There are numerous causes of restrictive cardiomyopathy (Table 35–21). This condition is characterized by restrictive diastolic filling of the left ventricle secondary to decreased left ventricular compliance. Systolic function is normal. Restrictive cardiomyopathy is a relatively rare condition.

Physical examination reveals signs of right-sided heart failure with elevated jugular venous pressures, hepatomegaly, ascites, and peripheral edema. The jugular venous pulse reveals a prominent *a* wave with rapid *x* and *y* descent. Sinus tachycardia is common. Heart sounds are often muffled. The chest radiography reveals the heart to be normal in size. ECG findings demonstrate diffuse, low-voltage, and nonspecific changes.

The gold standard of diagnosis is cardiac catheterization. This reveals elevated left ventricular end-diastolic pressures greater than the right ventricular end-diastolic pressure. There is a characteristic "dip and plateau" configuration, resembling a square root sign. Right atrial pressures are elevated and have characteristic rapid *x* and *y* descent. Echocardiography reveals typically normal left ventricular volumes and mildly increased wall thickness with normal systolic function. Diastolic flow abnormalities are detected across the mitral and tricuspid valve with Doppler echocardiography. Endomyocardial biopsy may be helpful in this situation to differentiate restrictive from constrictive diseases.

The mainstay of therapy for restrictive cardiomyopathy remains restriction of dietary salt and the judicious use of diuretics. Occasionally, vasodilator therapy is helpful. Digitalis is prone to proarrhythmic effects in this condition.

TABLE 35–21. ETIOLOGIES OF RESTRICTIVE CARDIOMYOPATHY

Infiltrative: sarcoidosis, ameboid infection, hemochromatosis
Endomyocardial fibrosis
Loffler's endocarditis
Scleroderma
Radiation

TABLE 35–22. ETIOLOGIES OF PERICARDITIS

Infectious
  Viral
  Bacterial (streptococci, staphylococci)
  Tuberculosis, fungal
  AIDS
Neoplastic
Postinfarction
Metabolic (uremia, myxedema)
Autoimmune (Dressler's syndrome, connective tissue disease)
Drug induced
Trauma
Radiation
Aortic dissection

Pericardial Diseases

Pericarditis can be the result of numerous etiologies (Table 35–22).

Acute Pericarditis

Acute pericarditis is characterized by chest pain, fever, and a pericardial friction rub. Chest pain is typically sharp or stabbing in nature and varies in intensity. This pain is typically worse with deep inspiration, positional changes, or coughing. Pain can radiate to any location within the chest wall. Patients frequently develop relief from the chest pain by leaning forward.

Pericardial friction rub is a one-, two-, or three-component friction rub characterized as a very scratchy noise. Not all components are heard. Often, the pericardial friction rub can be intermittent. The rub is heard best during expiration with the patient leaning forward. A pericardial friction rub is found in only 70 per cent of patients with acute pericarditis.

Fever is found commonly, although it is not diagnostic of acute pericarditis. The ECG is remarkable for ST segment elevation in multiple leads in early stages of acute pericarditis. This ST segment elevation can be differentiated from that of myocardial infarction by multiple nonterritorial lead involvement. As acute pericarditis progresses, the ST segments return to baseline. This is followed by diffuse T wave inversion. Another ECG hallmark of acute pericarditis is the presence of P-R interval depression in the inferior leads.

Therapy for acute pericarditis requires observation for development of concomitant myocarditis and ventricular arrhythmias, observation for the development of pericardial effusions, determining the underlying etiology, and treatment with anti-inflammatory medications. Most patients recover quickly with aspirin or nonsteroidal anti-inflammatory medications. Corticosteroid therapy is used only in severe cases.

Pericardial effusions may occur with acute pericarditis. Compression of the right ventricle may occur with pericardial effusion accumulation, with an accelerated rate in the pericardial sac. Slow accumulation of fluid allows the pericardial sac to stretch. When there is rapid accumulation of fluid, cardiac tamponade may result. The amount of pericardial effusion can be documented with two-dimensional echocardiography. Progression of fluid accumulation also can be followed using serial echocardiography. Therapy for pericardial effusion includes treatment of the underlying condition and judicious use of diuretic therapy.

Cardiac tamponade is an accumulation of fluid in the pericardial space in sufficient amount to cause severe restriction of diastolic filling, with resultant diastolic collapse of the right atrium and right ventricle. The development of cardiac tamponade is dependent on the ability of the pericardial sac to stretch and accommodate the given amount of fluid, as well as the rate of fluid accumulation. Prior episodes of pericarditis with resultant inflammation and thickening may restrict the ability of the pericardial sac to distend to accommodate fluid. Massive effusions may be present without tamponade, whereas relatively small amounts of fluid may collect quickly, resulting in cardiac tamponade.

Patients with cardiac tamponade are symptomatic secondary to low cardiac output and elevated venous pressure. Physical characteristics include signs of systemic hypotension and right heart failure. Pulsus paradoxus (a greater than 10-mm Hg drop in systolic pressure with inspiration) is a common sign in cardiac tamponade. Auscultation frequently reveals tachycardia. The heart sounds may be faint. A pericardial friction rub may be present. Echocardiography is the hallmark for diagnosis of pericardial tamponade. This demonstrates diastolic collapse of the right ventricular outflow tract and right atrium. This signifies a hemodynamically significant pericardial effusion. Sensitivity and specificity of right ventricular collapse for cardiac tamponade are 90 per cent. Cardiac catheterization is not necessary for the diagnosis of cardiac tamponade, unless the diagnosis is unclear or if pericardial constriction is suspected.

Treatment for pericardial tamponade includes relief of the high intrapericardial pressures. Percutaneous techniques or surgical techniques are both useful for management of pericardial effusion. Heart rate, arterial pressures, and central venous pressures should be monitored continuously. Serial echocardiograms should be performed to detect any changes in accumulation of pericardial fluid. Intravenous fluids are administered on an emergency basis in the presence of pericardial tamponade to sustain ventricular filling volumes, despite venous congestion. However, volume expansion alone is not adequate to treat this condition.

Pericardiocentesis often is performed in the cardiac catheterization laboratory under either fluoroscopic ECG or echocardiographic guidance. It is useful for the relief of cardiac tamponade or relief of symptoms in patients with large pericardial effusions, even in the absence of pericardial tamponade. Open surgical drainage is an alternative treatment strategy with very little risk. The pericardial fluid can be characterized as a transudate (protein less than 3 gm/dL) or an exudate.

Chronic Constrictive Pericarditis

Chronic constrictive pericarditis occurs when the healing of the pericarditis is followed by intense scar formation with subsequent restriction of diastolic filling. Constrictive pericarditis may follow any inflammatory reaction of the pericardium. With restriction of diastolic filling, stroke volume is diminished. Right atrial and systemic venous pressures are elevated.

Clinical manifestations of constrictive pericarditis include shortness of breath and exertional dyspnea. Jugular venous distention is characteristic on physical examination. Congestive hepatomegaly, splenomegaly, and ascites often occur.

Pericardial calcification may be detected on chest radiograph. Computerized tomography and magnetic resonance imaging are useful in identifying pericardial thickness. It is more difficult to determine pericardial thickness on echocardiography. Doppler echocardiography may be of assistance in determining flow patterns characteristic of constrictive pericarditis. Cardiac catheterization reveals elevation of ventricular end-diastolic pressures. The wave form and the amplitude of left ventricular diastolic pressure are identical to those of the right ventricle. Diastolic equilibration of the pulmonary artery, right ventricle, and left ventricle are common. Cardiac catheterization is useful in differentiating constrictive pericarditis from restrictive cardiomyopathy and cardiac tamponade.

Pericardial resection is the treatment of choice for symptomatic cases of pericardial restriction. Long-term results are very good, with operative mortality of less than 5 per cent. Following surgical removal of the pericardium, recurrence of constriction is very rare.

CONGESTIVE HEART FAILURE

Despite advances in therapy, heart failure has become a more common condition in clinical cardiology. In the Framingham heart study, 50 per cent of patients with the New York Heart Association classes II to IV heart failure died within 4 years of diagnosis. Even with recent advances in treatment for this condition, including the widespread use of ACE inhibitors, 40 per cent of these patients die within 4 years of therapy. Heart failure affects approximately 3 million patients in the United States and occurs in approximately 400,000 patients per year. This clinical syndrome is secondary to an inability of the heart to meet the metabolic demands of the tissues or an inability of the heart muscle to relax appropriately, leading to pulmonary edema.

Congestive heart failure can be secondary to a structural abnormality of the heart, such as valvular heart disease, ischemia, and myocardial infarction, or may be a primary myocardial cell abnormality. The precise mechanism for myocardial cell dysfunction in congestive heart failure is not clear. Unfortunately, cardiac dysfunction and symptoms of congestive heart failure tend to worsen independently of the underlying myocardial disease process. Therefore, various strategies are used in the treatment of congestive heart failure depending on the stage of progression.

Pathophysiology

Heart failure is regarded as two pathologic processes. The first is congestive heart failure, which develops as a consequence of impaired left ventricular function. The other is myocardial failure, in which there is dysfunction of the myocardial cells of the left ventricle. Characteristics of congestive heart failure include pulmonary congestion, peripheral edema, hepatomegaly, and a clinical syndrome associated with fatigue, anorexia, and progressive shortness of breath. In this clinical syndrome, neurohumoral mechanisms are activated with subsequent elevations of peripheral catecholamines.

Myocardial failure can occur as a result of various mechanisms. It may be caused by a quantitative loss of functioning myocardial cells secondary to myocardial infarction. It may be a poor adaptation by functioning myocardial cells to pressure overload situations, such as hypertension or aortic stenosis. The pressure overload is associated with an increase in wall tension, resulting in ventricular hypertrophy in order to normalize wall tension. Hypertrophy, to a certain extent, is beneficial to the myocardium. Hypertrophy is able to distribute the demand of mechanical work among a larger number of contractile cells and causes more effective cardiac output. In response to hypertrophy, functional adaptations of the myocardium occur, with a slowing of calcium-activated ATPase activity as well as slowing of the calcium pumps of the sarcoplasmic reticulum. Therefore, hypertrophy slows rates of contraction and slows the rate of relaxation. The slowing of the rate of relaxation affects diastolic function and thereby impairs filling of the left ventricle during diastole. Systolic function and left ventricular ejection fractions are still maintained in this clinical situation.

With sustained hypertension or aortic stenosis, hypertrophy of the left ventricle eventually will deteriorate into poor systolic function. This occurs when hypertrophy of the myocardial cells can no longer occur. The left ventricle then dilates to maintain cardiac output, which further increases left ventricular filling pressure and end-diastolic left ventricular volumes. This causes even further rise in diastolic wall tension. As diastolic volumes increase, myocyte enlargement proceeds. No further left ventricular hypertrophy can occur, and wall tension increases as myocytes are stretched. Eventually, all compensatory mechanisms for maintenance of cardiac output are lost and frank congestive heart failure ensues. Any further events, such as myocardial ischemia with resultant infarction or the occurrence of mitral insufficiency, worsen the already poor left ventricular function.

Compensatory Mechanisms

The first of several compensatory mechanisms for maintenance of left ventricular output is the Frank-Starling mechanism (Fig. 35–5). This demonstrates that the extended shortening of the myocardial cell is dependent on the initial muscle length. When the muscle length is increased by an increase in preload to maximize overlap between the thick (myosin) and the thin (actin) filaments, cardiac performance is enhanced. Factors that affect the left ventricular end-diastolic volume (preload) include total intravascular volume, body position, and intrathoracic pressures. Factors that alter the contractile state of the myocardium include neurohumoral influences such as catecholamines as well as medications (digitalis, dobutamine).

Other factors that negatively influence the contractile state are acidosis, hypoventilation, myocardial ischemia, and negative inotropic agents. Therefore, patients with depressed myocardial function must rely on an elevated left ventricular end-diastolic volume and subsequently increase wall tension to maintain an adequate cardiac output.

Neurohumoral mechanisms that are activated during congestive heart failure include an elevation of systemic catecholamines with stimulation of the contractile state of the myocardium. Also, the renin–angiotensin system is activated, resulting in an increased production of antidiuretic hormone. These influences are important in the maintenance of adequate systemic blood pressure. However, they also result in increased systemic vascular resistance, with promotion of water retention. This ultimately can result in worsening of the congestive heart failure. Atrial natriuretic peptide is elevated. This peptide has been shown to reduce pulmonary capillary wedge pressures and promote diuresis.

Short-term compensatory mechanisms for congestive heart failure work very well. However, long-term compensatory mechanisms are less than adequate.

Etiology

There are numerous causes of congestive heart failure, with the most common underlying cause in the United States being coronary artery disease. Right-sided or left-sided symptoms can predominate, with the etiologies being somewhat different depending on the type of symptoms. Table 35–23 depicts the different etiologies.

Clinical Presentation

Patients with congestive heart failure present with symptoms of right-sided heart failure or left-

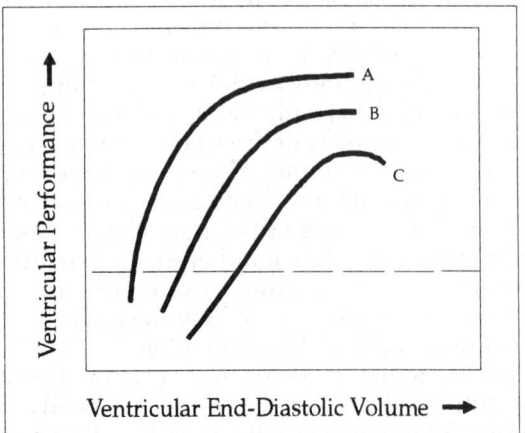

FIGURE 35–5. Frank-Starling curve. *A*, Increased contractile state. *B*, Normal curve. *C*, Reduced contractile state.

TABLE 35–23. ETIOLOGIES OF CONGESTIVE HEART FAILURE

Left Sided
Primary Myocardial Failure (idiopathic, myocarditis)
Structural abnormalities
    Valvular regurgitation (aortic insufficiency, mitral regurgitation)
    Congenital heart disease
    Pericardial disease
    Ischemic heart disease
Secondary etiologies
    Viral
    Hypertension
    High-output failure (e.g., thyrotoxicosis)
    Toxins (e.g., cobalt, lead)
    Cardiac depressants (e.g., disopyramide)
    Drugs (e.g., Adriamycin)

Right Sided
Primary pulmonary hypertension
Cor pulmonale
Congenital heart disease
Collagen vascular diseases (e.g., systemic lupus erythematosus, scleroderma)
Tricuspid regurgitation or stenosis
Right ventricular infarction
Secondary to left ventricular failure

sided congestive heart failure. When right heart pressures (pulmonary capillary wedge pressure, right ventricular pressure, and right atrial pressure) are elevated, liver congestion, elevation of neck veins, and peripheral edema occur. Pleural effusions and ascites also may occur.

Congestive heart failure secondary to inabilities of the heart to meet the metabolic demands of the body can produce renal insufficiency with subsequent water retention and elevation of the blood urea nitrogen and creatinine. This involves activation of the renin–angiotensin system. Decreased left ventricular systolic function also results in shortness of breath with exertion, as well as fatigue. In many patients, both right-sided and left-sided heart failure symptoms occur.

High-output cardiac failure also can occur. This is secondary to diseases such as Paget's disease, thyrotoxicosis, anemia, and beriberi. This results in intense peripheral vasodilation with warm extremities. There is a large arteriovenous oxygen difference. In these situations, the metabolic demands of the body are extremely demanding, exceeding even that of the high-output state.

Clinical Evaluation

Symptoms of congestive heart failure include exertional dyspnea, paroxysmal nocturnal dyspnea, dyspnea at rest, exercise intolerance, weakness, and fatigue. These symptoms are mainly due to poor left ventricular systolic function. Nausea and right upper quadrant pain can occur secondary to distention of the liver. Leg pain can occur secondary to peripheral edema.

Dyspnea is the result of increased elevation of left atrial pressure and pulmonary capillary wedge pressure producing a sensation of breathlessness. Because of the interstitial fluid accumulation, the work of breathing is increased. Dyspnea occurs first with exertion and progresses to the point at which it can occur at rest. Orthopnea is dyspnea occurring with the patient in the supine position. This is secondary to redistribution of fluid to the thorax. Paroxysmal nocturnal dyspnea occurs when a patient awakens from sleep with a sense of breathlessness. This is associated with interstitial pulmonary fluid. Breathlessness at rest also is associated with interstitial pulmonary edema and can be life threatening.

The New York Heart Association has devised a functional classification of heart disease according to the level of exertion required to produce symptoms:

Class I: No limitation of physical activity, no dyspnea, fatigue, or palpitations.
Class II: Slight limitation of physical activity, with dyspnea with ordinary physical activity. There is no dyspnea at rest.
Class III: Marked limitation of physical activity. Mild exercise results in symptoms. There is no dyspnea at rest.
Class IV: Severe limitation of physical activity and dyspnea is present at rest.

Physical Signs

Breathlessness is a hallmark of congestive heart failure. Depending on the level or severity of congestive heart failure, the patient may be breathless at rest or breathless only on maximal exertion.

Examination of neck veins is helpful to determine the level of the volume overload state. Right atrial pressures can be estimated by the distention of the neck veins. Examination of the lungs often reveals rales at the bases of the lungs. Severe congestive heart failure will result in rales throughout the entire lung fields. Pleural effusions may be detectable on physical examination by percussion of the bases of the lungs with the patient in the upright position.

The cardiac evaluation may give clues to enlargement of the left ventricle by displacement of the apical impulse downward and toward the axilla. Depending on the ventricular chamber involved, a heave may be detected either at the apex secondary to left ventricular enlargement or along the right sternal border secondary to right ventricular enlargement.

Pulmonary hypertension may result in accentuation of the pulmonic component of the second heart sound. If the left ventricular hypertrophy is secondary to aortic stenosis, the murmur of aortic stenosis may be apparent. A third or fourth heart sound can be present as a sign of congestive heart failure. The third heart sound is secondary to increased left ventricular end-diastolic pressures with further resistance to early atrial filling of the left ventricle. The fourth heart sound is associated with forceful contraction of the atrium into a noncompliant ventricle. This may be secondary to hypertrophy conditions of the left ventricle and/or severe distention of the left ventricle. Murmurs of mitral regurgitation may be detectable as the mitral annulus expands during left ventricular dilation.

Tachycardia may result as a compensatory mechanism in congestive heart failure to maintain cardiac output. Other signs of right ventricular heart failure may be apparent. Ascites, hepatomegaly, and peripheral edema are often common signs of volume overload. Anorexia and weight loss tend to be very late signs of severe left ventricular dysfunction.

Laboratory Evaluation

The chest radiograph can give helpful clues to the presence of pulmonary edema. As pulmonary capillary wedge pressures extend beyond 20 mm Hg, upper lobe pulmonary veins become more prominent. With pulmonary capillary wedge pressures exceeding 25 mm Hg, interstitial pulmonary edema and interlobular edema (Kerley's B lines) occur. Pleural effusions tend to occur with pulmonary capillary wedge pressures exceeding 25 mm Hg.

The ECG is helpful in delineating causes of left ventricular failure. Ischemia and left ventricular hypertrophy are seen easily on ECG. Echocardiographic evaluation is helpful in determining left ventricular systolic function and any structural abnormalities of the heart, such as valvular heart disease. Regional wall motion abnormalities can be correlated with coronary artery disease. Nuclear imaging can be used for direct assessment of left ventricular ejection fraction. Echocardiographic and nuclear imaging techniques can be repeated after therapy is instituted to determine improvement of left ventricular function.

Blood chemistries are often abnormal in congestive heart failure, including elevations of liver enzyme levels secondary to hepatic congestion. With reduced renal perfusion, the blood urea nitrogen becomes elevated. Serum electrolytes may become abnormal in severe congestive heart failure, with resultant hyponatremia.

Treatment

The initial step in approaching therapy for congestive heart failure is determining etiology and correcting the underlying condition (Table 35–24). Therefore, when ischemia is present, revascularization or medical therapy is necessary. Those in whom aortic stenosis is the etiology, surgical correction is necessary. Treatment of hypertension, abstinence from alcohol, and therapy for anemia or thyrotoxicosis is essential. After the underlying etiologies are removed, several general treatment measures are instituted. These include salt restriction and weight loss, as well as a reduction in excessive, strenuous, physical activity.

Patients with minimally symptomatic or asymptomatic congestive heart failure tend to need less therapy than those with symptomatic congestive heart failure. A major clinical trial has been designed to test efficacy of ACE inhibitors in patients

TABLE 35–24. APPROACH TO CONGESTIVE HEART FAILURE

Delineate the etiology
Evaluate diastolic function
Revascularization when appropriate
Salt restriction, moderation of physical exertion
Pharmacologic therapy
Consider cardiac transplantation, when appropriate

with left ventricular dysfunction in the asymptomatic state. In the prevention arm of the Studies of Left Ventricular Dysfunction (SOLVD), patients were enrolled with ejection fractions of 35 per cent or less. Patients were treated with either placebo or enalapril. The end point of these trials was death. In the prevention trial of SOLVD, total mortality risk was reduced by 8 per cent, which was not statistically significantly different than that of patients taking placebo; however, those receiving ACE inhibitors for minimally symptomatic or asymptomatic congestive heart failure did have fewer hospitalizations and fewer episodes of congestive heart failure (SOLVD Investigators, 1992a).

In the treatment arm of SOLVD, in which patients were symptomatic on initial enrollment, the mortality risk was reduced by 16 per cent compared to placebo, which was a statistically significant difference. Despite this therapy, more than one third of all patients died within 4 years (SOLVD Investigators, 1992b).

There are three broad classifications for pharmacologic therapy of congestive heart failure: diuretics, vasodilators, and inotropic agents. Often, all three drug classifications are used together. There is no set pattern for which drug classification should be used first. All medications can be added in sequence or they may be started together depending on the severity of the patient's clinical symptomatology. Patients with severe congestive heart failure may require hospitalization with intravenous infusion of diuretics and inotropic agents initially. In special incidences in which diastolic relaxation abnormalities occur, calcium antagonists may be of particular benefit.

Vasodilator Therapy

The target of vasodilator therapy in the treatment of congestive heart failure is minimizing afterload. Afterload is the tension generated in the left ventricle necessary to open the aortic valve and eject blood into the systemic circulation. Factors that are important in afterload determination include systemic arterial pressure, left ventricular end-diastolic volumes, and system vascular resistance. As congestive heart failure progresses, vascular resistance increases as a compensatory mechanism. The sympathetic and renin–angiotensin systems are helpful in maintaining systemic vascular resistance; however, this increase in systemic vascular resistance is an impairment to left ventricular ejection.

Vasodilators diminish left ventricular wall tension by reducing systemic vascular resistance and decreasing aortic impedance of left ventricular ejection. Some peripheral vasodilators also may cause venodilation, thereby reducing preload. Therefore, left ventricular ejection will be improved, as well as achieving a reduction in pulmonary venous congestion.

There are several choices for vasodilator therapy. Arterial vasodilators are extremely important in patients with low cardiac output or patients with congestive heart failure secondary to mitral or aortic regurgitation. Venodilators predominantly improve pulmonary venous congestion and reduce preload. They are often very helpful in patients who are receiving diuretic therapy.

ACE INHIBITORS. ACE inhibitors have been shown to improve mortality in patients with symptomatic congestive heart failure and yield very minimal improvement in patients with asymptomatic congestive heart failure. In The Survival and Ventricular Enlargement Trial (SAVE), early treatment with captopril was instituted in patients who were survivors of acute myocardial infarction. Patients had left ventricular ejection fractions that were less than 40 per cent but did not have symptomatic congestive heart failure. Reduction of mortality was 19 per cent with ACE inhibitor therapy (Pfeiffer et al., 1992). The rationale of the study was based on an observation that captopril may reduce left ventricular dilation following acute myocardial infarction.

In the Cooperative North Scandinavian Enalapril Survival Study II (CONSENSUS II), enalapril or placebo was started within 24 hours of acute myocardial infarction combined with standard medical therapy for acute myocardial infarction. Early mortality, at 6 months, was not changed (CONSENSUS Trial Study Group, 1987). Changes in mortality accomplished by ACE inhibitors after acute myocardial infarction in patients with reduced left ventricular function may require longer follow-up to be apparent.

ACE inhibitors tend to be arteriolar and venous vasodilators. Major complications of ACE inhibitors include skin rash, renal insufficiency in patients who are dependent on the renin–angiotensin system to provide adequate urinary outflow, hypotension, and a nonproductive cough. The cough caused by ACE inhibitors can be quite disturbing and may necessitate discontinuing this medication.

Inotropic Agents

In chronic congestive heart failure, positive inotropic agents appear to be indicated when ACE inhibitors and diuretics are no longer controlling symptoms. The three types of inotropic agents in this group are digitalis, dobutamine, and amrinone. The effect of *digitalis* on the heart is not completely understood. Its mechanism of action is inhibition of Na^+/K^+-ATPase. This leads to an increase in calcium influx into the myocardial cell. Digitalis also has direct and neurally mediated effects on the cardiac conduction system. Eighty per cent of oral digoxin is absorbed and excreted via the kidneys. The average half-life of digoxin is 36 hours. The typical loading dose of this medication is 1 mg, which is given as divided doses over 6- to 8-hour intervals.

Digitalis increases contractility in both the failing heart and the normal left ventricle. The patients who benefit most from digoxin have more chronic and severe heart failure, greater dilation of the left ventricle, and reduced global ejection fractions. Digoxin is very useful in patients with congestive heart failure accompanied by atrial fibrillation.

Digoxin is of no use in patients with right ventricular failure secondary to cor pulmonale. Only measures that improve hypoxemia and reduce pulmonary vascular resistance are helpful in this condition. Digoxin is also of no use in patients with mitral stenosis unless the condition is accompanied by atrial fibrillation and rapid heart rates. In this case, it is useful for controlling heart rate. Digoxin is contraindicated in patients with HCM. It may increase the outflow obstruction in this condition. Digoxin also is contraindicated in patients with the Wolff-Parkinson-White syndrome, especially in the presence of atrial fibrillation. In this instance, digoxin shortens the refractory period of the accessory pathway, resulting in rapid increases in ventricular response rates.

Digitalis toxicity is common, especially in hospitalized patients. Conditions predisposing to digitalis toxicity include renal insufficiency and electrolyte disturbances such as hypokalemia, hypocalcemia, and hypomagnesemia. The noncardiac manifestations of digitalis toxicity include nausea, vomiting, fatigue, psychosis, and yellow vision. The cardiac manifestation of digitalis toxicity include any rhythm abnormality. It may cause depression of conduction, with second- and third-degree heart block present. It may increase automaticity of ectopic pacemakers, causing ventricular tachycardias, or it may result in a combination of the above, with resultant paroxysmal atrial tachycardia with AV block. Atrial fibrillation or atrial flutter, as well as supraventricular premature beats, is usually not a manifestation of digitalis toxicity.

Intravenous inotropic agents are often necessary in patients with pulmonary edema who require hospitalization. In this clinical setting, *dobutamine* tends to be the first agent of choice. Dobutamine is a synthetic sympathomimetic agent capable of stimulating β_1-, β_2, and α-adrenergic receptors. Dobutamine has differing effects at various dosing levels. At low doses, it causes slight vasoconstriction and stimulates myocardial contractility. Larger doses may induce vasodilator response with improved inotropic activity; however, dobutamine causes moderate arrhythmogenic and mild chronotropic effects on the myocardium. Dobutamine is most useful in the situation of acute congestive heart failure with the addition of diuretics and afterload-reducing agents.

Dobutamine is an intravenous medication. Infusion of dobutamine for up to 72 hours can be associated with several weeks of sustained clinical benefits. Some patients frequently are given intravenous dobutamine infusions on an outpatient basis to enhance clinical benefit. However, this has been shown to have a slightly worsened mortality rate, probably secondary to arrhythmogenic effects. Home infusion of dobutamine has been advocated by some.

The last group of agents in the inotropic drug category are the phosphodiesterase inhibitors. These agents increase levels of cyclic AMP in the myocardium and vascular smooth muscle. This acts to increase inotropic action of myocardial cells, as well as to decrease peripheral vascular resistance. The prototype phosphodiesterase inhibitor is *amrinone*, which is given by intravenous infusion. The predominant mechanism of improvement in left ventricular function appears to be direct arterial and venous dilation, with a lesser contribution produced by positive inotropic effects. The PROMISE (Prospective Randomized Milrinone Survival Evaluation) trial demonstrated negative impact on mortality secondary to proarrhythmic effects of the oral phosphodiesterase inhibitor milrinone in patients with functional class IV congestive heart failure (Packer et al., 1991). Therefore, the use of oral phosphodiesterase inhibitors in chronic congestive heart failure is less clear. Only a very small number of patients are candidates for cardiac transplantation, so the development of safe and effective agents for treating congestive heart failure is necessary.

VALVULAR HEART DISEASE

The management, diagnosis, and primary cause of valvular heart disease have undergone considerable change. No longer is rheumatic heart disease the most common etiology of valvular abnormalities. Echocardiography is now becoming the mainstay for diagnosing valvular heart disease.

Rheumatic fever is a generalized inflammatory disease affecting the upper respiratory tract. It is secondary to group A β-hemolytic streptococci. Rheumatic fever occurs approximately 10 to 21 days after infection, commonly affecting young people 5 to 15 years of age. It is very uncommon in adults. The mechanism of tissue damage is unknown. The Jones' criteria (Table 35–25) are used to establish the diagnosis of acute rheumatic fever. The presence of two major criteria indicate a high probability of the presence of acute rheumatic fever as long as evidence of a preceding group A streptococcal infection is present. During the initial attack of rheumatic fever, the incidence of carditis is nearly 40 to 60 per cent. The diagnosis of carditis requires one of the following four clinical manifestations: organic heart murmur, pericarditis,

TABLE 35–25.   RHEUMATIC FEVER—REVISED JONES CRITERIA*

Major Criteria	Minor Criteria
Carditis	Fever
Polyarthritis	Arthralgia
Chorea	Previous rheumatic fever
Erythema marginatum	↑ Erythrocyte sedimentation rate or positive C-reactive protein
Subcutaneous nodules	
	Prolonged P-R interval

* Plus evidence of previous streptococcal infection (i.e., recent history of scarlet fever, positive throat culture for group A streptococci, increased ASO titer).

congestive heart failure, and/or cardiomegaly. A murmur is almost always present.

Therapy for acute rheumatic fever is supportive. Antibiotic therapy does not alter the course of rheumatic fever or the development of carditis; however, it is useful to eradicate the streptococcal infection, thereby limiting long-term sequelae and valvular involvement secondary to prolonged inflammation. Penicillin continues to be the antibiotic of choice. Aspirin and prednisone occasionally are used as supportive agents. Long-term prophylaxis prevents recurrent attacks of rheumatic fever. The most effective regimen appears to be 1.2 million units of benzathine penicillin G monthly.

Valvular heart disease warrants prophylaxis against endocarditis. Procedures requiring prophylaxis and current recommendations are described in Tables 35–26 and 35–27.

Aortic Stenosis

There are three major varieties of aortic stenosis: rheumatic, senile calcific (degenerative), and congenital bicuspid aortic valve disease. Rheumatic aortic stenosis involves fusions of the leaflet commissures, with secondary thickening and fibrosis. Symptoms typically do not become apparent until the patient is greater than 50 years old. Patients with senile calcific aortic stenosis tend to have calcium deposits near the annular area of the valve leaflets. Eventually, progressive calcification and fibrosis limits valvular movement. Symptoms typically begin when the patient is greater than age

TABLE 35–26.   PROCEDURES REQUIRING ENDOCARDITIS PROPHYLAXIS

Dental procedures
Genitourinary procedures
   Cystoscopy, prostatectomy
   Vaginal delivery
   Indwelling bladder catheter
Gastrointestinal surgery
Upper respiratory tract surgery
Rigid bronchoscopy

TABLE 35–27. RECOMMENDATIONS FOR ENDOCARDITIS PROPHYLAXIS

Type of Procedure	Therapy	Alternate (Penicillin Allergy)
Dental or upper respiratory tract	*Oral:* Penicillin V 2 gm 1 hr before procedure; 1 gm 6 hr later	*Oral:* Erythromycin 1 gm 1 hr before procedure; 500 mg 6 hr later
	Parenteral: Penicillin G 2 million U I.V. or I.M. 30–60 min before procedure; 1 million U 6 hr later	*Parenteral:* Vancomycin 1 gm IV over 1 hr before procedure; repeat dosage not necessary
	Maximal protection (prosthetic valves): Ampicillin 1–2 gm I.V./I.M. plus gentamicin 1.5 mg/kg I.V./I.M. 30 min before procedure; 8 hr later, repeat this regimen, or use penicillin V 1 gm P.O. 6 hr later	
Gastrointestinal and genitourinary	Ampicillin 2 gm I.V./I.M. plus gentamicin 1.5 mg/kg I.V./I.M. 30–60 min before procedure; repeat once 8 hr later	Vancomycin 1 gm I.V. over 1 hr plus gentamicin 1.5 mg/kg I.V./I.M. 30–60 min before procedure; repeat once 8 hr later
	Low-risk procedures: Amoxicillin 3 gm P.O. 1 hr before procedure; 1.5 gm P.O. 6 hr later	

60. Congenitally bicuspid aortic valves tend to experience early calcification, and symptoms are present usually before the age of 50.

Aortic stenosis presents an obstruction to left ventricular outflow. The compensatory mechanism of the left ventricle is hypertrophy, which ultimately results in decreased left ventricular compliance and increased left ventricular end-diastolic pressures. Myocardial oxygen consumption is increased secondary to greater wall tension and to increased cardiac muscle mass. Because of the greater thickness of left ventricular wall, subendocardial coronary blood flow may be compromised, causing angina pectoris even without significant coronary artery disease. Fifty per cent of patients with severe aortic stenosis demonstrate angina. A life expectancy of 5 years following the onset of angina is expected in patients with untreated aortic stenosis.

Syncope is a frequent exertional symptom secondary to aortic stenosis. This occurs when peripheral vasodilation occurs with a fixed cardiac output. Other causes of syncope in patients with aortic stenosis include atrial and ventricular arrhythmias. Syncope is associated with an overall survival of 3 years in patients with untreated aortic stenosis.

Congestive heart failure is the third most common presenting symptom. It is associated with a very poor survival. It occurs as an end stage to severe left ventricular hypertrophy or as a result of multiple infarcts. Physical examination of patients with aortic stenosis demonstrates delayed carotid upstrokes. There is often a prominent apical impulse and an ejection systolic murmur heard beginning after the first heart sound. The murmur is typically harsh and crescendo–decrescendo. The intensity and duration of the murmur correlates with the severity of aortic stenosis. A coexistent aortic regurgitant murmur also can be found in

many instances. The fourth heart sound is common. Chest radiographs and ECGs demonstrate left ventricular hypertrophy.

The single most important diagnostic study in aortic stenosis is the echocardiogram. Echocardiography demonstrates the characteristics of the valve abnormality and the mobility of the leaflets. Left ventricular wall thickness, left atrial size, left ventricular size, and other valvular abnormalities also can be determined. Doppler echocardiography, with the use of the modified Bernoulli equation, is used to calculate the maximum instantaneous transvalvular pressure gradient. This valvular gradient tends to be slightly higher than the "peak-to-peak" gradient obtained at cardiac catheterization. Aortic valve area then can be calculated via echocardiography using the continuity equation. The resulting valve area, as calculated by Doppler echocardiography, correlates very closely to that determined by cardiac catheterization.

Cardiac catheterization had been the basis for diagnosis of aortic stenosis prior to sophisticated echocardiography. It is still useful when coronary anatomy must be defined prior to surgical repair of the aortic valve. When the aortic valve area is less than 0.7 cm^2, this is considered to be severe aortic stenosis. Valve areas between 0.7 cm^2 and 1 cm^2 are considered to have moderate aortic stenosis. Severe aortic stenosis usually is associated with transvalvular gradients of greater than 50 mm Hg when the cardiac output is normal.

In patients older than 60 years of age, the incidence of significant coronary artery disease is greater than 45 per cent. Therefore, coronary angiography is necessary in older patients requiring surgical repair of the aortic valve.

Surgical replacement of the aortic valve has been the mainstay of therapy. Even elderly patients tend to do very well with aortic valve replacement. Left ventricular function tends to improve after aortic valve replacement, with left ventricular hypertrophy tending to regress over time. Percutaneous balloon valvuloplasty is an option in patients who are not surgical candidates. Final valve area in most series has been reported to be 0.9 to 1 cm², suggesting a moderate residual aortic stenosis is present. Fifty per cent of patients undergoing balloon valvuloplasty tend to have restenosis within 9 months. Therefore, this procedure is considered only to be palliative.

Aortic Regurgitation

Aortic regurgitation is caused by dilation of the aortic root or primary disease of the leaflets. Causes of primary valvular disease include rheumatic fever, congenital bicuspid aortic valve, infective endocarditis, and leaflet involvement in ventricular septal defects. Diseases causing distention of the ascending aorta, thereby causing regurgitation, include long-standing systemic hypertension, connective tissue diseases, and ascending aortic aneurysms. Dissection of the ascending aorta also causes aortic regurgitation. Aortic regurgitation can be acute when secondary to dissection of the ascending aorta or in bacterial endocarditis. More commonly, it is chronic.

Aortic regurgitation results in volume distention of the left ventricle. The left ventricle undergoes gradual hypertrophy and dilation to accommodate further volume expansion. During diastole, the rapid runoff of blood volumes into the left ventricle causes low diastolic systemic blood pressures.

Patients with chronic aortic regurgitation tend to remain asymptomatic for long periods of time. When symptoms do occur, they are related to exertional dyspnea and orthopnea. There is typically a wide pulse pressure as a result of elevated systemic pressures secondary to enhanced stroke volume. This creates a number of physical characteristics, such as water hammer pulses. This is secondary to rapid upstroke and collapse of the pulse. The aortic component of the second heart sound is often diminished. The diastolic murmur heard in chronic aortic regurgitation is high frequency and decrescendo, beginning just after the second heart sound. The more severe the regurgitation, the longer the murmur persists in diastole. The best examining position for patients with aortic regurgitation tends to be with the patient sitting upright and leaning forward. The murmur is heard best along the left sternal border.

An Austin Flint murmur often is heard in patients with aortic regurgitation secondary to the diastolic inflow causing turbulence across the mitral valve. The chest radiograph and ECG often show left ventricular hypertrophy.

The most useful diagnostic test in determining aortic regurgitation is echocardiography. Severity of aortic regurgitation can be quantified with color-flow Doppler techniques. Doppler techniques alone are able to quantify the severity of aortic regurgitation. Cardiac catheterization also can determine left ventricular end-diastolic pressure and quantify aortic regurgitation by supravalvular aortography.

Immediate surgical intervention is required for acute, unstable aortic regurgitation because mortality is extremely high. However, chronic aortic regurgitation requires different therapy. Asymptomatic patients with mild aortic regurgitation usually need no therapy other than routine follow-up echocardiographic examination. They also require antibiotic prophylaxis against bacterial endocarditis. Symptomatic patients with less severe aortic regurgitation require medical therapy, usually in the form of afterload reduction and diuretics. ACE inhibitors tend to be the mainstay of afterload-reducing agents. Symptomatic patients with severe aortic regurgitation require aortic valve replacement.

Mitral Stenosis

The most common etiology of mitral stenosis is rheumatic heart disease. Rheumatic fever results in fusion of the valve leaflet cusps, with thickening and shortening of the chordae tendineae. As valve area decreases, elevations of left atrial pressures occur. This translates into elevated pulmonary capillary wedge pressure. Persistent elevation of pulmonary capillary wedge pressure results in increased pulmonary artery pressures and pulmonary edema. Persistent elevation of left atrial pressure results in left atrial distention and the occurrence of atrial fibrillation. The occurrence of atrial fibrillation in patients with mitral stenosis often results in a sudden increase in symptomatology as a result of rapid heart rates. Mitral stenosis is more common in women and often is exacerbated by pregnancy and atrial fibrillation.

Symptoms of mitral stenosis are typically those of dyspnea, with worsening of dyspnea on physical exertion. Advanced mitral stenosis may result in symptoms of right heart failure. Distention of the left atrium can cause hoarseness by compression of the left recurrent laryngeal nerve.

Physical examination often reveals rales secondary to elevated pulmonary capillary wedge pressures. Cardiac auscultation demonstrates a loud first heart sound and often a loud pulmonary component of a second heart sound. A low-pitched diastolic rumbling may be heard beginning with the opening snap. A murmur becomes loudest just before the first heart sound if the patient is in sinus rhythm. The shorter the interval between the second heart sound and the opening snap, the more severe the mitral stenosis. The longer the duration of the diastolic murmur, the more severe the mitral stenosis. Other signs of right ventricular failure also may be present on physical examination.

Electrocardiographic findings often include atrial fibrillation, right ventricular hypertrophy, and right axis deviation. Left atrial abnormalities also may be present. The chest radiograph may indicate interstitial edema and a large right ventricle. A dilated left atrium on the chest radiograph also may indicate the presence of concomitant mitral regurgitation.

The most important diagnostic technique is echocardiography. Thickened mitral leaflets with doming and reduced motion are the hallmarks of this process; often they are accompanied by an enlarged left atrium. The mitral valve half-time is a technique used for calculation of the mitral valve area. Transesophageal echocardiography is helpful for identifying thrombi in the left atrial appendage, as well as determining extent of calcification of the mitral valve leaflets and subvalvular apparatus.

Cardiac catheterization is often helpful to rule out concomitant coronary artery disease. Right heart pressure measurements, along with left ventricular end-diastolic measurements, are useful in determining mitral valve area.

Medical therapy is the mainstay of mitral stenosis management. Antibiotic prophylaxis is essential. Atrial fibrillation is controlled with digitalis or β blockade. Class IA antiarrhythmics may be necessary to restore normal sinus rhythm. Diuretics are helpful when right-sided heart failure or pulmonary congestion are present. Oral anticoagulation is indicated for congestive heart failure or atrial fibrillation.

Surgical intervention is necessary for patients with moderate or severe mitral stenosis who are symptomatic. Patients who have very little calcification of the mitral valve leaflets or valvular apparatus, trivial or mild mitral regurgitation, and no left atrial appendage thrombus are candidates for percutaneous balloon mitral valvuloplasty. The success rate of percutaneous balloon mitral valvuloplasty is greater than 90 per cent.

Mitral Regurgitation

Mitral regurgitation is the result of significant systolic backflow from the left ventricle into the left atrium. It may be the result of leaflet or annular abnormalities. It may be the result of chordae tendineae or papillary muscle defects. *Acute* mitral regurgitation is tolerated poorly. There is typically a normal-sized left atrium, which results in acute elevations of left atrial pressures and the onset of pulmonary edema. This type of mitral regurgitation is caused by trauma, endocarditis, ruptured

chordae, or ruptured papillary muscle. Acute myocardial infarction or ischemia often is responsible for rupture of the chordae or papillary muscles.

Chronic mitral regurgitation, in contrast, is tolerated well, with less pulmonary congestion. Causes of chronic mitral regurgitation include mitral valve prolapse, rheumatic heart disease, endocarditis, papillary muscle dysfunction, or severe left ventricular dilation. Dyspnea is the most common symptom of chronic mitral regurgitation. Left ventricular ejection is often hyperdynamic because of the low pressure of the left atrial cavity. Dilation of the left atrium and left ventricle eventually ensues.

The murmur of mitral regurgitation is holosystolic and most prominent at the apex, radiating to the axilla. It is typically high pitched. The chest radiograph demonstrates enlargement of the left atrium and left ventricle. The ECG often demonstrates left atrial enlargement and occasionally atrial fibrillation.

Echocardiography demonstrates an enlarged left atrium and is able to quantify the severity of mitral regurgitation by color-flow Doppler techniques. The etiology of the mitral regurgitation often is discerned. Flared leaflets, endocarditis vegetation, or mitral valve prolapse are easily detectable. Angiographic correlation with echocardiographic color-flow mapping is excellent in quantitating mitral regurgitation.

The end stages of severe mitral regurgitation include elevated pulmonary capillary wedge pressures, dilation of the left ventricle, and poor left ventricular ejection fraction.

Medical management is the mainstay of treatment for mitral regurgitation, with the target being afterload reduction. Severe acute mitral regurgitation may require intravenous nitroprusside and an intra-aortic balloon pump, with subsequent surgical intervention. Chronic mitral regurgitation often requires afterload reduction with ACE inhibitors and preload reduction with diuretics. Digitalis is helpful when atrial fibrillation is present or if left ventricular ejection is poor.

When surgical intervention is necessary, repair of the mitral valve is performed to preserve the native mitral valve apparatus and to maintain left ventricular geometry; otherwise, prosthetic valves are necessary. Oral anticoagulation is necessary for prosthetic valves or if atrial fibrillation occurs. Transesophageal echocardiography is a useful intraoperative technique in guiding surgical repair of the mitral valve. Endocarditis prophylaxis is necessary in all patients.

AORTIC AND PERIPHERAL ARTERIAL DISEASE

Most commonly diseases of the aorta and peripheral vasculature are acquired diseases, primarily the result of degenerative changes in the vascular wall. Prominent factors contributing to this degeneration are arteriosclerosis, hypertension, aging, and inflammatory and autoimmune processes. Arteriosclerosis is important in the pathogenesis of aortic aneurysms. Hypertension leads to structural changes in the arterial wall, especially involving medial degeneration. Aneurysms may occur at any location along the aorta from the sinus of Valsalva to the terminal bifurcation of the iliac arteries. Three common conditions affecting the aorta include abdominal aortic aneurysms, thoracic aortic aneurysms, and aortic dissection.

Abdominal Aortic Aneurysms

Greater than 90 per cent of aneurysms of the abdominal aorta are caused by atherosclerosis. These typically begin beyond the takeoff of the renal arteries. These aneurysms are a source of emboli to the distal extremities, as well as a persistent risk for aortic rupture. Most abdominal aortic aneurysms are asymptomatic. Any time an elderly person complains of dull abdominal or back pain, consideration of abdominal aortic aneurysm should be given. Physical examination characteristics typically demonstrate a pulsatile abdominal mass or audible bruit. Abdominal aortic aneurysms often are detected on routine radiographs of the abdomen, demonstrating calcification of the aneurysmal atherosclerotic plaque. Abdominal ultrasound is the most viable means of detecting and following abdominal aortic aneurysms.

The incidence of rupture of aneurysms larger than 6 cm in diameter approaches 50 per cent; however, the incidence of rupture of aneurysms 4 to 5 cm in diameter is only 23 per cent. Therefore, it is recommended to perform revascularization on patients with aortic aneurysms exceeding 5 cm in diameter. The 5-year survival rate in patients with repaired large abdominal aortic aneurysms is significantly better than that for those in the unoperated group. The major cause of mortality in performing surgery for abdominal aortic aneurysms remains cardiovascular complications.

Thoracic Aortic Aneurysms

The three most common causes of thoracic aortic aneurysms include atherosclerosis, cystic medial necrosis of the abdominal aortic wall consistent with Marfan's syndrome, and syphilis. Up to 20 per cent of patients have thoracic aortic aneurysms secondary to connective tissue diseases. Thoracic aneurysms typically produce more symptoms than abdominal aortic aneurysms. Presenting symptoms include pain, cough, dysphagia, and dyspnea, as well as hoarseness. All of these symptoms are secondary to impingement of the aneurysm on the tracheobronchial tree, esophagus, or recurrent laryngeal nerve. Aortic insufficiency is a common finding in patients who have thoracic aortic aneurysm associated with connective tissue abnormalities.

Thoracic aneurysms greater than 7 cm in diameter are more prone to rupture than smaller ones. The aggressiveness of surgical repair is dependent on the general condition of the patient. Surgical results have improved considerably in recent years, with greater than a 90 per cent survival rate for elective resection of ascending and descending thoracic aortic aneurysms. Major complications of repair of the aorta are technical, including hemorrhage from the tearing of the aorta. A particularly troublesome complication is paraplegia resulting from interruption of spinal cord arterial blood supply. Myocardial infarctions, cerebral infarcts, and peripheral emboli are also complications of this surgery. In patients who are not operative candidates, reduction of blood pressure and decreasing left ventricular wall tension are essential medical therapy.

Aortic Dissection

Aortic dissection is caused by a tearing of the aortic medial wall by a dissecting hematoma. Degenerative changes in the medial aorta are at fault. The rate of propagation of dissection is dependent on the rate of rise of arterial pressure, as well as the level of systemic blood pressure. Untreated dissections usually progress to rupture and death.

The most common clinical manifestation is severe pain. The pain is usually sharp and may mimic that of myocardial infarction, and may be located in the anterior chest as well as the interscapular area. Physical examination usually demonstrates elevated blood pressure at the time of presentation. The murmur of aortic regurgitation is detected in approximately one third of patients. The ECG is usually nonspecific and often may demonstrate only left ventricular hypertrophy. Chest radiographs can be helpful when mediastinal widening and a double density at the site of the aortic knob are present. Aortic dissection can be diagnosed definitively by the use of aortography or transesophageal echocardiography. Computerized tomographic scanning and magnetic resonance imaging are also useful techniques in the assessment of patients with aortic dissection.

There are two classifications of aortic dissection. The first was devised by DeBakey in 1955. According to this classification, type I dissections begin at the ascending aorta and extend to the abdominal aorta, type II dissections are localized to the ascending aorta and aortic arch, and type III dissections begin distal to the left subclavian artery and extend below the diaphragm. The second classification is the Stanford classification, in which type A dissections originate in the ascending aorta and type B dissections begin after the left subclavian artery. Two thirds of aortic dissection tend to be type A.

Much progress has been made in the treatment of aortic dissections, with nearly a 70 to 80 per cent survival rate for this once-fatal disease. Surgery is the treatment of choice for proximal or type A aortic dissections. With ascending aortic dissections, the potential for retrograde dissection and pericardial tamponade is very great. Patients with type B dissections have a slightly better prognosis with medical therapy. This therapy is intended to reducing arterial pressure and minimizing heart rates. The mainstay of medical intervention has been β blockade therapy.

Peripheral Arterial Disease

Atherosclerosis is the most common condition predisposing to peripheral vascular disease. This results in lower limb ischemia. The occurrence of pain is dependent on the severity of peripheral occlusive disease, as well as the development of collateral channels. When oxygen utilization exceeds that of oxygen supply, pain is produced.

Discomfort in the limbs occurring with exercise and relieved by rest is typically the first symptom of chronic occlusive arterial disease. It usually indicates multisegmental peripheral vascular disease. Intermittent claudication does not alter mortality. However, it may become so disabling as to limit activity and limit quality of life. Numbness and tingling may be other manifestations of severe peripheral vascular occlusive disease. The most severe manifestations include the occurrence of ischemic ulcerations of the lower extremities.

Noninvasive assessment of arterial inflow to the distal extremities is made via Doppler-determined systolic pressures in the posterior tibial and dorsalis pedis arteries. Comparison of the systolic blood pressure between the dorsalis pedis Doppler-derived pressure and the brachial arterial pressure is the hallmark of peripheral vascular diagnosis. Normally, secondary to peripheral augmentation of systolic blood pressures, the systolic pressure in the dorsalis pedis pulse should be greater than that of the brachial pulse by at least 10 mm Hg. When the ankle-to-brachial index is less than 0.8, significant peripheral vascular disease is usually present. Angiography is then needed to locate the site of stenosis in the peripheral vascular system.

When revascularization is considered in patients with peripheral vascular disease, it is important to consider the cardiovascular implications. Patients with ischemic peripheral vascular disease often have coexistent coronary artery disease. Therefore, screening for coronary artery disease is often necessary prior to lower extremity revascularization. Cigarette smoking is strongly contraindicated because this imparts a tenfold increase in amputation rates of patients with chronic occlusive peripheral vascular disease. Pentoxifylline may increase red cell deformability and may improve claudication in patients with intermittent claudication. Arterial reconstructive surgery is important to improve rest pain and to prevent tissue necrosis and amputation. Percutaneous transluminal angioplasty is an excellent alternative therapy to surgical bypass. Long-term patency rates for peripheral angioplasty are greater with stent placement and with larger diameter vessels.

REFERENCES

Brown MS, Kouanen PT, Goldstein JL: Regulation of plasma cholesterol by lipoprotein receptors. Science 212:628, 1981.

Bulkley BLT, Weisfeldt ML, Hutchins G: Idiopathic hypertrophic subaortic stenosis: Myocardial disarray with isometric contraction. N Engl J Med 296:135, 1971.

Califf RM, Topol EJ, Stack RS, et al for the TAMI Study Group: Evaluation of combination thrombolytic therapy and timing of cardiac catheterization in acute myocardial infarction: Results of Thrombolysis and Angioplasty in Myocardial Infarction: Phase 5 randomized trial. Circulation 83:1543, 1991.

CONSENSUS Trial Study Group: Effects of enalapril on mortality in severe congestive heart failure: Results of the Cooperative North Scandinavian Enalapril Survival Study (CONSENSUS). N Engl J Med 316:1429, 1987.

Hubert HB, Feinleib M, McNamara PM, et al: Obesity as an independent risk factor for cardiovascular disease: A 26 year follow up of participants in the Framingham Study. Circulation 67:968, 1983.

ISIS-I (First International Study of Infarct Survival) Collaborative Group: Mechanism for the early mortality reduction practiced by beta-blockade started early in acute myocardial infarction: ISIS-I. Lancet 1(8591):921, 1988.

Packer M, Carver JR, Rodeheffer RJ, et al: Effect of oral milrinone on mortality in severe, chronic heart failure. N Engl J Med 325:1468, 1991.

Perloff J: Physical Examination of the Heart and Circulation. Philadelphia, WB Saunders Company, 1982.

Pfeiffer MA, Braunwald E, Moye LA, et al: Effect of captopril on mortality and morbidity in patients with left ventricular dysfunction after myocardial infarction: Results of the Survival and Ventricular Enlargement Trial. N Engl J Med 327:669, 1992.

SOLVD Investigators: Effect of enalapril on mortality and the development of heart failure in asymptomatic patients with reduced left ventricular ejection fractions. N Engl J Med 327:685, 1992a.

SOLVD Investigators: Effect of enalapril on survival in patients with reduced left ventricular ejection fractions and congestive heart failure. N Engl J Med 327:669, 1992b.

Task Force on Blood Pressure Control in Children: Report of

the Second Task Force on Blood Pressure Control in Children—1987. Pediatrics 79:1, 1987.

Taylor RB: Patient profiling: Individualization of hypertension therapy. Am Fam Physician 42(suppl):295, 1990.

The fifth report of the Joint National Committee on Detection, Evaluation and Treatment of High Blood Pressure. Arch Intern Med 153:154, 1993.

Topol EJ for the GUSTO investigators: An international randomized trial comparing four thrombolytic strategies for acute myocardial infarction. The GUSTO investigators. N Engl J Med 329:673, 1993.

Topol EJ, Califf RM, Kereiakis DJ, et al: Thrombolysis and angioplasty in myocardial infarction trial. J Am Coll Cardiol 10(5, suppl B), 65B–74B, 1987.

Topol EJ, Califf RM, Vandormael M, et al: The Thrombolysis and Angioplasty in Myocardial Infarction-6 Study Group: A randomized trial of later reperfusion therapy for acute myocardial infarction. Circulation 85:2090, 1992.

SUGGESTED READINGS

Abbotsmith CW, Topol EF, George BS, et al: Fate of patients with acute myocardial infarction with patency of the infarct related vessel achieved with successful thrombolysis versus rescue angioplasty. J Am Coll Cardiol 16:770, 1990.

Abelmann WH: Myocarditis. N Engl J Med 275:832, 1966.

Abelmann WH, Lorell BH: The challenge of cardiomyopathy. J Am Coll Cardiol 13:1219, 1989.

ACC/AHA Task Force on Assessment of Diagnostic and Therapeutic Cardiovascular Procedures: ACC/AHA guidelines for the early management of patients with acute myocardial infarction. Circulation 82:664, 1990.

ACC/AHA Task Force Report: Guidelines for the early management of patients with acute myocardial infarction. J Am Coll Cardiol 16:249, 1990.

Anderson DW, Virmani R, Reilly JM, et al: Prevalent myocarditis at necropsy in the acquired immuno-deficiency syndrome. J Am Coll Cardiol 11:792, 1988.

Appleton CP, Hatle LK, Popp RL: Demonstration of restrictive ventricular physiology by Doppler echocardiography. J Am Coll Cardiol 11:757, 1988.

Benotti JR, Grossman W, Cohn PF: Clinical profile of restrictive cardiomyopathy. Circulation 61:1206, 1980.

Bolognese L, Sarasso G, Bongo AS, et al: Stress testing in the period after infarction. Circulation 83(suppl III):III-32, 1991.

Bonow R, Rosmg D, McIntosh C, et al: The natural history of asymptomatic patients with aortic regurgitation and normal left ventricular function. Circulation 68:509, 1983.

Braunwald E: Examination of the patient. *In* Braunwald E (ed): Heart Disease: A Textbook of Cardiovascular Medicine, 4th edition. Philadelphia, WB Saunders Company, 1992, pp 1–41.

Braunwald E, Kloner RA: The stunned myocardium: Prolonged post-ischemic ventricular dysfunction. Circulation 66:1146, 1982.

Coffman JD: New drug therapy and peripheral vascular disease. Med Clin North Am 72:1, 1988.

Cohn JN, Johnson G, Zeische S, et al: A comparison of enalapril with hydralazine-isosorbide dinitrate in the treatment of chronic congestive heart failure. N Engl J Med 325:303, 1991.

Cohn PF: The role of noninvasive cardiac testing after an uncomplicated myocardial infarction. N Engl J Med 2:90, 1983.

Committee on Rheumatic Fever, Endocarditis and Kawasaki Disease: Guidelines for the diagnosis of rheumatic fever: Jones criteria 1992 update. JAMA 268:2969, 1992.

Cooke JP, Safford RE: Progress in the diagnosis and management of aortic dissection. Mayo Clin Proc 61:147, 1986.

Cristicva TF, Schwartz RS, Gibbons RJ: Determinants of infarct size in reperfusion therapy for acute myocardial infarction. Circulation 86:81, 1992.

DeBusk RT: Specialized testing after recent acute myocardial infarction. Ann Intern Med 110:470, 1989.

DeJaegere PP, Arnold AA, Bald AH, Simoons ML: Intracranial hemorrhage in association with thrombolytic therapy: Incidence and clinical predictive factors. J Am Coll Cardiol 19: 289, 1992.

Dennis CA, Houston-Miller N, Schwartz RG, et al: Early return to work after uncomplicated myocardial infarction: Results of a randomized trial. JAMA 260:214, 1988.

Devereaux R: Diagnosis and prognosis of mitral valve prolapse. N Engl J Med 320:1077, 1989.

Epstein SE, Palmeri ST, Patterson RE: Evaluation of patients after acute myocardial infarction: Indications for cardiac catheterization and surgical intervention. N Engl J Med 307: 1482, 1982.

Faster V, Badimon L, Badimon JJ, Chesebro JH: The pathogenesis of coronary artery disease and the acute coronary syndromes: Part I. N Engl J Med 326:242, 1992a.

Faster V, Badimon L, Badimon JJ, Chesebro JH: The pathogenesis of coronary artery disease and the acute coronary syndromes: Part II. N Engl J Med 326:310, 1992b.

Feldman AM: Classification of positive inotropic agents. J Am Coll Cardiol 22:1223, 1993.

Fortin DF, Califf RM: Long-term survival from acute myocardial infarction: Salutory effect of an open coronary vessel. Am J Med 88:1–9N, 1990.

Fuster V, Gersch BJ, Guilianni ER, et al: The natural history of idiopathic dilated cardiomyopathy. Am J Cardiol 47:525, 1981.

Gibbons RJ, Holmes DR, Reeder GS, et al: Immediate angioplasty compared with the administration of a thrombolytic agent followed by a conservative treatment for myocardial infarction. N Engl J Med 328:685, 1993.

Gore JM, Sloan M, Price TR, et al: Intracerebral hemorrhage, cerebral infarction, and subdural hematoma after acute myocardial infarction and thrombolytic therapy in the Thrombolysis in Myocardial Infarction Study: Thrombolysis in Myocardial Infarction, Phase II, Pilot and Clinical Trial. Circulation 83:448, 1991.

Grines CI, Browne KF, Marco J, et al: A comparison of immediate angioplasty with thrombolytic therapy for acute myocardial infarction. N Engl J Med 328:673, 1993.

Gruppo Italiano per lo Studio della Streptochinas; Nell'infarto Miocardico (GISSI-I): Effectiveness of intravenous thrombolytic treatment in acute myocardial infarction. Lancet 1: 397, 1986.

ISIS-2 Collaborative Group: Randomized trial of intravenous streptokinase, oral aspirin, both or neither among 17,187 cases of suspected acute myocardial infarction: ISIS-2. Lancet 2:349, 1988.

ISIS-3 (Third International Study of Infarct Survival) Collaborative Group: ISIS-3: A randomized comparison of streptokinase vs. tissue plasminogen activator vs. anistreplase and of aspirin plus heparin vs. aspirin alone among 41,299 cases suspected acute myocardial infarction. Lancet 339:753, 1992.

Isner JM, Rosenfield K: Redefining the treatment of peripheral artery disease: Role of percutaneous revascularization. Circulation 88:1534, 1993.

Kalbfleisch SJ, Morady F: Therapy of arrhythmias in acute myocardial infarction. *In* Bates ER (ed): Thrombolysis and Adjunctive Therapy for Acute Myocardial Infarction. New York, Dekker, 1992, pp 352–387.

Kalon KLH, Pinsky JL, Kannel WB, Levy D: The epidemiology of heart failure: The Framingham Heart Study. J Am Coll Cardiol 22(A):6A, 1993.

Kennedy JW, Ritchie JI, Davis KB, et al: The Western Washington Randomized Trial of Intracoronary Streptokinase in Acute Myocardial Infarction. N Engl J Med 312:1073, 1985.

Kereiakes DJ, Parmley WW: Myocarditis and cardiomyopathy. Am Heart J 108:1318, 1984.

Kessler KM, Rodriguez D, Rahem A, et al: Echocardiographic observations regarding pericardial effusions associated with cardiac disease. Chest 78:736, 1980.

Krone RJ, Gillespie JA, Weld FM, et al for the Multicenter Postinfarction Research Group: Low-level exercise testing after myocardial infarction: Usefulness in enhancing clinical risk stratification. Circulation 71:80, 1985.

Krone RJ, Greeberg H, Dwyer EM, et al: Long-term prognostic significance of ST-segment depression during acute myocardial infarction. J Am Coll Cardiol 22:361, 1993.

Levine SA, Harvey WP: Clinical Auscultation of the Heart. Philadelphia, WB Saunders Company, 1959.

Lewis BS: Real time two-dimensional echocardiography in constrictive pericarditis. Am J Cardiol 49:1789, 1982.

Lewis H, Davis J, Archibald G, et al: Protective effects of aspirin against acute myocardial infarction and death in men with unstable angina. N Engl J Med 309:396, 1983.

Lipids Research Clinics Program: The Lipid Research Clinics Coronary Primary Prevention Trial Results 1: Reduction in incidence of coronary heart disease. JAMA 251:351, 1984.

Litwin SE, Grossman W: Diastolic dysfunction as a cause of heart failure. J Am Coll Cardiol 22(A):49A, 1993.

Lombard J, Selzer A: Valvular aortic stenosis: A clinical and hemodynamic profile of patients. Ann Intern Med 106:292, 1987.

Lorell B, Lembach RC, Pohost GM, et al: Right ventricular infarction: Clinical diagnosis and differentiation from cardiac tamponade and pericardial constriction. Am J Cardiol 43:465, 1979.

Lowe HW, Laks H, Migatter E, et al: Ischemic cardiomyopathy: Criteria for coronary revascularization and cardiac transplantation. Circulation 84(suppl III):III-290, 1991.

Mannering D, Cripps T, Leech G, et al: The dobutamine stress test as an alternative to exercise testing after acute myocardial infarction. Br Heart J 59:521, 1833.

Middlekauff HR, Stevenson WG, Stevenson LV: Prognostic significance of atrial fibrillation in advanced heart failure: A study of 390 patients. Circulation 84:40, 1991.

Muller DWM, Topol EJ: Selection of patients with acute myocardial infarction for thrombolytic therapy. Ann Intern Med 113:949, 1990.

Multicenter Diltiazem Post Infarction Trial Research Group: The effect of diltiazem on mortality and reinfarction after myocardial infarction. N Engl J Med 319:385, 1988.

O'Rourke R: Risk stratification after myocardial infarction: Clinical overview. Circulation 84(suppl I):I-177, 1991.

Otto C, Pearman A, Gardner C: Hemodynamic progression of aortic stenosis in adults assessed by Doppler echocardiography. J Am Coll Cardiol 13:545, 1989.

Packer M: Combined beta-adrenergic and calcium entry blockade in angina pectoris. N Engl J Med 320:709, 1989.

Parker JO: Nitrate therapy in stable angina pectoris. N Engl J Med 316:1635, 1987.

Parker JO, Farrel B, Lahey LA, Moe G.: Effects of intervals between doses on the development of tolerance to isosorbide dinitrate. N Engl J Med 316:1440, 1987.

Picallo G, Pirelli S, Marsa D, et al: Value of negative predischarge exercise testing in identifying patients at low risk after acute myocardial infarction treated by systemic thrombolysis. Am J Cardiol 70:31, 1992.

Report of the National Cholesterol Education Program Expert Panel on Detection, Evaluation, and Treatment of High Blood Cholesterol in Adults. Arch Intern Med 148:36, 1988.

Rermer KA, Lowe JE, Rasmussen MM, Jennings RB: The wave front phenomenon of ischemic cell death: I. Myocardial infarct size versus duration of coronary occlusion in dogs. Circulation 56:786, 1977.

Rezkalla S, Kloner RA: Management strategies in viral myocarditis. Am Heart J 117:706, 1989.

Rutherford J, Braunwald E: Chronic ischemic heart disease. *In* Braunwald E (ed): A Textbook of Cardiovascular Medicine, 4th edition. Philadelphia, WB Saunders Company, 1992, pp 1292–1364.

Ryan T, Armstrong WF, O'Donnell JA, Feigenbaum H: Risk stratification after acute myocardial infarction by means of two-dimensional echocardiography. Am Heart J 114:1305, 1987.

Sandler G: The importance of the history in the medical clinic and the cost of unnecessary tests. Am Heart J 100:923, 1980.

Sapira JD: The History, Art and Science of Bedside Diagnosis. Baltimore, Urban & Schwartzenberg, 1990, pp 9–45.

Shah PK, Cercek B, Lew AS, Granz W: Angiographic validation of bedside markers of reperfusion. J Am Coll Cardiol 21:55, 1993.

Skjaerpe T, Hegremaes L, Hatle L: Noninvasive estimation of valve area in patients with aortic stenosis by Doppler ultrasound and two-dimensional echocardiography. Circulation 72:810, 1985.

Sonnenblick EH, LeJemtel TH, Anversa P: Heart failure: Etiological models and therapeutic challenges. *In* Lewis BS, Kimchi A (eds): Heart Failure Mechanisms and Management. New York, Springer-Verlag, 1991, pp 33–41.

Spodick DH: The normal and diseased pericardium: Current concepts of pericardial physiology, diagnosis, and treatment. J Am Coll Cardiol 1:240, 1983.

Stevenson LW, Peeloff JK: The limited reliability of physical signs for the estimation of hemodynamics in chronic heart failure. JAMA 261:884, 1989.

TIMI Study Group: Comparison of invasive and conservative strategies after treatment with intravenous tissue plasminogen activator in acute myocardial infarction: Results of the Thrombolysis in Myocardial Infarction (TIMI) Phase II Trial. N Engl J Med 320:618, 1989.

Tumulty PA: Obtaining the History: *In* The Effective Clinician. Philadelphia, WB Saunders Company, 1973, pp 17–28.

Uretsky BF, Young JB, Shahide FE, et al: Randomized study assessing the effect of digoxin withdrawal in patients with mild to moderate chronic congestive heart failure: Results of the PROVED Trial. J Am Coll Cardiol 22:955, 1993.

U.S. Department of Health and Human Services: The Health Consequences of Smoking: Cardiovascular Disease. A Report of the Surgeon General. Rockville, MD, U.S. Department of Health and Human Services, 1983.

Van de Weaf, Arnold AER: Intravenous tissue plasminogen activator and size of infarct, left ventricular function, and survival in acute myocardial infarction. BMJ 297:300, 1988.

Waters DD, Bosch X, Bouchard A, et al: Comparison of clinical variables and variables derived from a limited predischarge exercise test as predictors of early and late mortality after myocardial infarction. J Am Coll Cardiol 5:1, 1985.

Widlus DM, Osterman FA: Evaluation and percutaneous management of atherosclerotic peripheral vascular disease. JAMA 261:3148, 1989.

Zijlstra F, De Boer MJ, Hoorntje JCA, et al: A comparison of immediate coronary angioplasty with intravenous streptokinase in acute myocardial infarction. N Engl J Med 328:680, 1993.

Diagnosis and Treatment of Arrhythmias

CARLOS VALLBONA

ELECTROPHYSIOLOGY

Automaticity, rhythmicity, conductivity, and contractility are four basic properties of all cardiac cells. The *automaticity* accounts for the capability of the cardiac cells to produce an electrical impulse that precedes the myocardial wall contraction. The fact that the atria and the ventricles contract according to a certain *rhythmicity* is due to the regular periodic occurrence of transmembrane action potentials (TAPs) in a special group of cells more susceptible than others to becoming depolarized. These cells become the cardiac pacemaker because they produce an electrical stimulus, which then is conducted to other parts of the heart. The most common pacemaker is located at the sinoatrial (SA) node, although the atrioventricular (AV) junction and, to a lesser extent, the bundle of His and Purkinje's fibers also may act as pacemakers. The usual rate of automatic depolarization of the SA node is 60 to 100 beats/min, whereas it is 40 to 60 beats/min at the AV junction and less than 40 beats/min at the bundle of His and Purkinje's fibers. This difference in rates accounts for the predominance of the SA node as the normal cardiac pacemaker.

The *conductivity* of special cells and fibers of the heart (e.g., atrial bundles and bundle of His) allows for rapid transmission of impulses through the atria and ventricles. The arrival of electrical impulses to the cardiac cells is necessary to allow these cells to display appropriate *contractility*.

The typical ventricular TAP occurs when an impulse arriving through Purkinje's network finds the ventricular cell with a transmembrane resting potential of -90 mV. At that threshold level, the impulse opens up the fast sodium channel and sodium (Na^+) ions enter the cell, which becomes depolarized rapidly, with a rebound reverse polarity of about $+20$ mV (phase 0). At that time, the sudden influx of Na^+ stops and there is a rapid drop of the potential (phase 1). The opening of a slow calcium channel allows for an influx of calcium (Ca^{2+}) ions, which maintain the cell in a relatively depolarized state for a while (phase 2). At the end of this phase, there is an efflux of potassium (K^+) ions to the outside of the cell, with rapid return to the resting potential of -90 mV (phase 3). However, this new state of repolarization is different from that before the onset of the TAP. The changes in intracellular Na^+ and K^+ concentration that have occurred in phases 0 through 3 must be restored to previous levels. This occurs during phase 4, thanks to a special pump mechanism that transports Na^+ ions from the inside to the outside of the cell and brings K^+ ions into the cell. The ionic flux during phase 4 does not alter significantly the transmembrane resting potential (Fig. 35–6A).

In the SA node, the ionic concentrations

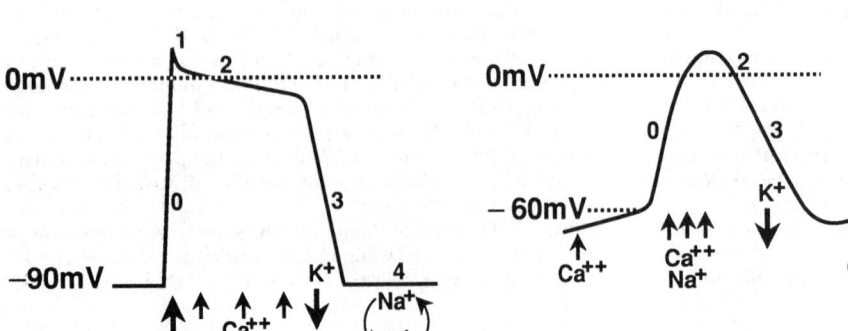

FIGURE 35–6. Transmembrane action potentials of the ventricle (*A*) and of the SA node (*B*).

A   B

throughout the cardiac cycle are different. During diastole, there is a gradual influx of Ca^{2+} and K^+ ions across the membrane, which causes the transmembrane resting potential during diastole to be less negative than in other cells. At the threshold level of -60 mV, there is a faster influx of Ca^{2+} and Na^+, causing a TAP whose rise and fall are not as steep as in the ventricular cells. Indeed, phase 0 is gradual, phase 1 is not noticeable, and phases 2 and 3 are also gradual and merged into one (Fig. 35–6B).

The ionic conditions across the cell membrane are critical determinants of the automaticity of all myocardial cells. This is the reason why arrhythmias may occur whenever the local extracellular or intracellular concentrations of Na^+, Ca^{2+}, or K^+ are different from normal. Sympathetic or parasympathetic tone, hypoxia, and certain drugs affect the rate of rise of the transmembrane resting potential during diastole, thus changing considerably the normal electrical conditions and eventually causing cardiac arrhythmias.

The conductivity of electrical impulses depends on the state of refractoriness of the conduction system. During phases 0, 1, 2, and the early part of 3, the cells cannot respond to any stimulus (absolute refractory period). However, in the latter stage of phase 3, the arrival of a strong impulse may produce a new TAP (relative refractory period). Thus, changes in conductivity may occur under pathologic circumstances if an impulse arrives at a portion of the conduction system earlier than normal in the cardiac cycle. If the cells are in the relative refractory period, the impulse may be transmitted, but if they are in the absolute refractory period, the impulse may be blocked.

Another important phenomenon that explains the genesis of some arrhythmias is the *re-entry* mechanism. Conduction through Purkinje's branches usually proceeds in anterograde fashion (Fig. 35–7A). Should an increase in refractoriness

occur in one branch (because of hypoxia or electrolyte changes), the anterograde conduction through that branch may be blocked but an impulse may arrive later and retrogradely via a connecting branch. The previously blocked area then may no longer be refractory, and thus allows repeated re-entry impulses in the conducting circuit (Fig. 35–7B). This re-entry phenomenon explains the ventricular tachycardias in myocardial infarction and the episodes of supraventricular tachycardia that are common in the pre-excitation syndromes of Wolff-Parkinson-White or Lown-Ganong-Levine syndrome.

ETIOLOGY

Cardiac arrhythmias may result from disturbances in (1) automaticity; (2) conductivity, including re-entry; and (3) both automaticity and conductivity. The following are common causes of arrhythmia:

1. *Changes in autonomic nervous tone.* The sympathetic system increases automaticity and conductivity. The parasympathetic system has opposite effects, but an increased vagal tone may slow down the SA node so much that a secondary pacemaker (in the AV node or even in the ventricle) may take over.

2. *Organic or functional lesions of the central nervous system.* These may affect the normal activity of the cardiac regulatory centers, disturb the balance between sympathetic and parasympathetic tone, and produce arrhythmias.

3. *Electrolyte disturbances.* Hyperkalemia, hypokalemia, hypomagnesemia, and hypocalcemia are the most common electrolyte disturbances that significantly alter the ionic conditions across the cell membrane and therefore enhance or suppress cardiac automaticity or conductivity or both.

4. *Myocardial disturbances.* Ischemia, hypoxia, injury, and inflammation may change automaticity, conductivity, or both. These lesions are not evenly distributed throughout the heart, so ectopic foci may produce TAPs unsynchronized with the pacemaker. Also, there may be localized areas of anterograde block, a condition that facilitates an abnormal re-entry process and subsequent tachycardia.

5. *Congestive heart failure.* In this condition, there are profound changes in oxygen concentration, pH, and electrolytes that alter the transmembrane resting potentials.

6. *Drugs.* Digitalis, antiarrhythmic agents, and sympathomimetic and psychotropic drugs cause changes in automaticity or conductivity or both. Excessive levels of these drugs in the blood may disturb the cardiac rhythm and cause undesirable arrhythmias.

7. *Endocrine disorders.* Thyrotoxicosis, myx-

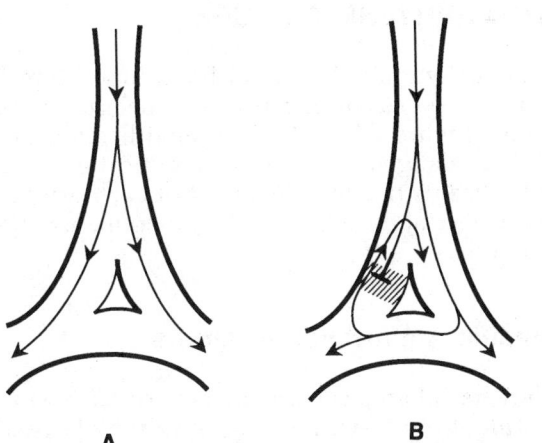

FIGURE 35–7. Re-entry mechanism in Purkinje's fiber. *A,* Normal anterograde conduction without reentry. *B,* Anterograde and re-entry conduction as a result of a block in one of the pathways.

edema, hyperparathyroidism, and pheochromocytoma are well-known causes of arrhythmia secondary to the extracellular metabolic changes that occur in these diseases.

8. *Miscellaneous causes.* Pulmonary embolism, hypertension, shock, anoxemia, anemia, and other conditions frequently cause arrhythmias because of secondary metabolic changes at the extracellular level. Also, the irritation of vagal receptors in the throat or in the tracheobronchial tree may explain the frequent occurrence of arrhythmias during bronchoscopy, gastroscopy, or nasopharyngeal suctioning in unanesthetized persons.

STEPS IN THE RECOGNITION OF ARRHYTHMIAS

Whenever an electrocardiogram (ECG) is obtained under usual circumstances, a strip of lead II is available for analysis of the rate and rhythm. In the case of patients who are monitored continuously in an intensive care unit or during regular activities by means of a Holter monitor, a beat-by-beat analysis of the cardiac rate and rhythm may be done from one of the selected chest leads. Regardless of the available lead, it is useful to analyze the ECG by answering the following questions:

1. *Heart rate:* Is it relatively constant or irregular?

2. *P-P and R-R intervals:* Are they consistently equal or variable from beat to beat? Are they identical to or different from each other?

3. *P-QRS-T sequence:* Is it normal? Is there a P wave not followed by a QRS complex and T wave, or, conversely, is there a QRS complex not preceded by a P wave?

4. *Atrial premature beats or premature atrial complexes:* Are there P waves that occur earlier than normal, and, if so, are they followed by the usual QRS complex and T wave or by an aberrantly conducted ventricular activation? Are they occurring at random or periodically?

5. *Ventricular premature beats, premature ventricular complexes, or extrasystoles:* Are there QRS complexes and T waves that occur earlier than normal in the cardiac cycle, are not preceded by a P wave, and have a configuration or duration that is different from the preceding or following beats? Are they occurring at random or periodically?

6. *Configuration of P waves, QRS complexes, and T waves:* Is the configuration of each one normal for the lead that is being monitored?

7. *Duration of the time intervals:* Are the standard time intervals normal for the prevailing heart rate?

Special analysis of arrhythmias with electrophysiologic stimulation (EPS) may be necessary in complex cases.

TABLE 35–28.   CLASSIFICATION OF ARRHYTHMIAS

Atrial Arrhythmias
Sinus bradycardia
Sinus tachycardia
Sinus arrhythmia
Sinus pause
Atrial standstill
Nonsinus atrial rhythm
Wandering atrial pacemaker
Atrial premature beats or premature atrial contractions
Multifocal atrial tachycardia
Paroxysmal atrial tachycardia
Atrial flutter
Atrial fibrillation

Junctional Arrhythmias
Junctional premature beats or premature junctional contractions
Junctional or nodal rhythm

Ventricular Arrhythmias
Ventricular premature beats, or premature ventricular contractions, or extrasystoles
Ventricular tachycardia
Ventricular fibrillation

Arrhythmias Caused by Atrioventricular Conduction Defects
First-degree AV block
Second-degree AV block
    Mobitz Type I (Wenckebach)
    Mobitz Type II
Third-degree AV block (complete) with AV dissociation

Rhythms Produced by Artificial Pacemakers

Special Clinical Syndromes That Predispose to Arrhythmias
Pre-excitation syndromes: Wolff-Parkinson-White and Lown-Ganong-Levine
Sick sinus syndrome
Mitral valve prolapse syndrome
Prolonged Q-T interval syndrome

CLASSIFICATION

Table 35–28 shows a classification of the typical patterns of arrhythmia.

ANTIARRHYTHMIC DRUGS

Antiarrhythmic drugs can be grouped into five basic classes according to their specific mode of action. Figure 35–8 shows a modification of the original Vaughan Williams classification system and presents the specific effect of each drug class on the TAP at the SA node, AV junction, or ventricular cells.

Specific Antiarrhythmic Drugs

Several pharmacologic agents are useful in the treatment of arrhythmias because they have a favorable influence on the slope or duration of the various phases of the TAP. Some antiarrhythmic drugs also may have a favorable influence on the refractory period of the conduction system. The ef-

Class I: Inhibit fast Na^{++} channel.
Reduce rate of rise of phase O.

I-A: **Widen TAP**

Disopyramide
Procainamide
Quinidine

I-B: **Shorten TAP**

Lidocaine
Mexiletine
Phenytoin
Tocainide

I-C: **Do not change TAP duration**

Flecainide
Propafenone

Other: **Slow conduction but not repolarization.**
Do not fit in IA,B, C above

Moricizine

Class II: Beta Adrenergic Blockers.
Decrease rate of slow repolarization
in phase 4.

Acebutolol	*Propranolol*
Atenolol	*Sotalol (Class III also)*
Esmolol	*Timolol*
Metoprolol	

Class III: Widen TAP duration like Class IA,
but do not affect fast Na$^+$ channel.

Amiodarone
Bretylium
Sotalol ** (Class II also)

Class IV: Ca^{++} channel blockers.
Slow rate of depolarization and
speed up repolarization.

Diltiazem
Verapamil

Class V: Other Agents

Glycosides:	*Magnesium sulfate*
Digoxin	*Anticholinergic and sympathomimetic drugs:*
Adenosine	*Atropine*
	Epinephrine

FIGURE 35–8. Vaughan Williams classification of antiarrhythmic drugs and mechanism of action. (Modified from Vaughan Williams EM: A classification of antiarrhythmic drug actions reassessed after a decade of new drugs. J Clin Pharmacol 24:129, 1984; *and* Sandóe E, Sigurd B: Arrhythmia: Diagnosis and Management, A Clinical Electrocardiographic Guide. St. Galen, Verlag für Fachmedien, 1984.)

fect of these drugs on various sites of the conduction system is shown in Figure 35–9.

Other Antiarrhythmic Drugs

Cardiac Glycosides

In addition to their positive inotropic effect (improved cardiac contractility), digitalis and other glycosides have important antiarrhythmic properties because they increase vagal tone and decrease sympathetic tone. As a result, there is a slow discharge rate of the SA node (bradycardia), a decrease in the automaticity of atrial and junctional pacemakers, and a prolongation of the refractory period at the AV node. This is usually manifested by a prolonged P-R interval. At therapeutic doses,

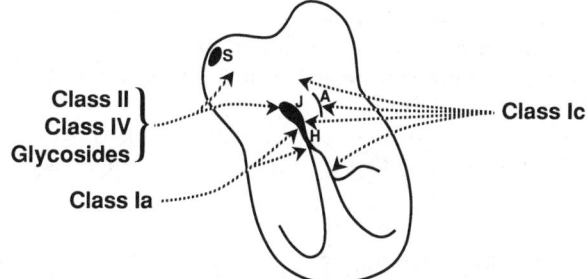

FIGURE 35–9. Site of action of antiarrhythmic drugs on conductivity. Class IC drugs are also effective in blocking re-entry through the aberrant pathway in preexcitation syndromes. S, sinoatrial node; J, atrioventricular junction; H, bundle of His and its branches; A, aberrant pathway in pre-excitation syndrome.

digitalis speeds up the repolarization process (short Q-T time and slight ST segment depression).

Adenosine

Adenosine is a highly effective antiarrhythmic drug because it terminates many re-entrant supraventricular tachycardias. It has fast action and disappears from the circulation within seconds.

Magnesium Sulfate

Magnesium sulfate is an antiarrhythmic agent that may be useful to control the ventricular tachycardia of the *torsades de pointes* type.

Anticholinergic and Sympathomimetic Drugs

Atropine and epinephrine are used widely to reestablish an adequate cardiac rhythm in cases of severe bradycardia, pulseless electrical activity (electromechanical dissociation), and asystole.

Dosage and Administration

Table 35–29 presents a summary of the drugs currently approved for the treatment of arrhythmias in the United States. Only the most common indications and recommended dosages for adults are listed. Some drugs, especially those of class IC, should be used with great caution by physicians who have limited experience with them. The administration of drugs for the treatment of severe arrhythmias should be done under careful monitoring and ready access to countershock or pacing equipment. The reader should be familiar with the most recent American Heart Association recommendations for advanced cardiac life support.

RECOGNITION OF SPECIFIC PATTERNS

Atrial Arrhythmias

Sinus Bradycardia

MECHANISM. The pacemaker is at the SA node, but the impulses are produced at a slow rate as a result of increased vagal tone, decreased sympathetic tone, or both.

ETIOLOGY. Sinus bradycardia is physiologically normal in athletes and in pregnant women.

In others, it may be due to increased intracranial pressure, lesions in the brain stem or medulla, coronary artery disease, myxedema, or jaundice. Episodes of sinus bradycardia may occur in the early stage of recovery from general anesthesia and during stimulation of vagal receptors of the throat or trachea.

CHARACTERISTICS. The heart rate is below 60 beats/min. The P-QRS-T sequence is normal. All complexes appear normal. The P-P and R-R intervals are equal. The P-R interval may be increased but is appropriate for the heart rate (Fig. 35–10). In many cases of bradycardia, the U wave is visible in practically all the leads.

SYMPTOMS. There are no symptoms, but dizziness or syncope may occur.

TREATMENT. If severe, sinus bradycardia may require atropine, or even pacing. Isoproterenol is no longer considered a drug of choice for the management of arrhythmias.

Sinus Tachycardia

MECHANISM. The impulses originate at the node at a rapid rate because of increased sympathetic tone, decreased vagal tone, or both.

ETIOLOGY. Sinus tachycardia occurs physiologically under the influence of exercise or emotion. It may be produced voluntarily by some persons. It occurs in febrile states, anemia, thyrotoxicosis, shock, congestive heart failure, hypoglycemia, and the adrenergic state of prolonged immobilization. It also may be a reaction to drugs such as atropine, nitrites, or quinidine, to alcohol, or to substances such as tobacco, caffeine, or cocaine.

CHARACTERISTICS. The heart rate is over 100 beats/min. The P-P and R-R intervals are equal. The P-QRS-T sequence is normal. All complexes appear normal. The P-R interval may be shortened but appropriate for the rate (Fig. 35–11).

SYMPTOMS. There are no symptoms except possibly a sensation of racing of the heart.

TREATMENT. Sinus tachycardia is treated by correcting the underlying cause. For example, use of sympathomimetic drugs or irritating substances should be discontinued.

Sinus Arrhythmia

MECHANISM. Impulses originate at the SA node at a varying rate because of cyclic changes in vagal tone.

ETIOLOGY. The most common cause of sinus arrhythmia is respiration. It may be normal in chil-

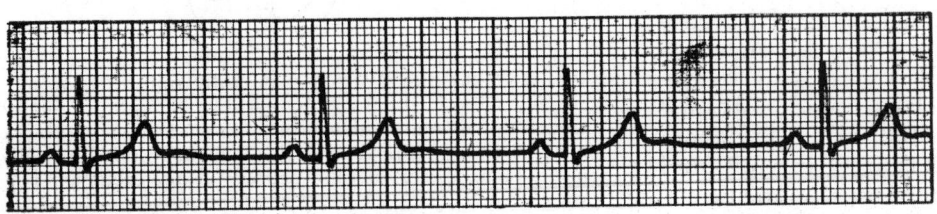

FIGURE 35–10. Sinus bradycardia.

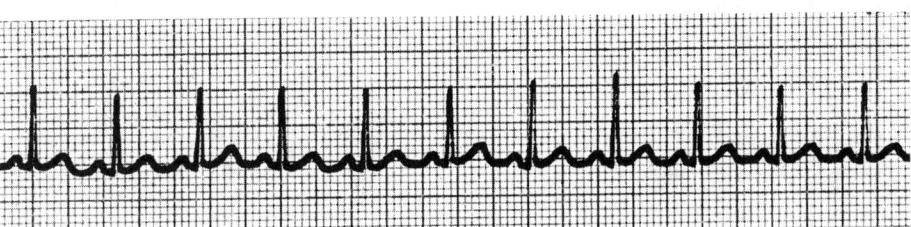

FIGURE 35–11. Sinus tachycardia.

dren and adolescents, as well as adults during sleep. It may be a pathologic manifestation of increased intracranial pressure or digitalis effect.

CHARACTERISTICS. The P-QRS-T sequence is normal. All complexes are normal. P-P and R-R intervals vary, becoming shorter during inspiration and longer during expiration. However, the P-P and R-R intervals of the same cardiac cycle are identical (Fig. 35–12).

SYMPTOMS. There are usually no symptoms. Physicians often unnecessarily request an ECG in a young, healthy person because of arrhythmic heart sounds. The respiratory origin of this arrhythmia may be detected easily by determining if the sounds speed up and slow down synchronously with respirations.

TREATMENT. No treatment is required.

Sinus Pause

MECHANISM. There is a transient inhibition of the SA node because of a sudden increase in vagal tone.

ETIOLOGY. Sinus pause may be noticeable during deep sleep. It may be due to stimulation of vagal receptors while gagging or during suction of the oropharynx or trachea. It may be a manifestation of a sensitive carotid sinus. Sometimes it is due to organic changes in the SA node, which then is not capable of regularly producing TAPs, as occurs in the sick sinus syndrome (see later).

CHARACTERISTICS. There are random episodes of prolonged P-P interval. The prevalent rhythm is of sinus origin, or there is a slight sinus arrhythmia (Fig. 35–13).

SYMPTOMS. Symptoms are frequently unnoticed by the patient, but there may be dizziness if the pause is long.

TREATMENT. No treatment is required if the pause occurs infrequently and is not long. If the pause is long, it may be treated in the same way as an atrial standstill.

Atrial Standstill (Sinus Arrest)

MECHANISM. In cases of sinus arrest because of vagal stimulation or an organic SA block, a nodal or ventricular pacemaker may take over and produce escape beats. Sometimes the escape beats occur at an accelerated rate.

ETIOLOGY. Atrial standstill is usually due to fibrosis of the SA node or to digitalis or quinidine intoxication. It may be a manifestation of sick sinus syndrome (see later).

CHARACTERISTICS. There are randomly occurring periods of absent P waves with junctional or ventricular escape beats (Fig. 35–14).

SYMPTOMS. There are usually no symptoms, although dizziness or blackout spells may occur.

TREATMENT. The patient eventually may require pacing. In case of sinus arrest, atropine or epinephrine may be effective in restoring pacemaker activity.

Nonsinus Atrial Rhythm

MECHANISM. There is a regularly activated low atrial pacemaker that is not at the SA node but is somewhat remote from the AV node. A common location is the coronary sinus.

ETIOLOGY. There is no specific cause, but nonsinus atrial rhythm may reflect an inability of the SA node to produce TAPs.

CHARACTERISTICS. The heart rate is normal. P waves in leads II, III, and often aVF are inverted. The P-R interval is usually normal. The QRS complexes and T waves are normal (Fig. 35–15).

SYMPTOMS. There are usually no symptoms.

TREATMENT. No treatment is required.

Wandering Atrial Pacemaker

MECHANISM. The pacemaker shifts from one atrial location to another sometimes in a cyclic pattern.

ETIOLOGY. Wandering atrial pacemaker may occur physiologically as a result of changes in vagal tone. It is more frequent in young people.

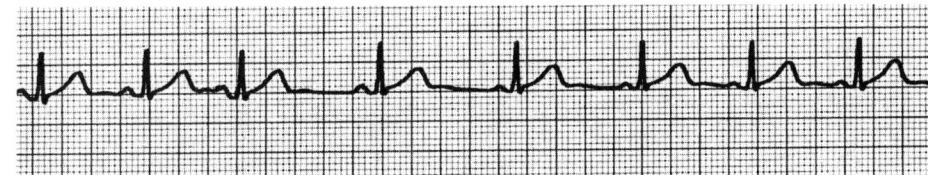

FIGURE 35–12. Sinus arrhythmia caused by respiration. Beats 1 through 3 and 7 and 8 coincide with inspiration. Beats 4 through 6 coincide with expiration.

TABLE 35–29. INDICATIONS, ROUTE OF ADMINISTRATION, AND DOSAGES OF ANTIARRHYTHMIC DRUGS*

Type of Drug	Primary Indication†	Secondary Indication†	Initial Dose‡	Maintenance Dose‡	Plasma Level (μg/mL)	Contraindications/Complications§
Class I						
Class IA						
Disopyramide	VPB, VT	Prophylaxis VPB	P.O.: 100–200 mg q 6 hr	P.O.: 100–200 mg q 6–8 hr	2–5	Congestive failure, conduction defects, prolonged Q-T interval, proarrhythmia (*torsades*), atropine effect
Procainamide	VPB, VT	Prophylaxis AF, AT, VT, AT in W-P-W	I.V.: 30 mg/min Max: 1200 mg or QRS 50% wider or Q-T prolonged	P.O.: 500–1000 mg q 4–6 hr	4–10	Prolonged QRS complex, proarrhythmia (*torsades*), hypotension, LE syndrome
Quinidine	APB, AF, VPB, VT	Prophylaxis AF	I.V.: 10 mg/kg P.O.: 250–500 mg q 4–6 hr	P.O.: 300–600 mg q 12 hr (gluconate) P.O.: 200–400 mg q 4–6 hr (sulfate)	2–5	Conduction defects, prolonged Q-T interval, proarrhythmia (*torsades*), idiosyncrasy, myasthenia
Class IB						
Lidocaine	VPB, VT, VF	Prophylaxis VPB, VT, VF	I.V.: 1.5 mg/kg bolus, repeat q 3–5 min Max: 3 mg/kg	I.V.: 2–4 mg/min	1.5–5	CNS effects and seizures
Mexiletine	VPB, VT	Prophylaxis VPB, AT in W-P-W	P.O.: 400 mg once P.O.: 100–200 mg q 8 hr	P.O.: 100–300 mg q 6–12 hr	0.5–2	CNS effects, liver dysfunction, GI upset
Phenytoin	VPB, VT (digitalis induced)	Prophylaxis VPB	I.V.: 50–100 mg q 5 min Max: 1000 mg	P.O.: 200–400 mg/day	5–20	CNS effects, blood dyscrasias, rash
Tocainide	VPB, VT	Prophylaxis VPB	P.O.: 200–400 mg q 8 hr	P.O.: 200–600 mg q 8 hr	3–10	CNS effects, blood dyscrasias, GI upset, interstitial pneumonitis
Class IC						
Flecainide	Prophylaxis AT	AT in W-P-W, AF Acute	P.O.: 50 mg q 12 hr Max: 150 mg q 12 hr	≤300 mg/day	0.2–1.0	Avoid long-term use Proarrhythmia effect, aggravates congestive heart failure, interaction with class II Do not use in asymptomatic ventricular arrhythmias post-MI
Propafenone	VPB, VT (sustained)		P.O.: 200 mg q 8 hr	150–300 q 8 hr	Not established	Avoid long-term use Proarrhythmia effect, aggravates congestive heart failure, interaction with class II Do not use in asymptomatic ventricular arrhythmias post-MI Metallic taste, dysgeusia, GI upset, bronchospasm
Class I—Other						
Moricizine	VPB, VT		P.O.: 200 mg q 8 hr	200–300 mg q 8 hr	Not established	Conduction defects, proarrhythmia, congestive failure, headache Do not use in asymptomatic ventricular arrhythmias post-MI
Class II						
Acebutolol	Prophylaxis ST, AT, VPB			P.O.: 200–400 mg q 12 hr Max: 600–1200 mg/day	Not established	Bradycardia, conduction defects, congestive failure, hypotension, bronchospasm, ANA formation, LE syndrome

Drug	Arrhythmia	Prophylaxis	I.V. Dose	P.O. Dose	Therapeutic Level	Toxicity / Side Effects
Atenolol		Prophylaxis ST, AT, VPB		P.O.: 50–100 mg q 12 hr		Bradycardia, conduction defects, congestive failure, hypotension
Esmolol	AT, AF, VT		I.V.: 0.5 mg/kg slowly + 0.025–0.05 mg/kg/min		0.15–2	Bradycardia, conduction defects, congestive failure, hypotension, bronchospasm, pain at infusion site
Metoprolol		Prophylaxis ST, AT, VPB		P.O.: 50–100 mg q 8–12 hr		Bradycardia, conduction defects, congestive failure, hypotension
Propranolol	VPB, VT	Prophylaxis ST, AT, AF, VPB	I.V.: 0.5–1 mg slowly + 1 mg q 2 min; Max: 5 mg	P.O.: 10–80 mg q 6 hr	Not established	Bradycardia, conduction defects, congestive failure, hypotension, bronchospasm
Sotalol (class III also)						
Timolol		Prophylaxis ST, AT, VPB		P.O.: 5–10 mg q 12 hr		Bradycardia, conduction defects, congestive failure, hypotension
Class III						
Amiodarone	Recurrent VT & VF	AT in W-P-W	P.O.: 800–1600 mg/day for up to 3 weeks	P.O.: 100–400 mg/day	Not established	Not first-line drug. Bradycardia, conduction defects, other severe side effects (pulmonary)
Bretylium	VF		I.V.: 5 mg/kg bolus + 10 mg/kg q 5 min; Max: 30 mg/kg		Not established	Hypotension, sensitivity to catecholamines
Sotalol (class II also)	VPB, VT	Prophylaxis VT		80 mg q 12 hr; Max: 480–640 mg/day	Not established	Same as class II drugs, prolonged Q-T interval, proarrhythmia (*torsades*)
Class IV						
Diltiazem	AT, AF with digitalis		I.V.: 20 mg slowly + 30 mg in 15 min	P.O.: 30–120 mg q 8 hr		Hypotension, congestive failure
Verapamil	AT, AF with digitalis		I.V.: 2.5–5 mg slowly + 5–10 mg in 15–30 min; Max: 20 mg	P.O.: 40–120 mg q 6–8 hr	0.1–0.3	Pre-excitation syndromes, 2nd degree AV block, VT, hypotension, congestive failure, Stevens-Johnson syndrome
Class V: Other Agents						
Digoxin	AT-AF	Congestive failure	I.V.: 0.5 mg slowly + 0.25 mg q 4–6 hr; Max: 0.75–1.5 mg	P.O.: 0.125–0.5 mg/day	0.001–0.002	AF pre-excitation syndromes in adults, proarrhythmia, GI effects, abnormal vision
Adenosine	AT		I.V.: 6 mg rapid + 12 mg in 1–2 min		Not established	Transient dyspnea, chest discomfort, hypotension
Magnesium Sulfate	VT (*torsades*)		I.V.: 1–2 gm			
Atropine	A		I.V.: 1 mg + 1 mg q 3–5 min; Max: 3 mg			
Epinephrine	A		I.V.: 1 mg + 1 mg q 3–5 min; Max: 3 mg			

*This table has been prepared according to recommendations published in *The Medical Letter* (1993:33 [Issue 846], 1993:34 [Issue 866], 1993:35 [Issue 893]) and the most recent Guidelines for Cardiopulmonary Resuscitation and Emergency Cardiac Care of the American Heart Association (JAMA 268:2171, 1992), with permission.

†A, asystole or pulseless electrical activity; AF, atrial flutter or fibrillation; APB, potentially lethal atrial premature beats; AT, supraventricular tachycardia; ST, sinus tachycardia; VF, ventricular fibrillation; VPB, potentially lethal ventricular premature beats; VT, sustained ventricular tachycardia; W-P-W, Wolff-Parkinson-White syndrome.

‡I.V., intravenous; P.O., oral; Max, maximum dose. CHILDREN: Doses should be calculated by body weight or body surface area. ELDERLY OR RENAL FAILURE PATIENTS: Usually will require 50 to 70 percent of adult doses.

§LE, Lupus erythematosus; CNS, central nervous system; GI, gastrointestinal; MI, myocardial infarction; ANA, antinuclear antibody.

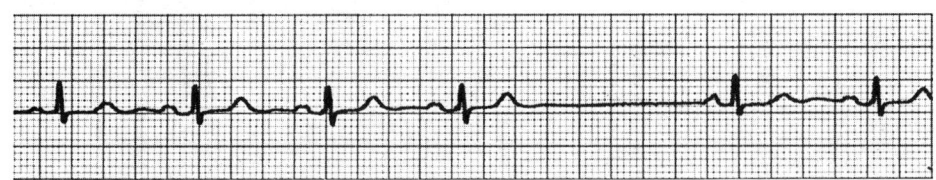

FIGURE 35–13. Sinus pause. The fourth beat is followed by a long pause before a return of normal sinus rhythm.

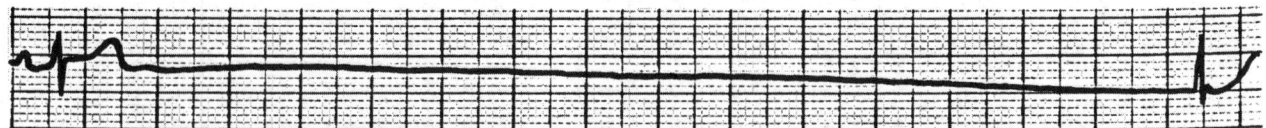

FIGURE 35–14. Atrial standstill (sinus arrest) followed by a junctional escape. (From Sandóe E, Sigurd B: Arrhythmia: Diagnosis and Management, A Clinical Electrocardiographic Guide. St. Galen, Verlag für Fachmedien, 1984, with permission.)

CHARACTERISTICS.   The P waves change in configuration. The P-R intervals vary from beat to beat. The P-P and R-R intervals vary also. The QRS complexes and T waves are normal (Fig. 35–16).

SYMPTOMS.   There are usually no symptoms.

TREATMENT.   No treatment is required.

Atrial Premature Beats or Premature Atrial Contractions

MECHANISM.   Random impulses are generated by one or more irritable atrial foci, sometimes with a re-entry phenomenon.

ETIOLOGY.   Atrial premature beats may be benign if they are due to emotion, fatigue, or central nervous system excitation. They may be due to the effects of alcohol, tobacco, caffeine, sympathomimetic drugs, or other stimulating substances. They also may indicate digitalis effect or the existence of foci of hypoxic myocardial cells.

CHARACTERISTICS.   There is random occurrence of abnormal P waves. The P-R interval in the premature beats is usually long. The QRS complexes are usually normal except when there is aberrant conduction to the ventricles. A compensatory pause (prolonged P-P interval) follows the atrial premature beat (Fig. 35–17).

SYMPTOMS.   There are usually no symptoms, although the patient may feel a thump in the chest.

TREATMENT.   No treatment is required if atrial premature beats are benign. If not, the cause of ectopic excitation should be eliminated. Occasion-

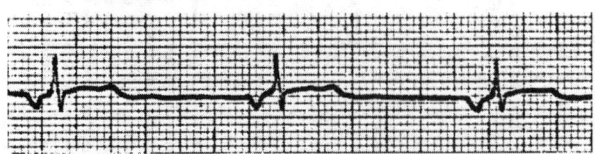

FIGURE 35–15. Nonsinus atrial rhythm. The pacemaker is located at the coronary sinus, causing the P waves on lead II to be negative.

ally there may be a need for treatment with a class I or III drug.

Multifocal Atrial Tachycardia

MECHANISM.   Random impulses originate irregularly and at a high rate in different points of the atria.

ETIOLOGY.   This arrhythmia occurs frequently in severe pulmonary disease.

CHARACTERISTICS.   There is a rapidly changing P wave configuration. The pattern resembles that of a wandering pacemaker, but the changes in P waves occur more randomly. The P-R, P-P, and R-R intervals are variable. The prevalent heart rate is fast (Fig. 35–18).

SYMPTOMS.   Symptoms of pulmonary disease are clinically evident.

TREATMENT.   It is necessary to correct the pulmonary condition. Digitalis may be tried cautiously. Other antiarrhythmic drugs are seldom effective, but a therapeutic trial with a calcium channel blocker may be warranted.

Paroxysmal Atrial Tachycardia (or Supraventricular Tachycardia)

MECHANISM.   TAPs are generated regularly and repeatedly in an ectopic focus at or near the AV node. They occur as a result of the re-entry phenomenon. Within the AV node, there is a longitudinal division of conduction fibers into α and β pathways. A block in the latter pathway causes re-entry of impulses within the node, with retrograde depolarization of the atria and anterograde depolarization of the ventricles through the normal conduction system. Patients with a pre-excitation syndrome (Wolff-Parkinson-White or Lown-Ganong-Levine) may have brief episodes of supraventricular tachycardia that require treatment if they persist for more than a few minutes.

ETIOLOGY.   This condition is usually pathologic. It may be congenital. Digitalis intoxication should be suspected if there is a block.

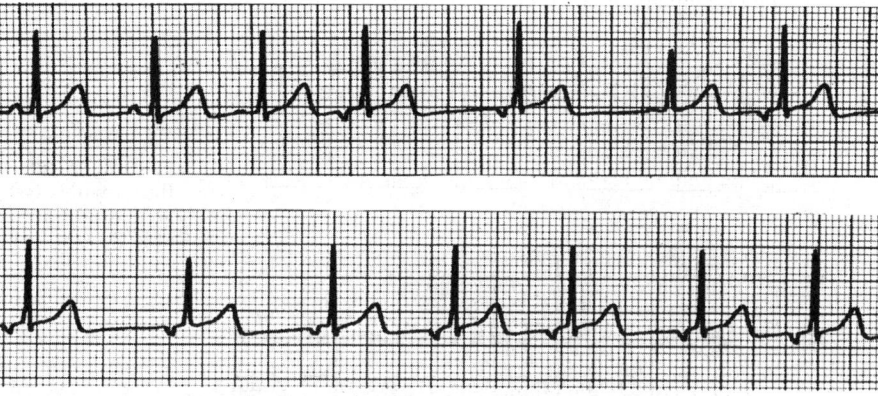

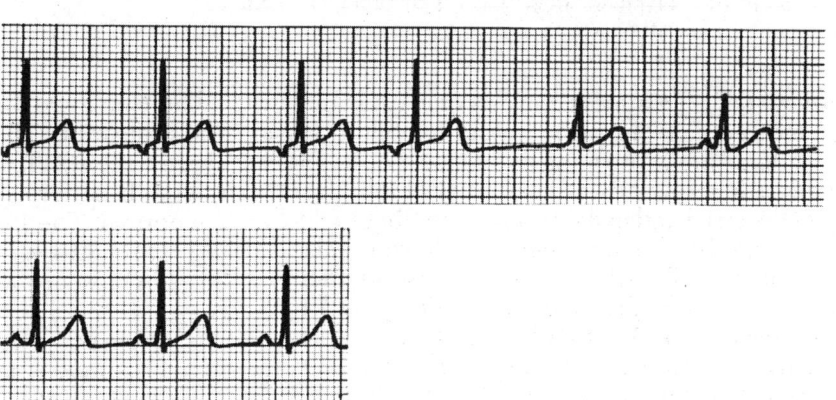

FIGURE 35–16. Wandering atrial pacemaker, shown on consecutive rhythm strip.

CHARACTERISTICS. The atrial rate is 160 to 220 beats/min. The P waves, if recognizable, are regular and often inverted. The QRS complexes are normal (except in cases of Wolff-Parkinson-White syndrome, in which the QRS complexes are wide and a Δ wave clearly is recognized). The R-R intervals are equal but short (Fig. 35–19).

SYMPTOMS. The patient notices thumping, fluttering, or palpitations that sometimes are associated with precordial pain, shortness of breath, or anxiety. Congestive heart failure precedes or follows the onset of paroxysmal atrial tachycardia.

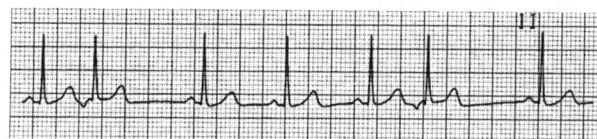

FIGURE 35–17. Atrial premature beats. The second and the sixth beats are produced by an ectopic atrial focus and are followed by a compensatory pause.

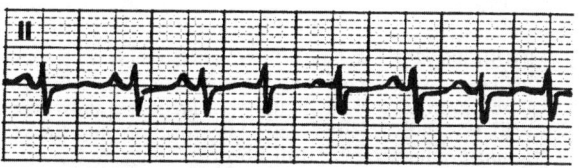

FIGURE 35–18. Multifocal atrial tachycardia. (From Sandóe E, Sigurd B: Arrhythmia: Diagnosis and Management, A Clinical Electrocardiographic Guide. St. Galen, Verlag für Fachmedien, 1984, with permission.)

A

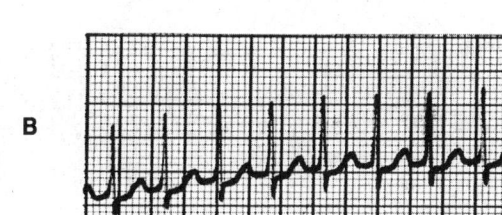

B

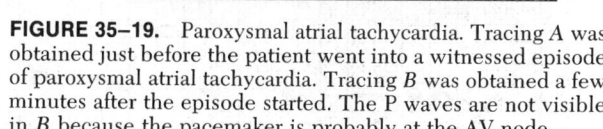

FIGURE 35–19. Paroxysmal atrial tachycardia. Tracing *A* was obtained just before the patient went into a witnessed episode of paroxysmal atrial tachycardia. Tracing *B* was obtained a few minutes after the episode started. The P waves are not visible in *B* because the pacemaker is probably at the AV node.

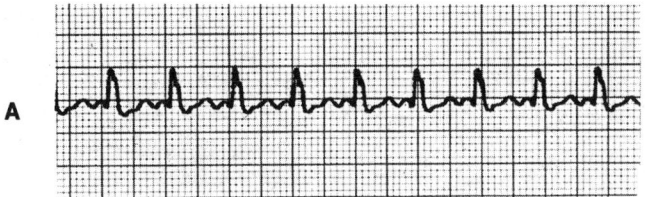
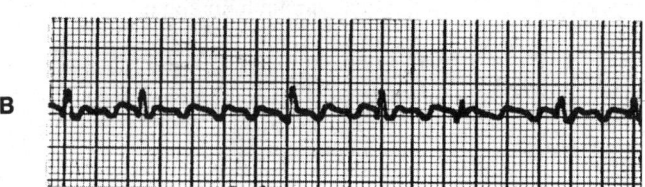

FIGURE 35–20. Atrial flutter. Tracing *A* shows a 2:1 atrial flutter with a fast ventricular rate. Tracing *B* shows a variable atrial flutter (4:1 or 3:1), which accounts for the variable R-R interval.

TREATMENT. Treatment consists of vagal stimulation and sedation. The first line of treatment includes adenosine intravenously because of its effectiveness in terminating the re-entry of impulses through the atrial and nodal conducting fibers. Calcium channel blockers (especially diltiazem) also may be used as first-line drugs because of their inhibition of AV node conduction. Verapamil is contraindicated in Wolff-Parkinson-White supraventricular tachycardia but may be used in cases of supraventricular tachycardia with narrow QRS complexes. Quinidine, procainamide, and disopyramide have been used effectively also. If there is no evidence of digitalis intoxication, digitalis may be indicated in cases of congestive heart failure or shock. If there is an acute myocardial infarction with a low or unstable blood pressure, synchronized cardioversion with a small energy current (100 to 300 joules) may be necessary.

Atrial Flutter

MECHANISM. An ectopic atrial focus produces rapid stimuli, which travel in circles in the atria. Only at the end of every second, third, or fourth atrial depolarization may the AV node be capable of conducting the impulse to the ventricles in a regular fashion.

ETIOLOGY. This process is usually pathologic and reflects organic heart disease.

CHARACTERISTICS. The atrial rate is fast (250 to 350 beats/min). The P waves are clearly visible and almost identical, and often produce the typical sawtooth pattern (F waves). The QRS complexes are normal. The P-P interval is very short, whereas the R-R interval is longer and regular (Fig. 35–20*A*), except when the ratio P:QRS varies between 4:1, 3:1, or 2:1 (Fig. 35–20*B*).

SYMPTOMS. There are usually no symptoms. If there are, they resemble those of paroxysmal atrial tachycardia if the ventricular rate is fast.

TREATMENT. The objective is to slow down the ventricular rate and convert to normal sinus rhythm or atrial fibrillation, which is more benign than flutter. This may be done with digitalis therapy, especially when there is congestive heart failure. One of the calcium channel blockers, such as diltiazem or verapamil, a β blocker, quinidine, or procainamide may be added to digitalis. If there is no change in 12 to 24 hours, cardioversion with a small energy current may be useful.

Atrial Fibrillation

MECHANISM. The atria depolarize from a variety of foci, which transmit impulses in a chaotic motion through random circular pathways.

ETIOLOGY. Atrial fibrillation frequently is associated with organic heart disease, but it may occur

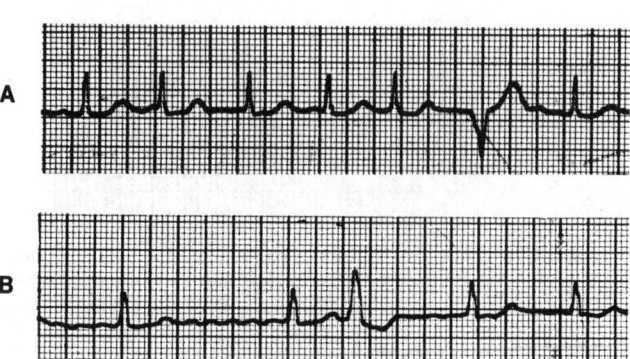

FIGURE 35–21. Atrial fibrillation. Tracing *A* shows atrial fibrillation with a fast ventricular response and one ventricular premature beat (sixth beat). Tracing *B* shows atrial fibrillation with a slower ventricular response and one ventricular premature beat (third beat).

as an occasional episode in young adults without demonstrated coronary artery disease.

CHARACTERISTICS. The P waves occur very rapidly and are not clearly identified or barely visible, and the baseline is irregular. The QRS complexes are normal, but sometimes there are randomly occurring abnormal QRS complexes resulting from transmission of atrial impulses through aberrant pathways. P-P intervals are not measurable, and R-R intervals are unequal. The predominant ventricular rate may be fast (Fig. 35–21A) or slow (Fig. 35–21B).

SYMPTOMS. Although sometimes the patient does not notice any symptoms, there may be a sensation of palpitations and, occasionally, dizziness and collapse. If there is associated congestive heart failure, the symptoms of this condition are obvious.

TREATMENT. The primary aim of treatment is to slow down the ventricular response. This may be accomplished with digitalis alone or in combination with either β blockers or calcium channel blockers. Digoxin may not be effective in patients in a hyperadrenergic state with congestive failure. In these cases, the first line of treatment is a calcium channel blocker. Class IA or IC drugs may be also used in combination with digitalis to reestablish a sinus rhythm. Cardioversion in a digitalized patient may be necessary to treat chronic fibrillation. It is important to administer anticoagulants to prevent the occurrence of emboli.

Junctional Arrhythmias

Junctional Premature Beats or Premature Junctional Contractions

MECHANISM. On a random basis, a premature beat may arise from the junctional (AV node) area. The location of the ectopic focus may be in the upper, middle, or lower portion of the junction.

ETIOLOGY. These arrhythmias are usually benign or an early manifestation of organic disease. They may be secondary to excitation or use of drugs or stimulating substances.

CHARACTERISTICS. An apparently normal or slightly abnormal QRS complex occurs earlier than usual in the cardiac cycle. The P wave is often inverted and precedes, is incorporated into, or follows the QRS complex, depending on the location of the ectopic focus. The P-P and R-R intervals are equal except in the prematurely occurring beat (Fig. 35–22).

SYMPTOMS. Symptoms are usually not noticeable except for a sensation of skipped beats.

TREATMENT. No treatment is required if the arrhythmias are benign.

Junctional or Nodal Rhythm

MECHANISM. The pacemaker is consistently at the AV junction, with retrograde conduction to the atria and antegrade transmission to the ventricles. The normal idiopathic junctional rhythm is slow, with a rate of 35 to 60 beats/min (junctional bradycardia). This rhythm may occur as an escape mechanism because of an extremely low or absent SA node activity. In some instances, there is an accelerated junctional rhythm at 60 to 100 beats/min because of enhanced junctional automaticity. In other instances, there is junctional tachycardia with a rate of 100 to 150 beats/min. If the rate is high, it may be difficult to distinguish junctional rhythm from atrial tachycardia because the P waves are not clearly seen in either case. Because of this, it may be preferable to use the nonspecific term *supraventricular tachycardia.*

ETIOLOGY. This rhythm is usually benign and may occur as a result of excitation.

CHARACTERISTICS. The rate may be slow, slightly accelerated, or tachycardic. All QRS complexes are normal. The P waves are negative in lead II and may precede, be incorporated into, or follow the QRS complex, depending on the location of the pacemaker within the junction. The P-P and R-R intervals are equal (Fig. 35–23).

SYMPTOMS. Symptoms are the same as those of bradycardia or tachycardia, depending on the predominant rate.

TREATMENT. No treatment is required except when there is tachycardia, in which case the treatment is similar to that of atrial tachycardia.

Ventricular Arrhythmias

Ventricular Premature Beats (VPBs), Premature Ventricular Contractions, or Extrasystoles

MECHANISM. An ectopic focus may randomly produce a TAP, which is transmitted throughout the ventricle outside of the regular conduction system. The so-called R-on-T phenomenon occurs when a VPB starts just before the preceding T

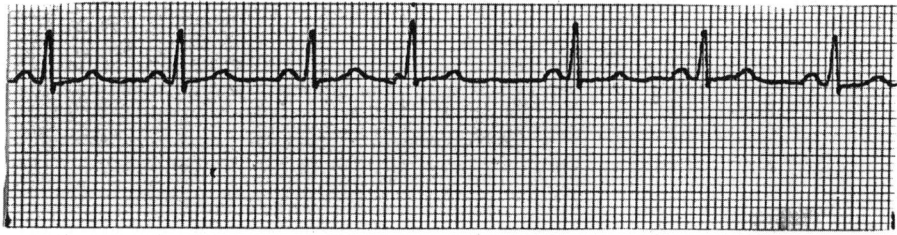

FIGURE 35–22. Junctional premature beat. The fourth beat originates at a middle nodal ectopic focus and it is followed by a compensatory pause.

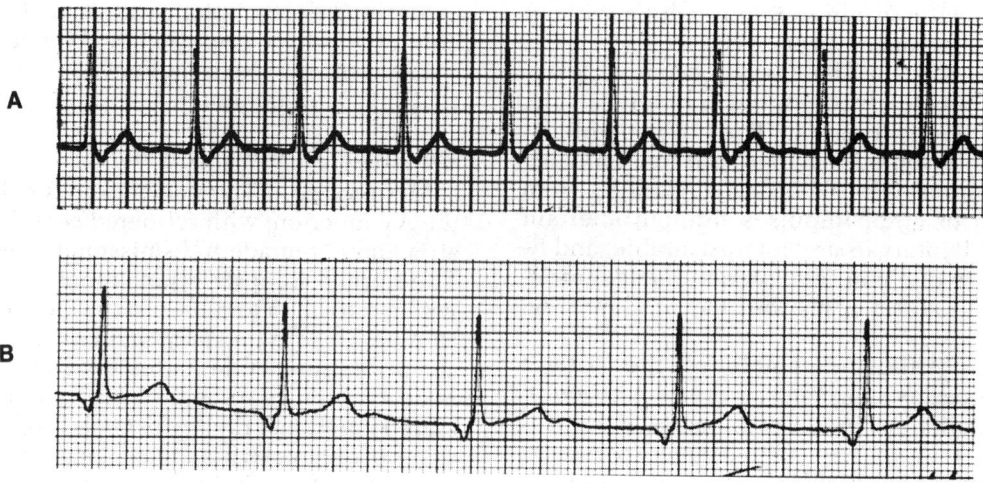

FIGURE 35–23. Junctional rhythm. Tracing *A* shows that the QRS complex has originated at the AV junction, and the P wave is produced in a retrograde fashion after the QRS complex. Tracing *B* shows a junctional rhythm with a pacemaker just above the AV node, causing an inverted P wave that precedes the QRS complex. The rate is slower in tracing *B* than *A*.

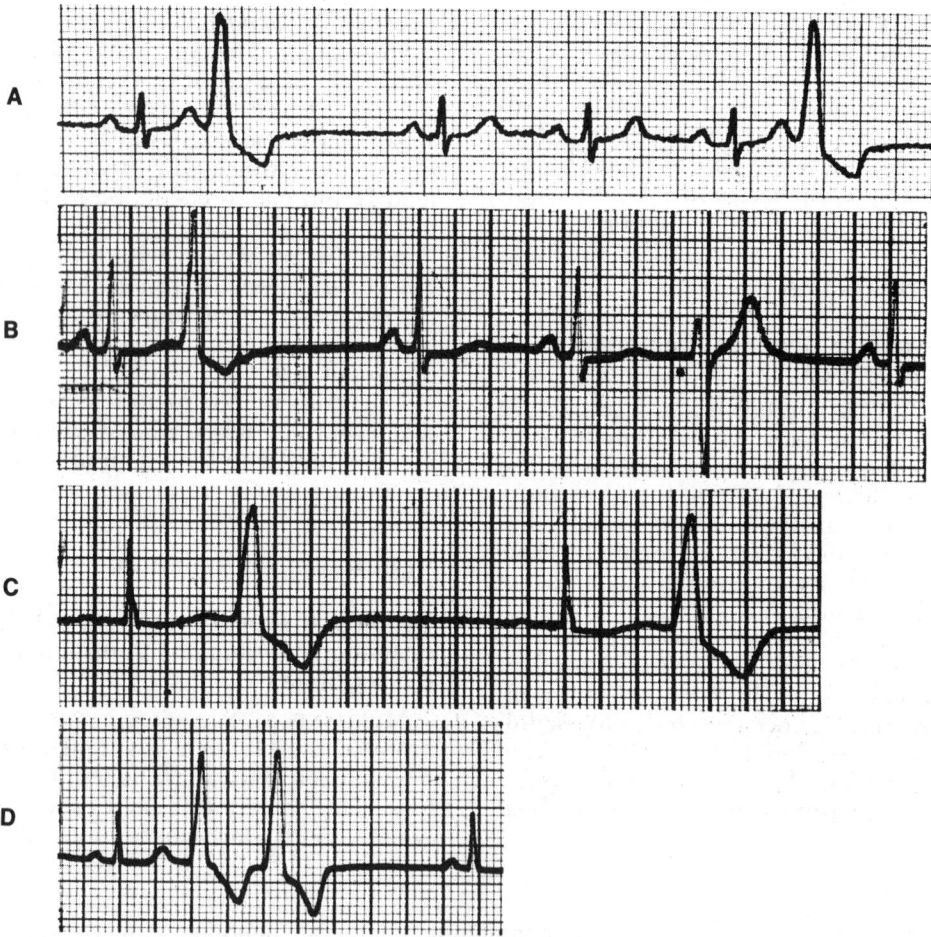

FIGURE 35–24. Ventricular premature beats. Tracing *A* shows two unifocal VPBs with a compensatory pause. Tracing *B* shows two VPBs that originate at different foci. Tracing *C* shows a bigeminal pattern with a normal QRS complex followed by a VPB (the prolonged P-R interval is probably due to digitalis). Tracing *D* shows a couplet of VPBs.

wave has returned to baseline. Sometimes two VPBs may occur in couplets or triplets, and it was previously thought that they heralded the imminent onset of ventricular tachycardia and fibrillation. However, there is no correlation between the so-called warning VPBs and the subsequent development of fibrillation.

ETIOLOGY. These arrhythmias may occur in otherwise healthy persons or during exercise. VPBs are considered benign if they are unifocal and occur at a rate of less than 1/min and 30/hr. If they are more frequent or if they are multifocal, occurring in couplets or triplets, they are considered to be potentially lethal. They actually may be produced by some antiarrhythmic drugs, which have a proarrhythmia adverse effect in some patients (especially class IC drugs and digitalis).

CHARACTERISTICS. The QRS complex is widened, notched, and slurred. There is no preceding P wave, but sometimes the P wave is seen following the QRS complex as a result of retrograde conduction. The T wave is usually opposite in direction to the QRS complex. The P-P and R-R intervals are equal and regular except at the prematurely occurring beat because of a compensatory pause. This pause is not seen when there is an underlying bradycardia, and the VPB may be interpolated within the regular cardiac cycle. Unifocal VPBs always have the same QRS configuration (Fig. 35–24*A*). Multifocal VPBs have varying configurations (Fig. 35–24*B*). In digitalis intoxication, the existence of a recurring pattern of a normal QRS complex followed by a VPB constitutes a pattern of *bigeminy* (Fig. 35–24*C*). Two consecutive VPBs occurring without compensatory pause are referred to as *couplets* (Fig. 35–24*D*).

SYMPTOMS. Symptoms are the same as in other premature beats.

TREATMENT. Treatment is the same as for atrial or junctional premature beats. The administration of a β blocker or one of the class IB, C, or A drugs (in that order of priority) may be effective.

Ventricular Tachycardia

MECHANISM. Ventricular tachycardia occurs when at least three rapid consecutive beats are produced by TAPs that originate at a ventricular ectopic focus. The ectopy may occur because of enhanced ventricular automaticity or a re-entry phenomenon through an area of Purkinje's network affected by a focal injury.

ETIOLOGY. Ventricular tachycardia is commonly associated with myocardial infarction, but it also is associated with other serious heart diseases, ventricular aneurysm, and digitalis intoxication.

CHARACTERISTICS. There are regularly occurring, broad QRS complexes, with T waves moving in the opposite direction from them. There are no visible P waves. The rate is faster than 120 beats/min, usually 160 to 250 beats/min (Fig. 35–25).

A special type of ventricular tachycardia is re-

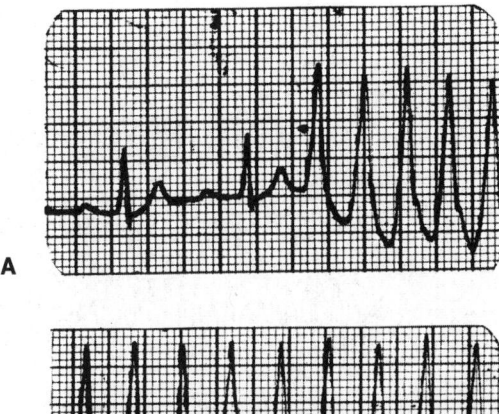

A

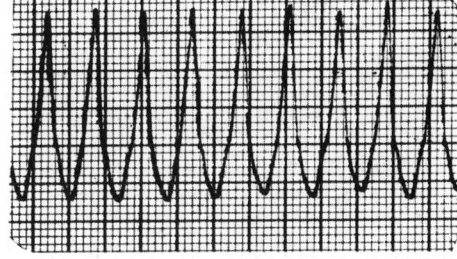

B

FIGURE 35–25. Ventricular tachycardia. Tracing *A* shows a normal sinus rhythm with a first-degree AV block followed by ventricular tachycardia. Tracing *B*, obtained 1 minute later, shows sustained ventricular tachycardia.

ferred to as *torsades de pointes,* which is characterized by cyclic changes in the polarity of the QRS complexes (Fig. 35–26). This ventricular tachycardia may occur in myocardial infarction or in patients with a congenital or acquired prolonged Q-T interval. Electrolyte disturbances or antiarrhythmic (class IA) or psychotropic drugs may cause severe prolongation of the Q-T interval. More recently, it has been reported that some antihistamines (terfenadine and astemizole) at very high doses or in conjunction with drugs that slow their metabolism may cause tachyarrhythmias, including *torsades de pointes.*

SYMPTOMS. The main symptom is a sensation of racing of the heart. There may be manifestations of unstable cardiac function.

TREATMENT. If the tachycardia is sustained but the patient is stable, an intravenous bolus of 60 to 100 mg of lidocaine, followed by a drip of 0.1% to 0.2% lidocaine solution, at 100 mL/hr, may be required. Thereafter, prevention with a β blocker is indicated. In the unstable patient, cardioversion may be necessary after appropriate sedation. The combination of a temporary pacemaker with an intravenous lidocaine drip may be necessary. *Torsades de pointes* tachycardia usually responds to the administration of magnesium sulfate (1 to 2 grams in 100 mL of 5% dextrose and water). If refractory, it may require the administration of isoproterenol intravenously (2 to 10 μg/min, titrated until there is a conversion to a supraventricular rhythm).

Ventricular Fibrillation

MECHANISM. A chaotic ventricular depolarization produced by multiple ectopic foci depolarizes

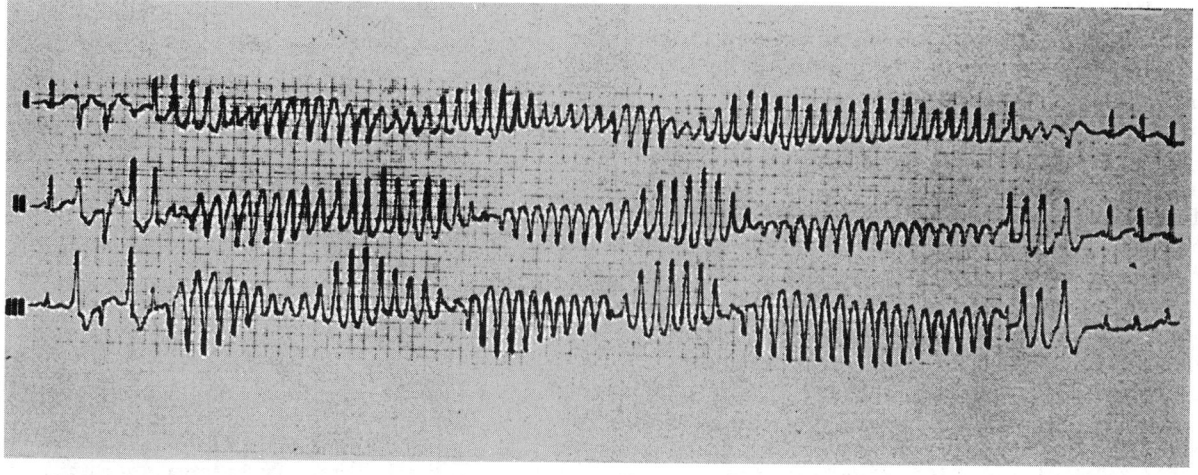

FIGURE 35–26. Ventricular tachycardia, *torsades de pointes*. At the beginning of this simultaneous recording of leads I, II, and III, several ectopic ventricular beats occur. A ventricular tachycardia with a rhythmic change in the QRS direction follows until the last few beats, which are of sinus origin. (From Krikler DM, Curry PVL: Torsade de pointes, an atypical ventricular tachycardia. Br Heart J 38:128, 1976, with permission.)

the surrounding areas in a random fashion in ventricular fibrillation. There is no emptying of the ventricles, and ventricular fibrillation is invariably fatal unless it is corrected by immediate defibrillation. Appropriately applied cardiopulmonary resuscitation maneuvers may empty the ventricles effectively and allow for survival until a countershock may be applied.

ETIOLOGY. Ventricular fibrillation occurs in severe myocardial disease. When it develops more than 48 hours after myocardial infarction, it has a very poor prognosis.

CHARACTERISTICS. There are erratic voltages without discernible P waves or QRS complexes. Whenever the voltage changes are of appreciable magnitude, the condition is referred to as coarse fibrillation (Fig. 35–27A), but when the voltage changes are small the condition is referred to as fine fibrillation (Fig. 35–27B).

SYMPTOMS. The patient is in a state of cardiogenic shock.

TREATMENT. Cardiopulmonary resuscitation and defibrillation with DC countershocks are needed immediately. A precordial thump may be an effective defibrillating maneuver in the case of a witnessed arrest (i.e., one that occurs while the patient is being examined or treated). Epinephrine, lidocaine, and bretyllium, when used in this sequential order, are useful intravenous pharmacologic adjuvants to DC countershocks.

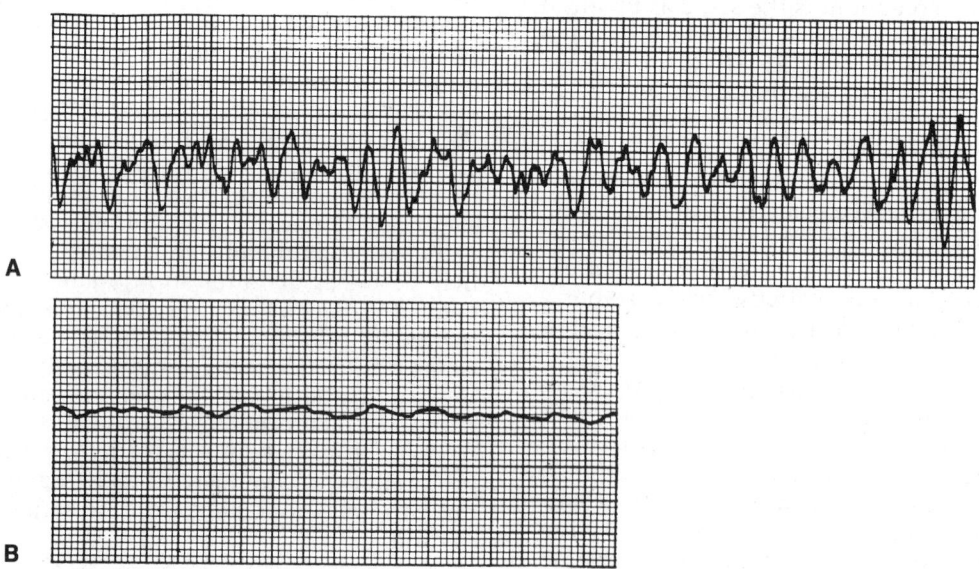

FIGURE 35–27. Ventricular fibrillation. Tracing *A* shows coarse ventricular fibrillation. Tracing *B* shows fine ventricular fibrillation. (From Textbook of Advanced Cardiac Life Support. Dallas, TX, American Heart Association, 1994, with permission. Copyright 1994 American Heart Association.)

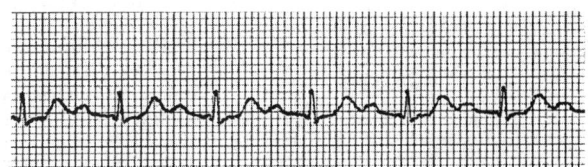

FIGURE 35–28. First-degree AV block. The P-R interval measures 0.24 second, which is too prolonged for a heart rate of 100/minute.

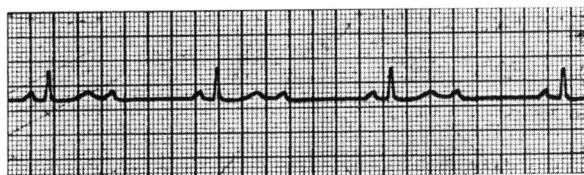

FIGURE 35–30. Second-degree AV block (Mobitz type II). The P wave is blocked every second beat (2:1 AV block).

Arrhythmias Resulting from Atrioventricular Conduction Defects

First-Degree AV Block

MECHANISM. A partial block at the AV junction delays transmission of impulses to the ventricles. However, all atrial impulses eventually are conducted through the normal pathways.

ETIOLOGY. Increased vagal tone may be the cause of a first-degree AV block in young persons. In the elderly, first-degree AV block may indicate digitalis effect or an organic lesion, such as stenosis of a small branch of the right coronary artery that irrigates the AV node.

CHARACTERISTICS. There are normally occurring P waves of SA origin. QRS complexes are normal. The P-R interval is longer than normally would be expected for the heart rate. A P-R interval greater than 0.20 seconds is indicative of first-degree AV block unless the heart rate is very slow, in which case a P-R interval of up to 0.24 seconds is considered normal. The P-P and R-R intervals are equal (Fig. 35–28).

SYMPTOMS. There are usually no symptoms.

TREATMENT. Usually no treatment is required. The physician may consider discontinuing digitalis if the patient is being treated with this drug.

Second-Degree AV Block, Mobitz Type I (Wenckebach Phenomenon)

MECHANISM. In a cyclic fashion, there is a progressive increase in the P-R interval until eventually a normal atrial impulse is completely blocked at the AV junction.

ETIOLOGY. Second-degree AV block may occur in adolescents as a result of autonomic lability. In older persons, it is not as severe as a second-degree AV block of the Mobitz II type.

CHARACTERISTICS. The P-R interval may start within normal limits, but it becomes progressively longer in the next few beats until there is a dropped QRS complex. The P-P intervals are gradually increasing. The R-R intervals become progressively shorter but, when the complete block occurs, there is a long R-R interval (Fig. 35–29).

SYMPTOMS. There are usually no symptoms, although the blocked P wave may cause a thumping sensation and slight dizziness.

TREATMENT. No treatment may be required.

Second-Degree AV Block, Mobitz Type II

MECHANISM. A complete AV block occurs at the AV junction or at the early portion of the bundle of His. This block occurs intermittently every other atrial beat or every two or three beats.

ETIOLOGY. Second-degree AV block is usually a manifestation of organic heart disease.

CHARACTERISTICS. The P waves occur regularly and are followed by normal QRS complexes, except when there is a dropped P wave. The P-P intervals are equal. The R-R intervals are equal, except in the blocked beat (Fig. 35–30).

SYMPTOMS. There are no symptoms if the ventricular rate is normal. The patient may experience dizziness or collapse if the ventricular rate is very slow.

TREATMENT. When this heart block occurs every other beat, it can lead to serious consequences and may require pacing. If pacing is not available and the patient's pulse rate is slow, it may be necessary to administer atropine or epinephrine.

Third-Degree AV Block (Complete) with AV Dissociation

MECHANISM. Impulses originate independently at the SA node and at the junction or ventricles.

FIGURE 35–29. Second-degree AV block (Mobitz type I). The first beat shows a P-R interval of 0.18 second. The second beat shows a P-R interval of 0.28 second. The third beat shows a blocked P wave. After a pause, the P-R interval begins at 0.18 second with a new sequence of gradual prolongation until a blocked P wave occurs.

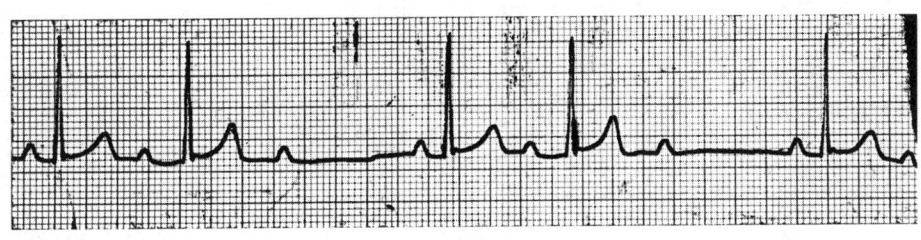

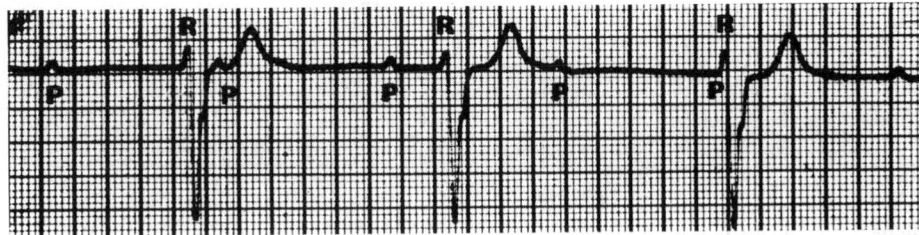

FIGURE 35–31. Third-degree AV block with AV dissociation. The P waves are identified by P. The QRS complexes are identified by R. In the last full beat, there is a P wave that coincides with the beginning of the QRS complex.

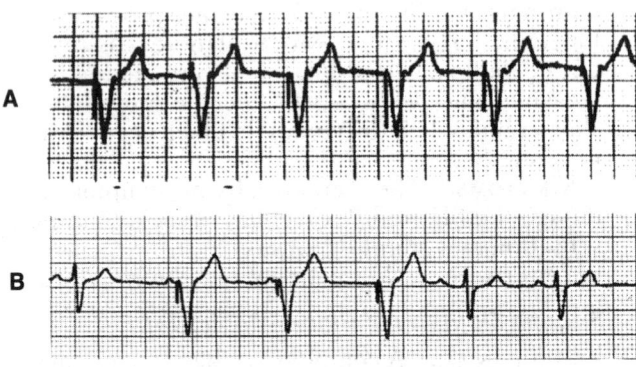

FIGURE 35–32. Artificial pacemaker. Tracing *A* shows an artificial pacemaker with a fixed rate. The sharp spike preceding each wide QRS complex is produced by the pacemaker. Tracing *B* shows a demand artificial pacemaker. The sharp spike downward precedes three wide QRS complexes (beats 2 through 4) while the other QRS complexes (beats 1, 5, and 6) are preceded by a P wave and are conducted through the bundle of His. The demand pacemaker was triggered by the fact that the ventricles did not receive an impulse at the prescribed minimum rate of 70 beats/min.

ETIOLOGY. Third-degree AV block indicates serious cardiac disease, usually coronary stenosis affecting the branch of the right coronary artery that irrigates the AV node.

CHARACTERISTICS. The P-P intervals are regular and equal. The R-R intervals are also regular and equal but usually longer than the P-P intervals because the ventricular rhythm is out of sequence with the atrial rhythm. If the ventricular impulses originate at the AV junction, the QRS complexes are narrow and the T waves are usually in the same direction. If the ventricular beats originate at the ventricle, the QRS complexes are wide and slurred, and the T waves are in the opposite direction to the QRS complexes (Fig. 35–31).

SYMPTOMS. Symptoms are usually those of either bradycardia or tachycardia.

TREATMENT. If the block is proximal (i.e., high in the junction) and accompanied by bradycardia or hypotension, it may be necessary to administer atropine or epinephrine. If the block is distal (i.e., low in the junction or in the bundle of His), it may be necessary to insert a transvenous pacemaker.

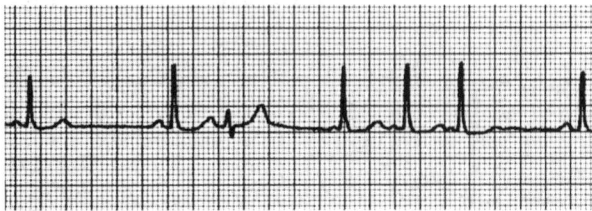

FIGURE 35–33. Sick sinus syndrome. The tracing shows an irregular heart rate with most beats of atrial origin. The third beat originated at the AV junction.

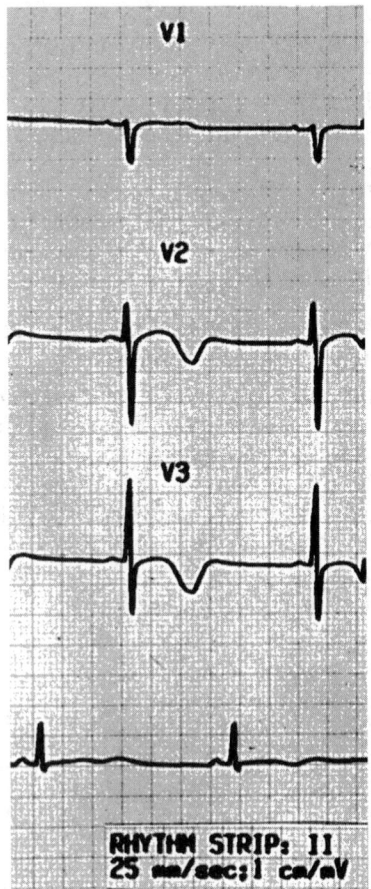

FIGURE 35–34. Prolonged Q-T syndrome.

RHYTHMS PRODUCED BY ARTIFICIAL PACEMAKERS

All well-functioning artificial pacemakers may be recognized by a sharp spike of voltage change that occurs just before a P wave or a QRS complex, depending on the location of the stimulating electrode. The permanent demand pacemakers are activated only when the patient's rate is lower than a pre-established threshold (Fig. 35–32).

SPECIAL CLINICAL SYNDROMES THAT PREDISPOSE TO ARRHYTHMIAS

Pre-excitation Syndromes

Both the Wolff-Parkinson-White and Lown-Ganong-Levine syndromes may cause recurrent supraventricular rhythms with very rapid ventricular rate. The tachycardia is due to re-entry of impulses from the conducting tissue to the atria via the aberrant pathway (Kent's bundle in Wolff-Parkinson-White syndrome or James' bundle in Lown-Ganong-Levine syndrome).

The required treatment is the same as that for supraventricular tachycardia, but verapamil, digoxin, and β blockers should be used with great caution or not used at all because, although they block conduction through the AV node, they facilitate re-entry through the aberrant pathway. In children, digoxin seems to be effective. In some cases, surgical ablation of the aberrant pathway is effective.

Sick Sinus Syndrome

This syndrome occurs whenever there is an organic lesion of the SA node. In this condition, there are periods of irregular sinus pause with recurrent episodes of supraventricular tachycardia, bradycardia, or VPBs (Fig. 35–33).

Usually, the best treatment for this syndrome is the establishment of a permanent demand pacemaker along with the administration of an antiarrhythmic drug, which should be selected according to the predominant heart rate and the most common type of ectopy.

Mitral Valve Prolapse Syndrome

In this condition, there is a myxoid change in the mitral valve with prolapse of one of the leaflets. In this syndrome, atrial premature beats, VPBs, or episodes of supraventricular tachycardia may be present. With rare exceptions, these arrhythmias are of benign course and usually respond well to β blockers.

Prolonged Q-T Syndrome

A prolonged Q-T interval may be congenital or acquired. There are two congenital syndromes that occur in families. One of them (Jervell and Lange-Nielsen syndrome) is accompanied by deafness, while the other (Romano-Ward syndrome) is not. An acquired prolonged Q-T interval (Fig. 35–34) may be due to electrolyte disturbances or drugs (especially tricyclic antidepressants, thioridazine, and, rarely, some antihistamines). Regardless of the cause, a prolonged Q-T interval is dangerous because it can lead to *torsades de pointes* tachycardia.

SUGGESTED READINGS

American Heart Association: Guidelines for cardiopulmonary resuscitation and emergency cardiac care of the American Heart Association. JAMA 268:2171, 1992.

American Heart Association: Textbook of Advanced Cardiac Life Support, 2nd edition. Dallas, TX, American Heart Assocation, 1990.

Chung EK: Electrocardiography, Part III: Complex Cardiac Arrhythmias. New York, MEDCOM Learning Systems, 1972.

Chung EK: Electrocardiography: Practical Applications with Vector Principles. Norwalk, CT, Appleton & Lange, 1985.

Jarris R (ed), Ezekowitz MD, Grauer K (consultants): Management of Chronic Atrial Fibrillation. Kansas City, MO, American Academy of Family Physicians, 1993.

Sandóe E, Sigurd B: Arrhythmia: Diagnosis and Management, A Clinical Electrocardiographic Guide. St. Galen, Verlag für Fachmedien, 1984.

Scheidt S: Basic Electrocardiography. West Caldwell, NJ: CIBA-GEIGY, 1986.

CHAPTER 36

EMERGENCY MEDICINE

Introduction to Emergency Medicine

JOHN L. LYMAN

The need for someone skilled in the practice of emergency medicine is not new, and medical emergencies requiring skill or knowledgeable intervention have been with us since recorded history. The Dead Sea Scrolls, dated thousand of years BC, describe interventions for closed head injuries and several other surgical procedures. Although even in the simplest of times the possibility of medical and surgical emergencies was very real, this reality has been enhanced manyfold by the evolution of our society. Consequently, medical emergencies have arisen because of our various mechanical means of transportation, our technologic advances with the prolongation of life, exposures to multiple environmental hazards, and so forth.

In addition to the daily preventive care and routine follow-up family physicians provide, they often are called on to provide urgent and emergent care for their patients. Furthermore, a measurable number of family physicians provide emergency medical services either as full-time employment or by rotating coverage through their local hospitals' emergency departments. Consequently, family physicians must be familiar with the broad range of life-threatening emergency conditions their patients may encounter.

In many ways family physicians are well suited to provide emergency care to their patients. Their training is generally broad based and multidisciplinary. Furthermore, if they are able to stay up to date with the latest emergency treatments, they often can provide quicker and more accurate diagnoses of problems because of their prior knowledge of their patients' health risks. In an emergency setting, this knowledge may make the diagnosis and treatment "easier" for the patient's personal family physician than for an emergency room doctor who has no such prior knowledge. This personal relationship, however, does not afford the family physician the luxury of a lackadaisical approach. Family physicians are held to the

same standard of care as their counterparts in full emergency practice, which is basically first to rule out life-threatening conditions and then to look for more benign causes of presenting signs and symptoms. Often this requires a rapid, algorithmic approach to these patients and problems. For example, although very few patients who present to the family physician's office with chest pain will have serious cardiac disease, the family physician working in the emergency department is under considerable medical–legal pressure not to miss any of these cases on the very first encounter. It is hoped that, in the future, with health care reform and further work in the area of practice guidelines, we will receive better guidelines for providing more cost-effective care in our emergency departments and private offices.

Family physicians are advised to stay abreast of the frequent changes and recommendations in basic (BCLS) and advanced cardiac life support (ACLS). In fact, most hospitals and emergency departments require physicians to provide proof of current certification in BCLS/ACLS to gain and maintain privileges. Family physicians also should consider certification in pediatric advanced life support (PALS) and advanced trauma life support (ATLS). This is particularly important if they intend to spend a significant amount of time in emergency medicine practice. Although this chapter will touch briefly on the important concepts of life support, the reader is advised to consult the specific manuals for each of these certifications to obtain the most up-to-date management recommendations.

INITIAL APPROACH TO EMERGENCY PATIENTS

As mentioned earlier, every emergency patient must be approached with the question of what potential life-threatening conditions could be present given the patient's presenting complaints, associated symptoms, and physical findings. Obviously, not all patients presenting to the emergency department have emergencies. Over the last two decades, we have seen a tremendous growth in emergency department patient visits. In 1971 there were approximately 55 million such visits, and that number increased in 1991 to over 93 million. It is estimated that less than 10 per cent of emergency department patients have true emergencies. Consequently, sifting through the large number of patients presenting to the emergency room to find the true emergencies has become a more difficult task. The number of physicians practicing in emergency departments is approximately 25,000, and less than half of these are board certified in emergency medicine. Nationwide, almost 40 per cent of hospital admissions come from patients evaluated first in the emergency department.

The time-honored concept of obtaining a complete history and then an appropriate physical is necessarily supplanted by the process of obtaining *sufficient* history and physical examination to work through the algorithm of life-threatening conditions and co-morbidity. For example, the physician evaluating the emergency patient with severe headache must obtain history and physical and possibly radiographic data appropriate to rule out subarachnoid hemorrhage or meningitis before assessing psychosocial stressors that may have triggered a severe tension or migraine headache.

Very often the conditions or problems leading to the emergency visit began or occurred at home. Consequently, the management of most emergency patients is a continuum of prehospital and hospital care. The treatment rendered and time elapsed before reaching the hospital is often critical to the patient's outcome. Consequently, the advice given to the family members and paramedics by the emergency physician can be critical to the eventual outcome. Furthermore, family physicians are often instrumental in recommending and obtaining the level of paramedical skills available to their communities and patients by being leaders in their respective medical communities. As shown by the research in prehospital care of acute myocardial infarction patients, the management in the field by trained emergency medical technicians under the guidance of a family physician or emergency room physician can significantly reduce morbidity and mortality.

Finally, a third, probably obvious, principle of emergency management is that of triage. Patients are treated on a first *need* basis and not on first come, first serve basis. In fact, by law, the initial encounter in the emergency setting must be with a medically trained person (i.e., nurse, nurse practitioner, physician assistant, physician) and not just a receptionist. It is this initial assessment of the severity of the patient's illness and its urgency that will triage the patient to the appropriate medial attention.

CARDIOPULMONARY ARREST

The patient who presents in cardiopulmonary arrest tries the mettle and expertise of any physician providing emergency care. Time is of the essence in the management of these patients, and the physician must work expeditiously and efficiently if there is to be a successful outcome. There is little room for error, so resuscitative efforts can be a trying experience for even the most practiced physician. Many times the physician has little or no information about the patient prior to his or her arrival in arrest. Consequently, because there are a myriad of etiologies for cardiopulmonary arrest, it is incumbent on the physician to consider at some level all potential possibilities.

To facilitate the approach to the patient in cardiopulmonary arrest, an organized process has been developed by the American Heart Association. This approach was developed in the 1950s and has subsequently been revised and refined multiple times. The American Heart Association's BCLS/ACLS approach allows every physician to deal with a cardiopulmonary arrest in an organized fashion. Consequently, the BCLS/ACLS approach is appropriate for the great majority of patients presenting with cardiopulmonary arrest.

The BCLS approach has its foundation in the mnemonic ABC. The "A" stands for assessment of the airway, and this directs the physicians attention toward establishing adequate airway control. The rationale is that, if the airway is not controlled and maintained, all subsequent procedures will be fruitless. There are a variety of ways to maintain a patent airway; the simplest and most effective is to simply lift the jaw of the patient forward, which lifts the tongue off the posterior larynx and has the effect of opening the airway. "B" in the mnemonic points to the need to establish some sort of breathing (ventilation). Once the airway has been secured, the patient sometimes will breath spontaneously. If this does not occur, then the physician or another attendant must provide breath to the patient via mouth-to-mouth resuscitation, bag-to-mouth resuscitation, or other variations. Finally, if these are not successful or the artificial ventilation will be required for a period of time, endotracheal intubation should be performed.

Once the airway and ventilation have been secured and initiated, the rescuer then must direct his or her attention toward circulation, the "C" component of the ABCs. If the patient is pulseless, chest compressions must be begun according to BCLS recommendations. This will provide circulatory support to vital organs, with the hope of continuing perfusion in spite of the cardiac arrest. Physicians are encouraged to follow the specific up-to-date recommendations of cardiac compressions because, even with the best of external cardiac massage, only 30 per cent of normal cardiac output or circulation can be achieved.

ACLS procedures are based on the same basic ABCs but also employ technologies that are advanced beyond the guidelines found in BCLS. Although ACLS continues to demand that the airway have primary attention, other techniques can be utilized to secure the airway, such as endotracheal intubation as mentioned earlier. Cardiac medications in cardiopulmonary arrest go beyond the basic BCLS protocols and will not be discussed in detail here. The use of pharmacologic interventions, electrical defibrillation, and other such techniques are part of the ACLS protocols, and practitioners are recommended to review the specific manuals for these procedures in order to know the most up-to-date recommendations for management. It is worth noting, however, that, for personnel with the equipment and expertise, defibrillation is the most important initial treatment for those patients with cardiopulmonary arrest secondary to recent or witnessed ventricular fibrillation.

The approach to the patient in cardiopulmonary arrest as devised by the American Heart Association is not foolproof and may need to be modified depending on the circumstances in which the patient presents. What is crucial, however, is that the patient presenting in extremis must be managed in an organized and rational fashion. Although some controversies may exist concerning various nuances and idiosyncrasies of the American Heart Association approach, to date it is by far the most efficient, reliable, and easily implemented approach to the general patient in cardiopulmonary arrest. It is imperative, therefore, that any physician who will be treating patients who may present with cardiopulmonary arrest be well versed in the American Heart Association approaches, namely BCLS and ACLS.

TREATMENT OF THE PATIENT WITH ALTERED LEVEL OF CONSCIOUSNESS

Treatment of the patient with altered mental status is not an uncommon circumstance in the emergency setting. In fact, any where from 2 to 3 per cent of patients presenting to a typical emergency department will have a problem with altered mental status. The reasons for altered mental status are many and varied, but by far the most common cause for this situation is metabolic problems.

As in other aspects of emergency medicine, it is incumbent on the physician to be able to diagnosis and treat simultaneously. Many of the causes of altered mental status may be treated in a slow and methodical way; for others, time is critical and seconds lost may be crucial to the final outcome. Most often the physician does not have the luxury of knowing immediately which treatment is appropriate for an individual patient because he or she may not have any prior knowledge of the patient or the patient's problems. Therefore, the physician's approach must be in a manner that assumes that time is of the essence for all patients.

To facilitate a rapid, timely approach to the patient, the physician must have a thorough understanding of all possible etiologies of altered mental status. A mnemonic has been developed to facilitate the recall of this wide variety of etiologies: AEIOU-TIPS. This mnemonic is deciphered as follows:

A—alcohols
E—endocrine, electrolytes, exocrine
I—insulin (diabetes)
O—opiates
U—uremia
T—trauma, temperature
I—infection
P—psychogenic, pulmonary embolism
S—stroke, subarachnoid hemorrhage, seizures, space-occupying lesions, shock

The physician treating the patient with altered mental status must consider at some level each of these possible etiologies and perform the history, physical, and laboratory testing along these lines.

One must have an appreciation for the normal physiology of consciousness to understand the alterations in level of consciousness. The brain depends on a real-time supply of substrate and has little substrate reserve, unlike other organs systems, so an interruption of any of the necessary substrates (i.e., oxygen or glucose) can result in an alteration of consciousness. A functional series of neurons and supporting structures in the midbrain, also known as the reticular activating system, serves another component of consciousness. Finally, a third component of consciousness relates to the activity of the cerebral hemispheres, which are aroused by the reticular activating system and allow us to be aware of our surroundings. Consequently, perturbations in the reticular activating system, cerebral cortex, or substrate supply to the brain can result in alterations in level of consciousness.

Physical examination at a basic level attempts to differentiate metabolic causes of altered mental status from structural lesions. Any patient with altered mental status requires attention to the basic ABCs of life support. The airway may need to be secured and endotracheal intubation provided, especially if respiratory difficulties are noted or a gag reflex is absent. Circulatory support may be needed in terms of fluids and/or pharmacologic agents. Examination of the pupils may be very important in the patient with altered mental status because they are relatively resistant to metabolic abnormalities. The reaction of the cornea to light and physical stimuli and the reaction of the eyes to caloric stimulation may provide clues to the etiology of the altered level of consciousness. Pupillary findings and their significance are discussed elsewhere in this text, particularly in the section on poisoning. The physical examination should pay further attention to the symmetry of reflexes and motor movements in the patient. Asymmetry of movement in response to noxious stimuli or the lack of voluntary movement or reflexes are significant findings in such patients.

Initial therapeutic interventions in the patient with altered mental status are generic and somewhat independent of the final etiology. Supplemental oxygen should be applied whenever possible and an intravenous access established. A rapid assessment of serum glucose should be made via bedside testing and, if necessary, intravenous glucose should be administered. Thiamine can be given empirically, 50 to 100 mg intravenously, particularly in patients suspected of alcohol abuse. Naloxone can be given empirically in any suspected drug overdose. Flumazenil, a new benzodiazepine antagonist, also can be administered to those patient suspected of ingesting such a drug. Caution should be used with flumazenil in patients who may have a potential withdrawal syndrome from benzodiazepines or have a underlying seizure disorder. The use of electrocardiography, computerized tomographic scanning, and multiple drug screening should be used as determined necessary by the evaluating physician. The major causes of death for patients with altered mental status include pulmonary insufficiency and aspiration, cardiac toxicity from toxic overdoses, hypotension and shock, uncal herniation from expanding intracranial masses or hemorrhage, and hepatic or renal toxicity from ingested toxins; the physician should consider these problems in life support of the patient with altered mental status.

THE PATIENT IN PAIN

If there is one thread that ties together the majority of patients presenting to the emergency department, it very well may be pain. The majority of patients presenting to an emergency department are experiencing some degree of pain and discomfort. Whereas 1 per cent of patients may present in cardiac arrest, and 3 per cent of patients may present with altered mental status, well over 50 per cent of an emergency physician's patients will present with painful conditions. It is incumbent on the emergency department physician that he or she be able to deal effectively with patients who are experiencing pain and discomfort.

In spite of the fact that persons with pain are common presenters to an emergency department, many studies have indicated that, in general, emergency medicine practitioners treat pain ineffec-

tively, inefficiently, or not at all. The reasons for such ineffectiveness are multiple, and include the following:

1. Little time is devoted to the training of a physician to effectively treating pain.
2. Relatively few studies have been undertaken in the study of pain in the emergency patient, and many of the studies that have been generated have dealt with chronic pain versus the acute pain that is common in emergency patients.
3. There is an unfounded fear, perpetuated by many of our colleagues, of the masking of an important diagnosis.
4. There is an inappropriate fear of side affects of analgesics, often reflecting an inadequate knowledge base.
5. There is a fear of creating drug dependency.

A clarification of the pain a patient is experiencing may be immensely helpful in delineating the disease process. One method of delineation follows the mnemonic PQRST:

P—palliation or provocation. What events or interventions provoke the pain and/or palliate the pain?
Q—quality. What is the nature of the pain: burning, aching, sharp, well defined?
R—region and radiation of the pain. Where on the body is the pain located, and does it radiate along any track?
S—severity of the pain. It is helpful to have each patient describe the amount of pain he or she is experiencing. One method is to have the patient to rate the pain on a scale of 1 to 10, with 10 being the most severe pain they have ever experienced and 1 being minimal pain.
T—timing. Are there any temporal events related to the pain, or any time-of-day notations?

A small amount of time spent delineating the pain that the patient is experiencing can be extremely helpful in defining the disease process that brought the patient to the emergency department. The classic example is a dull, achy, ill-defined periumbilical pain that over time translates into a sharp, well-defined, right lower quadrant pain, which is almost pathognomonic of appendicitis. If we were to ignore this temporal development of pain, the diagnosis of appendicitis would be made much more difficult. While the small amount of time spent delineating the pain can be helpful in terms of diagnosis, the additional small amount of time spent in providing treatment for the pain can be overwhelmingly rewarding.

A wide variety of methods to control pain are available to the emergency medicine practitioner. Pharmacologic interventions for generalized pain control are employed most commonly, and most often include oral or parenteral narcotics and nonsteroidal anti-inflammatory agents. Nitrous oxide, an inhalation analgesic with sedative and anxiolytic properties, is employed in many facilities. Local anesthetics are utilized to effect anesthesia in a specific region of the body. Nonpharmacologic interventions also are employed in many settings, and the emergency physician should at the very

least be aware of these alternatives to pain control. Such alternative approaches to pain control include hypnosis, acupuncture, and acupressure. Vocal anesthesia, in essence, is a simple action and gives assurance to the patient; it is an integral part of any form of pain control.

Trauma

ROBERT E. KYNERD

In the United States, injuries are the fourth leading cause of death for all ages, behind heart disease, cancer, and stroke; accidents are the leading cause of death for those between the ages of 1 and 37 years (National Safety Council, 1992). In many places throughout this country primary care physicians in general, and family physicians in particular, are the physicians responsible for the initial evaluation and management of these patients. In 1978 the American College of Surgeons developed the Advanced Trauma Life Support (ATLS) courses to assist physicians who do not deal with trauma on a frequent basis, from which the current standard of care for many areas has been derived. A 3-day course of instruction in the form of lectures, practical demonstrations, and role playing of scenarios, these courses provide practical instructions, guidelines, and hands-on experiences to assist the physician in acquiring the knowledge and skills necessary for the initial evaluation and management of severely injured patients (Collicott, 1992; Committee on Trauma, 1988; Schmidt and Moore, 1993).

EVALUATING THE SERIOUSLY INJURED PATIENT

Proper care of a multiply injured patient requires a coordinated team approach. Liberal consultation, ranging from a general surgeon to a trauma referral center, should be initiated early to prevent delays between evaluation and possible treatment.

The initial evaluation of the multiply injured patient, called the primary survey, is directed toward the identification and treatment of life-threatening

conditions (see Table 36–1). Subsequent efforts, called the secondary survey, are directed toward more detailed evaluations of the patient in a head-to-toe fashion, while continuing to reassess the patient for changes in condition. As part of the evaluation, various rating systems have been developed and adopted to aid in communication among health care workers, as well as to simplify ongoing evaluation of the patient's condition (Table 36–2).

Primary Survey

The algorithm ABCDE summarizes the primary survey. A patent *airway* is established and/or maintained while cervical spine control is obtained. Intubation may be necessary to relieve obstruction, protect the airway, or assist ventilation. Some authors advocate intubation if moderate to severe shock persists (defined as a systolic blood pressure less than 85 mm Hg). Which method of securing the airway is chosen will vary depending of the injuries identified in the patient and the expertise of the medical personnel. Potential methods include orotracheal intubation if cervical spine injuries are unlikely or midfacial or basilar skull fractures are suspected, blind nasotracheal intubation

TABLE 36–1. CAUSES OF MORTALITY IN MAJOR TRAUMA

Airway obstruction	Tension pneumothorax
Ongoing hemorrhage	Tension hemothorax
Transtentorial brain stem herniation	Open pneumothorax
Pericardial tamponade	Flail chest

TABLE 36–2. TRAUMA RATING SYSTEMS

A. Glasgow Coma Scale* (GCS)

Eye Opening		Best Motor Response		Verbal Response	
Spontaneous	E4	Obeys commands	M6	Oriented	V5
To speech	E3	Localizes	M5	Confused	V4
To pain	E2	Withdraws	M4	Inappropriate	V3
None	E1	Abnormal flexion	M3	Incomprehensible	V2
		Extension	M2	None	V1
		None	M1		

B. Revised Trauma Score† (RTS)

Coded Values	4	3	2	1	0
Glasgow Coma Scale score	13–15	9–12	6–8	4–5	3
Systolic blood pressure	>89	76–89	50–75	1–49	0
Respiratory rate	10–29	>29	6–9	1–5	0

* Determined by checking three items; correlates with the severity of injury to the brain. (From Jennett B, Teasdale G: Aspects of coma after severe head injury. Lancet 1:878, 1977, with permission.)

†Determined by evaluating three measurements; correlates with the severity of multiple injuries and need to transfer an RTS ≤ 11 or GCS ≤ 10 to a specialized treatment facility. (From Champion HR, Sacco WJ, Copes WS, et al: A revision of the trauma score. J Trauma 29:623, 1989, with permission.)

if cervical spine injuries are likely, and cricothyrotomy if maxillofacial and cervical spine injuries are present. The spine is protected and stabilized as needed. Patients suspected of having cervical spine injuries should remain in a hard collar until full evaluation can be completed. Similar precautions should apply to suspected thoracic or lumbar injuries, keeping the patient on a firm surface and "log rolling" when position changes are necessary.

Adequate *breathing* is ensured, whether spontaneous or assisted. For most patients, this means symmetric respirations with good air movement in all lung fields at rates of 10 to 30 breaths/min, which will achieve greater than 90 per cent oxygen saturation with normal Pco_2 and pH. In patients with head injuries, hyperventilation to decrease Pco_2 to less than 25 to 30 mm Hg will produce cerebral vasoconstriction and thereby diminish cerebral swelling and reduce intracranial pressure.

Circulation is restored while bleeding is controlled. Pulse and blood pressure should be assessed, cardiopulmonary resuscitation (CPR) performed when indicated, two (or more) large-bore intravenous lines established, and obvious hemorrhages controlled with direct pressure. Blood samples can be obtained and sent to the laboratory as the lines are established. Also, remember that even a blood clot can be used to determine a blood type and screen. Fluid resuscitation traditionally is begun with crystalloid fluid administration; colloid solutions can be used as an adjunct. If necessary, type-specific or O-negative blood can be given; with massive hemorrhage into the thoracic cavity, autotransfusion can be performed.

To prevent or minimize permanent *disability* from neurologic injuries, a brief neurologic examination is performed. Patients with evidence of either significant trauma to the head or brain stem dysfunction thought to be secondary to uncal herniation (abnormal pupillary light reflexes, depressed consciousness, and asymmetric motor responses) should have immediate neurosurgical consultation.

Complete *exposure* in preparation for a quick but comprehensive secondary evaluation of injuries is performed, while ongoing resuscitation continues.

Secondary Survey

A detailed physical examination is conducted, proceding in an orderly head-to-toe fashion. Special attention must be paid to the neurologic, cardiovascular, abdominal, and musculoskeletal systems. Laboratory studies should include blood type and crossmatch, complete blood cell count, coagulation studies, arterial blood gases, electrolytes, blood urea nitrogen, creatinine, lactate, and amylase. A nasogatric tube can decompress the stomach in patients requiring assisted ventilation and those with chest or abdominal injuries. If no blood is noted at the urethral meatus and no "highriding" prostate is noted on rectal exam of males (suggesting disruption of the urethra), a Foley catheter will provide urine samples for study and assist in assessment of adequacy of perfusion. Particular attention should be paid to the possibility of life-threatening injuries. At the same time, initial radiologic examinations are performed. In many institutions these routinely include a cross table lateral radiograph of the cervical spine, an anteroposterior chest radiograph, and an anteroposterior pelvic radiograph.

Medical history can be obtained from patients, family, friends, and paramedical personnel. Attempts should be made to obtain information about the mechanism of injury, chronic medical problems, current medications, and use of alcohol or other drugs. Allergies and tetanus immunization status also should be determined when possible.

Life- and Limb-Threatening Injuries

In assessing for head trauma, the physician should attempt to identify evidence of facial and skull fractures by careful palpation and inspection. A thorough cranial nerve examination should be performed, and the Glasgow Coma scale score determined early for serial monitoring and for communication with other health care professionals (see Table 36–2). If significant injury is suspected, early neurosugical consultation is adviced. The computerized tomographic (CT) scan has become the diagnostic procedure of choice. Hyperventilation may assist in controlling swelling and increased pressure, because reducing arterial PCO_2 to 25 to 30 mm Hg will reduce cerebral blood volume by producing vasoconstriction. Administration of corticosteroids has become controversial in trauma patients.

In evaluating for trauma to the neck, if a cervical spine injury is suspected, the neck must remain in a hard cervical collar until fractures are ruled out or other treatment initiated. In penetrating injuries (those that breach the platysmus), bear in mind that crepitus, swelling, and upper extremity neurologic deficits should suggest the possibility of injury to the trachea, the esophagus, and/or major neurovascular structures.

THORACIC TRAUMA

Thoracic trauma may be from blunt trauma or penetrating injuries.

Blunt Trauma

Blunt trauma to the chest is most commonly the result of motor vehicle accidents and falls. A high morbidity and mortality are associated with this type of trauma for several reasons: a high frequency of multiple system damage, multiple intrathoracic injuries, and some severe injuries that are initially silent clinically but rapidly produce deterioration in the patient if not treated.

Injuries result from two types of forces. Some intrathoracic structures are anchored; shearing forces at these points lead to tissue disruption of the heart, aorta, tracheobroncheal tree, and esophagus. Blunt impact forces can affect the sternum, ribs, lungs, and diaphragm.

Initial evaluation of the chest-injured patient often proceeds simultaneously with resuscitative therapy. Adequate respiration must be assured; large-bore intravenous access, including central venous pressure determinations (if indicated) begun; blood sent for type and crossmatch and other studies; and a thorough systematic examination completed. Blood gases, an electrocardiogram (ECG), and chest radiographs are minimum required studies.

Color, chest wall motion, and nature of respiration are vital in assessing for life-threatening injuries. Note the patient's neck veins. Shock with distended neck veins suggests tension pneumothorax or cardiac tamponade as an etiology. Flat-neck-vein shock suggests hemothorax or an extrathoracic cause for the shock.

Paradoxical chest wall motion represents a *flail chest,* common after steering wheel injury, that is caused by multiple two-point rib fractures. Large flail segments make adequate gas exchange impossible and mandate intubation and positive-pressure ventilation.

Absent breath sounds represent pneumothorax or hemothorax. The amount of respiratory distress seen with *pneumothorax* is a function of pulmonary reserve; young, otherwise healthy patients may have little distress with a complete unilateral pneumothorax. Tracheal deviation suggests tension pneumothorax; progressive mediastinal displacement acutely leads to compression of the great veins with loss of venous return to the right heart and eventual cardiovascular collapse. The patient with tension pneumothorax and cardiopulmonary compromise should receive immediate decompression with a large-bore needle in the second intercostal space at the midclavicular line. This usually affords enough improvement so that tube thoracostomy can proceed at a reasonable pace.

Respiratory distress without absent breath sounds or tracheal deviation may represent a ruptured diaphragm, an often-missed serious injury that requires a high index of suspicion for diagnosis. There will be fuzziness of the hemidiaphragm on the portable chest radiograph. Because the left hemidiaphragm is the one usually involved in blunt thoracic injuries, a nasogastric tube in the stomach may be seen in the hemithorax. Endotracheal intubation and nasogastric intubation may be helpful.

Tracheobronchial disruption may present in several ways, ranging from a mediastinal crunch or subcutaneous emphysema to complete unilateral atelectasis, mediastinal emphysema, pneumothorax with or without tension but with persistent air leak on chest tube drainage, or bronchiectasis. Hemoptysis varies from absent to massive.

The clinical relevance of a *hemothorax* depends on its magnitude, continued accumulation sufficient to cause signs of blood loss, and the degree of respiratory embarrassment caused by compression atelectasis. Lacerations of the heart and great vessels that cause hemothorax lead to death rapidly.

Injuries to pulmonary parenchyma are less rapidly lethal because the low-pressure pulmonary circulation tends to bleed more slowly, and the high thromboplastin levels in pulmonary tissue promote clot formation. Clinically significant hemothorax usually is due to disrupted intercostal or internal mammary arteries. The unclotted blood in a hemothorax may be drained via chest tube into an autotransfusion apparatus and returned to the patient.

Pulmonary contusion occurs commonly in the patient with blunt chest trauma and should be suspected particularly in patients with rib fractures or flail chest. Damage to tissue causes interstitial pulmonary hemorrhage with impairment of gas exchange. Blood gases and portable chest radiographs are vital to diagnosis but may be unrevealing soon after the injury. Assisted ventilation may be required if contusion is severe or reserve marginal.

Three types of *cardiac injury* are seen in blunt chest trauma: myocardial contusion, pericardial tamponade, and cardiac rupture. The mechanism of injury is a swinging disruptive force. The heart is tethered at its base, and there is a direct impact of the heart against the sternum.

Myocardial contusion may mimic infarction on an ECG, and enzyme elevations, arrhythmias, and congestive heart failure or shock may be seen. These should be treated in the usual fashion. The clinical course of myocardial contusion is generally more benign than that of infarction; histologically, a contusion resolves into tiny areas of fibrosis, which are scattered among normal parenchyma, rather than a single focal scar.

If pericardial tamponade is suspected after blunt trauma (narrow pulse pressure, high central venous pressure, distant heart sounds, low voltage on the ECG, possibly with electrical alternans of the QRS complex), pericardiocentesis may be a useful temporizing measure (Fig. 36–1). Open pericardiotomy by a qualified surgeon is the definitive treatment (Calhoon et al., 1992).

Cardiac rupture from blunt trauma is usually rapidly lethal; only the rare patient will survive the trip to hospital to undergo emergency thoracotomy.

Aortic disruption most often occurs at the ligamentum arteriosum, just distal to the left subclavian artery. A wide mediastinum on the chest radiograph, blood pressure differential between the upper extremities, and a positive aortogram mandate surgical repair.

Esophageal rupture, although rare in blunt chest trauma, must not be missed, because fatal mediastinitis will ensue within hours while diagnosis is delayed. Unexplained mediastinal air requires a Gastrografin swallow and/or endoscopy. Surgery is mandatory to avoid a fatal outcome.

Associated injuries must not be missed. The trauma victim's neck should be stabilized with a rigid collar or sandbags at the start if a neck injury

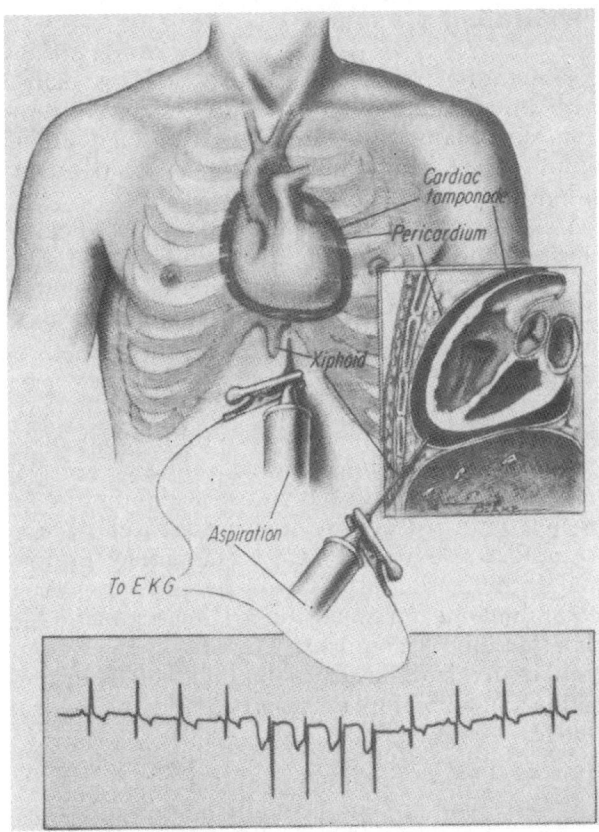

FIGURE 36–1. Technique of pericardiocenteses (see text for full description). (From Ebert P: The pericardium. *In* Sabiston DC, Spencer FC [eds]: Gibbon's Surgery of the Chest, 4th edition. Philadelphia, WB Saunders Company, 1983, p 996, with permission.)

is suspected. If intubation or cricothyrotomy is necessary, the possibility of cervical spine instability must be considered. The abdomen must be evaluated carefully, and, if there is any sign of serious injury, the general surgeon must be made aware of this also. Peritoneal lavage may be required in questionable cases (see later). Foley catheterization may be diagnostic of urinary tract injury (hematuria) in these patients or may be required to relieve bladder distention, especially in the patient with a spinal injury.

Simple rib fractures, probably the most common injury with blunt chest trauma, are managed with analgesia, rest, and careful outpatient follow-up. Fractures of the lower left ribs may be associated with splenic injury, and liver–spleen scan, CT scan, or inpatient observation may be wise. Fractures of any of the first four ribs should make one highly supicious of associated visceral or vascular injury requiring observation and possibly aortography. In spite of optimal therapy of blunt chest trauma, complications are not infrequent, including adult respiratory distress syndrome resulting from diffuse pulmonary contusion or associated injuries.

Penetrating Trauma

Penetrating trauma to the chest also is associated with pneumothorax, hemothorax, cardiac laceration, and many of the injuries discussed under blunt trauma. The same general resuscitative considerations apply.

In addition, open pneumothorax ("a sucking chest wound") can be produced. When respiration and circulation are assured, the chest wound should be covered with an occlusive dressing, such as Vaseline-impregnated gauze, to prevent ingress of air. In general, these wounds should never be probed; one can convert an innocuous injury to a dangerous one by injudicious probing. An open pneumothorax, with the lack of effective ventilation that accompanies it, must at minimum be treated with an occlusive dressing and a chest tube in rapid succession. Usually, emergency intubation of the patient also is required.

As blunt chest trauma, penetrating trauma to the chest may be accompanied by abdominal and/or renal injury, and these must be ruled out by examination and laboratory data, and possibly peritoneal lavage.

Tube Thoracostomy Drainage (Chest Tube Drainage)

Pneumothorax is the accumulation of intrapleural air as the result of a break in either the visceral or parietal pleura, whether from a spontaneous or traumatic etiology. Those resulting from trauma may be further classified as open, closed, tension, or hemopneumothorax (Kirby and Ginsberg, 1992). Pneumothorax is the most common entity managed by chest tube drainage (Fig. 36–2). Radiographic diagnosis of pneumothorax ideally requires posteroanterterior (PA), lateral, and expiratory views of the chest. From the PA chest film, the percentage of the pneumothorax may be estimated (Fig. 36–3) as the area of the hemithorax minus the area of collapsed lung divide by the area of the hemithorax.

The ECG in the patient with pneumothorax may demonstrate many changes resulting from intrathoracic air, cardiac rotation, right ventricular dilation, and altered coronary blood flow; the QRS axis shifts rightward, R wave voltage may decrease, the overall amplitude of the QRS complex may decrease, and the precordial T waves may become inverted, simulating ischemia.

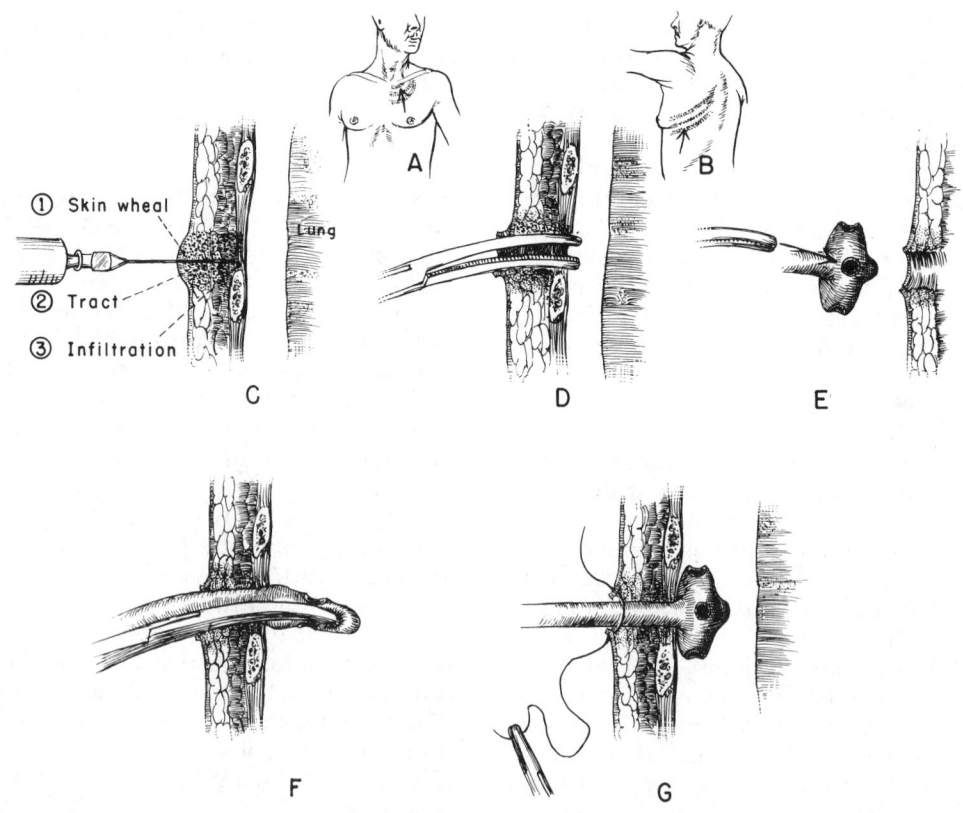

FIGURE 36–2.   The major steps in chest tube insertion (see text for details). After the tube is sutured securely, wrap the wound with petrolatum gauze to decrease air leakage. (From Rutherford RB, Campbell DN: Thoracic injuries. *In* Zuidema GD, Rutherford RB, Ballinger WF [eds]: The Management of Trauma, 4th edition. Philadelphia, WB Saunders Company, 1985, p 418, with permission.)

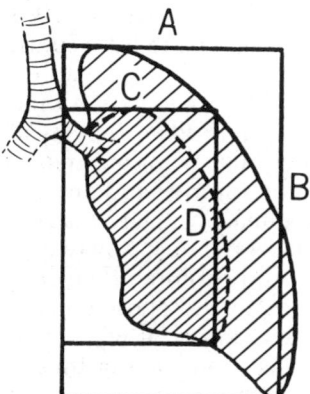

FIGURE 36–3.   Method of calculating percentage of pneumothorax: AB = area of hemithorax; CD = area of collapsed lung; (AB − CD)/AB = per cent pneumothorax. (From Donovan JW: Pneumothorax. Curr Top II Emerg Med 2(7). Philadelphia, Medical College of Pennsylvania, 1982, with permission.)

There is fairly general agreement on the need for tube drainage of any traumatic pneumothorax. Controversy exists, however, over the management of spontaneous pneumothorax.

Chest tube insertion is not a benign procedure. In order of frequency, its complications are the following (Curtis, 1978): hemothorax, pulmonary edema, bronchopleural fistula, pleural leaks, subcutaneous emphysema, and contralateral pneumothorax. Several techniques are available for chest tube insertion; one may use a trocar, finger dissection, or a large Kelly clamp or hemostat to enter the pleural space. For spontaneous pneumothorax, a 22 French chest tube is adequate. For draining a hemothorax, a 32 French tube should be used.

For all indications, the tube may be inserted in the fourth or fifth intercostal space at the anterior axillary line.

In the Kelly clamp method, with the patient supine, the skin is prepped and draped, and the skin over the sixth rib is anesthetized down to the periosteum. A 3-cm horizontal incision is made down to fat, and a clamp is used to extend a tract to the next interspace above (avoiding the neurovascular bundle that runs under the rib). The clamp then is pushed into the pleural space, and the hole is dilated. A check should be made for adherent lung using the gloved finger. The chest tube is grasped with the Kelly clamp. The skin-to–lung apex distance is measured on the chest tube and the end point marked on the tube with a small clamp. The tube then is placed in the chest with the Kelly clamp, directing it posteriorly and cephalad. The tube is secured with 0 wire or silk, a petrolatum-soaked gauze dressing is applied, the tube is connected to suction, and the small clamp removed. Tube placement should be verified with a chest film (Fig. 36–4).

Large hemothoraces, if unclotted, can be salvaged via chest tube drainage and the blood returned to the unstable patient using an autotransfusion technique (Davidson, 1979, 1981). The apparatus is simple, readily obtainable, functions in place of the water-seal Pleurevac unit, and accommodates a 32 French chest tube.

Emergency Thoracotomy

In rare cases, it may be necessary to do an emergency thoracotomy to resuscitate the chest-injured

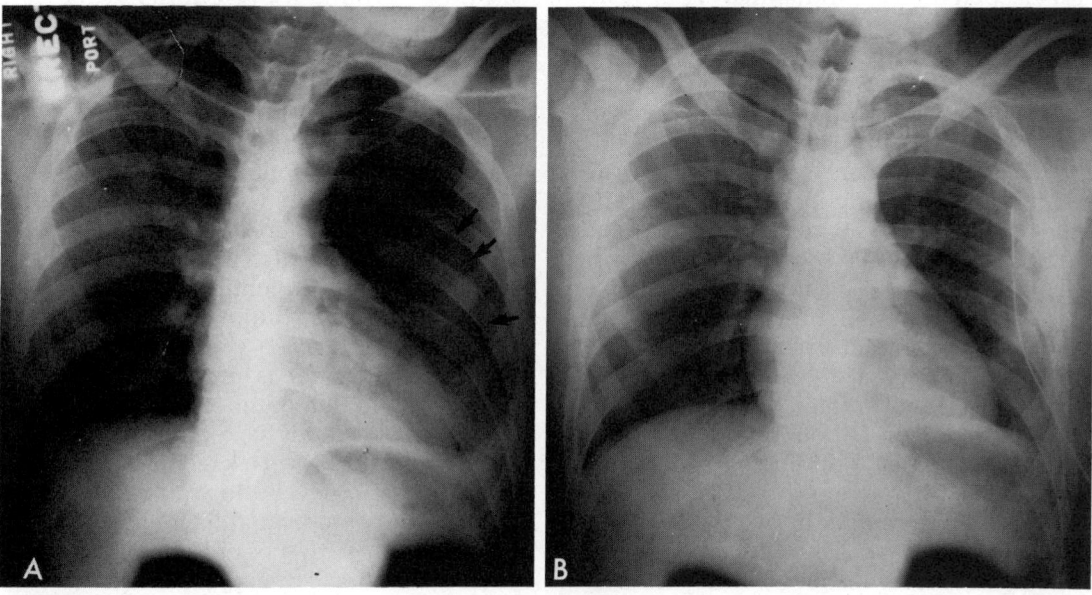

FIGURE 36–4.   Pneumothorax (*A*) with subsequent chest tube re-expansion (*B*). (From Morse SD, Rial WY: Emergency medicine. *In* Rakel RE, [ed]: Textbook of Family Practice, 4th edition. Philadelphia, WB Saunders Company, 1990, p 964, with permission.)

(or abdomen-injured) patient, but only if the patient is moribund, will not respond to other forms of therapy, and has had tension pneumothorax ruled out. There should be a reasonable chance of helping the patient specifically, such as releasing cardiac tamponade unresponsive to percardiocentesis attempts, controlling a bleeding point, or cross-clamping the descending thoracic aorta in cases of exsanguinating hemorrhage below the diaphragm.

Generally, emergency thoracotomy is only of utility in penetrating thoracic injury. It is most helpful in myocardial stab wounds with cardiac tamponade in which the tamponade is released readily with pericardial incision and the myocardial lacerations oversewn with silk sutures. Gunshot wounds of the heart are generally less salvageable.

Thoracotomy is required in only 10 per cent of major thoracic trauma overall, so emergency department thoracotomy is not a common procedure in most centers. Intubation and intravenous access are mandatory prior to actual thoracotomy. If possible, it is best to leave this procedure to a trained surgeon (Boyd et al., 1992; Wasserberger et al., 1989).

ABDOMINAL TRAUMA

Abdominal examination, which must be repeated at intervals, focuses on signs of peritoneal irritation. Absent bowel sounds, progressive distention, the presence of severe tenderness on palpation, rebound tenderness, and guarding are all suggestive of intra-abdominal injury. (However, these are initially absent in up to one third of patients with visceral injury.) Abdominal rigidity, involuntary on the part of the patient, is unequivocal evidence of peritoneal irritation, and the presence of rigidity or progressive development of other listed signs mandates laparotomy in the blunt or penetrating trauma victim.

A high index of suspicion is necessary to find abdominal trauma in many patients, especially those with blunt trauma. The peritoneal cavity can extend up to the fourth intercostal space anteriorly and the seventh intercostal space posteriorly on expiration, so that blunt or penetraiting chest trauma easily may have concomitant abdominal injury. Abdominal visceral injury also can occur in stab wounds of the back and in flank wounds.

Whether the abdomen is penetrated by stab or gunshot wounds (the major etiologies of penetrating trauma) affects the rate of visceral injury. Stab wounds enter the peritoneum in two thirds of victims but cause visceral damage in less than half of these cases. In contrast, gunshot wounds penetrate the peritoneal cavity over 80 per cent of the time and, in those cases, cause an almost 100 per cent rate of visceral injury as a result of both direct injury and a blast effect (Moore, 1981). Because of these data, there has been little controversy regarding mandatory exploratory laparotomy for a gunshot wound to the abdomen, although, if the patient is stable, there is an increasing tendency to consider abdominal CT scanning prior to surgery to delineate the injuries and any associated retroperitoneal trauma. A negative scan does not rule out hollow visceral injury, however; thus, most surgeons still would explore all such patients.

Stab wounds to the abdomen have been managed in a wider variety of ways. Perhaps the most common means of managing these wounds is by selective observation (often accompanied by CT scan). In the patient with no signs of instability or peritoneal irritation on physical examination, many surgical authors have recommended either local wound exploration under local anesthesia to exclude peritoneal entry or even a "stabogram" using radiologic contrast medium (although this has fallen into a large measure of disuse). To perform a stabogram, contrast medium such as Gastrografin is injected into the stab wound tract under moderate pressure and radiographs taken. Documentation of communication of the wound tract with the peritoneal cavity mandates laparotomy.

Most surgeons, at centers where CT scanning is available, currently would recommend abdominal scans for most abdominal stab wound victims, especially those without instability or local findings suggesting visceral injury, which would mandate rapid laparotomy. CT scanning would demonstrate occult or tamponaded solid visceral trauma or intraperitoneal fluid or blood. Injury to hollow organs might be missed, and thus admission and observation, supplemented with lavage, other studies, and even exploration, as appropriate, still would be required, even in the face of a negative scan.

Peritoneal Lavage

If local exploration, CT scanning, or other techniques cannot exclude peritoneal entry or if other indications exist, peritoneal lavage should be performed. Lavage is also useful in instances of blunt trauma in which abdominal findings are equivocal and radiographic studies unrevealing or contraindicated (such as early pregnancy).

Peritoneal lavage is an extremely sensitive technique for the detection of intra-abdominal injury; its overall accuracy is reported to range from 90 to 100 per cent. Prepackage lavage kits containing anesthetic, drapes, tubing, and multiply holed trocar-catheters are available commercially.

There are many possible indications for lavage. These include: (1) a trauma victim with an equivocal abdominal exam and hypotension or signs of blood loss not otherwise explained, (2) multiple injuries with altered mental status from any source (including alcohol), (3) an injured spinal cord, (4) fractures of the lower ribs or pelvis, (5) the presence of discontiguous injuries, and (6) cases in which emergency surgery under general anesthesia is required for nonabdominal injuries, to avoid deterioration in the operating suite from unsuspected intraperitoneal injury.

Absolute contraindications to lavage include a prior decision to perform laparotomy and a full bladder (always insert a Foley catheter first). Relative contraindications include prior abdominal surgery and midline scars and abdominal wall hematomas (may give a false positive). The presence of a gravid uterus requires using a higher site than usual for lavage but does not absolutely contraindicate the procedure. Some authorities also suggest a higher lavage site in patients with pelvic fracture or hematoma to attempt to decrease false positives.

The increased availability and use of CT scanning in abdominal trauma has led to a more thoughtful and selective approach to peritoneal lavage in recent years but has not rendered the procedure obsolete. CT scanning and lavage are regarded best as complimentary techniques in the evaluation of these patients. If CT scanning is performed after lavage, the presence of intra-abdominal fluid from the procedure may suggest hemorrhage and confuse the clinician; therefore, CT scanning is best performed first if it is readily available and the patient is stable. Prior lavage will not obscure occult solid visceral intraperitoneal injury in the face of a negative lavage. The scan may, in addition, demonstrate unsuspected retroperitoneal damage that the lavage fails to show or demonstrate intact solid intraperitoneal viscera and the presence of pelvic fracture or hematoma, causing falsely positive lavage results. It is important to emphasize that the scan may not reveal injury to hollow organs, such as the gut or bladder; hence, positive lavage results of any sort not explained by the scan will require further study (cystogram, gastrointestinal studies) or laparotomy, dependent on clinical context and patient condition.

The reported rates of complication from lavage range from 0.9 to 6.0 per cent (Lazarus and Nelson, 1980). Possible complications include hematomas, separation or infection of the abdominal incision, incisional hernia, vascular lacerations, omental lacerations, and bowel perforations.

The technique of peritoneal lavage (Fig. 36–5) begins with Foley catheterization of the bladder and nasogastric intubation. The area between the umbilicus and pubic symphysis is shaved, prepped with Betadine, and draped. A site in the midline, one third the distance from the umbilicus to the pubis, is anesthetized using lidocaine with epinephrine for hemostasis. A scalpel (no. 11 blade) is used to make a vertical incision several millimeters long through the skin and subcutaneous tissue. The trocar-catheter assembly is introduced into this incision. If awake and cooperative, the patient is asked to tense his or her abdominal musculature. Using two-hand control of the trocar (with one hand at the skin surface to avoid overpenetration of the catheter into the abdomen), pressure is applied until the trocar is felt to pop into the perineal cavity. The catheter should slide easily into the cavity; if it does not, extraperitoneal insertion is a possibility. In this case, the catheter must be removed and re-inserted. The catheter is slid toward the right colic gutter. Once it is in place, gentle aspiration is applied with a syringe. A return of 10 mL of nonclotting blood is a positive test and mandates laparotomy.

If no blood is aspirated, Ringer's lactate is infused through the catheter (20 mL/kg in children and 1 liter in adults), and the patient is moved gently from side to side and the fluid allowed to drain by gravity. Pink fluid through which newsprint cannot be read is a positive lavage; there is a 94 per cent chance of finding lesions requiring surgical correction (Parvin et al., 1975).

Aliquots of lavage fluid should be sent for red blood cell (RBC) count, white blood cell (WBC) count, amylase level, and Gram's stain. Greater than 100,000 RBCs/mm^3 in the lavage fluid is an absolute indication for surgical exploration, and it provides an overall diagnostic accuracy of 93 per cent, a sensitivity of 91 per cent, a specificity of 94 per cent, and a false-negative rate of only 4 per for stab wounds of the anterior abdominal wall (Thompson et al., 1980). RBC counts of 50,000 to 100,000 are equivocal, and the decision for laparotomy is individualized and often aided by other studies, such as CT scan. Less than 50,000 RBCs requires immediate observation only, unless chest wounds are present. In such patients, as few as 5000 RBCs require surgical intervention. At minimum, a diaphragmatic rent requiring repair will be found (Kessler and Stein, 1971). If tangential gunshot wounds are lavaged, an RBC count of 5000 or more also warrants laparotomy to assess damage to a hollow viscus. Such patients are often studied by thoracoabdominal CT scanning preoperatively to delineate trauma as fully as possible prior to exploration and repair.

A lavage fluid WBC count of 500/mm^3 or higher in blunt abdominal trauma suggests significant intra-abdominal injury; this is not the case in penetrating injury, in which the WBC count is far less useful (Mueller et al., 1981).

A lavage fluid amylase level of over 400 units or the presence of bacteria, feces, or bile in the fluid also indicates a positive lavage and mandates laparotomy, with or without further radiographic study as appropriate to the individual case.

As already mentioned, retroperitoneal injury, including genitourinary tract damage, colon injury, or pancreaticoduodenal trauma, may not be diagnosed by lavage. Accordingly, many authorities have suggested aggressive exploration of all back or flank gunshot wounds unless obviously superfi-

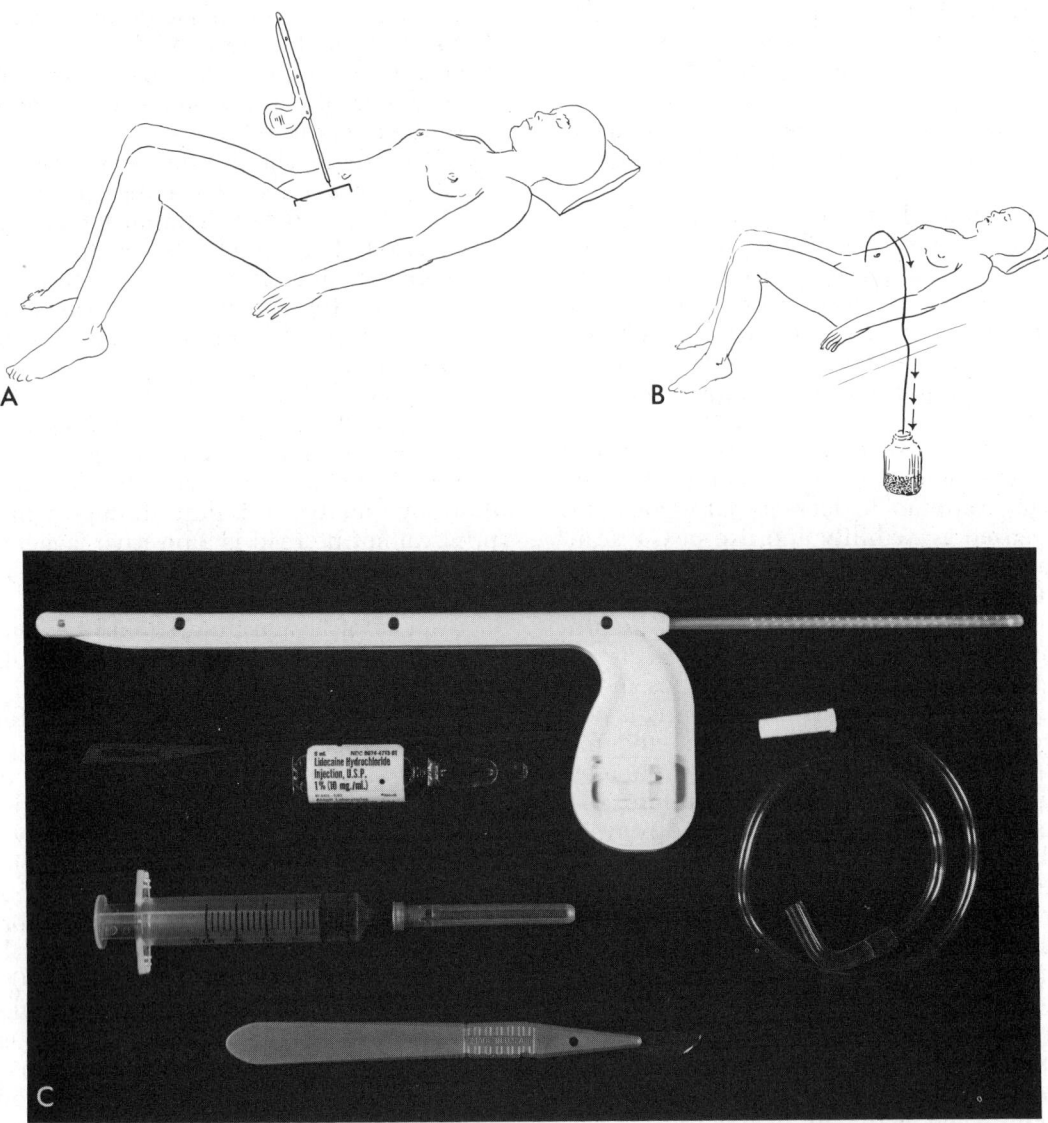

FIGURE 36–5.   Peritoneal lavage. *A,* An infraumbilical entry with a twisting or cautious pushing motion (if a trocar technique is used) is preferred. *B,* After fluid instillation and after the patient is shaken gently, drain the fluid by gravity. *C,* Representative equipment for catheter instillation. (From Morse SD, Rial WY: Emergency medicine. *In* Rakel RE [ed]: Textbook of Family Practice, 4th edition. Philadelphia, WB Saunders Company, 1990, p 968, with permission.)

cial; a more selective policy is used in stab wound management in these areas. The potential use of CT scanning techniques in both these patient groups is now widely recognized, and this modality is used in most stable patients if available. If there is any question as to genitourinary injury, an injected CT scan will be of great utility. If this is unavailable or not desired, or the patient may not be moved to the radiology suite, an infusion urogram may be performed in the emergency department with a portable technique, using 1 to 2 mL/kg of 50% Renografin dye given rapidly intravenously followed by an abdominal flat plate after 5 minutes to view the upper urinary tracts in any case of

trauma (even with hypotension, this technique is efficacious and usually not associated with subsequent renal failure). Renografin diluted with sterile saline (to a total volume of 250 to 300 mL in the adult) also may be placed in the bladder via Foley catheter to rule out bladder rupture via flat plate. This will not diagnose urethral injury, however. Urethrography will do so but should be performed in concert with urologic consultants. Note that peritoneal lavage fluid may be recovered by Foley catheter in large quantity during the lavage in the face of bladder disruption, and this may be the first or only clue to lower genitourinary tract injury.

After peritoneal lavage is completed, the catheter is removed, and the abdominal wall is closed with interrupted sutures. Patients with negative lavage may be discharged (rarely), subjected to further study (including CT scanning) as appropriate, and (in most cases) admitted for observation.

TRAUMA TO THE EXTREMITIES

During the primary and secondary surveys, many extremity injuries can be identified. Bleeding is controlled best initially by compression dressings. Lacerations can be repaired later, when the patient's more serious injuries have been managed. Fractures initially are treated by simple splinting. In most patients, it is recommended that definitive stabilization by external or internal fixation be performed within the first 24 hours, because this can reduce the incidence of pulmonary and other complications (Phillips and Contreras, 1990).

Tendon Repair

Lacerations of flexor tendons and most extensor tendons of the hand are considered complex injuries, and are best referred to hand specialists. Physicians with prior experience or special training may elect to repair some extensor tendons that are not under tension, utilizing one of several techniques. If tendon repair is not carried out, irrigation, débridement, loose primary skin closure, and splinting are recommended (Hart and Kutz, 1993; Hart and Uehara, 1993).

Amputations and Replantations

Since the 1960s, technical and instrument improvements have made possible the replantation of complete and incomplete amputations for patients with access to qualified surgeons. Injuries that qualify for consideration include: (1) multiple digits, (2) the thumb, (3) the wrist or forearm, (4) sharp amputations with minimal avulsion proximal to the elbow, (5), single digits at the middle phalanx, and (6) all children. Contraindications exist for some injuries: (1) patients unstable secondary to other life-threatening conditions, (2) crush injuries, (3) multiple-level amputations, (4) self-inflicted amputations, (5) serious underlying vascular disease, (6) age extremes, and (7) single-digit amputations at the proximal phalanx (Schlenker and Koulis, 1993).

Initial management consists of controlling hemorrhage with pressure dressings, cleaning the wound with irrigation using lactated Ringer's solution and gentle mechanical débridement, and irrigating and preserving the amputated part. The amputated part is wrapped in saline-soaked gauze and placed in a dry plastic bag, then placed on ice as soon as possible to cool it as close as possible to 4° C.

A trained surgeon should be contacted early, either at your facility or at a referral center. The ultimate decision whether to attempt replantation or not will be made by the surgeon; if an attempt is to be made, it should be within 6 hours of warm ischemia or 12 hours of cold ischemia to avoid irreversible myonecrosis of involved muscle tissue, or within 8 to 12 hours of warm ischemia or 24 hours of cold ischemia for bone, tendon, and skin.

PRINCIPLES OF WOUND CARE

The few fundamental principles of wound care necessary to prepare and suture lacerations adequately are straightforward but of great importance. All wounds must be cleansed. Initially, scrubbing with a sponge or soft brush and antiseptic solution will provide débridement. For large lacerations, high-pressure copious irrigation with 150 to 300 mL of saline solution using a 30- to 35-mL syringe and an 18- to 20-gauge needle also is advised to reduce bacterial counts in wounds and decrease the risk of infection. Hydrogen peroxide and detergents probably should be avoided because they have been shown to have deleterious effects on healing tissues (Chisholm, 1992). When possible, tissue that is crushed or devitalized should be excised prior to wound closure.

Once the wound is irrigated, the patient draped and anesthetized, and débridement completed, the wound may be closed. For optimal scar formation, wound margins must be free of undue tension. A layered closure of lacerations is helpful to achieve reduction of tension for skin closure in deep lacerations. Ideally, each layer of subcutaneous tissue should be sutured separately, but, in practice, all that often is needed is to assure eversion of wound edges and release of surface tension by sutures placed at the dermal–fatty junction of subcutaneous tissues (Moy et al., 1991).

Initial sutures should divide a laceration evenly in half, then into quarters, and so forth. Entry and exit of sutures should be equally distant from wound margins. Usually sutures placed every 5 mm will allow approximation without tension. Placing sutures too tightly will lead to increased scarring from the subsequent swelling of wound edges; leaving sutures in place longer and using larger "bites" for each suture also will create a more prominent scar. The factors involved in permanent scar formation are listed in Table 36–3.

Eversion of wound edges produces a better scar. This can be accomplished by making sutures that are deeper than they are wide. Angle the needle back away from the wound edge, making a bottle-shaped entry, and scrape the needle under the skin

TABLE 36–3. FACTORS IN SCAR FORMATION IN SUTURED WOUNDS

Tension on sutures
Length of time sutures in place
Amount of tissue held by suture (bite)
Region of body (face, hands, soles of feet less likely to railroad-track)
Infection
Keloid formation

From Morse SD, Rial WY: Emergency medicine. *In* Rakel RE (ed): Textbook of Family Practice, 4th edition. Philadelphia, WB Saunders Company, 1990, p 958, with permission.

TABLE 36–4. SUTURE REMOVAL

Face	3–5 days (subsequent reinforcement with benzoin tincture and microporous adhesive tape [Steri-strips] advised)
Scalp	7–10 days
Extremity	
Not over joint	7 days
Over joint	10–14 days (augment with splinting)
Feet	10–14 days (only sew feet if absolutely necessary)
Trunk	
Anterior	7 days
Back	10–14 days

From Morse SD, Rial WY: Emergency medicine. *In* Rakel RE (ed): Textbook of Family Practice, 4th edition. Philadelphia, WB Saunders Company, 1990, p 959, with permission.

on the way out to ensure everted edges. Vertical mattress sutures also may be used to the same purpose (Fig. 36–6).

For skin closure, practical differences between nonabsorbable sutures are slight. Synthetics (nylon or Dermalon, polypropylene or Surgilene, and so on) are stronger but harder to manipulate than silk or cotton. The braided structure of silk sutures makes them prone to infection, in theory, in comparison to monofilament synthetic sutures.

For routine wound closure, 4-0 suture usually will be adequate. Cosmetic repair requires 6-0 suture material. Sutures of 3-0 material may be required at some sites, such as the scalp or over major joints, to provide additional strength (Markovchick, 1992).

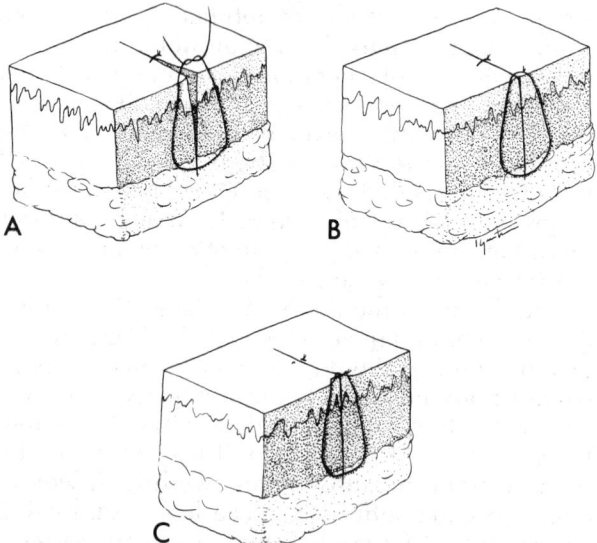

FIGURE 36–6. Good eversion of wound edges is crucial to subsequent cosmetic results. Make sutures deeper than they are wide, and wider at bottom than top to produce this result (*A, B*). A vertical mattress suture (*C*) is a simple variation that achieves good eversion and assures minimal tension on wound edges. (From Morse SD, Rial WY: Emergency medicine. *In* Rakel RE [ed]: Textbook of Family Practice, 4th edition. Philadelphia, WB Saunders Company, 1990, p 959, with permission.)

A useful schedule for suture removal is listed in Table 36–4 these represent general guidelines to be tempered by experience and individual preference.

Several areas of the body require attention to a few special principles. The scalp is very vascular and bleeds profusely; shock caused by extensive blood loss may be seen with large lacerations, and rapid closure may be advisable. Clamping of vessels is usually an inappropriate maneuver unless a major proximal artery has been transected and is identifiable. Hemostasis otherwise can be obtained first by direct pressure and then by either interrupted, vertical mattress, or running lockstitch sutures. It is wise, after anesthetizing the wound, to probe with the gloved finger and rule out an associated skull fracture (usually skull radiographs will not be required). Do not mistake the torn edges of the galea aponeurotica of the scalp for a bony defect; this is a common error. If at all possible, the edges of the torn galea should be reapproximated. Use large sutures, such as 3-0, on a large strong needle for scalp closure. If oozing persists, apply direct pressure. The patient can wash the area normally in 24 to 48 hours, as with any other uncomplicated laceration.

Eyebrow lacerations should be managed without shaving the brow; it may not grow back, and shaving it causes loss of a landmark to judge the cosmetic results of the repair (Berk et al., 1992).

The vermilion border of the lip requires special attention in closure of lacerations; the first suture placed should exactly reapproximate the edges at this border because a defect of only 1 to 2 mm is obvious (Fig. 36–7). In through-and-through lip lacerations, close the muscular tissues first with 4-0 or 5-0 chromic sutures, then the vermilion and external tissues with synthetic sutures. Some authorities close mucosal lacerations in the mouth with silk sutures, arguing for less hypertrophic scar formation and morbidity with this approach. However, doing so raises the potential for infection in

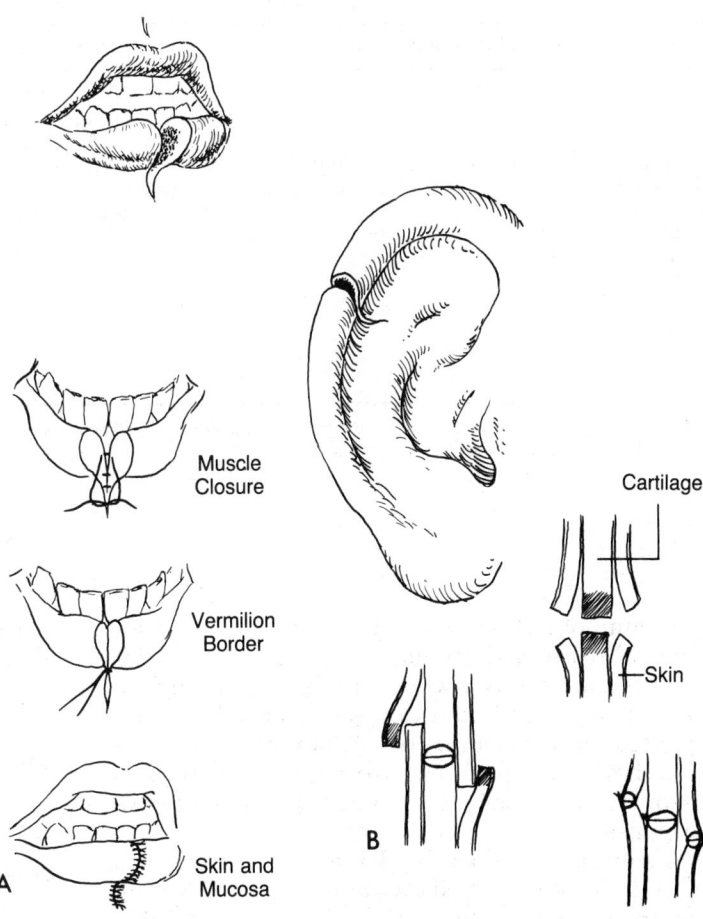

FIGURE 36–7. Ear and lip repairs require some special care. *A*, Close through-and-through lip lacerations in a layered fashion; the first surface suture must exactly reapproximate the torn vermilion border. *B*, The ear requires closure of cartilage and perichondrium with absorbable sutures; stagger the skin suture closure as shown to avoid a "pitting" deformity when the pinna heals. Anesthetize the pinna using plain lidocaine and injecting all the way around the base of the ear a full 360 degrees subcutaneously. (From Morse SD, Rial WY: Emergency medicine. *In* Rakel RE [ed]: Textbook of Family Practice, 4th edition. Philadelphia, WB Saunders Company, 1990, p 960, with permission.)

the wound, particularly if tissue is contused, because the mouth is never sterile. If closure is performed, oral penicillin coverage is advisable while the sutures are in place. Careful attention to oral hygiene is mandatory during healing in either event. Remove the sutures in 5 days.

Lacerations of the tongue rarely require suturing. However, a laceration of the tip longer than 1 cm will heal with a forked tongue deformity unless reapproximated.

Intraoral lacerations in children can be closed with absorbable suture material. This will obviate the need for subsequent removal and lessen the child's ordeal.

Lacerations seen more than 8 to 12 hours after injury, not caused by bite wounds, may be cleaned, dressed, and followed. If no infection is present by the third to fifth day after injury and closure is mandatory, secondary closure can be done.

Ear lacerations require closure of the perichondrium over any exposed cartilage to avoid necrosis from devascularization. The skin may be closed thereafter, and a pressure dressing may be applied to prevent hematoma and a cauliflower ear deformity. Anesthesia is obtained by intradermal and subcutaneous injection of agents free of epinephrine around the base of the pinna for a full 360 degrees.

ANESTHESIA TECHNIQUES

In general, whichever anesthetic is used, "use the smallest effective amount of the least toxic substance in the safest possible manner" (Ervin, 1978, p. 392).

Local anesthetics in common use today consist of either an ester (procaine-type) or amide (lidocaine-type) linkage joining an aromatic, lipophilic chain to a hydrophilic, tertiary amine. Table 36–5 lists representative drugs for local anesthesia. These medications are weak bases, prepared as hydrochloride salts to increase their shelf-life. The acidic pH causes most of the pain associated with injection, and can be decreased dramatically by buffering with 1 mL sodium bicarbonate to 10 mL anesthetic without decreasing efficacy (Arpey and Lynch, 1992; Norris, 1992).

True allergic reactions are uncommon; when they occur, they are usually in response to the

TABLE 36–5. LOCAL ANESTHETIC AGENTS

Chemical Class	Agent Commonly Used	Comment
Para-aminobenzoic acid (ester)	Procaine (Novocain) Tetracaine (Pontocain) Chloroprocaine (Nesacaine)	
Diethylamino-2′,6′-acetoxylidide (amide) *dl*-N-methylpipecolic acid 2,6-dimethylanilide (amide)	Lidocaine (Xylocaine) Mepivacaine (Carbocaine) Bupivacaine (Marcaine)	Marcaine is very long acting (up to 24 hours) Useful in toothache analgesia
Benzoic acid (ester)	Cocaine	Cocaine approved only for use in epistaxis Cocaine is the only local anesthetic that is a vasoconstrictor Appears useful for wounds topically with tetracaine and adrenaline (topical TAC therapy)

From Morse SD, Rial WY: Emergency medicine. *In* Rakel RE (ed): Textbook of Family Practice, 4th edition. Philadelphia, WB Saunders Company, 1990, p 961, with permission.

para-aminobenzoic acid metabolite of an ester agent. Cross-reactivity does not occur, but a concomitent allergy is always possible, so the physician must be prepared to treat major allergic responses and perform resuscitation in such a situation. Toxic reactions are more common, and vasovagal reactions are the most common adverse response.

A solution of lidocaine, 1% to 2% is used most often in local anesthesia. When working in vascular areas, such as the face, solutions containing 1:100,000 epinephrine will aid in hemostasis as well as help to prolong duration and minimize toxicity of anesthetics. Remember that epinephrine must never be used in anesthetizing end organs (digits, nose, ears, or penis) because it can cause ischemic gangrene.

A wound should be approached from its cut margin, placing a sufficient quantity of anesthetic into the dermal layer to provide the desired result. Introducing the needle into the wound is less painful than placing it through intact skin. Anesthesia should be provided before any vigorous cleansing or débridement; this has not been shown to increase rate of wound infection.

A 25-gauge needle should be used, raising a skin wheal and then advancing, aspirating each time before injection to avoid an inadvertent intravascular injection. In an adult, up to a maximum of 300 mg of lidocaine may be used in one local application; this must be scaled down appropriate to body weight in children.

Sedation of children before suturing is occasionally helpful, although a restraining papoose board or blanket is often equally useful. If sedation is used, one useful regimen is meperidine (Demerol), 0.5 to 1.0 mg/kg, and promethazine (Phenergan), 0.2 to 0.5 mg/kg, intramuscularly (the addition of chlorpromazine [Thorazine] in doses of 0.1 to 0.2 mg/kg produces even more profound sedation).

Nerve Block Techniques

Regional anesthetic techniques are many and varied. The most useful for laceration repair are digital blocks and regional facial blocks.

Digital nerves in the hand may be anesthetized before they divide at the metacarpal heads or selectively at the base of a finger. To perform transmetacarpal block, a 25-gauge needle is inserted perpendicular to the skin of the dorsum of the hand at the level of the metacarpal head (distal palmar crease) and advanced laterally to the same depth as the middle of the metacarpal head. Two or three milliliters of anesthetic is placed and the needle withdrawn. This is repeated on the other side of the digit. Anesthesia is obtained in less than 5 minutes.

More selective digital nerve block again uses a 25-gauge needle, placing anesthesia at the base of the proximal phalanx on both sides, both dorsally and ventrally. A quantity of local anesthetic that is too large can induce vascular compression with this technique and result in gangrene, so care is required (Fig. 36–8).

Facial sensation may be blocked selectively at the foraminal exits of each of the three trigeminal nerve divisions. The foramina for the supraorbital, infraorbital, and mental nerves lie in a nearly vertical line that lies just medial to the patient's cornea in the position of forward gaze (Fig. 36–8). Infiltration over the eyebrow and glabella blocks the supratrochlear and supraorbital nerves, to anesthetize the forehead and anterior scalp. Injection around the infraorbital foramen blocks the infraorbital area and the upper lip. Infiltration at the mental foramen blocks the lower lip and chin.

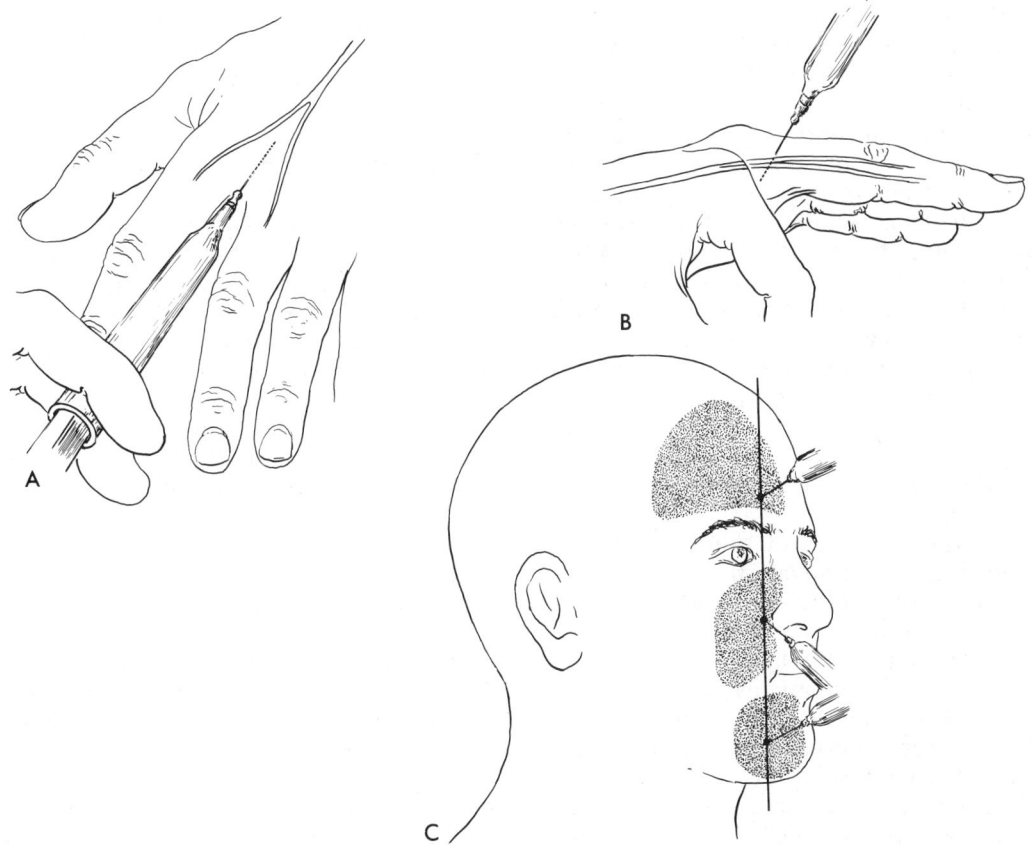

FIGURE 36–8. Regional blocks. *A,* Dorsal fingerweb entry is used for transmetacarpal block. *B,* A more distal site and arc-like pattern of injection provide a digital block. *C,* The branches of the trigeminal nerve, blocked in facial blocks, enter the face through foramina that lie in a straight line. (From Morse SD, Rial WY: Emergency medicine. *In* Rakel RE [ed]: Textbook of Family Practice, 4th edition. Philadelphia, WB Saunders Company, 1990, p 962, with permission.)

SPECIAL SITUATIONS

Trauma in the Geriatric Patient

Trauma accounts for 2 per cent of elderly deaths but 28 per cent of all injury fatalities in the United States (DeMaria, 1993). Mechanisms of injury include (1) motor vehicle accidents, (2) falls, (3) pedestrian accidents, and (4) stab and gunshot wounds (Levy et al., 1993). Under normal conditions, most elderly patients maintain internal homeostasis; however, their impaired response to the stress of trauma results in increased mortality for a given level of injury severity compared with younger persons. Complications play an important role in mortality; deaths after 24 hours result from multiple conditions, including respiratory complications, infections, cardiac complications, and multiple organ failure (Pellicane et al., 1992).

Trauma in the Pediatric Patient

In the United States, almost half of the deaths in children ages 1 to 14 result from trauma (Schafer-

meyer, 1993). Etiologies include (1) motor vehicle accidents, (2) poisonings, (3) fires, (4) falls, (5) homicides and suicides, and (6) pedestrian injuries. Thirty per cent have head injuries. Lacerations and abrasions are the most common injuries for children under 17, followed by fractures and dislocations, ingestions, and bites (Gratz, 1979). A special training course for those who will be dealing with pediatric trauma has been developed, called Pediatric Advanced Life Support (PALS) (Thompson et al., 1984).

Physiologic differences exist in the child (Rouse and Eichelberger, 1992). The younger the child, the more prominent the occiput. Cervical vertebral facets are flatter and oriented horizontally, while ligaments are more flexible. There is a greater body surface area–to–weight ratio. Acute blood loss is responded to by increasing heart rate (rather than stroke volume) and systemic vascular resistance, often maintaining blood pressure until blood loss exceeds 25 per cent of blood volume. Causes of death include airway compromise, hypovolemic shock, and central nervous system injury. Hypothermia is an important complication.

Several other special considerations should be

made in pediatric patients. Use uncuffed endotracheal tubes in children less than 8 years of age to avoid pressure necrosis. If peripheral access cannot be obtained, intraosseous access is the procedure of choice, although central access through the femoral vein or a venous cutdown may be attempted by those trained in these techniques.

Diaphragmatic hernia is increasing in incidence as a part of the lap belt complex of injuries. Blunt abdominal injuries in stable children often are evaluated and followed with CT scanning rather than by peritoneal lavage. Organs often injured include spleen, liver, pancreas, and a hollow viscous (especially in lap-belted children).

Trauma in the Obstetric Patient

The most frequent causes of blunt abdominal trauma requiring hospitalization of pregnant women are falls, motor vehicle accidents, and direct blows to the abdomen (Neufeld, 1993; Pearlman and Tintinalli, 1991). Continuous external fetal monitoring of pregnancies greater than 24 to 26 weeks' gestation should be instituted as soon as feasible. Vigorous maternal resuscitation is the first priority and ultimately results in the best fetal outcome. The most common causes of fetal death in blunt trauma are maternal death, maternal shock, and placental abruption. The most common obstetric problem caused by trauma is uterine contractions; 90 per cent stop spontaneously. Abruptio placentae, an important cause of fetal death, usually is associated with frequent uterine activity (more than eight uterine contractions per hour) during the first 4 hours of monitoring.

Any viable fetus with a gestational age of 24 or more weeks requires monitoring after a trauma event. Ultrasonography to assess the fetus is a valuable adjunct. Fetomaternal hemorrhage is detected by the Kleihauer-Betke acid elution technique on maternal blood. All Rh-negative mothers who present with a history of abdominal trauma should receive one 300-μg prophylactic dose of Rh immune globulin (Dudley and Cruikshank, 1990).

During pregnancy, several physiologic parameters undergo changes that must be kept in mind. Maternal blood volume increases, cardiac output increases unless the inferior vena cava is compressed by the uterus in the supine position, and blood pressure decreases while heart rate increases during the second trimester (Pearlman and Tintinalli, 1991).

Diagnostic peritoneal lavage by the open technique above the uterine fundus is safe. Bowel injury is more likely with penetrating injuries to the upper abdomen. Gunshot wounds should be explored; stab wounds in stable patients may be evaluated with diagnostic peritoneal lavage.

With injuries to the uterus, a viable fetus in distress is grounds for immediate cesarean section and exploration with any penetrating wound. In most patients having surgery for trauma, cesarean delivery is not necessary.

Falls from Heights

Significant falls from heights, while not generally common, are the second leading cause of trauma deaths in the United States. The abrupt vertical deceleration on impact results in injury as the body absorbs the kinetic energy accumulated during the free fall. The probability of death abruptly increases at seven stories with solid surfaces and at 130 feet with displaceable surfaces such as water, and is usually due to uncontrollable shock and lethal head injuries (Buckman and Buckman, 1991).

In urban free falls, patients who survive long enough to reach the hospital frequently have multiple injuries of the head, torso, and extremities. Head injuries, present in 10 to 20 per cent of these patients, are often the result of secondary impacts. Thoracic injuries are also common, as are intraperitoneal injuries. The latter are usually the result of shearing forces on a hollow viscera, such as the duodenum.

The most frequent impact pattern is a feet-first landing, resulting in multiple fractures of the lower extremities as well as burst fractures of the vertebral bodies. Three patterns of vascular injuries have been described: (1) rupture of the thoracic aorta (uncommon in patients who survive to reach the hospital), (2) peripheral vascular disruptions from fractures and dislocations, and (3) rupture of lumbar and hypogastric vessels.

Bicycle Injuries

Serious bicycle injuries often result from being struck by a motor vehicle, falling from a bicycle, or being struck by a bicycle, with most fatalities occurring in those under age 19 (Tucci and Barone, 1988). Injuries to the upper extremities are common, as are head and neck injuries; the types of injuries reported include contusions, fractures, and lacerations (Björnstig et al., and Friede et al., 1985). Many areas are instituting laws mandating the use of equipment such as safety helmets in an attempt to decrease the serious morbidity and mortality associated with these injuries (Stylianos and Eichelberger, 1993).

Dental Injuries

Patients with dental injuries frequently will present to acute care settings seeking assistance. While unfamiliar procedures should not be attempted by untrained individuals, knowing how to perform an appropriate examination can help determine the nature of the problem (Klokkevold, 1989).

Three techniques are employed routinely in the emergency setting. Percussion of teeth by tapping the crown with a blunt instrument detects the condition of the periodontal ligament; sensitivity suggests periapical inflammation. Transillumination of enamel with a high-intensity light can detect cracks as a break in the light transmission. Probing the gingival sulcus with a dental probe can detect periodontal disease.

A special situation occasionally encountered is the total dislocation (or avulsion) of a tooth. This is best treated by replantation in less than 2 hours. If immediate replantation is not possible, the tooth should be transported in a suitable transport medium; normal saline is ideal, milk is also good, and saliva (i.e., in the mouth) is an alternative option. Water should be avoided because its hypotonicity will lyse periodontal ligament cells.

Wringer Injuries

Wringer-type injury may be seen in children who put their hands between the rollers of older washing machines still in use. More commonly, adults will present with such an injury from an industrial accident, because mechanical devices using rollers or other rotating surfaces produce a similar shearing and compressive injury (Palmaccio and Greenberg, 1982).

The initial appearance of a wringer injury may be very benign. However, three major types of force have injured tissue, and injuries may be clinically manifest after some delay: compressive force leads to soft tissue edema with potential loss of vascular supply as a result of a compartment symdrome; frictional force generates heat and may lead to full-thickness burns; and shearing force can separate the dermis from deeper tissue and cause a delayed necrosis. Severe injury to hands and fingers, with permanent functional loss or amputation, is not uncommon.

About half the wringer-type injuries seen will have some significant complication. Most common are soft-tissue injuries, ranging from abrasion to full-thickness skin loss. Fractures or dislocations of phalanges may be present, but long bones are usually spared. Peripheral nerve injuries are common but usually incomplete and temporary.

The wringer injury's severity is classically difficult to assess in its early stage. Edema may not be clinically obvious for 48 hours, and devascularization may be relatively inapparent for up to a week.

Initial evaluation of wringer injury includes determination of the presence of edema and neurovascular status and search for fractures and dislocations. Good wound care should be performed, but lacerations should not be closed primarily until it is clear from history and examination that the injury is trivial, because these are really burst and crush injuries of uncertain viability (Proust, 1993).

Treatment is expectant in these injuries; a soft compression dressing and elevation using stockinette and an intravenous solution pole are good maneuvers, and neurovascular status must be followed. Most physicians advise that all patients with wringer injury, regardless of initial physical examination, be admitted to the hospital for 24 hours for elevation and observation, unless the duration and extent of injury are clearly trivial by history. Evidence of progressive neurovascular deterioration mandates fasciotomy.

High-Pressure Injections (Grease Gun Injury)

First reported in the literature in 1937, high-pressure injection injuries often occur in the work place in association with grease guns, spray guns, and diesel injectors that have become blocked. Typically, an inexperienced worker attempts to clear the blockage by wiping the nozzle with his or her finger and receives an injection of grease, paint, solvent, or other toxic material. Initially there may only be a small puncture wound and few symptoms. However, if aggressive treatment is not undertaken, within several hours extensive tissue swelling, tenderness, and pain will ensue, accompanied by tissue necrosis secondary to the toxic effects of solvents, the associated thrombosis of arteries and/or veins, and neurovascular compression in closed spaces. Grease injections do not cause large inflammatory responses unless a secondary bacterial infection occurs. They most frequently are associated with fibrosis, oleomas, and draining sinus (Booth, 1977; Silsby, 1976).

Injected materials tend to spread along fascial planes and tendon sheaths, as well as through soft tissues. Higher pressures are associated with greater dispersion of the material.

The initial history obtained from these patients should include hand dominance, occupation, material injected, time and pressure of injection, any previous therapy, and circumstances of the injury. The motor and sensory status of the injured extremity, and the vascular status, must be determined. At no time should the patient be given local anesthesia for pain relief, because this could increase tissue pressure and worsen necrosis (Proust, 1993).

Many injected materials will be radiopaque. Radiologic studies of the injured extremity should be obtained to assess the extent of spread of the injection. These patients must be told of the serious nature of their innocuous-looking injury at once and rapidly referred to a hand surgeon. Wide decompression and débridement usually are required, and often the wounds must be left open for copious irrigation and further débridement. Elevation, antibiotics, steroids, and tetanus toxoid are important adjuncts. Prolonged disability and slow healing are common with these injuries, which require prolonged follow-up and intense rehabilitative efforts.

Fishhooks (and Other Impalements)

Impalement, especially of the hand, by fishhooks is common in warm months. If the hook is caught in the soft fleshy part of the skin, with the point tenting up, the area should be anesthetized (either locally or by digital block in the finger), the hook pushed gently through, and the barb cut off; the shaft then may be withdrawn without further tissue damage (Fig. 36–9A). Antibiotics, tetanus toxoid, and observation thereafter are appropriate (Doser et al., 1991).

If the hook is pointing toward deeper structures, one can insert an 18-gauge needle adjacent to the barb so its bevelled open end fits over the barb; the needle and hook then are backed out together (Fig. 36–9B).

In some regions, the "string technique" is used for superficial unbarbed fishhooks. A filament is wrapped around the bend of the hook and the free ends are held in one hand. Gentle downward pressure on the shank of the hook disengages the tip, allowing retrograde extraction by gently tugging the filament (Fig. 36–9C) (Lantsberg et al., 1992; Terrill, 1993).

Foreign Bodies

Inquisitive children, perverse or retarded adults, and seriously suicidal patients may use any bodily

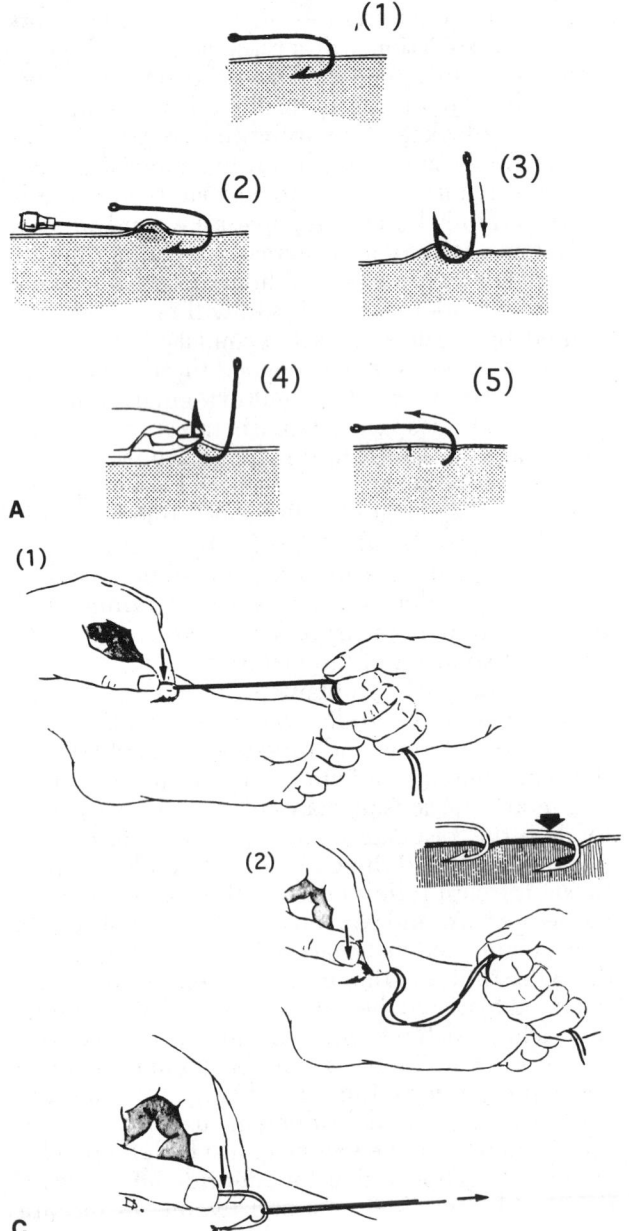

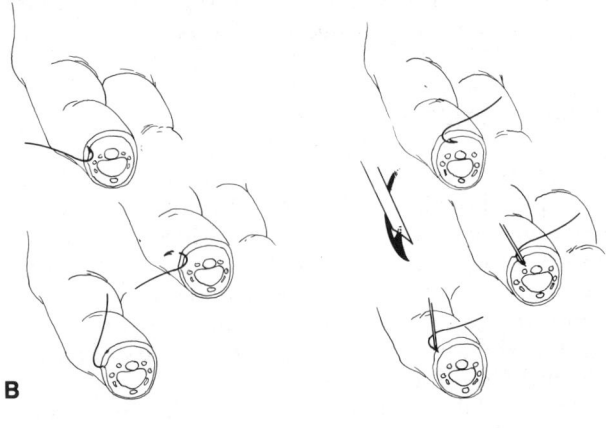

FIGURE 36–9. Techniques of fishhook extraction. Either push the barb through and cut it off (A), cover the barb with the bevel of a hypodermic needle and extract the two together (B), or try the "string" technique (C). (A from Tischler CD, Swan KG, Norton LW. Trauma. In Hill GJ [ed]: Outpatient Surgery, 3rd edition. Philadelphia, WB Saunders Company, 1988, p 64, with permission; B from Morse SD, Rial WY: Emergency medicine. *In* Rakel RE [ed]: Textbook of Family Practice, 4th edition. Philadelphia, WB Saunders Company, 1990, p 971, with permission; C from Tischler CD, Swan KG, Norton LW: Trauma. *In* Hill GJ [ed]: Outpatient Surgery, 3rd edition. Philadelphia, WB Saunders Company, 1988, p 63, with permission.)

orifice for the insertion of a wide variety of foreign materials. In initial evaluation, there are two questions of major importance. First, what is the chemical and physical nature of the object? Second, exactly what is it? Answers to these questions allow an appropriate clinical response for management.

Hydrocarbons, caustics, contaminated objects, wood, and organic fibers are highly reactive, inducing a marked foreign body reaction. Metal, glass, and uncontaminated inert objects, in contrast, are rather nonirritating unless their physical shape is jagged or their location is an already irritated region of the body.

Regions of the body where foreign objects lodge can be grouped by the danger level the foreign object's presence produces. Tracheobronchial, intravascular, and intraocular foreign bodies are all highly dangerous threats to life or organ function. Objects lodged in solid viscera, bodily orifices, the esophagus, and joints and cavities are potentionally dangerous. Obstruction to drainage or tissue contamination may lead to sepsis, and erosion or perforation of structures may occur with jagged objects. Minimal danger is present when objects lodge in skin, subcutaneous tissue, or muscle or enter the stomach and intestines. Specific situations will be examined below. Figure 36–10 demonstrates some representative radiopaque foreign bodies.

Tracheobronchial foreign bodies may be radiopaque or radiolucent. Coughing, choking, transient cyanosis, and an inspiratory wheeze over the involved bronchus should suggest this entitiy. If the object is made of organic vegetable material, it may absorb water and enlarge, producing progressive obstruction. Proximal migration may lead to acute subglottic obstruction and respiratory arrest if therapy is not undertaken rapidly.

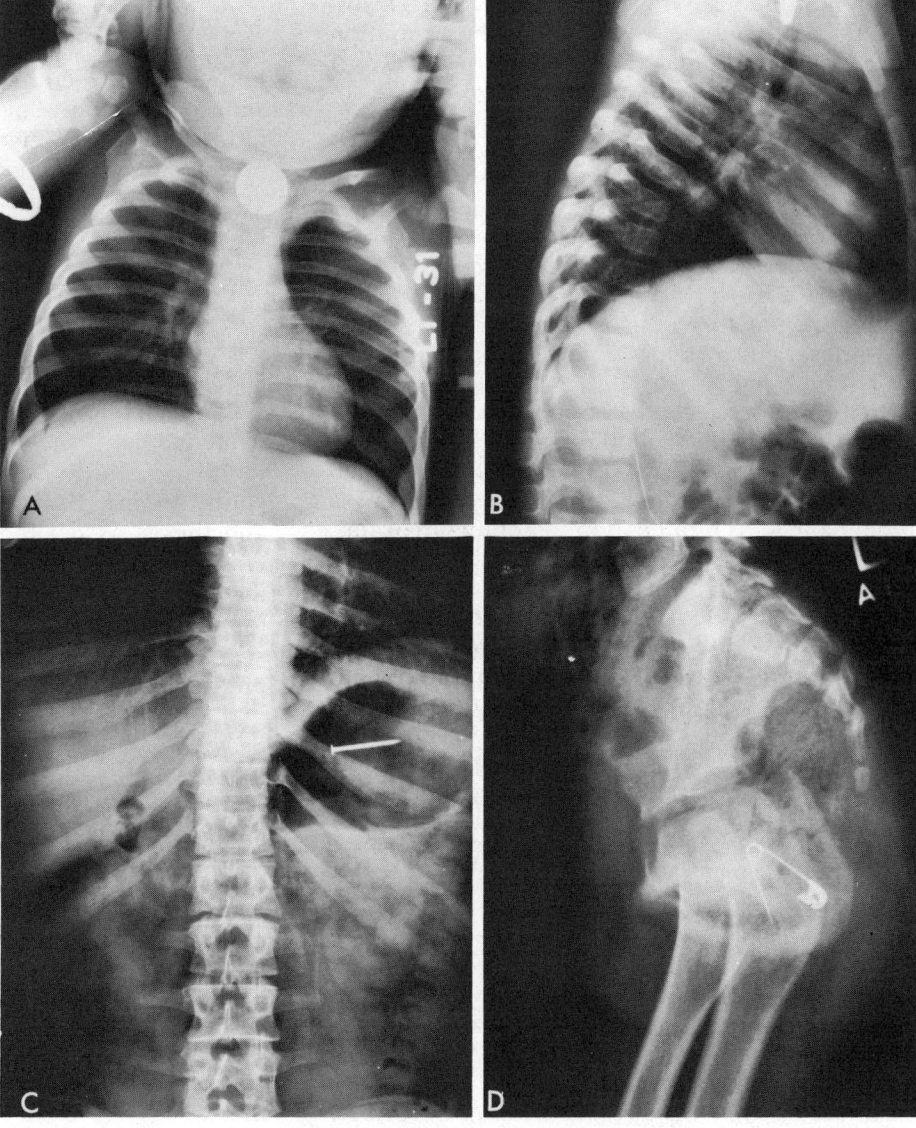

FIGURE 36–10. Multiple examples of foreign bodies. The swallowed coin (*A, B*) is classically caught at the thoracic inlet and is in the coronal plane. Even very sharp objects (*C*) usually pass once the stomach is entered and should be expelled from the rectum blunt end first. Thus, the safety pin (*D*) is atypical and may have been inserted via the anus; consider child abuse. (From Wagner DK: Ingestions and foreign bodies. Curr Top II Emerg Med 4(2). Philadelphia, Medical College of Pennsylvania, 1982, with permission.)

Inspiratory and expiratory films of the chest or bilateral decubitus films should be obtained. Patients with radiolucent foreign bodies show the following:

1. Early hyperaeration on the involved side.
2. No loss of volume when the involved side is dependent.
3. Mediastinal shift away from the involved side.
4. Delayed atelectasis and pneumonia.

Bronchoscopy is indicated as quickly as possible for removal.

Esophageal foreign bodies are common, and three locations are characteristic. Most commonly, the ingested object rests at the esophageal inlet as a result of the actions of the cricopharyngeus muscle sphincter, and, if it is smooth and flat, it rests in the coronal plane (Fig. 36–10). Smooth, nonreactive objects can be removed at this area by use of a Foley catheter, if the patient is cooperative or easily restrained. The procedure should be done under fluoroscopy with the patient in the semiprone Trendelenburg position to avoid aspiration and with contrast material instilled in the Foley balloon. The catheter is advanced beyond the object, the balloon inflated, and the catheter withdrawn. Sharp objects should be removed endoscopically to avoid perforation and its sequelae.

Esophageal foreign bodies also occur at the middle third of the esophagus where it abuts mediastinal structures and at the gastroesophageal junction. Glucagon (1 mg intravenously or intramuscularly) and other agents have been suggested for esophageal relaxation to promote passage of foreign objects.

Nonreactive objects that enter the *stomach* will be passed spontaneously 95 per cent of the time, including sharp objects (Fig. 36–10). Owing to peristaltic activity, these objects invariably pass through the anus blunt end first. Follow-up examination and radiographs are required to document passage.

Rectal foreign bodies are of concern because, if perforation occurs, invasive infection will occur. Attempts to remove large objects from the rectum produce a suction effect. A 30-mL Foley catheter passed proximal to the object will aid in extraction and break the vacuum. Occasionally, general anesthesia may be necessary. A sharp object in the rectum, which has its point directed toward the anal verge, probably was instilled through the anus. In the child, consider abuse (Fig. 36–10).

Nasal foreign bodies may present as a malodorous discharge with obstruction. After cocainizing the nostril, the child can be laid supine and mouth-to-mouth breathing used with a single forceful breath, closing the unobstructed nostril. The foreign object usually will be expelled. Alligator forceps also may be used for extraction.

Children commonly present with *aural foreign bodies*. Irrigation, directing the water stream upward and backward, can remove many inanimate objects, but should be avoided if vegetable matter is present because such objects can expand and become painful; with vegetable matter it is better to use a fine forceps or spoon, under anesthesia if necessary. Insects should be killed immediately, using mineral oil or ether, to prevent further local pain and trauma. Objects beyond the isthmus of the auditory canal can be difficult to access and, if not easily removed, are best left to more experienced hands (Bear, 1991).

Button batteries have been reported as foreign bodies in the ear, nose, and esophagus. These are dangerous situations because of the frequency with which local tissue necrosis occurs, and require close follow-up (Friedman, 1989; Holinger, 1990; McRae et al., 1989; Tong et al., 1992).

Foul vaginal discharge in a child means a *vaginal foreign body* until proved otherwise. Rectal examination usually allows palpation of the object through the rectovaginal septum. Extraction can be carried out using a nasal speculum and a fine forceps, or under anesthesia if necessary. Foreign bodies in the rectum or vagina or children always should raise the issue of child abuse in the mind of the examining physician.

Ocular foreign bodies are usually conjunctival, corneal, or intraocular. Conjunctival foreign bodies usually lodge under the upper lid beneath the tarsal plate. Pulling the upper lid over the lower usually will sweep the plate clean and clear the object. The lid can be everted for direct inspection. Whenever a foreign body is found, the cornea must be stained with fluorescein to look for an abrasion.

Corneal foreign bodies often can be removed using topical anesthesia and irrigation, or, if lodged, a sterile large-bore needle or a corneal spud (Augeri, 1991). Small children may require anesthesia. Associated abrasions must be followed closely and should be at least 50 per cent healed in 24 hours and totally healed in 48 hours. Mydriatics, topical antibiotics, patching, and systemic analgesia often are employed. Topical anesthetics should not be prescribed for home use.

If any possibility exists that an ocular injury has occurred while high-velocity fragments were generated (such as during grinding or hammering), or if slit-lamp examination reveals scleral laceration, an intraocular foreign body must be suspected. This demands orbital ultrasound and ophthalmologic consultation.

The hands and feet are prone to receive *implanted foreign bodies*. If visible or palpable, extraction can be immediate. Otherwise, the object should be allowed 3 to 5 days to encyst in the soft tissues. Removal then can be carried out easily (under fluoroscopy if necessary) with local anesthesia.

REFERENCES AND SUGGESTED READINGS

Trauma

Collicott PE: Advanced trauma life support (ATLS): Past, present, future—16th Stone Lecture, American Trauma Society. J Trauma 33:749, 1992.

Committee on Trauma, American College of Surgeons: Advanced Trauma Life Support Course, 1988 Core Course. Chicago, American College of Surgeons, 1988.

National Safety Council: Accident Facts. Itasca, IL, National Safety Council, 1992.

Schmidt J, Moore GP: Management of multiple trauma. Adv Trauma 11:29, 1993.

Trauma Indices

Champion HR, Sacco WJ, Copes WS, et al: A revision of the trauma score. J Trauma 29:623, 1989.

Jennett B, Teasdale G: Aspects of coma after severe head injury. Lancet 1:878, 1977.

Chest Trauma

Boyd M, Vanek VW, Bourguet CC: Emergency room resuscitative thoracotomy: When is it indicated? J Trauma 33:714, 1992.

Calhoon JH, Grover FL, Trinkle JK: Chest trauma: Approach and management. Clin Chest Med 13:55, 1992.

Curtis P: Spontaneous pneumothorax: A dilemma of management. J Fam Pract 6:367, 1978.

Davidson SJ: Autotransfusion from hemothorax. Curr Concepts Trauma Care 2:2, 1979.

Davidson SJ: Correct use of autotransfusion in the emergency patient. ER Rep 2:73, 1981.

Kirby TJ, Ginsberg RJ: Management of the pneumothorax and barotrauma. Clin Chest Med 13:97, 1992.

Wasserberger J, Ordog GJ, Dang C, Schlater TL: Emergency department thoracotomy. Emerg Med Clin North Am 7:103, 1989.

Abdominal Trauma

Drost TF, Rosemurgy AS, Kearney RE, Roberts P: Diagnostic peritoneal lavage: Limited indications due to evolving concepts in trauma care. Am Surg 57:126, 1991.

Feliciano DV: Diagnostic modalities in abdominal trauma. Surg Clin North Am 71:241, 1991.

Gay SB, Sistrom CL: Computed tomographic evaluation of blunt abdominal trauma. Radiol Clin North Am 30:367, 1992.

Henneman PL: Penetrating abdominal trauma. Emerg Med Clin North Am 7:647, 1989.

Kessler E, Stein A: Diaphragmatic hernia as a long-term complication of stab wounds of the chest. Am J Surg 132:34, 1976.

Lazarus HM, Nelson JA: Refining the technique of diagnostic peritoneal lavage. ER Rep 1:111, 1980.

Lucas CE: Second annual W. R. Ghent Lecture on Trauma. Abdominal organ injury: Diagnosis, treatment, and education. Can J Surg 33:189, 1990.

Moore EE: Evaluating and managing penetrating abdominal injuries. ER Rep 2:85, 1981.

Mueller GL, Burney RE, Mackenzie JR: Sequential peritoneal lavage and early diagnosis of colon perforation. Ann Emerg Med 10:131, 1981.

Parvin W, Smith DE, Asher WM, Virgilio RW: Effectiveness of peritoneal lavage in blunt abdominal trauma. Ann Surg 181:255, 1975.

Root HD, Hauser CW, McKinley CR, et al: Diagnostic peritoneal lavage. Surgery 57:633, 1965.

Smedira N, Schecter WP: Blunt abdominal trauma. Emerg Med Clin North Am 7:631, 1989.

Thompson JS, Moore JE, Van Duzer-Moore S, et al: The evolution of abdominal stab wound management. J Trauma 20:478, 1980.

Extremity Trauma

Phillips TF, Contreras DM: Timing of operative treatment of fractures in patients who have multiple injuries. J Bone Joint Surg 72-A:784, 1990.

Tendon Repair

Hart RG, Kutz JE: Flexor tendon injuries of the hand. Emerg Med Clin North Am 11:621, 1993.

Hart RG, Uehara DT: Extensor tendon injuries of the hand. Emerg Med Clin North Am 11:637, 1993.

Amputations

Schlenker JD, Koulis CP: Amputations and replantations. Emerg Med Clin North Am 11:739, 1993.

Wound Management

Berk WA, Welch RD, Bock BF: Controversial issues in clinical management of the simple wound. Ann Emerg Med 21:72, 1992.

Chisholm CD: Wound evaluation and cleansing. Emerg Med Clin North Am 10:665, 1992.

Markovchick V: Suture materials and mechanical after care. Emerg Med Clin North Am 10:673, 1992.

Moy RL, Lee A, Zalka A: Commonly used suture techniques in skin surgery. Am Fam Physician 44:1625, 1991.

Analgesia

Arpey CJ, Lynch WS: Advances in local anesthetics. Clin Dermatol 10:275, 1992.

Berman D, Graber D: Sedation and analgesia. Emerg Med Clin North Am 10:691, 1992.

Ervin ME: Minor surgical procedures. *In* Schwartz GR, Safar P, Stone JH (eds): Principles and Practice of Emergency Medicine. Philadelphia, WB Saunders Company, 1978, pp 386–398.

Norris RL: Local anesthetics. Emerg Med Clin North Am 10:707, 1992.

Geriatrics

DeMaria EJ: Evaluation and treatment of the elderly trauma victim. Clin Geriatr Med 9:461, 1993.

Levy DB, Hanlon DP, Townsend RN: Geriatric trauma. Clin Geriatr Med 9:601, 1993.

Pellicane JV, Byrne K, DeMaria EJ: Preventable complications and death from multiple organ failure among geriatric trauma victims. J Trauma 33:440, 1992.

Pediatrics

Gratz RR: Accidental injury in childhood: A literature review on pediatric trauma. J Trauma 19:551, 1979.

Rouse TM, Eichelberger MR: Trends in pediatric trauma management. Surg Clin North Am 72:1347, 1992.

Schafermeyer R: Pediatric trauma. Emerg Med Clin North Am 11:187, 1993.

Thompson BM, Rice T, Jaffe J, et al: 'PALS for Life!' A required trauma-oriented pediatric advanced life support course for pediatric and emergency medicine house staff. Ann Emerg Med 13:1044, 1984.

Pregnancy

Dudley DJ, Cruikshank DP: Trauma and acute surgical emergencies in pregnancy. Semin Perinatol 14:42, 1990.

Neufeld JDG: Trauma in pregnancy, What if . . . ? Emerg Med Clin North Am 11:207, 1993.

Pearlman MD, Tintinalli JE: Evaluation and treatment of the

gravida and fetus following trauma during pregnancy. Obstet Gynecol Clin North Am 18:371, 1991.

Falls

Buckman RF, Buckman PD: Vertical deceleration trauma: Principles of management. Surg Clin North Am 71:331, 1991.

Bicycling Injuries

Björnstig U, Öström M, Eriksson A, Sonntag-Öström E: Head and face injuries in bicyclists—with special reference to possible effects of helmet use. J Trauma 33:887, 1992.

Friede AM, Azzara CV, Gallagher SS, Guyer B: The epidemiology of injuries to bicycle riders. Pediatr Clin North Am 32:141, 1985.

Stylianos S, Eichelberger MR: Pediatric trauma: Prevention strategies. Pediatr Clin North Am 40:1359, 1993.

Tucci JJ, Barone JE: A study of urban bicycling accidents. Am J Sports Med 16:181, 1988.

Dental Trauma

Klokkevold P: Common dental emergencies: Evaluation and management for emergency physicians. Emerg Med Clin North Am 7:29, 1989.

Wringer Injuries

Palmaccio AJ, Greenberg MD: Wringer Injury. In Greenberg MI, Roberts JR (eds): Emergency Medicine: a clinical approach to challenging problems. Philadelphia, FA Davis, 1982, pp 11–15.

Injections

Booth CM: High pressure paintgun injuries. BMJ 2:1222, 1977.

Proust AF: Special injuries of the hand. Emerg Med Clin North Am 11:767, 1993.

Silsby JJ: Pressure gun injection injuries of the hand. West J Med 125:271, 1976.

Fishhooks

Doser C, Cooper WL, Ediger WM, et al: Fishhook injuries: A prospective evaluation. Am J Emerg Med 9:413, 1991.

Lantsberg L, Blintsovsky E, Hoda J: How to extract an indwelling fishhook. Am Fam Physician 45:2589, 1992. (see comments)

Terrill P: Fishhook removal. Am Fam Physician 47:1372, 1993. (letter; comment)

Foreign Bodies

Augeri PA: Corneal foreign body removal and treatment. Optom Clin 1(4):59, 1991.

Bear VD: The ear: "Dos" and "don'ts". Med J Aust 154:603, 1991.

Friedman EM: Caustic ingestions and foreign bodies in the aerodigestive tract of children. Pediatr Clin North Am 36:1403, 1989.

Holinger LD: Management of sharp and penetrating foreign bodies of the upper aerodigestive tract. Ann Otol Rhinol Laryngol 99:684, 1990.

McRae D, Premachandra DJ, Gatland DJ: Button batteries in the ear, nose and cervical esophagus: A destructive foreign body. J Otolaryngol 18:317, 1989.

Tong MCF, van Hasselt CA, Woo JKS: The hazards of button batteries in the nose. J Otolaryngol 21:458, 1992.

Poisoning

WILLIAM FULCHER

Modern technology has joined hands with nature to provide a seemingly endless list of substances for ingestion, inhalation, or continuous exposure by patients. Nearly any substance taken in excess may exert some toxic effect, and some substances, prescribed with the best of intent, may be harmfully synergistic or antagonistic when taken closely together.

Poisonings may occur because of suicidal intent, manipulative behavior, accidental occurrence, homicidal intent, or, in children, out of sheer curiosity. The workplace, the home, and the hobbyist's bench are all sources for acute or chronic exposure to toxic agents.

Thousands of pharmaceutical products are available for use; however, less than 20 of these agents are responsible for 90 per cent of accidental toxic ingestion. Thus, some syndromes are common and others, while uncommon, can be considered classic enough to merit some discussion (Table 36–6).

Eight-five per cent of all poisoning cases involve children, more than 70 per cent under 5 years of age. Children are more susceptible to the effects of toxins and poisons because of their smaller body size; therefore, prevention should be paramount in poisoning management. Education of parents about the risks of poisoning is an important activity.

Federal law requires that hazardous household products be safely packaged and be labeled so as to

TABLE 36–6. COMMON DRUG INGESTION SYNDROMES

Antidepressants (e.g., amitriptyline, doxepin, amoxapine)
Anticholinergic features common; dilated pupils, tachycardia, hot dry skin, decreased bowel sounds.
The "three Cs"; Coma, convulsions, and cardiac problems are the most common causes of death.
A major diagnostic feature is widening of the QRS complex greater than 0.1 s on ECG (*not* seen with amoxapine).
Hypotension and ventricular arrhythmias are common.

Key interventions: Control seizures, correct acidosis with ventilation and HCO_3. Avoid use of ipecac and physostigmine.

Antimuscarinic drugs (e.g., atropine, scopolamine, antihistamines, tricyclic antidepressants, jimsonweed, *Amanita muscaria* mushrooms)
Hallucinations, delirium, coma.
Seizure may occur with tricyclic antidepressants, antihistamines.
Tachycardia, hypertension.
Hyperthermia with hot, dry skin.
Mydriasis.
Decreased bowel sounds, urinary retention.

Key interventions: Control hyperthermia. Physostigmine is of limited value.

Cholinomimetic drugs (e.g., organophosphate and carbamate insecticides)
Anxiety, agitation, seizures, coma.
May see bradycardia (muscarinic effect) or tachycardia (nicotinic effect).
Pinpoint pupils.
Excessive salivation, sweating.
Bowel sounds hyperactive, with abdominal cramping, diarrhea.
Muscle fasciculations and twitching followed by flaccid paralysis.
Death due to respiratory muscle paralysis.

Key interventions: Respiratory support, atropine, pralidoxime (2-PAM). Remove clothes, wash skin, follow ECG, check other workers.

Opioid drugs (e.g., morphine, heroin, meperidine, codeine, methadone)
Sleepiness, lethargy, or coma, depending on dose.
Blood pressure and heart rate usually decreased.
Hypoventilation or apnea.
Pinpoint pupils.

Skin cool; may show signs of intravenous drug abuse with associated infectious disease complications.
Bowel sounds decreased.
Muscle tone flaccid; occasionally see twitching, rigidity.
Clonidine may present with identical syndrome.

Key interventions: Airway support. Frequent use of naloxone may be necessary because of its short half-life.

Salicylates
Confusion, lethargy, coma, seizures.
Hyperventilation, hyperthermia.
Anion gap metabolic acidosis.
Dehydration, potassium loss; hyper- or hypoglycemia.
Acute overdose: 6-hour level over 100 mg/dL (1000 mg/L) very serious.
Chronic or accidental overdose: level not reliable; more severe toxicity; often mistakenly diagnosed as upper respiratory infection or gastroenteritis.

Key interventions: Make the diagnosis; correction of acidosis and fluid and electrolyte abnormalities; hemodialysis if pH or CNS symptoms cannot be controlled.

Sedative-Hypnotics (e.g., barbiturates, diazepam, ethanol)
Highly variable depending on stage of intoxication; initially disinhibition and rowdiness, later lethargy, stupor, coma.
With deep coma: hypotension, somewhat small pupils.
Nystagmus common with moderate intoxication.
Bowel sounds decreased in deep coma.
Muscle tone usually flaccid; if increased, suspect PCP, methaqualone.
May be associated with hyperthermia (do not administer room temperature fluid).

Key interventions: Airway and respiratory support. Avoid fluid overload.

Stimulant drugs (e.g., amphetamines, cocaine, PCP)
Agitation, psychosis, seizures.
Hypertension, tachycardia, arrhythmias.
Mydriasis (usually). Vertical and horizontal nystagmus are common with PCP poisoning.
Skin warm and sweaty.
Muscle tone increased; muscle necrosis is possible.
Hyperthermia may be major complication.

Key interventions: Control seizures, blood pressure, and hyperthermia.

From Katzung BG (ed): Basic and Clinical Pharmacology, 5th edition. Norwalk, CT, Appleton & Lange, 1992, p 845, with permission.

---

bear information to protect and warn users against accidental ingestion, especially by children. Labeling must include the common, usual, or chemical names of hazardous ingredients and a single word such as "poison," "danger," "warning," or "caution" depending on the ingredients degree of toxicity. Also required is some statement of the principle hazard, such as "causes burns on contact," and precautionary measures to be taken. Listed also may be first aid instructions and some statement to reinforce the warning that the product must be kept out of the reach of children.

Child-proof containers should be used for medications, and parents or other adults should not put medications in inappropriate or unlabeled containers. Hazardous products should be kept in a designated storage area that is locked or securely out of reach of children.

Medications or other drugs should be administered seriously to children and never as a game. Drugs should never be referred to as candy, and this includes vitamins. Adults should take their own medication out of sight so as to minimize risk of imitation by young children.

Nearly one of every two children who have ingested poison will do so again within 1 year. If this occurs, in spite of precautionary measures, families should have a bottle of ipecac *syrup* available to induce vomiting en route to the hospital. (Ipecac fluid extract is also available and, although ten times more potent, generally is not recommended.) Individuals should be educated in the use of ipecac as well as the uselessness of other home remedies. The universal home remedy of burnt toast, tea, and milk of magnesia has no place in the modern management of poisoning.

Because many toxins are absorbed rapidly, vomiting performed at home or in route to the hospital has the best chance of removing the largest amount of toxin from the patient's stomach.

IMMEDIATE MANAGEMENT

The measures used for managing poison patients that are most responsible for survival are the nonspecific and supportive measures. All physicians must remember to maintain airway patency, breathing, and circulation of poisoned patients (Roberts, 1979). Advance resuscitation techniques, as well as control of body temperature and seizure activity and the prevention of infection from skin breakdown, should be instituted when indicated. In patients who present with coma or uncontrolled seizures or are obtunded, it is imperative to secure a good airway. A cuffed endotracheal tube will allow the physician to provide adequate ventilation to the patient and prevent aspiration or other pulmonary complications should the patient vomit or during procedures of gastric lavage and irrigation. Arterial blood gases should be measured in such patients, a large-bore intravenous line established, and, generally, a complete blood count and chemistry profile obtained. Patients who present in coma also should be treated with the standard coma protocol, which includes 50 mL of 50% dextrose over 3 to 4 minutes, naloxone (Narcan), and, if alcoholic, thiamine, 100 mg intramuscularly. Flumazenil, the benzodiazepine antagonist, also may be considered in the appropriate patient (Votey et al., 1991).

Once vital functions are secure, further absorption of toxic substances should be prevented. Ingested poisons often can be removed by inducing vomiting if the patient is awake and the airway protected by a good cough and gag reflex. Vomiting might be very helpful in removing substances that slow gastric emptying, such as opiates, some tricyclic antidepressants, and other anticholinergic substances.

Syrup of ipecac, which contains an emesis-inducing alkaloid, is the emetic of chose. It is given orally in dosages of 5 to 15 mL for small children and 30 to 60 mL for adults. Previously, it has been recommended that a patient drink several glass of water to induce gastric distention; however, this is not generally required. Some patients may need to walk around if possible to induce vomiting. If there is no vomiting in 20 to 30 minutes, the ipecac should be repeated and 240 mL of water given. In most cases, this will induce vomiting within 1 hour. However, ipecac may have decreased efficacy in patients who have ingested antiemetics, such as phenothiazines. It may be contraindicated to some degree in ingestions in which vagal tone is already markedly increased and, consequently, in which vomiting may lead to severe brachycardia (e.g., digitalis ingestion).

Vomiting should not be induced if the patient is stuporous or comatose. It should not be used for caustics, or for low-viscosity hydrocarbons unless these have sufficient *known* systemic toxicity to outweigh the potential for aspiration. It should not be used for rapid-acting convulsants (amphetamines, camphor, clonidine, cocaine, some antidepressants, isoniazid, lindane, nicotine, or strychnine). These are better removed by gastric lavage. Some studies demonstrate that induced vomiting removes only 30 to 40 per cent of gastric contents (less than 15 to 20 per cent if induced beyond 1 hour after ingestion), and some authorities recommend that gastric lavage follow vomiting in all significant ingestions. The side effects of ipecac (drowsiness and diarrhea) are minor but include cardiotoxicity and arrhythmia; consequently, if vomiting does not occur, the drug should be removed by gastric lavage.

In the past, apomorphine has been recommended to induce vomiting if ipecac fails. Although it induces vomiting quite rapidly, it has unpredictable narcotic-like depressant effects on the central nervous system (CNS). Although these can be reversed with naloxone, apomorphine is considered more difficult to use and also can induce hypotension.

As referred to later in this chapter, gastric decontamination should be undertaken in almost all poisoning. This involves induced emesis in appropriate situations, gastric lavage, and, if necessary, whole bowel irrigation. Gastric lavage should be performed when the patient meets several criteria. The airway should be protected by either a good gag reflex or a cuffed endotracheal tube. Patients seen within 4 to 6 hours of a large ingestion (or longer if there is decreased bowel motility), with no vomiting or with incomplete vomiting, should be lavaged. The technique should be performed *routinely* in the comatose patient without a *clearly negative ingestion* history. Lavage is performed with the patient in the left lateral decubitus position with the head down. In adults, a large-bore 36 French Ewald tube, and in children a 24 French tube, should be passed into the stomach orally (Lanphear, 1986). Standard nasogastric tubes often are used routinely in smaller children, but the Ewald tube's size and large-bore lateral holes make it superior for rapid lavage and removal of particulate matter (pill fragments) (Fig. 36–11).

Lavage may be performed with tap water or normal saline in the adult, but saline should be used in children to avoid hyponatremia. Lavage should be continued until the return is clear. Initial lavage returns should be saved for formal toxicologic analysis.

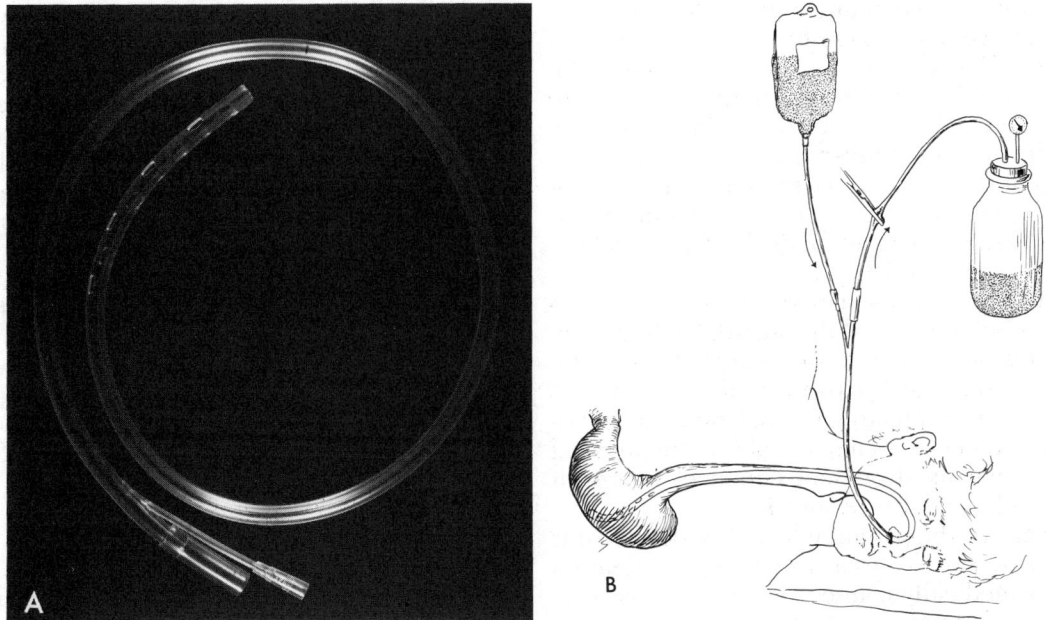

FIGURE 36–11. Perform nasogastric or orogastric lavage with an Ewald tube (*A*); its large caliber and multiple side-holes allow rapid, copious lavage and recovery of large pill fragments. Put the patient in the left lateral decubitus position (*B*); this minimizes loss of lavage through the pylorus. Drain the lavage by either wall suction or gravity. (From Morse SD, Rial WY: Emergency medicine. *In* Rakel RE [ed]: Textbook of Family Practice, 4th edition. Philadelphia, WB Saunders Company, 1990, p 945, with permission.)

After gastric lavage or vomiting, activated charcoal should be administered in a dose of 1 gm/kg of body weight and should be instilled into the stomach. Activated charcoal can absorb most poisons, and the principle is to attempt to give ten times the amount of activated charcoal by weight as the estimated toxin ingested. Exceptions to this include alcohols, potassium, lithium, and iron, which are not absorbed by activated charcoal. Charcoal should not be given before ipecac because it will absorb ipecac; however, it can be given before and should be given after gastric lavage. Usually a 50- to 100-gram slurry is administered. This can be flavored for oral administration and may be mixed with 1 mL/kg of 70% sorbitol, which improves its cathartic action. Finally, teaching in the past has recommended that charcoal not be given with a known or suspected acetaminophen ingestion because it will absorb the *N*-acetylcysteine (NAC; Mucomyst) antidote. Although it may absorb up to 30 to 40 per cent of the NAC, it also will absorb the acetaminophen and, as discussed later under acetaminophen toxicity, some authorities merely increase the dose of NAC to overcome this (Olson and Becker, 1992). Consequently, activated charcoal is no longer considered to be contraindicated absolutely in acetaminophen poisoning.

In many cases, saline cathartics such as Fleet Phospho-Soda or magnesium citrate can be instilled with charcoal to increase the transit time of ingested material. Magnesium citrate can be given in a dose of 250 mg/kg body weight. As mentioned earlier, sorbitol also may be used for this purpose.

FURTHER MANAGEMENT

Further management of the poisoned patient includes maintaining effective circulation. Vasopressors should be used to maintain effective circulating blood pressure if response to initial volume expansion with crystalloids (normal saline or lactated Ringer's solution) is inadequate. Seizures resulting from the poisoning may be controlled with diazepam or lorazepam; diazepam may be given in a dose of 0.1 to 0.2 mg/kg. Phenobarbital is also useful in a 15-mg/kg loading dose given intravenously at a rate not to exceed 50 mg/min. Phenytoin (DPH) may be given in a dose of 15 to 18 mg/kg intravenously at a rate no greater than 50 mg/min.

It is important to monitor the severely poisoned patient with an ECG and cardiac monitor. The ECG may be the quickest way to detect tricyclic antidepressant (TCA) overdose, especially in the comatose patient with anticholinergic signs (dry armpits) (Groleau et al., 1990). The physician should obtain sufficient history to know if the patient has had a concomitant illness and to get a better idea of what and how much was ingested. If the physician is not thoroughly familiar with the treatment for the specific poison, he or she should contact the local poison control center.

The physical examination should be preceded

by removing any contaminated clothing and removing skin contamination by washing with soap and water. Dry chemicals, however, should be brushed off. These materials should be put into proper containers to prevent poisoning or toxicity to other health care workers. The physical examination should search for associated illness or injury, such as head trauma, hemorrhage or shock, evidence of infection, metabolic disorders, and hypothermia (Arena, 1979).

Patients may hide substances in body orifices to avoid their detection, and the suicidal patient may insert drugs or toxins into these areas for self-destructive intent. This possibility always must be kept in mind in evaluating the poisoned or intoxicated patient, because an oversight in the physical exam may have disastrous consequences as a result of continued avoidable absorption.

It is clear that the patient who delibertly poisons himself or herself deserves psychiatric evaluation as soon as medically stable. The psychiatrist may be vital in setting up supports to aid the patient in avoiding recurrent ingestion. Furthermore, if the self-poisoned patient refuses medical treatment, psychiatric evaluation will be necessary in determining whether the patient is mentally competent. Determining that the patient is incompetent to make such a decision will allow for medically indicated, involuntary therapy.

The well-being of the vast majority of poisoned patients depend on relatively simple interventions along with highly skilled nursing care and close observation to detect complications. More sophisticated procedures, such as forced diuresis, hemoperfusion, or hemodialysis, are needed only occasionally.

Complete *quantitative* toxicologic analysis is often not necessary in the mildly poisoned patient; however, qualitative screens of gastric contents, urine, and serum should be made available. Each practitioner should know what the local lab can do, how rapidly, and whether results will be qualitative or quantitative.

New rapid detection kits for multiple drug testing of the urine may decrease the time required for drug screens from several hours to minutes. (One example is the *TRIAGE* monoclonal antibody kit from Biosite [Buechler et al., 1992]). It should be kept in mind that, although classic toxicologic syndromes exist, many poisoning cases will represent multiple ingestions. Often this can be delineated only by formal toxicologic screening in the face of a classicly incomplete or deliberately incomplete history. Despite these potential problems, urine screening and history are often sufficient to begin the emergency management of poisoned patients. Consequently, serum for quantitative toxicology evaluations is best drawn but held, to be analyzed only if needed later. Obvious exceptions to this rule are medications or toxins for which the specific quantity in the serum is important for therapy.

These include acetaminophen, carboxyhemoglobin, digoxin, ethylene glycol, iron, lithium, methanol, salicylate, and theophylline. These drugs should have urgent quantative serum concentrations determined.

In addition to the above-listed general activities for all poisoned patients, there are specific antidotes for specific poisons or syndromes. Many of these will be discussed in more depth later. For complete, up-to-date information for any potential poisoning, contact your local poison control center (Table 36–7).

SPECIFIC TOXICOLOGIC SYNDROMES

Aspirin

Ubiquitous and often candy flavored, aspirin is a common source of pediatric poisoning. The acutely toxic dose is around 150 mg/kg, with severe toxicity in the 300 to 500-mg/kg range. About 20 per cent of aspirin is oxidized in tissue and 70 per cent is excreted in the urine.

Aspirin toxicity can be acute or can result from chronic use. Patients at risk for chronic aspirin toxicity include the chronically ill and the elderly with decreased albumin levels and renal insufficiency.

Diagnosis

The early manifestations of salicylate toxicity include nausea, vomiting, tinnitus, listlessness, and hyperventilation. An increase in respiratory rate will result in a respiratory alkalosis in adults and some children. No other derangement may occur in mild toxicity. In infants and in older patients ingesting very large doses of aspirin, a metabolic acidosis may supervene, probably as a result of incomplete intermediary metabolism. Metabolic acidosis may be the sole disturbance in children under 3 years of age. Severe hypoglycemia can be seen in salicylate poisoning because salicylates reduce liver glycogen and deplete ATP, which leads to impairment of glucose production. A depression of the synthesis of vitamin K–dependent clotting factors may lead to a prolonged prothrombin time. Inhibition of platelet function may add to this process and produce a bleeding diathesis. In severe intoxication, noncardiogenic pulmonary edema may occur. Seizures, coma, and hyperpyrexia also may result.

In acute ingestion, a blood salicylate concentration is useful. One should refer to a Done nomogram for categorization of the severity of intoxication (Done, 1981). Blood salicylate levels are not as useful in subacute or chronic intoxication, but levels greater than 30 mg/dL (300 mg/liter) are significant (Dugandzic et al., 1989).

TABLE 36–7. AMERICAN ASSOCIATION OF POISON CONTROL CENTERS: 1991 CERTIFIED REGIONAL POISON CENTERS

Alabama
Children's Hospital of Alabama Regional
  Poison Control Center, Birmingham
800-292-6678 (in-state only)
205-939-9201
205-933-4050

Arizona
Arizona Poison and Drug Information
  Center, Tucson
800-362-0101 (in-state only)
602-626-6016

Samaritan Regional Poison Center,
  Phoenix
602-253-3334

California
Fresno Regional Poison Control Center,
  Fresno
800-346-5922 (in-state only)
209-445-1222

Los Angeles County Medical Association
  Regional Poison Center, Los Angeles
800-777-6476
213-664-2121
213-484-5151

San Diego Regional Poison Center,
  San Diego
800-876-4766 (in-state only)
619-543-6000

San Francisco Bay Area Regional Poison
  Control Center, San Francisco
800-523-2222 (northern California only)
415-476-6600

Santa Clara Valley Medical Center
  Regional Poison Center, San Jose
800-662-9886 (in-state only)
408-299-5112

University of California-Davis Medical
  Center Regional Poison Control
  Center, Sacramento
800-342-9293 (northern California only)
916-734-3692

Colorado
Rocky Mountain Poison and Drug
  Center, Denver
800-332-3073 (in-state only)
303-629-1123

Florida
Florida Poison Information Center,
  Tampa
800-282-3171 (in-state only)
813-253-4444

Georgia
Georgia Regional Poison Control Center,
  Atlanta
800-282--5846 (in-state only)
404-589-4400

Indiana
Indiana Poison Center, Indianapolis
800-382-9097 (in-state only)
317-929-2323

Kentucky
Kentucky Regional Poison Center of
  Kosair Children's Hospital, Louisville
800-722-5725 (in-state only)
502-589-8222

Maryland
Maryland Poison Center, Baltimore
800-492-2414 (in-state only)
301-528-7701

Massachusetts
Massachusetts Poison Control System,
  Boston
800-682-9211 (in-state only)
617-232-2120

Michigan
Blodgett Regional Poison Center, Grand
  Rapids
800-632-2727 (in-state only)

Poison Control Center, Detroit
800-462-6642 (in-state only)
313-745-5711

Minnesota
Hennepin Regional Poison Center,
  Minneapolis
612-347-3141

Minnesota Regional Poison Center,
  St. Paul
800-222-1222 (in-state only)
612-221-2113

Missouri
Cardinal Glennon Chidren's Hospital
  Regional Poison Center, St. Louis
800-366-8888
314-772-5200

Montana
Rocky Mountain Poison and Drug
  Center, Denver
800-525-5042 (in-state only)

Nebraska
The Poison Center, Omaha
800-955-9119
402-390-5555

New Jersey
New Jersey Poison Information and
  Education System, Newark
800-962-1253 (in-state only)
201-923-0764

New Mexico
New Mexico Poison and Drug
  Information Center, Albuquerque
800-432-6866 (in-state only)
505-843-2551

New York
Long Island Regional Poison Control
  Center, East Meadow
516-542-2323

New York City Poison Control Center,
  New York City
212-340-4494
212-764-7667

Ohio
Central Ohio Poison Center, Columbus
800-682-7625 (in-state only)
614-228-1323

Regional Poison Control System,
  Cincinnati Drug and Poison
  Information Center, Cincinnati
800-872-5111 (in-state only)
513-558-5111

Oregon
Oregon Poison Control Center, Portland
800-452-7165 (in-state only)
503-494-8968

Pennsylvania
The Poison Control Center, Philadelphia
215-386-2100

Pittsburgh Poison Center, Pittsburgh
412-681-6669

Rhode Island
Rhode Island Poison Center, Providence
401-277-5727

Texas
North Texas Poison Center, Dallas
800-441-0040 (in-state only)
214-590-5000

Utah
Intermountain Regional Poison Control
  Center, Salt Lake City
800-456-7707 (in-state only)
801-581-2151

Washington, D.C.
National Capital Poison Center,
  Washington, D.C.
202-625-3333

West Virginia
West Virginia Poison Center, Charleston
800-642-3625 (in-state only)
304-348-4211

Wyoming
Rocky Mountain Poison and Drug
  Center, Denver
800-442-2702 (in-state only)

From Johnson CA: Management of snake bite. Am Fam Physician 44:174, 1991, with permission.

Treatment

Treatment should include intensive vital sign support and gastrointestinal decontamination. One should correct dehydration, hypoglycemia, and hypokalemia. Severe acidosis can be corrected with sodium bicarbonate. Hemodialysis should be considered for critically ill patients (those with seizures, unresponsive acidosis, or salicylate levels greater than 120 mg/dL, or elderly patients with levels greater than 60 mg/dL). One should measure salicylate levels every 4 to 6 hours during hospital management. If evidence of hypoprothrombinemia develops, one should give vitamin K, 10 mg intramuscularly.

Acetaminophen

A dose of acetaminophen (Tylenol, Daytril) of 150 mg/kg or greater should be considered toxic. The threshold for toxicity may be lower in alcohol abusers, patients with liver disease, or those with induced liver enzymes. Gastric emptying should be undertaken within 8 to 12 hours after ingestion (Temple, 1981). Cathartics may be useful and, although charcoal has been avoided in the past if sufficient NAC (Mucomyst) is given, it may aid in decreasing toxicity. A plasma level of acetaminophen should be obtained, but not earlier than 4 hours after ingestion, and a Rumack-Matthew nomogram consulted (Fig. 36–12).

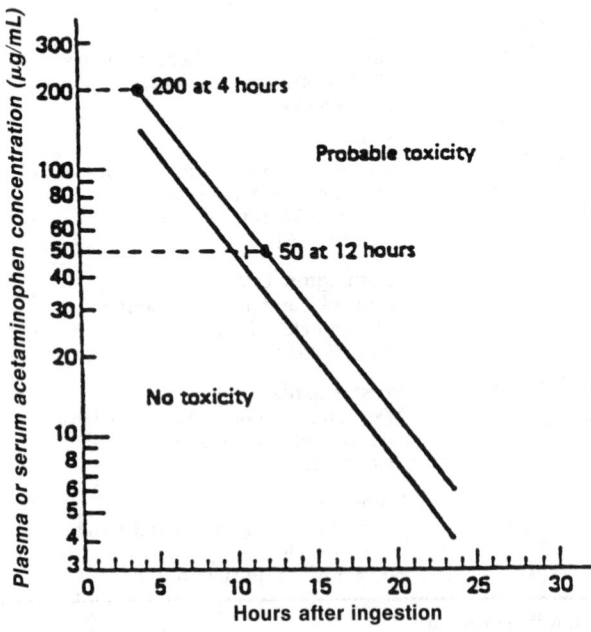

FIGURE 36–12. Nomogram for acetaminophen toxicity. The upper line represents concentrations causing hepatoxicity, while the lower line represents a value 25 per cent lower (a prudent level to begin therapy). (From Rumack BM, Matthew M: Acetaminophen poisoning and toxicity. Pediatrics 55:871, 1975, with permission.)

Diagnosis

Early signs and symptoms of acetaminophen overdose include anorexia, nausea, vomiting, pallor, and diaphoresis (Rumak et al., 1981). These resolve and, in untreated patients, an elevation of liver enzymes occurs in 1 to 4 days. In severe toxicity, this may be followed by eventual hepatic failure; in 1 per cent of adults although rarely in children.

Treatment

Antidotal therapy within NAC (Mucomyst) administered within 16 hours of ingestion reduces hepatic damage and fatality and has been reported useful if given before 24 hours (Smilkstein et al., 1988). NAC given orally is an effective agent when given in a loading dose of 140 mg/kg. The 10% to 20% NAC solution is diluted to 5% with juice or soda to make it more palatable. This should be followed by repeated doses of NAC at 70 mg/kg every 4 hours for up to 18 doses or until the acetaminophen level is zero. Nausea and vomiting are the major side effects of NAC, and they may require redosing if the patient vomits less than 1 hour after a dose. As mentioned earlier, charcoal can absorb up to 30 per cent of NAC given, but it is not considered an absolute contraindication by some toxicologists (Olsen and Becker, 1992). To overcome this absorption, some toxicologists recommend using a higher loading dose of NAC (190 mg/kg) as the loading dose. Furthermore, considerable favorable experience (especially in Great Britain) with intravenous NAC soon may result in this route becoming the standard therapy in the United States.

Iron

Each year about 2000 cases of iron toxicity are reported in children in the United States. Ferrous sulfate, the cheapest and most common iron preparation, is also the most frequently involved in overdoses. Any patient who has ingested excessive iron should be considered for hospitalization and observed for at least 24 hours.

Diagnosis

The serum iron concentration is usually maximal 4 hours after ingestion. Elemental iron equivalent should be calculated to determine the degree of toxicity: 33 per cent of ferrous fumarate, 20 per cent of ferrous sulfate, 10 per cent of ferrous gluconate. Ingestion of 20 to 30 mg/kg is considered toxic, and over 60 mg/kg elemental iron potentially lethal. In general, toxicity is expected when the serum iron level is greater than 500 μg/dL or when it exceeds the total iron-binding capacity (Proudfoot et al., 1986).

There are four clinical stages in the evolution of

TABLE 36–8. STAGES IN IRON TOXICITY

First Stage (1–6 hours): Local Toxicity
  Nausea
  Vomiting
  Hematemesis
  Abdominal pain
  Diarrhea
  Melena
Second Stage (10–14 hours): Latent Period
  Deceptive improvement
Third Stage (4–40 hours): Systemic Toxicity
  Fever
  Bleeding diathesis
  Hyperglycemia
  Hepatic failure
  Hematochezia
  Myocardial toxicity with T wave inversion
  CNS toxicity—lethargy, restlessness, seizures, coma
  Shock
  Acidosis
  Death
Fourth Stage (2–5 weeks): Late Complications
  Pyloric obstruction
  High small bowel obstruction

From Morse SD, Rial WY: Emergency medicine. *In* Rakel RE (ed): Textbook of Family Practice, 4th edition. Philadelphia, WB Saunders Company, 1990, p 946, with permission.

iron toxicity (Table 36–8). Iron salts are directly corrosive to mucosal surfaces and hepatotoxic. Iron absorption may be increased dramatically by its corrosive action on the gastrointestinal tract. Derangement of normal hepatocellular oxidative mechanisms by free iron leads to a buildup of organic acids and acidosis. Additionally, release of hepatic ferritin into circulation can reflexly cause shock and lactic acidosis. Healing of ulcerated gastrointestinal lesions can lead to late complications of cicatrix.

Treatment

Treatment of iron ingestion involves intensive support and gastrointestinal decontamination, including vomiting, lavage, and whole-bowel irrigation. Gastric lavage can be performed with 5% bicarbonate or Fleet Phospho-Soda diluted 1:4 with saline, because this produces an insoluble carbonate or phosphate iron salt. Charcoal is not effective in iron ingestion.

In the past, some have recommended that an estimate of the magnitude of recent iron ingestion can be made by using an abdominal flat plate because undissolved tablets of iron and other drugs may be identified by plain radiographs. The mnemonic CHIPS is helpful in reminding the physician of the drugs that may be detectable by this technique (*c*hloral hydrate, *h*eavy metals such as iron or arsenic, *i*odine, *p*sychotropics, *s*odium). The physician must remember that these may be visible only if they are *not* dissolved, and consequently radiography is useful only if it is positive. Significant ingestion can occur in the face of a negative abdominal radiograph.

Specific treatment of iron poisoning with deferoxamine intravenously or intramuscularly should begin when the serum iron level exceeds 400 μg/dL 4 to 5 hours after ingestion. Deferoxamine also should be used in any patient with severe clinical signs or those who have ingested more than 500 mg of elemental iron. Patients with shock or acidosis should receive deferoxamine 40 mg/kg intravenously over 4 hours and then 20 mg/kg intravenously or intramuscularly every 3 to 12 hours depending on the individual clinical picture, serum iron level, and response to therapy. The drug increases urinary iron excretion 100-fold and imparts a rose color to the urine. The complex is excreted in the urine, so an inadequate urine output will result in ineffective response to deferoxamine, and dialysis should be considered. Hypotension can occur with too-rapid infusion of deferoxamine.

Most patients without shock or coma who are treated properly survive iron ingestion. The overall mortality rate is 2 to 3 per cent but, with shock or coma, this can rise to 10 per cent.

Caustics

A caustic is any chemical causing tissue injury to the gastrointestinal tract when it is ingested. Caustics may be divided into alkalis and acids. Commons sources of caustic agents are listed in Table 36–9.

Acids produce coagulation necrosis of the gut mucosa and, unless the agent is unusually strong or the contact prolonged, the formation of eschar limits the damage to superficial layers. Alkali caustics, in contrast, produce liquefaction necrosis and saponification of tissue. This results in deep penetration and injury that is often extensive and ongoing (Howell, 1986). Solid agents produce the

TABLE 36–9. SOURCES OF CAUSTIC INGESTION

Acids	Cause eschar formation and
Toilet bowl cleaners	coagulation necrosis
Swimming pool cleaners	
Disinfectants	
Battery acid	
Metal cleaners	
Permanent wave neutralizers	
Alkalis	Cause saponification and
* Bleaches	liquefaction necrosis:
Disinfectants (ammonia)	deep penetrating burns
Drain cleaners	
Toilet bowl cleaners	
Clinitest tablets	
Paint removers	
Oven cleaners	
* Dishwashing detergents	

Adapted from Morse SD, Rial WY: Emergency medicine. *In* Rakel RE (ed): Textbook of Family Practice, 4th edition. Philadelphia, WB Saunders Company, 1990, p 946.
* Usually cause mild surface irritation/burns.

greatest damage in the oral pharynx and upper esophagus, while gastric damage from liquids is more extensive. The esophagus is damaged more readily by alkali than by acids because the squamous epithelium is relatively resistant to acid. The reverse is true for the stomach.

The pH of the caustic agent ingested is significantly related to the damage caused. The higher or lower the pH, the greater the chance of harm. Ingestion of alkali, for example, with pH under 12.5, may not cause esophageal ulceration or irritation.

Diagnosis

Once the patient is stabilized, determine the substance taken, the intervals since ingestion, the quantity taken, whether vomiting has occurred, and the pH of the caustic. One should determine whether there is pain, dysphagia, dyspnea, or hematemesis.

The physical exam should center on evidence of respiratory distress and oral or gastrointestinal irritation. One should look for burns, drooling, and signs of gastrointestinal irritation or perforation. One third of patients with oral burns will have associated esophageal burns, but up to 15 per cent of patients with esophageal injury may have no oral lesion.

Treatment

The treatment of caustic ingestion involves rapid dilution with water, normal saline, or milk. One should not attempt to neutralize acids or alkali because the heat produced by the chemical reaction may produce greater damage to the mucosa and the gas generated may potentially lead to rupture of a weakened hollow viscus. Induced emesis, gastric lavage, charcoal, and saline cathartics are generally contraindicated. Patients should be provided with potent analgesia, volume repletion, transfusion if necessary, and definitive therapy for bleeding or perforation. Nothing should be allowed by mouth other than the diluent used in the acute management, and this may be instilled by a nasogastric tube that has been placed carefully.

Fiberoptic endoscopy is vital to guide therapy and to delineate prognosis. The risk of endoscopy is low if the procedure is stopped at the beginning of the first area of internal third-degree burn. No stricture formation occurs from first-degree burns; however, 15 to 30 per cent of second-degree burns and nearly 100 per cent of third-degree burns will result in stricture. Endoscopy should be performed in any *symptomatic* patient with or without oral burns (Ferguson et al., 1989). Considerable controversy exists at this time as to whether endoscopy is indicated for *asymptomatic* patients *without* oral burns.

Corticosteroids have a controversial role in the management of caustic ingestion. To date, no studies have supported the efficacy of steroids in reducing the development of stricture. They currently are used when patients are too unstable for endoscopy or in patients who have circumferential burns and no other contraindications to their use. They generally are contraindicated in esophageal or gastric perforation. If used, the recommended dosage of steroid is 40 mg of methylprednisolone every 8 hours in adults and children over 2 (20 mg per dose in children under 2).

Antibiotic therapy in this setting is also controversial. Prophylactic antibiotics have not been proven to decrease complications of caustic ingestion unless the endoscopy or exam clearly indicates the presence of perforation. In the presence of perforation, most authorities recommend prophylactic use of a broad-spectrum antibiotic effective against gram-positive organisms and other oral flora.

Cocaine

Cocaine use in its many forms has resulted in an epidemic of morbidity and mortality. The number of reports of known and suspected deaths caused by acute cocaine intoxication increases each year. Cocaine is a local anesthetic and sympathomimetic that is abused in the form of snorting, smoking, or injecting. Persons who inject cocaine intravenously or smoke freebase (crack) develop rapidly toxic blood levels of cocaine. The use of cocaine has been reported to cause a "kindling" effect in which the continued self-administration of the drug causes greater and greater euphoria (Spotts and Shontz, 1984). This results in users self-administering increasing amounts of cocaine and often grossly exceeding the estimated "safe" levels of cocaine, which are thought to be 2 to 3 mg/kg or less.

Diagnosis

Symptoms of cocaine use and intoxication include euphoria, excitement, restlessness, and toxic psychosis. Continued use and toxic levels may result in hypertension, tachycardia, arrhythmia, seizures, hypothermia, myocardial infarction, and stroke.

Treatment

Treatment of the acutely intoxicated patient should include intensive support and gastrointestinal decontamination if appropriate. One should treat sympathetic hyperactivity like that for all stimulant drugs (amphetamines, phencyclidine). Diastolic blood pressure greater than 120 mm Hg or hypertensive encephalopathy can be treated with nitroprusside. Tachycardia and ventricular tachyarrhythmia may respond to intravenous Inderal. Patients complaining of chest pain should have an ECG, and one should strongly consider instituting a "rule-out" myocardial infarction admission or observation because patients with cocaine intoxication may develope myocardial infarction despite initially normal ECGs. Seizures require evaluation for intracranial hemorrhage and consequently may warrant CT scan. Seizures are usually transient because of the rapid metabolism of cocaine; however, if they persist, diazepam may be useful for seizure control. Cocaine is a short-acting drug, so, very often, supportive therapy is all that is required for mild to moderate intoxication. Psychiatric referral should be recommended and made because these patients need intensive detoxification and may require drug therapy and psychotherapy for depression after discontinuing their cocaine use.

Hydrocarbons

Commercially available hydrocarbons are usually a mixture of organic compounds. Most cases of hydrocarbon ingestion are accidental, with rarely more than a taste (5 to 10 mL) being ingested; however, 1 to 2 mL of many hydrocarbons can cause severe pneumonitis if aspirated into the lungs. The risk of toxicity and complications from exposure to these agents correlates with their physical properties. Of these properties, viscosity is most important because it directly relates to the risk of pulmonary aspiration. The volatility and the presence of nonhydrocarbon additives also has an impact on toxicity (Kulig and Rumack, 1981).

Viscosity is quantified using the Saybolt Seconds universal (ssu) unit, which measures the seconds it takes for a quantity of liquid to flow through a standard aperture (Fig. 36–13). Low-viscosity hydrocarbons possess the greatest risk of aspiration because of the ease of spread over mucous membranes, which most commonly occurs at the time of initial ingestion. Volatile hydrocarbons such as kerosene and mineral spirits pose special aspiration risks because they fume when in contact with the warm environment of the pharynx.

Additives and contaminants impart their other special toxicities to ingested hydrocarbons. The general classes of additives may be recalled by using the mnenomic CHAMP for *c*amphor, *h*alogenated hydrocarbons, *a*eromatics, *m*etals, and *p*esticides. Consequently, low-viscosity hydrocarbons can be separated into those that have no systemic toxicity, those that have known systemic toxicity, and those with unknown toxicity based on additives. A comprehensive text of toxicology or the local poison control center should be consulted about hydrocarbons and their additives.

Diagnosis

The larger the volume of hydrocarbon ingested, the higher the risk of vomiting and aspiration. Patients who do not vomit have the lowest risk of pneumonitis. Symptoms of aspiration may be delayed for up to 6 hours, but there is usually some immediate distress. Immediate symptoms include gagging, coughing, and choking. Most hydrocarbons are extremely irritating to the gut, so they cause nausea, vomiting, diarrhea, and pain in many cases. Contaminated skin and clothing must not be overlooked in protecting the patient from further systemic absorption and protecting staff from exposure.

Fever is common after hydrocarbon ingestion, and it usually resolves in a day or two. Marked CNS dysfunction or cardiac dysfunction in hydrocarbon ingestion is usually due to toxic additives or to pulmonary aspiration with hypoxia and acidosis.

Treatment

The treatment of hydrocarbon ingestion is controversial in some areas, and general guidelines are offered below. Hydrocarbons of high viscosity usually need no treatment. This includes products such as diesel and fuel oil, grease, and petroleum jelly. It is hydrocarbons of low viscosity that constitute the greatest risk to patients. Low-viscosity hydrocarbons *without known* systemic toxicity should *not* be removed from the stomach unless patients are having severe gastrointestinal symptoms or CNS distress (Arena, 1987). Activated charcoal is probably not helpful in these patients; saline cathartics may be of help if very large quantities have been ingested. Thankfully, most hydrocarbons do possess some intrinsic cathartic properties.

Patients who ingest low-viscosity hydrocarbons with unknown or clear systemic toxicity should have vomiting induced if greater than 15 to 30 mL

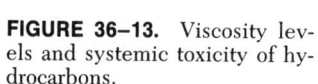

FIGURE 36–13. Viscosity levels and systemic toxicity of hydrocarbons.

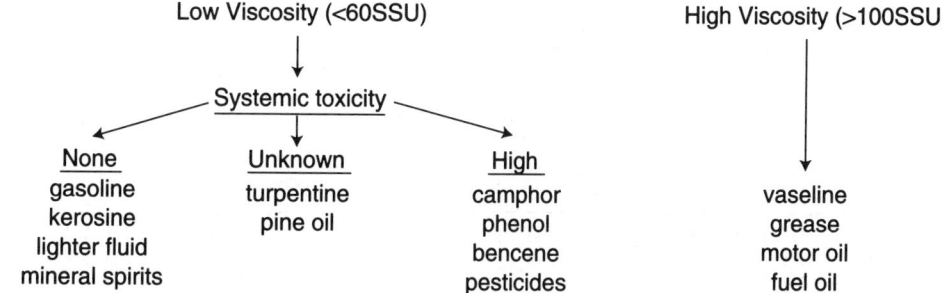

of the agent was ingested. Ipecac should not be administered to those patients who have ingested toxins that can cause rapid onset of seizures (i.e., camphor). Gastric lavage should be performed, and activated charcoal can be used to absorb the toxic additives. Oil demulcents (mineral oil) are contraindicated because their use increases the frequency of pulmonary complications. Prophylactic steroids and antibiotics have not been shown to be of benefit in reducing complications of hydrocarbon ingestion.

Patients who ingest significant amounts of hydrocarbons should be admitted to the hospital for observation and, if respiratory distress occurs, a chest radiograph should be obtained. Respiratory distress, hypoxemia, or abnormal chest radiographs are also reasons for admission and observation in the hospital.

Opiates

The CNS contains stereospecific opiate receptors concentrated in areas concerned with pain transmission and pain perception. In these areas, high concentrations of enkephalins have been found. The pituitary also contains high concentrations of another type of peptides, β-endorphins. These peptides function as neurotransmitters in areas of opiate receptors, inhibiting neuronal activity. Thus, they behave in some manner as antagonist narcotics and are known opiate neurotransmitters.

Narcotics may have pure agonist, pure antagonist, or mixed agonist and antagonist properties (Table 36–10). Agonist narcotics work like opiate neurotransmitters binding to receptor sites to decrease sodium permeability and inhibit neuronal activity. Antagonist binding produces opposite actions and also probably alters receptor structure so

TABLE 36–10. NARCOTIC AGENTS

Drug	Dose (mg)	CNS Respiratory Depressant
Pure Antagonist		
Naloxone (Narcan)	0.8–2.0	No
Naltrexone		No
Mixed Agonist/Antagonists		
Nalorphine (Nalline)	10–15	Yes
Levallorphan (Lorfan)	5–10	Yes
Pentazocine (Talwin)	30–50	Yes
Pure Agonists		
Morphine		Yes
Codeine		Yes
Heroin		Yes
Others		Yes

From Morse SD, Rial WY: Emergency medicine. *In* Rakel RE (ed): Textbook of Family Practice, 4th edition. Philadelphia, WB Saunders Company, 1990, p 948, with permission.

TABLE 36–11. SYMPTOMS OF NARCOTIC INJECTION OR INGESTION

Organ System	Effect
Central nervous system	Analgesia
	Progressive obtundation
	Respiratory depression
	Vomiting
	Hypothermia
	Impaired cough reflex
	Seizures (high doses)
Gastrointestinal tract	Ileus and constipation
	Increases sphincter tone
	Biliary spasm
	Risk of hepatitis
Cardiovascular system	Infectious risks; endocarditis, valve disease, embolization
	Orthostatic hypotension
Lungs	Bronchospasm
	Pulmonary edema
	Emboli
Genitourinary system	Urinary retention
	Glomerular disease
Eyes	Miosis
Skin	Cellulitis
	Ulcers
	Abscesses
	Lymphedema
Musculoskeletal system	Rhabdomyolysis
	Osteomyelitis
	Septic arthritis
Endocrine system	Hypoglycemia
	Amenorrhea
	Sterility ($\downarrow$ testosterone)

From Morse SD, Rial WY: Emergency medicine. *In* Rakel RE (ed): Textbook of Family Practice, 4th edition. Philadelphia, WB Saunders Company, 1990, p 948, with permission.

that fewer receptors are available for agonist binding. Agonist-induced inhibition of enkephalon production may explain the hyperexcitability seen in sudden narcotic withdrawal, when neither endogenous or exogenous opiates are present.

All narcotic agents, whether natural (morphine, codeine), semisynthetic, or synthetic, have similar effects, potential for addiction, and cross tolerance. The physiologic effects of narcotic agents are listed in Table 36–11. Table 36–12 records the clinical signs of opiate withdrawal.

TABLE 36–12. NARCOTIC WITHDRAWAL

Mild	Moderate	Severe*
Mydriasis	Agitation	Insomnia
Rhinorrhea	Hypertension	Diarrhea
Yawning	Tachycardia	Vomiting
Piloerection		Hypotension
Cramps		Seizures
Tearing		

* Emergency treatment should be undertaken in a patient only when severe manifestations are present.

From Morse SD, Rial WY: Emergency medicine. *In* Rakel RE (ed): Textbook of Family Practice, 4th edition. Philadelphia, WB Saunders Company, 1990, p 948, with permission.

Diagnosis

Emergency management of the comatose patient who has taken an overdose of opiates begins with assessment of airway patency, respiratory activity, and circulatory status. Intubation and mechanical ventilation and establishment of a vascular access are necessary. Other etiologies for the coma state should not be overlooked and, because trauma and infection are also common in these patients, findings suspicious for them also should be sought aggressively (Goldfrank et al., 1981).

Treatment

Venous blood should be obtained for appropriate toxicologic analysis, electrolytes, blood sugar, and blood counts. The patient should receive 1 or 2 ampules of 50% dextrose and water followed by 0.8 to 2.0 mg of naloxone (Narcan) intravenously. Narcan can be repeated in 5 minutes. If a response is achieved, 10 ampules of naloxone can be placed in 1 liter of intravenous solution and infused at 100 to 200 mL/hr. Physicians should be aware that clonidine intoxication can appear very similar to opiate intoxication, but will have no response to naloxone. Propoxyphene can be particularly resistant to Narcan reversal, and physicians should watch patients carefully for even the slightest improvement before they give up on this therapy (Olsen and Becker, 1992). Naloxone can be given intramuscularly to continue therapy if intravenous access is accidentally lost.

Because of their effect on gastric motility, opiates can be recovered from the stomach by lavage many hours after ingestion. Gastrointestinal decontamination by lavage may be very useful even many hours after ingestion.

Ninety per cent of opiate overdoses involve abuse of some other agent. Often these are barbiturates, benzodiazepine, alcohol, or TCAs. This is another reason why incomplete response to naloxone may be seen and another good reason for gastric lavage. There is no cross tolerance between these other depressants and narcotics; therefore, during management, simultaneous or sequential withdrawal syndromes may become evident and require medical management. Because of the high rate of recidivism and repeated overdose in these patients, management can be highly frustrating. The general approach to acute management is similar to that in patients who ingest other CNS depressants.

Sedative-Hypnotics

The use (and abuse) of sedatives to treat anxiety and other related conditions is widespread. Patients can develop tolerance to these drugs and may take higher doses to achieve the same initial relaxation they were seeking. Furthermore, most sedative-hypnotics will "unmask" depression by suppressing the anxiety features with which these patients often present. The co-consumption of other drugs or alcohol with sedative-hypnotic use (intoxication) is common; consequently, the physician should expect a mixture of physical findings and possibly withdrawal symptoms when treating these patients.

Diagnosis

The patient with sedative-hypnotic overdose presents with the signs and symptoms of increasing lethargy, ataxia, and dysarthria, which can progress to stupor and coma. Frequent physical findings include nystagmus, ophthalmoplegia, hypotension, respiratory depression and arrest, and hypothermia. As mentioned previously, patients also may present with signs and symptoms of other drugs taken (e.g., narcotics, ethanol, acetaminophen). With severe sedative overdose and resulting coma, the patient may have fixed pupils and a flat electroencephalogram, both of which can return to normal after recovery.

Urine and serum drug screens may be useful in determining which categories of drugs were taken; however, the elimination of most sedative-hypnotics varies so greatly from person to person that drug levels will provide only gross predictions of the duration of sedation.

Treatment

The physician must provide aggressive support of ABCs. Severe hypotension and shock should respond to crystalloid (normal saline), with vasopressors reserved for those who do not respond to fluid challenge.

Gastric decontamination procedures should be employed as described earlier. Protect the airway with a cuffed endotracheal tube if the gag reflex is depressed and gastric lavage is attempted. Activated charcoal with sorbitol should be given.

Hypothermia should be checked for and corrected if found. Flumazenil (Romazicon) is now available to reverse the effects of benzodiazepine overdose. Given intravenously in doses of 0.2 mg slowly over 5 to 10 minutes, flumazenil may be repeated as it wears off (1 to 3 hours) up to a total dose of 3 to 5 mg. Caution should be exercised in using flumazenil in patients with history of seizures, suspected benzodiazepine addictions or tolerance, and TCA overdose (Votey et al., 1991).

Tricyclic Antidepressants

According to the 1991 American Association of Poison Control Centers report, the TCAs still account for the highest number of *fatal* medication ingestions in the United States, with over 500,000 TCA overdoses reported and a 2 per cent mortality for overdoses (Litovitz et al., 1991). TCAs possess

TABLE 36–13. SIGNS AND SYMPTOMS OF CENTRAL ANTICHOLINERGIC SYNDROME

Central	Peripheral
Agitation	Mydriasis
Disorientation	Tachycardia/hypertension
Hallucinations	Vasodilation
Seizures	Fever
Coma	Urinary retention
Respiratory failure	Ileus
Circulatory collapse	Saliva production
	Sweat production
	Bronchial secretion
	Lacrimation

From Morse SD, Rial WY: Emergency medicine. *In* Rakel RE (ed): Textbook of Family Practice, 4th edition. Philadelphia, WB Saunders Company, 1990, p 949, with permission.

three major pharmacologic activities: sedation, mood elevation, and peripheral and central anticholinergic actions. They share the latter property with phenothiazines and the belladonna alkaloids (Table 36–13). Tricyclic agents are metabolized almost exclusively in the liver, and there are many active intermediary metabolites. Most of the circulating drug is protein bound. Because of lipid solubility, the volume of distribution in the body is very large. In overdose patients, the half-life of these agents can be greater than 24 hours; thus, high levels of active drug can remain at tissue sites for days. Tissue levels may have no relation to measure blood levels, and small changes in the percentage of drug bound to protein can represent a major change in unbound and active drug.

Diagnosis

The initial history may be unreliable in determining the true magnitude of ingestion. In fact, any patient with coma, seizures, hypotension, arrythmia, and anticholinergic signs (mydriasis, dry armpits) should be considered for a possible TCA overdose. The initial presence of peripheral anticholinergic signs does not correlate with the later development of major toxic symptoms (Crome, 1986). Furthermore, some of the newer antidepressants, such as amoxapine and the antipsychotic loxapine, can cause seizures without associated anticholinergic signs or cardiotoxicity.

Treatment

Initial emergency management of the patient includes the usual intensive stabilization of airway, breathing, and circulation. Arterial blood gases and venous blood samples for analysis should be obtained, and an ECG obtained to evaluate for cardiotoxicity. One should not induce vomiting because these drugs may lower the seizure threshold. Activated charcoal is useful for TCA overdose. The patient should be monitored by ECG for at least 6 hours, looking for evidence of widened QRS complex and the development of other CNS signs.

Acute plasma levels of TCA greater than 100 ng/mL are related to higher risks of coma, seizure, hypotension, cardiac arrhythmia, and respiratory failure (Groleau et al., 1990). Lower levels are no guarantee of lack of tissue toxicity. Few data exists to date on toxic levels in children; however, greater than 20 mg/kg is considered serious (the equivalent of two 100-mg tablets in a 10-kg child) (Braden et al., 1986).

As mentioned earlier, initial management should include gastric lavage because of the drug-induced gastric delay in emptying. Activated charcoal should be mixed with a cathartic to aid in removal from the lower gastrointestinal tract. Hypotension should be treated with normal saline, and often sodium bicarbonate can be useful as well. If a vasopressor is needed, norepinephrine can be used. If seizures develop, diazepam or phenytoin should be useful.

In the past, physostigmine, an anticholinesterase, had been recommended for general treatment of TCA poisoning. Although it is no longer recommended for routine use in seizure management, physostigmine can be quite useful for many other aspects of tricyclic ingestion, specifically, the anticholinergic symptoms. The drug may be given in a dose of 1 to 4 mg over 60 seconds and repeated every 20 to 30 minutes as needed. In children over 6 months old, 0.5 mg can be given every 5 minutes, with a maximum dose of 2 mg or evidence of toxicity. Side effects of physostigmine can be reversed with atropine. Physostigmine can be useful as a diagnostic tool in coma related to TCA ingestion. It can be used, if necessary, for cardiac depression and hypotension; however, other agents are available. It is not risk free because it can itself induce bradycardia and seizures. It should be reserved for acute management of life-threatening symptoms resistant to other measures.

Alkalinization of the blood is probably second only to gastric decontamination in importance in the patient with significant TCA poisoning. Alkalinization of the blood with sodium bicarbonate (an initial bolus of 0.5 to 3.0 mEq/kg body weight and subsequent doses to keep arterial pH at 7.50 to 7.55) is useful in the treatment of arrhythmias induced by TCAs and phenothiazines. Continuous infusion of intravenous fluids with 1 to 2 ampules of sodium bicarbonate per liter can be used to titrate blood pH to around 7.50. Controversy exists as to whether the effectiveness of bicarbonate is due to a change in protein binding with alkalosis or a direct result on the heart of the reversal of acidosis. It is not of use in the CNS manifestations of toxicity, nor has it been shown useful in *prophylaxis* for cardiotoxicity (Guzzardi, 1981).

Ventricular arrhythmia may respond well to bicarbonate; however, phenytoin and lidocaine also may be useful. Lidocaine may be used at a dose of 1 to 2 mg/kg. Phenytoin in low-dose aliquots may improve cardiac arrhythmia and myocardial toxicity when bicarbonate and lidocaine have failed. Phenytoin may be given at 15 to 18 mg/kg intravenously, not to exceed 50 mg/min; phenytoin itself can precipitate heart block and hypotension. Quinidine and procainamide should not be used because they may worsen the cardiotoxicity of TCA overdose.

Propranolol has been utilized in the management of tricyclic-induced arrhythmias and is efficacious. Because of its depression of atrioventricular conduction and its myocardial depressant and β-blockade effects, it is a third-line drug when used. Careful monitoring is essential, and small doses must be given (i.e., 0.5 to 1.0 mg intravenously every 5 minutes, not to exceed 5 mg).

Hemodialysis is not efficacious in treating TCA ingestion because of the large volume distribution of these drugs and their high degree of protein binding.

All patients with signs of serious toxicity, including Q-T interval prolongation greater than 0.10 second on ECG, or with an uncertain magnitude of ingestion should be hospitalized in an intensive care setting and monitored until signs of toxicity have been absent for 24 hours. With aggressive support and specific therapy, the central anticholinergic syndrome and the cardiotoxicity of the TCA can be reduced markedly.

Phencyclidine

Phencyclidine (PCP) has been replaced by cocaine as the drug intoxication most frequently seen presenting to the emergency room. PCP, a powerful, easily synthesized, low-cost agent, was one of the most widely available and abused drugs in recent years. It has many street names (angel dust) and often is used with other agents to enforce their potency (Doweiko, 1979). The drug is related closely to the anesthetic ketamine.

Phencyclidine's primary effects are on the cardiovascular and central nervous systems. They are dose related, with mixed stimulant and depressant properties that correlate with its complex action on membrane receptors at various sites in the brain.

Diagnosis

The major subjective effects of PCP include difficulty thinking, depersonalization, altered sensory perceptions, and deranged body image. The user becomes inattentive and emotionally labile. In most cases, the major toxic behavioral effect is a wildly agitated state with aggressive and violent behavior. Additional side effects include fever, hypertension, seizures, rhabdomyolysis, myoglobinuria, respiratory depression, and vasodilation. Overdose patients often present in an acute confusional state associated with aggressive behavior. Patients may have dilated or constricted pupils. They may have hypertension, hyperther-

mia, and tachycardia. There is often both vertical and horizontal nystagmus, with the former nearly pathognomonic in the conscious intoxicated patient. Often there is sensory gait ataxia, a blank facial stare, and increased muscle tone. As the drug is hepatically metabolized and cleared in the bile and urine, symptoms resolve. At higher doses, the drug induces an immobile coma of unpredictable duration associated with seizures. Hypertension may give way suddenly to cardiovascular collapse and apnea (Burns et al., 1981).

Chronic abuse of PCP can lead to a paranoid schizophrenia–like illness with auditory hallucinations and violent behavior. In this respect, the drug shares many characteristics of cocaine and amphetamines. Specific evaluation and therapy for PCP intoxication begins by obtaining a blood and urine sample for toxicologic analysis. The drug is concentrated heavily in urine and most easily found there.

Treatment

PCP is a weak base, so acidification of the urine could markedly enhance its excretion. There is great controversy regarding this treatment, however, because PCP intoxication may result in rhabdomyolysis, and acidification of the urine could result in greater myoglobin deposition in renal tubules and potential renal shutdown. Consequently, acidification of the urine is not recommended. In fact, if rhabdomyolysis occurs or is strongly suspected, one should ensure good urine output and *alkalinize* the urine.

There is no specific antagonist for PCP, and presently symptomatic therapy is best. Patients should be observed in a quite, supportive setting. Diazepam, 2 to 5 mg intravenously every 30 minutes, or Haldol, 5 to 10 mg, may be used to control agitation or psychosis. Seizures and hypertensive crisis respond to usual pharmacologic agents. Usually patients with mild cases of PCP ingestion are behaving normally within 6 hours and may be discharged after 2 to 3 hours of normal behavior. Suicidal risk should be assessed before discharge. Occasionally, a confused patient will not clear for 1 to 3 days and will require psychiatric hospitalization (such patients may be poor metabolizers of the drug).

Organophosphates and Carbamates

Organophosphates and carbamates, two distinct chemical compound groups, are found in insecticides and other commercial products. Both produce inhibition of acetylcholinesterase, accounting for their toxicity resulting from a buildup of acetylcholine at cholinergic synapses. Organophosphate compounds may be absorbed by virtually any route: skin, conjunctiva, lung, or gastrointestinal tract.

Diagnosis

The signs and symptoms of organophosphate poisoning may be classified into three categories (Table 36–14). Patients exposed to organophospates will present with classic symptoms that can be remembered by the mnemonic DUMBELS (*d*iarrhea, *u*rination, *m*iosis, *b*ronchospasm, *b*radycardia, *e*xcitation, *l*acrimation, *s*alivation). Miosis is found in almost all patients with moderately severe poisoning, but its absence should not delay treatment following exposure. Most organophosphate insecticides have a garlicky odor that the patient may exhibit.

The onset of symptoms of organophosphate poisoning is most rapid following inhalation and least rapid after percutaneous absorption. Symptoms most always begin within 24 hours of exposure. Carbamate compounds do not penetrate the CNS effectively and, thus, have a more limited toxicity. In all other respects, the symptoms are the same as those of organophosphate poisons.

Lab confirmation of exposure to organophospates should be sought by measuring RBC cholinesterase or plasma pseudocholinesterase levels and by screening body fluids for organophospates and their metabolites. The urine can be tested for paranitrophenol in the case of exposure to parathion or chlorothmon.

In acute poisoning, clinical manifestations generally occur only after more than 50 per cent of serum cholinesterase is inhibited. In mild poisoning, cholinesterase activity is 20 to 25 per cent of normal. It is less than 20 per cent of normal in moderate poisoning and less than 10 per cent in severe cases. If the depression of cholinesterase activity occurs slowly and gradually, minimal symptoms may be present even with very low levels of serum or RBC cholinesterase.

Treatment

Specific pharmacologic interventions should not be delayed pending determination of cholinesterase levels when there is a strong suspicion of exposure to these agents. Pharmacologic management is one portion of the total management (Table 36–15) and involves two complimentary drugs: atropine for muscularinic and CNS manifestations, and pralidoxime for nictonic manifestations. Cyanosis should be corrected before atropine is given to avoid hypoxia-related ventricular arrhythmias. If atropine is given, observation is recommended for at least 24 hours.

Initial treatment should involve intensive support and gastric decontamination. The management of the airway should take into account the increase in secretions that occurs with organosphosphate exposure. Clothing should be removed and placed in a safe container so that further exposure of the patient and staff is avoided. Atropine should be given for muscarinic symptoms at 1 to 2 mg intravenously, repeating with 2 to 4 mg every 4 to 10 minutes until signs of atropinization occur (flushing, mydriasis, dry mouth, tachycardia). Some cases may require 40 to 50 mg of atropine over 24 hours.

Pralidoxime (PAM) is a specific antidote that restores acetylcholinesterase activity by prevention

---

TABLE 36–14. SIGNS OF ORGANOPHOSPHATE POISONING

CNS Manifestations
Agitation
Emotional lability
Headache
Tremor
Slurred speech
Generalized weakness
Ataxia
Seizures
Coma
Respiratory and cardiovascular depression

Nicotinic (Sympathetic and Somatic Motor) Symptoms
Fasciculations
Cramps
Weakness
Areflexia
Hypertension
Tachycardia
Pallor

Muscarinic (Parasympathetic) Manifestations
Salivation ⎫
Lacrimation ⎬ SLUD syndrome
Urination ⎥
Defecation ⎭

Miosis
Bronchospasm

From Morse SD, Rial WY: Emergency medicine. *In* Rakel RE (ed): Textbook of Family Practice, 4th edition. Philadelphia, WB Saunders Company, 1990, p 950, with permission.

TABLE 36–15. MANAGEMENT OF ORGANOPHOSPHATE POISONING

General Support
Especially respiratory, with good toilet

Decontaminate
Removal of contaminated clothing
Copious skin washing
Emesis/lavage/charcoal/cathartic

Pharmacologic Management
Atropine—slowly I.V., every 15 min until atropinization (dry mucous membranes, dilated pupils, tachycardia)
    2–4 mg in adults/dose
    0.05 mg/kg in children/dose
    Adjust subsequent doses to maintain therapeutic effect for next 24 hr
Pralidoxime (PAM)—only for organophosphates—must give within 24 hr of exposure, given slowly I.V.
    1 gm for adult
    10–12 mg/kg for children
    Repeat dose in 1–2 hr for persistent weakness or tremors

From Morse SD, Rial WY: Emergency medicine. *In* Rakel RE (ed): Textbook of Family Practice, 4th edition. Philadelphia, WB Saunders Company, 1990, p 951, with permission.

and reversal of phosphorylation of this enzyme, but only *before* the complex undergoes the gradual change to an irreversibly bound state. Thus, the drug should be used as early as possible and is generally useless after 24 hours. Improvement in muscle weakness usually occurs over 10 to 40 minutes. Giving PAM and atropine together may increase the side effects of atropine, so close observation is required. PAM is given in a dose of 1 to 2 grams in normal saline over 5 to 10 minutes. This may be repeated in 3 to 4 hours or given as a constant infusion. The dose for children is 25 to 50 mg/kg. Patients must have adequate renal function and urine output to benefit from PAM (Zwiener and Ginsberg, 1988).

Carbamate inhibition of acetylcholinesterase is reversed spontaneously and rapidly by hydrolysis, so PAM is not required. PAM may even increase cholinesterase inhibition in this context and reduce the efficacy of atropine. It is contraindicated, therefore, in carbamate poisoning.

CNS depressants may worsen coma in these patients and should not be used. Phenothiazines and theophylline derivatives have anticholinesterase activity also and are contraindicated, as are succinylcholine, physostigmine, and any other parasympathomimetic agents.

Death from organophosphate poisoning usually results from respiratory failure (within 24 hours in untreated severe cases). With good treatment, complete recovery can be expected within 10 days. Following exposure, patients should not return to contact with these agents until their cholinesterase levels have returned to at least 75 per cent of normal.

Occasionally, long-term sequelae may occur, lasting weeks to months. These include peripheral neuropathy, personality change, memory impairment, confusion, depression, and thought disorders.

Carbon Monoxide

Carbon monoxide is a tasteless, odorless, colorless, nonirritating gas produced by incomplete combustion of carbonaceous material. The most common sources are automobile exhaust; illuminating and heating gases (except natural gas); cigarettes; insufficiently ventilated furnaces, stoves, and chimneys; and the indoor use of charcoal grills. The major toxic properties of carbon monoxide result from its propensity to combine with hemoglobin to form carboxyhemoglobin, which is unable to transport oxygen to tissues. Carbon monoxide has an affinity for hemoglobin that is 250 times that of oxygen. The gas also may bind to enzymes in the respiratory chain of mitochondria and to myoglobin, producing direct muscle hypoxia. Although the reduction in the oxygen-carrying capacity of blood is proportional to the amount of carboxyhe-

TABLE 36–16. SYMPTOMS OF CARBON MONOXIDE POISONING

Carboxyhemoglobin Concentration (%)	Symptoms and Signs
0–10	None
10–30	Progressively severe headache
30–40	Headache
	Nausea and vomiting
	Weakness
	Visual complaints
40–50	Syncope
	Tachycardia
	Tachypnea
50–60	Coma*
	Seizures
	Cheyne-Stokes breathing
60–70	Severe compromise of cardiopulmonary function
70–80	Death

* If carboxyhemoglobin level rises extremely rapidly, coma may occur before other symptoms become manifest.

From Morse SD, Rial WY: Emergency medicine. *In* Rakel RE (ed): Textbook of Family Practice, 4th edition. Philadelphia, WB Saunders Company, 1990, p 952, with permission.

moglobin, oxygen delivery to tissues is reduced further by a left shift of the oxyhemoglobin dissociation curve. Symptomology correlates with carboxyhemoglobin level (Table 36–16).

Diagnosis

The earliest consistent symptom of carbon monoxide poisoning is headache. Cerebral and myocardial hypoxia account for the major toxicity of carbon monoxide. Cerebral edema and increased intracranial pressure may occur as a result of hypoxia-induced capillary leak. In carbon monoxide poisoning, the globus pallidus often is affected profoundly.

Myocardial toxicity, which does not correlate well with carboxyhemoglobin levels, may be apparent immediately or require several days to evolve. ECG findings include ischemic ST segments, T wave changes, arrhythmias, and conduction blocks. Congestive heart failure may supervene.

A variety of skin changes have been reported, including edema, erythema, and bulla formation. Initial arterial blood gas evaluation may reveal a normal Po_2 but mild acidosis. Measurement of only Po_2 or following the clinical course with pulse oximeters can give incorrect estimates of the oxygen-carrying capacity of the blood and, consequently, underestimate the severity of carbon monoxide poisoning. Clinicians are recommended to request carboxyhemoglobin levels and consult a chart or nomogram for expected signs and symptoms (Table 36–16). Carboxyhemoglobin levels greater than 25 per cent are considered serious, with levels greater than 80 per cent being rapidly fatal.

Treatment

Therapy for carbon monoxide poisoning requires immediate removal of the patient from the contaminated environment and treatment with high flow 100% oxygen therapy via endotracheal tube if necessary (Norkool and Kirkpatrick, 1985). Oxygen therapy should be provided with a well-fitted, nonrebreathing mask and not loose facial masks or nasal prongs.

In patients breathing room air, the half-life of carbon monoxide is 5 to 6 hours. This decreases to 40 to 90 minutes with 100% oxygen therapy and is reduced even further when hyperbaric oxygen is administered. Hyperbaric oxygen therapy is not widely available and it is not clear or proven that this slightly more rapid reduction of carbon monoxide justifies transport of all patients to facilities with hyperbaric capabilities.

Clinical instability is characteristic of carbon monoxide intoxication. A severe clinical relapse may occur after an apparent full recovery, correlating with extensive demyelination of the cerebral hemispheric tissue. Deterioration often is noted after increased physical activity, so restricted physical activity and bed rest are indicated following severe carbon monoxide poisoning, especially with neurologic symptoms. The only permanent long-term sequelae recognized from carbon monoxide poisoning are parkinsonism and mental status changes of varying severity.

Noxious Gases

Carbon monoxide, hydrogen cyanide, and hydrogen sulfide may be considered examples of the noxious gases. Further categorization by chemical properties and pathophysiology determines patient symptoms. Noxious gases are of three types: biologically inert gases that harm by hypoxia caused by oxygen displacement, systemic toxins with specific (usually CNS) actions, and agents that act as mucosal irritants. Some noxious agents are both toxins and irritants (Hedges, 1978).

Diagnosis

Local irritants produce injury proportional to their concentration, the duration of exposure, water content of exposed tissue, and water solubility of the gas. Common symptoms of exposure to noxious gases include burning eyes and mouth, sore throat, cough, shortness of breath, and headache. Table 36–17 lists some common gases by type, and the symptom complex is seen with each.

Treatment

Table 36–18 lists some specific treatments available for a variety of systemic gaseous poisons. The production of methemoglobinemia, in which a portion of the circulating hemoglobin iron is in the

TABLE 36–17. NOXIOUS GASES

Gas	Symptom Complex Mechanism
Biologically Inert	
Carbon dioxide	Hypoxia/narcosis
Hydrocarbons	Hypoxia/narcosis
Systemic Poisons	
Carbon disulfide	CNS stimulation, then depression
Carbon monoxide	Tissue hypoxia due to COHgB
Hydrogen cyanide	Inhibition of cytochrome oxidase
Mucosal Irritants	
Ammonia*	*All may produce the following:*
Halogens*	Keratoconjuctivitis
Hydrogen halides* (symptoms may be delayed)	Pharyngitis/rhinitis
	Laryngeal edema
	Tracheobronchitis
Oxides of nitrogen	Bronchospasm
Phosgene	Pulmonary edema
Sulfur dioxide	Nausea/vomiting
Combined Irritant/Toxin	
Hydrogen sulfide	Blocks cellular oxidations
Methylated halogens	CNS depression
	Organ injury by blocking oxidation pathways in lung, heart, liver, kidney

* Skin injury.
From Morse SD, Rial WY: Emergency medicine. *In* Rakel RE (ed): Textbook of Family Practice, 4th edition. Philadelphia, WB Saunders Company, 1990, p 952, with permission.

ferric state, is certainly of use in treating cyanide poisoning because *methemoglobin* binds the cyanide ion tightly. The hepatic enzyme rhodanese then uses thiosulfate as a cofactor to degrade the

TABLE 36–18. SPECIFIC THERAPY FOR SYSTEMIC POISONS

Poison	Therapy
Carbon disulfide	Sedation
	?Methemoglobinemia*
Carbon monoxide	100% oxygen
Hydrogen cyanide	100% oxygen
	Methemoglobinemia*
	?Hydroxocobalamin
Hydrogen sulfide	100% oxygen
	?Methemoglobinemia*
Methylated halogens	Wash skin/clothing
	Sedation
	Bicarbonate for acidosis
	Dialysis for renal failure
	?Penicillamine
	Observe for delayed symptoms

* Production of methemoglobinemia (prepackaged kits may be obtained from Eli Lilly Co. [Lilly cyanide kit]):

1. Inhalation of 1 ampule amyl nitrate every 5 min until I.V. is established.

2. Three per cent nitrate intravenously: adult, 10 mL over 2 to 4 min; children 0.33 mL/kg (10 mg/kg) then 5 mg/kg every 30 min to maintain 30 per cent methemoglobin.

3. Sodium thiosulfate, 25% solution, 50 mL I.V. over 15 min.
From Morse SD, Rial WY: Emergency medicine. *In* Rakel RE (ed): Textbook of Family Practice, 4th edition. Philadelphia, WB Saunders Company, 1990, p 953, with permission.

cyanide moiety and detoxify it. In the United States, the only available cyanide antidote kit is the Lilly cyanide kit, and the instructions for dosage of amyl nitrate pearls, sodium nitrite, and sodium thiosulfate should be followed. In hydrogen sulfide exposure, sodium nitrite should be used, not sodium thiosulfate, because rhodanese is not involved in the reaction.

Methemoglobin therapy should be stopped if hypotension supervenes or the methemoglobin level exceeds 40 per cent. In the case of nitrite poisoning, it is possible to reverse excessive levels of methemoglobinemia if necessary by the use of methylene blue. Methylene blue acts to generate reducing equivalents in the RBCs that convert the methemoglobin iron to its reduced or ferrous state, permitting oxygen transport again. Methylene blue is given in a dose of 1 to 2 mg/kg of a 1% solution over 5 to 15 minutes. It may be repeated in 30 to 45 minutes if no improvement is evident (Schimelman, 1981).

Methemoglobin levels are followed easily by most blood gas laboratory machines. The classic clinical sign of methemoglobinemia is cyanosis unresponsive to supplemental oxygen and chocolate brown arterial blood that does not change on exposure to air, but has normal oxygen tension on arterial blood gas determination. The patient is often more blue than sick.

The irritant effects of noxious gases usually can be treated symptomatically on an outpatient basis. Patients with dyspnea while breathing room air should be observed carefully. Pulmonary edema usually is not delayed with exposure to noxious gases, except in the case of phosgene. These patients should be admitted for 24-hour observation after a significant exposure, even if no symptoms are present.

If therapy is prompt and vigorous, the prognosis after inert or local irritant gas exposure is often good. Patients exposed to systemic poisons have a more guarded prognosis and persistent mental and neurologic deficits are not uncommon.

Poisonous Mushrooms

Increasing interest in natural plant foods by many persons and the search for mood-altering mushrooms (psilocybin) has increased the potential for ingestion of poisonous mushrooms. With over 500 species of mushrooms identified, only about 100 are considered poisonous to humans; however, some are potentially lethal. The adage among mushroom collectors and experts that, "if you can't positively identify it, you should not bet your life on eating it," should be adopted by all persons interested in mushrooms.

Although most poisonous mushrooms cause only gastrointestinal disturbances, some (*Amanita* species) can be fatal (Pond et al., 1986). Mushrooms possess toxins with muscarinic, anticholinergic, and local irritative properties. The *Amanita* and *Gyromitra* groups contain toxins that result in delayed (24 to 72 hours) hepatic and renal failure. Although most mushroom poisoning results in prompt onset of symptoms (30 to 90 minutes), one should not be fooled by the normal delay of *Amanita* poisoning, which often begins 6 to 8 hours after ingestion.

A suspected toxic mushroom ingestion should receive the usual intensive support and gastric decontamination as for all poisoning. In fact, because there are no specific antidotes to the hepatic and renal failure of some mushroom toxins, gastric decontamination becomes very important. One should induce emesis and provide gastric lavage, charcoal and, perhaps, whole-bowel irrigation to decrease toxin absorption. If multiple types of mushrooms are ingested, one should treat as if the worst possible type was ingested. Muscarinic symptoms may be treated with atropine and anticholinergic symptoms with physostigmine. Fluid replacement should proceed aggressively in the face of gastroenteritis, and one should be prepared to manage hypoglycemia and support the renal and hepatic function if they deteriorate.

Poisonous Plants

Many times physicians are consulted about the ingestion of plants that may be hazardous. Young children often consume leaves and flowers of potentially toxic plants. The major types of irritants found in plants are as follows: oxalates, cyanogenic glycosides, cardiac glycosides, anticholinergics, nicotine-like chemicals, solanine, and toxalbumins. If the identity of the plant is not known, this can be determined by consulting textbooks or gardening guides, or by contacting nursery experts or a local poison control center.

Rarely do plant ingestions cause fatal reactions, but children are more susceptible to smaller amounts of toxin. If any doubt exists regarding the amount ingested, it is best to observe the patient closely. Emesis should be induced and activated charcoal with cathartic given.

TABLE 36–19. COMMON TOXIC AND NONTOXIC PLANTS

Toxic	Nontoxic
Azalea	African violet
Caladium	Baby tears
Delphinium	Coleus
Mistletoe	Fuchsia
Pits: cherry, apricot, peach	Gardenia
Hydrangea	Jade plant
Mountain laurel	Begonia
Philodendron	Spider plant
Poinsettia	Wandering Jew

Oxalate-containing plants (caladium, philodendron) usually cause irritation of the mucous membranes and other symptoms. Oral and pharyngeal edema may accompany drooling and dysphagia. Cyanide-containing plants (elderberry) or pits (peach, cherry, apricot) can produce symptoms of cyanide poisoning, but rarely is enough ingested to be serious. Nicotine-containing plants (azalea, tobacco) cause nausea, vomiting, salivation, diarrhea, restlessness, seizures, and mydriasis. It is not uncommon for tobacco pickers to get mild "nicotine sickness" from the resin absorption through their sweating skin in the summertime.

Solanine-containing plants may have nicotinic and atropinic symptoms, and the response to ingestion is unpredictable. Toxalbumin-containing plants (castor beans) result generally in gastroenteritis and irritation of mucous membranes. Large ingestion may result in dehydration and shock.

In general, one should treat based on the observed symptoms or predicted effects of the toxin ingested. Charts are available that describe various common plants and types of reactions if ingested, as well as several common nontoxic plants (Table 36–19).

REFERENCES AND SUGGESTED READINGS

Arena JM: Poisoning. Springfield, IL, Charles C Thomas, 1979.

Arena JM: Hydrocarbon poisoning—current management. Pediatr Ann 16:879, 1987.

Braden NJ, Jackson JE, Walson PD: Tricyclic antidepressant overdose. Pediatr Clin North Am 33:287, 1986.

Buechler KF, Moi S, Noar B, et al: Simultaneous detection of seven drugs of abuse by the TRIAGE PANEL for drugs of abuse. Clin Chem 38:1678, 1992.

Burns RS, Lerner SE, Linder RL: The clinical picture of phencyclidine intoxication. Curr Top II Emerg Med 3(10), 1981.

Crome P: Poisoning due to tricyclic antidepressant overdosage: Clinical presentation and treatment. Med Toxicol 1:261, 1986.

Done AK: Salicylate poisoning. Curr Top II Emerg Med 3(2), 1981.

Doweiko H: Identifying street names of drugs. J Emerg Nurs 5:44, 1979.

Dugandzic RM, Tierney MG, Dickinson GE: Evaluation of the validity of the Done nomogram in the management of acute salicylate intoxication. Ann Emerg Med 18:1186, 1989.

Ferguson MK, Migkiore M, Staszak VM, Little AG: Early evaluation and therapy of caustic esophageal injury. Am J Surg 157:116, 1989.

Goldfrank L, Bresnitz E, Weissman R: Opioids and opiates. Curr Top II Emerg Med 3(8), 1981.

Groleau G, Joffe R, Barish R: The electrocardiographic manifestations of cyclic antidepressant therapy and overdose: A review. J Emerg Med 8:597, 1990.

Guzzardi LJ: Tricyclic antidepressant overdose. Curr Top II Emerg Med 3(7), 1981.

Hedges JR: Acute noxious gas exposure. Curr Top Emerg Med 2(10), 1978.

Howell JM: Alkaline ingestions. Ann Emerg Med 15:820, 1986.

Kulig K, Rumack BH: Hydrocarbon ingestion. Curr Top II Emerg Med 3(4), 1981.

Lanphear WF: Gastric lavage. J Emerg Med 4:43, 1986.

Litovitz TL, Bailey KM, Schmitz BF, et al: 1990 Annual Report of the American Association of Poison Control Centers: National Data Collection System. Am J Emerg Med 9:461, 1991.

Norkool DM, Kirkpatrick JN: Treatment of acute carbon monoxide poisoning with hyperbaric oxygen: A review of 115 cases. Ann Emerg Med 14:1168, 1985.

Olsen KR, Becker CE: Poisoning. *In* Saunders CE, Ho MT (eds): Current Emergency Diagnosis and Treatment, 4th edition. Norwalk, CT, Appleton & Lange, 1992, pp 730–768.

Pond SM, Olson KR, Woo OF, et al: Amatoxin poisoning in Northern California: 1982–1983. West J Med 145(2):204, 1986.

Proudfoot AT, Simpson D, Dyson EH: Management of acute iron poisoning. Med Toxicol 1(2):83, 1986.

Roberts J: Drug overdose in the emergency room. Curr Top Emerg Med 3(1), 1979.

Rumack BH, Peterson RC, Koch GC, Amara IA: Acetaminophen overdose. Arch Intern Med 141:380, 1981.

Schimelman M: Nitrate/nitrite poisoning. Curr Top II Emerg Med 3(5), 1981.

Smilkstein MJ, Knapp GL, Kulig KW, Rumack BH: Efficacy of oral and acetyl cysteine in the treatment of acetaminophen overdose: Analysis of the National Multi Center Study (1976–1985). N Engl J Med 319:1557, 1988.

Spotts JV, Shontz FC: Drug induced ego states. I. Cocaine: phenomenology and implications. Int J Addict 19:119, 1984.

Temple AR: Emergency treatment of acetaminophen overdose. Curr Top II Emerg Med 3(3), 1981.

Votey SR, Bosse GM, Bayer MJ: Flumazenil: A new benzodiazepine antagonist. Ann Emerg Med 20(2):181, 1991.

Zwiener RJ, Ginsberg CM: Organophosphate and carbonate poisoning in infants and children. Pediatrics 81:121, 1988.

Bites, Stings, and Other Envenomation

WILLIAM FULCHER

ANIMAL BITES

Traumatic wounds constitute a large percentage of emergency department visits, and animal bites constitute a large proportion of these wounds. National estimates range from 300 to 700 bites per 100,000 population. Increasing contact between and exposure to animals through human occupation and recreation seem to ensure the fact that physicians will continue to see a variety of bites from both common and exotic animals. Bite wounds require, in addition to basic wound management, an understanding of the oral bacterial flora particular to the animal involved, a consideration of envenomation, and, finally, the problem of tetanus and rabies prevention. Consequently, the family physician must assess the following in all bites to provide effective care: type of bite, severity, and location; the origin of bite (type of animal) and possibility of rabies; time since the bite; the first aid administered; associated injuries; evidence of infection; pre-existing illness in the victim; and tetanus status.

The most important initial first aid for animal bites is copious irrigation. Without question, the most useful management for *contaminated* wounds (soil, feces) is irrigation with normal saline using a large 30 to 50-mL syringe and an 18- or 19-gauge needle. This will provide an irrigating pressure that will significantly clean debris from wounds and consequently reduce the risk of infection.

Depending on the type of bite described below, the physician will need to explore the wound, débride devitalized tissue, achieve good hemostasis, decide on proper surgical repair, and apply adequate dressing to achieve immobilization. Cosmetic concerns that should be considered include the location of the wound (face or hand), age of the wound (old versus "fresh" [less than 6 to 8 hours]), and signs of infection (clean versus contaminated), which will dictate who should repair the wound and when and where the repair should take place (Connolly and Kilgore, 1979). Prophylactic antibiotics for animal bites have been shown to be useful in animal models only if administered *before* the bite occurs; this is obviously rarely possible in the real world. *Prophylactic* cultures of animal bites are likewise not very useful; however, cultures of infected draining wounds are helpful in guiding subsequent antibiotic use. The physician must decide on the need for tetanus prophylaxis or immunization as well as the risk of rabies in each particular bite and treat as outlined later.

The postemergency treatment disposition will depend on the assessment described here and specifics outlined in the syndromes discussed later. Patients released from the emergency department or office must have well-documented and specific instructions for follow-up and possible wound complications. Explicit instructions for local wound care, signs of infection, and time for suture removal should be given to the patient and possibly an accompanying family member or friend. Patients should be instructed in writing that all wounds may heal with scars, may get infected, and may have undetectable foreign bodies at the time of initial assessment. This not only will ensure some uniform standard of care for bite wounds but, it is hoped, will reduce medicolegal risk for family physicians providing emergency care for bites.

Tetanus and Tetanus Prophylaxis

Tetanus has become rare with the routine use of tetanus toxoid in pediatric immunizations and with boosters following most traumatic skin injuries and many types of surgery. In fact, tetanus has a predicted incidence of less than 1 case per 1 million in the United States, with approximately 100 cases reported yearly. There still remains a significant reservoir for tetanus in the unimmunized (e.g., migrant workers) and the underimmunized (elderly). In 10 to 20 per cent of tetanus cases, no wounds or skin lesions are present. Neonatal tetanus can occur in infants born to mothers not adequately immunized because the mothers cannot confer passive immunity transplacently. Finally, narcotic addicts also have an increased risk of developing tetanus.

Tetanus is caused by the anaerobic, gram-positive rod *Clostridium tetani*. The spores of this organism are ubiquitous in nature and, although the organism itself is quite susceptible to killing by heat, the spores are extremely resistant to destruction. Consequently, these spores can enter a wound through soil contamination and lead to the germination and multiplication of *C. tetani*, with consequent toxin production that leads to tetanus. "Tetanus-prone" wounds are wounds that produce anaerobic conditions, such as deep puncture wounds, crush injuries, burns, and wounds contaminated with soil or feces.

Tetanus develops usually within 10 to 14 days of injury, and the symptoms emerge over 2 to 5 days. Patients initially present with trismus and occasionally dysphagia. They complain of increasing pain in the injury site and may develop a stiff, painful neck. The symptoms then progress to include diffuse spasms of skeletal muscle; spasms of the paraspinal muscles may lead to opisthotonos. These spasms also may cause vertebral body fractures, respiratory insufficiency (a frequent cause of death), and rhabdomyolysis. Death in developed countries is now usually due to hyperpyrexia and cardiac arrhythmias.

Treatment for suspected tetanus should include immediate administration of tetanus immunoglobulin (TIG), 1000 units intravenously and 2000 units intramuscularly to bind circulating toxin (Matthews, 1991). Surgical débridement of the involved wound should be scheduled, and patients should be given penicillin, 1 million units every 6 hours, or erythromycin, 500 mg every 6 hours, if penicillin allergic. The support of airway, breathing, and circulation is mandatory. If vital capacity is less than 50 per cent of predicted, the physician should consider paralysis and mechanical ventilation. If vital capacity is greater than 50 per cent but trismus interferes with the airway, an endotracheal tube or tracheostomy should be employed. For mild disease, the physician may find lorazepam or diazepam useful for muscle spasms (Matthews, 1991).

Tetanus Prophylaxis

There is no natural immunity to tetanus toxin. Appropriately timed toxoid injections are mandatory to protect all age groups. The toxoid is highly effective in promoting active immunity for at least 10 years after adequate immunization series.

Tetanus boosters, if even for wound management, need be given only every 10 years unless a wound is considered tetanus prone (see earlier). In those cases, tetanus toxoid should be given if the patient has not received a dose in 5 years. Patients who have never had primary tetanus immunization may require toxoid and TIG at initial management (Immunization Practices Advisory Committee, 1981).

Patients 7 years and older should receive active immunization with tetanus–diphtheria toxoid (Td) (containing diphtheria toxoid in a reduced dose). This decreases local and systemic reactions to the immunization and also provides enhanced diphtheria protection, which many adults require. Pa-

TABLE 36–20. IMMUNIZATION SCHEDULE

History of Adsorbed Tetanus Toxoid (Doses)	Tetanus-Prone Wounds		Nontetanus-Prone Wounds	
	Td†	TIG	Td*	TIG
Unknown or fewer than 3	Yes	Yes	Yes	No
3 or more†	No§	No	No‡	No

Verify a history of tetanus immunization from medical records so that appropriate tetanus prophylaxis can be accomplished.
Td: Tetanus and diphtheria toxoids adsorbed (for adult use)
TIG: Tetanus immune globulin (human)
* For children less than seven years old: DTP (DT, if pertussis vaccine is contraindicated) is preferable to tetanus toxoid alone. For persons seven years old and older, Td is preferable to tetanus toxoid alone.
† If only three doses of fluid toxoid have been received, a fourth dose of toxoid, preferably an adsorbed toxoid, should be given.
‡ Yes, if more than 10 years since last dose.
§ Yes, if more than five years since last dose. (More frequent boosters are not needed and can accentuate side effects.)
From the Committee on Trauma, American College of Surgeons. Guide to Prophylaxis Against Tetanus. Chicago, American College of Surgeons, 1987, with permission.

tients under age 7 should receive routine diphtheria–pertussis–tetanus (DPT) vaccine. In all cases in which inadequate primary immunization is likely (the required regimen is four primary injections and a preschool booster between ages 4 and 6), a primary immunization sequence should be completed.

If passive immunization is needed, human TIG is used in a dose of 250 mg intramuscularly; extremely "dirty" wounds may justify 500 mg. This must be injected at a site distant to the tetanus toxoid injection site to avoid neutralizing the toxoid. Because this is human immunoglobulin, the risk of adverse reaction is minimized. Table 36–20 provides a summary of the use of Td and TIG in wounds.

Rabies Prophylaxis

Of the potential zoonotic disease complications from animal bites, rabies is one of the most rare but dreaded in the United States. A disease of warm-blooded animals, rabies is common in South America, Africa, Asia, and continental Europe. Human rabies cases are common in many areas of the world, with nearly 1000 fatal cases reported annually to the World Health Organization. The incidence of rabies in the United States has decreased considerably since the near-universal immunization of the dog population. Rabies in wildlife, particularly carnivores and bats, constitutes the largest source of infection for humans and domestic animals in the United States. Dog bites are the most common bite in which rabies prophylaxis is considered; however, there is an extremely low incidence of rabies in dogs now (Doan-Wiggins, 1988).

The most difficult question in rabies prophylaxis is when to treat. In the United States, wild carnivores (skunks, coyotes, raccoons, bobcats, bats) are more likely to be infected than other animals and have been the cause of most human rabies cases since 1970. Unless the animal is captured and shown not to be rabid, rabies prophylaxis is required. Significant exposures include scratches, abrasions, open wounds, or mucous membrane contact with saliva or other infectious material from a rabid animal. When the animal is not available for observation, the decision to institute rabies prophylaxis may be delayed up to 48 hours while attempts are made to locate the animal. If the animal is not located or if the animal exhibited abnormal behavior before the bite, one is wise to begin rabies prophylaxis (Fig. 36–14). Unprovoked attacks are considered more likely to indicate a rabid animal. Bites sustained while attempting to feed or handle apparently healthy animals, including dogs, should be considered unprovoked (Doan-Wiggins, 1988).

The type or location of exposure is important. Deep puncture wounds or bites of the head, neck, face, hands, and fingers should be considered serious exposures in the appropriate animal. If the animal can be captured, it should be observed for 10 days. Most animals will exhibit signs of rabies, if infected, during this time. Bats are an important exception to this and may harbor active rabies infection for months without exhibiting signs of infection. If the animal exhibits signs of rabies, the animal should be killed in a manner that does not destroy the head. Examination of the brain is essential for determining whether the animal indeed is infected with rabies. The brain of the animal should be transported promptly to a facility that can test it with fluorescent antibody techniques, to confirm rabies infection.

As mentioned in the previous discussion of general bite wounds, irrigation of saliva containing rabies virus is a crucial part of rabies management. This is perhaps the most effective rabies prevention for even high-risk bites. Rabies immunoglobulin (RIG) should be infiltrated into and around the animal bite. A dose of 20 units/kg of body weight should be divided, with half used in the local injection and half given at other sites intramuscularly. Human RIG has eliminated the serum sickness reactions that followed the old equine antirabies serum. Local pain and low-grade fever may follow the use of RIG; however, such minor reactions should not interrupt the postexposure prophylaxis for rabies (Corey, 1980).

Human diploid cell vaccine (HDCV) for rabies was developed in the 1960s and provides an anti-body response in nearly 100 per cent of recipients. Current World Health Organization recommendations for postexposure prophylaxis include five 1-mL doses of HDCV on days 0, 3, 7, 14 and 28 in conjunction with passive RIG on day 0. Serum for rabies antibody determination should be collected 2 to 3 weeks after the last dose and, if no response is noted, an additional booster should be given.

Corticosteroids and other immunosuppressive agents may interfere with the development of activity immunity. Pregnancy is *not* considered a contraindication to postexposure prophylaxis for rabies.

Specific Bite Syndromes

Dogs

Dog bites are probably the most common animal bites seen by emergency and family physicians. They involve laceration, avulsion, and crush injury to tissue and introduction into the various tissue planes of a variety of bacterial organisms with increased potential for infection. Dog bites are quite common in children and result in a high incidence of facial and extremity injuries. Physicians should remember the ABCs of resuscitation when treating facial and neck injuries from dog bites. Treatment of dog bites includes acute wound management as described earlier, tetanus prophylaxis, consideration of rabies prophylaxis, and surveillance for wound infection (Callahan, 1978). Acute wound management does not differ from management of other complicated, contaminated lacerations. Wounds should be irrigated copiously as described earlier. Débridement of devitalized tissue can be undertaken if necessary unless it would produce difficulty with cosmesis or function. Dog bites have, despite their associated crush component, a low incidence of infection (2 to 5 per cent on average). There are no data to suggest that prophylactic antibiotic therapy decreases the infection rate of dog bites as long as they have been well cleaned and débrided (Goldstein et al., 1980). A patient should be followed closely for signs of infection, however, and should be treated with antibiotics if one supervenes. Sutures used for initial repairs also should be removed if infection results and it is cosmetically feasible.

Infections from dog and other animal bites are more common in patients over 50 years old, diabetics, wounds that are greater than 24 hours old before evaluation, and patients with immune suppression. The oral flora of dogs includes *Escherichia coli*, *Staphylococcus aureus* (32 per cent average), *Streptococcus*, *Pasteurella*, and other gram-negative organisms. Ten to 15 per cent of organ-

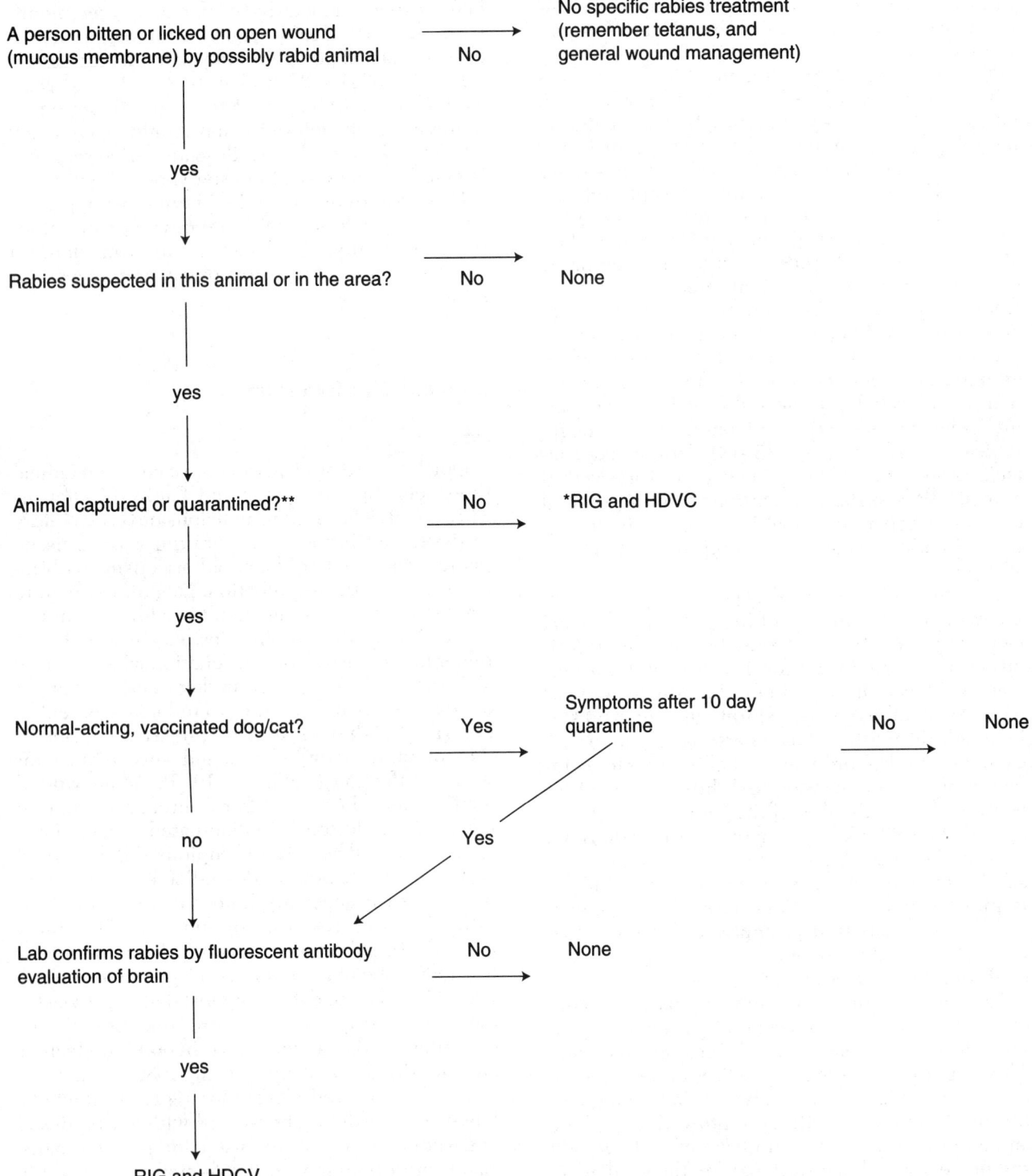

FIGURE 36–14. Postbite rabies management. *Rabies immunoglobulin and human diploid cell vaccine. **Treatment may be delayed up to 48 hours to capture animal and observe behavior. (Adapted from Corey L, Hattwick MAW: Treatment of persons exposed to rabies. JAMA 232:272, 1975.)

isms are penicillin resistant; consequently, the choice of a penicillinase-resistant penicillin or cephalosporin would be prudent in the infected dog bite (Goldstein et al., 1978). Wounds of the hand should be given special consideration be-

cause of the multiple tissue planes and tendon structures that may be involved with the deep penetration of dog bites. Finally, unprovoked attacks are considered more likely to indicate a rabid dog, as described earlier. Individuals bitten while feeding an otherwise apparently healthy dog should consider this an unprovoked attack. Although the incidence of rabies in domestic dogs is very low, the physician should attempt to quarantine the dog for observation and contact the local health department for information on the prevalence of rabies in dogs in the area.

Cats

Cat bites usually are seen on the extremities and hands. Scratches also may produce infection. The long, slender teeth of cats deeply inoculate bitten tissues with the multiple organisms in their oral flora. These include anaerobic bacteria, streptococci, coagulase-positive staphylococci, and, very often, *Pasteurella multocida,* a highly penicillin-sensitive, gram-negative rod that can cause early local wound infection. This organism is seen in dog bites as well but is less often a cause of infection after dog bites. Clinical infection with *P. multocida* usually presents within 24 hours of the bite and includes inflammation, pain, and swelling around the bite, with a grey serosanguinous discharge. The discharge may show few organisms on Gram's stain. Regional lymph nodes may enlarge in one third of infections, but fever is present in less than 20 per cent. This infection can be slow to heal even with proper therapy. Penicillin is considered the drug of choice unless other organisms are believed to be involved in the infection. A penicillinase-resistant penicillin or cephalosporin would be an acceptable alternative, especially if the infected site is more than 24 to 48 hours old. Although *Pasteurella* has been considered sensitive to a wide variety of antibiotics, failures have been reported with erythromycin.

Wild Carnivores

The wild carnivores are the largest source of rabies infection in the United States. Small carnivores such as fox, bobcat, skunk, raccoon, and coyote should be considered high risk for carrying rabies. General antibiotic requirements for infected bites should follow those recommendations for dog or cat bites. Large carnivore bites or attacks may involve more serious trauma, such as large crush wounds or lacerations. Excessive evisceration of the victim may be the most important and morbid injury for bites or attacks from bears, mountain lions, or other large zoo carnivores. The emergency physician should employ the basic support of ABCs and major trauma protocols in these cases.

Rodents

Rodent bites, which include bites from mice, gerbils, squirrels, chipmunks, and rabbits, are common but often minor. These animals are not considered sources of rabies. Some of these animals, such as rabbits, may have *P. multocida* in their oral flora. Copious irrigation and cleansing with soap and water should be adequate for most rodent bites. If signs of infection develop, the physician should obtain a culture of any discharge and treat appropriately. A broad-spectrum cephalosporin or penicillinase-resistant penicillin would be prudent until culture reports return.

Humans

Human and other primate bites are considered the most dangerous bites that the emergency physician will deal with because these bites often involve more virulent bacteria than other animal bites. The mixture of aerobic and anaerobic flora in the human bite, along with the often complex deep structure injury to hands and other anatomic structures involved, leads to high rates of infection and infectious complications. Human bites are often the result of violence, and the embarrassment surrounding the bite or the injury usually leads to a delay in treatment. Many times human bites involve extremities, the face, and ears, and injury to these structures may make management more difficult. A classic human bite injury occurs when persons punch opponents in the teeth, which then may cause a deep inoculation of organisms into the soft tissue around the metacarpal head and occasionally even into the extensor tendons or metacarpophalangeal joints. This may result in tenosynovitis, septic arthritis, or osteomyelitis. Human bites or lacerations in these areas must be examined with the joint in extension and flexion to reproduce the position of injury. Deep penetration otherwise may be missed, with a subsequently deforming infection of tendon or joint space (Martin, 1987).

Human bites of the hand should never be closed primarily. After good wound cleansing and débridement, the hand should be splinted a position of safe immobilization (Fig. 36–15), elevated, and watched closely for infection. If delayed closure is anticipated, oral antibiotics may be given (Malinowski et al., 1979).

If infection occurs in a human bite, antibiotic therapy following cultures can be initiated with an agent possessing broad-spectrum activity against gram-positive organisms, such as a cephalosporin. Coverage against anaerobes and gram-negative rods also may be needed. One of the second- or third-generation cephalosporins may be particularly useful with its added gram-negative and anaerobic spectra. Augmentin and clindamycin are also reasonable alternatives, as is the use of multiple other agents as dictated by initial clinical impression. These considerations hold for all infected animal bites as well.

Monkeys and Other Primates

Primate bites may be an important source of injury in research, university, or zoo environments. There is a high incidence of infection, with greater than 25 per cent of such bites becoming infected. Like human bites, other primates may infect their wounds with multiple organisms. Vigorous and co-

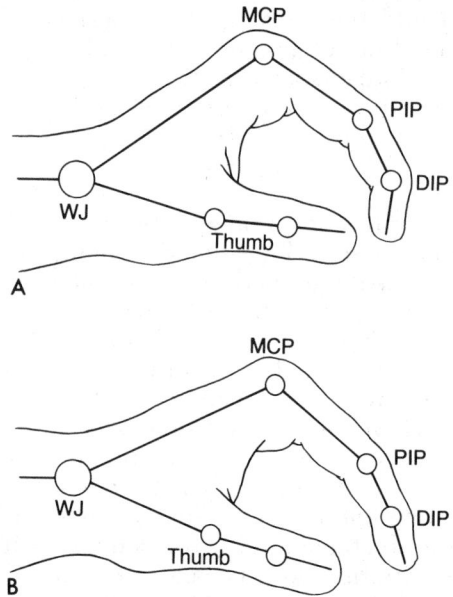

FIGURE 36–15. Splinting the injured hand. The two most common positions are those of function (*A*) and safe immobilization (*B*) (see text). WJ = wrist joint, MCP = metacarpophalangeal joint, PIP = proximal interphalangeal joint. (From Morse SD, Rial WY: Emergency medicine. *In* Rakel RE [ed]: Textbook of Family Practice, 4th edition. Philadelphia, WB Saunders Company, 1990, p 954, with permission.)

pious irrigation is the most important way to decrease infection. Antibiotic selection and use should follow recommendations under human bites.

Livestock

Livestock such as cows, pigs, and horses can be a source of bite wounds; however, more common is trauma caused by hoofs, horns, or heads. Livestock bites should be thoroughly irrigated, especially if contaminated with feces. The crush component of large livestock bites may increase the risk of infection, so such wounds should be thoroughly cleaned, dressed with bulky absorptive dressings, and immobilized as needed. If signs and symptoms of infection develop, cultures for identification and antibiotic sensitivity of involved organisms should be performed and a broad-spectrum antibiotic regimen implemented. One should remember that contaminated wounds are a source of tetanus in the underimmunized, so the tetanus status of the infected individual is important to ascertain.

Snakes (Ophidism)

Each year in the United States, about 45,000 persons are bitten by snakes, although only 6000 to 7000 bites are from poisonous snakes (Blackmon and Dillon, 1992). Worldwide, 40,000 persons die from snake bites each year, although the U.S. average is around 10 to 20/year. There are at least 19 venomous species of snake in the United States.

The two main types are crotalids, or pit viper (rattlesnakes, cottonmouths, copperheads), and elapids (coral snakes). Among poisonous snake bites in the United States, 95 per cent are from pit vipers, mostly rattlesnakes (Otten, 1988).

Envenomation occurs in only 15 to 20 per cent of poisonous snake bites (Russell, 1980). In the spring, when snakes first emerge from hibernation with full poison glands, a snake bite is generally more severe and more common. The fangs of poisonous snakes produce two distinct fang puncture marks, while the teeth of nonpoisonous snakes only produce two rows of similar scratches. As mentioned earlier, the majority of U.S. poisonous snakebites are from pit vipers, which can be distinguished from nonpoisonous snakes by several features (Fig. 36–16). Table 36–21 lists major poisonous snake species, their geographic location, and the major venomous syndrome they produce.

The coral snake is a small elapid with bands of black, yellow, and red. It has a blunt snout that is always black. Several harmless species of snake resemble the coral snake, but their snouts are usu-

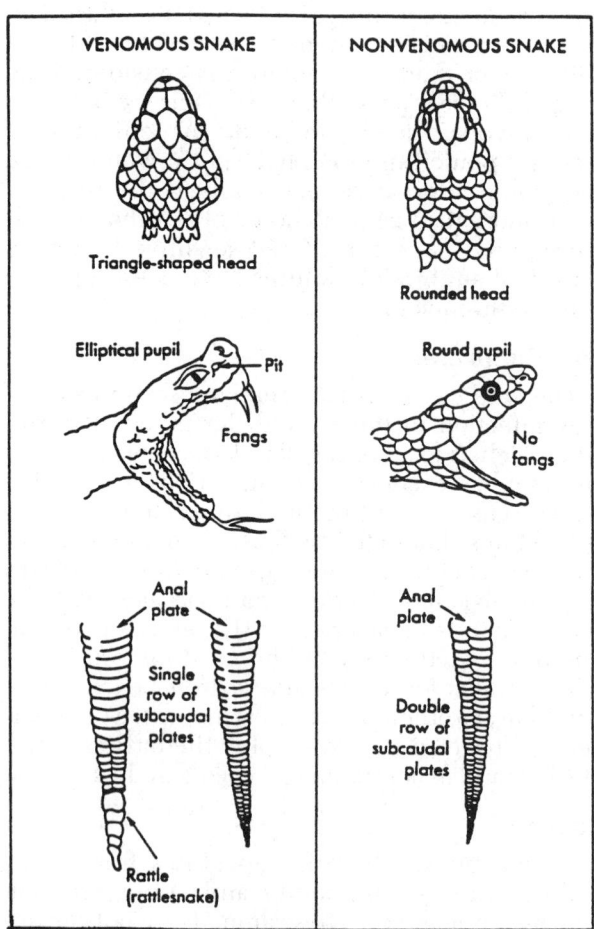

FIGURE 36–16. Features of poisonous and nonpoisonous snakes. (From Otten EJ: Venomous animal injuries. *In* Rosen P et al [eds]: Emergency Medicine: Concepts and Clinical Practice. St. Louis, CV Mosby, 1988, p 878, with permission.)

TABLE 36–21. MAJOR POISONOUS SNAKES IN UNITED STATES

Snake	Geographic Location	Syndrome
Florida diamond-back rattler (*Crotalus adamanteus*)	North Carolina south, west to the Mississippi	Hemotoxic
Texas diamond-back rattler (*C. atrox*)	Arkansas to Southern California	Hemotoxic
Timber rattler (*C. horridus*)	Entire East Coast, west to Minnesota through Texas	Hemotoxic
Prairie rattler (*C. viridis*)	Great Plains to Rockies	Hemotoxic
Pacific rattler (*C. oreganus*)	Pacific Coast, Idaho, Arizona	Hemotoxic
Pigmy rattler (*Sistrurus miliarius*)	Carolinas south, west to Texas	Hemotoxic
Massasauga (*S. catenatus*)	New York through Great Plains to Texas and Arizona	Hemotoxic
Copperhead (*Agkistrodon moreson*)	Massachusetts to Florida, Great Plains, south to Texas	Hemotoxic
Water moccasin (*A. piscivorus*)	Virginia to Florida, Gulf States, Midwest, and Texas	Hemotoxic
Coral, or harlequin, snake (*Micrurus fulvius*)	Southeastern United States	Neurotoxic

From Morse SD, Rial WY: Emergency medicine. *In* Rakel RE (ed): Textbook of Family Practice, 4th edition. Philadelphia, WB Saunders Company, 1990, p 956, with permission.

ally red or grey. The coral snake is very secretive and will, on rare occasions, produce a poisonous bite; however, it prefers to retreat. It may be confused with other similarly colored snakes and has such small fang marks that they may not be identifiable on the victim (Norris and Dart). Although the coloration method of identification is not infallible, the following rhyme has been used to identify the coral snake from others: "Red on yellow, kill a fellow; red on black, venom lack."

NONPOISONOUS SNAKES. Although traditional dogma has held that the typical nonpoisonous snake bite is no more serious than its local wound requirements, recent reports have indicated that the bites of some snakes, heretofore considered "harmless," can provoke serious systemic symptoms. For example the red-neck keelback (*Rhabdophis subminatus*) has been reported to cause life-threatening symptoms, presumably from its toxin-containing saliva (Cable et al., 1984). This should not come as a surprise, however, because many of the snake and reptile predecessors, the dinosaurs, where thought to use the same mechanism to incapacitate bitten prey. It would seem prudent, therefore, for physicians to consider any modern-day snake or reptile bite with systemic symptoms as potentially serious and consult a local poison control center for advice.

DIAGNOSIS. Snake venom is a mixture of proteolytic enzyme and toxic protein. Crotalid venom is mainly cytolytic and elapid is mainly neurotoxic. Cytolytic venom causes cell lysis, enhances spread of venom, causes hemolysis, increases capillary permeability, and alters hemostasis. Neurotoxic venom disrupts neuromuscular activity, causing paresthesia, weakness, and respiratory paralysis.

If at all possible, the snake should be identified or captured. If the nature of the snake or its identification is not clear to the physician, a local herpetologist or poison control center should be consulted. Care should be taken to avoid another bite. Decapitated heads of poisonous snakes are able to exhibit reflex biting reactions for up to 1 hour after being removed from the body.

Marked local symptoms may appear rapidly following a poisonous bite. Pain is prominent, followed by edema that progresses proximally from the bite. An entire extremity may become massively swollen within 1 hour. Local hemorrhage with bloody oozing and tissue necrosis may both be prominent, particularly with hemotoxin venom. Systemic symptoms, including nausea, vomiting, hemorrhage, cardiorespiratory distress, coma, and collapse, can follow significant envenomation in the absence of therapy. Elapids and the Mojave rattlesnake have been reported to produce few or no early local signs of envenomation, but bite victims may develop neurologic symptoms such as paresthesia, blurred vision, dysphagia, ptosis, and hypersalivation after a delay of 2 to 6 hours (Jansen et al., 1992). Often a metallic taste in the victim's mouth can be an early sign of envenomation (Snyder and Knowles, 1988). Table 36–22 delineates the clinical signs of the two major syndromes.

TREATMENT. The single undisputed vital course of action following poisonous snakebite is rapid transport to an emergency facility capable of administering antivenin for definitive therapy. The bitten part should be immobilized as if it were a fracture and at a level below the heart. All constrictive rings and other items should be removed. The patient should be kept as absolutely calm as possible. There should be no exertion on the vic-

TABLE 36–22. MAJOR SNAKEBITE SYNDROMES

Neurotoxic	Hemotoxic
Drowsiness	Local hemorrhagic necrosis
Bradycardia/hypotension	Petechiae due to
Muscle weakness	thrombocytopenia
Ptosis	Parenchymal hemorrhages
Difficulty swallowing	Fibrinolysis
Respiratory failure	Disseminated intravascular
Trimus	coagulation (DIC)
Nausea/vomiting	Hemolysis
Coma/seizures	
Cardiorespiratory collapse	

From Morse SD, Rial WY: Emergency medicine. *In* Rakel RE (ed): Textbook of Family Practice, 4th edition. Philadelphia, WB Saunders Company, 1990, p 956, with permission.

tim's part. The use of tourniquets, incision and suction, and ice for the treatment of most snakebites has been questioned seriously by authorities dealing with snakebites (Stewart et al., 1981). It is clear that a loosely fitting venolymphatic occlusive constriction band applied proximal to the bite may retard the absorption of venom into the systemic circulation. This type of tourniquet should be applied loosely enough that the finger of the rescuer or physician can slip easily underneath the band. Rescuers and emergency physicians should not apply ice directly to the bite site nor pack the extremity in ice. In most cases this will increase local damage (Johnson, 1991).

If the distance to a source of antivenin is more than 2 hours away, the snake has been identified as venomous and, the victim is very young, elderly, or infirm, incision and suctioning may be considered as first aid by rescuers who have no open cavities or oral mucosal lesions that would put them at risk of absorbing toxin or infecting the wound (Smith and Figge). There is some evidence that commercial venom extractors that can be used without incising the bite wound, if used within 5 minutes of the bite, may remove up to 25 per cent of venom (Blackmon and Dillon).

Polyvalent antivenin for the treatment of pit viper bites is available from numerous sources and prevents death, relieves pain, aborts serious effects, and shortens convalescence. The initial dose of antivenin is administered depending on the severity of symptoms, lapse of time since the bite, size and age of patient, and size of the snake (Table 36–23). Antivenins are heterologous sera (horse) and their use should be preceded by conjunctival and or skin testing for allergy. Evidence of skin allergy to antivenin does not constitute a contraindication to the administration of antivenin but does indicate that it will require more careful observation and management. Likewise, negative skin testing for allergy does not guarantee against anaphylaxis during subsequent utilization of antivenin. When sera are given, equipment and personnel to manage anaphylaxis and cardiopulmonary collapse should be on hand. Usually this requires admission to an intensive care or other unit for appropriate management.

Antivenin should be given by slow intravenous drip. It generally should not be given intramuscularly or into the bite area. Several charts are available to guide the physician in the appropriate use of adequate amounts of antivenin for progressive degrees of envenomation. For severe envenomation, more than 20 vials of antivenin may be necessary. One of the more common errors in treatment of severe snakebites is the use of too *little* antivenin. If, during the emergency room or hospital evaluation, the hematocrit falls below 30 per cent, transfusion may be required. It is prudent to draw blood early for crossmatching because snake venom may interfere with crossmatching if it is delayed.

An antivenin index center (405-271-5454) exists in Oklahoma providing emergency information 24 hours a day on antivenins available for all snakes that are stocked in zoos, labs, and other institutions in North America. The scientific and common names of the snake involved should be ascertained. Most snake antivenin can be obtained from the Centers for Disease Control and Prevention (404-633-3311).

INSECT BITES AND STINGS

Hymenoptera Stings

Bees and Wasps

Stings from bees and wasps are common occurrences requiring acute care in the United States. These insects kill more Americans annually than snakes as a result of anaphylactic reactions.

Bee stingers are hooked and remain in tissue after their insertion. This leads to evisceration and death of the stinging bee, but also to a continued pumping of venom into the wound. Wasps lack a hook on their stinger and can sting multiple times, which makes them potentially more dangerous. Their stings are also more tetanus prone that those

TABLE 36–23. ENVENOMATION SYNDROMES AND TREATMENT

Grade	Signs and Symptoms	Antivenin Dose (Vials)
0	No envenomation; fang punctures present; no local or systemic signs	No antivenin; local wound care
I	Mild envenomation; fang punctures present; local pain and swelling; no systemic signs	3–5
II	Moderate envenomation; fang punctures present; severe pain; swelling 6–12 inches; some abnormal systemic or laboratory findings	6–10
III	Severe envenomation; fang punctures present; severe pain; swelling more than 12 inches; petechiae and bullae present; severe systemic reaction; bleeding and/or disseminated intravascular coagulopathy; markedly abnormal laboratory findings	15 or more
IV	Multiple envenomations; markedly abnormal signs and symptoms in all categories; life-threatening	25 or more

Adapted from Christopher DG, Rodning CB: Crotalidae envenomation. South Med J 79:159, 1986, with permission.

of bees because many species of wasps or hornet are saprophytic and feed on excrement.

Hymenoptera venom resembles mild snake venom, having both hemotoxic and neurotoxic properties. It has strong histamine-like action on tissue. A local pruritic wheal is the most common reaction, which usually requires only cold compresses and occasionally antihistamines, local wound care, and, if necessary, tetanus prophylaxis.

A delayed syndrome of local allergy is not uncommon, with progressive localized heat, redness, and swelling of tissue around the sting, often with low-grade fever. This may be difficult to differentiate from infection when it occurs 1 or more days after the sting. The presence of intense pruritis and absence of lymphangitis or adenopathy suggest an allergic reaction. These patients are best treated initially with antihistamines, ice, elevation, splinting, and careful observation, with antibiotic use reserved for further progression of signs (Toewe, 1980).

The anaphylactic response to hymenoptera stings, which includes cardiovascular collapse, bronchospasm, diarrhea, and urticaria, can be dramatic and life threatening. It often requires the use of such agents as epinephrine (which may be injected sublingually in profound collapse if no intravenous or endotracheal route is available), antihistamines, corticosteroids, oxygen, intravenous fluids, and on occasion complete cardiopulmonary resuscitation (Auerbach, 1987). This response most always warrants hospitalization, if only for short-term observation (Table 36–24).

Further management of the sting should include removal of remaining stingers by gentle scraping. Use of forceps may cause further injection of the venom into the wound. Topical cold or ice packs may reduce swelling and pain. Applying a paste or poultice of meat tenderizer may decrease local symptoms. Oral intramuscular or intravenous diphenhydramine may be given in mild sting reactions, and intravenous steroids such as hydrocortisone (2 mg/kg) should be administered in moderate to severe envenomation.

Recovery from anaphylaxis caused by stings is usually complete within 48 hours. All patients subsequently should carry a kit with them that contains epinephrine, such as the ANA-Kit from Holister Stier Labs, wear a Medic-Alert bracelet documenting their sensitivity, and consider undergoing desensitization therapy.

Fire Ants

The fire ant is another unwelcome insect member of the order Hymenoptera that is harmful to humans. The most clinically important species, *Solenopsis invicta*, was brought into Alabama from Brazil in the 1930s. It is now found in several southern states and seems to be replacing many native species. The only limiting factor to its spread seems to be cold winters. The venom of this fire ant is unique in the animal world in that it is 95 per cent alkaloid. This venom may induce hemolysis, depolarization of cell membranes, activation of the alternate compliment pathway, and general tissue destruction (Otten, 1988). The ant produces the sting after biting the victim; while holding with its jaws, it rotates around the bite, stinging the victim several times. Over the next 24 hours, a sterile pustule develops with local burning, redness, and itching. Up to 10 per cent of victims may have some degree of hypersensitivity, and symptoms of urticaria, angioedema, nausea and vomiting, dyspnea, wheezing, dizziness, and respiratory arrest have been reported. Ice applied to the area of the sting usually relieves pain and swelling. In the event of a hypersensitivity reaction, first aid and emergency treatment should be provided similar to that for other Hymenoptera stings.

Spider Bites

All spiders inject venom when they bite, but only two species of spider in the United States routinely cause serious envenomation syndromes: the black widow spider (*Lactrodectis mactans*) and the brown recluse spider (*Loxosceles* species) (Pennell et al., 1987).

Black Widow Spider

The black widow spider is found in nearly all states of the continental United States. The adult female has a globular black body about one-half inch long with an orange–red hourglass figure on its ventral surface; the male is about one half the size of the female. The web usually looks disordered and is out-of-doors or in outhouses. This spider often is not seen during the day.

The initial sharp pain of the black widow spider's bite usually fades rapidly. The patient develops local muscle cramps 15 minutes to 2 hours later. The neurotoxic venom causes muscle pain, contraction, and ascending motor paralysis. The abdomen may become board-like and serious systemic symptoms may follow, including delirium, seizures, shock, cyanosis and, in occasional cases, death. In nonfatal cases, symptoms peak in 3 to 24 hours and then gradually resolve over several days.

TABLE 36–24. ANAPHYLAXIS MANAGEMENT

Epinephrine: 0.3–0.5 mL of 1:1000 solution S.Q., I.M., or sublingual injection; I.V. more cautiously
Corticosteroids: 100 mg hydrocortisone I.V.
Antihistamines: 25–50 mg diphenhydramine I.V.
Oxygen
Trendelenburg, fluids, pressors, CPR as needed

From Morse SD, Rial WY: Emergency medicine. *In* Rakel RE (ed): Textbook of Family Practice, 4th edition. Philadelphia, WB Saunders Company, 1990, p 958, with permission.

After the diagnosis is made, the patient should receive 1 ampule of Lyovac antivenin intramuscularly after conjunctival and/or skin testing for horse serum sensitivity. Lyovac antivenin is a horse-derived heterologous antiserum produced using black widow spider venom. It is specific for the management of black widow spider bites and has no use in brown recluse bites or snake bites. One or two doses of Lyovac usually resolve symptoms in 1 to 3 hours by counteracting the neurotoxic venom.

Victims of black widow spider envenomation should be admitted to a hospital for good nursing care and ancillary therapy. Muscle pain responds to heat and infusion of 10 per cent calcium gluconate. Sedatives, muscle relaxants, and adrenocorticoids are also efficacious in managing muscular symptoms. Respiratory status must be observed carefully. Local therapy at the bite site is of no value, nor are tourniquets or suction.

Brown Recluse Spider

The brown recluse spider's venom is cytotoxic and hemotoxic, causing local progressive tissue necrosis and systemic syndromes, including disseminated intravascular coagulation. This spider is brown with a violin-shaped dark area on its dorsal thorax. Its body is about 1 cm long. The spider lives indoors, in cellars, and in other areas, and is even found in shoes and bedding. It cannot live at temperatures less than 40°F; therefore, it generally is found in the southern states. On initial envenomation, this spider injects a venom rich in protease, hyaluronidase, and esterase. Mild pain becomes progressively more severe. A blister forms and then escharifies by the end of the first week after the bite. A typical bull's-eye lesion is created when the red blister is encircled by a pale, irregularly shaped, ischemic halo, which in turn is surrounded by extravasated blood. Over the next 2 to 5 weeks, the eschar becomes loose, leaving a necrotic ulcer that heals poorly and in some cases requires skin grafting.

In some cases, arthralgia, rash, and prolonged high fever may occur, with weakness and prostration. Hemolysis and hemoglobinuria may be seen, with shock and renal derangement.

For years the best and only early therapy was considered to be total excision of all involved tissue with primary closure, if less than 24 hours had elapsed since the bite occurred and there were strong signs or suspicion of envenomation. Other treatments have included local infiltration of phentolamine, thought to decrease ischemia from the norepinephrine in the venom. Intralesional and high-dose systemic corticosteroid have been other therapies. Opioids may increase toxicity of brown recluse venom.

Studies done at Vanderbilt University have developed another effective treatment approach (King and Rees, 1983). Patients strongly suspected of sustaining a brown recluse spider bite are tested for glucose-6-phosphate dehydrogenase (G6PD) deficiency and started on Dapsone, 50 mg twice daily for 10 days. Dapsone may begun while testing for G6PD is underway. This particularly useful in children with severe envenomation and hemolysis. If the individual is found to be G6PD deficient, then Dapsone is stopped because of its potential for hemolysis. Ice applied to the local bite site and the use of erythromycin, 250 mg four times a day for 10 days, also may be beneficial. Exercise of the affected extremity or the application of heat may increase the activity of enzymes in the venom and consequently is not recommended. Reportedly, there is an antivenin in development being produced from rabbits.

Scorpion Bites

There are many species of scorpions in the United States, and most are relatively harmless, producing only local reactions to bites. One species, *Centruroides exilicauda*, can produce a severe local reaction and systemic neurotoxicity. It is found in the southwest United States; it is approximately 1 to 3 inches long and yellowish in color, with a prominent tubercle at the base of the stinger. Patients who are stung experience intense pain at the site of the sting with little or no immediate swelling. Often light touch or percussion of the sting site is excruciatingly painful. Pain and paresthesia at the site may disappear quickly but other systemic symptoms may subside more slowly. Systemic symptoms include restlessness, uncontrolled jerking, excessive sweating, incontinence, increased salivation, wheezing, and elevated blood pressure. Recovery without treatment usually occurs in 10 to 12 hours. Children under 10 years of age may have a more severe reaction. Treatment involves using cool compresses but not excessive cooling to the sting site. Supportive care is provided for vital signs. Unnecessary drugs should be avoided and, if possible, nonopioid pain medications should be used. Diazepam may be useful for seizure control. An antivenin made from goat serum is available in Arizona only for *C. exilicauda*, although it is not approved by the Food and Drug Administration. Further information may be obtained from Poison Control in Arizona (602-626-6016).

MARINE ENVENOMATION

Stingrays

Stingrays are the most common fish likely to injure humans, with approximately 2000 stings annually. Stingrays are members of the shark family and consequently have a cartilage skeleton. Spines at the base of the stingray tail comprise the stinger, which is surrounded by an integument sheath that encloses the poison gland. The spine may inflict mechanical trauma as well as a poisoning. Often these injuries are inflicted on bathers or fisherman when they step on submerged stingrays or when they try to handle them either in nets or fishing lines.

Stingray injuries are intensely painful and develop early swelling with moderate bleeding. The pain begins to radiate centrally and can be so excruciating as to lead to disorientation. Systemic symptoms begin within 30 to 60 minutes and include nausea, vomiting, weakness, sweating, vertigo, cramps, and tachycardia. More severe reactions may include syncope, paralysis, hypotension, arrthymia, and death. Treatment of stingray injuries includes immediate irrigation with sterile saline. The injury should be soaked in water as hot as the victim can stand because heat rapidly deactivates the toxin. The physician then should remove any obvious foreign bodies in the wound or pieces of the stinger; radiographs may be useful because often these are radiopaque. It may be useful to débride the injury if devitalized or dirty tissue is present. Plain lidocaine can be applied to the wound to decrease pain and facilitate exploration, or a nerve block of the affected area may be provided. Antibiotic treatment should be given and may include one of several choices: trimethoprim-sulfamethoxazole, 160 mg/800 mg, respectively, twice daily; ciprofloxin, 500 mg twice daily; or tetracycline, 500 mg four times a day for 7 days (Otten, 1988).

Portuguese Man-of-War/Jellyfish

These beautiful but harmful (deadly at times) animals are those seen by bathers that have floating bodies filled with gas and trailing tentacles loaded with poisonous, stinging cells (nematocysts). The jellyfish and man-of-war tentacles may reach astounding lengths of 50 to 100 feet and contain hundreds of thousands of nematocysts. Tentacles detached from the parent body may retain their stinging ability for weeks, even when washed up on to the beach. Injuries occur when bathers, swimmers, or divers come in contact with the tentacles and stinging cells.

Contact with jellyfish and man-of-war tentacles causes a release of venom and a localized burning skin, paresthesia, and red–violet rash in the pattern of the tentacle. More severe envenomation results in blistering, edema, and severe extremity pain. Systemic systems may develop over 4 to 8 hours and include headache, lethargy, vertigo, syncope, ataxia, seizures, coma, dysphagia, muscle spasm, arrythmia, respiratory arrest, and death (Stein et al., 1989). Erythema nodosum has been noted to occur after resolution of initial envenomation in affected extremities.

Initial treatment of envenomation involves rinsing with salt water or saline because fresh water may cause more cells to sting. One should not rub the area of the tentacles because this will cause more nematocysts to discharge their venom. One should attempt to detoxify the remaining venom using alcohol, ammonia, or vinegar as a rinsing solutions. One then may apply shaving cream to the affected area and gently scrape off the cream and any adherent remaining tentacles with a knife. After this is done, the affected extremities again should be washed or irrigated with one of the above-selected solutions. A 1% hydrocortisone cream can be applied for local care and oral steroids given for systemic or severe local reactions. Other more severe disturbances of basic vital signs should be dealt with as in all serious trauma or poisoning. Recent developments in antivenins may allow specific therapy for various jellyfish envenomations if the offending species can be identified (Burnett and Carlton, 1987).

Ciguatera Poisoning

Ciguatera poisoning is caused by ingesting tropical or semi-tropical coral reef fish, which accumulate and concentrate a toxin that originates in the plankton/dinoflagellate *Gambierdiscus toxicus*. Frequently eaten offenders are barracuda, jack, snapper, and grouper; larger and older fish are more likely to poison the person who eats them.

Symptoms of ciguatera poisoning generally begin within 15 to 60 minutes of ingestion but may be delayed for up to 12 hours. Initial symptoms include abdominal pain, nausea, vomiting, diarrhea, chills, paresthesia, pruritis, dysphagia, fatigue, ataxia, vertigo, and headache. The reversal of hot and cold sensation is often stated to be pathognomonic of ciguatera poisoning (Hashmi et al., 1989). Other alterations of vital signs should be treated with supportive therapy. The gastrointestinal symptoms resolve most often in 1 to 2 days. Severe hypotension should be managed with crystalloid intravenous therapy. Cardiac and central nervous system depression may be reversed using intravenous mannitol. In fact, intravenous mannitol, 1 gm/kg, has been shown to reverse many of the symptoms of ciguatera poisoning quickly, although the mechanism for its effectiveness is unknown (Pearn et al., 1989). Myocardial failure is reported to respond to calcium gulconate, which presumably interferes with the toxin's alteration of calcium receptor sites. Serious reactions and death in response to ciguetera are more common in individuals who have had previous ciguatera poisoning. Death is reported in 0.1 to 10 per cent of cases.

Scombroid Poisoning

Scombroid poisoning is a pseudoallergic reaction to the histamine-like toxins released after ingestion of improperly preserved or stored dark-fleshed fish. This can occur after ingestion of fish in the families that include albacore, tuna, mackerel, bonito, kingfish, and wahoo. Dolphins, sardines, anchovies, amberjack, and ocean salmon also have been implicated. In Hawaii, the most implicated culprit is the dolphin, and, in the northeast United States, it is the bluefish. Histidine in the dark muscle flesh of these fish presumably is transformed into histamine via bacterial proliferation after improper handling and storage of the fish. Because much of the histamine is converted to an inactive form in the human gut, other toxins are suspected in this syndrome also.

The symptoms of scombroid poisoning begin within 15 to 90 minutes of eating a meal with affected fish. The symptoms of histamine release include face and neck flushing, generalized warm sensation, urticaria, pruritis, angioneurotic edema, abdominal pain and cramps, nausea, vomiting, diarrhea, headache, bronchospasm, hypotension, and tachycardia. Left untreated, the symptoms usually resolve in 6 to 12 hours.

Most patients require only supportive therapy and diphenhydramine for the histamine-related symptoms. Severe reactions that include hypotension and bronchospasm may require epinephrine treatment. Nausea and vomiting often respond to typical antihistamine therapy. However, intravenous ranitidine and cimetadine may be necessary to control nausea and headache. Finally, if the patient presents to the emergency room within 1 hour of consuming a meal that is highly suspicious of containing scombroid fish, induced emesis and activated charcoal with sorbitol may be useful.

REFERENCES

Auerbach PS: Bee, wasp and spider envenomation. *In* Callaham ML (ed): Current Therapy in Emergency Medicine. Toronto, Brian C. Decker, 1987, pp 919–921.

Blackmon JR, Dillon S: Venomous snake bite: Past, present and future treatment options. J Am Board Fam Physicians 5(4): 399, 1992.

Burnett JW, Carlton GJ: Jellyfish envenomation syndromes updated. Ann Emerg Med 16:1000, 1987.

Cable D, McGehee W, Wingert WA, et al: Prolonged defibrination after a bite from a "non-venomous" snake. JAMA 251: 925, 1984.

Callaham ML: Treatment of common dog bites: Infections risk factors. J Am Coll Emerg Physicians 7:83, 1978.

Connolly WB, Kilgore ES: Hand Injuries and Infections. Chicago, Year Book Medical Publishers, 1979, pp 17–18.

Corey L: Rabies and other rhabdo viruses. *In* Isselbacher KJ, Adams RD, Braunwald E, et al (eds): Harrison's Principles of Internal Medicine. New York, McGraw-Hill, 1980, pp 818–821.

Doan-Wiggins L: Animal bites and rabies. *In* Rosen P, Baker FJ, Braen GR, et al (eds): Emergency Medicine: Concepts and Clinical Practice. St. Louis, CV Mosby, 1988, pp 665–676.

Goldstein EJC, Citron DM, Finegold SM: Dog bite wound and infection: A prospective clinical study. Ann Emerg Med 9: 508, 1980.

Goldstein EJC, Citron DM, Wield B, et al: Bacteriology of human and animal bite wounds. J Clin Microbiol 8:667, 1978.

Hashmi MA, Sorokin JJ, Levine SM: Ciguatera fish poisoning. N J Med 86:469, 1989.

Immunization Practices Advisory Committee, Centers for Disease Control: Diphtheria, tetanus and pertussis. Ann Intern Med 95:723, 1981.

Jansen PW, Perkin RM, Vanstralen D: Mojave rattlesnake envenomation: Prolonged neurotoxicity and rhabdomyolysis. Ann Emerg Med 21:322, 1992.

Johnson CA: Management of snake bite. Am Fam Physician 44(1):174, 1991.

King LE, Rees RS: Dapsone treatment of a brown recluse bite. JAMA 250(5):648, 1983.

Malinowski RW, Strate RG, Perry JF Jr, Fischer RP: The management of human bite injuries of the hand. J Trauma 19: 655, 1979.

Martin LT: Human bites: Guidelines for practical management. Postgrad Med 81:221, 1987.

Matthews JJ: Tetanus. *In* Harwood-Nuss A, Linden C, Luten RC, et al (eds): The Clinical Practice of Emergency Medicine. Philadelphia, JB Lippincott, 1991, pp 1031–1032.

Norris RL, Dart RC: Apparent coral snake envenomation in a patient without visible fang marks. Am J Emerg Med 7:402, 1989.

Otten EJ: Venomous animal injuries. *In* Rosen P, Baker FJ, Braen GR, et al (eds): Emergency Medicine: Concepts and Clinical Practice. St. Louis, CV Mosby, 1988, pp 677–694.

Pearn JH, Lewis RJ, Ruff T, et al: Ciguetera and mannitol: Experience with a new treatment regimen. Med J Aust 151: 77, 1989.

Pennell TC, Babu SS, Meredith JW: The management of snake and spider bites in the southeastern United States. Ann Surg 53:198, 1987.

Russell FE: Snake venom poisoning in the United States. Annu Rev Med 31:241, 1980.

Smith TA, Figge HL: Treatment of snake bite poisoning. Am J Hosp Pharm 48:2190, 1991.

Snyder CC, Knowles RP: Snake bites: Guidelines for practical management. Postgrad Med 83:52, 1988.

Stein MR, Marraccini JV, Rothschild NE: Fatal Portuguese man-of-war (Physalia physalias) envenomation. Ann Emerg Med 18:312, 1989.

Stewart ME, Greenland S, Hoffman JR: First aid treatment of poisonous snake bite: Are currently recommended procedures justified? Ann Emerg Med 10:331, 1981.

Toewe CH: Bug bites and stings. Am Fam Physician 21:90, 1980.

Thermal and Environmental Injuries

WILLIAM FULCHER

BURNS AND SMOKE INHALATION

Burns are extremely common injuries, with between 2 and 3 million people per year burned in the United States seriously enough to need medical attention. About 12,000 people per year die from their burns or the complications, and scores of thousands are partially or totally disabled for various periods of time (Demling, 1985). Patients with severe burns require extensive and expensive medical care, usually in specialized regional burn centers.

Most burn injuries are minor, however, and manageable by the family physician with little need for consultation. Approximately 90 per cent of burns are due to thermal injuries such as flames or scalds. Chemical burns and electrical burns, while less common, deserve special attention regarding their management.

Pathophysiology

The epidermis, or outer layer of the skin, acts as a barrier to the entry of bacteria and the egress of moisture and electrolytes. These functions are lost in the area of a burn wound. The stratum germinativum, or germinal layer, of the epidermis provides cellular replacement for the elements that constantly are being shed during normal skin growth. Below the epidermis lies the dermis, the deeper layer of skin, within which lie nerve endings, blood vessels, collagen, elastin fibers, and other elements, of which the hair follicles and sweat glands are of particular importance in burn repair. Hair follicles and sweat glands have epidermal linings that permit regeneration of epithelium for resurfacing of partial-thickness (second-degree) burns. Full-thickness burns, by definition, destroy all of these structures and, hence, destroy the skin's natural, spontaneous regeneration (Fig. 36–17).

Burns are described as either superficial (first degree), partial thickness (second degree), or full thickness and deeper (third degree). First-degree burns are superficial and involve the epidermis. They are red, hypersensitive, warm, tender, painful to the touch and, often, swollen. There is no blistering. Healing is usually spontaneous within about 1 week, and there is often some degree of

desquamation of the damaged skin. A classic example of first-degree burn is most sunburn.

Partial-thickness or second-degree burns involve destruction of the epidermis and the dermis of varying levels. Partial-thickness burns can be either superficial or deep. Deep partial-thickness burns can be difficult to differentiate from full-thickness burns. Varying levels of the dermis, with its follicles, sweat glands, and other structures, can be damaged; however, by definition, a partial-thickness burn (even a deep partial-thickness burn) will permit some spontaneous repair and regeneration. These burns usually have some measure of blister formation, and healing may require 2 to 3 weeks or longer. They can be quite painful, as are first-degree burns; however, edema formation within a *deep* partial-thickness burn may decrease its pain sensitivity and make it appear to be a full-thickness burn. If secondary trauma or infection develops, further tissue destruction may occur and a longer healing time may result (Braen and Jelenko, 1988).

Full-thickness or third-degree burns involve the total epidermis and sometimes deeper structures. The dermal structures, including nerves, are destroyed, so this burn is usually hard, thick, and anesthetic. The classic appearance of a full-thickness burn is thrombosed blood vessels in a translucent surface with little or no pain. No spontaneous regeneration is possible because the full dermis has

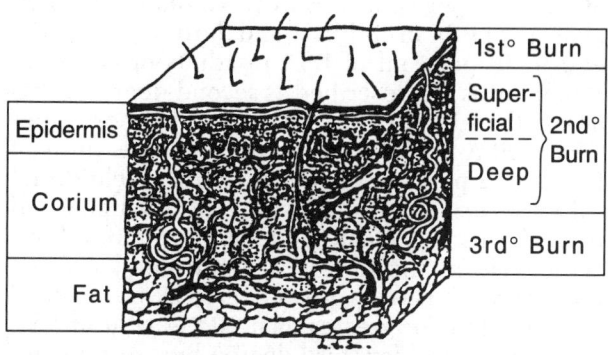

FIGURE 36–17. Layers of skin and the associated depth from various degree burns. (From Demling RH, Way LW: Burns & other thermal injuries. *In* Way LW [ed]: Current Surgical Diagnosis & Treatment, 10th edition. Norwalk, CT, Appleton & Lange, 1994, p 242, with permission.)

been destroyed. Skin grafts usually are needed for eventual repair, except in the most trivial cases.

Assessment and Management

The initial assessment of burns includes a determination of the type and surface area of a particular burn. The initial evaluation also should include the burn size, depth, site, presence of circumferential burns, inhalation injuries, electrical injuries, patient's age and comorbid illness, and, finally, any associated injuries or smoke inhalation. The "rule of nines" is a useful way to estimate the surface area of cutaneous burns in adults. In adults, the surface of the body is divided into areas that are a multiple of 9 per cent. This is altered in the child because of the relatively larger size of the head, and therefore the percentages of the extremities, trunk, and other areas are age dependent (Fig. 36–18). Another useful guideline that can be used in adults and children is to note the area of the patient's palm because this represents approximately 1 per cent of the body surface area. It can be used as a quick estimate of the extent of irregular burns during the initial assessment.

Initial management and decisions about further treatment and triage depend on the extent and degree of the burn and the age of the patient. The American Burn Association considers the following burns to be major burns, most of which should be referred to a major burn center for management: third-degree burns of greater than 10 per cent of body surface area (BSA) in adults or children; second-degree burns of greater than 25 per cent of BSA in adults or 20 per cent of BSA in children; burns involving hands, face, eyes, ears, feet, and/or perineum; and burn patients with inhalation injuries, major trauma, electrical injuries, or other serious comorbid disease.

Moderate burns, many of which are better managed in a major burn center but can be managed by physicians in hospitals with experience with burns, include the following: second-degree burns of 15 to 25 per cent of BSA in adults or 10 to 20 per cent of BSA in children, and third-degree burns of 2 to 10 per cent of BSA in adults or children. Minor burns are described as second-degree burns of less than 15 per cent of BSA in adults or 10 per cent of BSA in children and third-degree burns of less than 2 per cent of BSA in adults or children.

Physicians should consider hospitalizing all major burns and many moderate burns in a burn center. Hospitalization is recommended for second-degree burns of greater than 15 per cent of BSA in adults or greater than 10 per cent of BSA in children, and for third-degree burns of greater than 5 per cent of BSA in adults or children (Meyer and Salber, 1991). Much more liberal policies should be followed in small children because of the added difficulty of burn toilet and protection.

Additionally, the possibility of child abuse should be kept in mind while examining all burned children. Punctate burns such as those inflicted by cigarettes, burns of the diaper area or genitalia, or any situation in which parental attitude or history do not seem to fit the clinical circumstances should prompt the consideration of protective admission to the hospital.

Minor Burns

Minor burns can be treated effectively on an outpatient basis with analgesics and topical therapy. Most first-degree burns can be treated with cool compresses, antihistamines, and at times a rapidly tapering dose of oral steroid for edema and pain (prednisone, 40 mg daily for 3 to 5 days, then 20 mg daily for 3 to 5 days). Initial first aid should include cold compresses for 15 to 20 minutes to stop further destruction of tissue. If bullae are present, they should be left intact. If they are already ruptured, loose dead tissue or debris should be gently and thoroughly débrided. It is extremely important to handle areas of second-degree burns in a very clean, aseptic manner. This should involve the use of sterile drapes and gloves when cleansing, handling, and dressing the wound. This will significantly reduce the chance of infection.

After cooling and débridement, a topical antibiotic preparation is applied to second- or third-degree burns but not necessary to most first-degree burns. Silvadene (silver sulfadiazine) cream is the most common agent used and is quite efficacious in the prevention of early burn wound infection and sepsis. Early burn wound infection is most often due to streptococci and, although sebum is streptococcicidal, this property is lost when serum leaks into the burn wound (Robson et al. 1979). Other antibiotics that sometimes are used include Sulfamylon (mafenide acetate), Betadine ointment, and silver nitrate. One should be careful with the use of Silvadene on the face because it may result in a cosmetically unappealing pigmentation as the wound heals (Meyer and Salber, 1991).

Patients often apply many types of home remedies to burns. There is no place for butter, petroleum jelly, or other creams in the initial therapy of the burn. These agents must be cleaned off the burn wound in order to assess it and provide proper treatment once the patient arrives in the office or emergency department. Physicians should attempt to educate their patients and local first aid or rescue personnel to avoid this practice.

After topical antibiotic therapy is applied, a nonadherent dressing is applied (either Telfa or petroleum-soaked gauze) followed by a sterile gauze wrap. Dressings should be changed daily if no antibiotic cream is used; however, they should be changed twice daily if using an antibiotic ointment to maintain its antibacterial properties. It is wise for the physician to inspect the burn every 1 to 2

Rule of Nines

Area	Age — Years					% 2°	% 3°	% Total
	0-1	1-4	5-9	10-15	Adults			
Head	19	17	13	10	7			
Neck	2	2	2	2	2			
Ant. Trunk	13	17	13	13	13			
Post. Trunk	13	13	13	13	13			
R. Buttock	2½	2½	2½	2½	2½			
L. Buttock	2½	2½	2½	2½	2½			
Genitallia	1	1	1	1	1			
R. U. Arm	4	4	4	4	4			
L. U. Arm	4	4	4	4	4			
R. L. Arm	3	3	3	3	3			
L. L. Arm	3	3	3	3	3			
R. Hand	2½	2½	2½	2½	2½			
L. Hand	2½	2½	2½	2½	2½			
R. Thigh	5½	6½	8½	8½	9½			
L. Thigh	5½	6½	8½	8½	9½			
R. Leg	5	5	5½	6	7			
L. Leg	5	5	5½	6	7			
R. Foot	3½	3½	3½	3½	3½			
L. Foot	3½	3½	3½	3½	3½			
					Total			

Weight _____
Height _____

Shade in

2° = Blue

3° = Red

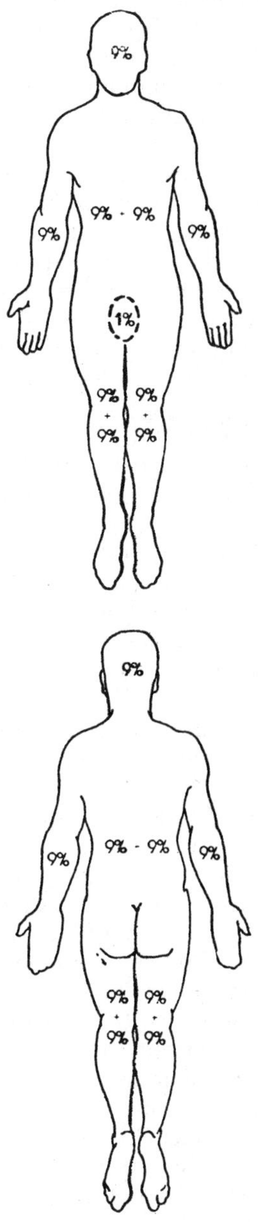

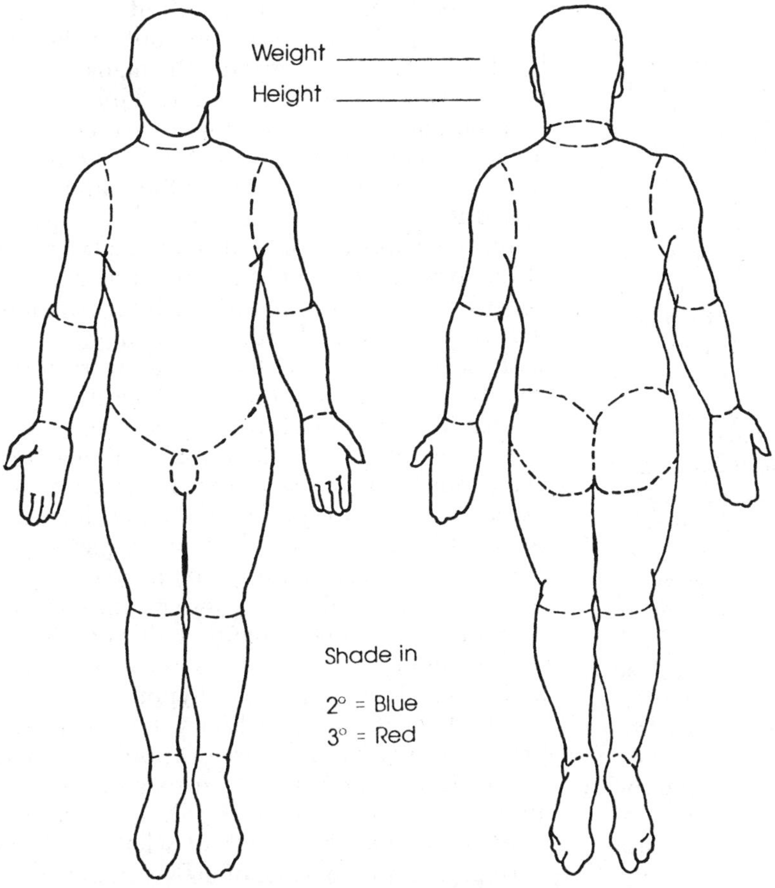

FIGURE 36–18. "Rules of nines" divides the body surface into areas of approximately 9 per cent or multiples of 9 per cent; the head and neck and an upper extremity each represent 9 per cent; a lower extremity and the front and back of the torso represents 18 per cent; the perineum 1 per cent. This method of estimation is sufficiently accurate for emergency situations. It is modified in children from birth to 1 year of age to allow 19 per cent for the head and neck and 13 per cent for each lower extremity. One per cent is subtracted from the head and neck and added to the lower extremities for each year from ages 1 to 10. (From Dimick AR: Emergency treatment of extensive burns. Curr Top II Emerg Med *1*(7). Philadelphia, Medical College of Pennsylvania, 1981, with permission.)

days at the beginning of therapy for evidence of proper healing and signs of infection, even with the most motivated patients. Further débridement or whirlpool treatments may be needed for good wound management and to abort early infection. If signs of infection develop, the physician is prudent to implement antibiotic treatment with a penicillinase-resistant penicillin or cephalosporin. If infection is extensive or the burn wound large, hospital management of the infection should be considered. Proper analgesia, elevation of the burn to reduce edema, and tetanus prophylaxis complete the outpatient regimen. When the physician feels comfortable with it, outpatient and home therapy are entirely justified with the motivated patient.

Major Burns

Serious and extensive burns require a systematic and thorough routine for evaluation and management. In all serious burns, the physician first should ascertain that airway, breathing, and circulation are adequate. If not already begun, one or two large-bore (16- to 18-gauge or larger), intravenous infusions should be started using normal saline or lactated Ringer's as the crystalloid solutions of choice.

In severely burned patients, there is a generalized increase in capillary permeability throughout the body, leading to fluid loss into the extravascular space and a state of hypovolemia, even shock. This begins within 6 to 8 hours of the burn and will last approximately 24 hours, and must be managed aggressively with fluid resuscitation. The managing physician should learn to expect "burn shock," although the exact mechanism(s) responsible for burn shock are controversial. Several factors can contribute to this process in the extensively burned patient: pain and psychological reactions leading to neurogenic shock, fluid transudation and hypovolemia, major electrolyte shifts, burn-related decrease in cardiac output, and acute erythrocyte hemolysis. If necessary, intravenous lines may be established through the eschar of the burn; however, they should be changed in 24 hours to decrease the rate of infection.

Routine insertion of central venous pressure (CVP) lines is controversial in the management of extensively burned patients because of the high rate of infection. The use of CVP lines should be reserved for patients who have significant underlying cardiovascular disease and who justify this level of monitoring. Most patients can be monitored quite well by clinical assessment during the initial 1 to 2 days of their fluid management.

Fluid administration, urinary output, and other vital clinical signs should be monitored closely. Initial fluid resuscitation is provided via one of several popular formulas (Dimick, 1981). The Parkland and Brooke formulas are perhaps the most commonly used ones. The Parkland formula estimates that a burn patient's acute volume requirements are approximately 4 mL of lactated Ringer's solution times the percentage of BSA burned times the patient's weight in kilograms. This volume is to be given over the first 24 hours after the burn, with half of this volume given in the first 8 hours and the remainder in the next 16 hours. The Brooke formula uses 2 mL/kg times BSA burned as the volume to be given; however, physicians using this formula should understand that many patients will require more volume than this based on their subsequent clinical assessments.

Patients should have routine blood studies, including complete blood count, electrolytes, glucose, blood urea nitrogen, creatinine, coagulation studies, and a type and crossmatch. Arterial blood gases should be obtained if there is any consideration of smoke inhalation or carbon monoxide intoxication. A 12-lead ECG should be obtained and cardiac monitoring provided. After initiating fluid resuscitation, the physician should evaluate the patient for associated injuries such as evidence of trauma, particularly if associated with the site of the burn injury. Up to 20 per cent of patients with major burns develop an ileus, so a nasogastric tube often is inserted routinely. A Foley catheter is inserted for monitoring urine output.

The physician then should contact the nearest local burn center and discuss the management and potential transfer of the patient. This will ensure that the patient gets the proper treatment, follow-up assessment, and resuscitation, as well as alerting the receiving physician of the patient's condition prior to arrival if transferred.

Seriously burned patients may incur a variety of other problems, including respiratory injuries, chest or extremity constriction from circumferential burns, myoglobinuria and hemoglobinuria with secondary renal failure, ileus resulting in vomiting and aspiration, and fractures or other trauma if the burn occurred in association with an explosion or fall. Table 36–25 summarizes the management of the severely burned patient. Because of these multiple potential problems and associated injuries, severely burned patients often are managed best in a regional burn center.

Physicians should not ignore or undertreat pain. Narcotics have been avoided during the initial management of burn patients because of their potential for worsening the hypotension of burn shock. After the first 24 hours, however, there is little reason to avoid the use of appropriate narcotic analgesics. It is clear that burns and their associated injuries then are painful; furthermore, we must remember that much of what we do to the burn patient in the name of management and treatment is also painful (i.e., débridement, whirlpool treatment, etc).

Finally, the physician also should remember to administer appropriate tetanus prophylaxis to every burn patient.

TABLE 36–25. MANAGING EXTENSIVE BURNS

1. Assure airway control. Intubate for suspected or definite airway edema. Provide supplemental oxygen.
2. Apply dry sterile dressings. Insulate with blankets to minimize heat loss. Avoid cold compresses with attendant risk of hypothermia and frostbite.
3. Aggressive volume resuscitation is necessary, owing to increased capillary permeability over the first 24–48 hours. Ringer's lactate may be given, in a dose of 4 mL/kg body weight/burn percentage. Follow central venous pressure and urinary output.
4. Paralytic ileus is common. Decompress the stomach via nasogastric tube.
5. Give tetanus toxoid and hyperimmune globulin for prophylaxis.
6. Don't miss other injuries, particularly if the history suggests blunt trauma, a fall, smoke inhalation, and so on.
7. Analgesia should be given intravenously in small doses. Morphine in small aliquots is the drug of choice.
8. Avoid topical creams prior to transfer to a burn facility.
9. Perform escharotomy for respiratory or neurovascular extremity compromise.

From Morse SD, Rial WY: Emergency medicine. *In* Rakel RE (ed): Textbook of Family Practice, 4th edition. Philadelphia, WB Saunders Company, 1990, p 973, with permission.

Chemical Burns

Chemical burns occur from strong acids or alkalis. The thrust of therapy is to remove the caustic agent quickly, usually by diluting with large quantities of water. All contaminated clothing must be removed without risking injury to other health care personnel. Chemical neutralization is contraindicated; the heat generated by this process increases tissue damage, and searching for such neutralizing antidotes wastes valuable time for initial treatment (Jelenko, 1971).

Acid caustics cause coagulative necrosis, and the damage they produce is generally more superficial than that produced by strong bases, which produces a liquefaction necrosis. Basic burns (strong alkalis such as lye) can be quite deep and penetrating if all the offending material is not quickly and adequately removed.

Eye exposure to caustic agents demands extensive irrigation with water, which ideally should begin *immediately* at the site of injury and continue en route to the hospital. Chemical burns of the eye should be irrigated with large amounts (2 liters or more) of sterile normal saline. Basic or alkali burns may require even more irrigation. The eye should be irrigated until the pH of the effluent is normal. After the irritant has been irrigated, the physician should examine the eye carefully for foreign bodies. An ophthalmology consultation is appropriate and particularly important for alkali burns.

Dry chemicals should be brushed off the body surface. They should not, if at all possible, be irrigated with water because this may increase their ability to cause a skin burn and penetrate through the skin.

Many chemical agents have specific therapy and antidotes recommended for them. Consequently, one should consult an up-to-date emergency medicine text or the local poison control center for the most current recommendations. For example, skin exposure to hydrofluoric acid reportedly responds to covering the wound or burn in dressings soaked with iced calcium gulconate solution. Deep or serious hydrofluoric acid burns may require subcutaneous injections of calcium salts to minimize the progressive necrosis that can result (Meyer and Salber, 1991).

Tar Burns

Tar burns are not unknown to the emergency physician. Tar is heated to 450° F and, although it cools rapidly, when it dries on the skin it often will cause a second-degree burn. The emergency physician should cool the tar burn if necessary with ice or cool compresses. There are many solvents that can dissolve the tar, but they can also cause more pain and tissue damage. Interestingly, Neosporin and other antibiotic ointments use a polyoxyethyline sorbitan base that can soften and dissolve the tar (Demling et al., 1980). This seems like a useful and humane way to remove tar and treat tar burns.

Smoke Inhalation

Smoke inhalation produces much of the morbidity and mortality caused by fires. Heated gases can lead to direct upper airway damage, with edema and airway obstruction. In addition, smoke is a combination of poisonous and noxious gases of variable composition depending on the material burned. Wood fires produce a large amount of carbon monoxide. The plastic polymers in many homes, when burned, can liberate a variety of gases, including hydrochloric acid, nitric acid, sulfuric acid, and hydrogen cyanide. These gases can produce severe airway and alveolar damage and systemic poisoning.

Smoke inhalation can cause thermal, chemical, systemic, or a combination of damages. Pulmonary damage caused by smoke inhalation seems to evolve in three distinct stages (Herndon et al., 1987). During the first 24 hours, bronchospasm, alveolar damage, and disrupted capillary membranes cause acute ventilatory insufficiency. This may progress to the second stage of noncardiogenic pulmonary edema. After about 72 hours, after loss of local infectious defense mechanisms, a pneumonitis caused by secondary infection can occur; many of these patients succumb.

The diagnosis of smoke inhalation requires a high index of suspicion. The physician should consider whether the patient was exposed to smoke or flames in a confined space, whether the patient lost consciousness, or whether the patient was a victim of an electrical fire, a steam explosion, or a natural gas explosion. Several findings on physical exam have been assumed to be presumptive of smoke inhalation. Notes should be made of cyanosis, respiratory distress, obtundation, singed nasal or facial hair, burns of the face or pharynx, rales or rhonchi, wheezes, and production of soot-stained sputum. Although these findings have been presumed to be fair predictors of smoke inhalation and carbon monoxide poisoning, they have not stood the test of time (Langford and Armstrong, 1989). Recent studies have indicated that they have a poor sensitivity and specificity for detecting patients with smoke inhalation and carbon monoxide injury. The physician is still left to the history and his or her best judgment in determining who should have arterial blood gases measured and who should be monitored closely for smoke inhalation injury. Those who are considered high risk should have a carboxyhemoglobin level drawn.

Victims of smoke inhalation require intensive management. Obviously, oxygen should be provided with adequate humidification. Intubation may be needed in victims with upper airway burns that interfere with good pulmonary toilet and secretion removal. Bronchospasm will respond to aminophylline and, as mentioned, serial blood gases, including carboxyhemoglobin levels, are required for management (Navar et al., 1985).

Chest radiographs are often normal in the early phases of smoke inhalation because the findings indicative of pulmonary edema and pneumonitis may lag behind the clinical picture by 24 to 48 hours. Victims of smoke inhalation should receive an ECG because myocardial infarction and other arrhythmias are not uncommon in adults, owing to hypoxia. Severely affected patients deserve admission to an intensive care unit or burn center. There is currently no role for *prophylactic* antibiotics or steroids in the smoke inhalation victim.

HEAT-RELATED ILLNESS

There are several minor and two major (serious and potentially life-threatening) heat-related illnesses. The minor forms are quite common and include heat syncope, heat tetani, heat edema, and heat cramps. The two serious forms of heat illness are heat exhaustion and heat stroke. Heat exhaustion is the more common of the major heat illnesses, while heat stroke, although less common (except in its epidemic form), is potentially more life threatening (Sine, 1979).

Acclimatization to heat usually results after 1 to 2 weeks of exposure to hot temperature. Even a fully acclimatized person or athlete can suffer a heat disorder, however, when the mechanism of heat removal or dissipation is exceeded by the rate of heat production. Patients who have chronic disabling diseases that reduce their circulatory response to heat exposure, who are elderly, or who are obese are more likely to succumb to serious heat illness. Furthermore, heat *exposure* can be made potentially more serious by its combination with fatigue, fever-producing infections, alcohol use, certain medications (especially those that interfere with sweating), and failure to maintain sufficient hydration or salt intake (Bareca, 1991).

Heat Edema

Heat edema is a benign swelling of the feet and ankles that is associated with prolonged sitting or standing during hot weather. It is not a result or complication of congestive heart failure or lymphatic disease. It is most likely a result of the vasodilation of skin and muscle vasculature combined with venous stasis in the lower extremities. It may have a component of salt and water accumulation from the increase in aldosterone that results from the body's adaptation to heat exposure. The difficulty in diagnosing and managing heat edema is in differentiating it from edema related to other illness. Treatment generally requires just rest in a cool environment, elevation of the lower extremities, and, sometimes, the use of support hose. Diuretics should not be used because "heat-stressed" patients often have mild intravascular volume depletion.

Heat Syncope

Heat syncope is a loss of consciousness (faint) that can occur after sudden exertion in the heat. It usually occurs in the well-trained and well-conditioned individual who must stand without moving in one spot in extremely hot weather. Excellent examples of this are military personnel forced to stand guard in a stationary position in the heat for long periods of time. Volume loss from sweating, and blood pooling in the lower extremities from the standing, contribute to an inadequate cerebral perfusion and syncope. Usually the core temperature is normal, although it may be mildly elevated. Patients can be managed by rest in a recumbent position, in a cool environment, and administration of plenty of water. Older patients should be evaluated after syncopal episodes for evidence of hypoglycemia, arrhythmia, or other common causes of syncope in this group.

Heat Cramps

Heat cramps are one of the most common, benign, and easily treated forms of heat illness. After a period of exertion, patients can experience painful cramps of the muscles used during that exercise or work. Cramps may be due either to a transmembrane imbalance of sodium or potassium or to the unopposed effect of calcium in the presence of salt depletion. Heat cramps are differentiated from heat *tetani* by the abscence of carpopedal spasm and by the typical delay of cramping of 6 to 12 hours after the patient's exposure to heat and exercise. Heat cramps respond to rest in a cool environment and to replacement of sufficient fluid and salt. The use of salt tablets is generally not recommended because liberal salting of the patient's diet usually will provide sufficient salt intake.

Heat Tetani

Heat tetani can follow brief, intense exposure to heat. The normal respiratory response to extreme heat is tachypnea, which can result in a symptomatic respiratory alkalosis brought on by hyperventilation. There is often carpopedal spasm, which differentiates this from heat cramps. Heat tetani also occurs during or immediately after exposure to intense heat and is not delayed, as is typical for heat cramps. Heat tetani can occur in sedentary or exercising persons, and it is treated by removing the patient from the source of extreme heat.

Heat Exhaustion

Heat exhaustion is a more profound clinical syndrome occurring in either a salt-depletion form or a water-depletion form (Table 36–26). Patients of both types may complain of weakness, fatigue, nausea, anorexia, lightheadedness, and muscle cramps. Patients with the water-depletion form of heat exhaustion are more likely to present with a slightly elevated temperature and more profound alterations of sensorium. They are also more likely to have tachycardia and slight hypotension. This subset of heat exhaustion patients, if not treated

TABLE 36–26. HEAT EXHAUSTION

	Salt-Depletion Type	Water-Depletion Type
Sweat losses	+ + + +	+ + + +
Water repletion	+	−
Still sweating	+	+
Hypotension	+	+ + +
Cramps	+	−
Neurologic symptoms	+	+ + +
Temperature	Normal	100–103° F
Leads to heat stroke	+/−	+ +
Nausea/vomiting	+	+
Serum sodium	+/−	+/−
Respiratory alkalosis	+	+

From Morse SD, Rial WY: Emergency medicine. *In* Rakel RE (ed): Textbook of Family Practice, 4th edition. Philadelphia, WB Saunders Company, 1990, p 974, with permission.

promptly, may proceed quickly to frank heat stroke. Patients with salt-depletion forms of heat exhaustion may present with symptoms of hyponatremia because they generally have ingested free water in excess of salt preceding their illness (weakness, nausea, dizziness, cramps).

Patients with either form of heat exhaustion usually respond rapidly to removal from the hot environment and to appropriate salt and water replacement as dictated by their clinical evaluation. Usually there are no sequelae to appropriately treated heat exhaustion. Most patients may be given salted fruit drinks or Gatorade orally. If they require intravenous therapy, normal saline or Ringer's lactate with 5 per cent dextrose usually quickly resolves their symptoms.

Heat Stroke

Heat stroke is an uncommon but true medical emergency, with a mortality rate reported in the literature varying from 10 to 80 per cent (Auerbach, 1992). There are two forms of heat stroke, but both are characterized by a core body temperature of 105° F or greater, profound neuropsychiatric symptoms, and, in most cases, anhidrosis. *Exertional heat stroke* usually occurs in the young, healthy athlete who is exercising inappropriately in an extremely hot environment. In this case, the heat production by the exercise exceeds the individual's ability to remove or shed the body heat. The *sedentary* or *"classic"* form of *heat stroke* usually involves elderly, chronic ill, sedentary patients whose age and/or medical conditions prevent them from shedding excess body heat when exposed to excessively hot environmental conditions. Finally, infants who are wrapped in too many blankets while suffering fever may experience a form of excessively elevated body temperature or heat stroke.

The development of heat stroke is more likely on hot, still, and humid days, when heat dissipation to the environment is limited. Losses via sweating and vaporization, the body's major cooling processes, are much less efficient in these conditions. An increased metabolic rate or increase in mechanical work will increase internal body heat generation and further predispose to marked and dangerous rises in core body temperature.

Many organ systems are affected by acute heat stroke, but the cardiovascular system is often the one most profoundly affected. Normal responses to heat exposure include vasodilation of the skin and an increase in cardiac output. Patients who are unable to increase their heart rate or cardiac output because of age or illness may suffer serious cardiovascular insufficiency. Acute circulatory failure causes death in over 80 per cent of heat stroke fatalities. Elderly patients are often hypovolemic, with hypotension and a low CVP (Tucker et al., 1985).

The young patient, in contrast, is usually in a hyperdynamic state with a high output failure and a low to normal CVP. On rare occasions in the young, healthy person, a *hypo*dynamic response occurs, with hypotension, low cardiac output, and *elevated* CVP. This latter situation may result from direct thermal toxicity to the myocardium and increased pulmonary vascular resistance with right ventricular overload. Intravenous isoproterenol has been reported to improve the hemodynamic picture dramatically in this subset of patients (O'Donnel and Clowes, 1972). Myocardial ischemia and infarction must be considered in many patients, particularly when they are elderly.

Diagnosis

Patients with heat stroke may present with headache, nausea, dizziness, diarrhea, visual changes, confusion, and, at times, seizures and coma. The skin is generally hot, flushed, and dry. Patients hyperventilate, which results in a respiratory alkalosis. Hypotension and poor cardiac output may result in a metabolic acidosis, coagulopathy, hematuria, hematemesis, easy bruising, petechiae, and oozing at venipuncture sites. The pulmonary complications of heat stroke include respiratory alkalosis, a high incidence of pneumonia resulting from aspiration, and spurious effects on arterial blood gas determinations (Table 36–27).

Mental status changes, including seizures, ataxia, and residual mental retardation in children, are not uncommon CNS effects of heat stroke. Acute renal failure occurs in approximately 25 to 30 per cent of exertional heat stroke cases, probably because of the concomitant myoglobinuria and rhabdomyolysis. Patients with "classic" heat stroke suffer closer to 5 to 10 per cent incidence of renal failure because they have a lower incidence of myoglobinuria (Clowes and O'Donnel, 1974). Rhabdmyolysis with myoglobinuria is not uncommon as a result of pressure necrosis of muscles, hypokalemia, relative hypoxia, and direct thermal toxicity to muscle. Intravascular hemolysis and hemoglobinuria also may lead to acute tubular necrosis. Hypoxia, thrombosis, parenchymal hemorrhage, renal vasoconstriction, direct thermal injury, and hyperuricemia all have been postulated as contributors to acute renal failure in heat stroke patients. Consequently, urinary output and renal

TABLE 36–27. VARIANCE OF BLOOD GASES WITH BODY TEMPERATURE

	↑ 1° C	↓ 1° C
pH	↓ 0.015	↑ 0.015
Pco_2 (mm Hg)	↑ 4.4%	↓ 4.4%
Po_2 (mm Hg)	↑ 7.2%	↓ 7.2%

* Departures from values at 37° C.
From Morse SD, Rial WY: Emergency medicine. *In* Rakel RE (ed): Textbook of Family Practice, 4th edition. Philadelphia, WB Saunders Company, 1990, p 975, with permission.

TABLE 36–28. MANAGEMENT OF HEAT STROKE

ABC still applies
Rapid cooling
Oxygen
CVP monitoring
Volume challenge for hypotension
Isuprel (1 μg./min.) for hypodynamic state
Foley catheterization
Steroids, antibiotics, anticonvulsants only for specific indications
Search for organ dysfunction, bleeding diathesis, precipitating illness
Prophylaxis for G.I. bleeding

From Morse SD, Rial WY: Emergency medicine. *In* Rakel RE (ed): Textbook of Family Practice, 4th edition. Philadelphia, WB Saunders Company, 1990, p 975, with permission.

function must be followed closely. If evidence of myoglobinuria ensues, one should use intravenous mannitol, 0.25 gm/kg, and bicarbonate to reduce the risk of myoglobin deposition in the renal tubules and renal failure.

Management

The thrust of managing heat stroke involves the standard techniques of CPR and rapid cooling. Immediate cooling, in fact, is perhaps the most important action to implement because the sooner the temperature is reduced, the lower the consequent morbidity and mortality (Vicario et al., 1986). Table 36–28 summarizes many of the management concepts for heat stroke.

Oxygen should be administered at 6 to 10 liters/min. Clothing should be removed and cold or ice packs applied to the axilla or groin. A cooling blanket may be used; however, spraying the body with cool (60° F) or tepid water and using fans to blow over the body to evaporate the water results in a more rapid body cooling. Body temperature should be measured by rectal probe, and cooling procedures halted when a core temperature of 100° to 101° F is reached. This will help avoid "overshoot hypothermia." If the core temperature begins to rise again, cooling procedures should be restarted. Patients who are initially unresponsive and have core temperature greater than 107° F should be

TABLE 36–29. RAPID COOLING FOR HEAT STROKE

Undress patient
Ice packs to pivotal points: neck, axillae, groin
Cool water (60° F) spray with fan evaporation
Ice gastric lavage
Hypothermic (relative) IV fluids, > room temperature
Control shivering
Lower core temperature to 100–101° (100.4°) as quickly as possible; question cooling procedure if temperature begins to rise
Avoid aspirin, Tylenol

Adapted from Morse SD, Rial WY: Emergency medicine. *In* Rakel RE (ed): Textbook of Family Practice, 4th edition. Philadelphia, WB Saunders Company, 1990, p 975, with permission.

considered for cold peritoneal lavage therapy. (Table 36–29). Shivering should be controlled because it may contribute to heat production. This may be accomplished with diazepam, 5 to 10 mg intravenously, or chlorpromazine, 12.5 to 25 mg intravenously.

It is important to maintain an adequate urine output during therapy. The presence of myoglobin in the urine may herald the onset of renal failure. As mentioned earlier, one should use intravenous mannitol, 0.25 gm/kg, and sodium bicarbonate to reduce the deposition of myoglobin in the renal tubules. Severe hypotension and poor cardiac output may be managed with dobutamine. Dobutamine is preferred over dopamine because of its lack of α-adrenergic effects on the kidneys with rapid and high-dose infusion (Bareca, 1991).

Aspirin and acetaminophen are not effective in lowering the temperature in hyperthermia caused by heat stroke. Aspirin may be contraindicated with heat stroke with concomitant bleeding diatheses, and acetaminophen may be contraindicated in the presence of hepatic damage.

Poor prognostic factors for recovery from heat stroke include temperature greater than 106° F, aspartate transaminase (glutamic-oxaloacetic transaminase) greater than 1000 IU, coma, rhabdomyolysis, renal failure, and hypotension. Education of the public to avoid unnecessary heat exposure, the use of appropriate clothing and fluid intake, and awareness of the effects of alcohol and various drugs on heat disposition will decrease the risk of systemic heat illness markedly. It should be the task of every family physician to educate his or her patients about the effects of heat illness during hot-weather months.

COLD-INDUCED ILLNESS

Cold-induced injury may be local in nature (frostbite, chilblains) or systemic (hypothermia).

Chilblains

Chilblains, or pernio, is a skin reaction/condition that results from repeated exposure to cold weather without actual tissue freezing or frostbite. Chilblains appear as reddish purple macular lesions on the face or exposed extremities and may progress to include edema and blistering. Protective covering of the skin in extremely cold, humid weather is an important primary prevention. Mild chilblains are managed by rewarming the affected area indoors at room temperature, careful handling (i.e., no massage) of affected tissue, and early treatment of secondary infection. Repeated cold exposure can lead to thick, ulcerated, scarring lesions that require extensive dermatologic treatment (Cooper and Danzl, 1991).

Frostbite

Frostbite injury may be thought of as superficial or deep. Superficially frostbitten tissue appears white and waxy acutely and, with thawing, becomes mildly hyperemic and vesiculated. Eventually the damaged area begins to reveal pink, somewhat cold-sensitive skin. Deep frostbite, which is a more severe injury, also looks white, waxy, and hard prior to thawing. With thawing, either the part remains cold and hard (an ominous sign of possible full-thickness tissue death) or massive swelling, large hemorrhagic bullae, and a black dry eschar eventually will form. Healing or mummification follows deep frostbite over the subsequent weeks. In general, the depth of tissue injury and tissue viability cannot be determined before 1 to 2 weeks after a frostbite injury (Kyosola, 1974). Consequently, a conservative approach to therapy is mandated, with early surgery being reserved only for uncontrolled secondary infection of the injured tissue.

Frostbite generally affects areas of endarterial flow, especially the hands, face, and feet. Cold exposure produces a reflex arteriolar spasm with cessation of capillary blood flow. Ice crystallization in the intracellular and extravascular spaces causes osmotic changes in interstitial fluid. Movement of water out of cells to maintain osmotic equilibrium is thought to produce intracellular dehydration and enzymatic dysfunction, leading to cell death. Only in the most severe cases does actual freezing of deep tissue occur. Nerves, blood vessels, and muscles are the most easily damaged tissues.

Table 36–30 summarizes the treatment for frostbite. The affected parts should never be rubbed or massaged to warm them up because this only adds mechanical damage to the thermal damage. A frostbitten or frozen part should never be rewarmed in the cold environment when there is a chance that it may be refrozen. Refreezing greatly increases the frostbite damage. Persons who have sustained frostbite outdoors should be brought to a safe area where frostbite can be managed effectively and refreezing prevented. Hikers have on occasion

TABLE 36–30.   TREATMENT OF FROSTBITE

Never rewarm outdoors or away from medical aid
No tobacco or alcohol
Rapid rewarming method of choice
Never rub
Keep warm, dry, open, or loosely dressed
Gentle cleansing, whirlpools, physical therapy, no early surgery
Leave bullae intact
Tetanus prophylaxis
Prevention with education and awareness of symptoms
Most cases heal without surgery, the worst in 6–12 months

From Morse SD, Rial WY: Emergency medicine. *In* Rakel RE (ed): Textbook of Family Practice, 4th edition. Philadelphia, WB Saunders Company, 1990, p 976, with permission.

walked to safety on frozen feet but been incapacitated by pain when rewarmed in the cold and then suffered subsequent refreezing (Auerbach, 1992).

Rapid rewarming is the method of choice in treating a frostbitten part, but a *point* source of heat (heater, oven, stove) should never be used because the rate of heat delivery to the frostbitten part is uneven and unpredictable. Furthermore, anesthesia of a frostbitten part often occurs, and this may predispose an extremity to superficial thermal burns when a point source of heat is used. Ideally, the frostbitten part should be immersed in water kept at 108° to 112° F for 20 to 30 minutes. This is generally water that is warm to the touch but not particularly hot. As thawing occurs, a significant degree of pain may be experienced in the frostbitten area; therefore, potent analgesia may be needed.

After rewarming, frostbitten digits or extremities should be left open to air or loosely dressed. Physical therapy, whirlpools, and gentle cleansing of skin and bullae may be required. Bullae should not be débrided if they are intact; however, if ruptured, the excess skin and devitalized tissue should be removed gently to decrease infection. Appropriate tetanus prophylaxis is mandatory. Most cases of frostbite either heal or mummify without surgery, although the worse cases can require up to 6 to 12 months to heal.

The sequelae of frostbite include parethesias, vasospasm on exposure to cold, periarticular osteoporosis, and, in children, loss of epiphyseal growth centers. Thin skin, hyperhidrosis, loss of skin appendages, and chronic pain also may be seen (Washburn, 1962).

Patient education regarding exposure protection and the early symptoms of frostbite (i.e., loss of discomfort in the cold, hardness and coldness of a distal part) is of paramount importance. Patients who have been frostbitten in the past are more prone to recurrent cold injury in the same part.

Hypothermia

Accidental hypothermia is defined as unintentional cooling of the body core temperature to less than 35° C or 95° F. This definition is used because metabolic heat production in response to cold stress peaks at a core temperature of 95° F and falls off at lower temperatures, leading to a progressively more severe clinical syndrome (Reuler, 1978).

A variety of clinical settings predispose individuals to hypothermia (Table 36–31). *Primary accidental hypothermia* involves accidental direct exposure to a cold environment without appropriate protection from the cold (O'Keefe, 1977). Many persons who are active in the outdoors must be informed that severe hypothermia can occur in temperatures well above freezing if they are not

TABLE 36–31. CLINICAL SETTINGS FOR HYPOTHERMIA

Inadequate Heat Production
Extremes of age
Inactivity, immobility (acute)
Inadequate food intake and malnutrition (chronic)
Endocrine disease or insufficiency (thyroid, adrenal pituitary)

Increased Heat Loss to Environment
Exposure (unprotected, unacclimated, wet)
Skin integrity disrupted by disease
Neonatal resuscitation

Impaired Heat Regulation
Drug and medication side effets
Trauma
Chronic diseases (diabetes)

Other Causes
Sepsis
Dehydration

appropriately dressed. The combination of wet clothing, heat loss resulting from wind and evaporation, and inadequate intake of fluid and carbohydrates has led to severe cases of hypothermia in temperatures as warm as the 50s (Farenheit).

Secondary hypothermia generally is seen in patients who are debilitated by chronic disease. Many diseases and changes caused by aging predispose persons to inadequate heat production in appropriate situations. Elderly patients, neonates, patients who are obtunded or physically immobile, and those who are intoxicated or on agents that impair heat generation are at higher risk for hypothermia. Persons who become exhausted and glycogen depleted in the cold are also at increased risk for developing hypothermia when cold stressed. Diseases such as cancer, severe trauma, vascular disease, cerebrovascular accidents, mental retardation, myxedema, and hypopituitarism all predispose patients to secondary hypothermia.

The major determinants of mortality in hypothermia are the presence and severity of associated disease states and the degree of presenting hypothermia. Reported mortality rates in large series of patients range from 10 to 80 per cent (Danzl, 1988). Only in myxedema coma is the actual depression of core temperature directly related to mortality, however.

Assessment and Clinical Features

Hypothermia has been categorized as mild, moderate, and severe based on initial core body temperature. Mildly hypothermic patients, with a temperature of 90° to 95° F (32.2° to 35° C) will often have associated CNS depression, increased shivering, and increased pulse and metabolic rate. These patients also often will have dysarthria, ataxia, and apathy. In most patients with mild primary hypothermia, active external rewarming will be sufficient to resolve their symptoms (Hamlet, 1987).

Moderate hypothermia is defined as a body core

temperature between 80° and 90° F (27° and 32.2° C). With moderate hypothermia, there is a progressive decrease in the level of consciousness and a decrease in vital signs. Shivering declines such that, as the body core temperature drops below 90° F, the body loses its ability to rewarm spontaneously. At this point the body is termed *poikilothermic*, meaning that it will assume the same temperature as the surrounding environment and will not (cannot) spontaneously warm to a higher temperature. The heart becomes progressively more irritable and, at temperatures around 82° F, the ventricular myocardium becomes so irritable that minimal stimulation of the patient can induce ventricular fibrillation. Rescuers and physicians therefore should take up to a full minute to assess for a spontaneous pulse before instituting CPR on "dead" patients with hypothermia (Perdue and Hunt, 1986). Arrhythmias are common, and ECG changes include lengthening of the Q-T interval and typical Osborne waves. Often there is a "cold diuresis" from an increased central volume and increased glomerular filtration rate resulting from progressively more severe peripheral vasoconstriction.

Finally, severe hypothermia is defined as a body core temperature less than 80° F (27° C). Patients are often comatose and areflexic. At a body core temperature of 77° F (25° C), hypotension develops. Myocardial irritability and sensitivity peaks at 77° to 70° F, and below 70° F asystole may supervene.

There is a 7 per cent decrease in cerebral blood flow for each 1° C decrease in core temperature. Mentation progressively deteriorates below 84° F (30° C), and the pupils may become dilated and fixed. At 66° F (20° C), the electroencephalogram becomes flat.

The cardiovascular and neurologic consequences of hypothermia as described above are often profound. Progressive bradycardia develops and all ECG intervals lengthen. Diffuse T wave inversion may occur and, with distention of the atria, atrial flutter and fibrillation may result. Although gross shivering may begin to disappear below 90° F, fine muscular tremor may be apparent on the ECG. The J-shaped Osborne waves on the ECG (Fig. 36–19) are pathognomonic for hypothermia.

Profound, severe hypothermia may clearly simulate death. The severely hypothermic patient is relatively protected from hypoxia, hypotension, and circulatory arrest because of the decreased metabolic rate. Prolonged resuscitative efforts are justified because complete neurologic and medical recovery can occur, particularly in the young and previously healthy patient. Consequently, the following clinical pearl should be observed: *"No one is dead until he or she is warm and dead."*

A variety of other organ dysfunctions occur in the hypothermic patient. Respiration may be compromised by aspiration and a "cold-induced" bronchorrhea. The latter results in a marked increase in tracheal and bronchial secretions. Hemoconcentration occurs as a result of fluid shifts into interstitial space. Anemia may be masked by this phenomenon because the hematocrit increases 2 per cent with each 1° C decrease in temperature. This hemoconcentration also may result in widespread thrombosis, and the WBC count may be altered by leukocyte sequestration. Ileus is common below 93° F (34° C). Hepatic function progressively declines, producing more pronounced and/or more prolonged effects from administered drugs. Protein binding is increased markedly as a result of the cold, so many drugs become ineffective in the hypothermic patient. This is compounded by a decreased receptor sensitivity to medications, making all but a few medications ineffective in the hypothermic patient. Finally, in some patients, pancreatitis and pancreatic necrosis have been reported (Reuler, 1978).

Renal blood flow and glomerular filtration fall with decreasing core temperature. In patients who become slowly hypothermic over several days, however, volume depletion may occur because a temperature-dependent decrease in enzyme function of the distal renal tubules leads to salt and water loss. This will contribute to the previously mentioned cold diuresis.

Glucose utilization is impaired in hypothermic patients, and hyperglycemia is not uncommon. The potent nature of insulin in the presence of decreased hepatic function, altered protein binding,

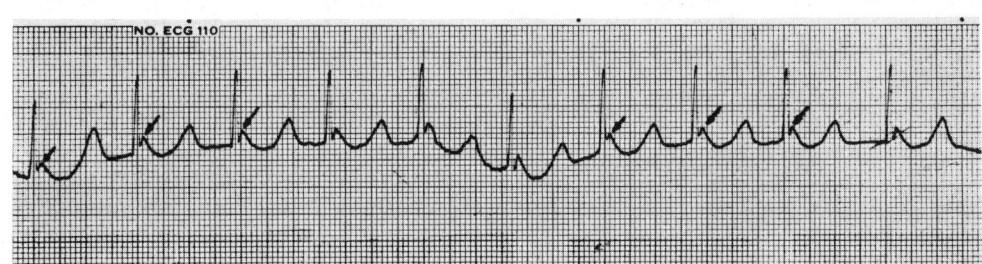

FIGURE 36–19.   Osborne waves (arrows) in an 80-year-old male with core temperature of 86° F (30° C). These waves disappeared with rewarming. (From Morse CD, Rial WY: Emergency medicine. *In* Rakel RE [ed]: Textbook of Family Practice, 4th edition. Philadelphia, WB Saunders Company, 1990, p 977, with permission.)

and altered receptor sensitivity should be kept in mind. Only extreme hyperglycemia should be treated actively with insulin. Occasionally, a diabetic ketoacidosis picture may be mimicked by hypothermia and should be managed with rewarming, fluid administration, and cautious insulin therapy.

Arterial blood gases are usually reported corrected to 37° C. The physician should use values corrected for actual body temperature because they will represent the actual pH, oxygen, and carbon dioxide content of the patient's blood. Table 36–27 also can be used to correct the arterial blood gases for hypothermia.

During the initial evaluation of the patient with hypothermia, the physician should be alert for physical findings that are not proportionate to the patient's body temperature. For example, abnormal vital signs for the degree of hypothermia may reflect hypoglycemia, hypovolemia, or other medication or drug use. Central nervous changes disportionate to the degree of body temperature may reflect CNS lesions, infections, or medication effects. An elevated respiratory rate that is not compatible with measured body temperature may suggest concomitant metabolic acidosis.

Treatment

Table 36–32 summarizes the therapeutic approach to systemic hypothermia. The treatment of hypothermia is oriented to the degree of hypothermia and comorbidity that the patient is experiencing. Rewarming can be passive or active. Passive rewarming involves the removal of the patient from the cold stress and the application of blankets or other insulation to allow the patient to rewarm himself or herself. This is quite efficacious in the

---

TABLE 36–32. THERAPY IN HYPOTHERMIA

1. Don't miss head trauma, frostbite, injection sites (e.g., insulin, opiates, and so on)
2. Hospitalize and monitor if temperature is less than 91° F (33° C)
3. Use glass thermometer that reads into *low* range, or electronic probe
4. Usual ABCs of CPR; handle cautiously to avoid cardiac arrest
5. Minimize drug use; avoid insulin when possible
6. Atrial arrhythmias revert with rewarming
7. PVCs—check Po_2, check pH, use lidocaine if needed, check electrolytes
8. Warm intravenous fluids with blood coils to 99°–112° F (37–43° C)
9. Heated oxygen, good pulmonary toilet
10. Thyroxine (400 µg) and steroids (300 mg hydrocortisone) for myxedema coma
11. Warm oral fluids if awake
12. Rewarming—active or passive
13. Prolong CPR—no one is dead until warm and dead

From Morse SD, Rial WY: Emergency medicine. *In* Rakel RE (ed): Textbook of Family Practice, 4th edition. Philadelphia, WB Saunders Company, 1990, p 977, with permission.

---

mildly hypothermic patient. One should remember, however, that, as body core temperature decreases below 90° F, the ability to spontaneously rewarm is lost. Active rewarming can be external or core, and involves the use of applied heat to provide an increase in body temperature. Active rewarming is warranted in all patients with a temperature below 90° F, patients at the extremes of the age spectrum, or those who have neurologic and endocrine disease or insufficiency preventing adequate response to hypothermia. External rewarming is most useful when it is applied to the trunk. A major concern in using active external rewarming is the phenomenon of the core temperature "afterdrop." This phenomenon occurs when the body core temperature continues to decline despite the application of external rewarming procedures. This is believed to be due either to an equilibration between the temperatures of various body tissues or a return of colder peripheral blood to the body core.

Core rewarming involves several methods of heating the body. Heated intravenous fluids and heated, humidified air are two of the most widespread and easily applied methods. Intravenous fluids can be heated safely to 40° to 42° C by microwave ovens (Leaman and Martyak, 1985). Humidified air can be applied, which will limit further heat loss via the respiratory system. Humidified oxygen at 20 liters/min can provide 30 to 40 kcal/hr, whereas warm intravenous fluids may provide 15 to 20 kcal/hr. Blood, if needed, also may be rewarmed by reconstituting with warmed normal saline. Heated blankets, as mentioned previously, may provide up to 600 kcal/hr and an increase in body temperature of 1° to 2° C/hr; however, they also may contribute to core afterdrop (Cooper and Danzl, 1991). In severely hypothermic patients, core rewarming with methods such as gastrointestinal lavage, dialysis, extracorporeal blood rewarming, and thoracic cavity lavage may be used. The latter may be particularly useful for warming the heart (Hall and Syverud, 1990). This method uses two thoracotomy tubes, one for inflow and one for drainage, and can warm the thoracic cavity and heart quickly, decreasing cardiac irritability. Heated peritoneal dialysis can provide up to 60 to 70 kcal/hr and is useful in the obtunded and severely hypothermic patient. Extracorporeal blood rewarming generally is limited to large medical centers but may be indicated for severely hypothermic patients.

As mentioned earlier, some controversy exists regarding active rewarming. Methods such as immersion in hot or warm water may limit access to the patient for CPR and, theoretically, all external rewarming methods may cause vasodilation and shock in volume-depleted patients. One also should be cautious not to apply heat to such a degree as to cause burns to the patient. Finally, as mentioned, the vasodilation of external rewarming may shunt cold peripheral blood back to the body's core suddenly, causing a core temperature afterdrop and increased cardiac irritability. The physician should use active external rewarming methods with a good understanding of their theoretical risk and be aware of the methods used for active core rewarming in severely hypothermic cases.

ELECTRICAL INJURY

Each year in the United States over 1000 people are killed in electrical accidents. Many electrical injuries occur in children, particularly under 6 years of age. Oral contact with electrical cords causes serious electrical injuries and burn damage. Adolescent risk-taking behavior around high-voltage fixtures is also a frequent source of injuries. Finally, carelessness or alcohol use in the workplace creates a risk for electrical injuries for many adults.

Heat generation is responsible for most of the burns seen with electrical injuries. The heat generation and damage caused by electrical injuries varies with respect to the voltage, amperage, tissue resistance, type of current, surfaces contacted, pathway of the current, duration of contact, and other associated trauma. Tissue resistance falls dramatically as the current exposure is prolonged (Cooper, 1981).

Volt for volt, direct current (DC) is less damaging than alternating current (AC). The former often produces major total body muscle contractions that repel the victim from the current source. AC current, in contrast, often produces tetani and (above 6 to 9 mA) prevents the victim from voluntarily letting go of the current source. This often will lead to clenching of the hands and a fixing of the patient to the current source. Consequently, AC current is considered to be about three times more dangerous than DC per volt.

AC voltage at 25 to 300 Hz and 25 to 220 volts is a common household current level and easily can cause ventricular fibrillation if the pathway of the current includes the heart. It quite often will cause respiratory paralysis as well. The pathway of the current usually determines the severity of tissue damage. Electrical burn damage is proportional to the current's density, and, as the cross section of an involved body part increases, the current and resistance decrease. Therefore, a finger will sustain greater damage than the trunk, all other factors being equal.

Heat damage is also proportional to tissue resistance. Bone is a poor conductor but retains heat a long time, often causing severe damage to deep tissues while surrounding superficial layers are less affected. Skin, when dry, has a very high current resistance, but, when wet, is markedly more conductive, which leads to increased electrical injury.

Neurovascular and muscle bundles are much more sensitive to current injuries than would be expected from their electrical and cellular properties. Thrombosis, neural damage, and myoedema with ischemia are all seen in a delayed fashion after electrical injury.

Several types of burns are seen with electrical injury: thermal burns from direct contact with current, deep electrical arc burns, and flash burns from ignited clothing. Always completely undress the patient and look for entry and exit wounds as well as other associated injuries when evaluating the person with an electrical injury.

Electrical injuries can be deceptive in their early appearance. Consequently, these patients should be admitted to the hospital for neurovascular checks of extremities and other cardiovascular monitoring as needed. When electrical current traverses the body, it can obliterate recent memory and cause transient neurologic deficits. This may make the patient's history unreliable. Always evaluate patients for associated cranial, spinal, or other trauma and initially treat the neck as unstable, particularly with DC voltage injuries.

The cause of immediate death in most severe electrical injuries is cardiac arrhythmia and/or respiratory arrest. Consequently, it is imperative that rescuers begin CPR immediately, especially if the patient appears "dead." Rescuers should be extremely careful to remove the victim from the source of the electrical injury. This may require turning off the current or carefully removing the victim from the source using a highly insulated or nonconductive material. The patient should be assessed in the field and, if necessary, CPR instituted. The patient also should be considered to have traumatic injuries and the neck stabilized. If necessary, intravenous fluids should be started in the field along with other resuscitative measures.

Victims of electrical injury should receive an ECG to evaluate for myocardial damage and should be monitored for 24 hours if the current passed through the heart. Other indications for admission in adults include high-voltage conduction injuries, documented loss of consciousness, cardiac arrest, ECG changes, arrhythmias, a history of or significant risk for coronary artery disease, chest pain, hypoxia, and myoglobinuria.

All patients should be evaluated for myoglobinuria or hemoglobinuria. Aggressive volume resuscitation may be needed to prevent pigment deposition in the kidneys and to replace burn-related third space losses. Urinary output generally should be maintained around 1 mL/kg/hr. Frequent neurovascular checks will help with the early detection of compartment syndromes caused by burn-related edema. When this is suspected, surgical consultation should be obtained to evaluate for fasciotomy.

The remainder of electrical burn management, especially when burns are severe, is similar to that for thermal burn management. If the current path involves the head and neck, an ophthalmology evaluation should be considered because cataracts can form up to 2 years after such injury.

As mentioned earlier, toddlers chewing on electrical cords may suffer lip and mouth burns, often at the commissure. These patients should be hospitalized and have surgical consultation. In up to 20 per cent of cases, the labial artery may be injured and produce delayed profuse bleeding, and surgical correction may be necessary.

LIGHTNING

Lighting is the most common lethal natural phenomenon. It is a massive, instantaneous DC countershock that causes 150 to 250 deaths per year in the United States, and four to five times more injuries. Twenty to 30 per cent of individuals struck by lighting die; however, 70 per cent of the survivors may suffer permanent sequelae. The incidence of lighting parallels the occurrence of thunderstorms in the United States, which are common in the south, southeast, Atlantic coast, Rocky Mountains, Appalachian range, and valleys of major river tidal basins. Sportsman, individuals with outdoor occupations (e.g., rangers, farmers, sailors), and construction workers are all at a increased risk for lighting injuries (Fontanarosa, 1993).

Lighting strikes may result in several mechanisms of injury. The most deadly and serious are direct strikes to the head or ground or step voltage injuries resulting in leg burns. Persons also may be injured by contact injury, which is voltage being transmitted to them from another object (tall tree) that has resulted in a lighting strike. There may be splash or "flash-over" injury and, finally, blunt trauma, which is associated with the extremely high DC voltage developed in lighting. A classic injury in lighting is the flash-over burn. The patient may have linear, punctate, feather-type burns that often are referred to as "Lichtenberg's flowers."

The voltage in a lighting strike is in the range of 10 million to 2 *billion* volts. The duration is so short (1/1000th to 1/10,000th of a second), however, that serious current injuries are uncommon. Most of the current passes over the victim, causing the flash-over burn phenomenon. Some internal current leak may cause arrhythmia, asystole, or respiratory arrest. There is seldom significant deep tissue destruction, deep burns, or myoglobinuria, as occurs with other electrical burns. However, there may be serious CNS injury, with subdural hematoma, subarachnoid hemorrhage, direct burns of the brain, intraventricular hemorrhage, seizures, and loss of consciousness (Ghezzi, 1989).

Rescuers should be aggressive with CPR. There is generally no need for excessive fluids, as required in other burns. All patients must be treated as if they have serious trauma. The neck should be stabilized and a thorough evaluation performed. All patients with cardiac or neurologic injuries should be admitted. Patients with associated trauma, burns, or rhabdomyolysis may need admission. Skin burns should be managed as outlined previously. Because of the associated CNS injuries, dilated pupils are not an accurate indicator of brain death in lighting strikes, and resuscitation should be continued if appropriate despite this finding. Respiratory paralysis is generally the cause of death in the field, as a result of hypoxia. Consequently, the triage rule from the field for multiple lighting casualties is to "resuscitate the dead" (Cooper, 1980).

Victims may require neurologic and cardiac monitoring after resuscitation. Many will have tympanic membrane rupture, which is often treated and resolves with conservative management. Cataract formation is not uncommon, so an ophthalmology consultation should be sought.

DROWNING AND NEAR-DROWNING

Drowning is described as death by asphyxiation after immersion. Near-drowning is, by definition, survival for 24 hours following an immersion event or injury. A postimmersion syndrome has been described that is a progressive deterioration and often death following immersion and initial survival. Approximately 8000 to 9000 individuals drown per year, and drowning is the third leading cause of accidental death for most age groups.

Teenagers and toddlers are the individuals most likely to be involved in drowning. Eighty per cent of the teenagers are male and 60 per cent of the drownings involve alcohol use. This also is true of adults who drown. Toddlers constitute about 40 per cent of the victims. The most commonly recognized cause of drowning in toddlers is leaving the victim unattended in an area or around a fixture that can cause drowning. This can include a bathtub, a basin of water, or a swimming pool. Placing a fence at least 1.5 m high around open pools has been recommended as a way to prevent accidental drowning (Webster, 1967). Situations to consider in a drowning case include (1) alcohol use; (2) the presence of fatigue; (3) hyperventilation before swimming or diving, causing shallow water "blackout" (4) a sudden illness, such as seizure or myocardial infarction; (5) a head and neck injury resulting from a dive; (6) venomous animal sting; and (7) decompression illness in divers (Auerbach, 1992).

The most commonly recognized sequence of events in drowning includes laryngospasm, hypoxia, aspiration, ineffective circulation leading to brain hypoxia, brain injury, and death. Irreversible brain injury and death can occur within 5 to 10 minutes. Laryngospasm is considered the predominant mechanism of hypoxia. Fifteen to 20 per cent of drowning victims have *no* water in their lungs ("dry" drownings) and the remaining majority have very little. Aspiration of fresh water versus salt water has been of major interest and concern in the pathophyiology of drowning. Both types of water dilute pulmonary surfactant and cause atelectasis, with resulting pneumonia and pneumonitis. Excessive fresh water aspiration may cause hemodilution and hemolysis in the vascular system. Excessive salt water in the lungs may cause a hemoconcentration. However, these phenomena are of less importance than the laryngospasm, hypoxia, and resulting cardiorespiratory insufficiency that results from drowning.

Near-drowning victims often are brought to the emergency room for evaluation. They may present with a constellation of symptoms ranging from completely asymptomatic to florid pulmonary edema. Most often, victims will have a mild cough, transient tachypnea, and quite often vomiting.

Patients who do not spontaneously recover from an immersion injury or appear to have drowned should have immediate, prolonged CPR and airway management instituted at the scene (Ornato, 1986). Adequate CPR cannot be provided in the water, so victims should be brought carefully to the shore, remembering that all such victims may have a neck injury or cervical spine damage. Patients who recover without CPR or have a near drowning and present with no pulmonary complaints have a favorable prognosis. Any patient with respiratory complaints, chest radiograph changes, or the need for oxygen as measured by arterial blood gases should be admitted for a minimum of 24 hours of observation.

Hospital or emergency room management of the drowning victim should include aggressive CPR. This should continue until the patient is normothermic and further CPR appears futile. The physician should remember that there have been some recoveries after prolonged resuscitation, especially in children even with fixed and dilated pupils.

Cerebral resuscitation to prevent severe brain injury may require intensive respiratory management. Intubation may allow for the hyperventilation necessary for cerebral protection. Sedation or paralysis may be required to reduce agitation. Seizures should be treated if they occur, and intravenous mannitol given along with cautious fluid management or restriction.

Near-drowning patients often are resuscitated only to succumb later to aspiration pneumonitis secondary to contaminated water. Secondary drowning is defined as death caused by aspiration-related complications of pneumonitis or pulmonary edema. Severe brain injury from the initial insult may either prevent successful resuscitation or result in the previously mentioned progressive deterioration (postimmersion syndrome) after initial resuscitation and stabilization.

Cold water drowning has received great interest recently. Theoretically, the induction of the mammalian diving reflex could serve to preserve the core circulation and cerebral perfusion. A decrease in metabolic rate is thought to possibly protect the individual from the immersion-related hypoxia; however, in most cases this is counterbalanced by an increase in cardiac irritability as a result of hypothermia. In summary, the most favorable prognostic signs for near-drowning are recovery without CPR, no pulmonary complaints, and near-drowning in clean, cold water.

REFERENCES

Auerbach P: Disorders due to physical and environmental agents. *In* Saunders CE, Ho MT (eds): Current Emergency Diagnosis and Treatment. Norwalk, CT, Appleton-Lange, 1992, pp 703–729.

Bareca RS: Heat illness. *In* Hamilton GC, Sanders AB, Strange GR, et al. (eds): Emergency Medicine: An Approach to Clinical Problem Solving. Philadelphia, WB Saunders Company, 1991, pp 394–408.

Braen GR, Jelenko C: Thermal injury (burns). *In* Rosen P, Baker FJ, Braen GR, et al. (eds): Emergency Medicine: Concepts in Clinical Practice. St. Louis, CV Mosby, 1988, pp 433–443.

Clowes GHA, O'Donnel TF: Current concepts: Heat stroke. N Engl J Med 291:564, 1974.

Cooper MA: Electrical injuries. Curr Top II Emerg Med 1, 1981.

Cooper MA: Lightening injuries: Prognostic signs of death. Ann Emerg Med 9:134, 1980.

Cooper MA, Danzl DF: Hypothermia. *In* Hamilton GC, Sanders AB, Strange GR, et al. (eds): Emergency Medicine: An Approach to Clinical Problem Solving. Philadelphia, WB Saunders Company, 1991, pp 409–423.

Danzl DF: Hypothermic syndromes. Am Fam Physician 37:157, 1988.

Demling RH: Burns. N Engl J Med 313:1389, 1985.

Demling RH, Buerstatte WR, Perea A: Management of hot tar burns. J Trauma 20:242, 1980.

Dimick AR: Emergency treatment of extensive burns. Curr Top II Emerg Med 1(7), 1981.

Fontanarosa PD: Electrical shock and lightening strike. Ann Emerg Med 22(2,part 2):378, 1993.

Ghezzi KT: Lightening injuries: A unique treatment challenge. Postgrad Med 85:197, 1989.

Hall KN, Syverud SA: Closed thoracic cavity lavage in the treatment of severe hypothermia in human beings. Ann Emerg Med 19:204, 1990.

Hamlet MP: An overview of medically related problems in the cold environment. Milit Med 152:393, 1987.

Herndon DN, Langner F, Thompson P, et al.: Pulmonary injury in burned patients. Surg Clin North Am 67:31, 1987.

Jelenko C: Chemicals that burn. J Trauma 14:65, 1971.

Kyosola K: Clinical experience in management of cold injuries: A study of 110 cases. J Trauma 14:32, 1974.

Langford RM, Armstrong RF: Algorithm for managing injury from smoke inhalation. BMJ 299:902, 1989.

Leaman PL, Martyak GG: Microwave rewarming of resuscitation fluids. Ann Emerg Med 14:876, 1985.

Meyer AA, Salber PA: Burns and smoke inhalation. *In* Hamilton GC, Sanders AB, Strange GR, et al. (eds): Emergency Medicine: An Approach to Clinical Problem Solving. Philadelphia, WB Saunders Company, 1991, pp 691–702.

Navar PD, Safel JR, Warden GD: Effect of inhalation injury on fluid resuscitation requirements after thermal injury. Am J Surg 150:716, 1985.

O'Donnel TF, Clowes GHA: The circulatory abnormalities of heat stroke. N Engl J Med 287:734, 1972.

O'Keefe K: Accidental hypothermia: A review of 62 cases. J Am Coll Emerg Physicians 6:491, 1977.

Ornato JP: The resuscitation of near drowning victims. JAMA 256:75, 1986.

Perdue GF, Hunt JL: Cold injuries: A collective review. J Burn Care Rehabil 7:331, 1986.

Reuler J: Hypothermia: Pathophysiology, clinical settings, and management. Ann Intern Med 89:519, 1978.

Robson MC, Krizek TJ, Wray RC: Care of the thermally injured patient. *In* Zuidema GD, Rutherford RB, Ballinger WF (eds): The Management of Trauma. Philadelphia, WB Saunders Company, 1979, pp 666–730.

Sine RJ: Heat illness. J Am Coll Emerg Physicians 8:154, 1979.

Tucker LE, Standford J, Graves B, et al.: Classical heat stroke: Clinical and laboratory assessment. South Med J 78:20, 1985.

Vicario SJ, Okabajue R, Haltom T: Rapid cooling and classic heat stroke: Effect on mortality rates. Am J Emerg Med 4: 394, 1986.

Washburn B: Frostbite. N Engl J Med 266:974, 1962.

Webster PP: Pool drownings and their prevention. Public Health Rep 82:587, 1967.

CHAPTER 37

SPORTS MEDICINE

JOE E. HIMES and DAVID C. CAMPBELL

In its simplest form, sports medicine is the medicine of motion, and the benefits of treatment have been noted from the earliest times. Herodicus, working during the fifth century BC, treated injured athletes and prescribed therapeutic exercises and diet to nonathletic patients. Aristotle and Suchruta, an Indian physician, recognized the benefits of exercise for treating diabetes; and Galen was appointed physician to the gladiators, a title that would be analogous to today's team physician (Campbell and Yetter, 1990).

During the twentieth century, Walter Meanwell opened dialogue on the role of the team physician and athletic trainer. In 1938 Augustus Thorndike published the first American text on athletic injuries, emphasizing prevention, diagnosis, and treatment. Since that time there has been extensive growth in the field of sports medicine as our society continues to become more sports and fitness conscious.

ORGANIZED SPORTS MEDICINE

Primary care sports medicine has recently come of age. In 1991 the American Medical Society for Sports Medicine (AMSSM) was formed to address issues relating to primary care and sports medicine. In 1993 the American Board of Family Practice, along with the Boards of Internal Medicine, Pediatrics, and Emergency Physicians, offered testing for a certificate of added qualification in sports medicine. By so doing, they have recognized the special body of knowledge and dedication necessary to provide quality care to athletes, teams, and active individuals.

HEALTH BENEFITS OF EXERCISE

Using the "healthy people by 2000" framework, McGinnis (1992) summarized much of what is known about the health benefits of exercise. Regular physical activity can reduce the risk of all-cause mortality by more than 25 per cent. The risk of coronary heart disease can be reduced by one-half owing to favorable changes in lipid profiles, diastolic blood pressure, and obesity. Life expectancy can increase by more than 2 years. Regular physical activity can help to regulate and manage non-insulin-dependent diabetes mellitus and osteoporosis. Additionally, there appears to be a decreased risk of stroke and possibly a decreased risk of colon cancer when regular exercise is performed. Clearly the health benefits of an active lifestyle far outweigh those of inactivity.

FITNESS

To attain and maintain fitness, one must have an operational understanding of what constitutes fitness. The definition of the American College of Sports Medicine is as follows.

A state characterized by (a) an ability to perform daily activities with vigor, and (b) demonstration of traits and capacities that are associated with low risk of premature development of the hypokinetic diseases. The components of fitness include cardiorespiratory endurance, muscular endurance, muscular strength, flexibility, and body composition.

Several methods, each with their own variations, have been devised for the measurement of each component and are discussed elsewhere (Mellion et al., 1990; Pollock et al., 1984).

PREPARTICIPATION PHYSICAL EVALUATIONS

Definition and Approach

The preparticipation physical evaluation (PPE) is a focused evaluation of athletes or potential athletes prior to practice and competition. The American Academy of Family Physicians and the American Academy of Pediatrics, along with the American Medical Society for Sports Medicine, the American Orthopedic Society for Sports Medicine, and the American Osteopathic Academy of Sports Medicine, released guidelines for PPEs (Bergfeld et al., 1992). Although selected populations require differing approaches, there are several primary and

TABLE 37–1. OBJECTIVES OF THE PPE

Primary objectives
Detect conditions that may limit participation
Detect conditions that may predispose to injury
Meet legal and insurance requirements

Secondary objectives
Determine general health
Counsel on health-related issues
Assess maturity
Assess fitness level and performance

From Swander H (ed): Preparticipation physical evaluation (monograph). Kansas City, MO: American Academy of Family Physicians, 1992, with permission.

secondary objectives that may be considered for all populations (Table 37–1).

Certain conditions may limit participation depending on the nature and condition of the sport and athlete. Some combinations of condition and sport result in relative or absolute contraindications to participation. To facilitate decision-making, the American Academy of Pediatrics (AAP) Committee on Sports Medicine (1988) classified many popular sports as contact or noncontact (Table 37–2). These categories are based not only on body contact but also on velocity and equipment considerations. Using these classifications, the AAP developed clearance recommendations for participation of high-risk individuals in competitive sports (Table 37–3). These recommendations serve as guidelines for the physician counseling an athlete or the parents prior to activity.

The PPE should serve to detect conditions that could predispose the athlete to injury. They include not only congenital or developmental conditions but also acquired deficiencies such as inadequately rehabilitated injuries, diabetes, arthritis, and heart disease.

Whether for organized sports or local health clubs, PPEs are often used to satisfy legal and insurance requirements. As such, the physician must

be aware of what is required during the examination, including the completion of proper forms and laboratory tests. One review summarized state requirements for PPEs in school-aged children (Feinstein et al., 1988).

Many athletes have the mistaken view that the PPE supplants a comprehensive physical examination. By identifying these athletes, the physician can direct the PPE to include general health maintenance issues, such as diet information, immunization updates, and social issues. However, the PPE does not substitute for full, in-office evaluations. If necessary, the athlete should be referred or rescheduled for testing any questionable areas.

Certain sports, such as football, involve athletes and projectiles colliding at high speeds. Controversy exists, but most observers believe that immature athletes are at greater risk for injury when they participate in such sports with larger, stronger, more mature athletes. Ideally, athletes would compete by level, as determined by sexual maturity and ability rather than chronologic age. Sexual maturation is assessed using Tanner staging. Self-rating of pubic hair and breast development has shown good correlation to physician-administered ratings without the embarrassment of disrobing in front of strangers (Duke et al., 1980).

With proper planning, the PPE can be utilized to assess performance. Information gained from an assessment of agility, body composition, flexibility, strength, and endurance can be useful to athletes and coaches. Performance testing can identify weaknesses that require attention, supply a baseline from which to measure progress, and provide a comparison when assessing return to play after injury.

Timing, Frequency, and Methods of Evaluation

For those who participate in organized sports, it is suggested that the PPE take place approximately

TABLE 37–2. CLASSIFICATION OF SPORTS

Contact		Noncontact		
Contact/Collision	Limited Contact/Impact	Strenuous	Moderately Strenuous	Nonstrenuous
Boxing	Baseball	Aerobic dance	Badminton	Archery
Field hockey	Basketball	Crew	Curling	Golf
Football	Bicycling	Fencing	Table tennis	Riflery
Ice hockey	Diving	Field (discus, javelin, shot)		
Lacrosse	Field (high jump, pole vault)	Running/track		
Martial arts	Gymnastics	Swimming		
Rodeo	Horseback riding	Tennis		
Soccer	Skating	Weight lifting		
Wrestling	Skiing			
	Softball			
	Squash/handball			
	Volleyball			

From American Academy of Pediatrics, Committee on Sports Medicine: Recommendations for participation in competitive sports. Pediatrics 81:737, 1988, with permission.

TABLE 37–3. RECOMMENDATIONS FOR PARTICIPATION IN COMPETITIVE SPORTS

Consideration in Patient	Contact		Noncontact		
	Contact/ Collision	Limited Contact/ Collision	Strenuous	Moderately Strenuous	Nonstrenuous
Atlantoaxial instability	No	No	Yes*	Yes	Yes
Acute illnesses	†	†	†	†	†
Cardiovascular system	No	No	No	No	No
Carditis					
Hypertension	Yes	Yes	Yes	Yes	Yes
Mild	‡	‡	‡	‡	‡
Moderate	‡	‡	‡	‡	‡
Severe	§	§	§	§	§
Congenital heart disease					
Eyes					
Absence or loss of function of one eye	‖	‖	‖	‖	‖
Detached retina	¶	¶	¶	¶	¶
Inguinal hernia	Yes	Yes	Yes	Yes	Yes
Kidney (absence of one)	No	Yes	Yes	Yes	Yes
Liver (enlarged)	No	No	Yes	Yes	Yes
Musculoskeletal disorders	‡	‡	‡	‡	‡
Neurologic entities					
History of serious head or spine trauma, repeated concussions or craniotomy	‡	‡	Yes	Yes	Yes
Convulsive disorder					
Well controlled	Yes	Yes	Yes	Yes	Yes
Poorly controlled	No	No	Yes‡‡	Yes	Yes**
Ovary (absence of one)	Yes	Yes	Yes	Yes	Yes
Respiratory					
Pulmonary insufficiency	††	††	††	††	Yes
Asthma	Yes	Yes	Yes	Yes	Yes
Sickle cell trait	Yes	Yes	Yes	Yes	Yes
Skin (boils, herpes, impetigo, scabies)	‡‡	‡‡	Yes	Yes	Yes
Spleen (enlarged)	No	No	No	Yes	Yes
Testicle (absent or undescended)	Yes‖‖	Yes‖‖	Yes	Yes	Yes

* Swimming (no butterfly, breast-stroke, or diving starts).
† Needs individual assessment (e.g., contagiousness to others, risk of worsening illness).
‡ Needs individual assessment.
§ Patients with mild forms can be allowed a full range of physical activities; patients with mild or severe forms or who are postoperative should be evaluated by a physician.
‖ Availability of American Society for Testing Materials approved eye guards may allow competitor to participate in most sports, but it must be judged on an individual basis.
¶ Consult ophthalmologist.
# No swimming or weight lifting.
** No archery or riflery.
†† May be allowed to compete if oxygenation remains satisfactory during a graded stress test.
‡‡ No gymnastics with mats, martial arts, wrestling, or contact sports until no longer contagious.
‖‖ Certain sports may require a protective cup.
From American Academy of Pediatrics, Committee on Sports Medicine: Recommendations for participation in competitive sports. Pediatrics 81:737, 1988, with permission.

6 weeks prior to the beginning of practice. This scheduling allows enough time to perform additional tests, complete rehabilitation, or obtain needed consultations.

How often the PPE should be repeated is often the subject of legislation. Many organizations, including most states, require annual evaluations. However, it has been suggested that complete evaluations be performed every other year or at a change of school classification (i.e., grade school to junior high). During the intermittent years, limited evaluations addressing previous injuries or weak areas of performance are sufficient. This program works especially well when the same physician handles total care for the athlete.

Once the PPE timing and frequency have been determined, the method of evaluation must be se-lected. Office-based PPEs and station screening PPEs are two choices available (Table 37–4). An office-based examination places the patient, often known to the physician prior to the examination, with a single physician in a quiet environment. Office-based examinations facilitate continuity of care and afford opportunities to discuss delicate issues. For adult athletes and athletes with complicated medical histories, the office-based PPE is ideal. Unfortunately, office-based PPEs are time-consuming and expensive. They also assume that athletes have a primary care physician, an assumption that is not always correct.

A second common method employed for PPEs, referred to as station screening, places personnel at separate stations. The athlete rotates from station to station. Often all athletes and coaches are gath-

TABLE 37–4. POTENTIAL ADVANTAGES AND DISADVANTAGES OF OFFICE-BASED AND STATION SCREENING PPEs

Office-Based PPE	Station Screening PPE
Advantages	Advantages
Physician-patient familiarity	Specialized personnel
Continuity of care	Efficient and cost-effective
Opportunity for counseling	Good communication with school athletic staff
	Opportunity for performance testing
Disadvantages	Disadvantages
Many athletes do not have a primary care physician	Noisy, hurried environment
Limited time for appointments	Lack of privacy
Varying knowledge of and interest in sports medicine problems	Difficulty following up on medical problems and concerns
Greater cost	Lack of communication with parents
Lack of communication with school athletic staff	

From Swander H (ed): Preparticipation physical evaluation (monograph). Kansas City, MO: American Academy of Family Physicians, 1992, with permission.

ered together while these evaluations take place. This gathering of parties facilitates good communication. Because nonmedical or paramedical personnel can perform many of the tasks, station screening PPEs are efficient and cost-effective. However, the loud, hurried environment and lack of privacy may compromise certain aspects of the evaluation. In addition, parents may not be readily accessible, and follow-up may be difficult. Ultimately, the choice of which method to use should be based on the physician, available resources, and time.

History

The PPE is a screening evaluation. The history portion of the evaluation should be constructed to identify known past and present conditions that place the athlete or any other participant at increased risk. Several formats have been proposed (Bergfeld et al., 1991; Fields and Delaney, 1990; Smith et al., 1991). What follows is our suggested format.

1. *Has anyone in the athlete's family (grandmother, mother, father, brother, sister, aunt, uncle) died suddenly, before the age of 50 years?* Approximately 95 per cent of the sudden deaths of athletes under age 35 are related to cardiovascular abnormalities. Two of these abnormalities—eccentric left ventricular hypertrophy and cystic medial necrosis (Marfan syndrome)—show hereditary tendencies. Other conditions that demonstrate hereditary predilection and have been associated with premature sudden death are atherosclerotic cardiovascular disease and hypertension. These associations are particularly valid when first degree blood relatives have suffered consequences prior to age 50 years.

2. *Has the athlete ever passed out during exercise or stopped exercising because of dizziness or illness?* Exertional syncope may indicate cardiopulmonary insufficiency and warrants further investigation.

3. *Does the athlete have asthma, wheezing, shortness of breath, hay fever, coughing spells, chest pain or heaviness, or a racing heart during exercise?* Asthma and other forms of pulmonary disease are not contraindications to vigorous exercise provided the condition is identified and controlled. Ten per cent of the general population and fifty per cent of those with environmental allergies suffer exercise-induced asthma. The symptom most commonly experienced during attacks of exercise-induced asthma is cough.

4. *Has the athlete ever broken a bone, had to wear a cast, or had an injury to a joint?* Incompletely or incorrectly healed fractures combined with incompletely rehabilitated muscles, ligaments, or tendons places athletes at increased risk for reinjury and suboptimal performance.

5. *Has the athlete ever had a concussion (been knocked out)?* Closed head injuries with alteration of sensorium, or concussions, occur most often with contact sports and may be classified from grade I to grade III (Table 37–5). It is important to identify those athletes with previous concussions and determine the severity of the concussion, as well as the time interval and symptoms since the incident. Note that the more severe the grade, the more likely it is there will be residual structural brain scarring and subsequent reinjury. No matter how long the time interval between the concussion and the examination, no athlete should be allowed to return to contact sports while continuing to experience symptoms, which may include exertional or positional headache, visual disturbances, nausea and vomiting, memory lapses, or loss of consciousness. Even if the athlete is allowed to return to competition after a concussion occurs during that event, the athlete and athlete's family should be informed of possible delayed hemorrhage. The athlete should be followed closely by the family (or in a college situation, at the infirmary) for at least 24 hours. Late development of the above symptoms should prompt immediate surgical evaluation.

6. *Has the athlete ever had heat stroke?* Whether as a result of selection or as a sequela of illness, athletes who suffer heat stroke have increased risk for future heat stroke, especially during the year after the most recent episode. It is unclear whether athletes are at increased risk over

TABLE 37–5.   GRADING CONCUSSIONS IN SPORTS AND GUIDELINES FOR RETURN TO PLAY*

Grading		Guidelines		
Severity	Signs/Symptoms	First Concussion	Second Concussion	Third Concussion
Grade I (mild)	Confusion without amnesia; no loss of consciousness	May return to play if asymptomatic§ for at least 20 minutes	Terminate contest/ practice; may return to play if asymptomatic§ for at least 1 week	Terminate season; may return to play in 3 months if asymptomatic§
Grade II (moderate)	Confusion with amnesia†; no loss of consciousness‡	Terminate contest/practice; may return to play if asymptomatic§ for at least 1 week	Consider terminating season but may return to play if asymptomatic§ for 1 month	Terminate season; may return to play next season if asymptomatic§
Grade III (severe)	Loss of consciousness	Terminate contest/practice and transport to hospital; may return to play 1 month after two consecutive asymptomatic§ weeks; conditioning allowed after one asymptomatic§ week	Terminate season; may return to play next season if asymptomatic§	Terminate season; strongly discourage return to contact/ collision sports

* These guidelines are not absolute and therefore should not substitute for the clinical judgement of the examining physician.

† Posttraumatic amnesia (amnesia for events after the impact) or more severe retrograde amnesia (amnesia for events preceding the impact).

‡ Some clinicians include "brief" loss of consciousness in grade II and reserve "prolonged" loss of consciousness for grade III. However, the definitions of "brief" and "prolonged" are not universally accepted.

§ No headache, confusion, dizziness, impaired orientation, impaired concentration, or memory dysfunction during rest or exertion.

Adapted from Colorado Medical Society. Report of the Sports Medicine Committee: Guidelines for the Management of Concussion in Sports (revised). Denver, Colorado Medical Society, 1991, with permission.

longer periods or if those athletes most susceptible move on to other endeavors.

7. *Does the athlete have any chronic illness for which he or she sees a doctor or takes medication?* Chronic illnesses seldom lead to disqualification, but, the existence of such illnesses should be documented. In addition, steps should be made to identify the medications, special equipment, and staff teaching that might be needed.

8. *Does the athlete take medication (prescription or otherwise)?* Medications, including the birth control pill, should be identified in order to consider their potential interaction with exercise conditions or future medication selections.

9. *Has the athlete had any surgery or been hospitalized?* It is important to detect conditions, surgeries, or hospitalizations that might preclude participation. In addition, recent or multiple hospitalizations may indicate poor control of chronic diseases.

10. *Is the athlete allergic to any medications or to bee stings?* Identifying medication allergies is important so those medications may be avoided. Outdoor athletic events place athletes at risk for bee stings, which are potentially life-threatening in allergic individuals.

11. *Does the athlete have only one of the following paired body parts: eyes, ears, kidneys, testicles, or ovaries?* Unpaired essential organs present a special challenge. When the unpaired organ can be protected and the athlete can function, he or she may participate. For instance, with the absence of one eye, or visual acuity of 20/200 or less in one

eye, binocular vision is lost. Additionally, the potential for blindness exists if there is injury to the normally functioning eye. Such an athlete should not be allowed to box, as boxing involves direct blows to the eyes, and protection is prohibited by the rules (Dorsen, 1986).

12. *Does the athlete use tobacco, alcohol, or street drugs?* The PPE is an opportunity to counsel patients on healthy lifestyles. Additional important topics that may be quickly addressed are sexual promiscuity, seat belt usage, and immunization status.

13. *Does the athlete have any concerns about which he or she would like to speak to the doctor?* This question leaves the door open for any other concerns the athlete might have. It is intentionally open-ended.

Physical Examination

The physical examination should be tailored to the athlete. What follows are recommendations for child and adolescent PPEs in apparently healthy populations. Additional information may be necessary in other populations of athletes. Table 37–6 lists components of the physical examination. Alterations may be made to accommodate any particular problems of the athlete.

Anthropometric measurements should include height and weight. Certain sports, such as ballet, wrestling, football, gymnastics, and cheerleading, emphasize body habitus. For these sports body

TABLE 37–6. COMPONENTS OF THE PHYSICAL EXAMINATION

Anthropometrics
  Height
  Weight
  Body composition (especially for weight class athletes)
Eye examination
  Visual acuity*
  Legal blindness in one eye*
  Protective eye wear†
  Glasses or contacts
  Document pupil size (anisocoria)
Cardiovascular examination
  Blood pressure
  Pulses (radial, femoral)
  Heart (size, rate, rhythm, murmurs)
Pulmonary examination
  Diaphragmatic excursion
  Breath sounds
  Chest wall shape/deformities
Abdominal examination
  Masses/organomegaly
Skin examination
  Skin‡
  Nails
  Suspicious nevi or lesions
Musculoskeletal examination
  Neck
  Shoulders
  Elbows
  Wrists/hands/fingers
  Back (including scoliosis)
  Hips
  Knees
  Ankles/feet
Genitalia (male)
  Single or undescended testicle
  Testicular mass
  Hernia
Maturity
  Tanner staging

* Legal blindness is 20/200. Refer for formal evaluation if acuity is worse than 20/50.
† Protective eyewear should be recommended to all athletes; however, protective eyewear should be *required* in athletes with poor vision in at least one eye. Polycarbonate lenses have been shown to protect eyes from high-velocity missiles such as bats and balls.
‡ Contagious skin conditions such as acne, impetigo, furuncles/carbuncles, herpes, scabies, lice, and molluscum contagiosum would preclude participation in direct contact sports such as wrestling until the condition is treated or clinically not active.
Modified from Swander H (ed): Preparticipation physical evaluation (monograph). Kansas City, MO, American Academy of Family Physicians, 1992.

TABLE 37–7. SUGGESTED UPPER LIMITS OF NORMAL BLOOD PRESSURE IN CHILDREN BY AGE

Age (Years)	Arterial Blood Pressure, Systolic/Diastolic (mm Hg)
14–18	<135/90
10–14	<125/85
6–10	<120/80
<6	<110/75

From the 1984 report of the Joint National Committee on Detection, Evaluation, and Treatment of High Blood Pressure. Arch Intern Med 144:1045, 1984.

from lightweight polycarbonate are available. Also during the visual examination, unusual pupil sizes or shapes should noted for future reference.

The cardiovascular examination is the single most important part of the physical examination. Attempts should be made to examine the athlete in a quiet environment in order to maximize results. Blood pressure should be measured in a calm setting and with an appropriately sized cuff. Normal blood pressure values vary with age (Table 37–7). When performing the cardiac examination, impulse size, rate, rhythm, and heart sounds should be delineated. Particular attention is paid to the detection of murmurs and to the clinical delineation of benign, physiologic, and pathologic murmurs. All diastolic murmurs, harsh or loud systolic murmurs, and pansystolic murmurs should be considered pathologic until proved otherwise. On the other hand, systolic murmurs may be physiologic or pathologic. Positioning maneuvers while listening to the heart aids the examiner to identify potentially harmful murmurs (Table 37–8).

In athletes younger than age 30, the three most common causes of sudden death are hypertrophic cardiomyopathy, idiopathic left ventricular hypertrophy, and coronary artery anomalies. With both hypertrophic cardiomyopathy and idiopathic left ventricular hypertrophy, myocardial mass is increased but overall cardiac dimensions may not change dramatically. The result is a thick, stiff heart with decreased chamber size. When preload

TABLE 37–8. PHYSIOLOGIC AND PHARMACOLOGIC MANEUVERS THAT AFFECT THE MURMUR OF HYPERTROPHIC OBSTRUCTIVE CARDIOMYOPATHY

Maneuver	Murmur Intensity	Effect of LVOT/Vol
Squatting	Decreased	Decreased/increased
Upright posture	Increased	Increased/decreased
Exercise	Increased	Increased/decreased
Amyl nitrate	Increased	Increased/decreased

LVOT = left ventricular outflow tract; Vol = Volume of blood leaving left ventricle.
From Strong WB, Stead D: Cardiovascular evaluation of the young athlete. Prim Care, 11:61, 1984, with permission.

composition may be added to the preseason evaluation as a means of determining lean body mass and the percentage of body fat. It should be recognized that many factors in addition to body composition affect performance, and that unusually high and low percentages of body fat are unhealthy. Lohman et al. (1988) have provided a comprehensive review on body composition.

Visual acuity should be evaluated in all athletes and corrected to 20/50 or better. Protective eyewear should be recommended for all participants of contact sports and required when vision is compromised in one or both eyes. Unbreakable, lightweight, fashionable goggles and face shields made is decreased—perhaps by dehydration, hyperdynamic states such as exercise, or fluid shifts such as positional changes—the left ventricular outflow tract obstructs ejection of blood. Clinically, the athlete experiences syncope or near-syncope.

Coronary artery anomalies account for 14 per cent of sudden deaths among those under 30 years of age. The anomalies include origin of the left coronary artery from the sinus of valsalva and origin of the right coronary artery from a single left trunk. In both instances, either the left or right coronary artery is forced to traverse between the aorta and the pulmonary trunk. With exercise, both major vessels dilate, impinging on the coronary artery, which itself is trying to supply needed blood to the myocardium. Clinically, the athlete may be asymptomatic, may experience chest pain or dyspnea on exertion, or may feel palpitations. In many instances, however, the first "symptom" is sudden death.

Unfortunately, screening examinations are insensitive for identifying any of these conditions. The diagnostic test of choice for detecting hypertrophic cardiomyopathy or idiopathic left ventricular hypertrophy is the echocardiogram, with or without stress testing. For coronary artery anomalies, the only reliable test available is the arteriogram.

The pulmonary examination includes inspection for such features as increased respiratory effort, breathlessness, chest deformities, cyanosis, and clubbing. Breath sounds should be clear in all lung fields.

Often overlooked during mass inspections, the abdominal examination is a rapid screening technique for organomegaly and does not require the athlete to disrobe. The renal, hepatic, and splenic beds should be palpated. In female athletes the adnexae and suprapubic regions should be palpated as well.

Preparticipation physical evaluations often involve children and adolescents. These age groups may demonstrate a host of dermatologic abnormalities, including acne, impetigo, herpes, scabies, and lice. Many of these conditions are considered contagious, preventing athletic participation until resolution of the offending skin condition. Certain conditions are common in certain sports. For instance, wrestlers have a high incidence of acne, impetigo, and herpes gladiatorium, which is herpetic skin involvement of the head, neck, or chest. These conditions are spread by skin-to-skin contact and can lead to substantial morbidity (Belognia et al., 1991). Wrestlers should not practice or compete until skin lesions are clearing and dry.

The male genitalia are examined for testicular presence, Tanner staging, scrotal masses, and inguinal hernias. Often during the genital examination there is opportunity for the examiner to reassure the athlete that development is normal and to counsel about sexually transmitted diseases, in-

TABLE 37–9. ORTHOPEDIC SCREENING EXAMINATION*

Athletic Activity (Instructions)	Observation
Stand facing examiner	Acromioclavicular joints: general habitus
Look at ceiling, floor, over both shoulders; touch ears to shoulders	Cervical spine motion
Shrug shoulders (examiner resists)	Trapezius strength
Abduct shoulders 90 degrees (examiner resists at 90 degrees)	Deltoid strength
Full external rotation of arms	Shoulder motion
Flex and extend elbows	Elbow motion
Arms at sides, elbows 90 degrees flexed; pronate and supinate wrists	Elbow and wrist motion
Spread fingers; make fist	Hand or finger motion and deformities
Tighten (contract) quadriceps; relax quadriceps	Symmetry and knee effusion; ankle effusion
"Duck walk" four steps (away from examiner with buttocks on heels)	Hip, knee, and ankle motion
Back to examiner	Shoulder symmetry; scoliosis
Knees straight, touch toes	Scoliosis, hip motion hamstring tightness
Raise up on toes, raise heels	Calf symmetry, leg strength

* The orthopedic screening examination, which may require a reflex hammer, tape measure, pin, and examination table, takes about 90 seconds. Time studies indicate it is most efficiently done one athlete at a time rather than in small groups. It is designed to reveal previous inadequately rehabilitated injuries or those few previously unrecognized orthopedic conditions that might be adversely affected by participation in a sports activity. Positive findings require a more extensive examination and history. A more detailed examination should not be attempted at the screening examination.

From Dyment MD (ed): Sports Medicine: Health Care for Young Athletes, 2nd edition. Elk Grove Village, IL, American Academy of Pediatrics, 1991.

cluding the human immunodeficiency virus (HIV). Older athletes may be taught testicular self-examination.

The screening musculoskeletal examination is designed to rapidly detect gross abnormalities that warrant further investigation or rehabilitation. Table 37–9 outlines the screening musculoskeletal examination. Smith et al. (1991) offered a pictorial summation of the PPE.

As previously stated, the examiner identifies those conditions that either presently or potentially pose increased risk for the athlete or the athlete's teammates. Every effort should be made to find ways in which the athlete can participate safely. At times it may involve encouraging the athlete to change positions, use prophylactic medications, don protective equipment, or consider a change in sports.

Laboratory Tests

Routine urinalysis, blood count, roentgenograms, and chemistry profiles in childhood and adolescent populations cannot be recommended at this time.

EXERCISE PRESCRIPTION

Whether a child or an adult, it is important to obtain adequate exercise. Many patients remain unaware of what constitutes adequate, appropriate exercise. To facilitate this understanding, the physician can issue an exercise prescription that fits an individual's needs. Such an exercise prescription can range from a simple outline to a complex regimen. All exercise prescriptions have five components in common: type (mode), duration, frequency, intensity, and progression of physical activity. A properly applied exercise prescription can lead to enhanced physical fitness, reduced disease risk, increased safety, facilitated compliance, increased or maintained functional capacity, and an improved sense of well-being.

The type, or mode, of activity refers to the activity itself. Appropriate types of exercise depend on the individual's abilities and goals. In general, to enhance cardiorespiratory fitness, one should select an activity that involves repetitive motions involving large muscle groups in weight-bearing or non-weight-bearing situations. Activities such as walking, running, swimming, and bicycling promote cardiorespiratory endurance. Muscular strength is facilitated via specific exercises involving high-intensity, low-repetition, resisted movements of specific muscle groups. Weight-lifting or pull-ups are examples.

The duration and intensity of exercise must be considered together. Anaerobic, high-intensity exercises are of short (seconds to minutes) duration, resulting in increased strength gains. Aerobic, low-intensity, long-duration activities promote improved endurance. In general, aerobic exercise at 60 to 70 per cent of the maximal heart rate for 30 minutes three times per week promotes cardiovascular health. Sessions of 40 to 60 minutes or longer five to seven times per week are often necessary for weight control. Maximal heart rate can be measured directly during a maximal exercise test, or it can be estimated using a formula: 220 minus the person's age in years. Some individuals are unable to achieve predicted heart rates because of genetics, disease, or medications. These patients may employ a practical guideline for intensity called the *talk test*, which is the intensity at which one can barely carry on a normal conversation without becoming unduly short of breath.

Intermittent, short-duration, low-intensity exercise is of little if any benefit to cardiorespiratory endurance or muscular strength. However, such activities may carry psychological benefits. An example would be browsing at the mall, an activity that many patients incorrectly identify as exercise.

The frequency of exercise refers to how many exercise sessions are performed within a given duration of time. Typically this time frame is 1 week. A regimen of three to five sessions per week meets the needs of most individuals. Frequency should be adjusted for special goals and functional capacities. Rest periods for the entire body or specific body parts should be built into the schedule.

Progression of activity is a portion of the exercise prescription that is frequently overlooked. During the first weeks of an exercise program, progression of duration or intensity may occur rapidly and represents improvements in neural recruitment and mechanics. Over a period of approximately 6 weeks the progression slows, eventually reaching a plateau stage. The challenge is to present the athlete with a progression that provides rapid advancement with minimal risk of physical injury or psychological burnout. One technique, called periodization, achieves it by intentionally overstressing the body for defined periods followed by periods of relatively light work. Specific recommendations are beyond the scope of this text; however, it is advisable to manipulate only one of the variables at a time and continue to monitor for altered mood, decreased appetite, increased resting heart rate, and impaired performance, which could signal overtraining.

Whereas most athletes safely participate in unsupervised activities, certain individuals should initially partake in supervised programs. Included are cardiorespiratory patients initiating exercise programs, patients with unstable clinical profiles, and patients with high risk, symptomatic, chronic disease.

In keeping with the overall definition of fitness, the exercise prescription should address general flexibility. In particular, the low back, quadriceps, hamstrings, and heel cords are areas of general concern. Exercise programs for the elderly should also address specific needs in the neck and hip regions. Flexibility exercises employing slow, sustained movements held at the point of resistance or initial discomfort for 10 to 30 seconds should follow a warm-up period. Anderson and Burke (1991) have provided an excellent review on stretching techniques and theory.

EXERCISE FOR SPECIAL GROUPS OF ATHLETES

Adolescents and Children

Adolescents and children represent the largest groups of organized athletes in the United States.

TABLE 37–10. BILL OF RIGHTS FOR YOUNG ATHLETES

Right to participate in sports
Right to participate at a level commensurate with each child's maturity and ability
Right to have qualified adult leadership
Right to play as a child and not as an adult
Right of children to share in the leadership and decision-making of their sport participation
Right to participate in a safe and healthy environment
Right to proper preparation for participation in sports
Right to an equal opportunity to strive for success
Right to be treated with dignity
Right to have fun in sports

From Bill of Rights for Young Athletes from Sports Medicine: A Practical Guide for Youth Sports Coaches and Parents. Canton, OH, Professional Reports Corporation, 1992, with permission.

However, not all young people mature at the same rate or have the same goals. In fact, the primary reason athletes quit organized sports in this age range is not that they are poor athletes or that they are on a losing team. Instead, they quit because they are not allowed to play or are not having fun. This situation has led to the development of a Bill of Rights for Young Athletes (Table 37–10).

Shields (1986) provided a synopsis of growth and development as they relate to sport. The period from birth through preschool age is a time to determine whether the child is developing normally. Physical activities are unstructured and are purely for fun. Varied activities should be employed and be aimed at developing gross motor function. Playground equipment should be safe, with level surfaces, minimal moving parts, and appropriately sized utilities. Trampoline and swimming pool use require strict supervision.

Early school years provide a major step in the socialization process. Children interact not only with family but with schoolmates and teachers. During the early elementary-school years, coeducational activities have become increasingly acceptable. Team sports should teach broad concepts and allow for a wide range of abilities. To promote healthy habits, emphasis should be placed on proper fit and use of safety equipment.

Peripubertal and early teenage years involve all of the biologic, emotional, and social changes that accompany passage into adulthood. All three may progress at different rates at different times in the same individual. Linear growth often occurs in spurts, with bone growth preceding muscle, tendon, and neuronal adaptations. As a result, poor performance and muscle strain injuries may occur in previously high performance athletes. This discrepancy can be psychologically damaging when the adolescent athlete has abnormally large amounts of self-worth invested in athletic prowess. Adolescent athletes have been shown to be high risk takers compared to their nonathletic counterparts (Fig. 37–1) (Nattiv and Puffer, 1991). Increased rates of smoking, alcohol, and drug use have been identified in this group, but cause and effect have not been established.

During the adolescent years, athletic activities become increasingly sophisticated and competitive. Adolescents are ready to undertake adult-type

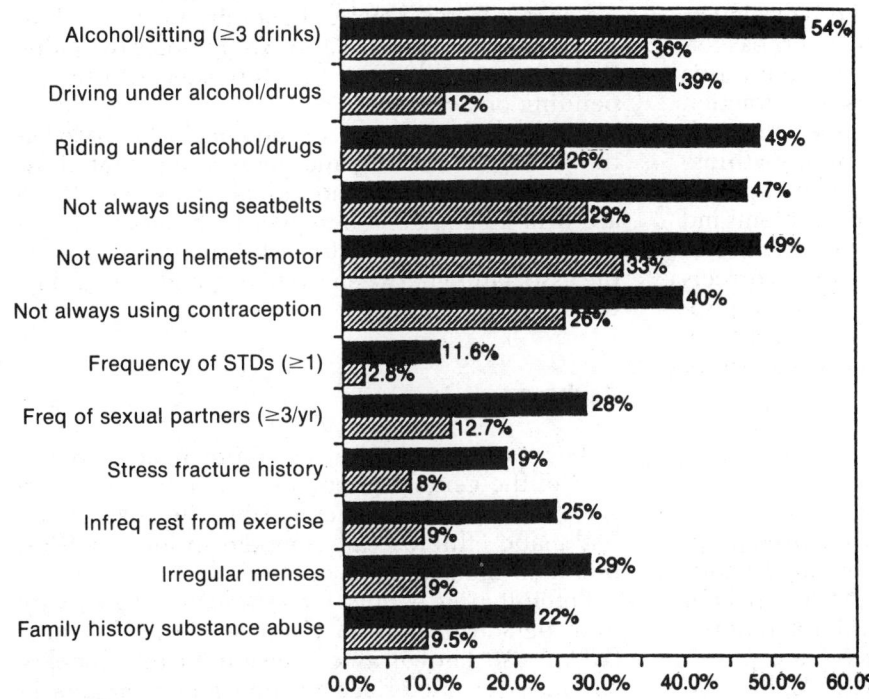

FIGURE 37–1. Lifestyle behaviors of athletes versus nonathletes. Athletes are represented by solid bars; nonathletes are represented by hatched bars. For all risk behaviors except Driving under alcohol/drugs, $p < 0.05$; for Driving under alcohol/drugs, $p < 0.001$. (From Nattiv A, Puffer JC: Life-styles and health risks of collegiate athletes. J Fam Pract 33: 585, 1991, with permission.)

Health Risks

Alcohol/sitting (≥3 drinks) — 54% / 36%
Driving under alcohol/drugs — 39% / 12%
Riding under alcohol/drugs — 49% / 26%
Not always using seatbelts — 47% / 29%
Not wearing helmets-motor — 49% / 33%
Not always using contraception — 40% / 26%
Frequency of STDs (≥1) — 11.6% / 2.8%
Freq of sexual partners (≥3/yr) — 28% / 12.7%
Stress fracture history — 19% / 8%
Infreq rest from exercise — 25% / 9%
Irregular menses — 29% / 9%
Family history substance abuse — 22% / 9.5%

play, and properly structured sports provide a structured avenue through which adolescents can find peer acceptance and self-esteem.

Weight training in pre- and postpubescent athletes has been found to increase strength and is thought to increase performance and protect against some types of injury (Tanner, 1993). However, the safety of weight training is directly dependent on proper instruction and supervision. It has been observed that low back strain is the most common injury associated with weight training, and it is recommended that prepubescent athletes not perform power clean, clean and jerk, squat lift, or dead lift maneuvers. Even so, weight training appears to be safer than many contact sports. When determining whether an individual should begin a weight training program, readiness to participate, emotional maturity, ability to follow instructions, and access to appropriate equipment must be taken into consideration. Exercise machines may hold an advantage over free weights because balance is not a factor and spotters are not required. However, most machines are sized for adults and may not provide for correct hand placement or resistance selection for children.

Today, many young people compete year-round; and as young people compete in more and more organized sports, overuse injuries have become more common. Increased repetition, decreased recovery time, poor equipment, improper technique, and abnormal mechanics contribute to overuse injuries. In the immature athlete, normal growth, with altered biomechanics resulting from rapid increases in height and weight and from decreases in flexibility, magnify the problem.

Examples of overuse injuries in immature athletes include spondylolysis of the lumbar spine in a gymnast, dancer, lineman, or basketball player; medial tibial stress syndrome in a runner, basketball player, or soccer player; rotator cuff tendinitis in a swimmer; Osgood-Schlatter disease (traction apophysitis of the tibial tubercle) in a volleyball player; and psychological burnout in any athlete who is pushed too hard. Strategies to combat overuse injuries involve identifying the problem and working with the athlete, parents, and coaches to develop a plan that allows relative rest, corrects biomechanical abnormalities, and improves equipment design and fit. At times it becomes necessary for the team physician to become an advocate for rules changes.

Arthritis

Despite evidence that exercise, when used properly, can become an adjunctive treatment of arthritis, Dexter (1992) reported that only 26 per cent of osteoarthritis patients had been informed of the benefits of exercise by their primary care physician. Exercises should include low loads, low impacts, and high repetitions, with goals being to reverse muscular atrophy, increase periarticular support, and increase intra-articular nutrient diffusion. Controlled repetition effectively stimulates cartilage regeneration and repair without promoting further damage. In view of these observations, Boulware and Byrd (1993) have presented strategies for optimizing exercise programs in arthritic patients.

Exercise programs should be balanced with isometric, isotonic, and aerobic exercises. Isometric exercises at multiple angles promote strength gains without the pain associated with joint movement, whereas aquatic exercises allow movement in a soothing, supportive environment. Rheumatoid arthritis, an inflammatory condition leading to joint hypomobility and destruction, benefits from active and passive range of motion exercises to help maintain or regain joint motion. Osteoarthritic individuals often have more pain in the afternoon; therefore they may tolerate exercise more in the morning. Patients with either rheumatoid arthritis or osteoarthritis may benefit significantly from braces, splints, and modified exercise equipment. Moist heat applied prior to exercise decreases joint fluid viscosity and increases joint capsule compliance. Icing after activity reduces pain and inflammation.

Arguments have been raised as to whether exercise causes osteoarthritis. McKeag (1992) pointed out that no prospective controlled study of the long-term effects of exercise on the musculoskeletal system exists. Such parameters as age, gender, ethnicity, geography, body habitus, bone density, hyperuricemia, hypertension, hypercholesterolemia, and trauma appear to be factors associated with the development of sports-related osteoarthritis. Trauma, whether clinical or subclinical, is a major risk factor, having the ability to change biomechanics adversely. Table 37–11 notes the joints that are more likely to develop osteoarthritis depending on activity.

To date, there has been no conclusive association between running and the development of osteoarthritis in normal individuals. However, there are firm associations between high-impact activities and subsequent osteoarthritis. An example is the association between skydiving and osteoarthritis of the spine.

Asthma

Asthmatics, representing approximately 3 per cent of the general population, benefit from exercise (Afrasiabi and Spector, 1991; Benatar, 1986). Asthmatic athletes can compete in all activities, provided the asthma is controlled.

Precipitating events for asthmatic attacks vary from person to person. Exercise-induced asthma (EIA), also known as exercise-induced bronchospasm, is characterized by transient increases in

TABLE 37–11. SPORTS PARTICIPATION AND ASSOCIATIONS WITH OSTEOARTHRITIS

Sport	Site (Joint)
Ballet	Talus Ankle Cervical spine Hip Knee Metatarsophalangeal
Baseball	Elbow Shoulder
Boxing	Hand (carpometacarpal)
Cricket	Finger
Football (American style)	Ankle Knee Spine
Gymnastics	Elbow Shoulder Wrist Hip
Lacrosse	Ankle Knee
Martial arts	Spine
Parachuting	Ankle Knee Spine
Rugby	Knee
Running	Knee Hip
Skiing (downhill)	Thumb
Soccer	Ankle/foot Cervical spine Hip Knee Talus Talofibular
Weightlifting	Spine
Wrestling	Cervical spine Elbow Knee

From McKeag DB: The relationship of osteoarthritis and exercise. Clin Sports Med. 11:471, 1992, with permission.

airway resistance in response to exercise. EIA has been observed in 10 to 15 per cent of the general population, in 50 per cent of those with allergic rhinitis, and in 80 to 90 per cent of persons with classic asthma (Mellion and Kobayashi, 1992). There are early forms (occurring at the time of exercise) and late forms (occurring up to several hours after the exercise session has been completed) of EIA. The mechanisms involved are not completely understood but are believed to be related to the changes in airway temperature and humidity that accompany ventilatory changes during exercise (Virant, 1992). Accordingly, EIA is noted more with high-intensity sports played in cool, dry environments, examples of which include ice hockey or cross-country skiing. Air pollution, in particular sulfur oxide, appears to exacerbate EIA.

Clinically, patients with EIA notice a cough, chest tightness, wheezing, and shortness of breath with physical exertion (McFadden and Gilber, 1992). By far the most noticeable symptom is cough during or following exertion.

The diagnosis of EIA can be made by demonstrating a 15 per cent decrease in the forced expiratory volume in 1 second (FEV_1) or peak expiratory flow rate (PEFR) or a 20 per cent decrease in the forced expiratory flow at 25 to 75 per cent of forced vital capacity (FEF_{25-75}) or maximum midexpiratory flow (MMEF) after a 3- to 8-minute bout of high-intensity exercise (Kyle et al., 1992). Flow measurements should be made prior to the exercise bout, immediately after exercise, and every 5 minutes thereafter for 30 minutes. Any associated changes should be reversible with use of an inhaled β-adrenergic agonist (McFadden and Gilber, 1992). Alternatively, it may be beneficial to undertake a therapeutic trial of inhaled β-agonist prior to exercise and watch for results empirically.

Treatment of EIA can be either nonpharmacologic or pharmacologic (Mahler, 1993). Nonpharmacologic treatment can be as simple as altering the type of exercise. Swimming, for instance, is performed in a warm, humid environment; therefore swimmers are more tolerant of EIA. Additionally, sports that require short bursts of activity, such as volleyball, may better suit the athlete with EIA. Another nonpharmacologic treatment utilizes the refractory period, a period characterized by attenuated bronchospastic responsiveness. Present in approximately 50 per cent of athletes with EIA, the refractory period begins about 20 minutes after exercise and continues for 4 to 6 hours. By performing high-intensity, short-duration warm-ups 30 minutes prior to practice or competition, athletes may be able to perform drug-free during this refractory period. Because of the refractory period, their performance is not affected by an exercise-induced bronchospastic event.

β-Adrenergic agonists are at the center of pharmacologic treatment of EIA (Grindel and McKeag, 1992; Morton and Fitch, 1992). Agents inhaled 30 minutes prior to exercise are not only efficacious but are accepted by all athletic governing bodies. If necessary, theophylline, cromolyn sodium, anticholinergics, terfenadine or astemizole, and calcium antagonists may be employed. Although inhaled corticosteroids are being recommended more for the treatment of asthma, their exact role in the treatment of EIA is incompletely understood. At this time, inhaled corticosteroids are recommended for the stabilization of classic asthma only.

Diabetes Mellitus

Type I diabetes mellitus (DM) is an autoimmune disorder resulting in absolute insulin deficiency and affecting 1 in 500 children under age 18. Type II DM, on the other hand, consists of insulin resistance and relative hyperinsulinemia. Between 10 million and 20 million adults suffer from type II DM, which has strong associations with obesity and family history (Landry and Allen, 1992). Aerobic exercise has been shown to potentiate hypoglycemic effects of both endogenous and exogenous insulin.

Insulin-dependent diabetics may participate in high-intensity exercise, provided precautions are taken to prevent hypo- and hyperglycemia. Prior to exercise, blood glucose levels and urinary ketones should be monitored. Elevation of blood glucose or urinary ketones at this time should lead to a postponement of the exercise session to avoid the possibility of severe hyperglycemia, ketosis, and dehydration during exercise. Exercise leads to vasodilation, resulting in an increased rate of insulin absorption. The latter is seen most often when insulin is injected at sites on exercising limbs. Therefore the abdomen is the preferred injection site in active diabetics. Postexercise hypoglycemia may result after intense exercise, which depletes glycogen stores, and can occur if blood glucose levels rise without a titrated supply of insulin. Thus care should be taken during the postexercise period as well as during the exercise period.

Type II diabetics benefit from the fact that exercise enhances insulin binding and reduces obesity. The net effect is to minimize or eliminate the need for hypoglycemic agents or even exogenous insulin.

Care should be taken when recommending exercise to diabetic patients, as many have concomitant diseases that limit exercise capacity. Special topics such as foot care, eye protection, and skin care should be undertaken at the onset of an exercise program and at regular intervals. Additionally, the physician should be cognizant of the fact that diabetics are more likely to demonstrate silent ischemia, prompting some to obtain graded-exercise treadmills prior to initiation of an exercise program and at regular intervals. Weight lifting with moderate resistance and increased repetitions is safe provided there is no retinopathy. Physically active diabetics should be empowered with glucose self-monitoring and diet and insulin education.

Elderly Individuals

Physical activity by elderly patients promotes many physiologic changes that increase quality of life, including increased work capacity, flexibility, strength, coordination, and mental outlook (Barry et al., 1993). Other changes may also lead to increased life expectancy. Such changes include decreased total cholesterol, increased high density lipoprotein, increased bone density, and increased insulin receptors. Increased strength and flexibility can significantly increase a patient's independence (Fiatarone et al., 1990).

Despite the benefits of exercise, elderly patients should use caution when embarking on or changing an exercise routine. Elderly patients have decreased blood volume and blunted baroreceptor reflexes, so they may be susceptible to orthostasis. Many elderly individuals must modify their programs to accommodate existing diseases. In addition, certain drugs modify and possibly limit normal responses to exercise. Examples include the blunted heart rate response while on β-blockers or calcium channel blockers, heat intolerance while taking phenothiazines, and hypotension from diuretics, vasodilators, antidepressants, sedative hypnotics, and nitroglycerin (Rousseau, 1991).

Epilepsy

Well controlled epileptic patients may safely participate in sports. High-velocity and high-contact sports should take into consideration frequency, time, and type of seizures, as well as level of control. Children or adolescents with frequent daytime seizures or psychomotor seizures should not participate in contact sports.

The issue of swimming remains unresolved. Decisions must be based on the level of supervision and the frequency and control of seizures. By increasing arterial pH, hyperventilation lowers the seizures threshold, and the practice of intentional hyperventilation prior to competition should be used cautiously, if at all, by swimmers with epilepsy.

All athletes on antiseizure medications should have levels checked often to ensure that they remain in the normal range. This safeguard is particularly important in rapidly growing children.

Female Individuals

The traditional view of athletes being male has changed dramatically. Female athletes are now competing successfully at all levels. Additionally, women are remaining active through their reproductive years and well past menopause. With changing patterns in participation, it has become clear that female athletes differ substantially from their male counterparts.

Prior to puberty, little difference exists between the male and female athlete. After puberty the male athlete, under the influence of male sex hormones, becomes larger and stronger. The female athlete is affected by puberty as well. It has been observed that girls undertaking strenuous, high-intensity exercise experience delayed onset of menarche and an increased incidence of secondary amenorrhea. Physiologically, amenorrheic athletes demonstrate a decreased luteinizing hormone

(LH) surge at midcycle as a result of decreases in gonadotropin-releasing hormone (GnRH) pulse generation at the hypothalamus. They also demonstrate less peripheral aromatization of dihydroepiandrosterone. Eumenorrhea can often be reestablished by subtle alterations in the exercise and diet regimens. Alternatively, hormone replacement therapy may be beneficial. It is important to educate these athletes, informing them that although the amenorrheic state may be convenient it represents an estrogen-deficient state, placing them at significantly increased risk for poor bone mineral accretion and stress fractures. Keep in mind that exercise-induced amenorrhea is a diagnosis of exclusion, and other causes of amenorrhea, including pregnancy, must be ruled out.

Since the early 1980s there has been a trend for pregnant women to remain active. The physiologic changes of pregnancy lead to enhanced maternal blood volume, oxygen consumption, heart rate, stroke volume, and uterine blood flow. At the same time there are decreases in peripheral resistance and physical work capacity. Maternal metabolism is increased, but the ability to eliminate excess heat is reduced. Current studies to determine the risks and benefits of exercise on the mother and fetus are ongoing, and most investigators have shown that moderate exercise does not alter outcome. Clapp and Dickstein (1984) demonstrated that exercising women gained less weight, delivered earlier, and had lighter offspring, none of which adversely affected the mother or the infant. Pregnant athletes should be advised to adjust exercise programs for fatigue, joint or ligament pain, nausea, and vomiting. The latter can lead to dehydration, which in turn can exacerbate heat intolerance and compromise uterine blood flow. Pregnant athletes should stop the exercise session if they experience pain, vaginal bleeding, shortness of breath, palpitations, rupture of membranes, regular uterine contractions, or dizziness. Scuba diving and high-velocity sports such as competitive bicycling should be avoided (Clapp et al., 1992) throughout the pregnancy, and supine activities should be avoided during the third trimester. In 1994, the American College of Obstetrics and Gynecology updated their recommendations for exercise during pregnancy and postpartum (ACOG, 1994). These recommendations are incorporated into Table 37–12.

Exercising women benefit from continuing exercise into the postmenopausal years. Weight-bearing exercise has been shown to have positive effects on bone metabolism, and exercise in general has favorably affected body composition, muscle strength, cardiovascular risk, and mental health (Shangold, 1990).

Hypertension

Hypertension affects 58 million adults and is a proved risk factor for cardiovascular mortality (Tanji, 1992). Physically active individuals, including athletes, are not immune; however, exercise plays a pivotal role in the nonpharmacologic treatment of essential hypertension.

Several mechanisms have been proposed to account for the success of exercise in the treatment of stage I hypertension. Reduction in catecholamines and associated adrenergic tone have been cited by some authors (Duncan et al., 1985; Hagberg et al., 1989). The *insulin hypothesis,* initially proposed by Krotkiewski et al. (1979) and later refined by Kaplan (1989) as the *deadly quartet,* notes the relation of obesity, hypertension, type II diabetes, and hypertriglyceridemia. Exercise has been shown to control each aspect of the quartet. Body composition alterations, including weight loss, have been shown to lower blood pressure. Other proposed mechanisms include attenuation of arterial baroreceptors, release of endogenous opioids, and alteration of systemic vascular resistance.

The American College of Sports Medicine (1990) recommended aerobic exercise at a frequency of three to five times per week for a duration of 15 to 60 minutes per session at an intensity of 55 to 90 per cent of maximal heart rate. This recommendation should be tailored to the individual's abilities and goals. In unfit and debilitated individuals, lower intensities of exercise for shorter durations can prove beneficial.

When medications must be used, note that antihypertensive medications such as β-blockers and calcium channel blockers blunt the heart rate response. In such cases, patients should be instructed on the use of perceived exertion to monitor exercise sessions. Diuretics may lead to hypokalemia and dehydration in active individuals and thus may not be good first-line antihypertensive agents. Angiotensin-converting enzyme (ACE) inhibitors and peripheral α-blockers such as prazocin and doxazocin carry few side effects and are excellent choices as first-line antihypertensive agents in active individuals.

Human Immunodeficiency Virus

The Centers for Disease Control estimates that there are between 1.0 million and 1.5 million HIV carriers in the United States. Six per cent of these cases are spread through heterosexual contact, although this percentage is increasing rapidly. HIV is present in low concentrations in tears, saliva, sputum, and urine; it is not found in sweat. Unfortunately, HIV is found in high concentrations in the blood of actively infected individuals.

So far, there has been no known transmission of HIV in the athletic setting; however, the fact that acquired immunodeficiency syndrome (AIDS) is now the second and fourth leading causes of death in males and females 25 to 44 years old, respectively, and that AIDs has no known cure has led

TABLE 37–12. AMERICAN COLLEGE OF OBSTETRICIANS AND GYNECOLOGISTS' GUIDELINES FOR EXERCISE DURING PREGNANCY AND POSTPARTUM

EXERCISE GUIDELINES. The following guidelines are based on the unique physical and physiological conditions that exist during pregnancy and the postpartum period. They outline general criteria for safety to provide direction to patients who are developing home exercise programs.

Contraindications to exercise during pregnancy
1. Pregnancy-induced hypertension
2. Preterm rupture of membranes
3. Preterm labor during the prior or current pregnancy, or both
4. Incompetent cervix/cerclage
5. Persistent second- or third-trimester bleeding
6. Intrauterine growth retardation

Exercise Guidelines
1. During pregnancy, women can continue to exercise and derive health benefits even from mild-to-moderate exercise routines. Regular exercise (at least three times per week) is preferable to intermittent activity.
2. Women should avoid exercise in the supine position after the first trimester. Such a position is associated with decreased cardiac output in most pregnant women; because the remaining cardiac output will be preferentially distributed away from splanchnic beds (including the uterus) during vigorous exercise, such regimens are best avoided during pregnancy. Prolonged periods of motionless standing should also be avoided.
3. Women should be aware of the decreased oxygen available for aerobic exercise during pregnancy. They should be encouraged to modify the intensity of their exercises according to maternal symptoms. Pregnant women should stop exercising when fatigued and not exercise to exhaustion. Weight-bearing exercise may under some circumstances be continued at intensities similar to those prior to pregnancy throughout pregnancy. Non-weight-bearing exercises such as cycling or swimming will minimize the risk of injury and facilitate the continuation of exercise during pregnancy.
4. Morphologic changes in pregnancy should serve a relative contraindication to types of exercise in which loss of balance should be detrimental to maternal or fetal well-being, especially in the third trimester. Further, any type of exercise involving the potential for even mild abdominal trauma should be avoided.
5. Pregnancy requires an additional 300 Kcal/d of energy to maintain metabolic hemeostasis. Thus, women who exercise during pregnancy should be particularly careful to ensure an adequate diet.
6. Pregnant women who exercise in the first trimester should augment heat dissipation by ensuring adequate hydration, appropriate clothing, and optimal environmental surroundings during exercise.
7. Many of the physiologic and morphologic changes of pregnancy last 4–6 weeks postpartum. Thus, prepregnancy exercise routines should be resumed gradually based on a woman's physical capability.

Adapted from The American College of Obstetricians and Gynecologists: Exercise During Pregnancy and the Postpartum Period. ACOG Technical Bulletin no. 189, Washington DC, © 1994, with permission.

to serious consideration regarding precautions in sport. Currently, each athlete should be considered a possible carrier, with universal precautions employed in the locker room and on the playing field. Players with open wounds should be removed from practice or competition until bleeding is controlled and the wound is occluded. Team physicians should instruct coaches and trainers on the current state of precautions, and gloves should be readily available at all times. A system for disposal of biohazardous waste should be in place and followed. Keeping in mind that the locker room is an extension of the workplace, current recommendations can be obtained from the Occupational Safety and Health Administration (OSHA) and the Centers for Disease Control and Prevention.

Finally, as many athletes are young and possibly promiscuous, it is advisable that regular team meetings be arranged. At these meetings the team physician can bring athletes, coaches, trainers, and even parents up to date on the current state of research, treatment, and prevention based on the rapidly changing information regarding this disease.

The effects of exercise on HIV patient outcome has been studied, and results have been favorable. Lapierre et al. (1990) reported that HIV patients who exercised demonstrated decreased levels of anxiety and depression while temporarily increasing natural killer cell activity. Rigsby et al. (1992) found that resistance and aerobic training significantly increased strength and cardiorespiratory fitness, but CD4 and CD8 cell counts were not significantly affected.

Physically Challenged Athlete

Spinal cord injury (SCI) below the first thoracic vertebra defines the condition of paraplegia (Davis, 1993). The physiologic sequelae include impaired motor function, poor bowel and bladder control, bone and muscle atrophy, decreased myocardial function, and vocational, marital, and social disharmony. As recently as World War II, 80 per cent of SCI patients died within 2 weeks of injury. Now, life expectancy may exceed 30 years, and paraplegic athletes have enjoyed improved access and increasing opportunities to engage in physical activity.

The level of spinal trauma dictates the tissues involved. In general, the higher the level of injury, the greater the disability and more somatic and autonomic dysfunction. When the injury is below T4, normal regulation of cardiac function is maintained. Higher level lesions disrupt sympathetic tone, resulting in lowered maximal heart rates, stroke volumes, and active muscle mass.

Advances in equipment have played a role in advancing our understanding of the physiology of SCIs. It is now possible to perform meaningful fitness testing and monitor the progression of fitness programs in paraplegic patients. It has been observed that elite wheelchair athletes attain cardiorespiratory fitness levels comparable to those of sedentary, nondisabled individuals despite having markedly smaller muscle mass available for exercise and reduced peak cardiac output. Wheelchair athletes also demonstrate cardiovascular drift, a condition in which the heart rate rises slowly after 20 minutes of continuous exercise.

Quadriplegia results when SCI occurs above T1. Quadriplegic athletes experience significantly greater loss of sympathetic and autonomic control than do paraplegic athletes (Figoni, 1993). There is a great challenge to find activities that exercise functioning muscles and stimulate motivation.

SOFT TISSUE INJURY AND REHABILITATION

Soft tissue injuries as they relate to sports medicine involve muscle–tendon units, ligaments, articular cartilage, and bursae. The injuries may be acute or chronic.

Acute Injury

Blunt force trauma to a muscle–tendon unit produces a *contusion,* defined as a crush injury that leads to a variable degree of muscle cell disruption and hematoma formation. Acutely, the athlete experiences pain, swelling, and dysfunction. Sequelae of contusions may include hematoma formation, scarring, inflexibility, weakness, and myositis ossificans. Contusions are treated with ice, compression, and elevation. The muscle should be rested in an elongated position. Return to play can be expected when the athlete regains full range of motion, equal strength, and agility.

Muscle–tendon units can also be acutely disrupted via tearing of the muscle, tendon, or muscle–tendon interface. Power for the tearing is supplied by the muscle actively contracting in an attempt to shorten or to resist lengthening. Such tears, or strains, are graded from first degree through third degree based on the extent of tissue damage, swelling, pain, and dysfunction. First-degree strains entail minimal cellular damage. Clinically, there is mild pain and stiffness. The athlete may be able to perform tasks but at a slightly lower level. Second-degree strains have moderate amounts of cellular damage with bleeding into the soft tissue spaces. There is mild to moderate ecchymosis, soft tissue swelling and tenderness, and

weakness. Palpation of the affected area may also reveal a focal muscle–tendon defect. The athlete has difficulty performing and may have difficulty bearing weight. A third degree strain is the most severe form and implies complete rupture of the muscle–tendon unit. Third degree strains are often preceded by first and second degree strains, which weaken the muscle–tendon unit. Strains are treated with ice, rest, compression, and elevation. Weight-bearing is as tolerated, with criteria for return to play being similar to those outlined for contusions, above.

An example of an acute third degree strain is the Achilles tendon rupture. The Achilles tendon, also known as the calcaneal tendon, is the common tendon of both the gastrocnemius and soleus muscles and is considered the strongest tendon in the body. With forced dorsiflexion of the foot against contracted soleus and gastrocnemius muscles, the Achilles tendon undergoes sudden strain and may rupture. Typically, rupture occurs approximately 4.5 cm proximal to the tendon's insertion onto the calcaneus. It is in the area of relative avascularity, and the poor blood supply is thought to predispose the tendon to injury in this area. Other conditions that may contribute to Achilles tendon rupture are pre-existing tendinitis, prior steroid injections, and shear stresses between the gastrocnemius and soleus tendons (Singer and Jones, 1986).

The diagnosis of Achilles tendon rupture is based on a history of a sudden "pop" in the area, local swelling and bruising, and weak push-off. The physical examination demonstrates a palpable tendon defect, tenderness, and a positive Thompson test (Fig. 37–2). The Thompson test is positive when the gastrocnemius muscle belly is firmly squeezed and the foot does not plantar-flex.

Treatment of Achilles tendon rupture may be surgical or conservative, with the objective being to restore the tendon to normal length and strength. Nonoperative treatment entails 3 weeks of cast immobilization with the knee flexed and the foot positioned in equinus, followed by another 8 weeks of short leg cast immobilization in equinus. Advocates for surgical treatment of Achilles tendon ruptures note that although the total recovery time is not significantly different between surgical and nonsurgical patients, some studies have noted lower reinjury rates in those treated surgically. This difference has not been demonstrated conclusively.

Acute ligament injuries result from tearing of the ligament substance fibers and are referred to as *sprains.* These injuries are graded from first degree through third degree based on the extent of pain, swelling, number of ligaments involved, and resultant joint instability. First degree sprains involve only one ligamentous structure and have no joint instability, whereas third degree sprains involve multiple ligamentous structures with resultant joint instability. Third degree sprains may rep-

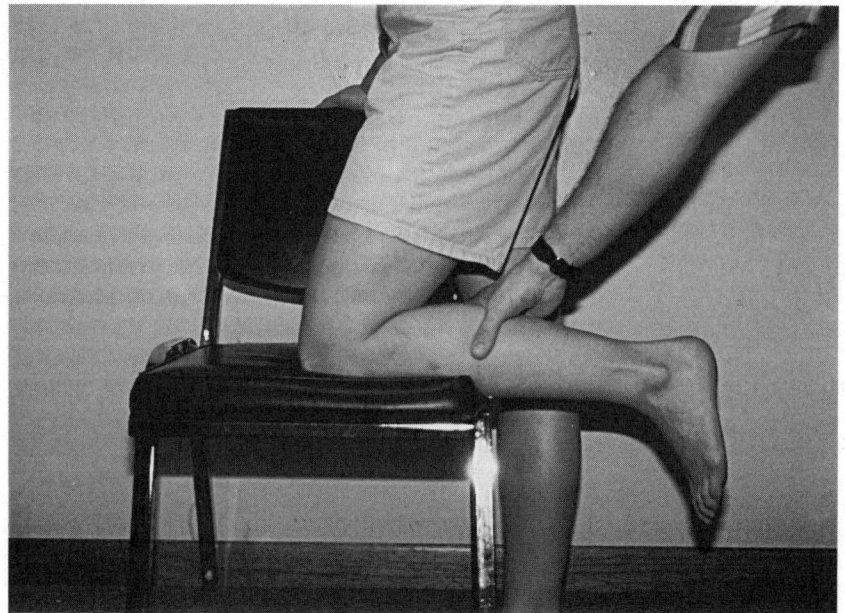

FIGURE 37–2. Thompson Test. Position patient so that heel cord is relaxed. Note position of foot. Grasp gastrocnemius muscle belly and squeeze firmly. Plantar flexion of foot indicates an intact Achilles tendon and is considered a negative Thompson test. Lack of plantar flexion indicates a complete Achilles tendon disruption and is considered a positive Thompson test.

resent complete ligament disruption and warrant more aggressive treatment to minimize chronic instability and dysfunction. Treatment of first and second degree sprains involves icing, splinting, compression, and relative rest. Weight-bearing is as tolerated. Third degree sprains can be treated with non-weight-bearing crutches, splinting, and temporary immobilization. Third-degree sprains can lead to chronic instability characterized by pain, swelling, and giving way; and they may require surgical reconstruction if initial conservative measures fail.

Acute injuries to bursae result in *traumatic bursitis,* a painful condition that involves swelling, tenderness, and warmth over the bursa. Swelling in the olecranon and prepatellar bursae can be impressive. Treatments of choice are aspiration, compression dressings, and protection. Corticosteroid injections into recurrent, sterile bursae can be rewarding. One must take care to differentiate traumatic bursitis from septic bursitis. Both septic and chronic forms of bursitis are best treated by excision.

Chronic Injury

Overuse injuries (Table 37–13) result from chronic, repetitive trauma with insufficient opportunity for healing between exercise sessions. The overuse itself can result from training errors, such as too much exercise, insufficient rest, inappropriate surfaces, or poor equipment. At times the athlete's own makeup contributes to the condition via poor flexibility, exercise addiction, or anatomic factors, all leading to biomechanical abnormalities.

Overuse of soft tissues results in microtrauma,

with the end result being chronic or acute muscle strain, tendonitis, ligamentitis, or chondromalacia. Tendons, ligaments, and articular cartilage are more susceptible to overuse injury because of their inherent lack of direct circulation, altered pH, low cell density, and low metabolic activity. Simply put, these tissues are made to be not injured; and once injury has occurred, they are slow to repair.

As a living entity, bone is subject to overuse injury. Immature bone can exhibit overuse at the growth plates. This injury is referred to as *apophysitis* and carries a host of eponyms, one of the most common being tibial tubercle apophysitis, also known as Osgood-Schlatter disease. Stress fractures are microfractures of bone resulting from chronic, repetitive stress and insufficient recovery. This combination inhibits the normal remodeling process. Stress fractures occur almost exclusively in weight-bearing bones of the spine, pelvis, and lower extremities (Fig. 37–3) and may precede complete fractures (McKeag, 1991). Stress fractures are more than 10 times commoner in female athletes, especially those individuals with inadequate diets or menstrual dysfunction. As a chronic process, stress fractures may require 2 weeks to visualize on plain film radiographs, as detection is not based on the fracture. Rather, visualization is based on the bone's sclerotic reaction. A high index of suspicion facilitates early detection. When plain film radiographs are negative and a stress fracture is strongly suspected, one should obtain a triple-phase bone scan. Triple-phase technetium phosphate bone scans have the ability to detect stress fractures at an early stage but at the expense of relatively high doses of radiation. An alternative method uses high-frequency ultrasound to vibrate the bone. When a stress fracture is present, the

TABLE 37–13. MUSCULOSKELETAL OVERUSE INJURIES: A CLINICAL GUIDE

Grade	History	Physical Examination	Pathophysiology	Diagnostic Aids	Treatment	Considerations
1	Transient pain after activity, usually lasts a few hours; soreness; duration of symptoms <2 weeks	Generalized tenderness	Increased lactic acid, muscle breakdown, minor inflammation	None	Ice if needed	Training regimen, new athlete, getting in shape
2	Longer-lasting pain late in activity or immediately after; duration of symptoms 2–3 weeks	Localized pain, but no discrete point tenderness	Mild musculotendinous inflammation	None	Ice, reduce training 10–25%	True overuse injury, wrong environment, wrong equipment, poor technique
3	Pain in beginning or middle of activity (getting closer to the start of activity); duration of symptoms 3–4 weeks	Point tenderness, percussion tenderness, pressure elsewhere produces pain at point, other evidence of inflammation (heat, erythema, swelling, crepitation)	Major musculotendinous inflammation, periostitis, bone microtrauma	Radiographs, bone scan is positive 75% of the time	Ice, reduce training 25–75%, initial rest period 5–7 days with concurrent nonsteroidal anti-inflammatory medication	"Prestress" fracture syndrome
4	Pain before or early in exercise, preventing or affecting performance; duration of symptoms >4 weeks	Same as grade 3, plus disturbance in function, decreased range of motion, muscle atrophy	Breakdown in soft tissue, stress fracture, compartment syndrome (especially if swelling is major finding)	Radiographs, bone scan is positive 95% of the time	Ice, rest from exercise, nonsteroidal anti-inflammatory medication	Immobilization (usually not necessary)

From McKeag DB: The concept of overuse. The primary care aspects of overuse syndromes in sports. Prim Care 11(1):43, 1984, with permission.

bone vibration increases, causing pain as the probe glides over the fracture site.

Treatment

Treatment of soft tissue injuries begins with prevention through education of coaches and athletes about proper training techniques, equipment, surfaces, and rules. Rest, absolute or relative, must be intentionally built into the schedule. Once an injury has occurred and is identified, the athlete should receive acute care and undergo rehabilitation with the goals of limiting pain, swelling, and total body detraining. Return of function involves restoration of full motion, strength, endurance, and proprioception. These goals are best accomplished by protecting involved areas with splints, braces, casts, or crutches, relative rest, ice, compression, elevation, and analgesic drugs. Though commonly employed, short-term use of anti-inflammatory agents has not been shown superior to simple analgesic agents. Physical therapy modalities may begin immediately, with more aggressive rehabilitation complementing the patient's condition, clinical course, and goals.

Patients may safely return to protected activities while continuing therapy. It is only after patients have regained full motion, strength, endurance, and proprioception that they should return to full, unrestricted activities.

Prevention

Prevention and rehabilitation of soft tissue injuries has traditionally included providing a foundation of strength and flexibility. The muscle–tendon unit is considered to possess viscoelastic properties that not only store and transmit energy but also "flow" to elongate and increase joint range of motion (Taylor and Dalton, 1990). Anderson and Burke (1991) proposed that increasing flexibility could provide injury prevention, reduce muscle soreness, enhance skill development, and promote muscle relaxation. Several studies have challenged the effectiveness of routine stretching to prevent injury and muscle soreness (Brunet et al., 1990; Smith et al., 1993; Van Mechelen, 1992; Van Mechelen et al., 1993); however, routine stretching continues to be recommended based on anecdotal cases and clinical experience. More studies are required to further delineate the precise role for stretching, particularly for runners (Knapik et al., 1992).

The amount of elongation obtained by stretching

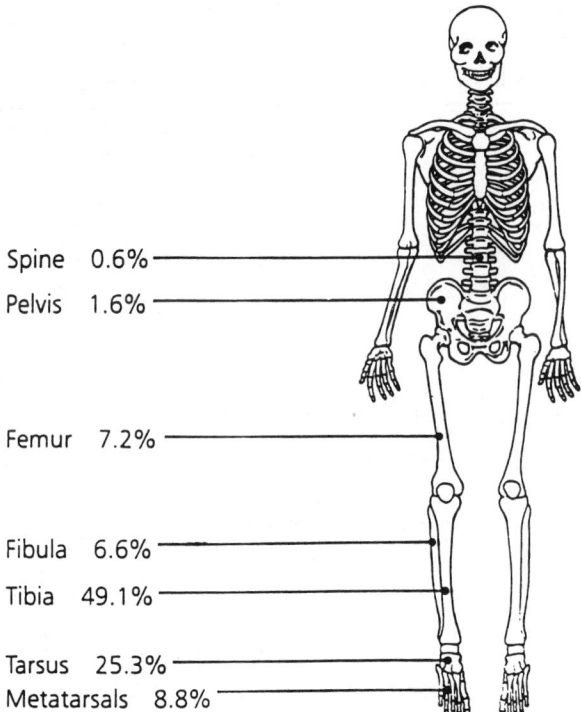

Spine 0.6%
Pelvis 1.6%
Femur 7.2%
Fibula 6.6%
Tibia 49.1%
Tarsus 25.3%
Metatarsals 8.8%

FIGURE 37–3. Locations of stress fractures in athletes. (From Matheson GO, Macintyre JG, Taunton JE, et al: Stress fractures in athletes: A study of 320 cases. Am J Sports Med 15(1):46, 1987, with permission.)

the muscle–tendon unit appears to be inversely related to the rate of stretch and directly related to the temperature of the tissue. Currently, the authors recommend a period of low-level activity that produces a light sweat. Activity should involve muscle groups to be used during sports participation or work. The presence of sweat indicates a rise in core temperature, increasing compliance of the muscle–tendon unit. The stretching exercises are then performed with slow, purposeful movements held at the end-range of motion for approximately 30 seconds. Each exercise is repeated two to four times. The athlete/worker then participates in their own particular activity with additional stretching after periods of rest (i.e., after half-time or being on the bench) and at the end of the practice session/game/work day. An excellent manual of basic stretching techniques for use by patients has been presented by Anderson (1980).

ATHLETIC NUTRITION

Elite and recreational runners alike benefit from sound nutritional practices. The focus should be to maintain or increase lean body mass and decrease total body fat in order to improve strength, endurance, and biomechanical performances. Balanced nutrition allows optimum performance during and recovery after exercise sessions by providing

proper amounts of water and nutrients at appropriate times. In general, these goals can be met by consuming a well balanced diet consisting of 60 to 70 per cent carbohydrates, 20 to 25 per cent fats, and 10 to 15 per cent proteins (Holt, 1993).

Food as Energy

Carbohydrates, fats, and proteins can all provide energy to the system; however, carbohydrates and fats provide the most usable energy during exercise. Carbohydrates in the form of blood glucose and hepatic and muscular glycogen stores provide relatively more energy during the early phases of exercise and during high-intensity, short-duration events. During long-duration, low-intensity activity, free fatty acids are preferentially used as an energy source. Although training does not alter fuel used by muscle, training does result in more efficient storage, retrieval, and utilization of substrates (Holt, 1993).

Carbohydrates are classified as simple or complex based on the complexity of the molecule. Complex carbohydrates must be broken down into simple units prior to utilization, providing slower, more predictable changes in blood glucose. High-carbohydrate diets increase glycogen stores and decrease recovery times.

Carbohydrate loading entails ingestion of a higher than usual carbohydrate diet. Classically, such loading would follow a period of carbohydrate depletion; however, classic carbohydrate loading can lead to nausea, vomiting, diarrhea, and bloating. Because each of these symptoms adversely affects performance and because carbohydrate loading offers no performance gains over continuous ingestion of a high-carbohydrate diet, classic carbohydrate loading is not recommended. Instead, the athlete is encouraged to taper exercise sessions and increase slightly the amount and percentage of carbohydrates ingested during the days or week prior to competition. It should be noted that high-carbohydrate diets are recommended for all athletes. If considered at all, carbohydrate loading is recommended for endurance athletes only and has no proved benefit in pure power sports.

With the ability to provide energy at 9 kcal/kg and a seemingly endless source of storage, fat provides a large amount of energy needs. Fat is utilized in the form of free fatty acids. However, fat must be retrieved from storage in adipose tissue, a process requiring time and oxygen. Therefore fat is utilized for energy in low to moderate level activities.

Proteins do not contribute significantly to short-term energy expenditure; proteins do contribute up to 10 per cent of energy during exercise sessions lasting over 2 hours. Such energy is provided when protein is transformed into glucose through gluconeogenesis. Proteins also provide essential amino acids necessary for muscle protein synthesis. The current U.S. recommended daily allowance (RDA) for protein is 0.8 gm/kg per day, but exact amounts of protein necessary for intensely trained athletes are unknown. Most research suggests that athletes undergoing intensive training benefit with up to 1.8 to 2.0 gm/kg per day. With the average American diet providing 1.5 gm/kg per day and the average athlete ingesting more than 2.0 gm/kg per day, protein supplements are not considered necessary unless nutritional practices are deficient (Mitchell et al., 1993).

Vitamins

Despite widespread practice, there appears to be no advantage for megavitamin replacement when compared to ingestion of a balanced diet (Singh et al., 1992). In fact, high-dose replacements may be harmful. Athletes on restricted diets benefit from replacement of specific deficiencies.

Fluids

Dehydration, or more properly hypohydration, is the condition of depleted body water. It may occur in hot or cold climates and is exacerbated by high-intensity activities and limited access to fluids. With sweat losses ranging from 1.5 to 3.0 liters per hour during heavy activity and increased insensible losses through increased ventilation, fluid intake is clearly important. As little as 2 per cent dehydration can result in impaired thermoregulation. Higher degrees of dehydration lead to progressively more dysfunction. Athletes often rely on thirst as an indicator for more fluids, but thirst often lags behind fluid needs (Greenleaf, 1992). Gisolfi and Duchman (1992) urged athletes to enter an event well hydrated and have provided guidelines for fluid replacement. For events lasting less than 1 hour, 300 to 500 ml of carbohydrate (CHO) beverage is recommended 0 to 15 minutes before the event and cool water as needed during the event. For events of 1 to 3 hours' duration, 300 to 500 ml of water should be ingested before the event followed by 800 to 1600 ml of a 6 to 8% CHO solution per hour (30 to 60 gm of CHO per hour) during the event. The addition of carbohydrates to the intraevent fluids provides a readily available energy source, and solutions containing up to 8% CHO do not alter fluid absorption. More concentrated forms rapidly lead to nausea, vomiting, diarrhea, and dehydration—all culminating in decreased performance. When the event planned is longer than 3 hours' duration, Gisolfi and Duchman recommend that the event fluid contain 6 to 8% CHO and 20 to 30 mEq sodium and be consumed at a rate of 500 to 1000 ml per hour. Sodium is added to fluids during long-duration events in order to replace sweat losses and as a guard against dilutional hyponatremia. During exercise, it is recommended that all fluids be consumed in frequent, small aliquots rather than all at once.

After events lasting more than 1 hour, recovery fluids should include 5 to 10% CHO with 30 to 40 mEq sodium. To optimize recovery, immediately after exercise the endurance athlete should ingest 0.35 to 1.50 gm CHO/kg body weight, followed by similar amounts at frequent intervals (Sherman, 1992). The timing of CHO ingestion is important, as residual increases in enzymatic activity leave the body more receptive to glycogen regeneration.

Because of the potential for dehydration during practice and gastrointestinal upset during initial exposure to any new hydration strategies, athletes are urged to make adjustments gradually during practice sessions.

ENVIRONMENTAL FACTORS IN SPORTS

Temperature

Homeostasis

Heat can be provided via internal (thermogenesis) and external means. Internally, heat is a by-product of metabolic reactions, which are only 25 per cent efficient. The core structures, including internal organs and deep muscles, produce 70 per cent of total body heat (Moss, 1986). Basal production, or the metabolic activity present when the body is at rest, is about 87 kcal per hour but is capable of increasing 20 to 25 times that level during periods of intense activity. External heat production is acquired passively through clothing, external heat sources, and the environment. Examples of the latter two factors include heaters and the sun.

Conservation

Body temperature can be conserved by superficial vasoconstriction, body insulation, and external measures. Superficial vasoconstriction shunts blood away from the skin and extremities, where heat is lost to the environment. Shunting maintains warm blood flow to the vital organs for as long as possible. The body insulation includes body fat and body hair. Both provide barriers to passive heat loss. External measures include proper clothing, campfires, warm foods and drink, and close body contact. These measures are highly refinable.

Elimination

In situations in which the body acquires too much heat, the body can utilize several mechanisms to eliminate excess heat. These mechanisms—radiation, conduction, convection, evaporation, and respiration—may lead to hypothermia

TABLE 37–14. WIND-CHILL INDEX (EQUIVALENT IN COOLING POWER ON EXPOSED FLESH)

Wind Speed* (mph)	Air Temperature (°F)																
	35	30	25	20	15	10	5	0	−5	−10	−15	−20	−25	−30	−35	−40	−45
4	35	30	25	20	15	10	5	0	−5	−10	−15	−20	−25	−30	−35	−40	−45
5	32	27	22	16	11	6	0	−5	−10	−15	−21	−26	−31	−36	−42	−47	−52
10	22	16	10	3	−3	−9	−15	−22	−27	−34	−40	−46	−52	−58	−64	−71	−77
15	16	9	2	−5	−11	−18	−25	−31	−38	−45	−51	−58	−65	−72	−78	−85	−92
20	12	4	−3	−10	−17	−24	−31	−39	−46	−53	−60	−67	−74	−81	−88	−95	−103
25	8	1	−7	−15	−22	−29	−36	−44	−51	−59	−66	−74	−81	−88	−96	−103	−110
30	6	−2	−10	−18	−25	−33	−41	−49	−56	−64	−71	−79	−86	−93	−101	−109	−116
35	4	−4	−12	−20	−27	−35	−43	−52	−58	−67	−74	−82	−89	−97	−105	−113	−120
40	3	−5	−13	−21	−29	−37	−45	−53	−60	−69	−76	−84	−92	−100	−107	−115	−123
45	2	−6	−14	−22	−30	−38	−46	−54	−62	−70	−78	−85	−93	−102	−109	−117	−125

* Wind speeds greater than 40 mph have little additional cooling effect. Example: A 30 mph wind, combined with a temperature of 30°F (−1° C), can have the same chilling effect as a temperature of −2° F (−19° C) when it is calm.

From U.S. Department of Commerce. National Oceanic and Atmospheric Administration.

if unchecked (Fritz and Perrin, 1989). The loss of heat by infrared rays to an object that is not in contact with the body is termed *radiation*. Radiation is normally the most significant form of heat loss, accounting for 50 to 75 per cent of heat loss. Conduction, the transfer of heat or cold by direct contact with an object, demonstrates a rate of heat transfer that is directly proportional to the temperature gradients and types of material. Denser materials, such as water or metal, are more efficient conductors. For instance, wet clothing conducts heat five times faster than dry clothing. Water immersion can increased heat loss 25 times. Convection involves the movement of air or water over the skin. This constant movement of wind or water greatly increases heat loss (Table 37–14). Typified by the sweating mechanism and respiration, evaporation is the body's major physiologic defense against overheating. Factors that modify evaporation include skin exposure, temperature, humidity, and convection. Finally, respiration involves the loss of heated air from the lungs or the inhalation of hot or cold air by the lungs via breathing. It utilizes evaporation and convection at the same time and is modified by mouth breathing, tachypnea, and dry environment.

Regulation

Normal body core temperature is 98.6° F (37° C). Variance is regulated at the hypothalamus, with the anterior hypothalamus monitoring heat loss and the posterior hypothalamus initiating conservatory responses.

Cold Injuries

Chilbains and Trenchfoot

Chilbains and trenchfoot are similar conditions that affect different body parts. Chilbains is a neurocirculatory skin disturbance that occurs most often on the feet, fingers, and ears when skin is exposed to cool temperatures and high humidity. Trenchfoot, also called immersion foot, follows prolonged exposure to temperatures of 0° to 10° C while feet are wet (Frey, 1992). Superficial capillary damage progresses to necrosis or gangrene of skin, muscle, and nerves. Symptoms include numbness, tingling, and burning. The skin is mottled, pale, and waxy. Treatment focuses on removal of wet clothing, cleaning and drying the area, and rapidly rewarming the tissues. Re-exposure should be prevented when possible (Dembert, 1982).

Frostbite

The term frostbite implies freezing of soft tissue, with the amount of damage dependent on temperature, wind-chill, and duration of freezing. Likely areas for frostbite are ears, nose, cheeks, fingers, and toes (McCauley et al., 1990). Frostbite should be treated with rapid rewarming in water at 104° to 108° F until the skin develops color, it is soft and pliable, and sensation begins to return to normal. Because refreezing of soft tissue can lead to extensive damage, avoid thawing the tissues until you are assured that refreezing can be prevented.

Hypothermia

Hypothermia, the lowering of body core temperature below 95° F (35° C), may be classified as mild, moderate, or severe, or as acute, subacute, or chronic (Table 37–15) (Dexter, 1990). Decreased cardiac output, loss of consciousness, carbon mon-

TABLE 37–15. CLASSIFICATION OF HYPOTHERMIA

Mild: rectal core temperature <98.6° F (37° C) and >95° F (35° C)

Moderate: rectal core temperature <95° F (35° C) and >90° F (32° C)

Severe: rectal core temperature <90° F (32° C)

Acute: those experiencing cold water immersion

Subacute: usually healthy people accidentally subjected to a cold environment without proper protection

Chronic: alcoholics and those suffering from old age, senility, or chronic metabolic disease

oxide exposure, endocrinopathies, central nervous system (CNS) disease, malnutrition, skin disease, or drugs may reduce the body's ability to compensate for heat loss.

Treatment of hypothermia begins with warm dry clothing, warm liquids, and carbohydrates. As the severity increases, warm fluids can be given intravenously, and shared body contact can be employed. Extreme cases may warrant trials of warm peritoneal lavage, gastric lavage, or extracorporeal bypass. All treatments should take into account the possibility of rewarming aftershock or "afterdrop," which occurs when cold, acidic blood rapidly returns to the central circulation as warm peripheral vessels dilate (Reed and Anderson, 1988). Afterdrop can lead to fatal dysrhythmia and is more likely to occur with whirlpool warming where extremities are held out of the water.

Poor prognostic indicators for severe accidental hypothermia include concomitant medical illness, long duration of cold exposure, low initial core temperature, altered mental status, absence of spontaneous respirations, altered cardiac rate or rhythm, and hypoxia. Profound hyperkalemia and elevated serum ammonia levels indicate cell lysis, and hypofibrinogenemia suggests intravascular thrombosis, all of which predict a dire outcome (Hauty et al., 1987). Keep in mind that in the face of severe hypothermia vital structures can remain well preserved for prolonged periods, and that all victims should be resuscitated until the core temperature has had an opportunity to reach near-normal. ("They're not dead until they're *warm* and dead.")

Heat Injuries

When heat regulation (see above) is overwhelmed, body core temperature increases. Those who are obese, unfit, dehydrated, young, old, or chronically ill are more likely to suffer hyperthermia (Sterner, 1990). A history of heat stroke within the past year also increases the chance of heat illness. Ambient conditions that favor the development of heat illness include a hot environment, high humidity, poorly ventilated areas, surface type, such as asphalt and artificial turf, and high levels of activity.

Acclimatization

Acclimatization is a 2- to 4-week adaptation process that enables humans to tolerate heat stress. It involves increased metabolic efficiency, improved sweating threshold and rate, improved myocardial efficiency, and increased sodium conservation.

Solar Damage

Skin cancer is the number one cancer by volume, with more than 300,000 cases per year (Potts, 1990). The development of skin cancer appears to be related to ultraviolet radiation exposure. Known risk factors for solar damage include the amount of sun exposure, number of serious sunburns, and skin type. Certain medications, including tricyclic antidepressants, antihistamines, diuretics, hypoglycemic agents, nonsteroidal anti-inflammatory agents, and antibiotics (especially tetracyclines), are likely to photosensitize skin and should be used with caution by athletes who perform outdoors.

The best treatment for solar damage is prevention through controlled exposure, clothing, and sunscreens. Sunscreens used by athletes should demonstrate good water immersion resistance. Even so, sunscreens should be used liberally and reapplied often.

Heat Edema, Tetany, and Syncope

Heat edema, a self-limited swelling of the hands and feet that lessens with acclimatization, is rarely serious. Heat tetany is carpopedal spasm resulting from hyperventilation, one mechanism employed by the body to eliminate excess heat. Heat syncope is postural hypotension, which occurs when blood is shunted from the central circulation to the peripheral circulation. Some degree of hypovolemia, absolute or relative, is often involved.

Treatment of heat edema, heat tetany, and heat syncope involves moving the athlete to a cooler environment, rest, and ingestion of cool fluids. Each of these heat-induced problems may be prevented by proper acclimatization, rescheduling exercise times to cooler times of the day, and maintaining adequate hydration.

Heat Cramps

Painful contractions of muscles after exertion, heat cramps may be related to hyponatremia (Knochel, 1989) or other electrolyte imbalances. Typically, the gastrocnemius and hamstring muscles are involved. Treatment of heat cramps involves passive muscle stretching, cessation of activities, transfer to a cooler environment, and ingestion of cool liquids. Electrolyte replacement may be beneficial.

Heat Exhaustion

With symptoms ranging from nausea, vomiting, headache, loss of appetite, and dizziness to irritability, weakness, tachycardia, orthostasis, hyperventilation, and muscle cramps, heat exhaustion is a more serious condition. There may be water and electrolyte depletion secondary to excessive sweating and inappropriate replacement. Although active cooling is seldom necessary, treatment should involve rest, rehydration, and replacement of electrolytes.

Heat Stroke

With elevated body core temperature and severe CNS dysfunction, heat stroke is the most severe form of heat injury, constituting a true medical emergency. The physical signs noted most often by Omri Inbar (1985) are coma (100 per cent), confusion/agitation (100 per cent), convulsion (72 per cent), vomiting (71 per cent), diarrhea (44 per cent), hypotension (35 per cent), and dry skin (26 per cent).

Heat stroke has been observed to occur in two forms: classic and exertional. Classic heat stroke is common in the elderly and those with chronic disease. It develops insidiously, with victims often dehydrated. The skin is noted to be hot and dry. Exertional heat stroke, on the other hand, occurs rapidly in young, motivated persons such as athletes. Its onset is rapid, and victims are noted to be profusely sweating 50 per cent of the time.

The *heat stress index* refers to the increased thermal stress placed on the body under conditions of increasing ambient air temperature or humidity (Table 37–16). This index recognizes the increasing inefficiency of the body to eliminate heat as a result of two processes. First, with higher air temperatures there is no temperature gradient for radiation and conduction. Second, the high humidity impedes evaporation.

On site treatment of heat stroke includes ensuring adequate airway patency, measuring the rectal core temperature, starting whole-body cooling, and initiating prompt evacuation. Whole-body cooling can be accomplished as simply as with a fan and water spray or as complexly as with an immersion bath. Once at the hospital, whole-body cooling should continue and any convulsions controlled. The acid-base status, cardiac function, and renal status should all be monitored.

Heat stroke can be prevented by holding practices and games during cooler parts of the day, adjusting activities to coincide with elevations of temperature and humidity, scheduling regular stops for fluids and rest, encouraging athletes to drink fluids, adhering to weight charts before and after practices, and using light-colored, loose clothing.

Prognosis after heat-related injury is related to the time it takes the core temperature to return to normal, the athlete's age, the presence of pre-existing diseases, and the degree of CNS dysfunction.

Air Pollution

Ozone

Ozone, produced by the interaction of atmosphere and sunlight, can lead to cough, chest pain, and throat discomfort. As little as 0.12 to 0.20 ppm, common in an urban environment such as Los Angeles, can decrease maximum inspiration and expiratory flow (Spektor et al., 1988). Densensitization occurs after exposure over 3 to 5 days for 1 to 2 hours each day. For unknown reasons, smokers appear to be less susceptible, and asthmatics are no more susceptible than the average population.

Sulfur Dioxide

Even though sulfur dioxide is an airway irritant that can impair ventilation and induce bronchoconstriction in asthmatic athletes, at urban levels sulfur dioxide has no ill effect on healthy individuals (Folinsbee, 1985). Bronchoconstriction can be prevented with prior administration of cromolyn sodium. Any tolerance that may result from prolonged exposure to sulfur dioxide is quickly lost.

Carbon Monoxide

With an affinity for hemoglobin 240 times that of oxygen, carbon monoxide interferes with intracellular transport and utilization of oxygen. Whereas a national standard has been set at 2 to 3 per cent, smokers often achieve levels greater than 4 per cent. Allred et al. (1989) measured carbon monoxide levels and exercise tolerance in men

TABLE 37–16. HEAT STRESS

Relative Humidity (%)	Apparent Air Temperature (°F)										
	70	75	80	85	90	95	100	105	110	115	120
0	64	69	73	78	83	87	**91**	**95**	**99**	**103**	**107**
10	65	70	75	80	85	90	**95**	**100**	**105**	**111**	**116**
20	66	72	77	82	87	**93**	**99**	**105**	**112**	**120**	**130**
30	67	73	78	84	90	**96**	**104**	**113**	**123**	**135**	**148**
40	68	74	79	86	**93**	**101**	**110**	**123**	**137**	**151**	
50	69	75	81	88	**96**	**107**	**120**	**135**	**150**		
60	70	76	82	**90**	**100**	**114**	**132**	**144**			
70	70	77	85	**93**	**106**	**124**	**144**				
80	71	78	86	**97**	**113**	**136**					
90	71	79	88	**102**	**122**						
100	72	80	**91**	**108**							

Danger Zone = −90° F (temperatures in bold-faced type).
From Mellion MB: Office management of sports injuries and athletic problems. Philadelphia, Hanley & Belfus, 1988 p 54; *and* The National Weather Service, with permission.

with known coronary artery disease. Exposure to as little as 2% carbon monoxide shortened the time to onset of angina and the length of time to ST changes. Each 1 per cent rise in carbon monoxide is equivalent to a 300-meter rise in altitude in terms of physiologic changes.

Travel

Modern athletes often travel great distances in pursuit of competition. In the process, they are exposed to rapid changes in time zones, foods, altitudes, and even depths. Prior to departure, the athlete's physician should review the athlete's immunization record and ensure that medications required by health organizations are supplied. Although exotic diseases are often the concern of all involved, the primary cause of death to world travelers is motor vehicle accidents (Birrer and Plotz, 1982).

Time Zone Changes

Jet lag, or *transmeridian desynchronism*, is a transitory disturbance between body and environment. As the number of time zones traversed increases, so does the severity of desynchronism. Disturbances in behavior, hormone levels, digestion, attention, visual acuity, memory, and physical fitness may be noticed (Rietveld, 1985). Resynchronization may take days to weeks. In general, resynchronization may be hastened in those who travel on a west-bound route, remain active, incorporate social cues such as meals, and are young (Suvanto et al., 1990). If possible, athletes should arrive at least 2 weeks prior to competition, live on the destination time schedule for 2 weeks prior to competition, deliberately increase social cues, especially meal times, upon arrival, establish an active routine, avoid caffeine and theophylline, and maintain a high-protein, high-carbohydrate diet (Kleiner, 1990; O'Connor and Morgan, 1990).

International Travel

International travel adds many concerns, chief among which are food safety and immunization status. Suggestions to prevent unnecessary gastrointestinal upset include avoiding tap water, raw meats, fish, and vegetables; eating hot foods while hot and cold foods while cold; peeling fruit; avoiding noncarbonated beverages, soups, and desserts; using insect repellents; and maintaining an adequate state of hydration (Birrer and Plotz, 1982).

Traveler's diarrhea, a self-limiting enteritis characterized by cramps and diarrhea, may be caused by *Escherichia coli*, *Shigella*, *Salmonella*, or *Campylobacter* (Dupont and Ericsson, 1993). Treatment depends on the degree of debilitation. Many athletes require no therapy or simple rehydration. Avery and Snyder (1990) have outlined simple, effective rehydration therapies. Bismuth subsalicylates reduce the number of unformed stools by 50 per cent and decrease associated symptoms. Loperamide decreases motility, decreasing diarrhea by up to 80 per cent. Antibacterial therapy is recommended if there have been (1) three unformed stools in a 24-hour period; (2) diarrhea associated with moderate to severe abdominal pain or cramps, fever, or dysentery; or (3) symptoms that recur when drugs that relieve them are discontinued. It should be noted that traditional antibacterial agents such as trimethoprim-sulfamethoxazole have become less effective with the development of drug-resistant organisms (Dupont and Ericsson, 1993; Advice for travelers, 1990).

Many countries recommend or require that visitors be immunized against diseases endemic in the country of origin or the country of travel. Requirements are updated often, and the most current source of information can be obtained from most state and local health agencies. When first notified that the athlete is to be visiting a foreign country, investigate the needed immunizations, as some immunizations require a series of boosters that must be given at specified intervals and completed prior to the date of departure.

Altitude

With increasing altitude, there is decreasing barometric pressure and partial pressure of oxygen at the alveoli. In the athlete, performance decreases are related to aerobic demands, with a 3 per cent decrease in myocardial oxygen consumption (MVO_2) for every 360 feet (100 m) rise over 5000 feet (1500 m). Anaerobic performance is not affected. Living and training at high altitude over a period of weeks to years can lead to physiologic adaptations such as increased capillary density, myoglobin concentration, mitochondrial density, and oxidative capacities. However, short-term exposure results in alterations in training, sleep, and general performance. One conservative method for calculating the time necessary for adaptation requires 14 days for the first 7500 feet (2300 m) above sea level and then 7 days for each additional 1000 ft (300 m) rise.

Acute mountain sickness (AMS) is a syndrome consisting of headache, nausea, anorexia, fatigue, dyspnea, periodic breathing, and sleep disturbances; it typically lasts 1 to 2 days upon arrival at a high altitude. Although not life-threatening, AMS is most likely to occur with rapid ascents over 9000 feet (3000 m) above sea level. Treatment includes rest, fluids, and nausea relief. Acetazolamide in doses of 250 mg three times daily beginning 2 to 3 days prior to ascent effectively alters periodic breathing and acid-base status, and has been proved effective for the prophylactic treatment of AMS (Ellsworth et al., 1987). Dexamethasone in doses 4 mg by mouth every 8 hours can reduce the symptoms associated with AMS.

High altitude pulmonary edema (HAPE), consisting of a constellation of symptoms including severe dyspnea, exhaustion, and dry cough, is a life-threatening condition that takes approximately 24 to 96 hours to develop (Schoene, 1987). Prevention involves a slow ascent, dexamethasone (Decadron; 4 mg q 6 hr), and continuous positive airway pressure (CPAP). Treatment focuses on recognition of the disorder and rapid descent, oxygen, dexamethasone, and nifedipine (Bartsch et al., 1991). A portable device resembling a large sleeping bag or small tent and working in such a way as to simulate descent has been used successfully to treat HAPE at high altitude prior to evacuation.

Yet another possible complication of traversing at altitude is *high altitude cerebral edema* (HACE). Generally occurring above 10,000 feet (3300 m), HACE is characterized by severe headaches, hallucinations, ataxia, weakness, impaired mentation, and stupor. HACE may progress rapidly and result in death. The only effective treatment is oxygen, evacuation, and hospitalization.

Depth

Both skin and scuba diving present potential risks associated with the water environment. Such risks include poor visibility, dangerous currents, seasickness, hypothermia, barotrauma, and soft tissue infections. Salt-water diving increases chances of an animal bite or envenomization because of the diverse nature of its inhabitants.

Barotrauma of the tympanic membrane, known as *barotitis media*, occurs when the diver does not equilibrate middle ear and outside hydrostatic pressures. In the dense underwater environment, it may require less than 5 feet of depth change. If the tympanic membranes has not ruptured, rest, analgesics, and decongestants are treatments of choice. Complete tympanic rupture requires full otologic examination. The canal is kept free from debris, but antibiotic drops are not indicated. If healing has not occurred within 10 to 14 days, the diver should be referred to a specialist.

Decompression sickness (DCS) is a complex entity that may occur as long as 36 hours after shallow or deep dives; it may be mild, moderate, or severe. Nitrogen gas is initially dissolved in the blood and body tissues under the high ambient pressures of the underwater environment. When the diver ascends too rapidly, the nitrogen gas in solution coalesces into tiny bubbles, which then cause symptoms based on their location. Although much more common after scuba diving, DCS can occur in deep water skin divers as well. Symptoms of DCS may include musculoskeletal pain ("bends"), cutaneous pruritus, anorexia, and fatigue. Severe forms of the disorder result when nitrogen bubbles block vital structures such as the lungs ("chokes"), CNS, and vestibular system. Prevention of DCS requires careful planning and adherence to dive schedules. Divers should follow recommendations regarding time intervals after the dive and air travel. Once DCS is suspected, divers should be placed on 100% oxygen and transported to the nearest hyperbaric chamber (Bove and Davis, 1990).

REFERENCES

American College of Obstetricians and Gynecologists. *ACOG Technical Bulletin: Exercise During Pregnancy and the Postpartum Period,* no. 198, Washington, DC, February 1994.

Advice for travelers. Med Lett 32:33, 1990.

Afrasiabi R, Spector, SL: Exercise-induced asthma. The Physician and Sports Med 19(5):49, 1991.

Allred EN, Bleecker ER, Chaitman BR, et al: Short-term effects of carbon monoxide exposure on the exercise performance of subjects with coronary artery disease. N Engl J Med 321:1426, 1989.

American Academy of Pediatrics Committee on Sports Medicine: Recommendations for participation in competitive sports. Pediatrics 81:737, 1988.

American College of Sports Medicine. Guidelines for Graded Exercise Testing and Exercise Prescription. Philadelphia, Lea & Febiger 1990, pp 95–96.

Anderson B: Stretching. Bolinas, Shelter Publications, 1980.

Anderson B, Burke ER: Scientific, medical, and practical aspects of stretching. Clin Sports Med 10(1):63, 1991.

Avery ME, Snyder, JD: Oral rehydration therapy for acute diarrhea: the underused simple solution. N Engl J Med 323:891, 1990.

Barry HC, Rich BSE, Carlson RT: How exercise can benefit older patients: a practical approach. Physician Sports Med 21(2):124, 1993.

Bartsch P, Maggiorini M, Ritter M, et al: Prevention of high-altitude pulmonary edema by nifedipine. N Engl J Med 325:1284, 1991.

Belognia EA, Goodman JL, Holland EJ, et al: An outbreak of herpes gladiatorium at a high-school wrestling camp. N Engl J Med 325:906, 1991.

Benatar SR: Fatal asthma. N Engl J Med 314:423, 1986.

Bergfeld J, Lombardo J, Nelson M, et al: Preparticipation Physical Evaluation. [A joint publication of the AAFP, AAP, AMSSM, AOSSM, and AOCSM, it is available directly from these academies.]

Birrer RB, Plotz C: Medical advice for international travelers. Am Fam Physician 25:155, 1982.

Boulware DW, Byrd SL: Optimizing exercise programs for arthritis patients. Physician Sports Med 21(4):104, 1993.

Bove AA, Davis JC: Diving Medicine. Philadelphia, WB Saunders Company, 1990.

Brunet ME, Cook SD, Brinker MR, Dickinson JA: A survey of running injuries in 1505 competitive and recreational runners. J Sports Med Phys Fitness 30:307, 1990.

Campbell DC, Yetter JT: Sports medicine. *In* Rakel RB (ed): Textbook of Family Practice, 4th ed. Philadelphia, WB Saunders Company, 1990.

Clapp JF, Dickstein S: Endurance exercise and pregnancy outcome. Med Sci Sports Exerc 16:556, 1984.

Clapp JF, Rokey R, Treadway JI, et al: Exercise in pregnancy. Med Sci Sports Exerc 24(suppl):S294, 1992.

Davis GM: Exercise capacity of individuals with paraplegia. Med Sci Sports Exerc 25:423, 1993.

Dembert ML: Medical problems from cold exposure. Am Fam Physician, 25:99, 1982.

Dexter PA: Joint exercises in elderly persons with symptomatic osteoarthritis of the hip or knee: Performance patterns, medical support patterns, and the relationship between exercising and medical care. Arthritis Care Res 5(1):36, 1992.

Dexter WW: Hypothermia: safe and efficient methods of rewarming the patient. Postgrad Med 88(8):55, 1990.

Dorsen PJ: Should athletes with one eye, kidney, or testicle play contact sports? Physician Sports Med 14(7):134, 1986.

Duke PM, Litt IF, Gross RT: Adolescents self-assessment of sexual maturation. Pediatrics 66:918, 1980.

Duncan JJ, Farr JE, Upton SJ, et al: The effects of aerobic exercise on plasma catecholamines and blood pressure in patients with mild essential hypertension. JAMA 254:2609, 1985.

Dupont HL, Ericsson CD: Prevention and treatment of traveler's diarrhea. N Engl J Med, 328:1821, 1993.

Ellsworth AJ, Larson EB, Strickland D: A randomized trial of dexamethasone and acetazolamide for acute mountain sickness prophylaxis. Am J Med 83:1024, 1987.

Feinstein RA, Soileau EJ, Daniel WA: A national survey of preparticipation physical examination requirements. Physician Sports Med 16(5):51, 1988.

Fiatarone MA, Marks EC, Ryan ND, et al: High-intensity strength training in nonagenarians. JAMA 263:3029, 1990.

Fields KB, Delaney M: Focusing the preparticipation sports examination. J Fam Pract 30:304, 1990.

Figoni SF: Exercise responses and quadriplegia. Med Sci Sports Exerc 25:433, 1993.

Folinsbee LJ: Air pollution and exercise. *In* Welsh RP, Shephard RJ (eds): Current Therapy in Sports Medicine 1985–1986. St. Louis, CV Mosby, 1985, pp 54–56.

Frey C: Frostbitten feet: steps to treatment and prevention. Physician Sports Med 20(1):67, 1992.

Fritz RL, Perrin DH: Cold exposure injuries: prevention and treatment. Clin Sports Med 8(1):111, 1989.

Gisolfi CV, Duchman SM: Guidelines for optimal replacement beverages for different athletic events. Med Sci Sports Exerc 24:679, 1992.

Greenleaf JE: Problem: thirst, drinking behavior and involuntary dehydration. Med Sci Sports Exerc 24:645, 1992.

Grindel SH, McKeag DB: Management of the athlete with exercise-induced asthma. Clin J Sports Med 2:208, 1992.

Hagberg JM, Montain SJ, Martin WH, et al: Effect of exercise training in 60 to 69 year old persons with essential hypertension. Am J Cardiol 64:348, 1989.

Hauty MG, Esrig BC, Hill JG, Long WB: Prognostic factors in severe accidental hypothermia: experience from the Mt. Hood tragedy. J Trauma 27:1107, 1987.

Holt WS: Nutrition and athletes. Am Fam Physician 47:1757, 1993.

Kaplan NM: The deadly quartet: Upper body obesity, glucose intolerance, hypertriglyceridemia, and hypertension. Arch Intern Med 149:1514, 1989.

Kleiner SM: Can't stomach long trips? Try these healthful tips. Physician Sports Med 18(8):41, 1990.

Knapik JJ, Jones BH, Bauman CL, Harris JM: Strength, flexibility and athletic injuries. Sports Med 14:277, 1992.

Knochel JP: Update on summer heat syndromes. Patient Care June:87, 1989.

Krotkiewski M, Mandronkas K, Sjöstrom L, et al: Effects of long-term physical training on body fat, metabolism and blood pressure in obesity. Metabolism 28:650, 1979.

Kyle JM, Walker RB, Hanshaw SL, et al: Exercise-induced bronchospasm in the young athlete: Guidelines for routine screening and initial management. Med Sci Sports Exerc 24:856, 1992.

Landry GL, Allen DB: Diabetes mellitus and exercise. Clin Sports Med 11:403, 1992.

LaPierre AR, Ironson G, Antoni M, et al: Exercise intervention attenuates emotional distress and natural killer cell decrements following notification of positive serologic status for HIV-1. Biofeedback Self Regul 15:229, 1990.

Lohman TG, Roche AF, Mastorell R, (eds): Anthropometric Standardization Reference Manual. Champaign, IL, Human Kinetics Books, 1988.

Mahler DA: Exercise-induced asthma. Med Sci Sports Exerc 25:554, 1993.

Matheson GO, Macintyre JG, Taunton JE, et al: Stress fractures in athletes: A study of 320 cases. Am J Sports Med 15:46, 1987.

McCauley RL, Heggers JP, Robson MC: Frostbite; methods to minimize tissue loss. Postgrad Med 88:6777, 1990.

McFadden ER, Gilber IA: Asthma. N Engl J Med 327:1928, 1992.

McGinnis JM: The public health burden of sedentary lifestyle. Med Sci Sports Exerc 24(suppl):S196, 1992.

McKeag DB: Overuse injuries: The concept in 1992. Prim Care 18:851, 1991.

McKeag DB: The relationship of osteoarthritis and exercise. Clin Sports Med 11:471, 1992.

Mellion MB, Kobayashi RH: Exercise-induced asthma. Am Fam Physician 45:2671, 1992.

Mellion MB, Walsh WM, Shelton GL: The Team Physician's Handbook. Philadelphia, Hanley & Belfus, 1990.

Mitchell MD, Dimeff RJ, Burns BL: Effects of supplementation with arginine and lysine on body composition, strength, and growth hormone levels in weightlifting. Med Sci Sports Exerc 25(suppl):S25, 1993.

Morton AR, Fitch KD: Asthmatic drugs and competitive sport—an update. Sports Med 14:228, 1992.

Moss J: Accidental severe hypothermia. Surg Gynecol Obstet 162:502, 1986.

Nattiv A, Puffer JC: Lifestyles and health risks of collegiate athletes. J Fam Pract 33:585, 1991.

O'Connor PJ, Morgan WP: Athletic performances following rapid traversal of multiple time zones: a review. Sports Med 10:20, 1990.

Omri Inbar: Exercise in the heat. *In* Welsh RP, Shephard RJ (eds): Current Therapy in Sports Medicine 1985–1986. St. Louis, CV Mosby, 1985, pp 45–49.

Pollock ML, Wilmore JH, Fox SM: Exercise in Health and Disease: Evaluation and Prescription for Prevention and Rehabilitation. Philadelphia, WB Saunders Company, 1984.

Potts JF: Sunlight, sunburn, and sunscreens. Postgrad Med 87(8):52, 1990.

Reed G, Anderson RJ: Management of acute hypothermia. Hosp Med 24:149, 1988.

Rietveld WJ: Time-zone shifts and international competition. *In* Welsh RP, Shephard RJ (ed): Current Therapy in Sports Medicine 1985–1986. St. Louis, CV Mosby, 1985, pp 56–58.

Rigsby LW, Dishman RK, Jackson AW, et al: Effects of exercise training on men seropositive for the human immunodeficiency virus-1. Med Sci Sports Exerc 24:6, 1992.

Rousseau P: Exercise prescription for the elderly patient. Fam Pract Recert 13(3):58, 1991.

Schoene RB: High-altitude pulmonary edema: pathophysiological and clinical review. Ann Emerg Med 16:987, 1987.

Shangold MM: Exercise in the menopausal woman. Obstet Gynecol 75(suppl):53, 1990.

Sherman WM: Recovery from endurance exercise. Med Sci Sports Exerc 24(suppl):336, 1992.

Shields CE: Physical activity in the young. Am Fam Physician 33:155, 1986.

Singer KM, Jones DC: Soft tissue conditions of the ankle and foot. *In* Nichols JA, Hershman EB (eds): The Lower Extremity and Spine in Sports Medicine. St. Louis, CV Mosby, 1986, pp 507–508.

Singh A, Moses FM, Deuster PA: Chronic multivitamin-mineral supplementation does not enhance physical performance. Med Sci Sports Exerc 24:720, 1992.

Smith DM, Lombardo JA, Robinson JB: The preparticipation evaluation. Prim Care 18:777, 1991.

Smith LL, Brunetz MH, Chenier, et al: The effects of static and ballistic stretching on delayed onset muscle soreness and creatine kinase. Res Q Exerc Sport 64:103, 1993.

Spektor DM, Lippman M, Thurston GD, et al: Effects of ambient ozone on respiratory function in healthy adults exercising outdoors. Am Rev Respir Dis 138:821, 1988.

Sterner S: Summer heat illness. Postgrad Med 87(8):67, 1990.

Suvano S, Partinen M, Harma M, Ilmarinen J: Flight attendants' desynchronosis after rapid time zone changes. Aviat Spac Environ Med 61:543, 1990.

Tanji JL: Exercise and the hypertensive athlete. Clin Sports Med, 11:291, 1992.

Tanner SM: Weighing the risks: Strength training for children and adolescents. Physician Sports Med 21(6):105, 1993.

Taylor DC, Dalton JD: Viscoelastic properties of muscle-tendon units: The biomechanical effects of stretching. Am J Sports Med 18:300, 1990.

Van Mechelen W: Running injuries: A review of the epidemiological literature. Sports Med 14:320, 1992.

Van Mechelen W, Hlobil H, Kemper HC, et al: Prevention of running injuries by warm-up, cool-down, and stretching exercises. Am J Sports Med 21:711, 1993.

Virant FS: Exercise-induced bronchospasm: epidemiology, pathophysiology, and therapy. Med Sci Sports Exerc 24:851, 1992.

CHAPTER 38

ORTHOPEDICS

O. MAX JARDON and MONTY S. MATHEWS

The most common reason for a patient to consult a physician is pain, either acute or chronic. The diagnostic skills of the family physician can readily be applied to the musculoskeletal causes of pain, and thus the cause and treatment found to alleviate the distress. Diagnosis depends in the main on accurate historical and physical assessment accompanied by minimal laboratory aids.

LACERATIONS AND CONTUSIONS

Lacerations

A leading cause of visits to a family physician are lacerations. These are best managed by cleansing and irrigation with antibiotic solution and usually primary suturing. If the wound is reasonably clean and less than 6 hours old, this will usually give a satisfactorily healed wound with a minimal scar and few complications. However, there are a number of wounds that preclude primary closure, are very hazardous, or have contraindications for primary closure. Some types of lacerations frequently involve deep structures and have severe complications.

Wounds Near Joints

Wounds near joints should be considered a major hazard and closed only after making certain that the joint space has not been violated or that major tendinous or ligamentous structures have not been interrupted.

A 6-year-old boy who sustained a nail puncture near the left patella was treated by superficial cleansing and primary closure. He later developed signs of joint sepsis from this undiagnosed penetration. (Some studies have reported an incidence of 70 per cent infections with untreated penetration wounds.) This sepsis was treated with antibiotics and no drainage. As a result, the patient developed osteomyelitis with growth arrest, a fused knee, and 6 inches of shortening of this extremity by maturity. These problems were later corrected by multiple operations that required 20 hospitalizations, and the patient ended up with a 1-inch shorter leg and a liability settlement.

MANAGEMENT BY THE FAMILY PHYSICIAN. Any wound adjacent to a joint should be assessed for penetration and contamination of the joint space. Penetration can often be detected by injecting 30 to 40 mL of sterile saline into a joint and observing the flow from the puncture. When in doubt, the best course is exploration to the depth of the wound under sterile conditions to see whether or not penetration has occurred. If penetration has occurred, then the joint must be explored, thoroughly irrigated, and débrided. Reliance on antibiotic coverage alone is usually a poor move and is not a substitute for appropriate surgical exploration and drainage. Signs of infection in a joint demand immediate surgical exploration and cleansing, not merely a change in antibiotics.

Cuts about the knuckles of the hand are prone to major complications, such as infection and tendon laceration, and these must be suspected in wounds or fractures over the proximal or distal interphalangeal joints. These may cause mallet finger or boutonnière deformity, which are discussed in the section on Jammed Finger or Finger Sprain.

Human Bite Injury

Human bites are most serious and have a high complication rate when they occur about the knuckles of the hand. Several serious complications can result from these apparently innocuous lesions. When the fist is clenched and strikes the teeth of an opponent in a fight, the joint is especially prone to penetration. All too often, the problem appears benign early on and treatment is delayed, only to have the patient return later with a severe complication. Human saliva contains millions of organisms per milliliter of about 42 different species, both aerobic and anaerobic. Mann (1981) and others reported complications in over 50 per cent of human bite injuries. These included permanent stiffness, amputation, or rapidly spreading infections requiring high amputation. At least eight deaths have been reported in cases of human bites. One should never consider this to be a minor injury.

MANAGEMENT BY THE FAMILY PHYSICIAN. Family physicians should treat such wounds with a high index of suspicion, even though the injury is denied by the patient. Human bites have a unique course and behave in a unique way, as contrasted with other wounds, especially in the hand. Wound material should be cultured for both anaerobic and aerobic bacteria. No culture is considered negative unless both of these have been done. A radiograph should be obtained to rule out osteomyelitis, fractures, retained teeth, or bone abscesses.

Mann (1981) has demonstrated that these wounds must be débrided and irrigated thoroughly. Broad-spectrum antibiotics such as gentamicin sulfate are used, and the patient is hospitalized. Débridement is necessary to convert an anaerobic environment to an aerobic one. All necrotic tissue is removed and all infected spaces are drained. These wounds must never be closed primarily but left open for drainage. These are best managed by a surgeon who is skilled in serious hand infections.

After drainage, the hand is splinted for 24 hours; then active motion is encouraged. Intravenous antibiotics are continued for about 5 days and, if all is well, the patient then is discharged on oral antibiotics and close supervision is continued until healing by secondary intention is complete.

Dog and Cat Bites

These types of bites occur over 2 million times per year and constitute about 1 per cent of emergency room admissions. Large dogs tend to lacerate when they bite, whereas small dogs avulse small pieces of tissue. Cats cause puncture wounds. Twenty per cent of the bites are caused by German Shepherds, and 63 per cent of victims are bitten by a family or a neighbor's dog. The average patient age is 5 years, with 92 per cent under 21 years of age (Zook et al., 1980).

MANAGEMENT BY THE FAMILY PHYSICIAN. Zook et al. (1980) have shown that meticulous débridement, irrigation, and antibiotic treatment reduce the complications of infection, scarring, and systemic symptoms for dog bites. Cat bites need only cleansing and an antibiotic effective against *Haemophilus*-type organisms.

Where rabies is a concern, the guidelines of the Public Health Service Advisory Committee, as described by Corey and Hattwick (1975), should be followed (Fig. 38–1). For most severe dog bite lacerations, the ampicillin or a cephalosporin should be started intravenously and the patient hospitalize for 48 hours for further therapy.

Small lacerations and minor avulsions can be managed under local anesthetic in the emergency room. More severe cases need general anesthesia in an operating room with thorough débridement. The wound must be copiously irrigated with water, preferably by some lavage system. The wound edges are sharply excised, and loose fat and foreign matter are removed. Subcutaneous sutures should be avoided. The wound edges should be closed with only minimal tension. A small pressure dressing to obliterate the dead space is utilized. Small, inert, nonreactive sutures are best. The sutures should be removed at 5 days and Steri-strips used to support the wound for a few more days.

This approach decreases the incidence of infection. The wound should be closely monitored for 3 to 5 days in case some infection develops.

Lacerations Prone to Clostridial Infection

Clostridial infections are life- or limb-threatening infections and are particularly prone to occur in certain types of wounds, such as small punctures over open fractures, wounds about the buttocks, and certain types of mass casualty wounds.

SMALL PUNCTURE OVER OPEN FRACTURE. These wounds do not appear severe and belie the extent of contamination. The bone ends can carry dirt and debris back in under the skin. Superficial irrigation will not cleanse these tissues, and serious infection is the consequence. Amputation all too often is necessary and is a common end result of only superficial débridement. Youngsters are particularly prone to this complication.

Management by the Family Physician. Undermanagement must be avoided. All open fractures require surgical exploration and thorough cleansing regardless of their benign appearance, and should never be closed primarily. They should be referred to an appropriate surgeon for management.

WOUNDING IN WATER. Lacerations occurring in water are most deceptive. They tend to look clean, yet the contamination and soft tissue damage can be extensive. Boat propeller injuries are often extensive and lead to muscle necrosis. Closure of such wounds creates an abscess, and dead tissue can create an anaerobic milieu for gas gangrene to develop. Brown and Kinman (1974) discussed ten cases of gas gangrene in survivors of an Everglades plane crash near Miami. They pointed out that primary closure of wounds incurred in water is inexcusable and is bad management.

Management by the Family Physician. Care is based on prompt and complete débridement and cleansing of the wound, with wound closure delayed because the amount and type of contamination is uncertain.

WOUNDS ABOUT THE BUTTOCKS. Although infrequent, wounds about the buttocks are apt to have a disproportionate number of septic complications, often are contaminated with feces, and may represent an open pelvic fracture. If these wounds communicate with the vagina or rectum, they are lethal injuries unless appropriately handled. The risk of death from sepsis or hemorrhage exceeds 50 per cent. Many cases require colostomy with rectal disimpaction and irrigation. All such wounds require specialized surgical management.

Management by the Family Physician. In this class of severe injuries, it is best to provide prompt referral to a specialist in surgical care.

MASS CASUALTY WOUNDS. Many of these wounds can be accompanied by clostridial infec-

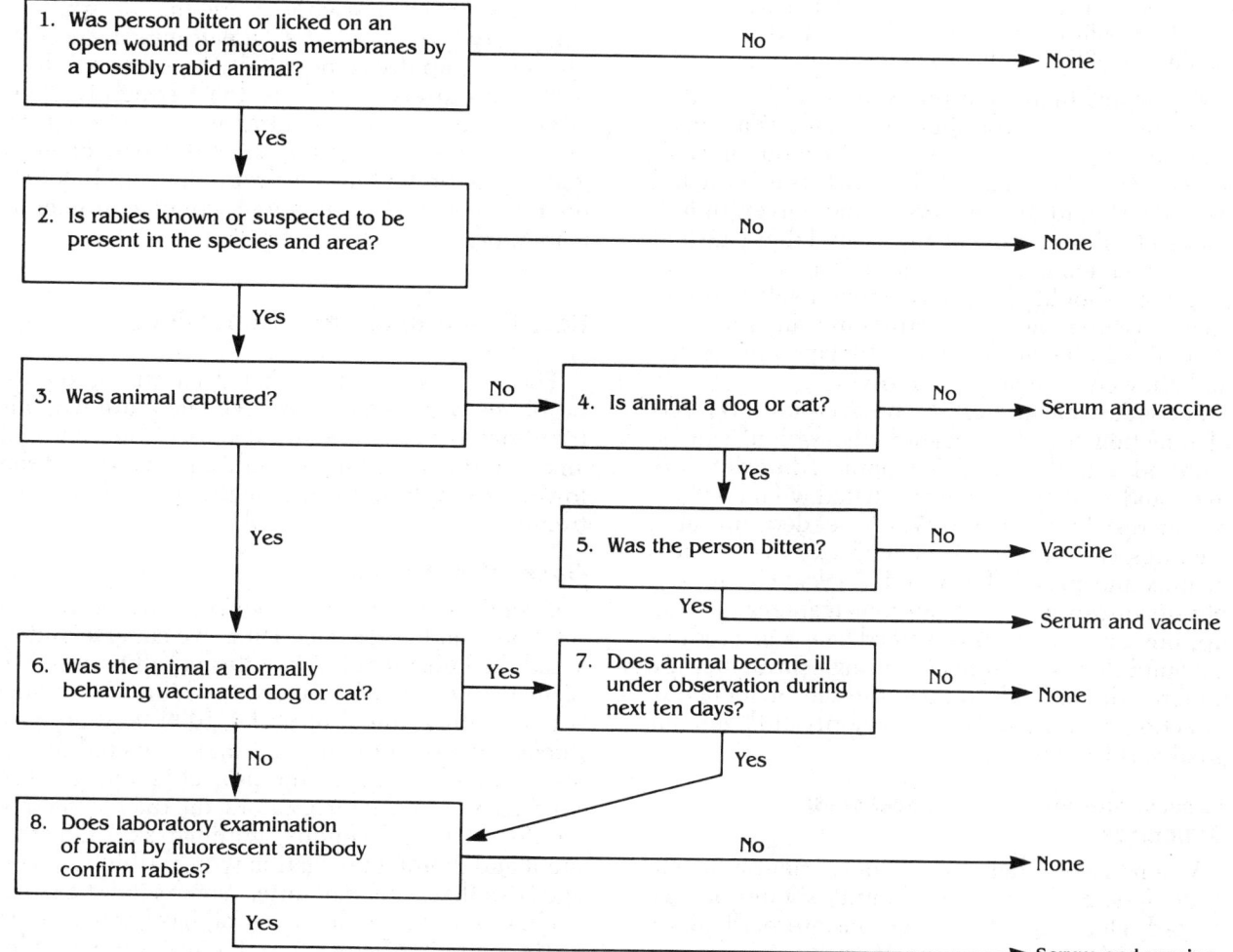

FIGURE 38–1. Postexposure rabies prophylaxis algorithm. (From Corey L, Hattwick M: Treatment of persons exposed to rabies. JAMA 232:272, 1975.)

tion or other overwhelming infection. The Texas City explosion and the Worcester, Massachusetts, and Flint, Michigan, tornadoes had an incidence of gas gangrene of 3 to 5 per cent in the wounds incurred. This is a frequency experienced in World War I battle injuries. Military surgery has improved and, in Viet Nam, the incidence of gas gangrene was down to 0.016 per cent, or only 22 cases. In this same period, Brown and Kinman (1974) reported 29 cases in a single metropolitan area.

Management by the Family Physician. Military surgeons have repeatedly urged that all wounds be promptly and thoroughly débrided and irrigated, and dressed and not closed. No contaminated wound should be closed primarily, especially in a mass casualty situation, and débridement and cleansing are often marginal because of the speed with which surgery must be carried out.

Débridement and irrigation should not be delayed in musculoskeletal wounds or open fractures because of some imagined need to observe for head and abdominal injuries. These patients must go to surgery and be débrided. Scanning techniques such as exist at the present time can pick up head and abdominal injuries and assess them well without prolonged observation. Poor débridement of open fractures often produces the most severe complications in multiply injured patients.

The word "débridement" originally was "debridlement," meaning the unleashing of all tight restrictions about a wound. In débridement, one should conserve skin, bone, and neurovascular structures while excising all damaged muscle and connective tissue. One leaves only muscle that is contractile and viable. Copious irrigation must be done utilizing 10 to 12 liters of antibiotic solution or a 50% Betadine solution. If all of this is unavailable, soap and potable water can suffice.

The poem of Sir James Learmouth summarizes débridement quite well.

On the edge of the skin take a piece very thin.
The tensor the fascia, the more you should slash'er.
Of muscles much more 'til you see fresh gore,
And the bundles contract at the least impact.
Hardly any of bone only bits quite alone.

Physicians in ancient times knew of the ability of wounds to close on their own and, as a consequence, never closed wounds. As modern caregivers, we often forget this. All contaminated wounds should be left open and never tightly packed to allow egress of any wound drainage and prevent contaminated material from being trapped. One should close only enough soft tissue to cover vascular and neural structures and no more. Wounds can be closed in 5 to 10 days when clean and allowed to heal secondarily.

Secondary closure can be delayed until the risk of infection has disappeared; the wound can be cultured and closed at that point. After débridement and irrigation, a contaminated wound is best put at rest in splintage. When needed, unstable fractures can be stabilized with external fixators or pins and plaster for 3 to 4 weeks. The most a physician can do in wound management is clean up, prevent sepsis and hemorrhage, and produce a wound that is capable of healing. Antibiotics are a mere adjunct and do decrease the incidence of infection somewhat, but the priority still remains good surgical practice.

Lacerations around Neurovascular Structures

When lacerations occur near neurovascular structures, nerve or arterial injury should be suspected. Deep forearm lacerations are particularly notorious for such complications.

The primary caregiver must assess motor function and sensation, but these can be unreliable in the acutely injured or inebriated patient, and assessment must be repeated. The only certain way to assess nerve laceration is exploration of the wound in an operating room. When a physician suspects such damage, the patient should be referred to an experienced surgeon.

Major damage to arteries can go unrecognized unless the physician is experienced or acutely aware of the possibility of this damage. Deep lacerations about the knee or elbow can be particularly confusing, as can supracondylar humeral fractures or dislocations of the knee and some shoulder dislocations. Multiple shoulder dislocations put a patient at risk for this problem (Jardon et al., 1973).

Puncture wounds in the vicinity of major vessels also need assessment. The presence or absence of a distal pulse is an unreliable sign. Any pulsatile swelling is usually the consequence of penetration into an artery or a blunt trauma that has resulted in a tear, and is usually a reliable indicator of arterial damage.

MANAGEMENT BY THE FAMILY PHYSICIAN. Evaluation of lacerations, fractures, and dislocations about joints requires alertness to possible vessel damage. Any doubts as to the integrity of distal circulation should prompt arteriographic study.

If injury is demonstrated, repair must be accomplished as rapidly as possible. In years past, ligation of an artery was done too frequently. This often led to ischemic contracture, severe sepsis, or amputation. Currently, arterial repair or even grafting is preferable. Appropriate, rapid (1 to 4 hours) referral to a competent vascular surgeon is mandatory.

Soft Tissue Injury and Contusions

The soft tissue injuries that are most apt to raise problems with regard to management are wounds from gunshots, severe contusions of the foot and ankle, and compartment syndrome, usually of the lower extremity but occasionally of the upper extremity.

Gunshot Wounding

Over the centuries, treatment of gunshot wounds has been modified somewhat as we came to understand the behavior of projectiles in soft tissues. We have learned that low-velocity wounding, which occurs with a speed of under 1000 feet/sec, produces a wound of entry and then a wound of exit about the same size as the projectile and tends to produce minimal damage along the tract of the projectile. In these wounds, minimal skin débridement and thorough irrigation with antibiotic coverage is all that is needed unless some vital structure, such as a nerve or blood vessel, has been severed or the bone has been injured. Once a bullet stops moving, the damage ceases. Therefore, the removal of the bullet is necessary only if the bullet is apt to produce some untoward side effect, such as mechanical irritation when it is in or near a joint or painful abrading when in some superficial location. Lead poisoning can occur in some instances of lead bullets in contact with body fluid (i.e., synovial fluid). Legal considerations must be kept in mind with regard to bullets and their fragments; these should be labeled as to location and kept separate, and all witnesses present at removal should be noted.

When wounding occurs from a high-velocity projectile (over 3000 feet/sec), there is usually a small entry wound with a very large exit wound. Considerable cavitation occurs within the wound, with a secondary shock wave produced and usually some tumbling of the projectile after it enters the tissue. This causes considerable damage and, when a bone is struck, there may be secondary muscle damage from bone fragments (Fakler and O'Benar, 1987). Cavitation is the development of a space around the bullet tract, which may be several times the diameter of the bullet. The pressure within this cavity is below atmospheric pressure, and clothing and debris can be pulled into the wound through this pressure differential. Such a bullet tract necessitates open débridement by a surgeon who is experienced in treatment of high-velocity wounds; the surgeon must be able to evaluate the total damage to skin, bone, vessels, and nerves.

Very-high-velocity wounds (usually over 5000 feet/sec) cause greater cavitation and secondary wound damage. Tissue death is greater and requires even more extensive open surgery for proper management.

Most of the characteristics of high-velocity wounds are also seen in shotgun wounds, which tend to blow tissue away and carry dirt into the wound. Often there are pieces of the shotgun load left in the depth of the wound, which contaminate it and lead to infection. Therefore, shotgun injuries require a thorough débridement much in the manner of that for high-velocity wounding.

MANAGEMENT BY THE FAMILY PHYSICIAN. Fractures and other injuries that are associated with gunshot wounds are treated by thorough débridement and open wound management. The only exception is that of a wound from a low-caliber handgun with a low velocity, which can be managed with local wound care at the entrance and exit with thorough irrigation. All wounds from either high- or low-velocity missiles that involve a joint should be explored by someone familiar with joint pathology to remove any potential foreign bodies. All penetrating wounds near vessels of importance require arteriography to demonstrate the integrity of the vessels. Wounds made by low-velocity pistol shots or standard .22 rifle shots require only minimal care, much in the manner of a puncture wound, if they are not in the proximity of some important structure. Any other gunshot wound needs specialized surgical care by someone with knowledge of the surgical problems these wounds can cause, which can vary in complexity. Any such wound does require antibiotic coverage. The interested reader is referred to Swan and Swann's (1980) monograph on gunshot wounds.

Contusions of the Hand and Wrist

Severe contusion and crush injury to the hand disrupt the soft tissues more than they do bone. The swelling subsequent to any such injury is a major concern and may compromise the circulation to the intrinsic muscles of the hand by virtue of a compartment syndrome around the smaller muscles. The edema that occurs can restrict motion and tends to stiffen the joints. The swelling that is noted is the biggest problem in any attempt to restore function to the hand after such injury. Many fractures of the hand and wrist develop problems from the swelling that are far more significant than the skeletal injury itself.

Edema and its complications cannot be ignored, because they can lead to severe consequences.

A construction worker sustained a fracture of his left wrist, which was reduced and immobilized in a snugly applied cast. The patient complained fairly rapidly of painful swelling and stiffness after the application of this cast. Unfortunately, his complaints were not taken seriously and the physician insisted the cast should stay on for 8 weeks until the fracture healed. Once the cast was removed, the patient was unable to move his painful, stiff fingers, and this stiffness persisted despite many months of physical therapy from several individuals. When seen 2 years after this injury, he had lost all motion of the metacarpophalangeal joints of the fingers and had permanent 50 per cent loss of function in this hand.

MANAGEMENT BY THE FAMILY PHYSICIAN. One must not concentrate solely on reducing the fracture; the soft tissue injury also must be considered. The edematous hand should be treated to eliminate the swelling as promptly as possible and the swollen hand should be wrapped in a compressive dressing and elevated in a comfortable position. If the cast appears to be too tight, it can be removed and reapplied at a later time. Failure to eliminate such swelling can produce ischemic necrosis of intrinsic muscles and cause permanent contractures of the hand.

Occasionally one sees compartment syndrome of the intrinsic muscles of the hand; this requires surgical release by a good hand surgeon. One must be cognizant of this possibility and refer appropriately when there is excessive pain in response to passive stretch of intrinsic muscles of the hand.

The position for immobilization of the hand is that in which the ligaments are kept on maximal tension, which is approximately 80 degrees flexion at the metacarpophalangeal joint and slight flexion of the interphalangeal joints. This position can be maintained in a boxing glove–type bandage (Fig. 38–2). The hand should be splinted in this position with elevation for 2 to 3 days until swelling subsides. After edema has diminished, one can then encourage active motion of all joints. Any injured extremity should be exercised at the proximal joints, such as the shoulder or hip, to prevent stiffness. Emphasis on combating complications of contusion and edema help the patient's recovery and avoid unsatisfactory results in many instances.

Contusions of the Foot and Ankle

BLUNT INJURY WITHOUT FRACTURE. Blunt injury without fracture often produces severe and permanent damage.

A 16-year-old girl twisted and severely bruised her ankle. She was seen several hours later by her physician, who wrapped her ankle in a rigid UNNA cast–type dressing. She was then placed on crutches but did not elevate the leg. The cast dressing became progressively tighter and for some reason her dressing was not removed until several weeks later. At this time, the patient had suffered a fixed equinovarus deformity of the foot and ankle.

The edema of the leg and rigid dressing applied to this limb combined to produce permanent damage re-

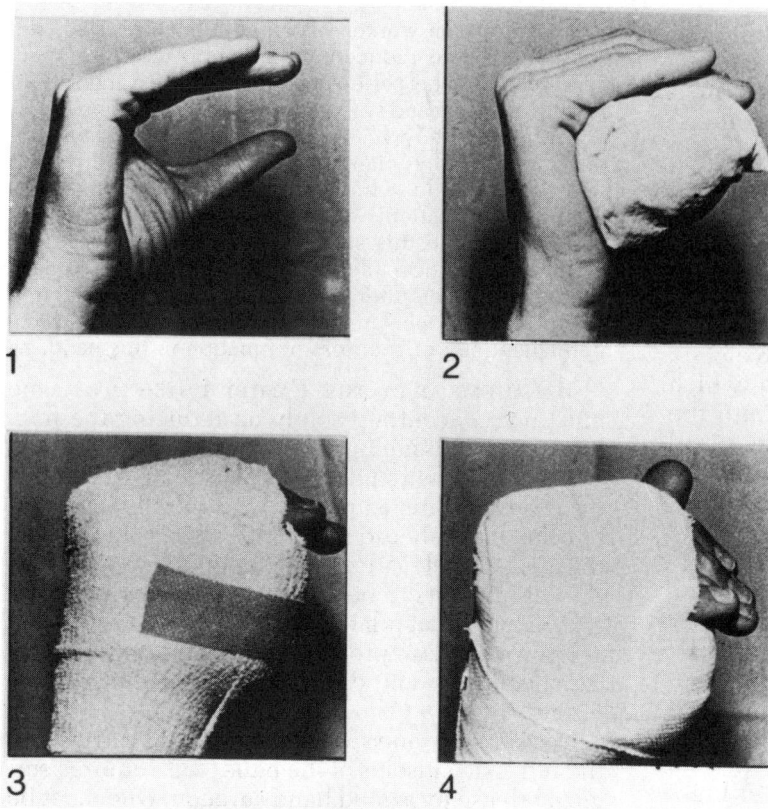

FIGURE 38–2.   Position of immobilization of the hand after injury as it should be, with metacarpophalangeal joints flexed maximally and the intraphalangeal joints slightly flexed. Thumb is abducted and opposed to the other fingers. Maintain this position by a firm ball dressing inserted into the palm to produce a "boxing glove bandage." (Courtesy Mr. J. Sikorski, Department of Surgery-Orthopaedics, University of Western Australia.)

sulting in inversion of the foot. This fixed contracture of the musculature and deep compartment left her with a permanent functional impairment (Fig. 38–3).

Management by the Family Physician.   Contusion and swelling about the ankle can cause permanent disability. One should avoid rigid dressings, elevate the leg, and be cognizant of the fact that edema is the enemy. Understanding the pathophysiology of compartment syndrome is essential to avoiding unfortunate complications in some relatively minor injuries.

COMPARTMENT SYNDROMES.   The so-called compartment syndrome is the result of increased pressure within a closed osteofascial space. As shown in Figure 38–4, the basic problem is that a decrease in local blood flow or perfusion when the pressure in the compartment is above perfusion pressure results in insufficient metabolic flow for muscles and nerves, leading to muscle necrosis.

The precipitating cause can be either hemorrhage within the compartment or edema developing after injury. Another cause can be decreased

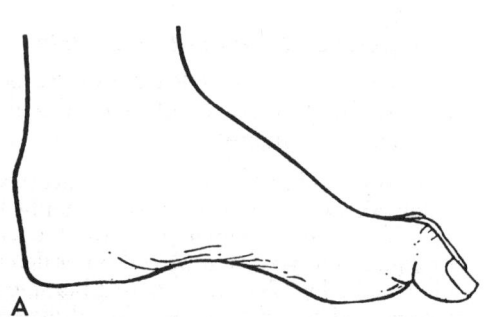
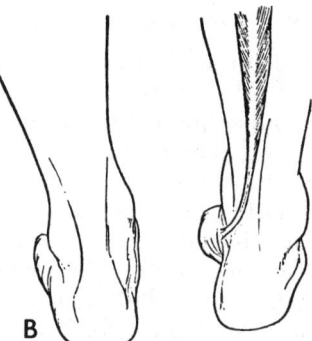

FIGURE 38–3.   *A*, Sprains, contusions, and fractures about the ankle may frequently produce extreme swelling that can develop into compartment syndromes, particularly if a rigid dressing is applied. *B*, Ischemic contractures of the posterior compartment muscles leave the patient with a fixed inverted deformity of the ankle with a painful high arch and clawtoes. (From Connolly JF: DePalma's The Management of Fractures and Dislocations: An Atlas, 3rd edition. Philadelphia, WB Saunders Company, 1981, with permission.)

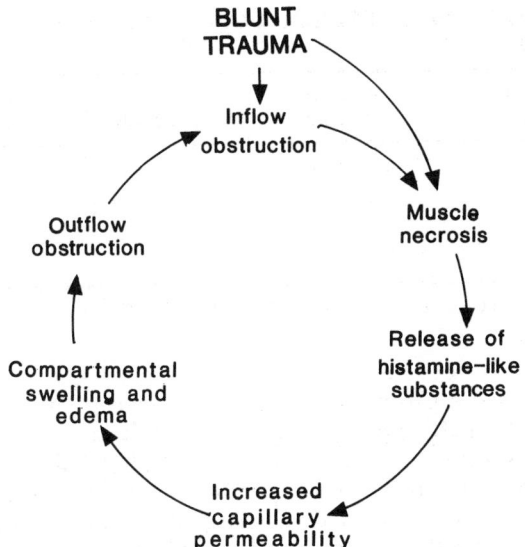

BLUNT
TRAUMA

Inflow
obstruction

Muscle
necrosis

Release of
histamine–like
substances

Increased
capillary
permeability

Compartmental
swelling and
edema

Outflow
obstruction

FIGURE 38–4. Pathology of compartment syndrome.

arterial flow from shock, with decreased venous return after injury or ligation. In some instances increased metabolic needs in an athlete can cause edema and result in a compartment syndrome. One must recognize the multiple etiologies of this syndrome in order to understand clearly the puzzling clinical findings and history (Table 38–1).

The syndrome does not necessarily result from arterial injury, so the distal pulses may be palpable despite a significant problem. The skin is not normally pallorous, as seen in arterial occlusion. The symptoms are extreme tenseness within the compartment, extreme pain on passive stretch of the muscles within the compartment, and gradual loss of motor function and sensation with eventual paralysis. This syndrome has been confused with arterial occlusion, phlebitis, and nerve injury. The findings listed in Table 38–2 should be helpful in differentiating compartment syndrome from conditions that have a similar presentation and therefore may be confused with it.

Accurate compartmental pressure measurements can be obtained by placing a cannula or needle into the compartment and attaching it to a saline-filled tube connected to a transducer that can read out the intercompartment pressure (Fig. 38–5). Normal arteriolar perfusion pressure is about 17 mm Hg. Pressures that are over 30 mm Hg are significant and associated with ischemia and permanent neuromuscular damage unless this pressure is relieved.

Management by the Family Physician. A compartment syndrome has been known to develop anywhere from 2 hours to 7 days after injury. Continued surveillance must be the rule for any limb that has considerable swelling, and must go on for several days. An ischemic event of 6 hours or so is sufficient to produce permanent muscle and nerve

TABLE 38–1. ETIOLOGIES OF COMPARTMENTAL SYNDROMES

Decreased compartmental volume	Closure of fascial defects
	Application of excessive traction to fractured limbs
Increased compartmental content	Bleeding
	Major vascular injury
	Coagulation defect
	Bleeding disorder
	Anticoagulant therapy
	Increased capillary filtration
	Reperfusion after ischemia
	Arterial bypass grafting
	Embolectomy
	Ergotamine ingestion
	Cardiac catheterization
	Lying on limb
	Trauma
	Fracture
	Contusion
	Intensive use of muscles
	Exercise
	Seizures
	Eclampsia
	Tetany
	Burns
	Thermal
	Electric
	Intra-arterial drug injection
	Cold
	Orthopedic surgery
	Tibial osteotomy
	Hauser procedure
	Reduction and internal fixation of fractures
	Snakebite
	Increased capillary pressure
	Intensive use of muscles
	Venous obstruction
	Phlegmasia cerulea dolens
	Ill-fitting leg brace
	Venous ligation
	Diminished serum osmolarity—nephrotic syndrome
	Other causes of increased compartmental content
	Infiltrated infusion
	Pressure transfusion
	Leaky dialysis cannula
	Muscle hypertrophy
	Popliteal cyst
Externally applied pressure	Tight casts, dressings, or air splints
	Lying on limb

From Matsen FA: Compartmental Syndromes, New York, Grune & Stratton, 1980, with permission.

degeneration. The only real answer to a compartment syndrome is a fasciotomy, which decompresses the compartment contents. Logically, because the basic problem is one of too much material in too small a space, and the solution is enlargement of that space. Delays in treatment increase the damage inflicted and increase the incidence of complications. The three most common compartment syndromes are noted in Figure 38–6.

The technique of fasciotomy is fairly simple, and this procedure must be done promptly once the

TABLE 38–2. CLINICAL FINDINGS OF COMPARTMENT SYNDROME, ARTERIAL OCCLUSION, PHLEBITIS, AND NERVE INJURY

	Compartment Syndrome	Arterial Occlusion	Phlebitis	Nerve Injury
Compartment pressure increased above 50 mm Hg	+	−	−	−
Pain on passive stretching	+	+	+	−
Paresthesia or anesthesia	+	+	−	+
Paresis or paralysis	+	+	−	+
Intact distal pulse	+	−	+	+

Modified from Mubarak SJ, Hargens AR: Compartment Syndromes and Volkmann's Contracture. Philadelphia, WB Saunders Company, 1981.

need is recognized. Matsen (1980) has demonstrated graphically how decompression can be accomplished through a parafibular incision that reaches all four compartments of the leg. Techniques of decompression of the forearm compartments are also discussed by Matsen.

In general, it is a good idea to obtain prompt surgical consultation when fasciotomy is deemed necessary. This prevents significant muscle loss or even loss of the limb. Associated problems, including renal damage similar to that seen in crush injury, can occur when the syndrome is fully developed and must be remembered when dealing with these cases.

AMPUTATIONS

Amputation is extremely frequent in the population, occurring in about 1 in 10,000 persons per year (Hansson, 1964). Therefore, the family physician will be involved with a fairly large number of amputee patients with a variety of problems over his or her career.

Rehabilitation Management

The most common cause of amputation is peripheral vascular disease, particularly that associated with diabetes (Hansson, 1964); this type of gangrene-producing vascular disease is the cause of about 85 per cent of lower limb amputations. This represents a change in etiology since the 1950s, when the most common cause was trauma. It also reflects an increasing life span and more active treatment of peripheral vascular disease as well as improved management of vascular injuries from trauma.

Proper planning of an amputation, even in an elderly patient, can maximize the patient's chance for the use of a prosthesis and restore some good function. In addition, it must be remembered that a unilateral foot problem in a diabetic or nondiabetic peripheral vascular disease patient will become bilateral more than half of the time (McCollough et al., 1972). Initial amputations in diabetic patients should be as conservative as possible, and proper management requires the understanding of the difference between a warm and a cold diabetic foot (Fig. 38–7). Slightly over half of diabetic gangrene occurs in a warm foot with intact major vessel flow; hence, a resection of a limited amount of the foot may give a satisfactory weight-bearing foot (Fig. 38–8).

If a high level of amputation is necessary because of major vessel disease, such as gangrenous cold foot, one should make every attempt to preserve the knee joint. The major criterion for the level of amputation is the vascularity of the skin flaps, which is evident at the time of surgery. If there is decent skin flap bleeding, there is usually

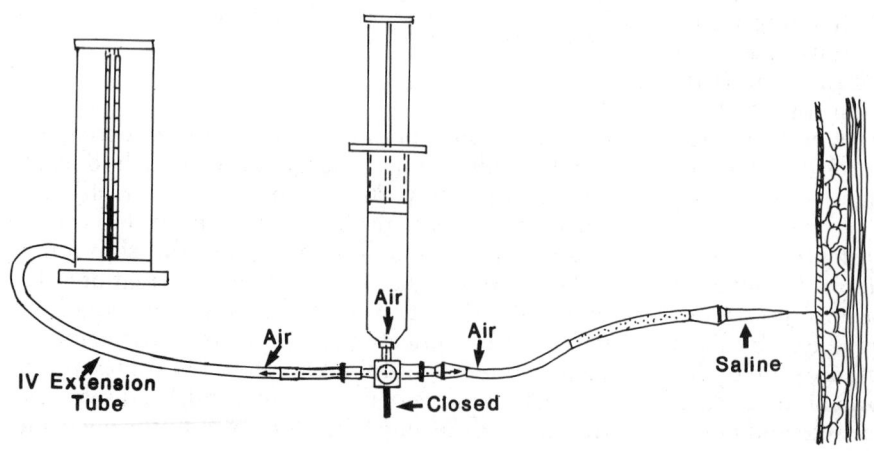

FIGURE 38–5. Measurement of compartment pressure.

ANTERIOR COMPARTMENTAL SYNDROME OF THE LEG

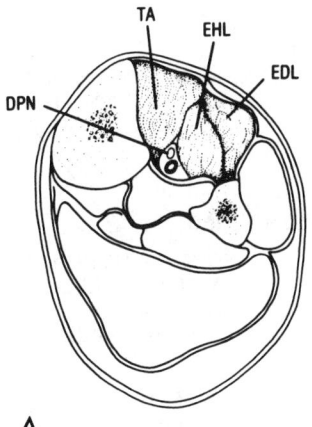

A

Symptoms and signs

- Weakness of toe extension and foot dorsiflexion
- Pain on passive toe flexion and foot plantar flexion
- Hypesthesia in the dorsal first web space
- Tenseness of the anterior compartmental fascia

VOLAR COMPARTMENTAL SYNDROME OF THE FOREARM

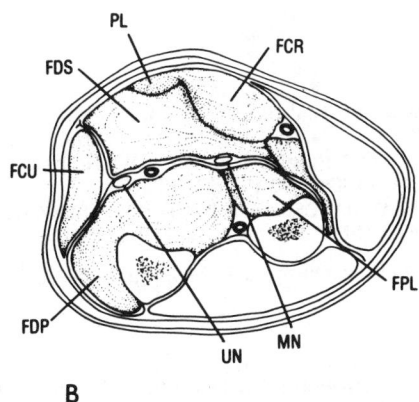

B

Symptoms and signs

- Weakness of finger and wrist flexion
- Pain on finger and wrist extension
- Hypesthesia of the volar aspect of the fingers
- Tenseness of the volar forearm fascia

DEEP POSTERIOR COMPARTMENTAL SYNDROME OF THE LEG

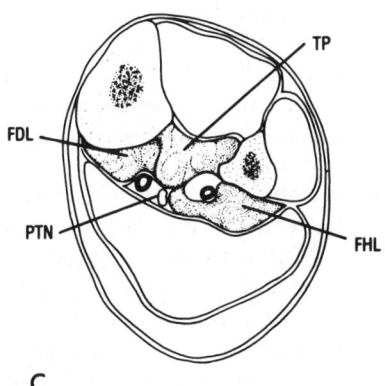

C

Symptoms and signs

- Weakness of toe flexion and foot inversion
- Pain on passive toe extension and foot eversion
- Hypesthesia of the plantar aspect of the foot and toes
- Tenseness of the deep posterior compartmental fascia (between the tibia and Achilles tendon)

FIGURE 38–6. Summary of symptoms and signs as well as a schematic of the anatomic lesion associated with the most common compartment syndromes. (From Matsen FA: Compartmental Syndrome. New York, Grune & Stratton, 1981, with permission.)

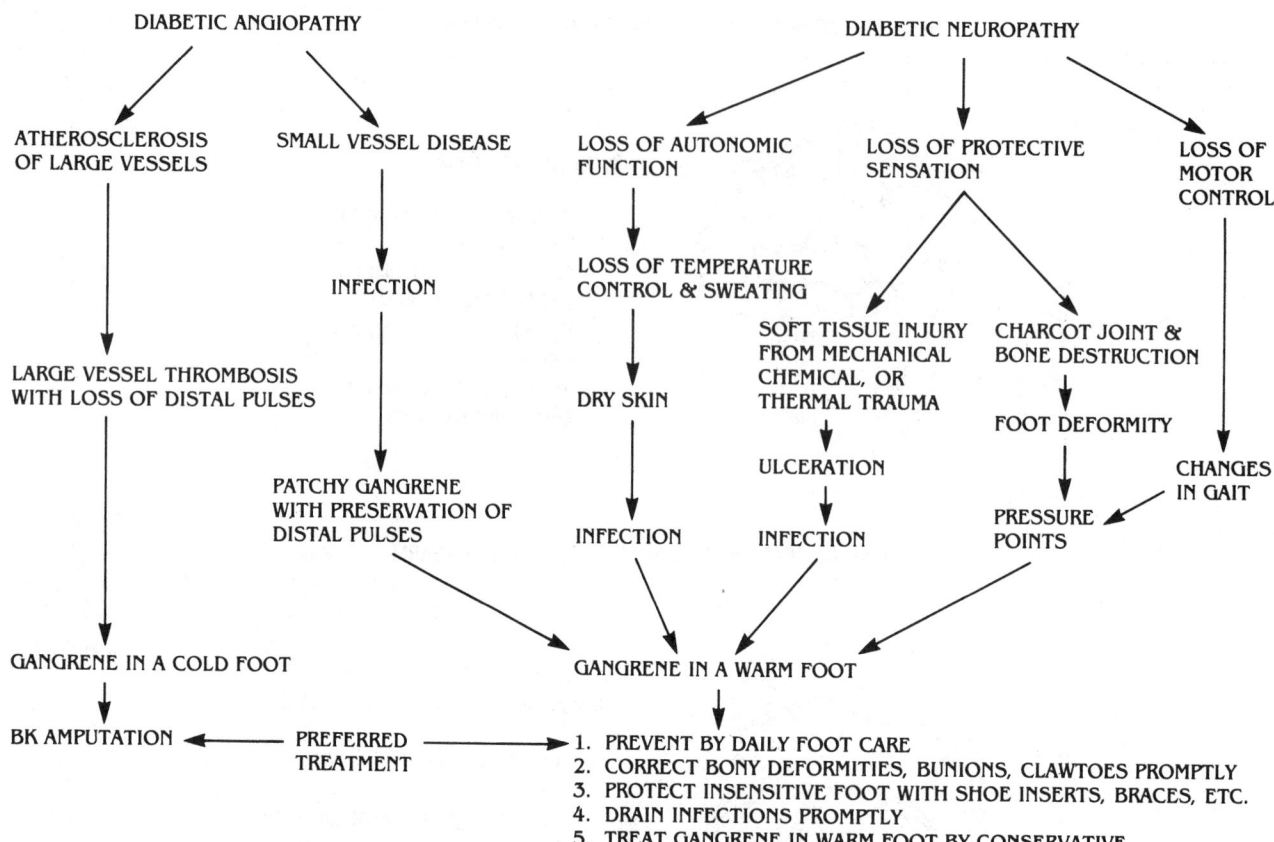

FIGURE 38–7. Etiologies of diabetic gangrene. BK, below the knee.

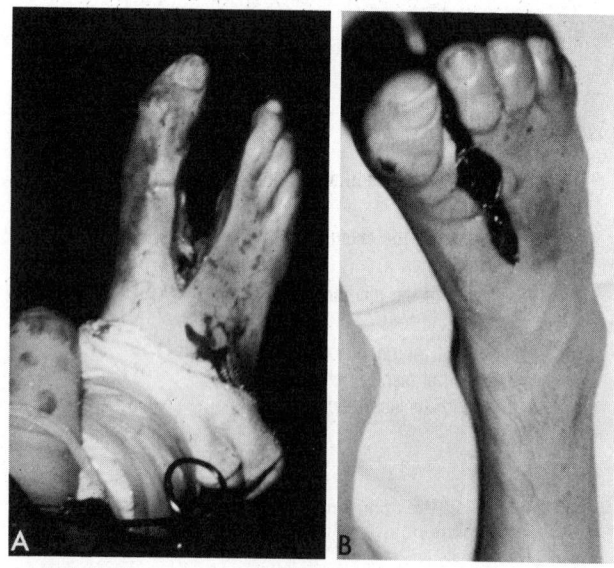

FIGURE 38–8. *A*, This patient suffered diabetic gangrene of the second toe with a warm foot. Resection of the ray proved to be the treatment of choice, because circulation to the remaining foot was normal. *B*, Two weeks following ray resection, the wound site was granulating satisfactorily. The patient had the benefit of a normally functioning and useful foot.

healing and closure. Transcutaneous oxygen levels above 30 to 35 per cent usually indicate there will be healing. The rehabilitation of the patient who has a below-knee amputation is much better, and a decent prosthesis gives better function than a persistently infected and painful ischemic limb. Figure 38–9 shows a radiograph of a patient who had suffered chronic osteomyelitis for 30 years, with a history of 27 operations. A below-knee amputation improved his function and eliminated the constant need for treatment. Conceivably, an amputation 20 years prior would have been of great benefit to this working man.

MANAGEMENT BY THE FAMILY PHYSICIAN. The family doctor should appreciate the importance of conservation of knee function in amputations and be aware of the differences between the warm and cold foot, as previously mentioned. In the warm foot, conservative drainage and other surgical treatment is indicated rather than below-knee amputation, and the patient who does require an amputation should be referred to an appropriate rehabilitative facility that is not interested solely in the removal of a limb. In other words, the surgery should be done by someone who is familiar with the rehabilitative phase.

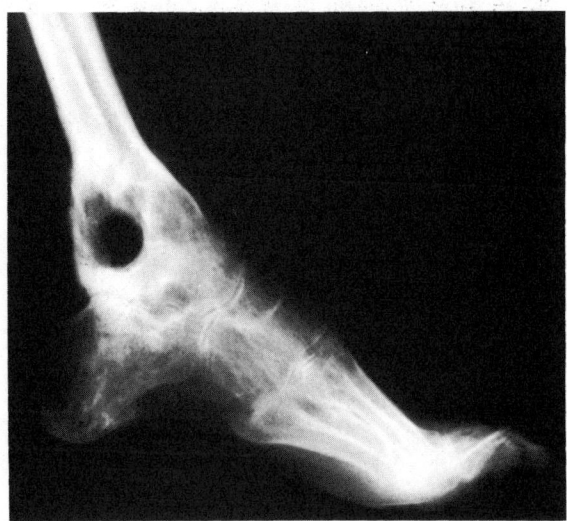

FIGURE 38–9. Lateral radiograph of a patient with a 30-year history of osteomyelitis and multiple operations. A below-knee amputation with prompt prosthetic fitting provided better function for the patient than did his chronically infected limb.

Reimplantations

Microvascular surgery has resulted in some salvage of digits, hands, and forearms. Unfortunately, inappropriate reimplantation has too often increased the period of disability and has not resulted in the function one would expect. Reimplantation is not always indicated, and considerations in deciding when it should be attempted include the work potential of the patient. In other words, will the potential benefit to the patient be worth the risk, expense, and loss of time and the costly rehabilitation, or is it better to go ahead with a definitive proper amputation and return the patient to useful life with rapidity? Another consideration is whether or not function will be improved or if there is a reasonable chance of function being returned. These decisions are best made by someone who is familiar with reimplantation and the risks and benefits. One should never promise the patient a reimplantation; this determination should be left to the surgeon who specializes in such work.

Indications that tip the decision in favor reimplantation are thumb amputation proximal to the interphalangeal joint, loss of multiple digits, one-digit amputation in a hand that is compromised by other injuries or prior injuries, transverse amputation between the metacarpophalangeal joints and the midportion of the forearm, and upper extremity amputations at more proximal levels in children (Phelps et al., 1978). In selected cases, reimplantation with the repair of arteries, veins, and nerves can have good success in the hands of an expert. Reimplantation of the lower extremity has not been justified except for foot amputations in the young child in most instances.

MANAGEMENT BY THE FAMILY PHYSICIAN. Many of these cases should be referred to someone familiar with reimplantation. Do not promise a reimplantation, but allow this decision to be made by the operating surgeon. The severed part should be placed in a cool, saline-soaked dressing, sealed in a plastic bag, and cooled on ice, being careful not to freeze the part. This is transported with the patient to a reimplantation center as rapidly as possible. Very often this can be done best by automobile rather than some elaborate means of air transportation. One should avoid unnecessary medications, excessive anticoagulants, or vasopressor agents. One can give appropriate antibiotics and intravenous fluids as needed prior to transportation.

Fingertip Amputations

Fingertip amputations can occur in a young child who catches the fingertip in a car door. This type of amputation usually goes through the nailbed into the pulp of the fingertip, and the distal phalanx may or may not be involved. Healing by secondary intention with frequent dressing changes is usually best in these cases, leading to a less sensitive scar. None of the elaborate skin grafts and flaps give as good a result as secondary healing.

MANAGEMENT BY THE FAMILY PHYSICIAN. Fingertip amputations are one type of injury that is frequently seen and can be very effectively managed by the family physician using the process of healing by secondary intention. One should cleanse the injured fingertip, leaving the nail in place to act as a splint. In the adult, any exposed bone may be cleaned off, but this is unnecessary in the child. After cleansing the wound, an occlusive dressing is placed over sterile gauze, with plaster over this, and appropriate antibiotics and tetanus prophylaxis are given. The hand is elevated in a sling and supported for 2 to 3 days. The cast dressing can be taken off at approximately 10 to 14 days. If the bone is exposed in the fingertip, about 3 weeks of casting is preferable treatment. This method of treatment maximizes finger length, gives the best possible scar, and keeps disability at a minimum in this common injury. This is considered the treatment of choice in most instances.

SPRAINS AND STRAINS

Many joints are affected by sprains and strains with relative frequency. These include the ankle, fingers, wrist, elbow, shoulder, and knee. Of particular interest is the so-called sprained wrist, because there are many pitfalls involved in the management of this injury.

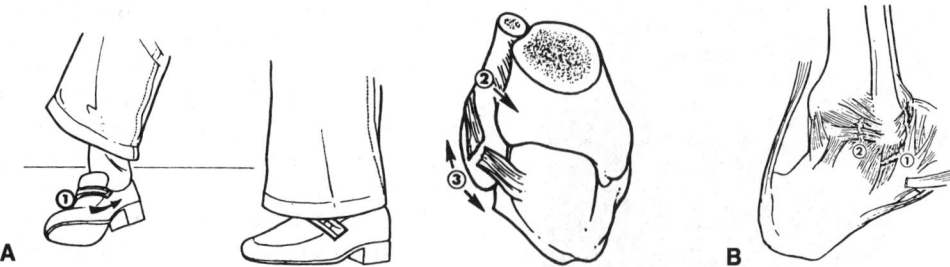

FIGURE 38–10.   *A,* Ankle sprain characteristically results from inversion injuries (1). This causes the fibula to abut against the anterior aspect of its groove in the tibia (2). The strain is absorbed by the anterior tibiofibular ligament, which ruptures (3). *B,* Most common sites of ankle sprains are the anterior fibulotalar ligament (1) and the posterior fibulotalar and calcaneofibular ligaments (2). (From Connolly JF: DePalma's The Management of Fractures and Dislocations: An Atlas, 3rd edition. Philadelphia, WB Saunders Company, 1981, with permission.)

Ankle Sprains

Ankle sprains produce the most common set of joint instability problems, depending on the mechanism of the injury. Sprains usually result from an inversion mechanism, whereas an eversion or external torsion usually produces a fracture. The ankle is essentially made up of three bones, including the lateral malleolus, which is elongated and sits in a groove along the lateral side of the tibia. When the ankle is forcefully inverted, the fibula rather rapidly abuts against the tibial tubercle and the resultant strain is absorbed by the anterior talofibular ligament. Continued overloading will disrupt the calcaneofibular and talocalcaneal ligaments (Fig. 38–10).

Estimates are that about one significant ankle sprain occurs per 10,000 population per day. Therefore, this represents one of the most frequent musculoskeletal problems to be treated by the family physician. The vast majority of these injuries are minor disruptions of the anterior talofibular ligament, and are best managed by minimal supervision. About one in four acute ankle sprains will have some recurrent episodes of instability. When this occurs, it should not be undertreated or ignored. These problems can be corrected by appropriate reconstructive procedures that give a good result, in contrast to many of the ligamentous injuries around the knee.

The ankle can be repaired late, as contrasted with the knee, which should be repaired acutely. In the initial evaluation, one must consider whether or not the patient has suffered any similar ankle problems in the past and keep in mind what level of function the patient needs for future demand on that ankle. A history of popping or a painful snap at the time of an ankle injury is usually indicative of a significant ligament injury. Examination should include direct palpation of the area for maximal tenderness, usually anterolaterally or posterolaterally and occasionally anteromedially. In addition, one should palpate to see if there is a tender sulcus along the anterolateral aspect of the ankle with inversion.

The amount of pain the patient has bears no relationship to the amount of anatomic disruption. In other words, a complete ligamentous tear can be relatively pain free when stress is placed on the ankle, despite considerable instability in the ankle.

A radiograph should be considered for every sprained ankle because it is so easy to confuse fracture with sprain, and there may be osteochondral fractures of the surface of the talus or other minor fractures. The Ottawa ankle rules were developed as guidelines to determine which cases of ankle sprain warrant radiographic evaluation. Briefly, these rules say that an ankle radiograph is needed if the patient has pain in the area of the medial or lateral malleolus and at least one of these findings at examination: 1) tenderness of bone at the back edge or tip of the lateral malleolus, 2) tenderness of bone at the tip or back edge of the medial malleolus, or 3) inability to bear weight immediately after the injury or later in the emergency room. Radiographic study of the foot is needed if the patient complains of midfoot pain and any one of the following: 1) tenderness of bone at the base of the fifth metatarsal, 2) tenderness of bone at the navicular, or 3) inability to bear weight immediately at injury or later in the emergency room.

A recent study has validated the Ottawa ankle rules as an accurate tool in the identification of ankle and midfoot fractures (Stiell et al., 1994). The 3-month study of over 500 ankle injuries correctly identified all malleolar and midfoot fractures. Cost and emergency room time were reduced and unnecessary radiographs were avoided.

Radiographs of the sprained ankle should not be coned down but should include the ankle, foot, and most of the tibia or fibula in order to not miss fractures higher up. Stress radiographs taken in forced inversion are sometimes helpful to demonstrate instability, but ankle instability can be present even with a normal stress radiograph. These are best done late, after recovery, to assess the chronic unstable ankle.

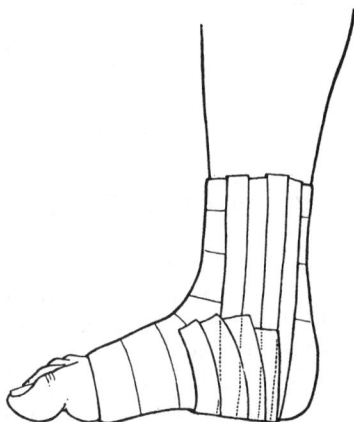

FIGURE 38–11. The most effective method of supporting most acute ankle sprains is by using an Ace wrap reinforced with 1-inch medial and lateral tape strips. The anterior and posterior aspects of the ankle are left free to allow the patient to flex and extend the ankle. The patient is encouraged to bear weight with crutches. (From Connolly JF: DePalma's The Management of Fractures and Dislocations: An Atlas, 3rd edition. Philadelphia, WB Saunders Company, 1981, with permission.)

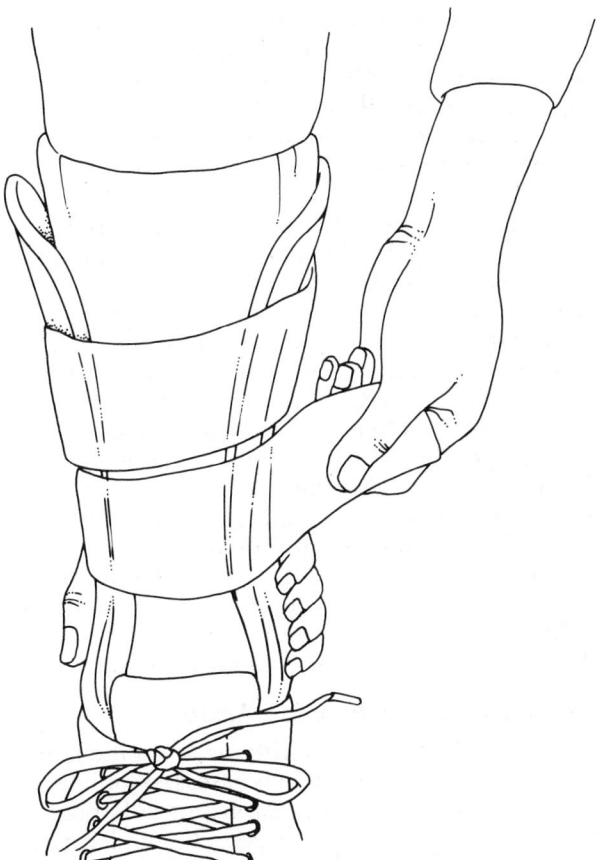

FIGURE 38–12. Diagram of an air splint. Straps are adjusted to heel size, and the lower straps wrapped about ankle and the side extensions are centered. The splint is then pressurized and straps adjusted until a comfortable support and pressure are attained.

MANAGEMENT BY THE FAMILY PHYSICIAN. The vast majority of ankle sprains can be treated with minimal external support, icing the wound down with ice bags, and elevation. The patient should be allowed partial weight bearing with crutches or a cane, because non–weight bearing tends to tighten the heel cord and calf muscles and lead to increased disability.

An effective method of supporting the ankle is to wrap an Ace bandage onto it acutely from the toes to just above the malleoli about mid-calf and reinforce this with a full roll of 2-inch tape applied medially and laterally (Fig. 38–11). Another good appliance is an air cast or splint (Fig. 38–12), which can give good support and be fitted with ease. These need a lace-up shoe to hold them in place. The straps can be adjusted for comfort. The ankle is wrapped mainly for comfort and, if the patient experiences too much swelling or irritation, the wrapping and support should be loosened in order not to injure the skin or lead to ischemic change. It is advisable for a patient to elevate the ankle for 2 to 3 days and apply ice to the painful areas and then begin ambulation when the pain has subsided somewhat.

Functional rehabilitation is encouraged because this is good for ligamentous structures and aids in proprioception about the ankle. Exercises on a balance board will help develop coordination (Fig. 38–13).

The patient's history and the degree of instability and pain on stressing and palpating for local defects of the capsule will determine clinically if the sprain is a minor grade I injury or if it is a complete grade III injury. The gray zone, or grade II injury, is difficult to ascertain acutely. This should

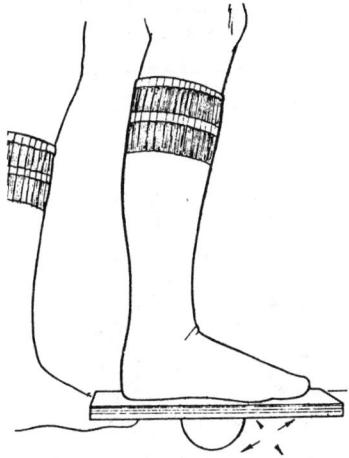

FIGURE 38–13. As the ankle pain subsides, about the third to the fifth day, balancing exercises can begin to allow the patient to regain ankle proprioception and to avoid recurrent instability problems. (From Connolly JF: DePalma's The Management of Fractures and Dislocations: An Atlas, 3rd edition. Philadelphia, WB Saunders Company, 1981, with permission.)

be treated initially as a grade I, or minor, strain, understanding that grade III injuries, with a palpable anterolateral sulcus on inversion stressing and injuries to anterofibular and posterior calcaneofibular ligaments, require more than just elevation and taping. In general these should be treated in a cast.

Overall, one does not treat all ankle sprains in a cast because this leads to severe stiffness and prolongs the disability to a much greater extent than managing the sprain with some motion. However, if the ankle is so unstable that taping does not provide total support, the ligament is best repaired acutely. This is particularly true with unstable ankles in young, active athletes. Individuals with recurrent problems of instability or an acute grade III problem should be offered an operative repair. Long-standing ankle instability leads to degenerative arthritis and other problems.

Avulsion fractures seen on radiographs should be evaluated by an appropriate orthopedics consultant to determine whether or not ligamentous damage warrants primary operative repair.

Recurrent Instability of the Ankle

Persistent ankle instability is a problem well known in sports. The ankle is assessed for instability by special stress radiographs, usually taken in inversion. The results of these radiographs are not always reliable, and should be used as adjunct information to the history and physical examination. In general, more than 10 to 15 degrees of tilt in comparison with the opposite ankle is considered evidence of significant instability. Patients with significant instability should probably be referred

for ligament reconstruction; although some patients will improve with an ankle rehabilitation program, this improvement usually is not significant.

Jammed Finger or Finger Sprain

Finger sprains can be treacherous, with a number of hidden injuries being possible. These injuries include tendon avulsions, such as mallet finger, boutonnière deformity, or flexor profundus avulsions; phalangeal fractures; and dislocations. A simple jammed finger is usually an unimpressive injury that produces a lot of disability but usually is not too serious. To detect and treat this injury and prevent potential problems, the physician should systematically evaluate the finger for the above injuries, no matter how unimpressive the sprain looks at first glance. This means a thorough palpation of all areas for tenderness, determination of active and passive range of motion, stress testing to evaluate for instability or loss of tendon function, and, of course, adequate anteroposterior and lateral radiographs centered on the finger to detect any fractures.

Tendon Avulsions

Mallet Finger. A mallet finger deformity is the most common injury to the tendon of the digit. It is usually caused by a blow to the end of the finger, producing pain, swelling, and deformity. The degree of deformity may vary, but the patient cannot actively extend the distal phalanx. The ten-

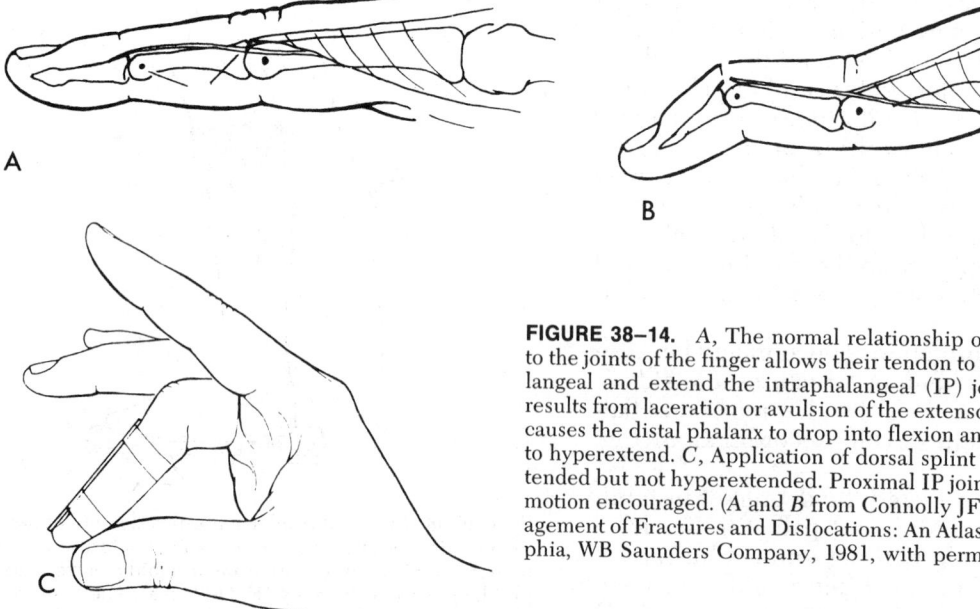

FIGURE 38–14. *A*, The normal relationship of the intrinsic muscles to the joints of the finger allows their tendon to flex the metacarpophalangeal and extend the intraphalangeal (IP) joints. *B*, Mallet finger results from laceration or avulsion of the extensor tendon insertion that causes the distal phalanx to drop into flexion and the proximal IP joint to hyperextend. *C*, Application of dorsal splint with distal IP joint extended but not hyperextended. Proximal IP joint is left free and active motion encouraged. (*A* and *B* from Connolly JF: DePalma's The Management of Fractures and Dislocations: An Atlas, 3rd edition. Philadelphia, WB Saunders Company, 1981, with permission.)

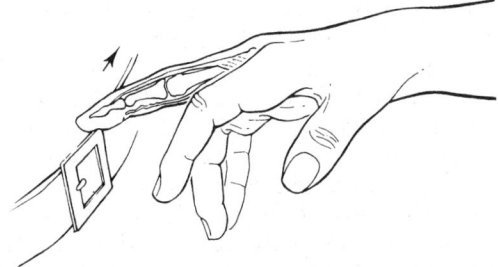

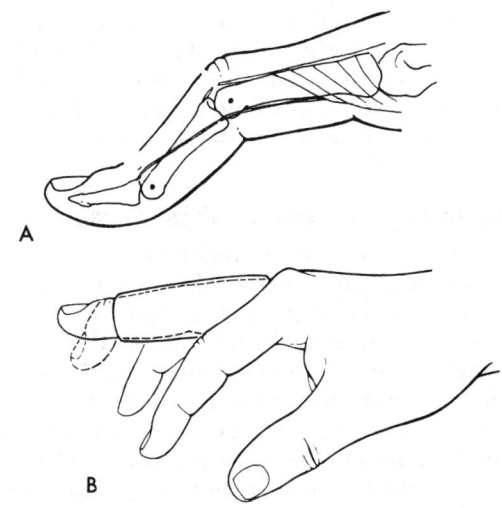

FIGURE 38–15. Flexor profundus tendon is avulsed during forceful flexion of the finger. The injury tends to pass unrecognized or will be dismissed as a "jammed" finger unless the patient's inability to flex the distal phalanx is recognized. The diagnosis becomes obvious once the patient is asked to move the distal phalanx. (From Connolly JF: DePalma's The Management of Fractures and Dislocations: An Atlas, 3rd edition. Philadelphia, WB Saunders Company, 1981, with permission.)

FIGURE 38–16. *A*, Disruption of the central slip insertion onto the middle phalanx leads to gradual displacement of the proximal phalanx dorsally, with flexion contracture of the proximal interphalangeal joint and extension contracture of the distal interphalangeal joint. *B*, If there is any suspicion of boutonnière deformity, the proximal interphalangeal joint must be immobilized in an extension splint. This is one of the rare indications for immobilization of a finger injury in extension. (From Connolly JF: DePalma's The Management of Fractures and Dislocations: An Atlas, 3rd edition. Philadelphia, WB Saunders Company, 1981, with permission.)

don may continue to retract, increasing the deformity (Fig. 38–14A, B).

Management by the Family Physician. Prompt recognition of the extensor tendon avulsion allows closed treatment with a dorsal splint, which is used for 5 or 6 weeks (Fig. 38–14C). Mallet finger deformities associated with fractures that cannot be reduced anatomically require referral for open reduction and internal fixation.

FLEXOR TENDON AVULSIONS. This injury occurs most often in the ring or small finger in a patient who forcibly grasped something like the shirt of a fellow football player as he lunged forward (Fig. 38–15). The flexor profundus avulsion also occurs in older patients who avulse this tendon while lifting heavy objects.

Too often the significance of this injury goes unrecognized. The profundus tendon then retracts proximally in its sheath and completely up into the palm in some instances. Physical examination will show the tenderness to be localized over either the proximal interphalangeal joint or in the palm, but usually not at the site of tendon insertion. The diagnosis is made readily by observing the patient's inability to flex the distal interphalangeal joint. Sometimes the radiograph will show a piece of bone lodged at one of the pulleys of the tendon in the finger or in the palm.

Management by the Family Physician. Prompt repair of the avulsed tendon restores normal grip to the injured finger. Successful repair can be accomplished up to about 3 weeks after injury. Delayed recognition may leave the patient with some degree of permanent functional impairment. To avoid missing this injury, it is necessary to assess the ability to flex and extends all joints of this "jammed finger." These patients should be promptly referred to a hand surgeon for repair.

BOUTONNIÈRE DEFORMITY. Boutonnière deformity usually results from a direct laceration over the proximal interphalangeal joint, involving the extensor slip that attaches to the middle phalanx.

This permits a progressive flexion contracture to develop. Another mechanism is a closed crush injury that can allow avulsion of this central slip. The flexion deformity begins to develop over several days and may not be noted initially. Thus, it is easy for this injury go unrecognized. Progressive disruption occurs and allows a buttonhole deformity, which then allows the disrupted tendon to retract below the mechanical center of the proximal interphalangeal joint. An extensor contractures develops of the distal interphalangeal joint then develops over a few weeks or months following the injury (Fig. 38–16A). This becomes a chronic problem.

Management by the Family Physician. If there is doubt about the integrity of the tendon, the joint should be immobilized in an extension cast for 3 to 6 weeks, which ensures adequate healing and prevents flexion contracture of the joint (Fig. 38–16B). Even in a patient seen 6 to 12 weeks after initial injury, a cast may be effective in correcting a boutonnière deformity. If an avulsion fracture is present, it is better to refer the patient for operative repair.

Wrist Sprains

Wrist sprains and carpal bone injuries are among the most likely to be misdiagnosed and are subject to frequent delayed diagnoses. Fractures of the carpal scaphoid are notorious for their tendency to pass as a wrist sprain, as are dissociations of the lunate scaphoid joint and other dissociations of the carpal bones. Fractures of the hamate and scapholunate separations also can mask as sprains of the wrist.

Radiographic Evaluation of Wrist Sprains

One common reason for misdiagnosis of wrist injuries is inadequate radiographic studies. Usual anteroposterior and oblique radiographs may not detect even a complete dislocation of the carpus. Evaluation of any seriously injured wrist should include anteroposterior radiographs of the wrist in maximum radial and ulnar deviation in particular to detect scapholunate dissociation or scaphoid fractures. Flexion also will show carpal instability in many instances. A supinated wrist view with the fist clenched can demonstrate mild carpal subluxations in many instances. Finally, a tunnel view may detect fractures of the volar aspect of the wrist, such as fractures of the hook of the hamate.

MANAGEMENT BY THE FAMILY PHYSICIAN. Even when the radiograph fails to demonstrate a fracture, if the patient has pain localized to the anatomic snuffbox, the injury should be treated as a fracture, with casting that immobilizes the thumb and wrist. This cast should be kept on for approximately 2 weeks and then removed, and the radiographs repeated. If at this time a vascular response has demonstrated a fracture line to be present, the wrist should be immobilized with a new cast until the fracture has healed. If no fracture is noted at 2 weeks and the patient still has pain, scapholunate subluxation should be considered and appropriate consultations or studies obtained. If the patient is pain free at the end of 8 to 10 weeks of cast immobilization, one can discontinue casting. Some scaphoid fractures will not achieve union; when this occurs, a hand surgeon should repair and graft the fracture.

Ganglions

Dorsal ganglions of the wrist present as a cyst-like herniation or ganglion cyst. These characteristically cause discomfort on the dorsal surface of the wrist, presenting as a firm mass that can enlarge to varying sizes. They also can occur on the volar surface.

Synovial ganglions of the fingers, similar to those that develop in the wrist, are quite common. They are usually about 5 mm in diameter and tender and may be disabling on strong grasp. These usually small synovial ganglia herniate through the tendon sheath of the finger. They can disappear as suddenly as they appeared simply by splinting.

MANAGEMENT BY THE FAMILY PHYSICIAN. The usual ganglion cyst can be aspirated of fluid content and immobilized in a cast for 3 weeks or so, holding the wrist in a slightly dorsiflexed position to encourage scar formation and healing in the capsular area of damage. If the ganglion recurs after this treatment, surgical excision is advised. The physician must keep in mind that wrist ganglion and synovitis from rheumatoid arthritis can be confused. Also, any progressively enlarging lump or bump belongs in a pathologist's bottle and not in the patient's body. One should get appropriate consultations or surgically remove these cysts.

A synovial ganglion can be palpated as a pea-sized lesion at the base of the finger. It usually can be ruptured with a 22-gauge needle through a small skin wheal raised with local anesthetic. One should try not merely to puncture the cyst but to tear its walls to stimulate repair after rupture. Relief is usually immediate and complete (Bruner, 1963). This technique is quite simple and can be performed in any office under sterile conditions; it should be tried in preference to surgical excision.

Acute and Chronic Scapholunate Subluxation or Dissociation

Scapholunate subluxation is noted as a widening of the joint space between the scaphoid and lunate on radiographs (Fig. 38–17A). It should not be dismissed simply as a wrist sprain. This injury also can manifest as a progressive dissociation over a period of some weeks, and persistent clicks with pain should be evaluated by a hand surgeon early on. This chronic dissociation of the scapholunate allows a proximal migration of the capitate and rapid progressive arthritis in the wrist joint, and can be severely disabling.

In the acutely sprained wrist, if no fracture of the carpal scaphoid is demonstrated, one should try to rule out subluxation of this joint with adequate radiographs. Obtaining a true lateral view of the wrist and a posteroanterior view with the fist clenched and wrist supinated will sometimes show widening of this joint. On a lateral radiograph, the axis of the radius, lunate, and capitate should form a straight line and the axis of the scaphoid should intersect the radiolunate axis at about a 30- to 60-degree angle. When subluxation occurs, the scaphoid rotates downward and the lunate tilts upward so that the intersection of these angles will exceed 70 degrees (Fig. 38–17B).

Scapholunate subluxation can occur in individuals such as carpenters, who subject their wrists to repeated heavy loading. The diagnosis is recognized by progressive pain in this region with a palpable click on extension of the wrist and loss of grip strength.

MANAGEMENT BY THE FAMILY PHYSICIAN. This is not an uncommon injury and should be suspected in cases of persistent wrist pain that mimics carpal scaphoid fracture, especially with a click present on palpation. This is an injury that requires

FIGURE 38–17. *A,* Disruption of the scapholunate and radiocarpal ligament leads to progressive dissociation between the scaphoid and the rest of the carpal bones. This injury is frequently mistaken for a persistent wrist sprain. *B,* Chronic dissociation of the scapholunate joint allows the scaphoid to rotate downward toward the palm. This increases the angle between the scaphoid axis and the radiolunate-capitate axis. The capitate then slowly migrates toward the radius, and osteoarthritis rapidly develops. (From Connolly JF: DePalma's The Management of Fractures and Dislocations: An Atlas, 3rd edition. Philadelphia, WB Saunders Company, 1981, with permission.)

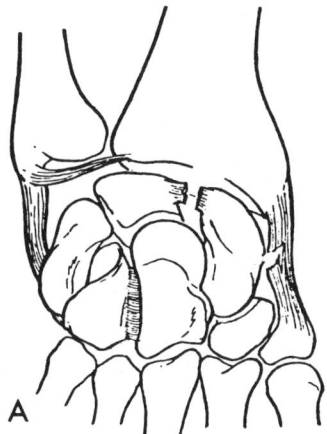 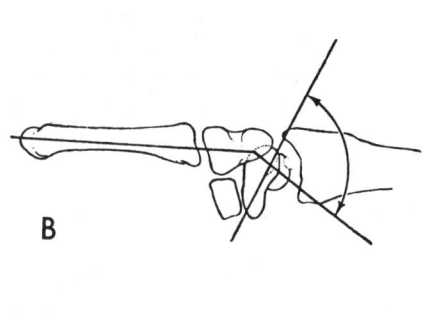

referral to a hand surgeon early on for appropriate reduction and repair.

Stenosing Tenosynovitis (De Quervain's Disease)

De Quervain's disease, or stenosing tenosynovitis at the base of the thumb, may be misdiagnosed as an acute wrist sprain. Characteristically this tendinitis is of the abductor pollicis longus and extensor pollicis brevis tendons around the distal base of the radius above the wrist, and can be diagnosed by history and physical examination.

The pain from this condition is felt usually down the thumb and up into the forearm. Tenderness may be evident at the level of the carpal bones or at the insertion of the abductor longus into the base of the first metacarpal.

The diagnosis of tenosynovitis of the thumb extensor and abductor tendon is made by testing the thumb for pain in resisted extension and abduction of the thumb. This necessitates gliding of the inflamed tendons and will produce pain. Radial deviation with a sudden flexion of the thumb will sometimes elicit such pain, termed "Finkelstein's sign."

MANAGEMENT BY THE FAMILY PHYSICIAN. Stenosing tenosynovitis is treated by injection of lidocaine (Xylocaine) or bupivacaine (Marcaine) mixed with triamcinolone hexacetonide, 1 to 2 mL, into the tendon sheath with a 25-gauge needle. This will usually relieve the symptoms. The wrist should be kept in a splint for several days and then motion allowed. If this does not suffice, one should refer the patient for the possibility of surgical release of the tendon sheath.

Carpal Tunnel Syndrome

The initial symptoms of this disease include numbness with characteristic paresthesias, or pins and needles sensation, in the radial three and one half digits of the hand. The causes may vary from overuse of the wrist to residual deformity of a Colles' fracture, pregnancy, rheumatoid synovitis, and particularly overuse. These paresthesias tend to waken the patient at night, and rest, elevation, and shaking of the wrist tend to bring some relief. The paresthesias are the result of too much pressure and represent the peripheral nerves' signals that a partial compression has occurred. The pins and needles sensation in carpal tunnel syndrome has been related by Flatt (1974) and others to anoxia. Nighttime inactivity tends to eliminate muscle pumping and thus leads to venous stasis and increased anoxia. Cyriax (1978) has pointed out the clinical significance of the pins and needles, which can be sensed only distal to the site of the nerve compression and which can be used to localize the site. Aching symptoms may be noted proximal to the site of compression, but paresthesias are always distal.

The differential diagnosis of carpal tunnel syndrome includes cervical lesions and thoracic outlet syndrome. Cervical disk lesions produce paresthesias but also involve more of the arm in general. Cervical disk paresthesias usually are not related to wrist function. Thoracic outlet syndrome may awaken the patient at night, but here again the paresthesias do not relate to wrist activity and tend to involve more of the arm and forearm than in carpal tunnel syndrome. Electromyographic study of nerve conduction is very important and can help differentiate these conditions.

MANAGEMENT BY THE FAMILY PHYSICIAN. When an electromyographic test shows impaired conduction of the median nerve at the wrist, operative decompression is advisable. The only exception is the carpal tunnel syndrome that develops in the last trimester of pregnancy and usually subsides after delivery. If clinical symptoms persist, then carpal tunnel release should be done after the delivery. Occasionally, injection of 1 mL triamcinolone hexacetonide or a similar cortisone into the area under the transverse carpal ligament parallel to the nerves and tendon can give relief. The nerve is located between the palmaris longus and the flexor carpi radialis tendon. One should be careful to avoid intraneural injection. If such injection relieves the symptoms, the diagnosis of carpal tunnel syndrome is confirmed. Relief may be permanent but usually is not. If it is not, decompression may become necessary. One should not delay recommending operative treatment because damage only progresses and there may be a loss of intrinsic muscle function that is rarely recovered. This has serious consequences for grip strength in the long term.

Elbow Sprains

As with other joints, pain in the elbow can arise from a number of causes and can originate in both the hard and the soft tissues.

Nursemaid's Elbow

This condition gets its name because it results from a forceful pull on the extended pronated elbow of a child, who is usually under the age of 4. Traction on the pronated arm produces a tear in the ligament. The pronated position then allows the overshaped radial head to slip partially in under the ligament, with the characteristic presentation of a child who refuses to move the elbow from the flexed pronated position. Radiographs of nursemaid's elbow or subluxed radial head usually show no abnormality at the elbow, and the diagnosis is usually purely clinical. One must be sure to rule out any undisplaced supracondylar fracture in the humerus before making a diagnosis of nursemaid's elbow. Occasionally, a supracondylar fracture may not be evident initially and can be seen only on lateral radiographs as a radiolucent line posterior to the distal humerus (so-called fat pad sign) that represents a hematoma from the fracture elevating the fat behind the elbow.

MANAGEMENT BY THE FAMILY PHYSICIAN. Treatment of nursemaid's elbow consists of gentle but firm supination of the child's forearm, flexing the elbow gently to 90 degrees. With one hand on the forearm and the other hand holding the humerus, the thumb is placed over the radial head and the child's forearm rapidly and firmly rotated into full supination. Reduction is usually achieved with a palpable click or pop, and the pain is immediately relieved. If the injury is of greater than 12 hours' duration, the relief of pain may not be quite as prompt. It is wise to immobilize the elbow in a sling for 5 to 7 days, and caution the parents about pulling on the child's forearm. If the problem is a recurrent one or treatment has been delayed greater than 12 hours, the elbow should be immobilized in a splint for about 2 weeks.

Little Leaguer's Elbow

This condition results from fatigue injuries in an adolescent who uses the elbow for throwing. It is most often seen in boys who practice baseball pitching to excess. The adolescent bone structure does not withstand the loading from repetitive

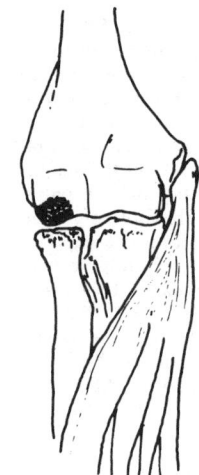

FIGURE 38–18.   Little Leaguer's elbow results from overuse of an adolescent's pitching elbow. Lesions may include fatigue fractures of the medial epicondyle, radial head, or capitate. (From Connolly JF: DePalma's The Management of Fractures and Dislocations: An Atlas, 3rd edition. Philadelphia, WB Saunders Company, 1981, with permission.)

hard throwing as well as does an adult elbow, and commonly the injury is an avulsion fracture of the medial humeral condyle (Fig. 38–18). One may also see fatigue fractures of the lateral humeral condyle or radial head on occasion.

MANAGEMENT BY THE FAMILY PHYSICIAN. The most effective management is prevention. The adolescent athlete should be warned to avoid excessive throwing and overuse of the elbow. If loose bodies develop in the elbow, surgical intervention is necessary to remove them.

Tennis or Golfer's Elbow

Tennis elbow is extremely common and results from small tears usually at the origin of the extensor carpi radialis longus, although other muscles in the extensor group may be involved. It occurs most often in a part-time or nonathlete in the 40-year age range. Golfer's elbow, arising on the common flexor surface or medial side of the elbow, is analogous to tennis elbow in nearly every way except that it is a tendinitis of the wrist flexors. The condition is seen less frequently than tennis elbow. Treatment of this condition is the same as that for lateral epicondylitis, and the response is usually better. However, it should be noted that only about 5 per cent of 1000 patients in a study by Coonrad and Hooper (1973) had actually played tennis or golf.

Many individuals with tennis elbow have never seen a physician and recover without treatment. When the patient does come to the attention of a physician, the usual complaint is pain down the back of the forearm and into the wrist and dorsum of the hand. The pain may also move upward toward the shoulder in some instances. The pain is made worse by any attempt to lift objects of any weight in extension, and twinges of pain may become so severe that the patient drops even relatively lightweight objects. Picking up a telephone may be particularly painful.

The patient may not recall a specific injury but only relate progressively increased pain with exertion.

The history and clinical course support the conclusions of Cyriax (1978) and Coonrad and Hooper (1973) in that tennis elbow results from scar formation in a partial tendon tear. At surgery one may occasionally see this scar. Repeated irritation from muscle pull prevents adequate healing and gives rise to pain. Physical examination of the active range of motion of the elbow is usually fairly painless, but forced extensor pressure against the examiner's hand with the arm flexed and supinated and the extensors put to full use is very painful over the lateral epicondyle. This wrist extension against resistance produces severe pain and re-creates the symptoms on the lateral condyle and forearm, and is specific for the condition.

MANAGEMENT BY THE FAMILY PHYSICIAN. Treatment of tennis elbow is primarily rest. If the symptoms have been present for less than 6 weeks, this may be the only treatment necessary, and is best accomplished with a dorsal plaster splint maintaining the wrist in extension for a couple of weeks. Often this is not possible or is it sufficient; in this instance, injection of triamcinolone hexacetonide mixed with bupivacaine (Marcaine) or lidocaine (Xylocaine) can be injected into the point of maximum tenderness with considerable relief. A small (25- or 22-gauge) needle can be utilized and, with slow injection, this will be quite painless. Following injection, the elbow should be kept at rest as much as possible, using a dorsal splint for about 7 days. Frequently a permanent cure is achieved with two to three injections.

Surgical treatment may be advised if the patient has had symptoms for a year or more with adequate treatment. A surgical release can be performed, with removal of any bursa or synovitis that might be a source of symptomatology. This is only necessary in a few patients, perhaps 1 in 50.

Ulnar Nerve Entrapment (Cubital Tunnel Syndrome)

The ulnar nerve runs behind the medial humeral condyle in a groove. There is an arcuate ligament that holds the nerve in its groove and subjects it to some compression with prolonged flexion. The result may be a complaint of pins and needles sensation in the fourth and fifth fingers after minor but prolonged activity requiring elbow flexion, such as holding a telephone receiver or newspaper or sleeping with the elbow flexed behind the head.

A permanent neuropathy can result from cast application holding the elbow in an excessively flexed position, or, if the ulnar nerve is prone to dislocation from its groove, a cast can trap it in dis-

location. One should avoid immobilizing the elbow in more than 90 degrees of flexion for even brief periods of time during surgical procedures or in casts because iatrogenic nerve injury is a serious and preventable cause of cubital tunnel syndrome.

A second common cause of ulnar entrapment at the elbow is a valgus deformity following a childhood fracture. This is known as tardy ulnar nerve palsy. Before diagnosing the cubital tunnel syndrome, one also should take care to rule out causes of ulnar compression proximal or distal to the elbow. This would include conditions such as thoracic outlet syndrome proximally or ganglion or other impingement of the nerve at the wrist.

Cyriax's (1978) rule that a pins and needles sensation always begins at the site of nerve entrapment and moves distally is helpful in differentiating the location of the entrapment. Nerve conduction studies are also helpful.

MANAGEMENT BY THE FAMILY PHYSICIAN. If electromyograms show a persistent impaired condition at the elbow, anterior transposition of the nerve should be recommended promptly and should be done by an experienced surgeon. If there is no demonstrable electromyographic abnormality, a trial therapeutic injection of triamcinolone can sometimes be diagnostic. This is placed within the nerve sheath and not in the nerve. About 1 mL of triamcinolone should be injected with a very small (25-gauge) needle just deep to the condylar groove between the nerve and the bone. Repeated injections are not recommended.

Pancoast's Tumor

This is a tumor at the pulmonary apex in a patient suffering with shoulder pain or forearm pain and some severe weakness of intrinsic muscles of the hand, which may develop quite rapidly. This rapidly progressive lesion is frequently mistaken for ulnar neuropathy or cervical disk syndrome, or perhaps even frozen shoulder. Horner's syndrome (ptosis, miosis, anhidrosis, enophthalmos, narrowing of the palpebral fissure, slight elevation of the lower lid, flushing of the affected side of the face) can be associated with this arm pain and indicates a need for thorough radiographic study of the lung and its apex.

Shoulder Pain, Sprains, and Stiffness

The symptoms of shoulder pain originate from the tendons and periarticular structures in most instances. The shoulder is designed for mobility rather than stability, and any stiffness in the joint may give considerable functional impairment. Because of the shallowness of the joint, it is most susceptible to dislocation or subluxation.

Chronic and Acute Tendinitis and Bursitis

Almost any tendon around the shoulder can be torn or is subject to painful scarring, depending on the activities of the patient. Athletic individuals suffer commonly from acute and chronic wear injuries. Tendon degeneration in most individuals occurs as a gradual wear process that involves the rotator cuff structures. The supraspinatus and the long end of the biceps are especially susceptible. This is because the mechanism of shoulder abduction requires that the humeral head externally rotate at about 70 or 80 degrees of elevation to clear from underneath the anterior acromion process and the coracoacromial ligament.

The primary symptom of tendon attrition is generally a painful, aching shoulder of rather nondescript type. Pain from supraspinatus tendinitis is not necessarily localized to the tendon but is generalized through the whole deltoid area. The aching from tendinitis frequently extends down to the forearm and wrist and consequently is really quite nonspecific. Such lack of specificity in shoulder pain is due to our interpretation of the source of pain as coming from the C-5 dermatome rather than any structure specifically at the shoulder. The same type of general aching is associated with arthritis, bursitis, adhesive capsulitis, and lesions at the apex of the lung.

Physical examination usually can differentiate these lesions by demonstrating whether or not the pain is aggravated when the tendon is stressed. Shoulder examination should not consist merely of poking the patient and finding a site of pain, or a "trigger point." To diagnose supraspinatus tendinitis, the pain should be exaggerated or aggravated when the shoulder is abducted and externally rotated against resistance. Bicipital tendinitis will give pain that is aggravated when the patient flexes forward against resistance. Tendon lesions will demonstrate a full range of passive motion and only active resisted motion seems to be impaired. Other conditions that give shoulder pain, such as arthritis or adhesive capsulitis, impair passive as well as active resisted motion.

Radiographs of the shoulder in painful tendinitis or bursitis are unrevealing but should be obtained to help differentiate other conditions, including chronic posterior shoulder dislocations, infections, tumor, and arthritides. About 10 to 15 per cent of shoulder radiographs will demonstrate some calcification of the supraspinatus tendon insertion. This calcification is usually inert, but occasionally requires surgical removal (Fig. 38–19) or treatment with ultrasound, which sometimes can resolve the problem.

MANAGEMENT BY THE FAMILY PHYSICIAN. The majority of conditions about the shoulder can be relieved by injecting 1% bupivacaine into the subacromial bursa or tendon region and applying ice. This also helps differentiate glenohumeral arthritis and subluxation from tendon problems. One should avoid injecting directly into a tendon because this can weaken the structure and lead to rupture.

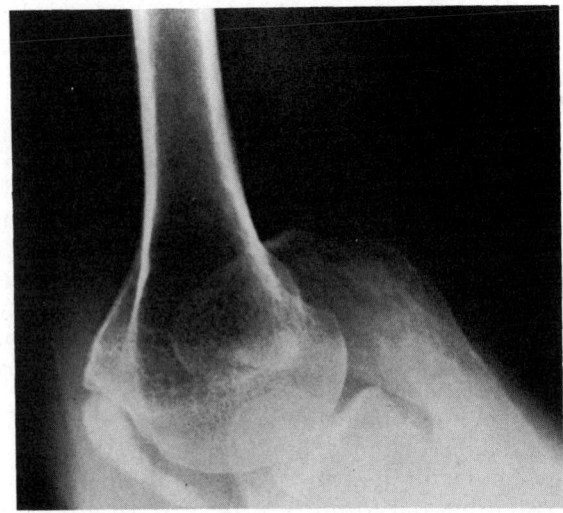

FIGURE 38–19. This chronic calcium deposit seen on an axillary view of the shoulder caused the supraspinatus tendon to be pinched between the coracoacromial ligament and the humerus during elevation of the arm. The calcium was removed and the coracoacromial ligament released to restore shoulder elevation and relieve the patient's painful impingement. Ordinarily, calcium deposits need not be removed unless they are causing mechanical impingement syndromes.

Overuse syndrome in the shoulder should be treated by anti-inflammatory medications and rest for 5 to 7 days. Baseball pitchers should avoid throwing overhead, and swimmers should alter their breathing style and avoid the type of swimming that precipitates trouble for a period of 7 to 10 days. Tennis players should rotate the body toward the net as they raise the arm above the horizontal. All of these actions help relieve symptoms.

For acute calcific bursitis in the middle-aged individual, more intensive therapy may be necessary, including local injection of triamcinolone or a similar corticoid process in an attempt to disperse calcific substances. This process can be assisted with several ultrasound treatments in many instances. Calcification around the shoulder may be thought of as analogous to uric acid deposits in a gouty joint. It causes inflammation, and the resultant degenerative enzymes tend to produce pain and degeneration of the tendinous tissue. Corticosteroids can diminish the intensity of the inflammatory response and hence the level of shoulder pain. Use of systemic anti-inflammatory medication for acutely inflamed shoulders is relatively ineffective compared to the prompt response one gets with an accurate injection of a corticosteroid. Surgical excision of calcium deposits is reserved for the more chronic, symptomatic conditions that are unresponsive to injection and other treatment.

Rotator Cuff Ruptures

Rupture of the supraspinatus tendon from the rotator cuff occurs in middle-aged people, usually when the shoulder has been subjected to a sudden

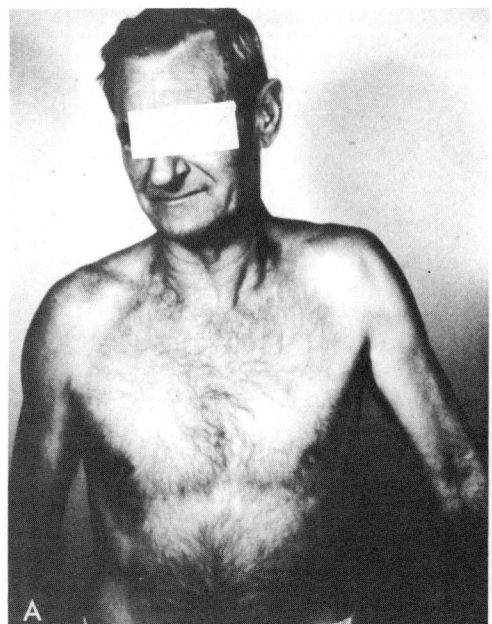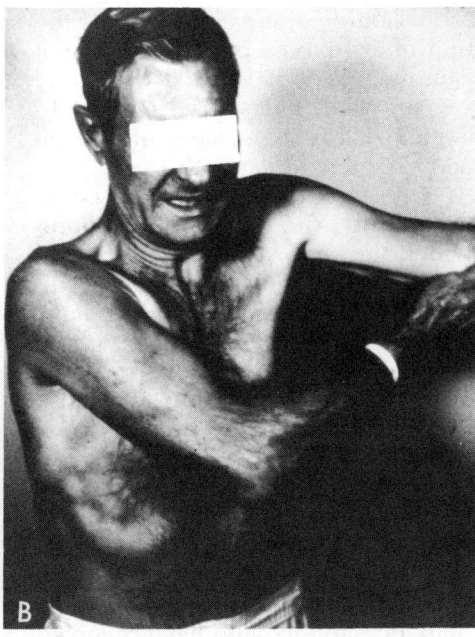

FIGURE 38–20. *A*, This 45-year-old house painter, in falling from a scaffolding, hung the weight of his entire body on his left shoulder. He felt a sudden "pop" and giving way of the shoulder. On examination 1 month later, as shown here, he had considerable deltoid atrophy and could only abduct to approximately 30 degrees without pain. *B*, Passive elevation of the shoulder between 30 and 90 degrees produces a painful arc. The pain comes from the torn rotator cuff being pinched between the anterior coracoacromial ligament and the head of the humerus. Prompt repair of this acute tendon injury is essential in the working person before permanent muscle atrophy complicates restoration of shoulder function. Chronic tendon degeneration in the elderly patient, however, does not usually require operative repair.

load. Typically this would be an individual who catches his or her body weight with one arm when falling or stumbling (Fig. 38–20). A sudden pull on the shoulder support muscles can cause a rupture of their tendinous attachment at the tuberosity of the humerus. The patient will relate feeling a sudden pop in the shoulder and then suffering severe pain. Subsequently, he or she is unable to elevate the arm.

On physical examination, the patient will demonstrate a painful arc within the shoulder's range of motion. There is no pain with passive abduction of the shoulder to 45 degrees, pain with abduction from 40 to 100 degrees, and no pain when the arm is passively raised overhead. This painful arc is indicative of a swollen, avulsed, and sensitive tendon being pinched between the humeral head and anterior acromion in the mid-range of motion.

MANAGEMENT BY THE FAMILY PHYSICIAN. Injection of the painful area with local anesthetic will help with some of the discomfort. Active abduction remains limited in most instances. The diagnosis is confirmed by magnetic resonance imaging or shoulder arthrogram, which will show communication between the glenohumeral and subacromial bursae through the tear of the rotator cuff.

Treatment of significant rotator cuff tears is usually surgical repair. Small tears are associated with degenerative change, and repair can be delayed for a period of some months. If these tears become

chronic and will not resolve, then late repair can be done.

Biceps Tendon Rupture

The long head of the biceps can rupture as a result of degenerative changes, and sometimes from an acute tear or from cortisone injections into the tendon groove. The patient initially notices a mass developing when the elbow is flexed, much like the so-called Popeye muscle.

MANAGEMENT BY THE FAMILY PHYSICIAN. Biceps ruptures that are seen early should probably be repaired. They may be asymptomatic in the older patient and not require repair. However, younger, more active, individuals or heavy laborers who have a rupture should be referred promptly for surgical repair. Delay past 2 or 3 weeks does not allow appropriate repair, and the patient will not regain function as well. Operative repair of the acute biceps tendon rupture is even more imperative if the tear is at the distal insertion into the radius.

Adhesive Capsulitis

Frozen shoulder, or adhesive capsulitis, restricts motion in all directions. This chronically stiff and painful shoulder generally begins without any significant trauma and is usually seen in middle age. The duration of symptoms may range from 6 months to several years. In a study of over 100 patients with frozen shoulders, it was found that the average duration of symptoms prior to treatment was about 8 months (Connolly et al., 1972). Only 7 per cent of the patients demonstrated any calcification on radiographs. Eight per cent of the patients developed symptoms bilaterally.

The etiology of this condition appears to be an alteration in the mobile axillary fold of the shoulder capsule, which thickens and shrinks and becomes a "checkrein." Motion is then limited in all directions. Biopsies from frozen shoulders have shown changes of fibrosis and fibroplasia without much evidence of inflammation (Lundberg, 1969). The chronic frozen shoulder, therefore, is a fibroplasia or alteration occurring in middle age associated with changes in the characteristics of the collagen content of the joint capsule.

The diagnosis of a frozen shoulder is common, but one should consider other possibilities and exclude them. One should always think of Pancoast tumor in these painful shoulders. Infection can be deceptive in diabetic patients who have received cortisone injections, and also should be kept in mind. A chronically locked posterior shoulder dislocation can be ruled out with appropriate radiographs. Rarely, a tumor of the scapula can be present and cause problems.

MANAGEMENT BY THE FAMILY PHYSICIAN. The management of the frozen shoulder is varied. The symptoms seem to last forever, responding minimally to standard physical therapy modalities. This is because the checkrein must be passively stretched out to regain the necessary external rotation in abduction. Once this is accomplished, the pain tends to subside rapidly.

Overcoming the restraint of the capsule to this motion is best achieved by an exercise program in which the patient brings clasped hands up behind the head, braces the scapulas against a wall, and forces the elbows back toward the wall (Fig. 38–21). In addition, active abduction exercises as prescribed by a knowledgeable physical therapist should be done. Persistence in a good exercise program several times per day is usually rewarded by prompt improvement in motion and diminution of pain in a 3- to 4-week period. If the patient does not improve symptomatically by 6 weeks, he or she should be referred to an orthopedist who can perform shoulder manipulation under anesthesia or prescribe special exercises that may be useful in controlling the symptoms.

Any manipulation should be done very carefully by someone who is familiar with the technique, because one can excessively torque the shoulder and inflict further damage, such as fracture.

Anterior Glenohumeral Joint Dislocation

The shoulder joint, because of its great mobility, is prone to dislocation. The usual mechanism is forced abduction and external rotation. Complete

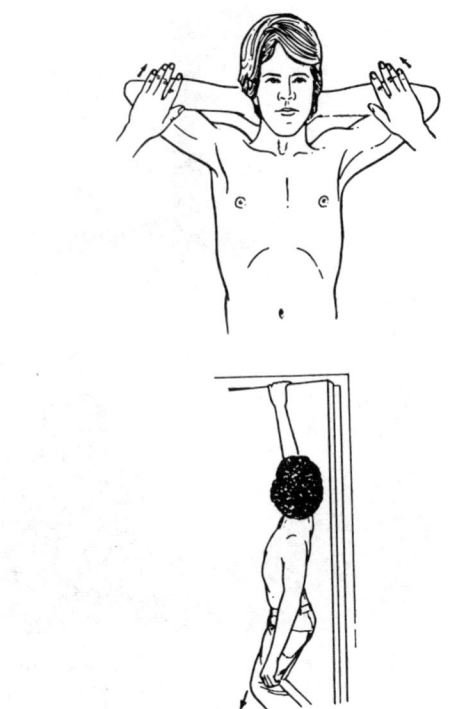

FIGURE 38–21. Abduction–external rotation exercises for the frozen shoulder will overcome the restriction by the axillary fold to shoulder motion. (From Connolly JF: DePalma's The Management of Fractures and Dislocations: An Atlas, 3rd edition. Philadelphia, WB Saunders Company, 1981, with permission.)

anterior shoulder dislocation is usually obvious to all observers and demands prompt reduction.

The standard reduction methods are the Stimson technique, the Hippocratic maneuver, and the Kocher maneuver (see Figs. 38–52 and 38–53 in Atlas of Fracture and Dislocation Management, later in this chapter (Connolly, 1981). One should avoid overvigorous attempts at manipulative reduction without adequate anesthetic, because it is easy to fracture the humeral head or avulse the axillary artery, as described in older patients (Jardon et al., 1973). Adequate anesthetics and muscle relaxants must be used to avoid these serious complications.

Some patients do not completely dislocate the shoulder but tend to subluxate the radial head in and out of the glenoid. This results in repeated episodes of sharp shoulder pain without a complete dislocation. The mechanism of subluxation is forceful external rotation and abduction that is sufficient to tear the capsule anteriorly. This allows the head to slide briefly over the rim of the glenoid without completely dislocating from the socket.

The diagnosis of recurrent glenohumeral subluxation is based on the mechanism of external rotation and abduction associated with sharp, sudden pain. Radiographs sometimes will show a small avulsion of the anterior rim of the glenoid. This condition can impair the patient's function considerably and is best referred to someone familiar with shoulder arthroscopy and shoulder surgery who can appropriately repair this instability.

Posterior Glenohumeral Dislocation

This dislocation may pass unrecognized because it tends to give a false appearance of normal on anteroposterior radiographs; an axillary view is required for diagnosis. It is not as clinically evident as an anterior dislocation. It is more common in epileptics and occurs occasionally in people who fall directly on the front of the shoulder. Patients with symptomatology of a posterior shoulder dislocation or a locked shoulder in internal rotation need to have appropriate reduction. The reduction of the acute posterior shoulder dislocation is carried out using the modified Hippocratic maneuver as described by Connolly (1981) (see Fig. 38–54 in Atlas of Fracture and Dislocation Management, later in this chapter).

Acromioclavicular Dislocations

Injury to the acromioclavicular joint causes shoulder disability of varying degree. This injury occurs as a result of force applied directly to the tip of the shoulder or upper arm. The force tears the acromioclavicular ligaments and frequently the coracoacromial ligaments, allowing varying degrees of upward displacement of the clavicle.

The completely dislocated clavicle in an individual with heavy shoulders frequently produces minimal acute symptoms and no long-term functional impairment (Fig. 38–22). A prominently displaced clavicle in a slender person with a torn trapezius and deltoid muscle usually has a great deal of symptomatology and may need operative repair.

MANAGEMENT BY THE FAMILY PHYSICIAN. Attempting to treat this type of dislocation with a harness or braces is usually ineffective. In some cases, one can provide no treatment other than a collar and cuff for 3 to 5 days and the patient will do quite well. If the patient desires operative repair, he or she should be referred to an orthopedic surgeon knowledgeable in the management of the completely dislocated acromioclavicular joint. In slender patients, a complete separation may present such a prominence of the clavicle that they may desire to have this repaired, even though long-term symptomatology may not be great (Fig. 38–23).

The individualized approach to acromioclavicular joint separations allows the patient to test the shoulder through a period of trial immobilization and determine whether or not the symptoms warrant operative repair. This is a good example of management tailored to symptoms and to the needs of the patient rather than a jump right to surgery.

Tietze's Syndrome

In 1921, Tietze described recurrent attacks of pain at the costochondral junction lasting for a min-

ute or so. A painful swelling at the costochondral junction is often palpable or visible, and coarse crepitation may be present with a scapulothoracic excursion.

MANAGEMENT BY THE FAMILY PHYSICIAN. This is a slowly recovering, self-limiting condition of vague etiology (likely trauma or stress on the junction of bone and cartilage). Treatment is supportive. Injection of a mixture of triamcinolone and local anesthetic into the area of maximal tenderness is often helpful. Heat and analgesics are useful (Connolly, 1981).

Knee Sprains and Injuries

Only the ankle is more vulnerable than the knee to both ligamentous and bony injury. The unstable knee produces even more functional impairment than does an unstable ankle. Effective reconstructive procedures are available for the unstable ankle. The chronically unstable knee is more difficult to correct. Early recognition and repair of the acute damage offers the best chance of retaining normal function.

Ligamentous Injuries

The family physician who first evaluates the patient with a knee injury has the best opportunity to determine the need for operative repair. He or she must learn to separate the major, or grade III, injury from the minor, or grade I, injury. There are also grade II injuries, but these are in a gray zone that may or may not prove to be of major significance. These grade II injuries require a judicious period of observation to determine the degree to which they will impair joint function. Understanding the mechanisms of injuries and the anatomic structures likely to be involved helps one to sort out those injuries.

MECHANISMS OF INJURY. Most ligamentous injuries result characteristically from twisting the knee with the foot fixed to the ground. Either a valgus–external rotational injury or a varus–internal rotational twist may be applied to the joint. Depending on the mechanism, the support structures on either the medial or the lateral side of the joint are then injured (Fig. 38–24).

Hyperextension or hyperflexion mechanisms can also disrupt knee ligaments. Most often the anterior cruciate ligament is torn with hyperextension overload, and the posterior cruciate is injured most commonly by hyperflexion (Fig. 38–25).

The Lachman test is a good test for anterior cruciate ligament laxity. To do this test, the knee is placed in a position of about 30 degrees of flexion. The femur is stabilized and an anteriorly directed force is applied to the proximal calf of the leg. The examiner should then estimate the displacement in millimeters and thus assess the firmness of the end point, which can be graded as firm (which is

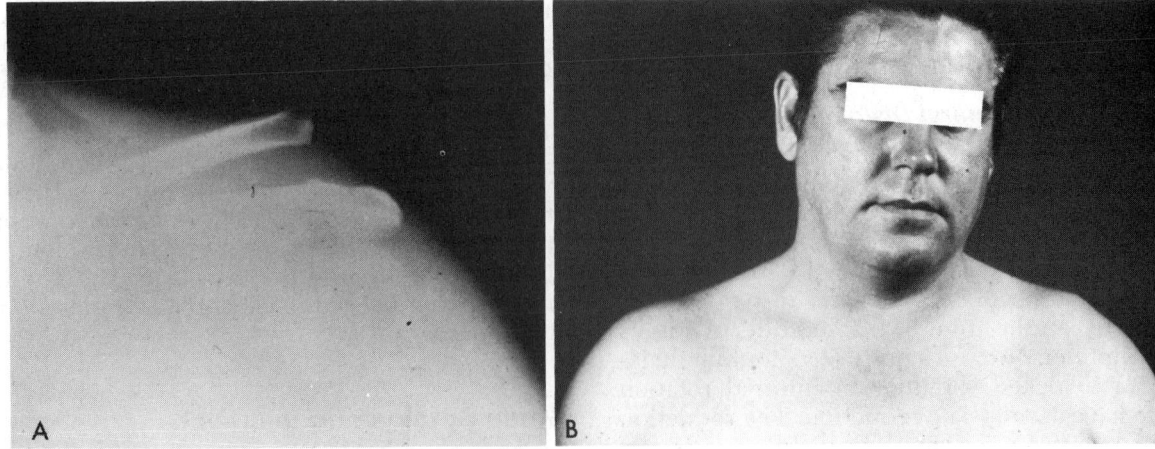

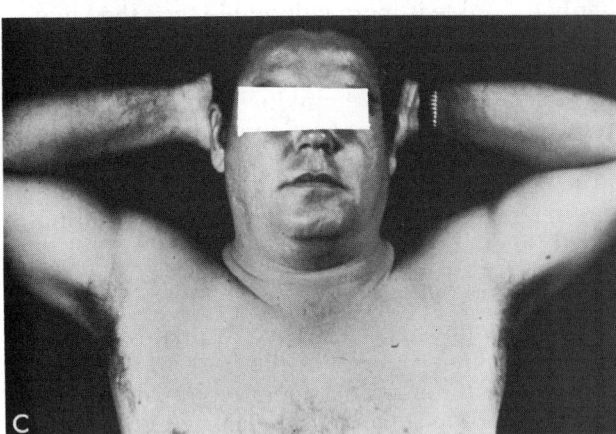

FIGURE 38–22. *A,* This anteroposterior view shows a complete acromioclavicular dislocation that occurred in a well-muscled laborer. *B,* The prominence of the dislocated clavicle in this patient was barely noticeable because of the thick shoulder musculature. The patient was treated symptomatically with ice applications and early shoulder motion exercises. *C,* At 2 weeks he had regained full range of shoulder motion despite the complete acromioclavicular dislocation. He was back to work considerably earlier than would have been possible had operative treatment been recommended.

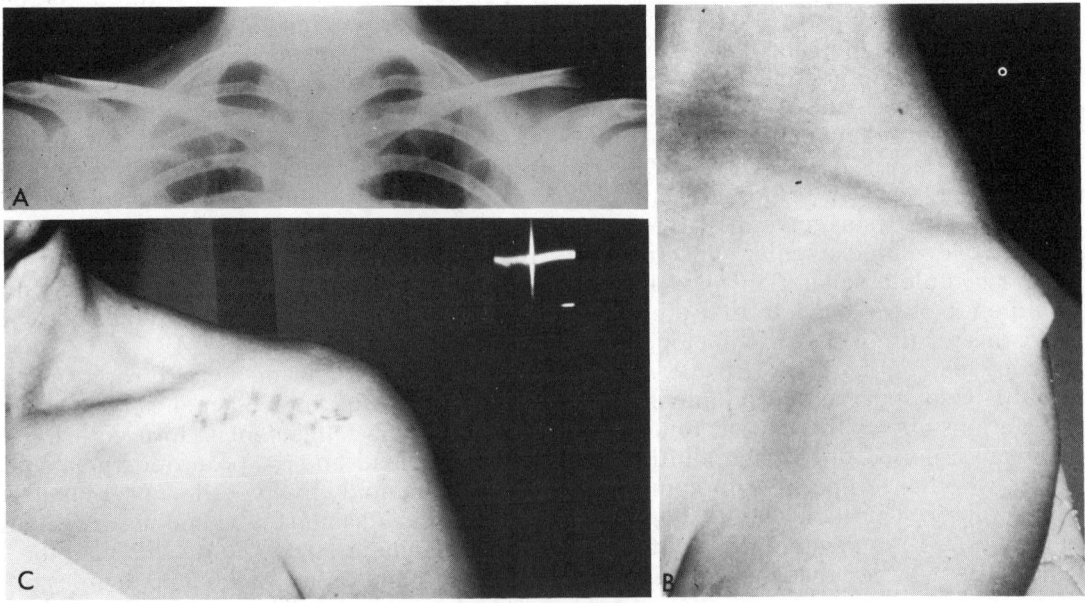

FIGURE 38–23. *A,* Anteroposterior radiograph showing complete dislocation of an acromioclavicular joint in a relatively asthenic woman. *B,* In contrast to the patient shown in Figure 38–22, this woman had little shoulder musculature and the upward displaced clavicle produced pain. *C,* The deformity was corrected by an elective repair of the coracoclavicular ligaments with resection of the distal 1 cm of the clavicle.

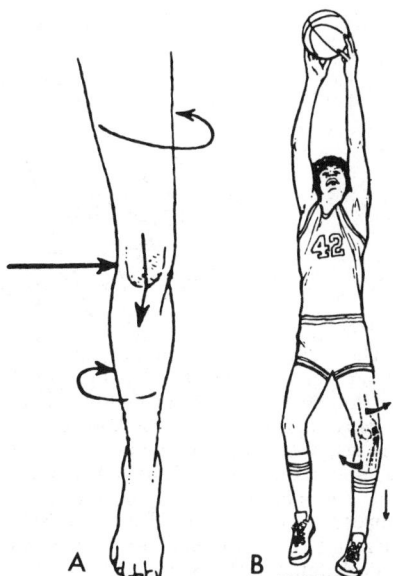

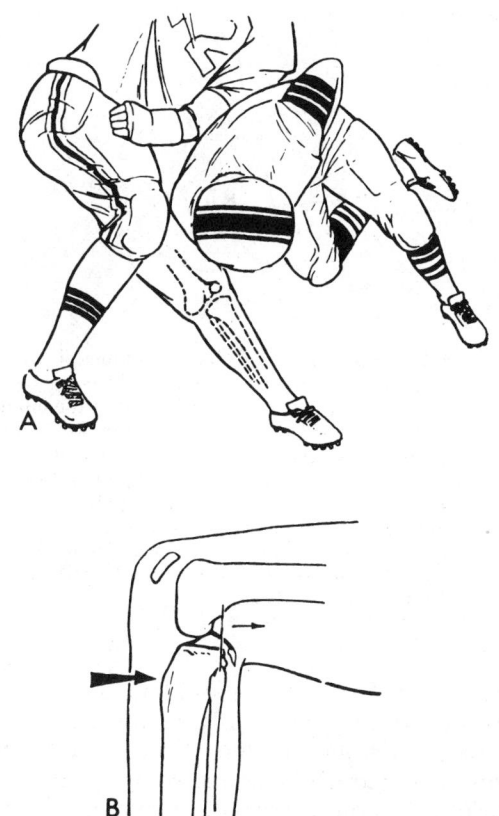

FIGURE 38–24. *A,* A valgus–external rotational injury to the knee disrupts the medial joint structures. *B,* A varus–internal rotational, torsion injury to the knee disrupts the lateral joint structures. Characteristically, this occurs as an individual lands off balance and applies a varus stress to the knee joint. (From Connolly JF: DePalma's The Management of Fractures and Dislocations: An Atlas, 3rd edition. Philadelphia, WB Saunders Company, 1981, with permission.)

FIGURE 38–25. *A,* A hyperextension injury to the internally rotated knee frequently causes disruption of the anterior cruciate ligament. *B,* A hyperflexion injury to the flexed knee jars the tibia's posterior relationship to the femur and disrupts the posterior cruciate ligament. (From Connolly JF: DePalma's The Management of Fractures and Dislocations: An Atlas, 3rd edition. Philadelphia, WB Saunders Company, 1981, with permission.)

normal), marginal, or soft (which is determined to be pathologic). Any perceived side-to-side difference is usually significant, if it is noted. The Lachman test essentially is a variation on the drawer sign and is much more reliable. The drawer sign itself is the least reliable of tests.

HISTORY AND PHYSICAL. The history usually is that the patient felt a "pop" at the time the knee was twisted and gave way. This always indicates significant structural disruption. It remains up to the physician to identify the anatomic area and the degree of involvement.

The knee must be inspected carefully for ecchymosis or localized swelling, and one should watch how the patient moves the knee actively. Particularly, one must determine if there is any limitation of motion from a mechanical obstruction or locking or loss of quadriceps function. Quadriceps tendon rupture and patellar dislocation are among the more commonly overlooked conditions presenting as common "knee sprains."

The knee must be felt carefully for areas of tenderness that indicate the site of torn muscle, ligament, or cartilage. One of the more specific signs of meniscal injury is point tenderness along the anteromedial and posteromedial joint lines.

If an effusion is palpable, its source should be determined precisely. Fluid that accumulates within 2 hours after injury indicates intra-articular bleeding. Marked effusion can be aspirated from the joint, as shown in Figure 38–26 (Connolly,

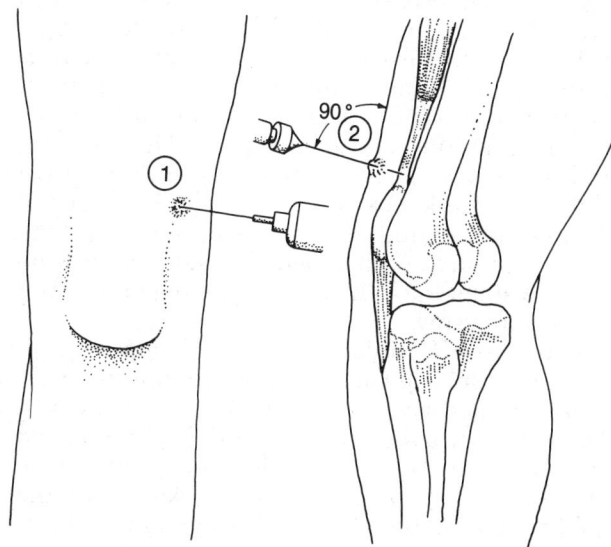

FIGURE 38–26. Aspiration of the knee joint is performed with strict aseptic precautions. *(1)* An intradermal wheal is raised, using local anesthetic and a fine hypodermic needle. *(2)* After a few minutes, a large-bore needle is passed into the joint at a right angle to the skin.

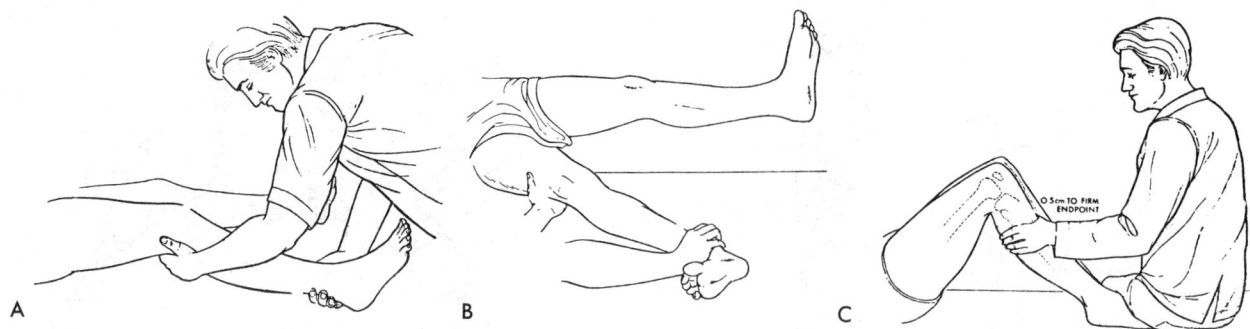

FIGURE 38–27.   *A,* Abduction-adduction stress test of knee ligaments. The patient must lie on the examining table with the hip extended over the edge to relax the hamstrings. The examiner places one hand on the lateral side of the thigh and one hand above the ankle. The uninjured side is tested first. *B,* The test should be done on the injured side with the knee in 30 degrees of flexion and in full extension. Instability of the knee in full extension is indicative of a serious ligamentous disruption (grade III injury). *C,* Anterior-posterior drawer testing for cruciate ligament injury. The patient lies with the hips flexed 45 degrees and the knees flexed 90 degrees. The examiner rests gently on the patient's feet and checks the uninjured side first. The tibia is drawn forward in external rotation, neutral rotation, and internal rotation. Forward displacement on the injured side of 0.5 cm more than on the uninjured side and without a firm end point is a positive result. (From Connolly JF: DePalma's The Management of Fractures and Dislocations: An Atlas, 3rd edition. Philadelphia, WB Saunders Company, 1981, with permission.)

1981). Fluid that becomes evident only 12 to 24 hours after the injury usually represents an irritative synovial reaction. One of the more common causes of hemarthrosis identified by arthroscopy is a tear of the anterior cruciate ligament.

Integrity of the knee ligaments can be assessed early (30 minutes) with no anesthetic. After this period, anesthetic is needed. The examiner should evaluate for both medial and lateral instability as well as for anterior and posterior drawer signs (Fig. 38–27). Such an assessment particularly depends on the examiner's tactile sense, which one should develop in order to assess the ligamentous injury with confidence.

GRADES OF INJURY.   The family physician who evaluates knee injuries should be capable of separating a grade I from a grade III injury. Grade I, or incomplete, injuries involve only a few fibers of the ligaments. There is usually no history of functional instability, of "giving way." The swelling and tenderness about the knee are minimal. On abducting the knees at both 0 and 30 degrees of flexion, the injured joint opens up no more than the uninjured joint. Radiographic studies show no fracture about the joint and no opening of the joint line on stressing.

With grade III injuries, there is complete rupture of capsular ligaments, either within the substance of the ligament or at its bony attachments. The patient usually gives a history of popping and gross functional instability after the injury. Some individuals may be able to lock the knee with the quadriceps and be fully weight-bearing in spite of their significant injury.

Pain with complete ligament injuries tends to be less than with incomplete injuries. That is because the blood from the completely torn ligament extravasates outside the joint. Partial ligament tears tend to bleed into the joint and produce painful capsular distention. The injury should be considered to be a grade III if the examiner feels the joint open more than 5 mm compared with the uninjured side with the knee in 30 degrees of flexion.

MANAGEMENT BY THE FAMILY PHYSICIAN.   Grade III injuries in most patients should be evaluated to rule out fracture and, if negative, immobilized and referred for operative repair. The family physician will often be faced with an acutely swollen knee and the dilemma of whether there is a grade III injury or not. In this instance, fracture should be ruled out and the patient placed on crutches and instructed to use ice until the swelling is resolved, then re-examined to assess more fully the degree of instability.

Lesser injuries should be treated nonoperatively. The more common acute partial ligament injuries can be treated by applying a compression dressing, rest, ice, and elevation to alleviate any swelling that will cause prolonged disability. Ice should be applied for 15 to 20 minutes three times a day to aid in resolving swelling and inflammation. The patient should also begin quadriceps strengthening exercises early.

A patient with any degree of ligamentous injury should be followed closely to be sure the injury is responding appropriately to treatment. Full extension of the knee should return by 7 to 10 days, and flexion should be close to normal by 2 weeks. The patient should be placed in a functional rehabilitation program that includes progressive activities that initially place little strain on the injured ligament, then progressively adds agility and simulated activities to return to participation in sports, which should be accomplished within a few weeks. Resolution of pain and swelling and progressive recovery of full motion are the determinants of recovery from a knee ligament injury.

Failure to follow the expected pattern of recovery within 7 to 10 days should make one consider an alternative diagnosis for a more severe injury. The family physician should consider referral to an orthopedic surgeon or, if available, obtain a magnetic resonance imaging examination.

Quadriceps Rupture

Other conditions are frequently confused with ligamentous injuries of the knee. One of the more common is disruption of the extensor apparatus, either from patellar dislocation or from tearing of the quadriceps.

Quadriceps rupture occurs most often in middle-aged and elderly patients who sustain a sudden hyperextension or flexion twist to the knee. This can be confused with ligamentous tears but should not be difficult to diagnose. These patients cannot extend the knee actively. The physician should never forget the importance of inspection. The patient should always move the joint actively before the examiner palpates or moves it passively.

Unlike the locked knee from a torn meniscus, passive extension with the torn quadriceps is full. However, a palpable gap is evident above the patella when the patient is asked to contract the quadriceps forcefully.

MANAGEMENT BY THE FAMILY PHYSICIAN. The disrupted quadriceps tendon apparatus should be repaired promptly.

Patellar Instability

Patellar instability is more common than is quadriceps rupture. It is seen most often in active young individuals, particularly teenage girls with knock-knees. It can occur from an injury to the knee that tears the medial patellar retinaculum and allows the patella to slide laterally over the femoral condyle.

Typically, the patient gives a history of coming down rapidly with the knee extended. A valgus and external rotatory strain then causes the patella to shift laterally; the patella quickly dislocates and causes the whole extensor support to give way. The patient falls to the ground and the patella may or may not then reduce spontaneously.

The diagnosis of patellar instability should be suspected by this somewhat bizarre history of a "drop attack." The suspicion is confirmed by a "fear" sign on physical testing. This apprehension sign is elicited with the patient's knee relaxed in a flexed position. The examiner then presses the patient's patella laterally and provokes the patient's fear of impending instability or patellar dislocation, proving there is pathologic laxity.

MANAGEMENT BY THE FAMILY PHYSICIAN. An acute patellar dislocation can be reduced by slowly placing the knee in extension and gently applying pressure along the lateral edge of the patella. This usually will reduce it without anesthesia. If this is the patient's first dislocation, he or she can then be managed with immobilization and full extension, with a foam pad over the vastus medialis obliquus and a lateral buttress holding the patella medially, using a long leg immobilizer. Three to 6 weeks is usually sufficient time for the medial patellar retinaculum to heal. Approximately 50 per cent of patella dislocations will recur, despite treatment.

Recurrent episodes of patellar instability are treated symptomatically with temporary immobilization and crutches followed by functional rehabilitation and braces to minimize lateral patellar tracking.

Patellofemoral Pain Syndrome

Patellofemoral pain syndrome, also known as extensor mechanism malalignment, is probably the most common anterior knee problem seen by the family physician. This condition is often referred to as "chondromalacia patella," a term that should be reserved for articular cartilage damage observed by arthroscopy or radiography.

The historical feature of this problem is that of anterior knee pain. It is often worse with sitting in a tight space with the knee flexed, or on descending stairs or slopes. Swelling is usually minimal, if present. The patient may complain of some snapping, popping, or crepitus about the patella.

Positive physical findings are usually localized to the patella. The patient has pain on patellofemoral compression, otherwise known as the shrug test. There is often crepitation about the patella on range of motion, and a palpable tenderness around the patella. The patient often has accompanying foot malalignment, such as pes planus or leg length discrepancies, which aggravate the symptoms. These patients often have a dysplastic vastus medialis obliquus and tight hamstring muscles. Patellar tendinitis, or "jumper's knee," is often just an extension of the patellofemoral pain syndrome, but more localized to the patellar tendon itself. The patient often has tenderness at the inferior pole of the patella with this condition.

Traditional radiographs of the knee are usually negative for this condition. However, one may see lateral displacement of the patellas on sunrise films.

Treatment is usually multimodal, involving functional rehabilitation, nonsteroidal anti-inflammatory medication, functional bracing of the patella, and orthotics for foot malalignment. Very few patients require surgical intervention, which is usually in the form of a lateral release or extensor mechanism reconstruction.

MANAGEMENT BY THE FAMILY PHYSICIAN. This problem is readily managed by the family physician in the form of medication, ice, and appropriate functional exercises that primarily include those that strengthen the medial quadriceps complex and stretch the hamstrings. This condition is often a chronic, intermittent disorder, and the patient should be counselled appropriately regarding recurrence of this problem.

Meniscal Tears

Medial meniscus tears are the most common cause of knee joint pain or sprain. The medial joint cartilage is torn by a twisting injury with the knee partially flexed. The meniscus in this position is forced toward the center of the joint and becomes caught between the femur and tibia. It is then torn longitudinally by shearing forces when the joint is suddenly extended. If the tear extends sufficiently anteriorly, the detached segment may catch in the intercondylar notch like the handle of a bucket. This obstructs normal articular gliding of the femur on the tibia and thereby locks the knee or prevents it from completely extending.

The medial meniscus is five to seven times more susceptible to such tears than is the lateral meniscus. Both medial and lateral meniscal tears produce the common medial joint line pain and the sensation of locking.

The clinical diagnosis of meniscal tears may be difficult for even an experienced orthopedic surgeon. The most consistent physical finding of meniscal tear is tenderness to palpation along the joint line anterior and posterior to the collateral ligament.

Reproducing a painful click during McMurray's test is diagnostic, but it cannot be done with the acutely tender knee. The patient lies supine with the hip and knee flexed acutely and maximally. The examiner palpates the posterior medial joint line with one hand and then externally rotates the foot and leg with the other as far as possible. The externally rotated and flexed knee is extended slowly. As the torn meniscus is caught between the femur and tibia, a click is felt that the patient describes as painful. Most often this results from posterior meniscal tears and consequently occurs with the knee going from complete flexion to approximately 90 degrees of flexion.

To examine for a lateral meniscal tear, the knee is flexed and the leg internally rotated. Then the leg is extended slowly while the examiner tries to produce the painful click.

A dynamic method of testing for meniscal injury is to have the patient walk in a duck waddle or squatting position. This maneuver applies an extreme compression load on the joint and is never possible when the patient has a torn meniscus. However, other conditions, including a ligamentous tear and patellofemoral arthritis, will produce pain on squatting and prevent the patient from carrying out this test. Nevertheless, if the patient is able to duck waddle without pain, the likelihood of internal derangement of the knee is extremely low.

MANAGEMENT BY THE FAMILY PHYSICIAN. The family physician can serve his or her patient best by identifying the individual with possible meniscal tear before further damage is inflicted on the knee. The patient who persists in daily activity with a locked knee is particularly likely to damage the anterior cruciate ligament adjacent to the torn meniscus. Abrasions of the femoral condyle and chondromalacia of the patella also occur with altered knee mechanics from meniscal injury. The sooner the pathology is recognized and corrected, the better is the long-term prognosis for the knee to remain free of arthritis.

If there is any diagnostic doubt, the patient should be referred for evaluation by magnetic resonance imaging or arthroscopy. The development of magnetic resonance imaging has considerably reduced the need for invasive diagnostic arthroscopy and has allowed for more accurate noninvasive diagnoses about the knee. Treatment of a torn meniscus is based on the location of the tear. Often the segment that is torn is removed; however, now with advent of the ability to do suturing through the arthroscope, some meniscal tears are repaired. Arthroscopy and magnetic resonance imaging have substantially reduced morbidity and recovery time for meniscal injuries.

Other injuries affecting extension of the knee include patellar fractures and Osgood-Schlatter's disease. Both can be managed by the family physician, who can distinguish the significant from insignificant consequences of these conditions.

Osgood-Schlatter Disease

Osgood-Schlatter disease results from repetitive hyperextension strain produced by the pull of the patellar tendon on the tibial tuberosity. The usual teenage patient presents with a chief complaint of a painful knob just below the knee. This prevents the young boy or girl from participating in vigorous sports. It is tender to direct palpation, and, frequently, a small mobile fragment can be felt, which also may be seen on a radiograph of the tibial tuberosity (Fig. 38–28).

Generally, the pain symptoms subside with rest but tend to return as the individual resumes sports or does much stair climbing. We physicians tend to dismiss the symptoms as "growing pains" or undertreat the lesions of the patellar tendon insertion. The young person usually learns to avoid sports and activities that bring on the symptoms. The result is that he or she tends to be labeled as a laggard.

Symptoms can persist and flare up in the active adult with a history of Osgood-Schlatter disease who attempts to participate in sports or is forced to do much marching during military training. A more specific treatment of this common disability in adolescence could avoid many of the recurring problems in the active individual.

MANAGEMENT BY THE FAMILY PHYSICIAN. The patient with Osgood-Schlatter disease should be managed initially with relative rest. These patients often benefit by hamstring stretching, heel cord

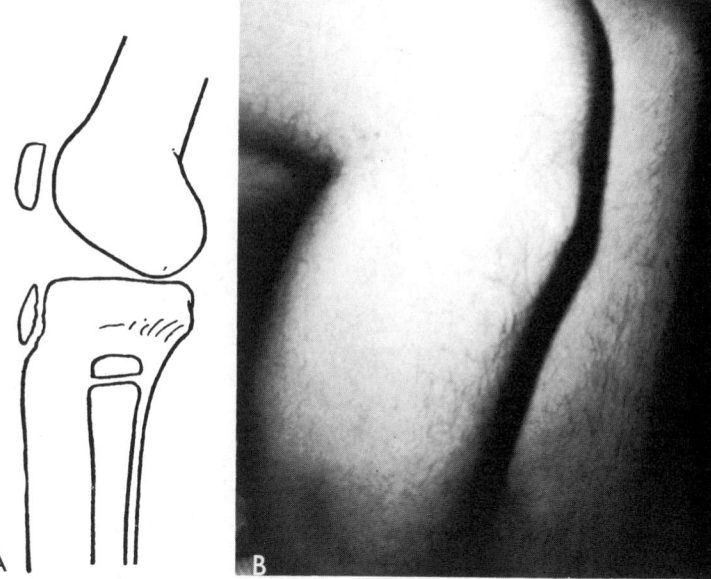

FIGURE 38–28. *A,* Osgood-Schlatter disease frequently produces a loose ossicle on the superior aspect of the tibial tuberosity, pulled loose by the patellar tendon. *B,* Persistent Osgood-Schlatter disease in a 25-year-old man prevented this patient from participating actively in sports for 10 years. The symptoms were relieved by simple excision of the loose ossicle in the tibial tuberosity.

stretching, and quadriceps stretching exercises. Activity modification is usually necessary. If the problem is exacerbated by direct pressure over the tuberosity, padding is sometimes helpful.

Patients who do not respond to this approach may benefit from a period of immobilization in a long leg knee immobilizer (Fig. 38–29). Active non–load-bearing exercises should be encouraged during the time of splinting. Rarely is surgical intervention needed. Surgery involves removal of the bony fragments, generally in a skeletally mature patient.

FRACTURES

In young, active people fractures are among the most common injuries. Elderly people with osteoporosis are also prone to fracture. Proper care of fractures depends on identifying the type and extent of fracture injury and applying the treatment that will maximize the normal healing process. Of major concern is avoidance of the complications of fractures and soft tissue injury.

In general, fractures that involve growth centers or joint surfaces, fractures that are open (through the skin), or fractures with which one is unfamiliar should be referred for care by an orthopedic surgeon. This admonition also is applicable to markedly displaced, badly comminuted, segmental, or unstable fractures (those that will not stay reduced).

The pattern of a fracture is determined by the directions and type of forces applied to cause this disruption. Age, resiliency of bone, and basic struc-

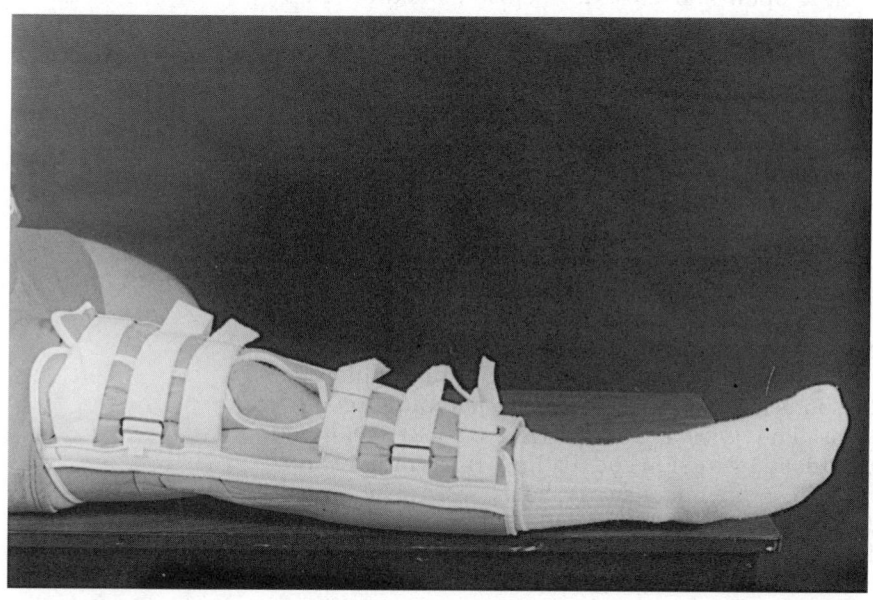

FIGURE 38–29. Long leg immobilizer is useful for stable patellar fractures, severe Osgood-Schlatter disease, and ligamentous injuries.

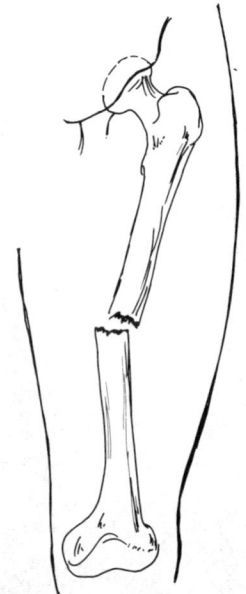

FIGURE 38–30.   Simple closed transverse fracture.

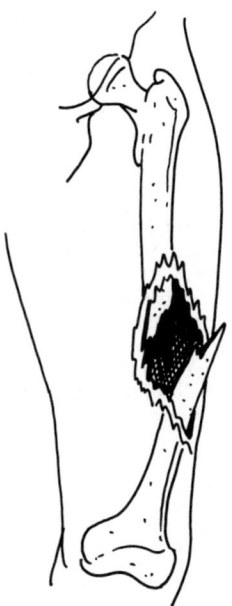

FIGURE 38–31.   Open fractures communicate with the atmosphere. They must be treated as infected from the moment of first contact. The size of the wound is no index of the amount of contamination. History of puncture in water or filthy surroundings often indicates the worst infections (See text for classification and detailed cases).

ture of the bone also play a role in the final pattern. The type of a fracture can give some index of the proper method of reducing it and the proper techniques of immobilization. The soft tissues around the fracture site are always injured to varying degrees, and thus require evaluation regarding circulation, motor, and sensory function and, in open fractures, some idea of the soft tissue damage as an index to likelihood of infection or other complications.

Types of Fractures

All types of fractures belong in one of two categories: open and closed. A closed fracture (Fig. 38–30) is a fracture that does not communicate with the outside environment. An open fracture (Fig. 38–31), which communicates with the external environment, is classified according to the extent of wounding and soft tissue damage into types I, II, and III, with subtypes A, B, and C (Gustillo and Anderson, 1976), which is helpful in determining the treatment and estimating the prognosis of the fracture (see discussion under Fracture Complications, later in this section).

The various types of fractures can be described as follows. *Transverse fractures* (see Fig. 38–30) usually occur by a bending force or direct blow to the bone and can occur in certain pathologic conditions. The *oblique fracture* (Fig. 38–32) usually is produced by torsion and loading. It has rather short fracture ends and usually heals well. The *spiral fracture* (Fig. 38–33) is produced in a similar fashion, with a twisting or rotatory force that is loaded and tends to break with sharp ends. This is an indi-

rect injury, usually with less damage to circulation, and usually heals fairly rapidly.

Compressive fractures are usually not markedly displaced and can be of the greenstick type (Fig. 38–34) or torus buckling of the cortex, which are often seen in children. These heal rapidly with good results. Compressive fractures seen in adults include compressions of vertebrae (Fig. 38–35), which are usually stable and can usually be handled quite nicely with bed rest and appropriate bracing. These are often seen in osteomalacia or

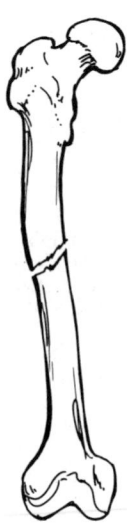

FIGURE 38–32.   Oblique fracture.

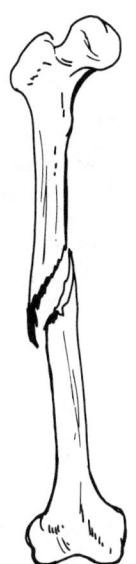

FIGURE 38–33.   Spiral fracture.

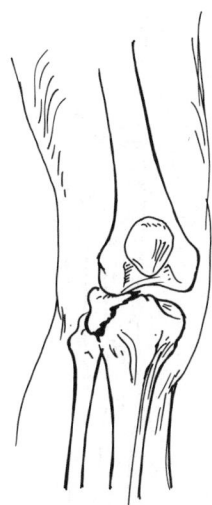

FIGURE 38–36.   Compression fracture of knee.

osteoporosis and certain pathologic conditions such as myeloma or metastases. Fractures of some joints can occur with compression (Fig. 38–36). These usually require consultation for open surgical reduction or evaluation to determine whether surgery is necessary.

Comminuted fractures are seen with associated soft tissue injuries that are sometimes severe (Fig. 38–37). These fractures are usually the result of direct violent blows that produce multiple fragments; reduction is sometimes very difficult to achieve and maintain. *Segmental fractures* (Fig. 38–38) can result in devitalization of a segment of bone. Reduction is quite difficult and union is slow; segmental fractures probably should be treated by a consultant. *Impacted fractures* (Fig. 38–39) are those that result from direct violent blows that drive bone fragments firmly together.

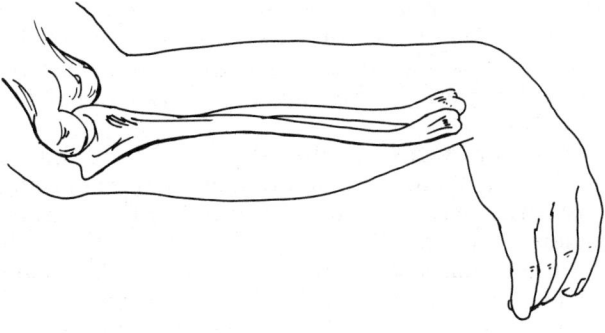

FIGURE 38–34.   Compression fracture of forearm in child.

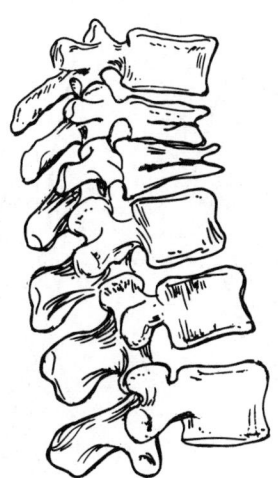

FIGURE 38–35.   Compression fracture of spine.

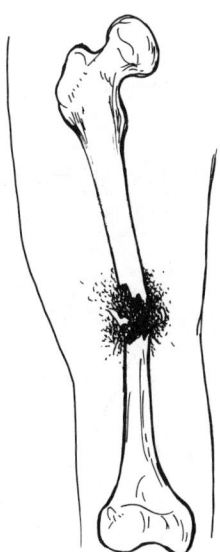

FIGURE 38–37.   Comminuted fracture.

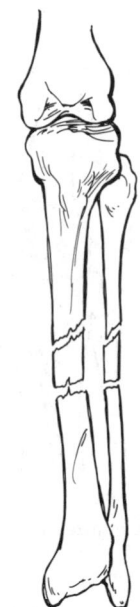

FIGURE 38–38. Segmental fracture.

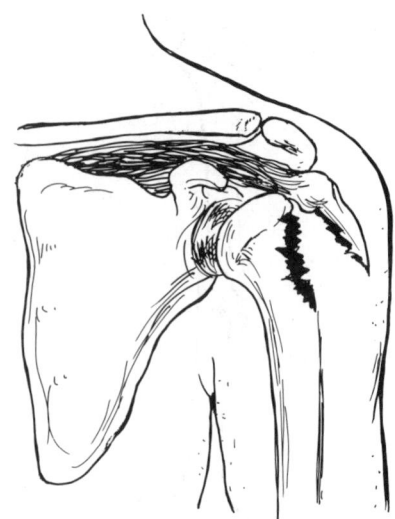

FIGURE 38–40. Avulsion fracture of greater tuberosity of shoulder.

These are seen quite often in the shoulder, and the impacted fragments usually move in unison. Healing is quite rapid. *Avulsion fractures* (Fig. 38–40) are those in which indirect force against a muscle mass pulls off a fragment of bone. These are often seen around the rotator cuff of a shoulder, occasionally in patellar tendon fractures, in hamstring fractures at the point where the hamstrings attach, and in fractures in which the Achilles tendon pulls loose. Finally, *fracture–dislocations* (Fig. 38–41) are fractures that occur with dislocations of the joint. These are always complex injuries that require consultation and good surgical care.

Fracture Repair

In general, bone usually heals by forming more of itself, eventually restoring the skeleton to full function. When this process fails (nonunion), the bone unites with scar tissue that is not strong enough to perform the usual normal function of the skeleton.

Most fractures of the shafts of long bones undergo a complex repairative process that occurs in a series of stages. The first stage is inflammation, wherein the torn periosteum and blood vessels form a hematoma (Fig. 38–42). A few days later this is infiltrated (Fig. 38–43) with macrophages and other cells that remove necrotic tissue and leave a delicate fiber network behind (Fig. 38–44). In the ensuing 1 to 2 weeks (the second stage), callus develops as the fiber network is replaced by collagen fibers that are then surrounded by a ma-

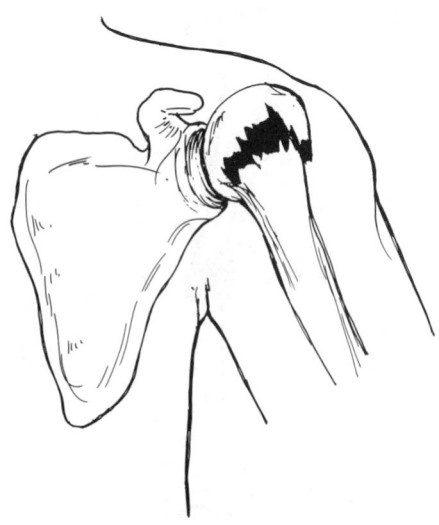

FIGURE 38–39. Impacted fracture.

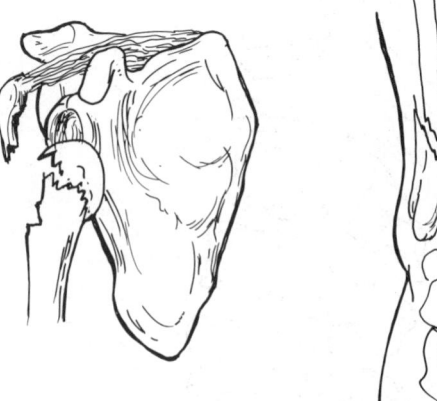

FIGURE 38–41. Fracture with dislocation of shoulder (left) and ankle (right).

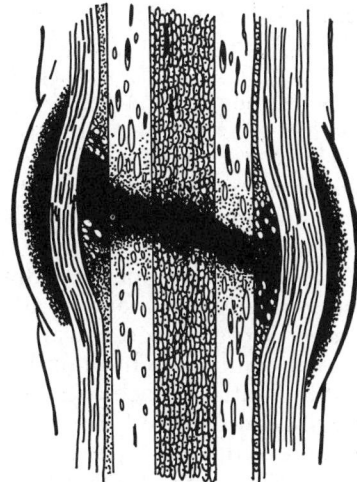

FIGURE 38–42. Fracture hematoma.

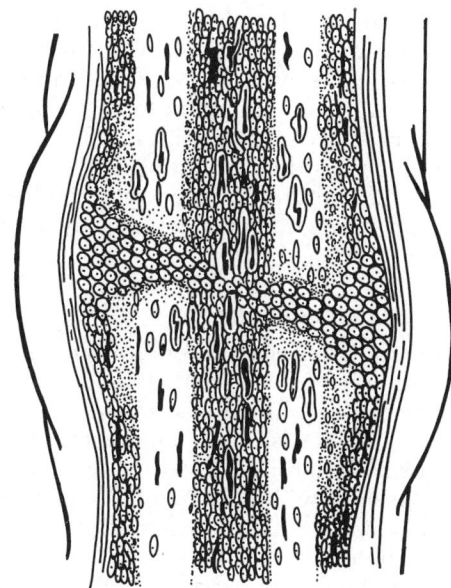

FIGURE 38–44. Fiber network and callus formation.

trix called osteoid. This eventually mineralizes into a woven bone pattern. The final stage is remodeling of this callus and reduction in its size to form lamellar (nonwoven) bone, which is the normal structure of the skeleton. After this stage is complete, the bone is as strong as it was prior to the fracture.

Fracture Complications

In dealing with fractures, one of the major objectives is to avoid the many known complications, as described here.

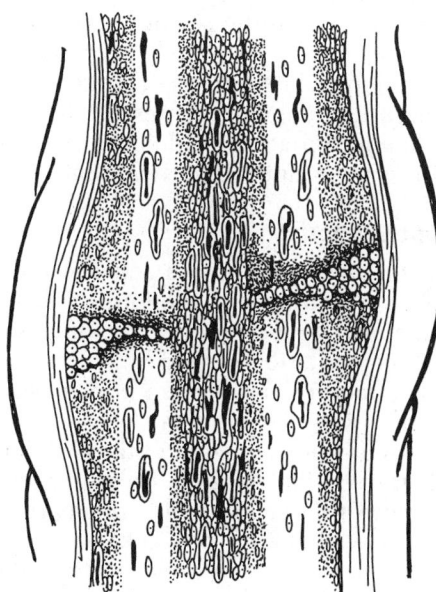

FIGURE 38–43. Infiltration of hematoma by cells.

Neurovascular Complications

At the time of an injury or during a reduction, the displaced fracture fragments or bone ends can trap or lacerate nerves or blood vessels. The radial nerve at the midshaft and upper end of the humerus is particularly prone to this, as is the median nerve and brachial artery near the elbow. The sciatic nerve can be injured with fractures around the hip or dislocations of the hip. Immediate reduction of dislocations about the hip will relieve pressure on the sciatic nerve, which is the best prevention of palsy, and about 60 per cent of these entrapments seem to respond to reduction. In the remaining 40 per cent of cases, the patient may sustain partial permanent loss of function.

Another common problem is compartment syndrome (see under Lacerations and Contusions, earlier in this chapter). Appropriate treatment for this situation is loosening of any dressings and fasciotomy to provide sufficient space to relieve the pressure and prevent permanent ischemic problems, with subsequent contracture and death of muscles and other contents in the compartment. A common site of ischemic contracture from arterial injuries is supracondylar fracture of the humerus. Both the radial and median nerves are in this area and are susceptible to injury, as is the brachial artery, which can be trapped or lacerated. If this occurs, the patient can develop a Volkmann's ischemic contracture with pulselessness, pallor, paralysis, and extreme pain. The family practitioner must have a clear mental picture of the difference between arterial interruption and compartment syndrome (see Table 38–2) in order to understand these conditions fully. Appropriate orthopedic and vascular consultations must be obtained early on when a compartment syndrome is present.

Again, neurovascular complications with some types of fractures can be severe and must be identified by a careful examination. This requires frequent re-evaluation and monitoring, especially during the first day or two, with fractures that are prone to give considerable problems, such as the supracondylar fracture, dislocation of the hip with fracture, and pelvic fractures, which may injury the bladder.

Pulmonary Complications

Postfracture pulmonary problems include pulmonary embolism, pulmonary edema from fluid overload or cardiac failure, gastric aspiration pneumonia, and atelectasis. A common complication is fat embolism, which can develop after long bone fractures, usually within 72 hours. Lodging of the fat embolus in the lung produces sudden-onset respiratory problems resulting in hypoxemia. Symptoms include fever, tachycardia, rapid respiration, and mental confusion. Petechiae can develop, especially in an antigravity distribution (e.g., chest and axillae). An arterial po_2 of 60 mm Hg or less is confirmatory. A progressive decrease in pulmonary compliance, arteriovenous shunting, and increased airway resistance are noted. These pulmonary alterations prevent normal oxygen perfusion through the alveolar capillary membrane, resulting in anoxia of severe degree. This respiratory distress syndrome must be treated with dispatch or death may result.

Embolus-induced respiratory distress syndrome can be prevented or reduced in severity by early mobilization of the patient, especially those with multiple fractures. Recovery is possible with intensive oxygen therapy. Correction of hypoxia and maintenance of an arterial oxygen tension above 70 mm Hg is the heart of treatment. If a mask will not maintain arterial oxygen tension of 70 mm Hg or more, then ventilatory assistance by closed system or even positive end-expiratory pressure assisted ventilation may be needed. This care may be necessary for days to weeks until the pulmonary lesion resolves and assisted respiration can be stopped.

Infection

All open fractures and dislocations are potentially infected. Open injuries can be assessed according to Gustillo's classification system, which is a useful treatment guide.

A type I open fracture has a laceration of 1 cm or less and is clean. A type II open fracture has a clean laceration of greater than 1 cm. A type III open fracture is comminuted and dirty, and may include partial to complete amputation. Type III wounds are subdivided into types III-A, III-B, and III-C. Type III-A is a severe wound with crushing. Type III-B connotes severe loss of coverage to bone and deep tissues. Type III-C fractures have loss of coverage plus vascular injury requiring repair. Type III-A fractures have about a 5 per cent infection rate, while that of type III-B fractures may be above 50 per cent. Arterial injuries with fracture have a high infection and amputation rate (approximately 50 per cent).

Types I and II open fractures can be treated with débridement and copious irrigation with immobilization or fixation and delayed primary closure and will do well. All type III open fractures require open surgical reduction and repair under anesthesia by a surgeon experienced in care of complex musculoskeletal injury. Such wounds should be cleansed and the patient placed on antibiotic prophylaxis after initial culture if there is more than minimal treatment delay. A patient with a dirty open fracture wound should never be transported without clean-up and dressing if a delay of 4 to 6 hours is expected.

An open fracture should never be closed primarily—even types I and II fractures can become infected, and the degree of soft tissue damage is proportional to the likelihood of infection. Injuries in water or potentially manure-contaminated environments are most apt to acquire clostridial infection. The best treatment of infection in open fractures is prevention, and débridement and irrigation within 4 to 6 hours is mandatory. After initial culture, broad-spectrum antibiotics should be given for at least 48 hours. Closure should be delayed for 5 to 7 days after injury, and then done only after cultures and the wound appearance indicate the wound is clean.

When a contaminated open fracture is not cleaned properly, acute or chronic infection is likely and can have severe consequences, including osteomyelitis, gas gangrene, and tetanus. Osteomyelitis is a chronic bone infection that can be controlled in many instances but can be cured only by amputation. When the serious complication of gas gangrene results, extremely aggressive treatment is needed. An experienced surgeon can save the patient's life, and sometimes the limb can be saved with appropriate débridement and systemic penicillin or other antibiotic treatment.

Late Complications

Post-traumatic arthritis can occur as a result of malunion or irregularity of the joints after interarticular fracture. Prevention is the only sensible treatment; consultation should be obtained for interarticular fracture and malunion or postfracture angular and rotary deformities. Anyone caring for fractures should be cognizant of these deformities and their prevention. When a fracture is not well reduced, consultation is mandatory early in the clinical course (first days or week).

Growth deformities can occur as a result of epiphyseal or metaphyseal fractures in growing children. Any fracture involving a growth plate should be considered a case for consultation and potential open reduction with appropriate fixation. If a growth plate injury results in a bony bridge and angular deformity in a child, early correction is needed with excision and interposition of fat or Silastic to allow proper growth. In some cases, arrest of the opposite side of the epiphysis is useful when little longitudinal growth remains.

Osteonecrosis (death of bone) from interruption of blood supply can occur following certain fractures. This is most commonly seen in fractures of the subcapital type in the femur, talar neck fractures, carpal scaphoid fractures, condylar fractures of the knee, and some metatarsal fractures. Radiographically, these can become apparent as increased bone density followed by creeping substitution (lysis of bone) and then remineralization; collapse of the bony architecture can occur and lead to osteoarthritis. Fractures of these types should be referred early for proper preventative or alternate treatment options.

Some limb injuries have persistent burning pain that is disproportionate for the injury and the time from injury. This may be typified by swelling, redness, or hypersensitivity to touch. When this occurs, one must consider *reflex sympathetic dystrophy* (Sudeck's atrophy) as a cause. This may be seen in 3 to 5 per cent of limb injuries. Treatment involves a structured rehabilitation program in the face of pain, sympathetic nerve block, pain medication, and emotional support. In any event, once reflex sympathetic dystrophy is diagnosed, help from a specialist in pain management is needed.

Fracture Care

Fracture treatment principles are not complex. If a fracture is at an angle or displaced, it is aligned (reduced). This restores normal configuration and reduces residual deformity to a minimum. Reduction can be open or closed. Closed reduction means manipulation of fragments into normal alignment with radiographic control and casting or splinting. If this is impossible, then open or surgical reduction is utilized to achieve alignment. When this is completed, fixation is accomplished either by internal (rods, plates, pins) or external (frames and pins or plaster cast) means. Immobilization, whether by casting, splinting, or fixation, is continued until the repair or healing is complete.

In trauma patients, specific fracture injuries are usually identified during the secondary survey. All limb injuries require neurovascular evaluation. Any vascular compromise or suspected ischemia remaining after alignment and splinting require appropriate consultation with vascular or orthopedic surgeons or both. All musculoskeletal injuries should be splinted prior to movement if possible. This will reduce further soft tissue damage, pain, and blood loss.

Open wounds with bleeding should receive a clean compressive sterile dressing before splinting. Splints must incorporate the joint above and below the fracture and, for dislocated joints, the entire bone above and below the joint. Fractures with significant deformity should be pulled into alignment with gentle longitudinal traction prior to splinting. Once a limb is splinted, neurovascular function is re-evaluated and documented. Pulse, capillary refill, and sensory integrity are evaluated frequently until the danger of complication has passed. Elevation will reduce swelling. Splinting is simple and effective and should reduce pain markedly. Severe pain after splinting may mean loss of circulation or compartment syndrome, which require vascular consultation.

Basic Principles of Fracture Reduction

When reducing a fracture, the reduction force must be in the opposite direction of the causal force. The first step is use of traction, either manual or with mechanical assist, to disimpact a fracture. Traction usually restores length and usually accomplished reduction. When that is not the case, proper manipulation can obtain reduction by increasing angulation to unlock the fracture and hook the fragments into proper alignment. The reduction can be checked by palpation, assessing restoration of length and lack of deformity, and finally by radiography.

For example, manipulative reduction of forearm fractures can be accomplished with the following steps (see Fig. 38–49 in Atlas of Fracture and Dislocation Management, later in this section).

1. Place the patient supine and suspend the forearm over the edge of the examining table with the fingers in finger traps.
2. Using a sling over a felt pad, apply countertraction just sufficient to maintain alignment once it is achieved.
3. Palpate the bone and align by feel. Rotation and manipulation will usually "hook" the fractured cortices. Neutral rotation is essential.

Reduction also can be obtained with an assistant providing countertraction and the operator applying traction to the thumb and forefinger.

A cast can then be applied, and should incorporate the wrist and elbow. The cast should have 90 degrees of elbow flexion and in most cases neutral rotation with slight wrist flexion and ulnar deviation (modified Cotton-Loder position).

Splints

Splints are of three kinds: rigid, soft, and traction. Rigid splints are applied to one or more sides of the broken bone and held with bandages or straps. Padded splints can be of the air filled, pillow, or swathe type. Inflatable splints are good only for fractures below the elbow or below the knee. Traction splints apply some longitudinal force and hold the bone fragments in alignment by countering large muscle pulls. These are usually used for fractures of the thigh and hip. Sling and swathe splints are utilized for all fractures of the upper extremity, from fingertip to clavicle. Lower leg splints of any of the three types named are useful. Hip and thigh fractures are best immobilized in traction splints, but, if not available, one can pad between the limbs and bind the fractured limb to the sound limb for emergency splintage.

Management of Some Specific Fractures

Greenstick fractures of the forearm in children should be completed by reversing the mechanism of injury. Total anatomic reduction is not necessary, but angular and rotational deformity must be eliminated. Bayonet or corner-to-corner apposition will give a satisfactory result. Fractures in the mid-forearm (i.e., those that are not in the proximal one fifth or the distal one third of the forearm) usually require open reduction.

Unstable fractures and intra-articular fractures in most cases require surgical exposure and some kind of internal fixation. For example, the Smith fracture is a comminuted fracture with volar displacement and usually is very unstable. It may need pin fixation through the radial styloid with casting (see Fig. 38–48 in Atlas of Fracture and Dislocation Management, later in this section). It must be remembered that all surgery introduces the risk of infection and potential osteomyelitis.

Fractures of the spine and neck require complete immobilization of the injured spine for transportation to the hospital and require appropriate consultation with radiology and persons knowledgeable in assessment of stability of the spine. Some stable fractures can be handled with appropriate bracing or no bracing at all and physical therapy, whereas others that are unstable require surgical stabilization in order to prevent the devastating complication of permanent spinal injury. This is particularly important during early transport, and such immobilization must be carried on until there has been an accurate assessment of the degree of stability. This can be accomplished using most litters or spinal fracture boards with the head in an extrication collar or sand bagged into position with appropriate fixation with tape or straps.

Fractures of the pelvis usually result in hypovolemia because there is generally significant associated blood loss. Pelvic fractures can rupture surrounding blood vessels and result in a large retroperitoneal hematoma with shock, and can also injure the urinary bladder or urethra. Multiple fractures may even need pneumatic antishock garments to control the blood loss and stabilize the pelvis. Fractures of the pelvis require evaluation of the degree of blood loss as well as injury to the urinary tract, and in general should be cause for consultation unless they are extremely simple. Appropriate consultative help should be obtained when dealing with these fractures.

FRACTURES OF THE HAMATE. Fractures of the hamate are notorious for going unrecognized. This fracture usually results from a direct blow from the handle of a tennis racket, golf club, or some similar piece of equipment during an unbalanced swing. Thus, they are seen frequently in athletes and people requiring strong grip for the activity in which they are engaged. The patient usually suffers pain localized to the dorsal ulnar region of the wrist rather than the palmar area, which is confusing. The diagnosis depends on the suspicion of the physician based on the history and physical examination. Carpal tunnel radiographs will demonstrate the fracture at the base of the hamate (Fig. 38–45).

Management by the Family Physician Although this fracture may unite if the hand and wrist are immobilized in plaster after the acute injury, in most cases it will need excision and therefore should be referred early on to a hand surgeon for appropriate care.

FRACTURES OF THE PATELLA. The usual mechanism of this injury is a direct blow to the front of the knee, which produces fracture with varying degrees of comminution and displacement. The prime consideration, therefore, should be not so much the fracture, but what the fracture has done to the patient's ability to extend the knee.

Occasionally, the patella retinaculum that surrounds the fracture maintains the integrity of the extensor apparatus and allows the patient to extend his or her knee fully despite the fracture. Knee flexion may then be possible to 45 degrees without evidence of fracture distraction. Such an obviously stable fracture requires only symptomatic treatment to relieve pain and temporary protective splinting to prevent further damage to the extensor mechanism.

Displacement of the fractured patella with knee flexion or inability of the patient to extend the knee actively indicates disruption of the extensor apparatus and the need for operative repair.

Management by the Family Physician The major component of the patient's pain symptoms comes not from the fracture but from the hemarthrosis distending the sensitive joint capsule. The hemarthrosis can be aspirated and the patient's range of motion can then be elevated better. If the patient can actively extend the knee with no lag, and flexion to 30 to 40 degrees causes no palpable opening of the fracture, the patella retinaculum has not been disrupted. These stable fractures require protective support.

Patella fractures can be immobilized by one of two methods depending on the compliance of the

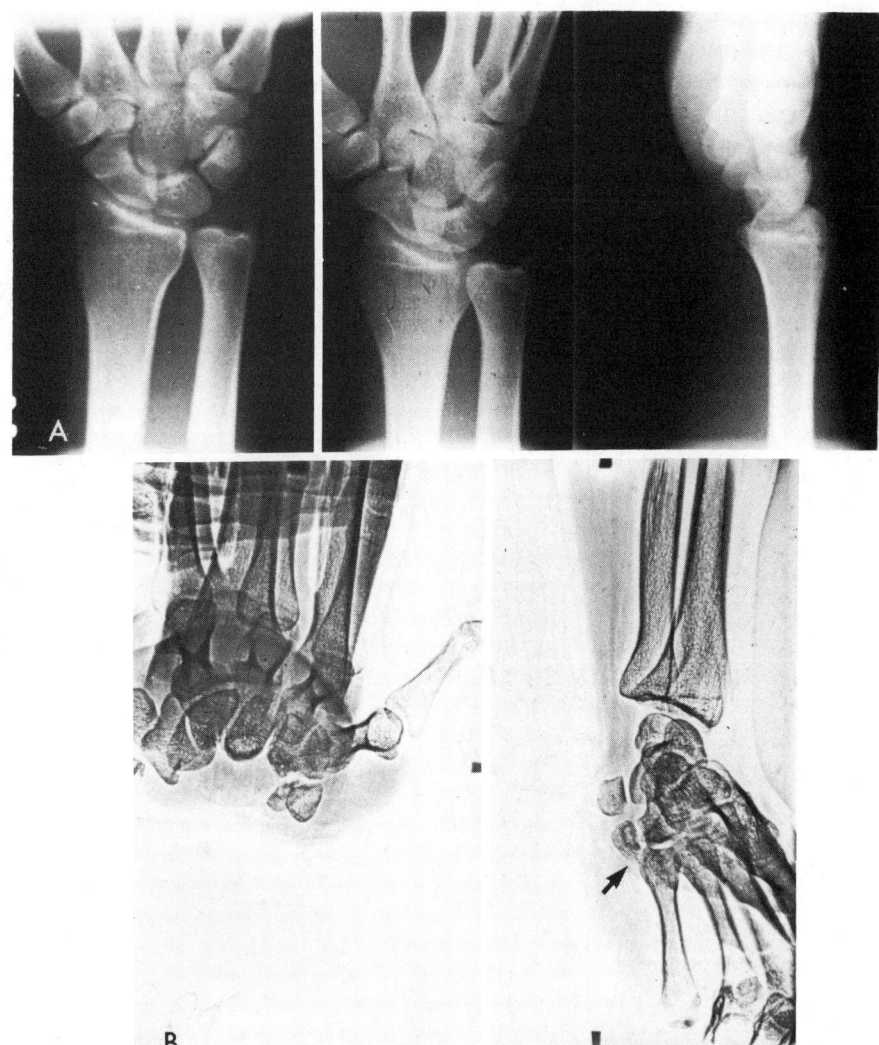

FIGURE 38–45. *A,* This patient had persistent wrist pain after a blow to the palm from the handle of a baseball bat. Standard radiographs of the wrist showed no fractures. *B,* His physician wisely suspected that the hamate was fractured. This could be demonstrated only on special carpal tunnel and oblique views of the hamate. He was treated by excision of the fractured process. (From Connolly JF: DePalma's The Management of Fractures and Dislocations: An Atlas, 3rd edition. Philadelphia, WB Saunders Company, 1981, with permission.)

patient. In a compliant patient, the use of a long leg knee immobilizer is recommended. The alternative is placing the patient in a long leg cylinder cast. Regardless of choice of immobilization, the patient should be encouraged to bear weight on the injured limb as tolerated.

Generally by the end of a week of immobilization, the patient has achieved pain relief sufficient to allow active knee exercises. When the patient is walking, he or she should continue to be splinted to protect against sudden flexion. When there is concern that the patient will not follow directions, it would be prudent to immobilize the leg for 6 weeks before removing the splint or cast. The drawback of this approach is that the patient will have a stiff knee when the splint or cast is removed. This stiffness requires a long rehabilitation period. An alternative operative treatment is internal fixation of the patella fracture followed by active exercise. Appropriate fractures for this type of management are displaced or comminuted patella fractures or a stable fracture in an unstable patient.

Atlas of Fracture and Dislocation Management

This short section of pictorial fracture and dislocation treatment is included for quick reference. It assumes some basic knowledge of fractures and dislocations and provides line drawings and brief explanations of methods of treatment. Admittedly, these descriptions are abbreviated and incomplete, but they do cover some of the more common fractures and dislocations. Readers who desire to study the management of these types of fractures and dislocations in greater depth are referred to the latest edition of *DePalma's The Management of Fractures and Dislocations: an Atlas,* edited by John F. Connolly.

The following fractures and dislocations are depicted:

Diplaced fractures of the thumb metacarpal, including Bennett's fracture (Fig. 38–46).

Fractures of the metacarpals other than the thumb,

which can be treated in a more simple fashion (Fig. 38–47).

Smith's-type fracture, which requires open reduction and internal fixation (Fig. 38–48).

Forearm fractures, including Colles' fracture, showing reduction using finger trap traction (Fig. 38–49).

Clavicle fractures and acromioclavicular separations (Fig. 38–50).

Fractures of the proximal humerus and avul-

sion fractures of the greater tuberosity (Fig. 38–51).

Various dislocations of the shoulder and appropriate methods of reduction (Figs. 38–52 through 38–55).

Fractures of the tibia with intact fibula (Fig. 38–56).

Both-bone fractures of the lower extremity (Fig. 38–57).

Ankle fractures (Fig. 38–58).

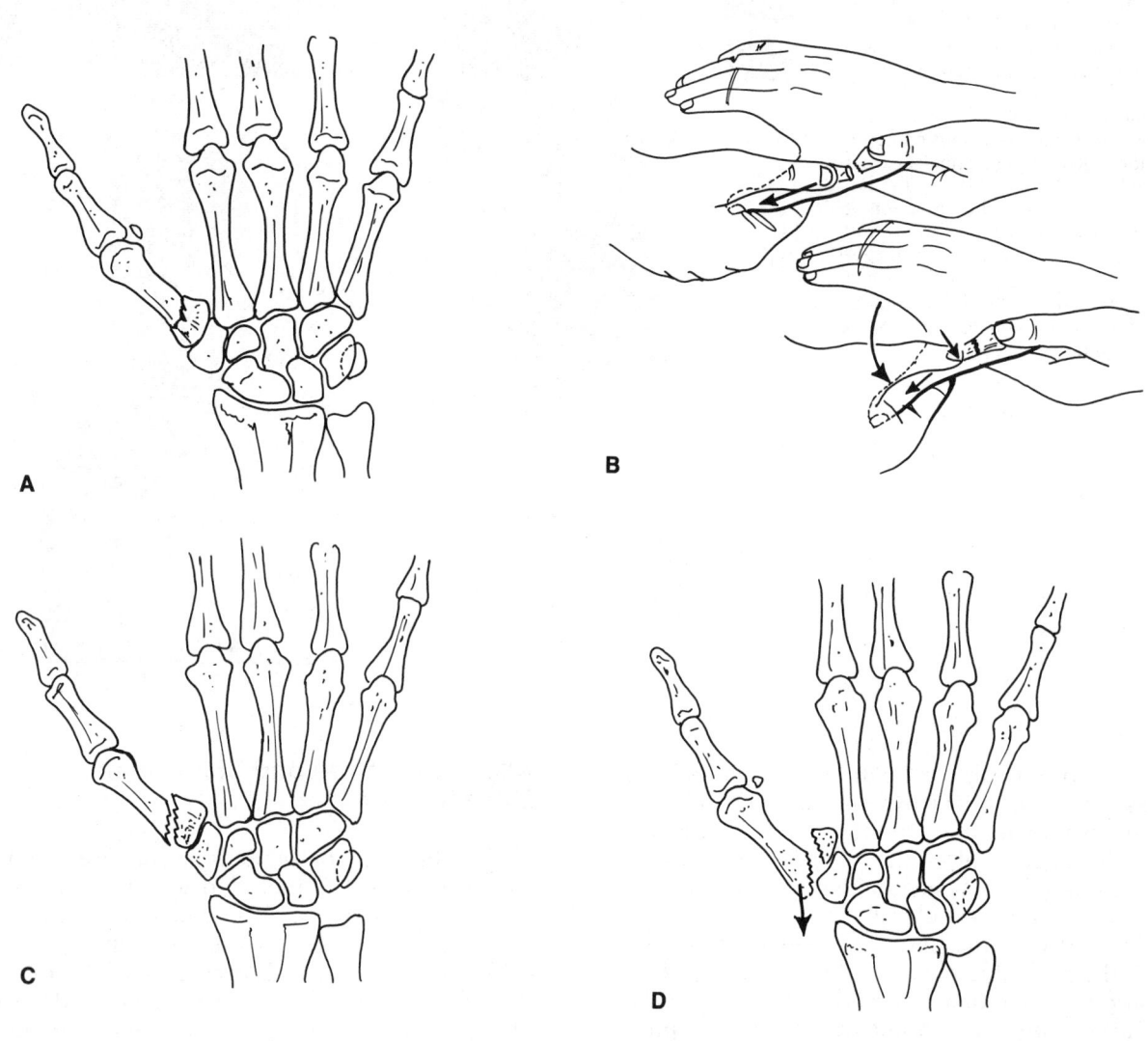

FIGURE 38–46. Displaced fractures of the thumb metacarpal. *A*, Stable displaced mid-metacarpal fracture. *B*, Manual reduction of fracture. *C*, Stable fracture of base of thumb metacarpal can be reduced and, if stable, placed in a thumb spica cast. *D*, Unstable fractures of the thumb metacarpal (Bennett's type) tend to displace in cast and need appropriate consultation and fixation. *E*, Application of thumb spica cast. *F*, Completed thumb spica cast is left on for 5 to 6 weeks. (From Connolly JF: DePalma's The Management of Fractures and Dislocations: An Atlas, 3rd edition. Philadelphia, WB Saunders Company, 1981, with permission.)

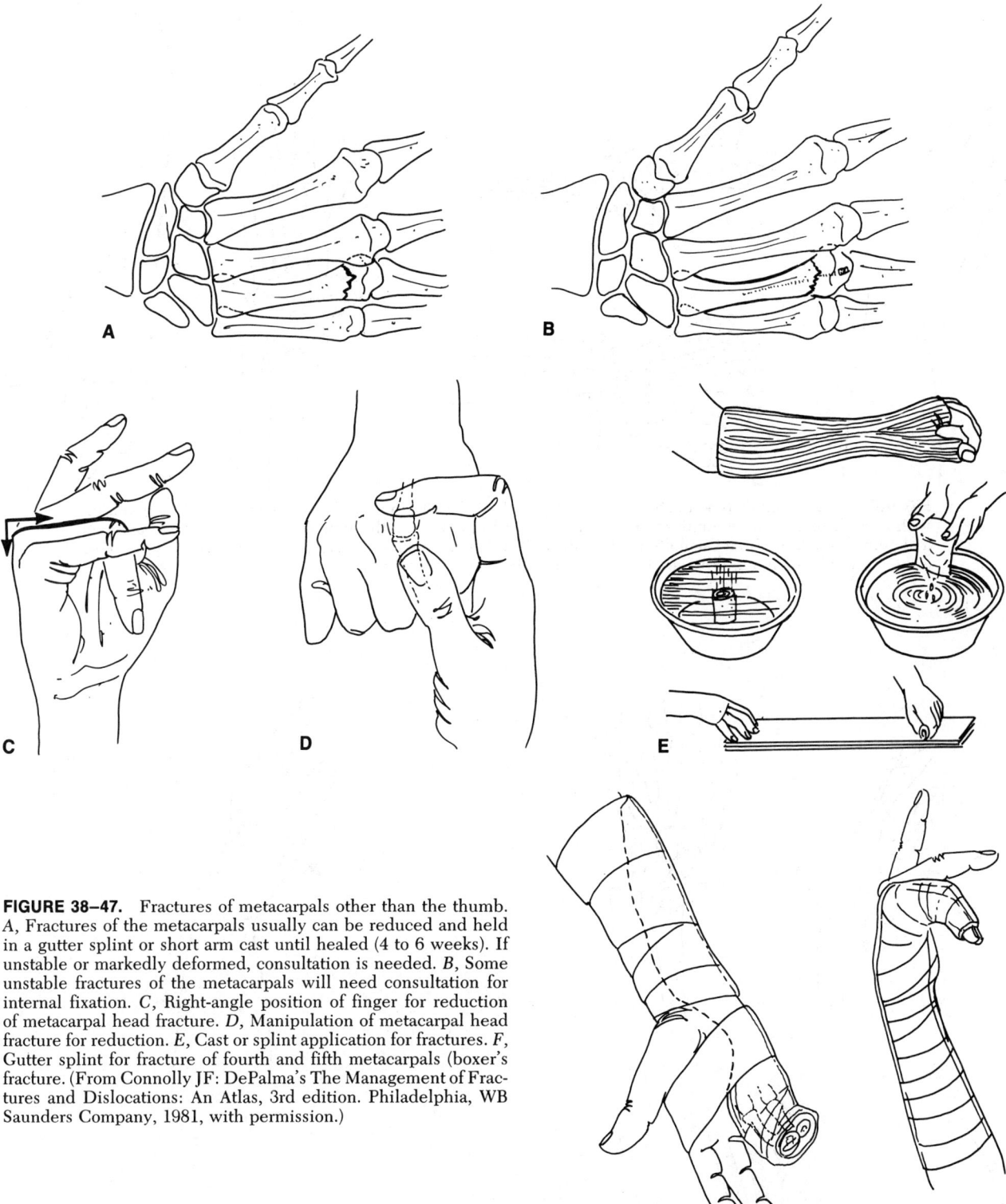

FIGURE 38–47. Fractures of metacarpals other than the thumb. *A*, Fractures of the metacarpals usually can be reduced and held in a gutter splint or short arm cast until healed (4 to 6 weeks). If unstable or markedly deformed, consultation is needed. *B*, Some unstable fractures of the metacarpals will need consultation for internal fixation. *C*, Right-angle position of finger for reduction of metacarpal head fracture. *D*, Manipulation of metacarpal head fracture for reduction. *E*, Cast or splint application for fractures. *F*, Gutter splint for fracture of fourth and fifth metacarpals (boxer's fracture. (From Connolly JF: DePalma's The Management of Fractures and Dislocations: An Atlas, 3rd edition. Philadelphia, WB Saunders Company, 1981, with permission.)

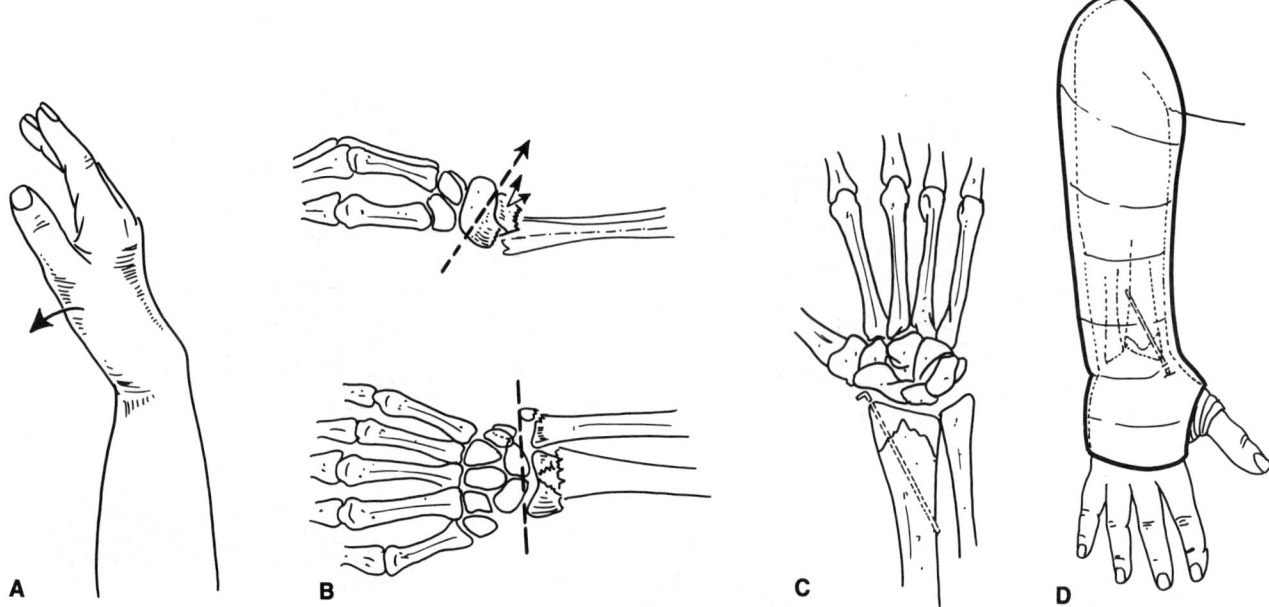

FIGURE 38–48. Smith's-type fracture. *A*, Garden spade deformity in Smith's-type fracture. *B*, Comminution with volar displacement in Smith's-type fracture. *C*, Pin fixation of Smith's-type fracture. *D*, Cast over reduced and pinned fracture. (From Connolly JF: DePalma's The Management of Fractures and Dislocations: An Atlas, 3rd edition. Philadelphia, WB Saunders Company, 1981, with permission.)

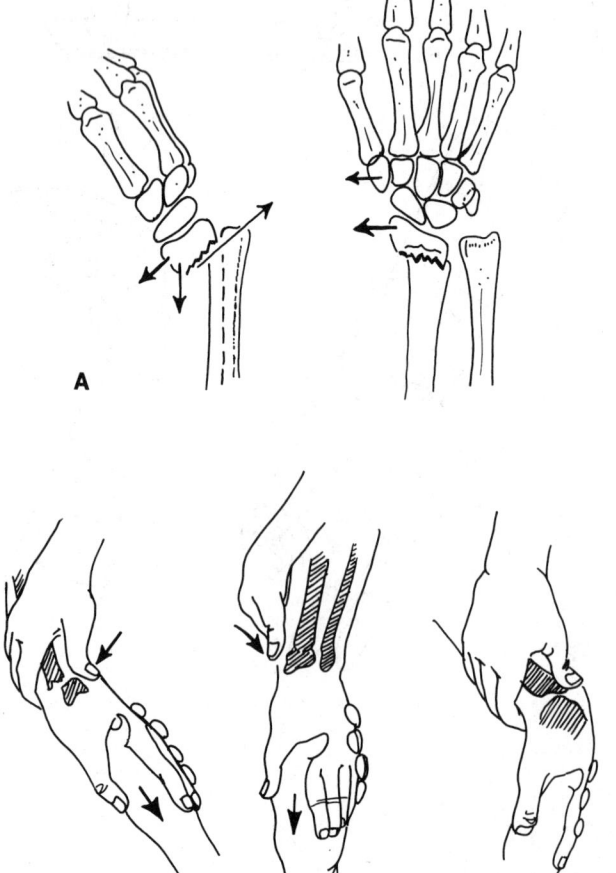

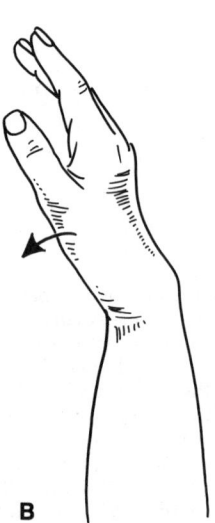

FIGURE 38–49. Forearm fractures. *A*, Colles' fracture. *B*, Silver fork deformity of Colles'-type fracture. *C*, Manual reduction of Colles' and similar forearm fractures. *Illustration continued on following page*

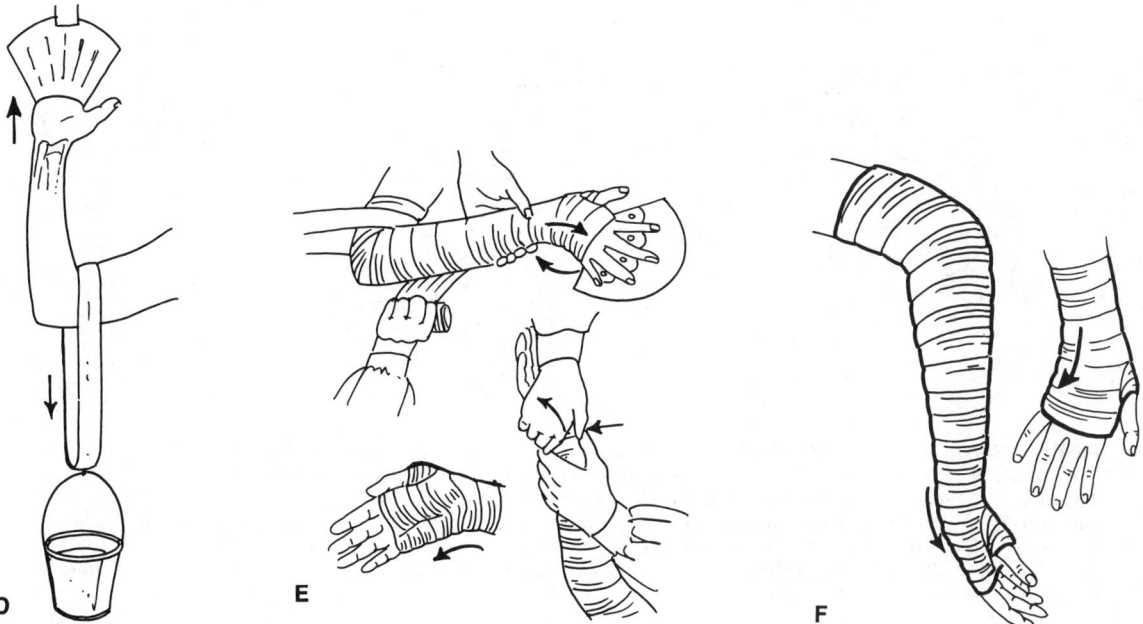

FIGURE 38–49. *Continued. D,* Finger trap reduction. *E,* Casting in finger trap traction. *F,* Modified Cotton-Loder position with cast incorporating both joints for forearm fracture. (From Connolly JF: DePalma's The Management of Fractures and Dislocations: An Atlas, 3rd edition. Philadelphia, WB Saunders Company, 1981, with permission.)

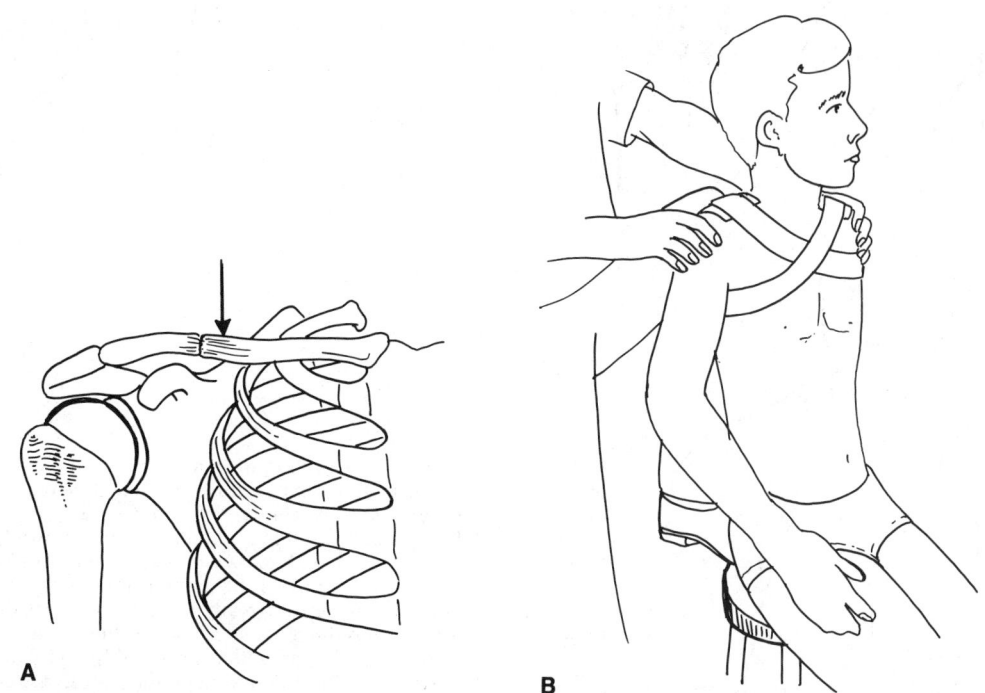

FIGURE 38–50. Clavical fractures and acromioclavicular separations. *A,* Clavical fractures that are not complex can be immobilized in a Meek brace, figure-of-8 bandage, or plaster figure-of-8 until healed (usually 6 to 8 weeks). *B,* Meeks brace. *Illustration continued on following page.*

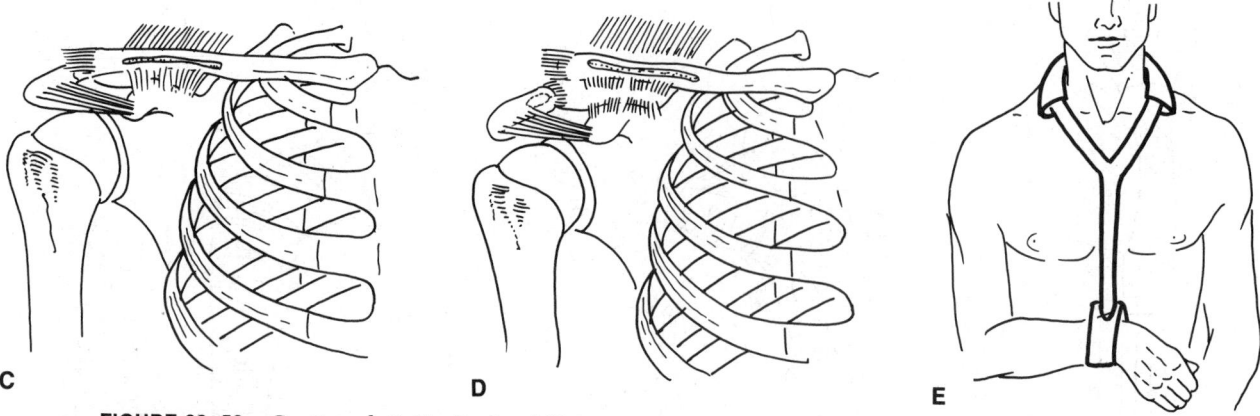

FIGURE 38–50. *Continued. C,* Grades I and II acromioclavicular separations can be handled in a collar and cuff. Grade II separations should be referred for possible surgical repair if the patient desires active treatment. This may reduce later arthritic changes. *D,* Grade III acromioclavicular separation can be handled with a collar and cuff if the patient does not mind a bump deformity. Patients who do not want a bump deformity should be referred for early repair. *E,* Collar and cuff for acute acromioclavicular separation. (From Connolly JF: DePalma's The Management of Fractures and Dislocations: An Atlas, 3rd edition. Philadelphia, WB Saunders Company, 1981, with permission.)

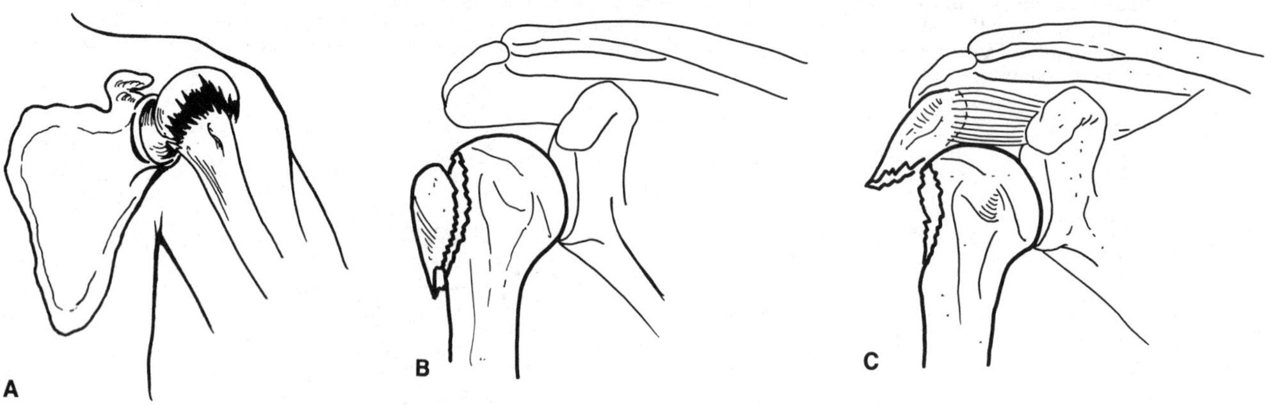

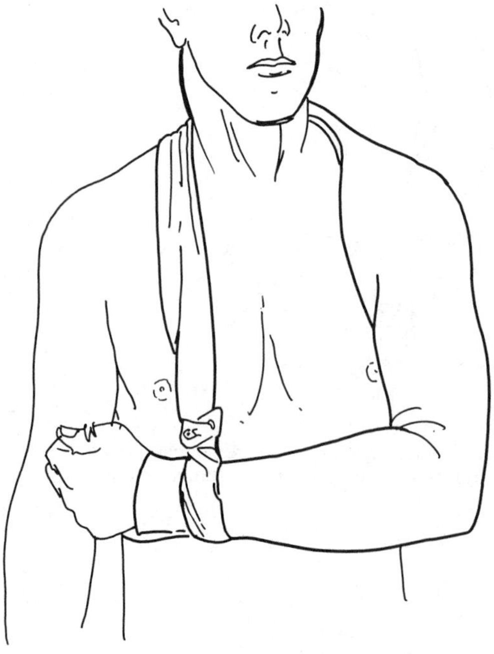

FIGURE 38–51. Fractures of the proximal humerus and avulsion fractures of the greater tuberosity. *A,* Fracture of the proximal humerus without dislocation usually can be treated by binding the arm to the body with a Velpeau dressing. Prolonged immobilization is not necessary. At 2 weeks, circumduction exercises can be started, with more vigorous exercises begun at 4 weeks. *B,* Undisplaced avulsion fracture of the greater tuberosity can be treated in a Velpeau dressing. *C,* Greater tuberosity avulsion fractures displaced more than 5 mm require open reduction and screw fixation. When displaced less than 5 mm, they are treated as any other proximal humerus fracture, with a Velpeau-type dressing. *D,* Stockinette support for control of shoulder. A bandage applied to the chest completes a Velpeau-type dressing. (From Connolly JF: DePalma's The Management of Fractures and Dislocations: An Atlas, 3rd edition. Philadelphia, WB Saunders Company, 1981, with permission.)

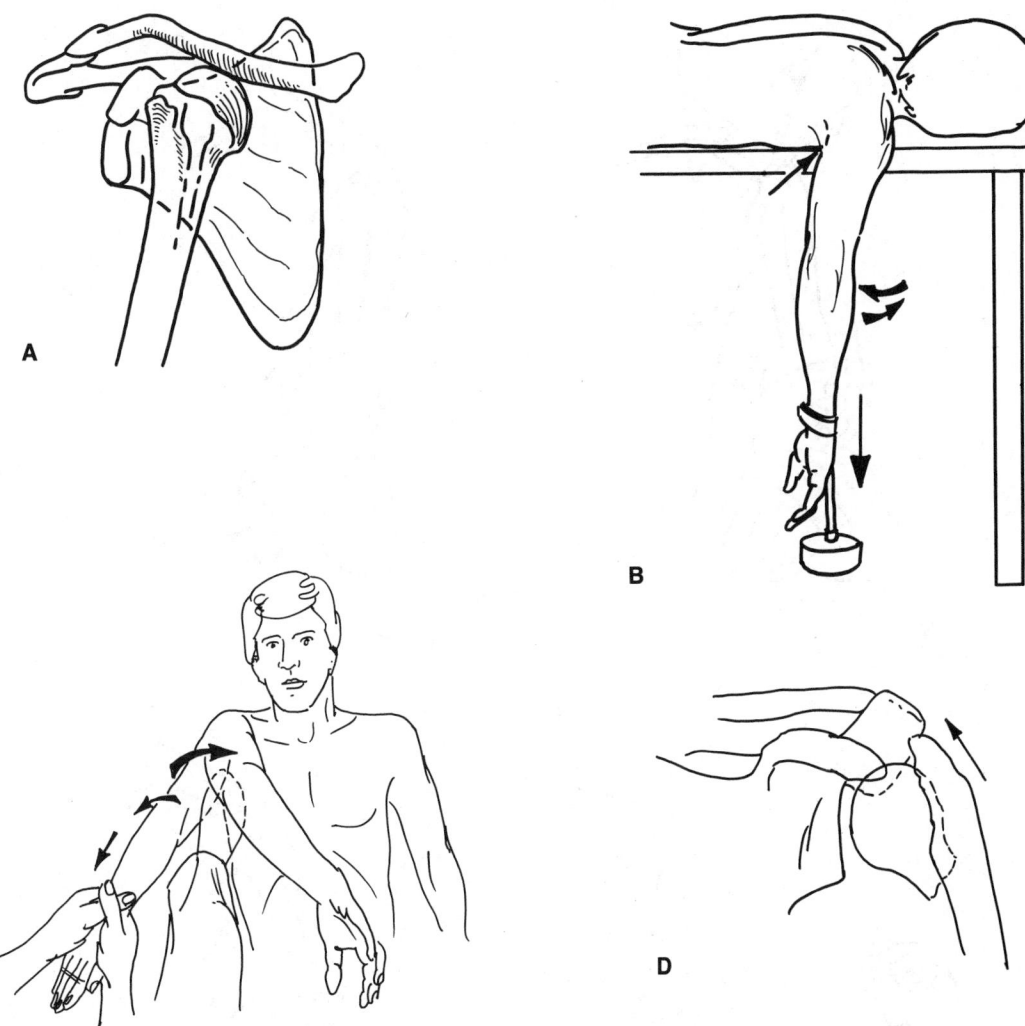

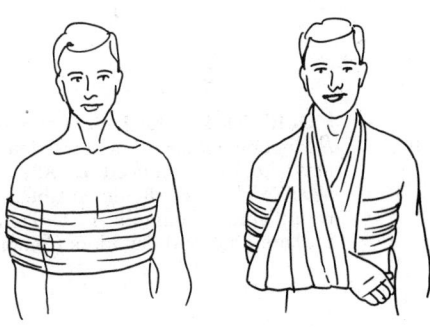

FIGURE 38–52. Anterior dislocation of the shoulder. *A,* Anteroposterior view of dislocation. *B,* Stimson technique for reduction. Ideally, this maneuver should be tried first because it is the least traumatic. The patient is placed prone on a table edge with the arm hanging down. Ten to 20 kg (22 to 25 pounds) of weight is applied to the arm for 10 to 15 minutes. If reduction does not occur, gentle external and internal rotation will aid the process. *C,* Hippocratic maneuver for reduction. As an alternative to the operator's foot, an assistant can apply countertraction with a folded towel or sheet. *D,* A fracture-dislocation sometimes can be maneuvered manually into a reduced position or carried into position with transcutaneous pins, but in general the patient should be referred to an orthopedist. *E,* Velpeau dressing for fracture or reduced dislocation of the shoulder. (From Connolly JF: DePalma's The Management of Fractures and Dislocations: An Atlas, 3rd edition. Philadelphia, WB Saunders Company, 1981, with permission.)

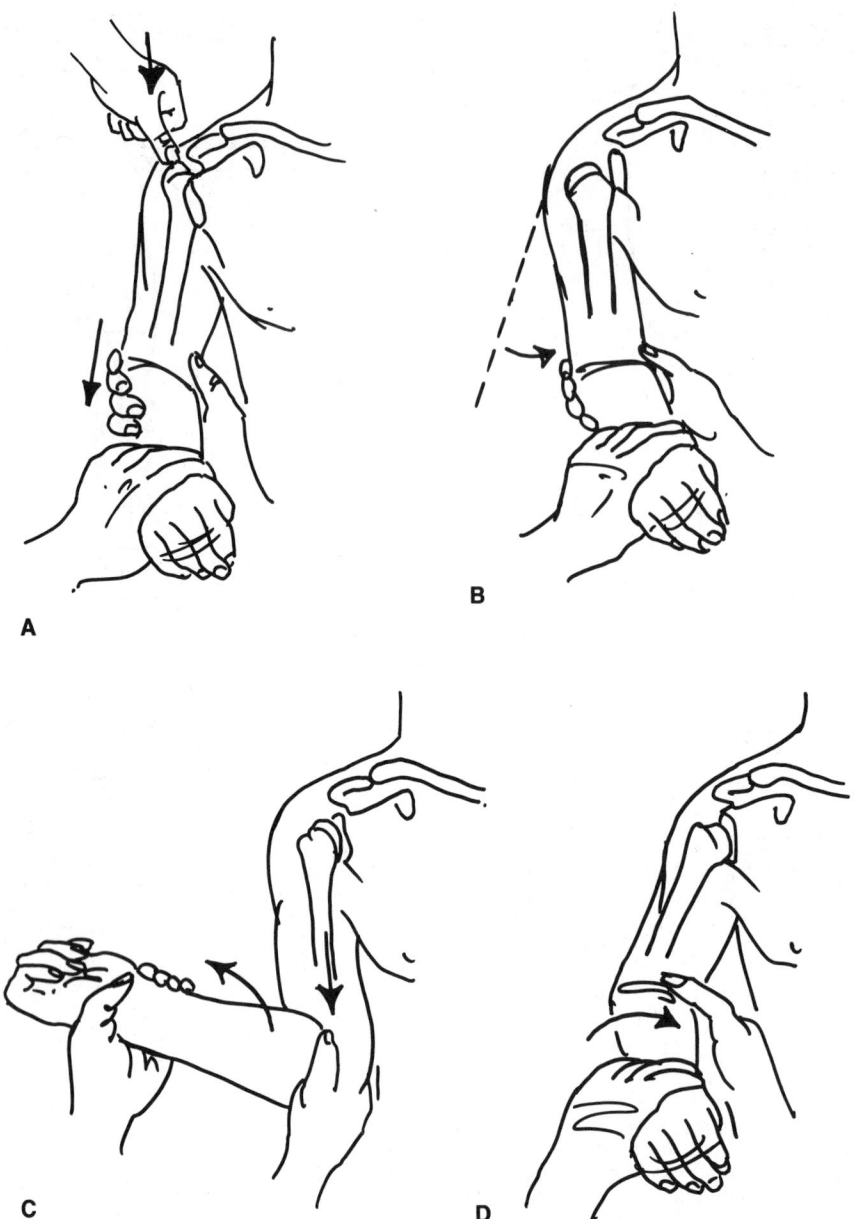

FIGURE 38–53. Kocher maneuver for reduction of anterior shoulder dislocation. *A,* Application of traction. *B,* Adduction with continued traction. *C,* External rotation with continued adduction and traction. The dislocation now should be reduced. *D,* After reduction, the arm is rotated internally and placed in a Velpeau dressing. *NOTE*: The arm should not be rotated internally if reduction is not accomplished because a fracture may result. (From Connolly JF: DePalma's The Management of Fractures and Dislocations: An Atlas, 3rd edition. Philadelphia, WB Saunders Company, 1981, with permission.)

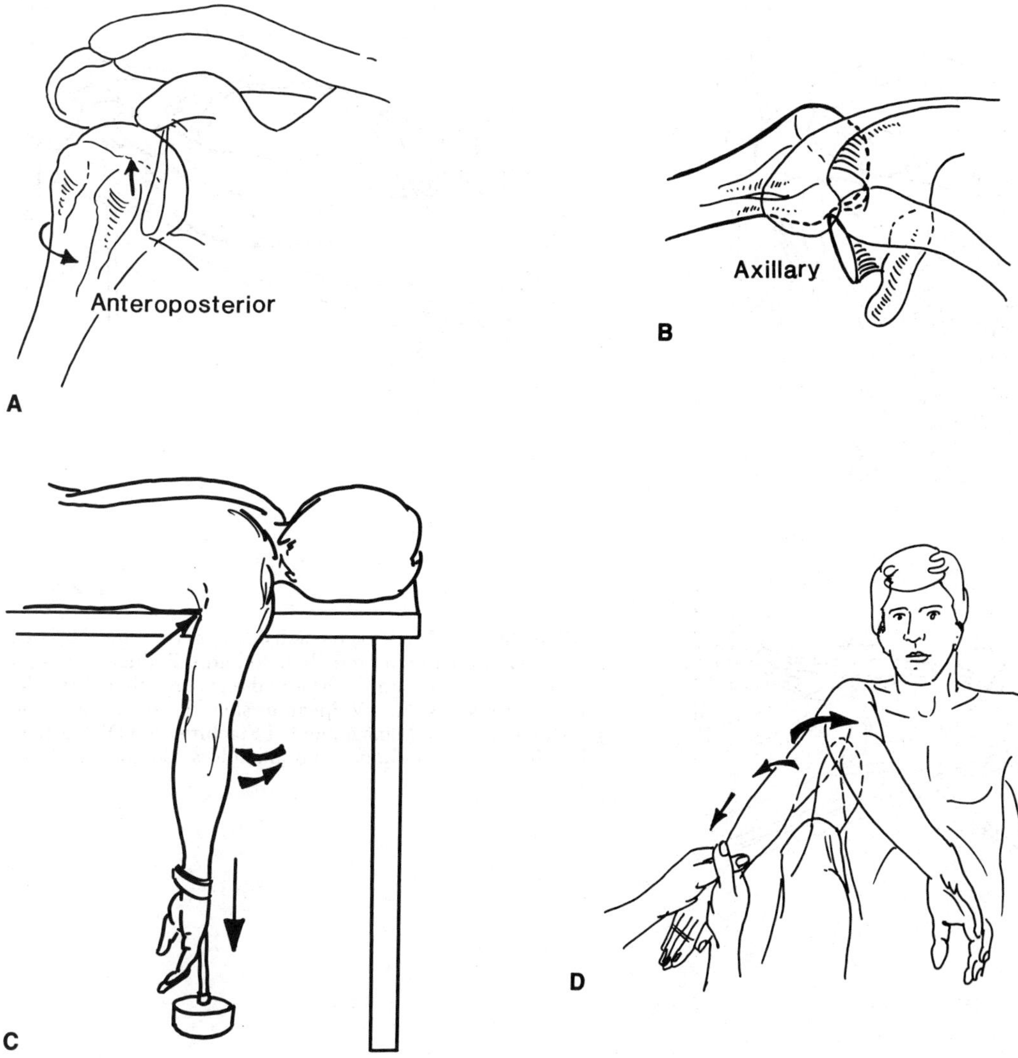

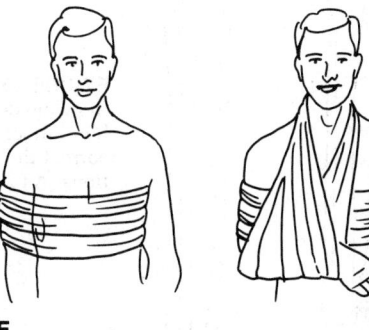

A

Anteroposterior

B

Axillary

C

D

E

FIGURE 38–54.   Posterior dislocation of the shoulder. *A,* Anteroposterior view. *B,* Axillary View. *C,* Stimson technique for reduction. *D,* Hippocratic maneuver for reduction. *E,* Velpeau dressing. The shoulder should be immobilized for 6 weeks, and then rehabilitation started with range-of-motion and strengthening exercises. (From Connolly JF: DePalma's The Management of Fractures and Dislocations: An Atlas, 3rd edition. Philadelphia, WB Saunders Company, 1981, with permission.)

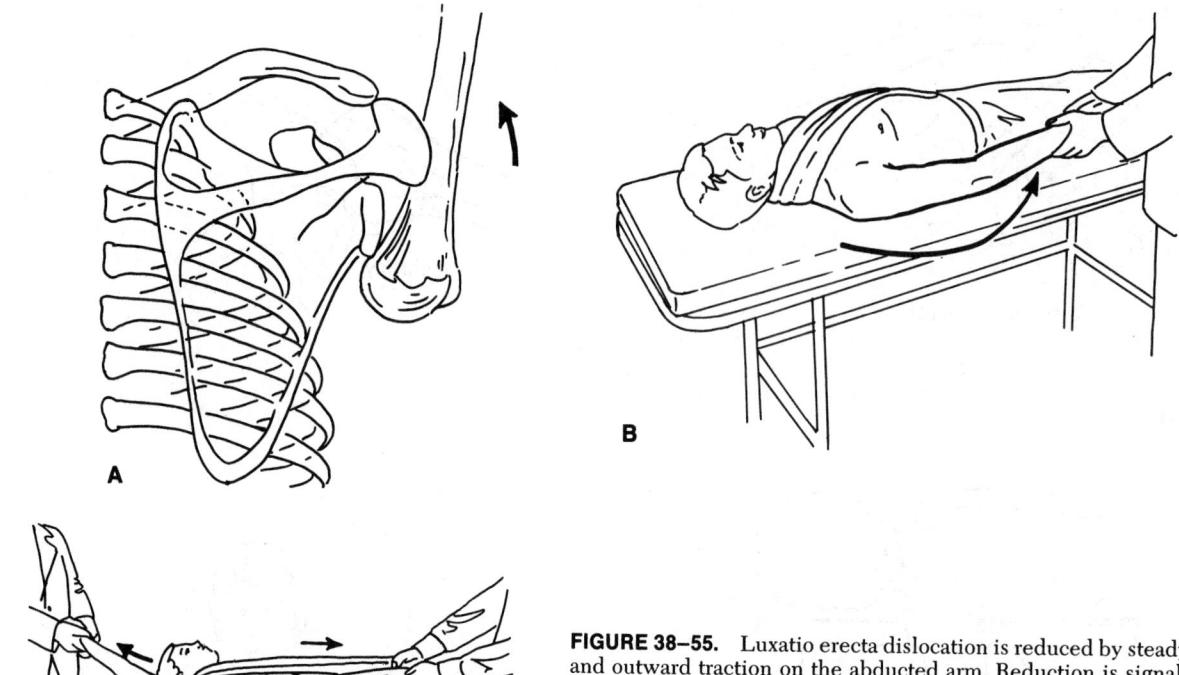

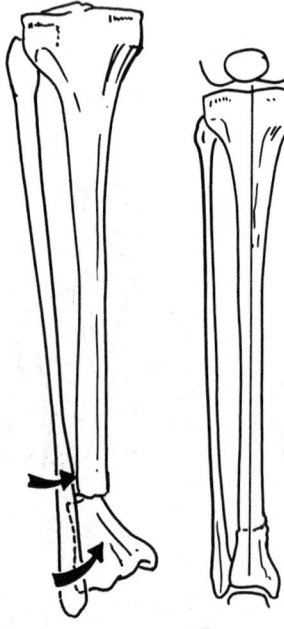

FIGURE 38–55.   Luxatio erecta dislocation is reduced by steady upward and outward traction on the abducted arm. Reduction is signaled by an audible or palpable clunk. The arm then is brought to the side and immobilized for 6 weeks in a Velpeau or shoulder dressing. (From Connolly JF: DePalma's The Management of Fractures and Dislocations: An Atlas, 3rd edition. Philadelphia, WB Saunders Company, 1981, with permission.)

FIGURE 38–56.   Fracture of the tibia with an intact fibula. These fractures are prone to varus (bowleg) deformity and must be monitored by radiographs taken every 2 weeks to detect the problem. Should it begin, immediate consultation is needed, and perhaps osteotomy of the fibula to correct the problem. (From Connolly JF: DePalma's The Management of Fractures and Dislocations: An Atlas, 3rd edition. Philadelphia, WB Saunders Company, 1981, with permission.)

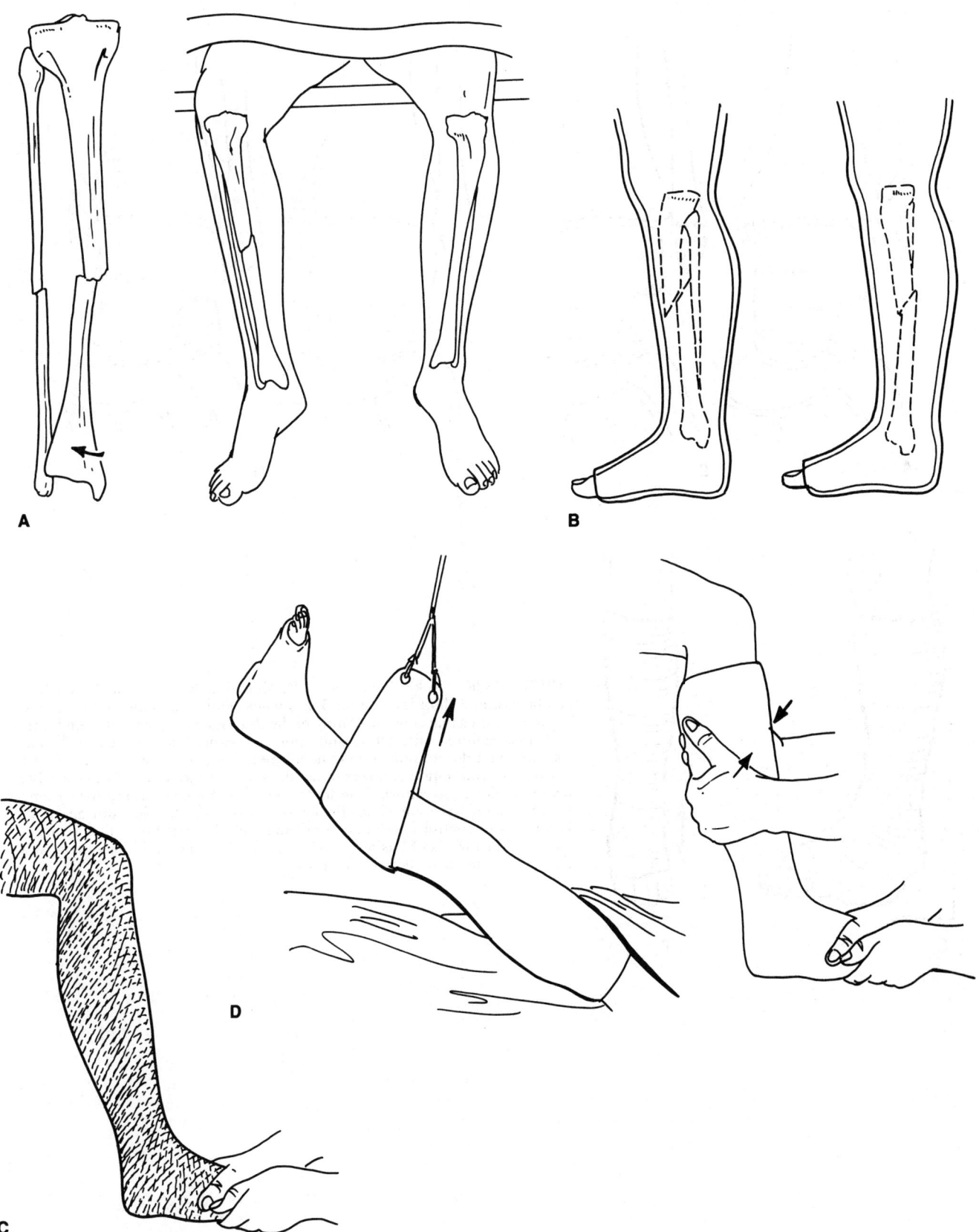

FIGURE 38–57. Both bone fractures of the lower leg. These fractures can be aligned with the legs hanging over the edge of an exam table and can be placed in a long leg cast, if stable. The patient should be hospitalized for 24-hour observation for compartment syndrome. When stable at 4 weeks or so these fractures can be recast in a short leg cast and weight bearing to tolerance allowed. (From Connolly JF: DePalma's The Management of Fractures and Dislocations: An Atlas, 3rd edition. Philadelphia, WB Saunders Company, 1981, with permission.)

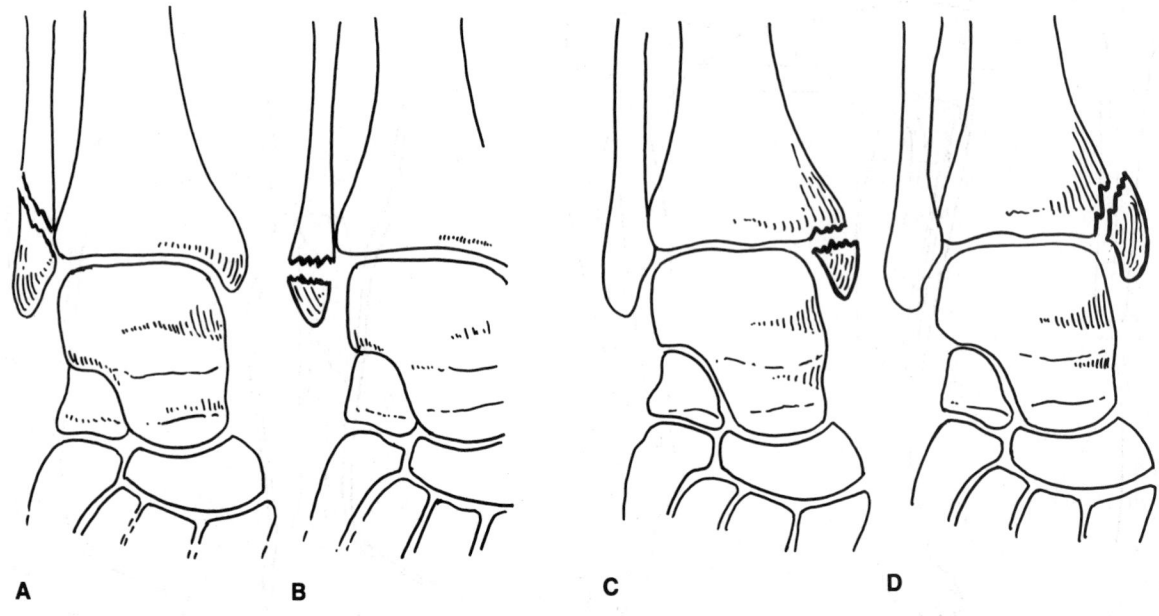

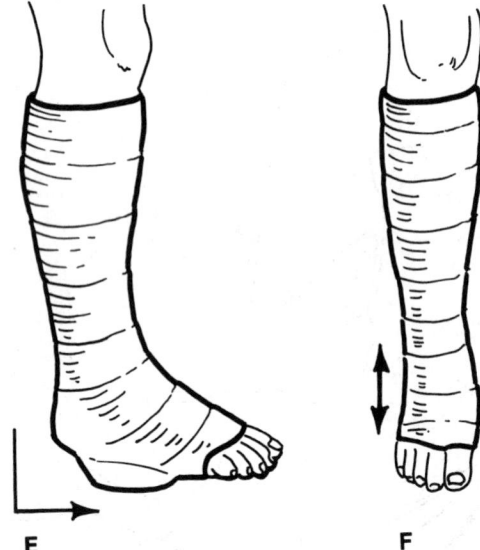

FIGURE 38–58. Ankle fractures. *A–D*, Medial or lateral malleolar fracture can be cast in a short leg cast for 5 or 6 weeks and then mobilized in an Ace wrap. Fractures that show widening of the interosseous space between fibula and tibia require consultation and open reduction. Some medial malleolar fractures that do not reduce may need open fixation. *E* and *F*, The leg cast consists of wrapping two layers of padding over stockinette with four or five layers of plaster, as shown. The foot should be in a neutral position. A long leg cast should have some knee flexion so the foot clear the floor during ambulation and to control rotation. (From Connolly JF: DePalma's The Management of Fractures and Dislocations: An Atlas, 3rd edition. Philadelphia, WB Saunders Company, 1981, with permission.)

MORTON'S NEUROMA

Morton (1876) described a type of severe pain in the forefoot. The history is that of a patient seized with pain necessitating standing still on the good foot and perhaps removing the shoe to rub the painful area. In a short time the pain will abate. Between bouts of pain the patient has no symptoms. The disorder usually is seen between ages 15 and 55 and is more common in females. The etiology may be mechanical irritation of the digital proper nerve between adjacent metatarsal heads (Betts, 1940). Most commonly affected is the nerve between the third and fourth toes, although the neuroma can occur between other toes. Direct compression of the interspace will elicit or reproduce the pain.

MANAGEMENT BY THE FAMILY PHYSICIAN. Initial treatment of Morton's neuroma should be with nonsteroidal anti-inflammatory medications and the use of a small metatarsal pad in the shoe. Occasionally, patients will benefit from a cortisone injection. Chronic conditions are best managed by surgical resection of the nerve, which will leave the patient with permanent anesthesia but no functional deficit.

DIABETES-RELATED ORTHOPEDIC PROBLEMS

Minor foot problems such as bunions or clawtoe can become limb-threatening or even life-threatening for the diabetic patient. Diabetes produces the majority of adult amputees today. This contrasts with the statistics prior to 1951, when most amputations followed trauma.

The major orthopedic problems resulting from diabetes that will be discussed in this section are diabetic vascular disease and diabetic neuropathy.

Diabetic Vascular Disease

The major difference between diabetic and nondiabetic peripheral vascular disease is that, in diabetes, the basement membrane of the capillaries and small vessels becomes pathologically thickened, thereby preventing profusion across the capillary wall. This thickening, at least in the mature diabetic patient, is a segmental lesion. It does not obstruct flow, but it does limit exchange across the vessel wall. This produces edema, local lymphatic obstruction, and an interstitial backwash, which makes an ideal medium for infection. Consequently, infection and subsequent gangrene is 40 times more common in the diabetic than in the nondiabetic patient with atherosclerosis. Diabetic infection with gangrene occurs in either a foot that is cold as a result of proximal obstruction without collateral distal flow or a foot that is warm or even hot, indicating adequate small vessel flow but impaired perfusion.

Approximately one third of diabetic gangrene occurs in the cold foot, and this is managed like any other atherosclerotic occlusion, either with arterial grafting or with amputation. The remaining two thirds of patients with diabetic gangrene usually have palpable major pulses and adequate peripheral flow. For these patients, drainage of infection, débridement of necrotic tissue, and conservative amputation are most successful. Distinguishing between the two types of diabetic gangrene is usually not difficult (see Fig. 38–7).

Diabetic Neuropathy

The basic problem producing the common neuropathic changes in the diabetic appears to be the alteration in metabolism of the Schwann cells in the nerve sheath, with resultant demyelinization of the nerve. As with angiopathic changes, the onset of clinical symptoms from diabetic neuropathy is not necessarily related to the duration or severity of the diabetes. A number of patients first find out that they have diabetes when they develop symptoms of neuropathy or distal gangrene.

Anatomic, sensory, and motor nerve fibers all are involved in the neuropathic process. The diabetic patient's loss of autonomic function causes inability to control body temperature and inadequate sweating mechanism. The result is dry, scaly skin, which makes wounds and abrasions of the patient's foot highly susceptible to infection. The loss of autonomic control may cause the patient's skin temperature in the foot to be 4° to 5° F less than the body's core temperature and results in the characteristic diabetic "cold foot." The unwary individual may sustain burns from keeping hot water bottles or other heating aids on cold feet while asleep.

Sensory neuropathy in diabetes can produce extremely painful paresthesias, which are sometimes described as dart-like or tabetic in nature. The paresthesias are worse at night, frequently are aggravated by cold, and are generally associated with decreased ankle jerk reflexes. This pain of neuropathy is generally relieved by walking, as opposed to the pain of angiopathy, which is made worse by walking. Diabetic "tabes" can be confused with disc disease.

The most devastating neuropathy of diabetes is that which results in the loss of protective sensation and causes the patient to continue to walk on injured pressure points, literally walking the protective skin off the sole (Fig. 38–59). The loss of protective sensation can break down the skeletal support of the foot from repetitive fatigue fracture. This neuropathic destruction of the bones in the diabetic foot is now the most common cause of Charcot's joint. Quite frequently, the radiographic changes of this neuropathic bone destruction are

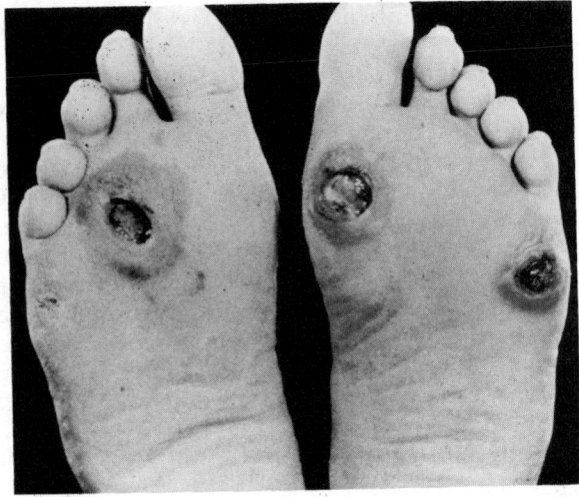

FIGURE 38–59. Typical multiple neurotrophic ulcers have developed in this diabetic patient as a result of loss of protective sensation over pressure areas.

confused with those of osteomyelitis (Fig. 38–60A). This is completely unnecessary and avoidable, because the differential diagnosis between osteomyelitis and Charcot's changes can be made by simple clinical observations. (Bone scans are no help; circulation is increased in both conditions.) Osteomyelitis is most often associated with abscess formation or draining infection. Charcot changes characteristically produce swelling, defor-

mity, and sometimes redness, but not drainage and other signs of acute infection (Fig. 38–60B).

Involvement of motor nerve fibers may result in paralysis, including footdrop or wristdrop. This does tend to improve with time and with control of the blood sugar. Weakness of the intrinsic muscles of the foot produces gait alteration and adds to the development of pressure points, abrasion, infection, and ultimate gangrene.

Management of Diabetic Problems

MANAGEMENT BY THE FAMILY PHYSICIAN. The family physician can play an important role in prevention of diabetic foot problems by encouraging self–glucose monitoring. Recent information has shown that frequent monitoring and tight control of blood sugar levels can reduce the incidence of angiopathy and neuropathy that can lead to gangrene. However, luck of the genetic draw and particularly the host response play major roles in the development of diabetic foot problems.

Host response may be altered with education. A self-evaluation program should be developed to remind the diabetic patient of the high likelihood of having vascular and neurologic disease. The patient must be reminded to pay proper attention to the care of feet and is encouraged to do so at each visit.

The diabetic foot must be inspected every day

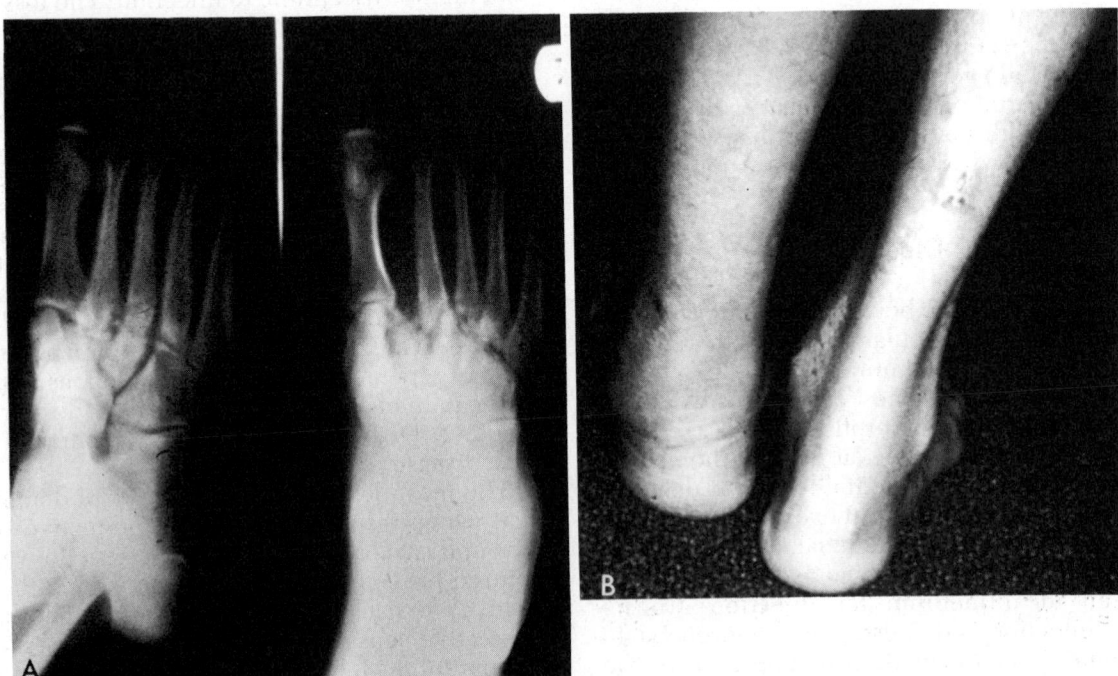

FIGURE 38–60. *A,* Neurotrophic changes led to this bone destruction (Charcot's joints), as seen on these radiographs of a diabetic patient. This should not be confused with osteomyelitis if the physician examines the foot as well as the radiograph. *B,* A patient with neurotrophic foot and ankle demonstrates swelling and warmth but no drainage or ulceration.

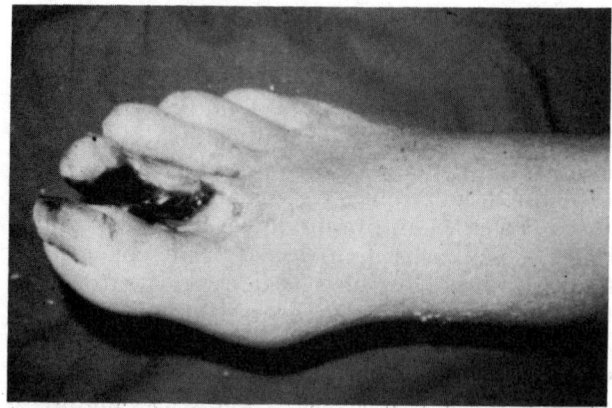

FIGURE 38–61. Failure of this patient to attend to proper nail and foot hygiene produced this infection and eventual diabetic gangrene.

either by the patient or, if the patient has poor vision, by a family member. Nails should be trimmed evenly so as to prevent ingrowth and infection of the nail edges. The diabetic patient should wash and carefully dry the feet each day and particularly avoid walking barefooted, hot water applications, and chemical treatment of calluses. Inadequate attention to foot care invariably leads to trouble (Fig. 38–61).

Bony prominences that cause calluses, bunions, or clawfoot are likely to produce pressure necrosis and infection of the skin. These should be corrected promptly by surgical procedures before the infection supervenes. Rather than being a contraindication to foot surgery, the diabetic state should be considered a prime indication for early surgical correction of foot deformities.

Shoes are extremely important and must be chosen carefully. We prefer thick-soled shoes or ripple shoes to relieve pressure points and absorb weight-

bearing forces. If necessary, a pressure area can be relieved by paring down the ripple of the sole over either the first or fifth metatarsal head.

Neuropathic bone destruction or Charcot's deformities are particular therapeutic problems in juvenile diabetics, who sometimes try to ignore their condition. These impressively damaged skeletal structures do heal when adequately protected with a cast and weight-bearing orthosis. A very effective orthosis is the "patellar tendon–bearing" type, which includes a rigid ankle and transfers the weight-bearing load to a custom-made socket contacting the proximal tibia and patellar tendon (Fig. 38–62).

SURGICAL MANAGEMENT OF DIABETIC GANGRENE. The source of most therapeutic indecision about diabetic care is the infected foot that has not responded to the usual modalities of bed rest, elevation, and antibiotics. In managing such a problem, a decision about surgical drainage must not be delayed more than 2 to 3 days. To persevere determinedly with antibiotic treatment of an abscessed foot will only convert a salvageable limb into a below-knee amputation.

The amputation, should it be necessary, must be as conservative as possible in the diabetic foot with warm gangrene. Soft tissue drainage (Fig. 38–63), a partial ray resection (see Fig. 38–8), or Syme's amputation work well in the foot with small vessel disease but adequate major arterial flow. If a complicating infection extends close to the site of amputation, the wound can be left open and closed secondarily.

There is very little justification today for automatically selecting an above-knee amputation level for diabetic gangrene, especially when one considers that 20 to 30 per cent of diabetic amputees will eventually require amputation of the opposite limb. Studies over the past 10 years have

FIGURE 38–62. *A*, This diabetic patient with neurotrophic fractures of her foot and ankle can be treated by well-padded, protective casts until the acute fractures subside. *B*, A weight-bearing orthosis can then be used to shift the weight off the neurotrophic foot and ankle to the proximal tibia.

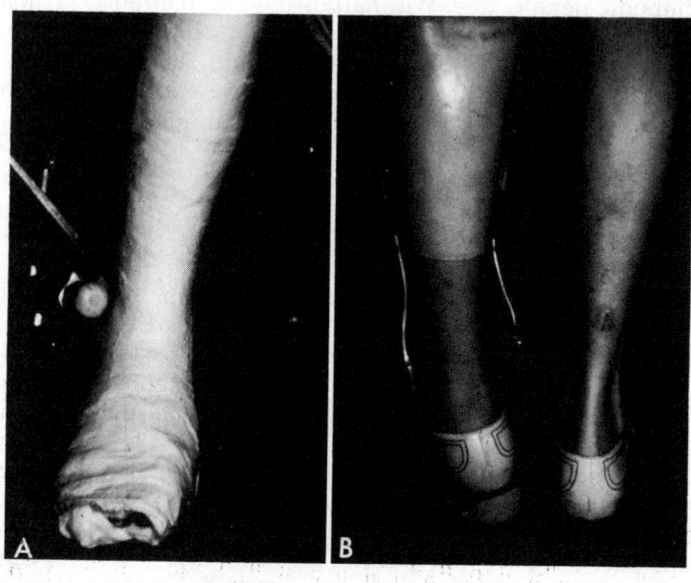

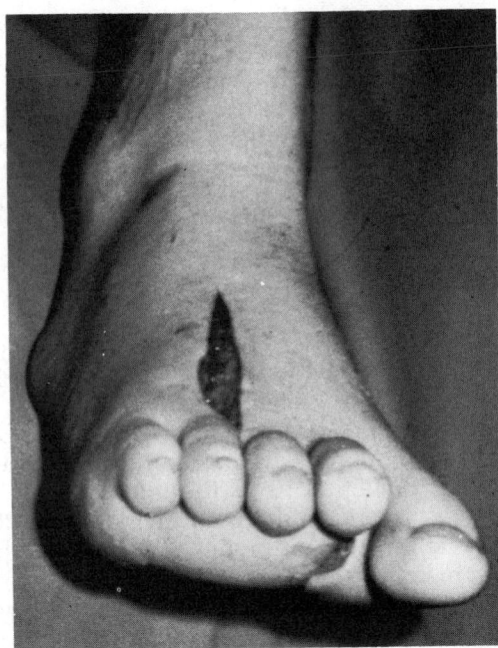

FIGURE 38–63. Prompt drainage of the dorsal and plantar abscesses of this diabetic patient's foot salvaged a useful weight-bearing extremity. Antibiotic treatment cannot be expected to cure diabetic foot abscesses.

shown that, in the elderly diabetic patient, below-knee amputation heals quite well. The rehabilitation potential is so much greater when the patient's knee is preserved that the lower level should be employed in almost every instances of diabetic gangrene.

ARTHRITIS

In this section, rather than skipping superficially through the arthritides, which are well covered in Chapter 39, we shall focus on them from an orthopedic perspective. We shall discuss fundamental concepts that have been useful for us to maximize the effect of both medical and surgical treatment. We shall also present a few common problems that both the family physician and the orthopedist tend to overlook or undertreat.

Traumatic Arthritis

Traumatic arthritis represents a common, but only vaguely understood disease that is particularly likely to afflict young, active individuals subject to injury. Arthritis secondary to trauma should be distinguished from osteoarthritis resulting from biochemical breakdown of cartilage matrix. The boundary between traumatic arthritis and osteoarthritis has been obscured by the tendency of patients to relate most joint diseases to a traumatic episode, either real or imagined.

Trauma sufficient to fracture the joint surface may or may not induce arthritis. This is beyond the control of the physician. Other factors, particularly the severity of joint stiffening and the degree of joint instability, are to a significant extent related to initial treatment.

In the upper limb, the major complication to avoid is a stiff joint. In the lower limb, joint instability as well as stiffening is of prime concern. In the upper limb, there is a tendency to overtreat the fracture by imposing unnecessary immobilization and inducing a stiff joint. In the lower limb, physicians are prone to undertreat articular fractures and accept joint instability, which could and should be avoided.

Upper Limb Problems

Techniques that are most likely to minimize traumatic arthritis in the upper limb include both appropriate fracture stabilization and emphasis on early restoration of joint motion. At one time, rest was considered essential for healing a diseased or injured joint. Despite occasional benefits in the past from prolonged and uninterrupted rest of diseased joints, the detrimental results of prolonged joint immobilization and the importance of motion for articular cartilage healing have been demonstrated repeatedly (Salter et al., 1980).

Avascular cartilage must be nourished by synovial fluid, which is "pumped" into the cartilage during motion. Complete immobilization of joints for only a few weeks produces measurable changes in the cartilage matrix and eventual breakdown of usually smooth articular joint surfaces. Immobilization also weakens the tensile strength of the ligaments supporting joints. Frequently the result is ligamentous laxity, induced by even brief periods of joint immobilization.

Examples of upper limb articular fractures in which joint motion should be emphasized over fracture reduction include fractures of the radial head and fractures of the surgical neck of the humerus. Radial head or neck fractures are best managed by aspirating the hemarthrosis and then encouraging the patient to move the elbow promptly. The major portion of pain after injuries to joints results from distention of the joint capsule. Aspirating the hemarthrosis in the elbow, which may amount to only a few cubic centimeters, does much to relieve the patient's acute discomfort (Fig. 38–64).

The elbow should not be immobilized in flexion for more than 2 or 3 days. The usual motion limited after radial head fractures is elbow extension. If necessary for patient comfort, apply a plaster-of-Paris splint to maintain the elbow in maximum extension at night. However, encourage active elbow flexion during daytime activities.

If, on moving the elbow, the radial head fracture fragment is found to block flexion, it can be removed surgically. This is best determined first by

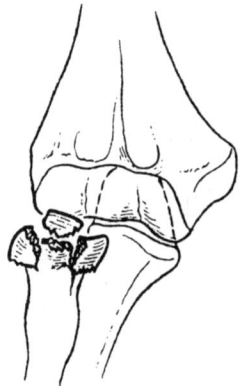

FIGURE 38–64. Radial head fractures should be treated by aspirating the elbow joint to relieve the pain from capsular distention. Then local anesthetic is injected and the range of elbow motion checked to determine whether any of the fracture fragments block flexion or extension. Surgical excision is necessary only if there is blockage of joint motion; otherwise, active range of motion of the elbow is encouraged.

a trial of motion. Such an approach allows the patient to return to most activities in 2 or 3 weeks. This contrasts with the 3 or 4 months or recovery necessitated by prolonged immobilization or inordinately aggressive surgical treatment.

Another common fracture of the upper limb for which treatment is likely to impair joint function is a fracture of the surgical neck of the humerus. Prolonged immobilization until there is radiographic evidence of fracture union neglects the rapid and detrimental effect of immobilization on joint function. The supraspinatus muscle, an important suspensory muscle of the shoulder, is particularly prone to rapid atrophy with disuse. The result is that the humeral head will subluxate or partially dislocate inferiorly and the shoulder will tighten in a "frozen" position (Fig. 38–65). The consequence is an injury that requires 6 months for recovery rather than 6 weeks, as it should.

To avoid this unnecessary sequence of joint mal-

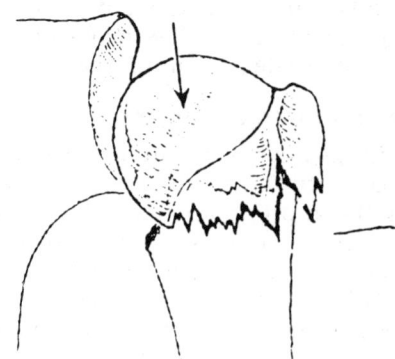

FIGURE 38–65. Prolonged immobilization of a surgical neck fracture of the humerus frequently causes inferior subluxation of the humeral head as a result of atrophy of the supraspinatus muscle. This can be combated by early range-of-motion exercises.

adies, the patient with a humeral neck fracture should be treated symptomatically and the radiograph ignored. These are usually stable injuries and invariably heal despite some shoulder motion. As soon as the patient's acute pain symptoms subside, usually within 3 to 7 days, he or she can begin a range-of-motion program, starting with circumduction. The program can be advanced over subsequent weeks to include external rotation and abduction exercises as illustrated in Figure 38–21.

This emphasis on restoring joint motion, however, depends on an adequate initial assessment that the articulation is stable. That is, one must be sure that the patient does not have a dislocation as well as a fracture.

A fracture that has caused joint instability mandates internal fixation prior to allowing the joint motion so necessary for articular healing. This is particularly true with articular fractures in the lower limb that alter weight-bearing mechanics of the joint.

Lower Limb Problems

Not all articular fractures involve weight-bearing portions of joints. Consequently, not all interarticular fractures invariably are followed by traumatic arthritis. The most common fracture of the acetabulum, the fracture of the central portion (Fig. 38–66A), rarely produces traumatic arthritis. However, fractures involving the superior weight-bearing portion of the acetabulum are very likely to impair hip function (Fig. 38–66B).

Although fractures of the lateral tibial plateau may be comminuted, incomplete reduction can be accepted without risking residual arthritis (Fig. 38–67A). This is because a good portion of weight is borne in the lateral compartment of the knee by the lateral meniscus rather than the fractured articular surface. In contrast, fractures of the medial tibial condyle carry a high risk of joint instability and subsequent arthritis when treated closed. Internal fixation with relatively simple percutaneous pins stabilizes these joint fractures and permits early restoration of motion (Fig. 38–67B).

Fractures of the ankle are among the most problematic for the family physician to treat. These have been indicated as a common cause of medical liability settlements among nonorthopedists who treat fractures. Ankle fractures may seem relatively innocuous, but slight displacement of the talus and the ankle mortise can lead to an unsatisfactory result (Fig. 38–68). Internal fixation and early mobilization of the ankle joint provides the most satisfactory answer to the bimalleolar fracture, which commonly causes ankle instability.

Management of Traumatic Arthritis

Management by the Family Physician. The optimum treatment of traumatic arthritis is preventive. Management of fractures about joints must in-

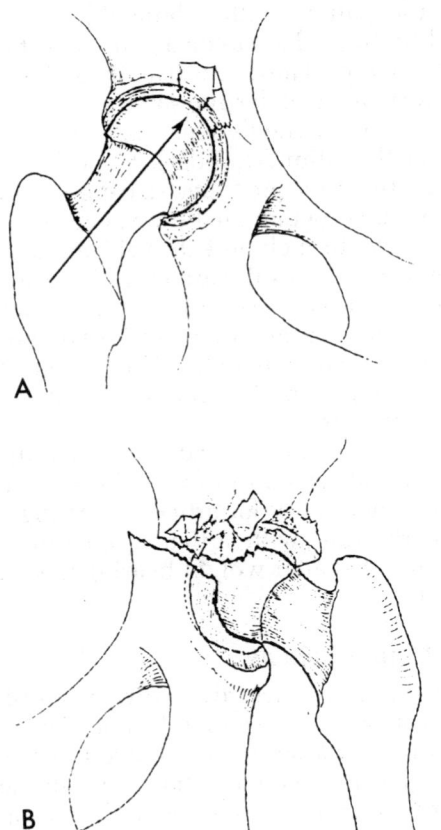

FIGURE 38–66. *A,* The most common acetabular fracture involves the central non–weight-bearing portion and can be treated symptomatically unless there is central protrusion. *B,* An acetabular fracture involving the weight-bearing portion commonly leads to traumatic arthritis.

corporate methods of relieving pain immediately by joint aspiration and should be directed at restoring joint motion promptly by either operative or nonoperative techniques.

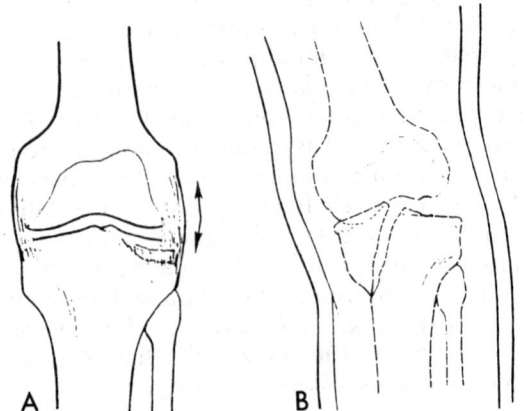

FIGURE 38–67. *A,* Lateral tibial condylar fractures do not require anatomic reduction because a good deal of the weight in the lateral portion is carried by the lateral meniscus. *B,* Medial tibial condylar fractures require anatomic reduction if progressive varus deformity and traumatic arthritis are to be avoided.

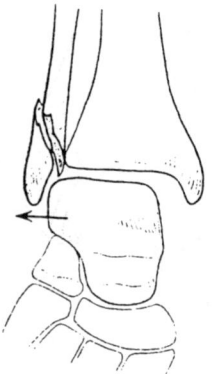

FIGURE 38–68. Ankle fractures are sometimes treacherous because the degree of lateral displacement may not be evident without careful assessment of radiographs. Generally, internal fixation is necessary to allow early mobilization of the ankle joint.

Osteoarthritis

This is by far the most common form of arthritis treated by either family physicians or orthopedists. The disease results from a combination of biochemical and biomechanical breakdown of articular cartilage, frequently superimposed on collapse of the subchondral joint support. Wear and tear is not the only factor producing osteoarthritis. Many patients also have genetically governed susceptibility to joint breakdown, as manifested by Heberden's nodes, the pathognomonic finding in osteoarthritis.

The symptoms from this disease may range from painless stiffening or crepitance of the joint to a constant joint ache that severely handicaps the patient. The degree of radiographic change does not necessarily correlate with the severity of pain symptoms. McCarty (1979) and others have pointed out that only 30 per cent of patients with radiographic evidence of osteoarthritis actually are symptomatic. Analogous to gout, it is the inflammatory response within the joint that, by releasing prostaglandins and inflammatory lysozymes, causes much of the pain. The major objective in treating the osteoarthritic patient is to relieve pain.

Management of Osteoarthritis

The family physician can aid his or her patients with osteoarthritis quite effectively by selecting and timing the appropriate medical, physical, and surgical therapies. He or she should be cognizant of the indications and contraindications for various modalities of treatment, including surgery, and should keep in mind that total joint replacement is not the only, nor always the most effective, solution to arthritic pain symptoms.

MANAGEMENT BY THE FAMILY PHYSICIAN. A basic approach to providing pain relief in most patients with osteoarthritis is to decrease the inflammatory intra-articular response. This may merely

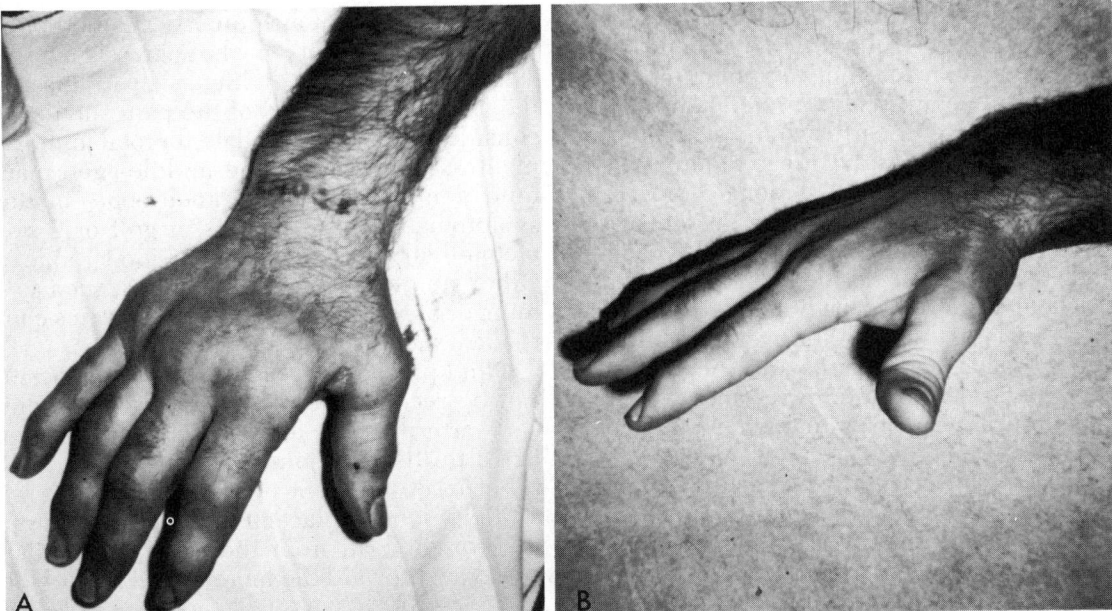

FIGURE 38–69. *A,* This patient had considerable pain and stiffening in the small metacarpophalangeal joints of his hand as a result of early synovitis. The synovitis was treated with a series of three intra-articular injections into all of the joints using cortisone preparations as described in the text. *B,* Synovitis cleared rapidly after a series of three cortisone injections, and mobility returned to near normal.

require rest and aspirin, the first line of treatment. Simmons and Chrisman (1965) have shown the beneficial effect of sodium salicylate in inhibiting cartilage degradation and promoting reconstitution of injured articular surfaces.

Nonsteroidal anti-inflammatory medication such as indomethacin and ibuprofen are well known to the family physician as the second line of defense against disabling joint pain. Steroidal treatment has a definite place as well in managing osteoarthritis. Intra-articular injections of triamcinolone or similar steroidal preparations, when used judiciously, can provide significant relief of arthritic pain. This joint injection technique should be used intermittently; a weight-bearing joint should not be injected more than three times a year. Intra-articular cortisone injections are most effective in non–weight-bearing joints such as the thumb metacarpal or carpometacarpal joints, the elbow, or the shoulder (Fig. 38–69).

Physical modalities are frequently overlooked in the medical management of early symptomatic arthritis. Use of walking aids at night or on weekends can diminish joint loading effectively. This is particularly ideal for relief of acute arthritic flare-ups.

Orthoses or braces offer another mechanical means for unloading painful weight-bearing joints. The patellar tendon–bearing orthosis mentioned in the treatment of diabetic joint disease (see Fig. 38–62) has been particularly helpful for unloading symptomatic arthritic ankles. Knee braces also may be useful, particularly for the patient whose pain results from ligamentous stretching of the unstable knee.

One of the most common areas where bracing can relieve arthritic pain symptoms is in the spine. Older patients whose spine has become unstable because of arthritic degeneration of the intravertebral and facet joints frequently experience symptoms of spinal claudication. This is because the back hurts with any prolonged standing or walking as a result of dural impingement by the narrowed lumbar spine. Frequently, these patients obtain relief only by lying down with the lumbar spine flexed. This contrasts with claudication symptoms from ischemia, which can be relieved by sitting or standing still. Lumbar arthritic symptoms can frequently be alleviated by flexion jackets made of light plastic material. These jackets maintain lumbar flexion and allow the patient to walk comfortably without impingement on the sensitive dura.

Exercise can be of definite therapeutic benefit if done to relieve joint contracture. For example, the patient who walks with the knee flexed because of a 15-degree flexion contracture at least doubles the load he or she must carry on the knee. This is because the muscles are constantly firing and loading the joint to prevent the knee from buckling. Effective therapy of an arthritic knee must work to eliminate such flexion contractures. The patient should be advised not to sleep with a pillow under the knee, because this only adds to the flexion deformity. When sitting, the patient should place the affected leg out on another chair with the knee maximally extended. He or she can then use gravity to obtain further extension and also actively contract the quadriceps in the extended position to stretch the posterior capsule and hamstrings.

In the hip, a common deformity is adduction and flexion. Such contractures concentrate loading on a narrow area of articular cartilage and accelerate joint breakdown. Exercises that range the hip passively using a skateboard or a stationary bicycle help distribute loading across the articular surfaces. Swimming is another excellent form of exercise therapy that can be prescribed for the arthritic patient without fear of overloading the diseased joints. By employing these well-proven therapies, the family physician can help the arthritic patient maximize the use of his or her own joint systems for many months or years prior to the need for any surgical treatment.

INDICATIONS FOR RECONSTRUCTIVE JOINT SURGERY. The ultimate mechanical solution to the arthritic problem is total joint replacement. Although this has proved to be a very useful technique, it is only a halfway solution to the problem of arthritis. The main indication is to relieve pain unresponsive to other therapies. Artificial joints, like any mechanical device, carry a risk of mechanical failure. The present estimate is that at least 20 per cent of total hip replacements can be expected to produce symptoms from loosening within 5 years after operation. Newer methods and techniques are being developed to diminish this complication rate, but mechanical failure will be intrinsic to any mechanical approach.

Joint replacements offer dramatic relief in many patients, so they tend to be recommended too freely. A total joint arthroplasty should not be recommended for a person who is grossly overweight. The active young individual who is apt to abuse the joint once relieved of the pain should also be considered a poor candidate for total joint replacement. Neither should the middle-aged man with mild genu varum and a knee ache, moderately symptomatic after 18 holes of golf or 2 hours of racquetball, be considered for joint replacement. Other simple treatment modalities, such as swimming or bicycle riding, should be given a complete trial by such patients.

Other procedures, such as high tibial osteotomy, can be recommended for the active patient with early arthritic symptoms. When employed for limited arthritis of the joint, this can provide good pain relief in 80 per cent or more of patients without artificial joint replacement. The technique shifts the weight load from the diseased medial joint space over toward the more lateral side of the joint (Fig. 38–70).

A previous history of joint infection is no longer considered an absolute contraindication to arthroplasty. A history of gram-negative sepsis should signal caution. Careful assessment of the joint for active infection based on sedimentation rate, bone scanning, and joint biopsy or aspiration can determine whether a total joint arthroplasty is likely to become infected. New techniques, such as biologic fixation and those incorporating an antibiotic into the cement, can permit reconstructive arthroplasty despite a previous but inactive joint infection.

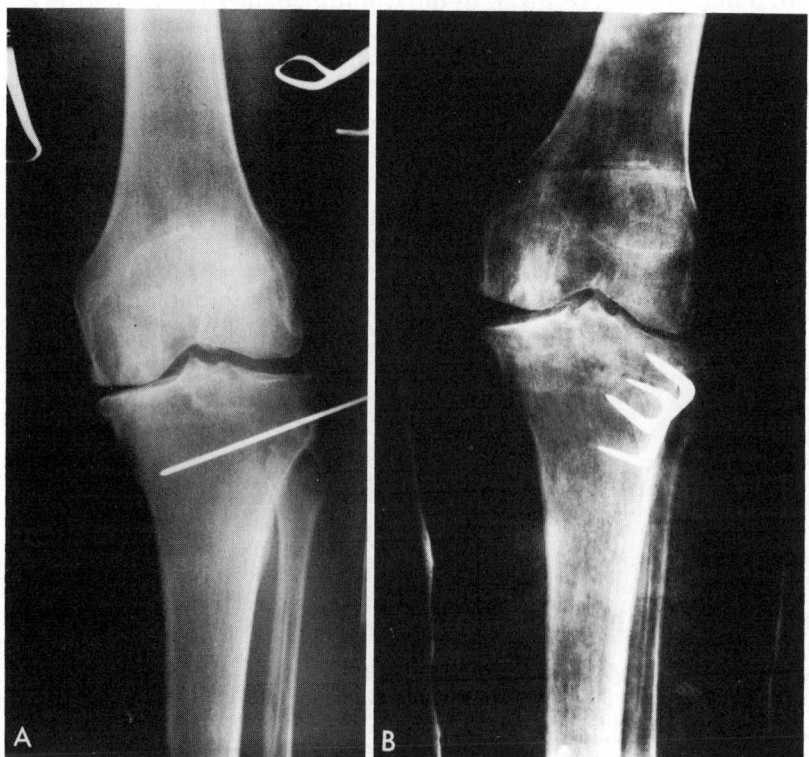

FIGURE 38–70. *A,* This is an intraoperative radiograph showing typical arthritic changes in the medial joint space but relative preservation of the lateral joint space of the knee. *B,* The high tibial osteotomy corrected the weight-bearing alignment and shifted the load of the knee toward the lateral side of the joint.

TABLE 38–3. RHEUMATOID ARTHRITIS DIAGNOSTIC CRITERIA*

1. Morning stiffness
2. Pain on motion or tenderness in at least one joint
3. Swelling (soft tissue thickening of fluid, not bony overgrowth alone) in at least one joint
4. Swelling of at least one other joint
5. Symmetrical joint swelling with simultaneous involvement of the same joint on both sides of the body; terminal phalangeal joint involvement will not satisfy the criterion
6. Subcutaneous nodules over bony prominences, on extensor surfaces, or in juxta-articular regions
7. Roentgenographic changes typical of rheumatoid arthritis (which must include at least bony decalcification localized to or greatest around the involved joints and not just degenerative changes)
8. Positive agglutination (anti-gammaglobulin) test
9. Poor mucin precipitate from synovial fluid (with shreds and cloudy solution)
10. Characteristic histologic changes in synovial membrane
11. Characteristic histologic changes in nodules

Categories	Number of Criteria Required	Minimum Duration of Continuous Symptoms
Classic	7 of 11	Six weeks (nos. 1–5)
Definite	5 of 11	Six weeks (nos. 1–5)
Probable	3 of 11	Six weeks (one of nos. 1–5)

* American Rheumatism Association 1958 revision.

Rheumatoid Arthritis

Rheumatoid arthritis begins in the joint's synovium. Its ultimate effect is to destroy the joint surfaces and the supporting ligaments via actively proliferating synovitis.

Diagnostic criteria for rheumatoid arthritis are constantly being re-evaluated. Not all patients who meet the American Rheumatism Association's criteria for definite rheumatoid arthritis (Table 38–3) actually prove to have the disease. The diagnosis does not hinge on merely one or two findings, particularly laboratory findings. The prevalence of rheumatoid arthritis in adults under 35 years is less than 0.3 per cent. This figure increases exponentially in subsequent decades and exceeds 10 per cent in patients over 65 years of age. Rheumatoid arthritis is infrequent in young adult males, as compared with other inflammatory arthritides, particularly ankylosing spondylitis.

The course of the disease is always variable and difficult to predict at its onset. A positive serum rheumatoid factor and erosive bone changes on radiographs imply poor prognosis. As a general rule, one third of patients will have some functional limitation and one third will become severely handicapped (see Tables 38–4 and 38–5). These statistics may not be entirely comforting to the patient, but they indicate that a majority of patients with rheumatoid arthritis do not, in fact, become severely crippled. The possibility of severe crippling should not be passed over lightly. Chronic rheuma-

TABLE 38–4. AMERICAN RHEUMATISM ASSOCIATION FUNCTIONAL CLASSES

Class	Function
I	Complete ability to carry on all usual duties without handicaps
II	Adequate for normal activities despite handicap of discomfort or limited motion at one or more joints
III	Limited only to little or none of duties of usual occupation or self-care
IV	Incapacitated, largely or wholly bedridden or confined to wheelchair; little or no self-care

toid arthritis is a very disabling and debilitating disease and needs constant care.

MANAGEMENT BY THE FAMILY PHYSICIAN. The aims of rheumatoid arthritis treatment are to (1) educate the patient and his or her family, (2) relieve pain, (3) suppress inflammation, and (4) prevent or correct deformities promptly. Treatment should be problem oriented, and the physician should know about the patient, the past treatment and response to therapy, and any complications or coexisting disease, including allergies, gastrointestinal diseases, renal disease, hepatic diseases, infection, and altered immunities.

The following is a brief outline of therapy based particularly on the American Rheumatism Association's functional classes (Table 38–4) and anatomic stages of disease (Table 38–5). These serve as helpful comparative tools for the family practitioner to select therapy and to evaluate response.

TABLE 38–5. AMERICAN RHEUMATISM ASSOCIATION ANATOMIC STAGES

Stage I: Early
*1. No destructive changes roentgenologically
2. Roentgenologic evidence of osteoporosis may be present

Stage II: Moderate
*1. Roentgenologic evidence of osteoporosis, with or without slight bone destruction; slight cartilage destruction may be present
*2. No joint deformities, although limitation of joint mobility may be present
3. Adjacent muscle atrophy
4. Extra-articular soft tissue lesions, such as nodules and tenovaginitis, may be present

Stage III: Severe
*1. Roentgenologic evidence of cartilage and bone destruction, in addition to osteoporosis
*2. Joint deformity, such as subluxation, ulnar deviation, or hyperextension, without fibrous or bony ankylosis
3. Extensive muscle atrophy
4. Extra-articular soft tissue lesions, such as nodules and tenovaginitis, may be present

Stage IV: Terminal
*1. Fibrous or bony ankylosis
2. Criteria of Stage III

* The criteria prefaced by an asterisk are those that must be present to permit classification of a patient in any particular stage or grade.

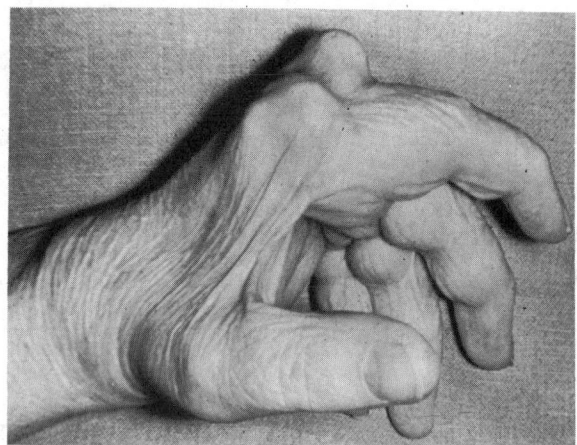

FIGURE 38–71. Long-standing rheumatoid arthritis destroys the metacarpophalangeal joints and produces volar subluxation of these joints and stiffening of the proximal interphalangeal joints. Of major concern is progressive deformity of the thumb, which may become superimposed on the severe finger deformities.

Stage I, Class I Patients. The single most important element in the management of rheumatoid arthritis is patient education. The patient must be reminded that symptoms do remit and fluctuate from day to day. The physician should help with the patient's psychological adjustment. He or she should advise reasonable rest and salicylates to control pain and encourage moderate, simple exercise therapy for these patients. The hands and feet must be observed carefully for progressive deformities.

Rheumatoid arthritis is primarily a disease of the small joints of the hands and feet. Intrinsic muscle tightness in the hands produces an unbalanced pull, which eventually dislocates the metacarpophalangeal (MCP) joints and subsequently stiffens the proximal interphalangeal (IP) joints (Fig. 38–71). Tightness of the intrinsic muscles that are the flexors of the MCP joints and extensors of the IP joints is tested by reversing the position of these joints. That is, with the MCP joint extended in a normal finger, the patient should still have the ability to flex the distal IP joint. If the patient's intrinsic muscles are tight, however, the stretching of the tendons of the MCP joint prevents any flexion of the distal IP joint.

A useful exercise when intrinsic muscle tightness first becomes evident is to have the patient hold a block in the hand to keep the MCP joints extended. By trying to grip around the block, the patient stretches out the tight intrinsics by active function of the extrinsic flexors, particularly the profundi, which tend not to be involved as severely as the intrinsic muscles.

The feet of a rheumatoid arthritis patient always must be carefully evaluated, just as for a diabetic patient. Simple methods such as metatarsal bars and appropriately placed pads in shoes can afford the rheumatoid arthritis patient considerable relief from common foot symptoms. Surgical correction should be recommended promptly for symptomatic bunions, clawfoot, or arthritis of the hindfoot. Concern for the large joints of the body should not be allowed to overshadow real problems in the small joints.

Stage II, Class II Patients. These patients require the same basic regimen of therapy and anti-inflammatory drugs as do patients in the early stage and class. However, as their disease progresses, they may require more potent medications. There are several classes of medications that can be used, including the antimalarial drugs, gold compounds, penicillamine, and immunosuppressive agents such as methotrexate, azathioprine, and others. These medications have many side effects and require close monitoring. It might be wise for the family physician to consult with a rheumatologist in the use of these medications.

Stage III, Class III Patients. These patients demand continued vigorous therapy. Steroids particularly can be of value here, not so much when given systemically but when injected intra-articularly (see Fig. 38–69). These intra-articular injections should be given over a month's time at biweekly intervals. Each inflamed joint should be injected separately with a small 25-gauge needle. In essence, this provides a chemical synovectomy, which is particularly valuable in the small joints of the hand.

If synovitis persists and remains unresponsive to chemical synovectomy and to systemic medical treatment for more than 6 months, surgical synovectomy should be advised. Stage III and Stage IV disease particularly demand contributions by the orthopedic surgeon in cooperation with the family physician or rheumatologist before the patient advances unnecessarily to a functional Class IV. Most family physicians are quite familiar with the frequently dramatic pain relief following total hip replacement in the rheumatoid arthritis patient. Many are unaware of or inattentive to problems in the small joints, particularly the hand and foot, that are equally amenable to appropriate treatment.

Some deformities in particular may be allowed to pass without adequate correction. The patient then progresses rapidly to a state at which he or she must hold cups or glasses with both hands in order to drink (Fig. 38–71). Correction of the deformities in the thumb joints, although seemingly a minor undertaking to offer patients, can provide significant functional improvement. Deformities of the thumb rank with foot problems as causes of persistent symptoms that can be readily alleviated by prompt attention.

A final area that tends to be undertreated or under-recognized in the rheumatoid arthritis patient is the cervical spine. This may frequently become of life-threatening significance. Synovitis attacks ligaments in the first and second cervical

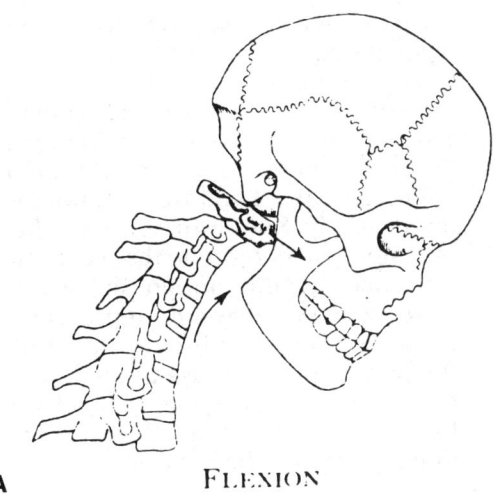

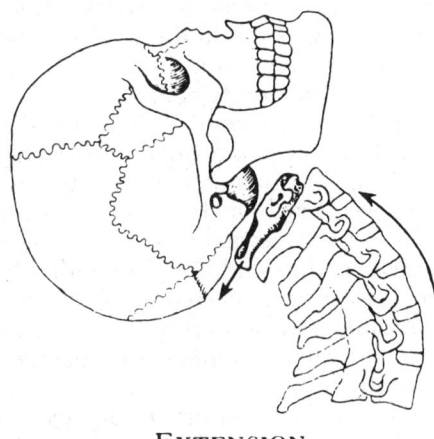

A   FLEXION   EXTENSION

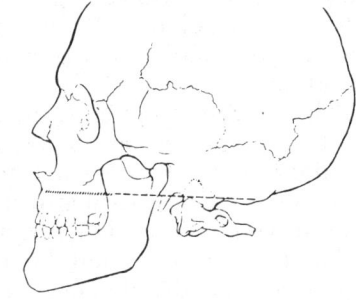

B

FIGURE 38–72. *A*, Rheumatoid arthritis commonly causes anteroposterior C1-2 instability in the chronic patient. This should be evaluated by flexion-extension radiographs prior to endotracheal intubation. *B*, A less frequent complication is upward migration of the odontoid through the base of the skull, producing cranial nerve symptoms.

vertebrae (Fig. 38–72). About 5 per cent of these patients actually go on to cord injury and myelopathy as a result of the cervical spine instability. This possibility must be kept in mind when a rheumatoid arthritis patient suddenly complains of weakness in the arms or legs. Generalized weakness is usually due to neurologic complications rather than to worsening of the rheumatoid process. Any rheumatoid arthritis patient who is to undergo a surgical procedure must be carefully evaluated by flexion-extension radiography. We were consulted on two patients in whom the unfortunate complication of quadriparesis could have been avoided if the rheumatoid disease of the cervical spine had been recognized and the cervical instability anticipated before induction of anesthesia.

Rheumatoid arthritis is a long-term problem that can be effectively managed by the family physician, particularly one who perceives the progressive functional and anatomic nature of the disease, is aware of appropriate therapies for each stage, and appreciates indications as well as contraindications for surgical management.

Septic Arthritis

In the preantibiotic era in the 1930s and 1940s, mortality from acute osteomyelitis and joint infections frequently exceeded 30 per cent. No development in orthopedics has produced more significant benefit to patients than has the effective treatment of septic arthritis and osteomyelitis. Many senior physicians can well remember orthopedic wards filled with patients suffering both acute and chronic symptoms of bone and joint infections.

Septic arthritis and associated osteomyelitis as seen today usually develop from direct penetration of the joint, from an open fracture; or by spread from contiguous infection, such as a diabetic foot or a pressure sore in a paralyzed patient. The source of a septic joint resulting from hematogenous spread seen most commonly today is gonococcal infection.

It is essential that the family physician appreciate these different etiologies of septic arthritis. Some infections, such as those produced by direct penetration of the joint or associated with an open fracture or spread from a contiguous infection, require prompt surgical drainage. Others, particularly those produced by hematogenous spread as from gonococcal infection, do not usually require surgical drainage.

Gonococcal Arthritis and Other Joint Infections Not Requiring Surgical Drainage

The gonococcus appears to have an unusually strong affinity for synovial tissue when gonococcemia occurs. Most patients are in the second or third decades, but newborn infants as well as elderly patients have been infected. The joint infection usually occurs 1 to 2 weeks after the urethritis, but as long as the individual is carrying the gonococcus in the genitourinary tract or rectal mucosa, spread to the joints is possible.

With gonococcemia, characteristic skin lesions develop. These are small hemorrhage-like spots 5 to 6 mm in diameter with 1 to 2 mm of central necrosis. Erythematous inflammation around tendon sheaths, particularly in the heel, also is characteristic of the condition. The individual with gonococcal arthritis usually presents with severe discomfort and a good deal more local pain to touch than do other patients with inflamed joints, except those with gout.

The major differential diagnoses when there is multiple joint involvement include acute rheumatic fever, infectious hepatitis B, and systemic lupus. In male patients, Reiter's syndrome must also be considered. Monoarticular involvement brings gout and pseudogout into the differential conditions.

The diagnosis depends on blood or joint fluid cultures of gonococcus. A positive culture from the genitourinary tract does not necessarily make the diagnosis of gonococcal arthritis in the absence of a positive blood or joint culture. The organism is relatively fastidious, and the joint fluid should be cultured immediately after aspiration. Most synovial fluid cell counts with gonococcal arthritis are over 50,000/mm^3. However, the cell count on the synovial fluid must be done properly and without glacial acetic acid, which, when mixed with the hyaluronidase of synovial fluid, will precipitate out the cells.

When joint fluid studies are unrevealing, the characteristic skin lesions of gonococcemia may be quite helpful for diagnosis, although these are also seen in infections caused by *Haemophilus influenzae* and *Neisseria meningitidis*, and other septicemias.

MANAGEMENT BY THE FAMILY PHYSICIAN. Gonococcal arthritis should be a prime diagnostic suspect in any acutely inflamed, painful joint. After appropriate diagnostic studies, including blood cultures and cultures of synovial fluid and any skin lesions, treatment is begun with cefotaxime, 25 to 50 mg/kg intravenously every 8 to 12 hours for 10 to 14 days. Increasing resistance to penicillin has been reported; however, it may be used as an alternative if sensitivity tests demonstrate coverage by penicillin. Treatment should not be delayed for results of the culture, however, because patients with gonococcal infections may not demonstrate a positive culture. Response to antibiotic therapy generally leads to relatively prompt relief of pain and inflammation. Surgical drainage of gonococcal arthritis is almost always unnecessary.

Other types of septic joints produced by hematogenous spread from organisms such as staphylococcus or streptococcus are also treated best by intravenous antibiotics when the diagnosis has been made promptly. The antibiotics should be administered in high doses and by the intravenous route to ensure adequate blood and synovial fluid levels. Surgical drainage is not ordinarily necessary for the usual septic knee—that in a child—that has been recognized and treated promptly and monitored closely. Knee aspiration should be performed repeatedly to determine the response to therapy as indicated by diminution in synovial fluid cell count. The synovial fluid represents a dialysate of blood, and, in most instances, antibiotic levels in the joint approach those in the blood. However, if the septic joint does not respond within 48 hours to adequate parenteral therapy, prompt surgical drainage should be advised.

Joint Infections Requiring Surgical Drainage

Although certain joint infections, such as gonococcal arthritis and staphylococcus and streptococcus infections in the knee, can be treated successfully by high-dose parenteral antibiotics, other infections, owing to their notorious effect on joints, demand surgical drainage.

Septic arthritis of the hip is one such joint infection for which prompt surgical drainage is essential (Fig. 38–73). Pus accumulating in the hip joint space rapidly displaces and then dislocates the young infant's hip. The common result is permanent deformity after the childhood infection resolves.

Diagnosis of the septic hip joint should be made first by aspirating pus from the hip. When a positive hip aspirate is obtained, surgical drainage should be carried out as soon as the patient can

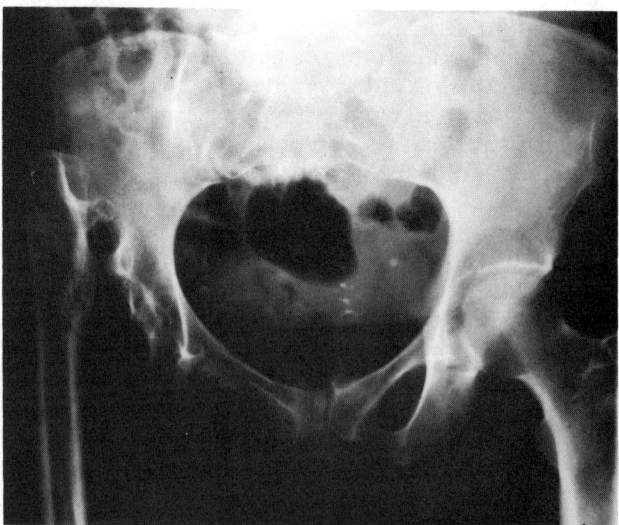

FIGURE 38–73. The residual effect of a septic joint in infancy resulted in this severely destroyed hip joint in the adult. (Courtesy of Dr. Walter W. Huurman, Department of Orthopaedic Surgery, University of Nebraska Medical Center, Omaha, Nebraska.)

tolerate anesthetic. The capsule should be opened widely for adequate decompression and the hip maintained in an extended position until the infection has been controlled.

Other infected joints that mandate prompt surgical drainage include those with a pre-existing chronic synovitis that prevents adequate antibiotic penetration. This is particularly true in the rheumatoid arthritis patient or the patient with chronic arthritis of the joint. Although virtually all antibiotics penetrate synovial membranes and reach therapeutic levels in joints equivalent to blood levels, if a tense, undrained effusion limits antibiotic access, the joint then becomes essentially a walled-off abscess rather than a true joint. This should be treated like an abscess anywhere in the body.

Certain gram-negative infections, such as those seen in drug addicts or in patients with poor circulation as a result of sicklemia, require open drainage more promptly than do the more usual gram-positive infections.

Joints that become infected postoperatively or even many years after arthroplasty require prompt drainage if the artificial joint is to be salvaged. Hematogenous spread from the genitourinary tract to a previously satisfactorily functioning joint has occurred 2 or more years postoperatively in our observation. Consequently, prophylactic antibiotics should be administered during any manipulative procedure, such as a tooth extraction or cystoscopy, that might cause bacterial septicemia and risk hematogenous infection of the prosthetic joint.

BACK PAIN

Back pain is responsible for vast numbers of patient visits, lost time, a large number of operations, and great amounts of litigation. About 120,000 discectomies are done per year, and many of these could be prevented by a knowledgeable primary care physician. Lower back pain can be caused by disorders of any of the structures making up the spinal column complex as well as problems remote to the spine (see Table 38–6).

The spinal column is a chain of vertebrae stacked on one another and held together by a ligamentous and muscular complex. There are essentially 24 vertebrae plus the sacrum and coccyx of fused elements, with interposed discs, two facet joints with interposed ligaments, and a neural foramen between the vertebrae.

A fairly large percentage of back pain results from degenerative disc disease, particularly at the L4-5–S1 levels. Only a small percentage is noted above this level. Thus, when making a diagnosis of disc pain at higher levels, one must look hard for other causes, such as malignancy, disc space infection, or trauma. The cervical and lumbar segments of the spine are highly mobile and hence prone to disc herniation at the C7, T1, and L4-5–S1

TABLE 38–6. DIFFERENTIAL ETIOLOGIC FACTORS IN BACK PAIN

1. Tumors
   a. Benign (such as meningiomas, neuromas, osteoid osteomas, Paget's disease)
   b. Malignant—primary bone or neural tumors and metastases
2. Trauma
   a. Acute sprain or strain
   b. Chronic sprain or strain
   c. Fractures
   d. Subluxated facet (facet syndrome)
   e. Spondylolisthesis with strain
3. Toxicities from heavy metals
4. Congenital asymmetries of facets or transitional vertebrae
5. Metabolic disorders—osteoporosis or osteomalacia
6. Inflammatory arthritis—rheumatoid and Marie-Strümpell's disease
7. Infections, acute and chronic
8. Degenerative disc or facet disease
9. Mechanical disturbance
   a. Poor muscle tone
   b. Poor posture
   c. Unstable vertebrae
   d. Scoliosis (severe)
10. Extrinsic disease such as aortic aneurysm, uterine fibroids, prostate disease, hip disease
11. Psychological, to include hysteria, malingering, and acute remunerative spinal pain (Green-Poultice disease)

levels, where flexion-extension loads are concentrated.

Most vertical (up and down) loading is absorbed by the annulus fibrosis, the casing of the disc (Fig. 38–74). When this structure is torn, the degenerated content of the nucleus pulposus may be allowed to impinge on sensitive adjacent structures. This will result in back pain without radiation down the legs.

Rupture of the annulus may also allow the central pulpy material to work out and impinge on the nerve structures located lateral to the disc. The result is a neurogenic pain or *sciatica* radiating down the leg. (This should be distinguished from back pain produced by the central protrusion of the disc). The roots usually involved in sciatica are those that exit below the level of the disc herniation—that is, the L5 root with L4-5 disc herniation and the S1 root with the L5-S1 herniation (Fig. 38–75).

The mechanism of disc rupture, either from a tear of the annulus or from nuclear displacement, is quite consistently a twist with the lumbar spine flexed. This may result as the patient simply bends forward over the sink to brush his or her teeth. Flexion makes the lumbar spine vulnerable because it produces lumbar kyphosis with a subsequent gap in the posterior aspect of the intervertebral joint (Fig. 38–76A). The body weight in the flexed position forces the intervertebral joint contents posteriorly. This contrasts with the normal position of lumbar lordosis, which narrows down

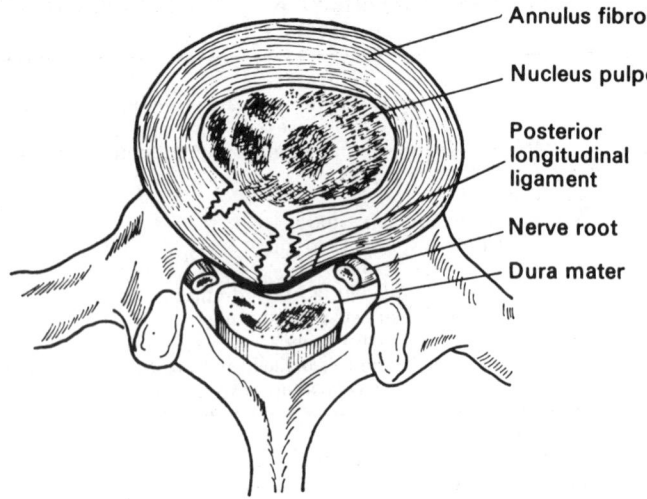

FIGURE 38–74. The disc structure includes an outer fibrocartilaginous annulus fibrosus and an inner, more fluid nucleus pulposus. Either of these structures may rupture and produce either lumbago or sciatica. (From Cyriax J: Orthopaedic Medicine, Vol. 1. London, Cassell, Ltd., 1978, with permission.)

the posterior aspect of the disc space (Fig. 38–76*B*).

Pain is produced by pressure on the sensitive dural sleeve that surrounds the root for about 2 cm as it exits the canal. A peripheral nerve itself is quite insensitive to pressure, as anyone who has sat on a hard theater seat for a few hours knows. Compression of the peripheral nerve characteristically produces paresthesias, or "pins and needles," distal to compression.

Any stretching of an entrapped dural sleeve with peripheral disc herniation produces a sharp pain radiating down the leg, frequently to the foot or ankle. In the absence of such positive nerve stretch symptoms, the diagnosis of disc herniation is not likely.

The other type of dural pain, *lumbago*, is associated with a central disc herniation, which also causes pain by stretching the dura. This dural pain may not follow any consistent pattern of reference, in contrast with that associated with peripheral dural and nerve root entrapment. Pain from central entrapment of the dura can be referred anywhere in the body between the waist and the feet. These

sites include the anterior abdominal wall, where the pain can be mistaken for appendicitis or an ovarian cyst. Entrapment may produce pain radiating into the groin, much like a hernia, or up the trunk toward the thorax, or down in the perineum toward the testicles or the coccyx. Pain from a central disc protrusion stretching the dura is a great mimic and always must be considered with the diagnosis of atypical abdominal, perineal, or thigh symptoms.

Diagnostic Considerations

History of Onset

Other causes of backache can range from "A" (ankylosing spondylitis) to "Z" (herpes zoster). Tumors, both primary and secondary, infections, and vascular disorders are particularly important differential diagnoses to be considered. To diagnose the common cause of back problems (i.e., disc disease) effectively and with reasonable assurance of not overlooking other causes, a systematic approach is absolutely essential. One must listen to and exam-

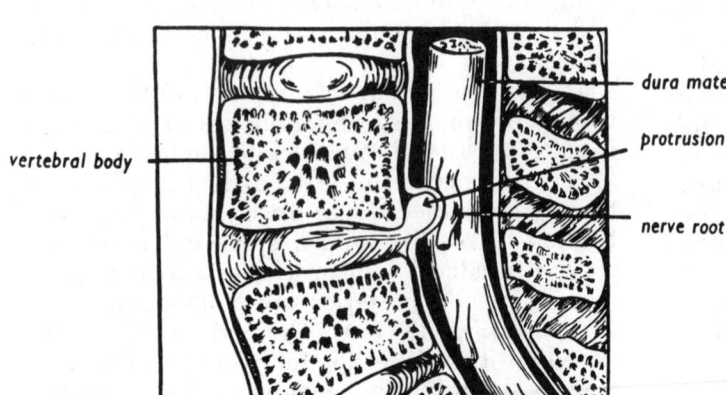

FIGURE 38–75. Herniation of the nucleus pulposus through the tear in the annulus produces a collar-stud abscess type of herniation that does not reduce spontaneously the way a moveable cartilaginous displacement reduces. (From Cyriax J: Orthopaedic Medicine, Vol. 1. London, Cassell, Ltd., 1978, with permission.)

FIGURE 38–76. *A,* Flexion of the lumbar spine produces most disc protrusions and herniations. When the spine is flexed forward in the standing position, the disc space is opened posteriorly and the cartilaginous portion of the annulus is pushed back toward the spinal canal. This may cause the lumbago associated with prolonged standing in this flexed position. *B,* With the lumbar spine in lordotic position, the disc space closes posteriorly. Treatment for lumbago should be directed, therefore, at increasing lumbar lordosis. (From Cyriax J: Orthopaedic Medicine, Vol. 1. London, Cassell, Ltd., 1978, with permission.)

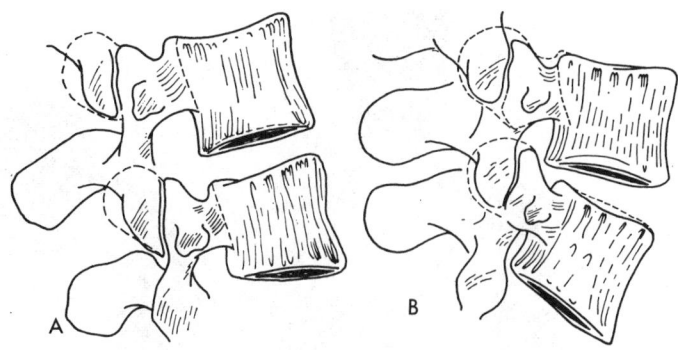

ine the backache patient as carefully as the patient with chest pain.

The patient's presenting history of symptoms may vary considerably because of the nature of the disc lesion, which can be either a cartilaginous loose body or a fluid gelatinous leak. The first type of lesion, the loose cartilage from the annulus, produces a sensation of the back suddenly going out. This usually occurs with a "click" as the patient moves into a flexed position and experiences a sharp pain. However, the annulus may also bulge out slowly and cause backache only after the patient stands for long periods in a slightly flexed position. Individuals who stand during work are quite familiar with this particular pain, which can generally be relieved by hyperextending the lumbar spine.

The second type of lesion, the slow leak of the nuclear material, alters the patient's history considerably. Leakage of the nucleus pulposus past the annulus results in a large mass that slowly pushes out through its narrow tract to impinge on the dura, much like a collar-stud abscess (see Fig. 38–75). For example, the patient may give a history of working in the garden, following which he or she experienced a slight backache. The next day, however, the patient could not get out of bed because of severe pain down the leg rather than in the back. This indicates that the nucleus pulposus has pushed through the torn annulus and is impinging on the dural sleeve around the nerve root rather than the central part of the canal.

The persistent location of this type of herniated pulpy nucleus is in the posterolateral aspect of the intervertebral joint, the weakest part of the system. This is also the location of the strong posterior longitudinal ligament, which is centrally located and turns the disc to one side or the other. The dural sleeve is most exposed to entrapment by the disc at this location. The universal symptom of pain down the leg is then from stretching of the dural sleeve. Such a peripheral herniation may not be sufficiently large initially to affect nerve conduction, and no neurologic deficit may be evident.

The motor and sensory components of the root emerge separately. Impingement from above impairs sensory conduction. As the disc material moves farther laterally on the peripheral nerve, it moves away from the sensitive dural sleeve and consequently the pain diminishes as the neurologic deficit worsens. Frequently the patient notices that, when footdrop occurs, the sharp pain down the leg goes away.

FACTORS AFFECTING HISTORY. Comprehending the variations and permutations in pathology is essential to appreciate the possible variations in the patient's history. A common symptom indicating dural irritation is pain on coughing or sneezing; however, this is not pathognomonic for disc disease. Neural tumors and occasionally sacroiliac joint disease may also be aggravated by sudden changes induced by coughing.

The position that brings on the back symptoms also reflects disc pathology. Disc pressures are greatest in the sitting position, followed by standing, with the least pressure in the lying position. The influence of poor sitting posture, resulting in lack of lumbar lordosis, also contributes to the possibility of pushing disc material posteriorly into the disc space.

Older patients suffering from disc disease associated with asymmetric narrowing of the spinal canal characteristically develop back symptoms during walking. This has been called "spinal claudication" but differs from the claudication of vascular origin in that the patient must lie down to relieve the pain. Vascular claudication, in contrast, is relieved by any kind of rest in any position. The back pain produced by walking in the elderly patient only remits when the sensitive dura is no longer stretched by the stenotic canal. The discogenic pain can be aggravated or even produced by sitting and is relieved only by the supine position.

Physical Assessment

Physical assessment of the patient with back pain begins with observation of the patient's entry, undressing, and movement to the exam table, as well as body habitus, posture, and obvious deformities. The combination of a good history before examination and then an examination as outlined here will usually give the diagnosis. Additional laboratory data and plain radiographs in anteropos-

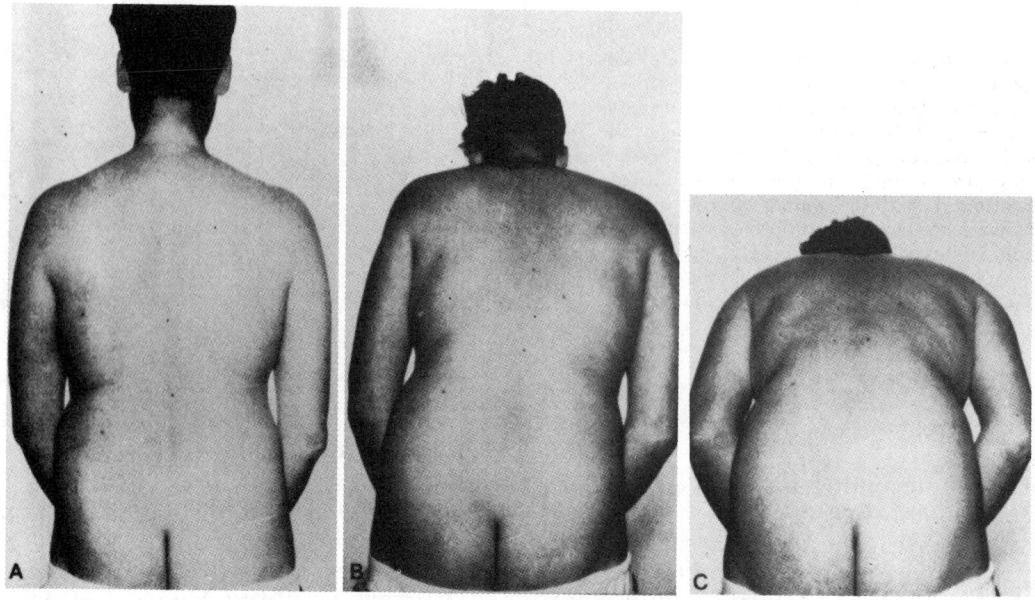

FIGURE 38–77. The sciatic list or a painful arc is characteristic of a herniated disc. The painful arc particularly is evident as a brief jog during certain ranges of flexion. (From Cyriax J: Orthopaedic Medicine, Vol. 1. London, Cassell, Ltd., 1978, with permission.)

terior, lateral, and both oblique planes will usually sort out the rest of the diagnostic problems.

The physical assessment proceeds with examination of leg length, ability to walk on heel and toe, pelvic obliquity, and any listing or flexion. The site of pain and extent of pain radiation, as well as active flexion, extension, rotation, and side-to-side motion, are also checked. With the patient supine, the true leg length (anterior superior spine to medial malleolus) is determined. All hip movements are checked and the straight-leg-raising test is done to see if hip disease is present. The abdomen is examined for tumor, aneurysm, gallbladder tenderness, and such. While the patient is sitting, a brief neurologic examination of motor power reflexes and sensory changes is done. Calf and thigh are measured for atrophy. Finally, a rectal examination is done on both sexes and a pelvic examination on female patients.

The architecture of the patient's spine is inspected carefully while he or she stands. A list to one side is quite typical of an acute disc herniation and indicates that the patient has tried to prevent nerve and dural stretch. A sciatic list is particularly pronounced in the younger individual with any L4-5 disc lesion (Fig. 38–77). Such a list may be confused with lumbar scoliosis. One should keep in mind that idiopathic scoliosis is never acutely painful by itself.

The best estimate of leg length discrepancy is made with the patient standing evenly on both legs while the physician palpates the top of the iliac crest. This allows direct visual and tactile estimation of the pelvic tilt. If one iliac crest is lower than the other, ¼-inch blocks are placed under the

shorter limb until the physician and the patient feel the crests to be even. This technique provides the most significant information regarding leg lengths (i.e., do both legs reach the ground without causing the pelvis to tilt?).

Muscle plantar flexion and dorsiflexion strength are tested by having the patient balance on the tiptoes and heels.

Spine motion is tested next, beginning with spine extension, then lateral bending, and finally, flexion, which is most likely to aggravate the patient's pain. One must keep in mind that the patient leans in the direction in which the nerve root is being pushed by the disc. A disc that protrudes lateral to the nerve root on the patient's right, for example, will cause him or her to lean to the left. A disc that protrudes central to the nerve root on the right side will cause the patient to lean toward the side of the lesion (i.e., the right side).

A frequently observed phenomenon during spine motion is a sudden deviation to one side as the patient reaches a half-flexed position. This is a significant manifestation of a painful arc whereby the patient experiences the dura's suddenly being stretched over a protruded disc in that particular part of the flexion arc (Fig. 38–77). The patient suddenly deviates laterally in this half-flexed position and may not even be aware that he or she does so.

This visible alteration in spine motion occurs as a loose disc fragment suddenly shifts position when the lumbar spine passes from a lordotic to a kyphotic shape. The painful arc, therefore, is pathognomonic of a disc lesion. The other differential conditions do not produce evidence so consistently

TABLE 38–7. LEVELS OF INNERVATION FOR MOTOR FUNCTION IN LOWER LIMBS

Nerve Level	Motor Function
L2,3	Hip flexion
L4,5	Hip extension
L3,4	Knee extension
L5-S1	Knee flexion
L4,5	Ankle dorsiflexion
S1-2	Ankle plantar flexion
L4	Foot inversion
L5-S1	Foot eversion

of a loose body shifting within the intervertebral joint and altering motion. Sensory loss is tested for by simply touching lightly and simultaneously over the patient's feet and inquiring about any differences in sensation to this slight touch stimulus. This sensory testing depends entirely on the patient's subjective response as well as his or her ability to answer accurately. Attempts at other sensory testing, such as pinprick or vibratory testing, equally rely on the patient's responses and are unnecessary for the usual disc evaluation.

After testing for patterns of cutaneous dysesthesia, the next step is careful assessment of motor function, beginning with the hip and working to the toes. A useful guide to the relationship of the nerve roots to muscle function is listed in Table 38–7. All these tests must be carried out against resistance and compared with the opposite limb function in order to detect subtle diminution of muscle strength. Careful motor testing, however, is a very useful diagnostic aid in localizing the site of the disc lesion.

A common finding may be a weakness of the big toe extensor. This should be checked carefully, because it may indicate an L4 or L5 nerve root lesion. If the peroneal everting muscles are also weak in conjunction with a weak toe extensor, the lesion would be at L5. If peroneal weakness is accompanied by a weak calf muscle, as seen on plantar flexion, an S1 nerve root lesion is involved. Weakness of the anterior tibial muscle most often indicates an L4 root lesion.

One should palpate for arterial pulses from the femoral artery downward. Claudication from iliac artery thrombosis can mimic sciatica and must always be ruled out, and not only in the elderly. We have seen several young patients referred with back and buttock symptoms produced by a Marfanlike disease of the aortoiliac arteries.

A diminished ankle jerk may be apparent only as a decreased push against the examiner's hand when the Achilles tendon is tapped. This most often indicates an S1 nerve root lesion.

The Babinski reflexes should be checked, particularly when the symptoms arise in the upper lumbar spine or are associated with diffuse muscle weakness or bilateral involvement. One should

keep in mind that a common cause of an upper motor neuron lesion in the elderly patient is a central protrusion of a disc in the cervical spine (see section on Neck Pain Cervical Disc Protrusion, later in this chapter).

To evaluate for sacroiliac pathology, the examiner presses down and out on the anterior superior iliac spine with the patient resting on the firm examining table. The patient should be advised that the object of this maneuver is not so much to produce pain localized to the sacroiliac joint as it is to determine whether this aggravates the lumbago or sciatica.

The final and most important test of the physical examination is the nerve stretch test. This is done with the patient's pelvis supported on the firm examining table. Begin with the uninvolved side first. Lift the limb with the knee extended in order to demonstrate the test. Then raise the limb on the symptomatic side, again with the knee extended. At the point at which the patient first notices pain beginning in the back, buttock, or leg, the leg is held steady. The patient then is asked to flex his or her neck. This should reproduce pain down the involved buttock and leg if there is disc impingement that prevents gliding of the dura.

This test is specific for dural entrapment and eliminates other diagnoses, such as sacroiliac strain or facet syndromes, that may confuse the clinical picture. Other than the dura, there is no structure between the head and the leg that could be stretched by this maneuver. This test is as specific for disc disease as Kernig's sign is for meningitis. One must always test carefully for this dural stretch sign, and suspect a diagnosis other than disc herniation if this test is negative. Children and older patients do sometimes prove exceptions to this rule.

The straight-leg-raising test may be positive without neurologic signs if there is only a small protrusion sufficient to interfere with dural gliding but not yet large enough to affect nerve conduction. Conversely, with severe sciatica, the disc may compress the nerve so firmly that it becomes insensitive. Muscle weakness and footdrop then develop. The ankle jerk is lost, and the skin in the foot becomes insensitive. The straight-leg-raising test will then become normal as the patient gains relief of the pain symptoms at the expense of neurologic impairment.

Other Diagnostic Tests: Radiographs, Myelography, and Scanning

The initial diagnosis of disc disease should be entirely a clinical one. Standard radiographs are of no value other than to rule out differential conditions such as fracture, spondylolisthesis, tumor, or occasionally a disc space infection.

Myelography or computerized tomographic (CT) or magnetic resonance scanning should not be done at the time of initial diagnostic evaluation.

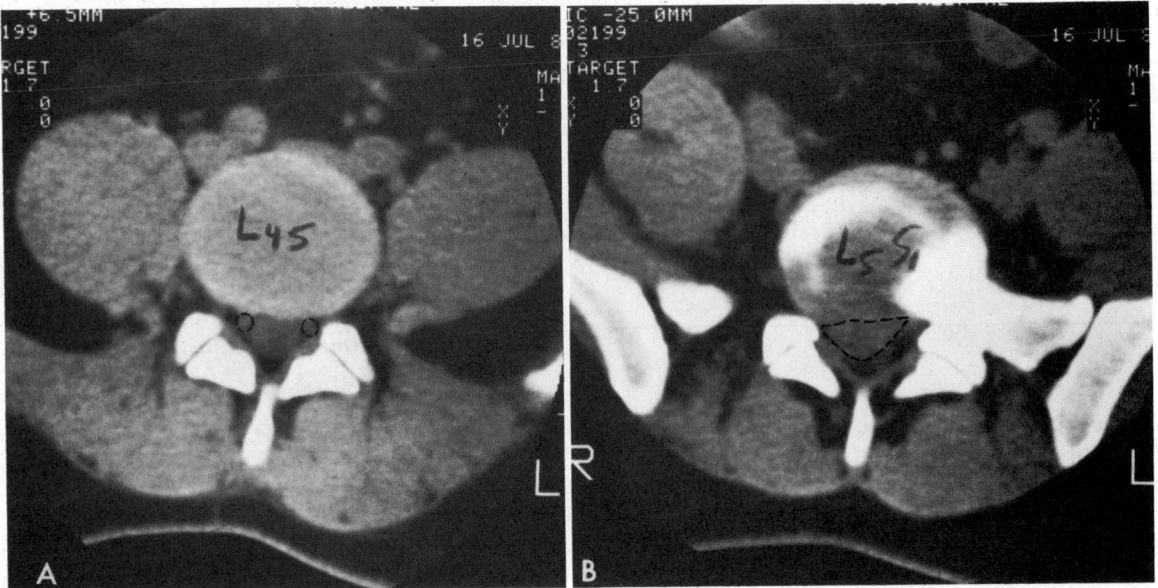

FIGURE 38–78. *A*, L4-5 interspace showing no compression and no bulging. *B*, Same patient showing L5-S1 interspace with central to right herniation of nucleus pulposus into the canal, displacing the right nerve root posteriorly and laterally, with some evidence of lateral movement of the dural contents to the left. At the time of surgical exploration, this patient was found to have a very large herniation onto the axilla of the S1 nerve on the right.

These are necessary only if the patient has not responded to the prescribed treatment as expected. Computerized tomographic scans are particularly useful in defining conditions such as arachnoidal adhesions, extradural infections, congenital anomalies, trauma to the spine, or degenerative joint or disc disease. Metastatic disease to the spine is also found earlier with the scanning technique.

Intraspinal tumors are best demonstrated by myelography, although the CT scan can assist in defining the exact extent of the lesion. Tethered cord, diastematomyelia, and meningocele are other conditions well defined by CT scan. The shape and the size of the canal are also determined best by this newer diagnostic method. In fact, assessment of back pain and back conditions has become the most widely accepted indication for body scanners since the introduction of this technology (Fig. 38–78). This technology should not be allowed to supplant careful physical assessment supplemented by diagnostic methods such as epidural and facet injections, which are discussed later in this section.

Management of Back Pain

MANAGEMENT BY THE FAMILY PHYSICIAN. The prime objective in treating disc disease is pain relief. Only infrequently is the neurologic deficit sufficient to be of concern. Occasional massive central defects that cause bilateral symptoms, weakness, and numbness, as well as bladder or bowel paralysis, are major exceptions. One must always be alert

to the infrequent patient with loss of sphincter control, which indicates a midline defect requiring immediate surgical decompression.

Controlled physical activity should be prescribed to the patient with back pain with or without mechanical obstruction. Recent studies show that there are positive benefits from shortened stays of bed rest and from increasing the patient's activity sooner. Bed rest should be limited to no more than 2 days, because longer periods result in the adverse effect of deconditioning. The patient should be instructed to lie with hips and knees in a flexed position to a moderate degree. As the discomfort diminishes, the patient should be encouraged to get out of bed and participate in aerobic activities such as walking, advancing this activity as tolerated. Periods of sitting should be discouraged.

Systemic analgesics and anti-inflammatory medications are often helpful in the treatment of low back pain. Narcotic analgesics should be used for brief periods until the specific therapy-directed mechanical back arrangement becomes effective. Nonsteroidal anti-inflammatory medications can be used for longer periods of time. Muscle relaxants have a very limited role other than their use for sedation. Local heat or ice application provides a temporary analgesic effect for pain symptoms but does not alter the underlying physical abnormality.

Mechanical correction of disc protrusion must constitute the main treatment. This can be done in several ways. For mild discogenic low back pain, treatment may simply require postural correction via education of the patient regarding habitual acts

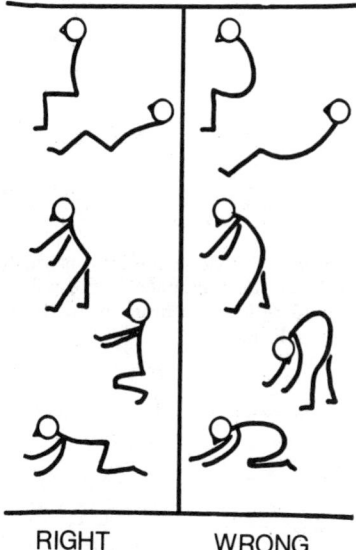

RIGHT   WRONG

FIGURE 38–79. Patient education is important and particularly should emphasize ways in which the patient can improve habitual actions that lead to back symptoms. On the left are schematic illustrations of the correct ways to sit, stand, lift, or bend, which maintain lumbar lordosis. On the right are the incorrect ways for carrying out these activities, which flex the lumbar spine, eliminate lumbar lordosis, and produce lumbago. (From Cyriax J: Orthopaedic Medicine, Vol. 1. London, Cassell, Ltd., 1978, with permission.)

likely to bring on the disc symptomology (Fig. 38–79). Particular emphasis should be placed on the importance of maintaining proper lumbar lordosis. The primary treatments for acute nuclear protrusions with neurogenic symptoms or paresthesias of the leg have been flexion exercises and traction. These methods are designed to open up the disc space posteriorly and gradually allow nuclear material to recede back into the disc space. Flexion exercises are used to open the intervertebral foramina facet joints, to stretch hip flexors and back flexors and extensors, to strengthen abdominal and gluteal muscles, and to mobilize the posterior fixation of the lumbosacral articulations. Wil-

liams exercises have been modified over the years but basically consist of partial situps in the hook-lying position (feet on the floor, knees flexed, head slightly raised) to strengthen abdominal muscles, pelvic tilts to flatten lumbar lordosis, and knees-to-chest exercises to stretch hip flexors (Fig. 38–80). Exercise therapy should be used primarily to make the patient comfortable and should not aggravate the symptoms of sciatica. The patient should be thoroughly instructed in these exercises and understand the reason for each. This is often accomplished most easily with consultation with a physical therapist.

There are many forms of traction. The rationale for this therapy is that stretching enables the disc space to open posteriorly and gradually allow the nuclear material to recede back into the disc space. In general, heavy traction is required (Fig. 38–81).

With a combination of traction and exercise therapy, more than 80 per cent of patients with disc lesions can be relieved of pain symptoms and returned to work activities within 4 to 6 weeks. To accomplish this, however, patient education is essential. The patient particularly must be educated in the mechanics of disc protrusion and the importance of lumbar lordosis in maintaining the disc space. Illustrative guides such as those shown in Figure 38–79 are helpful. This information must be discussed with the patient, rather than merely handed to him or her like a political flyer as he or she goes out the door.

Reassure the patient that this is not a crippling disease. Discuss seating posture in detail, because this is the major culprit causing backache in today's sedentary age. Encourage the patient to participate in a regular sport that maintains lumbar lordosis, such as swimming, golf, or even horseback riding. Discourage activities that require a good deal of lumbar flexion, such as gardening, racquetball, or tennis. A return to a full range of vocational or avocational activities without pain and without surgical intervention should be the norm in most patients with back pain of lumbar disc origin.

FIGURE 38–80. A pelvic traction apparatus must be sufficiently strong to support the patient and apply several hundred pounds of traction across the pelvis. Ordinary sling traction in bed does nothing more for the patient than enforce immobilization.

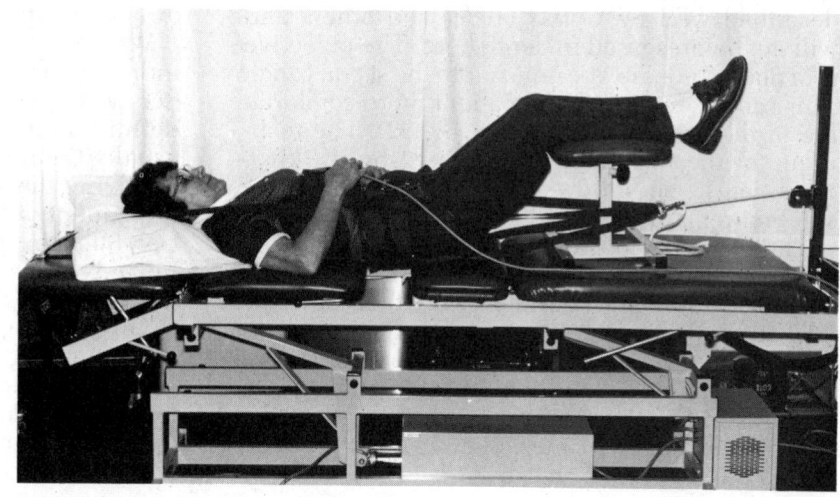

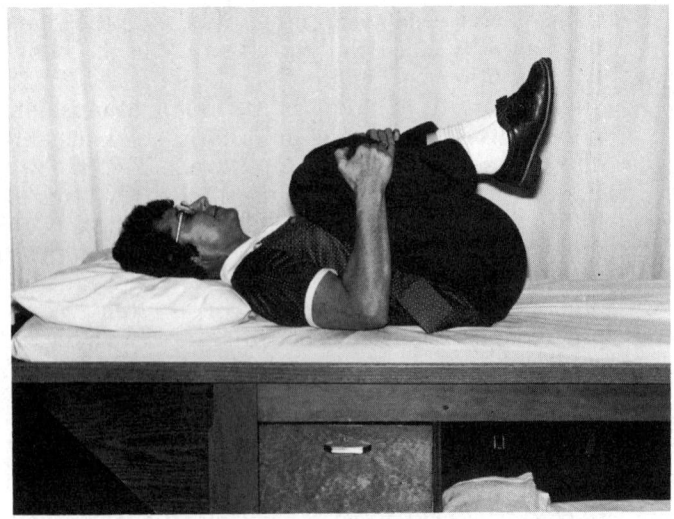

FIGURE 38–81. Flexion exercises, as illustrated here, are very useful to open the space in the posterior portion of the spine and relieve entrapment of the dura from herniated disc material.

If the described therapies, including manipulation, traction, and exercises, do not relieve the patient's symptoms, the next step should be epidural injection. This technique can be valuable both diagnostically and therapeutically. Epidural injections help to ensure that the back pain is dural and not coming from articular facets or the sacroiliac joint. They help isolate pain referred from some other unusual condition, such as chronic appendicitis or an ovarian cyst. They also differentiate the myelopathy associated with a disc at a higher level, particularly the cervical spine.

The technique of epidural injection may be helpful in the backache developing in the last trimester of pregnancy. It can also be helpful in distinguishing cases of coccygodynia resulting from sacral nerve root involvement. Epidural injection is indicated for root pain of sciatica with or without neurologic signs. It should be tried before advising laminectomy, because it does not work well after laminectomy.

The technique is simple and is suitable for outpatients. It should be thoroughly described to the patient and distinguished from a lumbar puncture, which many patients fear. The method has been described well by Cyriax (1978) and others and will not be presented in depth here. The objective is to place a needle or cannula into the sacral canal. This can be done with the patient quite comfortable in the prone position (Fig. 38–82). The technique of the injection, as described by its advocates, must be followed carefully so that the solution remains epidural and is not intrathecal.

The response to the epidural injection may be variable. Some patients experience increased pain for 1 to 2 days and then improve. Others relapse. The dural stretch test (i.e., straight leg raising with neck flexion) is a useful index of response. If pain symptoms improve but the patient does not return to normal after the injection, one can repeat the injection one or two times. Many patients require two to three epidural injections over a 4- to 7-day interval to relieve symptoms. If the pain and dural stretch signs persist, laminectomy should be advised.

INDICATIONS FOR LAMINECTOMY. The main indication for laminectomy and disc excision is to relieve leg and back pain. The worst results from laminectomy are with those done for pain in the patient without definite neurologic or myelographic finds. Myelogram, CT scan, or magnetic resonance imaging is now always performed preoperatively to confirm the clinical diagnosis of a disc herniation and to define the level.

The second indication for laminectomy is persistence of a gross lumbar list despite adequate therapy. This generally indicates a disc sufficiently large to be resistant to closed methods.

A relative indication is limited neurologic deficit, such as weakness of the foot. If the patient notices progressive inability to control the foot, he or she may be suffering from involvement of two nerve roots, and the foot weakness can become permanent. The pain may be relieved as the neurologic deficit worsens, but complete paralysis is likely to persist. This should be explained to the patient and disc removal advised promptly if foot-drop develops.

Whereas weakness of the foot is not an absolute indication for laminectomy, weakness of the bladder with incontinence or retention of urine is a definite indication for early laminectomy. This is usually the result of a massive midline herniation involving the sacral nerve roots, which can leave the patient with permanent loss of sphincter control. Such an acute paresis from disc lesions is fortunately quite infrequent, occurring in less than 2 per cent of disc herniations.

Discectomy, when advised for the proper indications, can be a very effective operation with gratifying results. However, it is employed far too often as a quick but inadequate solution to disc problems. The patient with severely disabling symptoms after laminectomy is far more common than

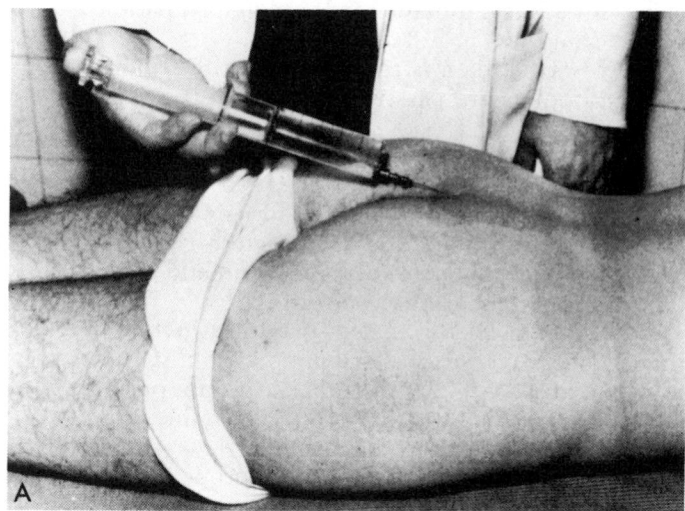

FIGURE 38–82. Epidural injection, as described by Cyriax, can be a useful diagnostic and therapeutic tool in managing acute disc herniations. The method should be considered prior to recommending surgical intervention. (From Cyriax J: Orthopaedic Medicine, Vol. 1. London, Cassell, Ltd., 1978, with permission.)

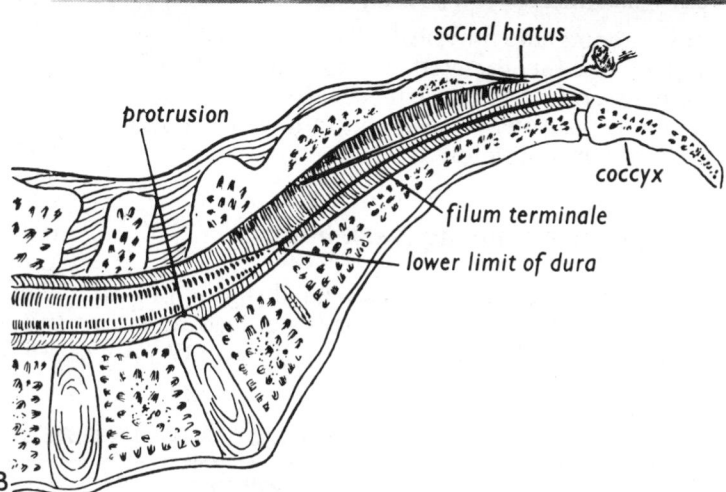

is the patient with a disabling result or intermittent backache after conservative treatment. By appreciating the mechanisms of backache as well as the rationale of treatment, the interested family physician can serve the patient with common low back problems quite effectively. He or she may even help the individual avoid induction into the growing army whose insignia is the laminectomy scar.

DIFFERENTIATING FUNCTIONAL AND ORGANIC BACK PAIN. One must certainly avoid cynicism, but the physician must recognize the great difficulties that workers' compensation and medical insurance create by encouraging the patient to stay ill rather than get healthy. The clinician will occasionally encounter the situation in which objective findings do not match the subjective complaints of the patient. These cases are termed "functional," which is used medically in distinction to "organic." In these functional cases, there is usually a psychological component as well as a secondary gain involved. Observing this patient is often all that is necessary to differentiate the functional from the organic by recognizing patterns of movement with varying types of organic disorders. For

example, when performing a situp, patients with discogenic disease have increased pain with flexion and will not assume an upright position without rolling to one side to get up. Conversely, patients with a functional disorder will generally have no difficulty with arising from a supine position. Functional patients often have exaggeration of symptoms, such as lurching from one piece of office equipment to another with pain greater than would be expected.

To evaluate these patients further, Waddell et al. (1980) developed a screening tool incorporating positive signs of functional pain. Finding three or more of these five signs is clinically significant:

1. *Tenderness*—nonorganic tenderness is nonspecific and diffuse:

(a) superficial—the skin is tender to light pinch over a wide area of lumbar skin.

(b) nonanatomic—deep tenderness is felt over a wide area and is not localized to one structure, often extending superiorly and inferiorly.

2. *Simulation Test*—these should not be uncomfortable:

(a) axial loading—complaint of low back

pain with vertical pressure on the skull of a patient who is standing.

(b) back pain is reported when the shoulders and pelvis are passively rotated in the same plane.

3. *Distraction Test*—when a positive finding is demonstrated on physical exam in the usual manner, the patient is rechecked for any disparity when his or her attention is distracted. Findings that are found only on the formal exam and not at other times are considered positive.

4. *Regional Disturbances*—findings involve a divergence from the accepted neuroanatomy, such as unexplained giving way of muscle groups or sensory abnormalities that fit "stocking" rather than dermatomal patterns.

5. *Over-reaction*—response disproportionate from what would be expected.

These nonorganic physical signs can easily be learned and incorporated, without the patient's awareness, into the routine physical exam. Patients screening positively should be followed up and dealt with appropriately.

Osteoporosis Causing Back Pain

Osteoporosis is a major skeletal disorder produced by too little or too porous bone, leading to a pathologic weakening and fracture deformity. In 26 per cent of women surveyed over the age of 60 (Urist et al., 1970), bone had progressed to this pathologic state.

The most common presentation is back pain from a compression fracture of the vertebral body. The most frequently compressed body is T12, which is also the most subject to flexion-extension overloading. Any fracture above T7 should generally be considered as resulting from trauma, electroconvulsive therapy, epilepsy, or metastatic tumor rather than a failure caused by osteoporosis. Other fractures related to pathologic failures in osteoporotic bone include Colles' fracture, femoral neck fractures, and proximal humeral fractures.

Osteoporosis can be confused with osteomalacia, in which the adult bone is not adequately mineralized. The osteomalacia seen today is most often the result of intestinal malabsorption or kidney disease, particularly that associated with renal dialysis. In younger epileptic patients, a frequent cause of osteomalacia is long-term anticonvulsant treatment. Anticonvulsant medications, particularly phenytoin (Dilantin), interfere with hepatic activation of vitamin D. The result is decreased calcium absorption from the gut, hypocalcemia, and osteomalacia with secondary hyperparathyroidism. Osteoporosis may be associated with osteomalacia, but the etiology and the contrast between these two conditions should be kept in mind (Table 38–8).

TABLE 38–8. CONTRAST BETWEEN OSTEOPOROSIS AND OSTEOMALACIA

	Osteoporosis	Osteomalacia
Definition	Too little bone	Abundant uncalcified osteoid
Mineralization	Normally calcified	Insufficiently calcified

Physical properties	Brittle
	    Leads to fracture
		Soft
		    Leads to bowing

Bone tenderness	Local at fracture site	Generalized
Serum calcium	Normal (upper limit)	Low or normal
Serum phosphate	Elevated (except in Cushing's disease)	Low or normal
Serum (Ca^{++} phosphate)	Normal	Low
Alkaline phosphatase	Normal	High
Parathyroid hormone	Normal	High

X-ray	Loss of spongiosa
	Thin but intact cortex
	Vertebral deformities
	    Biconcave
	    Wedge
	    Collapsed
		Loss of cortex, often eroded

Biopsy	Sparse, thin trabeculae	Osteoid seams and secondary hyperparathyroidism
Candidate	Postmenopausal women, not black Immobilized person Corticoid excess Thyroid excess Chronic alcoholic (?)	Intestinal malabsorption Uremia Tubular effects Familial vitamin D–resistant rickets Anticonvulsant therapy Cirrhosis
Reversibility	Usually *not*	Yes

From Gordon G, Vaughan C: Clinical Management of the Osteoporoses. Chichester, England, John Wiley & Sons, Ltd., 1976, p. 10, with permission.

The most common type of osteoporosis is that induced by immobilization, either localized to a fractured bone or generalized in a bedridden patient. This complication from immobilization is frequently forgotten, particularly in young patients. The result may be massive mobilization of calcium from the bone and hypercalcemia complicated by renal stones. The tendency of young patients to drink a great deal of milk in the misbelief that this helps fracture healing aggravates the metabolic imbalance.

The second most common type of osteoporosis is the hypogonadal type, which includes postmenopausal and senile osteoporosis. A third type of osteoporosis results from excessive catabolic agents, particularly hypercortisolism, hyperthyroidism, and cytotoxic chemotherapy.

History

The usual presentation of a pathologic osteoporotic fracture is typically in a postmenopausal, fair-skinned, lightweight woman of Northern European descent who experiences pain localized to the site of a recent thoracic fracture. Usually this patient presents 10 years after menopause or 3 to 4 years after hysterectomy and oophorectomy. Generalized bone tenderness is not characteristic of osteoporosis but does occur with osteomalacia and myeloma.

The acute fracture pain should subside in a few weeks. Persistence or worsening of the pain should cause one to suspect an underlying malignancy rather than osteoporosis. Also, bone pain from osteoporotic fracture should be relieved by rest, in contrast with pain from malignancy. Not all compression fractures from pathologic osteoporosis produce symptoms. Painless vertebral compression can cause considerable loss of height, particularly in the postmenopausal woman or in a patient with Cushing's syndrome.

Physical Examination

On physical assessment of the patient with back pain suspected of being caused by an osteoporotic fracture, one must look for stigmata of Graves' and Cushing's diseases as well as of renal, gastrointestinal, and liver dysfunction. Most important, the common differential diagnoses of carcinomatosis and myeloma must be considered. These possibilities should be suspected in patients with too much osteoporosis too soon after menopause. Five per cent of patients initially diagnosed as having osteoporotic fractures prove to have these more serious underlying conditions (Gordon and Vaughan, 1967).

Another consideration is the possibility that the elderly patient's pain results from arthritis of the spine rather than from osteoporosis. These two conditions are mutually exclusive. The bone mass that increases in osteoarthritis prevents the diminution of bone associated with osteoporosis. The presence of osteophytes, particularly the pathognomonic Heberden's nodes on the distal IP joints, shifts the diagnosis to osteoarthritis.

Careful assessment of the patient with symptomatic osteoporosis should also include accurate measurement of the individual's height. Osteoporotic compression fractures invariably lead to thoracic kyphosis and loss of height. The best indicator of the patient's response to treatment is whether or not the height is stabilizing. The standing height must be measured accurately at each visit and compared with baseline measurements to evaluate the course of the pathologic osteoporosis as well as the response to treatment. A loss in height of 6 mm or more indicates a new fracture and failure of treatment for some reason.

Laboratory Findings

The initial laboratory assessment of the patient suspected of having pathologic osteoporosis (i.e., the patient with symptomatic fracture) should include serum calcium, phosphate, and alkaline phosphatase levels and electrophoretic protein pattern. All of these studies should be normal or in the normal range with osteoporosis. Abnormal levels in these studies help to detect the most common differential diagnoses, including osteomalacia, metastatic malignancy, myeloma, and osteitis fibrosa.

Hypercalcemia occurs in most conditions of rapid bone turnover: malignancy, hyperparathyroidism, thyrotoxicosis, acromegaly, and acute disuse osteoporosis in children but not in adults. Consequently, hypercalcemia in an osteoporotic patient should cause the physician to consider conditions other than the garden-variety postmenopausal osteoporosis.

An elevated serum phosphate level is also usually a good indicator of osteolysis. However, it may be lowered if the condition responsible for the lysis also decreases tubular reabsorption of phosphate. The conditions most likely to cause this include hyperparathyroidism, hypercorticism, and myeloma producing an acquired Fanconi's syndrome.

Serum alkaline phosphatase is of particular importance in the differential diagnosis of osteoporosis. In the absence of liver disease or pregnancy, alkaline phosphatase reflects osteoblastic activity. The most marked elevations occur in osteitis fibrosa (Paget's disease), osteomalacia, polyostotic fibrous dysplasia, and metastases. Long bone fractures elevate the alkaline phosphatase level only transiently, and vertebral body fractures have no effect at all. Consequently, an elevated alkaline phosphatase level on repeated careful determinations indicates an underlying cause other than the usual hypogonadal osteoporosis.

Radiographic Findings

Radiographs of the osteoporotic spine show the characteristic loss of bone tissue, with disproportionate loss of trabecular bone relative to cortical bone. However, by the time these changes become evident on standard radiographs, the pathologic process is far advanced.

The pathognomonic radiographic finding is eburnation or thickening of the superior-inferior end plates. This gives a false appearance of increased cortical density that is relative because of excessive loss of trabecular bone, which is the primary bone that becomes porotic. In using radiographs, one must ensure that overpenetration has not produced artifactual osteoporosis.

Compression of the vertebral body in the osteoporotic spine occurs most often at the T12 level (Saville, 1970). A single fracture at T7 or above should always be evaluated for causes other than osteoporosis. Any osteoporotic atraumatic-type compression fracture in a man under age 60 should also prompt a search among the differential conditions, particularly myeloma.

Differential Diagnosis

Myeloma, the most common of all malignancies of bone, radiographically mimics osteoporosis. Chemically it simulates hyperparathyroidism. Myeloma may present in its early states as painless vertebral fractures. Most typically, however, the patient suffers a generalized and persistent bone tenderness and malaise. The alkaline phosphatase level tends to be low as a result of crowding out of osteoblasts by myeloma cells in the marrow. Although a myeloma spike on the serum electrophoresis pattern can be demonstrated in 70 to 80 per cent of cases, the diagnosis depends on bone marrow histology. This can usually be done by sternal aspiration.

Waldenström's macroglobulinemia closely resembles osteoporosis and multiple myeloma. Metastatic breast carcinoma is another cause of back pain that must be distinguished from osteoporosis. The lung, kidney, ovary, thyroid, and gastrointestinal tract must also be considered as primary sources for metastases to the spine. A careful history, particularly of a primary tumor elsewhere and persistent back pain unrelieved by rest, is most helpful in the differential diagnosis.

Alkaline phosphatase levels are elevated with metastases, in contrast with the normal levels in osteoporosis. Radiographs may show cortical erosion with progressive destruction of the vertebrae, which would be more consistent with metastases than with osteoporosis. Bone scans can be particularly helpful in differentiating between these two conditions, especially when done sequentially (Galasco and Sylvester, 1978). Needle biopsy is rarely indicated for this differential diagnosis. When in doubt about the cause of an isolated compression fracture of a vertebral body, procrastination is in order. Metastasis, particularly from the breast, soon becomes evident elsewhere. In contrast, the pain from an osteoporotic fracture improves within 3 to 4 weeks.

If the patient manifests any neurologic changes, the differential diagnostic consideration should not delay the urgently needed treatment. Operative biopsy and stabilization of the spine become mandatory.

Management of Osteoporotic Backache

MANAGEMENT BY THE FAMILY PHYSICIAN.   Treatment of symptomatic osteoporosis of the spine should be based on what we know at present about its etiology. The underlying cause (i.e., increased bone absorption relative to bone formation) ultimately results in an overall decrease in bone mass in the postmenopausal woman (Heaney and Recker, 1975).

This sudden loss of bone tissue appears to be related directly to the abrupt depletion of gonadal hormones at menopause. Estrogen therapy can prevent these changes and can restore normal premenopausal values for calcium balance and bone turnover. This is well worth considering, not only because of an overall fracture rate in osteoporotic patients of 5 per cent per annum more than in nonosteoporotic patients.

Conjugated estrogen, 0.065 mg, should be given for 25 days of each month combined with progesterone, 5 to 10 mg, on days 16 through 25 concomitantly with the conjugated estrogen. The patient should then have a 5- to 7-day hormone-free period to allow for the shedding of the endometrial lining to diminish risk of endometrial hyperplasia or cancer. A patient who has had a previous hysterectomy would not require the progesterone therapy. Some physicians are now using continuous estrogen and progesterone therapy and finding that the endometrial cavity becomes atrophic. The woman eventually discontinues having menses, which is obviously appealing to many postmenopausal women with this schedule of replacement.

Calcium intake should be increased to at least 1000 mg/day. Vitamin D supplementation in the form of 50,000 units twice weekly aids in calcium absorption from the gut. The principle effect of calcium and vitamin D therapy may be to decrease bone turnover and increase intestinal absorption. Vitamin D does not increase bone mass or decrease fracture rates. If a patient continues to have osteoporotic fractures, sodium fluoride and calcitonin should be added. Sodium fluoride increases skeletal mass by boosting osteoblastic activity. Calcium supplementation must be given with fluoride to ensure adequate bone mineralization. The usual daily dose of sodium fluoride is 40 to 65 mg. Calcitonin, a hormone produced in the thyroid gland that suppresses bone reabsorption, is injected muscularly or can be given intranasally.

Other medical measures that have proven beneficial in the prevention of further bone loss include regular exercise against gravity that must be performed at least 3 times per week and avoidance of excessive protein, alcohol, smoking, and caffeine.

Patients who sustain an acute compression fracture experience severe pain and require bed rest until the discomfort associated with physical activity is alleviated. The period of bed rest should kept to a minimum, however, because mobilization speeds bone reabsorption. Analgesics in the form of salicylates or other nonsteroidal anti-inflammatory drugs are useful in controlling pain. Mobile sacral corsets increase interabdominal pressure and provide comfort but are usually poorly tolerated and tend to weaken abdominal muscles. The back pain usually resolves over 3 to 4 months, and patients are encouraged to participate in non–weight bearing exercises, such as swimming initially, and to resume normal weight-bearing activity as soon as possible.

No single therapeutic modality, but rather a combination of treatments, will best aid patients suffering from this common and perplexing disease of bone.

NECK PAIN AND CERVICAL DISC PROTRUSION

Neck pain is secondary only to backache in the list of universal musculoskeletal afflictions. Not everyone with a "pain in the neck" consults a physician, but those who do should receive the benefit of effective therapy from an interested physician. Unfortunately, too often all that physicians offer is reassurance that symptoms will subside with passive resignation.

As in the lumbar spine, the vast majority of cervical spine pain results from disc disease. Very often much of the mechanical derangement from cervical disc disease persists or progresses. Cervical myelopathy from chronic disc disease is among the most common spinal cord diseases in middle-aged and elderly patients (Wilkinson, 1964). This disease can and does progress to the point of cord damage and frequently is mistaken for amyotrophic lateral sclerosis or progressive muscle atrophy, both of which are much less common conditions.

Although management of cervical disc disease is controversial and sometimes marked by unprofessional casuistry, the pathophysiology is fairly well understood.

History of Neck Pain

Cervical disc protrusion generally progresses in easily recognized stages throughout life. A young person in the teens or 20s may wake up once or twice a year with severe unilateral neck pain, wryneck, or acute torticollis. This pain lasts for 2 or 3 days but recovers spontaneously in 7 to 10 days. Such acute torticollis, or "cervicago," is quite analogous to the acute lumbago described previously. It represents a sudden displacement of a cartilaginous fragment of the disc with spontaneous repositioning back into the disc space (Fig. 38–83).

Subsequently, the patient in the late 20s or 30s will begin to experience intermittent attacks of scapular pain. These attacks last 2 to 4 weeks and are usually unilateral; however, they may involve

FIGURE 38–83. *A,* "Cervicago," analogous to lumbago, is the result of disc impingement on dura. Characteristically, the pain radiates to the neck, trapezius, and occipital and interscapular areas without radiation down the arm. *B,* With a protruded disc sensitizing the dura, flexion, extension, rotation, or lateral bending of the neck will worsen pain symptoms. This relationship to neck motion is as important for the diagnosis of the cervical disc disease as is a positive straight-leg-raising test for lumbar disc disease.

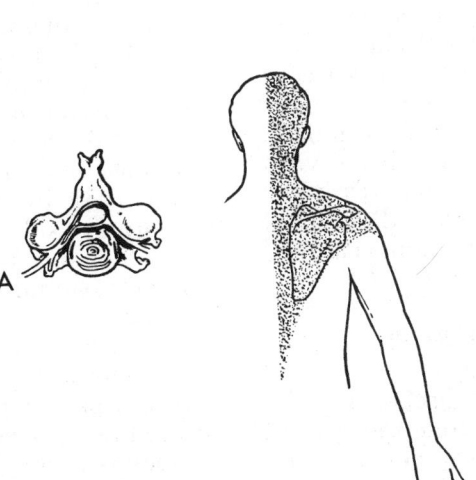

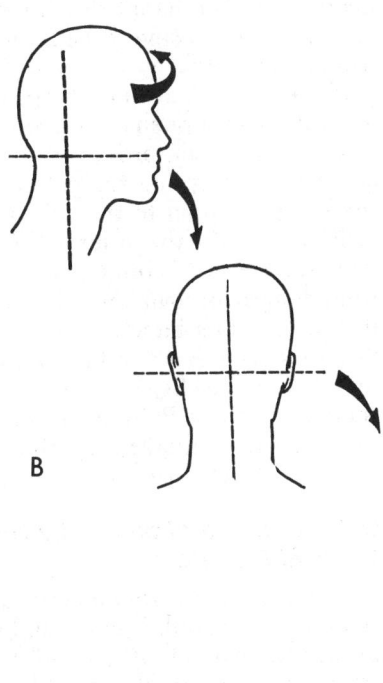

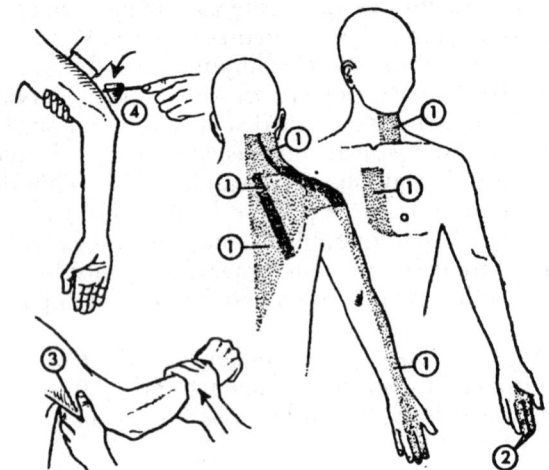

FIGURE 38–84. Should the disc cause entrapment of the seventh cervical nerve root, pain will radiate into the neck, trapezius region, vertebral border of the scapula, anterior chest wall, outer aspects of the arm, and index and middle fingers (1). The patient will experience paresthesias of the index and middle fingers particularly (2). There will be diminished muscle power evident, particularly in the triceps (3). The triceps reflex tends to be diminished (4).

alternating sides of the neck. Once again, this represents a loose disc fragment that eventually returns to its intervertebral position. However, the symptoms may at any time become much worse and progress to severe unilateral pain from compression on the dural sleeve of the root (Fig. 38–84). Such root pain is characterized by brachial or arm radiation that is much worse at night and may or may not be associated with "pins and needles" in the hands. Such nerve root symptomatology remains severe for 2 to 3 months and then usually subsides.

If the disc continues to protrude centrally, it eventually will push out the posterior longitudinal ligament and compress the dura. The result is a constant aching that the patient experiences from the occiput down to the scapula. This is particularly common in the older patient with chronic disc disease. Chronic compression of the spinal cord from central protrusion will produce paresthesias in the patient's hands or feet and can eventually progress to paresis or total paraplegia. This cervical myelopathy has been mentioned previously in the section on Back Pain as an important differential diagnosis in evaluating a patient for lumbar as well as cervical disc disease.

Other Considerations in the History of Cervical Disc Pain

The usual pain from a cervical disc lesion is located in the scapular region and is referred upward toward the ear (see Fig. 38–83). It is generally not aggravated by coughing. This contrasts with the pain from thoracic and lumbar disc lesions, which

characteristically are worsened by increased intradural pressure during coughing.

In the elderly patient, the disc pain will frequently persist as a severe occipital/cervical headache. This is particularly likely to awaken the individual from sleep in the morning, and is resistant to most analgesics.

Differential considerations are numerous, but one particularly should exclude metastatic lesions to the spine. Symptoms from metastases come on much more rapidly and are associated with more marked limitations of neck motion than is seen in cervical spine disease.

In the younger patient the possibility of ankylosing spondylitis should be considered as the cause of neck pain and stiffness. Cervical stiffness may sometimes present as a first complaint of this condition. However, further evaluation will always demonstrate diminished chest expansion and lumbosacral as well as cervical spine stiffness.

Physical Examination

To evaluate a patient with neck pain adequately, the physical examination should be as systematic as it would be for any patient with chest pain. Full examination of a patient with neck and scapular pain begins with inspection for any asymmetric posture—for example, stiffness, torticollis, or muscle asymmetry.

Range of Motion Testing

With the patient sitting on an examining stool, neck motion is evaluated, including flexion, extension, rotation, and lateral flexion to both sides (see Fig. 38–83). The motion that reproduces the pain is noted particularly. The patient should move the neck actively, and then the physician should move the patient's neck passively through all six dimensions. One must be sure to evaluate for scapular motion, which includes shoulder elevation and forward and backward movement. One can check for scapular winging by have the patient press against a wall with arms held forward.

Interpretation of range of motion tests should be based on the fact that neck flexion stretches the dura in the cervical and thoracic regions. Typical findings in a patient with cervical disc disease include gross limitation of side flexion and rotation toward one side. Motion on flexion and rotation to the other side is usually full, although it may be slightly painful. If side flexion of the neck away from the painful side produces pain, there may be a tumor in the apex of the lung. In this case, pain results from passive stretching of the lung apex. Also, if pain is produced by scapular approximation, the thoracic region rather than the cervical region is implicated.

Arthritis in the cervical spine of an older patient generally causes painless stiffening. Pain caused by motion of the arthritic neck would indicate disc disease as well as arthritis. Marked limitation of motion coming on quickly and associated with steadily increasing severity of pain suggests metastases.

Gross limitation of passive motion in a young person is characteristic of ankylosing spondylitis. Also, symptoms of a cervical disc lesion with radiating pain down the arm usually do not present under the age of 30 to 35. Any patient in the 20s with severe neck and arm or brachial pain should be considered to have a neuroma or tumor in the neural foramen. If the patient complains of pain on coughing, if the nerve root pain lasts for more than 3 to 4 months, if there is unusual weakness, or if long track signs are evident in the young person, a neuroma is a very likely diagnosis.

Testing for Nerve Function

Following the assessment of neck and scapular motion, the patient is evaluated for muscle strength in the neck, shoulder, and arm to detect any evidence of nerve root paresis. Most patients with cervical disc protrusions do not present with root paralysis. Rather, as mentioned above, the major presentation from the disc is neck and shoulder pain reproduced in testing of neck motions (see Fig. 38–83). One should not wait for neck movements to produce pain radiating down the arm or for clear root palsy to appear in order to diagnose a cervical disc protrusion. By the time these occur and make the diagnosis obvious, the chance for simple, effective treatment has passed.

Motor function must be tested against resistance. This can be done expeditiously in the same systematic manner in which one tests for neck motion. A particular weakness of motor function implicates a certain root level, as outlined in Table 38–9.

The patient must also be examined carefully for cutaneous analgesia. Numbness in the thumb and index finger would indicate a C6 level; numbness in the index, long, and ring fingers, C7; and numbness in the midring and small finger, C8.

The deep tendon reflexes must be checked. Remember that the biceps is innervated by C5 and

C6, the brachioradialis by C5, and the triceps by C7 (see Fig. 38–84).

By far the most common root involvement likely to result from disc disease is C7. The explanation is, as in the lumbar spine, the abrupt transition from a thoracic kyphosis to a cervical lordosis that concentrates the flexion-extension loading on the C7-T1 disc.

A final but important part of the physical assessment is to look for evidence of upper motor neuron lesions. No examination of the cervical spine is complete without checking for this. Similarly, no assessment of myelopathy is adequate unless the possibility of a central disc protrusion at the cervical level is considered. Examine the patient for spasticity, hyperactive reflexes, and positive Babinski reflexes in the lower limb, as a final part of the cervical spine evaluation.

Other Considerations: Whiplash Injuries

The term "whiplash" carries with it a certain opprobrium in the minds of physicians, but we should not forget that real pathology may be present. Invariably, the neck is injured in a rear-end collision in which the occupant in the front seat of a car receives an unexpected hyperextension-hyperflexion overload to the cervical spine. The result may rarely cause rupture of the anterior longitudinal ligament and backward subluxation of one vertebra on the other, producing quadriplegia and sudden death; or it may produce the usual lesion, which is a cervical disc protrusion with symptoms causing progressive pain and aching from dural stretch.

Because the emphasis too often is placed on radiographic rather than physical examination, the problem becomes a frustrating one for physicians, patients, attorneys, and insurance carriers alike. Quite frequently, the compensation aspects overshadow the patient-physician relationship and cloud the issue. The pain symptoms are real and are frequently amenable to treatment, as with any other disc lesion.

Most patients prefer prompt treatment of the disc lesion even though this might diminish their insurance settlement. Treatment should be based on the pathology and in particular derived from adequate physical examination. It should not be merely an overly optimistic hope, based on a "negative" radiograph, that strained muscles and ligaments will heal provided the patient is given a cervical collar and enough time.

Radiographic Evaluation of Cervical Disc Lesions

The expense of radiographs far exceeds any benefit they are likely to provide in the diagnosis of cervical disc disease. The only real help from radiography is a negative one—that is, a radiograph

TABLE 38–9. LEVELS OF INNERVATION FOR MOTOR FUNCTION IN THE UPPER LIMB

Nerve Level	Motor Function
C1	Neck rotation
C2,3,4	Shoulder shrugging
C5	Abduction and lateral rotation of shoulders
C5,6	Elbow flexion
C6	Wrist extension
C7	Elbow extension
C7	Wrist flexion
C8	Ulnar deviation at wrist
C8	Thumb extension and adduction
T1	Approximation of 4th and 5th fingers

should be taken to rule out conditions such as tumor or infection.

It must be kept in mind that narrowing of a disc space is commonly seen in a painless necks. Osteophytes are virtually universal in cervical spines after the age of 30. Usually, disc lesions occur in joints where the space has not decreased in size. It is essential to remember that radiographic diagnosis must always be subject to the findings of the physical examination and not the insurance coverage.

Management of Neck Pain

MANAGEMENT BY THE FAMILY PHYSICIAN. Prophylactic treatment is the first consideration in this common source of progressive spinal and neurologic disease. Patients should be advised to avoid sleeping prone, and in particular to sleep without a pillow or with a very low one. Heat in the form of moist heat via a hot water bottle or a hot shower may also relieve a neckache. Massage may be helpful for any associated spasm.

If a patient works at a desk, requiring long periods of neck flexion, the cervical posture should be corrected (Fig. 38–85). A few simple techniques can help typists and others avoid this common source of cervical disc disease.

The protruding disc that recurs and causes repeated neck problems eventually may not reduce spontaneously. After the age of 35, a protruding disc may well incapacitate the patient and cause severe nerve root symptoms. Osteophytes then develop as the bulging disc lifts up ligament and periosteum. Nerve root or cord signs may then follow.

This sequence is not inevitable and should not be accepted with passive resignation. Early manipulative treatment can reduce disc fragments quite readily and should be considered the treatment of choice for acutely symptomatic patients. This holds true despite reports of occasional complications, particularly cerebrovascular accidents, occurring from inappropriate chiropractic manipulation. Manipulation must be done by individuals who are knowledgeable about the cervical lesions.

During manipulation, the patient should be fully awake and cooperative so as to be able to inform the manipulator regarding any change for better or worse after each maneuver. Manipulation done in this safe manner can be effective in relieving neck pain of years' duration as well as of recent onset.

Cervical manipulation by an expert proves safer by far than most surgical procedures such as discectomy or fusion, which are well known to produce their share of death and quadriplegia. The patient may need a series of such manipulations but usually leaves the physician's office considerably improved following this technique.

SUBSEQUENT FOLLOW-UP. The patient should be advised that recurrent attacks may be expected unless he or she is careful about the posture of the neck, particularly at night. If the disc displaces again, it should be reduced as promptly as possible.

The patient should be reminded about sleeping posture and to avoid the use of a pillow. A bathtowel type of collar should be recommended for support at night. Exercises are inadvisable for cervical discs. They may actually produce recurrent displacement of the disc cartilage.

If a patient is subject to frequent recurrence of the disc protrusion, he or she should be advised to use a home traction apparatus. This allows the individual to exert heavy traction on the neck via a pulley system that can be extended over a door. It is important that the individual apply sufficient traction to the neck to lift the buttocks off the seat of a chair (Fig. 38–86). While traction is applied and the disc space is open, the patient can find a position of lateral flexion or rotation that is corrective of the disc displacement.

Failure to respond to this approach should prompt a diligent search for destructive processes in the cervical spine, particularly if there are nerve root problems. Discogenic pain that fails to respond to manipulation should be referred for consideration of an anterior cervical fusion or possibly for removal of an osteophyte stretching adjacent nerve roots. Once again the physician who appreciates the pathomechanics of disc disease and the simple but important mechanical methods of therapy can best serve patients.

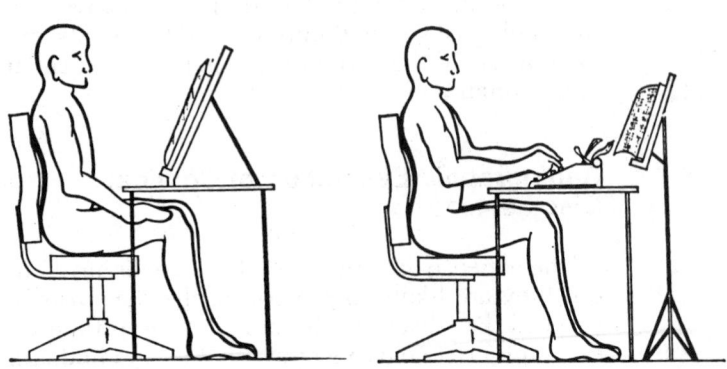

FIGURE 38–85. Habitual positioning of the neck in certain occupations is a great cause of cervical disc problems; for example, working at a desk with the neck flexed can produce "cervicago." The patient must be educated about the need to improve neck posture and use simple supports to avoid neck flexion as illustrated here. (From Cyriax J: Orthopaedic Medicine, Vol. 1. London, Cassell, Ltd., 1978, with permission.)

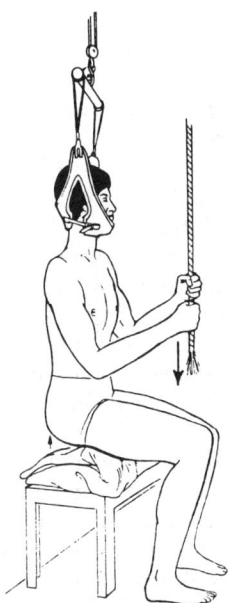

FIGURE 38–86. A cervical traction apparatus can be quite helpful for the patient with recurrent disc symptoms and can be used at home. The patient should apply traction with sufficient vigor to lift the buttocks from the stool. (From Connolly JF: DePalma's The Management of Fractures and Dislocations: An Atlas, 3rd edition. Philadelphia, WB Saunders Company, 1981, with permission.)

CHILDHOOD ORTHOPEDIC PROBLEMS

Limp and Clumsiness

Congenital Dislocation of the Hip

Congenital hip dislocation remains a common cause of limp in childhood. Despite the well-documented advantages of early detection in routine perinatal examinations, a large portion of initial diagnoses are still made by the mother or grandmother. The parent's suspicion is usually aroused by a previous history of congenital dislocation of the hip (CDH) in a relative or by the observation that the infant's hip has become stiff when the diapers are changed.

A family physician can do much to improve the outcome in treating CDH by understanding the differing modes of presentation and the pitfalls in diagnosis, particularly overreliance on radiography.

Congenital hip dislocation occurs in approximately 1 per cent of live births, but varies among ethnic groups and geographic areas. Risk factors include female sex, particularly first born; family history of CDH; breech presentation; and other associated musculoskeletal abnormalities. The hip should be examined in every newborn infant and re-examined at every well-baby check-up until the first birthday.

Congenital dislocation may develop in utero, in which case it is usually more resistant to treatment;

however, instability may develop after birth as well. The position the child assumes could encourage complete dislocation in an infant with dysplastic or subluxating hips. Positioning with the hip in flexion and abduction encourages normal develop of the acetabulum in a stable hip. In an infant with unstable hips detected in the normal newborn nursery, this position can be maintained with a Pavlik harness (Fig. 38–87). Three to 4 months is the usual time period for development of a stable acetabulum in infants in a Pavlik harness. Unstable hips detected after 6 months require longer and more aggressive treatment.

Hip instability or hip stiffness is the key physical finding in the diagnosis of CDH (Fig. 38–88). The examiner will not commonly encounter a clicking sensation during the examination of the hips. This and the absence of other signs of instability are usually insignificant and will resolve within a few weeks, and may not be reproducible by other examiners. In contrast, the palpable sensation of a clunk of dislocation during flexion and abduction and then again as the hip reduces in abduction (Ortolani's maneuver) is diagnostic. Treatment without further delay or debate is essential.

Hip stiffness in an infant is abnormal. A normal newborn hip can be abducted to lie flat on the examining table. Asymmetric abduction is diagnostic of unilateral CDH. One third of congenital dislocations occur bilaterally; therefore, any abduction limitation to less than 50 degrees should be considered abnormal.

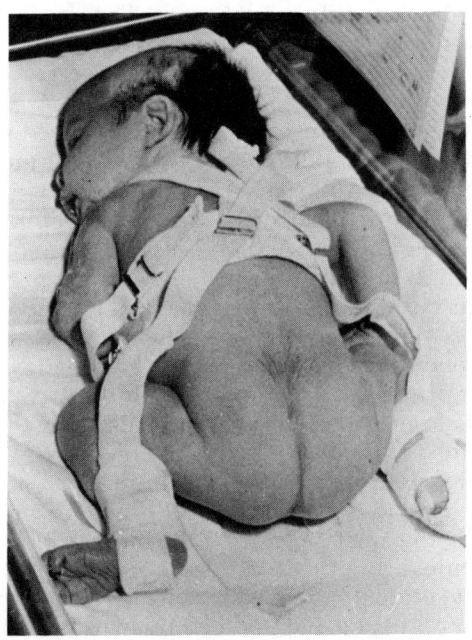

FIGURE 38–87. Any unstable hip in the newborn should be positioned with hips flexed maximally and in slight abduction (the human position). Double or triple diapers are ineffective for this purpose. A simple harness (Pavlik's harness) works quite well.

EXAMINATION FOR CONGENITAL DISLOCATED HIP

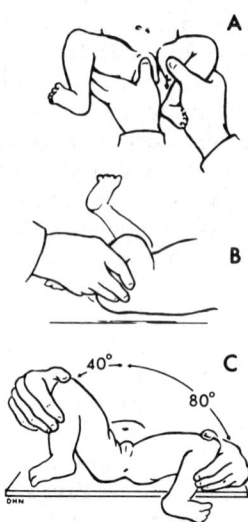

1. Test all babies at birth, repeat at 3 and 6 month check up

2. Look for instability and/or stiffness

3. Be sure baby is on a firm surface and not crying

TO EXAMINE FOR INSTABILITY:

(Figures A & B)

Fix pelvis between thumb and fingers of left hand. Flex hips and bring to midabduction. Press thumb on lesser trochanter to cause femoral head to move out over acetabulum. Release of thumb pressure causes femoral head to slide back into acetabulum.

(Figure C)

Unilateral or bilateral limitation of hip abduction to less than **50°** is indicative of **C.D.H.** and warrants treatment.

FIGURE 38–88. The diagnosis of congenital hip dislocation in the newborn is entirely clinical. The tests for hip dislocation include palpable instability of the hip or limitation of abduction.

Reliance on radiographs alone should be discouraged. Lack of ossification of the femoral head makes imaging of the femoral head in the acetabulum difficult in the newborn. Ultrasound has become a more valuable adjunctive diagnostic tool in the evaluation of CDH. Ultrasonography allows evaluation in a dynamic manner. One can repeat the physical exam with ultrasound and obtain images of the femoral head actually subluxating or dislocating over the acetabulum. The depth of the acetabulum can also be evaluated by ultrasound.

MANAGEMENT BY THE FAMILY PHYSICIAN. The family physician should develop a habit of examining every newborn for CDH. This should be repeated at every normal newborn exam until the first birthday. Any suspicion of instability or stiffness in the neonate's hip warrants treatment by positioning in a Pavlik harness. Radiographic and ultrasound examinations may help confirm the diagnosis but should not rule out CDH if the physical exam is positive. Treatment should be instituted early enough to improve long-term prognosis.

The principle of treatment with the Pavlik harness is to maintain the fetal position long enough to induce normal development of the hip joint. Double or triple diaper therapy has been advocated by some; however, we do not recommend this for the unstable hip. This intervention does not achieve the desired degree of flexion during the first critical months after birth. This method is also more expensive and compliance is less than with the Pavlik harness.

Cerebral Palsy

Cerebral palsy is a nonprogressive abnormality in motor function that may also affect intellect, emotional behavior, speech, sight, hearing, and touch. This diagnosis represents a spectrum of all nonprogressive conditions in which damage occurs to the upper motor neurons during the prenatal or neonatal period.

The main types are spastic and athetoid palsy. The degree of affliction can vary from barely perceptible to vegetative, immobile, and institutionally dependent. The severity can be described in part by the terms monoplegia (one leg), diplegia (both legs), hemiplegia (arm and leg on same side), and tetraplegia (all four limbs).

Birth trauma is the most common cause and includes precipitous or prolonged labor, fetal distress, asphyxia, or kernicterus (usually athetoid in type, resulting from basal ganglia damage). Neonatal head injury, anoxia, or viral encephalitis can be a cause. Such damage results in spasticity in coordination and muscle agonist-antagonist imbalance. These imbalanced forces can lead to fixed and severe orthopedic deformities.

Spastic cerebral palsy is characterized by increased muscle tone, exaggeration of tendon reflexes, a tendency to contractures, clonus, reflex hyperexcitability, and abnormal persistence of neonatal reflexes. A persistent Babinski's sign is helpful to make the diagnosis after 2 years of age. As the child matures, spasticity and rigidity become more evident and often lead to abnormal posturing and contractures. Pseudobulbar palsy presents when the spasticity is bilateral, accounting for swallowing difficulties and drooling of involved children (Eigher, 1993).

The athetoid type has a writhing or continuous abnormal movement pattern, with speech difficulty in the presence of a fully functional intellect. Severely affected children can be detected in the neonatal period as floppy, spastic children with a feeble cry or poor sucking reflex, an exaggerated startle reflex, or an abnormally persistent grasping reflex. Milder cases may not be noted until later in development as incoordination or clumsiness is noted.

MANAGEMENT BY THE FAMILY PHYSICIAN. The family physician should recognize the prevalence of cerebral palsy and its various manifestations. Early detection is not as essential as it is for congenital hip dislocation, for example. Therefore, when in doubt about the nature of a gait or posture abnormality in an infant or child, it is usually prudent to wait and see. As the child matures, the true nature of any neurologic deficit will become evident.

Keep in mind that cerebral palsy is a nonprogressive disease of childhood. Paraparesis without involvement of the upper limb or progressive worsening of the neurologic deficit should cause one to look for treatable conditions, particularly spinal cord lesions.

The aims of treatment are to maximize function through prevention or correction of fixed deformities and the teaching of compensatory skills. Orthotics and bracing are very useful in conjunction with therapy and surgery in the prevention and correction of gross deformity. Programmed approaches to the problem that preclude the judicious use of surgical procedures or orthotics are not realistic in practice. Many of these youngsters are surprisingly independent, bright, and communicative after an effective multidisciplinary approach to therapy.

Muscular Dystrophies

The dystrophies are a group of rather rare hereditary myopathies of a progressive nature. Several types are described, with variable ages of onset, sex-linked character, hereditary patterns, and different rates of progression, and patterns of afflicted muscle may vary. Other conditions of myopathy that involve the limb girdle regions or the shoulder and pelvic muscles come on slowly and progress less rapidly than does the most common, pseudohypertrophic form.

DUCHENNE'S MUSCULAR DYSTROPHY. Duchenne's, or pseudohypertrophic, dystrophy is inherited most often as a sex-linked recessive pattern. Hence it afflicts males. Age at onset is about 3 to 5 years, presenting as a weakness of the calf muscles with an apparent hypertrophy of the muscles. Characteristically the boy's calves become enlarged and doughy to palpation. However, the diagnostic physical test is the child's inability to raise himself from the floor without bracing his knees with his hands (Fig. 38–89). This is due to weakness beginning primarily in the quadriceps and hip extensor muscles.

The diagnostic laboratory findings include elevated creatine phosphokinase (CPK) and aldolase levels. Any male child seen because of a complaint of clumsiness, leg weakness, or easy fatigability should be screened by these laboratory tests.

Management by the Family Physician. The possibility of muscular dystrophy should be suspected in any "clumsy boy." A CPK determination should be obtained promptly in any such child. In some areas, CPK studies are recommended in newborn boys routinely, much in the way that phenylketonuria screening has been accepted. Female members of the family should also be evaluated with CPK studies when an affected boy is detected. Carriers of the condition should be so informed and given genetic counseling.

Treatment of the condition can only be supportive, not curative. Therapy should concentrate on stretching tight muscles and strengthening whatever remains of the diseased muscles. Lightweight orthotic support of the ankles is particularly useful in preventing equinovarus deformity. Surgery should be recommended with extreme caution, because it may occasionally aggravate the child's problem rather than help if it is not appropriately timed.

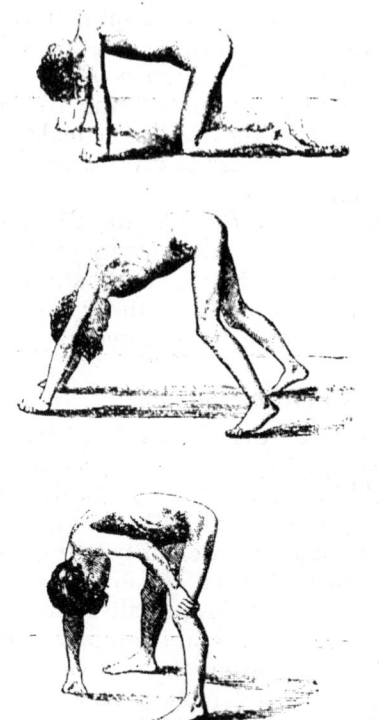

FIGURE 38–89. Illustration of Gower's sign from Gower's original text shows the process by which the boy with muscular dystrophy must raise himself from a crouched position using his arms and hands rather than the weakened thigh muscles. (From Gower WR: Pseudohypertrophic Muscular Paralysis. London, Churchill, 1879, with permission. Courtesy of B. Kakulas, Professor of Neuropathology, University of Western Australia.)

As the disease progresses, the spine tends to collapse, requiring constant adjustment of wheelchairs and spinal orthoses. The spinal deformity contributes significantly to the young man's ultimate demise from respiratory insufficiency.

To manage the multiple problems of these severely handicapped individuals, a well-run rehabilitative facility or clinic is quite essential. As these boys grow into young adulthood, they become progressively weaker and are more difficult to care for at home.

Unfortunately, present attempts to treat this progressive disease can be considered only halfway solutions, and we anxiously await developments from fundamental research studies.

LIMB GIRDLE AND FASCIOSCAPULOHUMERAL DYSTROPHIES. The limb girdle type of muscular dystrophy may be inherited as a dominant or recessive gene. Presentation is usually during adolescence or early adulthood, with weakness and wasting of the shoulder pectoral muscles. Usually the presentation is weakness in reaching above the head. The progression is one of slow deterioration that can cripple in 10 to 20 years and is not often fatal.

Fascioscapulohumeral dystrophy is an autosomal dominant inherited genetic myopathy of incomplete penetrance. The onset is during adolescence, with facial muscle weakness (e.g., the patient cannot whistle). Soon, wasting of the shoulder girdle muscles is noted (the patient cannot raise the arms over the head). The malady is slowly progressive, with years of mild involvement, and life expectancy is normal.

Management by the Family Physician. The family physician should be aware of all of the dystrophies and their inheritance patterns. Referral should be made early for definitive diagnosis and effective counseling and treatment.

Legg-Calvé-Perthes Disease

Legg-Calvé-Perthes disease, an avascular necrosis of the capital femoral epiphysis, is a condition that should be high on the list of differential diagnoses when there is a childhood limp. The disease consists of impaired vascularity to the femoral epiphyseal growth center, generally occurring between ages 3 and 10. Eventually a mechanical collapse occurs in the subchondral bone on the weight-bearing portion of the head of the femur. The result is considerable anatomic distortion of the proximal epiphysis. Children at this age are capable of reconstituting the shape of the femoral head provided it is contained well within the acetabulum, and therefore the prognosis is not as dire as it would be in an adult.

The characteristic presentation is a history of a limp with pain in the knee for 1 or 2 months. If the examining physician overlooks the referred pattern of pain from the hip to the knee, the condition may go unrecognized and be dismissed a growing pains, sometimes with dire results.

The most effective method of detecting early stages of Legg-Calvé-Perthes disease is by physical examination. The patient is generally a boy around 6 years of age who points to the knee as a source of his problem, with tenderness to palpation on the anterior and posterior aspects of the hip when examined.

The first sign of pathology is limitation of joint rotation, internal and external. This can be elicited when the child lies on his back with the hips extended. The hip is rotated gently internally while the physician feels the soft tissue resistance and observes the child for signs of pain during hip rotation. Abduction of the hip also elicits similar feelings of resistance and pain, although they may be mild.

The radiographs in early Legg-Calvé-Perthes disease must be carefully evaluated for signs of capsular swelling, widening of the joint space, and early demineralization of the femoral metaphysis and femoral neck immediately adjacent to the growth line. Only in the later stages of the disease does the femoral epiphysis develop the increased density and signs of collapse that occur as the disease progresses.

MANAGEMENT BY THE FAMILY PHYSICIAN. First, one must be cognizant of the pathology and the association of knee pain with a hip problem; the complaint must be taken seriously when there is a problem with knee pain. If an underlying cause cannot be found, the patient should be referred for other ideas and full assessment. Usually the clinical and graphic diagnosis is evident. Occasionally there is a possibility of tuberculosis or some pyogenic hip infection, and this can usually be ruled out by appropriate aspiration.

One must check for an insidious limp and pain at the groin and anteromedial thigh. About 17 per cent of the patients may give a history of related trauma, and may have limited abduction and internal rotation in particular, a positive Trendelenburg sign, and a sense of limb length discrepancy usually resulting from an adducted appearance. The clinical signs of risk are significant loss of motion, joint contracture, and pain. Treatment is not indicated if there is an absence of clinical risk signs, absence of radiographic risk signs, and presence of Catterall stage 1 or 2 or Salter A types already in the reossification stages.

Anteroposterior radiographs should be taken in the frog lateral position. Plain radiographs can usually determine the extent of the epiphyseal involvement, as described by Catterall (1971) and Salter et al., (1980). A bone scan may be helpful in the early stages of the disease when the diagnosis is in doubt. Magnetic resonance imaging is extremely sensitive in detecting infarction, although not as accurate in portraying the stages of healing as are plain radiographs. Arthrography is used primarily to determine and demonstrate flattening of the femoral head, which cannot be seen on plain films. Arthrography is also useful in determining the best position of containment when attempting to position the limb so that the hip is in an ideal position for healing.

The primary goal in the treatment of Legg-Calvé-Perthes disease is to prevent the deformity and altered growth disturbances that occurs, thereby preventing degenerative disease later in life. Up to 60 per cent of patients do not need any particular special treatment, but, in general, it is suggested that the opinion of a pediatric orthopedic surgeon be obtained with regard to the most appropriate method of treatment. The cornerstone of modern-day treatment is proper containment of the femoral head in the acetabulum.

One of the first principles of treatment is motion in a position in which the femoral head is contained within the acetabulum. Return to full or partial range of motion from previous contractures is obtainable with physical therapy in 7 to 10 days. Containment can be accomplished by nonoperative means, including casts of a Petrie type or the Atlanta Scottish Rite orthosis, or one can perform surgical containment with early mobilization and thus avoid prolonged bracing and achieve permanent containment. This is done with a varus osteotomy in some instances. The prerequisites for this are full range of motion, good hip congruency, and an ability to contain the full femoral head in abduction and internal rotation.

The second choice for surgical containment is an innominate osteotomy, as described by Salter (1961). Its prerequisites are a full range of motion, a fully rounded femoral head, and hip joint congruency. This operation will give better anterolateral coverage than the other operative procedure. When the patient has late Legg-Calvé-Perthes disease and needs a salvage procedure, Chiari osteotomy, cheilectomy and abduction-extension osteotomies can be performed, but these procedures are normally selected by an orthopedic surgeon to whom the patient is referred.

Slipped Capital Femoral Epiphysis

Slipped capital femoral epiphysis may present as a painless progressive childhood limp or as an acute femoral neck fracture. This entity results from a gradual fatigue failure occurring through the growth plate of the proximal femur. It generally occurs during the preadolescent period of rapid growth. It is more common in boys and the overweight, and occurs in the age range of 10 to 17 years, slightly older than patients with Legg-Calvé-Perthes disease. Ten to 15 per cent of patients present with an acute failure similar to a femoral neck fracture. Twenty per cent of patients also have the problem on the contralateral side.

There are two primary pitfalls in the diagnosis of slipped femoral epiphysis. First, the problem often presents initially as knee pain. The patient with a spilled epiphysis will often assume a position slightly abducted and externally rotated and be unable to flex the hip without those prior maneuvers (Fig. 38–90A and B). Second, incomplete radiographic evaluation may miss a slipped femoral epiphysis. The standard anteroposterior view may not visualize the displacement of the femoral epiphysis in a posterior and inferior direction. Widening of the epiphyseal line and demineralization of the metaphysis may be evident. A lateral view is usually necessary to recognize an early slip. The step-off between the femoral neck and the bony epiphysis may be obvious (Fig. 38–90C).

MANAGEMENT BY THE FAMILY PHYSICIAN. The family physician should have a heightened awareness of the individuals who are at risk for this problem who present with a limp. Diagnosis is confirmed by radiography. Treatment should not be delayed. The patient should be placed in skin traction with the hip in abduction, with an internal rotation strap applied to the thigh (Fig. 38–91). The patient should then be referred for pinning to prevent further slippage. Multiple pins are preferable to a single nail to prevent displacement and to encourage closure of the epiphyseal plate. Deformity can often be corrected by the time the child reaches bony maturity.

Patients with this problem should be counseled regarding the possibility of chondrolysis or avascu-

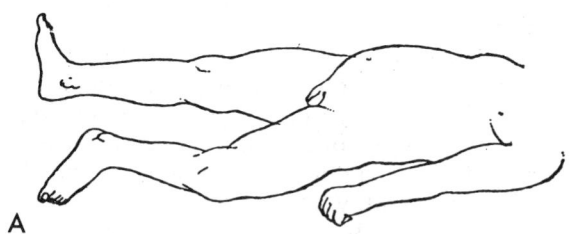
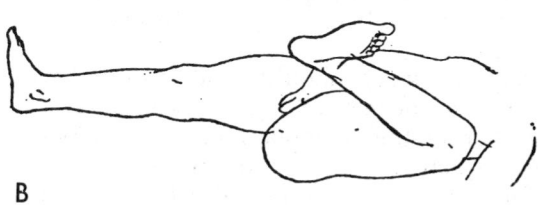
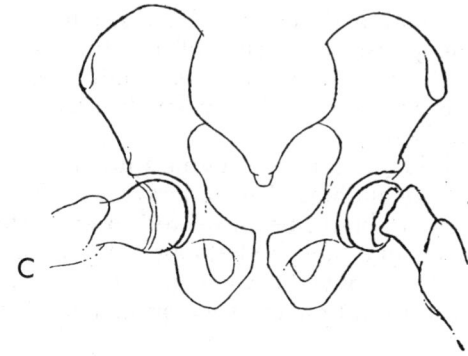

FIGURE 38–90. *A*, Characteristically, the adolescent with acute slipped capital femoral epiphysis maintains the leg in a shortened, abducted, externally rotated position like an adult with a femoral neck fracture. *B*, The characteristic sign of a chronic slipped capital femoral epiphysis is the tendency of the hip to rotate markedly externally during flexion. *C*, A radiograph—in particular, a frog-leg lateral view—shows widening of the epiphyseal line and displacement of the bony epiphysis.

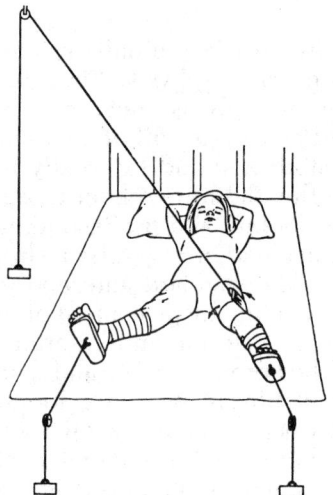

FIGURE 38–91. The acute slipped capital femoral epiphysis should be protected in skin traction, with an internal rotation strap applied to the thigh.

lar necrosis of the articular cartilage, which could lead to early osteoarthritis regardless of the time of initiation of treatment. They should also be reminded of the increased chance of bilateral involvement until they achieve skeletal maturity.

Common Foot Problems

The two most common foot problems in children are pigeon toes and flat feet. A number of these feet merely represent variants within the range of normal development that will correct with time. Overtreatment of these normal variants can be worse than the disorder. A percentage of these deformities do persist into adulthood and cause disability that might have been prevented by more vigorous treatment.

The family physician should be alert to the pathomechanics of these problems in order to determine whether treatment by reassurance of the parents, by corrective splints and exercise, or by referral for more vigorous orthopedic management is indicated.

Examination of the Infant's or Child's Foot

When examining the foot of an infant or child, the examination should not be restricted to the foot. The physician must look carefully for any signs indicating a more serious problem, particularly muscle weakness or spasticity as the child stands or lies.

The child should be examined unencumbered by diapers or clothing. The undersurface of the foot in particular should be inspected to evaluate for deformities in either the forefoot or hindfoot. The foot should be moved in inversion and eversion to detect rigidity or limitation of motion. Examination should continue up the legs to note torsion or bowing of the tibia or knee motion and particularly hip abnormalities.

A similar complete examination should be carried out in the older child seen for the first time for foot problems. Walking should be observed with the shoes on and off. The shoes should be inspected for abnormal wear. A normal heel-toe gait wears the shoes more on the outer border of the heel and inner border of the toes. Abnormal wear may indicate a spasticity or some mechanical deformity in the foot. The child's feet must be checked carefully for blisters or calluses reflecting abnormal gait or poorly fitting shoes.

The arches of the feet should be examined while the child is both standing and sitting. The common flexible flatfoot appears to have a normal arch when the patient does not bear weight. Flattening becomes evident only with weight bearing. Rigid flat feet, in contrast, are flat and everted whether or not the patient is bearing weight. The range of both eversion and inversion of both feet must be checked to determine any rigid limitation. Also, heel cord tightness should be sought by holding the foot inverted to control motion of the subtalar joint and then maximally dorsiflexing the ankle with the knee extended.

One must palpate for peroneal muscle tightness around the lateral malleolus as the foot is inverted. This tightness is frequently secondary to conditions such as congenital coalitions of joints. Peroneal muscle spasm may also indicate early rheumatoid arthritis of the hindfoot joints.

Finally, the child's spine and hips must be evaluated. Quite frequently major problems, including scoliosis, diastematomyelia, and CDH, present only as an initial complaint of "peculiar gait."

Pigeon Toes

Toeing-in is a very common problem that both the orthopedist and the family physician manage. It results from conditions in either the foot, the tibia, the femur, or a combination of these three. These include metatarsus adductus, tibial torsion, and femoral anteversion.

METATARSUS ADDUCTUS. The characteristics of this deformity are (1) adduction of the tarsometatarsal joint, causing the individual to walk on the lateral side of the foot (adductovarus); (2) an increase in the height of the longitudinal arch; and (3) an increase in the space between the first and second toes (see Figs. 38–92 and 38–93).

Infants normally tend to turn their forefoot inward in response to any plantar stimulus. The most reliable method to decide whether the forefoot is fixed in adduction is to inspect the lateral border of the foot from the undersurface (see Fig. 38–92A). In the normal infant's foot, there is a definite concavity felt and seen along the lateral border at the base of the fifth metatarsal. If the forefoot is adducted, this concavity becomes a convexity

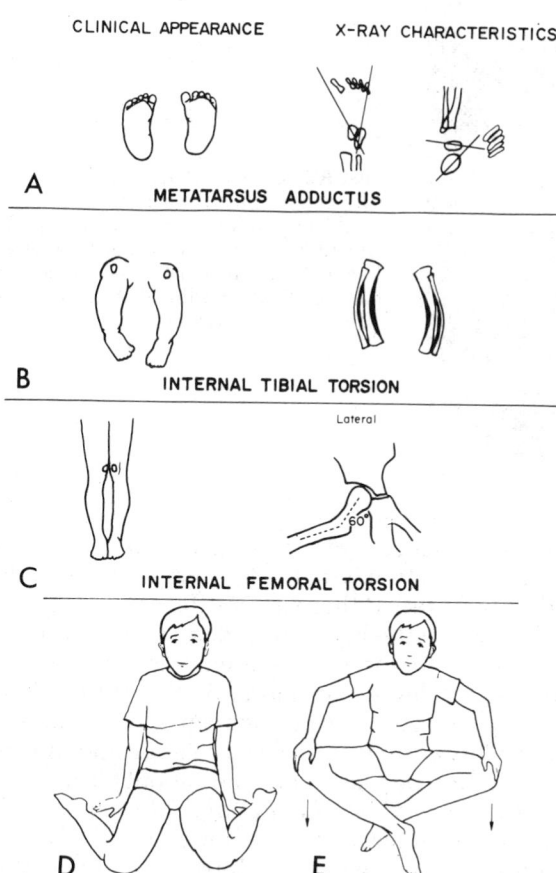

CLINICAL APPEARANCE   X-RAY CHARACTERISTICS

A   METATARSUS ADDUCTUS

B   INTERNAL TIBIAL TORSION

Lateral

C   INTERNAL FEMORAL TORSION

D   E

FIGURE 38–92. *A,* Pigeon toes caused by metatarsus adductus are characterized by a convex lateral border of the foot and prominent base of the fifth metatarsal. Anteroposterior radiographs show adduction of the forefoot and widening of the space between the first and second metatarsals. The talocalcaneal angle is increased as the calcaneus is turned out from under the talus, while the talus remains relatively fixed by the ankle. On lateral films, the metatarsals appear to be stacked on one another as a result of the turned in position of the forefoot (adductovarus). *B,* Toeing-in from tibial torsion is characterized by a posterior position of the medial malleolus relative to the lateral malleolus. Radiographs frequently show bowing of the tibia, which magnifies the apparent internal rotation. Increased medial cortical density seen as bowed tibia and fibula is due to compressive stress. *C,* Femoral torsion is characterized by an inward turning of the patellas with the hips in full extension. Lateral radiographic views show an increased angle of anteversion between the femoral neck and shaft. *D,* Children with excessive internal femoral torsion tend to sit with legs tucked under thighs and hips rotated inward. *E,* An effective method of decreasing internal femoral rotation is to have the child regularly sit "Indian style." While sitting in this position, the child can then push the thighs and hips out into external rotation, stretching out the iliofemoral ligament.

associated with a prominent base of the fifth metatarsal.

Management by the Family Physician. The majority of cases of pigeon toes resulting from forefoot adduction will correct spontaneously by 2 to 3 years of age, provided the child's foot is flexible. This flexibility can be demonstrated by stroking along the lateral border of the child's foot and ankle so as to stimulate the peroneal musculature. If the

child is able to straighten out the forefoot adduction, generally the problem will correct spontaneously. Further treatment is not required.

If there is a question about the flexibility of the foot, the child should be referred for treatment as soon as possible. The parents should not be advised to apply a regular shoe to the opposite foot (e.g., to put the right shoe on the left foot). This is actually harmful because it tends to flatten the longitudinal arch of the child's foot.

The treatment for the inflexible metatarsus adductus or one that does not completely correct with peroneal muscle action is a series of casts applied over a 2- to 4-month period. These can be molded firmly around the lateral border of the foot to restore the natural concavity and eliminate the convexity. The result is usually a satisfactory correction with two to three cast changes.

Failure to correct metatarsus adductus does not cause a great deal of disability for the patient, although it can result in discomfort and painful calluses. These are most likely to occur under the first and fifth metatarsals in association with a structurally inefficient high arch or cavus foot (Fig. 38–93).

TIBIAL TORSION. In a normal fetus, the tibia is internally rotated so that the medial malleolus is posterior relative to the lateral malleolus. At birth, the malleoli become even. When the child starts walking, the medial malleolus is about 20 degrees anterior to the lateral one. The habit of laying the infant prone with the feet turned in slows this normal external rotational process of the ankle. However, the need to externally rotate the feet becomes inevitable as the child starts walking and needs a stable base of support.

Clinical assessment is made by inspecting the alignment of the knee and ankle with the knees flexed (see Fig. 38–92*B*). Invariably, tibial torsion is evident in any child who first starts walking. This will correct spontaneously in a normal child who is not overweight or rachitic. The fact remains that the parents may be concerned about the child's bowlegs and tendency to turn the feet inward.

The usual approach to tibial torsion is to correct the in-turning by simple splintage. This can be done effectively with a device such as an extra shoelace or key chain run through holes at the back of the infant shoes (Fig. 38–94). This maintains the child's legs in external rotation during sleep. If a more rigid device is needed, a bar attached to the shoes will hold the feet externally rotated. In addition, the bar stimulates the everting muscles of the child's foot as he or she tries to kick off the splint.

FEMORAL TORSION. Another common cause of in-toeing evident in the older child who has been walking is internal femoral torsion or anteversion. Femoral anteversion is the degree to which the head of the femur lies anterior to the transcondylar axis of the shaft (see Fig. 38–92*C*).

At the 30th week in utero, this angle is about 60 degrees and results from the fetus being positioned

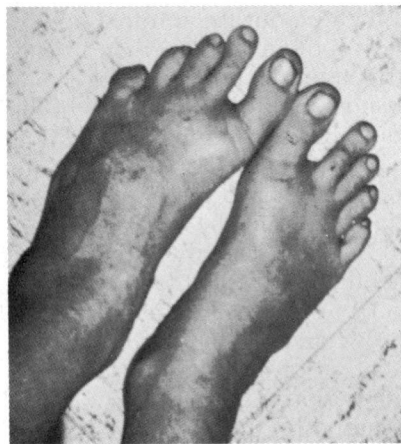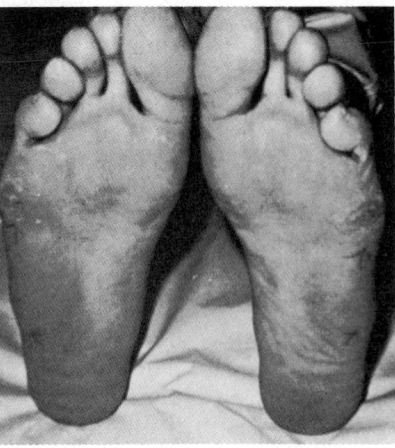

FIGURE 38–93. Persistent metatarsus adductus in this 21-year-old man has resulted in painful calluses under the first and fifth metatarsals. (From Connolly J, Regen E, Hillman JW: Pigeon-toes and flat feet. Pediatr Clin North Am 17:295, 1970, with permission.)

with the lower limbs fully flexed onto the abdomen. After birth, the neck-shaft angle decreases to 40 degrees as the limbs are brought down into extension, although full hip extension is not possible in the newborn. As the hips continue to extend, the neck angle is remolded by the force of the tight anterior hip capsule ligament and the response of growing bone to applied forces. The anterior angle of the femoral neck continues to decrease until in the adult it is only about 12 degrees.

Physical Examination. Femoral anteversion causes in-toeing as a result of the forces from the tight capsule and the anterior iliofemoral ligament in full extension. As the child walks with the hip fully extended, this ligament forces the femur to rotate internally. The patient's knees then characteristically face one another in the weight-bearing phases of gait (see Fig. 38–92C).

A simple method for detection of femoral ante-

version is to measure the range of external and internal hip rotation with the hip both fully extended and fully flexed. If there is significant femoral anteversion when the hip is extended, external rotation is zero while internal rotation may measure as much as 60 degrees or more. As the hip flexes toward 90 degrees, the anterior capsule becomes relaxed. Consequently, external rotation and internal rotation then become equal (i.e., about 60 degrees).

Management by the Family Physician. The child with femoral anteversion generally is more comfortable sitting with the hips internally rotated. Consequently, he or she assumes a position with the legs tucked under the thighs and the hips turned in while doing things like watching television (see Fig. 38–92D). This adds to the tightening of the hip capsule and its tendency to perpetuate the torsional deformity. Persistent anteversion of the femur may cause the child to compensate by turning the tibia externally, producing a flatfooted gait.

To avoid this problem, it is best to treat femoral anteversion by simple external rotational exercises. The child should sit with the legs externally rotated and be encouraged to force the knees downward toward the floor (see Fig. 38–92E). Attempted correction by twister cables or bars is worse than the disease. These devices tend to rotate the limb at the knee rather than at the hip. This is particularly a problem if there is any spasticity of the muscles producing the internal femoral torsion.

Operative correction by derotational osteotomy is not indicated for femoral torsion in the otherwise normal child. Derotational osteotomy may prove a useful procedure if the child has cerebral palsy with muscle spasticity. If spasticity is suspected as a cause of gait abnormality or femoral anteversion, the child should be referred for orthopedic evaluation.

Flat Feet

The majority of flat feet are of the flexible type; that is, flattening is evident only as the individual loads the arch during standing. Approximately 2

FIGURE 38–94. A simple inexpensive method of maintaining a child's legs externally rotated for treating "tibial torsion" is to run an extra lace between slits in the backs of the shoes. (From Connolly J, Regen E, Hillman JW: Pigeon-toes and flat feet. Pediatr Clin North Am 17:297, 1970, with permission.)

FIGURE 38–95. Radiographic findings in flat feet. *A*, Radiographs of the normal child's foot are characterized by a talocalcaneal angle between 30 and 50 degrees in anteroposterior and in weight-bearing lateral views. *B*, Radiographs of flat feet show an increased talocalcaneal angle as the calcaneal support is lost and the calcaneus turns out from under the talus. In the weight-bearing lateral view, the talus is pointing into the sole of the foot in the flexible flatfoot, while in true, congenital vertical talus, both the talus and calcaneus are directed toward the sole of the foot and the talus no longer articulates with the navicular. *C*, Calcaneonavicular bars frequently are detected only on special views.

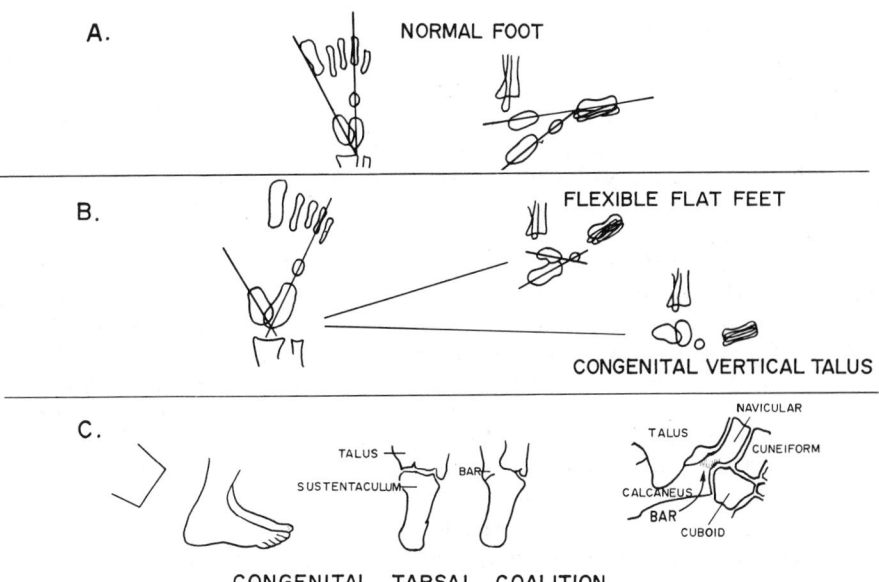

per cent of flat feet are classified as rigid, resulting from severe bony alterations. In these rigid flat feet, the foot remains flat whether or not the patient is bearing weight.

Common causes of rigid flat feet include congenital vertical talus or talonavicular dislocation, congenital coalitions or bars between the bones of the hindfoot, and accessory navicular bones (Figs. 38–95 and 38–96). Those flatfoot conditions that producing a rigid flattening, particularly congenital vertical talus or congenital tarsal coalition, require orthopedic correction.

FLEXIBLE FLAT FEET. Flattening of the arch of the foot occurs when the talus loses its base of sup-

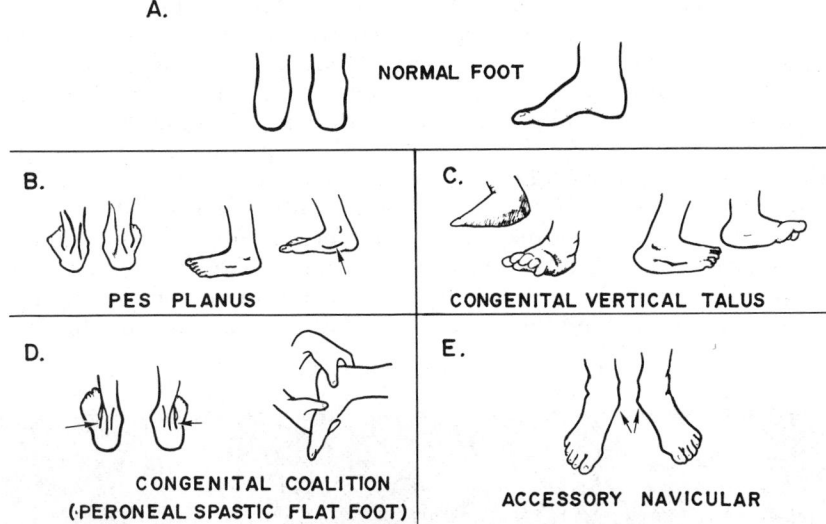

FIGURE 38–96. Clinical appearance of flat feet. *A*, In the normal foot, weight is borne slightly on the medial side of the heel, as seen from the rear. On side view, the normal arch has adequate talar support from the calcaneus, and weight is transmitted to the os calcis and metatarsal heads. *B*, Flat feet are characterized by a turning out of the calcaneus from under the talus as seen from the rear. On side view, the loss of talar support *(arrow)* is evident as weight is borne on the entire medial side of the foot. *C*, Congenital vertical talus in infancy appears as a rigid calcaneovalgus foot but characteristically has a concavity on the dorsolateral border of the foot. If the deformity is untreated, with weight bearing the foot takes on a "rocker-bottom" appearance as the heel goes into equinus and the forefoot dorsiflexes. *D*, Congenital coalitions are associated with a valgus heel position and a tendency to symptomatic muscle spasm *(arrows)*. These rigid flat feet have limitation of subtalar motion as a result of the bony block. *E*, Accessory navicular bones *(arrows)* occasionally may become sufficiently symptomatic in the older child or adult to benefit from surgical removal (From Connolly J, Regens E, Hillman JW: Pigeon-toes and flat feet. Pediatr Clin North Am 17:300, 1970, with permission.)

port and is depressed medially. The result is a grossly evident, prominent medial talus with weight bearing (Figs. 38–95*B* and 38–96*B*).

Most of the support for the talus is provided by the anterior end of the calcaneus or the sustentaculum talus. It is actually the loss of support as the calcaneus drifts into a valgus or turned-out position that is the basic problem in the flexible flatfoot.

Adding to the valgus tendency of the heel is a tight Achilles tendon. The Achilles normally is a weak foot inverter as well as a plantar flexor. However, as it displaces laterally with the calcaneus, it tends to pull the heel further out from under the talus.

The valgus position of the heel causes the forefoot to twist out into an abducted position. Consequently, the bones on the medial side of the foot become separated, while those on the lateral side of the foot are compressed. The medial border becomes convex and elongated. The lateral border appears concave and shortened. The intrinsic plantar muscles become stretched and lose their strength, reducing the contribution these muscles make to normal foot architecture.

The result of these mechanical alterations is that the talus must be supported by ligaments rather than bone. The normally strong ligaments of the foot are stretched and ultimately become lax. The muscles of the foot and calf must then support the talus and the other components of the longitudinal arch. Consequently, symptoms from flat feet in the older child or adolescent begin with aching of the calf muscles with prolonged standing. The arch of the foot also hurts from overstretching the ligaments.

Conditions that should be differentiated from the usual flexible flatfoot include congenital vertical talus (Figs. 38–95*B*, 38–96*C*, and 38–97), congenital coalitions (Figs. 38–95*C* and 38–96*D*), and accessory navicular problems (Fig. 38–96*E*).

Not infrequently, flattening of the foot may result from muscle imbalance, either as a result of paralysis or injury to the posterior tibial muscle, or as a result of peroneal spasticity in cerebral palsy

(Fig. 38–96*D*). The everting peroneal muscles overpull in relation to the inverting muscles. The result is that the calcaneus is pulled out from under the talus, causing an unstable, severe flatfoot.

All of these conditions should be kept in mind as one evaluates the individual patient's symptoms and physical findings, as described previously in this section.

Management by the Family Physician. Most infants are flatfooted when they first start to walk. They develop an arch by around the second or third year of life as they gain balance and muscle control of the foot. The status of the infant's arch can be determined on physical examination by palpating the medial border of the foot and feeling the relationship of the talus and the calcaneus. The stability of the talus is the key physical finding in judging the need for active treatment of the infant's flatfoot. In general, no corrective treatment is necessary for the usual infant's flatfoot. Special shoes are usually more of a detriment than a value in this age group.

"Corrective shoes" are of no value in actually correcting foot deformities. They offer only static support to the foot, and they do little to alter any architectural instability. When a child reaches adolescence and becomes symptomatic from flat feet, arch supports or inserts may be useful to relieve mild aching.

CONGENITAL VERTICAL TALUS. Congenital vertical talus in infancy appears as a rigid calcaneovalgus foot but characteristically has concavity on the dorsal lateral border of the foot (see Fig. 38–96*C*). The head of the talus can often be felt in the foot as the examiner traces the child's arch with his or her thumb. Most calcaneovalgus feet in the newborn correct spontaneously.

Walking is usually not delayed with congenital vertical talus, but, as the child stands to walk, the deformity is worsened and the foot then develops a "rocker-bottom" appearance, with the midfoot resting on the ground. The heel and forefoot become suspended off the ground (see Fig. 38–96*C*).

Radiographic evaluation is often difficult be-

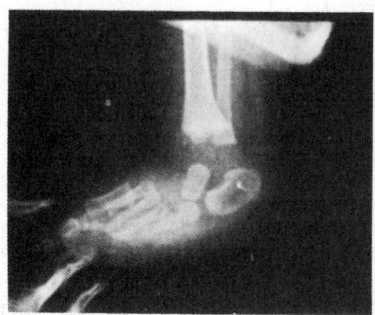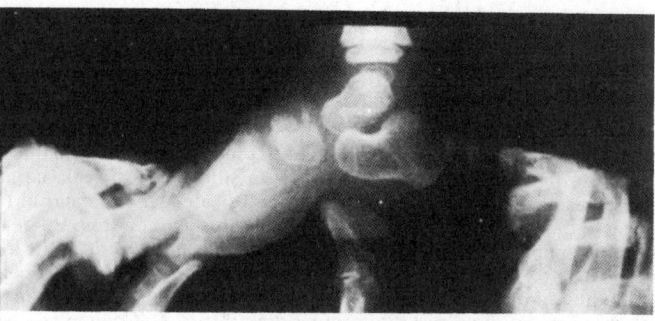

FIGURE 38–97. Congenital vertical talus deformity in a 1-year-old girl. The talus does not line up with the forefoot on plantar flexion. After 2 years of treatment with Denis Browne splints, the vertical talus has been corrected and the talonavicular relationship is normal. (From Connolly J, Regens E, Hillman JW: Pigeon-toes and flat feet. Pediatr Clin North Am 17:301, 1970, with permission.)

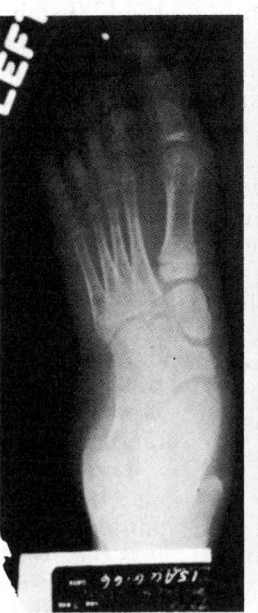 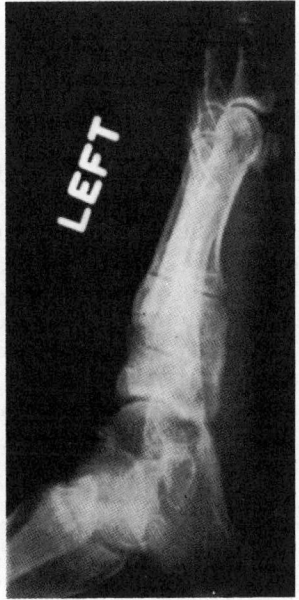 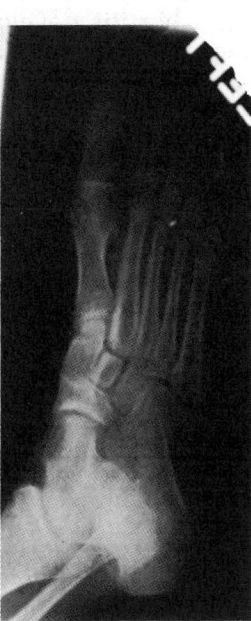

FIGURE 38–98. Multiple similar tarsal coalitions in a 7-year-old girl *(left)*, her 35-year-old father *(center)*, and her 5-year-old sister *(right)*. These include the calcaneocuboid, the talocalcaneal, and the naviculocuneiform joints. The break seen on the dorsal surface of the talus in the father's foot frequently is associated with talocalcaneal and calcaneonavicular fusions as a result of alternations in the normal gliding of the navicular on the talus. (From Connolly J, Regens E, Hillman JW: Pigeon-toes and flat feet. Pediatr Clin North Am 17:305, 1970, with permission.)

cause of the failure of ossification of the navicular until age 3 to 5 years.

Management by the Family Physician. Congenital vertical talus or calcaneovalgus deformity is treated with a rigid bar that keeps the feet inverted and allows the child to walk.

CONGENITAL TARSAL COALITION. The most frequent congenital coalitions, or fusions, are those between the talus and calcaneus and between the navicular and calcaneus. All varieties of single or multiple coalitions have been noted in the foot. There have been several familial reports indicating that multiple tarsal coalitions run in families (Fig. 38–98).

Congenital coalitions can cause rigid flat feet that may be completely asymptomatic. Pain usually develops if the congenital bar fractures as the child becomes active in preadolescence. The result then is symptomatic strain and spasm in the peroneal and extensor muscles of the foot.

Rigid flat feet from congenital coalitions remain flat whether or not the patient remains weight bearing. There is considerable limitation of motion, particularly inversion and eversion, caused by the bony block of the subtalar joint.

The patient will usually have no complaints until near adolescence, when he or she begins to stand for prolonged periods. He or she then may be bothered by aching in the medial aspect of the foot and ankle and note pain in the lateral peroneal and calf region from muscle overstrain.

To add to the predicament, the radiographs of the foot may appear normal unless the possibility of congenital coalition is considered. An oblique view of the subtalar joint must be obtained to visualize the more subtle coalitions. Tomograms or CT scans may also be necessary.

A frequent finding in a more mature foot is lip-ping of the superior margin of the head of the talus. This is due to the alterations imposed by the congenital coalition on the gliding motion in the talonavicular joint (Fig. 38–98).

If the calcaneal or navicular bar is recognized early, the symptoms may be relieved by excision of the bar. If the symptoms are allowed to persist and structural changes of the talus to develop, a triple arthrodesis may be required.

Management by the Family Physician. The majority of patient with coalitions do not require treatment. If a well-defined calcaneonavicular bar is evident on radiographs and is causing peroneal spastic flatfoot, surgical excision of the bar should be recommended.

Ideally, early detection by the family physician may allow treatment by less extensive methods than triple arthrodesis. However, the possibility of triple arthrodesis should not be excluded for patients with recurring, persisting symptoms of a rigid flatfoot.

ACCESSORY NAVICULAR BONES. A common and undertreated cause of flatfoot, particularly seen in the preadolescent, is a sesamoid bone situated along the medial arch. This accessory navicular bone, the most frequent sesamoid in the foot, is located on the medial side of the navicular in close proximity to the posterior tibial tendon. It may cause enough of a prominence to be termed a "double ankle" (Fig. 38–96E).

Like symptoms from congenital coalitions, accessory navicular bone symptoms may not be noticeable until adolescence or young adulthood. The bony prominences then become quite tender, especially along the medial arch. There may also be associated muscle contracture and pain with prolonged standing.

The pain is the result of several factors, including a bursitis developing over the bony prominence. There is also a tendency for the accessory bones to overcrowd the soft tissues and tendons on the medial side of the foot. The altered pull of the posterior tibial tendon impairs the mechanics of the foot.

Management by the Family Physician. Mild symptoms may be relieved by inversion exercises and longitudinal arch support in the young individual. However, one should not persist in these methods if they are not completely successful. The patient should be referred for removal of the accessory bone or the navicular prominence, a procedure that is quite successful in relieving the annoying and persisting symptoms of these conditions.

HIP FRACTURE IN THE ELDERLY

About 250,000 hip fractures per year are seen in the United States. The incidence doubles each decade after age 50, so that by the ninth decade about 30 per cent of women and 16 per cent of men will have had at least one hip fracture.

The major cause of these fractures is decreased strength of the femur secondary to senile osteopenia. Other factors, such as poor balance, poor motor control, impaired reflexes and mentation, and sometimes drug use in this age group, are contributory.

Fractures can be intracapsular or extracapsular and hence will require different treatments. A few intracapsular fractures can be handled conservatively if stable and in good position. Most will require orthopedic intervention.

The best means of evaluation is the use of standard radiographs. Clinically, most patients will be in pain and unable to ambulate. Inspection usually shows an externally rotated, shortened extremity with pain on motion.

MANAGEMENT BY THE FAMILY PHYSICIAN. Management of the elderly patient with a hip fracture is based on the patient's overall health and functional status. Generally, the patient would be hospitalized unless he or she is essentially bedbound and has an impacted fracture. Preoperatively, the patient should be placed in Buck's traction with 4 to 5 pounds of weight applied and sand bags placed medially and laterally to immobilize the limb.

The patient should be well hydrated and evaluated by an anesthesiologist as well as an orthopedic surgeon in preparation for operative treatment. Unless the patient has major medical problems, it is ideal to provide surgical intervention early. Elderly patients with fractures are at high risk of developing thromboembolic problems, urinary problems, skin breakdown, and pulmonary and cardiac problems with delays in operative stabilization.

Postoperatively, early mobilization and ambulation are very important in the elderly to increase their prognosis for a more active recovery and reduce the incidence of complications. Prevention of osteoporosis (as outlined in the section on Osteoporosis Causing Back Pain) can reduce the incidence of hip fracture in the elderly. Progressive physical therapy with use of assistive devices can help patients with hip fracture become more functional.

REFERENCES

Allen MJ: Conservative management in fingertip injuries in adults. Hand 12:250, 1980.

Betts LO: Morton's metatarsalgia: neuritis of the fourth digital nerve. Med J Aust 1:514, 1940.

Borenstein DG: Low Back Pain. Philadelphia, WB Saunders Company, 1989.

Brown P, Kinman P: Gas gangrene in a metropolitan community. J Bone Joint Surg 56A:1445, 1974.

Bruner J: Treatment of sesamoid synovial ganglia of the hand by needle rupture. J Bone Joint Surg 45A:1689, 1963.

Catterall A: The natural history of Perthes disease. J Bone Joint Surg 53B:37, 1971.

Connolly JF: DePalma's The Management of Fractures and Dislocations: An Atlas, 3rd edition. Philadelphia, WB Saunders Company, 1981.

Connolly JF: Early diagnosis and mis-diagnosis of congenital dislocated hip. Nebr Med J 60:471, 1975a.

Connolly JF: Perils and pitfalls of open tibial fractures. Am Fam Physician 11:64, 1975b.

Connolly JF: Wound management and the legacy of H. Winnett Orr. Nebr Med J March: 60, 1982.

Connolly JF, Brooks AL: Vascular problems in orthopaedics. Instr Course Lect 22:12, 1973.

Connolly JF, Regen E, Evans OB: The management of the painful stiff shoulder. Clin Orthop 84:97, 1972.

Connolly JF, Regen E, Hillman J: Pigeon-toes and flat feet. Pediatr Clin North Am 17:291, 1970.

Coonrad RW, Hooper W: Tennis elbow: Its course, natural history, conservative and surgical management. J Bone Joint Surg 55A:1177, 1973.

Corey L, Hattwick M: Treatment of persons exposed to rabies. JAMA 232:272, 1975.

Curtiss P, Collins W: Spinal cord tumor—a cause of progressive neurological changes in children with scoliosis. J Bone Joint Surg 43A:517, 1961.

Cyriax J: Orthopaedic Medicine. London, Cassell, Ltd., 1978.

Eigher PS: Cerebral palsy. Pediatr Clin North Am 40(3):537, 1993.

Einhorn TA: Hip fractures in the elderly. Resident and Staff Physician 34(9):97, 1988.

Fackler ML, O'Benar JD: Letter to the editor on ballistics. Milit Med 192:531, 1987.

Flatt A: The Care of the Rheumatoid Hand. St. Louis, CV Mosby, 1974.

Foster BK: Pediatric hip and pelvis disorders. Curr Opin Pediatr 5:356, 1993.

Galasko G, Sylvester B: Back pain in patients treated for malignant tumors. Clin Oncol 41:273, 1978.

Goldray D, Merdler C, Weisman Y: Vitamin D deficiency and osteopenia in the elderly. Geriatr Med Today 7(7):49, 1988.

Gordon G, Vaughan C: Clinical Management of the Osteoporoses. Bucks, England, HM&M Publishers, 1976.

Gustillo RB, Anderson JT: Prevention of infection in the treatment of one thousand and twenty-five open fractures of long bones. J Bone Joint Surg 58A:453, 1976.

Hansson J: The leg amputee. Acta Orthop Scand Suppl 69:112, 1964.

Heaney RP, Recker RR: Estrogen effects on bone remodeling at menopause. Clin Res 23:535, 1975.

Heyse-Moore G: A rational approach to the use of epidural medication in the treatment for sciatic pain. Acta Orthop Scand 49:366, 1978.

Hoehler FK, Tobias JS, Buerger AA: Spinal manipulation for low back pain. JAMA 245:1835, 1981.

Jardon OM: Physiologic stress, heat stroke, malignant hyperthermia—a perspective. Milit Med 147:8, 1982.

Jardon OM, Wingard D, Barak AJ, et al: Malignant hyperthermia. J Bone Joint Surg 61A:1064, 1979.

Jardon OM, Hood LT, Lynch RD: Complete avulsion of axillary artery as a consequence of anterior shoulder dislocation. J Bone Joint Surg 55A:189, 1973.

Kevnohan WG, Nugent SRN, Haugh PE, et al: Sensitivity of manual palpation in testing the neonatal hip. Clin Orthop 294:211, 1993.

Larsson U, Choler U, Lidstrom A, et al: Auto-traction for treatment of lumbago-sciatica: A multicentre controlled investigation. Acta Orthop Scand 51:791, 1980.

Levin ME, O'Neal LW: The Diabetic Foot. St. Louis, CV Mosby, 1973.

Lundberg BJ: The frozen shoulder. Acta Orthop Scand Suppl 119:5, 1969.

Mann RJ: Human bites of the hand. Am Fam Physician 23:110, 1981.

Matsen FA III: Compartmental Syndromes. New York, Grune & Stratton, 1980.

McCarty DJ: Arthritis and Allied Conditions. Philadelphia, Lea & Febiger, 1979.

McCullough N, Jennings J, Sarmiento A: Bilateral below-the-knee amputation in patients over fifty years of age. J Bone Joint Surg 54A:1217, 1972.

McRae R: Practical Fracture Treatment, 2nd edition. New York, Churchill Livingston, 1992.

Miller RG, Burton R: Stroke following chiropractic manipulation of the spine. JAMA 229:189, 1974.

Mooney V, Robertson J: The facet syndrome. Clin Orthop 115:149, 1976.

Morton TG: A peculiar and painful affection of the fourth metatarophalangeal articulation. Am J Med Sci 71:37, 1876.

Mubarak SJ, Hargens AR: Compartment Syndrome and Volkmann's Contracture. Philadelphia, WB Saunders Company, 1981.

Nachemson A, Morris J: In vivo measurements of intradiscal pressure. J Bone Joint Surg 46A:1077, 1964.

Newman J: Non-infective disease of the diabetic foot. J Bone Joint Surg 63B:593, 1981.

Phelps D, Lilla J, Boswick J: Common problems in clinical replantation and revascularization in the upper extremity. Clin Orthop 133:11, 1978.

Salter RB: Innominate osteotomy in the treatment of congenital dislocation and subluxation of the hip. J Bone Joint Surg 43B:518, 1961.

Salter R, Bell R, Keely F: The protective effect of continuous passive motion on living articular cartilage in acute septic arthritis. Clin Orthop 159:223, 1981.

Salter RB, Simmonds DF, Malcolm BW, et al: The biological effect of continuous passive motion on the healing of full-thickness defects in articular cartilage. J Bone Joint Surg 62A:1232, 1980.

Sarmiento A, Warren D: A re-evaluation of lower extremity amputations. Surg Gynecol Obstet 129:799, 1969.

Saville P: Observations on 80 women with osteoporotic spine fractures. *In* Barzel U (ed): Osteoporosis. New York, Grune & Stratton, 1970, p 3.

Simmons D, Chrisman D: Salicylate inhibition of cartilage degeneration. Arthritis Rheum 8:960, 1965.

Soboleski DA, et al: Sonographic diagnosis of developmental dysplasia of the hip: Importance of increased thickness of acetabular cartilage. Am J Radiol 161:839, 1993.

Stiell IG, McKnight RD, Greenberg GH, et al: Ottawa ankle rules. JAMA 271:827, 1994.

Stulberg SD, Cooperman DR, Wallensten R: The natural history of Legg-Calvé-Perthes disease. J Bone Joint Surg 63A:1095, 1981.

Swan KG, Swan RC: Gunshot Wounds: Pathophysiology and Management. Littleton, MA, PSG Publishing, 1980.

Urist M, Gurvey M, Fareed D: Long-term observations on aged women with pathologic osteoporoses. *In* Barzel U (ed): Osteoporosis. New York, Grune & Stratton, 1970, pp 3–32.

Waddell G, McCullogh JA, Kummel E, Renner RM: Nonorganic physical signs in low back pain. Spine 5:117, 1980.

Weiss NS, Uve CL, Ballard JH, et al: Decreased risk of fractures of the hip and lower forearm with postmenopausal use of estrogen. N Engl J Med 303:1195, 1980.

Wenger DR, Ward WT, Herring JA: Current Concepts Review: Legg-Calvé-Perthes disease. J Bone Joint Surg 73A:778, 1991.

Whitesides TE, Haney TC, Mormoto K, et al: Tissue pressure measurements as a determinant for the need of fasciotomy. Clin Orthop 113:43, 1975.

Wilkinson M: Anatomy and pathology of cervical spondylosis. Proc R Soc Med 57:159, 1964.

Zook E, Miller M, Van Beek A, Wavak P: Successful treatment protocol for canine fang injuries. J Trauma 20:243, 1980.

CHAPTER 39

RHEUMATIC DISEASE

JOHN G. FORT and ROBERT L. PERKEL

The field of rheumatology encompasses a wide variety of disorders. A common feature is involvement of the musculoskeletal system, although rheumatology includes such diverse diseases as rheumatoid arthritis (characterized by a proliferative synovitis), scleroderma (characterized by fibrosis), and polyarteritis (characterized by vasculitis). The underlying theme of many of these diseases is the presence of an abnormal immune response that leads to an inflammatory process with diverse manifestations. Other rheumatic problems are related to injury or degeneration and are not immune-mediated. Regardless of the nature of the process or the presenting complaint, the physician should proceed with a careful history and physical examination, develop and prioritize a comprehensive differential diagnosis, and devise a diagnostic and treatment plan.

Familiarity with rheumatology is important for any primary care provider. Musculoskeletal complaints are common and can lead to significant morbidity and disability in all age groups. These complaints also constitute a frequent reason for an office visit. Among them, back, knee, and neck symptoms are among the 20 principal reasons for a physician office visit (Rakel, 1990).

Some rheumatic complaints are short-lived and cause no sequelae, but many are chronic in nature and can lead to serious disability. These disorders require that the physician provide continuing and comprehensive care not just for the medical problem but also for the emotional and psychological consequences of the disease. In addition, the potentially serious functional consequences of some rheumatic disorders place stress on the patient's spouse, children, and other family members. Family members may be required to provide physical and emotional support to the affected members and thus must also be familiar with the disease.

Physicians treating such patients may avail themselves of the services of other health care providers including rheumatologists. Initial and ongoing consultation with a rheumatologist should be sought for the management of some patients especially if certain therapeutic interventions are contemplated. In addition, consultation with physical and occupational therapists, orthopedic surgeons, neurologists, and others may be needed depending on the course and nature of the disease. Other supportive care may be necessary, and the family physician should be prepared to coordinate the patient's needs, thereby ensuring continuing, comprehensive care for the patient.

COMMON MUSCULOSKELETAL SYMPTOMS

Patients visiting a physician for musculoskeletal problems usually have a number of typical complaints, including pain, stiffness, or swelling of the affected joints. Pain is the most frequent cause of an office visit. The pain may be described as sharp or dull, the nature of the pain depending on the cause. The intensity of the pain varies, affected by the patient's past experiences and tolerance to pain. Patients may confuse the intensity of the pain with its character, so it is important to question patients carefully. Pain may be localized to the affected joint(s), or it may be poorly localized—the patient complaining of limb pain or diffuse pain. A careful attempt must be made to localize the area of pain. An understanding of the anatomy and careful attention during the physical examination frequently help to identify the probable site of pain. In addition, it is important to determine the factors that relieve the pain and those that worsen it, as these factors provide clues as to the nature of the problem. Care must be taken to distinguish musculoskeletal pain from vascular or neurologic pain. Vascular pain (e.g., intermittent claudication) is typically brought on by activity and is described as a deep muscle ache that resolves quickly with rest. Neurologic pain, as with nerve root compression, may radiate and is often associated with paresthesia. The vascular and neurologic examinations often point to these causes of pain.

Stiffness is another frequent complaint and is described as an inability to move a joint with ease; joint movement is often painful as well. Typically, joint stiffness is most pronounced upon arising from sleep but may occur to some extent after prolonged sitting. It is important to elicit from the patient information about the duration and location of the stiffness, as it provides clues as to the diagnosis and the joints involved. Joint stiffness typically lasts longer with the more inflammatory arthritides. For instance, with osteoarthritis it typically lasts less than 15 minutes, whereas with rheumatoid arthritis it generally remains more than an hour. Prolonged back stiffness that is relieved with motion suggests the presence of ankylosing spondylitis rather than the more common mechanical back pain.

Joint swelling may be due to a number of factors. It may be caused by soft tissue proliferation as in rheumatoid arthritis, where there is proliferation of synovium; or it may be due to bony overgrowth, typically seen with osteoarthritis. In addition, a joint may appear swollen because of an effusion. Most joint swelling is readily identifiable. With more subtle swelling, comparison with the contralateral joint may be helpful. In some joints, such as the hip, swelling cannot be visualized.

The primary function of joints is, of course, to provide movement; and with many rheumatic disorders this function is seriously compromised. Patients perceive this dysfunction as an inability to walk, to climb stairs, and so on. Restricted motion is often due to pain but may also be due to structural joint problems such as muscle or tendon contractures. A careful, complete joint examination with attention to range of motion is important in patients suspected of having a musculoskeletal disorder. It is best to be systematic in the approach to the joint examination beginning with the head and working down to the toes. Although many examiners are unfamiliar with the degrees and planes of motion that are to be expected, several rules of thumb are helpful. First, always compare the left and right sides. Restricted motion is often apparent if one side is normal. Second, comparison with a control is helpful: A good approximation may be made with the examiner, for instance.

Three factors—the number of joints involved, the symmetry of the joint involvement, and the presence of systemic features—are important and useful when formulating a differential diagnosis. With regard to the number of joints involved, diseases can be classified as mono- (one), oligo- (several), or poly- (many) articular. Their differential diagnoses are shown in Table 39–1. Joint symmetry refers to involvement of the same joints on the right and left side of the body. It is important to remember that this involvement need not be to the same degree. Thus diseases are referred to as either symmetric or asymmetric with respect to joint involvement. Rheumatoid arthritis and systemic lupus erythematosus (SLE) are typically symmetric, whereas the joint involvement of ankylosing spondylitis is typically asymmetric. Lastly, the presence or absence of systemic features is an important finding when establishing the diagnosis. Features such as weight loss, fever, and malaise signal the presence of a systemic process such as rheumatoid arthritis or SLE. Other rheumatic diseases, such as osteoarthritis, characteristically lack these findings. Systemic features need not be constitutional or nonspecific. Patients with rheumatoid arthritis may develop an episcleritis or interstitial lung disease; patients with SLE may develop seizures or pleuritis. Thus there is a need to proceed carefully with a complete history and physical examination in patients with musculoskeletal complaints.

FURTHER EVALUATION OF PATIENTS

When evaluating a patient with a rheumatic complaint it is important to consider both articular and nonarticular manifestations. The initial evaluation should concentrate on the chief complaint, although it is important to assess all joints clinically and functionally to detect the presence of subclinical disease. Care should be taken to evaluate the signs and symptoms discussed above. Other aspects of the evaluation of patients include the use of laboratory tests, radiography, and functional assessment.

Laboratory Studies

The evaluation of patients with musculoskeletal pain often includes laboratory studies. Laboratory tests are helpful for establishing a diagnosis, monitoring disease activity, and monitoring drug reactions. Laboratory tests, however, cannot substitute for a careful history and physical examination. Important tests include those of a general nature, such as a complete blood count (CBC), urinalysis, and multichemistry panels, as well as more specific tests for rheumatologic conditions such as antinuclear antibody (ANA) or rheumatoid factor (RF). For example, with a CBC one can determine the presence of anemia due to a chronic disease in a patient with rheumatoid arthritis or a hemolytic anemia in someone with SLE, the presence of thrombocytopenia in SLE, or the presence of lymphopenia also seen in SLE. With the urinalysis one can determine the presence of renal involvement in SLE or drug toxicity in patients with rheumatoid

TABLE 39–1. CLASSIFICATION OF COMMON ARTICULAR DISEASE ON THE BASIS OF THE JOINTS MOST COMMONLY INVOLVED

Monarticular	Oligoarticular and Asymmetric	Polyarticular and Symmetric
Septic arthritis	Ankylosing spondylitis	Rheumatoid arthritis
Osteoarthritis	Psoriatic arthritis	Systematic lupus erythematosus
Gout	Reiter's syndrome	
Pseudogout	Osteoarthritis	
Trauma		
Hemarthrosis		
Avascular necrosis		
Tumors		
Osteoarthritis		

arthritis on gold therapy. Chemical analyses can detect an elevated uric acid level in someone with gout or even renal insufficiency in a patient with SLE.

Measurement of acute-phase reactants is important for determining disease activity. The two tests most frequently done are the erythrocyte sedimentation rate (ESR) and the C-reactive protein (CRP) assay. Both tests are nonspecific and may be elevated in patients with infections, tumors, or other inflammatory diseases as well as in those with rheumatic diseases. The ESR is a simple, inexpensive, albeit incomplete way to monitor disease activity. These tests do not always parallel disease activity, however, a fact that should be kept in mind.

The RF test is reported either as a tube dilution titer or in enzyme-linked immunosorbent assay (ELISA) units. In the proper setting, it can be used to confirm the clinical diagnosis of rheumatoid arthritis. It is not always present, however, especially early in the disease course when the clinical picture may not be clear. Moreover, the RF assay may be positive in other disorders as well. Generally, the higher the RF titer, the more specific the test is for rheumatoid arthritis.

The detection of ANA is frequently useful in patients with rheumatic complaints. These antibodies represent a portion of the autoantibodies found in patients with rheumatic diseases and are found in a number of such disorders. It should be noted that the ANA assay detects not a single antibody but a family of related antibodies, some of which have been characterized. The group includes antibodies to double-stranded DNA (nDNA), to ribonuclear protein U1 (RNP), the so-called Smith antigen (anti-Sm), Sjögren syndrome antibodies SSA and SSB, anti-centromere antibodies (ACA), and antibodies against topoisomerase 1 (Scl-70), among others. ANA antibodies are usually detected by indirect immunofluorescence tests using human cell lines. The ANA test is performed by doubling dilutions of the patient's serum, and the result is reported as a titer, with most laboratories considering titers of 1:160 or more as positive. Generally, the higher the titer, the more significant are the results. Today, many specific ANAs are detected by ELISA. These tests are generally more sensitive to low levels of antibodies than previous methods, a point that should be kept in mind when confronted with low positive values.

The ANA assay is often used as a screening test for SLE and other rheumatic disorders. Several facts must be remembered: The ANA assay should not be done routinely in patients; there should be a high index of suspicion before ordering the test. Often the test is ordered without good reason and is positive, especially at a low titer. Such positive tests may be due to drugs, age, or other causes and may induce a great deal of anxiety in both patient and physician. A positive test in and of itself does not constitute a diagnosis of rheumatic disease. The diagnosis can be established only in the context of the proper clinical picture. In addition, interpreting changes in ANA titers as an indication of a change in disease activity is not always accurate.

Synovial Fluid Analysis

Obtaining synovial fluid (SF) for analysis is often critical to the diagnosis and treatment of patients with joint disease. The technique for obtaining SF is discussed later (see Arthrocentesis). A number of studies can be performed on SF, and on the basis of these tests SF can be classified into three broad categories that help with the differential diagnosis (Table 39–2). Noninflammatory SFs usually have low cell counts, have generally intact mucopolysaccharide (normal viscosity), and are clear owing to low cell counts that typically comprise a large percent of mononuclear cells. Noninflammatory SF is commonly seen in patients with osteoarthritis or osteonecrosis. Inflammatory SFs, which tend to

TABLE 39–2. SYNOVIAL FLUID CHARACTERISTICS

Parameter	Noninflammatory	Inflammatory	Purulent
Clarity	Clear	Slightly turbid	Tubid
Viscosity	Very good	Good to fair	Low
WBCs/mm^3	< 3,000	> 50,000	3,000–50,000
PMNs (%)*	< 5	> 70	> 90
Disease states	Osteoarthritis	Rheumatoid arthritis	Septic arthritis
	Osteonecrosis	Gout	Gout
	Polymyalgia rheumatica	Pseudogout	Pseudogout
	Systemic lupus erythematosus†	Psoriatic arthritis	
	Scleroderma	Reiter's syndrome	
	Trauma	Viral arthritis	
	Polyarteritis nodosa	Behçet disease	

* Polymorphonucleated cells.
† Occasionally inflammatory.
Adapted from McCarty DJ: Synovial fluid. *In* McCarty DJ, Koopman WJ (eds): Arthritis and Allied Conditions, 12th edition. Philadelphia, Lea & Febiger, 1993, with permission.

have a higher cell count and thus appear more turbid, typically are seen in patients with rheumatoid arthritis, psoriatic arthritis, and occasionally gout or pseudogout. Purulent SFs have high cell counts (causing the turbidity) comprised mostly of polymorphonuclear cells. Purulent SFs are seen with bacterial infectious arthritis and crystal arthropathies.

Crystal analysis of SF is important, especially if one suspects a crystal arthropathy. To adequately view crystals, the microscope must be equipped with a polarizer. Urate can be distinguished from calcium pyrophosphate (CPPD) crystals on the basis of birefringence and morphology, although, this distinction is occasionally misleading. The best method for distinguishing these two crystals is through the use of a compensator, which allows color to appear in the polarized field (Gater, 1984; Owen, 1971). Urate crystals are characteristically bright yellow when parallel to the optical axis of the compensator and blue when perpendicular. CPPD crystals have the exact opposite color characteristics.

If an infectious process is suspected, the SF should be subjected to appropriate stains and cultures. Other tests, such as complement levels and protein and glucose assays, can be performed on SF but are generally not helpful and should be used only under special circumstances.

Radiology

Radiographic studies form an important aspect of a patient's evaluation. The radiographic findings vary depending on the diagnosis. Keep in mind that early in the disease course the findings may be subtle or absent. Proper views and technique are important for obtaining the most information from the films. Radiographs are also important for monitoring the patient's progress and response to therapy. Periodic assessment is usually indicated but should play an adjunctive role to the clinical evaluation. Radiographic techniques such as magnetic resonance imaging (MRI) have greatly increased our ability to see soft tissue elements such as ligaments, menisci, and cartilage and to examine the spine and its neurologic content in detail. Care must be taken when assessing a patient not to rely solely on radiographic findings, however. Careful attention to the clinical history and the physical findings is essential in order to place radiographic findings in their proper context.

Functional Assessment

Many rheumatic disease can produce significant functional impairment. Basic activities of daily living and higher level functioning may be affected. These areas are often overlooked when evaluating patients, yet for the patient these aspects of their disease are most important. Functional assessments have been standardized and disease-specific methods developed, and they have proved valuable especially in controlled trials that have evaluated the efficacy of therapeutic agents. Some, such as the Health Assessment Questionnaire (HAQ) and the Arthritis Impact Measurement Scales (AIMS), have a broader scope. In addition, joint counts, range of motion, grip strength, and other parameters have been used. Functional assessment is often performed in a less systematic, simpler manner. It may consist of determining how many blocks the patient can walk without pain or how many stairs the patient can climb. Whatever method is used, the impact of the disease on the patient's function should not be overlooked.

ARTHROCENTESIS

Joint aspiration, an important procedure in rheumatology, is used for diagnostic and therapeutic purposes. Although there is some variation depending on the joint to be aspirated, the technique is generally the same. The knee is the easiest joint to aspirate and the one with which most physicians are familiar. There are few absolute contraindications to a joint aspiration. Care should be taken when performing this procedure in a person with a bleeding diathesis because of the concern for excessive bleeding. Caution must be exercised when inserting a needle through an infected area of skin because of the danger of introducing an infection into the joint. The skin should be prepared cleanly and gloves used. Careful attention must be paid to maintaining sterility at the site of arthrocentesis. A local anesthetic can be used in the skin and subcutaneous tissue to minimize patient discomfort. Once the needle is in the joint, fluid is aspirated and sent for appropriate analysis. The tests ordered are determined in part by the differential diagnosis. Certain aspects of synovial fluids help categorize the process into subgroups (Table 39–2). Generally a cell count and differential count are helpful. If the differential diagnosis includes gout or pseudogout, the fluid should be sent for crystal analysis. If it includes a septic process, appropriate stains and cultures are prepared.

The procedure is similar if intra-articular steroids are to be given during arthrocentesis. It is generally helpful to drain the joint as dry as possible before injecting the medication, as it reduces the distention of the capsule, which can lead to pain and instability. Many steroid preparations are used that vary from short-acting to long-acting. The amount injected in large part depends on the potency of the preparation used and the size of the joint (smaller joints requiring less). Many rheumatologists mix steroids and a local anesthetic (e.g., lidocaine 1%) in equal parts to instill into the joint.

There is a concern over the potential of flocculation of the steroid preparation when it is mixed with local anesthetics that contain preservatives. Whether this problem is clinically significant is not established (Owen, 1993).

The response to injections varies and is difficult to predict. Generally, the more advanced the joint process, the less satisfactory is the response. The procedure can be repeated after 2 to 4 weeks if the response is suboptimal. If again no significant response is obtained, additional injections are not likely to be helpful. In some individuals, symptoms can be alleviated for a variable amount of time, usually weeks to months. The procedure can be repeated should symptoms recur. There is a theoretic concern that too frequent instillation of steroids may cause damage to the cartilage and ligamentous structures of the joint. In large joints such as the knee, injections should be limited to three or four a year. The same general rules should be applied to other joints.

USE OF NSAIDs IN RHEUMATIC DISEASES

Nonsteroidal anti-inflammatory drugs (NSAIDs) are among the most widely used drugs in the world. They appear in prescription and nonprescription forms and are used as analgesics for a number of conditions ranging from musculoskeletal complaints to headaches to surgical pain. They are also widely used as anti-inflammatory agents primarily for musculoskeletal disorders. NSAIDs come in a number of preparations that seem to proliferate each year. Physicians and patients alike are bewildered by the choices available, the differing dosing schedules, and the conflicting reports on efficacy and side effects of the various agents.

NSAIDs exert their effect presumably by suppression of prostaglandin synthesis, although other mechanisms may also be important. The inflammatory reactions that accompany rheumatic disease are complex, and prostaglandin production may not be the most important element in those processes. Moreover, inflammatory reactions may vary depending on the stage or activity of the disease even in individuals with the same rheumatic disease. This point may help explain the clinical observation that some patients respond well to a particular NSAID, whereas others with the same disease do not. It is usually not possible to predict a given individual's response to a particular NSAID. On the other hand, large studies suggest that most NSAIDs have comparable efficacy, and so most NSAIDs are generally equally effective at comparable doses.

In Table 39–3 NSAIDs have been classified on the basis of their chemical structure, dosing schedule, and dosing range. Because it is not possible to predict an individual's response to an NSAID, the prescribing process often becomes one of trial and error. For patients on chronic NSAID therapy, it may be best to use a preparation with once- or twice-a-day dosing. There are two strategies regarding the dose: Start low and build up as needed, or start with the maximum dose and reduce the dose to the smallest effective dose. In either case, it is important to allow an adequate therapeutic trial, usually at least 2 weeks, although patients may

TABLE 39–3. CLASSIFICATION OF NSAIDs

Class	Available Preparations*	Trade Name*	Dosing Schedule†	Dosage Range†	Comments‡
Salicylates	Aspirin	Various	q.i.d.	2.4–3.6 gm	Use salicylate level**
	Diflunisal	Dolobid	b.i.d.	500–1500 mg	Tinnitus
Phenylacetic acids	Diclofenac	Voltaren	b.i.d.	100–200 mg	Hepatitis
Carbo- and heterocyclic acids	Etodolac	Lodine	b.i.d. to q.i.d.	800–1200 mg	
	Indomethacin	Indocin	b.i.d.	75–200 mg	CNS problems
	Sulindac	Clinoril	b.i.d.	150–400 mg	Renal sparing?
	Tolmetin	Tolectin	t.i.d.	600–1800 mg	Pseudoproteinuria
Propionic acids	Ibuprofen	Motrin	q.i.d.	0.8–3.2 gm	Aseptic meningitis
	Naproxen	Naprosyn	b.i.d.	500–1000 mg	Allergic pneumonitis
	Ketoprofen	Orudis	t.i.d. to q.i.d.	150–300 mg	
	Oxaprozin	Daypro	q.d.	600–1200 mg	
	Flurbiprofen	Ansaid	b.i.d. to q.i.d.	200–300 mg	
	Fenoprofen	Nalfon	t.i.d. to q.i.d.	1.2–3.2 gm	Nephritis
Fenamic acids	Meclofenamate	Meclomen	t.i.d. to q.i.d.	200–400 mg	Diarrhea
Oxicams	Piroxicam	Feldene	q.d.	10–20 mg	
Nonacidic compounds	Nabumetone	Relafen	q.d.	1–2 gm	

* Lists only the most common preparations and trade names. Many are available as generic drugs.
† Recommended dosing schedule and dosages. They may vary depending on several factors, such as disease, age, renal function, and weight. Doses and schedule should be individualized.
‡ Special considerations or unusual side effects reported. Similar side effects may have been reported for other NSAIDs.
** Dose adjusted to attain salicylate level of 20 to 30 mg/dL, if tolerated, for anti-inflammatory effect.

continue to experience improvement beyond that time frame. If the therapeutic response is suboptimal, another NSAID, from a different class, may be tried. Some patients try several NSAIDs before finding one that helps. If a patient has failed five or six NSAIDs, he or she is not likely to respond to the others. At this point, patients may be frustrated and not wish to try other preparations. Persistence, though, may pay off.

The NSAIDs should not be used indiscriminately. They are associated with many side effects and drug interactions that should be kept in mind when prescribing them. Indeed, the widespread use of NSAIDs, prescription and nonprescription, has initiated a debate regarding their overuse and abuse. Careful consideration should be given to the expected benefits versus the potential side effects before prescribing these medications. Simple analgesics, such as acetaminophen, may be preferable, especially in elderly patients, patients with a history of significant intolerance to NSAIDs, those with a history of peptic ulcer disease, and those with renal dysfunction. Moreover, while on chronic NSAID therapy patients should have periodic laboratory tests including a CBC, urinalysis, and renal function assessment. Some NSAIDs require periodic monitoring of liver function tests as well, especially during the early stages of use.

Patients should be provided with clear instructions on the proper use of NSAIDs, and they should be reinforced at each visit. Most if not all of these drugs should be taken with food. It is important to define what constitutes food, as some patients take medication with coffee or a similar beverage. In addition, if a medication dose is forgotten, the stomach is usually empty several hours after a meal, so it may be preferable to simply skip the dose or take it with a light snack.

The most common side effects associated with these drugs are gastrointestinal and include stomach pain, indigestion, nausea, and reflux. The more serious complications include mucosal erosions and bleeding peptic ulcers. The true incidence of serious gastrointestinal complications is difficult to determine, but a number of studies have linked NSAIDs with an increased risk for these complications. Several medications have been used to decrease the gastrointestinal side effects, including sucralfate, H_2-blockers such as cimetidine and ranitidine, and more recently misoprostol. Studies indicate that misoprostol is effective, especially at full doses (200 μg q.i.d.), although at full doses patients may experience side effects (Agrawal et al., 1991; Graham et al., 1993).

Other side effects of these drugs include renal dysfunction, usually in the form of decreased renal function. It may manifest as a rise in serum creatinine, particularly in elderly patients, those with existing renal impairment, or those on diuretics (Sandler, 1991). Some patients experience sodium retention and edema, and others may develop new-onset hypertension or an exacerbation of heretofore controlled hypertension. Skin reactions, which are uncommon, include photosensitivity and erythema multiforme. Hematologic manifestations are primarily cytopenias. Hepatic effects include transaminase elevation and rarely hepatitis. Central nervous system involvement may include headache, dizziness, or aseptic meningitis.

RHEUMATIC DISEASES

Osteoarthritis

Osteoarthritis (OA) is characterized by changes in cartilage, bone, and synovium of joints. The cause of OA is unknown, but the disease appears to be multifactorial, leading to a common reaction in joint tissues (Hough, 1993). The main site of pathology appears to be the articulating cartilage, which undergoes degeneration. This change may lead to a low-level, secondary inflammatory process. OA is the most common joint problem. Affected joints include those of the hand (proximal interphalangeal joints (PIPs) or distal interphalangeal joints (DIPs), large weight-bearing joints such as the knee and hip, and the spine, especially the cervical and lumbar areas.

The incidence of OA clearly increases with age and appears to be more common in women than men. Other risk factors are less well defined. The issue of exercise as a cause for OA is not resolved. It appears that normal joints of individuals of all ages can tolerate exercise without leading to OA. On the other hand, people with abnormal joints, including those with injuries to ligaments, tendons, or menisci, may develop OA even in the absence of exercise (Lane and Buckwalter, 1993). The role of obesity is also unclear. Some studies suggest a relation between obesity and OA of the knee and the hands. It is not clear, though, that the mechanism involved is mechanical in nature (Felson, 1993). Regardless of the individual factors that can lead to OA, the pathogenic findings are similar and include cartilage degeneration, bone changes including osteophytes, and synovial changes usually in the form of localized synovitis.

Osteoarthritis is typically classified as primary (when no cause can be found) or secondary (when there is an identifiable underlying systemic or local process) (Table 39–4). It is always important to consider a systemic or neuropathic process as a cause of osteoarthritis because a different treatment plan may be required. Whether the process is primary or secondary, the joint symptoms are similar. The onset of symptoms is usually insidious. Initially, the symptoms tend to be episodic and are brought on by a change in the normal pattern of activity. As the disease progresses, symptoms become more persistent and include pain with activity and morning stiffness of the affected

TABLE 39–4. CLASSIFICATION OF OSTEOARTHRITIS

Primary or idiopathic OA
Peripheral joints
Spine
Other forms
  Erosive inflammatory osteoarthritis
  Chondromalacia patellae
  Diffuse idiopathic skeletal hyperostosis

Secondary OA
Trauma
Crystal deposition disease
  Calcium pyrophosphate disease (pseudogout)
  Monosodium urate (gout)
Neuropathic conditions
  Diabetes or tabes dorsalis
Systemic metabolic or endocrine disorders
  Hyperparathyroidism
  Acromegaly
  Hemochromatosis
  Wilson's disease
  Ochronosis
Underlying joint disease
  Rheumatoid arthritis
  Infection
  Fracture

From Mascots RW: Clinical and laboratory findings in osteoarthritis. *In* McCarty DJ, Koopman WJ (eds): Arthritis and Allied Conditions, 12th edition. Philadelphia, Lea & Febiger, 1993, with permission.

joint(s). Later, the pain may increase in intensity and can be brought on by minimal activity. There may be periods of exacerbation followed by more quiescent, though rarely asymptomatic, intervals. This pattern is accompanied by a progressive decline in joint mobility and in the patient's functional capacity. Patients may begin to experience rest pain especially at night. Swelling of the joint(s) appears and is usually due to bone proliferation about the joint or to joint effusions. Deformities may develop as the disease progresses. Patients may also develop crepitation, a sensation of grating that accompanies joint movement.

Clinical Pattern

The clinical pattern of OA varies. It may present as a monarticular process especially in the hip. OA may alternatively present as an oligoarticular disease with involvement of large weight-bearing joints and hands. In some patients the presentation is generalized (Fig. 39–1). Some specific sites of note are described in the following sections.

HAND INVOLVEMENT. Hand involvement in OA is common. There appears to be a hereditary component to OA of the hand. The most commonly involved joints are the DIPs, the PIPs, and the first carpometacarpal joint (Fig. 39–2). The metacarpophalangeal (MCP) joints are typically spared in OA. With hand OA, cysts begin to form over the lateral and medial aspects of the DIPs (called Heberden nodes) and the PIPs (called Bouchard nodes). Often this process begins in only one or two joints, although over a period of years many of the remaining DIPs and PIPs become involved. Deformities develop as the disease progresses. Despite these obvious deformities, hand function remains good.

HIP INVOLVEMENT. Osteoarthritis of the hip may develop as a monarticular process. The most common complaint is pain brought on by walking. The pain may be felt anteriorly over the groin but occasionally is referred to the knee or buttock. This point should be kept in mind especially in patients with knee symptoms. Stiffness of the joint is common. On examination there may be limited range of motion, especially internal rotation.

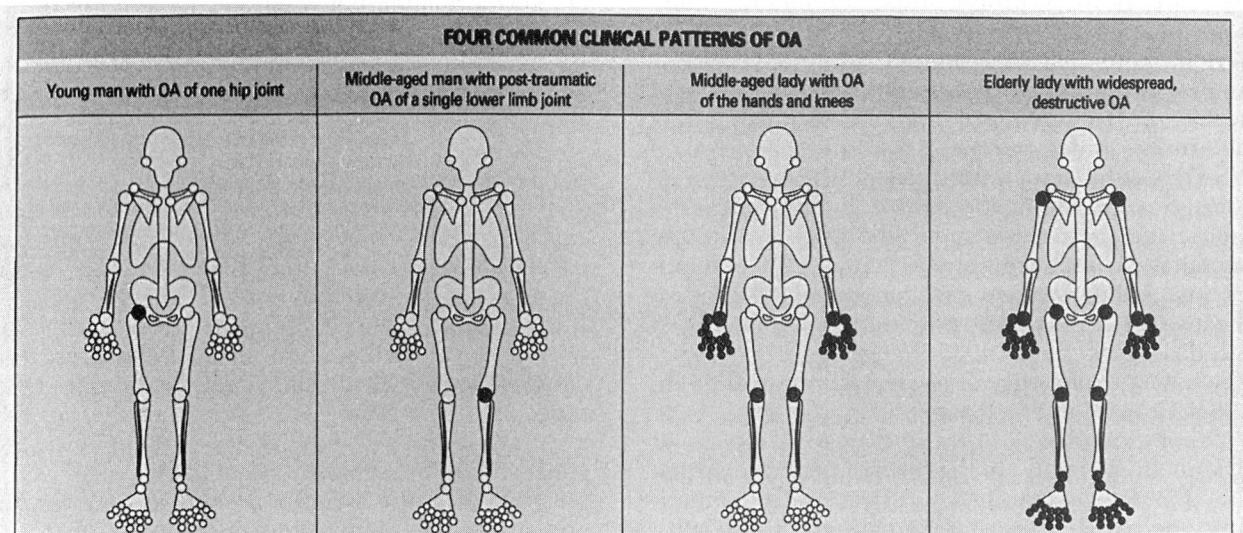

FIGURE 39–1. Four common clinical patterns of osteoarthritis. (From Dieppe P: Osteoarthritis: Clinical features and diagnostic problems. *In* Klippel JH, Dieppe, PA, eds: Rheumatology. London, CV Mosby, 1994, with permission.)

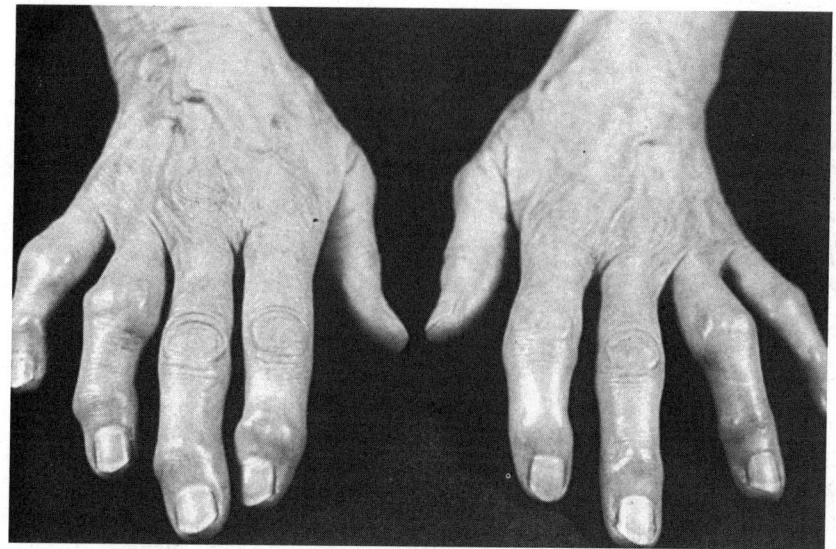

FIGURE 39–2. Osteoarthritis of the hands. Bony enlargement can be seen in the DIP and PIP joints in patients with osteoarthritis. (From the Clinical Slide Collection on the Rheumatic Diseases. Copyright 1991 by the American College of Rheumatology, with permission.)

KNEE INVOLVEMENT. The knee is comprised of three compartments—medial, lateral, and patello-femoral—and one or more of these compartments may be affected. The most common involvement is of the medial compartment. The clinical findings vary slightly depending on the compartment(s) involved. The typical presentation begins with pain on walking and morning stiffness. There may be accompanying quadriceps muscle atrophy, limitation of motion (especially full extension), and crepitation. Deformity may also be evident: Medial compartment disease may lead to a varus deformity and lateral compartment disease to a valgus deformity.

Diagnosis

No specific laboratory test exists for OA. In the absence of other conditions, laboratory tests are essentially normal. The ESR is normal except in patients with erosive OA, in which case it may be moderately elevated. The RF assay is negative. Because OA occurs primarily in the older age group, the ANA assay may be weakly positive. The latter is a nonspecific finding that does not suggest a connective tissue disease such as rheumatoid arthritis or SLE. Radiographs are helpful. The characteristic radiographic changes of OA include joint space narrowing and bony sclerosis. Osteophyte formation is also characteristic of OA and does not occur in rheumatoid arthritis (Fig. 39–3).

Treatment

The management of OA is directed at controlling the pain and maintaining joint function. It is not clear that any of the currently available forms of therapy halt disease progression. There is no known therapeutic agent that can reverse the process, although spontaneous regressions have been documented. Despite this fact, it would be wrong to conclude that nothing should be done.

Physical therapy and joint protection are important components of therapy. It is important to reverse muscle atrophy and maintain muscle groups about the affected joints. This point is important for maintaining joint stability and improving function, especially range of motion. The exercise regimen need not be grueling; on the contrary, it should be designed to gently increase muscle tone and joint range of motion without jarring the affected joints. It is important that the patient realize the importance of this aspect of care. Exercise should be reviewed with the patient at each encounter to reinforce this message. Devices such as slip-on-braces or splints may be used to help stabilize affected joints.

Medications are used primarily for two reasons: to control pain and to fight inflammation. The most commonly used analgesic is acetaminophen. This medication is well tolerated, has few side effects, and appears to be effective, at least for the short term (Bradley et al., 1991). NSAIDs are also commonly used to control pain and fight inflammation. Although anti-inflammatory agents are used, it is not clear that inflammation is important in the pathophysiology of OA. The use of NSAIDs for OA is widespread but not without detractors. There is a theoretic concern that the use of NSAIDs may accelerate the disease process. Yet there is little doubt that NSAIDs effectively control the symptoms of OA and improve a patient's functional status (Brandt, 1993). The choice of one class of medication over another depends on a number of factors. One must carefully compare the risks of NSAID toxicity with the expected benefit. In the elderly, in those with renal disease, or in those with a history of gastrointestinal intolerance to NSAIDs, the use of analgesics alone may be preferable. When possible, the patient should participate in the decision regarding therapy.

For patients with significant disability or signifi-

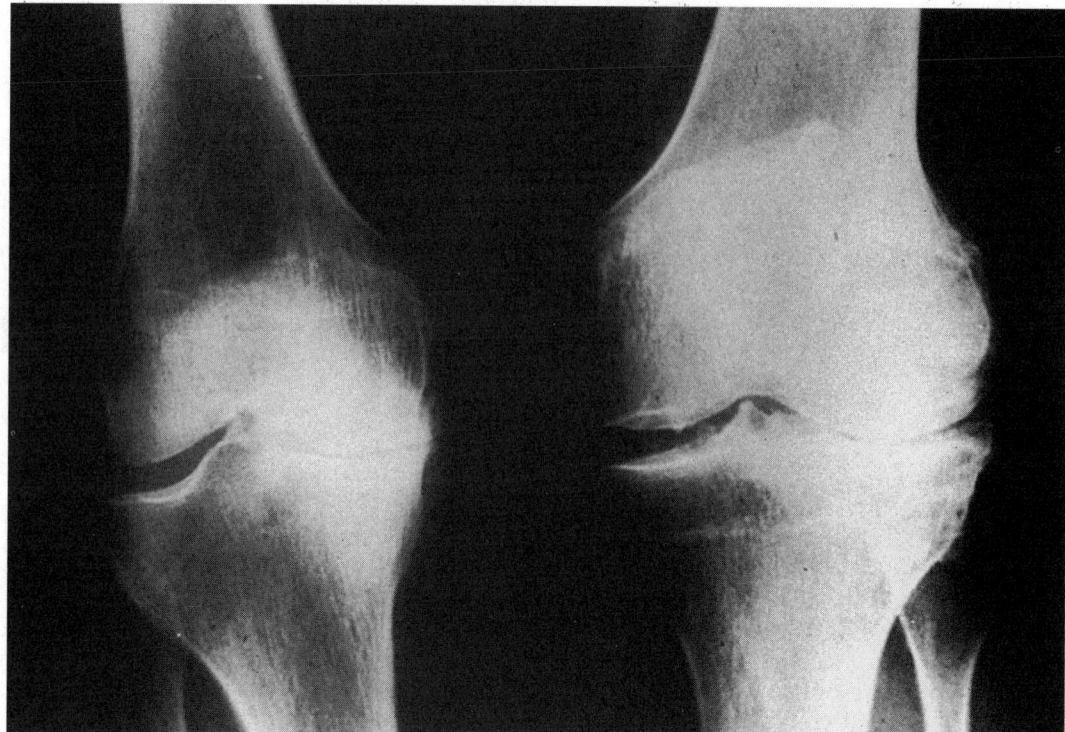

FIGURE 39–3. Osteoarthritis of the knees. In the left knee there is joint space narrowing of the lateral compartment; in the right knee narrowing is seen in the medial compartment. In addition, bony sclerosis of adjacent bony margins is evident. Unicompartmental joint space narrowing and the reactive bony changes (osteophytes) help differentiate osteoarthritis from rheumatoid arthritis. (From the Clinical Slide Collection on the Rheumatic Diseases. Copyright 1991, by the American College of Rheumatology, with permission.)

cant pain not responsive to medical treatment, surgical options should be discussed, most commonly partial or complete joint replacement. Surgery is likely to bring about significant pain relief. Functional improvement is more difficult to predict and depends in part on postoperative attention to physical therapy.

Rheumatoid Arthritis

Rheumatoid arthritis (RA) is characteristically a symmetric, polyarticular disease. Although its name clearly points to the main site of pathology—the joints—the disease is a systemic process that frequently causes constitutional symptoms and may involve other organ systems. The cause of the disease is unknown. The main pathologic finding is proliferative synovitis. Although arthritis is frequently thought of as a disease of the elderly, RA belies this misconception. It can be seen in adults of any age but has its peak onset during the fourth and fifth decades. In the United States the prevalence appears to be around 1 per cent in the white population, and similar rates have been reported among African-Americans. The disease is more common in women with a female/male ratio of around 3:1. A frequently overlooked fact is that

severe RA is associated with decreased life expectancy when compared to controls or the general population. Patients with mild disease have a life expectancy similar to that of the general population (Lawrence, 1994).

The disease may present in a number of ways. The most common presentation is gradual. Initially symptoms are mild and may involve only a few joints, especially in the hands. Symptoms may be intermittent but become persistent and increase in severity over a period of weeks to months. Typically, patients seek help after many weeks of discomfort. Occasionally, other presentations supervene. Some patients present with an abrupt onset of symptoms and many joints involved. Rarely, patients present with a monarticular process especially involving large joints before involving the others.

Whatever the presentation, there are features of the process that point to the diagnosis. The American College of Rheumatology has developed useful criteria that focus on the salient features of RA (Table 39–5). Joint stiffness is a characteristic clinical finding in patients with RA; it is most pronounced in the morning and usually lasts more than an hour although in some patients it persists all day. The stiffness is alleviated by movement and heat.

TABLE 39–5.   1987 REVISED CRITERIA FOR THE CLASSIFICATION OF RHEUMATOID ARTHRITIS*

Morning stiffness of at least 1 hour†
Arthritis in at least three joint areas simultaneously due to swelling or joint fluid†
Arthritis of the hand or wrist joints†
Symmetric arthritis†
Subcutaneous rheumatoid nodules
Radiographic changes typical of RA in hands and wrists
Positive serum rheumatoid factor

* For classification, a patient is said to have RA if at least four criteria are satisfied.
† Must be present at least 6 weeks.
From Arnett FC, Edworthy SM, Bloch DA, et al: The American Rheumatism Association 1987 revised criteria for the classification of rheumatoid arthritis. Arthritis Rheum 31:315, 1988, with permission.

The arthritis is typically characterized by swelling, tenderness, and warmth. These symptoms are due to the proliferative synovitis. There is swelling of soft tissues that tends to be soft or "boggy," in contrast to the swelling of OA, which is firm and "bony." Palpation of the joint elicits tenderness. The arthritis should involve at least three joints, such as knees, wrists, ankles. In addition, involvement of the hand is particularly helpful to the diagnosis and for distinguishing RA from OA. Involvement of the PIPs, MCP, and wrist is typical of RA; the DIPs are typically spared (Fig. 39–4). The presence of simultaneous symmetric involvement of right and left joints is also important. It should be noted that this symmetry need not be absolute. Additionally, patients may be unaware of subclinical involvement, so it is always important to do a full joint examination on patients suspected of having RA. If allowed to progress, RA may produce significant and characteristic deformities and disability. Ulnar deviation of the fingers is characteristic. Other changes include subluxations, tendon

contractures, atlantoaxial subluxation, and varus or valgus joint deformities.

Other criteria point to the systemic nature of RA. Rheumatoid nodules are firm and frequently develop over pressure areas. They are most frequently seen over the extensor surface of the arms, over the Achilles tendon, and the fingers and toes. They can be detected in as many as 20 per cent of RA patients, usually in those who are RF-positive. They are most frequently seen in patients with severe disease and may regress with treatment (Matteson et al., 1994). The presence of serum RF is also a classification criterion. The test may be negative in patients with clinical RA especially during the early stages of disease. A small percentage of patients remain RF-negative despite longstanding clinical evidence of RA.

Radiographic evaluation of patients suspected of RA is important. Radiographic changes typical of RA are considered important for establishing the diagnosis, deciding therapeutic intervention, and monitoring disease progression. The best places to observe these changes are the hands and wrists if there is clinical involvement. Changes considered typical of RA are marginal bone erosions and periarticular osteopenia (Fig. 39–5).

The clinical course of RA is highly variable. In some patients the disease is monophasic with active clinical symptoms being present for weeks or months followed by a remission that may be permanent. Other patients experience progressive disease characterized by increasing symptoms and additive joint involvement. The most common clinical course, however, is polycyclic, which is characterized by intermittent disease without complete remissions.

Extra-articular features include the presence of rheumatoid nodules. Other features include vascu-

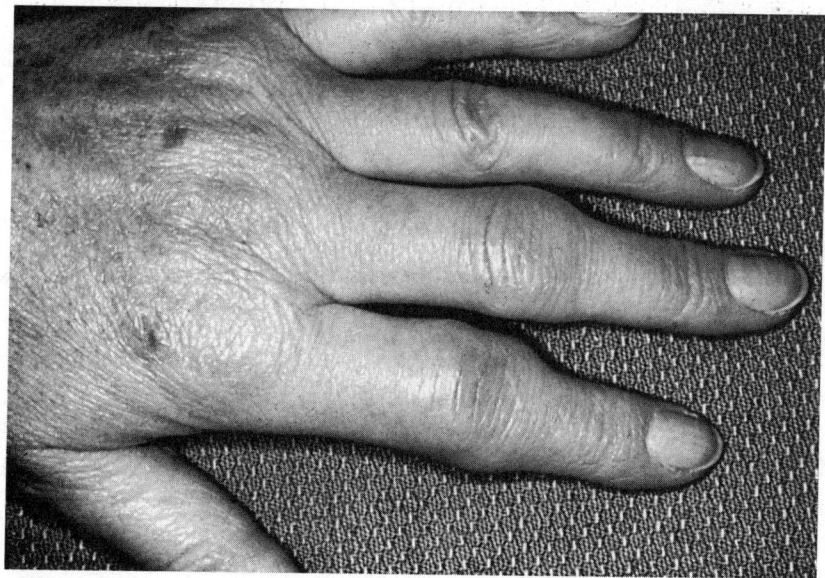

FIGURE 39–4. Hand involvement in rheumatoid arthritis. Soft tissue swelling is evident in the PIPs. The DIPs are spared. (From the Clinical Slide Collection on the Rheumatic Diseases. Copyright 1991, by the American College of Rheumatology, with permission.)

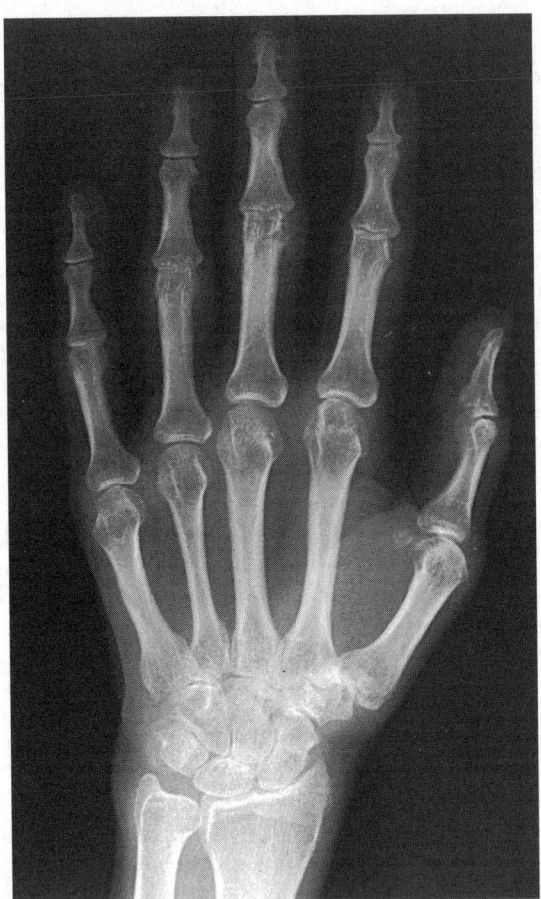

FIGURE 39–5. Radiographic changes of early RA of the hand showing soft tissue swelling and periarticular osteoporosis around the PIPs and MCPs (top). Joint space narrowing and an early erosion can be seen in the PIP of the fourth finger (bottom). (From Dieppe PA, Bacon PA, Bamji AN, Watt I: Rheumatoid arthritis of the hands and feet. *In* Slide Atlas of Rheumatology. London, Gower Medical Publishing, 1987, with permission.)

litis, especially of the digits, and interstitial pneumonitis. Felty syndrome consists of RA in the presence of splenomegaly and neutropenia. Many extra-articular features tend to be prominent after years of disease activity.

The treatment of RA should be multifaceted and multidisciplinary. The major goals of therapy are to control the synovitis and pain and to restore or maintain the functional status of the patient. Rheumatologists have for years used a treatment pyramid to outline the steps in the treatment process. This pyramid provides for a stepwise progression in the treatment plan based on the clinical course of the disease and the response to treatment. Although still widely used, since the 1980s there have been many challenges to this approach (Pincus and Wolfe, 1991). Although often not emphasized, the base of the pyramid incorporates many crucial aspects of care, including proper education of the patient and family as to the nature of the disease. Upon initial diagnosis patients are

often frightened and usually expect the worst outcome. With education and time, patients understand that they have a measure of control over their disease and can actively participate in its management. It is therefore important to obtain patient understanding and approval of the treatment plan. Only then can the best possible outcome be attained. Many patients require counseling and benefit from talking and meeting with other RA patients. Additionally, rest should be emphasized as important. Although rest may seem impossible for a busy mother or others with equally demanding vocations, patients should attempt to modify their work-without-rest habits to any extent possible. Physical therapy and joint conservation are also important aspects of care and are needed throughout the course of the disease. By emphasizing this conservatism constantly, patients recognize the importance physicians place on this aspect of care, the goals being the maintenance or restoration of function and the prevention of joint deformities.

Pharmacologic treatment begins with anti-inflammatory agents. For many years aspirin was the medication of choice. However, plain aspirin is poorly tolerated because of gastrointestinal irritation at the required anti-inflammatory doses. Aspirin is associated with other side effects as well, including tinnitus and hearing loss. Enteric-coated aspirin as well as nonacetylated forms such as choline magnesium trisalicylate (Trilisate) or salsalate (Disalcid) produce fewer gastrointestinal problems than plain aspirin and may be used. During treatment with aspirin products, salicylate levels should be checked periodically and the patient's hearing closely monitored. Today NSAIDs are used more frequently. Virtually all of the currently available NSAIDs have been used to treat RA. Because treatment is prolonged, it is generally best to use a long-acting agent that is given once or twice a day. It is preferable to start with the maximum dose and to make sure the patient is on the proper dose for at least a 2- to 4-week period before evaluating the efficacy of the drug. If there is a good response, the dose can be adjusted downward, symptoms permitting. It is also important for the physician to give proper instruction on how to take the medication, discuss the side effects, and re-enforce these issues at each visit.

The use of steroids for treatment of RA is controversial (Weissman, 1993). Physicians should resist the temptation to use steroids, instead of NSAIDs, as the first anti-inflammatory agent. RA patients requiring steroids should have active disease, and treatment options should be planned in consultation with a rheumatologist. Prednisone may be used at low doses (5 to 15 mg/day) in an attempt to bring symptoms quickly under control. In this setting, prednisone is used in conjunction with disease-modifying antirheumatic drugs (see below) until the latter have had a chance to exert their beneficial effect. Once clinical improvement has been observed, the dose of prednisone should be tapered. Even at these low doses, the use of prednisone is associated with side effects. The concomitant use of both NSAIDs and steroids, however, raises the risk for gastrointestinal problems (Piper et al., 1991). To reduce the osteopenic effects, patients should attempt to maintain some level of activity and take supplemental calcium and vitamin D (Lukert and Raisz, 1990).

The use of disease-modifying antirheumatic drugs (DMARDs) constitute the next tier of the treatment pyramid. They consist of a group of unrelated medications that seem to have a more profound effect on the disease course than do NSAIDs. These medicines include gold (either intramuscular or oral preparations), D-penicillamine, hydroxychloroquine, sulfasalazine, and methotrexate. In controlled studies these drugs have proved to be superior to placebo for alleviating the signs and symptoms of RA. There are some difficult questions regarding these medications: When should these drugs be started? Which drug should be used first? There are no easy answers, and consultation with a rheumatologist and input from the patient may be required.

The current inclination is to start these drugs earlier in the disease course than past practice has dictated. The goal is to control the synovitis before it can cause irreversible damage to the joints. Also, combination therapy with two or more DMARDs is currently being advocated. DMARDs should be considered for the patient with relatively recent onset of disease who is showing radiographic changes, such as erosions or joint space narrowing. For patients with more advanced but still active disease, these drugs may still be helpful for preventing additional joint damage, but they do not reverse existing damage. Factors that should be weighted when deciding which DMARD to use include the course of the disease, the potential benefit versus the toxicity of the drug, and the patient's own comfort with and understanding of the expected benefits and side effects of these medications. Treatment of extra-articular features is essentially similar to treatment of the underlying RA. Patients with resistant features may benefit from more aggressive therapy with cytotoxic agents.

Surgical therapies are of benefit in some patients. Surgical synovectomy should be considered in patients who, despite adequate medical treatment, have persistent localized synovitis. For example, synovectomy may be useful in the hands and wrist where persistent disease may lead to tendon rupture. In patients with joint destruction and pain not responsive to medical management, joint replacement should be considered. The main indication for surgery is pain control. Functional improvement depends on a number of factors including postoperative physical therapy.

Crystal Arthropathies

The presence of crystals in the joint space can under certain circumstances activate inflammatory mediators, resulting in joint swelling and pain. The crystals most commonly encountered clinically are monosodium urate, which leads to gouty arthritis, and calcium pyrophosphate (CPPD), which leads to pseudogout, so called because clinically it resembles gout. The best way to distinguish the two is by direct examination of synovial fluid for crystals. Certain optical properties readily distinguish one crystal from another (see Synovial Fluid Analysis, above).

Gout

Gout generally affects men more frequently than women especially in the younger age groups. The peak age of onset in men is 40 to 50 years; in women it usually is age 60-plus. Gout has three stages: (1) asymptomatic hyperuricemia; (2) acute gout; and (3) tophaceous gout. Hyperuricemia antedates the clinical manifestations of gout by many years. Generally, the higher the serum uric acid level, the earlier the clinical manifestations appear. During this time patients have no complaints referable to the hyperuricemia. Some patients, however, experience urolithiasis with uric acid stones. The first bout of gouty arthritis is monarticular in most individuals. Usually, it occurs at the first metatarsophalangeal joint, constituting classic podagra, which is characterized by an acute onset of pain, swelling, redness, and warmth. The symptoms tend to reach maximum intensity quickly, usually within 24 hours. The pain is typically described as intense, and the area tends to be sensitive to even the lightest touch. There may be constitutional symptoms, such as low grade fever, and laboratory results may indicate an elevated white blood cell count.

After the first gouty attack, patients typically experience a disease-free interval. The likelihood of a subsequent attack depends on a number of factors including the serum uric acid level. Subsequent episodes are similar to the initial presentation, and frequently patients recognize the onset of a new attack much earlier in the clinical course. Gouty arthritis may appear in other joints of the lower extremity with more frequency than in joints of the upper extremity. As the disease progresses, large collections of monosodium urate, called tophi, develop especially around the fingers and toes and over the olecranon bursae. Patients develop persistent joint symptoms and on examination have chronic synovitis that is polyarticular and symmetric; it may be confused with rheumatoid arthritis.

Because gout usually presents as a monarticular arthritis the differential diagnosis should include other monarticular processes, such as trauma and septic arthritis. The diagnosis of gout is best confirmed by the presence of hyperuricemia and gouty crystals in synovial fluid. Synovial fluid stains and cultures are negative. A radiograph of the affected joint is helpful for excluding significant trauma and may reveal findings typical of gout, such as erosions or opacities due to tophi. However, these signs may be absent especially early in the disease course.

Treatment of gout depends on the clinical stage (Table 39–6). In patients with asymptomatic hyperuricemia, no specific treatment is recommended. Dietary changes may help but are seldom followed. Patients should refrain from foods high in purine, such as organ meats and some seafood. Excessive alcohol ingestion, including beer, should be avoided. Medication that can increase the serum uric acid, such as diuretics, should be avoided if possible.

Patients who present with acute gouty arthritis can be managed in a number of ways. The goals of treatment are to control the inflammatory process and avoid alterations of serum uric acid. The most commonly used agents are NSAIDs and colchicine. It is important to start treatment as soon as possible to ensure a prompt response. NSAIDs are used more frequently and are effective. Although many of the initial studies on the use of NSAIDs for gout were done with indomethacin, most of the newer NSAIDs are equally effective. It is important to use an agent that has a rapid onset of action, and high doses should be given initially. The duration of treatment is generally about a week—less if the attack subsides sooner. Colchicine can also be used for acute gout. Oral and intravenous preparations are available. When using colchicine it is important to remember that treatment should continue until one of three endpoints is reached: (1) resolution of the gouty arthritis; (2) development of side effects; or (3) the maximum dose of colchicine is reached. The usual oral dose is 0.5 mg initially, followed by 0.5 mg every hour until the attack resolves, the patient develops side effects such as nausea or diarrhea, or a maximum dose of 6 mg is reached. The use of intravenous

colchicine is controversial, and it should be used only by those familiar with the drug.

The treatment of gout between episodes of arthritis varies. Although the disease continues to progress unless the hyperuricemia is corrected, some patients may not experience a new attack for months or even years. Patients can be instructed to take NSAIDs at the first sign of a new attack so that new attacks of gout may be successfully aborted by the patient. For patients with more frequent attacks, colchicine is effective in reducing the frequency of gouty episodes. The usual dose is 0.5 mg once or twice a day.

Some patients, particularly those with tophaceous gout, benefit from correction of hyperuricemia. There are two types of drug used for this purpose: drugs that enhance renal excretion of uric acid (uricosuric agents) and those that decrease uric acid production (xanthine oxidase inhibitors). During induction of normal uricemia, patients are at increased risk for bouts of gouty arthritis. Thus it is usually necessary to keep patients on colchicine 0.5 mg once or twice a day to prevent these bouts. Once the desired serum uric acid level is reached, colchicine therapy should continue for several months. The treatment of gouty attacks during this stage is similar to the treatment outlined above. Again, care must be taken to avoid changes in the patient's serum uric acid during the acute attacks.

Uricosuric agents should be avoided in patients who excrete excessive amounts of uric acid or those with a history of uric acid stones, as their use increases the risk for such stones. In addition, patients with impaired renal function or decreased renal clearance may not benefit from these agents. If uricosuric agents are used, high fluid intake should be maintained. The goal is to decrease serum uric acid levels to less than 7 mg/dL. The most commonly used uricosuric drug is probenecid, and the usual starting dose is 250 mg twice a day. The dose can be slowly increased every 2 to 4 weeks. Most patients achieve target serum uric acid levels on a dose of 1 gm daily, but higher doses may be needed. Another uricosuric agents is sulfinpyrazone. The starting dose is 50 mg twice a day, gradually increasing it to 300 to 400 mg in three or four divided doses.

Allopurinol is the only xanthine oxidase inhibitor available in the United States. It blocks the conversion of xanthine and hypoxanthine to uric acid and thus lowers serum uric acid. The usual starting dose is 100 mg daily. The dose can be increased by 50 to 100 mg every 2 to 4 weeks depending on the serum uric acid level. Most individuals require 300 mg a day to achieve a target serum uric acid level less than 7 mg/dL. Patients with renal disease should receive smaller doses.

Pseudogout

The term pseudogout refers to an acute monarthritis that clinically resembles gout but is

TABLE 39–6. TREATMENT OF GOUTY ARTHRITIS

Stage of Disease	Treatment Options
Asymptomatic hyperuricemia	Dietary changes including no excessive alcohol ingestion
	Avoidance of drugs that increase serum uric acids
Acute gouty arthritis	NSAIDs
	Colchicine
	Avoidance of changes in serum uric acid
Tophaceous gout	Uricosuric agents
	Allopurinol
	Colchicine prophylaxis
	NSAIDs as needed
	Dietary changes

TABLE 39–7. COMPARISON OF GOUT AND PSEUDOGOUT

Parameter	Gout	Pseudogout
Male/female ratio	2:1 to 7:1	4:1
Peak age (years)	40–50	>60
Most common joint	First MTP	Knee
Serum urate	Elevated	May be normal
Radiology	Erosions	Chondrocalcinosis
Crystals		
Type	Monosodium urate	Calcium pyrophosphate
Shape	Thin needles	Small, rod-shaped
Birefringence	Strong	Weak

Adapted from Cohen MG, Emmerson BT: Gout. *In* Klippel JH, Dieppe PA (eds): *Rheumatology.* London, CV Mosby, 1994, with permission.

caused by CPPD crystals and not uric acid crystals (Table 39–7). The etiology of this disease is unknown. There is a strong association between pseudogout and osteoarthritis. Certain metabolic states such as hyperparathyroidism may predispose to this disorder. The disease is more common in the elderly and most frequently involves the knee joint followed by the wrist, shoulder, and ankle. Like gout, the onset is sudden, with peak intensity usually reached within 24 hours. The involved joint is swollen, painful, and tender to palpation. It may also be accompanied by systemic features such as a low grade fever; and as in the case of gout, the differential diagnosis should include septic arthritis. Diagnosis is based on the finding of CPPD crystals on synovial fluid examination. Radiographs may demonstrate chondrocalcinosis (Fig. 39–6).

Treatment of pseudogout is best accomplished by aspirating the synovial fluid from the involved joint and injecting the joint with steroids, which usually results in prompt relief. For patients in whom a relative contraindication exists for arthrocentesis or if the patient refuses, NSAIDs are used with success. However, care should be exercised with the use of NSAIDs especially in the elderly, those with renal impairment, or those with a history of peptic ulcer disease due to side effects. In such cases, analgesics may be used until the attack subsides.

Spondyloarthropathies

The spondyloarthropathies constitute a group of related disorders characterized by an inflammatory arthritis of the spine associated with a peripheral oligoarthritis. These entities are compared in Table 39–8. These diseases appear to have a striking association with the HLA-B27 haplotype. This relation is clearly important, but testing for HLA-B27 is rarely necessary and should be done only if the clinical and radiographic findings are not diagnostic. Spinal involvement is characterized by sacroiliitis, an inflammatory arthritis of the sacroiliac joint leading to chronic low back pain. Radiography may demonstrate joint erosions that lead to an apparent widening of the joint (Fig. 39–7). As the disease progresses, bony bridges form that eventually lead to complete ankylosis of the joint. Another characteristic feature of this group of diseases is the presence of an enthesopathy (an enthesis is the site of insertion of a tendon, ligament, or articular capsule). Patients with spondyloarthropathies may develop an inflammatory enthesopathy that leads to many of the spinal, articular, and periarticular symptoms common in these disorders. Calcification may occur at these sites, producing the characteristic radiographic changes: syndesmophytes, calcaneal spurs, and ossification near joints and around the pelvic area.

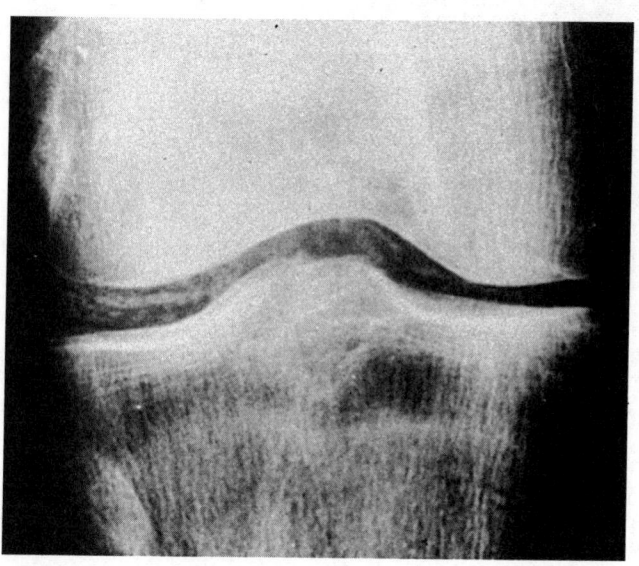

FIGURE 39–6. Radiography of knee showing chondrocalcinosis. There are calcifications of the menisci and articular cartilage. The calcifications, though linear, are not smooth and continuous but interrupted by multiple focal deposits. (From the Clinical Slide Collection on the Rheumatic Diseases. Copyright 1991, by the American College of Rheumatology, with permission.)

TABLE 39–8.   SPONDYLOARTHROPATHIES

Characteristic	Ankylosing Spondylitis	Reiter Syndrome	Psoriatic Arthritis	Enteropathic Arthopathy
Age of onset	Young adult to middle age	Young to middle age	Young to middle age	Young to middle age
Male/female ratio	3:1	4:1	1:1	1:1
Sacroiliitis or spondylitis	Almost 100%	< 50%	~ 20%	< 20%
Peripheral arthritis	~ 25%	~ 90%	~ 95%	15–20%
HLA-B27 (Whites)	~ 90%	~ 75%	< 50%*	~ 50%*
Eye involvement†	25–30%	~ 50%	< 20%	~ 15%

* HLA-B27 positivity higher in those with sacroiliitis or spondylitis.
† Predominantly conjunctivitis in Reiter syndrome and psoriatic arthritis; uveitis in the other disorders.
Adapted from Arnett FC, Khan MA, Wilkens RF: A new look at ankylosing spondylitis. Patient Care 23(19):82, 1989, with permission.

Ankylosing Spondylitis

With ankylosing spondylitis the musculoskeletal involvement is usually spinal with a typical presentation being a young man with chronic low back pain. Because the underlying process is inflammatory, patients often complain of stiffness of the lower back that improves with activity. Other areas of the spine may be involved as the disease progresses. Thus patients may develop thoracic and cervical spine symptoms often associated with a decreased range of motion of the affected areas. The most commonly tested anatomic sites for decreased range of motion are lumbar spine flexion and expansile chest diameter during inspiration. Lumbar motion can be measured using the Schober test done with the patient standing erect. One mark is placed midline over the back at the level of the fifth lumbar vertebrae and another mark 10 cm above it. The patient is asked to flex at the hips without bending the knees. For normal individuals the distance between the two lines should increase to 15 cm or more. An abnormal value is a distance less than or equal to 14 cm (Kahn, 1994). In addition to spinal involvement, patients may experience an asymmetric oligoarthritis often characterized by pain associated

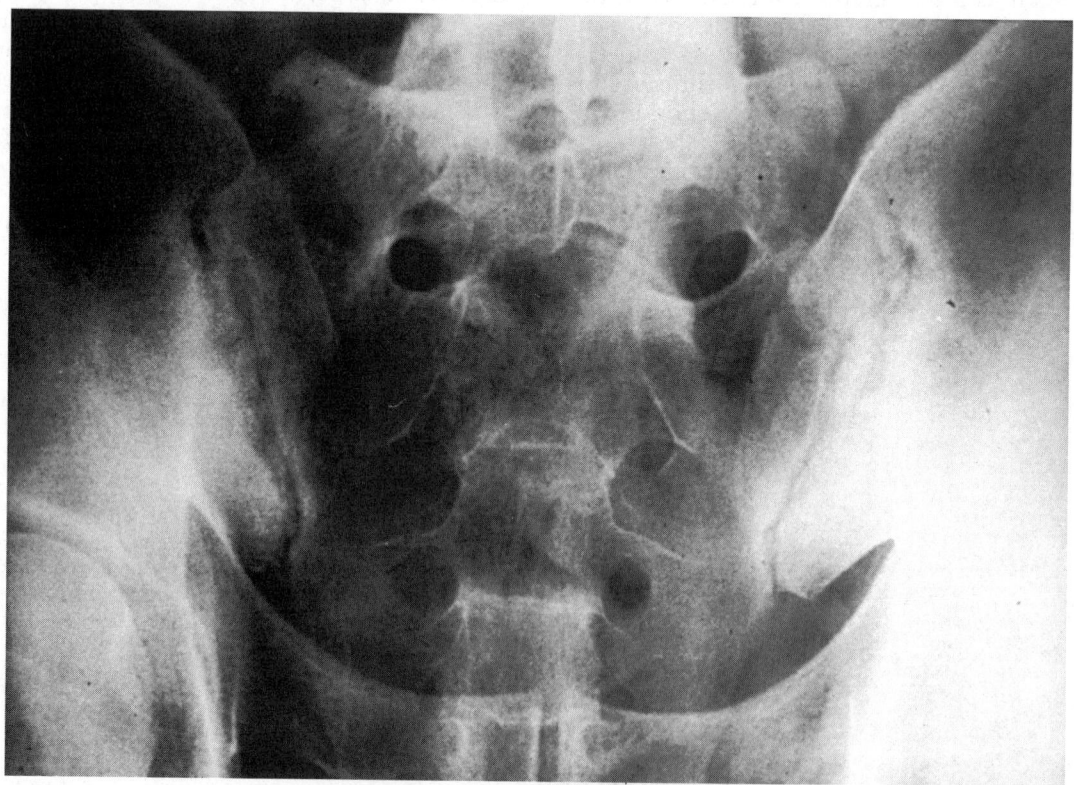

FIGURE 39–7.   Radiographs of sacroiliac joints. Subchondral bone resorption and irregularity of the joint space has given rise to pseudowidening. Increased sclerosis is present around the sacroiliac joint. These changes occur relatively early. (From the Clinical Slide Collection on the Rheumatic Diseases. Copyright 1991, by the American College of Rheumatology, with permission.)

with swelling and stiffness of the involved joint. The most commonly involved joints are the large joints of the lower extremity, such as the hip or knee. The most common nonarticular problem encountered in these patients is anterior uveitis.

The diagnosis is based on the constellation of symptoms, demonstration of reduced motion of the lumbar spine or chest wall, or radiographic evidence for sacroiliitis. Treatment is directed at controlling the symptoms and maintaining range of motion of the affected areas. No medication exists today that can effectively stop radiographic progression of the disease. Physical therapy, especially of the back, is important, and a physical therapist should be included as a part of the patient's health team. Therapeutic goals include maintaining range of motion and proper posture. The most commonly used medications are NSAIDs, which can provide symptomatic relief of the pain and stiffness and allow for more pain-free physical therapy. Treatment of the uveitis should be accomplished via an ophthalmology referral.

Psoriatic Arthritis

The association between psoriasis and arthritis is well documented. This diagnosis should be considered in patients with psoriasis who present with arthritis. However, patients with psoriasis may also develop osteoarthritis or other forms of arthritis. Five distinct patterns of psoriatic arthritis have been described, not all of which have spinal involvement: (1) DIP-predominant disease characterized by involvement of the DIPs; (2) polyarticular disease characterized by a symmetric polyarthritis similar to rheumatoid arthritis; (3) arthritis mutilans characterized by a destructive process involving the hands; (4) asymmetric oligoarticular pattern; and (5) spondylitis. In any given patient there may be an overlap of patterns (Moll and Wright, 1973). Clinical findings depend on the pattern of involvement. The peripheral arthritis is inflammatory in nature and is associated with joint swelling, warmth, and tenderness. Symptoms usually include stiffness, pain, and loss of function; but patients may also experience periarticular pain as well as pain about the pelvis, chest wall, and shoulders. These symptoms are due to the enthesopathy typical of this disease. Symptoms of spinal involvement are similar to those of ankylosing spondylitis.

The diagnosis is based on clinical evidence of psoriasis, including nail changes and an inflammatory peripheral or spinal arthritis (or both). Laboratory testing may reveal an elevated ESR, and radiographs may document the presence of sacroiliitis, erosive arthritis, or periostitis. Patients are typically RF- and ANA-negative.

Management is directed at controlling the inflammation and maintaining function. Additionally, the skin disease may require treatment with topical medications, including tar, anthralin, and corticosteroids. For more severe cases, a dermatologist should be consulted to consider oral methoxsalen plus ultraviolet light (PUVA) or other systemic forms of therapy. The musculoskeletal complaints are usually treated initially with NSAIDs. The choice of NSAID depends on the patient's response and tolerance to the medication. Some reports suggest that NSAIDs exacerbate the psoriasis. If so, the NSAID should be changed to a different class. In patients with refractory peripheral arthritis unresponsive to NSAIDs, DMARDs may be used. The most commonly used DMARDs for psoriatic arthritis are methotrexate and gold, although others have been used successfully. There is a concern that antimalarials exacerbate the psoriasis and are thus generally avoided. Methotrexate has the added advantage of alleviating the skin disease as well (Gladman, 1992).

Reiter's Syndrome

Also termed reactive arthritis, Reiter's syndrome consists of an asymmetric predominantly lower limb oligoarthritis. Other manifestations include tendinitis such as of the Achilles tendon. Reiter's syndrome is frequently associated with conjunctivitis, urethritis, or both; and there may be other extra-articular features such as keratoderma blennorrhagia. These characteristic hyperkeratotic skin changes may occur in the plantar areas (Fig. 39–8). The syndrome typically follows an infection, usually of the gastrointestinal or genitourinary system (Kingsley and Panayi, 1992). It has also been seen in association with acquired immunodeficiency syndrome (AIDS), and consideration should be giving to testing high risk patients for the presence of antibodies to human immunodeficiency virus (HIV).

The articular manifestations are treated primarily with NSAIDs. Because treatment duration is generally prolonged, once or twice a day NSAID dosing is preferred. Intra-articular steroids can also be used for the involved joints (see Arthrocentesis, above). For refractory cases other drugs, such as sulfasalazine, azathioprine, or methotrexate, have been used with some success. Although infections seem to precipitate Reiter's syndrome, at the time of diagnosis there is often little clinical evidence for such an etiology. The role of antibiotics in the treatment and prevention of new attacks is controversial. Some studies suggest a potential role for tetracycline (Lauhio et al., 1991). Cutaneous manifestations are generally responsive to keratolytic agents or topical steroids.

Arthritis Associated with Inflammatory Bowel Disease

Ulcerative colitis and Crohn's disease are associated with peripheral and spinal arthritis. The peripheral involvement is in the form of an oligoarthritis that frequently involves large joints particularly of the lower extremity. Articular mani-

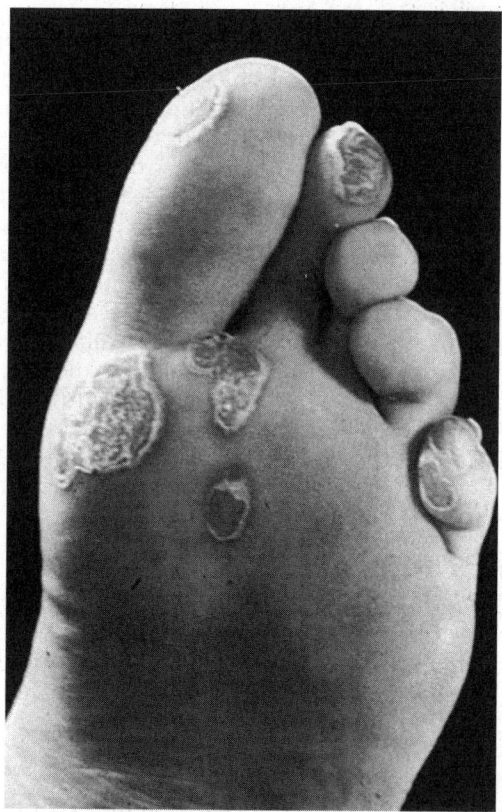

FIGURE 39–8. Discrete, circinate, scaly, and plaque-like lesions on the foot are due to Reiter's syndrome and may resemble psoriasis. (From the Clinical Slide Collection on the Rheumatic Diseases. Copyright 1991, by the American College of Rheumatology, with permission.)

festations tend to correlate with periods of active bowel disease. Sacroiliitis and other spinal involvement may also occur, though tending to be independent of the activity of the bowel disease. Occasionally, articular manifestations occur in the absence of intestinal symptomatology. Thus a search for occult inflammatory bowel disease is necessary in some patients.

Treatment is directed against the underlying bowel disease. NSAIDs have been used for the articular manifestations but should be used cautiously in light of the bowel disease. Spinal involvement can be treated as in patients with ankylosing spondylitis.

Septic Arthritis

Infections of the joint space constitute one of the few true rheumatologic emergencies. Proper consideration of this diagnosis and timely treatment reduces the likelihood of a poor outcome. Septic arthritis is usually bacterial in origin but may be due to viruses or fungi. Viral arthritides do not require specific therapy and resolve with few if any sequelae. Fungal joint infections are rare and diffi-

cult to treat. They can be seen in patients who are HIV-positive (see HIV Rheumatic Manifestations, below). The risk for septic arthritis is related to the size of the joint, with larger joints such as the knee or hip most commonly involved. The presence of any underlying joint disease such as rheumatoid arthritis or osteoarthritis appears to predispose the joint to an infection.

The usual presentation of septic arthritis is that of a monarthritis with an acutely swollen, painful joint. Systemic features such as fever, chills, and malaise often are present. The most common source of the infecting organism is hematogenous; therefore one should seek evidence for infection at some other site(s). The most likely specific bacterial etiology is age-dependent. In young, sexually active adults, *Neisseria gonorrhoeae* is the most common organism. Other common pathogens include *Staphylococcus aureus* and *Streptococcus pneumoniae*. Septic arthritis caused by *N. gonorrhoeae* usually has a unique clinical picture. Often this arthritis is not monarticular but, rather, presents as a migratory polyarthritis with polyarthralgia. The clinical picture may also include tenosynovitis and skin changes consisting of macules, papules, or vesicles, which are usually few in number and asymptomatic.

The initial diagnosis is based on the typical clinical presentation of a monarthritis associated with signs of systemic illness. This picture, however, is not always the presentation. Regardless of the clinical or laboratory findings, if septic arthritis is suspected patients should be treated accordingly. Blood, urine, and if indicated gonococcal cultures should be prepared. Synovial fluid analysis is critical in any patient suspected of a septic arthritis. Typically, the synovial fluid appears purulent with a white blood cell (WBC) count higher than 50,000/mm³. One cannot rely solely on the cell count, however, because in the elderly or the immunocompromised individual the count may be substantially lower. Synovial fluid should also be subjected to the appropriate stains and cultures and should be examined for crystals, as gouty arthritis can clinically mimic septic arthritis. Radiographs of the affected joint may exclude the possibility of osteomyelitis, which if suspected may be better delineated with either a three-phase bone scan or MRI.

Treatment of septic arthritis includes control of pain, rest of the involved joint during the acute stage, joint drainage, and appropriate antibiotic therapy (Table 39–9). If the bacteriologic stains are negative, initial antibiotic therapy should be broad and directed against the most likely organism given the clinical setting. If the stain is positive, one can initiate antibiotic therapy accordingly. If cultures become positive, the antibiotic regimen is adjusted accordingly. A critical aspect of treatment is joint drainage. If an easily accessed joint such as the knee (relatively simple to perform

TABLE 39–9.   TREATMENT OF SEPTIC BACTERIAL ARTHRITIS

Synovial Fluid Findings	Likely Organism Coverage for Adults	Possible Antibiotic	Comment
Positive Gram stain Gram-positive cocci In clusters	*Staphylococcus aureus* *Streptococcus epidermitis*	Nafcillin, cefazolin, or vancomycin	If methicillin resistance suspected, use vancomycin.
In chains Gram-negative cocci	*Streptococcus* species *Neisseria gonorrhoeae*	Third generation cephalosporin (e.g., ceftriaxone), penicillin	Use ceftriaxone if penicillinase-resistant *N. gonorrhoeae* is suspected.
Gram-negative bacilli	*Escherichia coli* and other Enterobacteriaceae	Third generation cephalosporin, an aminoglycoside or a quinolone	
Negative Gram stain	*S. aureus, Streptococcus* species or *N. gonorrhoeae*	Cefazolin or nafcillin	For suspected *N. gonorrhoeae*, use ceftriaxone. For suspected methicillin resistance, use vancomycin.

arthrocentesis) is involved, it should be drained as often as the effusion accumulates: usually once or twice a day for the initial few days of treatment during which time careful recording of synovial fluid volume, white cell count, and cultures is important. Ideally, rapid sterilization of the synovial fluid accompanied by a significant drop in the WBC count should occur. If it does not or the involved joint is the hip or other joint not readily accessible to arthrocentesis, surgical drainage may be required. An orthopedic surgeon should be consulted from the onset of care, so if surgical drainage is needed the surgeon is already familiar with the case and can proceed quickly. After the initial few days of management, treatment should focus on restoring joint function, which can best be accomplished with early joint mobilization and physical therapy.

The duration of antibiotic therapy varies depending on the organism involved and the immune status of the patient. Current technology permits intravenous treatment at home after the initial hospital course. Patients with gonococcal septic arthritis should probably be treated intravenously for 1 to 2 weeks followed by 1 to 2 weeks of oral antibiotics. Patients with nongonococcal bacterial septic arthritis uncomplicated by osteomyelitis or the presence of a joint prosthesis should be treated for a minimum of 2 weeks intravenously followed by 2 weeks of oral antibiotics. Patients with osteomyelitis or joint prostheses, or who are immunocompromised, should receive a minimum of 4 weeks of intravenous antibiotics. Because of the generally worse prognosis, patients with *S. aureus* or gram-negative bacilli should receive a minimum of 4 weeks of intravenous antibiotics. In all these scenarios, the duration of therapy may need to be prolonged if clinically the patient does not respond satisfactorily. A worse outcome can be expected when treatment is delayed or in those cases causes by *S. aureus*.

Lyme Disease

Lyme disease is caused by the tick-borne spirochete *Borrelia burgdorferi*. The disease is characterized by multisystem involvement including skin, joints, nervous system, and heart. Most patients do not recall a tick bite. The first manifestation of the disease may be the characteristic skin changes, erythema migrans, appearing usually as red macules or papules that often expand into a red rim with central clearing. Multiple lesions may appear. Constitutional symptoms may be present at this time and include headaches, fever, chills, myalgias, or arthralgia. These symptoms eventually disappear. Joint involvement usually begins later in the disease course. Typically, articular manifestations are monarticular or oligoarticular. The most commonly involved joint is the knee; but other joints, large and small, may be affected. Joint disease is associated with swelling, warmth, and tenderness of the joint. In children Lyme arthritis may be confused with juvenile rheumatoid arthritis (see Pediatric Rheumatic Diseases, below). Other late manifestations include meningitis, facial palsy, and atrioventricular blocks.

Treatment of Lyme disease depends in part on the stage of disease. During the early stages, tetracycline 250 mg q.i.d. for 2 to 4 weeks is usually sufficient. In children, amoxicillin 250 mg t.i.d. for 2 to 4 weeks is preferred. Patients with more advanced stages of Lyme disease, such as arthritis, usually require intravenous antibiotic therapy. A third generation cephalosporin, such as ceftriaxone 2 gm daily for 2 to 4 weeks, should be used. The efficacy of long-term antibiotic therapy for the treatment of persistent nonspecific symptoms attributable to Lyme disease has not been demonstrated (Lightfoot et al., 1993).

Prevention of Lyme disease is important and consists primarily in avoiding tick bites especially during the warm months when exposure is most likely. Many areas of the United States are endemic for Lyme disease. Adults should closely examine their skin and that of their children for evidence of tick bites whenever exposure has been likely. In addition, proper clothing and insecticides help reduce the risk of exposure.

Systemic Lupus Erythematosus

Systemic lupus erythematosus (SLE) is a chronic autoimmune disease characterized by multiorgan involvement. The cause of this disease is unknown, but host genetic factors play an important role in disease susceptibility and expression. A positive family history exists in about 10 per cent of cases (Arnett and Reveille, 1992). External factors also appear to be important as evidenced by the existence of drug-induced lupus, which can mimic many of the serologic and clinical manifestations of the disease (Stratton, 1985). SLE is not a common disease, with most studies suggesting prevalence rates below 1 per cent for the general population. SLE is a disease primarily of young women, affecting women on average ten times more frequently than men, although it has been described in men, the elderly, and children.

The American College of Rheumatology has established classification criteria for the disease (Table 39–10) that clearly outline the most common and specific signs and symptoms of SLE. Because many organ systems may be involved, clinical manifestations are varied. Thus in patients suspected of SLE, a careful history and physical examination are needed, and ongoing surveillance for systemic involvement is required. All new symptoms as well as changes in existing symptoms should be carefully evaluated.

The relative frequency of organ involvement at onset and in general is clinically relevant (Table 39–11). The most common symptoms at onset are constitutional and include malaise, fatigue, fever, and weight loss as well as arthralgia. Arthritis, which is usually polyarticular and symmetric, is also a frequent clinical manifestation. Symptoms include joint pain, swelling, stiffness, and tenderness. Thus the articular manifestations may mimic those of rheumatoid arthritis. Although the arthritis of SLE is not a destructive arthritis as in rheumatoid arthritis, deformities may develop especially in the hands. Skin changes are also common and appear in a number of forms. The characteristic "butterfly" rash is a facial erythematous, sometimes elevated lesion that appears over the malar area (Fig. 39–9). It may be precipitated by exposure to sunlight and may last for weeks. Discoid lesions are erythematous, scaly plaques that frequently occur over the scalp, face, and neck area but may appear on the extremities as well (Fig. 39–10). These lesions may heal with scar tissue

TABLE 39–10. 1982 REVISED CRITERIA FOR SLE*

Criterion	Definition
Malar rash	Fixed erythema, flat or raised, over malar eminences sparing nasolabial folds
Discoid rash	Erythematous raised patches with adherent keratotic scaling and follicular plugging
Photosensitivity	Skin rash as a result of unusual reaction to sunlight, by patient history or physical examination
Oral ulcers	Oral or nasopharyngeal ulcerations, usually painless and observed by the physician
Arthritis	Nonerosive arthritis involving two or more peripheral joints, characterized by tenderness, swelling, or effusion
Serositis	Pleuritis: convincing history of pleuritic pain or rub heard by physician or evidence of pleural effusion *or* Pericarditis: documented by ECG or rub or evidence for pericardial effusion
Renal disorder	Persistent proteinuria > 0.5 gm/day or > 3+ if quantitation not done *or* Cellular casts: may be red blood cell, hemoglobin, granular, tubular or mixed
Neurologic disorder	Seizures or psychosis in the absence of offending drugs or known metabolic derangement (e.g., uremia, ketoacidosis, or electrolyte imbalance)
Hematologic disorder	Hemolytic anemia with reticulocytosis *or* Leukopenia: < 4000/mm^3 on more than two occasions *or* Lymphopenia: < 1500/mm^3 on more than two occasions *or* Thrombocytopenia: < 100,000/mm^3 in the absence of offending drugs
Immunologic disorder	Positive LE cell preparation *or* Anti-DNA antibodies in abnormal titer *or* Anti-Smith antibodies present *or* False-positive serologic test for syphilis known to be positive for at least 6 months and confirmed by *Treponemia pallidum* immobilization or fluorescent treponemal antibody test
Antinuclear antibodies	Abnormal titer of antinuclear antibody by immunofluorescence or an equivalent assay at any point in time in absence of drug

* A person is said to have systemic lupus erythematosus if any 4 or more of the 11 criteria are present, serially or simultaneously, during any interval of observation.
From American College of Rheumatology, 1982, with permission.

TABLE 39–11. FREQUENCY OF SLE MANIFESTATIONS

Manifestation	At Onset (%) (n = 108)	Anytime (%) n = 605	Anytime (%) n = 520
Arthralgia	77	85	92
Constitutional	73	84	86
Skin	57	81	72
Arthritis	56	63	92
Renal	44	77	46
Raynaud's phenomenon	33	58	18
Lymphadenopathy	25	32	59
CNS	24	54	26
Pleurisy	23	37	45
Gastrointestinal	22	47	49
Pericarditis	20	29	31
Mucous membranes	18	54	9
Vasculitis	10	37	21
Lung	9	17	—
Myositis	7	5	—

From the University of Toronto: at onset, based on 108 patients; at any time, based on 605 patients diagnosed before 12/90. From the University of Southern California at Los Angeles: anytime, based on 520 patients.

Adapted from Gladman DD, Urowitz MB: Systemic lupus erythematosus: Clinical features. *In* Klippel JH, Dieppe PA (eds): Rheumatology. London, CV Mosby, 1994.

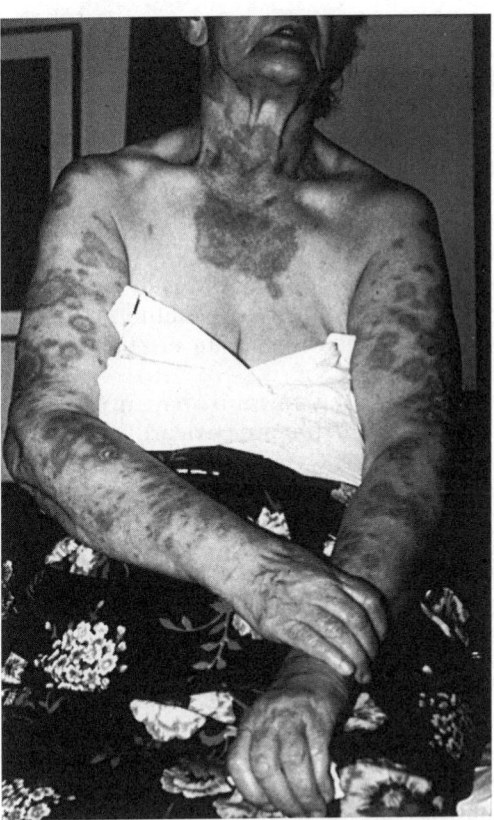

FIGURE 39–10. Multiple discoid lupus lesions. (From Dieppe PA, Bacon PA, Bamji AN, Watt I: Systemic lupus variants. *In* Slide Atlas of Rheumatology. London, Gower Medical Publishing, 1987, with permission.)

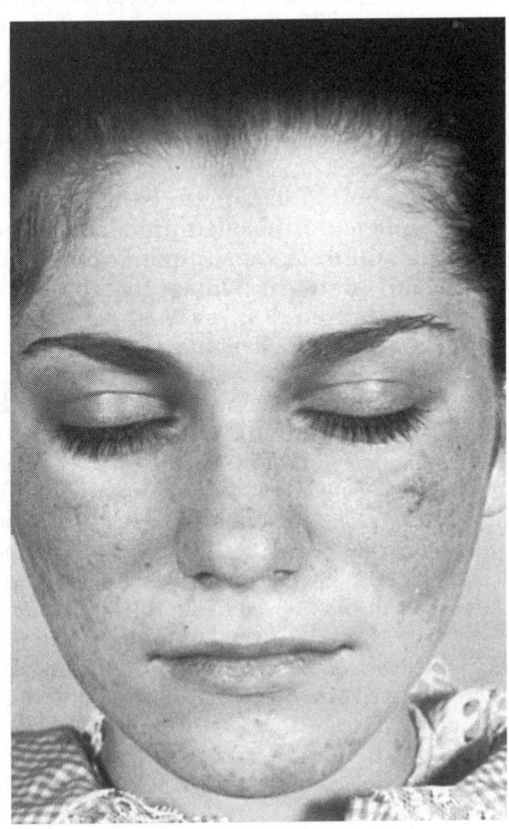

FIGURE 39–9. Typical butterfly rash in a patient with systemic lupus erythematosus. (From the Clinical Slide Collection on the Rheumatic Diseases. Copyright 1991, by the American College of Rheumatology, with permission.)

and loss of skin pigment. One form of SLE is primarily a skin disease in the form of discoid lesions and is termed discoid lupus; it is generally not associated with other system involvement and has a better prognosis than SLE. Other skin lesions include urticaria, livido reticularis, and subacute cutaneous lesions.

Renal involvement appears at the onset in approximately half of individuals with SLE and may eventually affect up to three fourths of all SLE patients (Table 39–11). Renal involvement is one of the most serious systemic sequelae, leading to significant morbidity and mortality in patients with SLE. Renal lesions vary but are almost always glomerular. New-onset hypertension may herald the onset of lupus nephritis. Some patients present with a nephrotic syndrome including peripheral edema, which may be secondary to a membranous glomerulopathy. Some patients have more serious disease in the form of a diffuse glomerulonephritis. Other renal lesions include mesangial glomerulopathy, focal segmental or focal proliferative glomerulonephritis, and sclerosing glomerulonephritis. Cytopenias are also common in SLE patients and include thrombocytopenia, which may be profound. Other causes, including drug-induced thrombocytopenia, should always be considered in such patients. Anemia is common in SLE patients due to chronic disease, renal insufficiency, or drugs. Less common is a hemolytic anemia due to autoantibodies directed against erythrocytes. Central nervous system (CNS) involvement may also occur, often leading to puzzling symptomatology, including manifestations such as seizures (of any type) or headaches. Psychiatric disorders in the form of organic brain syndrome, psychosis, or neurocognitive dysfunction may also develop. Less common CNS manifestation include strokes and a transverse myelitis (Adelman et al., 1986; Kovacs et al., 1993).

Serositis is common and may involve several sites including the pleura, pericardium, and peritoneum. Pleural involvement usually takes the form of chest pain, with patients giving a history of pleuritic-type pain. Some patients may develop pleural effusions. On examination a pleural rub may be heard. Pericarditis occurs less frequently, although patients may present with classic symptoms of pericarditis including chest pain. Often, however, the pericarditis is clinically silent and detectable only by echocardiography. Cardiac tamponade is a rare complication in SLE patients. Involvement of the peritoneum may present as abdominal pain and may be associated with anorexia and nausea or vomiting. It is important in any case of serositis to keep in mind that there are other potential causes for the symptoms. Of most concern is the possibility of an infectious process. Patients should be carefully evaluated before attributing symptoms of serositis to SLE.

Infections constitute a serious diagnostic challenge to physicians treating SLE patients in whom serious infections are a leading cause of mortality. The use of immunosuppressants contributes to this increased risk of infection. Physicians treating SLE patients should be cognizant that any or all symptoms may not simply be related to SLE activity. This recognition is of particular concern in patients with fever, which may be a constitutional sign of SLE but more often than not signals the presence of infection. A careful clinical search for infection including bacteriologic cultures is necessary to ensure that this possibility is evaluated.

Laboratory studies are important for the diagnosis, for monitoring disease activity, and for evaluating the effect of medications. A positive ANA assay is important for establishing the diagnosis, although there is a small percentage of individuals (fewer than 5 per cent) who are ANA-negative despite frequent testing (Reichlin and Harley, 1993). The diagnostic criteria for SLE do not specify a particular titer. Most laboratories consider a titer of 1:160 or higher as positive, although the higher the titer the more confirmatory is the test. Nevertheless, the ANA assay is not specific for SLE, and high titers are seen with a number of connective tissue disorders. Antibodies to native or double-stranded DNA are highly specific for this disease

but appear in only 70 per cent of untreated SLE patients.

Other autoantibodies, such as anti-Smith (anti-Sm) antibodies, may be present and help support the clinical diagnosis of SLE. The ESR is frequently elevated in patients with SLE and may be used as an indicator of disease activity. The ESR, however, is not a substitute for a careful history and physical examination. Antibodies against phospholipids may also be present in SLE patients. These antibodies are associated with a number of clinical phenomena including pregnancy loss and thrombotic states, both arterial and venous. Phospholipid antibodies can be detected using a number of techniques including the VDRL, anti-cardiolipin antibodies, and lupus anticoagulant tests. SLE patients may develop a false-positive VDRL because specific treponemal antibodies tests are negative. Anti-cardiolipin antibodies are typically detected by ELISA. There are a number of tests used to detect the presence of a lupus anticoagulant including the partial prothrombin time (PTT) and the Russell viper venom time (dRVVT).

Kidney disease is usually detected by urinalysis, which may demonstrate cellular or granular casts, red or white blood cells, or proteinuria. It is also important to monitor the creatine clearance and the serum creatinine. The level of serum complement components C3 and C4 appear to parallel renal disease activity, with reduced concentrations noted in patients with active disease. In most SLE patients with renal involvement, a kidney biopsy is necessary to define accurately the type of renal lesion present. This definition is important because certain lesions, such as diffuse proliferative glomerulonephritis, indicate a worse prognosis and often require more aggressive therapy than other renal lesions.

The treatment of SLE is multifaceted. The diagnosis of SLE is often accompanied by confusion and concern on the part of the patient. Considerable anxiety exists regarding a future with this disease that for many patients is viewed as serious. Although the potential for serious involvement exists in all SLE patients, many affected individuals lead fairly normal lives without serious impediment. Discussing these and other issues (e.g., pregnancy and genetic counseling) is important. Patients usually benefit from speaking with other people who have SLE. It is critical to involve the patient's spouse and family in discussions regarding diagnosis, treatment, and prognosis. This important support and social network for the patient should be considered part of the management team.

Pharmacologic treatment varies depending on the major site(s) of involvement. Patients with serositis may respond to NSAID therapy, and articular symptoms improve with NSAIDs. Minor skin involvement may be treated with topical steroids.

Patients with more serious joint or skin involvement may benefit from hydroxychloroquine (Plaquenil) at a dose of 200 to 400 mg/day in conjunction with NSAIDs. Patients with major organ involvement or those with significant constitutional symptoms unresponsive to NSAID therapy benefit from steroids. The dose of steroids should be commensurate with the severity of the symptoms and the degree of organ involvement. For example, patients with severe thrombocytopenia may require high doses of steroids, such as 60 mg of prednisone daily. Patients with serious kidney involvement, especially those with diffuse proliferative glomerulonephritis, also require high doses of steroids and even cytotoxic agents such as cyclophosphamide. Major organ involvement other than kidney disease unresponsive to steroids has been likewise treated with cytotoxic agents. Additional forms of therapy used include intravenous pulse steroids, plasmapheresis, and intravenous γ-globulin infusions.

Patients should be carefully followed during induction of remission with immunosuppressants. Once clinical remission is achieved, the dose of such medication should be tapered slowly and clinical and laboratory parameters monitored closely for signs of reactivation. A commonly encountered problem is too fast a steroid taper, often leading to a "roller coaster ride" of steroid dosing. To mitigate this problem, the steroid taper should be less dramatic. The goal is to find the lowest dose that can keep the patient's disease in remission. For individuals requiring continued use of steroids, alternate-day regimens may help reduce the side effects.

Sjögren's Syndrome

Sjögren's syndrome is an autoimmune disorder characterized by a chronic inflammatory process of certain exocrine glands. The syndrome may appear as a primary disorder, but more frequently it is associated with other connective tissue disorders such as rheumatoid arthritis or SLE. The cause of the disease is unknown. It is more prevalent in women.

The most commonly involved areas are the lacrimal and salivary glands, but other areas may be involved including the pancreas, lung, and kidney. Lacrimal gland involvement leads to a decrease in tear production. Clinically, patients experience a dry, gritty sensation in their eyes. In advanced cases this sicca syndrome may lead to corneal ulcerations and even visual loss. Involvement of the lacrimal gland can be demonstrated in a number of ways. Schimmer's test, which measures tear production on a strip of absorbent paper, detects decreased tear production. Ophthalmologic examination may reveal keratoconjunctivitis. A rose bengal test can detect small ulcerations in the cornea. Sali-

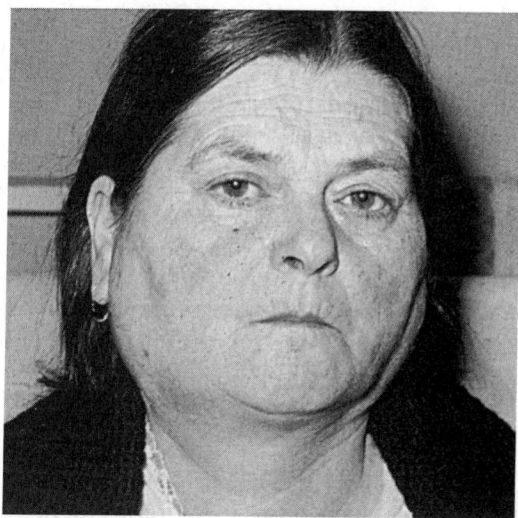

FIGURE 39–11. Patient with Sjögren's syndrome associated with parotid gland swelling. (From Moutsopoulos HM, Tzioufas AG: Sjögren's syndrome. *In* Klippel JH, Dieppe PA, eds: Rheumatology. London, CV Mosby, 1994, with permission.)

vary gland involvement may lead to periodic or persistent swelling of salivary glands, most commonly the parotids, and to decreased production of saliva (Fig. 39–11). Patients typically complain of a dry mouth, eventuating in difficulty chewing certain foods such as meats or dry food. Patients may also experience swallowing difficulties. Moreover, loss of saliva can lead to accelerated tooth loss due to decay. There may also be associated lymphadenopathy especially of the head and neck. Rarely, patients with Sjögren's syndrome develop lymphomas.

The diagnosis is generally based on the appearance of dry eyes, dry mouth, or both, usually in the context of another connective tissue disease. Laboratory testing may reveal the presence of autoantibodies known as SSA and SSB (Sjögren's syndrome antibodies A and B, also known as anti-Ro and anti-La). In uncertain cases biopsy of minor salivary glands usually in the inner lip may reveal findings typical of this disorder (Daniels, 1984).

Treatment of Sjögren's syndrome is essentially symptomatic. Artificial tears often relieve uncomfortable dryness. For more advanced cases, goggles may be required to minimize tear evaporation. For the dry mouth, frequent fluid intake is helpful. Artificial saliva is also available. Patients should carefully maintain oral hygiene and have frequent follow-up visits with the dentist. Steroids and other immunosuppressants are generally used in patients with significant renal, pulmonary, or CNS involvement.

Vasculitic Syndromes

The term vasculitis refers to a group of disorders characterized by an inflammatory process involving blood vessels. Vasculitis can be seen in association with other connective tissue diseases, such as rheumatoid arthritis or SLE, or it can be idiopathic. There are several classification schemes, but the one most often used and the one most useful for the clinician is based on the size of the vessels involved (Fig. 39–12). Vasculitic syndromes seem to have a predilection for affecting certain size vessels. Nevertheless, in many syndromes a variety of vessel sizes may be involved, thereby leading to an "overlap syndrome" in the size of vessels affected. The inflammatory vasculitic process causes luminal narrowing of the blood vessel, resulting in ischemia and eventually necrosis of that vessel's territory. Because any blood vessel can be involved, the manifestations of these diseases are protean. Nevertheless, there are typical areas that are more frequently implicated, serving as clues to the diagnosis. The American College of Rheumatology has published classification criteria for many vasculitic syndromes that are helpful in the diagnosis of these complex diseases. Moreover, recent studies confirm the usefulness of detecting serum anti-neutrophilic cytoplasmic antibodies (ANCAs) to confirm the clinical diagnosis of certain vasculitic syndromes such as polyarteritis nodosa and Wegener's granulomatosis (Falk et al., 1990).

Polymyalgia Rheumatica and Giant Cell Arteritis

Polymyalgia rheumatica (PMR) and giant cell arteritis (GCA) often occur together. Approximately 15 per cent of patients with PMR also have GCA, and about half of all GCA patients have concurrent PMR. These two entities may represent different spectrums of the same process, although the exact nature of their association in unknown.

PMR is commonly seen in elderly patients, with women affected twice as often as men. As the name implies, there are both muscular and articular symptoms. Typically, patients experience pain, achiness, and stiffness about the shoulder, pelvic, and neck areas. Symptoms are generally symmetric. Frequently morning stiffness and nighttime symptomatology dominate the clinical picture. Symptoms are generally poorly localized anatomically and develop gradually. Systemic features such as malaise, weight loss, and low grade fever commonly accompany joint symptoms. Physical examination usually reveals diffuse tenderness over involved joints and muscles. Range of motion may be reduced owing to pain. There is generally little evidence for inflammation, although some patients experience joint swelling and effusion. Lab-

STRATIFICATION OF VASCULITIS SYNDROMES

Type of vasculitis	Aorta and its branches	Large and medium-sized arteries	Medium-sized muscular arteries	Small muscular arteries	Venules, arterioles
Takayasu's arteritis	●				
Temporal arteritis	●	●			
Polyarteritis nodosa		●	●	●	
Churg–Strauss arteritis		●	●	●	
Isolated CNS vasculitis			●	●	
Wegener's granulomatosis			●	●	●
Vasculitis associated with connective tissue diseases				●	●
Leukocytoclastic vasculitis: Henoch–Schönlein purpura Hypersensitivity vasculitis Others				●	●

FIGURE 39–12. Common vasculitic syndromes stratified by the size of the vessels most commonly involved. (From Lightfoot RW: Overview of the inflammatory vascular diseases. *In* Klippel JH, Dieppe PA, [eds]: Rheumatology. London, CV Mosby, 1994, with permission.)

oratory studies are usually normal except for mild anemia and a characteristically elevated ESR.

Treatment depends in part on the severity of symptoms. Patients with mild disease may be started on NSAIDs. For those who do not respond or those who have more severe symptoms, oral steroids are useful. Prednisone in doses between 10 and 20 mg usually provides rapid relief of symptoms, and the ESR generally returns to normal. The prednisone can then be slowly tapered to the smallest dose needed to control symptoms. Patients usually require treatment for a year, although some require longer courses of treatment (Chuang et al., 1982).

A large-vessel vasculitis known as giant cell arteritis, or temporal arteritis, is often associated with PMR. The first name refers to the typical pathologic giant multinucleated cells found in affected vessel walls. The second name refers to the vessel most commonly involved, although any vessel may be involved including the vertebral artery or the external and internal carotid arteries. GCA is almost exclusively a disease of the elderly with most cases reported in individuals over 60 years of age. Like PMR, it is more common in women.

Typical symptoms include headaches that are usually located over the temporal area and are described as dull and different from the patient's usually headaches (if any). There may be associated scalp tenderness upon hair-combing or scalp touching. Visual problems, including sudden loss of vision, are serious, concerning symptoms. Usually due to involvement of a blood vessel of the orbit or retina, acute visual loss constitutes a medical emergency. Prompt consideration of the diagnosis and immediate treatment are important if permanent visual loss is to be avoided. Other symptoms include jaw claudication, hearing loss, loss of taste, and pain in the throat as well as peripheral manifestations such as hemiparesis and peripheral neuropathies. Articular symptoms are similar to those described for PMR. Physical findings may include a prominent temporal artery that is tender to palpation. The pulse may be absent if the vessel is occluded at that level. Other findings include diffuse scalp tenderness, optic nerve ischemia on funduscopic examination, and absent peripheral pulses. The most striking laboratory abnormality is a markedly elevated ESR, often at a level higher than 100 mm/hr.

The diagnosis is based on clinical findings in the presence of a markedly elevated ESR. Histologic confirmation of the diagnosis usually should be sought. The temporal artery is often the most successful biopsy site, but site location must be dictated by clinical symptoms. Patients with visual symptoms or advanced disease should be treated immediately. In this instance, the clinician should not postpone treatment until a biopsy is performed. Although treatment may alter subsequent histologic findings, minimal if any changes are expected

within the first 48 hours of treatment, which consists in corticosteroid therapy at high doses. This high dose regimen may present to the clinician a rather daunting prospect in a frail, elderly patient. The initial starting dose is controversial. The goal is to control symptoms and prevent catastrophic complications such as blindness. An acceptable starting dose is 60 mg of prednisone. Patients should be closely monitored for side effects from the medication including hyperglycemia, mental status changes, and gastrointestinal upset. Prophylaxis for osteoporosis should also be instituted. Most patients report significant improvement on prednisone. The ESR should be monitored and often shows a dramatic drop to normal within a few weeks. The prednisone can be tapered following clinical remission and normalization of the ESR. Initially, the drug can be tapered in 10-mg increments every 2 weeks. As the dose is reduced, the incremental changes should be smaller. The patient's clinical course and ESR must be closely monitored for signs of reactivation. Too rapid tapering may lead to disease recrudescence. The duration of treatment varies depending on the patient's response, but it usually lasts 1 to 2 years.

Another large-vessel inflammatory syndrome is Takayasu's arteritis, a rare vasculitic syndrome that primarily affects the aorta and its major branches. It is a disease with a variegated presentation that affects mostly young women. It progresses through several phases. Initially, Takayasu's arteritis is characterized by constitutional symptoms such as fever, malaise and weight loss. As the disease progresses, vessels become occluded and signs of vascular ischemia become apparent. Visual symptoms may appear, and cardiac or pulmonary manifestations secondary to systemic or pulmonary hypertension may develop. On physical examination, the most striking features include absent pulses and the presence of vascular bruits.

The diagnosis is usually established with arteriography of the aorta and its major branches, both thoracic and abdominal. Findings include segmental narrowing, aneurysms, or vessel occlusion.

Treatment consists in high dose prednisone, usually 1 mg/kg/day. If clinical remission is achieved, the dose can be tapered. If steroids alone are unsuccessful, cytotoxic agents such as cyclophosphamide have been used.

Polyarteritis Nodosa

Polyarteritis nodosa (PAN), another form of vasculitis, affects small and medium-size muscular arteries (Lightfoot et al., 1990). Pathologically characterized by a necrotizing vasculitis that affects the entire vessel wall, any vessel may be involved. The manifestations of PAN are therefore varied. The most common sites of involvement are the skin and kidneys.

Diagnosis usually requires a high index of suspicion and subsequent confirmatory testing, including tissue sampling, radiographic procedures, or both. Biopsy of an involved area may lead to the demonstration of a necrotizing vasculitis. Arteriograms may demonstrate aneurysmal, fusiform dilatations, or segmental narrowing suggestive of a vasculitic disorder. In patients with evidence of kidney disease, a renal arteriogram will likely confirm the diagnosis. In some patients, no obvious site is evident, and several strategies have been proposed to help confirm the diagnosis, including abdominal arteriography or a blind biopsy of muscle, sural nerve, or testis (Dahlberg et al., 1989).

Treatment consists in high dose prednisone, usually 40 to 80 mg daily. Once clinical remission is achieved, the dose may be tapered. For patients with extensive disease or in those unresponsive to prednisone, cytotoxic agents such as cyclophosphamide have been used in conjunction with steroids. Cyclophosphamide can be given orally (1 to 2 mg/kg/day) in conjunction with prednisone. Treatment duration should be for at least a year.

Wegener's Granulomatosis

Wegener's granulomatosis, (WG), a vasculitis, often involves the upper and lower respiratory tract and the kidneys. Other associated manifestations include arthritis, skin rash, and constitutional symptoms such as fever, malaise, and weight loss. The characteristic pathologic finding is a granulomatous vasculitis. Characteristic lung involvement is defined by the formation of multiple, often bilateral nodular infiltrates that may cavitate. Sinus involvement usually develops into a chronic sinusitis with superimposed recurrent infections. As the disease progresses, nasal septal perforation may develop. Renal involvement can be severe and includes a diffuse necrotizing glomerulonephritis (Hoffman et al., 1992). Patients with clinical evidence of WG are often serology-positive for ANCAs.

Treatment of WG depends in part on the extent of organ involvement. Medications used include antibiotics, steroids, and cytotoxic agents. Some forms of limited WG may be treated less aggressively. There are reports regarding the efficacy of trimethoprim-sulfmethoxazole in such patients. Patients with major organ involvement, such as lung or kidney, usually require high dose steroids and immunosuppressants such as cyclophosphamide (Hoffman et al., 1992).

Churg-Strauss Syndrome

The Churg-Strauss syndrome (allergic angiitis and granulomatosis) is a rare vasculitic syndrome that affects small and medium-size arteries. It is characterized by asthma, peripheral eosinophilia, and granuloma formation. Typical lung involvement includes multiple and bilateral nodules, changing pulmonary infiltrates, or interstitial pneumonitis. Constitutional symptoms may also figure prominently in this syndrome. Diagnosis is

accomplished via a biopsy of an involved site, usually the lung. Treatment consists in high dose prednisone.

Behçet's Disease

Behçet's disease is a systemic vasculitic syndrome characterized by mucocutaneous involvement associated with ocular and musculoskeletal symptoms. Although the disease is rare in the United States, high prevalence rates have been reported among peoples of Turkey, Iran, and Japan.

The diagnosis is often difficult and is based solely on clinical findings. To sustain this diagnosis, clinical findings should include recurrent oral ulceration (aphthous or herpetiform). These lesions should be observed by the physician and be of a recurrent nature (at least three bouts over a 12 month period). Additionally, patients may demonstrate recurrent genital ulcers: In men they are most common on the scrotum and in women on the labia. Ocular lesions consist of uveitis or retinal vasculitis. Patients may also develop skin lesions, pathergy, or arthritis/arthralgia. Joint symptoms are usually monarticular or oligoarticular. Neurologic complications are uncommon but can be devastating, including stroke or transverse myelitis.

Treatment usually consists in immunosuppressants. Steroids are often used early in the disease. Other drugs such as chlorambucil, azathioprine, and cyclosporin A appear to be more useful for long-term treatment, especially in patients with major organ involvement such as CNS or ocular vasculitis (Yazici, 1994).

HIV Rheumatic Manifestations

Rheumatic syndromes have been identified in patients with HIV infection. The most commonly described syndromes in this group of patients are the spondyloarthropathies. HIV infection should be considered in patients with a spondyloarthropathy, particularly in light of the fact that the clinical manifestations may be indistinguishable from those in patients who are not HIV-positive. In selected patients, articular complaints are the presenting manifestations of HIV infection.

Reiter's syndrome is the most common syndrome reported in HIV-positive individuals. Patients experience an asymmetric oligoarthritis as well as skin changes, and they may report antecedent urinary or gastrointestinal infections similar to those in other Reiter's syndrome patients. Back symptoms attributable to sacroiliitis have been reported, but radiographic evidence of sacroiliitis has been rare. The clinical course of Reiter's syndrome in HIV-positive patients is variable. Some HIV-positive individuals develop frank psoriasis associated with arthritis that is usually asymmetric and oligoarticular—and thus similar to HIV-negative psoriatic arthritis. Other rheumatic conditions reported include septic arthritis, Sjögren syndrome, vasculitis, and myopathies.

Treatment of HIV-positive rheumatic manifestations is complicated by the coexisting HIV infection. The clinical manifestations and severity of the rheumatic disease as well as the immune status of the individual must be considered carefully. Most articular symptoms can be managed with the use of NSAIDs. Methotrexate has been used in Reiter's syndrome and psoriatic arthritis patients with more active disease. Septic arthritis should be treated no differently than in other septic arthritis settings. The infectious agents responsible likely include opportunistic organisms such as fungi or mycobacteria not typically seen in HIV-negative patients (Calabrese, 1993; Kaye, 1989).

Pediatric Rheumatic Diseases

The pediatric age group is also affected with the spectrum of rheumatic diseases. Although these diseases are similar to their adult counterparts, there are some important distinctions with which the primary care physician should be familiar. Moreover, the impact of these diseases on children and their families can be profound, requiring the coordinating physician to be a source of education, support, and guidance.

Juvenile Rheumatoid Arthritis

Juvenile rheumatoid arthritis (JRA) consists of a chronic inflammatory synovitis that usually presents as one of three distinct subtypes: systemic, polyarticular, or pauciarticular. These different forms of JRA usually develop before the age of 16 years and, with the exception of the systemic type, are more prevalent in girls. The systemic subtype is characterized by features such as high fevers, rash, lymphadenopathy, and hepatosplenomegaly. The joint disease is usually polyarticular and symmetric. The polyarticular subtype also describes symmetric polyarticular joint involvement but lacks many of the systemic features. Some patients with the polyarticular form experience systemic symptoms, but they are generally mild. Pauciarticular JRA, the most common presentation of JRA, is characterized by an oligoarthritis that is generally asymmetric. This subtype is also characterized by a high prevalence of uveitis, which may be asymptomatic.

Laboratory studies usually reveal an elevated ESR. Many patients have a positive ANA assay. RF is generally absent in patients with JRA, with the exception of a subgroup with a polyarticular presentation who have clinical disease indistinguishable from rheumatoid arthritis.

Treatment considerations include the special circumstances called for when dealing with a chronic debilitating disease in a child. Growth, development, and education issues must be addressed in an ongoing manner by the primary care physician in conjunction with a team approach that includes educators, therapists, and family. Additionally, patients should be examined periodically by an ophthalmologist to check for the development of uveitis. Pharmacologic treatment of JRA has generally been conservative, although there has been a recent emphasis on more aggressive management earlier in the disease course. Anti-inflammatory agents should be used initially. For many years aspirin was the preferred drug, but the possible linkage of Reye syndrome and aspirin has caused decreased use of the drug in favor of other NSAIDs. Some of these drugs, including ibuprofen, naproxen, and tolmetin, have been approved for use in children and come in liquid preparations. For children who do not respond to NSAIDs, DMARDS (including gold, methotrexate, and hydroxychloroquine) have been used (Athreya and Cassidy, 1991).

Systemic Lupus Erythematosus

Systemic lupus erythematosus is uncommon in children. Nevertheless, it is important to consider this diagnosis if symptoms and signs warrant. The most common clinical manifestations are constitutional and include fever and malaise. As in adults, the disease is typically multisystemic, with organ involvement similar to that in adults. The familiar butterfly rash is present in only one third of cases. Arthritis is common and usually polyarticular. SLE may present as thrombocytopenia and can be confused with idiopathic thrombocytopenic purpura (ITP). Renal involvement occurs in up to two thirds of children with SLE; and as with the adult disease, renal lesions vary. A kidney biopsy may be required to confirm the specific type of renal pathology. The diagnosis of the pediatric disease is based on the same criteria as are used for the adult disease. Children frequently have a positive ANA assay.

Treatment is also similar to that in adults with the proviso that there are special concerns regarding the effect of steroids on growth and development. The use of cytotoxic drugs is also a potential problem in children because of the concerns regarding the risk of sterility and malignancies. These concerns must be balanced against the potential benefit these medications confer. Parents should be made fully aware of the benefits and short- and long-term risks so an informed decision can be made regarding therapy (Lehman, 1993).

Other Rheumatic Diseases

Children develop other rheumatic diseases as well. *Spondyloarthropathies* including ankylosing spondylitis occur in children. They may present as an asymmetric oligoarthritis and thus mimic JRA. Radiography is usually not helpful for distinguishing these disorders, as bony maturity has not been reached and sacroiliitis may not be apparent.

Inflammatory muscle disease also develops in the pediatric age group. Juvenile dermatomyositis includes muscle weakness with skin changes, differing from the adult variety in that vasculitis is prominent (Ansell, 1991). Treatment of juvenile *dermatomyositis* is similar to that in adults (see Inflammatory Muscle Disease, below). *Scleroderma* may also develop in children, but localized forms are more common, including morphea, which presents as indurated waxy lesions of the skin that may be single or multiple. Similar lesions that appear as bands constitute linear scleroderma and may affect an extremity. The affected limb may undergo deformity and growth retardation.

The most common vasculitic disease process in children is *Henoch-Schönlein purpura*. The characteristic purpuric lesions usually appear in dependent areas such as the lower extremities and buttocks. Other clinical manifestations include arthritis, abdominal pain, and renal involvement.

Treatment is supportive, and the disease is usually self-limited. Steroids are required in some children with abdominal or other organ involvement.

Acute Rheumatic Fever

Rheumatic fever is a systemic inflammatory process, the result of an immunologic reaction to group A β-hemolytic streptococci. Symptoms of this disease usually appear several weeks after an infection with this organism, usually pharyngitis. For obscure reasons, the disease has dramatically decreased over the last few decades in the United States. Sporadic cases are still reported, but we seem to be witnessing an increase in disease prevalence due to largely unknown reasons. The disease primarily strikes children between the ages of 5 and 10 years, although it has been reported in teenagers and young adults as well.

Initial symptoms include high fevers associated with other constitutional symptoms. Arthralgia is common but may be fleeting and migratory. Arthritis may develop with joint pain, swelling, and erythema, usually starting as a monarthritis; as articular manifestations are additive, however, it may evolve into a polyarticular, symmetric arthritis. Other manifestations include carditis, which is present in as many as three fourths of all affected children. Cardiac findings include new-onset murmurs, pericarditis, cardiomegaly, or congestive heart failure. A characteristic rash called erythema marginatum may appear as an evanescent rash with a "chicken wire" appearance, but this sign is rarely encountered in the United States today. Subcutaneous nodules may develop and persist for weeks. These nodules are small and appear over the extensor surfaces or the occiput (or both). The nodules are rarely present early in the disease course and are uncommonly associated with rheumatic fever today. Chorea is an uncommon and often subtle manifestation of acute rheumatic fever. More extensive choreiform movements involving the entire limb, face, or trunk have been described.

The diagnosis is based on the characteristic constellation of symptoms noted above. These symptoms have been grouped into the major and minor Jones criteria for diagnosis of the disease (Table 39–12). Laboratory tests are helpful primarily for establishing antecedent streptococcal infection. Such tests include detection of antibodies to streptolysin O (ASO titer), streptokinase, and deoxyribonuclease B. A throat culture should be done, although most patients are likely to be negative. A positive throat culture may, however, identify carrier states. The ESR is usually elevated, as is the C-reactive protein level. Synovial fluid analysis usually reveals an inflammatory fluid without crystals and negative bacteriologic stains and culture.

Therapy has two main goals: control the acute inflammatory process and eradicate and prevent further streptococcal pharyngitis. During the acute stage anti-inflammatory agents are helpful for controlling many of the symptoms. Aspirin has been the drug of choice and is dosed at 80 to 100 mg/kg/day in children and 4 to 6 grams or more a day in adults. Salicylate levels should be monitored to determine the dose, with therapeutic levels between 20 and 30 mg/dL. NSAIDs are probably equally effective, but there are few published data to support their use instead of aspirin. Steroids have been used in patients unresponsive to aspirin or in those with carditis. Additional supportive care is important and includes bed rest, especially for those with carditis, and adequate hydration. The duration of disease is variable, but it generally lasts 6 to 8 weeks. Anti-inflammatory therapy can be tapered gradually after this period.

If a throat culture demonstrates active streptococcal infection, oral penicillin should be adminis-

TABLE 39–12. JONES CRITERIA FOR THE DIAGNOSIS OF RHEUMATIC FEVER

Major Manifestations	Minor Manifestations
Polyarthritis	Fever
Carditis	Arthralgia
Erythema marginatum	Previous history of rheumatic
Subcutaneous nodules	fever or rheumatic heart
Chorea	disease

Diagnosis of rheumatic fever is based on
 Two major criteria *or*
 One major and two minor criteria
  plus
 Evidence of an antecedent streptococcal infection.

Evidence for previous streptococcal infection includes the following.
  Increased ASO titer or other streptococcal antibodies
  Throat culture positive for group A β-hemolytic streptococcus
  Recent scarlet fever

Adapted from Williams RC: Acute rheumatic fever. *In* Klippel JH, Dieppe PA (eds): Rheumatology. London, CV Mosby, 1994, with permission.

tered for 10 days. Alternately, long-acting benzathine penicillin may be administered intramuscularly. Erythromycin may be given to children allergic to penicillin. Continued prophylaxis against streptococcal infections is required (Williams, 1994).

Nonarticular Rheumatic Complaints

Nonarticular rheumatic complaints are common in children. Limb pain, also known as growing pains, is one such complaint. The cause of these symptoms are unknown. Typically, the discomfort begins at night; it is usually quite painful but lasts only a few hours. The physical examination is unremarkable, and treatment is symptomatic. Growing pains are benign and typically disappear with time.

Hypermobility syndrome is a common cause of extremity pain in children. These children typically have joint range of motion that exceeds that of other children. It is believed that this excessive range of motion leads to injury and thus pain around the joints. There is often a positive family history of hypermobility syndrome. Treatment is primarily education and restriction of an offending activity if it can be identified. These children require only reasonable restriction of their activities.

Inflammatory Muscle Disease

Inflammatory myopathies accompany a number of connective tissue diseases, such as scleroderma, SLE, and rheumatoid arthritis. They also can occur as primary processes, such as polymyositis (PM) and dermatomyositis (DM), which are discussed together in this section. Both PM and DM are characterized by a chronic inflammatory process that affects striated muscle. DM also possess a characteristic skin involvement that distinguishes it clinically from PM. The cause of PM/DM is unknown. These diseases are uncommon and occur primarily in adult women (3:1 female predominance), although they are also seen in children. In some patients, especially in the elderly, there is a clear association with malignancy.

The most common clinical complaint is weakness, usually insidious in onset and affecting the upper and lower extremities and the neck. Typically, patients experience difficulty with proximal muscle weakness and complain that it is difficult to perform activities of daily living such as stair-climbing, combing hair, or even raising their heads from a pillow. Physical examination usually reveals weakness of several proximal muscle groups. Patients may also evidence muscle tenderness, areas of muscle swelling, and even areas of muscle atrophy in more advanced cases. DM is also associated with skin changes, typically found over the face and neck area as well as over the upper back. Areas of involvement are usually erythematous or violaceous (the heliotrope rash) and scaly (Fig. 39–13). Skin changes may also occur over the dorsal aspect of the PIPs, DIPS, or MCPs of the hand and are referred to as Grotton's papules.

The association of DM/PM with malignancies is well documented. It most commonly occurs in elderly patients but should be considered in all patients. There is controversy regarding the extent to which a search for malignancy should reach. The work-up for a malignancy should be guided by clinical symptoms, physical findings, or laboratory findings. Additionally, patients should have appropriate cancer screening based on age and sex. The yield of further search for hidden malignancies is likely to be low and is not indicated.

The diagnosis of PM/DM is based on the clinical finding of proximal muscle weakness associated with elevated muscle enzymes, especially creatine kinase and aldolase. Also, certain autoantibodies,

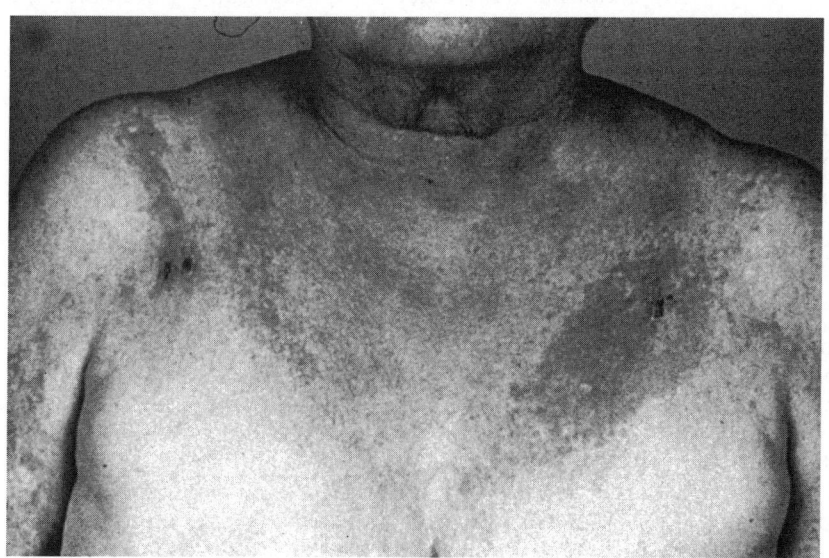

FIGURE 39–13. Dermatomyositis with a prominent erythematous eruption over light-exposed areas. (From Revised Clinical Slide Collection on the Rheumatic Diseases. Copyright 1991, by the American College of Rheumatology, with permission.)

such as anti-Jo-1, have been described in these patients but are positive in only a small percentage of cases. An electromyogram may reveal characteristic changes such as increased irritability, but these findings are not specific. Muscle biopsy should be performed in all patients suspected of this disorder to confirm the diagnosis and exclude other conditions. It is important that the specimen be handled by someone knowledgeable with muscle pathology.

The usual form of treatment is oral steroid therapy, usually at doses of 60 to 100 mg/day (Plotz et al., 1989). Patients should also begin prophylaxis against osteoporosis. The clinical response is often slow, and patients may worsen before improving. It is best to follow the patient's muscle strength as an indicator of disease activity and response to treatment. Serum muscle enzyme concentrations can also be followed and generally normalize with treatment. Patients usually require 6 to 8 weeks of high dose steroids, at which time if the disease is still active steroid-sparing agents can be used. Among the most commonly used such drugs are azathioprine and methotrexate, either of which may be added to the treatment regimen while the steroids are gradually reduced to an alternate-day schedule. Patients often require treatment for many months before a complete remission can be obtained. Treatment should continue for at least 1 year, at which point medication can be slowly tapered with careful attention to the patient's strength and muscle enzyme levels. Relapse can occur. Other important aspects of care include physical therapy, which should begin as soon as possible during the course of treatment. The goal of physical therapy is to maintain and gradually increase the patient's strength. It is important to remember that patients may not fully recover to their preillness levels of strength. Patients with rheumatologic symptoms of DM/PM-associated malignancies often benefit from treatment of the underlying malignancy.

Fibrosing Conditions

Several disorders are characterized by an excessive production of collagen that leads to fibrosis of the skin and other organs. Among this group of diseases are scleroderma, morphea, and eosinophilic fasciitis.

Scleroderma

Scleroderma is characterized by an inflammatory reaction that leads to fibrosis at multiple sites. This fibrosis is most visible in the skin, but other areas such as the lung and gastrointestinal tract may be involved. Scleroderma is also associated with vascular changes that consist of intimal hyperplasia associated with fibrosis. Raynaud's phenomenon is common in patients with scleroderma but may be seen with other connective tissue diseases as well (e.g., SLE). This phenomenon is characterized by episodes of blanching or cyanosis of digits following cold exposure or after emotional stress. Sclerodermatous skin changes usually begin as edema, especially of the digits, that subsequently evolves into a thickened skin that is bound to subcutaneous tissues. Skin involvement is variable and may be limited to distal areas such as fingers or may be widespread involving the trunk and face. Articular symptoms include the more characteristic tendon rubs and less common polyarthritis syndrome. Tendon rubs are coarse, palpable nodules over tendons, especially those in the extremities. The most common gastrointestinal finding is dysfunction of the lower esophageal sphincter, frequently associated with retrosternal burning discomfort and other gastroesophageal reflux symptoms. Two other areas of sclerodermatous involvement lead to significant morbidity and mortality. Kidney involvement can lead to a scleroderma renal crisis characterized by malignant hypertension, renal failure, and microangiopathic hemolytic anemia. Prompt recognition and control of this hypertension is imperative. Lung involvement usually takes the form of an interstitial pneumonitis, but pulmonary hypertension may develop. The most common respiratory symptoms are dyspnea and a chronic, nonproductive cough. Lung involvement is the most common cause of disease-related death in patients with scleroderma.

The diagnosis of scleroderma is made on the basis of the characteristic skin changes that occur (Fig. 39–14). If any clinical doubt exists, a skin biopsy reveals extensive fibrosis of subcutaneous tissue. Studies of the distal esophageal sphincter also reveal characteristic changes. Pulmonary function testing typically shows decreased diffusion capacity. Abnormal laboratory studies include a positive ANA assay, usually with a nucleolar pattern. Patients with the CREST form of scleroderma (scleroderma with *c*alcinosis, *R*aynaud's phenomenon, *e*sophageal, *s*clerodactyly, and *t*elangiectasia) have anti-centromere antibodies that are specific for this disorder.

Treatment generally consists in supportive and symptomatic care. Physical therapy helps limit deformities, and careful attention to skin injury is important especially for the toes and fingers. To diminish the frequency of Raynaud's phenomenon, it is important that patients protect and warm their digits especially during winter. Calcium-channel blockers may effectively control Raynaud's phenomenon as well. Effective treatment of the underlying fibrosing condition is not available, although D-penicillamine has been shown to be effective in some patients (Jimenez and Sigal, 1991; Steen et al., 1982). Steroids do not appear to have a role in the treatment of fibrosis but may be helpful in patients with an associated inflammatory myositis. Scleroderma renal crisis should be treated with ag-

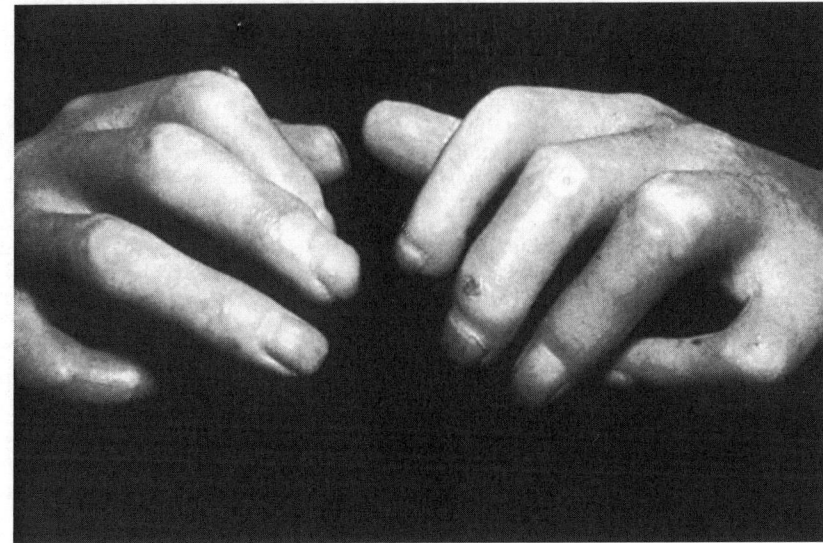

FIGURE 39–14. Sclerodermatous changes of the hand. Flexion contractures have occurred in the fingers secondary to skin tightening. Areas of increased and decreased pigmentation are also visible. (From the Clinical Slide Collection on the Rheumatic Diseases. Copyright, by the American College of Rheumatology, with permission.)

gressive control of hypertension and other supportive measures, such as restoration of circulating volume. The use of angiotensin-converting enzyme (ACE) inhibitors, sometimes in high doses, is critical to the successful treatment of scleroderma renal crisis (Steen et al., 1990). Patients with lung disease should be given vaccines for influenza and pneumococcal pneumonia. Prompt antibiotic treatment of bacterial bronchitis or pneumonia is also important. D-Penicillamine may be effective in patients with sclerodermatous lung disease. Supplemental oxygen may be required in hypoxic patients.

There are several forms of localized scleroderma, including morphea and linear scleroderma. These disorders are not associated with the systemic features of scleroderma. Morphea usually appears as small or large patches of scleroderma-like skin changes. Lesions typically have a hypopigmented center with erythematous borders. Morphea may appear as a single lesion or multiple lesions over the trunk or extremities. Linear scleroderma appears as a band of thickened and hyperpigmented skin over the face or an extremity. In children it can lead to growth problems of the affected extremity (see Pediatric Rheumatic Disease, above).

Eosinophilic Fasciitis

Eosinophilic fasciitis is a rare disorder characterized by peripheral eosinophilia, pain, and swelling of extremities, followed by progressive induration of skin and subcutaneous fat. Skin changes are not those of scleroderma, but the affected skin may appear shiny with an orange-peel appearance. The diagnosis is established by the results of a deep biopsy at affected sites that should include skin, subcutaneous fat, fascia, and muscle. Prednisone is usually helpful for controlling the symptoms.

Fibromyalgia

Fibromyalgia, or fibrositis as it is also known, consists of a constellation of symptoms associated with few physical findings and essentially normal laboratory tests. The disease affects primarily women but has been described in men and children. The cause of this disorder is unknown. The main complaints are joint and muscle pain and stiffness, easy fatigability, and difficulty with sleep. The symptoms appear insidiously, although some patients may recall a precipitating physical or emotional event. There usually exists a significant degree of functional impairment with inability to work or difficulty with chores at home. Patients report a lack of energy and diffuse pain as the main reason for their impairment. Stiffness appears worse in the morning upon arising and may last hours; in some patients it is present all day. Patients frequently complain of joint swelling, particularly in the hands, although there is no objective evidence for this edema found on examination. Sleep disturbances vary, but most patients admit to a lack of nonrestorative sleep; that is, they awake from sleep not feeling refreshed. Most patients report either frequent nocturnal awakening or difficulty falling asleep. A detailed, complete history often reveals concomitant psychological factors including depression and anxiety.

Physical examination of these patients is characterized by the absence of findings. The most common abnormality is the presence of tender points. These points are located about joints or over the axial skeleton and are characteristic of the disease (Fig. 39–15). Often patients are unaware of these points. The number of tender points varies among patients. For classification purposes, the American College of Rheumatology recommends a minimum of 11 tender sites from a total of the 18 sites typi-

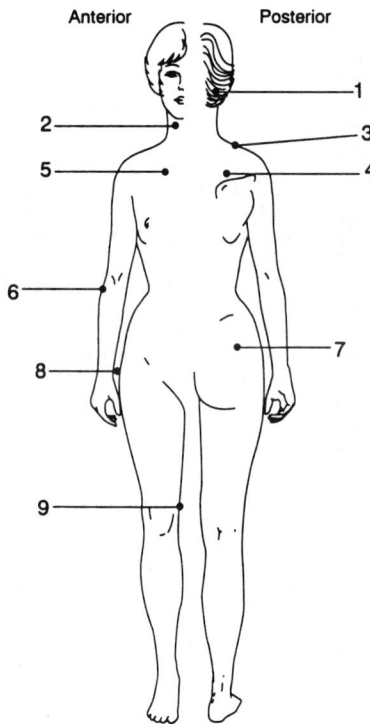

FIGURE 39–15. Location of bilateral tender point sites in patients with fibromyalgia. (From Yunus MB, Masi AT: Fibromyalgia, restless leg syndrome, periodic limb movement disorder and psychogenic pain. *In* McCarty DJ, Koopman WJ, [eds]: Arthritis and Allied Conditions, 12th edition. Philadelphia, Lea & Febiger, 1993, with permission.)

cally involved (Wolf et al., 1990). Laboratory studies are used to exclude other diagnoses and are essentially normal including the ESR and RF.

Treatment is often symptomatic. Patients are generally apprehensive about the nature of their symptoms and the degree of functional impairment with which they live. Frequently patients have seen a number of physicians without a satisfactory outcome. The treatment plan is outlined in Table 39–13. Treatment can be frustrating for both patient and physician. Immediate results are unlikely, and the therapy should focus on long-term goals. Confirmation of this diagnosis can be reassuring to patients who often believe they may have a life-threatening disease. Patient education as to the nature of the disorder and the expected outcome is important. Physical therapy, including exercises, is an important aspect of care. Analgesics can be used to control pain. NSAIDs are used extensively, but patient response is variable. It is sometimes difficult to obtain significant relief of symptoms. This potential benefit should be weighed against the potential complications associated with the chronic use of NSAIDs. Psychotropic drugs such as amitriptyline and other tricyclic antidepressants are used at bedtime. Small doses of amitriptyline (10 to 50 mg h.s.) may be used. Depression often accompanies fibromyalgia,

TABLE 39–13. MANAGEMENT OF FIBROMYALGIA

1. Exclude other diagnoses and confirm diagnosis of fibromyalgia.
2. Assure patient as to diagnosis.
3. Educate patient as to nature of disease and the expected benefits from therapy.
4. Prescribe physical therapy including exercise.
5. Inject trigger points with local anesthetics and steroids (practical in patients with a limited number of well localized tender points).
6. Give analgesics: acetaminophen or NSAIDs. Avoid addictive or narcotic drugs.
7. Give psychotropic drugs, such as amitriptyline. Use in low dose at bedtime.
8. Manage psychological factors with possible referral to a psychiatrist.
9. If the above measures are unsuccessful, refer to a chronic pain center.

Adapted from Yunus MB, Masi AT: Fibromyalgia, restless leg syndrome, periodic limb movement disorder and psychogenic pain. *In* McCarty DJ, Koopman WJ (eds): Arthritis and Allied Conditions, 12th edition. Philadelphia, Lea & Febiger, 1993, with permission.

and such patients may benefit from antidepressant doses of these drugs.

Low Back Pain

Low back pain is a common cause for a visit to a physician and a common cause of disability in the United States. The causes of back pain are many and include structural problems such as a herniated disk, inflammatory diseases such as ankylosing spondylitis, or even pain referred from abdominal viscera. Structural problems are probably the most common cause and include pain due to trauma or overuse.

The evaluation of someone with back pain should be systematic and thorough. A history of the onset and nature of the pain is important. In one scenario the onset of pain is sudden, related to trauma, and of recent origin, suggesting a mechanical etiology. In another situation the pain may have a gradually onset, lack a precipitating event, and be more chronic in nature. This picture suggests a nonmechanical cause of the pain. The quality and the location of the pain may provide insight to the cause (Table 39–14). Radiation of pain down to the leg suggests a radicular problem. Coughing or sneezing may exacerbate radicular pain. Aggravating factors are also important to consider. Mechanical back pain typically worsens with activity, whereas inflammatory back pain improves. Patients with spinal stenosis may develop pseudoclaudication, so called because it mimics the pain of vascular claudication. These patients develop back and gluteal pain with walking. They may develop bilateral leg pain even when standing still, which is uncommon with vascular claudication.

Examination of the patient should be complete

TABLE 39–14. CATEGORIES OF LOW BACK PAIN

Category	Source	Quality	Process
Superficial somatic	Skin, subcutaneous tissue	Sharp, burning	Cellulitis, herpes zoster
Deep somatic	Muscles, periosteum, joints, ligaments, fascia, vessels	Sharp, boring, dull ache	Compression fractures, trauma
Radicular	Spinal nerves	Radiating, tingling, shooting	Herniated disk, spinal stenosis
Neurogenic	Motor-sensory nerves	Burning	Femoral neuropathy
Visceral or referred	Abdominal or pelvic viscera, aorta	Colicky, boring, tearing	Aortic aneurysm, pancreatitis
Psychogenic	Cerebral cortex	Variable	Depression, somatization

Adapted from Borenstein DG: Spinal disease: Low back pain. *In* Klippel JH, Dieppe PA (eds): Rheumatology. London, CV Mosby, 1994, with permission.

as well as focused on the back. The back is inspected for abnormal curves or postural deformities that are secondary to the pain. There may be a scoliosis or an accentuation of the normal lumbar lordosis. It is important to check the three planes of motion of the back. Flexion and extension of the back may be limited especially in patients with mechanical problems. Pain with flexion suggests problems with the anterior elements of the spine, and pain with extension suggests problems posteriorly. The other planes of motion include lateral motion and rotation of the lumbar spine. Pain on these planes suggests a muscular or ligamentous origin. Examination of the paraspinal muscles may reveal the presence of muscle spasms as well as areas of muscle tenderness. It is also important to perform a complete neurologic examination. Reflexes of the lower extremity may be affected in patients with root compression: The knee jerk usually tests the lumbar roots L3 or L4, and the ankle jerk tests the sacral root S1. The neurologic examination should also include a check for sensory changes along dermatomes of the lower extremities. It is important to check the strength of muscle groups as well, both distal and proximal. A positive straight-leg-raising test suggests sciatic nerve irritation. The test, done with the patient lying supine, consists in raising the leg with the knee extended. A positive test occurs when the patient's radicular symptoms are reproduced, which should occur when the leg is raised 30 to 70 degrees off the table. Symptoms outside this range are generally not related to sciatic irritation.

Further testing depends largely on the clinical findings. Plain radiographs are usually the best place to start. However, many asymptomatic individuals have advanced osteoarthritic and degenerative disk disease of the lumbar spine. Thus care should be taken to correlate clinical findings with radiographic findings. MRI or computed tomography (CT) is used to define more accurately the anatomic structures present. These studies are expensive, however, and not always needed. They are best used in cases where the cause of pain is not clear, the pain is intractable, or neurologic changes are progressive. As with plain radiographs, care

must be taken to correlate these more sophisticated radiographic results with clinical findings. If serious root entrapment is suggested by motor or sensory abnormalities, an EMG/NCS (nerve conduction study) may help determine the chronicity and extent of the problem.

Treatment of low back pain includes several modalities: physical measures, medication, and injections and nerve blocks. Physical measures are important: rest, physical therapy, support, and heat therapy. Rest is difficult for most patients because of busy schedules. It is best accomplished with a person lying on his or her back with the hip and knees slightly flexed. Patients should also avoid lifting or bending. Physical therapy includes back exercises. The goals may include simple stretching of back muscles during the acute pain to more vigorous exercise programs to strengthen muscles once the back symptoms have improved. Application of heat using a heating pad for about 30 minutes three or four times a day often provides symptomatic relief. Support measures may include back braces or corsets, which are used primarily during the acute phase of the pain.

Medications used in patients with low back pain include analgesics, NSAIDs, and muscle relaxants. Analgesics include non-narcotic preparations (e.g., acetaminophen) and narcotics. Generally non-narcotics are used first and in full doses. In patients with more severe pain, narcotics may be used for a short period in conjunction with other therapeutic modalities. NSAIDs are frequently prescribed for patients with back pain and are used for both analgesia and their anti-inflammatory effect even though inflammation may not play an important role in the pathogenesis of pain. Muscle relaxants are also used primarily in patients with muscle spasms or a significant muscular component.

Injections of localized, tender areas around bony structures, ligaments, or muscles may be helpful. Sites for treatment are identified by careful palpation of areas of tenderness. Reproducibility of the patient's symptoms at the sites of injection is important. A combination of a local anesthetic with a steroid preparation may provide significant relief.

Other forms of therapy include nerve blocks.

The nerve block is usually performed in patients with persistent root symptoms. Patients are given epidural injections of a local anesthetic and steroids.

Surgery is rarely needed. Many back pain syndromes resolve or significantly decrease with time. Surgical options may need to be considered in patients with intractable back pain or those with progressive neurologic dysfunction including limb weakness.

REFERENCES

Adelman DC, Saltiel E, Klineberg JR: The neuropsychiatric manifestations of systemic lupus erythematosus: An overview. Semin Arthritis Rheum 15:185, 1986.

Agrawal NM, Roth S, Graham MD, et al: Misoprostol compared with sucralfate in the prevention on nonsteroidal anti-inflammatory drug-induced gastric ulcer. Ann Intern Med 115:195, 1991.

Ansell BM: Juvenile dermatomyositis. Rheum Dis Clin North Am 17:931, 1991.

Arnett FC, Reveille JD: Genetics of systemic lupus erythematosus. Rheum Dis Clin North Am 18:865, 1992.

Athreya BH, Cassidy JT: Current status of the medical management of children with juvenile rheumatoid arthritis. Rheum Dis Clin North Am 17:871, 1991.

Bradley JD, Brandt KD, Katz BP, et al: Comparison of an anti-inflammatory dose of ibuprofen and acetaminophen in the treatment of patients with osteoarthritis of the knees. N Engl J Med 325:195, 1991.

Brandt KA: Should osteoarthritis be treated with nonsteroidal anti-inflammatory drugs. Rheum Dis Clin North Am 19:697, 1993.

Calabrese LH: Human immunodeficiency virus (HIV) and arthritis. Rheum Dis Clin North Am 19:477, 1993.

Chuang TY, Hunder GG, Ilstrup DM, et al: Polymyalgia rheumatica: A 10 year epidemiologic and clinical study. Ann Intern Med 97:672, 1982.

Dahlberg PJ, Lockhart JM, Overholt EL: Diagnostic studies for systemic necrotizing vasculitis. Arch Intern Med 149:161, 1989.

Daniels TE: Labial salivary gland biopsy in Sjögren's syndrome. Arthritis Rheum 27:147, 1984.

Falk RJ, Hogan S, Carey TS, et al: Clinical course of anti-neutrophil cytoplasmic autoantibody-associated glomerulonephritis and systemic vasculitis. Ann Intern Med 113:656, 1990.

Felson DT: Epidemiology of the rheumatic disease. In McCarty DJ, Koopman WJ (eds): Arthritis and Allied Conditions, 12th edition. Philadelphia, Lea & Febiger, 1993.

Gater RA: A Practical Handbook of Joint Fluid Analysis, Philadelphia, Lea & Febiger, 1984.

Gladman DD: Psoriatic arthritis: Recent advances in pathogenesis and treatment. Rheum Dis Clin 18:247, 1992.

Graham DY, White RH, Moreland MD, et al: Duodenal and gastric ulcer prevention with misoprostol in arthritis patients taking NSAIDs. Ann Intern Med 119:257, 1993.

Hoffman GS, Kerr GS, Leavitt RY, et al: Wegener granulomatosis: An analysis of 158 patients. Ann Intern Med 116:488, 1992.

Hough AJ: Pathology of osteoarthritis. In McCarty DJ, Koopman WJ (eds): Arthritis and Allied Conditions, 12th edition. Philadelphia, Lea & Febiger, 1993.

Jimenez SA, Sigal SH: A fifteen year prospective study of treatment of rapidly progressive systemic sclerosis with D-penicillamine. J Rheumatol 18:1496, 1991.

Kahn MA: Ankylosing spondylitis: Clinical features. In Klippel JH, Dieppe PA (eds): Rheumatology. London, CV Mosby, 1994.

Kaye BR: Rheumatic manifestations of infection with human immunodeficiency virus (HIV). Ann Intern Med 111:158, 1989.

Kingsley G, Panayi G: Antigenic responses in reactive arthritis. Rheum Dis Clin North Am 18:49, 1992.

Kovacs JAJ, Urowitz MB, Gladman DD: Dilemmas in neuropsychiatric lupus. Rheum Dis Clin North Am 19:795, 1993.

Lane NE, Buckwalter JA: Exercise: A cause of osteoarthritis. Rheum Dis Clin 19:617, 1993.

Lauhio A, Leirisalo-Repo M, Lähdevirta J, et al: Double-blinded, placebo-controlled study of three-month treatment with lymecycline in reactive arthritis, with special reference to Chlamydia arthritis. Arthritis Rheum 34:6, 1991.

Lawrence RC: Rheumatoid arthritis: Classification and epidemiology. In Klippel JH, Dieppe PA (eds): Rheumatology. London, CV Mosby, 1994.

Lehman TJA: Systemic lupus erythematosus in children and adolescence. In Wallace DJ, Hahn BH (eds): Dubois' Lupus Erythematosus, 4th edition. Philadelphia, Lea & Febiger, 1993.

Lightfoot RW, Michel BA, Bloch DA, et al: The American College of Rheumatology 1990 criteria for the classification of polyarteritis nodosa. Arthritis Rheum 33:1088, 1990.

Lightfoot RW, Luft BJ, Rahn DW, et al: Empiric parenteral antibiotic treatment of patients with fibromyalgia and fatigue and a positive serologic result for Lyme disease. Ann Intern Med 119:503, 1993.

Lukert BP, Raisz LG: Gluco-corticoid induced osteoporosis: Pathogenesis and management. Ann Intern Med 112:352, 1990.

Matteson EL, Cohen MD, Conn DL: Rheumatoid arthritis: Clinical features: systemic involvement. In Klippel JH, Dieppe PA (eds): CV Mosby, London, 1994.

Moll JMH, Wright V: Psoriatic arthritis. Semin Arthritis Rheum 3:55, 1973.

Owen DS: A cheap and useful compensated polarizing microscope [letter to the editor]. N Engl J Med 285:1152, 1971.

Owen DS: Aspiration and injection of joints and soft tissues. In Kelly WN, Harris ED, Ruddy S, Sledge CB (eds): Textbook of Rheumatology, 4th edition. Philadelphia, WB Saunders Company, 1993.

Pincus T, Wolfe F: Treatment of rheumatoid arthritis: challenges to traditional paradigms. Ann Intern Med 115:825, 1991.

Piper JM, Ray WA, Daugherty JR, Griffin MR: Corticosteroid use and peptic ulcer disease: Role of nonsteroidal anti-inflammatory drugs. Ann Intern Med 114:735, 1991.

Plotz PH, Dalakas M, Leff RL, et al: Current concepts in the idiopathic inflammatory myopathies: Polymyositis, dermatomyositis and related disorders. Ann Intern Med 111:143, 1989.

Rakel RE: The family physician. In Rakel RE (eds): Textbook of Family Medicine, 4th edition. Philadelphia, WB Saunders Company, 1990.

Reichlin M, Harley JB: Antinuclear antibodies: An overview. In Wallace DJ, Hahn BH (eds): Dubois' Lupus Erythematosus, 4th edition. Philadelphia, Lea & Febiger, 1993.

Sandler DP, Burr FR, Weinberg CR, Nonsteroidal anti-inflammatory drugs and the risk of chronic renal disease. Ann Intern Med 115:165, 1991

Steen VD, Medsger TA, Rodnan GP: D-Penicillamine therapy in progressive systemic sclerosis (scleroderma). Ann Intern Med 97:652, 1982.

Steen VD, Costantino JP, Shapiro AP, Medsger TA: Outcome of renal crisis in systemic sclerosis: Relation to availability of angiotensin converting enzyme (ACE) inhibitors. Ann Intern Med 113:352, 1990.

Stratton MA: Drug-induced systemic lupus erythematosus. Clin Pharm 4:657, 1985.

Weissman MH: Should steroids be used in the management of rheumatoid arthritis. Rheum Dis Clin North Am 19:189, 1993.

Williams RC: Acute rheumatic fever. *In* Klippel JH, Dieppe PA (eds): Rheumatology. London, CV Mosby, 1994.

Wolfe F, Smythe HA, Yunus MB, et al: The American College of Rheumatology 1990 criteria for the classification of fibromyalgia. Arthritis Rheum 33:160, 1990.

Yazici H: Behçet's syndrome. *In* Klippel JH, Dieppe PA (eds): Rheumatology. London, CV Mosby, 1994.

CHAPTER **40**

EVALUATION OF SKIN LESIONS

SHELLEY P. ROATEN, Jr, M. BASEM CHAKER,
and AMIT G. PANDYA

When a skin condition is the patient's primary complaint, many experienced clinicians begin the evaluation with inspection of the skin, followed by the history, remainder of the physical examination, and tests. This approach satisfies the urge to look and avoids potential bias in the history that might erroneously limit diagnostic possibilities.

HISTORY AND EXAMINATION

Although there are reasonable exceptions for dermatoses of limited distribution, the most thorough skin examination is accomplished with the patient disrobed and then covered with appropriated gowns and drapes. The examiner first seeks an overview of the arrangement and distribution of the dermatosis followed by inspection of individual lesions. Understanding the vocabulary of these descriptions is essential for documentation, follow-up of progress, and communication of findings to other physicians.

Just as a knowledgeable botanist might identify a geographic area from a description of its forest and trees, the observant physician can often identify a rash from an accurate description of its lesions and their distribution. It is important to remember that only a differential diagnosis may be possible at the initial visit, which is then clarified by later visits. Physicians must also accept that there is an occasional condition that resolves spontaneously without an accurate label or specific treatment.

Arrangement and Distribution of Lesions

Attention is first focused on the arrangement and distribution of lesions. *Arrangement* refers to the groupings or relations among lesions, many of which are associated with specific diagnoses (Table 40–1). Melanoma, for example, is typically solitary, whereas groups of vesicles suggest herpes virus infection. *Distribution* (Table 40–2) refers to the predilection of many skin disorders for specific locations. Atopic dermatitis usually involves the

antecubital and popliteal fossae, and psoriasis typically appears on the opposite sides of the elbows and knees. Bilaterally symmetric eruptions suggest an "endogenous" cause, such as a viral exanthem or drug eruption. Photosensitivity reactions favor extensor surfaces of the extremities and spare areas covered by clothing. In some cases the reason for a particular distribution is unknown, but it may still be a valuable diagnostic clue.

Primary Lesions

After noting general appearance and patterns, the examiner shifts attention to visual inspection and palpation of individual lesions. The lesions sought are traditionally referred to as *primary* and *secondary*. Although they are not well standardized, these descriptive categories facilitate our ability to diagnose and communicate findings. Primary lesions (Fig. 40–1) are defined as those arising de novo in the skin, without an antecedent visible lesion. *Macules* and *patches* are flat, nonpalpable areas of skin that differ in color from the surrounding skin; patches are larger than macules. *Papules, nodules,* and *tumors* are solid elevated lesions of respectively larger sizes, and *plaques* are only slightly elevated relative to their large surface area. *Vesicles, bullae,* and *pustules* are raised, fluid-filled lesions that differ in size and fluid composition. *Wheals* are elevated lesions that are edematous and transitory. *Petechiae* and *purpura* are circumscribed deposits of blood or blood pigments, the latter being larger. A *cyst* is an epithelium-lined fluid or semisolid filled space, often with an overlying punctum.

Some authorities also recognize a subcategory of "special" primary lesions that are particularly characteristic of a few diseases. Acne, for example, is easily recognized by its open and closed *comedones.* Typical *burrows* help identify scabies and cutaneous larva migrans. A discrete, globular, *umbilicated papule* is virtually diagnostic of molluscum contagiosum. The *iris* or *target* lesions of erythema multiforme appear as erythematous wheals or plaques with a purple, gray, necrotic, or vesicular center.

TABLE 40–1.   ARRANGEMENT OF LESIONS

Arrangement	Examples
Isolated	Melanoma, keratoacanthoma
Scattered	Molluscum contagiosum, common warts
Grouped	Verruca plana, lichen planus, insect bites
Herpetiform (grouped vesicles)	Herpes simplex, herpes zoster
Zosteriform (dermatomal)	Herpes zoster
Annular (ring)	Tinea corporis, erythema multiforme (iris lesions), drug eruptions, lupus erythematosus, secondary syphilis, pityriasis rosea
Linear	*Rhus* contact dermatitis, linear scleroderma, Kaposi sarcoma
Reticular (lacy, net-like)	Livedo reticularis, oral lichen planus

Secondary Lesions

Secondary lesions evolve from a preceding visible lesion. *Scales* and *crusts* are actually superficial to the skin; the former are flakes composed of aggregates of shedding epidermal cells, and the latter are masses that result from the drying of exudates. *Excavations* of the skin are areas where superficial skin layers are interrupted, including *ulcers, fissures,* and *excoriations.*

TABLE 40–2.   DISTRIBUTION OF LESIONS

Site	Lesion
Generalized	Secondary syphilis, viral exanthems, some drug eruptions
Acral	Dyshydrotic dermatitis, plantar warts, tinea pedis
Intertriginous	*Candida* infections, erythrasma
Palms and soles	Secondary syphilis, erythema multiforme, dyshydrotic dermatitis
Extensor	Psoriasis, solar keratosis, ichthyosis, lupus erythematosus
Flexor	Atopic dermatitis
Dermatomal	Herpes zoster
Circumscribed	Herpes simplex, contact dermatitis, erysipelas
Truncal	Tinea versicolor, pityriasis rosea
Hair-bearing areas	Psoriasis, tinea capitis, pediculosis
Lower extremities	Erythema nodosum, stasis dermatitis
Mucous membranes	Lichen planus, aphthous ulcers, thrush, erythema multiforme
Sites of pressure	Urticaria
Sites of trauma	Psoriasis, lichen planus, molluscum, warts
Unilateral	Herpes zoster, lichen simplex chronicus
Follicular	Acne, bacterial folliculitis, some fungal infections, pityriasis rubra pilaris

PRIMARY LESIONS

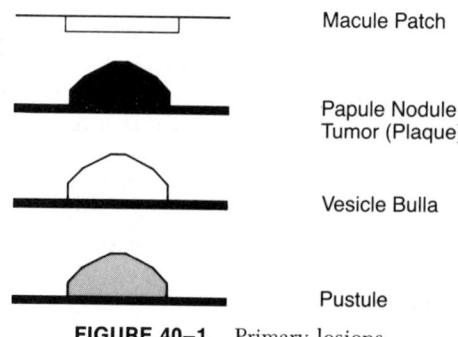

FIGURE 40–1.   Primary lesions.

Lichenification is an area of skin that is thickened, with increased prominence of skin lines. *Scars* are indicative of deep involvement or trauma, with subsequent repair that incompletely restores normal skin architecture. If scars are hypertrophic, they are called *keloids.* *Atrophy* of the epidermis or dermis may have several clinical manifestations, most often appearing as depressions below the level of surrounding skin.

Often primary and secondary lesions are intermingled on the skin of a single patient, requiring "selective vision," or attention to each type of lesion. Each patient may have all the lesions that occur during the natural evolution of his or her disease, for which the history can establish the appropriate sequence of events.

History

The complaints of a dermatologic patient are rather limited; he or she itches, has a rash or discrete lesion, or occasionally has pain, anesthesia, or a burning sensation. Our task is to discover the temporal characteristics, precipitating or palliative factors, and related personal or family history. Most of this information is obtained with a few simple questions.

1.   How long has the rash or itching been present?
2.   How has the appearance changed?
3.   Is it constant or recurrent?
4.   Are there factors that seem to make it better or worse?
5.   Has a similar problem occurred in a family member?
6.   Has it been treated at home or by another physician?
7.   Are any drugs being taken, either prescription or nonprescription?

If not already known, questions regarding the patient's age, occupation, habits, and physiologic state (menses, pregnancy) may also be indicated.

The history or examination may lead to specific additional questions, but generally the history obtained with these few questions is complete. Most errors occur by omission of the general drug history and the previous treatment of the skin condition.

We should not, of course, allow the ease of the dermatologic history to divert our attention from the patient as a whole. In the first place, the complaint may be only a means of entry into the office, with a more important agenda awaiting discovery. Second, the skin may be one of several organs affected by an underlying disease or condition. Either of these situations indicates the need for a more general medical history.

Microscopic Examinations

Microscopic examinations are most often used to support the diagnosis of common dermatophytes. Scale, hair, vesicles, and nail scrapings can be examined by this method. Slide preparation time limits usefulness in a busy office, but knowledge of the techniques is valuable for unusual lesions; other patients can be examined while slides macerate for the appropriate length of time.

Specimens from scaly lesions or from fingernails are most easily obtained by scraping the material onto the center of a microscope slide. The fungal organisms are found in the hyperkeratotic material under the free edge of an affected nail. A vesicle roof can be removed with a scalpel, whereas hairs are removed by plucking them with tweezers or similar instrument. A drop or two of 10% to 20% potassium hydroxide (KOH) and a coverslip are added, and light pressure is applied to the coverslip to "flatten" the scales. Gently heating the slide hastens maceration. Scales and hair are generally readable within 10 to 15 minutes, but nail scrapings may take several hours. Solutions of KOH with dimethylsulfoxide (DMSO) are available and greatly reduce maceration time. Microscopic examination reveals characteristic spores and hyphae or budding yeast forms. The key maneuver is moving the microscope condenser up and down under a likely looking fragment until the light causes maximum contrast between the fungus and its surroundings. Usually, the low-power objective ($10 \times$) is the best choice for detection, with the medium-power objective used for confirmation.

Sometimes the examiner finds a lesion that "looks fungal," but the KOH preparation appears to be negative. For superficial fungi, no harm results if the examination is repeated after the patient applies 1% hydrocortisone cream to the lesion for 1 week. This maneuver is particularly helpful if lesions have been partially treated prior to the first examination; hyphae are more evident at the next visit.

Examination of smears prepared with Gram's stain is occasionally indicated to distinguish bacterial from fungal skin infections or to establish tentative identity of a bacterium. Staining is also helpful to confirm the presence of herpes virus. For that purpose the base of a vesicle is scraped with a scalpel, and the material is placed on a slide and stained with Wright's or Giemsa's stain (referred to as a Tzanck preparation). Multinucleate giant cells are characteristic of herpes infection, including varicella and shingles.

Microscopic examination can sometimes confirm a resistant or atypical case of scabies by scraping the mite onto a slide with mineral oil or microscope immersion oil. Admittedly, the examination is almost superfluous if the burrow is typical.

Biopsy

Biopsy is most often indicated for those lesions that may be malignant (exhibiting a change in color or growth) and for chronic lesions for which the diagnosis is imprecise or unknown.

Immunofluorescence techniques are valuable for identification of bullous disease and suspected lupus erythematosus. The most popular methods for obtaining tissue are excisional biopsy, shave biopsy, and punch biopsy, each of which can ordinarily be accomplished with simple local anesthesia.

Excisional biopsy is indicated for the best cosmetic result and when removal of the entire lesion is desired. Full-thickness excisional biopsy also is necessary for the most accurate histologic diagnosis. Shave biopsy easily removes small elevated lesions, and the bleeding is stopped with light electrocautery. Shaving is quick and simple and is useful in areas where the cosmetic result is less important. Punch biopsy also yields excellent tissue specimens easily. Both reusable and disposable punches are available. The punch instrument is rotated into the skin to the desired depth, the cylinder of skin excised, and the bleeding stopped with pressure, sutures, or Monsel's solution (ferrous subsulfate). A specimen obtained by any of these biopsy methods should be placed immediately in a labeled specimen container with formalin or another suitable preservative. Complete removal of pigmented lesions is desired, as it is not possible to stage a melanoma or accurately diagnose an atypical mole from a portion of the lesion. Biopsies of suspected inflammatory disorders, such as lupus, should include some subcutaneous fat in the specimen; shave biopsy is not indicated.

If excisional biopsy is indicated, an ellipse of skin is ordinarily removed. For best closure, the length of the ellipse should be at least 2.5 to 3.0 times its width. The long axis is oriented parallel to natural skin lines, so a less noticeable scar results. Punch biopsy can also result in a small ellipse if the skin is stretched *perpendicular* to skin lines while the instrument is being inserted.

Cultures

Practically speaking, bacterial and fungal cultures are neither necessary nor cost-effective for most typical skin infections encountered in the family physician's office. For lesions that are uncommon, are clinically atypical, or fail to respond to standard therapy, accurate identification of the organism is indicated. Initial cultures for bacteria are usually performed on blood agar or a reliable transport medium, and suspected fungal organisms are inoculated in Sabouraud's agar or similar medium. If oral therapy for fungal infection is contemplated, a documented positive culture or KOH examination is important because of the cost and potential side effects of treatment.

Other Diagnostic Tests

Obviously, a wide variety of blood or radiologic examinations are appropriate when skin disease is potentially related to abnormalities of other organ systems, such as cutaneous lupus, sarcoidosis, or suspected secondary syphilis. Cytologic imprints, viral cultures, and cell cultures are helpful in some special situations.

GENERAL MANAGEMENT

Hydration

Probably the oldest rule of dermatology is "if it's wet, dry it; and if it's dry, wet it." Wet dressings and soaks paradoxically cause drying of the skin by their application and therefore are considered useful for moist, weeping, or encrusted lesions. Although water is probably the active ingredient, a mild astringent or antibacterial agent is often included to perform those respective additional functions. Useful astringents include *Burow's solution* (one Domeboro tablet per pint of water) and weak solutions of white *vinegar* (1 or 2 ounces per pint of water), applied as dressings or soaks several times daily. Hydrogen peroxide (2%) may be used if there is an infection present, and it is useful for removing crusts. Powders might seem to be useful for their drying effect, but they have disadvantages. Talc, for example, serves fairly well as a dry lubricant but is totally nonabsorbent. Starch absorbs moisture well but tends to aggregate into irritating clumps and can serve as a nutrient for bacteria and yeast.

The moistening of dry, scaling lesions is usually accomplished through the occlusive effect of ointments or pastes, which increase relative hydration of the skin by reducing water loss. If the area is soaked in water for a few minutes immediately before application, considerable moisture is retained.

Frequently used preparations are *zinc oxide ointment* and plain white *petrolatum.*

Management of Itching

Itching alone or in association with various visible lesions often responds to nonspecific antipruritic measures. Orally administered antihistamines can be given two to four times daily, using a slightly larger dose at bedtime to promote sleep. *Diphenhydramine* (Benadryl) is safe and reliable; some authorities prefer *hydroxyzine* (Atarax, Vistaril) for the itching associated with urticaria and similar lesions of presumed allergic etiology. The newer antihistamines, such as terfenadine (Seldane) or astemizole (Hismanal), offer reduced sedation. Several proprietary topical preparations containing camphor, menthol, or phenol are useful for relief of itching confined to small areas. Calamine lotion is popular and safe, but many physicians avoid Caladryl because of the risk of cutaneous sensitization to the additional antihistamine. If the itching is more widespread, some patients obtain temporary relief from cool or tepid baths without soap. Others find the addition of a package of Aveeno colloidal oatmeal to the bath water soothing. (*Note:* Caution patients or their parents that the tub becomes slippery.)

The itching associated with dry skin (xerosis) deserves special emphasis because it is so common, especially among the elderly. It is easily the most common cause of itching seen in a primary care office and must be considered before a complicated work-up is begun for the differential diagnosis of itching. It occurs more often during cold, dry weather and is exacerbated by the use of strong alkaline detergent bath soaps. Xerosis responds to simple hydration and to the avoidance of various factors that result in dehydration of the skin. In particular, patients should use mild soaps (Dove, Basis) sparingly and should avoid excessively hot water. A few people try to treat itching with alcohol rubdowns, which temporarily cools the skin but actually exacerbates the problem of dry skin by removing protective lipids.

Pruritus ani, itching of perianal skin, is probably just a puzzling symptom rather than a distinct clinical or pathologic entity. No lesion is customarily seen, but there may be localized chronic lichenification, redness, edema, or fissures. There is no clear etiology, but there are associations with emotional stress, fecal residue on the skin, diabetes mellitus, overzealous cleansing, and other conditions. The most important task is to discover and treat any of the specific diseases that are accompanied by perianal itching, such as pinworms, fungal infections, contact dermatitis, colitis, and Hodgkin's disease. If no cause can be found, local application of a low-potency nonhalogenated topical steroid cream or lotion can help control the itching.

Cleansing gently with a mild liquid soap (Cetaphil) is a helpful adjunctive treatment.

Avoidance of Causative Agents

Perhaps because the principle seems obvious, physicians may spend too little time explaining the avoidance of causative factors or suspected causes. Allergic contact dermatitis is a particularly good example, and its cause should be discussed with the patient. Appropriate avoidance may follow easily after identification of the allergen or may require more complicated general advice about clothing, gloves, jewelry, cosmetics, and other environmental factors. It may be necessary to eliminate possible causes sequentially.

Skin lesions associated with the ingestion of medications often pose a greater problem. Should the offending drug be discontinued, continued with close observation, or exchanged for another drug of similar purpose? The questions usually yield to common sense, with the answer derived from the importance of the drug relative to the severity of the skin reaction. Although the skin reactions and drugs are too numerous for discussion here, we must point out that any drug should be suspected when a rash follows its ingestion.

Corticosteroids

Dermatoses generally responsive to topical corticosteroids are the following.

1. Eczema (contact and irritant dermatitis, neurodermatitis, atopic dermatitis, some photosensitivity reactions)
2. Psoriasis
3. Seborrheic dermatitis
4. Types of pruritus ani, especially in association with psoriasis

A few other dermatoses that respond less predictably include lichen planus, granuloma annulare, pemphigus, and some lesions that respond to intralesional steroid injections.

These lists are limited, and the clinician's first obligation is to be reasonably certain that he or she is treating a lesion likely to respond. The second step is selection of the appropriate steroid from a staggering list of commercially prepared alternatives. Finally, an infectious etiology that might be exacerbated by potent topical steroids must be ruled out. Topical steroid selection depends on relative steroid potency, side effects, vehicle, and cost.

Clinical potency and potential side effects of topical steroids are directly related; no steroid preparation offers greater strength without a parallel increase in the probability of side effects and cost. Systemic side effects are rare but can occur with widespread application to abnormal skin, especially in children. Local effects include striae, skin atrophy, hypopigmentation, and acneiform eruptions. Both potency and side effects are greater for fluorinated steroids than for nonfluorinated steroids. The correct steroid is the *least* potent one that can reasonably be expected to achieve results. Results can often be predicted from a knowledge of the usual natural history of the disease or from the patient's previous response to steroids used for the condition. As a general rule, no fluorinated steroid should be applied to the face or to the axillary, vaginal, or anal areas; hydrocortisone is a safer alternative.

The vehicle in which the steroid is incorporated affects potency and convenience of application. Vehicles vary in their ability to cause percutaneous absorption; more steroid absorption into the skin means more clinical potency (and more side effects). With some unavoidable oversimplification, vehicles can be ranked in the order of their ability to promote absorption as follows, in decreasing order: gels and ointments, creams, lotions, and sprays.

Naturally, the ease of application is represented approximately in reverse order, which probably helps explain why creams are a popular compromise. The rank also suggests, for example, that an inadequate response to a steroid cream might improve with a change to an ointment formulation of the same steroid. Ointments are usually undesirable on the face and in intertriginous areas, but they are particularly useful for dry, scaly dermatoses such as psoriasis. Gels and lotions are usually most desirable in hair-bearing areas.

Apart from the effect of vehicles, steroids vary in their inherent potency *as formulated*. They also differ drastically in cost. The information in Table 40–3 is intended as a guide to the selection of corticosteroids based on potency groups. The examples were selected as relatively low cost representative choices in their groups. Note that knowledge of a few alternatives covers the entire spectrum of potency, and that generic preparations are available for most strengths (Table 40–3).

Although Table 40–3 was prepared with attention to low cost, wholesale costs vary substantially. The *Drug Topics Red Book* (Medical Economics Data, Montvale, NJ, 1994) or a similar source is suggested. Patients should be told that hydrocortisone 0.5% or 1% (e.g., Cort-Aid) for topical use is available without a prescription for treatment of relatively mild skin conditions.

The use of occlusive materials, such as plastic wrap, over areas of topical steroid application is a method of dramatically increasing absorption and potency. Disadvantages are the inconvenience and the higher risk of adverse effects. Occlusion may be best tolerated with nighttime use; it should be used only for resistant conditions and for a few days at a time. Often the change from a cream to an oint-

TABLE 40–3. TOPICAL CORTICOSTEROIDS

Potency	Steroid/Strength	Trade Names
Lowest	Hydrocortisone 0.5–1.0%	Several, nonprescription: Penecort, Cort-Dome
	Methylprednisolone acetate 1%	Medrol
Low	Desonide 0.05%	Desowen, Tridesilon
	Fluocinolone acetonide 0.1%	Synalar
	Triamcinolone acetonide 0.025%	Aristocort, Kenalog
Intermediate	Betamethasone valerate 0.1%	Valisone
	Halcinonide 0.025%	Halog
	Triamcinolone acetonide 0.1%	Aristocort, Kenalog
High	Betamethasone diproprionate 0.05%	Diprosone, Alphatrex
	Desoximetasone 0.25%	Topicort
	Triamcinolone acetonide 0.5%	Aristicort, Kenalog
Highest	Betamethasone diproprionate 0.05%	Diprolene
	Clobetasol proprionate 0.05%	Temovate

Adapted from Topical steroids. Med Lett 33:857, 1991.

ment or gel provides sufficient "occlusion." Although intralesional steroid injections are indicated for some diseases, cautious use is in order owing to the atrophy and other complications that may result.

Application of Medications

As for other medications, writing a prescription for the appropriate amount of a topical medication requires attention to the area of coverage, the frequency and expected duration of treatment, and the appointment schedule. As a rough rule of thumb, approximately 30 gm of a cream or ointment is required to cover the skin of an average adult. By estimating surface areas in a manner similar to estimating the area of skin burns, one can roughly predict the amount required per application. Coverage of an entire arm, for example, requires about 3 gm (9 to 10 per cent of 30 gm). An expected treatment course of 20 applications over 10 days for one arm would therefore require about 60 gm.

The pharmacokinetics of topical application are not well established; it has been empirically determined that application two or three times daily is sufficient for most medicines. Evidence suggests

that a single application each day may be just as effective for most topical steroids. A good general rule is to attempt to reduce the frequency after a beneficial effect is achieved.

Treating the Whole Person

A methodical scientific approach to the treatment of specific diseases is desirable but not to the extent that we ignore the impact of disease on the patient and his or her social environment. The physical disabilities and the emotional or social consequences of skin disease vary depending on the individual and the disease involved. Each patient has his or her own perception of the problem; and to the extent that skin is a "public organ," those around the patient may have reactions that range from curiosity to actual fear. Obviously, skin diseases can impair health, job performance, and relationships with family and friends.

The mere fact that a knowledgeable physician can touch, critically inspect, and discuss the lesions without evidence of avoidance is reassuring to the patient. An important early step is to explore the patient's understanding of his or her own disease briefly and to dispel myths associated with such conditions as acne, warts, and leprosy. A perceptive physician not only helps the patient understand the disease and its management, it also helps the patient deal with the confusion, anger, frustration, helplessness, and withdrawal that may accompany severe skin disorders. Finally, a positive approach includes methods of reducing the physician's own potential frustration during management of difficult problems.

SPECIFIC SKIN LESIONS AND DISORDERS

Eczemas

Contact Dermatitis

Allergic eczematous contact dermatitis is a cutaneous immune response that lends itself to interesting diagnostic exercises. It responds dramatically to appropriate therapy. It is primarily a cell-mediated hypersensitivity reaction but may involve other immune responses as well. The eruption is characterized by papules, vesicles, excoriation, erythema, and sometimes edema (Fig. 40–2). Especially in its early stages, the rash involves mainly the skin sites contacted by the allergen (hapten). If exposure is chronic, the skin may become lichenified, hyperpigmented or hypopigmented, and erythematous, with only occasional vesicles (Fig. 40–3).

The classic "acute" reactions occur 1 to 3 days after contact with the oleoresin of poison ivy (Fig.

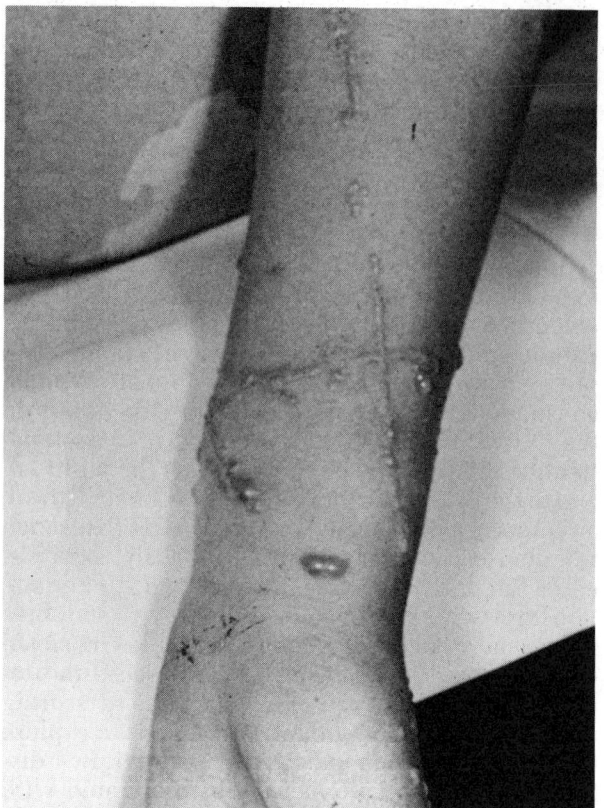
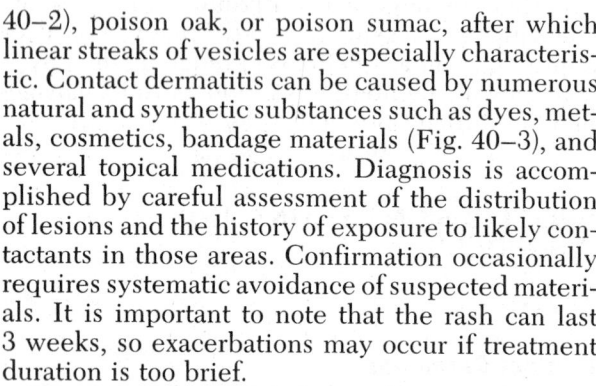

FIGURE 40–2. Contact dermatitis.

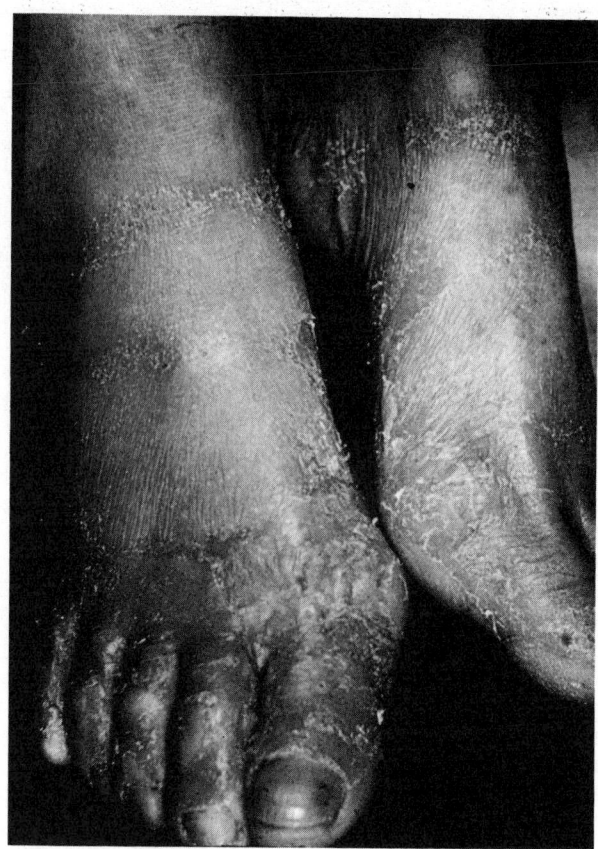

FIGURE 40–3. Contact dermatitis.

40–2), poison oak, or poison sumac, after which linear streaks of vesicles are especially characteristic. Contact dermatitis can be caused by numerous natural and synthetic substances such as dyes, metals, cosmetics, bandage materials (Fig. 40–3), and several topical medications. Diagnosis is accomplished by careful assessment of the distribution of lesions and the history of exposure to likely contactants in those areas. Confirmation occasionally requires systematic avoidance of suspected materials. It is important to note that the rash can last 3 weeks, so exacerbations may occur if treatment duration is too brief.

Physicians should be alert to the contact dermatitis that can occur with topical medications. Notable examples are reactions to topical antibiotics, anesthetics, antiseptics, antihistamines, and even corticosteroids. If the original rash being treated fails to respond or changes in character, contact dermatitis should be considered.

Patch tests are occasionally indicated for diagnosis of a mystifying case, subject to the limitations of examiner experience, cost, and the risk of further sensitization to the testing materials.

TREATMENT. The treatment of contact dermatitis naturally includes cessation of contact. Victims of poison ivy contact, for example, should learn what the plant looks like and where it grows. The relation of skin lesions to other contactants should

be explained in enough detail so patients can eliminate contact in the future.

During its early weeping stages, the typical papulovesicular eruption responds to wet dressings or soaks. Patients may also obtain minimal relief from the itching by using oral antihistamines, especially at bedtime. After the weeping subsides, topical steroids are applied at a strength consistent with the estimated severity of the rash. Particularly severe reactions can be treated with a short, tapering course of a steroid, such as prednisone, given orally in the appropriate dosage. A typical regimen for an adult is prednisone 60 mg administered orally daily in divided doses, then tapered gradually. Exacerbation may occur if the steroid is discontinued too quickly, and tapering the dosage over 2 to 3 weeks is customary. A parenteral steroid such as triamcinolone (Kenalog) may be administered intramuscularly for sustained effect; adult dosage is 40 mg, repeatable once weekly.

Neurodermatitis (Lichen Simplex Chronicus)

The term neurodermatitis can lead to some confusing searches through textbook indexes. Some authors use the term neurodermatitis, or disseminated neurodermatitis, in reference to the adult form of atopic dermatitis. Others use neurodermatitis to refer to circumscribed neurodermatitis, or

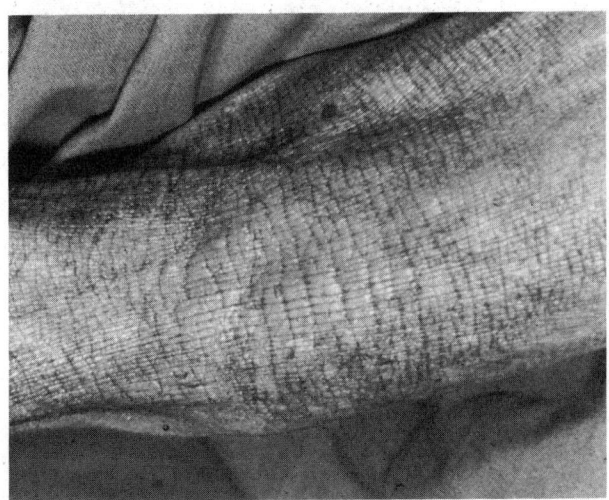

FIGURE 40–4. Neurodermatitis.

lichen simplex chronicus, which is the usage intended here.

Lesions of neurodermatitis appear as poorly circumscribed patches of excoriation and lichenification that may be chronic (Fig. 40–4). The lesions are thought to be the skin's response to repeated scratching; because they itch, the lesions are self-perpetuating. The initial event may have been a minor irritant, but chronicity and recurrence are due to scratching. Patients with xerosis often have associated neurodermatitis. Lesions are most often seen in adults on the posterior neck, wrists, ankles, ears, and perianal areas.

TREATMENT. Effective treatment of neurodermatitis logically includes an explanation to the patient of the probable etiology and a request that scratching be avoided. An Unna boot or similar protective dressing may be useful for lesions on the extremities. In the anal or genital area, gentle cleansing followed by application of hydrocortisone cream is safe and effective; the more potent fluorinated steroids may be used for other areas. It is sometimes clear that the lesions are at least partly related to emotional stress, for which counseling and short-term psychotropic medication might be indicated. Hydroxyzine (Atarax) and doxepin (Sinequan) are popular choices.

Atopic Dermatitis (Atopic Eczema)

Eczema is a rather vague morphologic term that describes a clinical picture of scaling, serous exudation, excoriation, erythema, and fissuring. Atopic dermatitis is often expressed as an eczematous eruption but tends to vary according to the patient's age. Itching is a common feature. In infants eczematous lesions tend to appear on the face, scalp, and extensor aspects of the extremities. During childhood papules, erythema, and lichenification tend to predominate on flexor surfaces, wrists, and neck. In adults the flexor surfaces, neck, scalp,

and chest frequently have scaly, lichenified, erythematous lesions. Especially for infants and children, the history often reveals hay fever, asthma, or allergic rhinitis in the patient or a family member.

TREATMENT. Patients with atopic eczema should use a mild bath soap, such as Dove or Basis. Treatment consists primarily in symptomatic relief (usually antihistamines for the itching) and topical corticosteroids. Weeping, moist lesions should be first treated with Burow's or 0.25% vinegar soak solutions (2 teaspoonfuls in 1 quart of water). Efforts to discover a particular food, inhalant, or other factor that leads to exacerbations should be attempted, especially in children, even though success is uncommon. General reduction of common allergens in the household may be helpful, but immunotherapy by desensitization has no proved benefit. Patients with atopic eczema should probably maintain a small amount of low-potency topical steroids in the home medicine cabinet in order to initiate therapy for exacerbations. Do not prescribe the more potent steroids on a long-term basis.

Diseases of Sweat Glands and Follicles

Acne Vulgaris

Acne vulgaris, a common disease usually seen in adolescents, consists of a variety of lesions including comedones, papules, pustules, cysts, and subsequent scars. The lesions occur primarily on the face but may involve the upper trunk and shoulders (Fig. 40–5). The condition is self-limited but may last for years and have significant social consequences for the patient. Diagnosis is usually simple, but some thought should be given to acne variants. Acne or similar lesions may occur, for example with drug ingestions (corticosteroids, iodides, bromides, isoniazid, phenytoin, lithium), occupational exposure (coal tar derivatives, some oils), and possibly use of some cosmetics and detergents.

Ordinary acne is a multifactorial disease of the sebaceous follicles; its occurrence is probably most dependent on genetic predisposition and the influence of androgens on the follicles. The most useful pathophysiologic model states that comedones begin with increased sebum production and altered keratinization. Keratinized cells sloughed into the follicular lumen are abnormally adherent to each other, thereby mechanically limiting the extrusion of lumen contents. The bacterial flora of the follicle, principally *Propionibacterium acnes,* causes breakdown of the sebaceous lipids to more inflammatory products, initiating the familiar sequence of papules, pustules, cysts, and scars. Diet, surface dirt, and sexual habits have generally been discredited as etiologic factors.

TREATMENT. Rational therapy can be based on the pathophysiologic model described earlier, keeping in mind that many patients with acne man-

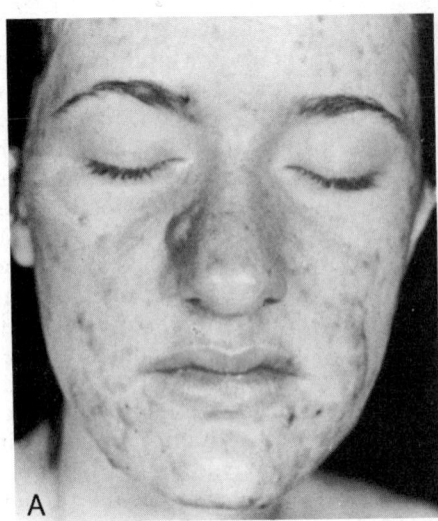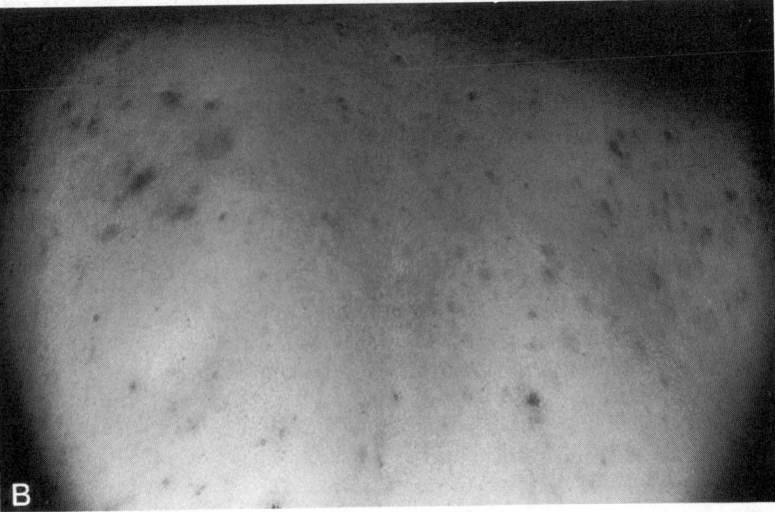

FIGURE 40–5. Acne vulgaris.

keeping in mind that many patients with acne manage well with no medical therapy at all. Table 40–4 summarizes a reasonable approach.

Tretinoin (Retin-A) is available in a cream (0.025%, 0.05%, 0.1%), a gel (0.025%, 0.01%), and a less desirable liquid form. Its chief action is to reduce adherence of keratinized cells, thereby discouraging comedogenesis, but it also has keratolytic properties. Because skin irritation causes some patients to abandon therapy, it is suggested that application of retinoic acid be started slowly, with a low-strength preparation applied once daily; 0.025% cream is a good first choice.

Significant irritation need not be incurred with retinoic acid for improvement of acne. Many patients tolerate application of a cream or a gel twice daily. An explanation of use should include the following.

1. Improvement is evident only after several weeks, and an *exacerbation* of acne may occur during the first month.
2. The eyes, mouth, and angles of the nose should be avoided during application.
3. Exposure to sunlight should be reduced to avoid sunburn.

TABLE 40–4. ACNE THERAPY GUIDE

Lesion/Stage	Therapy
Primarily comedones	Retinoic acid cream/gel
Mildly inflammatory: comedones and papules	Topical antibiotic *or* benzoyl peroxide lotion or gel (sometimes retinoic acid)
Moderate or severe inflammatory: many papules and pustules, some cysts	Benzoyl peroxide *and* oral or topical antibiotic (sometimes retinoic acid) Referral of treatment failures
Conglobate abscesses, severe scarring	Referral

4. Abrasive soaps and cleansers should not be used.

Benzoyl peroxide is available in several strengths of cream, gel, or lotion. It acts primarily as an antibacterial agent to reduce the population of *P. acnes* and has a keratolytic effect. Application usually begins once daily, and some patients tolerate twice-daily use. If irritation can be avoided, combined therapy with tretinoin and benzoyl peroxide is rational, provided they are applied at different times of the day. The precautions about irritation, abrasive soaps, and avoidance of mucous membranes are similar to those for tretinoin.

Some antibiotics are also useful for controlling inflammatory acne. Tetracycline is the one most often administered orally, with minocycline (Minocin) a popular choice for resistant cases. Tetracycline should not be prescribed for children or for pregnant women because of its staining effect on developing teeth. Topical antibiotics are effective alternatives, including erythromycin (T-Stat, Benzamycin, Emgel, EryDerm) and clindamycin (Cleocin T) preparations.

Routine cases of acne are inappropriate indications for estrogen therapy. Patients who are already taking an oral contraceptive for another indication often display improvement of their acne with a highly estrogenic preparation, but that approach incurs the risk of other side effects of estrogen administration. The potential benefits and risks must be weighed carefully.

Cis-retinoic acid (isotretinoin, Accutane) can be given orally for severe cystic, scarring acne. It has serious potential side effects, however, and should be prescribed only by those who are experienced with its use.

Rosacea

Rosacea is a chronic condition of insidious onset that affects the facial skin of adults, particularly

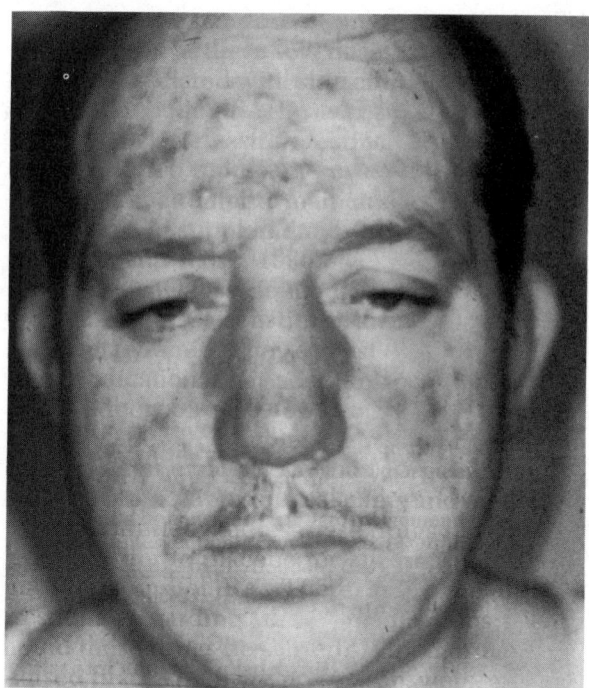

FIGURE 40–6. Rosacea.

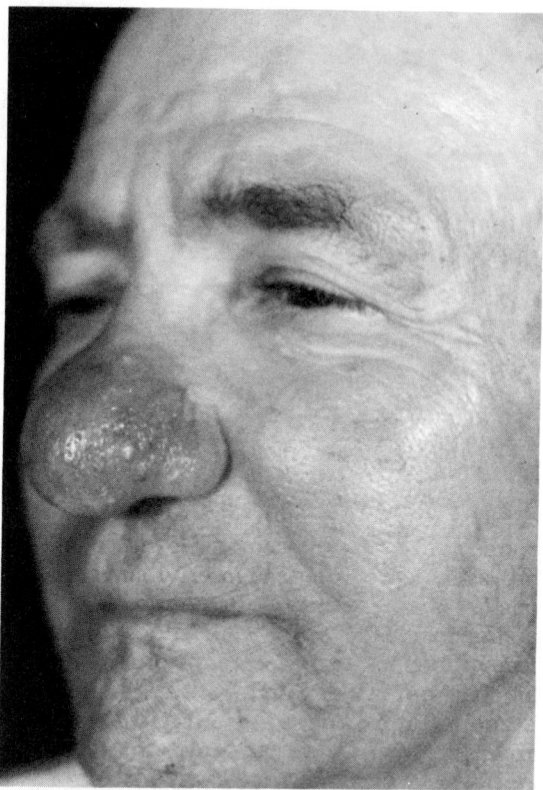

FIGURE 40–7. Rosacea/rhinophyma.

around the nose. It manifests as hyperemia and telangiectases (Fig. 40–6), sometimes with papules, pustules, or nodules. Rosacea occurs most often in adults between the ages of 30 and 50 years; women are affected more frequently, but men typically have the more severe cases. It may ultimately lead to rhinophyma (Fig. 40–7), a hyperplasia of the nasal soft tissues with enlargement and deformity. The red-nosed appearance, reminiscent of W. C. Fields, is a significant cosmetic and social problem.

The etiology of rosacea is unknown but probably is related to dysfunction of the sebaceous glands. Seborrheic dermatitis is commonly coexistent. Associations are also known to exist with some ocular lesions, including blepharitis and conjunctivitis, and with migraine headache. In addition to the cosmetic consequences, patients may be stigmatized by the presumed relation of "rum nose" to alcohol consumption and dietary indiscretions. No causative relations have been established, and the disease occurs in nondrinkers. An existing case of rosacea, however, can be exacerbated by excessive sun exposure or ingestion of alcohol, caffeine, or hot liquids.

The differential diagnosis includes seborrheic dermatitis, acne vulgaris, cutaneous tuberculosis, halogen acne, and eczema. Inappropriate use of fluorinated topical steroids on the area may also lead to a similar appearance; questions about steroids must be a part of the initial history.

TREATMENT. Treatment of the acne-like component of the condition is similar to that for acne vulgaris. Oral tetracycline is reported to control the acneiform lesions and to reduce the hyperemia or erythema by unknown mechanisms. Topical metronidazole (Metrogel) is also effective. Other treatments include electrodesiccation or laser surgery of the telangiectases and surgical repair of the nasal hyperplasia. It also seems logical to avoid stimuli that may increase cutaneous vasodilation, such as heat, cold, excessive sunlight, alcohol, caffeine, highly seasoned foods, and avoidable emotional stress.

Seborrheic Dermatitis

Seborrhea and seborrheic dermatitis (Fig. 40–8) are the major clinical expressions of an ill-defined disorder of the sebaceous glands. The conditions are typically chronic or intermittent, and all age groups are affected. In infants it appears as "cradle cap," as diaper-area dermatitis, and sometimes as a generalized erythematous eruption. Adults may suffer only from occasional dandruff or may have associated scaly, red skin lesions on hairy areas of the body. Typical locations are the scalp around the ears and eyebrows, in the nasolabial folds, along the sternum, and near the pubis. The distribution is bilaterally symmetric. Individually, the lesions are poorly circumscribed patches of erythema with yellowish, greasy-looking scales. Facial seborrheic dermatitis is the most common cause of a "butterfly rash" and should be considered before systemic lupus erythematosus.

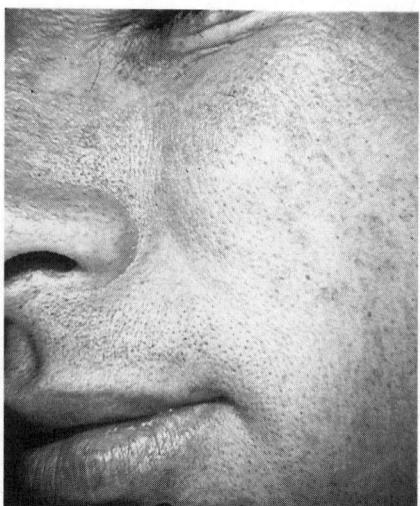

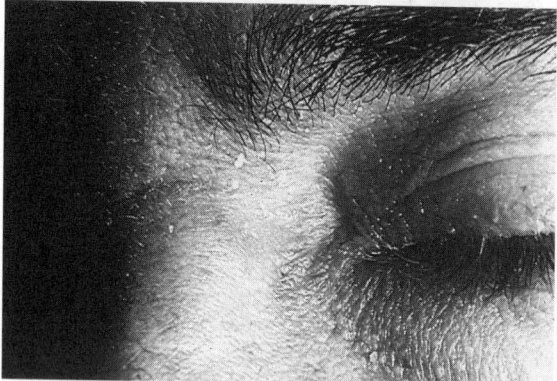

FIGURE 40–8. Seborrheic dermatitis.

TREATMENT. Seborrhea of the scalp (dandruff) usually responds to selenium sulfide (Selsun), tar (e.g., Pentrax), or ketoconazole (Nizoral) shampoos used two or three times weekly. Daily use is sometimes necessary at the beginning of therapy. Severe cases benefit from an occasional application of Synalar, Lidex, or Temovate liquid to the scalp. Patience and regular use of standard baby shampoos usually suffices for cradle cap.

Seborrheic skin lesions in adults respond to topical steroids applied sparingly to the affected area. Hydrocortisone is often effective and is probably the only reasonable choice for facial lesions but may require application several times daily. Topical ketoconazole (Nizoral) cream has also been shown to improve the skin lesions of seborrhea.

The infantile forms of seborrhea are usually self-limited and therefore best "treated" with nonmedical measures such as dry diapers and clean skin. For severe cases short-term application of hydrocortisone produces a dramatic response. In infants seborrheic dermatitis can be confused with atopic eczema or early manifestations of Letterer-Siwe disease.

Miliaria (Heat Rash)

Miliaria is a common skin condition in infants, and almost half of adults retain the tendency. It results from obstruction of the sweat pores, rupture of the duct wall, and retention of sweat within the skin. Recognized subtypes are called miliaria crystallina, rubra, and profunda when sweat retention occurs at successively greater depths. Miliaria crystallina is characterized by tiny vesicles on normal-appearing skin without inflammation, usually in the intertriginous areas. Miliaria rubra, the most common type, often known as prickly heat, consists of small erythematous papules with a minute central vesicle. Pustules may develop in chronic cases. Miliaria rubra occurs most often on the trunk and neck, consistently sparing the face and volar surfaces. Itching or burning of the affected areas is common. Miliaria profunda produces papular lesions without itching or burning.

Patients are predisposed to miliaria in a hot, humid environment, especially when clothing is occlusive. Infants and the bedridden elderly are most susceptible. Miliaria is the most prevalent form of anhidrosis, as the normal functions of sweat production are lost in the affected areas. Patients with extensive miliaria rubra can suffer hyperpyrexia or heat exhaustion if they remain in the environment.

The only effective treatment is to place the patient in a cooler environment, where the sweat pore obstructions gradually resolve over several days. Mild benzoyl peroxide creams and cleansers may yield some improvement. No topical therapy has proved to have value, and many exacerbate the problem.

Dyshidrosis (Pompholyx, Dyshidrotic Eczematous Dermatitis)

Dyshidrosis, of unknown etiology, usually is found in areas of hyperhidrosis. It is probably a simple eczema promoted by moist conditions. The lesions are small, tense vesicles seen on the palms and soles, lateral surface of digits, and interdigital spaces (Fig. 40–9). There is itching and sometimes

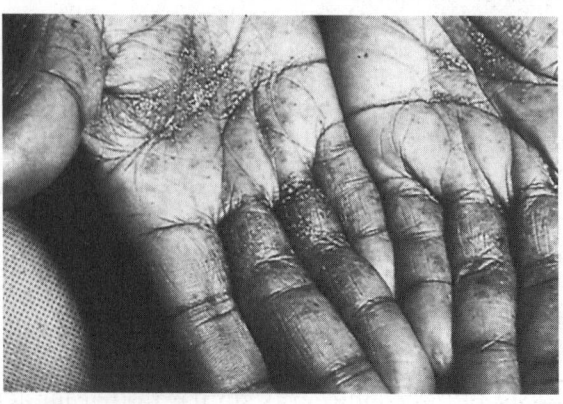

FIGURE 40–9. Dyshidrosis.

a burning sensation. Secondary bacterial infection may ensue.

The principal conditions to be distinguished from dyshidrosis are fungal infections and contact dermatitis, either of which can produce vesicles in a similar distribution. Some authorities believe that the disease can be a precursor of psoriasis.

TREATMENT. Management starts with attempts to control the hyperhidrosis or secondary infections, as necessary. Topical steroids are used as for other kinds of eczema. A search for a topical sensitizer should be undertaken for chronic cases. The patient should reduce contact with harsh cleansers and water. Immediate use of skin moisturizers is appropriate after contact with water or soap.

Hyperhidrosis

To a large extent, the existence of hyperhidrosis is in the eye of the beholder; if the patient perceives excessive sweating, he or she has it. Typical locations for hyperhidrosis are the palms and soles or the axillae, but it may occur almost anywhere on the body and may even be unilateral. The clearest association is with anxiety and stress, exacerbated by hot weather. Areas of excessive perspiration may be observed during the examination (Fig. 40–10). If palms and soles are involved, the skin may appear pink, soft, and waterlogged. Tenderness of the feet may be found.

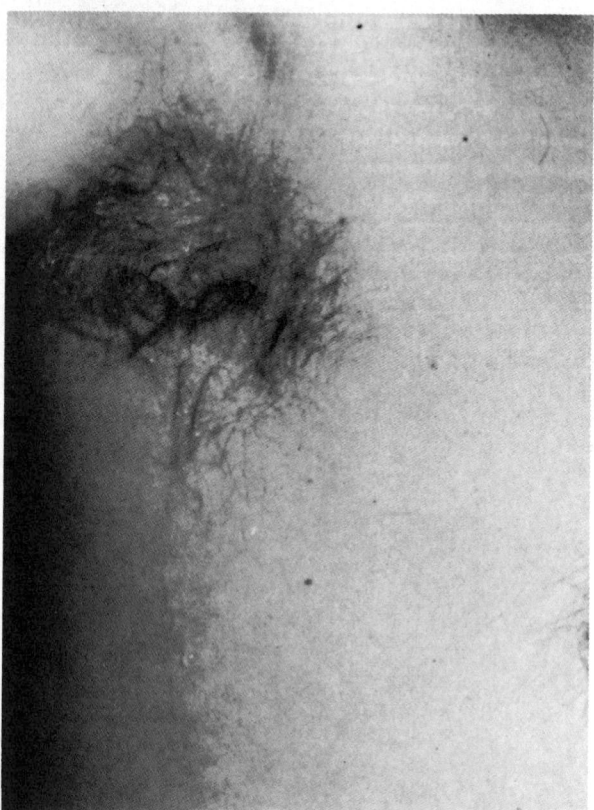

FIGURE 40–10. Hyperhidrosis. (From Hurley HJ: Diseases of the apocrine and eccrine sweat glands. *In* Moschella SL, Hurley HJ [eds]: Dermatology, 3rd edition. Philadelphia, WB Saunders Company, 1992, p 1518, with permission.)

Causes of secondary hyperhidrosis should be sought during the initial evaluation, especially if the sweating is generalized, the onset is relatively sudden, or anxiety does not seem to be a factor. The major diseases include hyperthyroidism, hypothalamic disorders, exposure to cholinergic agents, lymphomas, defervescence of fever, hypoglycemia, syncopal episodes, pheochromocytoma, Horner syndrome, drug withdrawal, tuberculosis, and others.

TREATMENT. The treatment of primary hyperhidrosis requires attention to the underlying anxiety as well as localized therapy for the affected areas. Several options are available for the hands and feet, with different options for the axillae. No treatment is uniformly successful, but the most popular is topical application of aluminum preparations. For hands, feet, or axillae, a solution of aluminum chloride in anhydrous ethanol (Xerac AC, Drysol) is used. The solution is applied to *thoroughly dry* skin at bedtime, and occlusion with plastic wrap increases its effectiveness. The frequency of application may be decreased for maintenance after the first few days. Sensible advice about selection of absorbent clothing and socks is also in order. Other alternatives used for hands and feet include systemic anticholinergic agents, topical methenamine, and iontophoresis.

When aluminum compounds are not successful in the axillary areas, other options or adjunctive methods include systemic anticholinergic agents, topical scopolamine hydrobromide, and surgical intervention for the most severe cases.

Perioral Dermatitis

Perioral dermatitis is a descriptive term applied to a papular, erythematous eruption around the mouth. It occurs most often in young women but is also occasionally described in men. Some regard the condition as a clinical variant of rosacea or seborrheic dermatitis. Associations have been suggested with the use of oral contraceptives, hormonal factors, and particularly potent topical steroids on the face. Contact dermatitis (due to toothpaste or mouthwash) must also be considered.

TREATMENT. Successful treatments have been reported with oral tetracycline, 250 mg two to four times daily. Topical erythromycin or clindamycin is also effective. Patients who have been using potent steroids can be weaned by applying 1% hydrocortisone for about 2 weeks. The stronger steroids should not be used.

Hidradenitis Suppurativa

Hidradenitis suppurativa, a chronic disease of the apocrine sweat gland areas, is characterized by infection, abscess formation, and scarring. It occurs most often in the axillae but at times involves the anogenital area or areolae of the breasts. It results from occlusion of the apocrine duct and bacterial colonization, principally by staphylococci, streptococci, or some gram-negative organisms. There may be an antecedent history of local trauma or irritation, and it is commonly associated with obesity.

Clinically, the established condition is seen as recurrent abscess formation with purulent drainage and the formation of sinus tracts and scars. The areas are painful and tender. The incidence is slightly higher in women, and exacerbations may be related to menses. Although the presentation is characteristic, early occurrences may be confused with carbuncles. The differential diagnosis of anogenital lesions includes lymphogranuloma venereum, granuloma inguinale, and ulcerative colitis.

TREATMENT. Early recognition is important, and systemic antibiotics are the principal method of therapy. Antibiotic selection should be based on culture and sensitivity tests. Incision and drainage of the fluctuant nodules is tempting but promotes the development of sinus tracts. Oral penicillin, erythromycin, and tetracycline are most often indicated, with other antibiotics for the less typical organisms. Some clinicians add systemic or intralesional injections of corticosteroids for the more severe cases. Adjunctive therapy includes the use of soothing compresses of Burow's solution and the avoidance of depilatories, commercial deodorants, shaving, and constrictive clothing. Bedtime applications of aluminum chloride in anhydrous ethanol (Xerac AC) can be used for its antiperspirant and antibacterial properties. Gentle cleansing of the area with an antibacterial soap is also reasonable (Betadine or Hibiclens). Failure of conservative management requires surgical exteriorization or excision of the areas involved. The uncontrolled disease can lead to limited limb mobility and disseminated infection.

Folliculitis

The term folliculitis generally refers to a bacterial infection localized to the hair follicle, most often due to *Staphylococcus aureus*. The everyday form of folliculitis is found in a hot, humid environment with the use of occlusive clothing. The lesions are small papules or pustules at the openings of hair follicles, identified by the protruding hair. Individual lesions are transient, but new ones tend to appear so long as the particular environmental conditions exist.

Similar lesions are observed following exposure to some hydrocarbons in industrial settings or ingestion of certain foods or medications containing halogens (iodide, bromide, chloride). Prominence of the hair follicles, with or without mild inflammation, is seen in malnourished adults.

Pseudofolliculitis barbae is a condition seen in black men. It is due to penetration of the skin by closely shaved hairs in the beard area, causing an inflammatory papule.

TREATMENT. Folliculitis often responds to cooler surroundings and lighter clothing. Individual lesions can be touched with a drop of benzoyl peroxide lotion (Benoxyl, Desquam-X), and oral antibiotics are occasionally indicated for the more severe cases. If needed, synthetic penicillins, tetracyclines, and erythromycin are appropriate choices. The regimen for pseudofolliculitis barbae may include a topical application of benzoyl peroxide prior to shaving, a topical steroid after shaving, and oral tetracycline. Growing a beard, avoiding close shaves, and the use of chemical depilatories (Magic Shave) are other alternatives.

Bacterial Infections

Impetigo

IMPETIGO CONTAGIOSA. Impetigo contagiosa is a type of superficial pyoderma with transient vesicular lesions followed by a characteristic "honey-colored" thick crust that appears to sit on normal or eroded skin (Fig. 40–11). Bacterial cultures yield mixtures of group A streptococcus and *Staphylococcus aureus*; some studies suggest a predominance of staphylococci. Typical impetigo occurs mostly in children, especially those of preschool ages, and is highly communicable. Spread to new areas of the body occurs by autoinoculation due to scratching. The peak seasonal incidence is summer, and lesions may occur and spread for weeks if untreated.

Treatment. Appropriate management of impetigo requires the use of antibiotics. Topical application of mupirocin (Bactroban) ointment three times daily is the preferred initial therapy. If topical therapy is ineffective, penicillin is the traditional choice; benzathine penicillin may be given intramuscularly, or penicillin V may be given orally four times daily for 10 days. Erythromycin may be used four times daily for 10 days in patients allergic to penicillin. Increased attention to skin hygiene is indicated, with gentle soap and water cleansing; vigorous scrubbing is unnecessary. Although antibiotics have not been proved to prevent poststreptococcal glomerulonephritis in the patient, they do hasten resolution of skin lesions and reduce transmission to contacts.

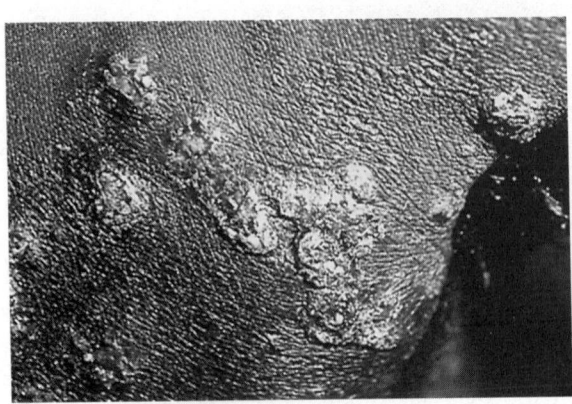

FIGURE 40–11. Impetigo.

BULLOUS IMPETIGO. Bullous impetigo, in contrast, is caused by group 2 staphylococci in infants and children. It is characterized by rapid evolution of a flaccid bullae without surrounding erythema, which rupture and leave a thin, light brown crust. The scattered, round lesions are thought by some observers to resemble cigarette burns, which must therefore be included in the differential diagnosis.

Treatment. Topical mupirocin is the initial form of therapy, but penicillinase-resistant penicillins, such as dicloxacillin, should be considered if the initial response is not prompt. Other expressions of staphylococcal skin infection include the scalded skin syndrome and scarlatiniform eruptions.

Ecthyma

Ecthyma is similar to impetigo contagiosa and is probably best thought of as "deep impetigo." It is caused by group A streptococci, sometimes with *Staphylococcus aureus,* and may result from poor hygiene or minor trauma. Children and neglected elderly patients are the usual victims, with lesions occurring on the lower extremities, buttocks, hands, or vulva. There is an initial transient vesicle or pustule, followed by a deep ulcer extending into the dermis, covered by an adherent brown or yellowish crust (Fig. 40–12). The lesion is best distinguished clinically from impetigo by a surrounding halo of erythema. Relations to poststreptococcal glomerulonephritis and autoinoculation are the same as for impetigo.

TREATMENT. Treatment requires the same antibiotics as for impetigo, but they usually are given for a longer time due to the depth or extent of infection.

Erysipelas (St. Anthony's Fire, Streptococcal Cellulitis)

Erysipelas is a superficial cellulitis due to group A streptococci, with marked involvement of the lymphatics. It occurs most often in infants, toddlers, and the elderly. The portal of entry for the organism may be a site of minor trauma, but it is seldom recognized at the time of diagnosis. In adults there is a predilection for the face and head; in infants the umbilical stump and anterior abdomen may be infected, with rapid progression to bacteremia. In addition to bacteremia, subsequent myocarditis, otitis media, and glomerulonephritis have been described. Patients with nephrotic syndrome are thought to be particularly susceptible to erysipelas.

The infection evolves rapidly, and the patient is generally acutely ill and febrile. The area is brawny red, edematous, tender, and warm, with a distinct, slightly elevated margin. There may be vesicles or bullae within the area of redness, and occasionally petechiae or ecchymoses. Local desquamation occurs with healing. Significant differential diagnoses include herpes zoster, osteomyelitis of the facial bones, contact dermatitis, and erysipeloid (an infection of seafood handlers).

TREATMENT. The infection can be self-limited, but it is lethal for some patients and thus demands antibiotic therapy, most often with appropriate dosages of penicillin or erythromycin. There is a tendency for the condition to recur in the same area, which can be attributed to damaged lymphatics.

Viral Infections

Warts

Warts are benign tumors of the skin caused by several DNA viruses of the papova group. The typical common wart is a rounded nodule or tumor with a velvety, rough, or vegetative surface. Warts have been given several descriptive names, depending on their appearance and location.

1. *Filiform warts,* usually on the face and the neck, have an exaggerated horn-like surface.
2. *Flat warts,* found on the face, arms, and knees, do not have a velvety surface. They are flesh-colored and flat.
3. *Common warts,* usually found on the hands, appear as rough or scaly papules (Fig. 40–13).
4. *Anogenital warts* (condylomata acuminata), found on the external genitalia or perianal area, have an exaggerated velvety surface (Fig. 40–14).
5. *Plantar warts,* found on the soles of feet, have a hyperkeratotic surface (Fig. 40–15).

TREATMENT. A brief explanation is required for the following descriptions of preferred therapy. Generally speaking, therapy for warts is based on an attempt to destroy the lesion, for which a variety of methods have been employed. A theory of "immune recognition" has been invoked with some support, but the basic fact is that warts tend to come and go with little explanation, and their disappearance sometimes follows treatment.

Flat warts on the face can be treated with keratolytic agents (benzoyl peroxide, salicylic acid, treti-

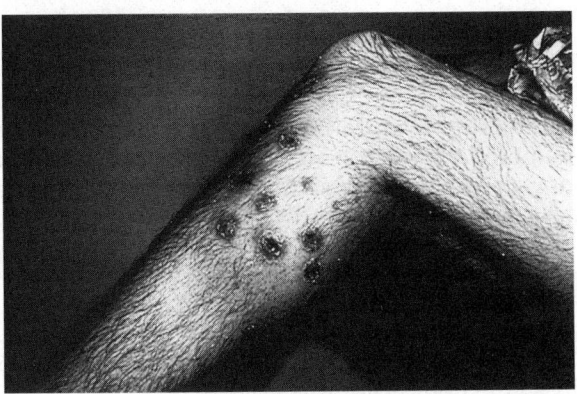

FIGURE 40–12. Ecthyma.

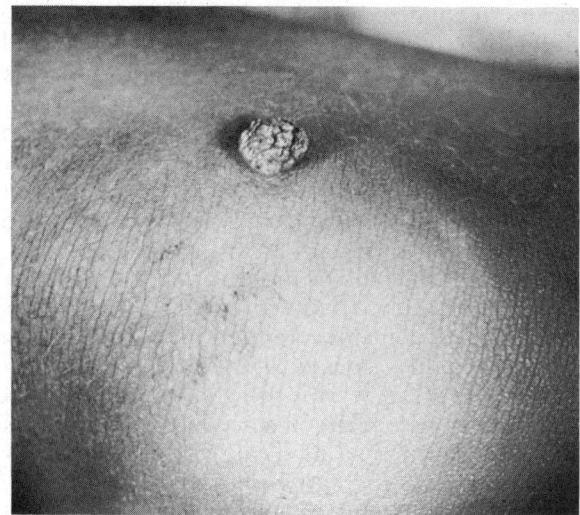

FIGURE 40–13. Common wart.

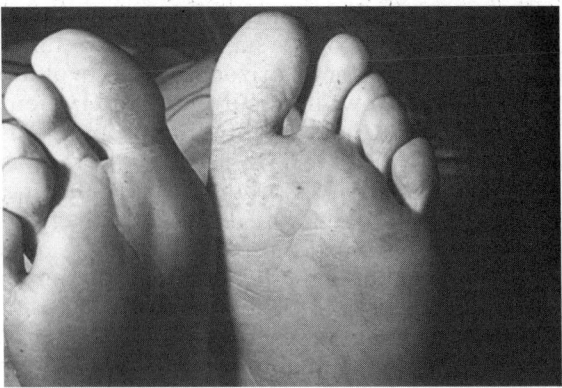

FIGURE 40–15. Plantar warts.

noin), topical 5-fluorouracil, or liquid nitrogen. Filiform warts are probably best treated by shave excision. Depending on the location, common warts can be treated with liquid nitrogen or carbon dioxide cryotherapy, or a variety of noxious chemicals can be applied. Patients have tried proprietary medications such as Compound W or Duofilm with some success. Chemicals for office use include

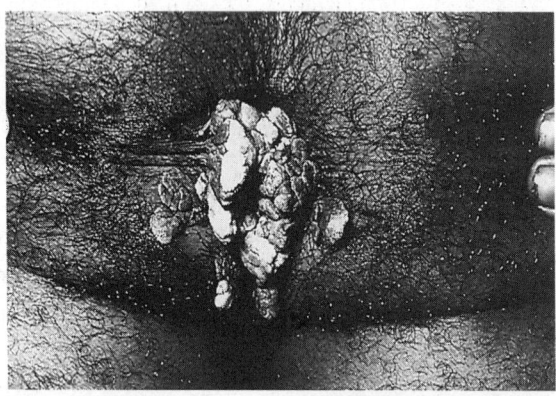

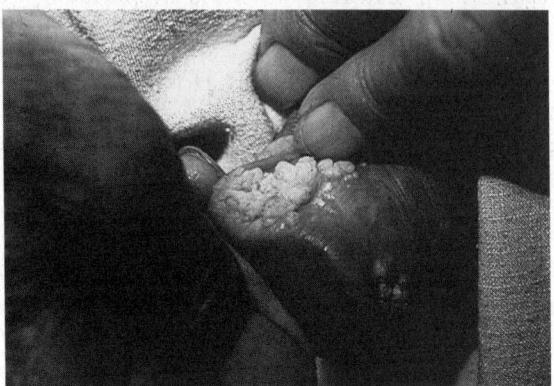

FIGURE 40–14. Anogenital warts.

trichloracetic acid. Because of the discomfort of freezing, periungual common warts are usually treated by painting the lesions with cantharidin or 20% to 50% salicylic acid. Anogenital warts are painted with 20% podophyllin in tincture of benzoin. Because podophyllin can cause severe local and systemic toxicity, it should be applied only to lesions of limited size and number and then washed from the skin within 2 to 6 hours. It should not be used for treatment in pregnant or nursing women. Never prescribe or dispense podophyllin for use at home. If application by the patient is desired, podofilox (Condylox) topical solution is an alternative; it is applied twice daily for three consecutive days each week for up to 4 weeks. Cryotherapy is another alternative, and surgical excision or carbon dioxide laser excision may be necessary for extensive anogenital lesions. Weekly follow-up is often desirable during therapy, especially for anogenital warts. Anoscopy is also advised when perianal warts are seen. Plantar warts may be painful and their removal difficult. Cautious treatment is necessary, as plantar scars are also painful in some cases. Various combinations of freezing or topical chemotherapy with gentle débridement are indicated. The topical agents include 50% salicylic acid in Vaseline, or other products with salicylic acid (e.g., Duofilm). Carbon dioxide laser surgery is available for resistant plantar warts.

Molluscum Contagiosum (Water Wart)

Molluscum contagiosum is a viral disease seen most often in children as umbilicated, discrete, flesh-colored papules (Fig. 40–16); most patients have multiple lesions. It can be transmitted sexually and is seen in adults. The papules are dome-shaped, with a central depression from which a yellowish-green material can be expressed. The head, eyelids, trunk, and genitalia are most often affected.

The lesions of molluscum contagiosum must be distinguished from warts, varicella, papillomas, and epitheliomas. If necessary, laboratory studies

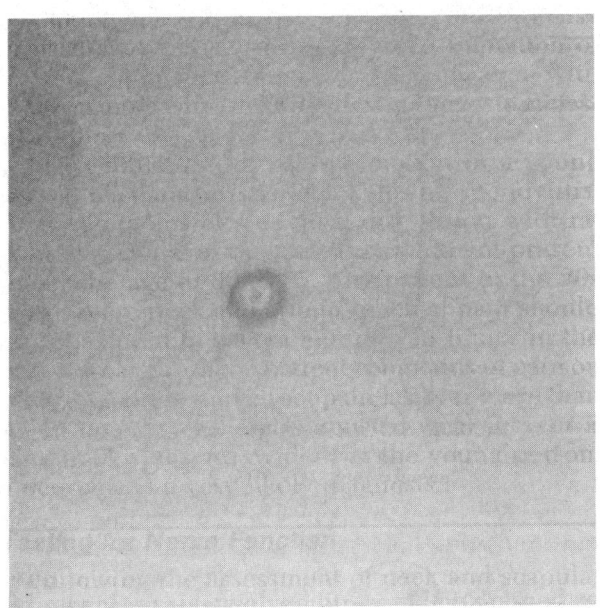

FIGURE 40–16. *Molluscum contagiosum.*

may be done. Stained smears of the central material show eosinophilic inclusion bodies. Also, biopsy is diagnostic.

TREATMENT. Individual lesions are self-limited, lasting about 2 to 4 months; but autoinoculation occurs, and crops of lesions may recur for years. Removal can be accomplished with a sharp curette or liquid nitrogen. Topical cantharidin is also effective.

Herpes Virus Infections

HERPES SIMPLEX. The herpes simplex virus (HSV) causes a variety of disorders, including lesions of the skin and mucous membranes, keratoconjunctivitis, and encephalitis. Complete discussion of the mucocutaneous lesions alone could fill a book, but some key clinical points deserve emphasis.

There are two types of virus: HSV-I and HSV-II. Generally, but not exclusively, type I produces lesions "above the belt," and type II infections are primarily genital. The primary lesion from the original infection is more severe than lesions that appear during recurrences. After the primary infection, the virus lies dormant in neural cells until it is reawakened spontaneously or by a precipitating factor. The usual precipitating factors are emotional stress, sunlight, fever, and surgical manipulation of the nerve ganglia. Most transmission occurs through direct mucocutaneous contact.

Clinical syndromes include primary herpes gingivostomatitis, recurrent herpes labialis, and herpetic whitlow. Primary herpes gingivostomatitis favors children and young adults, especially those aged 1 through 5 years. Manifestations are fever and sore throat, with painful vesicles on the

tongue, palate, gingiva, buccal mucosa, or lips. The vesicles tend to be found in clusters, in contrast to aphthous ulcers, which are usually fewer in number and more widely scattered. Vesicles coalesce into plaques covered with a gray exudate. Tzank stains and cultures may be needed to differentiate herpes from other causes of sore throat pain. Treatment is symptomatic. Acetaminophen or aspirin may be given for fever and discomfort. Some practitioners use mouth rinses made from extemporaneous blends of acetaminophen syrup, liquid antacids, viscous lidocaine, and Benadryl.

Recurrent herpes labialis (cold sore, fever blister) occurs at the junction of the lip and contiguous skin (Fig. 40–17). About one third of the U.S. population have recurrent cold sores; the factors determining individual susceptibility are unknown. Ulcers found entirely on the oral mucosa are more likely to be aphthous ulcers or erythema multiforme than herpes lesions. Symptomatic remedies are used.

Primary genital herpes erupts as a group of small vesicles, followed by ulcers, 3 to 14 days after contact (Fig. 40–18). Tender inguinal lymph nodes, malaise, and dysuria are common, and aseptic meningitis is seen more often among infected women. Cervical herpes may be seen without external herpetic lesions; features are mucopurulent discharge, friability, and ulceration. Recurrences are more frequent after type II infection; approximately 20 per cent of primary infections are due to type I. The differential diagnosis includes syphilis, chancroid, lymphogranuloma venereum, and granuloma inguinale. Recurrences are described as more likely to be painful in women but more frequent in men. Many patients report a prodrome of burning, itching, or dysesthesia, at which time oral acyclovir might be considered.

Herpetic whitlow is a primary or recurrent

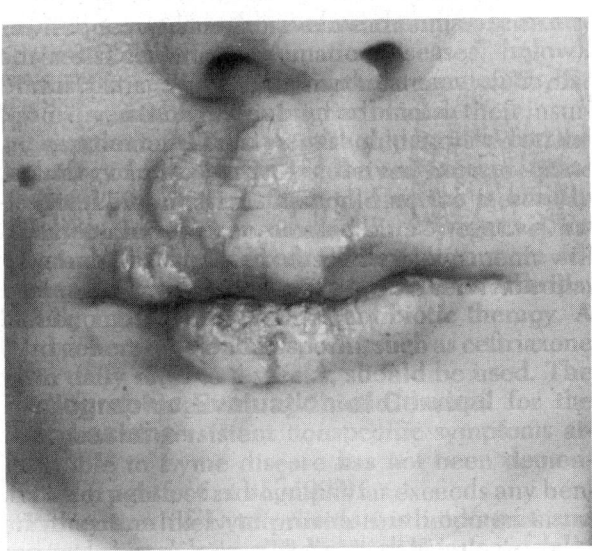

FIGURE 40–17. Herpes simplex of the lip.

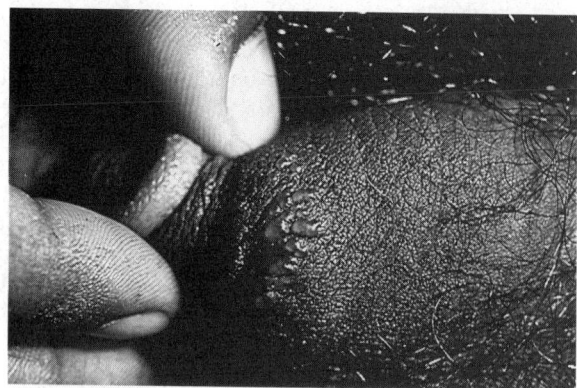

FIGURE 40–18. Herpes simplex of the penis.

herpes infection of the fingers and hands. Those at greatest risk are dentists, physicians, and dental technicians. The infection causes localized vesicles, erythema, edema, and pain and may last 2 to 6 weeks. It is essential to differentiate herpetic whitlow from a bacterial infection; microscopic identification of multinucleated giant cells is helpful (Tzanck preparation).

Other important factors to note in herpes infections include the following:

1. Herpes keratoconjunctivitis is a leading cause of infectious blindness in the United States. The superficial corneal ulcer is characteristic. Ophthalmologic evaluation and early treatment are essential.

2. Eczema herpeticum is widely disseminated herpetic lesions associated with atopic dermatitis.

3. Herpes simplex encephalitis is a highly lethal sporadic disease that is unrelated to previous herpes infection.

Treatment. Acyclovir (Zovirax) is the first relatively nontoxic, effective agent for treatment of herpes simplex, but clinical benefits are limited. If used for facial or oral lesions, acyclovir has been shown to hasten negative results on viral cultures but produces no significant change in the clinical course or recurrences. The picture is more promising for genital lesions. There is more rapid healing of primary lesions when acyclovir is applied topically, but no change occurs in recurrence rates. Topical acyclovir has little benefit when used for a recurrent eruption. Oral acyclovir, 200 mg five times daily for 5 days, can shorten the course of recurrences if it is begun during the prodromal phase. The long-term use of oral acyclovir, 400 mg twice daily, has been shown to reduce or eliminate recurrences of genital herpes. Because chronic use is expensive and entails the risk of side effects, it is generally recommended only for those who experience at least three or four episodes per year. It is also indicated for those patients whose herpes outbreaks are associated with erythema multi-

forme. The use of intravenous acyclovir for herpes encephalitis appears to improve survival.

Herpes Zoster (Shingles, Zoster)

The varicella/zoster virus produces a primary infection called varicella (chickenpox) and recurrent skin eruptions called herpes zoster or shingles. Like its cousin herpes simplex, the virus resides in nerve cells until reawakened. The time between the onset of chickenpox and the onset of herpes zoster is ordinarily many years, but primary infection at an early age is thought to shorten the average time for recurrence.

Chickenpox is characterized by a generalized rash with successive crops of lesions beginning on the face and spreading to the trunk, with relatively few lesions on the extremities. Individual lesions progress rapidly from macules and papules to vesicles, pustules, and crusts. Vesicles and shallow ulcers are seen on the oral mucosa. Pruritus is often intense, and older children and adults with the disease may have fever, chills, headache, and other constitutional symptoms.

Herpes zoster (shingles) is a delayed expression of the same virus that originally caused chickenpox, although the original infection may have been mild or even unnoticed. The dormant virus resides in sensory nerve ganglia for a variable time. Some reversions of the latent virus to an active and infective state are halted by immune responses. When a reversion overcomes the immune reaction, the virus first multiplies within the ganglion, leading to neuritis and neuralgia. Then viral particles are released into skin at the nerve endings, yielding characteristic clusters of vesicles (Fig. 40–19). A syndrome of radicular pain without cutaneous lesions has been reported when immune mechanisms are able to recover in the middle of the process.

Clinically, patients with herpes zoster experi-

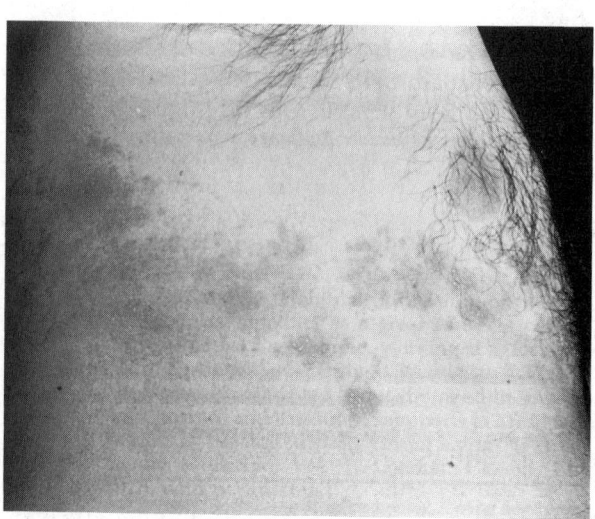

FIGURE 40–19. Herpes zoster.

ence segmental pain and paresthesia, followed within hours or days by the appearance of grouped vesicles on an erythematous base. The rash is typically unilateral and does not cross the midline, although patients occasionally have some hematogenous spread resulting in lesions at other locations. Crusting occurs as the vesicles resolve.

Herpes zoster is more common in patients with cancer, acquired immunodeficiency syndrome (AIDS), and other immunosuppressed states, but the converse relation is not established; that is, the occurrence of herpes zoster, in itself, does not justify a search for malignancy or immune defects.

The most common complication is persistent pain (postherpetic neuralgia), particularly in older patients. Other complications include localized hypesthesia or anesthesia, secondary bacterial infections, ophthalmic zoster, and disseminated zoster. Immunocompromised hosts are at much greater risk for complications.

TREATMENT. Treatment for most cases of varicella is symptomatic, with more specific treatments reserved for the complications. Aspirin must be avoided in patients with chickenpox because of the association with Reye syndrome, but acetaminophen may be used for fever. The pruritus usually responds to cool compresses, calamine lotion, or tepid baths with 0.25 cup of baking soda added. Simple antihistamine medications, given orally, also appear to be safe. Another popular alternative is to give the patient baths with colloidal oatmeal, in which case ensure that parents or patients know that the bathtub becomes slippery and potentially dangerous with this method.

Immunocompromised patients with herpes zoster may be treated with antiviral agents, including acyclovir and vidarabine. Immunocompetent patients younger than 50 years of age generally experience a benign course that does not justify the use of either antiviral or corticosteroid therapy. Immunocompetent patient over age 50 have a greater risk of postherpetic neuralgia. They may benefit from antiviral therapy, and some authorities advocate systemic corticosteroids. For these patients, acyclovir is given at a dosage of 800 mg five times daily for 10 days. Oral prednisone, if used, is given in a tapering course over 3 weeks. When postherpetic neuralgia occurs, it may persist for months and may be difficult to control effectively. Analgesics are fairly helpful, but they must be used with care to avoid habituation or addiction. Tricyclic antidepressants or chlorprothixene (Taractan) in small doses reduce pain for some patients. Sublesional corticosteroid injections, transcutaneous nerve stimulation, and other methods have proponents. An occasional patient with intractable pain is treated with neurosurgery.

Superficial Fungal Infections

The common superficial fungi of skin are *Candida albicans*, tinea versicolor, and the dermatophytes called tinea. Except for *Candida*, these fungi affect only the skin, hair, and nails. In this discussion, the term "topicals" or "topical antifungal agents" refers to medications that include clotrimazole (Lotrimin), miconazole (Micatin), econazole (Spectazole), ketoconazole (Nizoral), sulconazole (Exelderm), oxiconazole (Oxistat), ciclopirox (Loprox), and others. Clotrimazole and miconazole preparations appear in some nonprescription preparations and perhaps offer a lower-cost treatment. The newer agents offer once-daily application and shorter duration of therapy. Topical nystatin (Mycostatin) is effective only for candidiasis. Products that combine a strong, fluorinated topical steroid with an antifungal agent (Lotrisone) are not recommended for diaper rash or for application to the face or genitalia.

Tinea Versicolor

Tinea versicolor is caused by *Malassezia furfur*, a fungus resistant to griseofulvin. The disorder occurs as scattered hypopigmented or hyperpigmented discrete plaques covered with fine scales located primarily on the trunk and proximal extremities. The plaques may coalesce over large areas (Fig. 40–20). The condition tends to be chronic with frequent recurrences. Itching is unusual but can be severe. The lesions often appear hypopigmented during the warm months (owing to a sunscreen produced by the organism) and darker than surrounding skin during the cool months—hence the name versicolor.

If necessary, a KOH preparation of superficial scales confirms the thin hyphae and clusters of spores, often described as "spaghetti and meatballs."

TREATMENT. The lesions respond gradually to 10- to 20-minute applications of selenium sulfide shampoo (Exsel 2% or Selsun 1%) to the affected areas; many authorities recommend daily application for 1 week, followed by weekly application for about 6 weeks. Topical antifungal agents, such as clotrimazole and miconazole, are effective but ultimately expensive for the large areas involved.

FIGURE 40–20. Tinea versicolor.

Probably the most important feature of management is to tell the patient that pigmentation normalizes slowly, recurrence is common, and lesions are solely a cosmetic problem. Some studies suggest that oral ketoconazole is effective for resistant cases of tinea versicolor.

Candida Albicans

Candida albicans, a yeast-like fungus, is an opportunist that causes lesions in a susceptible host involving mucous membranes or moist areas of skin. Growth is encouraged by diabetes mellitus, oral contraceptives, broad-spectrum antibiotics, and immunosuppression. Examination of KOH preparations confirms the presence of budding yeast-like cells. The major clinical syndromes associated with *C. albicans* are oral moniliasis, monilial vaginitis, monilial paronychia, and monilial intertrigo.

Oral moniliasis (thrush) occurs most often in infants. When it occurs in an adult, some thought must be given to the possibility of immunosuppression. It is seen as white, curd-like plaques on the oral mucosa or tongue (Fig. 40–21), sometimes accompanied by fissures at the corners of the lips (perlèche). Thrush is treated most often with nystatin oral suspension (Mycostatin, Nilstat) placed in the mouth four times daily. A dosage of 2 ml for infants is used, or 4 to 6 ml for children and adults. Treatment is continued until 48 hours after the visible lesions are gone. For adults and older children, oral clotrimazole lozenges (Mycelex) are effective when dissolved in the mouth four times daily.

Monilial vaginitis is seen as white, curd-like plaques on a red base in the vagina, occasionally accompanied by lesions of the perineal skin. Nystatin vaginal tablets may be inserted once daily for 14 days. Clotrimazole (Gyne-Lotrimin), miconazole (Monistat), and terconazole (Terazol) offer a shorter duration of therapy. The vaginal cream formulations are especially helpful if there are lesions outside the vagina, as creams can be applied to both mucosa and skin.

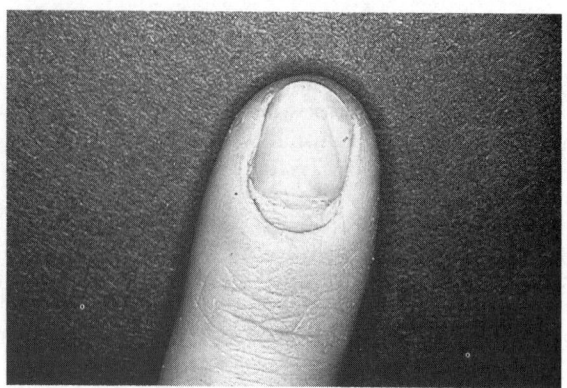

FIGURE 40–22. Monilial paronychia.

Monilial balanitis occurs most often in the moist, protected area under uncircumcised foreskin and manifests as erythematous plaques, small pustules, and thick white exudate. It usually responds to application of topical antifungal agents and correction of any predisposing conditions. Concomitant treatment of an infected sexual partner may be necessary in recurrent cases. A 2-week course of oral nystatin or ketoconazole can be used for men with repeated infections.

Monilial paronychia involves the nail folds; there is chronic but relatively painless redness and swelling from which a thick, yellowish fluid can sometimes be expressed (Fig. 40–22). The condition should be distinguished from bacterial paronychia, which is more acute, painful, and purulent. The most effective therapy consists of rubbing an antifungal liquid such as clotrimazole solution (Lotrimin, Mycelex) into the nail folds twice daily, often for several months. Patients should also make a special effort to keep the hands dry.

Monilial intertrigo consists of beefy red, fairly well circumscribed patches with satellite pustules in moist areas of the groin, perineum, and axillae and under the breasts. A topical antifungal agent, such as clotrimazole or econazole, may be used successfully, and the area should be kept dry.

Diaper Rash

There are four common causes of diaper rash, but an individual patient may have a combination of causative factors. Most rashes in this area are due to *Candida* infection, irritant or contact dermatitis, or bacterial infection. A few are due to seborrheic dermatitis, which is usually recognized by its coexistence in other typical areas such as the scalp (cradle cap) and face.

Irritant or contact dermatitis is a reaction to diaper material or urine and appears as simple redness in the area, with distinct borders at the diaper edges and sparing of the skin folds. *Candida* infections are characterized by a dark intertriginous red rash including satellite papules and pustules, with the skin folds likely to be involved. The differen-

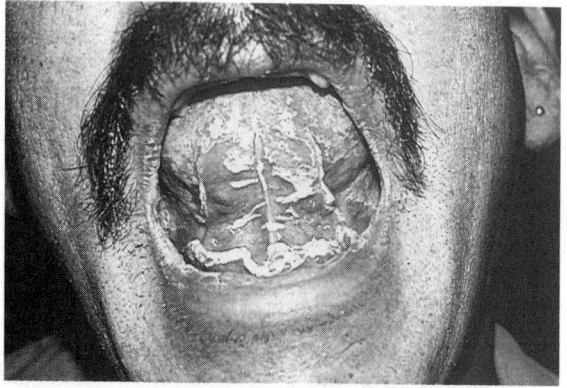

FIGURE 40–21. Oral moniliasis/thrush (HIV-positive).

tiation of *Candida* infections from atypical cases of seborrheic dermatitis may require KOH preparations or fungal cultures. Bacterial infections are often a complication of other causes but may also represent a localized occurrence of impetigo contagiosa or bullous impetigo.

TREATMENT. In general, the treatment of diaper rash should include frequent diaper changes, careful cleansing to remove urine and feces, drying the area thoroughly, and the avoidance of plastic pants or other occlusive clothing. For irritant or contact dermatitis, those simple measures may suffice. Though true contact dermatitis is probably uncommon, a change in the type of diapers or laundering method is worthwhile for resistant or recurrent episodes. Some physicians recommend a brief course of hydrocortisone cream (0.5% or 1.0%) or a protective agent such as zinc oxide ointment, Desitin, or A & D Ointment. Those with bacterial infections should also receive an appropriate antibiotic, such as topical mupirocin or systemic penicillin or erythromycin. Those with *Candida* are treated with topical nystatin (Mycostatin) cream. If irritation and *Candida* both appear to be involved, nystatin cream and hydrocortisone cream 1% can be combined in equal parts.

Dermatophytes

Lesions caused by the dermatophytic fungi are most often referred to by the name tinea, followed by a word that denotes the area of the body affected. They rarely cause infection of tissues other than the skin, hair, and nails.

Tinea Capitis. Tinea capitis is characterized by circular patches of fine scale and hair loss on the scalp, usually in prepubertal children (Fig. 40–23). The lesions in some patients exhibit greenish fluorescence when examined with a Wood's lamp; those that do not fluoresce can be diagnosed with a KOH preparation. The topical antifungal preparations are not ordinarily effective, and treatment with oral griseofulvin (Grifulvin V, Grisactin, Gris-PEG) is required. The dosage should be determined with care, as "microsize" and "ultrami-

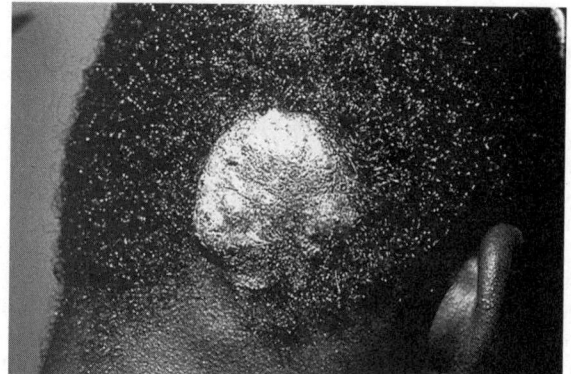

FIGURE 40–24. Kerion.

crosize" formulas are available, with considerable variation in strength. For adults a daily dose of 500 mg of the microsize type is effective; for children the dosage is 5 mg per pound. The ultramicrosize preparations, such as Gris-PEG, require only about two thirds of that dosage. The medication should be taken with food. Resistant cases may require higher doses; oral ketoconazole (Nizoral) is an alternative. Treatment of tinea capitis takes about 4 to 6 weeks.

Kerion (Fig. 40–24) is a deep inflammatory variation of tinea capitis. Because of the inflammatory component, it is sometimes necessary to add an oral steroid, such as prednisone, to the antifungal therapy.

TINEA BARBAE. Tinea barbae (tinea sycosis) is a fungal infection of the beard and mustache areas in men. It is seen most often in rural areas, associated with exposure to cattle and dogs. *Microsporum* and *Trichophyton* species are common causes. Clinical presentations include circinate lesions similar to those of tinea corporis, superficial ones resembling folliculitis, and an inflammatory type similar to kerion of the scalp (Fig. 40–25). Majocchi's granuloma is another name for a deep follicular lesion.

Wood's lamp examination is helpful with *M.*

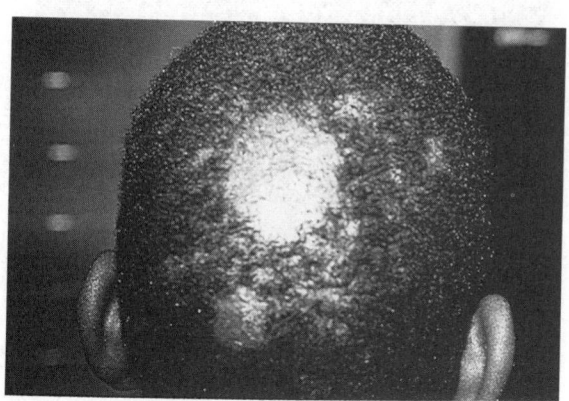

FIGURE 40–23. Tinea capitis.

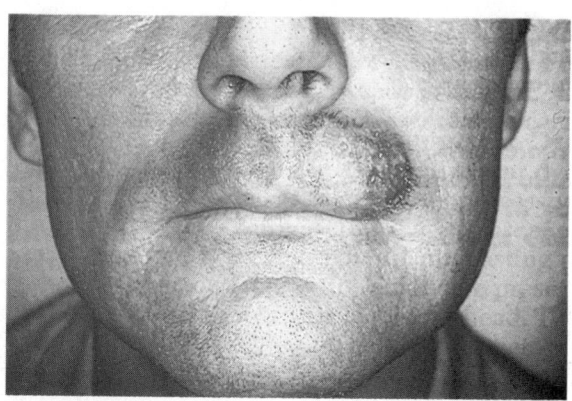

FIGURE 40–25. Tinea barbae, inflammatory.

canis infections, and KOH examination or culture on Sabouraud's medium is required to confirm other types of infection. The differential diagnosis includes bacterial folliculitis, perioral dermatitis, contact dermatitis, *Candida* infection, and herpes simplex infection; additional diagnostic aids include bacterial or viral cultures, Tzanck smears, and contact allergy testing.

Treatment. Though most lesions of tinea barbae resolve spontaneously within weeks or months, oral griseofulvin hastens resolution. Warm compresses with Burow's or saline solution may provide some symptomatic relief, and systemic antibiotics are indicated for bacterial superinfection.

TINEA CORPORIS. Tinea corporis (ringworm) results in persistent oval or round plaques with central clearing and a red, scaly or vesicular border (Fig. 40–26); it is seen most often in children. In adults it may be associated with diabetes mellitus or immunosuppression. The lesions may be single or multiple, with no particular grouping or pattern. They can be distinguished from other papulosquamous eruptions by scraping a few scales onto a microscope slide and undertaking a KOH examination to observe the characteristic hyphae. Lesions in reasonable numbers respond to a topical antifungal agent, such as clotrimazole or miconazole, within 2 to 4 weeks. Widespread or resistant lesions are treated with oral griseofulvin for the same period. Treatment should be continued for a few days after clinical resolution.

TINEA CRURIS. Tinea cruris, or "jock itch," occurs in the genital intertriginous areas with similar morphology and treatment as described for tinea corporis. Rather than discrete small lesions, though, there tends to be a large erythematous plaque (Fig. 40–27) with characteristic central clearing and a distinct scaly or vesicular border. Monilial intertrigo is associated with satellite pustules and causes more involvement of the scrotum than is seen with tinea cruris.

Treatment. Topical antifungal agents work well for tinea cruris and have the additional advantage of being effective against *Candida*.

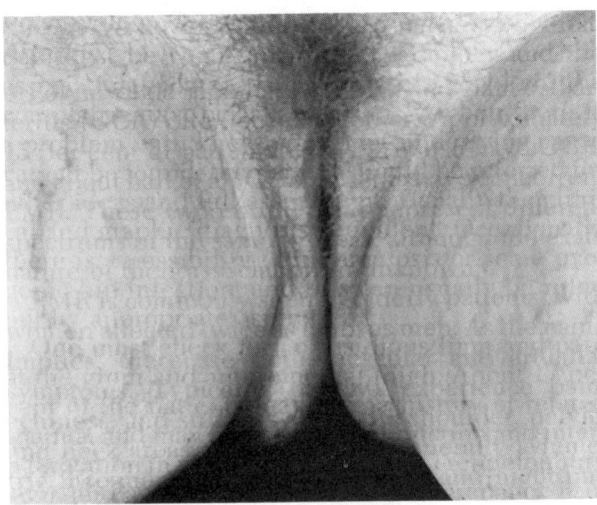

FIGURE 40–27. Tinea cruris.

TINEA PEDIS. Tinea pedis (athlete's foot) most often causes cracking and maceration between the toes (Fig. 40–28) and scaling along the lateral edges of the feet; it may also manifest as an acute vesiculobullous eruption of the plantar surface. Lesions are often secondarily infected by bacteria, and tinea infection of the toenails also may be present. Tinea pedis can usually be distinguished clinically from contact dermatitis, psoriasis, and other foot conditions, with a KOH preparation used as needed.

Treatment. Topical antifungal agents are often used, with adjunctive soaks or antimicrobials as indicated by the presentation. Topical terbinafine

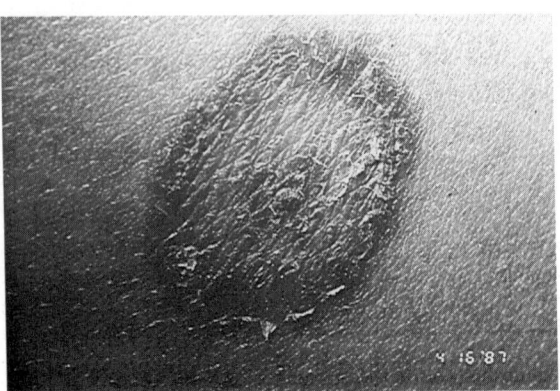

FIGURE 40–26. Tinea corporis.

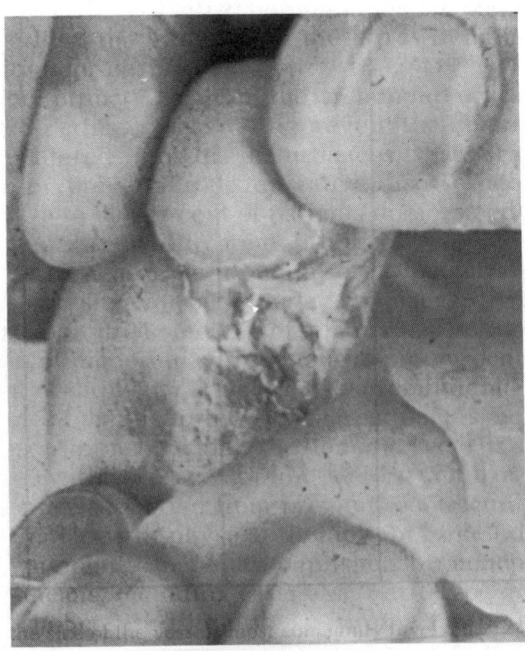

FIGURE 40–28. Tinea pedis.

(Lamisil) is a particularly good choice for this indication, as it is often effective within 1 week. Oral griseofulvin is sometimes necessary, often for as long as 3 months. Recurrence is common, and preventive measures include absorbent socks and the use of antifungal powders (e.g., Tinactin, undecylenic acid). Hyperhidrosis may also be present and should be treated concurrently.

TINEA MANUUM. Tinea manuum is fungal infection of the hand (Fig. 40–29) often found in association with tinea pedis. *T. rubrum* causes the "one hand, two feet" variant, where one palm is spared. There is scaling and slight redness, particular along skin lines.

Treatment. Griseofulvin is usually necessary for several weeks until the lesions clear.

TINEA UNGUIUM. Tinea unguium is a specific term that refers to dermatophytic infection of the nail plate, whereas the term onychomycosis includes nail infection by any fungus or yeast. Onychomycosis is the most common disorder of nails and is frequently associated with a fungal infection elsewhere on the body.

There is a rather complicated system for clinical classification of onychomycosis into subtypes, with each a clinical presentation characteristic of certain organisms. Specific diagnosis by means of KOH preparations and fungal or mold cultures is problematic but should be done if oral therapy is contemplated. It is important to distinguish these infections from some other nonfungal causes of nail destruction. Ordinarily, clinical distinction is possible because the associated skin lesions are characteristic (i.e., distorted nails associated with psoriasis, hand eczema, Darier's disease, or lichen planus).

Probably the most characteristic clinical presentation of tinea unguium is a process of insidious onset that results in a thick, discolored nail (white, brown, yellow) with a ragged edge and accumulated keratotic debris under the end of the nail (Fig. 40–30). The process may involve some or all of the fingernails and toenails. There are no other symptoms unless secondary infection occurs.

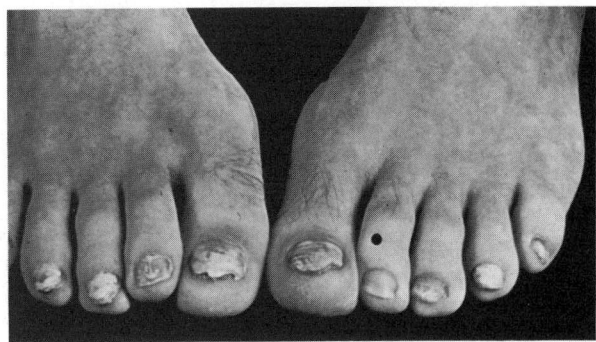

FIGURE 40–30. Tinea unguium.

Treatment. Systemic therapy with griseofulvin (Grifulvin-V, Grisactin, Gris-PEG) requires at least 4 to 6 months for fingernails and 12 to 18 months for toenails; recurrences are common, especially for toenail infections. Many clinicians are reluctant to recommend griseofulvin for toenail infections. Because griseofulvin is not free of cost or side effects, patients should be well informed and may choose to live with ugly nails until secondary infection or ingrown nails force treatment. Surgical avulsion of the nail may be necessary, sometimes in combination with administration of griseofulvin or a topical agent. Some authorities report success in chemical avulsion of the nail using a 40% urea preparation, with or without antifungal agents. Use of topical antifungal agents alone is not usually effective, but a trial may be justified if the other methods are inappropriate or contraindicated. Oral ketoconazole is slightly more effective than griseofulvin but must be given for long periods. The newer oral agents such as terbinafine or fluconazole show promise when used as pulse therapy (i.e., 1 week per month).

Sporotrichosis

The cutaneous form of sporotrichosis is a chronic, progressive disease resulting from implantation of *Sporothrix schenkii*, a fungal saprophyte found on thorns, splinters, or other plant materials. It is commonly associated with occupational exposure or cultivation of rose bushes. The disease is spread by the lymphatics from the original site, and the same fungus can invade the viscera. The characteristic appearance is a roughly linear spread of lesions along the lymphatics from a primary lesion on the hand (Fig. 40–31). Individual lesions are indurated papules or nodules with central ulceration; they are painless unless secondarily infected. The differential diagnosis includes tularemia, staphylococcal lymphangitis, and mycobacterial infection.

TREATMENT. Treatment of the localized disease is with a saturated solution of potassium iodide, administered orally at a daily dosage of 2 to 6 gm. A typical starting dosage is 10 drops three times

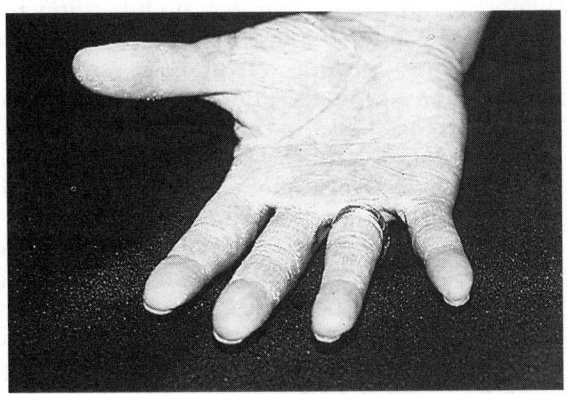

FIGURE 40–29. Tinea manuum.

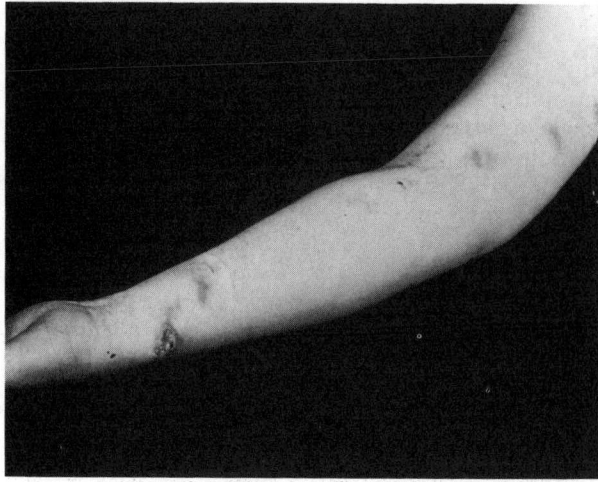

FIGURE 40–31. Sporotrichosis.

daily after meals. Intravenous sodium iodide is an alternative. Patients intolerant to the iodides or with disseminated disease are treated with intravenous amphotericin B.

Syphilis and Other Sexually Transmitted Diseases

Syphilis

PRIMARY SYPHILIS. Syphilis results from infection with *Treponema pallidum*, a spirochete. The classic lesion of primary infection is the chancre, a single, relatively painless ulcer with raised, indurated borders and a scant serous exudate (Fig. 40–32). Less common presentations include multi-

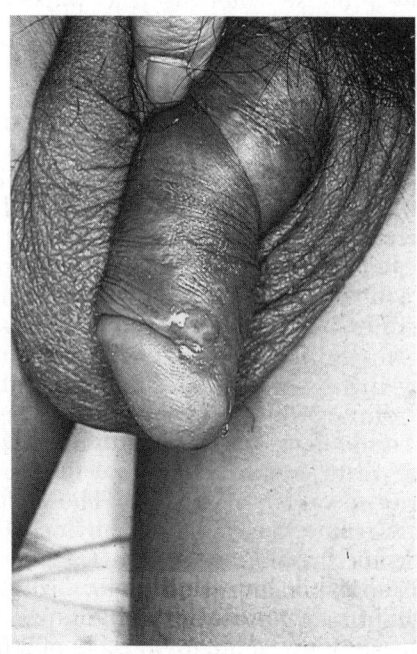

FIGURE 40–32. Primary syphilis.

ple erosions and ulcers, exudative balanitis, and edematous phimosis. There is usually a painless regional adenopathy. Though ordinarily seen on the genitalia, chancres have been found around the anus, mouth, lips, tonsils, tongue, fingers, toes, axillae, umbilicus, eyelids, breasts, and even colostomy sites.

Particularly when there are multiple ulcers, the differential diagnosis includes genital herpes, chancroid, granuloma inguinale, lymphogranuloma venereum, and other causes of balanitis or vulvitis. The diagnosis of primary syphilis is best established by darkfield microscopy. If darkfield examination is not available, slides can also be prepared and sent by mail for direct immunofluorescence examination. Serology (Venereal Disease Research Laboratory [VDRL] test or rapid plasma reagin test) may be positive on initial presentation, but conversion may not occur until 2 to 3 months after the chancre appears. With the appropriate risk factors and clinical presentation, a serology test that had negative results must be repeated to exclude syphilis.

SECONDARY SYPHILIS. Secondary syphilis develops 6 weeks to 6 months after infection. The primary chancre may still be present when secondary lesions erupt. With the onset of lesions, the VDRL or rapid plasma reagin test is reliably positive. The more specific fluorescent treponemal antibody absorption test is then used for verification. The lesions reflect dissemination via blood or lymph circulation, and each is loaded with spirochetes.

The rash of secondary syphilis is a great mimic and may resemble a wide variety of other skin diseases. The classic lesions are papulosquamous, with a predilection for the head, neck, palms (Fig. 40–33), and soles. Most of these lesions do not itch, but itching does not eliminate the possibility of secondary syphilis. Even this characteristic presentation requires differentiation from other common papulosquamous eruptions, including superficial fungi, pityriasis rosea, drug eruptions, and psoriasis. In addition to the typical lesions, secondary syphilis may also produce macules, papules, follicular lesions, nail changes, nodules, mucous membrane lesions, "moth-eaten alopecia" of the scalp, and rarely pustules. There may also be systemic signs or symptoms reflecting involvement of other organ systems, harbingers of the consequences of late syphilis. The multiple complications and delayed consequences of untreated syphilis are beyond the scope of this summary.

TREATMENT. The treatment of primary or secondary syphilis is two intramuscular injections of 2.4 million units of benzathine penicillin 1 week apart. An alternative regimen is available for aqueous procaine penicillin. Patients sensitive to penicillin may be treated with tetracycline or erythromycin 500 mg four times daily for 15 days.

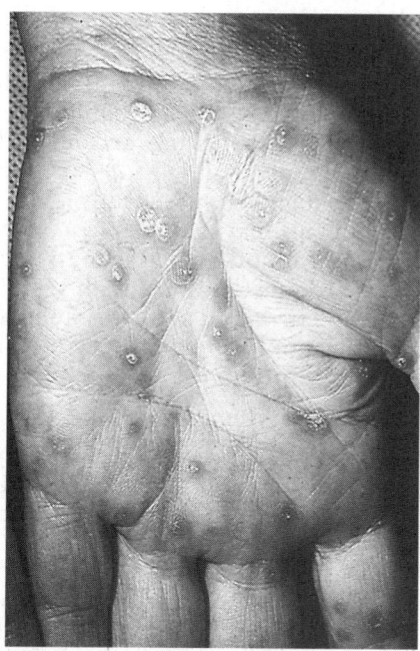

FIGURE 40–33. Secondary syphilis on the palm.

Chancroid

Chancroid is an infectious, autoinoculable disease caused by *Hemophilus ducreyi*, a gram-negative bacillus. It is characterized by a small, soft, round ulcer with an erythematous halo. In contrast to the chancre of syphilis, lesions are usually tender and often multiple (two to six lesions). Typical locations are genital and perianal. About half of the patients have tender, enlarged regional lymph nodes that may form inguinal abscesses with spontaneous drainage. Confirmation of the clinical diagnosis is aided by stained smears or cultures of exudates, but exclusion of syphilis and other etiologies is essential.

TREATMENT. Chancroid was formerly treated with tetracycline or sulfonamide prior to the emergence of resistant strains. The current recommendations are trimethoprim/sulfamethoxazole 320/1600 mg daily, or erythromycin 2 gm daily, for 1 week. Some effectiveness has been demonstrated for single-dose regimens.

Lymphogranuloma Venereum

Lymphogranuloma venereum is caused by *Chlamydia trachomatis*. The primary lesion is a soft, painless genital ulceration, followed within 1 to 2 weeks by tender inguinal lymph nodes. The nodes tend to coalesce into a fixed inguinal mass and may lead to drainage and chronic sinus formation. Red or purple discoloration of the skin develops over the mass of lymph nodes. The diagnosis is accomplished by a complement-fixation test or by culture.

TREATMENT. Standard treatment is oral tetracycline 500 mg four times daily for 3 weeks; minocycline (Minocin) is an alternative.

Granuloma Inguinale

Granuloma inguinale results from infection by *Calymmatobacterium granulomatis*, a gram-negative rod. The primary lesion may be a papule, subcutaneous nodule, or ulcer on the genitalia or other locations. The subcutaneous nodule may be mistaken for a lymph node, but true adenopathy is rare. A smear prepared with the Wright or Giemsa stain is examined for characteristic Donovan bodies, which are safety pin-shaped dark bacilli in the cytoplasm of macrophages. The infection responds to tetracycline 500 mg four times daily for 3 to 4 weeks. Some resistance occurs, and alternative regimens include ampicillin and other choices.

Benign Neoplasms

Nevi (Moles)

Moles, common benign lesions of skin, are composed of collections of nevus cells within the skin. The nevus cells are of neuroectodermal origin, some resembling melanocytes and some similar to Schwann cells. The traditional histologic classification is junctional, intradermal, or compound depending on whether the predominant location of the cells is in the epidermis, the dermis, or both sites, respectively. The lesions first appear during early childhood, increase in number through early adulthood, and then usually resolve with advancing age. Pigmented nevi may be flat, dome-shaped, pedunculated, or verrucous, with great variation in size and surface characteristics. Some are hairy, and others are hairless. For the experienced examiner, there are some correlations between appearance and histologic type.

If moles are benign and virtually ubiquitous, why pay attention to them? Moles earn most of their importance from their relation to cutaneous melanoma. Many melanomas arise from pre-existing nevi, so there is some degree of malignant potential, and the appearance of melanoma and nevi can be similar. The assessment of malignant potential or the differentiation of melanoma from an atypical mole on clinical grounds may be difficult. There are not enough physicians, time, or money to remove all the moles from humankind, but there are some reasonable guidelines for excision that have met the test of time.

1. *Removal for cosmetic reasons or due to irritation*: Patients may desire removal for cosmetic reasons or when contact by clothing causes chronic irritation of the mole.

2. *Atypical appearance or change in appearance*: Worrisome features include dark pigmentation, irregular distribution of pigment, irregular borders, "satellite" lesions, asymmetry, and large size (5 mm or more). Inflammation, infection, bleeding, and sudden onset of growth of a stable mole are also cause for excision and biopsy.

3. *Specific lesions with increased malignant potential:* These lesions include dysplastic nevi, some nevi present from birth, and those on acral and mucosal surfaces.

4. *Removal from sites that are difficult to monitor:* Patients are advised to observe pigmented nevi for change, particularly when there is a personal or family history of melanoma. It is probably wise to offer to excise lesions that are difficult to see, such as those on the scalp or perianal areas.

Complete removal by some method of excision is the acceptable treatment; destructive methods should not be employed. The safest course is pathologic examination of *every* specimen, regardless of benign appearance. Preliminary incisional biopsy is justified for lesions in difficult locations.

Seborrheic Keratoses

Seborrheic keratoses are benign lesions of purely cosmetic significance that tend to occur after the fourth decade of life and are unrelated to seborrheic dermatitis. There are often multiple lesions, each one of which starts as a flat tan or brown lesion and grows slowly to produce a raised, thick superficial brown or black scaly papule. Each keratosis is 2 mm to 2 cm in size, with a surface characterized by tiny pits and furrows (Fig. 40–34). Reassurance may be the only management required, but lesions can be removed easily by electrodesiccation and curettage or with liquid nitrogen cryotherapy.

Skin Tag (Achrocordon)

Most people develop at least a few skin tags during middle or late adulthood. Most lesions are small, pedunculated, flesh-colored, and soft, but some can be several centimeters in size, and a few are darkly pigmented. They are commonly located on the face, upper chest, and intertriginous areas.

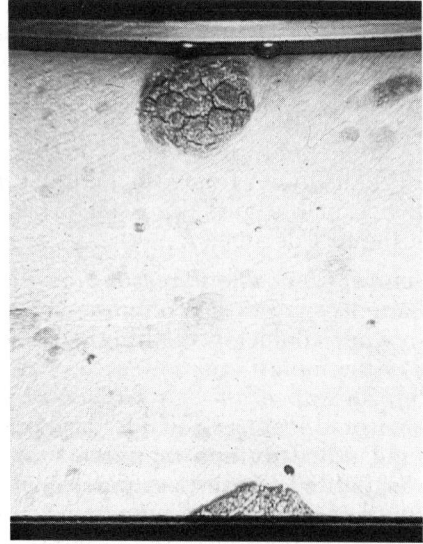

FIGURE 40–34. Seborrheic keratoses.

The tags are completely asymptomatic unless they become irritated by clothing, or when the pedicle twists and causes infarction. Sometimes, they fall off spontaneously or may be accidentally removed by the patient during shaving or some other activity.

Although the diagnosis is usually evident, the pigmented skin tags may cause some concern, and biopsy can confirm and reassure the patient. Patients may also request removal of the skin tag because of repeated irritation or for cosmetic reasons; options include simple amputation at the base, excision, and liquid nitrogen.

Dermatofibroma (Histiocytoma)

Dermatofibroma, a benign nodule usually found on the leg, is more common in women. The lesion is usually firm, round, and less than 1 cm in diameter; it ranges in color from pink to red or purple. It is fixed to the skin but not to underlying tissues. The lesions tend to be stable for many years and are often mentioned by patients as an afterthought. They are thought to be due to an abnormal scar reaction after incidental trauma, such as an insect bite or folliculitis. Occasionally it is confused with a mole, wart, or keloid, a question easily resolved by biopsy.

Senile Hemangioma (Senile Angioma, Cherry Angioma, Cherry Spot)

Senile hemangiomas are small (2 to 4 mm), raised, red or purple lesions that occur primarily on the trunk of middle-aged and older adults. They are usually multiple and may be associated with tiny petechia-like spots. They persist indefinitely but are completely benign and do not require treatment. If removal is desired for cosmetic reasons, desiccation and curettage, destruction with liquid nitrogen, or laser treatment may be used.

Pyogenic Granuloma

Pyogenic granuloma is a pedunculated or sessile, red or purple, polypoid benign tumor composed of highly vascular granulation tissue. It often occurs at sites of trauma or infection; despite the name, however, no infectious etiology is proved. Although it is benign, pyogenic granuloma grows rapidly and bleeds easily with minor trauma. Clinically, it may be confused with Kaposi sarcoma, metastatic renal cell carcinoma, or malignant melanoma. Surgical excision is the treatment of choice.

Lipoma

A lipoma is a benign tumor composed of mature adipose cells. It is flesh-colored, soft or rubbery in consistency, and sometimes lobulated. Lesions may be single or multiple. A neurofibroma may have a similar appearance but is usually distinguished by other clinical features of Von Recklinghausen's disease. If removal is justified owing to sudden enlargement or pain, or for cosmetic reasons, excision is used. If the tissue does not look like normal fat on gross examination, it should be submitted for histologic examination.

Epidermoid Cyst (Sebaceous Cyst, Epidermal Cyst)

A sebaceous or epidermal cyst is a fairly firm, smooth, flesh-colored nodule with a small central pore. The cyst may be found almost anywhere on the body but most often on the face, scalp, neck, and back. The size ranges from a few millimeters to more than 5 cm. The cyst is filled by a foul-smelling, semisolid keratin material surrounded by a cyst wall. The lesion is normally asymptomatic, but it may become red and tender with infection.

TREATMENT. Treatment is incision and removal of the entire cyst and its contents. All of the cyst wall and the overlying tissue must be removed to ensure a cure. Depending on the degree of past and present inflammation, that feat may not be as easy as it sounds. One suggested method is to use a narrow skin ellipse that includes the pore, followed by sharp and blunt dissection to remove the cyst and its contents en bloc. Others favor the use of a 4-mm skin punch to remove a plug of skin containing the pore, expression of the contents, and then sharp curettage to remove the cyst wall. If the cyst is obviously infected, it may be more prudent to incise and drain it, pack it temporarily with Iodoform gauze, and consider definitive removal after the inflammation subsides.

Keratoacanthoma

Keratoacanthoma is a common benign tumor that is thought to arise from hair follicles. It occurs primarily on the face and hands as a solitary, dome-shaped flesh-colored or red growth with a depressed central crust (Fig. 40–35). There may be fine blood vessels just underneath the surface. The central keratotic plug may grow into a horn, or it may disintegrate, leaving a lesion that resembles a dry ulcer crater with an elevated border. Its size ranges from 2 mm to 1 cm or more at diagnosis, and the growth rate is rapid. Clinically and histo-

logically, a keratoacanthoma can be confused with squamous cell carcinoma. The rapid growth adds to the fear of malignancy.

TREATMENT. Because the lesion is considered benign and usually resolves spontaneously over several weeks or months, the experienced and courageous clinician might advocate observation at frequent intervals. Because of the differential diagnosis and cosmetic considerations, however, complete excision is advised, with histologic examination performed to exclude the possibility of malignancy.

Malignant Neoplasms

Certain malignancies merit description by virtue of their frequency of occurrence and their potential seriousness. With few exceptions, the basic message is that any skin lesion with features suggestive of malignancy deserves a biopsy. General features of malignancy include rate and type of growth, color change, ulceration, bleeding, and loss of skin markings within the lesion. If malignancy is suspected, the best biopsy technique is usually excision. New evidence of patient concern about an old lesion should arouse suspicion that the lesion is changing.

Basal Cell Carcinoma (Basal Cell Epithelioma)

Basal cell carcinoma is a serious disease. Although it rarely metastasizes, untreated local spread can be destructive. Morphologically, the most common basal cell carcinoma is the noduloulcerative type. It begins as a whitish or pinkish papule with telangiectasia and then evolves into a sessile nodule with a raised, translucent, pearl-colored, telangiectatic border, with central ulceration and crusts (Fig. 40–36). The center often bleeds when crusts are removed. Occasionally,

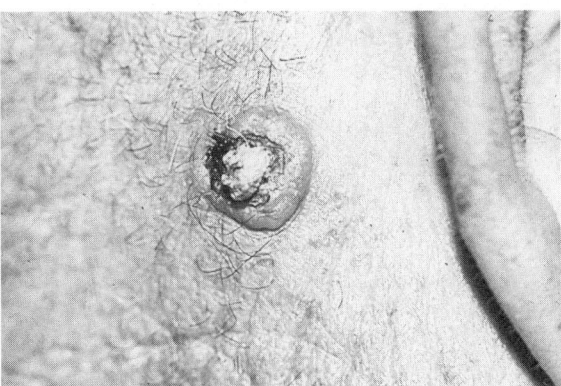

FIGURE 40–35. Keratoacanthoma.

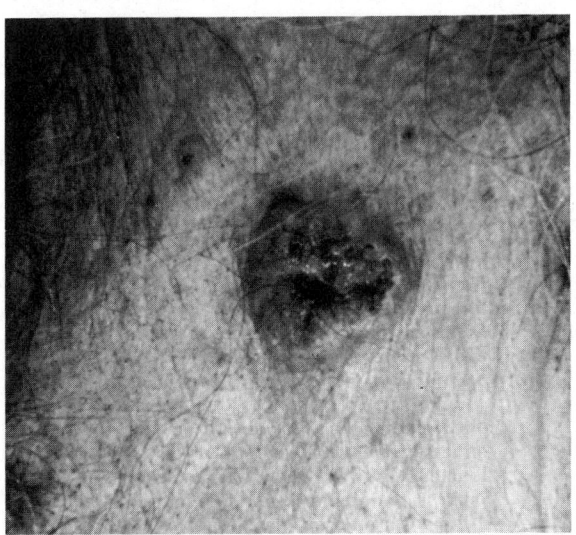

FIGURE 40–36. Basal cell carcinoma.

basal cell carcinoma is flat, resembling a persistent plaque of neurodermatitis or eczema.

TREATMENT. All suspected lesions should be biopsied before treatment; small lesions may be easily excised, but incisional biopsy is sufficient for the diagnosis of larger ones. Excision is a standard method of therapy by family physicians, but some physicians are also experienced in electrodesiccation and curettage. The need for plastic surgery or for more extensive chemosurgery or x-ray therapy usually indicates consultation with someone experienced in these techniques. Appropriate situations for consideration of Mohs micrographic surgery include lesions near the eyes, nose, ears, and mouth, lesions larger than 1 cm, and lesions that recur after excision.

Squamous Cell Carcinoma

Squamous cell carcinoma is a more treacherous lesion than basal cell carcinoma because of its faster growth rate, greater tendency for metastasis, and its variability of appearance. It may arise from actinic keratoses, leukoplakia, or chronic ulcers and may first look like a benign nodule or papilloma. An important diagnostic feature is the increase in size. Lesions may have a raised border and a central ulcer like basal cell carcinoma (Fig. 40–37) or may be fungoid in appearance. The most common locations are the lips, ears, tongue, and dorsal surface of the hands. The incidence increases with the patient's age.

TREATMENT. The preferred treatment is excision, radiation therapy, or both, provided by an experienced professional.

Actinic Keratoses

Actinic keratoses, premalignant lesions related to excessive sunlight exposure, may transform over time into squamous cell carcinomas. They may be single but are more often multiple, occurring primarily in the same age group as seborrheic kerato-

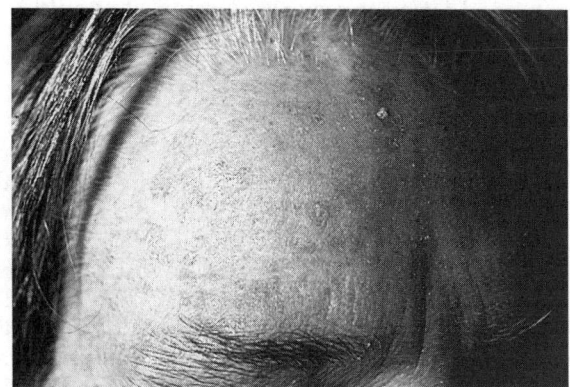

FIGURE 40–38. Actinic keratoses.

ses but favoring sun-exposed areas of fair-skinned individuals (Fig. 40–38). Individual lesions of 2 mm to 1 cm diameter appear as flat, gray tan, or brown spots, with adherent scale and mild surrounding erythema. If the scale is scraped away, the lesion usually bleeds. If only a few are present, liquid nitrogen application is effective, or electrodesiccation and curettage may be used. A more practical treatment for multiple lesions is topical 5-fluorouracil cream (Efudex) or masoprocol cream (Actinex). Treatment with 5-fluorouracil causes a violent inflammatory response, which must be explained carefully to the patient. Some authorities recommend application to separate areas sequentially or alternative applications of a topical steroid to control the inflammation. For resistant lesions on the back of the hands, some add nightly application of retinoic cream to the usual regimen of 5-fluorouracil. Masoprocol causes less inflammation and removes most actinic keratoses within 1 month. Patients with actinic keratoses obviously should limit subsequent exposure to sunlight by avoidance with appropriate clothing and sunscreen preparations.

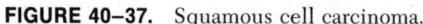

FIGURE 40–37. Squamous cell carcinoma.

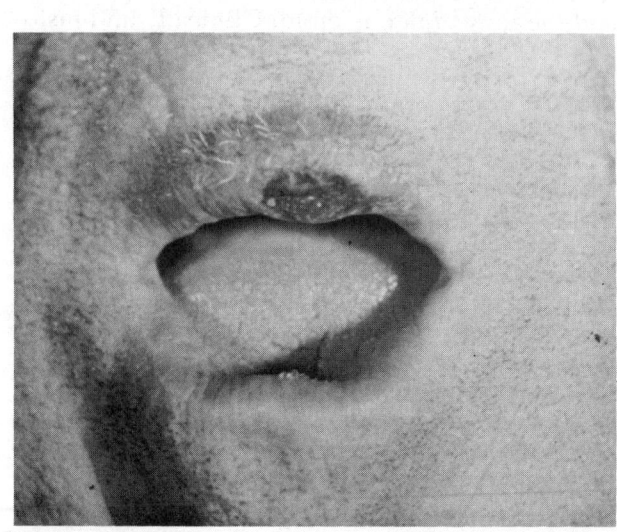

Melanoma (Malignant Melanoma)

Melanoma is the most feared of the cutaneous malignancies, but early recognition can save the patient's life. Metastasis is erratic, but it is fairly common and lethal. There are four recognized histopathologic types of melanoma: lentigo maligna melanoma, superficial spreading melanoma, nodular melanoma, and acral-lentiginous melanoma.

Features of pigmented lesions that should prompt biopsy are as follows.

1. Variegation of color is probably the single most important feature. In addition to brown and tan, look for admixtures of blue, red, white, pink, purple, and gray.

2. Irregularity or notching of the tumor border is also characteristic of melanoma.

3. Rapid growth is commonly observed.

4. Loss of skin markings within the lesion is a common finding, but this characteristic also is seen with benign lesions.

TREATMENT. Because there is no substantial evidence that biopsy increases the risk of metastasis, either incisional or excisional biopsy is acceptable. Of the two extremes, reluctance to biopsy a lesion has more serious consequences than does performing unwarranted biopsy. Reluctance is particularly common when pigmented lesions are under the nail; such lesions must be biopsied or referred for biopsy. Definitive treatment includes wide excision and other measures, which are beyond the scope of this discussion.

Cutaneous T Cell Lymphoma

The term cutaneous T cell lymphoma (CTCL) includes disorders formerly known as mycosis fungoides, Sezary syndrome, reticulum cell sarcoma, lymphoma cutis, and histiocytic lymphoma. CTCL is a neoplasm of helper-T cells that initially manifests as skin disease and later involves other organs. The cutaneous lesions may be single or multiple and have a highly variable appearance; for each lesion there is typically a slow progression from macule through plaque to nodule or tumor. CTCL should be suspected and a biopsy performed when a patient with chronic dermatitis fails to respond to conventional therapy (e.g., contact dermatitis, atopic dermatitis, neurodermatitis, psoriasis, tinea corporis). Because biopsy specimens early in the course of disease may show only "nonspecific chronic dermatitis," it may be necessary to repeat the biopsy every 3 to 4 months for persistent or growing lesions.

After biopsy confirmation of CTCL, a comprehensive investigation of blood, lymphoid tissue, and other organ systems is undertaken to establish the extent of disease. The evaluation includes thorough physical examination, review of systems, complete blood count, renal and liver function tests, biopsy of any enlarged lymph nodes, and other tests as indicated by the initial results. Treatment is based on extent of disease at the time of diagnosis and includes topical nitrogen mustard, oral psoralen plus ultraviolet A (UVA) light, electron beam irradiation, and photopheresis.

Psoriasis and Other Papulosquamous Eruptions

Psoriasis

Psoriasis is a chronic or recurrent papulosquamous eruption in which discrete areas of skin develop an increased mitotic rate and increased capillary blood supply. Clinically, the result is multiple irregular plaques with a red base and superimposed silvery-white thick scales. Psoriasis is most often recognized in adults, although it also occurs in children. A familial predisposition to the disease is known. The lesions of psoriasis commonly appear on the scalp, elbows, and knees, but they may be seen anywhere on the skin (Fig. 40–39). They exhibit the Koebner phenomenon, as they tend to appear in scar tissue following injury.

Another clue to diagnosis is Auspitz' sign, which means that a punctate bleeding site appears when a scale is plucked from the lesion. Ridges or pits may be seen in the nails. Psoriasis tends to be worse during the winter. Only a few patients have itching, but the cosmetic and psychological impairment can be severe.

Psoriasis occasionally causes confusion with other skin diseases, including tinea corporis, seborrheic dermatitis, pityriasis rosea, secondary syphilis, and lichen planus. In the appropriate circumstances, biopsy, KOH preparation, blood serology, or dermatologic consultation may be indicated.

TREATMENT. Multiple therapies have been used for psoriasis. Topical steroid application is by far the most often used therapy for limited or localized disease. Many patients respond best to the potent ointment or gel steroid preparations and may require occlusion intermittently. Coal tar

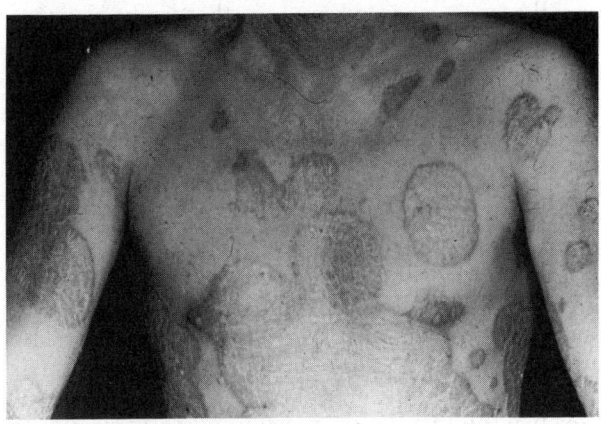

FIGURE 40–39. Psoriasis.

shampoos are useful for scalp lesions, and new gel forms of coal tar derivatives are less messy for use on the skin. Recalcitrant scalp lesions may also be treated with a topical steroid lotion: Triamcinolone acetonide (Kenalog) and betamethasone valerate (Valisone) are popular. The general rules for steroid use are especially important for patients with chronic, widespread lesions. Recall that fluorinated steroids should not be used for facial lesions; a second prescription for 1% hydrocortisone cream may be given for use on the face. Patients with widespread or recalcitrant disease are best treated with exposure to ultraviolet light, such as the Goeckerman regimen (tar compounds with UVB) or PUVA (oral psoralen with UVA). Patients generally benefit from the use of skin lubricants or bath oils.

Methotrexate can be administered orally for control of resistant cases when the physician is thoroughly familiar with its use; most family physicians initiate this therapy through consultation. Many authorities recommend that a liver biopsy be obtained and be proved normal before methotrexate therapy is begun. Isotretinoin and etretinate are other options with substantial risks and strict guidelines for appropriate use.

Pityriasis Alba and Pityriasis Rosea

PITYRIASIS ALBA. Pityriasis alba is a mild, chronic, self-limited disease of prepubescent children and teenagers. It appears as irregular, well circumscribed ovoid patches on the face with extremely fine scales and hypopigmentation.

Treatment. Some authorities believe the condition is a minor form of atopic dermatitis and advocate use of a skin lubricant such as petrolatum. Others recommend 0.5% or 1.0% hydrocortisone plus sun exposure to repigment the areas. It should be differentiated from tinea versicolor and vitiligo, and an explanation to the patient may be sufficient treatment.

PITYRIASIS ROSEA. Pityriasis rosea is a self-limited papulosquamous eruption that occurs at all ages but is most common among young adults. An initial single plaque, called the herald patch, is usually seen somewhere on the body days or weeks before the generalized eruption. The subsequent rash consists of multiple tan or fawn-colored oval plaques covered with fine scales, arranged with their long axes along skin cleavage lines (Fig. 40–40). Lesions are commonly confined to the trunk and proximal extremities but may also be seen on the face, especially in children. New lesions may appear for a week or two, but the rash usually disappears entirely within 5 to 6 weeks.

Treatment. Itching is sometimes an associated feature, requiring only symptomatic therapy. The most important aspect of management of pityriasis rosea is consideration of the differential diagnosis. Because the lesions are morphologically similar to those of some cases of secondary syphilis, serologic

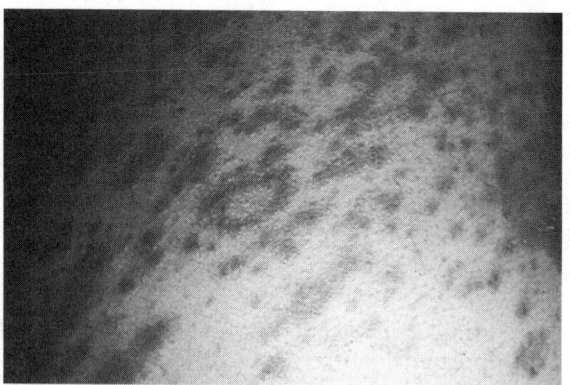

FIGURE 40–40.   Pityriasis rosea.

examination is prudent, especially if a herald patch was not seen. Drug eruptions, psoriasis, and lichen planus should be considered. The herald patch suggests tinea corporis, a problem resolved by KOH preparation.

Lichen Planus

The eruption of lichen planus consists of small, angular, shiny, flat-topped, violaceous or purple-hued papules. Lesions usually appear in ill-defined groups with a predilection for flexor surfaces, mucous membranes, and genitalia. The eruption is often pruritic, sometimes intensely so. The isomorphic (Koebner) phenomenon may result in a distribution of lesions along lines of injury due to scratching. Lesions with lichen-like appearance have been observed in response to several medications including antimalarials, gold, furosemide, and captopril.

TREATMENT. Lichen planus is a self-limited process; two thirds of cases resolve within 1 year. Many treatments have been used, without striking success. Symptoms may be improved with oral antihistamines, topical steroids, or other antipruritic lotions. Persistent cases or those unresponsive to symptomatic therapy may require consultation.

Urticaria and Erythema Multiforme

Urticaria

Urticaria is an eruption of skin characterized by a typical primary lesion called a wheal. The wheal is a circumscribed, raised, edematous, red lesion that itches. Individual lesions are transitory but may last minutes or hours. There may be pallor of the surrounding skin. Multiple lesions are the rule (Fig. 40–41).

Wheals are an end result of a variety of immunologic and nonimmunologic processes that lead to localized release of histamine and other vasoactive substances from mast cells of the skin. An abbreviated list of precipitating factors includes food, venoms, drugs, pollens, heat, cold, light, blood prod-

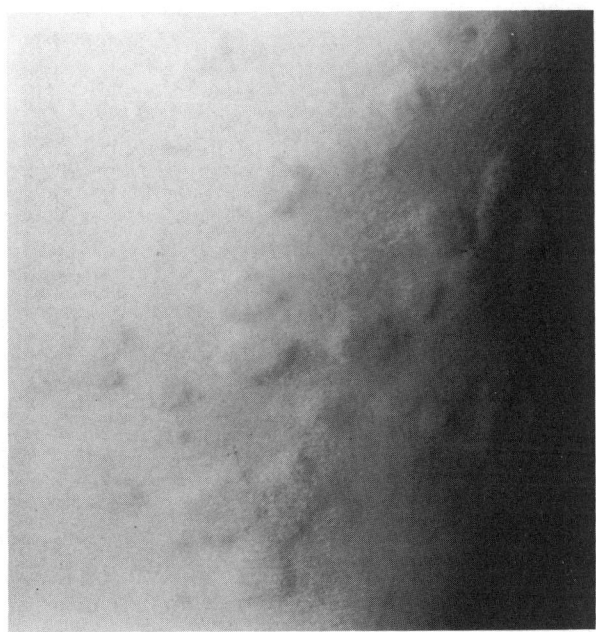

FIGURE 40–41. Urticaria.

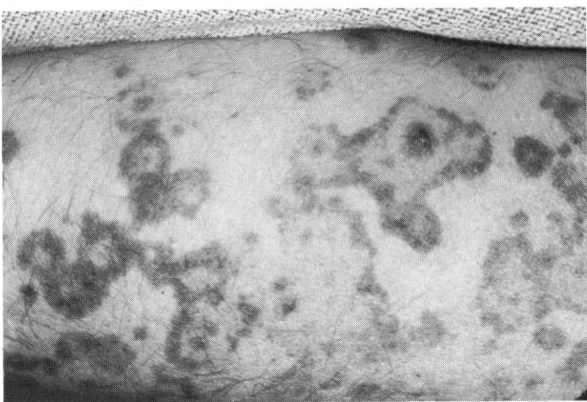

FIGURE 40–42. Erythema multiforme.

ucts, radiocontrast agents, helminths, pressure, emotional stress, and chronic infections.

It should be apparent that recognition of urticaria is simple, but the etiologic diagnosis can be difficult or impossible. A thorough history and examination are indicated when urticaria is persistent or chronic (arbitrarily, longer than 4 to 6 weeks). If the etiology is still unknown, a reasonable evaluation might include a complete blood cell count with differential count, urinalysis, chest radiographic study, and stool examination for parasites. Special cases may require immunologic investigation, which is beyond the scope of this summary.

TREATMENT. Parenteral epinephrine is indicated for acute urticaria associated with anaphylaxis or angioedema. Ordinarily, acute urticaria or chronic urticaria is treated with an antihistamine, of which the most effective is hydroxyzine (Atarax, Vistaril). A brief course of oral steroids is used occasionally for persistent cases. Although not approved for this indication, experienced clinicians sometimes use doxepin (Sinequan) for its antihistaminic properties.

Erythema Multiforme

Erythema multiforme is an acute or recurrent rash that occurs through immune mechanisms, either in response to known precipitating factors or of idiopathic cause. The most convincing causative associations have been established with herpes simplex and *Mycoplasma* infection and with sulfa drugs, particularly the sulfonamides. In about half the cases, no precipitating factor can be identified. More cases are seen during the spring and fall than in other seasons.

The lesions may be widespread on skin and mucous membranes and are occasionally accompanied by itching or burning. Some patients have fever with or without an associated infection or source of inflammation. Typically there are multiple, symmetrically distributed target (iris) lesions that have a predisposition for acral areas (Fig. 40–42). There may also be urticarial plaques, which are more persistent than the wheals seen with urticaria. Favored locations include flexor surfaces of the extremities, palms and soles, genitalia, and lips. The development of vesicles or bullae in pre-existing lesions signals a more severe course. The most severe form of the disease is known as the Stevens-Johnson syndrome, which is characterized by significant constitutional signs and symptoms and by multiple inflammatory bullae on the mucous membranes.

Although typical cases are rather easily identified, the differential diagnosis of atypical cases includes urticaria, necrotizing vasculitis, secondary syphilis, septicemia, Rocky Mountain spotted fever, viral exanthems, lichen planus, and bullous impetigo.

TREATMENT. Treatment of milder cases is generally symptomatic, with antihistamines, salicylates, and other anti-inflammatory agents employed with varying degrees of success. More severe cases require additional supportive care and attention to the metabolic consequences and specific organs affected. Probably the most difficult task is judging the appropriate methods and extent of a search for occult causes. As for urticaria, the search most often depends on a thorough history and examination. A typical eruption subsides within 2 to 3 weeks, but recurrences are fairly common.

Selected Alopecias

See "tinea" descriptions for hair loss due to fungi.

Androgenetic Alopecia (Male-Pattern Baldness)

Men are affected more often than women by androgenetic alopecia. In men the typical pattern is recession in the parietal areas and on the crown, leaving behind scalp of normal appearance. In women, diffuse loss on the crown is typical. If the process occurs in a woman under 50 to 60 years of age, endocrinologic evaluation should be considered, seeking a source of excessive androgens, especially if there are other signs of virilization.

TREATMENT. Hair transplantation and cosmetic remedies (hair styling and wigs) have been the mainstays of legitimate therapy. Topical minoxidil (Rogaine) is the first medication approved by the U.S. Food and Drug Administration (FDA) for the treatment of male baldness, although it is not for everyone. The best candidates are men under 40 years of age whose balding has progressed for less than 10 years. The presence of remaining "peach fuzz" hairs seems to be the most important single factor predictive of success. The treatment is fairly expensive and requires a long-term commitment; the hair growth is lost a few months after the applications are stopped.

Telogen Effluvium (Febrile Alopecia, Toxic Alopecia)

A large number of hair follicles enter the telogen (resting) phase in unison, with resultant hair loss. The loss is usually diffuse rather than patchy and follows a stressful event by 2 to 4 months. Postpartum telogen effluvium is a common example, and others include occurrences following a severe infection, fever, or adverse drug reaction.

TREATMENT. Hair regrowth usually occurs within a year, and no specific treatment speeds recovery.

Traumatic Alopecia (Traction Alopecia, Trichotillomania)

Trichotillomania results from repetitive, often subconscious, manipulation of hair by the patient. The typical presentation is a well circumscribed area of absent and broken hairs without evidence of scalp involvement (Fig. 40–43); the diagnosis is confirmed primarily by history. A similar pattern of traumatic hair loss results from damage by rollers and some other hair styling methods, typically around the hairline.

TREATMENT. Treatment consists in management of the underlying psychopathology or avoidance of the hair styling methods that cause damage.

Alopecia Areata

The general term alopecia areata refers to single or multiple patches of well demarcated hair loss from the scalp (Fig. 40–44). Alopecia totalis is the total or near-total loss of scalp hair, and alopecia universalis is generalized loss of body hair. Men

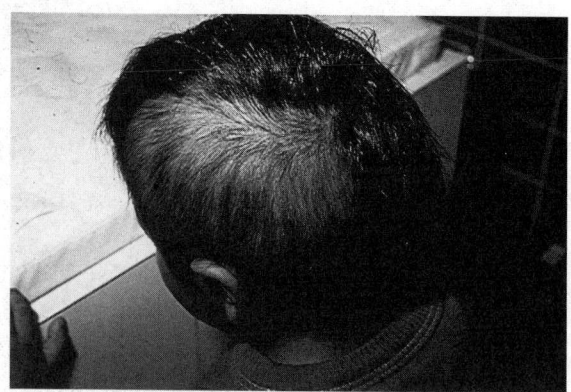

FIGURE 40–43. Trichotillomania.

and women are affected about equally, with the peak incidence occurring at ages 40 through 60. The underlying skin appears normal. If present, "exclamation point hairs" are pathognomonic; they are short, stubby hairs tapered at the proximal end. Spontaneous regrowth usually begins at the periphery and spreads centrally, but recurrences are common. Although the etiology is unknown, suggested contributing factors include genetic predisposition, stress, and disorders of immune regulation. Associated findings are nail dystrophies, cataracts, atopy, and pernicious anemia.

Diagnosis on clinical grounds is the rule, but biopsy may be necessary. Fungal tests are appropriate if there are signs of inflammation, and serologic tests for syphilis may be in order.

TREATMENT. No treatment is entirely satisfactory, and these efforts should probably be left to physicians who have considerable experience with the condition. Alternatives include systemic and local injections of steroids, topical irritants, and PUVA therapy. Topical minoxidil may also prove useful for this condition.

Parasitic Infestations

Scabies

Scabies results from parasitic infestation of the skin. The disease is highly contagious on close contact and is seen most often in crowded conditions, such as nursery schools and in large families in a single household. The incidence is increased among patients with AIDS. It also occurs as a contemporary form of venereal disease. The cause is the bite of a mite called *Sarcoptes scabiei*, the female of which burrows into the skin and lays her eggs.

The primary lesion of scabies is a tiny burrow 2 to 3 mm in length. It is frequently hidden within the secondary eruption, and few mites are actually present in a single patient. Secondary lesions are minute reddish papules and excoriations of the fin-

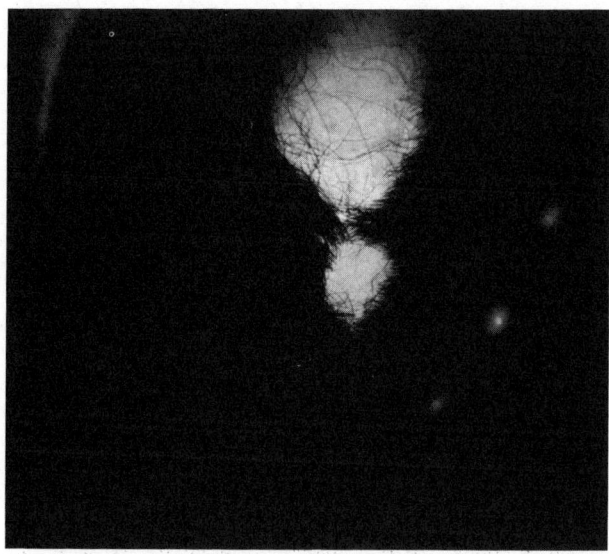

FIGURE 40–44. Alopecia areata.

ger webs, forearms, axillae, lower abdomen, and genitalia, which probably represent a hypersensitivity reaction to a small number of bites (Fig. 40–45). The face is rarely involved, except in infants. Itching is intense and is particularly noticeable at night. With some skill and luck, the mite can be recovered from a burrow for microscopic confirmation of the diagnosis. Burrows are most often found on the forearms and finger webs.

TREATMENT. A single application of permethrin 5% cream (Elimite) is effective for adults and children more than 2 months of age. The cream is massaged into the entire skin surface from head to toe, then washed off after 8 to 14 hours. Persistent pruritus for several days is not an indication of treatment failure; a topical steroid could be used for temporary relief of itching. Persistent or recurrent rash after 2 to 3 weeks is a reasonable cause for repeat application. Treatment alternatives for adults and older children include lindane 1% lotion (γ-benzene hexachloride, Kwell), 10% crotamiton (Eurax), and nonprescription preparations based on pyrethrin insecticides (Rid, A-200). Con-

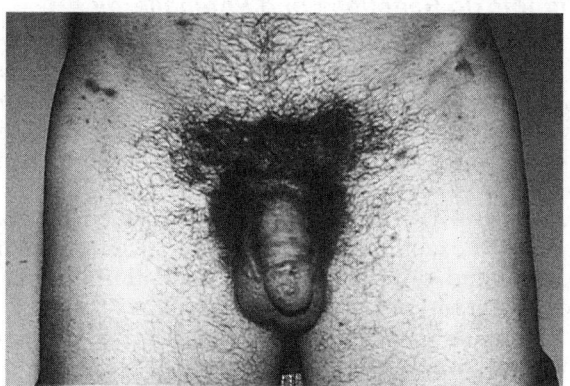

FIGURE 40–45. Scabies.

currently with treatment, clothing and bed linens should be laundered and dried with heat.

Pediculosis (Lice)

PEDICULOSIS CAPITIS. Pediculosis capitis (head lice) is a condition associated with crowded conditions and long hair, often seen among children in schools or day-care centers. It is transmitted by shared combs, hats, and pillows. The lice are sometimes seen, but diagnosis is usually made by observing the tiny, pearl-colored nits (ova) attached to hair shafts. Grayish fluorescence under a Wood's light can accentuate the nits, if necessary; and they are more evident when the hair is wet. In fact, the diagnosis is frequently made by the patient's mother, barber, or teacher or as an incidental finding by the physician.

Treatment. The usual treatment is γ-benzene hexachloride (lindane, Kwell); agents containing pyrethrins (e.g., A-200) are probably safer for children under 5 years of age. Kwell is used as a shampoo and then is reapplied as an overnight lotion after the hair is dry. Ordinarily, only one application is necessary, but it may be repeated in a week or so as needed. Although it is not necessary to remove all the nits to achieve a cure, removal can usually be accomplished with a fine-toothed comb as desired for aesthetic reasons. Removal is made easier if the hair is covered for a few hours with a towel soaked in white vinegar to soften the cement that holds the nits to the hair shafts.

PEDICULOSIS CORPORIS. The body louse, pediculosis corporis, is seen less often than the head louse. Lice and ova may be seen on skin or hair but are found most easily in the seams of clothing. Itching and scattered erythematous macules are typical.

Treatment. The customary treatment is lindane (Kwell) applied as a body lotion, followed by improved hygiene. Clothing should be washed and dried, as dry heat is effective against the lice and eggs.

PHTHIRIASIS PUBIS. Phthiriasis pubis (crab louse) is often transmitted by sexual contact but may also be obtained via shared clothing. Despite its name, the louse may be found in hair-bearing areas elsewhere on the body. Itching is common, and the diagnosis may be obscured by secondary infection of the excoriations. There may be a scattered macular rash and occasionally other allergic responses.

Treatment. Lindane (Kwell) is used as for pediculosis corporis, with attention to secondary infections or allergic sequelae as needed.

Paronychia

Fungal Paronychia

Paronychia results from infection of the nail fold with bacteria or yeast. Some clinical features help distinguish the cause, with bacterial or yeast cultures for confirmation. Paronychia due to *Candida* (monilia) is characterized by a relatively insidious onset, with redness, some tenderness, and swelling of the skin just proximal to the nail and along its lateral margins. Thick cheese-like material can be expressed in some cases, and there may be some green or brown discoloration of the nail. Chronic cases lead to distortion and discoloration of the nail. The condition is more likely to occur in those who frequently immerse their hands in water, particularly if detergents are used. Involvement of multiple fingers or toes is common. Diagnosis is confirmed by culture on Sabouraud's agar.

TREATMENT. Treatment includes avoidance of or protection from water and harsh detergents plus topical application of an antifungal agent, such as clotrimazole solution (Mycelex) or sulconazole solution (Exelderm). If inflammation and pain are prominent, fluocinonide solution (Lidex) can be applied before the antifungal liquid. If nail damage occurs, it resolves slowly or incompletely over 4 to 6 months.

Bacterial Paronychia

Bacterial paronychia, in contrast to fungal paronychia, ordinarily has a more acute onset, is accompanied by more pain and tenderness, and may be attended by localized vesicles or pustules. If material can be expressed from underneath the edge of the skin, it is frankly purulent. Involvement of only one finger is typical. The introduction of bacteria into the nail fold often results from traumatic removal of a hangnail. The diagnosis is confirmed and antibiotic sensitivity determined from the exudate.

TREATMENT. Treatment includes administration of a systemic antibiotic and may require inci-

sion and drainage; lack of treatment can result in a closed-space infection or osteomyelitis.

Because the paronychias may lead to some destruction or distortion of the nail, they may be confused with other causes of nail dystrophy, such as tinea (onychomycosis). The other causes of nail changes are not accompanied by tenderness, redness, or edema unless there is coexistent paronychia.

Sunlight and Its Consequences

Acute Reactions to Sunlight (Sunburn and Photosensitivity Reactions)

The most common reaction to acute sunlight exposure is sunburn, characterized by erythema on the exposed areas and sometimes accompanied by pain, swelling, and the formation of vesicles or bullae as occurs with first and second degree burns due to other causes. The injury results from ultraviolet radiation from any source, especially the ultraviolet B and C spectrums. Relative susceptibility is in part determined by genetic factors, and some additional protection from sunburn is afforded by induced pigmentation, or tanning. Particularly when the sunburn does not fit the previous pattern for an individual, some thought should be given to the possibility of photosensitivity, phototoxicity, and photoallergy.

TREATMENT. In view of the self-limited nature of simple sunburn, it is essential that treatments cause no additional harm. Many commercial remedies fail that requirement owing to their high cost and the potential for sensitization. Reasonable therapy for mild cases of sunburn includes avoidance of further acute exposure, soothing compresses with tap water or Burow's solution, and emollients for dry skin. Steroid lotions or sprays may also be used when justified by the symptoms present at the early stages of the burn. Protection from recurrence depends on reduced exposure, controlled exposure to induce tanning, and the use of sunscreens or other barriers.

Phototoxic Reactions and Photoallergy

Phototoxic reactions refer to the hastening or exacerbation of sunburn due to the combined action of sunlight and a chemical applied to the skin or ingested. These reactions are said to be reproducible in almost anyone if the dosage of chemical and sunlight is sufficient. Examples of the offending substances are certain plants, tetracycline, psoralens, hexachlorophene (used in some bath soaps), and unfortunately the para-aminobenzoic acid esters found in some sunscreens.

Photoallergy is an immune-mediated process requiring sensitization to the causative agent. Sulfonamides, thiazides, and chlorpromazine (Thorazine) are examples. The resulting rash may have eczematous and papular components and may involve areas of the skin not exposed to sunlight. For clinical purposes, the distinction between photoallergy and phototoxicity is not critical.

TREATMENT. Therapy is based on avoidance of the offending agent and treatment of the eczematous component.

Porphyria Cutanea Tarda

Porphyria cutanea tarda might be considered photoallergy to endogenous agents (i.e., the circulating porphyrins), leading to a bullous eruption and characteristic urinary findings (dark discoloration and red fluorescence under Wood's light).

Repeated or Chronic Sunlight Exposure

Prolonged exposure to sunlight or to ultraviolet radiation from artificial sources can produce skin damage, which is ameliorated to some extent by the natural protection of skin pigments. The damage falls into two broad categories: carcinogenesis and the conditions called dermatoheliosis.

Skin cancer
  Basal cell cancer
  Squamous cell cancer
  Melanoma
Dermatoheliosis
  Solar keratoses
  Solar lentigo
  Aging, wrinkles, telangiectasia

The cumulative effects of exposure to ultraviolet light are *directly* related to the intensity and duration of the exposure and *inversely* related to the effectiveness of natural protection due to skin color, tanning ability, and mechanisms of skin repair.

TREATMENT. Logical measures to reduce the lifetime burden of radiation include avoidance of midday sun, use of protective clothing, and controlled exposure to increase protective tanning. Consistent use of sunscreens is also helpful. The simplest agents are the physical barriers, including combinations of titanium oxide, zinc oxide, iron oxide, or red veterinary petrolatum. They offer effective protection for small areas but are usually less acceptable cosmetically than the transparent sunscreens. The new commercial preparations in bright colors may help solve the problem with cosmetic appearance and acceptance.

The chemical sunscreens are colorless or invisible on the skin and reduce the penetration of ultraviolet radiation. The relative effectiveness of these preparations is stated numerically as a sun protection factor (SPF); these SPF ratings have been adopted by the FDA for comparisons; a higher number means greater protection. The sun protection factor for a given product is determined by comparing the dosage of sunlight required to produce erythema with the product and without it. In addition, other properties of importance for the sunscreens include resistance to sweating and water immersion, ease of application, and propensity to cause phototoxicity or other adverse reactions. As a rule of thumb, fair-skinned individuals should probably use a product with a high number (SPF 15 to 30), whereas those with darker skin who tan more easily can use a lower number (SPF 4 to 10). Adverse reactions should prompt change to another agent with different ingredients.

AIDS-Associated Conditions

Patients with human immunodeficiency virus (HIV) infection or AIDS can have a variety of immunologic defects, which in turn can result in several abnormalities of the skin and mucous membranes. Most of these problems are infectious, but some other dermatoses are promoted by AIDS. The following discussion emphasizes key clinical features and recognition of the more common manifestations, which indeed may be early clues that the syndrome exists.

Kaposi Sarcoma

Kaposi sarcoma (idiopathic hemorrhagic sarcoma) is a multifocal neoplasm with vascular tumors in the skin and other organs. The variety associated with AIDS is sometimes called "epidemic" Kaposi sarcoma to distinguish it from the classic form described in elderly patients of eastern European or Jewish origin. It begins as a violaceous or reddish-pink macule that develops quickly into a nodule or plaque-like tumor 1 to 3 cm in diameter. There are usually multiple lesions located on the face or trunk; the extremities are less often involved (Fig. 40–46). Lesions sometimes become confluent and may ulcerate. Discomfort is uncommon unless there is irritation by clothing. Affected extremities may be enlarged owing to edema. Biopsy can distinguish the lesions from other tumor-like growths. Several treatment methods are used, depending on the clinical circumstances. Recurrences are common.

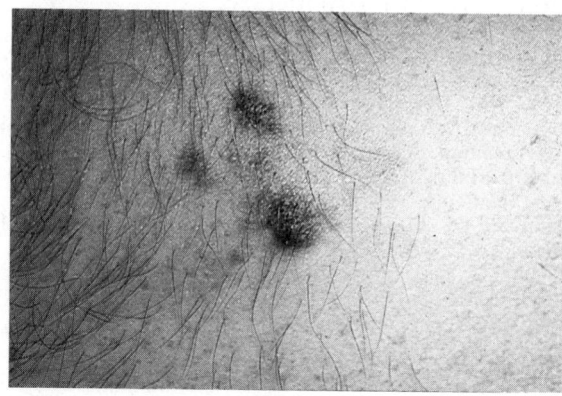

FIGURE 40–46. Kaposi sarcoma.

Although melanoma and some other tumors have been found in AIDS patients, no pathophysiologic relations have been established.

Dermatoses

Seborrheic dermatitis is found in more than three fourths of patients with AIDS late in the course of the disease, and it is frequently severe and generalized. Generalized redness of the skin and xerosis are also common. Psoriasis is seen in about 10 per cent of patients, either as a new occurrence or as a florid exacerbation of old disease. Pityriasis rubra pilaris and ichthyosis have been reported less often. Reported vascular manifestations include angiomas, petechiae, telangiectases, purpura, and splinter hemorrhages of the nail beds. Drug eruptions are common, including a morbilliform reaction to trimethoprim–sulfamethoxazole (Bactrim, Septra) and hyperpigmentation associated with zidovudine (AZT, Retrovir).

Fungal Infections

Candida infections may be found in multiple locations, the most common of which is the mouth, descending into the esophagus (Fig. 40–21). Typical white plaques are seen on the tongue and oral mucosa, with sore throat and dysphagia. If necessary, esophagoscopy can confirm the esophageal component. As the number of T-helper cells decreases, *Candida* lesions increase in severity. Treatment with topical agents such as miconazole or nystatin is effective for the milder cases, with systemic ketoconazole used for the difficult cases.

Tinea versicolor and the superficial fungi commonly affect AIDS patients and may be relatively resistant to standard therapy. Cryptococcosis, histoplasmosis, sporotrichosis, and other fungi have also been identified, fairly often in disseminated form or with atypical presentations. There should be a high index of suspicion and a low threshold for obtaining diagnostic biopsy specimens or cultures for these infections, as they are life-threatening. Prompt initiation of therapy is essential.

Viral Infections

Herpes simplex infections are present in most patients with AIDS. They tend to exhibit erosion and ulceration rather than the classic vesicular eruption. Lesions tend to be widespread and commonly involve the perirectal and oral areas. Intravenous or oral acyclovir may be indicated.

Both chickenpox and herpes zoster are common occurrences, with relative severity paralleling the decreasing number of T-helper cells. The onset of herpes zoster in an unusually young patient justifies obtaining, at least, a thorough history of AIDS risk factors.

Molluscum contagiosum is also common in the oral, genital, and rectal areas. Confirmation by culture and biopsy is probably appropriate, as similar lesions due to histoplasmosis and cryptococcosis have been reported. Anogenital warts are often a problem, but the specific role of immunodeficiency states is not known.

Bacterial Infections

Bacterial skin infections are common, particularly in those AIDS patients who are intravenous drug abusers. Localized infections are seen, with staphylococci or streptococci as leading causes, although some unusual organisms also may be seen. Of recent interest is an entity called bacillary angiomatosis, which results from infection by a rickettsia-like organism, *Rochalema hensle*. The infection promotes a vascular proliferation that manifests as widespread erythematous-violaceous papules similar in appearance to Kaposi sarcoma. The lesions respond to erythromycin or doxycycline.

Syphilis is common in patients with HIV infection; as many as 25 per cent of syphilis cases are reported to be associated with HIV. HIV-infected individuals respond well to standard CDC-recommended antibiotic therapy, but those with neurosyphilis may suffer an increased incidence of subsequent relapses.

SUGGESTED READINGS

Abramowicz M: Sunscreens. Med Lett 30:768, 1988.

Ashton R, Leppard B: Differential Diagnosis in Dermatology. New York, JB Lippincott, 1990.

Champion RH, Burton JL, Ebling FJG: Textbook of Dermatology. London, Blackwell Scientific, 1992.

Fitzpatrick TB, Eisen AZ, Wolff K, et al: Dermatology in General Medicine. New York, McGraw-Hill, 1993.

Lookingbill DP: Principles of Dermatology. Philadelphia, WB Saunders Company, 1986.

Moschella SL, Hurley HJ: Dermatology. Philadelphia, WB Saunders Company, 1992.

Photoplex—a broad spectrum sunscreen. Med Lett 31:794, 1989.

Sauer GC: Manual of Skin Diseases. New York, JB Lippincott, 1991.

Topical corticosteroids. Med Lett 33:857, 1991.

CHAPTER 41
ENDOCRINOLOGY

DAVID R. RUDY and MANUEL TZAGOURNIS

DIABETES MELLITUS

Diabetes mellitus is a clinical entity with abnormalities related to hyperglycemia and an absolute or relative insulin deficiency. It is common and can affect virtually any organ system, manifesting diverse symptoms and signs. Some of the complications that accompany the diabetic state may be considered a syndrome. Carbohydrate, protein, and lipid metabolism are involved that directly or indirectly produce structural changes in blood vessels, nerves, and other tissues.

Although type I (insulin-dependent) diabetes differs from type II (non-insulin-dependent) diabetes, the two can result in classic clinical manifestations, the best known of which are polyuria, poldydipsia, and polyphagia with weight loss. These classic findings are related to hyperglycemia and related diuresis when the renal threshold for glucose reabsorption is exceeded. Loss of calories, fluids, and electrolytes in the urine ensue. However, there is a vast spectrum of clinical manifestations ranging from an asymptomatic state to coma due to diabetic ketoacidosis.

Diabetes mellitus is not a single disease but, rather, is heterogeneous. The classification advocated by the World Health Organization Expert Committee is summarized in Table 41–1. Of greatest clinical importance are type I and type II diabetes. The individual with type I diabetes requires exogenous insulin to survive or to avoid ketoacidosis. Genetic factors interact with autoimmune reactions often stimulated by viral infections. On the other hand, the individual with type II diabetes may have insulin resistance as well as insulin secretory abnormalities, and usually the islet cells are not destroyed as in type I.

The "other" types are secondary to certain identifiable factors that damage the islet cell or interfere with the normal functions of insulin, such as antibodies directed against the receptor for insulin. *Impaired glucose tolerance* exists when glucose concentrations are above normal but do not meet the criteria for the diagnosis of diabetes. *Gestational diabetes* occurs in a person who develops glucose abnormalities while pregnant. Most women with this type revert to normal after delivery, but they are at high risk for diabetes later in life. *Potential abnormality of glucose tolerance* is a category that is meant to alert the clinician to the likelihood of a person becoming diabetic. Examples might be a homozygous twin of a patient with type II diabetes or a nondiabetic mother of an infant weighing more than 9 pounds at birth.

Insulin-Dependent Diabetes

Type I diabetes or insulin-dependent diabetes (IDDM) has been called early-onset, juvenile, and autoimmune diabetes. Patients have an absolute deficiency of insulin; and in almost all circumstances there is destruction of islet cells in the pancreas.

Epidemiologically, type I diabetes is found throughout the world, but with certain geographic and ethnic predispositions. The incidence is high in Scandinavian countries and the United States and low in Japan (Krolewski and Warram, 1985). The incidence of IDDM in children is outlined in Table 41–2. White children tend to have a higher frequency of type I diabetes than do black children. A great deal of information has accumulated elucidating genetic and environmental factors in the etiology of type I diabetes.

When a genetically susceptible individual is exposed to an environmental influence such as certain viral infections, type I diabetes may develop acutely or after a relatively long time. An autoimmune reaction involving the islet cells leads to progressive loss of insulin secretory capacity and ultimately clinical diabetes. Islet cell antibodies (ICAs) are autoimmune markers present in most of the children diagnosed with type I diabetes. In one report the ICAs found in adult patients classified as type II at diagnosis were associated with beta cell functions, which progressively failed. After a few years they were similar to type I patients (Gottsater et al., 1993). Type II diabetic patients without ICAs showed no such progression.

Genetic susceptibility to type I diabetes is dependent to a great extent on the inherited major histocompatibility system. Human lymphocyte antigens (HLA), encoded in any given individual, vary in their ability to induce autoimmunity to islet cells. The class II proteins, particularly DR and

TABLE 41–1. WHO COMMITTEE CLASSIFICATION OF DIABETES AND OTHER DEGREES OF GLUCOSE INTOLERANCE

Clinical types
  Diabetes mellitus
    Type I: insulin-dependent
    Type II: non-insulin-dependent
      Nonobese
      Obese
    Other types, including diabetes associated with certain
      conditions and syndromes
      Pancreatic disease
      Disease of hormonal etiology
      Drug or chemically induced conditions
      Insulin receptor abnormalities
      Genetic syndromes
      Miscellaneous
  Impaired glucose tolerance
    Nonobese
    Obese
    Impaired glucose tolerance associated with certain condi-
      tions and syndromes
  Gestational diabetes
Normal glucose tolerance but substantially increased risk of developing diabetes
  Previously abnormal glucose tolerance
  Potential abnormality of glucose tolerance

DQ, seem to influence susceptibility to diabetes profoundly, increasing the risk tenfold with the right combination. On the other hand, aspartate at position 57 of the DQ β-chain is protective against type I diabetes. Thus environmental agents may trigger an immune reaction or otherwise injure beta cells if the appropriate genetic background is present. An explanation of how this interaction might occur is suggested by the following model (Robinson et al., 1993): An antigenic peptide is bound by class II dimers differentially depending on the HLA proteins in that individual. A lack of

TABLE 41–2. INCIDENCE OF IDDM IN CHILDREN AGES 0–14

Country	Incidence/100,000/Year
Japan	0.6
Dominican Republic	1.7
Cuba	2.3
Yugoslavia	2.7
France	3.7
Italy	4.7
German Democratic Republic	7.4
Canada	9.0
New Zealand	9.0
USA (nonwhites)	9.7
Denmark	13.7
Scotland	13.8
Norway	17.6
USA (whites)	18.2
Sweden	22.6
Finland	29.2

From Krolewski AS, Warram JH: Epidemiology of diabetes mellitus. *In* Marble A, Krall LP, Bradley RF, et al (eds): Joslin's Diabetes Mellitus, 12th ed. Philadelphia, Lea & Febiger, 1985, p 2, with permission.

tolerance to the protein can develop, and immune responses are directed to self-proteins in the beta cell. A reaction to a peptide in bovine serum albumin may explain why early exposure to cow's milk in an immature gut might trigger an immune response that results in islet cell damage. Viruses can infect beta cells and destroy them in a susceptible host or stimulate the development of antibodies leading to autoimmune type I diabetes.

Measurements of ICAs are currently used to screen individuals who might participate in studies for the prevention of type I diabetes by immune intervention therapy. Determining HLA type is warranted currently only in the context of defined research studies.

Clinical Manifestations

The clinical presentation of type I diabetes is similar to that of type II, but it is more abrupt and more severe. Symptoms are secondary to the hyperglycemia but also may result from specific organ involvement such as neuropathy. The onset of symptoms such as polyuria, polydipsia, and polyphagia with weight loss may occur within hours or may progress over a period of weeks or even months. Glucose levels that exceed the renal threshold for glucose reabsorption result in an osmotic diuresis with relatively more loss of water than electrolytes initially as well as a loss of calories (glucose). Thus diabetes is one of the relatively few diseases in humans that can result in weight loss despite adequate caloric intake. The other diseases are thyrotoxicosis and gastrointestinal losses of calories, as seen with malabsorption or parasitic infestation.

A host of other symptoms may be present. Fatigue is prominent along with weakness, blurred vision, nausea, and monilial infection of the vagina and pubic areas or upper thighs of men. The neuropathic symptoms of painful feet or numbness may be among the presenting clinical manifestations, as may abdominal pain due to an enlarged liver. Unusual symptoms such as a painful mass due to infarction of muscle (Rocca et al., 1993) or those associated with a carpal tunnel syndrome are challenging to the clinician.

Major features of types I and II diabetes are contrasted in Table 41–3. With symptomatic type I diabetes one may see a patient clinically dehydrated with a fast pulse rate, low blood pressure, and deep prolonged respirations with a fruity odor to the breath if ketoacidosis is present. The patient may be alert and anxious or comatose. Patients who are already on insulin therapy and who present with uncontrolled diabetes usually have some precipitating cause, and the clinician must be alert to the possibility of infection, stroke, emotional distress, myocardial infarction, renal failure, or simply the omission of insulin.

TABLE 41–3. FEATURES OF IDDM AND NIDDM

Feature	IDDM	NIDDM
Age of onset	Usually <30	Usually >40
Rate of onset	Rapid	Slow
Body weight	Thin	Obese
Ketosis	Common	Rare
Prevalence	<0.5%	>2%
HLA association	Present	Absent
Concordance—identical twins	<50%	>95%
Islet cell mass	Greatly reduced	Slightly reduced
Insulitis	50–70% at onset	Not seen
Association with endocrinopathies	Occasional	Rare

Diagnosis and Management

It is usually not difficult to diagnose type I diabetes. A single criterion of unequivocal elevation of plasma or serum glucose above 200 mg/dL is almost always associated with the classic symptoms. Rarely, if ever, is a glucose tolerance test necessary. A person below the age of 20 years who presents with hyperglycemia and ketoacidosis is presumed to have type I diabetes and to be in need of insulin therapy. The patient might enjoy a "honeymoon" period after the initial insulin therapy and be controlled without insulin for a time, but the need for insulin invariably returns. Individuals who developed mild diabetes early in life and do not need insulin are said to have maturity-onset diabetes of youth. Preventive measures to preserve islet cells with immunosuppression or other means are still experimental and require entry into an established clinical research trial.

The distinction between types I and II diabetes becomes more troublesome when a patient presents later in life. A person who has an episode of ketoacidosis is likely to be a type I diabetic irrespective of age. The presence of islet cell antibodies might be of assistance, as may proof that insulin secretion is inadequate by measuring serum insulin or C-peptide concentrations.

It is generally worthwhile to obtain a consultation with an endocrinologist at the time of diagnosis. Diabetes is a chronic disorder with acute and long-term complications, some of which are preventable. Standards of medical care for patients with diabetes are published and may be obtained from the American Diabetes Association. Briefly, the initial visit should include a history and physical examination with special attention to patient education, determination of other vascular risk factors, and complete ophthalmoscopic, neurologic, vascular, and foot examinations. Baseline laboratory evaluation includes glucose levels, glycosylated hemoglobin, lipids, urinalysis, serum chemistries, and an electrocardiogram (ECG) in adults. A management plan is then implemented with certain goals, nutritional advice, self-monitoring of glucose, and contraceptive advice. The patient must be able to distinguish between hypoglycemia and symptoms of uncontrolled diabetes. Proper techniques to inject insulin and to make minor adjustment in the dosage must be practiced. The better the patient understands the disease, the better he or she copes with it in an independent and helpful way.

We prefer to admit a patient for initial insulin therapy even if it is for a brief time, but most insurance companies are reluctant to reimburse for inpatient services. Thus an efficient outpatient environment must be made available. Habits of self-management should be established early. Such training, encouragement, and education about the disease serve to promote self-confidence for the long-term care of the diabetes.

Initially, it is necessary to provide regular insulin, fluids, and electrolytes to normalize the person who has marked hyperglycemia and dehydration. Normal saline can be infused with the addition of 15 mEq of potassium chloride when adequate urine flow is ensured. If more than 1 liter of fluid is necessary, Ringer's lactate solution may be used or 1 liter of 0.5 N saline that contains 5% glucose and potassium chloride.

Regular insulin must be provided. The continuous intravenous infusion of insulin is convenient and effective. An infusion pump is helpful for achieving smooth control of glucose concentration and permits dose adjustments. One liter of 0.5 N saline containing 100 units of regular human insulin is infused initially at a rate of 10 ml per hour (providing 1 unit per hour) or at 20 ml per hour (providing 2 units per hour). About 10 ml of the fluid is permitted to run out of the needle in order to coat the tubing with insulin. A 5% glucose solution should be infused simultaneously to provide 100 gm of glucose per 24 hours until the patient is comfortable and stable. Glucose concentration is measured by Dextrostix or Chemstrip bG every 2 to 4 hours. The insulin dosage can easily be adjusted to more or fewer units per hour if needed.

Intramuscular insulin can be given at dosages of 5 or 10 units every 1 or 2 hours with glucose monitoring by fingersticks. When glucose levels reach a reasonable range (between 100 to 225 mg/dL [5.6 mmol/L to 12.5 mmol/L]) diabetic control can be achieved by giving supplemental regular insulin subcutaneously every 4 to 6 hours as indicated by glucose monitoring.

Virtually all type I patients should take at least two injections of insulin per day. A great deal of individual variation exists, so it might be necessary to use different types of insulin and times of injection. A popular regimen involves a mixture of intermediate-acting insulin (e.g., NPH or Lente) plus a quick-acting insulin (e.g., Semilente or regular) before breakfast and before dinner. Human insulin is preferred. The initial doses should be low and then gradually adjusted. For example, one can begin with 10 units of NPH plus 5 units of regular insulin in the morning and approximately half of that dose (5 units of NPH plus 2 or 3 units of regular insulin) before dinner. A common proportion of the mixture is two thirds and one third, respectively. Gradual increases can be made until the afternoon glucose level is in the normal range and the fasting level is satisfactory. The peak action of NPH occurs about 8 to 10 hours after injection. Once a glucose level of about 100 mg/dL is achieved in the afternoon, further increases in the NPH insulin might produce hypoglycemia. It is important to teach the patient to make 1- to 2-unit adjustments in insulin by home glucose monitoring before meals and at bedtime. The adjustments are based on when the insulin preparations begin to act and peak. A diabetic diet should aim for consistency in total calories and carbohydrate portions. The traditional diabetic diet with its exchanges is helpful when teaching the family and patient how to handle regular food intake. Adjustments must be made for a regular exercise program and in unusual circumstances such as stressful situations, infections, or injuries. More detailed discussion of diet and exercise can be found in the section on type II diabetes. Table 41–4 presents examples of the time of action of some commonly used insulin preparations.

For many years experts disagreed about the importance of good control of glucose levels. Recently, a multiple center study of type I diabetics supported by the National Institutes of Health, the Diabetes Control and Complications Trial (DCCT) reported its findings on the effect of glucose control on chronic complications. This well designed trial concluded that individuals who achieved normoglycemia by frequent glucose monitoring, extra

TABLE 41–4.   TIME COURSE OF ACTION OF COMMON INSULIN PREPARATIONS*

Insulin Preparation	Onset of Action	Peak Action (hr)	Duration of Action (hr)
Short-acting			
Regular Iletin II (crystalline zinc)	15–30 min	2–4	5–7
Novolin R	30 min	2.5–5.0	5–8
Humulin R	30 min	2–4	6–8
Intermediate-acting			
Lente	1–2 hr	6–12	18–24
NPH	1–2 hr	6–12	18–24
Novolin L	2.5–5.0 hr	7–15	18–24
Humulin N	1–3 hr	6–12	14–24
Novolin 70/30	30 min	7–12	24
Long-acting			
Ultralente (beef/ pork)	4–6 hr	14–24	28–36
Humulin U	4–6 hr	8–20	24–28

* Average values are given. Considerable variation is found in individual diabetic patients.

supplemental insulin injections, or continuous subcutaneous insulin infusions by insulin pumps had significantly fewer complications than those less well controlled. Retinopathy, neuropathy, and nephropathy were less frequent and severe in patients who were treated intensively rather than traditionally with one or two injections per day. Glycosylated hemoglobin determinations were useful for determining if euglycemia was achieved. Hypoglycemic reactions were more frequent in the closely controlled patients, but apparently severe problems did not arise (Reichard, 1993). That trial will surely result in new and stricter standards of diabetic control in the future. Consultation with experts is warranted when control is difficult in a type I diabetic person.

Acute Complications of Diabetes

Diabetic ketoacidosis is the most dramatic complication of insulin deficiency. Coma or diminution in mental status may result from ketoacidosis or other metabolic disturbances, such as hyperosmolar coma, lactic acidosis, or hypoglycemia. Coma or lethargy may be due to nondiabetic causes such as alcohol, head trauma, drug overdose, stroke, or other conditions that impair consciousness. Significant mortality still exists with diabetic ketoacidosis, often because of underlying precipitating causes such as stroke, infection, or myocardial infarction. Insulin deficiency results in impaired glucose transport to insulin-sensitive tissues. An osmotic diuresis occurs with loss of fluids and electrolytes. Simultaneously, insulin is no longer sufficient to inhibit the release of free fatty acids (FFAs) from fat stores, and FFAs become excessive. The liver fails to oxidize them completely, and products of incomplete oxidation accumulate. Acetoacetic acid and β-hydroxybutyric acid lower the pH, and acidosis occurs when buffering capacities are overwhelmed. Structural proteins break down, and glucogenic amino acids are converted to additional glucose by a liver lacking the inhibiting effect of insulin on gluconeogenesis.

The clinical manifestations of ketoacidosis are predictable. Dehydration is evident, as are rapid deep (Kussmal) respirations. A fruity odor due to ketones may be present. Nausea and gastric distention prevent adequate fluid or food intake. Weakness and mental confusion ensue. A tender abdomen and enlarged liver are not unusual. Table 41–5 summarizes the symptoms and signs encountered in patients presenting with diabetic ketoacidosis compared with those found in nonketotic hyperosmolar hyperglycemia.

The *diagnosis* should be confirmed quickly. The glucose level is usually over 250 mg/dL, and acetoacetate is positive in its reaction to sodium nitroprusside powder or a crushed Acetest tablet. If a

TABLE 41–5. PRESENTING FINDINGS IN DIABETIC KETOACIDOSIS COMPARED TO THOSE IN NONKETOTIC HYPEROSMOLAR COMA

Signs and Symptoms	Ketoacidosis	Hyperosmolar Coma
Dehydration	+ + + +	+ + + +
Stupor, coma, convulsions	±	+ + + +
Kussmaul breathing	Present	Absent
Glucose (mean)	475 mg/dL (26 mmol/L)	1166 mg/dL (65 mmol/L)
Osmolality	310	384
Ketosis	Present	Not present
Serum sodium	132 mEq/L	144 mEq/L
Acidosis	+ + + +	±

Based on data from Unger and Foster (1992) and Siperstein (1992), with permission.

strongly positive change is seen in serum diluted by an equal amount of saline, diabetic ketoacidosis is almost certain. The arterial blood pH confirms acidosis.

Treatment should be initiated as soon as the diagnosis is made. Underlying disease or other reasons for ketoacidosis must be clarified so potential life-threatening conditions can be addressed. Baseline glucose, bicarbonate, and electrolyte levels should be measured and then repeated at about 2-hour intervals initially. Continuous intravenous insulin administration at rates of about 5 units per hour is a reliable and convenient way to provide insulin. Another acceptable regimen is regular insulin 10 to 20 units injected intravenously, followed by insulin every 2 to 4 hours subcutaneously if the patient is not hypotensive. Normal saline is usually the first fluid given. One liter over about 2 hours is usually well tolerated; then fluid can be given at a rate of about 200 or 300 ml per hour for 12 to 24 hours or until volume appears to be replenished. Urine output is a helpful guide once excessive glucose levels begin to decrease. Hypotonic fluids such as 0.5 N saline can be used after the initial 2 liters of fluid. Sodium bicarbonate is recommended only if the initial arterial pH is below 7.0. Unless the ketoacidosis is severe and prolonged, the serum potassium level is elevated or normal despite total body depletion. Thus potassium supplements should be initiated after urinary output is certain, or if there is initial hypokalemia. One liter of 5% glucose containing 1000 mg of phosphate and 40 mEq of potassium is a good replacement solution a few hours after saline and insulin therapy have been instituted. There is no substitute for close observation and anticipation of problems.

Hypoglycemia is the other major and common acute complication of type I diabetes. Nearly every patient who requires insulin experiences hypoglycemia some time during the course of the disease. Rarely, hypoglycemia is sufficiently severe to

cause death or permanent neurologic abnormalities.

The clinical manifestations of hypoglycemia are explained either by the responses to counterregulatory hormones or the consequences of neuroglycopenia. When glucose falls to 40 to 50 mg/dL, epinephrine, growth hormone, glucagon, and cortisol are secreted to counter the hypoglycemia. Perspiration, tremors, hunger or nausea, tachycardia, pallor, and irritability occur, typical sympathetic nervous system effects. The central nervous tissue depends on oxygen and glucose to maintain the active metabolic processes of nerve cells. If glucose becomes too low or hypoglycemia is prolonged, symptoms of neuroglycopenia occur: headache, lethargy, confusion, bizarre behavior, blurred vision, and disorientation. Paralysis, coma, seizures, permanent neurologic impairment, and even death may result. The diagnosis is suggested by the characteristic symptoms and signs and is confirmed by fingerstick or venous blood glucose determination.

Therapy consists in ingesting rapidly absorbed food such as fruit juices, candy, or a packet of "instant glucose," which can be applied to the oral mucosa. Severe hypoglycemia is treated by infusing a solution of 25 gm of glucose or 10% dextrose in water. Insulin-dependent patients should have glucagon vials at home and a trained family member to mix and administer 1 mg intramuscularly in hypoglycemic emergencies.

Long-Term Complications

The chronic complications related to microvascular diseases (particularly retinopathy and nephropathy) and neuropathy remain major problems in the care of diabetic patients. Type I diabetics also are at high risk for developing atherosclerotic complications such as coronary disease or stroke. These complications occur with any form of diabetes, but they are more prevalent and somewhat more severe with type I diabetes. Hyperglycemia appears to be the common underlying metabolic abnormality that causes the development of microvascular complications. Patients with acquired diabetes due to chronic pancreatitis or hemochromatosis are vulnerable to these complications given a long enough bout of hyperglycemia. The microvascular lesions are not limited to the retina and glomerulus; they are noted in capillaries throughout the body as well. The exact mechanism of microvascular damage is unknown, but glycosylation of proteins and excessive use of certain metabolic pathways (e.g., sorbitol) have been implicated as damaging to certain tissues.

RETINOPATHY. The leading cause of blindness in the United States is diabetic retinopathy. It is rare to see retinopathy before puberty or until diabetes has been present for approximately 5 years. More than 90 per cent of people with type I diabetes have retinopathy after 20 years, and the cumula-

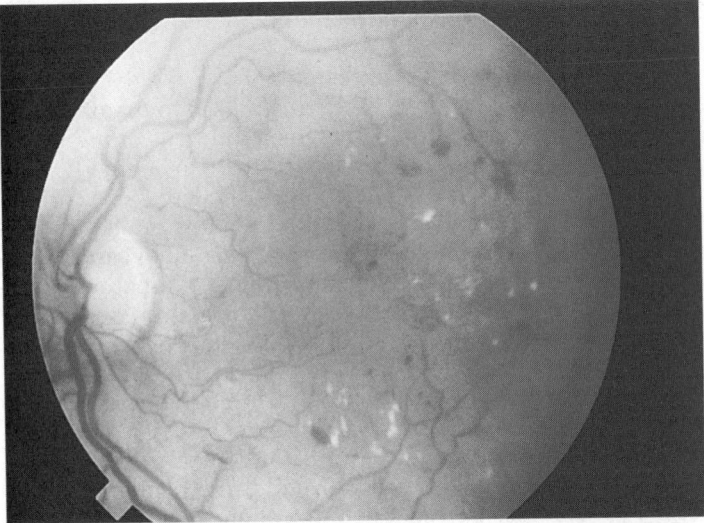

A

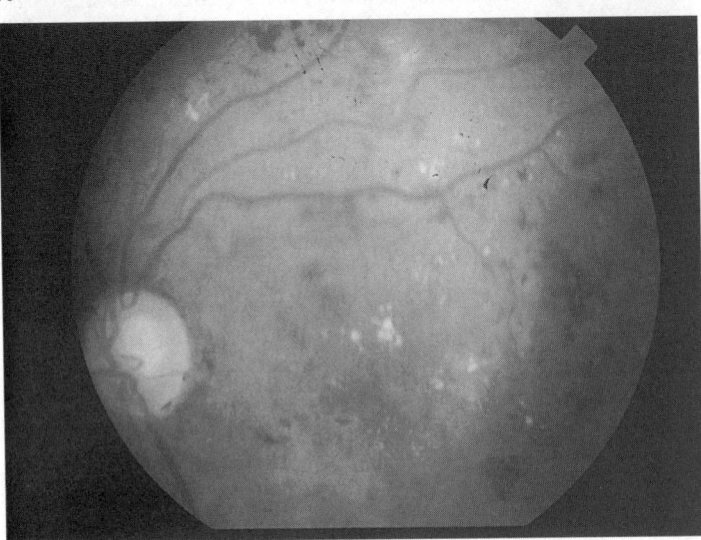

B

FIGURE 41–1. A, Background diabetic retinopathy. Scattered hard exudates, dot/blots, hemorrhages, and microaneurysms. B, Proliferative diabetic retinopathy. Note the extensive neovascularizations along vessels. (Courtesy of Dr. A. W. Fryczkowski, The Ohio State University.)

tive prevalence of blindness is 16 per cent among those followed for 40 years (Nathan, 1993). There are two types of diabetic retinopathy: background retinopathy and proliferative retinopathy. Background diabetic retinopathy occurs after 5 years and consists of microaneurysms, intraretinal dot hemorrhages, and serous fluid that leaks from abnormal retinal vessels (hard exudates). Cotton-wool exudates represent infarctions in the inner retinal layers. Proliferative retinopathy refers to new vessel formation in response to ischemia that extends from the retina into the vitreous cavity. These vessels are fragile, bleeding easily and promoting retinal detachment. Examples of background retinopathy and neovascularization are shown in Figure 41–1.

It is imperative that retinas of type I diabetics be examined by an ophthalmologist on an annual basis after about 4 years of diabetes, if new retinal changes are discovered, or if visual symptoms appear acutely. The therapy of choice for prolifera-

tive retinopathy or macular edema is xenon or argon laser treatment. This technique has dramatically altered the course of diabetic retinopathy since the 1970s. The Diabetic Control and Complication Trial convincingly showed that excellent control of glucose levels decreases the frequency and severity of eye complications of diabetes. Vitrectomy has been beneficial for severe retinopathy associated with hemorrhage, scarring, and retinal detachment. Treatment of hypertension may alleviate or slow the progression of the retinopathy.

NEPHROPATHY. Diabetic nephropathy is a much higher risk in type I than type II diabetes. Microalbuminuria, or loss of 30 to 300 mg of albumin per day, is an early sign of this complication. Hyperfiltration and intrarenal hypertension are key factors in the development of nephropathy. Hypertension accelerates the renal disease. Glomerular basement membrane thickening and increased mesangium are early histologic changes from which are formed typical nodular and intracapillary glomerulosclerosis among other changes. Proteinuria higher than 300 mg per day is noted about 15 years after the onset of type I diabetes in those in whom nephropathy occurs. Hypertension secondary to the nephropathy develops, as does the nephrotic syndrome. The glomerular filtration rate decreases, heralding end-stage renal disease.

A urinalysis should be done and a serum creatinine level determined yearly when following type I diabetics. Detection of microalbuminuria alerts the clinician that nephropathy is developing. Consultation should be requested when a patient's serum creatinine reaches about 3 mg/dL. A diabetologist and nephrologist should work with the family physician to delay the progression of renal failure and to prepare for dialysis or renal transplantation.

As with retinopathy, the DCCT showed that intensive therapy of diabetes can delay or improve diabetic nephropathy in its early stages. There is evidence that with good control of hypertension (Nathan, 1993) proteinuria can be reduced and the expected decline in the glomerular filtration rate can be slowed. Angiotensin-converting enzyme (ACE) inhibitors may be effective in decreasing urinary excretion of albumin even in normotensive diabetic patients (Mathiesen et al., 1991). Urinary infections should be treated quickly and obstruction of urine flow corrected. Furosemide or other loop diuretics are effective in renal failure, but large doses are sometimes needed. Dietary restriction of protein to 0.6 gm/kg of ideal body weight per day and of phosphorus to 500 to 1000 mg per day can retard the progression of renal failure in type I diabetics (Zeller et al., 1991). Insulin requirements change as renal failure progresses, and it is not unusual to see more frequent hypoglycemic reactions. The outlook for end-stage renal disease has improved greatly in recent years.

Renal transplantation has been highly beneficial to diabetics with renal failure. Combined pancreas/kidney transplantation is a dramatic example of the progress that has transpired in this field during a brief period. Pancreas transplantation is discussed separately. Renal transplantation effectively corrects end-stage renal disease for many years.

NEUROPATHY. Diabetic neuropathy is common in both type I and type II diabetics. It can occur early in diabetes or years after the onset of hyperglycemia. There is still disagreement regarding the pathogenesis of diabetic neuropathy. Proponents of the metabolic theory of damage to nerves argue that excessive glycosylation of nerve proteins, abnormal sorbitol metabolism, and myoinositol defects affecting the sodium pump and ATPase activity result in neuropathy. Others implicate neural ischemia through microvascular disease of the vasonervosum, particularly with mononeuropathies. It is likely that metabolic and microvascular factors interact to produce this common complication.

The most frequent clinical manifestation of diabetic neuropathy is peripheral, symmetric involvement of the sensory nerves. The earliest sign of diabetic neuropathy is loss of the ankle reflex. In fact, it is rare to have diabetic neuropathy if the ankle reflex is intact. A simple classification of the neuropathies in diabetes includes (1) peripheral polyneuropathy, (2) mononeuropathy, and (3) autonomic neuropathy.

The clinical symptoms of peripheral polyneuropathy are primarily sensory, but motor fibers are affected as well. Paresthesias—expressed as burning feet, tingling, and numbness—are characteristic manifestations. Infrequently, fairly severe pain is present, and anesthesia may develop in the affected area. Motor manifestations such as muscle atrophy, weakness, footdrop, and weakness of grasp may accompany advanced disease. The neuropathic foot is a serious consequence of this complication. Insensitivity to mild trauma or compressive shoes may result in a foot ulcer, most commonly on the plantar aspect of the distal metatarsal. These lesions are usually painless, making it important to teach the patient to look at the feet each day. Infected foot ulcers account for amputations in diabetics. Continuous trauma to an insensitive foot also produces structural changes in joints of the feet. The most common etiology of Charcot's joints is no longer syphilis but diabetes.

Mononeuropathy usually has a sudden onset and can involve a cranial nerve, the femoral nerve, or almost any other nerve in the body. The loss of both sensory and motor function is typical. There is evidence that this type of neuropathy is due to an ischemic episode of a segment of nerve. The prognosis for mononeuropathy is better than for polyneuropathy. Diabetic amyotrophy, a variant that involves more than one nerve, is characterized by muscle wasting and profound but reversible weakness.

Autonomic neuropathy can be extensive and a great burden to the patient. Impotence is a distressing manifestation in men, estimated to affect one half of all male diabetics over age 50. Retrograde ejaculation and hypotonicity of the bladder are other genitourinary manifestations of autonomic neuropathy. The gastrointestinal system is involved mainly by gastroparesis, which delays gastric emptying and complicates good control of the diabetes. Also, diabetic diarrhea may result in frequent stools, incontinence, or nocturnal symptoms. Autonomic neuropathy also affects the vascular and cardiac reflexes. Painless myocardial infarction is not uncommon in diabetics, nor are orthostatic hypotension and resting tachycardia.

The *diagnosis* of neuropathy is made by a careful history and neurologic examination. The absence of ankle reflexes is an early sign. Decreased vibratory sensation can be shown by examination with a manual or an electronic tuning fork. Confirmation is required in some cases by electrophysiologic studies of motor and sensory nerves. Barium swallow roentgenography is useful for diagnosing delayed gastric emptying. Penile plethysmography is valuable for differentiating diabetic impotence from that due to psychological causes. Sometimes angiography is necessary to rule out ischemic or vascular causes of impotence.

Therapy of the neuropathies is limited and discouraging. Strict control of hyperglycemia had been shown by the DCCT to improve neuropathies. However, most treatments are directed to the alleviation of symptoms. Fortunately, painful neuropathies frequently subside spontaneously with time. Mild analgesics can be used, and the peripheral neuropathies might respond to a topical application of capsaicin ointment. Some individuals are relieved with amitriptyline (Elavil) 25 or 50 mg at bedtime. Metoclopramide (Reglan) is helpful for gastric paresis. Antibiotics and cholestyramine (Questran) relieve diabetic diarrhea. Various devices are available for impotence, for example a hydraulic implantable penile pump that transfers fluid from a reservoir to inflatable chambers in the corpora. Urologic consultation is necessary to help with this problem. Penile injections with papaverine by the patient have been successful in some. Severe orthostatic hypotension can be alleviated by support hose and fludrocortisone (Florinef) 0.1 mg per day. Prevention of, or more accurately retarding the progression of, neuropathy is certainly preferable, and this goal is possible to some degree with good control (Reichard et al., 1993).

DIABETIC DERMOPATHY. Commonly, "shin spots" are seen in type I diabetics; they are atrophic scars on the anterior part of the lower extremities that have resulted from slow healing of common trauma. Necrobiosis lipoidica diabeticorum is a lesion that is more extensive, ulcerating, and necrotic, occurring more commonly in female type I diabetics. The involved area has an atrophic erythematous appearance with yellowish exudate, ulceration, and scarring. The lesion should be kept clean with warm soapy washings, and neomycin-corticosteroid cream can be applied with occlusive dressings. Type I diabetics also have cutaneous symptoms related to moniliasis, furuncles, and eruptive xanthomas secondary to hypertriglyceridemia. Nystatin is prescribed for fungal infections including vaginitis, and bacterial infections are treated with local cleansing and topical or systemic antibiotics.

Diabetes as a Surgical Disease

Pancreatic transplantation is a dramatic example of of new advances in treating diabetes. It is gratifying to witness an insulin-dependent patient—who for years has had to inject insulin daily, carefully monitor food intake, and worry about hypoglycemic reactions—awaken from a pancreatic transplant procedure and be free of the need for insulin. From its innovation in 1966 until the past few years, the results of pancreatic transplantation were poor, and only a few institutions in the world were doing them. In 1992 approximately 50 combined pancreas–kidney transplantations were performed at The Ohio State University Medical Center. A single cadaver donor provides both a pancreas and kidney to the recipient. The procedure utilizes the entire pancreas with renal drainage to the bladder and is usually completed within 5 to 6 hours. The average hospital stay is about 2 weeks.

Pancreatic transplantation can restore glucose metabolism to normal. Some patients with successful transplants have even experienced hypoglycemic reactions. The harvested organs are transplanted within approximately 12 hours. The recipient's pancreas is left intact. The entire cadaveric pancreas is placed in the iliac fossa and revascularized using iliac vessels. The exocrine drainage is directed into the urinary bladder. The use of cyclosporin and urinary exteriorized drainage (instead of the enteric drainage used previously) revolutionized this procedure. One-year patient survival and pancreatic graft functional rates approximate 90 and 70 per cent, respectively. Hyperinsulinemia is present and due to direct systemic venous drainage from the transplanted pancreas rather than the insulin entering directly into the liver via the portal veins as is the case under normal circumstances. Rejection is signaled by a decrease in urinary amylase concentration and a blunting of the acute, or first, phase of insulin release. Improved techniques and modern laboratory capabilities have enhanced the safety and efficacy of such procedures in high-risk diabetics.

Non-Insulin-Dependent Diabetes Mellitus

Epidemiology

Non-insulin-dependent diabetes mellitus (NIDDM, type II diabetes mellitus, nonautoimmune diabetes mellitus) does not usually lead to diabetic ketoacidosis. It is associated with insulin resistance and is treatable by diet and oral hypoglycemic agents. Some patients are placed on insulin to control the hyperglycemia. The proximate cause of the hyperglycemia is the *ineffectiveness of insulin* and delayed secretion from islet cells as contrasted with the paucity (or absence) of insulin found in type I diabetes. In fact, it is characteristic early during the course of the disease and with far-reaching consequences to have hyperinsulinemia in combination with insulin resistance, resulting in a constellation of clinical manifestations known as syndrome X.

Depending on the source, its prevalence in the United States is 2.7 to 4.4 per cent. According to the Framingham Study, the incidence of type II diabetes in the 40- to 49-year decade is 230 per

100,000, increasing with age to 939 per 100,000 by the 70- to 79-year decade. It has a strong genetic basis, with obesity being a precipitating factor. It varies across races, having a prevalence of about 1 to 2 per cent in white (European) peoples and 1 per cent in the Japanese. It is twice as prevalent among black Americans as among white Americans. Pima Indians (aboriginal Americans) of Arizona show a prevalence of 40 per cent or more and Micronesians of Nauru 34 per cent. Other racial predispositions include Black African, Polynesian, Melanesian, and Mexican American. In this respect it contrasts with type I diabetes, which is found in higher incidence and prevalences in northern Europeans.

More than 80 per cent of type II diabetics are obese at the time of diagnosis, and more than two thirds are over the age of 40 (Tzagournis and Skillman, 1989). The incidence is increased by a factor of 2.3 in obese individuals when obesity is defined as 120 per cent of ideal weight. Some type II patients may be in a transient phase of type I, exhibiting hypoinsulinemia and a thin habitus, manageable for the time being without insulin. Whereas the type I diabetic apparently requires an external assault in addition to an inherited susceptibility (only 50 per cent concordance in twins), type II displays nearly 100 per cent concordance in twin studies. About 38 per cent of offspring and 33 per cent of siblings of individuals with type II diabetes demonstrate degrees of glucose intolerance, in sharp contrast to those with type I diabetes in whom only 4 per cent of parents and 6 per cent of siblings of diabetics develop diabetes.

Type II diabetes mellitus manifests all the complications of IDDM associated with hyperglycemia but at a lower risk ratio and after a longer duration of disease. They include the sequelae of microangiopathy (retinopathy, nephropathy), neuropathy, and cataracts as well as the manifestations of macroangiopathy: coronary artery, cerebrovascular, and peripheral vascular disease. This picture can be deceiving to the primary care physician, who may associate such complications with IDDM. However, the odds of a case of diabetic glomerulopathy being found in one's practice do not particularly favor type I diabetes over type II. Although a patient with type I diabetes faces a 40 per cent chance of developing diabetic glomerulopathy and type II patient only a 5 to 10 per cent risk, the prevalence of type II in the U.S. population is about 11 million versus about 2 million for type I. Thus there are roughly equal chances of glomerulopathy in patients presenting in the health care system.

Clinical Manifestations

Type II diabetes exhibits classically the same triad of polyuria, polydipsia, and polyphagia as does IDDM. However, most of the time it is much less dramatic, presenting with symptoms and signs of infections common to chronic hyperglycemia, an increased incidence of urinary tract infections and candidiasis, vaginitis in female NIDDM diabetics, and infections in the intertriginous areas in both sexes (under the breasts, between folds of redundant skin in the obese, crural zones). Because NIDDM patients seldom present with urgent symptoms of their diabetes, it is important to be alert to subtle and insidious findings of neuropathy, nephropathy, and retinopathy of which the patient is unaware.

Nonautoimmune Diabetes and Syndrome X (Insulin Resistance Syndrome)

Type II diabetes is known to the practitioner as much for its vascular complications as for the hyperglycemia and direct sequelae thereof. Syndrome X is the name given to the constellation of conditions that includes adult-onset nonautoimmune diabetes mellitus as the central focus. In the face of insulin resistance, insulin levels rise owing to a compensatory response. Insulin's other actions may lead to "essential" hypertension, coronary artery disease, or cerebrovascular disease before or even in the absence of the onset of hyperglycemia (Karam, 1992). These sequelae account for most of the associations of type II diabetes and other atherosclerotic risk factors and for the independent atherosclerotic risk status of diabetes mellitus.

Even normally glucose-tolerant people who are hyperinsulinemic have higher blood pressures, higher triglyceride levels, and lower high density lipoprotein (HDL) cholesterol levels than do those without hyperinsulinemia. Many are obese, aggravating or precipitating insulin resistance.

Glucagon, produced in the alpha cells of the islets of Langerhans, normally rises in response to insulin and counteracts hypoglycemia. The effect of insulin on glucagon is not blunted in the insulin resistance syndrome. Thus hyperinsulinemia causes increases in levels of glucagon.

The proliferative effects of insulin are detrimental to cells in the intima and arterial media. Insulin has a direct proliferative effect on the vascular intima, which abets the atherosclerotic occlusive process.

Type II diabetic persons have a prevalence of *hypertension* of almost 50 per cent, compared to 15 to 20 per cent for the entire U.S. population, and those with hypertension have a prevalence of glucose intolerance of 15 to 18 per cent (Kannel et al., 1991) compared to about 4.4 per cent of the U.S. population. Most hypertensives, particularly the obese, exhibit insulin resistance and hyperinsulinemia. Reduction of insulin levels in obese diabetics results in a reduction of blood pressure in a significant proportion of patients (DeFronzo and Ferrannini, 1991; Reaven, 1991). Whereas the risk of atherosclerosis increases with increasing blood pressure levels, the presence of diabetes increases the risk by a factor of 1.2 to 1.5 times that of hypertension alone.

The effect of insulin on blood pressure may be explained by its ability to increase renal tubular reabsorption of sodium (volume enhancement) and directly stimulate sympathetic activity (increasing peripheral resistance). Most prospective studies of hypertension treatment fail to show a reduction in coronary heart disease events after lowering the blood pressure, although clearly reducing the number of cerebrovascular events. Some postulate that failure to remediate underlying hyperinsulemia may be an important factor in explaining these findings. Hyperinsulinemic normotensive patients have higher mean pressures than those with normal insulin levels.

Hyperinsulinemia contributes to *dyslipidemia* by promoting increased hepatic production of very low density lipoprotein (VLDL) and hence triglyceride. The metabolic "delipidation" of VLDL results in an increase in circulating low density lipoprotein (LDL) and a decrease in HDL cholesterol.

Obesity, particularly of the truncal type, is associated with insulin resistance. Obesity-related insulin resistance is not infrequently accompanied by hyperglycemia and a decrease in insulin receptors on peripheral tissues. Insulin resistance occurs in direct and dynamic relation to the blood glucose level, abating as blood glucose control is effected, whether by diet, sulfonylurea treatment, or insulin therapy.

Effects of Stress

The role of stress in the control of NIDDM has been appreciated anecdotally by family physicians and their patients for years. Patients have explained lapses in blood glucose control on the basis of emotional stress and tension. Hyperglycemia is aggravated by release of glucocorticoids and by sympathetic discharge during the stress response. Catecholamines, engendered by hyperinsulinemia and by stress, result in impairment of pancreatic beta cells, which results in further hyperglycemia and further desensitization of beta cells. Sympathetic stimulation also results in activation of the renin-angiotensin system, further raising blood pressure. Depending on a person's patterns of eating or not eating in response to emotional stress, compliance with the diet may suffer because of stress.

Diagnosis

The diagnosis is made by finding a fasting blood glucose (FBS) level higher than 140 mg/dL (7.8 mmol/L) on two determinations, a random blood glucose (RBS) level over 200 mg/dL (11.1 mmol/L), or an RBS level over 200 mg/dL at any point after a standard glucose tolerance load (75 gm) and classic symptoms. Once diagnosed, education, instruction, and spurring of motivation must begin. This phase must not be put off, lest the patient be lulled by a perceived benign attitude on the part of the physician.

Management and Follow-up

The complications of diabetes type II are aggravated, if not caused, by hyperglycemia. Therefore home blood glucose monitoring is taught and put into operation immediately. The patient should determine blood glucose levels four times per day for the first several weeks. The best schedule is before meals and at bedtime. After stabilization, most type II patients who are not on insulin and their doctors are content to monitor twice per day (in the morning and before the evening meal).

Urine glucose monitoring is not as accurate for obvious reasons of the varying renal threshold, leading to mistaken impressions of blood glucose levels. In addition, if the mean renal threshold is around 180 mg/dL, a negative urine glucose test does not reveal how far under the threshold is the glucose level. Maintenance under 150 mg/dL is the ideal.

Figure 41–2 plots a stepwise therapeutic approach to the initial and follow-up management of type II diabetes. After the initial examination and orientation of the patient, the patient's measurable atherosclerosis risk factors are ascertained and discussed. The weight loss that is usually indicated in the treatment of diabetes type II is also beneficial for control of hypertension, hypercholesterolemia, and reduced HDL cholesterol. Salt restriction to 4 gm/24 hr (2 gm sodium) is invoked if hypertension is present. Cholesterol content of the diet and optimization of dietary saturated fatty acid content is controlled if these lipids are abnormal. Elevation of the triglyceride level is a prominent finding in syndrome X, and it may be further elevated as a result of hyperglycemia. In the case of triglycerides, simple weight loss is beneficial in correcting them.

If the FBS is less than 200 mg/dL (11.1 mmol/L), the patient is placed on a diabetic diet without medication, plus exercise. If after 2 to 3 months the FBS is still greater than 150 mg/dL (8.3 mmol/L), an oral hypoglycemic agent (OHA) is added. To take the latter step in the absence of weight loss or convincing evidence of compliance is to admit defeat.

If the baseline FBS is higher than 200 mg/dL (11.1 mmol/L), diet and exercise may need to be supplemented with insulin at least temporarily. Then an OHA is added as insulin is withdrawn on trial. In general, FBS levels in excess of 300 mg/dL (16.7 mmol/L) do not respond to OHAs. Conversely, most patients with FBS levels less than 250 mg/dL (14 mmol/L) exhibit at least partial responsiveness, and most respond to OHAs if the FBS is 200 mg/dL (14 mmol/L) or less. Overall, about 85 per cent of type II diabetics respond to OHAs initially, but 25 per cent fail secondarily. Secondary failures may be only temporary and are

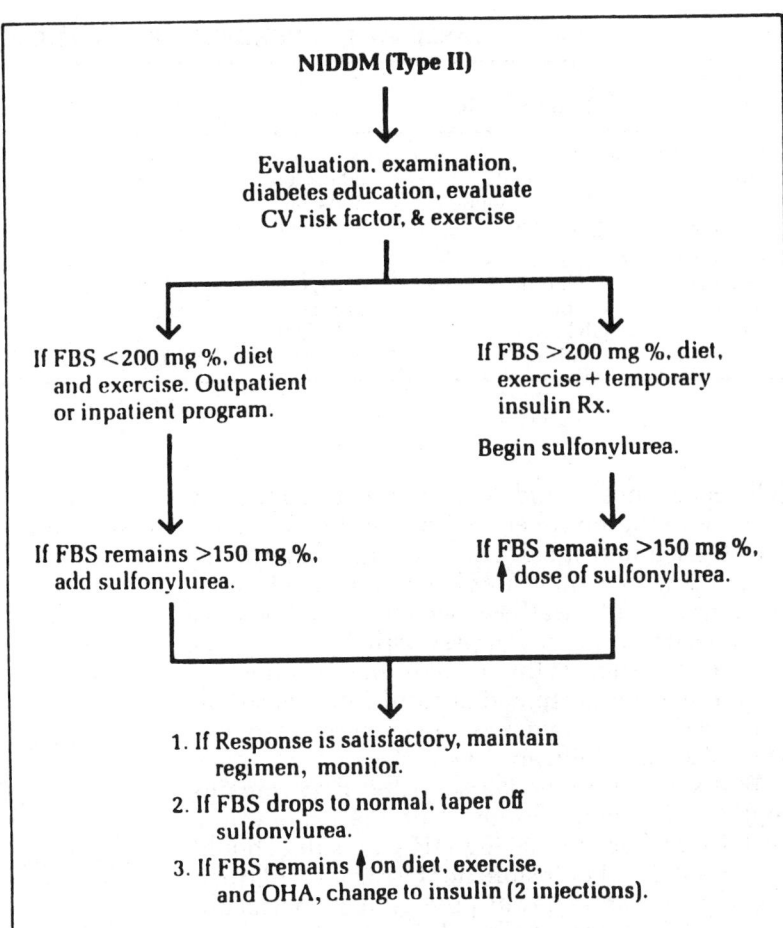

FIGURE 41-2. Algorithm for management of type II diabetes mellitus.

due to infection, surgery, or other acute stress. If after 2 to 3 months the FBS is still higher than 150 mg/dL (8.3 mmol/L) but less than 200 mg/dL (11.1 mmol/L), the OHA is increased.

FREQUENCY AND CONTENT OF FOLLOW-UP VISITS. If the FBS falls below 150 mg/dL (8.3 mmol/L), the patient should continue to be monitored by home blood glucose tests at least twice a day for the foreseeable future and to be seen by the physician monthly to quarterly. Visits should include a minimum of interval history; blood pressure determination; examination of the eyes, heart, lung fields, peripheral pulses, and Achilles tendon reflex; inspection of the feet; and minimal laboratory determinations. The FBS (or 2-hour postprandial blood glucose level), weight, and glycosylated hemoglobin should be determined. Hemoglobin A_{1C} values vary among laboratories but should be close to normal.

If the FBS falls to normal over several months, monitoring is maintained while the OHA is tapered off. The diet and exercise regimen must continue. If this program is successful the patient has probably complied with the diet and exercise program, and if the patient was obese (80 per cent of patients) he or she has almost certainly lost weight. One of the challenges to the physician is to con-

vince the patient that the diabetes is not "cured"—that a return to the former lifestyle will assuredly bring a return of the disease.

CHOOSING AN ORAL HYPOGLYCEMIC AGENT. Table 41–6 lists the OHAs in use in the United States; they presently comprise only sulfonylureas. They act by stimulating the beta cells and increasing insulin receptors; some of the second generation agents may cause a decrease in glycogenolysis as well. The main difference of clinical interest between the first generation (tolbutamide, chlorpropamide, acetohexamide, tolazamide) and second generation (glyburide, glipizide, glibornuride) sulfonyl ureas is potency on a milligram by milligram basis. In addition, the second generation group may be taken on a once-per-day schedule.

The biguanides are currently receiving attention in the United States. The only drug of that category in the United States had been phenformin, which was removed from the U.S. market because of the risk of lactic acidosis. However, metformin has undergone U.S. trials and has also been found to be effective in other parts of the world. Encouraging for its implications for syndrome X, its action is not on the beta islet cells; hence it does not aggravate hyperinsulinemia. It functions to reduce intestinal absorption and hepatic glucose output

TABLE 41–6. APPROVED ORAL ANTIDIABETES AGENTS

Trade Name	Generic Name	Dosage (mg)	Unit Size	Doses/Day	Relative Potency (mg)	Duration (hr)
First generation agents						
Orinase	Tolbutamide	500–3000	500	2 or 3	1000	6–12
Diabinese	Chlorpropamide	100–500	100, 250	1	250	36–72
Tolinase	Tolazamide	100–1000	100, 250, 500	1 or 2	250	12–24
Second generation agents						
Diabeta	Glyburide	1.25–20	1.25, 2.5, 5.0	1 or 2	5	24
Micronase	Glyburide	1.25–20	1.25, 2.5, 5.0	1 or 2	5	24
Glynase	Glyburide	0.75–12.0	1.5, 3.0	1 or 2	5	24
Glucotrol	Glipizide	2.5–40.0	5, 10	1 or 2	10	12–24

(gluconeogenesis) and to increase utilization of glucose in the peripheral tissues. Side effects are mostly gastrointestinal. There are new experimental drugs with actions unrelated to beta cell function, for example acarbose, which slows digestion of disaccharides and complex carbohydrates. Recent studies suggest this agent is directly effective in limiting the postprandial insulin response engendered by sulfonylureas and even the response after placebo (Hoffman, 1994).

WHEN TO START INSULIN. If the FBS remains high (> 200 mg/dL fasting) with the patient on a diet, exercising, and taking OHAs, insulin should be started. Neither insulin nor OHAs is ideal treatment. Each may aggravate preexisting hyperinsulinemia. Often the threat of insulin "shots" is enough to inspire the patient to new heights of compliance.

Once started, insulin should be given as twice-daily doses. As an initial trial, two thirds of the daily requirement can be given in the morning and one third in the afternoon.

For most type II patients, a surrender to insulin is usually a surrender to noncompliance. For consideration of discontinuing insulin in order to try OHAs or, better, diet and exercise, the following criteria portend success: duration of diabetes less than 5 years, present dosage of insulin less than 40 units, age 40 years or more, and FBS level less than 200 mg/dL.

DIET. Details of the diabetic diet are contained in Chapter 42. Briefly, there are certain principles that are helpful to keep in mind. First, the ideal diet is virtually the same for type I as for type II, though lapses from the diet generally carry fewer consequences for type II diabetics in the short run. Second, for hour to hour control, restriction of free glucose and other simple carbohydrates is perhaps more critical than for complex carbohydrates. However, day to day control is more related to daily calories. Third, in most type II diabetics, calorie and fat control translate into weight loss, which improves glycemic control in the obese type II diabetic. In fact, many patients' diabetes disappear after as little as a 10 per cent weight loss, even in those who were as much as 30 per cent overweight at the time of diagnosis.

The following guidelines allow rapid initial estimates of proteins, fats, and carbohydrate requirements based on ideal weight estimation in diabetes.

1. Ideal weight is estimated by the patient's height and sex: For females, it is 100 lb for 60 inches and 5 lb for every inch over 60 inches (5 feet). Ten per cent may be added or subtracted for frame. For males, it is 106 lb for 60 inches and 6 lb for every inch over 60 inches (5 feet). Ten per cent may be added or subtracted for frame.

2. A preliminary estimate of *caloric needs* may be based on the ideal weight in pounds multiplied by 10. For example, a man who is 5 ft 11 in should weigh 172 lb, and his estimated caloric requirement is 1720 calories. Caloric requirements may be increased by 15 to 20 per cent for the physical laborer or competitive athlete. Medical applications of diets are discussed in terms of *proportions of calories*, before being translated into weight. For example, the American Heart Association recommends that fat content be limited to 30 per cent of calories supplied, not weight.

3. *Carbohydrates* should supply 50 to 60 per cent of this requirement, or 946 calories. At 4 calories per gram, this amount is 237 gm of CHO. Free sugars influence blood glucose out of proportion to the calorie content. In practice, up to 25 per cent of CHO calories may be in mono- and disaccharides, preferably from fruits and vegetables. The remainder are in the form of complex carbohydrates.

4. *Protein* content of the diet is prescribed at about 15 per cent of daily calories ingested. For this hypothetical patient the calorie allowance is 258. At 4 calories/gm these calories are supplied by 64.5 gm. About 25 per cent of protein must be "complete" or "adequate" (i.e., supplying all the essential amino acids). Patients with renal disease can be maintained in nitrogen balance on as little as 0.25 to 0.35 gm per pound of ideal weight.

5. The *fat* content of the diet is 30 per cent of calories. For the 172 lb patient with caloric needs

of 1720, it is 516 cal ÷ 8 kcal/gm = 64.5 gm. The quality of fatty acids ideally is one third each of saturated, monounsaturated, and polyunsaturated fat.

FIBER. Research has shown an ameliorating effect on the severity of hyperglycemia of increased fiber in the diet; it is associated with reduced insulin and OHA requirements. The greatest therapeutic effects apparently come with amounts near 70 gm per day, far in excess of the average daily American diet, which contains 10 to 15 gm per day. To maintain even the latter amount requires more than one bowl of a high bran cereal and several fruit exchanges from among high fiber-containing fruits.

EXERCISE. In type I diabetes, exercise is a factor to consider when estimating insulin requirements and a cause for closer follow-up and frequent adjustments of insulin dosage. *For type II diabetes exercise is an essential part of therapy.* Because it potentiates insulin, exercise has an alleviating effect on hyperinsulinemia with all the redeeming effects on syndrome X (reduction of blood pressure, reductions of total and LDL cholesterol, and elevation of HDL cholesterol) in addition to lowering hyperglycemia. Patients should be told that exercise may be life-saving, adding years through prevention of coronary artery disease, strokes, and peripheral vascular disease as well as mitigating the complications of neuropathy, nephropathy, and retinopathy. Table 41–7 shows calories burned for various levels of exercise at three divergent weights.

Patients who have not been recently athletic are the rule and an ECG stress test would not be unreasonable in this moderately high-risk group. According to the Framingham Study tables, diabetes in men and women confers risk of coronary disease equal to 5 years additional age by the age of 45. They should be instructed to begin exercise modestly, in stepwise fashion.

1. Walk one-half mile daily the first week, one mile the second week, and two miles the third week; then the distances depend on the time available.

2. The value of exercise in calories burned is placed in perspective: about 100 calories per mile on foot, regardless of the pace, whether running or walking, for a 150 kg person, adjusted upward or downward for weight above or below 150 kg. This may be refined as follows: calories burned per unit time are increased in proportion as average heart rate during exercise is related to average heart rate while walking for the same amount of time. For example, if one burns 100 calories while walking one mile in 20 minutes with an average pulse rate of 82, then if one exercises for 20 minutes with an average pulse rate of 123, then he/she burns 100 × 123/82 = 150 calories in that amount of time, regardless of the distance covered.

TABLE 41–7. REPRESENTATIVE CALORIES BURNED PER HOUR FOR WEIGHTS AND ACTIVITIES

Exercise	Calories Burned per Hour, by Subject's Weight		
	110 lb	154 lb	198 lb
Martial arts	620	790	960
Racquetball (two people)	610	775	945
Basketball (full-court game)	585	750	910
Skiing			
Cross country (5 mph)	550	700	850
Downhill	465	595	720
Running			
8 Minute mile	550	700	850
12 Minute mile	515	655	795
Swimming			
Crawl, 45 yards/min	540	690	835
Crawl, 30 yards/min	330	420	510
Stationary bicycle, 15 mph	515	655	795
Aerobic dancing			
Intense	515	655	795
Moderate	350	445	540
Walking			
5 mph	435	555	675
3 mph	235	300	365
2 mph	145	185	225
Calisthenics			
Intense	435	555	675
Moderate	350	445	540
Scuba diving	355	450	550
Hiking			
20 lb pack, 4 mph	355	450	550
20 lb pack, 2 mph	235	300	365
Tennis			
Singles, recreational	335	425	520
Doubles, recreational	235	300	365
Ice skating	275	350	425
Roller skating	275	350	425

From *Prevention's Giant Book of Health Facts,* Emmaus, PA, p. 567, with permission. Copyright 1991 Rodale Pres, Inc.

3. Jogging would be good as aerobic exercise and has a definite beneficial effect on total cholesterol and HDL cholesterol.

Management of Nonglycemic Complications

The pathophysiology of the sequelae of syndrome X (degenerative complications) has been discussed. These sequelae are hypertension, dyslipidemia (elevated total cholesterol, elevated LDL), unfavorably low levels of HDL, and their sequelae: coronary artery disease, cerebrovascular disease, and peripheral vascular disease.

Essential hypertension and elevated blood pressure secondary to nephropathy are common in type II diabetes. There is evidence to suggest that *low renin hypertension* is usual in diabetes type II, a state shared by 30 to 35 per cent of persons with essential hypertension. Although a good response to diuretics would be expected, thiazides have a tendency to aggravate hypertriglyceridemia, lower HDL, and raise LDL cholesterol (MRFIT Research Group, 1982); the same aberrations are found in syndrome X.

Pharmacologic issues in diabetic patients should be considered. Thiazide diuretics elevate blood glucose and triglycerides and precipitate frank diabetes. β-Adrenergic blockers aggravate cholesterol dyslipidemia and may cause hyperglycemia. They also blunt the gluconeogenic response to hypoglycemia and may mask the symptoms of hypoglycemia, depriving insulin-dependent diabetics of important protection.

α-Adrenergic blocking agents have no known effect on carbohydrate metabolism and may have a slightly beneficial effect on serum lipids. ACE inhibitors have no adverse effect on carbohydrate metabolism and may improve glucose tolerance. ACE inhibitors seem to decrease proteinuria in diabetic glomerulosclerosis. However, because syndrome X hypertension tends to be a low renin hypertension, ACE inhibitors may be of limited value alone in blood pressure control. In practice, calcium channel blocking agents, ACE inhibitors, and α-adrenergic blockers are reasonable first-step drugs for type II diabetes.

The *dyslipidemia* of type II diabetes and syndrome X is commonly seen in private practice. Mild to moderate elevations of triglycerides, total cholesterol, and LDL cholesterol and suboptimal HDL cholesterol are frequently seen together. Obviously, that combination adds to the atherosclerosis risk status of the diabetic. The best approach, assuming the patient is overweight, is diet for weight loss and correction of insulin resistance. A diabetic diet with calories estimated at a deficit until ideal weight is attained is appropriate for correction of the lipid abnormalities as well. If the patient fails to adhere over time despite adequate insistence by the doctor, medication may be used. Acceptable choices in the diabetic are probucol (Lorelco) and lovastatin (Mevacor). If hypertriglyceridemia is not a significant problem, cholestyramine (Cholybar) and colestipol (Colestid) may be used.

Preventive care and heightened alertness to *coronary artery disease* (CAD) must be practiced in diabetics. Established CAD is diagnosed, treated, and followed the same in diabetics as in nondiabetics. The doctor must be alert to the increased incidence of silent myocardial infarction in diabetics, a matter relevant during the preoperative evaluation and long-term follow-up.

The same is said for *cerebrovascular disease*, keeping in mind that the most powerful risk factor for strokes is hypertension. Special attention is paid to the carotid pulses at the times of follow-up. *Peripheral vascular disease* is present in many diabetics. Amputations are five times as frequent in diabetics as in nondiabetics. A careful history looking for claudication, palpation of pulses, and inspection of the skin are mandatory in type II as well as type I cases.

Glycemic Complications

IMMEDIATE COMPLICATIONS. The symptoms of hyperglycemia are polyuria, polydipsia, and polyphagia, though polyphagia is unusual in type II diabetes. Blurred vision is a prominent symptom due to the refractive error caused by hyperglycemia. Correction of the hyperglycemia results in abeyance of these symptoms.

Increased susceptibility to infections, *Candida* in particular, is a manifestation of hyperglycemia. Candidiasis is evident in such areas as the vagina, under pendulous breasts, under uncircumcised foreskins, between heavy thighs, and sometimes in the mouth.

NONKETOTIC HYPEROSMOLAR HYPERGLYCEMIA. A manifestation of decompensation in type II diabetes is hyperosmolar hyperglycemia, which can lead to hyperosmolar nonketotic coma. Ordinarily, hepatic production of glucose via glycogenolysis and gluconeogenesis results in a maximum plateau of 300 to 500 mg/dL (17–28 mmol/L). Decreased renal excretion and decreased tissue utilization result in glucose entry into the extracellular space at a rate that exceeds removal, and the blood glucose level then rises above 500 mg/dL. The condition is more likely to occur when an increase in the insulin requirements (as during acute infections) combines with decreased oral intake of fluids and compromised renal function. It is found in sick older type II diabetics but occurs at times with type I diabetics as well (diabetic ketoacidosis [DKA] and nonketotic hyperosmolar hyperglycemia [NKHH] may coexist). The result is a cycle of increasing dehydration, rising osmolality, and decreasing ability to excrete glucose through the kidneys. Hyperosmolar hyperglycemia may coexist with DKA, but when this association occurs the coma is nearly always due to the hyperosmolar hyperglycemia. Siperstein (1992) stated that DKA itself does not cause coma, and that there is little or no relation between the level of mental function and pH.

As many as one half of type II cases are previously undiagnosed before presenting with NKHH. The NKHH may have been precipitated by a medication that decreases glucose tolerance, such as thiazide diuretics, glucocorticoids, phenytoin, furosemide, and cimetidine. Other patients, regardless of whether they are known diabetics, present with the clinical picture of a serious acute condition that has precipated hyperglycemia, such as stroke or myocardial infarction. Other precipitating conditions include pneumonitis, heat stroke, burns, pancreatitis, and urinary sepsis. The possibility of stroke, head injury, or brain tumor should be investigated if no other precipitating cause is apparent. Hypokalemia aggravates insulin resistance and inhibits secretion of insulin, so it may be a contributing precipitant of NKHH.

The pathogenesis of NKHH begins with an insufficiency of *effective* insulin, resulting in increased liver production of glucose. The increased blood glucose cannot be utilized normally by cells, resulting in rising glycemia and osmolality. An osmotic diuresis results in excessive water loss. The body reaches a state of sodium and potassium deficiency, although serum concentrations may be normal or high. The response of the central nervous system (CNS) to this state is obtundation and lowered seizure threshold.

Polydipsia may be conspicuously absent in an older patient, and lack of appropriate thirst contributes to the cycle of dehydration. If the patient is in coma, the chances are high that the hyperosmolar state is present with or without DKA. For NKHH to account for coma, the serum osmolality ordinarily exceeds 340 mOsm/L, or a blood glucose of about 800 mg/dL (44 mmol/L). Obtundation and convulsions are caused by the hyperosmolar state; Kussmaul breathing and a pH below 7.2 may be due to DKA or lactic acidosis. Neither DKA nor hyperosmolar hyperglycemia cause fever, so its presence demands a search for the cause. Table 41–5 illustrates the laboratory findings of NKHH compared with those in diabetic ketoacidosis. The prominent laboratory finding is the blood glucose level, which can reach incredibly high levels, up to 4000 mg/dL (222 mmol/L).

Treatment. After the diagnosis is made, a precipitating cause is sought even as aggressive corrective therapy begins. Careful cardiorespiratory and neurologic histories are obtained, along with probing for focal and constitutional symptoms of sepsis and other infectious disease. If a precipitating cause is not readily apparent, computed tomography (CT) or magnetic resonance imaging (MRI) of the head is often indicated, especially if the sensorium fails to clear as the hyperosmolality recedes. Antibiotic therapy should be started on any patient with fever while blood, urine, and other cultures are incubating, looking especially for gram-negative organisms.

Coma and death are caused by hyperosmolality and dehydration. Although insulin is a prerequisite of management for lowering the blood glucose, intravenous fluid therapy is the mainstay. There are two reasons for the reticence of physicians to be aggressive with fluid therapy: fear of congestive heart failure and fear of cerebral edema. Congestive heart failure is not common in the absence of severe acidosis. Cerebral edema is a complication of treatment of DKA (< 1 per cent risk) and is unusual in hyperosmolar coma. The cause of this feared complication was once thought to be over-aggressive correction of blood glucose or rapid rehydration, but the incidence correlates with neither of these factors (Rosenbloom, 1990).

Adequate fluid replacement is considered to be one half of the water deficit during the first 5 hours. The average deficit is 10 per cent of the total body weight. Assessing the weight in kilograms allows quick conversion to liters. The 60 kg person would require 6 L, the 80 kg person 8 L, and so on, half of the deficit to be repleted during the first 5 hours. In the case of a 60 kg woman the rate would be 6 × ½ × ⅕ = 0.6 liter per hour for the first 5 hours. Normal saline is recommended if the patient is hypotensive or the sodium is less than 140 mmol/L; otherwise 0.5 N saline is recommended. The solution can be changed from normal saline to 0.5 N saline as blood pressure recovers, assuming the sodium concentration is normal as well.

Insulin therapy is based on the same criteria as for treatment of DKA, generally being initiated as a bolus of 10 to 30 units regular type insulin followed by 2 to 10 units per hour by continuous intravenous drip, as discussed in the section on DKA and type I disease. As insulin is given and the glucose level begins to fall, potassium is driven rapidly back into the cells from the extracellular fluid. Thus 20 to 40 mEq of KCl is given per hour after urine flow is ensured, unless the initial potassium is 4.5 to 5 mmol/L. Phosphate is given if the initial PO_4 concentration is below 1 mmol/L: 20 mmol for every 40 mmol K^+. As soon as the patient has had 24 hours of a normal blood glucose level and normal intake and output, he or she may be allowed near-normal activity and resumption of usual medications and diet.

Hyporeninemic Hypoaldosteronism

Hyporeninemic hypoaldosteronism is infrequent but may be found in diabetics with nephropathy and rarely in those with normal renal function. The renin response is interrupted at one of several points in its production. These patients exhibit hyperkalemic hyperchloremic acidosis and a relative hypotension with clinical orthostatic hypotension. They exhibit great amounts of prorenin, which correlates with glycemic control. Occasionally, exogenous mineralocorticoids are needed to treat orthostatic hypotension and hyperkalemia.

Diabetes and Pregnancy

Pregnancy presents a special challenge to the patient and clinician. Extraordinary care is required to protect the mother and fetus. Close follow-up is usually needed via consultation of the family physician with a diabetes specialist or an obstetrician familiar with treating a high-risk pregnancy (or both). The infant of the diabetic mother has an increased chance of having anomalies, macrosomia, prematurity, respiratory distress syndrome, and death. One of the most characteristic congenital anomalies of diabetes is sacral agenesis or caudal dysplasia. It is found more than 200 times more frequently in offspring of diabetic mothers as in those born to nondiabetics. Spontaneous abortions are more prevalent among diabetic pregnancies. The mother faces a higher risk of ketoacidosis as well as acceleration of retinopathy and nephropathy. The key message in the care of the diabetic who is pregnant is to maintain normoglycemia and a normal glycosylated hemoglobin level. Ketoacidosis is detrimental to both mother and fetus.

All pregnant women should be screened for diabetes between the 24th and 28th week of pregnancy. A 50 gm oral glucose load is given and a glucose level measured 1 hour later. If the glucose is 140 mg/dL or greater, a 3-hour glucose tolerance test should be done. About 25 per cent of women with gestational diabetes develop permanent diabetes mellitus within 10 years of delivery. Perinatal mortality rates increase with increasing severity of diabetes, but they have decreased dramatically with improved prenatal care (Gabbe, 1986). Although White's classification of diabetes during pregnancy is not as widely used as previously, it is still useful for anticipating maternal and fetal problems (Table 41–8).

Strict control of hyperglycemia is imperative throughout the pregnancy. It is desirable to maintain fasting glucose concentrations at 100 mg/dL or less and the 2-hour postprandial value at approximately 120 mg/dL. Home glucose monitoring is necessary and helpful. Oral hypoglycemic agents are not recommended during pregnancy. Thus if a woman's blood glucose exceeds desirable levels, insulin is used. Frequent injections of regular insulin can supplement the usual doses of the morning and evening insulin regimen. In a few patients it is necessary to use an insulin pump with continuous subcutaneous insulin infusion. The first 2 months of pregnancy are important in respect to prevention of malformations by correcting maternal hyperglycemia and metabolic abnormalities.

Insulin-requiring diabetic mothers should be seen in the outpatient setting at 2- to 3-week intervals or more frequently if control is not satisfactory. A diabetic diet consisting of approximately 30 to 35 kcal/kg ideal body weight is appropriate. Hypertension is frequent during the third trimester, and infections should be treated early. Ultrasonography is performed at approximately 6-week intervals to evaluate fetal growth and to detect malformations. Contraction stress tests and determination of the lecithin/sphingomyelin ratio may be necessary.

Immediately after delivery the absence of regulatory hormones of the placenta creates a situation in which hypoglycemia is more apt to occur. Thus 5% dextrose in water should be in place. Insulin might not be required for several hours after delivery. The newborn should be examined for fetal anomalies, which are more common than in a newborn of a nondiabetic mother. Hypoglycemia occurs in almost half of the newborns of diabetic mothers compared to a few per cent of newborns generally. Higher than normal maternal glucose, some of which may cross the placenta, can result in high fetal insulin secretion and islet cell hyperplasia. That response normalizes a few days after birth. Macrosomic infants (4000 gm or more) are still common, although good control during pregnancy has made this condition less frequent. Hypocalcemia and hyperbilirubinemia are also more common than in infants of nondiabetic mothers. There is no substitute for an experienced team consisting of the family physician, obstetrician, diabetologist, and neonatologist to achieve optimal results for the mother and infant.

Management of the Surgical Patient with Diabetes

Advances in glucose monitoring and fluid infusion pumps have facilitated the treatment of diabetes under stressful circumstances. For elective surgery, planning should occur among the patient, surgeon, anesthesiologist, and diabetologist. The patient must be motivated to achieve good metabolic control for several days prior to the procedure. A history, physical examination, and screening laboratory tests, including an ECG, should be obtained prior to admission. Diabetics are more likely than nondiabetics to have silent myocardial infarctions. We prefer to admit the patient 1 day prior to surgery to ensure adequate control of glucose, electrolytes, and hydration. Nothing is given by mouth for 12 hours before surgery. Tests for ketones are conducted during the preoperative period in type I diabetics using Acetest tablets (Miles Laboratories). Long-acting insulin or oral hypoglycemic agents are withheld the evening prior to surgery in favor of the use of regular insulin when necessary. An accurate preoperative weight is helpful for subsequent follow-up.

Wound healing is improved with proper glucose control. Hyperglycemia is known to inhibit phagocytosis and impede responses to infectious agents.

TABLE 41–8. WHITE'S CLASSIFICATION OF DIABETES DURING PREGNANCY

Class	Type of Diabetes	Major Determinants
A	Gestational	Chemical diabetes, asymptomatic
B	Overt	Onset after age 20 or <10 years' duration
C	Overt	Onset before age 20 or 10–19 years' duration
D	Overt	Onset before age 10 or >20 years' duration and retinopathy (nonproliferative)
F	Overt	Diabetic nephropathy
H	Overt	Cardiac involvement
R	Overt	Retinopathy (proliferative)

Modified from White F: Classification of obstetric diabetes. Am J Obstet Gynecol 130:228, 1978, with permission.

Maintaining glucose concentrations between 100 and 200 mg/dL (5.6 and 11.1 mmol/dL) enhances immune system function and minimizes the risk of acute metabolic complication.

The effect of most uncomplicated surgical procedures on glucose levels is surprisingly small. One can expect an average elevation of about 37 mg/dL (2.1 mmol/L). A long procedure in an acutely ill patient, however, can produce more severe hyperglycemia.

Several treatment regimens during the perioperative period have been used satisfactorily over the years. Patients who are well controlled by diet alone or oral hypoglycemic agents primarily require observation by a knowledgeable clinician. If glucose levels exceed 225 mg/dL (12.5 mmol/L), small doses of regular insulin ranging from 3 to 10 units, may be given subcutaneously or intravenously. If there is any concern about hypotension, intravenous insulin is preferred, so absorption is not a factor. Postoperatively, glucose should be monitored at the bedside every 4 to 6 hours and about 5 units of regular insulin administered subcutaneously if the glucose exceeds 225 mg/dL (12.5 mmol/L).

For type II diabetics who are not well controlled and for all insulin-dependent diabetics, two options are offered. The continuous intravenous infusion of insulin is preferred. An infusion pump is helpful for achieving smooth control of glucose levels by gradual and frequent insulin dose adjustments. The insulin infusion can be started the evening before surgery and continued until the patient can take food by mouth or at least 1 day postoperatively. One liter of 0.5 N saline containing 100 units of regular human insulin is infused initially at a rate of 10 ml per hour (providing 1 unit per hour). Glucose concentration is measured by Dextrostix or Chemstrip bG every 2 to 4 hours preoperatively and every 1 to 2 hours during the surgical procedure. Fingerstick glucose values may not be accurate in severely hypotensive patients, but venous blood tested by the reagent strip is acceptable. The insulin dose can easily be adjusted to more or fewer units per hour if needed. The inclusion of KCl 20 mEq/L is optional. About 10 ml of the fluid is allowed to run out of the needle in order to coat the tubing with insulin. A 5% glucose solution in a separate bottle should be infused simultaneously to provide 100 to 150 gm of glucose per 24 hours. Tests for ketones by Acetest tablets can be performed during the operative procedure if it extends beyond 3 to 4 hours or if the patient has unstable diabetes.

If the patient is expected to take fluids or food within several hours after the surgical procedure, a 5% glucose solution may be infused at a rate of about 100 ml per hour prior to surgery. Two-thirds of the usual insulin dose is given prior to a morning surgical procedure. Glucose is monitored during the operative and postoperative periods at approxi-

TABLE 41–9. PERIOPERATIVE MANAGEMENT OF THE DIABETIC PATIENT

Preoperative management
All patients
Discontinue long-acting insulin and oral hypoglycemic agents the evening prior to surgery.
Achieve satisfactory glucose control and hydration.
Well controlled type II patients
Monitor glucose concentrations.
Use regular insulin only if glucose exceeds 225 mg/dL (12.5 mmol/L).
Type I and unstable type II patients
Monitor for plasma ketones.
Monitor glucose concentrations.
Use continuous insulin infusion or small doses of regular insulin injections every 4 hours.

Operative and postoperative management
Well controlled type II patients
Monitor glucose concentrations every 2 to 4 hours during surgery and 4 to 6 hours postoperatively.
Use small doses of regular insulin intravenously if warranted.
Type I and unstable type II patients
Use infusion pump for insulin administration beginning 12 hours before surgery. Adjust insulin dose and glucose infusions by glucose determinations every 2 to 4 hours.
or
Give two thirds of usual dose of insulin on the morning before surgery and give supplemental regular insulin if needed according to glucose monitoring.
Monitor for plasma ketones.
Infuse glucose solution (about 5 gm per hour).

mately 2-hour intervals. The glucose infusion can be increased if the concentration falls below 100 mg/dL (5.6 mmol/L), or small doses of insulin (about 5 units) can be administered intravenously for glucose levels above 225 mg/dL (12.5 mmol/L). Postoperatively, diabetic control can be achieved by giving supplemental regular insulin subcutaneously every 4 to 6 hours as indicated by glucose monitoring (Table 41–9).

Maintaining normal electrolytes and proper hydration are essential elements of a successful postoperative recovery. Attention to urinary output and the cardiac status is, of course, necessary in patients who are prone to heart or kidney problems. Anticipation of vascular and metabolic complications so they can be treated quickly and effectively is the key to preventing a prolonged, complicated postoperative course.

HYPOGLYCEMIA

Hypoglycemia can be categorized in two main divisions: postprandial and postabsorptive hypoglycemia. Postabsorptive hypoglycemia is also called fasting hypoglycemia, or organic hypoglycemia.

Glucose counterregulatory mechanisms, mainly glucagon and epinephrine, are activated at glucose levels below 65 to 70 mg/dL (3.6 to 3.9 mmol/L).

Symptoms develop at 50 to 55 mg/dL (2.8 to 3.0 mmol/L). Between 45 and 60 mg/dL (2.5 and 3.3 mmol/L) symptoms, when present, tend to be those of sympathetic nervous system discharge, diaphoresis, palpitations, tremor, and weakness. At levels below 45 mg/dL, symptoms are due to CNS glucose deprivation (neuroglycopenia) and consist of diplopia/blurred vision (85 per cent) confusion or abnormal behavior (80 per cent), unconsciousness or amnesia (53 per cent), and grand mal seizures (12 per cent) as found in insulinoma (Cryer, 1992).

Postprandial (Reactive) Hypoglycemia

By definition, postprandial (reactive) hypoglycemia occurs within 4 hours after a meal or glucose load. Glucose levels rarely fall lower than 45 mg/dL (2.5 mmol/L). In practice, the most common complaints leading to evaluation of this syndrome are symptoms of sympathetic discharge, such as tremulousness, inability to concentrate, sweating, and mental irritability after meals. Preceding meals tend to be rich in carbohydrate (particularly simple carbohydrates) and devoid of protein. Postgastrectomy alimentary hypoglycemia is due to rapid emptying with resultant rapid insulin release. When the mechanism cannot be explained by preceding surgery, it is called functional alimentary hypoglycemia.

If the diagnosis of reactive hypoglycemia is made only by satisfying Whipple's triad (appropriate symptoms related temporally to a mixed meal, a blood glucose level in the low range, and recovery as blood glucose recovers), the syndrome occurs in only about 5 per cent of the cases with suggestive symptoms. The rate of fall of the blood glucose level is now said not to be a determinant of hypoglycemic symptomatology. The syndrome's existence, however, is not in doubt, to which any primary care physician can attest. It is possible that the levels at which patients develop symptoms and the rates of fall in blood glucose level vary so much from one individual to another that diagnostic criteria are not adequate. It has been renamed idiopathic postprandial syndrome for that reason. Postprandial hypoglycemia is generally overdiagnosed, and "hypoglycemia" is a ready culprit to cite for all manner of patients' functional complaints. A reactive hypoglycemia may be seen with early diabetes due to the delayed and elevated insulin levels.

The syndrome is still treated by diets low in simple carbohydrates and high in protein, along with avoidance of caffeine. (Caffeine produces similar symptoms owing to its direct sympathomimetic action.) Of the few drugs suggested for symptomatic relief, β-blockers (usually propranolol) may offer relief, as the symptoms are those of sympathetic autonomic discharge. The fear of masking hypoglycemic symptoms would not apply here, as the level of blood glucose is benign, if it is low at all. Frequent small meals rather than a few large meals can be helpful.

Alimentary hypoglycemia may be severe enough to cause neurologic symptoms and occurs 1.5 to 3.0 hours after a meal. It may be confused with the dumping syndrome, an effect due to the rapid entry of large volumes of food and fluid into the gut. Congenital enzyme deficiencies that result in hypoglycemia (hypoglucosemia) include galactosemia and hereditary fructose intolerance.

Postabsorptive Hypoglycemia (Fasting Hypoglycemia, Organic Hypoglycemia)

Postabsorptive hypoglycemia is defined as clinically low plasma glucose levels during the 12-hour postabsorptive period. The diagnosis is definite when the FBS is less than 45 mg/dL (2.5 mmol/L) and strongly suggested when levels are between 45 and 60 mg/dL (2.5 to 3.3 mmol/L).

Common to most of the causes of organic hypoglycemia is a disorder in glucose counterregulatory mechanisms, i.e., glucagon and epinephrine. Usually a dysfunction in both is required for symptoms to be produced, unless hyperinsulinemia is the primary cause.

The causes of postabsorptive hypoglycemia are drugs, critical organ failure, hormonal failure, nonbeta cell tumors, endogenous hyperinsulinism, sepsis, and disorders peculiar to childhood. In emergency departments most hypoglycemic patients have diabetes, acute alcoholism, or combinations of the two. Sepsis is the third most common cause, and hypoglycemia in these patients too appears often to be precipitated by alcohol.

The causes of hypoglycemia in diabetics are insulin and sulfonylureas. Alcohol has an important role in aggravating hypoglycemia of any cause. Insufficient glucagon response to falling plasma glucose occurs in IDDM patients about 3 years after onset. Physical exercise potentiates the action of insulin. The vagaries of insulin dosing in coordination with diet and exercise levels are the precipitants of hypoglycemia in many cases. Hypoglycemia due to oral hypoglycemic agents is characterized by persistence owing to the long half-lives of the OHAs compared with regular or even NPH insulin.

Ethanol inhibits gluconeogenesis, even in the noncirrhotic liver. To exhaust otherwise intact regulatory mechanisms (glucagon, glycogenolysis, growth hormone), a full binge is required (up to a full day without significant food intake). There are drugs in addition to insulin, alcohol and sulfonylureas that can cause hypoglycemia. Included among the proved causes are quinine, salicylates, and sulfonamides.

Organ failures as a cause of postabsorptive hypoglycemia include that of the liver (but only with near-complete destruction), the heart in congestive failure, and cachectic renal failure. Sepsis is associated with hypoglycemia, probably through continued glucose consumption as hepatic production decreases Likewise, starvation leads to hypoglycemia via the mechanism of glucose utilization. Hormonal deficiencies that lead to hypoglycemia include cortisol (adrenal insufficiency) and somatotropin.

Insulinoma, the quintessential paradigm for postabsorptive hypoglycemia, has long directed the student to look for beta cell pancreatic insulinomas first, assuming that the obvious hypoglycemic reactions to insulin in diabetics has been ruled out. In fact, the incidence of insulinoma is rare, 1 in 1 million, but the tumor accounts for 66 to 85 per cent of all endogenous hyperinsulinism. During 40 years of primary care practice, while looking for a first case, a practitioner sees 2000 ostensible and 100 actual cases of idiopathic reactive hypoglycemia. A low fasting glucose concentration accompanied by an inappropriately high insulin level establishes the diagnosis, although confirmatory tests are needed.

The differential diagnosis is the same in the pediatric group as for adults, with some special additions. Neonates, though tolerant of plasma glucose levels, are particularly vulnerable to hypoglycemia during the transition from maternal energy sources to their own hepatic energy intake and glucose production that occurs during the first 72 hours. Maternal diabetes confers degrees of insulinism, beginning with hyperglycemia when the mother is poorly controlled at delivery. Hypoglycemia in immature neonates probably results from impaired gluconeogenesis in the liver. Sepsis causes hypoglycemia based on utilization of glucose, which is faster than liver production and calorie intake can replete.

Ketotic hypoglycemia of childhood is a usually benign, short-term starvation phenomenon associated with intercurrent illness, often gastroenteritis. It is characterized by acetone smell on the breath in the absence of hyperglycemia. The child is often not "ill" and responds to fluid and calorie intake.

THYROID DISORDERS

Thyroid disorders are common in clinical practice, second in frequency only to diabetes among endocrine illnesses. As with most hormonal diseases, clinical manifestations result from excessive thyroid hormone (hyperthyroidism) or inadequate secretion (hypothyroidism). The thyroid gland weighs 20 to 25 gm in the normal state and consists of two lobes, an isthmus, and a small pyramidal lobe extending from the isthmus. The gland is constituted by cells surrounding follicles that contain colloid. Parafollicular or C cells, the source of the hormone calcitonin, also reside in the thyroid gland. Enlargement of the gland is termed a goiter. It can be inflamed (thyroiditis) and develop benign and malignant tumors.

Thyroid hormones phylogenetically are important regulators of morphologic changes and basic cellular metabolic processes. The thyroid has the ability to avidly concentrate iodine from extracellular fluids. Dietary sources provide about 0.5 mg daily in geographic areas that are not iodine-deficient. The thyroid has the ability to metabolize iodine and incorporate it into organic compounds. Iodination of tyrosine to form monoiodotyrosine and diiodotyrosine are early steps leading to coupling to form tetraiodothyronine (T_4) and triiodothyronine (T_3). The hormones are held in thyroglobulin in the follicles. The T_4/T_3 ratio of secreted hormone is approximately 10:1. Once in the plasma, thyroid hormone is bound mostly to a protein called thyroid-binding globulin (TBG) and to a lesser extent to a prealbumin binding protein. A single iodine atom is removed from T_4 in peripheral tissue to produce the active form of the hormone. TBG is altered in various situations. It is increased with estrogen administration, contraceptive pills, pregnancy, and certain liver diseases. It is decreased by androgens, the nephrotic syndrome, and major systemic illnesses.

Thyroid function is mediated by thyrotropin (thyroid-stimulating hormone, TSH), a pituitary hormone. Thyrotropin-releasing hormone (TRH), of hypothalamic origin, modulates TSH activity. A finely regulated feedback system exists normally. Low concentrations of T_4 and T_3, sensed by the pituitary gland and the hypothalamus, results in increased TRH secretion. Somatostatin, another hypothalamic factor, inhibits TSH secretion. As T_4 and T_3 levels increase, TRH and TSH are inhibited (Fig. 41–3). TSH enhances iodine uptake by the thyroid and increases all the steps leading to the synthesis and secretion of thyroid hormones. The entire system is delicately balanced, so thyroid hormone in appropriate concentrations can modulate critical cellular oxidation and metabolic processes throughout the body.

Thyroid Function Tests

Many laboratory tests are available to measure specific aspects of thyroid function. The metabolic state correlates best with free T_4 or T_3 hormone concentrations. However, technical difficulties and expense associated with determining free hormone levels have resulted in other, less direct measurements. Thus commonly used and practical tests for thyroid function in clinical practice are described (Kaye, 1993). Accurate methods are available to measure the total circulating concentrations of T_4, T_3, and reverse T_3. Bound and unbound fractions of the hormones are included in

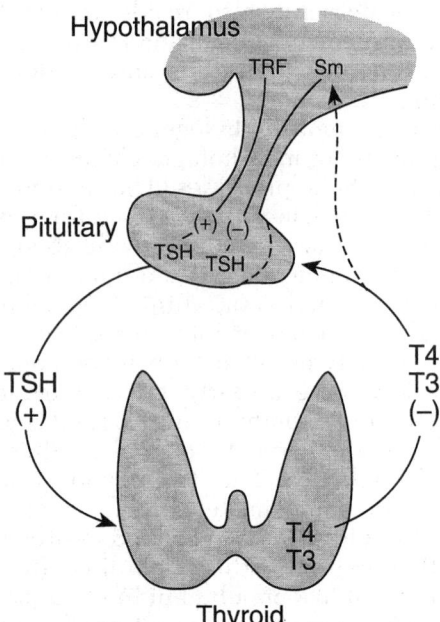

FIGURE 41–3. Finely regulated feedback system that controls thyroid hormone secretion. TRF = thyrotropin; TSH = thyroid-stimulating hormone; Sm = somatostatin.

the measurement. For that reason the thyroid-binding proteins must be simultaneously estimated in order to interpret the results properly. The direct measurement of T_3 by radioimmunoassay is helpful in certain circumstances, such as T_3 thyrotoxicosis, when T_4 levels are normal. The normal T_3 concentration ranges from 70 to 190 ng/dL. It decreases slightly with aging.

Serum T₄ Concentration and Thyroid Hormone-Binding Ratio

Measurement of the total serum T_4 and thyroid-binding proteins are the common tests ordered by clinicians to assess thyroid function. Such a combination along with a serum TSH level is sufficient to diagnose virtually all of the common cases of hyperthyroidism and hypothyroidism.

The serum T_4 concentration, measuring bound and unbound T_4, ranges between 5 and 11 μg/dL in most laboratories. A high concentration of iodine does not increase these values as it did protein-bound iodine in the past. Serum T_4 levels are high in the presence of hyperthyroidism and low with hypothyroidism. When TBG is elevated, as during pregnancy or with the use of estrogens, the T_4 level is also high, even though the patient is euthyroid. Accordingly, a test for hormone binding to proteins is ordered simultaneously.

The thyroid hormone-binding ratio is determined by an in vitro uptake test usually using tracer quantities of radioactively labeled T_3. These techniques have been called T_3 resin uptake tests, but that terminology can be confusing now that serum T_3 levels can be measured. The tracer T_3 is

bound to thyroid-binding protein. The proportion of labeled hormone that is not bound to TBG is measured after a standard time and obviously varies with the number of unoccupied sites for hormone. The results of a specific test can be compared with those obtained in a standard control serum, and a ratio can be determined. Multiplying the ratio by the serum T_4 concentration yields a satisfactory estimate of the free thyroid hormone concentration, termed the *free T_4 index*.

Serum TSH Concentrations

The ability to measure serum TSH by radioimmunoassay has given clinicians an exquisitely sensitive test of thyroid function. With primary hypothyroidism, TSH concentration rises early during the course of the disease. In fact, the diagnosis of hypothyroidism by TSH elevation has been made in a patient with no thyroid enlargement, normal routine thyroid function tests, and no discernible clinical manifestations (Herrold and Tzagournis, 1971). An elevated value can confirm that the problem resides in the thyroid instead of the pituitary gland. Thyroid hormone replacement alone in a patient with pituitary insufficiency can result in adrenal insufficiency. The clinician should know if other critical endocrine testing is needed.

Modern testing of TSH is highly sensitive and can determine when thyroid hormone is excessive also. Thus it is useful for diagnosing hyperthyroidism and for follow-up of patients taking thyroid hormone as replacement therapy or for suppression of a goiter. The normal range of serum TSH is 0.5 to 5.0 mU/L, although there are variations among laboratories.

Thyroid Radioactive Iodine Uptake and Scintiscanning

The radioactive iodine uptake test is not used as commonly as in the past. It is a direct physiologic test of thyroid uptake using tracer doses of inorganic radioiodine. In the past iodine 131 (^{131}I) was used, but ^{123}I is now used primarily because of its short half-life and the much lower radiation dose delivered to the thyroid gland. The tracer dose mixes with iodide normally present in extracellular fluid. The proportion of isotope that accumulates in the thyroid gland can easily be counted at certain intervals and reflects the rate of clearance. The normal range is 5 to 25 per cent in 24 hours. Increased uptake is seen with hyperthyroidism or in unusual situations in response to iodine deficiency, with thyroid biosynthetic defects, or with conditions that cause excessive loss of binding proteins. Decreased uptake is associated with hypothyroidism, thyroiditis, increased iodine, exogenous thyroid intake, or ingestion of antithyroid agents. It is prudent to order an uptake test prior to treating thyrotoxicosis with ^{131}I therapy to ensure adequate uptake of the iodine. Some cases of subacute thyroiditis are associated with hyperthyroidism but do not take up increased tracer isotope. Factitious hyperthyroidism would show virtually no radioactive iodine uptake.

External scintiscanning with a rectilinear scanner or stationary camera produces an image of the thyroid that is helpful. The ^{131}I isotope previously used for this purpose, has been replaced by ^{123}I with its shorter half-life and absence of beta radiation, or with technetium 90 (^{90}Tc) pertechnetate. The images help the clinician define areas of increased or decreased function, evaluate size and location (e.g., a mediastinal location of thyroid tissue), and identify "cold" nodules suspicious for cancer. Total body scans are usually performed for identifying metastatic thyroid cancer with the ^{131}I isotope.

Other Relatively Common Thyroid Tests

Ultrasonography has improved our ability to image the thyroid. Cystic lesions are sonolucent, whereas solid lesions produce multiple echoes. This technology has improved in recent years and is helpful during the work-up of thyroid nodules.

The *thyrotropin-releasing hormone* (TRH) test has some limited value. TRH 400 μg is infused intravenously, and TSH is determined 30 minutes later. The normal peak value is approximately 5 to 30 mU/L. The response is accentuated in patients with primary hypothyroidism and tends to be flat in those with hyperthyroidism. Its main value is that it can distinguish between pituitary or hypothalamic causes of secondary hypothyroidism. If the pituitary is diseased, TRH stimulation results in a subnormal response.

Serum *thyroglobulin* measurements are of value primarily for the follow-up of people treated for differentiated thyroid carcinomas. Elevations are noted in the presence of those cancers and of hyperthyroidism, goiters, and thyroiditis as well.

Thyroid *antibodies* to thyroglobulin or to thyroid microsomes are useful for diagnosing Hashimoto's thyroiditis. They are also elevated in Graves' disease or in patients with transient thyrotoxicosis due to chronic autoimmune thyroiditis.

Fine-needle aspiration of a thyroid nodule via a percutaneous route is best performed with the help of a consultant. Other thyroid tests are available, but their indications are limited.

Thyrotoxicosis

Excessive thyroid hormone has profound effects on virtually every organ system in the body. Thyrotoxicosis, or hyperthyroidism, can be a dramatic disease with life-threatening implications or a subtle disorder lasting many years with few manifestations. It is more common in women than in men. In the United States the prevalence of Graves' disease, the most common form of thyrotoxicosis, is approximately 0.4 per cent. In addition to Graves'

disease, there are several other causes of the hyperthyroid state. Toxic multinodular goiters, thyroid adenomas, thyroiditis, autonomous secretion of TSH, and ectopic thyroid tissue may result in a hyperthyroid state. Exogenous thyroid intake, iatrogenic or surreptitiously ingested, can produce thyrotoxicosis (factitious thyrotoxicosis).

Graves' disease is an autoimmune disease. Immunoglobulin G reacts with the thyroid cells, especially the TSH receptor, and mimics the action of the TSH hormone. In its simplest terms, Graves' disease is caused by an antibody that stimulates the thyroid to produce excessive amounts of hormone. Thyroid-stimulating immunoglobulin (TSI) and TSH displacing antibody can be measured and are elevated in many patients with Graves' disease. Thyroid antibodies are diverse. They may cause inflammation (as in autoimmune thyroiditis), stimulate the gland (as in Graves' disease), or block the binding of TSH by the receptor (producing hypothyroidism). In addition to the physiologic changes that one sees in all hyperthyroid states, Graves' disease is commonly associated with infiltrative ophthalmopathy and infrequently with infiltrative dermopathy (pretibial myxedema).

Thyrotoxicosis secondary to autonomously functioning nodules in a multinodular goiter is less common than Graves' disease. An adenoma of the thyroid may also function autonomously and produce excess thyroid hormones. These nodules or adenomas do not recede with TSH suppression and are not dependent on some substance from the serum to stimulate hormone production. However, normal surrounding thyroid tissue is suppressed, often by the negative feedback from excess hormone produced by the nodule. A scintiscan of the thyroid might show a nodule or an adenoma taking up an increased amount of radioactive iodine, whereas the remainder of the thyroid gland is taking up little or no tracer radioiodine.

Other forms of thyrotoxicosis are seen less frequently in clinical practice or are not as readily recognized. Subacute thyroiditis may for a period of time cause the release of excessive thyroid hormone. Thyrotoxicosis can be associated with a painless thyroiditis. It is usually transient but can recur. Excessive TSH secretion due to a pituitary tumor or disorder of the hypothalamus is a rare cause of hyperthyroidism. In this situation, T_4 and T_3 concentrations are high and fail to suppress the TSH level. Excessive iodine intake can induce hyperthyroidism in people who have underlying thyroid abnormalities (e.g., iodine-deficient goiters or multinodular goiters). Ectopic thyroid tissue present in teratomas or factors secreted by choriocarcinoma or hydatidiform mole that stimulate the thyroid are rare causes of thyrotoxicosis. Exogenous intake of hormone should not be overlooked as a cause of thyrotoxicosis. Patients who take thyroid hormone have changing requirements over the years, and mild thyrotoxicosis may go unnoticed for a long time. Osteoporosis may be accelerated by mildly elevated levels of thyroid hormone in the elderly. Factitious thyrotoxicosis can be a challenging problem because the patient usually denies taking the hormone; frequently these individuals are knowledgeable about health care or are in some allied health profession. They would have high T_4 and T_3 levels, low TSH levels, usually a nonpalpable thyroid gland, and virtually no radioactive iodine uptake. Emotional or psychiatric symptoms are invariably present.

Clinical Manifestations

The clinical symptoms and signs of thyrotoxicosis are predictable based on organ responses to excessive thyroid hormone. However, rapidity of onset, intensity of the disease, age of the patient, concomitant illnesses, and the underlying cause of the thyrotoxicosis modify clinical manifestations.

Symptoms common in thyrotoxic patients are nervousness, heat intolerance, fatigue, increased perspiration, and rapid heart rate. Other common complaints are weight loss, more frequent bowel movements or diarrhea, emotional lability, and weakness. Many of these symptoms are nonspecific. Certain symptoms, however, are highly specific for thyrotoxicosis. Loss of weight despite a good appetite and adequate caloric intake is an excellent clue, as is heat intolerance. Relatively few other diseases present with such complaints. Hyperthyroid patients may complain of thinning and loss of scalp hair, erythema of the palms, amenorrhea or hypomenorrhea, and changes in the appearance of the nails. In the elderly the classic symptoms are found less frequently. They tend to have subtle manifestations and symptoms related to the cardiovascular system, such as angina, irregular heart action, and manifestations of osteoporosis. Long-standing relatively mild hyperthyroidism, usually found in the elderly, has been termed *silent thyrotoxicosis*. Most patients who have Graves' disease or toxic multinodular goiter notice enlargement of the neck or a shirt size increase. In patients with Graves' disease early symptoms may be related to infiltrative ophthalmopathy or dermopathy. One or both eyes may protrude, eye muscle abnormalities may cause diplopia, or periorbital edema may be noted. A patchy or confluent erythematous infiltration of the skin, usually in the pretibial area, is occasionally seen with Graves' disease.

Because of a certain overall appearance thyrotoxicosis is sometimes one of those diseases that you diagnose as you enter the examining room. The patient is fidgety, agitated, and anxious. There is tachycardia or atrial fibrillation. The systolic blood pressure is high and the pulse pressure wide. The skin in thyrotoxicosis patients is characteristic. It is warm, silky, moist, and thin, resembling the skin of a baby. Areas of vitiligo when present are typically symmetric. The nails might show a separation

TABLE 41–10. AMERICAN THYROID ASSOCIATION SUMMARY OF EYE CHANGES IN GRAVES' DISEASE

Class	Definition
0	No symptoms or signs
1	Upper lid retraction, stare, lid lag
2	Soft tissue involvement, symptomatic
3	Proptosis >22 mm
4	Extraocular muscle involvement
5	Corneal involvement
6	Optic nerve affected with visual loss

of the distal part from the nail bed extending more proximally than normal (onycholysis). Occasionally, the digits show clubbing or thyroid acropachy. The eyes appear to stare at you, and there is less blinking than normal. Lid retraction is common, as is lid lag (the jerky lagging of the lids as the globe follows a finger slowly downward). In those with Graves' disease infiltrative ophthalmopathy can precede but more commonly accompanies or follows the hyperthyroid state. Table 41–10 summarizes the eye findings in Graves' disease. Proptosis may be unilateral or bilateral (Fig. 41–4). Extraocular muscle involvement is manifested by restricted movements, particularly in the superior lateral direction, producing diplopia.

Unless the cause of the thyrotoxicosis is exogenous thyroid hormone or ectopic thyroid production, thyromegaly is virtually always present. The thyroid in Graves' disease enlarges symmetrically, and sometimes a pyramidal lobe can be palpated arising superiorly from the isthmus. A venous hum can be heard, and sometimes a thrill can be palpated. The gland can enlarge to four to five times normal size. Toxic nodular goiters are irregularly increased, or a single nodule may be palpated. The

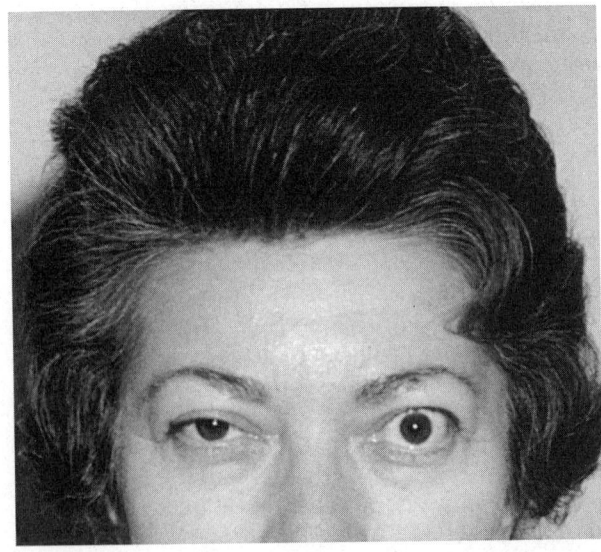

FIGURE 41–4. Unilateral exophthalmos in a woman with Graves' disease.

precordium is active, and tachycardia can be accompanied by a systolic flow murmur. The tip of the liver or spleen occasionally can be palpated because of the congestion and lymphocytic infiltration in the organ. Lymph nodes may also be palpable. There is a fine to coarse tremor usually present that can be demonstrated by placing a Kleenex on the dorsum of the outstretched hand. Tendon reflexes are brisk and increased. Infiltrative dermopathy in the pretibial skin or foot areas are *pathognomonic* of Graves' disease. Muscle weakness is not unusual, and the patient has difficulty standing from a squatting position. In the elderly the cardiovascular signs are present, as is thyromegaly and typical skin changes. Tremor is also present in most elderly patients.

Diagnosis

Thyrotoxicosis is ordinarily detected by the clinical manifestations of the patient. Several other disorders should be considered in the differential diagnosis, including marked anxiety, mitral valve prolapse, diabetes mellitus, pheochromocytoma, and malignancies associated with weight loss. The most common etiology of unilateral proptosis is Graves' disease, but obviously local causes such as neoplasm, an arteriovenous fistula or a cavernous sinus thrombosis must be considered. A CT scan in patients with unilateral proptosis is worthwhile. The clinical diagnosis is easily confirmed by excellent laboratory tests.

The combination of an elevated free thyroxine index and a suppressed TSH concentration confirms the diagnosis of thyrotoxicosis arising from the thyroid gland. The free T_4 measurement is increasingly available and accurate. It is, of course, elevated in the patient with thyrotoxicosis. The rare exception to TSH suppression in hyperthyroid patients is a pituitary tumor that is secreting TSH or ectopic TSH production. Radioactive iodine uptake is increased in patients with Grave's disease, toxic nodules, or adenoma. With factitious hyperthyroidism the uptake is near zero, and is usually low with thyroiditis. In rare cases the thyrotoxicosis may be due to increased secretion of T_3, whereas T_4 levels are normal (T_3 thyrotoxicosis). However, it is not cost-effective to order a free T_3 test unless the initial standard tests are inconsistent with the clinical picture.

Treatment

It is important to include the patient in the discussion on therapy, as options are truly available. Each of three of the most commonly used treatments have certain advantages and disadvantages. Radioiodine, surgery, and antithyroid drugs have been widely used for many years, and their effects are well known. β-Adrenergic blockers produce symptomatic relief in almost all patients with thyrotoxicosis. Propranolol has been used most widely at a dose of 10 to 40 mg four times a day, titrating it so tachycardia, tremor, and restlessness are alleviated.

Radioiodine, specifically ^{131}I, is the most commonly used treatment in adults. It becomes concentrated in the thyroid and produces injury to the cells over a period of weeks to months. It is simple, inexpensive, effective therapy. Its disadvantages are the theoretic future influence it might have on tumor formation or genetic changes and the high incidence of hypothyroidism it induces. ^{131}I should not be used in pregnant women because it crosses the placenta readily and can be concentrated by the fetal thyroid. Most clinicians avoid its use in children, although genetic damage or an increased incidence of leukemia or other cancers has not been shown to occur. Hypothyroidism has not been a major concern so long as a patient is reliable and willing to be followed and treated.

The dose of ^{131}I usually ranges between 2 and 20 mCi by mouth. Various tactics have been suggested to determine the correct amount to produce euthyroidism without relapses or hypothyroidism—but to no avail. A 10 mCi dose results in 90 per cent of patients with Graves' disease becoming euthyroid or hypothyroid (Caruso and Mazzaferri, 1992). Relapses require additional treatment. The patient begins to notice improvement in about 2 weeks, and the peak effect occurs within 2 to 3 months. Hypothyroidism can occur many months after treatment. Some clinicians believe that ^{131}I worsens the infiltrative ophthalmopathy seen with this disease, but that issue is still unclear.

The mean dosage of L-thyroxine in patients with Graves' disease made hypothyroid is somewhat lower than the average daily replacement dosage of 1.6 μg/kg of ideal body weight (Mandel et al., 1993). It is likely due to the continuous production of thyroid hormone from areas not completely destroyed by the ^{131}I.

Antithyroid drugs for treatment of hyperthyroidism have been effective and relatively safe. The thionamides propylthiouracil and methimazole (Tapazole) are the agents used in the United States. They inhibit thyroid hormone synthesis by interfering with iodine metabolism and coupling of iodotyrosines. Propylthiouracil has the additional action of inhibiting peripheral conversion of T_4 to T_3 at the higher range of dosage. The disadvantages of using the antithyroid drugs are the adverse reactions they engender, which occur in fewer than 5 per cent of treated patients. The most serious of these reactions is agranulocytosis, which occurs in about 1 of every 250 patients treated. It is almost always reversible if the drug is discontinued at an early stage of suppression. The blood count must be checked intermittently especially during the first several weeks of treatment when leukopenia is most apt to occur. A baseline white blood cell (WBC) count is useful because in Graves' disease it is frequently lower than normal. Other adverse reactions to thionamides include allergies, skin rash, liver reactions, musculoskeletal pains, and fever. Propylthiouracil is given in doses of 100 to 300 mg q 12 hr, and methimazole is given as 10 to 20 mg q 12 hr. Larger dosages are sometimes needed. As the hyperthyroid state improves, the dosage is decreased gradually. TSH levels are helpful for following patients. The thyroid gland becomes less vascular and decreases in size to a variable degree; paradoxically, however, it can increase if the thyroid is blocked excessively and TSH increases in the blood. Propylthiouracil is preferred in pregnant women because it is thought to cross the placental barrier less readily than methimazole. An endocrinologist should be consulted for patients with special problems such as pregnancy or childhood thyrotoxicosis. The onset of action of the antithyroid drugs is more rapid than with radioiodine treatment, showing clinical effects within 2 weeks of treatment. The usual recommendation is to treat the patients for approximately 1 year, then withdraw the drug. Approximately one half of Graves' disease patients have a remission of the disease by then. If the hyperthyroid state relapses, the patient may want to consider surgery or radioiodine therapy. Individuals with mild disease or small goiters are more likely to obtain a remission on these drugs.

Surgery remains an option for the thyrotoxicosis due to Graves' disease or toxic nodules. It is used less frequently than in the past. The surgeon leaves about 5 to 8 gm of the gland behind. The advantage of this option is rapid correction of the underlying problem. The disadvantages include the need of a major surgical procedure, a small risk of recurrent laryngeal nerve damage or hypoparathyroidism (about 1 per cent), thyroid storm if the patient is not well blocked, and formation of hematomas or infections in the surgical field. A β-adrenergic blocker is used during preoperative preparation of the patient, preferably along with antithyroid drugs. Potassium iodide, or SSKI, 5 drops three times a day, is helpful for decreasing thyrotoxicosis and reducing the vascularity of the gland. Unfortunately, there can be relapses of thyrotoxicosis postoperatively, and hypothyroidism occurs as well, albeit at a lesser prevalence than with radioiodine therapy. During pregnancy, thyroid surgery should be planned for the second trimester.

β-Adrenergic blockade is a helpful adjunct to any of the more definitive treatment options. In mild cases a β-blocker alone may suffice to control the symptoms. Iodine can be useful for acute treatment. It inhibits hormone release and synthesis of T_4, but there is an initial stimulation of organic iodination and T_4 synthesis. The therapeutic effect is lost with chronic use. Therefore iodine is used mainly in urgent situations or preoperatively.

Thyroid storm is a dramatic, life-threatening increase in thyrotoxic symptoms and signs. It is usually precipitated by stress, surgery, or infection; and fever is present. The cardiovascular manifestations are prominent and include marked tachycardia or even heart failure. Treatment should be instituted with antithyroid drugs, iodine or iopanoic acid (Telepaque), β-adrenergic blockers, and glucocorticoids. Propylthiouracil is probably the preferred antithyroid drug because of its additional effect in decreasing peripheral T_3 conversion from T_4. Large doses of approximately 1000 mg per day in divided doses are given initially. Intravenous prednisone 60 mg per day is infused to counter relative adrenal insufficiency, but the evidence that steroids are helpful is not proved. Propranolol can be given intravenously if it is not contraindicated (e.g., in patients with asthma) in small doses of 5 to 10 mg every few hours, titrating it as needed to slow the heart rate or control arrhythmias. Oral doses of 40 to 80 mg q 6 hr can be given if the patient is able to take medications by mouth or by a tube to the stomach.

Special circumstances in patients with thyrotoxicosis necessitate the help of a consultant. Pregnant women are prone to abortions and fetal complications. Neonatal Graves' disease may be present in a newborn of a mother with the same disease. Autoimmune antibody crosses the placenta and stimulates the infant's thyroid. The infant may need antithyroid drugs and supportive care for several weeks until the abnormal protein is catabolized. It is also important to recognize hypothyroidism in the infant whose mother took antithyroid drugs so therapy can be initiated quickly.

Infiltrative ophthalmopathy can become a troublesome complication causing muscle dysfunction with diplopia, severe proptosis, or loss of vision. Supportive treatment includes artificial tears, a diuretic such as Diamox used 4 or 5 days of the week, and elevating the head of the bed at night to diminish the orbital and periorbital edema. Prednisone in large doses, 60 to 80 mg per day tapering over a period of 3 to 4 weeks, is often effective in decreasing optic nerve pressure and the swelling and irritation associated with the eye manifestations of Graves' disease. Orbital irradiation has been used successfully to relieve the severe forms of the eye disease, but surgical decompression is a more common definitive treatment for severe cases. The patient should be counseled that the eye manifestations tend to remain active for up to 2 years, after which the infiltrative process tends to become quiescent. Some regression of the proptosis is possible as the active disease subsides. It is unwise to attempt surgical correction of the extraocular muscle abnormalities while the eye disease is active because further fibrosis or inflammation necessitates additional surgical procedures. Surgical intervention is needed in fewer than 10 per cent of cases, so most cases of infiltrative ophthalmopathy can be treated supportively while the disease process subsides.

TABLE 41–11. TYPES OF HYPOTHYROIDISM

Primary hypothyroidism
  Conditions characterized by lack of thyroid tissue
    Primary idiopathic hypothyroidism
    Athyreotic cretinism
    Postablative hypothyroidism
  Goitrous hypothyroidism
    Hashimoto's thyroiditis
    Defects in hormone synthesis
    Iodine deficiency
    Drug-induced (antithyroid and other goitrogenic agents)
    Iodide-induced goiter

Secondary hypothyroidism (relative lack of TSH)
  Pituitary destructive processes (e.g., Sheehan syndrome)
  Infiltrative disorders of pituitary
  Defective production or delivery of TRH (tertiary hypothyroidism)

Relative or Absolute Insufficiency of Thyroid Hormone

Thyroid hormone insufficiency causes a group of disorders that can be categorized as hypothyroid states and euthyroid goitrous states. The hypothyroid conditions can be further categorized into those characterized by lack of thyroid tissue, lack of thyrotropic hormone (or of TSH-releasing hormone), and goitrous hypothyroidism. These disorders are outlined in Table 41–11.

Clinical Manifestations

The insufficiency of thyroid hormones affects all tissues. Subjectively, the patient may or may not complain of lack of energy. Fatigue, cold intolerance, dry skin, mild overweight, and inability to eat the same amounts of foods as before without gaining weight) are well known to the clinician. Patients who are elderly or unaccustomed to seeing doctors may present with any or all of the above plus somnolence and lethargy.

Patients who labor physically for their living complain of fatigability. In patients with white collar or managerial jobs it is surprising how seldom hypothyroidism is diagnosed as a result of the patient's complaints, though fatigue is a common complaint in that setting. The patient may complain of cold intolerance. More often, thyroid function tests routinely ordered unveil the diagnosis.

The cardiovascular system findings include a narrowed pulse pressure and bradycardia. Pericardial effusion of a proteinaceous and mucopolysaccharide-rich fluid contributes to an enlarged silhouette. Dyslipidemia is present, but angina pectoris is surprisingly infrequent until thyroid hormone is given and the heart's demands increase to normal.

Shortness of breath occurs, especially if there is pleural effusion. Myxedematous infiltration of intercostal muscles and of the hypopharynx contribute to alveolar hypoventilation, obstructive sleep apnea, and ultimately coma.

Mild weight gain is common. Far more common are euthyroid obese people seeking an acceptable cause by suggesting to the doctor that their thyroid function be tested. Much of the weight gain in hypothyroidism is fluid, as judged from the diuresis that occurs soon after treatment is begun. Hyponatremia is explained by secondary antidiuretic hormone excess, which results in water retention out of proportion to salt retention. Constipation is a common complaint and is caused by the slowed peristalsis. Achlorhydria occurs in about one half of patients with primary hypothyroidism and overt pernicious anemia in 12 per cent.

Hypothyroidism is a cause of anovulation, infertility, and menorrhagia. Testosterone metabolism is altered, and cortisol and aldosterone turnover are decreased although their levels are normal.

Concomitant psychiatric symptoms include paranoia and depression. The extreme state, *myxedema madness*, is characterized by agitation. Headaches are common, and patients may have syncopal attacks whose prolonged duration may presage the onset of myxedema coma. Deep tendon reflexes are characteristically slow and, more strikingly, slow during the recovery phase.

Myxedema consists of the above problems in extreme degrees. Often patients manifest a typical appearance: slow raspy voice, slurred speech (due to lingual myxedema), dry skin, and a round, puffy face; they may be diagnosed by the physician at the door of the examining room. Other findings include absence of the lateral portion of the eyebrows, although this absence occurs in euthyroid states as well. The thyroid may or may not be palpable or enlarged, depending on the type of thyroid disease. Ultimately, coma results, usually in the aged. At that point the patient manifests bradycardia and hypothermia.

It is crucial to recognize hypothyroidism in the newborn. Newborn hypothyroidism in the extreme is cretinism and leads rapidly to retarded mental and physical development. It can be diagnosed only if it is considered on the basis of soft signs, such as a bulging fontanelle, delayed meconium passage, or persistent neonatal jaundice. There is an adage for such situations: "If you think about it, order it!" T_4 and TSH assays are thus undertaken. If diagnosis is delayed, the stigmata of cretinism appear, and growth retardation occurs. Childhood and adolescent hypothyroidism result in delayed puberty, developmental retardation, and dwarfism. Hypothyroidism is a cause of reversible dementia in the aged.

Subclinical hypothyroidism—defined as a TSH level of 5 to 20 μU/mL in the absence of symptoms, signs, and T_4 or T_3 abnormalities—is more common in older people and in women. These individuals have an 8 per cent chance of developing clinical hypothyroidism within 5 years, (the risk increasing in the presence of antimicrosomal antibodies and in persons over 65 years of age). Many who seem to have "subclinical" cases, in the final analysis, do not. As many as 32 per cent of treated "subclinical" hypothyroid cases have alleviation of symptoms of hypothyroidism.

HYPOTHYROIDISM CHARACTERIZED BY PAUCITY OR ABSENCE OF THYROID TISSUE (THYROPRIVIC HYPOTHYROIDISM). Thyroprivic hypothyroidism includes postablative hypothyroidism (postexcision or destruction by ^{131}I therapy), primary idiopathic hypothyroidism, and thyroid aplasia or dysplasia (including sporadic athyreotic cretinism). Postablative hypothyroidism occurs eventually in 30 per cent of patients after (subtotal) thyroidectomy, usually within the first year but sometimes much later. In addition to the clinical features and laboratory findings of hypothyroidism, they display, of course, the relevant surgical scar. Hypothyroidism after ^{131}I therapy for thyrotoxicosis may emerge within a few weeks or appear years later, so patients must be followed for life. Postablative hypothyroidism should not be diagnosed too hastily after surgery, as it may occur temporarily, and function may rebound after 1 to 2 months.

Primary idiopathic hypothyroidism is the second most common diagnosis in the thyroprivic category. Women outnumber men, and the incidence is highest during the fifth and sixth decades of life. Most are probably "burned out" autoimmune processes.

ENDEMIC GOITER (IODINE-DEFICIENCY GOITER). Endemic goiter is caused virtually always by dietary iodine deficiency. It has occurred in all parts of the world throughout history, although it is worst in mountainous areas, sparing the sea coasts, where natural sources of iodine exist in seafoods. That only a small number of the population in endemic areas develop the disease suggests that an inherited defect of iodine incorporation in hormone synthesis is an underlying factor in goiter formation. Endemic cretinism occurs in areas where endemic goiter is found. Iodine deficiency may be a cause of *nontoxic goiter,* and individuals may be euthyroid or hypothyroid. Iodization of salt has virtually abolished the disease in North America.

The development of a goiter in association with iodine deficiency comprises the same stages as for other goiters of relative hypothyroidism, beginning with diffuse (hyperplastic) enlargement and proceeding to colloid and multinodular goiter. Early repletion of iodine results in disappearance of the hyperplastic goiter but causes little or no regression of the multinodular goiter.

GOITER DUE TO GOITROGENIC AGENTS. Several drugs in the standard armamentarium are antithyroid and hence goitrous in their effects. They include those designed for the purpose of treating hyperthyroidism (propylthiouracil, methimazole [Tapazole]) as well as lithium, phenylbutazone, topical resorcinol, and the antituberculous drugs para-aminosalicylic acid and ethionamide. Naturally occurring agents may be ingested accidentally but are of little importance except as aggravating factors in areas of iodine deficiency.

THYROID APLASIA/DYSPLASIA. Sporadic cretinism due to congenital athyreotic cretinism is relatively rare. Other cases of congenital hypothyroidism are goitrous and may occur secondary to maternal medication, such as iodine-containing preparations, or as endemic cretinism. The diagnosis must be made during the neonatal period in order to forestall the complete expression of cretinism.

HYPOTHYROIDISM CHARACTERIZED BY DEPRIVATION OF THYROTROPIN (TROPHOPRIVIC). The most common causes of trophoprivic hypothyroidism are postpartum pituitary necrosis (Sheehan syndrome) and other situations of destruction of the pituitary due to hypotension or tumor. The critical factor in making the differentiation between primary and secondary hypothyroidism is the unfailing ordering of TSH whenever hypothyroidism is suspected. Treatment of hypothyroidism without treating the underlying pituitary insufficiency would precipitate adrenal insufficiency.

Laboratory Studies

Table 41–12 enumerates thyroid function tests and their normal ranges. The earliest abnormality in primary hypothyroidism is TSH elevation. Many patients never manifest hypothyroidism but show only an elevated TSH level, stimulating the gland enough to produce adequate thyroid hormone. Some of these patients eventually manifest nontoxic (euthyroid) goiter and others subclinical hypothyroidism. The T_4 test may be elevated and T_3 uptake depressed in the absence of thyroid pathology if any factor increases the thyroxine-binding globulin (TBG), such as estrogen or progesterone therapy and pregnancy. Testosterone, glucocorticoids, cirrhosis, and the nephrotic syndrome have the opposite effect. The measurement of free T_4 avoids these spurious alterations. Radioactive iodine (RAI) uptake varies depending on the type of hypothyroidism. Thyroprivic hypothyroidism shows a depressed RAI uptake. With goitrous hypothyroidism the defect is not a lack of glandular tissue but the blockade of hormone synthesis, and the RAI uptake is normal or even elevated.

If the TSH is not appropriately elevated, pituitary-based or trophoprivic hypothyroidism must be considered. CT scan of the sella turcica would be appropriate to gain circumstantial evidence of pituitary disease along with primary assessment of the remainder of the pituitary-endocrine axis, including a serum prolactin level. Most family doctors prefer to consult an endocrinologist at this point, sending a complete report of the problem and an updated work-up.

Thyroid tests, indeed thyroid function, are subject to the vagaries of medications due to their effects on TBG, TSH, and true thyroid function.

TABLE 41–12. THYROID FUNCTION TESTS

Test	Description and Use
Sensitive TSH (immunoradiometric)	Lower limit of detection, 0.1 μU/mL; test of choice in management of hypothyroidism
Conventional TSH (radioimmunoassay)	Lower limit of detection, 1 μU/mL
Total T$_4$	Measures all T$_4$ bound to plasma proteins; concentration varies with changes in plasma proteins
Free T$_4$ index	Estimate of free T$_4$, calculated by multiplying RT$_3$U by total T$_4$; corrects for variations in thyroxine-binding globulin
RT$_3$U	Indirect measurement of thyroxine-binding globulin (the main protein that binds T$_4$)
Free T$_4$ (immunometric techniques)	Influenced by serum levels of lipids, proteins, and certain drugs; some researchers believe it is superior to free T$_4$ index
Free T$_4$ (equilibrium dialysis)	"Gold standard" of free T$_4$ assays
TRH challenge	Measures TSH after thyrotropin-releasing hormone is injected; test has been replaced by the sensitive TSH assay for most purposes
T$_3$ radioimmunoassay	Rarely used in management of hypothyroidism
Antithyroid antibodies, antimicrosome antibodies	Neither sensitive nor specific; used to help determine likelihood of autoimmune thyroiditis and conversion from subclinical to overt hypothyroidism

T$_3$ = Triiodothyronine; T$_4$ = thyroxine; RT$_3$U = resin T$_3$ uptake; TRH = thyrotropin-releasing hormone; TSH = thyroid-stimulating hormone.
From Martinez M, Derksen D, Kapsner P: Making sense of hypothyroidism. Postgrad Med 93(6):135, 1993, with permission.

Table 41–13 lists the more common of these effects.

Management

The preparation most commonly used for thyroid replacement is the synthetic L-thyroxine (Levoxine, Synthroid). It has a half-life similar to that of thyroxine (tetraiodothyronine, T$_4$), requiring about 4 weeks for full effect and about that long to abate. When it was first marketed during the 1960s, 100 μg (0.1 mg) was said to be equal to 1 grain of natural thyroxine. At that time endocrinologists taught that the average thyroid gland produced the equivalent of three grains per day, and that most patients would require about 2 grains to treat hypothyroidism and to suppress TSH in nontoxic nodular goiters. However, both estimates have been revised downward to 2.5 grains of desiccated thyroid and less than 0.15 mg of synthetic T$_4$ in most cases. The older, natural preparation is Thyroid USP (desiccated thyroid) from beef and pork thyroid glands. It is a mixture of T$_3$ (9 μg) and T$_4$ (38 μg) in 65 mg.

Triiodothyronine (liothyronine) is a synthetic preparation that is rapidly absorbed and has a "short" half-life of 2.5 days (Cytomel, Triostat, Thyrar). This preparation is suited to situations in which it may be unsafe to commit the patient to a long-acting preparation from which it would be impossible to quickly withdraw, as for those with angina pectoris. Liothyronine is seldom used for maintenance. Its dosage is up to 75 μg per day—divided in to 12.5- to 25.0 μg increments for a replacement dosage.

For young people with no suspicion of heart disease, treatment is usually initiated with 0.05 mg T$_4$ and raised to 0.10 to 0.15 mg. Rarely is it urgent to achieve the euthyroid state. Table 41–14 lists conservative recommended starting dosage schedules for age and medical conditions, allowing 2

TABLE 41–13. DRUGS THAT AFFECT THYROID FUNCTION TEST RESULTS

Drug	Mechanism
Amiodarone HCl (Cordarone)	Induces hypothyroidism and hyperthyroidism; interferes with T$_4$ metabolism
Corticosteroids	Suppress TSH; decrease thyroxine-binding globulin; block conversion of T$_4$ to T$_3$
Cough medications	Can induce hypothyroidism if preparation contains iodine
Dopamine HCl (Dopastat, Intropin)	Suppresses TSH
Estrogens	Increase thyroxine-binding globulin, falsely increasing total T$_4$ level
Lithium (Eskalith, Lithane, Lithobid)	Induces hypothyroidism by blocking secretion of T$_4$ and T$_3$
Phenytoin sodium (Dilantin)	Interferes with binding of T$_4$ to plasma proteins; decreases total T$_4$ level; may decrease free T$_4$ level
Salicylates	Interfere with binding of T$_4$ to plasma proteins when given in high doses; decrease total T$_4$ level but not free T$_4$ level

T$_3$ = triiodothyronine; T$_4$ = thyroxine; TSH = thyroid-stimulating hormone.
From Martinez M, Derksen D, Kapsner P: Making sense of hypothyroidism. Postgrad Med 93(6):135, 1993, with permission.

TABLE 41–14. RECOMMENDED STARTING DOSES OF L-THYROXINE FOR HYPOTHYROIDISM

Criteria	Initial Dose (μg/day)
Age <50 with primary hypothyrodism	100
Age 51–65 without coronary artery disease	50
Age <50 with secondary hypothyroidism	50
Age >65 and all patients with coronary artery disease	25

From Drug Therapy Newsletter (Carolinas Medical Center, Department of Family Practice) 5(26):2, 1993, with permission.

weeks between increments of 25 μg. Because 3 weeks or more are required for full absorption, the therapeutic effect is gradual. Dosage is titrated to normalization of the T_4 level and ultimately to TSH. The capability of lower limit TSH assay allows close observation for subclinical iatrogenic hyperthyroidism, most important in older patients and those with conditions such as CAD, heart failure (CHF), angina, and osteoporosis.

Thyroid hormone is cleared more rapidly as metabolism increases with treatment, so the dosage required may increase. T_4 should be remeasured after several months in order to keep abreast of such requirements. Elderly people clear thyroxine slowly and should be started on lower dosages and reassessed every 2 months during the first 6 months of therapy. Early responses to therapy are increased energy, increased mentation, diuresis, return of reflex speed, and recovery.

Rapid treatment is necessary only in patients with myxedema or severe hypothyroidism and acute infection. The latter may lapse into coma when sepsis supervenes. When haste is necessary, liothyronine (T_3) may be used at a schedule of 25 μg q 8 hr. Alternatively, 500 μg of L-thyronine is given intravenously. In these circumstances, glucocorticoid support is given, as chronic low metabolism has often resulted in a sluggish TSH response to stress, and adrenal insufficiency may intervene.

Key to the treatment of cretinism of the newborn is rapid correction of the serum T_4 level to 10 μg/dL (130 nmol/L) and maintenance of this level for the first 4 years in order to avoid permanent mental retardation. Of course the treatment should be maintained indefinitely. An acceptable starting dosage is 50 μg of T_4 per day.

Nontoxic Goiter (Euthyroid Goiter, Simple Goiter)

The toxic goiters are a fascinating group of disorders that share a variety of causes of inefficient (not deficient) hormone production or trophic stimulation, which causes hyperplasia of the thyroid without stimulating excessive hormone production. Many are characterized by defective conversion (iodination) of T_3 to T_4. The conditions included here are those for which there are no known external agents. They occur overwhelmingly in women, in a ratio of 8:1.

Most simply stated these goiters begin with a phase of hyperplasia in response to TSH stimulation, responding in turn to a relative lack of thyroxine. A diffuse goiter forms that enlarges with time but regresses when TSH is suppressed by thyroid hormone. Patients presenting with diffuse enlargement are more likely to be in their twenties or thirties.

After a variable time areas of hyperplasia develop into nodules that are hyperplastic and actively produce hormones. Patients presenting with nodular goiter are likely to be over 50 years old and may have had undetected diffuse goiters for long periods. Up to this point the patient is eumetabolic but goitrous, and TSH may be elevated. Later, degrees of autonomy may develop within certain nodules, but the gland remains generally under the control of the pituitary. Most patients remain stable at this stage, but some fall behind in thyroxine production, becoming hypothyroid (goitrous hypothyroidism). There may be a further stage of development wherein a hyperplastic nodule or nodules develop autonomy (adenomatous hyperplasia) and, producing thyroid hormone in excess, result in toxic nodular goiter.

Physical examination reveals diffuse or nodular thyromegaly. There is much inaccuracy in the description of the thyroid by palpation when findings are compared to those at surgery. A diffuse goiter can be confused not only with a nodular goiter but with Graves' disease, especially if the latter is not in toxic exacerbation and does not have ophthalmic manifestations. The best differentiating factor is the laboratory finding of TSH receptor antibodies. Individuals with Hashimoto's thyroiditis exhibit antithyroid antibodies.

Laboratory Findings

Serum T_3 and T_4 concentrations are normal. RAI uptake is generally normal but may be slightly elevated despite other indications of a euthyroid state. TSH may be elevated in the young person with simple diffuse goiter but is usually normal with nontoxic nodular goiter.

Treatment

For the young person with *diffuse goiter* and elevated TSH, thyroid therapy alone (0.1 to 0.15 mg daily) suffices to reduce TSH to normal and effects regression of the goiter. With *nontoxic nodular goiter*, suppression can be tried, particularly if the TSH level is higher than 0.5 mU/L. Follow-up is necessary to observe the status of metabolism and goiter size. If the goiter is a problem of space occupancy (airway, comfort), of cosmetic significance, or found to be autonomous, ^{131}I may be the treatment of choice. Situations requiring differentiation of these finer points are infrequent in primary care practice and may warrant endocrinologic consultation.

Thyroiditis

Thyroiditis is classified differently by different authorities. The following categorization facilitates differentiation of these conditions clinically and pathologically.

Acute Thyroiditis

Acute thyroiditis (acute pyogenic thyroiditis), a bacterial infection, is a rare condition usually found in women ages 20 to 40. Only 224 cases had been reported as of 1983. The gland is normally resistant to bacterial infection, and these cases are associated with nodular goiter (50 per cent), thyroglossal duct, internal fistulas, external wounds, or perhaps immune compromise. The symptoms and signs are those of suppurative disease (acute onset, dolor, tumor, rubor, calor, fluctuance, leukocytosis). Transient measurable elevations of T_4 or RAI uptake may occur. Treatment is antibiotics and incision and drainage if needed.

Subacute Thyroiditis

Subacute thyroiditis occurs in two varieties. One is a viral disease, which often has an acute and painful course. Called granulomatous thyroiditis, painful thyroiditis, or de Quervain's thyroiditis, it has been associated with a variety of viruses, including mumps. There appears to be a genetic predisposition to an abnormal immune response. Two thirds of white and Chinese patients share the HLA type Bw-35. Eighty per cent of those affected are women (Singer, 1991). A key difference between acute and subacute thyroiditis is the occurrence of hypermetabolism in 50 per cent of cases of subacute granulomatous thyroiditis due to release of preformed T_4, which is elevated out of proportion to T_3. RAI uptake is depressed during the period of inflammation owing to failure of iodine incorporation. The erythrocyte sedimentation rate is elevated, as a sine qua non, usually above 50 mm per hour. The course is 2 to 4 weeks of varying severity and up to 6 months of less severe symptoms. Five per cent of these patients may be left with hypothyroidism. The treatment is salicylates, other nonsteroidal medications, and sometimes glucocorticoids. The severely hypermetabolic individuals tend to be those who progress to hypothyroidism. However, only 2.5 per cent in one series were left with a goiter.

The other subacute thyroiditis is called by some painless thyroiditis. Most cases occur postpartum, but a few are sporadic. Postpartum painless thyroiditis is probably autoimmune in origin, manifesting an 80 per cent prevalence of autoimmune microsomal antibodies. Many patients present with thyrotoxicosis, and this entity accounts for up to 20 to 30 per cent of the incidence of thyrotoxicosis (Singer, 1991). As with painful subacute thyroiditis, severe cases are apt to progress all the way through the stages that lead to hypothyroidism. Goiter is a more common residuum with the painless than with the painful form, being present in up to 48 per cent, and recurrent hyperthyroidism is found in 11 per cent. Differentiation from Graves' disease is accomplished by finding a depressed RAI uptake in the face of hypermetabolism. The course is self-limited and amenable to treatment with β-adrenergic blocking agents during the hypermetabolic phase and thyroxine replacement if hypothyroidism occurs.

Chronic Thyroiditis

Chronic thyroiditis occurs in two main varieties. *Hashimoto's disease* (struma lymphomatosa) is a common disease that is autoimmune in causation and occurs in subclinical variants (as defined by the presence of autoantibodies); it affects up to 10 per cent of the English population (Singer, 1991). A defect in hormone synthesis results in TSH elevation, which produces glandular hyperplasia similar to other goiter formations. The most common antibodies are thyroglobulin and microsomal antibodies. A genetic tendency is evidenced by associations with HLA B-8, HLA DR-3, HLA DR4, and HLA DR5, as reported by various investigators. The disease may be precipitated by a variety of environmental assaults, including viral infection (as in type I diabetes), bacterial infection (*Yersinia enterocolitica*), and, surprisingly, iodine when it is excessive. Occasionally iodine-induced myxedema occurs with Hashimoto's disease. Ninety-five per cent of patients are women between the ages of 30 and 50 years. Patients usually present with goiter, hypothyroidism (20 per cent), and autoantibodies, though clinical manifestations may be announced more acutely with hyperthyroidism (5 per cent) and autoantibodies.

Early in the course of the disease, RAI uptake might be elevated as a result of the dysfunctional TSH effect of the antithyroglobulin antibodies, though the patient is eumetabolic with normal T_3 and T_4. TSH itself is elevated as a sign of incipient hypothyroidism. Examination reveals most often a firm goiter, usually involving the gland diffusely but on occasion a single lobe or nodule. A rare path of development is Graves' disease. Euthyroid or hypothyroid patients warrant thyroid treatment to suppress TSH and arrest the growth of the goiter. Shrinkage to normal size occurs in only a few cases.

Riedel's thyroiditis (Riedel's struma; "woody thyroid"), is a rare chronic thyroiditis that affects women more often than men (3:1) and presents with a hard consistency and symptoms of unilobar or bilateral mechanical interference with swallowing or the airway. The patient may be euthyroid or hypothyroid, and the cause is unknown. Treatment is surgical if mechanical problems occur. Follow-up in goitrous cases includes determination of TSH to detect incipient hypothyroidism. Riedel's thyroiditis is now thought to be an expression of the group of multifocal idiopathic fibrosis (also called idiopathic inflammatory fibrosclerosing) syndromes, including retroperitoneal and mediastinal fibrosis, sclerosing cervicitis and cholangitis, and orbital pseudotumor ("cerebri"). As such, rarely it has a progressive and even fatal course.

Thyroid Neoplasms

Benign Neoplasms

Nodules may be found during evaluation of a solitary thyroid nodule and are discussed in a later section. They include microfollicular adenoma, macrofollicular adenoma, embryonal adenoma, fetal adenoma, and Hürtle cell adenoma.

Papillary hyperplasia is included for taxonomic reasons. It is essentially the lesion of Graves disease: a diffuse response to thyrotrophic immune globulins that attach to TSH receptors.

Malignant Neoplasms

Although carcinoma of the thyroid is the most common endocrine cancer, it comprises only 1 per cent of the incidence of cancer in the United States, with an overall case fatality rate of about 10 per cent. Table 41–15 lists the properties and distinguishing characteristics of thyroid carcinomas.

PAPILLARY CARCINOMA. Papillary cancer is the most common of the thyroid carcinomas, accounting for 80 per cent. Women are affected more commonly than men (3:1), but the prognosis is worse in men. Those characteristically affected are 20 to 50 years of age, with a worse prognosis during the sixth decade. The risk in children is increased in those who have undergone irradiation to the neck area. The tumors are slowly growing; and though regional node metastasis is present in 30 to 50 per cent at the time of presentation, only 5 to 7 per cent of the tumors metastasize distantly. The prognosis is a more than 95 per cent 20-year survival (or longer). This cancer is commonly found incidentally, is multicentric (or spreads within the gland to many lymphatics before metastasizing), and may be labeled occult when foci are less than 5 mm in diameter. The clinical presentation is usually an asymptomatic euthyroid patient with a self-discovered or incidentally discovered palpable nodular thyroid, thyroid nodule, or cervical lymph node. The RAI uptake discloses a "cold" nodule. Variants of papillary carcinoma according to cell type, architecture, and aggressiveness include columnar cell carcinoma, diffuse sclerosis, and encapsulated papillary carcinoma.

FOLLICULAR CARCINOMA. The follicular variant is often found within elements of papillary carcinoma and appears to arise from that tumor. The female/male ratio is similar to that for papillary carcinoma, and there are several histopathologic characteristics that suggest development from papillary carcinoma. Patients are older at the time of presentation, and there is less regional lymph node spread but more likelihood of hematogenous spread—hence a greater tendency for distant metastases and a poorer prognosis. If categorized according to histologic aggressiveness, the aggressive types have only a 44 per cent 10-year survival, whereas those not as invasive have an 86 per cent survival rate. Again, elderly patients have the worst prognosis. Follicular carcinoma also exhibits a cold nodule on RAI uptake scintiscan, but it does take up some iodine. It manifests TSH responsiveness to a greater degree than papillary carcinoma.

Treatment of Papillary and Follicular Carcinomas. Most of these tumors are treated by thyroidectomy. To the extent that it can be shown that the tumor is TSH-responsive and subject to calculated RAI uptake, it is amenable to therapeutic ^{131}I (100 to 150 mCi). Rarely, L-thyroxine suppression of TSH is the sole treatment and is a necessary part of long-term therapy.

ANAPLASTIC CARCINOMA. The anaplastic tumors are highly aggressive and confer a poor prognosis—a matter of months. Many arise in long pre-existing goiters. They comprise 10 per cent of all thyroid cancers and present with irritative and space-occupying symptoms. Treatment is limited to palliative surgery, irradiation, and experimental chemotherapy.

MEDULLARY CARCINOMA. Medullary tumors constitute 5 to 10 per cent of all thyroid cancers. As a familial condition, it is a concomitant of multiple endocrine neoplasia (MEN): MEN 2A (associated with pheochromocytoma and hyperparathyroidism) and MEN 2B (marfanoid habitus and a variety of neuromas, as well as pheochromocytoma). It also occurs as a non-MEN autosomal dominant disease and as a sporadic type. Arising from parafollicular C cells, it elaborates calcitonin, a normal product of C cells that also serves as a tumor marker. Numerous other substances may be produced, including 5-hydroxytryptamine, adrenocorticotropin, somatostatin, prostaglandins, and carcinoembryonic antigen (CEA). They present with symptoms of a growing space-occupying goiter. Patients should

TABLE 41–15. PROPERTIES AND CHARACTERISTICS OF THYROID NEOPLASMS

Neoplasm	Proportion (%)	Gender Prevalence	Age Range (years)	Prognosis
Papillary Ca	50–80	3:1 F > M	20–60	90% at 20 years
Follicular Ca	10–15	3:1 F > M	40–60	44–80% at 10 years (< aged)
Anaplastic Ca	10	F ≥ M	>50	Poor (months)
Medullary Ca	2–10	F ≥ M	>40	67% to 10 years*

* Eighty per cent of medullary carcinomas occur in sporadic form, 20 per cent are familial, including MEN-2A and MEN-2B.

be evaluated for MEN and relatives screened for calcitonin levels. Treatment is total thyroidectomy.

LYMPHOMA. Lymphoma of the thyroid is rare. It tends to arise within a gland involved with Hashimoto's thyroiditis. The chances of it occurring with Hashimoto's disease are about 0.5 per cent. The presentation is likely to be based on the space-occupying properties, as the tumor is metabolically nonfunctional.

Evaluation of the Solitary Thyroid Nodule

An approach to the solitary nodule encompasses the diagnosis of thyroid carcinoma in general. Fine-needle aspiration biopsy (FNAB) has replaced the large needle biopsy for diagnosis, as the latter is fraught with a high complication rate. Most thyroid diseases can present as a solitary nodule, and many may prove to be the most prominent nodule of a multinodular gland. Although cold nodules (nonfunctioning on RAI uptake scans) are more likely to be carcinoma, only 16 per cent prove to be so. Furthermore, 9 per cent of "warm" nodules (showing the same degree of uptake as the surrounding gland) and 4 per cent of "hot" nodules (taking up iodine and hyperfunctioning to the point where TSH suppression renders the surrounding gland hypoactive) are malignant. The following were the results of 9119 FNABs, which were performed based on the indications recommended in this section: benign tumor 74 per cent, malignant tumor 4 per cent, indeterminate 11 per cent, biopsy inadequate 11 per cent (Mazzaferri, 1993). The use of FNAB as an initial test has reduced the number of surgically explored cases by one half and increased the prevalence of cancer at surgery by 100 per cent. At the Mayo Clinic the sensitivity of FNAB was shown to be 93.5 per cent and the specificity 87 per cent if positive is defined as both frankly malignant and suspicious. Malignant findings are more likely to occur in men than in women (2:1), though women are four times as likely to have goiters. Patients under age 30 and over age 50 are more prone to thyroid cancer than those in the 30- to 50-year age group (2:1 in the younger age and 2.5 rising to 6:1 as age progresses from 50 to 70 years of age). Patients who have a history of irradiation to the neck have a 25 per cent lifetime risk of nodular goiter, of whom 25 per cent develop carcinoma, for a lifetime risk for cancer of 6 per cent. From a different vantage point, risk status of patients with nodular thyroid disease may be categorized as follows, by frequency with chances of malignant tumor.

1. *Low risk*: no suspicious findings, female sex. Proportion of nodular thyroid cases 44 per cent. Chance of malignancy 11 per cent.

2. *Moderate risk*: age less than 20 years or over 60 years, male sex, history of neck irradiation, questionable fixation to tissues or nodule larger than 4 cm. Proportion of nodular thyroid cases 38 per cent. Chance of malignancy 14 per cent.

3. *High risk*: rapid tumor growth, strikingly firm nodule, fixation to local tissues, vocal cord paralysis, or enlarged lymph nodes. Proportion of nodular thyroid cases 18 per cent. Chances of malignancy 71 per cent.

Still, FNAB poses problems when the result is indeterminate, there is insufficient tissue, or the result is normal in the presence of a definite nodule. These findings comprise the category of nondiagnostic results. The dilemma is eased by the use of isotopic scanning and repeated biopsies. Ultrasonography is of greatest help when monitoring the nodularity during suppression treatment with thyroid hormone. The following is a verbal algorithm for management of the solitary thyroid nodule.

I. Solitary (predominant) nodule
   A. If the patient is of moderate or high risk: FNAB
   B. No risk factors: radioisotopic imaging
      1. If nodule is cold or warm: FNAB
      2. If nodule is hot: treat if toxic (hypermetabolic), observe if euthyroid.

II. Results of FNAB
   A. Frankly malignant: surgery
   B. Suspicious: radioisotope imaging (if not already accomplished [see step IB]). If warm or cold: surgery. If hot: treat or observe
   C. Frankly benign
      1. Cystic nodule: if disappears with aspiration, observe; if persists and is more than 4 cm in diameter, surgery; if less than 4 cm, observe
      2. Solid nodule: suppressive therapy, periodic physical examination, repeat FNAB at 1 year
   D. Indeterminate (after immediate repeat with several aspirations in different areas of the nodule)
      1. Option 1: if low risk status, suppressive therapy and repeat FNAB in 6 months
      2. Option 2: if high or moderate risk, surgical exploration
   E. Insufficient material (or normal tissue): repeat within a brief time period. If repeats show "normal" tissue on three occasions: suppression therapy for 6 months and re-evaluate if low risk; exploration if high or moderate risk.

Euthyroid Sick Syndrome

"Euthyroid sick syndrome" is a semijargon term for the combination of aberrated thyroid function tests in various states of illness or with medication in euthyoid individuals. It occurs because of such factors as a change in secretion, distribution, and metabolism of thyroxine and subnormal fractions of thyroxine-binding proteins with the illness. Up to 70 per cent of euthyroid patients have depressed T_3 (which may also be normal in 20 to 30 per cent of hypothyroid patients). The T_4, free T_4, and free T_4 I index are often affected and may be spuriously slightly elevated with mild illness and are mildly depressed in 50 per cent of patients with critical illness. TSH may be elevated in chronic illness or during the recovery phase of acute illness. The negative thyroid diagnosis is elucidated by the discordance of TSH and T_4 findings for either hyper- or hypothyroidism.

DISTURBANCES IN CALCIUM AND PHOSPHATE

Ninety-nine per cent of total body calcium is contained within the bones in a dynamic state of equilibrium; the extracellular and cellular fluids make up the remainder. Serum calcium is controlled by bone metabolism, intestinal absorption, and renal excretion as orchestrated by $1,25(OH)_2$ cholecalciferol (vitamin D_3), parathormone (PTH), and calcitonin. PTH affects each of the foregoing in a manner that raises serum calcium with vitamin D as an agent. Calcitonin operates to lower serum calcium, particularly in favor of bone formation. PTH operates mainly by feedback in response to a falling serum calcium level and a rising serum phosphate.

Hypercalcemia

The most common causes of hypercalcemia are primary hyperparathyroidism and hypercalcemia due to malignant disease. Together they comprise 68 per cent of the cases of hypercalcemia. Table 41–16 lists the main causes of hypercalcemia and their relative proportions.

TABLE 41–16. CAUSES OF HYPERCALCEMIA

Diagnosis	Percent of Cases
Malignancy	34.4
Hyperparathyroidism	34.2
Hypervitaminosis D	12.2
Hyperthyroidism	3.9
Milk-alkali syndrome	3.9
Immobilization	2.3
Idiopathic	0.9
Sarcoidosis	0.9
Dysproteinemias	0.6
Addison's disease	0.6
Laboratory error	13.4

From Schmidt N: Hyperparathyroidism: A review. Am J Surg 139:657, 1980, with permission. Published by American Family Physician, Kansas City, Missouri.

Clinical Manifestations

As the calcium level rises to 20 per cent above normal (13 mg/dL [3.24 mmol/L]), patients complain of nonspecific symptoms such as fatigue, difficulty in mental concentration, headache, depression, muscle weakness, and constipation. As the calcium rises to 14 to 15 mg/dL (3.5 to 3.7 mmol/L), psychiatric symptoms, nausea, vomiting, stupor, and coma may occur. Also there are complaints of myalgias; and the more direct sequelae of hypercalcemia give rise to polyuria (leading to renal insufficiency), polydipsia, nephrolithiasis, and bony pain symptoms. Gastrointestinal symptoms associated with peptic disease can occur.

HYPERCALCEMIA DUE TO MALIGNANT DISEASE. With cancer, hypercalcemia is due to one of the following mechanisms: (1) lytic bone metastases, with or without a humoral factor causing increased bone resorption (e.g., breast, renal cortical carcinoma, lung); (2) hematologic dyscrasias (e.g., multiple myeloma, certain lymphomas and leukemias), resulting in either or both "punched-out" lytic lesions of bone or osteoporosis; or (3) humorally mediated bone resorption (humoral hypercalcemia of malignancy [HHM]). The latter occurs in the absence of bone metastases and is due to a PTH-related protein (PTH-RP) elaborated by the tumor. These patients may present with symptomatic hypercalcemia as the main problem. The serum calcium rises faster and higher than in primary hyperparathyroidism. Hypercalcemia of malignancy is likely to present with (total) serum calcium of 14 mg/dL (3.5 mmol/L) or higher.

Table 41–17 gives a helpful breakdown of historical and laboratory findings in cancer versus PHPT. Hypercalcemia due to malignancy is favored by several findings: a more acute onset, an elevated alkaline phosphatase, and hypochloremic alkalosis (hyperchloremic acidosis favors primary hyperparathyroidism).

PRIMARY HYPERPARATHYROIDISM. Primary hyperparathyroidism (PHPT) is characterized by hypercalcemia, hypophosphatemia, and osteitis fibrosa cystica caused by autonomously secreted excess PTH, reflected in an elevated PTH assay. It occurs much more commonly than was believed 25 years ago. Some now cite a figure of 100,000 new cases per year, about twice the incidence cited 10 years ago. Hypercalcemia diagnosed as PHPT was found in 1 per 1000 of 26,000 consecutive serum calcium measurements (Aurbach et al., 1992), which would constitute 248,000 cases in the United States. Women outnumber men 2:1. Much of the recent increase in this disease is probably due to asymptomatic cases picked up incidentally as hypercalcemia on multiple-channel chemical profiles.

About 80 per cent of cases are caused by solitary adenomas; 15 per cent by hyperplasia, 4 per cent by parathyroid carcinoma, and 1 per cent from

TABLE 41–17. DIFFERENTIAL DIAGNOSIS OF HYPERCALCEMIA: MAJOR CONSIDERATIONS

Parameter	Malignancy	Hyperparathyroidism
Duration	Acute (recent onset)	Chronic (long history)
Serum calcium	Frequently >14 mg/dL	Usually <14 mg/dL
Serum chloride	Usually <103 mEq/dL	Usually >103 mEq/dL
Anemia	Frequent	Unusual
Serum PTH	Slightly high for calcium level	Quite high for calcium level
Urinary calcium	>400 mg/day	<400 mg/day
Sedimentation rate	Increased	Normal
Alkaline phosphatase	Increased	Usually normal
Weight loss	Marked	Minimal
Serum phosphate	Low, normal, or high	Usually low
Renal stones	Uncommon	Common
Response to steroids	Sometimes effective	Not responsive
Radiographic study	Soft tissue lesions, metastatic lesions	Subperiosteal bone resorption
HCO_3	Normal, high	Normal, low

water cell hyperplasia. Hyperplasia cases are often associated with MEN-I syndrome. Familial cases, with or without the MEN-I syndrome, are associated with hyperplasia in all glands rather than adenoma. Of the MEN-I cases found among those with hyperplasia, Zollinger-Ellison syndrome with hypergastrinemia, gastric hypersecretion, and intractible peptic ulcer disease constitute a small percentage.

The diagnosis is made by the laboratory findings of hypercalcemia, hypophosphatemia, elevated PTH assay, hypercalciuria, and increased urinary cAMP. The symptomatic cases present with an insidious and lengthy onset of weakness, fatigue, headache, weight loss, or depression, perhaps interrupted by an attack of nephrolithiasis or an acute onset of any combination of debility, bone pain, pathologic fracture, or even polyuria, polydipsia, pruritus, anorexia, and vomiting. Rarely an adenoma presents with a nodule in the neck that can be mistaken for a goiter. The presence of hypercalciuria excludes familial hypocalciuric hypercalcemia, a benign condition for which surgery is not indicated.

Treatment comprises surgery to remove the adenoma or all but half of one of the four (or more) hyperplastic parathyroid glands. Several approaches to localize the glands have been tried. Preoperative imaging studies have not proved helpful thus far owing to poor sensitivity and mediocre specificity, though ultrasonography may be helpful. The preponderant opinion of surgeons is that initial surgery is 95 per cent successful. Recurrence of symptoms invokes the difficult decision for re-exploration or exploration of the mediastinum.

OTHER CAUSES OF HYPERCALCEMIA. *Neonatal PHPT* is rare and usually occurs in the presence of familial hypercalcemic syndromes. There exists also idiopathic hypercalcemia of infancy, which tends to be associated with various congenital anomalies.

Secondary hyperparathyroidism is the term given to elevation of PTH secondary to chronic hypocalcemia or hyperphosphatemia. It occurs most frequently in association with renal insufficiency. With renal failure, the syndrome of renal osteodystrophy may include osteitis fibrosa, osteosclerosis, osteomalacia, and osteoporosis. There is a combined effect of elevated PTH, persistent hypocalcemia due to skeletal resistance to PTH, and impaired production of $1,25(OH)_2$ cholecalciferol. Treatment is directed at calcium repletion by exogenous calcium carbonate, use of calcitriol (vitamin D metabolite) to enhance calcium absorption from the intestine, and restriction of phosphates in the diet.

Other nonparathyroid conditions associated with hypercalcemia, such as thyrotoxicosis, vitamin D excess, adrenal insufficiency, milk alkali syndrome, and sarcoidosis, present varying laboratory findings and clinical manifestations as would be expected. Thyroid function tests are elevated in patients with thyrotoxicosis; vitamin D assay is elevated in the presence of hypervitaminosis D (also in PHPT); and serum cortisol depression and hyperkalemia are seen with adrenal insufficiency. The milk alkali syndrome is associated with azotemia, a lack of hypercalciuria, and a history of excessive intake of sodium bicarbonate. Thiazide diuretics may cause hypercalcemia.

Neonatal hyperparathyrodism is often associated with a family history of familial hypocalciuric hypercalcemia and is due to hyperplasia of the parathyroids. It must be considered in infants with failure to thrive (hypotonia, poor feeding, constipation, and respiratory distress). Failure to diagnose the disorder results in 50 per cent first-year mortality. *Idiopathic hypercalcemia of infancy* presents with hypotonia and constipation. It may result in nephrocalcinosis and renal failure.

Treatment

Laboratories vary in methodology and stated limits of normal. This discussion uses normal limits of the total (in contrast to ionized) serum calcium level of 9.0 to 11.0 mg/dL (2.2 to 2.74 mmol/ L). Ionized serum calcium concentrations are useful if hypoalbuminemia is present. Note that Table 41–16 indicates that laboratory error accounts for 13.4 per cent, thereby warranting repeated testing of all newly discovered elevated levels. In a hospitalized population, the most common cause of hypercalcemia is cancer, whereas in an outpatient population it is PHPT. The former is chiefly a therapeutic problem, whereas the latter is one of diagnosis.

The cancer patient with hypercalcemia presents a therapeutic challenge, often an emergency. The polyuria of hypercalcemia is secondary to the effects of calcium on the kidney and leads to relative dehydration. The mainstay of emergency treatment of this condition is rehydration/diuresis, employing up to 3000 ml normal saline or more given intravenously per day along with the diuretic furosemide. Other measures suited to the acute situation include glucocorticoids for treating some tumors, myeloma, hypervitaminosis D, sarcoidosis, milk-alkali syndrome, and of course Addison's disease; indomethacin for certain prostaglandin-secreting tumors, calcitonin, and mithramycin. These measures can reduce the serum level by 1 to 2 mg/dL per day and can have dramatic effects on the patient's clinical condition. Table 41–18 outlines the main tenets of therapy.

The underlying cancer must be treated appropriately. The hypercalcemia can be managed during the acute phase while efforts are made to treat the underlying cancer. The long-term treatment of hypercalcemia involves biphosphonates (i.e., etidronate [Didrone]) or judicious use of the medications previously mentioned.

Hypocalcemia

The symptomatology of hypocalcemia is due to a paucity of ionized calcium (4.0 to 4.6 mg/dL, 1.0 to 1.5 mmol/L). Hypocalcemia is caused by: (1) failure of stimulus for maintenance of serum calcium (insufficiency or ineffectiveness of PTH or vitamin D); (2) losses from the serum exceeding the capacity of PTH and vitamin D to reverse; or (3) decreased capability of bone, via resorption, to respond to the maintenance stimuli of PTH or vitamin D.

Clinical Manifestations

The most sensitive and earliest *symptoms and signs* of hypocalcemia are usually neuromuscular, and they rarely occur unless the ionized calcium level drops below 3.2 mg/dL, usually equivalent to a total calcium level of 7.5 mg/dL, unless they are due to hyperventilation. In the latter case the total calcium may be normal but shifted from ionized to bound based on alkalosis. Paresthesias and muscle spasms and weakness are followed by tetany. The Chvostek and Trousseau signs are positive at this point, and reflexes are hyperactive. These two signs may be positive in the face of hypokalemia as well as hypocalcemia, and they may be the presenting picture of such syndromes as primary aldosteronism (discussed under Disorders of the Adrenal Glands, below). It is important to know the baseline status of the patient, as some manifest Chvostek's sign as a normal variant. Psychiatric symptoms of irritability, anxiety, depression, confusion, psychosis, and dementia may intrude. Seizures occur with severe or prolonged hypocalcemia.

TABLE 41–18. TREATMENT OF HYPERCALCEMIA

Therapy	Usual Dose	Indication	Comment
Fluids	3000 ml/day or more	Serum calcium greater than 12.0 mg/dL; give rapidly I.V. if stuporous	Use 0.9% NaCl if given I.V.; monitor cardiac status and electrolytes, especially serum K
Furosemide	80 mg q 2 hr	Add when fluids given rapidly	
Phosphate	Oral: Neutraphos 2 caps q.i.d. IV: 1500 mg P over 6–8 hr	Serum calcium >12 mg/dL in symptomatic patient with normal renal function and serum P < 5 mg/dL	Keep P > 5.5 mg/dL. May take several days to show maximum effect: poor gastrointestinal tolerance
Prednisone	10–60 mg/day	Responsive tumor or sarcoidosis	May take a week for response
Indomethacin	25 mg q.i.d.	Responsive tumor	Effective in 8 hours. May be ineffective after two or more doses.
Calcitonin	2 μg/kg SC	Acute hypercalcemia	Effective within 8 hours
Mithramycin	25 μg/kg I.V.	Failure of or contraindication to other therapies	Effect may last for days. Effective in 48 hours. Monitor renal and liver function, WBC, BUN, SGOT, platelets
Hemodialysis		Renal failure	

At the severe end of the spectrum, cardiovascular signs become significant and may be life-threatening: hypotension, bradycardia, QT and ST prolongation, impaired contractility, digitalis insensitivity, and cardiac arrest. These sequelae usually do not appear until the hypocalcemia is well below 3.2 mg/dL.

Lowered or ineffective PTH results in less resorption of calcium from bone, decreased reabsorption from the renal tubules, and inadequate intestinal calcium absorption. Though primary (idiopathic) hypoparathyroidism is rare (usually due to an autoimmune process), the identical picture develops after extirpation of the glands. Furthermore, the parathyroid glands fail to function in the face of *hyper-* or *hypomagnesemia* (reversible by treatment of the magnesium aberration), sepsis, burns, and pancreatitis. It may be present after parathyroidectomy, intentional or accidental. Pseudohypoparathyroidism is an example of ineffective PTH action (abnormal receptors). Most of the findings of hypoparathyroidism are due to the combination of hyperphosphatemia and hypocalcemia, irrespective of the PTH level. A characteristic of hypoparathyroidism, primary or secondary, is soft tissue calcifications, which can ultimately involve ocular lenses, causing cataracts, or the basal ganglia, resulting in extrapyramidal symptoms. A diagnosis of *primary hypoparathyroidism* is based on the findings of hypocalcemia, hyperphosphatemia, and normal renal function; and it is confirmed by abnormal PTH assays.

The actions on the gut of *vitamin D* and related metabolically active products (calciferols) are complementary to PTH and more powerful, causing increased calcium absorption. Thus hypovitaminosis D is a potent cause of hypocalcemia. In bone the action of the calciferols contrasts with that of PTH in that it effects mineralization (calcification) of osteoid (PTH causes calcium to depart from bone via resorption). Lack of vitamin D is the specific cause of the unique bone disease, rickets in children, and osteomalacia in adults. Impairment of vitamin D (production or effectiveness) may be due to renal disease—(lack of conversion from 1-OH-cholecalciferol to 1,25-$(OH)_2$-cholecalciferol, by far the most active calciferol), a nutritional cause (intake or malabsorption), liver disease, sepsis, or hypomagnesemia.

Loss of calcium from serum in excess of the capacity for correction by PTH and calciferols occurs in *clinical situations of precipitation of calcium*. It may be caused by citrate in blood (chelation), pancreatitis (which impairs PTH as well), hyperphosphatemia (which produces its reciprocal effect on calcium partly by driving it into nonosseous tissues), or rhabdomyolysis, which results in release of phosphate. Hypocalcemia due to decreased bone resorption occurs with hypothyroidism and after the pharmacologic effects of calcitonin, *cis*-platinum (which induces hypomagnesemia), diphosphonates, and mithramycin.

Neonatal hypocalcemia is an acute condition of the first few days of life, associated most often with immaturity. Hypocalcemia during the second week of life is also associated with prematurity and is caused by hyperphosphatemia secondary to immature kidneys retaining phosphates ingested in cow's milk.

Treatment

For purposes of following hypocalcemia in the hospital, it is best for calcium to be measured as the ionized form. Hypocalcemia can be divided into mild (3.2 to 3.9 mg/dL [0.8 to 0.9 mmol/L]) and severe (<3.2 mg/dL [<0.8 mmol/L]). Some believe there are theoretic reasons *not* to treat mild hypocalcemia. They have to do with the vulnerability of tissues to calcium in the presence of ischemia or sepsis. Patients at this level are usually asymptomatic.

Patients who are symptomatic or have levels of ionized calcium below 3.2 mg/dL should be treated by intravenous infusion of 100 mg elemental calcium within 5 to 20 minutes. This dose is followed by a continuous infusion of 0.5 to 2.0 mg/kg per hour (35 to 150 mg per hour for the average adult). Oral intake of calcium tablets and vitamin D or calcitriol is appropriate for long-term use.

Hypophosphatemia

Hypophosphatemia is defined as serum levels of *inorganic phosphorus* below 0.8 mg/dL (0.26 mmol/L). Clinical features include muscle weakness, paresthesias, cranial nerve palsies, tremors, and confusion. Chronic hypophosphatemia is defined as inorganic phosphorus levels below 1.5 mg/dL (0.5 mmol/L). It occurs in situations of severe illness and rapid influx of phosphate into the cells, such as occurs in acute diabetic acidosis under treatment or remineralization of "hungry bone" after treatment of hyperparathyroidism.

PITUITARY DISORDERS

The pituitary gland represents a magnificent coordinator of external signals and internal responses to those influences. It closely interacts with the nervous system. In turn, the pituitary controls many hormonal responses that regulate biochemical and metabolic activities throughout the body. An efficient feedback control system exists under normal circumstances. The pituitary receives neurosecretory signals directly or via the hypophyseal portal system.

Neurosecretory cells in the hypothalamus secrete a variety of peptides and neurohormones that reach the pituitary. Clinically, the important ones include vasopressin, a nonapeptide with water-conserving activity; oxytocin, which stimulates uterine and mammary duct contractions; and specific factors that induce anterior pituitary cells to secrete hormones. Thyrotropin-releasing hormone, for example, stimulates the secretion of thyrotropin. Likewise, corticotropin-releasing factor, luteinizing hormone releasing hormone (LHRH), and growth hormone-releasing hormone (GHRH) control secretion of specific anterior pituitary hormones. Inhibitory peptides also are released that depress hormone secretion, such as prolactin-inhibiting factor, or somatostatin.

The posterior lobe of the pituitary is associated with the control of water excretion because of the presence of vasopressin or antidiuretic hormone. It also contains oxytocin. The anterior lobe of the pituitary gland contains the cells that synthesize and secrete the major hormones, corticotropin (ACTH), thyrotropin, luteinizing hormone, follicle-stimulating hormone, and prolactin. ACTH and related products are responsible for melanocyte stimulation. Obviously, deficiency of these hormones, an excess of one or more of them, or abnormalities in the region of the pituitary can cause clinical manifestations. Those likely to be encountered in clinical practice are discussed primarily.

Hypopituitarism

A variety of pathologic changes can result in deficient pituitary hormone production. They include head trauma, genetic disturbances, tumors, infections, histiocytosis, granulomas, autoimmune processes, and vascular incidents.

Clinical Manifestations

The clinical features are dependent on which hormones are affected, the age of the patient, and the anatomic area of involvement. An anterior pituitary tumor or peripartum hemorrhage with hypotension causing Sheehan syndrome does not often cause diabetes insipidus. Likewise, lesions in the posterior pituitary or the hypothalamus that result in diabetes insipidus may not affect the trophic hormones at all. Hypothalamic disorders may have little or no effect on usual endocrine functions but may present with hyperphagia, obesity, anorexia, emotional symptoms, somnolence, hypothermia, or hyperthermia.

The classic clinical manifestations of deficient pituitary hormone production relate to a lack of major hormonal effects. A mother may find that she cannot nurse her infant after Sheehan syndrome because of prolactin deficiency. Clinical features of growth hormone deficiency are dependent on the age of the patient. Idiopathic or GHRH deficiency presenting at birth results in decreased *velocity* of growth. The infant has a normal birth weight because growth hormone is not needed in utero for growth and development. Delayed bone age is observed. The child has normal proportional extremity to body height. If the growth hormone deficiency occurs after growth is completed, there are relatively few symptoms. Some patient have decreased muscle mass, and symptoms of hypoglycemia may more easily occur.

Gonadotropin deficiency results in symptoms and signs in both children and adults. Kallmann syndrome, which is present at birth, represents a condition of isolated LHRH deficiency, hyposmia, and usually incomplete formation of the olfactory lobe. Growth progresses normally, but there is delayed bone maturation and epiphyseal closure. Thus the extremities become longer relative to the total body height. There is delayed or arrested pubertal changes with gonadotropin deficiency. If gonadotropin deficiency occurs after puberty, clinical features in women include amenorrhea, infertility, decreased libido, and atrophic vaginal and breast changes. If gonadotropin deficiency is secondary to a prolactin-producing tumor, breast tissue is preserved or increased. In men the clinical manifestations are more subtle and gradual. Facial hair growth decreases; impotence, complete or partial, occurs; there is fine wrinkling of the skin; and the testicles become softer and smaller than normal. The man tends to become passive, and muscle mass may decrease.

Lack of thyrotropin and ACTH results in symptoms similar to those described for hypothyroidism and adrenal insufficiency. With ACTH deficiency, however, the hyperpigmentation seen with Addison's disease is absent. Also, body fluid volume and blood pressure are better preserved because mineralocorticoid secretion is maintained by other stimuli. Women tend to lose their secondary sexual hair, and both sexes may have pale complexions.

Other clinical manifestations may accompany pituitary insufficiency. General weakness, fatigue, and lack of energy are relatively common complaints. If a mass is responsible for the disease, the patient may have headaches, cerebrospinal fluid rhinorrhea, visual field defects, and cranial nerve palsies.

Diagnosis

The principal diagnostic issue is to differentiate between primary or secondary hormonal deficiency. The clinical presentation is helpful in most cases, but testing for specific hormones is necessary. The common approach in endocrinology (i.e., if a hormone deficiency is suspected) is to measure the hormone, stimulate it, then measure it again; this approach is particularly appropriate here.

A combined anterior pituitary test has been developed based on intravenous injection of several releasing factors sequentially over about 20 seconds. The respective trophic hormones are measured, as are the hormones from the target organ. It is an expensive test and best performed with a consulting endocrinologist. Pituitary imaging by CT or MRI is helpful. Skull films, which were used formerly to measure sella enlargement, are simply not adequate today. Visual field examination can detect defects that are not obvious by the usual physical examination.

Human growth hormone (hGH) concentrations fluctuate and preclude an accurate diagnosis by a random measurement. There is considerable overlap between normal and abnormally low values. hGH levels increase during deep sleep and in response to exercise, estrogen, hypoglycemia, and amino acid stimuli. Several provocative tests can be used to compare a basal hGH concentration with a stimulated level. An insulin tolerance test utilizing 0.1 unit/kg body weight is infused, and a blood sample is obtained every 15 minutes over the next hour. hGH concentrations normally peak at approximately 45 to 60 minutes. Failure to stimulate hGH is good evidence for pituitary insufficiency. Glucose levels and close clinical monitoring are needed to avoid marked hypoglycemia. Many clinicians avoid ordering this test if plasma cortisol levels are less than 5 μg/dL. Arginine 0.5 g/kg or 30 gm for adults infused over 30 minutes also normally produces a peak hGH value at about 1 hour. Levodopa by mouth, clonidine, glucagon, or exercise are other provocative tests. Insulin-like growth factor 1 may be low in hGH deficiency, but it is also low in the presence of malnutrition.

The hypogonadotropic state is confirmed by finding low luteinizing hormone (LH) and follicle-stimulating hormone (FSH) levels in the presence of low testosterone or estradiol concentrations. In the untreated postmenopausal woman it is easy to estimate pituitary function because the LH and FSH levels should be elevated. Stimulation by LH releasing factor results in an increase in LH and FSH if the pituitary cells are functional, but that test does not rule out a deficiency of hypothalamic releasing hormone as the etiology of the hypogonadotropin hypogonadism. Clomiphene (Clomid) has been used to stimulate LH and FSH levels. Gonadotropin measurements are variable in premenopausal women, and the phase of the menstrual cycle must be known to properly interpret test results. Hyperprolactinemia may depress gonadotropin levels; therefore prolactin should also be measured.

Whenever hypothyroidism is diagnosed, one should measure the thyrotropin (thyroid-stimulating hormone, TSH) level to determine whether it is primary or due to TSH deficiency. Low T_4 and TSH levels are virtually diagnostic of a hypothalamic or pituitary cause of the disease. Thyrotropin-releasing hormone stimulation with measurements of TSH and T_4 concentrations provide additional information. A low plasma cortisol level accompanied by a decreased ACTH concentration is also good evidence of a hypothalamic or pituitary cause of adrenal insufficiency provided the person

is not taking steroids. The metyrapone test is commonly used to test for ACTH reserve. Metyrapone 750 mg q 4 hr for 1 day in adults blocks an enzymatic step in cortisol production, thereby causing the pituitary to increase ACTH production if it is capable of doing so. Measurement of 17-OH steroids or compound S shows an increase with an intact pituitary adrenal axis (17-OH steroids increase at least twofold). If the pituitary is abnormal, the increase does not occur. The adrenal itself must be functioning normally, which can be confirmed by an ACTH stimulation test as described in the section on Addison's disease.

Treatment

Adequate replacement therapy exists to treat hypopituitary states. Either the deficient pituitary hormone or the hormone that it stimulates is replaced. Commercial growth hormone is now synthesized in contrast to previously pooled hormone from human pituitaries. Thus it is relatively safe and effective. A dose of 0.3 mg/kg per week is injected as 0.1 mg/kg three times a week. After the first couple of years, it is often necessary to give the hormone more frequently to sustain normal growth. It has not been customary to give growth hormone to adults as replacement therapy.

Treatment of hypogonadotropic hypogonadism depends on the circumstances of the patient. A man who is not interested in fertility may be given testosterone enanthate 100 to 200 mg IM every 3 weeks. A woman may be given cyclic therapy with an estrogen such as Premarin (conjugated estrogens) 0.6 mg, plus medroxyprogesterone 5 to 10 mg during the third week, or a contraceptive tablet containing ethinyl estradiol 30 μg. These treatments produce pubertal changes, maintain secondary sexual characteristics, and allow normal sexual functions. If fertility is required, hormones that stimulate the testes or ovary must be used after sexual maturation has been achieved. Human chorionic gonadotropin (hCG) is available in vials of 5000 IU or 20,000 IU. Therapy is individualized preferably with the help of an endocrinologist, and then menotropin (Pergonal: 75 IU of FSH plus 75 IU of LH) is added to promote spermatogenesis or ovulation. Long-term pulsatile administration of LHRH with a portable infusion pump or LHRH intranasally is best monitored by a specialist. Bromocriptine therapy is frequently effective in patients who have elevated prolactin levels with secondary gonadotropin deficiency. Adrenal insufficiency secondary to ACTH deficiency is treated with steroid replacement: hydrocortisone 20 mg in the morning and 10 mg in the evening or prednisone 5 mg in the morning and 2.5 mg in the evening. For stressful events, supplemental doses should be given, or 100 mg of hydrocortisone intramuscularly can be used. It is prudent to recommend that the patient wear a MedicAlert bracelet. Likewise, thyroid replacement is recommended rather than TSH injections for thyrotropin deficiency. The average dose in adults is approximately 0.1 to 0.125 mg per day, or 1.6 μg/kg ideal body weight.

Diabetes Insipidus

A deficiency or absence of vasopressin results in polyuria and the inability to adequately concentrate the urine. Most of the fluid presented to the proximal convoluted tubule of the kidney is reabsorbed without change in osmolality. In the loop of the Henle the tubule is impermeable to water. As the hypotonic fluid enters the distal convoluted tubule and the collecting duct, water is reabsorbed if vasopressin (antidiuretic hormone, ADH) is present. If not, dilute urine is excreted. Thus the kidney must be responsive and the thirst mechanism intact to maintain normal water homeostasis (Baylis, 1992). Urine output by the normal kidney can increase to almost 20 liters per day.

Vasopressin secretion is stimulated mainly by an increasing plasma osmolality. Specialized osmoreceptors in the hypothalamus sense change in the osmolality and initiate signals for thirst as well as vasopressin release. The syndrome of diabetes insipidus occurs when vasopressin is deficient. There are many causes, including head trauma, idiopathic, genetic, and destructive lesions.

The diabetes insipidus may be transient (e.g., after trauma or surgery). If the hypophyseal stalk is disrupted relatively low, vasopressin can maintain water balance even if the posterior pituitary is entirely destroyed.

Clinical Manifestations

The onset of symptoms is frequently abrupt, occurring spontaneously or after some trauma. There is great polyuria, nocturia, and thirst. A patient a The Ohio State University vividly described his severe thirst, which had its onset during an automobile trip. Normal at the beginning of the trip, he noted that he had to stop almost every hour to urinate and drink any type of fluid that he could get. Ice cold water satisfied him the most. He completed his hunting trip ingesting large amounts of water, beer, and soft drinks. Milder forms of the disease exist. Cortisol or thyroid hormone deficiency may ameliorate symptoms because of changes in glomerular filtration rate or vasopressin release by nonosmotic signals. Growth can be impaired in children if they learn that eating less than normal amounts of food reduces the solute load to the kidney and lessens symptoms of diabetes insipidus.

Diagnosis

One must differentiate excessive water intake and nephrogenic diabetes insipidus from the true form. The diagnostic work-up need not be complicated. If a 24-hour urine output is less than 3 liters and the plasma osmolality and sodium level are normal, diabetes insipidus is unlikely. A history of emotional illness or neurologic disorders suggests polydipsia as the cause of symptoms.

If necessary, a dehydration test is done followed by an injection of vasopressin to assess renal responsiveness. A reasonable protocol may consist of the following: The patient is weighed, and the basal plasma and urine osmolality are determined. Fluid is withheld for 8 hours, and the patient is weighed every 1 to 3 hours; the plasma and urine osmolality determinations are then repeated. If weight loss exceeds 5 per cent of basal body weight, the test is stopped. An injection of vasopressin or 2 μg of desmopressin is given intramuscularly, and the plasma and urine osmolalities are measured at 8 and 16 hours. The patient is permitted to eat and drink reasonable amounts after the injection. Most individuals with excess water intake reach plasma osmolalities of almost 300 mosm/kg and show some rise in urine osmolality before the injection. If urine osmolality after dehydration is 300 mosm/kg or less and does not rise after vasopressin, nephrogenic diabetes is diagnosed. A response to vasopressin of 600 to 800 mosm/kg indicates diabetes insipidus. Plasma vasopressin is measured if the test is available, with a rise after dehydration favoring a normal reaction or a nephrogenic etiology and subnormal levels suggesting diabetes insipidus. In patients with long-standing excess water intake, the results may be ambiguous and require additional testing.

Treatment

So long as a person has an intact thirst mechanism and water is available, treatment may not be necessary. However, severe polyuria requires therapy simply to improve the quality of life and for convenience. Desmopressin is much more potent than the vasopressin previously used. It can be given intranasally 10 μg per day or less frequently. Correction of nephrogenic diabetes insipidus requires correction of the underlying condition (e.g., hypokalemia or hypercalcemia). A thiazide diuretic or indomethacin may decrease urinary output in patients with nephrogenic diabetes insipidus of unknown etiology.

Hyperpituitarism

Excessive production of pituitary hormones is mainly due to an abnormal negative feedback involving the hypothalamus, pituitary tumors, or ectopic hormone production. Most clinical entities are due to macroadenoma or microadenoma ($<$ 10 mm diameter). It is convenient to consider these endocrinopathies by the hormone that is secreted excessively.

Hyperprolactinemia

Prolactin measurement has been possible only since the 1970s. Hyperprolactinemia is therefore a relatively recently recognized disorder; it is the most common disorder of pituitary hormones. Prolactinoma comprises more than one fourth of tumors found in the pituitary. Women are more apt to have a prolactinoma than men. Other causes of elevated prolactin levels include drugs, especially dopamine receptor antagonists, renal failure, liver disease, manipulation of the nipples, and diseases of the hypothalamus-pituitary region that disrupt normal control by prolactin-inhibiting factors.

Clinical manifestations are variable and depend on the cause, the degree of excessive secretion of prolactin, and the age and sex of the patient. Drug-induced elevation of prolactin may be associated with galactorrhea, or it may be asymptomatic. Prolactinomas may cause a mass effect with headaches, or visual field defects may be present. Galactorrhea occurs in more than half of patients with adenoma. Women may have amenorrhea or other symptoms related to estrogen deficiency. In men there can be decreased libido, infertility, and rarely galactorrhea. Impotence is common with prolactinoma, and a small percentage of impotent men are found to have a prolactinoma upon investigation.

DIAGNOSIS. One or several samples of blood can be obtained to measure the prolactin level. If it is elevated, the clinician must determine if the etiology is a prolactinoma, idiopathic, or secondary to other causes. Values of prolactin higher than 200 ng/ml favor a prolactinoma, but patients with idiopathic hyperprolactinemia or those with the empty sella syndrome may have similar levels. A good history and physical examination helps rule out other causes. Imaging the pituitary gland with MRI or CT is valuable. Some microadenomas cannot be visualized, but most are. The MRI is more efficient for visualizing tissues surrounding the pituitary, but either technique seems adequate.

TREATMENT. Treatment most frequently is pharmacologic, although irradiation or surgery is needed in some people. Obviously, if the hyperprolactinemia is drug-induced or due to neurogenic stimuli, proper advice can be offered. Bromocriptine 2.5 mg three times a day has been proved to give gratifying results—decreasing the prolactin levels, reducing the size of some tumors, and restoring gonadal function. Higher doses of the drug are sometimes needed. Surgical treatment, if required, is best performed by a transsphenoidal approach. Good results can be expected, particularly if there is a microadenoma present. Large tumors are more difficult to cure, and a greater chance of postoperative hypopituitarism exists. Radiotherapy is an option that is not used as frequently as in the past.

Acromegaly

Growth hormone excess is almost always due to a pituitary adenoma. These lesions comprise about 13 per cent of pituitary tumors. A few cases of acromegaly are due to hypersecretion of GHRH; rarely is ectopic GH secretion the cause. The incidence of acromegaly is about 3 per million. It is a slowly progressive disease causing features to change and producing disability by its effects on virtually all organs and tissues. GH secretion is pulsatile, with values tending to peak during sleep. It increases the production of insulin-like growth factor (IGF-1).

Clinical manifestations appear gradually, and they are striking. Headaches, visual field defects, and symptoms related to a pituitary mass may develop if the tumor is large. More often there is a gradual onset of coarse facial features, an increase in glove and foot size, prognathism, separation of the front teeth, arthralgias, and thickened tissues. Later the patient notes a deepening of the voice, spade-like hands, thickened heel pads, exaggerated nasolabial folds, increased sweating, and fatigue. Nerve entrapment syndromes are common; and amenorrhea, impotence, galactorrhea, and infertility may appear as other anterior pituitary functions become impaired.

Hypersecretion of hGH during the growth years results in gigantism. Remarkable heights result from years of hGH stimulation before epiphysial closure take place. hGH causes insulin resistance, and about one fourth of acromegalic patients also develop diabetes mellitus. Hypertension is common.

DIAGNOSIS. The characteristic appearance of a person with acromegaly should lead to prompt biochemical confirmation of the disease. hGH concentrations are usually elevated, but they may also be within the normal range. A 24-hour sampling should reveal that hGH levels are increased at least twofold. Glucose normally suppresses hGH secretion. The failure of hGH to decrease to less than 2 μg/L in response to a glucose tolerance test is highly suggestive of acromegaly. Serum IGF-1 concentrations are consistently elevated in acromegalic individuals. Radiographic imaging with CT or MRI is valuable for the diagnostic work-up. The adenomas tend to be large and may extend beyond the sella.

TREATMENT. Treatment is directed toward removing the adenoma, reducing hGH secretion to normal or below, and preserving anterior pituitary function. It is desirable to remove the adenoma by a transphenoidal surgical approach, but it is not always possible to do so. It is important to refer the patient to an experienced neurosurgeon. Cure rates have been less than 50 per cent with large adenomas extending beyond the sella. Irradiation by a proton beam using heavy particles has produced encouraging results, but only a few medical centers have the equipment and facilities for that therapy. Irradiation by a linear accelerator delivering about 4500 cGy is an option, but reduction of hGH is slow, pituitary insufficiency is relatively common, and hGH remains higher than desirable in some patients. Somatostatin given two or more times per day at doses of 50 to 100 μg (Sandostatin) can produce beneficial responses in almost one half of patients, but it is an expensive treatment.

Responses to treatment can be monitored by measuring IGF-1 levels. Early treatment is desirable because it may produce regression of the coarse features. Untreated or undertreated acromegaly places the person at risk for hypertension, congestive heart failure, diabetes, other tumors, and progressive musculoskeletal disabilities.

Cushing's Disease and Other Pituitary Adenomas

Corticotropin-producing adenomas account for about 10 per cent of pituitary tumors. Approximately 25 per cent of tumors are nonfunctional and are mainly chromophobe adenomas. Gonadotropin-secreting adenomas account for fewer than 10 per cent of pituitary adenomas, and thyrotropin-secreting tumors are rare.

Craniopharyngioma is not a tumor arising from pituitary cells. It is an embryonic Ratheke's pouch tumor derived from cell rests of the craniopharyngeal canal. In addition to growth failure, symptoms arise from increased intracranial pressure with headaches and visual symptoms. Like other masses in the region of the pituitary, it can produce hormone deficiencies. Craniopharyngioma is an infrequent cause of sexual precocity during childhood. The usual recommended treatment of craniopharyngioma is surgical removal via craniotomy.

Corticotropin-secreting tumors are usually associated with abnormal corticotropin-releasing hormone (CRH) stimulation. The clinical manifestations of this disease are discussed under Disorders of the Adrenal Gland, below. Transphenoidal surgery to resect the adenoma is usually recommended. Irradiation of the adenoma over a 5-week period, delivering about 4500 Gy, is prudent if adrenalectomy has been done to relieve the Cushing syndrome. This regimen diminishes the probability that Nelson syndrome will develop. The syndrome is characterized by an aggressive pituitary tumor developing in about 20 per cent of patients with Cushing's disease presumably by the continued stimulation of pituitary cells by CRH. Symptoms and signs of a mass appear with local extension and a characteristic pigmentation due to high ACTH levels. The diagnosis is confirmed by imaging with MRI or CT and a markedly elevated ACTH concentration. A few such patients respond to bromocriptine, but surgery or irradiation is usually required.

Gonadotropin-secreting adenomas have been described only since the 1970s. Some chromophobic adenomas thought to be non-hormone-producing have been shown to produce gonadotropin. Adenomas have developed secondarily in patients with untreated hypogonadism. LH and LHRH are inhibited by estrogen (in women) and testosterone (in men). In women FSH is inhibited by progesterone and in men by inhibin, secreted by the testes. LHRH, if uninhibited, stimulates gonadotropin-secreting cells, producing hyperplasia or an adenoma. Clinical features are primarily related to the mass, with headaches, visual symptoms, and the crowding out of other trophic cells. Testicular size and consistency are normal or increased, which would be unexpected if the patient had hypogonadism. The diagnosis is established by imaging techniques as well as finding FSH, LH, or both elevated in the presence of normal testosterone or estrogen levels.

Thyrotropin-producing adenoma is a rare cause of hyperthyroidism. Treatment is surgical if the mass effect produces symptoms. Rarely a hypothyroid individual who is untreated or undertreated may develop an adenoma of thyrotopin-producing cells, but replacement thyroid hormone therapy can reduce the tumor.

Syndrome of Inappropriate Secretion of Antidiuretic Hormone

The syndrome of inappropriate secretion of ADH (SIADH) is not necessarily due to an abnormally high vasopressin or ADH level. If even low secretion of ADH continues despite hypotonicity of plasma, it is "inappropriate" or unregulated secretion (Bartter, 1973). The syndrome is one of hyponatremia and hypotonicity of plasma, with continued action of vasopressin on renal tubules resulting in water reabsorption. In that circumstance ADH should be almost completely inhibited, so hypotonic fluids are excreted as urine.

The clinical features of SIADH are lethargy, headache, and weakness developing when the serum sodium declines below approximately 120 mEq/L. As hyponatremia worsens, profound disorientation, seizures, and coma may develop.

The diagnosis depends on finding hyponatremia, low plasma osmolality, and relative hyperosmolality of the urine. Urine sodium is inappropriately high for the abnormally low levels in the plasma. The differential diagnosis includes ectopic production of ADH or similar peptides by a tumor, administration of such drugs as chlorpropamide, or a variety of conditions involving the central nervous system (CNS), lungs, or hormonal deficiencies such as Addison's disease and hypothyroidism. Trauma or hemorrhage also can stimulate vasopressin secretion.

Restricting water intake to about 500 ml per day is usually sufficient to gradually improve plasma sodium concentrations and osmolality. A *slow* infusion of 3% sodium chloride solution can be infused if cerebral symptoms and signs are worsening and if hypervolemia is not present. Treatment of the underlying disease, if present, is the definitive approach.

DISORDERS OF THE ADRENAL GLANDS

Adrenal Cortex

The adrenal gland is at least two functional endocrine organs that happen to exist within the same capsule, the cortex and the medulla. The cortex consists of three functional units that are related intimately by virtue of their overlapping control mechanisms emanating from the pituitary. The zonae fasciculata and reticularis synthesize glucocorticoids and androgenic steroids, respectively. These zones, fasciculata more than reticularis, are under the direct control of the anterior pituitary and adrenocorticotropic hormone (ACTH). Negative feedback from rising cortisol levels has most of its direct effect on the hypothalamus to produce less corticotropin-releasing hormone (CRH), which is the main driving force on the pituitary to produce ACTH. Cortisol produces a lesser degree of negative feedback on ACTH. Stress results in stimulation of ACTH production independent of CRH.

The zona glomerulosa comprises the outermost 15 per cent of the cortex and produces aldosterone, the main mineralocorticoid, which is responsible for maintaining blood volume through sodium and hence water retention in the renal tubule. Histologically, it is interdigitated with, rather than clearly demarcated from, the fasciculata, which forms 75 per cent of the cortex and where occurs the production of cortisol, the main glucocorticoid. The remaining 10 per cent of the cortex is constituted by the reticularis, which is clearly separated from the fasciculata and which produces the minor adrenal androgens dehydroepiandrosterone (DHEA), its sulfate DHEAS, androsterone, and small amounts of the estrogens estrone and estradiol. The anatomic intimacy of the three layers is germane when one considers that primary adrenal insufficiency or excess is usually caused by conditions that affect all three layers. Secondary adrenal insufficiency or excess is due to pituitary or hypothalamic processes that affect mainly the fasciculata or reticularis (or both), leaving aldosterone virtually unaffected. Inborn errors of metabolism tend to involve any combination of the three functions, as most of the enzymes are involved in hormone production in all three zones. Figure 41–5 shows the enzymes involved in the production of the adrenocortical hormones.

Aldosterone production is normally controlled by the renin-angiotensin system activated by volume/pressure and sodium concentration sensors in the juxtaglomerular apparatus as well as by neurogenic influences. Mineralocorticoid sequelae may result from abnormal cortisol or androgen synthesis, and cortisol itself has a weakly mineralocorticoid effect.

Cortisol production is controlled by ACTH and other by-products of its precursor, all of which have melanocyte-stimulating capabilities. They are subject to negative feedback from serum cortisol levels and positive feedback from falling cortisol levels, and they are in turn stimulated by CRH and arginine vasopressin.

Control of the production of sex steroids in the

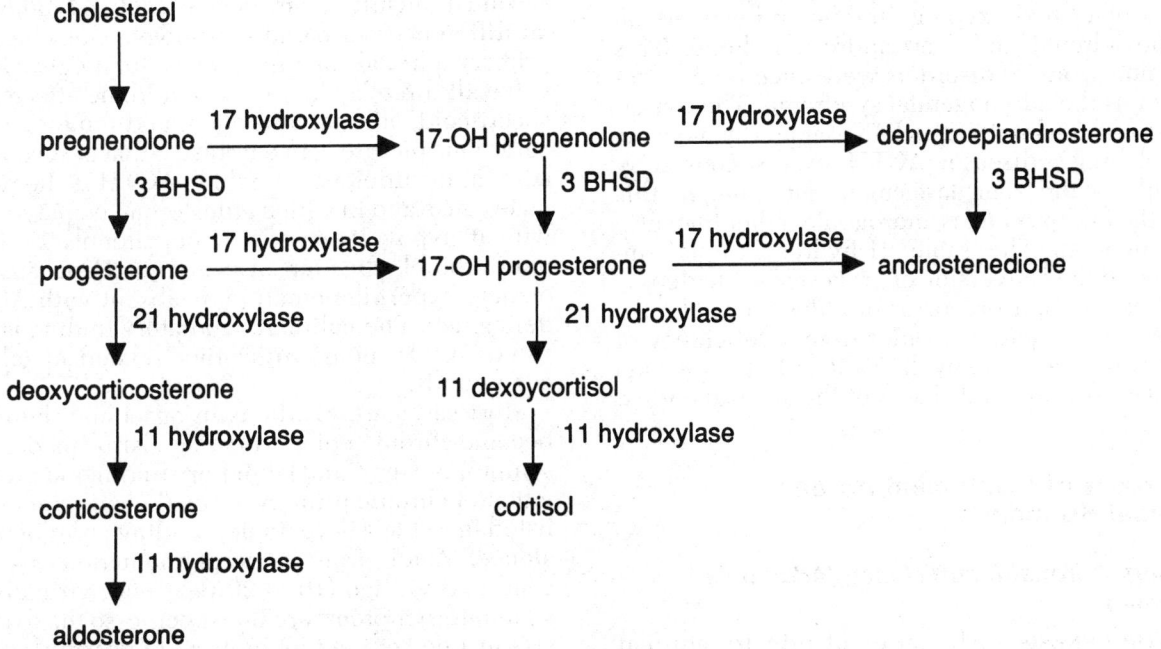

FIGURE 41–5. Production pathways for adrenocortical steroids. (Modified from Orth DN, Kovacs WJ, DeBold CR: Williams Textbook of Endocrinology, 8th edition. Philadelphia, WB Saunders Company, 1992.)

TABLE 41–19. CLASSIFICATION OF DISEASES OF THE ADRENAL CORTEX

Disorders of insufficiency of adrenal cortical hormones
  Primary adrenal insufficiency due to destructive processes (Addison's disease)
  Secondary adrenal insufficiency due to insufficiency of ACTH; aldosterone unaffected
  Tertiary adrenal insufficiency (due to decreased CRH effect on pituitary ACTH production)
  Isolated aldosterone deficiency (inborn metabolic errors; hyporeninemic hypoaldosteronism; as acquired primary aldosteronism of many types)

Disorders of excess of adrenal cortical hormones
  Cushing syndrome
    ACTH-dependent (Cushing's disease and ectopic ACTH syndrome)
    ACTH-independent (adrenal adenoma and adrenal carcinoma)
    Medication-induced
  Primary hyperaldosteronism
  Congenital adrenal hyperplasia

reticularis is less well understood, but ACTH plays a role, as do other pituitary hormones. Most virilizing effects of the adrenals are a result of metabolic errors of glucocorticoid production.

The cyclopentano-perhydrophenanthrene, or "steroid," nucleus promulgates overlapping clinical syndromes when their products are involved in metabolic errors. An example is congenital adrenal hyperplasia due to deficiency of 21-hydroxylase resulting in the defective conversion of 17-hydroxyprogesterone to 11-hydroxycortisol, the precursor of cortisol. This form of congenital hyperplasia results in virilization. The lack of adequate cortisol production results in stimulation of ACTH production, which in turn promotes buildup in the fasciculata of 17-hydroxyprogesterone and conversion to the adrenal androgen androstenedione. This common group of disorders were once lumped together as the adrenogenital syndrome. The hyperplasia comes about in much the same way it occurs in Cushing's disease: ACTH excess constantly stimulates the zona fasciculata, although in this case the end-product is androgenic rather than glucocorticoidal. The same 21-hydroxylase is employed in the conversion of progesterone to deoxycorticosterone, a precursor of aldosterone; hence some of these patients suffer from a deficiency of mineralocorticoid as well. Table 41–19 presents the classification of diseases of the adrenal cortex.

Disorders of Insufficient Adrenal Cortical Hormones

Primary Adrenal Insufficiency (Addison's Disease)

PATHOGENESIS. All causes of primary adrenal insufficiency are necessarily bilateral. From the time of its first description by Thomas Addison in 1849 until tuberculosis was brought under control, bilateral involvement by this infectious disease was the most common cause of adrenal insufficiency. As tuberculosis prevalence waned, so did the incidence of primary adrenal insufficiency; and the relative proportion of cases caused by autoimmune processes assumed the majority position, around 75 per cent. Tuberculosis declined to 20 per cent of cases (Orth et al., 1992). The remaining 5 per cent are due to malignant tumors (bilateral metastases) or hemorrhage. About 50 per cent of autoimmune cases are associated with other autoimmune endocrinopathies. The more common constellation of these endocrinopathies, polyglandular autoimmune syndrome II (PGA II), is one which the associated syndromes tend to be diabetes type I and Hashimoto's thyroiditis (sometimes Graves' disease). The female/male prevalence is nearly 2:1. PGA I is rare, begins during childhood, and includes hypoparathyroidism. The essential pathologic picture is that of lymphocytic infiltration.

Bilateral involvement with infectious agents or cancer is not unusual because of the rich blood supply, which accommodates blood-borne pathologic processes. However, because of the ability of the cortices to function with only little of their original volume of tissue, the clinical significance of such involvement is not as prominent as in autoimmune disease, which indeed may destroy the cortices entirely. The opportunistic infections of acquired immunodeficiency syndrome (AIDS) are now included in the infectious causes of adrenal insufficiency.

CLINICAL MANIFESTATIONS. The symptoms and signs of this disorder are different from those of secondary insufficiency because of two fundamental differences in pathophysiology. The causes of primary adrenal insufficiency virtually always involve all three layers, so the syndrome affects glucocorticoid, adrenal androgen, and mineralocorticoid. This picture is in contrast to that of secondary adrenal insufficiency in which ACTH is the proximate cause and in which aldosterone is spared, and with it hypovolemia and hyperkalemia. Furthermore, the classic sign of primary adrenal insufficiency, hyperpigmentation, is absent with ACTH deficiency. The hallmark laboratory finding is elevated ACTH along with other related metabolic compounds.

Most cases are insidious in onset and therefore become chronic before the diagnosis is made. The symptoms, signs, and laboratory findings at presentation of chronic primary adrenal insufficiency are listed in Table 41–20, in descending order of prevalence. Aside from hyperpigmentation (94 per cent) and vitiligo (10 to 20 per cent), virtually all signs and symptoms are nonspecific, so the diagnosis must be kept in the forefront of possible causes in all chronically ill patients. On the other hand, sensitivity is near 100 per cent for decreased en-

TABLE 41-20. MAJOR SYMPTOMS, SIGNS, AND LABORATORY FINDINGS IN PATIENTS WITH CHRONIC PRIMARY ADRENAL INSUFFICIENCY

Parameter	Frequency (%)
Symptom	
Weakness, tiredness, fatigue	100
Anorexia	100
Gastrointestinal symptoms	92
Nausea	86
Vomiting	75
Constipation	33
Abdominal pain	31
Diarrhea	16
Salt craving	16
Postural dizziness	12
Muscle or joint pains	6–13
Sign	
Weight loss	100
Hyperpigmentation	94
Hypotension (systolic blood pressure <110 mm Hg)	88–94
Vitiligo	10–20
Auricular calcification	5
Laboratory Finding	
Electrolyte disturbances	92
Hyponatremia	88
Hyperkalemia	64
Hypercalcemia	6
Azotemia	55
Anemia	40
Eosinophilia	17

From Orth DN, Kovacs WJ, DeBold CR: The adrenal cortex. *In* Williams Textbook of Endocrinology, 8th ed., Philadelphia, WB Saunders Company, 1992, with permission.

ergy, anorexia, and weight loss so these characteristics may be viewed as essential to the diagnosis, with pigmentary changes being nearly so. Therefore anyone in whom pigmentary change is coupled with fatigability, anorexia, and weight loss should be seen as having primary adrenal insufficiency until proved otherwise.

A low physiologic threshold results in pigmentation more on sun-exposed zones, rubbed areas such as under belts and brassiere straps, dorsi of flexed joints such as the knees and elbows, and areas of chronic inflammation. The latter accounts for hyperpigmentation in the oral mucosa at sites of gingivitis. In dark-skinned people mucosae may darken without physiologic provocation. The seeming ironic occurrence of vitiligo signifies the autoimmune form of adrenocortical destruction.

Variable gastrointestinal symptoms are proportionate to the severity and acuteness of the disease. Vomiting and abdominal pain are relatively common. Hypovolemia due to sodium loss as a result of hypoaldosteronemia is the basis for orthostatic lightheadedness and hypotension and occurs before the onset of persistent hypotension. Salt or ice craving is common, but only 16 per cent are sensitive (Table 41–20); nor is this sign specific, being present with other causes of chronic hypovolemia and anemia.

LABORATORY FINDINGS. Laboratory and other ancillary findings begin with the definitive abnormally low level of cortisol (normal 8 to 24 μg/dL [220 to 660 nmol/dL]), which in primary adrenal insufficiency is unresponsive to ACTH stimulation. A fasting level of cortisol below 10 μg/dL is suspicious, and 5 μg/dL or lower is presumptive of adrenal insufficiency. Given the width of diurnal variations in cortisol under physiologic conditions, a screening serum level alone may not be definitive for ruling out the disease unless a morning specimen shows a level of 25 μg/dL or above; otherwise, the 1-hour ACTH stimulation test is necessary. One hour after obtaining blood for basal (morning) cortisol and ACTH levels, 0.25 mg ACTH is infused intravenously. The cortisol level should rise by more than 10 μg/dL or any value be equal to 25 μg/dL in order to rule out adrenal insufficiency. If the cortisol level fails to rise by 10 μg/dL, adrenal insufficiency is present; based on this test alone it may be judged to be either primary or secondary, as atrophic adrenals (e.g., in long-standing secondary insufficiency) do not reliably respond to this dose of ACTH. However, if the corticotropin level in the basal sample was higher than 100 pg/dL (20 to 100 pg/dL, 4 to 22 pmol/L) the diagnosis is primary insufficiency. If cortisol levels rise only moderately, one can resort to much longer ACTH stimulation tests to stimulate secondarily atrophic adrenal cortices and differentiate them from primarily deficient adrenals.

Hyponatremia and hyperkalemia are present in most cases of primary adrenal insufficiency (Table 41–20) as a result of aldosterone deficiency. Hyperkalmia does not occur as a result of secondary adrenal insufficiency. Azotemia is of the prerenal pattern, the blood urea nitrogen being elevated out of proportion to serum creatinine, as a result of hypovolemia. Adrenal insufficiency is a cause of organic hypoglycemia, so unexplained fasting hypoglycemia should raise the suspicion. CT scanning may show normal or small adrenals bilaterally in autoimmune disease or enlargement in granulomatous or malignant processes.

TREATMENT. The acute syndrome may be precipitated in previously undiagnosed chronic patients by stress or surgery, or the chronically ill undiagnosed patient may slip into adrenal crisis "announced" by hypotension and abdominal pain. Emergency treatment consists of replacement with intravenous glucocorticoid, four doses repeated every 6 to 12 hours depending on the preparation, and infusion of normal saline as dictated by blood pressures and cardiac status. Dexamethasone 4 mg IV has the virtue of not interfering with cortisol measurements. This is important because the evaluation of adrenal function includes the measurement of cortisol before and after ACTH administration. We recommend that hydrocortisone not be given intramuscularly, as it is absorbed erratically.

Though mineralocorticoid is started early, it does not affect volume repletion for the first few days.

Maintenance therapy for Addison's disease consists in an equivalent of cortisone acetate 25.0 to 37.5 mg daily. It may be hydrocortisone 20 to 30 mg per day, prednisone 5.0 to 7.5 mg per day, or dexamethasone 0.5 to 0.75 mg per day, given in divided doses. Some clinicians give a higher dose at bedtime to effect most closely the early morning peak level. Dosage is adjusted upward for heavy patients, failure of symptom response, failure to reverse pigment changes or situations of increased metabolism due to certain drugs such as phenytoin, barbiturates, and rifampin, which inhibit ACTH synthesis.

Mineralocorticoid maintenance, necessary in all patients with primary adrenal insufficiency, is accomplished by fludrocortisone (9α-fluorohydrocortisone), given as 0.1 mg tablets, one daily, titrated against blood pressure, serum potassium, symptoms of postural hypotension, and causes of dehydration (e.g., heat-induced salt and water loss).

In the past Addison's disease was fatal within 2 to 3 years. However, since the availability of hydrocortisone during the 1950s the prognosis of adrenal insufficiency is a normal quality of life and longevity so long as the patient is given maintenance therapy, assuming a treatable underlying cause.

Secondary Adrenal Insufficiency

Secondary adrenal insufficiency is defined as deficiency of ACTH. It is brought about by any destructive process in the pituitary. The most insidious cause is that of a slowly growing pituitary adenoma, previously undiagnosed, that has assumed space-occupying proportions and begins to affect the remaining pituitary hormones. Clinical features and diagnosis are discussed under Pituitary Disorders, above, as well as here.

CLINICAL MANIFESTATIONS. Symptoms vary significantly from those of primary adrenal insufficiency. First, there are no mineralocorticoid sequelae, as the glomerulosa is driven by the renin-angiotensin system rather than the pituitary-adrenal axis. Second, there are no pigmentation changes because such signs are due to ACTH-related pituitary hormones, which, rather than present in excess as in primary insufficiency, are lacking. Third, panhypopituitarism involves, by definition, other trophic hormones such as TSH, FSH, LH, prolactin, and hGH. Therefore patients who are severely weak, with abdominal pain, weight loss, menstrual dysfunction in females (nonspecific to be sure), and typical hypothyroidism, without pigmentary changes, should be evaluated for panhypopituitarism.

DIAGNOSIS AND LABORATORY FINDINGS. The diagnosis is virtually always based on the results of the 1-hour ACTH stimulation test. Baseline cortisol levels are less than 10μg/dL; and if ACTH is less than 20 pg/dL (4 pmol/L), the diagnosis is sec-

ondary or tertiary adrenal insufficiency. If the plasma cortisol level is equal to or more than 20 μg/dL (550 nmol/L) or more at any time in the test, including at baseline evaluation, adrenal insufficiency is ruled out. A basal ACTH level higher than 100 pg (20 to 100 pg, 4 to 22 pmol/L) virtually rules out secondary or tertiary adrenal insufficiency. A CRH stimulation test should differentiate between a pituitary problem (secondary) and a hypothalamic problem (lack of CRH, tertiary adrenal insufficiency). In this test CRH 1 μg/kg body weight is injected intravenously after a 4-hour fast. Blood for cortisol and ACTH assays is obtained at baseline and at intervals of 5, 10, 15, 30, 45, 60, 90, and 120 minutes after the injection. The normal response is ACTH levels that increase twofold to fourfold within 15 minutes after injection and cortisol levels that increase to high normal values (up to 24 μg/dL) at 30 to 60 minutes after injection. Those with adrenal insufficiency secondary to ACTH deficiency have little or no increase in ACTH or cortisol. Those with tertiary adrenal insufficiency have low or inconclusive baseline ACTH levels that increase in exaggerated fashion within 15 minutes after injection and remain elevated longer. Cortisol levels, however, are sluggish in their response owing to a greater degree of atrophy than is found with secondary disease.

TREATMENT. Treatment is the same as for primary adrenal insufficiency except for mineralocorticoid, which is not needed, and attention to the other pituitary-dependent endocrine glands as needed.

Isolated Aldosterone Deficiency

The most common form of isolated aldosterone deficiency is hyporeninemic hypoaldosteronism. By definition, the level of aldosterone is due to low renin levels. Patients present with hyperkalemia or hypovolemia (or both), weakness, and discernible renal failure. The cause has remained elusive. About 50 per cent of patients are diabetic, and 50 per cent are hypertensive. Treatment is oriented to the hyperkalemia and is conservative, attending to diet and medications that do not elevate potassium. Fludrocortisone is reserved for those who are symptomatic, hyperkalemic, and unencumbered with hypertension. The congenital form of hypoaldosteronism, due to an inborn enzyme deficiency, is rare. It is treated with fludrocortisone in the standard doses used for primary adrenal insufficiency.

Disorders of Excess Adrenocortical Hormones

CUSHING'S SYNDROME. Cushing's syndrome is the constellation of symptoms and signs caused by an excess of glucocorticoid hormone. Unless stated otherwise in this discussion, all statistics apply to the Cushing's syndrome that is not induced by medication. If the syndrome is caused by excess

ACTH from the pituitary, the patient has *Cushing's disease,* constituting 70 per cent of Cushing's syndrome. Other causes are ectopic ACTH syndrome (8 to 15 per cent), adrenal adenoma (7 per cent), adrenal carcinoma (8 to 15 per cent of Cushing's syndrome), or factitious or iatrogenic disease (Baker and McFarland, 1990). A reliable screen for virtually ruling out Cushing's syndrome of any cause is a plasma cortisol level 1 hour after sleep equal to less than 5 μg/dL.

Medication-Induced Cushing's Syndrome. Experience from family practice tells us that by far the most common Cushing's syndrome encountered in primary care is iatrogenic. This conclusion is based on the records of patients who have been given therapeutic glucocorticoids such as prednisone or dexamethasone at 5 to 10 times physiologic replacement dosages. Typical indications for such medications are cancer (carcinoma and leukemias) and severe connective tissue diseases (e.g., rheumatoid arthritis, periarteritis, and lupus erythematosus). In these instances the cause is known, the syndrome is immediately recognized, and the symptoms and signs are those of pure glucocorticoid excess, unmixed with effects of androgen trophic hormones from the pituitary.

These cases are of glucocorticoid excess without hyperpigmentation or virilization. The long-term physiologic effects of excess glucocorticoid are net protein catabolism, glucose intolerance, sodium and water retention, and suppression of the inflammatory response. These effects determine the clinical manifestations. History reveals the use of glucocorticoid medications for at least several weeks. The symptoms and signs are truncal obesity with a "buffalo hump" (an effect of the obesity and osteoporosis), relatively spindly extremities (due to muscle wasting), ruddy complexion, moon-like (round) face, thin skin (atrophy due to protein catabolism), and purple striae ("stretch marks" due to weight gain, in about half of patients). Complicating conditions are non-insulin-dependent diabetes mellitus (frequent), hypertension (frequent), and nonhealing infections and abscesses. The laboratory findings are the expected suppression of CRH and ACTH along with occasional hypokalemia and lymphopenia. All medication-induced cases, including that in the uncommon malingerer, manifest these laboratory findings along with a physical absence of androgenizing effects such as hirsutism.

Cushing's Syndrome Due to Neoplasm of the Adrenal Cortex. Adrenal adenoma producing Cushing's syndrome consists of one cell type and as such causes a pure glucocorticoid syndrome as in medication-induced disease. Thus hirsutism and pigmentary findings are absent. Less commonly, the cell type may produce androgenic effects without glucocorticoid excess. Females are more often affected than males. Carcinoma and ad-

enoma are responsible for 22 per cent of cases of Cushing's syndrome (Miller and Crapo, 1993).

Adrenal carcinomas develop rapidly and cause a variety of endocrine changes, ranging from no effect to Cushing's syndrome, virilization, feminization, and mineralocorticoid effects. Virilizing effects include hirsutism and frequent polycythemia. Females are more often affected than males. In children, approximately one half of the cases of Cushing's syndrome are caused by carcinoma.

The laboratory findings are those of plasma cortisol excess, which occurs irrespective of normal diurnal variation and autonomy. Autonomy is demonstrated by failure of cortisol or urinary 17-ketosteroid suppression by dexamethasone and unresponsiveness to physiologic rises in ACTH in the metyrapone test. Carcinomas and adenomas may produce similar test results, but the ACTH stimulation test can help to distinguish between the two. Whereas 60 per cent of adenomas respond to such maximal stimulation by an increased output from baseline plasma cortisol levels, carcinomas do not (Orth et al., 1992).

The metyrapone test is based on the blocking effect of metyrapone on the final step of production of cortisol, resulting in a great increase of the precursors 17-OH-corticosterone and 11-deoxycortisol. The falling cortisol levels normally feed back positively to stimulate ACTH production, resulting in accelerated but side-tracked steroidogenesis and increased plasma precursors. Ectopically produced ACTH does not increase in response to metyrapone. With Cushing's syndrome caused by adrenal tumors, pituitary ACTH is already maximally suppressed, the adrenal tumors would be insensitive to ACTH if it were to rise, and the remaining cortical tissue is likely to be atrophic. Therefore there is no increase in corticotropin or plasma cortisol precursors, except in about half of patients with adrenal adenomas. Thus with CT or MRI evidence of a unilateral adrenal tumor and flat levels of plasma precursors or falling urinary 17-OH-corticosterone in the metyrapone test, the diagnosis is most likely adrenal carcinoma. If other evidence points to hypercortisolism and suppressed ACTH, and if cortisol precursors are increased in the metyrapone test, the diagnosis is probably solitary adrenal adenoma (i.e., ACTH is not maximally suppressed by the tumor and normal cortical tissue or the adenoma is not totally autonomous). Endocrinologic consultation is virtually mandatory at this point, as there is no single test that can in every case differentiate malignant from adenomatous primary adrenal hypercortisolism in the face of dormant ACTH and atrophic adrenal cortical tissue. Urinary 17-ketosteroids tend to be extraordinarily high in patients with adrenal carcinoma.

Radiographic modalities may be helpful. Bilateral adrenal enlargement may be due to hyperplasia, be ACTH-dependent, or be caused by a pituitary or ectopic source. The presence of adrenal

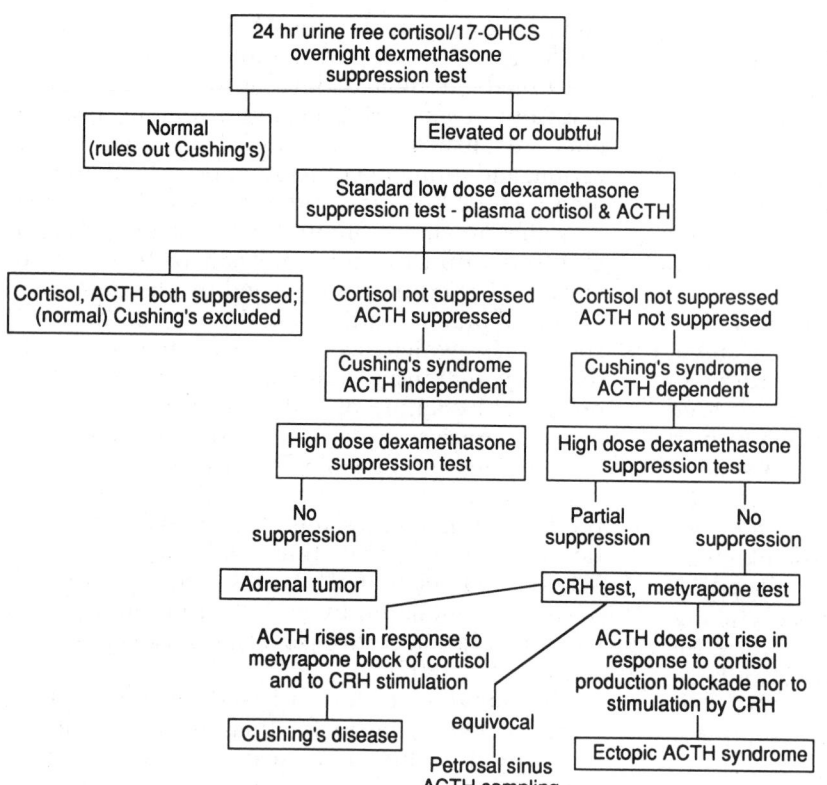

FIGURE 41–6. Evaluation for suspected Cushing's syndrome.

tumor is diagnosable by CT and MRI, but the function (or malignant or benign nature) is often left to surgical exploration and pathologic examination. Figure 41–6 outlines the work-up of suspected Cushing's syndrome.

Surgical resection is the goal. Adenomas—perhaps responsible for more than one third of cases of primary adrenal tumors causing Cushing's syndrome—are virtually always curable. For those with carcinoma, the adrenolytic agent mitotane is initiated prior to surgery to minimize perioperative complications. For those who do not achieve remission, an enzyme inhibitor such as aminoglutethimide or metyrapone is instituted and maintained.

CUSHING'S DISEASE. Cushing's disease is ACTH-dependent Cushing's syndrome caused by excess, inappropriate corticotropin from the pituitary. The oversecretion of ACTH and related products is typically low grade and chronic. It is due most often to microadenomas; fewer cases are due to macroadenomas, and only 4 per cent are associated with diffuse hyperplasia. CRH from the hypothalamus and "intermediate lobe" adenomas are likely causes of hyperplasia (Miller and Crapo, 1993). The symptoms and signs are virtually the same as for other forms of Cushing's syndrome except for statistically increased chances of hyperpigmentation, hirsutism, and virilization.

Laboratory Diagnosis. The earliest plasma cortisol and ACTH findings may be afternoon elevations, even when morning levels remain normal, a departure from the physiologic diurnal variation. The standard screening test continues to be the *overnight dexamethasone suppression test*. Dexamethasone 1 mg is given at midnight, and a blood sample for a plasma cortisol assay is obtained at 8 a.m. If ACTH is suppressible by this amount of dexamethasone, the morning cortisol level is 5 µg/dL or less (140 nmol/L), and the ACTH level is below 20 pg/mL (4.4 nmol/L); ACTH-dependent Cushing's syndrome can then be ruled out. The sensitivity is excellent, but specificity is only 85 to 88 per cent.

If Cushing's disease is suspected and the cortisol level on the overnight dexamethasone suppression test is higher than 5 µg/dL, a 2-day *"low dose" dexamethasone suppression test* should be done. This test consists of administration of 0.5 mg every 6 hours for 2 days. A 24-hour urine specimen is collected for 17-hydroxysteroid, cortisol, and creatinine assays for baseline values and then again after the first 24 hours. The last specimen is to authenticate the 24-hour collection. Normally, the measured ACTH level should be suppressed. The potency of dexamethasone is so great and so little is required that it contributes an insignificant amount to the metabolic breakdown products of cortisol; hence the 17-hydroxysteroids reflect cortisol output. A positive test is failure of 17-hydroxysteroid suppression to less than 4 mg per 24 hours (11 µmol) or a urine free cortisol level of less than 25 mg per 24 hours (68 nmol). A positive (for failure of ACTH suppression) 2-day low dose test virtually ensures the presence of ACTH-dependent hypercortisolism or autonomous adrenal secretion, except for rare false-positive results, which may be due to diabetic states, malnutrition, or emotional or physical stress.

In the case of positive tests, the *high dose dexamethasone suppression test* (2 mg every 6 hours) is used to help differentiate between a pituitary source and an adrenal tumor. ACTH is already maximally suppressed in the presence of an adrenal tumor or an ectopic ACTH source that is unsuppressible. The common Cushing's disease with high but partially suppressible ACTH secretions usually demonstrates 24-hour hydroxysteroid values suppressed to 50 per cent or less of the baseline 24-hour collection.

The preponderance of microadenomas are less than 10 mm in diameter and therefore not seen in plain films of the sella turcica, unlike other clinically significant pituitary tumors. CT scans detect about one third of these adenomas, and MRI does better. Bilateral diffuse adrenal enlargement when present favors ACTH dependence caused by secondary hyperplasia.

Treatment. Once Cushing's disease is diagnosed, 80 per cent of the cases are cured by subtotal transsphenoidal hypophysectomy, with the best statistical results for microadenomas and in children. There is only a 50 per cent cure rate with macroadenomas and an overall 15 per cent cure rate in adults. After initial failure, an additional 8 per cent are cured by irradiation. Mitotane, an adrenolytic agent, controls an additional 10 per cent. The remainder are controlled by adrenal enzyme inhibitors or finally adrenalectomy. Medical treatment of Cushing's disease has been studied, appearing most promising as a combination of pituitary irradiation followed by mitotane maintenance therapy for periods of up to 2 years. "Sustained" remissions (>3 years) have been achieved in approximately 62 per cent. This rate is less favorable than results with surgery but has a place in the management of poor surgical candidates and in the 8 per cent of surgically explored patients who show no evidence of adenoma in the pituitary, 41 per cent of whom do not obtain a cure by subtotal hypophysectomy.

CUSHING'S SYNDROME DUE TO ECTOPIC ACTH. Ectopic ACTH constitutes roughly 15 per cent of cases with Cushing's syndrome. Malignant tumors cause more than 90 per cent these cases. About 50 per cent of the malignant tumors are small cell carcinoma, and the remainder are preponderantly thymomas, pancreatic islet cell carcinomas, medullary thyroid carcinomas, and neural crest tumors. They are typified by high levels of cortisol, metabolic effects including salt retention, and high and unsuppressible ACTH levels. The onset of these symptoms is relatively rapid, per-

haps explaining the fact that the full-blown habitus is unusual.

In the laboratory the 24-hour urine free cortisol level is elevated; the morning ACTH is elevated above 100 pg/mL (not in itself diagnostic); the overnight 1 mg dexamethasone test shows elevated cortisol that is not suppressed; and the elevated 8 a.m. plasma cortisol level is not suppressed on the standard "low dose" or high dose dexamethasone suppression tests. These patients tend to show day to day variations of cortisol and basal plasma ACTH concentrations, overlapping those with Cushing's disease. Metyrapone does not cause an increase in ectopically produced ACTH as it would in pituitary-produced ACTH. CRH does not stimulate an increase in production of ACTH in ectopic ACTH syndrome as it would in Cushing's disease.

Surgical resection of the source of ectopic ACTH is the goal, but most of these tumors are unresectable. They are controlled to varying degrees by adrenal enzyme inhibitors, and most survive only about 1 year. If the patient has a slowly progressive tumor, enzyme inhibitors may be combined with adrenalectomy, and survival may be as long as 10 years.

Primary Aldosteronism

Primary aldosteronism is one of the types of secondary, or nonessential, hypertension, accounting for 0.1 to 1.0 per cent of cases. About 70 per cent are caused by a solitary adrenal adenoma and the remainder, in descending order, are due to bilateral adrenal hyperplasia, rarely unilateral adrenal hyperplasia, and even more rarely adrenal carcinoma (Greenspan and Baxter, 1994). The hallmark of the disease is volume-dependent hypertension (characterized by sodium retention, suppressed renin level, responsiveness to diuretic therapy) with associated hypokalemia.

DIAGNOSIS. The proper initiation of therapy of any kind for hypertension is preceded by several tests and considerations to rule out secondary forms of hypertension. It includes testing the serum electrolytes preferably after discontinuing diuretics for a couple of weeks before determination of serum potassium (K^+). Under these conditions, assuming no other cause for hypokalemia, a cut off point of 4.0 mmol/L is said to be 100 per cent sensitive but only 64 per cent specific (Orth et al., 1992). A cutoff of 3.5 mmol/L is much more specific but purportedly only 85 per cent sensitive (Grekin, 1986), 15 per cent showing K^+ levels between those two limits. Many cases of essential hypertension responsive to diuretics are controllable cases of primary aldosteronism. Specificity is improved by repeated measurement under correct conditions and finding urinary K^+ excretion inappropriately high (> 30 mEq per day). The next screening step is determination of plasma aldosterone and renin levels at 10 a.m. With primary aldosteronism the plasma aldosterone level is elevated and renin is low and unresponsive to low salt diet (< 50 mmol per day). Near confirmation may be accomplished by showing the plasma aldosterone level to be elevated (> 20 ng/dL, 555 pmol/L) and unsuppressed by 5 days of a high salt diet (> 100 mmol per day = 4 gm salt per day).

Adenomas must be differentiated from hyperplasia, as the former can be cured by adrenal resection. Adenomas cause more severe hypokalemia and hypertension, but they cannot be recognized by that alone. They are physiologically unresponsive, whereas hyperplasia is somewhat responsive, showing an increase in aldosterone in response to increased renin, as is produced by upright posture for 3 hours. CT and MRI may elucidate an adrenal mass. Adrenal vein catheterization for lateralization of aldosterone output is one of several measures that can be undertaken with the help of a subspecialist.

TREATMENT. Adrenal adenomas causing primary aldosteronism are treated by resection, whereas the hypertension and hypokalemia associated with primary adrenal hyperplasia respond less well to even total adrenalectomy. If evidence fails to confirm an adenoma, the patient is treated empirically for hyperplasia by the sole use of the aldosterone antagonist spironolactone (Aldactone) at 25 mg q.i.d.

Congenital Adrenal Hyperplasia

Congenital adrenal hyperplasia is a collection of syndromes of adrenal cortical metabolic arrests due to specific enzyme deficiencies. It was once called the adrenogenital syndrome. The first cases were recognized for their in utero virilizing effects on female newborns and their response to treatment (restoration of normal negative feedback to suppress ACTH). In boys they cause precocious puberty, except for those with the rare cytochrome P-450$_{c17}$ (17-hydroxylase) deficiency whose metabolic error causes androgen deficiency, resulting in pseudohermaphroditism. These defects are rare, each inherited as a separate autosomal recessive trait in 1 per 5000 or more births. Deficiencies of three enzymes are discussed: 21-hydroxylase, 11-hydroxoylase, and 17-hydroxylase. A fourth, 3β-hydroxysteroid dehydrogenase (3β-HSD), is rare and usually fatal during infancy.

21-Hydroxylase Deficiency (P-450$_{c21}$ Deficiency)

21-Hydroxylase deficiency is the most common form of congenital adrenal hyperplasia, comprising 90 per cent of this group. The deficiency of 21-hydroxylase results in deficient production of both cortisol and deoxycorticosterone (DOC), a precursor of aldosterone that itself has weak mineralocorticoid activity (Fig. 41–5). The effect is to shunt metabolism toward the androgenic products and to increase production of the progestational precursors of cortisol and aldosterone. It is inherited as

an autosomal gene carried on chromosome 6, so it is associated with certain HLA types. Virilization of female infants results in pseudohermaphroditism ranging from ambiguuous genitalia to incorrect sex assignment. Males may be normal, albeit precocious, or infertile. Milder versions result in adult infertility in women due mainly to gonadotropin suppression by excessive progestogen, which is amenable to hormone therapy. The metabolic blockade is apparently incomplete as the insufficiency of glucocorticoid tends not to be significant. In the severe form there is mineralocorticoid deficiency and salt wasting or hypotension. The diagnosis is made by evaluating patients with the foregoing clinical picture for 17α-hydroxyprogesterone (pregnanetriol) under either basal or ACTH-stimulated conditions. Refinements of diagnosis are left to endocrinologic texts and consultation.

Treatment consists in glucocorticoid therapy exceeding normal adult replacement dosages to suppress ACTH plus mineralocorticoid when it is clinically necessary to address the salt wasting and hypotension. An example is hydroxycortisone 25 mg/m² in divided doses or dexamethasone 0.5 mg/m² nightly to recreate the normal diurnal distribution of glucocorticoid output. Genital malformations are corrected surgically. The main challenge occurs in children and at the transition to adulthood, requiring careful titration of dosages against hormonal and clinical indicators.

11-Hydroxylase Deficiency (P-450$_{c11}$ Deficiency)

11-Hydroxylase deficiency is the second most common form, comprising 5 per cent of congenital adrenal hyperplasia. It is inherited as an autosomal recessive gene. As can be seen from Figure 41–5, cortisol and aldosterone production are blocked when this enzyme is lacking. Again ACTH is relatively free from negative feedback, and the aldosterone precursor deoxycorticosterone builds up. The amount of this weak mineralocorticoid is high enough to produce hypertension. Diagnosis is made by demonstrating elevated plasma 11-deoxycortisol levels. Treatment is similar to that for 21-hydroxylase deficiency except that the precursor to be followed is plasma 11-hydroxycortisol.

17-Hydroxylase Deficiency (P-450$_{c17}$ Deficiency)

17-Hydroxylase deficiency is inherited as a single autosomal recessive trait and is rare. Because this enzyme is required for the production of the adrenal androgenic steroids DHEA and androstenedione, infants are born with androgen deficiency, which takes the form of sexual infantilism in females and pseudohermaphroditism in males. Most of these infants exhibit a mineralocorticoid-generated hypertension, apparently as a result of the increased precursors of aldosterone in the DOC–corticosterone–aldosterone pathway. Diagnosis is based on finding elevated plasma DOC and corticosterone levels and low levels of cortisol and adrenal androgens. Treatment is glucocorticoid suppression of ACTH and estrogen plus progesterone replacement at puberty.

Adrenal Medulla

Pheochromocytoma

Pheochromocytomas are tumors of chromaffin cells that produce epinephrine or norepinephrine, catecholamines that cause the symptoms and signs of adrenergic discharge. Most secrete norepinephrine (NE) despite the fact that 85 per cent of the catecholamine of the normal adrenal is epinephrine. NE-secreting pheochromocytomas tend to stimulate α_1-receptors and cause sustained hypertension. Epinephrine-secreting tumors tend to stimulate α_2-receptors and cause the classic paroxysms of hypertension, headache, and tachycardia. Pheochromocytomas are relatively rare, comprising 0.1 to 0.4 per cent of the causes of hypertension, though epinephrine-secreting tumors may present without hypertension. Ninety per cent of pheochromocytomas occur in the adrenal medulla. Many other statistics fit the "rule of tens": 10 per cent of the total are bilateral, 10 per cent extra-adrenal, 10 per cent familial, 10 per cent malignant. A significant percentage of the familial cases are a part of multiple endocrine neoplasia (MEN) syndromes. MEN-2A is the association of pheochromocytoma, medullary carcinoma of the thyroid, and hyperparathyroidism. MEN-2B is the association of pheochromocytoma, medullary carcinoma of the thyroid, and mucosal neurofibromatosis. Pheochromocytoma is associated also with neurofibromatosis and with retinal cerebellar hemangioblastosis (Von Hippel Lindau disease). Extra-adrenal pheochromocytomas are found in chromaffin tissue, such as the paravertebral ganglia, mostly within the abdomen. However, sites may include pericardium or the bladder, the latter presenting as micturition-precipitated paroxysms of catecholamine symptoms. Extra-adrenal pheochromocytomas produce NE and have a slightly greater probability of malignancy than intra-adrenal tumors.

CLINICAL MANIFESTATIONS. The most common presentations are (1) sustained hypertension; (2) paroxysms consisting of headache, anxiety, tremulousness, tachycardia, and diaphoresis with occasional hypotension; and (3) cardiovascular emergencies including accelerated and malignant hypertension; hypertensive encephalopathy, and symptoms suggestive of myocardial infarction. Orthostatic hypotension or paradoxical recumbent hypotension occurs as a manifestation of hypovolemia, refractoriness of overstimulated α_1-receptors, or vasodilatation caused by α_2-stimulation. Complications include lactic acidosis, myocarditis, and pulmonary edema.

DIAGNOSIS. Pheochromocytoma should be considered but not necessarily screened for whenever hypertension is first diagnosed. Suspicion is heightened if hypertension is present in a setting atypical for essential hypertension, such as young age of onset, lack of a family or personal history of hypertension or diabetes, difficulty of control, presence or family history of any of the MEN-II constellation of diseases, café au lait spots, retinal angiomas, neuromas, or neurofibromas, and the presence of paroxysms as described. *One should not dismiss the possibility of pheochromocytoma in the absence of paroxysms.* Once suspected, a single 24-hour urine specimen is obtained to assay free catecholamines, metanephrines, and the metabolite vanillylmandelic acid (VMA); these tests are reliably sensitive and specific. An exception is the paroxysmally symptomatic case in which the collection may have to be repeated for the 24 hours following a paroxysm if an initial screen was negative. Testing for all three agents diminishes the chances of false values. Normal values may vary with each laboratory, but typically they are as follows: free catecholamines 100 to 150 μg (590 to 890 nmol per 24 hours; metanephrines less than 1.3 mg (7 μmol per 24 hours; VMA 7.0 mg (35 μmol per 24 hours (Wilson and Foster, 1992). For these assays the patient should be devoid of stress (i.e., at rest) and taken off all medication if possible, particularly sympathomimetic drugs and monoamine oxidase inhibitors, to avoid false-positive reactions. Antihypertensive agents are less likely to cause false-negative results. The urine must be kept cold and acidified, and it is tested for creatinine to confirm the 24-hour production.

Provocative tests are no longer used because of the risk of precipitating attacks. Plasma and other blood tests offer poor specificity. Pharmacologic tests such as adrenolytic tests are not applicable in primary care.

Once pheochromocytoma is confirmed, the tumor must be located. CT or MRI of the abdomen is the first step. Other modalities likely to be used in the event the adrenals are normal on CT and MRI are arteriography, venography, and scintigraphy.

TREATMENT. The therapeutic goal is surgical removal after 2 to 4 weeks of control of hypertension and volume repletion. For the 90 per cent that are benign, the cure rate is excellent and survival approaches normal. Care must be taken to avoid β-adrenergic blockade until after α-adrenergic blockade has been achieved in order to avoid precipitation of hypertensive crises due to compensatory α discharge. α-Blockade is effected with phenoxybenzamine (Dibenzyline) 10 to 20 mg t.i.d. to q.i.d., titrating to blood pressure control at or below 160/90 mm Hg and higher than 80/45 mm Hg orthostatically (Bravo and Gifford, 1993). An alternative is the α-adrenergic blocker prazosin (Minipres) 1 to 5 mg t.i.d. to q.i.d.; prazosin causes less reflex tachycardia and orthostatic hypotension. Labetalol and calcium channel blockers may also be used.

Control throughout the perioperative period is critical and involves close invasive monitoring, control of dysrrhythmias throughout induction (often with propranolol), and ensurance of volume replacement, including preoperative whole blood. A nitroprusside drip is commonly used during surgery. It is crucial to control the pheochromocytoma in pregnant women before delivery.

OVARIAN AND TESTICULAR DISORDERS AND RELATED SYNDROMES

Normal Sexual Development

The gonadal ridge gives rise to a primitive gonad by 1 month of gestation. Histologically, the testis is recognizable in the medulla by 7 weeks and the ovary not until 3 months in the cortical portion. The primitive testis produces the antimüllerian factor (AMF) and testosterone. AMF inhibits development of the müllerian ducts, and testosterone promotes development of the wolffian ducts into the vasae deferentiae and the epididymi. Along with the other critical factors intra-abdominal pressure is a requirement for final descent of the testicles into the scrotum during the second and third trimesters. In the absence of AMF, the müllerian ducts persist and develop into the upper third of the vagina, paired uterine horns, and oviducts. In male fetuses Sertoli cells of the testes are under the influence of FSH and are involved in spermatogenesis and inhibin, whereas Leydig cells are controlled by LH and produce testosterone. In the female, oocytes in the developing follicles, under the stimulus of FSH, are surrounded by granulosa cells, which elaborate estrogen and develop after ovulation into the corpus luteum, which produces both estrogen and progesterone during the second half of the cycle under the influence of both FSH and LH.

Adrenarchy, with production of adrenal androgens by a proliferating zona reticularis under the influence of ACTH, precedes gonadarchy and is largely independent. Puberty is initiated by reactivation of the LHRH pulse generator in the hypothalamus, which was last active during fetal and neonatal life. It constitutes an increase in the amplitude and frequency of LHRH up to 60-minute cycles in girls and 120-minute cycles in boys. Gonadotropins from the pituitary respond to the LHRH stimuli and initiate increased production of the sex hormones in the gonads that cause secondary sexual development. Girls begin sexual maturation first with development of breast buds and pubic hair at about 10 to 12 years of age. Menarche follows about a year later. Growth accelerates and peaks between 10.5 and 14.0 years, during which

TABLE 41–21. STAGES OF PUBERTAL DEVELOPMENT IN GIRLS AND BOYS AND THE AGES AT WHICH THEY NORMALLY OCCUR (WESTERN SOCIETY)

Stage	Girls' Ages (years)	Boys' Ages (years)
Growth spurt	10.5–14.0 (peak 12.0)	12.5–16.0 (peak 14)
Menarche	10.0–16.5 (mean 13.0)	—
Breast development		
Thelarchy	8–13	—
Completion	13–18	—
Pubic hair	11–14	12–16
Testicular growth		
(Tanner stage 2) (>2 cm)	—	9.5–13.0
Completion	—	13.5–17.0

Based on data from Slap GB: Normal Physiological and Psychosocial Growth in the Adolescent. J Adolesc Health Care 7:135, 1986. Copyright 1986 by the Society for Adolescent Medicine.

period pubic hair attains the adult female pattern. Male development begins with corrugation of the scrotum followed shortly by testicular enlargement. Pubic hair growth is initiated 2 years later in boys than in girls as is the growth spurt, which otherwise lasts for the period between 12 and 16 years of age and results in greater total growth. Axillary hair in boys starts soon after it does in girls. Testosterone rises and peaks during the second trimester of fetal development, subsides at birth, rises again during the second to fourth months of life, subsiding again until the rapid rise at the age of about 12. It reaches the adult high plateau at 17 years, from which it gradually subsides for the remainder of adult life. Table 41–21 shows stages of maturation matched with the approximate ages of occurrence in boys and girls.

There are several problems of reproductive physiology that present to the family practitioner. It is useful to be able to diagnose and manage the most common ones and to refer the less usual ones in an informed fashion.

Precocious Puberty

Precocious puberty is defined as the onset of increased testosterone and all its sequelae of secondary sexual development and spermatogenesis before age 9 in boys or before estrogen production, breast development, or menarche before age 8 in girls. It occurs 10 times more commonly in girls than in boys. It may be classified according to whether it is initiated by and dependent on LHRH or initiated by gonadotropin or sex hormone release independent of LHRH. By definition, when the syndrome is LHRH-dependent and the effect of the resultant gonadotropin is brought to bear on normal gonads, which then produce hormones appropriate to the gender, these children are *isosexual* in their development.

True Sexual Precocity

True sexual precocity is caused either by a disruption that triggers activation of the hypothalamic LHRH pulse generator or by some mechanism that cannot be found (idiopathic true isosexual precocity). It occurs five times as frequently in girls as in boys (Grumbach and Styne, 1992). About 80 per cent of girls and only 50 per cent of boys with true isosexual precocity fall into the category of idiopathic true sexual precocity after an evaluation to rule out causes. The remainder have a neurologic cause, seemingly nonspecific, for premature activation of hypothalamic LHRH, ranging from head trauma, meningitis, and epilepsy to CNS tumors in the region of the hypothalamus, such as hamartoma, glioma, or astrocytoma.

DIAGNOSIS. The diagnosis is made by finding measured LH levels in appropriate pulses, a pubertal LH response to LHRH, pubertal testosterone values in boys or pubertal estradiol values in girls, MRI or CT findings of a CNS tumor, or a history of another cause for reactivation of the LHRH pulse generator.

Treatment. Treatment is aimed at definitive management of the underlying cause, arrest of symptoms and signs of precocity and regression of those already in evidence, control of height (prevention of premature closure of long bone epiphyses), and prevention and management of the vast potential of biopsychosocial sequelae of sexual precocity. The favored endocrinologic approach has changed gradually from FSH suppression to the prevention of developmental and growth-stimulating effects of estrogen by administering progestional agents (medroxyprogesterone acetate and cyproterone, which is also antiandrogenic) to LHRH agonism in constant (nonpulsed) fashion. LHRH given on a constant schedule has the paradoxical effect, through binding with gonadotropic cells of the pituitary, of suppressing the gonadotropins FSH and LH. Resumption of puberty occurs within weeks of discontinuing this therapy.

Incomplete Isosexual Precocity

Incomplete isosexual precocity is the name given to the same clinical picture as true sexual precocity but when it is caused by gonadotropin-secreting tumors or by conditions of premature primary production of androgens in boys or estrogens in girls. The causes of incomplete isosexual development are different for boys and girls. For boys they include gonadotropin (hCG)-secreting tumors, adrenal hyperplasia of the 11- and 17-hydroxylase deficiency types, other adrenal neoplasms (previously described), Leydig cell adenomas of the testicle, and familial testotoxicosis. Aberrant hCG has no appreciable effect on the immature female. The causes of incomplete isosexual precocity in girls are estrogen-producing tumors in the adrenals and ovaries, follicular cysts incidental to LHRH dependent or independent stimulation, and unusual conditions such as juvenile hypothyroidism and premature adrenarche. The latter rarely causes significant symptoms. Incomplete isosexual precocity, which occurs more often in girls than in boys, may be a part of the McCune-Albright syndrome, which otherwise affects both boys and girls and is characterized by café au lait spots and polyostotic fibrous dysplasia. Peutz-Jeghers syndrome may be associated with gonadal tumors secreting hormones of both the same and opposite sex.

The more likely causes of isosexual precocity are diagnosed as follows. Gonadotropic hormone-secreting tumors demonstrate elevated hCG in boys along with a normal prepubertal response of LH to LHRH and prepubertal testosterone levels. Leydig cell adenomas show higher than expected pubertal testosterone levels in the face of prepubertal LH activity and LH responses to LHRH in boys. High estradiol levels are found in the face of low gonadotropin and a prepubertal LH response to LHRH in girls with granulosa cell tumors (estrogen-secreting) and follicular cysts, the two being differentiated by CT scan. Feminizing adrenal tumors manifest the same picture as granulosa cell tumors and follicular cysts with the addition of abnormally elevated DHEA levels.

Treatment of these disorders depends on treatment of the underlying cause.

Accidental Sexual Precocity

Accidental sexual precocity usually results from unknown ingestion of androgenic or estrogenic substances in foods by children. Iatrogenic sexual precocity may occur incidental to androgenic treatment of conditions such as undescended testicles with hCG or by estrogenic creams in girls.

Contrasexual Precocity

Contrasexual precocity is prepubertal feminization in boys and masculinization in girls. Rare in boys, it is caused by such conditions as unusual variations of congenital adrenal hyperplasia and chorioepithelioma. In girls the most common cause is congenital adrenal hyperplasia. Other causes are arrhenoblastoma and adrenal carcinoma. Evaluation for this problem is covered under amenorrhea and hirsutism.

Delayed Puberty

A frequent complaint in family practice, usually initiated by a concerned parent, is apparent delayed puberty. The normal age of puberty in the United States, defined as for 95 per cent of the population, is 12 years for girls and 14 years for boys. Unlike precocious puberty this complaint occurs more often in boys, estimated at 3:1, possibly influenced by greater cultural tolerance for late maturing girls than for boys. Once confronted, it is more likely to yield an organic cause if the patient is a girl than if a boy. Organically induced delay is due to central (hypophyseal or pituitary) factors or to primary gonadal factors. With constitutional delayed puberty, pubic hair development (pubarche) consequent to adrenarche is also likely to be delayed, and bone age is likely to be younger than the chronologic age, commensurate with the state of delayed sexual development. The patient tends to achieve pubarche, albeit delayed, at an appropriate bone age (i.e., before the 12 and 14 year bone age marks in girls and boys, respectively). With organic delayed puberty due to central failure of gonadotropin (hypogonadotropic hypogonadism) where CRF and ACTH are functioning normally, pubarche and bone maturation are more likely to occur at the expected chronologic age, whereas voice deepening, phallus and testicular size, or breast and vulvar development and menarche in girls, are delayed or are not forthcoming. *Sexual infantilism* is the term that describes indefinitely delayed development of secondary sex characteristics, which might well also be called uninitiated or failed puberty.

Hypogonadotropic hypogonadism of various types have in common low measured levels of FSH or LH (or both). Idiopathic hypopituitary dwarfism may occur with or without gonadotropin deficiency. LHRH pulsation can be interrupted by anorexia nervosa and by excessive weight loss in athletics. Acquired causes are tumors and other lesions exerting a mass effect on the hypophyseal-pituitary area. There may be a thin line between sequelae of certain assaults resulting in precocious puberty versus delayed puberty. The most common mass effect to cause centrally delayed puberty is due to craniopharyngiomas, and prolactinomas may also be a cause. Other causes are infiltrative, such as the storage diseases, postinfectious states, and occasionally irradiation.

Primary gonadal failure is known as *hypergonadotropic hypogonadism*. It causes delayed puberty as well and is discussed separately.

In girls the complaint may be focused on the lack of menarche. If pubic hair and breast development are appropriate for age, an evaluation should be delayed for at least 6 months. The initial evaluation of delayed puberty after a detailed neurologic history is measurement of FSH and LH to determine whether one is dealing with hypo- or hypergonadotropic hypogonadism. If gonadotropins are elevated, the patient should be evaluated for primary hypogonadism (discussed below).

Couple Infertility

The approach to couple infertility in family practice is to consider the least expensive and most likely causes first. It means first getting a thorough history of the couple's relationship and sex life and determining if the couple's expectations are realistic: Have they attempted pregnancy long and intently enough to be able to say they have an infertility problem? Relationship and sexologic problems are covered in Chapters 32 and 49. Once the complaint is validated, a sperm count is indicated, as 40 per cent of couple infertility is due to aspermia or azospermia. The causes of male infertility include hypogonadism, as described, and other disorders.

Treatment of the male partner with testosterone enanthate 200 mg IM every 2 or 3 weeks has been tried with the hope that sperm counts will rebound when it is stopped. For the female partner clomiphene 50 mg may be given for 5 days beginning on day 5 of the cycle to stimulate ovulation. This dose can be increased during subsequent months.

Insemination with donor spermatozoa is indicated for couples with unresponsive azospermia. Technologies and options for in vitro fertilization are increasing rapidly. Another procedure entails recovery of oocytes, usually by laparoscopy, after ovarian stimulation. A wide range of procedures can then be used to achieve fertilization of the oocytes and implantation in the uterus.

Problems of the Testicle and of Virilization

Testicular and virilization problems may be divided into problems of fertility and of testosterone production. In turn, they may be primary (caused by testicular failure or dysfunction) or secondary to hypothalamic–pituitary dysfunction.

Male Hypogonadism (Hypergonadotropic Hypogonadism)

LACK OF VIRILIZATION. Men with hypogonadism are likely to present with impotence, lack of libido, or gynecomastia, or earlier during their boyhoods with delayed puberty. Though most hypogonadal men have problems of libido and potency, the converse is not true; vascular and functional problems far outrank endocrine causes of impotence. Problems of virilization virtually always include infertility, though many of these men, such as those with the Kallmann syndrome, can be made fertile during the course of treatment. Their disorder is generally classified as primary or secondary to a pituitary or hypophyseal etiology.

Klinefelter syndrome, a form of primary hypogonadism, is the most common cause of male hypogonadism if it is defined as failure of both spermatic function and virilization. It is caused by a chromosomal abnormality in which the karyotype is 47,XXY (or up to 47,XXXXY); it occurs in 1 in 500 to 1 in 1000 births, possibly caused by meiotic nondysjunction in the XX or XY chromosomes of either parent. It produces a testicular developmental abnormality consisting of small testicular size (< 2 cm), hyalinization of the seminiferous tubules, and compromised Leydig cells, which are found in clumps. Patients are chromatin-positive because of the presence of two or more X chromosomes. LH levels are elevated in response to lower than normal testosterone or if testosterone is normal as a result of elevated LH, the result may be increased production of estradiol by the testis, the cause of gynecomastia in 85 per cent of cases and an increased incidence of breast carcinoma that is as high as 20 per cent of that in females. Puberty is not delayed but incomplete, in that secondary characteristics are not attained to optimal degree. The typical patient is tall by virtue of a long lower segment, and most patients identify as males; they have problems with fertility, an invariable and immutable problem of Klinefelter syndrome. Treatment is testosterone if needed and mastectomy for the gynecomastia.

The *Kallmann syndrome* (primary isolated gonadotropin deficiency) is not nearly as common as Klinefelter syndrome. It is, however, the second most common cause of male hypogonadism. It is an inherited deficiency of FSH or LH (or both) with some variability. It is transmitted by X linkage or autosomeal inheritance, perhaps subject to mutations. It has been mentioned in the section on the pituitary gland.

Other cases of primary hypogonadism are secondary to trauma, chemotherapy, irradiation, castration, or systemic diseases such as sickle cell disease, hemochromatosis, hyper- and hypothyroidism, Cushing's disease (secondary to the relative depression of LH by cortisol), and chronic liver disease. Their presentation, course, and potential reversibility depend on the remediability of the underlying conditions. In addition to Kallmann syndrome, Cushing's disease, and isolated FSH deficiency, another cause of secondary hypogonadism is hyperprolactinemia due to micro- or macroadenoma. Its endocrine effects disrupt the pulsatile LH and FSH release. Its space-occupying effect may include compression and disabling of gonadotropic cells of the pituitary. Either event leads to relative impotence by lowering the testosterone levels or azospermia. These problems are remediable to the extent that such treatment as bromocriptine may lower the prolactin levels, or surgery may relieve the space-occupying effects of the adenoma.

MALE INFERTILITY. Unless otherwise stated, this section deals with male infertility without problems of virilization. After prostatitis and possibly problems of potency, the most common male genital problem presented to the family physician is infertility. The normal sperm count is over 20 million per milliliter, with motility of more than 60 per cent, and normal morphology in at least 60 per cent. Spermatogenesis requires FSH stimulation of Sertoli cells, ideal temperature during stor-

age in the seminiferous tubules, and intact transport from testicle to recipient, which requires LH to stimulate testosterone production in the Leydig cells in order to effect sexual potency. Those causes of infertility that are part of the hypogonadism syndrome have been briefly covered. About 40 per cent of all cases of infertility are due to varicocele, of which about half respond to surgical repair. Obstruction of the epididymis or vas deferens accounts for about 5 per cent and occurs in association with local infection, subtle developmental abnormalities, cystic fibrosis, and diethystilbestrol progeny. An additional 6 per cent are due to cryptorchidism (discussed later). One to two per cent each may be attributed to Klinefelter syndrome and viral orchitis. Mumps is the preponderant cause of viral orchitis; is present in 25 per cent of patients with mumps and is bilateral in 10 per cent, of whom one third fail to recover fertility and have associated with bilateral testicular atrophy but with adequate androgenization. Hypogonadotropic hypogonadism accounts for fewer than 1 per cent of cases. Table 41–22 lists causes of infertility

TABLE 41–22. MALE DISORDERS OF INFERTILITY CLASSIFIED ACCORDING TO WHETHER ANDROGENIZATION IS ADEQUATE

Insufficient Androgen	Normal Virilization
Hypothalamic/pituitary factor-induced infertility	
Defective LH/LHRH pulse (Kallmann syndrome)	Isolated FSH deficiency
Cushing's disease	Congenital adrenal hyperplasia
Hyperprolactinemia	Hyperprolactinemia
Hemochromatosis	Exogenous androgen
Panhypopituitarism	
Testicular factor-induced infertility	
Structural defects	*Structural defects*
Chromosomal abnormalities (e.g., Klinefelter's)	Germinal cell aplasia, cryptorchidism, varicocele, other
Acquired defects	*Acquired defects*
Viral orchitis	*Mycoplasma* infection
Trauma	Radiation
Radiation	Drugs (cyclophosphamide; sulfasalazine)
Drugs (spironolactone, alcohol; ketoconazole; cyclophosphamide)	Environmental toxins
Environmental toxins	Autoimmunity
Autoimmunity	Systemic disease
Granulomatous disease	Febrile illness
Associated systemic disease	Celiac disease
Liver	Neurologic cause: paraplegia
Renal failure	Androgen resistance
Sickle cell disease	
Neurologic causes	
Myotonic dystrophy	
Paraplegia	
Androgen resistance	
Sperm transport defect-induced infertility	
—	Obstruction of epididymis or vas

Modified from Griffin JE, Wilson JD: Disorders of the Testes and the Male Reproductive Tract. In Williams Textbook of Endocrinology, 8th edition. Philadelphia, WB Saunders Company, 1992, with permission.

in men according to the presence or absence of virilization.

GYNECOMASTIA. Gynecomastia is an enlargement of the male breast involving proliferation of glandular tissue. Enlargement of male breasts commonly occurs at puberty. Virtually all such cases resolve without treatment. The same is true of breast enlargement in the newborn, which subsides with maternal and placental estrogen stimulation. A small percentage of men after age 70 may have gynecomastia secondary to decreased testosterone levels and relatively higher estrogen levels. These conditions usually require no treatment. Palpation of a firm disk of tissue underneath the areolar area indicates that glandular tissue is present, distinct from fatty enlargement.

Drugs such as estrogens, spironolactone, digitalis, and cimetidine among others can cause gynecomastia. Hypogonadism, liver disease, hyperthyroidism, and ectopic production of gonadotropins also may produce gynecomastia. Men with Klinefelter syndrome develop breast enlargement that persists. Approximately one fourth of patients with the complaint have idiopathic gynecomastia, and one fourth have puberty-associated gynecomastia (Braunstein, 1993). Drugs, liver disease or malnutrition, hypogonadism, testicular tumors, and other systemic conditions comprise the other causes of gynecomastia.

Treatment is limited to plastic surgery for cosmetic and psychological reasons if the enlargement is severe enough. Discontinuing a drug known to produce gynecomastia usually relieves the condition. Breast carcinoma, although rare in men, must be ruled out because it is usually an aggressive tumor that metastasizes readily. Clomiphene 50 to 100 mg per day for up to 6 months or tamoxifen 10 mg b.i.d. have been used with fair success as antiestrogenic agents to reduce gynecomastia.

Cryptorchidism

The prevalence of cryptorchidism is 0.5 to 0.75 per cent of adult men, including those treated and untreated. Though a 3 per cent incidence exists at birth, 50 per cent resolve (the testicles descend) by 1 month and 80 per cent by 1 year of life. The condition occurs in 20 per cent of premature male births and is otherwise more likely to occur in association with problems of chromosomal abnormality (e.g., Klinefelter syndrome) and other types of congenital hypogonadotropic hypogonadism, such as the Kallmann and Prader-Labhart-Willi syndromes. Infertility occurs in 90 per cent of those with uncorrected bilateral disease and one half of those with uncorrected unilateral disease. Treatment before age 3 to 4 years results in reduction of infertility rates to about 40 per cent and 25 per cent, respectively. Ten per cent of testicular cancers occur in postpubertal undescended testicles (ten times their representation in the population), usually in the 10 per cent of cases in which the testicles are or were located intra-abdominally. Orchiopexy, if done before the age of adolescence, remediates the cancer risk but not completely. The annual incidence of testicular cancer in the U.S. population is 5300 to 5700. It may be translated into a lifetime cumulative incidence of 0.22 per cent. The risk of cancer in uncorrected undescended testes may then be calculated to be 3.5 per cent, although some have stated the risk to be as high as 5 per cent. Maldescent of testicles is virtually a type of gonadal dysgenesis. Given the history of maldescent of a testicle, a normally descended contralateral testicle is at higher than expected risk for cancer and manifests a lower mean sperm count. Only 10 per cent of undescended testicles are intra-abdominal, the site of highest risk of cancer; and 60 per cent are to be found in the inguinal canal or high in the scrotum. The remainder are located out of the normal path of descent; rarely, the empty scrotum is due to anorchia. Anorchia, or disappearing testes, occurs in 1 per 20,000 births, thus comprising 0.5 to 1.0 per cent of undescended testes. Recognition of this condition is important because it is associated with lack of virilization and attendant secondary developmental abnormalities. Anorchia is diagnosed by finding elevated FSH and LH levels and an abnormally low testosterone level, which responds to 2000 units of hCG by rising within 72 hours. In the event of anorchia a buccal smear should be prepared to rule out female genotypia with severe adrenal hyperplasia wherein external genitalia may be indistinguishable from male genitalia with an empty scrotum.

An important part of well-baby care is the monitoring of maldescended testicles. Generally there is no great urgency in this follow-up so long as the child is examined frequently and a point in time is chosen after which endocrinologic or surgical consultation is elected; most physicians believe the best time for re-evaluation is between the ages of 3 and 5. No benefit is gained by waiting until after the age of 1 year except for technical facility during surgery. Descent can be effected by medical administration of hCG as well as by surgical orchiopexy. hCG given as 250 to 2000 units (depending on age) intramuscularly three times per week may result in descent within 2 weeks. If hCG fails to effect descent but the testosterone level rises, undescended testicle(s) are confirmed. Orchiopexy may then be elected. If there is no rise in the testosterone level, the diagnosis is disappearing testes. Patients with a history of treated undescended testes must be examined frequently for the rest of their lives and educated early about self-examination.

Male Climacteric

Belief in the existence of the male climacteric, analogous to female menopause, is not unanimous. Certainly some aged men have suggestive symptoms, such as mild hot flashes and evidence of hypogonadism. During the late teens and early twenties young men reach a peak in regard to degree of erections, intensity of ejaculation, and brevity of their refractive periods. Gradually these characteristics wane with age but do not end abruptly. Plasma testosterone levels remain within normal levels for men well into the eighth or ninth decade of life. However, relatively more protein binding occurs so there is less free testosterone available. Seminiferous tubule reduction also occurs, and FSH and LH levels may rise somewhat in the aged man. It is likely that only infrequently does the clinician encounter a male climacteric. If hypogonadism is appropriately diagnosed in the aged man, replacement therapy may be cautiously used to alleviate the condition, as described in the section on hypogonadism.

Osteoporosis in Men

Men suffer clinically significant effects of osteoporosis with aging but at a substantially lower rate than women. Most importantly, they have a lifetime cumulative hip fracture probability of 17 per cent (Table 41–23). Risk factors are the same as for women except that, of course, the male anabolic steroid testosterone does not fall off precipitously at a set period in life as estrogen does for women. Furthermore, hormone replacement is not an option, as it is in women, owing to the detrimental effects of testosterone on blood pressure and serum lipids. Thus prevention of osteoporosis in men is limited to maintenance of exercise, calcium supplementation, and cessation of smoking (see osteoporosis in women, below).

Problems of the Ovary and Related Syndromes

Primary Amenorrhea

Primary amenorrhea is defined as failure of onset of menses by the age of 16 years, regardless of the state of development of secondary sexual characteristics. It may be the presenting complaint of de-

TABLE 41–23. CUMULATIVE LIFETIME INCIDENCE OF FIVE FRACTURE LOCATIONS IN WOMEN AND MEN

Fracture Site	Incidence (%)	
	Women	Men
Hip	33	17
Distal radius	24	5
Humerus	12	4
Pelvis	9	3
Spine	46	—

From Gallagher JC, Melton LJ, Riggs BL, et al: Epidemiology of fractures of the proximal femur. Clin Orthop Relat Res 150:163, 1980 *and* Melton LJ, Kan SH, Frye MA, et al: Epidemiology of vertebral fractures in woman. Am J Epidemiol 129:1000, 1989, with permission.

layed puberty. In practice, this term is applied to those who are adequately estrogenized. Anovulation may be primary (i.e., never having occurred) or acquired. The latter cases are discussed under secondary amenorrhea. Chronic anovulation, with polycystic ovary syndrome being the most common cause, may be associated with adequate estrogen, in which case menses may be induced by progesterone administration and withdrawal. Anovulation without estrogen does not yield uterine bleeding with withdrawal of administered progesterone and hence indicates the existence of hypo- or hypergonadotropic hypogonadism. Ovarian failure (primary hypogonadism) presents as primary amenorrhea. Gonadal dysgenesis is the most common form of primary ovarian failure presenting with primary amenorrhea and is discussed separately, along with Turner syndrome. Anatomic problems include müllerian agenesis, imperforate hymen, labial agglutination, and various defects of uterine fusion. These defects generally cause pelvic pain or, if communicating, dysmenorrhea. Constitutional delayed puberty accounts for a significant number of cases.

If secondary sex characteristics are normal, the evaluation should be put off for at least 6 months. Thin girls menstruate later than heavy girls (Baker and McFarland, 1990), presumably due to lack of the critical adipose mass needed for ovulation, a cause for secondary amenorrhea in athletes and anorectic girls. A pelvic examination is necessary to rule out anatomic defects and is supplemented as needed with pelvic ultrasonography to help evaluate the internal anatomy. After pregnancy is ruled out, thyroid function tests should be done along with a buccal smear for chromatin, which is negative in Turner syndrome except in cases of mosaicism (46,XX/45,XO). Prolactin levels are important for ruling out prolactinoma. If the patient is virilized, plasma testosterone levels and urinary 11-hydroxysteroids and 17-ketosteroids should be measured. A separate discussion of hirsutism can elucidate this condition. If there is a lack of secondary sex characteristics, LH and FSH levels are determined to exclude hypogonadotropic hypogonadism (or hypergonadotropic hypogonadism). Those who have sexual ambiguity should be evaluated for chromosomal abnormalities as well. Treatment depends on the underlying cause and may include surgery. Figure 41–7 is a brief decision guide to the evaluation of secondary amenorrhea. The evaluation is the same for primary as for secondary amenorrhea, though congenital conditions such as gonadal dysgenesis and agenesis obviously are found with secondary amenorrhea. Briefly, after pregnancy is ruled out, physical examination elucidates most cases of gonadal dysgenesis (physiognomy) and müllerian agenesis (pelvic findings). Withdrawal bleeding after progesterone administration (10 days of medroxyprogesterone acetate) allows presumption of the presence of es-

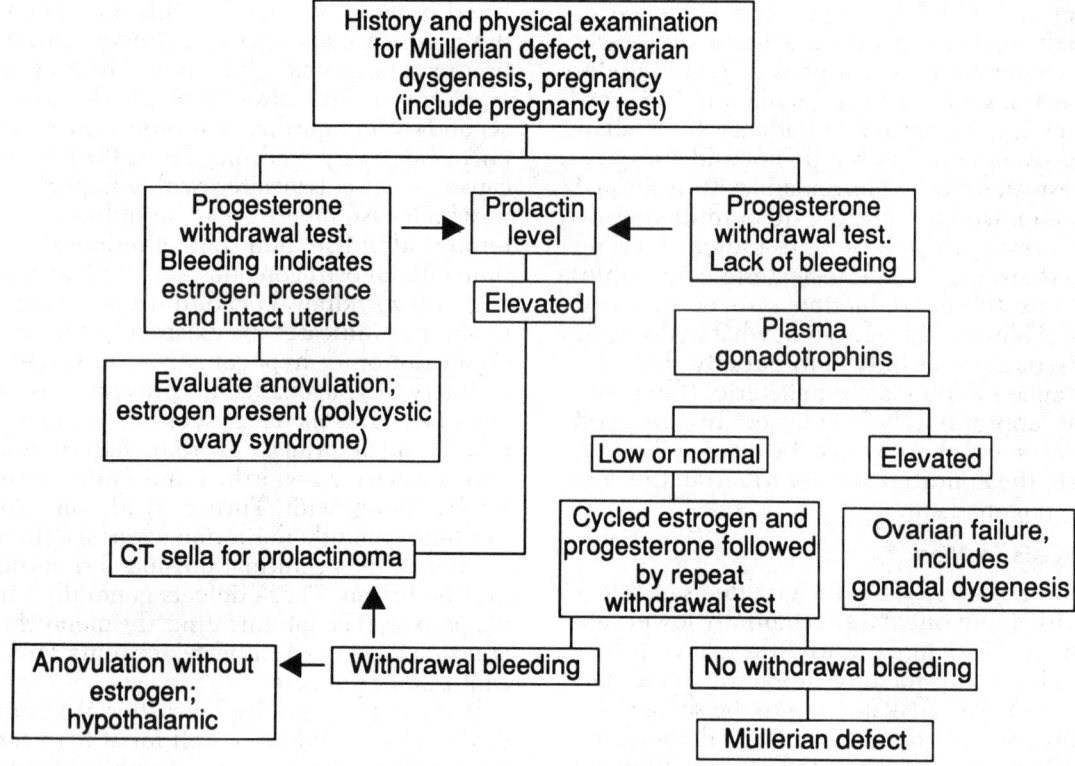

FIGURE 41–7.   Diagnostic algorithm for amenorrhea. (Modified from Carr BR: Disorders of the Ovary and Female Productive Tract. *In* Williams Textbook of Endocrinology, 8th edition. Philadelphia, WB Saunders, 1992.)

trogen with the likely diagnosis of polycystic ovary syndrome. A serum prolactin level may be desirable to exclude hyperprolactinemia. Lack of withdrawal bleeding mandates serum prolactin, FSH, and LH determinations. If the prolactin level is elevated, the patient should be evaluated for prolactinoma. If prolactin is normal, the gonadotropins may be low, indicating the need for a test of estrogen priming (e.g., 30 days of conjugated equine estrogens), followed by medroxyprogesterone acetate 10 mg daily overlapping the last 10 days of estrogen. If withdrawal bleeding results, the diagnosis is hypogonadotropic hypogonadism. If gonadotropins are lower than normal and withdrawal does not occur after estrogen priming and progestogen, the patient must be assumed to have müllerian dysgenesis. If gonadotropins are high, the diagnosis is gonadal dysgenesis. Chromatin testing or chromosome studies (or both) are then indicated.

Female Hypogonadism

Hypogonadotropic hypogonadism has been discussed as a cause of delayed puberty and of sexual infantilism. Hypergonadotropic hypogonadism in women, excluding secondary failure (premature and normal menopause, surgical menopause), is virtually always due to gonadal dysgenesis.

TURNER SYNDROME.   Turner syndrome is one of X monosomy (45,XO), wherein the child is born with only one sex chromosome or mosaicism with the normal 46,XX. The child is a phenotypic female (the default phenotype where the Y chromosome is absent). The result is gonadal dysgenesis, short stature (mean height 54 inches [Baker and McFarland, 1990]), sexual infantilism, and a strong association with widely spaced nipples, shield-like chest, webbed neck, short fourth metacarpals, low hairline, lymphedema in the newborn, and aortic coarctation. Milder versions of the foregoing apparently depend on incomplete expression of X monosomy by virtue of the mosaicism or the presence of critical parts of a second X chromosome. Sources differ as to the frequency of Turner syndrome among live births probably because as many as 10 per cent of abortuses have the 45,XO pattern and as many as 60 per cent of those with Turner syndrome may be lost at birth (Grumbach and Styne, 1992). Thus frequency estimations vary from 1 in 3000 to 1 in 10,000. Unlike Klinefelter syndrome, parental age seems not to be a factor in the production of this abnormality.

It is diagnosed based on the evaluation as described above.

Treatment is generally managed by an endocrinologist but can be effected by a knowledgeable and motivated family physician alone or working closely with the subspecialist. It consists in cycled estrogen and progestogen beginning at the time of normal puberty. Dosages and scheduling are similar to those employed for postmenopausal replacement therapy (described below) except that estrogen may be given in smaller dosages than in the adult (e.g., 0.3 mg CEE).

Secondary Amenorrhea

Secondary amenorrhea is defined as failure of menstruation after normal establishment of menses at an earlier age. The most common cause of asymptomatic amenorrhea is pregnancy. Many brief intervals of secondary amenorrhea are encountered in primary care practice that resolve spontaneously. Missed periods may occur because of rapid weight loss, anemia, or other systemic illnesses. Missed ovulation may be due to the presence of a persistent follicle or a persistent corpus luteum, which may persist as cysts, causing intervals of amenorrhea eventually interrupted by irregular breakthrough bleeding. Therefore although a pelvic examination or an ultrasonographic study may be indicated early, secondary amenorrhea should be diagnosed and investigated endocrinologically after three or four missed periods. Oral contraceptives cause lightening of the menses, which can diminish to amenorrhea, rarely resulting in endometrial fibrosis. Acquired hypergonadotropic hypogonadism before age 40 is called secondary ovarian failure; after age 40 it is called menopause.

Pregnancy can be excluded by serum hCG determination after a pelvic examination, during which the adnexae are evaluated for a mass or cystic lesions. Findings are confirmed by ultrasonography. A progestogen withdrawal test may be done as described for primary amenorrhea. Estrogenized women respond by withdrawal bleeding within 3 days of progestogen priming as outlined above. If there is no withdrawal bleeding, depending on the patient's age and whether there are symptoms of estrogen deficiency, an FSH level may be determined at this time. If it is determined to be above 40 mIU/mL, secondary ovarian failure or menopause is diagnosed. If no diagnosis is made after three missed periods, the evaluation is done as described for primary amenorrhea and in Figure 41–7.

Female Infertility

Infertility is the inability to conceive despite attempting to do so for 1 year. The cause lies in the male partner as frequently as it does in the female partner. Prior to embarking on an expensive workup, semen should be examined for abnormalities of sperm numbers, motility, and morphology. Causes of infertility in men have been discussed. Failure to ovulate and tubal abnormalities are the major problems encountered in women. A gynecologist with experience evaluating these problems should help with the work-up for infertility.

Presenting complaints may include only an inability to conceive with normal menses and normal sex steroid production, although other findings may exist, such as abnormal menses, amenorrhea, hirsutism, and hypogonadism. A complete history should explore psychological factors, pelvic infections, and previous procedures that might have affected the cervix, uterus, or tubes. Many women who are ultimately found to have tubal disease or adhesions give no history of previous infections.

A history and physical examination helps evaluate the general health of the patient as well as any specific genitourinary abnormalities that are present. Systemic illnesses affecting the hormonal cycle must be considered. Verification of ovulation by documenting a basal body temperature rise of 0.4° F in midcycle should be done early in the investigation. A progesterone level above 3 ng/ml indicates that ovulation has occurred. A postcoital test is done by aspirating mucus from the cervix about 8 hours after coitus. The elasticity should be about 8 cm, and it should form a ferning pattern when dried on a slide. At least five motile sperm per high power field are seen in most normal specimens.

If anatomic abnormalities and endometriosis are not found, endocrine studies should be undertaken, including gonadotropin, androgen, estrogen, and adrenal steroid assays. Hysterosalpingography, endometrial biopsy, and laparoscopy require the help of a specialist.

If a specific condition is found, therapy should be directed to that problem. For example, hyperprolactinemia may be treated with bromocriptine and *Chlamydia* infection with antibiotics. Likewise, microsurgery may be successful in restoring tubal integrity, and a small dose of prednisone may suppress ACTH-dependent androgen secretion from the adrenal glands.

Galactorrhea

Secretion of milk or milk-like fluid from the breast 1 year or more after the last pregnancy or discontinuation of nursing is termed galactorrhea. It is rare in men but can occur especially with a prolactinoma. Galactorrhea may accompany a large number of disorders, both endocrine and nonendocrine.

An important condition to consider is pituitary tumor, which may also cause amenorrhea. Prolactinoma is the most frequent pituitary tumor associated with galactorrhea, but growth hormone-secreting tumors and other adenomas can also cause the condition. A large number of cases of galactorrhea are classified as idiopathic. Usually the menses and endocrine studies are normal. Important causes include hypothyroidism, a large number of drugs, the empty sella syndrome, and neurogenic stimulation (suckling, manipulation of the nipples, emotional stress). Other symptoms suggestive of a pituitary mass, such as headaches and visual field defects, may accompany galactorrhea. Imaging with CT or MRI is indicated in these circumstances. Prolactin levels are valuable not only for diagnosis but for follow-up of these individuals.

Treatment is directed to the underlying cause whenever possible. Mild cases of galactorrhea need not always be treated. Bromocriptine 2.5 mg b.i.d. is effective when hyperprolactinemia is present. Tumors also have been reported to shrink with bromocriptine treatment. Many drugs, such as methyldopa, benzodiazepines, phenothiazines, and estrogens, can be discontinued long enough to alleviate the galactorrhea. Symptoms do not necessarily reappear if the provoking drug is used again after some time. It is important to be certain that infection is not an aggravating influence, and certainly appropriate antibiotic therapy is indicated if a culture is positive.

Hirsutism

Hirsutism is a common condition characterized by male-type sexual hair distribution. Certain ethnic groups, such as those from southern European countries, have more body hair than others and do not have a medical problem. The increased body hair appears on the upper lip, chin, chest, midline of the lower abdomen, and extremities. The Ferriman and Gallwey scoring system estimates the degree of hirsutism (Ferriman and Gallway, 1961) and is commonly used to evaluate treatment responses.

Hirsutism is the result of increased androgen levels. The sources of the increased androgens are fairly equally divided from the adrenal gland and ovary. Exogenous androgens, tumors that secrete androgens, or increased peripheral conversion of weak androgens to more potent ones also cause hirsutism. Hirsutism can exist with or without other signs of virilization, such as balding, acne, clitoral enlargement, and loss of breast tissue.

Clinical Manifestations

Increased body hair usually develops gradually during the second and third decade of life. Young women are self-conscious about it. Menstrual abnormalities or amenorrhea may accompany the hirsutism. Other features of virilization are present in women who have relatively large increases in androgen production, as in those with tumors or Cushing syndrome. Facial hair tends to be the most troublesome to women, but sometimes the major increase in hair is found in the periareolar areas or as a typical male pattern extension from the pubic area to the umbilicus. Other presenting features may include infertility, acne, obesity, and acanthosis nigricans. Hirsutism that develops during middle age or later suggests that androgen production may be originating in an adrenal or ovarian tumor or from late-onset congenital adrenal hyperplasia.

Diagnosis

The fine hair found in a familial or ethnic pattern is not usually associated with increased androgen levels. Women with true hirsutism commonly have subtle defects in adrenal steroidogenesis (Siegel, et al., 1990). ACTH stimulation by 100 units of cosyntropin revealed enzyme deficiencies that were not evident when DHEA was measured in the basal state. Thus mild forms of congenital adrenal hyperplasia and ovarian disorders, particularly polycystic ovaries, are the common causes of hirsutism. Diagnostic studies need not be extensive in women with mild hirsutism and normal menses. A plasma testosterone level, plasma DHEA assay, and a 24-hour urine specimen for 17-ketosteroid assay should suffice as reliable screening tests. An elevated 17-ketosteroid level that returns to normal with low-dose dexamethasone (Decadron; 0.5 mg q.i.d. for 2 days) strongly suggests an adrenal source of androgens. An elevated plasma 17-hydroxyprogesterone value suggests 21-hydroxylase deficiency, the most common enzyme abnormality in the pathway of cortisol production. Further studies with ACTH stimulation are helpful mainly for differentiating the location and type of enzymatic errors. Ultrasonography or imaging by CT or MRI usually detects adrenal or ovarian masses. An androgen-secreting tumor is associated with greatly elevated plasma testosterone levels (170 ng/dl or 6 nmol/L). Ovarian secretion of excessive androgen can be estimated by measuring 17-hydroxyprogesterone after stimulation by nafarelin, a long-acting gonadotropin-releasing hormone.

Treatment

For mild cases of hirsutism no treatment is necessary, or hair removal by mechanical means can be initiated. (Electrolysis, bleaching, or depilatory creams are effective, contrary to popular beliefs.) Patients with late-onset congenital hyperplasia can be given low-dosage steroids in the evening to suppress androgen secretion from the adrenals. The dose of prednisone is 5 mg or of dexamethasone 0.5 mg at night. Spironolactone has well recognized antiandrogenic properties. It can be used in doses of 50 to 100 mg per day to block the biologic action of androgens by competing for their receptors. Oral contraceptive pills effectively reduce body hair growth by suppressing gonadotropin secretion and to some extent ACTH secretion. Nonandrogenic progestogens, such as desogestrel, should be used rather than those with androgenic properties. Obesity is fairly common in women with hirsutism, and weight loss should be encouraged. If a tumor is causing increased androgens, surgical removal is the treatment of choice.

Menopause

Menopause is defined as permanent cessation of menses due to hypergonadotropic ovarian failure after age 40. Clinically acceptable definitions of menopause include typical symptoms in the appropriate setting, such as age, associated vasomotor and emotional symptoms, and cessation of menses, even for only a few months, with the corroborating finding of elevated FSH level (> 40 mIU/mL; > 40 IU/L), 1 year of amenorrhea in the appropriate clinical setting, or increased FSH level (> 40 mIU/mL) in an atypical setting. In the latter case, even if menses resume, menopause is imminent. If amenorrhea exists for less than 6 months, there should be confirmation by FSH; and pregnancy must be ruled out before instituting hormone replacement therapy. The changes wrought by the rapid fall in estrogen include thinning and drying of mucosa, especially in the vaginal area; loss of beneficial effects on cholesterol; loss of protein anabolic effects, which contributes to osteoporosis by reducing the osteoid matrix of cancellous bone; reduction in the conversion of hydroxycholecalciferol to the much more potent form of vitamin D 1,25-dihydroxycholecaliferol (vitamin D^3), which results in decreased intestinal absorption of calcium; and loss of parathormone-inhibiting effect, which results in still more calcium loss from bone.

Acutely, amenorrhea may be sudden in onset, but it is preceded by a 5-year premenopausal period of waning ovarian function; usually it is heralded by 3 to 12 months of irregular menstrual periods. Vasomotor instability is expressed as hot flashes (subjective and objective heat sensation, drop in body temperature, and diaphoresis) in attacks lasting 5 to 10 minutes; such attacks are reversible with modest dosages of estrogen such as conjugated equine estrogens (CEE, Premarin) 0.3 mg daily. Atrophy of urogenital epithelium leads to local irritation, dysuria, and dyspareunia. Psychological instability takes the form of lability, anxiety, depression, or rapid changes of mood. There may be confusion and memory loss. Insomnia occurs in 46 per cent of climacteric women and fatigue in 38 per cent. Urogenital atrophy may lead to pelvic relaxation, prolapse, and urinary incontinence; and there may be a steady decline in libido.

The chronic effects of menopause are increasingly significant, as women born in the United States now have a life expectancy of 80 years and menopause occurs at an average age of 51.4 years; people over age 65 will comprise 20 per cent of the population by the year 2025. With more than one third of adult life spent in a state of estrogen deficiency, women face problems of chronic estrogen deficiency, consisting of osteoporosis and ac-

celeration of atherosclerosis. Menopause and the postmenopausal state are best approached holistically, wherein mental and sexual health, osteoporosis, and cardiovascular disease can often by treated (secondarily prevented) by a unified broad approach. For discussion purposes, the two main long-term organic sequelae of menopause, atherosclerosis and osteoporosis, are treated separately.

Atherosclerosis

Cardiovascular effects of menopause emanate from the loss of favorable effects of estrogen on serum lipids and other cardiovascular risks. Postmenopausal women have more atherosclerotic cardiovascular disease than do age-matched premenopausal women, as well as higher serum cholesterol and LDL cholesterol levels and a lower HDL cholesterol level. Estrogen treatment of the estrogen-deficient individual results in a decrease in total and LDL cholesterol and an increase in HDL cholesterol. Table 41–24 illustrates that coronary artery disease (CAD) is the major cause of death in postmenopausal women. Some of this benefit may be lost when a progestogen derived from 19-nortestosterone (e.g., norethindrone) is cycled with estrogen in hormone replacement therapy (HRT) in women who have a uterus. It appears not to be the case with C-21-derived progestogens, such as medroxyprogesterone acetate, which have a neutral effect on serum lipids. It is estimated that HRT or estrogen replacement therapy (ERT—used in those who have no contraindication to unopposed estrogen) can prevent roughly half of the CHD deaths in postmenopausal women. Whatever rela-

TABLE 41–24. CUMULATIVE MORTALITY DUE TO FOUR CONDITIONS PER 100,000 POPULATION FOR WOMEN (TO AGE 75): EXPECTED AND PREDICTED AFTER POSTMENOPAUSAL HRT

Condition	Mortality Expected (no.)	Projected Mortality from HRT (no.)	Relative Risk from HRT
Coronary artery disease	10,500	5,250	0.5
Osteoporosis—fractures	938	419	0.5
Endometrial carcinoma	188	37	0.2
Carcinoma of breast (postmenopause)	1,406	2,250	1.6
Total (Net relative risk)	13,032	7,956	0.61

HRT = hormone replacement therapy with estrogen cycled with a progestogen.

Compiled from the following sources: Henderson BE, Ross RK, Paganini-Hill, A: Estrogen use and cardiovascular disease. J Reprod Med 30(10 suppl):814, 1985; Barrett-Connor E, Bush TL: Estrogen and coronary heart-disease in woman. JAMA 265:1861, 1991; Gambrel RD: The Menopause (Review). Invest Radiol 21:369, 1986; Riggs BL: Effect of the flouride/calcium regimen on vertebral fracture occurrence in post menopausal osteoporosis. NEJM 306:446, 1982.

tive risk for CAD is conferred by a woman's baseline blood pressure, glycemic state, and smoking status is multiplied by the relative risk attached to her lipidemic status.

Osteoporosis

Because of the diversity of pathophysiology alluded to above, of which the increasing size of the intertrabecular spaces of bone are but one part, it may be appropriate to refer to this process as *osteopenia*. However, most writers use the term osteoporosis generically to cover the whole process of osteopenia of age. Bone density decreases well before and accelerates during the menopause so that 50 per cent of cancellous bone and 5 per cent of cortical bone are lost between the ages of 40 and 80. Eleven per cent of women incur vertebral fractures between the ages of 45 and 65, with a cumulative lifetime risk of 46 per cent for this fracture. Colles fractures pose a 24 per cent lifetime risk for women and fractures of the pelvis 9 per cent (Table 41–23). The incidence of hip fractures accelerates beginning at about age 65. Osteoporosis confers a lifetime risk of 33 per cent for hip fracture in untreated women who live to age 85, and the fracture carries a 20 per cent first-year mortality. Other risk factors for osteoporosis are small body build (strongly associated with northern European or Oriental racial extraction), smoking (as strong a risk factor as estrogen is protective), sedentary lifestyle, poor nutrition (particularly calcium intake less than 1.5 gm per day), and underlying medical conditions that have in common immobility (e.g., rheumatoid arthritis), certain medications, and hypercortisolism (e.g., Cushing's disease or iatrogenic glucocorticoid). Table 41–25 lists risk factors for osteoporosis.

The best estimates are that the foregoing fracture incidences can be reduced by 50 per cent through the use of HRT, which would have the effect of reducing the lifetime cumulative mortality due to hip fracture from 6 per cent to 3 per cent. Though screening modalities such as single and dual photon absorptiometry exist, they are best used as research tools or as demonstrations to motivate high risk patients. Patients are best chosen for secondary preventive treatment by their risk status based on race, body build, physical activity, and smoking status. Except for contraindications to estrogen and obvious low risk status, including obesity or large-boned build, all patients should be given consideration for hormone replacement. Regardless, patients should be placed on supplemental calcium unless contraindicated by a history of calcium oxalate kidney stone formation.

Treatment

Relief from the acute symptoms of menopause can be obtained by modest estrogen dosages, such as 0.3 mg CEE. This dosage does not prevent osteoporosis. Mild tranquilizers can be used but are

TABLE 41–25. RISK FACTORS FOR OSTEOPOROSIS

Factor	Definition
Gender	Female
Race	Northern European
Body Build	Small boned
Diet	Calcium intake <1.5 gm/day Vitamin D <1000 U/day
Exercise	None
Smoking	Yes
Underlying medical conditions	Hypercortisolism Thyrotoxicosis Intestinal malabsorption Systemic mastocytosis Adult hypophosphatasia Drug treatment with hydantoin, heparin, methotrexate Waldenström's macroglobulinemia
Other systemic disorders	Rheumatoid arthritis, diabetes mellitus, chronic liver disease, alcoholism, Down syndrome, chronic lung disease

Modified from Rudy DR, Falko JM: Osteoporosis in primary care. Ohio State Med J 81(3):209, 1985, with permission.

not physiologically directed to the base problem of estrogen deficiency. Furthermore, they are inappropriate if the predominant mood is depression. Estrogen creams can effectively treat atrophic vaginitis and are absorbed to the extent that they can give systemic relief from the acute symptoms as well. Because of systemic absorption of vaginal estrogen creams, however, they should not be prescribed when estrogen is contraindicated.

Oral calcium is the most conservative regimen that can be employed for long-term prevention of osteoporosis, at dosages that ensure a total intake of 1.5 gm per day. Given the average daily dietary consumption of 600 mg by the American woman, most clinicians prescribe 1 gm per day. It is best given in the form of calcium carbonate as 250 mg or 500 mg tablets (e.g., Oscal) or in a chewable antacid form such as Tums, which contains 200 mg, the latter requiring five chewable tablets per day. This regimen alone is not nearly as potent as estrogen replacement for prevention of osteoporosis and obviously has no beneficial effect on atherosclerotic cardiovascular disease. In the face of contraindications to estrogen or patient resistance to estrogen therapy, oral calcium may be the sole preventive therapy.

The most potent available postmenopausal regimen for osteoporosis prevention and reversal of the detrimental lipid effects of estrogen deficiency is estrogen replacement therapy (ERT). Many of the doubts regarding the safety of estrogen replacement have been settled. ERT does not cause blood pressure elevation, and it is not a risk factor for endometrial carcinoma, unless administered in unopposed fashion (i.e., not cycled with a progestogen). Therefore in the presence of an intact uterus, a progestogen is given along with estrogen, overlapping the last 10 of 25 days each month or at a lower dosage along with estrogen every day of the month. When estrogen and progesterone are both used, the term hormone replacement therapy, rather than estrogen replacement therapy, is appropriate.

There has been considerable controversy regarding the question of whether ERT or HRT increases the risk of breast cancer. The strongest case for ERT as a contributing cause of breast cancer comes from a Swedish study by Bergquist (1989) in which patients who had taken estrogen had a higher rate of breast cancer than those who had not. All but a small cohort of that study group had taken ethinyl estradiol, which is much more potent than CEE, the preparation most often used in the United States, even after correction for the smaller milligram dosages employed with ethinyl estradiol. Others have found no increased risk in users of the potent contraceptive pills even among those with family histories of breast cancer (Murray, 1989). Table 41–26 lists the commonly used estrogen preparations and their relative potencies. When the potency per unit weight and the vagaries of absorption and metabolism are taken into account, oral contraceptive effective estrogen dosages are on the order of five to eight times those normally prescribed for postmenopausal replacement.

A liberal estimate of the relative risk for breast cancer mortality in women with postmenopausal hormone replacement is 1.6 across all ages after menopause. If atherosclerosis mortality can be reduced by 50 per cent and hip fracture mortality by 50 per cent by the use of ERT or HRT, the saving

in mortality favors estrogen replacement by nearly 2:1 (Table 41–24).

Before embarking on an ERT or HRT program, not only must the patient be well informed and motivated, but precautions must be observed and baseline measurements carried out. Pregnancy is to be ruled out regardless of menstrual status; a baseline mammogram should be ordered or have been accomplished within the previous year; standard pelvic examination and Papanicolou smears are done to establish normal anatomy; endometrial biopsy is done if history or findings suggest a possibility of endometrial carcinoma; thyroid function tests are done if treatment is for systemic symptoms of the climacteric, which may be mimicked by thyrotoxicosis.

By the current U.S. definition, HRT means cycled or daily estrogen, usually CEE 0.625 mg daily for 25 days per month or daily without break and, in the presence of the uterus, a progestogen overlapping the last 10 days of a 25-day estrogen cycle or simultaneously daily (e.g., medroxyprogesterone 5 mg daily for 10 to 14 days per month or 2.5 mg daily). Withdrawal bleeding with the 25-day cycle or breakthrough bleeding with the unbroken daily schedule generally ceases by the end of 6 months, reassurance of which may go a long way toward gaining acceptance by patients reluctant to tolerate a return of menstrual periods. A regimen of growing popularity is transdermal estrogen. It may be given daily, but progestogen must still be given orally when the uterus is present. A disadvantage is that it misses the first pass through the liver and consequently lacks the lipid-remediating effects. The other estrogens listed in Table 41–28 may be used in cyclic regimens in their recommended dosages. Rarely, estradiol levels may be utilized to assess therapeutic success. If bleeding continues beyond 6 months, an endometrial biopsy is indicated to rule out endometrial carcinoma.

The ERT or HRT should be started as soon as menopause is iminent. The first 3 years appears to be crucial. The answer to the question as to how long to continue hormonal therapy has evolved. Until recently, the recommended upper limit of age for therapy had climbed steadily to 75 years, although some favor no upper limit. One report (Felson et al., 1993) indicated that advantages in bone preservation become less important after the age of 75, but much work needs to be done before such a conclusion can be justified.

Continuation of exercise is important for prevention of osteoporosis, as bed rest results in a rapid loss of bone mass. Good protein nutrition is crucial, and smoking cessation is mandatory.

Atrophic vaginitis and symptoms of bladder and urethral irritation occasionally require a temporary program in a woman who is not a candidate or who refuses long-term estrogen replacement. Systemic symptoms respond to vaginal estrogen, and the contraindications apply as with oral therapy. Simi-

TABLE 41–26. BIOLOGIC POTENCIES AND DOSAGES FOR ESTROGEN PREPARATIONS USED FOR LONG-TERM HRT

Preparation	Relative Biologic Potency	Range of Typical Dose (mg)
Piperazine estrone sulfate (Ogen)	1.0	0.35–1.50/day
Estradiol, oral, micronized (Estrace)	1.2	1–2/day
Estradiol, transdermal (Estraderm)	10.0	0.05 or 0.10 twice weekly
Conjugated estrogens (Premarin)	2.6	0.625–1.250/day
Esterified estrogens (Estratab, Menest)	2.6	0.625–1.250/day
Ethinyl estradiol* (Estinyl, Feminone)	496.5	0.02–0.05/day

* Also used in multiple contraceptive combinations.
From Rudy DR: Hormone replacement therapy. Postgrad Med 88(8): 159, 1990, with permission.

larly, limited periods of oral estrogen may be employed to relieve acute menopausal symptoms, even before the cessation of menses if estrogen deficiency is confirmed by an FSH level of more than 40 mIU/mL. After 6 months a commitment should be made to institute a full HRT regimen or to discontinue estrogen therapy.

Contraindications to estrogen therapy are unexplained vaginal bleeding; chronically impaired liver function; acute vascular thromboemolic disease, including acute myocardial infarction and stroke; a history of thromboembolic disease if the patient was taking hormones at the time, including contraceptives; and a history of breast or endometrial carcinoma. It is now well appreciated that unopposed estrogen, given long term, constitutes a risk of endometrial carcinoma; and, equally, that when opposed by overlapping progestational agents, there is no such risk. Carcinoma of the breast and estrogen therapy have been discussed. ERT and HRT are associated with a two- to three-fold increased risk of cholecystitis.

Other Modes of Treatment

Other treatments for osteoporosis include the diphosphonates (e.g., etidronate [Didronel]), which are approved for treatment of Paget's disease of bone. They may be used for prevention of osteoporosis in a regimen consisting of pulsed etidronate at 400 mg per day for 2 weeks followed by calcium 500 mg per day for the balance of 3 months (Watts et al., 1990). In that study the fracture rate was reduced by 50 per cent, comparable to the success found with HRT. It has the advantage of not being contraindicated in breast cancer. Calcitonin is effective but must be given intramuscularly. It has been used for Paget's disease of bone and is utilized mostly in "pathologic" states, in which medical conditions such has glucocorticoid use have resulted in osteoporotic fractures. Fluoride has been shown to increase bone density but is fraught with gastrointestinal and arthralgic side effects. Moreover, it causes bone fragility along with increased density.

Future Developments

An interesting development for prevention of osteoporosis is the consideration of tamoxifen, an estrogen receptor (ER) blocking agent used for treatment of ER-positive breast carcinoma, as a preventive agent against osteoporosis. Its competitive inhibition/blockading action requires molecular similarity to estrogen. In this case the result is that it has the bone mass-saving and lipid-remediating effects of estrogen while lacking the ability to stimulate ER-positive carcinoma. Thus it appears to be protective against the osteoporosis and atherosclerosis of menopause and estrogen-positive breast cancer as well. It has not been studied extensively to determine if it has beneficial effects on lipids and bone comparable to those of estrogen.

OTHER ENDOCRINE AND METABOLIC DISORDERS

Ectopic Hormone Production

A cell has the genetic material to produce any hormone or protein that can be synthesized, but regulatory processes designate certain functions to specialized cells. When malignant changes occur, many abnormal and normal substances are produced in an uncontrolled fashion.

The earliest ectopic hormone to be recognized from a tumor source was ACTH and ACTH-like hormones, most notably from oat cell carcinomas of the lung. The onset of Cushing syndrome can be abrupt and severe, but features such as the round facies may not have had time to become typical. PTH or PTH-related peptides cause hypercalcemia in the presence of certain malignancies. Vasopressin, calcitonin, GHRH, prolactin, insulin and insulin-like growth factors, and the gonadotropins are other ectopic hormone syndromes that have been described. The clinical manifestations are similar to those produced by excessive secretion of the natural hormone. Therapy is directed to the underlying tumor, but supportive therapy is frequently all that can be offered.

Multiple Endocrine Neoplasia

The occurrence of two or more endocrine tumors in the same patient is referred to as multiple endocrine neoplasia (MEN). The two major forms are type 1 and type 2. Both types are familial, and inheritance is thought to be autosomal dominant.

The MEN-1 syndrome consists mainly of parathyroid, pancreatic, and pituitary adenomas. Lipomas are also associated with this syndrome, as are carcinoid and adrenal cortex tumors. Hyperparathyroidism is the most common manifestation of MEN-1. The glands are hyperplastic, but they can be discrete adenomas. They are difficult to treat because if the surgeon leaves even a small portion of one gland in the neck hyperparathyroidism can recur. Removing all the glands and transplanting a small portion of one to the antecubital space is sometimes attempted. Pancreatic tumors can secrete excessive gastrin (Zollinger-Ellison syndrome), insulin, or glucagon. Each has its characteristic clinical features. Gastrinoma is associated with severe recurrent ulcers and increased acid secretion. Insulinomas produce fasting hypoglycemia and sometimes metastasize to the liver. Glucagonomas secrete glucagon in excess and are associated with a migratory skin rash, glucose elevations, and weight loss. They frequently metastasize before a diagnosis is established. They can sometimes be controlled successfully by somatostatin or streptozotocin. The pituitary tumors are mostly prolactinomas, but growth hormone- and ACTH-secreting tumors are found. Family testing should be done so early endocrine diseases can be recognized and treated.

The MEN-2 syndrome is associated with medullary carcinoma of the thyroid (MTC) and pheochromocytoma. MTC is a cancer of the C cells, which secrete calcitonin. Most MTCs are not hereditary but occur sporadically. MCT presents as a neck mass and occasionally with diarrhea and systemic symptoms. Baseline calcitonin levels are usually elevated, but pentagastrin or calcium given intravenously causes a rapid, marked increased in plasma calcitonin. Pheochromocytoma tends to be multiple and to produce typical clinical symptoms and signs. It may or may not be present when MCT

is diagnosed; however, MCT is almost always present when pheochromocytoma is diagnosed.

Autoimmune Endocrine Disorders

Endocrine glands seem to be particularly susceptible to autoimmune reactions. Addison's disease, Grave's disease, thyroiditis, insulin-dependent diabetes, and pituitary disorders are examples of autoimmune involvement of hormone-producing cells. Autoantibodies can be measured for many of the entities. There is also a tendency for autoimmune reactions to affect more than one gland. Addison's disease is commonly associated with thyroid disease (Schmidt syndrome), and insulin-dependent diabetes is also found frequently with Addison's disease.

REFERENCES

Aurbach GD, Marks SJ, Spiegel AM: Parathyroid hormone, calcitonin and the calciferols. *In* Williams Textbook of Endocrinology. Philadelphia, WB Saunders Company,, 1992.

Baker C, McFarland KF: Endocrinology. *In* Rakel R (ed): Textbook of Family Practice. Philadelphia, WB Saunders Company, 1990.

Bartter FC: The syndrome of inappropriate secretion of antidiuretic hormone (SIADH) in Disease-a-Month. HP Dowling (ed). Dis Mon. November, 1973.

Baylis PH: Disorders of water balance. *In* Grossman A (ed): Clinical Endocrinology. Oxford, Blackwell Scientific, 1992, pp 238–255.

Bergkvist L, Adami HO, Persson I et al: The risk of breast cancer after estrogen and estrogen-progestin replacement. N Engl J Med 321(5):193, 1989.

Braunstein GD: Gynecomastia. N Engl J Med 328:490, 1993.

Bravo EL, Gifford RW: Pheochromocytoma. Endocrinol Metab Clin North Am 22:329, 1993.

Caruso DR, Mazzaferri EL: Intervention in Graves' disease. Postgrad Med 92:8, 1992.

Catherino WH, Jordan VC: A risk-benefit assessment tamoxiphen therapy. Drug Saf 8:381, 1993.

Cryer PE: Glucose homeostasis and hypoglycemia. *In* Textbook of Endocrinology, 8th edition. Philadelphia, WB Saunders Company, 1992.

DeFronzo RA, Ferrannini E: Insulin resistance: A multifaceted syndrome responsible for NIDDM, obesity, hypertension, dyslipidemia, and atherosclerotic cardiovascular disease. Diabetes Care 14:173, 1991.

Felsen DT, et al: The effect of postmenopausal estrogen therapy on bone density in elderly women. N Engl J Med 329:1141, 1993.

Ferriman DM, Gallway JD: Clinical assessment of body hair growth in women. J Clin Endocrinol Metab 21:1440, 1961.

Gabbe SG: Diabetes mellitus: obstetric management. *In* Davidson J (ed): Clinical Diabetes Mellitus. New York, Thieme, 1986, p. 38.

Gottsater A, Landin-Olsson M, Fernlund P, et al: Beta-cell function in relation to islet cell antibodies during the first 3 years after clinical diagnosis of diabetes in type II diabetic patients. Diabetes Care 16:902, 1993.

Greenspan FS, Baxter JD: Basic and Clinical Endocrinology, 4th ed. East Norwalk, CT, Appleton & Lange, 1994.

Grekin R: The adrenal gland. *In* Mazzaferi EL (ed): Endocrinology, 3rd edition. New York, Elsevier Science Publishing, 1986.

Grumbach MM, Styne DM: Puberty, Ontogeny, Neuroendocrinology, Physiology and Disorders. *In* Williams Textbook of

Endocrinology, 8th edition. Philadelphia, WB Saunders Company, 1992.

Herrold J, Tzagournis M: Diagnosis of early hypothyroidism by TSH measurement. Am J Med Sci 262:333, 1971.

Hoffmann J: Efficacy of 24 Week Monotherapy with Acarbose, Glibenclamide, or Placebo in NIDDM Patients. Diabetes Care 17(6):561, 1994.

Kannel WB, Wilson PWF, Zhang TJ: The epidemiology of impaired glucose tolerance and hypertension. Am Heart J 121:1268, 1991.

Karam JH: Type II diabetes and syndrome X. Endocrinol Metab Clin North Am 21(2):32, 1992.

Kaye TB: Thyroid function tests: Application of newer methods. Postgrad Med 94:1, 1993.

Krolewski AS, Warram JH: Epidemiology of diabetes mellitus. *In* Marble, Krall, Bradley, Christlieb, Soeldner (eds): Joslin's Diabetes Mellitus, 12th edition. Philadelphia, Lea & Febiger, 1985, p 2.

Laakso M, Lehtos S, Pentillo I: Lipids and lipoproteins predicting coronary heart disease in patients with noninsulin-dependent diabetes. Circulation 88(4.1):1421, 1993.

Malarkey WB: Prolactinomas. *In* Mazzaferri EL, Samaan, NA (eds): Endocrine Tumors. Oxford, Blackwell Scientific, 1993, pp 124–135.

Mandel SJ, Brent GA, Larsen PR: Levothyroxine therapy in patients with thyroid disease. Ann Intern Med 119:492, 1993.

Mathiesen ER, Hommel E, Giese J, Parving H: Efficacy of captopril in postponing nephropathy in normotensive insulin dependent diabetic patients with microalbuminuria. BMJ 303:81, 1991.

Mazzaferri EL: Current concepts: Management of a solitary nodule. N Engl J Med 328:553, 1993.

Merli GL, Bell RD: Preoperative management of the patient with neurologic disease. Med Clin North Am 71:511, 1987.

Miller JF, Crapo L: The medical treatment of Cushing's syndrome. Endocr Rev 14:443, 1993.

Multiple Risk Factor Intervention Trial Research Group: Multiple risk factor intervention trial: Risk factor changes and mortality results. JAMA 248:1465, 1982.

Murray PP, Stadel BV, Schlesselman JJ: Oral Contraceptive Use in Women with a Family History of Breast Cancer. Obstet Gynecol 73(6):977, 1989.

Nathan DM: Long-term complications of diabetes mellitus. N Engl J Med 328:1676, 1993.

Orth DN, Kovacs WJ, DeBold CR: The adrenal cortex. *In* Textbook of Endocrinology, 8th edition. Philadelphia, WB Saunders Company, 1992.

Reaven GM: Insulin resistance and compensatory hyperinsulinemia: Role in hypertension, dyslipidemia and coronary artery disease. Am Heart J 121:1283, 1991.

Reichard P, Nilsson BY, Rosenqvist U: The effect of long term intensified insulin treatment on the development of microvascular complications of diabetes mellitus. N Engl J Med 329:304, 1993.

Report of the US Preventive Services Task Force: Guide to Clinical Preventive Services. Baltimore, Williams & Wilkins, 1989.

Robinson BH, Dosch HM, Martin JM, et al: A model for the involvement of MHC class II proteins in the development of type 1 (insulin-dependent) diabetes mellitus in response to bovine serum albumin peptides. Diabetologia 36:364, 1993.

Rocca PV, Alloway JA, Nashel DJ: Diabetic muscular infarction. Semin Arthritis Rheum 22:280, 1993.

Rosenbloom AL: Intracerebral crises during treatment of diabetic ketoacidosis. Diabetes Care. 13:22, 1990.

Rudy DR: Osteoporosis: Overcoming a costly and debilitating disease. Postgrad Med 86(2):151, 1989.

Rudy DR: Hormone replacement therapy: How to select the best preparation and regimen. Postgrad Med 88(8):157, 1990.

Siegel SF, Finegold DN, Lanes R, et al: ACTH stimulation tests and plasma dehydroepiantrosterone sulfate levels in women with hirsutism. N Engl J Med 323(13):849, 1990.

Singer PA: Thyroiditis: acute, subacute and chronic. Med Clin North Am 75:(1):61, 1991.

Siperstein MD: Diabetic ketoacidosis and hyperosmolar coma. Endocrinol Metab Clin North Am 21(2):415, 1992.

Skillman TG: Diabetic acidosis. Heart Lung 7:594, 1978.

Tzagournis M, Skillman TG: Diabetes Mellitus: An Overview. Monograph. Kalamazoo, MI, The Upjohn Company, 1989.

Unger RH, Foster DW: Diabetes. *In* Williams Textbook of Endocrinology, 13th edition. Philadelphia, WB Saunders Company. 1992.

Watts NB, Harris ST, Genant HK et al: Intermittent Cyclical Etidronate Treatment of Postmenopausal Osteoporosis. New Engl J Med 323(2):73, 1990.

Weitz HH, Goldman L: Cardiac surgery in the noncardiac patient. Med Clin North Am 71(3):413, 1987.

Wilson JD, Foster DW (eds): Williams Textbook of Endocrinology, 8th edition. Philadelphia, WB Saunders Company. 1992.

Women's Health in the Perimenopause: Implications for Clinicians. Clinical Proceedings of The Association of Reproductive Health Professionals. July 1993.

Zeller K, Whittaker E, Sullivan L, et al: Effect of restricting dietary protein on the progression of renal failure in patients with insulin-dependent diabetes mellitus. N Engl J Med 324:78, 1991.

CHAPTER 42

NUTRITION AND FAMILY MEDICINE

SUSAN J. SPEER and EUGENE A. FELMAR

The integration of nutritional care into medical practice is essential to quality patient care. A patient's nutritional status is a "vital sign" of health as important as blood pressure and pulse (Report, 1991). Physicians integrate nutritional care into medical practice in two broad areas: health promotional nutrition and therapeutic nutrition. The role of nutrition in health promotion includes not only diet and disease prevention but also the changing nutritional needs and special concerns associated with normal growth and aging. The role of dietary modification as an adjunct to medical therapy is of equal importance. Illness and injury affect the patient's nutritional status by directly altering nutrient requirements or by affecting the ability to ingest, digest, absorb, or metabolize nutrients.

Routine nutritional assessment is a logical first step in integrating nutritional care into everyday medical practice. Nutritional assessment is the requisite in determining the need for nutritional intervention. Nutritional intervention is any action taken to decrease the risk of or to treat existing poor nutritional status (AAFP, 1992). Because nutritional problems are often multifactorial, nutrition interventions may be multidisciplinary including medical and dental care, mental health services, social services, nutrition education and counseling services, and specialized nutritional support.

NUTRITIONAL STATUS ASSESSMENT

Nutritional assessment is the process of determining an individual's nutritional status: the degree to which nutrient intake is adequate for health and appropriate for optimal health maintenance. Ideally every patient is screened for possible nutritional problems. Populations at increased nutritional risk include patients with increased nutritional requirements (e.g., growing children or trauma patients), decreased ability to fulfill nutritional needs (e.g., the poor or chronically debilitated person), or nontraditional food practices (e.g., food faddist or recently immigrated person).

Nutritional assessment should be tailored to fit the patient and the setting. In practice, a brief nutritional assessment of the basically healthy adult takes less than 5 minutes. The patient's medical history is reviewed to determine the presence of illnesses or use of medications that could decrease nutrient availability or increase nutrient need. Readily available blood chemistries and the patient's clinical appearance are evaluated for obvious indicators of poor nutritional status, such as low hemoglobin or wasted appearance. Body weight is evaluated. Weight stability over time is assessed. Questions focused on lifestyle and eating habits complete the nutritional screen. They include inquiries about economic security, recent changes in functional status or dependence, appetite and eating difficulties, regularity of meals, any diet restrictions, and use of nutrient supplements. This abbreviated approach is appropriate for screening children when modified by additional attention to growth velocity, parental feeding concerns, and more quantifiable dietary information.

Those patients identified to be at nutritional risk or who present with more detailed medical problems require a more complete nutritional assessment. This assessment includes the detailed clinical, laboratory, psychosocial, and dietary information required to characterized the presence, nature, and extent of possible nutritional problems (LSRO, 1989). The more complete assessment is designed to provide the information necessary to individualize the nutrition intervention plan according to the patient's life habits, educational level, economic status, cultural food practices, food preferences, and health requirements.

Nutritional assessment can be integrated into the routine of the physician's history and physical examination. Indicators of poor nutritional status are generally quantifiable factors (e.g., pounds underweight), which provide evidence that poor nutritional status is present. These factors are perhaps easiest to identify; and if abnormal to a certain defined extent, they mandate consideration of nutritional intervention (AAFP, 1992). Risk factors are those characteristics, such as inappropriate dietary intake or dependence, that increase the likelihood of poor nutritional status developing over time. The physician must be alert to these definite, though perhaps less quantifiable, risk factors if poor nutritional status is to be consistently detected, or detected as early as possible, in the individual patient (Report, 1991).

Patient History

Key areas to assess include conditions that (1) increase nutritional requirements; (2) affect the patient's ability to obtain, digest, absorb, or normally metabolize nutrients; (3) signal occult nutritional compromise; and (4) require dietary modification as an adjunct to medical treatment.

Surgery, trauma, fever, and systemic infection increase nutritional demands. Prior hospitalization for these condition should alert the physician to the possibility that the patient's nutritional status may be compromised or that the nutritional store may be inadequate.

Poverty and reliance on economic assistance programs indicate a risk for obtaining adequate or appropriate food. Social isolation or dependence on others for cooking, shopping, or feeding place the patient at risk for inadequate or inappropriate dietary intake, as do mental health problems, alcoholism, and drug addiction. Seemingly unrelated conditions, such as arthritis of the hands, may physically compromise a patient's ability to obtain adequate nutrition. Family dynamics such as marital instability or poor parenting behaviors are risk factors that may affect the dietary adequacy of children in particular.

Complaints of anorexia, early satiety, nausea and vomiting, problems with chewing or swallowing, or changes in bowel habits alert the physician to possible problems with nutrient intake. Chronic vomiting or diarrhea or other conditions that affect nutrient absorption (e.g., pancreatitis or colitis) have obvious nutritional implications. A concomitant change in the usual weight, or the growth velocity in children, increase the likelihood of malnutrition.

Many medications affect nutritional status (1) directly by altering nutrient absorption, metabolism, or excretion, or (2) indirectly through changes that affect the ingestion of food. Drug-induced changes in taste and smell acuity, appetite, and gastrointestinal function can affect food intake. Older persons, debilitated patients, children, pregnant or lactating women, anyone on a marginally adequate diet, and patients on long-term drug therapy are particularly at risk. Specific recommendations for nutrient supplementation during drug therapy can be found in Table 42–1. Additionally, dietary intake may affect drug action in clinically important ways. For exam-

TABLE 42–1. DRUG–NUTRIENT INTERACTIONS

Therapeutic Class	Drug — Proprietary Examples	Drug — Generic/Active Compound	Recommended Daily Vitamin/Mineral Supplement or Restriction During Drug Therapy*
Anticonvulsants	Dilantin	Phenytoin†	Vitamin D 400–800 IU‡ Vitamin K 1–5 mg Folic acid 0.4–1.0 mg (not > 2.0 mg/day)
Anti-inflammatory agents	Mysoline Azulfidine Bayer aspirin Bufferin Other aspirin Indocin	Primidone Sulfasalazine Aspirin Indomethacin	Vitamin K 1–5 mg‡ Folic acid 0.4–1.0 mg Ascorbic acid 50–100 mg Folic acid 0.4–1.0 mg Iron 20–50 mg Iron 20–50 mg
Antilipemic agents	Questran Colestid	Cholestyramine Colestipol	Vitamin A 2000–5000 IU Vitamin D 200–800 IU Vitamin K 2–25 mg Folic acid 0.4–1.0 mg
Antituberculous agents	INH Rifamate	Isoniazid Rifampin-isoniazid	Vitamin B_6 25–50 mg Niacin 15–25 mg Vitamin D 400–800 IU
Hypotensive drugs	Apresoline	Hydralazine	Vitamin B_6 25–100 mg
Oral contraceptives	Norinyl Demulen Ovral Ortho-Novum Modicon and others	Estrogen/progestin	Vitamin B_6 1.5–5 mg Folic acid 0.4–1.0 mg Avoid high doses of vitamin C (i.e., ≥1000 mg)
Tranquilizers	Thorazine Mellaril	Chlorpromazine Thioridazine Other phenothiazines	Riboflavin 2–5 mg

Pregnant or lactating women should consult their physicians for specific micronutrient recommendations.
* Short-term drug therapy may or may not necessitate specific vitamin/mineral supplementation.
† Calcium-containing foods and supplements should be given 2 hours or more away from drug dose.
‡ If Dilantin (phenytoin)-induced demineralization is identified, give vitamin D 2000 IU/day. Pregnant women on Dilantin or Mysoline should receive vitamin K 5 mg/day for 3 days prior to delivery, and neonates should receive 1 mg.
From Roe DA: Drug-Induced Nutritional Deficiencies, 2nd edition. New York, Van Nostrand Reinhold, AVI Publishing, 1985, with permission.

TABLE 42–2. FOOD GROUP PLAN

Food Group	Recommended No. of Servings				
	Child	Teenager	Adult	Pregnant Woman	Lactating Woman

Dairy
  1 cup milk or yogurt *or*
  Calcium equivalent: 1½ slices (1½ oz)
    cheddar cheese*
  1 cup pudding
  1¾ cups ice cream
  2 cups cottage cheese*
	3	4	2	4	4

Meat
  2 oz cooked lean meat, fish, or poultry *or*
  Protein equivalent
    2 eggs
    2 slices (2 oz) cheddar cheese*
    ½ cup cottage cheese*
    1 cup cooked dried beans or peas
    4 tbsp peanut butter
    4 oz tofu
	2	2	2	3	2

Fruit/vegetable
  ½ cup cooked or juice
  1 cup raw
  Portion commonly served, such as a
    medium-size apple or banana
	5–9	5–9	5–9	5–9	5–9

Grain (whole grain, fortified, enriched)
  1 slice bread
  1 cup ready-to-eat cereal
  ½ cup cooked cereal, pasta, grits, or rice
	6–11	6–11	6–11	6–11	6–11

* Count cheese as a serving of milk or meat but not both simultaneously.

ple, the antithrombotic action of warfarin is antagonized by a high intake of green leafy vegetables, which are rich sources of vitamin K.

Changes in functional and cognitive status (including depression) are potential signals of a declining nutritional state. Disabling physical or mental conditions similarly affect and are affected by nutritional status.

Dietary history completes the information obtained during the patient interview. Information about dietary intake can be obtained by a variety of methods depending on time and purpose. Abbreviated questions are sufficient for nutritional screening. A complete assessment includes investigations into cultural and religious food practices, personal preferences, attitudes and beliefs, and food allergies or intolerances, as well as dietary modifications (medically prescribed or self-imposed) and nutritional supplementation. Detailed information about meal schedule and the quantity and quality of food intake is usually obtained with a 24-hour activity-associated dietary recall. A diet recall is a verbal report of food and beverage intake over the past 24 hours, or "yesterday." Asking the patient to recall the day's activities along with food intake provides a structure for recall and reveals eating patterns and lifestyles that may play a role in developing a nutrition intervention.

A simple test of nutritional adequacy can be performed by comparing daily food intake information to the number of servings recommended in the Food Group Plan (Table 42–2). Figure 42–1 illustrates this type of simple analysis. Dietary intakes that meet the minimum recommended number of servings are minimally adequate in key nutrients such as protein, iron, calcium, vitamin C, vitamin A, niacin, thiamine, and riboflavin. Lack of day-to-day variety and heavy reliance on processed foods can lead to nutrient deficiencies even while satisfying the serving recommendations. Calories, fat, sugar, and sodium intake vary, depending on food choices and preparation methods. Occasionally, when assessing difficult dietary problems or monitoring adherence to prescribed dietary modifications, a diary of food intake recorded for a specified period of time is necessary.

Physical Examination

The clinical examination may reveal physical signs of excessive (e.g., obesity) or inadequate nutrient intake (e.g., cheilosis and B vitamins). Table 42–3 lists the clinical signs of nutrient deficiency and toxicity. The physical examination also includes anthropometric determinations that can be used for initial nutritional status assessment and, in some cases, to monitor the effectiveness of long-term nutritional support.

Height and weight in both children and adults, and head circumference in children, are the most common physical measurements utilized for assessing nutritional status in office practice. The

Obtaining a 24-hour dietary recall can be time-consuming, but it is the easiest method for evaluating possible dietary deficiencies and excesses. Remember that this information is only a "window" on the patient's eating behaviors and food intake. Cross-questioning for usual intake extends the usefulness of the information.

Jot down everything the patient recalls eating the previous day. Do not "lead" the patient by asking about breakfast, lunch, and dinner. Instead ask: What did you eat first, next . . . ? After posing the initial questions, go back and ask for specifics such as: How much? What kind? How was it prepared? Determine whether this day's intake is typical. If not, how is it different? If necessary, alter the information to reflect a more representative day.

Next, using the serving sizes listed in Table 42–2, compare the patient's intake to the recommended number of servings, as shown below. In the example below of an adult woman, the diet contains inadequate dairy products; thus her diet is probably low in the major nutrients offered by this food group—calcium and riboflavin.

	Food Groups			
Food	**Dairy**	**Grain**	**Vegetable/Fruit**	**Meat**
½ cup 2% milk	½			
1 cup cereal		1		
1 slice toast		1		
1 orange			1	
1 sandwich				
2 slices bread		2		
2 slices lunch meat				1
1 apple			1	
3 oz chicken breast				1
1 cup rice		2		
½ cup broccoli			1	
tomato salad			1	
1 peach			1	
Total	½	6	5	2
Recommended	2	6	5–9	2

FIGURE 42–1. Analysis of daily food intake. (Modified from Coombs JB, Speer SJ: *Nutrition I/II.* Monograph, edition no. 129/130. Kansas City, MO, American Academy of Family Physicians, 1990.)

standards for evaluating anthropomorphic measurements in children are the National Center for Health Statistics (NCHS) Growth Grids, although other grids are available for use with special populations such as premature infants or children with Down syndrome (AAP, 1993a). Measurements of recumbent length are used on the infant grids (birth to 36 months) and standing height on the grids for children (age 2 to 18 years). Weight-for-height greater than the 95th percentile indicates obesity, and that less than the 5th percentile indicates underweight. Evidence of excessive or inadequate dietary intake helps confirm a nutritional etiology. A height-for-age less than the 5th percentile or a nonconsistent head circumference measurement may indicate chronic undernutrition (Robbins, 1984).

Serial measurements can indicate nutritional risk before weight and length become abnormal. Failure to thrive is indicated by a precipitous drop in growth velocity (e.g., a decrease of 20 percentile points over a 3- to 6-month period) (Berwick, 1988). Approximately 50 to 90 per cent of failure to thrive cases are caused by improper feeding (Hockelman et al., 1987). A rise in weight-for-height channel may predict developing obesity.

In adults, a relative weight (actual weight divided by desirable weight) of 85 per cent or a history of weight loss indicates nutritional risk. A relative weight of 120 per cent is mild overweight, and 140 per cent is considered severely overweight (DHHS, 1988). Unintentional loss of 10 per cent of body weight over 6 months or a recent loss of more than 10 pounds is associated with decreased functional ability and increased nutrition-mediated complications, such as infection or poor wound-healing (Alpers, 1988; Heymsfield et al., 1994; Jensen et al., 1983)—even if the patient's current weight is not less than the desirable weight (Alpers, 1988).

Desirable weights have traditionally been those weights-for-height associated with the greatest longevity based on actuarial data from the Metropolitan Life Insurance Company (MLIC) (Table 42–4). The 1983 MLIC weights are generally higher than those for 1959, but still significantly lower than the average weights measured in population surveys such as the National Health and Nutrition Examination Survey (NHANES). The midpoint of the weight range for a given height is commonly used as the standard. The following formula approximates the desirable weight for a given height: to a base of 120 pounds for a woman (or 130 pounds for a man), add 3 pounds for every inch of height over 5 feet.

Although relative weight is a more accessible term for patient counseling, the currently preferred definition of obesity is the body mass index (BMI). This index, calculated by dividing body weight in kilograms by height in square meters, correlates more closely with total body fat (DHHS, 1988). Figure 42–2 is a nomogram that facilitates calcula-

TABLE 42–3. ESSENTIAL VITAMINS AND MINERALS

Nutrient	Major Body Functions	Rich Food Sources	Signs and Symptoms of Deficiency	Signs and Symptoms of Toxicity
Fat-Soluble Vitamins				
Vitamin A (retinol)	Constituent of rhodopsin (visual pigment); maintenance of epithelial tissues; role in mucopolysaccharide synthesis, bone and tooth formation	Provitamin A (carotenes): dark green leafy vegetables (e.g., spinach, chard); yellow/orange vegetables and fruits (e.g., carrot, sweet potato, mango, cantaloupe) Retinol: liver, whole milk, butter, cheese, fortified milk, margarine, breakfast cereal	Nightblindness, xerosis, Bitot's spot, keratomalacia, perifollicular hyperkeratosis, anorexia, bone changes	Anorexia, headache, blurred vision, dry skin, pruritus, painful extremities, hepatomegaly, splenomegaly
Vitamin D	Increases calcium absorption; promotes growth and mineralization of bones	Egg yolk, liver, fatty fish (i.e., salmon and fish oils); fortified milk and margarine	Children: rickets Adults: osteomalacia	Hypercalcemia; anorexia, nausea, vomiting, constipation, polydipsia, polyuria, renal stones, hypertension Infants (severe): mental retardation, aortic stenosis, *elfin facies*
Vitamin E	Antioxidant, protects cell membranes	Vegetable oils, wheat germ, fish liver oils, nuts and seeds, green leafy vegetables, whole grains	Neurologic syndromes: areflexia, gait disturbances, paresis of gaze	Fatigue, headache, delayed wound healing, increased bleeding, muscle weakness LBW infants: hepatosplenomegaly, azotemia, thrombocytopenia
Vitamin K	Important in blood clotting (formation of active prothrombin)	Green leafy vegetables; cabbage family vegetables (e.g., cauliflower); tomato, beef liver	Hypothrombinemia and hemorrhagic disease	Hemolytic anemia, hepatotoxicity LBW infants: jaundice, lethargy, hypotonia
Water-Soluble Vitamins				
Vitamin C	Collagen synthesis neurotransmitter synthesis; antioxidant: protects vitamins A and E; functions in wound healing and immune response	Citrus fruits; green leafy vegetables (e.g., broccoli, asparagus); cabbage family vegetables; cantaloupe, strawberries, mango, peppers, tomato	Scurvy Infants and elderly: bone changes, bleeding gums, anemia Adults: fatigue, aching bones, joints, and muscles, perifollicular hemorrhages, bleeding gums, failed wound healing	Nausea, abdominal cramps, diarrhea
Thiamine (vitamin B_1)	Coenzyme for removal of carbon dioxide (thiamine pyrophosphate)	Pork, legumes, green peas, tofu; whole grain and enriched breads and cereals; nuts and seeds	CV (wet) beriberi: edema, heart failure Neurologic (dry) beriberi: Wernicke's encephalopathy, peripheral neuropathies, lactic acidosis with carbohydrate loading	Anaphylactic shock with large IV doses
Riboflavin (vitamin B_2)	Cofactor in energy metabolism (FAD, FMN)	Dairy products, green leafy vegetables, whole and enriched grains, meats, liver, poultry, fish	Reddened, greasy scaly, puritic skin in the oroaculogenital area; dyssebacea (*shark skin*), angular stomatitis, cheilosis, magenta tongue	No cases reported
Niacin	Cofactor in glycolysis and fat metabolism (NAD, NADP)	Meat, poultry, fish, peanuts, legumes; whole and enriched grain products; milk, eggs, nuts, and seeds (can be formed from tryptophan)	Pellagra: photosensitive dermatitis, diarrhea, mucosal inflammation, dementia, beefy red tongue	Release of histamine: severe flushing, pruritus, GI disturbances, elevated serum uric acid and glucose, hepatic toxicity
Vitamin B_6	Coenzyme in amino acid metabolism (pyridoxal phosphate)	Meat, poultry, fish, legumes, potato, green leafy vegetables, whole grain products, banana, nuts, and seeds	Seborrheic dematitis, glossitis, cheilosis, angular stomatitis, peripheral neuropathy	Peripheral sensory neuropathy, ataxia, perioral numbness
Folate	Coenzyme in amino acid metabolism (pyridoxal phosphate)	Liver, dark green leafy vegetables, legumes, peanuts, wholegrains	Megaloblastic anemia, glossitis	None reported in humans; masks vitamin B_{12} deficiency
Vitamin B_{12} (cobalamin)	Coenzyme in nucleic acid metabolism	Foods of animal origin: meats, poultry, fish, eggs, dairy products	Megaloblastic anemia, glossitis anorexia, sensory neuropathy, dementia	No clear toxicity reported

Table continued on following page

TABLE 42–3.   ESSENTIAL VITAMINS AND MINERALS (Continued)

Nutrient	Major Body Functions	Rich Food Sources	Signs and Symptoms of Deficiency	Signs and Symptoms of Toxicity
Biotin	Coenzyme in fat synthesis, amino acid metabolism, and glycogen formation	Legumes, vegetables, meats	Scaly dermatitis, alopecia	None reported
Pantothenic acid	Constituent of coenzyme A involved in energy metabolism	Widely distributed in food; nutritional yeast	Burning feet syndrome; fatigue	Diarrhea, water retention
		Minerals		
Calcium	Bone and tooth formation, blood clotting, nerve condition	Dairy products; small fish with bones; dark green leafy vegetables; tofu; unhulled sesame seeds	Hypocalcemia: tetany, depression, psychosis, osteoporosis, rickets	Constipation, hypercalciuria, hypercalcemia
Phosphorus	Bone and tooth formation; acid-base balance	Meats, dairy products, grains	Hypophosphatemia: bone loss (rickets), weakness, anorexia, pain	Hypocalcemic: tetany (infants)
Potassium	Acid-base balance, water balance, nerve function	Milk, fruits especially citrus, prunes, apples, pear, peach, banana, vegetables especially green leafy, potato, carrot, tomato, meats, legumes, whole grains	Hypokalemia: weakness, anorexia, nausea, irrational behavior, cardiac dysrhythmias	Hyperkalemia: cardiac toxicity
Sodium	Acid-base balance, water balance, nerve function	Salt, soy sauce, processed foods	Hypovolemia, muscle weakness	Edema, hypertension
Chloride	Formation of gastric juice, acid-base balance	Salt, natural waters	Infants: hypochloremic metabolic acidosis	Hypertension
Magnesium	Activates enzymes involved in protein synthesis	Seeds, nuts, legumes, whole grains, dark green leafy vegetables, bananas	Hypomagnesemia, hypokalemia, hypocalcemia, nausea, weakness, mental derangement	Hypermagnesemia: nausea, vomiting, hypotension
Iron	Constituent of hemoglobin and enzymes involved in tissue respiration	Liver, red meats, poultry, eggs, legumes, green leafy vegetables, whole and enriched grain products, nuts, dried fruits	Fatigue, anemia, glossitis	Acute: vomiting, cyanosis, diarrhea, shock Chronic: hepatomegaly, slate-gray skin, cardiomyopathy, arthropathy, diabetes
Zinc	Constituent of enzymes involved in nucleic acid, protein, and alcohol metabolism		Anorexia, growth, retardation, hypogonadism, hypogeusia, poor wound healing	Acute: vomiting Chronic: hypocupremia, microcytosis, impaired immune response, low HDL levels
Iodine	Constituent of thyroid hormone	Iodized salt, shellfish, and marine fish, dairy products, eggs, some vegetables	Endemic goiter, cretinism	Iodide goiter, myxedema
Selenium	Antioxidant (functions with vitamin E)	Seafood, organ meats, other meats, some grains and seeds	Muscle pain, cardiomyopathy	Alopecia, fingernail changes, garlic odor, nausea, diarrhea, periperal neuropathy
Copper	Hemoglobin synthesis, connective tissue, metabolism, bone development	Organ meats, seafood, nuts, seeds, drinking water	Hypochromic anemia, neutropenia, osteoporosis, growth retardation	
Manganese	Constituent of enzymes involved in fat metabolism	Nuts, dried fruit, whole grain products, tea	Weight loss, dementia, N/V, changes in hair color	
Fluoride	May be important in maintenance of tooth structure	Seafood, tea, cereal, drinking water	Not an essential nutrient	Mottled, pitted teeth; impaired bone health; kidney, nerve, and muscle dysfunction
Chromium	Involved in glucose metabolism	Brewer's yeast; meat products; dairy products; eggs	Weight loss, peripheral neuropathy, glucose intolerance	
Molybdenum	Xanthine metabolism	Legumes, grains, organ meats	Irritability, coma	Gout-like syndrome

LBW = low birth weight; CV = cardiovascular; FAD = flavin adenine dinucleotide; FMN = flavin mononucleotide; NAD = nicotinamide adenine dinucleotide; NADP = nicotinamide adenine dinucleotide phosphate; HDL = high density lipoprotein.
Note: Essential fatty acids are linoleic and linolenic acids. Signs of deficiency are scaly dermatitis, alopecia, impaired wound healing.
Essential amino acids are isoleucine, leucine, lysine methionine, phenylalanine, threonine, tryptophan, valine, and histidine.
Cobalt is essential as a component of vitamin B$_{12}$ and sulfur as a constituent of sulfur-containing amino acids. Silicon, vanadium, tin, nickel, boron, and arsenic are also essential trace minerals.

TABLE 42–4. DESIRABLE WEIGHTS: METROPOLITAN LIFE INSURANCE (1983)

Height (Feet and Inches)	Weight (Pounds)		
	Small Frame	Medium Frame	Large Frame
Men			
5 Feet			
2 Inches	128–134	131–141	138–150
3	130–136	133–143	140–153
4	132–138	135–145	142–156
5	134–140	137–148	144–160
6	136–142	139–151	146–164
7	138–145	142–154	149–168
8	140–148	145–157	152–172
9	142–151	148–160	155–176
10	144–154	151–163	158–180
11	146–157	154–166	161–184
6 Feet			
0 Inches	149–160	157–170	164–188
1	152–164	160–174	168–192
2	155–168	164–178	172–197
3	158–172	167–182	176–202
4	162–176	171–187	181–207
Women			
4 Feet			
10 Inches	102–111	109–121	118–131
11	103–113	111–123	120–134
5 Feet			
0 Inches	104–115	113–126	122–137
1	106–118	115–129	125–140
2	108–121	118–132	128–143
3	111–124	121–135	131–147
4	114–127	124–138	134–151
5	117–130	127–141	137–155
6	120–133	130–144	140–158
7	123–136	133–147	143–163
8	126–139	138–150	146–167
9	129–142	139–153	149–170
10	132–145	142–156	152–173
11	135–148	145–159	156–176
6 Feet			
0 Inches	138–151	148–162	158–179

Note: Weights at ages 25 through 59 are based on lowest mortality. Weight (in pounds) is according to frame (in indoor clothing weighing 5 lb for men and 3 lb for women; shoes with 1-inch heels).

Courtesy of *Statistical Bulletin*, Metropolitan Life Insurance Company, New York.

individuals. Depending on the skill and experience of the clinician, arm anthropometry may be useful when body weight is not obtainable or invalid owing to edema or massive tumor burden (Heymsfield et al., 1994).

Laboratory Investigations

Determination of red blood cell indices, lipid levels, and fasting blood glucose levels are the only diet-related indices used in routine office practice that have obvious implications for nutritional status. Tests for vitamin and mineral levels are generally reserved for confirming specific deficiencies suspected from clinical or dietary information. However, low serum vitamin C, vitamin A, and zinc levels have been suggested as routine indicators of poor overall dietary quality (Report, 1991).

Because measurable body changes are usually late manifestations of malnutrition, especially in adults, biochemical indices have been investigated for use as early markers of protein–calorie malnutrition. Circulating proteins such as albumin, transferrin, prealbumin, retinol-binding protein, and GF-1 are sensitive to dietary protein and energy intakes. There is substantial evidence that low serum albumin predicts increased morbidity and mortality (Heymsfield et al., 1994). In hospitalized patients hypoalbuminemia is directly correlated with prolonged hospital stays and increased mortality (Heymsfield et al., 1994). Decreased serum albumin levels have also been associated with increased mortality in nonhospitalized patients (Heymsfield et al., 1994). Progressively lower levels of albumin and transferrin are sometimes used to rank nutritional status. Albumin and transferrin levels of 2.1 to 2.7 gm/dL and 100 to 150 mg/dL, respectively, signal moderate malnutrition. Lower levels are associated with severe deficit (Alpers, 1988).

Determination of serum protein levels adds to the clinical picture but must be interpreted with caution during nutritional assessment of the acutely sick patient. Albumin (and other circulating liver proteins) are discrete markers of protein nutriture only in the absence of other clinical factors that influence metabolism and serum levels (Heymsfield et al., 1994). Albumin is reduced by many conditions, including zinc deficiency, hypothyroidism, liver disease, renal disease, malignant diseases, radiation therapy, protein-losing enteropathy, and acute physiologic stress such as injury or infection (Heymsfield et al., 1994).

In summary, there is no single nutritional measure, or group of measures, that can be relied on solely for determining nutritional status. Anthropometric determinations are useful for identifying both chronic and recent nutritional problems in growing children. Undernutrition that results in underweight or decreased growth velocity in chil-

tions of BMI. A BMI between 20 and 25 is considered desirable, and BMIs of 27 and 31 are approximately equivalent to relative weights of 120 per cent and 140 per cent, respectively. A BMI below 18.5 is considered underweight (Heymsfield et al., 1994).

Measurement of the waist and hip circumference allows calculation of the waist-to-hip ratio (WHR). The WHR estimates abdominal adiposity. An increased WHR (greater than 0.9 in men and 0.8 in women) increases medical risk independently of obesity and in addition to it (Kissebah et al., 1989).

Other measures of body composition, such as measures of subcutaneous fat (e.g., triceps skinfold thickness) or estimates of muscle mass (e.g., midarm muscle circumference), are poorly reproducible and have limited usefulness when assessing

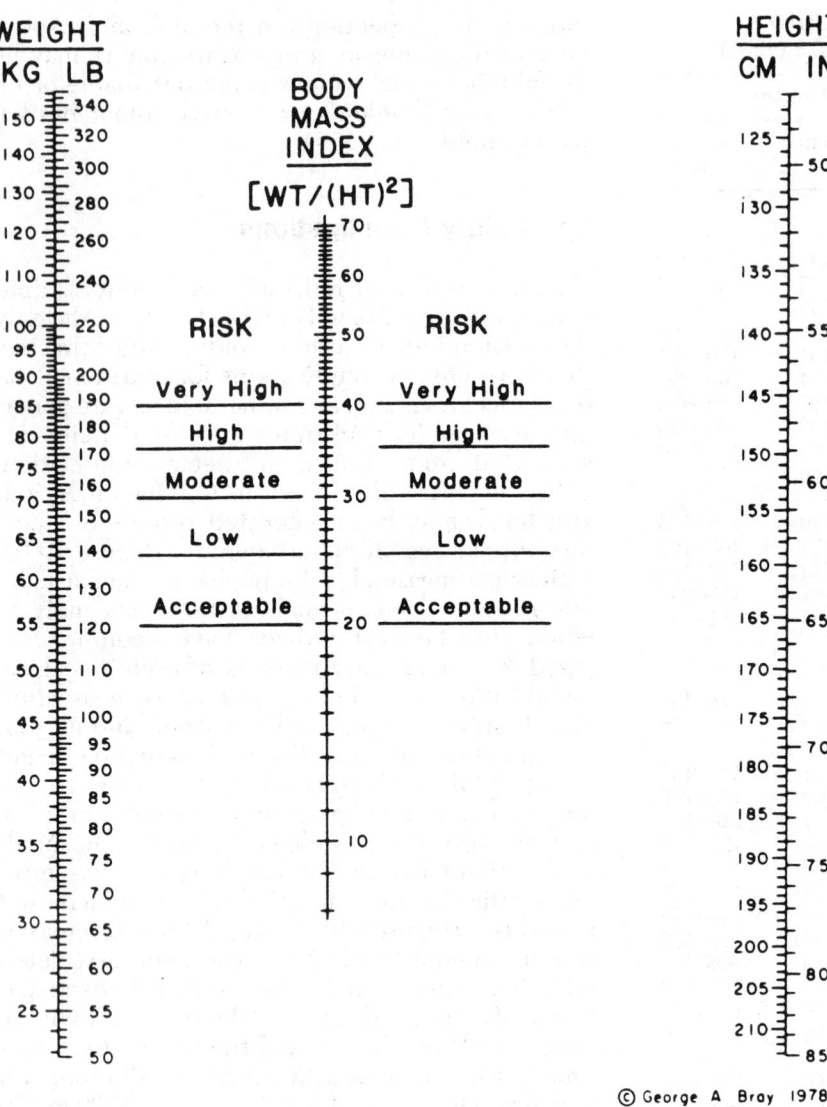

FIGURE 42–2. Nomogram for determining body mass index (BMI). To use this nomogram, place a ruler or other straight edge between the body weight in kilograms or pounds (without clothes) located on the left-hand line and the height in centimeters or inches (without shoes) located on the right-hand line. The body mass index is read from the middle of the scale and is in metric units. (From Bray GA: Classification and evaluation of the obesities. Med Clin North Am 73:161, 1989, with permission.)

© George A Bray 1978

dren also increases susceptibility to such nutrition-mediated complications as infection (Jeejeebhoy, 1990b). By contrast, the functional changes that affect risk of morbidity and mortality or quality of life in adults generally precede measurable body changes. In adults, anthropometry is less sensitive, especially to mild or recent deterioration of nutritional status relative to other indicators such as circulating protein levels. Unfortunately, as discussed above, biochemical indices are often difficult to interpret especially in the acutely ill patient. This point underscores the need to evaluate a variety of risk factors and indicators, including medical history and dietary and psychosocial information, before arriving at a decision about an individual's nutritional status.

NUTRITION AND HEALTH PROMOTION

Health promotional nutrition counseling provides patients information on ensuring dietary adequacy without excess. To effectively promote an optimal diet the family physician must understand the role of nutrition in health maintenance, know the various dietary components and their food sources, and be able to communicate this information to the patient in the form of simple dietary advice. This simple advice is embodied in the ten dietary guidelines discussed below.

Dietary Guidelines

The basic dietary guidelines promoted by various health organizations in the United States are remarkably similar to each other and to guidelines that have been prepared independently in more than 20 other industrialized countries (Table 42–5). Some sets of guidelines include recommendations for adequate intake of specific nutrients (i.e., calcium, iron, fluoride), but the focus of most guidelines is on avoiding the excessive calorie, fat, saturated fat, cholesterol, sodium, and alcohol intakes that are associated with the development of chronic degenerative diseases. Five of the ten leading causes of death (coronary heart disease, some types of cancer, stroke, diabetes mellitus, and atherosclerosis) are associated with diet (DHHS, 1988). The dietary guidelines presented here are a combination of those guidelines for general wellness and disease prevention promoted by the U.S. Department of Agriculture (USDA), Department of Health and Human Services (DHHS), and National Research Council (NRC).

1. *Eat a nutritionally adequate diet from a variety of foods.* This principle is basic to a healthful diet. Eating a variety of foods maximizes the probability of eating adequate amounts of essential nutrients, defined and still to be defined, as well as dietary factors that are not considered essential but that may have a beneficial effect on body functioning (e.g., fiber). Our standards of dietary adequacy for defined nutrients are represented by the Recommended Dietary Allowances (RDAs). These standards are established by the National Research Council and are updated every 5 to 10 years (Table 42–6).

The RDAs are set at levels that incorporate margins of safety. They are intended to be sufficiently generous to encompass the presumed variability in requirements among individuals and to account for variations in the efficiency of utilization and biologic availability of nutrients in the context of the typical American diet. Thus the RDAs exceed the actual requirements for most nutrients with the exception of energy. Energy (expressed as calories) recommendations are set at the average population requirement for each age and gender group based on the actual median weights for the U.S. population (Table 42–7). Estimated safe and adequate daily dietary intakes (ESADDIs) are ranges of safe intake established for seven nutrients for which there were insufficient data to develop a defined RDA (NRC, 1989b) (Table 42–8).

The RDAs were originally intended for use in estimating adequate intakes for population groups. However, an individual's intake, averaged over a sufficient length of time, may be compared to the RDAs to estimate the risk of developing nutritional deficiencies (NRC, 1989b). The probability of malnutrition in the individual becomes progressively greater as nutrient intake becomes lower. Note that the RDAs are intended to be sufficient to prevent the impairment of normal physiologic functioning that may be caused by nutrient deficiency in an otherwise healthy person. They do not address special nutritional needs arising from metabolic disorders, chronic disease, trauma, premature birth, and other medical conditions (e.g., fever, infection) and drug therapies that may change nutrient requirements by altering nutrient absorption, metabolism, or excretion (NRC, 1989b).

Practical advice to patients on how to meet the RDAs in everyday diet takes the form of the Food Group Guide. (Table 42–2). Consuming the recommended number of servings from each food group, selected from a variety of foods within each group, helps ensure that the RDA will be met over time. Altering the serving sizes (e.g., half-portions for young children) makes the Food Group Guide applicable to all age groups. Replacing meats in the protein category with servings of legumes, nuts, or eggs makes the Guide useful for ovo-lacto vegetarians.

Nutrient deficiencies are rare in the United States. Clinical evidence of malnutrition or specific nutrient deficiencies are generally found in vulnerable groups, such as those who are unable or unwilling to obtain enough food (e.g., low income populations or chronic dieters) or a sufficient variety of foods (e.g., food faddists), or those with increased nutritional needs due to growth (e.g., pregnant women) or repair (e.g., surgery patients). Evidence of nutrient deficiencies from national nutrition surveys help physicians direct abbreviated dietary evaluations at reported at-risk nutrients and their food sources. Deficiencies of iron and calcium pose the most serious public health problems because population surveys have detected both low dietary intake of these nutrients and evidence of specific nutrition-related health problems (e.g., calcium and osteoporosis) or biochemical evidence of impaired status in some groups (DHHS, 1986; LSRO, 1989).

One of five young, low-income children are iron-deficient. The National Health and Nutrition Examination Survey also found low iron intakes in all income groups for women (LSRO, 1989). Impaired vitamin C levels were found in 15 per cent of low-income adult males. Ten percent of Mexican-American preschoolers had low serum vitamin A levels, but levels were not excessively low in the general population (DHHS, 1986; LSRO, 1989). There is evidence of impaired zinc, magnesium, folate, and vitamin B_6 status in some groups, but these nutrients have not been sufficiently monitored in the past (DHHS, 1986). Food sources of these nutrients are listed in Table 42–3.

Problems with excessive intake of vitamins and minerals are usually not found except in instances of oversupplementation. Hypervitaminosis is more likely to be associated with the fat-soluble vitamins. Adverse reactions to excessive intakes of water-soluble vitamins, which are rapidly excreted, are less common but not unknown (e.g., vitamin B_6 and peripheral neuropathy). Hazards from excessive mineral intake usually are due to acute poisoning (a child consuming iron supplements intended for parents), chronic excessive intake (iodine excess from chronic kelp ingestion), or product contamination (lead and arsenic contamination of herbal products) (Dubick and Rucker, 1983; Roe, 1989).

The use of vitamin and mineral supplements is

TABLE 42–5.   DIETARY RECOMMENDATIONS

Type of Recommendation Reference	Maintain Appropriate Body Weight, Exercise	Limit or Reduce Total Fat (% kcal)	Reduce Saturated Fatty Acids (% kcal)	Increase Polyunsaturated Fatty Acids (% kcal)	Limit Cholesterol (mg/day)	Limit Simple Sugars
General Health Maintenance						
U.S. Senate (1977)	Yes	27–33	Yes	Yes	250–350	Yes
USDA/DHHS (1990)	Yes	Yes	Yes	No	Yes	Yes
DHHS (1988)	Yes	Yes	Yes	No	Yes	Yes
NRC (1989a)	Balance energy intake and expenditure	≤30	<10	Up to 10	<300	Yes
Heart Disease						
NIH (1985)	Yes	<30	<10	Up to 10	250–300	NC
AHA (1988)	Yes	<30	<10	Up to 10	<300	NS
Cancer						
ACS (1984)	Yes	~30	Yes	No	NC	NC
NCI (1987)	Yes	Yes	Yes	No	NC	NC

Adapted from National Research Council, Committee on Diet and Health: Diet and Health: Implications for Reducing Chronic Disease Risk. Washington, DC, National Academy Press, 1989. Copyright 1989 by the National Academy of Sciences.

not necessary for most healthy persons consuming adequate, balanced diets (see the section on vitamin and mineral supplementation below).

2. *Maintain desirable body weight.* Mortality and morbidity are increased in people who are too thin or too fat (Truswell, 1994). Overweight is the greater problem in the United States with more than 25 per cent of American adults overweight and 9 per cent severely overweight (DHHS, 1988). Overweight is defined as a BMI corresponding to the 85th percentile of weight for young American adults (about 27) and severe overweight by a BMI corresponding to the 95th percentile (greater than 31). Obesity is defined as excessive body fat. Most overweight persons are obese (NIH, 1993).

Overweight is associated with non-insulin-dependent diabetes mellitus, hypertension, coronary heart disease, gallbladder disease, osteoarthritis, gout, and breast and endometrial cancer (NIH, 1993). Increased abdominal fat (defined by a waist/hip ratio higher than 0.9 in men and 0.8 in women) carries an even higher risk for non-insulin-dependent diabetes, hypertension, stroke, and heart disease and an increased overall mortality rate (NRC,

1989a; VanItallie and Lew, 1993). Weight reduction has been shown to improve control of type II diabetes, decrease high blood pressure, and improve cholesterol profile by decreasing total and LDL cholesterol (DHHS, 1988). Whether weight reduction among the overweight population decreases overall mortality remains to be seen (NIH, 1993).

Although evidence suggests that genetic influences in the individual response to food and physical activity have an impact on the development of obesity, patterns of caloric intake and energy expenditure play an important role (DHHS, 1988). Exact energy requirements are dependent on age, body size and composition, and physical activity. The energy expended by a person at rest (resting energy expenditure, or REE) accounts for the largest proportion of daily energy needs (60 to 70 per cent), and differences in physical activity account for much of the individual variation in energy requirements. Table 42–7 may be used for calculating individual energy needs. For example, multiplying body weight in kilograms by a factor of 35 estimates the daily energy needs of an average-

TO THE U.S. PUBLIC

Increase Complex Carbohydrates (% kcal from total carbohydrates)	Increase Fiber	Restrict Sodium Chloride (g)	Moderate Alcohol Intake	Other Recommendations
Yes	Yes	8	Yes	Reduce additives and processed foods
Eat adequate starch and fiber		Yes	Yes	Variety in diet
Yes	Yes	Yes	Yes	Fluoridation of water, adolescent girls and women increase intake of calcium-rich foods; children, adolescents, and women of childbearing age increase intake of iron-rich foods
(At least 55); five daily servings of vegetables and fruit; ≥ six daily servings of cereals, breads, and legumes	Directly through vegetables, fruits, and cereals	≤6 g/day with a goal of 4.5 g/day	If you drink, limit to <1.0 oz alcohol or <2 drinks/day	Avoid dietary supplements, especially in excess of RDAs; drink fluoridated water; limit protein intake to moderate levels (less than twice the RDA)
Increase to make up caloric deficit	NC	NC	NC	Specific recommendations for high-risk groups; also physicians, public, and food industry
(50 or more)	NS	≤3 g/day of sodium	1–2 oz ethanol/ day	Protein to make up remainder of calories; wide variety of foods
Through whole grains, fruits, and vegetables	Yes	By limiting intake of salt-cured, pickled, smoked foods	Yes	Emphasize fruits and vegetables; avoid high doses of supplements; pay attention to cooking methods
Yes, more whole grains, fruits, and vegetables	20–35 g	NC	Yes	Variety in diet; avoid fiber supplements

weight woman aged 25 to 50 years engaged in light to moderate activity (e.g., carpentry work, housecleaning). Subtract 5 points from the factor given (e.g., 30) to estimate energy needs for sedentary adults engaged in seated and standing activities only.

Energy is measured in kilocalories, commonly referred to as calories. One kilocalorie represents the amount of heat energy necessary to raise the temperature of 1 kg of water from 15° C to 16° C under standard pressure conditions (NRC, 1989b). The caloric contribution per gram of carbohydrate, protein, fat, and alcohol is 4, 4, 9, and 7 (kilo)calories, respectively. Although only total diets containing calories in excess of needs can truly be called "fattening," calorically dense high fat and high sugar foods (and alcohol) are easily overeaten. A diet composed of the minimum number of adult servings in the Food Group Plan, using only nonfat items and excluding additional sugars and fats, totals approximately 1200 kcal and is marginally adequate in iron, folacin, vitamin B_6, and zinc (Pi-Sunyer, 1994).

In the United States and other westernized countries, body weight has been increasing while overall caloric intake has been decreasing, pointing to sedentary lifestyle as a factor in weight gain (NRC, 1989a). A pound of adipose tissue is estimated to be equivalent to 3500 kcal. A daily reduction in food intake of 500 kcal, or an increase in physical activity requiring 500 kcal, or a combination of the two theoretically results in 1 pound of weight lost per week. Moderate regular physical activity such as daily walks or jogging, bicycling, or swimming a minimum of three times per week for at least 20 minutes is also associated with decreased risk of coronary heart disease (DHHS, 1988; NRC, 1989a).

3. *Eat less fat, saturated fat, and cholesterol.* There is strong and consistent evidence for the relation between dietary saturated fat, high blood cholesterol, and increased risk of coronary heart disease (CHD) (DHHS, 1988). Excess saturated fat is the major dietary contributor to high blood cholesterol, and dietary cholesterol increases blood cholesterol though the effect is weaker and more variable (DHHS, 1988). Although the effect of dietary cholesterol on low density lipoprotein (LDL) cholesterol is variable, increased intakes may re-

TABLE 42–6. FOOD AND NUTRITION BOARD, NATIONAL ACADEMY OF SCIENCES—NATIONAL RESEARCH
Nutrition of Practically All Healthy

Age (years) or Condition	Weight†		Height†		Protein g	Fat-Soluble Vitamins			
	kg	lb	cm	in		Vitamin A (µg RE)‡	Vitamin D (µg)§	Vitamin E (mg α g-TE)‖	Vitamin K (µg)
Infants									
0.0–0.5	6	13	60	24	13	375	7.5	3	5
0.5–1.0	9	20	71	28	14	375	10	4	10
Children									
1–3	13	29	90	35	16	400	10	6	15
4–6	20	44	112	44	24	500	10	7	20
7–10	28	62	132	52	28	700	10	7	30
Males									
11–14	45	99	157	62	45	1000	10	10	45
15–18	66	145	176	69	59	1000	10	10	65
19–24	72	160	177	70	58	1000	10	10	70
25–50	79	174	176	70	63	1000	5	10	80
51+	77	170	173	68	63	1000	5	10	80
Females									
11–14	46	101	157	62	46	800	10	8	45
15–18	55	120	163	64	44	800	10	8	55
19–24	58	128	164	65	46	800	10	8	60
25–50	63	138	163	64	50	800	5	8	65
51+	65	143	160	63	50	800	5	8	65
Pregnant women					60	800	10	10	65
Lactating women									
1st 6 months					65	1300	10	12	65
2nd 6 months					62	1200	10	11	65

* The allowances, expressed as average daily intakes over time, are intended to provide for individual variations among most normal persons as they live in the United States under usual environmental stresses. Diets should be based on a variety of common foods in order to provide other nutrients for which human requirements have been less well defined.

† Weights and heights of reference adults are actual medians for the U.S. population of the designated age, as reported by NHANES II. The median weights and heights of those under 19 years of age were taken from Hamill et al. (1979). The use of these figures does not imply that the height-to-weight ratios are ideal.

‡ Retinol equivalents. 1 retinol equivalent = 1 µg retinol or 6 µg β-carotene.

§ As cholecalciferol. 10 µg cholecalciferol. 400 IU of vitamin D.

‖ α-Tocopherol equivalents. 1 mg D-α tocopherol = 1 α-TE.

¶ 1 NE (niacin equivalent) is equal to 1 mg of niacin or 60 mg of dietary tryptophan.

From National Research Council, Subcommittee on the 10th Edition of the RDAs. *Recommended Dietery Allowances*, 10 edition. Food and Nutrition Board, Commission on Life Sciences, National Research Council. Washington, DC, National Academy Press, 1989. Copyright 1989 by the National Academy of Sciences.

sult in denser, more atherogenic postprandial lipoproteins (NRC, 1989a).

Restricting total fat intake facilitates a reduction in dietary saturated fat. Diets high in total fats are also linked to an increased incidence of obesity and some types of cancer (colon, prostate, breast). The current American diet derives 36 to 37 per cent of total calories from fat, 13 per cent from saturated fat, and has a cholesterol intake ranging from 435 mg daily for men to 304 mg for women (DHHS, 1988). This amount is about one-third more than the recommended intake, which limits total fat to less than 30 per cent of calories, saturated fat to less than 10 per cent, and cholesterol to less than 300 mg daily (Table 42–5). Further reductions in total fat intake and saturated fat intakes (e.g., total fat 20 per cent and saturated fat 5 to 7 per cent of total calories) would likely produce even greater health benefits (NRC, 1989a).

Most dietary fats are triglycerides. Triglycerides are esters of glycerol and fatty acids. Fatty acids are categorized as saturated or unsaturated depending on the presence of doubly bonded carbons. These double bonds prevent the chain from being fully "saturated" with hydrogen. Depending on the number of double bonds present, unsatu-

rated fatty acids are further divided into mono- and polyunsaturated fatty acids. In naturally occurring unsaturated fatty acids, hydrogens are configured in the *cis* formation (same side) around the carbon double bonds. The process of hydrogenation, used to harden vegetable oils for products such as margarine and shortening, converts some polyunsaturated fatty acids to *trans* monounsaturated fats.

Unsaturated fatty acids are grouped according to the first doubly bonded carbon counted from the methyl (omega) end of the fatty acid. Thus the essential polyunsaturated fatty acid linoleic acid is designated an omega-6 fatty acid, and linolenic acid is designated an omega-3 fatty acid. These fatty acids are found in abundance in vegetable oils. The longer chain omega-3 fatty acids eicosapentanoic (EPA) and docosahexanoic (DHA) are found predominantly in the fat of cold water fish such as salmon and, to a lesser extent, in some vegetables.

The saturated fatty acids (with the exception of stearic acid) are powerful inducers of elevated serum total and LDL cholesterol levels. Some have demonstrated that the *trans* fatty acids are as potent as saturated fats in raising serum cholesterol levels (NCEP, 1993). Saturated fats predominate

COUNCIL: RECOMMENDED DIETARY ALLOWANCES, Revised 1989*: Designed for the Maintenance of Good People in the United States

Water-Soluble Vitamins							Minerals						
Vitamin C (mg)	Thiamine (mg)	Riboflavin (mg)	Niacin (mg NE)¶	Vitamin B_6 (mg)	Folate (µg)	Vitamin B_{12} (µg)	Calcium (mg)	Phosphorus (mg)	Magnesium (mg)	Iron (mg)	Zinc (mg)	Iodine (µg)	Selenium (µg)
30	0.3	0.4	5	0.3	25	0.3	400	300	40	6	5	40	10
35	0.4	0.5	6	0.6	35	0.5	600	500	60	10	5	50	15
40	0.7	0.8	9	1.0	50	0.7	800	800	80	10	10	70	20
45	0.9	1.1	12	1.1	75	1.0	800	800	120	10	10	90	20
45	1.0	1.2	13	1.4	100	1.4	800	800	170	10	10	120	30
50	1.3	1.5	17	1.7	150	2.0	1200	1200	270	12	15	150	40
60	1.5	1.8	20	2.0	200	2.0	1200	1200	400	12	15	150	50
60	1.5	1.7	19	2.0	200	2.0	1200	1200	350	10	15	150	70
60	1.5	1.7	19	2.0	200	2.0	800	800	350	10	15	150	70
60	1.2	1.4	15	2.0	200	2.0	800	800	350	10	15	150	45
50	1.1	1.3	15	1.4	150	2.0	1200	1200	280	15	12	150	45
60	1.1	1.3	15	1.5	180	2.0	1200	1200	300	15	12	150	50
60	1.1	1.3	15	1.6	180	2.0	1200	1200	280	15	12	150	55
60	1.1	1.3	15	1.6	180	2.0	800	800	280	15	12	150	55
60	1.0	1.2	13	1.6	180	2.0	800	800	280	10	12	150	55
70	1.5	1.6	17	2.2	400	2.2	1200	1200	320	30	15	175	65
95	1.6	1.8	20	2.1	280	2.6	1200	1200	355	15	19	200	75
90	1.6	1.7	20	2.1	260	2.6	1200	1200	340	15	16	200	75

TABLE 42–7.   MEDIAN HEIGHTS AND WEIGHTS AND RECOMMENDED ENERGY INTAKE

Age (years) or Condition	Weight		Height		REE* (kcal/day)	Average Energy Allowance (kcal)†		
	kg	lb	cm	in		Multiples of REE	Per kg	Per Day‡
Infants								
0.0–0.5	6	13	60	24	320		108	650
0.5–1.0	9	20	71	28	500		98	850
Children								
1–3	13	29	90	35	740		102	1,300
4–6	20	44	112	44	950		90	1,800
7–10	28	62	132	52	1,130		70	2,000
Males								
11–14	45	99	157	62	1,440	1.70	55	2,500
15–18	66	145	176	69	1,760	1.67	45	3,000
19–24	72	160	177	70	1,780	1.67	40	2,900
25–50	79	174	176	70	1,800	1.60	37	2,900
51+	77	170	173	68	1,530	1.50	30	2,300
Females								
11–14	46	101	157	62	1,310	1.67	47	2,200
15–18	55	120	163	64	1,370	1.60	40	2,200
19–24	58	128	164	65	1,350	1.60	38	2,200
25–50	63	138	163	64	1,380	1.55	36	2,200
51+	65	143	160	63	1,280	1.50	30	1,900
Pregnant								
1st trimester								+0
2nd trimester								+300
3rd trimester								+300
Lactating								
1st 6 months								+500
2nd 6 months								+500

* Calculation based on FAO equations, rounded.
† In the range of light to moderate activity, the coefficient of variation is ±20 per cent.
‡ Figure is rounded.

TABLE 42–8. ESTIMATED SAFE AND ADEQUATE DAILY DIETARY INTAKES OF SELECTED VITAMINS AND MINERALS*

Age (years)	Vitamins		Trace Elements†				
	Biotin (μg)	Pantothenic Acid (mg)	Copper (mg)	Manganese (mg)	Fluoride (mg)	Chromium (μg)	Molybdenum (μg)
Infants							
0–0.5	10	2	0.4–0.6	0.3–0.6	0.1–0.5	10–40	15–30
0.5–1	15	3	0.6–0.7	0.6–1.0	0.2–1.0	20–60	20–40
Children and Adolescents							
1–3	20	3	0.7–1.0	1.0–1.5	0.5–1.5	20–80	25–50
4–6	25	3–4	1.0–1.5	1.5–2.0	1.0–2.5	30–120	30–75
7–10	30	4–5	1.0–2.0	2.0–3.0	1.5–2.5	50–200	50–150
Adults							
11+	30–100	4–7	1.5–2.5	2.0–5.0	1.5–2.5	50–200	75–250
	30–100	4–7	1.5–3.0	2.0–5.0	1.5–4.0	50–200	75–250

* Because there is less information on which to base allowances, these figures are not given in the main table of RDA and are provided here in the form of ranges of recommended intakes.

† Because the toxic levels for many trace elements may be only several times the usual intakes, the upper levels for the trace elements given in this table should not be habitually exceeded.

From National Research Council, Subcommittee on the 10th Edition of the RDAs: Recommended Dietary Allowances, 10th edition. Food and Nutrition Board, Commission on Life Sciences, National Research Council. Washington, DC, National Academy Press, 1989. Copyright 1989 by the National Academy of Sciences.

in foods of animal origin (meat, poultry, dairy products, and eggs) and in the tropical oils (coconut, palm, and palm kernel oils).

Unsaturated fatty acids (and carbohydrates), when substituted for saturated fats in the diet, decrease serum total cholesterol, lowering both the LDL and high density lipoprotein (HDL) subfractions (DHHS, 1988). Because there are no naturally occurring diets high in polyunsaturates and high levels have been associated with enhanced tumor growth in animals, intake of polyunsaturated fat should be held at the current level of 7 per cent or limited to no more than 10 per cent of total calories (NRC, 1989a). Safflower, sunflower, soybean, and corn oils are all high in polyunsaturates. The average American intake of linoleic acid is 6 per cent of calories, well above the requirement of 1 to 2 per cent of calories (NRC, 1989b), or the amount in about 1 tablespoon of safflower oil.

The omega-3 fatty acids, chiefly EPA and DHA, lower serum cholesterol and have an antithrombotic effect at relatively high doses (NRC, 1989a). Smaller doses (5 to 10 grams) have been shown to lower triglyceride levels significantly in patients with hypertriglyceridemia (Davidson et al., 1991a). Lack of data on the long-term effect of ingesting concentrated sources of these fatty acids recommends against their routine use (NCEP, 1993; NRC, 1989a).

Monounsaturated fats are as effective as polyunsaturated fats in lowering serum total and LDL cholesterol levels (NRC, 1989a). They may have an advantage over polyunsaturated fats, as they have been shown by some to spare HDL (NRC, 1989a). Thus they may improve the total cholesterol/HDL risk ratio. Current recommendations are to hold monounsaturated fatty acid intake at 10 to 15 per cent of total energy intake. Currently, most of the

monounsaturated fat content in the American diet is derived from animal sources. A low saturated and cholesterol diet, necessarily limited in animal foods, would be in balance with the addition of the highly monounsaturated plant oils, such as olive and canola oils (NRC, 1989b).

Cholesterol is a fat-like substance found only in animal products (meat, fish, poultry, milk products, and eggs). A single egg yolk contains approximately 215 mg of cholesterol, and the American Heart Association (1988) recommends no more than three or four egg yolks per week. Organ meats (e.g., liver) and shrimp are also high in cholesterol and should be consumed in limited quantities. The average cholesterol content of beef and light poultry meat is nearly equivalent (70 to 80 mg per 3 ounce serving), and red meat has two to three times the total and saturated fat content of light poultry meat and lean fish.

Dietary counseling to reduce the intake of fats and cholesterol focuses on decreasing intakes of the major sources of fat in the American diet: meat, poultry, fish, dairy products, and added fats and oils (e.g., butter, margarine, and cooking oils). Animal products (meats and dairy products) tend to be higher in both total and saturated fats than most plant foods and provide two-thirds of the saturated fat in the American diet. The remaining amount comes from various plant products, including the highly saturated tropical oils found in many commercial baked products (e.g., donuts, cakes, cookies, crackers) and snack items (e.g., chips) (NCEP, 1993). Intake of meats, poultry, and fish should be limited to no more than 6 ounces per day. Substituting lower-fat meat and dairy products, instead of eliminating these groups, helps ensure an adequate calcium and iron intake, two nutrients of special importance to women and children. Replacing high-fat snack foods and baked products with plain whole grains, fruits, and vegetables reduces fat and saturated fat intake and improves overall dietary quality.

4. *Eat more food containing complex carbohydrates and fiber.* Complex carbohydrates and fiber are principally found in whole grains, legumes, vegetables, fruits, nuts, and seeds—foods that are generally low in fat (with the notable exception of nuts, coconut, and avocado). Complex carbohydrate is defined as those plant foods high in starch and naturally occurring sugars. Fiber is defined as those plant materials that are resistant to digestion by human digestive enzymes. Plant foods are not only excellent sources of complex carbohydrates and fiber but are also excellent sources of vitamins and minerals.

Lower incidences of heart disease, diabetes mellitus, some types of cancer, and diverticulosis are found in populations who habitually consume diets high in complex carbohydrates and fiber. The typically lower intake of energy and fats, especially saturated fat and cholesterol, associated with diets high in carbohydrates and fiber may also influence the risk of CHD and diabetes (NRC, 1989a).

There are several components of plant foods that may be responsible for their beneficial effects. The action of fiber in diluting potential carcinogens and speeding intestinal transit time might function to decrease the risk of colon cancer (NRC, 1989b). There is some clinical evidence that diets high in certain fiber components, characterized as soluble fiber, found in whole grains (especially oat, rice bran, and barley), legumes (mature bean and peas), and certain fruits and vegetables decrease blood cholesterol and postprandial glucose and insulin levels (NRC, 1989a). Fiber-rich foods, including those containing the insoluble fibers such as cellulose found in wheat bran, add bulk to the stool and are beneficial in the management of constipation and the prevention of diverticulosis (Cerda, 1993; DHHS, 1988).

Increased consumption of fruits and vegetables, including the cruciferous vegetables (e.g., cabbage and broccoli) lowers cancer rates of the lung, bladder, and gastrointestinal tract through protective factors and mechanisms not fully established (DHHS, 1988; NRC, 1989a). The antioxidant effect of vitamin A, or its precursors the carotenes (contained in dark green leafy and deep yellow and orange fruits and vegetables), has been associated with a decreased incidence of cancer, particularly of the lung, larynx, and bladder (NRC, 1982). Vitamin C (contained in dark green leafy vegetables, citrus fruits, cantaloupe, mango, peppers, and strawberries) has similarly been associated with protection against cancers of the stomach and esophagus (NRC, 1982).

Antioxidants (vitamins A, C, and E, carotenes, and selenium) have also been associated with reduced cardiovascular risk and cataract prevention.

Increased β-carotene intake has been associated with reduced rates of major vascular events including myocardial infarction and stroke (Gaziano et al., 1990). Evidence from epidemiologic studies find inverse relations between cardiovascular mortality and plasma levels of antioxidants, particularly vitamin E (found in whole grains and green vegetables) (Grey et al., 1991). A role for antioxidants in cataract prevention is also supported by epidemiologic evidence (Robertson et al., 1991). The limited data available on selenium precludes firm conclusions on its role in the prevention of heart disease, but there is some evidence that selenium protects against cancer (Diplock, 1991). Increasing intake of fruits and vegetables also increases potassium intake, a nutrient associated with reduced prevalence of hypertension and stroke (NRC, 1989b) (see below).

Increasing the carbohydrate intake from the current 48 per cent of calories to the recommended level of 55 to 60 per cent of calories can be accomplished by eating the recommended five or more servings of fruits, vegetables, and legumes and six or more servings of whole grains, breads, and cereals daily. There is no RDA for carbohydrate, but a minimum intake of 50 to 100 grams daily is necessary to prevent ketosis (NRC, 1989b).

The recommended daily intake of 20 to 30 grams of fiber would double the current average fiber intake of 12 grams (NRC, 1989b). Concerns that high fiber intakes may substantially decrease the bioavailability of minerals such as calcium, iron, and zinc is not supported by nutritional status assessment of persons following high fiber diets (NRC, 1989a). An increased consumption of naturally occurring fiber-rich foods is generally preferable to concentrated fiber supplementation. Caution is indicated when adding concentrated fiber supplements to marginally adequate diets. High fiber diets should also be cautiously recommended for those patients with compromised gastrointestinal motility (Cerda, 1993).

5. *Limit consumption of foods high in sugars.* Limited consumption of dietary sugars, regular oral hygiene, and fluoridation of drinking water are the most important measures for prevention of dental caries. All dietary carbohydrate is substrate for the acid-producing bacteria responsible for tooth decay, but sucrose (common table sugar) is particularly cariogenic. Added sweeteners, mostly sucrose and high-fructose corn syrup, account for 11 per cent of calories in the typical American diet, nearly one-fourth the total carbohydrate intake (NRC, 1989b). Because newly erupted teeth are most vulnerable, children are susceptible to the cariogenic effects of simple carbohydrates (DHHS, 1988).

Dietary strategies for reducing tooth decay are directed at decreasing the amount and frequency of sugar-rich foods in the diet. The longer the cariogenic food remains in the oral cavity, the more potential it has to cause tooth decay. Sticky sweets, such as dried fruits or caramel candies, pose a greater threat than sweets that wash off quickly (DHHS, 1988). Allowing a child to sleep with a baby bottle allows pooling of juice, milk, or formula on the upper teeth for extended periods. This practice results in a distinctive pattern of tooth decay called "nursing bottle syndrome."

Foods that have an acid-buffering effect protect against tooth decay. Such foods include those with relatively high protein and fat content, such as meats, nuts, and cheese. The "toothbrush" effect of crisp raw foods such as apples and celery is ineffective for plaque removal but does stimulate salivary flow. This can buffer up to 90 per cent of acid production, thereby helping to prevent tooth decay (AAP, 1993a).

6. *Reduce salt intake.* High salt intake is positively correlated with increases in mean systolic and diastolic blood pressure and with the age-related rise in blood pressure seen in both men and women (DHHS, 1988; ICRG, 1988; NRC, 1989a). Because a substantial proportion of the individuals in the United States develop hypertension with age, a moderate reduction in salt intake to 6 grams daily (2.3 mg of sodium) appears justified. The current average *sodium* intake of adults is 4 to 6 grams per day, much greater than the estimated safe minimum sodium intake of 500 mg (DHHS, 1988).

Two-thirds of dietary sodium intake comes from salt added by manufacturers during food processing and by the consumer when cooking and at the table. The remaining one-third is contributed by the naturally occurring sodium in foods (DHHS, 1988). Removing the salt shaker from the table and using less salt when cooking reduces sodium intake by only 1 to 2 grams. Further reductions in sodium intake call for the elimination of obviously salted foods, such as potato chips, and limited use of high-sodium processed foods such as lunch meat and canned soups.

Potassium may also be a factor in the development of high blood pressure and the incidence of stroke. Potassium intake is inversely correlated with blood pressure, and a high sodium/potassium ratio is positively correlated with increased blood pressure (DHHS, 1988; Knapp, 1990). Increasing daily potassium intake by 400 mg (the amount found in one to two servings of fruits or vegetables) has been associated with a decreased incidence of stroke, independent of a blood pressure effect (NRC, 1989a). The average adult potassium intake approximates 2.5 grams per day, an amount that barely achieves the minimum requirement of approximately 1.6 to 2.0 grams per day (NRC, 1989b). Compliance to recommendations for increased intake of fruits and vegetables would raise the potassium intake of adults to about 3.5 grams (90 mEq) per day, the amount associated with a beneficial effect (NRC, 1989a, 1989b).

7. *Take alcohol only in moderation, if at all.*

Many health organizations recommend limiting alcohol intake to no more than two drinks per day (DHHS, 1988; NRC, 1989a; USDA/DHHS, 1990). One drink is 12 ounces of beer, 5 ounces of wine, or 1.5 ounces (1 jigger) of distilled spirits. Each of these drinks contain approximately 0.5 ounce of pure alcohol.

At least 9 per cent of the population consumes two or more drinks daily (DHHS, 1990). This level of alcohol consumption is directly associated with high blood pressure (DHHS, 1988). Although moderate alcohol consumption has been associated with lower CHD risk, perhaps because of beneficial effects on HDL cholesterol levels (Gaziano et al., 1993), even moderate alcohol consumption poses certain other well known risks, including cancer and liver disease (DHHS, 1990). A threshold level of safe alcohol consumption during pregnancy has not been established (AAP, 1993b).

8. *Maintain adequate iron intake.* Children, adolescents, and women of childbearing years, especially from low income families, are the most vulnerable to iron deficiency (DHHS, 1988). Dietary iron deficiency results not only in the most prevalent form of anemia in the United States but also in reduced work capacity, depressed immune function, changes in behavior, and impaired intellectual performance (DHHS, 1988). The prevalence of iron-deficiency anemia is highest among children ages 1 to 2 years (9.3 per cent). Adolescent girls have the next highest prevalence (7.2 per cent) followed closely by women age 20 to 44 years (6.3 per cent) (NRC, 1989a).

Breast-feeding or the use of iron-fortified formula is the most important nutritional safeguard against iron deficiency in infants. Older children and adults can improve their iron intake by increasing consumption of lean meats, chicken, fish, legumes, dark green leafy vegetables, and iron-enriched and whole grain breads and cereals. Factors in meat improve iron absorption. Concomitant consumption of vitamin C also increase the bioavailability of iron from plant foods. Foods cooked in iron pots absorb variable amounts of iron.

9. *Maintain adequate calcium intake.* Chronically low calcium intake, particularly during the first two to three decades of life, may compromise the development of peak bone mass and increase the risk of developing osteoporosis later in life (NRC, 1989a). Osteoporosis occurs in both men and women, but postmenopausal women are two times more likely to have severe osteoporosis leading to bone fracture. Other factors, including alcohol intake, cigarette smoking, and a low level of physical activity, are implicated in the development of osteoporosis (DHHS, 1988).

Women, because of their low energy intake, and adolescents, because of increased nutrient requirements, often have diets insufficient in calcium intake. The RDA for calcium in adolescents and adults to 25 years is 1200 mg per day (NRC, 1989b).

Only adolescent boys approach this level of intake. Ninety per cent of boys regularly consume the RDA for calcium, whereas only about 75 per cent of girls had intakes at or above the calcium RDA (NRC, 1989a). The average calcium intake of adult women is 530 mg, well below the recommended 800 mg per day (NRC, 1989b).

Consumption of two to three servings of nonfat milk each day provides 600 to 900 mg of calcium. Individuals with lactase deficiency can often tolerate yogurt, acidophilus milk, hard cheeses, or lactose-reduced fluid milk products (Cerda, 1993). Other calcium-rich foods include dark green leafy vegetables (e.g., broccoli and kale), lime-processed tortillas and tofu, unhulled sesame seeds, and enriched breads and cereals.

The bioavailability of calcium from calcium supplements varies among brands and calcium salts (Harward, 1993). Chewable calcium tablets are readily solubulized and efficiently absorbed (Harward, 1993). Calcium supplements are more efficiently absorbed when taken with meals, especially in patients with achlorhydria (Wood and Serfaty-Lacrosniere, 1992).

Estrogen replacement therapy is thought to be the most effective way to decrease the rate of bone loss and risk of fracture in postmenopausal women. Calcium supplementation alone has been shown to delay bone loss in women with low dietary calcium intakes (less than 400 mg per day) who were 5 years postmenopausal, a time when the effect of hormone changes on bone loss has decreased (Dawson-Hughes et al., 1990). The beneficial effects of calcium supplementation appear to be greater in cortical bone (predominating in the hip) than in trabecular bone (spine) (Harward, 1993). However, the role of isolated calcium supplementation in the treatment of osteoporosis remains controversial. Adequate calcium and vitamin D intake and regular physical activity, combined with estrogen replacement therapy in postmenopausal women, provides the most effective therapeutic regimen for the prevention and treatment of osteoporosis. Calcium intakes of 1 gram per day are recommended for women undergoing estrogen replacement and 1500 mg per day in the estrogen-deficient woman (NIH, 1984).

10. *Maintain optimal intake of fluoride.* Fluoride is not an essential nutrient but has been proved beneficial in reducing the incidence of dental caries. Consumption of optimally fluoridated water by children during years of primary and secondary tooth formation has been shown to reduce the prevalence of dental caries by more than 50 per cent (DHHS, 1988). Supplemental fluoride is recommended for children living in areas with inadequate concentration of fluoride in the water supply (Table 42–9). There is no evidence that the recommended fluoridation levels adversely affect health (NRC, 1989a).

11. *Maintain protein intake at moderate levels.*

TABLE 42–9. SUPPLEMENTAL FLUORIDE DOSAGE SCHEDULE

Age	Dosage (mg/day), by Concentration of Fluoride in Drinking Water*		
	< 0.03 ppm	0.3–0.6 ppm	> 0.6 ppm
6 months to 3 years	0.25	0	0
3–6 Years	0.50	0.25	0
6–16 Years	1.00	0.50	0

* A dose of 2.2 mg sodium fluoride contains 1 mg fluoride.
From the Council on Dental Therapeutics, American Dental Association, ADA News, May 16, 1994, with permission.

The National Research Council recommends that levels of protein intake be lower than twice the RDA for all age groups (NRC, 1989a). The major source of protein in the typical American diet is animal protein. There are no known benefits, and possibly some risk, in regularly consuming high levels of animal protein. Some epidemiologic studies have found an association between diets high in meat (and consequently animal protein) and increased risk of certain cancers and CHD (NRC, 1989a). High protein intakes have also been shown to increase the glomerular filtration rate and age-related progression of renal disease, although the effect of high dietary protein on the risk of chronic renal disease is not certain (NRC, 1989a).

The average American protein intake exceeds the adult RDA of 0.8 gm/kg of desirable body weight, especially in young men. Protein intakes average 95 to 100 grams per day in men and approximately 65 grams per day in women (LSRO, 1989). Eating lean meats less frequently and in smaller portions (2 to 3 ounces) would decrease the protein, saturated fat, and cholesterol intake of the U.S. population (NRC, 1989a).

NUTRITION THROUGHOUT THE LIFE CYCLE

The increased nutritional demands secondary to growth and development during infancy, childhood, adolescence, pregnancy, and lactation and the changing physiologic needs of the older person make these age groups particularly vulnerable to nutritional problems. The great importance of adequate nutrition for optimal growth, health, and quality of life is reflected in the numerous nutrition-related community services available to aid the family physician in nutritional care of these groups. The poor, homeless, and disabled also have needs that may similarly benefit from such services. A guide to locating local nutrition-related community services is shown in Table 42–10.

TABLE 42–10. NUTRITION-RELATED COMMUNITY SERVICES*

Program	Provision	Eligibility	Local Contact
Food Stamps	Coupons to purchase food	Low-income households	County Welfare Office
Federal Commodities Program	Federally donated surplus foods	Low-income households	Distributing agent
Congregate Meals Program	Low-cost meals and nutrition education	Needy older persons	Local Agency on Aging
Home-Delivered Meals	Low-cost meals (may provide modified diets)	Needy older persons	Local Agency on Aging
Special Supplemental Food Programs for Women, Infants, and Children (WIC)	Nutrition education and coupons to purchase specific supplemental foods providing at-risk nutrients (protein, iron, calcium, vitamin C)	Pregnant/postpartum/ breast-feeding women and infants and children up to age 5 years with nutritional and financial need	County Health Department
Headstart	Health and nutritional service including meals	Needy preschool children	Local Headstart Office
Child Care Meals Program	Free or reduced-price meals	Needy children in participating centers	Facility administration
School lunch and Breakfast Programs (including summer program)	Free or reduced-price meals	Needy children in participating schools	School administration
Special Milk Program	Free milk	All children attending a school or institution meeting poverty guidelines	School/institution administration
Food banks/pantries/ kitchens, etc.	Foodstuffs or meals	Determined by local distributing agent	Various distributing agents such as churches
Homemaker/Chore Service	Cooking and shopping assistance	Private-party or various assistance programs	County Welfare Office or various private agencies
In-Home Health Aide/ Personal Care	Feeding assistance	Private-party or various assistance programs	County Welfare Office or various private agencies

* Services vary at different sites.

Pregnancy

The U.S. Surgeon General's inclusion of maternal nutrition as a risk factor in the incidence of low infant birth weight and infant mortality rate, and the continued prevalence of nutritional anemias, especially in some subgroups, underscores the importance of nutritional care during pregnancy (DHHS, 1990). The goal of nutritional care during pregnancy is to ensure appropriate nutritional intake for optimal fetal growth and maternal well-being.

Nutritional risk assessment of the prepregnant state is critical to determining appropriate nutritional recommendations during pregnancy. Maternal risk factors for pre-existing or continuing nutritional problems include economic insecurity, alternative food practices, drug or alcohol abuse, or evidence of diet-related complications during previous pregnancies (e.g., low-birth-weight infant or maternal anemia). Prepregnancy weight is a gross indicator of prepregnancy energy stores and the basis for weight gain recommendations during pregnancy. Table 42–11 gives a more complete list of nutritional risk factors and indicators that signal the need for complete nutritional assessment and counseling.

Maintenance of appropriate weight gain is an important aspect of nutritional care. Adequate pregnant weight gain decreases the risk of delivering a low-birth-weight infant and the attendant complications (IOM, 1990). However, gains at the higher end of recommended may increase the incidence of fetal macrosomia. In addition, the problem of postpartum weight retention may be exacerbated. On average, each successive birth adds approximately 1 kg of postpartum weight above that which is normally gained with advancing age (IOM, 1990). The residual gain is likely to be surpassed in women with high gestational weight gains.

Table 42–12 lists recommendations for maternal weight gain based on prepregnancy weight classification. In general, women who gain less than 21 pounds during pregnancy are more than twice as likely to deliver low-birth-weight infants than women who gain more (DHHS, 1990). The effect of gravid weight gain is weakest in the obese woman (prepregnancy BMI higher than 29), who may do well with a gain of less than 15 pounds (IOM, 1990). Inadequate weight gain (less than 2

TABLE 42–11. NUTRITIONAL RISK FACTORS DURING PREGNANCY

Factors Present at the Onset of Pregnancy
Age
  18 Years or younger at last menstrual period or reproductive
    age <3 (chronological age minus menarchal age)
  35 Years or older at last menstrual period
Weight
  Pregravid underweight (90% of desirable body weight)
  Pregravid obesity (>120% of desirable body weight)
Obstetric history
  Previous LBW, SGA, or premature infant
  Previous high-birth-weight infant
  Neonatal death, fetal loss, stillbirth, congenital anomaly
  Preeclampsia, gestational diabetes, anemia, inadequate
    weight gain (<21 lb total)
Frequent pregnancies (two during the last 12 months)
High parity (more than five previous deliveries)
Chronic illness
Low socioeconomic status
Abuse of nicotine, alcohol, drugs
Bizarre food practices
Recent rapid weight loss, surgery, or trauma

Factors Occurring During Pregnancy
Multiple pregnancy
Intrauterine growth retardation
Breast-feeding during pregnancy
Hyperemesis gravidarum
Inadequate weight gain
  Less than 2 lb per month
  Less than 1 lb per month (pregravid weight more than 130%
    desirable)
Excessive weight gain (>6 lb per month)
Gestational diabetes
Pregnancy-induced hypertension
Anemia
Vitamin/mineral megadoses; herbal remedies
No cooking facilities; food access problems
Strict vegetarianism
Bizarre food practices or food faddism
Avoidance of an entire food group (e.g., milk intolerance)
Mental health problems (e.g., depression, mental retardation)

pounds per month by the normal-weight woman or less than 1 pound per month in the obese woman) or excessive weight gain (more than 6 pounds per month) requires nutritional investigation (IOM, 1990).

During pregnancy, energy needs and recommended intakes for all nutrients (vitamins and minerals) are increased. Adhering to the general meal pattern for pregnant women described in Table 42–2 ensures that the physiologic requirements for most nutrients can be met. The exception is iron (see below). Additional servings of recommended foods or moderate amounts of added fats and sugars are necessary to meet the increased energy (calorie) needs during the last 5 to 6 months of gestation. Pregnant teenagers should increase the recommended dairy servings to five daily to provide extra calcium and protein intake.

The increased requirement for iron during pregnancy cannot be met by diet alone. Recent recommendations for prenatal vitamin and mineral supplementation call for a low dose (30 mg elemental) iron supplement for all pregnant woman (IOM, 1990). Additional nutrient supplementation is recommended only when indicated by individual dietary assessment and risk determination (Table 42–13) (IOM, 1990). Although vitamin and mineral supplementation is not a replacement for nutritional assessment or a well balanced diet, routine prenatal supplementation remains inexpensive, safe nutritional protection for all pregnant women. If intake of dairy products is absent or restricted, additional supplementation with at least 600 mg of calcium is warranted.

Periconceptual supplementation with folate has been shown to reduce the incidence of spina bifida and other neural tube defects (NTDs). Supplementation with 4 mg of folate daily is recommended for all women planning to become pregnant who

TABLE 42–12. RECOMMENDED WEIGHT GAINS FOR PREGNANT WOMEN* BY PREPREGNANCY BODY MASS INDEX

Body Mass Index	Recommended Total Gain		Recommended Rate of Gain	
	kg	lb	First Trimester (total kg/lb)	Second/Third Trimester (rate per week, kg/lb)
Low (<19.8 or weight for height <90% desirable)	12.5–18.0	28–40	2.3 (5)	0.49 (1)
Normal (19.8–26.0)	11.5–16.0	25–35	1.6 (3.5)	0.44 (1)
High† (>26.0–29.0 or weight for height 120–130% desirable)	7.0–11.5	15–25	0.9 (2)	0.3 (2/3)

* Young adolescents and black women should strive for gains at the upper end of the recommended range. Short women (151 cm or 62 inches) should strive for gains at the lower end of the range. Total gain for women carrying twins is 35 to 45 pounds.
† The recommended target weight gain for obese women (BMI >29.0) is at least 6.0 kg (15 pounds).
From U.S. Institute of Medicine. Subcommittee on Nutritional Status and Weight Gain During Pregnancy, Subcommittee on Dietary Intake and Nutrient Supplements During Pregnancy. Nutrition During Pregnancy. Part I: Weight Gain. Part II: Nutrient Supplements. Committee on Nutritional Status During Pregnancy and Lactation, Food and Nutrition Board, Institute of Medicine, National Academy of Sciences. Washington, DC, National Academy Press, 1990. Copyright 1990 by the National Academy of Sciences.

TABLE 42–13.   RECOMMENDATIONS FOR NUTRIENT SUPPLEMENTATION DURING PREGNANCY

Nutrient	Candidates for Supplementation	Level of Nutrient Supplementation
Iron	All pregnant women (second and third trimesters)	30 mg ferrous iron daily
Folic acid	Pregnant women with suspected dietary inadequacy of folate	300 μg/day
Vitamin D	Strict vegetarians and others with low intake of vitamin D-fortified milk and inadequate exposure to sunlight	10 μg/day
Calcium	Women under age 25 whose daily dietary calcium intake is less than 600 mg	600 mg/day
Vitamin B_{12}	Strict vegetarians	2 μg/day
Zinc/copper	Women receiving iron therapy for iron-deficiency anemia	15 mg Zn/day, 2 mg Cu/day
Multivitamin–mineral supplements	Pregnant women with poor diets and for those who are considered high risk: multiple gestation, heavy smokers, alcohol or drug abusers	Preparation containing iron 30 mg, zinc 15 mg, copper 2 mg, calcium 250 mg, vitamin B_6 2 mg, folate 300 μg, vitamin C 50 mg, vitamin D 5 μg

From U.S. Institute of Medicine, Subcommittee on Nutritional Status and Weight Gain During Pregnancy, Subcommittee on Dietary Intake and Nutrient Supplements During Pregnancy. Nutrition During Pregnancy. Part I: Weight Gain. Part II: Nutrient Supplements. Committee on Nutritional Status During Pregnancy and Lactation, Food and Nutrition Board, Institute of Medicine, National Academy of Sciences. Washington, DC, National Academy Press, 1990. Copyright 1990 by the National Academy of Sciences.

have had a previous NTD-affected pregnancy (CDC, 1991). Supplementation should begin 1 month prior to conception and continue through the first trimester. Studies have also shown a decreased incidence in NTDs in primagravidas taking between 0.4 and 1.0 mg of folate periconceptually. All women of childbearing years who are capable of becoming pregnant should consume at least 0.4 mg of folate daily (CDC, 1992). Carefully selected diets may contain 0.4 mg of folate. Rich sources of folate include liver, legumes, leafy green vegetables such as spinach and asparagus, peanuts, sunflower seeds, and oranges. Over-the-counter prenatal supplements generally contain 0.4 mg of folate. A prescription is required for prenatal agents containing 1 mg of folate.

Some special considerations of dietary counseling during pregnancy include information on caffeine intake, use of sugar substitutes, alcohol, and the dietary effects of cigarette smoking. Coffee and caffeine intake has been associated with an increased incidence of low birth weight and fetal loss (Infante-Rivard et al., 1993; IOM, 1990). The level at which adverse effects have been reported range from 150 mg of caffeine (1.5 cups of coffee) to seven or more cups of coffee per day. We recommend that pregnant women keep their caffeine intake from all sources, including teas and sodas, to a minimum (FDA, 1980).

Safe levels of alcohol intake during pregnancy have not been defined. As little as one or two alcoholic drinks per day has been associated with a substantially increased risk of giving birth to a growth-retarded baby, and chronic intake of 3 ounces of alcohol per day (six drinks) is associated with fetal alcohol syndrome (AAP, 1993b; Williams et al., 1992).

Women who do not quit smoking during preg-

nancy should receive special attention to dietary adequacy. Maternal weight gains at the higher end of the recommended range may offset the low infant birth weights seen in this cohort (Williams et al., 1992). Although there is no evidence that sugar substitutes such as saccharin and aspartame (Nutrasweet) cause problems during pregnancy in humans, it appears prudent to limit excessive use.

The role of diet in the treatment of disease states during pregnancy is beyond the scope of this text; however, a brief summary of nutritional care during gestational diabetes can be found in the section Diet and Diabetes Mellitus, below. Dietary treatment for some of the common discomforts of pregnancy are given in Table 42–14 (Coombs and Speer, 1990).

Nutritional care for the postpartum, nonlactating woman focuses on restoration of depleted maternal reserves and weight loss if needed. It is reasonable to continue vitamin and mineral supplementation for at least 6 weeks postpartum. Women who did not gain adequate weight or who had a multiple pregnancy, frequent pregnancies, or anemia should continue vitamin and mineral supplementation for an extended period, at least 2 to 3 months. If postpartum weight reduction is attempted using a diet of fewer than 1200 calories, extended nutrient supplementation is also advised. A less restricted diet (e.g., the Food Group Guide with reduced consumption of high fat, high sugar "extras") combined with regular physical activity is a more healthful approach to postpartum weight loss.

Lactation

The goals of nutritional care during lactation are to provide the calories and nutrients necessary for

TABLE 42–14. COMMON COMPLICATIONS OF PREGNANCY AND POSSIBLE DIETARY SOLUTIONS

Problem	Possible Solutions
Nausea/vomiting	Small, frequent feedings No missed meals Carbonated beverages and belching Night or early morning snack before rising Bland, soft food Avoid heat and aroma of cooking food Lie down and rest after eating
Constipation	Fluid, 8 cups per day Increased fiber: whole grains, bran, vegetables, and fruit, especially prunes and figs
Heartburn	Small, frequent feedings Avoid spicy, rich, or greasy foods Avoid caffeine, chocolate, and alcohol Eat slowly Remain semiupright at least 1 hour after eating
Underweight or inadequate weight gain	Address any underlying cause such as nausea/vomiting, poor appetite, financial difficulties, stress, or desire to lose weight (if obese) Assess dietary adequacy and include missed servings or increase use of calorie-dense foods, such as milkshakes Stress frequent meals and nutritional snacks Illustrate adequate gain and discuss importance
Obesity or excessive gain	Evaluate diet and ensure adequate intake and use of prenatal supplements Eliminate high calorie foods while maintaining nutritional adequacy Exercise as tolerated Illustrate desirable pattern of gain (2–3 pounds per month during last two trimesters) Acknowledge need for weight loss postpartum
Toxemia (pregnancy-induced hypertension)	Prevention: adequate diet and appropriate weight gain, especially in poor, underweight, or overweight women Treatment: as above Sodium intake no less than 2 gm per day
Iron-deficiency anemia	Iron supplementation (take with meals or slow release) Counsel on food sources of iron Cook in iron pots
Pica (unusual craving and consumption of nonfood substances)	Counsel against the ingestion of dirt, clay, starch, or other substances that may damage the GI tract, interfere with nutrient absorption, or replace more nutritious foods Iron supplementation

Modified from Coombs JB, Speer SJ: *Nutrition I/II.* Monograph, edition no. 129/130. Kansas City, MO, American Academy of Family Physicians, 1990.

sufficient production of nutritionally adequate milk and to maintain or replenish maternal nutritional stores. Attention is also given to avoidance of substances that may contaminate the milk and affect the health and well-being of the infant. Breast-feeding women, like many postpartum women, may also be concerned about returning to prepregnancy weight status.

Dietary intake similar to the prenatal diet pattern (Table 42–2) supplies sufficient nutrients to meet the needs of the lactating woman. Quality and quantity of human milk remains surprisingly stable over a wide range of nutrient intakes. Supplementation is not necessary to improve the quality of milk in an otherwise adequately nourished woman, although postpartum supplementation with prenatal vitamins and minerals for a period of a few weeks to several months is recommended to help replenish maternal reserves.

Breast-feeding women studied in the United States support their lactation with an average intake of 2200 calories (less than is recommended) and an average weight loss that would indicate mobilization of approximately 300 calories from maternal fat stores (Williams et al., 1992). Lactating women typically lose about 0.6 to 0.8 kg per month during the first 4 to 6 months. After this period they may experience continued weight loss but at a slower rate (IOM, 1991). Approximately 20 per cent of women do not lose weight or even gain weight while breast-feeding (IOM, 1991).

Women who currently choose to breast-feed tend to be older, well educated, and white—women generally characterized as well nourished. This paradigm may not be valid for all groups. Newly immigrated women, groups who restrict their eating patterns, teenagers, and low income women require special attention to avoid nutritional problems in themselves and their infants (IOM, 1991). Diets of complete vegans should be supplemented with 2.6 μg of vitamin B_{12}. Women who avoid dairy products should be advised to consume lactose-reduced milk or a supplement with at least 600 mg of calcium daily. Women avoiding vitamin D-fortified milk, combined with limited exposure to sunshine (ultraviolet light), should be supplemented with 10 μg of vitamin D per day. Nutrient supplementation at levels above RDA amounts can result in unusually high levels of some nutrients in maternal milk (i.e., vitamin B_6, vitamin D, iodine, and selenium). The possible adverse consequences of these excesses is undetermined (IOM, 1991).

Moderate ingestion of caffeine-containing products (e.g., one to two cups of coffee) need not be prohibited. Higher caffeine intakes may result in an irritable, wakeful infant (Williams et al., 1992). Similarly, occasional consumption of small amounts of alcohol need not be prohibited, but intakes greater than 0.5 g/kg of body weight (about 1 ounce of pure alcohol, or two drinks) may decrease the milk ejection reflex, increase the alcohol content of the milk, and result in lethargic nurslings (IOM, 1991). Timing the ingestion of alcohol immediately after nursing is the safest time for the infant (Williams et al., 1992).

The implications that components of the maternal diet may contribute to the development of colic in the infant by passage of food allergens, especially from cow's milk, is not well supported (IOM, 1991). Some mothers do complain of adverse infant reactions to foods in the maternal diet. Four to six hours is generally required before food components or metabolites appear in breast milk (Williams et al., 1992). Suspected offending food can be omitted from the diet to see if relief ensues, real or imagined (Williams et al., 1992). In our experience, most foods that are well tolerated by the mother when eaten in moderation are tolerated by the infant during lactation.

Excessive maternal weight loss indicates inadequate maternal diet and may adversely affect milk volume. This point is especially true during the first 4 to 6 weeks when lactation is becoming established (Williams et al., 1992). In an overweight lactating woman a loss of more than about 1 pound per week may affect milk volume (IOM, 1991). Attention to adequate weight gain and signs of contentment in the infant are instructive.

Although it is important to provide adequate fluids, increasing the fluid intake over the demands of thirst does not increase milk volume (IOM, 1991). Maternal stress and the nursing behavior of both mother and infant (i.e., demand feeding and a vigorous nursling) are potentially the most important determinants of milk volume (IOM, 1991). Increased maternal rest, a diet adequate in both calories and nutrients, and increased frequency and duration of nursing generally increase milk supply within 24 to 48 hours (Williams et al., 1992). Infant appetite spurts and an increased demand for nursing are common at about 3 and 6 weeks of age and again between 2.5 and 3.0 months and 4.5 and 6.0 months of age (Huggins, 1990).

Infant Nutrition

Infant nutritional care begins during pregnancy with a discussion on the choice of bottle feeding or breast-feeding and instruction on appropriate parental feeding skills. This care continues with routine assessment of infant nutritional status and anticipatory guidance on progressive changes in dietary intake. The focus of nutritional care during infancy is adequate calories and nutrients for optimal growth and well-being.

Breast milk alone is nutritionally adequate to supply the needs of healthy full-term infants to the age of 4 to 6 months. Investigation of maternal nutritional status is imperative when assessing the adequacy of dietary intake for the breast-fed baby. Adequacy of intake can be gauged by adequate growth and weight, frequency and duration of feeding, and eight to ten wet diapers per day. Breast-fed babies generally nurse more frequently than bottle-fed babies, nursing every 1 to 2 hours (8 to 15 times daily) during the newborn period (IOM, 1991). This demand gradually declines to about every 2 to 3 hours (six to eight times daily) at age 4 months.

At 4 to 6 months the introduction of iron-fortified cereals followed by the gradual addition of a complete range of solid foods is sufficient to meet the increasing iron needs of most infants. Infants of iron-deficient mothers, premature infants, and small-for-gestational age (SGA) infants benefit from earlier iron supplementation.

Recommendations on the need for vitamin D supplementation vary. If maternal vitamin D intake is questionable or adequate exposure to sunlight (about 2 hours per week clothed) is not reliable, supplement the breast-fed infant with 10 IU vitamin D daily. Babies who are exclusively breast-fed (i.e., no supplemental formula) beyond 1 year of age (when most babies would be offered vitamin D-fortified cow's milk) should also receive vitamin D supplementation. Both the mother and infant of a complete vegan (no animal products) require supplementation with vitamin B_{12}. The schedule for fluoride supplementation is shown in Table 42–9.

Standard iron-fortified infant formula is recommended for bottle-fed babies throughout the first year (AAP, 1993a). No further supplementation for the healthy term infant is necessary, with the exception of fluoride, if adequately fluoridated water is not used to mix the infant formula. A simple rule-of-thumb for calculating adequate formula intake in the infant, prior to addition of solids, is 2 to 3 fluid ounces per pound. Under normal conditions no additional fluid is necessary for breast or formula-fed babies (Williams et al., 1992).

Table 42–15 shows a common schedule for introducing solid foods to infants. Developmental signs of readiness for the introduction of solid foods include a decreased extrusion reflex, ability to sit upright with some back support, and sufficient con-

TABLE 42–15. SCHEDULE OF INTRODUCTION OF SOLIDS

Timing	Approximate Total Daily Intake of Solids	Comments
Four to five months	Dry cereal: start with ½ tsp (dry measurement), gradually increase to 2 to 3 tbsp Vegetables: start with 1 tsp, gradually increase to 2 tbsp Fruit: start with 1 tsp, gradually increase to 2 tbsp Divide food among 3–4 feedings per day	Cereal: offer iron-enriched baby cereal first; begin with single grains (rice, barley, corn); mix cereal with an equal amount of breast milk or formula. Vegetables: try a mild-tasting vegetable first (carrots, squash, peas, green beans); stronger-flavored vegetables (spinach, sweet potatoes) may be tried after the infant accepts some mild-tasting ones. Fruits: mashed ripe banana and unsweetened, cooked bland fruits (apples, peaches, pears) are usually well liked; apple juice and grape juice (unsweetened) may be introduced; initially, dilute juice with an equal amount of water. Introduce one new food at a time and offer it several times before trying another food. Give a new food once daily for 1–2 days; increase to twice daily as the infant begins to enjoy the food; watch for signs of intolerance. Include some foods that are good sources of vitamin C (other than orange juice).
Five to six months	Dry cereal: gradually increase to 4 tbsp Fruits and vegetables: gradually increase to 3 tbsp of each Meat: start with 1 tsp, gradually increase to 2 tbsp Divide food among 3–4 feedings per day	Meat: offer pureed or milled poultry (chicken or turkey) followed by lean meat (veal, beef). Continue introducing new cereals, fruits, and vegetables as the infant indicates readiness to accept them, but always introduce one at a time.
Six to eight months	Dry cereal: up to ½ cup Fruits and vegetables up to ¼ to ½ cup of each Meats: up to 3 tbsp Divide food among 3–4 feedings per day	Soft table foods may be introduced (e.g., mashed potatoes, squash, small pieces of soft peeled fruits). Toasted whole-grain or enriched bread may be added when the infant begins chewing. If introduction of solids is delayed until now, it is not necessary to use strained fruits and vegetables. Continue using iron-fortified baby cereals.
Eight to twelve months	Dry cereal: up to ½ cup Bread: about 1 slice Fruits and vegetables: up to ½ cup of each Meat: up to ¼ cup Divide food among 3–4 feedings per day	Table foods may be added gradually; cut table foods into small pieces. Start with foods that do not require too much chewing (cooked cut green beans and carrots, noodles, ground meats, tuna fish, soft cheese, plain yogurt). If fish is offered, check closely to be sure that there are no bones in the serving. Mashed cooked egg yolk and orange juice may be added at about 9 months. Occasionally offer mashed tofu or thoroughly cooked dried peas and beans in place of meat.

Modified from Suitor CW, Hunter MF: Nutrition: Principles and Application in Health Promotion. Philadelphia, JB Lippincott, 1980.

trol of head and neck to indicate refusal (Fomon, 1993). Introduction of solids delayed beyond 6 to 9 months may decrease later acceptance (Williams et al., 1992).

Infants demonstrating slow growth, particularly those less than 4 months of age, require increased frequency and duration (amount) of milk feeding, not early introduction of solids. Infants decrease their milk intake when solids are introduced, and milk is calorically more dense than all solids with the exception of pureed meat and egg yolk, solids typically introduced later. Although obesity during infancy does not correlate well with adult obesity, it is an indicator of possible dietary problems (Williams et al., 1992). See Table 42–16 for solutions to this and other common diet-related problems of infancy.

Childhood and Adolescence Nutrition

Routine nutritional assessment and counseling remain important throughout the growing years.

Nutritional care continues to focus on adequate calories and nutrients for optimal growth and well-being. With the emergence of self-feeding skills some attention is turned to laying the foundation for chronic disease prevention. Lifelong eating habits are established during this period. Some chronic illnesses, such as cancer, atherosclerosis, and obesity, are thought to be influenced by early food intake (AAP, 1993a; DHHS, 1988). Most dietary guidelines call for reduced intakes of fat, saturated fat, cholesterol, and sodium for children over the age of 2 years. A prudent low fat diet need not sacrifice adequate nutrition, although occasional overzealous application of these principles has led to failure to thrive of some young children (Williams et al., 1992).

During the preschool years, growth slows and the child's appetite and attention to food become more variable. Food refusals, food jags, bizarre food combinations, and rituals are common but usually self-limiting. They do not pose a serious threat to the child's nutritional status provided par-

TABLE 42–16. COMMON DIET-RELATED PROBLEMS OF INFANTS

Problem	Possible Cause(s)	Solutions
Spitting-up; regurgitation	Immature gut Improper feeding technique	No formula change Feeding technique: 40–60 degree feeding position; frequent burping; upright burping; no large nipple hole; gentle handling
Colic-like symptoms	Unknown cause Improper feeding technique Inadequate breast milk production	Crying and comforting techniques No formula change unless other allergy symptoms Feeding technique: small, frequent feeding; better feeding position; frequent burping; longer sucking; pleasant environment Build up breast milk supply: more frequent, longer duration nursing; adequate maternal rest
Failure to thrive	Underfeeding	Increase frequency and amount of milk feedings Ensure proper formula preparation Instruct caretaker in proper feeding technique and parenting behavior Improve child's psychosocial environment: financial/food/housing assistance; parental/marital counseling
Obesity	Overfeeding	Decrease quantity of formula to 24–32 oz/day; introduce solids if delayed Ensure proper formula preparation; do not superdilute formula Change composition of diet: eliminate or decrease sweets, sweetened beverages, and fatty foods Proper feeding technique: spoon-feeding only; no solids in the bottle; attention to infant cues of satiation; eliminate multiple night feedings in older infant; encourage defined feeding schedule
Constipation	Inadequate fluids Inadequate fiber	Increase fluids; decrease solids if too rapidly introduced Add bulk: whole grains and bran, fresh fruits and vegetables, legumes if age-appropriate Try apple and pear juices Discontinue cow's milk if early introduction
Diarrhea	Short duration: gastroenteritis Chronic: postgastroenteritis Nonspecific infantile diarrhea Food intolerance or allergy	Acute: maintain fluid and electrolyte balance with breast milk or increasing concentrations of dilute formula Do not use more than 2–3 oz/lb body weight of oral rehydration solution; add water or breast milk to satisfy thirst Lactose-free diet not necessary Slow reintroduction of bland solids: rice cereal, banana, potato—not delayed longer than 24 hours Lactose-free diet; discontinue pear/apple juice and other high sugar beverages; dilute formula initially Balanced diet with adequate fat; limit excessive fluid or sweet beverages as above Omit offending food Consider protein hydrolysate formula if coexisting cow's milk and soy allergy Check tolerance by age 3–4 years
Vomiting	Gastroenteritis	Omit 1–2 feedings Maintain fluid and electrolyte balance with 1–2 teaspoons of water each 5 minutes until vomiting ceases, then 1–2 oz each 10–15 minutes; slow reintroduction of bland solids
Food allergy/ intolerance	Cow's milk, wheat, citrus, soy, egg white, peanuts	Eliminate and challenge with offending food; check for immunologic basis with skin test Design restrictive diet with help of a registered dietitian to ensure adequacy
Iron-deficiency anemia	Inadequate iron intake Iron loss	Acute: iron supplementation 6 mg Fe/kg/day Increase dietary iron intake: iron-fortified formula and infant cereal; high-iron solids such as meat, egg yolks, legumes Increase bioavailability: serve with vitamin C source Decrease iron loss; decrease cow's milk if early introduction or excessive intake

Modified from Coombs JB, Speer SJ: *Nutrition I/II.* Monograph, edition no. 129/130. Kansas City, MO, American Academy of Family Physicians, 1990.

ents continue to offer a variety of nutritious foods at meal and snack times. Studies have demonstrated that children self-select a nutritiously adequate diet over time and do not include offerings of the low-nutrient snack foods and desserts that are common in many American homes (Williams et al., 1992).

In the school-age child growth proceeds at a steady pace, and children become more settled in their eating habits. With the child's greater willingness to eat a variety of foods and greater capacity for intake, nutritional problems become less critical. Greater attention can be given to health promotional dietary changes at this age.

As the child matures, food choices are increasingly influenced by television, peers, school lunch offerings, day-care situations, and family interactions. The development of a comprehensive nutritional care plan for the at-risk child requires exploration of the child's eating environment. Table 42–17 lists solutions to some of the common diet-related problems of childhood. By altering the portions sizes (e.g., one-third portions for toddlers, one-half portions for preschool children) the Food Group Plan (Table 42–2) can be used as a basis for evaluating dietary adequacy or advising parents on nutritionally adequate meal planning.

The nutritional concerns of childhood extend into adolescence. Iron continues to be the nutrient most often found deficient, with some surveys finding low vitamin B_6 status and problems with adequate calcium, zinc, and folacin intakes (Carruth, 1990). Children and adolescents identified with hyperlipidemia or hypertension, who are otherwise healthy, are subject to dietary treatment protocols similar to those used for adults, but always with careful attention to maintain nutritional adequacy for growth.

Nutrition counseling and changing habits in adolescents and young adults can be difficult. This age group is increasingly independent, and eating habits may deviate considerably from family habits. One method to achieve good dietary practice is to relate suggested dietary changes to daily concerns, such as physical appearance, beauty, or athletic prowess. Food changes should be discussed keeping in mind the adolescent's familiar settings (e.g., healthy fast-food dining). Table 42–18 outlines common diet-related problems of adolescence.

Obesity during childhood and adolescence can be a particularly troublesome problem. Forty per cent of obese 7-year-olds become obese adults, compared to 10 per cent of nonobese children. The relative risk of obesity increases with age, and 70 per cent of preadolescent children (10- to 13-year-olds) remain fat into adulthood (Epstein, 1993). The treatment of obesity in children and teenagers should be as comprehensive as that described for adult obesity (see Dietary Treatment of Adult Obesity, below). Excessively restricted diets in prepubertal children should be avoided. Research on the treatment of obesity in children has repeatedly demonstrated the importance of exercise (Epstein, 1993). Parent and family involvement appears critical to successful outcomes (Epstein, 1993; Mellin, 1987).

Care should be taken when approaching teenagers who are overweight or perceive themselves to be overweight. The onset of eating disorders (anorexia nervosa and bulimia) often begins during adolescence with efforts to lose weight that escalate into a preoccupation with food and body size (Herzog and Copland, 1985).

Adolescent girls and athletes, particularly in weight-related sports, are most susceptible to anorexia nervosa and bulimia. Signs of developing eating disorders in this age group are a weight below 15 per cent expected for height, overweight but with rapid weight fluctuations, history of constant dieting or excessive exercise, statements about feeling "too fat" when actually underweight, reported episodes of "binge" eating, evidence of self-induced vomiting (erosion of tooth enamel, esophagitis), laxative (complaints of constipation and cramping), or diuretic use (hypokalemia), cessation of menses, or obsession with body shape and weight (Simko et al., 1989).

The anorectic may appear to be a "model" child, somewhat rigid and perfectionistic, with high academic achievement. Bulimia is more often associated with impulsive behavior and substance abuse (Lucas and Huse, 1994; Williams et al., 1992). The anorectic is usually thin, whereas the bulimic may be of normal weight or slightly overweight (Lucas and Huse, 1984).

Treatment of eating disorders involves medical care, psychotherapy, and nutrition intervention and education. See the section Eating Disorders, below.

Nutrition in the Older Adult

The rate of the aging is influenced by genetic, environmental, and lifestyle factors. Specific individuals differ in terms of physiologic, psychological, and social changes at a given chronologic age. The goals of nutritional care in the healthy elderly are maintenance of health and optimal physical and mental condition. In the elderly with health problems, nutritional care also includes dietary modifications for disease management, prevention or treatment of nutrient deficiencies, and avoidance of drug–nutrient interactions.

Dietary inadequacies are most common among ethnic minorities, chronically ill or dependent persons, the poor, and the institutionalized elderly (DHHS, 1986). Despite the fact that both the physiologic and social changes associated with aging tend to have an adverse effect on nutritional status, it is a mistake to consider all elderly individuals as nutritionally deficient. The nutritional quality of the average diet of older persons per 1000 kcal is better than that of adolescents. The elderly eat less (Williams et al., 1992), however and the decline in lean body mass and reduction in metabolic rate that accompany aging makes consumption of a nutrient-dense diet more important.

The available data on specific requirements for essential nutrients in the older person is limited. Most nutrient recommendations are extrapolated from younger age groups. There is some indication

TABLE 42–17. COMMON DIET-RELATED PROBLEMS OF CHILDREN

Problem	Possible Cause(s)	Solutions
Picky eater/food jags	Growth slowed/varied and appetite follows Greater awareness of outside world/distraction Asserting independence	Guidelines for adequate diet Small servings, proper texture for age Parents choose what to eat, child chooses how much Avoid mealtime battles Offer more frequent, nutritious snacks Prophylactic vitamin/mineral supplements
Overweight	Overfeeding Lack of physical activity (too much television viewing)	No restrictive diet Eliminate or decrease high fat, high sugar, low-nutrient foods Plain food preparation More exercise Explore issues of self-esteem, outside activities, and family dynamics
Failure to thrive or underweight	Underfeeding	As for picky eater Encourage use of nutritious higher calorie foods (whole milk, milkshakes, cheese, nuts, meats) If severe, consider short-term use of protein-calorie supplements (e.g., Instant Breakfast) Improve child's psychosocial environment: financial/food/housing assistance; parenting/marital counseling
Chronic diarrhea	Postgastroenteritis syndrome Food allergy or intolerance Excessive intake of sweet beverages	Maintain fluid and electrolyte balance with more than usual fluid intake and gradually increase concentrations of dilute milk feedings and soft, bland foods Eliminate offending food Discontinue use of soda or fruit juice, especially pear or apple juice
Constipation	Recent weaning to cow's milk Inadequate fluid intake Inadequate fiber intake	Increase water and juice intake, especially pear and apple juices Add bulk with whole grain breads and crackers, bran cereals and muffins, fresh and dried fruits, starchy vegetables and legumes
Iron-deficiency anemia	Excessive cow's milk (>40 oz/day) Inadequate intake of iron-containing foods	Wean to cup Increase high iron foods such as red meats, iron-fortified cereals, legumes, nuts, dark green leafy vegetables, eggs Feed vitamin C food with plant sources of iron Cook in iron pots
Lactose intolerance	Lactase deficiency: primary or postenteritis	Calcium, riboflavin, protein, and calories are at risk when dairy foods are eliminated Use calcium-fortified soy milks (not creamers) in place of cow's milk Yogurt and aged cheese may be tolerated Other sources of calcium and riboflavin: tofu, unhulled sesame seeds, and dark green leafy vegetables Consider calcium supplements
Dental caries	Poor dental hygiene Frequent intake of cariogenic foods (high sugar, sticky foods): dried and fresh fruits and juices, candies, pastries, breads, crackers, cereals, and milk	Better dental hygiene and fluoride treatments Decrease frequency of between meal snacking and bedtime snacking Increase use of low cariogenic snacks: meats, nuts, cheese Combine low cariogenic foods with high cariogenic foods
Hyperactive-like symptoms	Poor family dynamics or parent–child interactions A small subgroup may be susceptible to food additives, colors, and naturally occurring salicylates Excessive caffeine intake	Explore family dynamics and parental expectations of childhood behavior—suggest family counseling Trial of additive and sugar-free diet If nutritionally adequate, does not pose burden, and family feels it helps—continue No more than 1 serving of chocolate or caffeine-containing soda per day
Vegetarianism	Various	Determine exact food restrictions Discuss vegetarian food guide Emphasize food sources of limited nutrients Grind or mash bulky foods for young child; use tofu, legumes, and nuts as protein sources Cook in iron pots; include vitamin C source with meals Make snacks and desserts count (i.e., nutrient-dense foods) If strict vegetarian, use vitamin D, calcium, and vitamin B_{12}-fortified soy milk or give supplements Refer strict vegetarian infant, child, pregnant, or lactating woman to a registered dietitian

Modified from Coombs JB, Speer SJ: *Nutrition I/II*. Monograph, edition no. 129/130. Kansas City, MO, American Academy of Family Physicians, 1990.

TABLE 42–18. COMMON DIET-RELATED CONCERNS OF ADOLESCENTS

Concern	Cause	Counseling
Obesity	Overeating Lack of exercise Other	Premenarche or growth spurt: improved eating habits, more exercise, no fewer than 1600 calories Postgrowth spurt: treat as for an adult with attention to motivators Explore issues of self-esteem, outside activities, and family dynamics Attention to signs of bulimia: see text
Underweight	Poor appetite Poor eating habits Restrictive diet Growth spurt	Assess dietary adequacy Increase intake high-calorie and nutrient-dense foods (nuts, dried fruit, dairy products, whole grains) Small, frequent feedings Attention to signs of anorexia nervosa: see text
Athletic diet regimens	Alteration of eating habits to enhance performance or meet performance criteria	Balanced adequate intake Attention to iron status No need for extra protein, vitamins, minerals, or ergogenic aids Advise against weight cycling Counsel on pregame meal, fluid, and electrolyte needs during activity One-day carbohydrate loading (75% of calories) is safe Attention to signs of eating disorders: see text
Vegetarianism or alternate diets	Various	Offer educational materials and menu plans

Modified from Coombs JB, Speer SJ: *Nutrition I/II*. Monograph, edition no. 129/130. Kansas City, MO, American Academy of Family Physicians, 1990.

that the elderly have an increased need for protein and vitamins B_6, B_{12}, and D than is currently indicated in the RDAs (Ausman and Russell, 1994). Surveys indicate low dietary intake of calcium and vitamin D, and biochemical tests indicate that 5 to 20 percent of the elderly population may be deficient in thiamine, riboflavin, iron, and folate (Ausman and Russell, 1994).

Nutritional status assessment of the older person requires attention to the conditions that commonly influence appetite and food intake in this age group: limited financial resources; difficulty with shopping, food preparation, or self-feeding; difficulty with chewing or swallowing; gastrointestinal changes or discomfort; and social isolation or depression. The potential for medication effects on appetite and mental status should not be overlooked nor should investigation into alcohol intake. Changes in appetite, food intake, weight status, and functional ability are key early warning signs of malnutrition. The Nutrition Screening Initiative has published a set of nutrition assessment forms and a nutritional care implementation manual that are appropriate for office use (AAFP, 1992).

Recommendations for nutrition care must take into account the individual's life habits, psychosocial status, economic condition, and physical abilities. It should not be assumed that the patient has knowledge of the principles of good nutrition and food preparation methods.

Medically prescribed and self-imposed dietary restrictions are common among older persons because of the frequency of chronic illnesses. While searching for relief from many of the common problems of aging, the elderly become targets of nutrition quackery and are perhaps more susceptible than other age groups to fad diets and nutrient sup-

plementation schemes. Each dietary restriction or modification limits the selection of available foods. The loss of favorite foods, changes in flavor, and alteration of cooking methods can adversely affect appetite and food intake. New dietary modifications should be recommended only when it is reasonably anticipated that they will result in a significant improvement in health status.

Many of the diet-related problems of the older person are associated with chronic illnesses that are treated elsewhere in this chapter. Other common problems and suggested solutions are listed in Table 42–19.

SPECIAL SITUATIONS

Vitamin and Mineral Supplementation

Surveys on food supplement usage show that three of every four Americans believe that taking extra vitamins can make them feel better or more energetic—regardless of the adequacy of their diets. Despite the fact that there are nearly 4000 cases of vitamin poisoning each year, 80 per cent among children (Dubick and Rucker, 1983), most people consider it safe to take vitamins in any amount.

The use of vitamin and mineral supplements is not necessary for most healthy persons consuming adequate, balanced diets. However, many people have poor eating habits, regularly skip meals, make limited food choices, or rely on highly processed convenience foods. Constant dieting, especially on diets of fewer than 1200 calories, may also result in nutritionally deficient intakes over time. The use of cigarettes, alcohol, recreational drugs, or se-

TABLE 42–19. COMMON DIET-RELATED CONCERNS OF OLDER ADULTS

Concern	Cause	Counseling
Constipation	Decreased GI motility Drug side effect Laxative abuse Inadequate fluid and fiber intake	Fluid, 8 cups per day Higher fiber intake: whole grains, bran, vegetables, fresh and dried fruits (prunes and figs) Ensure adequate diet or advise vitamin/mineral supplementation when increased fiber Encourage exercise Regular bowel habits
Flatulence	GI changes Drug side effects Dietary factors (e.g., lactose intolerance)	Eat small, frequent meals Well cooked foods; cut small or shred; chew thoroughly Treat constipation: increase fiber gradually Eat gas-forming foods sparingly: legumes, cabbage family vegetables, melons, dried fruits Avoid greasy and spicy foods Trial of lactose-free diet Exercise as tolerated
Fluid balance/ dehydration	Unconscious, confused, depressed, disabled, or anorectic persons Laxative abusers Diuretic users Persons with diarrhea or vomiting	Encourage 6–8 cups of fluid per day: sipping throughout the day If patient cannot serve self, address problem to caregiver Keep a record
Malnutrition	Inadequate intake (may not be voluntary)	Address any underlying cause such as economic difficulties, physical barriers, poor mental health, medication interactions, dental problems, or restrictive diet prescriptions Assess current intake and plan adequate meal pattern according to preferences and abilities Refer to community resources, such as congregate meals, home-delivered meals, food stamps, commodity programs, shopping and cooking assistance
Osteoporosis	Primary/involutional Postmenopausal	Ensure adequate calcium and vitamin D intake Exercise Avoid medicines that increase calcium excretion As above Supplement with: 1 gm calcium during estrogen replacement therapy or 1.2–1.5 gm calcium without estrogen

Modified from Coombs JB, Speer SJ: *Nutrition I/II.* Monograph, edition no. 129/130. Kansas City, MO, American Academy of Family Physicians, 1990.

lected prescription medications may also adversely affect nutritional needs.

Infants, menstruating women, pregnant and lactating women, the elderly or debilitated, or people whose diets are restricted for weight loss or other reasons may benefit from vitamin and mineral supplementation. In general, prophylactic supplements should be balanced and comprehensive, providing those nutrients most likely to be deficient: vitamins C, A, and B$_6$, folate, calcium, iron, zinc, and magnesium. Supplements should also be low potency, providing supplemental nutrients at levels approximating only 100 per cent of the RDA.

Single supplementation should be avoided except when specifically indicated therapeutically or when multivitamins do not provide a large enough dose of the required nutrient (e.g., calcium). Megadoses generally refer to amounts at least ten times greater than the RDA. At this level vitamins and minerals act more like drugs than nutrients, with all the risks of medication overdose and undesirable side effects (Dubick and Rucker, 1983). Large doses of zinc, for instance, can result in a relative deficiency of copper (NRC, 1989a). Minimum toxic doses for vitamins and minerals are listed in Table 42–20.

Evaluating Nutritional Claims

The public and physicians may have difficulty evaluating the validity of nutritional claims. The nutrition department of a local university or public health department or a registered dietitian in private practice or community education can be a local resource for help in evaluating unfamiliar nutrition products or claims. The National Council Against Health Fraud (800-821-6671) or the NIH's Office of Alternative Medicine (301-402-2466) are potential resources of accurate information on alternative nutritional practices. The U.S. Food and Drug Administration's magazine, the *FDA Consumer,* frequently carries articles and editorials that discuss health fraud and nutrition quackery. If no other resources are available or acceptable as discussed above, it may prove helpful for the physician to request the patient to bring the sup-

TABLE 42–20. VITAMIN AND MINERAL SAFETY INDICES

Nutrient	Estimated Daily Adult Oral Minimum Toxic Dose (mg)
Vitamin A	25,000–50,000 IU
Vitamin D	50,000 IU
Vitamin E	1,200 IU
Vitamin C	1,000–5,000
Thiamine	300
Riboflavin	1,000*
Niacin (nicotinamide)	1,000
Pyridoxine	2,000†
Folacin	400
Biotin	50
Pantothenic acid	1,000
Calcium	12,000
Phosphorus	12,000
Magnesium	6,000
Iron	100
Zinc	500
Copper	100
Fluoride	4 to 20
Iodine	2
Selenium	1

* However, only about 25 mg of riboflavin can be absorbed in a single oral dose given to an adult.

† More recent data suggest that the toxic dose of pyridoxine for some individuals is much lower.

Modified from National Research Council, Committee on Diet and Health: Diet and Health: Implications for Reducing Chronic Disease Risk. Washington, DC, National Academy Press, 1989. Copyright 1989 by the National Academy of Sciences.

porting literature on the product or nutritional claim so the two can analyze it together.

People are often emotionally or philosophically attached to their nutritional practices and beliefs. The medical community is sometimes painted as disinterested, ignorant, or secretive about "alternative" nutrition practices. Under these circumstances, advising patients can be difficult. The physician must demonstrate open-mindedness and establish a rapport with the patient before challenging beliefs. Beware of an authoritarian, dismissive, or confrontational attitude, which may cause the patient to withhold information about life practices that could be critical to the medical decisions about health care. Try to establish how the patient hopes to benefit or gain from a dubious practice. Be prepared to suggest alternatives. Avoiding alcohol, tobacco, street drugs, dietary imbalances, stress, and physical inactivity are proved health-promoting activities.

Alternative Diets: Vegetarianism

Vegetarianism is not necessarily a harmful practice against which the patient must be persuaded. Indeed, vegetarians have lower rates of hypertension, non-insulin-dependent diabetes, gallbladder disease, and obesity; they also have lower mortality rates for cardiovascular disease and are at decreased risk for breast, lung, and colon cancer compared to nonvegetarians (ADA, 1993). These effects may be attributable to other lifestyle characteristics that are sometimes associated with vegetarianism, such as regular physical activity and abstinence from smoking, alcohol, and illicit drug use.

The term vegetarian describes a variety of eating practices that rely mainly on plant foods. The strict vegetarian, or vegan, diet relies solely on plant foods (fruits, vegetables, legumes, grains, nuts, and seeds). The lacto-vegetarian diet adds dairy products and the ovo-lacto-vegetarian diet adds eggs. Even within these classifications, however, there is considerable variation in the nature and extent animal products are excluded in the diet. Individual evaluation is necessary to assess dietary adequacy. Some persons describe their eating habits as "vegetarian" simply because they avoid meat from four-legged animals but continue to consume limited quantities of poultry or fish as well as dairy products and eggs.

Plant proteins are considered "incomplete" because they are generally limited in one or more essential amino acids when compared to the more "complete" animal proteins. Combining plant foods with complementary amino acid patterns, such as legumes with grains, nuts, or seeds, results in a higher quality complete protein. Although complementary proteins do not have to be eaten in the same meal, many traditional meal patterns provide these combinations, e.g., peanut butter (legume) and bread, tofu (soybean) and rice, pinto beans and corn tortillas (grain).

Nutritionally adequate ovo-lacto and lacto-vegetarian diets can be planned by replacing animal protein selections in the Food Group Plan (Table 42–2) with an equal number of servings of legumes, nuts, and seeds (and eggs). Although strict vegetarian diets can be more limited in high quality protein, vitamin B_{12}, calcium, vitamin D, iron, riboflavin, and zinc than vegetarian diets that include some animal products, most nutrient requirements can be met with careful food selection. The exception is vitamin B_{12}.

Strict vegetarians may derive vitamin B_{12} from microorganism contamination of food products (e.g., surfaces of unwashed fruits and vegetables or contamination of spirulina, seaweed, tempeh, or other fermented products), but as much as 80 to 90 per cent of the vitamin assayed in these products may be inactive analogs (ADA, 1993). More reliable sources of vitamin B_{12} for the strict vegetarian are fortified cereal products, fortified soy milk and meat analogs, and some brands of nutritional yeast. Vitamin B_{12} is found in all animal products. Diets that contain at least two to three servings of milk or eggs approach the adult RDA of 2 μg. Sources of other nutrients at risk in the strict vegetarian diet are listed in Table 42–3.

Iron supplementation is recommended for vegetarians and nonvegetarians during pregnancy. Both pregnant and lactating strict vegetarian women and their infants require supplementation with vitamin B_{12}. Vitamin B_{12} deficiency has been identified in nurslings of vegan mothers even though the mothers did not demonstrate signs of B_{12} deficiency (Frader et al., 1978). If exposure to sunlight is limited, vitamin D supplementation is recommended for all members of vulnerable groups. Two hours of sun exposure per week while clothed, or 0.5 hour per week of full body exposure, has been shown to produce sufficient endogenous vitamin D to meet the needs of infants (Specker et al., 1985).

Adequate protein and calories may be a concern in the strict vegetarian diets of children and pregnant and lactating women. Strict vegetarian children demonstrate slower growth and are generally shorter and lighter than their nonvegan counterparts (Jacobs and Dwyer, 1988). The vegetarian diet is bulky, and care must be taken to offer well cooked foods and age-appropriate textures (e.g., ground, mashed, chopped) to ensure an adequate energy intake. Including vitamin B_{12}, vitamin D, and calcium-fortified soymilk as a substitute for the dairy group is strongly recommended for strict vegetarians, especially nutritionally vulnerable groups. During periods of physiologic risk, such as infancy, childhood, adolescence, pregnancy, lactation, and illness, total vegetarians should be referred to a registered dietitian for assessment of dietary adequacy and assistance in dietary planning if necessary.

Sports Nutrition

A variety of regular foods can satisfy the energy and nutrient needs of both the professionally competitive and recreationally active person. Recommended dietary composition for athletes follow the same guidelines as for general wellness (Table 42–5). Contrary to popular thought, weight training does not increase protein requirements (Hultman et al., 1994). Only athletes engaged in endurance training require more protein than sedentary individuals (up to 1.4 gm/kg body weight per day). The typical American diet contains 10 to 15 per cent of total energy as protein, so increased food intake sufficient to meet energy needs is sufficient to provide the extra protein. Extra intake of protein in the form of protein drinks and pills is unnecessary.

Athletes anticipating competition involving prolonged exercise of more than 90 minutes may benefit from modified carbohydrate loading starting 3 to 4 days prior to the event. A carbohydrate-rich diet (75 to 80 per cent of calories) is consumed while progressively decreasing training time and resting the day before the competition. Endurance athletes and those training in sports requiring repeated maximal burst of effort (i.e., football, soccer) may benefit from routinely consuming high carbo-hydrate diets (70 to 80 per cent of total calories) to prevent glycogen depletion during training (Coleman, 1991; Hultman et al., 1994).

The precompetition meal should be eaten at least 2 hours before the start of the event. Easily digested and absorbed foods such as breads and cereals, fruits and juices, skim milk, and yogurt are appropriate. Intake of rapidly absorbed sugars 30 to 45 minutes preceding the event may impair performance in some athletes by stimulating the release of insulin and resulting in hypoglycemia. The rise in exercise hormones (epinephrine and norepinephrine) blunts the insulin response to the sugar consumed a few minutes before exercise (Coleman, 1991). Carbohydrate feedings taken during exercise lasting 90 minutes or more protects glycogen stores and may enhance endurance (Coleman, 1991). Large intake of carbohydrate (e.g., drinks containing more than 10 per cent carbohydrate or 100 grams per liter) can delay gastric emptying and cause discomfort (Coleman, 1991).

Hydration is vitally important during exercise. The athlete should drink 3 to 6 ounces of water (or other fluid) every 15 to 20 minutes during exercise. Replacing each pound of body weight lost during exercise with 16 ounces of water ensures continued hydration. Electrolyte replacement during ultraendurance events (e.g., 50-mile runs or 100-mile bike rides) may be necessary. Drinking 100 to 200 ml of a solution containing 50 to 100 gm/L of carbohydrate and 10 to 30 mM salt (concentrations found in many sports drinks) every 15 to 20 minutes provides optimal rates of gastric emptying and efficiency of rehydration. Chilled solutions empty more quickly and can reduce body temperatures (Lyle and Forgac, 1991). Drinking 400 to 500 ml of fluid 10 to 15 minutes before the event helps maintain water balance but superhydration 40 to 80 minutes before the event can precipitate diuresis (Hultman et al., 1994).

Tremendous individual variation exists in the ability to tolerate pre-event meals and rehydration solutions during strenuous exercise. Each individual must experiment before the competition to develop an effective individual strategy.

The ability to exercise and perform well is clearly reduced by deficient nutritional intake, but there is little documentation that vitamin and mineral supplementation improves performance in athletes who are not deficient. Indeed, excessive intake may impair performance (e.g., excessive niacin intake inhibits free fatty acid release) (Whitmire, 1991). The increased need for energy-associated vitamins (thiamine, riboflavin, and niacin) and trace minerals can be met by the increased food intake necessary to meet calorie needs. Athletes who restrict intake (e.g., gymnasts, dancers, divers, wrestlers) to control body weight may not be consuming an adequate diet. A daily multivitamin and mineral supplement is reasonable in this instance or any case where there is doubt about dietary adequacy.

In most athletes the low hemoglobin concentration termed "sports anemia" is a result of training-induced hemodilution. True iron deficiency anemia may be found in 10 per cent of athletes, confirmed by low serum ferritin levels and transferrin saturation (Hultman et al., 1994).

NUTRITIONAL MANAGEMENT OF SELECTED DISEASE STATES

Although routine nutritional counseling and health promotion has a place in nearly every patient contact, more detailed nutrition intervention plans frequently accompany the medical management of illnesses. The nutrition intervention plan includes outcome goals, a diet prescription, a list of nutritional problems to be addressed, strategies for change, and referrals for further assistance as needed.

For example, a middle-aged overweight woman who is moderately hypertensive may have outcome goals of (1) loss of 10 pounds and (2) normalized blood pressure. Her diet prescription might be for a calorie-controlled, low sodium, low fat diet. Her nutritional problems could be excessive intake of empty calorie snack foods and reliance on high sodium processed foods. Nutritional counseling should address these problems with a personalized diet plan and ideas for acceptable snack foods and substitutes for high sodium processed foods. Handing the patient a preprinted diet sheet with little or no explanation usually results in confusion, frustration, poor adherence, and lack of success for both the patient and physician.

Patient adherence to nutritional recommendations is enhanced by individualizing the intervention plan. Problem behaviors that have been specifically identified through nutritional assessment must be addressed and changes proposed in small, manageable steps (i.e., behavior shaping). This stepped approach can be implemented by focusing on short-term behavioral goals instead of global outcome goals (e.g., focus on designing an acceptable walking schedule rather than give a general recommendation to "lose weight."). Additional steps can gradually be added at each regular medical care visit until these small changes combine to produce improved life habits. Ask patients to formally contract and commit to specific goals. Patients who have given their word expect to be held accountable and will have an increased likelihood of success (Moore et al., 1991).

Community resources for nutrition education and counseling offer the physician support for this type of in-depth nutrition intervention. Nutrition education is giving information or teaching about food and diet. Nutrition information is available from a variety of community resources or may be provided by the physician or office staff.

Nutrition counseling refers to individualized guidance on appropriate diets and nutrient intakes taking into consideration health, cultural, socioeconomic, functional, and psychological factors. Nutrition counseling includes an in-depth nutritional assessment followed by development of a nutritional care plan. This plan may include recommendations for food selection to increase or decrease specific nutrients or nonnutrients in the diet; changes in the timing, size, or composition of meals; modified food textures; and in some instances recommendations to change the route of nutrient administration from oral to feeding tube or intravenous nutrition (AAFP, 1992). Table 42–21 offers assistance in locating local community resources, such as registered dietitians in private practice, who provide nutrition education and counseling.

DIETARY MANAGEMENT OF HYPERLIPIDEMIA

Hypercholesterolemia

The National Cholesterol Education Program recommends dietary therapy as the first line of treatment for elevated blood cholesterol. Dietary therapy is designed to reduce intake of saturated fatty acids and cholesterol and to promote weight loss in patients who are overweight. Appropriate physical activity is considered an essential element in the nonpharmacologic treatment of elevated blood cholesterol (NCEP, 1993).

Patients with high LDL cholesterol levels (higher than 160 mg/dL) and those with borderline high LDL cholesterol levels (130 to 160 mg/dL) but with two other risk factors for CHD are candidates for dietary intervention. For secondary prevention in those patients with known CHD or other atherosclerotic disease, dietary therapy should be initiated if LDL cholesterol levels are above 100 mg/dL. Patients with borderline high cholesterol (200 to 240 mg/dL) or LDL cholesterol levels and fewer than two other risk factors for CHD should be given instruction in dietary modification and physical activity and reevaluated at 1 year.

The recommended dietary therapy for elevated blood cholesterol occurs in two steps, the Step-One and Step-Two Diets. This stepped approach restricts total fat intake and progressively lowers saturated fat and cholesterol intakes. The Step-One Diet calls for a total fat content of less than 30 per cent of calories, saturated fat intake less than 10 per cent of calories, and less than 300 mg of cholesterol daily. The Step-Two Diet, used if the response to the Step-One Diet is insufficient, involves a further reduction in saturated fat intake to less than

TABLE 42–21.   CONTACT GUIDE FOR LOCAL NUTRITION EDUCATION AND COUNSELING SERVICES*

Source	Contact	Provisions
USDA Cooperative Extension Services	County Agricultural Service: Food and Nutrition Specialist (or call 312-647-1200 for master list of extension agents)	Information on food, shopping, and cooking
County, city, and local health departments	Nutritionist/public health dietitian	Publications on a variety of nutrition and diet topics; location and description of local nutrition education programs and nutrition-related social services, individual nutrition counseling
Local affiliates of the large national health associations	White pages listing in local phone book; call national office, below	
American Heart Association	214-373-6300	Nutrition and diet publications and education programs; referral list of dietitians in private practice
American Diabetes Association	703-549-1500	Nutrition and diet publications and education programs; referral list of dietitians in private practice
American Cancer Society	404-329-7647	Nutrition and diet publications and education programs; referral list of dietitians in private practice
National Dairy Council	800-426-8271	Publications on a variety of nutrition and diet topics; group nutrition education materials
American Dietetic Association	312-899-1979	Referral list of dietitians in private practice who offer individual nutrition counseling and education
Community colleges	Department of nutrition or community outreach/adult education department	Classes on diet and nutritional science; community classes on nutrition, diet, cooking, and shopping
Hospitals	Foodservice or nutrition service	Individual nutrition counseling for inpatients; outpatient nutrition counseling and community nutrition education or weight control classes
Health Maintenance Organization (HMO)	Department of patient education or health education or nurse/dietitian educator	Individual nutrition counseling and group nutrition education for HMO members
Dietitians in private practice	Local phone book; local American Dietetic Association affiliate; national office above	Individual nutrition counseling and group education
Other nutrition-related organizations (see Nutrition-related community services) (Table 42–10)		

* Services vary at different sites.

7 per cent of calories and in cholesterol to less than 200 mg daily. Because the Step-One Diet is essentially the same diet as that advocated for general wellness many patients have already adopted this dietary pattern (NCEP, 1993). If so, the Step-Two Diet comprises the first phase of therapy. Patients with established CHD should begin immediately on the Step-Two Diet. The contents of both diets are shown in Table 42–22.

A minimum of 6 months of intensive dietary therapy and counseling generally should be carried out before considering drug therapy. Shorter periods can be considered in patients with severe LDL cholesterol elevations (higher than 220 mg/dL) or known CHD (NCEP, 1993). Drug therapy should be added to, not substituted for, dietary therapy (NCEP, 1993). Involvement of a registered dietitian is recommended, particularly for intensive di-

etary therapy, such as a retrial of the Step-One Diet or progression to the Step-Two Diet (NCEP, 1993). Long-term adherence through permanent changes in eating behavior requires individualization of dietary therapy.

The view that dietary modification is impractical or ineffective for most patients is not justified (NCEP, 1993). The response to dietary modification shows considerable individual variation primarily reflecting differences in the content of baseline diets, baseline cholesterol levels, dietary adherence, and inherent biologic responsiveness. The expected reduction in serum cholesterol with dietary modifications similar to the Step-One Diet is 3 to 24 per cent (NCEP, 1993). In general, patients with higher serum cholesterol levels and higher consumption of saturated fat and cholesterol experience greater absolute reductions in

TABLE 42–22.   STEP 1 AND STEP 2 DIETS FOR TREATMENT OF ELEVATED CHOLESTEROL

Food Group	Step 1 Diet	Step 2 Diet
Meat, poultry, seafood	Fish or poultry without skin; lean cuts of beef, lamb, pork, well trimmed ≤5–6 oz Shellfish eaten only occasionally Organ meats limited Extra lean (15% fat) ground meats Lunch meat: 10% fat or 3 gm fat/oz	Organ meats, shrimp, and crayfish limited Lean cuts of meats; trim and have ground Lunch meat: 2 gm fat/oz
Eggs	Egg yolks, ≤4 per week	Egg yolks, ≤2 per week
Dairy products	Skim or 1% milk Nonfat or low-fat yogurt Cheese: <6 g fat/oz Frozen low-fat yogurt, ice milk or sherbet (3 gm fat/serving)	Cheese: <2 gm fat/oz Frozen low-fat yogurt, sherbet (2 gm fat/serving)
Fats and oils	Unsaturated vegetable oils: safflower, corn, sunflower, soybean, cottonseed, olive, canola, peanut Margarine Salad dressings Shortenings Nuts, seeds, olives, avocados	No shortenings
Breads and cereals	Fat, 1 gm/serving Homemade baked goods made with allowed ingredients Low-fat crackers Cereal, rice, pasta	No change
Fruits and vegetables	Fresh, frozen, canned, or dried fruits and vegetables	No change
Desserts	Homemade baked goods made with allowed ingredients Hard candy, angelfood cake, gingersnaps, fruit ice, sorbet, fig bars, fat-free cookies	No change

LDL cholesterol levels. A doubling of the blood lipid response may be achieved by concomitant weight loss (by the overweight) (NCEP, 1993).

The addition of soluble fibers to the diet may produce an additional 5 to 15 percent reduction in serum cholesterol beyond that achieved with the Step-One Diet (Davidson et al., 1991b). About 25 per cent of the recommended total dietary fiber intake of 20 to 30 grams daily for adults and should be soluble fiber (6 grams) (NCEP, 1993). This level of fiber intake can be achieved with the recommended five or more servings of fruits and vegetables and six or more servings of whole grain products per day. Rich sources of soluble fibers are oat bran, barley, legumes, root vegetables, apples, pears, figs, and berries.

Dietary therapy and increased physical activity may decrease the risk for CHD through means other than their effects on LDL cholesterol. Weight reduction and exercise not only promote reduction of cholesterol levels; they also reduce triglycerides, increase HDL, reduce blood pressure, and improve glucose tolerance. Low saturated fat and cholesterol intakes decrease the risk for CHD independently of effects on LDL cholesterol. In addition, an increased intake of fruits, vegetables, whole grains, and legumes appears to supply substances that protect against CHD. This effect may be mediated through agents such as the antioxidant vitamins and fiber (NCEP, 1993). Similarly, increased physical activity reduces the CHD-

caused mortality rate unrelated to the effects of exercise on serum lipids. This benefit may be a result of exercise-induced increases of vascularization to the heart (NCEP, 1993). For these reasons it is advisable to continue with the recommended dietary modifications and increased physical activity as appropriate regardless of whether the specific goals of LDL cholesterol lowering are achieved.

Hypertriglyceridemia

Obesity and excess calories, dietary fat, alcohol, and carbohydrates are associated with hypertriglyceridemia. Because the benefits of lipid-lowering therapy is most firmly rooted in changes in LDL cholesterol levels, therapy to lower triglycerides should not increase LDL levels and ideally should raise HDL cholesterol levels. The NCEP Step-One Diet is recommended for all patients with elevated triglycerides, with a progression to the Step-Two Diet as indicated in order to achieve further modification in plasma lipids. These diets are effective in lowering total and LDL cholesterol, facilitate weight loss, and aid in lowering serum triglycerides (NIH, 1992). Very low fat diets (10 to 20 per cent) are useful for treating exogenous hypertriglyceridemia (chylomicronemia) and disturbances of remnant metabolism (type III hyperlipoproteinemia) (Feldman, 1994; NCEP, 1993).

Excessive calorie intake and obesity are frequently associated with hypertriglyceridemia and low HDL cholesterol levels. In these instances weight loss alone may normalize serum triglycerides. When weight loss is combined with regular exercise, HDL cholesterol levels may increase 10 to 20 per cent (NIH, 1992). Although triglyceride levels change immediately with calorie restriction, HDL cholesterol levels may fall during weight reduction and then rise over a 3- to 6-month period after weight stabilization (Denke, 1994).

Alcohol increases plasma triglycerides in some patients, especially overweight patients with high baseline triglycerides levels (Denke, 1994). Alcohol intake should be reduced or eliminated in those patients consuming more than two drinks per day or those with high triglyceride levels (Denke, 1994; NIH, 1992).

Although high carbohydrate, very low fat (less than 25 per cent of total calories) diets tend to raise triglyceride levels and lower HDL cholesterol levels, population studies do not support an increase in CHD risk with these diets (Denke, 1994; NIH, 1992). Some investigators find the increased triglycerides to be a transient effect, and studies of lipoprotein composition suggest that high carbohydrate, very low fat diets produce large triglyceride-rich very low density lipoprotein (VLDL) particles that are less atherogenic than the dense, cholesterol-rich VLDL observed in some states of abnormal triglyceride metabolism (Denke, 1994; NCEP, 1993). Many patients with hypertriglyceridemia have impaired glucose tolerance or diabetes mellitus. In these patients the underlying disease must be controlled before effecting a decrease in plasma triglycerides (Feldman, 1994). Restriction of the use of added sweeteners may decrease plasma triglycerides, aid in glucose tolerance, and facilitate calorie reduction and weight loss.

Long-chain omega-3 fatty acids (chiefly eicosapentanoic and docosahexanoic acids) in doses of 5 to 10 grams may decrease plasma triglyceride levels by as much as 1200 mg/dl (Denke, 1994). Although omega-3 fatty acids administered in capsules may reduce very high triglyceride levels that do not respond adequately to other dietary modifications, their use is not recommended. Omega-3 fatty acids tend to worsen diabetic control and may raise LDL cholesterol and apolipoprotein B levels (NCEP, 1993; NIH, 1992).

DIET AND HYPERTENSION

The Report of the Expert Panel on the Detection, Evaluation, and Treatment of High Blood Pressure advocates the initial use of nondrug therapy for at least 3 to 6 months after the diagnosis of hypertension. The following modifications are practical and safe for most hypertensives and within the guidelines for general health promotion diets.

1. If the patient is overweight, *weight reduction* should be the primary goal. Individuals with high waist/hip ratios (central obesity) have a greater prevalence of hypertension than those with lower body obesity (Stein and Black, 1993). The average effect of each 2 pound decrease in body weight is 1.6/1.3 mm Hg fall in systolic and diastolic pressures (Kaplan, 1994). The addition of sodium restriction to weight loss may be additive (Stein and Black, 1993). Exercise used as an adjunct to weight loss has a direct positive effect on blood pressure and reduces overall cardiovascular mortality (Kaplan, 1994).

2. *Alcohol intake* should be limited to no more than 30 ml of ethanol per day (8 ounces wine, 24 ounces beer, or 2 ounces 100 proof spirits) (NHBPEP, 1993). Intake of more than four alcoholic drinks per day increases blood pressure by an average of 5 to 6 mm Hg systolic and 2 to 4 mm Hg diastolic pressure (Stein and Black, 1993).

3. Dietary *sodium intake* should be restricted to no more than 2.3 grams per day (NHBPEP, 1993). Although there are no good clinical predictors of the best candidates for sodium restriction, hypertensives in general show a greater "salt sensitivity," as do African Americans, older persons, obese persons, and those with a family history (Kotchen and Kotchen, 1994; NHBPEP, 1993). Hypertensives with low plasma renin levels may derive the greatest benefit from sodium restriction (Stein and Black, 1993). Sodium restriction shows a linear dose-response relation to blood pressure. Restriction of dietary sodium intake to about one-half the mean American intake (from 5 grams to about 2 grams per day) lowers blood pressure an average of 8 mm Hg systolic and 5 mm Hg diastolic (Kaplan, 1994). Sodium restriction reduces the potential for diuretic-induced hypokalemia and may improve the effectiveness of most antihypertensive drugs. Ad libitum salt intakes of 15 to 20 grams per day may overcome the antihypertensive effect of diuretics (Kaplan, 1990).

Approximately 1.5 to 2.0 grams of sodium occurs naturally in a 2000 kcal diet composed of unprocessed foods. A 2 gram sodium dietary restriction requires the use of special unsalted canned and commercially prepared products and a limited amount of low sodium luncheon meats and cheese. The diet may include regular fluid milk, regular bread and cereals, and small amounts of regular condiments such as catsup, mayonnaise, and salad dressings. Dining out poses a significant problem, as most restaurant fare is liberally salted (fast food is notably high).

4. *Potassium, magnesium,* and *calcium intakes* should be monitored for adequacy. Potassium intakes greater that 3.5 grams per day may be protective against sodium-induced blood pressure elevations and decrease stroke mortality independently of a blood pressure effect (NRC, 1989a). Low sodium diets that replace high sodium processed

foods with unprocessed fruits, vegetables, and whole grains are naturally higher in potassium.

Use of potassium-containing salt substitutes or supplements should be avoided in patients with renal insufficiency or those using potassium-sparing diuretics. However, potassium supplementation may be necessary for those on potassium-wasting diuretics. Magnesium deficiency may also develop as a result of increased urinary excretion with the use of thiazide and loop diuretics (Roe, 1985). Although supplementation magnesium in the nondepleted patient does not lower blood pressure, magnesium supplementation of patients taking diuretics may lower blood pressure (DHHS, 1988). The role of dietary calcium in the development and treatment of high blood pressure is uncertain (Knapp, 1990). Recommending calcium supplementation for the treatment of high blood pressure is premature, but ensuring an adequate calcium intake is important for health maintenance and the prevention of osteoporosis.

5. Reduce *dietary fat, saturated fat,* and *cholesterol intake.* These dietary modifications are advocated to reduce general coronary heart disease risk; and low fat diets may also facilitate weight loss. The lower average blood pressures found in many vegetarian groups is probably not a direct effect of lower fat and saturated fat but may be attributable to a combination of factors including lower protein and higher fiber intakes (Kaplan, 1994).

Because most Americans with elevated blood pressure have stage 1 or mild hypertension, the modest blood pressure reductions achieved with nondrug therapies should be sufficient to reduce the blood pressure to safe levels in many hypertensives (NHBPEP, 1993). For those with more severe hypertension that requires drug therapy, lifestyle therapy can decrease the amount of medication needed and reduce the potential for drug side effects. The lack of data demonstrating a clear cardiac benefit derived from the drug treatment of mild blood pressure elevations underscores the need to optimize lifestyle change for treatment of hypertension (Knapp, 1990).

DIET AND DIABETES MELLITUS

Diet remains the cornerstone of therapy for all types of diabetes mellitus: insulin-dependent (IDDM), non-insulin-dependent (NIDDM), and gestational diabetes mellitus. Achieving normal metabolic control while avoiding hypoglycemia and minimizing the potential for developing the long-term complications (vascular disease, neuropathy, and nephropathy) are the goals of nutritional care in diabetes (ADA, 1984). Generally these goals are best achieved by controlling blood glucose and lipid levels (DHHS, 1988).

The preliminary results of the Diabetes Control and Complications Trial (DCCT) demonstrate a 60 per cent reduction in the risk of diabetic retinopathy, nephropathy, and neuropathy between the intensive treatment and standard treatment groups of IDDM patients (ADAPS, 1993). Although mean blood glucose values were above normal limits in the experimental group, this trial underscores the long-term benefit of blood glucose control. Care must be taken when generalizing the results of this trial to all patients. In these trials there was also a greatly increased incidence of hypoglycemia resulting from attempts to achieve normal blood glucose levels ("tight control"), and presumption that tight control similarly benefits non-insulin-dependent diabetics remains to be demonstrated.

The principles of dietary treatment are similar for both major types of diabetes (IDDM and NIDDM) but with slightly different emphases for each. For the 5 to 10 per cent of diabetics who have IDDM, the focus of dietary management is coordination of dietary intake with exogenous insulin administration and adequate dietary intake for the maintenance of normal growth and weight. Therefore day-to-day consistency in total intake of food, composition of meals, and timing of meals and snacks are important. Additional foods to compensate for delayed meals and special attention to feeding during illness are critical.

When meals are delayed, the IDD patient should take 10 grams of carbohydrate (about one fruit exchange) for every 0.5 hour the meal is late. Similarly, to prevent hypoglycemia, the patient with IDDM who is ill and unable to eat regular meals should take 50 grams of carbohydrate, in whatever form is most acceptable to the patient (e.g., fruit juice, crackers, soup), during each 8 hour period (West, 1980).

The foundation of any treatment plan for the 80 to 90 per cent of diabetics who are type II and obese is weight reduction. Weight loss reduces insulin resistance and can normalize fasting and postprandial blood glucose levels. In fact, simple calorie restriction reduces blood glucose levels before actual body weight change (Quinn, 1993). A modest weight loss of 10 to 20 pounds improves diabetes control even if ideal weight is not achieved (ADA, 1994). Regular meals and consistency of intake is desirable for coordination with oral hypoglycemics and for the development of good eating habits in the aid of weight reduction.

Regular physical activity as tolerated is beneficial for treatment of all types of diabetes. Exercise improves glycemic control by increasing insulin sensitivity, reducing cardiovascular risk factors, and aiding weight loss (ADA, 1988; DHHS, 1988). Coordination of dietary intake with an exercise schedule is most important in IDDM. An additional 15 grams of carbohydrate (one starch exchange) is recommended for each hour of unusual physical activity of moderate intensity (e.g., jogging, tennis) and 25 grams per hour of strenuous

TABLE 42–23. ADA DIETARY RECOMMENDATIONS FOR PERSONS WITH DIABETES

Dietary Factor	Recommendations
Calories	Should be adequate to maintain reasonable weights for adults or normal growth in children, or increased metabolic needs during pregnancy and lactation or recovery from catabolic illness; reasonable weight is that weight acknowledged as achievable and maintainable and may not be the same as traditionally defined ideal body weight
Protein	Should be the same as the average intake for the general population: 10–20% of daily calorie intake; with the onset of nephropathy protein intake should be restricted to no more than the adult RDA: .8 gm/kg body weight or ~10% of daily calories
Carbohydrate	Dietary carbohydrate and fat should make up the remaining 80–90% of daily non protein calorie intake; the percentage of calories from carbohydrate should vary based on the patient's eating habits and blood glucose and lipid goals; individuals who have normal blood lipid levels and maintain a desirable weight may implement the US Dietary Guidelines recommendations of 30% or less of calories from total fat and 50–60% of calories from dietary carbohydrate
Fat	Less than 10% of calories should be derived from saturated fats and up to 10% of calories from polyunsaturated fat leaving the remaining 60–70% of total daily calories from monounsaturated fats and carbohydrates; the NCEP Step II dietary guidelines (<30% of calories from total fat, <7% saturated fat, and <200 mg/day dietary cholesterol) should be implemented if elevated LDL cholesterol is a primary problem; if elevated triglycerides is the primary problem, an increase in monounsaturated fat intake (to 20% of calories) and a more modest carbohydrate intake may be beneficial
Cholesterol	Should be restricted to 300 mg/day or less to reduce cardiovascular risk.
Fiber	Should be the same as that recommended for the general population: 20–35 g dietary fiber from a wide variety of food sources
Alternative sweeteners	Both nutritive (e.g., sucrose, fructose) and non-nutritive sweeteners (e.g., saccharin, aspartame, acesulfame K, sorbitol) are acceptable in diabetes management
Sodium	Should be the same as that recommended for the general population: no more than 2400–3000 mg/day; those with hypertension should restrict their intake to no more than 2400 mg/day
Alcohol	Should be moderate and may need to be restricted entirely in persons with a history of alcohol abuse, medication-induced hypoglycemia, pancreatitis, or poor control of blood sugar or blood lipids
Vitamins and minerals	Supplementation is generally not needed when dietary intake is adequate; there is no evidence that persons with diabetes will benefit from supplementation with chromium or magnesium unless they are demonstrably deficient in these minerals

From Nutrition Recommendations and Principles for People With Diabetes Mellitus. Diabetes Care 17(5):519, 1994, with permission.

exercise if the pre-exercise blood glucose level is 100 to 180 mg/dl. If pre-exercise blood glucose levels are between 80 and 100 mg/dL it is necessary to double the recommended carbohydrate intake to prevent exercise-induced hypoglycemia. No extra food is necessary if blood glucose levels are higher; but if they are over 250 to 300 mg/dL, exercise should be delayed until control is better. Some patients experience hyperglycemia if pre-exercise blood glucose values are over 250 mg/dL and ketosis is present (Krall and Beaser, 1989).

Gestational diabetes occurs in 2 to 5 per cent of all pregnancies. Initially, dietary management is the same as for NIDDM, but the index of acceptable metabolic control is lower (i.e., fasting blood glucose below 105 mg/dL or 2-hour postprandial blood glucose of 120 mg/dL) (ADAPS, 1992). If this level of control cannot be consistently maintained, insulin therapy is recommended. The dietary treatment emphasis then shifts to concerns of the type I diabetic. The diet prescription for pregnant diabetics must be altered to allow extra protein (a total of about 75 grams) and calories (2000 to 2200) to support fetal growth.

The current American Diabetes Association's nutrition recommendations emphasize individualized nutritional therapy based on patient-specific treatment goals and assessment of the patient's lifestyle, cultural, ethnic, and financial considerations (Table 42–23). The idea of a single ADA diet for persons with diabetes is obsolete. Although the nutrition recommendations are still loosely based on the prudent diet recommendations for the general population there are important differences. The observation that diets containing nearly 60 per cent carbohydrate may result in elevated triglyceride and reduced HDL-cholesterol levels has led to the recommendation to vary the exact percentage of carbohydrate and fat in the diet of susceptible individuals. A low saturated fat, moderate carbohydrate diet may be achieved by replacing saturated fat calories with monounsaturated fat calories through the addition of avocado, nuts, and oils to the diet. The recommendation for high monounsaturated fat diets may be premature and the higher total fat intake (40 per cent) may exacerbate the problem of obesity and would not be appropriate for those patients with severely elevated triglycerides (<1000 mg/dL) and hyperchylomicronemia.

The "glycemic index" of foods attempts to quantify the blood glucose and insulin responses to different types of carbohydrate. The idea that higher fiber foods would have a lower glycemic potential was not borne out. The variability in glucose response as a result of the form of the food (e.g., ground or whole), the preparation method (e.g., canned or home-prepared), and the influence of food combinations makes the glycemic index unreliable as a basis for therapy (DHHS, 1988; Jenkins and Grundy, 1989). It is useful for identifying some foods that would not be recommended as frequent snacks or single item meals because of their high glycemic potential (e.g., bananas or baked potatoes).

Although various starches and sugars do produce different glycemic responses, simple sugars have not been consistently shown to aggravate hyperglycemia. The use of caloric sweeteners such as sucrose (white table sugar) need not be strictly prohibited. Intake should be limited to no more than 5 per cent of carbohydrate intake (about 1–3 teaspoons) and permitted only in those patients with good blood glucose and lipid control (DHHS, 1988). The use of fructose, or sorbitol, results in a

lower blood sugar response when substituted for table sugar in food products. Both sweeteners are equicaloric with sucrose, however, and their use does not necessarily result in a lower calorie product. Saccharin and Equal (Nutrasweet) are virtually calorie-free.

The traditional approach to dietary management of diabetes involves calculating a daily calorie allowance, adjusting it for weight loss or gain, and selecting an exchange list diet that provides the proper number of calories, with meals and snacks scheduled to coincide with medication peaks.

The exchange lists are groups of foods classed together according to similar composition and origin. The exchange list system is similar to the Food Group Plan (Table 42–2), but portion sizes are specified for each food so one serving can be "exchanged" for another within the same group and kilocalorie and carbohydrate intake remain essentially the same. For example, 0.5 cup of orange juice is roughly equivalent in calories (60 kcal) and carbohydrate (15 grams) to one medium apple (Table 42–24).

TABLE 42–24. ABBREVIATED EXCHANGE LIST

Exchanges and Examples of Portion Sizes	Average Composition per Exchange			
	CHO (gm)	Protein (gm)	Fat (gm)	kcal
Starch/Bread ½ cup pasta ⅓ cup rice or cooked dried beans ½ cup starchy vegetables (corn, peas, potatoes, or winter squash) 1 slice of bread ½ English muffin, bagel, or hamburger/hotdog bun ½ cup cooked cereal ¾ cup dry, unsweetened cereal 4–6 crackers 3 cup air-popped popcorn	15	3	—	80
Meat and Substitutes 1 oz cooked poultry, fish, or meat ¼ cup cottage cheese or tuna 1 egg 1 oz cheese 1 tbl peanut butter ⅓ cup cooked dried beans or peas	—	7	3–8	55–100
Vegetables ½ cup cooked or juice 1 cup raw	5	2	—	25
Fruits 1 medium piece 1 cup berries or melon ½ cup juice or canned fruit ¼ cup dried	15	—	—	60
Milk 1 cup nonfat milk or yogurt	12	8	—	90
Fats and Oils 1 tsp margarine, oil, mayonnaise 2 tsp diet margarine or mayonnaise 1 tbl salad dressing 2 tbl reduced-calorie salad dressing	—	—	—	45

CHO = carbohydrate; tsp = teaspoon; tbl = tablespoon.

Although not all patients are candidates for a written exchange list diet, the exchange list plan is a powerful tool for teaching food composition and portion control. Intensive education is necessary for effective use of the exchange list diet, and possible benefits include better blood sugar control and greater patient self-reliance. This approach may be necessary for the difficult-to-control IDDM or the obese diabetic in need of a structured weight control diet. Shared care with a registered dietitian is strongly encouraged for such patients.

A phased approach may be more useful for the newly diagnosed, young, resistant, or unmotivated patient. Begin with a "no added sugar" diet, that is, eliminating obvious sources of sugar such as pies, cakes, pastries, candies, sweetened cereals and beverages, and fruit juices. Discuss the importance of regular meal and snack times in the context of coordination with medication or development of sound eating habits. Next, dietary counseling for a low fat, low saturated fat diet decreases cardiovascular risk and helps lower calorie content of the diet. The concept of balanced meals (i.e., a variety of foods) and standard serving sizes often flows naturally from patient questions about which foods and how much of certain foods are allowable. This approach allows a comfortable introduction to the "exchange lists" and the idea that foods within each list (e.g., the fruit list) contain about the same nutrients and calories when eaten in the serving sizes given.

Eventually, the exchange lists can be used to plan diets, either for weight control or consistency of intake. Patients generally accept the exchange list diet more readily when it is introduced in this gradual fashion, and they can see the benefit of knowing that nearly all foods are "okay" when eaten within their diet plan. The exchange list then becomes the vehicle for adding variety to the diabetic diet by using it as the basis for information on shopping and label reading, cooking and recipe modification, and tips on dining out.

Limit dietary changes to those specific to the individual patient's need for improved cardiovascular risk and to meet the patient/physician-defined limits of metabolic control. A simple low fat, "no added sugar" diet may be the limit of the patient's interest and sufficient for blood sugar control.

The use of home blood glucose monitoring helps make the patient a partner in dietary planning and reinforces beneficial dietary changes. The home monitor permits both the patient and the physician to quantify the success of the dietary, exercise, and medication prescription. There is little controversy regarding the use of the home glucose monitor for IDDM. However, the role of the monitor is not as well defined for the management of NIDDM.

DIETARY TREATMENT OF ADULT OBESITY

Current theories on obesity treatment are evolving into two camps: (1) the nihlists, who believe we should not continue to attempt treatment of obesity as all weight reduction efforts have proved dismally ineffective, and (2) the optimists, who believe that some success is better than none, and the benefit to the few outweighs the discouragement of the many.

The role of the family physician in the treatment of obesity lies mainly in counseling and guidance about (1) setting reasonable weigh loss goals; (2) selecting an appropriate weight loss program for the patient; and (3) referring the patient (when it is appropriate) to reputable adjunct health professionals such as registered dietitians, exercise physiologists, or mental health professionals.

The following guide should help the family physician care for those patients who both need and want weight reduction therapy. It is designed to help the patient avoid the psychological and physical harm of repeatedly failed weight loss attempts.

1. *Do not address the issue of body weight unless the patient voices a concern or there is a true medical necessity for weight loss.* Determining medical necessity involves reviewing the patient's history for the presence of conditions related to obesity (i.e., hypertension, diabetes, arthritis, congestive heart failure, hyperlipidemia). Evaluate the degree of overweightedness by comparing the presenting body weight to standards of desirable body weight for height or classifications of body mass index. Measure regional fat distribution (abdominal versus peripheral). A more aggressive approach is indicated when (1) there is a medical condition present that is exacerbated by overweight, (2) the degree of overweight is severe, or (3) the weight is centrally distributed. Even then, treatment recommendations and goals must be individualized.

2. *Establishing a reasonable weight loss goal is critical.* It involves more than choosing the midpoint of the desirable weight range for height on the MLIC tables of desirable weight (Table 42–4). Consider the patient's weight history. Patients who have been heavy since childhood or those who have failed repeated attempts at weight loss with reputable programs have less chance of weight loss maintenance. As a goal for these patients, weight maintenance may be more reasonable than weight loss. Because people commonly gain body weight with advancing age, weight maintenance may represent weight loss over several years. In addition, there is some evidence that weight fluctuations (the "yo-yo" syndrome) have a negative impact on body composition and overall mortality (Blair et al., 1993; Lissner et al., 1991; Rodin et al., 1990).

Determine desirable body weight and the limits of medical risk for the patient (e.g., the risk of diabetes mellitus rises at 20 per cent overweight and the risk of heart disease at 30 per cent) (DHHS, 1988). Use these ranges along with the lifetime weight to set reasonable weight loss goals. For instance, many patients may have an idea of a body weight that is more "usual" or a weight that is most easily maintained. Even though it may be above the standard desirable weight range, it is sometimes sufficient to improve their medical conditions.

3. *Establish medical goals for weight loss* and tie the success of weight loss to these endpoints. For example, a 1 kg weight loss may result in a 2- to 3 mm Hg drop in blood pressure. For many patients with high blood pressure, a 10 pound weight loss may be sufficient to control blood pressure without medication and, with a moderately low sodium diet, may prevent the age-associated rise in blood pressure (Kaplan, 1990).

4. *Educate the patient about what is known about the etiology and treatment of obesity.* Genetic influences account for 40 per cent of the individual differences in response to eating and exercise and 25 to 30 per cent of individual differences in percent body fat (Bouchard, 1989). The theory of the "set point" of body weight results in what may be termed a "controlled obesity" where a reduction in resting metabolic rate defends the overweight (Keesey, 1993). This point emphasizes the need for exercise to increase maintenance calorie needs and offset the factors encouraging weight regain.

In addition, current data about control of food intake is provocative in that it indicates poor control of fat intake in relation to fat oxidation (Ravussin and Swinburn, 1993). It has implications for recommending a low fat diet for treatment of obesity instead of focusing solely on control of total calories. A positive approach that emphasizes improvements in health and fitness with exercise and low fat diet, instead of a focus on fatness and restrictive diets, is generally more readily accepted by the patient.

5. *Guide the patient in designing a weight loss program.* Table 42–25 can help the physician guide the patient to select an appropriate weight loss program. Group commercial weight loss programs recommending low calorie diets (1000 to 1200 kcal) are most effective for those with only 20 to 30 pounds to lose. Very low calorie diets (VLCDs) are often indicated if the patient needs to lose more than 50 pounds. Surgery (gastric restriction or bypass) may be a consideration for patients with clinically severe obesity (BMI higher than 40) that have repeatedly failed nonsurgical treatment (NIH, 1991).

The most effective weight loss programs combine nutrition education, exercise, and behavior modification that involves techniques in stimulus control (e.g., keep food out of sight, eat only at the table), eating management (eat slowly), behavior substitution (exercise instead of eating when angry), self-monitoring (food and exercise diaries), reward, relapse prevention, and cognitive restructuring (positive self-talk that focuses on progress rather than failure) (DHHS, 1988). The combination of lifestyle change therapy and 1000- to 1200-kcal diets consistently produces losses of 1 pound per week or more, with losses of as much as 30 pounds in 25 weeks (Smoller et al., 1988).

Very-low-calorie diets provide 300 to 600 kcal per day in high quality protein foods or liquid meal replacements. These diets must always be provided under a physician's direct supervision and should be accompanied by the type of comprehensive program described above that teaches strategies for weight loss maintenance during the refeeding phase. These programs can result in an average weight loss of 20 kg in 12 weeks and as much as 41 kg in 24 weeks (Smoller et al., 1988). Evidence indicates that 800 kcal formula diets result in weight losses similar to those seen with the standard 400 kcal formula (Foster et al., 1992). VLCDs are contraindicated in pregnant women and patients with cancer, hepatic disease, renal failure, or psychological disturbances, including depression (Smoller et al., 1988). Complications include fatigue, dizziness, muscle cramping, headache, gastrointestinal distress, cold intolerance, dry skin, hair loss, and an increased risk of symptomatic gallstone formation (Foster et al., 1992; Wadden, 1993a).

If the patient refuses a group program or needs special help with multiple dietary problems, refer the patient to a registered dietitian. Some registered dietitians specializing in weight reduction can teach basic behavioral and cognitive modification techniques that aid in permanent changes in eating and exercise behavior.

6. *The patient must include increased physical activity as part of her or his weight reduction program.* In our experience, brisk walking or bike riding can serve as an effective adjunct to weight loss if the patient can achieve 10 to 20 mile-equivalents per week (divide miles biked by 3 to find the equivalent of walking 1 mile at a 4 mph pace). This exercise regimen is not appropriate for all patients, but any amount of exercise results in improved self-esteem and well-being, and it increases calorie output (Grillo et al., 1993). Increased physical activity combined with diet restriction produces larger weight losses than either approach alone and is critical to long-term weight control (Wadden, 1993a).

Individualization of the exercise program is critical. The family physician may choose to refer to a sports medicine clinic, exercise physiologist, or ACSM certified fitness specialist or personal trainer who can help the patient design an appropriate exercise regimen.

7. Depending on the patient's self-assessed problems with uncontrolled eating (binge eating), body image, family dynamics, self-efficacy, self-image, or usual practices of self-sabotage, *the patient may benefit from referral to a mental health professional experienced in issues related to*

TABLE 42–25. ANALYSIS OF SOME POPULAR WEIGHT-LOSS PROGRAMS

Diet	Entry Criteria	Cost	Medical Supervision	Nutrition Education, Behavior Modification, Exercise Included?	Description, Comments
< 600–800 kcal/day *Reasonable*					
Health Management Resources (HMR)	20% above ideal body weight or 40 lb overweight for VLCD diet	$115/week for medically supervised program, $90/week for moderate program	Yes	Yes	Medically supervised VLCD (520–800 kcal) program and moderate program with less intensive supervision (800–1000 kcal); Available in 3 phases: Weight loss Refeeding Maintenance Use of liquid formula diet and/or HMR frozen entrees (150–230 kcal)
Medifast	20% above ideal body weight	$62.50 to $75/week	Yes	Prescribed but not necessarily provided by a multidisciplinary team of professionals	4-Phase program: Medical evaluation Weight reduction (450 kcal liquid diet for women; 480 kcal for men) Realimentation Maintenance
Optifast	30% above ideal body weight; 20% if medically at risk or 50 lb overweight	$100/week	Yes	Yes	4-Phase program Modified fast (420–800 kcal liquid diet) Refeeding Stabilization Maintenance (optional)
Unreasonable Total fasting	Not appropriate for anyone	—	No	No	Not advised due to high loss of lean body mass, vitamin and mineral deficiencies, and other complications
800–1,200 kcal/day *Reasonable* Diet Center	Physician approval needed for individuals more than 40% or 50 lb overweight or who have preexisting health problems	$50/week for reducing phase; less for other phases	? (Nurse travels to different sites)	Prescribed, but not necessarily provided by a multidisciplinary team of professionals	4-Phase program Conditioning (unlimited kcal) Reducing (minimum of 1000 kcal) Stabilizing Maintenance Individual differences in caloric needs are taken into consideration for all phases. Vitamin/mineral supplement taken daily: 1000 mg of vitamin C is recommended daily, which seems excessive
Diet Workshop	Physician approval needed for individuals with preexisting health problems	Registration fee of $14 and then $9/week	No	Prescribed but not provided by a multidisciplinary team of professionals	Based on system of food "units" Reducing phase (900–1000 kcal increased gradually to 1200 kcal until goal weight is achieved) Maintenance (kilocalories according to individual needs) Vitamin/mineral supplement recommended
Jenny Craig Weight Loss Centers	Physician approval needed for individuals with preexisting medical conditions	$185 for membership; $60 to $70/week for food	No	Prescribed but not provided by a multidisciplinary team of professionals	2 Phases: Reducing (about 1000 kcal for women; 1200–1400 kcal for men) Maintenance (kilocalories according to individual needs) Complete reliance on packaged foods initially

Table continued on opposite page

TABLE 42–25. ANALYSIS OF SOME POPULAR WEIGHT-LOSS PROGRAMS *(Continued)*

Diet	Entry Criteria	Cost	Medical Supervision	Nutrition Education, Behavior Modification, Exercise Included?	Description, Comments
Nutri/System	Physician approval needed for individuals more than 100 lb overweight or who have preexisting medical problems	Variable according to location and goal weight; $60 to $69/week for food	No	Prescribed but not provided by a multidisciplinary team of professionals	2 Phases: Weight loss (minimum 1000 kcal for women; 1200 kcal for men) Maintenance (kilocalories according to individual needs) Complete reliance on packaged foods until maintenance phase; low-fat (14%), high-carbohydrate (61%) diet; special diet modifications for medical conditions
Weight Watchers	More than 10 lb overweight	$12–20 registration fee, $7–9/week	No	Prescribed but not provided by a multidisciplinary team of professionals	Based on system of food exchanges Weight loss (1040–1450 kcal for women; 1440–1910 kcal for men) Maintenance (kilocalories according to individual needs)
Not recommended Slim Fast/Ultra Slim Fast	Physician approval recommended for individuals who are pregnant, nursing, under 18 years old, have health problems, or who want to lose more than 30 lb or more than 15% of their body weight	$8–12/week	No	Limited	Over-the-counter meal replacement is mixed with low-fat milk (Slim Fast) or water (Ultra Slim Fast). Slim Fast is 190 kcal/serving, Ultra Slim Fast is 220 kcal/serving. 2 Phases: Weight loss (2–3 formulas, 1 fruit, 1 meal of 410 kcal; 1100–1200 kcal/day) Maintenance (1–2 formulas, 2 meals; 3 fruits; 6 oz milk; 1450–1520 kcal/day) Frozen entrees (230–400 kcal) also available. This diet can be dangerous if instructions are not followed properly

From Dwyer JT, Lu D: Popular diets for weight loss. In Stunkard AJ, Wadden TA (eds): Obesity: Theory and Therapy, 2nd edition. New York, Raven Press, 1993, with permission.

weight loss. Studies indicate that 25 to 45 per cent of persons entering weight loss programs suffer from binge eating disorder (Wadden and Stunkard, 1993b). Sufferers report eating "more food than most people would eat" during a discrete period of time coupled with a sense of being out of control. This behavior is similar to bulimia nervosa but lacks the purging phase. A psychiatric referral may be indicated, and cognitive therapy and antidepressant medication are currently being explored as treatment for this disorder (Stunkard, 1993).

8. Just as with treatment for hypertension or diabetes, *treatment of obesity requires lifelong therapy.* Patients who participate in formal weight-loss maintenance programs, who exercise regularly, or who do both are most likely to achieve long-term weight loss maintenance (Wadden, 1993a). The role of the family physician in continued positive encouragement and support in monitoring the related medical condition and helping the patient to re-set goals as needed cannot be overlooked.

Evaluating popular weight loss programs and books is important. Unproven, potentially harmful, and sometimes down-right ridiculous weight loss diets and schemes abound. The estimated sales of weight reduction pills and diets is $5 billion to $6 billion yearly (DHHS, 1988).

Review of the unending list of fad weight loss diets is beyond the scope of this text and would quickly become outdated. The *Diet Therapy/Obesity Update* supplement to *Nutrition and the M.D.* occasionally includes critical reviews of popular weight loss diets (see reference list).

Following the principles that any recommended diet must be nutritionally adequate and provide the minimal number of recommended servings from all food groups, and that permanent weight loss requires habit retraining and lifelong change, the family physician is prepared to evaluate any weight loss protocol presented. Maintenance of weight lost in any treatment program varies with the extent to which the intervention strategies themselves are implemented and result in behavior changes that can be maintained for a lifetime (Rock and Coulston, 1988).

EATING DISORDERS

Anorexia nervosa (self-starvation) and bulimia nervosa (binge–purge syndrome) are disorders characterized by grossly disturbed eating behavior that eventually leads to disease or disability (Lucas and Huse, 1994). Usual onset of anorexia nervosa is between 13 and 20 years of age, occurring 8 to 12 times more often in females than males (DHHS, 1988; Herzog and Copeland, 1985; Lucas and Huse, 1994). Prevalence is stable at approximately 1 per cent in the general population, but the incidence of eating disorders among athletes and dancers may be as high as 30 per cent (Taylor, 1988). Bulimia is more common than anorexia nervosa, with the reported incidence varying between 2 and 9 per cent depending on the strictness of the diagnostic criteria used (Lucas and Huse, 1994). In its strictest diagnosis bulimia is virtually nonexistent in males (Lucas and Huse, 1994). The onset of bulimia is later, 17 to 25 years; and it is not uncommon for a bulimic woman to present for the first evaluation at age 30 or 40 (Herzog and Copeland, 1985). Family, social, cultural, psychological, and perhaps physical factors combine to cause these problems in vulnerable individuals (DHHS, 1988; Herzog and Copeland, 1985).

Early diagnosis is key to successful treatment of these disorders. Anorexia nervosa should be suspected when significant weight loss cannot be explained by physical illness, especially in adolescent girls (Lucas and Huse, 1994). Low weight is secondary to restrictive caloric intake sometimes coupled with excessive exercise and purging behavior similar to that seen in bulimia (Edwards, 1993). In its later stages anorectics present with classic symptoms of starvation: emaciation, thin dry skin, bradycardia, hypotension, hypothermia, and cold intolerance (Edwards, 1993; Lucas and Huse, 1994). Constipation is common, as is amenorrhea in females and loss of sexual interest in males (Lucas and Huse, 1994). Anorectics can be subdivided into two groups that each represent about half the sufferers and have implications for management (DHHS, 1988; Edwards, 1993): "restricters," who confine their disorder to restricted food intake; and "bulimics," who also engage in binge–purge cycles.

Bulimics are more difficult to diagnose. Bulimia may be associated with wide fluctuations in weight

and occurs in both normal and overweight individuals. The patient suffering from bulimia may complain of constipation, bloating, and abdominal pain, and may feel weak and lethargic (Taylor, 1988). Signs of self-induced vomiting (skin lesions on the knuckles, hypertrophy of the salivary glands, erosion of tooth enamel, esophagitis) or laxative–diuretic abuse (hypokalemia) may be evident, but often the physical examination is unremarkable (Edwards, 1993; Taylor, 1988). The physician must maintain a high index of suspicion. No laboratory profile is diagnostic for either anorexia nervosa or bulimia, and abnormalities may not be observed until the illness is in its advanced stage (Lucas and Huse, 1994).

Personality features of bulimics differ from those with anorexia nervosa who restrict their intake. Anorectics often present with rigid, unspontaneous demeanor. They are unusually serious and polite but inhibited and brief in response. By contrast, bulimics often have impulse control problems that manifest as shoplifting or other forms of stealing, as well as substance abuse and alcoholism. Depressive symptoms are common, and suicide attempts are frequent in patients with bulimia (Lucas and Huse, 1994).

The role of the family physician in the management of these disorders is to diagnose the condition and coordinate the treatment. Anorectics often resist treatment, whereas bulimics are usually more motivated (Herzog, 1985). Mildly affected patients may respond to concerned counseling about normal body changes in adolescent growth, nutrition, and the consequences of starvation, bingeing, and purging (Lucas and Huse, 1994). Severe cases are best viewed as chronic illnesses that require multidisciplinary management using medical, psychiatric, nutritional, and other supportive resources (Edwards, 1993).

Specific pharmacologic therapy for anorexia nervosa is not well established. The use of antidepressants has shown promise in decreasing the frequency of bingeing and purging in both depressed and nondepressed patients with bulimia (Edwards, 1993). Depending on the severity of malnutrition and medical complications, and the inability to control purging behaviors or other self-destructive behaviors, intensive hospital treatment may be required. Referral to treatment centers or psychotherapists and nutritionists specializing in eating disorders is often recommended.

Dietary treatment for anorexia nervosa focuses on weight stabilization and improved nutritional status followed by gradual weight gain through normal self-feeding. Small, frequent feedings individualized to patient preferences (e.g., vegetarianism or low fat diets) are used initially to reduce sensations of fullness and meet the psychological needs of the patient, who is fearful of gaining weight rapidly and becoming fat. As the patient becomes less fearful, phased goals for caloric intake or weight gain are set. Registered dietitians often function to educate patients on nutritional needs and food composition. They also assist in designing an appropriate diet plan that includes gradual progression to meet calorie or weight gain expectations.

Dietary treatment for bulimia is directed toward encouraging regular eating habits. This practice minimizes the likelihood of binges and purges, which are often triggered by periods of fasting. Definition of desirable body weight and what constitutes well balanced meals are key issues in the education of this patient. Initial emphasis is placed on weight stabilization until the patient feels more confident with her ability to control eating behaviors when the need for weight loss can be reassessed.

The overall mortality rate for anorexia nervosa is 15 to 21 per cent, among the highest levels for psychiatric disorders (DHHS, 1988). Outcome studies of bulimia nervosa are rare, but in one study after short-term follow-up approximately two-thirds of patients no longer had symptoms of the disorder (Lucas and Huse, 1994). As with anorexia nervosa, the outcome likely varies greatly, with many patients recovering fully whereas others develop severe chronicity and complications.

NUTRITION AND CANCER THERAPY

Weight loss and malnutrition frequently accompany many cancers (Clifford and Barnett, 1993; Ohnuma, 1993). Oncology therapy commonly continues to compound and increase the nutritional deficit. Early malnutrition is more commonly associated with certain cancers and sites (e.g., leukemia, lymphomas, oat cell cancer of the lung, gastrointestinal malignancies) but becomes nearly universal in the presence of disseminated metastatic disease. Pretreatment weight loss and malnutrition often lead to poor tolerance of surgery, chemotherapy, or radiotherapy. Weight loss and survival are negatively correlated for almost all cancer types (Ohnuma, 1993). Children appear to be at even greater nutritional risk than adults for obvious reasons.

The symptom complex of anorexia, weight loss, tissue wasting, asthenia, and impaired organ function has been termed *cancer cachexia*. Several factors, such as anorexia, dysphagia, gastrointestinal dysfunction, altered intermediate metabolism, the effect of tumor metabolites, and competition of the tumor for available nutrients, act simultaneously or sequentially to produce the end result of tissue wasting (Daly and Torosian, 1993; Ohnuma, 1993).

Maintenance of good nutritional status is a significant challenge for the physician managing the cancer patient. The well nourished patient not only fares better throughout treatment but generally has an improved sense of well-being (Clifford

and Barnett, 1993). Encouraged oral intake is the first line of defense but generally is not effective in repleting the malnourished patient owing to the many factors that work to prevent adequate nutritional intake and absorption (e.g., the anorexia of depression or treatment-induced nausea and vomiting) (Clifford and Barnett, 1993). The common problems of nausea and vomiting, anorexia, early satiety, altered taste and smell sensation, stomatitis, and diarrhea may be alleviated with alterations in the texture, temperature, and composition of the diet, the use of bland foods, small frequent meals, minimizing food odors, individualizing the meal schedule, providing a cheerful and relaxed feeding atmosphere, and the use of high calorie, high protein nutritional supplements. A concerted effort at increased dietary intake between therapy cycles may help. The use of megestrol acetate has produced weight gain in a variety of cachectic cancer patients by stimulating appetite and food intake and decreasing nausea and vomiting (Ohnuma, 1993).

Tube feeding, often used in patients undergoing head and neck surgeries or experiencing upper gastrointestinal obstruction, can effectively improve or maintain nutritional status (Ohnuma, 1993). Patients who cannot tolerate use of the gastrointestinal tract because of nausea, vomiting, or other complications may benefit from parenteral nutrition. Total parenteral nutrition (TPN) appears justified in surgical patients who are at high risk (e.g., severely malnourished patients who are expected to develop prolonged inadequacy in nutritional intake such as patients with gastrointestinal obstruction or fistula, evisceration, or intra-abdominal infection) (Ohnuma, 1993; Sax and Souba, 1993). TPN has not consistently proved to augment the response rate or survival of adult patients treated with radiotherapy, although there may be some benefit in the case of radiation enteritis (Clifford and Barnett, 1993; Ohnuma, 1993).

Parenteral support during chemotherapy does not provide clear benefits, and the American College of Physicians has concluded that in these patients parenteral nutritional support was associated with net harm (Clifford and Barnett, 1993). Its use during chemotherapy should be strongly discouraged. In contrast, TPN and combined TPN and enteral support have proved beneficial in children treated with chemotherapy and radiotherapy (Ohnuma, 1993). Nutritional support in patients with terminal cancer must be decided on a case-by-case basis.

Specific nutrient deficiencies may occur as a side effect of cancer treatment, especially chemotherapy. Clinical manifestations of folic acid deficiency are frequently seen in patients treated with methotrexate. Vitamin K deficiency occurs in patients with intestinal malabsorption or obstructive jaundice and after long-term treatment with antibiotics (Ohnuma, 1993).

DIETARY MANAGEMENT OF RENAL DISEASE

Chronic Renal Insufficiency

The goal of nutritional care in patients with chronic renal insufficiency is to slow the progression of kidney disease and delay the need for dialysis while maintaining an adequate nutritional status. The diet is mainly restricted in protein and phosphorus. Specific restrictions in sodium, potassium, fluid, and calories are based on individual need.

A common predialysis diet consists of 60 grams of protein per day (0.55 to 0.60 gm/kg body weight), with at least 60 per cent high biologic value protein (protein from animal sources) (CDA, 1992; Kopple, 1994). Phosphorus is restricted to about 600 to 800 mg per day (5 to 10 mg/kg body weight) (CDA, 1992). This restriction is facilitated by the protein restriction that limits milk products and meats. This level of phosphorus intake is approximately one-third to one-half the usual adult intake (NRC, 1989b). Calories should be sufficient to maintain protein stores and body weight.

If serum potassium is elevated, potassium is restricted to 40 to 70 mEq per day (CDA, 1992). The upper end of potassium restriction (70 mEq, or 2700 mg of potassium) may represent only a modest reduction in usual intake. Sodium is restricted to 1 to 3 grams per day if needed to control serum levels or prevent edema. Fluid is generally not restricted. Calcium supplementation is usually necessary to achieve the 1200 to 1600 mg recommended calcium intake required to achieve calcium balance (CDA, 1992).

High protein intakes are implicated in the acceleration of renal insufficiency and mild protein restriction (to no more than the RDA of 0.8 gm/kg body weight in adults) may benefit persons such as diabetics who have an increased risk of developing renal disease (ADA, 1992). Emerging evidence also indicates that low phosphorus diets may retard the progression of renal disease. The evidence does not warrant dietary restriction of either protein or phosphorus until the glomerular filtration rate drops below 70 mL/1.73 m^2 per minute (Kopple, 1994).

Nephrotic Syndrome

Optimal levels of dietary protein intake for treatment of nephrotic syndrome have not yet been identified. Current recommendations suggest a dietary protein intake of 0.7 gm/kg of desirable body weight (DBW) plus a one-to-one replacement of each gram of protein lost in the urine (CDA, 1992; Kopple, 1994). Urinary protein losses in adults usually range from 3 to 16 grams per day, whereas children may lose protein in amounts up to 50 mg/kg

of body weight daily (CDA, 1992). High protein diets are implicated in the progression of renal failure, and there is some evidence that lower protein diets (0.8 gm/kg of DBW) may decrease urinary protein loss and help maintain or slightly increase serum albumin levels in patients with nephrotic syndrome (Kopple, 1994).

NUTRITION AND LIVER DISEASE

The goal of nutritional care in patients with liver disease (hepatitis, alcoholic liver disease, and hepatic cirrhosis) is to provide sufficient calories and nutrients to support liver cell regeneration without precipitating hepatic encephalopathy. Protein restriction to 60 grams per day (0.6 to 0.8 gm/kg DBW) is commonly indicated. Sodium is restricted to 2 grams per day if edema is present and occasionally limited to as little as 500 mg per day if ascites is severe. Deficiencies of water-soluble vitamins (folic acid, thiamine, vitamin B_6) and zinc are most likely to occur in the malnourished alcoholic with advanced liver disease (Korsten and Lieber, 1994). Small, frequent feedings and supplementation with high calorie enteral products may help ensure adequate intake in the patient experiencing nausea and anorexia.

The conventional approach to dietary treatment of hepatic encephalopathy is a temporary reduction in protein intake. The initial diet prescription allows 0.5 gm/kg body weight but is further reduced to 10 to 20 grams of high biologic value protein per day if symptoms are not alleviated (CDA, 1992). The observation of an increased ratio of circulating aromatic amino acids to branched-chain amino acids, which increases the aromatic amino acids available to the brain, has led to the development of both enteral and parenteral products high in branched-chain amino acids. However, relief of encephalopathy is not consistently observed with the use of these products (Korsten and Lieber, 1994; Rudman and Feller, 1990).

NUTRITION IN THE MANAGEMENT OF GASTROINTESTINAL DISEASES

Peptic Ulcer

A bland diet and increased consumption of milk is no longer indicated for treatment of peptic or duodenal ulcers. Milk is not only a weak antacid, but the high calcium and protein content contributes to rebound hyperacidity (ADA, 1992; Cerda, 1993; Meyer, 1994). Similarly, a low fiber diet has not been shown to speed healing (ADA, 1992; Meyer, 1994). Current recommendations are to eat a well balanced diet, eliminating foods known to increase acid production or cause discomfort in the individual patient. Alcohol, caffeinated beverages (coffee, tea, cola), decaffeinated coffee, pepper, and caffeine-free carbonated beverages have all been shown to stimulate gastric acid secretion or irritate a raw ulcer (ADA, 1992; Meyer, 1994). This diet is sometimes referred to as the "CAPS-free" diet: no caffeine, coffee, alcohol, pepper, or spices.

Hiatal Hernia

The benefit of a bland diet in the treatment of hiatal hernia or peptic and duodenal ulcers has never been scientifically proved (ADA, 1992). Certain foods recur on patient lists of offending foods, and it is often recommended that these foods be omitted. Omission of spicy foods, citrus fruits and their juices, tomato and its juice, and raw onions probably helps to relieve direct chemical irritation on the esophageal mucosa. Eliminating coffee, caffeine, and alcohol eliminates gastric acid stimulants. Fatty foods, chocolate, and peppermint, as well as alcohol and smoking, relax the lower esophageal sphincter pressure and allow the gastric contents to irritate the esophageal mucosa (ADA, 1992; Cerda, 1993; Meyer, 1994). Weight reduction in the obese, remaining in an upright position for several hours after eating, raising the head of the bed, and loosening tight clothing are also recommended for management of hiatal hernia.

Bowel Disease

An individualized approach to the dietary management of gastrointestinal diseases is important. The recommendations listed here are a starting place for patient counseling. Many patients discover foods that idiosyncratically relieve or exacerbate symptoms. Every effort should be made to tailor the diet to the patient's tolerances, avoiding undue restrictions when possible. Long-term use of fiber- and residue-restricted diets are generally not recommended because they may actually aggravate symptoms during nonacute phases of the disease (CDA, 1992). Patients are encouraged to resume a more liberal diet as tolerated when symptoms subside.

High fiber diets are recommended for the treatment of constipation, some phases of irritable bowel syndrome, and the prevention and treatment of the nonacute phase of diverticular disease. Nonsoluble fibers, such as wheat bran, are particularly effective for treatment of constipation. They absorb water, increase stool weight, and accelerate intestinal transit time. Both soluble and insoluble fibers (e.g., psyllium hydrophilic mucilloid) are useful for treating the nonacute phases of irritable bowel syndrome and diverticular disease. However, foods that offer small particles that can be sequestered in the segmented colon, such as seeds, nuts, legume casings, the small seeds of strawber-ries and other berries, popcorn, corn kernels, and raw carrots, should be avoided by those with diverticular disease.

Irritable bowel syndrome is often characterized by alternating bouts of constipation and diarrhea (Cerda, 1993). Some find that high fiber diets, particularly the soluble fibers, can stabilize stools, alleviating both constipation and diarrhea. However, the usefulness of high fiber diets depends on the severity of symptoms. In our experience, patients who are experiencing increased flatulence, pain, and excessive diarrhea do better on self-selected diets often low in fiber and similar to a soft, bland diet. Antidiarrheal medication is occasionally necessary to control the diarrhea.

Diets low in fiber and residue are recommended for use during the acute phases of ulcerative colitis, diverticulitis, and Crohn's disease (CDA, 1992; Rosenberg and Mason, 1994). A fiber-restricted diet limits the intake of indigestible carbohydrate by using only limited amounts of well cooked or canned vegetables, and canned, cooked, or overripe peeled fruits, and replacing whole-grain bread and cereal products with refined products. Legumes, seeds, and nuts are omitted. A low residue diet further restricts the intake of foods that act as a laxative or increase the fecal output, such as milk and milk products (limited to 2 cups per day), prune juice, and meat and shellfish with tough connective tissue (CDA, 1992). Additional dietary modifications may be needed if fat malabsorption or lactose intolerance is present.

Continued omission of milk products or strict reductions in fruits and vegetables may require supplementation with calcium, riboflavin, vitamin C, and folate. Patients with extensive disease or resection of the terminal ileum may become deficient in vitamin B_{12}. Patients with persistent watery diarrhea may have decreased zinc status, and iron deficiency may result from blood loss or absorption problems. Malabsorption can also affect vitamin D and calcium status (Rosenberg and Mason, 1994).

NUTRITION AND THE HOSPITALIZED PATIENT

Appropriate nutrition support for the hospitalized patient is critical to recovery. Malnutrition is associated with increased length of stay, increased morbidity and mortality, and increased costs (Glassman, 1986; Willmore, 1991). The history and physical examination are the two most important tools used to identify those hospitalized patients at risk of nutrition-mediated morbidity and mortality who would most benefit from aggressive nutritional support. A limited number of laboratory tests and measurement of body weight are of value when assessing a patient's nutritional status. Determination of the albumin level in combination

SELECT APPROPRIATE CATEGORY WITH A CHECKMARK, OR ENTER NUMERICAL VALUE
WHERE INDICATED BY A "#")

A. History
   1. Weight change and height
      Overall loss in past 6 months: Amt. = # _____ kg; % Loss = # _____ Height = # _____ cm
      Change in past 2 weeks: _____ increase, _____ no change, _____ decrease.
   2. Dietary intake change (relative to normal)
      _____ No change.
      _____ Change _____ duration = # _____ weeks.
      Type: _____ suboptimal solid diet, _____ full liquid diet,
      _____ hypocaloric liquids _____, starvation.
      Supplement: (circle) nil, vitamin, minerals, # _____ frequency/week.
   3. Gastrointestinal symptoms (that persisted for >2 weeks)
      _____ none, _____ nausea, _____ vomiting, _____ diarrhea, _____ anorexia.
   4. Functional capacity
      _____ No dysfunction (e.g., full capacity).
      _____ Dysfunction: duration # _____ weeks.
          type: _____ working suboptimally, _____ ambulatory, _____
          _____ bedridden.
   5. Disease and its relation to nutritional requirements
      Primary diagnosis (specify) _____
      Metabolic demand (stress): _____ no stress, _____ low stress, _____ moderate stress,
      _____ high stress.
B. Physical (for each trait specify: 0 = normal, 1+ = mild, 2+ = moderate, 3+ = severe)
   #_____ Loss of subcutaneous fat (triceps, chest)   #_____ Ascites
   #_____ Muscle wasting (quadriceps, deltoids,   #_____ Mucosal lesions
         temporalis)
   #_____ Ankle edema   #_____ Cutaneous lesions
   #_____ Sacral edema   #_____ Hair change
C. SGA rating (select one)
   _____ Well nourished.
   _____ Moderately (or suspected of being) malnourished.
   _____ Severely malnourished.

FIGURE 42–3. Subjective global assessment. (Adapted from Detsky AS, McLaughlin JR, Baker JP, et al: J Parenter Enteral Nutr 11:8, 1987 by Jeejeebhoy KN: Clinical and functional assessments. *In* Shils ME, Olson JA, Shike M [eds]: Modern Nutrition in Health and Disease, 8th edition. Philadelphia, Lea & Febiger, 1994, with permission.)

with a clinical evaluation currently provides the best measure of nutritional status in the ill or hospitalized patient (Jeejeebhoy, 1990b).

A validated clinical examination format termed the Subjective Global Assessment (SGA) has been developed by Detsky and colleagues for the hospitalized patient (Detsky et al., 1987; Jeejeebhoy, 1994). The physician can use the SGA format to prompt review of the (1) adequacy of past nutritional intake, (2) catabolic effects of the basic disease, and (3) patient's current physical state as indicated by functional status and clinical indicators of nutritional deficiency or excess. In category A (Fig. 42–3), evaluation of unintentional weight loss is modified by the pattern of loss as well as the absolute amount. Losses of less than 5 per cent of previous weight are considered small, whereas losses of more than 10 per cent are "definitely significant." If the weight loss is stabilized or partially corrected, the patient is considered better nourished than if he or she continues to lose. Significant gastrointestinal symptoms are those that have persisted on almost a daily basis for 2 weeks or more. An example of a high-stress disease is a severe flare of ulcerative colitis with high volume bloody diarrhea on a daily basis. A low stress disease might be a limited malignant tumor.

During the physical examination (category B), loss of subcutaneous fat is merely a subjective impression of the degree of fat loss in the triceps region and the midaxillary line at the level of the lower ribs. Muscle wasting is determined by loss of bulk and tone detectable by palpation. A coexisting disease such as congestive heart failure or hepatic cirrhosis modifies the weight placed on the finding of edema or ascites. Evaluation of hair change includes the color, appearance, and pluckability of the patient's hair. Mucosal and cutaneous lesions refer to the presence of glossitis or skin rash suggestive of nutrient deficiency (Jeejeebhoy, 1990a). (See Table 42–3 for a complete list of the clinical signs of nutrient deficiencies and excess.)

Arriving at a rank of nutritional status (category C) is based on the clinician's subjective weighting of the variables reviewed, with most of the judgment based on evidence of weight loss, poor diet, loss of subcutaneous tissue, and muscle wasting. Assignment of rank should be based on unequivocal information, assigning a higher rank when in doubt (Jeejeebhoy, 1994). Patients rated as severely malnourished are most likely to benefit from aggressive nutritional support.

The decision to initiate nutritional support depends not only on nutritional status assessment but overall assessment of the patient's clinical status and probable clinical outcome. Nutritional support is most likely to improve the clinical outcome of a malnourished patient in a hypercatabolic state who is suffering from a potentially reversible disease process (Schlichtig and Ayres, 1988). A general rule of thumb is "7 days or 7 per cent weight loss"; that is, if a patient has not been able to eat for 7 days or has lost 7 per cent of body weight since admission, nutritional support should be considered (McClave et al., 1990). Patients with severe malnutrition and a positive outlook for success of treatment should receive immediate nutritional support even if the patient might eat better tomorrow. The benefit of delaying medical treatment in order to improve nutritional status is unclear. At least 7 to 10 days is necessary to achieve marginal improvement in nutritional status with total parenteral nutrition or tube-feeding (Bozetti, 1987).

The first step in the initiation of nutritional support is calculation of nutritional needs. Daily calorie needs for the nonambulatory hospitalized patient can be estimated by multiplying the patient's body weight in kilograms by the following factors depending on metabolic needs and clinical status: 25 to 30 kcal for the mildly stressed, malnourished patient; 35 to 40 kcal for moderate stress or malnutrition; 40 to 45 kcal for the severely stressed, malnourished patient.

The requirement for protein in the well nourished relatively unstressed adult is approximately 0.8 to 1.0 gm/kg body weight. Protein needs increase to 1.0 to 1.5 gm/kg in the moderately stressed patient (e.g., fever, fracture, infection, wound healing) and up to 1.5 to 2.0 gm/kg for protein repletion or more severe stress (CDA, 1992). A nitrogen/calorie ratio of 1:150 (nitrogen = protein ÷ 6.25) is sufficient for most acutely stressed patients (Shils, 1994).

Nutritional support in the hospitalized patient takes three forms: (1) encouraged oral intake; (2) enteral hyperalimentation by tube-feeding; (3) total parenteral nutrition or a combination enteral and parenteral intake. Methods for encouraging oral intake include catering to patient food preferences, changing food texture (e.g., chopped), arranging feeding assistance, and adding concentrated sources of calories, protein, or other specific nutrients. Additional calories and protein are often provided as regular between-meal "snacks" (e.g., sandwich and milk), liquid high calorie and protein supplements (e.g., Carnation Instant Breakfast, Ensure, or Sustacal), or nutrient modules added to regular foods (e.g., protein powder added to milkshakes or glucose polymers added to soup).

Enteral Nutrition

When patients are unable to ingest adequate nutrients by mouth and the gastrointestinal tract can be safely and effectively used, enteral nutrition by tube-feeding is the preferred method (ASPEN, 1987). Safe and effective use of the gastrointestinal (GI) tract is defined by the absence of dysfunction, such as gastroparesis, complete intestinal obstruction, paralytic ileus, high output enteric fistulas, severe diarrhea, extreme malabsorption, and the initial phase of short bowel syndrome (ASPEN, 1987; Shike, 1994). Even if the GI tract is not entirely whole, a sufficient length may be available for absorption of a defined formula diet (i.e., 100 to 150 cm of functioning jejunum or ileum), and the hypertrophy of this remaining bowel is aided by enteral intake (Rombeau and Kripke, 1991). Advantages of enteral feeding over the alternative of parenteral nutrition include preservation of the structure and function of the GI tract (which includes its role in host defense by preventing bacterial translocation and sepsis), more efficient utilization of nutrients, fewer infectious and metabolic complications, greater ease of administration, and lower cost (Sax and Souba, 1993; Shike, 1994).

Access by nasogastric or enteric tube is generally preferred in patients who require short-term feeding (e.g., less than 4 to 8 weeks). For longer-term tube feeding, tube enterostomy is the preferred access (Rombeau and Kripke, 1991). Feedings are commonly delivered by continuous infusion at rates of 150 mL/hr, although higher rates (to 250 ml/hr) are sometimes tolerated. When feeding into the stomach, bolus feedings of 500 mL over 10 to 15 minutes are usually well tolerated (Shike, 1994). The feedings are started at an initial rate of 30 to 50 mL/hr (or a bolus of 150 ml) and gradually increased, as indicated by residual volume or the development of diarrhea, until the final rate is achieved (Schlichtig and Ayres, 1988).

More than 100 commercial enteral solutions are available for use in tube-feeding. Most hospital formularies list specific product availability and indications for use. Hospital nutrition services usually maintain literature comparing the ingredients and nutrient compositions of available formulas from a variety of manufacturers. Composition varies according to intended use. Standard commercial solutions contain carbohydrate at 40 to 60 per cent of total calories, fat 30 to 40 per cent, and protein 12 to 18 per cent, with a calorie/nitrogen ratio of 150:1 (Shike, 1994). Solutions are generally designed to provide the RDA for vitamins and minerals in 1500 to 2000 calories.

The requirement for water is commonly calculated at 1 ml/kcal (or 30 to 35 mL/kg body weight). Standard enteral formulas are approximately 75 per cent free water, so multiplying the volume by a factor of 0.25 estimates additional water necessary (Gottschlish et al., 1993). This extra water can be added to the formula with a concomitant increase in flow rate, or it can be added as the water used to flush the tubing each shift.

An isotonic, 1 kcal/ml solution (e.g., Osmolite or Isocal), with approximately 35 to 40 grams of protein per liter is appropriate for most patients. Volume-restricted patients or those with elevated calorie and protein needs require the solutions with 1.5 to 2.0 kcal/ml. The increased osmolarity of these solutions can be offset by initially using them as diluted feedings. No clear advantage has been demonstrated for use of the "elemental" formulas in patients with impaired digestion or absorption, and the higher osmolality presents a disadvantage for osmotic diarrhea (Shike, 1994). Benefits from the use of specialty formulas for stress or respiratory, hepatic, or renal failure have not been consistently shown (Rombeau and Kripke, 1991). Fiber-containing formulas may be useful for normalizing bowel function for patients with diarrhea or those requiring long-term tube-feeding. Fiber has important trophic effects on the mucosa of the large bowel (Shike, 1994). Blenderized foods are more appropriately delivered through the larger-bore enterostomy tubes.

Nausea, vomiting, constipation, and diarrhea are common complications of tube-feeding. Nausea and vomiting are usually caused by too rapid an infusion or by an underlying intestinal disorder. Constipation occurs in as many as 15 per cent of patients receiving long-term enteral feedings, and there is no clear evidence that fiber-containing formulas consistently relieve this problem. Diarrhea has been reported in 5 to 30 per cent of patients and is more prevalent in the critically ill (Rombeau and Kripke, 1991; Shike, 1994). It can result from decreased absorptive capacity (e.g., fat malabsorption, celiac sprue, lactase deficiency), formula hyperosmolality, bacterial contamination of formula or delivery system, or by enterally administered medications including antibiotics, hyperosmolar drug solutions, and magnesium-containing antacids (Rombeau and Kripke, 1991; Shike, 1994). In some reports as many as half of the patients receiving enteral feedings and antibiotics develop diarrhea (Shike, 1994). When there is no clearly identifiable cause of the diarrhea, decreasing the delivery rate or the osmolality of the solution may be helpful. Nonspecific treatment with an antidiarrheal agent can be tried cautiously, and the addition of a bulking agent may help solidify the stool (Rombeau and Kripke, 1991). There is some evidence that tube feeding is poorly tolerated when serum albumin levels fall to less than 2.5 gm/dl (Gottschlish et al., 1993).

Aspiration is potentially the most serious complication of enteral feeding but occurs in as few as 1 per cent of patients (Shike, 1994). It is most likely to occur in patients with impaired gastric emptying, when the tip of the tube is misplaced in the upper stomach or esophagus, or when the patient's upper body is not elevated to 30 to 45 degrees for feeding (Shike, 1994). In patients with impaired gastric emptying, feedings are best delivered into the jejunum.

Parenteral Nutrition

When the GI tract cannot be safely or effectively used for feeding, parenteral nutrition (PN) is indicated. Figure 42–4 outlines the selection process for choosing the route of nutrition support. Once nutritional support, either enteral or parenteral, is initiated, it should be continued until the patient is taking at least 60 per cent of caloric needs through ad libitum oral intake (Sax and Souba, 1993).

The components of PN are dextrose, amino acids, lipids, electrolytes, vitamins, and trace minerals. The dextrose monohydrate used in PN yields 3.4 kcal/gm and is commonly available in initial concentrations of 30 to 70 per cent. The higher dextrose concentrations are generally used when fluid restriction is required. Maximal glucose clearance rates are up to 14 mg/kg/min in the healthy adult, but tolerance is less than half that figure (5 to 7 mg/kg/min) in the critically ill patient (Shils, 1994). Infusion above the limiting rate results in hyperglycemia and glycosuria, which may lead to dehydration, increased production of carbon dioxide and a resultant increase in minute ventilation, and the conversion of excess glucose to fat resulting in fatty liver (Shils, 1994). If calculated total calorie needs are greater than 35 calories per kg of body weight, solutions relying solely on dextrose to supply energy needs may provide an excessive carbohydrate load.

Amino acid solutions are available in initial concentrations varying from 3.5 to 15.0 per cent. Calories contributed by protein are generally not considered available for meeting total energy needs. Mixed-fuel formulas that provide nonprotein calories from both carbohydrate and fat (usually in a carbohydrate/fat ratio of 70:30 or 60:40) are preferable. Lipid emulsions are available in 10 or 20 per cent solutions, contributing 1.1 and 2.0 calories per milliliter, respectively. Maximal lipid clearance rates are figured at 3 gm/kg/24 hr or 1 mL/kg/hr for a 10 per cent solution or 40 to 60 mL/hr for a 20 per cent lipid solution (McClave et al., 1990; Pursell and Turner, 1990). Infusion of two 500 mL bottles of 10 per cent fat emulsion weekly is necessary to prevent essential fatty acid deficiency.

Multivitamin and trace mineral (zinc, copper, manganese, chromium) solutions are commercially available in standard amounts based on the guidelines of the Nutrition Advisory Board of the American Medical Association. These substances should be added to the PN solution daily. Evidence suggests that the recommended copper and manganese levels in these solutions is too high. Both

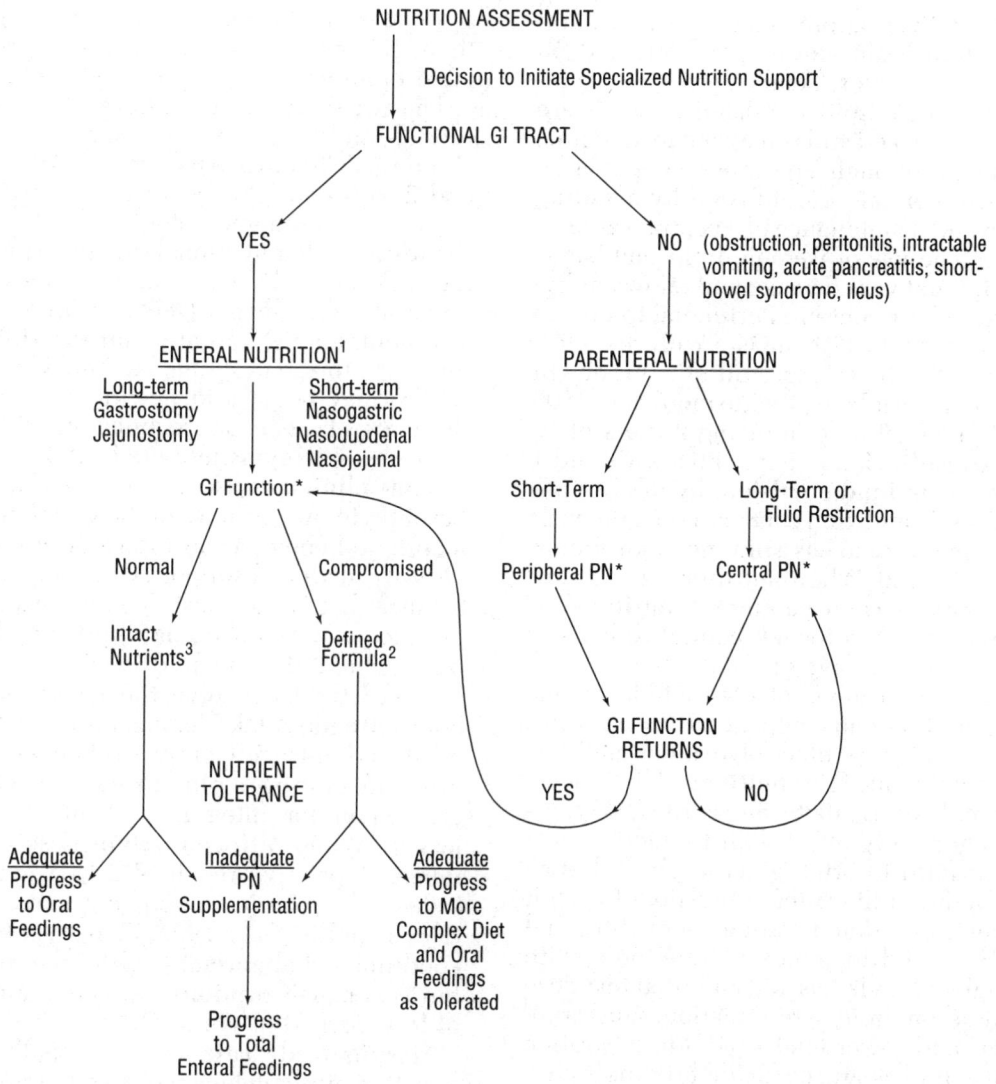

FIGURE 42–4. Clinical decision algorithm: route of nutrition support. GI: gastrointestinal; PN: parenteral nutrition. * Formulation of enteral and parenteral solutions should be made considering organ function (e.g., cardiac, renal, respiratory, hepatic). [1] Feedings may be more appropriate distal to the pylorus if the patient is at increased aspiration risk. [2] Elemental, low/high fat content, lactose-free, fiber-rich, and modular formulas should be provided according to the patient's GI tolerance. [3] Polymeric, complete formulas, or pureed diets are appropriate. (Reprinted from the American Society for Parenteral and Enteral Nutrition (A.S.P.E.N.). From Guidelines for the use of parenteral and enteral nutrition in adult and pediatric patients. JPEN 17(4), (suppl) July-August: 1SA to 52SA, 1993, with permission. A.S.P.E.N. does not endorse this material in any form other than its entirety. For information on ordering a complete set of guidelines, contact A.S.P.E.N., 8530 Fenton Street, Suite 412, Silver Spring, MD 20910; 301/587-6315.)

these elements are excreted in bile, and long-term administration in the presence of obstructive jaundice may pose a significant risk (Shils, 1994).

Neither selenium nor vitamin K is included in the standard preparations and must be administered separately. Selenium (40 to 80 μg) can be added to the PN solution daily. Vitamin K 5 mg administered intramuscularly once per week is generally sufficient to meet nutritional needs (Shils, 1994). Iron is administered as needed by evidence of iron deficiency. Iodide is needed only in the occasional depleted adult. Calcium, phosphorus (as inorganic phosphate), and magnesium are added within the recommended ranges of 10–25, 300–450, and 12–20 mEq per day, respec-

tively, with appropriate changes as evidenced by excessive losses or retention from the intestine or kidney (Shils, 1994). Electrolytes (sodium, chloride, potassium) are added individually as required.

Most hospital pharmacies prepare three or four standard PN solutions with fixed dextrose and amino acid concentrations. The caloric value of the dextrose solution is equal to the volume of the solution × final dextrose concentration) × 3.4 kcal. The number of grams of protein contained within a standard solution is equal to the volume of the solution × final amino acid concentration.

Common central line solution with final concentrations of 35 per cent dextrose and 5 per cent amino acids deliver approximately 1.2 kcal/ml (1190 nonprotein kcalocalories per liter) and 50 grams of protein per liter. Total calories can be increased with added lipid emulsions, which are generally piggy-backed and run over 8 to 12 hours. Parenteral access through a peripheral vein has an advantage over central vein infusion by avoiding the insertion and maintenance of a central catheter (Shils, 1994). The use of isotonic lipid emulsions reduces peripheral vein damage and allows delivery of a larger caloric content. Peripheral tolerance to osmolality is 900 to 1100 mOsm with the addition of 1 unit of heparin per 1 ml of solution. In general, it is not feasible to provide more than 1800 kcal and 85 grams of protein (using 2 liters of 10 per cent dextrose/4.25 per cent amino acids and 1 liter of 10 per cent lipid emulsion) by the peripheral route. This formulation contributes 60 per cent of calories from lipid and has a nitrogen/nonprotein calorie ratio of 1:130. When nutritional needs are high or the outlook is for parenteral nutrition administration longer than 1 week, central venous access is preferred (McClave et al., 1990).

Metabolic complications of PN include hyperglycemia, hyperlipidemia, hepatic steatosis, azotemia, respiratory distress, electrolyte abnormalities, and occasionally specific nutrient deficiencies (Schlichtig and Ayres, 1988; Shils, 1994). Hyperglycemia is generally offset with the addition of exogenous insulin to bring glucose levels below 150 mg/dL or the addition of fat emulsions to result in lower dextrose administration (Schlichtig and Ayres, 1988). Lipid tolerance is monitored with baseline triglyceride levels and an initial test dose followed by serum lipid determination. Longer infusion times and lower total lipid administration may improve lipid clearance (Schlichtig and Ayres, 1988). Liver enzyme abnormalities have a number of etiologies, the most common probably being the administration of large amounts of dextrose resulting in fatty liver infiltrates. Respiratory distress may also be attributed to excessive dextrose administration as discussed above. Azotemia may be the result of excessive protein administration but is more likely caused by an underlying abnormality such as dehydration or low cardiac output (Schlichtig and Ayres, 1988). The requirement for thiamine is increased with the use of high glucose solutions. Several cases of deficiency and death have been reported with rapid onset (1 to 2 months) of the characteristic metabolic changes of thiamine deficiency (i.e., lactic acidosis and peripheral neuropathy) (Shils, 1994).

Nutrition monitoring in the hospitalized patient undergoing relatively short-term nutritional support is difficult. The SGA method, because of its reliance on changes in body composition, is not sensitive enough to be used for monitoring nutritional progress (Detsky et al., 1987). Serial body weights generally serve to monitor fluid balance, and several weeks of adequate nutritional support are necessary to demonstrate weight gain. Even then, gain in adipose tissue is not necessarily related to improved nutrition-mediated function.

The circulating proteins transferrin, prealbumin, retinol-binding protein, and somatomedin C have shorter half-lives (8 to 9 days, 2 to 3 days, 12 hours, and 2 to 6 hours, respectively) than the 18 to 20 days for albumin and are attractive for monitoring the response to nutritional therapy. However, they are influenced by many of the same factors that affect albumin levels (see Nutritional Status Assessment, above) and are similarly difficult to interpret in the acutely sick patient. Somatomedin C (GF-1) may be a valid nutritional marker during the acute-phase response, but more clinical studies are needed (Heymsfield et al., 1994).

Some clinicians use a 10 per cent increase over baseline in one or more of the circulating proteins mentioned above as an indicator of the effectiveness of nutritional support. Currently, the nitrogen balance test is the most effective way of gauging the adequacy of nutritional support in the hospitalized patient (Heymsfield et al., 1994). Nitrogen balance studies involve the measurement of 24-hour nitrogen intake (grams of protein divided by 6.25) and nitrogen output (obtained as 24-hour urine urea nitrogen plus an additional 3 to 4 grams to account for integumental and fecal nitrogen losses). When nitrogen output is subtracted from intake, a positive result of 2 to 4 grams per day indicates protein adequacy and anabolism (Heymsfield et al., 1994). This test is invalid in conditions of abnormally high protein losses (i.e., burns or malabsorption) and a creatinine clearance of less than 50 mL/min (CDA, 1992).

Hospitalized patients occasionally remain in negative nitrogen balance despite implementation of nutrition support. The goals of nutritional therapy during the acute phase of critical illness or hypermetabolic state is nutritional stability. If nitrogen balance remains markedly negative despite seemingly adequate therapy, consider (1) increasing protein intake to as much as 2.5 gm/kg; (2) increasing total calories provided (higher calorie intakes ensure that protein is spared for anabolism); (3) adding exogenous insulin to maintain glucose levels below 150 mg/dL; and (4) checking for adequacy of electrolyte and trace minerals provided (insufficient quantities of phosphorus, sodium, potassium, and zinc may produce suboptimal nitrogen balance) (Schlichtig and Ayres, 1988).

Occasionally a specialized nutrition support team, including physician, nurse, pharmacist, and dietitian, are available to provide consultation when enteral and parenteral hyperalimentation is needed. Even in the absence of a specialized support team, the hospital nutrition service frequently offers assistance in nutritional status assessment, development of an intervention plan, and nutritional status monitoring by a registered dietitian.

REFERENCES

AAFP (American Academy of Family Physicians), American Dietetic Association, National Council on Aging: Nutrition Interventions Manual for Professionals Caring for Older Americans: Executive Summary. Washington, DC, Nutrition Screening Initiative, 1992.

AAP (American Academy of Pediatrics), Committee on Nutrition; Barness LA (ed): Pediatric Nutrition Handbook, 3rd edition. Elk Grove Village, IL, American Academy of Pediatrics, 1993a.

AAP (American Academy of Pediatrics), Committee on Substance Abuse and Committee on Children With Disabilities: Fetal alcohol syndrome and fetal alcohol effects. Pediatrics 91:1004, 1993b.

ACS (American Cancer Society): Nutrition and Cancer: Cause and Prevention. American Cancer Society Special Report. New York, American Cancer Society, 1984.

ADA (American Diabetes Association): Physician's Guide to Type II Diabetes (NIDDM): Diagnosis and Treatment. New York, American Diabetes Association, 1984.

ADA (American Diabetes Association): Physician's Guide to guide to Insulin-Dependent (Type I) Diabetes: Diagnosis and Treatment. Alexandria, VA: American Diabetes Association, 1988.

ADA (The American Dietetic Association): Handbook of Clinical Dietetics, 2nd edition. New Haven, Yale University Press, 1992.

ADA (The American Dietetic Association): Position of the American Dietetic Association: vegetarian diets. J Am Diet Assoc 93:1317, 1993.

ADA (The American Diabetes Association): Nutrition recommendations and principles for people with diabetes mellitus. Diabetes Care 17(5):519, 1994.

ADAPS (American Diabetes Association Position Statement): Gestational diabetes mellitus. Diabetes Care 15(2, suppl):5, 1992.

ADAPS (American Diabetes Association Position Statement): Implications of the diabetes control and complications trial. Diabetes Spectrum 6:225, 1993.

AHA (American Heart Association): Dietary guidelines for healthy American adults: A statement for physicians and health professionals by the Nutrition Committee, American Heart Association. Circulation 77:721A, 1988.

Alpers DH, Clouse RE, Stenson WF: Manual of Nutritional Therapeutics, 2nd edition. Boston, Little Brown, 1988.

ASPEN (American Society for Parenteral and Enteral Nutrition). Board of Directors: Guidelines for the use of enteral nutrition in the adult patient. J Parenter Ent Nutr 11:435, 1987.

Ausman LM, Russell RM: Nutrition in the Elderly. *In* Shils ME, Olson JA, Shike M (eds): Modern Nutrition In Health and Disease, 8th edition. Philadelphia, Lea & Febiger, 1994.

Berwick D: Failure to thrive. *In* Dershewitz RA (ed): Ambulatory Pediatric Care. Philadelphia, JB Lippincott, 1988.

Blair SN, Shaten J, Brownell K, et al: Body weight change, all-cause mortality, and cause-specific mortality in the Multiple Risk Factor Intervention Trial. Ann Intern Med 119:749, 1993.

Bouchard C: Genetic factors in obesity. Med Clin North Am 73:67, 1989.

Bozetti F: Nutritional assessment from the perspective of a clinician. J Parenter Ent Nutr 11(5, suppl):115S, 1987.

Carruth BR: Adolescence. *In* Brown ML (ed): Present Knowledge in Nutrition. Washington, DC, International Life Sciences Institute-Nutrition Foundation, 1990.

DCA (Chicago Dietetic Association), South Suburban Dietetic Association: Manual of Clinical Dietetics, 4th edition. Chicago, American Dietetic Association, 1992.

CDC (Centers for Disease Control): Use of folic acid for prevention of spina bifida and other neural tube defects: 1983–1991. 40:513, 1991.

CDC (Centers for Disease Control): Recommendations for the use of folic acid to reduce the number of cases of spina bifida and other neural tube defects. MMWR 41:1, 1992.

Cerda JJ: Diet and gastrointestinal disease. Med Clin North Am 77:881, 1993.

Clifford C, Barnett K: Diet as risk and therapy for cancer. Med Clin North Am 77:725, 1993.

Coleman E: Carbohydrates: the master fuel. *In* Berning JR, Steen SN (eds): Sports Nutrition for the 90s. Gaithersburg, MD, Aspen Publishers, 1991.

Coombs JB, Speer SJ: Nutrition I/II. Monograph, edition 129/130. Home Study Self-Assessment Program. Kansas City, MO, American Academy of Family Physicians, 1990.

Daly JM, Torosian MH: Nutritional support. *In* Devita VT, Hellman S, Rosenberg SA (eds): Cancer: Principles and Practice of Oncology, 4th edition. Philadelphia, JB Lippincott, 1993.

Davidson MH, Burns JH, Subbaiah PV, et al: Marine oil capsule therapy for the treatment of hyperlipidemia. Arch Intern Med 151:1732, 1991a.

Davidson MH, Dugan LD, Burns JH, et al: The hypocholesterolemic effects of β-glucan in oatmeal and oat bran. JAMA 265:1833, 1991b.

Dawson-Hughes B, Dallai GE, Krall EA, et al: A controlled trial of the effect of calcium supplementation on bone density in postmenopausal women. N Engl J Med 323:878, 1990.

Denke MA: Diet and lifestyle modification and its relationship to atherosclerosis. Med Clin North Am 78:197, 1994.

Detsky AS, Mclaughlin JR, Baker JP, et al: What is subjective global assessment of nutritional status? J Parenter Ent Nutr 11:8, 1987.

DHHS (U.S. Department of Health and Human Services, U.S. Department of Agriculture): Nutrition Monitoring in the United States: A Progress Report from the Joint Nutrition Monitoring Evaluation Committee. Public Health Service. DHHS Publication no. (PHS) 86-1255. Washington, DC, US Government Printing Office, 1986.

DHHS (U.S. Department of Health and Human Serivces, Public Health Service): The Surgeon General's Report on Nutrition and Health. DHHS (PHS) Publication no. 88-50210. Washington, DC, US Government Printing Office, 1988.

DHHS (U.S. Department of Health and Human Services, Public Health Service): Healthy People 2000: National Health Promotion and Disease Prevention Objectives. DHHS Publication no. (PHS) 91-50213. Washington, DC, US Government Printing Office, 1990.

Diplock AT: Antioxidant nutrients and disease prevention: an overview. Am J Clin Nutr 53(1, suppl):189S, 1991.

Dubick M, Rucker R: dietary supplements and health aids—a critical evaluation. Part 1. Vitamins and minerals. J Nutr Educ 15(2):47, 1983.

Edwards KI: Obesity, anorexia, and bulimia. Med Clin North Am 77:899, 1993.

Epstein LH: New developments in childhood obesity. *In* Stunkard AJ, Wadden TA (eds): Obesity: Theory and Therapy, 2nd edition. New York, Raven Press, 1993.

FDA (Food and Drug Administration, US): Caffeine and pregnancy. FDA Drug Bull 10:19, 1980.

Feldman EB: Nutrition and diet in the management of hyperlipidemia and atherosclerosis. *In* Shils ME, Olson JA, Shike M (eds): Modern Nutrition In Health and Disease, 8th edition. Philadelphia, Lea & Febiger, 1994.

Fomon SJ: Recommendations for feeding normal infants. *In* Fomon SJ (ed): Nutrition of Normal Infants. St. Louis, Mosby-Year Book, 1993.

Foster GD, Wadden TA, Peterson FJ, et al: A controlled comparison of three very-low-calorie diets: effects on weight, body composition, and symptoms. Am J Clin Nutr 55:811, 1992.

Frader J, Reibman B, Turkewitz D: Vitamin B-12 deficiency in strict vegetarians. N Engl J Med 299:1319, 1978.

Gaziano JM, Manson JE, Ridker PM, et al: Beta carotene therapy for chronic stable angina. Circulation 82:III-201, 1990.

Gaziano JM, Buring JE, Breslow JL, et al. Moderate alcohol intake, increased levels of high-density lipoprotein and its subfractions, and decreased risk of myocardial infarction. N Engl J Med 329:1829, 1993.

Glassman RG: Nutrition assessment: a critical review. Top Clin Nutr 1(4):16, 1986.

Gottschlish MM, Matarese LI, Shronts EP: Nutrition Support Dietetics: Core Curriculum, 2nd edition. Silver Spring, MD, American Society for Parenteral and Enteral Nutrition (ASPEN), 1993.

Grey KF, Puska P, Jordan P, Moser UK: Inverse correlation between plasma vitamin E and mortality from ischemic heart disease. Am J Clin Nutr 53(1, suppl):326S, 1991.

Grillo CM, Brownell KD, Stunkard AJ: The metabolic and psychological importance of exercise in weight control. *In* Stunkard AJ, Wadden TA (eds): Obesity: Theory and Therapy, 2nd edition. New York, Raven Press, 1993.

Hamill PV, Drizd TA, Johnson RD, et al: Physical growth: National Center for Health Statistics percentiles. Am J Clin Nutr 32:607, 1979.

Harward MP: Nutritive therapies for osteoporosis: the role of calcium. Med Clin North Am 77:889, 1993.

Herzog D, Copeland P: Eating disorders. N Engl J Med 313:295, 1985.

Heymsfield SB, Tighe A, Zi-Mian W: Nutritional assessment by anthropometric and biochemical methods. *In* Shils ME, Olson JA, Shike M (eds): Modern Nutrition in Health and Disease, 8th edition. Philadelphia, Lea & Febiger, 1994.

Hockelman RA, Blatman S, Friedman SB, et al: Primary Pediatric Care. St. Louis: CV Mosby, 1987.

Huggins K: The Nursing Mother's Companion, revised edition. Boston, Harvard Common Press, 1990.

Hultman E, Harris RC, Spriet LL: Work and exercise. *In* Shils ME, Olson JA, Shike M (eds): Modern Nutrition in Health and Disease, 8th edition. Philadelphia, Lea & Febiger, 1994.

Infante-Rivard C, Fernandez A, Gauthier R, et al. Fetal loss associated with caffeine intake before and during pregnancy. JAMA 270:2940, 1993.

IOM (U.S. Institute of Medicine), Subcommittee on Nutritional Status and Weight Gain During Pregnancy, Subcommittee on Dietary Intake and Nutrient Supplements During Pregnancy: Nutrition During Pregnancy. Part I. Weight Gain. Part II. Nutrient Supplements. Committee on Nutritional Status During Pregnancy and Lactation, Food and Nutrition Board, Institute of Medicine, National Academy of Sciences. Washington, DC, National Academy Press, 1990.

IOM (Institute of Medicine), Subcommittee on Nutrition During Lactation: Nutrition During Lactation. Committee on Nutritional Status During Pregnancy and Lactation, Food and Nutrition Board, Institute of Medicine, National Academy of Sciences. Washington, DC, National Academy Press, 1991.

IRCG (Intersalt Cooperative Research Group): Intersalt: an international study of electrolyte excretion and blood pressure: Results for 24 hour urinary sodium and potassium excretion. BMJ 297:319, 1988.

Jacobs C, Dwyer JT: Vegetarian children: appropriate and inappropriate diets. Am J Clin Nutr 48:811, 1988.

Jeejeebhoy KN: Assessment of nutritional status. J Parenter Ent Nutr 14(5, suppl):193S, 1990a.

Jeejeebhoy KN: Assessment of nutritional status. *In* Rombeau JL, Caldwell MD (eds): Enteral and Tube Feeding, 2nd edition. Philadelphia, WB Saunders Company, 1990b.

Jeejeebhoy KN: Clinical and functional assessments. *In* Shils ME, Olson JA, Shike M (eds): Modern Nutrition In Health and Disease, 8th edition. Philadelphia, Lea & Febiger, 1994.

Jenkins DJ, Grundy S: Current issues in nutrition and metabolism. Diabetes Spectrum 2:123, 1989.

Jensen TG, Englert DM, Dudrick SJ: Nutritional Assessment: A Manual for Practitioners. Norwalk, CT: Appleton-Century-Crofts, 1983.

Kaplan NM: Clinical hypertension, 6th edition. Baltimore, Williams & Wilkins, 1994.

Keesey RE: Physiological regulation of body energy: Implications for obesity. *In* Stunkard AJ, Wadden TA (eds): Obesity: Theory and Therapy, 2nd edition. New York, Raven Press, 1993.

Kissebah AH, Freedman DS, Peiris AN: Health risks of obesity. Med Clin North Am 73:111, 1989.

Knapp HR: Hypertension. *In* Brown MI (ed): Present Knowledge in Nutrition, 6th edition. Washington, DC, International Life Sciences Institute—Nutrition Foundation, 1990.

Kopple JD: Nutrition, diet, and the kidney. *In* Shils ME, Olson JA, Shike M (eds): Modern Nutrition In Health and Disease, 8th edition. Philadelphia, Lea & Febiger, 1994.

Korsten MA, Lieber CS: Nutrition in pancreatic and liver disorders. *In* Shils ME, Olson JA, Shike M (eds): Modern Nutrition In Health and Disease, 8th edition. Philadelphia, Lea & Febiger, 1994.

Kotchen TA, Kotchen JM: Nutrition, diet, hypertension. *In* Shils ME, Olson JA, Shike M (eds): Modern Nutrition in Health and Disease, 8th edition. Philadelphia, Lea & Febiger, 1994.

Krall LP, Beaser RS: Joslin Diabetes Manual, 12th edition. Philadelphia, Lea & Febiger, 1989.

Lissner L, Odell PM, D'Agostino RD, Stokes J III, et al: Variability of body weight and health outcomes in the Framingham population. N Engl J Med 324:1039, 1991.

LSRO (Life Sciences Research Office, Federation of American Societies for Experimental Biology): Nutrition Monitoring in the United States—An Update Report on Nutrition Monitoring. Prepared for the U.S. Department of Agriculture and the U.S. Department of Health and Human Services. DHHS Publication no. (PHS) 89-1255. Washington, DC, US Government Printing Office, 1989.

Lucas AR, Huse DM: Behavioral disorders affecting food intake: Anorexia nervosa and bulimia nervosa. *In* Shils ME, Olson JA, Shike M (eds): Modern Nutrition In Health and Disease, 8th edition. Philadelphia, Lea & Febiger, 1994.

Lyle BJ, Forgac T: Hydration and fluid replacement. *In* Berning JR, Steen SN (eds): Sports Nutrition for the 90s. Gaithersburg, MD, Aspen Publishers, 1991.

McClave SA, Short AF, Mattingly DB, Fitzgerald PH: Total parenteral nutrition. Postgrad Med 88:235, 1990.

Mellin LM: Shapedown: Just for Teens. Larkspur, CA, Balboa Publishing Co., 1987.

Meyer J: The stomach and nutrition. *In* Shils ME, Olson JA, Shike M (eds): Modern Nutrition in Health and Disease, 8th edition. Philadelphia, Lea & Febiger, 1994.

Moore SA, Nagle JP, Streiffer RH: Nutrition counseling: healthy people. American Academy of Family Physicians. HELP Newsletter 5(1):1, 1991.

NCEP (National Cholesterol Education Program): Second Report of the Expert Panel on Detection, Evaluation, and Treatment of High Blood Cholesterol in Adults (Adult Treatment Panel II). National Institutes of Health, National Heart, Lung, and Blood Institute NIH Publication no. 93-3095. Washington, DC, US Government Printing Office, 1993.

NCI (National Cancer Institute): Diet, Nutrition, and Cancer Prevention: A Guide to Food Choices. National Institutes of Health, Public Health Service, U.S. Department of Health and Human Services. NIH Publication no. 87-2878. Washington, DC, US Government Printing Office, 1987.

NHBPEP (National High Blood Pressure Education Program). The Fifth Report of the Joint National Committee on Detection, Evaluation, and Treatment of High Blood Pressure. Bethesda, MD, US Department of Health and Human Services, National Heart, Lung, and Blood Institute. NIH Publication no. 93-1088. Washington, DC, US Government Printing Office, 1993.

NIH (National Institutes of Health): Osteoporosis. NIH Consensus Statement 5(3), 1984.

NIH (National Institutes of Health): Lowering blood cholesterol to prevent heart disease: consensus conference. JAMA 253:2080, 1985.

NIH (National Institutes of Health): Gastrointestinal Surgery for Severe Obesity. NIH Consensus Statement 9(1):1, 1991.

NIH (National Institutes of Health): Triglyceride, high density lipoprotein, and coronary heart disease. NIH Consensus Statement 10(2):1, 1992.

NIH (National Institutes of Health), Technology Assessment Conference Panel: Methods for voluntary weight loss and control. Ann Intern Med 119:764, 1993.

NRC (National Research Council), Committee on Diet, Nutrition, and Cancer: Diet, Nutrition, and Cancer. Washington, DC, National Academy Press, 1982.

NRC (National Research Council), Committee on Diet and Health: Diet and Health: Implications for Reducing Chronic Disease Risk. Washington, DC, National Academy Press, 1989a.

NRC (National Research Council), Subcommittee on the Tenth Edition of the RDAs: Recommended Dietary Allowances, 10th edition. Food and Nutrition Board, Commission on Life Sciences, National Research Council. Washington, DC, National Academy Press, 1989b.

Nutrition and the M.D.: A Continuing Education Service For Physicians and Nutritionists. [For subscriptions write P.O. Box 2468, Van Nuys, CA 91404].

Ohnuma T: Cachexia, malnutrition and nutritional support. *In* Holland J, Frei E III, Baast RC, et al (eds): Cancer Medicine, Vol 2. Philadelphia, Lea & Febiger, 1993.

Pi-Sunyer FX: Obesity. *In* Shils ME, Olson JA, Shike M (eds): Modern Nutrition in Health and Disease, 8th edition. Philadelphia, Lea & Febiger, 1994.

Pursell TA, Turner WW: Pocket Manual of Intensive Nutritional Care, 3rd edition. Philadelphia, BC Decker, 1990.

Quinn S: Diabetes and diet: we are still learning. Med Clin North Am 77:773, 1993.

Ravussin E, Swinburn BA: Energy metabolism. *In* Stunkard AJ, Wadden TA (eds): Obesity: Theory and Therapy, 2nd edition. New York, Raven Press, 1993.

Report of Nutrition Screening 1: Toward a Common View. A Consensus Conference. Washington, DC, Nutrition Screening Initiative, 1991.

Robertson JM, Donner AP, Trevithick JR: A possible role for vitamins C and E in cataract prevention. Am J Clin Nutr 53(1, suppl):346S, 1991.

Robbins GE, Trowbridge FL: Anthropometric techniques and their application. *In* Simko MD, Cowell C, Gilbride JA (eds): Nutrition Assessment: A Comprehensive Guide for Planning Intervention. Rockville, MD, Aspen Systems Corp., 1984.

Rock CL, Coulston AM: Weight control approach: a review by the California Dietetic Association. J Am Diet Assoc 88:44, 1988.

Rodin J, Radke-Sharpe N, Rebuffe-Scrive M, et al: Weight cycling and fat distribution. Int J Obes 14:303, 1990.

Roe DA: Drug-Induced Nutritional Deficiencies, 2nd edition. Westport, CT, AVI Publishing, 1985.

Roe DA: Diet and Drug Interactions. New York, Van Nostrand Reinhold, 1989.

Rombeau JL, Kripke SA: Enteral nutrition. *In* Fischer JE (ed): Total Parenteral Nutrition, 2nd edition. Boston, Little, Brown, 1991.

Rosenberg IH, Mason JB: Inflammatory Bowel Disease. *In* Shils ME, Olson JA, Shike M (eds): Modern Nutrition in Health and Disease, 8th edition. Philadelphia, Lea & Febiger, 1994.

Rudman D, Feller AG: Liver disease. *In* Brown ML (ed): Present Knowledge in Nutrition, 6th edition. Washington, DC,

International Life Sciences Institute-Nutrition Foundation, 1990.

Sax HC, Souba WW: Enteral and parenteral feedings: guidelines and recommendations. Med Clin North Am 77:863, 1993.

Schlichtig R, Ayres SM: Nutritional Support of the Critically Ill. Chicago, Year Book Medical Publishers, 1988.

Shike M: Enteral feeding. *In* Shils ME, Olson JA, Shike M (eds): Modern Nutrition in Health and Disease, 8th edition. Philadelphia, Lea & Febiger, 1994.

Shils ME: Parenteral nutrition. *In* Shils ME, Olson JA, Shike M (eds): Modern Nutrition in Health and Disease, 8th edition. Philadelphia, Lea & Febiger, 1994.

Simko MD, Cowell C, Hreha MS: Practical Nutrition: A Quick Reference for the Health Care Practitioner. Rockville, MD, Aspen Publishers, 1989.

Smoller JW, Wadden RA, Brownell KD: Popular and very-low-calorie diets in the treatment of obesity. *In* Frankle RT, Yang M (eds): Obesity and Weight Control. Rockville, MD, Aspen Publishers, 1988.

Specker BL, Valanis B, Hertzberg V, et al: Sunshine exposure and serum 25-hydroxyvitamin D concentrations in exclusively breast-fed infants. J Pediatr 107:372, 1985.

Stein PP, Black HR: The role of diet in the genesis and treatment of hypertension. Med Clin North Am 77:831, 1993.

Stunkard AJ: Talking with patients. *In* Stunkard AJ, Wadden TA (eds): Obesity: Theory and Therapy. New York, Raven Press, 1993.

Taylor CB: Eating disorders in athletes and dancers. Nutrition and the M.D. 14(7):1, 1988.

Truswell SA: Dietary goals and guidelines: National and international perspectives. *In* Shils ME, Olson JA, Shike M (eds): Modern Nutrition in Health and Disease, 8th edition. Philadelphia, Lea & Febiger, 1994.

USDA/DHHS (U.S. Department of Agriculture, U.S. Department of Health and Human Services): Dietary Guidelines for Americans, 3rd edition. Home and Garden Bulletin no. 232. Washington, DC, USDA, November 1990.

US Senate: Dietary Goals for the United States, 2nd edition. Report of the Select Committee on Nutrition and Human Needs. Stock no. 052-070-04376-8. Washington, DC, U.S. Government Printing Office, 1977.

VanItallie RB, Lew EA: Estimation of the effect of obesity on health and longevity. *In* Stunkard AJ, Wadden TA (eds): Obesity: Theory and Therapy, 2nd edition. New York, Raven Press, 1993.

Wadden TA: The treatment of obesity: an overview. *In* Stunkard AJ, Wadden TA (eds): Obesity: Theory and Therapy, 2nd edition. New York, Raven Press, 1993a.

Wadden TA, Stunkard AJ: Psychosocial consequences of obesity and dieting. *In* Stunkard AJ, Wadden TA (eds): Obesity: Theory and Therapy. New York, Raven Press, 1993b.

West KM: Recent trends in dietary management. *In* Podolsky S (ed): Clinical Diabetes: Modern Management. East Norwalk, CT, Appleton-Century-Crofts, 1980.

Whitmire DA: Vitamins and minerals: A perspective in physical performance. *In* Berning JR, Steen SN (eds): Sports Nutrition for the 90s. Gaithersburg, MD, Aspen Publishers, 1991.

Williams SR, Worthington-Roberts BS, Schlenker ED, et al: Nutrition Throughout the Life Cycle, 2nd edition. St. Louis, Mosby-Year Book, 1992.

Willmore DW: Catabolic illness: strategies for enhancing recovery. N Engl J Med 325:695, 1991.

Wood RJ, Serfaty-Lacrosniere C: Gastric acidity, atrophic gastritis, and calcium absorption. Nutr Rev 50(2):33, 1992.

CHAPTER 43

GASTROENTEROLOGY

Wm. MACMILLAN RODNEY

Study the past, diagnose the present, foretell the future. Practice these acts. As to disease, first of all, do no harm.—Hippocrates

In the adult office practice of many family physicians, gastrointestinal (GI) illnesses rank among the ten most common complaints. Questions relating to the GI system occur each and every practice day. Furthermore, repeated surveys have documented the high prevalence of GI complaints that go unreported (Table 43–1).

This high prevalence of GI illness is becoming more and more important as the percentage of patients over age 50 increases. These prevalence studies identify only a few patients as truly asymptomatic. This factor causes confusion as family physicians attempt to implement early detection and prevention of colorectal cancer. Hiatal hernia, constipation, and diverticulosis exist in 50 percent or more of patients 65 years of age and older. The family physician must integrate those findings into the context of chief complaint, present illness, primary diagnosis, secondary diagnoses, therapy, and prognosis.

This chapter proposes that the family physician can greatly benefit from an integrated overview of common GI symptoms, signs, and disorders. Powerful new tools are emerging for use within the office setting. For example, the development of flexible sigmoidoscopy during the 1970's created a generation of office-based primary care endoscopists during the 1980's, and these physicians are examining, photographing, obtaining biopsy specimens, and video recording GI pathophysiology on a daily basis. In addition to improved early detection of colorectal cancer, these tools enhance patient care via improved information management and more accurate diagnosis in the office. Remote and real-time consultation, similar to that seen by remote computer-assisted electrocardiogram (ECG) interpretation, will become available. Family physicians of the 1990s can routinely apply office-based diagnostic methods that were available only in university medical centers during the 1970s (Rodney, 1993a; Rodney et al., 1993b).

This chapter begins with an examination of emergency conditions that are not common but are absolutely necessary to identify immediately, followed by the less urgent, though more common, chronic disorders.

ACUTE ABDOMINAL PAIN

In 1921 Sir Zachary Cope published the first edition of his classic text *Early Diagnosis of the Acute Abdomen*. Using only the history and physical examination, the author sought to assist readers such that disease requiring surgery could be identified rapidly and accurately. "The general rule can be laid down that the majority of severe abdominal pains which ensue in patients who have been previously fairly well, and which last as long as six hours, are caused by conditions of surgical import" (Cope, 1972).

Abdominal pain is the fifth most common presenting complaint of adult medical patients. Although renal colic and pelvic inflammatory disease are examples of non-GI illness that may be exhibited as abdominal pain, most abdominal pain is due to a GI disorder. In Adelman's study of family practice patients presenting with abdominal pain, 9 per cent were admitted to the hospital for evaluation or surgery (Adelman, 1987a). The final diagnoses of 556 ambulatory patients presenting over a 2-year period (Table 43–2) suggested that a large percentage of these patients have a self-limited illness that eludes a definitive diagnosis.

Because the identification of illnesses requiring urgent intervention is paramount, this chapter begins with descriptions and definitions of the acute abdominal pain syndromes. These disorders are used as "learning examples." Mastery of these approaches is useful for the diagnosis and management of the disorders that follow. Usually it is the patient who defines his or her pain as being "acute." One working definition for acute abdominal pain is when the patient cannot wait until tomorrow or next week for an appointment.

The history, physical examination, laboratory tests, and imaging studies form the foundation for the diagnostic process. First and foremost, the diagnosis is best served by a rigorous history. In 85 per cent of patients, the experienced physician can make the correct diagnosis in this fashion by systematically using the "attributes of pain" mnemonic $(PQR)^2ST^3$ (Table 43–3) and a uniform review of systems (DeGowin and DeGowin, 1981). The diagnosis can be missed simply by underemphasizing this first important step. This diagnostic

TABLE 43–1. PREVALENCE OF GI CONDITIONS IN ADULTS

Condition	%
Hemorrhoids	50–80
Dyspepsia	50–80
Abdominal pain	30–70
Diverticulosis	30–50
Hiatal hernia	20–50
Unreported symptoms of IBS	14–17
Gallstones	10–32
Constipation	9–30
Colonic polyps	8–40

Utilizing questionnaires, interviews, autopsy data, and symptom diaries, numerous studies have documented substantial numbers of illness in a variety of populations. As age increases, the prevalence increases.

IBS = irritable bowel syndrome.

tool therefore bears repeating. An accurate, systematic, thoughtful description of the presenting complaint is the hallmark of excellence in the differential diagnosis.

APPENDICITIS

Identification of appendicitis was one of the first benefits of a revolution that transformed all of medicine. This revolution was the application of the scientific method. It allowed pathologist-physician

TABLE 43–2. FINAL DIAGNOSIS FOR THE PRESENTING SYMPTOM OF ABDOMINAL PAIN (ACUTE AND CHRONIC) IN FAMILY PHYSICIANS' OFFICES

Diagnosis	Frequency	%*	Cumulative %
Abdominal pain, etiology undocumented	280	50.4	50.4
Acute gastroenteritis	51	9.2	59.5
Urinary tract infection	37	6.7	66.2
Irritable bowel syndrome	32	5.8	71.9
Pelvic inflammatory disease	21	3.8	75.7
Hiatal hernia or reflux	13	2.3	78.1
Diverticulosis	12	2.2	80.2
Diarrhea, cause undetermined	9	1.6	81.8
Cholelithiasis	9	1.6	83.5
Tumor, benign	8	1.4	84.9
Duodenal ulcer	8	1.4	86.3
Urolithiasis	7	1.3	87.6
Appendicitis	6	1.1	88.7
Ulcerative colitis	5	0.9	89.6
Muscular strain	5	0.9	90.5
Other†	53	9.5	100.0

* Does not total 100 per cent because of the rounding-off error.

† Includes pyelonephritis, endometriosis, malignant tumors, esophagitis, gastritis, gastric ucler, hepatitis, spontaneous abortion, anixiety, depression.

Adapted from Adelman A: Abdominal pain in the primary care setting. J Fam Pract 25(1):27, 1987. Reprinted by permission of Appleton & Lange.

TABLE 43–3. ANALYSIS OF A SYMPTOM: ABDOMINAL PAIN (PQR²ST³)

Provoking—What makes your pain worse? Does it hurt more when you move, take a deep breath, or cough?
Palliating—What makes your pain improve?
Quantity—On a scale of 1 to 10, how bad is the pain?
Quality—Could you describe what this pain feels like?
Region—Where is the pain located?
Radiation—Does the pain radiate (e.g., back, shoulders, genitals)?
Severity—Is the pain sufficiently severe to disrupt activities of daily living?
Temporal issues
  Was the onset sudden or gradual?
  Does the pain come and go or is it constant?
  Is this the first time you have had this pain?

These 11 questions are the foundation of rational inquiry regarding the etiology of abdominal pain. Although there are variations and disease-specific augmentations, this initial foundation should be established during the diagnostic process.

Fitz to propose in 1886 that the common and usually fatal disease of perityphlitis was actually appendicitis. In a controversial paper, Fitz advocated that surgery could cure appendicitis (Fitz, 1886). One hundred years have passed, but Fitz' special new tool—the scientific method and its system of logic—remains underutilized in the day-to-day practice of medicine.

Clinical Epidemiology

Appendicitis occurs most frequently between the ages of 10 and 30. However, 7 per cent of patients are under age 5, and 5 per cent are over age 60. Appendicitis, diverticulosis, hemorrhoids, hiatal hernia, and irritable bowel syndromes have been described as diseases of Western civilization. An association with low fiber, high fat diets exists for all of these diseases. Although the lifetime risk of appendicitis is projected at 7 per cent, appendectomy is no longer among the ten most frequent operations in the United States. In centers utilizing sensitivity and specificity theory to derive improved predictive value from physical findings and laboratory values, negative surgical exploration rates have dropped without a corresponding increase in the frequency of perforation (Malt, 1986; Schwartz, 1987).

Present Illness

Because the bowel is mobile and anatomy varies, the location of the appendix is not constant, which explains the number of signs and symptoms that have been associated with acute appendicitis. In particular, this variability explains the fact that fewer that 50 per cent of patients with the disease follow a "textbook" clinical course. Nevertheless, the textbook description is useful for emphasizing another traditional strong point of clinical medicine (i.e., serial observations of the patient as an important diagnostic tool). Generally, patients initially report a malaise that may be attributed to indigestion. Common first symptoms include mild epigastric pain, colicky periumbilical pain, and some irregularity of bowel habit (constipation or diarrhea). During the initial stages, anorexia, nausea, and vomiting are common. Within hours or during the course of the day the pain may shift to the right lower quadrant (McBurney's point). If not reported, tenderness on deep palpation may be elicited. A low grade fever may be reported by the patient. When the condition is untreated perforation may occur, leading to a generalized peritonitis; and in some cases a tender mass may develop in the right lower quadrant (a periappendiceal abscess).

Careful clinicians formulate the differential diagnosis on the basis of the history alone, so it is appropriate to itemize considerations in the differential diagnosis of acute abdominal pain (Table 43–4). At this point, items in the differential diagnosis are reinforced, excluded, or de-emphasized depending on the results of the physical examination, laboratory studies, and further observations. The differential diagnosis list is comprehensive; therefore the consideration of acute appendicitis serves as a useful clinical template for many GI disorders.

TABLE 43–4. STRUCTURAL APPROACH TO THE DIFFERENTIAL DIAGNOSIS OF ACUTE ABDOMINAL PAIN

Thoracic Structures
Cardiac (e.g., myocardial infarction)
Pulmonary (e.g., pneumonia)
Esophageal
Vascular (e.g., aneurysm)

Abdominal Structures
Liver
Gallbladder
Pancreas
Stomach
Small intestine
Large intestine
Kidneys, ureters, bladder
Female reproductive organs
Blood vessels
Rectum
Musculoskeletal system
Vascular—aneurysm
Others

Miscellaneous
Psychogenic
Metabolic (e.g., diabetes)
Abscess
Infectious
Neoplastic
Trauma/obstruction
Others

Review of Systems

In addition to a rigorous symptom analysis (Table 43–3), the family physician must deal with a constellation of personal, family, and community issues associated with each case. Common errors of omission are the medical history including allergies, medications, previous surgeries, previous hospitalizations, family history, social history, and the use of social drugs. For women, the obstetric history and the date of the last normal menstrual period are critical. The temporal sequence of positive items within the review of systems should be described in detail. This sequence is important for distinguishing appendicitis from the other possible conditions within the differential diagnosis.

Physical Examination

The diagnostic process cannot succeed without knowing the vital signs and performing abdominal, pelvic, and rectal examinations. The principles of inspection, auscultation, palpation, and percussion are particularly important during examination of the abdomen. At this point, some of the confirmatory special examinations can be utilized when appropriate. The right lower quadrant is frequently tender over a small area, and rebound tenderness can be elicited. Confirmatory signs such as the iliopsoas sign, the obturator sign, and Hoover's sign are beyond the scope of this chapter. The digital rectal examination may be valuable for diagnosing acute appendicitis. Some examiners have noted that tenderness on the right side is the single most useful diagnostic sign of acute appendicitis. When considering a rigid abdomen with no bowel sounds, one may assume that generalized peritonitis is present and surgical consultation is urgently needed.

Diagnostic Plan

Although hemograms, urinalyses, and radiographs have generally been ordered for investigation of acute abdominal pain, none of these items is diagnostic. A negative laboratory examination in conjunction with a strongly suggestive clinical history merits serious observation. White blood cell counts above $15,000/\mu L$ should raise the suspicion of a perforated appendix, but this finding is also consistent with mesenteric adenitis. The finding of some white blood cells and red blood cells in the urine is entirely consistent with appendicitis, but it is nonspecific. The finding of more than 30 red blood cells or more than 20 white blood cells in the urine suggests a primary lesion in the urinary tract. In selected instances, chest and abdominal radiographs are helpful, and the same may be said for intravenous pyelograms, barium enemas, and ultrasound examinations. Physicians who consider these examinations realize that each case must be individualized and that such studies need not be done routinely.

Psychosocial Aspects and Special Considerations

Because most patients who present with acute abdominal pain do not have an abdominal problem requiring surgery, the negative predictors of appendicitis are frequently more helpful than the textbook descriptors of classic appendicitis. Symptoms lasting more than 72 hours with pain in locations other than those stipulated suggest that appendicitis is not the diagnosis. If the patient has no anorexia and the temperature is below 37.5° C or above 38.6° C, appendicitis is less likely. Exceptions exist, but they are uncommon.

Recent Literature and New Directions

(1) Women surviving a perforated appendix have a fivefold increased risk of infertility (Mueller et al., 1986). (2) Ultrasonography is a relatively inexpensive, noninvasive, nonirradiating modality that has been added to the nonspecific diagnostic armamentarium, but operator-dependent false negatives and availability limit its use (Siegel et al., 1991). (3) Laparoscopy, which is rarely indicated, may evolve as a useful tool with which to confirm the diagnosis or prevent unnecessary surgery in patients with suspected appendicitis (Paterson-Brown et al., 1988). (4) Amylase is elevated in at least 10 per cent of patients with appendicitis, but this finding does not help with the diagnosis. Therefore amylase, electrolytes, glucose, creatinine, and calcium assays are examples of biochemical tests that should be carefully individualized to each situation.

In conclusion, if the family physician suspects appendicitis after the initial evaluation, consultation with a colleague in general surgery is frequently helpful.

CHOLECYSTITIS AND CHOLELITHIASIS

Cholecystectomy is one of the four most frequently performed operations in the United States, and family physicians are frequently involved in the initial care of patients with acute cholecystitis. The advent of potential medical therapy and the understanding that most gallstones exist asymptomatically were major developments during the 1980s. Although gallstone dissolution is a promising and U.S. Food and Drug Administration (FDA)-approved therapy, cholecystectomy remains the definitive treatment, except for a few patients who could be candidates for dissolution. The dissolution drug, ursodiol (Actigall) has some side effects. Moreover, the drug must be taken daily for years, possibly indefinitely, for dissolution to occur. Diagnostically, modern additions have been ultrasonography, cholescintigraphy, endoscopic retrograde cholangiopancreatography, and others. Each development has yielded useful new knowledge but at the cost of increased complexity. Although diagnostic yield (sensitivity) has improved, controversy over elective cholecystectomy in asymptomatic gallstone patients reflects the unresolved predictive value of early diagnosis. We advise against elective surgery in the asymptomatic patient unless there are individual mitigating circumstances.

The differential diagnosis of acute cholecystitis is straightforward most the time. Chronic cholecystitis is a histologic disease. There are no symptoms unless a stone blocks the cystic duct. Once blockage occurs, acute biliary colic ensues.

Clinical Epidemiology

The prevalence of gallstones between the ages of 55 and 65 is 23 per cent for women and 10 per cent for men. Most gallstones are derived from cholesterol. A traditional clinical picture of a patient likely to have gallstones relied heavily on the four Fs (female, fat, forty, and fertile). Autopsy studies have demonstrated that the prevalence of cholelithiasis increases with age, and female patients predominate. The prevalence in the age group 60 to 79 is 23 per cent, with a prevalence of 32 per cent in those over age 80. Groups with a high prevalence of gallbladder disease include women who have been pregnant, diabetics, American Indians, and women who are overweight. Rare causes of pigmented stones are hemolytic disease, longstanding cirrhosis, and disorders of the ileum (e.g., regional enteritis, obesity bypass surgery, and others). Although birth control pills have been linked to a higher prevalence, this association is not clinically important. Because cholecystitis is so common, many patients do not fall into the high risk group.

Present Illness

Among the group treated with a placebo in the National Cooperative Gallstone Study, 305 patients were followed for 2 years. The chief conclusions drawn were from this study were as follows.

1. Most patients without a history of biliary tract pain remain asymptomatic.
2. A history of biliary tract pain is highly predictive of future episodes of pain.
3. Gallstones do not grow rapidly but rarely dissolve or pass spontaneously.

Family physicians frequently encounter patients with biliary tract pain. A stone blocking the cystic duct results in acute biliary colic, which if it continues for a prolonged period can evolve into acute suppurative cholecystitis.

The pain is abrupt, frequently causing the patient to double over with a "10 out of 10" severity. (The patient reports the pain to be 10 on a scale of 1 to 10, where 1 is mild and 10 is most severe or terrible). Much of the time, the colic is steady, and the pain is most commonly epigastric. It may radiate along the right upper quadrant around to the back, straight through to the back, or even up to the shoulder.

The patient frequently rolls around to obtain relief, whereas a patient with coronary ischemia does not. Patients are nauseated, and they sometimes vomit. The attacks commonly awaken people from their sleep between 1 to 3 a.m. The pain may resolve with in a few hours or within 8 to 12 hours; or it is not quelled until the patient receives a narcotic. Usually injection of a narcotic relieves the pain. When the pain does subside, it does so rapidly. Attacks of biliary colic rarely lead to cholecystitis and urgent surgery. When a stone is not blocking the cystic duct, chronic cholecystitis and cholelithiasis are asymptomatic entities. These gallbladder disorders are *not* responsible for flatulence or indigestion.

Review of Systems

The onset of pain is rarely related to meals or the type of food eaten. Many patients with postprandial abdominal pain believe they have gallbladder disease, but many of them suffer from one of the dyspepsia or chronic abdominal pain syndromes (described later in the chapter). Acute surgical cholecystitis becomes a consideration when pain persists or worsens. Surgical consultation may be considered when the pain is associated with fever, there is increasing leukocytosis, and there is a worsening response on physical examination. Most patients with acute cholecystitis have had abdominal pain that has persisted for at least 4 to 6 hours and was unrelieved by narcotic injections.

Physical Findings

The gallbladder is rarely palpable in patients with severe acute cholecystitis. As biliary colic leads to acute cholecystitis, there is increasing localized tenderness that spreads and is associated with muscle guarding or rigidity, or both, in the right upper quadrant. Right-sided pain, which worsens with deep inspiration, may appear. Murphy's sign has been defined as an right upper quadrant tenderness in the midclavicular line that worsens during deep inspiration. This finding suggests acute cholecystitis. Murphy's sign can be elicited with an ultrasound transducer placed directly over the gallbladder. Family physicians with obstetric–gynecologic ultrasound skills have been able to acquire this ultrasound skill rapidly, thereby increasing the specificity of Murphy's sign. Mild jaundice has been found in as many as 20 per cent of patients.

Diagnostic Plan

A hemogram usually reveals an increased white blood cell count. Although serum amylase and lipase values are usually normal, they may be elevated if there is associated pancreatitis. Serum alkaline phosphatase and bilirubin levels are rarely elevated. Sometimes the transaminases—serum glutamic oxaloacetic transaminase (SGOT) and serum glutamic pyruvic transaminase (SGPT) —are as high as 100 units/mL or more and the bilirubin as high as 4mg/dL with an uncomplicated attack of acute cholecystitis. Unless the white blood cell count is high, laboratory tests frequently lack predictive value.

Only 10 to 15 per cent of gallstones are visible on plain x-ray studies, so abdominal films are rarely helpful. Ultrasound imaging has evolved as the procedure of choice. When calculi, gallbladder wall thickening, and gallbladder sludge are found, the diagnosis of acute cholecystitis is reinforced. The presence of stones by itself does not ensure the diagnosis of acute cholecystitis. To make this diagnosis, technetium 99m image display and analysis scans have been invaluable. After intravenous injection, images are obtained within the first 60 minutes and repeated at 3 to 6 hours. The isotope is excreted with the bile and fills all ducts as well as the gallbladder unless the cystic duct is obstructed. When the gallbladder does not appear on the image, it is presumed that gallbladder duct obstruction is present. Oral cholecystography is not indicated as a test for acute cholecystitis, but it is valuable in regions where ultrasonography is not available. There is no longer any need for intravenous cholangiography. Ultrasonography can be used in acute situations because it takes little time. It is noninvasive, emits no radiation, and is not disturbed by high bilirubin levels. It can also be used for pediatric and pregnant patients. At the same time, other abdominal contents can be visualized (e.g. kidney, liver, and pancreas). Technical difficulties may occur in grossly obese patients, and occasionally overlying bowel gas interferes. Nevertheless, the overall sensitivity for sonography has been calculated at 85 to 94 per cent with a positive predictive value of more than 90 per cent.

Management and Therapy

Upon hospitalization or in the emergency room, an intravenous line is established and patients are given nothing by mouth. Hydration and electrolyte balance are maintained. Nasogastric suction is rarely necessary, although it is sometimes helpful if the patient is vomiting. Meperidine can be used every 2 to 3 hours in a dosage of 75 to 100 mg intramuscularly for pain. Intravenous injection avoids the pain of an intramuscular injection. Morphine-type drugs are generally avoided because of the theoretic spasm in the sphincter of Oddi, which is believed to worsen the pain. If the pain does not resolve after several hours, an emergency operation may be indicated, as it may be if the physical findings are worsening and the white blood cell count is increasing. If an initial dose of meperidine does not relieve the pain, surgical consultation should be sought. If too much time is allowed to elapse, gangrene and perforation or abscess may occur. Thus during the routine course of events the diagnosis of acute cholecystitis provides sufficient indication for emergency cholecystectomy. Under emergency circumstances, cholecystectomy can be a life-saving measure.

Summary and Special Considerations

Guidelines for the management of gallbladder disease are fairly discrete when the condition is exhibited asymptomatically as biliary colic or acute cholecystitis. It is less clear how to manage patients with "asymptomatic" gallstones that have been found coincidentally (Laupacis et al., 1988). The fear that future attacks of biliary colic may occur have led to a large number of elective cholecystectomies. Most patients with asymptomatic gallstones remain asymptomatic, whereas those with attacks are likely to continue with attacks. Therefore surgery is generally indicated for symptomatic patients but usually not for asymptomatic patients.

New treatments are emerging with some promise. For example, ursodiol (Actigall), taken orally, dissolves stones. However, the patient must have cholesterol gallstones and a functioning gallbladder to be a candidate for this therapy. Furthermore, the patient may need to take the drug daily for 2 years with full knowledge of a 40 per cent fail rate, and the drug is costly. Laparoscopic cholecystectomy has emerged as the intervention of choice.

The phenomenon of phantom pain after cholecystectomy is particularly difficult. Usually, we obtain a second opinion and consider psychometric evaluation for a somatis disorder if no organic causes can be found. Among women of reproductive age with negative imaging studies but with clinical syndromes similar to acute and chronic cholecystitis, treatment for anterior perihepatitis, known as Fitz-Hugh–Curtis syndrome, has resulted in cure (Shanahan et al., 1988). These authors suggested that all sexually active patients with suspected acute cholecystitis and a normal ultrasound scan be screened for *Chlamydia trachomatis*.

DIVERTICULOSIS–DIVERTICULITIS

Diverticulosis is the presence of saccular outpouchings from the large intestine. They occur most commonly in the sigmoid colon. Once regarded as a pathologic curiosity, the low fiber, high fat dietary environment of the civilized twentieth century has been associated with an autopsy-confirmed prevalence as high as 60 per cent of patients over age 60. The hypothesis of the relation between dietary fiber and diverticulosis has been supported by multiple studies, including a prevalence study of Oxford vegetarians (12 per cent) and matched controls (33 per cent) (Gear et al., 1979). The widespread diagnosis of diverticulosis and the frequent application of accurate imaging studies—x-ray studies, computed tomography (CT), and endoscopy—among the large number of family practice patients presenting with symptoms of abdominal pain reflects the high prevalence of the condition.

As with gallstones and hiatal hernia, the presence of the condition does not necessarily mean it is the cause of the patient's pain. Most patients with diverticuli do not have symptoms, although few have perforation, hemorrhage, and subsequent complications. In a tertiary care setting, 294 selected patients were prospectively followed for 15 years. During the follow-up period, clinical diverticulitis developed in 25 per cent, perforation in 5 per cent, substantial hemorrhage in 5 per cent, and obstruction in 5 per cent (Boles and Gordon, 1958). Having come under medical observation for one reason or another, these patients probably represent a select group. This phenomenon is also known as referral bias. Therefore in most patients diverticulosis is an incidental finding that may reflect many years of a Western diet and lifestyle. At this point, it is only speculation on our part that lifestyle modifications can prevent the development of diverticulosis-associated morbidity.

Diverticulitis begins with the inflammation of one or more diverticuli. If it is not known why the inflammation occurs. Clinical pain arises from inflammation of the colon wall and the adjacent peritoneal surface. Most of the time the inflammation is confined to the bowel wall, resulting in the most common entity (i.e., diverticulitis). If the inflammation continues, an abscess may arise; and perforation or obstruction may follow. These complications are uncommon.

Diverticular hemorrhage is a probable cause in some 20 to 40 per cent of adults who present with lower GI bleeding. It should be noted that diverticular hemorrhage does not occur as part of the clinical syndrome of diverticulitis. Most often diverticular hemorrhage appears suddenly in an asymptomatic patient.

Present Illness

A syndrome attributed to diverticuli has been called painful diverticular disease. This syndrome may be exhibited as a generally constant left lower quadrant pain. The pain may be perceived in the right lower quadrant or the suprapubic area. Patients may complain of associated constipation or diarrhea, or both, but it is difficult to know whether this finding represents a coincidental event or a true association. Sometimes the pain is made worse by the passage of a bowel movement. The pain may be intense with localized tenderness, but the white blood cell count is normal. Acute diverticulitis could be suspected in these cases, but it is not likely when pain has been present for weeks to months without signs of inflammation.

Acutely ill patients who present with the rapid development of fever and acute, severe abdominal pain in the left lower quadrant merit immediate attention. Depending on the severity of the findings, an outpatient or a hospital setting is chosen.

Review of Systems

At one time diverticulitis was described as a left-sided appendicitis because patients can present with pain in the left lower abdomen. There is historical merit for this concept. A previously documented attack of diverticulitis is historically helpful. The patient with diverticulitis usually reports a severe, steady left lower quadrant pain that is frequently associated with urinary frequency. The pain becomes worse when the patient walks, coughs, or moves around.

Physical Findings

The most common finding is abdominal tenderness that localizes to the left lower quadrant. Sometimes a palpable mass is found. Even if the palpable mass is not present, there usually is exquisite tenderness in the left lower quadrant. Bowel sounds are generally present. Rectal examination may reveal tenderness high on the left side. If the severity of the inflammation worsens, a tender mass may be palpable, the abdominal signs may worsen, and the bowel sounds may disappear. With extreme cases peritoneal signs are evident, and sepsis may be the presenting syndrome. With acute diverticulitis, the oral temperature is usually 38.0° C (100.4° F) or lower. As inflammation spreads, the fever and white blood cell count increase.

Diagnostic Plan

The history and physical examination usually establish the diagnosis. The laboratory tests are generally of little value unless the white blood cell count goes above 15,000/mm^3. If the white blood cell count and the temperature are elevated and abdominal findings are present, surgical consultation should be requested without delay. Most patients with acute diverticulitis can be managed as outpatients. Patients with diverticulitis who have more advanced findings may require hospitalization. CT is now the test of choice (Lefrink and Miedema, 1992).

In one series of hospitalized patients with severe diverticulitis, physical findings were tabulated to reveal the following: abdominal tenderness 67 per cent; palpable pelvic mass 27 per cent; palpable abdominal mass 26 per cent; signs of generalized peritonitis 14 per cent; shock 4 per cent. Eighteen per cent of the patients had negative physical findings (Walker et al., 1977).

Flexible sigmoidoscopy, colonoscopy, or barium enema should not be used in these cases because a considerable risk of perforation exists with instrumentation if acute diverticulitis is present. Therefore a period of observation during medical therapy is preferred prior to any invasive studies. In those cases in which the differential diagnosis includes ischemia or colitis, gentle, limited sigmoidoscopy can be performed. Excessive air insufflation and forceful manipulation should be avoided while performing this procedure. Once the patient is identified as possibly having a severe case of diverticulitis, hospitalization, intravenous antibiotics, and consultation are rapidly undertaken. Management is individualized at that point.

Differential Diagnosis and Therapy

For those who are hospitalized, the family physician and consultant team usually work through the clinical course. If the patient deteriorates (i.e., has more pain, increasing fever, and worsening physical examination despite antibiotic therapy), surgery should be considered to avoid perforation, full-blown peritonitis, or both. For those who have had previous attacks of diverticulitis, surgery should be considered earlier because they are more likely to have attacks in the future. Usually the sigmoid colon alone is removed. Patients who must be emergently decompressed may require a colostomy with resection. If the attack of diverticulitis can be stabilized medically, an elective sigmoid resection is preferred. An elective resection is performed only if the patient is repeatedly symptomatic or develops a fistula to the bladder (or other organs).

For those patients who are not hospitalized, there are many management issues. The differential diagnosis for mild left lower quadrant abdominal pain includes, but is not limited to, irritable bowel syndrome, inflammatory bowel disease, carcinoma, ischemic colitis, radiation colitis, infectious colitis, and others. More information follows in specific sections dealing with each of the common entities.

Psychosocial Aspects and Special Considerations

Although hospital services and surgical operations for diverticulitis and its complications are reported commonly in the literature, the need for operative intervention has been reported to be 0.4 per cent (Horner, 1958). Many of the cases previously described as diverticulitis may actually have been intermixed with irritable bowel syndrome, self-limited gastroenteritis, and other conditions. There seems to have been a high natural remission rate, and it should be noted that most patients with incidentally noted diverticulosis are free from acute diverticulitis and the severe complications described above. These individuals can be safely managed as outpatients. Because abdominal pain unassociated with any anatomic or inflammatory abnormality is so common, previous associations between diverticular disorders and the various other irritable bowel syndromes have been difficult to establish (Drossman et al., 1982).

Treatment of Acute Diverticulitis

The patient with localized left lower quadrant pain and a temperature below 38.9° C (102° F) (who does not have abdominal distention) can be managed as an outpatient with the concurrence of the surgical consultant. These outpatients should receive liquids only. Bed rest and antibiotics such as the oral cephalosporins can be prescribed. Oral codeine may be used for pain. While at home, the patient should be advised to report worsening pain, spreading pain, abdominal distention, vomiting, or temperature spikes. These features would reflect a worsening course. In such a case the physician must be notified and hospitalization considered urgently.

Diet and Drug Therapy

Previously recommended bland low fiber low seed diets for diverticulosis are no longer indicated. After the acute attack, recommendations now include a high fiber, low fat diet. The chapter on nutrition may describe these diets more fully. Anticholinergic drugs, antispasmodic drugs, sedatives, and tranquilizers may be used for patients

who have concurrent irritable bowel syndrome unspecified colonic spasm.

There are no direct clinical data indicating that a high fiber diet prevents the development of either diverticuli or diverticulitis. However, the epidemiologic data are convincing in the minds of some, but not all, experts. A study of 100 patients who had been discharged with confirmed diverticular disease compared those patients who complied with the recommendation of 40 gm of fiber per day with those who did not comply with the diet. The high fiber diet was associated with a 91 per cent probability of being symptom-free. Only 80 per cent of the patients who did not follow the high-fiber diet were symptom-free, and all major complications occurred in this group as well (Hyland and Taylor, 1980). In any case, it seems reasonable to recommend high fiber diets: They are healthy. For patients who dislike raw dietary bulk, hydrophilic colloids (Metamucil, Konsyl, Modane bulk, and others) may be prescribed, recommending one heaping tablespoon once or twice a day. Rapid initiation of large amounts of fiber can cause flatulence, distention, and discomfort. Therefore a gradual buildup to the desired amount is recommended. Anticipatory guidance regarding the side effects should also be given.

Clinical Suggestions

As for the irritable bowel syndrome, the opportunity to explore lifestyle issues and dietary considerations is important here. It may be useful to create a "grocery store" quiz regarding equivalent weights of dietary products that are required to produce 20 grams of fiber per day. This amount of fiber intake approximately doubles the daily fecal weight. For example, it would require 22 ounces of whole carrots, 49 ounces of fresh apples, 13 ounces of whole meal bread, or 4.5 ounces of commercial bran cereal. The equivalent amount of unprocessed bran would be 1.5 ounces. Another equivalent would be approximately two bowls of commercial cereals such as Allbran or Bran Buds. There are many choices. Any of the many good diet books available make the above calculations and food choices as simple as looking at a table. Although data are incomplete, diet seems to help alleviate some symptoms of the condition.

ACUTE PANCREATITIS

Acute pancreatitis is a logical fourth element in this overview of acute abdominal pain syndromes in which early identification is the key to appropriate hospital therapy and consultation. Appendicitis, cholecystitis, diverticulitis, and pancreatitis are diseases with degrees of clinical severity ranging from mild to severe. When severe, each condition may be exhibited as a potential acute surgical abdomen. The family physician must be aware of these life-threatening illnesses, even though most patients with abdominal pain do not require hospitalization.

Because the clinical presentation of acute pancreatitis may vary from acute abdominal pain to episodes of excruciating abdominal pain and vascular collapse, pancreatitis is included within the broad differential diagnosis of abdominal pain. Regardless of the underlying cause, the common pathway in the pathogenesis of pancreatitis is the liberation of corrosive pancreatic enzymes. Local pancreatic digestion and possible hemorrhage ensue. There is massive third spacing with subsequent hypovolemia. When there is severe massive tissue destruction adjacent to the pancreas, organs that are distant to the pancreas can be affected as well.

Clinical Epidemiology

Most patients (65 to 90 per cent) with acute pancreatitis have either chronic alcoholism or gallstones. Perforated peptic ulcer disease, trauma, neoplasms, hypercalcemia, hyperlipidemia, drugs, viral infections, and other conditions account for a small percentage of cases. The condition may be idiopathic in as many as 25 per cent of cases. The disease may occur at any age, but it is most frequently seen between the ages of 40 and 60. Acute pancreatitis typically occurs in a man in his thirties or forties who has been drinking heavily for 6 to 10 years. For alcohol abuse of this degree, the estimated pancreatitis risk is 5 to 10 per cent. Gallstone pancreatitis, the more dangerous of the two types, occurs at a later age.

Chronic pancreatitis indicates that there has been some permanent and progressive damage to the pancreas. In some cases this damage leads to diabetes, malabsorption, or both. Patients with chronic pancreatitis present with repeated attacks of abdominal pain.

Present Illness and Review of Systems

The patient presents with a history of deep, gnawing, constant epigastric pain that radiates to the back in 50 per cent of patients. In some patients the pain is substernal, generalized to the left upper quadrant, right upper quadrant, or even to the lower abdomen. Most often the pain has been present for more than 24 hours. This pain is worsened by food or alcohol intake and, in an alcoholic, may be precipitated by binge drinking. Sometimes the pain is less severe when the patient leans forward. In advanced stages, movement worsens the pain, as it does in any of the previously discussed acute abdominal pain syndromes. The onset of pain is usually gradual with a plateau being reached within several hours.

Physical Findings

A low grade fever 37.8° to 38.9° C (100° to 102° F) may be present; a temperature in excess of 38.9° C (102° F) suggests another diagnosis or a complication. Because hypovolemia is a common complication, orthostatic vital signs should be recorded. Regulation of an appropriate fluid intake is essential. Urinary output must be monitored carefully. Even when blood pressure is normal, a mild tachycardia may reflect worsening hypovolemia.

The patient with pancreatitis is in severe distress due to the abdominal pain. A stoic acceptance of discomfort suggests other diagnoses. The abdomen is tender but not rigid. Distention and decreased bowel sounds may be evident when ileus results from the diffusion of inflammatory fluid around the pancreas. The purplish discoloration of extravasated pancreatic hemorrhages (i.e., Grey Turner's sign in the flanks and Cullen's sign in the periumbilical area) are rarely seen.

Diagnostic Plan

Elevated serum amylase concentration continues to be the sine qua non of acute pancreatitis, although a perforated viscus or bowel obstruction can also cause elevated amylase levels. Other causes of high amylase include tubal pregnancy and parotiditis. Serum amylase levels return to normal within 1 to 3 days, and so abnormal values are sometimes missed. The serum lipase level remains elevated for 7 to 14 days or more, a finding that is occasionally helpful. Although the amylase level and the creatinine clearance ratio were widely acclaimed during the late 1970's, their usefulness has not survived the test of time (Moosa, 1984).

The hematocrit temporarily may be high as a secondary effect of hypovolemia. When rehydrated, patients with a low hematocrit may be suffering from acute hemorrhagic pancreatitis. If the bilirubin, SGOT, SGPT, and alkaline phosphatase rise, a common duct stone may exist. This possibility could be further explored with an abdominal ultrasound scan and possibly endoscopic retrograde cholangiopancreatography. Hypocalcemia, hypoalbuminemia, hyperglycemia, and leukocytosis in the range of 15,000 to 20,000 white blood cells (WBCs)/μl are frequently found. Leukocytosis above 20,000/μl suggests more severe disease. Because "shock lung" may ensue, chest radiographic studies, pulse oximetry, and blood gas assays should be considered. In severe cases, renal failure may appear despite adequate fluid intake. Urinary output should be monitored with care.

There have been a variety of promising laboratory assays directed at improving the clinical diagnosis of pancreatitis, but none has established a clear advantage over the serum amylase test (and clinical evaluation). The lipase assay is believed to be a highly sensitive, specific test for pancreatic disorders, although this belief has been questioned. Using a cutoff for amylase about 1.5 times the upper limit of normal, a sensitivity of 99.9 per cent and a specificity of 98.4 per cent were found. Some authors concluded that total serum amylase is the initial assay of choice for diagnosing acute pancreatitis (Steinberg et al., 1985).

Although other abdominal diseases can cause the amylase to be elevated, a patient with an acute attack of abdominal pain and an elevated serum amylase level probably has acute pancreatitis. Hospitalization and consultation would be justifiable even under the most stringent criteria. Although some have questioned the acquisition of routine chest and abdominal films for these patients, the absence of free air in the abdomen remains one reassuring sign that a large perforated viscus is unlikely. Furthermore, some radiographic findings help to re-enforce the diagnosis. Such findings include an absent left psoas shadow, calcifications in the region of the pancreas, and an isolated air-filled loop of small bowel that cuts off in the area of the transverse colon (i.e., the sentinel loop). There have been dramatic improvements with the utilization of ultrasonography, endoscopic retrograde cholangiopancreatography, and computed tomography. Nevertheless, with the laboratory tests and evaluations discussed to this point, the family physician should have sufficient diagnostic information to warrant an appropriate disposition for the acutely ill patient.

Differential Diagnosis

Because the presentation of acute pancreatitis may be similar to that of many other entities that present with diffuse upper abdominal pain, all of the other causes of acute abdominal pain must be considered. The diseases most commonly confused with pancreatitis are acute cholecystitis, choledocholithiasis, perforated peptic ulcer, and ruptured abdominal aneurysm. Pancreatitis may present with diffuse upper abdominal pain, back pain, left upper quadrant pain, and right upper quadrant pain. Therefore all of the causes of acute abdominal pain should be considered.

Psychosocial Aspects and Special Considerations

Prognostically, a 10 per cent mortality rate continues to exist for acute pancreatitis. Almost all cases resulting in death are associated with acute necrotizing or hemorrhagic pancreatitis. Another 40 per cent of patients become quite ill but survive their attack. The remainder have relatively mild, self-limited disease. Medical therapy is primarily supportive, with the major objective being stabilization.

Permanent pathologic damage to the pancreas results in chronic pancreatitis. In addition to exocrine deficiency (with malabsorption, diabetes, or both), a chronic pain syndrome may be present that is difficult to manage. Many of these patients suffer from substance abuse and other behavioral problems that require time, patience, compassion, and skill to resolve. Those patients who continue drinking are more likely to have recurrent attacks. In patients who can stop drinking, the frequency of attacks may decrease. This area is one in which the family physician can apply basic preventive principles to counsel his or her patients with the hope of reducing the number of future attacks. Exocrine deficiency may be treated with supplementation of pancreatic enzyme preparations with each meal. Chronic pancreatitis also leads to the need for diabetic management (discussed in Chapter 41).

Patients with chronic pancreatitis frequently have complex symptoms, and it is best for them to be referred to a gastroenterologist. Depending on the results from the consultation, some of these patients can then be successfully followed by their family physician.

Special Clinical Questions

When biliary tract disease is believed to be the cause of pancreatitis and the pancreatitis is stabilized, surgery (cholecystectomy) should be scheduled during the next several weeks if no other contraindications exist. Presumably, additional gallstones can migrate, causing more episodes of pancreatitis. Therefore surgery usually should be performed quickly.

Diabetes associated with chronic pancreatitis is often brittle. In these instances, the follow-up is most helpful when daily monitoring is utilized to the extent to which the patient complies. Hypoglycemia is a real risk, and frequently tight control is not possible.

Pancreatic enzymes can be administered clinically, with the physician determining the dose by monitoring the steatorrhea and the patient's weight. Tablets must be given before, during, and after eating until the stool volume and stool fat visibly decrease.

OBSTRUCTION AND DISTENTION SYNDROMES

The family physician cannot diagnose and manage the remainder of the GI disorders without a

TABLE 43–5. ETIOLOGIES FOR BOWEL OBSTRUCTION AND ABDOMINAL DISTENTION SYNDROMES

Cardiovascular Conditions
Cardiac low output—congestive heart failure
Thromboembolism
Mesenteric ischemia
Others

Medication
Anesthetics
Narcotics
Anticholinergics
Others

Neuromuscular Conditions
Multiple sclerosis
Parkinson's disease
Paraplegia
Others

Endocrine Conditions
Diabetes
Hypothyroidism
Others

Abdominal Inflammatory Conditions
Appendicitis
Cholecystitis
Diverticulitis
Pancreatitis
Pelvic inflammatory disease
Crohn's disease
Ulcerative colitis
Toxic megacolon
Others

Miscellaneous Conditions
Ascites
Aerophagia

Mechanical Obstruction Abnormalities
See Table 43–6

TABLE 43–6. MECHANICAL CONSIDERATIONS IN THE DIFFERENTIAL DIAGNOSIS OF THE BOWEL OBSTRUCTION AND ABDOMINAL DISTENTION SYNDROMES

Luminal Lesions
Cancer
Foreign bodies
Bezoars, gallstones
Intussusception
Fecal impaction
Inflammation
Others

Extrinsic Lesions
Adhesions
Abscess
Extrinsic tumors
Other

Strangulating Lesions
Adhesions
Hernias
Volvulus
Others

working knowledge of these acute conditions that require hospitalization and urgent consultation. It is not essential to achieve an instantly accurate diagnosis in each case; however, the key is generic recognition of the cases in which delay would be harmful for the patient. A tabular classification of intestinal obstruction and distention syndrome etiologies should assist in this task (Tables 43–5, 43–6). Furthermore, approaches to these conditions may be considered building blocks for following patients with gastroenteritis, GI bleeding, and inflammatory bowel disease.

Silen (1979) compiled the overall causes of intestinal obstruction from 13 reported series comprising a total of 12,731 patients. The differences in the distribution of etiologies between adults and children are outlined in Table 43–7.

ACUTE DIARRHEAL SYNDROMES

Diarrhea has been defined in many ways. Some believe it means more frequent bowel movements, whereas others have defined it as being the passage of formless stools. Pathophysiologically focused investigators believe that stool weight per day is the most reliable definition. Hence a good working definition of diarrhea is "having more and looser bowel movements than usual."

The clinical questions in an office practice may include, but not necessarily be limited to, the following: How sick is this patient? Is he or she febrile? Is the patient toxic, with dehydration or hypotension (or both)? Is it an illness that requires hospitalization or consultation? If it is an illness suitable for ambulatory management, is it self-limited? Should an antibiotic be prescribed, or is the best treatment supportive?

Acute gastroenteritis occurs frequently among

TABLE 43–7. ETIOLOGIES OF MECHANICAL INTESTINAL OBSTRUCTION: ADULTS AND CHILDREN

Etiology	%
Adults	
Hernia	41
Adhesions	29
Intussusception	12
Cancer	10
Volvulus	4
Miscellaneous	4
Children	
Hernia	38
Pyloric stenosis	15
Ileocecal intussusception	15
Atresia	14
Anular pancreas	14
Adhesions	7
Miscellaneous	4

Adapted from Silen W (ed): *Cope's* Early Diagnosis of the Acute Abdomen, 15th edition. New York, Oxford University Press, 1979, with permission.

adults and children. The likelihood of dehydration sufficiently severe to merit hospitalization is more likely among children of developing countries. Several family physicians (such as Mull and Smilkstein) are internationally prominent for their work in oral rehydration therapy and international health. In the United States most of these diarrheal illnesses are self-limited and require merely reassurance, dietary counseling, occasional antibiotics, and a watchful eye for complications. Rehydration solutions are not commonly required.

Clinical Epidemiology and Differential Diagnosis

Exceeded only by upper respiratory infections, gastroenteritis is the second most frequent illness in the United States. Viral infections are the most common cause of gastroenteritis. Acute diarrheal syndromes are generally defined as being of abrupt onset and usually lasting less than 2 to 3 weeks, although some believe that pediatric acute diarrheal syndromes may last 4 weeks or more (Bruckstein, 1988). This section focuses on the infectious etiologies, which include viral, bacterial, and parasitic infections.

Rotavirus, Norwalk-like agents, other small viruses, and enteric adenoviruses cause many of the viral gastroenteritis syndromes. Stool viral cultures are not indicated. Virus identification does not make a clinical difference, and the tests themselves are difficult and expensive. These viral illnesses are self-limited, and aggressive diagnostic workup is not indicated.

Special situations include traveler's diarrhea, food poisoning, diarrhea in the elderly and in children in day care centers, and antibiotic-associated colitis. New office laboratory methods, such as an enzyme-linked immunoassay for rotavirus (Rotazyme) and latex agglutination for *Clostridium difficile* (Marion Labs), will continue to be developed. Decision analysis is combining probability theory with clinical observations to produce a new set of management strategies by which physicians can learn and teach. For example, stool cultures represent the gold standard for the diagnosis of bacterial infection. Because the likelihood of bacterial infection is less than 50 per cent and stool cultures require time and expense, it is not clear when the physician should order stool cultures, particularly for infants who are at risk for severe complications.

Using regression analysis techniques, the clinical history, and a stool smear for leukocytes, the presence of five or more leukocytes per high powered field has provided a positive predictive value of 59 per cent and a negative predictive value of 97 per cent for a bacterial etiology of acute childhood diarrhea. Three historical questions have emerged as being helpful: Was the onset abrupt? Were there

---

TABLE 43–8. COMMON ACUTE DIARRHEA SYNDROMES

Fecal Leukocytes Often Present (Inflammatory)
  Salmonella
  Shigella
  Campylobacter
  C. difficile
  Invasive *E. coli*
  Entamoeba histolytica
  Yersinia
  Crohn's disease*
  Ulcerative colitis*
  Others
Fecal Leukocytes Usually Absent (Noninflammatory)
  Viral infections
  Giardia lamblia
  Cryptosporidium
  Vibrio cholerae
  Toxigenic *E. coli*
  Lactose intolerance
  Sprue
  Staphylococcal food poisoning
  Many others

In the correct setting, the use of a methylene blue stain on a liquid stool specimen can provide strong, but not pathognomonic, presumptive evidence for a bacterial infection. Note that some parasitic and idiopathic inflammatory conditions may also produce fecal leukocytosis.

* Does not commonly present as acute diarrhea.

---

more than four stools per day? Did the diarrhea start before the vomiting? Positive answers to these three questions provided a powerful predictor (7:1) of bacterial etiology compared to when even one of the questions was answered negatively (DeWitt et al., 1985). This type of study should be modified to suit various family practice questions and should be replicated.

A reasonable work-up can be better understood if the diarrhea syndromes' etiologies are classified as inflammatory and noninflammatory (Table 43–8). Other diarrheal classifications have been based on osmotic, malabsorptive, and structural factors. For family physicians, Table 43–8 is useful, as it demonstrates that most (but not all) of the diseases that are treatable with antibiotics are inflammatory. Because clinical findings are similar for the various types of inflammation, a set of simple steps should quickly answer the major questions.

Present Illness

Most of these disorders induce some combination of abdominal pain, diarrhea, nausea, vomiting, fever, and tenesmus. Rotavirus presents most frequently in infants and children. After an incubation period of several days, the affected children present with an initial temperature of 37.8° to 38.9° C (100° to 102° F). There is associated respiratory distress, vomiting, and some degree dehydration. The syndrome usually lasts 7 to 10 days; and the stools are generally watery without blood, pus, or mucus. Some clinicians have found it useful to investigate these cases initially via an enzyme-linked immunoassay (Rotazyme), which is 97 per cent accurate for identifying rotavirus.

The Norwalk agents are the most common causes of diarrhea among adults, whereas rotavirus affects mainly infants and children. The Norwalk virus usually causes a low-grade fever that arrives abruptly and lasts 1 to 3 days. The patient may feel terrible, and the WBC count may be variable. Nevertheless, in most cases resolution can be expected within 3 days. The rotavirus illness usually lasts 5 to 6 days and is accompanied by more extensive vomiting and diarrhea. The second most common causes of pediatric viral gastroenteritis are the enteric adenoviruses. The illnesses they produce typically last 5 to 12 days (Blacklow and Greenberg, 1991).

These distinctions are useful only in a retrospective manner. The physician should advise the patient that the course of viral gastroenteritis is likely to be 14 days or more. In the cases that last longer, further evaluation is usually necessary.

When the present illness is characterized by diarrhea that contains blood, the probability of such agents as *Shigella, Salmonella, Escherichia coli, Campylobacter,* and *Yersinia* being responsible is increased. *Entamoeba histolytica* can produce symptoms ranging from mild to severe dysentery, but it is rare in most parts of the United States. *Yersinia* has been known to mimic acute appendicitis, but fortunately it is uncommon. Nevertheless, *Yersinia* infection, which can mimic appendicitis, highlights the variability of the syndromes and the need for ongoing observation of patients with severe acute diarrheal syndromes.

Physical Findings

The pediatric literature has reinforced the value of "soft data" (i.e., the observational gestalt) acquired by the experienced clinician as he or she scans the general appearance of the patient and derives an impression regarding toxicity. Hydration is assessed by observing the mucous membranes and estimating volume depletion. Orthostatic blood pressure and pulses should be noted. Weight is the most important estimate in children, and it is particularly useful for the family physician, who is responsible for continuity of care. The degree of fever is an important indicator for continuing hydration needs. Capillary refill times are not reliable.

The abdominal examination generally reveals diffuse tenderness with normal or increased bowel sounds. Findings of focal tenderness, rigidity, and peritoneal signs are not consistent with viral gastroenteritis. These factors are covered in more detail in the section of acute abdominal pain syndromes. Digital rectal examinations are generally not helpful in adults or children.

Abnormal orthostatic hemodynamic measurements may be more prevalent than previously believed. Among 281 adult patients discharged with the diagnosis of acute gastroenteritis, 27 per cent had positive orthostatic vital sign changes (defined as a pulse increase of 30 beats per minute on standing) (Olshaker and Mason, 1988).

Diagnostic Plan

The initial work-up requires few studies. A hemogram is usually not necessary. A methylene blue stain of the stool should be obtained and cultures obtained when the stain reveals positive results. Occasionally, it is wise to obtain stool cultures despite the absence of fecal leukocytes, but these situations are rare. Although many diarrhea algorithms exist, numerous laboratory tests are not necessary. Some of the information that follows may be useful in those rare cases where additional studies have been obtained. For example, eosinophilia on a hemogram is rarely found with protozoan infestation, such as with *E. histolytica* or *Giardia lamblia*. Peripheral eosinophilia usually indicates the presence of helminthic infestation, such as with *Ascaris lumbricoides*. The travel history may suggest the need for stool samples for ova and parasites. In cases of suspected ambebiasis, a positive indirect hemagglutination titer higher than 1:256 is helpful.

Cryptosporidium has been implicated as a pathogen in humans. The diarrhea it causes is usually self-limited but may persist for a month. Because no therapy has been effective in immunocomprised patients (who are at greatest risk) and no treatment is necessary for immunocompetent individuals, testing is not advised.

Dehydration and toxicity are the critical criteria for hospitalization. Most frequently these conditions occur at the extremes of age (i.e., among infants and the elderly). Patients presenting with delirium clearly should be admitted for further work-up and management. Findings consistent with an acute surgical abdomen should be admitted. Patients with serious underlying illness, such as severe organic heart disease, malignancy, or vascular disease, may be special cases in which the threshold for hospitalization is lower. As a general rule, the clinician should otherwise accept the wide margin of safety associated with these self-limited illnesses.

Diet and Therapy

Therapeutic considerations for viral illness generally focus on patient comfort and dietary therapy. Even in those cases where a bacterial agent is strongly suspected, culture results are not available until 2 days later. Initial oral fluid and electrolyte replacement may include carbonated beverages and commercially available drinks such as Gatorade. When nausea and vomiting continue to prohibit adequate replacement therapy, hospitalization and intravenous therapy should be considered. Once the appropriate rehydration therapy is tolerated, dietary considerations include food selection, feeding intervals, and meal quantity. It is not necessary to completely rest the bowel, and so far as possible the patient should be allowed to select his or her own foods. Transient secondary lactase deficiency is common in diarrheal states, so milk products are generally avoided. Among infants, reintroduction of lactose-containing substances such as milk, may be monitored by testing for stool pH. The presence of a reducing substance or the lowering of stool pH to 4 or 5, as found by using Clinitest tablets or Nitrazine sticks, suggests a continuing disaccharidase deficiency.

In developing countries, diarrhea is a major cause of death and malnutrition in children. The World Health Organization (WHO) has stated, "Oral rehydration therapy (ORT) is the keystone of all diarrheal disease control programs because it is simple, highly effective, inexpensive, and technologically appropriate. A solution prepared from oral rehydration salts is used both to treat clinically evident dehydration and to prevent dehydration by replacing losses early in the course of disease." The solution recommended by the WHO (Table 43–9) contains, in grams per liter: NACI 3.5, KCI 1.5, trisodium citrate 2.9 (or $NaHCO^3$ 2.5), and glucose 20. Home-based ORT therapy can be given at the onset of diarrhea to minimize dehydration (Avery and Snyder, 1990; Mull and Mull, 1988).

Although highly effective for treating dehydration, ORT does not diminish the amount of diarrhea. Appropriate drug therapies are useful adjuncts. Even without drugs, approximately 90 per cent of children with watery diarrhea who visit a health care facility can be successfully and optimally treated solely with ORT and continued feeding. In these developing world situations, antibiotic or antiparasitic therapy should be reserved for patients with dysentery, proved or presumed cholera, or proved infection with *E. histolytica* or *G. lamblia*.

"Currently available adjunct agents, including antimotility and antisecretory agents, exogenous aciduric flora, and absorbents, have no practical value and increase both the cost of treatment and the risk of adverse reactions. The practice encountered in many countries of routinely treating episodes of diarrhea with multiple adjuncts and antibiotics, sometimes available as combination agents, is to be deplored." Oral rehydration therapy is the only proved cost-effective method of treating routine self-limited diarrhea, and the economic savings from treating the disease in this way can be considerable (World Health Organization, 1988).

For children, clear liquids do not include caffeinated colas. Increasing the number of small feedings may be an effective replacement (i.e., 30 to 60 ounces every 60 minutes) for two or three large meals. Some have recommended that fruit juices be withheld because of their high osmolality and their inherent fruit juice malabsorption potential (Hayms, 1988). In that study, evidence of carbohydrate malabsorption was accompanied by symptoms in only 30 to 40 per cent of subjects. Therefore diet therapy is highly variable and must be individualized. Adequate caloric intake is important in all cases. Even adults can benefit from variations of the so-called BRAT (*b*ananas, *r*ice, cooked *a*pple, and *t*oast) diet for achieving a return to a regular diet as soon as possible. The return to a nearly normal diet can be accomplished even though the stools may remain loose for several days to several weeks or more. In some cases, children may have an altered bowel habit that persists for the remainder of their toddlerhood. In these cases, appropriate growth and development should be monitored. Usually the child continues to do well (Bezerra, 1992).

TABLE 43–9. ORAL ELECTROLYTE SOLUTIONS

Product	Conc. When Diluted (mEq/L)				Glucose (gm/L)	Form	$ Cost per Quart†	mOsm/L
	Na	K	Cl	Base*				
WHO Oral Rehydration Salts	90	20	80	30	20	Powder	0.35	333
Rehydralyte (Ross)	75	20	65	30	25	Liquid	40.8	305
Infalyte (Penwall)	50	20	40	30	20	Powder	2.88	251
Lytren (Mead Johnson)	50	25	45	30	20	Liquid	3.35	220
Pedialyte (Ross)	45	20	35	30	25	Liquid	2.81	250
Resol (Wyeth)	50	20	50	34	20	Liquid‡	2.52	330
Gatorade	20	3						

* HCO, or derived from citrate.
† Cost to the pharmacist, based on the average wholesale price (*Drug Topics Red Book 1987* and June 1987 *Update*).
‡ Also contains 4 mEq each of Ca and Mg, and 5 mEq of PO.
Modified from Rakel RE (ed): Conn's Current Therapy. Philadelphia, WB Saunders, 1988, p 12, with permission.

TABLE 43–10. ANTIBIOTICS FOR SPECIFIC DIARRHEA SYNDROMES

Specific Pathogen or Condition	Drug	Adult Dosage
Salmonella	Drugs usually not indicated due to prolongation of carrier state	1 tablet b.i.d.
	When absolutely needed TMP-SMX (Bactrim DS, Septra DS).	
	Alternative: ciprofloxacin	500 mg b.i.d.
Shigella species	TMP-SMX	800/160 b.i.d. × 5–7 days
	Alternative: ciprofloxacin	500 mg b.i.d. × 5–7 days
	Alternative for severe cases (pediatric): ceftriaxone—parenteral	50 mg/kg daily × 5 days
Campylobacter	Erythromycin	500 mg q.i.d. × 5–10 days
C. difficile	Metronidazole	250 mg t.i.d. × 7 days
	Oral vancomycin	125 mg q 6 hr × 1 week
	Adjunctive: cholestyramine (binds toxin)	4 gm q.i.d.
Food poisoning due to *Staphylococcus aureus*	No antibiotic	
Giardiasis	Atabrine (quinacrine)	100 mg t.i.d. × 7 days
	Alternative: metronidazole (Flagyl)	250 mg t.i.d. × 7 days
Amebiasis	Metronidazole	750 mg t.i.d. × 10 days
	Intraluminal phase: iodoquinol (Yodoxin)	650 mg t.i.d. × 20 days
	Pepto-Bismol	30/60 ml q.i.d.
Yersinia enterocolitica	Sensitive to many drugs, but none alter the course	
Traveler's diarrhea	TMP-SMX	800/160 b.i.d. × 5 days
	Doxycycline	100 mg b.i.d. × 5 days
	Alternative: ciprofloxacin	500 mg b.i.d. × 5 days

The most common indication for empiric antibiotic therapy is traveler's diarrhea. A treatment regimen usually consists in sulfamethoxazole-trimethoprim taken twice daily for 3 days or until symptoms resolve.

Although physicians are asked to prescribe antibiotics and antidiarrheals empirically, they should resist. Drugs that are effective for one disease may exacerbate another. For instance, antibiotics effective for shigellosis may enhance the carrier state of salmonellosis. Opiate-containing agents such as diphenoxylate hydrochloride (Lomotil) may convert a nonbacteremic dysentery into sepsis or produce serious problems such as toxic megacolon. Opiates and anticholinergics also carry with them the risk of side effects such as ileus, dry mouth, blurred vision, drowsiness, urinary retention, and insomnia. The psychological benefits of simply prescribing a medication are acknowledged. Compounds such as Kaopectate and Pepto-Bismol can confer this psychological benefit and are generally safe. Wait for culture results before starting antibiotics (Table 43–10). Certain exceptions exist, such as treating antibiotic-associated colitis when the history is appropriate. For example, antibiotics may be started during septic shock in an elderly patient with adherent yellowish plaques on the bowel wall, as seen on endoscopy.

There are many other causes of infectious diarrhea, including *Clostridium perfringens*, *Listeria monocytogenes*, *Aeromonas*, *Hydrophilia*, and *Bacillus cereus*. Each family physician must decide the point at which consultation, hospitalization, or referral is indicated. Symptoms such as nocturnal diarrhea, weight loss of 10 to 20 per cent, and progressive abdominal pain are important clues that indicate the need for further evaluation. It should be emphasized that most acute diarrhea syndromes are self-limited.

Among adults, sporadic idiopathic chronic diarrhea has been recognized as a specific syndrome that can last many months. In the presence of a negative work-up, however, most cases are self-limited (Afzalpurkar et al., 1992).

GASTROINTESTINAL BLEEDING SYNDROMES

Upper GI hemorrhage most frequently presents as *hematemesis* (the vomiting of blood or a darker coffee-ground-like material). Initially, it may or may not be associated with melena, a black, tarry, sticky substance with a sickly sweet odor. *Hemorrhoidal bleeding* is characterized by the passage of bright red blood after the bowel movement with soiling of the toilet tissue and toilet water with blood and streaks of bright red blood on the stool. In contrast, *hematochezia*, or lower GI hemorrhage, manifests as the passage of large amounts of bright red to burgundy-colored stool.

Because hematemesis, melena, or hematochezia due to any cause is associated with significant blood loss, patients with this condition merit hospitalization. Unwitnessed or dubious self-reports of bleeding should be evaluated on an urgent basis.

Ninety per cent of patients with GI hemorrhage admitted to the hospital stop bleeding within 24

TABLE 43–11. DIFFERENTIAL DIAGNOSES FOR GI BLEEDING

Upper GI Tract
  Esophageal lesion
    Varices
    Mallory-Weiss syndrome
    Cancer
    Erosive esophagitis
  Gastric lesion
    Erosive gastritis
      Gastric ulcer
      Cancer
      Varices
    Duodenal ulcer
  Epistaxis

Lower GI Tract
  Diverticulosis
  Angiodysplasia
  Cancer
  IBD
  Ischemic disease
  Coagulopathy
  Radiation
  Colitis
  Polyps
  Hemorrhoids
  Other

Rectum
  Hemorrhoids
  Fissure
  Cancer
  Polyp
  IBD
  Other

IBD = inflammatory bowel disease including Crohn's disease, ulcerative colitis, and many of the infectious diseases such as those caused by *Shigella, Yersinia, Campylobacter,* and others.

hours. Rapid diagnosis is advisable in order to plan treatment and to perform intervention endoscopy with coagulation of bleeding sites where appropriate. Whereas most patients with upper GI bleeding have hematemesis, melena, or both, about 15 per cent of these patients have only hematochezia with a negative nasogastric aspirate.

False alarms that mimic melena can be caused by iron, bismuth preparations, or certain fruits, such as blackberries or cherries. A fecal occult blood test quickly tells the story. For patients who are found to be anemic, a stool guaiac test (the most popular of which is Hemoccult) may be positive when there is no physical evidence of GI bleeding.

The differential diagnosis of the most common causes of GI bleeding is outlined in Table 43–11.

Clinical Epidemiology

In one study 351 patients admitted over a 10-year period with a diagnosis of acute GI hemorrhage were classified by bleeding location as follows: stomach/duodenum 57 per cent, esophageal varices 33 per cent, lower GI source 10 per cent.

Emergency surgery was required in almost one fourth of the cases (Greenberg, 1985). This report reflects a fairly typical experience of hospitals serving patients with GI hemorrhage, although the rate of emergency surgery is high.

Once patients have been documented to be experiencing GI hemorrhage, it is crucial that they be hospitalized as soon as possible. Immediately upon admission to the emergency facility, they should be assessed for evidence of hypovolemia and at least two large-bore intravenous catheters placed. A blood specimen should be sent to the laboratory for type and cross-match as well as coagulation factor assays. As soon as possible, surgical consultation should be requested.

According to the surveys, 87 per cent of practicing family physicians maintain intensive care unit privileges and therefore remain involved in the management of hospitalized patients with acute GI bleeding. Most family practice training programs have been able to secure hospital privileges in these areas, and most patients continue to expect and value involvement by the family physician.

Upper GI Bleeding

In the office or over the phone, the guiding principle is urgent evaluation of upper GI bleeding. The patient is usually directed to the emergency room if there is any doubt in the physician's mind. After vital signs have been recorded, intravenous lines established (wide open with normal saline), and blood sent to the laboratory for type and cross-match and coagulation studies, the history-taking process and thorough physical evaluation may begin. A nasogastric tube is placed to observe if any blood is present in the stomach and if it can be cleared with cool saline. Testing nasogastric aspirate that has no visible evidence of blood seems to be a worthless endeavor. If hypotension continues before the blood is ready, the lower part of the body should be elevated, and in some instances, a MAST suit (military antishock trousers) can be utilized.

The patient is asked if he or she has ever had bleeding before and if so what kind. The patient is quizzed about the presence of symptoms of peptic ulcer disease and if nonsteroidal anti-inflammatory drugs (NSAIDs) have been taken recently. The knowledge of a history of alcoholism is useful, as is a description of easy satiety and prolonged weight loss. These few simple questions cover the most common causes of upper GI hemorrhage: esophageal varices, peptic ulcer disease, erosive gastritis, and tumor. Physical examination may reveal the stigmata of chronic liver disease, an abdominal mass, hepatosplenomegaly, and ascites. In most instances, endoscopy is carried out once the patient has been stabilized. If lesions such as bleeding esophageal varices or a vessel in a peptic ulcer are seen, they are treated. Sclerotherapy of varices can stop bleeding but does not affect the patient's life course overall. The value of coagulating bleeding ulcers is still unknown, but the vast literature amassed on the subject seems to favor the procedure.

Lower GI Bleeding

Lower GI bleeding can be roughly divided into two vastly different types: (1) hematochezia and massive lower GI hemorrhage; and (2) minimal lower GI bleeding, which is seen with perianal disease and is probably the most common cause of bright red blood per rectum. It is rare for the bleeding of hemorrhoids to lead to anemia.

Patients presenting with large amounts of bright red blood per rectum or maroon stools must be stabilized as described in the previous section on upper GI hemorrhage. When the patient is stable, a nasogastric tube is placed to determine if the source of the blood is the upper GI tract. The bleeding in 10 to 15 per cent of patients with hematochezia has an upper GI source.

Patients with lower GI bleeding frequently have no history of their condition. The most common causes are diverticulosis, angiodysplasia, carcinoma, and ischemic colitis. The list of less common causes is vast (Cello, 1985).

Not only do patients with lower GI bleeding have no history of the disorder, but many have no current symptoms other than GI hemorrhage. The most common causes, namely diverticular disease and angiodysplasia, are asymptomatic. Patients with colon cancer and ischemic colitis may have had a change in their bowel habits and cramping.

Once again, as soon as two large-bore intravenous catheters have been inserted and blood has been sent for type and cross-match and measurement of coagulation factors, discussion with a consultant is helpful. For patients who have massive bleeding and who have been stabilized by blood transfusion, abdominal angiography is done to determine the site of bleeding. In the colon, embolization sometimes stops or slows the bleeding. If the patient is bleeding at a rapid rate, a technitium 99m-tagged red blood cell study that can reveal the bleeding site may be appropriate. This determination is important because if emergency surgery is required the surgeon must know the part of the bowel that is affected so it can be resected. Angiodysplasia and diverticuli bleed predominantly from the right side of the colon, but some actively bleeding lesions frequently stop bleeding when the patient is anesthetized and the abdomen is opened. At the time of surgery, it may be impossible to find the source of the hemorrhage. If the bleeding has slowed or stopped, the patient may then be given a balanced electrolyte purge (Golytely) and colonoscopy performed. The site of

TABLE 43–12. DIAGNOSTIC GRADING SYSTEM FOR HEMORRHOIDS

Degree	Criteria
First	No prolapse, usually asymptomatic
Second	Prolapse during defecation that later reduces spontaneously
Third	Prolapse that requires reduction but allows simple manipulation by the patient
Fourth	Prolapse that cannot be easily reduced by the patient

This hemorrhoidal classification system utilizes the degree of prolapse and is based on a description by Bedell AW: Thrombosed hemorrhoids. *In* Mayhew HE, Rogers LA (eds). Basic Procedures in Family Practice. New York, Churchill Livingstone, 1984, p 243, with permission.

bleeding can thus be determined in many patients, and sometimes treatment is definitive, such as when an angiodysplastic lesion of the right colon is cauterized.

PERIANAL DISEASE AND HEMORRHOIDS

Hemorrhoids are defined as varicosities arising from the hemorrhoidal veins in the perianal area (Table 43–12). This affliction of civilization may occur in 50 per cent or more of the population in the United States. Many are fortunate enough not to suffer from hemorrhoids, whereas some suffer from hemorrhoids repeatedly.

External hemorrhoids originate distal to the dentate line and drain via the inferior hemorrhoidal plexus to the iliac veins. Internal hemorrhoids are located proximal to the dentate line. These vessels come from the superior hemorrhoidal venous plexus, and they drain through the inferior mesenteric veins. Both internal and external hemorrhoids communicate with one another.

Both types of hemorrhoid may be asymptomatic. Some patients have no other discomfort than soiling of their underclothing because the hemorrhoids do not allow a hermetic seal of the anus. This situation may lead to perianal itching and burning due to the irritating fecal liquid. The most common presentation of hemorrhoids is asymptomatic bleeding. Most commonly, the person notices blood streaking the stool, and when they wipe themselves they find blood on the toilet tissue. If the bleeding is more active they may see blood in the toilet bowl.

For unknown reasons, hemorrhoids thrombose periodically. If the hemorrhoids are internal, the patient may just notice the prolapsing of tissue with the bowel movement; whereas if the hemorrhoids are external, extreme pain is felt, especially when the patient moves the bowels or even touches the swollen perianal area.

If the patient has acutely thrombosed *external* hemorrhoids (i.e., turgid, blue, and extremely tender), under the proper circumstances and with local anesthesia the physician can make a nick over the hemorrhoid. Removal of the clot affords the patient some relief. However, if the hemorrhoid has been thrombosed for several days and is "not ripe," the procedure only increases the pain.

When the patient has an acutely thrombosed external hemorrhoid, pain is the most difficult problem. Most salves and ointments are not helpful. Sometimes treatment with an anesthetic ointment is helpful. The most soothing therapy is for the patient to stay off the feet as much as possible to decrease the pressure of gravity and to take sitz baths throughout the day. In this instance, analgesics may be necessary. If a patient has recurring episodes of thrombosis that interfere with the quality of his or her life, local surgical treatments are available. Prior to surgery these patients should avoid constipation by using bulk agents, and if they feel tissue prolapsing after a bowel movement they should gently push the hemorrhoids back where they belong.

Ligation (or banding) is a simple, quick method used to relieve *internal* hemorrhoids in the office. It is not appropriate for external hemorrhoids because of the painful nature of the procedure when squamous epithelium is entrapped by the rubber bands that are applied. Specific instruments such as the McGiveny Hemorrhoid Ligator are available from surgical supply houses.

The patient need not be in a knee-chest position. The hemorrhoidal complex is visualized using a slotted anoscope, and the hemorrhoid is grasped with forceps (Fig. 43–1). Once stabilized, the barrel of the ligator is placed down over the hemorrhoidal complex, and a rubber band is mechanically displaced. It is this band placement that ligates the blood supply to the hemorrhoidal complex. When the patient experiences immediate severe pain, it usually indicates that the band has been placed below the pectinate line. In such cases, the rubber band should be snipped off and reapplied. Removal of an inappropriately placed band should be attempted even though there may be difficulty doing so.

The patient should be advised that a dull ache will ensue immediately after application of the ligation. Later in the day, the patient may have a feeling of fullness or an urge to defecate, which should be resisted. The discomfort is rarely severe enough to cause the patient to be absent from work, but symptoms persist at a low level over the next 2 to 3 days. Stool softeners and analgesics are usually prescribed, depending on the judgment of the physician. It is recommended that not more than one hemorrhoid be ligated every 3 weeks. Hundreds of thousands of these procedures have been performed in offices, although it should be noted that some specialists have stopped performing hemorrhoidal banding. In May 1985 four case reports described death following rubber band ligation of internal hemorrhoids. These reports underline the fact that increasing pain following hemorrhoidal banding should not be ignored as an insignificant symptom. These reports emphasize that "the combination of urinary hesitancy, perianal pain, and systemic symptoms shortly after ligation of hemorrhoids should alert the physician to a potential life threatening condition requiring immediate evaluation and therapy" (Russell and Donahue, 1985).

There are options for nonmedical treatment of hemorrhoids in the office. Ligation has been described, and sclerotherapy and cryosurgery have their proponents. The equipment for ligation and sclerotherapy is relatively inexpensive. Family physicians with cryosurgery units in the office can adapt them to many uses, one of which is the treatment of hemorrhoids. An infrared coagulator is another option that produces good results. Although the equipment is more expensive, the infrared coagulation method has emerged as the easiest to learn and use.

ANAL FISSURE

The anal tissue is closely related to that of the hemorrhoid. A fissure, which is a crack that occurs in the mucocutaneous line, is painful, especially with defecation, and it frequently leads to blood on the surface of the stool. Constipation results because of fear of pain with defecation. One may see the fissure during physical examination of the area, although many of these patients are almost impossible to examine in this area because of discomfort. They may respond to analgesic ointments, but many who continue with chronic symptoms do well with a surgical consultation. With the patient under anesthesia, the surgeon stretches the muscles of the anal opening, a method that frequently results in healing of the fissure.

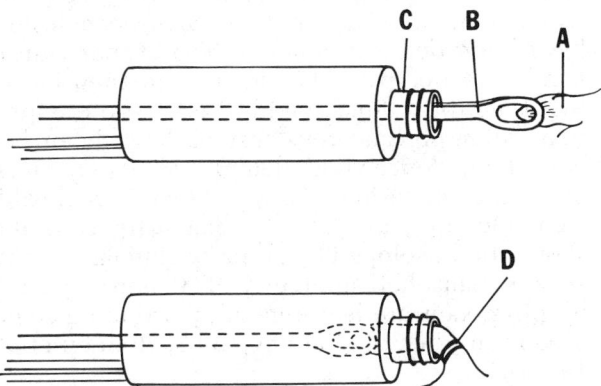

FIGURE 43–1. Rubber band ligation of an internal hemorrhoid. A = hemorrhoid; B = ring; C = double-banded ligator; D = double bands. See text for discussion of the procedure. (From Mayhew HE: Basic Procedures in Family Practice: An Illustrated Manual. New York, Churchill Livingstone, 1984, p 247, with permission.)

COLORECTAL CANCER

Approximately 150,000 Americans are diagnosed with colorectal cancer each year, one half of whom die within 5 years. Most of these patients come to the physician after symptoms have occurred. It is now clear that for colon cancer the earlier the stage and the more limited to the bowel wall is the lesion, the more promising is the 5-year survival rate. Whereas 50 per cent of patients who appear with symptoms die within 5 years, 80 to 90 per cent of patients with tumors detected with screening programs and whose tumors are localized to the bowel wall survive. Because the main risk factor in the United States is age, the best way to save people from this disease is to detect it in its early stages by screening the asymptomatic individual over age 50.

Screening is especially valuable, as it appears that colon cancers take many years to grow and become invasive. Many of them, if not most, arise from colorectal polyps.

The American Cancer Society Guidelines of 1980 were established on the basis of sophisticated mathematic modeling techniques that have been endorsed by the American Academy of Family Physicians and other institutions. These recommendations include annual rectal examinations starting at age 40 and three fecal occult blood tests annually starting at age 50. Sigmoidoscopic examinations are recommended every 3 to 5 years starting at age 50. In clinical practice, the major barriers to early detection have been patient and physician noncompliance.

Diagnostic Yield of Screening

The diagnostic yield of the rectal examination for cancer is low (3 to 5 per cent). Compliance with fecal occult blood tests ranges from 22 to 80 per cent (Rodney and Ruggerio, 1985c). Elderly patients, with the greatest age-related risk, report a reluctance to lean down into a toilet bowl and attempt to retrieve, with a small wooden stick, a fresh stool specimen to be smeared on a small card. The card is then stored in their house, pending transport by them to their physician at a later time. Many of the recommendations regarding avoidance of false positives such as those due to red meat, aspirin, and peroxidase-containing foods (beets, radishes, turnips) are usually ignored. The low sensitivity for polyps (5 to 20 per cent) and cancer (25 to 70 per cent) has raised serious doubts about the wisdom of mass screening for fecal occult blood. However, it is the best test physicians have at present and should be offered to the patient with enthusiasm until we have something better to suggest. Only 3 to 5 per cent of patients over age 50 are found to have a positive fecal occult blood test. About 15 per cent of those individuals have polyps,

and 2 to 3 per cent of the latter patients have cancer, most often in an early stage. It is important that the fecal occult blood test card be developed as soon as possible after collection, as the true positive rate diminishes with time. If even one of the three specimens is positive for blood, the patient must be evaluated. A repeat examination is not indicated: A single positive stool is a beacon for carcinoma. Unless there are mitigating circumstances, a positive fecal occult blood test should lead to colonoscopy. There is debate about whether the patients should have only sigmoidoscopy and barium enema, as the yield is low for treatable lesions such as polyps. Considering cost restraints, the performance of an air contrast barium enema and sigmoidoscopy is a legitimate option for patients with positive stools. Colonoscopy is emerging as the most sensitive and specific examination. Family physicians are encouraged to develop these skills (Rodney 1993a).

Poor acceptance of rigid sigmoidoscopy had been recorded in multiple studies. The 1980s, however, witnessed the introduction of flexible endoscopy into the office of the family physician. Diagnostic yields became higher, patient comfort was improved, and the technique was teachable (Rodney, 1992; Rodney and Felmar, 1984). Sensitivity was 40 to 80 per cent, depending on the depth of insertion, and the predictive value of a positive test was nearly 100 per cent. Videoendoscopy and image processing allowed documentation, remote consultation, patient education, and a variety of powerful information management techniques that could be performed at relatively low cost in the office (Rodney, 1985a). A 5-year longitudinal study suggested that flexible sigmoidoscopy in the office was associated with positive changes in the behavior of physicians and patients for all of the colorectal cancer screening tests (Rodney, 1985b; Rodney and Albers, 1986; Rodney et al., 1985d). It should be pointed out that in this series and most others most procedures were performed in patients with two or more GI symptoms. Significant lesions have been detected among 10 to 20 per cent of family practice patients who are screened for the first time (prevalence yield). Follow-up examinations after precancerous lesions have been harvested (incidence yield) detect a lower percentage of significant lesions. New data support flexible sigmoidoscopy as a basic diagnostic skill that should be developed by all practicing family physicians (Ransohoff and Lang, 1993); and some family physicians are learning and performing colonoscopy in practice (Rodney, 1988; Rodney et al., 1993a).

Patients over age 50 should have a yearly fecal occult blood test; and starting at age 50 patients should have flexible sigmoidoscopic examinations every 3 years. If an adenomatous polyp is seen on fibersigmoidoscopy colonoscopy is indicated, because in 20 to 30 per cent of the patients more polyps appear proximally. The battle against colorectal cancer, one of the most common cancers in the United States, must be fought at the family physician's office where the physician must convince his or her asymptomatic patients who are 50 years of age and older to do uncomfortable things such as collect stools for blood and present themselves for sigmoidoscopy and colonoscopy.

JAUNDICE SYNDROMES

For purposes of clarity, there are two categories of jaundice in clinical use. The first category includes patients who have no symptoms other than jaundice. The other category includes patients who are symptomatic, usually with anorexia, nausea, and fatigue, and who are usually suffering from parenchymal liver damage. In contrast, the first group may have anything from cholestatic jaundice to carcinoma of the pancreas. In either of the two cases, the jaundice is not a medical emergency. Patients may be jaundiced as long as 6 months due to an obstructed common bile duct before evidence of fibrosis appear. There are a few circumstances where early diagnosis and treatment are necessary, such as the patient with ascending cholangitis and sepsis or the one with acute pancreatitis caused by a stone in the common bile duct. Thus for the most part the work-up can take place thoughtfully and in an unhurried manner.

Neonatal Jaundice

In 1975 the purpose of identifying neonatal jaundice was to prevent kernicterus, a brain damage syndrome associated with a bilirubinemia of at least 20 mg/dL, leading to seizures and mental retardation. Since that time millions of infants in the United States have been placed under "bili lights" as prophylaxis for this serious disease. In retrospect, physicians have overexercised the strategy of catastrophic expectations. The major problem has been in the definition of risk for kernicterus. The initial definitions were based on the study of a few infants, with little or no thought given to the effect of the baby's race, feeding habits, and the natural history of physiologic jaundice (Newman and Maisels, 1992).

Kernicterus is real, and the differential diagnosis of neonatal jaundice is substantial. Benign physiologic jaundice is the most common type of jaundice. Certain clues alert the physician to the possibility of abnormal jaundice when jaundice is evident during the first 24 hours of life. When these clues are present, infection or isoimmunization should be considered. Physiologic jaundice rarely increases by more than 5 mg/dL during any one day. Physiologic jaundice is not associated with a direct bilirubin level of more than 1 to 2

mg/dL. Finally, physiologic jaundice usually resolves by 1 week in the term neonate or within 10 days in the premature infant. When neonatal jaundice exhibits unusual characteristics, a working differential diagnosis should include hemorrhage (e.g., cephalhematoma), isoimmunization (e.g., ABO incapability or Rh disease), infection, polycythemia, and congenital liver damage.

Useful historical items when assessing risk include the mother's gestational history and a description of the events surrounding the birth. A normal comprehensive neonatal physical examination should be performed, but laboratory studies define the syndrome. In the United States, screening is now legislated for hypothyroidism, phenylketonuria, and galactosemia. In addition, most hospitals have a protocol for the acquisition of cord blood while the mother and child are in the delivery room. All infants born to O-positive women must have their blood type determined. If the infant is type A, B, or AB, a Coombs test is done. When the Coombs test is positive, additional tests include direct and total bilirubin assays on the cord blood, as well as a hemogram with peripheral smear and a reticulocyte count. When the cord blood bilirubin level is 4 mg/dL or more, assays are done at 4, 8, 12, 18, and 24 hours of age. Additional assays are performed as indicated. If the bilirubin level is rising rapidly or phototherapy has been instituted, the assays are performed more frequently.

For the term infant, phototherapy rarely begins unless the bilirubin rises to 10 mg/dL before 12 hours of age, 12 mg/dL before 18 hours of age, and 14 mg/dL before 24 hours of age. Exchange transfusions are rarely initiated unless the bilirubin rises to 20 mg/dL or more. In the United Kingdom with certain age- and maturity-adjusted guidelines, phototherapy is rarely instituted before the bilirubin rises to 18 mg/dL, and exchange transfusions usually do not start until it is 23 mg/dL. It should be noted that Oriental, Indian, and Hispanic infants normally have a higher level of bilirubinemia. Among breast-fed infants, 63 per cent demonstrate a serum bilirubin level of 12 mg/dL or more at some time. Aggressive treatment strategies have led to a significant decline in the ability of some mothers to continue breast-feeding their infants. This factor is of concern, as breast-feeding has documented benefits and the benefits of zealously applied hospital phototherapy have not been documented. Furthermore, the financial costs of phototherapy are significant.

A number of investigators have pointed out the need to redefine physiologic jaundice and study more closely the natural history of neonatal jaundice in a variety of settings and ethnic phenotypes. Other investigators have pointed out that contemporary definitions of normal serum bilirubin have falsely labeled a group of healthy jaundiced babies with no disease (Maisels et al., 1988). Most frequently, a review of the mother's history, the mother's blood type, and a careful physical examination of the newborn are sufficient to rule out disease and act on significant data. Repeat serum bilirubin determinations, when indicated, can easily be obtained in the office or during a home visit. Rarely, hospitalization, consultation, or both are required. Jaundice that lasts beyond 1 week and a bilirubin level increasing beyond 17 mg/dL in the outpatient setting may merit consultation and serial observations on a day-to-day basis.

Jaundice in the Adult

For the purposes of clinical discussion, the topic of jaundice may be divided into two types: (1) jaundice with few other symptoms; and (2) jaundice with marked constitutional symptoms. The patients with few symptoms frequently present with obstructive jaundice or complicated parenchymal disease. The family physician should complete a full history and physical examination. The usual liver tests include bilirubin, SGOT, SGPT, and alkaline phosphatase assays and a prothrombin time. These tests are followed by an ultrasound examination of the liver to demonstrate if obstruction is present. With this baseline information, the patient with a clearly complicated case may be referred for consultation. The consultant recommends or engages in invasive studies. Most of the time the patient presenting with constitutional symptoms and jaundice is suffering from hepatitis.

Viral Hepatitis

In the United States, the most common causes of jaundice are hepatitis A, hepatitis B, and hepatitis non-A non-B. Hepatitis types C, D, and E have emerged as additional distinct, but not fully analyzed, subsets of viral hepatitis (Lee, 1993). There are small percentages of hepatitis secondary to mononucleosis, toxoplasmosis, and cytomegalovirus infection, but they are rare. Rarely, toxic poisoning (e.g., with carbon tetrachloride) or an allergic reaction to drugs mimics hepatitis. It is important to ask about drug exposure with any patient presenting with hepatitis, as certain drugs, such as isoniazid (INH), may destroy the liver if not stopped immediately.

Most patients with hepatitis present with lethargy, fatigue, anorexia, and possibly nausea and vomiting. Some have right upper quadrant pain and discomfort as well as yellow skin and dark urine. The presence of a high fever, above 38.3° C (101° F) is not uncommon.

Hepatitis A is common in industrialized populations and spreads readily when there is a breakdown in hygiene, such as in less developed countries. This illness, after an incubation period of 2 to 6 weeks, may result in a severe viral hepatitis syndrome, although most patients recover within several weeks. There is no chronic carrier state of hepatitis A, so once the patient acquires the disease immunity follows. Unfortunately, a small percentage of patients develop fulminant hepatic necrosis. At present, there is no way to identify these patients, nor is there any way to prevent their downhill course. The antibody that develops after infection is anti-HAV-IgG. Table 43–13 describes the current serologic markers for hepatitis. It is important to do some investigating to find the patient's contacts so that those exposed during the 2 weeks prior to the discovery of the patient's illness may be passively immunized with immune globulin.

Hepatitis B is a burden in our society. Ten per cent of those who are infected have evidence of chronic infection. This disease has been spread by sexual contact, especially among homosexual men, and by sharing of needles by drug users. In the hospital environment, the virus may be transmitted by needlestick. Prior to screening blood for transfusions for hepatitis B markers, hepatitis B was the most common cause of post-transfusion hepatitis. Now it accounts for fewer than 10 per cent of cases. See Figure 43–2 for the course of acute hepatitis B.

Hepatitis C usually follows transfusion up to 6 months later, or it may appear as a sporadic infection. Research studies now under way are isolating the actual virus particles, and soon more will be known about this disease that, up until now, has defied intensive epidemiologic investigation.

Hepatitis D virus (delta hepatitis) usually occurs in intravenous drug users—but only in former carriers of hepatitis B. Hepatitis E is a recently identified enteric virus that has only rarely been identified in the United States. Non-A non-B hepatitis remains as the description of those in whom no viral markers are detected and in whom no history of toxin or drug exposure can be found.

Acute viral hepatitis (A, B, or non-A non-B) frequently manifests as anorexia, malaise, nausea, vomiting, and the appearance of jaundice and dark urine. Some patients have a rash, and some have arthralgias and myalgias. Physical examination usually reveals an unhappy individual who appears jaundiced. The abdomen may be tender, especially in the right upper quadrant, where the liver is tender. Gentle percussion tenderness may be elicited as well.

The bilirubin, SGOT, SGPT, and alkaline phosphatase levels are elevated. The bilirubin level during an attack of acute viral hepatitis may go as high as 30 mg/dL. Patients have been reported with acute viral hepatitis who have had serum enzyme levels in the thousands. An elevation of the alkaline phosphatase level usually suggests a cholestatic phase. If the patient has a high grade fever and an alkaline phosphatase level 10 to 20 times

TABLE 43–13.   VIRAL HEPATITIS SEROLOGIC TESTS AND KEY DEFINITIONS

Test	Description
Hepatitis A	
Anti-HAV-IgM	IgM antibody to hepatitis antigen. The antibody of the IgM class signifies a recent acute infection. It develops at the onset of symptoms and resolves in less than 1 year.
Anti-HAV-IgG	IgG antibody to hepatitis A antigen. In the presence of a negative anti-HAV-IgM, it indicates a past HAV infection, which in turn indicates that the patient is immune. It appears 1–2 weeks after the IgM antibody.
Hepatitis B	
HBs/Ag	Hepatitis B surface antigen is the earliest indicator of the presence of acute hepatitis B infection. It can be present for several months before symptoms and may remain detectable for up to 6 months. Persistence past 6 months may indicate a chronic carrier state.
Anti-HBs	Antibody to hepatitis B surface antigen is an indicator of clinical recovery and subsequent immunity. It appears 1–2 months after HBsAg disappears, and it may be present for life.
HBcAg	No clinical significance; not readily available.
Anti-HBcIgG	Antibody to hepatitis B core antigen is an early indicator of acute infection. It is also a lifelong marker that represents past exposure. It may precede the detection of HBsAg. It persists for years but does not necessarily confer immunity.
IgM Anti-HBc	It is an early indicator of acute active infection and is usually short lived (3–6 weeks). Persistence of e antigen suggests progression to a chronic carrier state.
HBeAg	Active infection is present and the patient highly contagious.
Anti-HBe	Seroconversion from antigen to antibody is prognostic for resolution of infection; in a carrier it means very low infectivity.
IgM anti-HBc	IgM fraction of antibody to hepatitis B core antigen is the test of choice to rule out acute hepatitis B infection. The IgM fraction disappears within the first few months.
Hepatitis C	
Anti-HCV	Antibody to hepatitis C virus that appears 3–12 months after exposure.
Hepatitis D	
Anti-HDV	This antibody is hepatitis D virus may appear late and be short-lived.
Hepatitis NANB	No markers detectable, epidemiology parallels that of hepatitis B.

normal, a common duct stone with cholangitis must be suspected. Serum enzyme levels cannot be used to prognosticate. In other words, patients with extremely high levels of SGOT, SGPT, and bilirubin are not less likely to have total resolution than the others. Therefore the liver tests do not need to be repeated as a means of determining general resolution of the illness. The danger symptoms of severe parenchymal destruction is an altered sensorium (in the form of hepatic encephalopathy),

liver flap, and prolongation of the prothrombin time.

Because most of these diseases resolve without complications patients can be managed as outpatients, which gives them the opportunity to rest when fatigued and to eat when hungry. However, patients must keep utensils and glassware separate and cleaned separately from those of other family members. The liver disease is improving when the patient notices a return of appetite and lessening

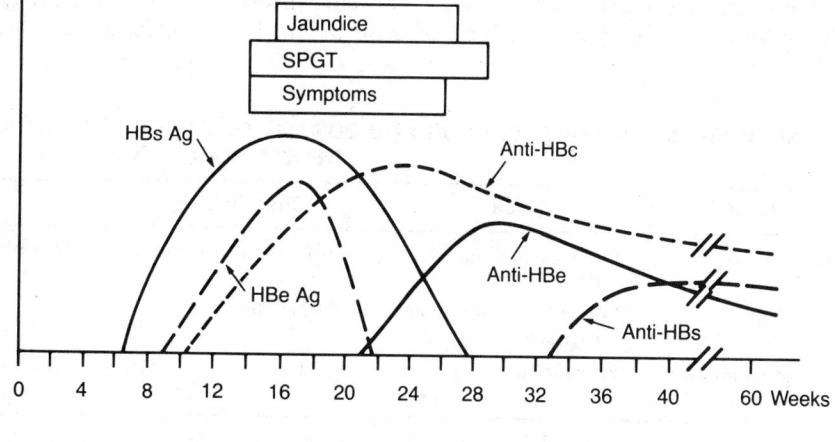

FIGURE   43–2. Course   of   acute hepatitis B.

Weeks After Exposure

TABLE 43–14. RECOMMENDATIONS FOR HEPATITIS B PROPHYLAXIS AFTER PERCUTANEOUS EXPOSURE

Source	Unvaccinated	Exposed Person Has Been Vaccinated
HBsAG-positive	HBiG (×1) immediately* Initiate HB vaccine† series	Test exposed person for anti-HBs‡ If inadequate antibody, HBIG§ (×1) immediately plus HB vaccine booster dose
Known source High risk Low risk HBsAg-positive	Initiate HB vaccine series Test source for HBsAg-positive, HBIG (×1) Initiate HB vaccine series	Test source for HBsAg only if exposed person is a vaccine nonresponder; if source is HBsAg-positive, give HBIG (×1) immediately plus HB vaccine booster dose Nothing required
Unknown source	Initiate HB vaccine series	Nothing required

* HBIG dose 0.06 mL/kg IM.

† HB vaccine dose 20 μg IM for adults; 10 μg IM for infants or children under 10 years of age. Give first dose within 1 week and second and third doses 1 and 6 months later.

‡ Unless the person has been tested within the last 12 months. If the exposed person has adequate antibody, no additional treatment is indicated.

§ Less than 10 standard reference units by radioimmunoassay, negative by enzyme linked immunoassay.

Adapted from MMWR 34:313, 1985.

of the fatigue. These signs appear before evidence of improvement of the liver on laboratory tests. Should the patient become confused and not be able to eat, hospitalization is indicated and consultation sought. If possible, it is beneficial to allow the patient to recover at home. Not only is this measure recommended for the patient's good, but when such patients are admitted to the hospital they become potential infective sources for hospital employees. Tables 43–14 and 43–15 contain recommendations for hepatitis immunization.

The clinical course of hepatitis is usually one of recovery over a period of weeks to months. The patient may return to physical activity when he or she feels ready. There is no evidence that premature exercising or physical activity prolongs or worsens acute viral hepatitis. However, if patients become physically active before being ready, they feel fatigued, worn out, and sometimes nauseated to the point of vomiting. Thus the best approach is to allow patients to resume their lives when they feel ready. If a patient with hepatitis does not recover as expected (i.e., exhibits persistently elevated liver tests and continuation of symptoms), referral to a gastroenterologist is indicated.

In many areas, subspecialists, such as gastroenterologists, are ready and willing to be consulted by telephone about a troublesome case a family physician is following. This contact is frequently helpful and sometimes makes a referral unnecessary. It must be mentioned parenthetically that there is no treatment that can reliably shorten the course of acute hepatitis or prevent chronicity, including the use of corticosteroids. These medications may make the patient feel better, but they have no effect on the disease. Steroids may even help lead to chronicity. Interferon has been approved for treatment of selected cases of chronic hepatitis B and hepatitis C. Most patients treated with interferon relapse and progress. Consultation or referral is recommended.

DYSPHAGIA SYNDROMES

Esophageal Disorders

Dysphagia describes the subjective report of having difficulty swallowing. Dysphagia is almost always due to anatomic constriction of the lumen of the esophagus caused by such diseases as peptic esophagitis with stricture, lower esophageal ring, and neoplasia. These lesions account for most of the patients who present with dysphagia. Much rarer diseases that cause difficulty swallowing are achalasia, scleroderma, and a vast number of sys-

TABLE 43–15. INDICATIONS FOR AND DOSAGE OF STANDARD HUMAN IMMUNE SERUM GLOBULIN FOR INTRAMUSCULAR USE

Illness	Goal	Dose (mL/kg)*	Comments
Hepatitis A	Prevention, single exposure	0.70 every 2–4 weeks	Use higher dose in adults or in those with heavy exposure
Hepatitis B	Prevention, continuous exposure	0.02–0.40	Repeat every 4–5 months if exposure continues
Hepatitis non-A, non-B	Prevention	0.12	Use with transfusions under special circumstances

* Immune serum globulin is a 16.5% solution (165 mg/mL) for intramuscular use, available only in 2- or 10-mL vials from several manufacturers.

Adapted from Anderson DC, Strohm R: Immunization. JAMA 258:3001, 1987, with permission. Copyright 1987, American Medical Association.

temic neurologic diseases including pseudobulbar palsy due to stroke. Even rarer causes include extrinsic compression of the esophagus by an enlarged atrium, aortic arch, aortic aneurysm, mediastinal tumors, or pulmonary cancer. Dysphagia should not be confused with *odynophagia,* which is defined as pain on swallowing.

The site of obstruction can usually be described easily by the patient by putting a finger over the area. The only exception is that some patients feel blockage at the gastroesophageal junction in their neck. A sense of obstruction in the neck may indicate *globus hystericus.* Patients with globus hystericus describe a lump or fullness in the throat that is present all of the time and yet does not impede swallowing. Globus hystericus is easily differentiated from dysphagia, and family physicians are aware of its frequent occurrence in response to psychosocial issues. When a patient presents with a description of dysphagia, globus hystericus cannot be easily ruled out; and a full evaluation is necessary. It should begin with upper GI tract endoscopy, although radiography may be an appropriate alternative initial test.

The terms *chalasia* and *achalasia* are related to the dysphagia syndromes; they describe mechanical problems of anatomy relating to the function of the lower esophageal sphincter. Achalasia is a rare cause of infant and adult regurgitation in which the lower esophageal sphincter remains closed, not relaxing so as to permit passage of food. Chalasia is seen in the more frequently observed infant regurgitation syndrome in which the lower esophageal sphincter does not close and the feedings are allowed to pass in a retrograde fashion from the stomach.

Clinical Epidemiology

The dysphagia syndromes are not frequent, although the family physician encounters several cases over the course of a year. Peptic esophageal stricture, lower esophageal rings, and cancer are diseases most prevalent in the middle-aged adult (40 to 60 years). Stroke patients and those with neurologically derived dysphagia represent a group of severely afflicted patients for whom pharyngeal dysphagia represents a special problem. Aspiration, chronic coughing, and decreased food intake are especially difficult problems for these patients. Consultation with specialists in rehabilitation medicine and nursing can be helpful. The geriatric literature points out that these stroke patients can rapidly develop nutritional depletion, aspiration pneumonia, and death (Detsky, 1994). Because there is no effective treatment for most patients with this condition, the use of percutaneous endoscopic gastrostomy has increased.

Useful Eponyms

Plummer-Vinson syndrome is characterized by iron deficiency anemia, atrophic gastritis, spoon nails, and upper esophageal webs. It is rare in the United States.

Barrett's esophagus describes the finding of columnar epithelium extending up into the esophagus, displacing the normal squamous epithelial covering. This condition results from chronic GI reflux and is frequently associated with esophagitis and stricture. The primary concern is that the metaplastic epithelium of Barrett's esophagus may be premalignant. Adenocarcinoma within the columnar line segment of the esophagus develops in 1 to 3 per cent of these patients over several years. Some physicians recommend repeated endoscopic evaluations with biopsies every 1 to 2 years to identify the dysplasia that is a forerunner of carcinoma.

Schatzki's ring, a circumferential band located at the squamocolumnar junction (lower esophageal ring), is characterized by the abrupt onset of food sticking in the esophagus. Eventually the food is regurgitated or passes on, and the patient can complete the meal without difficulty. As the ring narrows, the attacks occur more often and the bolus of food required to cause the obstruction is smaller. Endoscopic dilatation of these rings precludes the need for surgery. The beneficial effects of this procedure are generally permanent, although some patients require repeat dilatation several years later.

Zenker's diverticulum is located in the proximal (pharyngoesophageal) portion of the esophagus. It is an outpouching that retains undigested food, thereby compressing the true esophagus and producing dysphagia through external compression. Regurgitation of undigested food may follow within a variable time, ranging from hours to days. This condition is also a rare cause of dysphagia.

Present Illness and Review of Systems

The history is helpful for determining causes of dysphagia. Once the diagnosis is established, all of these patients require upper endoscopy. Some physicians recommend initial investigation with barium swallow x-ray studies.

A benign narrowing such as Schatzki's ring may present with acute distal esophageal obstruction when a large piece of food that has not been chewed thoroughly is swallowed. Such individuals then suddenly feel as though they are going to choke. They may salivate and tear and move around rapidly to obtain relief, and they sometimes try to drink a carbonated beverage. Eventually, they regurgitate the food, resulting in complete relief. When these patients do not have an acute obstruction from a large bolus of food, they rarely experience any dysphagia whatsoever.

Constant, progressive, rapidly evolving dysphagia without previous esophageal symptoms suggests carcinoma of the esophagus or gastric cardia. Intermittent dysphagia, similar to that occurring in the lower esophageal ring, may be seen in less dramatic form in patients suffering from motility disorders of the esophagus. Chronic dysphagia, described as being of waxing and waning intensity but sustained over the years, is more consistent with some of the neurologic motor disorders or with peptic esophageal stricture. If a long history of heartburn (pyrosis) has preceded the development of dysphagia, a benign esophageal stricture is likely to be the cause.

Regurgitation of undigested food with postprandial gurgling in the neck several hours after eating is suggestive of Zenker's diverticulum, a rare problem. In the patient who has sustained a stroke and has difficulty with speech as well as coughing after eating, oral pharyngeal dysphagia must be suspected.

Physical Findings

For most patients with dysphagia, three physical findings are particularly valuable. The most common finding is weight loss if the dysphagia is especially severe. Patients with carcinoma may have palpable supraclavicular nodes from metastatic disease or upper abdominal masses. Other than these few exceptions, the physical examination is not helpful. For those few patients who have neuromuscular dysphagia, glaring neurologic abnormalities are usually evident, or the patient has presented with dysphagia after having been diagnosed with a disabling neurologic disease. For patients who have sustained large strokes and experience difficulty swallowing, giving them a glass of water to drink is helpful. If the patient starts coughing and liquid comes through the nose, the diagnosis is almost certain. If the patient does not have a gag reflex when a tongue blade is inserted deeply, the diagnosis of pseudobulbar palsy is likely.

Diagnostic Plan

Initially, the best test is esophagoscopy, which is used to uncover any evidence of luminal obstruction. The only contraindication to the use of this test is the patient who has a severe neurologic disorder and in whom oropharyngeal dysphagia is suspected. In these patients a cine-esophagram with Gastrografin is most helpful.

If an esophageal stricture or a lower esophageal ring is seen at the time of endoscopy, it can be treated immediately with endoscopic dilation. Any tumors should be biopsied. Achalasia has a typical endoscopic appearance. The esophageal lumen is widely distended, with few or no contractions. The lower esophageal sphincter is tight, but once intubated the sphincter pops open.

If the results of endoscopy are negative, the next step is to obtain a cine-esophagram, with or without the patient swallowing a bolus of food. From that point, decisions can be made by the consultant for further work-up. Esophageal manometry can be a helpful test, but it is not available in all areas. Moreover, it requires a great deal of care and informed interpretation. The manometric study con-

firms the diagnosis in patients with achalasia, scleroderma, and many neurologic disorders.

Psychosocial Aspects and Special Considerations

In office practice, the evaluation of dysphagia is frequently straightforward. Most patients with this condition have lower esophageal rings or peptic esophageal strictures that can be treated by endoscopic dilatation.

Less frequently, this common complaint is the tragic precursor to terminal esophageal carcinoma, metastatic carcinoma, or both. With the appropriate consultation for definitive treatment of the primary cancer, the family physician becomes a provider of care and manager of resources during the terminal phase of these illnesses. He or she is equally responsible for the care and management of patients with irreversible neuromuscular disorders.

Chest Pain of Noncardiac Etiology

Some patients present with chest pain that suggests coronary ischemia, yet the results from a cardiac work-up are negative. Some of these patients are thought to have esophageal spasm. Frequently, they are difficult to evaluate. For such cases, consultation with a gastroenterologist or cardiologist for diagnostic evaluation may be helpful.

DYSPEPSIA SYNDROMES

This section deals with the most common causes of dyspepsia encountered in an ambulatory practice. They include nonulcer dyspepsia, peptic ulcer disease, and gastroesophageal reflux disease. Each of these conditions causes symptoms that are usually localized to the upper abdomen and lower mid-chest area.

Nonulcer Dyspepsia

Most agree that nonulcer dyspepsia is a variable, vaguely described feeling of upper abdominal discomfort that is related to the ingestion of food or drink. During the 1800s it was viewed as a symptom of overindulgence and is sometimes still viewed in this way. Patients usually complain that immediately after eating they notice bloating, distention, belching, flatulence, heartburn, or most often just a mild upset in the upper abdomen. This condition can be described as upset stomach, nausea, or even pain. Some emphasize one or all of the aforementioned symptoms. Many of these patients describe their discomfort as "my ulcer," although peptic ulcer disease has not been diagnosed. Only a small number of these patients have organic disease, and among those who do it is frequently due to a peptic ulcer or ingestion of NSAIDs.

Clinical Epidemiology

The extraordinary frequency of this generally noninfectious, non-neoplastic disorder is due to the dietary excesses and physical deconditioning of the twentieth century. In addition to adiposity, this condition is associated with tobacco and alcohol abuse. Stress is often closely related to the symptoms. In most patients these symptoms represent some of the manifestations of the irritable bowel syndrome, which affects 20 per cent of the population. Although stress plays a dominant role, a reduction of fatty, greasy foods and spices in the diet, sometimes in conjunction with taking an antispasmodic drug or antispasmodic–sedative combination, may result in marked relief. No organic disease is found even when these patients undergo extensive diagnostic evaluations. Indeed, they never develop organic disease such as peptic ulcer. This information is valuable to the patient because the worry engendered by their abdominal symptoms frequently adds to their overall stress.

Nonulcer dyspepsia may also be caused by medications that lower the pressure of the lower esophageal sphincter, such as nitrites, anticholinergics, some tranquilizers, and β-adrenergic agents (e.g., theophylline). Common dyspepsia-producing drugs are the NSAIDs (e.g., aspirin and ibuprofen).

Pregnancy is a self-limited condition that has been associated with decreased pressure of the lower esophageal sphincter. In any female of childbearing age with the recent onset of dyspepsia, the absence of pregnancy should be confirmed before any medication is prescribed.

In practice, fewer than 1 per cent of patients who present with dyspepsia have serious organic disease. However, it is the fear of serious illness that frequently causes the patient to seek an appointment. This fear may invoke the ordering of multiple radiologic and endoscopic investigations to rule out cancer. Most dyspepsia problems nevertheless remain idiopathic and self-limited.

Treatment

Because the symptoms of nonulcer dyspepsia and peptic ulcer disease can be similar, most physicians suggest that the patient be placed on a 8-week course of H_2 blockers. If the patient does not improve, endoscopy should be performed. If the patient does not respond to H_2 blockers or worsens after 7 to 10 days, re-evaluation should include endoscopy. In some patients a trial of sedative antispasmodic drugs for another 7 to 10 days may confirm the presence of nonulcer dyspepsia. If the symptoms resolve while the patient is on H_2 blockers, further diagnostic studies are unnecessary, as the diagnosis of peptic disease is likely. If the symptoms return when the H_2 blockers are stopped after 8 weeks of treatment, endoscopic evaluation should be considered.

Peptic Ulcer Disease

Benign gastric ulcers, pyloric channel ulcers, and duodenal ulcers are considered in this section. Esophageal ulcers are dealt with in the section on reflux esophagitis.

Peptic ulcer disease is frequently seen in the family physician's office. Most patients with this condition, unlike the patients with nonulcer dyspepsia, have a fairly straightforward history. They describe epigastric discomfort as covering a small or large area and describe the pain with varying adjectives, such as emptiness, burning, heaviness, and bloating. The finding that is suggestive of peptic ulcer disease, however, is that the onset of discomfort occurs 30 minutes to 2 hours after a meal and is relieved by eating. Some patients are also awakened at 2:00 to 3:00 a.m. and likewise find relief by eating or drinking. The recurring postprandial nature of the symptoms, with complete relief or almost complete relief after eating or drinking, is almost as good as a diagnostic study. When asked, many of these patients describe previous episodes that lasted weeks or months interspersed with periods that were totally symptom-free. This pattern is classic for peptic ulcer disease.

The only positive physical finding may be mild epigastric tenderness. Carcinoma of the stomach is suspected when patients in their late forties or fifties present for the first time with dyspepsia, anorexia, and coexisting weight loss. Table 43–16 depicts a risk scoring system for malignancy.

The American College of Physicians created a formal policy statement in response to the perceived overapplication of diagnostic testing for the dyspepsia syndromes (Kahn and Greenfield, 1985).

TABLE 43–16. RISK SCORING SYSTEM FOR GASTRIC MALIGNANCY AS THE CAUSE FOR DYSPEPSIA

Parameter*	Risk Multiplier
Age (years)	
50–59	2×
60–69	3×
>70	4×
Vomiting	2×
Male sex	2×
Smoking	3×
Previous ulcer	3×
Hiatal hernia present	3×

* These six historical items created a weighted score that correctly identified all malignancies in a group of 1600 patients presenting to a referral center in the United Kingdom.

From Holdstock G, Harmon M, Machin D, et al: Perspective testing of a scoring system designed to improve case selection for upper gastrointestinal investigation. Gastroenterology 90:1164, 1986, with permission.

Physicians were urged to utilize clinical judgment, technologic restraint, and where appropriate empiric therapy. Thus with dyspepsia or suspected peptic ulcer disease, therapy should precede laboratory investigations. The following statement by Kahn and Greenfield (1985) is a useful rule of thumb for sequencing most diagnostic strategies of the various dyspepsia syndromes: "Endoscopy is reserved for two subsets of patients: for those that have no response or minimal response to empirical therapy after 7 to 10 days; and for approximately 30 per cent of patients whose symptoms persist (improved, but not resolved) after a 6 to 8 week period of empirical therapy. If all dyspeptic patients are treated empirically, considerable diagnostic resources will be saved." Some physicians elect to treat dyspeptic patients who seemed to have the irritable bowel syndrome with a 2-week trial of sedative antispasmodics rather than H₂ blockers.

A wide variety of therapeutic agents are available (Table 43–17). Note that most of the agents have received FDA approval on the basis of proved effectiveness for documented dyspepsia due to peptic ulcer disease. It is acknowledged that many of these drugs are prescribed for nonulcer dyspepsia, even though the agents have not proved helpful in clinical trials of nonulcer dyspepsia (Nyren et al., 1986). Regimens that call for medication once a day at bedtime or twice a day are equally effective and can replace the initially recommended four times a day protocols. Furthermore, there has been evidence supporting maintenance therapy at reduced dosages (e.g., cimetidine 400 mg qhs, ranitidine 150 mg qhs, famotidine 20 mg qhs). Antacids continue to be an approved modality, but usually

patients prefer the ease and convenience of pills. Although side effects are sometimes associated with the H₂-receptor antagonists, they are rare. The margin of safety is judged to be so large that some predict over-the-counter status for cimetidine during the 1990s. Although there is much discussion regarding the relative advantages and disadvantages of the four widely available h₂-receptor antagonists, these agents are probably equivalent for most noncomplicated cases. Patients frequently notice some improvement within 1 to 3 days, in contrast to the more prolonged symptom resolution phases seen with sucralfate and antacids.

For patients taking many drugs, such as the elderly, cimetidine is most likely to produce drug interactions. Theoretically, the other H₂-receptor antagonists would be a better choice in the elderly, although it has not been proved by clinical trials. Another special situation among elderly patients is upper GI bleeding secondary to NSAID usage. A prostaglandin-type drug known as misoprostol (Cytotec) has been approved for the prevention of NSAID-induced gastric ulcers in patients at high risk of complications (e.g., the elderly, those with debilitating disease, and those with proved NSAID-related bleeding). Although legitimate for selected cases, misoprostol has not been proved to reduce symptoms associated with NSAID use or ulcer complications when NSAID therapy is continued (Feldman et al., 1992). Overall, prophylactic misoprostol is rarely indicated.

Omeprazole (Prilosec) is the first of a new class of antisecretory agents. These agents bind the proton pump of the parietal cell, inhibiting the final step in the secretion of hydrogen ions into the gastric vesicles. Omeprazole is potent, and one dose acts for more than 24 hours. Omeprazole is approved to treat refractory gastroesophageal reflux and acute duodenal ulcers. It provides good, fast symptomatic relief, but it is not approved for maintenance therapy. Most physicians reserve it for patients who do not respond to the H₂ blockers (Maton, 1991).

A problem does arise in pregnant women who have peptic ulcer disease. None of the H₂-receptor antagonists has been shown to be free of teratogenic effects in humans. Therefore these patients must tolerate unwieldy antacid regimens or use Sucralfate. Misoprostol is clearly contraindicated.

Once a therapeutic agent is selected, it seems reasonable to treat the patient for 6 to 8 weeks and then stop. If the symptoms do not return, no further investigation or treatment is necessary. More than half of such successfully treated patients, though, have a recurrence. It seems reasonable to reinitiate therapy when a recurrence is brought to the attention of the physician. A re-evaluation at that time is necessary to determine if aggressive invasive diagnostic studies should be carried out. Once again, there are well respected experts on both sides of this decision. One study followed a group of pa-

TABLE 43–17. COMMONLY PRESCRIBED AGENTS FOR EMPIRIC THERAPY OF PRESUMED DYSPEPSIA DUE TO PEPTIC ULCER DISEASE

Agents	Dosage Schedule
H₂-receptor antagonists	
Cimetidine (Tagamet)	400 mg b.i.d. or 800 mg q.h.s.
Ranitidine (Zantac)	150 mg b.i.d. or 300 mg q.h.s.
Famotidine (Pepcid)	20 mg b.i.d. or 40 mg q.h.s.
Nizatidine (Axid)	300 mg q.h.s. or 150 mg b.i.d.
Sucralfate (Carafate)	1 gm q.i.d. or 1–2 gm b.i.d.
Antacids	
Liquid	140 mEq (usually 30 mL); 1 and 3 h pc and q.h.s. *or*
Tablet	120 mEq tablet q.i.d.
Omeprazole (Prilosec)	20 mg daily (not approved for long-term maintenance; a second-line drug)

A variety of other drugs, such as anticholinergics, tricyclic antidepressants, bismuth preparations, and prostaglandin analogues, have been widely tried outside the United States but have not been proved to be as effective as H₂-blockers for the treatment of peptic ulcer disease. There is little evidence that combined therapy accomplishes more than the administration of individual agents.

tients with duodenal ulceration for 5 years. Half of the patients were randomized to receive cimetidine continuously, and the others received it intermittently (i.e., for symptoms only). At the end of 5 years, the patients receiving maintenance therapy had a 24 per cent probability of remaining symptom-free, whereas none of the patients receiving intermittent therapy had remained symptom-free (Wade and Roley-Jones, 1988). This study points out that any patient who has had two or more relapses within 2 years probably is a candidate for maintenance on a continuous h2-receptor antagonist (or equivalent). Some patients prefer to wait for symptoms to appear and then initiate a full therapeutic program. This choice is acceptable, as symptoms are usually obliterated within 2 to 5 days and in the early stages are not severe. The optimum duration and long-term effects of these treatment strategies are unknown.

If a patient fails the trial period H2 blockers and a gastric ulcer is found through endoscopy, multiple biopsy specimens from around the rim are obtained to determine whether the lesion is benign or malignant. It appears that waiting 2 to 4 weeks on an empiric H2-blocker regimen would not affect the outcome of a gastric carcinoma.

Patients with nonulcer dyspepsia and peptic ulcer disease are best cared for by a primary care physician. By seeing the patient in continuity with full understanding of the patient's family history, lifestyle, personal values, and medical history, this physician is most effective. In selected cases, the family physician may request advice from a consultant. When the consultation is completed, the patient should return to the care of the family physician.

After a decade of debate, several studies show that eradication of *Helicobacter pylori* reduces both ulcer-healing time and the ulcer-recurrence rate (Graham et al., 1991; Hentschel et al., 1993). In a study by Graham et al., duodenal and gastric ulcers healed more quickly when treated with metronidazole (Flagyl) 250 mg tid, tetracycline 500 mg qid, and bismuth subsalicylate (Pepto-Bismol) 1 to 2 tablets with each meal and 2 tablets at bedtime. This triple therapy was given for 2 weeks. Simultaneously, ranitidine (Zantac) 300 mg qhs was given for 16 weeks. In addition to ranitidine, Hentschel et al., used metronidazole 500 mg tid and amoxicillin 750 mg tid. They provided concomitant therapy with an H2 blocker.

Although the diagnosis of *H. pylori* infection can be confirmed by the C13 urea breath test, family physicians are more likely to utilize tests of biopsy specimens. Biopsy specimens can be cultured or stained. Some family practice offices are using the *Campylobacter*-like organism (CLO test) test because of its accuracy, accessibility, and low cost. This development is important as more family physicians are performing esophagogastroduodenoscopy (Hocutt et al., 1994).

Confounding variables include the high prevalence of *H. pylori* among large groups of asymptomatic patients. Serology testing for IgG antibodies to *H. pylori* is of limited value for this reason. Studies are lacking on nonulcer dyspepsia patients, and most family practice dyspepsia patients do *not* have ulcers. Although physicians differ in opinion, *H. pylori* eradication therapies seem reasonable in infected patients refractory to other standard treatments (Rodney, 1993).

Gastroesophageal Reflux Disease

Gastroesophageal reflux is common. Symptoms of gastroesophageal reflux disease (GERD) occur daily in 7 per cent and every 3 days in 33 per cent of the population. As many as 44 per cent of the people have symptoms of GERD on a monthly basis. Indigestion aids are used two or more times a week by 13 per cent of the population. Most of these individuals have never discussed dyspepsia with their physicians. GERD is almost always associated with a hiatal hernia. Approximately 50 per cent of people over 50 years of age have a hiatal hernia, as do up to 84 per cent of patients with erosive esophagitis.

The most common symptom is substernal burning after eating, with the patient describing the sensation as rising from the epigastric area up to the neck. It is made worse by fatty foods, spicy foods, and large meals, especially if accompanied by alcohol or caffeine. When these patients do heavy lifting or bending, they may feel food or liquid rising into their throat; and some are awakened at night with a suffocating cough as acid and gastric contents rise up into the throat. The substernal burning is frequently relieved by drinking fluids, especially antacids. When the pain is intense, it may mimic coronary heart disease and may even radiate up into the jaws and down both arms.

Most patients with reflux esophagitis do not have visible abnormalities on endoscopy. Endoscopy has a sensitivity of about 50 per cent and a specificity of nearly 100 per cent. The barium esophagram has a sensitivity of 40 per cent and a specificity of 95 per cent for GERD, but the radiographs cannot detect mucosal damage. Histologic study can increase sensitivity and specificity, but the biopsy specimens must be obtained more than 2.5 cm proximal to the gastroesophageal junction (because transient reflux occurs in normal subjects). Interpretation requires a well oriented specimen. The characteristic findings are a thickened basal layer (comprising more than 15 per cent of the thickness of the mucosa) and relative lengthening of the papillary projections of the lamina propria (comprising more than two thirds of the total thickness of the epithelium) (Fennerty and Sampliner, 1993).

The physician cannot tell by history alone whether the patient has ulcerative esophagitis with peptic ulcerations or just symptoms of acid reflux. The main complication of reflux esophagitis is peptic ulceration and stricture, which is uncommon. The risk of cancer is increased only when a Barrett's esophagus arises as a result of chronic reflux.

It is unclear why GI reflux is symptomatic in some patients and not in others. Common findings in the asymptomatic group are obesity and dietary indiscretion, possibly combined with smoking.

Diagnosis

When patients present with typical symptoms of reflux esophagitis, a therapeutic trial is in order. Endoscopy is not necessary at this stage, nor is an upper GI series. First, patients are instructed carefully about their diet. They are told to avoid greasy foods, fatty foods, and spicy foods because they enhance reflux. The size of the meals should be diminished, and the patient should have nothing to eat for at least 3 to 4 hours before bedtime. Caffeinated beverages are allowed in moderation and are not harmful. Decaffeinated beverages frequently produce more symptoms because of the way they are prepared. It is known that spicy foods cause symptoms but do not physically harm the mucosa. The reaction is similar to pouring alcohol over a cut. It hurts, but the cut is not made larger and the healing is not affected. If patients smoke, they are encouraged to stop. If unable to stop, they should be asked carefully about the use any of irritant drugs, such as NSAIDs.

Treatment

If overweight, patients are encouraged to reduce, as even a 5 to 10 per cent loss of weight may result in tightening of the lower esophageal sphincter and decreased reflux. Patients are also advised to place a 3 to 4 inch block under the bedpost at the head of the bed, so when they are sleeping at night there is encouragement for the acid and reflux material to stay below the sphincter. For patients with mild symptoms, antacid tablets or liquid may be used. For those with severe symptoms, H_2 blockers are prescribed and continued sometimes for many months. If the patient does not experience improvement or has any symptoms of dysphagia whatsoever, the family physician should consider endoscopy, a consultation, or both.

GASTROPATHY DUE TO INTAKE OF NSAIDs

Although cited as having fewer side effects than aspirin, NSAIDs produce gastric ulceration and hemorrhage in a small number of patients. Some patients who have symptoms when taking the drugs have no ulcers on endoscopy. Other patients who have GI hemorrhage without prior symptoms are found to have ulcerations in the stomach or duodenum, or both. Thus the endoscopic appearance may be totally unrelated to the symptoms.

If the patient who is taking these drugs develops symptoms, the drug is suspended and an H_2 blocker is started. Depending on the severity of the condition, enteric-coated aspirin (Ecotrin) may be used, or the physician may choose one of the nonacetylated salicylates such as Trilisate, Salsalate, or Dilazid. If symptoms recur or continue despite the administration of H_2 blockers and the drug must be continued, consultation may be requested for evaluation and possible endoscopy at this time. It is important to note that patients who have a history of an ulcer while taking aspirin in the past should be taking H_2 blockers while they are taking the NSAIDs, even if the administration takes place over a prolonged period.

Cisapride is approved by the FDA for the symptomatic treatment of patients with nocturnal heartburn due to GERD. Because GERD is a chronic disease, most patients use a variety of medications to keep their symptoms in check. Although studies have been inconclusive, many have prescribed metoclopramide (Reglan) 5 to 20 mg taken before meals and at bedtime. One disadvantage of this drug has been the occurrence of lethargy, fatigue, psychotropic side effects, and extrapyramidal side effects, which occur in 10 to 30 per cent of patients. Some physicians recommend against long-term maintenance therapy.

By contrast, the adverse effects associated with cisapride have been few and mild. Generally, fewer than 2 per cent of patients stop therapy because of side effects. The recommended dose is 10 mg four times daily (15 minutes before meals and at bedtime). Some patients require adjustment to 20 mg qid to obtain satisfactory results. The duration of therapy is generally 8 to 12 weeks, but some believe cisapride has a great potential for "off-label" indications, such as long-term maintenance therapy.

CHRONIC ABDOMINAL PAIN AND DIARRHEA

Many patients who come to the family physician complain of chronic abdominal pain and diarrhea. The task is to differentiate functional from organic disease and then to be able to apply proper therapy. Most of these patients are suffering from irritable bowel syndrome. The following discussion should help the physician arrive at the correct diagnosis.

Inflammatory Bowel Disease

History of Present Illness and Pathophysiologic Correlations

The two major categories of inflammatory bowel disease—ulcerative colitis and Crohn's disease—

have several unique pathologic features and some distinct clinical differences that help distinguish them.

There is no known cause for these diseases. Ulcerative colitis is limited to the colon and rectum, whereas Crohn's disease may involve any part of the GI tract from the mouth to the anus. Five per cent of patients with either of these disorders may have extraintestinal manifestations. Ulcerative colitis, which also includes proctitis and proctosigmoiditis, involves the rectum in more than 95 per cent of cases; and if there is proximal spread, the involvement is continuous and symmetric. Crohn's disease, on the other hand, involves the rectum in fewer than 50 per cent of cases; and the mucosal abnormalities are discontinuous, asymmetric, and patchy. With ulcerative colitis the mucosa is primarily involved, whereas with Crohn's disease the entire thickness of the bowel wall is affected by the inflammatory reaction, explaining the obstruction, abscesses, and fistula seen with Crohn's disease. These lesions are rarely seen in patients with ulcerative colitis. Multiple granulomas are found in the diseased tissue in 60 per cent of patients with Crohn's disease, whereas there are none in ulcerative colitis. With irritable bowel syndrome, the mucosa and biopsy specimens of the wall of the bowel are normal. The finding of a severe perianal fistula with burrowing and abscesses are hallmarks of Crohn's disease.

Clinical Epidemiology

The incidence of idiopathic inflammatory bowel diseases crosses racial and ethnic barriers. In the United States, irritable bowel disease seems to be much more common among Whites than Blacks, and among females than males. The median age at presentation is approximately 30 years, with about 25 per cent of patients being teenagers. Although there are no genetic markers, disease clusters in families have been noted in approximately 30 per cent of the cases. Although some have speculated that there is a male predominance for Crohn's disease and a female predominance for ulcerative colitis, these distinctions are not useful in clinical practice. It should be noted that there have been secondary peaks in the incidence of ulcerative colitis and Crohn's disease during or beyond the sixth decade. Utilizing data from the Mayo Clinic Epidemiology Project, the prevalence of chronic ulcerative colitis among residents of Rochester, Minnesota during the 19-year period from 1960 to 1979, was 225 per 1 million population (Treacher et al., 1986).

History of Present Illness and Review of Systems

Most patients with inflammatory bowel disease present with chronic diarrhea that may not be different in any way from the diarrhea of patients with irritable bowel syndrome. However, when diarrhea is bloody, inflammatory bowel disease is more likely. A history of weight loss and awakening in the middle of the night because of diarrhea almost guarantees the diagnosis of organic disease. In youths, retarded growth or delayed puberty is common with Crohn's disease. Other symptoms such as fever, anorexia, and weight loss are common with inflammatory bowel disease. Extraintestinal manifestations such as iritis, nondeforming arthritis, ankylosing spondylitis, erythema nodosum, pyodermic gangrenosum, and aphthous ulcerations can occur in 2 to 5 per cent of patients with inflammatory bowel disease but never with the irritable bowel syndrome.

Most patients with ulcerative colitis present with diarrhea that is mild to moderate and without constitutional symptoms. The more severe the illness, the greater the number of stools and the more likely it is they are accompanied by constitutional symptoms such as fever, fatigue, and weight loss. The course of ulcerative colitis can be intermittent with flare-ups, and remission can occur without therapy. A few patients with ulcerative colitis present with severe or fulminant panniculitis, ranging from an acute abdomen to toxic megacolon; and there is little doubt that these patients require urgent hospitalization. During an exacerbation, patients with ulcerative colitis and Crohn's disease can look and feel ill, yet if the disease is mild they can appear normal except for the complaint of diarrhea.

When Crohn's disease primarily involves the colon, it may be indistinguishable from ulcerative colitis. Because Crohn's disease frequently affects the terminal ileum or the terminal ileum and the right side of the colon, patients with this condition may have steady right lower quadrant pain due to transmural inflammation. The pain may worsen with movement. Sometimes abscesses develop because of the microperforations in the area of disease, and sometimes acute small bowel obstruction appears because of cicatricial narrowing and the injudicious ingestion of high-residue food. Some of these people develop painful perianal fissures and fistulas that are diagnostic of Crohn's disease.

Physical Findings

The patient with ulcerative colitis or Crohn's disease may exhibit weight loss and anemia. Oral aphthous ulcers may be present. Less frequent findings are erythema nodosum, iritis, and asymmetric nondeforming arthritis. With Crohn's disease a tender mass may be felt in the right lower quadrant, and during the illness the abdominal examination may reveal mild to severe tenderness. However, during remissions the results of the physical examination may be entirely negative. When a mass is palpated, the possibilities are matted, inflamed loops of small bowel versus an abscess. Bowel sounds are not helpful unless the patient presents with severe cramping abdominal pain and distention. In this severe setting, a lack of bowel sounds suggests obstruction. Positive fecal occult blood in a patient with chronic diarrhea changes the diagnosis from functional to organic disease, requiring a full evaluation. Pelvic examination should be performed in all female patients. At the bedside of patients with irritable bowel syndrome, the tenderness of muscle spasm-related pain tends to diminish with persistent palpatory pressure, whereas the inflamed bowel causes pain that does not diminish and frequently becomes more uncomfortable.

Endoscopic Examination

Sigmoidoscopic examination and fecal occult blood testing should be part of the examination in patients presenting with chronic diarrhea. Colonoscopy of the cecum is not always required, but flexible sigmoidoscopy is essential for initial evaluation.

Endoscopically, the findings of confluent erythematous inflammation of the rectum is most consistent with ulcerative colitis and infectious colitis. Pseudopolyp formations indicate chronic inflammatory colitis. Solitary aphthous ulcers, rake-like lesions, strictures, and rectal sparing are consistent with Crohn's disease. In cases in which severe inflammation is seen, the physician should perform a simple biopsy and then leave the area because the risk of iatrogenic perforation is high. Once the endoscope is inserted, it is appropriate to obtain biopsies underneath the peritoneal reflection, even if no abnormalities are seen. Frequently neutrophilic infiltration is seen in mucosa that appeared normal to the observer's eye. Thus biopsy of normal mucosa may be helpful if the clinical history is strongly suggestive.

The finding of anal or perianal lesions, such as sinus tracts, rectovaginal fistula, and abscesses, is consistent with Crohn's disease but not with ulcerative colitis. The mucosa in a patient with Crohn's disease may appear cobblestoned or nodular. Pseudopolyps may appear in patients with Crohn's disease and ulcerative colitis. Loss of haustra, distortion of normal architecture, or both may be found. Light reflection patterns and subtle signs of edema (loss of vascularity) may be helpful for directing the clinician to biopsy certain affected areas.

Diagnostic Plan

Fecal occult blood testing and fecal leukocyte smears are obtained from patients presenting with diarrhea. Positive results merit stool cultures for pathogens and stool smears for ova and parasites when applicable. Flexible sigmoidoscopy could be done at the time of biopsy. When inflammatory bowel disease is suspected, consultation with a gastroenterologist is usually sought. Recent developments in therapy are beyond the scope of this chapter.

Among patients presenting with diarrhea, fatigue, anemia, loss of skin turgor, weight loss, and positive orthostatic measurements, hospitalization is ordered and a consultation requested. Most patients with inflammatory bowel disease initially consult their family physician and are worked up as outpatients. Few patients have clear-cut cases of inflammatory bowel disease, and it is up to the family physician to distinguish them from the many patients with irritable bowel syndrome.

For patients with chronic intermittent abdominal pain and alternating diarrhea and constipation, and for those with chronic diarrhea who lack any constitutional symptoms, it may be appropriate to order no studies and simply advise them to follow a low fat, low residue diet with the addition of a bulk agent, sedative-antispasmodic drug, or both. The patient with irritable bowel disease usually is markedly improved within a 2-week period, whereas the patient with inflammatory bowel disease has no significant recovery. Patients who experience prolonged diarrhea for the first time at the age of 40 or older require intestinal evaluation with endoscopy, air contrast barium enema, or both to rule out colorectal cancer.

Endoscopic biopsy results consistent with nonspecific inflammation are not helpful. The patient's presentation determines the need for consultation. When the endoscopic findings are clearly abnormal or if biopsy specimens of normal tissue demonstrate significant polymorphonuclear cell inflammation, consultation is recommended.

Because of the increasing risk of cancer in patients with ulcerative colitis over time, those who have had ulcerative pancolitis should undergo colonoscopic surveillance at regular intervals. The detection of high grade dysplasia mandates colectomy (Lashner, 1992).

Irritable Bowel Syndrome

The irritable bowel syndrome, a common malady, exists in 10 to 22 per cent of the population, most of whom do not seek medical care (Lynn and Friedman, 1993). It is by far the most common cause of chronic abdominal pain, diarrhea, or constipation. It is second only to the common cold in terms of causing loss of time from work, and patients with this condition account for 50 per cent of all patients seen by gastroenterologists.

Irritable bowel syndrome is a functional disorder that has no evidence of structural abnormalities; it never becomes an organic disease, although many patients who have it are concerned about the development of carcinoma or colitis. The syndrome appears during the late twenties, although it may occur in teenagers and patients as old as age 40. Beyond that time, the physician must suspect organic disease. In the United States females with the condition predominate over males, whereas in

India the opposite is the case, so there must be some type of culturally dictated difference relating to the cause of irritable bowel syndrome.

The syndrome can be roughly broken down into four types, although many patients have mixtures of the types.

1. *Alternating diarrhea with constipation.* These patients may continue for several days with no bowel movements and then awaken early in the morning and pass a formed stool. They may need to return several more times to pass increasingly soft stools. They then may continue throughout the day without bowel activity, or they may move their bowels once or twice after a meal. The onset of diarrhea may occur after severe lower abdominal cramping in the midline or the left or right lower quadrant.

2. *Nervous diarrhea.* These patients have diarrhea frequently after meals as well as after stress. The onset of diarrhea may occur suddenly and with little cramping pain.

3. *Constipation* is a common malady in the United States. These patients complain of an inability to defecate and have difficulty moving their bowels when the delayed urge arises. This pattern does not relate to those patients who have the wrong conception about bowel activity, namely, that they should have a bowel movement every day.

4. *Upper GI distress with bloating, distention, and discomfort after eating.* This type has been described with the upper GI dyspeptic syndromes and is known as nonulcer dyspepsia.

Pathophysiology

Patients with irritable bowel syndrome are hypersensitive to bowel stimulation. Many studies have been done to demonstrate this hyperreaction. When their bowel is distended with a nasogastric tube, patients with the irritable bowel syndrome experience discomfort and pain long before a control patient with no such syndrome. These patients are most sensitive to food and emotional distress. If these patients are given spicy foods or large amounts of roughage, they frequently complain of abdominal distention, cramping, and sometimes diarrhea. If the patients are under stress, their symptoms may become markedly intensified, and they are even more sensitive to food. An analogy that may be pointed out to them is the albino person for whom normal sunlight can cause skin burning, whereas normal sunlight has no effect on someone else without the problem. There is an increased incidence of the condition in families of patients with the irritable bowel syndrome, and that information may be helpful.

On physical examination, the only findings may be a tender left lower quadrant, sometimes with a rope-like loop of tender colon. Results of diagnostic studies such as sigmoidoscopy, barium enema,

stool cultures, and occult blood tests are negative. Sometimes sigmoidoscopy with air insufflation reproduces the patient's pain and discomfort. This reaction may help the family physician determine the patient's response to noxious stimuli.

Differential Diagnosis

The differential diagnosis of irritable bowel syndrome includes the inflammatory bowel diseases, as described in the previous section. Lactose intolerance may mimic the irritable bowel syndrome and can easily be discovered by having the patient avoid milk totally for a period of 3 to 5 days. If the symptoms markedly improve or cease altogether, the diagnosis is established.

Treatment

It must be emphasized that patients with irritable bowel syndrome are not malingering. They have true pain and discomfort secondary to the hypersensitivity—just as some people blush and perspire more easily than others. The patient must understand that the family physician is aware that the condition is a true physical problem and not an imaginary illness. In these patients acute or chronic emotional stress may bring on or enhance the irritable bowel syndrome. Thus one of the first issues that must be addressed is the possibility of any stress that occurred at the time the disease appeared or intensified. It is at this point that family physicians must explain to the patient that they are looking for a cause of increased sensitivity of the bowel, and that the patient's conscious mind has no control over the condition. If the physician is able to identify psychosocial issues, these issues should be addressed on an individual basis. The patient, however, should not be probed aggressively for causes of stress, as it increases their stress. At this point, treatment of the physical symptoms should be attempted. With time, the patient may be willing to talk about stress or may become aware of it. The patient's diet should not include spicy foods, fried foods, or fatty foods. Likewise, the patient should not eat large meals or raw roughage in large quantities, such as fruits, vegetables, or salads. Certainly, one salad and one fruit a day is fine. The patient is advised to take a bulk agent. Usually psyllium seeds are recommended because this bulk agent seems to be much better tolerated by these patients. The dosage can start out as 1 heaping tablespoon a day in a glass of juice or water, which can be taken at any time. If no improvement occurs after 1 or 2 weeks, an antispasmodic agent may be added; and if the patient is exceptionally stressed or anxious, a sedative-antispasmodic drug may be used. Table 43–18 describes various medical therapies that have been recommended. If the patient does not get better with one of these regimens, consultation with a gastroenterologist is appropriate.

TABLE 43–18. ORAL THERAPY FOR SYMPTOMS OF IRRITABLE BOWEL SYNDROME

Agent	Dosage	Comments
Constipation (Predominantly Irritable Bowel Syndrome)		
Cathartic Agents		
Psyllium agents (e.g., Metamucil, Konsyl, Modane)	1 tablespoon daily t.i.d.	Usually with meals or in juice; start low to avoid gas; encourage at least 8 glasses H₂O daily; avoid other cathartics
Lactulose (Chronulac)	15–30 mL daily t.i.d.	Individually titrated to desired bowel pattern
Cisapride (Propulsid)	5–10 mg t.i.d.	Unlabeled use
Diarrhea (Predominantly Irritable Bowel Syndrome)		
Constipating Agents		
Psyllium agents	As above	As above
Loperamide (Imodium)	Initial 4 mg followed by 2 mg for each unformed stool	Average daily dose 4–8 mg; now available over the counter
Diphenoxylate HCl (Lomotil)	2.5–5.0 mg after each unformed stool	Maximum daily dose 20 mg, average dose 2.5–5.0 mg b.i.d.
Codeine phosphate	7.5–30.0 mg daily b.i.d.	Not recommended: risk for addiction
Aluminum hydroxide gel (Alugel)	30 ml every 3–4 hr pm	Use with caution for chronic renal failure
Cholestyramine (Questran)	0.5–1.0 pack 1–6 times daily	Unlabeled use
Anticholinergic-Antispasmodic Agents		
Dicyclomine (Bentyl)	10–20 mg b.i.d.–q.i.d. before meals	Not proved by clinical trials
Clidinium (Quarzan)	2.5–5.0 mg a.c. and q.h.s.	Not proved by clinical trials
Propantheline bromide (Probanthine)	15 mg a.c. q.h.s.	Not proved by clinical trials
Glycopyrrolate (Robinul)	1–2 mg a.c.	Not proved by clinical trials
Anisotropine (Valpin 50)	50 mg a.c. q.h.s.	Not proved by clinical trials
Tincture of belladonna	4–20 gm Hs a.c. q.h.s.	Not proved by clinical trials
Anticholinergic/Antispasmodic Drugs with Sedatives		
Librax	1–2 days a.c., q.h.s.	Not proved by clinical trials
Donnatal	1–2 tabs a.c. q.h.s.	Not proved by clinical trials
Combid spansules	1 cap b.i.d.	Not proved by clinical trials
Pathibamate	1–2 tabs a.c. q.h.s.	Not proved by clinical trials
Low dose antidepressants	q.h.s.	Unlabeled use
Amitriptyline	25–50 mg q.h.s.	Unlabeled use
Desipramine	25–50 mg q.h.s.	Unlabeled use
Miscellaneous Agents		
Simethicone (Mylicon, Silain)	2–4 tabs p.c. and q.h.s.	For gas
		Not proved by clinical trials
Activated charcoal	2–4 tabs p.c., q.h.s.	Not proved by clinical trials

These options reflect the poorly understood multifactorial pathophysiology of irritable bowel syndrome. The medications usually represent only one aspect of a coordinated therapeutic approach, which should include patient education, diet, counseling, and regularly scheduled follow-up visits. A therapeutic trial should last at least 3 weeks before being labeled unsuccessful. The antidyspepsia agents are helpful in selected patients.

If the patient is amenable, some form of psychotherapy may be beneficial. One study showed that even a short course of ten psychotherapy sessions improved the treated group when compared with a control group who received no psychotherapy (Svedlund et al., 1983).

Patient Education

It should be pointed out that excellent patient education materials are available from the National Foundation for Ileitis and Colitis, which has an office in New York City. Two excellent resource books are *The Crohn's Disease and Ulcerative Colitis Fact Book* and *People Not Patients*. An excellent four-page handout entitled *Coping with Irritable Bowel Syndrome* was published in the August 1982 issue of *Drug Therapy* (Freedman, 1986; Schuster, 1987), and some excellent dietary tips are available in the literature (Freedman, 1986; Schuster, 1987) and from commercial sources, such as the Patient Information Library. Some family phy-

sicians believe that the use of videoendoscopy may be an important patient education technique that allows the patient and family to visualize the intestinal mucosa (Rodney, 1987).

ENDOSCOPIC DIAGNOSIS AND THE ROLE OF BIOPSY IN THE OFFICE

Since the late 1970s new perspectives on colorectal disease have developed from multiple studies describing office-based flexible sigmoidoscopy. Relatively low-priced video and computer enhancement techniques allow physicians to recognize and understand colorectal lesions in an improved way. In particular, videoendoscopy has provided a new dimension—information management. This dimension of image processing can be manipulated by the physician to improve diagnostic skill. Case management, patient education, and compliance issues also appear to be improved by the use of this increasingly available office procedure.

Tissue diagnosis remains the gold standard, but not all lesions can be biopsied or excised with equally low morbidity. This fact remains true despite the improved design of biopsy equipment and flexible endoscopes. Modern flexible biopsy forceps operate with a biting mechanism that penetrates less deeply into the mucosa, which lowers the risk of perforation or hemorrhage after the procedure. Tissue specimens obtained with these biopsy forceps appear miniscule compared with those taken with the methods used previously. These tissue amounts remain sufficient for histologic analysis. Specimens returned as being inadequate in amount should be discussed individually with the pathologist. Specimens of this nature were not common in pathology training programs prior to 1973. Some pathologists have fixative preferences, whereas others accept the standard 10% formalin preservative.

As with previous biopsy techniques, tissue obtained from a fibrinous plaque or a necrotic ulcer base rarely yields an acceptable diagnosis. Biopsy of vascular structures is contraindicated. Relatively contraindicated is the biopsy of lesions for which management is obvious; polyps on a stalk, in most cases, are an example. On the other hand, endoscopists should be encouraged to biopsy abnormal lesions for which the diagnosis is not clear. With experience, the need for biopsy should diminish. Hypertrophied papillae, skin tags, endoscope-induced trauma, and fecal debris variants may be biopsied by the neophyte. With experience, these items are noted and left alone.

Hyperplastic polyps are a special problem. Large numbers of these lesions are found. Hyperplastic polyps should not be diagnosed without some tissue analysis. Hyperplastic polyps are not neoplastic, and they do not carry an increased risk of cancer for their bearer (Fenoglio-Preiser and Hutter, 1985). Unfortunately, sampling is not perfect, and multiple biopsies are time-consuming. Some physicians initially biopsy several of these lesions and return to the others only if the biopsy results are neoplastic (adenoma or carcinoma). Other physicians compulsively remove all lesions and perform annual surveillance colonoscopy. This practice remains controversial, with the current trend favoring a less invasive, more conservative approach. On this issue, Hippocrates' axiom regarding the difficulty of decision ("Life is short and the art long. . . . ") timelessly applies to the need for individualized clinical judgment by the managing physician.

Not all anorectal lesions are apparent to the naked eye, and biopsy is helpful with many nonvascular lesions. Although some specialists have advocated against biopsy of obviously malignant lesions, biopsy can be helpful even in these cases. Immediate biopsy greatly assisted in the diagnosis and management of one of our patients: a case of anorectal melanoma. A metastatic work-up was performed prior to referral. Tragically, metastasis had occurred, but this information obviated further invasive procedures. Health care fragmentation was minimized, and family support was mobilized in a timely fashion.

Suggestions for the Acquisition and Maintenance of Endoscopic Skills

Skills in GI endoscopy have at least six major dimensions. The first of these dimensions is demonstration of the mechanical skills for manipulating and relating to the equipment. It should include the ability to maintain and disinfect the equipment. Second, there must be the ability to obtain and record diagnostic information. Skills in recognition, documentation, and tissue confirmation of pathology are desirable (Silverstein and Tytgat, 1987). Appropriate use of other diagnostic assistance and consultation deserve mention and further study. Third, the ability to effectively manage the diagnostic information obtained should be demonstrated. Fourth, there should be a commitment to an ongoing analysis of outcomes. Continued professional growth is not possible without study and self-inspection. A database that systematically records the indications, diagnoses, and outcomes of the first 100 endoscopic procedures is an example. It is not necessary to perform 10 procedures a day to remain capable. Large numbers of endoscopies are not necessary so long as there is rational thought, prudent judgment, and good management. The fifth component is the incorporation, or synthesis, of new knowledge as the physician gains experience. It is the professional responsibility of a physician to follow and contribute to the progress of medical knowledge. Finally, a teacher learns twice. Meaningful participation in an ongoing educational program can help a good physician become even better.

REFERENCES

Adelman A: Abdominal pain in the primary care setting. J Fam Pract 25:27, 1987a.

Adelman A: Management of dyspepsia. Am Fam Physician 35: 222, 1987b.

Afzalpurkar RG, Schiller LR, Little KH, et al: The self-limited nature of chronic, idiopathic diarrhea. N Engl J Med 327: 1849, 1992.

Avery ME, Snyder JD: Oral therapy for acute diarrhea: The underused simple solution. N Engl J Med 323:891, 1990.

Bedell AW: Thrombosed hemorrhoids. In Mayhew HE, Rogers

LA (eds): Basic Procedures in Family Practice. New York, Churchill Livingstone, 1984, p 243.

Bezerra JA: Treatment of infants with acute diarrhea: What's recommended and what's practiced. Pediatrics 90:1, 1992.

Blacklow NR, Greenberg HB: Viral gastroenteritis. N Engl J Med 325:252, 1991.

Boles RS, Gordon SM: The clinical significance of diverticulosis. Gastroenterology 35:579, 1958.

Bruckstein AH: Acute diarrhea. Am Fam Physician 38:217, 1988.

Cello JP: Diagnosis and management of lower gastrointestinal tract hemorrhage—medical staff conference, University of California, San Francisco. West J Med 143:80, 1985.

Cope Z: The Early Diagnosis of the Acute Abdomen. London, Oxford University Press, 1972, p 3.

DeGowin EL, DeGowin RL: Bedside Diagnostic Examination. New York, Macmillan, 1981, p 32.

Detsky AS, Smalley PS, Chang J: Is this patient malnourished? JAMA 271:54, 1994.

DeWitt TG, McCarthy PL, Humphrey KF: Who should have stool cultures? Pediatrics 76:551, 1985.

Drossman DA, Sandler RS, McKee DC, et al: Bowel patterns among subjects not seeking health care: Use of a questionnaire to identify a population with bowel dysfunction. Gastroenterology 83:529, 1982.

Feldman M, Maton PN, McCallum RW, et al: Treating ulcers in reflux: What's Patient Care 26(13):53, 1992.

Fennerty MD, Sampliner RE: Gastroesophageal reflux disease. Hosp Med, April:28, 1993.

Fenoglio-Preiser CM, Hutter RVP: Colorectal polyps: Pathologic diagnosis and clinical significance. Cancer 35:322, 1985.

Fitz RH: Perforating inflammation of the vermiform appendix: With special reference to its early diagnosis and treatment. Am J Med Sci 92:321, 1886.

Freedman G: The role of fiber and other dietary factors in IBS. Pract Gastroenterol 10(2):51, 1986.

Gear JSS, Ware A, Fursdon P, et al: Symptomless diverticular disease and intake of dietary fibre. Lancet 1:511, 1979.

Graham DY, Lew GM, Evans DG, et al: Effective triple therapy (antibiotics plus bismuth), on duodenal ulcer healing: A randomized controlled trial. Ann Intern Med 115:266, 1991.

Greenburg HI: Changing patterns of gastrointestinal bleeding. Arch Surg March:341, 1985.

Hayms JS: Carbohydrate malabsorption following fruit ingestion in young children. Pediatrics 82:64, 1988.

Hentschel E, Brandstatter G, Dragosics B, et al: Effect of ranitidine and amoxicillin plus metronidazole on the eradication of Helicobacter pylori and the recurrence of duodenal ulcer. N Engl J Med 328:308, 1993.

Hocutt JE, Rodney WM, Zurad E, et al: Esophagogastroduodenoscopy for the family physicians. Am Fam Physician 49: 109, 1994.

Holdstock G, Harmon M, Machin D, et al: Prospective testing of a scoring system designed to improve case selection for upper gastrointestinal investigation. Gastroenterology 90: 1164, 1986.

Horner JL: Natural history of diverticulosis of the colon. Am J Dig Dis 3:343, 1958.

Hyland JMP, Taylor I: Does a high fibre diet prevent the complications of diverticular disease? Br J Surg 67:77, 1980.

Kahn H, Greenfield S: Position paper: Endoscopy in the evaluation of dyspepsia from the Health and Public Policy of the American College of Physicians. Ann Intern Med 102:266, 1985.

Lashner BA: Recommendations for colorectal cancer screening in ulcerative colitis: A review of research from a single university-based surveillance program. Am J Gastroenterol 87: 168, 1992.

Laupacis A, Sackett DL, Roberts RS: An assessment of clinically useful measures of the consequences of treatment. N Engl J Med 318:1728, 1988.

Lee WM: Acute liver failure. N Engl J Med 329:1862, 1993.

Lefrink RJ, Miedema BW: Colonic diverticuli: When complica-

tions require surgery and when they don't. Postgrad Med 92(6):97, 1992.

Lynn RB, Friedman LS: Irritable bowel syndrome. N Engl J Med 329:1940, 1993.

Maisels MJ, Gifford K, Antle CE, et al: Jaundice in the healthy newborn infant: A new approach to an old problem. Pediatrics 81:505, 1988.

Malt RA: The perforated appendix. N Engl J Med 315:1546, 1986.

Maton PN: Omeprazole. N Engl J Med 324:965, 1991.

Moosa AR: Diagnostic tests and procedures in acute pancreatitis. N Engl J Med 311:639, 1984.

Mueller BA, Daling JR, Moore DE, et al: Appendectomy and the risk of tubal infertility. N Engl J Med 315:1506, 1986.

Mull JD, Mull DS: Mothers' concepts of childhood diarrhea in rural Pakistan: What ORT program planners should know. Soc Sci Med 27(1):53, 1988.

Newman TV, Maisels MJ: Evaluation and treatment of jaundice in the term newborn: A kinder, a gentler approach. Pediatrics 89:809, 1992.

Nyren O, Adami HO, Bates S, et al: Absence of therapeutic benefit from antacids or cimetidine in non-ulcer dyspepsia. N Engl J Med 314:339, 1986.

Olshaker JS, Mason JD: The usefulness of serum electrolytes in the evaluation and treatment of acute adult gastroenteritis. Ann Emerg Med 17:423, 1988.

Paterson-Brown S, Thompson JN, Eckersley JRT, et al: Which patients with suspected appendicitis should undergo laparoscopy? BMJ 296:1363, 1988.

Ransohoff DF, Lang CA: Sigmoidoscopic screening in the 1990's. JAMA 269:1278, 1993.

Rodney WM: Videosigmoidoscopy in a family medicine residency. Prim Care 5(6):41, 1985a.

Rodney WM (ed): Flexible Sigmoidoscopy for the Family Physician. Kansas City, MO, American Academy of Family Physicians and the American Society for Gastrointestinal Endoscopy, 1985b.

Rodney WM: New uses for videoendoscopy in the office: Patient education. Diagnosis 9(5):52, 1987.

Rodney WM: Procedural skills in flexible sigmoidoscopy and colonoscopy for the family physician. Prim Care 15:79, 1988.

Rodney WM: Flexible sigmoidoscopy and the despecialization of endoscopy: an environmental impact report. Cancer 70: 1266, 1992.

Rodney WM: Peptic disease syndrome: Should we treat H. pylori? Am Fam Physician 47:742, 1993.

Rodney WM, Albers G: Flexible sigmoidoscopy: Primary care outcomes after two types of continuing medication education. Am J Gastroenterol 81:133, 1986.

Rodney WM, Felmar E: Why flexible sigmoidoscopy instead of rigid sigmoidoscopy? J Fam Pract 19:471, 1984.

Rodney WM, Ruggerio C: The Coloscreen self-test for detection of fecal occult blood. J Fam Pract 21:200, 1985c.

Rodney WM, Beaber RJ, Johnson RA, et al: Physician compliance with colorectal cancer screening (1978–1983): The impact of flexible sigmoidoscopy. J Fam Pract 20:265, 1985d.

Rodney WM, Dabov G, Orientale E, et al: Colonoscopy in FP: Sedation as associated with a more complete exam. J Fam Pract 36:394, 1993a.

Rodney WM, Weber JR, Swedberg JA, et al: Esophagogastroduodenoscopy by family physicians phase II: A national multisite study of 2,500 procedures. J Fam Pract 13:121, 1993b.

Russell TR, Donahue JH: Hemorrhoidal banding: A warning. Dis Colon Rectum 28:291, 1985.

Schuster MM: What to feed the patient with irritable bowel syndrome. Pract Gastroenterol 11(1):13, 1987.

Schwartz S: Tempering the technological diagnosis of appendicitis. N Engl J Med 3127:703, 1987.

Shanahan D, Lord PH, Grogono J, et al: Clinical acute cholecystitis and the Curtis-Fitz-Hugn syndrome. Ann R Coll Surg 70:44, 1988.

Siegel MJ, Carel C, Surratt S: Ultrasound sonography of acute abdominal pain in children. JAMA 266:187, 1991.

Silen W: Cope's Early Diagnosis of the Acute Abdomen, 15th edition. New York, Oxford University Press, 1979.

Siegel MJ, Carel C, Surratt S: Ultrasound sonography of acute abdominal pain in children. JAMA, Oxford University Press, New York 266:187, 1991.

Silverstein FE, Tytgat GNJ: Atlas of Gastrointestinal Endoscopy. Philadelphia, WB Saunders Company, 1987.

Steinberg WM, Stafford GS, Davis ND, et al: Diagnostic assays in acute pancreatitis. Ann Intern Med 102:576, 1985.

Svedlund J, Ottson J, Sjodin I, et al: Controlled study of psychotherapy in the irritable bowel syndrome. Lancet 1: 589, 1983.

Treacher DF, Barkes DJP, Hutton JP, et al: Irritable bowel syndrome: Is a barium enema necessary? Clin Radiol 37:87, 1986.

Wade AJ, Roley-Jones D: Long-term management of duodenal ulcer in general practice: How best to use cimetidine? BMJ., 296:971, 1988.

Walker JD, Gray IA, Polk HC: Diverticulitis in women: An unappreciated clinical presentation. Ann Surg 1985:402, 1977.

World Health Organization: Diarrhoeal Disease Control Programme: Drugs in the Management of Acute Diarrhoea in Infants and Young Children. Geneva, World Health Organization, 1988.

Space limitations prohibit a comprehensive listing of all worthwhile publications on this topic. Therefore I have created a comprehensive bibliography of the resource material on which this chapter was based. It is available upon request.

The author wishes to acknowledge the invaluable contributions to the previous (4th edition) chapter by Marvin Derezin, M.D.

CHAPTER 44

ONCOLOGY

VIRGINIA RHODES, LORI A. WHITTAKER, and RICHARD PAZDUR

Family practice physicians have become increasingly involved in the field of oncology. As primary care providers, they are involved in cancer screening and early detection of malignancies and are becoming increasingly involved in the care of patients undergoing chemotherapy and radiation treatment. An understanding of the basic science of oncology and the recent advances in the clinical fields of medical, radiation, and surgical oncology specialties is necessary to this participation. An understanding of palliative care medicine is a requisite to those physicians who are involved in bringing comfort, dignity, and acceptable quality of life to patients who are beyond curative measures.

CARCINOGENESIS

Carcinogenesis is the process by which cells gain malignant potential. To understand this process, we must understand the cellular, molecular, and biochemical changes involved in the transformation of a normal cell to a tumor cell. We must then understand the complex tumor–host interaction that allows that cell to proliferate, invade, and metastasize.

Carcinogenic Agents

Since the eighteenth century, when John Hill (1759) proposed that tobacco snuff was a cause of oral cancer and Percival Pott (1775) identified a relation between soot and scrotal cancer in chimney sweeps, many other substances have been implicated in human carcinogenesis. Such agents, or carcinogens, include not only exogenous or environmental factors but also endogenous substances. An important group of endogenous carcinogens are the oxyradicals, or activated oxygen species. These species are formed during normal cellular pathways, such as lipid metabolism, and their rate of production may be increased by processes such as inflammation or by the action of certain carcino-

gens. Other carcinogens, such as ionizing radiation, benzopyrene, benzene, cigarette smoke, and asbestos, can induce free radical formation. Oxyradicals bind to DNA and induce a variety of genetic alterations that may play a role in the carcinogenic process. Table 44–1 lists examples of some known carcinogens.

Common to most carcinogens is their ability to cause DNA damage. Such agents are referred to as *mutagens* or *genotoxic carcinogens*. There is another, less well characterized group of carcinogens, the *nongenotoxic carcinogens*, which act by mechanisms other than direct DNA damage. A subgroup of these agents induce cell proliferation and growth and are referred to as *mitogens*.

In general, chemical carcinogens do not act directly to cause DNA damage but must be activated by endogenous mechanisms. The most common mechanism of activation involves the cytochrome P450 system. This system comprises a group of enzymes, designated CYPs, whose main function is to metabolize and detoxify harmful compounds. During the metabolic process, however, they may alter the structure of potential carcinogens to render them electrophilic and capable of binding to DNA. Individual variations in the metabolic phenotypes of the cytochrome p450 enzymes are the cause of the observed variations in susceptibility to certain carcinogens. For example, a four- to sixfold increased lifetime risk of lung cancer has been observed in individuals who express the extensive metabolic phenotype CYP-2D6. Other enzymes involved in the activation of carcinogens include the acetyltransferases and the glutathione transferases. These enzymes too exist as genetic pleiomorphisms. Moreover, individual variations in DNA repair mechanisms have been associated with varying susceptibilities to cancer (Poulsen et al., 1993; Sheilds and Harris, 1991).

We have recently begun to understand the changes that occur at the molecular level during carcinogenesis. Carcinogens, through their action on the cell's genetic material, may turn on or turn off important regulatory genes, thereby establishing a cascade of events resulting in tumorigenesis.

TABLE 44–1. CARCINOGENS

Exogenous Factors

Chemical agents—e.g., components of tobacco smoke, food additives, air pollutants, industrial chemicals

Physical agents—e.g., radiation (ionizing and nonionizing), asbestos

Viral agents—e.g., hepatitis B virus (hepatocellular carcinoma), Epstein-Barr virus (Burkitt's lymphoma and nasopharyngeal cancer), human papilloma virus (cervical cancer), human T cell leukemia/lymphoma (HTLV-I)

Endogenous Factors

Hormones—e.g., estrogens (breast and endometrial cancers), androgens (prostate cancer)

Activated oxygen species and oxygen radicals

Oncogenes

In 1910 Rous identified an RNA virus as the causal agent in sarcomas in chickens. This virus, called Rous sarcoma virus, was the first in a series of oncogenic animal viruses to be recognized. Although viruses play a role in only a few human cancers, it was the study of animal tumor viruses that led to dramatic discoveries in tumor biology.

Since Rous' work, more than 20 other oncogenic RNA viruses and a few DNA viruses have been discovered. With the advent of molecular biology, single genes responsible for conferring malignant potential on infected cells have been isolated from these simple viral genomes. These genes were termed *oncogenes* (Heubner and Todaro, 1969) and were named with three-letter codes after the virus in which they were discovered (e.g., *src* for Rous sarcoma virus).

Animal tumor viruses provided a model system for the study of oncogenic processes but were thought to have little direct relevance to human cancer until viral oncogenes were discovered to be homologous to genes found in normal mammalian cells (Stehelin et al., 1976). These normal cellular genes were referred to as *proto-oncogenes*; and although not intrinsically oncogenic, they could be "activated" to become oncogenic by point mutation, translocation and gene rearrangement, or amplification. Their relevance to human cancers was revealed in a landmark study in which Weinberg and coworkers identified a gene in human bladder cancer that was homologous to a viral oncogene (Shih et al., 1981). Using a method of DNA transfer developed during the 1970s, this group transfected DNA from a human bladder cancer cell line into recipient mouse cells. After several rounds of transfection, a single human gene responsible for the malignant phenotype was identified and found to be highly homologous to the viral oncogene of the Harvey murine sarcoma virus (H-*ras*) and related to the oncogene of the Kirsten sarcoma virus (K-*ras*). Since then, many other viral oncogenes have been found to have homologues in human tumors. Transfection studies have also allowed the detection of human oncogenes not found in animal viruses.

Important inroads to the understanding of the oncogenic process on a cellular level were made through the study of oncogene protein products and the elucidation of their functions (Bishop, 1987, 1991). These functions can be divided into several broad categories, all of which are involved in the regulation of cell growth and proliferation. Selected oncogene protein products, their functions, and their methods of activation are summarized in Table 44–2.

Certain oncogenes play a role in a wide variety of

TABLE 44–2. HUMAN ONCOGENES AND THEIR FUNCTIONS

Oncogene	Associated Cancers	Function	Activation
Growth Factors			
sis	Sarcomas	PDGF	?
Growth Factor Receptors			
erbB/neu	Breast, ovarian, stomach, neuroblastoma	EGF receptor	Amplification
hst	Gastric		Rearrangement
ret	Papillary thyroid		Rearrangement
Nonreceptor Kinases			
abl	CML	Tyrosine kinase	Translocation
src	Colon	Tyrosine kinase	?
raf	Papillary thyroid	Serine/threonine kinase	Rearrangement
Signal Transducers			
ras	Colorectal, lung, bladder, kidney, breast, skin; leukemias; others	GTP binding	Point mutation
gsp	Pituitary tumors	GTP binding	Point mutation
Transcription Factors			
myc	Lung, breast, colorectal; leukemias; lymphomas; neuroblastoma		Amplification Translocation
myb	Myeloid leukemias		Translocation

CML = chronic myelogenous leukemia; PDGF = platelet-derived growth factor; EGF = epidermal growth factor; GTP = glutamyl transpeptidase.

human cancers. One such group is the *ras* family. Mutated *ras* oncogenes have been found in cancers of the gastrointestinal tract, urogenital tract, breast, lung, and thyroid and in leukemias, neuroblastomas, and melanomas. The *ras* oncogenes seem to have a strong association with adenocarcinomas.

The *myc* family of oncogenes is likewise prevalent in a wide variety of cancers. It was first identified in Burkitt's lymphoma, but amplifications of c-*myc* have also been identified in lung, breast, colorectal, and other gastrointestinal malignancies; urogenital cancers, including bladder, prostate, and testicular tumors; and neuroblastomas. It is not clear exactly what part these oncogenes play in the development of these disparate malignancies. In some cases their activation may be a function of the oncogenic process rather than a cause of it.

Tumor Suppressor Genes

Another group of genes that have profound implications in the carcinogenic process are tumor suppressor genes. The first of these genes to be discovered was the retinoblastoma (*Rb*) gene. Retinoblastoma is a childhood malignancy of embryonic retinal cells that occurs in both hereditary and much rarer sporadic forms. Through the study of chromosomal banding patterns in children with retinoblastoma, it was observed that one band of chromosome 13 was occasionally missing, suggesting the loss of one or more critical genes in this chromosomal region. Subsequently, a specific deleted gene, *Rb*, was identified and cloned.

For retinoblastoma to develop, both copies of the *Rb* gene must be inactivated. The event that deletes the second copy of the *Rb* gene is usually chromosome loss, deletion, or recombination. It results in a loss of heterozygosity or "reduction to homozygosity" for genes flanking the *Rb* locus. Studies on the loss of heterozygosity of chromosomal regions in other tumors led to the identification of additional tumor suppressor genes, such as *p53* and *DCC*. Other tumor suppressor genes were identified by family linkage studies in inherited cancer syndromes such Wilms' tumor (*WT-1* gene), neurofibromatosis (*NF-1* gene), and familial adenomatous polyposis (*APC* gene) (Marshall, 1991). Table 44–3 lists some of the known tumor suppressor genes and the malignancies with which they are associated.

Certain tumor suppressor genes are associated with only one or a few types of cancer, whereas others seem to play a role in a large number of malignancies. The most common tumor suppressor gene, and indeed the most frequently mutated gene in human cancer, is *p53*. Somatic mutations of *p53* have been found in a wide variety of sporadic cancers, including those of the breast, adrenal gland, lung, colon, brain, and other sites. Germ line

TABLE 44–3. TUMOR SUPPRESSOR GENES IN HUMAN MALIGNANCIES

Locus	Chromosome	Associated Malignancies
APC	5p	Familial adenomatous polyposis; colorectal cancer
MLM	9p13	Familial melanoma
WT-1	11p	Wilms' tumor; hepatoblastoma; breast, bladder, and lung cancers
MEN-1	11q	Multiple endocrine neoplasia type I
Rb-1	13q	Retinoblastoma; breast and bladder cancer; osteosarcoma
p53	17p	Lung, colorectal, and breast cancer; osteosaroma; others
NF-1	17q	Neurofibromatosis type 1
BRCA-1	17q	Familial breast and ovarian cancers
DCC	18q	Colorectal cancer
NF-2	22q	Neurofibromatosis type 2

Data obtained from Harris and Hollstein (1993) N Engl J Med, King et al. (1993) copyright 1993 Scientific American, Weinberg (1993) copyright 1993, American Medical Association, with permission.

mutations of *p53* are responsible for the rare Li-Fraumeni cancer family syndrome (Milkin et al., 1990). Mutations at any of the more than 100 sites of the *p53* gene can render it tumorigenic. The *p53* gene appears to be an important growth regulator in many cell types, which helps to explain its role in such a large number of malignancies (Chang et al., 1993; Harris and Hollstein, 1993; Levine, 1992).

Hereditary Cancer Syndromes

Certain families have been observed to have a high propensity for the development of specific malignancies. Pedigree analysis of some of these families identified a usually autosomal dominant pattern of inheritance and a tendency for earlier age of onset than is seen with sporadic cancers. The identifiable inherited defect in these syndromes has always been a mutated or absent tumor suppressor gene. So far, no dominant oncogenes have been implicated as the heritable agents in cancer family syndromes, although oncogenes certainly play a role in the carcinogenic process of many of these cancers (see the discussion of the colorectal cancer model below). Certain tumor suppressor genes, such as *APC*, *p53*, and *Rb*, have been associated with both sporadic and inherited malignancies. Some inherited cancer syndromes, such as retinoblastoma, Wilms' tumor, and familial melanoma, are associated with a single tumor type. In others there is an inherited propensity for groups of tumors. These hereditary cancer syndromes are outlined in Table 44–4.

TABLE 44–4. CANCER FAMILY SYNDROMES

Syndrome	Associated Tumors
Associated with Multiple Malignancies	
Hereditary breast–ovarian cancer syndrome	Breast and ovary
Lynch II syndrome	Breast, ovary, prostate, colon
Cancer family syndrome	Breast, colon, endometrial
Li-Fraumeni syndrome	Sarcomas, breast, brain, lung, laryngeal, adrenocortical, leukemia
Multiple endocrine neoplasia	
Type I (MEN-I)	Pituitary, parathyroid (benign), pancreas
Type IIa (MEN-IIa)	Thyroid, parathyroid (benign), pheochromocytoma
Type IIb (MEN-IIb)	Thyroid, parathyroid, neuromas
Neurofibromatosis	
Type I	Optic gliomas, neurofibrosarcomas, neurofibromas
Type II	Acoustic neuromas, neurofibrosarcomas, neurofibromas
von Hippel-Lindau syndrome	Kidney, adrenal (usually benign), CNS angiomas, cysts in multiple organs
Associated with Single Malignancies	
Wilms' tumor	
Retinoblastoma	
Familial adenomatous polyposis and colon cancer	
Gardner syndrome (colon cancer)	
Hereditary nonpolyposis colon cancer (Lynch I syndrome)	
Familial melanoma	

Multistep Carcinogenesis

Many years ago it was proposed on the basis of epidemiologic data that cancer develops in a multistep fashion, that is, as a result of a series of events occurring over a lifetime (Armitage and Doll, 1957). There is generally a long latent period between exposure to a given carcinogen and the development of cancer, and not everyone exposed to the carcinogen develops disease.

Early studies with chemical carcinogens supported this hypothesis. The classic example is derived from experiments on the induction of murine skin tumors (Berenblum, 1941). It was noted that papillomas could be induced to form on the skin of mice by a single application of 3-methylchlorantrene (3-MC), followed by repeated application over a period of weeks of the irritative substance croton oil, which contains tetradecanoyl phorbol acetate (TPA). If TPA application was continued, eventually a few of the papillomas developed into invasive squamous cell carcinomas. Growth of these carcinomas was independent of further stimulation by TPA. On the basis of these experiments, the chemical 3-MC was termed an *initiator and TPA a promoter* of carcinogenesis. Many other chemical carcinogens have since been classified as either initiators or promoters. Initiators were found to be mutagenic and to require only one exposure to cause a tumor. Promoters were found to act as growth stimulators. The critical event in the transformation of a benign cell into a cell with malignant potential was termed *conversion,* and the clonal expansion of that malignant cell and the development of invasive and metastatic characteristics was referred to as *progression* (Hathway, 1986; Varmus and Weinberg, 1993).

The identification of oncogenes has led to a better understanding of the nature of the genetic events occurring during the initiation–promotion–conversion–progression model of carcinogenesis. It is now apparent that several oncogenes may be activated, or tumor suppressor genes inactivated, to generate an individual cancer. The actual genetic sequence of events has been studied extensively in several tumors.

The best known example of the multistage nature of carcinogenesis in humans is colon cancer, as described by Fearon and Vogelstein (1990). Colon cancer provides an excellent model system with which to study carcinogenesis, as colon carcinomas are known to develop from identifiable premalignant adenomatous polyps. Individuals with familial adenomatous polyposis syndrome carry alterations in the tumor suppressor gene *APC* (chromosome 5), resulting in the formation of hundreds of colonic polyps. The *APC* gene has also been found to be altered somatically in sporadic colon cancers. Loss of a functioning *APC* gene results in hyperproliferation of the colonic epithelium and the early appearance of adenomas. This phase is accompanied by hypomethylation of DNA and resulting genetic instability. A mutation of K-*ras* on chromosome 12 then occurs in a cell of a small adenoma, causing it to undergo clonal expansion and develop into a larger, more dysplastic lesion. This phase is followed by deletion of the *DCC* gene, a putative tumor suppressor gene on chromosome 18 and by loss of *p53* on chromosome 17. The loss of these tumor suppressor genes appears to be associated with the transition from late adenoma to invasive cancer.

In addition to these fairly well defined events, other known oncogenes may play a role in colon carcinogenesis. More than 70 per cent of colon cancers overexpress the *myc* oncogene, and the tyrosine kinase activity of the protein product of the *src* oncogene increases in proportion to the stage of progression. Another gene, *MCC*, closely linked to the *APC* gene on chromosome 5, is also mutated in most sporadic colon cancers (Carney and Sikora, 1990; Hunter, 1991).

Dysplasia and Preneoplasia

There are numerous other examples, especially in tumors arising from epithelial or endothelial surfaces, of a stepwise progression through various histologically identifiable preneoplastic phases to invasive cancer. The preneoplastic lesions are confined to the epithelial surface and do not extend through the underlying basement membrane, lacking the invasive characteristics of cancer cells. They exhibit histologically dysplastic features. Preneoplastic lesions may progress to invasive cancer, remain stable, or regress spontaneously. In lung cancer, for example, fiberoptic bronchoscopy has enabled identification of a series of histologic changes of the bronchial mucosa, from hyperplasia and metaplasia, through dysplasia and carcinoma in situ, to frankly invasive cancer. Multiple oncogenes and tumor suppressor genes have been implicated along this pathway, including *ras, myc, erb-B, Rb,* and *p53.* Similar changes have been observed in other parts of the aerodigestive tract, such as the dysplastic changes seen as leukoplakia in the oral cavity.

Cervical cancer arises from a progression of preneoplastic changes that are detectable by the cervical Papanicolaou (Pap) smear. At least some of the dysplastic changes seen on the cervix are thought to be attributable to the sequestering and inactivation of *p53* by the E6 protein of the human papillomavirus. Preneoplastic lesions have also been identified in breast cancer, bladder cancer, and squamous cell carcinoma of the skin.

Field Cancerization

A concept that was originally proposed 40 years ago and has recently re-emerged in discussions of multistep carcinogenesis is *field cancerization* (Lippman et al., 1993; Slaughter et al., 1953). It refers to the multicentric nature of premalignant lesions in a field of tissue exposed to common carcinogens, such as the bronchial mucosa of smokers. A number of cells are initiated by a carcinogen and then stimulated to proliferate by promoting agents, forming preneoplastic lesions. Eventually one cell in one lesion suffers a critical genetic event and is converted to a malignant phenotype. This cell then undergoes clonal expansion and progression to eventually become an invasive cancer. At the same time, however, other cells, having been exposed to the same carcinogens, are at various stages of the carcinogenic pathway and could be induced to progress and become new primary tumors. This model helps explain the increased risk of second malignancies observed in individuals with certain primary tumors and emphasizes the importance of primary prevention strategies for dealing with human cancer.

Invasion and Metastases

Cancer mortality is due in large part to the ability of cancer cells to invade surrounding tissues, disseminate throughout the body, and form secondary tumors at distant sites. An understanding of the complex processes of invasion and metastases is crucial to the understanding of carcinogenesis in general.

Tissue stroma is separated from epithelial or endothelial surfaces and organ parenchyma by the basement membrane, a dense continuous barrier composed of collagen, glycoproteins, and proteoglycans. It is invasion of tumor cells through the basement membrane that signals the transition from a premalignant to a malignant state. Invasion may be thought of as occurring in three phases: adherence of tumor cells to the basement membrane; disruption of the basement membrane by proteolytic digestion; and migration of cells through the basement membrane into the underlying stroma (Kim et al., 1993; Liotta et al., 1991; Varmus and Weinberg, 1993).

Once tumor cells have invaded the underlying tissue stroma, they grow and proliferate. Continued growth, however, is limited by blood supply; and development of this blood supply, or *angiogenesis*, becomes critical for continued proliferation. Tumor cells develop the ability to secrete angiogenesis factors, such as fibroblast growth factor, angiogenin, and transforming growth factors. The newly formed blood vessels are thin-walled and provide clusters of tumor cells with access into the circulation. Lymphatic vessels, which lack basement membranes, also provide a conduit for dissemination of tumor cells.

Fewer than 0.01 per cent of circulating tumor cells eventually form metastases. The processes governing metastatic potential are poorly understood. Circulating tumor cells must first evade the host's immune system, which requires escape from both the specific T cell-dependent immune response and nonspecific mechanisms such as macrophage-mediated or natural killer cell-mediated killing. One mechanism of escape seems to involve the production of protective fibrin cocoons around tumor cells in the circulation. Another mechanism may involve blocking antibodies.

The next step in the metastatic process involves extravasation from blood vessels in a distant tissue.

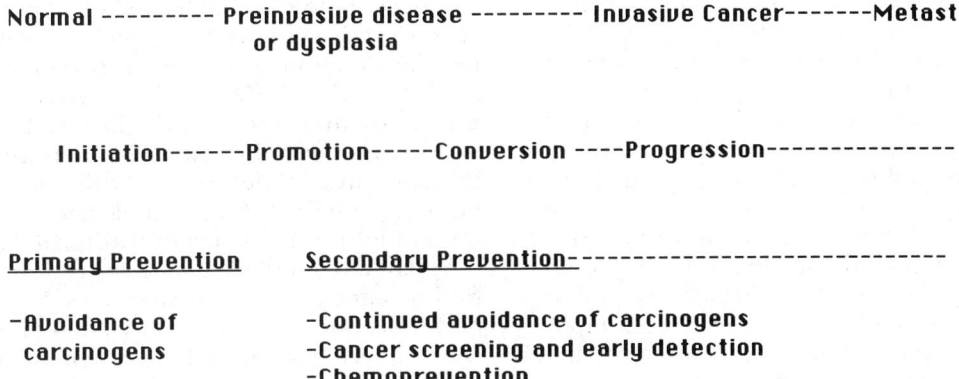

FIGURE 44–1. Cancer prevention strategies for multistep carcinogenesis.

What signals a given tumor cell to invade a particular tissue is unknown, although it is clear that many tumors have a predilection for specific metastatic sites. For example, breast and prostate cancers typically metastasize to bone, lung cancer to the brain and adrenals, and colorectal tumors to the liver and lung. Study of these tropisms may yield important clues to the metastatic process.

CANCER PREVENTION

One of the most important roles played by the family physician in the field of oncology is in the area of cancer prevention. As we begin to understand the carcinogenic process, we can identify factors that place patients at increased risk for cancer and so develop interventional strategies to avoid or counteract these risks (Fig. 44–1). Cancer risk assessment and prevention should be a routine part of the health maintenance program for every family practice patient (Table 44–5).

When discussing cancer prevention, we must consider individual variations in disease risk. Variables include exposure to carcinogens, detoxification, and carcinogen-activating mechanisms, DNA repair mechanisms, absent or mutated tumor suppressor genes, and activated proto-oncogenes.

TABLE 44–5. SUMMARY OF AMERICAN CANCER SOCIETY RECOMMENDATIONS FOR THE EARLY DETECTION OF CANCER IN ASYMPTOMATIC PEOPLE

Test or Procedure	Population		
	Sex	Age	Frequency
Sigmoidoscopy, preferably flexible	M & F	50+	Every 3–5 years
Fecal occult blood test	M & F	50+	Every year
Digital rectal examination	M & F	40+	Every year
Prostate examination*	M	50+	Every year
Papanicolaou test	F		All women who are or who have been sexually active, or have reached age 18, should have an annual Pap test and pelvic examination. After a woman has had three or more consecutive satisfactory normal annual examinations, the Pap test may be performed less frequently at the discretion of her physician.
Pelvic examination	F	18–40	Every 1–3 years with Pap test
		>40	Every year
Endometrial tissue sample	F	At menopause if at high risk†	At menopause and thereafter at the discretion of the physician
Breast self-examination	F	20+	Every month
Breast clinical examination	F	20–40	Every 3 years
		>40	Every year
Mammography‡	F	40–49	Every 1–2 years
		50+	Every year
Health counseling and cancer checkup§	M & F	>20	Every 3 years
	M & F	>40	Every year

* Annual digital rectal examination and prostate-specific antigen assay should be performed on men age 50 and older. If either is abnormal, further evaluation should be considered.
† History of infertility, obesity, failure to ovulate, abnormal uterine bleeding, or unopposed estrogen or tamoxifen therapy.
‡ Screening mammography should begin by age 40.
§ To include examination for cancers of the thyroid, testicles, ovaries, lymph nodes, oral region, and skin.
From Mettlin C, Jones G, Averette H, et al: Defining and updating the American Cancer Society guidelines for the cancer-related checkup: prostate and endometrial cancers. CA Cancer J Clin 43:45, 1993, with permission.

However, because many of these variables cannot be easily screened for, cancer risk is most easily assessed by determining known carcinogen exposure and family history.

Primary prevention refers to the avoidance of risk factors in an attempt to prevent the occurrence of disease. Many of the variables discussed above are intrinsic to a given patient and cannot be changed. However, exposure to carcinogens is one factor that can be altered and should be the focus of patient education and counseling strategies. For example, cigarette smoking alone has been implicated in up to 30 per cent of all cancer deaths, and family physicians should be active in initiating and encouraging smoking cessation in all their patients who smoke. Advice on healthy low fat, high fiber diets, sun-exposure protection, and safe sexual practices should also be routine. Some patients may be exposed to particular occupational or environmental carcinogens, and this information should be elicited and acted upon.

Secondary prevention involves the early detection of disease that is already present. Cancer is much more readily treated and cured if detected in its early stages, before wide local invasion or metastases has occurred. Certainly, detection during the premalignant phase offers an even better prognosis. Chapter 11 outlines in detail the recommendations for cancer screening and early detection. We reproduce here the American Cancer Society (ACS) guidelines for cancer screening (Table 44–5). The ACS is only one of several agencies that issues cancer screening guidelines; other groups, such as the National Cancer Institute, American Association of Family Physicians, and United States Preventive Services Health Task Force, differ in some of their recommendations.

Not all cancer sites are amenable to cost-effective routine screening examinations or tests. Currently targeted are breast, cervical, colorectal, head and neck, penile, prostate, testicular, and skin cancers. Certain other cancers, such as ovarian, endometrial, and lung, may be screened for in individuals at high risk. Individuals at high risk for cancer, especially in terms of family history or predisposing disease conditions, must be identified because the screening guidelines may differ for those individuals. Table 44–6 lists high-risk cancer screening guidelines for selected malignancies.

Molecular markers may lead to future innovations in cancer screening strategies. Mutated forms of the *ras* oncogene have now been found in stool specimens of patients with early colorectal cancers (Sidransky et al., 1992). Thus screening for activated proto-oncogenes in blood or body fluids may prove worthwhile. In families with a high prevalence of cancer, screening for mutated or absent tumor suppressor genes may identify those individuals at risk.

Chemoprevention

Chemoprevention refers to the use of chemical compounds to halt the carcinogenic process before the development of invasive cancer. Studies on the multistep nature of carcinogenesis suggest the possibility of blocking tumor progression at various stages. Compounds that have antioxidant effects, stimulate DNA repair mechanisms, shield DNA structures, stabilize membranes, or act as scavengers of mutagens or mitogens could theoretically have chemopreventive properties. Compounds currently undergoing investigation include polyphenols, thiols, carotenoids and retinoids, carbohydrates, trace metals, terpenes, tocopherols, indoles, and isothiocyanates. Clinical trials with isotretinoin (13-*cis*-retinoic acid) have shown regression of oral leukoplakia and reduction of the incidence of second primary tumors in patients

TABLE 44–6. SUGGESTIONS FOR HIGH-RISK CANCER SCREENING

Cancer Site	High-Risk Criteria	Screening Guidelines
Colon	Family history* Familial polyposis coli Ulcerative colitis Previous colonic polyps	Colonoscopy beginning at least 5 years before earliest familial cancer or at time of diagnosis of related condition Repeat every 1–5 years Fecal occult blood test during intervening years
Breast	Family history* History of lobular carcinoma in situ or atypical hyperplasia on biopsy Previous breast cancer	Baseline mammogram at age 25 or at diagnosis, then every 2–3 years to age 40 and annually thereafter Yearly clinical examination Monthly breast self-examination
Lung	Exposure to asbestos Smoking > 2–3 packs per day	Chest radiograph and sputum cytologic analysis every 4 months†
Ovary	Family history*	Pelvic ultrasonography, color flow Doppler of ovarian vessels, and Ca-125 assay annually†

* Family history refers to two or more first-degree relatives or one first-degree relative and two or more second-degree relatives. Also includes multiple cancer family syndromes.
† Experimental protocols only—not current standard of care.

with head and neck cancer (Lippman et al., 1993). Studies are currently under way using oral and topical retinoids for treatment of cervical dysplasia; oral retinoids for treatment of bronchial metaplasia; topical retinoids for treatment of premalignant skin lesions; calcium and nonsteroidal anti-inflammatory agents (NSAIDs) for prevention of colorectal cancer; and tamoxifen for prevention of breast cancer in high-risk patients.

DIAGNOSIS OF CANCER

Before the treatment of malignancy can be undertaken, an accurate pathologic diagnosis must be established. Although most diagnoses can be established by morphology alone, the advent of immunohistochemical studies, flow cytometry, monoclonal antibody technology, cytogenetic techniques, and molecular biologic techniques have allowed a more precise, thorough characterization of tumors. These advances in the ability to diagnose and characterize tumors and to follow cancers after diagnosis have advanced the treatment of malignant disease.

Staging

Selection of the appropriate treatment for a patient with cancer requires detailed knowledge of the extent of disease. Diagnostic imaging, physical examination, and laboratory tests must be performed to determine whether disease is localized or has metastasized. A staging system that groups patients according to the extent of disease allows consideration of prognostic information associated with the natural history of the disease and guides therapeutic choices.

The International Union Against Cancer (UICC) and the American Joint Committee on Cancer Staging and End Stage Reporting (AJCCS) together have developed the TNM system now used routinely for solid tumors. With this system, T characterizes the extent of the primary tumor, N describes the status of regional lymph nodes, and M denotes the presence or absence of distant metastases. The TNM characterizations are classified into groups that represent the stages from limited to extensive disease. In general, early stage disease is amenable to regional therapy given with curative intent, whereas advanced disease requires systemic therapies for control or cure.

PRINCIPLES OF THERAPY

Radiotherapy

The goals of radiotherapy are to provide the maximum energy to the target tumor in a homogeneous fashion so as to provide uniform cell kill while minimizing absorption and toxicity to the intervening normal tissues. Hyperfractionation (multiple fractions given on a single day) or accelerated fractionation are currently under investigation for their ability to improve local tumor control.

The interaction of radiation with matter is described as the amount of energy absorbed per unit mass. A commonly used unit of measure of the absorbed dose is the Gray (Gy), which is equal to 1 joule/kg, or 100 rad.

One of the two radiotherapy techniques most frequently used is *external beam therapy*, in which the source of radiation is located outside the patient. External beam therapy is delivered in discrete fractions, usually on a daily basis. Before treatment, the patient must undergo a simulation in which superficial radiation is used to plan the beam location. The patients usually are marked and immobilized to ensure reproducible ports.

The second technique, *brachytherapy*, uses a source of radiation that is implanted within or near the tumor. The source emits continuous rays with limited penetration, destroying tumor cells, with minimal absorption and toxicity to normal tissues. The catheters used to introduce the radiation source may be placed with precision by endoscopic procedures. This modality is useful for treating obstructing lesions in the bronchial tree or esophagus.

Chemotherapy

Neoadjuvant Chemotherapy

The concept of neoadjuvant chemotherapy arose from the recognition that many tumors at diagnosis have invaded tissues beyond their primary site. Neoadjuvant chemotherapy is administered before definitive local therapy (surgery or irradiation). The potential benefits of neoadjuvant chemotherapy include the ability to improve local control before resection, allowing more conservative surgery and preserving function. Also, the response of the tumor to chemotherapy can be accurately assessed by examining the specimen after surgical resection. The type of chemotherapy administered after surgery can be based on the response of the tumor to presurgical chemotherapy. Finally, neoadjuvant chemotherapy provides for early control of systemic disease.

Adjuvant Chemotherapy

Adjuvant chemotherapy involves the administration of chemotherapeutic agents after removal of the primary tumor, when there is no evidence of residual gross disease. Drugs used in the adjuvant setting are those that have been effective against advanced disease. The principles of dose intensity and maintaining a rapid repetitive schedule of

TABLE 44–7. COMMON TOXIC EFFECTS OF CHEMOTHERAPEUTIC AGENTS

Toxic Effect	Chemotherapeutic Agents
Neurologic	Vincristine,* asparaginase,* procarbazine, vinblastine, intrathecal methotrexate, intrathecal cytarabine
Pulmonary	Bleomycin,* busulfan, carmustine, cyclophosphamide, methotrexate, mitomycin, chlorambucil, melphalan, mercaptopurine, cytarabine, procarbazine, vinblastine
Otologic	Cisplatin*
Renal	Cisplatin,* streptozotocin,* methotrexate, mitomycin
Hemorrhagic cystitis	Cyclophosphamide, ifosfamide
Hepatic	Methotrexate, 6-mercaptopurine, azathioprine, asparaginase, mithramycin, nitrosoureas, streptozotocin, chlorambucil, dacarbazine
Cardiac	Daunomycin,* doxorubicin,* rubidazone,* amsacrine, bleomycin, cyclophosphamide, cytarabine, etoposide, 5-fluorouracil, vincristine, vinblastine
Emesis	Cisplatin, dacarbazine, dactinomycin, mechlorethamine, cyclophosphamide, carmustine, lomustine, doxorubicin, daunorubicin, cytarabine, procarbazine
Stomatitis	Mechlorethamine, cytarabine, fluorouracil, mercaptopurine, methotrexate, thioguanine, bleomycin, daunorubicin, doxorubicin, mitomycin, vinblastine, vincristine, procarbazine
Gonadal dysfunction	Chlorambucil, cyclophosphamide, busulfan, nitrogen mustard, procarbazine, doxorubicin, vinblastine, cisplatin, cytarabine
Myelosuppression	Mechlorethamine,* melphalan,* busulfan,* carmustine,* lomustine,* semustine,* cytarabine,* etoposide,* vinblastine*

* Dose-limiting effect.

drug administration are important for prolonging patient survival.

Chemotherapy for Advanced Malignancy

Chemotherapy for advanced malignancy, although often not given with curative intent, is documented to control disease-related symptoms and to prolong survival in a subset of patients. It may be combined with surgery and radiotherapy. The response to chemotherapy is measured by defined criteria and designated as complete response, partial response, minimal response, or progression. Complete response is defined as the disappearance of all evidence of disease with no reappearance of the disease for a specified time period (usually 4 weeks). Partial response is defined as reduction by at least 50 per cent in the sum of the products of the two longest diameters of all lesions, maintained for at least one course of therapy with no new appearance of disease. Minimal response describes any tumor reduction less than a partial response.

The toxic effects of chemotherapy can be varied and involve many organ systems; they are outlined in Table 44–7. Toxic effects may limit the chemotherapy dose and the schedule of drug delivery.

Biologic Therapy

Biologic agents have a wide variety of clinical actions. Some, such as interferons, have a direct antiproliferative effect. Others can activate or influence effector cells of the immune system. Some biologic agents now under clinical investigation may possess antimetastatic or antiangiogenic actions. Others, acting on the cellular level, regulate gene activation or cellular differentiation.

Biologic agents have proved to be useful for treatment of hairy cell leukemia, myeloma, renal cell carcinoma, and melanoma. The most widely used of these agents are the interferons and interleukin-2, with or without lymphokine-activated killer cells or tumor-infiltrating lymphocytes. The toxic effects of biologic agents include fever and flu-like symptoms, fatigue, central nervous system (CNS) effects (interferon), and capillary leak syndrome (most commonly associated with interleukin-2).

Hormonal Therapy

Orchiectomy, the first hormonal treatment, has long been a standard therapy for prostate carcinoma. Newer hormonal agonists and antagonists are used for breast cancer and prostate cancer and are being investigated for their therapeutic role in other malignancies. Luteinizing hormone releasing factor agonists are being employed for prostate cancer. Tamoxifen (an antiestrogen) has been active against advanced breast cancer and is now being investigated for its role in preventing breast cancer in women at high risk of developing the disease.

Drug Resistance

Drug resistance may have pharmacologic, kinetic, or genetic causes. Dose-response curves have been developed for many agents, and cellular killing may depend on achieving a dose of the drug that approaches the maximum tolerated dose. The *maximum tolerated dose* is defined in phase I clinical trials as the dose at which a predefined proportion of patients experience unacceptable toxic effects. Failure to deliver the maximum tolerated dose may prevent chemotherapy from reaching a sanctuary site, such as the CNS.

Chemotherapeutic agents are most effective against actively proliferating cells and less effective against cells in the resting phase of the cell cycle (G_0). Kinetic resistance to chemotherapeutic agents is inherent in resting cells and in proliferating cells that do not match the cell cycle selectivity of the particular chemotherapeutic agent.

Genetic drug resistance has been shown to occur by spontaneous mutations as the tumor clones expand. In addition, genetically mediated resistance to multiple drugs has been associated with the *MDR-1* gene, which codes for a P-glycoprotein product in the cell membrane that acts as an efflux pump to drive drugs out of the cell.

Strategies to overcome drug resistance are being investigated, and several have been employed clinically. At present, however, combination chemotherapy with non-cross-resistant drugs is the most successful way to avoid drug resistance.

BREAST CANCER

Epidemiology and Risk Factors

Breast cancer is the most common malignancy among women in North America, and its incidence is increasing steadily. It is second only to lung cancer as a cause of cancer death among women.

The cumulative (lifelong) risk for a U.S. woman of developing breast cancer is approximately 10 to 11 per cent. The risk of dying of breast cancer is smaller: only 3 to 4 per cent.

Factors associated with an increased risk of developing breast cancer include family history of breast cancer in primary or secondary relatives, early menarche, delayed menopause, few or late pregnancies, excessive alcohol intake, obesity, and radiation exposure. Approximately 70 per cent of patients have no identifiable risk factors (Henderson, 1990).

Oral contraceptives and fibrocystic breast disease are controversial risk factors. The risk of developing breast cancer after oral contraceptive use is small: approximately twice that of the general population. There is no significant evidence that oral contraceptive use should be avoided. Fibrocystic lesions that are proliferative or display atypical hyperplasia are associated with an increased risk of malignant transformation. No significant modifications of diet or lifestyle have been proved to decrease the risk of developing breast cancer, but modifications of dietary patterns, such as fat consumption, are being examined.

Evaluation of Palpable Masses

Palpable masses in postmenopausal women must be regarded with suspicion, as benign cysts are uncommon in this age group. A negative mammogram does not exclude the possibility of breast cancer in a woman presenting with a palpable mass. The patient should undergo prompt evaluation by fine-needle aspiration or excisional biopsy. In women older than 35 years, diagnostic mammography is performed before biopsy. Fine-needle aspiration should be performed only by experienced cytologists. If this expertise is not available, an excisional biopsy is recommended. Incisional biopsies are done only if the mass is too large to be completely excised or in the presence of metastatic disease.

Premenopausal women with a mass that persists throughout the menstrual cycle may first be evaluated by aspirating the lesion to ascertain whether it is cystic or solid. A cytologic examination of the aspirated fluid should be performed. If the palpable defect persists after aspiration or recurs, or if the aspirated fluid is bloody, the patient should be referred for mammography and biopsy. Paget's disease of the nipple is associated with invasive breast carcinoma. Any woman exhibiting nipple discharge or eczematous nipple changes should be referred for mammography and biopsy.

Evaluation of Nonpalpable Mammographic Abnormalities

Stereotactic needle localization and an aspiration cytologic examination may be performed with sensitivity and specificity approaching 90 per cent. Simple needle or dye localization and biopsy followed by radiography of the removed sample is used to document removal of microcalcifications. Only 15 to 30 per cent of these lesions are malignant.

Pretreatment Evaluation and Staging

Once the diagnosis of breast cancer is established, the clinical stage must be determined. Routine staging evaluation is outlined in Table 44–8. Breast cancer is initially staged on a clinical basis with evaluation of the extent of primary tumor, the involvement of lymph nodes, and the presence of distant metastases. The TNM system for breast cancer is outlined in Table 44–9.

TABLE 44–8. STAGING EVALUATION OF ADULT SOLID TUMORS

Study	Tumors						
	Breast	Lung	Colon	Prostate	Testicular	Ovarian	Cervical
Chest radiograph	*	*	*	*	*	*	*
Mammogram	*					*	**
Barium enema						*	*
Proctoscopy						*	*
Cytoscopy							
Computed tomography							
Chest		*			*		
Abdomen	**		*	*	*	*	*
Pelvis			*	*	*	*	*
Brain	**	**					
Bone scan	*	*			*		
Lymphangiogram						*	**
IVP						*	*
CBC	*	*	*	*	*	*	*
SMA	*	*	*	*	*	*	*
Liver function	*	*	*	*	*	*	*
Renal function				*	*	*	*
Bone marrow		†					
CEA	*	*	*			*	
AFP					*	*	
β-hCG					*	*	
CA-125 antigen						*	*
PAP				*			
PSA				*			
CSF	**	**					

IVP = intravenous pyelography; CBC = complete blood count; SMA = sequential multiple analysis; CEA = carcinoembryonic antigen; AFP = α-fetoprotein; β-hCG = β-human chorionic gonadotropin; PAP = prostatic alkaline phosphatase; PSA = prostate-specific antigen; CSF = cerebrospinal fluid.

* Study performed for routine staging evaluation.
** Study performed only if symptoms suggest disease in this area.
† Study obtained only for small-cell lung cancer.

Prognostic Factors

The number of axillary lymph nodes involved with metastatic disease is the most important prognostic variable. Increasing numbers of positive axillary nodes are associated with progressive increases in the percentage of treatment failures. Survival was markedly shorter in patients with four or more positive nodes than in their counterparts with fewer than four (Fisher et al., 1983). Because subsequent studies have confirmed these findings, patients are classified according to the number of histologically positive axillary nodes: node-negative, one to three positive nodes, four to nine positive nodes, or ten or more positive nodes.

Other factors that connote a poor prognosis include large primary tumor size, negative estrogen (ER) and progesterone (PR) receptor status, high histologic grade, high proliferative rate as expressed by the S-phase fraction, certain histologic subtypes, and overexpression of oncogenes such as *erb*-B-2, *EGF-r*, and *myc* (Clark and McGuire, 1988).

Therapy of Breast Cancer

Local Therapy

The standard method of local control has been the modified radical mastectomy with axillary node dissection. The pectoralis minor muscle is preserved with this technique. Similar survival rates have been reported for radical and modified radical mastectomies (Fisher et al., 1985).

Radiotherapy may be administered after mastectomy. Postoperative irradiation is recommended to enhance local control in node-positive patients and in patients with large tumors that have a high probability of local recurrence (McCormick, 1991). Radiation is conventionally administered after adjuvant chemotherapy.

For patients with stage I and II disease, lumpectomy is an alternative to mastectomy. Lumpectomy involves removal of the tumor plus a margin of normal tissue and preservation of the remaining breast tissue. An axillary lymph node dissection should always be performed to adequately stage the disease. Radiotherapy is added later with the goal of eradicating any residual foci of cancer. Prospective randomized trials that have compared modified radical mastectomy with lumpectomy followed by radiotherapy have demonstrated similar overall survival rates (Fisher et al., 1989c). Patients with advanced disease (stage III or IV), diffuse microcalcifications seen by mammography, two or more cancers located in different breast quadrants, tumors that are large compared to the overall breast size, or certain collagen-vascular diseases are not candidates for breast-conserving surgery (NIH Consensus Conference, 1991).

TABLE 44–9. TNM STAGING OF BREAST CANCER

Primary Tumor (T)

TX	Primary tumor cannot be assessed
T0	No evidence of primary tumor
Tis	Carcinoma in situ: intraductal carcinoma, lobular carcinoma in situ, or Paget's disease of the nipple with no tumor
T1	Tumor 2 cm or less in greatest dimension
T1a	0.5 cm or less in greatest dimension
T1b	More than 0.5 cm but not more than 1 cm in greatest dimension
T1c	More than 1 cm but not more than 2 cm in greatest dimension
T2	Tumor more than 2 cm but not more than 5 cm in greatest dimension
T3	Tumor more than 5 cm in greatest dimension
T4	Tumor of any size with direct extension to chest wall or skin
T4a	Extension to chest wall
T4b	Edema (including peau d'orange) or ulceration of the skin of the breast or satellite skin nodules confined to the same breast
T4c	Both (T4a and T4b)
T4d	Inflammatory carcinoma

Note: Paget's disease associated with a tumor is classified according to the size of the tumor.

Regional Lymph Nodes (N)

NX	Regional lymph nodes cannot be assessed (e.g., previously removed)
N0	No regional lymph node metastasis
N1	Metastasis to movable ipsilateral axillary lymph node(s)
N2	Metastasis to ipsilateral axillary lymph node(s) fixed to one another or to other structures
N3	Metastasis to ipsilateral internal mammary lymph node(s)

Distant Metastasis (M)

MX	Presence of distant metastasis cannot be assessed
M0	No distant metastasis
M1	Distant metastasis (includes metastasis to ipsilateral supraclavicular lymph node(s)

Stage Grouping

Stage 0	Tis	N0	M0
Stage I	T1	N0	M0
Stage IIA	T0	N1	M0
	T1	N1	M0
	T2	N0	M0
Stage IIB	T2	N1	M0
	T3	N0	M0
Stage IIIA	T0	N2	M0
	T1	N2	M0
	T2	N2	M0
	T3	N1	M0
	T3	N2	M0
Stage IIIB	T4	AnyN	M0
	AnyT	N3	M0
Stage IV	AnyT	AnyN	M1

From Beahrs OH, Henson DE, Hutter RVP, et al (eds): Manual for Staging of Cancer, 4th edition. Philadelphia, JB Lippincott, 1992, with permission.

Chemotherapy

Numerous trials have demonstrated that adjuvant therapy can prolong disease-free survival and improve the overall survival rate in node-positive women. Several adjuvant chemotherapy regimens are detailed in Table 44–10. The toxic effects of adjuvant therapy include hair loss, weight loss or gain, emesis, fatigue, and premature menopause.

Endocrine manipulation may also be used as an adjuvant therapy. The antiestrogen tamoxifen effectively reduces the rate of mortality in postmenopausal women with receptor-positive tumors (Early Breast Cancer Trialists' Collaborative Group, 1988).

ADJUVANT THERAPY IN NODE-POSITIVE WOMEN. Premenopausal women with positive axillary lymph nodes, regardless of their hormone receptor status, should receive combination chemotherapy for six cycles. Postmenopausal women with positive nodes but negative hormone-receptor status should also receive combination chemotherapy. Postmenopausal women with positive nodes and positive hormone-receptor status should received adjuvant hormonal therapy with tamoxifen, currently recommended to continue for 5 years (Consensus Conference, 1985).

ADJUVANT THERAPY IN NODE-NEGATIVE WOMEN. The use of adjuvant chemotherapy in patients with

TABLE 44–10. COMBINATION CHEMOTHERAPY REGIMENS FOR BREAST CANCER

Acronym and Drugs	Dose (mg/m²), Route, Schedule	Cycle Frequency
CMF ± P		
Cyclophosphamide	100 PO days 1–14	28 days
Methotrexate	40 IV days 1, 8	
5-Fluorouracil	600 IV days 1, 8	
Prednisone	40 PO days 1–14	
CMF		
Cyclophosphamide	600 IV day 1	21 days
Methotrexate	40 IV day 1	
5-Fluorouracil	600 IV day 1	
CMFVP		
Cyclophosphamide	60 PO daily	NA
Methotrexate	15 IV weekly	
5-Fluorouracil	400 IV weekly	
Vincristine	0.625 IV weekly × 10 weeks	
Prednisone	30 PO daily × 14 days	
	20 PO daily × 14 days	
	10 PO daily × 14 days	
FAC		
5-Fluorouracil	500 IV days 1, 8	21 days
Doxorubicin	50 IV day 1	
Cyclophosphamide	500 IV day 1	
CAF		
Cyclophosphamide	100 PO days 1, 14	28 days
Doxorubicin	30 IV days 1, 8	
5-Fluorouracil	500 IV days 1, 8	
AC		
Cyclophosphamide	600 IV day 1	21 days
Doxorubicin	60 IV day 1	

Adapted from Osborne CK: Breast cancer. *In* Wittes RE (ed): Manual of Oncologic Therapeutics 1991/1992. Philadelphia, JB Lippincott, 1991, with permission.

axillary node-negative disease is controversial. These women have a good prognosis: Most are cured by surgery alone. However, long-term follow-up of these patients has demonstrated that disease recurs in 10 to 40 per cent, suggesting that patients may benefit from adjuvant therapy. Both chemotherapy and hormonal therapy are effective in prolonging disease-free survival of patients with node-negative disease (Fisher et al., 1989a,b). Patients with tumors smaller than 1 cm, a low S-phase fraction, diploid DNA, nuclear grade classification I, and positive hormone-receptor status have the best prognosis and require no additional therapy. In contrast, patients with tumors larger than 3 cm, nuclear grade classification III, negative hormone-receptor status, and high S-phase fraction are at higher risk for tumor recurrence. It has been suggested that these women should receive adjuvant therapy (McGuire and Clark, 1992). Premenopausal women and women with receptor-negative tumors should receive chemotherapy, and postmenopausal patients with receptor-positive tumors should receive tamoxifen (Harris et al., 1992).

Therapy for Metastatic Breast Cancer

Patients with hormone receptor-positive tumors should receive sequential therapy with tamoxifen followed by second- and third-line endocrine therapies, including progestins (megestrol acetate), aminoglutethimide, and androgens (fluoxymestrone). Approximately 50 to 65 per cent of patients respond to the first hormonal therapy, with a median response duration of 8 to 12 months. Patients whose disease progresses on tamoxifen have an approximately 50 per cent probability of responding to second-line endocrine therapies.

Patients with metastatic disease who have hormone receptor-negative tumors should receive combination chemotherapy. Between 45 and 85 per cent of patients have an objective tumor response (Buzdar, 1988). The recently introduced agent paclitaxel (Taxol) has promising activity as a single agent: More than 50 per cent of patients experience clinical responses.

LUNG CANCER

Epidemiology and Risk Factors

During the twentieth century, lung cancer has risen to epidemic proportions; it is the leading cause of cancer deaths in the United States, where approximately 150,000 new cases of lung cancer are diagnosed yearly. Screening asymptomatic patients who are in groups at high risk for lung cancer has not significantly altered the rates of morbidity or mortality of the disease (Eddy, 1989). Unfortunately, only 13 per cent of patients diagnosed with lung cancer survive 5 years.

The most important risk factor for the development of lung cancer is tobacco use. Evidence linking smoking to lung cancer was presented more than 40 years ago, and support for this link has grown steadily.

Other risk factors for the development of lung cancer include passive exposure to tobacco smoke; exposure to chromium, nickel, inorganic arsenic compounds, asbestos, or radon; altered expression of tumor suppressor genes; and diets poor in antioxidants.

Histologic Types of Lung Cancer

Lung cancer comprises small-cell and non-small-cell types. This distinction is based on differing tumor characteristics and biologic behaviors. The non-small-cell lung tumors include squamous cell carcinoma (also known as epidermoid), adenocarcinoma, and large-cell carcinoma.

Non-Small-Cell Lung Carcinoma

Symptoms

The symptoms of lung cancer include new or progressive cough, localized wheezing or stridor, hemoptysis, pleuritic chest pain, recurrent pulmonary infections, hoarseness, superior vena cava syndrome, and the Pancoast syndrome of lower brachial plexopathy, Horner's syndrome, and shoulder pain. Patients with advanced disease may present with neurologic symptoms, bony pain, weight loss, or failure to thrive.

Evaluation and Staging

The goal of diagnostic evaluation and staging of lung cancer is to identify patients who are candidates for surgical resection, as surgery is the primary curative modality. However, only 20 to 30 per cent of lesions are resectable at diagnosis. The staging evaluation is outlined in Table 44–8. Computed tomography (CT) of the chest should be extended to include the liver and adrenal glands, as these organs are often sites of metastases.

A tissue diagnosis may be obtained by sputum cytologic analysis, bronchoscopy with brushings or washings if lesions are endobronchially or centrally located, or bronchoscopic biopsy. Bronchoscopy provides poor diagnostic yield (less than 20 per cent) for lesions smaller than 2 cm or located in the periphery. Peripheral lesions may be evaluated by transthoracic needle biopsy under fluoroscopic or CT guidance or thoracotomy. More than 95 per cent of tumors may be diagnosed without thoracotomy. Mediastinoscopy or mediastinotomy is often performed before definitive pulmonary resection to exclude the involvement of mediastinal nodes, which may preclude curative resection. The TNM staging system is used for non-small-cell lung cancer with provisions for inclusion of pleural and pericardial effusions as outlined in Table 44–11.

Once the tumor is deemed operable by clinical staging and mediastinoscopy, the patient should be evaluated physiologically for the ability to tolerate resection of pulmonary parenchyma. Preoperative assessment should include spirometry, arterial blood gas analysis, split-perfusion lung scanning, or exercise testing with measurement of maximal oxygen uptake. Right-heart catheterization and measurement of pulmonary artery pressure may help assess the operative risk (American College of Physicians Position Paper, 1990). Testing cardiac function, including electrocardiogram (ECG), nuclear ventricular function analysis (MUGA), and echocardiogram, is required in some patients.

Therapy

Patients with stage I or II disease should undergo surgical resection with curative intent. If patients are unable to tolerate surgery because of poor cardiopulmonary function or other comorbid conditions, radiotherapy may be used as the primary therapeutic modality. Postoperative radiotherapy reduces the rate of local recurrence in patients with nodal involvement and is recom-

TABLE 44–12. COMBINATION CHEMOTHERAPY PROGRAMS FOR NON-SMALL-CELL LUNG CANCER

Cisplatin plus vindesine
  Cisplatin 120 mg/m^2 days 1, 29; then q 6 wk
  Vindesine 3 mg/m^2 days 1, 8, 15, 22, 29; then q 2 wk

Cisplatin plus vinblastine
  Cisplatin 120 mg/m^2 days 1, 29; then q 6 wk
  Vinblastine 5 mg/m^2 days 1, 8, 15, 22, 29; then q 2 wk

Cisplatin plus etoposide
  Cisplatin 60 mg/m^2 day 1; then q 3–4 wk
  Etoposide 120 mg/m^2 days 4, 6, 8; then q 3–4 wk

Mitomycin plus vindesine
  Mitomycin 10 mg/m^2 days 1, 22; then q 6 wk
  Vindesine 3 mg/m^2 days 1, 8, 15, 22, 29; then q 2 wk

Cisplatin plus vindesine plus mitomycin
  Cisplatin 120 mg/m^2 days 1, 29; then q 6 wk
  Vindesine 3 mg/m^2 days 1, 8, 15, 22, 29; then q 2 wk
  Mitomycin 8 mg/m^2 days 1, 29, 71 only

Cisplatin plus vinblastine plus mitomycin
  Cisplatin 120 mg/m^2 days 1, 29; then q 6 wk
  Vinblastine 4 mg/m^2 day 1
         2 mg/m^2 day 8
         4.5 mg/m^2 days 15, 22, 29; then q 2 wk
  Mitomycin 8 mg/m^2 days 1, 29, 71 only

Adapted from DeVita VT Jr, Hellman S, Rosenberg SA: Principles and Practice of Oncology, 4th edition. Philadelphia, JB Lippincott, 1993, p 711, with permission.

TABLE 44–11. TNM STAGING SYSTEM FOR LUNG CANCER

Stage	Description	5-Year Survival Rate (%)
I	T1–2N0M0	60–80
II	T1–2N1M0	25–50
IIIA	T3N0–1M0	25–40
	T1–3N2M0	10–30
IIIB	Any T4 or any N3M0	< 5
IV	Any M1	< 5

Primary Tumor (T)	
TX	Positive malignant cell; no lesion seen
T1	< 3 cm diameter
T2	> 3 cm diameter
	Distal atelectasis
T3	Extension to pleura, chest wall, diaphragm, or pericardium
	< 2 cm from carina or total atelectasis
T4	Invasion of mediastinal organs
	Malignant pleural effusion

Regional Lymph Nodes (N)	
N0	No involvement
N1	Ipsilateral bronchopulmonary or hilar
N2	Ipsilateral or subcarinal mediastinal
	Ipsilateral supraclavicular
	Contralateral mediastinal, hilum, or supraclavicular

Distant Metastasis (M)	
M0	None
M1	Metastases present

Adapted from DeVita VT Jr, Hellman S, Rosenberg SA: Principles and Practice of Oncology, 4th edition. Philadelphia, JB Lippincott, 1993, p 682, with permission.

mended for patients with node-positive disease or positive margins.

Surgical resection is also the procedure of choice for stage IIIA disease, but advanced N2 disease (see Evaluation and Staging, above) as visualized on CT is generally considered inoperable. These patients, along with those with stage IIIB disease (locally advanced disease that is confined to the chest), receive radiotherapy.

Adjuvant chemotherapy has produced prolonged disease-free survival after complete resection of the tumor, but no benefit in overall survival has been consistently documented. The role of adjuvant chemotherapy after complete resection remains undefined (Green, 1993; Holmes, 1993).

Combination chemotherapy is used in patients with stage IV cancers. There is no standard chemotherapy program for this disease. Regimens containing cisplatin have response rates of 20 to 40 per cent. Commonly used regimens are listed in Table 44–12. Agents being investigated for non-small-cell lung cancer include the taxoids (paclitaxel and docetaxel), gemcitabine, topotecan, and long-term oral etoposide (Lilenbaum and Green, 1993).

Small-Cell Lung Cancer

The epidemiology and risk factors of small-cell lung cancer are similar to those of non-small-cell lung cancer. Small-cell lung cancer is an aggressive malignancy with early metastases. This aggressive biologic behavior is manifested clinically by a short symptomatic period and abrupt presentation with extensive disease. The median survival of untreated patients is only 4 to 6 weeks.

Paraneoplastic syndromes can be associated with lung cancer and may be the initial presenting symptom or a manifestation of progressive disease. These syndromes are more frequently associated with small-cell lung cancers. They include ectopic ACTH and Cushing syndrome and ectopic antidiuretic hormone (ADH) and the syndrome of inappropriate antidiuretic hormone (SIADH). Neurologic syndromes can include encephalomyelitis and the Eaton-Lambert syndrome, which is characterized by muscle weakness and fatigue, most pronounced in the pelvic girdle and thighs. This syndrome is similar to myasthenia gravis in that it may also include dysarthria, dysphagia, blurred vision, diplopia, ptosis, and paresthesia; but in contrast to myasthenia, muscle strength improves with exercise, as documented by electromyography (Richardson and Johnson, 1992).

Evaluation and Staging

Patients with small-cell lung carcinoma are considered to have systemic spread of their disease at the time of diagnosis. Thus surgery is not routinely employed for this disease.

The staging system for small-cell lung cancer, proposed by the Veterans Administration Lung Cancer Study Group during the 1960s, categorizes small-cell lung cancer into limited disease and extensive disease. *Limited disease* is defined as disease confined to one hemithorax and its regional lymph nodes with or without local extension or involvement of ipsilateral supraclavicular nodes. *Extensive disease* encompasses any disease beyond these limits (Table 44–13). The goal of staging is to identify patients with limited disease who can be treated with additional radiotherapy.

The staging evaluation reflects the rapid and widespread dissemination of small-cell disease. Routine staging for small-cell carcinoma includes the studies obtained for non-small-cell lung cancer

TABLE 44–13. TWO-STAGE CLASSIFICATION SYSTEM FOR SMALL-CELL LUNG CANCER

Limited disease (30%)*
  Primary tumor confined to hemithorax
  Ipsilateral hilar lymph nodes
  Ipsilateral and contralateral supraclavicular lymph nodes
  Ipsilateral and contralateral mediastinal lymph nodes

Extensive disease (70%)*
  Metastatic lesions in the contralateral lung
  Distant metastatic involvement (e.g., brain, bone, liver)
  Pleural effusion†

* Approximate percentage of patients with this extent of disease at the time of diagnosis.
  † Currently, the presence of a malignant pleural effusion denotes T4, or extensive disease.
  Adapted from Patel AM, Dunn WF, Trastek VF: Staging systems of lung cancer. Mayo Clin Proc 68:475, 1993, with permission.

TABLE 44–14. COMMONLY USED COMBINATION CHEMOTHERAPY PROGRAMS FOR SMALL-CELL LUNG CANCER

Acronym and Drugs	Dose, Route, Schedule	Cycle Frequency (days)
CAV		
Cyclophosphamide	1000 mg/m^2 IV day 1	21
Doxorubicin	45 mg/m^2 IV day 1	
Vincristine	2 mg IV day 1	
CAE		
Cyclophosphamide	1000 mg/m^2 IV day 1	21
Doxorubicin	45 mg/m^2 IV day 1	
Etoposide	50 mg/m^2 IV days 1–5	
CAVE		
Cyclophosphamide	1000 mg/m^2 IV day 1	21
Doxorubicin	50 mg/m^2 IV day 1	
Vincristine	1.5 mg/m^2 IV day 1	
Etoposide	60 mg/m^2 IV days 1–5	
EP		
Etoposide	100 mg/m^2 IV days 1–3	21
Cisplatin	25 mg/m^2 IV days 1–3	
CMCcV		
Cyclophosphamide	700 mg/m^2 IV day 1	28
Methotrexate	20 mg/m^2 PO days 18, 21	
Lomustine	70 mg/m^2 PO day 1	
Vincristine	1.3 mg/m^2 IV days 1, 8, 15, 22 first cycle; then day 1	
CAV and EP		
As above	As above, alternating	21

Adapted from DeVita VT Jr, Hellman S, Rosenberg SA: Principles and Practice of Oncology, 4th edition. Philadelphia, JB Lippincott, 1993, p 736, with permission.

(Table 44–8) and others. CT of the brain is more frequently used for small-cell disease, because approximately 30 per cent of patients have brain metastases at presentation and up to 80 per cent have brain metastases at some point in their disease. Patients should also undergo bone marrow biopsy and aspiration if other studies do not identify extensive disease; in 5 to 15 per cent of patients, the bone marrow is the only site of advanced disease.

Therapy

Chemotherapy is the primary treatment for both limited and extensive disease. Patients respond quickly and exhibit maximal response within four to six cycles. There is no benefit to prolonged chemotherapy. Widely used chemotherapy regimens are outlined in Table 44–14.

Limited small-cell lung cancer is characterized by micrometastases that require chemotherapy for control. However, because the primary tumor site is the site of progression or relapse in 80 per cent of patients, combined radiotherapy and chemotherapy is the standard approach to treating limited disease (Aisner, 1992). Patients who respond completely to chemoradiotherapy are then candidates for prophylactic cranial irradiation to reduce the risk of developing brain metastases (Abner, 1993).

Extensive small-cell lung cancer is treated with chemotherapy with regimens similar to those used for limited disease. The optimum duration of therapy is undefined, but most patients do not benefit from prolonged therapy.

Palliative radiotherapy to the brain or spinal cord or for symptomatic bone disease may be used. Intrathecal administration of chemotherapy (usually preservative-free methotrexate) for leptomeningeal disease rarely relieves symptoms completely or prolongs survival. The median duration of survival from the diagnosis of leptomeningeal disease is less than 2 months.

COLON CANCER

Epidemiology and Risk Factors

Recent data reveal that approximately 1 person in 20 is diagnosed with colorectal carcinoma, and approximately 155,000 new cases are diagnosed yearly. The disease is slightly more prevalent in men than women.

A progressive increase in the risk of developing colon cancer from the second to the ninth decade of life is acknowledged. Environmental factors that promote colon cancer include diets rich in fats and low in fiber, vegetables, folate, and calcium (Levin, 1992b). Genetic heritable syndromes also increase the risk of developing colon cancer. Such syndromes include familial adenomatous polyposis, Gardner syndrome (multiple colonic and duodenal adenomatous polyps with benign soft tissue tumors and osteomas), and Turcot syndrome (colonic polyposis with CNS tumors). These syndromes are inherited in an autosomal dominant or recessive fashion. Other heritable syndromes not associated with adenomatous polyps include hereditary nonpolyposis colorectal cancer, Lynch I syndrome with early onset of colon carcinoma in several generations of family members, and Lynch II syndrome with early onset of colon, breast, ovarian, pancreatic, biliary, ureteral, and renal malignancies. The risk of developing colon cancer is higher than normal in patients with long-standing inflammatory bowel disease (Levin, 1992a). Finally, family members of patients with colon carcinoma have a higher risk than the general population of developing colon cancer and require regular screening.

Screening

Colon cancer is the second leading cause of cancer death in the United States, and its incidence appears to be increasing. Reviews by Eddy (1990) and Ransohoff and Lang (1991) include current recommendations for screening patients at average and high risk and note the limitations of the current screening modalities (covered in Chapter 11).

Management of Colonic Polyps

There are several histologic types of polyps, some of which confer an increased risk of developing colon cancer (Table 44–15). All adenomas contain some degree of dysplasia or cellular or glandular atypia, but they do not invade the muscularis mucosa as carcinomas do.

Many polyps are amenable to endoscopic removal. A laparotomy is infrequently required to remove polyps. Because patients who have a documented adenoma have a 30 to 50 per cent chance of having a synchronous polyp at another site in the colon, the entire colon must be visualized. If full colonoscopy is not possible, an air-contrast barium enema must be performed to evaluate the right colon. Because barium enema alone does not adequately visualize the rectum, flexible sigmoidoscopy should also be done.

The risk of a malignancy developing from an adenomatous polyp is proportional to the per cent of the villous component of the polyp (tubulovillous, 25 to 75 per cent villous component; villous, 75 to 100 per cent villous component) and to the size of the polyp. A size larger than 2 cm confers an increased risk; but because malignancy can develop in polyps less than 1 cm in size, all polyps should be removed when they are visualized.

Other than removal, benign adenomas and adenomas with a focus of carcinoma in situ require no more immediate evaluation. Because of the risk of recurrent metachronous polyps, patients should undergo repeat colonoscopy within 1 to 3 years. Patients with invasive cancer (through the muscularis mucosa into the submucosa) in a sessile adenoma or with invasion of lymphatic or vascular

---

TABLE 44–15. CLASSIFICATION OF POLYPS

Neoplastic Polyps
    Adenomas
        Tubular
        Tubulovillous
        Villous

Nonneoplastic Polyps
    Hyperplastic
    Inflammatory
    Hamartomas
    Juvenile
    Peutz-Jegher
    Other (normal mucosa)

Adapted from Hornsby-Lewis L., Winawer SJ: Natural history and current management of colorectal polyps. Oncology 4:140, 1990, with permission.

spaces, deep stalk invasion, or positive margins at the cautery line have an increased risk of regional nodal involvement, colonic wall involvement, or distant metastatic disease and require surgical removal of a segment of colon. These patients should then undergo more frequent surveillance—once yearly.

Symptoms

Patients with colorectal carcinoma may experience intermittent abdominal pain or vague discomfort that is occasionally difficult to localize. Patients may have occult bleeding (associated with right-sided lesions) or gross bleeding mixed with stool. Rectal bleeding should not be attributed to hemorrhoidal lesions without more definitive investigation. Patients may also have symptoms of anemia, including fatigue, weakness, and dyspnea on exertion. Symptoms of advanced disease include change in the caliber of stools, nausea and vomiting suggestive of obstruction, acute abdomen with perforation, and painful liver metastases.

Preoperative Evaluation and Staging

The goal of evaluation and staging is to identify patients whose disease is potentially curable by resection. The presence of an isolated focus of metastatic disease does not necessarily preclude curative surgery. Several clinical trials have documented that 25 per cent of patients who have isolated liver metastases can be cured by resection of the solitary lesion. The staging evaluation is outlined in Table 44–8. The evaluation should include full colonoscopy or barium enema to rule out synchronous neoplasms (present in 3 to 5 per cent of patients). Patients with localized disease should immediately undergo resection. All patients should be counseled before surgery regarding the possibility of the need for colostomy, either temporary or permanent.

The staging system most commonly employed in colorectal carcinoma is the Dukes' system, which is compared with the TNM system in Table 44–16. Colorectal cancer is unique in that the size of the tumor is not included in the staging system as a prognostic factor.

Follow-Up After Curative Resection

The primary goals of follow-up are to monitor patients for metachronous colon or rectal lesions and to detect recurrent or metastatic disease. Most tumors that recur do so within 2 years after surgery. The risk of recurrence is approximately 25 per cent for stage II (Dukes' B) lesions and 50 per cent for stage III (Dukes' C) lesions. Follow-up includes (1) a physical examination; (2) laboratory evalua-

TABLE 44–16. COMPARISON OF STAGING SYSTEMS FOR COLON CANCER

Primary Tumor (T)

TX	Primary tumor cannot be assessed
T0	No evidence of tumor in resected specimen (prior polypectomy or fulguration)
Tis	Carcinoma in situ
T1	Invades submucosa
T2	Invades muscularis propria
T3–T4	Depends on whether serosa is present

    Serosa present:

T3	Invades through muscularis propria into subserosa
	Serosa (but not through)
	Pericolic fat within the leaves of the mensetery
T4	Invades through serosa into free peritoneal cavity or through serosa into a contiguous organ

    No serosa (distal two thirds of rectum, posterior left or right colon)

T3	Invades through muscularis propria
T4	Invades other organs (vagina, prostate, ureter, kidney)

Regional Lymph Nodes (N)

NX	Nodes cannot be assessed (e.g., local excision only)
N0	No regional node metastases
N1	Presence of 1–3 positive nodes
N2	Presence of 4 or more positive nodes
N3	Central nodes positive

Distant Metastases (M)

MX	Presence of distant metastases cannot be assessed
M0	No distant metastases
M1	Distant metastases present

Astler-Coller Modification of Dukes' Staging

A	Mucosal lesion
B1	Extension into but not through, muscularis propria
B2	Extension through muscularis propria; no nodal involvement
B3	Involvement of adjacent structures; no nodal involvement
C1	No penetration through muscularis propria; nodal involvement
C2	Penetration through bowel wall; nodal involvement
C3	Involvement of adjacent structures; nodal involvement
D	Distant metastases

Dukes' Staging System Correlated with TNM

Dukes' A	= T1N0M0
	= T2N0M0
Dukes' B	= T3N0M0
	= T4N0M0
Dukes' C	= T (any) N1M0, T (any) N2M0
Dukes' C2	= T (any) N3M0
Dukes' D	= T (any) N (any) M1

Modified Astler-Coller (MAC) System Correlated with TNM

MAC A	= T1N0M0
MAC B1	= T2N0M0
MAC B2	= T3N0M0, T4N0M0
MAC B3	= T4N0M0
MAC C1	= T2N1M0, T2N2M0
MAC C2	= T3N1M0, T3N2M0
	T4N1M0, T4N2M0
MAC C3	= T4N1M0, T4N2M0

Adapted from Beahrs OH, Henson DE, Hutter RVP, et al: Manual for Staging of Cancer, 4th edition. Philadelphia, JB Lippincott, 1992, p 77. *and* DeVita VT Jr, Hellman S, Rosenberg SA: Principles and Practice of Oncology, 4th edition. Philadelphia, JB Lippincott, 1993, p 941, with permission.

tions, including complete blood count, liver functions, and carcinoembryonic antigen (CEA) level; and (3) diagnostic imaging, including serial chest radiographs and CT scans of the abdomen and pelvis. Patients also undergo regular colonoscopy to detect anastomotic recurrences, polyps, or second primary tumors.

Adjuvant Therapy of Colon Cancer

The combination of 5-fluorouracil (5-FU) plus levamisole administered for 1 year has been established as a standard adjuvant treatment for stage III (Dukes' C) colon cancer (Laurie et al., 1989). A later trial confirmed that 5-FU and levamisole reduced the risk of cancer recurrence by 41 per cent and the overall death rate by 33 per cent in these patients (Moertel et al., 1990). The NIH Consensus Conference (1990) concluded that all stage III patients should receive adjuvant therapy with 5-FU and levamisole for 1 year. Adjuvant chemotherapy has not proved beneficial for any other stage of colon cancer.

Treatment of Advanced Colon Carcinoma

Approximately 50 per cent of patients with colorectal cancer develop liver metastases. Isolated liver metastases may be considered for resection or hepatic arterial chemotherapy. Intra-arterial treatment entails considerable expense and was not demonstrated by a randomized, controlled study to confer a survival advantage.

Palliative chemotherapy for recurrent or advanced disease is characterized by an overall response rate of approximately 20 to 30 per cent. Most regimens contain 5-FU; and no single schedule, combination, or dosing scheme is accepted as standard. Frequently used regimens are detailed in Table 44–17. Calcium leucovorin (folinic acid) is frequently used in conjunction with 5-FU as a

biochemical modulator of the drug. The effectiveness of salvage chemotherapy is limited, and patients in whom the standard regimens fail should be referred for investigational therapies in clinical trials.

RECTAL CANCER

Clinical Evaluation

Rectal cancers are more likely than colon cancers to be symptomatic before diagnosis, with bleeding, pain, tenesmus, or obstipation. Stage for stage, rectal cancers are characterized by a poorer prognosis and greater number of local recurrences than colon cancers. As for colon cancers, evaluation is directed at identifying patients who are candidates for surgery. Rectal cancers may not be visualized on barium enema examinations; patients should also undergo an endoscopic procedure (usually flexible sigmoidoscopy) to visualize the rectum. Transrectal or intrarectal ultrasonography may demonstrate penetration of the tumor through the rectal wall and can identify lymph node metastases (Hawes, 1993).

Treatment of Resectable Rectal Cancer

Patients with cancers of the upper and middle thirds of the rectum usually have an anterior or low anterior resection with restoration of bowel continuity. Cancers of the lower one third of the rectum, however, usually require abdominoperitoneal resection, which necessitates permanent colostomy. The choice of surgical procedure is influenced by the need for adequate distal margins.

Complications of radical surgery have included infection, bleeding, neurogenic bladder, sexual dysfunction, and colostomy. Clinical trials have examined more conservative surgical approaches aimed at sphincter preservation. Preoperative ra-

TABLE 44–17. 5-FLUOROURACIL: SCHEDULES AND DOSES FOR COLON CANCER

Dose	Schedule	Route	Toxicity
500 mg/m^2	Days 1–5 every 4 weeks	IV	GI, myelosuppression
600 mg/m^2	Every week	IV	GI, myelosuppression
1000 mg/m^2/day	Continuous infusion until toxicity (7–10 days)	IV	Stomatitis
200–300 mg/m^2/day	Continuous infusion via catheter and pump	IV	Stomatitis, dermatitis (hand–foot syndrome)
600 mg/m^2 + leucovorin 500 mg/m^2	Weekly × 6	IV	Diarrhea, mucositis, myelosuppression
425 mg/m^2 + leucovorin 20 mg/m^2	Days 1–5 every 4–5 weeks	IV	Mucositis, diarrhea, myelosuppression
750 mg/m^2 + α-Interferon 9 × 10^6 units	5-Day loading 3 Times weekly	IV SC	Myelosuppression Fever, mucositis, neurologic

Adapted from Wittes RE (ed): Manual of Oncologic Therapeutics 1991/1992. Philadelphia, JB Lippincott, 1991, p 170, with permission.

diotherapy or chemoradiotherapy can also be used to reduce local tumor size and allow a more conservative surgical approach.

Adjuvant therapy for patients who have had a curative resection and have stage II or III (Dukes' B or C) rectal cancer comprises a combination of pelvic irradiation and chemotherapy. For early stage rectal cancer (stage I, Dukes' A), no adjuvant therapy is recommended (NIH Consensus Conference, 1990).

PROSTATE CANCER

Epidemiology and Risk Factors

Prostate cancer is the most common cancer among U.S. men and is second only to lung cancer in terms of the number of cancer deaths. Approximately 130,000 new cases were diagnosed in 1992, and 32,000 men died of the disease. The mortality rate due to the disease in black men is nearly twice that of white men. The overall incidence increases with age more rapidly that any other malignancy.

The natural history of prostate cancer is one of slow but progressive disease. Several studies that have followed untreated patients have confirmed an orderly progression, with local disease leading to distant metastases.

Risk factors for prostate cancer include family history, race, exposure to cadmium and nitrates, diets high in animal fat and low in fiber, altered steroid hormone metabolism, and vasectomy. Vasectomy confers only a minimally increased risk, related to increased levels of circulating testosterone. Benign prostatic hypertrophy may be associated with an increased risk of malignancy (Pienta and Esper, 1993).

Screening

Yearly digital rectal examination starting at age 40 and prostate specific antigen (PSA) testing beginning at age 50 are recommended. Patients with a family history of prostate cancer should initiate screening at an earlier age. A second marker of established disease, prostatic acid phosphatase (PAP), is not useful as a screening test because its elevation denotes advanced disease.

Symptoms

Nearly 70 per cent of patients present with progressive symptoms of urinary tract obstruction: urgency, hesitancy, nocturia, or frequency. Patients may have pain due to urinary retention. Pain in the perineum or rectum or constipation suggests locally advanced disease. Patients may also have painful coitus or new onset of erectile dysfunction and urinary tract bleeding. Advanced disease can

first appear as abdominal pain, bone pain, neurologic deficits related to cord compression, lymphedema, or constitutional symptoms such as weight loss or anorexia.

Evaluation and Staging

Patients who have the symptoms listed above, a nodule detected on rectal examination, or elevated PSA are candidates for prostate biopsy. Biopsies may be guided by digital examination or ultrasound scans, which identify hypoechoic areas. If biopsy specimens are collected randomly (no obvious lesion identified), core biopsies should be obtained from at least six areas of the prostate (Andersson, 1992). Needle biopsy is preferred. Patients with obstructive symptoms should not undergo transurethral prostatic resection but, rather, proceed to definitive therapy.

Once the diagnosis of cancer is established, patients with localized disease who may be candidates for surgery or radiotherapy should be identified. Routine staging is outlined in Table 44–8.

Patients who are candidates for prostatectomy by clinical staging (A2, B1, B2, and some patients with C disease) should have their lymph nodes sampled by either an open procedure or laparoscopy before radical prostatectomy. Detection of involved nodes allows potentially morbid surgery to be avoided in the presence of disseminated disease (Middleton, 1988).

Two staging systems are commonly employed for prostate cancer. The TNM and the American Urological Association (AUA) systems are compared in Table 44–18.

TABLE 44–18. STAGING SYSTEMS FOR PROSTATE CANCER

TNM	AUA	Criteria
T1	A	Tumor is incidental histologic finding.
T1A	A1	Three or fewer microscopic foci are present.
T1B	A2	More than three microscopic foci are present.
T2	B	Tumor is present clinically or grossly and is limited to the prostate
T2A	B1	Tumor is < 1.5 cm, with normal tissue on at least three sides.
T2B	B2	Tumor is > 1.5 cm or in more than one lobe.
T3	C	Tumor invades the prostatic apex or is found in or beyond the prostatic capsule, bladder neck, or seminal vesicle but is not fixed
T3	C1	There is no invasion of seminal vesicles.
T3	C2	There is invasion of seminal vesicle.
T4	C2	There is pelvic wall fixation.
N	D	Lymph node metastasis is present.
M	D	Distant metastasis is present.

Adapted from DeVita VT Jr, Hellman S, Rosenberg SA: Principles and Practice of Oncology, 4th edition. Philadelphia, JB Lippincott, 1993, p 1087, with permission.

Prognostic Factors

Histologic appearance is the most significant independent prognostic factor. Grading systems include the Broder, Mostofi, Brown, and Gleason systems. The Gleason system, which is most widely used, recognizes five histologic patterns, represented in a standardized drawing. In general, tumors with a Gleason score of 2 to 4 have a good prognosis, those with a score of 5 to 7 have an intermediate prognosis, and those with a score of 8 to 10 have the worst prognosis.

Therapy

Cancer Confined to the Prostate

Patients with localized prostate cancer have a choice of two therapeutic options: surgical prostatectomy or radiotherapy. In a 1987 National Institutes of Health Consensus Development Conference, the two therapies were acknowledged to be equally effective (NIH Consensus Development Panel, 1988).

Patients with stage A or B cancer and some with stage C and negative lymph nodes are surgical candidates. Prostatectomy provides the advantage of immediate relief of obstructive symptoms. Patients who undergo prostatectomy have a survival rate of 74 per cent at 10 years and 55 per cent at 15 years—rates similar to those of age-matched controls. Radiotherapy spares the patient anesthesia and a potentially morbid procedure and yields comparable survival rates, although in patients with obstructive symptoms who opt for radiotherapy the symptoms may worsen initially. The overall incidence of impotence and incontinence as complications is not significantly different for the two modalities. Adjuvant radiotherapy or chemotherapy after prostatectomy is currently recommended only for patients with positive surgical margins or a PSA that fails to normalize after surgery.

Advanced Disease

Advanced disease requires systemic chemotherapy or hormonal manipulation. Hormonal manipulation is tried initially and consists of surgical orchiectomy or medical castration with luteinizing hormone-releasing hormone (LHRH) agonists or antiandrogens. Estrogen therapy is no longer used because of its thrombotic and cardiovascular risks. This therapy is palliative: quality of life is a significant therapeutic goal, and pain is relieved in 60 to 80 per cent of the patients who undergo this therapy.

The LHRH agonists provide continuous rather than pulsatile stimulation to LHRH receptors, which reduces the rates of secretion of follicle-stimulating hormone (FSH) and luteinizing hormone (LH). During the initial phase of this therapy, the LH level can increase briefly, leading to an elevated testosterone level and the "flare" phenomenon characterized by increased bone pain. Testosterone is reduced to castrate levels within 3 to 4 weeks. In selected patients, such as those with large metastases to the spine, LHRH agonists should not be used as monotherapy. These patients should receive concomitant antiandrogens for the first 2 to 4 weeks to block the flare phenomenon, which could result in neurologic deterioration. The LHRH agonists include leuprolide and goserelin and are administered by monthly subcutaneous depot injections.

Flutamide is a nonsteroidal antiandrogen that acts peripherally to block androgen uptake and receptor binding. The side effects of hormonal therapy are minimal, and the duration of response is typically about 1 year.

Patients whose disease progresses on front-line hormonal therapy may be administered second-line therapy, such as the adrenal blocking agents aminoglutethimide and ketoconazole. In contrast to breast carcinoma, in which second-line hormonal therapies are highly effective, only 20 per cent of patients whose prostate cancer progresses on initial hormonal therapy respond to a second-line therapy; the response duration is approximately 6 months.

Chemotherapy is reserved for disease that is refractory to hormone therapy. Standard chemotherapy that consistently elicits a response or improves survival has not been defined. Approximately 15 to 30 per cent of patients respond. The median survival is 30 to 40 weeks.

Active agents include doxorubicin, cyclophosphamide, 5-FU, methotrexate, and vindesine. Estramustine is a unique agent that combines nitrogen mustard with estradiol phosphate and is used in combination with vinblastine. Investigational agents include paclitaxel, gallium nitrate, pamidronate sodium, liarozole, and suramin, which acts as an adrenocorticolytic and antiproliferative agent (Dawson, 1993). Strontium 89 has been approved for the therapy of painful bone lesions (Mertens et al., 1993).

TESTICULAR CANCER

Epidemiology and Risk Factors

Testicular cancer is the most common malignancy of men in the 15 to 35 year age group and the second most common malignancy of men in the 35 to 39 year age group. There are approximately 5500 new cases per year in the United States, and about 2 to 3 per cent of the cancers are bilateral.

This disease has a characteristic age distribution, with a small peak at around age 2 years and a large peak during young adulthood. There is also a modest peak and plateau at around age 65. Most tumors in young adults are of germ cell origin, with their incidence peaking at ages 25 to 29, or seminomas, whose incidence peaks at ages 35 to 40.

The most specific risk factor for the development of testicular cancer is cryptorchidism. The risk for patients with this condition is 3 to 14 times higher than that of the general population. Five to ten per cent of patients with a history of cryptorchidism develop malignancy in the contralateral descended testis.

Other risk factors associated with testicular cancers include testicular torsion, hydrocele, inguinal hernia, testicular atrophy, mumps orchitis, XY gonadal dysgenesis, XXY Klinefelter syndrome, and abnormalities of chromosome 12 (isochromosome 12p).

Classification of Tumors

Ninety-five per cent of all primary testicular tumors arise from germinal elements and are malignant. The nongerminal Sertoli and Leydig cell lesions account for the other 5 per cent. Testicular tumors are divided into seminomas and nonseminomatous tumors (Table 44–19).

Screening

Testicular evaluation should be included in any physical examination. The U.S. Preventive Health Services Task Force recommends regular screening for testicular cancer in men with a history of cryptorchidism, orchiopexy, or testicular atrophy.

Symptoms and Preoperative Evaluation

The most common presenting symptom is a painless swelling or nodule in the testis. Patients may also note a heaviness in the scrotum or pain related to secondary torsion. Patients occasionally present with the complaint of infertility. Patients with retroperitoneal adenopathy may present with abdominal or back pain. Other symptoms include dyspnea related to mediastinal or lung disease and gynecomastia secondary to increased levels of human chorionic gonadotropin (hCG).

The initial physical examination should include careful examination of the testes for masses. The differential diagnosis of scrotal masses includes epididymitis, inguinal hernia, hydrocele, spermatocele, and testicular torsion. All masses should be considered malignant until malignancy is excluded. Tumor marker analysis and bilateral ultrasonography to distinguish masses from cystic lesions are included in the initial evaluation. The definitive diagnosis of testicular cancer is made by radical inguinal orchiectomy. *Transscrotal orchiectomy is contraindicated*, as this procedure increases the incidence of local recurrence and may lead to inguinal nodal dissemination.

Tumor Markers

The markers most often used to detect testicular tumors are the β-subunit of hCG (β-hCG), α-fetoprotein (AFP), and lactate dehydrogenase (LDH). Levels of these markers are obtained initially to aid in the diagnosis of tumor type, as a prognostic indicator of tumor burden, and as a baseline to monitor the effectiveness of subsequent therapy.

The level of β-hCG is elevated in 40 to 60 per cent of patients with testicular cancer, including all patients with choriocarcinoma, 80 per cent of patients with embryonal carcinoma, and 10 to 25 per cent of patients with pure seminoma. An elevated β-hCG level suggests the presence of syncytiotrophoblastic elements in the tumor (Klein, 1993).

Luteinizing hormone cross-reacts in some assays for hCG and so inaccurately suggests recurrent cancer. This cross-reactivity can be distinguished from true elevations in hCG by administering 200 mg of testosterone to suppress LH production and retesting the patient within 48 hours.

The AFP level is elevated in 50 to 70 per cent of patients with testicular cancer, including patients with yolk sac carcinoma, mixed tumors such as teratocarcinoma, and embryonal carcinoma. Patients with pure seminoma and choriocarcinoma do not

TABLE 44–19.   HISTOLOGIC CLASSIFICATION OF PRIMARY TUMORS OF THE TESTIS

Germinal Neoplasms (demonstrating one or more of the following components)
Seminoma
    Classic (typical) seminoma
    Anaplastic seminoma
    Spermatocytic seminoma
Embryonal carcinoma
Teratoma (with or without malignant transformation)
    Mature
    Immature
Choriocarcinoma
Yolk sac tumor (endodermal sinus tumor; embryonal adenocarcinoma of the prepubertal testis)

Nongerminal Neoplasms
Specialized gonadal stromal neoplasms
    Leydig cell tumor
    Other gonadal stromal tumors
Gonadoblastoma
Miscellaneous neoplasms
    Adenocarcinoma of the rete testis
    Mesenchymal neoplasms
    Carcinoid
    Adrenal rest "tumor"

From Richie JP: Detection and treatment of testicular cancer. CA Cancer J Clin 43:153, 1993, with permission.

TABLE 44–20. CLINICAL STAGING SYSTEMS FOR SEMINOMA

Boden-Gibb Stage	Memorial Sloan-Kettering Cancer Center	TNM
A (I): tumor confined to testis	A	I Negative II Positive
B (II): spread to regional nodes	B1 > 5 cm	N1: metastasis in a single lymph node ≤ 2 cm in greatest dimension N2: metastasis in a single lymph node ≥ 2 cm but not > 5 cm in greatest dimension or multiple lymph nodes, none > 5 cm in greatest dimension
	B2 > 5 cm	N3: metastasis in a single lymph node > 5 cm in greatest dimension
	B3 > 10 cm (bulky)	
C (III): spread beyond retroperineal nodes	C	M1 Distant metastasis

From Richie JP: Detection and treatment of testicular cancer. CA Cancer J Clin 43:159, 1993, with permission.

have elevated AFP levels. An elevation in AFP level in patients with these histologic types implies the presence of mixed tumors with embryonal or yolk sac elements. These tumors behave as nonseminomatous tumors (Klein, 1993).

Evaluation and Staging

Local staging is performed at orchiectomy. Routine staging studies are outlined in Table 44–8. Several systems are used to stage testicular tumors. Seminomas are staged primarily by the Boden and Gibb system. This system is compared to the Memorial Sloan-Kettering Cancer Center staging system and the TNM system in Table 44–20. The staging system for nonseminomatous germ cell tumors is depicted in Table 44–21.

Therapy

Seminomas

EARLY DISEASE. Testicular seminomas are sensitive to both radiotherapy and chemotherapy. The

TABLE 44–21. PATHOLOGIC STAGING SYSTEMS FOR NONSEMINOMATOUS GERM CELL TUMORS

Skinner	Walter Reed	TNM
A: confined to testis	I	N0
B: spread to retroperitoneum	IA	N1
B1: < 6 positive nodes; no node > 2 cm; no extranodal extension	IA	N1
B2: < 6 positive nodes; any node > 2 cm	IIB	N2
B3: massive retroperitoneal disease	IIC	N3
C: metastatic	III	M1

From Richie JP: Detection and treatment of testicular cancer. CA Cancer J Clin 43:160, 1993, with permission.

established therapy for early disease (stages I and IIA) is radical orchiectomy followed by adjuvant radiotherapy. Patients with stage I disease receive external beam radiation (2500 to 3000 cGy) with shielding of the remaining testicle. Patients with stage IIA disease receive this radiation as well as a boost to the involved nodes (total dose 3600 cGy). Patients with stage I disease may be treated with orchiectomy alone provided the patient adheres to a surveillance schedule of physical examination, imaging studies, and tumor markers.

ADVANCED DISEASE. Treatment of advanced disease (stages IIB, IIC, and III) consists of cisplatin-based chemotherapy. The current accepted regimen is three to four cycles of chemotherapy with bleomycin, etoposide, and cisplatin. Other regimens are detailed in Table 44–22. No additional therapy is recommended for patients who respond completely after the three or four cycles. Patients who have normalization of markers but residual abnormalities on radiography or CT scans are referred for surgical resection and histologic examination. These radiologic abnormalities may be residual disease, mature teratoma, or fibromas. Patients with residual disease are referred for salvage chemotherapy.

Nonseminomatous Germ Cell Tumors

EARLY DISEASE. Patients with clinical stage I nonseminomatous germ cell tumors are treated with radical inguinal orchiectomy and retroperitoneal lymph node dissection. Although a morbid procedure, retroperitoneal lymph node dissection is the standard for staging because other techniques understage 20 to 25 per cent of tumors. Retroperitoneal lymph node dissection is increasingly being replaced by a modified procedure that preserves fertility in a larger proportion of patients. Patients with negative or minimally involved nodes at dissection require no further therapy (stage A and B1). Patients with more advanced nodal disease (stage B2) benefit from two cycles of

TABLE 44–22. CHEMOTHERAPY OF TESTICULAR TUMORS

Acronym and Drugs	Dose (mg/m²), Route, Schedule	Cycle Frequency (days)
BEP		
Cisplatin	20 mg/m² IV 5 consecutive days	21
Etoposide	100 mg/m² IV days 1–5	
Bleomycin	30 units IV days 2, 9, 16	
PVB		
Cisplatin	20 mg/m² IV 5 consecutive days	21
Vinblastine	0.15 mg/kg IV days 1, 2	
Bleomycin	30 units IV days 2, 9, 16	
Triple Therapy		
Initial		
Methotrexate	5 mg PO for 16–25 days	
Chlorambucil	10 mg PO for 16–25 days	
Dactinomycin	0.05 mg IV days 3–7, 12–16, 21–25	
After 2-week rest period		
Methotrexate	5 mg PO × 7 days	21
Chlorambucil	10 mg PO for 16–25 days	
Dactinomycin	0.5 mg IV days 3–7	
VAB-6		
Vinblastine	4 mg/m² IV day 1	21
Dactinomycin	1 mg/m² IV day 1	
Bleomycin	30 units IV push; then 20 units/m²/day IV days 1–3	
Cisplatin	120 mg/m² IV day 4	
Cyclophosphamide	600 mg/m² IV day 1	
VIP		
Vinblastine	0.11 mg/kg days 1, 2*	21
Ifosfamide	1.2 gm/m² daily × 5	
Cisplatin	20 mg/m² daily × 5	

* Etoposide (VP-16) 75 mg/m² daily × 5 may be substituted for vinblastine.
Adapted from Perry MC (ed): The Chemotherapy Source Book. Baltimore, Williams & Wilkins, 1992, pp 762–763, with permission. Copyright 1992, Williams & Wilkins Co.

adjuvant postoperative chemotherapy (Williams et al., 1987).

ADVANCED DISEASE. Three or four cycles of a cisplatin-based combination regimen is the therapy of choice. Complete responders require no further therapy. No benefit is derived from maintenance chemotherapy (Einhorn et al., 1981). Patients whose markers do not normalize or whose disease progresses radiographically are referred for salvage therapy with a regimen that includes ifosfamide. Again, residual radiologic abnormalities are resected, and the need for further therapy is determined by the results of a histologic examination.

RECURRENT DISEASE. In contrast to other solid tumors, recurrent germ cell tumors are highly responsive to salvage chemotherapy; the goal is cure. Combination chemotherapy regimens containing cisplatin and medications not previously used to treat the patient's tumor (e.g., ifosfamide and etoposide) are usually employed.

Extragonadal Germ Cell Tumors

Extragonadal germ cell tumors arise in midline body structures such as the mediastinum, retroperitoneum, and pineal gland. When an extragonadal primary germ cell tumor is suspected, a meticulous search must be performed to exclude an occult primary testicular tumor. Because the testicle is a sanctuary site for chemotherapy, occult tumors of the testicle may not be cured by this modality.

These tumors usually present in a relatively advanced stage with symptoms specific to their site of origin. Treatment for localized seminomatous extragonadal tumors includes radiotherapy, whereas patients with distant disease receive cisplation-based chemotherapy. All extragonadal nonseminomatous germ cell tumors are treated with chemotherapy. Cure rates are lower than for the testicular counterparts, which may be related to the difficulty of resecting residual disease (Hainsworth and Greco, 1992).

OVARIAN CANCER

Epidemiology and Risk Factors

Ovarian cancer is the fourth most common cause of cancer deaths in women in the United States and is the leading cause of death due to gynecologic malignancies. In 1992 approximately 21,000 new cases and 13,000 deaths related to the disease were reported. The incidence of epithelial tumors increases steadily with age, reaching a peak in the 70- to 79-year-old group. In contrast, germ cell tumors are most common in children and young women.

The risk of developing ovarian cancer is increased in women who have had no or a few pregnancies, a history of breast cancer, a diet high in fat, regular alcohol consumption, or exposure to asbestos or talc. Ovarian cancer is hereditary in approximately 5 per cent of cases. The use of oral contraceptives appears to be protective, with the reduction in risk directly proportional to the duration of use (Daly, 1992).

Types of Ovarian Carcinoma

Eighty to ninety per cent of all ovarian malignancies are epithelial carcinomas. The remaining tumors are derived from germ cells or stromal elements. The WHO classification of ovarian tumors is depicted in Table 44–23. A unique subclass of epithelial tumors is the "borderline" tumors, which express cells that appear neoplastic but grow and metastasize slowly; the 5-year survival rates for these patients exceed 90 per cent. The 5-year survival rate for other epithelial tumors is 25 to 30 per cent.

Symptoms

Patients may present with symptoms of lower abdominal discomfort, nausea, increased abdominal girth related to ascites, vaginal bleeding, and rarely acute pain related to ovarian torsion or hemorrhage. Because symptoms are vague, most patients present with advanced disease: In 75 per cent the disease has spread beyond the ovary, and in 60 per cent metastases are found beyond the pelvis at diagnosis.

Evaluation and Staging

All women with abdominal or pelvic symptoms should have a thorough pelvic examination on initial presentation before other diagnostic testing. The differential diagnosis of an adnexal mass includes endometriosis, fibroma, functional cyst, extrauterine pregnancy, and tumors.

Adnexal masses in premenarchal girls or postmenopausal women are suggestive of neoplasm and usually indicate the need for exploratory surgery. Functional cysts do not occur in these age groups. Ultrasonography can differentiate cysts from complex masses, but even cysts should be evaluated by surgery in these age groups.

Ovarian enlargement in women of reproductive age is usually benign and related to functional cysts. Patients should have a pelvic examination and ultrasonography every 4 to 6 weeks. Indications for surgery include masses that do not regress after three menstrual cycles or with the use of oral contraceptives, masses larger than 8 cm, complex

TABLE 44–23. WORLD HEALTH ORGANIZATION* CLASSIFICATION OF MALIGNANT OVARIAN TUMORS

Common Epithelial Tumors
Malignant serous tumors
  Adenocarcinoma, papillary adenocarcinoma, papillary cystadenocarcinoma
  Surface papillary carcinoma
  Malignant adenofibroma, cystadenofibroma
Malignant mucinous tumors
  Adenocarcinoma, cystadenocarcinoma
  Malignant adenofibroma, cystadenofibroma
Malignant endometrioid tumors
  Carcinoma
    Adenocarcinoma
    Adenoacanthoma
    Malignant adenofibroma, cystadenofibroma
  Endometrioid stromal sarcomas
  Mesodermal (Müllerian) mixed tumors: homologous and heterologous
Clear cell (mesonephroid) tumors; malignant carcinoma and adenocarcinoma
Brenner tumors, malignant
Mixed epithelial tumors, malignant
Undifferentiated carcinoma
Unclassified

Sex Cord-Stromal Tumors
Granulosa-stromal cell tumors
  Granulosa cell tumor
  Tumors in the thecoma-fibroma group
  Fibroma
  Unclassified
Androblastomas: Sertoli-Leydig cell tumors
  Well differentiated
    Tubular androblastoma, Sertoli cell tumor (tubular adenoma of Pick)
    Tubular androblastoma with lipid storage, Sertoli cell tumor with lipid storage (folliculome lipidique of Lecene)
    Sertoli-Leydig cell tumor (tubular adenoma with Leydig cells)
  Leydig cell tumor, hilus cell tumor
  Intermediate differentiation
  Poorly differentiated (sarcomatoid)
  With heterologous elements
Gynandroblastoma
Unclassified

Lipid (Lipoid) Cell Tumors
Germ cell tumors
  Dysgerminoma
  Endodermal sinus tumor
  Embryonal carcinoma
  Polyembryoma
  Choriocarcinoma
  Teratomas
    Immature
    Mature dermoid cyst with malignant transformation
    Monodermal and highly specialized
      Struma ovarii
      Carcinoid
      Struma ovarii and carcinoid
      Others
  Mixed forms
Gonadoblastoma
  Pure
  Mixed with dysgerminoma or other form of germ cell tumor

* With permission of WHO, Geneva, Switzerland.
From DeVita VT Jr, Hellman S, Rosenberg SA: Principles and Practice of Oncology, 4th edition. Philadelphia, JB Lippincott, 1993, p 1229, with permission.

cysts with septations on ultrasonography, fixed or painful masses, or any mass presenting with ascites.

Presurgical evaluation is outlined in Table 44–8. The staging laparotomy is the definitive diagnostic and staging procedure for ovarian carcinoma. It includes removal of the tumor-involved ovary, contralateral ovary (spread occurs in 6 to 13 per cent), uterus, fallopian tubes, and omentum; lymph node sampling; and random peritoneal biopsies, including the underside of the diaphragm. Ascitic fluid or abdominal washings are also sent for cytologic analysis. The tumor is usually aggressively debulked, as patients with minimal residual tumor have a better prognosis than women with macroscopic residual disease (de Souza and Friedlander, 1992). The International Federation of Gynecology and Obstetrics (FIGO) staging of ovarian cancer is outlined in Table 44–24.

The most important prognostic factor for ovarian cancer is the stage at presentation. The 5-year survival rates are 50 to 85 per cent for stage I, 37 to 79 per cent for stage II, 7 to 18 per cent for stage III, and 2 to 8 per cent for stage IV.

Therapy

Stages I and II

The only patients likely to be cured by surgery alone are those with stage IA tumors of histologic grade 1 or 2. These women, along with stage IB patients, require no further therapy after a staging laparotomy. Patients with grade 3 tumors or stages IC or II tumors require postsurgical adjuvant therapy. Although the optimum adjuvant chemotherapy regimen has not been defined, alkylating agents and cisplatin are commonly prescribed. The Gynecologic Oncology Group (GOG) favors intraperitoneal phosphorus 32 or three courses of cisplatin plus cyclophosphamide (Deppe and Malviya, 1991).

Stages III and IV

Therapy for advanced disease involves initial cytoreductive surgery followed by radiotherapy or chemotherapy. Chemotherapy has become the preferred modality and usually involves a carboplatin- or cisplatin-based regimen. Widely used regimens are outlined in Table 44–25. Responses may vary by age and the general medical status of the patient. Carboplatin is less nephrotoxic, neurotoxic, emetogenic, and ototoxic than cisplatin and may be used to replace cisplatin in combination regimens. There is no difference in survival between patients treated with cisplatin and those treated with carboplatin (Ozols, 1992). Regimens containing paclitaxel are now being examined in clinical trials.

Second-Look Laparotomy

The most reliable method of assessing response to chemotherapy is the second-look laparotomy. Patients who have no evidence of disease radiographically are surgical candidates. Second-look surgery allows for discontinuation of therapy if no residual disease is seen or for planning salvage therapy for women with residual disease. Approximately 55 per cent of patients have identifiable tumor at the second look procedure. Patients with residual disease may benefit from a second debulking procedure. An elevated preoperative level of the marker CA-125 predicts residual tumor.

Salvage Therapies

Paclitaxel has been approved for use in ovarian cancer patients whose disease is refractory to platinum-based treatments. More than 30 per cent of these women respond to paclitaxel. Toxic effects include neutropenia, neuropathy, and allergic reactions. Other investigational modalities being

TABLE 44–24. FIGO STAGE GROUPING FOR PRIMARY CARCINOMA OF THE OVARY (1987)

Stage I: Growth limited to the ovaries
  IA: Growth limited to one ovary; no ascites. No tumor on the external surface; capsule intact.
  IB: Growth limited to both ovaries; no ascites. No tumor on the external surfaces; capsules intact.
  IC: Tumor either stage IA or IB but with tumor on the surface of one or both ovaries, or with capsule ruptured, or with ascites present containing malignant cells, or with positive peritoneal washings.

Stage II: Growth involving one or both ovaries with pelvic extension
  IIA: Growth involving one or both ovaries with pelvic extension.
  IIB: Extension and/or metastases to the uterus and/or tubes.
  IIC: Tumor either stage IIA or IIB but with tumor on the surface of one or both ovaries, or with capsule(s) ruptured, or with ascites present containing malignant cells, or with positive peritoneal washings.

Stage III: Tumor involving one or both ovaries with peritoneal implants outside the pelvis and/or positive retroperitoneal or inguinal nodes. Superficial liver metastases equal stage III. Tumor is limited to the true pelvis but with histologically verified malignant extension to small bowel or omentum.
  IIIA: Tumor grossly limited to the true pelvis with negative nodes but with histologically confirmed microscopic seeding of abdominal peritoneal surfaces.
  IIIB: Tumor of one or both ovaries with histologically confirmed implants of abdominal peritoneal surfaces, none exceeding 2 cm in diameter; nodes negative.
  IIIC: Abdominal implants > 2 cm in diameter and/or positive retroperitoneal or inguinal nodes.

Stage IV: Growth involving one or both ovaries with distant metastasis; if pleural effusion present, there must be positive cytologic test results to allot a case to stage IV; parenchymal liver metastasis equals stage IV.

From DeVita VT Jr, Hellman S, Rosenberg SA: Principles and Practice of Oncology, 4th edition. Philadelphia, JB Lippincott, 1993, p 1234, with permission.

TABLE 44–25. CHEMOTHERAPY FOR OVARIAN CANCER

Acronym and Drugs	Dose (mg/m²), Route, Schedule	Cycle Frequency (days)
CHAD		
Cyclophosphamide	600 mg/m² IV day 1	28
Hexamethylmelamine	200 mg/m² PO days 8–22	
Doxorubicin	25 mg/m² IV day 1	
Cisplatin	50 mg/m² IV day 1	
CHAP		
Cyclophosphamide	150 mg/m² PO days 2–8	28
Hexamethylmelamine	150 mg/m² PO days 2–8	
Doxorubicin	30 mg/m² IV day 1	
Cisplatin	50 mg/m² IV day 1	
CP		
Cyclophosphamide	1000 mg/m² IV day 1	21
Cisplatin (platinum)	50 mg/m² IV day 1	
Hexa-CAF		
Hexamethylmelamine	150 mg/m² PO × 14 days	28
Cyclophosphamide	150 mg/m² PO × 14 days	
Methotrexate	40 mg/m² IV days 1, 8	
5-Fluorouracil	600 mg/m² IV days 1, 8	
PAC-1		
Cisplatin (platinum)	50 mg/m² IV day 1	
Doxorubicin	50 mg/m² IV day 1	
Cyclophosphamide	750 mg/m² IV day 1	
VAC		
Vincristine	1.5 mg/m² IV weekly × 10–12 weeks	28 (up to 2 years)
Dactinomycin	0.5 mg/m² IV × 5 days	
Cyclophosphamide	5–7 mg/kg/day IV × 5 days	

Adapted from Perry MC (ed): The Chemotherapy Source Book. Baltimore, Williams & Wilkins, 1992, pp 761–762, with permission. Copyright 1992, Williams & Wilkins Co.

used to treat ovarian cancers include administration of topotecan or tetraplatin and immunotherapy.

Ovarian Germ Cell Tumors

Dysgerminomas are the female equivalent of testicular seminomas. Limited disease can be treated with radiotherapy, whereas advanced disease is treated with chemotherapy. Germ cell tumors other than dysgerminoma are treated with cisplatin-based chemotherapy (Williams, 1991).

CERVICAL CANCER

Epidemiology and Risk Factors

Cancer of the cervix is the third most prevalent genital cancer in women in the United States, with approximately 13,000 new cases reported in 1992. It is the second most common cause of death due to gynecologic cancers in the Western world and is the leading cause of death among women in many developing countries.

The average age of onset is 50 years for invasive cancer, 35 years for carcinoma in situ, and 25 years for cervical dysplasia. The incidence of the disease has been decreasing since the introduction of the Pap smear in 1941.

Risk factors for cervical cancer include low socioeconomic status; early onset of sexual activity; multiple sexual partners; exposure to herpes virus 2 or human papilloma virus types 16, 18, 31, 33, 34, or 35; cigarette smoking; and nutritional deficiencies.

Screening

The American Cancer Society recommends screening with the Pap smear in low-risk women starting at age 20 or earlier if the woman is sexually active. Patients should have a Pap smear annually for two consecutive years, and if both are negative screening can continue once every 3 years until the age of 65. Women at high risk should have annual Pap smears.

Management of abnormal smears first entails treatment of any infections. The Pap smear is repeated after the infection has resolved. Pap smears suggesting dysplasia or human papilloma virus infection should be followed up with colposcopy and biopsy of any abnormal sites.

Symptoms

Many lesions detected by Pap smear are asymptomatic. Early invasive carcinoma may produce vaginal discharge or bleeding, especially postco-

TABLE 44–26. STAGING OF CARCINOMA OF THE UTERINE CERVIX

AJCCS	FIGO	Criteria
Primary Tumor (T)		
TX		Primary tumor cannot be assessed
T0		No evidence of primary tumor
Tis	0	Carcinoma in situ
T1	I	Cervical carcinoma confined to uterus (extension to corpus should be disregarded)
T1A	IA	Preclinical invasive carcinoma, diagnosed by microscopy only
T1A1	IA1	Minimal microscopic stromal invasion
T1A2	IA2	Tumor with invasive component 5 mm or less in depth taken from the base of the epithelium and 7 mm or less in horizontal spread
T1B	IB	Tumor larger than T1A2
T2	II	Cervical carcinoma invades beyond uterus but not to pelvic wall or to the lower third of the vagina
T2A	IIA	Without parametrial invasion
T2B	IIB	With parametrial invasion
T3	III	Cervical carcinoma extends to the pelvic wall and/or involves lower third of vagina and/or causes hydronephrosis or nonfunctioning kidney
T3A	IIIA	Tumor involves lower third of the vagina, no extension to pelvic wall
T3B	IIIB	Tumor extends to pelvic wall and/or causes hydronephrosis or nonfunctioning kidney
T4	IVA	Tumor invades mucosa of bladder or rectum and/or extends beyond true pelvis

Regional Lymph Nodes (N)
Regional lymph nodes include paracervical, parametrial, hypogastric (obturator), common internal and external iliac, presacral, and sacral

NX		Regional lymph nodes cannot be assessed
N0		No regional lymph node metastasis
N1		Regional lymph node metastasis

Distant Metastasis (M)

MX		Presence of distant metastasis cannot be assessed
M0		No distant metastasis
M1	IVB	Distant metastasis

AJCCS = American Joint Committee on Cancer Staging and End Stage Reporting; FIGO = International Federation for Gynecology and Obstetrics. From DeVita VT Jr, Hellman S, Rosenberg SA: Principles and Practice of Oncology, 4th edition. Philadelphia, JB Lippincott, 1993, p 1174, *and* Beahrs OH, Henson DE, Hutler RVP et al.: Manuel for Staging of Cancer, JB Lippincott, with permission.

ital spotting. Late symptoms suggesting advanced disease include pain in the pelvis, rectum, vagina, or urinary tract or rectal symptoms.

Evaluation and Staging

Once the diagnosis of invasive cancer is established, patients require a full evaluation, including pelvic examination under anesthesia to assess the extent of tumor involvement. Additional staging studies are outlined in Table 44–8. In contrast to ovarian carcinoma, the staging of cervical cancer is purely clinical. The FIGO and AJCCS staging systems for cervical cancer are presented in Table 44–26.

Therapy

Stage IA

Women with microinvasive IA1 carcinoma should undergo hysterectomy. If further childbearing is desired, patients can be treated with conization followed by careful monitoring.

The incidence of lymph node involvement increases with depth of invasion and the presence of lymphovascular invasion. Lesions invasive to less than 3 mm with no lymphovascular involvement can be treated with hysterectomy. Patients with invasion greater than 3 mm require pelvic lymph node dissection as well. Patients who are poor surgical candidates can be treated with intracavitary irradiation.

Stages IB and IIA

Because 15 to 25 per cent of stage IB and IIA patients have positive nodes, surgical management includes pelvic lymph node dissection. Radical hysterectomy with lymph node dissection and definitive irradiation are equally effective therapies for these stages. For younger women in whom preservation of ovarian function is desired, surgery may be preferred. There is no consistent benefit to adjuvant radiotherapy or chemotherapy in women with positive nodes at lymphadenectomy.

Stages IIB, III, and IV

The standard therapy for advanced disease is radiotherapy alone. Occasionally, patients are considered for radical pelvic exenteration. The intracavitary therapy is administered with a cylindrical applicator placed in the uterine cavity and ovoids placed at the cervix and fornices. The applicator is then afterloaded with the radioactive agent. As tumors reach more advanced stages this technique is less effective for delivering a uniform dose; external beam therapy then becomes the procedure of choice.

Recurrent Cervical Cancer

Patients who develop local recurrence may be considered for salvage radiotherapy or radical surgery such as pelvic exenteration. Most palliative chemotherapy regimens contain cisplatin; the optimum treatment duration is unclear, but usually four to six courses are administered (Omura, 1992). Investigational therapies include intralesional or topical interferon and differentiating agents such as the retinoids (Lippman et al., 1992).

PEDIATRIC MALIGNANCIES

Although pediatric malignancies are rare, cancer is the second leading cause of death among children younger than age 15. In the United States approximately 11,000 to 12,000 children and adolescents under age 20 are diagnosed with cancer each year.

Because the signs and symptoms of malignancy may be subtle in children, tumors often present in advanced stages. With a few exceptions, screening for cancer in children is ineffective and less practical than for adults, as standard screening techniques are not available.

In general, pediatric malignancies are more responsive to therapy than adult tumors. Hence cure can often be the therapeutic aim.

Acute Lymphoblastic Leukemia

Childhood acute lymphoblastic leukemia (ALL) is the most common malignancy in children in the United States, with approximately 2500 new cases annually. The peak incidence is between the ages of 2 and 6 years, and the disease is generally more common in boys. Nearly two thirds of children with ALL are now cured with conventional chemotherapy.

Risk factors for childhood ALL include early radiation exposure, Down syndrome (trisomy 21), Fanconi syndrome, Bloom syndrome, Rubinstein-Taybi syndrome, Poland syndrome, Schwachman syndrome, neurofibromatosis, and childhood immunodeficiency diseases such as Wiscott-Aldrich syndrome, congenital hypogammaglobulinemia, and ataxia-telangiectasia.

The clinical presentation may include pallor, fatigue, petechiae, purpura, bleeding, and fever. Patients may also present with extramedullary symptoms such as lymphadenopathy, hepatomegaly, and splenomegaly. Anorexia and bone pain are common. The differential diagnosis includes infectious mononucleosis, idiopathic thrombocytopenic purpura, acute infectious lymphocytosis, pertussis and parapertussis, viral illnesses, and aplastic anemia.

Bone marrow aspiration with biochemical, immunologic, and cytogenetic studies establish the diagnosis. Most lymphoblasts are positive for terminal deoxynucleotidyl transferase (TdT), which allows them to be distinguished from myeloblasts. The cytogenetic analysis shows abnormalities in two thirds of the patients, including pseudodiploidy or hyperdiploidy, the Philadelphia chromosome [t(9;22)], and translocations t(8;14) and t(4; 11). The translocation t(8;14) is specific for B cell ALL. Immunologic studies have demonstrated ALL to have three distinct subsets. Twenty per cent are of T cell lineage and 80 per cent of B cell lineage. The B cell leukemias are then further classified as pre-B or early pre-B. Most cases of childhood ALL express the common ALL antigen (CALLA, CD10).

Poor prognostic variables include high white blood cell count at diagnosis, very young age or older age at presentation, L_2 morphology (more abundant cytoplasm and more variation in size and shape of cells), male sex, severe thrombocytopenia, CNS leukemia, lymphadenopathy or organomegaly, and T cell disease.

This leukemia is treated with combination chemotherapy with or without radiotherapy to sanctuary sites. Induction therapy consists of a four-drug regimen of vincristine, prednisone, L-asparaginase, and daunorubicin. Patients who do not achieve remission after induction chemotherapy have a poor prognosis (Poplack, 1985).

The CNS is a major sanctuary site and is a site of relapse in 75 per cent of patients who do not receive prophylactic therapy. Prophylactic therapy includes (1) craniospinal irradiation with or without methotrexate or (2) triple-drug intrathecal therapy with methotrexate, cytosine arabinoside, and prednisone.

Consolidative or intensification therapy, aimed at increasing leukemic cell kill, can be given concurrently with CNS prophylactic therapy and uses drugs not previously administered for induction, including cyclophosphamide and cytosine arabinoside.

Maintenance therapy is employed to lengthen the duration of remission. It usually requires administration of methotrexate and 6-mercaptopurine on a weekly basis for 2 to 3 years.

Relapsing patients may be candidates for allogeneic bone marrow transplantation. Patients for whom HLA-matched donors are not available are treated with reinduction chemotherapy.

Wilms' Tumor

Arising in the kidney from embryonal renal cells, Wilms' tumor is the most common childhood abdominal tumor. Approximately 500 new cases are seen yearly in the United States. The tumor is limited to infants and preschool children and is bilateral in 5 per cent of cases.

A large flank mass or generalized abdominal enlargement is the most common presentation of Wilms' tumor. Pain occurs in 25 per cent of cases. Gross hematuria is rare, as the tumor usually distorts but does not invade the caliceal system. Other presenting symptoms include fever, vomiting, anorexia, anemia, weakness, and weight loss. Congenital abnormalities, such as hemihypertrophy, aniridia, and genitourinary anomalies, may be associated with Wilms' tumor.

Evaluation includes careful physical examination, CT of the abdomen, intravenous pyelogram (IVP), and abdominal ultrasound scans to evaluate the renal vein and vena cava. If there is suspicion that the tumor extends up the vena cava, an echocardiogram should be obtained to evaluate the right atrium. The system used for staging Wilms' tumor is provided in Table 44–27.

TABLE 44–27. NATIONAL WILMS' TUMOR STUDY CLINICOPATHOLOGIC STAGING SYSTEM

Stage I

Tumor limited to kidney and completely excised. The surface of the renal capsule is intact. Tumor was not ruptured before or during removal. There is no residual tumor apparent beyond the margins of resection.

Stage II

Tumor extends beyond the kidney but is completely removed. There is regional extension of the tumor (i.e., penetration through the outer surface of the renal capsule into the perirenal soft tissues). Vessels outside the kidney substance are infiltrated or contain tumor thrombus. The tumor may have been biopsied, or there has been local spillage of tumor confined to the flank. There is no residual tumor apparent at or beyond the margins of excision.

Stage III

Residual nonhematogenous tumor confined to the abdomen: (1) lymph nodes on biopsy are found to be involved in the hilus, the periaortic chains, or beyond; (2) there has been diffuse peritoneal contamination by tumor, such as by spillage of tumor beyond the flank before or during surgery or by tumor growth that has penetrated through the peritoneal surface; (3) implants are found on the peritoneal surface; (4) the tumor extends beyond the surgical margins either microscopically or grossly; and/or (5) the tumor is not completely resectable because of local infiltration into vital structures.

Stage IV

Hematogenous metastases. Deposits beyond stage III (e.g., lung, liver, bone, and/or brain).

Stage V

Bilateral renal involvement at diagnosis. An attempt should be made to stage each side according to the above criteria on the basis of the extent of disease before biopsy.

From Holland JF, Frei E III, Bast KC, et al: Cancer Medicine, 3rd edition. Philadelphia, Lea & Febiger, 1993, p 2209, with permission.

Management of Wilms' tumor involves a combined modality approach. The tumor is initially resected to determine the pathologic stage. In addition to radical nephrectomy, limited para-aortic lymph node dissection is performed. Surgery for bilateral tumors is conservative, with preservation of as much renal parenchyma as possible.

Current chemotherapy regimens involve the combination of dactinomycin, vincristine, doxorubicin, and cyclophosphamide, with more intense therapy delivered to patients with advanced disease. Therapy duration varies from 10 weeks to 6 months. Chemotherapy is followed by radiotherapy in stages III and IV. Preoperative chemotherapy is being investigated for large tumors that are not easily resectable. The overall 5-year survival rate is 90 per cent (Ganick, 1987).

Osteosarcoma

Osteosarcoma is the most common primary bone malignancy in children and adolescents. Approximately 500 to 900 new cases are diagnosed each year in the United States. The peak incidence occurs during the second decade of life, and there is a male predominance.

Patients often present with painful or massive lesions at the ends of long bones. Lesions are most common in the distal femur, proximal tibia, and proximal humerus. One to three per cent of patients have multifocal tumors, and 15 to 20 per cent have metastatic disease, most commonly to the lungs, at presentation.

Diagnostic evaluation includes radiography of the affected bone and chest, CT or magnetic resonance imaging (MRI) of the affected limb for surgical planning, CT of the chest to assess for occult metastases, and a bone scan. Initial laboratory work includes a complete blood count, liver function tests, and alkaline phosphatase level. Osteosarcomas have a characteristic permeative radiographic appearance and are characterized by production of osteoid, which may extend into soft tissues (seen on radiographs). The definitive diagnostic procedure is needle biopsy.

Management of osteosarcomas involves surgery and chemotherapy. Although cure is the primary therapeutic objective, limb preservation is a secondary goal. Contraindications to limb-sparing surgery include large tumors in which a clear surgical margin cannot be achieved, neurovascular involvement, and growth in children who have not reached full adult height.

In patients for whom limb-sparing surgery is not possible, the standard surgical procedure is amputation of the limb above the affected area. Because approximately 80 per cent of patients treated with surgery alone relapse at a site distant from the primary site, adjuvant chemotherapy has become part of standard therapy. Frequently employed agents include doxorubicin, cisplatin, high-dose methotrexate, bleomycin, cyclophosphamide, ifosfamide, and actinomycin D. The use of preoperative chemotherapy has evolved from successful adjuvant chemotherapy and provides early control of systemic disease, allowing limited resection with potential sparing of the affected limb (Meyer and Malawer, 1991).

Ewing's Sarcoma

Ewing's sarcoma is a rare pediatric primary bone tumor. Fewer than 200 new cases per year are diagnosed in the United States. The incidence is slightly higher in males than females.

Patients with Ewing's sarcoma characteristically present with painful lesions, usually at the midshaft of a bone. An associated mass may be present. The most frequently involved bony sites include the femur, tibia, fibula, and pelvis.

Diagnostic evaluation includes radiographs of the involved bone, which often show a patchy, moth-eaten pattern of bony destruction at the diaphysis with elevation of the periostium and a lamellar or "onion-skin" appearance. Further evaluation includes a bone scan, chest radiograph, bone marrow aspirate and biopsy at a site distant from the primary tumor; laboratory tests include an alkaline phosphatase assay. The definitive diagnostic procedure is biopsy.

Therapy is directed toward control of both the local tumor and distant metastatic disease. Nearly all patients have micrometastatic disease at diagnosis; and adjuvant chemotherapy with vincristine, actinomycin D, cyclophosphamide, and doxorubicin has become standard. Local control is achieved with surgery or radiotherapy (Meyers, 1987).

Neuroblastoma

Neuroblastoma is the most common pediatric extracranial solid tumor, with an incidence of 1 per 7000 children under age 15. The tumors originate from pluripotent neural crest cells and are characterized by unpredictable behavior and resistance to therapy.

The malignancy is associated with fetal hydantoin syndrome, von Recklinghausen's disease, Hirschsprung's disease, and alterations in chromosomes 1 and 11. A two-mutation model similar to that for retinoblastoma is postulated to explain both familial and sporadic cases.

Clinical presentation varies with the site of the primary tumor. The tumor can arise wherever sympathetic nervous tissue is present, including the sympathetic side chain, visceral ganglia, paraganglia, adrenal medulla, bladder, and genitalia.

There tumors, characterized by neuroendocrine granules, often produce active catecholamines and other hormones. Symptoms may be related to hormone production and may include diarrhea or hypertension that does not respond to therapy.

Diagnostic evaluation includes physical and neurologic examinations, complete skeletal survey, bone scan, bone marrow aspirate and biopsy, IVP for tumors in the abdomen, and CT of the chest or abdomen. Laboratory evaluation should include evaluation of a 24-hour urine collection for catecholamine levels. Carcinoembryonic antigen (CEA), serum ferritin, chromogranin A, ganglioside G_{D2}, and neuron-specific enolase serve as tumor markers. A complete blood count and liver and renal function tests are also performed. The staging systems currently employed for neuroblastoma are outlined in Table 44–28.

Therapy is directed by stratifying patients into low and high risk groups. Stages I and II have a high probability of cure with surgery alone (85 to 95 per cent); the addition of chemotherapy does not improve the prognosis. More advanced disease can be treated with surgery after reducing the tumor size by chemotherapy or irradiation. Chemotherapy then follows surgery and includes cyclophosphamide, doxorubicin, etoposide, and cisplatin. Radiotherapy is administered to residual tumor masses. The prognosis for patients with advanced stage disease is poor.

Rhabdomyosarcoma

Rhabdomyosarcoma is the most common pediatric soft tissue sarcoma in children under age 15. It has a bimodal age distribution, with the first peak at ages 2 to 6 and a second peak during adolescence. Rhabdomyosarcoma is associated with several congenital disorders, including neurofibromatosis, Gorlin's basal cell nevus syndrome, and the fetal alcohol syndrome.

The sites most typically involved are the head and neck, genitourinary tract, extremities, trunk, and retroperitoneum. Evaluation includes laboratory work: assays that reflect liver and renal functions as well as LDH and calcium levels. Imaging includes a chest radiograph, CT or MRI for extremity or craniofacial primary tumors, bone marrow aspirate and biopsy, bone scan, skeletal bone survey, and CT scans of the chest or abdomen. Tumors of the head and neck should also be evaluated with cerebrospinal fluid cytologic analysis.

Therapy of rhabdomyosarcoma is determined by the site of involvement, histologic type, and extent of tumor involvement. Limited primary tumors of

TABLE 44–28. CLINICAL STAGING SYSTEMS OF NEUROBLASTOMA: EXTENT OF DISEASE AT DIAGNOSIS

Stage	Criteria
Evans/CCSG Staging System	
I	Tumor confined to the organ or structure of origin.
II	Tumor extending in continuity beyond the organ or structure of origin but not crossing the midline. Regional lymph nodes on the homolateral side may be involved.
III	Tumor extending in continuity beyond the midline. Regional lymph nodes bilaterally may be involved.
IV	Remote disease involving bone, parenchymatous organs, soft tissues or distant lymph node groups, or bone marrow.
IV-S	Patients who would otherwise be stage I or II but who have remote disease confined to one or more of the following sites: liver, skin, or bone marrow (without evidence of bone metastases).
St. Jude/POG Staging System	
A	Complete gross excision of primary tumor, margins histologically negative or positive. Intracavitary lymph nodes not intimately adhered to and removed with resected tumor are histologically free of tumor. If primary is in abdomen (including pelvis), liver is histologically free of tumor.
B	Incomplete gross resection of primary tumor. Lymph nodes and liver histologically free of tumors as in stage A.
C	Complete or incomplete gross resection of primary tumor. Intracavitary nodes histologically positive for tumor. Liver histologically free of tumor.
D	Disseminated disease beyond intracavitary nodes (i.e., bone marrow, bone, liver, skin, or lymph nodes beyond cavity containing primary tumor).
International Neuroblastoma Staging Systems (INSS)	
1	Localized tumor confined to the area of origin; complete gross excision, with or without microscopic residual disease; identifiable ipsilateral and contralateral lymph nodes negative microscopically.
2A	Unilateral tumor with incomplete gross excision; identifiable ipsilateral and contralateral lymph nodes negative microscopically.
2B	Unilateral tumor with complete or incomplete gross excision; positive ipsilateral regional lymph nodes; identifiable contralateral lymph nodes negative microscopically.
3	Tumor infiltrating across the midline with or without regional lymph node involvement; *or* unilateral tumor with contralateral regional lymph node involvement; *or* midline tumor with bilateral regional lymph node involvement.
4	Dissemination of tumor to distant lymph nodes, bone, bone marrow, liver, and/or other organs (except as defined for stage 4-S).
4-S	Localized primary as defined for stage 1 or 2 with dissemination limited to liver, skin, and/or bone marrow.

From Holland JF, Frei E III, Bast KC, et al: Cancer Medicine, 3rd edition. Philadelphia, Lea & Febiger, 1993, p 2175.

the trunk, extremity, or paratesticular regions can be treated with surgery followed by adjuvant chemotherapy and irradiation if residual disease exists. The benefit of adjuvant chemotherapy is well established. Combinations of vincristine, dactinomycin, cyclophosphamide, and doxorubicin are used. Primary tumors involving the orbit, parameningeal region, and prostate are managed by chemotherapy and irradiation alone.

Late Consequences of Treatment

Because children with cancers now survive longer, the incidence of long-term sequelae related to antineoplastic therapy have been increasingly recognized. Side effects may be seen in many organ systems and can have a significant impact on the quality of life of cancer survivors.

The most frequent late consequences of antineoplastic therapy include cardiomyopathy with congestive heart failure, endocrine hormone deficiency, gonadal failure and hormonal dysfunction with amenorrhea or sterility, growth retardation or asymmetric growth, alterations in neuropsychiatric and intellectual functioning, encephalopathy, pul-

monary fibrosis, and an increased incidence of secondary malignancies (Byrd, 1985).

ONCOLOGIC EMERGENCIES

Oncologic emergencies are defined as any acute, potentially life-threatening events directly or indirectly related to a tumor or its treatment. If not quickly recognized and treated, these conditions may result in significant morbidity or death. Occasionally these emergent conditions are the presenting symptoms of a previously undiagnosed neoplasm. The differential diagnosis for any cancer patient presenting with such an acute condition must also include medical emergencies unrelated to the cancer.

Malignant Pericardial Tamponade

Malignant pericardial effusions are the most common cause of cardiac tamponade. Cancers of the lung, breast, and esophagus as well as lymphoma and leukemia often cause significant effusions. Pericardial tamponade and constrictive pericarditis may also be caused by irradiation of the mediastinum.

Symptoms can include dyspnea, chest tightness or pain, nausea, vomiting, wheezing, or acute hypotension and circulatory collapse. On examination, patients may be tachycardic or hypotensive, and have muffled heart tones. A pulsus paradoxus of more than 10 mm Hg is suggestive of the diagnosis. Echocardiography can confirm the diagnosis, and therapy includes pericardiocentesis or pericardial window.

Superior Vena Cava Syndrome

Superior vena cava syndrome is characterized by rapid progression of facial and upper body edema. Severe episodes may involve compromise of the airway and respiratory collapse. Increased intracranial pressure may lead to death. Tumors responsible for superior vena cava syndrome include bronchogenic cancer, breast cancer, lymphomas, mediastinal germ cell tumors, and thymomas.

Physical findings include venous distention in the neck and chest, facial edema and plethora, cyanosis, arm and hand edema, tachypnea, stridor, papilledema, lethargy, and confusion. The diagnosis is made by CT with rapid contrast injection.

Therapy is directed at the specific malignancy. Although mediastinal radiotherapy has been the treatment most frequently used, systemic chemotherapy, especially in patients with chemotherapy-sensitive tumors who have never received chemotherapy, is increasingly recommended. Temporizing measures such as airway control, oxygen, head elevation, and steroids are used until definitive therapy is initiated.

Bleeding

Bleeding may be due to direct tumor invasion into vascular structures, abnormalities in plasma clotting factors, or thrombocytopenia. Epistaxis and oral mucosal bleeding are common but rarely life-threatening. Patients with predisposing lesions such as peptic ulcer disease should be treated with prophylactic H_2 blockers. Aspirin and NSAIDs should be avoided. Chemotherapy with cyclophosphamide or ifosfamide predisposes to hemorrhagic cystitis. In these cases, irrigation of the bladder with saline, steroids, or formalin is the initial treatment; if bleeding is persistent, cystoscopy and fulguration are performed. Bleeding can be minimized by administering the missing factors and platelets, as well as topical thrombin and tranexamic acid.

TABLE 44–29. CLASSIFICATION OF VESICANT, IRRITANT, AND NONVESICANT CANCER CHEMOTHERAPEUTIC AGENTS*

Agent
Vesicants
Actinomycin
Daunorubicin
Doxorubicin
Epirubicin
Idarubicin
Mechlorethamine
Mitomycin
Vinblastine
Vincristine
Irritants
Carmustine (BCNU)
Dacarbazine (DTIC)
Etoposide (VP-16)
Mithramycin
Streptozocin
Teniposide (VM-26)
Nonvesicants
Asparaginase
Azacytidine
Bleomycin
Carboplatin
Cisplatin
Corticosteroids
Cyclophosphamide
Cytarabine (Ara-C)
5-Fluorouracil (5-FU)
Floxuridine (FUDR)
Ifosfamide
Interleukin-2
Interferons
Methotrexate
Mitoxantrone
Thioguanine
Thiotepa (TSPA)

* Vesicants are cancer chemotherapeutic agents capable of forming a blister or causing tissue destruction. Irritants are cancer chemotherapeutic agents capable of causing pain at the injection site or along the vein, with or without an inflammatory reaction.

From Holland JF, Frei E III, Bast KC, et al: Cancer Medicine, 3rd edition. Philadelphia, Lea & Febiger, 1993, p 2455, with permission.

Extravasation

Chemotherapeutic agents are classified as nonvesicants, irritants, or vesicants (Table 44–29). By definition, vesicant agents can cause necrosis if extravasation occurs. Once it does, the drug should be immediately discontinued. The treatment of extravasation caused by daunorubicin, doxorubicin, epirubicin, achromycin, or mitomycin involves cooling the site with ice packs for approximately 24 hours and elevating the limb. For that caused by the vinca alkaloids vinblastine and vincristine, warm compresses and local injection of hyaluronidase are initiated. In any case of extravasation, a plastic surgeon should be consulted immediately, as rapid débridement may minimize injury.

Chemotherapeutic drugs should be administered by health care professionals who have a thorough understanding of venous access and treatment of extravasation.

Tumor Lysis Syndrome

Tumor lysis syndrome is associated with rapid killing of neoplastic cells and the subsequent release of large quantities of intracellular ions and products into the circulation, which may result in significant metabolic derangements and acute renal failure. Tumor lysis is most frequently seen in rapidly growing tumors such as leukemias and lymphomas.

Metabolic derangements include hyperuricemia, oliguric renal failure with increased BUN and creatinine levels, hyperkalemia, hypocalcemia, hyperphosphatemia, and systemic acidosis. Patients may develop clinical symptoms such as oliguria, fluid overload, seizures, cardiac arrhythmias, muscle cramps, tetany, nausea, vomiting, or lethargy.

Patients at high risk for development of the syndrome should receive prophylactic allopurinol and hydration with alkalinization of the urine. Tumor lysis syndrome should be treated with vigorous diureses and, if necessary, hemodialysis.

Hypercalcemia

Hypercalcemia is the most frequent metabolic emergency in oncology. Tumors most commonly associated with hypercalcemia include breast, lung, hypernephroma, multiple myeloma, squamous cell carcinoma of the head and neck, and parathyroid cancer. Symptoms include fatigue, anorexia, nausea, polyuria, polydipsia, and constipation. Neurologic symptoms are common and include muscle weakness, lethargy, and hyporeflexia.

Evaluation includes calcium, alkaline phosphatase, and electrolyte assays and measures of renal function. Therapy includes hydration, steroids, and administration of intravenous bisphosphonates (etidronate or pamidronate), gallium nitrate, mithramycin, or calcitonin. Agents such as thiazide diuretics and vitamins A and D, which increase calcium levels, should be avoided.

Hyponatremia and the Syndrome of Inappropriate Antidiuretic Hormone

Hyponatremia is observed in conjunction with the syndrome of inappropriate antidiuretic hormone (SIADH). Before being diagnosed as having SIADH, patients must be proved to have normal renal, thyroid, and adrenal functions. The hallmark of SIADH is urine inappropriately concentrated with a high level of sodium in the face of low plasma osmolality. This syndrome is often seen in patients with small-cell carcinomas.

Symptoms include anorexia, nausea, myalgias, lethargy, and seizures. Certain chemotherapeutic agents, such as vincristine and cyclophosphamide, can decrease the sodium level. Evaluation of patients suspected of having SIADH includes measurement of serum and urine electrolytes and osmolality, a creatinine assay, and tests of thyroid and adrenal functions. Therapy includes fluid restriction, demeclocycline, and infrequently administration of 3% hypertonic saline.

Spinal Cord Compression

Metastases to the spine may extend to the epidural space and cause spinal cord compression. Metastases from breast, lung, and prostate cancers are the most frequent neoplastic causes of cord compression. Patients may present with back pain, radicular pain, weakness, sensory loss, or change in bowel or bladder habits.

Therapy must be instituted immediately to avoid progression of symptoms. Dexamethasome with a large initial bolus (10 to 100 mg) and continued regular doses is the initial treatment, which should be instituted while diagnostic tests are being performed. Definitive therapy is usually radiotherapy, which should be initiated on an urgent basis. Decompressive laminectomy has also been performed, usually in patients in whom cancer had not been diagnosed or in those whose disease progressed even while on radiotherapy.

Neutropenic Fever

Fever is common in cancer patients and can result from tumor necrosis, inflammation, transfusions, or chemotherapeutic or antimicrobial drugs. Most fevers (55 to 70 per cent) are caused by infections, especially in patients with neutropenia (absolute neutrophil count fewer than 500 polymorphonuclear cells). Infections in such cases of severely compromised immunity can become life-threatening within hours, and urgent therapy with empiric antibiotics is the standard practice.

Classic signs and symptoms of infection may be absent in neutropenic patients. The physical examination should meticulously evaluate all possible sources of infection. Initial evaluation should include a chest radiograph, urinalysis and culture, sputum culture, two sets of preantibiotic blood cultures, and culture of an aspirate or biopsy specimen from any accessible site suggesting infection. Initial empiric therapy should cover gram-positive and gram-negative organisms with emphasis on *Pseudomonas aeruginosa*. Patients who do not defervesce on the initial regimen should receive additional therapy with vancomycin and antifungal agents.

REFERENCES

Abner A: Prophylactic cranial irradiation in the treatment of small-cell carcinoma of the lung. Chest 103:445S, 1993.

Aisner J: Treatment of limited-disease small cell lung cancer. Semin Oncol 19:51, 1992.

American College of Physicians Position Paper: Preoperative pulmonary function testing. Ann Intern Med 112:793, 1990.

Andersson L: Indications and techniques of prostate biopsies. Prostate (suppl 4):115, 1992.

Armitage P, Doll R: A two-stage theory of carcinogenesis in relation to the age distribution of human cancer. Br J Cancer 11:161, 1957.

Beahrs OH, Henson DE, Hutter RVP, et al (eds): Manual for Staging of Cancer, 4th edition. Philadelphia, JB Lippincott, 1992.

Berenblum I: The mechanism of carcinogenesis: A study of the significance of cocarcinogenic action and related phenomena. Cancer Res 1:807, 1941.

Bishop JM: The molecular genetics of cancer. Science 23:305, 1987.

Bishop JM: Molecular themes in oncogenesis. Cell 64:235, 1991.

Buzdar AU: Chemotherapeutic approaches to advanced breast cancer. Semin Oncol 15:65, 1988.

Byrd R: Late effects of treatment of cancer in children. Pediatr Clin North Am 32:835, 1985.

Carney D, Sikora K: Genes and Cancer. Chichester, John Wiley & Sons, 1990.

Chang F, Syrjanen S, Kurvinen K, Syrjanen K: The p53 tumor suppressor gene as a common cellular target in human carcinogenesis. Am J Gastroenterol 88:174, 1993.

Clark GM, McGuire WL: Steroid receptors and other prognostic factors in primary breast cancer. Semin Oncol 15:20, 1988.

Cohen AM, Minsky BD, Schilsky RL: Colon cancer. *In* DeVita VT, Hellman S, Rosenberg SA (eds): Cancer: Principles and Practice of Oncology, 4th edition. Philadelphia, JB Lippincott, 1993, pp 929–977.

Consensus Conference: Adjuvant chemotherapy for breast cancer. JAMA 254:3461, 1985.

Daly MB: The epidemiology of ovarian cancer. Hematol Oncol Clin North Am 6:729, 1992.

Dawson NA: Treatment of progressive metastatic prostate cancer. Oncology 7:17, 1993.

Deppe G, Malviya VK: Ovarian cancer advances in management. Hematol Oncol Clin North Am 5:1285, 1991.

De Souza PL, Friedlander ML: Prognostic factors in ovarian cancer. Hematol Oncol Clin North Am 6:761, 1992.

DeVita VT Jr, Hellman S, Rosenberg SA: Principles and Practice of Oncology, 4th edition. Philadelphia, JB Lippincott, 1993.

Early Breast Cancer Trialists' Collaborative Group: Effects of adjuvant tamoxifen and of cytotoxic therapy on mortality in early breast cancer. N Engl J Med 319:1681, 1988.

Eddy DM: Screening for lung cancer. Ann Intern Med 111:232, 1989.

Eddy DM: Screening for colorectal cancer. Ann Intern Med 113:373, 1990.

Einhorn LH, Williams SD, Troner M, et al: The role of maintenance therapy in disseminated testicular cancer. N Engl J Med 305:727, 1981.

Fearon ER, Vogelstein B: A genetic model for colorectal tumorigenesis. Cell 61:759, 1990.

Fisher B, Bauer M, Wickerham L, et al: Relation of number of positive axillary nodes to the prognosis of patients with primary breast cancer. Cancer 52:1551, 1983.

Fisher B, Redmond C, Fisher ER, et al: Ten-year results of a randomized clinical trial comparing radical mastectomy and total mastectomy with or without radiation. N Engl J Med 312:674, 1985.

Fisher B, Costantino J, Redmond C, et al: A randomized clinical trial evaluating tamoxifen in the treatment of patients with node-negative breast cancer who have estrogen-receptor-positive tumors. N Engl J Med 320:479, 1989a.

Fisher B, Redmond C, Dimitrov NV, et al: A randomized clinical trial evaluating sequential methotrexate and fluorouracil in the treatment of patients with node-negative breast cancer who have estrogen-receptor-negative tumors. N Engl J Med 320:473, 1989b.

Fisher B, Redmond C, Poisson R, et al: Eight-year results of a randomized clinical trial comparing total mastectomy and lumpectomy with or without irradiation in the treatment of breast cancer. N Engl J Med 320:822, 1989c.

Ganick DJ: Wilms' tumor. Hematol Oncol Clin North Am 1: 695, 1987.

Ginsberg RJ, Kris MG, Armstrong JG: Non-small cell lung cancer. *In* DeVita VT, Hellman S, Rosenberg SA (eds): Cancer: Principles and Practice of Oncology, 4th edition. Philadelphia, JB Lippincott, 1993, pp 673–723.

Green MR: New adjuvant strategies for the management of resectable non-small-cell lung cancer. Chest 103:352S, 1993.

Hainsworth JD, Greco FA: Extragonadal germ cell tumors and unrecognized germ cell tumors. Semin Oncol 19:119, 1992.

Hanks GE, Myers CE, Scardino PT: Cancer of the prostate. *In* DeVita VT, Hellman S, Rosenberg SA (eds): Cancer: Principles and Practice of Oncology, 4th edition. Philadelphia, JB Lippincott, 1993, pp 1073–1113.

Harris CC, Hollstein M: Clinical implications of the p53 tumor suppressor gene. N Engl J Med 329:1318, 1993.

Harris JR, Lippman ME, Veronesi U, Willett W: Breast cancer. N Engl J Med 327:473, 1992.

Hathway DE: Mechanisms of Chemical Carcinogenesis. London, Butterworth, 1986.

Hawes RH: New staging techniques: Endoscopic ultrasound. Cancer 71:4207, 1993.

Henderson IC: What can a woman do about her risk of dying of breast cancer? Curr Probl Cancer 14:165, 1990.

Heubner RJ, Todaro GJ: Oncogenes of RNA tumor viruses as determinants of cancer. Proc Natl Acad Sci USA 64:1087, 1969.

Holland JF, Frei E III, Bast KC Jr, et al: Cancer Medicine, 3rd edition. Philadelphia, Lea & Febiger, 1993.

Holmes EC: Postoperative chemotherapy for non-small-cell lung cancer. Chest 103:30S, 1993.

Hornsby-Lewis L, Winawer SJ: Natural history and current management of colorectal polyps. Oncology 4:139, 1990.

Hoskins WJ, Perez CA, Young RC: Gynecologic tumors. *In* DeVita VT, Hellman S, Rosenberg SA (eds): Cancer: Principles and Practice of Oncology, 4th edition. Philadelphia, JB Lippincott, 1993, pp 1152–1225.

Hunter T: Cooperation between oncogenes. Cell 64:249, 1991.

Ihde DC, Pass HI, Glatstein EJ: Small cell lung cancer. *In* DeVita VT, Hellman S, Rosenberg SA (eds): Cancer: Principles and Practice of Oncology, 4th edition. Philadelphia, JB Lippincott, 1993, pp 723–758.

Kim YS, Liotta LA, Kohn EC: Cancer invasion and metastases. Hosp Pract May 15:92, 1993.

King MC, Rowell S, Love SM: Inherited breast and ovarian cancer: What are the risks? What are the choices? JAMA 269:1975, 1993.

Klein EA: Tumor markers in testis cancer. Urol Clin North Am 20: 67, 1993.

Laurie JA, Moertel CG, Fleming TR, et al: Surgical adjuvant therapy of large-bowel carcinoma: An evaluation of levamisole and the combination of levamisole and fluorouracil. J Clin Oncol 7:1447, 1989.

Levin B: Inflammatory bowel disease and colon cancer. Cancer 70:1313, 1992a.

Levin B: Nutrition and colorectal cancer. Cancer 70:1723, 1992b.

Levine AJ: The p53 tumor suppressor gene. N Engl J Med 326: 1350, 1992.

Lilenbaum RC, Green MR: Novel chemotherapeutic agents in the treatment of non-small cell lung cancer. J Clin Oncol 11:1391, 1993.

Liotta LA, Steeg PS, Stetler-Stevenson WG: Cancer metastasis and angiogenesis: An imbalance of positive and negative regulation. Cell 64:327, 1991.

Lippman SM, Kavanagh JJ, Paredes-Espinoza M, et al: 13-cis-retinoic acid plus interferon alpha-2a: Highly active systemic therapy for squamous cell carcinoma of the cervix. J Natl Cancer Inst 84:241, 1992.

Lippman Sm, Benner SE, Hong WK: Chemoprevention strategies in lung carcinogenesis. Chest 103(suppl 1):15S, 1993.

Marshall CJ: Tumor suppressor genes. Cell 64:313, 1991.

McCormick B: Radiotherapy in breast cancer. Curr Opin Oncol 3:1002, 1991.

McGuire WL, Clark GM: Prognostic factors and treatment decisions in axillary-node-negative breast cancer. N Engl J Med 326:1756, 1992.

Mertens WC, Stitt L, Porter AT: Strontium-89 therapy and relief of pain in patients with prostatic carcinoma metastatic to bone: A dose-response relationship? Am J Clin Oncol 16:238, 1993.

Mettlin C, Jones G, Averette H, et al: Defining and updating the American Cancer Society guidelines for the cancer-related checkup: prostate and endometrial cancers. CA Cancer J Clin 43:42, 1993.

Meyer WH, Malawer MM: Osteosarcoma clinical features and evolving surgical and chemotherapeutic strategies. Pediatr Clin North Am 38:317, 1991.

Meyers PA: Malignant bone tumors in children: Ewing's sarcoma. Hematol Oncol Clin North Am 1:667, 1987.

Middleton RG: Value of and indications for pelvic lymph node dissection in the staging of prostate cancer. Monogr Natl Cancer Inst 7:41, 1988.

Milken D, Li FP, Strong LC, et al: Germ line p53 mutations in a familial syndrome of breast cancer, sarcomas and other neoplasms. Science 250:1233, 1990.

Moertel CG, Fleming TR, MacDonald JS, et al: Levamisole and fluorouracil for adjuvant therapy of resected colon carcinoma. N Engl J Med 322:352, 1990.

NIH Consensus Conference: Adjuvant therapy for patients with colon and rectal cancer. JAMA 264:1444, 1990.

NIH Consensus Conference: Treatment of early stage breast cancer. JAMA 265:391, 1991.

NIH Consensus Development Panel: Consensus statement: the management of clinically localized prostate cancer. Monogr Natl Cancer Inst 7:3, 1988.

Omura GA: Current status of chemotherapy for cancer of the cervix. Oncology 6:27, 1992.

Ozols RF: Chemotherapy for advanced epithelial ovarian cancer. Hematol Oncol Clin North Am 6:879, 1992.

Patel AM, Dunn WF, Trastek VF: Staging systems of lung cancer. Mayo Clin Proc 68:475, 1993.

Perry MC (ed): The Chemotherapy Source Book. Baltimore, Williams & Wilkins, 1992.

Pienta KJ, Esper PS: Risk factors for prostate cancer. Ann Intern Med 118:793, 1993.

Poplack DG: Acute lymphoblastic leukemia in childhood. Pediatr Clin North Am 32:669, 1985.

Poulsen HE, Loft S, Wasserman K: Cancer risk related to genetic polymorphisms in carcinogen metabolism and DNA repair. Pharmacol Toxicol 72(suppl 1):93, 1993.

Ransohoff DF, Lang CA: Screening for colorectal cancer. N Engl J Med 325:37, 1991.

Richardson GE, Johnson BE: Paraneoplastic syndromes in lung cancer. Curr Opin Oncol 4:323, 1992.

Richie JP: Detection and treatment of testicular cancer. CA Cancer J Clin 43:151, 1993.

Sheilds PG, Harris CC: Molecular epidemiology and the genetics of environmental cancer. JAMA 266:681, 1991.

Shih C, Padhy LC, Mureray M, Weinberg RA: Transforming genes of carcinomas and neuroblastomas introduced into mouse fibroblasts. Nature 290:261, 1981.

Sidransky D, Tokino T, Hamilton SR, et al: Identification of ras oncogene mutations in the stool of patients with curable colorectal tumors. Science 256:102, 1992.

Slaughter DB, Southwick HW, Smejkal W: "Field cancerization" in oral stratified squamous epithelium. Cancer 6:963, 1953.

Stehelin D, Varmus HE, Bishop JM, Vogt PK: DNA related to the transforming gene(s) of avian sarcoma viruses is present in normal avian DNA. Nature 260:170, 1976.

Varmus H, Weinberg RA: Genes and the Biology of Cancer. New York, Scientific American Library, 1993.

Weinberg RA: Oncology. II. Molecular mechanisms of carcinogenesis. In Rubenstein E, Federman DD (eds): Scientific American Medicine. New York, Scientific American, 1993.

Williams SD: Chemotherapy of ovarian germ cell tumors. Hematol Oncol Clin North Am 5:1261, 1991.

Williams SD, Stablein DM, Einhorn LH, et al: Immediate adjuvant chemotherapy versus observation with treatment at relapse in pathological stage II testicular cancer. N Engl J Med 317:1433, 1987.

Wittes RE (ed): Manual of Oncologic Therapeutics 1991/1992. Philadelphia, JB Lippincott, 1991.

Young RC, Perez CA, Hoskins WJ: Cancer of the ovary. In DeVita VT, Hellman S, Rosenberg SA (eds): Cancer: Principles and Practice of Oncology, 4th edition. Philadelphia, JB Lippincott, 1993, pp 1226–1263.

CHAPTER 45
HEMATOLOGY

ALAN K. DAVID

Hematology is the study of the cellular elements of the blood—their origins, functioning, and disorders. The family physician orders and reviews blood counts on a daily basis for a wide variety of purposes. Understanding the reasons for an elevated or diminished count or a qualitative abnormality is essential for the diagnosis and treatment of patients in the family physician's practice. The development of a simple classification system for use as an organizational framework in the approach to problems found in the cellular elements of the blood is an important tool. That framework helps one formulate a diagnostic and treatment plan and assess the success of treatment of any of these abnormalities. The finding of a low white blood cell count, a decreased red blood cell count, or an excessive platelet count is often unexpected. By themselves, these findings do not always constitute a diagnosis, much like finding a fever in a patient. Instead, they require investigation, further testing, and an organized approach. Such investigation can be conceptually and practically implemented in the framework of a busy family practice.

PREVALENCE AND INCIDENCE

The classic study of what constitutes the content of family practice was well documented in a study done by the Medical College of Virginia in 1976 in which 526,000 patient encounters with family physicians were diagnostically categorized. A number of common abnormalities of the hematopoietic system were found among the top 250 diagnoses, such as iron deficiency anemia (29th), other anemias (112th), megaloblastic anemias (153rd), leukemia (189th), and lymphadenopathy (240th). It has been estimated that as many as 25 per cent of infants, 6 per cent of all children, 30 per cent of pregnant women, and 50 per cent of all menstruating women may be iron-deficient at one level or another due to inadequate dietary intake and physiologic blood loss. With conditions such as alcoholism, 50 per cent of individuals are iron-deficient, and 90 per cent are folate-deficient because of poor nutrition. Lymph node enlargements are seen most commonly in response to localized infection. However, systemic diseases, malignancies, collagen-

vascular diseases, and even skin disorders may cause generalized lymphadenopathy. Platelet disorders are both quantitative and qualitative by definition, but they occur relatively infrequently in the family physician's patient population, ranking 479th in the Virginia study.

HISTORY AND PHYSICAL EXAMINATION

The symptoms of a low grade or chronic anemia may be vague, particularly when compared to the anemia of an individual who has developed the problem suddenly from blood loss or acute hemolysis. Patients with chronic or low grade anemia may complain only of easy fatigability, weakness, some shortness of breath, and dizziness on exertion. Occasionally they may note pallor. The acute onset of anemia may bring about headache, postural hypotension, jaundice, discolored urine, decreased ability to think clearly, and marked fatigability. When a patient complains only of fatigue, it is more likely caused by other abnormalities, such as depression or thyroid disease. Eliciting a family history of anemia or a personal history of recurrent anemia in an individual is an excellent clue to a genetic or chronic ongoing condition. A history of easy bleeding or bruising suggests a platelet disorder. If symptoms or signs such as pallor or fever are found with easy bruising, more bone marrow elements may be involved, as with aplastic anemia or leukemia. Fever, weight loss, anorexia, and fatigue in the presence of anemia may indicate a systemic infection or abnormalities of white blood cells or lymph nodes (such as with a malignancy).

Physical abnormalities may be found by careful observation. Pallor may be seen particularly in the nail beds and sclera. Examining the patient carefully for petechiae, evidence of jaundice, and enlargement of the liver or spleen may be important clues to the etiology of anemia or a white blood cell problem. Cardiovascular symptoms such as marked orthostasis or the development or intensification of heart murmurs may indicate the acute development of anemia. Careful examination of the reticuloendothelial system, particularly the liver and spleen, lymph node regions, and the mouth and posterior pharynx are helpful for ascertaining the extent and involvement of a hematologic problem. In the time-limited realm of the ambulatory practice of the family physician, the examination should focus on careful observation and an otherwise good screening physical examination. Finding occult blood in the stool is also helpful as part of the physical examination process to check for gastrointestinal blood loss.

NORMAL GROWTH AND DIFFERENTIATION

Hematopoiesis

The bone marrow is the site of hematopoiesis after the seventh month of intrauterine life and remains so unless there is life-threatening illness. The marrow has a volume of approximately 1.7 liters with 1×10^{12} hematopoietic cells that rest on a framework of fat, fibroblasts, blood vessels, macrophages, and a sinusoidal network with a venous drainage system. Hematopoietic cells must pass through the sinusoidal walls in order to enter the circulation. To do so they must be able to change their shape. The most immature cells cannot make such a change and are retained in the marrow until they fully develop. This is why immature forms are not seen in the peripheral blood unless there is marked stress systemically and particularly to the marrow. Elements of the blood undergo growth, differentiation, maturation, or self-renewal from a pluripotent stem cell. These pluripotent stem cells can be pure or mixed in terms of their ability to produce colonies of red blood cells, white blood cells, megakaryocytes, or even lymphoid cells. Stem cells have also been called colony-forming units–blasts (CFU-blasts). Stem cells can undergo differentiation, or self-renewal. In cases of obliteration of the bone marrow for bone marrow transplantation, only about 5 per cent of normal marrow stem cells are required to repopulate an entire bone marrow. The stem cell can give rise to lymphoid clones and myeloid clones. Figure 45–1 demonstrates the evolution of a pluripotent stem cell into the major lines produced by the bone marrow.

Erythropoietin

Erythropoietin is a humoral protein mediator and stimulator of red blood cell growth and differentiation. It is coded on a single gene on the long arm of chromosome 7 and has been synthesized so it is commercially available. In the body it is synthesized primarily in the kidney and is released by a sensor in the kidney that senses tissue oxygenation. Its circulating half-life is approximately 5 hours. It stimulates erythropoiesis in the presence of a factor called burst-promoting activity, which stimulates the erythroid stem cells to undergo differentiation. It also enhances hemoglobin synthesis and can increase the total number of precursors undergoing development. Release of reticulocytes from the marrow is under its control. Recombinant erythropoietin is particularly useful to treat the anemia of end-stage renal disease when there is a marked lack of erythropoietin due to malfunctioning kidneys.

As erythrocytic precursors develop, there are approximately four doublings between the proerythroblast stage and the normoblast stage, which results in a 16-fold increase in the number of total cells. Approximately 10 per cent of erythroid precursors die in the marrow. Reticulocytes are those red blood cell precursors that have just had their nucleus extruded after the orthochromatic normoblast stage. They can be identified by supravital staining with new methylene blue, which stains them a deeper blue. This staining is caused by residual RNA on ribosomes left over from the process of manufacturing hemoglobin. Reticulocytes spend 4 days before becoming normal red blood cells: 3 days are spent in the marrow and 1 day in the peripheral blood.

Red Blood Cells

The average red blood cell (RBC) has a life-span of 120 days. There are approximately 2.5 liters of

---

FIGURE 45–1. The most primitive pluripotent stem cells ultimately give rise to granulocytes, macrophages, erythroid cells, and platelets. They probably can also differentiate along the lymphoid line (dotted line) to produce B and T cells. This pluripotent hematopoietic stem cell—either colony-forming unit-blast (CFU-blast) in human marrow culture or colony-forming unit-spleen (CFU-S) in the rodent spleen colony-forming assay—has impressive self-renewal capacity; however, its first recognizable descendant, the colony-forming unit-granulocyte-erythroid-macrophage-megakaryocyte (CFU-GEMM), has much less self-renewing capacity and instead differentiates into granulocytes, erythrocytes, monocytes, and megakaryocytes. Although the initial choice of lineage seems to be random, growth factors such as erythropoietin (EPO), thrombopoietin, interleukin-3 (IL-3), interleukin-5 (IL-5), granulocyte-macrophage colony-stimulating factor (GM-CSF), granulocyte colony-stimulating factor (G-CSF), and macrophage colony-stimulating factor (M-CSF) play a major role in controlling the subsequent differentiation of hematopoietic cells. (Adapted from Rubenstein EH, Federman D: Hematology (Chapter 5). New York, Scientific American Medicine, 1993, with permission. Copyright 1988 Scientific American, Inc.)

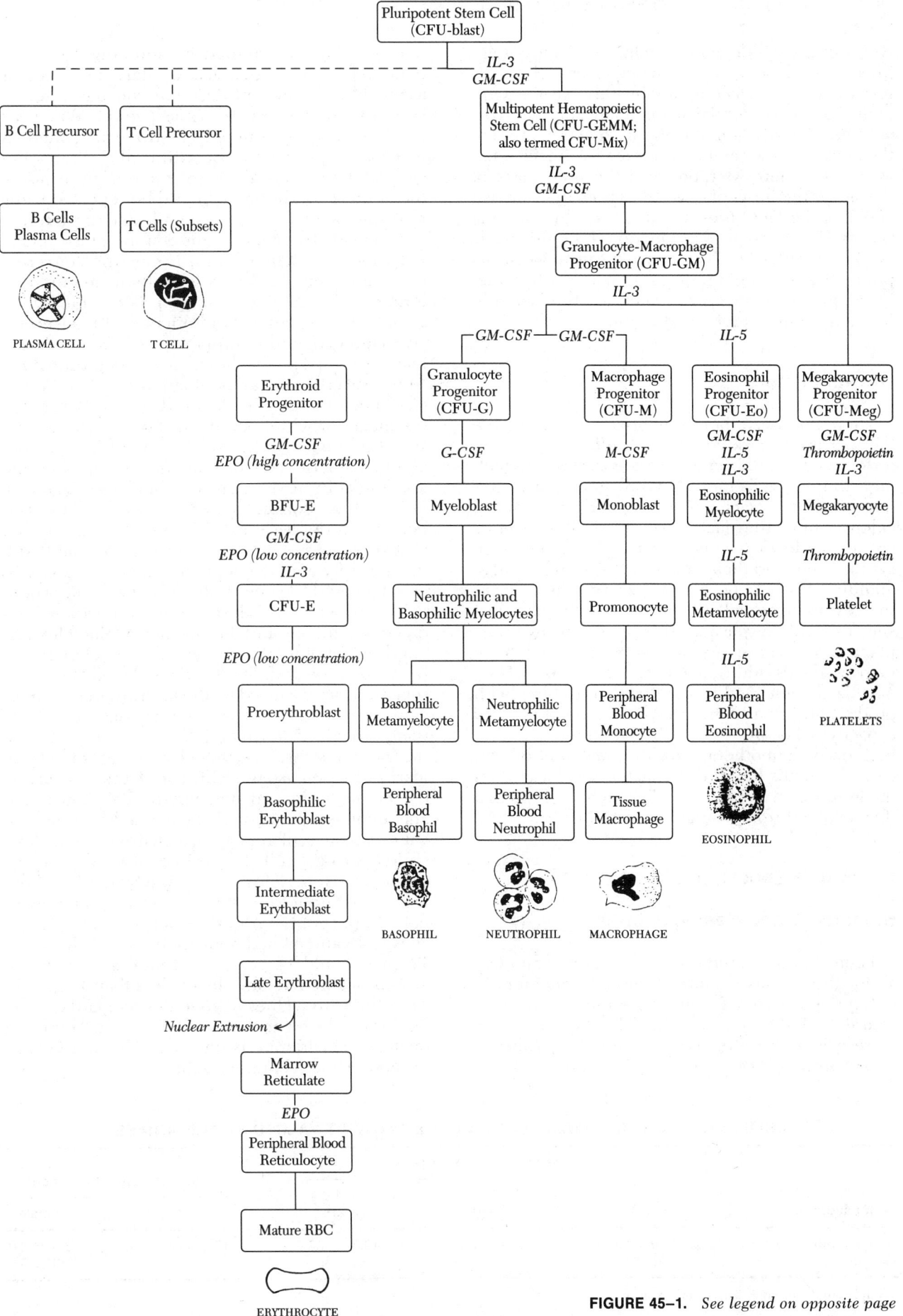

FIGURE 45–1. *See legend on opposite page*

RBCs in the average adult man, representing approximately 3 per cent of lean body mass. The bone marrow must replace approximately 0.8 per cent of the RBC mass per day to maintain a normal RBC volume. The relation of RBCs in the circulation to the bone marrow can be expressed by the formula: $M = IT$, where M represents the total mass of RBCs, I is the input of new RBCs from the marrow, and T is the RBC life-span in days. Thus anemia is caused by decreased production (I) or hemolysis or loss of RBCs (T). The marrow can increase its production six to eight times normal if it has adequate precursor materials, such as iron, vitamin B_{12}, folic acid, protein, and so on.

Growth Factors

There are four other growth factors that enable the marrow to produce its multiple products: interleukin-3 (IL-3), granulocyte-macrophage colony-stimulating factor (GM-CFS), granulocyte colony-stimulating factor (G-CSF), and macrophage colony-stimulating factor (M-CFS). These factors are available in commercial forms, having been synthesized; and they enhance the proliferation of granulocytes, monocytes, megakaryocytes, erythrocytes, and mast cells. They are used for disorders such as myelodysplasia and in bone marrow transplant cases where the newly transplanted bone marrow needs additional stimulus to grow. They have also been used to stimulate white blood cell production in patients with limited bone marrow capacity who are susceptible to infection after high-dose chemotherapy for the treatment of cancer. The genes for all these factors are located on the long arm of chromosome 5, which suggests that they evolved from a single ancestral gene.

NORMAL HEMATOLOGIC VALUES

Hematocrit and Hemoglobin

There is no absolute test that defines anemia, although the most commonly used parameters to determine whether anemia is present are the hematocrit and the hemoglobin. The hematocrit is more accurately defined as the packed cell volume, or that portion of the blood made up of RBCs. If the hematocrit is determined by spinning the blood obtained by fingerstick in a capillary tube, there is as much as a 4 per cent variation from one determination to another in the same patient. When the hematocrit is determined electronically, there is less than 1 per cent error. Clinically, when a fingerstick hematocrit does not seem to fit or match the clinical condition, it should be repeated using a peripheral venous blood sample and the determination made by an electronic counting instrument.

To measure hemoglobin, it must be converted to cyanmethemoglobin which is then measured calorimetrically to give an appropriate value. Delusional errors, excessive protein in the blood, excessive jaundice, and improper lysis of the cells can lead to errors in the hemoglobin determination. The African-American population may have levels of hemoglobin that are 0.5 to 1.0 gm/dL lower than the mean for white populations of similar age and sex. Table 45–1 outlines the normal hemoglobin and hematocrit values for infants, young children, and adults by sex within two standard deviations. During the neonatal period, the hemoglobin and hematocrit decrease over the first 6 weeks of life to levels that remain fairly constant for the first 2 years of life: average hemoglobin about 12 gm/dL and average hematocrit about 36 per cent. These values are of course dependent on nutrition, adequate iron intake, and the absence of blood loss. As children get older, the hemoglobin level increases because of the shift of the oxygen hemoglobin dissociation curve caused by the high circulating inorganic phosphate levels seen during periods of bone growth. Entering adolescence, boys secrete increased testosterone, which stimulates the bone marrow to increase the RBC count, thereby raising the hemoglobin and hematocrit. The hematocrit and hemoglobin in women has a lower normal value because of repeated menstrual blood loss, child-bearing, and borderline iron deficiency. When determinations were made by the U.S. Public Health Service on samples from normal individuals, 10 per cent of American women between the ages of 18 and 44 had hemoglobin levels less than 12 gm/dL, and 11 per cent of men of similar age groups had hemoglobin levels less than 14 gm/dL. Thus there are values beyond the standard two deviations of the mean that may be normal. This point must be considered as one evaluates individuals for borderline laboratory values.

TABLE 45–1.   NORMAL HEMOGLOBIN AND HEMATOCRIT VALUES BY AGE AND SEX

| Measurement | Normal Value, By Age | | | Normal Value, by Gender | |
	1–3 Days	1 Month to 2 Years	3–12 Years	Male	Female
Hemoglobin (gm/dL)	19.0 ± 2.2	12.0 ± 1.5	12.5 ± 1.5	15.5 ± 2.0	13.5 ± 2.0
Hematocrit (%)	61 ± 7.4	36 ± 4	38 ± 4	46 ± 5	40 ± 5

Values are the mean ± 2 SD from the mean.

White Blood Cell Count

The white blood cell (WBC) count is measured electronically by the electrical impedance the WBCs cause as they disrupt an electronic charge. These counts are accurate, with normal values being 4500 to 10,500/mm^3. Equally important to the total WBC count is the absolute count of neutrophils. Neutrophils have a half-life of about 6.5 hours and a total life-span of about 10 hours. They are distributed equally in the circulating pool and the marginal pool of the bone marrow, spleen, and remaining reticuloendothelilial system. The lower limit for the absolute neutrophil count is about 1500 to 1800 cells/mm^3 with the lower value more appropriate for African-Americans. Neutrophils are important for the resolution of bacterial infections and prevention of septicemia. Errors may be caused by inappropriate sampling of the diluted blood and incorrect identification of all the cells that can be counted. Blood from a normal individual has an RBC/WBC ratio of approximately 500:1.

TERMINOLOGY; ADDITIONAL USEFUL TESTS

Blood Smear

The peripheral blood smear is often neglected today in clinical medicine. Many times a blood smear is not examined by laboratory personnel or physicians because the WBC differentials are often performed electronically. However, with a puzzling hematologic picture, examination of the peripheral blood smear under the microscope can still be helpful. A drop of blood is placed near the end of a glass slide and smeared with another slide held perpendicularly; the cells are thus spread in a single layer at the "feather" edge so they are contiguous and do not touch. This area is examined microscopically under a oil immersion lense.

Red blood cells should be examined for their variations in color, size, and shape. *Target cells* may be seen in the presence of thalassemia and other hemoglobinopathies. *Howell-Jolly bodies* are remnants of DNA found in new cells just pumped out of the bone marrow or in cells that remain in the circulation in patients who have had their spleen removed. *Heinz bodies* are small bits of oxidized hemoglobin seen on the peripheral smear after staining with methylviolet. The presence of Heinz bodies indicates decreased enzyme reducing power of the RBC, as is seen with some hemoglobinopathies and in problems such as glucose-6-phosphate dehydrogenase (G-6-PD) deficiency.

White blood cell abnormalities, such as hypersegmented neutrophils, are seen with production defect anemias caused by deficiencies in vitamin B$_{12}$ or folic acid. Toxic granulations in neutrophils may indicate infection.

Platelets can be seen in the peripheral smear as small blue 1- to 2-μm diameter objects with small granular inclusions. There are usually 5 to 10 platelets per high power oil field or 1 platelet for every 10 to 20 RBCs.

Reticulocyte Count

Red blood cells newly released from the bone marrow contain residual RNA and ribosomes left over from the manufacturing process of hemoglobin. A peripheral blood smear stained with new methylene blue detects reticulocytes, which have a bluish cast. The normal reticulocyte count is 0.5 to 1.5 per 100 RBCs counted and is expressed as a per cent. Reticulocytes are larger than mature RBCs, being 10 to 15 μm compared to the 7 μm diameter of a normal mature RBC. Reticulocytes persist in the bone marrow for up to 3 days and then 1 day in the circulation before they lose their reticular RNA and become normal RBCs.

Reticulocytosis occurs in acute situations such as blood loss, marked hemolysis, or when replacement of a previously deficient factor such as iron, vitamin B$_{12}$, or folate occurs in a patient who has a production deficit anemia. The *absolute reticulocyte count* can be measured by taking the reticulocyte per cent × the total RBC count determined from a routine complete blood count. Neither the reticulocyte per cent nor the absolute reticulocyte count completely reflects whether the bone marrow is responding appropriately to the degree of anemia seen in a particular patient. If the bone marrow is unable to produce appropriate reticulocytes, the reticulocyte percentage or absolute number may appear appropriate when in fact there is a suboptimal response. The degree of reticulocytosis can be then corrected by taking into consideration the hematocrit of the patient. This value is a *corrected reticulocyte count.* The lower the hematocrit, the more immature reticulocytes are pumped into the peripheral circulation. They then remain there longer, accounting for the increase in the reticulocyte percentage and absolute count. The following numbers indicate the correlation of the peripheral circulation maturation time of reticulocytes with the hematocrit:

Hematocrit (%)	Time (days)
45	1.0
35	1.5
25	2.0
15	2.5

With a hematocrit of 45 per cent the normal maturation time for a reticulocyte is 1 day. For each 10 points that the hematocrit drops, the maturation time increases by one-half day; thus a hematocrit of 25 per cent would have a reticulocyte maturation time of 2 days. The absolute reticulocyte count should have a range of 25,000 to 75,000 cells/mm^3 with a mean of approximately 50,000 cells/mm^3. If one takes a 1 per cent reticulocyte count $\times$ 5 $\times$ 10^6 RBCs/mm^3, it would equal 50,000 reticulocytes as an absolute reticulocyte count. Let us now take an example of a patient who is anemic. If the patient's hematocrit is 25 per cent and the RBC count is 2.5 $\times$ 10^6 with an uncorrected reticulocyte count of 5 per cent, the absolute reticulocyte count is 125,000. This figure appears to indicate a good response by the bone marrow at 2.5 times normal. On the other hand, if one takes that figure and divides by the maturation time because the more immature reticulocytes stay in the circulation longer, the 125,000 may be an inappropriately high number. When one divides the 125,000 by the maturation time of 2.0 days, the corrected reticulocyte count is 62,500, which is just barely above the mean of 50,000.

Corrected absolute reticulocyte count =

reticulocyte % (5%) $\times$ RBCs (2.5 $\times$ 10^6)

= 125,000/2 days^7 maturation = 62,500

In this case, then, the bone marrow response is inadequate and is probably caused by a production deficit.

Red Blood Cell Distribution Width

The RBC distribution width (RDW) is a measure of the variation in size of different populations of RBCs. It is not a measure of mean RBC size, such as the mean corpuscular volume. It is a calculated number that indicates the coefficient of variation of RBC sizes spread over an entire population. The amount of variation between the 20th and 80th percentiles of RBC sizes in the population is calculated. An average coefficient of variation might be 10.0 $\pm$ 1.5. A number larger than this one indicates that more than one population of RBCs exists. This point is demonstrated by the curves in Figure 45–2. Here a homogeneous population of RBCs has one hump in the curve and a heterogeneous population of RBC sizes produces two humps. The wider variation with two populations gives a larger number for the coefficient of variation. This value may be helpful for diagnosing anemias such as that due to early iron deficiency, where there is a small population of RBCs and a normal size population of RBCs.

If there has been acute blood loss with new large RBCs being pumped in the circulation, the RDW is elevated. The RDW is normal and useful for distinguishing the anemia of chronic disease, which has a homogeneous population of microcytic cells,

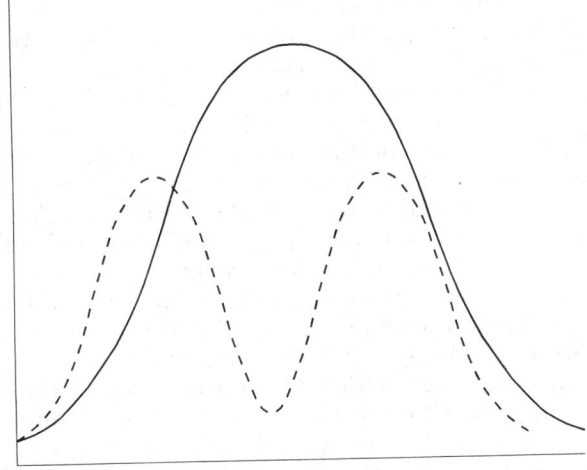

 # RBCs

Distribution by Size

— **One Population**
-- - **Two Populations**

FIGURE 45–2. Red blood cell distribution width.

as do the thalassemias, which have a uniform microcytic cell population. There are several conditions that can falsely elevate the RDW: (1) In leukemias with high WBC counts, the WBCs may be so small they are measured as RBCs. (2) Some inflammatory diseases cause RBCs to clump, and they are then measured as a single cell. (3) Patients with cardiac valves may produce fragmented RBCs. (4) Patients who have had significant RBC transfusions may have falsely elevated RDWs.

CLASSIFICATION SCHEMES OF DISORDERS

Many textbooks of internal medicine and hematology have detailed, lengthy listings of all the possible diagnoses of anemia, WBC disorders, and so on. These lists are impossible to memorize and often have an extensive framework that is not useful in the clinical setting. The simplest conceptual framework that helps one sort out where a particular disorder or abnormality might fall and how to begin to approach it is what is needed for the family physician. The fundamental question to ask in each case—whether it is RBCs, WBCs, or platelets—is whether there is an excess, a deficiency, or a qualitative problem with regard to the problem encountered. Table 45–2 has a classification scheme that we follow in general in this chapter. It delineates simply the major considerations of RBC disorders, WBC disorders, and platelet disorders.

TABLE 45–2. HEMATOPOIETIC DISORDERS CLASSIFICATION SYSTEM

Red Blood Cell Disorders	Leukocyte Disorders	Platelet Disorders

Anemia
  Blood loss
  Impaired
    production
  Hemolysis
	Leukopenia	Thrombocytopenia

Polycythemia	Leukocytosis	Thrombocytosis

	Qualitative
	  disorder
		Qualitative
		  disorders

TABLE 45–3. RED BLOOD CELL DISORDERS CLASSIFIED BY KINETIC ANALYSIS

Anemia
Actual anemia
  Blood loss (acute/chronic)
  Defective red blood cell production
    Cell line failure
    Aplastic anemia
    Red blood cell aplasia
    Chronic renal failure

    Defective DNA synthesis
    Vitamin B_{12}/folic acid deficiency

    Defective hemoglobin production
    Iron deficiency

    Miscellaneous
    Sideroblastic anemias
    Bone marrow infiltration
    Anemia of chronic disorders
  Hemolysis
    Extrinsic causes
      Antibody formation: drugs, viral, autoimmune
      Infection
      Mechanical: microangiopathic hemolysis
    Intrinsic causes
      Membrane defects: spherocytosis
      Globin defects: thalassemia, sickle cell
      G-6-PD deficiency
      Metabolic defects
      Porphyria
Apparent anemia
  Dilutional (i.e., pregnancy or macroglobulinemia)
  Splenomegaly

Polycythemia

RED BLOOD CELL DISORDERS

Red blood cell disorders may be classified as the RBCs being excessive, which is polycythemia, or deficient, which defines anemia. However, anemia is really best defined as the condition of reduced oxygen-carrying capacity of the blood, resulting in tissue hypoxia. Hemoglobin is the best test to determine anemia, and the hematocrit is the best reflection of polycythemia. RBC disorders have been classified by the mean corpuscular volume (MCV), a morphologic RDW/MCV system, or a kinetic system. For our purposes, the kinetic classification system is useful; it is represented by the formula $M = IT$, where M is the mass of the RBCs, I is the input of the RBCs, and T is the length of time the cells' survive. All elements of anemia can fit into this equation in which the input of RBCs represents production defects, and the transit time or the life-span of RBCs can be affected by blood loss or hemolysis (or both). A detailed classification of RBC disorders by kinetic analysis is outlined in Table 45–3. This system is simple enough to remember in terms of the major categories of blood loss, hemolysis, or impaired production. The dynamic state of the RBCs, how they are produced, and how they are lost is the basis for this system. Many family physicians have found this system easier to remember than the typical classifications using the MCV, RDW, or some complicated schematic.

Apparent Anemia

On occasion, the laboratory values of patients reflect reduced hemoglobin or low hematocrit in a situation in which the patient actually has adequate oxygen-carrying capacity. Such a situation obtains when the relation of the RBC mass to the plasma volume is altered. For example, a pregnant woman may expand her plasma volume by 50 per cent, which would then reduce the proportion of RBCs in terms of the plasma volume so the hematocrit falls without an actual reduction in the total amount of hemoglobin. However, a dilutional phenomenon on occasion also reduces the hemoglobin concentration. Many patients who are pregnant are treated unnecessarily with large doses of iron plus prenatal vitamins when they are physiologically normal and not anemic. The normal hematocrit and hemoglobin values for a pregnant woman after the 12th week of gestation are 33 ± 3 per cent and 11 ± 1.5 gm/dL, respectively. Athletic individuals who are well trained, particularly long distance runners or swimmers, may develop what appears to be an abnormally low hematocrit level while the RBC mass is appropriate. This is due to an expansion of plasma volume and does not represent anemia. Some patients have an inherited abnormal hemoglobin called Kansas, which unloads oxygen far more readily than normal hemoglobin. Therefore a hemoglobin Kansas level of 8 gm/dL is sufficient to carry oxygen to the tissues; yet the patient's laboratory values are at levels defining anemia. Patients who have developed macroglobulinemia also have increased plasma volume and a dilutional effect on the hematocrit level. Thus they may appear anemic but have a normal number of RBCs. Asynchrony of the hematocrit and hemoglobin levels or abnormal hematologic values in a patient who is apparently normal should be investigated and explained.

Actual Anemia

Anemia of Blood Loss

Acute blood loss is often easy to diagnose when there is major trauma, upper gastrointestinal (GI) bleeding, or profound lower GI bleeding. More obscure causes of acute blood loss may be retroperitoneal bleeding from an abdominal aorta that has leaked, intra-abdominal bleeding from an ectopic pregnancy, or deep tissue bleeding into muscle in a person with a fractured pelvis or other trauma. It is important to remember that a patient who has lost 2 liters of blood in an acute hemorrhagic situation and is showing signs of shock may have a normal hematocrit and hemoglobin because the blood volume has been lost in a proportional manner; that is, both RBCs and plasma volume have been lost equally. Thus the concentration of hemoglobin and the percentage of RBCs relative to the blood volume is appropriate. It may take up to 72 hours for the situation to equilibrate and the level of anemia actually quantitated.

The symptoms of acute blood loss are usually postural hypotension, an increased heart rate, and signs of shock if blood loss exceeds 1 liter. Reduced central venous pressure and cool extremities may also develop. The body compensates to a degree for acute anemia by increasing the cardiac output to keep RBCs moving to peripheral tissues at a rate that compensates for the reduced number of RBCs. It also keeps oxygen pressure high in the venous bed, which reduces the likelihood of tissue hypoxemia. The hemoglobin must reach a level of 7 gm/dl before cardiac output changes significantly. Heart murmurs may appear or intensify, and bruits may even be heard over the skull. Decreased perfusion of the kidneys from acute blood loss increases the erythropoietin level and stimulates increased production of RBCs. Patients with coronary artery disease may develop angina, and those with peripheral vascular disease may develop muscle cramps in the extremities due to decreased perfusion.

Acute blood loss must be treated quickly and promptly with crystalloids and packed RBCs when appropriate. The appropriate volume must be calculated to avoid fluid overload. In situations where shock is present, volume expanders may be more appropriate. One principle of fluid replacement is that the volume of crystalloids must be three times that of the colloid volume to achieve the same effect. Once blood pressure and fluid volume are restored, packed RBCs should be administered in appropriate quantities to bring the hematocrit back to a level of at least 30 per cent and the hemoglobin to 10 gm/dl.

Chronic blood loss is most commonly caused by GI tract polyps, neoplasms, inflammation, or recurrent menstrual loss in women during the reproductive years. Patients with previous gastric surgery often are not able to absorb iron appropriately or may have recurrent gastritis and sustain blood loss as well. Other forms of chronic blood loss that occur less frequently are chronic intravascular hemolysis seen with paroxysmal nocturnal hemoglobinuria with hemoglobinemia, blood loss in idiopathic pulmonary hemosiderosis into the lungs, and recurrent bleeding episodes that are factitious in mentally disturbed patients. Athletes such as swimmers and long-distance runners have reduced iron body stores, and anemia that results from plasma volume expansion, possible traumatic hemolysis of RBCs in muscles, and occult GI bleeding. The use of aspirin and nonsteroidal anti-inflammatory drugs (NSAIDs) may significantly increase the likelihood of the latter problem. The search for blood loss is most likely to be successful when utilizing a detailed history and tests of organ systems that might be involved in chronic blood loss. More information about the effects of chronic blood loss and iron deficiency is given in the section on iron-deficiency anemia.

Anemia of Defective RBC Production

CELL LINE FAILURE. The bone marrow carefully regulates the growth and differentiation of stem cells in order to provide the normal cellular elements of the blood. The major finding in a production deficit is the decrease or near absence of one or more of the normal cellular elements with a low reticulocyte count when the RBC line is primarily affected. Production deficits may be associated with failure of one or more bone marrow cellular lines, defects in hemoglobin synthesis, insufficient nutrients for the bone marrow, and a host of miscellaneous causes. When a patient is found with a significant deficiency of bone marrow elements in their blood, the first task is to differentiate between deficient production and increased peripheral destruction. Production deficits due to infections, autoimmune diseases, tumors, drugs, toxins, and specific systemic illnesses may account for partial or complete bone marrow failure.

APLASTIC ANEMIA. Aplastic anemia is caused by a decreased number of functioning pluripotent stem cells, which results in a marked deficiency of all three cell lines of the bone marrow: RBCs, WBCs, and platelets. The causes of aplastic anemia are many; Table 45–4 lists them primarily in the categories one must consider most often. A congenital form, otherwise called Fanconi's anemia, often has other associated abnormalities, such as hypoplasia of certain bones, the spleen, and the kidney; microcephaly; and mental retardation. Almost half the cases of aplastic anemia occur later in life with an unknown etiology. The most likely common pathway of aplastic anemia is a mechanism of immune suppression of pluripotent stem cells. Bone marrow transplantation tends to be the best treatment when there is pretransplantation immunosuppressive therapy. The use of antithymocyte or

TABLE 45–4. ETIOLOGIES OF APLASTIC ANEMIA

Toxins: benzene, glues
Radiation
Drugs: anticancer, chloramphenicol, gold, antiepileptics, certain NSAIDs, arsenic
Infections
Immune disorders
Paroxysmal nocturnal hemoglobinuria
Malignant disorders
Fanconi's anemia
Infections: parvovirus
Infectious mononucleosis
Non-A non-B hepatitis

antilymphocyte globins with or without bone marrow transplantation produces marked improvement in many patients with aplastic anemia, providing further evidence to support an immunosuppression etiology. Causes of aplastic anemia that must be carefully sought are the use of anticancer or immunotherapeutic drugs, inflammatory drugs (particular antibiotics such as chloramphenicol and sulfonamides), anticonvulsant drugs, and toxins such as glues, insecticides, paint thinners, and benzenes. More recent knowledge of the effects of viruses has indicated that hepatitis (particularly non-A non-B), Epstein-Barr virus, and parvovirus may cause aplastic anemia. Diseases that may present a confusing picture that resembles aplastic anemia are bone marrow replacement by myelofibrosis, cancer, granulomatous disease, or necrosis of the bone marrow. Hypocellular leukemias, paroxysmal nocturnal hemoglobinuria, and anorexia may also present with similar pictures.

The clinical features of a person with aplastic anemia are marked anemia with reticulocytopenia, increased susceptibility to actual infection, and easy bruising or bleeding tendencies. The history is particularly important, as removal of a toxin, chemical, or drug from the patient's therapeutic regimen or environment may result in improvement and resolution of the condition. Patients with aplastic anemia are more likely to have bleeding tendencies at lower platelet count levels (20,000 platelets/mm^3) because the platelets are old, less functional, and less active in hemostasis. Splenomegaly or lymphadenopathy are not hallmarks of aplastic anemia, and other diagnoses must be entertained if these conditions are noted. Severe cases of aplastic anemia are associated with a platelet count less than 20,000/mm^3, a neutrophil count of less than 500/mm^3, and an absolute reticulocyte count of less than 50,000. The MCV may be moderately to significantly elevated, but an MCV higher than 120 μm^3 with hypersegmented neutrophils may indicate a megaloblastic condition of folate or vitamin B$_{12}$ deficiency. In cases of pancytopenia with an increased reticulocyte count, paroxysmal nocturnal hemoglobinemia may be the cause. The

bone marrow aspiration is usually unproductive. The bone marrow biopsy reveals a severely hypocellular marrow with replacement primarily by fat cells.

Treatment calls for a careful investigation of the history in order to remove any possible etiologic agents, such as drugs, toxins, or exposure to chemicals. Infections must be treated vigorously, and antibiotics are instituted after appropriate cultures but without waiting for the culture results. Bleeding tendencies can be managed with platelet transfusions, particularly when the platelet count is below 20,000/mm^3. However, after several weeks of platelet transfusions, sensitivity and antibodies to platelets develop, particularly to HLA antigens. Further transfusions of platelets are then increasingly less effective. Minimal transfusions of RBCs is an important consideration for decreasing the likelihood of sensitization: It increases the success of bone marrow transplantation should it be needed. Bone marrow transplantation tends to be used more often in patients less than 40 years of age because of the long-term complications of graft-versus-host disease, which increase with the age at transplantation. Bone marrow transplants are most effective when they are obtained from identical twins or HLA-matched siblings. Pretransplantation immunosuppressive therapy increases the likelihood of bone marrow transplantation success. Patients who are not good candidates for bone marrow transplantation may be treated with antithymocyte globulin or antilymphocyte globulin manufactured in horses. Sensitivity to horse serum, such as serum sickness, and other problems may occur. Antiviral agents and immunosuppressive doses of steroids have not been particularly helpful. Bone marrow growth factors, such as interleukins and the colony-stimulating factors, have been tried and may be useful for helping the bone marrow recover after transplantation or after immunosuppressive therapy has shown some degree of success.

MYELODYSPLASIA. Myelodysplasia is a group of abnormalities of the bone marrow in which there is a marked decrease in one or all three cell lines characterized by abnormal cell morphology, macrocytic anemia, and a low reticulocyte response. Myelodysplasia is primarily a disease of older persons and is thought to be the result of the neoplastic transformation of a pluripotent stem cell. Abnormalities on chromosome 5 or 7 are often found in these individuals. Marrow replacement and fibrosis are neoplastic proliferation patterns, including myelofibrosis, polycythemia vera, chronic myelogenous leukemia, and essential thrombocytosis. The treatment of myelofibrosis and myelodysplasia is supportive, with transfusions of RBCs and platelets when absolutely necessary. If the abnormalities evolve into acute leukemia, it can be treated with appropriate chemotherapy.

RED BLOOD CELL APLASIA. Patients with RBC aplasia are significantly anemic. There is no reticulocyte response, and the erythroid precursors in bone marrow are depleted or virtually absent. These findings suggest that the pluripotent stem cells are intact because WBCs and platelets exist in normal numbers. After erythroid precursors differentiate from the pluripotent stem cell, they appear to be attacked by immune mechanisms. Some work has suggested an autoantibody to erythropoietin as well. A congenital form of RBC aplasia called the Diamond-Blackfan anemia is a genetic defect of erythroid stem cells. Some limited forms occur in children with chronic hemolytic anemia caused by human parvovirus infection, otherwise known to be the cause of fifth disease. Other etiologies in children are hereditary spherocytosis, sickle cell disease, and thalassemia. The acquired adult form has an association with thymoma about 50 per cent of the time. Anywhere from 30 to 50 per cent of cases of adult acquired RBC aplasia may involve a thymoma, so a computed tomography (CT) scan of the chest is a necessary part of the evaluation of a patient with pure RBC aplasia. Secondary causes of RBC aplasia may be other kinds of neoplasms such as Hodgkin's disease, chronic leukemias, rheumatoid arthritis, systemic lupus erythematosus, antiviral drugs, trimethoprim, sulfamethoxazole, infectious mononucleosis, and hepatitis. Because the etiology involves mechanisms of immunosuppression, thymectomy may be curative. In patients without this or another treatable etiology, immunosuppressive therapy with steroids and in some cases cytotoxic therapy may be helpful. If patients become less responsive to immunosuppressive therapy, splenectomy plus immunosuppression may resolve or alleviate the problem.

ANEMIA OF RENAL FAILURE. Because erythropoietin is produced in the kidney, it decreases markedly in chronic renal failure and end-stage renal disease. The decline in hematocrit occurs most often after the creatinine clearance becomes less than 40 ml/min. Other contributing factors may be chronic inflammatory disease leading to the anemia of chronic disorders, folic acid deficiency, frequent blood removal for tests, hemodialysis, blood loss, and the effect of uremia itself. In addition, aluminum toxicity due to antacids has been suggested as a possible cause of the anemia found in patients with severe renal disease. Clinically, the peripheral smear demonstrates Heinz bodies and a picture of a microangiopathy, with hemoglobin levels of 5 to 8 gm/dL in hemodialysis patients and 10 gm/dL in peritoneal dialysis patients. Today erythropoietin, manufactured by the recombinant DNA process, is the treatment of choice for the anemia of renal disease. It can be used on patients who are on dialysis and those who have not yet reached that stage.

ERYTHROPOIETIN. Erythropoietin is produced by a recombinant DNA process and is exactly identical to the naturally produced 165 amino acid sub-

stance. It is derived from mammalian cells in which the DNA gene for erythropoietin has been inserted. Levels of erythropoietin can be commercially measured and range from 0.01 to 0.03 units/ml. Erythropoietin is generally given with a subcutaneous injection at a rate of 50 to 300 units/kg spread over a three times per week injection schedule. Generally, one sees a reticulocytosis within 10 days and an increase in hematocrit and hemoglobin within 2 to 6 weeks. The target level is a hematocrit of 30 to 33 per cent. A maintenance level of approximately 100 units/kg can be used on a three times per week schedule. The contraindications to erythropoietin are untreated or uncontrolled hypertension, a sensitivity to mammalian cells, and allergic sensitivity to serum albumin from humans. Reasons for an inappropriate or inadequate response to erythropoietin are iron deficiency (serum ferritin levels should be checked prior to the institution of erythropoietin therapy), a serious underlying infection or inflammatory process, occult blood loss, hemoglobinopathies, myelodysplastic disorders, other deficiencies such as folic acid and vitamin B_{12}, chronic hemolysis, and aluminum intoxication.

Patients with human immunodeficiency virus (HIV) disease are often treated with AZT (zidovudine), which tends to suppress erythropoiesis and lower erythropoietin levels. Erythropoietin has been used on a similar schedule of three injections per week at a dosage of 100 to 200 units/kg spread over the three injections. This regimen has markedly increased the hematocrit and reduced the transfusion requirement in these patients. Once a response and an adequate hematocrit have been achieved, a maintenance dose of 100 units/kg spread over three injections per week can be used to maintain appropriate hemoglobin and hematocrit levels.

The cost of this therapy is not insignificant, but transfusion therapy, its complications, and the effects of the anemia are far more severe and costly than the use of this recombinant DNA erythropoietin therapy.

Megaloblastic Anemias

Megaloblastic anemias are the primary examples of ineffective erythropoiesis. The classic examples are megaloblastic anemias, sideroblastic anemias, thalassemia, and myelodysplasia. Physiologically, there is a decreased reticulocyte count, erythroid hyperplasia in the marrow with abnormal large forms, and decreased delivery of RBCs to the peripheral circulation. In some megaloblastic anemias, 90 per cent of RBCs die before they can leave the marrow. The primary defect is a lack of DNA synthesis, but there is adequate RNA production. The exact mechanisms are still unclear. It can be caused by a deficiency of folic acid or vitamin B_{12}, by drugs that block DNA synthesis, or by drugs that block the actions of vitamin B_{12} or folic acid.

The clinical picture is classically an anemic patient with macrocytic RBCs, an elevated MCV, and hypersegmented neutrophils with five or six lobes. Vitamin B_{12} deficiency causes this kind of anemia in a secondary manner because this vitamin is necessary to convert the inactive form of folic acid to an active, usable form. Thus when vitamin B_{12} is deficient it causes the same problems as a deficiency in folic acid and neurologic complications as well. The human body does not produce folic acid or vitamin B_{12} in sufficient quantities internally, so diet and supplementation are necessary.

FOLIC ACID. Folic acid is found in leafy green vegetables, meat products, and dairy products; 0.1 to 0.2 mg of folic acid is necessary per day. The average dietary intake is approximately 0.4 mg per day. Unfortunately, folic acid is labile; and cooking vegetables, fishes, and meat destroys 50 to 90 per cent of the available folic acid. Once it reaches the intestinal tract, however, 60 per cent of it is absorbed unless blocked by a drug such as ethanol or phenytoin. The blood level reflects only recently absorbed folate. The RBC folate level is a reflection of the body stores and can be useful for the diagnosis. The primary metabolic roles of folic acid are an amino acid conversion of homocysteine to methionine and, in purine metabolism, producing thymidine. Deficiency of folate prevents the activation of thymidine, which is thought to lead to deficient DNA synthesis.

VITAMIN B_{12}. Vitamin B_{12} is essentially cobalamin, which is a porphyrin with a cobalt atom and a cyanide molecule. It is produced by bacteria. Sources for human consumption are primarily animals in terms of meats, seafood, dairy, and eggs, as they have the bacteria necessary to produce vitamin B_{12}. A total of 1 to 5 μg per day is necessary, and cooking foods high in vitamin B_{12} does not significantly reduce the content in those foods. Dietary vitamin B_{12} is bound primarily by a salivary R protein, with the remainder bound in the stomach by intrinsic factor protein manufactured by parietal cells of the stomach. The R protein binding does not make vitamin B_{12} available to the circulation, but the R-bound vitamin B_{12} is released from the R protein by pancreatic enzymes in the small intestine. Much of it is then bound by the intrinsic factor protein. The villi of the terminal ileum cells have receptors that then enable the intrinsic factor-bound vitamin to be absorbed into the circulation. Because vitamin B_{12} facilitates the demethylation of methyltetrahydrofolate to tetrahydrofolate, which is the active form of folic acid, vitamin B_{12} deficiency is considered the folate trap. In essence, if a person has vitamin B_{12} deficiency and is treated with folic acid alone, there is some initial improvement; but tissue levels continue to fall even though serum levels may seem adequate owing to the inadequate levels of vitamin B_{12} needed to activate folate in the cell. The anemia and all its consequences and associated symptoms thus continue.

CLINICAL PICTURE. Folic acid deficiency has a direct effect on the synthesis of DNA in cells, and vitamin B_{12} has an indirect effect because of its role in the conversion of folic acid to its active forms. With the loss of either or both of these elements, there is a build-up of immature cells in the bone marrow resulting in erythroid hyperplasia. These cells do not produce adequate DNA. Many of the cells die without ever reaching the peripheral circulation. In the peripheral circulation, one sees macrocytes and ovalocytes. Erythroid precursors and giant metamyelocytes have an abnormal nuclear/erythroplasmic ratio. Hypersegmented neutrophils are the most sensitive index of megaloblastic anemia clinically. There may also be pancytopenia because of the problem of making DNA that affects other bone marrow elements. Hemolysis may occur, as the cells that are sent into the peripheral circulation are inadequate, defective, and rapidly removed. This sequence results in decreased haptoglobin levels, urine hemosiderin, and elevated liver enzymes. Folic acid deficiencies produce a mild to moderate anemia, although sometimes it is severe. In pregnant women, folic acid deficiency may result in neural tube defects. Central nervous system (CNS) signs of irritability and memory loss occur. The neurologic symptoms that are found with vitamin B_{12} deficiency are not present with folic acid deficiency alone.

Vitamin B_{12} deficiency creates the same hematologic picture, but glossitis of the tongue and paresthesia beginning in the thoracolumbar region and extending in the lower extremities are common. The anatomic effects are found in the lateral and dorsal columns of the spinal cord, with vibration and position sense affected. The deep tendon reflexes may at first be decreased. As the neurologic defects progress, Babinski reflexes develop, with ataxia and a positive Romberg test following. Later spasticity, increased deep tendon reflexes, clonus, and even paraplegia can occur. Systemic symptoms of the CNS include depression and memory impairment. The neuropathy is thought to be due to impaired methionine synthesis.

The classic picture is rarely seen today. In fact, a small percentage of individuals may have megaloblastic anemia without significant macrocytosis. Other causes of macrocytosis include liver disease, alcohol intake, increased reticulocytosis, anticonvulsant drugs, and AZT. The classic picture may also be masked by profound iron deficiency in conditions such as thalassemia. Blood levels of folate or vitamin B_{12} are not diagnostic in all cases of megaloblastic anemia.

Anti-intrinsic factor antibodies can be found in about 70 per cent of patients with pernicious anemia. The Schilling test is performed with a radioactive dose of vitamin B_{12} given orally and a larger dose of unlabeled vitamin B_{12} given parenterally. The parenteral dose saturates the transport mechanisms, so a large proportion of vitamin B_{12} is excreted in the urine. If less than 10 per cent of the oral radioactive dose is excreted in the urine, there is poor absorption. The test can be repeated adding intrinsic factor, which should correct the results. However, there are false positives and false negatives, and the test cannot be considered 100 per cent reliable.

MANAGEMENT. Patients with folic acid deficiency must undergo a meticulous history, with inquiry into the use of alcohol, the use of drugs, and the presence of other anemias. Sideroblastic anemias, iron deficiency, thalassemia, and hemolysis may be confusing factors. Malabsorption causing folic acid deficiency is not common but may account for 10 to 15 per cent of cases. Diagnosing the malabsorption phenomenon diagnosis folic acid deficiency.

Treatment is oral folic acid at a dose of 1 mg per day. A reticulocytosis is seen within 1 to 3 days, peaking at 5 to 7 days. Hypersegmented neutrophils may persist for weeks. Treatment should be continued indefinitely as long as the underlying cause persists. Prophylaxis in pregnancy is treated with 1 mg of folic acid per day even though 0.4 mg with a good diet is probably sufficient.

Megaloblastic anemia with neurologic deficits should not be treated with folic acid alone, as the neurologic deficits do not resolve. Because vitamin B_{12} deficiency usually relates to malabsorption, the need for lifelong maintenance should be conveyed to the patient. The usual dose is 1 mg intramuscularly (1000 μg). The same response is seen with vitamin B_{12} as with folic acid: improvement in the hematologic picture within a matter of days and weeks. Once an adequate hematologic response has been obtained, monthly maintenance injections can be given at the same dose of 1000 μg intramuscularly per month. Neurologic symptoms of vitamin B_{12} deficiency do not disappear with folate even though there may be a transient improvement in the hematologic picture. Mild to moderate neurologic symptoms may start to improve within the first week, but more often than not more time is necessary. Sensory changes may resolve within several weeks and are usually fully reversible. Serious problems such as ataxia, spasticity, and paraplegia may take much longer, require rehabilitation therapy, and may never completely resolve. The goals of therapy in either case are to reverse the abnormalities, prevent relapse, and build up tissue and body stores as a reserve. Folic acid therapy is usually not needed indefinitely so long as dietary, drug, alcohol, or other problems can be resolved. When the terminal ileum is absent or intrinsic factor cannot be produced by the stomach, vitamin B_{12} therapy must be continued for life.

Iron-Deficiency Anemia

A lack of iron available to the bone marrow produces a anemia characterized by small hypochromic cells with a slightly decreased life-span. Although many cases of iron deficiency are related to inadequate amounts of iron, the inadequate iron supply is often caused by chronic blood loss. For purposes of this discussion, this disorder is considered a production deficit anemia even though its ultimate etiology may be related to chronic blood loss.

BIOCHEMISTRY OF IRON. Iron is an essential element in hemoglobin and myoglobin (referred to as heme iron) and is necessary for many chemical reactions in the body. Iron metabolism is controlled by the iron content of the diet, the availability of this iron, the substances in which the iron is found, the body's need for iron, and the effectiveness of erythropoiesis. Iron found in grains and cereals can be absorbed at a rate of only 5 per cent. In contrast 34 per cent of heme or myoglobin-bound iron found in animal proteins can be absorbed. When dietary deficiency is causative, it is most likely to be a deficiency in animal protein. About 1 to 2 mg of iron can be absorbed per day from a diet in which 6 mg of iron per 1000 calories are found. The average diet of 1600 to 1800 calories contains 10 to 12 mg of iron per day in the United States. If this iron is present as nonheme iron, it is not readily available. The absorption and availability of heme iron are not affected by hydrochloric or gastric acid, whereas nonheme iron is bound to a protein in the intestinal tract. Tea and coffee tend to reduce the absorption of nonheme iron, whereas ascorbic acid, amino acids, and sugar stimulate nonheme iron absorption. Ascorbic acid reduces the ferric iron (Fe^{+3}) to ferrous iron (Fe^{+2}), which is the preferable ionic form for iron absorption. The average absorption of iron by the intestinal tract is about 12 per cent of the dietary intake, whereas in iron deficiency states it can rise to 34 per cent.

Transferrin is the protein that transports iron in the plasma. It can be measured by its iron-binding capacity or by transferrin saturation. When the body is deficient in iron, with decreased plasma iron, iron is transferred to the bone marrow from hematopoietic storage cells by transferrin. Increased iron-binding capacity and low transferrin saturation are hallmarks of iron deficiency.

The storage form of iron is ferritin, which is a protein shell that holds approximately 4500 iron atoms. Ferritin is found most commonly in liver muscle and the rest of the reticuloendothelial system. Ferritin can be measured clinically and reflects the state of body iron stores. Hemosiderin is another form of storage iron that can be seen only after staining the bone marrow and other biopsied organs with Prussian blue. Conditions such as cancer, infection, inflammation, and liver disease can elevate the serum ferritin level despite inadequate total iron body stores, thereby masking the iron-deficiency anemia.

Iron can be found in the storage forms of hemosiderin and ferritin and in myoglobin, hemoglobin, and transferrin. Women tend to have a lower iron stores than men because of their chronic reproductive menstrual blood loss and the loss of iron and blood as a result of repeated pregnancies. Women lose about 2 mg of iron per day and men about 1 mg in the stools, urine, skin, and nails. As noted previously, the GI tract can absorb 1 to 2 mg of iron from a diet with 10 mg of elemental iron present. Thus simply adding more iron to the diet in a nonheme iron manner is not always an appropriate way to resolve iron deficiency. Older individuals tend to absorb iron at about the same rate but have a lower rate of incorporation of iron into RBCs than younger subjects. Iron deficiency is often confused with the anemia of chronic disorders, which results from chronic disease and inflammation. The hematologic pictures may appear to be similar, but iron is trapped in macrophages and is not available to RBCs in the bone marrow for their development.

CLINICAL PICTURE. Iron deficiency in adults is most often caused by chronic blood loss either from the GI tract or during menstruation in women. Patients who have had gastric surgery may have iron deficiency because of recurrent blood loss, malabsorption, or a poor dietary intake. As body stores of iron are depleted, the body attempts to absorb more iron but can do so only marginally from a normal diet; it also mobilizes iron from all storage sites. Iron-deficient RBCs are subject to a degree of hemolysis and a decreased life-span as a result. Gradually, the RBCs become smaller, although microcytic, hypochromic cells are seen only with significant, long-standing iron deficiency. Iron deficiency during pregnancy may cause prematurity and perinatal mortality, as well as decreased mental and motor function during infancy and early childhood. Iron is also necessary for intestinal flora to grow. Individuals with severe iron deficiency may have blue sclera, nail changes, atrophy of the GI mucosa, gastric achlorhydria, thrombocytosis, and pica (compulsive eating of ice, clay, or other substances to compensate for the lack of iron).

CLINICAL DIAGNOSIS. Other entities that sometimes mimic the hypochromic, microcytic picture of classic iron deficiency include the thalassemias, the anemia of chronic disease, and sideroblastic anemias. The anemia of chronic disease and iron deficiency both have low RBC counts, whereas the thalassemia syndromes have high RBC counts. The RDW tends to be normal with the thalassemia syndromes and is increased in the presence of iron deficiency because of the wide variation of cell size. Table 45–5 lists the significant laboratory findings of early and late iron deficiency anemia. In the United States most iron deficiency is of a mild variety, with hemoglobin values of 9 to 12 gm/dL. The MCV may be normal to borderline with normal-appearing cells. By the time the classic picture is apparent, the anemia is profound. A low plasma iron, increased plasma iron-binding capacity, or transferrin saturation of less than 15 per cent

TABLE 45–5. DIAGNOSIS OF IRON-DEFICIENCY ANEMIA

Measurement	Early Stages	Late Stages
Hemoglobin/hematocrit	Normal to slightly reduced	8–11 gm/dL (24–33%)
Red blood cell distribution width index	Slightly increased	Elevated to normal
Serum iron	Normal to borderline	Below normal
Iron-binding capacity	Normal to increased	Increased
Ferritin level	Decreased	Decreased

usually establishes the diagnosis. The gold standard is the evaluation of iron stores using a Prussian blue stain of the bone marrow to determine the presence or absence of iron. Plasma ferritin levels relate directly to iron stores but, as noted before, may be falsely elevated in patients with cancer, infection, inflammation, or liver disease. This situation may mask an iron-deficiency anemia. Moreover, the serum ferritin level normally decreases during the second and third trimesters of pregnancy. The diagnosis is tentatively made by treating the patient with iron and observing the response. With significant reticulocytosis and an increase in the hemoglobin and hematocrit levels within 3 weeks, a presumptive diagnosis of iron deficiency may be established.

TREATMENT. It is necessary to determine whether the iron deficiency is related solely to inadequate dietary intake, decreased absorption, or chronic blood loss. The blood loss must be detected by a solid history of GI or gynecologic symptoms. Tests for occult blood in the stools should be performed in all patients suspected of having iron-deficiency anemia. Iron therapy should be prescribed with the simplest, most straightforward, inexpensive iron preparations available. Liquid preparations are reasonable and may provide the iron more directly for absorption. Iron should be taken about a half-hour to an hour prior to meals. Most doses of liquid or tablet iron contain 45 to 50 mg of elemental iron per dose. If the dose is taken with an ascorbic acid preparation (e.g., orange juice), it is in the most advantageous form (Fe^{+2}) for absorption. One dose per day should be given for the first week, increased to two doses per day during the second week and to three doses per day the third week and thereafter. This regimen allows the patient's system to become accustomed to the medication, thereby avoiding side effects such as constipation or gastric upset, which is why 80 to 90 per cent do not take the medicine fully or at all. This regimen should be continued for at least 2 months until the hemoglobin and hematocrit levels return to normal. It results in approximately a 1-gram increase in the iron supply, which in turn results in a net increase in hemoglobin of about 300 grams. About 80 to 90 per cent of patients tolerate this regimen well. If constipation is a problem, addition of a simple over-the-counter stool softener can inexpensively counteract this barrier to compliance.

When the hemoglobin and hematocrit do not rise appropriately (2 gm/dL in 3 weeks) with an early reticulocytosis, other issues should be considered. For example, the patient may continue to have blood loss; the diagnosis of the anemia is wrong or inappropriate; there is an inflammatory process; there are other causes for ineffective erythropoiesis, such as a lack of folic acid or vitamin B_{12}; the patient is taking the iron inappropriately with foods or drinks that might block its absorption; or the patient is not taking the medication.

In rare instances where there is an urgent need to replace iron stores prior to surgery or where oral iron replacement cannot be tolerated orally because of side effects or other GI conditions, it may be helpful to give iron parenterally. It can be given intramuscularly several times a week, with the calculations based on information in the *Physician's Desk Reference*. It can also be given intravenously in the form of iron dextran diluted in isotonic saline after a test dose is administered to look for any possible reactions. Because of possible anaphylactic reactions, the test dose is given for about 2 minutes, and the patient is watched for an hour. The infusion may then continue until the entire dose is given. The need to given iron parenterally is a rare phenomenon, and the family physician probably should consult appropriate medical resources before carrying it out because of its infrequency and the need to appropriately calculate a correct dosage. First, the deficit between the patient's hemoglobin level and the level needed is calculated. This figure is then multiplied by the weight of the patient (in kilograms), which in turn is multiplied by 65 ml/kg, which is the blood volume per kilogram. This calculation gives the total hemoglobin deficit. Each gram of hemoglobin contains 3.4 mg of iron. The hemoglobin deficit in grams is multiplied by 3.4 mg/gm, which gives the total milligrams of iron needed for replacement. This iron deficit is then multiplied by the formulation of iron one wishes to give in parenteral fashion to determine the appropriate dosage mechanism and frequency.

14 gm/dL (normal) − 7 gm/dL (actual) = 7 gm/dL

deficit × 70 kg × 65 ml blood/kg = 318.5 gm

× 3.4 mg Fe/gm = 1082 mg Fe needed

Iron-deficiency anemia is the most common anemia presenting to the family physician. It can be diagnosed easily with good clinical suspicion and treated effectively and inexpensively with regimens as outlined previously. Follow-up of the problem is important. Consideration of medication side effects, patient compliance, and other diagnoses is necessary when iron therapy is not remarkably successful within a short time.

Anemia of Chronic Disease

The anemia associated with chronic disease is a hypoproliferative anemia with a low reticulocyte count, hematocrits ranging from 27 to 35 per cent, a normal RDW, elevated serum ferritin level, and a slightly shortened RBC survival time. The iron levels are low, as are the iron-binding capacity and the transferrin saturation levels. Increased or normal bone marrow iron stores are a diagnostic feature of this entity. This anemia fits into the category of impaired production because RBCs cannot be produced adequately owing to altered iron metabolism and storage in reticuloendothelial cells. This anemia counts for approximately 25 per cent of the anemias found in a primary care practice. It is associated with chronic disease conditions such as neoplasia, inflammation, chronic infections, patients with chronic liver disease, chronic congestive heart failure and coronary artery disease, chronic renal failure, diabetes, collagen vascular disease, chronic fungal infections, and tuberculosis.

A number of mechanisms are reported to be operative in the etiology of this anemia. First, the bone marrow's response to erythropoietin is believed to be suppressed perhaps due to inhibitory factors produced by the chronic inflammatory conditions associated with the anemia. Interleukin-1 is produced in inflammatory conditions and may inhibit the effects of erythropoietin on the bone marrow. Second, when old RBCs are destroyed, the iron molecules are degraded, removed from the RBC, and either stored in macrophages or returned rapidly by transferrin to the bone marrow for reuse. With this anemia the transferrin pathway back to the bone marrow is markedly underutilized. Most of the iron enters the reticuloendothelial storage system, where it is essentially trapped and unable to be used by the bone marrow. This mechanism accounts for the increased ferritin level and the stainable iron found in bone marrow. Third, GI iron absorption is decreased, and RBC survival is modestly reduced.

Clinically, patients with anemia of chronic disease are usually asymptomatic with a mild to moderate anemia (hemoglobin levels of about 7 to 11 gm/dL). The anemia is usually normocytic normochromic, although occasionally it reaches levels where the cells are hypochromic microcytic. Serum iron and total iron-binding capacity (TIBC) levels are markedly reduced. As noted previously, the serum ferritin level is usually increased, and the RDW is normal. These two features distinguish this anemia from iron-deficiency anemia along with the reduced TIBC level, which is markedly elevated in iron deficiency. If the clinical picture is that of a hypochromic microcytic anemia, differentiation must be made between iron deficiency anemia, thalassemia, sideroblastic anemia, anemia of renal disease, and a primarily myeloproliferative disorder. The major features that distinguish the anemia of chronic disease from iron deficiency are the normal RDW, elevated ferritin level, the low iron-binding capacity, and the presence of stainable iron in the bone marrow.

The treatment of this anemia is supportive and should be directed at the underlying inflammatory, neoplastic, or chronic disease for the anemia to be resolved. Injections of erythropoietin aimed at a bone marrow that cannot respond to erythropoietin are not helpful. Iron therapy is not indicated and may, over a long period, cause iron overload.

Anemia Due to Hemolysis

The fundamental mechanism leading to hemolysis of RBCs is an alteration of the RBC membrane, which results in either its removal by the reticuloendothelial system or intravascular rupture, spilling hemoglobin and membrane fragments into the plasma. The two major contributors to RBC survival are its flexible shape and its internal biochemical mechanisms for membrane maintenance and the stabilization of hemoglobin. The RBC is one of the few cells in the body that during development extrudes its nucleus and then becomes a reticulocyte with residual RNA. The reticulocyte normally spends 3 days in the bone marrow and 1 day in the circulation. It has the biconcave, or cup, shape of the mature red blood cell. The biconcave shape allows the cell to change its shape and to pass through capillaries as small as 3 μm in diameter and to make its length five to six times greater than its width. The RBC is about 7 to 10 μm in diameter, whereas the reticulocyte is approximately 9 to 10 μm in diameter. The life-span of the RBC is 115 to 120 days. During that life-span it progressively loses water and surface area. Roughly 0.8 per cent of the total number of RBCs are lost and replaced each day.

A 70-kg man produces 50 ml of whole blood per day to maintain homeostasis, which requires the manufacture of 7 grams of hemoglobin each day. Hemoglobin normally comes in three forms: hemoglobin A, which is composed of two α- and two β-chains; hemoglobin A_2, composed of two α- and two γ-chains; and hemoglobin F, which is two α- and two δ-chains. The α-chains are constant in virtually all forms of hemoglobin, and it is the β-chains that have amino acid substitutions or are replaced. α-Chain production is governed by an area of DNA on chromosome 16 where the β-, δ-, and γ-chains are all controlled by DNA on chromosome 11. The remarkable fact about hemoglobin manufacture is that the chains must be matched in terms of production quantities, joined in the cytoplasm, and then a heme entity added from the mitochondria, where they are constructed. Hemoglobin exists in two states: relaxed and tense. In its re-

laxed state it is bonded to oxygen. In its tense state it is deoxygenated and admits a 2,3-diphosophgylcerate (2,3-DPG) molecule to stabilize it. The function of the cytoplasm in the RBC is to provide reducing power to prevent oxidation of the hemoglobin to keep 2,3-DPG generated, which keeps the hemoglobin, sodium, and water levels stable. The high concentration of hemoglobin in the RBC at a level of about 33 to 35 gm/dL as measured by the mean corpuscular hemoglobin concentration (MCHC) means that the liquid within the RBC is viscous. The usual size reflected by the MCV is 80 to 90 femtoliters (fL), with a femtoliter being 10^{-15} liters.

BLOOD FLOW. Those factors that determine blood flow are the deformability of RBCs, plasma protein concentrations, hematocrit, caliber of the vessels, and flow rate in a particular size tube. When the flow rate is low, RBCs tend to clump, blood viscosity increases, and the resistance to flow increases as well. This situation can cause a variety of changes that can be destructive to RBCs.

MECHANISMS OF HEMOLYSIS AND ANEMIA. The presence of anemia in a hemolytic state depends on the rate of destruction of RBCs versus the production of new RBCs by the bone marrow. The bone marrow, given adequate nutrients, can increase normal production of RBCs six- to eightfold and thus compensate for an ongoing hemolysis or blood loss problem. The life-span of RBCs may be one-sixth of normal, or approximately 20 days, and the bone marrow may compensate for a time with an appropriate reticulocytosis. When destruction exceeds the productive capacity of the bone marrow, anemia ensues with jaundice, decreased haptogobin levels, perhaps hemoglobinuria, elevated liver enzymes due to hemoglobin and bilirubin being metabolized and hemosiderinuria, which results from iron depositing in renal tubular cells as hemoglobin travels through the kidney. The two major sites for hemolysis are extravascular or intravascular. Extravascular hemolysis occurs when the RBC membrane is changed enough to have it detected and removed by the reticuloendothelial system. When the change in the RBC is acute and sudden, as during an antibody-mediated attack or when the reticuloendothelial system cannot compensate for damaged RBC membranes, intravascular hemolysis occurs. In this situation, the RBCs rupture and leak their hemoglobin and membrane components into the plasma circulation. The hemoglobin forms into dimers, which are then attached to haptoglobin, the protein transport molecule, which carries it to the liver and kidneys. A low unbound haptoglobin level is indicative of hemolysis. When the haptoglobin-carrying capacity is exceeded, hemoglobinuria ensues. After several days of hemoglobinuria, iron is deposited in renal tubular cells and is then excreted by the kidney and urine, resulting in hemosiderinuria. The membranes of RBCs that undergo intravascular hemoly-

TABLE 45–6. CLASSIFICATION OF HEMOLYTIC ANEMIAS

Extracorpuscular mechanisms
  Microangiopathic hemolysis
  Immune hemolysis
  Autoimmune mechanisms
  Drug-induced
  Cold agglutinin disease
  Hypersplenism

Intracorpuscular mechanisms
  Membrane defects: spherocytosis, paroxysmal nocturnal hemoglobinuria
  Metabolic defects: G-6-PD deficiency
  Hemoglobinopathies: sickle cell disease, thalassemia

sis also may stimulate disseminated intravascular coagulation.

Table 45–6 provides a specific classification system for hemolytic anemias. The two major categories are intracorpuscular defects and extracorpuscular defects. In the intracorpuscular system are membrane defects, metabolic defects, and hemoglobin defects that cause hemolysis of RBCs. Only one of the problems in this category is not inherited: paroxysmal nocturnal hemoglobinuria. In the extracorpuscular category elements attack, damage, or destroy RBCs often, but not always, within the circulation. Microangiopathic hemolysis, autoimmune hemolysis, drug-induced hemolysis, cold agglutinin disease, and hypersplenism belong in this category.

INTRACORPUSCULAR HEMOLYSIS: MEMBRANE DEFECTS. The cellular membrane of the RBC carefully regulates sodium, potassium, and water concentrations in the cell to maintain shape and cell function. When defects in the membrane allow sodium to enter more rapidly than is appropriate, water follows and the cell gains volume and loses its flexibility and deformability. Changes in metabolic activity that result lead to further cell swelling until the cell is removed by the reticuloendothelial system. If the membrane defect causes a loss of potassium, water follows and the cell becomes dehydrated and smaller with a rise in the MCHC. The cell again loses its deformability and is rapidly removed.

HYDROCYTOSIS. In patients with hydrocytosis, an inherited disorder, the sodium and potassium concentration in the RBCs increase osmotically, attracting water and resulting in larger cells and a change in the surface/volume ratio. This condition usually presents early in life as a compensated hemolytic anemia with a palpable spleen in many cases. Splenectomy helps to decrease the early removal of RBCs, resulting in less severe anemia. The problem can not be cured, as it is inherited and persists throughout life.

HEREDITARY SPHEROCYTOSIS. A cell membrane disorder, hereditory spherocytosis is inherited as an autosomal dominant; it affects about 2 of 1000 people. A deficiency in the membrane decreases membrane stability, leading to less surface area and smaller cells. It results in microspherocytes, that are rigid and that become trapped in the spleen and are removed. One-fourth of patients with hereditary spherocytosis are not anemic because there is a compensated, low grade hemolysis that is undetectable until a severe infection or stress on their system such as pregnancy increases the hemolysis. Alternatively, when the marrow's capacity to produce adequate RBCs to compensate for the low grade hemolysis is compromised, anemia becomes noticeable.

The peripheral smear in clinical spherocytosis reveals microspherocytes, a significantly increased MCHC (35 gm/dL or higher), increased reticulocytosis, splenomegaly, mild levels of jaundice, and generally a positive family history. If the Coomb's antibody test is negative and there is a positive family of this phenomenon, other considerations such as an autoimmune hemolytic process can be eliminated. The diagnosis is often confirmed by a osmotic fragility test, which can be positive. Complications of ongoing anemia may be cholelithiasis, a splenic rupture, and aplastic anemia. Aplastic anemia is often brought on by a respiratory infection instigated by viruses. Fortunately, aplastic anemia is a rare complication of spherocytosis.

Treatment of the disorder is surgical splenectomy, which eliminates most of the illness manifestations and all but eliminates the possibility of aplastic crisis. However, RBCs still do not survive as long as normal, lasting perhaps only 85 to 90 days after splenectomy instead of the 115 to 120 days, the normal RBC life-span.

PAROXYSMAL NOCTURNAL HEMOGLOBINURIA. Paroxysmal nocturnal hemoglobinuria (PNH) is the only intracorpuscular defect in hemolytic anemias that is *not* inherited. The defect is a mutation of a marrow stem cell that produces a line of RBCs that are highly susceptible to complement-mediated lysis. The cell line produced by the somatic mutation requires only one-fifth to one-twenty-fifth the amount of complement to cause cell lysis. Additionally, PNH red blood cells have a deficiency of decay-accelerating factor (DAF) which means that six to eight times the normal amount of complement is deposited on the PNH cell membrane, making it more susceptible to lysis. Patients with PNH do not have a positive family history for the disease, which again indicates that it is a mutation and not an inherited genetic disorder. PNH patients also have RBCs that are deficient in acetylcholinesterase, which increases their likelihood of complement lysis as well. Other cell lines may be affected, resulting in neutropenia and thrombocytopenia, again suggesting that PNH is a mutation of a stem cell that leads to abnormalities not only of RBCs but occasionally of other cell lines.

Patients most often present with coffee- or coca cola-colored urine at their first morning emptying of the bladder. Acute episodes of hemolysis are precipitated by infection or stress; or they have no known antecedent cause and are simply spontaneous. The intravascular hemolysis precipitates an increased coagulation state that can lead to blood clots in large venous drainage beds of the body, such as mesenteric veins, hepatic veins, large veins of the proximal lower extremity, and the pelvic area. Small infarcts in kidneys, liver, and other organs may lead to organ dysfunction, painful episodes of renal disease, splenic infarcts, and even Budd-Chiari syndrome, which comprises a blood clot of the hepatic vein obstructing the venous drainage of the liver into the inferior vena cava. Long-term complications may include the development of aplastic anemia and on occasion acute myelogenous leukemia. Although reported in some series of patients, they occur relatively infrequently.

In patients who have chronic hemolysis with acute episodic crises of hemolysis or recurrent thromboembolism, the diagnosis of PNH should be strongly considered. A chronically low level of serum haptoglobin and evidence of hemoglobinuria or hemosiderinuria can also be found if one takes a careful history and looks for hemolysis and venous occlusive symptoms. The diagnosis is made by documenting hemolysis and then detecting increased susceptibility to complement-mediated lysis using the HAM test in which complement-mediated hemolysis is increased in an acidic medium. The sucrose hemolysis test can also be used but is somewhat less reliable. The peripheral smear does not show any remarkable or unusual findings, and the bone marrow may show hypoplasia or hyperplasia.

The treatment of PNH patients calls for the use of regular transfusions to maintain the hematocrit above 30 per cent if possible. To avoid future transfusion reactions and sensitization, which would likely increase lysis of RBCs over time, the use of leukocyte-poor units are especially helpful. Steroids in the form of an androgen such as fluoxymesterone at 20 to 30 mg per day may increase RBC production, and occasionally corticosteroids in the form of prednisone may help reduce the frequency and severity of acute hemolytic episodes. This therapy should be used sparingly with rapid tapering. Because there is chronic blood loss, the patients are usually iron-deficient. However, the administration of large doses of iron with an ensuing reticulocytosis of new RBCs simply provides new cells for complement-mediated lysis. Therefore iron should be used sparingly and may be provided from repeated transfusions. Iron is not the mainstay of therapy but must be considered and administered in a low dose regimen. Painful episodes of hemolysis are managed with colloid infusions, which expand the plasma and perhaps reduce the rate of hemolysis. Patients who have major venous occlusion of the inferior vena cava

or other large vessels may be treated with heparin and in some cases thrombolytic therapy for a period of 24 to 72 hours using streptokinase or urokinase. Thrombolytic therapy is indicated in cases where heparin and routine anticoagulation does not stop the progress of a thrombus or in a situation in which a major vein occlusion causes significant dysfunction.

The long-term course of PNH is variable. Most often these patients have years of chronic hemolytic anemia with episodes of acute hemolytic crisis. On occasion, however, the PNH is aggressive and patients die within a matter of 6 to 12 months. Other patients appear to be cured after a lengthy period with the assumption that the abnormal clone of RBCs simply dies out and disappears. Many patients die of the complications of neutropenia and infection or serious venous occlusion in major organs such as the liver, brain, or kidney. Complications such as aplastic anemia and acute leukemia also can be terminal events for patients with this illness. Most patients, however, learn to live with the illness and to compensate fairly well so long as there are not many acute hemolytic episodes and other serious complications.

Hemolytic Anemia Due to Metabolic Defects

Red blood cells have a number of mechanisms to protect themselves from premature oxidation because hemoglobin and RBC function depends on a reduced metabolic state. When glutathione and reduced nicotinamide adenine dinucleotide (NADH) and NADH phosphate (NADPH) are deficient, hemoglobin and proteins associated with hemoglobin are easily oxidized, causing the production of Heinz bodies. These bodies are attached to the membrane of the RBC and are the products of hemoglobin oxidation. They can be seen after staining with methyl violet on a routine peripheral blood smear. The cells have lost their normal deformability and their ability to roll. Consequently, they are identified by the spleen and other portions of the reticuloendothelial system for removal. There are rare metabolic defects of reducing chemicals that occur in families who have chronic hemolysis and Heinz bodies. A classic and much more common metabolic deficiency leading to hemolysis is described below.

GLUCOSE-6-PHOSPHATE DEHYDROGENASE DEFICIENCY. Glucose-6-phosphate dehydrogenase (G-6-PD) is an enzyme that functions as a powerful reducing agent in the RBC and keeps the cell from being easily oxidized. Deficiency of G-6-PD affects approximately 10 per cent of African-American males in the United States, some individuals of Mediterranean ancestry, and a significant portion of the black African population. Manufacture of this enzyme is controlled by a gene on the X chromosome, and so it appears to be sex-linked. One affected X chromosome in a male individual produces signs and symptoms of the deficiency, whereas it would take two affected X chromosomes in the female individual. However, females do have a variable degree of G-6-PD deficiency. One theory suggests that they may have a line of RBCs with the unaffected X chromosome that predominates and another line of RBCs with the X chromosome that is deficient. Hence they may have two populations of RBCs: one with healthy amounts of G-6-PD and another that is G-6-PD deficient. There are three major classes or varieties of G-6-PD deficiency, although many forms have been described: Class I, or the congenital, chronic non-spherocytic hemolytic anemia form, is uncommon. Class II comprises those cases in which the enzyme deficiency is marked and hemolysis tends to be episodic. The most common variant, Class III, occurs in individuals in which the enzyme is measurably low but not severe, and hemolysis is infrequent and is usually caused by oxidative substances.

Oxidizing agents may be found in food, drugs, and the environment. As an example, fava beans can lead to oxidation of RBCs and subsequent hemolysis but usually only in individuals with the Mediterranean familial variety. A number of drug classes can produce oxidation and therefore chronic hemolysis in patients with G-6-PD deficiency. Some examples are nitrofurantoin, analgesics such as phenacetin or aspirin, dapsone (which belongs to the sulfone group), sulfonamides such as sulfamethoxazole, chloramphenicol, quinine, and anti-malarial drugs such as primaquine and chloroquine. Severe infections, problems such as diabetic ketoacidosis, and organ failure may also precipitate hemolysis in these patients.

A patient who has recurrent or low grade hemolysis should be screened with a G-6-PD enzyme screening test with follow-up confirmation made by a direct enzyme assay. Hemoglobinopathies and other enzyme deficiencies necessary for maintaining appropriate reducing power of the RBC may be considered part of the differential diagnosis.

Patients with G-6-PD usually do well so long as they are kept away from drugs that lead to increased oxidation in the RBC. There are some reports that vitamin E in high doses, approximately 800 IU per day, may stabilize the RBC membrane and protect the cell so the level of hemolysis is slowed and hemoglobin levels improve. Acute hemolytic crisis related to increased oxidation in patients with the G-6-PD deficiency can be managed with transfusions of G-6-PD-rich RBCs. Disseminated intravascular coagulation is a complication of acute hemolysis. Patients who have a similar picture but who are not G-6-PD-deficient may be deficient in pyruvate kinase, which functions in the Embden-Meyerhof chemical pathways that are important to the production of adenosine triphosphate (ATP). Patients with pyruvate kinase deficiency have congenital hemolysis of a low grade

nature. When hemolysis necessitates transfusions on a repeated basis, splenectomy may be considered as the treatment of choice.

HEMOLYTIC ANEMIAS: DEFECTS IN HEMOGLOBIN. Hemoglobin is composed of two pairs of protein chains: one pair labeled α and one pair β. The designation given hemoglobin A = $\alpha 2$, $\beta 2$. Hemoglobin cannot be made without two α-chains, and the hemoglobinopathies are characterized by abnormalities in the β-chains. Either they are replaced with γ- or δ-chains, or amino acid substitutions in the β-chains occur that change the character, function, and stability of the hemoglobin molecule itself. Abnormal hemoglobins may function in ways that are helpful to the RBC and the patient. The chains may be synthesized in unequal amounts, resulting in lower functional hemoglobin production. The abnormal hemoglobin may abnormally bind oxygen, be unstable, tend to form a gel or crystal, or be easily oxidized inappropriately. Sickle cell anemia and thalassemia are discussed as examples of hemoglobin disorders that cause an unstable RBC resulting in hemolysis.

Sickle Cell Anemia. Sickle cell anemia is an inherited autosomal condition in which glutamic acid in the sixth position on the β-chain is replaced by a valine amino acid resulting in a different kind of hemoglobin: hemoglobin SS in the homozygous condition and hemoglobin AS in the heterozygous condition. Patients who are hemoglobin AS have 50 per cent of their hemoglobin in the S form, whereas homozygotes with sickle cell anemia have 70 to 98 per cent of their hemoglobin in the SS form. Sickle cell trait, or hemoglobin AS, is found in 8 to 10 per cent of black individuals in the United States. Persons of Mediterranean descent from India or Saudi Arabia have varying percentages of hemoglobin AS. Sickle cell anemia occurs in about 0.2 per cent of African-Americans in the United States. Sickle cell anemia is distributed in a worldwide fashion but predominates in the Mediterranean, Saudi Arabian, and Indian populations. This distribution appears to be caused by independent mutations in these geographic groupings. People with hemoglobin AS and SS have a protective advantage against malaria: RBCs with these hemoglobins are resistant to invasion by malarial parasites. In fact, if the parasite infects the cell, the rate of sickling increases, causing the cell with the infected parasite to be removed from the circulation sooner. Resistance to invasion by the parasite and enhanced removal of infected cells contribute to a relative resistance to infection by *Plasmodium falciparum* malaria.

The pathophysiology of the sickle cell is such that when it loses its oxygen content or becomes relatively dehydrated the hemoglobin tends to polymerize into long tube-like fibers. This phenomenon then causes an elongated cell that is subject to hemolysis and trapping in the microcirculation, resulting in vaso-occlusive crises. Hypoxemia, acidosis, RBC dehydration, hyperosmolality of the renal medulla (which dehydrates RBCs), and viral infections can play a role in increasing the sickling phenomenon. Sickled RBCs are more adhesive to endothelial cells; and when those endothelial cells are infected with a virus it significantly increases adhesiveness. When the conditions causing sickling are corrected, the sickled cell may return to a more normal shape and function. However, some cells are irreversibly sickled, indicating that the membrane cytoskeleton has been damaged. Heinz bodies are found to occur spontaneously, indicating oxidation of hemoglobin resulting from decreased reducing power of the cell to maintain itself normally. These irreversibly sickled cells are generally removed in the sinusoidal networks of the reticuloendothelial system, but approximately one third may be hemolyzed intravascularly, causing jaundice and anemia with a reduced level of free haptoglobin. Patients with sickle cell anemia often have a low hematocrit, which helps to reduce blood viscosity deoxygenation, thereby decreasing the likelihood of polymerization of hemoglobin to its abnormal form.

The microvascular capillaries, capillary bed, and veins become occluded when there is microvascular disease or if the pH falls, the MCHC increases, capillary transit time is prolonged, or infection ensues. Increased numbers of sickled RBCs occlude small vessels, which can lead to ischemic infarction, pain, and reduced organ function over time. Particularly affected areas are (1) the portal circulation in which oxygen tension is low; (2) the kidney in which the renal medulla is hyperosmolar and dehydrates RBCs, increasing the MCHC; (3) the lung; and (4) the brain. It is not clear why some patients have severe frequent episodes and others do not. Avascular necrosis of the bone marrow is usually the cause of severe pain. Risk factors include a hemoglobin level higher than 8.5 gm/dL, cold weather, deoxygenation, infection, pregnancy, and a high reticulocyte count. Individuals with α-thalassemia comprise about 30 per cent of the black population in the United States. Persons with α-thalassemia plus sickle cell anemia have a lower MCHC, lower reticulocyte counts, yet higher hemoglobin levels than those with sickle cell anemia alone. The lower MCHC usually benefits the patient because the lower hemoglobin viscosity leads to a reduction in sickle cell crises.

Clinical Diagnosis. A patient with sickle cell disease usually has chronic hemolysis, producing a moderate anemia, intermittent jaundice, and a marrow cavity with a thinned cortex. Vascular occlusive episodes (which produce pain) and the appearance of Howell-Jolly bodies (indicating ischemic splenic infarction) occur by the time the patient becomes an adult.

The diagnosis can be made by finding sickled cells on the peripheral smear and Howell-Jolly bodies, which are cytoplasmic remnants of the nucleus normally removed by the spleen but not when the spleen has been infarcted by repetitive sickle cell crises. The marrow is moderately hypoplastic. For a sickle cell preparation blood is mixed with 2% sodium metabisulfite, which produces sickling. The proportion of sickled cells is measured at once and then 1 hour later to make the diagnosis. The gold standard of diagnosis is hemoglobin electrophoresis, which shows the relative proportion of hemoglobin forms.

Patients with long-standing sickle cell anemia may have pain syndromes related to bone marrow vaso-occlusive crises and aseptic necrosis of the femoral head. Cholelithiasis occurs in 40 to 60 per cent of patients. Liver and heart complications may also develop. Other associated problems include vascular occlusions in the pulmonary bed, localized infections, chronic renal infarctions leading to papillary necrosis, renal tubular acidosis, and declining renal function with age. Priapism may occur with vaso-occlusive crises and may require exchange transfusions. In the eye, conditions such as neovascularization, vitreous hemorrhage, and retinopathy are often found as well. Patients with sickle cell anemia are susceptible to *Salmonella* infections owing to decreased complement activation activity. Osteomyelitis secondary to *Salmonella*, and pneumococcal sepsis secondary to autosplenectomy are seen fairly often. Patients with sickle cell anemia should be given pneumovax vaccine to prevent streptococcal pneumonia and sepsis. *Hemophilus influenzae* today causes a high percentage of pneumonia in sickle cell anemia patients. Neurologically, these patients are subject to stroke. Thrombosis peculiarly is more common in children, whereas hemorrhage is largely confined to adults. The rationale for this phenomenon is thought to be the occlusion of small vessels in hypoxic situations. Additionally, there is an increased attraction of sickle cells to the endothelium, causing proliferation of the endothelial intimal membranes and vascular occlusion. There is a high rate of recurrence of stroke within 36 months of the initial event. Parvovirus infections can also cause aplastic anemia in a crisis situation.

Treatment

Patients with sickle cell anemia should have their hemoglobin and hematocrit levels maintained at a moderately low level because it is in fact protective for some of the vaso-occlusive infarctive complications related to viscosity. When there is a painful crisis, the patient should be placed at rest, hydrated, given oral analgesics (e.g., oral morphine), and have the blood alkalinized mildly with an intravenous bicarbonate solution. Oxygen should be given to keep the hemoglobin well oxygenated; the amount of deoxyhemoglobins must be kept low. Parenteral narcotics are rarely necessary, especially if large volumes of liquids, oxygen at least 3 to 5 liters per minute, and oral morphine or similar preparations are used to control pain.

Treatment with drugs that increase the proportion of hemoglobin F, which does not polymerize and so cause a cell to sickle, has been shown to be helpful. Azacitidine increases the proportion of RBCs with fetal hemoglobin but is an anticancer agent with significant toxicity. Hydroxyurea also increases fetal hemoglobin. The goal is to raise fetal hemoglobin levels to about 20 per cent of the total hemoglobin to obtain a desirable result. Complications associated with hydroxyurea are significant, however, and it should not be used for routine therapy.

Patients undergoing surgical operations with general anesthesia are at increased risk of hypoxemia, sickling, and sickle cell crises. They should be transfused with approximately 1 unit of packed RBCs that have high proportions of hemoglobin A once a week for 4 to 5 weeks prior to surgery. This measure raises the hemoglobin A level to 50 per cent, which decreases the likelihood of sickle cell episodes. The hematocrit should be kept below 35 per cent to keep the MCHC from reaching a level where increased sickling is likely to occur in the hemoglobin S cells.

Pregnancy definitely increases the risk of vaso-occlusive crises in the mother. There is a high incidence of fetal loss among women who have sickle cell anemia. Vaso-occlusive episodes in the placenta may result in lower birth weights and fetal deaths.

Sickle Cell Trait

Patients with sickle cell trait are heterozygous for the autosomal gene and have a far lower likelihood of sickling than those who are homozygous. Most of these people are asymptomatic throughout their entire life. Within each RBC 50 per cent of the hemoglobin is hemoglobin S and 50 per cent is hemoglobin A. Patients with sickle cell trait may develop complications when they encounter environments with low oxygen saturations such as high mountain environments, incompletely pressurized high altitude airplanes, heat stroke and dehydration, and major muscle trauma resulting in rhabdomyolysis. Basic training in the military with its emphasis on prolonged exertion, dehydration, and possible heat stroke is a risk factor for individuals with sickle cell trait. On the other hand, African-American football players who are in good condition and have sickle cell trait have no higher rates of complications from that sport than do other African-American men.

Thalassemias. The thalassemia anemias are caused by an abnormal or unsynchronized rate of synthesis of the normal α- or β-chains. The designation of the kind of thalassemia, such as β-thalassemia, indicates which chain is being produced in markedly diminished amounts. For instance, α-thalassemia indicates there is a marked reduction in the production of α-chains with a resultant excess of β-chains. In β-thalassemia, β-chains are not produced in normal amounts. The unmatched excessive number of α-chains accumulate in the RBC, precipitate, and damage the membrane, causing leakage and decreased ATP; the result is a rigid RBC. The decrease in the normal amounts of hemoglobin results in a misshapen hypochromic RBC that is small and has a target cell appearance. Likewise, in α-thalassemia the decreased α-chain production leads to excessive β-chains, which gather in groups of four called tetrads and form a molecule called hemoglobin H. This hemoglobin has a high affinity for oxygen and is markedly unstable. In either scenario, there is ineffective erythropoiesis, with many of the cells being abnormal and dying in the bone marrow or being removed from the circulation at an early point, which results in a reduced RBC life-span. Patients have varying degrees of anemia. Some individuals are hypoxic, which results in an enlarged marrow cavity, extramedullary erythropoiesis, cholelithiasis, and liver enzyme abnormalities. The genetic location for all non-α-chains is found on both chromosomes 11 and 16. It is thought that *both* gene deletions and genetic production of an unstable messenger RNA causes the defects described above.

β-*Thalassemia.*   The most common form of thalassemia is a deficiency in the production of β-chains, resulting in β-thalassemia. There are three variants, or three clinical syndromes: β-thalassemia major, β-thalassemia minor, and thalassemia intermedia.

1.   β-*Thalassemia major (Cooley's anemia).* The most severe thalassemia is the homozygous form with virtual absence of β-chains. It presents as a severe anemia during the first several months to 1 year of life. The peripheral smear has markedly abnormal RBCs with basophilic stippling representing aggregates of RNA and excess unmatched α-chains. There are nucleated RBCs, hypochromic, microcytic RBCs, and a severe anemia requiring blood transfusions to prevent complications of congestive heart failure and skeletal deformities. The parents of such an infected child both carry the β-thalassemia gene. In the most severe form, no β-chains are synthesized.

A less severe form is characterized by small numbers of β-chains, but the predominant hemoglobins produced are hemoglobin F and hemoglobin A_2. Most children with this illness live only until early adulthood and die of heart problems related to iron overload. There is also an increased susceptibility to infection. Hypersplenism occurs and can lead to pancytopenia. When these patients are splenectomized, pneumococcal vaccine is necessary to avoid pneumococcal sepsis.

Treatment to date is with agents that increase the proportion of hemoglobin F RBCs. Azacitidine can accomplish this increase, but it is an antileukemic agent and its toxicity is too severe to be used routinely. Hydroxyurea also increases the proportion of hemoglobin F RBCs and F reticulocytes and is used more commonly. A number of series have now been reported in which bone marrow transplantation has been used to replace the patient's stem cells with new stem cells capable of producing adequate amounts of normal hemoglobin. Unfortunately, 15 to 25 per cent of these transplant patients have died from infection and other complications. Of those who have survived, more than 95 per cent produce normal hemoglobin and no longer have thalassemia.

Another method of therapy being explored is altering the genes of stem cells. A normal gene for β-chain synthesis can be transferred to stem cells removed from the bone marrow, inserted into these cells, and then placed back in the bone marrow. This technique works well in mice but has had variable success in humans. Other studies have used erythropoietin to stimulate the bone marrow to produce more cells that have hemoglobin F and thus compensate for the cells that have the thalassemia hemoglobin.

2. *β-Thalassemia minor (β-thalassemia trait).* The heterozygous form of β-thalassemia presents with a hypochromic microcytic picture but mild or virtually no anemia. Patients tend to have elevated levels of hemoglobins A_2 and F. Patients with the highest hemoglobin F levels have the least severe anemia. Patients may present with what resembles iron deficiency. However, with iron deficiency there is hypoproliferation of the bone marrow and reduced numbers of RBCs, whereas patients with β-thalassemia trait have adequate to normal number of RBCs. Thus a person with a hypochromic microcytic anemia and a normal number of RBCs has at least an 85 per cent chance of having thalassemia trait, not iron deficiency. Iron studies such as a serum iron level, iron-binding capacity, and ferritin level should be determined to eliminate the possibility of a concomitant iron deficiency as well.

3. *Thalassemia intermedia.* Because of variable genetic penetration and expression, a thalassemia form intermediate between thalassemia minor and thalassemia major has been found with varying clinical manifestations. Patients with this thalassemia intermedia may have significant anemia (hemoglobin as low as 6 to 7 gm/dL), but it may be higher than that also. The patients are not so sick that they require regular transfusions unless they have severe infections or other illness. Hemoglobin F levels may be in the 30 to 50 per cent range, with hemoglobin A levels somewhat above that. The patients usually do not require vigorous treatment and can be monitored and treated conservatively.

α-Thalassemia. When α-thalassemia presents, it is important to remember that there are no substi-

tutes for the α genes or the α-globin chains, as the gene for α-chains is present only on chromosome 16. There are four α-globin genes, two on each chromosome inherited from each parent. α-Thalassemia and its varieties are seen most commonly in patients of Asian descent. Complete absence of the genes for α-globin chain production in which the patient is homozygous for α-thalassemia is called hemoglobin bart. These children make δ-chains, which then form tetrads. Small numbers of β-chains are also produced, and they form tetrads. Neither of these hemoglobins can release oxygen, and the children are born hydropic. Hemoglobin H disease is an example where β-globin chains are formed in adequate amounts, but there are no α-chains for them to be matched with, or at least not in significant numbers. This situation brings about a picture of a hemolytic anemia, occurring most often in patients of Asian, Middle Eastern, or Mediterranean origin. These patients have a moderate anemia and usually do not require transfusions unless there are significant infections or stresses of reduced oxygen content in their environment.

Although β-thalassemia can be diagnosed easily by hemoglobin electrophoresis demonstrating increased hemoglobins F and A_2, the diagnosis of α-thalassemia can be obtained only in laboratories dedicated to the study of such a disease. Patients who have mild to moderate anemia, an MCV of less than 75 μm^3, and an RBC count higher than 5 $\times 10^6/mm^3$ have a significant chance of having a thalassemia syndrome.

Genetics. The thalassemia syndromes are found throughout the world in a variety of forms and degrees of severity. Because they produce high levels of hemoglobin F, which persists early in life, hemoglobin F retards the growth of malaria and thus is a protective mechanism against this parasite. Parents who have had a child with Cooley's anemia or have thalassemia in the family should undergo prenatal diagnosis and counseling. The use of hemoglobin electrophoresis and nucleotide probes can provide a definitive diagnosis in most cases where thalassemia is present.

HEMOLYTIC ANEMIAS: EXTRACORPUSCULAR DEFECTS. Hemolytic anemia can also present with problems external to the RBC, such as microangiopathic hemolysis, immune hemolysis, autoimmune hemolysis, or hypersplenism; hemolysis caused by drugs, toxins, infections, or physical agents; and hemolysis associated with rare diseases.

MICROANGIOPATHIC HEMOLYTIC ANEMIAS. Trauma to RBCs in the form of stretching or shearing forces causes a traumatic hemolytic anemia. Some of the causes of this phenomenon are vasculitis, infection such as meningococcemia, disseminated intravascular coagulation, hemodynamic jets, thrombocytopenic purpura, metastatic cancers, and even subclavian catheters. Two drugs that are particularly known to cause hemolytic anemia are (1) mitomycin, an anticancer drug that can cause traumatic hemolysis with an associated disseminated intravascular coagulation; and (2) cyclosporin, an immunosuppressive agent used in transplant patients. Turbulent or jet-like flow of RBCs caused by deformed aortic valves, ventricular-septal defects, the Starr-Edwards valvular prosthesis, and large hemangiomas may also cause this phenomenon. Essentially, the RBCs are subjected to either a shearing or stretching force that they cannot withstand. Such forces may be either vascular jets or fibrinous strands that partially plug small vessels such that the RBC is damaged; some of its contents leak, and its membrane is damaged. The cells may rupture intravascularly or may be damaged and then removed by the reticuloendothelial system. Some patients have a well compensated anemia, and others may become acutely anemic when a sudden event precipitates this phenomenon. When the etiologic event is discovered, the underlying disease or illness should be addressed. Treating an infection, removing a drug, giving cancer therapy, or revising or replacing a heart valve, an arteriovenous malformation, or a kidney dialysis shunt may be needed. Patients usually require iron and folate replacement as well.

A variant of this condition is noted in individuals who run long distances or who play an instrument such as the bongo drums where there is trauma to the muscular tissues of the body. This repetitive trauma destroys RBCs circulating near the surface and causes traumatic hemolytic anemia.

IMMUNE HEMOLYSIS. Immune hemolysis occurs basically in two forms. In one form, an antibody to RBCs (usually immunoglobulin G [IgG]) enters the circulation and attaches itself to the RBCs. These cells then become bound to macrophages or monocytes, which digest portions of the RBC membrane. The changed RBC is returned to the circulation and is then removed by the reticuloendothelial system. The classic example is Rh incompatibility between an Rh-negative mother and her Rh-positive infant. In this case, the D-antigen from the infant crosses the placenta into the mother and stimulates the IgG antibody, which crosses back into the infant and attaches itself to the fetal RBCs, which are then partly digested by macrophages and subsequently destroyed in the reticuloendothelial system. The infant becomes progressively anemic, jaundiced, and may in severe cases become hydropic.

With the second form of immune hemolysis, antibodies to a particular RBC type are already in the circulation. When that cell enters the circulation, antibodies attach themselves to it, complement is activated, and intravascular hemolysis occurs. This reaction is mediated by IgM antibodies and is usually more sudden and more devastating in its acuity than the previously described form. The classic example takes place when an individual with type O blood receives type B blood with the B-antigen on its RBCs. The person who receives the blood has a circulating antibody that is an anti-B IgM. The antibody attaches to the RBC, activation of complement occurs, and the extensive hemolysis that results may be severe enough to precipitate disseminated intravascular coagulation.

Methods for detecting the kind of hemolysis that is occurring are the direct and indirect Coombs' tests. The Coombs' tests are outlined in Figure 45–3. The direct Coombs' test detects the presence of RBCs that already have an antibody attached to their surfaces. In essence, an anti-human-globulin antibody to IgM is incubated with the patient's RBCs. If the cells clump, the reaction is considered positive, proving the binding of the RBCs by antibody. For the indirect Coombs' test, the patient's serum is mixed with human RBCs of a specific antigenic character. The human anti-globulin is then added. In this situation, clumping occurs only if the serum of the patient tested had antibody to a specific RBC type and was then clumped by anti-human globin antibody added to the mixture. The direct Coombs' test detects antibody already attached to RBCs, as is found with Rh incompatibility between mother and newborn. The indirect Coombs' test detects antibodies that are present in the serum and can react with a specific RBC antigenic type.

AUTOIMMUNE HEMOLYTIC ANEMIA. Autoimmune hemolysis is usually found secondary to other disorders, such as systemic lupus erythematosus, certain cancers particularly non-Hodgkin's lymphoma, Hodgkin's disease, myeloma, and chronic ulcerative colitis. It can also appear as an idiopathic form without other disease. The mechanism is usually the production of an IgG antibody that attaches to RBCs, causing an attack by macrophages and neutrophils, which then changes the RBC, causing it to be removed by the spleen and other portions of the reticuloendothelial system. Occasionally, a much more acute phenomenon occurs, causing rapid intravascular hemolysis, but for the most part autoimmune hemolytic anemias are

---

Direct Coombs' Test
Patient's RBCs (washed)–attached IgG antibody + Anti-human IgG antibody → Clumping of RBCs

Indirect Coombs' Test
Patient's serum with IgM
antibody to an RBC antigen + Specific RBC antigenic type + Anti-human IgG antibody → Clumping of RBCs

FIGURE 45–3. Coombs' test. RBCs = red blood cells.

extravascular, taking place primarily in the reticuloendothelial system. Sensitized RBCs that have an attached IgG molecule give a positive direct Coombs' test, even though there may not be active hemolysis evident in the clinical and laboratory picture of the patient. The severity of hemolysis is directly related to the number of IgG molecules attached to the RBCs. The cause of these autoimmune disorders is not clearly understood. The specific disease process produces abnormal immune cells that manufacture abnormal IgG molecules, which then attach to RBCs and make them sensitive to hemolysis.

The clinical picture is usually that of a chronic hemolysis, but acute episodes may occur with a sharp drop in hematocrit. Patients may be moderately or severely anemic and may have jaundice, lymphadenopathy, or an enlarged liver or spleen. The direct Coombs' test is positive and should be titered. Leukopenia and thrombocytopenia are often present, and the peripheral blood smear shows a macrocytic polychromatic picture with much rouleaux formation.

The patient who is found to have an autoimmune hemolytic anemia should have the underlying cause treated vigorously. The immune system must be suppressed so there are fewer abnormal IgG molecules produced that can attack the RBCs. This therapy includes high doses of prednisone (60 to 100 mg a day). The response is measured by a rise in the reticulocyte count, improvement in hematocrit and hemoglobin, and cessation of other symptoms. A decrease in antibody titer as measured by the Coombs' test is an important means of monitoring therapy. If hematologic parameters are improving and if the Coombs' titer is decreasing, which is a significant measure of reduced abnormal antibody production, the medication can be tapered. Some patients are able to be completely removed from any immunosuppressive therapy. Almost all patients must be treated with folic acid and iron. A few patients require maintenance on low-dose alternating-day steroids, and others suffer a chronic, relapsing hemolytic process with acute exacerbations. If corticosteroids are helpful but cannot be reduced, a splenectomy may be considered. Removal of the spleen simply reduces the number of IgG antibodies produced against the RBCs, as the spleen is a prime site for antibody manufacture. Splenectomy also reduces the rate of removal of RBCs from the circulation. This measure may allow the prednisone dose to be reduced to a tolerable level, although it cannot always be completely discontinued. If corticosteroids and splenectomy do not resolve the hemolytic process, immunosuppressive agents, such as azathioprine (Imuran) or cyclophosphamide (Cytoxan), can be used. These drugs elicit a less dramatic, slower response but can be helpful.

Patients with autoimmune hemolytic anemia who require blood transfusion may be difficult to crossmatch. The antiglobulin tests may remain positive despite trying to match them with a number of units. There may be positive direct and indirect Coombs' tests, with free antibodies in the circulating plasma. In an acute situation, one must choose the least reactive units to transfuse into the patient.

Patients who have solid cancers other than lymphoma or Hodgkin's disease do not do well with the usual treatments for hemolytic anemia unless the tumor itself is surgically removed. On occasion, a dermoid cyst can produce an autoimmune hemolytic anemia, and removal often resolves the problem.

DRUG-RELATED IMMUNE HEMOLYSIS. There are three types of drug-related hemolysis, each of which has a positive direct Coombs' test: a hapten type, an immune complex type, and an autoimmune hemolytic type. The degree of severity varies significantly from very mild to severe hemolysis associated with intravascular coagulation.

With the *hapten type* of immune hemolysis, antibiotics such as penicillin or cephalosporin are tightly bound to the RBC membrane. The binding occurs with a protein that attaches the drug to the RBC. This complex causes an antibody response directed against that complex on the RBC, inducing hemolysis. Other drugs involved in such reactions are tolbutamide and cisplatin. The direct Coombs' test in which an anti-IgG is used to detect the presence of IgG on the RBC is positive, whereas the indirect Coombs' test is negative. Discontinuing the drug in question and changing to a drug of another class usually stops the immune hemolysis of the hapten type.

With the *immune complex type*, the drug elicits an antibody response with a IgG or IgM molecule, which is then attached to RBCs, activating a complement-induced lysis. (Drugs that are commonly associated with causing immune hemolysis are the sulfonamides, sulfonylureas, quinidine, chlorpropamide, antituberculosis drugs such as rifampin and isoniazid, aspirin, and phenacetin.) The direct Coombs' test is again positive, particularly with an anticomplement reagent. Most of the hemolysis is extravascular, but if complement is activated in great amounts intravascular lysis may result as well. Discontinuing the drug, supporting the patient, and treating any complications usually alleviates the problem.

Autoimmune hemolytic anemia is most often induced by drugs such as methyldopa, procainamide, levodopa, and certain nonsteroidal anti-inflammatory drugs (NSAIDs). These drugs appear to inhibit certain aspects of the immune system, which then allows B lymphocytes to produce autoantibodies. These autoantibodies, usually of an IgG nature, attach themselves to RBCs and cause hemolysis. Many patients on these drugs have a positive direct Coombs' test, but fewer than 1 per cent ever develop significant hemolysis. For example, 21 per cent of patients on procainamide have a positive direct Coombs' test, but only 3 per cent have evidence of hemolysis. Removal of the drug remedies the problem.

HYPERSPLENISM. A chronically enlarged spleen is somewhat rare but may cause significant amounts of hemolysis. Spleen enlargement may be due to cirrhosis of the liver, sarcoidosis, tuberculosis, some infectious diseases, connective tissue disorders, lymphoma, rheumatoid arthritis, among others. Physiologically, blood must go through small spaces in the spleen. Blood flow is often slowed in patients with these conditions, resulting in decreased oxygen, reduced glucose, and damage to the cell if the spleen is not functioning appropriately. RBCs are then exposed to macrophages, which remove defective areas of the cell and even whole cells. Thus an enlarged spleen has a significantly greater blood volume, reduced flow rates, and a greater reserve of blood cells than normal; and it quantitatively removes more cells from the circulation than one would expect.

Hypersplenism is difficult to diagnose, and the diagnosis usually is based on clinical suspicion and its association with other illnesses. Other cell lines may be affected, and the bone marrow is usually hyperplastic.

If the underlying disease cannot be resolved and the patient has significant hematologic distress, splenectomy is indicated. In some patients the presence of a large spleen may also enlarge the plasma circulation, resulting in a dilutional anemia even when the spleen is not over-functioning in terms of trapping and destroying RBCs. This situation can best be assessed by looking at the total RBC mass using a chromium 51 isotope. If a hemodilutional anemia has occurred, removal of the spleen reduces the plasma volume to normal values, and the RBC indices and hematocrit and hemoglobin levels return to normal.

INFECTIOUS CAUSES OF HEMOLYSIS. Specific infectious agents have some predilection for causing hemolysis by a variety of mechanisms. *Mycoplasma* pneumonia can cause hemolysis by producing cold agglutinins. *Hemophilus influenzae* produces substances that lead to a complement-induced hemolysis. *Clostridia* releases destructive enzymes into the circulation that digest RBCs, producing a devastating acute hemolysis in the face of sepsis from this organism. Malaria organisms parasitize RBCs, leading to their destruction in increasing numbers. Septic situations such as meningococcemia or other gram-negative septicemia can produce disseminated intravascular coagulation, which produces fibrin strands in small vessels, inducing a microangiopathic hemolytic picture. Parvovirus infections cause hemolysis and inhibit production of erythroid precursor cells. This reaction continues for approximately a week to 10 days; it is usually self-limited and disappears when the viral infection and its sequelae have resolved. Patients who have a chronic or underlying hemolytic disorder and become infected with some of these organisms may develop an acute, more devastating form of hemolysis that can lead to an aplastic crisis. Awareness of underlying chronic hemolytic disorders and the effects of infection on them is therefore important.

Polycythemia

Polycythemia is defined as an absolute increase in the mass of circulating red blood cells and comes in both a primary and a secondary form. There is also spurious polycythemia in which the plasma volume is constricted, giving rise to a falsely elevated RBC count, although the RBC mass is normal. The reasons for this type are not clear, and it is fairly rare. The classification of polycythemia is outlined in Table 45–7.

Primary polycythemia is an absolute increase in the RBC mass. For example, in neonates the RBC mass is physiologically increased but rapidly declines after birth. In the familial type the RBC mass is increased owing to enzyme deficiencies or altered hemoglobins. Finally, an autonomous increase in the RBC mass is found in polycythemia vera.

Most secondary polycythemias are due to cellular hypoxia, which is the initiating event that stimulates increased erythropoietin production. This increase in turn stimulates increased production of RBCs, so more oxygen can be carried to hypoxic cellular sites. Conditions that predispose to cellular hypoxia are high altitudes (where there is decreased oxygen tension), pulmonary diseases, cardiovascular shunts, elevated levels of carboxyhemoglobin, altered hemoglobins that have high oxygen affinity and do not release oxygen appropriately to the tissues, and declining erythropoietin production (found with chronic renal disease and certain kinds of liver and adrenal problems). Elevated erythropoietin levels then commit increased numbers of precursor RBCs into

TABLE 45–7. CATEGORIZATION OF POLYCYTHEMIA

Primary polycythemia
  Neonatal
  Familial
  Polycythemia vera

Secondary polycythemia
  Cellular hypoxia
    High altitudes
    Pulmonary disease
    Shunts
    Decreased oxygen-carrying capacity
    Decreased oxygen delivery
    Inappropriate erythropoietin production

a maturation cycle that increases the total RBC mass.

Clinically, polycythemia does not become recognized in most patients until their adult years, even in cases when there is a family history. The RBC mass can most accurately be measured using chromium 51 (^{51}Cr)-labeled RBCs. When the hematocrit is higher than 60 per cent this radioisotope measurement is unlikely to add to the diagnostic accuracy. It is also important to measure arterial blood gases to determine the oxygen saturation and the oxygen content of the blood as well as carboxyhemoglobin levels. If there are no defective hemoglobins in the individual's RBCs, if enzyme systems such as 2,3-DPG are normal, and no secondary causes are found to stimulate increased secretion of erythropoietin, polycythemia vera (an out-of-control set of stem cells producing increased numbers of RBCs) is the most likely the diagnosis. Most situations, seen by the family physician, however, are secondary or acquired cases of polycythemia relating to lung disease and other hypoxic stimuli leading to an increased RBC mass as compensation.

The erythropoietin level can now be clinically measured by laboratories, but there is a fairly broad range of normal values and the test results may not be absolutely diagnostic of secondary polycythemia. Patients complain of headaches, vertigo, mental confusion, dizziness, visual disturbances, and other symptoms related to the increased RBC mass, which leads to hyperviscosity of the blood. Alterations in the WBC or platelet count may occur, but they are more often found with polycythemia vera. The RBC mass should be determined by ^{51}Cr studies when the hematocrit in a nonsmoking man is higher than 51 per cent and in a nonsmoking woman is higher than 48 per cent. Hypoxia is defined as an arterial oxygen saturation less than 92 per cent or a partial pressure of oxygen of less than 60 mm Hg.

Spurious Polycythemia

Patients with spurious polycythemia or a reduced plasma volume are often middle-aged men who are obese, smoke, drink significant amounts of alcohol, and have high blood pressure. The cause for this spurious polycythemia is not known; but reduced alcohol consumption and elimination of smoking, control of blood pressure, and weight reduction are important when managing this problem.

Secondary Polycythemia

Patients with secondary polycythemia must undergo a detailed investigation as to the etiology. The causes of hypoxia should be dealt with and alleviated when feasible. Patients with chronic obstructive lung disease (COPD) and polycythemia should be instructed about techniques to cease smoking, and phlebotomy should be done to reduce the hematocrit to a level of 48 per cent or less.

Improved work capacity occurs when the hematocrit is reduced to 48 to 50 per cent, and cardiopulmonary function is maximized when the hematocrit ranges from 47 to 52 per cent. RBC production in these hypoxic states overcompensates for the physiologic needs of the body and causes problems for the patient with increased viscosity and blood flow difficulties. Patients with COPD who have had repeated phlebotomy to keep their hematocrits at a high normal level have reduced pulmonary artery pressure, pulmonary vascular resistance, and ventricular work. Thus phlebotomy has been shown to be helpful in keeping these patients maximally functional. It is not a substitute, however, for addressing the primary problem that has led to the cellular hypoxia.

Polycythemia Vera

Polycythemia vera is a myeloproliferative disorder in which a clone of pluripotent stem cells autonomously proliferates, leading to an absolute increase in the RBC circulating mass. It is autonomous because there are no physiologic or secondary mechanisms other than spontaneous proliferation of stem cells leading to this phenomenon. Because it is a stem cell undergoing uncontrolled proliferation, there is a high likelihood of eventual leukemic transformation. Polycythemia vera occurs most commonly in the 50- to 70-year age group, although individuals as young as teenagers have been found with this process. The incidence is approximately five cases per million with a slight male predominance and a slight predominance among individuals of Caucasian or European extraction. Some patients have abnormal appearing B lymphocytes, granulocytes, and megakaryocytes that seem to be derived from the abnormal stem cell clone that is proliferating large numbers of RBCs. However, the predominant disturbance is an increased production of RBCs from the stem cell clone. The proliferation of RBCs is independent of erythropoietin stimulation. Most likely there is a mutation in a stem cell that causes this process.

Four stages are described in the natural history of polycythemia vera: preerythrocytic phase, erythrocytic phase, proliferative phase, and "spent" or postpolycythemic, myeloid metaplasia phase. The pre-erythrocytic phase is often asymptomatic and may be heralded only by the incidental finding of splenomegaly, pruritus after bathing, or burning and erythema of the palms and soles. The RBC mass is mildly increased. The second, or erythrocytic, phase results in ischemic episodes secondary to vascular occlusions due to the expanded RBC mass and hyperviscosity. Patients may present with cyanosis, plethora, and bleeding episodes often related to abnormal platelet function, even though there are increased numbers of platelets found in the circulation. If there are bleeding episodes, the RBC mass, hematocrit, and hemoglobin may not be as elevated as one would expect. The blood loss masks the laboratory appearance of the disease. Splenomegaly is found in 90 per cent and an enlarged liver in 50 per cent of patients at this stage. Bleeding becomes more prominent with bruising and hemorrhage during the proliferative phase. Here leukocytosis is also noted, and the splenomegaly is consistent and progressive. About 20 per cent of patients reach the fourth, "spent," phase in which there may be severe anemia, mild hemorrhagic findings, and continued splenomegaly. Myelofibrosis may be occurring during this phase, as the abnormal stem cell clone has burned itself out and either leukemia or fibrosis replaces the normal bone marrow.

Laboratory findings reveal an increased absolute RBC mass and elevated hemoglobin and hematocrit levels corresponding to the levels discussed previously. If bleeding occurs, iron deficiency, folate deficiency, and microcytosis may also become apparent. Thrombocytosis is common in at least 50 per cent of cases, and there are wide variations in platelet size causing an increased mean platelet volume (MPV). The platelets have a shortened survival time and functional abnormalities that allow the hemorrhagic phenomena to occur. The WBC count may be elevated with an increased percentage of basophils; and there may be an increase in the leukocyte alkaline phosphatase levels. The bone marrow is usually hypercellular with panymyelosis, and marrow iron is often absent. Whole blood viscosity increases, plasma viscosity is normal, and hyperuricemia may occur owing to an increased turnover of cellular material. There are no diagnostic chromosomal abnormalities, and erythropoietin levels are decreased. The median survival is approximately 18 months, according to studies performed during the 1950s and 1960s in untreated patients. The erythrocytic (second) phase may last anywhere from 5 to 20 years in treated patients. Frequent phlebotomy is performed to maintain high-normal hematocrit and hemoglobin levels. Aspirin and antiplatelet therapy have not been found to reduce the likelihood of complications such as thrombic events. Approximately 20 per cent of patients reach the fourth, or "spent," phase. It takes approximately 10 years to progress from phase III to phase IV. Many of these patients die of complications within 3 years of reaching the fourth phase, especially from conversions to an acute leukemia. Patients who have been treated with anticancer agents or radioactive phosphorus are much more likely to convert to a leukemic picture if they reach the final phase of the illness than if they have not been treated with these agents previously. The symptoms of itching and burning during the first two phases can be treated with a histamine blocker such as cimetidine.

As the second phase progresses, phlebotomy is probably the best overall treatment on a longitudinal basis. Younger patients do better over the long run with simple phlebotomy. If it is necessary to withdraw more than 6 units of blood per year from them, the risk of thrombosis increases. In this event, alkalating or myelosuppressive agents may be helpful. Hydroxyurea is capable of maintaining the hematocrit below 50 per cent and the platelet count at a level below $1 \times 10^6/mm^3$. Older patients may benefit from radioactive phosphorus or other alkalating agents, as they are unlikely to live 20 years or longer and thus have less long-term risk for leukemia.

In conclusion, individuals with polycythemia vera can be managed symptomatically and have their risk of thrombosis and complications reduced through careful monitoring of their RBC mass hemoglobin and hematocrit with repetitive phlebotomy. Agents such as hydroxyurea do not seem to increase the risk of leukemia and should be used in younger patients. Anticancer therapy may be an excellent choice for patients over age 70.

Lymphadenopathy

Enlarged lymph nodes, single or multiple, are a common problem seen by the family physician in ambulatory practice. They may be a result of a reactive phenomenon to infection, inflammation, malignancy, or systemic generalized disease. Most enlarged lymph nodes seen in younger individuals are benign. Table 45–8 demonstrates that the four major determinants of significant lymphadenopathy are the age of the patient, location of the adenopathy, character of the lymph node, and clinical

TABLE 45–8. LYMPHADENOPATHY

Considerations	Significance
Age of patient	
<30 Years of age	80% Lymphadenopathy benign; most often infectious
>50 Years of age	40% Benign probability
Location of node enlargement	
Cervical nodes, axillary nodes, epitrochlear nodes, bilateral hilar adenopathy	Benign/infectious
Generalized; unilateral, jugular, or mandibular areas; supraclavicular/scalene nodes; Virchow's node; femoral triangle nodes; thoracic/retroperitoneal; unilateral hilar adenopathy	Malignant
Characteristics of the node enlargement	
Rubbery, soft, mobile, tender, matted	Benign
Hard, nontender, fixed	Malignant
Clinical setting of patient: solitary, nontender, enlarged cervical node	
Elderly, smoker	Malignant
College student	Infectious with pharyngitis and fever

setting in which this enlarged lymph node(s) occurs. For example, a relatively soft, small (less than 1 cm), movable node may be found in the submandibular or anterior cervical region in as many as 50 to 60 per cent of individuals less than 50 years of age. Inguinal nodes up to 1 to 2 cm may be found in normal, healthy adults. The significance of an enlarged lymph node or lymph node group depends on the patient's age, location, character of the lymph node enlargement, and the clinical setting.

The age of the patient is important in that those individuals who are less than 50 years old are much more likely to have a benign or infectious process causing the lymphadenopathy than are patients over age 50, in whom only 40 per cent of the cases are of a benign or infectious nature. Thus, the age of the patient is important in the differential consideration of malignant disease, serious systemic disease versus infection, or reactivity of a lymph node group.

Nodal location is also important and indicative of the kind of process one must consider. Enlarged lymph nodes in younger persons found in the anterior or posterior cervical regions or the occipital regions are generally benign, but this consideration is also dependent on the character of the node and the clinical setting in which this enlargement occurs. If two distinct, but separate, lymph node groups are enlarged, a hematologic malignancy is more likely, such as chronic lymphocytic leukemia or lymphoma. Infectious processes such as infectious mononucleosis, viral hepatitis, secondary syphilis, histoplasmosis, toxoplasmosis, or cytomegalovirus infection are more probable when generalized lymphadenopathy is found. If one-sided lymph node enlargements are discovered in the neck, mandibular region, and in older patients in the anterior scalene node regions, a malignancy deserves much greater consideration.

Virchow's node is defined as an enlarged left supraclavicular node usually infiltrated with a metastatic tumor from below the diaphragm, especially of gastrointestinal origin. A matted node that is enlarged could be due to a local phenomenon such as an infection, bite, or trauma to the arm, but it may also represent a melanoma, a lymphoma, or metastatic breast cancer in a young woman. Bilateral hilar adenopathy and enlargement of nodes in the femoral triangle are more likely to be seen with systematic disease, generalized infection, or on occasion with lymphoma. The character of the node, overall size, and relation to other lymph node groups have a bearing on whether biopsy is indicated. When there is thoracic adenopathy, unilateral hilar adenopathy, or mediastinal adenopathy particularly in older adults, systemic disease such as sarcoid or lymphoma must be considered strongly as must lung cancer depending on the clinical setting. Mediastinal adenopathy in young persons may, however, may be associated with sarcoidosis or infectious mononucleosis. Bilateral chest node enlargement would indicate something more systemic or a lymphoma, whereas a unilateral enlargement would indicate a carcinoma of the lung or a metastatic cancer. Enlarged nodes found in the abdomen or retroperitoneal space are much more likely to be malignant and are characteristic of lymphomas or germ cell tumors in men.

The characteristics of the nodes that are enlarged are important in helping to determine whether they represent a reactive process to infection or systemic illness or they are involved in tumor spread. Nodes that are enlarged, well circumscribed, rubbery, firm, mobile, and not particularly tender are more likely to be reactive lymph nodes or involved in a lymphomatous process. Some may also be painful, particularly if the rate of growth has been rapid due to inflammation. Lymph nodes that are hard, nontender, nonmovable, and fixed to the underlying tissues are much more likely to be infiltrated with metastatic tumor from a regionally proximate cancer.

The clinical setting is important. An elderly individual who smokes and has an enlarged supraclavicular or cervical lymph node may be much more likely to have a cancer in the mouth, head and neck, or lung than a younger individual who has enlarged cervical lymph nodes accompanied by a fever and sore throat indicative of infectious mononucleosis. Patients with acquired immunodeficiency syndrome (AIDS) may have generalized lymphadenopathy indicative of either a severe systemic infection or lymphoma.

When one encounters an enlarged lymph node or lymph node group that does not have striking hallmarks of malignancy and there are no other symptoms, it is appropriate to watch and observe the patient over several weeks. Nodes that do not become smaller or revert to a more benign appearance should be biopsied. Biopsy of nodes result in about a 40 to 50 per cent yield in terms of a positive diagnostic result. Nodes that are difficult for the pathologist to read as reactive and those lymph nodes diagnosed with follicular hyperplasia may have an occult lymphoma, and a second opinion might be beneficial. For a patient with repeated lymph node enlargements that have no clearly infectious etiology, repeat lymph node biopsies are indicated and may establish a diagnosis. Most lymph node enlargements found by the family physician are benign and resolve within a short time. Those that do not resolve require further investigation and ultimately biopsy if no cause can be found.

WHITE BLOOD CELL DISORDERS

Physiology and Function

White blood cells play a major role in defending the patient's system against infection. The phagocytic role belongs primarily to the neutrophils, monocytes, and macrophages; lymphocytes have a larger role in delayed response to infection and in the production of antibodies and other proteins important in defense against infectious agents. All WBCs in the marrow are derived from the pluripotent stem cell described earlier in this chapter. Interleukin-3 and GM-CSF are the primary determinants of the ability of the pluripotent cell to proliferate and differentiate to produce the various WBC entities.

The bone marrow contains a proliferating pool of granulocytic precursors and a developed pool of granulocytic precursors that serve an emergency reserve. They are commonly known as the proliferating pool and the marrow granulocytic reserve (MGR) pool. The mean generation time of marrow WBCs in the proliferative pool is 24 hours. The MGR has at least ten times the number of neutrophils that are produced on a daily basis and contains a much larger number of neutrophils than exist in the circulating pool measured by the typical WBC count. The MGR is important to the ability of a patient to respond to infection or to chemotherapy. Bone marrow is a reasonable reflection of the MGR. If neutrophilic precursors do not comprise more than 25 per cent of the total WBC precursors, the patient's marrow reserve may be in danger. Once mature neutrophils leave the bone marrow, they survive about 10 hours and are divided between two interchangeable pools: the marginating granulocytic pool found in the reticuloendothelial system (e.g., the spleen) and the circulating granulocytic pool measured in the plasma. Once neutrophils leave the circulation, they do not return. The relation between these pools of WBC are shown in Figure 45–4.

Eosinophils, basophils, and mast cells all arise from the same pluripotent stem cell precursor. Eosinophil production is stimulated by eosinophilopoietin. T lymphocytes play an important role in the body's eosinophil response. When T cells are depleted, the body is unable to mobilize enough eosinophils to respond to parasitic infections. The eosinophils have a marrow transit time of about 9 days and a half-life in the blood of about 5 hours. Most eosinophils are found in the tissues, and the ratio of tissue to blood eosinophils is 100:1.

Monocytes and macrophages have a generation time of 48 hours and a marrow transit time of 6 days—in contrast to the transit time for neutrophils in the marrow, which is 12 to 14 days. There is no monocyte or macrocytic reserve. These cells circulate in the peripheral blood and then enter the tissues, where they can become pulmonary macrophages, Kupffer cells in the liver, and macrophages in other areas such as the brain, abdominal cavity, and bone.

Neutrophils act primarily by phagocytosis of invading bacteria and then destroy these abnormal elements through the use of enzymes found in their granules. Eosinophils act to kill parasites by bombarding the parasite with peroxidasas and toxic proteins from their granular elements. T cells stimulate their development and migration to areas where they are needed. Monocytes and macrophages secrete a number of chemicals that activate lymphocytes. They are specifically active against organisms that are intracellular or encapsulated, such as *Mycobacterium tuberculosis*, *Listeria*, *Cryptococcus*, *Salmonella*, and *Toxoplasma*. Macrophages may also secret interleukin-1, tumor necrosis factor, and other interferons.

Normal WBC Values

It is important to know not only the total WBC count but the absolute count of specific WBCs, such as neutrophils, eosinophils, and lymphocytes. Table 45–9 presents the normal white cell values and ranges found in the peripheral blood. These values may vary among races and people of different geographic origins. A given patient might have leukopenia, but if it is balanced among all elements it may not be as severe as the leukopenia in a person who has a normal WBC count but severe neutropenia with a neutrophil count of less than $500/mm^3$. Approximately 6 per cent of the total WBCs are located in the peripheral blood, and WBCs spend only 2 per cent of their life cycle in the peripheral circulation. Thus it is but a single measure of the functional capability of the body to fight off infection.

Neutropenia

Neutropenia is defined as an absolute neutrophil count that is less than $1800/mm^3$. The total WBC

Proliferating WBC $\rightarrow$ Marrow granulocytic $\rightarrow$ Marginating granulocytic $\rightarrow$ Circulating granulocytes
precursors   reserve   pool

FIGURE 45–4. White blood cell kinetics.

TABLE 45–9. NORMAL LEUKOCYTE VALUES IN PERIPHERAL BLOOD

Cell Type	Cells/mm³*		Percent of Total Differential Count
	Median	Range	
All leukocytes (WBCs)	7000	4,300–10,000	100
Total neutrophils	4000	1800–7200	55
Band neutrophils	500	100–2000	10
Segmented neutrophils	3500	1000–6000	45
Lymphocytes	2500	1500–4000	36
Monocytes	450	200–900	6
Eosinophils	150	0–700	2
Basophils	30	0–150	1

* To calculate the number of cells per liter, multiply by 10^6.
Adapted from Rubenstein EH, Federman D: Hematology (Chapter 5). New York, American Scientific Medicine, 1993, with permission. Copyright 1989 Scientific American, Inc.

count is multiplied by the percent of neutrophils to obtain the absolute neutrophil count. Although neutrophil counts as low as 1000/mm³ do not predispose greatly to infection, counts less than 500/mm³ are much more serious, as they do predispose to a life-threatening infection.

Neutropenia is caused by three major phenomena: (1) defective neutrophil production; (2) accelerated neutrophil removal; and (3) neutrophil redistribution. This kinetic categorization is similar to that used for the study of RBC disorders.

Most often neutropenia is discovered because the patient has an infection and a WBC count is ordered. Attention should be directed to a history of drug utilization, a family history of infectious problems, and problems such as hemorrhage, anemia, and inflammation. The physical examination should focus on whether the liver and spleen are enlarged, the discovery of enlarged lymph nodes, evidence of bleeding, bone marrow abnormalities, and systemic diseases such as connective tissue disorders. Bone marrow aspiration and biopsy can provide significant information regarding the etiology and extent of the neutropenia. Some conditions cause a maturation arrest, in which neutrophilic precursor development is arrested at the myelocyte stage, and more mature forms are virtually absent. A drug might be implicated in this situation. The marrow granulocytic reserve (MGR) can be estimated from the bone marrow or by giving the patient a dose of corticosteroids, etiocholanolone, or endotoxins. For example, 40 mg of prednisone elevates the neutrophil count by approximately 4000/mm³ in about 4 to 6 hours. This "test" is not needed routinely for investigating causes of neutropenia unless the bone marrow reveals no clues as to the cause of the depressed neutrophilic count.

TABLE 45–10. CAUSES OF PRODUCTION DEFICIT NEUTROPENIA

Drug-induced
Immune mechanisms
Infection
Ineffective granulopoiesis
Starvation
Cyclic neutropenia
Hereditary neutropenia
Myelodysplasia
Felty's syndrome
Chronic idiopathic neutropenia

Neutropenia Caused by Production Deficits

Table 45–10 lists the major causes of production deficit neutropenia. Production deficit neutropenia has three postulated mechanisms of action. One mechanism is direct myelosuppression by such agents as anticancer drugs, benzene, and irradiation. A second mechanism is nonimmune effects on the bone marrow due to drugs such as analgesics (i.e., phenylbutazone, phenacetin, indomethacin), phenothiazines, tranquilizers, sulfonamide, anticonvulsants such as phenytoin, antibiotics such as chloramphenicol and penicillin derivatives, and histamine-blocking agents such as cimetidine or ranitidine and procainamide. There is also an immune effect that some agents and drugs cause in which they are either attached to a neutrophil, rendering the neutrophil immunologically different, which leads to an immunologic attack; or they may form a drug–antibody immune complex that is absorbed onto the neutrophil membrane, which then induces an antibody–antigen reaction that removes the WBC. Drugs that are particularly implicated in this class are aminopyrine, antithyroid drugs, antiplatelet drugs, aspirin, quinine and its derivatives, and celphasporins or β-lactam antibiotics.

Pure WBC aplasia is a rather severe form of immune neutropenia. Granulocytic colony-forming units are suppressed by a complement-fixing IgG. In some situations the IgG antibody is directed against metamyelocytes, bands, or mature neutrophils, and the bone marrow demonstrates a myeloid hyperplasia. Here moderate neutropenia occurs. In other situations the antibody is directed against earlier granulocytic forms, such as promyelocytes and myelocytes, producing myeloid hypoplasia and severe neutropenia. Occasionally, lymphocytes in other diseases, such as Felty's syndrome with rheumatoid arthritis, produce antineutrophil antibodies, and suppressor T cells may inhibit the colony-forming units of granulocytes as well.

In most cases neutropenia is discovered incidentally when a severe infection is investigated by a blood count. Absolute neutropenia must be followed up with a bone marrow examination. In the case of drug-induced neutropenia, the most important part of the management is to obtain a detailed history and withdraw any possible causative drugs or agents. Androgens have been tried in some situations but do not seem to increase neutrophil production or resolve neutropenia. Steroids may be helpful in those patients in whom there is an autoimmune mechanism particularly suggested by finding large granular lymphocytes. Lithium, which has been known to increase the neutrophil count, can shorten the duration of neutropenia secondary to any of the above-noted mechanisms. The therapeutic dose is 300 mg three or four times a day, with the lithium blood level equaling about 1.0 mEq/L. Response to this regimen is variable and may be used for up to 6 weeks if toxic side effects do not occur. When patients are infected or septic in a neutropenic state, bactericidal antibiotics should always be used in preference to bacteriostatic agents, as the body's ability to fight infection is severely compromised.

Infections can cause neutropenia by inducing a production deficit. With infectious mononucleosis, 20 to 30 per cent of patients have a mild neutropenia related to a production deficit induced by the virus itself. HIV infection is associated with a profound neutropenia and may be related to a production deficit because giving GM-CSF produces an increase in neutrophils. Some infections are simply so overwhelming that the marrow cannot keep up with the demand for neutrophils and their increased destruction, resulting in a relative to absolute neutropenia. Gram-negative sepsis is often associated with neutropenia because of toxins that inhibit neutrophil production or significant margination of neutrophils. When the spleen is enlarged, neutrophils may be sequestered there, which would fit into a redistribution category of neutropenia.

Patients with deficiencies in vitamin B_{12} or folic acid may have ineffective granulopoiesis similar to that found with megaloblastic anemia associated with the deficiencies of those important nutrients. The serum lysozyme level is high, indicating that WBCs are being produced but are dying rapidly in the marrow.

Some families in ethnic groups have hereditary neutropenia. With this disorder there seems to be adequate numbers of marrow stem cells, but they are deficient in their ability to develop appropriately.

Starvation syndromes often result in both leukopenia and neutropenia. Patients with anorexia nervosa in particular may have neutropenia plus leukopenia. This condition rarely reduces the neutrophil count to levels where infections are serious or common. When the nutritional status returns to normal, so does the neutrophil count.

Cyclic neutropenia is seen when the absolute neutrophil count varies significantly over periods of time, sometimes reaching an absolute neutrophil count of 500/mm³ or less. Patients may then have repeated infections with fever approximately every 3 to 4 weeks. The MGR is also reduced, and the patient cannot respond appropriately to infection. There is no known cause, but lithium has been found helpful in some of these cases.

Dysplastic syndromes otherwise known as myelodysplasia or hematologic malignancies often are associated with neutropenia. It often coincides with marked anemia and thrombocytopenia. Conditions in this classification may be preleukemia and include paroxysmal nocturnal hemoglobinuria (PNH). Neutrophils in PNH are highly susceptible to complement lysis, which may be the mechanism inducing the neutropenia.

Another entity, chronic idiopathic neutropenia, is often mild to moderate in severity. Patients rarely have significant infection because the phagocytic function of other cells is generally preserved. When a patient is discovered with a consistent neutropenia without severe infection, it is still important to discover the cause. A detailed history of drug and toxin exposure, study of the bone marrow, and examination of the reticuloendothelial system are helpful. Most patients are not severely impaired and can fight off reasonable infections. On occasion when infections arise, treatment of the infection with appropriate bactericidal antibiotics and use of prednisone in an alternate-day fashion may be helpful.

Felty's syndrome is the condition in which rheumatoid arthritis is associated with an enlarged spleen, neutropenia, weight loss, anemia, enlarged lymph nodes, and recurrent fevers. The bone marrow reveals the absence of maturing neutrophils. Because it is an autoimmune connective tissue disease problem, there is speculation that T cell suppression of WBC development is part of the etiology; other patients have antineutrophil antibodies. There are few infectious problems clinically so long as the neutrophil count does not drop below 500/mm³. The neutropenia can cause trouble and should be monitored closely, with appropriate antibiotic therapy given when the neutropenia reaches dangerously low levels. Steroid therapy is sometimes helpful. Controversy exists as to whether splenectomy is effective. When it works well, it reduces the anti-neutrophil antibody titer, which is probably being manufactured in the spleen itself.

Increased Removal of Neutrophils

Two major situations exist in which an immune mechanism causes increased neutrophil removal or destruction. In the first scenario, anti-neutrophil antibodies are produced in patients with Felty's syndrome or when certain drugs (e.g., aminopyrine) are prescribed. There are usually no RBC abnormalities, and the diagnosis must be one of exclusion—ruling out other causes of the neutropenia. In the other situation, accelerated neutrophil removal by activated complement may occur when blood is exposed to dialysis coils or fibers in a cardiopulmonary bypass machine. Donors whose blood is filtered for apheresis may also develop complement-activated processes in which the pulmonary capillary bed may be occluded by sticky globs of neutrophils. The absolute neutrophil count drops, and those neutrophils that remain do not respond normally to infection. In these situations, patience and support of the patient usually allows the problem to be alleviated over a period of time. Additional procedures that may cause this problem should be avoided or minimized.

Neutrophil Redistribution

Neutrophils may be shifted out of the peripheral circulation into the reticuloendothelial system for a number of reasons. One example is gram-negative sepsis. The diagnosis is made when the patient has fever, positive blood cultures, hypotension, and thrombocytopenia in addition to marked neutropenia. In another case, sometimes the spleen simply gobbles up neutrophils and shortens their life-span. It may also store them after having removed them from the circulation. The usual causes are a premalignant syndrome, a malignancy, or a connective tissue disease.

Neutrophilia

Four basic mechanisms exist to increase the neutrophil count in patients: (1) increased production of neutrophils by the bone marrow; (2) impaired exit of neutrophils from the blood; (3) decreased neutrophils in the MGR; and (4) enhanced release of neutrophils from the MGR. Situations that can cause neutrophilia are exercise and the administration of epinephrine or corticosteroids, all of which produce a movement of neutrophils from the MGR to the peripheral circulation. Steroids increase the half-life of neutrophils from approximately 6.5 hours to almost 16.0 hours. In situations where sepsis causes neutrophilia, endotoxin has been shown to cause a total WBC count elevation within as short a time as 4 to 6 hours. A peripheral blood smear that has toxic granulations and demonstrates a significant shift to the left, with the presence of 6 to 10 per cent band forms, characterizes an infection rather than exercise- or corticosteroid-induced neutrophilia. Lithium has been described previously as a treatment for neutropenia and can indeed raise the neutrophil and total WBC count significantly after several weeks of therapy. Both lymphocytes and neutrophils increase in total numbers, but the increase in neutrophils predominates.

Exceedingly high WBC counts with increased numbers of neutrophils can occur with malignancies. Some tumors may produce GM-CSF, resulting in a leukemoid reaction. Measurement of neutrophil alkaline phosphatase levels reveals normal or elevated levels in contrast to reduced levels found with a leukemic process such as chronic myeloid leukemia.

Eosinophils

A marked decrease in eosinophils may occur with some infectious processes, but it is rare and is not as clinically significant as eosinophilia. Eosinophilia is defined as an absolute eosinophil count higher than 500/mm^3. Eosinophilia can be associated with a number of chronic skin disorders, such as eczema, contact dermatitis, mycosis fungoides; allergic problems such as asthma, hives, hay fever, and angioneurotic edema; administration of any number of drugs; connective tissue diseases; parasitic and certain fungal infections, such as aspergillosis and coccidioidomycosis; sarcoid; hemodialysis; malignant disorders of the reticuloendothelial system; and some unusual syndromes in which pulmonary infiltrates and elevated eosinophil counts occur. The two most prominent examples are Löffler syndrome, which is relatively mild, and pulmonary infiltrates with eosinophilia (PIE), in which cough, fever, sweats, shortness of breath, eosinophilia, and infiltrates predominate. This syndrome usually responds to steroids and may last several years.

Lymphocyte Abnormalities

A reduction in lymphocyte counts below 1500/mm^3 is significant and is found with severe infections, uremia, and Hodgkin's disease. It may also be related to irradiation or chemotherapy, aplastic anemia, and immunodeficiency states. One of the most well known causes of decreased lymphocyte counts is HIV infection, in which T cells with the CD4 marker are decreased. The latter is a measure of the severity of the disease and patient susceptibility to infection. Some experts believe that the absolute lymphocyte count can also be a marker for the nutritional status of severely ill, hospitalized patients. If the lymphocyte count is reduced to 1500/mm^3 or less, the patient may be in a severe nutritional deficiency state, which must be corrected.

It is quite uncommon for lymphocytes to increase to an absolute number of 5000/mm^3 or more. Infections such as brucellosis, tuberculosis, and in young adults measles and chickenpox may be causative. If the high lymphocyte count is chronic and stable, lymphocytic leukemia is a more likely consideration. When there is an absolute lymphocytosis and more than one third are atypical, other disease processes should be considered. Atypical lymphocytes have more cytoplasm, more DNA synthesis, and more capacity for protein synthesis. Infectious mononucleosis, hepatitis, cytomegalovirus (CMV) infection, toxoplasmosis, and typical childhood viral illnesses may cause an atypical lymphocytosis, as may certain allergic reactions to drugs and serum sickness. If an infectious or allergic cause is not found in a case of marked typical lymphocytosis, strong consideration should be given to the diagnosis of lymphoma. Appropriate studies including bone marrow aspiration and biopsy should be carried out.

Splenomegaly

As many as 3 per cent of patients in the United States may have a palpably enlarged spleen. Most of these people do not develop any significant disease in long-term follow-up studies. In fact, 30 per cent have a palpable spleen 3 years later without evidence of disease or important associated phenomena. The most appropriate approach is to obtain a detailed history, perform a thorough physical examination, and personally examine the blood smear. If the patient is systemically ill with weight loss, anorexia, fever, chills, sweats, and itching, more detailed laboratory tests (e.g., bone marrow biopsy and aspiration) are indicated. Travel history, exposure to people with infection, the use of alcohol and drugs, and other important sociodemographic data are necessary. In addition, a urinalysis and a chemical screening panel are helpful. If a patient is not symptomatic, does not feel ill, has no lymphadenopathy, does not have any blood count or peripheral smear abnormalities, has no evidence of renal disease and normal liver function, the work-up may stop and the patient can be followed at regular intervals (months). Tests such as a tuberculin skin test and biopsy of abnormal skin or lymph node areas may also be helpful. The differential diagnosis, which is rather long, includes such entities as infectious mononucleosis, CMV infection, typhoid, malaria, tuberculosis, systemic fungal infections, connective tissue diseases, hemolytic disorders, alcoholic liver disease, chronic active hepatitis, and neoplasia, specifically lymphoma.

If the spleen is chronically enlarged and must be removed, certain hazards present themselves. Patients who are immunized after removal of a spleen do not respond as appropriately with IgM and IgG antibodies, particularly to pneumococcal vaccine, meningococcal vaccines, and *Hemophilus influenzae* vaccinations. Splenectomized patients are also susceptible to infection, particularly sepsis due to *Salmonella* and/or pneumococcus. Thus in patients for whom splenectomy is planned, it is important to immunize them ahead of time and place the patient on penicillin prophylaxis for 6 months to 1 year postsplenectomy to protect them from early and repetitive bouts of infection.

PLATELETS AND PLATELET DISORDERS

Platelets are produced by megakaryocytes, which are under the control of a colony-stimulating factor and thrombopoietin. The same pluripotent stem cells that produce WBCs develop under these stimuli into megakaryocytes, which are large cells with abundant cytoplasm. They undergo divisions of the nucleus without concomitant cell division. As the cytoplasm of the cell matures, it develops a bluish-gray, sometimes vacuolated appearance with beaded strands. These beads gradually pinch off from the cytoplasm and become platelets. Large platelets, in most situations, are thought to be the youngest with the most enzymatic activity, whereas small platelets are older and have less activity. Platelets survive 8.5 to 10.0 days in the circulation with a half-life of 4 days. The bone marrow can increase its production of platelets seven- to eightfold above normal. There is no pool of reserve platelets in the bone marrow, but about 30 to 40 per cent of the platelets are in the spleen and freely interchange with the circulation as needed. Platelets are important to the first phase of blood clotting because they adhere to damaged endothelium and release enzymes that activate clotting factors such as fibrinogen and von Willebrand factor. Platelet activity occurs as a first aggregation wave, which is then followed by a second phase in response to the need for clotting. Platelets facilitate clot retraction and maintain the integrity of small vessels in the capillary bed as they prevent RBCs from leaking through single-cell-thick blood vessel walls.

Thrombocytopenia

Table 45–11 outlines the three major causes of decreased platelets: decreased production, increased platelet destruction, and sequestration. The most common clinical finding due to a low platelet count is petechiae. Petechiae are probably due to microscopic bleeding at the capillary level where there is increased vascular pressure. Exam-

TABLE 45–11. CLASSIFICATION OF THROMBOCYTOPENIA

Decreased Platelet Production
Congenital or acquired deficits
Ineffective production: $\downarrow$ vitamin B_{12}, folate; $\uparrow$ alcohol
Marrow dysfunction: aplasia, hypoplasia, infiltration, cancer

Increased Platelet Destruction
Immune: idiopathic thrombocytopenic purpura, infection, drug, human immunodeficiency virus
Nonimmune: disseminated intravascular coagulation, vasculitis, drug

Sequestration
Hypersplenism

ples are seen in the lower extremities, the oral mucosa of the cheeks because of chewing and the force of that activity, and where there are pressure points from clothing such as belts or the tops of tight socks. At extremely low platelet counts, there may be ecchymoses, bruising, and mucosal bleeding. There is no absolute low platelet count at which bleeding is guaranteed to occur. Generally, patients with a platelet count of less than 20,000/mm^3 are more likely to bleed than those who have counts higher than that. Additionally, patients with idiopathic thrombocytopenic purpura (ITP) bleed less at a given low platelet count than patients with aplastic anemia. If patients have a platelet count that is low, with small platelets and thus small mean platelet volume (low MPV), they are more likely to bleed because the platelets are older and less functional. In contrast, an individual with a low platelet count and a large MPV is less likely to bleed. Low platelet volumes are indicative of reduced production; whereas low platelet counts but a large platelet volume indicate rapid replacement of platelets with new platelets, although they maybe dysfunctional platelets. The differential diagnosis of a low platelet count requires a good history considering drug use, the possibility of HIV-related activity, transfusions, lymphoma, autoimmune disease, connective tissue disease, the size of the spleen, and treatment for hematologic disorders in the past. The laboratory work-up requires at a minimum a complete blood count, platelet count, reticulocyte count, and bone marrow aspiration to examine the production characteristics or lack thereof of megakaryocytes.

Decreased Production of Platelets

Production deficits may range from a congenital inability to produce adequate numbers of platelets to replacement of the marrow or aplasia of the marrow due to irradiation or cytotoxic drugs. If the bone marrow is basically normal except for a decreased number of megakaryocytes, it is likely that the patient has been affected by a drug such as ethanol or gold. If the bone marrow is generally hypoplastic or aplastic, it is more likely that irradiation, cytotoxic drugs, or an infiltrating cancer or fibrosis has impaired the marrow's inability to produce not only platelets but other normal cell lines as well. If there are an adequate number of megakaryocyte precursors but an inability of megakaryocytes to develop appropriately, deficiencies of vitamin B_{12} or folic acid or excess amounts of alcohol may be affecting megakaryocyte development.

The treatment of thrombocytopenia due to decreased production is to first identify the cause and then to alleviate or remediate it if possible, particularly in the case of a drug or cancer etiology. If the platelet count is extremely low (less than 20,000/mm^3) or the patient has evidence of bleeding, the platelet count must be restored with platelet packs to stop the blood loss. Generally, each platelet pack

raises the platelet count by 10,000/mm^3/m^2 of body surface area. A general rule of thumb is to use six platelet packs, which should increase the platelet count by 40,000 to 50,000/mm^3. Transfused platelets should last at least 24 to 48 hours, with a slow decline over that time. Platelet transfusions several times a week may be necessary until the patient develops autoantibodies to the platelets or the condition resolves and platelet production ensues in a more normal fashion.

Increased Platelet Destruction

IMMUNE MECHANISMS. Two basic observations confirm the diagnosis of increased platelet destruction. One is the finding in the bone marrow of normal or increased numbers megakaryocytes, with the peripheral circulation demonstrating a low platelet count. This discrepancy suggests increased platelet removal or destruction. Alternatively, when platelet packs are infused into a thrombocytopenic patient with only slight or no elevation noted in the platelet count or return to the pretransfusion level within 24 hours, increased platelet destruction or removal is likely. As an example, in patients with ITP platelets may survive only 30 to 60 minutes. The mechanisms for immune destruction may involve the use of a drug setting up an antibody-coated platelet to septicemia, infection with infectious mononucleosis, HIV or varicella, disseminated intravascular coagulation, or hematologic malignancies.

Idiopathic Thrombocytopenic Purpura. Patients with ITP have an immunoglobulin attached to the platelets called the platelet-associated IgG (PA-IgG). If one takes plasma with ITP and transfuses it into a compatible individual without ITP, a major drop in the platelet count occurs, indicating that there is an anti-platelet immunoglobulin in the plasma. In addition, pregnant women with ITP have babies who have depressed platelet counts, indicating transplacental transfer of an anti-platelet factor. The spleen recognizes platelets with these antibodies attached to them and destroys them because they are abnormal. The marrow responds with increased platelet production but only two to five times normal instead of the seven- to eightfold increase expected. Thus immunoglobulins affect the development of platelets as well as increasing production. Generally, the platelets of ITP are large and do not have functional abnormalities. Bleeding does not occur so long as there are adequate numbers. On rare occasions, patients with ITP have platelets that do not function well. Prolonged bleeding time and an increased bleeding diathesis occurs at higher platelet counts because of the functionally disabled platelets.

Idiopathic thrombocytopenic purpura occurs most often in young women, but an increase has been seen in HIV-positive men in recent years. Patients with infectious mononucleosis and autoimmune thyroid diseases such as Graves' disease and Hashimoto's thyroiditis may also have ITP. Generally, the spleen is not palpable. If the spleen is palpable, diagnoses such as systemic lupus erythematosus, lymphoma, infectious mononucleosis, and a hematologic malignancy should be suspected. Generally, bleeding is not a serious problem, but uterine bleeding might be voluminous in some women and CNS bleeds are dangerous. Acute ITP is often preceded by a viral illness in children and young adults. Generally, it remits spontaneously within less than 3 months. Adults are more likely to get chronic ITP, which persists through spontaneous remissions and relapses over a longer period. Clinically, most patients do well without significant bleeding. However, intracranial bleeding can occur and leads to a mortality rate of 1 to 5 per cent. Therapy is applied according to the degree of bleeding, which is related to the severity of the platelet count reduction and other illnesses causing the problem in the first place.

Treatment. Patients who simply have small numbers of petechiae or occasional bruising but no significant bleeding rarely require significant therapy. They should be advised to avoid aspirin, and in the case of infection the platelet count should be monitored carefully until the infection is resolved, as it may induce a lower platelet count.

When patients develop mucosal bleeding, usually from the GI tract, definitive therapy should be started. Prednisone is started at 60 to 100 mg per day; and aspirin and other antiplatelet drugs are avoided or discontinued. Activities where muscle trauma, bleeding, or valsalva maneuvers may occur should be discouraged particularly as the latter may increase the likelihood of intracranial bleeding. The mechanism of action of steroids involves interference with the ability of macrophages to destroy platelets. In addition, steroids reduce the immune system's ability to make the antiplatelet antibody. Steroids can be tapered carefully over the course of 4 to 6 weeks when the platelet count has returned to normal and is stabilized. In a patient who has been stable with low or no steroid therapy and then sustains a recurrence of ITP with falling platelet counts, splenectomy should be considered. This measure generally produces a lengthy remission in 65 to 80 per cent of patients. The platelet count should be close to 50,000/mm³ or higher when the splenectomy is performed to avoid complications of bleeding just from the surgery. Splenectomy usually works because it eliminates the destruction of many of the platelets in the spleen and diminishes the body's ability to produce platelet antibody because the lymphoid cells in the spleen are a factor in antibody production. Patients who cannot withstand a splenectomy, such as the elderly, debilitated, or immunosuppressed, may respond to chemotherapeutic agents such as vincristine or vinblastine. Danazol may also be effective and helps reduce the steroid dose. It takes 2 to 3 months of therapy to determine if it is effective. Patients undergoing a splenectomy should be given pneumococcal vaccine prior to surgery, as administration of the vaccine afterward does not generate as good a response and may induce reactivation of the ITP.

The patient who presents with active bleeding from the mucosal linings of the body or in the CNS must be hospitalized and treated vigorously. High doses of prednisone should be administered orally and intravenously, platelets should be given in 6- to 12-platelet-pack units every 6 to 12 hours with RBCs as needed. If bleeding cannot be managed, emergency splenectomy can be performed. In this case, platelet packs are given at the beginning, during, and after surgery, with high doses of steroids preoperatively and postoperatively. On occasion, plasmapheresis or the use of human γ-globulin given intravenously may be helpful. Plasmapheresis removes the anti-platelet antibody, and human γ-globulin binds the anti-platelet antibody, rendering it ineffective. Platelet transfusions then produce higher counts and prevent or stop active bleeding. If a patient has had a splenectomy, Howell-Jolly bodies should be present in their red blood cells. A patient who is not responding to splenectomy and in whom Howell-Jolly bodies disappear may have an accessory or regenerated spleen. Repeat splenectomy may be indicated.

In the pregnant woman with a low platelet count, the differential diagnosis must include ITP versus preeclampsia. Once preeclampsia has been eliminated, steroids may be used to treat the ITP in the pregnant woman. Another concern is that the infant may have an increased risk of bleeding due to low platelet levels because the anti-platelet antibody can cross the placenta. Pregnant women with active ITP benefit from treatment with prednisone 20 to 30 mg per day 2 weeks before their expected date of delivery. At the time of labor, fetal venous scalp blood should be obtained to determine the platelet count of the infant. If the infant platelet count is less than 50,000/mm³, plans for a vaginal delivery should be stopped and an immediate cesarean section undertaken. If the infant is thrombocytopenic, prednisone 2 mg/kg should be given in the immediate neonatal period until the platelet count rises.

Other Immune Causes of Thrombocytopenia. Other immune etiologies for thrombocytopenia are systemic lupus erythematosus, Hodgkin's disease, non-Hodgkin's lymphoma, and Evan syndrome in which ITP is associated with an autoimmune hemolytic anemia. On occasion, patients have a significant drop in platelets 2 to 10 days after they have been transfused with whole blood. This problem affects primarily women over age 40 and produces low platelet counts (10,000/mm³). This process suggests exposure to other kinds of platelet antigens from previous transfusions or pregnancy. The platelets in the recent blood transfusions have generated an immune response. The administration of human γ-globulin intravenously and prednisone may be effective in preventing or resolving this problem.

Drug-induced immune problems may also occur as the result of administration of quinidine or quinine, heparin, and gold.

NONIMMUNOLOGIC CAUSES OF INCREASED PLATELET DESTRUCTION. Nonimmunologic mechanisms for increased platelet destruction include damaged endothelial cells that induce platelet aggregation, platelet-activating factors, increased thrombin levels, and intravascular coagulation with platelet consumption. More recently described phenomenona are thrombotic thrombocytopenic purpura (TTP) and adult hemolytic-uremic syndromes (HUS). These entities are difficult to distinguish, although they have five major hallmarks: (1) severe hemolytic anemia; (2) severe thrombocytopenia with shortened platelet survival and increased number of megakaryocytes; (3) fever; (4) CNS abnormalities and signs; and (5) renal disease that is much more significant in HUS patients than in TTP patients. TTP tends to occur more often in adults, usually with a median age of about 25 years, whereas the HUS is found more often in children and adolescents. Renal disease is much more severe in HUS, but TTP has more CNS complications.

Several mechanisms of disease have been proposed. One theory postulates endothelial damage with platelet activation, fibrin strand formation, followed by thrombocytopenia, and finally microangiopathic hemolysis. Causes of these syndromes include pregnancy, pre-eclampsia, drugs, infections such as Legionnaire's disease, toxigenic *Escherichia coli*, cancer, and anticancer drugs. It is a life-threatening illness with a mortality rate of 60 to 80 per cent. Fatal outcomes usually occur within 10 days of the onset of the illness. Principles of therapy include corticosteroids, use of antiplatelet drugs to inhibit aggregation, infusion of plasma and plasma exchange. Splenectomy has been used and on occasion has been remarkably successful.

Other causes of non-immunologic platelet destruction include disseminated intravascular coagulation and viral, parasitic, fungal, and bacterial infections. Specific illnesses are rubella, varicella, infectious mononucleosis, dengue fever, malaria, sepsis secondary to *E. coli* infection, hypothermia, massive transfusion secondary to bleeding, and pregnancy.

PLATELET SEQUESTRATION. Enlargement of the spleen predisposes to increased trapping of platelets. Normally, 20 to 30 per cent of the circulating platelets are confined to the spleen. With an enlarged spleen, 50 to 80 per cent of the total platelet number are sequestered in the spleen.

With hypersplenism the vascular bed increases and traps approximately 50 to 80 per cent of the total platelets, rendering the patient thrombocytopenic. In addition, survival time of platelets is reduced to about 2.5 days, and the bone marrow increases its output only 1.5 to 2.0 times instead of the usual sevenfold increase. The bone marrow apparently senses the total number of platelets available in the spleen *and* in the circulation and does not increase its production to correct the relative deficiency of platelets available to the circulation to stop hemorrhaging.

Diseases that can cause hypersplenism and thrombocytopenia are hemolytic anemias, hemoglobin C disease, hereditary spherocytosis, autoimmune hemolytic anemia, infections such as tuberculosis, connective tissue disease, infiltrative diseases of the spleen such as lymphoma, myeloproliferative diseases, Gaucher's disease, and congestive splenomegaly caused by cirrhosis, portal vein obstruction, or congestive heart failure. Management in this condition should be directed toward the process causing the enlarged spleen. Splenectomy is indicated only if it assists in the correction of the original disease process or if bleeding situations cannot be controlled adequately with platelet therapy.

Thrombocytosis

Platelet counts elevated above 500,000/mm³ are most often a reaction to another process. Platelet function is normal, and the likelihood of hemorrhage or thromboembolism does not increase even if the platelet count is higher than 1×10^6/mm³. Platelet counts may increase in response to cancers (particularly Hodgkin's disease), cessation of alcohol ingestion (which may have suppressed platelet production), infections such as osteomyelitis or tuberculosis, inflammatory diseases of the bowel, vasculitis, surgery, blood loss, or splenectomy for hemolytic anemia. No complications usually result from these elevated platelet counts, so no specific therapy is necessary.

Thrombocythemia

Platelet counts that increase autonomously in response to the myeloproliferative disorders are labeled essential thrombocythemia. Platelet counts in myeloproliferative disorders or essential thrombocythemia may range from 1×10^6 to 3×10^6/mm³. Here platelet function is usually abnormal, leading to the increased likelihood of hemorrhage and thromboembolism. The absolute platelet level does not accurately reflect a propensity to bleeding or the development of thrombotic episodes. Patients with polycythemia vera and elevated platelet counts may have itching and burning sensations in the extremities (fingers and toes). It can be relieved with aspirin or indomethacin in small doses. Asymptomatic patients can be managed with either alkylating agents or with hydroxyurea at a dose of

15 mg/kg per day. Hydroxyurea has the benefit of not predisposing to a secondary malignant disorder, but the WBC count must be monitored carefully. Aspirin may also be helpful in low therapeutic doses, such as one adult aspirin every other day. The use of these therapeutic agents is complicated and depends on the clinical condition, history, and symptoms of the patient with regard to hemorrhage or thrombotic phenomena.

HEMATOLOGIC MALIGNANCIES

Hematologic malignancies come from the unregulated proliferation of a pluripotent stem cell clone that suppresses normal marrow cell growth by using space and nutrients reserved for normal cell growth. It is characterized by growth that is unregulated and abnormally differentiated. Malignancies of the hematopoietic system are named for the cell type involved; for example, lymphocytic leukemia involves lymph cells, myeloid leukemias arises from myeloid stem cells, and lymphomas arise from lymphocytes. Until recently the mechanism for leukemia was thought to be unregulated, rapid replication of an abnormal tumor cell with no control or regulation. Current evidence suggests that normal marrow cells undergo cell division up until the myelocyte stage and then differentiate and mature into the circulation until they expire. In contrast, malignant cells found in myeloid leukemia differentiate poorly, retaining many immature characteristics, and do not lose the ability to undergo repeated cell division and multiplication once out of the marrow. Leukemic cells may in fact leave the marrow, enter different portions of the body, replicate themselves in the circulation or other organs, replicate again, and so on. Normal cells reach a point at which cell division no longer occurs, whereas malignant hematopoietic cells retain the capacity to continually divide and remain in an immature stage. Further evidence for this phenomenon suggests that normal myeloblasts are generated within 24 to 48 hours, whereas leukemic myeloblasts take 15 to 60 hours. Thus there is not a great deal of difference in the actual generation time. As the abnormal cells expand in number, they take over the bone marrow space and nutrients, excluding the normal series of RBCs, WBCs, and platelets, which gradually disappear, rendering the patient functionally aplastic. Approximately 2×10^{12} malignant leukemic cells can cause death. This number can be expressed as a weight of 1 to 2 kg of malignant cells occupying a volume of 1.7 liters. It takes approximately 10^9 leukemic cells for a leukemia to be detected. The difference between early detection at 10^9 and lethality at 10^{12} is only a 1000-fold difference.

The causes of hematologic malignancies are numerous and not totally known. RNA viruses may transform cells into malignancies, and ionizing radiation exposure can do likewise. Certain drugs, among them chloramphenicol and phenylbutazone, produce aplastic or hypoplastic marrow, which makes the patient more susceptible later on to leukemia. Cytogenic abnormalities are found in most leukemias, suggesting that either the result or the cause has something to do with chromosome abnormalities.

The diagnosis is made by finding immature and abnormal cells in the blood smear and malignant cells replacing normal components of the marrow. With acute myelogenous leukemia, cytoplasmic Auer rods occur, which are immature granules found in the myeloblasts. Leukemic cells from the myeloid series are myeloperoxidase-positive, and some lymphoid malignancies exhibit immunoglobulin patterns on the cell receptors that are specific for a malignant process. In addition, monoclonal antibodies to T and B lymphocytes and to myeloid cells may help establish the diagnosis as well.

Treatment

Treatment regimens in the past focused on inducing a remission, whereas treatment today focuses on cure by eliminating all the malignant cells. Such elimination can be accomplished in some situations by repeated cycles of chemotherapy and in others by bone marrow transplantation. Most chemotherapy is organized into four phases: (1) an induction phase to eliminate most detectable malignant cells; (2) a phase wherein several more courses of chemotherapy are added to reduce the abnormal cell population further; (3) a third phase consisting of repeated, intensive combinations of therapeutic agents while the patient is in clinical remission in order to destroy remaining malignant cells so they can no longer differentiate and reproduce; and (4) a maintenance phase that keeps any residual leukemic cells from multiplying and developing further.

Patients undergoing chemotherapy have multiple side effects, are subject to infection and bleeding, and must be supported to prevent these complications from occurring and becoming lethal. The patients must also be given psychological support during this long-term therapeutic journey. As malignant cells are destroyed, uric acid levels become elevated and are usually treated with allopurinol. Patients often require nutritional support, which can be done orally or parenterally with hyperalimentation. Because the specific treatment regimens change frequently with new data, this information is not discussed in detail here.

Therapy today focuses on bone marrow transplantation. This process replaces the abnormal bone marrow elements with new functional bone marrow, which takes over and produces all the normal elements of the blood from a new stem cell series. Autologous transplants are from the patients themselves; isogeneic transplants are from identical twins; and allogeneic transplants are from a histocompatible donor (most often a blood relative). Allogeneic transplants are the ones most likely to undergo rejection. Thus the immune response must be suppressed in order for the bone marrow transplant to "take" appropriately. The volume of bone marrow transplanted is approximately 750 ml. If the bone marrow is donated from a histocompatible donor, the recipient's bone marrow must be killed with radiation and alkalating or other chemotherapeutic agents. During this time the patient is aplastic and is susceptible to bleeding and severe infection. Prevention of rejection long term is usually accomplished with azathioprine and steroids. Autologous marrow from the patients themselves is used frequently when there is a hematologic malignancy, particularly for the lymphomas and acute leukemias. When the patient's marrow is obtained, the leukemic stem cells are killed using monoclonal antibodies or alkalating agents to kill the abnormal stem cells and not the normal stem cells. The treated marrow is then reinfused into the patient, and graft-versus-host disease is not a problem. A response, if successful, usually appears within 2 to 4 weeks—measured by an increase in the WBC count and the platelet count.

Chronic Myelogenous Leukemia

Chronic myelogenous or myelocytic leukemia (CML) arises from a malignant stem cell and produces a clone of myelogenous cells that have delayed maturation, decreased aging, and the capability for continuous cell division. Three phases of the disease occur: a chronic phase, an accelerated phase, and a blast crisis phase. About 90 to 95 per cent of the cases are positive for the Philadelphia chromosome, which is a reciprocal translocation involving chromosomes 9 and 22.

During the chronic phase of the disease, which generally lasts approximately 3 to 5 years, the patient is usually not particularly ill but has splenomegaly, intermittent weight loss, and hepatomegaly. The WBC count is markedly elevated (50,000 to 300,000/mm^3) with a normal maturation sequence from blasts through mature neutrophils. Anemia is mild to moderate, and platelets are usually more than adequate. Acute treatment of an elevated WBC count, which may cause thrombosis in patients in this stage, consists of leukopheresis or intravenous daunorubicin (or both) to acutely reduce the WBC count. During such treatment, the patient must be well hydrated and receive allopurinol to prevent hyperuricemia. Chronic therapy uses busulfan, which is an alkalating agent that reduces the WBC count but also has the potential to destroy normal stem cells and cause an aplastic marrow. Hydroxyurea is also effective in reducing

the WBC count. There is some evidence that it may delay the second and third phases. However, survival time is not any longer than with busulfan. Other treatments have been tried, and the most promising therapy for individuals under age 50 is an allogeneic bone marrow transplant in which total body irradiation combined with chemotherapeutic agents eliminates all or most of the malignant stem cells in the patient's marrow. This regimen works best when there is an HLA-identical sibling donor of bone marrow. Survival increases up to 9 to 12 years in 70 per cent of the cases.

The accelerated phase of the disease is characterized by increasing spleen and liver enlargement, more severe anemia, and decreasing platelet counts. The patient is more symptomatic, with systemic symptoms of weight loss, fevers, night sweats, and pain particularly related to extramedullary hematopoiesis. A blood count often demonstrates increased numbers of basophils, immature myeloid forms, and eosinophils. The blast phase simply induces an increase in the systemic symptoms, significant anemia, thrombocytopenia, and an increase in the peripheral blast count. The patients begin to look clinically as if they are having an acute myelogenous leukemia attack. Approximately one fourth of the patients with CML have what appears to be a lymphocytic blast crisis. Treatment of these two phases is much less successful. Hydroxyurea and busulfan may help decrease the WBC count but do not prolong survival; they simply buy time. Bone marrow transplantation is much less successful: Fewer than 25 per cent of patients are cured. Newer chemotherapeutic agents, as well as hydroxyurea and prednisone, may be helpful during this stage.

Acute Myeloblastic Leukemia

Acute myeloblastic leukemia (AML) is a rapidly progressive malignancy of a clone of stem cells of myeloid origin that can kill a patient within 1.5 to 3.0 months from the time of discovery if not treated. The primary form of AML arises from a transformed malignant stem cell, and the secondary form occurs in patients who have received chemotherapy particularly with alkalating agents. Patients treated with chemotherapy for Hodgkin's disease, multiple myeloma, ovarian cancer, and others are at increased risk for AML. Patients with AML are often discovered because of a profound infection with fever or the acute onset of a bleeding problem with petechiae or easy bruisability. Patients also relate symptoms of profound weakness, fatigue with exercise, dizziness on exertion, fever with and without infection, and bleeding diathesis. The physical examination may reveal enlarged lymph nodes, an enlarged spleen, hepatomegaly, and on occasion testicular, cutaneous or meningeal infiltration. Meningeal involvement occurs in about 7 to 10 per cent of patients, which is a much lower incidence than is seen among patients with acute lymphoblastic leukemia (more than a 40 per cent incidence). The diagnosis is established when the peripheral smear showing undifferientiating myeloid blasts is confirmed with a bone marrow examination in which malignant myeloblasts infiltrate and replace the entire bone marrow. The patients are functionally aplastic and subject to infection, hemorrhage, and profound anemia. A number of variants of AML have been described, most of which have chromosomal abnormalities.

Current therapy is moving dramatically toward bone marrow transplantation, particularly if the patient is less than 50 years old. Older patients are less likely to obtain a remission with chemotherapy but should be given a trial of induction anyway, even though it is expensive, time-consuming, and fraught with dangers of anemia, hemorrhagic complications, and infections. Once older patients have been induced into complete remission (which may last 18 to 24 months), bone marrow transplant may be considered, although 20 per cent of these patients remain in remission for up to 3 years. Some programs induce a remission in all patients and then offer younger patients (under age 50 to 60) a bone marrow transplantation from a matched allogeneic source or their own autologous bone marrow that has been treated. Unfortunately, 20 to 30 per cent of patients receiving a bone marrow transplant die of complications during the first year. Complications consist of fever from bacterial sepsis, infection of indwelling catheters, herpes or yeast infections, and opportunistic organisms infections. CNS leukemic infiltrates are treated with intrathecal methotrexate.

In patients with AML that occurs secondary to treatment of a prior malignancy, it is much more difficult to induce a complete remission, and the survival rate is poor. As many as 10 to 15 per cent of patients with Hodgkin's disease treated with alkalating agents may develop AML as long as 10 years after treatment has ceased. Abnormalities on chromosome 5 or 7 are usually associated with this therapy and the subsequent AML. Fewer than 40 per cent of the patients achieve a complete remission. Allogeneic bone marrow transplants are having greater success in eliminating evidence of the disease for a longer time than traditional chemotherapy and radiation.

Chronic Lymphocytic Leukemia

Most chronic lymphocytic leukemia (CLL) arises from a stem cell that normally produces B lymphocytes but in this situation undergoes malignant transformation. Approximately 5 per cent of CLL comes from a stem cell that would normally produce T lymphocytes. CLL, then, is a disease process in which malignant lymphocytes most often replace normal B lymphocytes, thereby inhibiting the production of normal immunoglobulins and causing impaired humoral defense mechanisms. It is interesting that although 25 per cent of patients with CLL have low immunoglobulin levels, 5 to 10 per cent may have elevated globulin levels similar to those found with plasma cell tumors.

Diagnosis

Patients with CLL demonstrate few systemic symptoms and are diagnosed by finding marked lymphocytosis on the blood smear, infiltrates of lymphocytes in the bone marrow, and an abnormal lymphomatous pattern in the biopsy specimens from lymph nodes. The bone marrow has focal replacement with a lymphocytic leukemic infiltrate that borders at times on the picture seen in a lymphoma. WBC counts are elevated because of the increased numbers of lymphocytes that apparently survive for extended periods. Prognostic factors relate to the degree of enlargement of the spleen and liver, how much marrow is replaced by lymphocytic infiltrates, the number and sites of nodal involvement, and the degree to which other cellular elements of the bone marrow have been crowded out causing anemia and thrombocytopenia. Poor prognostic factors are low γ-globulin levels (less than 700 mg/ml) and an absolute lymphocyte count in the peripheral blood of more than 60,000/mm^3.

Therapy

For patients who do not have widespread disease or significant systemic symptoms, the drug of choice is still chlorambucil at a dose of 0.1 mg/kg per day or on occasion cyclophosphamide at a dose of 2 mg/kg per day. However, some patients at early stages might be harmed by early treatment, and therapy should probably be withheld until there are systemic signs and symptoms along with anemia and thrombocytopenia of mild degree. Steroids are not helpful in this illness because they simply redistribute lymphocytes and do not destroy abnormal cells. If patients with this illness have an autoimmune hemolytic anemia, corticosteroids might be helpful. Infectious complications can be treated with antibiotics, but patients with low γ-globulin levels should be treated with intravenous IgG on a repetitive, every-3-week schedule. Splenectomy is indicated if there is a significantly enlarged, painful spleen, marked anemia secondary to hemolysis, and low platelet counts predictive of bleeding episodes. Morbidity is approximately 20 per cent with a mortality of 5 per cent so this surgery is reserved for those patients with significant disease involvement. Chronic systemic therapy should be withheld until there is evidence of progressive involvement of lymph nodes and infiltration of the bone marrow rendering the patient pancytopenic.

Acute Lymphoblastic Leukemia

Acute lymphoblastic leukemia (ALL) accounts for 10 to 15 per cent of all cases of acute leukemia in adults and a greater percentage in children. ALL is a high risk malignancy because the incidence of CNS involvement is approximately 40 per cent (much higher than that in AML). Findings suggestive of a poor prognosis are an age older than 30 years, blast count higher than 20,000/mm^3 in the peripheral blood, and a period of more than 4 weeks before remission begins.

Therapy consists of four agent chemotherapy programs designed to induce remission. Studies suggest that about 95 per cent of patients achieve a complete remission, and 5-year survival may be as high as 35 per cent. Bone marrow transplantation has been used, but may not be as successful as for other hematologic malignancies, although not enough data have been accumulated to study this treatment form versus others.

Personal and Family Care of Patients with Hematologic Malignancies

The family physician of a patient with a hematologic malignancy plays a vital role in honest, open discussions about the disease, its prognosis, and treatment options with the patient and family. The patient should always be given as much information as is known and should always be told first about the disease, its prognosis, treatment options, and so on. In many cases, this information must be discussed more than once because patients can absorb only a certain amount of emotionally charged information at any one time. Issues of pain control and continuing care of patients regardless of their decision to continue or stop treatment during the course of the illness must be brought up in an anticipatory fashion. Patients benefit from reassurance that their pain will be controlled using the best and most potent regimens available, and that despite the patient's choice of therapy or lack thereof the family physician will remain with them throughout the course of the illness.

The course of an illness, the patient's response to treatment, and the ultimate outcome are individualized features for each patient and each disease process. If the patient decides to terminate therapy, it should be discussed directly with the patient; the pressures and wishes of other family members must remain secondary to the patient's direct wishes. Patients must be given as much control and choice in their illness as possible, and several options can be made available to provide them with a sense of empowerment. Finally, death is an unpredictable event that may come sooner or later during the course of one of these illnesses. The family physician who has been with the patient throughout the illness is a crucial factor in the patient's dying and in the resolution of this event for the family. The family physician's presence at the bedside is crucial, important, and helpful to the entire therapeutic process.

SUGGESTED READINGS

Conley CL: Anemia: accurate diagnosis and appropriate therapy. Hosp Pract 4:57, 1984.

Kelley WN: Textbook of Internal Medicine, 2nd edition. Philadelphia, JB Lippincott, 1993.

Marsland DW, Wood M, Mayo F: A data bank for patient care, curriculum, and research in family practice. J Fam Pract 3: 25, 1976.

Rubenstein EH, Federman D: Scientific American Medicine. New York, Scientific American, 1993.

Wexler MM, Shapiro S, Mitchell A: Periconceptional folic acid exposure and risk of occurrent neural tube defects. JAMA 269:1257, 1993.

CHAPTER 46
URINARY TRACT DISORDERS

S. LANE BICKNELL, OSCAR McCALLUM,
and LUCIUS F. WRIGHT

Abnormalities of urination include complaints such as pain on urination (dysuria), frequency, urgency, incontinence, hesitancy, hematuria, and pneumaturia. Definitions of these disorders follow.

Dysuria: Pain on urination is most frequently caused by acute or chronic infections of the lower urinary tract including infection of the urethra, bladder, and prostate gland in men and the bladder and periurethral area with associated vaginitis and vulvitis in women.

Frequency: Frequency is a relative phenomenon. It is necessary to inquire into the actual number of urinations as well as the patient's subjective assessment. Small-volume frequency may be due to outflow obstruction with overflow phenomenon, as is seen in the individual with benign prostatic hypertrophy. The presence of frequency, urgency, and dysuria with small volume voidings should be considered to indicate a bladder inflammation until proved otherwise.

Nocturia: Nocturia, frequent urination at night interrupting sleep, is usually due to outflow obstruction, diabetes mellitus, or inflammatory conditions of the bladder.

Urgency: Urgency, the immediate need to void, is most often caused by bladder inflammation. Incontinence associated with urgency indicates urinary infection, neurogenic etiologies, or outflow tract obstruction.

Polyuria: True polyuria is increased frequency with increased volume, such as occurs with diabetes mellitus and diabetes insipidus.

Incontinence: Incontinence is loss of urinary control per urethra; it is differentiated from loss of urine from a point other than the urethra (e.g., a fistula), which should be termed leakage. Bladder abnormalities causing incontinence include infection, chronic outflow tract obstruction, extrinsic and intrinsic masses, and interstitial cystitis. Urethral obstruction can be caused by strictures, congenital urethral valves (usually found during childhood), and benign prostatic hypertrophy.

Hesitancy: Hesitancy, waiting for the stream to start, is usually indicative of bladder outlet obstruction and is associated with straining.

Retention: Retention, total or partial inability to empty the bladder with voiding, is found most frequently with outlet obstruction, neurogenic injury, and diabetes mellitus.

Hematuria: Hematuria, gross or microscopic urinary bleeding, may be initial, total, or terminal. It may or may not be associated with pain. Causes of hematuria are covered separately.

Pneumaturia: Pnematuria, air in the urine, is due to enterovesical fistula and is often accompanied by vegetable particulate matter.

SYMPTOMS

Flank Pain

Urologic causes of flank pain include obstruction, infection, and vascular occlusion. The patient with flank pain needs careful attention and evaluation, as both the urologic and nonurologic causes are clinically significant.

Obstruction

Ureterolithiasis is the most common cause of obstruction. Pain with ureteral obstruction is due to the stretching of the renal capsule by edema and swelling. The pain of ureterolithiasis is sudden, unilateral, and colicky in pattern. The pain radiates from the costovertebral angle toward the inguinal ligament and into the scrotum or labia majora and is severe. The patient is usually active and unable to sit or lie quietly (unlike those with severe pain caused by the nonurologic causes of flank pain). There may be associated sweating and nausea with vomiting.

Infection

Flank pain and pyuria (especially with white blood cell casts), chills, fever, and signs of systemic infection point to pyelonephritis. Patients with pyelonephritis may have obstruction causing their infection. The pain of pyelonephritis is usually unilateral. It may radiate from the costovertebral angle toward the epigastric area. Pyelonephritis in children under the age of 10 may not be evidenced by genitourinary tract symptoms.

Thrombosis

Renal vein thrombosis may mimic pyelonephritis or ureterolithiasis. If obstruction is acute and extensive, hematuria, flank pain, fever, and leukocytosis develop rapidly. Findings that differentiate this condition from infection or stones include gross hematuria, massive proteinuria, edema of the lower extremities, and oliguric renal failure. A blood clot from the renal vein and the inferior vena cava may propagate centrally with pulmonary embolization. Hypertension is usually not noted with renal vein thrombosis. Tumor thrombus may be seen with renal cell carcinoma. Thrombosis can also occur spontaneously in an infant who has become severely dehydrated secondary to diarrheal disease. Intravenous pyelography demonstrates a persistent nephrogram effect. Renal venogram in the hands of an experienced venographer usually yields the diagnosis. Ultrasonography or computed tomography (CT) are noninvasive means to demonstrate renal vein thrombosis.

Scrotal Pain

Clinical evaluation of the patient with scrotal pain begins with the history. Pain associated with a mass is helpful, as is a recent history of trauma, prostatitis, or mumps.

Torsion

Torsion of the testes (actually torsion of the spermatic cord) was first described in 1840. It is a condition *not* to be misdiagnosed. Torsion usually occurs before the age of 20. There are two categories of testicular torsion. Torsion occurring outside the tunica vaginalis tends to occur before the first birthday. It is usually found by a physician's examination in the nursery or as an incidental finding reported by the parent. This extravaginal torsion results in scrotal erythema and swelling and a firm, swollen mass palpable within the sac.

The other common time for torsion of the spermatic cord to occur is around puberty. This torsion occurs inside the tunica vaginalis. There is the sudden onset of pain with a firm, tender mass palpable in the scrotum. The pain may be so intense that it is associated with nausea and vomiting. There may be no history on antecedent trauma, although torsion can cause acute testicular pain and swelling similar to that due to trauma or intrascotal infection. A history of severe testicular pain with spontaneous remission should alert the physician to the possibility of torsion. One useful clinical tool is elevation of the involved testis with the patient in the upright position. This maneuver generally causes relief of the pain of epididymitis but exacerbates the pain due to torsion.

With torsion, palpation above the testes often demonstrates a cord twisted and thickened beyond its normal anatomic dimensions. The involved testicle may be elevated and retracted within the scrotum because of cord shortening. With intravaginal torsion (at puberty), the cremasteric muscles contract to cause abrupt twisting of the spermatic cord.

The appendix testes and the appendix epididymis (both called the hydatid of Morgagni) can torque to cause symptoms similar to torsion of the spermatic cord. Such symptoms are characterized by sudden onset and point tenderness. A localized ecchymosis may be noted on the scrotal sac. Frequently, a secondary hydrocele forms, making palpation of scrotal contents difficult.

Bacterial Infection

Epididymitis and epididymo-orchitis are bacterial infections of the contents of the scrotal sac and cause intense scrotal pain. These patients may have a history of antecedent urethritis. The first genitourinary symptom may be inguinal soreness, but the epididymis rapidly becomes exquisitely tender to palpation. With epididymitis, the testis is of normal size and consistency and is easily palpated as being anterior to the swollen, tender epididymis. Epididymitis may progress to epididymo-orchitis within 1 to 2 days, with the development of testicular swelling three to four times normal size. Follow-up examination after the resolution of these is definitely indicated to check for hidden malignancy, as these conditions may be the presenting finding in testicular carcinoma.

The sudden onset on testicular pain in an individual younger than age 20 requires urgent urologic consultation. Epididymitis in a patient younger than 20 is rare, and the diagnosis probably should not be made without urologic consultation. It is sometimes difficult for even the most experienced clinician to distinguish torsion from epididymitis or epididymo-orchitis on clinical grounds, and surgical exploration is often necessary.

Viral Infection

Orchitis usually follows a systemic viral infection. Within 7 to 10 days after the beginning of mumps parotitis, the testes may become swollen and uncomfortable. Orchitis rarely causes pain as severe as epididymitis or epididymo-orchitis. The discomfort associated with orchitis is due to swelling and edema of the testes, which are enclosed in the relatively nondistensible tunica albuginea. Mumps orchitis is usually unilateral. Occasionally, parotitis is absent; however, an elevated serum amylase indicates that mumps is the cause.

Tumors

Testicular cancers may present with pain if there is a sudden hemorrhage into the malignancy, causing testicular swelling. This disorder may be difficult to differentiate from epididymitis or epididymo-orchitis.

Abdominal Pain

Abdominal pain associated with genitourinary disorders may be due to infection, obstruction, or tumor. More commonly, pain is suprapubic and associated with bladder dysfunction (i.e., inflammation or retention). Renal or ureteral obstruction may cause referred pain to the ipsilateral lower quadrant or suprapubic area. Recurrent upper quadrant pain may be secondary to ureteropelvic junction obstruction or to renal calculi. Mild, dull upper quadrant pain may be associated with renal tumor.

Perineal Pain

Perineal pain is often due to acute or chronic prostatitis. The male patient claims it feels like "sitting on a tennis ball". There is usually low back pain as well. Female patients with cystitis or vaginitis may complain of perineal discomfort, but it is rarely the presenting complaint. Invasive bladder tumors may be associated with perineal pain; but again, other signs or symptoms generally dominate.

PHYSICAL EXAMINATION

1. *Kidneys:* Normal kidneys are rarely palpable. Lower pole renal tumors and cysts are palpable unless the patient is obese. It is helpful to elevate the flank with one hand while palpating with the other as the patient takes a deep breath. Renal masses are not tender unless associated with obstruction or infection. A tender mass is found with perirenal abscess.

2. *Ureter:* The ureter is not palpable. Tenderness may be noted with an acutely obstructing stone, but there is no associated rebound tenderness because peritoneal irritation is absent.

3. *Bladder:* The empty bladder is not palpable, but there may be tenderness in the suprapubic area on bimanual examination. When the bladder is distended, it presents as a midline, smooth, firm mass without tenderness. Manual pressure increases the desire to void and causes discomfort when there is urinary retention.

4. *Penis:* The penile shaft should be palpated for masses, localized induration (Peyronie's disease), and skin lesions. The foreskin should be retracted to examine the glans.

5. *Urethra:* The male urethra should be palpated from perineum to meatus. Areas of fibrosis (stricture), fistula, or abscess can be discovered. Urethral discharge can be seen by "stripping" the urethra. All discharges should be examined microscopically. The female urethra should be evaluated during the pelvic examination. The size and pliability of the meatus should be noted. Pressure on a urethral mass may cause pus to issue from the meatus, indicating a urethral diverticulum.

6. *Scrotum and contents:* The scrotal skin may exhibit cysts or excoriation (associated with incontinence). The epididymis is situated posterolaterally on the testis beginning superiorly with the head of the epididymis and ending inferiorly where it becomes continuous with the vas. Cord structures are easily palpable, with the vas being most prominent. It is helpful to evaluate the testicle and surrounding area by holding the cord firmly with one hand while palpating with the other. Men should be taught self-examination.

7. *Prostate:* Examination of the prostate requires the patient to bend over the examining table with his elbows and forearms on the table. The gloved examining finger should be well lubricated. Gentle pressure on the anus with the examining finger relaxes the sphincter and allows more comfortable examination for the patient.

The examination is started at the base and continued down each lateral border. The borders should be smooth and well defined. The size of the gland is estimated next (a Foley balloon filled with 30 mL of water serves as the baseline). The prostate should be symmetric from the midline laterally. Firmness should be uniform and without hardness or nodularity.

SCROTAL MASSES

Scrotal masses may be hard or soft. Hard masses include epididymitis, epididymo-orchitis, testicular torsions, torsion of the appendix testis, tuberculous epididymitis, post-traumatic hematocele formation, tumors of the spermatic cord, and testicular tumors. Soft masses include hydroceles, spermatoceles, varicoceles, indirect inguinal hernias, lipoma, and gummas of the cord.

Tumor

Intrascrotal malignancies are usually firm to hard, nontender masses that do not transilluminate. Most cancers present as painless, heavy feelings of increased tissue mass that are often found by the patient during manipulation of the scrotum during bathing. The presence of a suspicious testicular mass necessitates referral for evaluation, including possible exploration and biopsy.

Tumors of the spermatic cord are rare. They are most frequently benign lesions, but a diagnosis is possible only by tissue examination after removal by radical orchiectomy.

Hydrocele

Hydrocele is the most frequent soft mass found in the scrotum and may occur at any age. Early in life, communicating hydroceles develop from a patent processus vaginalis, which connects the tunica vaginalis to the peritoneal cavity. A free flow of fluid into the scrotal sac causes the hydrocele, which disappears when the patient lies down. Surgical repair may be necessary after the first year of life.

The more common noncommunicating hydrocele is an accumulation of fluid between the visceral and parietal layers of the tunica vaginalis, usually anterior to the testes. Except in the rare instance of a thickened tunica vaginalis, hydroceles always transilluminate. They are smooth and nontender unless associated with an inflammatory process or malignancy. Noncommunicating hydroceles may be due to lymphatic obstruction and may be either post-traumatic, postinfectious, infectious, or malignant in origin. They may be confused with scrotal hernia; however, palpation of a normal cord above the hydrocele makes this differentiation easy.

Hernia

Indirect inguinal hernias may present as scrotal masses and may even transilluminate similar to a hydrocele. The patient may present with the signs and symptoms of intestinal obstruction or simply with a nontender mass in the scrotum. A normal testis and epididymis in these individuals are usually easily palpated. The mass extends from the external inguinal ring into the scrotum. Bowel sounds may be heard on auscultation of the scrotum. A plain film of the lower abdomen may show dilated loops of small bowel inside the hernia sac. Irreducible scrotal hernias necessitate immediate surgical consultation because of the possibility of obstruction, incarceration, and strangulation.

Varicocele

Varicoceles are composed of dilated, tortuous, and redundant veins within the cord and are due to incompetent venous valves. Variococeles occur much more commonly on the left side than the right because of the acute angle the left spermatic vein makes when entering the renal vein. The right spermatic vein empties directly into the inferior vena cava. Sudden development of a varicocele should make the physician concerned about the possibility of retroperitoneal tumors or (in the case of left-side varicocele) obstruction from a renal vein tumor. Varicoceles are usually nontender and chronic and frequently disappear when the patient is supine. The diagnosis of a varicocele is made by palpation, and they are typically described as "a bag of worms." Unless associated with infertility, they have no other clinical consequence. Surgical correction of the varicocele may be attempted when fertility is in question.

Spermatocele

Spermatoceles are retention cysts of the epididymis or the rete testes. They may transilluminate and are nontender and smooth. They may be differentiated from hydroceles, as they are usually palpated as distinct from the testes. They are found in the upper portion of the junction between the testes and the epididymis.

Hematocele

Hematoceles are post-traumatic collections of blood inside the tunica vaginalis. They may be associated with testicular rupture. If a hard mass persists after the acute process is resolved, testicular cancer must be considered a possibility.

PENILE LESIONS

Cutaneous lesions of the external genitalia in male patients gain the attention of both patient and physician because of the possibility of venereal or malignant causes. Referral and possible biopsy are indicated if the diagnosis is not readily apparent or if the lesion fails to heal within 2 to 4 weeks.

Balanitis

Inflammatory lesions of the external genitalia include bacterial and viral infections and cutaneous mycoses. Balanitis and balanoposthitis are specific cutaneous infections of the external genitalia. Balanitis is an inflammation of the glans penis and is generally seen only in uncircumcised individuals. It is an intertriginous syndrome (i.e., a condition where apposed damp areas of skin develop localized inflammation). Such infection is usually due to poor personal hygiene. Occasionally, secondary infections including those due bacteria and fungi, can complicate this picture. Balanoposthitis is the extension of balinitis to the undersurface of the foreskin.

The treatment of both these conditions is essentially the same, that is, appropriate hygiene. Steroid creams may be used to decrease inflammation. The use of topical preparations containing steroid, antifungal, and antibacterial agents is indicated if secondary infection is a problem.

Syphilis

Solitary painless ulcers on the external genitalia are assumed to be primary chancres of syphilis until proved otherwise. The lesion may range from pinhead size to 0.5 inch or larger. The ulcer has a clean base and sharp borders, and usually there is a nontender inguinal adenopathy. The incubation from exposure to chancre formation is usually 3 to 6 weeks.

Chancroid

A bacterial infection that usually results in multiple ulcerations, chancroid becomes more infected and the lesions appear shaggier than leutic chancres. Extremely tender inguinal adenopathy occurs with this condition. Purulent adenopathy may be present. Darkfield examination is necessary to differentiate syphilis from chancroid.

Warts

Condyloma accuminata (warts) may occur anywhere on the external genitalia. In women they are seen on the labia majora and minora and the vagina mucosa. They are of viral etiology and are "heaped-up" (cauliflower)-appearing lesions. They are venereal in origin. Incubation may be from a few weeks to as much as a year, making the lesions particularly difficult to treat. Continuing appearance of new lesions may be due to incubating virus not seen during earlier examinations or to reinfection by contact with a sexual partner who has the disease. Treatment of the male patient includes painting the warts with podophyllin in benzoin. The patient should wash the medication off within 1 to 2 hours lest normal tissue be destroyed along with the warts. Repeated applications may be necessary. Lesions within the urethra should not be treated with podophyllin, as these lesions tend to heal by scar formation and a urethral stricture might ensue. Cystoscopic examination and fulguration of the base is necessary in this situation. Carbon dioxide lasering is a more effective treatment but should only be done by physicians experienced in the use of lasers.

Women with genital condyloma should be referred to a gynecologist.

Tumor

Penile cancer is rare. The reader is referred to the section on penile cancers for further discussion. Conditions such as erythroplasia of Queyrat and Bowen's disease are considered premalignant, and referral is indicated.

Phimosis

Phimosis and paraphimosis are seen in uncircumcised men and may cause considerable difficulty. With phimosis, the penile foreskin cannot be retracted because of adhesions of the foreskin to the underlying glans (balanoposthitis). Treatment is circumcision. Paraphimosis results when a retracted foreskin cannot be reduced over the glans. It results in edema of the glans, making reduction even more difficult. If untreated, vascular insufficiency of the glans may result. Reduction of the foreskin may be attempted in the physician's office; if unsuccessful, immediate referral is necessary. If reduction is accomplished, circumcision is indicated when the inflammatory response has resolved.

URINALYSIS

Urinalysis is the least expensive, most available, most significantly sensitive test used by clinicians for evaluating diseases of the genitourinary system. Urinalysis, however, is only as good as the collection technique used for procuring the sample and the scrupulousness with which the test is performed. A clean-catch specimen is recommended for urinalysis and for bacteriologic culture.

1. *Appearance:* Normal, freshly voided urine is transparent. Bile may cause brown urine, blood or myoglobin red or rust-colored urine, and porphyrins a port-wine color upon standing in natural light. Various foods or medicines may cause abnormal urine colors, for example, reddish-orange after rifampin or phenazopyridine (Pyridium), a reddish color after beet ingestion, and blue-green urine after ingestion of methylene blue.

2. *Concentration:* The specific gravity of the urine measures tubular concentrating function. Random urine samples do not give an accurate reflection of this capability. An early morning voided urine, especially with some degree of dehydration provides the best and simplest assessment of concentrating ability.

3. *pH:* The pH of normal urine is somewhat acidic (6.0) An alkaline pH may indicate infection by urea-splitting organisms (usually *Proteus* and sometimes *Pseudomonas*) or a systemic metabolic or respiratory alkalosis.

4. *Glucose:* Dipsticks with test materials impregnated with glucose oxidase are best for detecting glucose in the urine. A positive test indicates significant amounts of urinary glucose. False-negative tests may result from the ingestion of large amounts of ascorbic acid, which inhibits the glucose oxidase reaction. Other tests measure reducing substances, which include a variety of materials, including salicylates, dextran, large amounts of penicillin, cephalosporin or streptomycin, excessive urate levels, and pentose sugars.

5. *Ketones:* Ketones in the blood result in a positive acetone test on urinalysis. It occurs with

diabetic ketoacidosis, starvation, fasting, methanol poisoning, and viral gastroenteritis with decreased oral intake.

6. *Nitrates:* A positive nitrate test evidences a possible urinary tract infection. The presence of phenazopyridine gives a false positive result.

7. *Sediment:* Urine sediment is examined for cells, casts, and bacteria. White blood cells (WBCs) or bacteria on the unspun sediment must be considered significant and indicative of genitourinary pathology.

8. *Pyuria:* Inflammation of the genitourinary system is indicated by pyuria. Fewer than four WBCs per high-powered filed in a spun sediment is within normal limits. The presence of pyuria without bacteruria may indicate interstitial nephritis or renal tuberculosis.

9. *Casts:* Casts may or may not indicate significant renal disease. These casts are mostly of the narrow hyaline type. Casts are molds of renal tubular lumen produced by the precipitation of protein. WBC casts unequivocably place the disease in the kidney, indicating a tubulointerstitial abnormality including but not limited to pyelonephritis. Granular casts may precipitate after exercise and during fever. Red blood cell (RBC) casts are pathognomonic for glomerulonephritis.

10. *Crystalluria:* Except when due to elevated levels of cystine, uric acid, or sulfonamide in the urine, crystalluria deserves little attention.

IMAGING

Imaging of the genitourinary system continues to be vital for evaluation of that system.

Intravenous Urography (Intravenous Pyelography)

Intravenous pyelography (IVP) occupies the basic position when imaging the genitourinary system. It displays not only the anatomy but also to some extent the functional integrity of that system.

Ultrasonography

Although ultrasonography offers little in terms of demonstrating functional activity, it is an important noninvasive (Pollack, 1992) study for differentiating cystic from solid masses. It has a prominent role in evaluating prostatic size and postvoiding residual urine volume. It allows more precise biopsying of the prostate to detect (Lee, 1989) cancer and can aid in local staging. Scrotal ultrasonography can differentiate solid from cystic testicular masses.

Nuclear Scanning

Bone scans are almost routinely done when evaluating urologic malignancies for evidence of metastasis. Renal scans give information concerning function, perfusion, and obstruction; and they therefore aid in decisions about surgical versus medical management. Renal scans have an indispensible role in the postoperative follow-up of renal transplants. Radionuclide cystograms of children allow evaluation of vesicoureteral reflux with minimal exposure to x-rays.

Computed Tomography

Computed tomography (CT) of the abdomen has important clinical application when evaluating renal masses. It is often useful for defining the level of urinary obstruction. It is sometimes helpful for finding enlarged (more than 1 cm) lymph nodes, aortic aneurysms, and other retroperitoneal diseases.

Retrograde Pyelography

Retrograde pyelograms are most frequently used to evaluate the genitourinary system in patients who are allergic to intravenous contrast media and those in whom the IVP has not provided adequate delineation of the genitourinary system. Cystoscopic examination is required to perform retrograde pyelography.

Antegrade Pyelography

Antegrade pyelograms are done via the percutaneous route by means of a Chiba (skinny) needle. They are usually considered when retrograde pyelography has been unsuccessful. They are routinely done prior to stone manipulation via the percutaneous route.

Cystography

Instillation of contrast medium into the bladder is useful for delineating the presence and extent of bladder injury after trauma and may aid in the decision between operative and conservative management. Intraperitoneal extravasation mandates operative management, whereas extraperitoneal extravasation may allow simply catheter drainage. Voiding cystograms allow demonstration of vesicoureteral reflux and urethral abnormalities, such as valves.

Magnetic Resonance Imaging

The present state of magnetic resonance imaging (MRI) and its expense offers no advantage over more conventional imaging studies and is not recommended at this time.

HEMATURIA

The presence of more than two RBCs per high-powered field in the clean-voided specimen of males and nonmenstruating females and in the catheterized specimen of menstruating females is a significant finding in need of evaluation. Patients with asymptomatic hematuria, documented with two specimens, have a high incidence of significant pathology of the genitourinary system. Hematuria is often the first sign of a significant systemic disease (e.g., Goodpasture syndrome, polyarteritis nodosa, infectious endocarditis, lupus erythematosus, and Henoch-Schönlein purpura). The only situation in which a patient with hematuria does not merit full and total evaluation is probably the first or second episode of acute hemorrhagic cystitis in a female under the age of 40. The differential diagnoses for gross and microscopic hematuria are shown in Tables 46–1 and 46–2. Table 46–3 lists the causes of gross hematuria by major disease categories.

TABLE 46–1. DIAGNOSIS IN 1000 CASES OF GROSS HEMATURIA

Diagnosis	Patients (%)
Kidneys	15.0
Tumor	3.5
Infection	3.0
Calculus	2.7
Trauma	2.0
Obstruction	1.5
Others	2.3
Ureters	6.5
Calculus	5.3
Tumor	0.7
Others	0.5
Bladder	39.5
Infection	22.0
Tumor	14.9
Others	2.6
Prostate	23.6
Benign hyperplasia	12.5
Infection	9.0
Tumor	2.1
Urethra	4.3
Stricture	1.7
Calculus	1.3
Others	1.3
Essential hematuria	8.5

From Lee LW, Davis E, Jr,: Gross urinary hemorrhage: A symptom not a disease. JAMA 153:783, 1953. Copyright 1953, American Medical Association.

TABLE 46–2. DIAGNOSES FOR 500 CASES OF ASYMPTOMATIC MICROSCOPIC HEMATURIA

Diagnosis	Patients (%)
Kidneys	6.2
Calculus	3.4
Cyst	1.2
Hydronephrosis	0.6
Tumor	0.4
Others	0.6
Ureters	0.8
Calculus	0.4
Ureterocele	0.4
Bladder	8.6
Infection	6.6
Tumor	1.8
Others	0.2
Prostate	23.6
Benign hyperplasia	23.6
Urethra	23.4
Infection	21.2
Calculus	1.8
Others	0.4
Essential hematuria	44.0

From Greene LF, O'Shaugnessy EJ Jr, Hendricks ED: Study of five hundred patients with asymptomac microhematuria. JAMA 161:610, 1956, with permission. Copyright 1956, American Medical Association.

Evaluation

Subjective information during evaluation of the patient with hematuria involves inquiry into the presence of trauma and, if trauma is absent, the presence or absence of pain associated with blood in the urine. Hematuria associated with trauma to the upper abdomen, back, lower thorax, or especially the flank areas requires prompt evaluation. The absence of hematuria does not eliminate significant trauma to the kidney. If trauma is suspected, infusion pyelography is indicated. Nonvisualization of the kidney on IVP in an individual suspected of trauma to the kidneys, with or without hematuria, is assumed to be an interruption of the renal blood supply and requires immediate referral. The other situation requiring immediate referral is extravasation of dye into the perinephric space, which is indicative of renal rupture or lacer-

TABLE 46–3. CAUSES OF GROSS HEMATURIA BY MAJOR DISEASE CATEGORIES

Category	No.	%
Trauma	2	1.8
Stones	15	13.5
Neoplasia	46	41.8
Infection and inflammation	29	26.4
Congenital	4	3.6
Unknown and miscellaneous	14	12.7

From Carter WC, Rous SN: Gross hematuria in 110 adult urologic hospital patients. Urology 18:342, 1981, with permission.

ation. Bladder integrity in the patient with suspected trauma to the genitourinary system can be evaluated at the completion of the IVP, or it may be done by fluid cystography through an indwelling Foley catheter. Fracture of the pubis in the male patient may result in disruption of the urethra, with resultant gross blood dripping from the urethral meatus. Bladder catheterization may be impossible and should not be attempted.

Pain associated with hematuria may indicate nephrolithiasis, renal tumor, renal vein thrombosis, or renal artery embolism. Painful hematuria associated with suprapubic discomfort or dysuria (or both) is more indicative of hemorrhagic cystitis, bladder stones, or prostatic infections.

Painless hematuria in children is considered to be due to a glomerular lesion until proved otherwise. In addition to childhood glomerulopathies, one must consider polycystic renal disease, sickle cell disease, porphyria, vitamin C deficiency (scurvy), and bleeding dyscrasia. If the mother reports blood on the child's diaper after urination, an examination of the genitalia usually reveals irritation of the urethral meatus (meatitis). Hematuria is a late finding in patients with a Wilms tumor.

Hematuria in adults under age 40 usually indicates genitourinary infection; in adults older than 40 it is frequently indicative of a bladder tumor. In the elderly population, stone disease and inflammatory disease are secondary considerations. Hematuria in men older than 60 years is commonly due to prostatic obstruction (benign or malignant), bladder stones, or cancer. Hematuria in women older than 60 years is consistent with a bladder malignancy.

Between 20 and 40 per cent of patients with renal cancer present with gross hematuria and flank pain as their chief complaints. Bladder cancer causes episodic, gross, total hematuria (see below) that is usually painless. Nonmalignant causes of painless hematuria in adults include vasculitides of the kidneys (polyarteritis nodosa), infectious endocarditis, systemic lupus erythematosus, or renal parenchymal infections such as are seen with syphilis or tuberculosis. Hematuria associated with fever, rash, or joint pain may be due to an underlying systemic connective tissue disorder. Iatrogenic causes of hematuria include long-term bladder catheterization and the prescription of anticoagulants, salicylates, or both.

Objective examination of the patient with hematuria must involve evaluation for other signs of systemic disease, including fever, elevated blood pressure, skin rashes, arthritis, pericarditis, and endocarditis. Abdominal examination should be done carefully to evaluate for enlargement of the kidneys, liver, or spleen. A prostate examination in the male patient and a pelvic examination in the female patient are essential.

Laboratory evaluation begins with an appropriately collected and examined urine sample. A urine culture should be done; and if tuberculosis is suspected, a culture for acid-fast bacilli is indicated. The *three-glass-test* may be used to check for the source of bleeding. Initial hematuria (first glass) may be indicative of a urethral lesion such as a foreign body, urethritis, or cancer. Terminal hematuria (third glass) requires the sample from the posterior urethra and bladder neck. Blood in this specimen may come from inflammatory lesions in these areas or from the prostate. Total hematuria (all glasses) is associated with lesions such as cancer and tuberculosis above the level of the bladder neck. The blood has mixed in the urine prior to voiding and is therefore present in all samples. The three-glass test is only a guide and is not specific for localizing the site of genitourinary bleeding.

Pseudohematuria occurs when the voided urine appears to contain blood but does not. Causes include the use of phenolphthalein laxatives, phenazopyridine, phenothiazines, and rifampin. Other causes include the presence of myoglobin (after vigorous exercise or crush injury), hemoglobin in the urine (after intravascular hemolysis), or porphyria. The ingestion of beets or rhubarb can cause urinary discoloration similar to hematuria.

False-positive tests for blood in the urine can be seen when vaginal bleeding contaminates a "clean voided" specimen obtained from a menstruating female. Such situations necessitate a catheterized specimen to rule out urinary tract bleeding. Hematuria is seen often in patients on anticoagulation agents. Genitourinary bleeding secondary to anticoagulant medication, however, should not be diagnosed until a complete urologic evaluation is completed because the presence of tumors in the genitourinary system may be unmasked by these medications.

False-negative tests for hematuria may occur when the urine specimen demonstrates a low specific gravity or is permitted to stand unrefrigerated for more than one-half hour before analysis. The resulting lysis of RBCs and release of free hemoglobin into the specimen may lead the clinician to wrongly diagnose the patient's problem as hemoglobinuria rather than hematuria.

Renal function should be assessed by creatinine clearance and 24-hour urinary protein determination. The presence of more than 1 gram of protein per day associated with hematuria points to a glomerular lesion. During renal colic, the urine should be strained to determine the presence of calculi. Chemical analysis of the stones may guide therapy aimed at preventing recurrences. Cytologic examinations on urine sediments to evaluate for neoplasia are recommended for individuals more than 40 years old.

A kidneys and upper bladder (KUB) film may identify calcified ureteral or renal stones and determines renal size. In the absence of myeloma or diabetic renal disease, an IVP should be done.

Nephrotomography, angiography, renal ultrasonography, or CT scanning with contrast may be necessary to evaluate further an abnormal IVP after renal trauma or after the discovery of an intrarenal mass. Angiography also may be indicated for the diagnosis of certain suspected vasculitidies (e.g., polyarteritis nodosa) or arteriovenous malformations.

If a systemic connective tissue disorder is suspected, immunologic evaluations ought to be performed, including tests for antinuclear antibody (ANA), anti-DNA, and serum complement, and a lupus erythematosus (LE) cell preparation. If the diagnosis is not evident at the completion of this evaluation, referral is indicated.

Asymptomatic Proteinuria

In healthy individuals the anatomic structure of the glomerulus serves to keep plasma proteins from appearing in the glomerular filtrate, and any molecules that do escape the sieving action are usually taken up and catabolized in the proximal tubule. Thus the normal urine protein excretion of approximately 150 mg/day represents protein mainly of tubular and lower urinary tract origin. In routine practice, the presence of proteinuria depends on dipstick testing of freshly voided urine. It is important to recognize that this approach is qualitative, not quantitative. Proteinuria may be reported for highly concentrated urine specimens that is actually physiologic proteinuria. Large amounts of blood may also cause the dipstick test to show a positive result for proteinuria when in fact there is little nonblood protein in the urine. Many processes, such as exercise or fever, may cause a transient disruption of the filtration barriers, causing an increase in quantitative protein excretion. Because transient proteinuria is rarely significant, the approach to the patient with a positive dipstick test for protein begins with an estimate of its persistence or recurrence followed by determination of the quantity of protein being excreted.

Proteinuria may be detected in the asymptomatic patient. In such cases, special attention should be placed on determining the presence of hypertension, signs of systemic disease, especially diabetes, and the presence of edema. Protein excretion should be done quantitated in all patients. Collecting 24 hour urine samples is cumbersome, so a variety of short-cut methods have been developed, although none has proved any more reliable. For all patients collecting a 24 hour urine specimen, measurement of urinary creatinine excretion is desirable, even when the creatinine clearance test is not needed. Healthy adult men excrete 20 to 25 mg of creatinine per kilogram of body weight per day, and healthy women excrete 15 to 20 mg/kg/day. If urinary creatinine excretion is determined routinely, it is possible to ensure that adequate urine collections have been obtained.

Most patients with asymptomatic proteinuria have less than 3 gm of protein per day in their urine, have normal renal function, and have no hypertension or systemic disease. Invasive testing such as renal biopsy is rarely indicated in such individuals.

Orthostatic proteinuria is a clinical syndrome that is relatively common in adolescents: Their protein excretion is increased, but only while they are upright. Thus in young patients determined to have significant proteinuria, it is desirable to obtain a "split" collection: The patient first stays in bed for 12 hours and collects urine without getting up (the "recumbent" specimen) and then collects a second specimen for the following 12 hours while staying upright, out of bed (the "upright" collection). If all the protein is obtained in the "upright" specimen, the patient is categorized as having orthostatic proteinuria. Renal biopsy in such patients rarely discloses significant abnormalities, and the long-term prognosis is excellent (Springberg et al., 1982). No therapy is needed, and the patient can be reassured.

URINARY TRACT INFECTIONS

Urinary tract infections (UTIs) are among the most common problems encountered by primary care physicians. They can range from simple acute cystitis to life-threatening septicemia. The patient with an occasional UTI needs only an inexpensive antibacterial agent for a few days. Patients with recurring infections and those complicated by anatomic abnormalities, calculi, resistance, and so on are best served by referral to a urologist for evaluation and can often be returned to the referring physician when the abnormality is corrected.

Antibiotic Choices

The ideal antibiotic would have the following characteristics:

Effective
Low levels of resistance
Unlikely to develop resistance
Well tolerated
Reasonable cost
Convenient dosage

Obviously, effectiveness is the most important consideration. As we move into an arena demanding cost-effectiveness as well as clinical effectiveness, we must know more about the economic considerations of the treatment choices. Depending on length of treatment, several antibacterials meet the above characteristics: Sulfa, trimethoprim-sulfamethoxazole (Septra, Bactrim), nitrofurantoin macrocrystals (Macrobid), and ampicillin. The longer the duration of treatment, the more likely is the development of resistance and the need to switch to second-line, more expensive antibacterials (e.g., quinolones, cephalosporins).

Specimen Collection

Urinalysis with microscopic examination of the sediment is valuable for evaluating urinary symptoms and diseases and can give presumptive evidence of infection. Cultures of the urine are appropriate in infants, men, and women with unresolved infection.

Collection of the specimen by the clean-catch technique has been preferred in women, although difficulties in compliance with the technique may limit its usefulness. The patient is instructed to spread the labia and sponge the periurethral area with tap water. The area is then dried with gauze pads. After a stream has started, the patient collects a sample in a sterile container.

Men may simple void into a sterile container. If the patient is uncircumcised, he should retract the foreskin, wash the glans with povidone–iodine (Betadine), rinse with tap water, and dry. A specimen is collected after the stream is started. The first 5 to 10 mL may be collected if urethral infection is suspected. If prostatitis is suspected, the patient is told to stop urinating after the midstream specimen is obtained. The prostate is then massaged from each lateral border toward the middle, and the next 10 to 15 mL is collected when voiding is resumed.

Suprapubic needle aspiration is the most accurate technique for obtaining a specimen for culture in neonates and young children. The child is hydrated, so the bladder is full. After cleaning with alcohol, a local anesthetic is used to raise a skin wheal 2 to 3 inches above the symphysis in the midline. A 3.5-inch 22-gauge needle is then inserted through the skin and plunged into the bladder. Urine is aspirated by means of a sterile syringe (Graef and Cone, 1974).

Approach to Urinary Tract Infections

Stamey (1980) has suggested the following clinical classifications for urinary tract infections: (I) first infections (symptomatic); (II) unresolved bacteruria during treatment; (III) bacterial persistence; and (IV) reinfections. Classes III and IV represent recurrent urinary infections. Stamey's classification permits more logical and accurate planning for the diagnosis, treatment, prevention, and radiologic investigation of urinary tract infections.

First Infections

First infections (class I) uncomplicated by high fever or flank or costovertebral angle pain are eas-

ily diagnosed by urinalysis and easily treated by sulfonamides for 5 to 10 days. Follow-up urinalysis should be done 5 to 6 days after initiation of treatment. If pyuria or bacteruria is still seen, culture and sensitivity tests should be done and treatment with a specific antibacterial agent started. Urinalysis, cultures, or both should be repeated in 5 to 6 days.

Unresolved Bacteriuria

If infection continues despite specific antibacterial therapy (class II), the culture becomes even more important. Resistant bacteria have been identified by the cultures mentioned above. The emergence of different bacteria indicate either that there were two bacteria originally and the sensitivities were exclusive, or that resistant bacteria developed during treatment. At this point, a blood urea nitrogen (BUN) assay and a plain film of the abdomen can help to identify azotemia and staghorn calculi, respectively. Papillary necrosis from analgesic abuse can be diagnosed by IVP.

Bacterial Persistence

If the urine has been sterilized for a few days only to become infected with the same organism, chiefly *Proteus* (but occasionally *Staphylococcus epidermidis*), the most frequent cause in women is a giant staghorn calculus. In men, chronic bacterial prostatitis is the most common cause of bacterial persistence (class III).

Reinfections

Probably 99 per cent of all urinary tract infections in women are reinfections (class IV). More than 80 per cent of infections are due to *Escherichia coli* and about 13 per cent are caused by *Proteus*.

Special Problems

Special problems are associated with certain categories of recurrent bacteriuria (Table 46–4).

TABLE 46–4. MAJOR CATEGORIES OF INCREASED RISK WITH RECURRENT BACTERIURIA

Urea-splitting organisms that cause "staghorn" calculi
Congenital anomalies that become secondarily infected
Bacteriuria in the presence of urinary tract obstruction, acute or chronic
Diabetes
Pregnancy
Perinephric abscess
Analgesic abuse
Neurogenic bladder

From Stamey TA: Pathogenesis and Treatment of Urinary Tract Infections. Baltimore, Williams & Wilkins, 1980, with permission.

Urea-Splitting Bacteria That Cause Staghorn Calculi

Urea-splitting organisms frequently cause recurring urinary tract infections. Because these organisms alkalinize the urine, the salts of magnesium, ammonium, phosphate, and calcium can precipitate, and large "staghorn" calculi may form. Suspicion should be aroused when there is recurrent infection caused by *Proteus mirabilis*. Renal tomograms confirm the diagnosis. Treatment demands surgical removal of all of the stone and fragments. Failure to remove all of the stone ensures recurrence of infection and calculus. Close follow-up with frequent urine cultures is essential to detect and treat early infection and prevent further stone formation.

Congenital Anomalies That Become Secondarily Infected

Occasionally, a congenital anomaly causes persistent infection. Examples are calyceal diverticula, duplication with a nonfunctioning upper segment, urachal cysts, ureteral strictures, or ureteropelvic junction obstruction on the affected side. Treatment is usually surgical.

Bacteriuria in the Presence of Acute or Chronic Urinary Tract Obstruction

Bacteriuria associated with an obstructing ureteral calculus is usually brought about by unsuccessful stone manipulation. Chronic obstruction may be due to scarring after ureterolithotomy or ureteral reimplantation.

Diabetes

Urinary tract infection is increased in diabetics and carries the possibility of papillary necrosis and perinephric abscess. Emphysematous pyelonephritis is an infection that occurs only in diabetics. Prompt surgical drainage can be life-saving.

Pregnancy

Ureteral dilation to the pelvic brim occurs with all pregnancies. The right ureter is usually more dilated than the left. Early treatment of bacteriuria prevents most acute pyelonephritis during the last trimester. Short-acting sulfonamides, nitrofurantoin, and penicillin can safely be used even during the first trimester, but sulfonamides are to be avoided during the last trimester.

Perinephric Abscesses

The symptoms of acute pyelonephritis and perinephric abscess are similar, but the duration of fever and other symptoms is longer. When symptoms last longer than anticipated (about 5 days), additional studies (CT or ultrasonography) are required. Treatment is surgical drainage if there is inadequate renal function or nephrectomy if renal function is adequate.

Other Infections

Fungal Infections

Fungal infections, usually candidiasis, are rare and are associated with other conditions, such as immunosuppression, foreign bodies within the urinary system (catheters, stents), and prolonged use of antibacterials. Diabetics are especially susceptible to fungal infections. Fluconazole (Diflucan) is effective for symptomatic patients. In patients with foreign bodies (catheters, stents), removal is virtually mandatory.

Tuberculosis

As travel has increased, so has exposure to tuberculosis, as the disease is still prevalent in many parts of the world. The acquired immunodeficiency syndrome (AIDS) epidemic has increased the prevalence owing to compromise of the immune system. Treatment of genitourinary tuberculosis requires 6 months of triple-drug therapy.

INFLAMMATORY CONDITIONS OF THE PROSTATE

Asymptomatic urinary tract infections are rare in young men. The incidence increases from about 1.5 per cent during the sixth decade to 4.0 per cent during the eighth decade.

Drach et al. (1978) classified inflammatory conditions of the prostate as follows: acute bacterial prostatitis, chronic bacterial prostatitis, abacterial prostatitis, and prostatodynia (formerly called prostatosis).

Acute Bacterial Prostatitis

Acute bacterial prostatitis is easy to diagnose. Systemic symptoms begin first with malaise and fever. Urinary frequency and pain with varying degrees of obstruction develop rapidly. The prostate is swollen, tender, and may be hot to the touch. Leukocytosis is seen, and the urine is infected. Hospitalization is often necessary. Aminoglycosides should be started while awaiting culture and sensitivity results. Urethral catheterization should be avoided. If complete obstruction occurs, it is better to use a "suprapubic punch" with a Supracath or larger-caliber Intracath.

If the infection does not require hospitalization, trimethoprim-sulfamethoxazole is the drug of choice, although quinolones (Cipro, Floxin) offer a wider spectrum of activity and quicker response. The oral antibacterial should be continued for 3 weeks at full dosage.

Chronic Bacterial Prostatitis

Chronic bacterial prostatitis is more difficult to diagnose than the acute type. Unless the urine is

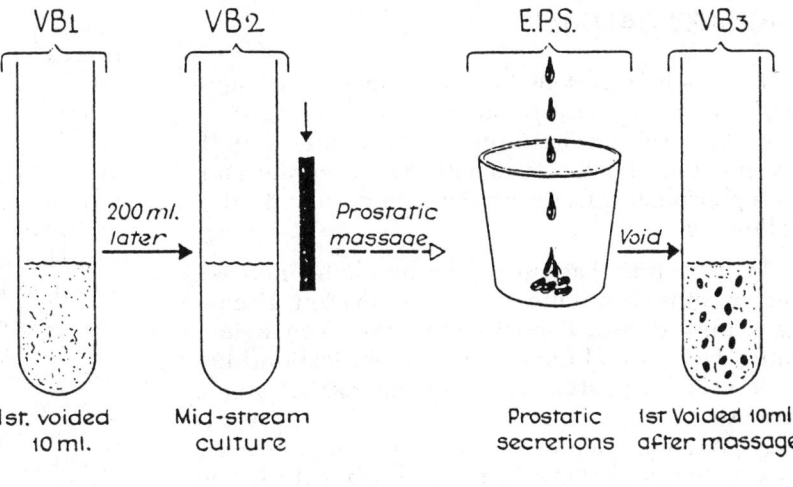

FIGURE 46-1. Cultures for suspected chronic prostatitis.

Urethral⟶Bladder⟶Prostate

infected, voiding symptoms are minimal. Mild low back and perineal discomfort are frequent complaints. The prostate feels normal on rectal examination. WBCs are seen in the prostatic secretions on microscopic examination. The diagnosis is dependent on culturing the organism from the urine after prostatic massage. If chronic prostatitis is suspected, VB1, VB3, and EPB cultures should be prepared on the first visit (Fig. 46–1).

Once infection is established in prostatic fluid, it may persist indefinitely. Part of the problem of eradicating the bacteria is due to the "barrier" between the blood and the prostatic fluid and the fact that many drugs that would be effective against those bacteria cannot cross the epithelial barrier.

A few patients can be cured of chronic bacterial prostatitis with long-term (3 to 4 months) full-dose therapy with trimethoprim-sulfamethoxazole or a quinolone. Suppressive therapy with trimethoprim-sulfamethoxazole 0.5 tablet daily or with a quinolone (Cipro 250 mg or Floxin 200 mg) prevents urinary symptoms. Because the bacteria are harbored in prostatic calculi and in corpora amylacea as well, their presence diminishes the possibility of cure. The presence of prostatic calculi suggests the need for suppressive therapy rather than curative regimens.

Urethritis

In men urethritis is either gonococcal or nongonococcal, and these two entities are often difficult to distinguish clinically. It is therefore important to use the Gram stain for differential diagnosis. There is a 98 per cent correlation between positive Gram stains and cultures for *Neisseria gonorrhoeae*. When the Gram stain is negative for gramnegative intracellular and extracellular diplococci, 98 per cent of cultures for *N. gonorrhoeae* are also negative. There is therefore a high confidence level with Gram stain alone when urethritis is present in the male patient (Bowie 1980).

Nongonococcal urethritis (NGU) may occur after successful treatment of gonococcal urethritis, but it often occurs alone. *Chlamydia trachomatis* has been implicated in this condition. Other organisms, such as *Ureaplasma urealyticum*, may also be important.

Both *C. trachomatis* and *N. gonorrhoeae* are susceptible to tetracycline, and it is the treatment of choice. Either tetracycline 500 mg twice daily or minocycline or doxycycline 100 mg orally twice daily for 7 days may be used.

The patient should be re-examined at 1 week; and if there is persistent discharge, the specimen should be smeared and cultured. If negative for *N. gonorrhoeae*, the tetracycline, minocycline, or doxycycline (1 gram tetracycline daily or 200 mg of either minocycline or doxycycline) is continued for 2 more weeks. If there is still discharge, consider noncompliance or reinfection. Culture of any specimen is helpful. For retreatment, use erythromycin 2 grams daily for a week and then 1 gram daily for 2 weeks.

If *N. gonorrhoeae* persists after 1 week of treatment with tetracycline, change to penicillin—either 4.8 MU, procaine penicillin G intramuscularly, amoxicillin 3.0 grams orally, or ampicillin 3.5 grams orally with probenecid 1.0 gram. Spectinomycin 2.0 gram intramuscularly should be used if there is suspicion that gonorrhea was acquired in Africa or Southeast Asia, as resistant organisms have originated there. It is imperative to treat the sexual partner. If there is persistence (failure) or recurrence despite specific treatment and compliance, and the partner(s) have been treated, investigation for prostatitis, urethral structure, foreign bodies, and so on should be instituted.

URINARY CALCULI

The etiology of stone formation depends on several factors. Urinary ribonucleic acid and glycosaminoglycan (normal urine constituents) inhibit sterile stone formation in vitro as do citrate and pyrophosphates. Contributing factors include the following.

1. Activities that cause dehydration by increasing sweating can promote stone formation. Examples are exercise, Turkish baths, and even swimming. Decreased fluid intake, immobilization, and sedentary occupation increase the risk of stone disease.

2. Anatomic abnormalities that cause urinary obstruction and stasis increase the possibility of stone formation by increasing the residence time for the urine. When the urine is supersaturated, there is more time for precipitation and stone growth to occur. Such abnormalities are prostatic obstruction, urethral stricture, neurogenic bladder with high residual urine, and ureteropelvic junction obstruction.

3. A normal diet may contain many elements implicated in stone disease. Oxalate is found in many vegetables (spinach, beets, greens), most berries, fruits and juices (grapes and citrus fruits), vitamin C, instant coffee, tea, and chocolate. Dietary vitamin D and acid ash are the most prominent regulators of intestinal calcium absorption. The main sources of acid ash are protein and soft drinks (weak phosphoric acid solutions). Carbohydrate, especially lactose, may increase the concentration of uric acid in urine. Meats, beer, and wine are high in purines.

4. Metabolic abnormalities such as primary hyperparathyroidism, renal tubular acidosis, and medullary sponge kidney are responsible for more than 90 per cent of so-called metabolic stones, but these cases account for fewer than 10 per cent of patients with recurrent stone disease.

5. Environmental climates that increase dehydration or that increase intestinal calcium absorption (increased sunshine increases vitamin D synthesis) also increase the propensity for stone formation. "Hard water" may bind oxalate in the intestine and reduce absorption, thereby decreasing stone formation.

6. The most common genetic cause of urinary lithiasis is gout. Twenty-five per cent of patients with gouty arthritis develop stones. Primary hyperoxaluria and cystinuria are rarer genetic causes.

7. "Infection stones" are phosphate calculi formed around a nidus of some other substance in persistently alkaline urine (pH above 7.0). The essential factor is a urease-producing bacterial infection splitting urea into ammonia, causing the persistently alkaline pH.

8. Medications can contribute to the development of stones. Antacids containing magnesium trisilicate may induce or accelerate growth of struvite stones or may induce silicon stones. Chemotheraputic agents that increase purine metabolism cause hyperuricemia and hyperuricosuria, especially in patients with myeloproliferative disease.

Evaluation

Evaluation of patients with their first episode of uninfected ureterolithiasis require stone analysis, urinalysis, and determinations of serum creatinine, calcium, and electrolytes. A complete evaluation should be done in all children and all patients with staghorn, cystine, uric acid, recurrent stone formation, or multiple stones at discovery. Table 46–5 outlines a method for evaluating patients after stone analysis. When these portions of the evaluation have been completed, patients with hypercalcemia and/or elevated serum proteins should undergo serum protein electrophoresis and urine examination for Bence Jones protein to detect multiple myeloma. Patients with hypercalcemia should also have an immunoreactive parathyroid hormone assay done to detect hyperparathyroidism.

Those patients who persistently have a urine pH above 5.5 and metabolic acidosis (carbon dioxide content less than 20mEq/L) should have an acid load test with NH_4Cl to exclude renal tubular acidosis. The test is contraindicated in the presence of overt acidosis.

Medical Management

Increased fluid intake is the single most effective method of treating stone disease, regardless of

TABLE 46–5. EVALUATION AFTER ANALYSIS OF URINARY TRACT STONES

Type of Stone Formed	10-Day Diet and Treatment Diary	24-Hour Urine Studies	Other Studies
Uric acid	X	Uric acid, creatinine	Serum uric acid, creatinine
Phosphate	X	Calcium, magnesium, phosphorus, uric acid, creatinine	SMA-12
Oxalate	X	Calcium, magnesium, phosphorus, uric acid, creatinine, sodium, oxalate	SMA-12

The pH of the first two voided urine specimens each day should be checked by nitrazine paper and recorded.

cause. In the absence of severely reduced renal function, a daily urine volume (output) of 3 to 4 liters is desired, and the 24-hour volume is measured to emphasize and assess intake.

Cystine Stones

At least 90 per cent of cystine stone-formers can be treated successfully with hydration. Continuous cooperation by the patient and support from the physician are necessary. If hydration therapy alone is ineffective, alkalinization of the urine is attempted. Sodium bicarbonate 2.5 grams is given every 6 hours. Additionally, protein intake should not exceed 56 grams per day. Urine pH should be monitored with each specimen the first week and then measured daily. The urine pH must be maintained above 7.5. Additional alkali may be required. If cystine excretion exceeds 1 gm/day, the patient may require penicillamine.

Uric Acid Stones

Hydration is the first step in the treatment of uric acid stones. Alkalinization of the urine with Polycitra or Urocit-K 1 or 2 tablespoons every 6 hours usually keeps the urine pH above 6.5 Nitrazine paper is used to monitor urine pH. Protein intake must be reduced to 56 gm/day.

When uric acid calculi recur despite this treatment, allopurinol 200 to 300 mg/day may be added. Among patients with uric acid stones, 75 per cent have a normal serum uric acid level and an elevated urine uric acid concentration.

Calcium Phosphate Stones

Most calcium phosphate stones are due to primary hyperparathyroidism. The treatment is therefore surgical excision of the parathyroid adenoma. When surgery fails or is not possible, hydration and orthophosphate administration may be beneficial. A dosage of 500 mg of orthophosphate every 4 hours is recommended, although a lower dose with gradual increases may be needed to prevent diarrhea. The patient should be observed for hypertension and for sodium and water retention.

Calcium Oxalate Stones

Patients who form calcium oxalate stones may have hyperabsorption of calcium from the intestine or renal tubular calcium leak in combination with high dietary oxalate, or primary or secondary hyperoxaluria. Hyperabsorption is more common than renal leak hypercalcuria and is differentiated by the patient having a normal urine calcium level during calcium fasting.

Hydration therapy is started along with dietary restriction of foods high in oxalate such as tea, instant and decaffeinated coffees, chocolate, citrus fruits and juices, berries, spinach, greens, beets, and nuts.

Hyperabsorbers of calcium are placed on neutral orthophosphate (Neutra-Phos 2 tablets three times a day). Hydrochlorothiazide 50 mg/day binds calcium in the intestine, decreases urinary calcium, and increases urinary pyrophosphate, a potent inhibitor of calculus formation in both absorbers and renal leak. Oral cellulose phosphate (Calcibind) may be given to bind calcium in the intestine. If there is concomitant evidence of hyperuricosuria, allopurinol 300 mg/day is given. The major side effect of both allopurinol and orthophosphate is diarrhea.

Renal Tubular Acidosis Type I

The common sign of renal tubular acidosis of (RTA) type I patients is calcium-containing calculi. Because type I RTA results from the inability of the distal nephron to maintain an adequate hydrogen ion gradient, patients have persistently high urinary pH. A recorded urinary pH of less than 5.3 makes it unlikely that the patient has type I RTA. (Finlayson, 1981)

Treatment requires daily ingestion of absorbable alkali. Urocit-K or Polycitra (1 or 2 tablespoons four times a day) usually restores urinary citrate levels. *Treatment is lifelong.* Types II and III RTA are rare and beyond the scope of this chapter.

Infected (Phosphate) Stones

The treatment of struvite stones is essentially surgical because the stones are too large to pass and the infection cannot be eradicated so long as the stone(s) are present. It is essential to remove all traces of stone and fragments in order to eliminate infection.

The most important aspect of long-term care is monitoring for reinfection and further stone formation. Monthly urine cultures are done for the first 6 months after surgery with KUB radiography every 3 months for the first year and then annually unless there is evidence of infection or rapid regrowth of the calculus. With evidence of regrowth, acetohydroxamic acid may be added to the treatment regimen.

Surgical Management

Urinary calculi managed surgically can be classified by anatomic location as renal, ureteral, or bladder calculi. Surgical decisions are based on location and size, and they are made more urgent by the presence of obstruction, persistent infection, refractory pain, or progressive loss of function.

Renal Calculi

Small calculi (less than 5 mm) that are attached to the papillae from which they originate do not require vigorous attention. In the absence of infection, only periodic follow-up by plain film of the abdomen and urinalysis is needed. For asymptomatic, slowly growing stones, semianual follow-up examinations for a year is adequate. If there is no progress even then, annual follow-up suffices.

For larger (more than 1.0 cm) asymptomatic calculi, extracorporeal shock wave lithotripsy (ESWL) offers the most practical means of elimination at present. Branched (staghorn) calculi require removal by extended pyelithotomy or nephrolithotomy. A renal scan should be done to assess function prior to surgery. All of the stone(s) and fragments must be removed. Appropriate antibiotics must be given pre- and postoperatively. Residual fragments may be eliminated by ESWL.

Ureteral Calculi

Prompt attention is required in cases of ureteral calculi. Small calculi (less than 5 mm) cause predictable obstructive symptoms (colic) at areas of anatomic narrowing (e.g., the ureteropelvic junction, the point at which the ureter crosses over the iliac vessels, and the ureterovesical junction). Sufficient analgesics must be given while waiting for the stone to pass.

Moderate-size stones (5 to 8 mm) may pass but are less likely to do so. They often travel into the distal ureter before impacting. At this location cystoscopic manipulation is possible, as is laser lithotripsy or electrohydrolic lithotripsy. ESWL is often effective in the upper ureter (Mobley et al., 1993).

Large stones (more than 1.0 cm) rarely pass. Usually they obstruct at the first area of anatomic narrowing, the ureteropelvic junction. Percutaneous manipulation and ESWL are equally effective.

Bladder Calculi

High residual urine content, fragments of ureteral stones, and prolonged catheter drainage are causes of bladder stones, which may reach impressive size. Bladder stones should be removed and the primary defect corrected if possible. Small stones can be washed out of the bladder through a cystoscope. Larger stones can be fractured by transurethral electrohydraulic lithotripsy and then washed out of the bladder. Renacidin irrigations have successfully dissolved large calculi. Suprapubic cystolithotomy is rarely required.

VASECTOMY

It is important to have an initial interview with the potential vasectomy patient and his wife to answer their questions, explain preoperative instructions and testing, inquire about allergies and bleeding problems, and inform them of possible complications. The family physician is advised to become acquainted with local requirements. The following three major concerns of the law may lead to adverse civil decisions involving vasectomy procedures (Mark, 1976): (1) negligence in the performance of the operation, postoperative instructions, or postoperative testing; (2) breach of warranty such as when a promised result fails to ensue; and (3) misrepresentation (when informed consent has not been secured).

Technique

Surgical technique begins with the preparation of the skin of the genitalia with an antiseptic solution such as povidone-iodine (Betadine). Alcohol solutions should not be used, as they may be irritating. Diazepam (Valium) 5 to 10 mg is commonly used intravenously for sedation.

The vas is found high in the scrotum and held in the subcutaneous position with the fingers while 1% lidocaine *without* epinephrine is injected into the skin and directly into the vas. An incision is then made in the skin directly over the vas and extended through the subcutaneous tissue, which is spread with a hemostat, permitting the vas to be picked up with a towel clip. Additional anesthetic may be injected into the sheath surrounding the vas, and a longitudinal incision is then made in the sheath to expose the vas. The vas itself should *not* be incised with this maneuver. The vas can be tented by the towel clip and a mosquito hemostat placed just underneath the vas in the tented area. The hemostat is spread open to separate the vas from its vessels and the sheath. With the sheath retracted by the hemostat, the vas is divided. The point of an electrocautery device is then placed in the lumen, and the mucosa is coagulated using low current because it is neither necessary nor desirable to destroy the muscular wall of the vas. Both lumens are coagulated separately. The urethral side of the vas is buried within its sheath and secured there with 4-0 chromic catgut stitch. The testicular end is left outside the sheath to retard recanalization should a sperm granuloma develop. The skin and dartos layers are then sutured as one with an absorbable stitch. The same technique is used on the opposite side to accomplish sterilization. It is safer to coagulate the vas rather than to ligate it. Ligation may lead to necrosis and sloughing at the site of the ligature, thereby exposing a patent lumen.

Postoperatively, the patient is instructed to go to bed for a few hours. An ice bag may be used to retard swelling and discomfort. He is advised to wear an athletic supporter for a few days. Semen specimens are obtained at 2 and 3 months after the procedure. Fresh specimens are not required, as total absence of sperm is expected in the second specimen. If dead sperm are seen at this time, a fresh specimen must be obtained and examined for live sperm. Contraception by other means is maintained until the physician is sure of complete aspermia.

Complications

The complications most frequently seen after vasectomy are bleeding, infection, and surgical failure. Bleeding shows up during the first day or two, whereas infection may take 4 or 5 days to appear. Surgical failure is not suspected until the first semen specimen is evaluated.

Sperm granulomas may form owing to spillage of sperm outside the vas. They rarely cause difficulty unless they involve the spermatic nerve, causing pain during intercourse or even with simple touching. These granulomas must be excised and the vas resealed. Congestive epididymitis may occur, but it usually responds quickly to heat and bed rest with scrotal elevation.

UROLOGIC CANCER

Renal Adenocarcinoma (Renal Cell Cancer, Hypernephroma)

As with most urologic malignancies, there are no pathognomic early symptoms or signs of the renal adenocarcinoma. The earliest symptoms may be vague flank or abdominal pain, loss of appetite and weight, or weakness. The classic triad of gross hematuria, flank pain, and mass is present in only 9 per cent of patients, and among those individuals almost half have metastasis at the time of diagnosis (Boileau, 1982).

Hematuria is the most frequent sign of renal cancer and should be investigated by IVP. A mass seen on IVP necessitates further evaluation by tomogram, ultrasonography, or abdominal CT. Percutaneous biopsy is rarely needed (Boileau, 1982).

Once the cancer has been diagnosed a systematic search for evidence of metastasis should be undertaken, including physical examination, chest radiography, radionuclide bone scanning, abdominal CT, and an SMA screen. The most frequent sites for metastasis, in decreasing order of frequency, are regional lymph nodes, lung, liver, and bone.

The treatment of choice is radical nephrectomy when there is no evidence of metastasis (Pritchett et al., 1988). In the presence of a solitary metastasis, nephrectomy and removal of the metastatic lesion can be accomplished, with longevity increased. In such cases, removal of a solitary bone lesion is associated with greater longevity than is the presence of a soft tissue lesion. When there are multiple lesions, nephrectomy is done only to relieve pain due to the expanding renal mass, or when hemorrhage threatens the patient's life.

There is no consistently beneficial chemotherapeutic agent, though interferon has shown promise. Interleukin-2 is less effective (Rosenberg, 1988).

Carcinoma of the Renal Pelvis

Carcinoma of the renal pelvis is a urothelial tumor. These tumors account for only 7 per cent of renal malignancies and fewer than 1 per cent of all genitourinary tumors (Johnson, 1982).

Painless hematuria, gross or microscopic, is the most frequent sign. An IVP usually demonstrates a filling defect. Cystoscopic examination is mandatory to rule out "seeding" of tumor into the bladder. Ureteroscopes can traverse the ureter into the renal pelvis to obtain a biopsy specimen. Cytology is sometimes helpful. The usual evaluation for metastatic lesions is done, including SMA, chest radiography, and bone scans. CT is sometimes helpful for evaluating the local extent of the lesion.

Nephroureterectomy is the treatment of choice for nonmetastatic tumors. Periodic cystoscopic examination and urinary cytology are mandatory, as recurrence in the bladder has been reported to be as high as 30 per cent (Murphy, 1990). Metastatic lesions have shown response rates as high as 50 per cent (one third of them complete responses) with platinum-based chemotherapy protocols (Johnson, 1982).

Carcinoma of the Ureter

Carcinoma of the ureter is rare. Hematuria is the most consistent finding. Flank pain is frequent, and there may be irritative bladder symptoms depending on the proximity of the tumor to the bladder (Johnson, 1982).

The IVP is almost always abnormal, demonstrating either an intraluminal filling defect with or without hydronephrosis or nonfunction of the kidney. Cystoscopy and retrograde urography should be done next. Cystoscopy may reveal synchronous bladder tumor(s), and sometimes the ureteral tumor protrudes from the orifice. Ureteroscopy may be possible with tumors higher up the ureter, and biopsy can establish the diagnosis. Evaluation for metastasis duplicates that for carcinoma of the renal pelvis.

Treatment is usually nephroureterectomy. Occasionally segmental resection is warranted, such as with small, low grade, low stage, distal-third ureteral tumors (without evidence of tumor anatomically higher in the ureter) (Johnson, 1982). Other considerations include patients with solitary kidneys, renal insufficiency, or bilateral tumors.

Platinum-based chemotherapy offers hope for locally extended or metastatic tumors. Follow-up requires frequent cystoscopic examination and urinary cytologic studies because recurrence due to seeding is high.

Bladder Cancer

The most frequent sign of bladder cancer is hematuria. As previously mentioned, an IVP should be done when there is gross hematuria; it is an integral part of the evaluation and may demonstrate a filling defect in the bladder. Cystoscopic examination and biopsy are necessary to establish the diagnosis. Staging procedures include bimanual pelvic or rectal examination (preferably with anesthesia at the time of cysto/biopsy), chest radiography, and SMA for superficial tumors. For invasive tumors, abdominal and pelvic CT are added.

Invasiveness determines the mode(s) of treatment. About 70 per cent present as superficial noninvasive tumors and are treated by transurethral resection and fulguration. The recurrence rate is high (60 to 70 per cent), and intravesical chemotherapy is usually indicated to prevent recurrence, delay progression, and improve survival. The drug of choice at present is BCG (bacillus Calmette Guérin) (Catalona et al., 1988). This agent, however, has worrisome side effects (e.g., drug-induced cystitis, bladder contracture, fever) that must be considered. It is never used in the presence of active urinary infection. Other drugs used for intravesical installation include thiotepa, doxorubicin, and mitomicin C. There is only limited experience with interferon. Frequent surveillance by urinary cytologic studies and cystoscopic examination is recommended.

Nonmetastatic invasive cancers are best treated by radical cystectomy or cystoprostatectomy and urinary diversion (Johnson and Boileau, 1982). Segmental resection is rarely done because of strict criteria. Platinum-based chemotherapy protocols are sometimes used as "sandwich therapy" given pre- and postoperatively. For metastatic disease, platinum-based chemotherapy continues to be useful, though not curative. Early results with paclitaxel (Taxol) have been encouraging.

Adenocarcinoma of the Prostate

Cancer of the prostate continues to be one of the most enigmatic tumors in humans. The more we have learned about the malignancy, the more controversial the subject has become. With an incidence of prostate cancer in the United States in 1993 of 165,000 new cases resulting in 35,000 deaths, its importance is beyond question and dialogue must continue (Boring et al., 1993).

The discovery and use of prostate-specific antigen (PSA), the most reliable predictor of prostate cancer, has been revolutionary. It has no peers in terms of aiding early diagnosis, staging, and monitoring of the results of therapy (Brawer and Lange, 1989). It is an indicator of progression as well. Though elevations of PSA are not specific for prostate cancer (PSA evaluations are seen with large benign glands, prostatitis, and prostate infarction), PSA elevations are found most frequently in patients with prostate malignancy. Cancers can and

do occur in the presence of a normal PSA assay and an abnormal prostate by digital rectal examination. Elevated PSA levels often precede development of a detectable tumor.

Transrectal ultrasonography has proved to be an invaluable tool for diagnosing prostate cancer. Imaging the prostate allows identification of hypoechoic areas within the prostate and precise biopsy of abnormal-appearing areas. With an elevated PSA and no definable hypoechoic area, sextant biopsies bring an increased yield of positive biopsies. Ultrasonography and possible biopsy are indicated when there is a palpable prostatic nodule or when there the PSA is elevated—and certainly when both conditions exist.

The rapid and multifold increase in diagnosing localized prostatic cancer has initiated controversies in treatment. Who should be treated? Who should be "watched"? Who makes the decision?

New treatments, improvements in traditional treatments, and combinations of treatments have made patient consultation more complicated. More time with patients and often with their families is required to present and explain all treatment options. Opinions on both well advised and poorly advised options are appropriate. Second opinions must not be refused. The goal is to find the best treatment plan for each patient, given that we all share some particular bias. Part of the uncertainty can be blamed on the protracted natural history of prostate cancer in many patients.

With the caveat that close follow-up (every 3 to 6 months) is mandatory, it is reasonable to offer "watchful waiting" to certain categories of patients. The best candidates for observation alone are the following.

1. Patients over 70 years of age
2. Patients with other major medical problems (e.g., coronary artery disease, insulin-dependent diabetes, chronic obstructive pulmonary disease)
3. Patients with low grade, low volume tumors
4. Patients with diploid tumors (Thompson, 1994)

"Watchful waiting" does not imply that no further treatment will be necessary or offered. Hormonal treatment may be offered as intervention for patients with rising PSA levels (above 30 ng/ml) and is certainly indicated when there is evidence of metastatic disease. Local progression almost always precedes metastatic disease (Fig. 46–2) and may require transurethral resection for relief of obstruction.

Definitive treatment is indicated for healthy patients below age 70 with stage A, B_1, or B_2 disease or with an aneuploid tumor. Radical prostatectomy, either perineal or retropubic, accompanied by bilateral pelvic lymphadenectomy is the traditional treatment of choice among urologists (Moore et al., 1988). The above age suggestion is often waived, and surgery is commonly done up to age 75. Usu-

STAGE A

(? OCCULT
    INCIDENTAL)

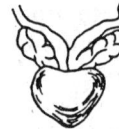

STAGE B

(NODULAR OR LIMITED
  WITHIN THE GLAND)

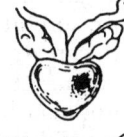

STAGE C

(LOCALIZED TO THE
  PERIPROSTATIC AREA)

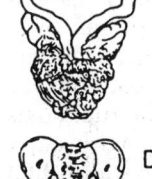

STAGE D

(D₁ REGIONAL METASTASES
  D₂ DISTANT METASTASES)

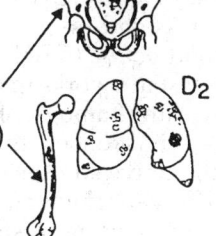

FIGURE 46–2. Clinical staging of prostatic cancer.

ally lymphadenectomy is done first and the specimen is examined immediately by frozen section while the patient is kept under anesthesia. If the lymph nodes are negative for metastatic tumor, the prostatectomy is accomplished. If the lymph nodes demonstrate tumor, the prostatectomy is abandoned.

In many locations, laparoscopic lymphadenectomy has replaced the open procedure (Danella et al., 1993). For some such instances perineal prostatectomy has regained popularity. This combination has reduced the hospitalization duration and in some series has reduced the rate of incontinence.

Development of the nerve-sparing technique has greatly enhanced the possibility of maintaining potency after prostatectomy. It has limitations, though, and impotence and incontinence remain the major postoperative sequelae. Impotence rates vary between 33 and 81 per cent (Catalona and Bigg, 1990) in reported series; continence rates reveal that 63 to 96 per cent of patients regain complete urinary control, 0 to 35 per cent have stress incontinence, and 0 to 17 per cent are totally incontinent (Steiner et al., 1991).

Radical prostatectomy remains the gold standard for potentially curable prostate cancer, although external beam radiation has its advocates and its place. Radiation therapy alters the biology of prostate cancer and, though not strictly curative, offers a noninvasive alternative in a defined patient population: primarily older patients and those desiring

nonsurgical treatment (Scardino and Wheeler, 1985).

Advances in technology, though still developmental, have made other options available for curative therapy. Cryoablation of the prostate is enjoying a resurrection after years of disuse because of complications. This resurrection has come about because of the development of transrectal ultrasonography and a more precise system for delivering liquid nitrogen to tissues (Onik et al., 1993). Ultrasound monitoring of the freezing process allows control, so injury to adjacent organs is prevented. Long-term results are unavailable for the new procedure, but survival rates for the older procedure have approximated those of radical surgery. The cost-effectiveness yields considerable savings over traditional procedures, but more time is needed to prove its clinical effectiveness.

Radiation therapy by implantable isotopes continues to improve owing to advances in technology, such as transultrasonography and percutaneous delivery systems via the perineal approach. Laser ablation of the prostate is also in its developmental stage, particularly in regard to prostate cancer.

For stage C disease, external beam radiation has been used to treat 40 per cent of patients, with survivorship at 5, 10, and 15 years of 62, 36, and 18 per cent, respectively (Bagshaw, 1988). Iodine 125 implantations result in similar survivorship (Paulson, 1988). Salvage surgery for irradiation failures is rarely indicated because of its surgical difficulty and increased complications. Onik et al (1993) has reported encouraging results with cryoablation of the prostate.

The mainstay of treatment for disseminated prostate cancer is hormone manipulation. The biologic goal is androgen deprivation, which can be accomplished simply by castration or by the use of luteinizing hormone-releasing hormone (LHRH) analogues, such as leuprolide (Lupron) or goserelin (Zoladex) given on a monthly basis. The advantage of castration is its cost-effectiveness and the advantage of LHRH analogues is the avoidance of surgery. Clinical effectiveness is equivocal. Diethylstilbestrol is not often used, despite its low cost, because of complications due to hypercoagulability (Byar, 1973).

Treatment of pain due to bony metastasis includes local irradiation, estramustine phosphate (Emcyt) (Murphy et al., 1984), and strontium 89 chloride (Metastron) (Porter et al., 1993).

Carcinoma of the Urethra

Carcinoma of the urethra is rare in both sexes. Most of these lesions are squamous carcinoma (male 78 per cent, female 68 per cent). In men urethral tumors are usually associated with stricture disease. Rapid recurrence of obstructive symptoms after dilation with increased or easy bleeding should raise a suspicion of malignancy (Johnson and Boileau, 1982). A mass may be felt in the perineal or pendulous urethra. Enlarged inguinal lymph nodes may be palpated. Endoscopic examination and biopsy confirm the diagnosis.

In women the most common sign is urethral bleeding or spotting. Irritative symptoms of dysuria and dyspareunia and symptoms of obstruction are frequent. Palpation may reveal a mass. Cystourethroscopy and biopsy confirm the diagnosis. Metastatic surveys include chest radiography, IVP, bone scan, SMA, and pelvic CT. Examination of the inguinal areas is important.

Treatment is both radiologic and surgical (Johnson and Boileau, 1982). Limited surgery (partial urethrectomy) may be employed, and interstitial implants have been effective in women. Urethrocystectomy and urinary diversion may be necessary and may be accompanied by inguinal lymphadenectomy.

Carcinoma of the Penis

Carcinoma of the penis is rare and seldom found in those circumcised during infancy (Crawford and Dawkins, 1988). The lesions are generally squamous in cell type and are easily palpable. Infection is usually found and must be vigorously treated prior to definitive therapy.

Surgical treatment depends on the extent and location of the disease. It may consist of circumcision or partial or total penectomy; and it may include inguinal lymphadenectomy.

Experience with Nd:YAG lasers has shown excellent functional results in selected (low-stage) cases without the need for partial amputation. Recurrence is rare, and the cosmetic results are satisfying. (Malloy, 1985)

Carcinoma of the Testis

Although a relatively rare group of tumors, testis cancers are the most frequent solid tumors in young men between the ages of 18 and 40. The emotional trauma and economic impact of young men afflicted early in their family lives and business or professional careers has attracted attention out of proportion to their incidence in the population (Damjanov, 1989). Despite spectacular therapeutic successes, testis tumors are the third leading cause of death in the affected age group.

The most common classification of testis tumors is from Dixon and Moore (1952):

I: seminoma alone
II: embryonal carcinoma, alone or with seminoma
III: teratoma, alone or with seminoma
IV: teratoma with embryonal carcinoma, choriocarcinoma, or both, and with or without seminoma
V: Choriocarcinoma alone or with embryonal carcinoma, seminoma, or both

Testis tumors usually present as a painless mass. Any intrascrotal or testicular mass should be considered cancer until proved otherwise (Johnson and Boileau, 1982). Germ cell tumors of the testis may produce beta human chronic gonadotropic hormone (β-hCG) or α-fetoprotein (AFP), or both. Symptoms of metastasis may be the presenting symptom and may include abdominal or back pain, nausea, vomiting, anorexia, and weight loss.

The diagnosis is confirmed by inguinal orchiectomy with early occlusion of the spermatic cord. Assays for β-hCG and AFP, chest radiography, urinalysis and pregnancy test, SMA, and a complete blood count (CBC) are done preoperatively. The metastatic work-up after diagnosis adds abdominal CT, lung tomography (if a mass or suspicion of a mass is seen on the chest radiograph), and IVP. Adjunctive studies may include bone scans and inferior venocavography.

The staging system described by Boden and Gibb (1951) works well in most clinical situations.

Stage I: tumor limited to testis without extension through the tunica albuginea or into the spermatic cord
Stage II: tumor extension beyond the testicle but not beyond the regional lymphatics
Stage III: distant metastases

Treatment depends on tumor type: seminomatous or nonseminomatous. Seminomatous tumors are treated by irradiation. Stage I tumors receive 2500 rad to the ipsilateral iliac nodes and periaortic nodes. Stage II tumors receive the same treatment plus 2500 rad to the mediastinal and supraclavicular areas. Patients with a stage III tumor undergo platinum-based chemotherapy and laparotomy for any residual mass.

Nonseminomatous tumors were listed above. Treatment of early-stage disease is retroperitoneal lymphadenectomy. Chemotherapy reduces the incidence of metastasis. A combination of *cis*-platinum, vinblastine, and bleomyin is used most frequently. Cures in excess of 95 per cent have been achieved. Some institutions advocate surveillance only for stage A tumors after orchiectomy, avoiding lymphadenectomy and its frequent side effect of retrograde ejaculation.

Follow-up is extensive for the first 2 years, with monthly chest radiography and β-hCG or AFP assays (or both), and quarterly abdominal CT scans and SMA screens.

Progress in the treatment of testis cancer has been nothing short of remarkable. Patients with testis tumors enjoy the highest cure rate of any solid tumor in humans (Skinner and Lieskovsky, 1988). The most common testicular neoplasms are malignancies of germ cell origin. They are the third most frequent malignancy in men during the third and fourth decades of life. The incidence increases in patients with a history of undescended testes. Twenty-five per cent of testicular tumors are misdiagnosed at the first visit to a physician.

Testicular tumors may appear as elevations on the surface of the testis or may replace the substance of the testis; they may feel like harder-than-normal tissue. Because lymphatic drainage from the testes is via the periaortic chain, inguinal adenopathy has no significance when diagnosing cancer of the testicle. With embryonal carcinoma and choriocarcinoma, gynecomastia may precede awareness of the scrotal mass. An inflammatory hydrocele may rapidly form, making examination difficult. Aspiration of this inflammatory hydrocele makes physical examination easier.

Advanced stage lesions, II and III, are treated primarily by *cis*-platinum-based chemotherapy. About 80 per cent of these patients become disease-free, and about 70 per cent are long-term survivors. The combination of *cis*-platinum, vinblastine, and bleomycin seems to be the most effective "cocktail," and initial chemotherapy is terminated within 9 to 12 weeks. Surgical intervention is reserved for patients with a residual mass that persists radiographically (Einhorn, 1988).

BENIGN PROSTATIC HYPERPLASIA

Progress and change have characterized the challenge of benign prostatic hyperplasia (BPH). Three separate areas of interest have developed. The first is the AUA Symptom Score, a cooperative study to bring uniformity to the evaluation of the symptoms of BPH. The second is successful medical therapy to relieve the symptoms and signs of BPH. Finally, technology has produced instruments capable of competing with the traditional surgical treatment of BPH; transurethral resection of the prostate (TURP).

The AUA Symptom Score Index (McConnell et al., 1994) asks seven questions pertaining to symptomatology (Table 46–6). Each question has six gradations of answers from 0 to 5 (Fig. 46–2). The questions are direct and easily answered. The numerical answers are then summated to arrive at the symptom score. It is a valid, reliable means of evaluating the severity of the symptoms given the subjective nature of most of the questions. Generally,

TABLE 46–6. INTERNATIONAL PROSTATE SYMPTOM SCORE (I-PSS)

Symptom	Score						Total Score
	Not at All	**Less Than 1 Time in 5**	**Less Than Half the Time**	**About Half the Time**	**More Than Half the Time**	**Almost Always**	
Incomplete emptying: Over the past month, how often have you had a sensation of not emptying your bladder completely after you finished urinating?	0	1	2	3	4	5	
Frequency: Over the past month, how often have you had to urinate again less than two hours after you finished urinating?	0	1	2	3	4	5	
Intermittency: Over the past month, how often have you found you stopped and started again several times when you urinated?	0	1	2	3	4	5	
Urgency: Over the past month, how often have you found it difficult to postpone urination?	0	1	2	3	4	5	
Weak stream: Over the past month, how often have you had a weak urinary stream?	0	1	2	3	4	5	
Straining: Over the past month, how often have you had to push or strain to begin urination?	0	1	2	3	4	5	
	None	**1 Time**	**2 Times**	**3 Times**	**4 Times**	**5 or More Times**	
Nocturia: Over the past month, how many times did you most typically get up to urinate from the time you went to bed at night until the time you got up in the morning?	0	1	2	3	4	5	
Total I-PSS score =							

a score of 7 or less is in the "mild" category. A score of 8 to 19 is intermediate, and patients with scores of 20 or higher are "severely" bothered by their symptoms (Barry et al., 1992). The Symptom Score augments, rather than replaces, objective studies such as uroflow, pressure flow, and SMA. It is useful as a clinical research tool, as well as for decision-making about therapy.

The second hurdle cleared is the reality of medical management for BPH. The two drugs approved for use are terazosin (Hytrin) and finasteride (Proscar). Terazosin is an α-$_1$-adrenergic antagonist. α-$_1$-Adrenergic receptors are found in abundance within the prostate, prostate capsule, and bladder neck (Lepor et al., 1993). By inhibiting these receptors, smooth muscle tone in these structures is decreased, as is resistance to the flow of urine. The patient is thus able to void better.

Side effects of terazosin are dizziness, headache, weakness, postural hypotension, and impotence. It only slightly affects blood pressure in nonhypertensive individuals; and as an antihypertensive it is effective in its own right. Because about 50 per cent of BPH patients are hypertensive, it is cost-effective in this population as well.

Dosage is usually started at 1 mg at bedtime for three nights, 2 mg for ten nights, and then 5 mg. Higher doses (10 mg) can be achieved within 2 weeks, if needed, with only a modest increase in side effects (Monda and Oesterling, 1993). The efficiency is dose-dependent, and improvement can be expected within a month. Other α_1-blockers such as doxazosin (Cardura) will be approved for use in BPH patients.

Finasteride is a 5α-reductase inhibitor. A brief survey of its mode of action is in order. The hypothalamus and pituitary gland control testicular androgen production. The hypothalamus secretes LHRH, which acts directly on the anterior pituitary to stimulate the release of luteinizing hormone (LH). LH binds to receptors in Leydig cells, stimulating the production and release of testosterone.

Testosterone circulates to the prostate, where it diffuses into prostate cells and is converted to dihydrotestosterone (DHT) by 5α-reductase. Testosterone and DHT then bind to a specific receptor protein, which enters the nucleus. The overall result is biosynthesis with cellular increase.

Finasteride directly inhibits 5α-reductase, thereby blocking the transcription of RNA and protein synthesis. Because finasteride acts only on testosterone-to-DHT conversion in prostate cells, it has no systemic androgenic or antiandrogenic effects.

The optimal dose of finasteride is 5 mg/day. Prostate volume as measured by ultrasonography begins to decrease within about 3 months. At 12 months, a 19 per cent decrease was noted in one study, and the peak urinary flow rate and Symptom Score improved (Gormley et al., 1992). The incidence of side effects of finasteride is low: decreased libido 4.7 per cent, decreased ejaculate volume 4.4 per cent, and impotence 4.4 per cent (Finasteride Study Group, 1993).

Finasteride lowers the PSA by about 50 per cent within 6 months. Prostate cancer surveillance should continue, and the PSA assay and digital rectal examination are mandated prior to starting finasteride. The PSA assay should be repeated 6 months later (for a new baseline level) and repeated annually. Serum PSA levels that do not decrease in 6 months should raise suspicion of prostate cancer, and evaluation should be initiated (Finasteride Study Group, 1993). The drug is continued indefinitely as discontinuance allows prostate growth and resumption of symptoms.

Urologists no longer have a monopoly on the treatment of BPH. Proper use of the AUA Symptom Score and approved medications allows primary care physicians an important new role in the treatment of BPH. Technologic advances such as transurethral incision of the prostate (TUIP), visual laser ablation of the prostate (VLAP), urethral coils and stents, and hyperthermia have created interesting new possibilities for treating BPH (McConnell et al., 1994). TUIP has had the most extensive trial use and is almost equivalent to TURP for prostates weighing 30 grams or less. It is cost-effective as well. VLAP may prove to be an effective treatment and can probably be done on an outpatient basis, further improving its cost-effectiveness.

TRAUMA

Renal Trauma

Renal injury may be due to blunt or penetrating injury. Such patients are usually seen in the emergency room. There is usually hematuria of some degree; though with shearing of the renal pedicle by rapid deceleration, there may be no hematuria. After blunt trauma, such as motor vehicle accidents, fractures of the 11th and 12th ribs, or injury to the transverse process of L_1 or L_2 may signal possible renal injury. An IVP or CT should be obtained, if possible. Arteriography is useful if the patient's condition permits. With major injuries involving the renal cortex and calyceal rupture, extravasation of contrast medium is seen; extravasation is not seen with less severe injuries. Likewise, severe penetrating injuries demonstrate extravasation, and less serious injuries do not.

Treatment of renal injuries depends on the extent of injury and the associated nonurologic injuries. Conservative therapy is the treatment of choice for contusions. Treatment of major renal injuries is usually surgical. If surgery is done, every effort must be made to control bleeding by clamping the renal hilar vessels and allowing more accurate evaluation and precise repair (McAninch, 1993).

Ureteral Trauma

Ureteral trauma is most often iatrogenic (e.g., surgery: gynecologic or general). The sooner it is recognized (e.g., at the operating table), the better. Repair is easier at that point than at any other time. Delayed recognition is usually unmasked by IVP. Fever, mass, ileus, or anuria may signal the need for IVP.

Bladder Trauma

Pelvic injuries with fracture may cause bladder injury due to penetration of bony fragments or sudden pressure on the distended bladder, causing rupture. Injuries may be extra- or intraperitoneal. The urine is grossly bloody. In the absence of a bloody urethral discharge, a catheter is placed and cystography is performed with 200 mL of diluted contrast material (Cystocon) dripped in. Cross-table lateral and anteroposterior films are obtained after the medium infusion has been completed. Drainage films are obtained when the bladder has emptied. The extraperitoneal versus intraperitoneal extent is differentiated. The extent of injury dictates the mode of repair. Most injuries—and all intraperitoneal injuries—require surgical repair. A suprapubic catheter and a urethral Foley catheter are left in place for a few days. The Foley catheter is removed first to minimize the development of stricture. When the patient can void normally, the suprapubic catheter is removed.

A small extraperitoneal injury may require 7 days of Foley catheter drainage. The catheter is then removed and most patients void normally.

Urethral Trauma

Significant urethral injuries occur mostly in men. The injuries may occur with crushing by straddle injury or by pelvic injuries in which the urethra is sheared off near the external sphincter.

If fresh blood is seen at the urethral meatus, *do not* attempt to insert a Foley catheter. Instead, obtain a retrograde urethrogram. It can be done by injecting contrast medium into the urethra with an irrigating syringe or Asepto syringe. Extravasation of medium indicates a need for urologic consultation.

The most common urethral injuries are caused by vigorous attempts at catheterizing a patient who has acute urinary retention. Patients most likely to have trouble being catheterized are those with a history of urethral disease (stricture) or previous transurethral resection. If several *gentle* attempts at catheterization fail, call a urologist.

Penile Trauma

The most common penile injury is "degloving" when clothes and penis are caught in power machinery. Urologic consultation is proper. If skin grafts are needed, the urologist may request plastic surgery consultation. Moist, sterile bandages should cover the penis until consultants arrive.

Mutilating injuries are rare. The dismembered penis should be kept in iced saline until repair can be accomplished.

Penile fractures during intercourse are also rare. When it does occur, there is localized swelling, pain, and hematoma. An ice pack should be kept in place to retard further bleeding until surgical repair can be accomplished. Surgical repair is mandatory.

Testicular Trauma

Significant trauma to the testicle is rare. Rupture of the tunica albuginea results in hematoma and extrusion of spermatogenic tissue. Prompt surgical repair is the treatment of choice and results in salvaging more spermatogenic tissue.

INCONTINENCE

Urinary incontinence is a common source of physical and social disability, resulting in an estimated direct cost of $10 billion per year in the United States. Stress urinary incontinence results in significant morbidity in one fourth to one third of middle-aged and elderly women (Wahle et al., 1994).

Evaluation of the incontinent patient begins with a complete examination, including a pelvic examination in women and palpation of the prostate gland in men. The autonomic arch innervating the bladder can be evaluated by testing the bulbocavernous reflexes. It involves squeezing the glans penis or clitoris, which normally causes contraction of the anal sphincter. An absent reflex suggests interruption of the normal neuronal arch. Neuronal competence can also be evaluated by checking rectal tone and by noting the individual's ability to contract the rectal sphincter voluntarily.

Evaluation of incontinence should include a postvoid residual catheterization. A residual volume of more than 30 mL is abnormal. IVP may detect outflow tract obstruction. A postvoid IVP film may demonstrate detrusor hypertrophy, bladder diverticuli, or intravesical prostatic enlargement. If discontinuation of any anticholinergic medication or treatment of infection does not result in alleviation of symptoms, referral is indicated.

There are three types of incontinence: stress, urgency, and overflow.

1. *Stress urinary incontinence* can be classified into two types: anatomic and intrinsic sphincter dysfunction. The main causes of anatomic incontinence are hysterectomy, hormone deprivation, and obstetric trauma. With stress incontinence there is hypermobility of the bladder neck and proximal urethra. Incontinence occurs with varying degrees of increased abdominal pressure (e.g., coughing, laughing, jogging, lifting). Physical findings most often demonstrate a cystocele and positive Marshall-Marchetti-Krantz (MMK) test. Surgical treatment results in a high (80 to 90 per cent) cure rate. The vaginal approach is preferable because of decreased morbidity. An abdominal approach is used when hysterectomy or other abdominal or pelvic surgery is planned. With intrinsic sphincter dysfunction, there is evidence of severe incontinence at low levels of activity (low intraabdominal pressure) and good pelvic support. Treatment is a "sling procedure" (McGuire et al., 1987) and sometimes periurethral injections of collagen (McGuire and Appell, 1994).

2. *Urgency incontinence* is a complaint wherein the patient has the urge to void but cannot reach the toilet in time. The problem may be due to neurogenic bladder instability, inflammatory conditions, or mobility problems (arthritis, parkinsonism). Bladder instability can be helped by anticholinergic agents such as oxybutynin (Ditropan) 5 mg every 12 hours. Inflammatory conditions can be improved by anticholinergic drugs but more importantly by treating the underlying disease, such as infection.

3. With *overflow incontinence* small amounts of urine are released every few minutes day and night. It occurs in conjunction with neurogenic disease caused by diabetes mellitus, stroke, spinal cord disease, and urinary obstruction. The bladder is distended, and there is a large amount of residual urine. If the obstruction can be surgically relieved, it is the most effective way to treat this condition. Intermittent catheterization is helpful, especially if the patient can do it. Often it is not possible, and an indwelling catheter is the last recourse. Behavioral training is helpful in some patients and should be tried if the patient can be motivated and encouraged.

CATHETER CARE

When catheters are left in place more than 72 hours, the urine tends to become colonized. If the catheter is left in place only temporarily and removed as quickly as the patient can void, no infection results. If left for a longer period with intermediate-term catheterization (5 to 10 days), antibacterial coverage is warranted. Antibacterials are also warranted in diabetics with short-term catheterization. Prophylactic use of antibacterials when there is long-term or permanent use of cathe-

ters is not indicated, as it leads to bacterial resistance. When patients are symptomatic (fever, bladder pain, gross hematuria), specific antibacterials based on sensitivity studies should be given for 7 days. Catheters should be changed once a month to prevent encrustation.

IMPOTENCE

Impotence is the consistent inability to attain and maintain erections sufficiently rigid enough for vaginal penetration and sexual satisfaction. An estimated 10 million men have erectile dysfunction, an age- and disease-dependent disorder with an incidence of 1.9 per cent at age 40 and 25 per cent at age 65. Diabetes mellitus is reported to have an incidence as high as 50 per cent. There are numerous causes of erectile dysfunction. The more widely recognized causes of the organic form of the dysfunction are listed in Table 46–7.

History

The patient complaining of impotence must be helped in the interview by asking pertinent questions to assist in defining the problem.

Does the penis ever get firm enough for penetration? When was the last time?
Does it detumesce prior to climax?
When was the last climax with intercourse? Masturbation?
Is there pain with climax? Bleeding?
Are there nocturnal erections? How often?
Are there other partners? Is the problem the same with all partners?
Is the marriage stable? Happy?
Does the wife contribute to the problem?

TABLE 46–7. CAUSES OF ORGANIC ERECTILE DYSFUNCTION

Vasculogenic Abnormalities	Arterial Insufficiency, Venous Incompetence
Neurogenic abnormalities	Somatic nerve neuropathy, CNS abnormalities
Psychogenic causes	Depression, performance anxiety, marital conflict
Endocrinologic causes	Hyperprolactinemia, hypogonadotropic hypogonadism, testicular failure, estrogen excess
Trauma	Pelvic fracture, prostate surgery, penile fracture
Systemic disease	Diabetes mellitus, renal failure, hepatic cirrhosis
Medications	Diuretics, tricyclic antidepressants, H_2 blockers, exogenous hormones, alcohol, antihypertensives, nicotine abuse
Structural abnormalities	Peyronie's disease

TABLE 46–8. TREATMENT OPTIONS VERSUS TESTS

Treatment	Test Required
Oral medication or vacuum erection device	None
Intracavernous injection therapy	Combined intracavernous injection and stimulation test
Penile prosthesis	Combined intracavernous injection and stimulation test or nocturnal penile tumescence
Venous surgery	Combined intracavernous injection and stimulation test Duplex scanning or cavernous arterial occlusion pressure test Cavernosometry, cavernosography
Arterial surgery (or mixed arterial and venous surgery)	Combined intracavernous injection and stimulation test Duplex scanning or cavernous arterial occlusion pressure test Cavernosometry, cavernosography Pharmacologic arteriography

From Lue TF: Impotence: A patient's goal-directed approach to treatment. *World J Urol* 8:67, 1990.

Organic impotence typically has a history of gradually declining performance that becomes consistently worse over time. Psychogenic impotence often has an abrupt onset, and performance may vary depending on moods, anxiety, partners, and so on. Impotence may coincide with the onset of medication or injury. When there is loss of interest in sex, the problem is frequently hormonal.

Laboratory testing is straightforward and rules out common problems, such as diabetes mellitus, renal failure, urinary infection, hormone imbalance. To that end, an SMA, CBC, and assays for uric acid, prolactin, and testosterone should be done routinely.

The patient's needs, desires, and thoughts must be acknowledged when selecting a treatment plan. By the same token, his or her goals affect the diagnostic plan. Lue (1990) proposed a goal-directed approach to testing that has been widely accepted (Table 46–8).

There are numerous treatment options available, from oral medication to reconstructive surgery. Yohimbine, one tablet three times a day is effective in 20 to 25 per cent of patients who have no immediate definable cause for impotence, such as diabetes mellitus, pelvic surgery, renal failure, and medications.

Vacuum erection devices work well in certain patients (Witherington, 1989). If patients decide on yohimbine or a vacuum erection device, no further testing is necessary.

Intracavernous injections are successful. When injections fail, they at least serve as a test. Currently, a three- to four-drug mixture is in use at various centers. The use of papaverine, phentolamine, and prostaglandin E_1 (PGE$_1$) allows dilution of each medication and fewer complications (e.g., pain, fibrosis, and prolonged erections). When increased medication is required, it is due to progression of the disease process (vascular, neurogenic) and not to the development of tolerance.

The more complicated, invasive studies are not universally available, are somewhat controversial, and are simply refused by some patients. Nevertheless, younger patients without an easily definable etiology should be referred to a urologist who has special interest in the treatment of impotence.

Penile prostheses have proved to be reliable, and their deimplantation rate due to infection or mechanical failure continues to decline with patient satisfaction increasing. At present, prostheses offer the most reliable of all the surgical procedures for the treatment of impotence.

PEDIATRIC ISSUES

Circumcision

Since the last edition of this book there have been a few changes in the fundamentals of newborn circumcision. Two changes in concepts that have been proposed are (1) anesthesia for newborn circumcision, and (2) the need for newborn circumcision. A discussion of the pros and cons of these two areas of controversy are beyond the scope of this presentation.

The instruments for newborn circumcision include the Plastibel, Gomco clamp, and Sheldon clamp. The baby should be restrained on a papoose board and the genital area prepared with povidone-iodine (Betadine) or another suitable agent. The child is then draped with a "peep" sheet and the adhesions between the glans penis and the foreskin are freed with a probe while holding the foreskin firmly with two mosquito clamps at 2 and 10 o'clock. At this point, the techniques vary, as follows.

1. *Plastibel.* The flexible Plastibel is inserted under the foreskin and tied securely in place with the supplied cord. This maneuver causes loss of blood supply to the foreskin, which is then excised. The handle to the bell is then broken off, and the parents are instructed that the bell and cord will fall off in several days.

2. *Gomco clamp.* A mosquito hemostat is used to clamp the dorsum of the foreskin to the area of the corona for 1 minute. A dorsal slit is then made with scissors, and the rigid bell of proper size is inserted over the glans penis and the clamp secured for 3 minutes. The foreskin is then excised.

3. *Sheldon clamp.* A mosquito hemostat is applied across the distal foreskin. The Sheldon clamp is slid into position over this mosquito hemostat. The jaws of the mosquito are closed sufficiently to prevent entrance of the tip into the urethra. The foreskin is then pulled through the jaws of the Sheldon clamp to the maximal amount of retraction, and the jaws of the Sheldon clamp are locked for 3 minutes. The foreskin is excised and the glans "popped" through the incision after removal of the Sheldon clamp.

After any of these procedures, the penis is wrapped with Vaseline gauze, and the parents are instructed to leave the dressing in place for 3 days.

Congenital Anomalies

The most frequent congenital anomalies are undescended testes and hypospadias.

Undescended Testis

Undescended testis must be differentiated from retractile testis. Undescended testis is noted at birth, whereas the retractile testis is not because the cremasteric reflexes are undeveloped at birth.

The room and the examiner's hands should be warm to examine the child who has an undescended testis. The child's legs are "frog-legged," and the examiner gently palpates the inguinal region by starting at the internal ring and sliding the finger toward the external ring. Retractile testes can be found and coaxed into the scrotum by this technique. True undescended testes may be palpated but cannot be manipulated into the scrotum.

Undescended testes occasionally can be stimulated to descend by the use of hCG. The dosage is 100 IU three times a week for 3 weeks for all age groups. Descent is much more likely when both testes are undescended.

Bilateral undescended testes require urologic consultation before a treatment regimen is formulated. Most undescended testes subsequently descend by the first birthday. Orchiopexy is planned later, as fewer than 1 per cent descend after age 1 year.

Orchiopexy should be accomplished before the boy is 6 years old. If orchiopexy has not been done by puberty, the unilateral undescended testes should be removed. The purposes of orchiopexy are to (1) promote normal development (spermatogenesis and hormone production), (2) prevent tumor formation, and (3) place the testis in a palpable location.

After orchiopexy, the patient should be examined annually until puberty. He should then be taught to examine his own testes in order to detect the development of a mass.

Hypospadias

Hypospadias with or without chordee (curvature) should be recognized at birth. Circumcision *should never be done*, as the consulting surgeon may need the prepuce to repair the defect. Consultation may be sought during the first year of life, although few attempts at correction are done that early. Ideally, surgical correction is undertaken by the time the child enters the first grade. When there is the combination of undescended testes and hypospadias, a buccal smear should be examined, along with blood karyotyping, serum electrolytes, and urine and plasma steroid determinations, to determine gender.

Enuresis

Before discussing the subject of enuresis several operational definitions are necessary.

Nocturnal enuresis: Enuretic events occur only during sleep
Diurnal enuresis: Enuretic events occur while the patient is awake.
Primary enuresis: Patient has never gained urinary control (may be nocturnal, diurnal, or both).
Secondary enuresis: There has been a period of urinary control.

EVALUATION. Evaluation of enuresis should begin with an interview that establishes the enuretic pattern of the patient. The family physician should inquire about symptoms of infection and prior or current enuresis in other family members, including the parents.

Physical examination emphasizes palpating the abdomen for masses or tenderness, palpating the genitalia for meatal stenosis or inflammation, bimanual rectoabdominal examination for anal sphincter tone, evaluation of the bulbocavernous reflex, and palpation for a bladder distended by a high residual urinary volume. Whenever possible, it is helpful to watch the patient void to assess the quality of the urinary stream.

Only urinalysis and urine culture need to be done as primary laboratory tests. A urine specific gravity higher than 1.024 rules out significant renal disease as a cause of obligatory polyuria. Patients with abnormal urinalysis or urinary tract infection should have blood urea nitrogen and serum creatinine assays, IVP, and voiding cystourethrography.

Patients with chemical or radiologic abnormalities should be referred to a urologist for further evaluation and cystoscopy. Children with daytime enuretic events should be referred before they begin school.

Patients with primary nocturnal enuresis who have a normal urinalysis without infection and a normal physical examination probably need no further evaluation. Most patients fall into this category. In patients with secondary enuresis, an inquiry should be made into the possibility of psychological trauma, such as the birth of a sibling, severe illness, moving to a new area, or death or divorce of the parents.

MANAGEMENT.   Management of enuresis is based on the reality that no one is more desirous of resolution of the problem than the patient. Judgmental or punitive attitudes of the parents or physician may be harmful. Although psychotherapy and dietary manipulation may have merit, there are four main forms of treatment that have found more success.

1. *Responsibility reinforcement* includes a progress record kept by the patient with a reward for each dry night. Patients and their families are encouraged to identify factors that may precipitate wet nights. Although this technique takes longer than others, the relapse rate is lower (Marshall et al., 1973).

2. *Bladder training* involves improving functional bladder capacity by increasing fluid intake and making a conscious effort to extend the interval between voidings. The investigation of Hagglund (1965) showed this procedure to have a better response rate than fluid restriction and night awakening or psychological management.

3. *Drug therapy* to correct enuresis has been improved markedly with the development of desmopressin (DDAVP). One spray in each nostril at bedtime carries an overall 75 per cent response rate. The response rate is above 90 per cent when there is a positive family history of nocturnal enuresis (Hogg and Husmann, 1994).

4. *Conditioning therapy* involves a signal alarm system triggered by the enuretic event. Results are said to be better than drug therapy. The apparatus, however, is cumbersome and requires considerable explanation and supervision. Moreover, "buzzer ulcers" are occasionally caused by weakened batteries leaking a constant low-voltage current to the wet skin.

Urinary Tract Infections

Symptoms of UTIs are vague from the neonatal period to about 2 years of age, consisting of fever, vomiting, and failure to thrive. After 2 years of age, the symptoms of dysuria, frequency, and abdominal or flank pain predominate (Govan et al., 1978).

Diagnosis depends on urinalysis and culture. Because of the possibility of fecal contamination, accuracy during the collection is important. When possible, a clean-catch midstream specimen is used. The most reliable method, however, is suprapubic aspiration (especially in the neonate). Catheterization is technically more difficult in the pediatric age group because of the small size of the urethra. Thus in septic infants or neonates the suprapubic route is preferred.

Investigation

Children should be thoroughly evaluated at the time of their first UTI. Initial tests include an IVP, voiding cystourethrogram, and creatinine clearance. Thirty to fifty per cent of these evaluations detect an anatomic abnormality that requires either surgical correction or frequent follow-up visits for evaluation with a urine culture. Waiting until a second infection is documented does not increase the diagnostic incidence of correctable abnormalities discovered by radiologic investigation. Furthermore, 80 per cent of those with first infections have another within 18 months. Deferring investigation is therefore justified.

Vesicouretal reflux is the most frequent abnormally found by *radiologic investigation*. There are usually three grades of reflux on voiding cystourethrogram:

Grade 1:   reflux into the ureter without extension into the renal pelvis
Grade 2:   reflux extending into the renal pelvis but without causing dilation of the calyces
Grade 3:   reflux into the renal pelvis causing dilation and distortion of the calyces

Additional evidence may be gained in the last instance by an IVP, which may show delayed excretion in addition to dilated and tortuous ureters. Cortical scars may also be demonstrated. Other abnormalities include obstruction at the ureteropelvic junction, ureterocele, ureteral duplication with ectopic orifice, and posterior urethral valves and urethral meatal stenosis in boys.

Creatinine clearance correlates well with the functional integrity of the kidneys. A 4-hour test is adequate, providing strict attention is given to the collection of the specimen. The first voided urine specimen is discarded and the exact time recorded. All urine specimens are then saved, including the final specimen, and the time of that voiding is accurately recorded.

Cystoscopic examination need not be done in all children with UTIs. It should be done when there is vesicoureteral reflux to assess the ureteral orifice and submucosal tunnel. It should also be done when there is hematuria or difficulty controlling infection or rapid reinfection.

Treatment

The treatment of choice for acute uncomplicated UTIs in children is oral sulfa for 7 to 10 days. There is no advantage to initiating long-term therapy at this point. Urinalysis and culture are required for follow-up at the end of the treatment period. Radiologic examination can be scheduled at this time. Almost all of the causes of treatment failure can be discovered in this way.

Ureteropelvic junction obstruction, posterior urethral valves, meatal stenosis, and severe vesicoureteral reflux may require surgical correction to gain control of infection or to prevent additional renal damage. Mild to moderate degrees of reflux can be treated prophylactically with antibacterials, as almost all cases of reflux of this grade resolve with age.

Reinfections are best treated with long-term, low-dose antibacterial agents after control of the acute phase. Either sufamethoxazole-trimethoprim, trimethoprim alone, or nitrofurantoin can be administered as a bedtime dose. Periodic urine cultures help ensure the effectiveness of the program. After three negative monthly urine cultures, increase the interval to 3 to 6 months.

If the patient is septic, tobramycin sulfate (Nebcin) should be started while awaiting the results of the urine culture and sensitivity tests, IVP, voiding cystourethrogram (VCU), and serum creatinine, which are ordered the day after admission. Tobramycin can be discontinued when fever has abated or when the sensitivity study indicates the effectiveness of less nephrotoxic drugs.

Effective treatment and follow-up help to achieve the long-term goal of UTI management. In that way progressive irreversible renal damage leading to renal failure is prevented.

Wilms' Tumor

The child with Wilms' tumor commonly presents to the primary physician with abdominal distention or an abdominal mass. Additionally, there may be fever, abdominal pain, or hematuria.

Finding an upper abdominal mass in a child indicates the need for abdominal ultrasonography in addition to a CBC, urinalysis, and serum electrolyte and chemical assays. If the mass is renal, further radiographic studies are necessary and should include at least an IVP and CT scan (Hardy, 1988).

Surgical removal is the cornerstone of treatment for management of this tumor. Pediatric urologists or surgeons are best qualified to perform this surgery. Multiple-agent chemotherapy (actinomycin D and vincristine) has been shown by the National Wilms' Tumor Study (NWTS) to be clearly superior to single-agent therapy. Additional protocols are in progress. There seems to be no advantage to radiation therapy for low stage tumors, and it is reserved for more advanced cases.

FEMALE UROLOGY

At some time during their lives, an estimated 10 to 20 per cent of women have a UTI. With most of these infections, the bacteria are confined within the bladder and are discomforting and inconvenient rather than life-threatening or even serious.

Severe morbidity does occur in association with certain conditions, such as pregnancy, diabetes mellitus, obstruction in upper tracts, vesicoureteral reflux, and immunosuppression. These entities must be recognized, as they require considerably more time, thought, evaluation, and perhaps more intensive or extensive therapy.

The pathogenesis of UTIs in women involves the interrelations between bacterial colonization of the vaginal mucosa and host susceptibility. There is abundant documentation demonstrating the correlation between increasing colonies of bacteria prior to the onset of acute urinary symptoms (Fowler and Stamey, 1977).

For adult women, Stamey's classification for bacteriuria is modified as follows:

1. First or occasional (occasional infections are always reinfections)

2. Frequent infections
   a. Reinfection
   b. Persistent infection

Reinfections account for about 99 per cent of frequent infections. During the interval between symptoms (infections), the urine is sterile. Frequent reinfections tend to increase with age.

Persistent infection means that the subsequent "frequent infection" is caused by the same organism. Between symptomatic events, the urine is not sterile. Urologic evaluation must be accomplished in these patients, as surgical intervention may lead to cure (e.g., removal of a calculus or correction of obstruction).

Acute Cystitis

Short-term therapy is now well accepted for patients with acute cystitis, provided they have no risk factors associated with more complicated conditions (e.g., diabetes mellitus, pregnancy, calculus, reflux, upper urinary tract obstruction, dysfunctional bladder, immunosuppression). Short-term (i.e., one time or 1 day) medications include amoxicillin 1.0 gram immediately and (possibly) at 12 hours, trimethoprim 100 mg once or twice, trimethoprim-sulfamethoxazole (double strength) once or twice, or tetracycline 1.0 gram once or twice for 1 day. The side effects of short-term therapy are significantly less than with more conventional therapy.

Recurrent Cystitis

The treatment of recurrent cystitis may be divided into two regimens: prophylactic and suppressive. Obviously, the acute phase must be treated at full doses before beginning the long-term dose form.

Prophylactic therapy is designed to prevent reinfection after the urine has been made sterile. The most successful medications used are nitrofurantoin 100 mg, trimethoprim-sulfamethoxazole (double strength) and trimethoprim alone (Fowler, 1986). Each is given once a day, usually at bedtime. Further reductions in therapy in sexually active women have included the use of these medications, or others, immediately after intercourse.

Suppressive therapy is used to treat persistent infections in an attempt to prevent flare-ups or to suppress bacterial growth. Once-a-day dosage is employed, and selection of the antibacterial agent depends on urine culture and sensitivity studies.

When the second documented infection is found within 6 months after a successfully treated infection, antimicrobial prophylaxis should be continued after the acute episode is treated. The drugs of choice are trimethoprim-sulfamethoxazole in combination, trimethoprim alone, or nitrofurantoin. One half (regular size) tablet of trimethoprim-sulfamethoxazole, one (100 mg) tablet of trimethoprim, or one (100 mg) tablet of nitrofurantoin macrocrystals (Macrobid) is given at bedtime for 6 to 12 months. If infections are less frequent than every 6 months, such long-term treatment is unnecessary. Postcoital use of an antibacterial drug often prevents acute cystitis.

The basis of recurrent UTIs in women involves colonization of the vaginal vestibule by Enterobacteriaceae from the fecal flora. Therefore it is helpful to understand the mechanism of action of each treatment regimen. Trimethoprim-sulfamethoxazole combination and trimethoprim alone work by eliminating most Enterobacteriaceae from the fecal flora and by being concentrated in the vaginal secretions in bactericidal concentrations, thereby killing the organisms before they can contaminate the urine. Nitrofurantoin, on the other hand, is either inactivated in the upper gastrointestinal tract or completely absorbed there. It has no influence on fecal flora or those in the vaginal vestibule. Its value lies in its effect on the organisms after they have entered the bladder.

Pregnancy

See page 541.

Stress Urinary Incontinence

See page 112, 712.

Urethral Syndrome

In addition to those patients who have documented UTIs, many women with symptoms of frequency, urgency, dysuria, suprapubic, and pelvic "pressure" or pain have a normal urinalysis or pyuria and sterile urine. Those with documented infection can be treated as previously described. If the urinalysis is normal or the culture negative, the following possibilities should be considered.

1. *Vaginitis* is almost always caused by *Candida albicans*, *Gardnerella vaginalis*, or *Trichomonas vaginalis*. *Candida albicans* is best diagnosed by Gram stain or potassium hydroxide preparation. Treatment is specific for each organism.

2. *Interstitial cystitis* is probably the most frequent cause of sterile pyuria. The etiology is unknown. Cystoscopy and biopsy are required for diagnosis. Symptomatic relief is often attained by the use of bladder instillations of dimethylsulfoxide (DMSO; Rimso) or Clorpactin WCS-90. Anticholinergics may be given in addition. Phenazopyridine (Pyridium) or Urised helps relieve symptoms.

3. *Carcinoma in situ* has no known etiology, although the incidence is higher in smokers. Cystoscopy and biopsy are required for diagnosis. Cytology is also helpful. Cystectomy is the current treatment of choice, although preliminary reports on the use of intravesical instillation of mitomycin C are encouraging.

4. *Spastic bladder* patients almost always have three characteristics: (1) symptoms only during waking hours, (2) normal urinalysis, and (3) negative urine cultures. It seems logical to assume that there are patients with the bladder counterpart to the "spastic colon," "nervous" stomach, and so on. They can best be treated by anticholinergics. Donnatal (which contains 15 mg of phenobarbital for anxiety) is useful, as is oxybutynin.

5. *Neurogenic bladder* patients have persistent, often progressive symptoms. They may have varying degrees of incontinence. Normal residual urine (30 mL or less) and normal bladder volume help to rule out neurogenic bladder dysfunction. Urodynamic studies may be indicated if there are abnormalities. Specific treatment is related to the type of dysfunction.

RENAL FUNCTION AND RENAL FAILURE

Normal Renal Function

The kidney performs a variety of excretory and endocrine functions, and in clinical practice these functions can be correlated with the glomerular filtration rate (GFR) as the single best indicator of overall function. GFR is not constant in health, varying in response to a number of stimuli including the amount of protein present in the diet. Furthermore, GFR increases from birth until 4 to 6 years of age, at which time it is proportional to body size. Thus the normal value for creatinine clearance may vary between 80 and 125 mL/min. Mean

GFR tends to decrease linearly with age, so a healthy 70-year-old has a GFR that is 70 per cent of normal. Because many drugs are cleared by the kidney, this physiologic aging of the kidney accounts for the frequency of adverse drug reactions at "normal" dosages when given to elderly patients.

The GFR is estimated in routine practice by use of the creatinine clearance test. The patient is asked to collect a timed (typically 24 hours) sample of urine. The volume and urine and serum creatinine levels are then measured and the clearance of creatinine calculated by dividing the amount of excreted creatinine by the plasma creatinine concentration. The results are usually expressed in milliliters per minute in the United States, so the amount is also divided by 1440, which is the number of minutes in the day. The amount of creatinine excreted is a function of muscle mass; the normal woman excretes 15 to 20 mg creatinine per kilogram body weight per day, and the average man excretes 20 to 25 mg/kg/day. When a creatinine clearance test is done it is useful to divide the amount of creatinine (in milligrams) by the patient's weight to determine that the collection was done properly.

When careful studies are done, it is clear that estimates of GFR determined from the creatinine clearance are variable, and that in both outpatient and inpatient settings accurate collections are difficult to complete. Thus the formula first developed by Cockcroft and Gault is widely used to estimate the creatinine clearance (Ccr) based on the patient's age, weight in kilograms, and serum creatinine in milligrams per deciliter.

$$Ccr = \frac{(140 - \text{patient's age})(\text{weight in kilograms})}{72 * (\text{serum creatinine})}$$

Oliguria and Azotemia

An abrupt decline in GFR may occur after a variety of insults. The clinical approach to the patient is largely determined by the severity of the underlying insult. In normal subjects with the ability to maximally concentrate the urine, a minimum of 400 mL of urine output per day is required to excrete the expected osmolar load resulting from the processes of intermediary metabolism. Thus a urine output less than 400 mL/day is defined as *oliguria*. *Anuria*, or the absence of urine output, is distinctly uncommon in the absence of urinary tract obstruction, and this finding demands prompt investigation of the urinary tract with ultrasonography, radionuclide studies, or direct examination via cystoscopy with retrograde urography where appropriate (Kaye and Pollak, 1982).

When renal function is impaired, azotemia de-

velops. When evaluating a patient with low urine output (less than 20 mL/hr), it is helpful to determine the presence of azotemia by measuring the BUN and serum creatinine concentrations. If the low urine output is secondary to poor renal perfusion—be it due to hypotension, heart failure, or other causes—the BUN increases disproportionately to the creatinine. Normally the BUN/creatinine ratio is less than 20:1; when it becomes more than 20:1, the patient is said to have prerenal azotemia. Postrenal azotemia may also be characterized by an increased BUN/creatinine ratio, but renal failure is usually characterized by a proportionate rise in both BUN and creatinine concentrations in the blood. The distinction is important because prerenal azotemia often indicates a serious disturbance in systemic hemodynamics, and if it is corrected promptly the development of acute renal failure is prevented.

In some cases it is difficult to determine if prerenal, or "renal," azotemia is associated with oliguria. In these patients, determination of urinary sodium excretion can be helpful, provided no diuretics have already been given. Patients with functional oliguria, where the kidney is responding as an intact organ to the perturbation in the patient's physiology, should have a spot urinary sodium concentration of less than 10 mEq/L. If the spot concentration is greater than 20 mEq/L, the odds favor intrinsic renal dysfunction. Routine measurement of sodium excretion and calculation of the fractional excretion of sodium is not necessary where diagnostic uncertainty does not prevail.

The differential diagnosis of azotemia is shown in Table 46–9.

When a patient presents without a clinical history that suggests the cause, a renal ultrasound scan is the safest way to exclude obstruction of the uri-

TABLE 46–9. DIFFERENTIAL DIAGNOSIS OF AZOTEMIA

Prerenal azotemia
  Decreased cardiac output states
  Hypovolemia
    External losses via kidney or intestine
    Internal losses ("third space")
      Nephrotic syndrome
      Cirrhosis
      Pancreatitis
      Intestinal obstruction
  Peripheral vasodilatation
    Sepsis
    Liver failure
    Antihypertensive medications

"Renal" azotemia (Table 46–10)

Postrenal azotemia
  Lower urinary tract obstruction
  Intraureteral obstruction
    Stones
    Tumors
  Extraureteral obstruction

TABLE 46–10.   MAJOR CAUSES OF ACUTE RENAL FAILURE

Hemodynamically mediated
  Hypovolemic shock
  Sepsis syndrome
  Hepatic failure

Nephrotoxic injury
  Antibiotics, especially aminoglycosides
  Allopurinol
  Cimetidine
  Radiocontrast media
  Myoglobin and hemoglobin
  Heavy metals, organic solvents, pesticides

Functional causes
  Angiotensin-converting enzyme inhibitors
  Nonsteroidal anti-inflammatory drugs

Rapidly progressive glomerulonephritis or interstitial nephritis

Vascular diseases, especially cholesterol emboli and malignant
  hypertension

Miscellaneous causes
  Hypercalcemia
  Hyperuricemia
  Oxalate nephropathy (ethylene glycol poisoning)
  Multiple myeloma

nary tract. Additionally, it provides useful information about kidney size, which helps to distinguish acute from chronic, irreversible renal failure. If the patient is not bleeding, the hemoglobin concentration may also help in that patients with acute renal failure should have near-normal values, whereas patients with chronic renal failure are usually anemic.

Acute Renal Failure

Acute renal failure is a clinical syndrome characterized by abrupt decline in GFR from normal to low levels. Severe cases are associated with oliguria, but less severe cases are associated with a urine output that remain between 800 and 1200 mL/day. The latter patient is said to have nonoliguric acute renal failure. The causes of acute renal failure are grouped as hemodynamically mediated, toxin-induced, and functional (Table 46–10) (Myers and Moran, 1986).

The clinical description of acute renal failure by Bywaters and Beall was based on observations of acute cessation of kidney function associated with a crush injury after air raids on London during World War II. Outside of earthquakes or similar major disasters, this form of acute renal failure is distinctly uncommon given the vigor and speed with which fluid volume resuscitation is usually achieved after major trauma (Better and Stein, 1990). Oliguric acute renal failure is now most commonly seen in septic patients with multiple organ failure syndrome.

Nonoliguric renal failure is common after toxic injuries, such as after exposure to radiocontrast medium or aminoglycoside antibiotics (Diamond and Yoburn, 1982). However, functional renal failure has become common as a result of widespread use of angiotensin-converting enzyme (ACE) inhibitor drugs and nonsteroidal anti-inflammatory drugs (NSAIDs). In healthy individuals the GFR is maintained within a fairly narrow range even as mean arterial pressure varies considerably, a phenomenon known as autoregulation. It is now apparent that both angiotensin II and prostaglandins are involved in this process. Administration of agents that block either of these metabolic pathways are likely to produce renal failure, especially when the patient is subjected to another physiologic stress. For instance, patients with significant congestive heart failure often demonstrate a reduced mean arterial pressure. If cardiac performance does not improve when ACE inhibitor drugs are given as afterload therapy for the failing myocardium, renal function may deteriorate as a result of blocking the angiotensin effect on intrarenal hemodynamics. Functional renal failure is so common that the first step for evaluating patients suspected of acute renal failure is to stop ACE inhibitors and NSAIDs. Management of acute renal failure is divided into two phases: conservative and dialytic. The goal of conservative management is to avoid the need for dialysis. To this end nephrotoxic drugs are discontinued, dosages for all medications are adjusted for a GFR less than 5 mL/min (*not* based on the current serum creatinine,) and fluid and potassium administration are limited.

A problem often encountered is that the fluid and electrolyte limits make it difficult to administer multiple intravenous medications and adequate parenteral nutrition. This situation indicates the need to initiate extracorporeal therapy. Other indications are intractable fluid overload, metabolic acidosis, and hyperkalemia. In the absence of these indications, the decision to start dialysis is based on the experience of the consulting nephrologist. Three options exist: hemodialysis, peritoneal dialysis, and continuous arteriovenous hemofiltration.

The prognosis in patients with acute renal failure of sufficient severity to require dialysis is poor, with an average mortality of 70 per cent despite full supportive therapy (Abreo et al., 1986). In patients with multiple organ failure syndrome the mortality rate approaches 100 per cent. Fortunately, patients with nonoliguric renal failure usually do not require dialysis, and the prognosis is determined by the underlying condition.

Chronic Renal Failure

Chronic renal failure is a clinical syndrome in which the patient's presentation may be bland initially but ultimately comes to dominate concern

TABLE 46–11. MAJOR CAUSES OF CHRONIC RENAL FAILURE

Primary renal diseases
    Chronic glomerulonephritis
    Chronic interstitial nephritis
    Polycystic kidney disease
    Alport syndrome

Systemic diseases
    Diabetes mellitus
    Hypertension
    Systemic lupus erythematosus
    Multiple myeloma and paraproteinemic states
    Systemic necrotizing vasculitis
    Hemolytic uremic syndrome and thrombotic thrombocytopenic purpura

Obstructive uropathy

Renovascular disease
    Atherosclerosis
    Cholesterol emboli

and if not treated leads to the patient's death. Patients rarely become symptomatic from chronic renal failure until the GFR is less than 10 mL/min, so most of the medical management must be done while the patient, and sometimes the physician, are not overly affected. Major causes of chronic renal failure are listed in Table 46–11.

The relation between the creatinine clearance (as a reflection of the GFR) and the serum creatinine (as a surrogate) is hyperbolic. Thus a 50 per cent reduction in the GFR, from a normal 100 mL/min to 50 mL/min, is associated with doubling of the serum creatinine, which might mean from a value of 0.7 mg/dL to 1.4 mg/dL. Both these values are within the "normal" range for many assays, so significant loss of GFR may not be readily apparent unless the patient has previous creatinine values in the medical record, or unless the relations outlined in the formula of Cockcroft and Gault are considered.

Diagnosis

Diagnosis of chronic renal failure first focuses on determining, if possible, the cause of the renal failure. Is the patient hypertensive? Is there a history of edema? Is there a family history of renal failure? Is there evidence for diabetes? Laboratory testing usually includes determination of creatinine clearance and 24-hour urine protein excretion plus visualization of the kidneys with renal ultrasonography. Specialized testing for markers of systemic diseases such as systemic lupus erythematosus is valuable on occasion. With these basic items of information it is usually possible to decide if the patient's problem is due to diabetes, hypertension, chronic glomerulonephritis, arteriolonephrosclerosis, chronic interstitial nephritis, or polycystic kidney disease. Some effort to make the correct diagnosis is useful, even though late management of patients with chronic renal failure does not depend on the cause of the renal failure.

Atherosclerotic renovascular occlusion has come to be recognized as an important cause of unexplained renal failure in elderly patients (Jacobson, 1988; Rimmer and Gennari, 1993). The role of revascularization therapy remains uncertain, as the risk of intervention in these patients is high, and in individual patients it is not certain that progression to renal failure is inevitable. Likewise, cholesterol embolization to the kidney is an important complication of angiography, especially when angioplasty of the renal artery is undertaken. In patients with significant atherosclerotic disease and progressive renal failure, though, further investigation may be warranted.

Treatment

Diabetes mellitus is the most common cause of renal failure likely to be encountered in routine office practice, and studies suggest two specific modes of therapy worthy of emphasis. First, it has now been shown that regulation of blood glucose, as reflected in the glycosylated hemoglobin level, to near-normal levels is effective in delaying the onset of proteinuria in type I diabetics. Because many of these patients are children or adolescents, attaining good control is a severe clinical challenge, but the data clearly show that the effort is worthwhile (DCCT Research Group, 1993).

In patients with established diabetic nephropathy, therapy with captopril, an ACE inhibitor, has been shown to delay the deterioration of renal function in a significant number of patients (Lewis et al., 1993). Diabetic nephropathy progresses inexorably if untreated, so these data support widespread use of these agents. ACE inhibitors are thought to be especially useful because of their effect on intrarenal hemodynamics; but as was pointed out earlier, this desired effect can become undesirable if acute renal failure supravenes. Close monitoring of renal function and potassium levels, as well as avoiding potentially nephrotoxic drugs such as NSAIDs, is essential to the safe use of these drugs.

In all patients with progressive renal failure aggressive blood pressure control and institution of a protein- and phosphorus-restricted diet is beneficial. Data suggest that the major limitation to the effectiveness of these therapies is the difficulty of obtaining patient compliance (Klahr et al., 1994). Even if these measures do not ultimately prevent the development of end-stage renal failure, they may help keep the patient asymptomatic longer, thereby delaying the need to start replacement therapy.

Renal Replacement Therapy

Hemodialysis, peritoneal dialysis, and renal transplantation are acceptable methods for replacing renal function in patients with renal failure, and all effectively prevent death due to uremia. Clearly, however, they do not prevent death. Selection of the appropriate mode of therapy is complex and involves considerable patient involvement and education. Early referral is imperative for all patients with progressive renal failure in whom replacement therapy is a reasonable consideration. In the United States the mean survival of patients requiring replacement therapy is 3 years. However, patients under the age of 70 who do not have clinically detectable disease other than renal failure do well, with a mean mortality rate of less than 10 per cent yearly (Wright, 1991). Unfortunately, patients referred for renal replacement therapy continue to get older and sicker, so the decision to pursue dialysis becomes progressively more complex. Primary care physicians have an important role to play in supporting patients and families as they deal with these complex end-of-life issues. For some, a decision to forego dialysis is clearly in the patient's best interests.

DISORDERS OF FLUID, ELECTROLYTES, AND ACID-BASE BALANCE

Dissection of disordered body fluid chemistry can be a satisfying exercise in applied physiology, provided a few key concepts are kept in mind. First, a laboratory report of an abnormal chemical test has no value independent of the patient from whom it was obtained. Second, the presence of an abnormality does not necessarily require correction. Third, the speed with which correction is attempted should be based on the severity of the patient's clinical condition; rapid correction should be reserved for those patients in whom the abnormality is associated with life-threatening manifestations.

Disorders of Sodium and Water Metabolism

Hyponatremia

Hyponatremia usually reflects an increase in plasma water, but it may reflect hyperglycemia or hyperlipidemia as well. Hyponatremia occurs in patients with an increased total body sodium content, the classic edema states of congestive heart failure, cirrhosis, and nephrotic syndrome because renal clearance of solute-free water is impaired. Hyponatremia occurs in patients with volume depletion in response to physiologic release of vasopressin (antidiuretic hormone, ADH). In euvolemic patients nonphysiologic release of vasopressin or potentiation of the hydro-osmotic effect of vasopressin at the level of the renal tubule, also known as the syndrome of inappropriate ADH (SIADH), is responsible for the development of hyponatremia. The diagnosis of SIADH, which

TABLE 46–12. DIFFERENTIAL DIAGNOSIS OF HYPONATREMIA

Patients with increased extracellular fluid volume
  Congestive heart failure
  Hepatic cirrhosis
  Nephrotic syndrome
  Renal failure

Patients with decreased extracellular fluid volume
  Gastrointestinal losses (vomiting, diarrhea)
  Renal losses (diuretics, adrenal insufficiency)
  "Third space" losses (peritonitis, pancreatitis, burns)

Patients with normal extracellular fluid volume
  Endocrine (hypothyroidism, glucocorticoid deficiency)
  Pain or trauma states
  Drugs (diuretics, chlorpropamide, clofibrate, cyclophosphamide, carbamazepine, nicotine, narcotics, antipsychotics)
  SIADH
    Malignancy (lung, lymphoma, pancreas)
    Pulmonary disorders (pneumonia, abscess, respiratory failure)
    CNS disorders (head trauma, stroke, acute psychosis, meningitis)

is one of exclusion, is the most commonly encountered cause of hyponatremia in hospitalized patients. The differential diagnosis of hyponatremic states is shown in Table 46–12.

The key to effective diagnosis and treatment is estimation of total body sodium content. The presence of dependent edema is usually apparent and generally reflects an increase in total body sodium content. A fall in systolic and diastolic blood pressures of more than 10 mm Hg associated with a rise in heart rate when going from the recumbent to the upright position usually indicates volume depletion. Patients with diabetes, the debilitated elderly, and those on antihypertensive medication may demonstrate orthostasis in the absence of volume depletion. Tissue turgor is a highly variable sign but is helpful in extreme cases. The greatest difficulty is usually encountered when deciding if a patient is euvolemic. In uncertain cases, determination of a "spot" urinary sodium concentration can be helpful, provided the patient has not been receiving diuretics. In patients with edema disorders and those with volume depletion, the value is often less than 10 mEq/L.

When hyponatremia develops rapidly, neurologic symptoms develop as a result of cerebral edema; but when the condition evolves slowly, the brain is able to adapt. Asymptomatic patients are encountered with strikingly low serum sodium concentrations. Correction of hyponatremia has been associated with an irreversible neurologic injury known as central pontine myelinosis (Ayus et al., 1987; Sterns, 1987). Because therapy is not always benign, use of hypertonic saline solutions should be reserved for those patients with neurologic symptoms. The goal of therapy is to raise the serum sodium concentration above 120 mEq/L and to correct the hyponatremia at a rate of 1 mEq/L/hr

TABLE 46–13. CLASSIFICATION OF DIURETIC DRUGS

Thiazides (hydrochlorothiazide, chlorthalidone, metolazone)
Loop agents (furosemide, bumetanide, ethacrynic acid)
Carbonic anhydrase inhibitor (acetazolamide)
Potassium sparing agents (spironolactone, triamterene, amiloride)
Osmotic diuretics (mannitol)

or less. Estimating the amount of hypertonic saline needed requires calculating the patient's total body water, which can be considered equal to 50 per cent of the patient's weight. The difference between the observed serum sodium concentration and the desired concentration multiplied by total body water yields an estimate of the amount of sodium (in milliequivalents) that should be given to the patient. In practice, the inability to measure total body water and the presence of urine and other fluid losses make the calculation only an approximation. Experienced clinicians recommend giving about half the estimated quantity of sodium and then rechecking the laboratory tests before proceeding further. In patients with volume depletion, use of normal saline, rather than hypertonic saline, is safer and equally effective. In patients without neurologic symptoms, restriction of fluid intake combined with therapy directed toward correcting the underlying disorder is usually all that is required.

Diuretics

Edematous patients with hyponatremia require both fluid restriction and administration of diuretics. The various types of diuretics are shown in Table 46–13.

Loop diuretics produce the greatest diuresis in the shortest time and are the mainstay in hospitalized patients. Lesser degrees of edema may respond to less potent agents such as thiazide diuretics. The aldosterone antagonists such as aldactone are especially useful for treating the edema of cirrhosis. It is important to remember that the loop diuretics produce their effect on the tubule only from the luminal ("urine") side of the renal tubular epithelium. In severely nephrotic patients or those with severe congestive heart failure, proximal reabsorption of filtrate may be so complete that inadequate quantities of diuretics are delivered to the loop of Henle, resulting in apparent resistance to the diuretic effect of the drug. In such patients, administration of metolazone, a thiazide diuretic with some activity in the proximal portions of the nephron, in conjunction with a loop diuretic may be needed to achieve adequate diuresis. Hypokalemia, hyponatremia, metabolic alkalosis, and volume depletion are recognized complications of diuretic use (Friedman et al., 1989; Johnson and Wright 1983; Tannen, 1985).

Hypernatremia

Maintenance of normal body fluid tonicity is critical to the function of biologic systems. The thirst sensation, which is driven by a variety of hormonal stimuli related to preservation of tonicity and volume of body fluids, normally prevents development of significant hypernatremia. Clinically significant hypernatremia is seen only in patients unable to verbalize thirst or unable to obtain fluids, such as the young, the debilitated elderly, those with neurologic disorders, and those with massive fluid losses such as that due to severe burn injury (Snyder et al., 1987).

Most patients with hypernatremia are not only dehydrated but also volume-depleted. Thus initial therapy consists in normal saline given intravenously. Normal saline has a sodium concentration of 154 mEq/L, so it is relatively hypernatremic; but with restoration of adequate circulating volume the kidney begins to excrete sodium in excess of water, leading to correction of the hypernatremia. Administration of free water, either orally or intravenously, must be slow. Abrupt lowering of plasma tonicity generates a gradient between the brain and the extracellular fluid favoring movement of water into the brain, resulting in significant cerebral edema. As in the case of the hyponatremic patient, final correction to normal tonicity is best done slowly after the initial resuscitation has been accomplished.

Polyuria

Lesser degrees of hypernatremia may be seen in patients with a variety of disorders characterized by loss of water in excess of loss of volume (Table 46–14). Polyuria is characteristic of those conditions in which the fluid loss is primarily a result of altered renal physiology, such as in the patient with hyperglycemia. Glucose is an osmotic diuretic, so once the filtered load exceeds the renal resorptive capacity glucosuria occurs with increased loss of water and electrolytes. Chronic renal failure is characterized by loss of both urinary concentrating and diluting capacity (isosthenuria)

TABLE 46–14. DIFFERENTIAL DIAGNOSIS OF HYPERNATREMIA

Patients with decreased extracellular fluid volume
  Renal losses (diuretics, glucosuria, postobstructive states, renal failure)
  Extrarenal losses (diarrhea, vomiting, burns, excessive sweating)
Patients with normal extracellular fluid volume
  Central diabetes insipidus
  Nephrogenic diabetes insipidus
Patients with increased extracellular fluid volume
  Hypertonic feeding in infants
  Administration of sodium bicarbonate intravenously

TABLE 46–15. DIFFERENTIAL DIAGNOSIS OF POLYURIA

Glucosuria
Central diabetes insipidus (post-traumatic, tumor, Guillain-Barré syndrome)
Nephrogenic diabetes insipidus
  Congenital (rare)
  Acquired (renal failure, hypercalciuria, hypokalemia, obstructive uropathy)
  Drug-induced (lithium, amphotericin, demeclocycline)
Psychogenic polydipsia

TABLE 46–16. DIFFERENTIAL DIAGNOSIS OF HYPOKALEMIA

Shift into the intracellular space
  Insulin
  β-Adrenergic receptor stimulation
  Alkalemia secondary to hyperventilation
Potassium depletion
  Gastrointestinal losses (diarrhea, laxative abuse)
  Renal losses (vomiting, diuretics, magnesium deficiency, hyperaldosteronism)

and may present as polyuria. The differential diagnosis is shown in Table 46–15.

Psychogenic polydipsia with secondary polyuria is particularly difficult to distinguish from the physiologic causes of polyuria shown in Table 46–15. Psychotic patients on neuroleptic drugs often ingest phenomenal quantities of fluid, and hyponatremia may be seen as a result (Goldman et al., 1988).

Disorders of Potassium Metabolism

Potassium is the principal intracellular cation; maintenance of a physiologic intracellular/extracellular potassium concentration ratio is crucial for the function of excitable tissue, especially cardiac muscle. It is therefore not surprising that a number of systems operate to maintain the serum potassium concentration within a narrow range. Insulin and epinephrine cause shifts of potassium into cells, and aldosterone facilitates excretion of potassium into the urine (Sterns et al., 1981). Changes in the measured serum potassium level may not reflect a change in total body potassium; they may instead reflecting a shift of potassium into or out of the cells. In those cases, addressing the underlying disorder is usually all that is required to correct the abnormality in the laboratory test. In patients with hyperkalemia and those with hypokalemia, the physiologic importance of the observed abnormality can be assessed by examining the electrocardiogram. In patients with hypokalemia U waves are seen, whereas those with hyperkalemia have a peaking of the T wave, prolongation of the PR interval to include third degree heart block, or ultimately the sine wave.

Hypokalemia

In most patients, hypokalemia reflects loss of potassium through gastrointestinal fluid losses, urinary potassium excretion, or a combination of the two (Table 46–16). Hypokalemia is seen occasionally in patients with extreme β-adrenoceptor stimulation induced by medications such as terbutaline.

Whereas diuretic- and diarrhea-induced hypokalemias are the most commonly encountered problems, spontaneous hypokalemia can be a clue to significant underlying metabolic disorders. Determining the presence of hypertension is helpful, as adrenal disorders are characterized by both hypertension and hypokalemia. However, the most common cause of spontaneous hypokalemia in a hypertensive patient is persistent high dietary sodium intake in the presence of a renovascular lesion, leading to sustained hyper-reninemia and hypertension.

Surreptitious laxative and diuretic use should be considered in patients in whom the cause of hypokalemia is not apparent from the routine history and physical examination. Diuretics are used more often by those working in medical occupations, and laxatives are more commonly used by the general population. Direct confrontation is generally to no avail, and confirming a clinical suspicion may require a variety of uncommon laboratory tests, conversations with significant family members, and indirect questioning of the patient (Wright and DuVal, 1987).

Potassium replacement is best done gradually and, if possible, orally. Concentrated intravenous potassium solutions are caustic and cause considerable discomfort when given by peripheral vein, so central administration is preferred. Aggressive intravenous potassium administration is variable in its effect of increasing serum potassium concentrations. In normal subjects, prompt internal distribution of the administered dose effectively buffers the rise in plasma potassium levels; but in ill patients, especially those with diabetes or renal failure, a catastrophic rise in potassium levels can be induced. Thus the rate of infusion should rarely exceed 10 mEq/hr. In most patients, provision of supplemental potassium 60 mEq/day should be sufficient to prevent hypokalemia. Failure to achieve a normal serum potassium level with this amount of replacement should lead to consideration of rarer diagnostic possibilities, such as magnesium depletion or renal tubular acidosis.

Hyperkalemia

The differential diagnosis of hyperkalemia is shown in Table 46–17. Perhaps the most commonly encountered cause of significant hyperkalemia is diabetic ketoacidosis. The etiology of the

TABLE 46–17. DIFFERENTIAL DIAGNOSIS OF HYPERKALEMIA

Renal failure
Aldosterone deficiency (Addison's disease)
Hyporeninemic hypoaldosteronism
Drugs
   Angiotensin-converting enzyme inhibitors
   Nonsteroidal anti-inflammatory drugs
   Heparin
   Cyclosporin A

TABLE 46–18. DIFFERENTIAL DIAGNOSIS OF HYPERCALCEMIA

Primary hyperparathyroidism
Malignancy (lung, breast, myeloma, renal cell, prostate)
Endocrine (thyrotoxicosis, Addison's disease)
Sarcoidosis
Paget's disease of bone
Drugs (vitamin A, vitamin D, thiazide diuretics, milk-alkali syndrome)

hyperkalemia in this condition is complex but reflects translocation of potassium from the intracellular to the extracellular space (Androgue and Madias, 1981). Thus the patient with ketoacidosis who presents with a normal serum potassium level reliably develops hypokalemia once therapy is instituted. In such patients potassium replacement should begin early in the course of treatment.

Diabetic patients are particularly prone to develop moderate hyperkalemia as a manifestation of diabetic nephropathy due to the predilection of the microvascular disease to involve the efferent arteriole and the juxtaglomerular apparatus. These patients develop a hyporeninemic hypoaldosteronism with hyperkalemia and often a mild metabolic acidosis. Administration of ACE inhibitor drugs such as captopril exacerbates this problem and can lead to the development of significant hyperkalemia. Because these drugs appear to have particular utility in slowing the progression of diabetic nephropathy, their use is encouraged, but both the physician and the patient must be alert to the dangers of hyperkalemia.

Life-threatening hyperkalemia is rare in patients with normal renal function, but recognition of the early electrocardiographic signs and prompt institution of therapy is imperative. In patients showing significant slowing of ventricular conduction, intravenous calcium is the most effective initial agent but reverses the changes only transiently. Intravenous glucose (with insulin in those suspected of impaired insulin response) is helpful because it forces increased translocation of potassium into cells. Intravenous sodium bicarbonate is commonly recommended but is not especially effective except in patients with concomitant severe metabolic acidosis. Ultimately, therapy must include removal of potassium from the body, either by dialysis or by administration of polystyrene resin (Kayexalate).

Disorders of Calcium, Phosphate, and Magnesium Metabolism

Calcium, phosphate, and magnesium metabolism are intimately tied to bone metabolism. A discussion of bone metabolism and metabolic bone diseases is outside the scope of this chapter. Instead, the focus is on those abnormalities likely to be encountered in daily practice.

Calcium

The causes of hypercalcemia are listed in Table 46–18.

Asymptomatic hypercalcemia appearing on a routine chemistry profile is most often due to hyperparathyroidism. Parathyroid hormone acts on the renal tubule to reduce urinary calcium excretion and increase urinary phosphate excretion; hence many patients have an accompanying low or low-normal serum phosphate level. The presence of a normal or high serum phosphate level in a patient with hypercalcemia should raise concern about an underlying destructive bone lesion from a metastatic lesion. The ease of measuring parathyroid hormone in clinical practice has reduced the diagnostic difficulty, but the decision to proceed with surgical exploration to excise the parathyroid gland is still difficult in asymptomatic patients (Lafferty and Hubay, 1989). In most instances, the decision hinges on the degree of elevation (with those having a value more than 1 mg/dL above the upper limit of normal more likely to need surgery), the compliance of the patient with prolonged medical follow-up, and the availability of a surgeon experienced in parathyroid surgery. Even experienced surgeons can have difficulty identifying the glands and determining which ones should be removed, so the patient's overall medical condition is also an important factor to consider before opting for surgery.

The symptoms of hypercalcemia range from constipation to weakness and in severe cases to lethargy, obtundation, coma, and death. Treatment of hypercalcemia begins with initiation of a saline diuresis by administering large amounts of intravenous saline followed by intravenous furosemide. Most patients with significant symptoms are volume-depleted, but a degree of renal failure is also common, so the goal of increasing urine output must be balanced with the risk of inducing pulmonary edema. If urine output can be sustained in excess of 150 mL/hr, improvement in serum calcium levels is likely. Use of other, more toxic measures, such as administration of mithramycin, calcitonin, or diphosphonates, is best done in conjunction with consultants familiar with their use, effects, and side effects.

True hypocalcemia is uncommon, but a low calcium level is seen in patients with hypoalbuminemia. Physiologic regulation of calcium metabolism is directed toward control of the ionized calcium, but the laboratory measures *total* calcium, which includes both free and bound portions. A reduction of 0.8 mg/dL can be expected for each 1 gm/dL reduction in serum albumin concentration. Hypomagnesemia, which is common in alcoholic patients, leads to hypocalcemia, often associated with resistant hypokalemia. Correction of hypomagnesemia leads to prompt correction of the hypocalcemia.

Hypocalcemia is treated by administering supplemental oral calcium and vitamin D. Selection of the form of vitamin D depends on considerations of cost and the desired result. Patients with chronic renal failure, for instance, are often given calcitriol. Use of this form results in replacement of the missing form of the active vitamin but is achieved at considerable expense. Iatrogenic hypercalcemia is the principal hazard of therapy.

Phosphate

Phosphates are important cofactors in glucose and energy metabolism as well as participants in bone formation. Hyperphosphatemia is a routine observation in patients with chronic renal failure, and the phosphate level in growing children is above that of the normal range in adults; otherwise, hyperphosphatemia is rare.

Hypophosphatemia is seen in alcoholics and other nutritionally depleted individuals (Knochel, 1985). Injudicious administration of glucose without adequate phosphate therapy in such patients can be fatal. Hypophosphatemia is also seen during the recovery phase from ketoacidosis, especially in those with a particularly severe case. Intravenous preparations of both sodium and potassium phosphate buffer solutions are readily available. The total daily dose in patients being repleted intravenously is 20 to 40 mmol of phosphate as the mixed buffer. Rapid administration is to be avoided because of the risk of hypocalcemia.

Magnesium

Hypermagnesemia is rarely seen except in patients with renal failure who receive magnesium-containing antacids or purgatives and in women being treated with parenteral magnesium for toxemia of pregnancy. The symptoms mimic those of hypercalcemia. Hypomagnesemia can cause both hypocalcemia and hypokalemia, and it is seen in alcoholic patients with significant nutritional depletion. Some drugs, notably diuretics and aminoglycoside antibiotics, also cause hypomagnesemia.

Acid-Base Disorders

In healthy individuals the pH of body fluids is closely regulated to 7.4 by the interaction of pulmonary excretion of carbon dioxide, renal conservation of filtered bicarbonate, and regeneration of the acid consumed by the processes of intermediary metabolism. Urinary excretion of acid is principally in the form of ammonium chloride and so-called titratable acid, which consists principally of phosphoric and sulfuric acids. Ingestion of the typical acid-ash meat diet of humans results in ingestion of quantities of inorganic phosphates and sulfates. Excretion of these compounds lowers the urinary pH, resulting in increased ammonium production and an increase in net acid excretion.

The chemical relations among bicarbonate, acid concentration, and carbon dioxide tension are described by the Henderson equation.

$$[H^+] = \frac{24 \times [CO^2]}{[HCO_3^-]}$$

This form of the equation is clinically useful, provided the relation between pH and hydrogen ion concentration can be remembered. For most purposes it is sufficient to remember that pH 7.4 equals a $[H^+]$ of 40 mEq/L, pH 7.2 equals a $[H^+]$ of 63 mEq/L, and pH 7.0 equals a $[H^+]$ of 100 mEq/L. With these rules of thumb, it is possible to calculate the value of any one variable provided the other two are known.

Clinical perturbations of acid-base balance occur mainly as a result of disordered respiration or metabolism, but combined disorders are not rare. The body attempts to compensate for a primary acid-base disturbance by altering the performance of either the lung or the kidney. Thus chronic respiratory failure results in increased urinary net acid excretion with a rise in serum bicarbonate concentration. These normal compensatory processes should not be mistaken for primary disturbances. Compensation is usually incomplete, and the degree of compensation can usually be predicted using the clinical rules shown in Table 46–19.

Respiratory Acidosis

Alveolar hypoventilation with acute retention of carbon dioxide leads to acute respiratory acidosis. Examination of the Henderson equation shows that doubling of the PCO_2 leads to doubling of the $[H^+]$. If the condition develops slowly and is chronic, however, serum bicarbonate increases and tends to bring the pH back toward 7.4.

Treatment of respiratory acidosis is directed at the underlying lung function disorder, when possible. A secondary goal of therapy must be to avoid inducing another disorder of acid-base metabolism. Administration of diuretics to patients with chronic hypercapnea and cor pulmonale, for exam-

TABLE 46–19. EXPECTED COMPENSATION IN PRIMARY ACID-BASE DISORDERS

Primary Disorder	Expected Range of Compensation
Metabolic acidosis	$PCO_2 = 1.5 (HCO_3^-) + 8 \pm 2$ PCO_2 = last two digits of pH
Metabolic alkalosis	$PCO_2 = 0.9 (HCO_3^-) + 9$
Acute respiratory acidosis	HCO_3^- increases 1 mEq/L for every 10 mm Hg increase in PCO_2
Chronic respiratory acidosis	HCO_3^- increases 3.5 mEq/L for every 10 mm Hg increase in PCO_2
Acute respiratory alkalosis	HCO_3^- decreases 2 mEq/L for each 10 mm Hg fall in PCO_2
Chronic respiratory acidosis	HCO_3^- decreases 5 mEq/L for each 10 mm Hg fall in PCO_2

ple, can lead to overt metabolic alkalosis in addition to the expected metabolic compensation. If the pH has returned to normal the patient has a mixed disorder. The rules shown in Table 46–19 can be used to determine whether the patient has a primary respiratory acidosis with expected compensation or has in fact developed a second disorder of acid-base balance. Likewise, when patients require mechanical ventilation after prolonged hypercapnea, care must be taken to avoid adjusting the settings so that the PCO_2 returns to 40 mm Hg. If the patient has compensated by raising the serum bicarbonate to 40 mEq/L, for instance, the Henderson equation shows that the $[H^+]$ would fall to 24 mEq/L (approximately pH 7.6), which would be termed posthypercapnic metabolic alkalosis.

Respiratory Alkalosis

Hyperventilation may be evident, as in the anxious patient with classic hyperventilation syndrome, or subtle, as in the patient with cirrhosis. The differential diagnosis of respiratory alkalosis is shown in Table 46–20.

Chronic respiratory alkalosis is unique in being the only disorder of acid-base metabolism in which compensation may be complete, and the pH may return to normal. Respiratory alkalosis can be associated with other primary disturbances of acid-base balance. The classic instance is aspirin overdosage, where the patient develops respiratory alkalosis due to central stimulation and metabolic acidosis due to the salicylic acid.

Metabolic Acidosis

Metabolic acidosis occurs when the acid load in the body is increased and the normal metabolic

TABLE 46–20. DIFFERENTIAL DIAGNOSIS OF RESPIRATORY ALKALOSIS

Anxiety
Fever, gram-negative sepsis
Hyperthyroidism
Pregnancy
Liver disease
Lung disease (asthma, early pulmonary edema, restrictive lung disease, pulmonary emboli, pneumonia)
Salicylates

acid load is not excreted properly, or when bicarbonate is lost. The differential diagnosis is facilitated by calculation of the "anion gap." Because electroneutrality is always maintained, the "gap" is a construct of the fact that only two major cations and two major anions are routinely measured in clinical practice. The sum of the chloride and bicarbonate concentrations is usually 12 to 16 mEq/L less than the sodium concentration. Because potassium concentrations do not vary much they are conveniently ignored. When a new acid is added to the system, consumption of bicarbonate occurs, but physiologic processes do not promptly eliminate the acidic anion and replace it with chloride, so the "gap" increases. The causes of metabolic acidosis with an increased anion gap are shown in Table 46–21. It is a short list and is worth committing to memory because virtually all life-threatening metabolic acidosis is of the increased anion gap variety.

Treatment of diabetic ketoacidosis, the most common form of increased anion gap metabolic acidosis, is discussed elsewhere (Chapter 41). It is important to recognize that ketoacidosis is also encountered in malnourished alcoholics and is frequently associated with nontraumatic rhabodmyolysis. Prompt therapy with fluids and glucose may prevent acute renal failure.

TABLE 46–21. DIFFERENTIAL DIAGNOSIS OF INCREASED ANION GAP METABOLIC ACIDOSIS

Ketoacidosis
  Diabetes
  Starvation
  Alcoholic
  Glycogenesis type I (von Gierke's disease)

Lactic acidosis
  Shock
  Respiratory failure
  Seizures
  Toxins (carbon monoxide, phenformin)
  Systemic diseases (liver failure, diabetes, malignancy, renal failure)

Toxins
  Methanol
  Ethylene glycol
  Salicylates
  Paraldehyde

Lactic acidosis usually occurs in settings where tissue oxygen delivery or utilization is impaired, mainly shock states. The other causes of lactic acidosis are rare. Ingestion of methanol or ethylene glycol should be suspected when unexplained metabolic acidosis is observed in alcoholic patients. Emergency therapy is directed toward blocking metabolism of the toxin by administering ethanol intravenously while arrangements are made to remove the methanol or ethylene glycol by dialysis.

Intravenous bicarbonate administration to treat acidosis is controversial (Narins and Cohen, 1987). Circulatory physiology is impaired when the pH is less than 7.1, regardless of the cause of the acidemia. Thus it has seemed logical to administer bicarbonate acutely. Unfortunately, this action is accompanied by a marked rise in plasma osmolality; and because penetration of bicarbonate into the brain and intracellular space is less rapid than into the extracellular space, paradoxical intracellular acidosis may occur. In view of these observations, the prudent course is to withhold bicarbonate therapy when rapid correction of the underlying disorder is anticipated, as would be the case in ketoacidosis, hypovolemic shock, or cardiopulmonary resuscitation.

Other forms of metabolic acidosis are accompanied by a compensatory rise in serum chloride concentrations and are therefore known as hyperchloremic metabolic acidosis (Batlle, 1981). The differential diagnosis of these disorders can be complex, as this disorder can develop as a result of inadequate urinary acidification, incomplete reclamation of the filtered load of bicarbonate, gastrointestinal losses of bicarbonate, or a combination of two or more mechanisms. Examination of the serum potassium level and determining the presence of hypertension are helpful steps in narrowing the differential diagnosis (Table 46–22).

Normally, net acid generation approximates 10 mEq/kg body weight per day, so administration of this amount of bicarbonate should result in normalization of the pH. Unfortunately, continued losses during replacement therapy makes it impossible to attain a normal pH in some patients. Alkali is available as sodium bicarbonate or, when sodium

TABLE 46–22. DIFFERENTIAL DIAGNOSIS OF HYPERCHLOREMIC METABOLIC ACIDOSIS

Hypokalemia states
  Renal tubular acidosis
  Diarrhea
  Ureteral diversion

Normal or hyperkalemic states
  Hydronephrosis
  Hyporeninemic hypoaldosteronism
  Plumbism
  Renal failure

TABLE 46–23. DIFFERENTIAL DIAGNOSIS OF METABOLIC ALKALOSIS

Chloride-responsive
  Gastrointestinal losses (vomiting, chloride-wasting diarrhea)
  Diuretic therapy
  Posthypercapnea

Chloride-resistant
  Adrenal hyperfunction
  Exogenous steroid administration
  Bartter syndrome

loading is undesirable, as a buffer solution (Shohl's solution.)

Metabolic Alkalosis

In euvolemic patients, bicarbonate resorptive capacity is saturated once the concentration exceeds 28 mEq/L. When bicarbonate is given to such patients the urine becomes alkaline and significant metabolic alkalosis does not develop. Thus for clinical metabolic alkalosis to occur, loss of hydrogen ion or gain of bicarbonate ions is necessary to generate the alkalosis, but the condition must be maintained by either volume depletion or mineralocorticoid excess. Because the former conditions are terminated by administration of intravenous normal saline, they are designated chloride-responsive metabolic alkalosis. The remainder are considered chloride-resistant (Table 46–23).

The chloride-responsive forms of metabolic alkalosis are far more common, and acidification therapy is rarely indicated. In patients with life-threatening metabolic alkalosis, administration of acetazolamide simultaneously with intravenous normal saline may speed the response by blocking reabsorption of bicarbonate by the kidney. Many patients with metabolic alkalosis are also hypokalemic, so replacement of potassium is often provided simultaneously with fluid administration. However, as the pH decreases, potassium leaks from the cells, so the total amount required to restore a physiologic potassium level is often much less than would be expected from analysis of the serum potassium level alone.

Mixed Acid-Base Disorders

Patients may have more than one disorder of acid-base balance (Narins and Emmett, 1980). As noted previously, aspirin overdosage is an example of a combination of metabolic acidosis and respiratory alkalosis. The presence of a mixed disorder can be suspected by the clinical history or when the degree of "compensation" anticipated is greater or less than predicted from the clinical rules shown in Table 46–19. Such patients are commonly encountered in the intensive care unit. Some care when analyzing the results of chemistry and arterial blood gas studies in acutely ill patients can prevent unanticipated failure of the patient to respond to the therapy selected.

CLINICAL NEPHROLOGY SYNDROMES

Nephrotic Syndrome

When protein excretion exceeds 3.5 gm/day, the patient is said to have nephrotic-range proteinuria. Usually such patients exhibit the full nephrotic syndrome, which includes edema, hypoalbuminemia, and hypercholesterolemia. In many patients the presenting complaint is dependent edema. Nephrotic syndrome is associated with significant damage to the glomerulus. Therapy and prognosis are best discussed in terms of the pathologic entities associated with nephrotic syndrome. Four lesions are commonly encountered in patients undergoing renal biopsy for evaluation of nephrotic syndrome: minimal-change disease, focal glomerulosclerosis, membranous glomerulonephritis, and membranoproliferative glomerulonephritis.

Minimal-Change Disease

Minimal-change disease, sometimes called lipoid nephrosis, is the most common form of nephrotic syndrome encountered in children, but it becomes less common as the age of the patient increases. The patient is usually normotensive and has normal renal function, and the urinalysis discloses no hematuria. Administration of high dose corticosteroids induces a prompt remission of the proteinuria and edema, usually within 7 to 14 days. Patients are customarily treated for several weeks and tapered off corticosteroids without reappearance of nephrotic syndrome (International Study of Kidney Disease in Children, 1981). Such patients are classified as steroid-responsive.

Minimal-change disease can relapse, with reappearance of the full-blown nephrotic syndrome in most patients. The older the patient at the time of onset, the higher the relapse rate tends to be. However, retreatment usually results in a prompt remission. With each relapse, the probability of another relapse after retreatment decreases, although a few patients have frequent relapses of nephrotic syndrome. Treatment of these patients with cytotoxic drugs such as chlorambucil has been successful in prolonging remission. Use of these drugs is controversial, as the long-term outlook for patients with frequently relapsing nephrotic syndrome is excellent and the toxicity of such drugs is often delayed. The decision to use these agents should be made in conjunction with expert consultants.

A few patients, especially those who are older, are cleared of their nephrotic syndrome in response to corticosteroids but relapse when the dose is tapered. Such patients are said to be "steroid-dependent." The prognosis in such patients is not as good, and many probably have a variant of

the disorder that produces focal glomerulosclerosis (Mendoza and Tune, 1992).

Focal Glomerulosclerosis

Focal glomerulosclerosis is a lesion that appears in a part of some glomeruli. Sampling error is always a concern in patients who do not follow the expected course of minimal-change disease. This lesion is common in adolescents and young adults but becomes more uncommon with advancing age. The lesion is also seen in association with human immunodeficiency virus (HIV) infection, heroin abuse, and a variety of clinical syndromes. Patients with nephrotic syndrome and focal glomerulosclerosis often have severe problems with edema and lose renal function rapidly, with a mean time from diagnosis to dialysis of 5 to 7 years. Drug therapy has not been successful in most of these patients, although scattered reports of success in a few patients continue to appear. The lesion tends to recur after renal transplantation but is not considered a contraindication to the procedure.

Membranous Glomerulonephritis

The lesion of membranous glomerulonephritis is seen most commonly in middle-aged patients and is seen in association with hepatitis B virus infection, malaria, and a number of other clinical disorders. The patient's presentation is variable but usually begins with edema. Hypertension is common but usually not severe, and renal function is usually normal. The urinalysis show minimal hematuria.

The natural history of membranous glomerulonephritis is as variable as the causes, but in general 25 per cent of cases spontaneously remit, 50 per cent have persistent nephrotic syndrome, and 25 per cent progress to end-stage renal disease over a mean of 7 to 10 years. Given the variability of outcome, the effect of treatment has been difficult to determine; most experts recommend a course of high dose corticosteroid therapy for at least 2 months. A variety of immunosuppressive regimens have been employed to treat patients with this disorder, but the results are often contradictory; aggressive therapy should therefore be reserved for those patients who present with renal failure or who demonstrate rapid loss of renal function (Collaborative Study of the Adult Idiopathic Nephrotic Syndrome, 1979; Falk et al., 1992; Ledingham, 1990; Ponticelli et al., 1992; Schieppati et al., 1993).

Membranoproliferative Glomerulonephritis

Membranoproliferative glomerulonephritis, subclassified as type 1 or type 2, is uncommon. The distinguishing characteristic is hypocomplementemia, usually reflecting activation of the alternate pathway, which often persists. Untreated, the disorder progresses to renal failure. Several corticosteroid-based regimens, with or without antiplatelet therapy, seem to be effective; but the sporadic appearance of this lesion has prevented a large-scale study of the best treatment protocols (Donadio and Offord, 1989).

Clinical Approach to the Patient with Nephrotic Syndrome

The approach to the patient with nephrotic syndrome begins with a thorough clinical assessment looking for signs of systemic disease. Diabetes mellitus is the most common cause of nephrotic syndrome. The clinical management of the patient with diabetic nephropathy is discussed in the section on chronic renal failure. In the absence of clinical indications, extensive laboratory testing is not cost-effective. Determining the predominant pattern of the proteinuria has not proved helpful. In patients with minimal-change disease, the measured protein is mainly albumin, whereas in most other conditions the measured proteins appear proportional to their concentrations in plasma. Measuring microalbumin and β-2-microglobulin excretion may have research value but is not part of routine practice. Urine protein electrophoresis is indicated mainly when excretion of Bence-Jones proteins is suspected. Although most patients with multiple myeloma excrete both light and heavy chains, an increasing number are encountered who preferentially excrete only the light chain portion of the immunoglobulin protein. Patients who overproduce kappa light chains seem particularly prone to develop rapidly progressive renal failure, but they usually do not have nephrotic syndrome.

In patients determined to have intrinsic, idiopathic renal disease, the main question revolves around the decision to perform a renal biopsy. Renal biopsy is the only way a specific histologic lesion can be defined. However, review of the foregoing discussion about these lesions shows that therapy in all cases is based on corticosteroids. Formal decision analysis using the best available data shows that empiric therapy with high dose prednisone is equal to biopsy-based treatment decisions. The choice is therefore a "toss-up" (Levey et al., 1987). For most patients, the decision to pursue a renal biopsy hinges on the need to estimate the prognosis more accurately. If there are no pressing decisions to make based on the results of the study, patients are likely to refuse. If new therapeutic strategies for the more aggressive lesions, such as focal glomerulosclerosis, are developed, though, the benefit of biopsy-directed therapy increases.

Most adults with idiopathic nephrotic syndrome do not respond to corticosteroid therapy and are left with persistent nephrotic syndrome. Hence the patient is exposed to the risks of sustained hypercholesterolemia, thrombosis of the renal vein, and infection—known complications of nephrotic syndrome (Bernard, 1988). Therapy with lipid-lowering drugs has been less than satisfactory to date, but the introduction of better tolerated agents may lead to the development of an effective strategy to combat the sustained hypercholesterolemia. Routine anticoagulation is not indicated, but the propensity to form thrombi should be taken into account whenever patients are at bed rest, such as following surgery, and appropriate prophylaxis with heparin is indicated (Llach, 1985).

Nephritic Syndrome

In contrast to the nephrotic syndrome, the nephritic syndrome is characterized mainly by hematuria with RBC casts and evidence of acute renal dysfunction in the form of edema, hypertension, or renal insufficiency. Poststreptococcal glomerulonephritis is the prime example of the acute nephritic syndrome but is rarely encountered in developed countries. Most patients with poststreptococcal glomerulonephritis recover, so management is primarily supportive with emphasis on controlling blood pressure.

Red blood cell casts after an upper respiratory infection in the absence of evidence of acute renal dysfunction is characteristic of immunoglobulin A (IgA) nephropathy, which is the most common form of "nephritis" encountered in routine practice. Once thought to be a benign disorder, it is now clear that it is a major cause of end-stage renal failure worldwide. A role for heredity has been defined in rural U.S. populations in Kentucky and Tennessee, where intermarriage among cousins is common (Julian et al., 1985; Wyatt et al., 1984).

A rare patient is seen who presents with an acute illness characterized by edema, hypertension, renal failure, and biochemical evidence of nephrotic syndrome. Urinalysis discloses RBC casts, WBC casts, and protein. Such patients usually have a course characterized by rapid loss of renal function. The syndrome is called rapidly progressive glomerulonephritis (RPGN). Patients with systemic lupus erythematosus, Goodpasture syndrome, and systemic necrotizing vasculitis present with RPGN. Aggressive therapy with immunosuppressive drugs, corticosteroids, and occasionally plasma exchange may be helpful (Balow, 1985; Bruns et al., 1989; Glassock, 1992). Renal biopsy with fluorescence microscopic studies to determine the immunopathology is essential for adequate diagnosis and therapy.

REFERENCES

Abreo K, Moorthy V, Osborne M: Changing patterns and outcome of acute renal failure requiring hemodialysis. Arch Intern Med 146:1338, 1986.

Androgue HJ, Madias NE: Changes in plasma potassium concentration during acute acid-base disturbances. Am J Med 71:456, 1981.

Austin J, Linas SL: Hypokalemia. *In* Jacobson HR, Striker GE, Klahr S (eds): The Principles and Practice of Nephrology. Philadelphia, BC Decker, 1991, pp 40–48.

Ayus JC, Krothapalli RK, Arieff AI: Treatment of symptomatic hyponatremia and its relation to brain damage: A prospective study. N Engl J Med 317:1190, 1987.

Bagshaw MA: Radiation therapy for prostate cancer. *In* Skinner DG, Lieskovsky G (eds): Diagnosis and Management of Genitourinary Cancer. Philadelphia, WB Saunders Company, 1988, pp 428–445.

Balow JE: Renal vasculitis. Kidney Int 27:954, 1985.

Barry JB, Fowler FJ, Leary MP, et al: The American Urological Association symptom index for benign prostatic hyperplasia. J Urol 148:1549, 1992.

Batlle DC: Hyperkalemic hyperchloremic acidosis associated with selective aldosterone deficiency and distal renal tubular acidosis. Semin Nephrol 1:260, 1981.

Batlle DC, Salem M, Levin M, et al: More on therapy for hyperkalemia in renal insufficiency. N Engl J Med 304:373, 1989.

Bernard DB: Extrarenal complications of the nephrotic syndrome. Kidney Int 33:1184, 1988.

Bersin RM, Arieff AI: Primary lactic acidosis. Am J Med 85:867, 1988.

Better OS, Stein JH: Current concepts: Early management and prophylaxis in acute renal failure in traumatic rhabdomyolysis. N Engl J Med 322:825, 1990.

Boden G, Gibb R: Radiotherapy and testicular neoplasm. Lancet 2:1195, 1951.

Boileau M: Cancer of the kidney: Overview. *In* Genitourinary Tumors Fundamental Principles and Surgical Treatment. Orlando, FL, Grune & Stratton, 1982, pp 293–320.

Boring CC, Squires TS, Tong T: Cancer statistics 1993. CA Cancer J Clin 43:7, 1993.

Bowie WR: Urethritis and infections of the lower urogenital tract. Urol Clin North Am 7:20, 1980.

Brawer MK, Lange PH: Prostate specific antigen: Its role in early detection, staging and monitoring of prostatic carcinoma. J Endourol 3:227, 1989.

Bruns FJ, Adler S, Fraley DS, Segel DP: Long-term follow up of aggressively treated idiopathic rapidly progressive glomerulonephritis. Am J Med 86:400, 1989.

Byar DP: Studies of cancer of the prostate: Proceedings of the Veterans Administration Research Group; studies of cancer of the prostate. Cancer 32:1126, 1973.

Cadnapaphonchai P, Dorman H, McDonald FD: Differential diagnosis of acute renal failure. *In* Jacobson HR, Striker GE, Klahr S (eds): The Principles and Practice of Nephrology. Philadelphia, BC Decker, 1991, pp 631–640.

Catalona WJ, Bigg SW: Nerve sparing radical prostatectomy: Evaluation of results after 250 patients. J Urol 143:538, 1990.

Catalona WJ, Dresner SM, Haaff OH: *In* Skinner DG, Lieskovsky G (eds): Diagnosis and Management of Genitourinary Cancer. Philadelphia, WB Saunders Company, 1988, pp 285–291, 1988.

Collaborative Study of the Adult Idiopathic Nephrotic Syndrome: A controlled study of short-term prednisone treatments in adults with membranous nephropathy. N Engl J Med 301:1301, 1979.

Crawford ED, Dawkins CA: Cancer of the penis. *In* Skinner DG, Lieskovsky G (eds). Diagnosis and Management of Genitourinary Cancer. Philadelphia, WB Saunders Company, 1988, pp 549–563.

Damjanov I: Tumors of the testis and epididymis. *In* Murphy WM (eds): Urological Pathology. Philadelphia, WB Saunders Company, 1989, pp 314–379.

Danella JF, Dekernion JB, Smith RB, Steckel J: The contemporary incidence of lymph node metastasis in prostate cancer: Implications for laparoscopic lymph node metastasis. J Urol 149:1488, 1993.

DCCT Research Group. The effect of intensive treatment of diabetes on the development and progression of long-term complications in insulin-dependent diabetes mellitus. N Engl J Med 329:977, 1993.

Diamond JR, Yoburn DC: Nonoliguric acute renal failure. Arch Intern Med 142:1882, 1982.

Dixon FH, Moore RA: Tumors of the male sex organs. *In* Atlas of Tumor Pathology, Second Series, Fascicle 8. Washington, DC, Armed Forces Institute of Pathology, 1952.

Donadio JV Jr, Offord KP: Reassessment of treatment results in membranoproliferative glomerulonephritis, with emphasis on life-table analysis. Am J Kidney Dis 14:445, 1989.

Drach GW, Meares EM, Fair WR, et al: Classification of benign disease associated with prostate pain: Prostatitis or prostatodynia? J Urol 120:266, 1978.

Einhorn L: Chemotherapy of disseminated testicular cancer. *In* Skinner DG, Liekovsky G (eds): Diagnosis and Management of Genitourinary Cancer. Philadelphia, WB Saunders Company, 1988, pp 526–531.

Falk RJ, Hogan SL, Muller KE, Jennette JC: Treatment of progressive membranous glomerulopathy: A randomized trial comparing cyclophosphamide and corticosteroids with corticosteroids alone. Ann Intern Med 116:438, 1992.

Finasteride Study Group: Finasteride (MK-906) in the treatment of benign prostatic hyperplasia. Prostate 22:291, 1993.

Finlayson B: Strategies for the medical management of patients with urinary stone disease. Monogr Urol 2:113, 1981.

Fowler J: Urinary tract infections in women. Urol Clin North Am 13:673, 1986.

Fowler JE Jr, Stamey TA: Studies of introital colonization in women with recurrent urinary infections. VII. The role of bacterial adherence. J Urol 117:472, 1977.

Friedman E, Shadel M, Halkin H, Farfel Z: Thiazide-induced hyponatremia: Reproducibility by single dose rechallenge and an analysis of pathogenesis. Ann Intern Med 110:24, 1989.

Glassock RJ: Intensive plasma exchange in crescentic glomerulonephritis: Help or no help? Am J Kidney Dis 20:270, 1992.

Goldman MB, Luchins DJ, Robertson GL: Mechanisms of altered water metabolism in psychotic patients with polydipsia and hyponatremia. N Engl J Med 318:397, 1988.

Govan DW, Fair WR, Friedland GW, et al: Management of children with urinary tract infections: The Stanford experience. Urology 6:273, 1975.

Gormley GJ, Stoner E, Bruskewitz RC, et al: The effect of finasteride in men with benign prostatic hyperplasia. N Engl J Med 327:1185, 1992.

Graef JW, Cone TE (eds): Manual of Pediatric Therapeutics. Boston, Childrens Hospital, 1974.

Hagglund TB: Enuretic children treated with fluid restriction or forced drinking: A clinical and cystometric study. Ann Paediatr Fenn 11:84, 1965.

Hardy BE: Wilms' tumor. *In* Skinner DG, Liekovsky G (eds): Diagnosis and Management of Genitourinary Cancer. Philadelphia, WB Saunders Company, 1988, 362–370.

Hogg RJ, Husmann D: The role of family history in predicting response to desmopressin in nocturnal enuresis. J Urol 150:444, 1993.

International Study of Kidney Disease in Children: The primary nephrotic syndrome in children: Identification of patients with minimal-change nephrotic syndrome from initial response to prednisone. J Pediatr 98:561, 1981.

Jacobson HR: Ischemic renal disease: An overlooked clinical entity? Kidney Int 34:729, 1988.

Johnson DE: Cancer of the female urethra: Overview. *In* Johnson DE, Boileau MA (eds): Genitourinary Tumors: Fundamental Principles and Surgical Techniques. Orlando, FL, Grune & Stratton, 1982, pp 267–274.

Johnson DE, Boileau MA: Genitourinary Tumors: Fundamental Principles and Surgical Techniques. Orlando, FL, Grune & Stratton, 1982.

Johnson JE, Wright LF: Observations on thiazide-induced hyponatremia. South Med J 76:1363, 1983.

Julian BA, Quiggins PA, Thompson JS, et al: Familial IgA nephropathy: Evidence of an inherited mechanism of disease. N Engl J Med 312:202, 1985.

Kaye AD, Pollak HM: Diagnostic imaging approach to the patient with obstructive uropathy. Semin Nephrol 2:55, 1982.

Klahr S, Levey AS, Beck GJ, et al: The effects of dietary protein restriction and blood pressure control on the progression of chronic renal failure. N Engl J Med 330:877, 1994.

Knochel JP: The clinical status of hypophosphatemia. N Engl J Med 313:447, 1985.

Lafferty FW, Hubay CA: Primary hyperparathyroidism: A review of long-term surgical and nonsurgical morbidities as a basis for a rational approach to treatment. Arch Intern Med 149:789, 1989.

Lanese DM, Teitelbaum I: Hypernatremia. *In* Jacobson HR, Striker GE, Klahr S (eds): The Principles and Practice of Nephrology. Philadelphia, BC Decker, 1991, pp 31–35.

Ledingham JGG: Immunosuppressive treatment in membranous nephropathy. Q J Med 74:117, 1990.

Lee F, Torp-Pedersen FT, Siders DB: The role of transrectal ultrasound in the early detection of prostate cancer. Cancer 39:337, 1989.

Lepor H, Tang R, Shapiro E: The alpha-adrenoreceptor subtype mediating the tension of human prostatic smooth muscle. Prostate 22:301, 1993.

Levey AS, Lau J, Parker SG, Kassirer JP: Idiopathic nephrotic syndrome: Puncturing the biopsy myth. Ann Intern Med 107:697, 1987.

Lewis EJ, Hunsicker LG, Bain RP, Rhode RD: The effect of angiotensin converting-enzyme inhibition on diabetic nephropathy. N Engl J Med 329:1456, 1993.

Llach F: Hypercoagulability, renal vein thrombosis and other thrombotic complications of nephrotic syndrome. Kidney Int 28:429, 1985.

Lue TF: Impotence: A patient goal-directed approach to treatment. World J Urol 8:67, 1990.

Malloy TR: Treatment of lesions of external genitalia. *In* Smith JA Jr (ed): Lasers in Urologic Surgery. Chicago, Year Book Medical Publishers, 1985, pp 30–32.

Mark DJ: Comment: Liability for failure of birth control methods. Columbia Law Review, 76:1187, 1976.

Marshall S, Marshall HH, Lyan RP: Enuresis and analysis of various therapeutic approaches. Pediatrics 52:813, 1973.

McAninch JW: Editorial: Renal trauma. J Urol 150:1778, 1993.

McConnell JD, Barry MJ, Bruskewitz RC: Benign prostatic hyperplasia: Diagnosis and treatment. Agency for Health Care and Research. Clin Pract Guideline. Quick Ref Guide Clin 1994, Feb(8):1–17.

McGuire EJ, Appell RA: Transurethral collagen injection for urinary incontinence. Urology 43:413, 1994.

McGuire EJ, Bennett CJ, Kohnak JA, et al: Experience with pubovaginal slings for urinary incontinence at the University of Michigan. J Urol 138:525, 1987.

Mendoza SA, Tune BM: Treatment of childhood nephrotic syndrome. J Am Soc Nephrol 3:889, 1992.

Mobley TB, Myers DA, Grine WB, et al: Low energy lithotripsy with the Lithostar: Treatment results with 19,962 renal and ureteral calculi. J Urol 149:1419, 1993.

Monda JM, Oesterling JG: Medical treatment of benign prostatic hyperplasia: E-alpha reductase inhibitors and alpha adrenergic antagonists. Mayo Clin Proc 68:670, 1993.

Moore MJ, O'Sullivan B, Tannock IF: How expert physicians would wish to be treated if they had genitourinary cancer. J Clin Oncol 6:1736, 1988.

Mundy GR, Reasner CA: Hypercalcemia. *In* Jacobson HR, Striker GE, Klahr S (eds): The Principles and Practice of Nephrology. Philadelphia, BC Decker, 1991, pp 110–118.

Murphy GP, Slack NH, Mittleman H: Use of estramustine phosphate by the National Prostatic Cancer Project and by Roswell Park Memorial Institute. Urology 23:54, 1984.

Murphy W: Urologic Pathology. Philadelphia, WB Saunders Company, 1990.

Myers BD, Moran SM: Hemodynamically mediated acute renal failure. N Engl J Med 314:97, 1986.

Narins RG, Cohen JJ: Bicarbonate therapy for organic acidosis: The case for its continued use. Ann Intern Med 106:615, 1987.

Narins RG, Emmett M: Simple and mixed acid-base disorders: A practical approach. Medicine (Baltimore) 59:161, 1980.

Onik GM, Cohen JK, Reyes G, et al: Transrectal ultrasound-guided percutaneous radical cryosurgical ablation of the prostate. Cancer 72: 1291, 1993.

Orwoll ES: The milk-alkali syndrome: Current concepts. Ann Intern Med 97:242, 1982.

Paulson DF: Surgical therapy for cancer of the prostate. *In* Skinner DQ, Lieskovsky G (eds): Diagnosis and Management of Genitourinary Cancer. Philadelphia, WB Saunders Company, 1988, pp 417–424.

Pollack HM: Imaging of the urinary tract. *In* Walsh PC, Retik AB, Stamey TA, Vaughan ED (eds): Campbell's Urology. Philadelphia, WB Saunders Company, 1992, pp 394–487.

Ponticelli C, Zucchelli P, Passerini P, Cesana B: Methylprednisolone plus chlorambucil as compared with methylprednisolone alone for the treatment of idiopathic membranous nephropathy. N Engl J Med 327:599, 1992.

Porter AT, McEwan AJB, Powe JE: Results of a randomized phase III trial to evaluate the efficacy of strontium-89 adjuvant to local field external beam irradiation in the management of endocrine resistant metastatic prostate cancer. Int J Radiat Oncol Biol Phys 25:805, 1993.

Pritchett TR, Lieskovsky G, Skinner DG: Clinical manifestations and treatment of renal parenchymal tumors. *In* Skinner DG, Lieskovsky G (eds): Diagnosis and Management of Genito Urinary Cancer. Philadelphia, WB Saunders Company, 1988, pp 337–361.

Rimmer JM, Gennari FJ: Atherosclerotic renovascular disease and progressive renal failure. Ann Intern Med 118:712, 1993.

Rombola G, Batlle DC: Hyperkalemia. *In* Jacobson HR, Striker GE, Klahr S (eds): The Principles and Practice of Nephrology. Philadelphia, BC Decker, 1991, pp 49–55.

Rosenberg SA: The development of new immunotherapies for the treatment of cancer using interleukin-2: A review. Ann Surg 208:121, 1988.

Scardino PT, Wheeler TM: Prostatic biopsy after irradiation therapy for prostate cancer. Urology 25:39, 1985.

Schieppati A, Mosconi L, Perna A, et al: Prognosis of untreated patients with idiopathic membranous nephropathy. N Engl J Med 329:85, 1993.

Skinner DG, Lieskovsky G (eds): Diagnosis and Management of Genitourinary Cancer. Philadelphia, WB Saunders Company, 1988.

Snyder NA, Feigal DW, Arieff AI: Hypernatremia in elderly patients: A heterogeneous, morbid, and iatrogenic entity. Ann Intern Med 107:309, 1987.

Springberg PD, Garrett LE Jr, Thompson AL Jr, et al: Fixed and reproducible orthostatic proteinuria: Results of a 20 year follow-up study. Ann Intern Med 97:516, 1982.

Stamey TA: Pathogenesis and Treatment of Urinary Tract Infections. Baltimore, Williams & Wilkins, 1980.

Steiner MS, Morton RA, Walsh PC: Impact of anatomic radical prostatectomy on urinary continence. J Urol 145:512, 1991.

Sterns RH: Severe symptomatic hyponatremia; treatment and outcome: A study of 64 cases. Ann Intern Med 107:656, 1987.

Sterns RH, Cox M, Feig PU, Singer I: Internal potassium balance and the control of the plasma concentration. Medicine (Baltimore) 60:339, 1981.

Tannen RL: Diuretic-induced hypokalemia. Kidney Int 28(6): 988, 1985.

Thompson I: Observation alone in the management of localized prostate cancer: The natural history of untreated disease. Urology 43:41, 1994.

Veis JH, Berl T: Hyponatremia. *In* Jacobson HR, Striker GE,

Klahr S (eds): The Principles and Practice of Nephrology. Philadelphia, BC Decker, 1991, pp 26–31.

Wahle GR, Young GPH, Raz S: Vaginal surgery for stress urinary incontinence. Urology 43:416, 1994.

Witherington R: A vacuum erection device for management of erectile impotence. J Urol 141:320, 1989.

Wright LF: Maintenance Hemodialysis. Boston, GK Hall, 1981.

Wright LF: Survival in patients with end-stage renal disease. Am J Kidney Dis 17:25, 1991.

Wright LF, DuVal JW: Renal injury associated with laxative abuse. South Med J 80:1304, 1987.

Wyatt RJ, Julian BA, Bhathena DB, et al: IgA nephropathy: Presentation, clinical course, and prognosis in children and adults. Am J Kidney Dis 4:192, 1984.

CHAPTER 47

OPHTHALMOLOGY

EARL R. CROUCH, Jr. and ALEXANDER BERGER

Patients present to the family physicians with a limited set of symptoms among which there may be subtle differences to indicate mild or serious ocular conditions. To be able to decide when to treat patients and when to refer them to an ophthalmologist, the family physician must possess a complete appreciation of the subtle differences in symptoms between serious and nonserious ophthalmologic diseases. Knowledge of the basic anatomy of the eye is essential in determining these diagnostic differences (Fig. 47–1).

RED EYE

The family physician frequently encounters patients who complain of a red eye. Usually, the condition causing the red eye is a simple disorder such as conjunctivitis or subconjunctival hemorrhage. These conditions improve spontaneously or are readily treated. A red eye, however, may be a symptom of a more serious disorder (i.e., herpetic dendritic ulcer, iritis, acute angle closure glaucoma, ophthalmia neonatorum, or congenital glaucoma). These conditions must be clearly distinguished from the much more common conjunctivitis and subconjunctival hemorrhage because immediate referral to the ophthalmologist is paramount.

To evaluate the red eye, the family physician needs to have available a penlight, magnifying glasses, a visual acuity chart, fluorescein dye, anesthetic drops, and a Schiotz tonometer.

Symptoms and Signs

Patients who complain of a red eye generally are able to tell the physician whether the eye became rapidly irritated or the irritation has progressed slowly. This information is important, as a small foreign body, such as a grain of sand, lodged in the conjunctival sac produces a rapid hyperemia, whereas a viral or allergic conjunctivitis, or an iritis, generally produces a slowly progressive redness.

Ocular pain is an important symptom (Table 47–1). Irritation of the superficial layer of the cornea, as is caused by a small foreign body, is accompanied by a superficial grain-of-sand sensation in the eye. Deeper inflammatory processes, such as iritis or iridocyclitis or a deeper penetrating foreign body in the cornea, present with more severe, dull pain in the eye.

Abnormal light sensitivity (photophobia) is a third danger symptom that must be elicited by the family physician. Photophobia occurs with corneal inflammation, iritis, and angle closure glaucoma. Patients who have conjunctivitis usually do not have abnormal light sensitivity (Table 47–2).

Patients who complain of a red eye often complain of discharge from the eye (Table 47–3). If they do not complain of eye discharge spontaneously, the physician must inquire into the presence, type, and quantity of discharge. Purulent (creamy white or yellow watery) discharge suggests a bacterial etiology. A serous or clear discharge suggests a viral cause. Scanty, white, stringy exudate occurs most commonly with allergic conjunctivitis. The absence of discharge indicates an unusual cause for a red eye, such as iridocyclitis, ultraviolet light keratitis (snow blindness), or acute angle closure glaucoma.

A complaint of diminished visual acuity is a serious danger sign and must be elicited in the history.

Physical Examination

It is important to examine both eyes, as many of the patients with conjunctivitis in one eye have clear signs of early conjunctivitis in the other. The type of injection must be closely inspected: conjunctival injection is characterized by clearly delineated, individually visible vessels in the conjunctiva that are branching from the sclera of the eye toward the cornea. Ciliary injection, on the other hand, appears as a red ring surrounding the cornea in which individual vessels are not clearly visible. The significance of ciliary injection is that the deep ciliary vessels are involved. Ciliary injection signifies a much more serious inflammatory condition of the eye, such as a deep corneal infection, iritis, or iridocyclitis. Inspect the palpebral conjunctiva carefully with magnification to determine if lymphoid hyperplasia (cobblestone appearance) exists. The type and quantity of dis-

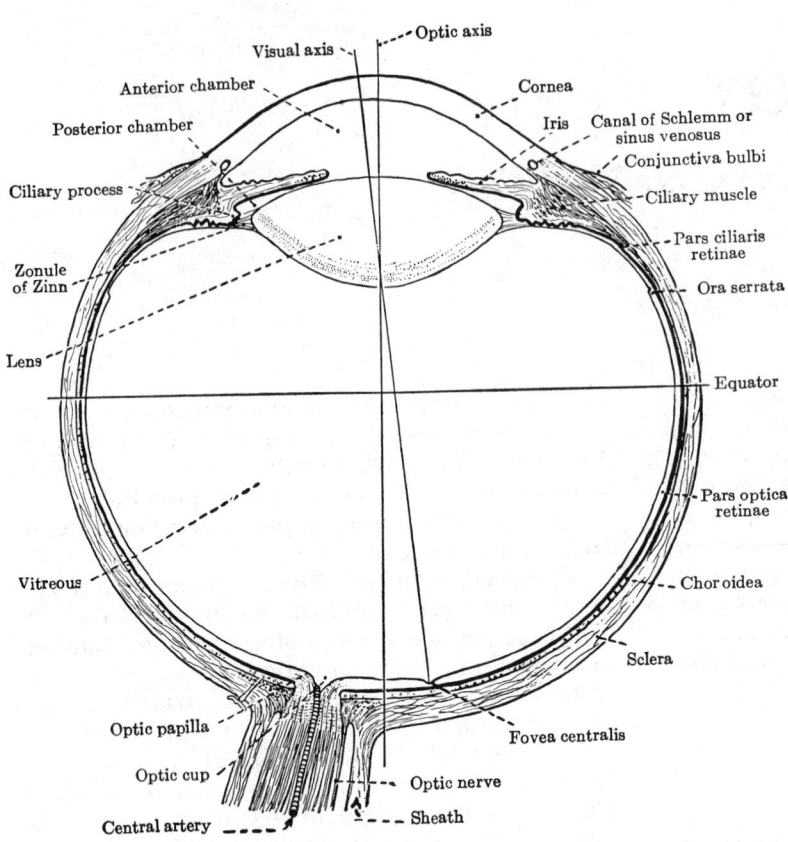

FIGURE 47–1. Anatomy of the right eyeball. (From Scheie HG, Albert DM: Textbook of Ophthalmology, 9th ed. Philadelphia, WB Saunders, 1977, with permission.)

charge is assessed by pulling down the lower lid. The appearance of the punctum—the entrance point of the tear duct—should be examined to determine if pus is coming out of the tear duct. Palpation of the tear sac on the upper portion of the nose (lacrimal crest) demonstrates tenderness in cases of acute dacryocystitis.

Carefully examine the cornea. Normally, the cornea is perfectly transparent. Excessive fluid within the stroma of the cornea results in partial opacification that can be observed by direct illumination with a penlight. A diffuse corneal haze can occur with congenital glaucoma and angle closure glaucoma. After inspection with a penlight under mag-

nification, perform corneal staining with fluorescein in the form of sterile filter paper strips. The stained part of the strip is moistened with water and touched to the conjunctiva away from the cornea. With blinking, the fluorescein spreads over the cornea. An ultraviolet light source enhances fluorescence. Areas of bright green staining denote absent or diseased epithelium. Corneal staining readily demonstrates a corneal abrasion and helps identify corneal foreign bodies and infectious epithelial defects such as herpetic, dendritic keratitis.

Examine the pupils carefully for size and shape. In most people, the pupils are of equal size. In a small percentage of people, there is congenital

TABLE 47–1. RED EYE: DIFFERENTIAL DIAGNOSIS

Parameter	Conjunctivitis, Bacterial	Iritis	Keratitis	Acute Glaucoma
Vision	Normal	Blurred	Blurred	Marked blurring
Pain	None	Moderately severe; intermittent stabbing	Sharp, severe	Severe; sometimes nausea and vomiting
Photophobia	None	Moderate	Moderate	Moderate
Discharge	Usually significant with crusting of lashes	None	None to mild	None
Conjunctival injection	Diffuse	Circumcorneal (surrounding the cornea)	Circumcorneal	Diffuse
Appearance of cornea	Clear	Clear	Cloudy	Cloudy
Pupil size	Normal	Constricted	Normal	Dilated
Intraocular pressure	Normal *Caution:* do not measure with discharge present	Normal or low	Normal	Elevated

From The Red Eye. American Academy of Ophthalmology, Professional Information Committee, San Francisco, 1986, with permission.

TABLE 47–2. APPROACH TO PATIENT PRESENTING WITH RED EYE (WITHOUT HISTORY OF TRAUMA)

1. Check for the following symptoms or signs
   a. Reduced vision
   b. Pain
   c. Photophobia
   d. Corneal staining
   e. Corneal edema
   f. Unequal pupils
   g. Elevated intraocular pressure
2. Refer to ophthalmologist if any of these signals are present.
3. If none of the above is present, the diagnosis is probably conjunctivitis.
4. The triad of a *red eye, pain,* and *loss of vision* should ALWAYS alert the examiner to a potentially blinding condition.

TABLE 47–3. CONJUNCTIVITIS CLUES

Discharge Type	Etiology
Purulent	Bacterial
Serous or clear	Viral
Stringy, white	Allergic
Preauricular lymph node enlargement	Viral

variation in the size of the pupils (anisocoria). In these cases, the patients are often aware of the fact that their pupils are unequal. In patients with previously equal pupils, inequality of the pupil may indicate iritis with which the affected pupil is typically partially constricted. In acute angle closure glaucoma, the pupil is usually partially dilated and may not be round. Unequal pupils is an important sign of significant ocular trauma.

Estimate the anterior chamber depth by side illumination with a penlight. If the anterior chamber is normal or deep, the entire surface of the eyes is then well illuminated. When the anterior chamber is shallow, the iris on the more distant side of the pupil is in shadow. A shallow anterior chamber in a red eye may indicate acute angle closure glaucoma or ocular trauma. The anterior chamber appears deep in patients with congenital glaucoma or trauma that results in a ruptured globe.

If the red eye does not have an obvious infection, measure the intraocular pressure by a Schiotz tonometer. The intraocular pressure is normal in most causes of the red eye with the exception of acute angle closure glaucoma. With iritis and trau-

matic perforating ocular injuries, intraocular pressure is generally low. Sterilize the tonometer before and after application to a red eye preferably by heat sterilization.

Preauricular lymph node enlargement is a frequent sign of viral conjunctivitis and usually is not present with acute bacterial conjunctivitis (Table 47–3).

Red Eye in Infants

Several conditions occur specifically during the first year of life. They include ophthalmia neonatorum, acute and chronic dacryocystitis, and congenital glaucoma.

Ophthalmia Neonatorum

Ophthalmia neonatorum is an inflammation of the conjunctiva that occurs during the first 4 weeks of life. Possible causes include chemical conjunctivitis, *Neisseria gonorrhoea* infection, nongonococcal bacterial conjunctivitis, and *Chlamydia* infection. The increased incidence of venereal disease and shortcomings of silver nitrate prophylaxis are significant factors in the constantly evolving clinical picture of ophthalmia neonatorum. Frequently, ophthalmia neonatorum is a manifestation of a systemic infection, indicating the need for precise etiologic diagnosis in all but the most transient cases. Table 47–4 outlines the management for the various types of ophthalmia neonatorum.

TABLE 47–4. MANAGEMENT OF OPHTHALMIA NEONATORUM

Disease	Diagnosis	Treatment
Gonococcal conjunctivitis	Gram-negative intracellular diplococci *plus* Growth on chocolate agar or Thayer-Martin *plus* Fermentation glucose and maltose negative	Topical tetracycline or erythromycin ointment q.i.d. for 2 weeks. Systemic aqueous procaine penicillin, 50,000 units/kg body weight/day IV for 7 days. Ophthalmology consultation
Other causes of bacterial conjunctivitis	Gram stain *plus* Growth on blood agar or chocolate agar	Gram positive: erythromycin ointment (0.5%) q.i.d. for 2 weeks. Gram negative: gentamicin ophthalmic (0.3%) solution q.i.d. for 2 weeks
Inclusion conjunctivitis (*Chlamydia*)	Giemsa stain: basophilic intracytoplasmic inclusion bodies *plus* Chlamydial culture	Tetracycline or sulfacetamide ointment q.i.d. for 4 weeks; with systemic involvement add systemic erythromycin for 3 weeks

CHEMICAL AND GONOCOCCAL CONJUNCTIVITIS. Chemical conjunctivitis is a condition resulting from the use of silver nitrate prophylaxis (Credé method). In recent years, silver nitrate has been replaced by erythromycin, so the incidence of chemical conjunctivitis has decreased significantly.

Prior to the Credé form of prophylaxis, gonorrhea was a common cause of ophthalmia neonatorum. Half of the patients with gonococcal conjunctivitis developed corneal clouding, a major cause of blindness. Gonococcal conjunctivitis still occurs despite erythromycin prophylaxis. Frequently, the infant with gonococcal conjunctivitis presents with swollen lids, purulent exudates, beefy red conjunctiva, and conjunctival edema. The gonococcal organism can penetrate the intact corneal epithelium and produce corneal perforation if recognition and treatment are delayed.

When gonococcal conjunctivitis is suspected, referral to an ophthalmologist is critical. Patients may also have systemic involvement with associated central nervous system (CNS) signs. Both parents should be examined for venereal disease and treated if necessary.

BACTERIAL CONJUNCTIVITIS. The most common gram-positive bacteria that are causative agents in conjunctivitis include *Staphylococcus aureus*, *Streptococcus pneumoniae*, and group A and B streptococci (Fig. 47–2). Gram-negative organisms include *Haemophilus influenzae*, *Escherichia coli*, and *Pseudomonas aeruginosa*. Bacterial conjunctivitis can occur at any age from the first day of life. Chemosis (edema of the bulbar conjunctiva), purulent discharge, lid edema, and injection are common signs. Associated systemic septicemia can occur, especially with *Pseudomonas* infection. Cultures should be prepared on blood and chocolate agar.

The best treatment prior to culture results is erythromycin ointment. Gram-negative organisms are best treated with gentamicin ophthalmic. Systemic antibiotics are recommended when there is evidence of systemic disease.

CHLAMYDIA INFECTION. *Chlamydia* infections are a leading cause of ophthalmia neonatorum. There is a high incidence of this type of infection because of the frequent exposure of the newborn to the organism during delivery and the lack of effective prophylaxis for *Chlamydia*. The onset of infection can occur at any time. The typical picture is a mild unilateral or bilateral mucopurulent conjunctivitis with moderate lid edema, chemosis, and conjunctival injection. Systemic involvement may include rhinitis, vaginitis, and otitis media.

Treatment is either tetracycline ointment or sulfacetamide ointment four times daily for 4 weeks. In addition, both parents should be treated with oral erythromycin or sulfacetamide for 3 to 4 weeks. Systemic tetracycline should be avoided in breast-feeding women who might transmit this organism to the newborn.

Acute Dacryocystitis

Neonates may present with acute dacryocystitis, an inflammation of the lacrimal sac (Fig. 47–3). Pain, tearing, redness, and discharge usually occur. If the child is febrile, cultures and Gram stains should be prepared. Pneumococcosis, *Staphylococcus aureus*, and *Streptococcus pneumoniae* are the most common organisms.

Systemic antibiotics are indicated for the acute stage. The ophthalmologist should be consulted immediately, because irrigation and probing may be necessary to establish drainage as quickly as possible.

Chronic Dacryocystitis (Partial Nasolacrimal Duct Obstruction)

Infants with chronic dacryocystitis usually present to the physician with a chronic history of tearing and crusting with a chronic yellow discharge. Topical antibiotics such as sulfacetamide four times daily should be employed. The mother should be taught to compress or massage the lacrimal sac four to six times a day. Approximately 80 per cent of these inflammations resolve spontaneously by 6 months of age. If treatment is not successful or if dacryocystitis persists, the patient should be referred for probing and irrigation of the nasolacrimal duct. Prior to age 14 months, a single probing is curative in most cases.

Congenital Glaucoma

Congenital glaucoma is a potentially blinding condition with an incidence of 1 per 10,000 births. It is often confused with chronic dacryocystitis.

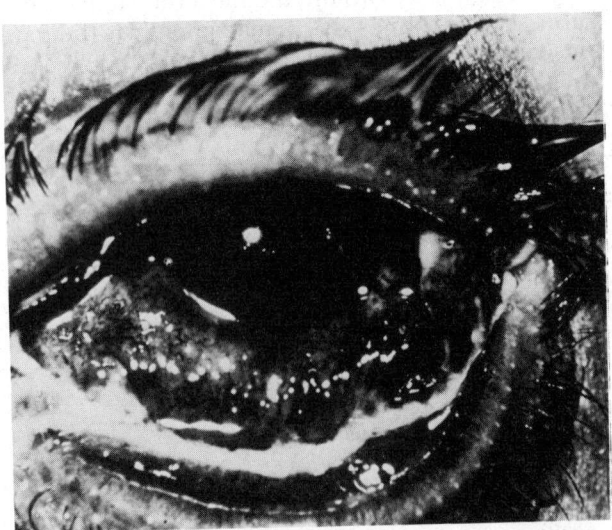

FIGURE 47–2. Purulent conjunctivitis may indicate infection with *Staphylococcus, Haemophilus influenzae, Streptococcus,* or *Pseudomonas.* (From The Red Eye. American Academy of Ophthalmology, Professional Information Committee, San Francisco, 1986, with permission.)

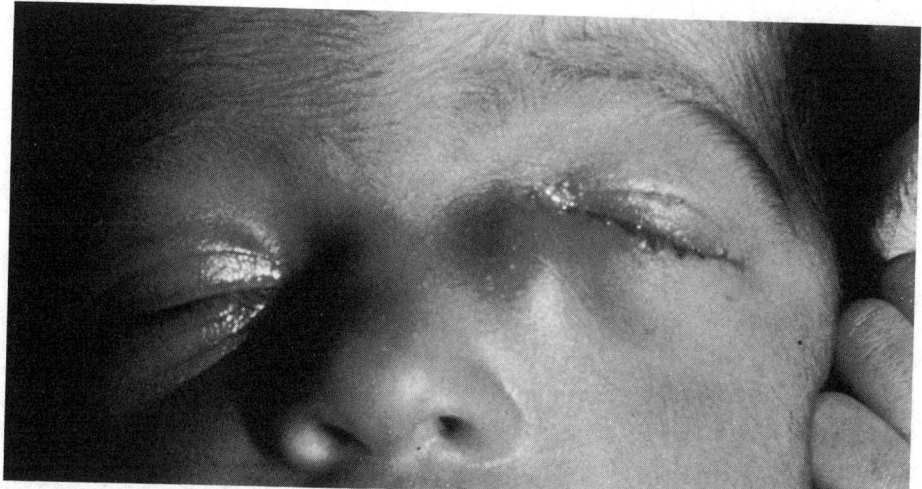

FIGURE 47–3. Acute dacryocystitis in a neonate with fever and malaise. Lacrimal sac massage and systemic antibiotics relieved the acute infection.

About two thirds of these cases are bilateral. These patients, like those with dacryocystitis, present with excessive tearing. The infants usually are light-sensitive (photophobic) and frequently bury their head in a blanket or pillow. These infants frequently have intense blinking or lid spasm (blepharospasm). An enlarged cornea or corneal clouding can be detected clinically (Fig. 47–4). Corneal edema is the result of elevated intraocular pressure, which causes breaks in the inner corneal layers (Descemet's membrane) and intrusion of anterior chamber fluid into the corneal stroma. Increased intraocular pressure causes significant optic nerve damage, which can lead to blindness.

Whenever glaucoma is suspected, immediate consultation is indicated. Surgical treatment of congenital glaucoma is successful in approximately 90 per cent of cases. These patients must be followed by an ophthalmologist for the rest of their lives as a precaution against recurrent elevations of intraocular pressure and amblyopia (lazy eye).

Red Eye in Adults and Older Children

Blepharitis

Blepharitis is a chronic lid inflammation that involves abnormalities of the glands surrounding the eyelashes. The two most common types are (1) chronic staphylococcal infections of the lid and (2) seborrheic blepharitis (Fig. 47–5). Staphylococcal blepharitis is the most common inflammation of the external eye. It is frequently asymptomatic initially, but as the disease progresses the patient complains of foreign body sensation, matting of the lashes, and burning. Lid crusting, discharge, redness, and loss of lashes are observed. Seborrheic

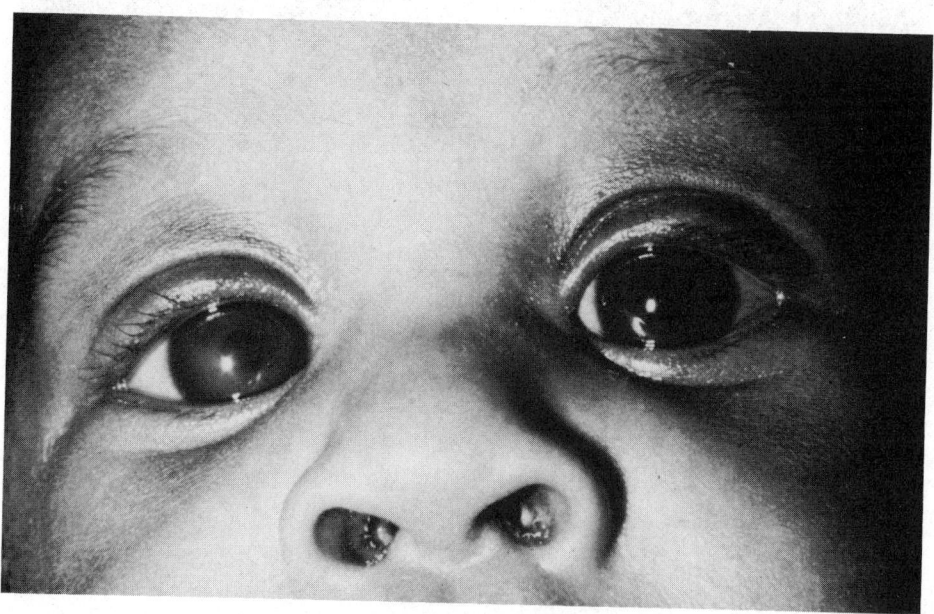

FIGURE 47–4. Congenital glaucoma in a 2-month-old infant who presented with a cloudy cornea involving the right eye. Intraocular pressure was elevated. The diagnosis was congenital glaucoma.

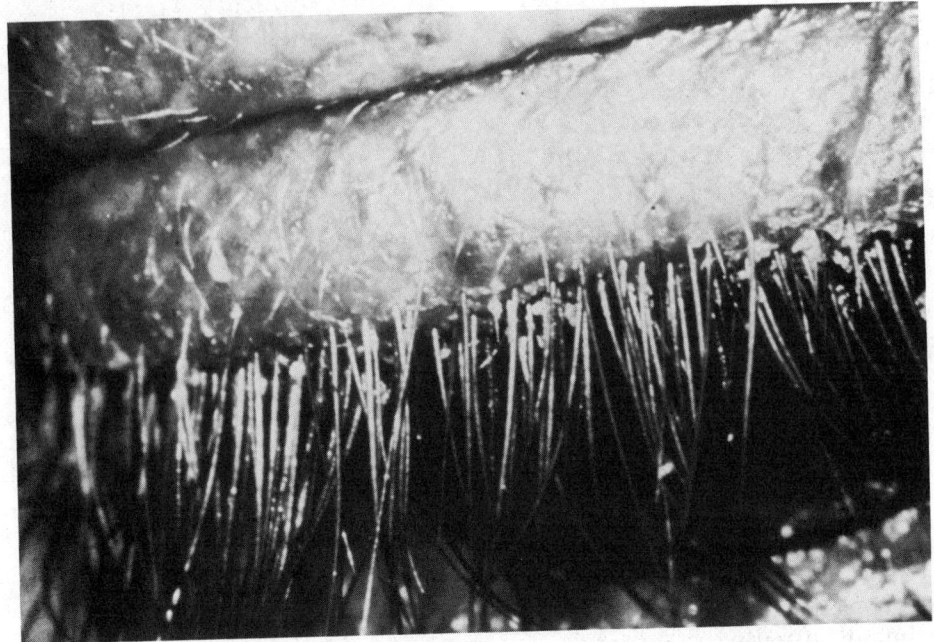

FIGURE 47–5. Seborrheic blepharitis is characterized by greasy, dandruff-like scales on the lashes. (From The Red Eye. American Academy of Ophthalmology, Professional Information Committee, San Francisco, 1986, with permission.)

blepharitis is associated with seborrhea of the scalp, lashes, eyebrows, and ears. It is characterized by greasy, dandruff-like scales on the lashes but no skin ulcerations.

Treatment of both these conditions is long and laborious. Lid hygiene is recommended for both conditions. Topical antibiotics are prescribed for staphylococcal blepharitis. Both conditions are recurrent and require repeated therapy.

Stye (Hordeolum)

A stye (Fig. 47–6) is the most common localized infection of one of the glands of the eyelids. It is an acute, boil-like lesion, and the patient usually has a swollen, tender, red eyelid. There may be a moderate amount of conjunctival injection.

Treatment includes warm compresses for 15 minutes four times a day and topical antibiotics. Systemic antibiotics are usually not indicated. Generally, the stye drains spontaneously within several days. If resolution does not occur within 2 weeks, the patient should be referred.

Chalazion

A chalazion (Fig. 47–7) is a chronic swelling of the eyelids not associated with conjunctivitis. The

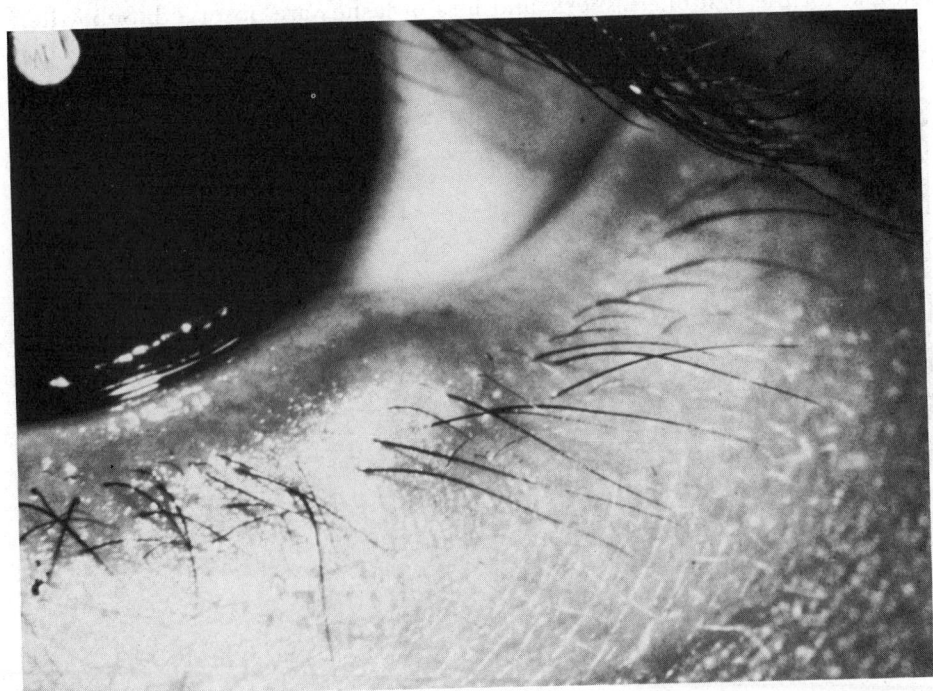

FIGURE 47–6. Acute hordeolum, or stye. The swollen, tender, red eyelid includes an acute, boil-like lesion. Treatment includes warm compresses and topical antibiotics. (From The Red Eye. American Academy of Ophthalmology, Professional Information Committee, San Francisco, 1986, with permission.)

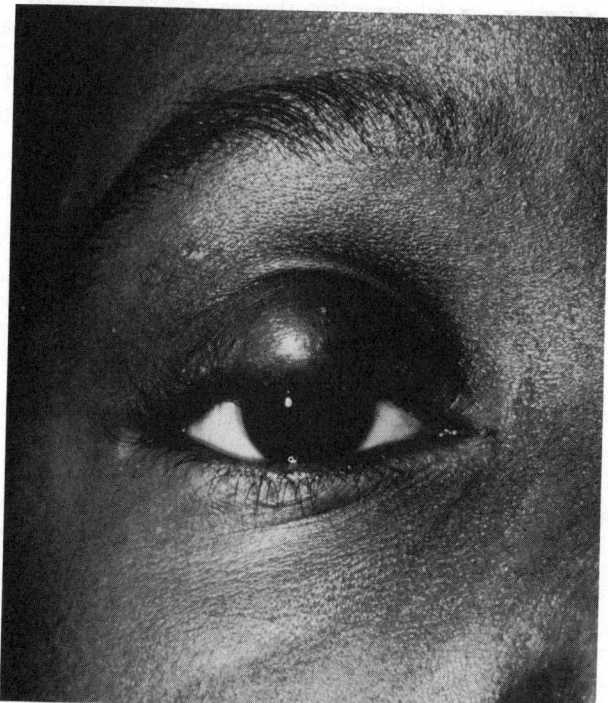

FIGURE 47–7. Chalazion of the right upper eyelid in a 10-year-old girl. (From The Red Eye. American Academy of Ophthalmology, Professional Information Committee, San Francisco, 1986, with permission.)

chalazion, a granulomatous inflammatory reaction, may persist for weeks or even months. Chalazia are usually rubbery, cystic, and nontender on palpation. When the upper lid is involved, vision is often temporarily blurred.

If the chalazion persists for more than 3 months, it may require incision and curettage. Recurrent chalazia may be caused by an underlying sebaceous gland carcinoma, so the lesion should be biopsied and sent to pathology.

Bacterial Conjunctivitis

All common bacteria may cause conjunctivitis. Presently, *Staphylococcus aureus, Diplococcus pneumoniae, Hemophilus influenzae,* and *Pseudomonas* are the most common organisms. In the presence of a severe purulent discharge, culture of the conjunctiva is mandatory (see Fig. 47–2). Subconjunctival hemorrhage can occur with bacterial conjunctivitis and is especially common with *H. influenzae* conjunctivitis.

Treatment of conjunctivitis is with a topical antibiotic, such as sulfacetamide, erythromycin, or neomycin–polymyxin B combination. Gentamicin or tobramycin ophthalmic should be reserved for unresponsive cases, especially when *Pseudomonas* or *Proteus* is cultured. Gonococcal and *Hemophilus* conjunctivitis require both systemic and topical therapy. If the conjunctivitis does not improve within 2 to 3 days, or the patient develops pain or reduction in vision, referral is indicated. Be certain *not* to use topical steroids or antibiotic–steroid combinations for conjunctivitis or other causes of red eye.

Topical corticosteroids have four potentially serious ocular side effects and are contraindicated for conjunctivitis.

1. Steroids can facilitate penetration of an undetected corneal herpetic infection to the deeper corneal layers and cause corneal perforation.
2. Prolonged local use of the corticosteroids (usually longer than 2 weeks) can cause chronic open angle glaucoma.
3. Prolonged use of topical corticosteroids can cause cataracts.
4. Topical corticosteroids are capable of potentiating the development of fungal corneal ulcers.

Viral Conjunctivitis

Viral conjunctivitis, in contrast to bacterial conjunctivitis, has a less prominent discharge that is usually watery. The condition is highly contagious, and hand washing is important to avoid infection. When infected, hospital personnel, day-care workers, and institutional personnel should avoid contact with others. Palpable preauricular lymph nodes frequently are present with viral conjunctivitis and comprise an important sign that can differentiate it from bacterial conjunctivitis. An associated upper respiratory infection may occur. In advanced cases, true photophobia and blurred vision caused by corneal involvement may be present and require consultation. However, most viral conjunctivitis is self-limiting, and no specific treatment is indicated. Topical steroids are contraindicated. Most viral infections resolve within 10 to 14 days, and specific serologic diagnosis is not necessary. If the conjunctivitis persists or there is any pain or change in vision, the patient should be referred.

Allergic Conjunctivitis

A number of antigens may give rise to superficial conjunctival reactions. Because of the elasticity of the conjunctival tissues, there may be considerable swelling. Allergic conjunctivitis patients have tearing and itching and present with redness and swelling of the conjunctiva and lids. A scant, white, stringy discharge occurs with allergic conjunctivitis. Allergic conjunctivitis frequently occurs in patients with hay fever, asthma, or eczema. The allergic condition of contact allergy commonly is associated with drugs, chemicals, or cosmetics coming in contact with the conjunctiva or eyelids.

The offending drug or allergens should be discontinued. The treatment of most allergic conditions includes oral antihistamines and occasionally topical antihistamines and vasoconstricting drops such as naphazoline.

Subconjunctival Hemorrhage

A patient may present with a bright red eye, normal vision, and no pain. Usually no obvious cause exists, but in some patients a history of coughing, sneezing, or straining prior to the hemorrhage is present. The patient should be reassured that it is nothing more than hemorrhage of the conjunctiva. There is no therapy, except reassurance that the blood will clear within 2 to 3 weeks. Hematologic or blood coagulation studies are usually of limited value in patients with subconjunctival hemorrhages unless there is a history of recurrence.

If trauma is suspected, the patient should be referred to an eye physician to rule out more serious injuries, such as perforation or severe contusion to the eye, causing damage to the intraocular structures. Subconjunctival hemorrhage may indicate that the patient is a battered child or adult, and other signs of bodily trauma should be investigated.

Corneal Herpetic Infections

Herpetic infections of the eye can produce conjunctivitis, corneal inflammation (keratitis), and uveitis (inflamed iris, ciliary body, and choroid). The herpes simplex virus is the most common cause of corneal opacification in temperate zone countries. The human is the only natural host for this DNA virus. Approximately 90 per cent of the population have systemic antibodies to the virus. Type 1 herpes simplex virus is the oral or labial type, and type 2 is the genital type. The incubation period of herpes simplex infection is 2 to 12 days. Herpes type 1 is the most common cause of ocular infection, but transmission of herpes type 2 also can occur.

PRIMARY HERPES SIMPLEX INFECTION. Primary ocular infection in a nonimmune subject usually presents as a conjunctivitis with a clear, watery discharge, skin vesicles on the lids, and preauricular nodes. Associated vesicles and ulcers on the oral mucosa and skin are common. Corneal involvement also may occur with single or multiple dendrites. If dendrites are present, the patient should be referred for treatment.

RECURRENT CORNEAL HERPES. At the time of the primary herpetic infection, the virus gains access to the CNS, where it resides in a latent state in the trigeminal and other ganglia. Recurrent attacks occur when the latent state is reversed. The virus travels via the sensory nerves to target tissues, one of which is the eye. Recurrent corneal involvement also includes the development of single or multiple dendritic ulcers. After a brief period the plaque of epithelial cells desquamates to form a linear branching ulcer (dendrite). When a corneal dendrite is detected by corneal staining with fluorescein, the patient should be referred.

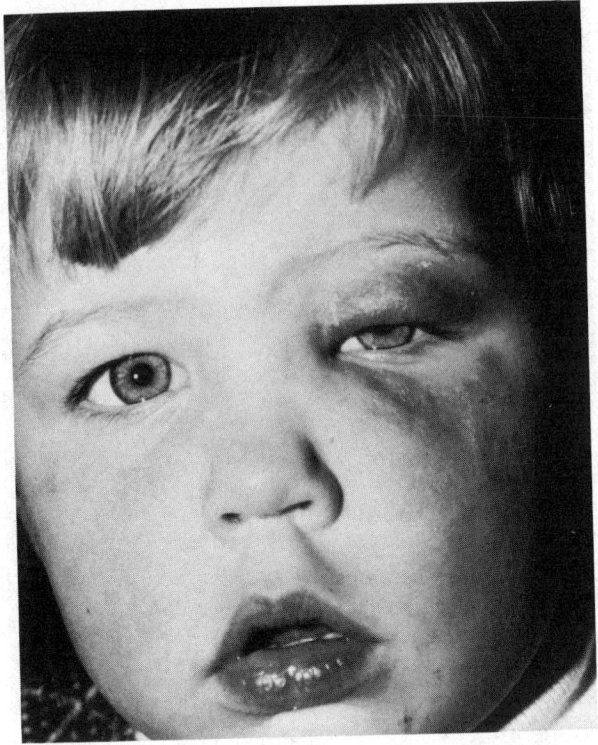

FIGURE 47–8. Orbital cellulitis in a 3-year-old patient. (From The Red Eye. American Academy of Ophthalmology, Professional Information Committee, San Francisco, 1986, with permission.)

Orbital Cellulitis

Orbital cellulitis (Fig. 47–8), most commonly caused by an extension of infection from the ethmoid sinus, can occur in both adults and children. It is the most common cause of exophthalmos (protruding eye) in children. Sometimes it is difficult to differentiate a periorbital or anterior lid cellulitis from a true posterior orbital cellulitis. With a true orbital cellulitis, the child or adult has pain on movement of the eye, conjunctival edema, and limited extraocular movements. The most common causative organisms are *Staphylococcus aureus*, *Streptococcus*, and *Haemophilus influenzae*. Cultures should be obtained from the nasopharynx, conjunctiva, and blood.

Immediate hospitalization and ophthalmologic consultation are necessary. Appropriate systemic antibiotic treatment depends on the causative organisms. Cavernous sinus thrombosis, meningitis, and blindness are serious complications of orbital cellulitis.

Iritis

Redness, pain, and photophobia occur with iritis. No discharge is seen, and the pupil is constricted. Circumcorneal (ciliary) injection may occur. Intraocular pressure is normal or low. Consultation should be obtained on all such patients.

Angle Closure Glaucoma

Acute elevations in intraocular pressure can occur when the outflow of aqueous humor is suddenly blocked. An acute angle closure attack may follow an episode of emotional or physical stress, dilation of the pupil in dim lighting, or rarely after the instillation of dilating eyedrops. A patient who is having an acute attack usually has symptoms that include severe ocular pain, redness, blurred vision, rainbow-colored halos around lights, and sometimes nausea and vomiting. On examination, the eye is usually red, the pupil in mid-dilation and oval, the cornea cloudy, and the intraocular pressure markedly elevated. Generally, only one eye is affected at a time.

An acute episode of angle closure glaucoma is an ocular emergency and requires immediate treatment to lower the intraocular pressure by medical treatment. Once the intraocular pressure is under control, YAG or argon laser peripheral iridectomy is performed.

OCULAR TRAUMA AND OTHER EMERGENCIES

Emergencies

True emergencies can be classified as those where therapy should be instituted within minutes. Two true emergencies in the eye include chemical burns of the cornea and central retinal artery occlusion.

Chemical Burns

Most acids produce the extent of their damage immediately upon contact. Of course, the more concentrated the acid, the more severe is the immediate effect. Alkali burns are more devastating to the eye, as they continue to cause damage long after the initial chemical contact. Corneal melting can lead to perforation; and severe, chronic glaucoma can occur as a later complication. Burns of the eye by acids or alkalis are true ocular emergencies. Alkali, such as lye, can cause permanent, irreversible blindness.

The immediate treatment of chemical burns must be continual irrigation of the eyes with up to 1000 mL normal saline or lactated Ringer's solution. If these solutions are not available, a shower, spigot, bathtub, or drinking fountain is appropriate. After initial ocular irrigation, ophthalmologic consultation must be immediate.

Central Retinal Artery Occlusion

Central retinal artery occlusion is generally not the result of trauma. However, prolonged intraorbital swelling can cause occlusion of the central retinal artery. Such situations occur particularly in patients who are having an operation in the face-down position. Characteristic fundus appearance with central retinal artery occlusion is narrow arterioles and a pale optic disk. In addition, there is a diffuse retinal whitening. A cherry-red spot occurs only several hours after the initial retinal artery occlusion. The treatment must be immediate, including breathing in a small paper bag as a means to increase the patient's carbon dioxide level. Emergency paracentesis is a rapid way to decompress the eye and may actually provide immediate restoration of vision. However, most physicians are reluctant to perform paracentesis on a patient within a few minutes. Ocular massage is another means of decompressing the eye.

Urgencies

Urgent situations include those where therapy should be instituted within several hours. They include penetrating injuries of the globe, acute narrow angle glaucoma, pupillary block glaucoma, orbital cellulitis, corneal ulcer, corneal foreign body, corneal abrasion, gonococcal conjunctivitis, ophthalmia neonatorum, and acute iritis. In addition, trauma with retinal tears, vitreous hemorrhage, retinal detachment, and hyphemas constitute urgent situations.

Ocular Foreign Body and Other Eye Injuries

The most common eye injury encountered in family practice is a foreign body in the eye. The most common causes of a foreign body in the conjunctival sac or one embedded in the cornea are particles blown in by the wind, occupational or work-related injuries, and metallic foreign bodies that may fly into the eye, such as after a person hits a metal object with a hammer. It is important to evaluate the location of the foreign body and, in the case of corneal foreign bodies, the depth of penetration. Symptoms may be helpful, as superficial foreign bodies in the cornea generally present with the complaint of a "dust particle" in the eye. Foreign bodies that have penetrated deeper into the corneal stroma produce a dull, aching pain perceived in or behind the eye.

On examination, it is important to look carefully at the inflammatory response of the eye. A purely localized conjunctival inflammation pattern is generally associated with superficial foreign bodies. Ciliary injection is a warning sign that a deep penetration may have taken place, and an ophthalmologic consultation should be sought immediately. Examine the eye after the instillation of ophthalmic local anesthetic in order to avoid blepharospasm and evasive eye movements. Inspect the cornea with a penlight or ophthalmoscope in a darkened room. Use of the slit on the ophthalmoscope may help visualize irregularities in the corneal surface. Staining with fluorescein demonstrates abrasions and helps identify otherwise transparent foreign bodies.

The family physician may elect to remove a foreign body in the conjunctival sac by irrigation with sterile solutions or after eversion of the upper lid with a moistened cotton swab. In the case of superficial corneal foreign bodies, attempt to remove it with a moist sterile swab.

Corneal Abrasions

Corneal abrasions are often due to foreign bodies underneath the upper lid. Evert the lid and examine for conjunctival foreign bodies. To evert the lid, the patient is seated and asked to look downward. The upper lid is grasped by its central lashes and pulled downward and slightly outward. The examiner then depresses the upper lid with a cotton applicator proximal to the upper tarsus margin. Gentle pressure is maintained until the upper lid is flipped into the everted position. Frequently, the foreign body is observed and can be removed with a cotton applicator. If the conjunctival or corneal foreign body is not easily removed with a cotton applicator, obtain ophthalmologic consultation. Corneal abrasions generally can be treated with an antibiotic ointment and patching.

Contact Lens Overwear

Contact lens overwear is managed similarly to corneal abrasion. Patients suffering from overwear syndrome have worn their lenses longer than usual and typically awaken during the early morning hours with severe pain and tearing. In response to prolonged wear, the cornea has become swollen (edematous) and has developed epithelial defects. Patients need reassurance that the condition is usually not serious even though the pain is severe. However, occasional contact lens-induced corneal abrasions, especially those associated with soft lenses, can rapidly progress to severe corneal in-

fection. Patients should be seen the next day and referred if they have not improved. Contact lens wear may be resumed only after the corneal epithelium is well healed.

Metallic Foreign Bodies

Metallic foreign bodies, if allowed to stay in the eye for a number of hours, frequently leave a rust ring that is clearly visible after removal of the foreign body. Rust rings irritate the cornea and result in long-lasting inflammatory changes in the eye. Follow-up should be at daily intervals with staining of the cornea to demonstrate the expected rapid healing. If healing does not take place over a period of 24 to 48 hours, suspect an infection in the corneal stroma and obtain consultation. Topical antibiotic ointments are used after removal of foreign bodies in an attempt to prevent this complication.

Corneal and Scleral Lacerations

Corneal and scleral lacerations fall within the realm of the ophthalmologist and should be referred immediately after a shield is placed on the eye. Frequently, signs of corneal and scleral lacerations include unequal pupils, hypotony (low intraocular pressure), or hyphema. Frequently, with a corneal laceration the lens is also involved. It is important to consider that there may also be posterior injuries to the globe, including retinal detachment, retinal tear, and vitreous hemorrhage (Fig. 47–9).

Blunt Eye Injuries

Blunt eye injuries are common. They may be the result of relatively trivial injuries or high velocity impact projectiles. An exact history of the trauma must be obtained in order to assess the velocity involved, which in turn may indicate the extent of ocular damage that may have occurred. Inquiry must be made to determine if visual acuity changes

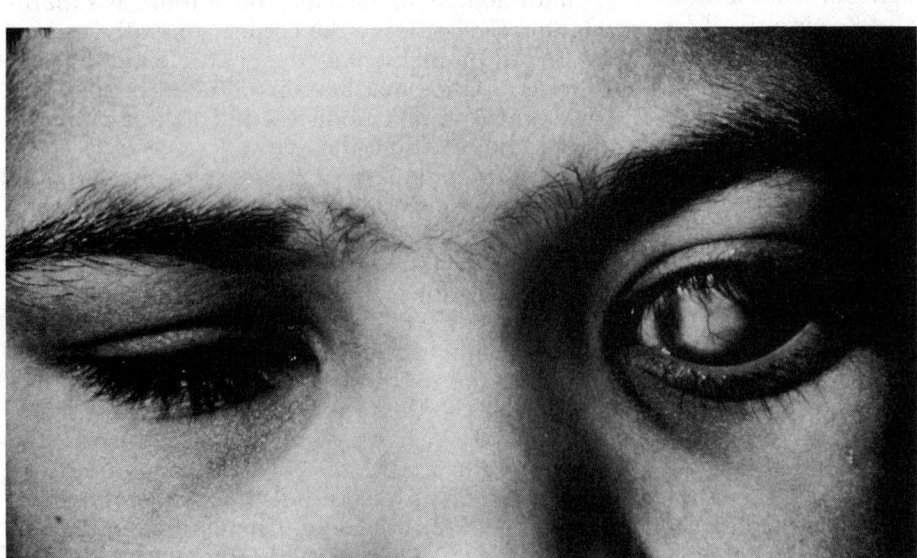

FIGURE 47–9. Corneal leukoma in a 6-year-old boy. The diagnosis was ocular trauma and penetrating corneal laceration.

occurred immediately after the injury. Flashing lights are often seen at the instant of injury and indicate irritation of the retina, as any message to the brain from the retina is perceived as light. Persistent blurred vision is indicative of a more serious injury. It may indicate blood in the anterior chamber that is suspended in the aqueous humor, refracting light and distorting the visual image. Free-floating blood in the anterior chamber cannot be appreciated by ophthalmoscopic examination, and a slit-lamp is necessary in order to observe the suspended red blood cells.

Black Eye (Bruised Eyelids)

A black eye may be serious or relatively minor. If accompanied by severe pain, bleeding, or constant blurred vision, more serious eye trauma must be considered.

Red Eye

Almost all ocular trauma cases include bleeding or dilation of blood vessels on the surface of the eye (subconjunctival hemorrhage). This sign may be observed with any degree of eye injury. For instance, a subconjunctival hemorrhage may be spontaneous or may indicate a mild or a serious injury.

Pupillary Change

Blunt trauma to the eye may result in lacerations of the sphincter muscle of the pupil. They are manifested by a so-called traumatic mydriasis. Unlike the unequal pupils seen with congenital anisocoria, traumatic mydriasis is characterized by recent onset of unequal pupils and by the irregularity of the dilated pupil. Although traumatic mydriasis by itself is not harmful, it suggests severe blunt trauma and is an indication for a careful assessment of other ocular structures, including the vitreous and retinal periphery.

Traumatic Hyphema

Blunt trauma to the eye may cause injury to the iris, angle structures, and other intraocular structures. Hemorrhage into the anterior chamber, or hyphema, is most often found in children. The agent producing hyphema is usually a projectile that strikes the exposed portion of the eye. A great variety of missiles and objects have been incriminated, including balls, rocks, projectile toys, air gun or BB pellets, and the human fist. With the increase of child abuse, fists and belts have started to play a prominent role. Boys are involved in three fourths of cases.

Rarely, spontaneous hyphemas occur and may be confused with traumatic hyphemas. Spontaneous hyphemas are secondary to neovascularization, ocular neoplasms (retinoblastoma), and vascular anomalies (juvenile xanthogranuloma). Vascular tufts that exist at the pupillary border have been implicated in spontaneous hyphema.

We prefer the following grading system for traumatic hyphemas: grade 1 hyphema, layered blood occupying less than one third of the anterior chamber; grade 2, blood filling one third to one half of the anterior chamber; grade 3, layered blood filling one half to less than the total anterior chamber; and grade 4, total clotted hyphemas, often referred to as blackball or eightball hyphema. A hyphema is an ocular emergency and should be referred immediately.

Secondary hemorrhage associated with traumatic hyphema results in a markedly worse prognosis. Eventual visual recovery to an acuity of 20/50 (6/15) or better occurs in approximately 64 per cent of patients with secondary hemorrhage compared with 79.5 per cent of those in whom no rebleeding occurred. True secondary bleeding into the anterior chamber is indicated by an obvious increase in the amount of blood in the anterior chamber. Secondary hemorrhage occurs in approximately 25 per cent of all hyphema patients (range 7 to 38 per cent). The incidence of secondary hemorrhage is higher in grade 3 and 4 hyphemas.

There are four complications of traumatic hyphema. They are directly attributed to the retention of blood in the anterior chamber and include posterior synechiae, peripheral anterior synechias, corneal blood staining, and optic atrophy. Optic atrophy may result from either acute, transiently elevated intraocular pressure or chronically elevated intraocular pressure.

Posterior synechiae may form in patients with traumatic hyphema. They are secondary to iritis or iridocyclitis. They are relatively rarely seen in patients treated medically but occur more frequently in patients who have had surgical evacuation of the hyphema. *Peripheral anterior synechiae* occur frequently in medically treated patients in whom the hyphema has remained in the anterior chamber for a prolonged period (9 days or more).

Corneal blood staining occurs primarily in patients who have a total hyphema and associated elevation of intraocular pressure. Factors that may increase the likelihood of corneal blood staining are (1) initial state of the corneal endothelium (decreased viability resulting from trauma or advanced age, e.g., cornea guttata); (2) surgical trauma to the endothelium; (3) a large amount of formed clot in contact with the endothelium; and (4) prolonged elevation of intraocular pressure. Each of these factors affects endothelial integrity. Corneal blood staining may occur with low or normal intraocular pressures; it may also occur in hyphemas that are less than total. Corneal blood staining has a larger potential for occurrence in patients who have a total hyphema that remains for at least 6 days with concomitant, continuous intraocular pressures above 25 mm Hg. Corneal blood staining may require several months or more to clear.

Nonglaucomatous *optic atrophy* in hyphema patients may be due either to the initial trauma or to transient periods of markedly elevated intraocular pressure. Diffuse optic nerve pallor (and not glaucomatous cupping) is the result of transient periods of markedly elevated intraocular pressure; it occurs with constant pressure of 50 mm Hg or higher for 5 days or 35 mm Hg or higher for 7 days. We have observed a number of patients with sickle cell trait who developed a nonglaucomatous optic atrophy with relatively small elevations of intraocular pressure (35 to 39 mm Hg) that lasted 2 to 4 days. Despite maximum medical therapy, final visual acuity was less than 20/400 in all patients. We continue to observe optic atrophy in sickle cell trait patients referred to our institution who have not had vigorous control of intraocular pressure and/or delay in paracentesis. Other studies indicate that patients with sickle cell hemoglobinopathies and anterior chamber hyphemas have more sickled erythrocytes in their anterior chambers than in their circulating venous blood. The sickled erythrocytes obstruct the trabecular meshwork more effectively than normal cells, and there is a concomitant elevation of intraocular pressure to higher levels with lesser amounts of hyphema. Moderate elevation of intraocular pressure in patients with sickle cell hemoglobinopathy may produce rapid deterioration of visual function due to profound reduction of central retinal artery and posterior ciliary artery perfusion.

PROGNOSIS AND TREATMENT. It is important to recognize that the prognosis for visual recovery from traumatic hyphema is directly related to three factors.

1. Amount of associated damage to other ocular structures (i.e., choroidal rupture or macular scarring)
2. Whether secondary hemorrhage occurs
3. Whether complications of glaucoma, corneal blood staining, or optic atrophy occur

Treatment modalities should be directed at reducing the incidence of secondary hemorrhage and the risk of corneal blood staining and optic atrophy. The success of hyphema treatment, as judged by recovery of visual acuity, is good in approximately 75 per cent of patients. Approximately 80 per cent of hyphema patients with less than one-third filling of the anterior chamber regain visual acuity of 20/40 (6/12) or better. Approximately 60 per cent of those with more than half but less than total hyphema regain 20/40 or better, whereas only approximately 35 per cent of those with initially total hyphema have good visual results. Approximately 60 per cent of hyphema patients below age 6 years have good visual results; older age groups have progressively higher percentages of good visual recovery.

It is important to recognize that the severity of the trauma is frequently related to the final visual outcome. Cataract, choroidal rupture, vitreous hemorrhage, angle recession glaucoma, and retinal detachment are commonly associated with traumatic hyphema, compromising the final visual result.

Retinal Detachment

Traumatic detachment of the retina can be observed after blunt eye injury, especially in older individuals. The patient may complain of reduced overall brightness in the involved eye or may have continuous light flashes, indicating retinal traction. After eye trauma it is imperative to inspect not just the central portions of the retina but, as far as possible, the peripheral portions as well. This examination should be performed in a darkened room and after instilling a short-acting mydriatic agent. Any questionable findings should be referred to an ophthalmologist immediately. Other serious post-traumatic injuries are traumatic tears of the iris, subluxation or dislocation of the lens that occasionally displaces into the anterior chamber, and blowout fracture of the orbit that presents with impaired eye movement in the upward direction because of entrapment of the inferior rectus muscle. Fortunately, these serious injuries are usually easy to recognize.

PEDIATRIC OPHTHALMOLOGY

Evaluation of Vision Within the First 4 Months of Life

Parents may report that their baby does not appear to look at them. This statement requires the physician to carefully document history of prematurity, fetal distress, anoxia, or birth trauma. A failure to reach developmental milestones may indicate neurologic abnormalities. A history of seizure disorder, cerebral palsy, or chromosomal abnormalities helps identify potential underlying causes. In this instance, visual acuity or the child's ability to fix must be assessed. Normal newborns follow faces. By the age of 2 or 3 months, infants normally follow light and high contrast toys. Assessment of vision can be achieved by using an optokinetic nystagmus drum. If vertical nystagmus can be obtained, visual acuity is 20/400 or better. Oculomotor disturbances may be the underlying etiology of the child's apparent visual inattention. Bilateral III nerve palsy, congenital fibrosis syndrome, or a partial III nerve paralysis may give this impression.

Nystagmus is an important sign of decreased vision, indicating visual acuity in the range of 20/200. The onset is usually at birth or shortly thereafter. The nystagmus can be a jerk or pendular nystagmus, and the direction should be characterized as horizontal, vertical, or rotary.

Abnormalities of the anterior portion of the eye can cause profound visual loss and are easily visible with a + 10.00 magnification. They include corneal opacities due to congenital glaucoma, Peter's anomaly (abnormal cornea and lens), and leukokoria related to congenital cataracts, inflammatory disease, or retinal abnormalities.

Evaluation of the posterior aspect of the eye, including examination of the red reflexes, may indicate an early retinal detachment or retinoblastoma. Optic nerve abnormalities may be associated with midline CNS defects, such as an absent septum velucitum, agenesis of the corpus callosum, or hypopituitarism. Computed tomography (CT) or magnetic resonance imaging (MRI) can identify these abnormalities. Electroretinography (ERG) may be helpful for determining the cause of decreased visual acuity. Abnormal ERG occurs with Leber's congenital amaurosis, congenital achromatopsia, and congenital stationary night blindness. Visual evoked potential testing may be necessary to determine whether vision is intact.

Some infants who have a completely normal eye examination but demonstrate poor fixation may actually have a delay in maturation of the visual system. Normally, the visual system matures by 4 to 6 months of age. Visual evoked potential acuities are in the range of 20/400 during the first few days of life and improve to close to a normal adult equivalent of 20/20 to 20/30 by 6 months of age. In some patients visual evoked responses and clinically assessed visual function may be abnormal, only to improve between 4 and 12 months of age. Delayed visual maturation is an incompletely defined syndrome; except for vision, the ocular examination is normal, including brisk pupillary response to light. Typically, there is no nystagmus, and ERG is normal.

Vision Screening and Ocular Examination

Appropriate vision screening is one of the most important factors in pediatric eye care. Because visual stimuli are critical to normal development, early detection and correction of problems can avoid serious vision impairment or blindness. The American Academy of Ophthalmology and the American Association of Pediatric Ophthalmology and Strabismus strongly support the goal of early detection and treatment of eye problems in children. In particular, vision screening is needed to detect four major conditions: strabismus, amblyopia, ocular disease, and refractive errors.

Family practice physicians are ideal vision screeners because of their ability to detect abnormalities at an early age. There are certain essential questions about vision screening: At what ages should it be performed? Which tests are recommended at each stage; how are they performed; and how useful is the information they provide? (3) What are the recommended referral criteria? On a practical level, vision screening must be cost-effective and time-efficient. The testing devices must be readily available and relatively easy to use. High sensitivity is essential to keep over- and under-referrals to a minimum.

The American Academy of Ophthalmology and the American Association of Pediatric Ophthalmology and Strabimus recommend that children be examined for eye problems in four stages.

1. In the newborn nursery. Physicians should examine all infants. Ophthalmologists should be consulted to examine patients at high risk for such conditions as retinopathy of prematurity (ROP), cataracts, and other ocular pathology.
2. At 6 months of age.
3. At 3 years of age.
4. At 5 years and older.

Table 47–5 summarizes these findings.

The Academy of Ophthalmology statement recommends that family physicians establish a close working relationship with a nearby ophthalmologist who is familiar with children's eye problems. The collaboration can help clarify questions about vision screening and the need for referral.

TABLE 47–5. RECOMMENDED VISION SCREENING BY FAMILY PHYSICIANS

Age	Examination	Referral Criteria
Newborn	Penlight examination of cornea Rule out nystagmus Red reflexes	Any ocular pathology Nystagmus Abnormal red reflexes or white reflex
6 Months	Fixation to light and small toys Penlight examination Corneal light reflex test, cover test Red reflexes	Object to occlusion Nystagmus; any ocular pathology Strabismus Abnormal red reflexes or white reflex
3 Years	Visual acuity: Snellen letters, tumbling E, or HOTV Corneal light reflex test, cover test Fundus examination	Acuity of 20/40 or less in one or both eyes Strabismus Any ocular pathology
5 Years or older	Visual acuity: Snellen letter, tumbling E, or HOTV (see text) Corneal light reflex test, cover test Fundus examination	Acuity of 20/30 or less in one or both eyes Strabismus Any ocular pathology

Newborn Screening

Vision screening of all infants in the newborn nursery should include two elements: (1) a penlight examination to inspect corneal clarity and evaluate for nystagmus; and (2) a simultaneous examination of both red reflexes. Infants at high risk for eye problems such as ROP, and those with a family history of congenital cataracts, retinoblastoma, and metabolic or genetic diseases should undergo a detailed ophthalmologic examination. Premature infants with a birth weight of less than 1700 grams and patients with respiratory distress syndrome are at greater risk of developing ROP. Each year, ROP causes some degree of visual loss in approximately 1300 infants in the United States and severe impairment in 400 to 800.

In most infants, ROP is a transient disease with spontaneous regression. Some patients, however, have progressive ROP. The current recommendation is that premature babies be examined between 6 and 9 weeks of age to rule out the development of ROP.

Cataracts are the most common cause of a white pupil (leukokoria) at birth (Table 47–6). The incidence may be as high as 1 in every 500 to 1000 live births in the United States. A positive family history of congenital cataracts is present in about 55 per cent of infants with congenital cataracts. Because they interfere with the normal development of the visual system, cataracts in infants must be approached differently from cataracts in adults. Some require no treatment, whereas others may require surgery within the first few weeks of life, followed by fitting of contact lenses or aphakic glasses and treatment for amblyopia.

Retinoblastoma is a life-threatening cause of leukokoria that may be detected within the first few weeks of life. It is the most common intraocular malignancy in children and occurs once in every 16,000 to 20,000 live births, resulting in 250 to 300 new cases annually in the United States. About 25 per cent of affected patients have a family history of retinoblastoma, usually bilateral. Some 60 per cent of patients with retinoblastoma present with a white fundus reflex, and 20 per cent present with strabismus. The prognosis for vision and life is directly related to the size and extension of the retinoblastoma.

TABLE 47–6. COMMON CAUSES OF LEUKOKORIA (WHITE PUPIL)

Cataracts (most common cause)
Retinoblastoma
Persistent hyperplastic primary vitreous (PHPV)
Retinal detachment
Vitreous hemorrhage (due to coexisting disease or ocular trauma)
Intraocular inflammation, as with *Toxocara canis* (less common)

Persistent hyperplastic primary vitreous is a congenital developmental abnormality that causes leukokia. It results from persistence of embryonic remnants of the eye's vascular system. The affected eye is often smaller than the other eye, and the lens may become opaque.

Other causes of leukokoria include retinal detachment and vitreous hemorrhage due to coexisting disease or ocular trauma. Intraocular inflammation such as that caused by *Toxocara canis* is an uncommon cause of leukokoria.

Screening at 6 Months

All infants should have a routine eye examination by a family physician at 6 months of age. The examination should assess the baby's ability to fixate on, and follow, a light or small toy, testing one eye at a time. It should also assess the infant's objection to occlusion of either eye. To screen for ocular alignment, the corneal light reflex test and cover test should be performed. Simultaneous examination of the red reflexes is useful to rule out abnormalities of the lens and retina. These and other tests are described in detail below.

By about 6 months of age, the infant's eyes reposition themselves with a jerking motion after following a series of presented objects to one side. This phenomenon, which has been called "railroad" or "telephone" nystagmus, is an entirely normal reaction. It can be elicited by having a subject watch a rotating drum that is painted with vertical stripes (optokinetic drum).

An optokinetic tape is useful for examining babies with possible diminished vision. The tape can be used to assess horizontal and vertical nystagmus. It is helpful for determining whether vision is present when the parents believe that the child may be blind.

Screening at 3 Years of Age

The early preschool years are the most important for detecting strabismus and amblyopia. A misalignment of the eye muscles is called *strabismus*. Adults who have strabismus frequently develop double vision, but children with strabismus quickly learn to ignore, or suppress, the image seen by the wandering eye. As a result of suppression, the straight eye takes over most of the work of seeing, and the crossed eye develops reduced central vision owing to lack of use. Loss of vision in the strabismic, or crossed, eye is called *amblyopia*. There are a number of conditions that can cause amblyopia, but the most common is strabismus (Fig. 47–10). Testing for visual acuity can detect amblyopia. As early as 3.0 or 3.5 years of age, visual acuity testing can be performed using Snellen ABCs or the tumbling E game. The child must identify every character on each line; if a child this

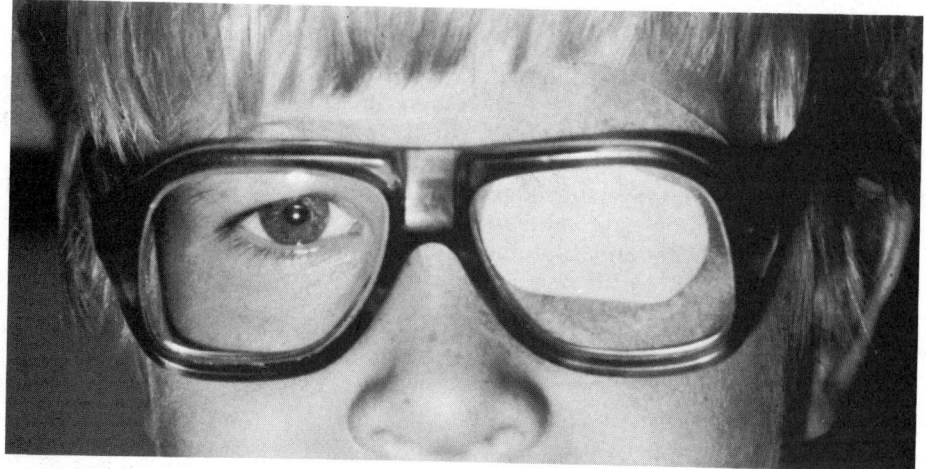

FIGURE 47–10. Amblyopia. This 5-year-old patient also required patching of the better-seeing eye to improve vision in the amblyopic eye.

age can read most of the characters on the line, it is considered acceptable. Other methods include HOTV matching letters (see below) and Allen picture cards. In addition to acuity testing, a fundus examination, cover test for strabismus, and corneal light reflex test should be performed.

Children with a visual acuity of 20/40 or less or a two-line difference in acuity between the two eyes (even within the passing range) should be referred for ophthalmologic examination. Children with strabismus or any ocular pathology should also be referred.

Screening and Eye Examinations at Age 5 and Older

The child should be screened prior to kindergarten, again in first grade (age 6), and every other year thereafter until 11 or 12 years of age. Visual acuity should be assessed, preferably with the Snellen acuity test. Family physicians have also used binocular instruments, including the Titmus and Telebinocular. Binocular instruments are used to test for visual acuity, hyperopia (farsightedness), and muscle balance. They take up little space and can be administered by one person. However, the child's eye cannot be observed during the screening process. Titmus testing is useful in children over age 5 years (Fig. 47–11).

In this age group, children with a visual acuity of worse than 20/30 or a two-line difference between the two eyes should be referred to an ophthalmologist, as should children with strabismus or any ocular abnormality.

Myopia, or nearsightedness, usually occurs by the third or fourth grade (ages 9 to 10). In patients

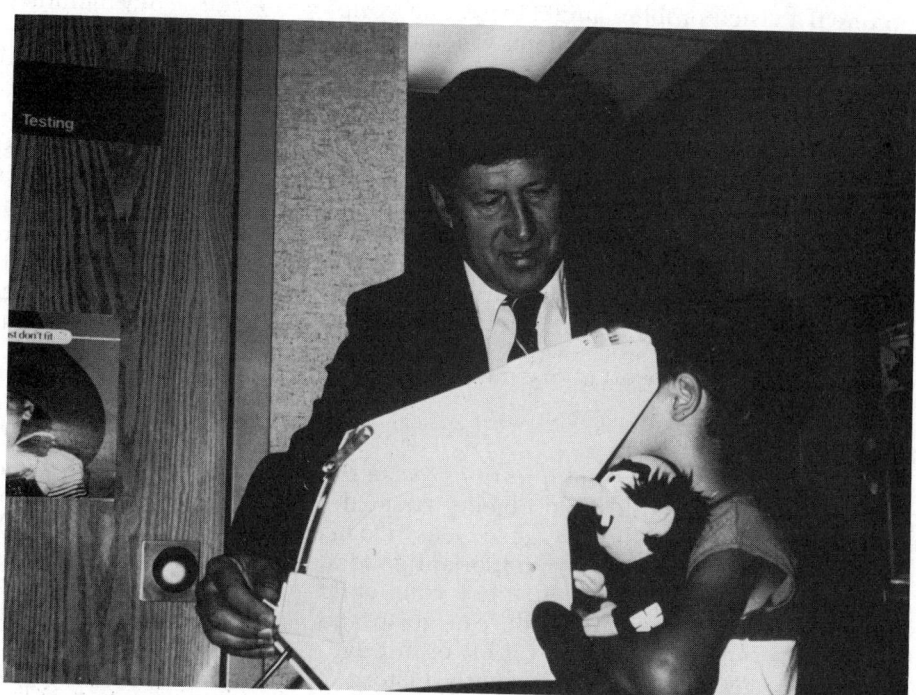

FIGURE 47–11. Titmus testing is an excellent way to screen children, particularly those older than 5 years.

with a family history of high myopia (more than −6 to −7 diopters), myopia may occur at birth. *Hyperopia*, or farsightedness, may not need to be corrected with glasses, particularly when it is +2.50 diopters or less. Glasses are usually prescribed, however, if hyperopia is more than +4.00 diopters. Glasses may also be needed to correct astigmatism, a common error in the focusing ability of the eyes. The Academy statement on vision screening indicates that 20 per cent of children need glasses before they attain full growth.

Special Groups Who Need Vision Screening

The following children should also be screened, even if they are not due to be examined by their age: (1) all children at high risk of having vision disorders, including those who are mentally retarded or who have trisomy 21 or cerebral palsy; and (2) all children who show signs or symptoms of visual problems, experience school failure, or have reading difficulties or other learning problems (including dyslexia). It is important to note, however, that children with learning disabilities such as dyslexia have the same incidence of ocular abnormalities (muscle imbalance, refractive errors) as children without such disabilities. Eye defects do not cause letter, number, or word reversal.

History as a Screening Tool

Before you begin objective testing of visual acuity, obtain an ocular history from the parents to determine if a visual problem might exist. The symptoms of potential eye problems include the following.

1. Rubbing the eyes
2. Shutting or covering one eye
3. Tilting or turning the head
4. Squinting
5. Being unable to see distant objects clearly
6. Bumping into objects.

The typical patients' complaints include the following.

1. Inability to see well at distance
2. Blurred vision
3. Double vision

There are several pertinent questions to ask the parents: Does your child hold objects unusually close to his or her face when trying to focus? Do his or her eyes appear to cross? An important general question is, How well do you think your child sees? Ask the parents if the child can grasp and pick up small objects easily and if his or her eyes follow them across the room. A family history of eye disease, including amblyopia and strabismus, is a particularly important clue.

Importance of the Family History

A positive family history can be an important clue for detecting vision problems in children. Charts of 500 randomized patients in a referral practice for pediatric ophthalmology were reviewed. Of the 500 patients reviewed, 220 had strabismus disorders that included exotropia (congenital and acquired) and esotropia (congenital, accommodative, and nonaccommodative). The study found that 42 per cent of esotropic patients and 39 per cent of exotropic patients had a positive family history of the condition in one or both parents.

Subdividing these patients into specific strabismus subgroups, there was a positive family history of strabismus in 57 per cent of patients with congenital esotropia, 34 per cent of patients with accommodative esotropia, 67 per cent of those with congenital exotropia, and 38 per cent of other exotropic patients. The one subgroup who did not have a positive family history were those with nonaccommodative esotropia that developed after 18 months of age.

Family history also figures prominently in the appearance of cataracts. A positive familial history of congenital cataracts occurs in up to 55 per cent of patients with congenital cataracts.

Testing Visual Acuity

Several diagnostic tests are used to detect strabismus, amblyopia, ocular disease, and refractive errors. They include visual acuity and fixation preference tests, the corneal light reflex test, the cover test, simultaneous red reflexes test, fundus examination, stereoscopic tests, and photorefractive techniques.

The best way to test for possible visual loss due to amblyopia is to measure the visual acuity or fixation preference of both eyes. Acuity testing must be geared to the patient's age. For children under 3 years, the ability to observe and follow small moving objects is critical. When there is no apparent sign of amblyopia, the only clue to poor vision may be an objection to having the better eye occluded when one eye is covered (fixation preference), or an inability to fix on distant objects. Both are common signs of amblyopia that may be due to a refractive error, media opacities, or an abnormality in the retina or optic nerve.

When testing children 3 to 4 years of age, symbols such as tumbling E's or Allen picture cards are appropriate. Equipment required for testing children over age 4 consists of standard wall charts containing Snellen letters, Snellen numbers, illiterate E's, and HOTV. Additional equipment needed includes some means of providing occlusion of the nontested eye. Ideally, it is in the form of occluder patches available from a medical supply house. The two brands on the market are Opticlude (3M Company) and Coverlet (Biersdorf).

Children 4 to 5 years old may not yet be able to perform vision testing by letters and numbers. For these children, the illiterate E test may be used. Literature is available for home use by parents to prepare children for the illiterate E test. This literature contains the practice E's, an illiterate E wall chart, and specific instructions for parents on their use. Another excellent test for this age group is the HOTV test. This test consists of a wall chart composed only of H's, O's, T's, and V's. The child is provided an 8.5 × 11.0 inch board containing a large H, O, T, and V. The examiner points to a figure on the wall chart and the child identifies the correct figure on the testing board. Both the illiterate E test and the HOTV test are excellent tests for this age group. Examiners may determine which test is most useful in their practice and utilize that test preferentially. Neither the illiterate E test nor the HOTV test should be used for children capable of being tested with letters and numbers. These tests may, however, be utilized as confirmation of a letter or number test in those circumstances where the examiner believes that poor performance on testing may be due to issues other than visual acuity. Some children between the ages of 3 and 4 years may not be able to perform the illiterate E or HOTV test. In these circumstances, a flash card-type picture test, such as the Allen card test, may be utilized.

The Allen card test consists in four flash cards containing seven figures. It is a good idea in a very young child to play with the cards initially and be certain that the child is able to identify all seven pictures. Sometimes the child may not know one or two of the figures. In this case, testing should be performed with the remaining figures.

All Allen figures are 20/30 size figures. The furthest distance at which the child is able to accurately identify the pictures becomes the numerator and 30 becomes the denominator. For example, if the child is able to accurately identify the pictures at 15 feet, the visual acuity would be recorded as 15/30. This vision would be equivalent to 20/40 or 10/20. The procedure is then repeated with occlusion, first of the left eye and then the right eye.

Stereoscopic and Photorefractive Tests

The visual acuity test is the most widely used vision screening test. Unfortunately, use of the visual acuity test may under-refer amblyopic children with strabismus in about 3 per cent of patients. Stereoscopic tests such as the random dot E stereogram are relatively inexpensive, relatively accurate, and easy to use.

The use of photorefractive apparatus is relatively new. Reproducible results of photography of the red reflex can screen the young, nonverbal infant or child. The sensitivity is high (95 per cent) for refractive error in the 1 to 2 diopter range. A problem with the technique is that cycloplegia is usually required to prevent false positives, especially for myopia. In addition, two photographs are needed to avoid missing an astigmatic refractive error. The technology offers great promise, but it must be cost-effective.

As new, more rapid and accurate vision tests evolve, they may be incorporated into the screening process.

Focusing on Strabismus and Amblyopia

Strabismus and amblyopia are two of the most common visual problems affecting children. Strabismus occurs in 4 per cent of the population and amblyopia in 2 per cent.

Movements of the eyes horizontally and vertically are controlled by the six muscles attached to the sclera. To see correctly, each extraocular muscle must work in the same direction. Movement of both eyes allows vision of single images. Through a blending process called fusion, the brain combines the two images into a single, three-dimensional image.

So long as the eye muscles are able to work together, the brain can process incoming visual information. When the eye muscles are not coordinated, one eye deviates inward, outward, or upward, and the other eye remains straight. When this occurs, the brain receives a different image from each eye and cannot combine the two disparate images into one.

Misalignment of the eye muscles results in strabismus. In addition to a breakdown or absence of fusion, the causes of strabismus may include refractive errors, anatomic anomalies, and abnormal tonic innervation. Adults who have strabismus frequently develop double vision, but children with strabismus quickly learn to ignore, or suppress, the image seen by the deviated eye. As a result of suppression, the straight eye takes over most of the work of seeing, and the crossed eye develops reduced central vision owing to lack of use.

Loss of vision in the strabismic or misaligned eye is called amblyopia, or "lazy eye." Amblyopia occurs in approximately 50 per cent of patients with strabismus. In children under 4 years of age, amblyopia is the most frequent cause of unilateral vision loss (Fig. 47–10). The condition is usually unilateral, though bilateral high myopia, hyperopia, or astigmatism may occur. Unless treatment begins early, loss of vision in the affected eye may be permanent.

Amblyopia is usually treatable if detected at 3 to 4 years of age but is generally irreversible after age

7. The primary treatment of amblyopia includes the use of patches, glasses, or both. The better-seeing eye is occluded, and underlying conditions such as cataracts or refractive errors are treated.

The corneal light reflex test, the cover test, and extraocular rotations are three basic tests for strabismus. To perform the corneal light test, project a penlight onto the cornea of both eyes simultaneously while the child looks straight ahead. Compare the placement of the two corneal reflections. When the eyes are straight, the light appears at the same point on each cornea. If a muscle deviation is present, the reflected light appears slightly off-center in one eye.

The strabismus drawing (Fig. 47–12) illustrates the placement of corneal reflections as they would appear for each direction of deviation. In the top example, note that the light is centered on the cornea of the left eye but is displaced laterally, or outward, on the right cornea, indicating that the right eye is turned inward or is esotropic. In the second illustration, the light is centered again on the left cornea but is displaced medially, or inward, on the right cornea, demonstrating an outward turning (exotropia) of the right eye. In the third example, the light indicates that the right eye is turned upward or is hypertropic, and the left eye is straight. The bottom illustration shows a hypotropic right eye; that is, the eye is rotated downward.

To perform the second diagnostic test for strabismus, the cover test (Fig. 47–13), have the child look straight ahead at an object 20 feet away. An eye chart is commonly used to test children over age 3. For younger children, it is helpful to use a colorful moving object, such as a noise-making toy. As the child looks at the distant object, cover the right eye and look for movement of the uncovered left eye. If the left eye does not move, there is no apparent misalignment of that eye. If the eye moves outward, the eye is esotropic. If it moves

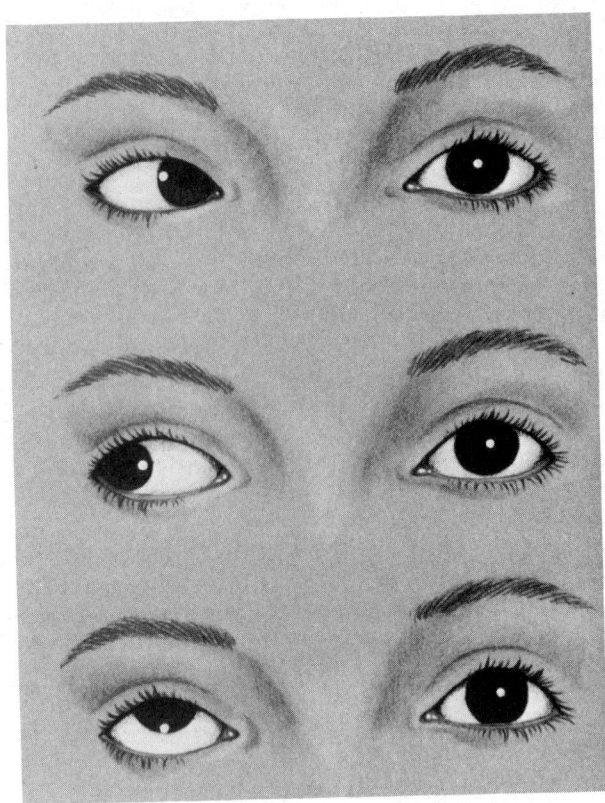

FIGURE 47–12.   Strabismus of right esotropia (top), right exotropia (middle), and right hypertropia (bottom). (From The Child's Eye: Strabismus and Amblyopia. American Academy of Ophthalmology, Professional Information Committee, San Francisco, 1982, with permission.)

inward, it is exotropic. After testing the left eye, repeat the same procedure with the right eye. A third test is to check extraocular movements in the cardinal positions of gaze (Fig. 47–14). The results of the corneal light reflex test, the cover test, and

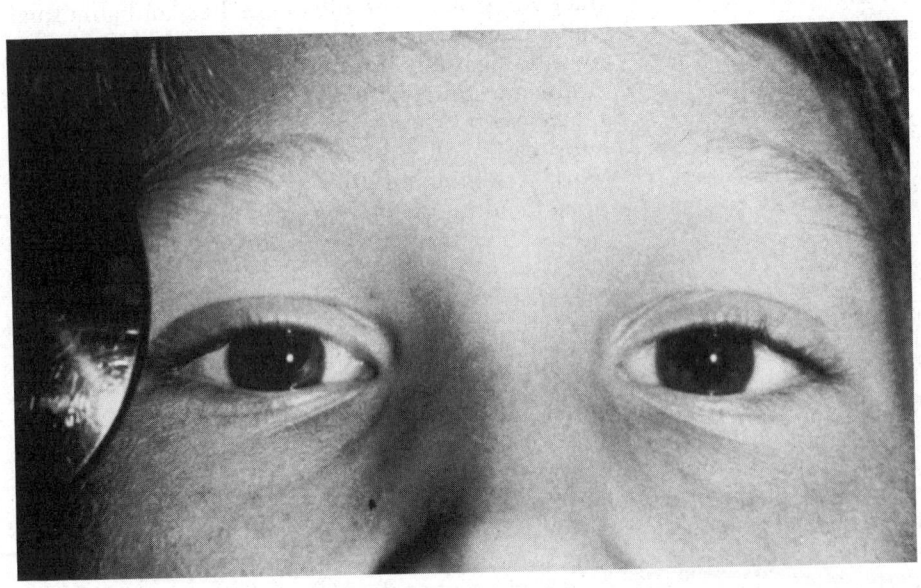

FIGURE 47–13.   Cover–uncover test. Evaluate the unoccluded eye for strabismus. (From The Child's Eye: Strabismus and Amblyopia. American Academy of Ophthalmology, Professional Information Committee, San Francisco, 1982, with permission.)

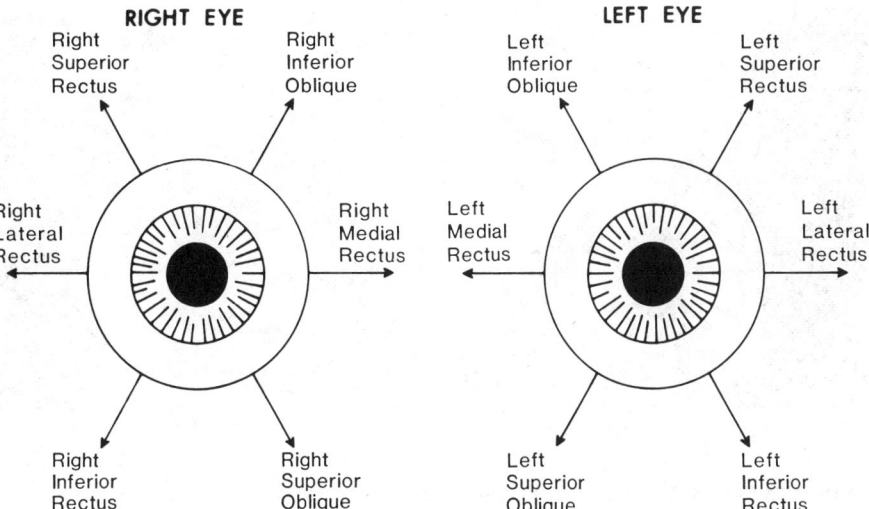

FIGURE 47–14. Ocular muscle movement in cardinal fields of gaze.

extraocular rotations provide a good basis for determining whether a misalignment is present.

Once you have performed the basic diagnostic tests for strabismus and amblyopia, use an ophthalmoscope to examine the red reflexes. Simultaneous examination of both retinal red reflexes is useful as a test of ocular alignment and to rule out abnormalities of the ocular media. This test is performed in a darkened room with the ophthalmoscope at maximum brightness. Once the child is properly positioned, the examiner should move back approximately 18 to 24 inches until both red reflexes are seen simultaneously through the ophthalmoscope. The two reflexes are compared. If an abnormality of the ocular media is present, such as a cataract or tumor, the red reflexes are asymmetric or a white reflex is present.

After examining the red reflexes, observe the ocular fundus, noting the size, shape, color, and cupping of the optic disk. Ophthalmoscopy permits direct visual examination of the retina, optic disk, and retinal vessels and may detect an underlying organic problem or disease condition.

Pseudostrabismus

A common misconception is that children with crossed eyes outgrow the condition. This belief stems from confusion between true strabismus and what is known as pseudostrabismus or false strabismus. A child with pseudostrabismus has broad folds of skin that partially cover the top of each eye and a flat nasal bridge that creates the illusion of crossed eyes. As the child gets older and the skin fold becomes less apparent, the condition becomes less noticeable.

When a child's eyes are truly crossed, it is always a serious condition and requires the care of an ophthalmologist.

Forms of Strabismus

Several forms of strabismus may occur (Table 47–7). Congenital or infantile esotropia accounts for nearly one fourth of all patients who present with strabismus. This condition is usually apparent shortly after birth or during the first 6 months of life. The deviation is generally constant and may be accompanied by a reduced ability to abduct (move the eyes outward). Babies with congenital esotropia usually do not have associated systemic findings. Surgery is the primary treatment to correct this condition (Fig. 47–15) and is performed at 6 months to 2 years of age.

Accommodative esotropia is the most common cause of esotropia and accounts for nearly one half of cases. This type of esotropia is due to excessive focusing or accommodation. Generally, accommodative esotropia is intermittent initially and gradually becomes constant. The age of onset is about 2 years, but it may occur as early as 6 months of age or as late age 7 years. Generally, patients with accommodative esotropia have a moderate amount of

TABLE 47–7. CLASSIFICATION OF STRABISMUS

Type	Percent of Cases	Age of Onset
Congenital or infantile esotropia	20	Birth to 6 months
Accommodative esotropia	45–50	6 months to 7 years (usually 2 years)
Nonaccommodative (acquired) esotropia	10	Variable, depending on etiology
Exotropia	20	Variable (usually during infancy to 4 years)
Hypertropia	<5	Variable, depending on etiology

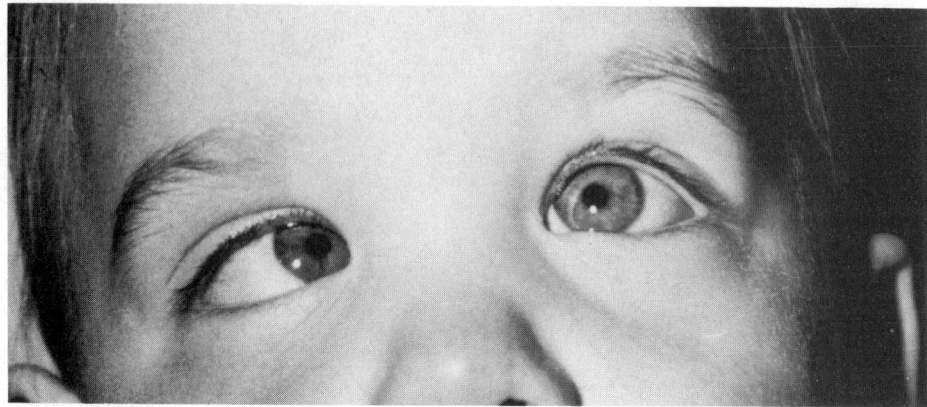

FIGURE 47–15. Congenital esotropia. With the right eye fixing, there is a left esotropia in this 12-month-old infant.

hyperopia (farsightedness). Glasses are commonly prescribed to relieve the eyes of the need to accommodate (Fig. 47–16). In this way, focusing is done by the glasses, enabling the eyes to straighten. Glasses are generally worn at all times to effectively straighten the eyes. If the inturning is greater at near than at distance, bifocals may be required (Fig. 47–17).

Nonaccommodative (acquired) esotropia is not caused by excessive accommodation. The most common causes of nonaccommodative esotropia include unequal refractive errors, cataracts, or corneal scars. Generally, the treatment is directed to the underlying condition, including the correction of amblyopia. Eye muscle surgery may be needed to correct the misalignment.

Exotropia accounts for approximately 20 per cent of strabismus cases. Eight per cent of cases of exotropia start out on an intermittent basis that may confuse or delay the diagnosis. Frequently, the parents note that the child closes one eye in bright sunlight or has an out-turned eye when fatigued or sick. It is important to test patients with exotropia at both near and distant positions when this condition is suspected. Other causes of exotropia include III nerve palsy, neurologic disease, and abnormalities in the bony orbit. Patients with Apert-Crouzon syndrome frequently present with exotropia. Small exotropic deviations are kept under observation. Larger deviations require surgery (Figs. 47–18 to 47–20).

Hypertropia, or vertical deviation, accounts for fewer than 5 per cent of patients with strabismus (Fig. 47–21). It can occur at any age. Vertical deviations are important because they frequently occur in conjunction with serious conditions such as trauma, tumors of the brain and orbit, and thyroid disease. A vertical deviation is usually named for the higher eye. Patients with vertical deviations may have a head tilt, which must be differentiated from ocular torticollis (Fig. 47–22).

Prisms are used to correct small hypertropic deviations, whereas surgery is indicated for large ones. Whenever diplopia (double vision) occurs with strabismus, it can be treated with glasses or prisms (or both).

Other Causes of Strabismus

Acute strabismus may be brought on by a viral upper respiratory tract infection, which can cause an acute VI nerve palsy. With the advent of antibiotics, middle ear infections with associated petrositis and VI nerve palsies are relatively uncommon. Sudden-onset strabismus may also indicate underlying neurologic disease. Another cause is spasm

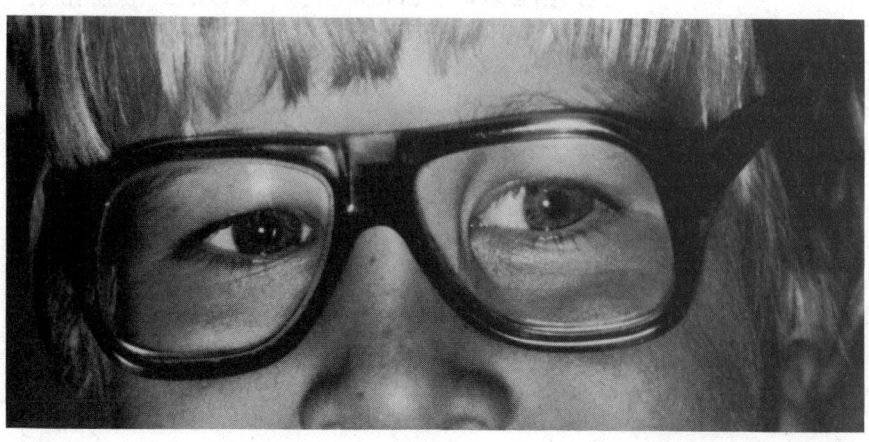

FIGURE 47–16. Accommodative esotropia and anisometropic amblyopia in a 5-year-old patient who has unequal refractive errors between the two eyes as well as accommodative esotropia.

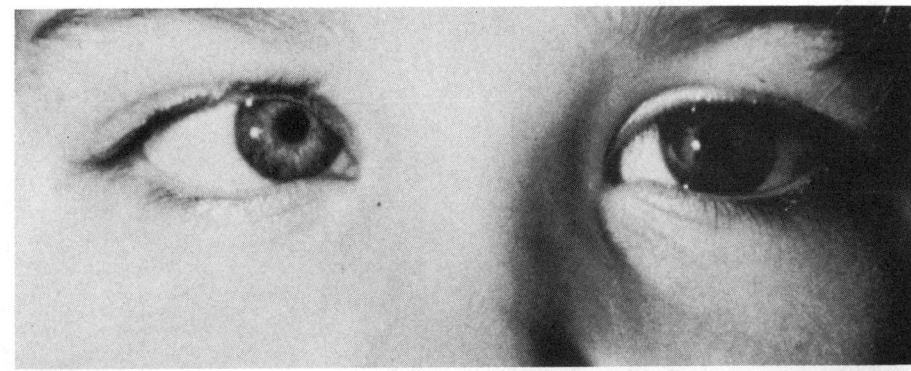
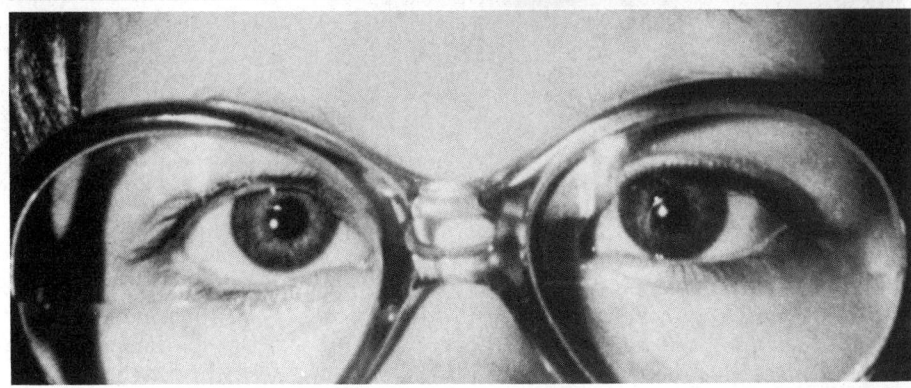

FIGURE 47–17. Accommodative esotropia in a 3-year-old patient uncorrected and corrected by hyperopic (farsighted) glasses. (From The Child's Eye: Strabismus and Amblyopia. American Academy of Ophthalmology, Professional Information Committee, San Francisco, 1982, with permission.)

of the near reflex. A hallmark of spasm of convergence is a miosis, or constricted pupil.

Paralytic and mechanical causes of strabismus occur with trauma and Duane syndrome. In addition, neurologic trauma accounts for paralysis to cranial nerves IV (innervates the superior oblique), VI (innervates the lateral rectus), and III (innervates all other extraocular muscles) (Fig. 47–23).

The proper corrective treatment for strabismus includes nonsurgical treatment, such as patching and eyeglasses. Eye muscle surgery is performed when it is clear that nonsurgical methods may not correct the misalignment. Four aspects of strabismus surgery should be stressed.

1.   The surgery is safe and effective.
2.   The eyeball is never removed to perform the surgery.

3.   More than one operation may be required to straighten the eyes.
4.   Both eyes may require surgery to correct the muscle deviation.

The goals when treating strabismus include the ability to provide and maintain equal vision in both eyes, to enable the eyes to work together, and to improve depth perception when possible.

Refractive Errors and Color Vision

Some eyes are either too long or too short and need help focusing light onto the retina. If an eye is too long, the light rays focus in front of the retina and the image on the retina is blurred. An individual with this condition can move things closer to

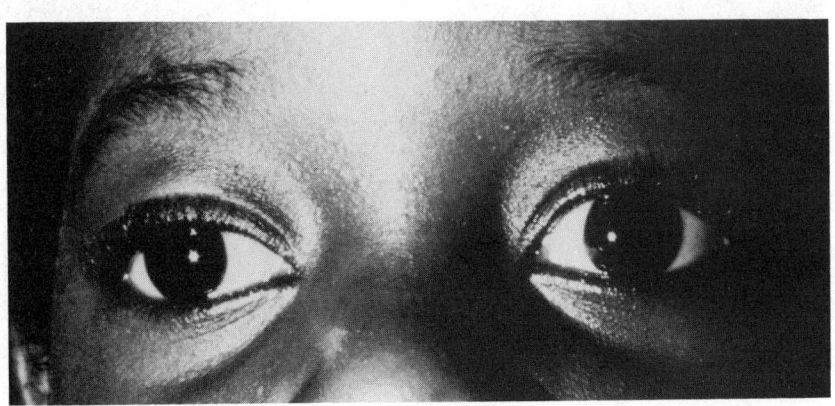

FIGURE 47–18. Exotropia in an 8-year-old patient with right exotropia.

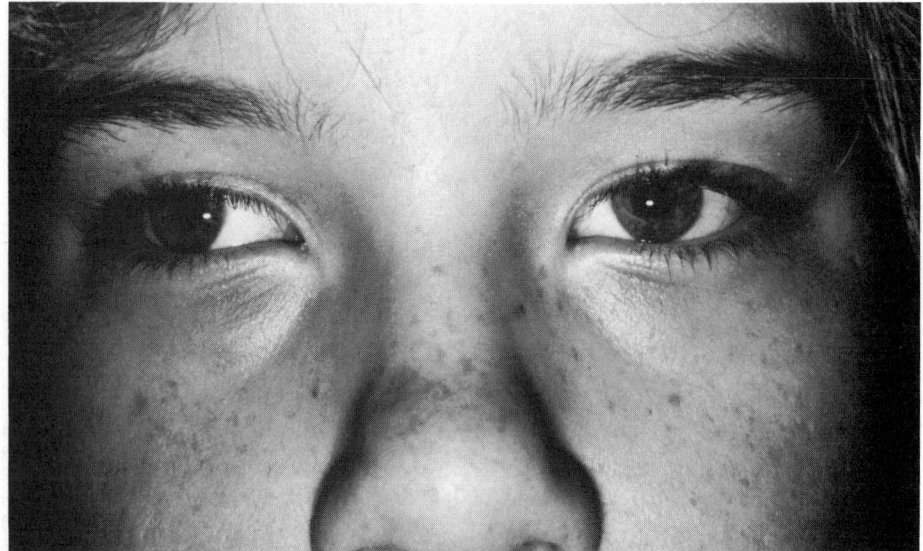

FIGURE 47–19. Positive angle kappa, which appears similar to exotropia, in an 8-year-old patient. Actually, this patient has retinopathy of prematurity with bilateral dragged maculas.

see better or can wear glasses. This condition is called *nearsightedness* (myopia). With *farsightedness* (hyperopia), the light focuses behind the retina because the eye is too short and causes a blurred image. Both conditions are corrected by glasses or contact lenses. *Astigmatism* is another common error in the focusing abilities of the eye. It is caused by an unequal curvature of the front surface of the cornea. Corrective eyeglasses are necessary if it causes blurred vision or discomfort. Unless there is a marked amount of myopia (nearsightedness), hyperopia (farsightedness), or astigmatism, or a significant refractive difference between the eyes, eyeglasses can adequately

compensate for these problems. Refractive errors requiring eyeglasses exist in nearly 20 per cent of the pediatric population prior to the attainment of full growth.

Color vision defects rarely result in significant visual difficulties. Eight per cent of white males have some red-green color deficiency, whereas fewer than 1 per cent of females are affected. In isolation, this defect rarely results in any real drawback to normal function, especially during childhood. We think that no special emphasis should be placed on the diagnosis of color blindness at early childhood examination. Although the identification of such defects can be helpful in a classroom

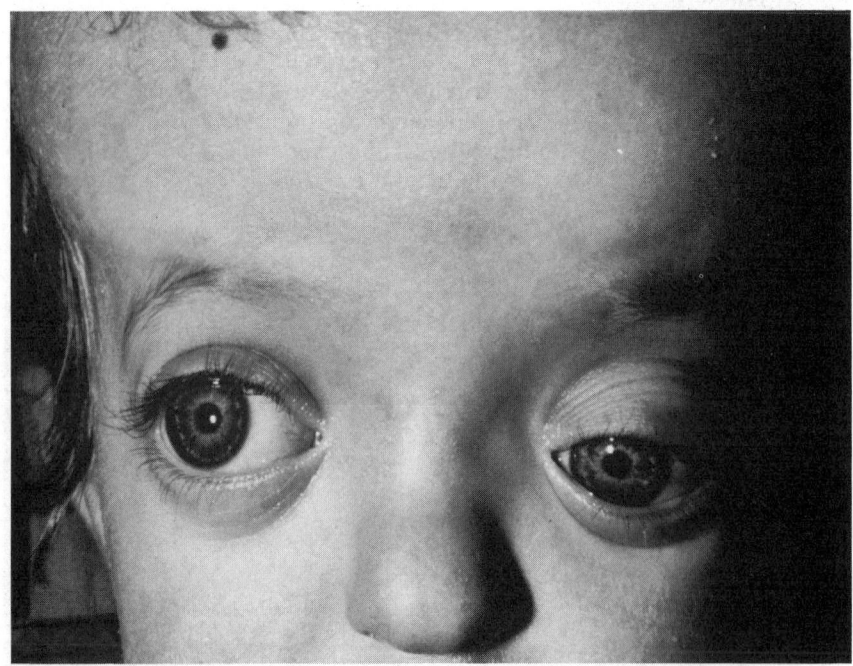

FIGURE 47–20. This patient presented with proptosis, amblyopia, and left exotropia. This patient had the diagnosis of Crouzon syndrome.

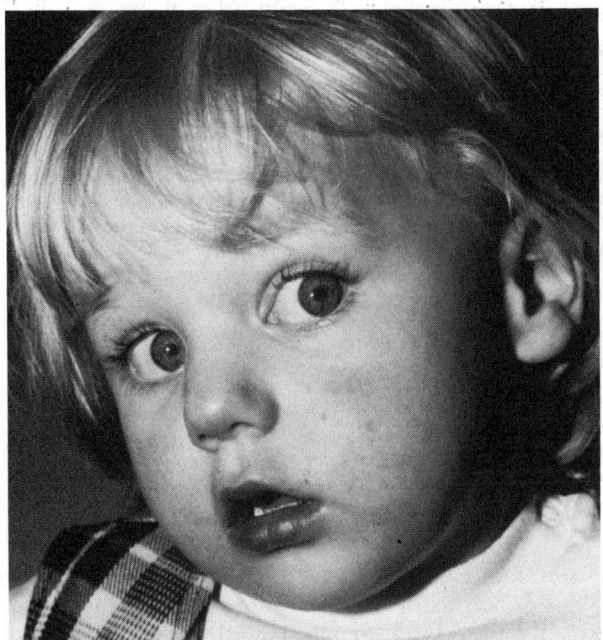

FIGURE 47–21. Positive head tilt in this 4-year-old can indicate a vertical deviation, especially a superior oblique palsy. (From The Child's Eye: Strabismus and Amblyopia. American Academy of Ophthalmology, Professional Information Committee, San Francisco, 1982, with permission.)

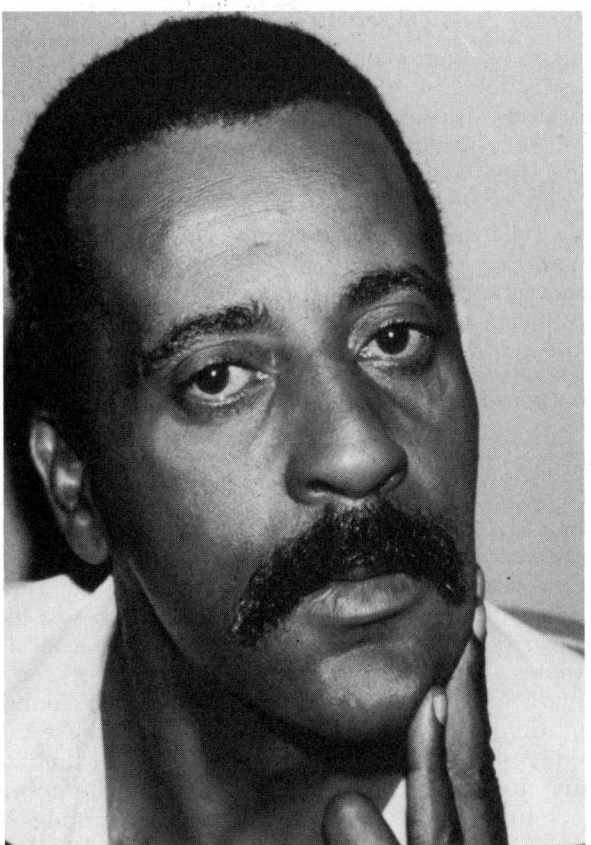

FIGURE 47–22. A 34-year-old patient with ocular torticollis. Note the abnormal head tilt.

situation, emphasis should not be placed on these minor abnormalities at this age. Color vision testing is not required unless a retinal dystrophy is suspected, the family history is positive, or the family specifically requests it.

Headaches

Headache is one of the most common conditions of humans, but children do not seem to have as many complaints about headaches as do adults. Most headaches are not serious and frequently are caused by tension. Many people believe incorrectly that eyestrain and the need for glasses are common causes of headaches.

Headaches caused by eye disease are usually felt in the eye or in the brow on the same side as the involved eye. Frequently, these headaches are associated with some other symptom, such as blurred vision, halos around lights, or extreme sensitivity to light. Most headaches are related to stress.

Learning Disabilities and the Eye

Although reading may be easier and faster when sight is clear, visual problems do not cause learning disabilities, and eye defects are not responsible for reversal of letters or other signs of reading disabilities. In the past, reading problems have been blamed on the eyes, though children with a learning disability have no greater incidence of eye problems than the rest of the population.

It is important that a thorough medical eye examination be performed. The presence or absence of visual defects can be diagnosed and corrected. Once vision is corrected, no other examinations or therapies involving the eyes diminish a learning disability. Visual training, muscle exercises, perceptual training, or hand–eye coordination exercises do *not* improve the child's learning abilities.

It is difficult to absolutely diagnose a learning disability before a child reaches the age of 6 to 7. However, once a diagnosis is made, educational assistance is needed promptly.

Pediatric Cataracts

Approximately 40 per cent of acquired pediatric cataracts are secondary to trauma, and as many as approximately one third of pediatric cataracts are inherited. The basic approach to the patient with pediatric cataracts is to determine whether the cataract is an isolated finding, part of a syndrome or other systemic abnormality, or associated with some other ocular disease (Table 47–8). When several members of the same family are affected by congenital cataracts, we may assume a hereditary origin. Autosomal dominant hereditary patterns

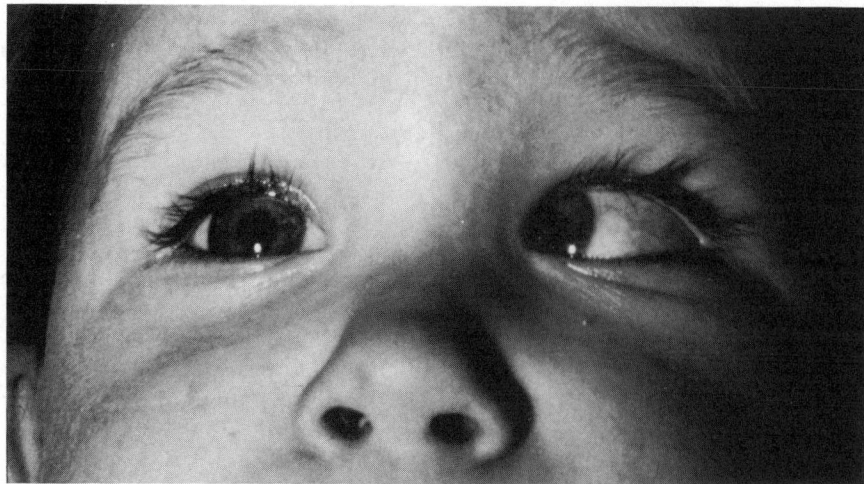

FIGURE 47–23. This 14-month-old patient presented with the chief complaint of underaction of the left lateral rectus muscle and left esotropia after an upper respiratory infection. This patient actually had a VI nerve palsy related to the viral syndrome.

are the most frequent mode of transmission. X-linked cataracts are rare and occur primarily with the oculocerebrorenal syndrome. Congenital or infantile cataracts have been described in association with a large number of congenital anomalies.

History and Ocular Examination

In patients with pediatric cataracts, the age when the cataract or decreased vision occurred should be determined. Detailed history of maternal intrauterine infections, including rubella, toxoplasmosis, herpes simplex, cytomegalovirus, and varicella, should be obtained. Drug and medication use during pregnancy and birth trauma should be ruled out.

A complete ocular examination should be performed including visual acuity assessment using fixation and following responses. Infants with complete bilateral congenital cataracts usually demonstrate decreased visual interest and may have delayed development. Nystagmus results from early visual deprivation and is an ominous sign of poor vision. Ocular fixation and following movements may be decreased or absent. In some cases, strabismus is a presenting sign, especially in children with monocular cataracts.

Glaucoma and other ocular disorders must be ruled out. Examination of the red reflexes by retinoscopy can reveal even minute lens opacities. Direct ophthalmoscopy or retinoscopy through the child's undilated pupil is helpful for estimating potential vision in an eye harboring a cataract. Any central opacity or surrounding cortical distortion larger than 3 mm has been shown to be visually significant. The presence of retinal detachment, retinoblastoma, or other ocular pathologies that preclude good visual outcome must be ruled out by indirect ophthalmoscopy or ultrasonography.

Most anterior polar cataracts are small, measuring less than 1 to 2 mm, and are usually not progressive. Surgery is seldom required, and the visual prognosis is excellent.

Nuclear cataracts are typically congenital, dense axial opacities of 3 mm or more. Nuclear cataracts are frequently associated with microphthalmos and are inherited as autosomal dominant traits. Visual results are generally only fair even if surgery is done early and poor if it is done late. Aphakic glaucoma has a much higher incidence in these patients. Rubella cataracts may occur as a manifestation of the classic rubella syndrome—the triad of cardiac defects, hearing impairment, and cataracts.

Partial Lens Opacities

The evaluation of partial lens opacities is related to the location of the cataract. Cataracts that are located anteriorly include anterior lenticonus, polar cataracts, persistent pupillary membrane opacities, and those occurring with anterior segment dysgenesis. Posterior cataracts include posterior polar, posterior lenticonus, and posterior subcapsular lens opacities. Posterior subcapsular cataracts are typically associated with corticosteroid use, atopic dermatitis, or inflammatory diseases, and they are generally bilateral.

Traumatic and Posterior Lenticonus

Traumatic cataract, the most common cause of unilateral cataract in children, is caused by penetrating or blunt trauma. Posterior lenticonus cataracts are the second most common cause of unilateral acquired cataract in children. Posterior lenticonus is a circumscribed oval or round bulge in the infant's or child's posterior lens capsule and cortex restricted generally to a 2 × 7 mm axial diameter. The bulge increases progressively, and cataractous changes occur in the cortex surrounding the posterior lenticonus. Generally, there is a reduced red reflex initially with posterior lenticonus; and cataractous changes occur in the cortex surrounding the posterior lenticonus. Among 21 patients with posterior lenticonus, only two had bilateral posterior lenticonus. The age at which posterior lenticonus was first detected varied from

TABLE 47–8. PEDIATRIC CATARACTS: CAUSES AND ASSOCIATED CONDITIONS

Intrauterine Infection
 Rubella
 Toxoplasmosis
 Herpes simplex
 Cytomegalovirus
 Varicella
Metabolic Disorders
 Galactosemia
 Galactokinase deficiency
 Hypoparathyroidism
 Pseudohypoparathyroidism
 Diabetes mellitus
 Hypoglycemia
 Hyperalimentation (vacuoles)
 Mannosidosis
Drug-induced
 Corticosteroids
 Chlorpromazine
 Ergot
 Naphthalene
 Triparanol
Inflammatory
 Juvenile rheumatoid arthritis
 Sarcoidosis
 Pars planitis
 Atopic dermatitis
Trauma
Genetic/Syndromes
 Autosomal dominant
 Autosomal recessive
 X-linked recessive
 Down syndrome (trisomy 21)
 Trisomy 13
 Trisomy 18
 Lowe syndrome
 Dubowitz syndrome
 Hallerman–Streiff syndrome
 Alport syndrome
 Cri du chat syndrome
 Cerebrotendinous xanthomatosis
 Marinesco-Sjögren syndrome
 Myotonic dystrophy
 Rothmund-Thomson syndrome
 Cockayne syndrome
 Incontinentia pigmenti
 Stickler syndrome
 Craniofacial syndromes
 Zellweger syndrome
 Wilson syndrome
 Hallgren syndrome
 Laurence-Moon-Bardet-Biedl syndrome
 Chondrodysplasia punctata
 Refsum disease
 Congenital ichthyosis
 Sclerodactyly
 G-6-PD deficiency
 Rubinstein-Taybi syndrome
Radiation Injury
Ocular Disease
 Retinitis pigmentosa
 Aniridia
 Persistent
  Hyperplastic
  Primary vitreous (PHPV)
 Leber congenital amaurosis
 Retinopathy of prematurity
 Retinoblastoma

3 months to 15 years. The interval between the oil-droplet posterior lenticonus and cataract development is variable. The eyes are normal in size, and visual results are good with surgery.

Posterior lenticonus cataracts occur as early as 3 months of age or as late as 15 years. If the vision becomes worse than 20/70 or 20/80, the cataract should be removed by specialized instrumentation followed by contact lens fitting.

Complete Lens Opacities

Work-up for complete cataracts includes systemic evaluation, ocular ultrasonography, metabolic evaluation, TORCH titers, and chromosomal analysis. Congenital cataract etiologies include intrauterine infection, metabolic disorders, chromosomal anomalies, or systemic syndromes. Work-up for congenital cataracts includes analysis of urine for reducing substances and amino acids. Serum chemistry for calcium, phosphorus, glucose, blood urea nitrogen (BUN), and TORCH titers should be obtained. When warranted, genetic and pediatric consultations should be requested. Radiologic imaging, including CT or MRI, may be warranted.

Surgical Issues Related to Pediatric Cataracts

Prompt clearing of the visual axis with immediate optical correction offers the best chance for visual recovery in pediatric patients with unilateral or bilateral cataracts. The surgical procedure recommended depends on the patient's age, risk of amblyopia and expected ocular growth, and reactivity to surgery. In patients younger than age 6 months to 2 years of age, the best option is to clear the visual axis and have it remain clear throughout the critical period of vision development with a lensectomy/vitrectomy procedure and 6-mm posterior capsulectomy with anterior vitrectomy. This procedure eliminates reopacification of the posterior capsule, which occurs in more than 90 per cent of pediatric patients under age 2 years. In children older than 2 years of age, lensectomy with vitrectomy and a 4-mm posterior capsulectomy is performed. Most of these children can be fitted with contact lenses, although an intraocular lens is indicated in some traumatic cataract patients. Traumatic unilateral cataracts present the least controversial situation in which intraocular lenses are considered in young children. However, we do not have a firm foundation of experience on which we can stand while assuring the parents that this form of optical correction—intraocular lenses—is best for their child. Advances in intraocular lenses and in surgical techniques have afforded improvements in pediatric intraocular implantation, particularly the use of Healon, vitrectomy instrumentation, and improvements in the lenses themselves, including surface passivated intraocular lenses. In the age group over age 8, lensectomy with insertion of intraocular lenses may be considered, but we do not have long-term follow-up studies for this age group.

The prognosis for children with monocular and binocular congenital and pediatric cataracts has improved markedly. Ongoing clinical studies will determine the best indications and procedures for use in pediatric cataract patients.

Retinoblastoma

Retinoblastoma is the second most common primary intraocular malignancy in all age groups (melanoma is most common in adults) and is the most common intraocular malignancy of childhood. Its incidence is approximately 1 in every 14,000 births. Generally, there are 250 to 300 new cases a year in the United States. A viral or oncogenic factor related to the environment may be associated with this condition.

The tumor occurs bilaterally in as many as one third of cases. It is generally diagnosed between 14 and 18 months of age, and more than 90 per cent of the tumors are diagnosed by age 3 years. Familial cases of retinoblastoma account for 6 per cent of patients. The disease is inherited through an autosomal dominant gene with incomplete penetrance. The remaining 94 per cent are sporadic cases that occur as a result of genetic mutation in 25 per cent and as a somatic mutation in about 75 per cent. It is difficult if not impossible to differentiate the genetic mutations clinically and to determine which tumors will be passed on to offspring. There are occasionally rare cases of retinoblastoma related to chromosomal abnormalities (partial deletion of the long arm of the 13 chromosome). It has also been associated with trisomy 21.

The diagnosis is made by the patient presenting with a white pupil (leukokoria) in 61 per cent of cases, strabismus in 22 per cent of cases, and sometimes with a retinal detachment, a red, painful eye, or spontaneous hyphema (Fig. 47–24). Generally, patients with small retinoblastomas have problems with vision or strabismus. More advanced lesions present with leukokoria and sometimes secondary glaucoma. The advanced lesions may metastasize to the orbit and produce proptosis through the orbital spread. In addition, patients with retinoblastoma may have systemic metastases to the CNS, skull bones, lymph nodes, and other organs.

The treatment of retinoblastoma is generally enucleation for the cases of advanced retinoblastoma involving more than 50 per cent of the eye. If the second eye is involved, treatment depends on the size of tumor and whether there is extraocular extension. External beam irradiation treatment may be performed on the second eye or bilaterally when necessary. Photocoagulation or cryotherapy are equally effective with small retinoblastomas confined to the retinal periphery. Systemic chemo-

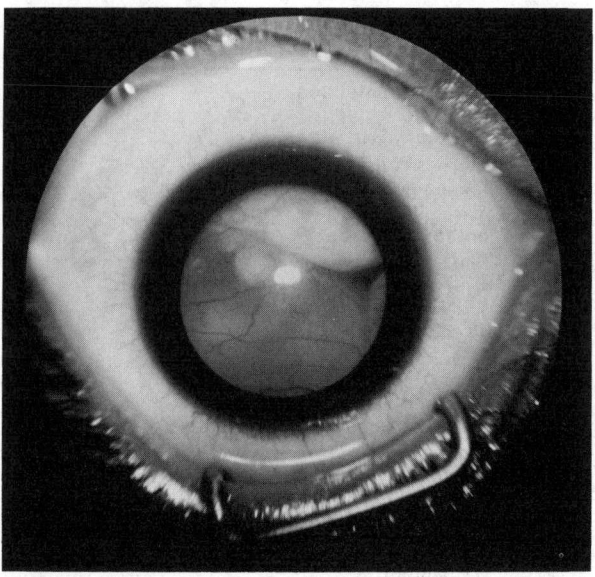

FIGURE 47–24. Total retinal detachment and advanced retinoblastoma in a 23-month-old infant who presented with leukokoria (white reflex).

therapy may be indicated after enucleation for advanced unilateral or bilateral cases.

CONTACT LENSES

A major use of contact lenses is to correct myopia, aphakia, and astigmatism. It is critical to have a well motivated patient in order to fit contact lenses successfully. Frequently, the patient is motivated by the cosmetic appearance. The aphakic patient may be motivated by the improvement of visual quality possible with contact lenses. There are many types of contact lenses, and they fall primarily into four groups.

1. Daily-wear hard lenses
2. Daily-wear soft lenses
3. Rigid, gas-permeable hard lenses (daily and extended wear)
4. Extended-wear soft lenses

Hard lenses have generally been constructed of polymethylmethacrylate (PMMA). This material minimally absorbs fluid compared to soft lenses, which may become 80 per cent hydrated. The main problems with hard lenses are discomfort associated with the use of the lens for at least 2 weeks after initial fittings. However, these lenses generally last more than 3 years. New materials for both hard and soft lenses continue to be developed, including the silicone lenses that are presently available. A major advantage of PMMA lenses includes the correction of corneal astigmatism up to 2 diopters.

Soft contact lenses do not require a prolonged adaptation period, nor is a rigid wearing schedule essential for successful use. The primary disadvantage of soft lenses is that visual acuity is decreased if the patient has a corneal astigmatism of more than 1 diopter. In addition, there are some fluctuations in visual acuity with blinking. The lens is easily damaged with handling, and the lenses have a short life-span compared to the conventional hard lenses. Generally, soft lenses last no longer than 1 year. The material used in soft lenses is generally hydrophilic material, such as hydroxyethylene methylmethacrylate (HEMA).

Rigid gas-permeable contact lenses are more comfortable than conventional PMMA hard contact lenses. In addition, they provide better visual acuity than soft lenses if astigmatism is present. Extended-wear hydrogel lenses are lenses that enable the eye to adapt to the lens for an indefinite time and provide stable visual correction if there is not significant astigmatism. We presently deal with a third generation of extended-wear hydrogel lenses. These extended-wear lenses can be used for diseased as well as aphakic eyes. Complications of extended-wear lenses include infection, ocular allergies, including enlargement of the follicles, contact lens opacification due to calcium deposits or lipoprotein coatings, corneal edema, and corneal vascularization. Therefore patients wearing extended-wear lenses should be treated with caution. Corneal ulcers are more common with extended-wear lenses than with daily-wear lenses. Careful patient hygiene and lens cleaning of both hard and soft lenses, and particularly of extended-wear lenses, cannot be overemphasized.

OCULAR MEDICATIONS

Ocular medications may have significant systemic side effects. Miotic eye drops, such as pilocarpine, are used for the treatment of chronic open angle glaucoma and may cause cholinergic effects on rare occasions with systemic absorption. Epinephrine eye drops can be absorbed in high enough concentrations to cause an acute elevation of blood pressure, headaches, and heart palpitations. Epinephrine should be used with caution in patients with systemic hypertension or coronary artery disease. Systemic absorption of timolol may exacerbate asthma. In addition, it may cause difficulty with breathing, brachycardia, and hypotension. This medication is contraindicated in patients with heart block, congestive heart failure, asthma, or obstructive lung disease. Other agents used for glaucoma include carbonic anhydrase inhibitors and oral medications to lower intraocular pressure and decrease aqueous production. Carbonic anhydrase inhibitors, such as acetazolamide (Diamox) or methazolamide (Neptazane), cause increased urination, decreased appetite, nausea, malaise, and kidney stones. Carbonic anhydrase inhibitors lower the serum potassium, particularly in patients

taking diuretics. Potassium supplements should be prescribed to prevent hypokalemia.

Unfortunately, at times patients are given an antibiotic–steroid combination that may increase intraocular pressure, cause cataracts, or potentiate fungal ulcers. Steroid glaucoma is a form of open angle glaucoma. If the condition is undetected and the patient continues to refill the medication, damage may occur to the optic nerve, including glaucomatous optic atrophy. Generally, the intraocular pressure is lowered once the steroids are discontinued. However, it may take several months for the pressure to return to normal levels. Vision loss that occurs during this period may be permanent. Because of the relative frequency of steroid glaucoma, cataract, and exacerbations of viral infections, topical corticosteroids should be avoided for minor ocular inflammations. It is important to emphasize that generally ocular conditions that warrant the use of topical steroids also warrant consultation with an ophthalmologist.

OPHTHALMIC CONDITIONS IN THE ADULT

The most important causes of central and peripheral visual impairment in the elderly include glaucoma, cataract, diabetic retinopathy, and macular degeneration. Most of these conditions can be controlled, or as in the case of cataracts vision can be restored to a significant level to improve the quality of life. Glaucoma and macular degeneration may be arrested with proper treatment. Regular eye examinations for the elderly can detect early signs of ocular abnormalities and ensure that proper treatment is initiated. Generally, adults after the age of 40 should have a complete examination at least every 3 years. After age 65, the examinations should be at 2-year intervals.

Diseases of the Eyelids

Entropion is a turning in of the eyelid margin so there is a rubbing of eyelashes or cilia with resultant ocular irritation. An *ectropion* is a turning out of the eyelid margin so the eye builds up excessive tears and becomes inflamed. Both conditions are more common in the aging population. Entropion and ectropion can cause symptoms of irritation and corneal changes.

Basal cell carcinoma is much more common in the elderly. The carcinoma occurs more commonly on the lower lid. Generally, basal cell carcinomas have pearly edges and a central depression that becomes ulcerated.

Dermatochalasis, or baggy eyelids, may interfere with vision, covering part of the eye. This condition is caused by atrophy of the skin of the lids

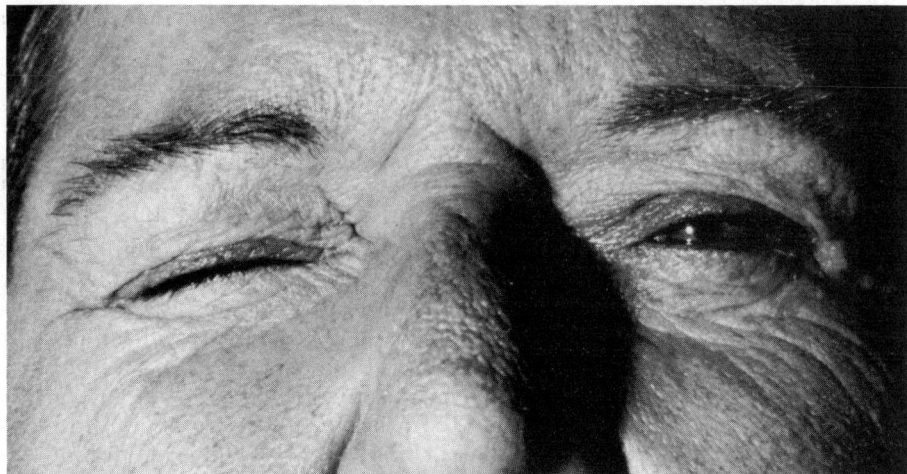

FIGURE 47–25. A 68-year-old woman with a history of lid spasm that was impossible to control. The blepharospasm caused her to be unable to drive.

resulting in loose skin. Dermatochalasis does not cause any permanent damage to vision.

Blepharospasm is a chronic spasm of the eyelids in older adults (Fig. 47–25). It may interfere with reading and driving. Botulinum injection in small doses is presently the treatment of choice.

Herpes Zoster and Herpes Simplex

Herpes zoster occurs more frequently in the aging population. When the skin lesions involve the eyelids and tip of the nose, the ophthalmologist should be consulted for evaluation. Corneal dendrites and ulcers can occur with herpes zoster and herpes simplex. Herpes simplex is more commonly associated with uveitis.

Ptosis

Ptosis can occur in a number of forms, including congenial ptosis, pseudoptosis, and acquired ptosis (Fig. 47–26). Congenital ptosis can occur as a bilateral ptosis or with a Marcus-Gunn jaw winking ptosis secondary to a misdirected III nerve. Acquired forms of ptosis include myogenic forms, including myasthenia gravis and progressive external ophthalmoplegia, and neurogenic forms, including Horner syndrome or III nerve palsy (Fig. 47–27). Pseudoptosis is due to conditions giving the appearance of a ptosis. Pseudoptosis is particularly common with microphthalmia (small eye) or phthisis bulbi. It may also be secondary to a hypotropia.

Congenital ptosis generally is corrected with a bilateral fascia lata brow suspension or a levator resection in instances where there is good levator function. Adult forms of ptosis include correction with a tarsoconjunctival resection, strengthening of the levator aponeurosis, or levator resection.

Dry Eye (Keratitis Sicca)

Tears, because of their lubricating and bacteriostatic properties, are essential for maintaining a

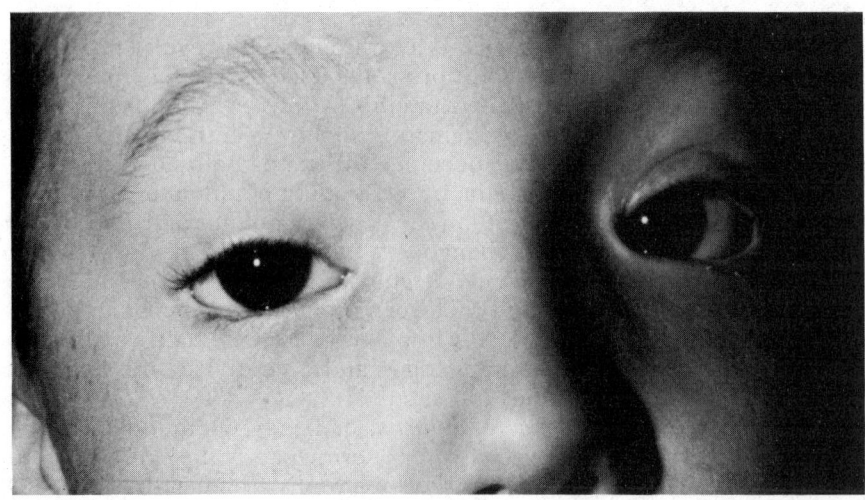

FIGURE 47–26. Congenital ptosis seen in a 4-year-old patient with bilateral ptosis of a congenital variety.

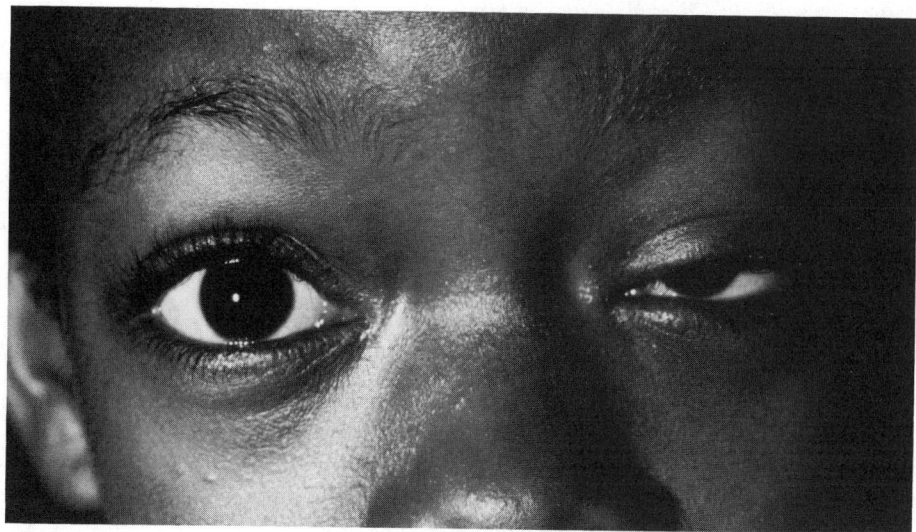

FIGURE 47–27. Ptosis of the left upper lid in an 8-year-old patient who had ocular myasthenia and subsequently developed ptosis of the right upper lid and exotropia.

healthy cornea and conjunctiva. A deficiency in tear production may result in a dry eye, also known as keratitis sicca. Keratoconjunctivitis sicca is an acquired disorder seen frequently during the fifth decade of life. The sexual predilection is toward women. Initial symptoms include a foreign body sensation, dryness, and burning, which often worsens as this condition progresses. Paradoxical tearing from reflex stimulation of the lacrimal gland occurs. Symptoms usually exceed the signs of this common condition. Examination reveals a lack of corneal and conjunctival luster with some dry spots being seen. With a decrease in aqueous tears, an attempt to compensate by an increase in mucin production occurs, leading sometimes to a stringy, rope-like discharge. Some cases of keratoconjunctivitis sicca are related to an autoimmune etiology, particularly those with dryness of other mucous membranes. It also occurs commonly with such conditions as rheumatoid arthritis (Sjögren syndrome).

Treatment of dry eyes includes artificial tears to replace the tear efficiency in symptomatic patients. At the time, the ophthalmologist is required to perform surgical closure of the punctum, tarsorrhaphy, and advocate goggles in severe cases. Topical antibiotics are required only if secondary infection occurs.

Exposure keratitis is a condition symptomatically similar to dry eyes that arises from incomplete eyelid closure during blinking or with sleep. It may result from Bell's palsy, scarred or malpositioned eyelids, or thyroid exophthalmos. Management involves the use of ophthalmic lubricating solutions and ointments. Mechanical measures designed to assist normal eyelid closure may be necessary, including frequent manual massage of the lids during the day to assist closure, "forceful blinking" exercises to elicit Bell's reflex, and taping the lids shut at night. Merely patching the eye is to be avoided because of an increased risk of corneal abrasion if the lids do not cover the eye underneath the patch. Severe cases and those requiring surgical correction, such as tarsorrhaphy, should be referred to an ophthalmologist.

Arcus Senilis

Arcus senilis, or corneal arcus, is a hazy white or yellow arc or deposit in the peripheral cornea. There are many causes of arcus senilis, and it is more common in the aging population. The deposit is composed of cholesterol and other lipids and does not generally indicate an underlying systemic abnormality in the elderly. It does not interfere with vision or function of the eyes.

Thyroid Myopathy

Hyperthyroidism is characterized by diffuse hyperplasia of the thyroid and infiltrative ophthalmopathy. The thyroid myopathy is seen in association with thyroid dysfunction, although thyroid function tests may be normal. With thyroid myopathy, the extraocular mechanism is unknown and the genetic predisposition uncertain.

Graves' ophthalmopathy occurs in approximately 95 per cent of patients with Graves' thyroid disease but is seen only rarely with Hashimoto's thyroid disease. The diagnosis of euthyroid Graves' ophthalmopathy is primarily a clinical diagnosis, confirmed with the assistance of CT.

Clinical characteristics include hypotropia, esotropia, or a combination of both vertical and horizontal muscle deviations. Almost always there is a positive forced duction test on examination. Many patients are euthyroid at the time of diagnosis, but there may have been a history of thyroid abnormalities. Thyroid myopathy is a common cause of acquired vertical deviation in adults but relatively uncommon in children.

Werner has classified eye involvement in Graves' disease by a NO-SPECS phenomenon:

No signs of symptoms
Only signs of lid retraction or gaze palsy with or without lid lag or proptosis
Signs and symptoms of soft tissue involvement
Proptosis
Extraocular muscle involvement
Corneal involvement with corneal drying
Sight loss with optic nerve involvement

The total muscle volume of the extraocular muscles increases as the disease worsens. The volume can be computed by averaging serial CT sections.

Indications for treatment of thyroid ophthalmopathy include diplopia, abnormal head position, a large horizontal or vertical strabismus, and loss of vision. Generally, the preferred treatment is orbital decompression if loss of vision is threatened. Nonsurgical management of the patient includes prisms to alleviate the diplopia in primary position or surgery, generally on adjustable sutures.

Cataracts

Cataract is a condition that affects a large percentage of the population. Generally, the normal aging and cataractous changes in the lens are related to its metabolic activity and changes in the concentration in various proteins and minerals. Posterior subcapsular cataracts often interfere with vision, whereas anterior cataracts may not.

Acquired cataracts may be due to penetrating trauma, irradiation, heat, or blunt trauma. Metabolic cataracts occur particularly in association with diabetes. Changes in the blood glucose may alter the refractive power of the lens. With hyperglycemia, there is an increased concentration of glucose in the anterior chamber aqueous humor. When the glucose enters the lens, water follows with resultant swelling.

Senile cataract (nuclear sclerosis) is the most common cause of lens opacity seen by the ophthalmologist. The most common type of cataract in older patients involves the lens nucleus. There is an increased density centrally in the lens that makes the lens focusing power stronger. As a result of this change in focusing power, frequent changes in glasses are required. This type of cataract develops slowly, and surgery may not be necessary for several months or even years.

Subcapsular cataract, particularly posterior subcapsular cataract, is an opacity just in front of the posterior capsule. It may be associated with reduced vision particularly with bright sunlight or night driving. The treatment for cataracts depends on whether vision is impaired or the patient's lifestyle is limited because of the cataracts.

Should cataract surgery be decided upon, the operation involves removal of the cataract, or cloudy lens material. Generally, the operation is performed under local anesthesia but may be done under general anesthesia. Formerly, the primary procedure for cataract removal was an intracapsular cataract removal (i.e., freezing of the entire lens and removing both the anterior and posterior capsule, the lens cortex, and lens nucleus).

At the present time, most ophthalmologists utilize an extracapsular cataract procedure. There are two forms of extracapsular cataract surgery. One is the aspiration technique and the other phacoemulsification.

The aspiration technique with instrumentation is utilized in adults as well as children. In children, the lens material is generally soft and can be removed by the aspiration technique. In the older patient, the hard nucleus is first removed, or expressed, and then the remaining soft cortex tissue is removed.

Phacoemulsification is an extracapsular technique that utilizes ultrasonic energy to break up the lens material so it may be withdrawn through a small needle. Unfortunately, phacoemulsification has been confused with a laser treatment for cataract removal. It is important to emphasize to patients that the laser is not used to remove the cataractous lens. Part of the confusion lies in the fact that secondary cataracts or opacification of the posterior capsule is eliminated with the use of the YAG laser. With the YAG laser there is photodisruption of the capsule, which produces an opening and provides good visual acuity.

Cataract removal is one of the most successful operations performed. Generally, adult patients are treated with intraocular lenses after cataract removal. If the patient has bilateral aphakia, contact lenses or cataract spectacles may be worn. However, there is a moderate amount of visual distortion that occurs with spectacle lenses as well as restriction of the peripheral field. An extended-wear contact lens is an alternative if an intraocular lens is contraindicated.

Glaucoma

Glaucoma is responsible for at least 10 per cent of blindness in the United States. With increased intraocular pressure, damage to the optic nerve and visual field abnormalities can occur.

Almost all elevated pressures are caused by an obstruction to the outflow of aqueous humor. Aqueous humor, formed inside the eye in the ciliary body, circulates around the lens and through the pupil into the anterior portion of the eye. It then exits through the anterior angle structures (the trabecular meshwork and Schlemm's canal),

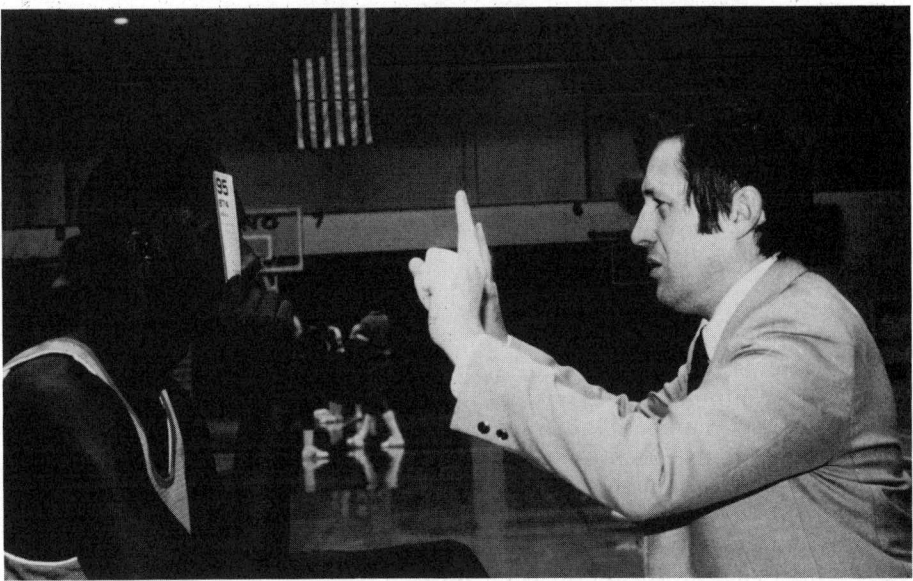

FIGURE 47–28. Testing peripheral fields by confrontation. (From The Athlete's Eye. American Academy of Ophthalmology, Professional Information Committee, San Francisco, 1986, with permission.)

moving through small vessels called aqueous veins and into the episcleral veins on the outside of the eye. If the flow of aqueous is obstructed, the pressure inside the eye increases. Occasionally, elevations result from back-pressure on the drainage system secondary to elevated venous pressure.

The most serious consequence of elevated intraocular pressure is damage to the optic nerve. As the pressure rises, retinal nerve fibers are destroyed at the optic nerve head, resulting in permanent visual loss. Peripheral vision usually is affected first, followed by progressive visual loss involving the entire field of vision.

The most common form of glaucoma is primary open angle glaucoma, which accounts for about two thirds of all cases. It tends to be familial, inherited multifactorially or as an autosomal recessive trait, and there is a high prevalence of carriers. The disease is bilateral and occurs predominantly after age 50, although there is a significant incidence among individuals in their thirties and forties; and it may even occur during the teenage years.

With open angle glaucoma there is a gradual increase in intraocular pressure causing a gradual loss of the peripheral (side) vision followed by reduction of the central field (Figs. 47–28, 47–29). Unfortunately, the damage to the vision caused by glaucoma is irreversible. If the glaucoma can be detected early, in most instances it is controlled and curable by medial treatment, laser surgery, trabeculectomy, or other filtering operations.

It is important to emphasize that glaucoma may occur at any age. Causes include congenital glaucoma, chronic open angle glaucoma, narrow angle glaucoma, or other forms of glaucoma including pigmentary glaucoma.

One of the most common forms of secondary glaucoma is steroid glaucoma, which occurs in a substantial number of patients who use corticosteroid eyedrops or ointments for several weeks or longer. This condition also may occur with oral or systemic corticosteroid use, although it is rare.

Steroid glaucoma is a form of open angle glaucoma and, like primary open angle glaucoma, can be effectively treated if detected early. If the intra-

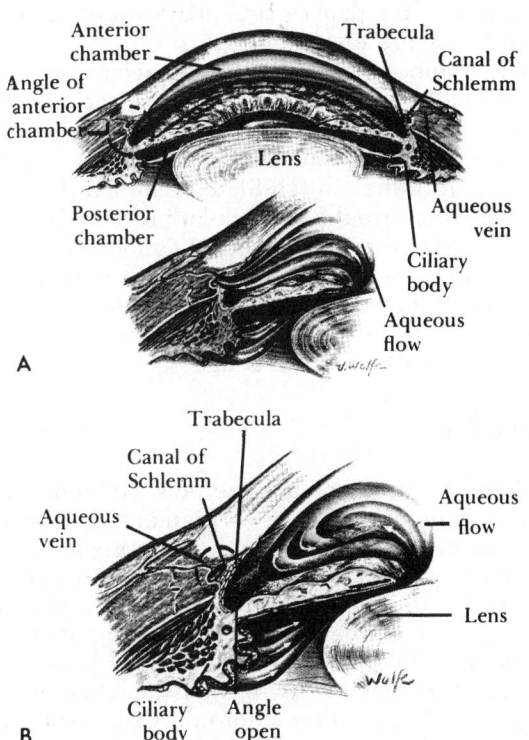

FIGURE 47–29. A, Flow of aqueous from the ciliary body, leaving the eye through the trabecula and canal of Schlemm via a normal open, wide angle. B, Chronic open-angle glaucoma. Arrows indicate obstruction to aqueous outflow in angle wall. (From Scheie HG, Albert DM: Textbook of Ophthalmology, 9th ed. Philadelphia, WB Saunders Company, 1977, with permission.)

ocular pressure is not lowered in time, there may be permanent damage to the optic nerve. Treatment for this type of glaucoma is discontinuation of corticosteroids, and initiation of topical glaucoma medications. The elevation of intraocular pressure is reversible once the steroids are discontinued, however, it may take 2 to 3 months or longer for the pressure to return to normal levels. Any visual loss that occurs in the meantime may be permanent.

Unfortunately, there is no reliably safe dose of topical steroids that can ensure the prevention of steroid glaucoma. Even topical medications that consist of a combination of steroids and antibiotics or other type of medication can cause elevated intraocular pressure. Because of the relative frequency of steroid glaucoma (and other ocular complications resulting from steroid use, such as cataract and exacerbation of viral infections), topical steroids should not be used for minor ocular inflammations, except in special circumstances.

Secondary glaucoma also may be caused by ocular trauma, retinal vein occlusion, intraocular inflammations (e.g., iritis), intraocular tumors, diabetes mellitus, and carotid vascular disease. No matter what the cause, any patient suspected of having secondary glaucoma should be referred to an ophthalmologist as soon as possible for further evaluation and therapy. Management depends on the cause of the disease and character of the intraocular pressure elevation.

The number of people with glaucoma increases dramatically with age, particularly after age 40; it is more severe in the African-American population. The incidence of glaucoma at the present time is 2 per cent in the United States. The family physician can measure the intraocular pressure by using tonometry to detect glaucoma. Tonometry can be used with a Schiotz tonometer held vertically or with a Goldman applanation tonometer held horizontally. This test should be performed at least every 3 years beginning at age 35 years.

Melanoma

Choroidal melanoma is the most common intraocular malignancy. It is a pigmented, elevated mass in the choroid. As the tumor spreads, it may produce a retinal detachment. In addition, retinal pigment epithelial alterations can occur in the form of drusen or as lipofuscin or orange pigment. The differential diagnosis of choroidal melanoma includes choroidal nevus, retinal detachment, and metastatic tumor to the choroid. All patients with intraocular tumors should have an extensive physical examination and laboratory testing to exclude metastatic spread of the neoplasm. Only 1 to 3 per cent of ocular melanomas have metastasized prior to the diagnosis of the eye lesion.

Most ophthalmologists recommend that enucleation as the preferred treatment for large lesions.

When a small melanotic lesion is detected, observation is indicated in older patients with slow-growing lesions.

Uveitis

A red eye, pain, photophobia, and increased tearing are the presenting symptoms of anterior uveitis. In addition, there may be decreased vision. Vascular injection, a circumcorneal injection involving the deep vessels of the sclera, is one of the key signs of anterior uveitis. Generally, uveitis patients are moderately light-sensitive. In addition, the inflammatory process may hinder aqueous production and reduce intraocular pressure. Patients suspected of an anterior uveitis should be referred to an ophthalmologist for consultation and treatment.

Patients with posterior uveitis usually present with a reduction in vision. There are many causes of posterior uveitis, which precludes extensive discussion here. Briefly, the most common causes of uveitis are sarcoidosis, ankylosing spondylitis, Reiter syndrome (urethritis, polyarteritis, and ocular inflammation), juvenile rheumatoid arthritis, ulcerative colitis, and ileocolitis.

One of the most common causes of posterior uveitis is toxoplasmosis, which accounts for up to 30 per cent of these cases. Toxoplasmosis may destroy the macula or other important visual structures in the eye. Characteristically, there is a exudation in the retina due to an inflammatory process. *Toxocara canis* may also present as uveitis.

Vitreous Floaters

The vitreous gel degenerates during middle age and forms microscopic strands within the eye. Vitreous shrinkages called posterior vitreous detachment are a common cause of vitreous floaters. The sudden onset of vitreous floaters can be alarming to the patient, particularly if they are of sudden onset. Generally, they are simply the result of the normal aging process. The sudden onset of flashes of light may indicate a retinal detachment. Additional symptoms, particularly loss of peripheral side vision, require repeat ophthalmologic examination. Vitreous floaters may interfere with clear vision, particularly reading. There is no treatment or cure for vitreous floaters, and they usually decrease over time.

DISEASES OF THE RETINA AND OPTIC NERVE

Retinal diseases account for 10 to 15 per cent of blindness. Included are such conditions as macular degeneration, diabetic retinopathy, retinal detachment, and retinal vascular disease.

Macular Degeneration

Age-related macular degeneration is the most common form of breakdown in the macular area, accounting for 70 per cent of all cases. Age-related maculopathy (formerly called macular degeneration) leads to loss of fine or central vision but not side vision. Laser treatment is of benefit in selected cases. However, most people with macular degeneration have an abnormality in size or position that precludes laser therapy for arresting progression. It is also important to emphasize that there is a 10 per cent chance of the condition occurring in the fellow eye within 1 year.

Another form of macular degeneration is exudative macular degeneration, which accounts for 10 per cent of cases. Normally, the macula is protected by thin tissue that separates it from the fine blood vessels that nourish the posterior aspect of the eye. When these blood vessels break or leak, scar tissue may form, often leading to abnormal growth of new blood vessels (neovascularization). These new vessels are particularly fragile, and leakage and bleeding may occur.

Most other forms of macular degeneration are inherited (including juvenile macular degeneration) or not associated with the aging process. Injury, infection, and inflammation may damage the macula. If macular degeneration involves both eyes, reading and close-up work becomes difficult. If an individual loses central vision related to macular degeneration, generally the peripheral vision is unaffected. The diagnosis of macular degeneration can be confirmed by an ophthalmologist, and testing includes color vision and fluorescein angiography when indicated.

There is no cure for the age-related involutional form of macular degeneration. However, ophthalmic laser surgery has been found to be beneficial in retarding the spread of the exudative form. However, it is successful only during the early stages of exudative macular degeneration. Laser is used to treat leaking membranes and destroy neovascularization.

Retinal Changes in Systemic Diseases

Routine ophthalmoscopy in hypertensive patients affords the physician a direct view of the arterioles and helps assess the long-term duration and severity of the hypertension as well as evidence of accelerated or malignant hypertension. In the vascular system, arterioles serve as the resistance vessels, and the overall cross section of the arteriolar bed determines peripheral resistance. With the fundus examination the physician has the ability to directly observe the degree of spasm in arterioles and the effects of long-term hypertension on the arteriolar wall.

The normal arteriolar wall is transparent, and the visible image is one of the blood column as it passes through the arteriolar lumen. An additional anatomic fact is that at the point of crossing of the arteriole and venule these vessels share a common adventitial layer. Hence when arteriolar thickening occurs, the venule is compressed, resulting in arteriolar-venous (A-V) nicking.

It is practical to divide the changes in the fundus seen in hypertension into two scales: a hypertensive scale and an arteriole-sclerotic scale. The hypertensive scale reflects a degree of spasm within the arteriolar system. There is no universally accepted classification of fundus changes in hypertension. Scheie's classification considers arteriolar vascular leakage changes and arteriolar sclerosis separately.

Hypertensive retinopathy is graded as follows:

Grade 1: generalized attenuation of retinal arterioles (particularly smaller branches)
Grade 2: more pronounced attenuation and focal arteriolar attenuation
Grade 3: generalized and focal arteriolar attenuation with retinal exudates, cotton-wool spots, and hemorrhages
Grade 4: grade 3 changes plus papilledema

Grading of the arteriolar changes is as follows.

Grade 1: broadening of the arteriolar reflex, minimal A-V crossing defects
Grade 2: increased arteriolar light reflex and A-V crossing changes
Grade 3: copper-wire arterioles and marked A-V crossing changes
Grade 4: silver-wire arterioles and severe A-V crossing changes

Diabetic Retinopathy

Diabetic retinopathy is the most common cause of blindness in Americans aged 20 to 74. Diabetics are at 25 times greater risk of becoming blind from diabetic retinopathy than are nondiabetics of becoming blind from all other causes. Diabetic retinopathy is more common in women, but men appear to develop a more complicated and severe proliferative retinopathy. Findings indicate that in type I diabetics it is unusual to detect diabetic retinopathy before 5 years after onset of the disease. At 15 years, most type I diabetics have some diabetic retinopathy, with the incidence of proliferative disease being higher than 40 per cent.

In type II diabetics, with onset after age 30 years, diabetic retinopathy is often detectable at the initial diagnosis. Diabetics requiring insulin have a higher incidence of diabetic retinopathy and proliferative disease.

The pathogenesis of diabetic retinopathy appears to be related to aldose reductase pathways and their inhibition. There is increased retinal blood flow, similar to the increased glomerular filtration in the kidneys. Following this development, there is breakdown of the blood–retina barrier, allowing large molecules to enter the extracellular space of the retina, causing macular edema.

It is important to emphasize that a high percentage of diabetic retinopathy is a background retinopathy, including microaneurysms, dot and blot hemorrhages, hard lipid exudates, and intraretinal microvascular abnormalities (IRMA). One of the major causes of visual loss due to diabetic retinopathy is macular edema, which is much more common in type II diabetics. In addition, vitreous hemorrhage, retinal detachment, and neovascular glaucoma occur with proliferative diabetic retinopathy. A diabetic retinopathy study has proved that laser photocoagulation can reduce the rate of severe visual reduction and proliferative disease.

At the present time, yearly ophthalmologic examinations are recommended for type I diabetics and more often if the disease is active. Yearly examinations are also recommended for patients with type II disease.

Retinal Detachment

Retinal detachment is separation of the retina from its blood supply. It usually follows a tear or hole in the retina. Retinal tears may be caused by trauma or retinal diseases, but the cause of most tears is not clear. When the retina is detached, vision is lost from the involved area of the retina. If the macula detaches, irreversible loss of vision may occur unless the detachment is treated within 24 hours. Anatomic reattachment of the retina is successful in up to 90 per cent of cases.

Giant Cell Arteritis (Temporal Arteritis)

Giant cell arteritis (temporal arteritis) is a generalized inflammatory process of medium-sized and large arteries. It generally occurs in patients over age 55, with no sex predilection. Involvement may occur in any organ system. Ocular involvement is generally associated with inflammation of the posterior ciliary arteries. Systemic features may include malaise, weight loss, fever, and tenderness of the scalp. In addition, there may be pain and tenderness of the muscles and joints and over the temporal arteries, ear, or jaw. The patient may have only a few of these symptoms. One of the presenting symptoms includes sudden visual loss (partial or complete), double vision, or amaurosis fugax. The visual loss is caused by an ischemic process in the optic nerve. Central retinal artery occlusion may also occur. It is important to diagnose giant cell arteritis as early as possible. Without corticosteroid treatment, patients may develop perma-

nent visual loss bilaterally. When one eye is involved with the giant cell arteritis, the second eye loses vision in 65 per cent of untreated patients. Generally, involvement of the second eye occurs within 10 days. When the diagnosis is suspected on the basis of clinical symptoms and signs, temporal artery biopsy may be necessary to confirm the diagnosis. The erythrocyte sedimentation rate (ESR) is often markedly elevated, although it may be normal for age. Patients with ischemic optic neuritis without signs or symptoms suggesting giant cell arteritis and a normal ESR may not require biopsy. However, when there is any question or doubt, temporal artery biopsy should be performed.

Once the diagnosis is established, steroid therapy should be instituted immediately. Up to 100 mg prednisone should be given orally plus intravenous corticosteroid therapy for the first 48 hours so the oral steroids can take immediate effect. The patient can be monitored by the symptoms that occur after the institution of treatment and by the ESR. Because of the severe systemic effects of giant cell arteritis, the patient should be followed closely.

Ischemic Optic Neuropathy

The clinical characteristics of ischemic optic neuropathy include an onset generally over age 60, a painless vision loss, and an afferent pupillary defect (Marcus Gunn pupil). In addition, there is usually a visual field abnormality. Examination of the optic disk reveals edema in virtually all cases. Pathology appears to be related to a diseased ciliary circulation. It is generally difficult to determine whether the disk edema will result in a mild peripheral (side) visual field defect and good visual acuity or reduced central acuity and a significant visual field defect.

It is important to emphasize that giant cell (temporal) arteritis must be ruled out in these patients. The ESR and a general physical examination are indicated. No treatment prevents the progression of ischemic optic neuropathy, including steroids and anticoagulants.

Transient Ischemic Attacks in Carotid Artery Disease

Transient ischemic attacks (TIAs) are neurologic deficits lasting less than 24 hours; they are reversible. The most common ophthalmologic TIA is amaurosis fugax—by definition, fleeting monocular blindness due to an embolic event. There is a sudden graying or reduction of vision often moving from the peripheral vision to the center to cover the entire visual field within a few seconds. After 1 to 5 minutes, the vision return starting with central vision. Other causes of TIAs include chronic disk edema (where vision loss lasts seconds not minutes), chronic papilledema with bilateral blackouts based on optic nerve disease (often also lasting a few seconds and due to postural changes), and basilar artery insufficiency. TIAs related to basilar artery insufficiency are usually bilateral blackouts lasting seconds or minutes, often with changes in the posterior circulation.

The most important mechanisms involving carotid TIAs with stroke are embolization from the carotid artery or its branches, reduced perfusion due to carotid stenosis or occlusion, or a combination of the two. In most patients (up to 90 per cent) the sight of the obstruction is the carotid sinus. Hollenhorst plaques are bright yellow cholesterol emboli that rarely occlude the retinal arterioles and may not produce visual symptoms. Fibrin platelet emboli can occur near retinal arterioles and produce visual symptoms. Either a cholesterol or fibrin platelet embolus is indicative of ulcerative disease in the carotid arteries and is associated with a high incidence of ischemic heart disease, peripheral vascular disease, and aortic abdominal aneurysms. A rarer form of carotid TIAs is related to valvular heart disease, particularly with a prolapsed mitral valve or cardiac arrhythmias. It is important to emphasize that approximately 50 per cent of patients with TIAs in the carotid have a major stroke within a month of the first attack.

SUGGESTED READINGS

American Academy of Ophthalmology Interprofessional Education Committee: The Child's Eye: Strabismus and Amblyopia. San Francisco, American Academy of Ophthalmology, 1982.

American Academy of Ophthalmology Professional Information Committee: The Aging Eye. San Francisco, American Academy of Ophthalmology, 1984.

American Academy of Ophthalmology Professional Information Committee: The Athlete's Eye. San Francisco, American Academy of Ophthalmology, 1986a.

American Academy of Ophthalmology Professional Information Committee: The Red Eye. San Francisco, American Academy of Ophthalmology, 1986b.

American Academy of Pediatrics Committee on Practice and Ambulatory Medicine: Vision Screening and Eye Examination in Children. Pediatrics 77:918, 1986.

Apple DJ: Ocular Pathology: Clinical Applications and Self-assessment, 3rd edition. St. Louis, CV Mosby, 1985.

Crouch ER, Goodrich KA: Practical aspects of pediatric vision screening. Am Orthop J 38:62, 1988.

Crouch ER, Williams PB: Trauma: ruptures and bleeding. In Duane TD (ed): Clinical Ophthalmology, Vol. 4. Philadelphia, Harper & Row, 1993, pp 1–17.

Ellis PP: Ocular Therapeutics and Pharmacology, 6th edition. St. Louis, CV Mosby, 1981.

Fraunfelder FT, Roy FH (eds): Current Ocular Therapy 2. Philadelphia, WB Saunders Company, 1985.

Grayson M: Diseases of the Cornea. St. Louis, CV Mosby, 1979.

Harley RD (ed): Pediatric Ophthalmology, 2nd edition. Philadelphia, WB Saunders Company, 1983.

Havener WH: Ocular Pharmacology, 5th edition. St. Louis, CV Mosby, 1983.

Helveston EM: Atlas of Strabismus Surgery. St. Louis, CV Mosby, 1985.

Henderson JW: Orbital Tumors. Philadelphia, WB Saunders Company, 1973.

Jaffe NS: Cataract Surgery and Its Complications, 4th edition. St. Louis, CV Mosby, 1984.

Kolker AE, Hetherington J Jr: Becker-Schaffer's Diagnosis and Therapy of the Glaucomas, 5th edition. St. Louis, CV Mosby, 1983.

Miller NR: Walsh and Hoyt's Clinical Neuro-Ophthalmology, 4th edition. Baltimore, Williams & Wilkins, 1982.

Moses RA, Hart WM (eds): Adler's Physiology of the Eye: Clinical Application, 8th edition. St. Louis, CV Mosby, 1987.

Newell FW: Ophthalmology: Principles and Concepts, 6th edition. St. Louis, CV Mosby, 1986.

Parks MM: Atlas of Strabismus Surgery. Philadelphia, Harper & Row, 1983.

Paton D, Goldberg MF: Management of Ocular Injuries. Philadelphia, WB Saunders Company, 1976.

Peyman GA, Sanders DR, Goldberg MF: Principles and Practice of Ophthalmology. Philadelphia, WB Saunders Company, 1980.

Scheie HG, Albert DM: Textbook of Ophthalmology, 9th edition. Philadelphia, WB Saunders Company, 1977.

Shields JA: Diagnosis and Management of Intraocular Tumors. St. Louis, CV Mosby, 1983.

Vaughan D, Asbury T: General Ophthalmology, 9th edition. Los Altos, CA, Lange Medical Publications, 1980.

CHAPTER 48

NEUROLOGY IN FAMILY PRACTICE

JOSEPH BRODERICK, ROBERT SMITH, WILLIAM CAHILL,
JEFFREY SHUREN, JOHN QUINLAN, and
FREDERICK SAMAHA

Patients with neurologic disease comprise a large part of a family physician's practice. Because the U.S. population is aging and neurologic diseases are more common in the elderly, family physicians see more and more patients with neurologic disease. This chapter is not meant to be a detailed compendium of neurologic diseases. Instead, our goal is to provide a practical and common sense guide to the patient with a neurologic problem. The family physician is often the front-line physician who should know when a neurologic disease is present, what part of the nervous system is likely affected, and when and how urgently to seek neurologic consultation. Because many neurologic problems require referral and are chronic in nature, the family physician should maintain contact with the patient throughout the referral phase and thereafter.

APPROACH TO THE NEUROLOGIC PATIENT

A physician evaluating a patient with a potential neurologic problem must try to answer three questions: Is there a neurologic problem? If so, where is the lesion in the nervous system? What is the underlying pathophysiology?

1. *Is there a neurologic problem?* The initial and often most difficult part of the diagnostic process is to determine if the presenting symptoms are due to a neurologic disorder or nonneurologic disease. The neurologic history is the most significant factor in making this determination. For instance, fatigue is a common presenting complaint that may be attributed by the patient or physician to dysfunction of the nervous system. However, fatigue without other neurologic complaints or findings is rarely due to an identifiable neurologic disease. This first question is particularly difficult because some patients with documented neurologic disease may also have functional (non-neurologic) complaints. Pseudoseizures, for example,

most commonly occur in patients with documented seizures. A good rule of thumb is always to give the patient the benefit of the doubt when deciding between functional and neurologic disease.

2. *Where is the lesion?* This question is actually composed of several questions: Is the neurologic problem in the central or peripheral nervous system? If central, does it involve the cerebral hemispheres, the posterior fossa structures (brain stem or cerebellum), or the spinal cord? Is the problem focal, multifocal, or diffuse? If monofocal, is it on the left, right, or middle?

3. *What is the underlying pathophysiology?* This question is the most difficult. However, if one knows the time course of the neurologic problem and can answer the second question (Where is the lesion?) the differential diagnosis can be narrowed considerably. Time course can be divided into three categories: acute (onset and evolution over minutes to hours), subacute (onset and evolution over days), and chronic (onset and evolution over months). In addition, one can characterize a disease as transient, progressive, or stable.

Neurologic diseases that are focal and sudden in onset include stroke and trauma. Neurologic diseases that are diffuse and sudden include toxic-metabolic diseases (e.g., hypoglycemia), global cerebral ischemia (cardiac arrest), and subarachnoid hemorrhage. Inflammatory and infectious diseases of the nervous system have a subacute time course. Two classic focal and subacute neurologic diseases are brain abscess and multiple sclerosis. The classic diffuse and subacute neurologic diseases are meningitis and encephalitis. Toxic and metabolic diseases can also have a diffuse and subacute presentation. The classic focal and chronic neurologic lesion is a neoplasm or something that acts as an enlarging mass, such as a subdural hematoma. Finally, chronic and diffuse deterioration usually represents a degenerative disease such as Alzheimer's disease. Figure 48–1 summarizes these diagnostic categories.

	Acute	Subacute	Chronic
Focal	Vascular (infarct or intraparenchymal hemorrhage) Trauma	Inflammatory (abscess, myelitis)	Neoplasm
Diffuse	Vascular (subarachnoid hemorrhage anoxia) Metabolic	Inflammatory (meningitis, encephalitis) Metabolic	Degeneration Metabolic

FIGURE 48–1. Most important temporal and spatial features of the major disease categories. (Modified from Daube J, Reagan TJ, Sandok BA, Westmoreland BF, [eds]: An Approach to Anatomy, Pathology, and Physiology by Systems and Levels. Boston, Little, Brown, 1986, with permission.)

NEUROLOGIC HISTORY

The neurologic history is the critical part of the neurologic evaluation. It is here where most of the answers to the three main questions lie. The physician should focus on the chief complaint and try to reconstruct a "videotape of the mind" concerning the sequence of events. The time course of events is critical to deciding the possible cause. Imprecise words, such as dizziness and numbness, must be clarified with other descriptors. If the patient has recurrent transient events or spells, one should ask the patient to describe in detail, from start to finish, a typical spell. Exact descriptions of the first and most recent spells may be helpful. Because neurologic disease often affects the patient's own awareness of his or her problem, it is essential that the family be interviewed whenever there is any question of cognitive or behavioral dysfunction. Many neurologic diseases have a profound effect on the daily life of family members, and they should be included in discussions with the patient.

NEUROLOGIC EXAMINATION

Cognition

Although much attention is directed to the evaluation of vision, strength, tactile sensation, coordination, and gait when performing a neurologic examination, it is important to remember that the most of the brain is devoted not to the above functions but to cognition. Evaluation of cognition begins with the history. Patients may report having memory loss, or they may be unaware of their deficit (anosognosia). By speaking with and observing the patient, evidence of the various cognitive deficits may be ascertained, such as aphasia (the patient makes paraphasic errors in spontaneous speech) or hemispatial neglect (the patient does not attend to objects in one-half of space).

There are several components to the cognitive or mental status examination (Table 48–1). Attention, memory, and language should be assessed early in the evaluation, as impairment of any of these functions may adversely affect the patient's ability to comply with subsequent testing. During the history the examiner should be able to determine the patient's appearance (neat, unkempt), behavior (appropriate, inappropriate), level of arousal (awake, lethargic), and awareness of his or her deficits.

Orientation is tested by asking the patient to state the date, month, year, season, time of day, name of the testing site, and its location. *Directed attention* (sustained attention) is the ability to persevere on a task—to "pay attention." Patients with poor directed attention are distractible. This factor can be assessed by testing digit span forward and backward. Strings of single digit numbers are spoken by the examiner at a rate of one per second, increasing the length of the string by one until the patient fails two attempts. The patient is asked to repeat the number string forward. On separate trials the patient is asked to repeat different number strings backward. Normal digit span is 7 ± 2 numbers forward and 5 ± 2 numbers backward.

Memory can be tested by giving patients three words, having them repeat the words, and then telling them to remember the words. The patient

---

TABLE 48–1. MENTAL STATUS EXAMINATION

Appearance/comportment/level of arousal/insight
Orientation
Directed attention
Memory
Language
Visuoconstructive skills
Visuospatial skills
Praxis
Executive function
Other (e.g., finger naming, right–left orientation, topographic orientation, calculations)

should then be distracted with another test. After a 5-minute delay the patient is asked to recall as many words as possible.

Language assessment is comprised of several components: fluency, verbal comprehension, repetition, naming, reading, and writing. Fluency is the ease with which speech is produced (articulation, initiation) and the number of words that can be spoken without pausing. Fluent speech is easily articulated with spoken phrases or sentences that are often composed of several words (at least six or more). Nonfluent speech is poorly articulated with slowed initiation and phrases or sentences composed of few words. Verbal comprehension is the ability to understand spoken language. The patient should be asked to perform tasks of increasing complexity (e.g., "point to the ceiling"; "before pointing to the door, point to the light"). Repetition is the ability to repeat sentences or phrases such as "no ifs, ands, or buts." In general, damage to the frontal lobe of the dominant hemisphere (anterior to the central sulcus) results in nonfluent speech with little impairment of comprehension, whereas damage to the parietal or temporal lobe (posterior to the central sulcus) results in fluent speech with marked impairment of comprehension. Repetition is often impaired when the locus of injury is near the sylvian fissure (perisylvian).

Reading and writing are impaired in most aphasia syndromes and may be tested by having the patient read a paragraph of text from a magazine or newspaper and then by writing two or more sentences spontaneously. Naming is tested by having the patient name objects and parts of objects in the room. Errors in naming (*anomia*) occur with all aphasia syndromes, although the types of error made may vary among syndromes. Naming errors are called *paraphasias*. Errors in producing the beginning of a word ("pable" for "table") are called phonemic paraphasias. Errors in which an item is identified by an incorrect but related name ("apple" for "orange") are called semantic paraphasias, and errors in which the word spoken is not a real word ("flig" for "dog") are called neologisms.

Visuospatial skills comprise the ability to perceive the environment and the relation of objects in the environment to one another and to the observer. *Neglect* (spatial inattention) is impaired ability to attend (attentional neglect) or respond (intentional neglect) to the environment, objects in the environment, or oneself that cannot be explained by primary sensory or motor deficits. Neglect is often for the side contralateral to the lesion (hemispatial neglect) though it may occur for multiple spatial planes (i.e., right versus left, near versus far, superior versus inferior). Patients with attentional neglect may fail to notice objects on one side of the room or food on one-half of the plate, whereas patients with intentional neglect may have problems initiating and maintaining visual or limb exploration in one-half of space. Though hemispatial neglect may occur secondary to lesions in either hemisphere, it is most often witnessed and more dramatic after right hemisphere damage (left hemispatial neglect).

For one test of neglect, the patient is shown a line drawn horizontally on a sheet of paper and asked to indicate its center (line bisection). Patients with neglect of the left side of the environment intersect the right side of the line. Another test is to have the patient draw a clock. Patients who neglect the left side often do not fill in the numbers on the left side of the clock or they crowd all of the numbers onto the right side of the clock.

Praxis, the ability to perform complex movements, is tested by asking patients to demonstrate how they would use various tools and how they would make various meaningful nontool gestures: "Show me how you would use a bread knife to cut a loaf of bread." "Show me how you would wave goodbye."

Executive function is the ability to manipulate information, select correct responses, inhibit incorrect responses, shift from one task to another, alternate or change responses, and make abstract judgments. Patients with deficits in executive function respond to the external environment rather than to their own internal directives and tend to have difficulty switching from one task or response to another. Often such patients continue to make the same response over and over again, even though the task or question has changed (*perseveration*). One way these skills can be assessed is by having both the patient and the examiner raise one hand and make a fist. The patient is instructed to raise two fingers when the examiner raises one finger and to raise one finger when the examiner raises two fingers. The examiner then raises one or two fingers in random order. Normal performance is eight of ten correct or better. Patients err if they raise the same number of fingers as the examiner (*echopraxis*), thereby mirroring what they see in the environment.

Gait and Posture

Watching a patient walk is the best overall screen for motor system problems, and it is a good screen for orthopedic problems as well. The patient should be encouraged to walk as quickly and smoothly as possible. Attention should be paid to the base of the gait, stride length, pace, arm swing, and overall stability. Toe-walking, heel-walking, and tandem walking are other components to the gait examination.

The patient's balance should be tested by having him or her put their feet as close together as possible. If the patient is not steady, the feet should be spread further apart. When steady, the patient should then close his or her eyes. If the patient begins to sway or fall, it is called a positive Romberg sign. It generally indicates a problem in sensory information from the legs and trunk due to a peripheral neuropathy or posterior column dysfunction in the spinal cord. Vestibular disease may also cause a positive Romberg sign. Cerebellar disease should not cause a positive sign, although a patient with cerebellar disease is often unsteady with his or her eyes open and becomes more so with them closed.

Cranial Nerves

The cranial nerve examination should include visual acuity, pupil size and response to light and accommodation, eye movements in all directions, visual fields, fundus examination, facial muscle strength and sensation, hearing, and speech. Visual acuity is the best overall screen for a problem in the visual system and should be tested using best corrected vision (glasses or contacts). Frequent causes of pupillary dysfunction in the elderly include past cataract surgery or glaucoma medications.

When testing eye movements, the patient should be asked if he or she experiences double vision. When the patient does see two images, the eye that sees the outer image or false image contains the weak muscle. For example, a patient has horizontal diplopia when looking to the left and reports that the outer image disappears when the left eye is covered. The left lateral rectus muscle is the weak muscle.

Facial weakness that is primarily limited to the lower face indicates an upper motor neuron lesion, whereas facial weakness that involves the upper and lower face points to a facial neuropathy. Speech may be tested by listening to the patient during the history and by having the patient repeat syllables rapidly such as "pa" (seventh nerve), "ta" (twelfth nerve), and "ka" (tenth nerve).

Motor Testing

The following muscles should be included in a general survey of muscle strength: deltoids, biceps, triceps, wrist flexors and extensors, interossei, hand grip, iliopsoas, quadriceps, hamstrings, foot dorsiflexors and plantar flexors. The nerves and nerve roots that supply these muscles are listed in Table 48–2. Weakness secondary to an upper motor neuron lesion tends to preferentially affect the extensors of the arm (deltoid, triceps, wrist extensors, finger extensors), intrinsic hand muscles such as the interossei, and flexors of the leg (iliopsoas, hamstrings, foot and toe dorsiflexors).

Reflex testing should include the biceps (C5,6, musculocutaneous nerve), triceps (C6–8, radial nerve), brachioradialis (C5,6, radial nerve), quadriceps (L2–4, femoral nerve), and achilles (S1, posterior tibial nerve) reflexes. Diminished or absent

TABLE 48–2. MAJOR MUSCLES: FUNCTION AND INNERVATION

Muscles	Function	Nerve	Plexus	Spinal Cord Segment or Root
Deltoid	Arm abduction	Axillary	Brachial	C5,6
Latissimus dorsi	Arm adduction	Thoracodorsal	Brachial	C6,7,8
Biceps	Flexion elbow	Musculocutaneous	Brachial	C5,6
Triceps	Extension elbow	Radial	Brachial	C6,7,8
Wrist extensors		Radial	Brachial	C6,7,8
Wrist flexors		Median and ulnar	Brachial	C6,7,8, T1
Finger extensors		Radial	Brachial	C6,7,8
Finger flexors		Median and ulnar	Brachial	C7,8, T1
Thenar	Abduction/adduction opposition thumb	Median and ulnar	Brachial	C8, *T1*
Interrossei	Spreading fingers apart	Ulnar	Brachial	C8, *T1*
Intercostals	Respiration	Intercostals	None	T1–11
Abdominals	Flexion spine	Intercostals	None	T6–L1
Iliopsoas	Flexion thigh at knee	Branch lumbar plexus and femoral	Lumbar	L2,3,4
Gluteus maximus	Extension	Inferior gluteal	Lumbosacral	L5, *S1*,2
Gluteus medius	Abduction of thigh	Superior gluteal	Lumbosacral	L4,5, S1
Quadriceps	Extension at knee	Femoral	Lumbar	L2, *3*,4
Hamstrings	Flexion at knee	Sciatic	Lumbosacral	L4,5, *S1*
Anterior tibial	Dorsiflexion of foot	Sciatic (peroneal)	Lumbosacral	L4,5, S1
Gastrocnemius	Plantar flexion	Sciatic (tibial)	Lumbosacral	L5, *S1*, S2
Toe extensors		Sciatic (peroneal)	Lumbosacral	L4,5, S1
Toe flexors		Sciatic (tibial)	Lumbosacral	L5, *S1*, S2
Peronei	Eversion foot	Sciatic (peroneal)	Lumbosacral	L5, S1
Post-tibial	Inversion foot	Sciatic (tibial)	Lumbosacral	L5, *S1*
Rectal sphincter	Continence of stool	Pudendal	Sacral	S3,4

reflexes usually indicate a problem in the motor or sensory nerve, whereas increased reflexes and clonus point to an upper motor neuron lesion. However, immediately after an acute spinal cord injury or cerebral injury (e.g., stroke) the reflexes may be diminished. It may be a week or longer before hyperreflexia begins to appear. The most important pathologic reflex is the Babinski sign, which is abnormal in adults and children older than 18 months. This reflex is tested by stroking the lateral sole with a sharp instrument such as the wooden end of a cotton-tipped stick. The abnormal response is for the toe to dorsiflex with fanning of the remaining toes and indicates a lesion of the corticospinal tract.

Tone can be tested passively by moving the arm at the elbow and the leg at the knee. The patient must be relaxed for accurate assessment. Resistance in both directions is most consistent with rigidity and is seen with disorders of the basal ganglia such as Parkinson's disease. Resistance to extension at the elbow or flexion at the knee that lessens with further passive movement (the clasp-knife response) is a sign of spasticity and indicates an upper motor neuron or corticospinal lesion. Another way to test for increased tone in the legs is to have the patient lie on his or her back and relax the legs. The examiner's hands are then placed under the knee, and the knee is lifted smoothly and quickly. With normal muscle tone, the heel of the foot should drag along the table or bed. In a patient with increased tone, the heel is lifted off the table before falling back to the table.

Coordination can be tested by finger-to-nose and heel-to-shin testing. Rapid tapping of the index finger on the thumb and tapping of the foot on the floor are other useful screening tests of motor system function. In some patients, the strength, coordination, muscle tone, and sensory function are normal, but the patient remains unable to do motor tasks upon command, such as using a key or brushing the teeth. This problem is called *apraxia* and indicates a problem in the dominant hemisphere.

Sensation

The screening sensory examination should include position sense testing at the toes, vibration testing at the toes and ankles, and pin sensation of the dorsum of the feet and hands. More detailed testing, including temperature sensation and light touch, should be done when the patient specifically complains of sensory loss or disturbance. If the patient reports a definite region of sensory loss, the physician should initiate pin testing within the area of decreased sensation and move toward the regions of normal sensation. This procedure can most clearly map the affected region.

Patients with lesions of the cortical sensory regions may have normal primary sensation but still have significant sensory problems. Tests of cortical sensation include *stereognosis* (identifying shapes such as a small key in the hand with the eyes closed), *graphesthesia* (identifying numbers traced on the palm or finger tip), *double-simultaneous stimulation* (lightly touching both arms, legs, or sides of the face), and *two-point discrimination*. NOTE: Cortical sensory testing is often abnormal if primary sensation is also affected.

Neurovascular Examination

The brain depends on adequate delivery of oxygenated blood. A good neurologic examination should include vital signs, heart and lung evaluation, and auscultation of the neck for bruits.

NEUROLOGIC DIAGNOSTIC TESTS

Diagnostic testing should be thought of as an extension of the neurologic examination in which hypotheses generated by the history are tested.

Brain and Spinal Cord Imaging Studies

Brain imaging has revolutionized the diagnosis and treatment of neurologic disease. The two major imaging studies are computed tomography (CT) and magnetic resonance imaging (MRI). CT imaging can easily distinguish different types of tissue (e.g., hemorrhage and fat) and localizes the region of brain pathology. The limitations of CT include (1) bony artifacts, which can obscure the temporal lobe, brain stem, and cerebellar pathology; and (2) inferior image resolution compared to MRI. MRI has no associated bony artifact and clearly images the temporal lobes, cerebellum, and brain stem. It detects demyelinating plaques in patients with multiple sclerosis better than CT. MRI with gadolinium contrast is the test of choice for patients with disease of the temporal lobes, brain stem, or cerebellum as well as patients with possible multiple sclerosis, new-onset seizures, and possible brain metastasis. Its sensitivity in detecting early infarction is greater than that of CT. In addition, advances in MRI technology have enabled excellent noninvasive imaging of extracranial and intracranial blood vessels. The drawbacks of MRI are cost (approximately three to four times the cost of noncontrast CT), claustrophobia (approximately 10 per cent of patients), and inferior visualization of acute hemorrhage compared to CT. MRI cannot image patients who are on a respirator, require electrical monitoring, or have a pacemaker or prior aneurysm clipping. Because MRI is more expensive than CT, neurologic consultation should be considered prior to ordering the MRI study to ensure that it is indicated.

Other imaging modalities include single photon emission computed tomography (SPECT) and positron emission tomography (PET), both of which can provide functional imaging of the brain. Both are useful as research tools and play little role, at present, in clinical decision-making for neurologic patients.

Magnetic resonance imaging or a myelogram followed by a CT are the best ways to image the cervical and lumbar spine in patients with a suspected spinal, spinal cord, or spinal root disease. Again, neurologic or orthopedic consultation should be obtained prior to obtaining the much more expensive imaging studies.

Electroencephalography

Electroencephalography (EEG) is a test that examines brain wave activity during awake and drowsy periods as well as during sleep. Its major use is to identify epileptogenic areas of brain that are responsible for a patient's seizures. It is also helpful in the comatose patient for looking for treatable causes of the coma, such as nonconvulsive status epilepticus. Finally, it is sometimes used as part of the brain death evaluation. The usefulness of the EEG is in direct proportion to the experience of the EEG technician and the neurologist interpreting the EEG. An EEG should be accompanied by neurologic consultation.

Electromyography

Electromyography (EMG) is a test composed of two parts: nerve conduction studies and a needle examination of selected muscles. The first part examines how quickly and well nerves conduct an electrical impulse. The second part examines whether the muscle fibers have been denervated by damage to motor neurons, motor nerves, the neuromuscular junction, or the muscles themselves. It also examines the size and shape of the motor units (muscle fibers supplied by one axon) to determine if any active or chronic damage to muscle or nerve is present. The usefulness of an EMG depends on the skill of the physician performing the examination.

Neurovascular Studies

See Cerebrovascular Disease, below.

Lumbar Puncture

To perform a lumbar puncture the patient is placed horizontally on his or her side with the body flexed. It is essential to position the spine parallel with the table and to maximize flexion. The space between the spinous processes should be palpated; and after local anesthesia a 20-gauge sterile needle is introduced just adjacent to the midline into the L4–5 intervertebral space using strict aseptic technique. A manometer is used to measure the opening pressure after the patient is relaxed. Normal cerebrospinal fluid (CSF) pressure is 70 to 200 mm H_2O (or 5 to 15 mm Hg). The procedure may also be performed with the patient sitting in a flexed position, which often provides a better view and feel of the lumbar spine anatomy. However, if this position is used, the patient must lie on his or her side before measuring the CSF pressure.

In the first tube, 2 mL of fluid is collected for glucose and protein determinations. The normal range for glucose is 48 to 85 mg/dL or more than 60 per cent of the serum glucose level. In patients with high serum glucose (e.g., 400 mg/dL), a lower percentage of CSF glucose is often normally seen. The normal range for CSF protein is 15 to 45 mg/dL. The second tube contains 5 mL of fluid for special protein studies such as immunoglobulin G (IgG) index and oligoclonal bands. In a third tube 1 mL is collected for a cell count. The color and clarity of the CSF should be recorded. The fourth tube is used for cytology or other studies, such as cryptococcal antigen, fungal cultures, viral cultures, or syphilis testing. Cytology as well as mycobacterial and fungal cultures require large amounts of CSF, and the laboratory should be contacted before the study to ensure the proper volume. Ideally, the CSF should be collected after the patient has fasted for at least 4 hours to allow equilibration between blood glucose and CSF glucose. If the CSF pressure is found to be unexpectedly high (greater than 250 mm Hg), only enough fluid to perform the necessary assays should be slowly removed, the stylet replaced, and neurologic assistance sought immediately. If the needle is removed, there will be leakage of CSF from the hole in the meninges into the extra-arachnoid space because of the pressure gradient between the CSF and this space. If the increased CSF pressure is due to an intracranial lesion, brain herniation can occur.

Frankly bloody CSF may be due to a "traumatic" tap. Even with a properly performed tap a small vessel may be punctured. In such cases the CSF clears as it is removed. If the CSF remains pink or yellow after centrifuging the red blood cells to the bottom of the tube, the sample is called xanthochromic. This situation indicates that the blood has been present at least some hours, such as with a subarachnoid hemorrhage, a high protein level, or increased levels of bilirubin.

Indications for lumbar puncture include suspicion of infection, possible cancer, inflammatory diseases such as multiple sclerosis, suspected subarachnoid hemorrhage when the CT or MRI studies are negative, symptomatic relief of headache in patients with pseudotumor cerebri or benign intracranial hypertension, and therapeutic delivery of anesthetics, antibiotics, and antineoplastic agents when indicated. Contraindications to lumbar puncture include tissue infection at the site of the puncture, the presence of a known or suspected intracranial mass lesion, or a bleeding tendency due to anticoagulation or thrombocytopenia.

The most common complication is postlumbar puncture headache. It may appear several hours to a day after the puncture. The incidence is 10 to 15 per cent and increases when the needle is left in place for a longer time, as with myelography. The headache is throbbing, bifrontal, and generalized; it is worse when the patient is upright and diminishes when the patient lies down. The headache is apparently due to loss of CSF, which results in displacement and stretching of pain-sensitive structures that surround the brain when the patient is upright. The condition usually responds to simple analgesics, hydration, and recumbency. If symptoms persist after conservative treatment, a "blood patch" is indicated.

A blood patch is performed by injecting 5 mL of the patient's own blood into the lumbar epidural space, where the blood clots and plugs the CSF leak. Unless experienced in this procedure, the family physician should request that it be performed by an anesthesiologist or neurologist.

GENERAL PRINCIPLES OF NEUROLOGIC DIAGNOSIS

The physician combines the results of the history and physical examination to form hypotheses about what is wrong with the patient. The following principles are good guidelines for neurologic diagnosis (Daube et al., 1986): (1) Always give the patient the benefit of the doubt when deciding between functional (non-neurologic) and organic (neurologic) disease (i.e., rule out organic disease). (2) Always try to rule out a focal disorder before deciding the problem is nonfocal. (3) Always try to rule out treatable/reversible disease before nontreatable disease. (4) Once having decided on an anatomic pathologic diagnosis, search for the underlying pathophysiologic mechanism (e.g., chemical, hematologic) that produced the lesion. (5) Always consider whether doing a study can benefit the patient, alter what you can do for the patient, or pose a risk to the patient greater than any benefit derived.

COMMON PATIENT COMPLAINTS AND PRESENTATIONS

Patients present to the family physician with one or several complaints rather than a disease. The following section deals with diagnostic and therapeutic approaches to common neurologic complaints and presentations.

Coma or Decreased Responsiveness

Coma results from impairment of the reticular activating system—the central control system that is involved with maintaining alertness. The reticular activating system has its origin in collections of neurons in the central upper pons and midbrain, which send fibers to the hypothalamus and thalamus. These fibers in turn send diffuse activating fibers to the cortices. Thus coma or decreased responsiveness to the environment indicates involvement of both cerebral hemispheres or the brain stem, or it is a unilateral hemispheric lesion with compression of deep midline cerebral structures bilaterally.

Because the patient cannot cooperate with the examination or history, examination of the comatose patient is pared down to five essential components: level of alertness, pupillary function, eye movements, respiratory patterns, and motor responses (Plum and Posner, 1980). Involvement of the cerebral hemispheres at the level of the thalamus is associated with small but reactive pupils. Midbrain damage is associated with fixed, dilated pupils, whereas pontine lesions are associated with pinpoint pupils. Unilaterally dilated and unresponsive pupils indicate involvement of the ipsilateral oculomotor nerve. Prior eye surgery can also produce a fixed pupil, and pharmacologic agents such as atropine (dilated pupils) or narcotics (pinpoint pupils) can also produce pupillary abnormalities in a comatose patient. Intact pupillary responses to light indicate that at least the upper part of the brainstem is functioning.

Eye movements should be examined first at rest. If spontaneous horizontal roving eye movements are seen, the part of the brain stem controlling eye movements is at least partially functioning. Sometimes in comatose patients with a pontine lesion, the eyes deviate downward, like the bobbing of a fishing bob. This "ocular bobbing" is associated with a poor prognosis. A patient may also have conjugate deviation of both eyes. If the eyes are looking away from the hemiplegic side, a cerebral lesion is present. If the eyes are looking toward the hemiplegic side, a pontine lesion is likely present.

If there are no spontaneous eye movements, the brain stem control of eye movements can be tested by the oculocephalic maneuver and calorics. With the oculocephalic maneuver, the head is turned quickly to one side. In the comatose patient with intact brain stem reflexes, the eyes move in the opposite direction and then slowly return to midposition in relation to the rest of the head (doll's-eyes response). In the comatose patient without brain stem reflexes, the eyes remain midposition and move en bloc with the head. In the alert patient, the response is variable.

Calorics should be tested with ice water with the head at about 30 degrees above the horizontal plane. The ears should be examined first to ensure that wax is not blocking the ear canal. The normal caloric response in an alert patient is nystagmus with the fast component of nystagmus in the direction of the opposite ear. In a comatose patient with intact brain stem reflexes, the eyes should slowly deviate to the side where the ice water is instilled. In a comatose patient with absent brain stem reflexes, the eyes do not move.

Cheyne-Stokes respiration is a distinctive pattern of respiration that indicates involvement of deeper midline cerebral structures and is exacerbated by congestive heart failure. In this pattern, hyperpnea cycles with apnea in a gradual sine wave fashion. Hyperventilation is almost always due to hypoxemia, sepsis, or metabolic acidosis and is rarely due to a central nervous system (CNS) lesion in isolation. A sustained inspiration without expiration for several seconds is occasionally associated with a pontine lesion.

The appropriate motor response in a comatose patient is pushing or grabbing toward a painful stimulus in a localizing fashion. A decorticate response is a patterned response consisting of flexion of the arms at the elbows and extension of the legs spontaneously or in response to a painful stimulus (Fig. 48–2). It indicates damage to the deep cerebral structures above the level of the red nucleus in the midbrain. A decerebrate response consists of extension of both arms and legs and indicates damage in the brain stem below the level of the red nucleus in the midbrain.

Localization of Process Causing Coma

Certain clinical features suggest a unilateral hemispheric lesion with subsequent brain herniation. If a history is available, the patient is often initially alert or sleepy with aphasia or unilateral motor or sensory findings, which subsequently progress to coma. The motor signs are often asymmetric (e.g., decorticate rigidity on one side and decerebrate on the other). Causes of coma that develop over several hours include hemorrhagic strokes and traumatic brain lesions. Coma due to a slower process, such as a brain tumor or brain abscess, is usually preceded by a focal neurologic problem over days to weeks or even months.

Diffuse or bilateral cortical and subcortical causes of coma are characterized by normal pupillary responses, an absence of focal motor findings, and occasional tremors or myoclonus. Bilateral cerebral hemispheric involvement is by far the most common cause of coma, and the differential diagnosis is broad: electrolyte abnormalities, organ failure, hypo- and hyperglycemia, infections, toxic substances such as alcohol, nutritional deficiencies such as thiamine deficiency (Wernicke-Korsakoff syndrome), hypoxia, anoxia, and subarachnoid hemorrhage.

Primary brain stem causes of coma are suggested by a history of diplopia, vertigo, bilateral limb weakness, ataxia, or occipital headache. Bilateral motor signs are usually present at onset, and ocular bobbing is a specific sign of a pontine lesion. The causes of acute coma include brain stem or cerebellar infarction or hemorrhage and head trauma. Abscesses or tumors usually present over days to weeks.

Diagnosis and Treatment

The first concern when evaluating the comatose patient is to ensure that the airway is secure and that breathing and vitals signs are stable. The physician should obtain a complete blood count (CBC); assays for electrolytes, creatinine, blood urea nitrogen (BUN), blood glucose, and ammonia; liver function studies; toxicology screen; urinalysis; arterial blood gas assays; and blood cultures if the patient is febrile. After these studies are done, the patient should receive thiamine 100 mg, 1 ampul of 50 % dextrose in water ($D_{50}W$), and 1 ampul of naloxone (Narcan) intravenously. An emergent CT scan of the head should then be obtained unless the cause of coma is absolutely clear (e.g., blood glucose of 20 mg/dL). If the CT is normal and no clear cause of coma is evident or if nuchal rigidity is present, a lumbar puncture should be done. If the CT, lumbar puncture, and laboratory studies are unrevealing, an EEG should be considered to rule out ongoing nonconvulsive status epilepticus. If all studies are negative, an MRI study can be done if the patient is stable and not intubated. For all patients with coma, a neurologic consultation should be obtained expeditiously unless the imaging studies demonstrate an intracranial mass lesion and the need for urgent neurosurgical consultation.

Speech Problems (Dysarthria and Aphasia)

It is important to determine if the patient is having difficulties with the pronunciation and mechanical production of speech (*dysarthria*), difficulties using or understanding language (*aphasia*), or both. Dysarthria can be due to a CNS problem, a peripheral neuromuscular problem, or a structural problem such as a cleft palate.

In 99 per cent of right-handers and 60 per cent of left-handers the left hemisphere is dominant for language function. Thus the presence of aphasia indicates a left hemisphere lesion more than 90 per cent of the time, even if the handedness of the patient is unknown. The classic aphasia syndromes are based on performance in speech production, comprehension, and repetition. Reading and writing tend to mirror speech production and comprehension. Aphasia classification is most useful for

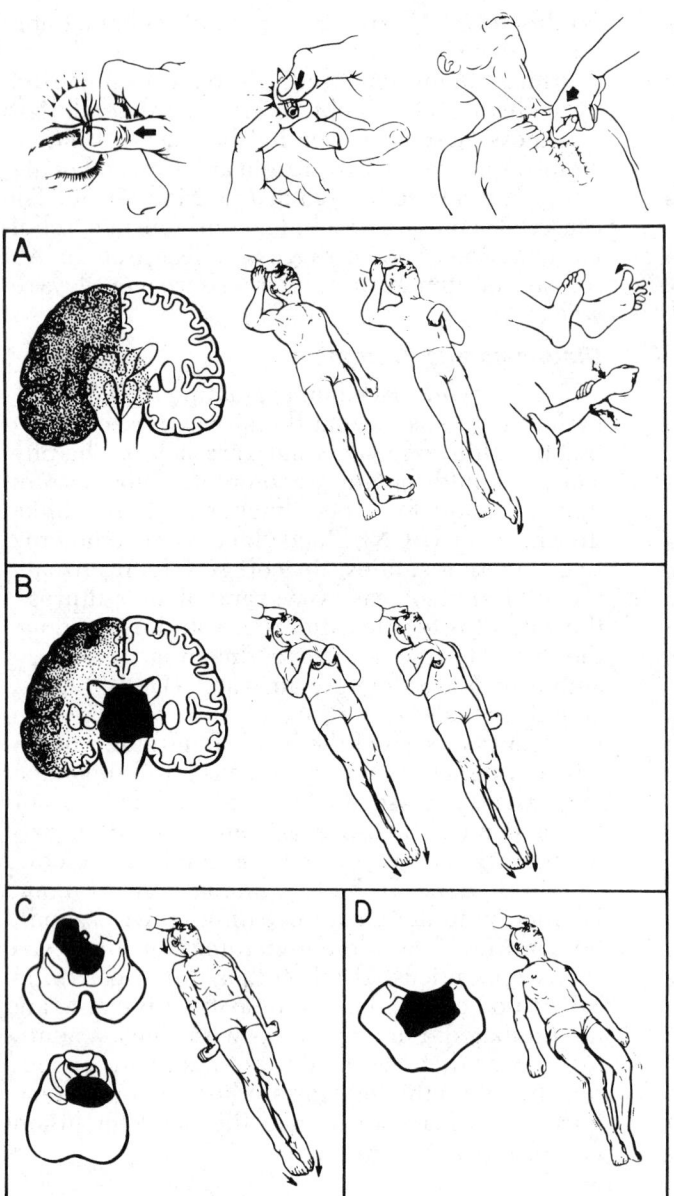

FIGURE 48–2. *A*, Left-sided decorticate posturing. *B*, The left drawing demonstrates bilateral decorticate posturing. The right demonstrates right-sided decorticate and left-sided decerebrate posturing. *C*, The left drawing demonstrates bilateral decerebrate posturing. (From Plum F, Posner JB: The Diagnosis of Stupor and Coma, 3rd edition. Philadelphia, FA Davis, 1980, with permission.)

anatomic localization when the patient is examined at least several days to weeks after the initial insult. During the acute event distant effects such as diaschisis (shutting down of connected brain areas) make anatomic localization difficult if not impossible. In general, however, the language system anterior to the central sulcus mediates speech production and the production and comprehension of syntax (the relation of words to each other within a sentence), whereas the language system posterior to the central sulcus mediates speech comprehension.

Broca's Aphasia

Patients with Broca's aphasia produce effortful, nonfluent, poorly articulated speech that is agrammatic (absence of prefixes and suffixes as well as of function words such as prepositions, conjunctions, and auxiliary verbs). Speech has a telegraphic quality (e.g., "I . . . go . . . store" instead of "I am going to the store"), and repetition is poor. Paraphasic errors are predominantly phonemic, and perseverations occur. Verbal and written comprehension of grammatic aspects of language are impaired. Most patients initially demonstrate global aphasia (see below), which improves over weeks to months. Patients often have a contralateral hemiparesis. Involved brain areas include the frontoparietal opercula, the insula, and the white matter deep to them. Patients with lesions isolated to Broca's area (posterior one third of the inferior frontal gyrus) are often mute, with rapid improvement of language over a few weeks with either no weakness or contralateral facial weakness.

Wernicke's Aphasia

Patients with Wernicke's aphasia produce fluent, often nonsensical speech composed of real words, phonemic and semantic paraphasias, and neologisms. Speech output may even be excessive and incessant (*logorrhea*). Verbal and written comprehension are poor, as is repetition. Writing parallels speech production. Hemiparesis is unusual, but a contralateral visual field defect is common. The posterosuperior temporal lobe is the brain region most commonly affected.

Conduction Aphasia

Patients with conduction aphasia produce fluent speech sometimes marked by paraphasic, predominantly phonemic errors. Verbal and written comprehension is relatively preserved, though difficulty may arise when trying to comprehend complex verbal or written material. The primary deficit is in repetition, which is poor. Conduction aphasia is usually observed in patients with Wernicke's aphasia as they recover. Hemiparesis is unusual, but a contralateral hemisensory loss is common. The inferior parietal lobe, posterior insula, and white matter deep to these structures are most commonly involved.

Global Aphasia

With global aphasia all aspects of language (speech production, comprehension, repetition, naming, reading, and writing) are profoundly impaired. Contralateral hemiparesis, hemisensory loss, and visual field defect are typical when global aphasia results from a single lesion. It may also result from two lesions, one involving the frontal lobe and one involving the posterior parietal/superior temporal lobe and sparing the primary motor and sensory cortex (e.g., an embolus that splits in two causing two strokes, i.e., double infarction). If the global aphasia reverses, the disorder tends to resolve into Broca's aphasia. A large perisylvian lesion is usually responsible.

Anomic Aphasia

Patients with anomic aphasia have difficulty finding words and produce paraphasias in spontaneous speech and on tests of confrontation naming. Other aspects of language are relatively preserved. Anomic aphasia may occur as the initial manifestation of a language disturbance or as a recovery stage for all subtypes of aphasia. Anomia can result from injury to any region of brain involved in language processing. When it occurs initially and in isolation it usually results from an insult to the mid-posterior middle temporal gyrus.

Other aphasic syndromes have been categorized (Albert et al., 1981), but all point to a problem in the dominant hemisphere. Occasionally, aphasia results from a lesion of the thalamus of the dominant hemisphere.

Memory Loss

Memory loss, or amnesia, may be anterograde (cannot form new memories), retrograde (cannot recall previously learned material), or both. In general, memory loss usually follows a gradient with recent memories lost to a greater degree than more remote memories (Ribot's law). The brain regions that function to encode and retrieve stored information are the medial temporal lobes (hippocampus, entorhinal cortex, parahippocampus, and possibly the amygdala), dorsal medial nucleus of the thalamus, and the basal forebrain (septal nuclei and the basal nucleus of Meynert). Information, however, is probably stored diffusely in the cerebral cortex and not within the above structures. The frontal lobes process temporal information (when something occurred) and are important for memory of self-generated responses.

Practically, most complaints of mild memory loss deal with an inability to remember names of people a patient should know, misplacing objects, and short-term memory lapses: "Did you remember to bring home a gallon of milk?" Some of these complaints are seen among otherwise normal adults. However, when short-term memory loss becomes severe, the problem may be incapacitating. Progressive difficulties with short-term memories and learning may be the first sign of a more generalized dementia (see Specific Neurologic Disorders, below) and should prompt neurologic consultation. Prominent memory complaints are also heard from patients with depression and anxiety disorders.

Vision Loss

Disorders of vision are discussed in Chapter 47. Vision loss falls into one of three primary categories: loss of vision in one eye, loss of vision in a field of vision on the same side (homonymous) in both eyes, and loss of vision in the temporal fields of both eyes (Fig. 48–3). Vision loss in one eye can be due to any problem from the cornea on the outer surface of the eye to the optic nerve, which carries information to the brain. Diagnostic evaluation should include a detailed ophthalmologic examination, including visual field testing to localize the problem further.

Unilateral vision loss due to optic neuritis may be accompanied by swelling of the optic nerve head on funduscopic examination. If the inflammation involves the optic nerve more proximally, the optic nerve may appear normal acutely. Some other causes of unilateral optic neuropathy include ischemia, a compressive tumor, and central vein occlusion. Papilledema is also associated with marked swelling of the optic nerve, although visual acuity in patients with papilledema usually remains good whereas patients with optic neuropa-

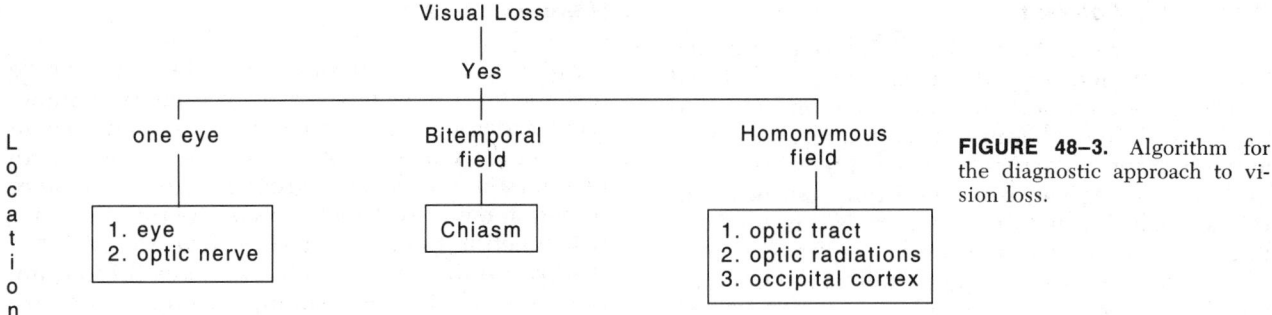

FIGURE 48–3. Algorithm for the diagnostic approach to vision loss.

thies often have substantial impairment of visual acuity.

Visual loss in the same visual field of both eyes indicates a problem in the opposite optic tract, optic radiations, or occipital cortex. A homonymous (same-sided) visual field loss without other neurologic signs usually indicates an occipital lobe lesion. Visual field testing and brain imaging should be performed in these patients. Vision loss in the temporal fields of both eyes indicates a lesion of the optic chiasm and is usually due to a sellar or suprasellar mass, such as a pituitary adenoma. MRI of the brain with contrast is the test of choice to image the pituitary and optic chiasm. If this test is not available, a CT scan with contrast and coronal cuts through the pituitary is the test of choice.

Double Vision (Diplopia)

Double vision, or *diplopia*, indicates that the eyes are not aligned properly so that one of the two retinal images does not fall on the macula. This condition can result from primary extraocular muscle weakness or fibrosis (e.g., thyroid disease); disorders of the neuromuscular junction (e.g., myasthenia gravis); a lesion of the third, fourth, or sixth cranial nerve; a lesion in the brain stem affecting systems that control eye movements; or anything that restricts movements of the eyes (e.g., an orbital mass). Double vision should resolve when one eye is closed. However, some patients may complain of diplopia that is localized to one eye, which usually indicates a problem in the ocular lens, cornea, vitreous, or retina. If the double vision is accompanied by other brain stem signs or symptoms such as vertigo, bilateral motor weakness, or sensory loss, the primary problem lies in the brain stem. The complaint of "double vision" should prompt ophthalmologic or neurologic consultation.

Rhythmic Eye Movements (Nystagmus)

Nystagmus is rhythmic, repetitive, alternating movement of the eyes that may be physiologic or pathologic. It may be fast in one direction and slow in the other (jerk type), or it may have equal speed in both directions (pendular). Nystagmus can be induced in normal people by caloric stimulation of the semicircular canals or by sustained circular rotation of a patient sitting in a chair. A common form of physiologic nystagmus on neurologic examination is called endpoint nystagmus because the patient has a few lateral jerky movements of the eyes on extreme lateral gaze. These movements usually quickly disappear after a few jerky movements. In contrast, with pathologic gaze-evoked nystagmus, the movements continue with sustained lateral gaze and are generally present in all directions of gaze. Drug toxicity, such as toxic levels of phenytoin or phenobarbital, are common causes of gaze-evoked nystagmus.

Pathologic nystagmus may or may not be associated with patient complaints of dizziness or vertigo. However, the presence of pathologic nystagmus indicates a problem in the eye control systems of the brain stem. Nystagmus that first appears during childhood is most commonly due to vision loss in both eyes and is often pendular and horizontal. Vertical nystagmus during primary gaze usually points to a focal lesion of the brain stem or midline cerebellum. Down-beating vertical nystagmus is even more specifically associated with lesions at the cervicomedullary junction. Nystagmus associated with positional vertigo is discussed below.

Disturbance of Pupillary Size and Function

Pupillary size is determined by a balance of input from the sympathetic (dilate) and parasympathetic (constrict) autonomic nervous system. Sympathetic input begins in the ipsilateral hypothalamus, descends in the ipsilateral brain stem and cervical spinal cord, exits via the cervical spinal roots, and ascends along the outer surface of the ipsilateral carotid artery to the orbit and then to the pupillary dilator muscles. The parasympathetic input begins in the midbrain in the ipsilateral Edinger-Westphal nucleus and exits with the ipsilateral third nerve on its way to the orbit and the pupillary constrictor muscles. The pupils constrict in response to light and accommodation.

Pupils in normal individuals may be slightly un-

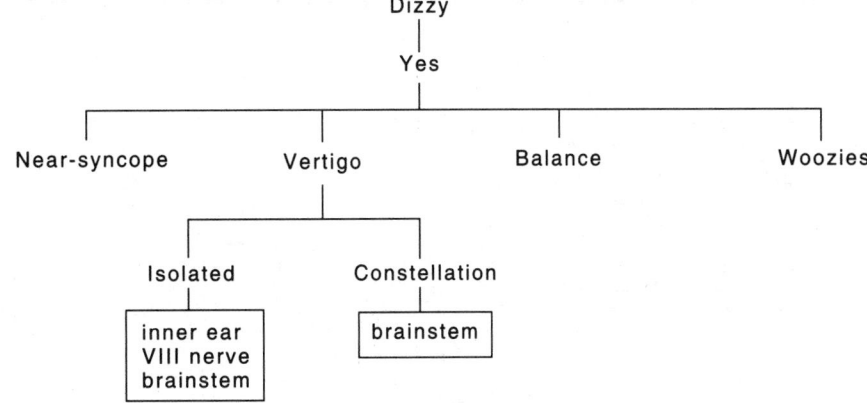

FIGURE 48–4. Algorithm for the diagnostic approach to dizziness.

equal in size but should respond equally to light and accommodation. A dilated, poorly responsive pupil usually points to a lesion of the third nerve somewhere between the brain stem and the orbit. Other causes include surgical trauma (e.g., cataract surgery), mydriatic agents, and an Adie's pupil. In the latter instance, the pupil is dilated and constricts poorly with light but better with accommodation. A unilaterally small pupil that is responsive to light and accommodation can result from disruption of the sympathetic input to the pupillary dilators (Horner syndrome). Ptosis of both the upper and lower lids also accompanies the small pupil. The responsible lesion can be in the ipsilateral brain stem, cervical spinal cord, cervical roots, sympathetic ganglia near the apex of the lung, carotid artery, or orbit. Classic Argyll Robertson pupils are bilaterally small and irregular and constrict better with accommodation than to light. They were first described in patients with neurosyphilis but may be seen in patients with diabetes.

Dizziness

"I was dizzy" is one of the most common patient complaints and one that requires detailed questioning to ascertain what the patient means (Fig. 48–4). It is useful to ask patients whether they felt that they or their environment were moving during the episode (vertigo), they felt lightheaded or were going to pass out (near-syncope), or that the primary problem was balance ("dizzy feet"). The physician should determine the time course of the dizziness (transient spell or permanent and the duration and frequency of spells); the relation of dizziness to activity, postural change, and head position; and other symptoms that accompany the dizziness. The more precise the description of dizziness, the more likely it is that a cause can be found.

Classification

VERTIGO. The major question is whether vertigo is due to a CNS disorder or a disorder of the end-organ or vestibular nerve. Hearing problems and tinnitus usually indicate a disorder of the peripheral end-organ or eighth cranial nerve. Isolated vertigo that typically occurs upon arising in the morning is more likely to have a peripheral cause. Complaints of accompanying double vision; motor weakness; sensory disturbance of face, arm, or legs; dysarthria; swallowing problems; and incoordination of the extremities point to a disorder of the brain stem or cerebellum, such as in patients with brain stem ischemia. Nausea and truncal instability can be seen with either brain stem and cerebellar or peripheral end-organ and eighth nerve disorders. Nystagmus is often seen in patients during acute vertigo.

The most common cause of isolated vertigo, with or without hearing difficulties, is a disorder of the vestibular end-organ or vestibular nerve. Acute vertigo generally has one of two time courses: acute episodes that gradually resolve over many hours or several days and briefer episodes lasting seconds to several hours. The common causes of prolonged vertigo include presumed viral inflammation ("vestibular neuronitis"), bacterial labrynthitis due to adjacent middle ear infections, and Menière's disease (Chapter 23).

The most common causes of brief spells of vertigo are benign positional vertigo and post-traumatic vertigo. These syndromes are thought to result from the dislodgement of tiny otoconia from the macula and saccule of the vestibular end-organ into the posterior semicircular canal. This process, called *cupolithiasis*, may occur spontaneously or be due to a significant insult such as trauma, infection, or ischemia. Patients with positionally induced vertigo complain of their vertigo after sudden head turning, sitting up, or lying down. The vertigo generally lasts only seconds to minutes, although patients may complain of longer periods of milder dizziness following the spells. The physician should ask any patient with positional vertigo about recent or remote head trauma.

As part of the neurologic examination, the physician should perform the Nylén-Bárány or Dix-Hall-

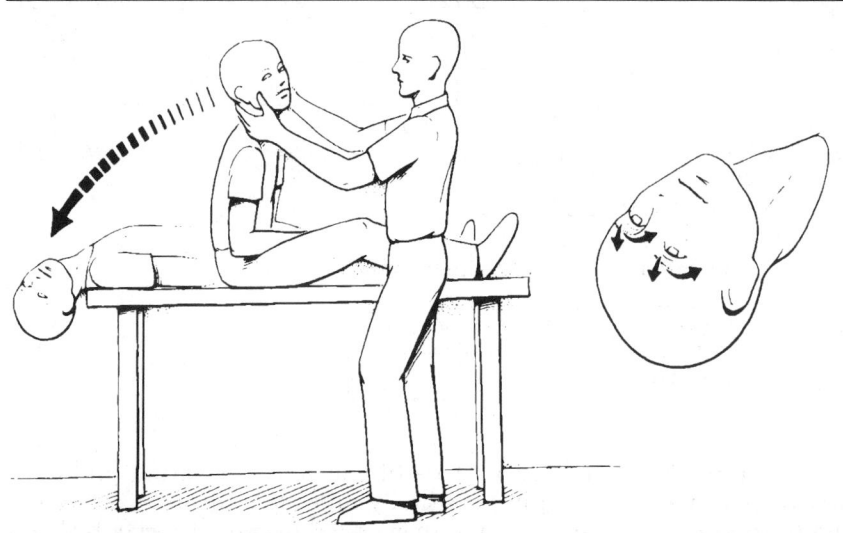

FIGURE 48–5. Dix-Hallpike or Nylén-Bárány maneuver. (From Mohr DN: The syndrome of paroxysmal positional vertigo: a review. West J Med 145:645, 1986, with permission.)

pike maneuver: The patient, who is seated at the end of the table, is asked to turn his or her head to one side and then recline quickly so his or her head hangs over the end of the table 30 degrees below the horizontal plane (Fig. 48–5). The patient must keep his or her eyes open. The physician observes the patient for 60 seconds for the development of dizziness and nystagmus. Characteristically, the nystagmus—a mixture of jerky, rotatory, vertical and horizontal movements—begins after a latency of several seconds and resolves within seconds to a minute. Repeating the maneuver fatigues the nystagmus and vertigo until no response is obtained. If there is no response, the patient should sit up quickly and be observed for about a minute. The procedure is then repeated with the head turned to the opposite side.

Rarely, disorders of the brain stem or cerebellum, such as demyelinating disease or tumors, can also be associated with positionally induced vertigo and nystagmus. However, in these cases, the nystagmus usually begins immediately without a latency period, is purely vertical or horizontal, and does not fatigue. The complaint of vertigo is usually less intense in these patients. Other causes of brief episodes of nonpositional or positional vertigo include Menière's disease, brain stem or cerebellar ischemia, otosclerosis, perilymphatic fistula, syphilitic infections, cholesteatomas, and tumors of the eighth nerve, cerebellum and brainstem (also see Chapter 23).

LIGHTHEADEDNESS (NEAR-SYNCOPE). Lightheadedness (near-syncope) generally indicates a problem with insufficient cerebral perfusion. It may be secondary to inadequate intravascular fluid volume (e.g., dehydration), inadequate or excessive autonomic control of blood pressure (e.g., medication effect, vasodepressor syncope, vasovagal syncope, diabetic autonomic neuropathy, Parkinson's

disease), inadequate cardiac output (e.g., heart failure, arrhythmias), or generalized cerebral vasoconstriction due to hyperventilation. Other symptoms that may accompany the lightheadedness include a darkening or graying of vision, mild nausea, and generalized paresthesias. All patients should have their blood pressure and pulse evaluated in the supine and erect positions to look for evidence of inadequate intravascular volume or insufficient autonomic regulation of blood pressure with postural change.

UNSTEADINESS OF GAIT. Some patients use the term "dizzy" to describe difficulties with balance while walking or standing. These patients often have some problem in the central motor control systems, such as the cerebellum or corticospinal pathways (see Central Disorders of Tone, Posture, and Movement, below) or a significant peripheral neuropathy that impairs sensory information from the lower extremities. Often in the elderly there is more than one cause of the unsteady gait.

DIZZINESS OF UNCLEAR CAUSE. Despite a physician's best efforts, a patient's complaint of dizziness or "wooziness" may defy accurate description. Patients in whom dizziness represents one of a large number of poorly defined complaints should be evaluated for signs of an anxiety disorder or depression.

Diagnosis

Patients with vertigo should undergo a formal audiometry evaluation in addition to complete neurologic and otoscopic examinations. The Nylén-Bárány maneuver should be performed. MRI or CT of the posterior fossa should be considered in all patients with recurrent vertigo with an unclear cause, in any person with other signs and symptoms of brain stem dysfunction, and in any person with significant unilateral or bilateral hearing loss. Referral to an otolaryngologist or neurologist should be obtained prior to imaging. Electronystagmographic testing and posturography by an experienced laboratory are indicated for some patients to document a lesion of the end-organ or nerve.

Patients with near-syncope should have an electrocardiogram and rhythm strip. A history of clear syncope may require 24-hour Holter or event monitoring. Other screening laboratory tests include a CBC, electrolytes and glucose assays, and thyroid function testing. Tilt-table testing can also be considered.

Treatment

Treatment of vertigo includes administration of meclizine (Antivert) and promethazine (Phenergan) for the nausea. Severe vertigo may require diazepam (Valium). Either of these therapies may result in sedation. Bacterial labrynthitis requires appropriate antibiotic therapy. Menière's disease may be treated symptomatically with diuretics. Endolymphatic shunts and destructive labrynthectomy are last resorts that should be considered only in cases with severe, long-standing disease. Perilymphatic fistulas may be corrected with repair of the fistula. Acoustic neuromas often require removal by an experienced team of neurosurgeons and otolaryngologists.

Benign positional vertigo is best treated with postural exercises of the head several times a day. Patients should move the head in all directions and hold each position for several seconds. This regimen initially may increase the patient's vertigo but over several weeks usually results in improvement of symptoms.

Hearing Loss

Hearing loss is discussed in Chapter 23. Without other complaints, it is due to a problem in the external canal (e.g., wax), middle ear (e.g., infection), inner ear (e.g., presbycusis), or the eighth cranial nerve (e.g., acoustic neuroma). Diagnostic evaluation should include otoscopic examination, hearing tests, and otolaryngologic consultation. Imaging of the eighth nerve is indicated in some patients, particularly if the cause of hearing loss (e.g., middle ear fluid) is not immediately evident. If the hearing loss is accompanied by vertigo, the problem is usually due to a disorder of the inner ear or eighth cranial nerve, and an imaging study is usually performed. Hearing loss associated with a brain stem lesion is almost always accompanied by other neurologic symptoms and signs.

Weakness

The most difficult task is to identify whether the patient who complains of "weakness" is referring to a loss of energy, fatigue, decreased daily performance, or true muscle weakness. If true muscle weakness is identified on neurologic examination, the pattern of weakness is used to determine the cause of the weakness.

Muscle weakness that involves only one side of the body (face, arm, and leg; face and arm; or arm and leg) indicates a problem in the CNS, usually in the opposite cerebral hemisphere (Fig. 48–6). Unilateral arm and leg weakness is usually due to a lesion of the opposite cerebral hemisphere but may also be due to a lesion in the opposite brain

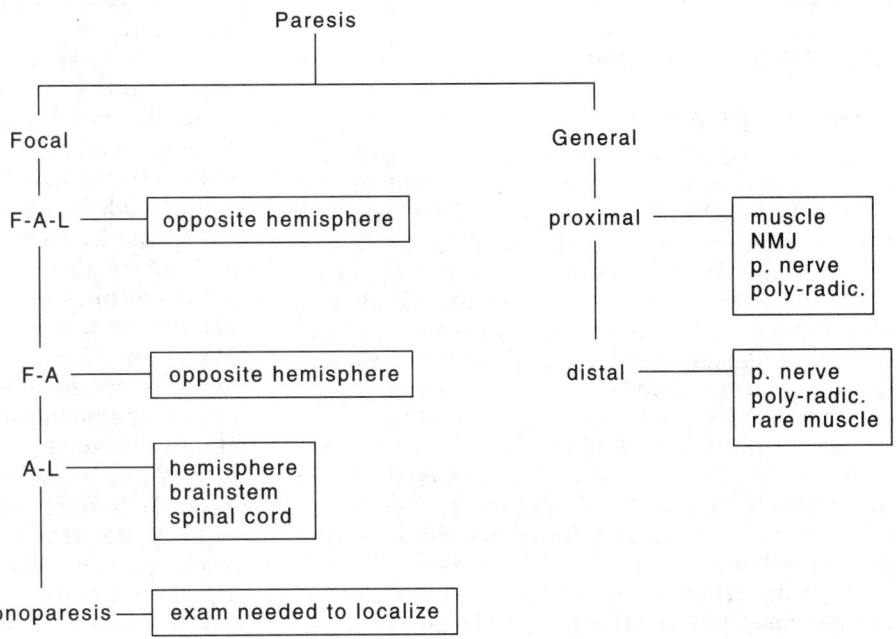

FIGURE 48–6. Algorithm for the diagnostic approach to motor weakness. F = face; A = arm; L = leg; NMJ = neuromuscular junction; p. nerve = peripheral nerve; poly-radic = polyradiculopathy.

stem motor pathways or the same side of the cervical spinal cord. Weakness isolated to one arm or leg requires more detailed knowledge of muscle and peripheral nerve anatomy.

Generalized weakness that is predominantly proximal or predominantly proximal or predominantly distal indicates a peripheral neuromuscular problem. Proximal patterns of weakness are characteristic of muscle and neuromuscular junction diseases or polyradiculopathies, whereas distal weakness is most consistent with peripheral nerve disorders and polyradiculopathies.

Brain or spinal cord imaging is often indicated for focal weakness involving more than an isolated arm or leg. EMG testing is commonly used in patients with generalized weakness. Early neurologic consultation is helpful for choosing the appropriate diagnostic test.

Loss of Feeling or Abnormal Sensation

Like the complaint of weakness, the pattern of sensory loss is critical for localizing the problem in the nervous system. Focal sensory loss involving one side of the body (face, arm, and leg; face and arm; arm and leg) point to a lesion in the opposite cerebral hemisphere or, less likely, the brain stem. Sensory loss in one arm or leg may be more difficult to localize, but a knowledge of the cutaneous distribution of peripheral nerves and nerve roots is needed. Diffuse "stocking–glove" sensory loss is consistent with a peripheral neuropathy or polyradiculopathy. Again, neurologic consultation is helpful when selecting the appropriate diagnostic test.

SPECIFIC NEUROLOGIC DISORDERS

Cerebrovascular Disease

Clinical Diagnosis

Stroke is the third leading cause of death and the leading cause of disability among adults in the United States. It also accounts for approximately half of all neurologic hospital admissions. *Stroke* is best defined as a brain injury due to one of two vascular causes: ischemia (inadequate blood supply) (Fig. 48–7A) or hemorrhage (leakage of blood through a damaged intracranial vessel). Hemorrhage can occur within the brain (intracerebral hemorrhage) (Fig. 48–7B) or in the subarachnoid space surrounding the brain (subarachnoid hemorrhage) (Fig. 48–7C). About 80 per cent of all strokes are ischemic, 14 per cent are due to intracerebral hemorrhage, and 6 per cent are due to subarachnoid hemorrhage.

Two main clinical features characterize a stroke: sudden onset and involvement of a focal part of the CNS. When seeing a patient with a possible stroke, the treating physician should ask the following questions (Broderick, 1993a): Is it a stroke? Is it an ischemic or hemorrhagic stroke? If the stroke is ischemic, what part of the brain and thereby what vascular distribution is affected? What is the origin of the thrombus occluding the affected artery: in situ thrombosis, artery-to-artery embolism, cardioembolism, or another more unusual cause? The history, physical examination, and laboratory tests try to answer these questions, and the answers often affect the choice of therapy.

1. *Is it a stroke?* Head trauma is the other common disease that can have a focal and sudden presentation like stroke, but a clear history and signs of head trauma are often evident. Focal seizures sometimes result in focal weakness or other focal neurologic dysfunction that may last for some time after the actual seizure has stopped (Todd's paralysis). If the seizure is unwitnessed, the diagnosis may not be suspected unless the patient has a known seizure disorder. These postseizure focal findings generally resolve within several hours. Rarely, hypoglycemia presents with a sudden onset of focal brain dysfunction. An accompanying history of insulin use and other hypoglycemic symptoms such as anxiety, change in level of alertness, shakiness, and sweating usually precede the focal neurologic findings. If the rapidity of the symptom onset is unknown, the differential diagnosis of a focal brain lesion becomes much broader.

2. *Is it an ischemic or a hemorrhagic stroke?* Focal brain infarction and brain hemorrhage may be difficult to distinguish clinically, even by the most skilled neurologist. This difficulty is particularly true for patients who have a small or moderate-size intracerebral hemorrhage that may present in the same manner as a similarly sized cerebral infarct. Larger intracerebral hemorrhages characteristically present with a focal deficit that progresses to marked obtundation or coma within several hours. Brain ischemia rarely progresses to coma this quickly. Nausea and vomiting are more common among patients with brain hemorrhage than patients with brain ischemia.

Subarachnoid hemorrhage presents most commonly as the sudden onset of a severe headache or syncope that is subsequently accompanied by a change in mental status and nuchal rigidity on physical examination. Although a decreased level of responsiveness is often seen with subarachnoid hemorrhage, focal findings are usually absent unless the hemorrhage extends into the brain parenchyma. Because of the limitations of the clinical history and examination, a CT scan of the brain is essential to differentiate between stroke subtypes.

3. *If the stroke is ischemic, what part of the brain, and thereby what vascular distribution, is affected?* Certain constellations of symptoms suggest ischemia in either the carotid or vertebral basi-

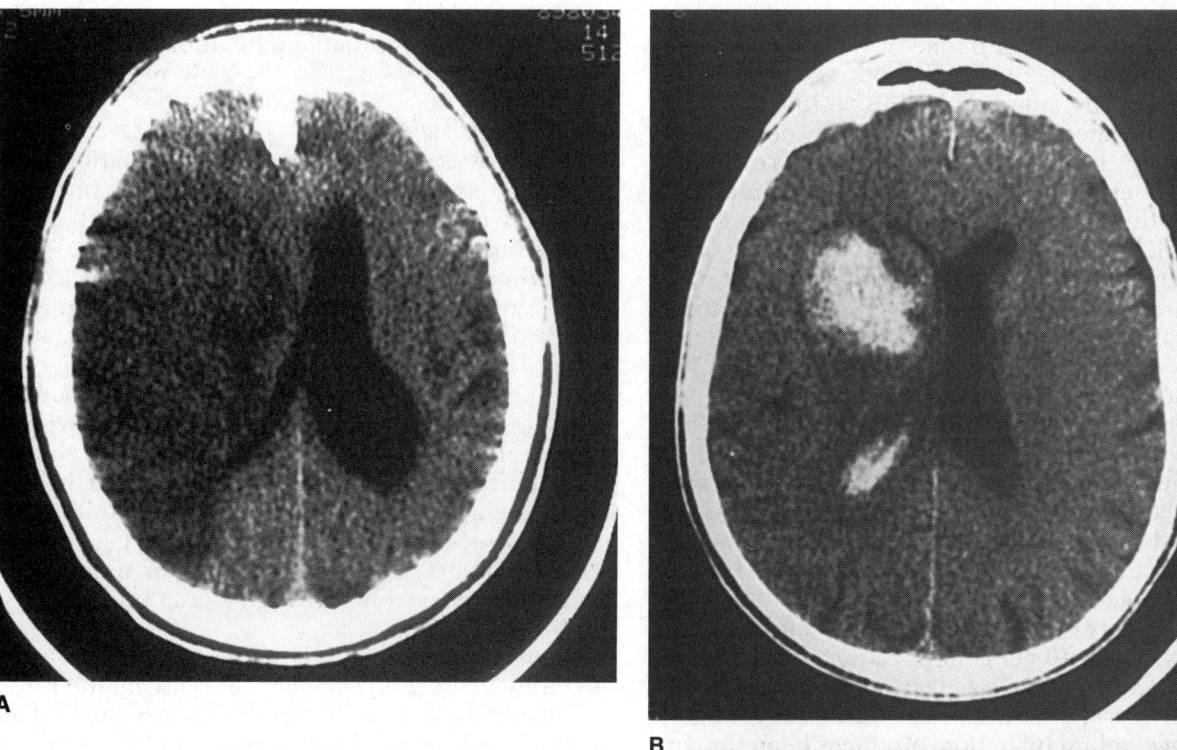

A

B

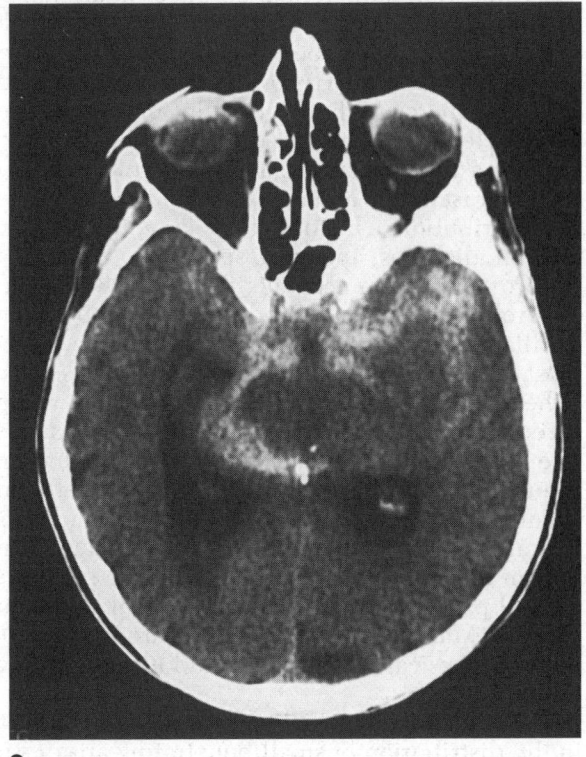

C

FIGURE 48–7. *A*, Acute large right cerebral infarct. *B*, Moderate-size right frontal intracerebral hemorrhage. *C*, Subarachnoid hemorrhage due to a ruptured aneurysm.

lar arterial systems. Signs referable to the carotid artery system include monocular blindness with or without cerebral signs; aphasia alone or combined with motor and sensory signs; or unilateral combined motor and sensory signs. Other "cortical" deficits seen with carotid system ischemia include apraxia (inability to perform motor functions de-

spite adequate strength and coordination), neglect (usually a right cerebral cortical lesion), constructional difficulties, and acalculia.

Signs referable to the vertebral basilar system include bilateral motor or sensory signs; right, left, or bilateral incoordination of the arms and legs; and vertigo, diplopia, dysphagia, or dysarthria accompanying motor, sensory, or cerebellar signs. Isolated loss of vision in one or both visual fields indicates a lesion in one or both occipital lobes that are usually supplied by the vertebral basilar system. Isolated vertigo more likely points to a problem in the vestibular end-organ or vestibular nerve rather than brain stem ischemia. Similarly, isolated diplopia usually points to a problem with the third, fourth, or sixth cranial nerves or the muscles they innervate. Isolated unilateral motor or sensory signs can represent ischemia within either the carotid or vertebral basilar systems, but more often within the carotid system, particularly if the face and arm are predominantly involved.

4. *What is the origin of the thrombus occluding the affected artery?* The four possible origins of thrombus occluding an artery include the vessel wall at the site of the occlusion (thrombosis), a proximal arterial wall (artery-to-artery embolus), the heart (cardiac embolus), or the venous system (transcardiac embolus). However, even after extensive laboratory evaluation, including cerebral angiography, about 40 per cent of patients with a cerebral infarct do not have a clear source of thrombus.

Large-vessel atherosclerosis, the most common cause of cerebral infarction, produces infarction by thrombotic occlusion of the artery at the site of atherosclerosis or by embolic occlusion of a smaller downstream vessel. Historical and physical findings that increase the probability of large-vessel atherosclerosis as the cause of an ischemic stroke include a neck or supraclavicular bruit, repeated transient ischemic attacks (TIAs) in the same arterial distribution, a history of smoking, prior hypertension, diabetes, and male sex.

Cardioembolism accounts for 20 to 23 per cent of cerebral infarctions (Broderick, 1993 a,b). Atrial fibrillation, either alone or in combination, is the most common potential cardioembolic source. Other cardiac conditions that have been recognized as major cardioembolic sources are congestive heart failure, acute myocardial infarction, rheumatic valvular disease, endocarditis, left ventricular aneurysm, and atrial myxoma. Conditions that are not as strongly associated with cardioembolism are mitral valve prolapse, aortic sclerosis, a small patent foramen ovale, and atrial septal aneurysm. Many of these diagnoses are evident by history, physical examination, and electrocardiography.

Lacunar infarcts, which are small, deep infarcts in the distribution of small penetrating arteries or arterioles, comprise 13 to 25 per cent of all ischemic strokes. Most of these infarcts are caused by primary thrombosis in small penetrating arteries or arterioles and are usually associated with prior hypertension or diabetes. However, cardioembolism and carotid artery-to-artery embolism can also cause lacunar infarcts. Less common causes of cerebral infarction include, but are not limited to, large-vessel arterial dissection, coagulo-

pathies, sickle cell disease, migraine, vasculitis, drug use (e.g., cocaine), and cerebral vein thrombosis.

Ischemic Stroke

DIAGNOSTIC EVALUATION. The evaluation of an ischemic stroke patient includes brain imaging, neurovascular examination, cardiac evaluation, and laboratory studies.

Brain Imaging. Every patient who has a new stroke or TIA should have either a CT or an MRI study of the brain. For a discussion of the relative merits of CT and MRI see the earlier section concerning diagnostic tests. If cost were not important and access unlimited, MRI would be the imaging test of choice for most stroke patients. MRI should be strongly considered in patients with suspected brain stem, cerebellum, or temporal lobe involvement. Also, if the physician wants to image the intracranial and extracranial arteries or intracranial veins noninvasively, MRI angiography is the best option.

Neurovascular Studies. Cerebral catheter angiography is the gold standard for imaging the intracranial and extracranial arteries. It provides excellent visualization of extracranial and intracranial arterial stenoses, aneurysms, vascular malformations, and the extent of collateral flow. Arterial ulcerations are less well visualized. Risks associated with cerebral arteriography include stroke (0.5 to 1.0 per cent) and death (0.1 per cent). The intravenous contrast material can precipitate severe allergic reactions or renal failure. Cerebral angiography is the best test to visualize cerebral aneurysms, vascular malformations, and the internal carotid artery prior to possible carotid endarterectomy. However, it is likely that MRI angiography (Fig. 48–8) will supplant catheter angiography for many indications as MRI technology continues to improve.

Carotid duplex ultrasonography is an excellent noninvasive test of the extracranial carotid arteries that uses two ultrasound techniques in combination: B-mode ultrasonography and pulsed Doppler ultrasonography. The B-mode technique provides anatomic images of the carotid arteries, and the Doppler technique calculates the velocity and turbulence of the blood flow. Higher velocities and turbulent flow are associated with greater degrees of carotid stenosis. Carotid duplex ultrasonography, performed by a good laboratory, is approximately equivalent to MRI angiography in terms of identifying high grade stenoses of the extracranial internal carotid artery. The cost of carotid duplex is about one fourth that for an MRI scan. The major limitations of carotid duplex are an inability to image the intracranial arteries, difficulty differentiating between severe carotid artery stenosis and occlusion, and an inability to clearly image 5 per cent of carotid vessels studied.

Transcranial Doppler ultrasonography is a newer technology that can visualize and record the

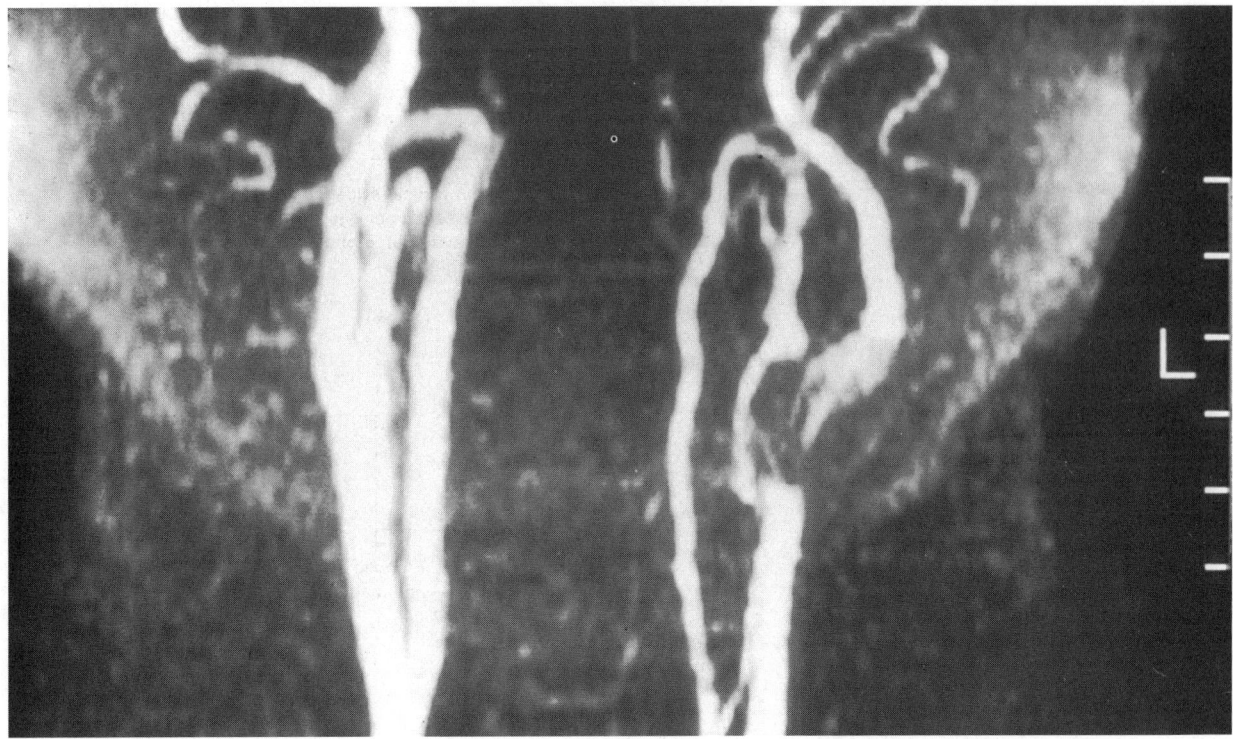

FIGURE 48–8. MRI angiogram of the carotid bifurcations showing a high grade stenosis of the left internal carotid artery near the carotid bifurcation.

velocities of blood flow in intracranial arteries. The major proved usefulness of transcranial Doppler at present lies in the detection and monitoring of arterial narrowing or vasospasm following subarachnoid hemorrhage.

Cardiac Evaluation. Every patient with a stroke or TIA should undergo a complete cardiac physical examination, electrocardiography, and chest radiography. Transthoracic echocardiography is another useful test in the ischemic stroke patient. More recently, transesophageal echocardiography has provided better imaging of the left atrium and associated thrombi. However, if the clinical history and examination electrocardiogram, and chest radiograph are negative for cardiac disease, even transesophageal echocardiography reveals an unsuspected thrombus in only 1 per cent of ischemic stroke patients. Figure 48–9 provides a decision tree regarding the use of echocardiography in stroke patients.

Laboratory Studies. Screening blood tests in stroke patients should include a CBC; erythrocyte sedimentation rate (ESR); assays for serum glucose, electrolytes, BUN, creatinine, creatine phosphokinase, and serum cholesterol (if not previously done); prothrombin time and activated partial thromboplastin time; and rapid plasma reagin for syphilis. Arterial blood gas assays should be added if the cardiopulmonary examination is abnormal. More detailed coagulation studies, such as those for protein C, protein S, anti-thrombin III, and anti-phospholipid antibodies, are others that are appropriate in some patients without a clear cause of their cerebral infarction.

MANAGEMENT AND TREATMENT. Modification of stroke risk factors is the safest and most effective way to prevent stroke for all asymptomatic and symptomatic patients. In particular, treatment of hypertension and efforts to stop smoking should be emphasized for all persons with and without clinically evident cerebrovascular disease.

Asymptomatic Carotid Artery Bruit or Stenosis. If transmitted cardiac murmurs are excluded, a carotid bruit is associated with an approximately 75 per cent chance of at least a 50 per cent diameter stenosis of the ipsilateral carotid artery. Patients with a carotid artery bruit should undergo a carotid duplex study to determine if a high grade stenosis exists. Patients with a high grade carotid artery stenosis have at least two to three times the risk of subsequent stroke compared to those who do not. Duplex ultrasonography allows documentation of changes in the carotid arteries over time, particularly if symptoms develop later.

There are two therapeutic options for patients with asymptomatic high grade carotid artery stenosis: medical management of stroke risk factors plus daily aspirin, or the first option plus prophylactic carotid endarterectomy. The first option is reasonable and safe, though not proved in this group of patients. The second option is also unproved but is associated with major perioperative morbidity

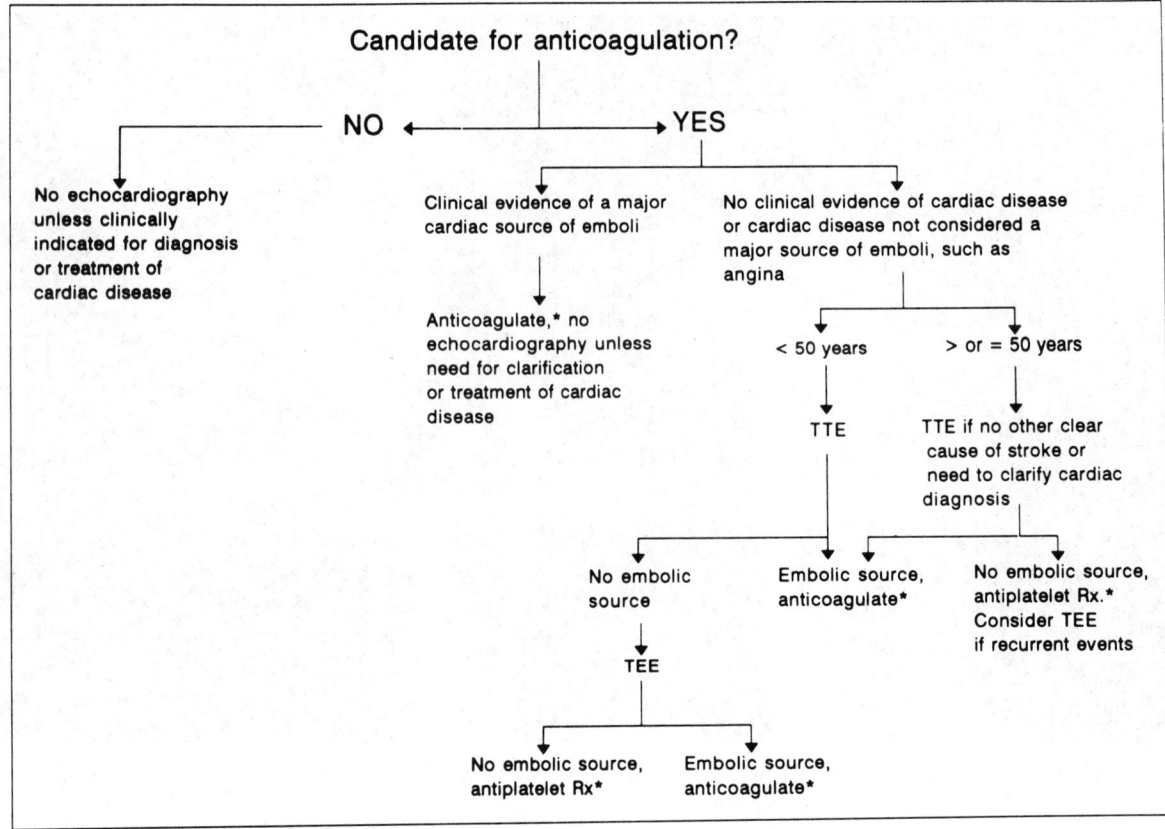

FIGURE 48–9. Decision tree for use of echocardiography in patients with TIA or stroke. TEE = transesophageal echocardiography; TTE = transthoracic echocardiography. (From Broderick J: Heart disease and stroke. Heart Dis Stroke 2:357, 1993, with permission. Copyright 1993 by American Heart Association.)

and a mortality of 4 to 7 per cent in controlled trials. A large multicenter study (the Asymptomatic Carotid Atherosclerosis Study Trial) is currently evaluating whether carotid endarterectomy is effective for patients with at least moderate stenosis of an asymptomatic carotid artery. Preliminary results suggest that carotid endarterectomy may be beneficial for some asymptomatic patients with a high grade stenosis.

Asymptomatic Patients with Atrial Fibrillation. Atrial fibrillation is present in almost 10 per cent of persons over age 65 and is associated with a fivefold stroke risk compared to persons without atrial fibrillation. Five large randomized studies have shown that warfarin can reduce the risk of stroke by 42 to 86 per cent with a low risk of major bleeding complications. The lowest effective anticoagulation regimen reported thus far was a prothrombin time that was 1.2 to 1.5 times the control value or a target International Normalized Ratio (INR) of 1.5 to 2.5. One study has also reported a benefit for aspirin as compared to placebo. A study comparing warfarin and aspirin has been completed but has not yet been published as of February 1994.

TIAs (Small Strokes). Management of patients with TIAs, or small strokes, depends on the sus-

pected vascular distribution, source of the thrombus, age, overall health of the patient, and the time since the onset of symptoms. The risk of stroke after a TIA is greatest during the first month. Patients seen several months after a TIA can be approached less emergently, whereas those seen within several days after onset should be treated with the same sense of urgency as an individual with unstable angina or acute stroke. Brain imaging, carotid duplex ultrasonography, and appropriate cardiac and laboratory screening tests should be done initially. Cerebral angiography should be considered if noninvasive testing demonstrates a probable carotid artery stenosis that may be related to the patient's symptoms and if the patient is an acceptable surgical candidate. Neurologic consultation should be obtained prior to angiography.

If the onset of the TIA was within several days and there are no contraindications (including hemorrhage seen by CT or MRI), heparin infusion can be considered while the investigations are in progress. The use of heparin in this situation is theoretically useful and reasonably safe but is controversial. All TIA patients should have long-term treatment for hypertension and smoking cessation as noted above. Other medical and surgical treatments depend on the general health of the patient and the results of brain imaging and other diagnostic testing.

The North American Carotid Endarterectomy Trial (NASCET) and the European Carotid Stenosis Trial have shown that carotid endarterectomy followed by low dose aspirin is effective for patients with a TIA who have an associated internal carotid artery diameter stenosis of 70 per cent or more. This conclusion assumes that a surgeon can perform the operation with low morbidity and mortality (less than 6 to 8 per cent) and that the patient has an acceptable operative risk in relation to other medical problems. Persons with a 30 per cent or less stenosis should be managed medically. The usefulness of carotid endarterectomy in patients with a 30 to 70 per cent stenosis is unknown and is currently being investigated by both the NASCET and European studies. Until these studies are completed, medical management of these patients is probably the best option.

Patients who have a probable cardioembolic source for their TIA, such as congestive heart failure, atrial fibrillation, or acute myocardial infarction, are probably best treated with low dose warfarin for prevention of recurrent strokes. The European Atrial Fibrillation Trial has clearly demonstrated that warfarin is more effective than aspirin for preventing recurrent strokes in patients with atrial fibrillation who have a TIA or minor stroke. However, for patients whose impaired cognition or risk of falling puts them at risk of hemorrhagic complications, an antiplatelet agent is appropriate. All other patients with a TIA who do not have a probable cardioembolic source should be treated long term with an antiplatelet agent.

Two antiplatelet agents have been shown to be effective in preventing recurrent stroke in patients with TIAs or strokes: aspirin and ticlopidine (Ticlid). In a head-to-head comparison, ticlopidine was a little more effective than aspirin in preventing recurrent strokes in patients with TIAs. Ticlopidine also effectively prevents recurrent strokes in patients with moderate or large strokes. Ticlopidine is clearly effective in women and men, whereas the benefit of aspirin in women is not as clear. The risks of aspirin include mainly gastrointestinal bleeding and allergic reactions; the risks of ticlopidine include rash (less than 5 per cent), diarrhea (10 per cent), and neutropenia (1 to 2 per cent). The latter side effect almost always occurs during the first 3 months and is reversible with stoppage of the drug. However, because of the side effects of ticlopidine, CBCs must be monitored every 2 weeks for 3 months. The cost of ticlopidine is approximately $1.00 a day, whereas aspirin costs only pennies a day.

The best use of ticlopidine and aspirin is evolving. Many neurologists use aspirin first for stroke prevention because of ease of use, lower cost, and the small risk of neutropenia with ticlopidine. Ticlopidine is the drug of choice for all patients who cannot tolerate aspirin or who have recurrent TIAs or strokes while on aspirin. However, an argument can be made that ticlopidine is another reasonable first choice for TIA and stroke patients, particularly women.

The best dose of aspirin is also controversial. All but one of the studies that have demonstrated the effectiveness of aspirin in patients with TIAs or mild strokes used three or four tablets a day (one tablet = 325 mg). A Swedish study showed that 75 mg a day is also effective in stroke prevention. Higher doses of aspirin are associated with a greater risk of bleeding than lower doses. Most neurologists who deal with stroke use one 325 mg tablet of aspirin a day for stroke prevention. However, a dose of three or four tablets a day is also reasonable based on the available evidence. If neither aspirin and ticlopidine can be used, low dose warfarin may be considered. The antiplatelet agent dipyridamole (Persantine) has not been shown to be effective in preventing strokes for any group of patients and is not recommended unless no other agent can be used.

Acute Ischemic Stroke. There is no proved effective therapy for acute ischemic stroke. However, a host of agents are currently being investigated and include thrombolytics (intravenous and intra-arterial), low-molecular-weight heparin, ancrod (a defibrinogenating agent), calcium channel blockers, NMDA receptor blockers, and free radical scavengers (lazaroid compound). Results of some of the thrombolytic trials should be available by 1995. Until any of these agents are proved to be safe and effective, none should be used by physicians outside of approved investigational protocols.

Present treatment of acute ischemic stroke should focus on maintenance of a adequate blood pressure, treatment of any active cardiac dysfunction such as congestive heart failure or dysrhythmias, prevention and treatment of complications such as pneumonia and deep venous thrombosis, and prevention of stroke recurrence. One common mistake made by physicians unfamiliar with treatment of acute stroke patients is overtreatment of elevated blood pressure. Cerebral arteries that are ischemic maximally dilate and lose their ability to autoregulate cerebral blood flow. Cerebral blood flow to the ischemic brain then becomes directly dependent on arterial blood pressure. In general, physicians initially should leave mild to moderate blood pressure elevations untreated, particularly because the blood pressure often falls spontaneously during the first hours after stroke onset.

The following guidelines can be used to control extreme blood pressure elevations. If the diastolic blood pressure is greater than 140 mm Hg on two readings 5 minutes apart, sodium nitroprusside can be infused at 0.5 to 1.0 μg/kg/min and then titrated upward if necessary. If the systolic blood pressure is higher than 230 mm Hg or the diastolic blood pressure is 121 to 140 mm Hg on two readings 20 minutes apart, labetalol (Normodyne) 20 mg can be given intravenously over 1 or 2 minutes. The labetalol dose may be repeated or doubled every 10 to 20 minutes until a satisfactory blood pressure reduction is achieved or until a cumulative dose of 300 mg has been administered. For patients with congestive heart failure or severe obstructive pulmonary disease, intravenous enalapril is a good antihypertensive agent. Alternative oral treatments include nifedipine (Procardia) 10 mg every 8 hours or captopril (Capoten) 12.5 mg every 8 hours. However, when the nifedipine is broken open in the mouth and applied sublingually, it leads to less predictable drops in blood pressure.

The target blood pressure range for patients with initially severe blood pressure elevations is a systolic blood pressure of 150 to 180 mm Hg and diastolic blood pressure of 90 to 105 mm Hg. Less severe elevations of blood pressure should be left untreated. Previous blood pressure medications or new oral agents can be started in patients with mild to moderate hypertension after the patient has been clinically stable for 1 to 2 days.

Vital signs and neurologic function should be monitored every hour for the initial 4 hours, every 2 hours for the next 8 hours, and every 4 hours thereafter. Initial laboratory studies are similar to those described for the management of TIAs and mild strokes. The intravenous solution should be either normal saline or Ringer's lactate, as glucose infusions theoretically can worsen cerebral infarction if hyperglycemia is present. Patients who are dehydrated clinically should be rehydrated, but large amounts of free water should be avoided to prevent exacerbation of brain edema. If possible, cardiac rhythm is monitored for at least 24 hours in the intensive care unit, and congestive heart failure is treated aggressively. The patient should be kept at bed rest and be given nasal oxygen at 2 L/ min unless oxygen is contraindicated. The patient should be given nothing by mouth until the neurologic deficit has been stable for at least 12 hours. Swallowing can be tested by having the patient quickly drink 6 to 8 ounces of water. If the patient gags during swallowing or coughs during the minute or so after drinking the water, the risk of aspiration is high. In these situations, a swallowing consultation may be useful, if available. In general, ischemic stroke patients who have a weak or paralyzed leg, or who have any degree of immobilization, should receive "minidose" heparin (5000 units subcutaneously every 12 hours) until he or she is ambulatory to prevent venous thromboembolism. Pressurized vascular boots are also helpful for preventing venous thromboembolism.

Good clinical care should also include proper positioning, a regular schedule of turning, good skin care, early attention to possible removal of an indwelling catheter, and establishment of a regular voiding and bowel evacuation pattern. Finally,

rapid involvement of physical, occupational, and speech therapy, if indicated, can help speed functional recovery and is often important emotionally for patients and families. For severely affected patients, range of motion exercises can be accomplished initially at the bedside.

The choice of agent to prevent stroke recurrence depends on the probably source of the thrombus and the patient's general medical condition as described for TIAs. If the cerebral infarction is large, heparin is not recommended during the first 1 to 2 weeks because of the increased risk of hemorrhagic transformation. Otherwise, indications for heparin use are controversial but are similar to those noted in the TIA section.

Intracerebral Hemorrhage

The most common cause of intracerebral hemorrhage is hypertension-associated damage to the media of the arteriolar wall and subsequent disorganization of small penetrating arterioles that supply the deep portions of the cerebral hemispheres, the pons, and the cerebellum. The most frequent location of "hypertensive" hemorrhages are the basal ganglia, deep cerebral white matter, cerebellum, thalamus, and pons. More superficial lobar hemorrhages can also be due to hypertensive vascular disease. In persons ages 65 and older, amyloid angiopathy has been increasingly recognized as a cause of superficial lobar hemorrhages. Other causes of intracerebral hemorrhage include aneurysms, vascular malformations, hemorrhage into an acute cerebral infarction, coagulation disorders, thrombolytic therapy, and cocaine use.

The 30-day mortality associated with intracerebral hemorrhage is 44 per cent with about 10 per cent of survivors having good functional recovery at 30 days. There is no proved operative or medical treatment of intracerebral hemorrhage. However, many neurosurgeons and neurologists recommend removal of large cerebellar or lobar hemorrhages associated with neurologic deterioration as well as hemorrhages associated with aneurysms or vascular malformations if the patient is not severely brain-damaged prior to operation. Medical therapy of intracerebral hemorrhage is limited to control of intracranial pressure and elevated blood pressure. Blood pressure elevations are often marked and require nitroprusside. Steroid therapy does not decrease morbidity or mortality. Neurologic and neurosurgical consultation should be obtained for patients with intracerebral hemorrhage unless the patient is clearly near death.

Subarachnoid Hemorrhage

Most nondramatic subarachnoid hemorrhages are due to one of three causes: aneurysm (Fig. 48–10), vascular malformation, and idiopathic. Over the age 20, aneurysm overwhelmingly is the most commonly identified cause. Approximately 10 per cent of patients with subarachnoid hemor-

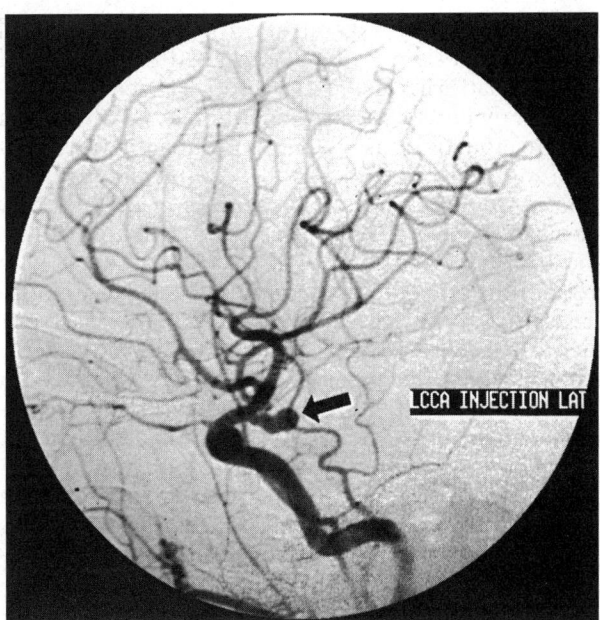

FIGURE 48–10.   Angiogram demonstrating a posterior communicating artery aneurysm (arrow).

rhage who undergo angiography have no underlying vascular pathology.

In patients with suspected subarachnoid hemorrhage, a CT scan and neurosurgical consultation should be obtained emergently. If the scan is negative for blood, CSF should be obtained and examined for blood and xanthochromia. Once subarachnoid hemorrhage has been diagnosed, subsequent management has three components: identification of the source of the bleeding, prevention of rebleeding, and prevention of brain infarction due to cerebral vasospasm. Identification of bleeding requires four-vessel cerebral angiography. If an aneurysm is identified and if the patient is alert or mildly lethargic, most experts suggest that the aneurysm should be clipped within the first 24 to 48 hours. However, the effectiveness of this strategy has not been proved by a randomized trial. For more severely affected patients, clipping the aneurysm is usually deferred 12 to 14 days until the risk of vasospasm has subsided. Arterial vasospasm refers to a narrowing of arteries in the subarachnoid space due to surrounding subarachnoid blood. The risk of vasospasm typically begins on about the third day after hemorrhage and peaks at approximately 1 week. Nimodipine (Nimotop), begun within 72 hours, and volume expansion (after aneurysmal clipping) have been shown to improve neurologic outcome in patients with subarachnoid hemorrhage. Subarachnoid hemorrhage is best managed by experienced neurosurgeons.

Epilepsy

Epilepsy is one of the more common neurologic conditions, affecting approximately 1 per cent of the population. Because it is often a neurologic condition that requires evaluation and treatment over a period of years, it is frequently seen in general medical practice. Many patients can be controlled with the limited number of medications available at this time. Some of these medications are associated with side effects, which may be subtle or prominent, limiting their use in a given patient. Many seizure patients are unemployed or underemployed and have decreased social contacts. Improving their seizure control while limiting toxic side effects can have a profound effect on their lives. Neurologic consultation should be obtained in the following situations: any patient with the new onset of seizures, poorly controlled seizures, or new type of seizures; treatment of epilepsy in situations such as pregnancy or status epilepticus; toxic side effects; and before stopping or changing antiepileptic medication. Many seizure patients who are well controlled can be handled on a routine basis by their primary care providers.

Classification

It is important to understand the protean nature of seizures. Not all seizures are associated with prominent motor activity such as jerking. In addition to the classic absence seizures of childhood, complex partial seizures in adults are frequently not associated with prominent jerking. Likewise, not all events with apparent alteration of consciousness are secondary to seizures. These nonepileptic events are discussed in greater detail below.

In an attempt to improve the understanding and treatment of epilepsy, the International League against Epilepsy published the updated classification of seizures in 1981. The first major distinction in this classification is between seizures that are *partial* in onset versus seizures that are *generalized* in onset. Partial seizures have a focal onset that can be demonstrated either clinically or by EEG to be localized to part of one cerebral hemisphere. Partial seizures can then be further classified as simple partial seizures or complex partial seizures.

Simple partial seizures have no associated alteration of consciousness. These seizures may be associated with a variety of signs and symptoms. They include isolated focal motor activity, focal somatosensory activity, or special sensory symptoms. Partial seizures can include formed or unformed visual hallucinations, auditory hallucinations, or tactile sensations. Simple partial seizures can be associated with autonomic signs and symptoms including piloerection, sweating, or pupillary dilation. Psychic disturbances can also be part of a partial seizure so long as no alteration of the patient's consciousness occurs. Such symptoms might include micropsia (objects appearing small), macropsia (objects appearing large), and teleopsia (objects appearing far away). The patient, however, is able to recognize that these disturbances are not real and maintains awareness throughout the partial seizure.

Complex partial seizures are focal-onset seizures that are associated with alteration of consciousness. These episodes may start with a simple partial seizure, called the aura, and then progress to alteration of consciousness. The alteration of consciousness may be subtle, so the patient is able to recall being spoken to or even able to reply but is not able to reply in an appropriate manner or fully recall the events later. Conversely, the alteration of consciousness may be so prominent that the patient has no recall of the time period during the seizure. Complex motor activity may occur during partial complex seizures. These automatic motor behaviors or automatisms consist of involuntary motor activity that may or may not be related to what the patient was doing prior to entering the seizure. Such automatisms might include simple eye blinking, lip smacking, or picking movements with the hands. On the other hand, the patient who was opening the refrigerator door at the onset of a complex partial seizure might continue to repetitively open the door during the period of the seizure itself. Sometimes these automatisms are associated with risk of injury, such as continued chopping movements with a knife or ironing movements in patients performing these tasks when they enter their seizures.

When a patient has a simple partial seizure that progresses to a complex partial seizure, they may recall the initial warning, or aura. In some cases patients who have auras may also have some of their complex partial seizures without auras. Partial seizures can evolve into *secondary generalized seizures* in which both hemispheres of the brain are involved with the seizure activity. A typical example of such a secondary generalized seizure is a grand mal seizure with tonic stiffening followed by generalized jerking. Certain focal features may be obtained from the history, including head turning to one side or posturing of one side of the body at the onset of the seizure. A difference in the amplitude of the jerking on one side of the body may be noted. Finally, postictal weakness (Todd's paralysis) is seen on one side. All these features are supportive of a focal onset to the seizures. It is important to note whether a seizure is focal in onset, as this information may lead to an evaluation for a focal brain lesion, such as a low grade tumor or vascular malformation. Moreover, some medications are more effective for partial onset seizures than for primary generalized seizures.

Primary generalized seizures have their onset diffusely over both hemispheres. Types of generalized seizures include classic absence seizures, atypical absence seizures, myoclonic seizures, clonic seizures, tonic seizures, tonic-clonic seizures, and atonic seizures. The classic absence seizure (petit mal) has its onset during childhood and often resolves or evolves into a different type of seizure pattern during the teenage years. Clinically, they consist of the abrupt onset of alteration of consciousness as well as the abrupt return of awareness at the end of the seizure. There is no aura or postictal period of confusion or lethargy. The patient is often unaware of these brief events, and they may occur hundreds of times a day. This frequent disruption of awareness can lead to a decrease in school performance. Motor automatisms, including eye blinking, may be associated with these absence seizures and are more likely with longer seizures. The drugs of choice for classic absence seizures are ethosuximide and valproic acid.

Myoclonic seizures consist of jerking movements that may be brief and abrupt. This type of seizure may be part of certain epilepsy syndromes, as is discussed below. Myoclonic activity may be initiated by certain situations, such as photic stimulation or with movement of an extremity. *Clonic seizures* consist predominantly of jerking movements without a tonic phase. Tonic seizures are generalized seizures of prominent stiffening that may be relatively short in duration. *Tonic-clonic seizures*, as the name suggests, start with a tonic phase and progress to clonic or jerking movements. Such seizures may be generalized from onset or generalize after an initial focal seizure. *Atonic seizures* are typically brief in duration and consist of the abrupt loss of muscle tone. These patients fall to the ground and may suffer a prominent injury, but they usually have a quick return of consciousness. Patients with this type of seizure often have other types of seizures as well.

It is important to distinguish between seizures and epilepsy. A seizure is a symptom or a sign that may be due to a variety of causes, including metabolic disturbances such as hyperglycemia or electrolyte imbalances, medication toxicity such as theophylline, alcohol toxicity or withdrawal, or acute head trauma. Epilepsy, on the other hand, is a syndrome associated with characteristic seizure activity. A variety of seizure types may be seen with a given epilepsy syndrome.

The epilepsies have been classified to improve understanding and treatment (Table 48–3). The major classification of epilepsy is whether they are focal (localization-related) or generalized epilepsy syndromes. Focal epilepsies may be idiopathic, or they may be symptomatic of some other condition. An example of a idiopathic focal epilepsy is benign childhood epilepsy with central temporal spikes. This syndrome typically affects the age group 3 to 13 years. It is associated with partial or generalized seizures that usually occur at night. Partial seizures may consist of sensory symptoms involving the tongue or mouth followed by difficulty with speech, salivation, tonic or jerking movements of the face, and possible secondarily generalized tonic-clonic seizures. This syndrome has a charac-

TABLE 48–3. INTERNATIONAL CLASSIFICATION OF EPILEPSIES AND EPILEPTIC SYNDROMES

Localization-related (focal, local, partial) epilepsies and syndromes
  Idiopathic with age-related onset: (a) benign childhood epilepsy with centrotemporal spike; (b) childhood epilepsy with occipital paroxysms
  Symptomatic (e.g., temporal lobe epilepsy, frontal lobe epilepsy)

Generalized epilepsies and syndromes
  Idiopathic, with age-related onset, listed in order of age: benign neonatal familial convulsions, benign neonatal convulsions, benign myoclonic epilepsy in infancy, childhood absence epilepsy (pyknolepsy), juvenile absence epilepsy, juvenile myoclonic epilepsy, epilepsy with grand mal seizures on awakening
  Idiopathic or symptomatic, in order of age of appearance: West syndrome (infantile spasms), Lennox-Gastaut syndrome, epilepsy with myoclonic-astatic seizures, epilepsy with myoclonic absences
  Symptomatic
    Nonspecific etiology: early myoclonic epilepsy
    Specific syndromes

Epilepsies and syndromes undetermined as to whether focal or generalized
  With both generalized and focal seizures: neonatal seizures, severe myoclonic epilepsy during infancy, epilepsy with continuous spike-waves during slow wave sleep, acquired epileptic aphasia
  Without unequivocal generalized or focal features (covers all cases with grand mal tonic-clonic seizures where clinical and EEG findings do not permit classification as clearly generalized or localization-related, e.g., seizures occurring during sleep)

Special syndromes
  Situation-related seizures: febrile convulsions, seizures related to other identifiable situations such as stress, hormonal changes, drugs, alcohol, or sleep deprivation
  Isolated, apparently unprovoked epileptic events
  Epilepsies characterized by specific modes of seizure precipitation
  Chronic progressive epilepsia partialis continua of childhood

Adapted from Commission on Classification and Terminology of the International League Against Epilepsy: Proposal for classification of epilepsies and epileptic syndromes. Epilepsia 26:268, 1985, with permission.

teristic EEG pattern of spike activity seen in the central-temporal brain region, which becomes more prominent during sleep. The seizures respond well to anticonvulsant therapy, such as carbamazepine, and the condition usually resolves spontaneously during the teenage years.

Epilepsy syndromes that are focal may also be symptomatic of other conditions. An example is epilepsia partialis continua, which is seen in the setting of Rasmussen's encephalitis affecting children 2 to 10 years of age. This rare syndrome is associated with partial seizures, progressive motor deficits, and mental deterioration. A viral cause is presumed, and the condition may respond to surgical removal of the affected brain region.

Generalized epilepsy syndromes may also be idiopathic or symptomatic. Childhood absence epilepsy, as described above, and juvenile myoclonic

epilepsy are two examples. In the latter epilepsy syndrome, myoclonic jerking may be prominent in the morning shortly after awaking. Absence seizures and generalized tonic-clonic seizure activity may be present and are seen more frequently with sleep deprivation or shortly after awakening. Photic stimulation may also elicit seizures. The characteristic age of onset is 13 to 19 years. The EEG consists of 4- to 6-Hz spike or polyspike wave activity, predominantly in the frontal regions. Unlike childhood absence seizures, most of these patients continue to have their seizures into adulthood. The drug of choice for this condition is valproic acid, although other medications such as primadone and clonazepam may be effective.

The Lennox-Gastaut syndrome is a generalized epilepsy syndrome that consists of multiple seizure types that are often difficult to control. Clinical features include drop attacks, atypical absence seizures, psychomotor retardation, and a characteristic EEG pattern of generalized slow spike-and-wave discharges. Felbamate (Felbatol) has been demonstrated to have some efficacy in this type of epilepsy.

Etiology

The relative frequency of the various causes of seizure disorders varies between children and adults. In children most seizures are thought to have a genetic, developmental, or idiopathic basis. Less frequently, the seizures are due to metabolic disturbances such as hypocalcemia, fever, infectious diseases, vascular insults, trauma, brain tumors, or toxins. Genetic conditions, however, comprise only a small portion of epilepsies with onset during adulthood. Stroke, tumor, trauma, infection, metabolic disorders, toxins, and degenerative diseases are the common causes. However, for many patients with epilepsy no cause is found.

Evaluation

It is important to obtain a history from the patient and from witnesses. Patients may be able to describe an aura or focal onset of jerking prior to alteration of consciousness. They can describe any perceived alteration of consciousness, which may conflict with the description of the witnesses. Finally, they can describe postictal symptoms and signs, such as focal weakness or language disturbances, which may aid in localization. Details of triggering events may help identify situations the patient should avoid.

Witnesses provide a different perspective. They may comment that the patient warned them of an impending seizure, although patients themselves may not recall an aura. Witnesses can also describe focal posturing or head-turning, or asymmetries of motor activity that support a focal onset. By specific examples, they may demonstrate that the patient had an alteration of consciousness of which the patient was unaware.

Detailed neurologic examination may elicit subtle deficits, such as focal weakness or posturing on gait testing that support focal cerebral dysfunction and a focal onset to the seizures. Birth marks, such as café au lait spots, may indicate a neurocutaneous syndrome as the underlying cause of a patient's seizures.

Laboratory studies are important to rule out the variety of toxic and metabolic disturbances that may be associated with seizure activity. Marked hyperglycemia may be associated with generalized seizures and is treated by correcting the blood glucose abnormality, not long-term anticonvulsive therapy. Hyponatremia, hypomagnesemia, and hypocalcemia are also associated with seizures that may respond simply to correction of the metabolic disorder. Renal disease can be associated with seizure activity and may increase the likelihood of seizures occurring with high levels of certain medications such as antibiotics. Seizures can occur with toxic levels of theophylline.

The EEG is important to the evaluation of a seizure disorder. Focal abnormalities including focal slowing or spike wave activity may help to define the seizure disorder as focal in onset (Fig. 48–11). This brain region should be further evaluated by radiologic studies to rule out a structural lesion.

Likewise, the EEG may define generalized discharges consistent with a primary seizure disorder (Fig. 48–12), allowing selection of an appropriate anticonvulsant. However, the EEG presents only a small temporal sample of the electrical activity of the brain. A single EEG has a low yield of detecting epileptiform activity in a patient with seizures. The yield can be increased, however, by repeating the study with sleep deprivation. Other procedures, such as hyperventilation and photic stimulation, can increase the yield of the study. Prolonged ambulatory EEG studies further enhance the detection of focal abnormalities and even typical clinical events. These systems may be worn comfortably for a day or longer and record eight to sixteen channels of EEG activity. Although these studies are more expensive than standard EEG, the improved yield is helpful in selected cases.

Video EEG telemetry monitoring is generally reserved for patients whose epilepsies are not responsive to major anticonvulsant therapy. At some centers, 20 per cent or more of patients who are thought to have medically intractable seizure disorders have their spells on a nonepileptic basis. These patients would not be expected to respond to anticonvulsant therapy. Video EEG telemetry monitoring is also important in those patients in

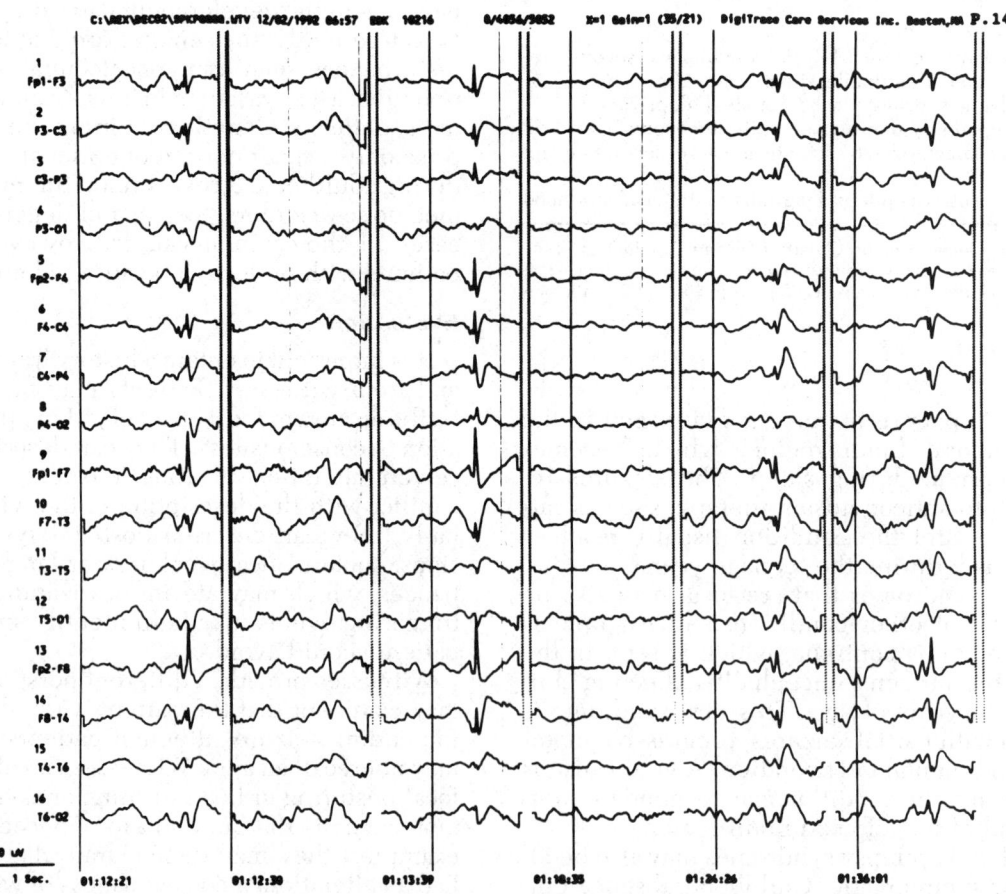

FIGURE 48–11. Patient with partial complex seizures who has intermittent right frontal spike discharges.

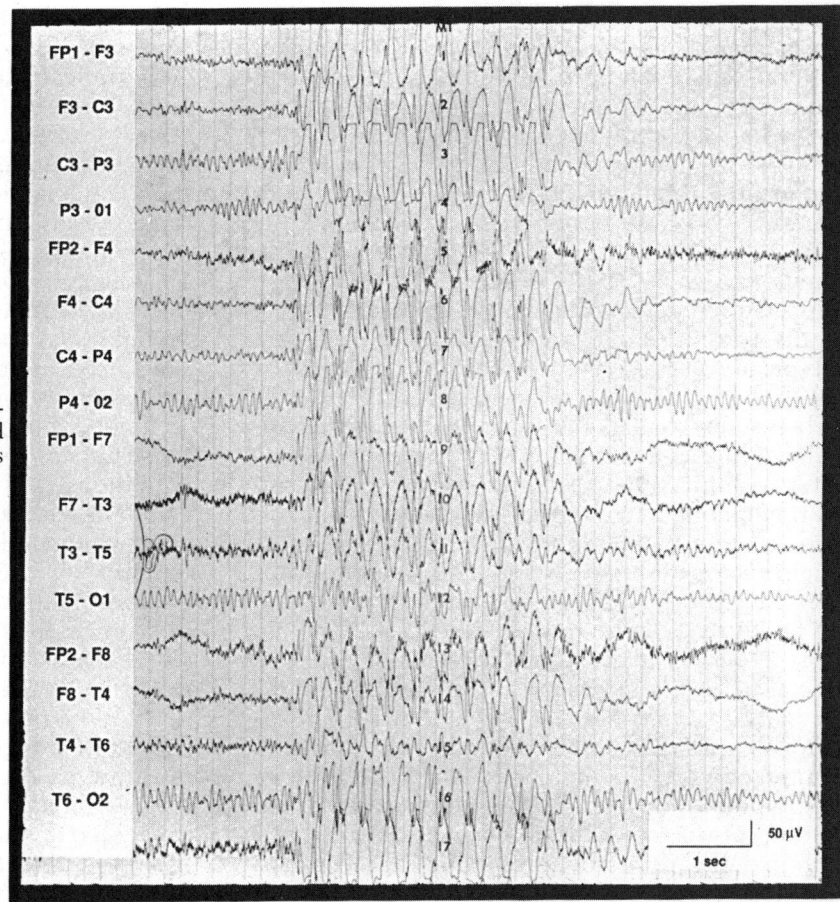

FIGURE 48–12. Patient with absence seizures who has a 3 second run of generalized three per second spike-wave discharges triggered by photic stimulation.

whom a focal onset can be defined, as these patients may be amenable to surgical therapy as discussed below.

A variety of radiologic studies are now available to evaluate patients with seizure disorders. CT is still helpful for ruling out structural lesions, but MRI has largely supplanted it. Most patients with focal epilepsy have the onset of their seizures in the medial aspect of their temporal lobes. This area is often difficult to evaluate by CT, but MRI provides excellent images of the temporal lobes, including the hippocampus and amygdala, in the axial and coronal planes. Asymmetries in the size of these structures may be helpful in localizing seizure onset during the presurgical evaluation.

Additional specialized techniques, such as PET scanning and SPECT studies, provide metabolic imaging of the brain. These images may be useful if surgery is being considered to control the patient's epilepsy but are not needed for the management of most patients with epilepsy. Lumbar puncture is sometimes indicated in patients with acute onset of seizure disorders. Its major value is to rule out meningitis or encephalitis.

Treatment

The goal of therapy for epilepsy is to control patients' seizures and allow them to return to their usual activities as much as possible. Because treatments may be associated with side effects that limit the daily performance of the patient, a therapeutic balance must be struck between efficacy and side effects.

MEDICAL THERAPY. Anticonvulsant medications remain the mainstay of treatment for epilepsy. Most of the major antiepileptic drugs used today have been available in some form since the 1970s or before. Two medications have recently been approved for use and others are in preliminary drug trials at this time.

Phenobarbital, which was introduced during the early 1900s, is effective in controlling generalized seizures and seizures with partial onset. It has several advantages. It is inexpensive compared to most prescription drugs and has a long half-life (3 to 5 days), allowing once-a-day dosing, thereby improving compliance. Its side effects of sedation and cognitive effects have prevented it from being the drug of choice for these types of seizure. It also induces production of hepatic enzymes and may affect the level of other medications given to the patient. It has comparatively low protein binding (approximately 50 per cent).

Primidone (Mysoline) is a barbiturate that has been shown to be effective against generalized seizures and seizures of partial onset. Its use is limited by its side effects of sedation, cognitive effects, and impotence. Primidone has a half-life of approximately 12 hours. One of its major metabolites is phenobarbital. The ratio of primidone and phenobarbital can be affected by other drugs, such as carbamazepine. When this medication is prescribed, both the primidone and phenobarbital levels should be checked at intervals. Primidone, like phenobarbital, is only about 50 per cent protein-bound.

Phenytoin (Dilantin) has been in use as an anticonvulsant since the 1940s. It has a half-life of approximately 1 day, which allows once-a-day dosing by the patient, improving compliance. However, it typically is prescribed three times a day. It is effective in controlling complex partial seizures as well as some generalized seizures. Its major disadvantage lies in its kinetics. Most patients on phenytoin exhibit zero-order kinetics through the typical therapeutic range. Small increases in dose can lead to large increases in the serum drug level, placing the patient at risk for toxic side effects. It does come in smaller dosing sizes, including a 50 mg tablet that can be broken in half and a 30 mg capsule. These smaller doses allow for small incremental increases in dose to titrate for clinical efficacy and to avoid toxicity. Phenytoin is approximately 90 per cent protein-bound, which can lead to interactions with other medications that are also highly protein-bound. The high degree of protein binding also presents problems in patients with protein deficiency states (e.g., kidney disease, malnutrition, pregnancy and burns). In this setting, measurement of the free phenytoin levels can be helpful for adjusting therapy. Common toxic side effects include ataxia, dizziness, and vision disturbances, which may include diplopia and oscillopsia (rapid eye movements).

Carbamazepine (Tegretol) has been used in the United States for more than 20 years and is effective in controlling partial onset and generalized tonic-clonic seizures. It is better tolerated than the barbiturates but has the disadvantage of a shorter half-life (approximately 12 to 17 hours and even shorter with some co-medication). Because of the short half-life, carbamazepine must be given more than once a day. Common side effects are similar to those of phenytoin and include ataxia, dizziness, and vision disturbances. Hyponatremia occurs in some patients, so the sodium level should be checked periodically, especially after dose increases. Leukopenia may also occur but is not a contraindication for continued carbmazepine use if it remains stable with an adequate number of granulocytes. However, the drug should be avoided in patients with bone marrow suppression or congestive heart failure. It is approximately 80 per cent protein-bound. Carbamazepine is metabolized to an epoxide with a relatively long half-life. This metabolite has anticonvulsant properties but may be associated with similar side effects. The epoxide level is not generally measured but must be kept in mind when patients report increased

side effects, especially in the setting of co-medication with valproate or felbamate.

Valproic acid (Depakene) has been available since the 1980s and is effective against partial onset seizures and for some primary generalized seizure disorders such as juvenile myoclonic epilepsy and classic absence seizures. It may be used to treat grand mal seizures associated with classic absence seizures. It has a half-life of approximately 12 hours, so most patients are dosed more than once a day. It is approximately 90 per cent protein-bound so, like phenytoin, protein-binding interactions may occur with other medications. Fatal hepatic toxicity has been a concern but occurs most commonly in children under age 10, especially those under age 2 with other medical or neurologic conditions. Gastrointestinal side effects are fairly common with valproic acid, but this problem has been alleviated with the new divalproex formulation.

Ethosuximide (Zarontin) has been considered by many as the drug of choice for treatment of classic absence seizures. It is not effective against grand mal seizures. Should these seizures occur in a patient on ethosuximide, a second medication should be added or the patient may be switched to valproic acid therapy. Ethosuximide has a relatively long half-life (2 days) but is generally given in divided doses. Side effects include gastrointestinal upset, sedation, headache, dizziness, and effects on the hematopoietic system. Because ethosuximide does not significantly bind to protein, it does not interfere with the protein binding of other medications.

Clonazepam (Klonopin) and other benzodiazepines have been used in some patients with seizures as a second line drug. It is beneficial in patients with certain primary generalized seizure disorders including those with myoclonic jerks or drop attacks. Its use is limited by sedation as well as tachyphylaxis, with benefit in many patients wearing off over a period of weeks to months. It has a half-life of approximately 1 to 2 days and is approximately 50 per cent protein-bound.

Felbamate (Felbatol), approved for use in the United States in 1993, is the first new major anticonvulsive drug introduced since the late 1970s. It has a long half-life (approximately 1 day) with side effects at peak levels, necessitating dosing three or four times a day. These side effects include a decrease in appetite, which may be associated with weight loss, insomnia, dizziness, and headache. Some patients note lack of sedation as a major benefit of its use compared to other antiepileptic drugs, but some develop significant insomnia. It is effective in controlling seizures with partial onset and has been demonstrated to improve control of seizures associated with the Lennox-Gastaut syndrome. Its disadvantage is a prominent interaction with the metabolism of other medications. When given as co-medication, it can elevate phenytoin and valproate levels. It lowers carbamazepine levels but elevates the carbamazepine 10,11-epoxide level. Dosages of co-medications must be adjusted when instituting felbamate therapy. During August 1994 the Food and Drug Administration (FDA) recommended that the use of felbamate be suspended, except in certain high risk patients, owing to reports of aplastic anemia in association with its use. The final assessment of this risk is pending at the time of this writing.

Gabapentin (Neurontin) is the most recently approved medication for the treatment of complex partial seizures. It is indicated as an add-on therapy for patients with poorly controlled partial seizures. Its major advantage is that it is not metabolized through the liver, decreasing the chances of drug interactions. The doses of concomitant antiepileptic medications do not need to be adjusted when instituting gabapentin therapy. It has linear kinetics and is not significantly protein-bound. Its renal clearance is similar to that of creatinine clearance, and the dose should be adjusted in the setting of renal disease. It has a short half-life (5 to 7 hours), so it is dosed three or more times a day. Cimetidine can lead to a rise in the gabapentin level, and antacids may interfere with its absorption. Side effects noted include fatigue, somnolence, dizziness, and ataxia.

SURGICAL THERAPY. Surgery can help control seizures that have failed to respond to major anticonvulsant therapy. Surgical therapy requires localization of the seizure focus to an area of the brain that can be resected without leaving significant residual deficits. In many operative candidates partial complex seizures originate in the unilateral hippocampus or amygdala of the mesial temporal lobe, but surgery can be performed on other locations as well. For those patients with medically intractable epilepsy but without a localized onset, corpus callosotomy may be considered. This procedure is most helpful in patients with severe atonic drop attacks, tonic seizures, or generalized tonic-clonic seizures.

The preoperative evaluation must define the epileptogenic focus. As with all epilepsy patients, a detailed history and physical examination is important. The neuroradiologic evaluation should include MRI, if possible with coronal cuts through the temporal lobes, to best image the mesial temporal structures. Asymmetry of temporal lobe structures may support the localization of seizure onset. Metabolic imaging studies are often helpful. A PET scan interictally may be able to define a region of hypometabolism in the area of the seizure focus, and the ictal PET or SPECT scan may demonstrate a hypermetabolic region there. Newer MRI techniques may be able to provide further information about local metabolism in the future. Neuropsychometric evaluation is also used to assess function attributed to various brain regions. The identification of brain regions with decreased cognitive performance can help identify the brain region that is the likely source of a patient's seizures.

A carotid amytal test may also be performed. This test involves carotid angiography with injection of a dose of amytal sufficient to sedate part of one hemisphere. It allows testing the opposite hemisphere in isolation. This test helps to determine the language dominant hemisphere, which may be important for defining the extent of the surgical resection. It may also be used to test the memory function of the temporal lobe opposite the one for which surgery is planned.

Video EEG telemetry monitoring with recording of the patient's typical seizures is helpful. It may be done by recording with electrodes in the standard sites over the scalp as well as by adding special electrodes to localize the onset of the seizure discharge. Patients whose seizure focus cannot be defined by the above studies may undergo phase two evaluation with intracranial electrodes. This procedure may involve depth electrodes placed within the brain itself or strips or grids of electrodes placed over the brain surface at selected locations. An additional advantage of using strip or grid electrodes is that cortical stimulation can be performed outside the operating room. This procedure can then map the functions of specific brain regions for a given patient. By mapping the seizure focus and functional brain areas, decisions can be made as to how much cortex can be removed to control seizure activity while avoiding postoperative functional deficits.

Using these techniques many centers in the United States have achieved success in patients who failed multiple medication trials. Such centers often report complete control of seizures in 50 per cent or more of their patients with 80 to 90 per cent of patients overall showing 90 per cent improvement in seizure control.

Special Issues

LABORATORY MONITORING. Carbamazepine has been associated with leukopenia, as noted above, and other medications including barbiturates and phenytoin may be associated with mild anemia. With the exception of gabapentin, currently available anticonvulsive medications are metabolized through the liver, and they may be associated with an elevation of hepatic enzymes. As noted above, carbamazepine may also be associated with hyponatremia. It is prudent to evaluate patients for these potential difficulties at intervals through easily available laboratory studies. Much has been written about the necessity and appropriate frequency of blood testing, noting the overall low incidence of significant toxicity. However, it is reasonable to begin the laboratory studies shortly after initiating therapy and repeating the studies at intervals that may be lengthened to a year if levels remain within acceptable limits and are stable.

Clinical judgment may indicate more frequent monitoring.

Evaluation of serum drug levels are important to the overall management of patients with epilepsy. However, the ranges described as therapeutic by a given laboratory cannot be used in isolation. Normal values reported by one laboratory may be different from those used by another laboratory, although the technique for measuring the drug may be identical. Typically, the lower end of the therapeutic range is defined as the point at which most patients begin to achieve improvement in seizure control. The upper limit is defined as a point where most patients begin to note unacceptable side effects. A great deal of individual variability exists. A given patient may have complete seizure control with a level below the usual range or above it. Some patients may develop unacceptable toxicity at levels below the usual therapeutic range, and others may tolerate levels above the therapeutic range. When the drug level is followed, the blood samples should be obtained at a consistent time of day and at a consistent time after the last dose. Morning trough levels are often monitored, but they may be difficult for a patient who is working. For such patients, late afternoon trough levels are more convenient and provide acceptable information. Doses of antiepileptic drugs should be adjusted based on the amount of seizure control and the side effects. The drug level and milligram per kilogram dosing should be used only as guidelines to help interpret the clinical response.

SAFETY ISSUES. Patients with seizures may develop sudden alteration of consciousness, often without warning. Even patients who usually have auras that precede their seizures may have seizures without an aura of sufficient duration to allow self-protection. Safety issues must be discussed frankly with patients who have seizures. Patients who have had a recent seizure should be advised to avoid all activities in which sudden loss of consciousness could lead to harm to themselves or others. Such situations include working at heights, working around heavy equipment with large moving parts, swimming alone, or bathing alone. Driving is a major safety issue with these patients. Even patients with auras may not have sufficient time to pull the car over to the side of the road prior to loss of consciousness, which can lead to injury to themselves or others as well as property damage. Most states define a period during which an individual must be seizure-free before resuming driving privileges. This period currently ranges from 3 months to 1 year. Some states require mandatory reporting. Information about a given state's requirements may be obtained by contacting the Department or Bureau of Motor Vehicles.

The longer seizures have been controlled, the lower is the likelihood that another seizure will occur during the performance of a given activity. Thus it is reasonable to return to proscribed activities when seizures are under control. Should a patient have a breakthrough seizure, restricting the patient's activities again must be considered for safety reasons. From a medical-legal point of view, it is important to document these discussions with the patients.

TREATMENT OF A SINGLE SEIZURE. Institution of anticonvulsant therapy after a single seizure is controversial. With adults the argument can be made that safety issues are paramount. Anticonvulsant therapy is appropriate after a single seizure if a structural lesion can be identified. There is a high likelihood of seizure recurrence in this setting. Institution of medication is generally avoided if a correctable precipitating factor is found, such as a metabolic derangement, medication toxicity, or the effects of alcohol. Many neurologists do not institute anticonvulsive therapy after the first unprovoked seizure, citing various studies that have reported a low incidence of recurrence of seizure activity in patients with a normal examination and a normal evaluation. Some studies of this group have reported recurrence rates as high as 50 per cent. Most neurologists institute therapy after a second unprovoked seizure.

WITHDRAWAL OF ANTIEPILEPTIC DRUG THERAPY. It is possible to discontinue antiepileptic drug therapy in patients who have remained seizure-free for a long period. Most of the work to support this position has been done in children who have been seizure-free for periods of 1 to 4 years at the time of attempted withdrawal. In such patients who have a normal neurologic examination and an EEG without epileptiform activity, the success rate for withdrawal of antiepileptic medication may be as high as 75 per cent.

The issues are more complicated in adults, as this age group has not been as well studied. Additionally, some children may have been included in earlier studies with seizure disorders that would be expected to remit on their own, such as benign rolandic epilepsy. A 25 per cent risk of failure is often not acceptable to an adult who is driving or whose career development may not tolerate a seizure at work. A patient who has been well controlled on an antiepileptic medication for a long time should be offered the opportunity to discontinue the medication to limit the possible side effects. From a practical point of view, however, many adults express a desire to continue on the medication if they have few medication side effects.

EPILEPSY AND PREGNANCY. A sizable number of epileptics are women of child-bearing potential. Until recently, such women often chose not to have children. It was even illegal in some states for women with epilepsy to marry. With changes in society's views and an improvement in therapy, more of these women are choosing to have children. Women considering pregnancy or who are pregnant often express concern regarding the likelihood of birth defects. There is a greater risk of fetal malformations in the offspring of women with epilepsy on any antiepileptic drug therapy. Epilepsy itself appears to increase slightly the risk of malformations, but risk is also associated with anticonvulsant medication. The risk increases further if polypharmacy is used to control the seizures. All the major antiepileptic drugs that have been available for a period of years are associated with an increased risk of fetal malformation. Some medications are associated with a higher risk of a given malformation. Valproic acid has been associated with an approximately 1 to 2 per cent risk of spina bifida, and carbamazepine has been associated with a 0.5 to 1.0 per cent risk. Valproic acid medication of pregnant patients represents an approximately 18-fold increase in risk compared to that in the average woman—comparable to the risk of a woman who had a previous child with spina bifida. The presence of this malformation can be detected in most pregnancies by level II ultrasonography and serum α-fetoprotein levels. Some centers substitute amniocentesis with measurement of α-fetoprotein in the amniotic fluid rather than serum measurements. Some women state that they would not consider an abortion even if they knew their child had spina bifida. If the women is at risk, it may still be a benefit to detect the spina bifida. Delivery by cesarean section can improve the neurologic outcome of such infants by avoiding the traumatic passage through the birth canal.

Other malformations, including cardiac defects, cleft lip, and cleft palate, may be seen in the offspring of mothers who are taking antiepileptic drugs. A variety of minor malformations have been described with maternal use of anticonvulsant medications, often combined under the heading of fetal anticonvulsant syndrome. Many of these minor malformations and dysmorphic anomalies do not significantly impair function of the offspring. Some abnormalities, such as impaired development of the distal phalanges, may not be detectable on re-examination of the child at 5 years of age. Studies on the cognitive outcome of infants born to mothers taking antiepileptic drugs during pregnancy have yielded conflicting results. Some studies demonstrate no detectable impairment.

The greatest risk for malformations is early in the pregnancy, during the period of major organogenesis. Spina bifida occurs if the posterior neuropore does not close normally at approximately day 28, and cardiac defects and cleft lip occur if the structures do not form normally at 6 weeks of age. Cleft palate occurs if normal development does not occur at 10 weeks of age. There is no indication that anticonvulsant use after these points produces these defects. It is of note that many women do not realize they are pregnant until well into or after this period of major organogenesis. If they are past this period, there is no reason to stop the anticonvulsant agent in an attempt to avoid the risk of major malformation.

Good seizure control during pregnancy is important, as the occurrence of grand mal seizures has been demonstrated to increase the risk of bleeding and fetal loss. Profound fetal bradycardia has been demonstrated with maternal grand mal seizures. Complex partial seizures may also place the woman at risk for injury, such as from a car accident. Thus a woman with an active seizure disorder should stay on antiepileptic therapy during the pregnancy, especially if she is already past the period of major organogenesis.

If a woman is planning to become pregnant, an effort should be made to place the woman on monotherapy to reduce the risk of malformation as much as possible. It may even be possible in some patients to withdraw the anticonvulsant prior to becoming pregnant. The risk of spina bifida may be lowered by preconceptual use of folate. If an anticonvulsant is used, it should be one that best controls the patient's seizures, as none of the current major medications is clearly safer than the others. These issues should be discussed extensively with the prospective mothers and documented in their medical records.

Major changes in antiepileptic drug metabolism occur over the course of a pregnancy. For example, levels of all commonly used medications fall. Again, the levels should be used together with the clinical course when making decisions concerning therapeutic adjustments. Once the woman delivers, the metabolic changes tend to reverse over the following weeks to months, so that doses that were increased during the course of pregnancy may need to be reduced during the postpartum period. In general, this reduction should be made gradually.

There is a risk of neonatal hemorrhage during the first day of life in infants born of mothers taking antiepileptic medications. This risk may be limited to the enzyme-inducing medications, including phenytoin, carbamazepine, and the barbiturates. The risk can be lowered by vitamin K supplementation during the last 2 weeks of pregnancy.

Breast-feeding issues are raised by many woman. Anticonvulsant medications cross into breast milk inversely proportional to their protein binding. A medication such as phenytoin, which is highly protein-bound, crosses into breast milk with a level only approximately 10 per cent that in the maternal serum. Ethosuximide on the other hand is present in breast milk at a concentration approximately equal to that in maternal serum. The baby's daily dose is not based just on this concentration but also on the amount of milk consumed per day. It is a relatively small amount compared to the placenta blood flow to which the fetus had been exposed over the previous 9 months. Additionally, the newborn is capable of metabolizing these medications. Studies have demonstrated that most infants do not achieve significant drug levels by breast-feeding alone. Additionally, for most of these medications, the level in the newborn is the same as that in the mother at the time of birth. These levels then gradually drop. Some medications, such as the barbiturates, may be associated with sedation of the infant, making the infant sluggish to feed. If this situation occurs, it may be best to limit breast-feeding in order to avoid further sedation. It should also be noted that if the mother was taking a barbiturate during pregnancy the infant is at risk to undergo barbiturate withdrawal. Such withdrawal may range from a subtle manifestation (e.g., a "jittery baby") to more severe symptoms including seizure activity. These withdrawal symptoms can be limited by keeping the infant in a quiet, darkened location. Breast-feeding allows administration of some barbiturate. Administration of barbiturate to an infant may also be used to help in the weaning process.

Birth control issues should also be discussed with these women. The enzyme-inducing antiepileptic drugs such as barbiturates, phenytoin, and carbamazepine can lead to stimulation of the hepatic metabolism of hormonal contraceptives. This situation leads to a decrease in their efficacy and breakthrough bleeding; hence pregnancy may occur. It is therefore important to advise women taking these medications to work with their gynecologist closely when choosing the proper oral contraceptive and to consider using a barrier method until seizures are controlled.

NONEPILEPTIC EVENTS.   As noted above, one of the reasons people fail to have their seizures controlled by major antiepileptic drugs is that their "seizures" or spells are not due to electrical seizure discharges in the brain. A variety of conditions can lead to events that clinically appear to be seizures. Other neurologic conditions include sleep disorders such as night terrors and rapid eye movement (REM) behavior disorder, myoclonus, paroxysmal dyskinesias, and migraine. Cardiogenic spells may be confused with epileptic seizures. Syncope may be difficult to discern from seizure activity by history alone. Convulsive syncope can occur with more prolonged hypoperfusion of the brain, which may be seen in the setting of blood-drawing or blood donation as well in the setting of routine syncope in which someone tries to protect the patient by holding them in an upright posture. Such patients would not be expected to respond to antiepileptic drug therapy. Psychiatric conditions may also be associated with spells that by history may be confused with seizure activity. They include fugue states, malingering, and a factitious disorder with physical symptoms. A variety of psychiatric conditions may be predisposing and a history of abuse is often elicited.

There may be clinical clues from observation of the seizures that point to a diagnosis of nonepileptic events due to a psychiatric cause. Such events often have a gradual onset and more discontinuous character with uncoordinated movements and dystonic posturing. Pelvic thrusting is seen more commonly, as is emotional crying. Lack of facial movements in the setting of a grand mal seizure is also supportive. Features often seen with grand mal seizures, such as incontinence or tongue biting, can be seen with nonepileptic events. None of these features can be used absolutely to decide which patient has epilepsy and which patient had a nonepileptic event. The greater the degree of stereotypic behavior, even if bizarre, the greater the likelihood that the events are epileptic in nature. Video EEG telemetry monitoring can be helpful for identifying an epileptic verses a nonepileptic cause. It is important to remove patients with nonepileptic events from antiepileptic therapy because of the potential side effects of the medications as well as to help them come to an understanding of the real nature of their events. However, nonepileptic events due to psychiatric causes may occur in patients with proved epilepsy. Thus a psychiatric cause of seizure-like events should always be diagnosed cautiously.

STATUS EPILEPTICUS.   Status epilepticus is variously defined as repeated seizure activity over a period of time without a return of awareness. It is a medical emergency with a mortality rate as high as 25 per cent. Among the variety of causes, medication withdrawal or noncompliance are two of the most common. These patients must be addressed aggressively, and emergent consultation with a neurologic specialist is appropriate.

The initial assessment of these patients includes protection of the airway and breathing as well as attention to other vital signs. Laboratory studies should be performed to rule out major metabolic disturbances as a precipitant of the status. Such tests include assays for potassium, sodium, calcium, magnesium, and glucose; a CBC; antiepileptic drug levels; and arterial blood gas assays. An intravenous line should be placed to allow administration of medications. An ampul of $D_{50}W$ with thiamine may be given pending measurement of the glucose level. If the patient is actively seizing, a benzodiazepine is used to provide a window of seizure control: Diazepam 10 to 20 mg or lorazepam up to 4 to 8 mg at a rate less than 2 mg/min. Phenytoin may then be instituted at a intravenous loading dose of 18 mg/kg at a rate of less than 50 mg/min. The blood pressure and electrocardiogram should be monitored. If seizures persist, phenobarbital may be added at 10 to 20 mg/kg at a rate of less than 100 mg/min. A combined respiratory depressant effect of the barbiturate and previously administered benzodiazepine is likely. Endotracheal intubation must be considered. If the patient continues to seize in the face of the above regimen, the patient may be placed in a medication-induced coma with a pentobarbital or diazepam drip or general anesthesia under the direction of an anesthesiologist. Such patients must be monitored in an intensive care setting. Monitoring the EEG may be helpful for maintaining the depth of medication-induced coma as well as assessing subclinical seizure activity.

Some patients present with nonconvulsive or subtle status epilepticus. These patients have alteration of responsiveness or awareness of abrupt onset that may be prolonged over hours to days. There may be subtle motor movements such as twitching of the extremities, facial muscles, or eyes. In such patients, the EEG is critical for the diagnosis. Administration of benzodiazepine should be considered during the course of the EEG in patients suspected of having nonconvulsive status to see if the seizure activity can be stopped.

FEBRILE SEIZURES. Febrile seizures generally occur between the ages of 3 months and 5 years in a patient with a febrile illness as the temperature is rising. They may be seen with any of the common causes of febrile illnesses in this age group, but if they occur in an infant less than 6 months old meningitis should be excluded by lumbar puncture. Occurrence in children over 5 years of age raises the concern for the development of nonfebrile seizures. There is often a positive family history for febrile seizures.

Febrile seizures may be classified as simple or complex. Simple febrile seizures last less than 15 minutes and are tonic, clonic, or tonic-clonic without focal features. EEG records add little to the management, especially if performed during the first 24 hours, as the findings may be nonspecific. Laboratory studies usually are of little help in ruling out other causes of seizures, especially if the child has recovered fully. Such studies should be selected based on the overall clinical appearance. Thus, while a lumbar puncture would not be indicated in most children with a simple febrile seizure, it should be done if meningitis is suspected clinically.

Complex febrile seizures may last longer than 15 minutes, have focal features, and occur repeatedly within a 24-hour period. The child may have an abnormal neurologic examination at baseline and may have a family history of epilepsy. These children have a greater risk for developing nonfebrile seizures, especially if more than one of these features is present. This risk approaches 50 per cent if the first three features listed above occur. These children warrant a more detailed evaluation. Infections and focal CNS lesions should be ruled out.

A second febrile seizure occurs in about one third of children, and about one in six have a third febrile seizure. The risk of recurrence is greater in children with a febrile seizure at less than 1 year of age. A history of a febrile seizure carries an increased risk for later development of epilepsy, but the risk appears to be less than 5 per cent. Thus management tends to be conservative.

Therapy begins with aggressive management of fevers including tepid baths and antipyretics such as acetaminophen. Antibiotics are used for suspected bacterial infections. Antiepileptic medications may be associated with prominent side effects such as sedation or hyperactivity. Antiepileptic medications are unproved for the control of simple febrile seizures or for the prevention of nonfebrile seizures. They may be warranted in selected cases, especially in the setting of complex febrile seizures.

TREATMENT OF EPILEPSY IN THE ELDERLY. Elderly patients are usually on several medications, leading to an increased chance of drug interactions. In addition, serum protein levels may be lower and the drug clearance rates may be slower in the elderly, which may lead to higher free levels of a medication for a given dose. Close monitoring of drug levels is important, particularly when a new medication is added. The elderly may also be more sensitive to the cognitive and sedating effects of antiepileptic medications as well as to the arrhythmogenic side effects of some of the medications. Initial doses should be small, and increases should be made gradually, as clinically indicated.

Disorders of Language and Cognition

Dementia

Dementia refers to a state in which the patient has intellectual impairment (deficits in two or more cognitive functions, e.g., language, spatial attention) that causes difficulties in carrying out activities of daily living, social skills, or a job. Using the term dementia does not indicate its cause, which may be static (does not change from the time of onset (e.g., stroke) or progressive (e.g., Alzheimer's disease), reversible (e.g., hypothyroidism, drug toxicity), or irreversible (e.g., head trauma). Table 48–4 is an abbreviated list of dementia etiologies.

Evaluation of the dementia patient should be directed at identifying treatable or reversible causes of dementia. After obtaining an in-depth history from the patient and caregivers, a physical examination, neurologic examination, and neuropsychological testing are performed. Laboratory studies should include serum electrolyte assays, CBC, test for fluorescent treponemal antibodies (FTA), vitamin B_{12}, and folate assays, thyroid function tests, electrocardiography, chest x-radiography, and brain imaging studies (CT or MRI). Further (e.g., spinal tap, EEG, brain biopsy) studies may be obtained depending on the physical examination findings and the laboratory results. It is important to remember that a dementia may be multifactorial. Patients with Alzheimer's disease can have worsened deficits secondary to infection, congestive heart failure, drug toxicity, hypothyroidism, and depression. Therefore all potential treatable

TABLE 48–4. ABBREVIATED LIST OF THE CAUSES OF DEMENTIA

Vascular disorders: multi-infarct dementia, vasculitis

Metabolic/toxic/inflammatory disorders: cardiac disorders, hepatic failure, renal failure, hypoglycemia, pulmonary disorders, hypothyroidism, vitamin B_{12} deficiency, drugs (e.g., ranitidine, propranolol, neuroleptics, alcohol), heavy metals (e.g., mercury, arsenic), industrial agents, systemic lupus erythematosus, multiple sclerosis

Infectious disorders: encephalitis (e.g., HIV), Lyme disease, Creutzfeldt-Jakob disease, syphilis

Neoplastic disorders: brain tumors, paraneoplastic syndromes (e.g., limbic encephalitis)

Hydrocephalus: normal-pressure hydrocephalus

Trauma: dementia pugilistica

Affective disorders: depressive pseudodementia

Genetic disorders: mitochondrial encephalopathies, Niemann-Pick disease, Wilson's disease, Kuf's disease, Huntington's chorea

Degenerative disorders: Alzheimer's disease, Pick's disease, Parkinson's disease, progessive supranuclear palsy

causes must be closely scrutinized. Finally, the underlying disease causing the dementia not only affects the patient but the caregivers as well. A dementia evaluation is not complete unless issues of short- and long-term management, legal matters, and caregiver stress are addressed.

ALZHEIMER'S DISEASE. Alzheimer's disease is a slowly progressive neurodegenerative disease (i.e., gradual loss of brain cells) in which characteristic histopathologic changes (i.e., senile plaques and neurofibrillary tangles) are found predominantly in the hippocampus, basal forebrain, and temporal, parietal, and frontal association cortices. It is by far the most common cause of dementia. Most patients are over age 65, and the incidence increases dramatically with age. The mean duration of the illness is 8 to 12 years, with the shortest time course being 1 year and the longest 25 years. Death usually results from physical immobility with intercurrent infection. There are three subtypes of initial presentation: (1) memory loss (most common and often seen in the over-65 age group); (2) language impairment (often occurs in the under-65 age group and in familial cases); and (3) visuospatial impairment (presents with deficits in spatial attention and visual perception).

The most common presentation of Alzheimer's disease begins with memory loss. Patients may forget appointments, people's names, where they left an item. As the amnesia worsens, patients develop difficulty finding words, and they make paraphasic errors. They become indifferent, less outgoing, and sometimes irritable. They may have trouble with topographic orientation and get lost when driving, first in unfamiliar surroundings and then in familiar surroundings. Patients lose insight into their deficits and develop problems with calculations,

making decisions, copying, and visuospatial processing. Apraxia is usually evident by the middle stages of the disease. Memory and all other cognitive functions continue to decline. Language impairment continues to progress from anomia to a transcortical sensory aphasia to Wernicke's aphasia and, in some patients, to a global aphasia. Late in the course of the disease patients demonstrate involvement of primary motor, sensory, and visual pathways with evident weakness, spasticity, numbness, and visual field defects as well as urinary and fecal incontinence. Depressive symptoms and depression are common in the early stages. Patients may develop hallucinations (more commonly visual) and delusions (e.g., paranoia, jealousy) at any stage of the disease, although more commonly in the middle stages. The presence of hallucinations, delusions, or parkinsonian features (rigidity, resting tremor, bradykinesia) usually signify a more rapid decline in function. Brain imaging studies (CT, MRI) may show cortical and subcortical atrophy, but the degree of atrophy does not correlate with cognitive function. Patients with Alzheimer's disease are more likely to have evidence of white matter ischemic changes on MRI than age-matched controls.

The drug tacrine has been approved by the U.S. Food and Drug Administration (FDA) for symptomatic treatment of patients with Alzheimer's disease. Tacrine is an acetylcholine esterase inhibitor that increases the availability of acetylcholine at the postsynaptic receptor. The benefit of the drug is mild at best and is associated with frequent elevation of liver enzymes, which requires stoppage of the medication. The medication has no effect on the course of the disease. No other medication is currently approved for treatment of Alzheimer's disease. Treatment should focus on contributing problems, removal of all nonessential medications, consistency in the daily routine and living environment, and emotional and logistical support of the primary caregivers.

PICK'S DISEASE. Pick's disease is a slowly progressive neurodegenerative disease that affects predominantly the frontal and temporal lobes, producing changes in personality, language, and memory. Alterations in personality tend to occur first (disinhibited or abulic), although in some cases a language disturbance precedes other deficits. Memory loss tends to occur later in the course. Patients with Pick's disease can be differentiated from those with Alzheimer's disease by: (1) onset prior to age 65; (2) early personality change; (3) disinhibition; (4) roaming behavior; (5) reiterative speech; and (6) hyperorality (the tendency to explore objects with one's mouth). Brain imaging studies may show prominent focal atrophy of the frontal and temporal lobes. There is no treatment for Pick's disease.

DEMENTIA ASSOCIATED WITH PARKINSON'S DISEASE. Parkinson's disease may be associated with three types of dementia: (1) Alzheimer's disease;

(2) diffuse Lewy body disease, which is clinically similar to Alzheimer's disease but at autopsy these patients have eosinophilic cytoplasmic inclusions (Lewy bodies) throughout the brain; and (3) a "subcortical" dementia. Subcortical dementia refers to a clinical syndrome in which the patient is distractible with poor concentration, forgetful rather profoundly amnesic, abulic, and slow to conceptualize and think; there is relatively normal language but hypophonic or dysarthric speech. Often gait, posture, and movements are abnormal as well. Subcortical dementia may occur with several diseases (e.g., Parkinson's disease, Huntington's disease), but the locus of injury usually extends beyond subcortical sites to cortical sites. The clinical manifestations of subcortical dementia are often observed after damage to the frontal lobe or basal ganglia, thalamus, or their connections.

One difficulty of treating patients with Parkinson's disease who are demented is that Sinemet or dopamine agonist drugs such as bromocriptine and pergolide often exacerbate patients' confusion and behavioral problems while improving their mobility. Often the physician must walk a fine line between maintaining a degree of mobility and creating confusion. This clinical problem is best managed by a neurologist experienced in caring for parkinsonian patients.

STROKE-ASSOCIATED DEMENTIA OR MULTI-INFARCT DEMENTIA. Stroke-associated dementia is the most common cause of dementia after that due to Alzheimer's disease. The hallmark of this disease is the onset of cognitive impairment with stroke. Sometimes there is no history of stroke. In patients without a stroke history, the cognitive impairment usually occurs in steps followed by plateaus. CT or MRI should show at least some evidence of ischemic brain damage. Patients with stroke-associated dementia, on average, have a shorter life expectancy than patients with Alzheimer's disease because of commonly associated coronary artery and other vascular disease. Because both Alzheimer's disease and stroke are common in the elderly, they often coexist. Thus elderly patients may have two factors contributing to their dementia.

The treatment of stroke-associated dementia is the same as for all patients with strokes or TIAs: control of hypertension and diabetes, smoking cessation, and antiplatelet agents.

NORMAL-PRESSURE HYDROCEPHALUS. Normal-pressure hydrocephalus is the clinical triad of a gait disturbance, dementia, and urinary incontinence; there may be parkinsonian features. Hydrocephalus is present with CSF pressures within the normal range (Fig. 48–13). The dementia is similar to other subcortical dementias. Disturbances in gait usually occur first. If cognitive deficits occur initially, the underlying cause is often a neurodegenerative disease. Some of these patients respond to ventricular shunting of the enlarged ventricles.

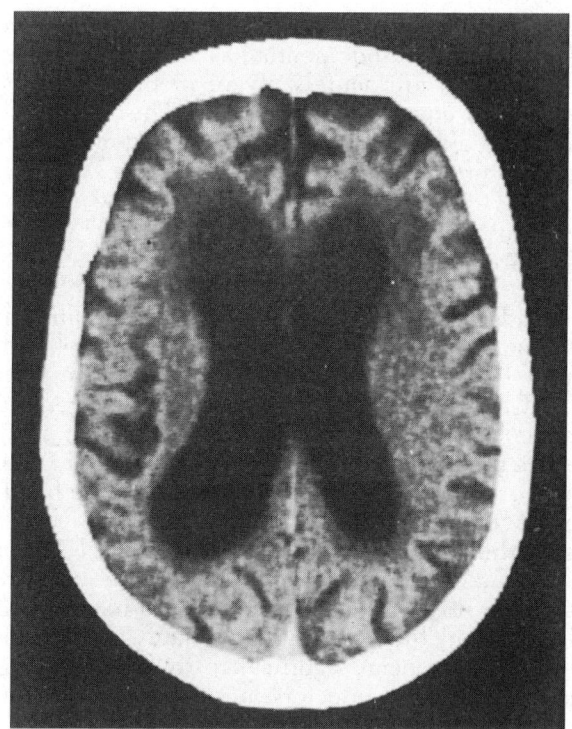

FIGURE 48–13. CT scan demonstrating enlarged lateral ventricles in a patient with normal-pressure hydrocephalus. (From Yock DH [ed]: Computed Tomography of CNS Disease. Chicago, Year Book Medical Publishers, 1985, with permission.)

METABOLIC DISORDERS. Metabolic disorders may produce dementia. Subjects with metabolic diseases may be apathetic, mentally slow, disoriented, somnolent, inattentive, emotionally labile, anxious, agitated, psychotic, and perseverative with dysarthric speech and decreased ability to generate speech. Impaired abstractions, poor memory, and sometimes myoclonus, asterixis, or reflex changes may also be present. Examples include hypothyroidism, vitamin B_{12} deficiency, hepatic or renal failure, repeated hypoglycemia, and medication effects. Treatment of the underlying disease may result in improvement.

DEPRESSIVE PSEUDODEMENTIA. Depressive pseudodementia is a syndrome in which depressed patients exhibit cognitive deficits on testing that respond to antidepressant therapy and are not the result of neuronal loss or brain injury. The disorder is commonly seen in patients with retarded depression and psychomotor slowing. Features of the patient's performance are similar to those seen with subcortical dementias and slowed responses, inattention, forgetfulness, and disturbed abilities to abstract, analyze detail, and elaborate. If errors in performance cannot be explained by poor concentration or lack of effort, the deficits are unlikely to be the result of an isolated depression. Typically subjects with pseudodementia respond with "I don't know" to direct questions including tasks of confrontation naming, or they fail to make or complete a response. In contrast to the degenerative dementias, pseudodementia has a subacute onset, and subjects are acutely aware of their deficits, tending to complain about them. They may also express feelings of guilt and shame and make self-deprecatory remarks.

Headache

Headache is an almost universal symptom, but for many it can become a debilitating problem. From 1980 to 1989, according to the Centers for Disease Control and Prevention, migraine, the commonest disabling headache, increased in prevalence from 25.8 per 1000 persons to 41.0 per 1000. Furthermore, it appears that many migraine headaches remain undiagnosed. In one multicenter headache study, 60 per cent of women and 70 per cent of men in a group of 23,611 migraine sufferers had clear migraine symptoms but had never been diagnosed by their treating physicians. These findings are of special significance to family physicians, who are the doctors most likely to be consulted first by a patient with headaches.

Diagnostic Classification

Headache patients are seen in family practice either between headaches when they want a prescription refilled or during an acute attack when a clear history may be difficult. In both circumstances, a definitive diagnosis may be elusive. Because headache may be a symptom of intracranial disease, the primary goal of the primary care physician should be to differentiate the benign headache from the one with a more serious cause.

In 1988 the International Headache Society (IHS) published a classification and criteria for 129 different types of headache and head and neck pain (Headache Classification Committee, 1988). The IHS classifies headaches into the categories listed in Table 48–5. Each category is subdivided into subtypes that include many types of headache that occur rarely in family practice, making the classification of more value to the headache specialist and

TABLE 48–5.   IHS HEADACHE CATEGORIES

Migraine
Tension-type headache
Cluster headache and chronic paroxysmal hemicrania
Miscellaneous headaches unassociated with structural lesion
Headache associated with head trauma
Headache associated with vascular disorders
Headache associated with nonvascular intracranial disorders
Headache associated with substances or withdrawal therefrom
Headache associated with noncephalic infection
Headache associated with metabolic disorder
Headache or facial pain associated with facial and cranial structures
Cranial neuralgias, nerve trunk pain, and deafferentation pain
Headache, not classifiable

TABLE 48–6.   IHS DIAGNOSTIC CRITERIA FOR MIGRAINE WITHOUT AURA (80 PERCENT OF MIGRAINE)

1. Lasting 4 to 72 hours
2. Two of the following: unilateral location,* pulsating quality, moderate or severe intensity, aggravated by routine physical activity
3. At least one of the following: nausea or vomiting, photophobia, phonophobia
4. At least five attacks fulfilling the first three criteria
5. No evidence of underlying disease

* Typically, the headache is located in one or the other temporal region, but it may also radiate to other areas of the head including the occipital area. The headache may eventually become global. Migraine without aura may also start in the occipital or frontal areas.

researcher than to the family physician. Headaches seen in family practice may be more simply classified into two main categories: primary and secondary. Primary headaches are migraine, tension-type, cluster, and other benign headaches listed in the first four IHS categories. Secondary headaches include all remaining headaches in the IHS classification and are associated with underlying diseases such as meningitis, tumor, hemorrhage, increased intracranial pressure, giant-cell arteritis, and others. Tables 48–6, 48–7, 48–8, and 48–9 list the distinguishing characteristics for each of the primary types of headaches. Table 48–10 lists the causes of secondary headaches. Because some secondary headaches have potentially life-threatening causes, the family physician should be particularly suspicious if any of the headache features in Table 48–11 are present.

In addition to the secondary causes of headache in Table 48–10, other conditions commonly seen in family practice may produce headache: diseases of the ear, nose, and teeth; glaucoma; refractive errors; and squint. Sinusitis of allergic nature causes a sensation of vague discomfort in the nasal, frontal, and periorbital areas. Many patients with common migraine headaches are incorrectly diagnosed as having sinus headaches. Sinus headaches should be accompanied by pain or discomfort when tapping the sinuses and usually are associated with a nasal discharge or stuffiness.

A few causes of secondary headache deserve

TABLE 48–7.   IHS DIAGNOSTIC CRITERIA FOR MIGRAINE WITH AURA (20 PERCENT OF MIGRAINE)

1. Headache similar to migraine without aura but is preceded by at least one of the following neurologic symptoms: visual (scintillating scotoma, fortification spectra, photopsia), sensory (paresthesia, numbness), unilateral weakness, speech disturbance (aphasia)
2. No evidence of organic disease

The neurologic symptoms progress from visual to sensory and fade in reverse order as the headache develops. The aura sometimes occurs without the headache and raises the possibility of a TIA.

TABLE 48–8. IHS DIAGNOSTIC CRITERIA FOR TENSION-TYPE HEADACHE

1. Headache pain accompanied by two of the following symptoms: pressing/tightening (nonpulsating), mild or moderate intensity, bilateral location, not aggravated by routine physical activity
2. Headache pain not accompanied by nausea or vomiting; and photophobia and phonophobia absent or only one present
3. Fewer than 15 days per month without headache
4. No evidence of organic disease

TABLE 48–9. IHS CRITERIA FOR CLUSTER HEADACHE

1. Severe unilateral orbital, supraorbital, and/or temporal pain lasting 15 to 180 minutes, often at night.
2. At least one of the following on the headache side: conjunctival injection, facial sweating, lacrimation, nasal congestion, ptosis, rhinorrhea, eyelid edema
3. No evidence of organic disease

Cluster headache occurs in middle-age men, and attacks usually cluster on a seasonal basis with 3- to 18-month periods of freedom from headache. The headaches of chronic paroxysmal hemicrania are similar in many respects to cluster headaches. However, these periodic unilateral headaches occur more frequently and are less severe than cluster headaches and are more common in women. These headaches respond dramatically to indomethacin.

TABLE 48–10. SECONDARY CAUSES OF HEADACHE

Head trauma
Vascular disorders (e.g., infarcts, TIAs, intracerebral hemorrhage, subarachnoid hemorrhage, aneurysm, arteritis)
High and low cerebrospinal fluid pressures (tumors, pseudotumor cerebri, postlumbar puncture headache)
Substances and their withdrawal (e.g., alcohol, nitrate/nitrite, carbon monoxide, analgesics, ergotamine, caffeine, birth control pills)
Viral and bacterial infections
Metabolic disorders (e.g., hypoxia, hypoglycemia)
Disorder of cranial structures (e.g., cervical spine, glaucoma, acute sinusitis, temporomandibular joint disease)
Cranial neuralgias (e.g., compression of cranial nerves and second and third cervical roots, herpes zoster)

TABLE 48–11. DANGEROUS HEADACHES IN FAMILY PRACTICE

New-onset headache in any patients over 50 years
Increasing intensity of headache after 24 hours from onset
Severe headache in migraine patient reported as "not my usual headache" or "my worst headache ever"
Major change in pattern of headaches
Onset with exertion
Change in cognition, level of alertness, or focal neurologic findings accompanying the headache
Nuchal rigidity
Unaccountable abnormality in vital signs

extra comments. Temporomandibular joint dysfunction is often seen as part of a stress syndrome and may accompany tension-type headaches. However, it is probably overdiagnosed as a primary cause of headache. Teeth grinding (bruxism) or tongue, cheek, or lip biting may be present. Pain worsens later in the day after chewing or talking. Movement of the jaw may be accompanied by noise, pain, or locking of the jaw. The joint may be tender to palpation. A well fitting bite plate used at night often improves matters.

Temporal arteritis or giant cell arteritis can produce unilateral, chronic, severe burning headaches in the temporal area where the artery is often prominent and tender. The syndrome occurs only in the elderly (over age 50) and may be accompanied by the symptoms of polymyalgia rheumatica, jaw claudication, and an elevated ESR. The most worrisome potential problems are ischemic optic neuropathy and, less commonly, stroke. For this reason, the diagnosis of temporal arteritis should always be considered in any elderly patient with a new headache syndrome. Arterial biopsy, which should include an adequate length of the superficial temporal artery, is the only certain means of diagnosis. The treatment of choice is steroids, which should be started whenever the disease is highly suspected, even when the confirmatory biopsy cannot be done for 1 to 2 days.

Benign intracranial hypertension or pseudotumor cerebri is characterized by chronic generalized headaches and papilledema due to increased intracranial pressure that may be accompanied by transient visual blurring and occasional diplopia due to sixth nerve palsy (due to stretching of the nerve). It most often occurs in overweight young women and is associated with pregnancy, steroid use, vitamin A, tetracycline use, and iron deficiency anemia. The most serious cause of this syndrome is a sagittal sinus thrombosis. For this reason, women with this syndrome should undergo an MRI of the brain with MRI venography or cerebral venous angiography. They should then undergo a lumbar puncture to document the degree of intracranial pressure elevation and to rule out any evidence of an underlying inflammatory process in the CSF. The protein level, glucose level, and cell count should be normal.

The most serious complication of this syndrome is optic nerve damage. Patients should have an ophthalmologic examination, including formal visual fields. If the visual fields indicate optic nerve dysfunction, optic nerve fenestration is the treatment of choice. Lumbar-peritoneal shunting is another option to salvage vision if the optic nerve fenestration is ineffective. Otherwise, the pressure elevations are treated with repeated lumbar punctures (draining of large amounts of fluid with a larger-gauge needle), acetazolamide, and a program of weight loss. Tricyclics may also be helpful for treating the headaches.

Headache after head injury usually subsides within a short time but may persist and become intractable even though skull damage is minimal. Such headaches are often accompanied by depression, dizzy spells, and vague muscle aches. Legal matters related to the injury can complicate matters. Early recognition of this condition and securing appropriate supportive treatment such as psychotherapy and physical therapy can help to avoid prolonged disability.

One type of head pain that is often included under the rubric of headache is trigeminal neuralgia or tic douloureux. The head pain consists of lightning-like jabs of pain in the distribution of the fifth cranial nerve, usually in the second or third division of the fifth nerve. The individual pain bouts last only a second or two but may come in volleys and are often precipitated by wind, eating, or touching an affected trigger zone. The neurologic examination is usually normal. Clear demonstration of sensory loss should prompt a search for a structural lesion affecting the fifth nerve, such as a tumor or multiple sclerosis. The cause of this pain syndrome is thought to be pulsation of a vascular structure (artery or vein) on the entry zone of the fifth nerve. All patients should have an imaging study (with contrast) that looks closely at the course of the fifth nerve (ideally an MRI study). Treatment consists in initial medical management with carbamazepine in doses used for seizures. The medication's benefit usually wanes, and a surgical procedure is then required. Surgical options include, among others, a radiofrequency lesion of the ipsilateral trigeminal nerve ganglion or intracranial exploration and separation of blood vessels that are touching the fifth nerve as it enters the brain stem.

Treatment

Although present-day medications have greatly improved headache treatment, nonpharmacologic therapy remains an essential feature of treatment. By keeping a daily diary the patient can identify and eliminate possible trigger factors, develop an insight into the nature of migraine, and create an incentive to make appropriate behavioral changes. Trigger factors include stress, anxiety, and depression; lack of sleep or too much sleep; hormonal changes (alterations associated with menstruation, menopause, estrogen therapy, and birth control pills); certain foods containing tyramine (cheese), phenylethylamine (chocolate), monosodium glutamate (Chinese food), or nitrates (preserved meats); caffeine overconsumption; red wine and beer; smoking; food aromas and perfumes; flickering light and high-pitched sounds; changes in barometric pressure; and travel.

Patients also learn that they must become personally involved in the management of their problem. Feelings of guilt are reduced when a physician explains the underlying pharmacologic nature of their headaches and that their problem is shared by millions of others. Books and audiotapes on relaxation help the patient cope with stress. Depression and headache may be closely related especially in those with intractable headache when the patient complains "no treatment has ever worked." Referral to a psychiatrist should not be delayed if such patients have suicidal thoughts because of their headache.

Drug treatment of headache falls into two categories: acute or abortive treatment for the headache attack and preventive treatment. These treatment categories can be used concurrently. Table 48–12 lists commonly used acute and preventive medications, recommended dosages, and adverse effects.

Over-the-counter analgesics are often self-administered by the patient before seeking treatment from a physician. Overuse may result in chronic daily headache. Nonsteroidal anti-inflammatory drugs (NSAIDs), when used in adequate dosages, can relieve acute migraine. When episodes are predictable, such as with menstrual migraine, these medications are given premenstrually as a prophylactic measure. Long-term NSAIDs should be monitored for reactivation of peptic ulcer disease by occult blood testing and for nephrotoxicity and hepatotoxicity.

Investigation into the role of serotonin (5-hydroxytryptamine, 5HT) in migraine has resulted in the production of the novel drug, the $5HT_{1D}$ agonist sumatriptan (Imitrex). This substance has been shown to be effective treatment for acute migraine in both subcutaneous (6 mg) and oral (100 mg) forms. Headache, nausea, and photophobia begin to be relieved within 10 to 15 minutes, and the maximum response occurs within about 1 hour. The response rate is about 70 per cent, and side effects are minimal. A feeling of pressure in the chest and throat occurs in a few cases. Contraindications are angina, hypertension, epilepsy, and pregnancy. The drug has not been studied in patients under 16 and over 65 years of age. The initial injection should be monitored by a physician. A second injection may be required should the headache return. Concurrent use of ergot preparations is contraindicated. The oral form of the medication is not yet approved for use by the FDA. One disadvantage of sumatriptin is the cost. One injection kit and two doses of drug cost more than $50. For patients with frequent migraines and poor or no insurance, the cost may be prohibitive.

Older, much less expensive, and somewhat less effective, the ergot preparations are available in various forms (suppository, sublingual, and inhalant). Overuse of ergots may lead to peripheral vasoconstriction or ergotism. Nausea associated with migraine or ergot medication may require an antinauseant such as promethazine (25 mg) or metoclopramide (10 mg). Dihydroergotamine (DHE-45) intramuscularly or intravenously after an intramuscular antinauseant is a good treatment for acute mi-

TABLE 48–12.　ANALGESICS AND ABORTIVE AND PREVENTIVE MEDICATIONS FOR HEADACHES

Medications	Dosage	Side Effects
Analgesics		
Aspirin (with/without caffeine)	60 mg q 4 hr	GI distress, dependency
Acetaminophen (with/without caffeine)	500–1000 mg q 4 hr	
NSAIDs		
Naproxen sodium (Anaprox DS)	550–1100 mg/day	GI distress
Flurbiprofen (Ansaid)	100–200 mg/day	GI distress
Ketorolac tromethamine IM (Toradol)	10–60 mg/day	GI distress
Ketorolac tromethamine tablets (Toradol)	10–60 mg/day	GI distress
Narcotic analgesics		
Fiorinal with/without codeine	1–2 tablets	GI distress
Aspirin 325 mg		
Caffeine 40 mg/codeine 30 mg		
Butalbital 50 mg		
Fioricet with/without codeine	1–2 tablets	GI distress
Acetaminophen 325 mg		
Caffeine 40 mg/codeine 30 mg		
Butalbital 50 mg		
Butorphanol tartrate nasal spray (Stadol NS)	1 mg (one spray in one nostril) Add 1 mg in 60–90 min q 3–4 hr as needed	Somnolence, dizziness, nausea/vomiting, dysphoria
Abortive preparations		
Serotonin agonist		
Sumatriptan 1 mg SC (Imitrex)	6–12 mg	Injection site reaction; warm sensation in head; flushing, tingling, pressure in chest/neck
Sumatriptan tablets* (Imitrex Tablets)	100–299 mg	
Ergot preparations		
Ergotamine tartrate Ergostat (sublingual)	2 mg	Nausea, vomiting, numbness, tingling, cramping pains in limbs, dependency
Ergotamine plus caffeine (Cafergot, Wigraine)	2 mg/100 mg	
Ergotamine suppository (Cafergot, Wigraine)	2 mg	
Dihydroergotamine IM	1 mg	
Dihydroergotamine IV (DHE 45)	0.5–1.0 mg	
Antiemetics		
Prochlorperazine (Compazine)	10 mg	Extrapyramidal reactions, parkinsonism, tardive dyskinesia, drowsiness, hypotension
Promethazine (Phenergan)	25 mg	
Chlorpromazine HCl (Thorazine)	10–25 mg	
Metoclopramide (Reglan)	10 mg	
Preventive medications		
β-Blockers		
Nadolol (Corgard)	10–240 mg/day	Bradycardia, hypotension, depression, weight gain, lethargy, bronchospasm, chest pain, insomnia
Propranolol HCl (Inderal LA, sustained released)	40–240 mg/day	
Calcium channel blockers		
Verapamil HCl (Calan, Isoptin)	120–480 mg/day	Hypotension, nausea, AV block, heart failure
Nifedipine (Procardia)	30–180 mg/day	
Diltiazem HCl (Cardizem)	120–360 mg/day	
Antidepressants		
Amitriptyline HCl (Elavil, Endep)	10–150 mg/day	Drowsiness, dry mouth, constipation, weight gain or loss
Nortriptyline HCl (Pamelor)	10–100 mg/day	
Fluoxetine HCl (Prozac)	20–80 mg/day	Sweating, dizziness, headache
Sertraline HCl (Zoloft)	50–200 mg/day	Sweating, dizziness, headache
Anticonvulsants		
Carbamazepine (Tegretol)	Follow serum levels	See text
Valproic acid (Depakene)	Follow serum levels	See text
Lithium carbonate (Lithobid)	Follow serum levels	See text
Ergot preparations		
Serotonin antagonist		
Methysergide maleate (Sansert)	1–8 mg/day	Nausea, weight gain, muscle cramps, peripheral arterial insufficiency, retroperitoneal and pericardial fibrosis

* Not yet available in the United States.

graine. Raskin (1986) and others have shown that repetitive intravenous dihydroergotamine can resolve chronic daily headache.

Narcotic-analgesic combination analgesics, such as those containing barbiturates and codeine should be used only on an intermittent basis for acute attacks. Opiates such as morphine should be used sparingly for headache (as rescue medicine) when all else has failed. Butorphanol tartrate (Stadol) is a nasal spray that has both agonist and antagonist narcotic properties and may be a safer potent analgesic for headache. Patients with a history of alcohol or drug abuse should not be treated with this group of drugs.

Preventive Treatment

Treatment with preventive drugs is required when acute treatment has not produced adequate results. Indications for preventive treatment include prolonged severe attacks, at least two or three incapacitating attacks per month or headache frequency that significantly affects a patient's life, and severe side effects of abortive treatments. Treatment with any agent should start with small doses, progress slowly, and be monitored for side effects. Medication should be maintained at the lowest dose that produces the desired effect. A partial initial response is often recognized as a decrease in severity and frequency of the headaches. Maximum response may require 2 to 3 months of continuous treatment. Alternative preventive medications may be required because of side effects or failure in response. Overuse of analgesics or abortive medication may reduce the effects of preventive medication. Tricyclics and β-blockers have been the most consistently successful preventive therapies.

Preventive medication may be maintained indefinitely. If there is a good sustained response, the medication can be tapered gradually after 9 to 12 months. Nonpharmacologic measures, which are an important addition to preventive management, may be the only treatment available during pregnancy, when drug therapy is best avoided.

Drug-Induced Headache

Drug overuse in headache patients should be suspected in patients who take 100 or more analgesics a month, use combination analgesics containing barbiturates or sedatives more than three times a week, or use an ergot preparation more than twice a week. Overuse can produce a throbbing global chronic daily headache that may be confused with chronic tension-type headache. Increasing ineffectiveness of analgesics results, and withdrawal symptoms including increased headaches appear when the medication is discontinued. The withdrawal symptoms of nausea and headache are often mistaken for migraine by the patient, who then takes more medication. To guard against this condition, all medication should be prescribed

within defined limits. Prescribing records should be maintained and care taken when prescribing medication over the phone.

This condition requires both pharmacologic and behavioral management. Matthew et al. (1990) recommended cessation of the offending agent and treatment with NSAIDs and 1000 mg of valproic acid daily. Raskin (1986) demonstrated that 0.5 to 1.0 mg of dihydroergotamine combined with 10 mg of metaclopropramide for nausea given intravenously at 8-hour intervals for 4 to 7 days can control the condition. Patients using narcotic analgesics should receive valproic acid for 2 weeks before admission to minimize withdrawal effects. During hospitalization patients require counseling to protect against the recurrence of drug overuse. More prolonged behavior modification programs including treatment of the attack with sumatriptan or dihydroergotamine may be required in inpatient units.

Myofacial "Trigger Points" and Headache

Palpation of the neck and shoulder in patients with cervicogenic headache may reveal localized tender areas and, in some cases, tender nodules suggesting myofascial disease. In a group of such patients Jaeger (1989) documented cervical spine disease. Infiltration of the tender area with local anesthetic, steroids, or both produces significant but often temporary relief.

Radiographic Diagnosis for Headache

One major diagnostic question for the primary care physician is when to perform brain imaging. If any of the conditions listed in Table 48–12 are present, the physician should obtain a CT scan of the head with contrast or an MRI scan. Usually, CT is sufficient. CT or MRI is probably not indicated when *all* the following are present in a patient with a headache: previous long-standing identical headaches; normal vital signs, alertness, and cognition; supple neck; no neurologic signs; improvement without analgesics or abortive medications.

Central Disorders of Tone, Posture, and Movement

The motor system provides us the ability to move our arms and legs and to maintain posture under a variety of circumstances. Patients with neurologic abnormalities of the central motor system have lesions located in any of five general areas: cortex, brain stem, spinal cord, cerebellum, basal ganglia (Kandel et al., 1991). A careful neurologic examination of a patient with motor abnormalities helps localize the area or areas of the causative lesion.

Cortex

The cortex has specific topographic distributions for motor neurons. The gyrus just anterior to the

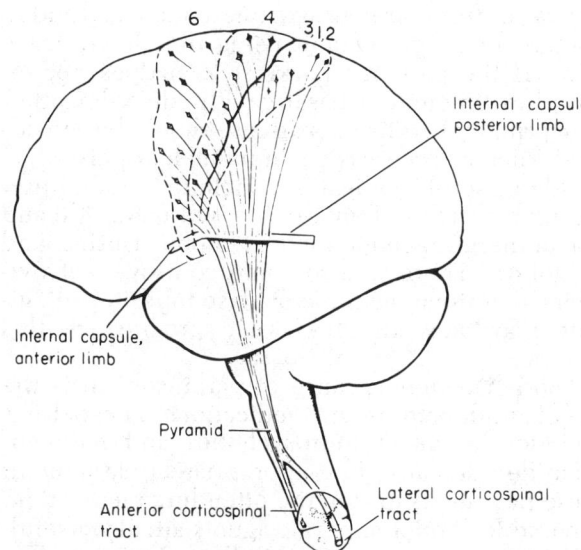

FIGURE 48–14. Course of corticospinal pathways from cortical motor neurons to spinal cord. (From Carpenter MB, [ed]: Core Text of Neuroanatomy, 2nd edition. Baltimore, Williams & Wilkins, 1978, with permission.)

central sulcus, the so-called motor area, has a topographic arrangement wherein the area controlling leg movement is located high on the cortex, the trunk motor area is in the intermediate area, and the arm, hand, face, and tongue areas are located lower in the motor cortical region. This cortical region is the area that controls voluntary movement. Planning for movement involves several other areas of the cortex called the supplementary, premotor, and posterior parietal cortices. This planning requires information from the parietal area about the environment outside the body and the position of various body parts in relation to each other and to the environment. Plotting the range, power, and attitudes of limbs to be moved occurs in the supplementary and premotor cortices.

Commands from the motor cortex are conveyed over two tracts: corticobulbar and corticospinal tracts. Both tracts course through the posterior limb of the internal capsule to the ventral portion of the brain stem (Fig. 48–14). The corticobulbar fibers control the muscles of the head, face, and throat and terminate in the motor and sensory nuclei of the brain stem. The corticobulbar connections to the facial nuclei are bilateral to the forehead area of the nucleus that innervates the forehead muscles, whereas the lower facial muscles are mostly innervated by contralateral fibers. Therefore lesions to one corticobulbar tract or cortical motor area causes weakness of the contralateral lower facial muscles, leaving the forehead muscles spared. Lesions of the peripheral facial nerve cause weakness in the ipsilateral upper and lower facial muscles equally.

After passing through the pons, most of the corticospinal tract fibers cross in the medullary area and enter the lateral column of the spinal cord (Fig. 48–14). Lesions of the motor cortical regions or the corticospinal tract tend to preferentially affect the abductor muscles of the shoulder, the extensor muscles of the elbow, wrist, fingers, and the intrinsic hand muscles in the upper extremity as well as the hip flexors, knee flexors, and foot dorsiflexors in the lower extremity. Thus the classic posture of a patient with a corticospinal lesion is a spastic upper extremity flexed at the elbow, wrist, and fingers and a spastic leg extended at the hip and knee.

Cerebellum

The medial portions of the cerebellum control motor activities of the proximal or balance muscles, and the lateral portions modulate finer movements of the distal musculature. The cerebellum receives sensory input from the spinocerebellar pathways and the contralateral motor cortex and vestibular nuclei. It also receives information about ongoing motor activity from the opposite cerebral motor regions. It exerts its motor influence through indirect connections with the frontal and parietal cortex as well as direct connections with the motor nuclei of the brain stem. The cerebellum adjusts ongoing movements to achieve better balance, if balance is in jeopardy, or adjusts fine coordinated movements to achieve a smoother motor performance. With a lateral cerebellar lesion, a simple finger-to-nose test results in missing the nose (dysmetria), falling short of the nose (hypometria), or overshooting the nose (hypermetria). A tremor appears at the end of the movement, known as a cerebellar intention tremor. The medial cerebellar lesions disrupt the coordination of the trunk muscles leading to truncal ataxia or staggering gait. Titubation or a truncal tremor may be present when the patient sits or stands. The patient's speech loses its normal inflection and rhythm and becomes monotonous and scanning in nature. Oscillatory movements of the eyes or nystagmus may also occur. The abnormalities of coordination in the arm and leg seen with cerebellar lesions occur on the same side of the body as the lesion. In summary, the clinical correlates of cerebellar pathology are incoordinated movements of the extremities, poor control of truncal balance and gait, and incoordination of speech.

Some diseases that diffusely affect the cerebellum include cerebellar alcoholic degeneration, inherited cerebellar ataxias, and paraneoplastic degeneration of the cerebellum associated with certain cancers. The most common structural causes of cerebellar dysfunction include strokes, tumors, and demyelinating disease. Patients with evidence of cerebellar dysfunction should have an brain imaging study to rule out a structural lesion of the cerebellum or cerebellar pathways.

Basal Ganglia

The basal ganglia system is composed of several interacting nuclei including the caudate, putamen, globus pallidus, substantia nigra, and subthalamic nucleus. The caudate and the globus pallidus, known as the striatum, receive input from most areas of the cortex; and their motor output goes through the thalamus to the premotor areas of the cortex. Lesions of the basal ganglia produce abnormal movements, slowness of voluntary movements, increased muscle tone, and loss of postural reflexes. The abnormal movements may be rhythmic, such as a resting tremor, writhing such as in athetosis, rapid such as in the choreiform movements of Huntington's chorea, or ballistic such as in the hemiballism that may be seen after an acute stroke of the subthalamic nucleus.

PARKINSONISM. The most common basal ganglia disorder is parkinsonism, which classically consists of a resting tremor, poverty of movement giving rise to a masked facies or maintenance of a posture for long periods, and rigidity. The tremor of parkinsonism is characteristically most prominent at rest and lessens with action or with sustained postures (e.g., outstretched hands). The normal righting reflexes of the body are also affected, and patients tend to lose their balance. The two most common causes of the syndrome of parkinsonism are Parkinson's disease and the use of antidopinergic medication, such as antipsychotic drugs. Other rarer neurodegenerative diseases (e.g., progressive supranuclear palsy), multiple strokes, brain trauma, normal-pressure hydrocephalus, toxic exposures (carbon monoxide and manganese), metabolic disorders (e.g., Wilson's disease or acquired hepatolenticular degeneration), or inherited disorders (e.g., olivopontocerebellar degeneration) also present with features of parkinsonism. All patients with parkinsonism should have general laboratory screening tests, a detailed family and medication history including past use of antipsychotic medications, and a brain imaging study.

With primary Parkinson's disease, there is a loss of dopaminergic neurons in the substantia nigra of the basal ganglia. Although the disease is slowly progressive, the symptoms of these patients can be considerably ameliorated by giving the neurotransmitter precursor L-dopa. The medication of choice for Parkinson's disease is Sinemet, which contains a combination of L-dopa and carbidopa. Carbidopa inhibits dopa decarboxylase, an enzyme that prevents peripheral metabolism of L-dopa. Sinemet comes in a shortacting and a slow-release form (Sinemet CR). Patients should be started initially at a low dose, for example, one tablet of Sinemet 25/100 twice a day or similar low dosage of Sinemet CR. The dosage should be gradually increased until the patient reports significant improvement to minimize the possible side effects or the medication, such as anorexia, nausea, and vomiting. The medication is adjusted for optimal clinical improvement with minimization of side effects. It is be taken at least a half-hour before meals to ensure its adequate absorption. The usual dosage varies from three to six tablets a day in divided dosages or its equivalent using the slow-release form. If the patient's parkinsonism does not respond to Sinemet, a basal ganglia disorder other than primary Parkinson's disease should be considered, such as progressive supranuclear palsy.

Other useful medications include anticholinergic agents such as benztropine hydrochloride and dopaminergic agents such as bromocriptine and pergolide. There is also some controversial evidence that the monamine oxidase inhibitor selegilene may slow the inevitable progress of this disease.

Another common cause of parkinsonism is the use of antidopaminergic medications. These drugs include the major antipsychotics and metoclopramide (Reglan). The appropriate treatment in these patients is to stop the offending medication, if possible. Anticholinergic agents are also useful.

ESSENTIAL, FAMILIAL, OR BENIGN TREMOR. Essential or familial tremor is a common movement disorder in adults. It is characterized by a tremor of the arms and sometimes the voice and head; the tremor is accentuated by action and sustained postures, such as having the patient hold his or her outstretched hands parallel to the floor. Unlike a parkinsonian tremor, the essential tremor diminishes at rest. Patients often have a family history of "the shakes"—hence the term familial tremor. The tremor can begin at any age and slowly but progressively becomes more marked with age. It is accentuated with emotional or physical stress and is characteristically improved with alcohol. Treatment of a tremor that affects a patient's daily motor functioning can include β-blockers and primidone. Starting doses of these medications, particularly primidone, should be low to guard against side effects.

HUNTINGTON'S CHOREA. Huntington's chorea is a rare but well known central motor system disease that is associated with abnormal extra movements. With this disease there is the onset of choreiform (quick, fluid, dancing-like) movements of the face, tongue, mouth, and extremities during young adulthood (twenties to thirties). These movements are eventually accompanied by progressive behavioral and cognitive changes. The disease is ultimately fatal. Huntington's disease has an autosomal dominant inheritance pattern. The genetic locus of the disease is on chromosome 4, and genetic testing is available for persons who are asymptomatic but have a positive family history. The major management of the disease involves genetic counseling of patients and their families. Incapacitating choreiform movements can be helped with haloperidol.

Disorders of the Peripheral Nervous System

When considering disorders of the peripheral nervous system, one must decide whether the patient has multiple symptoms (weakness with pain and numbness) or pure symptoms, such as weakness only. Because the peripheral nerve and nerve root carry motor, sensory and autonomic signals, the common peripheral nervous system diseases (sensorimotor peripheral neuropathies, compressive neuropathies, and radiculopathies) cause multiple symptoms. Pain is infinitely more commonly seen with peripheral nervous system diseases than with CNS diseases. Rarer peripheral nervous system diseases cause selective symptoms, such as weakness without pain (i.e., myopathies and motor neuron disease) or painless numbness/paresthesia without weakness (i.e., pure sensory neuropathies). EMG is often needed to confirm whether only one modality is affected. For example, with mild peripheral neuropathies, early symptoms are sensory but there may be subclinical motor involvement on needle examination.

The time scale in peripheral nerve system disease is an "order of magnitude" slower than in the rest of neurology. An acute peripheral neuropathy (Guillain-Barré syndrome) progresses over days. A subacute progressive myopathy (myositis) weakens the patient over weeks. Chronic radiculopathies afflict patients with pain for years. Though these diseases advance at slower rates than CNS diseases, patients can die suddenly of respiratory failure if the disease has severely weakened the patient and the treating physician is unaware (or unfamiliar) with the clinical risks. Guillain-Barré syndrome and myasthenia gravis continue to kill even young, otherwise healthy patients. Clinicians specializing in neuromuscular diseases use extreme vigilance and wariness when managing these cases.

Consideration of particular patterns of disease help us construct the most useful differential diagnosis. Bilaterally symmetric symptoms and signs are considered diffuse. In general, diffuse peripheral nervous system diseases affect the lower extremities more often than the upper extremities. Given this predilection, one must guard against missing the less common spinal cord pathology, which also affects the legs preferentially. Spinal cord disease must always be considered when symptoms and signs are restricted to the legs. Bladder and bowel dysfunction is often seen with spinal cord disease and is less commonly part of a peripheral nervous system disorder. Proximal/distal gradients of weakness are also important for determining which part of the peripheral nervous system is the cause of weakness. Peripheral neuropathies weaken distal muscles, myopathies commonly affect proximal muscles, and radiculopathies can affect proximal or distal strength.

Peripheral Neuropathies

Chronic Sensorimotor Peripheral Neuropathies. Symmetric sensory complaints (numbness, tingling, or pain) of both feet are commonly seen with peripheral neuropathies. If there is associated distal weakness, the patient may complain of ankle instability with difficulty walking on uneven ground and a tendency to twist an ankle. Walking in a dark room is impaired if there are problems with proprioception. Older patients who complain of unsteadiness or imbalance may be manifesting a mild peripheral neuropathy in addition to mild visual and vestibular impairment.

The clinical examination for mild peripheral neuropathies shows absent ankle reflexes and absent vibratory sensation at the toes. With advanced peripheral neuropathies there is wasting of foot muscles, and with severe peripheral neuropathies there is wasting of calf muscles and intrinsic hand muscles. With rare exception, peripheral neuropathies affect the lower extremities to a greater extent than the upper extremities. If patients have mild symptoms in the feet and major symptoms in the hand(s), they probably have a mild peripheral neuropathy and superimposed (possibly treatable) mononeuropathies of the arms (see below).

Chronic sensorimotor (usually axonal type) peripheral neuropathies are seen most often in clinical practice, have the broadest differential diagnosis, and are least likely to be responsive to treatment. The onset is usually during mid to late adulthood, and the most frequent identifiable causes in general practice are diabetes mellitus and alcoholism. Thyroid disease, vitamin B_{12} deficiency, vasculitis, Lyme disease, sarcoidosis, and heavy metal intoxication are rare causes of peripheral neuropathy but have great importance for the individual patient because they are treatable.

Guillain-Barré Syndrome. Guillain-Barré syndrome is a rare, potentially lethal acute peripheral neuropathy. Unlike most peripheral neuropathies, the patient complains more of leg weakness than sensory complaints in the feet. Another unusual feature is that the ascending (legs first) weakness progresses quickly over a matter of days. All patients lose their reflexes in the lower extremities, and in most cases of Guillain-Barré syndrome all reflexes are lost. CSF protein elevation is seen 5 to 15 days after the onset of symptoms in Guillain-Barré syndrome. This life-threatening peripheral neuropathy requires hospitalization, as intensive care support may be needed and the treatment (plasmapheresis or high dose intravenous immunoglobulin) is specialized.

Chronic Inflammatory Demyelinating Polyneuropathy. Chronic inflammatory demyelinating polyneuropathy may present as rapidly as Guillain-Barré syndrome, but it more commonly progresses over weeks to months. Weakness is a chief complaint and it usually involves the legs more than the arms. Almost all patient have absent reflexes. These patients have strikingly slowed conduction velocities on EMG nerve conduction studies (a marker of demyelination) and an elevated CSF protein level without pleocytosis. Chronic inflammatory demyelinating polyneuropathy is treatable, but the therapies are complicated (prednisone, plasmapheresis, or intravenous immunoglobulin) and should be managed by a specialist.

RARE PERIPHERAL NEUROPATHIES. Rare peripheral neuropathies include pure sensory neuropathies, pure motor neuronopathies, and "small fiber" neuropathies. Pure sensory neuropathies with subacute onset are seen as a rare paraneoplastic syndrome (usually with small-cell lung cancer), as a complication of chemotherapy (especially *cis*-platinum), or after pyridoxine overdose (vitamin enthusiasts who are looking for a "natural"—but neurotoxic in high doses—diuretic). Pure motor neuronopathies are considered with motor neuron disease below. So-called small fiber neuropathies cause burning distal pain, orthostatic symptoms, and impotence. The most common causes of a small fiber neuropathy are diabetes and amyloid neuropathies. Surprisingly, small fiber neuropathies cause impaired pain (pin) and temperature sensation with preservation of vibratory and light touch sense and reflexes.

HEREDITARY SENSORIMOTOR PERIPHERAL NEUROPATHIES. Hereditary sensorimotor peripheral neuropathies are distinct in that the earliest symptoms and signs appear during childhood and progress insidiously over the years. In mild forms, patients think the numbness and atrophy are unimportant traits "that run in the family." The term Charcot-Marie-Tooth disease is commonly used to mean hereditary, slowly progressive, sensorimotor peripheral neuropathies. In fact, there are many rare specific neuropathies, each defined by their inheritance pattern, clinical picture, neurophysiology, and in some cases specific genetic markers. Despite the fact that many diseases exist where few were thought to exist only a decade ago, no new treatments have been uncovered. These patients should be referred to neuromuscular clinics where they can be accurately categorized as we await the discovery of cures.

Mononeuropathies

Sensory complaints (numbness, tingling, or pain) primarily affecting the hand(s) are most commonly caused by mononeuropathies (i.e., carpal tunnel syndrome, ulnar neuropathy). The *carpal tunnel syndrome* (median neuropathy at the wrist) is the most common mononeuropathy. Patients complain of numbness over the palmar aspect of the thumb and second and third digit, aching in the hand, wrist, or forearm, and a tendency to drop items. Symptoms often worsen with repetitive hand movements, holding onto the steering wheel while driving longer periods, and awakening the patient at night. It is not uncommon for symptoms to fluctuate or even to resolve for months only to return with greater severity and disability.

The median nerve (Fig. 48–15) and finger flexor tendons pass through a canal at the wrist that has bony confines on three sides and a thick restrictive ligament (flexor retinaculum) on the fourth side. Work that requires repetitive wrist rotation while maintaining a firm grip on tools (boning meats, housekeeping work) predisposes to carpal tunnel syndrome. The carpal tunnel syndrome is a common, major cause of disability. If untreated, patients lose the ability to perform fine work due to the lack of sensitivity or, in severe cases, due to the loss of thumb abduction.

On examination there is decreased sensation (pin or two-point discrimination) over the palm side of the second and third digit when compared to the fifth finger. Thenar atrophy and definite weakness is a late sign of severe nerve injury; patients' complaints should be diagnosed and treated well before this sign occurs. Tinel's sign (tingling over the distribution of the nerve with tapping of the nerve over the carpal tunnel) is absent in many patients with carpal tunnel syndrome. Diabetes, thyroid disease, pregnancy, the use of crutches or a wheel chair, and certain arthritic conditions are other causes of carpal tunnel syndrome.

Night-time or full-time wrist splints and steroid injections are often tried but have their best effect in cases where the predisposing factors change (i.e., delivery of a baby, treatment of hypothyroidism). Otherwise, surgery performed by an experienced team is the most effective approach to eliminate pain, stabilize or improve strength, and prevent progressive nerve injury. In cases where management is unclear, the nerve function may be followed periodically with targeted nerve conduction studies to identify ominous trends prior to irreversible damage.

Ulnar neuropathy at the elbow is the second most common mononeuropathy of the upper extremity (Fig. 48–16). Patients often complain of numbness and tingling of the fifth and fourth fingers; aching pain in the elbow, forearm, or wrist; and weakness or clumsiness of the affected hand. Some patients have shallow ulnar grooves at the elbow on a hereditary basis that predisposes to repeated minor trauma or frequent ulnar nerve subluxation. A history of elbow trauma is most often lacking, and occupational causes probably play a secondary role to individual anatomy.

On examination, there is decreased sensation over the palmar aspect of the fifth digit and medial aspect of the fourth digit. Weakness when spreading the fingers and wasting the first dorsal interosseous muscle (seen best on the dorsum of the hand, between the first and second metacarpal bones) is seen in many patients with ulnar neuropathies.

Bending the elbow places stretch on the ulnar nerve (it takes the "long-way-around"). Patients should be advised to avoid prolonged elbow flexion, resting on a flexed elbow, and placing the hand under the pillow when they sleep. Surgical

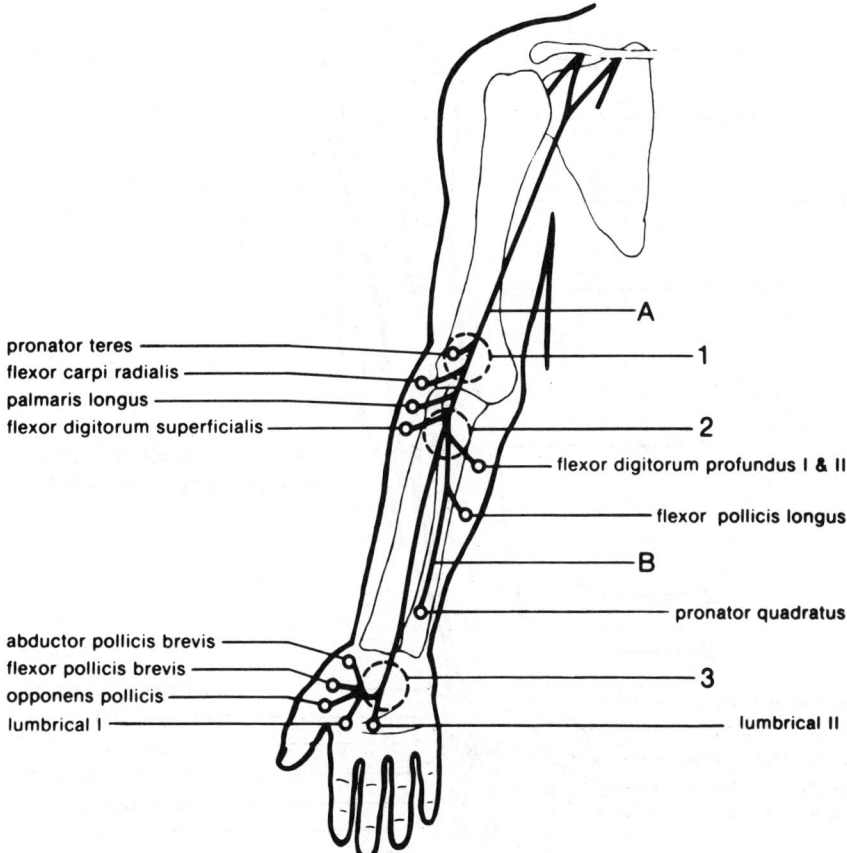

FIGURE 48–15. Median nerve (A) with its branch, the anterior interosseous nerve (B), and the muscles they supply. The nerve may undergo compression at the elbow between the two heads of pronator teres (1), or slightly distally (2) as in the anterior interosseous syndrome, or at the palm (3) as in the carpal tunnel syndrome. (From Kimura J: Electrodiagnosis in Disease of Nerve and Muscle: Principles and Practice, 2nd edition. Philadelphia, FA Davis, 1989, with permission.)

pronator teres
flexor carpi radialis
palmaris longus
flexor digitorum superficialis

A
1
2
flexor digitorum profundus I & II
flexor pollicis longus
B
pronator quadratus
3

abductor pollicis brevis
flexor pollicis brevis
opponens pollicis
lumbrical I
lumbrical II

therapy of the ulnar nerve is more complex than carpal tunnel surgery, and the results are less predictable.

Radial neuropathies usually cause more prominent weakness than sensory symptoms. Weakness in wrist extension and finger extension and normal elbow extension occur with radial neuropathies in the region of the spiral groove. This entity is often caused by prolonged compression due to a variety of causes. Radial nerve compression in the axilla can be caused by improper use of crutches. This problem is distinguished from involvement of the radial nerve at the spiral groove by the presence of triceps weakness. Paresthesias, when present, are located over the dorsum of the hand.

Peroneal neuropathy at the head of the fibula is the most common significant mononeuropathy of the lower extremity. It can occur with habitual leg crossing or leaning the lateral aspect of the leg against a firm object for prolonged periods (e.g., improper positioning during an operation), among other causes. The patient notes a "foot-drop" and varying degrees of numbness over the anterolateral aspect of the leg. If the nerve injury is severe and long-lasting, an ankle foot orthosis can provide excellent ankle stability and greatly improve walking efficiency.

Meralgia paresthetica is abnormal sensation or sensory loss in the distribution of the lateral femoral cutaneous nerve of the lateral thigh. It is due to stretching of the nerve as it courses under the inguinal ligament. This condition is most commonly seen in obese or pregnant patients and usually responds to weight loss or delivery of the baby.

Mononeuritis multiplex describes multiple mononeuropathies. The most common cause is diabetes. Less common, but more important in terms of intervention, are vasculitic neuropathies, particularly polyarteritis nodosa, systemic lupus erythematosus, and Wegener's granulomatosis.

Radiculopathies

Lumbosacral radiculopathies cause leg pain and paresthesias associated with back pain. With more severe radiculopathies, the patient may have specific complaints of weakness: foot slap when walking (L5), knee buckling (L2, L3, or L4), or inability to rise up on toes (S1). More often the severity of pain is the limiting factor with regard to activities. It is important to determine if there is urinary or fecal incontinence or urinary retention, which would be indicative of cauda equina (multiple bilateral lumbosacral roots) or conus medularis (terminal portion of the spinal cord) involvement. Both of these neurologic/neurosurgical emergencies require rapid, specific diagnosis.

Examination of leg muscle strength and reflexes are important for determining management strate-

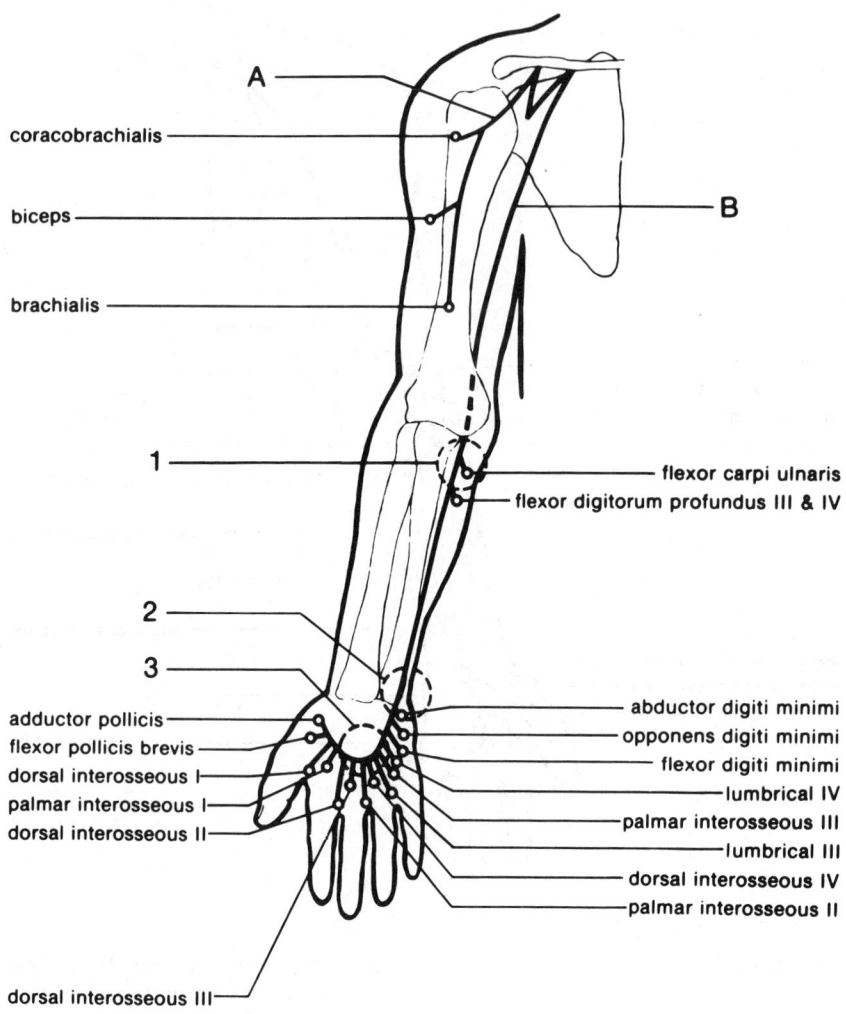

coracobrachialis

biceps

brachialis

A

B

1 — flexor carpi ulnaris
— flexor digitorum profundus III & IV

2

3

adductor pollicis
flexor pollicis brevis
dorsal interosseous I
palmar interosseous I
dorsal interosseous II

abductor digiti minimi
opponens digiti minimi
flexor digiti minimi
lumbrical IV
palmar interosseous III
lumbrical III
dorsal interosseous IV
palmar interosseous II

dorsal interosseous III

FIGURE 48–16. Musculocutaneous nerve (A), ulnar nerve (B), and the muscles they supply. The common sites of a lesion include the ulnar groove and cubital tunnel (1), Guyon's canal (2), and midpalm (3). (From Kimura J: Electrodiagnosis in Disease of Nerve and Muscle: Principles and Practice, 2nd edition. Philadelphia, FA Davis, 1989, with permission.)

gies. Several points bear emphasis: (1) The patient has difficulty or is unable to rise up on his or her toes with S1 radiculopathies, and the ankle reflex is decreased or absent. (2) Severe L5 radiculopathies cause dorsiflexor and hip abductor weakness, but there is no consistent change in reflexes. (3) L2–4 radiculopathies cause a decrease in the knee reflex and weakness when the patient squats on one knee.

Manual muscle testing of leg muscles is difficult because of the remarkable strength of most normal muscles. It is important to use the patient's weight to test leg muscles adequately. Having the patient repeatedly rise up and down on his or her toes (one side at a time) reveals significant weakness that could not have been found with normal manual muscle testing. Likewise, a single leg (half-depth) deep knee bend reveals weakness in the quadriceps muscles that were judged "normal" by normal manual muscle testing. Remember, if you have not overcome a muscle, you have not assessed its maximum strength. Match proximal and distal muscle groups to confirm root involvement: (1) S1 involvement, foot plantar flexor and hip extensor (or knee

flexor) weakness; (2) L5, foot dorsiflexor and hip abductor weakness; (3) L2–4, knee extensor weakness and knee adduction.

Diabetic polyradiculopathy causes severe leg pain and paresthesia usually without back pain. The onset of symptoms occurs typically over several days to a few weeks. Pain is often most prominent at the onset, whereas weakness becomes more prominent as the pain lessens. Quadriceps weakness is common and can cause falls or difficulty climbing steps. Mild to moderate weakness of the ankle dorsiflexor muscles is also often seen.

Malignant (carcinomatous) polyradiculopathy is a rare but ominous cause of back pain and bilateral (often asymmetric) leg pain. Most of these cases appear in patients with a known cancer history who also have spinal metastases.

Cervical radiculopathies cause arm (or shoulder) pain, paresthesias, neck pain, and in severe cases arm or hand weakness. The neck pain is severe, often radiates to the scapular region, and is deep and aching in character. Like lumbosacral radiculopathies, the pain usually overshadows any weakness. Hand paresthesias may occur when the neck, scapular, and arm pain intensifies. The distribution of paresthesias can help localize the affected root: lateral arm in C5, thumb and index finger in C6, middle finger in C7, little finger in C8, and medial arm in T1 root disease. Reflex loss (or decrease) can also localize the affected root: biceps reflex in C5 and triceps reflex in C7. Searching for weakness in certain muscles is useful: deltoids and biceps are weak in C5, wrist extensors and flexors in C6, triceps in C7, finger extensors and flexors in C8, and intrinsic hand muscles (interossei and thenar muscles) in C8-T1 radiculopathies.

Diabetes and Peripheral Nervous System Disease

Diabetes is the most common cause of peripheral nervous system injuries seen in primary care. Diabetes can affect all levels of the peripheral nervous system, including root, plexus, mononeuropathies, and generalized peripheral neuropathy. The most common manifestation of diabetes affecting the peripheral nervous system is a chronic, mild, sensorimotor, axonal-type peripheral neuropathy. It presents as foot numbness and tingling, and it may progress to cause significant wasting and weakness of distal leg muscles and even intrinsic hand muscles. The only known treatment that improves the diabetic peripheral neuropathy is strict control of the serum glucose concentration or pancreas transplantation.

Diabetes can cause a mononeuritis multiplex and or a syndrome like a chronic inflammatory demyelinating polyneuropathy. In both cases the presence of diabetes nearly eliminates the chance of a response to immunosuppressive therapy (i.e., prednisone). Furthermore, the use of prednisone in these patients often plays havoc with diabetes control, and other immunosuppressive medications expose the patients to still higher risk of infectious disease. Because of the bleak risk–benefit picture in patients with diabetes who present with chronic inflammatory demyelinating polyneuropathy and mononeuritis multiplex, the general practitioner should not treat the patients with immunosuppression without involvement of a neurologic specialist.

Mononeuropathies, particularly the median neuropathy of the wrist (carpal tunnel syndrome), ulnar neuropathy of the elbow, and peroneal neuropathy of the head of the fibula are more commonly seen in patients with diabetes than in the general population. If these mononeuropathies are much more severe than the underlying peripheral neuropathy, they respond nearly as well to conventional therapies (i.e., carpal tunnel decompression) as in patients with compressive mononeuropathies without diabetes.

A rather common manifestation of diabetes is a subacute onset of pain involving one or both legs with weakness involving the quadriceps muscles primarily. It may be the manifestation of a mid to low lumbar polyradiculopathy or a lumbar plexopathy. Most often this entity is self-limited and has a delayed, though often incomplete, recovery occurring over the next 6 to 12 months after onset.

Diabetes also causes radiculopathies or polyradiculopathies with more common (L5 and S1) root distributions. In this situation, discogenic causes must be evaluated as well as diabetic causes. Sometimes two processes are active (disk disease and diabetes), and by no means does the presence of diabetes eliminate the possibility of a surgically correctable lesion.

Tests for Nerve and Root Disease

Electromyography should be considered an adjunct to the clinical examination when evaluating patients with presumed peripheral neuropathies. The EMG nerve conduction studies are the best way to categorize peripheral neuropathies as being demyelinating (often treatable) or axonal (less likely treatable). Never order a sural nerve biopsy to make this distinction. In older patients with spondylosis, the symptoms and signs may suggest peripheral neuropathy in a patient with chronic back pain, whereas the EMG shows chronic multiple lumbosacral radiculopathies. This finding obviates an extensive peripheral neuropathy workup. If a patient with a peripheral neuropathy has prominent hand symptoms, the cause is usually mononeuropathies superimposed on a peripheral neuropathies. The EMG can identify if a mononeuropathy is likely to be responsive to treatment (i.e., decompression).

Cervical radiculopathies and mononeuropathies can be difficult to distinguish clinically. In fact, the two commonly coexist. It is important to sort out which symptoms are caused by which process so therapies can be stratified. For example, it would be better to have a carpal tunnel release performed first in a patient with hand paresthesias and forearm and neck pain who has EMG evidence of a severe carpal tunnel syndrome and a mild chronic C6 radiculopathy.

For first-time, acute (less than 4 weeks) lumbosacral radiculopathies, the EMG has little value. If the patient has a reliable strength examination that reveals a root weakness pattern with appropriate reflex changes, the clinical examination is more revealing than the EMG. It may take 4 weeks for fibrillation to develop after nerve injury. In certain common situations, the EMG can help determine how patients can be most safely stratified. In patients with an unreliable or pain-limited (inconsistent or variable) strength examination, the EMG can determine whether prominent weakness is due to severe denervation or poor effort. Patients with previous radiculopathies requiring surgical or prolonged medical therapy may also need EMG studies to distinguish old from new nerve injuries and to estimate the extent of previous damage.

Magnetic resonance imaging of the cervical and lumbosacral regions should be performed in patients with such significant neurologic symptoms or signs that they may be surgical candidates. Critical neurologic deficits include new-onset or progressive weakness; new onset or progressive severe, bilateral leg pain; bladder or bowel dysfunction; or leg spasticity. Patients with a history of cancer must be evaluated carefully to exclude meningeal metastases and epidural cord compression.

Myopathies

Muscular dystrophies cause slowly progressive symmetric weakness that usually affects the proximal muscles first. Patients often complain of difficulty rising from the floor and arising from low chairs or from a toilet seat. Upper extremity weakness is manifested by trouble raising objects over the patient's head. With most muscular dystrophies loss of function progresses gradually over many months or years. The various dystrophies can be distinguished by age of onset, pattern of weakness, associated symptoms, and hereditary pattern.

Duchenne's muscular dystrophy is often diagnosed when affected boys (2 to 3 years old) tend to fall when they try to run. The weakness progresses steadily to the point that the child is wheelchair-bound by age 10 in most cases. Even with excellent supportive care, patients die usually between the ages of 18 to 25. This muscular dystrophy is the most devastating of the common dystrophies. It affects only males (an X-linked recessive pattern). In all cases of Duchenne's muscular dystrophy there is an underlying cardiomyopathy, which is often the cause of death.

Becker's muscular dystrophy is genetically related to Duchenne's muscular dystrophy but is both much milder and more variable. This dystrophy usually appears during the adolescent or young adult years. The typical patient initially has difficulty rising from low positions and eventually has proximal arm weakness. The course of the disease is highly variable. Some patients remain ambulatory for their entire lives, whereas others are wheelchair-bound in their thirties. In some, but not all, cases of Becker's muscular dystrophy there is prominent cardiomyopathy. Surprisingly, the cardiomyopathy and the severity of skeletal muscle disease do not go hand in hand. Cases have been reported where the skeletal myopathy is relatively mild, but the cardiomyopathy progresses to the point of frank heart failure. Another unusual aspect of Becker's muscular dystrophy is that in some cases there is little cardiac or skeletal muscle destruction, but the skeletal muscles are painful. Unlike metabolic myopathies, the muscle pain in these cases is not tightly linked to the exercise intensity. Becker's muscular dystrophy, like Duchenne's muscular dystrophy, has an X-linked recessive inheritance pattern.

Myotonic dystrophy is the most common muscular dystrophy. It usually affects adolescents or young adults, although mild cases may not manifest symptoms until much later in life. The pattern of weakness in myotonic dystrophy is different than the other dystrophies. Distal muscle weakness involving ankle dorsiflexor, plantar flexor, and hand muscles can be seen early in the disease. Often the patients complain of muscle stiffness or incoordination, which is the result of the myotonia (uncontrolled electrical discharges that cause persistent muscle contraction). Facial muscle weakness with ptosis is seen commonly with myotonic dystrophy (Fig. 48–17). Myotonic dystrophy is associated with potentially life-threatening cardiac arrhythmias. Frontal balding, cataracts, mild diabetes, and a blunted personality are seen in varying combinations. This disease has a dominant inheritance pattern.

Fascioscapulohumeral muscular dystrophy, which initially involves proximal shoulder muscles and facial muscles, is a slowly progressive disease. The disease first appears in adolescents or young adults. To make this diagnosis, there should be definite facial muscle weakness, particularly involving the orbicularis oris and orbicularis oculi. Fascioscapulohumeral muscular dystrophy has a dominant inheritance pattern and carries a good prognosis. Two thirds of the patients are still ambulatory by the age of 40, there is no cardiomyopathy, and life expectancy is not reduced.

In the past, *limb-girdle muscular dystrophy* was considered one of the major dystrophies. However, it may represent more of a syndrome than a specific disease. Studies have failed to show sharply defined inheritance patterns. Diagnostic testing advances have shown that many male patients with so-called limb-girdle muscular dystrophy have Becker's dystrophy.

Myositis, the most common muscle disease, causes a painless progression of symmetric weakness over weeks to months. Although the rate of progression is more rapid than that for the muscular dystrophies, the complaints and the pattern of weakness seen in patients with myositis are similar. Most often, there is difficulty arising from chairs, going up and down stairs, and raising the arms over the head to comb or shampoo hair. The difference lies in the speed of progression. The changes that take place over years in muscular dystrophies occur over weeks in myositis. There are three major types of myositis: dermatomyositis, polymyositis, and inclusion body myositis.

Dermatomyositis can affect any age group and sex. The patient has progressive weakness with associated skin rash. A purplish rash around the eyelids is highly specific for dermatomyositis but is unfortunately not the most common rash. More often there is an erythematous, almost sun-burned

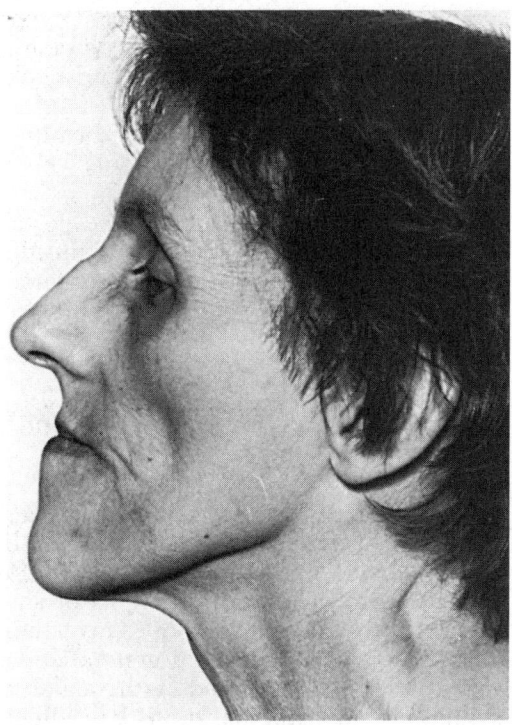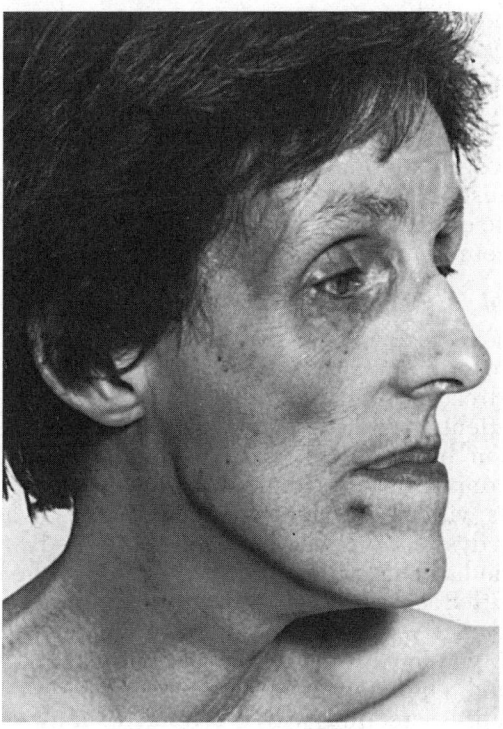

FIGURE 48–17. Patient with the classic facial appearance of myotonic dystrophy. (From Kimura J: Electrodiagnosis in Disease of Nerve and Muscle: Principles and Practice, 2nd edition. Philadelphia, FA Davis, 1989, with permission.)

appearance over the cheeks and over the extensor aspects of the arms, legs, and back. The rash can cause skin breakdown over the knuckles.

Polymyositis manifests as a subacute onset of weakness; there is no skin rash. Sometimes polymyositis is subcategorized depending on whether there is an underlying connective tissue disease or other associated illness. The subcategories are probably not important to remember, as polymyositis and associated diseases are diagnosed and treated independently.

Inclusion body myositis presents with weakness progressing over months. This disease is by far the slowest progressing myositis, in some cases weakness increases over several years. An important distinction between the clinical picture of inclusion body myositis and that of muscular dystrophies is that there is no family history of muscle disease in cases of inclusion body myositis. Inclusion body myositis is also unusual because distal muscle weakness (especially finger flexor weakness) is prominent in some cases.

There have been reports of myositis being associated with occult underlying malignancies. The more carefully this issue has been evaluated, the weaker is the connection. After diagnosing myositis, the malignancy search should follow American Cancer Society screening recommendations that are appropriate for the patient's age and sex. Workup beyond this level is not justified.

Rare muscle diseases have a wide variety of presentations. Metabolic myopathies, for example, cause primarily diffuse muscle pain and secondarily diffuse muscle weakness. Metabolic myopathies, in general, can be categorized as having abnormalities in glycogen metabolism or mitochondrial myopathies. Most myopathies that cause muscle pain have elevations in creatine kinase levels and include myophosphorylase deficiency, phosphofructokinase deficiency, and Becker dystrophy.

Patient Evaluation

Measurement of serum creatine kinase is the most important single test for evaluating patients with muscle disease. All cases of Duchenne's muscular dystrophy and Becker's muscular dystrophy and almost all cases of myositis have significant elevations in the creatine kinase level.

Electromyography is essential for evaluating patients with peripheral nervous system disease. For instance, patients with myotonic dystrophy display myotonic discharges on needle examination. Patients with myositis often exhibit "myopathic" motor unit potential changes and fibrillation when the disease is active. The EMG identifies motor neuron diseases, which also cause slowly to moderately progressive diffuse weakness.

As myopathies or motor neuron disease are relatively rare, these conditions are most accurately and economically worked up by referral to a neuromuscular clinic. The Muscular Dystrophy Association supports a large number of clinics throughout the United States. Muscle biopsies should be performed at neuromuscular clinics. If the biopsy specimen is not of proper size and from the correct location, frozen correctly, and kept from thawing, adequate evaluation may not be possible, and the biopsy must be repeated. It is beyond the scope of this text to discuss specific biopsy findings for the various neuromuscular diseases.

Treatment

There are presently no cures for muscular dystrophy. Some clinicians, however, do use prednisone to treat Duchenne's muscular dystrophy. These patients may have a slowing in the rate of progression, but it is unclear if the overall risks of using prednisone are worth the benefits obtained.

Patients with Becker's muscular dystrophy and myotonic dystrophy have significant cardiac disease. Periodic echocardiographic evaluation of the patient with Becker's muscular dystrophy is important, particularly if symptoms of heart failure are present. Myotonic dystrophy patients can have malignant and potentially life-threatening arrhythmias. Routine screening with electrocradiography for arrhythmias should be performed on a yearly basis. Also patients with myotonic dystrophy should be questioned with regard to symptoms suggestive of syncope, cardiac palpitations, or presyncopal symptoms. Significant conduction blocks are effectively and properly treated with cardiac pacing.

Myositis treatment should start out with a prednisone dosage of 1 mg/kg and the treatment continued for a surprisingly long time. The most common mistake made when treating myositis is to taper the prednisone too rapidly. In general, prednisone is maintained at the starting dose (1 mg/kg/day) for 1 to 2 months and thereafter reduced by 5 mg/day per month. Hence even for the most easily controlled case of myositis, the patient is on a significant dose of prednisone for approximately 1 year. If the patient does not respond to simple treatment with prednisone, additional agents may be needed. Azathioprine (Imuran) is the most commonly used adjuvant at this time. The establishment and modification of treatment programs should always be done in consultation with clinicians specializing in the care of neuromuscular diseases.

Other Considerations

Patients who have neuromuscular diseases should be considered at high risk for adverse operative and perioperative events. Some patients have elevated creatine kinase levels and do not have a clearly categorized muscle disease. In these patients, there should be particular caution with regard to general anesthesia. A proportion of these patients have a condition called malignant hyperthermia, where lethal reactions can occur when potent inhalant anesthetics and depolarizing muscle relaxants are used. Fatal "malignant hyperthermia-like" reactions can occur with other muscle diseases, such as the Duchenne's and Becker's muscular dystrophies.

Anesthetics and sedating medications require special consideration with patients who have myotonic dystrophy. These patients are especially sensitive to sedating medications and postanesthesia recovery may be delayed. An anesthesiologist should be consulted well before surgery, and drug selection should be weighed carefully in these individuals.

Myasthenia Gravis and Myasthenic Syndrome

Myasthenia gravis causes fluctuating, fatigable weakness; and it usually presents with diplopia or ptosis. The second most common manifestation is speech and swallowing problems or shortness of breath. Only exceptionally does myasthenia gravis present with complaints of generalized tiredness without being associated with ocular or bulbar symptoms. Myasthenia gravis can affect any age group. The symptoms can fluctuate initially so that on early examinations the patient complaining of double vision or ptosis may have a normal neurological examination. Symptoms may worsen during the latter part of the day and improve after rest, but this pattern is not a universal finding.

There is a multilevel grading system for myasthenia gravis, but to a large extent this disease can be categorized as ocular myasthenia gravis and generalized myasthenia gravis. The distinction between ocular myasthenia gravis and generalized myasthenia gravis is important because ocular myasthenia gravis carries no measurable mortality rate, whereas the patients with generalized myasthenia gravis are at risk of dying from respiratory failure. Because of the different prognoses, treatment and management strategies for the two types of myasthenia gravis vary somewhat. If speech, swallowing, breathing, or truncal and extremity weakness is documented, the patient is categorized as having generalized myasthenia gravis. Unfortunately, a proportion of patients who eventually are diagnosed as having generalized myasthenia gravis present with purely ocular findings. If symptoms remain restricted to the eyes for 2 years, the disease has a higher than 95 per cent chance of remaining restricted to the eyes for the life of the patient. During the first 2 years after diagnosis, all patients should be considered to have potentially generalized myasthenia gravis and should be instructed to contact their treating physician without delay for any symptoms of deteriorating respiratory function.

The most important initial focus in patients with the diagnosis of myasthenia gravis is to determine if there is any respiratory compromise and if their swallowing difficulty is sufficiently severe to place them at risk for aspiration. It is important to perform pulmonary function tests, particularly those focused on the mechanics of ventilation, early after the diagnosis of myasthenia gravis. If patients have a forced vital capacity that is below 80 per cent of the predicted value, they should be presumed to have generalized myasthenia gravis with at least some compromise of their respiratory strength.

Although Lambert Eaton myasthenic syndrome (LEMS) and myasthenia gravis are both immunologically mediated neuromuscular diseases, the clinical presentations are strikingly different. LEMS causes leg weakness that progresses over weeks to months and never causes ptosis or diplopia. Oddly enough for a neuromuscular disease, the patients also have areflexia. A little more than half of the patients have an underlying (often occult) small-cell lung cancer, whereas the other half have no associated malignancy. Probably 1 to 3 per cent of all the patients with small-cell lung cancer have LEMS. A treatment is now available that reverses much of the weakness and has acceptable side effects.

Diagnosis

Myasthenia gravis may be diagnosed by measuring the serum acetylcholine receptor antibody level. This test is highly specific and fairly sensitive. Among the patients with generalized myasthenia gravis, 80 to 90 per cent have antibodies to acetylcholine receptors. Only 50 per cent of patients with ocular myasthenia gravis have serum antibodies to acetylcholine receptors.

Electromyographic testing with repetitive nerve stimulation and single-fiber EMG for the diagnosis of myasthenia gravis is usually performed at specialty clinics. Neurophysiology testing is particularly important in patients who do not have antibodies to the acetylcholine receptor or who are suspected to have LEMS. However, in terms of prognosis and response to treatment, these antibody-negative patients are indistinguishable from patients with similar symptoms who have elevated antibodies.

Management

Some cases of mild ocular myasthenia gravis may be treated with pyridostigmine (Mestinon), an acetylcholine esterase inhibitor. Most cases of generalized myasthenia gravis, however, do not respond satisfactorily to this medication. In these cases a combination of surgical therapy (thymectomy) and prednisone treatment may be required to achieve complete remission (approximately 60 to 80 per cent of all cases).

The most important primary care consideration in patients with myasthenia gravis is the risk for respiratory failure. In patients with neuromuscular disorders at risk for respiratory failure and death, chest radiographs and arterial blood gas assays do not provide adequate warning. Monitoring the mechanics of ventilation (particularly forced vital capacity) provides the best warning of impending respiratory failure. Patients with myasthenia gravis who complain of shortness of breath should be taken seriously: They should be directed immediately to an emergency room where forced vital capacity and inspiratory and expiratory pressures can be measured. Patients with a forced vital capacity of less than 50 per cent of the predicted value should be monitored overnight in the hospital and evaluated by a neurologist with neuromuscular expertise prior to discharge. Respiratory failure is the most common cause of death for patients with myasthenia gravis. Patients with marginal respiratory function can be returned to normal neurologic function over several days with plasmapheresis. The dramatically beneficial effects of plasmapheresis last several weeks to several months.

Approximately 10 to 15 per cent of patients with myasthenia gravis have underlying thymomas. These lesions, much more common in the elderly, are a locally invasive, though not metastatic, tumor. Thymomas can be missed on regular chest radiographs, and for this reason chest CT scans are essential for properly evaluating patients with myasthenia gravis. In younger patients who do not have thymomas, thymic pathology, usually thymic hyperplasia, is a common finding. Patients with thymic hyperplasia do better with a thymectomy over the long run. The presence of a thymoma is a definite indication for thymectomy. These two factors mean that surgical removal of the thymus gland is a strong consideration for most patients with generalized myasthenia gravis.

Motor Neuron Disease

Patients with amyotrophic lateral sclerosis (ALS) may present with disturbance of speech and swallowing. Unlike those with myasthenia gravis, which is associated with a flaccid dysarthria, patients with ALS and bulbar symptoms usually have a spastic, as well as a flaccid, dysarthria. Spastic dysarthria causes a slow rate of consonant pronunciation. It is not uncommon to think that these patients have had a stroke because their voice is slowed dramatically. ALS does not, however, present with sudden changes in speech as do stroke syndromes. This disease has an insidious onset that progresses gradually over months. As distinct from myasthenia gravis, ALS never causes ptosis or diplopia. These symptoms would automatically lead one to consider myasthenia gravis rather than a progressive motor neuron disease.

Amyotrophic lateral sclerosis can present in several ways. Aside from the slowly progressive spastic and flaccid dysarthria, frequent manifestations are foot drop or hand weakness. These symptoms are usually worse on one side at initial presentation and affect the contralateral side some weeks to months later. ALS is therefore a strong consideration when patients note slowly progressive asymmetric weakness without significant sensory complaints. Also, patients with ALS usually do not have significant pain in the back or neck regions unless they have additional cervical and lumbar spine disease as well. These pain complaints are common in patients with cervical or lumbar radiculopathies who have asymmetric weakness. A certain degree of achiness is not uncommon in the limbs in patients with ALS.

Another important feature seen in most cases of ALS is spasticity and hyperreflexia involving the limbs. The combination of atrophy and spasticity raises the question of a cervical myelopathy (spinal cord lesion) in patients who have bilateral hand and arm weakness and hyperreflexia in the legs. In these cases imaging of the cervical cord must be performed to rule out a structural lesion causing a compressive myelopathy and multiple radiculopathies. An important distinguishing feature in patients with myelopathy as compared to ALS is the presence of bladder and bowel dysfunction. Incontinence is never caused by ALS, whereas it is a common manifestation of myelopathy.

When working up patients with ALS, it is important to obtain an MRI scan of the brain and brain stem if bulbar symptoms are the presenting cause, of the cervical cord region in patients presenting with hand or arm atrophy, and of the lumbosacral region in patients with weakness and atrophy of the leg muscles. An EMG is also helpful in these cases because it can identify the widespread denervation and reinnervation that is characteristic of ALS. Rarely, immunologically based diseases of the motor neuron can imitate ALS. These motor neuronopathies can be distinguished from ALS by finding conduction block on motor nerve conduction studies. This factor is another important reason for performing EMGs in patients with symptoms suggestive of ALS.

Treatment

Although there is no cure for ALS, there is much important care to be given. Most patients live for at least 2 to 3 years and during this time can be helped with a variety of aids. In patients with early-onset swallowing trouble, a gastrostomy tube can provide months of good health and well-being by maintaining good nutrition. Mobility assists allow the patients to leave their homes and keep in touch with life-long interests. Patients have great need of a physician's care as they approach respiratory failure. They require frank discussions as to what a ventilator can or cannot do and what help medications can provide if they decide not to go on a ventilator. The primary care doctor and neuromuscular doctor often work closely to help comfort these patients with this difficult disease.

Infectious and Inflammatory Disorders

The hallmark of the infections/inflammatory diseases is a subacute onset of signs and symptoms. The classic infectious diseases are bacterial meningitis and viral encephalitis. Classic inflammatory disorders include multiple sclerosis and sarcoidosis.

Bacterial Meningitis

Bacterial meningitis is also covered in Chapter 20. The classic features of meningitis are severe headache, fever, nuchal rigidity, photophobia, vomiting, altered mental status, and an ill-appearing patient. Seizures occur in 20 to 50 per cent of patients at some time during the course of the meningitis (Bharucha et al., 1991a). A patient may also manifest signs of generalized sepsis. Bacterial meningitis has a more fulminant course over one to several days. Seventy per cent of meningitis occurs in children less than 5 years of age. Viral meningitis is often less severe and may have a more subacute time course. Tuberculous and fungal meningitis generally has a subacute course of days to weeks.

The three most common responsible organisms in developed countries are *Hemophilus influenza* (most common in young children), *Neisseria meningitidis* (most common in young adults), and *Streptococcus pneumoniae* (most common in the elderly). *Myobacterium tuberculosis* is a common cause in developing countries and more recently in patients with acquired immunodeficiency syndrome (AIDS). Other, less common causes include gram-negative bacteriae, *Listeria monocytogenes* (particularly in immunosuppressed hosts and neonates), group B streptococci (neonates), and staphylococci (patients with head trauma, cranial surgery, and shunts).

Patients with suspected bacterial meningitis should undergo a detailed physical examination to look for potential sources of infection, such as the middle ear, skin, heart, or lungs. The key to diagnosis, however, is prompt lumbar puncture. If a CT scan can be obtained immediately (within 10 minutes) in a patient with suspected bacterial meningitis, it should be done prior to the lumbar puncture to rule out an associated brain abscess. If it cannot and there is no papilledema or focal neurologic findings on examination, the lumbar puncture should be performed without waiting for CT. Antibiotics should be ordered and be started as soon as possible when the diagnosis is suspected.

The CSF cell count, glucose level, and gram stain are the most helpful tests initially because they are available quickly. A low serum glucose level (see section on lumbar puncture) indicates a typical bacterial, tubucular (TB), or fungal infection until proved otherwise. Uncommonly, CSF glucose may be low or low normal in patients with herpes encephalitis, subarachnoid hemorrhage, or sarcoidosis. However, a glucose level near zero almost always indicates a bacterial infection. The CSF cell count in typical bacterial meningitis is usually in the thousands and consists of mostly

TABLE 48–13. PRINCIPLES OF THERAPY FOR BACTERIAL MENINGITIS

1. Treat as quickly as possible, before lumbar puncture results are available.
2. The drug should penetrate easily into the cerebrospinal fluid.
3. A high drug concentration is necessary.
4. If the causative organism is unknown initially, broad coverage is required.
5. Use the appropriate antibiotic.
6. Antibiotics must be given in maximum possible doses intravenously for the full duration of treatment. Two to three weeks are needed for treating group B streptococci and *Listeria monocytogenes*, and 3 weeks for Enterobacteriaceae.
7. Contacts of the patients and the patient with meningococcal or *Hemophilus* infections should receive chemoprophylaxis.

Adapted from Whitby M, Finch R: Bacterial meningitis: rational selection and use of antibacterial drugs. In Bradley WG, Daroff RB, Genichel GM, et al (eds). Neurology in Clinical Practice. Stoneham, MA, Butterworth-Heinemann, 1991, p 1056.

granulocytes. The cell count in TB and fungal meningitis patients is often in the hundreds and comprises mostly lymphocytes. The CSF cell count in viral meningitis is often in the low hundreds or less than a hundred and consists of mostly lymphocytes, although early in viral meningitis a higher proportion of granulocytes may be seen. The glucose level should be normal. Immunosuppressed patients, including those with AIDS, may have a bacterial meningitis with only a mild pleocytosis.

Other tests that may be helpful in the identification of the responsible organism include bacterial antigen immunoassays. These tests can be performed quickly but are not always positive, even in proved cases of bacterial meningitis. Bacterial and viral cultures are useful for determining the adequacy of treatment several days into the course of the illness but do not contribute to early treatment. The physician should repeat the lumbar puncture in cases where the initial results are confusing and to monitor the effectiveness of the therapy.

The principles of treatment are summarized in Tables 48–13 and 48–14. Antibiotic treatment should be accompanied by aggressive life support measures, as appropriate. In addition, there is evidence that intravenous steroids reduce morbidity in children with meningitis. Unfortunately, despite adequate therapy, the overall fatality rate due to bacterial meningitis is 10 per cent, and neurologic morbidity is 20 per cent (Bharucha et al., 1991a). Hydrocephalus and fluid collection in the extra-axial spaces are common sequelae in children. Because hearing loss is not uncommon in children, a formal hearing test should be performed in all children who recover from bacterial meningitis. Viral meningitis (except for that due to herpes simplex or cytomegalovirus) is treated by controlling the fever, hydration, and good nutrition.

Brain Abscess

The clinical signs of brain abscess include a subacute course of headache, nausea, vomiting, altered mental status, and focal findings on neurologic examination. Headache occurs in 75 per cent of patients, and a source of infection is present in 70 per cent (Bharucha et al., 1991a). Nuchal rigidity is seen in one fourth of patients. Lumbar puncture is contraindicated because of the risk of brain herniation. CT or MRI studies with and without a contrast agent should be done quickly. The characteristic CT finding is a ring-enhancing low density region with surrounding edema. In the early stages, only a small degree of central contrast enhancement may be present.

Treatment of brain abscess includes use of the appropriate antibiotic, surgical drainage of the abscess, and treatment of increased intracranial pressures and seizures. The choice of antibiotics is similar to that for bacterial meningitis. Before the organism is identified, broad-spectrum coverage should be used, such as cefotaxime and metronidazole. Infectious disease and neurosurgical consultation should be undertaken promptly. Antibiotic treatment should be continued for at least 6 to 8 weeks. Although the mortality rate is 5 to 15 per cent, 25 to 50 per cent of survivors have sequelae (Bharucha et al., 1991a).

Viral Infections of the Nervous System

Viral infection can affect the meninges (meningitis), brain (encephalitis), spinal cord (myelitis), and nerves (herpes zoster). Viral meningitis is less severe than bacterial meningitis. It is usually self-limited, but it is also a potentially life-threatening disorder. Like meningitis, encephalitis has a subacute course of hours to days. In patients with encephalitis, an altered mental state or focal neurologic findings almost always accompanies the headache and fever that is also seen with viral meningitis. The CSF findings are often similar to those of viral meningitis. Viral encephalitis may have a sporadic cause (e.g., herpes encephalitis, influenza) or an epidemic cause (e.g., the arboviruses). A physician should suspect an arbovirus infection (e.g., La Cross encephalitis) if there is a known epidemic during the late spring, summer, or early fall. However, one should always consider herpes simplex as the cause of a patient's encephalitis because it is treatable, and a delay in treatment may be disastrous.

Herpes encephalitis may present as a subacute personality change over days as an abrupt onset of mental status change over hours. Any neurologic findings or symptoms that suggest involvement of the frontal or temporal lobe make the diagnosis more likely. New onset of repeated partial complex seizures in a patient with evidence of encephalitis on CSF studies point strongly to the diagnosis of herpes encephalitis. The EEG may show charac-

TABLE 48–14. COMBINATION THERAPY FOR EARLY TREATMENT OF BACTERIAL MENINGITIS

Clinical Setting	Organism	Initial Treatment
Newborn to 29 days	Group B streptococcus E. coli L. monocytogenes	Ampicillin + gentamicin *or* Ampicillin + cefotaxime/ceftriaxone
Infants, 1–2 months	Transition between preceding group and subsequent group	Ampicillin + chloramphenicol *or* Ampicillin + cefotaxime/ceftriaxone
3 Months to 9 years	H. influenzae N. meningitidis S. pneumoniae	Ampicillin + chloramphenicol *or* Ampicillin + cefotaxime/ceftriaxone
10–29 Years	N. meningitidis S. pneumoniae H. influenzae	Penicillin + chloramphenicol *or* Penicillin + cefotaxime/ceftriaxone
30 years–59 years	S. pneumoniae N. meningitidis H. influenzae	Penicillin + chloramphenicol *or* Penicillin + cefotaxime/ceftriaxone
60+ Years	S. pneumoniae N. meningitidis Gram-negative bacilli	Ampicillin + chloramphenicol *or* Ampicillin + cefotaxime/ceftriaxone
Immunocompromised host	L. monocytogenes Enterobacteriaceae S. pneumoniae H. influenzae Nocardia asteroides M. tuberculosis	Ampicillin + third-generation cephalosporin + aminoglycoside If *Pseudomonas* suspected, use antipseudomonal penicillin + aminoglycoside For *N. asteroides*, use sulfadiazine or cotrimoxazole. For tuberculosis, see section on tuberculosis meningitis
Skull fracture with CSF leak	S. pneumoniae	Penicillin
Penetrating injury, or depressed fracture	S. aureus Enterobacteriaceae	Antistaphylococcal penicillin + chloramphenicol + aminoglycoside + antipseudomonal penicillin
Shunt infections	S. epidermidis S. aureus Enterobacteriaceae	Antistaphylococcal penicillin + chloramphenicol + aminoglycoside + antipseudomonal penicillin + removal of infected shunt
Other neurosurgery	S. aureus	Antistaphylococcal penicillin

Adapted from Bharucha NE, Bhabha SK, Bharucha EP: Infections of the nervous system: A. Bacterial infections. *In* Bradley WG, Daroff RB, Genichel GM, et al (eds). Neurology in Clinical Practice. Stoneham, MA, Butterworth-Heinemann, 1991, pp 1049–1084.

teristic periodic lateralized epileptiform discharges (PLEDs). The MRI scans show changes consistent with inflammation in the temporal or inferior frontal lobes but may not be positive until several days into the illness. If herpes simplex is suspected to be the cause of the patient's encephalopathy, acyclovir should be started (30 mg/kg/day for 10 days). The question of when to perform a brain biopsy is still controversial, but an argument can be made to defer brain biopsy unless the patient worsens on therapy, has atypical features (e.g., low CSF glucose), or has imaging findings not consistent with the diagnosis (Bharucha et al., 1991b).

Human immunodeficiency virus (HIV) infection frequently involves the nervous system. Presentations may include dementia, myelopathy, or peripheral neuropathy secondary to infection by HIV itself or encephalitis, meningitis, brain abscesses, or myelitis due to secondary infections from immunosuppression. The most common presentation related to primary HIV infection is HIV-related dementia, which occurs in 50 to 75 per cent of AIDS patients in clinical series. Treatment with zidovudine (azido thymidine, AZT) may help improve cognitive status in some patients with early cognitive changes. Any young patient with new-onset dementia should be investigated for HIV infection.

The most common secondary infection associated with AIDS is toxoplasmosis, which affects 28 per cent of AIDS patients (Tucker, 1991). Toxoplasmosis can present as a diffuse encephalitis or as a focal or multifocal brain abscess. The appropriate treatment is pyrimethamine and sulfadiazine; resolution of the brain lesions can be followed on CT or MRI. Other important secondary infections include cryptococcal meningitis; cytomegalovirus encephalitis, myelitis, or radiculitis; progressive multifocal leukoencephalopathy (progressive white matter disease secondary to a papova virus infection); herpes infections; and neurosyphilis (uncommon).

Multiple Sclerosis

Multiple sclerosis is characterized by multiple inflammatory lesions of the white matter in the CNS that result in demyelination (loss of myelin that surrounds axons) or destruction of axons if the inflammatory response is sufficient. The classic clinical definition of multiple sclerosis is a disease that produces multiple lesions of the CNS separated in space and time. In other words, it takes more than one lesion at one location and at one time to attribute a patient's clinical symptoms definitively to multiple sclerosis. For instance, a person with one isolated episode of optic neuritis would not meet the clinical definition of multiple sclerosis. However, if this same person develops a transient myelopathy 2 years later, the clinical diagnosis is much more definite.

Multiple sclerosis can present at any time in life, but the mean age of first symptoms is age 25 to 30; only 15 per cent of patients present after age 55. The most common clinical course is one of alternating exacerbations and remissions, with progressive deterioration in baseline neurologic function over time. Some patients present with a progressive course without remissions, and some may have only a few mild episodes over many years. In one recent population study in Rochester, Minnesota, 53 per cent of patients were working full-time at 15 years from onset; 61 per cent were ambulatory without aids; 39 per cent required gait aids, orthoses, or wheelchair for locomotion; and 62 per cent were driving with no or minor difficulties without the need for hand controls (Rodriguez, 1994).

The most common presenting symptoms are visual (optic neuritis), sensory (abnormal or decreased sensation over part of the face or body), and gait disturbances. However, other presenting symptoms include weakness of an arm or leg, bowel and bladder disturbances, incoordination of the extremities, vertigo or dizziness, diplopia, and behavioral or mild cognitive changes. The hallmark of the disease is the development of signs and symptoms of a focal CNS lesion over days to weeks. Sometimes the progression of a severe focal problem over several days suggests a stroke. The diagnosis of multiple sclerosis should always be considered in any young patient with a stroke-like presentation, particularly if the symptoms progress over several days.

The diagnosis of multiple sclerosis is aided greatly by imaging and CSF studies. The imaging study selected should focus on the part of the nervous system most likely affected as determined by the neurologic history and examination. MRI of the brain or spinal cord with gadolinium contrast is the test of choice in a patient with suspected multiple sclerosis, as it is clearly superior to CT for detecting the white matter lesions associated with multiple sclerosis (Fig. 48–18). CSF testing should be part of the diagnostic evaluation and include cell count, protein, glucose, and special protein studies, such as the IgG index and oligoclonal bands. CSF glucose is always normal in patients with acute multiple sclerosis, and the white blood cell count in the CSF is less than 50 cells in more than 90 per cent of patients. White blood cell counts higher than 50 cells are atypical and should prompt a search for an alternative diagnosis. Oligoclonal bands (two more than in the serum) and an elevated IgG index (more relative production of immunoglobulins in the CSF than in the serum) are consistent with the diagnosis of multiple sclerosis. However, these special protein tests are positive in only 70 per cent of cases. Moreover, other diseases, such as syphilis, sarcoidosis, cancer, and infections, may be associated with an elevated IgG index or oligoclonal bands.

Until 1993 treatment of multiple sclerosis consisted in high dose steroids for acute exacerbations, baclofen (Lioresal) or diazepam (Valium) for excessive spasticity and spasms, physical therapy to prevent contractions and maximize function, and symptomatic treatments such as treatment of urinary tract infections. In 1993, however, subcutaneous interferon β (Betaseron) was approved by the FDA for treatment of multiple sclerosis. This approval was based on a single moderate-sized randomized study that indicated that interferon β decreases the frequency of exacerbations in patients with the relapsing-remitting type of multiple sclerosis. The degree of neurologic disability was not significantly different, however, in the interferon β and placebo groups. The immunologic mechanism by which interferon β decreases the rate of exacerbation is currently unknown. There is a moderate rate of associated side effects, including a flu-like syndrome and pain at injection sites. The medication is also expensive. Because of the expense, side effects, and ongoing controversy concerning its degree of efficacy, treatment should be initiated only by an experienced neurologist.

Sarcoidosis

Sarcoidosis is an systemic granulomatous inflammatory disorder that affects the peripheral or central nervous system in 10 to 15 per cent of patients. The most common presentations include headache, unilateral or bilateral facial neuropathies, optic neuropathy, and diabetes insipidus; but any part of the central or peripheral nervous system may be affected. Patients usually have known sarcoidosis prior to involvement of the nervous system, but sarcoid patients may initially present with isolated neurologic complaints and findings. MRI with gadolinium contrast is the procedure of choice in any patient with suspected neurosarcoidosis. CSF examination should also be performed. A serum angiotensin-converting enzyme assay and chest radiograph should be obtained in any patient with suspected neurosarcoidosis without other systemic manifestations. The treatment of choice is

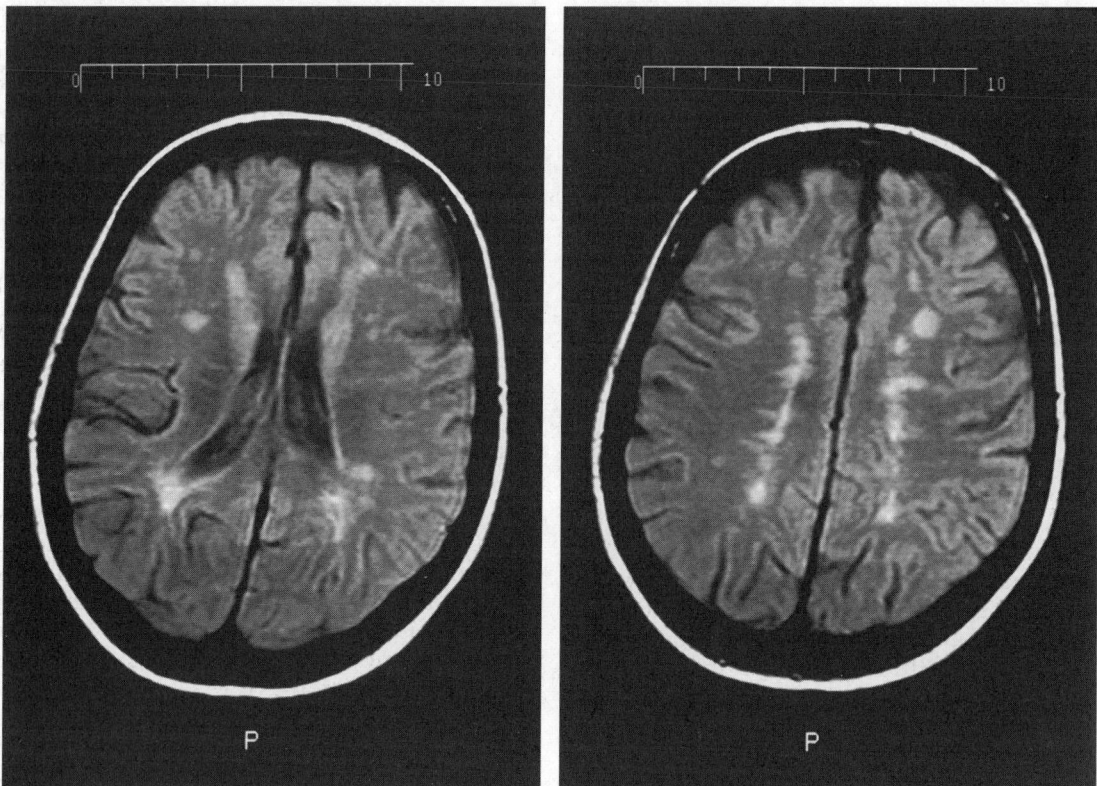

FIGURE 48–18.   MR image of a patient with multiple sclerosis.

high-dose steroids with slow tapering of the steroids after a clinical response. Other immunosuppressive agents are also used in selected patients.

Neuro-oncology

The clinical hallmark of the intracranial or intraspinal neoplasm is a focal neurologic deficit that progresses over weeks to months. Sometimes in slow-growing neoplasms the progression is over years. Three important clinical presentations are an intracranial mass or masses, spinal cord compression, and leptomeningeal cancer.

Intracranial Tumors

One major question the clinician must answer is whether an intracranial neoplasm is benign or malignant; and if it is malignant, whether it is a primary or metastatic tumor. The second question is whether the neoplasm is intra-axial (within the substance of the brain) or extra-axial (arises from tissues surrounding the brain, such as the meninges or cranial nerves). The clinical presentations of extra-axial and intra-axial tumors may be similar in that both may present with headaches, seizures, altered mental status, focal brain dysfunction such as hemiparesis or aphasia, nausea and vomiting, or papilledema. Generally, malignant tumors have a subacute presentation (weeks to several months),

whereas benign tumors have a slower evolution of symptoms. Patients with a suspected intracranial tumor should have a neurologic consultation to investigate the possibility of other diseases that could cause the patient's symptoms and mimic the findings of a brain tumor on brain imaging (e.g., granuloma, acute demyelinating disease, or a brain abscess).

The most common primary intra-axial tumor is an astrocytoma. The astrocytoma may be "benign" pathologically (e.g., grade I or grade II astrocytoma) or "malignant" (e.g., grade IV astrocytoma or glioblastoma multiforme). Other brain neoplasms that originate from the brain tissue itself include medulloblastoma (occurs primarily in the cerebellum in children), primary CNS lymphoma, oligodendrogliomas, mixed gliomas, and ependymomas. Primary brain lymphoma is the most common cause of a brain neoplasm in AIDS patients.

Brain metastases are another common cause of an intra-axial brain lesion and are probably the most common cause of an intra-axial cancer in the population as a whole. The most common sources of brain metastasis are lung cancer, breast cancer, and melanoma. Less common sources include renal, colon, ovarian, and testicular cancer.

Because clinical symptoms do not differentiate between types of brain tumor, clinicians must rely on brain imaging and other diagnostic tests. Characteristics that indicate a malignant intra-axial

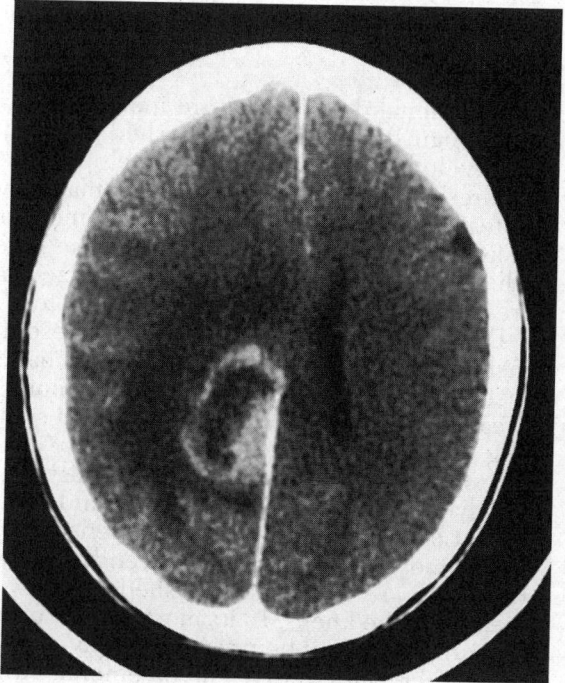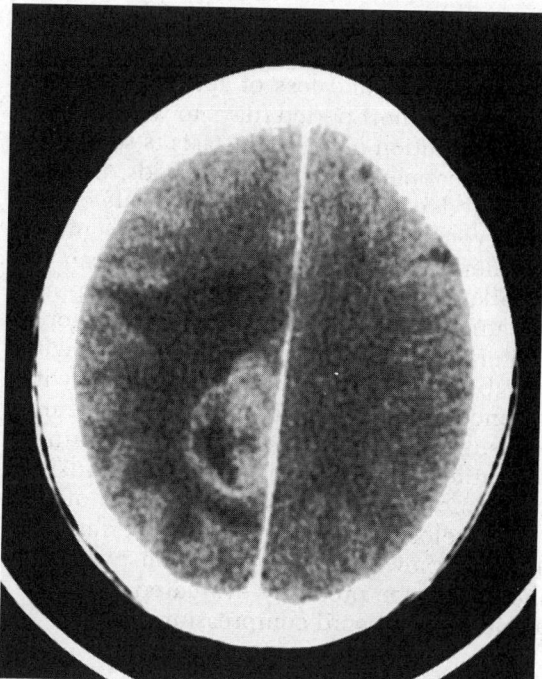

FIGURE 48–19. CT image of a patient with a glioblastoma multiforme.

tumor on brain imaging include marked enhancement of the tumor with intravenous contrast, irregular ring enhancement (Fig. 48–19), and multiple lesions. However, even brain imaging such as MRI cannot reliably differentiate between a malignant glioma, a solitary brain metastasis, or an abscess.

Patients who have a solitary brain lesion without known systemic cancer must have a thorough evaluation for an unsuspected primary cancer including a complete physical examination, mammography, chest radiograph, and stool hemoccult test. If pathologic examination of the removed tumor indicates a metastasis, further evaluation with CT scanning of the chest and abdomen or bone scanning should be done under the direction of an oncologist to look for evidence of other metastases and to identify the primary lesion if possible.

Initial treatment of brain tumors may include high dose steroids if the tumor is associated with marked edema and mass effect. Treatment of low grade gliomas includes surgical removal and possibly radiation therapy. Treatment of high grade gliomas include surgical removal when appropriate, radiation therapy, and chemotherapy in some patients. Treatment of brain metastases depends on the type of tumor. Single metastases are usually removed, followed by radiation therapy, if the patient's systemic cancer is under control. Multiple brain metastases are treated with irradiation and chemotherapy if appropriate.

The three most common extra-axial brain tumors are pituitary adenomas, meningiomas and acoustic neuromas. Pituitary adenomas may present with problems related to hormonal control, such as ga-

lactorrhea in a patient with a prolactinoma. They may also present with visual disturbances due to compression of the optic chiasm or optic nerve by the adjacent adenoma.

Meningiomas, which are thought to arise from arachnoidal elements in the meninges, account for 10 to 15 per cent of all intracranial tumors but are most common in adults after age 50. Because of their slow growth meningiomas may grow to a large size before causing clinical symptoms. Treatment consists in surgical removal when indicated. The meningioma may recur after surgical resection, particularly those located in the base of the skull. Radiation and hormonal therapies are used in selected patients. Small meningiomas without clinical symptoms may be seen incidentally on brain imaging obtained for other indications. These tumors do not need to be removed if there is no accompanying clinical symptoms, but follow-up is necessary.

Acoustic neuromas are discussed in Chapter 23. These tumors are generally benign and by definition involve the eighth cranial nerve. Neurofibromatosis is a dominantly inherited disease that may be associated with acoustic neuromas. Thus patients with a proved or suspected acoustic neuroma, particularly bilateral acoustic neuromas, should have a detailed skin examination for the presence of café au lait spots. Definitive treatment of these tumors is surgical removal.

Spinal Cord Compression

One of the most important syndromes to identify in a patient is spinal cord compression by a metastatic tumor. These patients often present with back pain that may progress to bilateral leg weakness and numbness and loss of sphincter control over a relatively short period (days to weeks). The reason identification of the metastasis is so important is that treatment (high dose steroids, irradiation, surgical decompression in appropriate cases) may preserve neurologic function. If the diagnosis and treatment are delayed until patients can no longer walk, they are unlikely to walk after appropriate treatment. Thus the syndrome of a myelopathy (bilateral leg weakness and numbness with bowel or bladder dysfunction) in a patient with known cancer is a neurologic emergency. Neurologic consultation should be promptly obtained and the patient started on high dose steroids; at the same time imaging of the spine, MRI of the spine, or myelography is emergently performed. Patients with known cancer and new onset of back pain should also be promptly evaluated for possible incipient spinal cord compression.

Leptomeningeal Cancer

Sometimes cancer does not present as a mass of tumor cells but, rather, as dissemination of tumor cells spread throughout the leptomeningeal space surrounding the brain, cranial nerves, spinal cord, and spinal roots. The clinical presentations in these patients is variable and include signs of dysfunction in the cerebral hemisphere (confusion or dementia), cranial nerves, spinal cord, or spinal nerves. It is the frequent involvement of multiple levels of the nervous system in a cancer patient that often suggests this diagnosis. The most common causes of leptomeningeal cancer are leukemia, melanoma, and lung and breast cancer; and lymphoma has a particular predilection for leptomeningeal spread. The diagnosis is made by cytology using large volumes of CSF. Often two or three CSF evaluations are necessary to make the diagnosis. Treatment is palliative with irradiation and occasionally chemotherapy, and the prognosis is poor.

Paraneoplastic Syndromes

Cancer can also affect the nervous system without discrete tumor cells affecting the nervous system but by a variety of mechanisms that usually involve an immunologic cause. These uncommon syndromes are referred to as paraneoplastic syndromes. The most well described syndromes include a cerebellar degeneration usually associated with lung or ovarian cancer in adults, a myoclonic encephalopathy associated with neuroblastoma in children, peripheral neuropathies seen with many types of cancer, and the myasthenic or Eaton-Lambert syndrome, a disease of the neuromuscular junction that may be associated with small-cell cancer.

Deficiency Diseases of the Nervous System

Nutritional deficiencies are important causes of neurologic disease in malnourished populations of undeveloped countries and in developed countries as a result of chronic alcoholism or malabsorption states. The most important and common vitamin deficiencies that affect the nervous system in adults and that are seen in industrialized nations are vitamin B_{12} and thiamine deficiencies.

Deficiency of vitamin B_{12} usually presents with insidious onset of paresthesias of the hands and feet that may be painful (So and Simon, 1991). Weakness, gait instability, and cerebral symptoms (e.g., confusion and mental slowing) are also seen. The neurologic examination classically indicates involvement of peripheral nerves and the spinal cord. Loss of vibration or position sense in the legs is the most common finding. Tendon reflexes at the ankle are usually diminished but may be increased at the knees. In its most severe form, spastic paraplegia may be present, as may signs of dementia or optic nerve involvement. Abnormal laboratory findings frequently include macrocytic anemia, although in some patients it is absent. A low serum vitamin B_{12} level with the appropriate clinical setting is diagnostic. Treatment is with intramuscular injections of vitamin B_{12} 100 μg daily or 1000 μg twice weekly for 2 weeks. This regimen is followed by weekly injections of 1000 μg for another 2 to 3 months. If a Schilling test demonstrates malabsorption of vitamin B_{12}, the patient should be placed on lifelong intramuscular maintenance therapy. Response to therapy depends on the previous duration of the disease, but most patients can expect at least some improvement.

Thiamine deficiency can result from inadequate intake (most commonly due to chronic severe alcoholism) or malabsorption. The acute manifestation of thiamine deficiency is Wernicke-Korsakoff syndrome. The clinical triad of Wernicke encephalopathy includes confusion, involvement of eye movements (nystagmus or lateral gaze impairment), and gait instability or ataxia. Most patients also present with signs of acute alcohol withdrawal including delirium, tachycardia, tremor, and sometimes seizures. Daily treatment with 100 mg of intravenous thiamine usually results in prompt improvement in the eye abnormalities and mental status. The gait improves more slowly, and patients are often left with some degree of short-term memory loss. Resulting severe impairment in short-term memory is referred to as Korsakoff syndrome and may be permanent.

ACKNOWLEDGMENTS

The authors thank Dr. Robert Albright and Ms. Susan Lannon for their helpful comments and Ms. Joan Mohlman for her assistance in the preparation of the manuscript.

REFERENCES

Albert ML, Goodglass H, Helm NA, et al: Clinical Aspects of Dysphasia. New York, Springer-Verlag, 1981.

Bharucha NE, Bhabha SK, Bharucha EP: Infections of the nervous system. A. Bacterial infections. *In* Bradley WG, Daroff RB, Fenichel GM, et al: Neurology in Clinical Practice, Vol. II. Boston: Butterworth-Heinemann, 1991a, pp 1049–1084.

Bharucha NE, Bhabha SK, Bharucha EP: Infections of the nervous system. B. Viral infections. *In* Bradley WG, Daroff RB, Fenichel GM, et al: Neurology in Clinical Practice, Vol. II. Boston, Butterworth-Heinemann, 1991b, pp 1085–1097.

Broderick J: Heart disease and stroke. Heart Dis Stroke 2:357, 1993a.

Broderick JP: Stroke and cerebrovascular disease. *In* Barclay L (ed): Clinical Geriatric Neurology. Philadelphia, Lea & Febiger, 1993b, pp 177–194.

Caplan LR: Stroke: A Clinical Approach, 2nd edition. Boston, Butterworth-Heinemann, 1993.

Commission on Classification and Terminology of the International League Against Epilepsy: Proposal for revised clinical and electroencephalographic classification of epileptic seizures. Epilepsia 22:489, 1981.

Commission on Classification and Terminology of the International League Against Epilepsy: Proposal for classification of epilepsies and epileptic syndromes. Epilepsia 26:268, 1985.

Cummings JL, Benson DF: Dementia: A Clinical Approach, 2nd edition. Boston, Butterworth-Heinemann, 1992.

Daube J, Reagan TJ, Sandok BA, et al: An Approach to Anatomy, Pathology, and Physiology by Systems and Levels. Boston, Little, Brown, 1986.

Edmeads J: Challenges in the diagnosis of acute headache. Headache 30(suppl):537, 1990.

Headache Classification Committee of the International Headache Society. Cephalalgia. 7(suppl):1, 1988.

Jaeger B: Are (cervicogenic) headaches due to myofacial pain and cervical spine dysfunction? Cephalalgia 9:157, 1989.

Kandel ER, Schwartz JH, Jessell TM: Principles of Neural Science, 3rd edition. New York, Elsevier, 1991.

Lipton RB, Stewart WF, Celentano DD, et al: Undiagnosed migraine headaches. Cephalalgia 11(suppl):89, 1991.

Matthew NT, Kurman R, Perez F: Drug induced refractory headache: clinical features and management. Headache 30:634, 1990.

Mayo Clinic and Mayo Foundation: Clinical Examinations in Neurology. Philadelphia, WB Saunders Company, 1976.

Mohr DN: The syndrome of paroxysmal positional vertigo: A review. West J Med 145:645, 1986.

Plum F, Posner JB. The Diagnosis of Stupor and Coma, 3rd edition. Philadelphia, FA Davis, 1980.

Raskin N: Repetitive intravenous dihydroergotamine as therapy for intractable migraine. Neurology 36:995, 1986.

Rodriguez M, Siva A, Ward J, et al: Neurology 44:28, 1994.

Smith R: Chronic headaches in family practice. J Am Board Fam Pract 5:589, 1992a.

Smith R: Refining the diagnosis and treatment of migraines. J Fam Pract Recertification. 14:12, 27–48, 1992b.

So YT, Simon RP: Deficiency diseases of the nervous system. *In* Bradley WG, Daroff RB, Fenichel GM, et al: Neurology in Clinical Practice, Vol. II. Boston, Butterworth-Heinemann, 1991, pp 1167–1184.

Strub RL, Black FW: The Mental Status Examination in Neurology, 2nd edition. Philadelphia, FA Davis, 1988.

Tucker T: Infections of the nervous system. C. Central nervous system manifestations of human immunodeficiency virus infection. *In* Bradley WG, Daroff RB, Fenichel GM, et al: Neurology in Clinical Practice, Vol. II. Boston, Butterworth-Heinemann, 1991, pp 1098–1106.

Weintraub S, Mesulam M-M: Mental state assessment of young and elderly adults in behavioral neurology. *In* Mesulam M-M (ed): Principles of Behavioral Neurology. Philadelphia, FA Davis, 1988, pp 71–123.

CHAPTER 49

SEXUAL HEALTH CARE BY THE FAMILY PHYSICIAN

CHARLES E. DRISCOLL

This chapter provides information to assist the family physician in delivering preventive and therapeutic care for patients troubled by sexual concerns. American sexuality has been reshaped by numerous forces, such as "free love", nude encounter groups, the new sexually transmitted diseases, and a commercialized, televised glitziness that sets an impossible standard for most to follow. During the 1990s there are many who are dealing with insecurity and conflict in their lives that centers on their sexuality. Helping patients to renegotiate an acceptable sexual adjustment for themselves is consistent with the goals of prevention and wellness common to the comprehensive practice of family medicine.

Sexual aberration or depravity is not within the realm of this discussion; rather everyday problems that affect most people are discussed. The key to successful sexual counseling is to attain comfort when speaking with patients about sexual matters so that nothing brings a look of shock to the face of the physician, nor is judgment intoned into his or her voice. With the human immunodeficiency virus (HIV) epidemic as yet unchecked, the primary care of sexual problems must always include a search for high risk sexual behaviors. Figure 49–1 provides a guide for working toward solutions to common sexual concerns. A solid basic knowledge of human sexual anatomy and physiology and effective relationship counseling skills are all that are necessary for the level of expertise required to initiate helpful interventions.

COMMON SEXUAL CONCERNS

Natural Response Cycle

The complete sexual response cycle can be divided into the following phases (American Psychiatric Association, 1987).

1. *Appetitive:* fantasies about and a desire for sexual activity.
2. *Excitement:* a subjective sense of pleasure and the accompanying physiologic changes. The major change in the man consists of penile tumescence leading to erection and the appearance of Cowper's glands secretion. The major changes in women are generalized vasocongestion in the pelvis, vaginal lubrication, and swelling of the external genitalia. The orgasmic platform is developed, that is, the narrowing of the outer third of the vagina by increased pubococcygeal muscle tension and vasocongestion, vasocongestion of the labia minora, breast tumescence, and lengthening and widening of the inner two-thirds of the vagina.
3. *Orgasm:* peaking of sexual pleasure with release of sexual tension in rhythmic contraction of the perineal muscles and pelvic reproductive organs. In the man, this stage is preceded by the sensation of ejaculatory inevitability, which is followed by emission of semen caused by contractions of the prostate, seminal vesicles, and urethra. In women orgasm is accompanied by contractions of the outer third of the vagina, although the contractions are not always subjectively experienced. Both men and women experience generalized muscular tension, contractions, and involuntary pelvic thrusting.
4. *Resolution:* a sense of general well-being and muscular relaxation. Men are physiologically refractory to further erection and orgasm for a period of time. In contrast, women may be able to respond to additional stimulation almost immediately.

The natural sequence typically develops out of desire and proceeds through phases of arousal and plateau (excitement), orgasm, and resolution. The length of time spent in the different phases of the sequence varies greatly from individual to individual, from one sex to the other, and from one occasion to another in the same person (Fig. 49–2).

On a physiologic level, the human sexual response is as natural a function as breathing or digestion. However, the cycle is sensitive to interference by what the individual thinks or feels. Inhibitions of clinical significance may occur at one or more phases in the response cycle.

Psychosexual Dysfunctions

Sex with a partner is the most intimate and vulnerable form of human communication because it

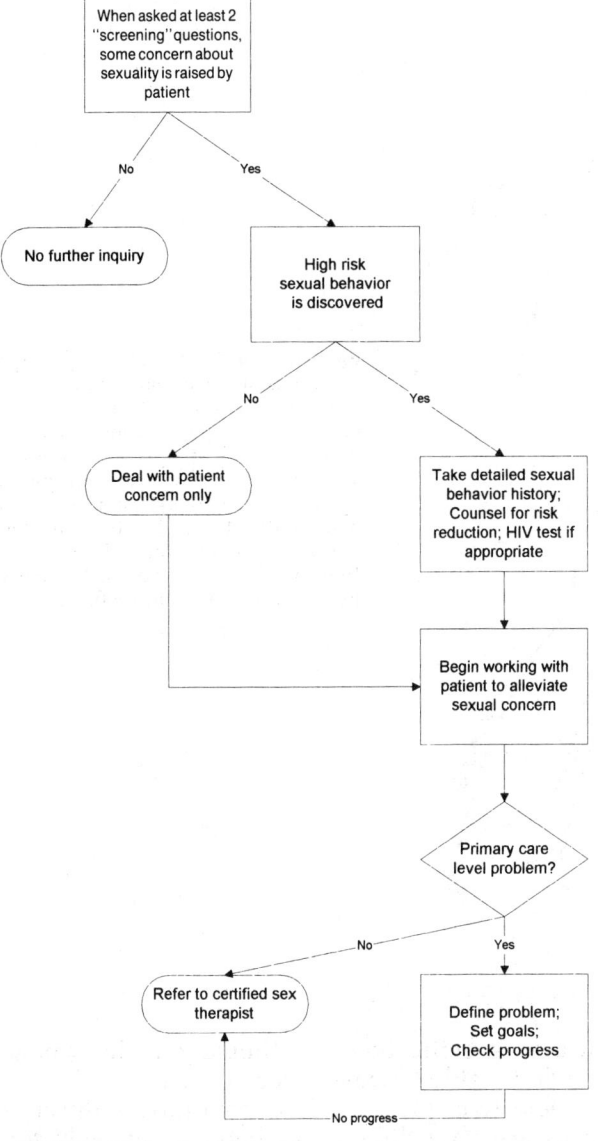

FIGURE 49–1. Sexual problems: primary care approach.

tors that contribute to the problem. In the relationship, there may also be physical factors, such as the lack of opportunity because of a separation due to illness or traveling. When the couple gets back together again, they must go through a period of adjustment. Adverse emotional factors include the conspiracy of silence, withdrawal from sexual contact, failure to express feelings, and perhaps a lack of affectionate touch. Interactional factors include power struggles, hurt and hostility, and perhaps a trade-off between control over money versus control over sex.

Performance anxiety is most commonly responsible for sexual dysfunction. When fears concerning sexual performance dominate a relationship, either or both of the partners sacrifice spontaneity and become careful observers of their own sexual behaviors, sometimes called "spectatoring." As they watch and measure their sexual response and look for physical signs of excitement, the experience ceases to be naturally occurring. The individual becomes unable to focus on pleasurable sensations, and the couple, instead of relating to each other in a warm and spontaneous way, becomes two actors attempting to carry out roles they expect of themselves. Unfortunately, spectatoring usually confirms the worst fears, short-circuiting the natural response. When both partners have previously been functional and performance anxiety is of short duration, the family physician may help by asking for a ban on intercourse and prescribing sensate focus exercises for nondemand pleasuring (Barbach, 1976). Encourage the couple to gently caress and pleasure each other in graduated stages, first by general body caressing and later genital caressing, but insist on the absence of pressure to go ahead to intercourse so there is time for the natural excitement response to return.

Eventually, when both partners feel secure in this exercise, the ban on intercourse is lifted. When one or both members of the couple have long-lasting problems with performance anxiety or deep-seated conflicts about closeness, intimacy, and pleasure, the couple needs more than this level of therapy, and referral to a qualified sex therapist who can devote more time to helping them work out their problems is indicated.

Disorders of Desire in Both Sexes

Inhibited sexual desire is the most common sexual complaint and is expressed as a problem by 30 to 40 per cent of patients seeking help for sexual problems (Kaplan, 1979). It may be a primary condition based on the individual's temperament (some people are simply at the asexual end of the continuum) or upbringing (which might have resulted in a fear of experiencing sexual pleasure). Secondary disorders of desire grow out of repeated disappointment and frustration during sexual en-

involves the sexual value system and self-esteem of two people. It requires the meshing of two sets of expectations, two sets of fears, and two sets of potential problems with communication. Sexual activity is supposed to be pleasurable, but sometimes it seems like a miracle that people ever manage to enjoy themselves. When a patient or couple present with complaints of sexual dysfunction, there is no uninvolved partner. Each person contributes to and is affected by what happens in the sexual relationship. It is not helpful to accept the statement of one partner that it is "all my fault." In fact, the superior stance of the "normal" partner may be part of the problem. The couple's relationship should be the focus of therapy, with collaboration between the partners to determine the desired outcomes. In either partner, there may be physical factors, psychological factors, and situational fac-

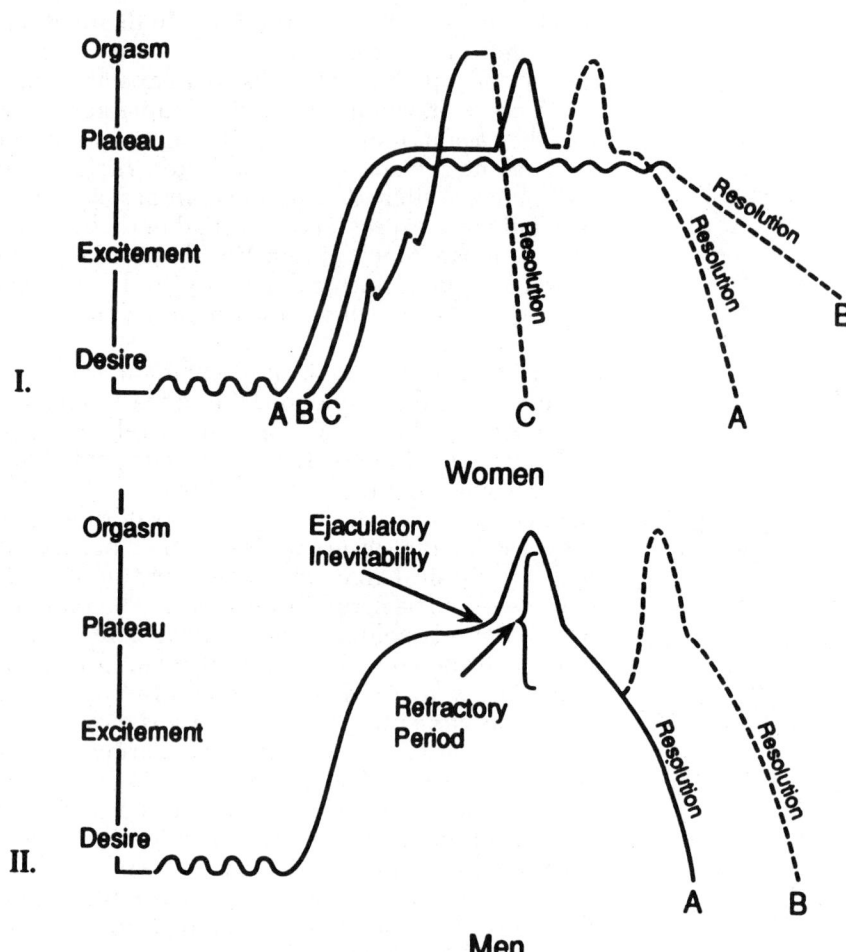

FIGURE 49–2. I. Three common variations of the sexual response cycle in women. A = arousal to one or more orgasms. B = pelvic congestion syndrome. C = "stuttering" pattern of arousal to rapid orgasm and resolution. II. A = arousal to orgasm. B = second orgasm after the end of the refractory period. (Adapted from Masters WH, Johnson V: Human Sexual Response. Boston, Little, Brown, 1966.)

counters, anger toward the partner, or fear of abandonment. Unless they are associated with readily identifiable conditions, such as anxiety, depression, problems with hygiene, or drug use, desire disorders are difficult for the family physician to treat with brief therapy and therefore merit referral.

Excitement Disorders in Women

General sexual dysfunction is a condition in which the woman derives slight or no pleasure from sexual stimulation. Erotic feelings and desire are not experienced; the typical physiologic signs of arousal (lubrication and development of the orgasmic platform) do not occur. These women are frequently anorgasmic but not necessarily so. Lack of pleasure in the experience is the key to diagnosis. These women rarely seek sexual activity of their own accord and may report experiencing irritation rather than pleasurable sensation on being touched. This may be a primary or secondary condition, absolute (with all partners), or situational (under specific conditions and with certain partners but not with others). Occasionally, with a partner of a different race or a different social class, or

with a specific type of stimulation, the woman might be able to experience arousal.

Objective evidence of this condition in the clinical situation is difficult to obtain. A sexual history can help to differentiate whether the condition is due to psychological conflict about sexual activity or about the particular partner or if there was inadequate sexual experience necessary to develop a natural response pattern. This condition may also result from repeated frustrating, unsatisfactory, or painful experience with sexual activity, so the body has simply "given up" trying to respond. Cases in which the woman has been able to become aroused in the past are associated with a better prognosis. The family physician can encourage the couple to place a ban on intercourse and to take part in the sensate focus exercises described previously. If the couple has attempted these exercises without any feeling of progress or if the couple has resisted doing the exercises, it would be wise to refer them to a sex therapist.

Excitement Disorders in Men

Excitement disorder in men is characterized by primary or secondary erectile dysfunction. It is estimated that 50 per cent of men have some period of erectile dysfunction during their lifetime (Kaplan, 1979).

Primary erectile dysfunction (never having been able to achieve erection sufficient for intercourse) is rare. In the absence of congenital, acquired physical, or endocrine factors, a psychogenic cause is most likely. Severe sexual anxiety may be related to religious beliefs, homosexual orientation, or traumatic failure at first coital attempts. It may occur in conjunction with vaginismus in a sexually anxious and inexperienced couple, producing an unconsummated marriage. The problem is of such complexity that referral to a sex therapist is appropriate.

Secondary erectile dysfunction is much more common, and transient episodes are considered normal. Fatigue, preoccupation with work, overeating, or drinking too much can easily cause a temporary problem. Because society puts enormous value on the man's ability to become erect, a single failure can produce performance anxiety that precipitates recurrences, establishing a pattern of dysfunction. If a man experiences erectile problems in 25 per cent or more of coital opportunities, the condition is defined as secondary erectile dysfunction (Masters and Johnson, 1970). It is important to assess the man for organic factors such as diabetes, circulatory inadequacy (atherosclerosis or venous insufficiency), lowered testosterone production, overuse of alcohol and nicotine, and drug use before concluding that a patient's erectile dysfunction is psychogenic in origin. Fifteen years ago it was believed that about 15 per cent of cases of erectile failure were organic; however, now that new technologies have improved diagnosis, the organic versus psychological causes are thought to be 75: 25. In most "psychological" cases of erectile failure, some organic factor can usually be identified as an initiating event. When the sex history suggests an organic cause for the dysfunction (e.g., vascular 50 per cent; endocrine 6 to 45 per cent; diabetes 2 to 20 per cent; drugs 2 to 25 per cent and neurologic 2 to 8 per cent) treatment for the specific cause should be instituted. All patients with a purely organic cause also have some degree of psychogenic potentiation of the disorder.

When the diagnosis of erectile failure is indeterminate or needs confirmation, erection capability can be tested by measuring nocturnal penile tumescence with sophisticated electronic equipment in a sleep laboratory. Two strain gauges on the penis (base of shaft and just below the glans) are used to check for normal nocturnal erections that cause an increase in circumference of more than 15 mm at both gauges. If it occurs, the erectile dysfunction is probably psychogenic (Baum, 1989). The family physician may make this determination using a commercially available product (Snap Gauge; Dacomed Corp., Minneapolis, MN), which measures erections by the breaking of several plas-

tic membranes that snap at different degrees of rigidity. Vasculogenic erectile failure can be suspected by measuring the penile systolic blood pressure via a Doppler probe. A penile artery pressure that is 70 per cent or less of brachial artery pressure suggests vascular insufficiency. This state can be confirmed by cavernosography, an invasive vascular radiographic study of penile circulatory adequacy. Performance anxiety and negative partner response may be a part of organic erectile failure as well. Therefore treatment may need to focus on the psychological as well as the organic components of the problem.

The treatment plan begins with a ban on intercourse, and the couple is instructed in nondemand pleasuring exercises. A man with erectile failure typically is so concerned with his partner that he does not readily allow himself to share in the pleasurable feelings. When asked how he feels about being caressed, a typical response is, "I don't think she likes doing this." The male needs to focus on himself and to let his partner feel and speak for herself. Many sexually dysfunctional people misread each other's nonverbal communication and tend to define their partner's reaction erroneously as negative. He fails to understand that the partner could enjoy touching his penis and so frequently does not allow the partner to fondle it.

A condition that may be confused with psychogenic impotence is the *external iliac steal syndrome* (Wagner and Green, 1981). The patient may achieve an almost normal erection but is not able to maintain it after coitus is initiated, particularly in the "missionary" position. Some patients may experience gluteal pain soon after their erection disappears. The condition is caused by restricted blood flow to the lower limbs and pelvic area. Measurement of penile blood pressure is a method frequently used to diagnose this condition. Angiography may be necessary to demonstrate stenosis or occlusion of the penile arteries. Surgical intervention is the treatment of choice for many of these men. For others, assurance that their condition has an organic basis, combined with instruction about alternative sexual activities or relief from performance anxiety, may be sufficient.

For the treatment of organic erectile dysfunction, mechanical aids to be tried include suction devices that draw blood into the penis and sustain erection by a constriction applied to the base of the shaft (Osbon ErecAid), and by external devices that can be worn to enhance rigidity (Synergist Erection System). Yohimbine hydrochloride blocks α-adrenergic receptors and is occasionally able to restore erectile function in cases of partial failure. Various vasoactive drugs (papaverine, phentolamine, prostaglandin E) have been utilized for intracavernosal injection of the penis. Blood flow into the penis increases by relaxing the smooth muscle in the spongy erectile tissue. A caveat about injection therapy is to expect some degree of fibrosis to develop in the shaft of the penis due to repeated needle injections. Prolonged erection (priapism) has also been noted as a complication of injection therapy. There are now multiple penile implant devices that offer an improvement over the perforated acrylic rods first used in 1960. The device has been continually modernized since 1973 when intermittent erections were accomplished with use of the Scott Inflatable Prosthesis.

The partner of a man with erectile dysfunction tends to be bewildered, blame herself, or attribute the man's erectile problems to: "He doesn't love me anymore." "I'm not attractive to him." "He's punishing me." "He must have another sexual partner." Although any of those factors may be involved, often they are not. The woman is disappointed, hurt, angry, frustrated, concerned, or possibly relieved, depending on how she feels about sexual activity. The family physician should determine what feelings are involved, allow their ventilation, and, if appropriate, help the couple begin to reinstitute successful communication with each other.

Orgasmic Phase Disorders in Women

Orgasmic dysfunction refers to the inability to experience orgasm after sexual stimulation. The stages of desire, excitement, and often plateau are experienced, but the woman is unable to break through into orgasm. This condition may be primary, secondary, or situational.

With *primary orgasmic dysfunction* (or primary anorgasmia), the woman has never experienced orgasm by any means, including self-stimulation, partner stimulation, fantasy, or dreams. However, when the woman's sex history is explored carefully and some descriptive assistance given, she may realize that she has, in fact, experienced orgasm, though not necessarily involving genital touching: for example, the little girl who has learned to squeeze her thighs together rhythmically and repeatedly while sitting in school and has experienced a rising, bubbling sensation in her genital area that is pleasurable and induces her to repeat this experience over and over. Any experience of orgasm precludes the diagnosis of true primary anorgasmia.

With true primary orgasmic dysfunction the physiological response pattern is underdeveloped or inhibited. For whatever reason, the woman has not learned to stimulate herself to orgasm, and she has not established her own reflex-response pattern to transfer to her partnership. When repeated arousal to the plateau level has taken place without orgasm, the woman tends to become frustrated at a certain point in the response cycle, and arousal is lost. The woman may begin to avoid the disappointment and physical discomfort of unrelieved pelvic congestion by avoiding sexual contact alto-

gether. The woman may not feel free to allow herself to reach orgasm because of negative content in her sexual value system, such as a prohibition against touching genitalia or the strong admonition to keep sexual feelings under control so as to avoid pregnancy or misuse by the man.

Research indicates that one effective treatment for primary anorgasmia is the use of directed masturbation exercises (Barbach, 1976; Heiman et al., 1976). It is not uncommon to encounter considerable firm resistance on the part of the woman who is being encouraged to utilize this technique. Yet she must, at her own pace, learn how to engage in self-exploration and lower her resistance. It is essential for her to assume responsibility for seeking and utilizing effective sexual stimulation, avoiding the common but erroneous belief that the man is responsible for "giving" her an orgasm. The woman first learns what kinds of stimulation are effective for her and then must be willing to teach her partner.

A negative body image often accompanies primary anorgasmia, and the woman is to look at herself nude in a mirror in the privacy of her home and carefully assess her feelings about each part of her body. She should note the correctable problems she sees and decide if it is worth the effort to correct them. Those that are uncorrectable must be accepted. Counsel the husband and wife together, suggesting the use of the guided-caress exercises and providing a prescription of reading for both partners (Barbach, 1976; Heiman et al., 1976). Their problem can perhaps be overcome with a relatively brief period of office counseling, but if resistances seem too high or the problems too pervasive, referral to a sex therapist is indicated.

With *secondary orgasmic dysfunction*, orgasm has been experienced in the past but is no longer. This condition may arise from decreased time and attention to courting as a preliminary to intercourse: "A kiss of the lips, a touch of the breast, and dive for the pelvis disease" (Masters and Johnson, 1970). Fatigue, the stress of raising young children, preoccupation with careers, and the allocation of too little time for intimacy are the most common contributing factors.

This problem is easiest to treat if it is discovered and dealt with before frustration, anxiety, and negative feelings have grown and before avoidance patterns have developed. Help the couple to discuss the problem openly; transmit information about the human sexual response cycle and development of the orgasmic platform; teach that sexual interaction need not cease with the man's orgasm and ejaculation; give permission to the woman to explore her own sexual sensations and to allow them to come into her partnership. If no progress is being made after several follow-up office visits, referral is indicated.

Situational orgasmic dysfunction refers to the occasional experienced orgasm, perhaps only with

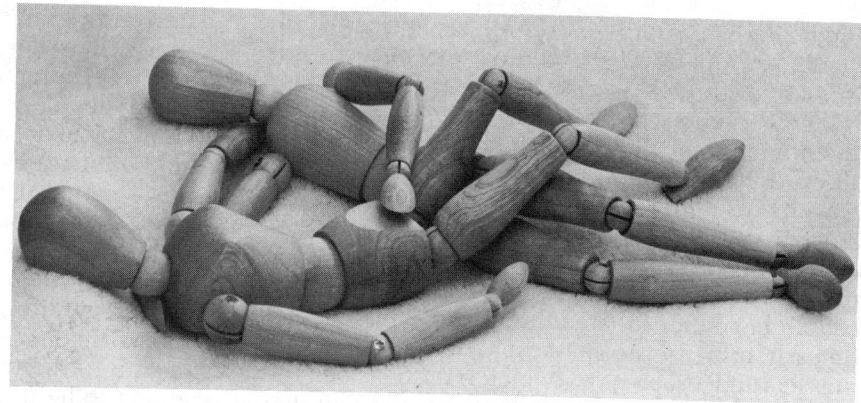

FIGURE 49–3. In this position, the man lies on his side and the woman lies on her back with both legs over his legs or with one leg over his side and the other leg between his legs. Both partners are supported by the bed, and the woman's breasts, abdomen, and clitoral area are accessible for additional stimulation. This position is useful for sexually dysfunctional couples and during advanced pregnancy or during times of illness or fatigue.

certain kinds of stimulation (for example, with self-stimulation but not with partner stimulation). Many authorities believe that this variation of female sexual response is normal.

The couple may be shown the special position that provides the greatest degree of access to the clitoral area while the penis is within the vagina (Fig. 49–3). It is a restful position for both partners. Intercourse can continue for a long time without strain, continued clitoral stimulation can easily be given by the man to his partner or by the woman to herself, or a vibrator may be used. Once the woman has had several successful experiences with orgasm in this fashion, she is usually able to utilize other positions. The man should be informed that a number of women benefit from continued clitoral stimulation during intercourse in order to reach orgasm, and that his partner can teach him how she likes to be touched in order to accomplish their mutual goal.

Orgasmic Phase Disorders in Men

The terms orgasm and ejaculation have traditionally been used interchangeably to describe the male experience of climax. Orgasm, however, can occur without ejaculation (some men in fact learn to have multiple orgasms), and ejaculation can occur with little or no sensation of pleasure or relief. Most notably this situation occurs when the man ejaculates before erection. These cases require referral.

Premature ejaculation is typified by the male becoming erect and ejaculating either just before intercourse or quickly after insertion. Contemporary society places too much emphasis on the importance of simultaneous orgasms, and so this situation becomes a problem for the man's self-esteem and for the woman's sexual satisfaction. In the past, premature ejaculation has been attributed to the presence of psychopathology or hostile feelings toward women. Now it is understood that control of the ejaculatory reflex is largely a matter of conditioning based on learning from early experiences.

The adolescent boy who learns to masturbate rapidly to ejaculation develops a rapid response pattern. Early experiences at intercourse where there is fear of discovery or the practice of ejaculating in the underwear during heavy petting sessions are precursors for difficulty in ejaculatory control.

The best treatment is a retraining process involving both partners whereby the man is encouraged to assume a passive role and to focus on his own sensations. After general body caressing the woman sits facing the man between or astride his legs and begins gentle manual pleasuring of his genitals to bring him erect. As he becomes aroused he thinks of a scale from 0 (no arousals) to 10 (the point of ejaculation). He analyzes his sensations of arousal and signals his partner as he approaches 7 or 8 on that scale (before the point of ejaculatory inevitability). At his signal the woman performs the *squeeze technique*, placing her thumb on the frenulum of the penis and her first and second fingers just above and below the coronal ridge on the opposite side of the penis. She may use both hands. She firmly grasps the penis for a count of ten so that the man's sense of ejaculatory urgency diminishes. His erection may or may not also diminish. Pleasuring resumes until he signals her again. This procedure is repeated three times per session; he is allowed to go on to ejaculation the fourth time. The couple is encouraged to repeat this exercise for two more sessions during week 1; during week 2 the use of a lubricant is introduced to approximate the feeling of being inside the vagina. The sessions are repeated as before.

As the man feels more confident with his ejaculatory control, the couple may next use the *stuffing technique*. They use the squeeze technique once but sufficiently to allow the penis to lose its erection; the man's flaccid penis is then stuffed inside the vagina with use of the female astride position. The female remains motionless until her partner gets used to being inside the vagina, then she begins to move slowly until he becomes erect. When he reaches the point he has learned to identify, he lets her know, and she disengages and uses the squeeze technique. This procedure of stuffing and squeezing is prescribed as three repetitions, with the fourth repetition proceeding to orgasm, and it is done for three sessions.

When vaginal containment can continue for about 5 minutes without ejaculation, the couple is allowed to initiate intercourse, using thrusting movements and allowing the man to ejaculate intravaginally. Whenever the man feels a need for assistance with ejaculatory control, he can ask his partner to use the squeeze technique again. If the couple has been separated for awhile, it is sometimes helpful to resume sexual activity by using this learned procedure. A pictorial and clear description of this procedure can be recommended for the patient's reading (Vandervoort and McIlvenna, 1972).

In place of the squeeze technique, other versions of treatment involve the *stop–start maneuver*, in which the couple simply stops moving when the man feels close to ejaculation. He then focuses thoughts on a distraction, such as a simple math problem, and rests until his desire to ejaculate is diminished.

Because the passive role for the man and the active role for the woman may be unfamiliar and anxiety-provoking to the couple, support and encouragement from the physician, as well as explicit instruction in procedures, are important. Make this treatment a playful and pleasurable exercise. When a good relationship exists between the couple, the woman often reports that she obtained considerable sexual arousal and a great deal of pleasure from giving to the man and assisting him in learning ejaculatory control. Because anorgasmia and premature ejaculation are a common combination, the treatment is a helpful experience for both partners.

When obtaining a sex history, it is not uncommon to discover that a man with secondary erectile failure has a history of premature ejaculation. The erectile dysfunction is treated first, and the ejaculatory control is dealt with later. The squeeze technique which includes body caressing and nondemand genital stimulation, may be the best treatment for both conditions.

As men become more willing to discuss their sexual practices, it appears that a number of men experience retarded ejaculation or difficulty ejaculating, particularly as they grow older. This problem should not be confused with retrograde ejaculation, which may result from diabetes, medications, or prior surgery. Anxiety about this normal development may cause even further difficulty and in some cases leads to erectile dysfunction. Some men report that they fake ejaculation on occasion in order to be able to stop the sexual interaction with which they have become tired or bored. If the man continues to pressure himself to ejaculate, performance anxiety tends to interrupt the natural response.

A small percentage of men are unable to ejaculate intravaginally—usually a primary condition. Some of these men can ejaculate with masturbation in private; others can ejaculate with manual or oral, but not coital, partner stimulation. A few are unable to ejaculate with any kind of stimulation. In a number of cases the condition is secondary to the use of drugs (Table 49–1). There are also many cases of psychogenic origin based on rigid religious beliefs, rejection of the spouse, severe hostility and negative feelings, homosexuality, or anxiety in regard to producing pregnancy.

Because the female partner is called upon to participate in the treatment of this disorder, it is important to help her understand the etiology of the dysfunction and to deal with any of her own hostility or distrust that has developed around this issue. The caress activities are employed to heighten the man's awareness of his physical sensations and to improve communication, particularly nonverbal communication patterns between the couple. The pressure to perform is eliminated. When genital pleasuring takes place, the woman stimulates the man's penis in the way he finds most arousing with the objective of producing ejaculation manually. The next step is to continue the sex play, keeping the man at a high plateau stage of arousal with the woman in the female astride position. As she excites him to the highest possible level of arousal before ejaculation, she then inserts the penis into the vagina rapidly, continuing penile stimulation with her hands if necessary or with her vaginal muscles. If ejaculation does not occur, the woman dismounts and continues manual stimulation until reinserting the penis at the point of ejaculatory inevitability (Kolodny et al., 1979). Often only one episode of intravaginal ejaculation is needed to reverse the dysfunction. If success is delayed, referral to a sex therapist is the best alternative.

Resolution Phase Disorder in Men

Priapism may result from systemic disease (sickle cell disorder, leukemia, metastatic cancer) or drug use (cocaine, papaverine, trazodone, and other psychoactive drugs; several antihypertensive agents; tolbutamide). Treatment should be emergent to provide detumescence of the erection, but eventual management is aimed at the underlying medical condition that triggers this abnormal response. Emergent treatment consists in aspiration of the corpora with a large-bore needle. Irrigation of the corpora with saline or 10% heparin solution may also be needed.

Vaginismus

The female dysfunction known as vaginismus is not easily classified according to the physiologic response cycle model and is considered separately.

TABLE 49–1. DRUG EFFECTS ON SEXUALITY

Drug	Desire (Libido)	Excitement (Erection/Lubrication)	Plateau (Delay of Orgasm)	Priapism	Orgasm (Ejaculation/Orgasm)
Hormones					
Androgens	↑	↑	–	*	↑
Progestins	↓	–	–	–	↓ M
Estrogens	↓ M ↑ ± F	↓ M	↑ M	*	↓ M
Corticosteroids	↓	–	–	–	Infertility
Cyproterone acetate	↓	↓ M	↑ M	–	Infertility M
Antihypertensives					
Spironolactone	↓	↓ M	–	–	–
Prazosin	–	↓	–	*	–
Diuretics	↓	↓	–	–	–
Methyldopa	↓	↓	↑	–	↓
α-Blockers (clonidine)	↓	↓	–	–	↓ Retrograde
β-Blockers (propranolol)	↓	↓	–	–	–
Guanethidine	↓	↓	↑	–	↓ Retrograde
Enalapril	–	↓	–	–	–
Hydralazine	–	–	–	*	–
Reserpine	↓	↓	–	–	↓
Nifedipine	–	–	–	*	–
Verapamil (others)	–	↓	–	–	–
Psychoactive agents					
Benzodiazepines	↓	↓	–	–	↓
Buspirone	–	–	–	*	–
Phenothiazines	↓	↓	–	*	↓ Painful
MAOIs	↓	↓	↑	–	↓
Fluoxetine	↓	–	–	–	↓
Tricyclics	↓	↓	↑	–	↓ Painful
Clomipramine	↓	↓	↑	–	↓ Painful
Lithium	↓	↓	–	–	–
Alcohol and sedative-hypnotics	↑ Low doses ↓ High doses	↑ ↓	↑ ↑	–	– ↓
Trazodone	–	↑	–	*	–
Stimulants	↑ Low doses ↓ High doses	↓	–	–	↑ ↓
Anticonvulsants	↓	↓	–	*	–
Miscellaneous					
Antihistamines	↓	↓	–	–	–
Cimetidine	↓	↓	–	–	Infertility M
Antiparkinsonian agents	↑ M	–	–	–	↓
Digoxin	↓	↓	–	–	–
Anticholinergics	–	↓	–	–	–
Omeprazole	–	Painful	–	–	–
Thyroxine	↑	–	–	–	–
Disulfiram	–	↓	↑	–	–
Timolol	↓	↓	–	–	–
L-Tryptophan	↓	↓	–	–	–
Ephedrine	–	–	–	–	↑
Naproxen	–	↓	–	–	↓
Clofibrate	↓	↓	–	–	–
Metoclopramide	↓	↓	–	–	–
Cocaine	–	–	–	*	–

↑ = enhanced/increased/shortened; ↓ = inhibited/decreased/lengthened; – = unknown/uncertain effect; M = male effect only; F = female effect only; * = documented effect; ± = variable effect.
Modified from The Medical Letter 34(876):74–76, 1992.

Vaginismus refers to involuntary spastic contraction of the muscles of the outer third of the vagina, occurring reflexively in response to imagined, anticipated, or real attempts at penetration. Vaginismus should be suspected from the sex history if the woman describes difficulty with tampon insertion, profound fears of pelvic examination, or inability to insert a diaphragm, contraceptive foam applicator, or vaginal suppository. This condition can effectively prevent intercourse, but it does not preclude orgasm for the woman. Many women with vaginismus are orgasmic with masturbation or oral stimulation by their partner. The most common presenting complaint is "no sex life."

Determine if the couple enjoys mutually pleasurable activities other than intercourse. The couple's self-esteem rises if they are, by a definition other than intercourse, having sexual activity with each other. Identifying the couple as sexually active with a problem that is usually treatable tends to be motivating.

Vaginismus may be a primary condition due to strict religious upbringing, fear of an alcoholic or incestuous parent, or fear of sexual abuse. This condition, occurring in combination with primary erectile dysfunction, results in an unconsummated marriage; it may be implicated in the development of secondary erectile dysfunction, as the male partner becomes frightened about causing pain for his female partner. Secondary vaginismus may be seen following attempted or completed rape, trauma, or any condition that causes dyspareunia. The most common cause of secondary vaginismus is the *vaginitis-vaginismus syndrome* (Sarrel and Sarrel, 1979). Monilial infections and vaginal herpes are so prevalent that many women are at risk for developing this condition if they continue to have intercourse while the infection is present and thus experience pain paired with sexual activity. Eventually the woman's vaginal muscles may learn to say "no" for her as a result of negative conditioning. Prevention requires that both the patient and her partner be given appropriate education and guidance, with a ban on intercourse until the infection is effectively eliminated.

Dyspareunia and vaginismus are distinct forms of female sexual dysfunctions that often occur together, although not always. Causes, in addition to infection, are lack of lubrication due to ineffective stimulation, fibrositis in the vaginal wall, traumatic conditions resulting from childbirth, or postmenopausal tetanic uterine contractions.

The physician must be unhurried and gentle in the sexologic examination, allowing the woman to be in control of the examination. A well lubricated examining finger is held at the introitus without insertion and the woman is asked is she is uncomfortable, avoiding the words "hurt" or "pain." Initial examination is done without the male partner present, but a nurse should be in attendance and she should talk with the woman while the examination is being conducted to allay her anxiety and to help distract her. Proceed slowly, always assuring the woman that she is in charge of what is going to happen, and attempt to insert one finger into the vaginal orifice to a depth of 1 to 2 inches using posterior pressure on the perineal body. If involuntary contraction of the vaginal muscles occurs, a diagnosis of vaginismus can be made.

This involuntary muscle contraction should be demonstrated to both partners after the woman has been seen alone. The man then realizes that the woman's reaction is not specific to him; it is not a

TABLE 49–2. KEGEL'S PUBOCOCCYGEUS MUSCLE EXERCISES

Women

The patient locates the correct muscle by sitting on the toilet with knees as far apart as possible and begins urination; contract perineum only to stop the flow.

Exercises should be practiced two to three times daily at varying intervals to avoid tenderness and fatigue.
1. Contract the pubococcygeus muscle and hold for a count of 3; relax. Begin with 10, work up to 30, at each practice.
2. Contract and release the pubococcygeus muscle as rapidly as possible in a flicking motion. Begin with 10, work up to 30 or more with each practice.
3. Breathe deeply and imagine drawing air in through the vagina, tightening the muscle as you inhale. Begin with 5, work up to 15, at each practice.
4. Bear down as if having a bowel movement or giving birth, relax, then tighten the pubococcygeus muscle. Begin with 5, work up to 15, at each practice. If done prior to intercourse, vasocongestion and arousal may be enhanced.

Once learned, these exercises may be done at any time, and if associated with things the patient does consistently, it is easier to remember to practice them. Regular practice over a period of months may be necessary before results are noted. Once good muscle tone is established, maintenance exercises of 10 to 30 contractions per day are usually sufficient.

Men

The patient locates the correct muscle by beginning to urinate and then stopping the flow. When the muscle is tightened, the penis lifts slightly.

Exercises 1, 2, and 4 above are recommended to enhance erections and ejaculatory control.

Adapted from Hartman WE, Fithian M: Treatment of Sexual Dysfunction. A Bio-Psycho-Social Approach. Long Beach, CA. Center for Marital and Sexual Studies, 1972.

voluntary refusal of intercourse. At this examination do not proceed with an attempt to insert a speculum. Instruct the woman in the Kegel exercises and prescribe a regimen for her to practice them (Table 49–2). Explain to the patient that doing these exercises will give her voluntary control over her vaginal muscles and she will eventually be able to relax the muscles enough to tolerate vaginal containment.

On the second appointment an examination is repeated to determine progress. If the examining finger can be inserted easily, instruct the woman to go through the Kegel exercises with the examining finger in place to be certain that she is exercising the muscle correctly. After the woman has practiced the exercises with the examining finger in place, the smallest of a set of well lubricated plastic dilators may be inserted in the vagina as the examining finger is withdrawn. When this step has been accomplished, the woman is given the dilator to insert herself, using lubrication and exercising her muscles before inserting. It is helpful to have her point the dilator toward her coccyx while inserting. When insertion has been accomplished fairly easily, she may go to the next size dilator. She is sent home with the dilators that she has used and is asked to practice inserting them during the coming week several times a day. She should hold them in place for 15 to 20 minutes while she performs the Kegel exercises. She is instructed to use this procedure when she can be comfortably alone and undisturbed; she may choose to self-stimulate her clitoris simultaneously.

When she has been able to progress to a no. 2 dilator comfortably, the pelvic examination is repeated using a pediatric speculum or a narrow-bladed Peterson speculum. If pelvic pathology is discovered, appropriate treatment is undertaken and the use of the dilators is restricted until recovery occurs. The purchase of an elaborate set of vaginal dilators is unnecessary. It is possible to use the plastic covers from disposable syringes as an inexpensive alternative, using the smallest size and following a progression as the woman is able to tolerate increasing diameters.

As the woman's comfort level increases, her male partner is included: first to watch, then to insert his finger, then the dilator, and finally his penis, with the woman in control in the female astride position. The woman may wish to reach orgasm first, before attempts at insertion of the penis are made, as the vaginal muscles relax after orgasm. Body caressing and nondemand pleasuring techniques are taught so treatment is set in the context of related mutual love-play. The treatment is highly successful when the female partner is motivated for intercourse. (If profound concern about pregnancy is one of the etiologic factors, reliable birth control must be prescribed and instituted before beginning treatment.) When the couple or the woman does not appear to be motivated for intercourse or if both partners have severe, long-standing sexual problems, referral to a sex therapist is indicated.

CARE OF THE HOMOSEXUAL PATIENT

Care for the homosexual patient does not differ significantly from that of the heterosexual patient. Much of what has been said about psychosexual dysfunction applies regardless of sexual orientation, although there are a few issues of special concern that pertain to homosexual behavioral practices. Although there are no "typical" homosexual patients or lifestyles, there is always some awakening of self-awareness that sexual preferences are different from most of the population. The process of acceptance and disclosure, or "coming out," with relatives and friends can be a stressful time in the life of a homosexual. There tends to be a sense of isolation; and with a number of questions that need answers, a support system is often painfully lacking. Homosexuals often conceal their true sexual orientation because of fear of reprisal but really prefer to have an honest relationship with their physician. The physician who is entrusted with this information must put aside value judg-

ments and give the patient an opportunity to ventilate his or her ideas. If a counseling session with other homosexuals is needed, the National Gay and Lesbian Crisisline can be consulted to locate local resource groups. A sensitive and caring family physician can assist the homosexual patient to develop a positive self-image, an understanding of safer sex practices, and a healthier overall lifestyle.

The sexual history is an important clue to potential biomedical issues. Lesbians have much less risk of contracting sexually transmitted diseases (STDs) than their homosexual counterparts; and gay men are more likely to have more STDs than heterosexuals. Moreover, they are also more likely to suffer traumatic complications of sexual intercourse. Enteric diseases and viral hepatitis are not uncommon. A significant health problem for many homosexual men is alcohol or other chemical abuse, often linked to the social environment that serves to bring homosexuals together.

In conclusion, if the physician is willing to listen and advise in a nonjudgmental fashion, a great deal of help can be given for the common problems with which homosexuals present. Sexuality is only a small part of a person's makeup, and their sexual orientation should not stand in the way of physicians providing excellent health care for the whole person.

SEXUAL ABUSE

Rape

Rape is an increasingly common crime of violence in which sex is utilized as one of the weapons; males as well as females are its victims. The true incidence of rape is unknown as most rapes go unreported. It is estimated that one in four adolescent girls are victims of molestation, forcible rape, or incest; and fewer than 50 per cent of these crimes are reported to law enforcement personnel or physicians (Woodline and Kossoris, 1981). Of those reported, the assailant goes unapprehended 50 per cent of the time. Males may be more reluctant to report sexual assault than females because of the connotation that if they have not been able to prevent the assault they are weak or unmasculine.

The age range for victims of rape extends from infancy to old age. The highest incidence of rape and other sexual assault occurs in the adolescent age group, but nearly 10 per cent are less than 10 years old and approximately 25 per cent are between 10 and 14 years of age. These data may be surprising to the physician who has rarely or never seen a rape victim, as most media dramatizations portray the victims as a young adult or middle-aged woman. Children rarely are portrayed as rape victims, although they may account for more than 60 per cent of them. Nearly half of female rape victims report voluntarily agreeing to go into a car, house, or apartment with a new male acquaintance; and one fourth volunteered excessive use of alcohol or drugs at the time of assault (Jenny, 1988). There may be some predisposing risk-taking behavior that can be modified by education for prevention of sexual assault.

Helplessness, humiliation, and fear of recurring attacks characterize rape victims; and in fact a high percentage of victims are raped more than once. Many rapes occur in the victim's own home, resulting in the feeling that "no place is safe." The perpetrator is more often than not known to the victim. The experience of rape produces an acute stress reaction known as the *rape trauma syndrome*, which is most severe 6 weeks to 3 months or more after the attack. The victim's initial feeling after escape is gratitude at being alive. Quickly, however, the survivor's feeling turns to self-blaming and preoccupation with the event, accompanied by a sense of loss of control over his or her life. Depression is a common sequela, and suicide attempts are fairly frequent. Somatic and sexual problems are also common, as anything that resembles the rape situation is likely to trigger the feelings connected with the initial trauma.

Counseling the victim requires a respectful, accepting, gentle approach. View the patient as a normal, healthy individual whose current emotional distress results from a serious life crisis, and communicate the conviction that the person will recover. The idea of being a survivor is important. If the physician is a man, it is reassuring to the female victim to have another woman present during the interview and examination after a rape. Many rape crisis centers can provide advocates who are trained to give both physical and emotional support to the victim during questioning and examination. Assist the victim to regain or maintain control of the situation by ensuring that he or she still has the ability and the opportunity to make choices. Goal-directed counseling, based on a series of graduated steps that delineate the victim's progress toward recovery, conveys an attitude of hopefulness and counteracts depression in rape victims.

The family physician can help the rape victim inform the spouse, partner, or parents about the rape, enlisting empathy and support. The partner or parents may also need help with their own reactions to the rape; rage and a desire for retaliation or revenge are common. Redirecting the focus of attention toward issues of personal safety and the need of the rape victim to retell the story over and over can be useful in the situation. The danger of suicide attempts after a rape, particularly among adolescents, must be recognized and measures taken to protect the person during the most stressful period after the attack. It is important to help the person re-establish and maintain a sense of self-esteem, which tends to be badly battered by this experience. If the partner or family is not sympathetic or supportive, put the patient in contact with other individuals who are able to serve in this role.

Sexual Abuse of Children

Physicians in all states are mandatory child abuse reporters; thus it is essential to be aware of the required procedure for the state in which one practices. Authorities agree that sexual abuse is probably the most underdiagnosed, and therefore under-reported, type of child abuse. Because it is a criminal offense for any adult to have sexual contact with a child, it is imperative that the physician cooperate in the investigative process.

A random survey from a population of 600 general practitioners and pediatricians in the State of Washington reveals that most sexual abuse relationships encountered are incestuous intercourse and molestation (Woodline and Kossoris, 1981). Father–daughter incest accounts for approximately 75 per cent of cases of incest; mother–son, father–son, mother–daughter, and brother–sister incest account for the remaining 25 per cent. Nearly 80 per cent of all father–daughter incest involved a stepfather or father-substitute, such as a live-in boyfriend. This statistic should alert the family physician to children who may be at higher risk, although incestuous relations can happen in all types of family.

Incest is a symptom of extreme family disorganization; the intergenerational boundaries have been broken, and there is confusion over power issues and a betrayal of trust by the caretaking adult. (Alcohol is a major factor in removing the restraints from adult sexual behavior that might otherwise be present.) Sibling or cousin incest may be somewhat less traumatic unless age disparity is present or force is used. When the behavior continues over time, there is always confusion between emotional closeness and sexual intimacy for the child, who is powerless and vulnerable. The child, usually female, who carries the guilty family secret comes to believe that the well-being and continuation of the family is her responsibility. The parental threat aimed at silencing the child enforces this belief. The mother, who may be withdrawn, depressed, or absent as a result of work, may collaborate consciously or unconsciously in the incestuous father–daughter relationship by absenting herself from sexual relations with her husband and ignoring signs of his inappropriate behavior. She may even insist that the child is lying if the girl comes to her for help—perhaps out of fear that the family will be destroyed economically and emotionally. The situation frequently does not come to light until the daughter is an adolescent and the father begins to overcontrol her social activities outside the family. In her anger the girl may then reveal the secret—her legacy of power over the parent she perceives as unjustly authoritarian and restrictive.

Obviously, a history of sexual abuse may not be offered by either child or parent because of fear or embarrassment. Therefore the physician must be alert to the possibility of abuse if there are such signs and symptoms as vaginal or penile discharge, genital trauma, lacerations, anal trauma, painful urination or defecation or the presence of gonorrhea, syphilis, *Trichomonas* infection, or genital warts. When these signs are present, smears obtained from the appropriate orifices should be examined for the presence of spermatozoa. If results are positive, there is strong evidence for the likelihood of sexual abuse. Colposcopic examination of the introitus is a helpful adjunct for detection. Vigorous follow-up should be instituted in such cases. The counseling required in cases of incest is time-consuming and more complex than the family physician can be expected to undertake. Preventive counseling might include attention to single-parent families where the adults may be isolated from a supportive network of other adult relationships. When children are visiting noncustodial parents under conditions of limited sleeping arrangements, encouraging the parents to have the children sleep in their own beds and discussing appropriate intimacy between parents and children could be helpful. Research findings suggest a link between childhood sexual abuse and later drug abuse, juvenile delinquency, and criminal behavior (Burgess et al., 1987). Psychiatric referral assists victims in dealing with their trauma and perhaps breaks the cycle of abused to abuser.

Medical Assessment and Care for the Sexual Abuse Victim

The medicolegal aspects of rape or sexual abuse require a methodical history, physical examination, and the collection of well documented laboratory evidence. Evidence collection and examination are best done in a hospital setting according to written protocol. From the moment the victim arrives at the hospital, at least one and preferable two of the health care team should remain with him or her at all times. The environment must seem safe to the victim; acceptance of the patient's story, provision of emotional support, and assurance of confidentiality are essential. All procedures that will follow should be fully described, and informed consent must be obtained in writing. Unless the victim of sexual abuse is a minor, reporting the incident and giving evidence to the police should be done only after obtaining the patient's permission. When the victim is a minor, the evidence should be collected and reported in accordance with existing state laws regarding child abuse.

A careful history should include the time, place, and circumstances of the rape or sexual abuse incident. The identity of the assailant, if known, should be recorded, as well as details of the type and amount of sexual contact. Hand-sewn dolls complete with genitalia and anal and oral openings can be used to help a child explain the occurrence more accurately. Physical force or injury should be documented, including the use or presence of weapons. Any witnesses should be identified. The type and degree of resistance employed by the victim should also be recorded. The occurrences that followed the abusive incident, including behavior that might alter or remove evidence (e.g., changing clothing, douching, bathing, or urinating) are important. The medical history and sexual history are also necessary, including date of last menstrual period and information about contraception and last sexual contact prior to the sexual abuse.

A thorough general physical examination to assess for trauma and to treat any injuries requiring immediate attention is performed next. Inspect the skin and clothing using a Wood's ultraviolet light, as semen shows up as a bright green fluorescence. A genital examination is performed to determine the condition of the hymen and the presence of genital injury; any secretions noted should be swabbed and examined for the presence of sperm. The pubic hair is inspected and combed into a plain white envelope. Add the comb to the envelope and seal it. Pubic hair plucked from the patient should be collected in a separate envelope and sealed. Fingernail scrapings labeled for each finger, should be obtained in a separate container. Smears should be taken from the vagina, anus, and cervix to be examined later for sperm, gonococci, and prostatic acid phosphatase. Vaginal and rectal specimens may be collected by aspiration after lavage with 10 mL of warmed physiologic sterile saline solution. A wet preparation should be examined immediately for the presence of motile sperm. A urine specimen is collected for examination for the presence of sperm and for a pregnancy test, and a blood specimen should be obtained for serology. All specimens should be labeled and submitted according to the clinical laboratory recommendations in the hospital, with signed receipts collected when specimens are transferred from one individual to the other in order to preserve the chain of evidence. Bimanual examination can be done to detect uterine size and perhaps preexistent pelvic pathology. After swabbing the anus for secretions to be examined for sperm, a rectal examination is done.

As additional evidence, vegetation and soil from the scene of a rape along with hair, clothing fibers, and blood samples of the suspect may be obtained. It is also customary to keep the victim's clothing that was worn at the time of the assault, particularly the underpants, and to seal them in an envelope as evidence.

Prophylactic treatment against venereal disease can be offered to the patient, as gonorrhea develops in 3 to 4 per cent of rape victims and syphilis develops in 0.1 per cent. The drug of choice for venereal disease prophylaxis is ceftriaxone sodium given intramuscularly at a dose of 250 mg. Oral tetracycline may also be prescribed for prophylaxis of *Chlamydia trachomatis* infection. When antibiotics are given, the patient should be warned that the normal bacterial flora may possibly be altered, causing an overgrowth of *Candida* with resultant vaginal discharge and itching. It is advisable to repeat venereal disease testing 6 weeks after the acute examination.

Female patients should be advised about the possibility of pregnancy. If an unwanted pregnancy is possible, the patient may be offered 5 days of postcoital estrogen therapy with ethinyl estradiol 5 mg per day or diethylstilbestrol 50 mg per day in divided doses.

INFLUENCE OF ILLNESS ON SEXUALITY

Speaking generally, sexuality may be either enhanced or distanced by any illness or disability; there may be increased harmony or increased discord. Illness can change sexuality for the better by creating greater closeness, as in cases of terminally ill patients who sense a limitation of time. However, all too often the effect is adverse.

Illness or disability may affect sexual functioning adversely in three ways. First, the illness may affect the somatic part of sexuality by creating pain, immobility, disfigurement, or a change in function. The psychological components of sexual functioning may be altered by fear, anxiety, moods, defensive behavior, or anger—all responses that can be triggered by illness. Finally, a combination of effects on the somatic and psychological systems may be produced when partial sexual dysfunction triggers a psychological response out of proportion to the event. For example, a partial erectile dysfunction secondary to drugs prescribed for hypertension may lead to a psychological reaction of anxiety and concern that further worsens the erectile dysfunction. Emotional responses to illness and disability, such as the fear of death, the embarrassment of disability, the need to be dependent, and the denial of illness, commonly alter an individual's feelings about intimacy and sexuality.

The physician who counsels an ill person about sexuality must remember that there is usually a change in motivation for sex following illness. Previous motivations may give way to increased needs to secure reassurance and to affirm masculinity or femininity. Sex may also be used to receive nurturing or other secondary gain. For example, a man may use sex as a symbolic test of potency, power, and affirmation of attractiveness. The sexual partner may become overprotective and parental, thereby restricting intimate behavior. (Misguided attempts to protect the partner are more likely to result when not enough information is present to encourage the normal emotional responses.) Anger or feelings of aversion may cause withdrawal of the sexual partner or even abandonment.

RESPONSE CYCLES

Either partner's sexual response cycle may be affected in any one of its phases. Common sexual dysfunctions that result from illness include diminished or abolished desire for sex, incomplete or prolonged excitement, prolongation of the plateau, inhibition or abolishment of orgasm, and prolongation of the resolution phase and refractory period.

Noted sex researcher Domeena Renshaw (Lief and Renshaw, 1981) has categorized eight common sexual difficulties in easy-to-remember fashion: the "four A's" (anxiety, anger, alcohol, aging) and the "four D's" (drug, depression, deliberate control, dissociation). Emotions that distress, such as anxiety and anger, activate the sympathetic system and preclude the occurrence of the normal parasympathetically controlled excitement phase. Alcohol has a paradoxical effect: In small amounts, it releases inhibitions and perhaps enhances sexuality; in larger amounts, sometimes as little as the content in two alcoholic beverages, it decreases the ability to perform. Aging and illness may interact to significantly alter sexual functioning in ways that may provoke psychological reactions that intensify the sexual failure.

The three main categories of drugs known to alter the sexual cycle are the antihypertensives (exerting adverse effects on desire, excitement, and orgasm); the antipsychotics and major tranquilizers (affecting primarily orgasm; one well known response is the retrograde ejaculation caused by Mellaril); and the antihistamines, including antiparkinsonian drugs. (See Table 49–1 for a summary of known drug effects on sexuality.)

Depression, a common sequela of myocardial infarction, often accompanies terminal illness and malignancy, and may occur as a primary endogenous disease. A cardinal symptom of depression is decreased libido. Deliberate control of sex may be exerted by the sexual partner of the ill patient, creating a gap in communication and intimacy. Fear of injuring the sexual partner may produce distancing; at the opposite extreme, fear of loss of the loved one may increase sexual demands. Dissociation is the psychotic condition in which there is loss of touch with reality and absent sexual drive.

BASIC RULES

There are six basic rules that physicians should keep in mind when they confront problems of sexuality resulting from illness.

1. *Obtain a sex history.* All patients deserve inquiry regarding their sexual functioning, but not

TABLE 49–3. ELEMENTS INCLUDED IN THE SEX HISTORY FOR PERSONS WITH ILLNESS

Preillness level of functioning
Present level of functioning
Medications being taken
Effects of illness on self-image
Part of the sexual cycle affected
Attitudes, fears, and communication of the couple
Desired outcome as a result of intervention

all patients require counseling or therapy. Illness may provide a legitimate, long-awaited excuse to discontinue sexual activity. When sexual partners are satisfied with the sexual pattern and indicate no desire to change, interference is unwarranted. It is especially important, however, to take a basic sex history of all ill and disabled patients. Patients who may be reluctant to volunteer such problems are then given an opportunity to do so. Table 49–3 suggests some areas for questioning.

2. *Give anticipatory guidance.* Anticipatory guidance may be important for preventing the occurrence of major dysfunction. This point is particularly true when surgical procedures are contemplated (Libman and Fichten, 1987). Giving basic information and expectations prior to the procedure usually prevents the sexual dysfunction that is predictable in certain instances. Referral to an expert is not commonly required.

3. *Learn from patients.* Learn from the patients themselves what works best for them. Ask those who have suffered some disability or illness about specific sexual problems they have encountered and how they have solved them; pass these useful tips on to other patients. It is often helpful to introduce a patient to someone who has suffered the same illness or disability and who has made a satisfactory adjustment.

4. *Increase the sexual repertoire.* Always attempt to widen the sexual repertoire of the patient; provide specific alternatives and suggestions for working around the disability.

5. *Perform a sexologic examination.* Provide an informative and educational examination for the patient. Use a semisitting position, a hand-held mirror, and a good deal of teaching-type communication. The patient then better understands what surgical procedures are about to be performed or how illness has affected the structure and function of the sex organs.

6. *Consultation.* The physician should recognize his or her limitations and seek additional consultation when necessary. An understanding and communicative sexual partner is important to the quality of the sexual adjustment after an illness. If a couple's problems involve more general areas of their relationship, someone better versed in handling sexual problems may be appropriate, or perhaps other types of counseling (e.g., marital, grief) need to be pursued.

COMMON SPECIFIC PROBLEMS

According to Alex Comfort (1978), problems of sexuality created by illness do not often involve major dysfunctions such as paraplegia or systemic disease. The three most common problems are interference with the patient's habitual behavior patterns, convalescence from myocardial infarction, and the sequelae of common surgical procedures such as mastectomy and prostatectomy.

Arthritis

To illustrate alteration of a sexual habit pattern, consider the arthritic patient who has problems with mechanical positioning of the hips. Often painful and contracted with muscular atrophy and weakness, the rheumatoid hip may create difficulties with coital positioning. In most patients arthritis produces fatigue and pain, each of which depresses sexual libido. Often the fingers and hands are severely affected, perhaps to the point of preventing sexual self-stimulation and stimulation of the partner. Stiffness, present in the mornings, generally improves toward noon, and the patient functions best at midday, tiring at night, with the greatest pain coming at bedtime. Also, some medications used for arthritis can produce depression (cortisone) and so depress sexual sensitivity even as they relieve pain (analgesics).

Counseling hints for the patient with arthritis include using a warm room with a warm bed, preferably a warm water bed, which reduces pressure on joints and decreases the need to expend work because of the self-propelling water wave. Pillows may be used to elevate joints that have contractures. If a pain medication does not decrease sexual sensitivity, it should be taken before sexual activity. When it does decrease sexual sensitivity, the pain medication should be taken immediately afterward. The patient may be advised that 2 to 4 hours of pain relief may be the resultant effect of orgasm. Sex is best tried when the patient is well rested; and arranging to be together at midday seems most reasonable. Hot baths and warmup exercises may limber the joints and at the same time provide sexual stimulation if they are given by the partner. Reduced weight-bearing may be accomplished by the use of side-to-side facing or rear entry positions. When Sjögren syndrome is present, additional vaginal lubrication is necessary and may be more sensual when applied by the partner. There may be a need for surgery in some joints, particularly the hips, to improve sexual functioning.

Diabetes

Approximately 30 per cent of diabetic women have some degree of sexual dysfunction. The female problems relate primarily to vaginal dryness, vaginal infections, decreased autonomic function, and atrophy of the vaginal epithelium. These problems lead to delayed arousal, painful or traumatic intercourse, decline in libido, or anorgasmia. Neurogenic bladder predisposes the woman to dribbling, incomplete emptying, or incontinence; infections are common. Embarrassment about wetness or odor may create an aversion to partner touch and orogenital contact.

To help the woman who has sexual difficulties related to diabetes, suggest that the couple regularly use vaginal lubrication to counteract dryness and prescribe topical estrogen therapy to preserve thickness of the vaginal epithelium. When vaginal infection occurs, promptly treat with appropriate agents (usually anti-*Candida* agents) and advise against intercourse until the vaginal lining has completely healed (usually 3 weeks). Instruct the couple about alternatives to penis–vagina intercourse for sexual pleasuring. The neurogenic bladder can be more completely emptied prior to intercourse by the Credé or Valsalva maneuver or intermittent self-catheterization. Drugs such as bethanechol 10 to 25 mg every 4 to 6 hours, may be used.

Sexual dysfunction may affect as many as 80 per cent of type I diabetic men after age 40. Commonly it is an organic form of erectile failure with a significant secondary psychological overlay of fear, guilt, or depression. The cause of erectile failure is thought to be secondary to autonomic and sensory neuropathy and perhaps vascular insufficiency. Temporary failure can result from poor diabetic control. Diabetics sometimes have failure of the internal bladder sphincter, leading to retrograde ejaculation. Usually erectile failure precedes the ejaculation disorder. Most male diabetics with sexual dysfunction related to erectile failure benefit from sex therapy and improved communication for reduction of performance anxiety. Erection may be improved by external suction devices (VED vacuum erection device or the Synergist Erection System). An empiric trial of therapy with yohimbine 5 mg three times per day may be tried in nonhypertensive diabetics to decrease outflow of blood from the penis. Zinc depletion has been implicated in this problem, particularly in the setting of renal disease with dialysis, and replacement with doses of 220 mg of zinc sulfate twice daily can be tried.

Intracavernous penile papaverine injections have produced good results for motivated patients who respond to its use. Neurologic erectile failure is more responsive than failure in men with vascular impairment. Papaverine is started at a dose of 7 to 8 mg injected shortly before intercourse once per 24 hours, increasing the dose as necessary up to a maximum of 30 mg (1 mL). Long-term complications include fibrosis of the corpora cavernosa, which may preclude later surgery. Urologic consultation is warranted before beginning papaver-

ine therapy. The surgical implantation of rigid or inflatable penile prostheses is reserved for those who fail conservative or medical therapy.

Heart Disease

Papadopoulos (1980) has reported on the sexual concerns and needs of postcoronary patients' wives. One hundred wives were interviewed, and nearly all wished that they could receive sexual instructions in the presence of their husbands. Many did not. It is wise to remember to include both partners in any sexual counseling in the context of illness.

Depression is nearly always present after myocardial infarction, and many men never return to their previous level of functioning. One third to one half experience a decrease in desire and frequency even up to several years after the myocardial infarction. Similar effects are noted in women following heart attack. A careful assessment of the patient for the presence of depression may reveal a treatable cause for sexual dysfunction.

The patient with heart disease should know that sexual activity up to and including orgasm requires approximately 5.5 metabolic units of energy expended. If a patient can climb two flights of stairs, the capacity to perform during sexual intercourse is present. The average heart rate at orgasm is 115 to 120 beats per minute. Most patients do not experience angina until the heart rate reaches a mean of 145 (+20) beats per minute. These averages indicate that sexual activity is usually safe. It is wise for the patient to undergo submaximal exercise testing prior to leaving the hospital in order to establish the presence of dysrhythmias or inability to perform at the required energy level.

Of 5559 sudden deaths in Japan, 18 (0.03 per cent) were related to coitus; but, 14 of the 18 were with extramarital partners (Ueno, 1969). It is advisable that the re-establishment of sexual activity occur with the usual and customary partner, whether within the marriage or without. In any case, sexual activity should be resumed by pleasuring without intercourse, with the introduction of sensate focus and relaxation techniques. These nondemand, nonstress activities allow the patient to resume intimacy immediately without the need for performance that may produce anxiety about angina or a second heart attack. The bedroom should be warm; a warmed water bed may reduce the work output needed for sexual intercourse. Long-acting nitrates may be taken prior to intercourse for prophylaxis of angina. Again, it is wise to avoid sex after meals, smoking, or argument. Where congestive heart failure may be a problem, the avoidance of orthopnea is accomplished through the use of the sitting position. In some cases of chronic heart disease with severe angina, coronary artery bypass surgery may be the only hope to offer resumption of normal sexual activity.

Cancer

A diagnosis of cancer constitutes a crisis that threatens mortality and may be assumed to affect sexuality in a variety of ways. When the diagnosis is superimposed on preexisting sexual problems, the impact can be devastating. Even in the case of a couple with an excellent sexual relationship prior to diagnosis, the insult to the patient's body of treatment, together with fatigue, emotional turmoil, depression, and pain, may severely damage the couple's sexual functioning. In addition to the patient's problems, partners have their own reactions and feelings that require attention. They may include fear of injuring the patient or of being injured themselves by the cancer or its treatment (especially radiation therapy) (Kudsk and Hoffmann, 1987).

Because most types of cancer and its treatment have an impact on body image and therefore on self-esteem, with concomitant effects on the patient's partnership, it is essential for the family physician to actively attend to the patient's concerns by introducing the topic of sexual health care even before treatment begins. This counseling may be the most important part of the process of identifying, evaluating, and remedying psychosexual dysfunction after treatment (Schain, 1988). For patients with committed partners, married or not, heterosexual or homosexual, the couple should be considered the unit of care.

The family physician's skill in listening to the patient and his or her partner, as well as individualizing the information given, is a vital factor in minimizing the impact of cancer and its treatment on the couple's sexual functioning. For the patient without a partner, the physician's reassurance that the patient is still a valuable person—in fact the "same" person as before diagnosis—can be greatly therapeutic. In all cases, preserving and enhancing the patient's self-esteem is a critical factor in promoting sexual rehabilitation. It is important for the physician to convey a message of hope; although patience and experimentation may be necessary, sexual healing can occur.

The specific suggestion to resume affectionate and intimate touch as soon as possible after surgery, with a return to intercourse as soon as physical healing has occurred, can help prevent a conspiracy of silence and a pattern of withdrawal from becoming established. Other sexual activities, such as oral or manual techniques, can be encouraged when intercourse is medically contraindicated for long periods. It can help to alleviate discouragement and provide comfort. The healing power of touch and the psychological effect of uninterrupted intimacy can hasten the patient's recovery and strengthen the relationship. The physician's active support of this process, combined with the invitation to voice concerns, ask questions, and reveal unspoken fears is an important part of the challenge of caring for the patient with cancer.

Because it is essential to avoid connecting pain with sexual activity, the active involvement of both partners in planning for optimal comfort and pleasure should be facilitated. For some couples, early viewing of the operative area is important for acceptance to occur. For others, "permission" to cover it in an attractive manner is paramount. Cleanliness of both partners is important to reduce the risk of infection. When vaginal lubrication has been compromised, a water-soluble lubricant such as Lubrin, Personal Lubricant, or Transi-lube can be recommended. Because semen may "burn" friable vaginal tissues (particularly after irradiation), the use of a condom can be helpful. A position that is restful for both partners, providing intromission without deep penetration and avoiding pressure on breast or abdominal incisions, is illustrated in Figure 49–3. Putting the patient in touch with people who have successfully recovered from a particular type of cancer can be helpful.

The most important part of counseling the cancer patient about sexuality is to preserve and protect the patient's sense of masculinity or femininity in the face of treatment procedures that may precipitate feelings of mutilation, repulsiveness, and desexualization. It is helpful to present alternatives to the couple's usual and habitual sexual pattern in order to accommodate their current needs. The information required is usually basic, and there may be simple solutions for what the couple deems a difficult problem. The physician's guidance and support for the patient's return to sexual functioning can help transform a potential tragedy into an experience of growth in communication and intimacy.

REFERENCES

References for Physician Use

American Psychiatric Association: Diagnostic and Statistical Manual of Mental Disorders, 3rd edition (revised). Washington, DC, American Psychiatric Association, 1987.

Antoniskis D, Sattler FR, Leedom JM: Importance of assessing risk behavior for AIDS—Why and how to obtain a relevant history. Postgrad Med 83:138, 1988.

Baum N: Impotence: Organic or psychogenic? Diagnosis 11(1): 37, 1989.

Bohlen JG, Held JP, Sanderson MD, et al: Heart rate, rate-pressure product, and oxygen uptake during four sexual activities. Arch Intern Med 144:1745, 1984.

Burgess AW, Hartman CR, McCormack A: Abused to abuser: Antecedents of socially deviant behaviors. Am J Psychiatry 144:1431, 1987.

Butler RN, Lewis MI: Sex After Sixty: A Guide for Men and Women for Their Later Years. New York, Harper & Row, 1976.

Comfort A (ed): Sexual Consequences of Disability. Philadelphia, George F. Stickley, 1978.

DeMoya D, DeMoya A, Lewis HR: RN's Sex Q & A—Candid Advice for You and Your Patients. Oradell, NJ, Medical Economics Books, 1984.

Doherty WJ, Baird MA: Family Therapy and Family Medicine: Toward the Primary Care of Families. New York, Guildford Press, 1983.

Fogel CI, Lauver D: Sexual Health Promotion. Philadelphia, WB Saunders Company, 1990.

Franger AL: Taking a sexual history and managing common sexual problems. J Reprod Med 33:639, 1988.

Goodwin JM: Sexual Abuse: Incest Victims and Their Families, 2nd edition. Chicago, Medical Yearbook Publishers, 1989.

Green R (ed): Human Sexuality: A Health Practitioner's Text, 2nd edition. Baltimore, Williams & Wilkins, 1979.

Haas K, Haas A: Understanding Sexuality, 3rd edition. St. Louis, Mosby-Year Book, 1993.

Hartman WE, Fithian MA: Treatment of Sexual Dysfunction. A Bio-Psycho-Social Approach. Long Beach, CA, Center for Marital and Sexual Studies, 1972.

Jenny C: Adolescent risk-taking behavior and the occurrence of sexual assault. Am J Dis Child 142:770, 1988.

Johnson LE, Morley JE: Impotence in the elderly. Am Fam Physician 38:225, 1988.

Kaplan HS: Disorders of Sexual Desire. New York, Brunner-Mazel, 1979.

Klein M: When talk is not cheap. New Physician 33:30, 1984.

Kolodny RC, Masters WH, Johnson VE: Textbook of Sexual Medicine. Boston, Little, Brown, 1979.

Kudsk EG, Hoffmann GS. Rehabilitation of the cancer patient. Primary Care 14:381, 1987.

Levenson A, Croft H: Patients' sexual problems: Aspects of physicians' qualifications and management. J Reprod Med 18:27, 1977.

Libman E, Fichten CS: Prostatectomy and sexual function. Urology 29:467, 1987.

Lief HI (ed): Sexual Problems in Medical Practice. Chicago, American Medical Association, 1981.

Lief HI, Renshaw DC: Primary Care of Common Sexual Problems: Diagnostic and Therapeutic Guidelines. American Medical Association Council on Continuing Physician Education, 1981.

Masters WH, Johnson VE: Human Sexual Response. Boston, Little, Brown, 1966.

Masters WH, Johnson VE: Human Sexual Inadequacy. Boston, Little, Brown, 1970.

Masters WH, Johnson VE, Kolodny RC: Crisis: Heterosexual Behavior in the Age of AIDS. New York, Grove Press, 1988.

Masters WH, Johnson VE, Kolodny RC: Human Sexuality, 4th edition. New York, HarperCollins Publishers, 1992.

Money J: Lovemaps: Clinical Concepts of Sexual/Erotic Health and Pathology, Paraphilia, and Gender Transposition in Childhood, Adolescence, and Maturity. New York, Irvington Publishers, 1986.

Money J, Ehrhardt A: Man and Woman, Boy and Girl: The Differentiation and Dimorphism of Gender Identity from Conception to Maturity. Baltimore, Johns Hopkins University Press, 1972.

Papadopoulos C: Sexual concerns and needs of the postcoronary patient's wife. Arch Intern Med 140:38, 1980.

Pomeroy WB, Flax CC, Wheeler CC: Taking a Sex History: Interviewing and Recording. New York, Free Press, 1982.

Quadagno DM: Update on the G-spot. Med Aspects Hum Sex 22(8):93, 1988.

Rekers GA, Milner GC: How to diagnose and manage childhood sexual disorders. Behav Med 6:18, 1979.

Ross MW, Channon-Little LD: Discussing Sexuality—A Guide for Health Practitioners. Sydney, MacLennan & Petty Pty, 1991.

Sarrel LJ, Sarrel PM: Sexual Unfolding: Sexual Development and Sex Therapies in Late Adolescence. Boston, Little, Brown, 1979.

Schain WS: The sexual and intimate consequences of breast cancer treatment. Cancer 38:154, 1988.

Sheehy G: Passages: Predictable Crises of Adult Life. New York, EP Dutton, 1974.

Sheehy G: The Silent Passage Menopause. New York, Random House, 1992.

Starr BD, Weiner MB: The Starr and Weiner Report on Sex and Sexuality in the Mature Years. New York, Stein & Day, 1981.

Trachtenberg DE, Bordeaux DR, Guilozet N, et al: Monograph No. 26: Sexual Maturation and Genital Problems. Home Study Self-Assessment Course. Kansas City, MO., American Academy of Family Physicians, 1981.

Ueno M: The so-called coition death. Nippon Hoigaku Zasshi 17:333, 1969.

Vincent CE: Sexual and Marital Health: The Physician As a Consultant. New York, McGraw-Hill, 1973.

Wagner G, Green R: Impotence: Physiological, Psychological, Surgical Diagnosis and Treatment. New York, Plenum Press, 1981.

Walz TH, Blum NS: Sexual Health in Later Life. Lexington, MA, DC Heath, 1987.

Wolman BB, Money J: Handbook of Human Sexuality. Englewood Cliffs, NJ, Prentice-Hall, 1980.

Woodline BA, Kossoris PD: Sexual misuse: rape, molestation and incest: Symposium on pediatric and adolescent gynecology. Pediatr Clin North Am 28:481, 1981.

References for Patient Use

A New View of a Woman's Body—A Fully Illustrated Guide. By the Federation of Feminist Women's Health Center. New York, Simon & Schuster, 1981.

AIDS: What Young Adults Should Know. Reston, VA, American Alliance for Health, Physical Education, Recreation and Dance, 1987.

An Intimate Parent-Child Talk. What Every 8–16 year old MUST know growing up in the 80's and 90's. Sexual information created by Daniel G. Amen, M.D. [115 minute videotape].

Barbach LG: For Each Other: Sharing Sexual Intimacy. New York, Signet, Doubleday, 1984.

Barbach LG. For Yourself: Fulfillment of Female Sexuality—A Guide to Orgasmic Response. New York, Anchor Press, Doubleday, 1976.

Bass E, Davis L: The Courage to Heal: A Guide for Women Survivors of Child Sexual Abuse. New York, Harper & Row, 1988.

Calderone MS, Ramey JW: Talking with Your Child About Sex. New York, Ballantine Books, 1982.

Comfort A, Comfort J: The Facts of Love. New York, Crown, 1979.

Hamilton E: Sex With Love: A Guide for Young People. Boston, Beacon Press, 1978.

Heiman J, LoPiccolo L, LoPiccolo J: Becoming Orgasmic: A Sexual Growth Program for Women. Englewood Cliffs, NJ, Prentice-Hall, 1976.

Johnson EW: Love and Sex in Plain Language, 3rd edition. Philadelphia, JB Lippincot, 1977.

Lewis HR, Lewis ME: The Parents' Guide to Teenage Sex and Pregnancy. New York, St. Martin's Press, 1980.

Masters WH, Johnson VE, Koldny RC: Masters and Johnson on Sex and Human Loving. Boston, Little, Brown, 1986.

Money J, Tucker P: Sexual Signatures: On Being a Man or a Woman. Boston, Little, Brown, 1975.

Mooney TO, Cole TM, Chilgren RA: Sexual Options for Paraplegics and Quadraplegics. Boston, Little, Brown, 1975.

Ralston A: What Do Our Children Need to Know About AIDS?

Guidelines for Parents. Novato, CA, Beneficial Publishing, 1988.

Sex: A Topic of Conversation for Parents of Young Children. Prepared by Sol Gordon, Mondell Productions [25 minute videotape].

Sex: A Topic of Conversation for Parents of Teenagers. Prepared by Sol Gordon, Mondell Productions [25 minute videotape].

Sex: A Topic of Conversation for Teenagers. Prepared by Sol Gordon, Mondell Productions [25 minute videotape].

Task Force on Concerns of Physically Disabled Women. New York, Human Sciences Press, 1978.

Vandervoort HE, McIlvenna T: The Yes Book of Sex: You Can Last Longer. San Francisco, Multimedia Resource Center, 1972.

Zilbergeld B: The New Male Sexuality: The Truth About Men, Sex, and Pleasure. New York, Bantom Books, 1992.

OTHER RESOURCES

AIDS Information Hotline
(800) 342-AIDS

Center for Marital and Sexual Studies
William E. Hartman and Marilyn A. Fithian, Co-directors
5199 East Pacific Coast Highway
Long Beach, CA 90804
(213) 597-4425

Impotence Information Center
PO Box 9
Minneapolis, MN 55440
(800) 843-4315

Kinsey Institute for Sex Research
416 Morrison Hall
Indiana University
Bloomington, IN 47401

Masters and Johnson Institute
4910 Forest Park Boulevard
St. Louis, MO 63108
(314) 361-2377

Multimedia Resource Center
1525 Franklin Street
San Francisco, CA 94109

National Center for the Prevention and Control of Rape
500 Fishers Lane
Room 6C-12
Rockville, MD 20857

National Gay and Lesbian Crisisline
(800) 221-7044

Sexual Attitude Reassessment Seminar
Program in Human Sexuality
Department of Family Practice and Community Health
University of Minnesota Medical School
Minneapolis, MN 55414

SIECUS (Sex Information and Education Council of the United States)
New York University
32 Washington Place
New York, NY 10003
(212) 673-3850

CHAPTER 50

CLINICAL GENETICS AND GENETIC COUNSELING

STUART K. SHAPIRA and MICHAEL A. CROUCH

The practice of clinical genetics involves the diagnosis of medical conditions that have an inherited basis for the purpose of providing appropriate medical care and family planning information. Genetic disease, considered in toto, is not a rare occurrence. Approximately 3 per cent of all infants are born with a major birth defect, most of which have a genetic basis. Additionally, approximately 7 per cent of all individuals manifest symptoms of a genetic disorder during childhood or adolescence. Finally, many adult conditions have a genetic basis, including hypertension, hypercholesterolemia, adult-onset diabetes, Alzheimer disease, psychiatric disorders, and numerous types of cancer. Indeed, the burden of genetic disease on general health is significant.

A large proportion of genetic diseases, specifically those in which birth defects are present, can be recognized during fetal life by prenatal ultrasonography or during the newborn period. The causes of various types of birth defects are summarized in Table 50–1. Though many birth defects have a primary genetic basis, it is important to differentiate these conditions from birth defects caused by fetal exposure to maternal factors. Such factors, which cause birth defects via teratogenic effects (Table 50–2), include certain viral infections during pregnancy, maternal exposure to alcohol, drugs, and certain medications, and various maternal medical conditions that predispose to fetal birth defects. These causes of birth defects would not be considered genetic but, rather, "environmental," as fetal development can be severely altered by many factors that perturb the normal fetal environment. It is important for the family physician to be aware of potential teratogenic agents and to advise their patients about the hazardous agents that should be avoided during pregnancy. Additionally, women with certain medical conditions that predispose to birth defects should be referred to obstetricians knowledgeable about high risk pregnancies and to prenatal genetics specialists prior to achieving a pregnancy.

In contrast to environmental and teratogenic effects, genetic causes of birth defects are far more prevalent and include numerous chromosomal abnormalities and deletions or duplications of small chromosomal segments not discernible by routine chromosome analysis (submicroscopic deletions or duplications). Additionally, many genetic conditions are caused by mutations within single genes or by mutations in several genes (polygenic or multifactorial inheritance). Therefore a fetus or newborn with birth defects should immediately alert the physician to the possibility of a genetic disease.

IDENTIFYING/RECOGNIZING AND EVALUATING THE DYSMORPHIC CHILD

Infants and children typically have physical features that resemble those of their parents or other family members. However, when children are born with birth defects or have physical features that substantially differ from those that are familial, they are considered "dysmorphic," or "distinctive," in their appearance. Dysmorphic features are not limited to the head and face, although approximately one half of all dysmorphic features occur in facial structures.

Dysmorphic features are often not noticed during the newborn period but may become apparent with growth and development of the child. Sometimes parents discount dysmorphic features as inconsequential, as a particular feature may seem similar to what they remember occurring in a distant relative. If on careful examination, however, a child has three or more dysmorphic features in association with psychomotor mental retardation or perhaps one or more birth defects, it is important to alert the parents about the possibility of a genetic or developmental problem, and that additional tests and evaluations are indicated. Primary care physicians may find it awkward to raise the possibility of genetic disease because the family often has numerous questions for which answers are best left to the genetics specialist. Calm reassurance that the specialist can evaluate for all possibilities is the course recommended for family physicians who mention the possibility of a genetic condition to the family.

Birth defects and dysmorphic features manifest

TABLE 50–1. CAUSES OF BIRTH DEFECTS

Cause	Incidence (%)
Chromosomal abnormalities	6–10
Single gene defects	3.0–7.5
Multifactorial inheritance (polygenic and environmental factors)	20–30
Environmental factors (maternal conditions and teratogens)	4–5
Unknown causes	50

as abnormal or altered development of body structures; they occur by the process of malformation, deformation, or disruption. *Malformations* are primary defects in morphogenesis of structures during embryonic or fetal development. The developmental program is either intrinsically abnormal because of genetic factors or is perturbed because of environmental factors, giving rise to abnormally developed body structures. Malformations are classified as major or minor, depending on whether the structural defect is of medical, surgical, or cosmetic importance. Major malformations include the congenital heart defects, ambiguous genitalia, neural tube defects (anencephaly, encephalocele, spina bifida), and cleft lip/cleft palate, while minor malformations include such features as up- or down-slanting eye fissures, abnormally positioned ears (e.g., low-set and posteriorly rotated), long philtrum, broadly spaced nipples, and short fingers. In fact, if any facial or body feature is either too large or small, long or short, or too wide or narrow compared to normal standard growth curves, that feature represents a minor malformation. Minor malformations may have no clinical significance, but approximately 20 per cent of infants and children with three or more minor malformations also have one or more major malformations. Therefore dysmorphic children require a thorough physical examination, and often additional radiographic, ultrasonographic, or magnetic resonance imaging (MRI) studies.

Deformations arise as defects in normally formed body structures that occur by the extrinsic force of compression, constriction, or immobility. The intrauterine environment can be deleterious to the developing fetus when there are uterine abnormalities (fibroids, bicornuate uterus, scarring), oligohydramnios, or multiple gestations. These factors can lead to mechanical forces causing deformations, such as clubfoot, joint contractures (arthrogryposis), or cranial distortions.

Disruptions, the third category of birth defects and dysmorphic features, occur by atrophy, breakdown, or amputation of previously normal body structures, primarily resulting when extrinsic compression or constriction leads to vascular insufficiency. Disruptions include amputation defects due to amnion rupture with amniotic band tissue wrapping around and constricting body structures, particularly portions of the extremities; amniotic

bands may also cause atypical facial clefts, ocular defects, exencephaly, encephalocele, and thoracogastroschisis.

Deformations and disruptions occur by an extrinsic process that is generally nongenetic in nature, and the recurrence in a future pregnancy would be unlikely, unless similar intrauterine environmental factors exist. Differentiating deformations and disruptions from malformations is crucial for optimal genetic counseling. Therefore a primary focus of the practice of clinical genetics is to identify and classify major and minor malformations occurring in an infant or child, most of which have a genetic basis. By recognizing a specific collection or pattern of malformations, the infant or child often can be assigned a genetic diagnosis or syndrome.

A syndrome is classified as a group of malformations due to a single or similar etiology; the cause(s) may or may not be known. For example, Down syndrome, which is known to be caused by three copies of chromosome 21 (trisomy 21), presents as a recognizable phenotype, usually consisting of some or all of the following features: flattened occiput and midface, brachycephaly, small ears, up-slanting palpebral fissures, Brushfield spots of the iris, high-arched palate, macroglossia, wide-spaced nipples, transverse palmar crease, abnormal dermatoglyphics, short fingers, fifth finger clinodactyly, increased spacing between the first and second toes, hypotonia, congenital heart defect (often of the atrioventricular canal), gastrointestinal defect (often duodenal atresia), developmental delay, and mental retardation. Essentially, recognizing the usual features of a particular syndrome aids in assigning a specific syndromic diagnosis, as would be the case for Down syndrome if a child had most of the features listed above. However, when the cause(s) of a syndrome is known, performing a specific laboratory test, such as a chromosome analysis for suspected Down syndrome, allows a definitive diagnosis or exclusion of particular conditions.

Many syndromes have, as yet, unknown causes, though several syndromes have recently been found to be caused in part by deletions or duplications of small chromosomal regions, often undetectable by standard chromosome analysis procedures. Examples include Prader-Willi syndrome, Angelman syndrome, Williams syndrome, Rubinstein-Taybi syndrome, DiGeorge syndrome, Schprintzen syndrome, and Langer-Giedion syndrome. Specialized laboratory techniques (fluorescent in situ hybridization, or FISH) utilizing fluorescent probes for detecting the deleted or duplicated chromosomal regions have been developed to diagnose these and other syndromes. However, without a specific test for diagnosing most syndromes and genetic conditions, the clinical geneticist must rely on past expertise and insight, as well as available clinical genetics databases and reference materials.

TABLE 50–2. TERATOGENIC AGENTS

Agent/Condition	Abnormalities
Viruses	
Rubella	Mental and growth deficiency; ocular and cardiovascular anomalies; deafness; microcephaly; immune and endocrine disturbances; delayed skeletal development
Cytomegalovirus	Mental and growth deficiency; ocular and cardiovascular anomalies; deafness; microcephaly; hydrocephalus; possible gastrointestinal anomalies
Herpes simplex	Mental deficiency and possibly growth deficiency; ocular anomalies; microcephaly; patent ductus arteriosus; hypoplastic distal phalanges
Varicella zoster	Growth and mental deficiency; ocular anomalies; microcephaly; limb hypoplasia; cutaneous defects; neurogenic muscular atrophy
HIV	Growth deficiency; 50% or more develop AIDS
Bacteria	
Syphilis	Growth and mental deficiency; ocular, dental, and skeletal anomalies; hydrocephalus; microcephaly; cutaneous lesions; nerve palsies; nephrosis
Parasites	
Toxoplasmosis	Growth and mental deficiency; ocular anomalies; microcephaly; hydrocephalus; deafness
Maternal Exposures	
Ethyl alcohol	Fetal alcohol syndrome; mental and growth deficiency; cardiac, ocular, CNS, and skeletal malformations; cleft palate; characteristic facies
Tobacco	Growth deficiency; no definitive association with human birth defects; increased risk of tubal pregnancy
Caffeine	No definitive association with human birth defects
Drugs	
Cocaine/crack	Mental deficiency; vascular disruption; possibly genitourinary tract anomalies
Other "street drugs" (e.g., marijuana, amphetamines, LSD)	No definitive association with human birth defects
Anticonvulsants	
Hydantoins (e.g., Dilantin)	Fetal hydantoin effects; growth and mental deficiency; cardiac, skeletal, and limb defects; cleft palate; characteristic facies
Oxazolidines (e.g., trimethadione)	Fetal trimethadione effects; growth and mental deficiency; characteristic facies; cardiac, CNS, gastrointestinal, genitourinary, and limb defects; cleft palate
Valproic acid	Fetal valproate effects; characteristic facies; cardiac and limb defects; spina bifida; cleft lip
Diazepam	Possibly low risk for facial clefts
Antibiotics	
Tetracyclines	Dental abnormalities
Streptomycin (and possibly other aminoglycosides)	Hearing loss
Chloroquine	Possibly ocular defects; possibly hearing loss
Other Prescription Medications	
Coumarin derivatives (e.g., warfarin)	Fetal warfarin effects; growth and mental deficiency; ocular, CNS, cardiac, and skeletal defects; microcephaly; characteristic facies; choanal atresia
Aminopterin	Fetal aminopterin effects; growth and mental deficiency; CNS, ocular, cardiac, and skeletal defects; characteristic facies; cleft palate; limb defects
Retinoic acid	Retinoic acid effects; growth and mental deficiency; CNS, cardiac, external ear, and thymic abnormalities; characteristic facies; cleft palate
Maternal Conditions	
Diabetes	Macrosomia; CNS, cardiac, skeletal, limb, and renal abnormalities; caudal regression
Phenylketonuria (PKU)	Maternal PKU effects; growth and mental deficiency; cardiac and vertebral defects; microcephaly; characteristic facies; cleft lip and palate
Heat or fever	Neural tube defects, possibly other CNS anomalies

GENETIC HISTORY AND PHYSICAL EXAMINATION

Infants and children with dysmorphic features and birth defects, as well as children with psychomotor retardation that may have a genetic basis, are approached by the clinician in a manner similar to the evaluation of all new patients. Detailed questioning and record keeping are necessary to explore all possible genetic and environmental causes. The medical history requires detailed assessment of the pregnancy history, as prenatal factors have obvious impact on fetal development. The specifics of the pregnancy should be compared with previous and subsequent pregnancies, particularly regarding fetal growth and parameters at birth, fetal activity, maternal weight gain, details of the labor and delivery, and neonatal complications. Full disclosure of possible teratogens (Table 50–2) is necessary, as is pinpointing the precise time the pregnancy was realized, and fully exploring any teratogenic exposures prior to that time.

A detailed family history is crucial for a genetic evaluation, as it may provide clues to the child's dysmorphic features, birth defects, or psychomotor retardation. It is essential to determine whether other family members have similar features or medical problems. Because specific genetic conditions occur more frequently in certain ethnic groups, assessing the ethnic background of the family is often helpful. Family history-taking represents an opportunity to screen for other unrelated health concerns for the family; therefore a complete family history requires determining if any family members are blood relatives, have had multiple miscarriages, died during early infancy or early childhood, were born with birth defects, have seizures, developmental delay, or mental retardation, and if any known genetic conditions have occurred in the family. The family history is recorded as a visual representation (the pedigree), which can depict family relationships that may otherwise be difficult to describe verbally (see Chapter 2).

A detailed physical examination requires careful observation and precise measurement of features. Often the clinical geneticist photographs or videotapes the patient in order to document dysmorphic features. Photographs or slides of the patient are useful for obtaining a "second opinion" by other geneticists. Additional family members may have to be examined. Photographs of relatives provided by the family or childhood pictures of the parents may be helpful.

Additional testing for the cause(s) of birth defects is crucial for making a specific syndromic diagnosis and for excluding all others. Infectious teratogens can be screened for with maternal and infant TORCH titers. A chromosome analysis screens for chromosomal abnormalities, and the FISH technique is useful for detecting specific microdeletion or microduplication syndromes. Many metabolic problems (inborn errors of metabolism) present with psychomotor retardation, dysmorphic features, or birth defects, so appropriate biochemical testing is often utilized to make a diagnosis. Endocrine testing may be useful for evaluating short stature, ambiguous genitalia, or disorders of sexual differentiation. A thorough search for additional malformations or medical problems generally requires radiologic and imaging studies, hearing and vision testing, and evaluation by other medical specialists (e.g., ophthalmologist, cardiologist, neurologist, endocrinologist).

A complete genetics evaluation is therefore an extensive undertaking that often results in answering the family's major question: "What is wrong with my child?" Common indications for obtaining a genetics evaluation are listed in Table 50–3. Once a diagnosis is established, a prognosis can be inferred based on similarly affected patients reported in the medical literature. Complications can be predicted, and appropriate medical management can be instituted. With a diagnosis in hand, appropriate genetic counseling can be provided, particularly regarding the recurrence risk in future pregnancies, prenatal diagnostic options (see below), and assessment of other at-risk family members.

TABLE 50–3. INDICATIONS FOR GENETIC EVALUATION

Multiple dysmorphic features
Birth defects (single or multiple)
Family history of similar birth defects or dysmorphic features
Features of an inborn error of metabolism (infantile metabolic crisis, hepatic dysfunction, neurologic dysfunction, storage disorder, metabolic acidosis, hypoglycemia, hyperammonemia)
Positive result on the State Newborn Screen
Psychomotor retardation
Movement disorders
Hyperactivity, attentional deficit disorder, tics, or other behavioral problems
Ambiguous genitalia
Abnormal sexual development
Short stature or other growth disorders
Familial cancer (e.g., retinoblastoma, Wilms tumor, renal carcinoma, optic glioma, acoustic neuroma, familial breast, colon, ovarian, and uterine cancer)
Multiple miscarriages
Infertility or sterility
Exposure to potentially teratogenic agents
Family history of a known genetic disorder

PRENATAL DIAGNOSIS

Couples who have had one child with a genetic condition and couples who are "at risk" for having children with genetic problems by virtue of a family history or by carrier testing for genetic disease may wish to undergo prenatal diagnosis. Prenatal diagnosis of birth defects or genetic conditions has become a routine part of comprehensive prenatal care. Several hundred fetal conditions, of which a few examples are listed in Table 50–4, can be identified with prenatal diagnostic techniques. Examination of the fetus for birth defects requires high-resolution ultrasonography by an experienced fetal ultrasonographer; other fetal imaging studies, such as fetal MRI and transvaginal fetoscopy, have also been utilized. Fetal tissue sampling for chromosome analysis, metabolic testing, DNA diagnostic testing, assessment of congenital infection, or testing for blood dyscrasias requires (1) obtaining placental tissue by chorionic villous sampling (CVS) at 9 to 10 weeks of pregnancy, (2)

TABLE 50–4. COMMON PRENATALLY DIAGNOSED DISORDERS

Chromosomal abnormalities
Submicroscopic chromosomal deletions or duplications
Birth defects
   Neural tube defects
   Many congenital heart defects
   Renal agenesis
   Body wall defects
   Thoracic and abdominal situs abnormalities
   Limb reduction defects
   Hydrocephalus
   Microcephaly
   Porencephalic cysts and some CNS malformations
Skeletal dysplasias
Metabolic disorders
   Phenylketonuria
   Galactosemia
   Amino acidopathies and organic acidopathies
   Urea cycle defects
   Storage disorders
   Mitochondrial myopathies
   Peroxisomal disorders
Single gene defects
   Cystic fibrosis
   Fragile X syndrome
   Duchenne-Becker muscular dystrophy
   Myotonic dystrophy
   Sickle cell disease and other hemoglobinopathies
   Hemophilia
Congenital infections

TABLE 50–5. INDICATIONS FOR PRENATAL DIAGNOSIS

Advanced maternal age ($\geq$ 35 years)
Previous child with a chromosomal abnormality
Previous child with a major malformation
Previous child with certain skeletal dysplasias
Previous child with a biochemical genetic disorder
Previous child with certain single gene disorders
High risk for certain genetic or biochemical disorders
Balanced chromosomal rearrangement in a parent
Abnormal maternal serum α-fetoprotein level (high or low)
Exposure to teratogenic agents

transabdominal or transvaginal amniocentesis at 3 to 5 months of pregnancy, (3) aspiration of fetal blood by periumbilical blood sampling (PUBS), or (4) fetal biopsy.

Measurement of maternal serum α-fetoprotein (MSAFP) has previously been recommended as a routine prenatal test. An elevated MSAFP level can indicate an open neural tube defect, abdominal wall defect, or other serious birth defect, and a low MSAFP level indicates an increased risk for Down syndrome or other chromosomal abnormalities. Advances in maternal serum testing have added human chorionic gonadotropin (hCG) and unconjugated estriol (uE3) to MSAFP testing, resulting in a triple screen. Women carrying Down syndrome pregnancies, in addition to more likely exhibiting low levels of MSAFP, more likely also have low uE3 and elevated hCG levels. Levels of these analytes may also show specific elevations or depressions in pregnancies with other chromosomal abnormalities, particularly trisomy 18 and trisomy 13. This technology screens most sensitively for neural tube defects, abdominal wall defects, and chromosome abnormalities between 16 and 18 weeks of pregnancy.

Common indications for prenatal diagnostic evaluation are listed in Table 50–5. Of course, the use of amniocentesis or CVS poses a risk to the pregnancy; the complication rate (infection, hemorrhage, cramping, preterm labor, miscarriage) associated with these procedures is 1:200 to 1:400. Other problems include failure of the fetal cell culture to grow and contamination of the fetal cells with maternal cells; in either case, a repeat amniocentesis procedure may be required. Unfortunately, normal results on fetal ultrasonography, a fetal chromosome analysis, or a triple screen do not completely eliminate the possibility that the infant will have a genetic condition. However, normal screening test results can be reassuring to the couple and the physician. If a genetic condition or particular birth defects are diagnosed prenatally, the family and physician have the option to modify the care of the fetus or newborn, to be psychologically and medically prepared for the birth of the affected child, and to discuss and possibly implement the option of pregnancy termination.

The failure to discuss prenatal diagnostic options with couples at increased risk for having children with genetic conditions or certain birth defects could result in the physician being medicolegally at fault. Legal action has been brought against physicians because of failure to counsel families appropriately, resulting in "wrongful birth", and courts are increasingly finding physicians responsible for the consequences of erroneous genetic counseling or counseling omissions.

Couples at high risk for having infants with genetic conditions or birth defects may decline prenatal diagnosis on moral, individual, or financial grounds. However, they may desire to decrease their risk of having an affected child utilizing other available reproductive options. Though some couples prefer to "take their chances," all couples must be informed of appropriate alternatives, including artificial insemination by donor sperm, surrogate motherhood, and in vitro fertilization with a donor egg, as well as the options of adoption, contraception, and sterilization. Advances have also been made in diagnosing certain genetic conditions before implantation. With this technique, a woman's eggs are fertilized in vitro; and once reaching the eight-cell blastocyst stage, a single blastomere is removed and studied for the presence or absence of certain genetic conditions. Only unaffected blastocysts are subsequently implanted in the mother. This technology has been successfully used for preimplantation diagnosis of embryos that are unaffected with cystic fibrosis, Tay-

Sachs disease, and Lesch-Nyhan syndrome; and it could potentially be used for prenatal testing for numerous single gene disorders as well as certain chromosomal abnormalities. However, this technology is new and expensive, and so far a rather low proportion of women undergoing the procedure actually achieve a viable pregnancy.

PATTERNS OF INHERITANCE AND COMMON GENETIC CONDITIONS

As listed in Table 50–1, most birth defects and genetic conditions with known causes are due to chromosomal abnormalities, single gene defects, or multifactorial inheritance. These categories of genetic conditions represent convenient groupings for additional discussion.

CHROMOSOMAL ABNORMALITIES

Disorders involving the chromosomes constitute a net gain or loss of genetic information within cells. From an evolutionary standpoint, cellular processes are finely tuned by the activity and influence of two copies of each gene (except for the sex chromosomes). When there is missing or extra chromosomal material, specific cell types can be irreversibly altered in their developmental program and physiologic function. Four types of chromosomal abnormality have been recognized: aneuploidy, cytogenetically visible structural rearrangements, submicroscopic deletions and duplications, and mosaicism. The clinical indications for performing a chromosome analysis are listed in Table 50–6. Though it is customary to perform routine and specialized chromosome analysis studies on a leukocyte culture from a heparinized blood sample, virtually any body tissue can be used. Specimens can even be collected postmortem or from aborted material, if death occurred less than 2 days previously; in these instances, skin or connective tissue is usually obtained for fibroblast culture and chromosome analysis. In the past a buccal smear was used to screen for abnormalities of sex chromosome number, but this screening test is rather crude. Most cytogenetic laboratories no longer offer buccal smear analysis, as leukocyte chromosome analysis is more accurate and can be performed in 48 hours on an immediate basis.

Aneuploidy

Chromosomal maldistribution during meiosis, leading to an altered number of chromosomes (aneuploidy), occurs in at least 4 per cent of recognized pregnancies. Often the genetic imbalances have such adverse effects on development that the conceptus does not survive. For this reason, aneuploid embryos constitute a major cause of first-trimester spontaneous miscarriage. However, a proportion of certain aneuploid conceptuses are viable, particularly those involving the sex chromosomes and autosomes 13, 18, and 21. Common aneuploid conditions and their features are listed in Table 50–7. Monosomy for the X chromosome (Turner syndrome) is viable despite the fact that 99.9 per cent of Turner syndrome conceptuses spontaneously miscarry. Monosomy for the autosomal chromosomes are rarely viable.

Polyploidy is the presence of more than two haploid sets of chromosomes and is generally another nonviable numerical abnormality of chromosomes that also results in first-trimester miscarriages. Polyploidy accounts for many cases of "blighted ovum" or "empty gestational sac" syndrome. However, one form of polyploidy—three haploid sets of chromosomes (triploidy)—may be viable to term (Table 50–7).

Cytogenetically Visible Structural Rearrangements

Gain or loss of segments of chromosomal material by chromosomal breakage are less frequent than numeric abnormalities of chromosomes. The diversity of chromosomal rearrangements is, however, more extensive. If a single chromosomal break occurs, the broken piece of chromosome may be lost from the cell (deletion). With more than one chromosomal break, rearrangements may occur within a chromosome (inversion, ring chromosome formation), between homologous chromosomes (duplication and deletion), or between nonhomologous chromosomes (translocation).

Many chromosomal deletion syndromes are relatively common and have specific features, such as partial deletion of the short arm of chromosome 4 (Wolf-Hirschhorn syndrome) or partial deletion of the short arm of chromosome 5 (cri du chat syn-

---

TABLE 50–6. INDICATIONS FOR PERFORMING A CHROMOSOME ANALYSIS

Features of a chromosomal syndrome
Multiple malformations ± mental retardation
Psychomotor or growth retardation (or both)
X-linked mental retardation (e.g., testing for fragile X syndrome)
X-linked disorder occurring in a female patient
Ambiguous genitalia
Hypogonadism, cryptorchidism, small testes
Primary amenorrhea
Multiple miscarriages
Infertility
Family history of a balanced chromosomal rearrangement
Prenatal diagnosis (advanced maternal age, positive family history, abnormal "triple screen and/or ultrasonography results)
Evaluation for a chromosomal breakage syndrome
Tumor tissue cytogenetic evaluation

TABLE 50–7. COMMON CHROMOSOMAL ANEUPLOID/POLYPLOID CONDITIONS

Condition	Designation	Features
Trisomy 21 (Down syndrome)	47,XX, +21 *or* 47,XY, +21	Growth and mental deficiency; characteristic facies; hypotonia; cardiac and gastrointestinal defects
Trisomy 18 (Edwards syndrome)	47,XX, +18 *or* 47,XY, +18	Severe growth and mental deficiency; characteristic facies; cardiac, renal, and skeletal defects; clenched hands; hypertonicity
Trisomy 13 (Patau syndrome)	47,XX, +13 *or* 47,XY, +13	Severe mental deficiency; scalp defects; CNS malformations; cleft lip and palate; polydactyly; cardiac and ocular defects
Turner syndrome	45,X	Short stature; nuchal webbing; broad chest; cubitus valgus; congenitally puffy hands and feet; cardiac and renal defects; amenorrhea; infertility
Klinefelter syndrome	47,XXY	Tall statute; gynecomastia; infertility; hypogonadism; occasional learning disabilities or behavioral problems (or both)
XYY syndrome	47,XYY	Tall stature; often behavioral problems; loose association with criminality
Triploidy	69,XXX *or* 69,XXY *or* 69,XYY	Growth and mental deficiency; characteristic facies; CNS, ocular, cardiac, and renal defects; spina bifida; omphalocele; cleft lip and palate; third and fourth finger syndactyly

drome). These and many other partial monosomy syndromes are more viable than monosomy for entire chromosomes. Approximately 2 to 8 per cent of undiagnosed children with psychomotor retardation and multiple minor malformations have a partial chromosomal deletion or a duplication. The family physician should always consider obtaining a chromosome analysis for the evaluation of such children.

Several chromosomal inversions (inverse rearrangement of an internal segment of the chromosome) are common in the general population and are of no clinical significance for the individual with the inversion. Inversions within chromosomes 1, 2, 9, and 16 occur most frequently. Similarly, translocations between chromosomes, in which no net chromosomal material is gained or lost during the rearrangement, generally do not adversely affect the individual with such a "balanced" translocation. In fact, approximately 1 in 500 normal individuals has a balanced structural chromosomal rearrangement. Individuals with balanced structural chromosomal rearrangements are, however, at high risk for producing gametes that are "unbalanced" regarding the usual haploid state of eggs or sperm. Thus fertilization with a normal egg or sperm results in an unbalanced conceptus, which may miscarry, or produce an infant with multiple malformations and psychomotor retardation. Multiple miscarriages or multiple children with birth defects and psychomotor retardation warrants further investigation of family members for balanced chromosomal rearrangements. Of children with trisomy 13, 18, or 21, about 1 to 6 per cent have 46 chromosomes (instead of 47), with the extra dose of their particular trisomy attached to another chromosome. These children are usually phenotypically indistinguishable from children with the typical trisomies. Therefore the major reason for performing a chromosome analysis on individuals with autosomal trisomy syndromes, other

than to confirm the diagnosis, is to determine if the child has a translocation chromosome rather than the usual trisomy state. One third of these children with a translocation chromosome have a parent with a balanced translocation, and these couples have a high risk of producing subsequent similarly affected trisomic offspring.

Submicroscopic Deletions and Duplications

It has been recognized that small segments of chromosomal material, containing 50 or fewer genes, can be deleted or duplicated on the chromosome and cause specific syndromes. Often these duplications or deletions are not visible by standard chromosome analysis. Because gain or loss of the same group of genes is the common mechanism for patients with each particular syndrome, these conditions have come to be known as "contiguous gene syndromes." Examples of contiguous gene deletion syndromes are listed above (see Identifying/Recognizing and Evaluating the Dysmorphic Child). Fewer contiguous gene duplication syndromes have been described; they include Cornelia deLange syndrome and Charcot-Marie-Tooth disease. Submicroscopic deletion and duplication syndromes are not generally diagnosed by routine chromosome analysis, and specialized testing must be utilized to confirm or exclude such diagnoses.

Mosaicism

Chromosomal mosaicism, or differing chromosomal complements within the cells of the same individual, arise by errors in the assortment of chromosomes during postzygotic (somatic) cell division. Mosaic individuals have at least two cell populations, from the standpoint of chromosome number. For example, individuals with Turner syndrome mosaicism, consisting of a normal cell line and an aneuploid cell line (e.g., 46,XX/45,X), have different proportions of normal versus aneuploid cells in each body tissue. Because of the possible varying proportions of normal to aneuploid cells, Turner syndrome mosaic individuals can exhibit every graduation, from typical Turner syndrome to near-normal appearance and reproductive function. In general, mosaic individuals often have less obvious clinical manifestations than nonmosaic affected individuals; but individuals identified because of clinical abnormalities most often have a sufficiently large population of chromosomally abnormal cells to be of serious consequence. The health care of such individuals is usually similar to that of individuals affected with the nonmosaic form of the chromosomal abnormality.

Genetic counseling issues for chromosomal mosaicism rely on the empiric observation that recurrence of mosaic chromosomal abnormalities in a family is usually low. However, clear data exist that gonadal mosaic cell lines in a parent (either for chromosomal abnormalities or for mutant genes) is an important reason for recurrence of apparently sporadic genetic disorders in families. For example, gonadal mosaicism has been shown to be the cause for noncarrier women of Duchenne muscular dystrophy (an X-linked recessive disorder) having multiple affected sons, or for normal parents to have multiple affected children with perinatal lethal osteogenesis imperfecta, type II (an autosomal dominant disorder). In each of these situations, a "normal" parent, with mosaicism likely limited to their gonads, produces gametes that contain the normal gene as well as a proportion of gametes with the corresponding mutant gene. This risk for recurrence in the family should be explicitly considered during genetic counseling.

SINGLE GENE (MONOGENIC) DEFECTS

Single gene (monogenic) defects are more common than chromosomal abnormalities as a cause of genetic disease. Monogenic disorders can be due to a qualitative or quantitative abnormality of gene function in that mutations within genes can alter the normal function of the protein produced by the gene, enhance the function of the protein, or completely eliminate any functional protein production by the gene. Therefore different mutations within a particular gene often have differing clinical effects. For example, the most common types of mutation that occur within the dystrophin gene (a gene on the X chromosome) are deletions or duplications of regions of the gene. Deletions or duplications in certain critical regions of the gene lead to features of Duchenne muscular dystrophy in affected boys who have the mutation; however, deletions or duplications in less critical regions of

TABLE 50–8. COMMON MONOGENIC DISORDERS

Autosomal Dominant
Charcot-Marie-Tooth disease
Huntington's chorea
Marfan syndrome
Myotonic dystrophy
Neurofibromatosis
Osteogenesis imperfecta
Tuberous sclerosis

Autosomal Recessive
Cystic fibrosis
Fanconi anemia
Galactosemia
Phenylketonuria
Sickle cell anemia
Tay-Sachs disease
Xeroderma pigmentosa

X-Linked Recessive
Duchenne-Becker muscular dystrophy
Fragile X syndrome
Hemophilia A and B
Hunter syndrome
Menkes syndrome
Testicular feminization
X-linked hydrocephalus

the gene lead to a milder form of the disease (Becker muscular dystrophy). Therefore the differing clinical features that exist among individuals affected with the same genetic condition often result from different types of mutation within the particular gene causing the disorder.

Each monogenic disorder generally follows a particular pattern of inheritance. These inheritance patterns are based on the dosage of mutant genes necessary to produce clinical manifestations of the disorder, as well as on whether the gene is located on an autosome or a sex chromosome. The three usual pattens of inheritance are autosomal dominant, autosomal recessive, and X-linked recessive; common disorders in each of these categories are listed in Table 50–8. X-linked dominant disorders are relatively infrequent. A pattern of inheritance, not related to the autosomes or sex chromosomes, is "mitochondrial inheritance."

Autosomal Dominant Inheritance

Autosomal dominant disorders occur when a single gene dose of a mutant gene is present on one of the autosomes. The risk of the single mutant gene being passed to a given offspring is 50 per cent, and the two sexes are equally likely to be affected. However, many autosomal dominant conditions are widely variable in expression among affected individuals, presumably owing to the effect on the protein molecule by the mutation, as well as by other differences in genetic or environmental background of the affected individual. Therefore there are varying degrees to which clinical signs of a particular autosomal dominant disorder are manifested in different individuals, even among affected individuals within the same family. Some individuals are so mildly affected they are not clinically recognizable; these individuals are said to lack penetrance. However, even mildly affected individuals have the same 50 per cent chance with each pregnancy of passing the mutant gene on to an offspring.

It often occurs in autosomal dominant disorders that no other family member, except the affected child, has features of the condition. In these cases, the child has a "new gene mutation" that occurred in one of the germ cells that formed the conceptus. Approximately 50 per cent of neurofibromatosis cases, 35 per cent of Marfan syndrome cases, and 85 per cent of tuberous sclerosis cases represent new mutations. The parents of a child with a new mutation generally have a low risk for recurrence in a future pregnancy, though the affected child has the 50 per cent chance of passing on the mutant gene to his or her children.

In addition to the autosomal dominant conditions listed in Table 50–8, most skeletal dysplasias (e.g., achondroplasia, many chondrodysplasias) and disorders of connective tissue (e.g., Stickler syndrome, some forms of Ehlers-Danlos syndrome) are due to mutations in autosomal dominant genes. Additionally, some neurodegenerative disorders (e.g., spinocerebellar ataxia, familial cases of Alzheimer disease, and multiple sclerosis) and familial cases of psychiatric disorders (some cases of schizophrenia and bipolar affective illness) are due to autosomal dominant genes. Familial cancers (e.g., breast, colon, retinoblastoma) are also due to the effect of an autosomal dominant mutant gene.

Autosomal Recessive Inheritance

Autosomal recessive conditions occur when both members of a gene pair have mutations that disrupt normal function. For an individual to inherit a double dose of the mutant gene, it is necessary that both parents have a single dose of the mutant gene, and they are designated "carriers." Carriers generally have no features of the particular genetic condition for which they carry a mutant gene because of compensation by the normal gene of the pair. However, when both parents are carriers, they have a 25 per cent risk with each pregnancy of having an offspring affected with the autosomal recessive condition. Relatives of known carriers also have a high risk to be carriers themselves and would have the same 25 per cent risk of having an affected child if their spouse were also a carrier; because some autosomal recessive conditions have a relatively high population carrier frequency, genetic counseling for relatives of known carriers is indicated. Additionally, consanguinity increases the risk that a couple will have a child with an autosomal recessive disorder; genetic counseling is indicated for such couples.

In addition to the conditions listed in Table 50–8, most enzyme defects are inherited in an autosomal recessive fashion. Examples include maple syrup urine disease, homocystinuria, defects in fatty acid metabolism, most glycogen storage diseases, most mucopolysaccharidoses (except Hunter syndrome), other storage disorders, most aminoacidopathies, organicacidopathies, and disorders of the urea cycle (except ornithine transcarbamylase deficiency, an X-linked recessive disorder). The hemoglobinopathies and other serum protein variants (e.g., α_1-antitrypsin deficiency) are also recessively inherited.

X-Linked Recessive Inheritance

Genes on the X chromosome in the normal male (46,XY) are present in but a single dose; hence a mutation in a gene on the male's X chromosome often produces a genetic condition. Because a female has two X chromosomes, a recessive mutant gene on one of her X chromosomes generally has little or no clinical effects; but she is a carrier for this mutation, and each of her male offspring has a 50 per cent chance of being affected with the X-linked recessive condition. In addition, each daughter of a female carrier has a similar 50 per cent chance to be a carrier. The following precepts are important for detecting X-linked recessive inheritance: (1) with rare exceptions, only males are affected, and the transmission is through unaffected or mildly affected carrier females; (2) there is no male-to-male (father-to-son) transmission, as a son receives his Y chromosome from his father; and (3) if an affected male is able to reproduce, none of his sons will be affected, but all of his daughters will be carriers for the condition.

Examples of typical X-linked recessive conditions are listed in Table 50–8. There are several X-linked disorders that cause preterm male lethality, but features of the condition occur in female carriers. Some of these disorders are recognized because of recurrent miscarriages and lack of males being born with the condition (e.g., incontinentia pigmenti, oral-facial-digital syndrome type I), and others occur by new gene mutation, whereby only affected girls are ever observed (e.g., Aicardi syndrome, Rett syndrome).

Mitochondrial Inheritance

Cellular mitochondria, in addition to containing the various enzymes of aerobic metabolism, fatty acid oxidation, and the respiratory transport chain, also contain circular strands of genetic information known as the mitochondrial DNA (mtDNA). Encoded within the mtDNA are several subunits of the respiratory chain enzymes, as well as a complete set of genes for producing mitochondria-specific transfer RNAs and ribosomal RNAs. Each mitochondrion contains 50 to 100 mtDNA molecules, and there may be thousands of mitochondria per cell. If a mutation exists within a gene encoded by the mtDNA, the severity of this mutation depends on (1) the fraction of mtDNA molecules within the mitochondrion that contain this mutation, (2) the fraction of mitochondria within the cell that contain mtDNA molecules with the mutant gene, and (3) the fraction of cells within a tissue that contain mitochondria bearing the mutation. Tissues with the highest rate of energy metabolism (skeletal muscle, cardiac muscle, brain, and liver) tend to exhibit the severest clinical features when mtDNA mutations are present.

The egg contributes essentially all the mitochondria to the conceptus; virtually none of the sperm's mitochondria are incorporated into the fertilized egg. Therefore mtDNA mutations show a pattern of inheritance known as "maternal inheritance." Essentially, all offspring (male or female) of a woman with a mitochondrial mutation have some proportion of cells containing varying proportions of the mutant mtDNA, whereas none of the offspring of a man with a mitochondrial mutation is affected. Because the fraction of mutant mtDNA molecules, "mutant mitochondria," and "mutant cells" vary from one individual to another, even within the same family, the variability of features in each condition is extensive, from severe to clinically undetectable.

Mitochondrial inheritance should be considered when all children of a woman have some degree of features of respiratory chain enzyme dysfunction (e.g., myopathy, neuropathy, seizures, encephalopathy, lactic acidosis). Examples of conditions due to mtDNA mutations include Kearns-Sayre syndrome, Leber optic atrophy, Pearson marrow-pancreas syndrome, MERRF syndrome, and MELAS syndrome.

MULTIFACTORIAL INHERITANCE

Many genetic conditions do not have a single gene or a chromosomal abnormality as the underlying cause but occur based on a combination of defects in several genes, known as polygenic inheritance. In addition, malformations and features of polygenic conditions may also be influenced by "environmental" factors in the uterus and fetal blood supply. Thus these conditions do not show a simple pattern of inheritance and so occur on a multifactorial basis. Examples of conditions with multifactorial inheritance include several major malformations (neural tube defects, some forms of cleft lip/cleft palate, some types of congenital heart disease, and pyloric stenosis), as well as diabetes, coronary artery disease, hypertension, epilepsy, and some types of cancer.

Empiric data collected from familial cases of conditions inherited in a multifactorial fashion indicate that the likelihood of a recurrence in a first-degree relative is higher than the general population rate, and is usually in the range of 3 to 5 per cent. For example, the general population rate of neural tube defects is approximately 0.1 per cent, whereas the recurrence risk for a couple who has had one child with spina bifida is approximately 3.0 per cent. Among more distant relatives, the likelihood of sufficient factors occurring within a particular individual to exceed the threshold of occurrence becomes progressively less. In fact, the incidence of affected individuals among third-degree relatives is similar to the low general population risk.

Multifactorial inheritance for the major malformations noted above applies only to the condition if it occurs on an isolated basis. If, for example, a type of congenital heart disease occurs as a component of Down syndrome, DiGeorge syndrome, or Turner syndrome, the mode of inheritance and the genetic counseling issues regarding recurrence would have to reflect the entire syndromic diagnosis. Similarly, if congenital heart disease is primarily due to an environmental teratogenic factor, as in maternal phenylketonuria effects or congenital rubella syndrome, the heart defect would have a low recurrence risk in a future pregnancy unless a similar environmental insult were to occur. Each of these various causes of congenital heart defect would have distinct genetic and health implications for the affected individual and other family members. Careful evaluation by trained genetics specialists can assist in appropriately diagnosing affected individuals, thereby providing optimal care to patients and their families.

CARE OF THE GENETIC DISORDER PATIENT AND FAMILY

The medical care of patients with genetic conditions generally should be organized by a "case coordinator" (usually a family physician or other primary care physician). Care for the patient with congenital malformations, psychomotor retardation, or complex medical issues should include the usual health care provided to all individuals, as well as specialized surgical management, medical therapy, and developmental/educational intervention as required by the special needs of each particular patient. It is often overwhelming to keep track of the array of medical specialists involved in each patient's care, and the appropriate recommendations for interventions at each stage of development. Often the family physician relies on the advice of genetics consultants, genetic syndrome networks, and medical or surgical subspecialists with particular expertise in caring for patients with genetic conditions.

Patients with genetic conditions require the same health care screening procedures provided to everyone. For example, children with Down syndrome require the usual immunizations and well-child care procedures recommended by the American Academy of Pediatrics. Similarly, adults with Down syndrome should have health evaluations using the standard accepted practices. Down syndrome patients do have special needs and the potential for a variety of additional medical and surgical problems, however, which should be attended to by their health care providers. Appropriate medical and surgical follow-up for Down syndrome patients often falls under the auspices of the primary care physician, so it is the obligation of the physician to become familiar with medical care recommendations for Down syndrome patients. This statement could be generalized to any child or adult with a genetic condition within a physician's medical practice. Advice and information regarding appropriate medical management for genetic patients can often be obtained from genetic consultants, syndrome networks, or family support groups. An example of a guide for practitioners that relates to the management of Down syndrome is described below (adapted from the Ohio/Western Pennsylvania Down Syndrome Network). The family physician should be aware that specific guides for patients with other genetic conditions (from neurofibromatosis, Marfan syndrome, and Turner syndrome to phenylketonuria, fragile-X syndrome, and sickle cell anemia) must be utilized in each case. Most guides would be developed in conjunction with advice from a genetics specialist. Each set of guidelines would supplement routine childhood and adult health care.

Down Syndrome Management Guide

Neonatal Period (Birth to 2 Months)

HISTORY. Document parental concerns and if there is vomiting or an absence of stools. Check for gastrointestinal (GI) tract obstruction. Review the feeding history to ensure adequate caloric intake.

EXAMINATION. Evaluate for cyanosis, irregular heart rate, cardiac murmur, cataracts, otitis media, intact hearing, normal hips, and normal fontanelles.

LABORATORY WORK-UP AND CONSULTATIONS. The following should be done: chromosome analysis, genetic counseling, thyroid function test (by State Newborn Screen), and evaluation by a pediatric cardiologist including an echocardiogram (even with absent murmur). Referral is made to a cardiac surgeon if a congenital heart defect is present. Consultation is undertaken with a GI and feeding specialist if feeding difficulties or gastroesophageal reflux exists, or with a general surgeon if there is evidence of GI obstruction.

DEVELOPMENT. Discuss early intervention and refer for enrollment in a local program.

Infancy (2 to 12 Months)

HISTORY. Question the parent about respiratory infections, otitis media, and constipation. (Use aggressive dietary management and consider Hirshsprung's disease if the infant is resistant to diet and laxatives.)

EXAMINATION. Check for hip dislocation. Visualize the tympanic membranes or refer to an otolaryngologist.

LABORATORY WORK-UP AND CONSULTATIONS. Test the auditory brainstem response by 12 months of age (earlier if there is a history of frequent otitis media). A pediatric ophthalmologic evaluation is done by 6 months of age (earlier if there is evidence of nystagmus, strabismus, or poor vision). A thyroid function test is done at 6 months of age. Refer for evaluation by an otolaryngologist if there is recurrent otitis media.

DEVELOPMENT. Occupational therapy evaluations are done for motor development and feeding, as is a generalized developmental evaluation (if not already done as part of an early intervention program).

Childhood (1 to 12 Years)

HISTORY. Review parental concerns and the current level of functioning. Assess the child for hearing problems, sleep problems (snoring: obstructive sleep apnea), and constipation. Review the ophthalmologic and dental care. Monitor for behavior problems. At puberty provide reproductive information. (Boys are generally sterile, but girls may be capable of reproduction. Because of their mental handicap, the girls may be taken advantage of sexually, so there is a need to discuss sexual abuse and birth control measures.)

EXAMINATION. General physical and neurologic examinations are undertaken at this time.

LABORATORY WORK-UP AND CONSULTATIONS. Thyroid function tests are done yearly to evaluate for hypothyroidism. Auditory testing is done yearly for the first 3 years of life and then every 2 years from age 3 to 13 years. Eye examinations are done every 2 years. Lateral cervical spine radiographs in flexion and extension are obtained to rule out atlantoaxial instability at 3 to 4 years of age. The initial dental evaluation is done at 2 years and then every 6 months. Orthopedic assessment is carried out at 2 to 3 years of age if flat feet and weak ankles are present. A diet/nutrition assessment is done if the child is obese.

DEVELOPMENT. The child is enrolled in an appropriate developmental or educational program with complete yearly educational assessment. Evaluations by speech and language pathologists are strongly recommended.

Adult

HISTORY. Question the patient about hearing or vision difficulties, behavioral problems, or memory loss. (There is an increased risk for the neuropathologic features of Alzheimer disease after age 40, although only a few patients show cognitive decline before age 60.) Note any sleep problems. Review the patient's current level of functioning and school or vocational plans. Review his or her reproductive plans, with counseling that women are at risk for having aneuploid offspring.

EXAMINATION. Conduct a general adult examination, including a gynecologic examination in women.

LABORATORY WORK-UP AND CONSULTATIONS. Thyroid function tests are done yearly and auditory and vision tests as needed. Conduct a diet/nutrition assessment if obesity is present.

DEVELOPMENT. A yearly educational assessment is done while the patient is still in school. Refer him or her for appropriate vocational training and to the appropriate agency for living quarters if necessary.

Comment

Providing medical care for genetic disorder patients and obtaining appropriate laboratory tests, referrals, and consultations can be challenging and rewarding. The family physician should make every attempt to become familiar with the special needs for each of these patients in the practice.

Care of the genetic disorder patient extends to the family, who initially may find it difficult to accept an "imperfect" child. Families should be allowed to express their grief and then be encouraged to move into a problem-solving mode. Most parents feel guilty and erroneously blame themselves or some event before or during the pregnancy for having caused the child's genetic problem. Repeated assurance that they did not cause the problem is necessary. Parents should receive genetic counseling and specific printed information about the genetic condition that covers health, social, and educational concerns. Often advice and support from other parents with similarly affected children is a valuable resource. Many local and national parent support groups exist. A list of organizations and agencies that may be of assistance to families with individuals affected with genetic conditions is available from the National Center for Education in Maternal and Child Health in Washington, DC (see Bibliography). Generally, the family physician is the "team leader" in terms of providing comprehensive care for the family and the affected patient.

TREATMENT OF GENETIC CONDITIONS

Effective treatments are available for numerous aspects of genetic conditions, though there are not yet any true cures for genetic problems. The closest thing to actual cures for genetic problems include surgical and cosmetic repair of malformations, dietary restriction in certain metabolic conditions, liver, kidney, or bone marrow transplantation for certain metabolic or immunodeficiency disorders, and enzyme replacement (currently used in a few metabolic disorders). On the horizon is gene therapy, whereby normal genes are inserted into the patient's cells to provide the deficient function; many research laboratories are evaluating the utility of gene therapy for the treatment of certain genetic immunodeficiencies, inborn errors of metabolism, thalassemias, hemoglobinopathies, cystic fibrosis, and muscular dystrophy. Many technical problems must be solved before gene therapy can be a reality.

Effective forms of treatment are already available for the medical and surgical complications in many genetic conditions. Examples of available treatments are summarized in Table 50–9. Appropriate medical management can improve the quality of life for most individuals with genetic conditions and their families.

TABLE 50–9. EXAMPLES OF TREATMENTS FOR GENETIC CONDITIONS

Dietary restriction
  Restrict galactose in galactosemia
  Restrict phenylalanine in phenylketonuria
  Restrict protein in urea cycle disorders

Replacement of missing physiologic substances
  Biotin in biotinidase deficiency
  Thyroxine in congenital hypothyroidism
  Factor VIII in hemophilia A

Medications to remove toxic substances
  Penicillamine in Wilson's disease
  Phenylacetate in urea cycle defects
  Carnitine in organic acidopathies

Avoidance of hazardous factors
  Fava beans in G-6-PD deficiency
  Halothane in malignant hyperthermia
  Barbiturates in porphyria

Surgical correction
  Repair of congenital heart defect
  Repair of cleft lip/cleft palate

Surgical management
  Colectomy in familial polyposis
  Ventriculoperitoneal shunt in spina bifida

Organ transplantation
  Bone marrow in immunodeficiency disorders
  Liver transplant in some urea cycle defects
  Kidney transplant in polycystic kidney disease

SUGGESTED READINGS

Beighton P: Heritable Disorders of Connective Tissue, 5th edition. St. Louis, Mosby-Year Book, 1993.

Brock DJH, Rodeck CH, Ferguson-Smith MA: Prenatal Diagnosis and Screening. New York, Churchill Livingstone, 1992.

Buyse ML: Birth Defects Encyclopedia. Cambridge, MA, Blackwell Scientific Publications, 1990.

Emery AEH, Rimoin DL: Principles and Practice of Medical Genetics, 2nd edition. New York, Churchill Livingstone, 1990.

Gorlin RJ, Cohen MM, Levin LS: Syndromes of the Head and Neck, 3rd edition. New York, Oxford University Press, 1990.

Hudis J: Teratogen Information Services. New York, March of Dimes Birth Defects Foundation, 1988.

Jones KL: Smith's Recognizable Patterns of Human Malformation, 4th edition. Philadelphia, WB Saunders Company, 1988.

McKusick VA: Mendelian Inheritance in Man: Catalogs of Autosomal Dominant, Autosomal Recessive, and X-linked Phenotypes, 10th edition. Baltimore, Johns Hopkins University Press, 1992.

National Center for Education in Maternal and Child Health: A National List of Voluntary Organizations in Maternal and Child Health. Washington, DC, 1985.

Scriver CR, Beaudet AL, Sly WS, et al: The Metabolic Basis of Inherited Disease, 6th edition. New York, McGraw-Hill, 1989.

Shepard TH: Catalog of Teratogenic Agents, 5th edition. Baltimore, Johns Hopkins University Press, 1986.

Stevenson RE, Hall JG, Goodman RM: Human Malformations and Related Anomalies. New York, Oxford University Press, 1993.

Thompson MW, McInnes RR, Willard HF: Thompson & Thompson: Genetics in Medicine, 5th edition. Philadelphia, WB Saunders Company, 1991.

Vogel F, Motulsky HG: Human Genetics: Problems and Approaches, 2nd edition. New York, Springer-Verlag, 1986.

Wiedemann H-R, Grosse K-R, Dibbern H: An Atlas of Characteristic Syndromes: A Visual Aid to Diagnosis for Clinicians and Practising Physicians. London, Wolfe Medical Publications, 1985.

CHAPTER 51

DIAGNOSIS AND TREATMENT OF ANXIETY DISORDERS

WAYNE KATON and JOHN P. GEYMAN

Whether viewed as mental illness, psychiatric problems, stress-related illness, or functional disorders, psychological dysfunction of individuals in our increasingly complex society may well be more frequent and more incapacitating than any other disease or disorder. Studies sponsored by the National Institute of Mental Health have shown that in the United States more than one half of all patients with mental health disorders are cared for solely by the primary care sector (Regier et al., 1984; Shapiro et al., 1984). Several studies have demonstrated that 25 to 33 per cent of primary care patients suffer from a *DSM-III* mental disorder (Hoeper et al., 1979). Moreover, primary care patients with mental disorder utilize approximately twice as much nonpsychiatric medical care (Hankin and Oktay, 1979). These patients also have a higher incidence of organic illness than patients without mental health problems (Eastwood, 1971). As a result of their long-term contact with all members of the family, family physicians have a special opportunity and responsibility to recognize and manage mental health problems.

Anxiety and depression represent the two most common mental health disorders encountered in everyday medical practice (Marsland et al., 1976). The Epidemiologic Catchment Area (ECA) Study, which measured the prevalence of mental illness in five major U.S. cities, found that anxiety disorders occurred in 15.4 per cent of the community, second only to disorders of substance abuse, which occurred in 16.7 per cent of the population (Yates, 1986). Anxiety has been found to be the fifth most common clinical diagnosis in primary care (Marsland et al., 1976; Vallbona, 1973). Moreover, the 1980–1981 National Ambulatory Medical Care survey (which gathered information on approximately 90,000 visits to a nationally representative sample of private physicians from nine specialty groups) determined that anxiety and nervousness accounted for 11 per cent of all visits to physicians (Schurman et al., 1985). Further evidence of the prevalence of anxiety was provided by a survey of 350 primary care physicians in which anxiety disorders were rated as the most common psychiatric problem seen in their clinics (Orleans et al.,

1985). Antianxiety agents in general and benzodiazepines in particular have been consistently the most prescribed medications in the United States since the 1970s, and primary care physicians wrote 85 per cent of these prescriptions (Mellinger et al., 1984).

Anxiety not only is caused by social problems but is frequently precipitated by medical illness. Thus Zung (1979) demonstrated that significant anxiety is found in 9 per cent of people in the community, in 32 per cent of people seeking primary care treatment, and in 52 per cent of patients with a known cardiologic illness. Anxiety frequently causes amplification of complaints of chronic medical illness and often worsens the pathophysiologic state in those illnesses (e.g., angina pectoris, asthma, peptic ulcer disease) that may be adversely affected by increased sympathetic nervous system arousal (Katon and Roy-Byrne, 1988).

DEFINITION

Anxiety has been described as a fearful emotion accompanied by certain physical symptoms. It may be of acute onset or of chronic nature as a long-standing problem featuring a variety of physical complaints. Rickels (1977) described anxiety in the following terms.

Anxiety is perceived as a subjective feeling of heightened tension and diffuse uneasiness defined as the conscious and reportable experience of intense dread and foreboding conceptualized as internally derived and unrelated to external threat. It is not merely fear because it lacks a specific object.

A major change precipitated by the development of the *Diagnostic and Statistical Manual of Mental Disorders* (*DSM-III*) in 1980 (American Psychiatric Association, 1980) is that anxiety is no longer considered to be a common unidimensional symptom often necessitating treatment with minor tranquilizers. Instead, advances in psychiatric nosology have developed specific identifiable diagnostic categories composed of carefully delineated clusters of symptoms (Friedman and Jaffe,

1983). Each of these categories or syndromes has differing etiologic, treatment, and prognostic implications. The *DSM-III* recognizes the following subclasses of anxiety disorders: phobic, obsessive-compulsive, panic, generalized, posttraumatic stress, and atypical anxiety. This chapter especially focuses on panic disorder and agoraphobia, which are the most common and severe anxiety disorders seen in primary care.

Anxiety disorders must be evaluated in a biopsychosocial framework. Thus genetic and biologic factors in anxiety must be evaluated within the social context in which the disorder began, taking into account the psychological strengths and vulnerabilities of the patient. These disorders occur in a wide variety of patients, from those with strong social support systems and many psychological strengths to patients who are devoid of social support and have many maladaptive personality traits.

DIAGNOSTIC APPROACHES

Panic Disorder

It is especially important to differentiate generalized anxiety disorder or transient states of anxiety associated with life stress from acute panic attacks. There are effective treatments for panic disorder, and accurate diagnosis and early aggressive treatment often decreases potential vocational and social disability.

The key distinguishing feature of panic disorder is the episodic nature of the panic attacks. Panic attacks manifest by the sudden onset of intense apprehension, fear, or terror and the abrupt development of at least four of the following symptoms, reaching a peak within 10 minutes: dyspnea (actually the patient often hyperventilates); palpitations; chest pain or discomfort; choking or smothering sensations; dizziness; a feeling of unreality or of being detached from one's self; paresthesia; diaphoresis; faintness; trembling or shaking; chills or hot flashes; nausea or abdominal distress; fears of dying; and a fear of going crazy or losing control during an attack (Table 51–1) (American Psychiatric Association, 1993).

In clinical samples the onset of panic disorder is generally between the ages of 17 and 30 years (mean 22.5 years) (Sheehan, 1979). In the ECA study, the highest 6-month prevalence was in the 25 to 44 year age group (Myers et al., 1984). In four epidemiologic studies the prevalence of panic disorder in women was 1.6 to 2.9 per cent and in men 0.4 to 1.7 per cent (Crowe et al., 1983; Myers et al., 1984; Uhlenhuth et al., 1983; Weissman et al., 1978). Several studies have found that patients with panic disorder are over-represented within the primary care medical system. Katon and colleagues (1986) randomly assessed 195 primary care patients, aged 17 years and older, with a structured

TABLE 51–1.   DEFINITION OF PANIC DISORDER WITHOUT AGORAPHOBIA

A. The following two conditions are present: (1) Recurrent unexpected panic attacks. (2) At least one of the attacks has been followed by a month (or more) of: (a) persistent concern about having additional attacks; (b) worry about the implications of the attacks or its consequences (e.g., losing control, having a heart attack, "going crazy"); or (c) a significant change in behavior related to the attacks.
B. There is an absence of agoraphobia.
C. The panic attacks are not due to the direct effects of a substance (e.g., drugs of abuse, medication) or a general medical condition (e.g., hyperthyroidism).
D. The anxiety is not better accounted for by another mental disorder, such as obsessive-compulsive disorder (e.g., fear of contamination), posttraumatic stress disorder (e.g., in response to stimuli associated with a severe stressor), separation anxiety disorder, or social phobia (e.g., fear of embarrassment in social situations).

psychiatric interview. A total of 6.5 per cent of patients met *DSM-III* criteria for panic disorder alone, and 6.5 per cent met criteria for major depression and panic disorder. Finlay-Jones and Brawn (1981), utilizing a structured psychiatric interview, found that 17 per cent of 164 female primary care patients suffered from anxiety neurosis (these patients have panic disorder, generalized anxiety, or both), with 8 per cent suffering from anxiety neurosis alone and 9 per cent having anxiety neurosis and major depression.

Three controlled studies have suggested that panic disorder is often precipitated by stressful life events. These studies suggested that patients with panic disorder often have a higher frequency than controls of (1) stressful life events that connote danger and threat (Finlay-Jones and Brawn, 1981); (2) events viewed as uncontrollable or undesirable and that cause severe lowering of self-esteem (Roy-Byrne et al., 1986); and (3) events that involve the death or severe illness of a friend or relative (Faravelli, 1985). Panic attacks have also been described after a physical illness, accident or trauma, rape or physical assault, and endocrinologic changes. Panic disorder is a familial disease, with controlled studies demonstrating that 18 to 40 per cent of first degree relatives of patients with panic disorder also suffer from this severe anxiety disorder (Cohen et al., 1951; Crowe et al., 1983; Noyes, et al., 1978). Moreover, a twin study demonstrated a significantly higher concordance for panic disorder in monozygotic twins versus dizygotic twins (Torgerson, 1983). Genetic studies have found that women are affected more frequently than men, the ratio approaching 2:1. More alcohol abuse is found in the male relatives of panic disorder patients than in control relatives (Cohen et al., 1951; Crowe et al., 1983; Noyes et al., 1978).

There has been an exponential growth in psychobiologic studies of panic disorder. These studies have demonstrated that patients with panic disorder are more susceptible to developing anxiety attacks than normal controls when challenged with specific provocative agents, including intravenous lactate, breathing air with increased carbon dioxide concentrations, isoproterenol, caffeine, and yohimbine (Roy-Byrne and Cowley, 1988). Whether these tests produce specific unique biochemical changes in patients with panic disorder or simply produce increased somatic sensations to which patients with panic disorder overreact is still controversial. Studies with position emission tomography (PET), magnetic resonance imaging (MRI), and brain electrical activity monitoring (BEAM) have implicated parahippocampal and temporal lobe abnormalities in panic disorder; these studies await replication (Katon et al., 1988; Roy-Byrne and Cowley, 1988). Abnormalities in the benzodiazepine γ-aminobutyric acid (GABA) system and the noradrenergic controls of the sympathetic nervous system have also been documented in panic disorder (Katon et al., 1988), but theories of the primacy of either of these systems in the causation of panic disorder remain controversial.

Table 51–2 shows the usual chronology in the development of panic disorder. Patients often experience the onset of the first panic attack, at times described as the worst experience in their life, after one or a series of life events overwhelm their coping mechanisms. Many patients are seen by a family physician after a first or second attack, and early intervention may arrest the syndrome at this point. Other patients go on to the second stage in which panic attacks become more frequent and the patient begins to develop anticipatory anxiety (i.e., anxiety between attacks because of the constant fear another will occur). During this second stage, the patient may begin to associate many environmental events with the anxiety and often develops multiple phobias and avoidance behavior. If patients have an attack while driving, they may avoid getting into the car; or if they have an attack while giving a speech, they may avoid public speaking. This pattern may culminate in the third stage, *agoraphobia*, which literally means "a fear of the marketplace" but actually describes the ultimate regressive behavior of being afraid to leave the house because of the association of panic attacks with

many environmental stimuli. In *DSM-IV* (American Psychiatric Association, 1993), agoraphobia refers to a fear of being in places or situations from which escape might be difficult or embarrassing, or help might be unavailable in the event of having an unexpected or situationally predisposed panic attack. Agoraphobic fears typically involve clusters of situations that include being outside the home alone, being in a crowd, standing in a line, being on a bridge, or traveling in a bus, train or car. Most patients with agoraphobia do leave the house and become involved in activities with a person they see as a protector. Agoraphobic patients often avoid being alone and regressively cling to significant others. Zitrin and coworkers (1978) have shown that almost all agoraphobics have panic attacks.

The patient with panic disorder has cognitive, affective, and somatic symptoms as well as social consequences to the development of the disorder (Grant et al., 1983) (Table 51–3). The patient often selectively focuses on the somatic components of the panic syndrome and attributes the increased anxiety and tension to the frightening nature of these somatic symptoms. Studies have demonstrated that the most common presenting somatic symptoms are cardiologic (chest pain and tachycardia), neurologic (headache, dizziness, faintness, paresthesia), and gastrointestinal (irritable bowel symptoms and epigastric pain) (Katon, 1984). The presentation of cardiologic symptoms may especially lead to costly and potentially dangerous medical tests in patients with panic disorder. Three studies have documented that nearly 50 per cent of patients with chest pain and negative angiographic studies suffer from panic disorder (Bass and Wade, 1984; Beitman et al., 1987; Katon et al., 1988). Some patients with panic disorder develop labile hypertension during an attack. The finding of labile hypertension with associated chest pain, flushing tachycardia, and shortness of breath often leads to an aggressive cardiac work-up as well as a potential work-up for pheochromocytoma. One study demonstrated that approximately 40 per cent of patients evaluated for pheochromocytoma suffered from panic disorder, compared with fewer than 5 per cent of hypertensive controls (Fogart

TABLE 51–2. THREE STAGES IN THE DEVELOPMENT OF PANIC DISORDER

Initial acute panic attack or cluster of attacks	→	Panic attacks increase in frequency	→	Agoraphobia
		Phobias develop		Increased dependence
		Anticipatory anxiety and avoidance behaviors develop		Dramatic changes in family system
		Medical care-seeking dramatically increases for somatic complaints		Chronic somatization develops

TABLE 51–3. COMPONENTS OF PANIC DISORDER

Cognitive
Worry
Sense of foreboding
Sense of impending doom or dread
Exaggeration of inocuous situations as dangerous
Exaggeration of probability of harm in specific situations
Tendency to be inattentive, distractible
Sense of unreality
Rumination
Loss of control

Affective
Anxiety or nervousness
Secondary depression
Irritability

Somatic
Tachycardia
Hyperventilation (patient complains of shortness of breath)
Tingling in hands and feet
Diaphoresis
Dizziness or syncope
Flushing
Muscle tension
Tremulousness
Restlessness

Social
Dependency
Vocational limitations
Isolation

Adapted from Grant B, Katon W, Beitman B: Panic disorder. J Fam Pract 17:909, 1983 with permission.

et al., 1994). These patients were generally studied because of labile hypertension or episodic symptoms such as tachycardia, flushing, and headache. Only 4 of more than 300 patients in this study who had a pheochromocytoma work-up were found to have this catecholamine-producing tumor. In patients with vague, ill-defined complaints, the physician must be alert to the possibility of panic disorder or major depression being the underlying etiology and must question the patient specifically about the somatic components of each syndrome.

Patients with panic disorder have been found to have an increased prevalence of mitral valve prolapse (MVP). A review of 17 studies found that 18 per cent of patients with panic disorder or agoraphobia met definite criteria for MVP, and 27 per cent met probable criteria for MVP versus an average rate of definite MVP of 1 per cent in normal controls and probable or definite MVP in 12 per cent (Margraff et al., 1988). These studies must be understood in the context of the current research on MVP. Wynne (1986) has suggested that there are two groups of subjects who carry the diagnosis of MVP. The first consists of persons in whom the disorder is primarily an echocardiographic finding. These people are no more symptomatic than controls, have no more arrhythmias, are often free of the typical auscultatory findings, and have a low risk of complications. The echocardiographic findings in this group are probably anatomic normal variants and reflect the technologic advances for defining valve motion but emphasize the difficulty of differentiating variants of normal valve mobility. The second group consists of patients who typically not only have evidence of prolapse on echocardiography but also have clinical findings of mitral valve regurgitation. These people have symptoms related to valvular insufficiency and appear to have an increased risk of infective endocarditis as well as progressive mitral regurgitation. Two useful markers have been identified to help differentiate between the first group (with trivial MVP) and the second group (with important MVP): (1) the degree of redundancy of the valve, a finding that can be defined echocardiographically; and (2) the presence of mitral regurgitation on physical examination. Nishimura and colleagues (1985) found that almost every patient with a complication of MVP had redundant valves, as indicated by an increase of mitral valve leaflet thickness of 5 mm or more.

Evidence from a study by Gorman and colleagues (1988) has determined that the MVP in patients with panic disorder was mild and not associated with thickened mitral valve leaflets (the high risk group of MVP patients described by Nishimura and colleagues in 1985). Patients with panic disorder and MVP have also been found to respond to treatment with imipramine as well as do patients with panic disorder alone (Gorman et al., 1981). Several cases have been described in which patients with panic disorder and echocardiographically proved MVP had normal echocardiograms after the panic attacks were successfully treated (Gorman et al., 1988). The findings suggest that panic disorder is associated with an increased prevalence of MVP, but it seems to be a mild type that is principally an echocardiographic finding of little relevance for treatment and not necessitating prophylactic antibiotic treatment.

Phobic Disorders

The essential feature of a phobic disorder is the persistent and irrational fear of a specific object, activity, or situation that results in a compelling desire to avoid the dreaded object, activity, or situation. The fear is recognized by the individual as excessive or unreasonable in proportion to the actual danger of the situation, object, or activity (American Psychiatric Association, 1993).

The phobic disorders are classified as *agoraphobia* (covered in the section on panic disorders), the most pervasive and severe form, which almost always occurs secondary to the onset of panic attacks; *social phobia*; and *specific phobia*. A specific phobia involves a persistent irrational fear of, and compelling desire to avoid, an object or a situation. Common specific phobias are fears of heights (acrophobia), animals, insects, airplanes, and closed-in spaces (claustrophobia).

With social phobia, there is a persistent fear of, and compelling desire to avoid, social or performance situations in which the individual is exposed to unfamiliar people or to possible scrutiny by others; the sufferer fears he or she may act in a way (or show anxiety symptoms) that will be humiliating and embarrassing (American Psychiatric Association, 1993). With both social and specific phobias, the person recognizes that the fear is excessive or unreasonable.

With specific phobias, psychosocial trauma can often be identified as the original precipitant; for example, being bitten by a dog as a child may lead to a phobia of all dogs. With both specific and social phobias, when the individual is exposed to the phobic stimulus he or she becomes overwhelmingly fearful and may experience symptoms identical to those of a panic attack. Individuals often have considerable anticipatory anxiety when they know they will be exposed to the phobic stimulus. Patients with specific and social phobias do not have panic attacks when *not* exposed to the specific phobic stimulus. Their phobias are circumscribed. In terms of patients seeking psychiatric treatment, almost 70 per cent have panic attacks and have developed multiple phobias, and 30 per cent have circumscribed social or specific phobias (Sheehan, 1979).

Generalized Anxiety Disorder

Patients with generalized anxiety disorder (GAD) have excessive anxiety and worry (apprehensive expectation), occurring more days than not for at least 6 months, about a number of events or activities (Table 51–4). The patient finds it difficult to control the worry. The anxiety and worry are associated with at least three of the following six symptoms: (1) restlessness or feeling "keyed up" or on edge; (2) becoming easily fatigued; (3) difficulty concentrating or the mind going blank; (4) irritability; (5) muscle tension; and (6) sleep disturbance (American Psychiatric Association, 1993). For some patients the symptoms of GAD are lifelong and persistent, whereas for others the symptoms are acute, intermittent, and closely related to environmental stressful events.

In primary care, most patients with symptoms of GAD develop their symptoms secondary to another major *DSM-IV* disorder, such as panic disorder, major depression, alcohol abuse, or an axis II personality disorder (Breslau and Davis, 1985; Katon et al., 1987a,b). These disorders and organic causes of anxiety must be screened for and ruled out before embarking on treatment of GAD. When the psychiatric and medical causes of GAD are indeed ruled out, only a small subset of patients remains with primary GAD.

Many other patients present with impairment in social relationships (marriage) or occupational functioning and symptoms of anxiety in response

TABLE 51–4. DEFINITION OF GENERALIZED ANXIETY DISORDER (INCLUDING OVERANXIOUS DISORDER OF CHILDHOOD)

A. Excessive anxiety and worry (apprehensive expectation), occurring more days than not for at least 6 months, about a number of events or activities (e.g., work or school performance)

B. Individual finds it difficult to control the worry.

C. The anxiety and worry are associated with at least three of the following six symptoms (with at least some symptoms present for more days than not for the past 6 months).
1. Restlessness or feeling keyed up or on edge
2. Being easily fatigued
3. Difficulty concentrating or mind going blank
4. Irritability
5. Muscle tension
6. Sleep disturbance (difficulty falling or staying asleep, or restless unsatisfying sleep)

D. The focus of the anxiety and worry is not confined to features of an axis I disorder; for example, the anxiety or worry is not about having a panic attack (as in panic disorder), being embarrassed in public (as in social phobia), being contaminated (as in obsessive-compulsive disorder), being away from home or close relatives (as in separation anxiety disorder), gaining weight (as in anorexia nervosa), or having a serious illness (as in hypochondriasis), and is not part of posttraumatic stress disorder.

E. The anxiety, worry, or physical symptoms cause clinically significant distress or impairment in social, occupational, or other important areas of functioning.

F. Not due to the direct effects of a substance (e.g., drugs of abuse, medication) or a general medical condition (e.g., hyperthyroidism) and does not occur exclusively during a mood disorder, psychotic disorder, or a pervasive development disorder.

Adapted from American Psychiatric Association: Diagnostic and Statistical Manual of Mental Disorders (revised). Washington, DC, American Psychiatric Association, 1987.

to a specific stressor or occurring within 3 months of the onset of the stressor. However, the patient does not have enough symptoms to fulfill criteria for GAD. According to the *DSM-III-R* (American Psychiatric Association, 1993) formulation, they are called adjustment disorders with anxious mood.

Post-traumatic Stress Disorder

Patients with post-traumatic stress disorder (PTSD) have experienced a severe catastrophic event that is outside the range of normal human experience and would be distressing to anyone (American Psychiatric Association, 1993). The patient frequently and persistently re-experiences the event by having recurrent, often intrusive images of the trauma and recurrent dreams or nightmares of the event, or by suddenly behaving or feeling as if the traumatic event were recurring. These behavioral abnormalities include illusions, hallucinations, or flash-back episodes and intense psychological or physiologic distress (or both) or reactivity when exposed to environmental stimuli

TABLE 51–5. DEFINITION OF POST-TRAUMATIC STRESS DISORDER

A. The person has been exposed to a traumatic event in which both of the following conditions have been met.
  1. The person has experienced, witnessed, or been confronted with an event or events that involve actual or threatened death or serious injury, or a threat to the physical integrity of oneself or others.
  2. The person's response involved intense fear, helplessness, or horror. *Note:* In children, it may be expressed instead by disorganized or agitated behavior.
B. The traumatic event is persistently reexperienced in at least one of the following ways.
  1. Recurrent and intrusive distressing recollections of the event, including images, thoughts, or perceptions. *Note:* In young children, repetitive play may occur in which themes or aspects of the trauma are expressed.
  2. Recurrent distressing dreams of the event. *Note:* In children, there may be frightening dreams without recognizable content.
  3. Acting or feeling as if the traumatic event were recurring (includes a sense of reliving the experience, illusions, hallucinations, and dissociative flashback episodes, including those that occur upon awakening or when intoxicated). *Note:* In young children, trauma-specific reenactment may occur.
  4. Intense psychological distress at exposure to internal or external cues that symbolize or resemble an aspect of the traumatic event.
  5. Physiologic reactivity upon exposure to internal or external cues that symbolize or resemble an aspect of the traumatic event.
C. Persistent avoidance of stimuli associated with the trauma and numbing of general responsiveness (not present before the trauma), as indicated by at least three of the following conditions.
  1. Efforts to avoid thoughts, feelings, or conversations associated with the trauma
  2. Efforts to avoid activities, places, or people that arouse recollections of the trauma
  3. Inability to recall an important aspect of the trauma
  4. Markedly diminished interest or participation in significant activities
  5. Feeling of detachment or estrangement from others
  6. Restricted range of affect (e.g., unable to have loving feelings)
  7. Sense of a foreshortened future (e.g., does not expect to have a career, marriage, children, or a normal life span)
D. Persistent symptoms of increased arousal (not present before the trauma), as indicated by at least two of the following.
  1. Difficulty falling or staying asleep
  2. Irritability or outbursts of anger
  3. Difficulty concentrating
  4. Hypervigilance
  5. Exaggerated startle response
E. Duration of the disturbance (symptoms in B, C, and D) is more than 1 month.
F. The disturbance causes clinically significant distress or impairment in social, occupational, or other important areas of functioning.

Specify if:
  Acute: if duration of symptoms is less than 3 months
  Chronic: if duration of symptoms is 3 months or more
Specify if:
  With delayed onset: onset of symptoms at least 6 months after the stressor

Adapted from American Psychiatric Association: Diagnostic and Statistical Manual of Mental Disorders (revised). Washington, DC, American Psychiatric Association, 1987.

that symbolize or resemble an aspect of the traumatic event (Table 51–5). Patients with PTSD persistently avoid stimuli associated with the trauma and experience numbing of general responsiveness as indicated by at least three of the following.

  1. Efforts to avoid thoughts, feelings, or conversations associated with the trauma
  2. Efforts to avoid activities, places, or people who arouse recollections of the trauma
  3. Inability to recall an important aspect of the trauma
  4. Markedly diminished interest or participation in significant activities
  5. Feelings of detachment or estrangement from others
  6. Restricted range of affect
  7. Sense of foreshortened future

Persistent symptoms of increased arousal are present, as indicated by at least two of the following: difficulty falling or staying asleep, irritability or outbursts of anger, difficulty concentrating, hypervigilance, exaggerated startle response.

Civilian cases of PTSD are occasionally seen in primary care, and these patients may have combinations of symptoms of PTSD, panic disorder, and major depression. Indeed, research experience has demonstrated that many PTSD patients have panic attacks during flashback phenomena (Mellman and Davis, 1985). Civilian cases are often precipitated by extreme trauma, such as a severe automobile accident, industrial accident, or national disaster. Many of these civilian cases become complicated by the legal and disability systems that may unwittingly lead to prolongation of disability. Early intervention with accurate diagnosis and aggressive treatment may prevent occupational and social disability secondary to this disorder.

MEDICAL DIFFERENTIAL DIAGNOSIS

Some studies have shown that among patients referred for mental health problems, such as anxiety, depression, and psychosis, 9 to 42 per cent had a medical illness that was at least partially responsible for their symptoms (Hall et al. 1978; Koranyi, 1979). Anxiety must be differentiated from a host of organic problems, including the various cardiovascular, respiratory, cerebral, metabolic, hormonal, and other disorders listed in Table 51–6. In a patient with a known medical ailment, that illness (including the symptoms, complications, and pharmacologic treatment) should always be suspected (Rosenbaum, 1982). For instance, the diabetic patient with hypoglycemic episodes, the asthmatic patient with a toxic aminophylline serum level, and the patient with recent myocardial infarction who is worried and concerned about resuming work and sexual relations may each suffer from symptoms of anxiety. The primary treatment

TABLE 51–6. ORGANIC DISORDERS SIMULATING ANXIETY SYNDROME

Cardiovascular
Ischemic heart disease
Valvular heart disease
Cardiomyopathies
Myocarditis
Arrhythmias

Respiratory
Emphysema
Occult pulmonary embolism
Hamman-Rich syndrome
Scleroderma

Cerebral
Transient cerebrovascular insufficiency
Psychomotor epilepsy
Essential tremor

Metabolic and Hormonal
Thyrotoxicosis
Pheochromocytoma
Adrenocortical insufficiency
Hypokalemia
Hypoglycemia
Hyperparathyroidism
Myasthenia gravis

Nutritional
Thiamine, pyridoxine, or folate deficiency
Iron deficiency anemia

Intoxication
Caffeine
Alcohol
Sympathomimetics
Amphetamines

From Walker JI: The anxious patient. J Fam Pract 12:733, 1981, with permission.

would be adjusting pharmacologic treatment or counseling about the illness and the limitations it imposes on that patient's life (Rosenbaum, 1982).

PSYCHIATRIC DIFFERENTIAL DIAGNOSIS

Patients with anxiety disorders have a high frequency of both current and lifetime histories of major depression. About 60 per cent of patients with major depression also have a concurrent anxiety disorder (GAD or panic disorder) (Leckman et al., 1983a). Approximately 20 per cent of patients with major depression have panic disorder (Leckman et al., 1983b).

Patients with panic disorder have been demonstrated to have a 50 to 90 per cent risk of having a major depressive episode at some point in their lifetime (Breir et al., 1984; Cloninger et al., 1981; Pariser et al., 1979; Raskin et al., 1982). In one primary care study 50 per cent of patients with panic disorder also suffered from major depression (Katon et al., 1986). Patients with panic disorder or agoraphobia with a history of major depression

have been shown to have a more severe anxiety disorder, greater levels of past impairment, and a longer duration of panic disorder or agoraphobia than do patients with panic disorder or agoraphobia with no history of depression (Breir et al., 1984).

The above data suggesting an overlap of panic disorder agoraphobia, GAD, and depression are supported by the report of Goldberg and colleagues (1979), who found that 67 per cent of patients with mental illness in primary care clinics have mixed symptoms of anxiety and depression. The implication of the above data is that a primary care patient with anxiety should be carefully screened for major depression and vice versa. The occurrence of both disorders frequently suggests that antidepressant medication is needed.

Anxiety is a frequent accompaniment of drug and alcohol abuse and withdrawal, and these problems must be suspected in patients with persistent requests for antianxiety medications. Moreover, patients with panic disorder, GAD, or social phobias often try to self-medicate with alcohol to modulate their anxiety (Quitkin et al., 1972). Although alcohol may temporarily decrease anxiety, the short half-life of this substance frequently leads to worsening anxiety as blood levels rapidly decrease. Moreover, alcohol may have a "kindling" effect on sympathetic nervous system tone, provoking long-lasting increases in arousal after a prolonged period of usage. Alcohol often upsets sleep cycles, which has also been found to worsen panic disorder (Roy-Byrne et al., 1988).

Several studies have documented that approximately one third of alcoholics have panic disorder or severe phobic behavior (or both) that often preceded this abuse (Bowen et al., 1984; Mullaney and Tripett, 1979; Smail et al., 1984). Longitudinal chronologic studies have revealed that self-medication with alcohol by these patients temporarily relieved phobic-anxiety but actually led to worsening social phobias; conversely, abstinence from alcohol led to improvement in phobic behavior (Stockwell et al., 1984).

History

A systematic approach is required for the accurate diagnosis of the underlying cause of anxiety. As for other clinical problems, this approach should place particular emphasis on the history and physical examination. Further laboratory and radiographic studies should be carefully selected on an individual basis and often have therapeutic as well as diagnostic value.

The history is probably the single best diagnostic tool in the work-up of the anxious patient, whether the anxiety is of acute or chronic nature. The history-taking process should be sufficiently open-ended and unhurried to elicit the patient's

TABLE 51–7. MOST FREQUENTLY REPORTED SYMPTOMS OF ANXIETY AND DEPRESSION

Symptom Category	Symptom Cues
Intellectual	Difficulty concentrating; poor memory
Anxious mood	Worries; anticipation of the worst; fearful anticipation; irritability
Tension	Feelings of tension, fatigability; startle response; moved to tears easily; trembling; feelings of restlessness; inability to relax
Fears	Of dark, of strangers, of being left alone, of animals, of traffic, of crowds
Depressed mood	Feelings of sadness, hopelessness; expresses pessimism, discouragement, and sadness; facial expression reflects despair or dejection
Feelings of guilt	Self-reproach; feels he/she has let people down; criticizes self to an unrealistic degree
Retardation	Slowness of thought and speech; impaired ability to concentrate; decreased motor activity
Work and activities	Thoughts and feelings of incapacity, fatigue, or weakness related to activities, work, or hobbies; loss of interest in activity, hobbies, or work—directly reported by patient or indirectly indicated by listlessness; indecision, and vacillation (feels he/she must push self to work or activities); decrease in actual time spent doing activities or decrease in productivity
Hypochondriasis	Patient absorbed in own physical ailments; preoccupation with health
Insomnia	Difficulty falling asleep; broken sleep; unsatisfying sleep and fatigue on waking; dreams, nightmares, night terrors; early awakening
Somatic	Pains and aches; twitching; stiffness; myoclonic jerks; grinding of teeth; unsteady voice; increased muscular tone; tinnitus; blurring of vision; hot and cold flushes; feelings of weakness; pricking sensation; easily fatigued; heaviness in limbs, back, or head; backaches, headaches, muscle aches; loss of energy; fatigability
Cardiovascular symptoms	Tachycardia, palpitations, pain in chest; throbbing of vessels; fainting feelings; missing beat
Respiratory symptoms	Pressure or constriction in chest; choking feelings; sighing; dyspnea
Gastrointestinal symptoms	Difficulty swallowing; wind; abdominal pain; burning sensations; abdominal fullness; nausea; vomiting; borborygmi; looseness of bowels; weight loss; constipation
Genitourinary symptoms	Frequent micturition; urgent micturition; amenorrhea; menorrhagia; frigidity; premature ejaculation; loss of libido; impotence
Autonomic symptoms	Headache; raising of hair; labile hypertension

Adapted from Goldstein BF, Brauger B: Pharmacologic considerations in the treatment of anxiety and depression in medical practice. Med Clin North Am 55:487, 1971, with permission.

concerns and fears, current life situation, family and other support systems, and concurrent medical problems. Table 51–7 presents a number of symptom cues related to anxiety and depression that are pertinent to a review of symptoms (Goldstein and Brauger, 1971). One particularly useful part of the history, especially in elderly patients with anxiety, is inquiry into the sleep–wake pattern of the patient. A sudden change in this 24-hour pattern frequently represents depression or situational anxiety, which often is related to alterations in a familiar environment (Gadge, 1976).

Physical Examination

A number of common physical findings of anxiety are well known to experienced clinicians. The patient looks worried and acts tense. The initial handshake often reveals a moist palm. Increased motor activity is often evident, such as frequent movements, crossing and uncrossing the legs while sitting, rearranging clothing, and nervous gestures. The facial muscles may show twitching or tics. Breathing is often rapid and superficial; and

with panic disorder frequent deep, sighing respirations are seen. Associated symptoms include mild tachycardia, muscular tension, and brisk but symmetric deep tendon reflexes. Other signs suggestive of anxiety include an unsteady voice, strained facies, grinding of teeth, dilated pupils, tremor of hands, flushing, and excessive perspiration and labile hypertension.

Additional Diagnostic Studies

It is important that a complete and adequate diagnostic work-up be carried out to elucidate the basis of anxiety, but the extent of this work-up should be individualized. The family physician may have known the patient well over a period of years and may have a good understanding of the patient's life situation, personality structure, concurrent medical problems, and previous laboratory and radiographic studies. Under these circumstances, it may be that no additional diagnostic studies are necessary to manage the patient's anxiety effectively. However, if the problem is a relatively recent complaint or if the patient is not well known to the physician or has not been fully worked up in the recent past, additional diagnostic studies are usually warranted. This work-up should be aimed at detecting previously unrecognized organic disease and assuring the patient that the problem is being taken seriously.

A variety of organic diseases should be considered when assessing the particular constellation of anxiety symptoms experienced by the individual patient. The patient with hyperthyroidism usually presents with tachycardia, palpitations, moist palms, tremor, weight loss, and subjective apprehension. Heart disease manifested by such events as angina, paroxysmal atrial tachycardia, and paroxysmal nocturnal dyspnea may require differentiation from an anxiety attack. Chronic anxiety may resemble other organic diseases, such as adrenal insufficiency, anemia, hypoglycemia, cerebral arteriosclerosis, and other forms of central nervous system (CNS) disease.

In view of the sizable differential diagnosis involved with a patient presenting with anxiety, further diagnostic work-up may require such studies as a complete blood count, urinalysis, an SMA-12 panel, thyroid function studies, electrocardiogram, chest roentgenogram, and more specific studies if indicated.

It is also helpful to obtain some assessment of the level of function in the patient's family. The Family APGAR score as developed by Smilkstein (1978) provides a valid and convenient diagnostic tool for this purpose. This screening questionnaire can be completed by the patient in less than 10 minutes and yields information that affords assessment of family function in terms of five components: adaptation, partnership, growth, affection, and resolve. An APGAR scoring system, which ranges from a highly functional family (APGAR 7 to 10) to a severely dysfunctional family (APGAR 0 to 3), is applied.

A family history of psychiatric problems, such as depression, anxiety, and substance abuse disorders, should be sought. Screening questions about childhood history of physical or sexual abuse are important. Both childhood physical and sexual abuse have been linked with an increased vulnerability to anxiety and affective disorders (Brown and Harris, 1993). These questions can be woven into the usual questions about familial chronic medical disorders such as hypertension or diabetes. Thus physicians can state to patients that they would like to draw a family tree of the patient's family. After initially screening for medical disorders in this family of origin, the physician should then screen for psychiatric disorders. Finally, the physician should question the patient about any experiences of childhood physical or sexual abuse.

MANAGEMENT

The family physician has several advantages over other therapists in terms of the management of clinical anxiety. Perhaps most important is the fact that the anxious patient usually perceives the problem as primarily medical rather than psychiatric. The family physician often has already established a strong physician–patient relationship, facilitating management, and often has seen the patient respond to previous stressful experiences, such as serious illness or death of another family member, divorce, or change of occupation. Knowledge of the patient's social, medical, and family history is likewise helpful. The family physician is generally the first to be consulted and often sees emotional problems in their early stages before fixed patterns of illness have been set.

General Principles

Management of clinical anxiety rests on the following guidelines.

1. *Prerequisites for the physician.* To manage the anxious patient effectively, physicians must understand their own feelings and reactions to patients presenting with this kind of problem. Patience and a nonjudgmental attitude are required of the physician together with the capacity to identify and encourage the particular interests and goals important to the individual patient.

2. *Adequate work-up.* The importance of an adequate diagnostic work-up has already been stressed as an essential foundation for effective management of the patient with anxiety. The patient must believe that the physician has gathered adequate information and understands the problem before any reassurance or counseling can be effective. There is no quicker way to create distrust than for the patient to believe that reassurance or advice is given lightly without sufficient work-up. Equally ineffective is the physician's continued ordering of laboratory tests or radiographic studies after the patient has been assured of the absence of organic disease.

3. *Treatment based on etiology.* Therapeutic intervention for the anxious patient requires precision during the diagnostic work-up, in terms of both identifying or ruling out organic disease and understanding the concerns of the patient as an individual. To be effective, management must be based to the greatest extent possible on the specific organic and psychiatric diagnosis of the patient.

4. *Development of a therapeutic plan.* A deliberate therapeutic plan must be developed as a joint effort involving the patient and the physician. This plan usually involves a series of office visits on a regular basis over time and may require specific therapeutic interventions, such as the use of counseling, psychotropic drugs, or both. Use of such a plan provides the physician the opportunity to periodically reassess the effectiveness and progress of management and to make changes in therapy if indicated.

5. *Education.* Most patients with anxiety disorders present to a clinic with physical symptoms, such as headache, epigastric pain, or palpitations. The patient is often fearful that the physical symptoms may be a harbinger of serious physical disease. It is essential that the family physician inquire about the patient's explanatory model for his or her symptoms. This inquiry, focusing on the medical disorder the patient is worried may be present, the patient's expectations regarding medical work-up, and his or her ideas about treatment, is helpful. It is also important that the physician not state that "Nothing is wrong with you" or give the patient the idea that it is "all in your head." Instead, the physician should provide a careful explanation about how the symptom cluster fits into a diagnostic category such as panic disorder. It is also helpful to mention that often there is a biologic predisposition to such a disorder that is provoked or expressed during periods of life stress. An explanation about the autonomic nervous system's control of the physiologic state of the body organs and that anxiety probably results from dysregulation of this involuntary component of the nervous system can provide the patient with an understanding of the link between anxiety and physical symptoms. An analogy suggesting that autonomic nervous system dysregulation is similar to a car alarm set at too low a threshold—so someone leaning against the car may set it off—naturally leads to explanations about both medications and stress reduction techniques (Roy-Byrne, 1992). Thus medication can reset the autonomic nervous system tone and restore to normal the "alarm" threshold to stimulation. Stress reduction techniques, such as psychotherapy, relaxation therapy, exercise, and avoidance of caffeinated beverages, may also assist in resetting this threshold.

6. *Building support mechanisms.* It is important to identify support mechanisms for patients, especially for those who are divorced, widowed, or elderly. Members of the extended family and friends are frequently helpful in this respect. The development of outside interests may help reduce patients' self-absorption with their own problems and is to be encouraged. It is often useful to involve other family members in the development of the therapeutic plan.

Specific Management Problems

It is essential to differentiate the subtype of anxiety the patient is suffering so as to prescribe specific effective treatment. Since the mid-1980s medication has been demonstrated to be effective in double-blind psychopharmacologic treatment trials for many of the subtypes of anxiety. Controlled clinical trials have also demonstrated efficacy of specific psychotherapies, such as cognitive–behavioral therapy.

Panic Disorder

Treatment of panic disorder depends to some extent on the stage of the syndrome. The family physician often sees the patient after the first panic attack or certainly during the first few months of the syndrome before multiple phobias, anticipatory anxiety, and avoidance behavior develop (stages 2 and 3). Studies of the general population have revealed that up to one third of the general population have had a panic attack at some point in their lifetime, but most people have never had a cluster of attacks in a short enough period to meet *DSM-III-R* criteria for panic disorder (Katon et al., 1987a,b; Norton et al., 1985). If the patient has had infrequent attacks without developing phobic behavior or has had a few attacks during severe stress over a period of years, often education by the family physician about anxiety and relaxation techniques is helpful, together with supportive psychotherapy aimed at helping the patient problem-solve in order to deal with these stressful life situations.

Once the panic attacks have begun to increase in frequency and the patient is starting to develop avoidant and phobic behavior, the following guidelines should be utilized (Katon, 1986, 1991).

1. Specific pharmacologic therapy should be initiated to completely block panic attacks.

2. Once the panic attacks have ceased, the patient should be encouraged to re-enter situations that he or she may have begun to avoid, such as crowds of people, parties, driving on freeways, going to movies. Many of these phobias involve social situations where the patient commonly had panic attacks.

3. The family physician should take a complete social and psychiatric history to address personality vulnerabilities, current life stress, and developmental problems that may have provoked the onset of panic attacks or made the person more vulnerable to life stress. Panic attacks develop in a broad range of individuals, from those with no prior psychiatric history to patients with severe personality disorders. Individuals who develop severe phobic behavior with panic attacks have been found to have more family problems in their family of origin and more maladaptive coping patterns as adults (Joyce et al., 1989; Vitaliano et al., 1987). For those patients whose attacks develop in the context of marital conflict, the family physician may need to refer the patient to marital therapy. For a patient with chronic problems with low self-esteem, rejection sensitivity, and poor interpersonal relationships, psychodynamic or family of origin therapy may be the treatment of choice.

4. Patients should be encouraged to read articles and books about panic disorder, and the family physician should educate the patient about the likely course of the illness. The length of pharmacologic treatment and relapse must be discussed.

5. For patients who elect not to have pharmacologic treatment, a specific type of psychotherapy, cognitive–behavioral treatment, has been developed. Cognitive–behavioral psychotherapy has been shown in controlled trials to be effective for patients with mild to moderate panic disorder. This type of psychotherapy provides extensive education about anxiety and the role specific thought patterns play in amplifying normal bodily sensation so they are experienced as frightening and uncontrollable (Roy-Byrne, 1992).

Double-blind, placebo-controlled studies have documented that there are four pharmacologic classes of medication that are equally effective and significantly more effective than placebo for treatment of panic disorder (Sheehan et al., 1980, 1984).

1. Tricyclic antidepressants
2. Serotonin reuptake inhibitors
3. High-potency benzodiazepines
4. Monoamine oxidase inhibitors

In primary care, the first-line treatment of choice for panic disorder should be the tricyclic antidepressants. These medications are safe, and studies of primary care patients have demonstrated that 50 per cent of patients with panic disorder also have a major depression (Katon et al., 1986). The tricyclic antidepressants are effective therapeutic agents for both disorders. Imipramine is the best studied drug for treatment of panic disorder with at least ten double-blind placebo-controlled studies demonstrating its efficacy (Roy-Byrne and Katon, 1987). Other studies have also documented that other tricyclics such as desipramine, nortriptyline, amitriptyline, clomipramine and doxepin are also effective (Lydiard, 1988).

The family physician should begin treatment with 10 to 25 mg of imipramine (or an alternative antidepressant), gradually increasing the dosage by 10 to 25 mg every 4 to 5 days until panic attacks cease. The ultimate dosage of medication needed is variable, with some patients responding at a low dosage (e.g., 25 to 50 mg) and others needing up to 300 mg. It is useful for the physician to have a guide to antidepressant side effects, such as that shown in Table 51–8 (Katon and Roy-Byrne, 1988). The physician can then rationally choose alternative antidepressants based on side effects. Thus if

TABLE 51–8. HETEROCYCLIC PROPERTIES OF ANTIDEPRESSANTS

Antidepressant	Potency of Reuptake Blockade		Dosage (mg)	H₁ Blocking	Anticholinergic Action	Sedation	Orthostatic Hypotension
	Serotonin	Norepinephrine					
Tertiary Amines							
Doxepin (Sinequan)	+++	++	100–300	Highest	Moderate	High	+++
Amitriptyline (Elavil)	++++	++	100–300	Moderate to high	Highest	High	+++
Imipramine (Tofranil)	++++	++	100–300	Low	Moderate	Moderate	++
Trimipramine (Surmontil)	+	+	100–300	High	Moderate	High	+++
Secondary Amines							
Nortriptyline (Pamelor)	+++	+++	50–125	Low	Low	Moderate	+
Protriptyline (Vivactil)	+++	++++	20–60	Low	High	Low	+
Desipramine (Norpramin)	++	++++	100–300	Low	Low	Low	+
Amoxapine (Asendin)	++	+++	100–300	?	Low	Low	++
Tetracyclic							
Maprotiline (Ludiomil)	+	+++	100–300	Moderate	Low	Moderate	++
Triazolopyridine							
Trazodone (Desyrel)	+++	+	150–500	Low	Lowest	High	+++
Serotonin Reuptake Inhibitors							
Fluoxetine (Prozac)	++++	0	20–80	0	Lowest	Low	0
Sertraline (Zoloft)	++++	0	50–200	0	Lowest	Low	0
Paroxetine (Paxil)	++++	0	20–50	0	Lowest	Low	0

0 = none; + = slight; ++ = moderate; +++ = marked; ++++ = pronounced.

anticholinergic side effects develop on imipramine, switching to a medication such as desipramine (which has fewer anticholinergic side effects) is helpful. Similarly, if the patient develops orthostatic hypotension secondary to treatment with imipramine, a switch to a medication with decreased orthostatic hypotensive side effects, such as nortriptyline, may be helpful.

Studies have found that fluoxetine has antipanic efficacy. However, one 20 mg capsule often causes jitteriness and overstimulation (Roy-Byrne, 1992). When prescribing the elixir (20 mg/5 mL), now in wide use, a starting dosage of 2 to 4 mg avoids the jitteriness. Increasing increments of 2 to 4 mg every 3 to 4 days are prescribed until panic attacks are alleviated. Usually an ultimate dosage of 20 mg is required. Other serotonin reuptake inhibitors (e.g., sertraline and paroxetine) are less well tested but should also have antipanic efficacy.

A subgroup of patients with panic disorder develop intolerable side effects on all tricyclic antidepressants or serotonin reuptake inhibitors. Some of these patients can be treated with low dosages of tricyclics, such as 5 to 10 mg initially, with a gradual increase in dosage. Another alternative is to couple a low dosage of alprazolam or lorazepam with the tricyclic, which often decreases the initial anxiety and jitteriness that may be a transient side effect of tricyclics.

A small subgroup of patients do not tolerate tricyclic antidepressants or serotonin reuptake inhibitors, and for these patients the high-potency benzodiazepines represent an effective second line of treatment. Alprazolam, lorazepam, and clonazepam have all been demonstrated to be more effective than placebo for treatment of panic disorders (Lydiard, 1988). Patients should be started on 0.5 mg of clonazepam b.i.d. with a gradual increase by 0.5 mg increments every 2 to 3 days until panic attacks cease. Dosages of lorazepam and alprazolam equalent to 0.5 mg of clonazepam are 1.0 mg lorazepam and 1.0 mg alprazolam (Roy-Byrne et al., 1988). One caveat is that patients with a history of polydrug or alcohol abuse, personality disorder, or chronic benign pain probably should not be treated with benzodiazepines owing to potential problems with abuse.

Monoamine oxidase inhibitors are potentially the most effective class of medications for panic disorder (Sheehan et al., 1984). However, the lack of familiarity of most family physicians with these medications and the potential hypertensive crisis that can ensue if the patient does not follow a low-tyramine diet preclude their regular use in primary care. For a patient who has not responded to a tricyclic antidepressant or benzodiazepine, psychiatric consultation may be helpful.

Generalized Anxiety Disorders

For GADs or less severe transient states of anxiety (adjustment disorder), the following modalities are often helpful.

PSYCHOLOGICAL SUPPORT. The process of psychological support by the family physician for patients with anxiety often involves a brief series of office visits to deal with the problem. In selected cases some kind of family counseling may also be indicated. In one study, for example, it was found that anxiety states in one or both parents were the most common psychosocial factor found in dysfunctional families with multiple health problems or exaggerated responses to organic illness (Schmidt, 1978).

At times it may be possible for the family physician to provide psychological support and counseling during a series of follow-up visits linked to other forms of treatment. A patient being treated for duodenal ulcer is a good example of a situation well suited to this approach. It takes little time to palpate for epigastric tenderness and evaluate the response to drug and dietary treatment during a series of follow-up visits. The remainder of each visit can be directed to identifying the sources of stress and concerns in the patient's life that may be subject to treatment through manipulation or counseling. Reassurance can be particularly effective for the anxious patient when combined artfully with treatment of concurrent medical problems.

Under other circumstances, it is preferable to schedule a brief series of formal sessions for counseling or supportive psychotherapy. Excellent results often can be obtained over a span of five or six visits, each as short as 20 to 30 minutes. Cathell (1968) suggested that the family physician should not imitate the psychiatrist's technique for treating emotional illness. He believed that the family physician tends to be more directive, authoritative, problem-oriented, and pragmatic than psychiatrists, and that the physician's methods should reflect such differences and the particular nature of the practice.

A study by Catalan and colleagues (1984) lent support to the effectiveness of brief, effective, problem-focused counseling for treatment of GAD by primary care physicians. In one study a group of family physicians who regularly prescribed benzodiazepines for the relief of anxiety were asked to participate in a randomized trial in which new patients with anxiety were treated. The intervention group was scheduled for brief supportive psychotherapy, and the controls were given the physician's usual prescription of a benzodiazepine. The patients were then followed at 3-month intervals. At 3 and 6 months there were no differences between the intervention patients and the controls in terms of psychiatric symptoms or distress. Moreover, the brief supportive counseling did not take significantly more physician time nor did the patients who received psychotherapy tend to self-medicate with drugs or alcohol. In this study one subgroup with more severe distress did benefit more from medication. In a second study, patients with this high level of distress were randomized to either benzodiazepine treatment by the family physician or to four to five sessions of problem-focused therapy by a psychiatrist (Gath and Catalan, 1988). The psychotherapy patients did as well as the patients treated with benzodiazepines at follow-up. This research team is now entering a third phase of the research in which the brief, problem-focused treatment will be taught to primary care physicians. The investigators will then measure the family physician's efficacy with problem-focused therapy versus treatment with benzodiazepines in a controlled clinical trial.

Anstett and Hipskind (1981) have described some useful criteria that assist in predicting successful outcomes of brief office counseling. They observed that successful counseling depends on agreement of the physician and patient on three issues: the nature of the problem, the goals of counseling and their respective roles during counseling, and the length and expertise of counseling. Table 51–9 lists the patient characteristics found to correlate with successful counseling outcomes. Relaxation techniques can help to decrease anxiety and are easily taught in two or three half-hour sessions by the family physician. Benson and Klipper (1976) provided a useful relaxation technique that can be mastered by most patients and elucidated a theoretic rationale that may add to patient motivation.

PSYCHOPHARMACOLOGY. The heterogeneous nature of GAD makes evaluation of treatment difficult. GAD is often associated with many other anxiety disorders, such as panic disorder, post-traumatic stress disorder and agoraphobia, as well as affective disorders such as major depression (Breslau and Davis, 1985; Katon et al., 1987a,b). In general, benzodiazepines, buspirone, β-blockers, and antidepressants have been found to be more effective than placebo in patients with GAD (Roy-Byrne and Katon, 1987).

TABLE 51–9. PATIENT CHARACTERISTICS CORRELATING WITH SUCCESSFUL COUNSELING OUTCOME

1. Demographic: relative youth, attractiveness, verbal ability, intelligence, success in other endeavors
2. Awareness that the problem is psychological in nature
3. Presence of "signal anxiety"
4. Personality traits: persevering, dependable, nonimpulsive, trusting
5. High motivation for change in self
6. Faith that counseling can be helpful
7. Awareness of how counseling works
8. Previous successful counseling experience
9. Personal resource system supportive of the aims of counseling
10. Absence of debilitating characterologic components in the patient's personality
11. Previous meaningful interpersonal relationships

From Anstett R, Hipskind M: Selecting patients for brief office counseling. J Fam Pract 13:195, 1981, with permission.

Numerous studies have demonstrated the efficacy of benzodiazepines in GAD. Concerns have centered not on efficacy but on the risks of the chronic use and abuse of benzodiazepines (Roy-Byrne and Katon, 1987). Table 51–10 lists the benzodiazepines available in the United States (Wesson, 1980). The major advantages of the benzodiazepines is their: (1) lower potential for dependence and abuse; (2) lower frequency of side effects and allergic reactions than antidepressants or phenothiazines; and (3) low lethality rate, even when taken in overdose. Moreover, they are thought not to activate liver microsomal enzymes and therefore do not alter the rate of metabolism of other drugs (Wesson, 1980).

In general, abuse of benzodiazepines by primary care patients is infrequent. Almost all abusers of benzodiazepines have had a history of polydrug or alcohol abuse; therefore patients with a history of substance abuse should probably not be prescribed benzodiazepines, especially long term (Roy-Byrne and Hommer, 1988). A larger concern for the primary care physician than abuse is the difficulty many anxious patients seem to have stopping these medications. Severe rebound anxiety and withdrawal symptoms can be moderate to severe (Pecknold et al., 1988). The benzodiazepines with a short half-life appear especially likely to precipitate rebound anxiety and withdrawal (Roy-Byrne and Katon, 1987). For most patients the symptoms experienced with drug discontinuation are not enduring, and the patient can be supported with brief, regular visits and reassured that the symptoms will subside. Several strategies to decrease rebound symptoms include tapering the medication slowly, converting short-acting benzodiazepines to long-acting benzodiazepines prior to tapering, and treating the patient with a tricyclic antidepressant before attempting to taper the benzodiazepine. Because of the problem with discontinuation of these medications, many authorities are recommending shorter-term treatment (i.e., several weeks to 6 months) (Roy-Byrne and Hommer, 1988).

One important development was the demonstration that tricyclic antidepressants are effective in the treatment of GAD (Kahn et al., 1986). This study demonstrated that imipramine was slightly more effective than chlordiazepoxide, although this increased efficacy did not become apparent for 3 to 6 weeks. Given the fact that many primary care patients with GAD also suffer from major depression and panic disorder, tricyclic antidepressants may be the safest, most effective treatment of GAD. Also, the antidepressants are much easier to taper, without the rebound anxiety and withdrawal problem seen with benzodiazepines.

A relatively new non-benzodiazepine alternative anxiolytic medication that appears effective in GAD is buspirone (Goa and Ward, 1986). This medication is non-sedating, does not cause any

TABLE 51–10.   BENZODIAZEPINES FOR TREATMENT OF ANXIETY

Benzodiazepine	Adult Dosages, Range (mg/day)*	Supplied as Tablet or Capsule (mg)
Alprazolam (Xanax)	0.25–4.00	0.25, 1.0, 2.0
Chlordiazepoxide hydrochloride		
Chlordiazachel	10–100	5, 10, 25
Librium	10–100	5, 10, 25
Librium Injectable	50–200	50 mg/ml ampul
Chlorazepate dipotassium		
Tranxene	15–60	3.75, 7.5, 15.0
Tranxene SD†	11.25–22.50	11.25, 22.5
Diazepam		
Valium	4–40	2, 5, 10
Valium Injectable	5–100‡	2-mg ampuls, 5 mg/ml
Flurazepam (Dalmane)	15–30	15, 30
Halazepam (Paxipam)	20–160	20, 40
Lorazepam (Ativan)	1–6	1, 2
Oxazepam (Serax)	30–120	10, 15, 30
Prazepam (Vestran)	20–60	10
Clonazepam (Klonopin)	1–6	0.5, 1.0

Modified from Wesson DR: Anxiety: its meaning and psychotropic drug treatment. In Buchwald D, et al (eds): Frequently Prescribed and Abused Drugs. Brooklyn, Career Teacher Center, State University of New York, 1980, p 25, with permission.

* Usually given in divided doses two to four times daily.

† Recommended as single daily dose.

‡ May be given intramuscularly or intravenously; usually not more than 20 mg in a single dose. Intravenous injection rate should not exceed 5 mg/min.

withdrawal symptoms when abruptly discontinued, has no synergistic effects with alcohol or other sedative hypnotic agents and appears to be as effective as benzodiazepines for GAD. Buspirone often takes two to three weeks to have an effect, and patients who have been treated previously with benzodiazepines tend to report this medication as less effective.

Finally, beta-blockers have been used to treat anxiety, but they generally have a less robust anxiolytic effect than the three classes of medication described above and have the added risk of precipitating a depression (Roy-Byrne and Katon, 1987).

Phobic Disorders (Specific Phobias, Agoraphobia, Social Phobias)

Specific phobias respond well to the behavior modification techniques of systemic desensitization (Wolpe, 1973) or in vivo exposure (Marks, 1987). For desensitization, the patient learns a relaxation technique and then, while in a relaxed state, is exposed to a gradual hierarchy of stimuli (through imagery or in vivo) that approaches the phobic object or situation. For instance, if a patient has a fear of dogs, after a relaxation technique is taught and mastered the patient may be exposed sequentially to a picture of a dog, a stuffed animal, or a dog in a cage; the next steps may be to hold a puppy and then to pet an adult dog. During each step of the hierarchy, if the anxiety of the patient becomes high the stimulus is withdrawn.

Marks (1987) demonstrated that in vivo exposure to the phobic stimulus, either gradually or all at once (flooding), is more effective for total efficacy and rapidity of cure than desensitization by im-

agery. Marks (1987) also showed that in vivo exposure may be an effective technique to treat agoraphobia. The therapist or physician develops a hierarchic list of phobias with the agoraphobic patient, with the weakest fears at one end and the most severe at the other. The patient then decides with the clinician what phobic situations he will "expose" himself to that week. Marks (1987) demonstrated that exposing the patient rapidly and for long periods to the phobic stimulus maximizes therapeutic efficacy.

For specific phobias, in vivo exposure alone is effective. For agoraphobia, evidence from two studies shows that imipramine in combination with exposure enhances the effects of exposure (Mavissakalian et al., 1983; Telch et al., 1985). It must be kept in mind that most patients with agoraphobia also have panic disorder; and although exposure therapy may decrease phobic avoidance, the patient may still be left with panic attacks. Thus the addition of imipramine may ameliorate the panic attacks, which often exacerbate phobic behavior. Monoamine oxidase inhibitors and high-potency benzodiazepines have also been shown to be effective for treatment of agoraphobia (Sheehan et al., 1984).

Exposure-based treatments have also been shown to be moderately effective (Alstrom et al., 1984) for social phobias. Studies have reported that monoamine oxidase inhibitors also are effective in 70 per cent of the cases of social phobia (M. Liebowitz, personal communication, 1987).

Post-traumatic Stress Disorder

Mellman and Davis (1985) have demonstrated that the recurrent intrusive images and feelings of intense autonomic arousal in individuals with PTSD are often similar to those of patients with panic attacks. Indeed, many patients with PTSD have both panic disorder and major depression, and they try to self-medicate their increased sympathetic nervous system tone with alcohol or sedative hypnotic agents.

Medications with a dampening effect on sympathetic nervous system tone have been found to be effective in PTSD patients. Reports have indicated that imipramine and monoamine oxidase inhibitors are effective in combat veterans with the disorder (Bleich et al., 1986). Also clonidine, an α-2-receptor agonist that diminishes release of norepinephrine (Kolb et al., 1984) and high-dosage propranolol have been found to be moderately effective (Van der Kolk, 1983).

Anecdotal, uncontrolled reports have suggested that behavioral, group, and psychodynamic therapy can be effective in PTSD patients (Fairbank and Nicholson, 1987). These therapies seem to have in common the reliving and continued exposure to painful thoughts and feelings, which may ultimately desensitize the patient to these images and the autonomic nervous system feelings evoked by them.

REFERENCES

Alstrom JE, Worklund CL, Persson G, et al: Effects of four treatment methods on agoraphobic women not suitable for insight-oriented psychotherapy. Acta Psychiatr Scand 70:1, 1984.

American Psychiatric Association: DSM-III criteria. Washington, DC, American Psychiatric Association, 1993.

Anstett R, Hipskind M: Selecting patients for brief office counseling. J Fam Pract 13:195, 1981.

Bass C, Wade C: Chest pain with normal coronary arteries: A comparative study of psychiatric and social morbidity. Psychosom Med 14:51, 1984.

Beitman BD, Basha I, Flaker G, et al: Atypical or nonanginal chest pain: Panic disorder or coronary artery disease. Arch Intern Med 147:1548, 1987.

Benson H, Klipper MZ: The Relaxation Response. New York, Avon Publishers, 1976.

Blazer DC: Psychopathology of Aging. Kansas City, MO, American Academy of Family Physicians, 1977, pp 15–16.

Bleich A, Siegel B, Garb R, et al: Posttraumatic stress disorder following combat exposure: Clinical features and psychopharmacologic treatment. Br J Psychiatry 149:365, 1986.

Bowen RC, Cipywny KD, D'Aray C, et al: Alcoholism, anxiety disorders and agoraphobia. Alcoholism Clin Exp Res 8:48, 1984.

Breir A, Charney DS, Heninger GB: Major depression in patients with agoraphobia and panic disorder. Arch Gen Psychiatry 41:1129, 1984.

Breslau N, Davis CC: DSM-III generalized anxiety disorder: an empirical investigation of more stringent criteria. Psychiatr Res 14:231, 1985.

Brown GW, Harris TO: Aetiology of anxiety and depressive disorders in an inner-city population. I. Early adversity. Psychol Med 23:143, 1993.

Catalan J, Gath D, Edmonds G, et al: The effects of nonprescribing of anxiolytics in general practice. I. Controlled evaluation of psychiatric and social outcome. Br J Psychiatry 144:593, 1984.

Cathell JL: Somehow, "GP style" psychotherapy works. Consultant 8:12, 1968.

Cloninger CR, Martin RL, Clayton P, et al: A blind follow-up and family study of anxiety neurosis: Preliminary analyses of the St. Louis 500. In Klein DF, Rabkin J (eds): Anxiety: New Research and Changing Concepts. New York, Raven Press, 1981, pp 137–148.

Cohen ME, Badal D, Kilpatrick A, et al: The high familial prevalence of neurocirculatory asthenia (anxiety neurosis, effort syndrome). Am J Hum Genet 3:126, 1951.

Crowe RR, Noyes R, Pauls DL, et al: A family study of panic disorder. Arch Gen Psychiatry 40:1065, 1983.

Eastwood MR: Screening for psychiatric disorder. Psychol Med 1:197, 1971.

Fairbank JA, Nicholson RA: Theoretical and empirical issues in the treatment of posttraumatic stress disorder in Vietnam veterans. J Clin Psychol 43:44, 1987.

Faravelli D: Life events preceding the onset of panic disorder. J Affect Disord 9:103, 1985.

Finlay-Jones R, Brawn GW: Types of stressful life events and the onset of anxiety and depressive disorders. Psychol Med 11:803, 1981.

Fogarty J, Engel C, Russo J, et al: Hypertension and pheochromocytoma testing: The association with anxiety disorders. Arch Fam Med 3:55, 1994.

Friedman D, Jaffe A: Anxiety disorders. J Fam Pract 16:145, 1983.

Gadge SW: Treating the aging patient. In Kelly JT (ed): Perspectives of Human Aging. Minneapolis, Craftsman Press, 1976, p 118.

Gath D, Catalan J: Evaluation of the outcome of brief psychological treatments in primary care. Presented at the Treatment of Mental Disorders in General Health Care Settings: A Research Conference. Pittsburgh, June 15–17, 1988.

Goa KL, Ward A: Buspirone: A preliminary review of its pharmacological properties and therapeutic efficacy as an anxiolytic drug. Drugs 32:114, 1986.

Goldberg D: Detection and assessment of emotional disorders in a primary care setting. Int J Ment Health 8:30, 1979.

Goldstein BF, Brauger B: Pharmacologic considerations in the treatment of anxiety and depression in medical practice. Med Clin North Am 55:487, 1971.

Gorman JM, Fyer AF, Gliklick J, et al: Effect of imipramine on prolapsed mitral valves of patients with panic disorder. Am J Psychiatry 138:977, 1981.

Gorman JM, Goetz RR, Fyer M, et al: The mitral valve prolapse–panic disorder connection. Psychosom Med 50:114, 1988.

Grant B, Katon W, Beitman B: Panic disorder. J Fam Pract 17:907, 1983.

Hall RC, Popkin MK, Devand RA, et al: Physical illness presenting as psychiatric disease. Arch Gen Psychiatry 35:1315, 1978.

Hankin J, Oktay JS: Mental disorder primary medical care. An analytic review of the literature. In: National Institute of Mental Health, Series D, No. 7, publication no. (ADM) 78-661, Rockville, MD, 1979.

Hoeper EW, Nyczi GR, Cleary PD: Estimated prevalence of RDC mental disorder in primary care. Int J Ment Health 8:6, 1979.

Joyce PR, Bushnell JA, Oakley-Browne MA, et al: The epidemiology of panic symptomatology and agoraphobic avoidance. Compr Psychiatry 30:303, 1989.

Kahn RJ, McNair DM, Lipman LS: Imipramine and chlordiazepoxide in depressive and anxiety disorders. II. Efficacy in anxious outpatients. Arch Gen Psychiatry 43:79, 1986.

Katon W: Panic disorder and somatization: a review of 55 cases. Am J Med 77:101, 1984.

Katon W: Panic disorder: Epidemiology, diagnosis and treatment. J Clin Psychiatry 47(10):21, 1986.

Katon W: Panic Disorder in the Medical Setting. Washington, DC, National Institute of Mental Health, 1991.

Katon W, Roy-Byrne PP: Antidepressants in the medically ill: Diagnosis and treatment in primary care. Clin Chem 34:829, 1988.

Katon W, Roy-Byrne PP: Panic disorder in the medically ill. J Clin Psychiatry 50:299, 1989.

Katon W, Vitaliano PP, Russo J, et al: Panic disorder: Epidemiology in primary care. J Fam Pract 23:233, 1986.

Katon W, Vitaliano PP, Anderson K, et al: Panic disorder: residual symptoms after the acute attacks abate. Compr Psychiatry 28:151, 1987a.

Katon W, Vitaliano PP, Russo J, et al: Panic disorder: Spectrum of severity and somatization. J Nerv Ment Dis 175(1):12, 1987b.

Katon W, Hall, ML, Russo J, et al: Chest pain: relationship of psychiatric illness to coronary arteriographic results, Am J Med 84:1, 1988.

Kolb LC, Burris BC, Griffiths S: Prapranolol and clonidine in the treatment of the chronic post-traumatic stress disorders of war. *In* Van der Kolk BA (ed): Post-Traumatic Stress Disorder: Psychological and Biological Sequelae. Washington, DC, American Psychiatric Press, 1984.

Koranyi EK: Morbidity and rate of undiagnosed physical illness in a psychiatric clinic population. Arch Gen Psychiatry 36:414, 1979.

Leckman JF, Merikangas KP, Pauls DL, et al: Anxiety disorders and depression: Contradictions between family study data and DSM-III convention. Am J Psychiatry 140:880, 1983a.

Leckman JF, Weissman MM, Merikangas KR, et al: Panic disorder and major depression. Arch Gen Psychiatry 40:1055, 1983b.

Lydiard RB: Panic disorder: pharmacologic treatment. Psychiatr Ann 18:468, 1988.

Margraff J, Ehlers A, Roth WT: Mitral valve prolapse and panic disorder: A review of their relationship. Psychosom Med 50:93, 1988.

Marks IM: Fears, Phobias and Rituals: Panic, Anxiety and Their Disorders. New York, Oxford University Press, 1987.

Marsland DW, Wood M, Mayo F: Content of family practice: a data bank for patient care curriculum, research family practice—526,196 patient problems. J Fam Pract 3:25, 1976.

Mavissakalian M, Michelson L, Dealy RS: Pharmacological treatment of agoraphobia: imipramine versus imipramine with programmed practice. Br J Psychiatry 143:348, 1983.

Mellinger GD, Balter MB, Uhlenhuth EH: Prevalence and correlates of long-term regular use of anxiolytics. JAMA 251:375, 1984.

Mellman TA, Davis GC: Combat related flashbacks in posttraumatic stress disorder: Phenomenology and similarity to panic attacks. J Clin Psychiatry 46:379, 1985.

Mullaney JA, Trippett C: Alcohol dependence and phobias: Clinical description and relevance. Br J Psychiatry 135:565, 1979.

Myers JK, Weissman MM, Tischler GE, et al: Six-month prevalence of psychiatric disorders in three communities. Arch Gen Psychiatry 41:959, 1984.

Nishimura RA, McGoon MD, Shub C, et al: Echocardiographically documented mitral-valve prolapse: Long-term follow-up of 237 patients. N Engl J Med 313:1305, 1985.

Norton RG, Harrison B, Hauch J, Rhodes L: Characteristics of people with infrequent attacks. Abnorm Psychiatry 94:216, 1985.

Noyes R, Clancy J, Crowe R, et al: The familial prevalence of anxiety neurosis. Arch Gen Psychiatry 35:105, 1978.

Orleans CT, George LK, Houpt JL: How primary physicians treat psychiatric disorders: A national survey of family practitioners. Arch Gen Psychiatry 42:52, 1985.

Pariser SF, Jones BA, Pinta EF, et al: Panic attacks: diagnostic evaluations of 17 patients. Am J Psychiatry 136:105, 1979.

Pecknold J, Swinson RP, Kuch K, et al: Alprazolam in panic disorder and agoraphobia: Results from a multicenter trial.

III. Discontinuation effects. Arch Gen Psychiatry 45:429, 1988.

Quitkin FM, Rifkin A, Kaplan J, et al: Phobic anxiety syndrome complicated by drug dependence and addiction: A treatable form of drug abuse. Arch Gen Psychiatry 27:159, 1972.

Raskin M, Peeke HVS, Dickman W, et al: Panic and generalized anxiety disorders: Developmental antecedents and precipitants. Arch Gen Psychiatry 39:687, 1982.

Regier DA, Myers K, Kramer M, et al: The NIMH epidemiologic catchment area (ECA) program: Historical context, major objectives, and study population characteristics. Arch Gen Psychiatry 41:934, 1984.

Rickels K: Drug treatment of anxiety. *In* Jarvik ME (ed): Psychopharmacology in the Practice of Medicine. East Norwalk, CT, Appleton-Century-Crofts, 1977, p 310.

Rosenbaum JF: The drug treatment of anxiety. N Engl J Med 7:401, 1982.

Roy-Byrne PP: Integrated treatment of panic disorder. Am J Med 92(suppl 1A):49S, 1992.

Roy-Byrne PP, Cowley D: Panic disorder: Biological aspects. Psychiatr Ann 18:457, 1988.

Roy-Byrne PP, Hommer D: Benzodiazepine withdrawal: Overview and implications for the treatment of anxiety. Am J Med 84:1041, 1988.

Roy-Byrne PP, Katon W: An update on treatment of the anxiety disorders. Hosp Comm Psychiatry 38:835, 1987.

Roy-Byrne PP, Uhde TW: Exogenous factors in panic disorder: Clinical and research implications. J Clin Psychiatry 49:56, 1988.

Roy-Byrne PP, Geraci M, Uhde T: Life events and the onset of panic disorder. Am J Psychiatry 143:1424, 1986.

Schmidt DD: The family as the unit of medical care. J Fam Pract 7:303, 1978.

Schurman RA, Kramer PD, Mitchel JB: The hidden mental health network: Treatment of mental illness by nonpsychiatrist physicians. Arch Gen Psychiatry 2:89, 1985.

Shapiro S, Skinner EA, Kessler LG, et al: Utilization of health and mental health services: Three epidemiologic catchment area sites. Arch Gen Psychiatry 41:971, 1984.

Sheehan D: The efficient treatment of phobic disorders. *In* Menschreck T (ed): Psychiatric Medicine Update. New York, Elsevier, 1979, p 189.

Sheehan DV, Ballenger J, Jacobsen G: Treatment of endogenous anxiety with phobic, hysterical and hypochondriacal symptoms. Arch Gen Psychiatry 37:51, 1980.

Sheehan DV, Claycomb JB, Surman OS: Comparison of phenelzine, imipramine, alprazolam and placebo in the treatment of panic attacks and agoraphobia. Paper presented at the American Psychiatric Association Annual Meeting, Los Angeles, 1984.

Smail P, Stockwell T, Canter S, et al: Alcohol dependence and phobic anxiety states. I. A prevalence study. Br J Psychiatry 144:53, 1984.

Smilkstein G: The family APGAR: A proposal for a family function test and its use by physicians. J Fam Pract 6:1231, 1978.

Stockwell T, Smail S, Hodgson R, et al: Alcohol dependence and phobic anxiety states. II. A retrospective study. Br J Psychiatry 144:58, 1984.

Telch MJ, Agras WS, Taylor CB, et al: Combined pharmacological and behavioral treatment for agoraphobia. Behav Res Ther 23:325, 1985.

Torgerson S: Genetic factors in anxiety disorders. Arch Gen Psychiatry 40:1085, 1983.

Uhlenhuth EH, Bolter MD, Mellinger GD, et al: Symptom checklist syndromes in the general population: corrections with psychotherapeutic drug use. Arch Gen Psychiatry 40:1167, 1983.

Valbona C: Monthly Statistical Report. Casa de Amigo Community Health Clinic, Houston, Texas, 1973.

Van der Kolk BA: Psychopharmacologic issues in posttraumatic stress disorder. Hosp Comm Psychiatry 34:683, 1983.

Vitaliano PP, Katon W, Russo J, et al: Coping as an index of illness behavior in panic disorder. J Nerv Ment Dis 175(2):78, 1987.

Weissman MM, Myers JK, Harding PS: Psychiatric disorders in a U.S. urban community: 1975–1976. Am J Psychiatry 135:459, 1978.

Wesson DR: Anxiety: its meaning and psychotropic drug treatment. *In* Buchwald C, et al (eds): Frequently Prescribed and Abused Drugs. Brooklyn, NY, Career Teacher Center, State University of New York, 1980, pp 21–34.

Wolpe J: The Practice of Behavioral Therapy, 2nd edition. Oxford, Pergamon Press, 1973.

Wynne J: Mitral valve prolapse. N Engl J Med 314:577, 1986.

Yates WR: The National Institute of Mental Health Epidemiologic Study: Implications for family practice. J Fam Pract 22:251, 1986.

Zitrin ZM, Klein DF, Woerner MG: Behavior therapy, supportive psychotherapy, imipramine and phobias. Arch Gen Psychiatry 35:307, 1978.

Zung WWK: Assessment of anxiety disorder: qualitative and quantitative approaches. *In* Fann WE, Karacan I, Pokorny AD, Williams RL (eds): Phenomenology and Treatment of Anxiety. New York, Spectrum Publications, 1979, pp 1–17.

CHAPTER 52
DEPRESSION

THOMAS L. SCHWENK and JAMES C. COYNE

Depression is an important concern in family practice because of its high prevalence, the key role played by family physicians in its assessment and management, and its powerful effect on health and medical care. Depressed persons are more likely to consult a primary care physician than a mental health specialist, and primary care physicians write more prescriptions for antidepressant medications than do psychiatrists (Regier et al., 1993; Sireling et al., 1985). Depression can be readily and effectively treated but is severely debilitating in the absence of effective treatment. Moreover, patients with major depression or subsyndromal depressive symptoms tend to be high utilizers of medical services (Regier et al., 1988). Misdiagnosis and lack of treatment may increase medical utilization and lead to unnecessary medical services and procedures. Yet the tasks facing family physicians in detecting and diagnosing depression in their practices and making appropriate treatment decisions are formidable, and the existing psychiatric literature and nosology are not as useful as they first appear.

Major depression has an estimated prevalence of 5 to 10 per cent, and two to three times as many patients have significant subsyndromal depressive symptoms (Katon and Schulberg, 1992). Depression is the most common psychiatric disorder in primary care, and it may even be the most common condition overall in primary care, exceeding even hypertension (Katon, 1987). The prescription of antidepressants and counseling for depression frequently occur in the absence of a recorded diagnosis of depression (Jencks, 1985), and many cases of depression presented to family physicians may remain undetected.

The efficacy of antidepressants and psychotherapy for depression is well established (Depression Guideline Panel, 1993) but most clinically significant cases of depression go untreated. The costs of untreated depression for the individual, the family, and society as a whole are high. It has been suggested that half of family practice patients with depression have serious difficulties maintaining their normal lives along with an increased risk of suicide. In general, depression and depressive symptoms are associated with more impairment of functioning than chronic medical illnesses such as arthritis, chronic lung disease, diabetes, and hypertension (Wells et al., 1989). Untreated depression has come to be viewed as a major public health problem, and better detection and treatment of depression by family physicians and other primary care providers has been proposed as its solution (National Institute of Mental Health, 1983).

Family physicians have been criticized for missing many cases of depression that are presented to them, including perhaps 30 to 50 per cent of all cases of major depression (Coyne and Schwenk, 1993; Freeling et al., 1985; Von Korff et al., 1987). Yet few family practice patients with significant depressive symptoms complain directly of depression or initially identify depression as their reason for the visit (Duer et al., 1988). Many patients deny that they are depressed even when asked directly. If they volunteer information on depressive symptoms at all, the symptoms often concern somatic complaints or fatigue rather than mood disturbance. The family physician must distinguish these symptoms from the acute and chronic health problems that occur concomitantly with depression in primary care and that serve as patients' stated reasons for the visit. It may require several patient visits and considerable vigilance and probing on the part of the family physician to detect the presence of significant depressive symptoms, distinguish them from other complaints, and make an appropriate diagnosis.

Undoubtedly, there are some depressed family practice patients with relatively unambiguous symptoms, or what has been termed "conspicuous psychiatric morbidity." These patients are similar to those seen by psychiatrists and would benefit from treatment, such that failure to diagnosis these patients represents a lost opportunity to improve their health and well-being. However, many depressed family practice patients present with strong somatic symptoms, are more mildly depressed even among patients with major depressive disorder, and have fewer neurovegetative features than patients found in psychiatric settings (Sireling et al., 1985). Depressed patients seen in family practice have a lower educational level, are less likely to have had past mental health treatment, are more likely to have lifetime histories of other psychopathology such as anxiety disorders and substance abuse, and have more physical symptoms and chronic health conditions that limit their mobility and exertion (Coyne and Schwenk, 1993). The dysfunctional and depressed condition of these patients has been found to persist for long periods in the face of nonrecognition. The relative benefit of treatment with antidepressants or psychotherapy (or both) in this type of family practice depressed patient is not known. There is a pressing need for diagnostic criteria, treatment guidelines, and medical education that deals with such patients. Family physicians must routinely make decisions without these aids for the present time.

It should be appreciated that depression, even when not present in the form of a complete syndrome, can have a significant impact on medical care and health outcomes. For instance, patients pejoratively labeled as malingerers on the basis of multiple, recurrent complaints without concurrent physical findings have been found to have significantly higher self-reports of depressive symptoms than controls (Katon et al., 1990). It is possible that detection and brief psychotherapeutic treatment of mildly depressed patients could reduce unnecessary outpatient visits, laboratory tests and x-ray studies, and hospitalizations. Furthermore, the patient's depressed mood and accompanying demoralization can also increase the perceived severity and medical intractability of an established chronic illness, as well as increase its impact on a patient's life; and it can decrease the patient's adherence to a long-term or involved regimen. Thus even when the issue is not one of a formally diagnosable depressive disorder, the suspicion of depressed mood can be important when managing patients who overutilize medical services or who have difficulties adapting to chronic illness.

CLASSIFICATION OF DEPRESSION AND DEPRESSIVE SYNDROMES

A major problem concerning the care of depressed patients by family physicians is the difficulty of classifying and labeling patients with varying degrees of depression and various types of symptom complexes. Ambiguous classification and labeling leads to inadequate treatment. Yet existing diagnostic criteria are largely derived from work with psychiatric populations in which the spectrum of depressive disorders is narrower than that encountered in family practice. Many family practice patients have chronic or intermittent depressive symptoms and yet are nonclassifiable according to the strict criteria proposed for major depression, dysthymia, adjustment disorder with depressed mood, and other depressive syndromes in the *Diagnostic and Statistical Manual of Mental Disorders* (DSM-IV, 1994).

The latest *DSM-IV* (1994) clarifies the situation to some extent by the proposed addition of a new

---

TABLE 52–1. DSM-IV CRITERIA FOR MAJOR DEPRESSIVE EPISODE

A. At least five of the following symptoms have been present during the same 2-week period and represent a change from previous functioning; at least one of the symptoms is either (1) depressed mood or (2) loss of interest or pleasure.
   1. Depressed mood most of the day, nearly every day, as indicated by either subjective report (e.g., feels sad or empty) or observation made by others (e.g., appears tearful). Note: in children and adolescents, can be irritable mood.
   2. Markedly diminished interest or pleasure in all, or almost all, activities most of the day, nearly every day (as indicated either by subjective account or observation made by others).
   3. Significant weight loss or weight gain when not dieting (e.g., more than 5 percent of body weight in a month), or decrease or increase in appetite nearly every day. Note: in children, consider failure to make expected weight gains.
   4. Insomnia or hypersomnia nearly every day.
   5. Psychomotor agitation or retardation nearly every day (observable by others, not merely subjective feelings of restlessness or being slowed down).
   6. Fatigue or loss of energy nearly every day.
   7. Feelings of worthlessness or excessive or inappropriate guilt (which may be delusional) nearly every day (not merely self-reproach or guilt about being sick).
   8. Diminished ability to think or concentrate, or indecisiveness, nearly every day (either by subjective account or as observed by others).
   9. Recurrent thoughts of death (not just fear of dying), recurrent suicidal ideation without a specific plan, or a suicide attempt or a specific plan for committing suicide.
B. Symptoms cause clinically significant distress or impairment in social, occupational, or other important areas of functioning.
C. Not due to the direct effects of a substance (e.g., drugs of abuse, medication) or a general medical condition (e.g., hypothyroidism).
D. Not occurring within 2 months of the loss of a loved one (except if associated with marked functional impairment, morbid preoccupation with worthlessness, suicidal ideation, psychotic symptoms, or psychomotor retardation).

Adapted from American Psychiatric Association: Diagnostic and Statistical Manual of Mental Disorders, 4th edition. Washington, DC, American Psychiatric Association, 1994, with permission.

---

criterion to the currently accepted list of criteria (Table 52–1). This new criterion addresses the issue of clinical or functional impairment caused by the depressive symptoms, thus providing slightly more latitude to primary care physicians attempting to classify depressed patients for the purpose of selecting effective treatment.

Even so, a careful review of the criteria for major depression (Table 52–1) suggests that this diagnosis fits more family practice patients than is generally appreciated. Misconceptions about these criteria are probably a source of the underdiagnosis of major depression by mental health professionals as well as family physicians. As can be seen, the criteria are based on symptoms and make no reference to precipitating stressors. Regardless of whether patients are facing a recent life change such as divorce or loss of employment that makes their mood state "understandable," if they meet these criteria they are to be considered depressed and appropriately treated. Mood disturbance is a requirement for diagnosis. Indeed, patients' reports of stressful life events should serve as a cue for further inquiry about symptoms of depression. The mood disturbance must persist most of the day, nearly every day, for 2 weeks, although a patient can fulfill this criterion and still have periods of a couple of hours at a time in which his or her mood is buoyed up. Sadness and dejection are not requirements, although many depressed patients report these feelings as their principal complaint. A loss of pleasure or interest in all or most usual activities is an alternate way of meeting the mood criteria, and persons having this type of mood disturbance may further complain that all emotional experience, including sadness, has been blunted or inhibited. In severely depressed patients, this inhibition of emotional expression may involve an inability to cry, even though mildly and moderately depressed persons readily cry.

The standard criteria for major depression also have some limitations. The criteria identify a heterogenous group of patients; two patients can be found to be depressed without having a single symptom in common. Furthermore, many patients in a typical family practice have significant depressive symptoms without ever meeting the criteria for this diagnosis. Dysthymia offers a possible diagnostic and therapeutic category for many depressed patients in family practice (see the diagnostic criteria in Table 52–2). Epidemiologic studies suggest that dysthymia is more prevalent than previously suspected, yet many patients who have persistent symptoms do not meet the criterion of a duration of two full years. Adjustment disorder with depressed mood is another relevant category and refers to symptoms such as depressed mood, tearfulness, and hopelessness that follow a stressful life event and persist no longer than 6 months. Yet appropriate therapeutic recommendations are not well established for dysthymia or adjustment disorder; and taken together with major depression, they still fail to accommodate the depressive features of many family practice patients. In particular, there is probably a considerable number of patients who suffer intermittent depressive symptoms chronically or episodically but who do not meet the criteria for any of these diagnoses. Recognition that these patients are prone to some mild mood disturbances can reduce the incidence of unnecessary laboratory tests and inappropriate treatment.

Figure 52–1 represents an effort to provide a classification that leads to treatment recommendations, capitalizes on strengths of the *DSM-III-R* criteria, and accommodates the broader range of depressive conditions encountered in family practice (Petty, 1987). Those diagnoses listed under major depression are more serious and are more deserv-

TABLE 52–2.   DSM-IV CRITERIA FOR DYSTHYMIA

A. Depressed mood (or can be irritable mood in children and adolescents) for most of the day, for more days than not, as indicated either by subjective account or observation made by others, for at least 2 years (1 year for children and adolescents).

B. Presence, while depressed, of at least three of the following:
1. Low self-esteem or self-confidence, or feelings of inadequacy.
2. Feelings of pessimism, despair, or hopelessness.
3. Generalized loss of interest or pleasure.
4. Social withdrawal.
5. Chronic fatigue or tiredness.
6. Feelings of guilt, brooding about the past.
7. Subjective feelings of irritability or excessive anger.
8. Decreased activity, effectiveness, or productivity.
9. Difficulty in thinking reflected by poor concentration, poor memory, or indecisiveness.

C. During the 2-year period (1 year for children or adolescents) of the disturbance, the person has never been without the symptoms in A and B for more than 2 months at a time.

D. No major depressive episode during the first 2 years of the disturbance (1 year for children and adolescents).

E. Has never had a manic episode or an unequivocal hypomanic episode.

F. Does not occur exclusively during the course of a chronic psychotic disorder, such as schizophrenia or delusional disorder.

G. Not due to the direct effects of a substance (e.g., drugs of abuse, medication) or a general medical condition (e.g., hypothyroidism).

Adapted from American Psychiatric Association: Diagnostic and Statistical Manual of Mental Disorders, 4th edition. Washington, D.C., American Psychiatric Association, 1994, with permission.

ing of intensive treatment such as combined psychopharmacology and counseling. Patients with diagnoses listed under minor depression generally respond to problem-solving, stress management, or supportive talk therapy. The physician should remain vigilant regarding the development of neurovegetative symptoms or more numerous or serious symptoms that signify that the patient has developed major depression, requiring more intensive and usually psychopharmacologic treatment.

Major Depression

The forms of major depression of greatest importance to family physicians are unipolar primary depressions and depression secondary to a major medical illness or an illness that requires surgery. Bipolar (manic-depressive) illness is considerably less common in primary care and usually requires joint care or care through referral to a psychiatrist, particularly regarding the subtleties of managing lithium administration and blood levels (unless the family physician has experience with these methods). Depressive conditions that are secondary to schizophrenia or substance abuse require attention

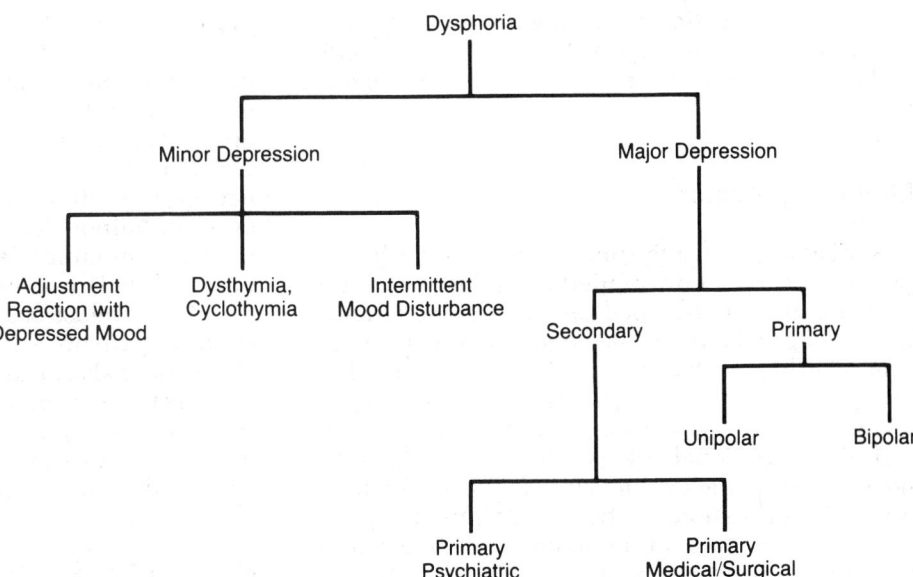

FIGURE 52–1. Classification of depressive syndromes. (Adapted from Petty F: Depression and medical/surgical illness: "Who wouldn't be depressed?" Prim Care 14:669, 1987, with permission.)

to the primary disorder, again often requiring psychiatric assistance or significant experience in dealing with patients with those major psychiatric diagnoses.

The diagnosis of unipolar, major depression is based on the *DSM-IV* criteria listed in Table 52–1. As discussed above, these criteria are relatively clear. One source of underdiagnosis is a low index of suspicion when dealing with patients who discount their feelings of apathy, anhedonia, or melancholic mood. Self-administered questionnaires can be used on a screening basis for sensitizing the physician to the need to consider the diagnosis of major depression, although these questionnaires err on the side of greater sensitivity at the expense of specificity. Even a single question inquiring about significant mood or motivational disturbance over the past year has been shown to be sufficiently sensitive to be useful in clinical practice (Froom et al., 1993), recognizing that such an approach has low specificity. False-positives that are likely to occur include patients with significant anxiety or neuroticism in the absence of a depressive syndrome. Questionnaires with studied validity in various primary care and medical settings include the Depression Inventory, Zung Self-Rating Depression Scale, General Health Questionnaire (GHQ), and Center for Epidemiologic Studies—Depression Scale (CES-D). A comparison of useful distinguishing features of these self-administered questionnaires is shown in Table 52–3.

Arriving at the diagnosis of major depression secondary to a significant medical illness or an illness that requires surgery depends on the physician's awareness of the numerous diseases and syndromes with which depression is associated. Many medical illnesses include symptoms of a psychomotor, cognitive, or neurovegetative type that are identical with those found with depression, making distinction difficult for treatment purposes.

TABLE 52–3. CHARACTERISTICS OF COMMONLY USED QUESTIONNAIRES FOR DIAGNOSIS OF DEPRESSION

Questionnaire/Instrument	No. of Items	Method of Administration	Characteristics and Use
Beck Depression Inventory (BDI)	21	Self-administered	Measures subjective experiences, psychological components of depression
Zung Self-Rating Depression Scale	20	Self-administered or by trained interviewer	Index of depression severity
Center for Epidemiologic Studies—Depression	20	Self-administered	Screening general or medical care populations
General Health Questionnaire (GHQ)	28	Self-administered	Screening for range of emotional distress in medical care population
Inventory to Diagnose Depression (IDD)	22	Self-administered	Useful for screening

(See the later section regarding a more complete discussion of inclusive versus exclusive methods of diagnosing depression in patients with biomedical illness.)

Minor Depression

A diagnosis of adjustment disorder with depressed mood can be applied to a patient with up to 6 months of mild mood disturbance, so long as his or her psychomotor and cognitive function continues fairly undisturbed. Dysthymic and cyclothymic patients are those with long-term personality styles including persistent or cyclical dysphoria, self-pity, irrational negativity, and "moodiness"—hence the previously used term "characterologic depression." Patients with this condition exhibit few or none of the neurovegetative symptoms that require psychopharmacologic treatment, nor are they cognitively impaired. These patients rarely respond to antidepressants or intensive psychotherapy but require the use of an interviewing style and a physician–patient relationship that support positive, constructive health behaviors. Some of these patients have a residual or an impending major depression or an attenuated form of another type of major depression, necessitating careful attention to the longitudinal course of the depressive symptoms, particularly the development of neurovegetative symptoms that would respond to psychopharmacologic therapy.

It should be noted that patients may suffer from an acute episode of major depression superimposed on a dysthymic condition. This phenomenon is more prevalent than once was thought and has been labeled "double depression." The fact that a patient has a history of dysthymia should not distract a physician from the possibility of the emergence of a full syndrome of major depression in the same patient. A primary care physician may have a particular disadvantage in this regard because of the familiarity with the patient that comes from a continuing relationship. Because of this familiarity, subtle changes in the patient's depressive symptomatology or severity may escape detection. The physician should maintain particular vigilance of the patient who is chronically depressed for signs that the depression is worsening and may respond to medication. Antidepressant medication is likely to prove effective for treating the major depression of such patients, in which case they may simply return to their baseline level of dysthymia.

As we have noted earlier, the criteria of DSM IV do not accommodate a group of patients who suffer episodic or chronic intermittent depressive conditions or who show recurrent but short-lived periods of lability of mood in the face of everyday life stress. In such states, the patients may be preoccupied with feeling of inadequacy, withdraw from their usual activities, complain, react with resentment and irritability, and otherwise prove demanding and difficult. An alternative to the criteria of the DSM IV that is widely used in psychiatric and epidemiologic research, the Research Diagnostic Criteria (Spitzer et al., 1978), acknowledges the existence of such persons with the classifications of episodic minor depressive disorder, chronic and intermittent minor depressive disorder, and labile personality. However, such diagnoses have served mainly as exclusion criteria for clinical studies, and so these patients are not well studied. The physician should also be alert to the possibility that what appears to be a minor condition actually may represent the onset of a more serious depressive disorder. A brief review of any history of depression can be revealing in this regard.

Masked Depression

Masked depression is a term that is subject to considerable misunderstanding and misuse. It has sometimes been used to broaden the category of depression to include patients who otherwise lack the required symptoms for diagnosis. Formally speaking, the diagnosis of depression requires the presence of mood disturbance. In psychiatric settings, this disturbance generally is the patient's presenting complaint. However, it is not always the case, particularly in family practice, and the physician may have to rely on inference and information from sources other than the patient to decide if mood disturbance is indeed occurring. For instance, the patient may vigorously deny sadness or loss of pleasure, yet a few questions reveal that he or she has largely withdrawn from family and friends and given up exercise and hobbies. In such an instance, a judgment of mood disturbance and therefore a diagnosis of depression may be justified.

From this perspective, masked depression refers to a presentation of depression rather than a distinct subtype. The diagnosis involves an often difficult judgment but one that is frequently required of family physicians. Moreover, because the diagnosis of this presentation of depression largely is based on somatic complaints, particularly chronic pain, this condition represents perhaps the largest reservoir of undiagnosed, treatable depression in the typical family practice.

Patients with masked depression initially present with a nearly inexhaustible list of somatic complaints, with particular emphasis on chronic pain (headache, chest pain, back pain, abdominal pain), gastrointestinal complaints (nausea, diarrhea, constipation, flatulence, bloating, belching, indigestion), neurologic complaints (fainting, fatigue, dizziness, visual blurring), and cardiorespiratory complaints (palpitations, dyspnea, syncope, hyperventilation). These patients appear to have an unexplained selective perception for the somatic manifestations of their psychological pain, with a corresponding denial of the psychological and neurovegetative symptoms. The association with panic attacks, hypochondriasis, or common somatoform disorders is unclear (Chapters 51 and 52), but differentiation from the last two conditions is critical for successful treatment. Depression that is described purely in the form of a list of somatic complaints is eminently more treatable than most somatoform disorders, whereas antidepressant therapy of even moderate dosage is often successful for panic attacks.

There are two techniques for differentiating depression from common somatoform disorders: (1) screening questionnaires and a careful inquiry about depressive symptoms in patients who have high scores (Table 52–3); and (2) empiric use of antidepressants when the index of suspicion is high. For example, in patients with a history of major depression or who describe under persistent questioning some component of neurovegetative, psychological, or cognitive dysfunction, a cautious trial of an antidepressant with a low incidence of serious side effects (Table 52–4) may have both diagnostic and therapeutic value.

EPIDEMIOLOGY AND NATURAL HISTORY OF DEPRESSION

The development of clearer diagnostic criteria, semistructured interview schedules, and rating scales has allowed a marked increase in information available on the epidemiology of depression. Current estimates of point prevalence for major depressive disorder are 2.3 to 3.2 per cent for men and 4.5 to 9.3 per cent for women. The prevalence among primary medical care patients is even higher, at least 5 to 10 per cent (Katon and Schulberg, 1992). The lifetime risk for major depressive disorder is 7 to 12 per cent for men and 20 to 25 per cent for women (Depression Guidelines Panel, 1993). Fewer than half of persons currently experiencing major depression seek professional help. Major depression is two to three times more com-

TABLE 52–4. SIDE EFFECT PROFILES AND THERAPEUTIC DOSAGE RANGES OF ANTIDEPRESSANT MEDICATIONS

| Drug | Anti-cholinergic* | CNS Effects | | Cardiovascular Effects | | | Weight Gain (over 6 kg [13 lb]) | Therapeutic Dosage Range (mg) |
		Drowsiness	Insomnia/Agitation	Orthostatic Hypotension	Cardiac Arrhythmia	GI Distress		
Amitriptyline (Elavil, Endep)	4+	4+	0	4+	3+	0	4+	75–300
Desipramine (Norpramin, Pertofrane)	1+	1+	1+	2+	2+	0	1+	75–300
Doxepin (Adapin, Sinequan)	3+	4+	0	2+	2+	0	3+	75–300
Imipramine (Janimine, Tofranil)	3+	3+	1+	4+	3+	1+	3+	75–300
Nortriptyline (Aventyl, Pamelor)	1+	1+	0	2+	2+	0	1+	40–200
Protriptyline (Vivactil)	2+	1+	1+	2+	2+	0	0	20–60
Trimipramine (Surmontil)	1+	4+	0	2+	2+	0	3+	75–300
Amoxapine (Asendin)	2+	2+	2+	2+	3+	0	1+	100–600
Maprotiline (Ludiomil)	2+	4+	0	0	1+	0	2+	100–225
Trazodone (Desyrel)	0	4+	0	1+	1+	1+	1+	150–600
Bupropion (Wellbutrin)	0	0	2+	0	1+	1+	0	225–450
Fluoxetine (Prozac)	0	0	2+	0	0	3+	0	10–40
Paroxetine (Paxil)	0	0	2+	0	0	3+	0	20–50
Sertraline (Zoloft)	0	0	2+	0	0	3+	0	50–150
Monoamine oxidase inhibitors	1	1+	2+	2+	0	1+	2+	Varies (usual dose 30–50)

0 = absent or rare; 2+ = in between; 4+ = relatively common.
* Dry mouth, blurred vision, urinary hesitancy, constipation.
Adapted from Depression Guidelines Panel. U.S. Department of Health and Human Services, Public Health Service, Rockville, MD. AHCPR Publication no. 93-0550, 1993.

mon in women than in men, with women 18 to 44 years of age having the highest rate. Depression is most common among persons aged 18 to 44, particularly between the ages of 25 and 34. Although the elderly have high rates of dysphoria, they do not have high rates of clinical major depression. Apparently, the rate of depression is increasing for persons born after 1935, and the age of onset is decreasing. The mean age of onset of a first episode of depression is now in the twenties. If current trends continue, family physicians can expect to see a higher number of young persons with major depression than in the past.

Although a person's morale or sense of well-being is predictably increased in association with higher income and education, increased rates of major depression apparently are not related to the absence of these benefits. Studies show that major depression affects equally the rich and poor, the educated and uneducated, blue collar and white collar workers, and persons of all races. Major depression is related to marital status, with single and formerly married individuals having higher rates than married individuals. Yet the highest rate of depression is found among persons who are married and are not getting along with their spouse. For both men and women, the risk of major depression in an unhappy marriage increases about 25-fold (Weissman, 1987). Major depression is consistently related to recent life events, particularly those involving a loss, with depressed persons having three to six times as many such events as nondepressed persons. Vulnerability to depression after a life event is substantially increased by having poor social relationships or low social support, particularly for women; for instance, a woman is three times more likely to become depressed after a stressful life event if she lacks a confiding relationship (Brown and Harris, 1978). Thus advances in our understanding of the biomedical aspects of depression should not distract us from its psychosocial dimensions (Coyne, 1987; Coyne and Downey, 1991).

The traditional view of major depression has been that it is a relatively benign condition, generally occurring in a single episode in a person's life and remitting without residual problems. However, it now appears that only about half of persons experiencing an episode of major depression suffer only a single episode. The emerging view of depression is that it is heterogeneous and highly variable in its course, but that it is basically a recurrent, episodic disorder with varying degrees of residual difficulties (Clayton, 1983). Episodes of major depression tend to last 4 to 8 months, although about 15 per cent of patients with major depression have a chronic course. Relapse after successful treatment is common, with about 50 per cent of patients relapsing within 2 years. This figure decreases with maintenance dosages of antidepressants. On average, persons who become clinically depressed can expect a mean of five to six episodes in their lifetimes. For the family physician, this fact suggests that knowledge of the patient's history can be important in detecting depression, and that inquiries about whether a patient has previously had periods in which he or she felt sad or blue every day for a couple of weeks can be crucial in resolving ambiguous cases.

A history of depression is a strong predictor of risk; and once it is taken into account, the predictive value of other risk factors is often eliminated. Comments in patients' charts about their history have been found to improve detection of new episodes of depression (Block et al., 1988). Although only about 25 per cent of depressed psychiatric patients and possibly fewer family practice patients have a clearly defined family history of depression, persons with a first-degree relative with major depression have a two- to threefold higher risk of major depression than the general population. Persons who become depressed earlier in life have stronger family histories of depression, and so family physicians should be alert to undetected depression in the parents of adolescents with major depression. Finally, assortative mating is high, with depressed men particularly likely to marry women who are vulnerable to depression.

Studies of dysthymia in the general population became available only during the late 1980s. A survey of five communities in the United States found rates from 2.1 to 4.2 per cent (Weissman et al., 1987). It is most prevalent among women under 65 years of age, in the unmarried, and in young persons with low income. It has a surprisingly high co-morbidity with other psychiatric conditions (70 to 75 per cent), particularly major depression, which raises questions as to whether it is a specific disorder. It may often represent the consequence of untreated or only partially remitted episodes of depression that have become chronic, or it may represent a milder manifestation of major depression.

Related Psychiatric Conditions

Major and minor types of depression have many features in common with other psychiatric conditions, and some overlap of diagnostic criteria can occur. The *DSM-IV* criteria for depression note the need for an absence of hallucinations and delusions and an absence of major psychotic disease. However, early and residual schizophrenia can be exhibited as depression owing to the ill-defined mood alterations and somatic preoccupations often present. The cognitive disturbances can masquerade as dementia, particularly in elderly patients in whom severe cognitive dysfunction is particularly common. In such cases, the symptoms suggesting dementia may disappear with appropriate treatment of the depression.

The *DSM-IV* criteria allow for the occurrence of major depression in patients who have a pre-existing personality disorder. Diagnosis can be difficult in that such patients' manipulative behavior, poor impulse control, and disordered interpersonal relationships may distract the physician from the presence of their depressive symptoms. Although treatment for depression is still indicated, persons with pre-existing personality disorders do not respond as well as other patients.

The somatic preoccupation of many depressed patients who are seen in primary care can be confused with hypochondriasis and common somatiform disorders. Patients who abuse alcohol, sedatives, or hypnotics can be depressed, as can patients who are withdrawing from cocaine or amphetamines. Accurate diagnosis may require that the patient first complete withdrawal from alcohol or abused drugs. Bereaved patients may pose some diagnostic problems. A patient who otherwise meets the criteria for major depression may still be thought to be experiencing uncomplicated bereavement when his or her condition is judged to be a timely and appropriate reaction to a loss. However, if these symptoms become prolonged or if marked psychomotor retardation or a morbid preoccupation with worthlessness develops, a diagnosis of major depression should be considered. Many depressed patients have significant anxiety symptoms and can be thought to have one of several anxiety disorders (Chapter 51). Depression and anxiety can best be distinguished by focusing on the neurovegetative and somatic components of depression, as the psychological symptoms of depression are often similar to those of anxiety.

BIOMEDICAL ASPECTS OF DEPRESSION

Neurobiology of Depression

Major depression requiring intensive psychopharmacology and psychotherapy is construed as ultimately being a neuroendocrinologic disorder. Irrespective of the presence of life stresses, major losses, or precipitating events, many patients with major depression have been shown to have major neurobiologic abnormalities. These abnormalities include an excess of 5-hydroxyindoleacetic acid (a serotonin metabolite); abnormalities in the hypothalamopituitary adrenal axis and the regulation of thyroid-stimulating hormone stimulation by thyrotropin-releasing hormone; and abnormal levels of melatonin, luteinizing hormone, growth hormone, and prolactin. For these reasons, previous distinctions between "exogenous," or "reactive," depression due to precipitating events and "endogenous" depression due to biologic abnormalities are considered unhelpful or irrelevant, as they neither clarify the etiology of the condition nor predict the

success of various therapies. In practical terms, patients can have a neurovegetative form of depression that responds well to antidepressants or requires more serious treatment such as electroconvulsive therapy irrespective of the presence or absence of significant life losses or precipitating events.

Defined in other ways, however, the notion of endogenous depression retains some validity. Reactivity to changes in life circumstances *while* patients are depressed has been found to predict the patient's response to biologically oriented treatment, with patients who are less responsive deriving greater benefit. Other predictors include (1) a distinct quality of mood and whether there has been a loss of the ability to experience pleasure; (2) psychomotor retardation; (3) feeling worse in the morning than in the evening; and (4) early morning awakening and appetite disturbance. These symptoms are related to measurable abnormalities in the neuroendocrine system and a variety of quantitative measures of sleep disturbance (Clayton and Barrett, 1983). Also, these symptoms have now replaced the absence of precipitating stress as the definitive criteria for endogenous depression. To reduce confusion, the term "reactive" has been abandoned in the United States in favor of "nonendogenous," and "melancholic" has replaced "endogenous." However, some cautions are in order. Most patients seen in family practice with major depressive disorder are not melancholic but nonetheless are responsive to antidepressants. The distinction is imprecise and its prediction of the patient's response to treatment is relative. Furthermore, many patients with melancholic symptoms face difficult psychosocial circumstances that require adjunctive psychotherapy for the alleviation of these symptoms.

Despite the assumption that major depression is ultimately a neuroendocrinologic disorder, in a carefully selected psychiatric research population only about 60 per cent of severely ill patients demonstrated any such neurohormonal abnormality with the methods that are currently available (APA Task Force, 1987).

The proportion of depressed patients seen in a family practice with such neuroendocrine abnormalities may be as low as 20 to 30 per cent. Furthermore, despite initial enthusiasm, efforts to diagnose pharmacologically treatable depression through biologic markers, such as the dexamethasone suppression test, have been relatively unsuccessful in primary care populations, particularly when compared with astute clinical diagnosis that allows recognition of the multiple forms of major depression that can appear in unselected populations.

The dexamethasone suppression test is conducted similarly to that for the diagnosis of Cushing syndrome, although the method differs somewhat. Despite encouraging results in tertiary populations, the test cannot be recommended in primary care populations because of its poor positive predictive value and an unacceptably high rate of false-positive results. It does distinguish between severe and mild depression, but one does not need the dexamethasone suppression test for this purpose, and exclusive reliance on it would cause many patients who would benefit from antidepressant medication to be missed. The dexamethasone suppression test and other neurohormonal tests, such as the thyrotropin-releasing hormone stimulation test, may be useful if done together, but no evidence exists regarding their usefulness in primary care. This point is particularly true for differentiating depressive patients who would benefit from antidepressant therapy or for distinguishing patients with depression in addition to a chronic illness from depression due to chronic illness. Although it is considered useful as a research tool, the dexamethasone suppression test has not proved to be the gold standard that it was hoped to be.

"Despite our burgeoning knowledge about neurotransmission, there are currently no reliable laboratory procedures that subtype depression clinically, guide the choice of antidepressant medication, or track treatment response" (Michels and Marzuk, 1993).

Depression and Biomedical Illness

As many as 60 per cent of depressed persons in the general population have another chronic medical condition, and the proportion among depressed family practice patients is likely to be higher. Depression and biomedical illness interact in several complex ways. Major depression may coexist in patients with severe medical illness and may be implicated as an increased risk for certain major illnesses. Chronically ill patients may be more likely to suffer from a secondary depression. Distinguishing depression coexistent with physical illness from depression due to physical illness represents one of the major challenges for the family physician. This distinction is critical for both diagnostic accuracy and treatment efficacy. Chronically ill patients suffer needlessly when major depression is underdiagnosed, usually owing to the physician's ascribing the depressive symptoms to the coexistent illness or dismissing the dysphoric and neurovegetative symptoms as inevitable (and therefore unimportant). Rehabilitation from a major medical illness, such as a myocardial infarction or a cerebrovascular accident, can be slowed tremendously by undiagnosed depression. Less-than-optimal results of rehabilitation can be accepted prematurely if the neurovegetative and psychological symptoms of depression are undetected, thereby allowing the patient's helpless and hopeless mood to sabotage rehabilitative efforts.

TABLE 52–5. ORGANIC ILLNESSES ASSOCIATED WITH DEPRESSION

Rheumatologic: systemic lupus erythematosus rheumatoid arthritis
Cardiac: mitral valve prolapse, myocardial infarction, hypertension
Endocrine: hyperthyroidism and hypothyroidism diabetes mellitus, hypercalcemia, Cushing syndrome, postpartum state
Gastrointestinal: cirrhosis, inflammatory bowel disease, pancreatitis, intestinal bypass
Hematologic: sickle cell anemia
Nutritional deficiencies: vitamin B_{12}, folate, iron, thiamine, niacin
Infectious: encephalitis, hepatitis, influenza, infectious mononucleosis, pneumonia, tuberculosis
Renal: renal transplant, uremia
Neoplastic: intracranial, leukemia, pancreatic, lymphoma
Neurologic: subdural hematoma, multiple sclerosis, CVA, Parkinson's, uncontrolled epilepsy
Miscellaneous: psoriasis, sarcoidosis, drugs (Table 52–6)

Finally, many organic illnesses can have depression as the presenting symptom or include depression as a significant component, and the physician must include these organic causes in any differential diagnosis for dysphoria.

Depression can be caused by dozens of organic illnesses, (Table 52–5), particularly those of the neurologic, metabolic, and endocrine types. Of particular importance for the family physician are diabetes mellitus, hyperthyroidism or hypothyroidism, postpartum state, cirrhosis, folate and iron deficiencies, infectious mononucleosis, influenza (particularly in the elderly), uremia, occult neoplasm, and the pseudodementia of the elderly with presumed Alzheimer's disease. Some studies suggest that 10 to 20 per cent of patients believed to have a major depression on initial presentation are found eventually to have an undiagnosed organic illness as the actual cause of the depressive symptoms. In addition, at least 200 medications have been implicated in causing depressive symptoms, including several drugs prescribed frequently for primary care (Table 52–6).

In addition to depression being the presenting symptom of severe underlying chronic illness,

---

TABLE 52–6. DRUGS COMMONLY ASSOCIATED WITH DEPRESSION

Amphetamines, other CNS stimulants
Barbiturates
Benzodiazepines
Cimetidine
Clonidine
β-Blockers
Corticosteroids
Indomethacin
α-Methyldopa
Oral contraceptives, estrogens
Reserpine, guanethidine
Sulfonamides

many common physical illnesses cause (or are associated with) depression. Twenty to thirty per cent of hospitalized patients suffer from major depression, with an additional 20 to 30 per cent suffering moderate depressive symptoms. This prevalence extends across disparate disease categories (e.g., patients with post-myocardial infarction, cerebrovascular accident, renal failure, and terminal cancer), suggesting a possible common neurobiologic pathway modified by psychosocial circumstances or pre-existing psychiatric morbidity. These patients present a diagnostic dilemma. Many of their symptoms satisfy the *DSM-IV* criteria for diagnosis (e.g., fatigue, loss of pleasure, sleep disturbance, appetite disturbance, and cognitive dysfunction), but it may be unclear whether the symptoms originated from the depression or the biomedical illness.

Guidelines are not well established for deciding whether symptoms that may originate from a concurrent biomedical illness should count toward a diagnosis of depression. The family physician can use either an *inclusive* or an *exclusive* approach to the evaluation of these patients. The inclusive approach attributes all symptoms of depression to the diagnostic criteria for depression, irrespective of whether the symptoms might actually be due to the associated physical illness. This method is conceptually "clean" because it is based on observable phenomenon but errs on the side of greater sensitivity than specificity, thus causing overdiagnosis of depression. This possibility must be remembered if the patient is exposed to potentially harmful therapies (e.g., antidepressants or electroconvulsive therapy) for an illness that may not exist.

The exclusive approach eliminates anorexia and fatigue from the list of possible depressive symptoms, as they are likely to be caused by an organic illness such as cancer. The diagnosis of depression must then be made from four of the remaining six *DSM-IV* criteria (assuming either depressed mood and loss of interest or pleasure are present). This approach leads to underdiagnosis, especially in patients with certain devastating systemic illnesses, such as cancer, who may benefit most from treatment for major depression. For purposes of greater sensitivity at the expense of specificity, the inclusive approach is recommended, but caution must be used to avoid excessive zeal in the aggressive treatment of every patient diagnosed in this fashion.

MANAGEMENT OF THE DEPRESSED PATIENT

Evaluation of Suicidal Risk

One of the critical objectives for the family physician caring for depressed patients is to assess sui-

---

TABLE 52-7. CORRELATES OF INCREASED SUICIDE RISK IN DEPRESSED PATIENTS

1. Increased age (peak risk in men is at 75; in women at 55 to 65)
2. Gender (women make more attempts; men are more often successful)
3. Marital status and social support (in order of decreasing risk: never married, widowed, separated or divorced, married without children, married with children)
4. Employment (greater in unemployed persons)
5. Presence of physical illness, especially chronic pain or terminal illness
6. Coexistent alcoholism or substance abuse
7. History of prior attempts
8. Communication to family, friends, or physician of intent, financial plans following death, or specific means of suicide.
9. Positive family history of successful suicide (especially that of parents)

---

cidal risk, at the initial diagnosis and during subsequent evaluations and continuing care. Studies suggest that most persons who commit suicide consult their family physician during the month prior to their death but do not receive treatment for depression. As many as 70 per cent of patients who commit suicide have one or more active physical illnesses; and these illnesses, rather than depression per se, may provide the reason for their visit.

The single best indicator of risk for suicide remains a direct or indirect statement of intent. Other correlates of increased suicidal risk are shown in Table 52-7. It is important to identify and refer patients at particularly high risk, such as a recently widowed elderly male patient who has coexistent alcoholism and a history of major depression or attempted suicide. Patients who have a major physical illness or a chronic debilitating condition for which there is little hope of improvement and who do not have significant family support are also at high risk. With malignancies and incurable conditions, the critical periods are when the diagnosis and prognosis have just been presented and when patients are coming to realize the seriousness of their condition.

The physician should take seriously any mention of suicide and not be deterred from inquiry by the fear that a frank discussion might lead to suicidal behavior. It is not unusual for even moderately depressed persons to have fleeting thoughts of suicide, and the physician's broaching of the topic may be appreciated by patients as a sign of the physician's recognition of their plight. The assessment of suicidal risk should focus on *intent* and *lethality*. Intent refers to a patient's commitment to an act that is expected to lead to death. Particular concern is warranted when the patient has a definite plan, considers using more than one method at a time, and has made preparations for death or has taken steps not to be discovered. Patients who do not have a well developed plan but who are impulsive, psychotic, or frequently intoxicated may pose similar risks. Lethality refers to the degree to which particular methods are likely to lead to death. As part of an assessment, the physician may ask outright if the patients are willing to make a commitment or contract not to kill themselves, and if they are what plans for help they have made if the urge worsens. Patients who cannot credibly make such a commitment should be considered at high risk.

Antidepressants

Whether major depression begins with precipitating psychosocial stresses or is an intrinsic neurochemical imbalance, the end result in patients with neurovegetative symptoms is a functional depletion of neurotransmitters. Controversy still exists regarding an exclusive and complete description of specific neurotransmitter deficiencies and neural synaptic locations of these deficiencies, but attention has shifted from the availability of neurotransmitters to the sensitivity of receptors, primarily histamine H_1, muscarinic and α-adrenoceptor receptor sites. Actions at these receptor sites are also responsible for the usual side effects of tricyclic and similar antidepressants: dry mouth, urinary retention, sedation and orthostatic hypotension. Studies documenting the effectiveness of antidepressant medication have mainly been conducted with psychiatric patients, but results are thought to apply to primary care patients with major depressive disorder as well. The Depression Guidelines Panel (1993) identified seven medication studies conducted in primary care settings and concluded that the overall efficacy of these drugs to be about 55 to 60 per cent. It recommended that all depressed patients be treated. Yet although antidepressants have been shown to be effective for mild as well as more severe depression (Paykel et al., 1988), the severity of depression found in many family practice patients falls below the threshold for which a response to antidepressants has been established. The most effective way to manage their illness is unclear, even though mild depression can be debilitating.

Drug selection depends on a number of special clinical situations as well as taking side effects into account (Table 52–4). For example, patients with a form of depression that has a significant component of anxiety, agitation, or sleep disturbance benefit from antidepressants with a significant sedative effect, such as amitriptyline, doxepin, or trazodone. Elderly patients prone to orthostatic hypotension would respond poorly to antidepressants that exacerbate this problem, such as amitriptyline or imipramine. Nortriptyline and desipramine are particularly good for elderly patients with orthostatic problems or prostatic hypertrophy. Patients without dominant neurovegetative symptoms would also benefit from a medication such as desipramine. Predicting the response of patients to one class of antidepressants is difficult, so lack of a response to therapeutic dosages should prompt the physician to check the blood level of the drug (for the purpose of checking patient compliance) or switch to a different antidepressant. In addition, the blood levels of four antidepressants—nortriptyline, desipramine, imipramine, and amitriptyline—have been shown to be somewhat more predictive of a dose-dependent response, or at least to have a threshold at which a response is expected.

The lethal dose of most cyclic antidepressants may be as low as 1000 to 1500 mg, so no single prescription should exceed this quantity, especially during the early phase of treatment when suicidal risk assessment is difficult and the risk of suicide may fluctuate. The use of fixed combination drug preparations is rarely if ever justified, especially as most combinations include minor or major sedatives that have little role in the treatment of depression.

Tricyclic antidepressants should be begun at a low dose (typically 25 mg) and increased to a therapeutic dose in 25- to 50-mg increments every 3 to 7 days. A convenient routine is to plan to see the patient weekly during the early stages of diagnosis and treatment for medication adjustment and supportive counseling (irrespective of referral for extended mental health care) and adjusting the dosage at each visit. Interim adjustments are useful as well. Compliance is markedly increased by giving the entire dosage of tricyclic antidepressant in the evening, specifically at dinner time, because peak blood levels are reached within 3 to 4 hours. Side effects should be assessed at each visit, distinguishing the "nuisance" effects such as dry mouth from more serious effects such as hypotension, palpitations, and urinary retention. Once an effective dosage is reached, treatment should continue for 6 to 12 months before withdrawal is even considered. Frequent courses of similar length or continuous treatment for more than a year are not uncommon owing to the relapsing nature of major depression.

Maintenance therapy at full dosage levels for periods of 1 year or longer are not unusual, especially for patients whose depression was not recognized for a considerable time. Some studies recommend maintenance treatment at full therapeutic antidepressant dosages when there is a personal history of a first severe depressive episode occurring at age 50 or older, two or more episodes of severe depression by age 40, or three or more episodes of depression occurring by any age (Greden, 1992). In addition, the Depression Guidelines Panel (1993) recommended consideration of full maintenance therapy if previous episodes were particularly severe or debilitating, involved suicidality, or were associated with a strong family history of recurrent depression.

Dosing with the newer selective serotonin reuptake inhibitors (SSRIs) is somewhat easier because dosage adjustments are few, although assessing response is more difficult because of the longer half-life and slower onset of action of these agents. These medications are best administered in the morning because of their potential to disrupt sleep. Patients should be assessed at 2 weeks for a response and dosages adjusted every 3 to 4 weeks depending on the response. The most frequent side effects are agitation, nervousness, gastrointestinal upset, and sexual dysfunction.

Assessing drug interactions is critical to the proper use of antidepressants, particularly because of their potentially widespread use. Important effects occur due to the activity of other drugs, such as clonidine (decreased effect), prazosin (increased effect), and anticoagulants (decreased metabolism). Agents that lower the activity of antidepressants include barbiturates, alcohol, oral contraceptives, and cigarette smoking. Increased antidepressant activity is caused by disulfiram (Antabuse), antiseizure medications, and amphetamine derivatives (presumably infrequently used).

The family physician needs to become familiar and comfortable with only a few of the many tricyclic drugs and related antidepressants, choosing those with complementary side effects. Monoamine oxidase inhibitors are used less often by family physicians because severe dietary restriction is necessary with their administration and they can be dangerous without meticulous attention to dietary details. Many family physicians believe that the need for switching from the usual antidepressants to monoamine oxidase inhibitors is an indication for referral of the patient to a psychiatrist.

Medication Versus Psychotherapy

Some controversy still surrounds the issue of whether to use antidepressants with psychotherapy or each method alone, but most evidence suggests that the two modalities are most effective when they are combined, especially for patients with severe depression. Psychotherapy may be most effective for mildly depressed patients, whereas medication is critical for patients who are more severely depressed and those with neurovegetative symptoms. Patients with major depression have at least a 70 per cent response rate to aggressive psychopharmacologic treatment, with or without psychotherapy. Patients with major depression, as measured by the presence of significant neurovegetative symptoms and standard *DSM-IV* criteria, are most likely to respond, whereas depression of a characterologic nature, such as cyclothymia or dysthymia, is less responsive. Some studies of family practice patients suggest that even patients with fairly mild depression, as measured by standardized questionnaires or structured interviews, respond well to short courses of antidepressants at less than the usual therapeutic dosage. This response is also seen in patients with chronic pain syndromes or masked depression. Even some patients with dysthymia who are developing major symptoms suggestive of major depression but do not yet fit the standard criteria may benefit from aggressive antidepressant therapy.

The superiority of antidepressant medication over placebo is well established, but there is still controversy surrounding the relative roles of psychotherapy and antidepressants. Some studies have shown medication to be superior to psychotherapy for the reduction of symptoms and prevention, but the same studies have also shown psychotherapy to be superior in its effect on social functioning. Antidepressant medication has little immediate effect on the interpersonal difficulties that accompany depression, and the effects of antidepressants are markedly reduced when patients are experiencing serious difficulties, such as intense marital conflict. Chronic interpersonal stress, particularly marital difficulties, has been shown to contribute to relapse. One study has shown that patients who have recovered from depression and who have had their medication terminated are more likely to remain free of depression if they have monthly opportunities to discuss and resolve interpersonal difficulties (Frank et al., 1990). Other studies have found psychotherapy to be superior to antidepressants. The most effective types of psychotherapy have some common features: They are relatively brief, are structured, and emphasize constructive changes in behavior rather than exploration of the past or the achievement of insight. One study in which such therapy was documented as being superior to antidepressants involved general practice patients in England (Blackburn et al., 1981).

Antidepressants are most effective in alleviating sleep disturbance, appetite disturbance, and other neurovegetative symptoms, whereas psychotherapy is most effective in dealing with suicidal feelings and interpersonal problems. However, there is considerable variability in patients' acceptance of treatment. An all-too-common situation is that of depressed women with marital difficulties being given only antidepressants, and the women then do not comply with treatment. If these patients are simply given time to talk about their problems, they are more willing to accept antidepressants.

Although absolute contraindications do not exist for the use of antidepressants during pregnancy and lactation, the physician should be cautious with their use, especially during the first trimester. The high prevalence of depression in women of childbearing years dictates that alternate nonpharmacologic treatment be considered. More generally, brief, structured, problem-solving therapies remain a viable option for both men and women in the treatment of depression. They are particularly indicated when patients report a positive response to previous psychotherapy, when they are failing to respond to medication alone, or when they just do not want to use pharmacologic treatments.

Contrary to popular belief, there is currently *no* evidence that antidepressant medication interferes with the effectiveness of psychotherapy. For moderate to severe depression, a combined approach is most effective. However, physicians have sometimes allowed psychotherapy to interfere with antidepressant therapy when they underprescribe or inappropriately reduce the dosage because a patient has initiated psychotherapy.

Psychological Management

Patients suffering from depression benefit from a clear, empathetic, confident style on the part of the physician. The physician should take care to grasp and acknowledge the nature and focus of the patient's distress. Attempts to minimize or deny this distress prove self-defeating and threaten the physician's rapport with the patient. However, without denying the reality of the patient's difficulties, it is useful to point out that a hopeless and pessimistic view is frequently a symptom of depression.

Patient Education

Both patient and family members need information about depression. They should recognize that it is not a matter of personal weakness or failure of will power. It should be pointed out that most episodes of depression resolve within 4 to 8 months. The expected loss of libido associated with depression should be explained to the patient and the spouse if there is conflict over sexual dissatisfaction. The patient and the family should be told when to expect the effects of both antidepressant medication and psychotherapy to appear. Specific side effects from antidepressant therapy should be construed as a sign that the drug is beginning to take effect.

Reducing Expectations

Depressed patients and family members should be instructed that depression can prove to be a tremendous drain on one's patience, morale, and energy level; and that all should appreciate that patients are not going to be at their best. Some activities can be put off or responsibilities reduced. Initiating an activity can prove particularly difficult for depressed persons. However, patients should be encouraged to consider whether they would feel better by initiating or deferring the activity, knowing that they have a greater risk of failure in not completing the activity despite their initial efforts.

Antidepressant Activities

Patients should be encouraged to undertake activities that provide some sense of mastery or pleasure. In particular, patients who see themselves as undeserving or self-sacrificing should be encouraged to view such suggestions as a prescription from the physician (Altrocchi et al., 1986). Patients benefit most if they are asked to commit themselves to specific activities and if the physician makes a follow-up inquiry as to whether the activities are actually being undertaken.

Contact with Family Members

The physician should acknowledge that depression is difficult for those who live with the patient. The family members should be encouraged not to take responsibility for the patient's mood but to take responsibility for their own behavior instead. Although family members should be encouraged to be supportive, they must avoid becoming overinvolved in miscarried efforts to prod or coerce patients into activities. "Constructive criticism" from family members is unlikely to be helpful to patients. Sometimes it is helpful for patients and family members to plan special activities or simple protected time together.

Physicians would do well to view depression as a marker for families with other difficulties. High levels of family stress, particularly marital discord, are common; and the children of depressed parents are at risk for a full range of other difficulties, including conduct problems, school refusal, and depression (Downey and Coyne, 1990). Spouses and children of depressed persons tend to have increased medical utilization with complaints of pain, minor ailments, and psychological distress.

Additional Treatment Approaches

Psychotherapy and antidepressants are the mainstay of treatment for depression. In addition to these major approaches, several additional approaches are available. The book *Feeling Good: The New Mood Therapy* (Burns, 1992) is an example of a self-help book that enhances positive thinking and provides a concrete plan for constructive action. Bibliotherapy may also include such books as *A New Guide to Rational Living* (Ellis & Harper, 1975), *Overcoming Depression* (Popolas and Popolas, 1987), *Control Your Depression* (Lewinsohn et al., 1979), or even a number of texts concerning assertion training. A prescription of relaxation exercise or more strenuous aerobic activity such as running, bicycling, swimming, or cross-country skiing may be helpful (Nicoloff and Schwenk, in press). Physical exercise not only may be a useful distraction from negative thinking but may enhance mood directly through poorly understood neurochemical changes. A prescription for

TABLE 52–8. INDICATIONS FOR REFERRAL TO A PSYCHIATRIST

1. Moderate or high suicidal risk (see Table 52–7)
2. Severe cognitive dysfunction with difficulty in daily living or nutritional deficiencies
3. Psychotic or delusional symptoms
4. Lack of family support for observation or care
5. Significant physical illness complicating antidepressant treatment
6. Uncertain diagnosis or complicating psychiatric diagnosis such as alcoholism
7. Bipolar disease
8. Lack of response to antidepressants (combined with severe neurovegetative symptoms, suggesting need for electroconvulsive treatment)

exercise similar to that used for cardiac rehabilitation is appropriate.

Indications for Referral

Several events or situations suggest the need for referral of depressed patients by family physicians to psychiatrists or more comprehensive mental health centers. Table 52–8 lists possible indications, none of which is necessarily absolute but all of which bear careful consideration by the family physician who does not have extensive training in caring for complicated depressed patients. The following indications should receive particular consideration: significant suicidal ideation or expressed intent; severe cognitive dysfunction, including self-care and nutritional deficiencies; severe bipolar disorder; and patients' failing multiple courses of antidepressants with documented compliance. Some of these circumstances require hospitalization (e.g., for electroconvulsive therapy), which usually requires referral to a psychiatrist.

DEPRESSION IN CHILDREN AND THE ELDERLY

Management of Depression in Children

The care of depressed children deserves special attention because of the increasing incidence of depression in children and adolescents, the apparently increasing incidence of suicide in adolescents, the devastating effects on families with depressed children, and the superior expertise required of physicians who care for these children. Depression is less common in prepubertal children than in adolescents or adults, but major depression in children can have serious developmental consequences. It is not a condition that children simply outgrow. Children meeting criteria for major depression are likely to suffer recurrences, and depression impedes the educational

progress and is linked to poor social competence and problems with peers and siblings.

When diagnosing depression, the family physician is in a crucial position to deal with the most common confounding situation: distinguishing depression from similar psychological characteristics that occur during the normal development of childhood. The family physician may understand the child's family environment to the extent that any change in behavior is more noticeable, family reaction to the depressed child is more visible, and features suggestive of depression are more detectable than when the case is evaluated by a consultant who has had limited contact with the patient and his or her family.

The incidence of depression, using standard *DSM-III-R* criteria, varies with age, from 1 to 4 per cent in children under 6 years of age to as high as 13 per cent in adolescents and preadolescents. Depression is almost impossible to diagnose in children under age 5 years because of the limited language and cognitive abilities of these patients. In older children, manifestations of low self-esteem, social isolation, sadness, anxiety, school problems, ill-formed suicidal ideation, and failure to make expected weight gains may signal depression. Adolescents show the same manifestations of depression as adults. However, these symptoms may not be apparent at first, and depressed adolescents may come to the attention of the family physician because of parents' complaints of their loss of interest in their appearance, sulkiness, withdrawal from family activities, and retreat to their rooms. Questionnaires and self-report inventories can be used in children older than 6 years who have age-appropriate verbal abilities. Children of this age group are thought to be reliable informants. If their report of mood and symptoms differs from that given by the parents, studies show that the children are ultimately more accurate. This fact strongly suggests that a child-centered approach to children with behaviors and mood suggestive of depression is appropriate despite the mood suggestive of depression is appropriate despite the possible protestations of parents. The use of antidepressants is sufficiently complex, particularly in prepubertal children, that referral is recommended. About 75 per cent of children with major depression respond to antidepressants, and improvement is usually seen first in school behavior and performance. A strong family-centered approach to counseling is best, and the family physician should play a strong role in coordinating and reinforcing such an approach. A comprehensive approach includes a detailed plan for altering the child's family and school environment, individual psychotherapy, psychopharmacologic interventions, attention to family members with associated depression or substance abuse problems, and a commitment to a long-term follow-up plan.

Management of Depression in the Elderly

Depression is a common psychiatric disorder in the elderly, with estimates of prevalence ranging from 5 to 50 per cent. A likely prevalence of dysphoric mood is 15 to 20 per cent and for major depression 3 to 5 per cent. The suicide rate increases with age, despite the declining incidence of depression with age. The presentation of the depressed elderly differs from that of other depressed adults by having a higher rate of somatization without mood alteration and by the common problem of depression presenting as dementia, the so-called pseudodementia syndrome. Patients with pseudodementia present with cognitive dysfunction, problems of self-care, and difficulties in concentration and memory. A relentless search for mood disturbance or neurovegetative symptoms is necessary to make the correct diagnosis of depression. The high rate of chronic and terminal illness in the elderly also causes a high rate of secondary depression. Depression associated with polypharmacy is a particular problem, with alcohol, sedatives, antihypertensives, and digitalis being the most common causes.

Treatment follows the recommendations for young adult patients, with a few important modifications. Pharmacokinetics differ considerably in the elderly owing to decreased gastrointestinal absorption, altered plasma protein binding, and decreased renal and hepatic clearance; and blood levels are often 50 per cent higher in the elderly for the same dosage given to younger patients. On the other hand, the elderly may be more sensitive to certain side effects of antidepressants, particularly orthostatic hypotension. Moreover, the elderly already may be taking other classes of medications, which may cause drug interactions. Cardiac effects and organic brain syndrome from the anticholinergic effects are particular concerns when managing elderly patients. For all of these reasons, an antidepressant with minimal anticholinergic and orthostatic side effects, such as desipramine, nortriptyline, trazodone, or the SSRIs, is frequently used in elderly patients. Severe depression may require electroconvulsive therapy, which is not contraindicated because of age. As in all depressed patients, psychotherapy should include attention to family and living environment and associated illness in family members.

REFERENCES

Altrocchi J, Antonuccio DO, Miller GD: Nondrug prescriptions for the depressed adult outpatient. Postgrad Med J 79:164, 1986.

APA Task Force on Laboratory Tests in Psychiatry: The dexamethasone suppression test: An overview of its current status in psychiatry. Am J Psychiatry 144:1253, 1987.

Blackburn IM, Bishop S, Glen AL, et al: The efficacy of cognitive therapy in depression: A treatment trial using cognitive therapy and pharmacotherapy, each alone and in combination. Br J Psychiatry 139:181, 1984.

Block M, Schulberg HC, Coulehan JC, et al: Diagnosing depression among new patients in ambulatory training settings. J Am Board Fam Pract 1:91, 1988.

Brown GW, Harris TL: Social Origins of Depression. New York, Free Press, 1978.

Burgin D: Depression in children and adolescents. Psychopathology 19(suppl 2):148, 1986.

Burns D: Feeling Good: The New Mood Therapy, 2nd edition. New York, William Morrow, 1992.

Clayton PJ: The prevalence and course of the affective disorders. *In* Davis JM, Maas JW (eds): The Affective Disorders. Washington, DC, American Psychiatric Press, 1983.

Clayton PD, Barrett JE (eds): Treatment of Depression: Old Controversies and New Approaches. New York, Raven Press, 1983.

Cohen-Cole SA, and Stoudemire A: Major depression and physical illness: Special considerations in diagnosis and biologic treatment. Psychiatr Clin North Am 10:1, 1987.

Coyne JC: Depression, biology, marriage and marital therapy. J Marital Fam Ther 13:393, 1987.

Coyne JC, Downey G: Social factors in psychopathology. Annu Rev Psychol 42:401, 1991.

Coyne JC, Schwenk TL: A follow-up study of depressed primary care and psychiatric patients. Presented at the Seventh Annual NIMH International Research Conference on Primary Care Mental Health Research, Washington, DC, 1993.

Depression Guidelines Panel: Depression in Primary Care.

Vols 1. Treatment of Major Depression. Vol 2. Clinical Practice Guideline. AHCPR Publication no. 93-0550 and 93-0551. Rockville, MD, US DHHS, PHS, AHCPR, 1993.

Diagnostic and Statistical Manual of Mental Disorders, 3rd edition (revised). Washington, DC, American Psychiatric Association, 1983.

Diagnostic and Statistical Manual, 4th edition. Washington, DC, American Psychiatric Association, 1994.

Downey G, Coyne JC: Children of depressed parents: An integrative review. Psychol Bull 108:50, 1990.

Duer S, Schwenk TL, Coyne JC: Medical and psychosocial correlates of depressive symptoms in family practice. J Fam Pract 27:609, 1988.

Ellis A, Harper RA: A New Guide to Rational Living. Englewood Cliffs, NJ, Prentice-Hall, 1975.

Finlayson RE, Martin LM: Recognition and management of depression in the elderly. Mayo Clin Proc 57:115, 1982.

Frank E, Kupfer DJ, Peral JM, et al: Three year outcomes for maintenance therapies in depression. Arch Gen Psychiatry 47:1093, 1990.

Freeling P, Rao BM, Paykel ES, et al: Unrecognized depression in general practice. BMJ 290:1880, 1985.

Froom J, Schlager DS, Steneker S, et al: Detection of major depressive disorder in primary care patients. JABFP 6:5, 1993.

Goldberg D, Huxley P: Mental Illness in the Community: The Pathways to Psychiatric Care. London, Tavistock Publications, 1980.

Goldberg ID: A scaled version of the General Health Questionnaire. Psychol Med 9:139, 1979.

Greden JF: Recurrent Depression: A Lifetime Disorder. New York, Dista Products, Division of Eli Lilly, 1992.

Hyman SE, Jenike MA: Approach to the patient with depression. *In* Goroll AH, May LA, Mulley AG (eds): Primary Care Medicine. Philadelphia, JB Lippincott, 1987.

Jencks SF: Recognition of mental distress and diagnosis of mental disorder in primary care. JAMA 253:1903, 1985.

Kamerow DB, Campbell TL: Is screening for mental health problems worthwhile in family practice? An affirmative view and an opposing view. J Fam Pract 25:181, 1987.

Katon W: The epidemiology of depression medical care. Int J Psychiatr Med 17:93, 1987.

Katon W, Schulberg H: Epidemiology of depression in primary care. Gen Hosp Psychiatry 14:237, 1992.

Katon W, Kleinman A, Rosen G: Depression and somatization: A review. Am J Med 72:127 (part 1), 72:241 (part 2), 1982.

Katon W, Von Korff M, Lin E, et al: Distressed high utilizers of medical care: DSM-III-R diagnoses and treatment needs. Gen Hosp Psychiatry 12:355, 1990.

Lewinsohn PM, Munoz RF, Youngren MA, et al: Control Your Depression. Englewood Cliffs, NJ, Prentice-Hall, 1979.

Michels R, Marzuk PM: Progress in psychiatry. II. N Engl J Med 329:628, 1993.

National Institute of Mental Health: Mental health services in primary care settings: Report of a conference 1983, April 2-3, 1979. Publication (ADM) 83-995, Series DN, no. 2. Rockville, MD, DHHS, 1983.

Nicoloff G, Schwenk TL: Exercise and depression. Physician Sports Med, in press.

Paykel ES, Hollyman JA, Frelling P, et al: Predictors of therapeutic benefit from amitriptyline in mild depression: A general practice placebo-controlled trial. J Affect Disord 14:93, 1988.

Petty F: Depression and medical/surgical illness: "Who wouldn't be depressed?" Prim Care 14:669, 1987.

Popolos D, Popolos J: Overcoming Depression. New York, Harper Collins, 1987.

Prestidge R, Lake R: Prevalence and recognition of depression among primary care outpatients. J Fam Pract 25:67, 1987.

Radloff LS: The CES-D scale: A self-report depression scale for research in the general population. Appl Psychol Meas 1:385, 1977.

Regier DA, Hirschfeld RMA, Goodwin FK, et al: NIMH Depression Awareness, Recognition, and Treatment Program: structure, aims, and scientific basis. Am J Psychiatry 145:1351, 1988.

Regier DA, Narrow WE, Rao DS, et al: The de facto US mental and addictive disorders service system. Arch Gen Psychiatry 50:85, 1993.

Richelson E: Pharmacology of antidepressants. Psychopathology 20(Suppl 1):1, 1987.

Rodin G, Voshart K: Depression in the medically ill: An overview. Am J Psychiatry, 143:696, 1986.

Rucker L, Dietch JT: Depression in primary care: Evolving concepts and approach to therapy. South Med J 79:215, 1986.

Schulberg H, McClelland M, Burns BJ: Depression and physical illness: The prevalence, causation, and diagnosis of comorbidity. Clin Psychol Rev 7:145, 1987.

Sireling LI, Paykel ES, Freeling P, et al: Depression in general practice: Case thresholds and diagnosis. Br J Psychiatry 147:113, 1985.

Spitzer RL, Endicott J, Robbins E: Research diagnostic criteria: Rationale and reliability. Arch Gen Psychiatry 35:773, 1978.

Von Korff M, Shapiro S, Burke JD, et al: Anxiety and depression in a primary care clinic. Arch Gen Psychiatry 44:152, 1987.

Weissman MM: Psychiatric epidemiology: Rates and risks for major depression. Am J Public Health 77:445, 1987.

Weissman MM, Leaf PL, Bruce ML, et al: The epidemiology of dysthymia in five communities: Rates, risks, comorbidity, and treatment. Am J Psychiatry 145:815, 1987.

Wells KB, Stewart A, Hays RD, et al: The functioning and well-being of depressed patients: Results from the Medical Outcomes Study. JAMA 262:914, 1989.

Yates WR (ed): Depression. Prim Care 14:657, 1987.

Zung WWK: A self-rating depression scale. Arch Gen Psychiatry 12:263, 1965.

CHAPTER 53

CRISIS INTERVENTION IN OFFICE PRACTICE

ROBERT E. FEINSTEIN and LAUREL CAREY

Routinely family physicians are faced with requests from their patients to solve a wide range of biopsychosocial problems. Many family doctors do not consider themselves competent to work with their patients to formulate the problem in a way that practical solutions can be developed within the time limitations of a general office medical practice. Crisis intervention provides a theory and treatment model that can be readily applied to helping patients with their biopsychosocial problems.

DEVELOPMENT OF CRISIS THEORY

During World War I Thomas Salmon (1917), a British military physician, was asked to evaluate severe "shell shock," which was producing a psychological paralysis in Allied soldiers. He discovered that the French suffered fewer psychological casualties from the horrors of war than did the British soldiers. The factors that seemed to account for the French advantage was that French soldiers were told that they could expect to recover from their psychological trauma. They received immediate psychological treatment for these traumas close to the front and were returned to battle as quickly as possible. These principles became the cornerstones of modern crisis treatment. Patients entering crisis treatment can expect that they will be treated immediately, recover from the crisis, are generally treated while living in their natural environment, and are returned to normal life as soon as possible.

Eric Lindemann (1944) applied and expanded Salmon's theories. He studied the acute grief reactions of many individuals who lost family members in the Coconut Grove fire, a disaster in Boston that claimed approximately 500 lives. Lindemann discovered that normal people, surviving such a horrific experience, develop an emotional crisis of pain, confusion, anxiety, and temporary difficulty in daily functioning. He found that these reactions are natural human states that last for about 6 weeks. He also noted that the psychological trauma caused by the crisis had little relation to pre-existing psychiatric illness. Instead, the outcome of the crisis was more closely related to the severity of the stressor, the personal reaction to the trauma, and the effect the trauma had on the person's support network of family and friends. Lindemann found that most survivors recovered spontaneously, and a smaller group seemed to decline to a low level of functioning.

Eric Erickson (1959) a sociologist, introduced the idea of a life cycle comprised of developmental stages and developmental crisis. He described eight periods throughout the life-span that involved age-specific psychological issues. For example, he described adolescence as a period where a normal individual seeks an adult identity with social roles that eventually permit autonomy, away from parents. Those who cannot successfully traverse this crisis period do not progress from their child-like dependence on parental figures. He described normal developmental crises throughout the life cycle that must be worked through and resolved if a person is to be able to progress successfully into the next life phase. His basic concept of "developmental crises" has been expanded to include crises such as leaving home for the first time, mid-life crisis, or parents experiencing the "empty nest syndrome." For many patients a crisis is experienced at transitional points between life phases, such as the crises of marriage, divorce, retirement, and death.

Gerald Caplan (1961, 1964) synthesized many of these earlier ideas into modern-day crisis theory and treatment. He defined the crisis state as a brief personal psychological upheaval precipitated by a stressor, or "hazard," that produces emotional turmoil such that persons are temporarily unable to cope, adapt, or function in their daily activities. He demonstrated that a crisis implies both potential for danger and an opportunity for growth. He subscribed to Lindemann's theories that how a crisis evolves depends on the severity of the trauma or precipitant, the personalized meaning of the event, and the effects of events on the support network of family and friends. He added that a crisis might also be based on failure of a person's individual coping style and ability to adapt. Unlike Linde-

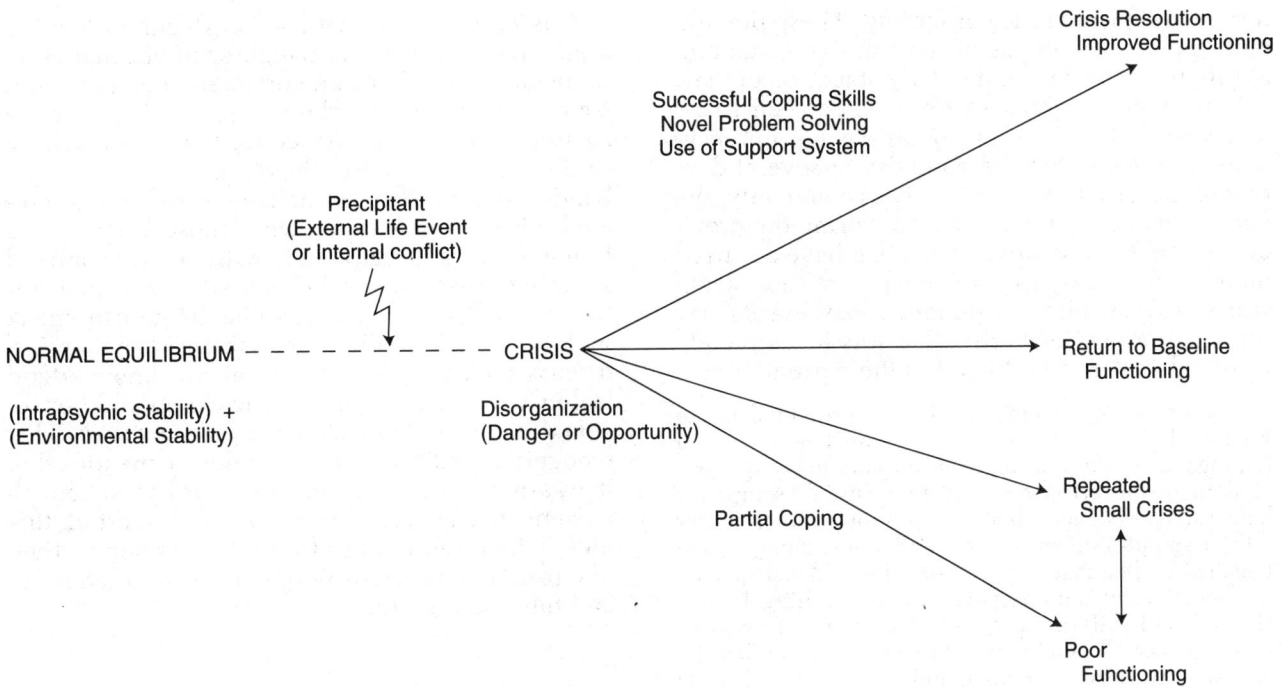

FIGURE 53–1. Crisis intervention theory.

mann, he thought that the pre-existing personality may also affect the development, evolution, and resolution of the crisis. Caplan confirmed that most crises resolve in about 6 weeks with four possible outcomes: (1) improved functioning; (2) functioning restored to precrisis levels; (3) incompletely restored functioning with a susceptibility to the development of future crises; or (4) a severely impaired, but stable, level of lower functioning. He confirmed Lindemann's findings that some individuals coped with a crisis by spontaneously and flexibly developing novel coping or problem-solving styles. He developed a crisis treatment that focused on developing better coping mechanisms and adaptations to life's traumas. An overview of a modern crisis theory is represented in Figure 53–1.

EVALUATING THE CRISIS

When a crisis develops, it may be evaluated and treated by understanding the interplay of the elements or the dynamics that contributed to its formation. These elements are the normal equilibrium state, the precipitant or stressor, the personalized interpretation or meaning of the events to the individual, the crisis state, the selective history, the system of social supports, and the preexisting personality or psychiatric condition.

Normal Equilibrium State and Stressors

Under normal circumstances, an individual has a sense of internal psychological equilibrium and

environmental support that generally permits daily activities of living, working, and having pleasure. Psychological equilibrium is determined by a delicate balance between the individual's internal wishes and fear, skills and capacities, and values and ideals. Environmental equilibrium refers to a stable balance between the basic need for food, shelter, physical comfort, and the social supports of job, family, religion, and society. A patient typically enters the emotional storm of a crisis after a stressor or acute precipitant disturbs the normal equilibrium. Stressors can be external life events, psychological events such as a disturbing dream or sudden anger, or developmental problems such as adolescence or a midlife crisis. Reality stressors frequently seen in a physician's office may include loss of health due to disease or the stress of coping with a death, divorce, marital separation, job loss, or financial loss. Holmes and Rahe (1967) developed a Social Readjustment Scale that lists 43 external life stressors that precipitate stress in most people. The events range in severity from death of a spouse (number 1) to divorce (number 2) through change to a different line of work (number 18) to change in social activities (number 36) to Christmas (number 42). Some common psychological stressors include loss of self-esteem, loss of love, sexual dysfunction, or sudden overwhelming emotions such as fear or rage. Common developmental stressors include latency, puberty, adolescence, marriage, birth of the first child, midlife crisis, chronic medical illness, or retirement.

Generally, most precipitants causing a crisis have components from a real life event and an internally disturbing idea or feeling. These precipitants produce emotional turmoil and a transient inability to adapt during the early stages of a crisis.

Most patients who seek treatment are surprised to discover that there has been a major unrecognized stressor either the same day or several days before the onset of the crisis. Less commonly, the stressor had occurred some time during the previous 6 weeks. Generally, events that have occurred more than 6 weeks previously are not acute stressors. Instead, these important past events may represent a previous crisis that was incompletely resolved and may be linked to the current crisis.

Susan is a 40-year-old woman who presented to the Family Medicine Center with worsening headaches and feelings of "shakiness" all over. Exploration of the precipitant of the crisis revealed that Susan's symptoms began 3 weeks ago, when her only daughter Jennifer left for an out-of-town college. With questioning, Susan began to realize that since her daughter's departure she has been tearful and upset over the tiniest thing. In fact, she recalled suffering the "worst migraine of my life" two nights ago, when her daughter informed her that she was so happy, loving school, and meeting new friends that she was not coming home for Thanksgiving.

Interpreting the Meaning of the Stressor

Whether precipitated by an external life event or an internal psychological thought or feeling, each individual interprets or adds meaning to the precipitant. For some people, as with Susan, an external life event may seem minor to others, but because of a the special meaning of the stressor to that individual it may produce a crisis.

Susan's perceived loss of her only child was a stressful precipitant that triggered a crisis. This initial precipitant gains significance because of the particular meaning she ascribed to this normal developmental crisis of leaving home. Susan became pregnant with Jennifer, her only child, before Thanksgiving of her first year in college. This event had "forced" Susan to marry Jennifer's father, drop out of school, and abandon her dream to be a teacher. Although she willingly had devoted her life to Jennifer, Susan became panic-stricken and developed "shakiness" and migraines out of a fear that her daughter was about to make this same mistake. Her daughter's departure for college was a painful reminder of Susan's lost career and triggered feelings of jealousy and anger toward Jennifer. "I began shaking with anger when Jennifer told me she wasn't coming home for Thanksgiving." This crisis was inadvertently heightened by her husband, who had recently been talking with her about her developing some outside interests. Susan felt angry and betrayed by her husband who had originally asked her to stay home.

This sequence of events—her daughter leaving home, her fear that the daughter might make the same mistake and become pregnant, her anger and jealousy over the daughter's opportunity to have a career, the missed chance for her own teaching career, and her unresolved anger at her husband—formed the personalized meaning that created this crisis for Susan. Once these events were formulated as precipitants with a personalized meaning, Susan could be helped to see that her life was not over. She was encouraged to speak with her daughter about the risk of pregnancy and discuss contraception. Susan also acknowledged jealousy of Jennifer's promising career and her residual blame and anger toward her husband. This recognition led to Susan's considering the idea that it was not too late for her to return to school to become a teacher. Her husband supported this idea, which helped her to see him as supportive. She resolved her crisis with improved functioning and the potential for a new career.

Crisis State

The crisis state has been defined as a brief psychological upheaval precipitated by a stressor. It produces an intense state of inner turmoil or disorganization that overwhelms a person's ability to cope and adapt. Patients who seek help while in a crisis have impaired normal functioning and may be in obvious psychological distress and pain. Typically, the pain of a crisis is so intense it is denied, unconsciously perceived as overwhelming distress, and may lead to an inability to cope. As with Susan, a crisis can be heralded by somatic complaints, or it may be expressed by crying, by becoming hysterical or mute, or by appearing confused, bewildered, severely anxious, depressed, suicidal, violent, or even occasionally psychotic. Typically, patients cannot explain why they are in crisis. A family physician can assist in such cases by becoming the detective of the "Why now?" aspect of the crisis. Answering this question initiates the crisis treatment and begins to facilitate resolution.

For example, a son who brought his dead father to the emergency room after a car accident appeared completely normal, with no apparent emotional awareness of the tragedy. The family physician asked the son to describe the specific events of the father's death—the "Why now?" This exercise produced brief hysteria in the son, moving him into an emotional crisis state and enabling him to cry and begin grieving.

Frequently, people in crisis do not seek help by themselves and, instead, are brought in by concerned family members, lovers, friends, or perhaps the police, ambulance, or other municipal personnel. In these cases, the crisis can be so intense that it may take hours until the specific causes and problems of the crisis can be identified.

Successful resolution of a crisis can be growth-promoting and can lead to improved functioning. For most patients, however, crisis resolution means a return to their normal baseline functioning. Other patients may "seal over" or deny any meaning of their behavior. For example, a patient who swallows pills and then denies any suicidal feelings has sealed over the crisis. Denial of the crisis and its causes can lead to partial crisis resolution and continuing poor adaptations. These patients then have a latent weakness, called a missed or unresolved crisis. Unresolved crises predispose a patient to future crises caused by even less stressful precipitants. In addition, these patients' stable functioning subsequently remains at a lower level. This group of patients may still have a future opportunity to be helped if the next crisis opens up the "sealed over" or unresolved crises, which can then be resolved more adaptively.

Selective History

From a crisis point of view, the patient's history is relevant only insofar as it can be utilized to help explain and resolve the current crisis. This telescoping and inquiring about how the patient's history relates to the current crisis may be difficult to untangle and understand. Many patients, wishing to avoid the pain of the current crisis, lead the physician "down the garden path" to chronic complicated problems that cannot be helped at a single office visit. To avoid this situation, the physician must first try to understand the dynamics of the current crisis and then look for similar events in the patient's past that are the same or have a configuration similar to that of the current situation. For example, a selective history that relates to a current suicide attempt might include the timing, circumstance, and effects of past suicide attempts or hospitalizations, or the past precipitants of such suicidal behavior. This selective history can then be utilized as a clue to making the current suicide attempt intelligible. Additional history, helpful for understanding a current suicide attempt, might be concerned with prior deaths, separations, severe medical illnesses, depression, alcoholism, or family suicides. Selective history that might be relevant for a violent crisis could include the timing and circumstances of past episodes of violence, childhood experiences of abuse or neglect, prior hospitalizations for violence, prior incarcerations, other legal problems, and the neurologic or medical history.

SOCIAL SYSTEMS

Every individual lives within a network of social interaction and social support. Most of our daily social interactions are with spouses, family, friends, lovers, work colleagues, neighbors, landlords, and so on. Each individual lives in a social network or society that enables one to obtain housing, food, clothing, work, school, finances, or medical care. In general, a stable, interested, helpful, available, social support system tends to prevent crises. Sometimes a dysfunctional support system produces or contributes to the crisis. When a patient is in a crisis, a family physician can help the patient choose and then mobilize the most helpful people in the support network. Such actions may include calling in a specific family member, speaking to a difficult boss, helping the patient obtain an attorney, or helping a patient access cost-effective medical care, economic assistance, food, clothing, or shelter.

Relative damage to a support network can have profoundly different effects. For example, an earthquake results in catastrophic destruction of the fabric of a society, which produces a sustained and prolonged crisis from which many never recover. The death of a spouse produces a more severe crisis if the deceased was also the sole financial provider. Even, a minor disturbance in a small or dysfunctional support network can produce a major crisis. For example, an elderly woman who is house-bound, without family, friends, or telephone, experienced a major crisis when her home health aide missed her appointed visit. To assess the support network, a family physician must consider if the network members are capable of helping, are interested, and are available.

PREVIOUS PERSONALITY OR PSYCHIATRIC DISORDER

For most people there is no correlation between a previous personality or psychiatric disorder and one's capacity to deal with a crisis. A schizophrenic may be just as able to handle an acute crisis as others who do not have psychiatric problems. How well an individual handles an acute crisis depends primarily on the variables previously discussed: the precipitant, the meaning of the events, the crisis situation itself, the patient's coping skills and styles, and the effect of the event on the patient's support system.

There are some cases where a preexisting psychiatric disorder may cause or influence the development of a crisis. Consider the case of a mentally retarded boy who became severely violent after his breakfast "farina" was not available to him. This situation would be a minor stressor for most people, but for him disruption of his daily routine and loss of his favorite food was perceived as catastrophic. His low intelligence and lack of verbal skills specifically related to his psychiatric condition predisposed him to the development of a crisis of violence.

Those with severe personality disorders and who have rigid coping styles are at risk for developing a crisis. They have less adaptive capacity to develop novel coping styles to aid in the resolution of a crisis.

CRISIS INTERVENTION TREATMENT IN THE OFFICE SETTING

Basic Approach

The focus of crisis intervention is evaluation of the precipitants of the crisis, the personal meaning of the events, the crisis state itself, the selective history, the support network, and the current psychiatric illness, if relevant. This information is used to formulate the causes of the crisis so specific problem-solving interventions may be used for crisis resolution.

A crisis treatment, consisting of a therapeutic contract for three to five sessions, can be offered to any patient with a biopsychosocial crisis. The time required for each session depends on the complexity of the case and the physician's skill. A family physician may begin the crisis therapy by exploring the "Why now?" (acute precipitant) of the crisis. If the crisis involves suicide, violence, or a life-threatening medical illness, these factors take priority over everything else and become the focus of the crisis treatment. The next priority level involves the immediate crises of a lack of food, clothing, shelter, or adequate medical care. Finally, the physician must examine the crises of everyday living.

The crisis treatment should focus on the dynamic interplay of recent events over the last few days to 6 weeks that have contributed to producing the crisis. Important aids that can guide identification of the crisis components and treatment of these specific elements are the time line, support network map, and wheel-and-spoke formulation of the crisis. Assessment and development of more adaptive coping styles follow. These elements lead to a general crisis resolution strategy.

Time Line

A time line is a pictorial representation of recent and past events that have led up to the crisis. A family physician can build a time line of events with the patient by discussing the immediate crisis and working backward over the last 6 weeks, looking for precipitants, contributing events, and the selective history that relates to the current crisis. Use of the time line is illustrated in the following case.

Mr. Jones, a 35-year-old obese man living with his mother, presented to his family physician with depression and anxiety. He had been anxious for the last month since his company announced the possibility of layoffs. He had become increasingly sleepless over the last week when thinking a job loss would create severe financial strain. He believed his job loss would also result in his having to postpone his marriage and would make it impossible for him to leave his mother's home. This patient had made a serious suicide attempt (by overdose) 1 year ago after a job loss and an argument with his mother where she humiliated him as an "inadequate provider." After his suicide attempt, he was briefly hospitalized and then placed on an antidepressant for 3 months. He did not seem to recover fully until he got his current job 6 months ago. Five months ago he became engaged and made plans to be married 8 months later.

A time line representing this case is shown in Figure 53–2. Developing such a time line with a patient helps focus on recent events and begins the process of formulating what can be done to help.

Support Network Map

A support network map may be organized around the genogram and immediate environmental supports. It may include one's immediate family, the family of origin for three generations, and all the people who are in the patient's immediate living environment, such as neighbors, landlord, and physician. In addition, it is helpful to include close friends and the religious or social agencies that are (or could be) involved for the benefit of the patient. With this map of the patient's support network, a family physician can help decide who needs to be more involved in the patient's care, who should be excluded, and what social, religious, legal, or economic agencies can be mobilized to assist the patient in crisis. To choose the most helpful participants, look for individuals and agencies that are interested, available, and capable

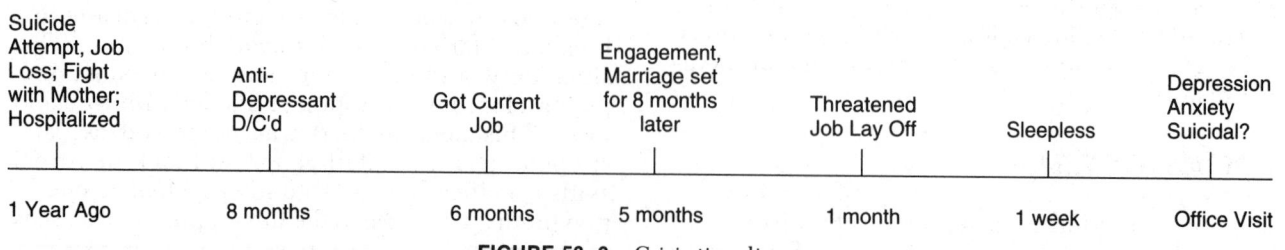

FIGURE 53–2. Crisis time line.

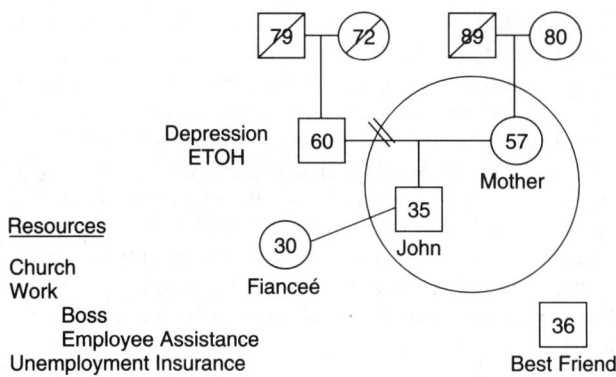

FIGURE 53–3. Support network map.

of assisting. Such a support network map is shown in Figure 53–3 with the case example from above.

John's support system reveals the potential resources that may be mobilized to help him in the resolution of the crisis. His fiancee, mother, grandmother, best friend, and boss could be called on to assist John or help develop a plan for crisis resolution. His church, the employee assistance program at work, and unemployment insurance are potential additional resources that could be utilized. The decisions about which support system elements to use should be negotiated in collaboration with the patient. John and his physician decided that his fiancee and the employee's assistance program would be the best choices for additional help. John also agreed to inquire about

obtaining unemployment insurance should he be laid off.

Wheel-and-Spoke Formulation of the Crisis

It is important to develop a formulation that specifies the multiple causes of the crisis. The wheel-and-spoke format helps the clinician and patient identify and formulate the crisis, as well as focus on setting the priorities for problem resolution. It can also be used to suggest any specific acute treatment required. A pictorial way to represent a case is to think of the acute crisis at the center of a metaphorical wheel. The spokes of the wheel are the problems that are thought to be causing, contributing, or feeding into the crisis. The physician can establish the priorities regarding the problems that are to be solved and in what order. This list of priorities can be indicated by numbers. For each problem listed, the family physician can recommend a specific assessment or evaluation, tests, or treatment approach that would be most helpful to the patient. Application of the wheel-and-spoke diagram for the case of John is shown in Figure 53–4.

COPING SKILLS, NOVEL PROBLEM-SOLVING, AND ADAPTATION

Fortunately, most individuals find ways to handle or cope with a crisis within 6 weeks. Crisis

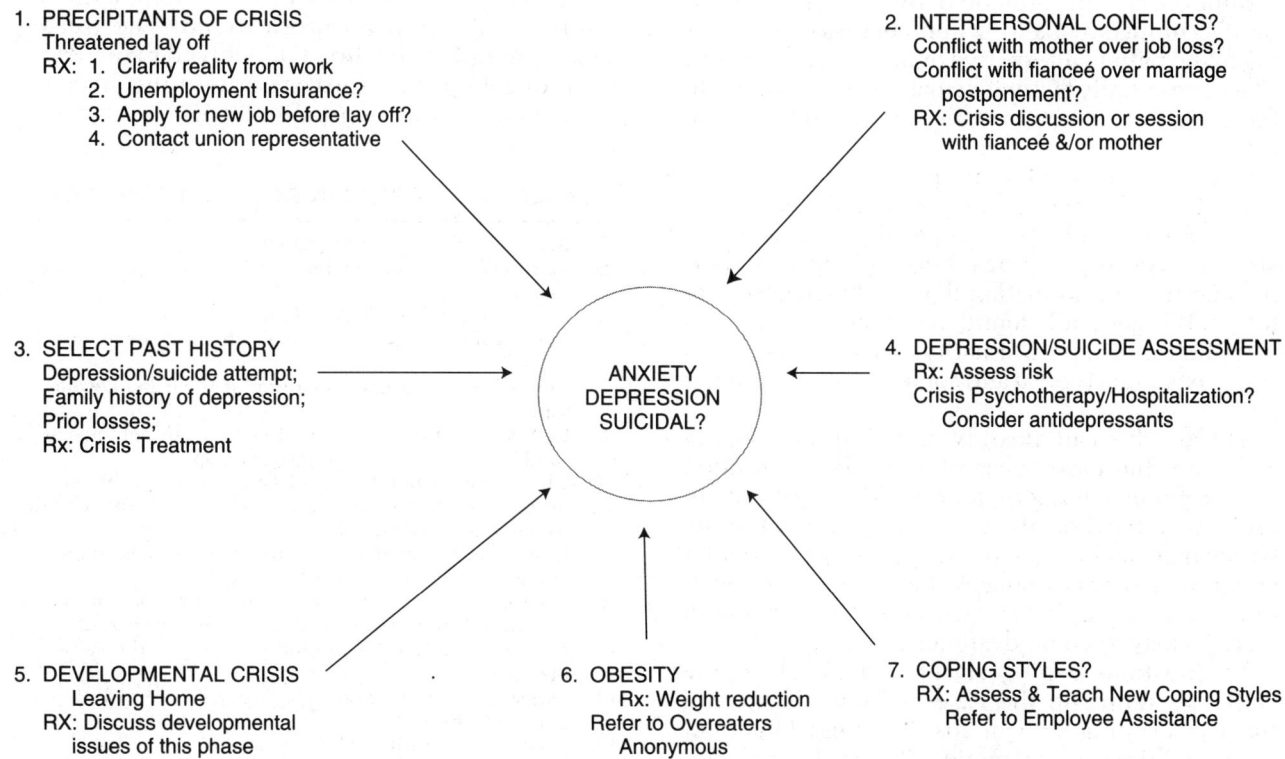

FIGURE 53–4. Wheel-and-spoke crisis formulation and treatment plan.

TABLE 53–1. COPING STYLES

Adaptive Coping Styles

Intuitive: using imagination, feelings, and perceptions to solve a problem

Logical/rational: carefully reasoned, logical, deductive style

Trial and error: trying a random solution and if it fails modifying it and trying again

Help-seeking: asking others for help

Informational: gathering information then deciding

Wait and see: allowing time or circumstance to determine the outcome

Action-oriented: taking an action to immediately rectify the problem

Contemplative: quietly thinking over the problem before action

Spiritual: asking for God's direction

Emotional: using emotion such as tears, anger, or fear to help solve the problem

Controlling: controlling people or oneself to gain the power to solve the problem

Manipulative: using a variety of manipulative styles to solve the crisis

Pathologic Coping Styles

Deceptive/antisocial: using dishonesty, lying, cheating, or stealing to solve a crisis

Suicidal: using the threat of suicide or suicide attempts to coerce someone or to solve a problem

Violent: using the threat of or actual violence to establish control and solve problems

Impulsive: unpredictable or impulsive responses without anticipation of possible outcomes

Random/chaotic: unproductive and extreme form of trial and error often seen in those with prolonged psychotic states

resolution can be promoted by evaluating a patient's coping style and, when necessary, suggesting to the patient alternative or novel coping styles. These new skills facilitate a patient's adaptation to the stressful life circumstances that produced the crisis.

Coping styles are the unique way patients deal with stress. Everyone has a repertoire of coping styles. For example, some cope with a stressful crisis by analyzing it, asking others for help, or gathering additional information that might suggest a solution. It is generally found that some coping styles work better in certain situations than others. Table 53–1 lists some typical and some pathologic coping styles.

Those who can flexibly use multiple coping styles are the most successful at crisis resolution and problem-solving in general. Many patients in crisis rely too heavily on a single coping style, which may not be the most adaptive for a particular situation. Patients who lack the capacity for developing a novel coping style, when confronted with a crisis, may become dysfunctional.

To illustrate coping styles and novel coping skills we return to the case of John. John has a history of coping with job loss by suicidal manipulation. In his current situation, it is a major concern that he not revert to this pathologic style of prob-

lem-solving. By discussing again his prior maladaptive style and by suggesting he could use a help-seeking and informational coping style, John came to believe he had new options. Using a help-seeking style, he asked his fiancee for her help. She was interested, willing, and able to pursue finding a job to help relieve the possible financial crisis. John used an informational style of coping to find out that he was eligible for unemployment insurance. This new information partially relieved the crisis. Furthermore, he began looking for new job opportunities.

CRISIS RESOLUTION STRATEGY

In addition to coping styles and coping skills, a family physician may teach a general strategy of crisis resolution. This crisis resolution strategy (Feinstein, 1992) is based on the crisis principles previously outlined and is summarized in Table 53–2. The family physician must walk through the steps with the patient several times, handling several crises, before encouraging the patient to attempt these steps as a self-help strategy. This approach has 14 steps.

1. Teach the patient to recognize early warning signs of crisis. Such signs are anxiety, occasional panic, regular feelings of being overwhelmed, a persistent sense of urgency, confusion, disorganization, and suicidal or homicidal feelings, thoughts, or actions.

2. Talk over the crisis or problem with the family physician or a trusted friend. The trusted person should not be directly involved in the crisis. For prevention of the next crisis, a family physician can develop with each patient a list of available

TABLE 53–2. CRISIS RESOLUTION STRATEGY

1. Recognize the early warning signs of a crisis.
2. Talk over the problem with a crisis practitioner or trusted friend.
3. Discuss painful feelings and emotions.
4. Identify the specific area of one's life most affected by the crisis.
5. Identify the stressors over the past 6 weeks. Develop a time line.
6. Decide who from the support system can help and who can hurt. Draw a support network map.
7. Obtain information that can help in crisis resolution.
8. Formulate the crisis and develop a problem list. Use the wheel and spoke technique.
9. Learn about the patient's coping style and suggest the use of a new or additional one that might help.
10. Make a specific plan based on new information, newly discovered feelings, and choose an effective coping style.
11. Implement a plan for resolution of one of the causes of the crisis.
12. Assess the results. If positive then go to step 13; if negative, go to step 14.
13. Tackle another cause of the crisis and so on.
14. Try again, get help, consult with a psychiatrist.

friends and practitioners, with their phone numbers, who may be reached as needed.

3. Crisis resolution begins by discussing the most painful feelings and emotions. One can suggest to a patient that discussing the areas of greatest pain has the potential for giving them the most relief.

4. Identify the specific area of the patient's life that is most affected by the crisis. Is the primary crisis located at work or at home; or is it an interpersonal, economic, or other crisis in one's life?

5. Identify the acute specific precipitants and other stressors that have emerged over the past 6 weeks that are currently contributing to the crisis. They can be identified by developing a time line with the patient. It is most likely that the acute precipitant occurred on the day of the office visit or within the last week. For example, one patient recognized from his time line that he had a crisis each time his wife left him to go on a business trip. He discovered the following repetitive pattern to his crises: Separation from his wife led to his feeling lonely, scared, abandoned. He dealt with these feelings by drinking and driving recklessly and by getting into frequent brawls at the local bars. His time line led the physician to suggest to this patient that during a separation he should call his wife regularly, not drink, and instead make arrangements to spend time with a trusted friend.

6. Teach patients to evaluate their own support system by drawing a support network map. Using this map, patients can be assisted in discovering who can help, who they are not calling on, and who makes things worse.

7. Obtain additional information that may help in crisis formulation and resolution.

8. The most difficult part of the crisis treatment, for both the physician and the patient, is developing the crisis formulation and problems list, setting the priorities of the treatment, and developing treatment options for each problem. Use of the wheel-and-spoke format can be helpful in this regard. With this approach the crisis is at the center of the metaphorical wheel, and the spokes represent the variety of factors that are causing or contributing to the symptoms. Treatment may be suggested for each problem identified.

9. Learn about the patient's current coping style and why it may not be working. Encourage the patient to use other coping styles he or she may have forgotten to use, or help the patient develop a new coping style.

10. Based on the new information, newly discovered feelings, and the crisis formulation, choose an effective coping style. The physician and patient should make a specific plan with a specific sequence of actions that will help the patient cope and resolve the crisis.

11. The patient should implement the plan. Initially, it may be less overwhelming if he or she tries to resolve one cause of the crisis at a time and is faithful to the plan.

12. Assess the results. Is the problem resolved?

13. If the answer to item 12 is yes, then tackle the next problem, and so on.

14. If the answer to item 12 is no, then try again. Go back to step 8 and try to reformulate the crisis or obtain additional psychiatric or other professional help.

REFERENCES

Caplan G: An Approach to Community Mental Health. Orlando, FL, Grune & Stratton, 1961.
Caplan G: Principles of Preventative Psychiatry. New York, Basic Books, 1964.
Erikson EH: Identify and the Life Cycle. New York. International Universities Press, 1959.
Feinstein RE: Emotional crises. *In* The Columbia University College of Physicians and Surgeons Complete Home Guide to Mental Health. New York, Henry Holt, 1992, pp 364–373

Holmes TH, Rahe RH: Social readjustment scale. J Psychosom Res 2:213, 1967.
Jacobson JF: Crisis-oriented therapy: symposium on brief psychotherapy. Psychiatr Clin North Am 2:1, 1979.
Lindeman E: Symptomatology and management of acute grief. Am J Psychiatry 101:141, 1944.
Salmon T: War neurosis (shell shock). Milit Surg 41:674, 1917.

CHAPTER 54
PERSONALITY DISORDERS IN OFFICE PRACTICE

ROBERT E. FEINSTEIN and SUSAN VANDERBERG

" 'Hateful' patient's are those whom most physicians dread" (Groves, 1978). They are objectively difficult and can elicit hate in many doctors. They are not patients "with whom a physician may have an occasional personality clash" (Groves, 1978). These difficult patients may mobilize intense feelings in a physician that may ultimately determine the quality of care the patient receives. "Hateful" patients often make physicians feel inadequate or impotent, elicit anger that is not adequately understood, or are sexually stimulating or arousing. They often develop an intense, aggressive, dependent clinging that can be exhausting for the physician. Unconscious physician anger toward such a patient ultimately results in a breakdown of patient–physician trust. The patient feels frustrated, unheard, not consulted, or angry with the physician; and the physician often feels misunderstood, devalued, or dissatisfied with his or her work. A dysfunctional patient–physician relationship contributes significantly to the deterioration of the medical experience and to poor quality medical care.

There are many causes of the dysfunctional patient–physician relationship. A leading cause not frequently discussed is the patient (or physician) with a personality disorder. Personality disorders often go unrecognized because those so afflicted may not verbalize or manifest the more typical psychiatric symptoms or complaints, despite the fact they may suffer from significant personal distress. Commonly, personality disorders can be secondarily recognized and experienced through the complaints of family, friends, or others who have had extended contact with the patient. It is easy to recognize the "personality disorder" when the individual suffers severe impairment in social, interpersonal, or occupational functioning. Patients and physicians have felt many disturbing emotions toward each other that are caused by the dysfunctional interaction of the patient with a personality disorder.

DEFINITION: PERSONALITY STYLE VERSUS PERSONALITY DISORDER

A *personality style* is the lifelong habitual way one thinks, feels, and behaves. This definition implies that each individual has a unique, enduring, slowly evolving organization of their perceptions, a typical style of thinking and fantasy, a hierarchy of emotional needs, a value system, and ideals. Personality style also implies a characteristic way in which one relates to oneself and manages internal conflicts, a typical way in which one relates to others, and a usual way of interacting and adapting to external reality.

The distinction between personality style and a personality disorder is a matter of degree. Personality styles that become rigid, extreme, maladaptively damaging to oneself or others or that lead to social or occupational impairment are called *personality disorders*. Although each person is unique, there seems to be a continuum of personality styles and disorders that are commonly encountered. We can recognize some personality disorders in characters from the movies: the hysteric in Scarlet O'Hara from "Gone with the Wind," the obsessive-compulsive in Felix Unger from "The Odd Couple," or the borderline portrayed by Glenn Close in the movie "Fatal Attraction."

CLASSIFICATION

Personality disorders are generally classified using a categorical or a dimensional approach. The *categorical system* describes individuals as having clusters of associated traits, symptoms, or behaviors that form discrete, separate personality disorders called prototypes. *DSM-III-R* (Spitzer and Williams, 1987) and DSM-IV (Frances et al., 1994) use a prototypic personality disorder classification and outlines diagnoses such as obsessive-compulsive and histrionic personality disorder. Categorical approaches have the advantage of colorfully describing personality styles and among physicians have been the most popular approach to classification.

Authors such as Cloninger (1987) and Siever and Davis (1991) have begun a trend toward a dimensional classification of personality disorders. The *dimensional system* describes personality traits as having measured variations along common dimensions. For example, Siever and Davis (1991) suggested a set of four personality dimensions: cognitive/perceptual, anxiety/inhibition, impulsivity/aggression, and affective stability. With the dimensional approach, a patient is classified along each dimension with gradations from high to low. This system accounts for a spectrum of personality traits that are observed in many patients who do not fit into the discrete prototypes.

Whereas the dimensional approach has promising biologic, research, and treatment links, the categorical approach follows the medical diagnostic thinking of physicians that organizes diseases into categories of illness. For this reason, this chapter focuses on categorical approaches.

To be classified as a prototypic personality disorder an individual must have a minimum number of traits. The primary care categorical approaches to personality disorders are exemplified by the descriptions of Groves (1978), Kahana and Bibring (1969), and *DSM-IV*. Groves described four categories of "hateful patients": dependent clingers, entitled demanders, manipulative help rejecters, and self-destructive deniers. Kahana and Bibring delineated seven categories of personality types and attitudes: (1) dependent, over-demanding; (2) orderly, controlled; (3) dramatizing, emotionally involved, captivating; (4) long-suffering, self-sacrificing; (5) guarded, querulous; (6) those with feelings of superiority; (7) patients who seem uninvolved and aloof.

TABLE 54–1. ABRIDGED SUMMARY OF DSM-IV

Cluster A (Odd or eccentric)
Paranoid: expects exploitation/harm; questions loyalty/fidelity; bears grudges; easily slighted
Schizoid: loner; aloof; indifferent to praise or criticism; social anxiety; constricted affect
Schizotypal: odd/eccentric; social anxiety; magical thinking; suspicious/paranoid ideation

Cluster B (Dramatic, emotional or erratic)
Antisocial: cruelty; problems with authority; unlawful behavior; dishonesty; irresponsibility; exploits others
Histrionic: overly emotional; seductive/sexual attention seeking; shallow/superficial
Borderline: unstable intense relationships; self-destructive/suicidal; impulsive; affect instability; identity disturbances
Narcissistic: grandiose; inflated self-importance entitled; exploits others; lacks empathy; needs admiration; hypersensitive to criticism
Self-defeating (DSM-III-R Appendix A): suffers; self-sacrificing; defeats others; self-destructive; cannot enjoy; easily hurt

Cluster C (Anxious or fearful)
Dependent: indecisive; lacks initiative; submissive; helpless; dependent; fears abandonment
Passive-aggressive: procrastinates; scorns authority; resents suggestions; superficially compliant; obstructs
Obsessive-compulsive: perfectionism; inflexibility; detail preoccupation; wishes to control others; stingy; overly conscientious; excessive morality or ethics
Avoidant: easily hurt; timid/fearful; social discomfort; avoids interpersonal interactions.

The *DSM-IV* is psychiatry's contributions to the categorical classification of personality disorders. This multiaxial system encourages physicians to consider personality variables for every patient. *DSM-IV* divides the personality disorders into three clusters. An abridged, compressed listing of these disorders appears in Table 54–1.

PHYSICIAN REACTIONS

Physicians working with patients who suffer from personality disorders seem to have specific, characteristic reactions to these patients that must be recognized, understood, and utilized for the patient's benefit. Typical subjective experiences and reactions to a patient should alert the doctor to the possible diagnosis of a personality disorder. These experiences and reactions include intense feelings, uncharacteristic fantasies, or atypical behaviors by the physician.

Intense Feelings

Intense feelings may comprise hate, fury, or frustration toward a patient. Feelings of love, sexual arousal, the desire to rescue the patient or give "exceptionally" good care may alternate with a wish to avoid the patient, terminate the relationship, or transfer the patient to the care of a colleague.

Physician Fantasies

Physicians may recognize they are interacting with a difficult patient by their own fantasies. Such fantasies might include excessive worrying about a patient after normal work hours, dreaming about a patient, or experiencing exaggerated or intrusive, angry, sexual, or curious fantasies about the patient during personal time.

Physicians' Atypical Medical Behaviors

A physician may also notice medical behaviors with a specific patient that are atypical to his or her customary medical practice. These unusual physician behaviors should trigger self-examination by the physician and evaluation of the possibility that the patient may have a personality disorder. Frequently, patients with a personality disorder are capable of arousing unconscious reactions that lead to new noncustomary physician behaviors.

Common atypical medical behaviors aroused in the physician may include the following: ordering of tests to placate a patient; asking for more than the usual number of consults on a patient whose case does not seem medically complicated; suggesting increasingly aggressive diagnostic testing or procedures when the yield of these tests is likely to be low; repeatedly extending the time spent with a particular patient or family; offering free samples of drugs; and lowering the customary fee or offering free treatment. A list of common physician reactions associated with specific personality disordered patients are summarized at the end of this chapter in Table 54–4. Recognition by the physician of his or her own unconscious and unanalyzed feelings, fantasies, and behaviors may aid in the diagnosis of the patient's personality disorder. More importantly, physicians who can recognize their own unusual reactions are better able to tolerate them, avert acting out their feelings with a patient, and thereby improve their medical decision-making.

PATIENTS' PSYCHOLOGICAL FEARS

Most patients are afraid when consulting a physician. The patient with a personality disorder may have fears that are exaggerated in their intensity and idiosyncratic in their quality. These fears, rooted in the patient's basic personality organization, are readily activated during a routine visit to the physician or when they feel sick and vulnerable. The capacity to delineate and empathize with the patient's fear and distorted world allows one to tailor the medical interaction to alleviating the patient's fears. This "tailoring" can dramatically improve interactions with the patient and thus improve the quality of medical care. For example, a patient with a paranoid personality is highly mistrustful and expects to be deceived or harmed by a dangerous world. When ill, he may become increasingly angry, suspicious, and mistrustful. Empathizing with the patient's paranoid world view may help the physician to realize that the patient requires an openness and honesty in all communications. The patient may also be helped by a comprehensive explanation of the physician's future medical intentions.

Patients with a borderline personality disorder fear separation, loss, or abandonment. When ill, they may cling to the physician and react to a separation (such as the physician's vacation) with anger, manipulative attempts, devaluing attacks, or panic. By understanding the patient's fears, it is possible to prevent worsening of his or her condition while the physician is away. This can be done by empathizing and discussing the patient's fears of separation or loss. The patient can be reassured of the physician's realistic medical availability and limits. In an effort to prevent a crisis from separation, prior to the physician's departure a patient can be scheduled for a meeting with the colleague who will be providing coverage. It may also be helpful to explore with this patient what he or she can do to cope while the physician is away (refer to Table 54–4).

PSYCHOPATHOLOGIC LEVEL OF PERSONALITY FUNCTIONING

A particularly useful model for describing level of personality organization was introduced by Kernberg (1975, 1984) and simplified by Goldstein, (1988). Kernberg assessed the psychopathologic level of personality organization as functioning on neurotic, borderline, and psychotic levels. These levels of functioning are determined by assessing reality testing, defenses, and identity diffusion (Table 54–2).

Neurotic Personality Organization

Patients with a neurotic personality organization have the capacity to differentiate what is real from what is not. When their reality testing is intact, patients can (1) differentiate their own thoughts from external sensory perceptions; (2) distinguish themselves from others; and (3) realistically evaluate how their own emotions, behaviors, and thoughts are perceived in relation to ordinary social norms. Neurotic patients typically use high level defense mechanisms centered on repression, including reaction formation, displacement, suppression, and inhibition, among others. They have stable, slowly evolving views of themselves and of others as having a mixture of both good and bad qualities.

Borderline Personality Organization

Patients with a borderline personality organization generally have intact reality testing that is, they can differentiate reality from fantasy, ideas from perceptions, and so on. However, the stress of an illness, extreme emotions, or drugs may pre-

TABLE 54–2. PERSONALITY ORGANIZATIONS*

Neurotic Personality Organization
Reality testing intact
Defenses: higher level; repression
Stable view of self and physician

Borderline Personality Organization
Reality testing generally preserved; loss of reality testing with stress
Defenses: splitting
Identity diffusion: changing views of self and physician

Psychotic Personality Organization
Reality testing lost
Defenses: primitive defenses and/or severe splitting
Identity diffusion prominent: chaotic or changing views of self and physician

* Adapted from Goldstein (1988) and Kernberg (1975, 1984, 1992).

cipitate transient breaks in reality that last seconds, minutes, or even hours. Breaks in reality often present as severe distortions of what the physician has said to them, transient misperceptions of reality events, feelings of unreality, depersonalization, and in the extreme case temporary hallucinations or changing delusions. Patients with borderline personality organization use defenses that are centered on splitting (all good or all bad thinking and feeling). Associated defenses include idealization, devaluation, and particular forms of projection. These patients suffer from an unstable identity (*identity diffusion*) that manifests as radically alternating and exaggerated views of self. For example, a patient may see himself as a kind, caring, giving person who is close to perfection. This perception oscillates within a brief time with a view of himself as a selfish, demanding, or hateful person. Patients who manifest identity diffusion see themselves and others in extremes of good and bad. There is memory for these alternating states, but the apparent contradictions seem to have no emotional relevance to the patient (i.e., splitting).

Psychotic Personality Organization

Patients with psychotic personality organization have a gross loss of reality testing that permits them to be differentiated from patients with borderline personality organization. They may have inappropriate or bizarre affect, behavior, and thought content; or they may suffer from hallucinations and delusions. They are frequently unable to empathize or clarify how others see them (Kernberg, 1984). They typically use primitive defenses (e.g., projection, incorporation, denial of reality) and have confused, blurred, or generally chaotic views of themselves and others. For example, they may see themselves as God at one time and the devil the next, or they may believe that they have both male and female sexual organs.

Variability in Personality Organizations

Personality organization levels are generally stable for each patient, although stress may cause the patient to vary within a limited range of personality organizations for each specific *DSM-IV* personality category. For example, patients with paranoid, schizotypal, or schizoid personality disorders generally function at a psychotic personality organization but, at their best, can function on a borderline level. Alternatively, patients with antisocial, histrionic, borderline, or narcissistic personality disorders typically function at a borderline level. With stress (such as the threat of abandonment) they may briefly lose reality testing and function on a psychotic level. Patients within cluster C (dependent, avoidant, passive-aggressive, obsessive-compul-

sive) typically can function at the neurotic or borderline level; it is only rarely, with extreme stress, do they function at a psychotic level (refer to Table 54–4).

PATIENT DEFENSES

Defenses are unconscious psychological processes used by the patient to help resolve internal conflicts, manage anxiety, or alleviate depression. They also help mediate external dangers and facilitate adaptations to reality. Different personality disorders use specific constellations of defenses. By understanding the constellation of defenses used with each personality disorder and when possible the specific defense mechanisms used, the physician may be able to modify the pathologic functioning of the defenses interfering with good patient–physician interaction. Patients functioning at the neurotic level use high level defenses centered on repression. Patients functioning at the borderline level use splitting defenses, and patients functioning on the psychotic level may use primitive defenses and severe forms of splitting (Kernberg, 1975, 1984).

High Level (Neurotic) Defenses

High level (neurotic) defenses are centered on repression. To repress is to exclude from awareness (or consciousness) any threatening impulses, feelings, memories, ideas, or experiences. A patient who uses repression fails to see, hear, or attend to threatening impulses, wishes, desires, or fears. Some high level defenses associated with repression are repression, displacement, and reaction formation (Table 54–3).

Splitting Defenses

The splitting defenses and related mechanisms observed with borderline personality functioning cause these patients to see themselves and others as "all good" or "all bad." In other words, there is no emotional experience of self and others as consisting of a realistic mixture of good and bad qualities. Hence they see the world as black or white, good or bad, and ideas as totally right or totally wrong. They alternate between these two feeling states at different times (Table 54–3).

Primitive Defenses and Severe Splitting

Primitive defenses can encompass projection, projective identification, denial, somatization, severe forms of splitting, and other defenses. These defenses help patients organize their psychotic

TABLE 54–3. DEFENSE MECHANISMS

Neurotic Personality Defenses: High Level (Repression Center)

Repression: involuntary forgetting of a painful memory, feeling, or experience

Controlling: manipulation or control of events or people to avoid unconscious anxiety or inner conflicts

Displacement: transferring one's feeling from one person to another

Reaction formation: unacceptable impulses expressed as attitudes and behaviors that are the direct opposite of those impulses

Intellectualization: unconscious replacing of feelings with facts or details

Suppression: conscious choice to put a disturbing experience out of one's mind

Ambivalence: coexistence of opposite feelings

Distortion: reorganization of external reality to fit internal needs and wishes

Phobia: attaching fear to an object or situation that is not objectively a source of danger

Inhibition: restricting thoughts, feelings, or behaviors for fear that unacceptable impulses will erupt and create anxiety or other damage

Rationalization: creating socially acceptable explanations for thoughts, emotions, or behaviors

Isolation: unconscious process by which thoughts and memories are stored without emotion

Sexualization: transformation of functions or objects into sexual symbols to avoid unconscious anxieties

Passive aggressive: superficial compliance and passivity disguising stubbornness and anger

Defenses of Borderline Personality Organization (Splitting Centered)

Splitting: dividing the view of self and others into "all good or all bad," (views that are often highly fantastic and distorted); defenses based on the use of splitting mechanisms:

Idealization: seeing self or others as powerful, ideal, or God-like

Omnipotence: seeing self or others as all-powerful

Devaluation: depreciating or exaggerating the badness of self or others

Projection: unconscious rejection of unacceptable impulses that are attributed (projected) onto others

Projective identification: projection of a part of oneself onto the other person, who one then fears and attempts to control (control of the other person psychically controlling the impulse in oneself)

Denial: refusal to acknowledge painful realities

Regression: unconsciously reverting to childlike thoughts, feelings, or behaviors

Hypochondriasis: irrational fears of having a physical illness (with a decreased threshold for pain and increased awareness of internal physiologic sensory perceptions) so as to avoid other unconsciously painful experiences

Defenses of a Psychotic Level of Functioning: Low Level (Primitive Defenses + Severe Splitting)

Splitting defenses: as listed above but becoming more extreme

Acting out: expressing in action or behaviors things that cannot be expressed in words or emotions

Incorporation: process of psychically taking something into oneself

Somatization: physical or medical symptoms caused by mental processes without known physical disease

Schizoid fantasy: retreat to idiosyncratic fantasy when faced with painful experiences

processes into a mode that allows them some adaptive functioning. Challenging these primitive defenses in the form of confronting the patient's reality distortions with other reality views of the same problem may reveal the underlying psychotic processes they help defend against. These defenses are defined in Table 54–3.

PSYCHOTHERAPEUTIC MANAGEMENT AND INTERVENTIONS

After several office visits with a patient, the physician may have a general idea of the patient's personality diagnosis, an understanding of the physician's likely reactions to that patient, a sense of the patient's typical fears, the level of personality functioning, the patient's main defenses, and some anticipation of problematic interactions that may arise during the process of delivering medical care (Table 54–4). With this information, the physician may be able to help the patient develop an alliance that allows good medical care. A physician cannot change the patient's personality disorder but may be able to help the patient function at a more adaptive level.

A review of the clinical management of a patient with a personality disorder involves establishing an alliance with empathy for the patient's fears, developing a therapeutic contract, agreeing on a focal problem to resolve, and promoting more adaptive functioning by using the psychotherapeutic techniques of confrontation, clarification, and interpretations.

Establish an Alliance

To establish a good patient–physician alliance, a physician should begin every patient encounter with a friendly, open, available attitude that conveys a willingness to listen and help. When beginning the interview, the patient is allowed to express any negative feelings about the physician or the medical care so far provided. The physician should listen to the patient's complaints without reacting defensively. The physician sometimes feels hurt, but it is important to realize that patients' complaints are often subjective feelings and do not necessarily represent any wrongdoing by the physician or a need for change. Listening with understanding to the patient's primary fears and with empathy for the patient's world view and then using commonly understood, simplified medical language can facilitate a good patient–physician interaction and working alliance.

Therapeutic Contract

During a regular office visit, the physician should alert the patient with a personality disorder

TABLE 54–4. PERSONALITY DISORDERS SCHEMA

DSM-IV	Common Physician Reactions	Patients Fear and Psychological Reaction	Neurotic Borderline Psychotic	Patient Defenses	Interventions
Cluster A Paranoid	Fearful, sense of danger, mistrust; feels accused or blamed	Fears being hurt, exploited, invaded; reacts with mistrust and anger; homosexual panic with invasive procedures	PPO or BPO	Primitive defenses Projection Projective-Identif. Denial Splitting defenses	Empathize with patient's fear of being hurt and acknowledge complaints without arguing or ignoring. Openly and honestly explain medical illness, nature of tests, etc. Correct reality distortions and do not confront delusions. If refuses care out of mistrust, ask if it is all right if you can disagree about the need for the test; do not insist. Interpret defenses, use counterprojection.
Schizoid	Detached or removed; "loner"; wish to involve patient with others or to break through the isolation	Fears intrusion or violation of privacy; then withdraws more from personal contact	BPO or PPO	Primitive defenses Denial Regression Splitting defenses	Empathize with patient's need for both privacy and contact. Accept the patient's unsociability. Neutrally impart medical information Do not demand involvement and do not permit total withdrawal. Reality test. Interpret specific defenses.
Schizotypal	Detached, removed; "Weird and alone" feelings; wish to involve or to break through the isolation	Fears intrusion or violation of privacy; may withdraw from personal contact	PPO or BPO	Primitive defenses Schizoid fantasy Regression Denial Splitting defenses	As above.
Cluster B Antisocial	Used/exploited; deceived causing anger and wishes to uncover lies; punish or imprison	Fears exploitation or sudden vulnerability; may lie, manipulate, cheat, exploit, steal, seek secondary gain	BPO with stress PPO	Acting out Somatization for secondary gain Splitting defenses	Empathize with the patient's fear of exploitation and low self-esteem. Are you being used for a secondary gain? If you suspect dishonesty, verify symptoms and illness progression with others. Do not moralize. Explain that deceiving results in your giving the patient poor care. Test reality. Interpret defenses.
Histrionic	Flattered or captivated, seduced, or sexually aroused; flooded by emotions; embarrassed; depleted	Loss of the care taker; loss of desirability, attractiveness or sexuality; seduces, flatters, or angrily devalues	BPO or NPO with stress PPO	Splitting defenses Sexualization Acting out Dissoc./Regress. Somatization, Repress. defenses	Empathize with patient's fear of losing love or care. Interact in a friendly way: not too reserved or too warm. Discuss patient's fears; reassure when possible. Limit-set if patient regresses. Correct reality distortions. Interpret specific defenses.

Table continued on following page

TABLE 54–4.   PERSONALITY DISORDERS SCHEMA (Continued)

DSM-IV	Common Physician Reactions	Patients Fear and Psychological Reaction	Neurotic Borderline Psychotic	Patient Defenses	Interventions
Borderline	Feel manipulated; fearful of anger; angry; impotent; depleted; self-doubting; wishes to rescue or get rid of the patient; guilty	Fears separations, loss, abandonment; may panic, be angry, impulsive, lose reality, reject help, devalue, manipulate, make suicidal gestures	BPO with stress PPO	Splitting defenses Projection Projective-identif. Idealize/devalue Omnipotence Acting-out Mini-psychotic	Empathize with patient's fear of abandonment and separation. Plan for absences. Express wish to help and satisfy reasonable needs. Set firm limits and do not punish. Reality test. Interpret splitting and other defenses. If suicidal, the patient must go to the emergency room. If the patient refuses, inform the patient of your wish to keep him alive, but that after the patient is safe, you will terminate the relationship.
Narcissistic	Devalued, inferior; fearful of patient criticism or anger; wish to retaliate with anger; devalue, or get rid of the patient	Fears loss of self-esteem or potency; acts entitled or viciously devalues, counterattacks, or idealizes physician	BPO or NPO with stress PPO	Splitting defenses Idealize/devalue Omnipotence Projection Projective-identif. Acting out Denial Regression	Empathize with the patient vulnerability and low self-esteem. Do not mistake patient's superior attitude for real confidence and do not confront entitlement. When you are devalued or attacked, acknowledge the patient's hurt, your mistakes, and express your continued wish to help. If devaluing continues, offer a referral as an option, not as punishment. Correct reality distortions. Interpret splitting and other defenses.
Self-defeating (DSM-III-R Appendix A)	Wish to rescue; sadistic fantasies that the patient will suffer or die; defeated, self-blaming, self-doubt, or hopeless	Loss of love, care; fears recovery; when improves may intensify complaint, depression, dependence; guilty, judgmental, harsh, self-destructive	BPO or NPO; rarely PPO	Splitting defenses Denial Projection Projective-identif. Idealize/devalue Repression React-formation	Empathize with patient's suffering and acknowledge and appreciate the difficulty of the illness or treatments. Emphasize that recovery may be a slow, steady process. The need for recovery can be presented as necessary to benefit others. Inquire about obviously self-destructive or self-defeating behaviors. Do not abandon. Interpret specific defenses.

PPO = psychotic personality organization; BPO = borderline personality organization; NPO = neurotic personality organization.

that a problem exists that is interfering with the patient's medical care. The physician may first ask for the patient's view of the present medical care. If the patient expresses the problem the physician can then begin discussing it. If time prohibits a discussion, a follow-up office visit can be scheduled. If the patient cannot identify the problem or the physician believes there is a different problem, the latter may say, "I believe that there is a [different] problem in my ability to help you to get the best medical care possible. I need to think about why this has happened, and I would like you to think about it also. I would like to see you next time for a longer office visit, when we can discuss your case in detail and find a better way to help you." With the patient's agreement, a time and future setting for a longer session can be established. Prior to the next visit, a focus can be chosen for that meeting.

Choosing a Focus for the Interview

Patients with severe personality disorders often experience common problems in terms of cooperating with their medical care. There may be a problem in the doctor–patient relationship or in the patient's understanding or acceptance of the medical diagnosis or treatment, which may include requests by the patient for help with a psychological, interpersonal, familial, or social problem. The physician must identify the focus of the session at the beginning of the interview. Resolving problems in the patient–physician relationship may need to take priority over other problem areas. When possible, it is best to focus on one problem area before working on others.

Psychotherapeutic Techniques

After a brief period of immersion in the patient's complaints, the physician should respond with empathic and reassuring responses addressed to the patient's fears. Initially, it may take the form of an educational or informational response to the patient. If this response is insufficient, as it usually is for personality disordered patients, it may be necessary to respond with an empathic confrontation, clarification, or an interpretation about the current problematic situation.

A *confrontation* is not a battle. It is an observation by the physician that is offered to a patient for his or her examination. It is usually a comment that draws attention to discrepancies or contradictions in the patient's perceptions or behaviors that are interfering with medical care. The physician may use confrontations in a nonjudgmental way and listen carefully for the patient's expanding self-awareness. Example: "I know that you want your medical condition to improve, yet your refusal to permit further diagnostic testing makes medical improvement unlikely."

A *clarification* is the doctor's request of the patient to add new information or perspective or to clarify misunderstandings, miscommunications, or information that seems vague or confusing. The need for repeated clarifications occur regularly with patients who have severe personality disorders. It is important to use clarifications before suggesting a new plan to correct the problem.

Interpretations are integrating comments that link confrontations and clarifications with a patient's current problem regarding the goal of complete medical care. Interpretations in the medical setting should generally be made about the immediate situation. They may address the patient's defenses, a difficulty in the doctor–patient interaction, or the external reality of the disease process, medical work-up, medical treatment, or the patient's life circumstances. For example, an interpretation offered to a borderline patient with chronic pain might be "I think you want relief from your pain. Yet your refusal to follow my recommendations makes relief from your pain unlikely [confrontation]. You then get angry with me because your pain is not relieved, and so you do not keep your scheduled appointments [clarification]. You do not use my help but then blame me and feel frustrated. Your anger with me helps you avoid the frustration you feel with your husband, who has become less than sympathetic toward your pain [interpretation]." Such interpretations take practice but can powerfully restore a realistic, helpful doctor–patient relationship.

GENERAL INTERVENTION

By establishing that a patient's personality organization is functioning at the neurotic, borderline, or psychotic level, it may be possible to intervene at that level to improve the patient's ability to function. Management strategies for patients functioning at the neurotic level involve correction of subtle distortions in reality perceptions and the use of psychotherapeutic interventions to deal with the specific high level defense mechanisms that are interfering with the patient's efforts to obtain optimal medical care.

Patients functioning at the borderline level frequently suffer from short-lived disturbances in reality testing. These disturbances may manifest as transient simple hallucinations, dramatic distortions of what has been said, transient misperceptions of reality events, misunderstanding of the physician's or patient's role, feelings of unreality, or depersonalization. Such reality distortions are not severe and can be helped by the use of confrontation, clarification, and interpretation.

The general strategy for managing splitting defenses involves intervening with the use of confrontations, clarifications, and interpretations: specifically, making patients aware that half of their emotional feelings have been split off or dissociated. This exercise involves reminding the patient who is currently loving and idealizing that last week he considered his physician much less competent and not helpful. Alternatively, the patient who hates the physician and tells him that he is all bad can be reminded of other good experiences he has had with the physician in the recent past. Other, more specialized techniques of dealing with the related splitting defenses are mentioned under specific personality disorders (see below).

Patients functioning at the psychotic level require primary interventions geared toward improving reality testing. Such intervention is necessary to preserve basic trust in the doctor–patient relationship. Explaining the current medical condition and correcting the patient's distortions of medical realities can be extremely useful. A patient suffering from hallucinations, delusions, or inappropriate or bizarre affect or behavior may require the use of medications, intervention with family members, or hospitalization. Occassionaly confrontations, clarifications, and interpretations may also be used to improve the patient's psychological functioning.

SPECIFIC INTERVENTIONS

A schema useful when working with personality disordered patients includes choosing the correct *DSM-IV* diagnosis, recognizing common physician reactions to each kind of personality disorder, understanding the patient's specific fears and reactions to those fears, and assessing the patient's level of personality functioning and main defenses. This conceptual framework may make it possible to formulate some helpful interventions for the specific personality disorder.

Paranoid Personality Disorder

When interacting with a paranoid patient, the physician commonly reacts with fear, and mistrust and has a sense of danger. The physician may also feel blamed or accused. Such patients may have a similar fear of being hurt, exploited, or invaded. They often react to suggestions for medical care with mistrust, excessive fault-finding, sensitivity to criticism, and hypervigilence; and they collect small insults that are used as proof of the world's injustices. When invasive procedures are performed, a male patient may react with full-blown panic and anxiety. This reaction may occur because many paranoid male patients unconsciously perceive invasive procedures as a homosexual assault.

Paranoid patients typically function at the level of a psychotic personality organization, as evidenced by severe, unwarranted suspiciousness of others. They rely most heavily on projection as their main defense. Using projection, they accuse the physician of a hurt that reflects their own aggressive style of hurting others.

A physician must empathize with the patient's mistrust and hypersensitivity and should avoid arguing or attempting to reason patients away from their paranoid world view. It is important to use confrontations and clarifications to help correct patients' distorted perceptions about their medical care. However, direct confrontation of a delusion or hallucination (their most troubling deficits in reality testing) often has the paradoxical effect of

making these patients more suspicious of the physician. Acknowledging that the patient's suspicion has an emotional reality can be helpful. Rather than confront mistrust or suspicions directly, it is helpful to acknowledge responsibility for any actions the patient might have perceived as mistakes. For example, "I did not appreciate how it might hurt you when I ordered that lab test." It may also help to openly express your understanding and concern for the patient's rights. If there is a medical need for special testing of which the patient is suspicious, acknowledge his or her fears; describe openly and honestly the details of the procedures, the potential for pain, and the likely risks and benefits. If the patient still refuses to comply, do not use direct persuasion. Ask the patient: "Is it alright with you if we have different opinions?" With the patient's consent to hearing a different opinion, openly discuss the medical need for the testing without trying to resolve the problem (Kernberg, 1984). At future office visits, attempt new and ongoing discussions of the patient's fears of complying with your request for specialized testing. It may take months for the paranoid patient to trust the physician enough to consent to the appropriate treatment.

Counterprojective statements by the physician can diffuse the projections and distortions directed at the physician. The doctor can use counterprojective remarks to help the paranoid patient access his or her feelings while focusing angry or suspicious feeling away from the physician toward others who are not present. For example, a physician harassed by an angry, suspicious, or blaming patient could use a counterprojective statement such as: "You felt angry and hurt when the lab technician drew your blood. You must have been hurt and perhaps you are also fearful of the results of these tests."

Schizoid and Schizotypal Personality

Physicians commonly feel uninvolved or detached, or they have a desire to break through the aloofness of both schizoid and schizotypal patients. Schizoid patients may give the physician the impression of the patient as a "loner." A common physician reaction to schizotypal patients is a feeling that the patient is both alone and "weird or strange." Patients with either diagnosis superficially fear personal contact and emotional involvement; and they fear that their privacy will be invaded. At the deepest levels, they long for emotional contact that is not overwhelming. In either situation they may react to suggestions for medical care with avoidance, withdrawal, apparent emotional detachment, or denial of the medical problem.

Schizotypal patients function at a psychotic level with impaired reality testing manifested by magical, odd, or psychotic modes of thinking. Schizotypal patients use regression to schizoid fantasy and to a lesser extent denial as their main defenses. They appear increasingly idiosyncratic and withdrawn when stressed.

Schizoid patients do not appear psychotic but, rather, more detached and alone. They often can function at a borderline level of personality organization. When stressed by a medical problem, schizoid patients use psychotic denial of their illness and withdrawal as their main defense.

Efforts to reach these patient are often perceived as intrusions into their privacy and actually may drive them away from their physician. They are relieved when the physician is not present and prefer fewer medical appointments and contacts. It may be helpful to accept their unsociability at a level that does not demand involvement or permit total withdrawal. Medical information that is presented in a neutral or unemotional manner is most likely to be heard and utilized.

Antisocial Personality Disorders

Common physician reactions to a patient with antisocial personality disorder are feelings of being used, exploited, or deceived. It leads to physician anger and a wish to be free of the patient, to uncover lies, and to punish or imprison the patient.

When ill, these patients fear they will become vulnerable, lose respect or admiration from others, and become easy prey to manipulation. They expect to be exploited, demeaned, or humiliated. Like the narcissistic patient, they often have low self-esteem, excessive self-love, compensatory feelings of superiority, grandiosity, recklessness, emotional shallowness, and a lack of concern for others. They often react to medical care with entitled demands for special treatment. When caught in dishonesty they may angrily attack or devalue the physician. They may resort to other psychopathic manipulations, such as deception, lying, cheating, or stealing.

They typically function at the borderline level of personality organization, and their reality testing appears intact. In fact, their friendly, facile, slick, superficial charm and intelligent appearance is often beguiling for the physician. When stressed by the potential of getting caught in their deceptive practices, they may lose reality testing, manifested by impulsive actions that can reveal severely impaired or even psychotic judgments. When they are receiving medical care for a bone fide illness, they typically function at the same level as those with a narcissistic personality disorder (Kernberg, 1992) and often can be managed similarly (see Narcissistic Personality Disorders, below).

To intervene with an antisocial patient, a physician must be alert and anticipate the possibility that the patient may be requesting unnecessary medical care. They may be seeking the secondary gain of illegal benefits or money or seeking to avoid work or legal problems. It is important not to inadvertently collude with the patient's plans for secondary gain. For example, if the physician thinks a patient's request for disability is fraudulent or unwarranted, the patient should not be referred for additional evaluations. If deception is suspected, the physician can ask for verification of symptoms from other reliable sources. Often there is dishonesty in a patient's communication in the form of partial truths or outright lying, cheating, or stealing. If it occurs, the physician must avoid the common reaction of moralizing. Instead, the patient is granted the reality that if he chooses to he can fool all his physicians. The patient can be told that the results of deception or giving false or inaccurate information is that the physician may make poorly informed medical decisions, which can ultimately result in the patient receiving inadequate or poor medical care. The physician can wonder with the patient why the patient needs to act self-destructively. Patients' may need to be reminded that the physician's role is to help the patient with medical problems and not to pass judgment.

Histrionic Personality Disorder

Patients with histrionic personality disorder have an emotionally expressive style, seek excessive attention, and are often dramatic. Physicians may feel flattered, captivated, seduced, or sexually aroused by these patients. Alternatively, the physician may feel overwhelmed by the patient's exaggerated or excessive emotions, embarrassed by their sexual overtures, or depleted. These patients recruit others, through use of their sexuality, to satisfy their needs to be romantically pursued and dependently taken care of and satisfied. They fear they are not desired and will lose the care of others.

There are two levels of functioning of patients with this personality disorder (Kernberg, 1984, 1992). Kernberg described a neurotically functioning hysteric who has intact reality testing, defenses centered on repression, and stable, mature relations with others. The female hysteric has a flirtatious clinging, child-like, dependence in intimate relationships but can function at mature levels in social and work situations (Kernberg, 1992). Male hysterics have similar psychological conflicts but may appear either as macho or effeminate (Kernberg, 1992). The hysteric of either sex often reacts to medical care with regression to a child-like, sexualized, dependent, clinging position. These individuals seek to gratify their wishes for dependent care by seducing or flattering others. Outside the physician's office, they typically function well.

By contrast, the histrionic patient who functions with a borderline personality organization (Kernberg, 1984, 1992) may display transient losses of reality testing, defenses centered on splitting, and chaotic sexualized relations with others. This patient is more self-centered and self-indulgent, with a pervasive child-like dependence that extends from intimate relationships into all aspects of social and occupational functioning. Female histrionics typically act flirtatious and may become indignant when a man shows sexual interest. Male histrionics also show a self-centered, dependent pattern but may additionally be severely hypochondriacal or have antisocial features (Kernberg, 1992). The histrionic of either sex may react to medical care with regression but, unlike the hysteric, uses defenses centered on splitting. These individuals may see the doctor as all good or all bad and can be devaluing. They may appear severely self-centered, attention-seeking, diffusely sexual, frequently hypochondriacal, somatic, and exploitative, with an exhausting dependence on their physicians.

When working with hysterics and histrionics, a physician must be friendly—not overly warm or reserved. Hysterics often benefit from some gratification of their dependent wishes and a free discussion of their fears and emotions. They can often be reassured by an educational, informational approach to their medical illness and are capable of expressing gratitude to the physician. The intense dependence of histrionics is often made worse when their needs are gratified. Offering excessive emotional care may make them greedy or demanding of need satisfaction. Histrionics benefit from firm, kind, limit-setting (especially to their sexual overtures), with neutral acknowledgment and gratification of their *reasonable* needs. They may be additionally helped by focusing on their distortions in reality perceptions and interpretations of the splitting mechanisms.

Borderline Personality Disorders

Borderline personality patients frequently become dependent on their physicians in a demanding, clinging, helpless, or self-destructive manner (Gunderson, 1984; Kernberg, 1975, 1984). Physicians typically feel manipulated, angry, depleted, exhausted, or self-doubting, with wishes to either get rid of the patient or rescue the patient from themselves.

These patients fear separation or abandonment and may react to potential losses with panic, emotional instability, anger, or impulsive (suicidal) actions. They often react to medical care by aggressively, dependently clinging to their physicians and other caretakers. When frustrated they may angrily devalue others and make entitled demands for special treatment. They tend to relate to others as all good or all bad, which generally accounts for their poor life functioning.

They function on the borderline level of personality organization, where reality testing is typically intact (Gunderson, 1984; Kernberg, 1975, 1984,

1992). However, under stress they may temporarily lose reality testing and manifest severe distortions in perception or sense of reality. They may misperceive the physician's intentions or instructions. They may also experience episodes of derealization, depersonalization, or brief psychotic episodes. Borderline patients have identity diffusion (extreme fluctuations from a grandiose perception of themselves to an excessively harsh underestimation of their abilities). They also suffer from stormy, chaotic relationships with others. They rely heavily on splitting, projective identification, projection, and devaluing.

Office management of these patients involves an empathic understanding of their feelings that their security is most threatened by fears of separation or abandonment and, secondarily, by rebuff or humiliation. They require firm limit-setting (e.g., what the physician can realistically offer). When the physician attempts to satisfy these patient's intense needs, it often results in an exhausted or angry physician. This situation can be avoided by setting realistic limits while offering the patient several ideas or options for more adaptive behaviors. Initial interventions should attempt to establish reality testing or correct distortions. If reality testing is intact, the most helpful interventions can be aimed at decreasing the pathologic splitting defenses by using confrontation, clarification, and interpretations of the problematic situation.

Narcissistic Personality Disorders

Physician reactions to the narcissistic patient are often difficult to manage. The superior, entitled, self-loving, arrogant attitude of these patients can be intimidating. They may elicit in the physician feelings of being devalued and inferior or fears of the patient's anger or criticism. Alternatively, the lack of empathy and interpersonal exploitation of these patients can readily provoke the physician to anger, a wish to retaliate with harsh criticism, or a wish to get rid of the patient.

The core fear of these patients is due to fragile self-esteem and their need for constant approval and praise from others. They fear loss of admiration, potency, and power and of being exploited when vulnerable. Any perceived insult to their "grandiose self" (Kernberg, 1984, 1992) makes them feel rejected, deflated, criticized, and frequently results in feelings of rage, shame, or humiliation.

The narcissistic patients who are most difficult to manage function at the level of borderline personality organization. Their reality testing is typically intact yet can undergo severe distortions when they perceive slights or rejection. Those narcissistic patients who have paranoid and antisocial features (Kernberg, 1992) have a worse prognosis.

They have a fragile identity that swings frequently from the grandiose to the worthless.

They rely heavily on splitting mechanisms to regulate their self-esteem. They portray themselves as grandiose and superior, which helps defend against split-off feelings of inadequacy and vulnerability. When they act self-importantly, they can devalue, viciously attack, or degrade those around them. Alternatively, as splitting operates, they may idealize and envy others who are for the moment seen as more powerful or successful. In this position their self-esteem plummets, as evidenced by their sense of worthlessness and their reports of deprecating and degrading self-attacks.

Office management of the narcissistic patient requires that the physician not mistake the patient's superior and entitled manner for genuine confidence. When being assaulted by a devaluing attack, it may help the physician see the attacking patient as a wounded child having a disruptive outburst. This recognition may prevent retaliation by the physician, which would only escalate a worsening situation. Intervention in the face of a devaluing attack involves acknowledging that the patient feels hurt and has a right to his or her opinions. If this patient can discuss the hurt feelings with a nonjudgmental, empathic physician, the problems generally resolve and a good–doctor patient alliance is restored. If it is not possible, the patient should be offered, without malice, defensiveness, or apology, the right to seek another expert for consultation. Such an offer may help the patient calm down and reconsider his or her position. In a long-term relationship with a narcissistic patient, the current splitting can be interpreted. It can be done by reminding the patient that in the recent past he or she has praised the skill and abilities of the physician. The patient can be asked why he or she is now so critical and angry. When this technique is effective, it allows patients to discuss their perceptions of insults to their self-esteem.

Self-Defeating (Masochistic)

Self-defeating patients are often suffering, depressed, and self-sacrificing (Spitzer and Williams, 1987). They repeatedly make poor choices that lead to failure or pain. A common physician reaction to these patients is a wish to rescue them from their own self-destructiveness. Trying too vigorously to help these patients frequently results in

worsening of the patients' complaints and symptoms, leaving the physician frustrated, angry, defeated, self-doubting, self-blaming, or hopeless. Alternatively, these patients can arouse sadistic fantasies in the physician, such as a wish that the patient would suffer or die.

Patients in this group are excessively dependent on love, support, and acceptance from others. They cannot directly express their anger and may be harshly self-judgmental. They fear recovery, which to them means losing love and care. Improvement of their medical condition can lead to the development of multiple new complaints that have no somatic basis.

Within this group, patients may function on either the neurotic or borderline level of personality organization. Neurotically functioning masochistic patients can make the physician feel mildly guilty that they are causing pain or suffering or are not adequately helping. The patient and physician both suffer. However, these patients ultimately can be helped and can express genuine gratitude toward the physician. Borderline functioning masochistic patients are passive-aggressive "help-seeking rejecters" (Groves, 1978) who make their physicians feel both helpless and responsible for their severe suffering or self-destructiveness.

Physicians can manage these patients by empathizing with the patient's realistic medical suffering, symptoms, or complaints due to the illness. It should not be suggested that the patient's symptoms are psychological or that the patient will improve or be cured quickly. Such misstatements may paradoxically increase the patient's symptoms, complaints, telephone calls, and office visits. Potential recovery can be presented as a likely but distant reality. If the patient cannot permit or admit relief of the symptoms or suffering, they can be asked to speak less about their symptoms for the benefit of other family members.

SCHEMA FOR PERSONALITY DISORDERS

The schema for office-based management of personality disorders that was presented in this chapter is summarized in Table 54–4, which outlines the *DSM-IV* classification of personality disorders, physician reactions to these patients, patient fears, psychopathologic level of personality functioning, patients' main defenses, and some interventions.

REFERENCES

Cloninger RC: A systematic method for clinical description and classification of personality variants. Arch Gen Psychiatry 44:573, 1987.

Frances A, Pincus HA, First MB (eds): Diagnostic and Statistical Manual of Mental Disorders. DSM-IV. Washington, DC, American Psychiatric Association, 1994.

Goldstein WN: Kernberg on the borderline: A simplified version. *In* Ross JM (ed): Concepts in Psychoanalytic Psychotherapy. Washington, DC, American Psychiatric Press, 1988.

Groves JE: Taking care of the hateful patient. N Engl J Med 298:883, 1978.

Gunderson JG: Borderline Personality Disorder. Washington, DC, American Psychiatric Press, 1984.

Kahana RJ, Bibring GL: Lectures in Medical Psychology: An Introduction to the Care of Patients. New York, International Universities Press, 1969.

Kernberg O: Severe Personality Disorders: Borderline Conditions and Pathological Narcissism. New York, Jason Aronson, 1975.

Kernberg O: Severe Personality Disorders: Psychotherapeutic Strategies. New Haven, Yale University Press, 1984.

Kernberg O: Aggression in Personality Disorders and Perversions. New Haven, Yale University Press, 1992.

Siever LJ, Davis KJ: A psychobiological perspective on the personality disorders. Am J Psychiatry 148:1647, 1991.

Spitzer, RL, Williams JB (eds): Diagnostic and Statistical Manual of Mental Disorders, 3rd edition (revised). DSM III-R. Washington, DC, American Psychiatric Association, 1987.

CHAPTER 55
SOMATIC PATIENT

ERICH E. BRUESCHKE and ROBERT E. ZITTER

Patients who present to the family physician with complaints for which no organic or physiologic basis can be found tend to be subjected to the extremes of medical attention. On the one hand they are frequently assigned labels such as hypochondriacs or somatizers, and on the other they are subjects of extensive tests, procedures, and pharmacologic treatment. Because the symptoms often mimic those of potentially serious disease but frequently no specific cause is found, this approach is a failure of the process used when approaching these patients and a lack of appreciation of the characteristics of such patient problems. Most importantly, these patients may receive less than optimal treatment and symptomatic relief, thereby enduring more suffering than is necessary.

This chapter delineates the various psychological and psychiatric conditions underlying the more common forms of somatization. Such discussion aids the primary care physician in more accurately diagnosing and effectively managing such cases rather than simply ruling out organic disease, an approach that by itself may even prolong somatization and increase the risk of iatrogenesis. The assessment should be aimed at ruling *in* the most probable causes for the observed problems rather than an exhaustive attempt to rule *out* all, frequently unlikely possibilities first.

PREVALENCE

Research consistently documents that as many as 50 per cent of patients coming to their primary care physician have psychosocial precipitants rather than medical problems (Stoeckle et al., 1964). Most of these individuals are experiencing depressive or anxiety disorders (or both) (Cadoret et al., 1980). Somatoform disorders as well as stress-related physician complaints without accompanying psychiatric diagnoses also account for large numbers of somatic patients.

Many patients suffering from an emotional disorder first present with physical symptoms and so consult their primary care physician rather than a mental health professional. Unfortunately, studies indicate that physicians identify depression, at best, in only one half of their patients. Cadoret et

al., (1980) found that nonspecific functional complaints, as well as pain and anxiety complaints, increased in number during the year prior to the diagnosis of depression and decreased to normal levels after the successful treatment of depression. Based on these and other studies, one can safely conclude that the typical somatic patient is not a malingerer; rather, this individual is likely to be truly in distress and to be experiencing any one of a number of psychiatric disorders or psychological influences or conditioning. The role of the family physician is to sort out these possibilities and to rule in anxiety or depression while using caution about selecting laboratory studies to identify specific problems for treatment.

SOMATIC COMPONENTS OF PSYCHIATRIC DISORDERS

Depression

The somatic components of depression may include fatigue, sleep difficulty, concentration impairment, poor appetite, increased agitation and anxiety, panic attacks, various pain states, poorly defined nonspecific physical complaints, and a general sense of not feeling well. Of course, any one of these problems may be the focus of the patient's concern and precipitate a visit to the doctor. Unfortunately, many depressed patients have little or no insight into their depressed state. Older persons, in particular, tend to focus more on somatic concerns than on affective states. A common mistake by the primary care physician is to treat an individual symptom (e.g., insomnia or chest wall pain) rather than diagnose the depression and treat this manageable condition. It is important to ask about all of the vegetative signs of depression as the patient may not volunteer this information.

Anxiety

Anxiety disorders, in particular panic disorders and generalized anxiety, have multiple somatic components. The *DSM-III-R* list of panic disorder symptoms include dyspnea, palpitations, chest

1523

pain, choking sensations, dizziness, unsteady feelings, paresthesias, hot and cold flashes, sweating, faintness, and trembling. Individuals with panic attacks often become progressively more disabled by their scary symptoms while going through the traditional medical systems, sometimes for years. They may become increasingly more hypochondriacal as they focus more and more on their somatic sensations. This heightened somatic concern, in turn, increases the level of anxiety, which is likely to lead to more physical symptoms, thereby feeding into the patient's hypochondriasis—a vicious cycle. The traditional medical approach may reinforce and strengthen this process rather than break it through proper education and therapy.

Patients suffering from generalized anxiety disorder usually experience similar automatic-mediated symptoms along with hypochondrical tendencies but without the acute panic attacks. It is important for the family physician to question the patient specifically about having panic attacks in the usual places (e.g., shopping malls, stores, church, and while driving), as the treatment of panic disorder (often antidepressants with supportive counseling) may be inappropriate for generalized anxiety disorder.

Somatoform Disorders

Patients diagnosed as having any one of the somatoform disorders share the common feature of presenting with physical symptoms suggestive of organic disease for which there are no demonstrable physical findings. With the exception of malingering or factitious disease, there is no conscious production of symptoms. Therefore these symptoms are "real" to the patient. Somatoform disorders include conversion disorder, hypochondriasis, somatoform pain disorder and somatization disorder. Most patients with somatoform disorders can be spotted by their thick charts. These patients, who often doctor-shop, have the greatest risk of undergoing needless medical tests and procedures and of becoming dependent on medication.

CONVERSION DISORDER

Conversion disorder refers to the loss or alteration of physical functioning that suggests physical disorder. "Classic" conversion symptoms include paralysis, paresthesias, blindness, and seizures. Such symptoms usually start suddenly during a time of acute stress or conflict and disappear quickly. The symptoms are involuntarily produced with no insight into the underlying conflict or secondary gain. The key here is for the physician to explore thoroughly the patient's life circumstances, not simply concentrate on the medical work-up or prematurely confronting the patient as to the lack of any "real" cause.

HYPOCHONDRIASIS

Hypochondriasis refers to the fear of having, or the belief that one has, a serious disease. This fear or belief is based on the patient's misinterpretation of various normal bodily sensations despite the attempts of others to convince the patient otherwise. Acquired immunodeficiency syndrome (AIDS) seems to be the most recent fear of hypochondriacal patients. Such individuals often come from alcoholic or dysfunctional families, sometimes with other hypochondriacal family members. They are generally anxious and do not directly address their real issues and anxieties.

SOMATIZATION DISORDER

Somatization disorder is characterized by recurrent, multiple somatic complaints over many years usually starting during young adulthood. These individuals may be the most difficult patients for the primary care physician to manage because of the breadth, number, and frequency of complaints across so many organ systems. The marked nature of this disorder should "tip off" the physician, who should be conservative with medications and diagnostic/treatment procedures.

SOMATOFORM PAIN DISORDER

Somatoform pain disorder refers simply to the preoccupation with pain in the absence of significant or anatomically consistent physical findings. Chronic back pain is probably the most common form of this disorder. Somatoform pain disorder may be the most disabling of the somatoform disorders, often resulting in significant time off from work. Once pain becomes chronic in nature, the prognosis for a successful outcome becomes much poorer because of conditioning factors (discussed later in the chapter). Unfortunately, as with many of the above problems, patients with chronic pain usually bounce around the medical system for several years before a mental health consultation is considered. Such individuals, owing to their increasing limitations, become clinically depressed at some point. It is of interest that biologic relatives of chronic pain patients have a much higher incidence of depression than is found in the general population. A fairly high percentage of chronic back pain is precipitated by a physical injury or trauma.

ADJUSTMENT DISORDER

Adjustment disorder with physical symptoms, in contrast to the somatoform disorders, describes those of us who experience stress-related physical symptoms without more global impairment or emotional dysfunction. Accounting for a large population, these patients may be easily diagnosed and managed. The primary care physician who asks about life stresses should find most patients with stress-related physical symptoms reasonably amenable to discussion, education, and if necessary short-term therapy, as the relationship between their symptoms and life circumstances can usually be made clear.

SUBSTANCE ABUSE

Substance abuse can lead to a host of physical problems, including gastrointestinal and liver disease, fatigue, and sleep difficulties. Withdrawal from alcohol or drugs, as well as from caffeine or nicotine, often causes increased anxiety and physical complaints. Excessive caffeine, particularly in sensitive individuals, may produce or exacerbate physical symptoms of anxiety such as trembling and anxiety attacks. Cocaine usage can trigger anxiety attacks. Periodically, substance abusers or dependent patients may present with physical symptoms for the underlying, sometimes subconscious purpose of obtaining additional prescriptions (e.g., tranquilizers or pain medications). Thus careful evaluation of alcohol, drug, and medication consumption and the history is mandatory for the assessment of somatic complaints.

PSYCHOTIC DISORDERS

Psychotic disorders—referring to those individuals with an underlying thought disorder—may be accompanied by intractable physical symptoms, sometimes of a bizarre or unusual nature (e.g., "It feels like water rushing through my stomach"). Such patients can be holding tenuously onto a marginal adjustment via somatization. If the physician senses oddities in the patient or finds a family history of more severe mental illness, it would be wise to refer the patient for a complete psychological evaluation.

PERSONALITY DISORDERS

Personality disorders, although not directly associated with somatic presentations, may play a role in the course and management of physical complaints. For example, a patient with an antisocial personality disorder may be more likely to abuse alcohol or drugs and display drug-seeking behav-

ior. Such an individual may also tend to be manipulative, to malinger, and to seek secondary gain via physical symptoms. Patients with borderline or histrionic personality disorders tend to experience periods of acute emotional distress, which may include a mixture of depressive or anxiety symptoms and somatic complaints. Often these episodes are short-lived and diminish when the acute stressor resolves. Borderline patients can be difficult to manage, as they often project great anger toward their caregivers, including physicians. Individuals with the more anxious personality disorders, such as dependent and avoidant personality disorders, may be more prone to mixed depressive and anxious symptoms along with concomitant physical complaints. These patients may also unknowingly receive significant reinforcement for physical complaints via attention or through avoidance of anxiety-provoking situations.

CONDITIONING FAMILY FACTORS

Operant conditioning is a powerful way in which physical complaints can develop, strengthen, and be maintained. Behavior followed by positive consequences (i.e., positive reinforcement) or by the removal of negative ones (i.e., negative reinforcement) increase as time goes by. Those behaviors that are consistently ignored or punished tend to extinguish or drop out. Almost any physical symptom or complaint can inadvertently be reinforced, albeit by caring persons with good intentions. Examples of reinforcement include attention, affection, and sympathy by family members, financial compensation, time off from work, avoidance of responsibility, addiction to pain medication, attention from health care professionals, and avoidance of focusing on other personal or family problems.

Adult patients most likely to have physical symptoms come under such contingencies are those with poor vocational or interactional skills. For example, a man with chronic back pain with few marketable job skills may not receive much less income on disability than working at a low-paying job. That patient who is not assertive in his marriage may have more of his psychological needs met via back pain behavior than through his usual marital interactions. Unfortunately, few patients initially have any insight into these patterns. Thus it is important for the physician to conduct a broad assessment of the patient's functioning in order to formulate workable hypotheses.

Children are susceptible to inappropriate contingencies operating within a dysfunctional family environment, particularly one with severe marital difficulties. A child may receive subtle or not so subtle reinforcement for sick behavior (e.g., abdominal complaints). This attention may allow the parents to avoid focusing on their own problems while everybody worries about the sick child. Such a scenario underlies many school phobias (e.g., the child with gastrointestinal difficulty every week-day morning). We saw a 14-year-old boy with "real" diarrhea every morning but not on weekends or vacations. He had missed many days of school and had been hospitalized twice with complete negative work-ups over a 2-year period. The pattern was obvious to the psychological consultant. The boy was fine during the rest of the day once it was too late to go to school. He spent much time with his mother during the day, thus receiving clear attention/reinforcement. The parents, clearly not emotionally close, denied marital problems, but the husband worked long hours and his wife appeared angry with him. She and her 14-year-old son were close despite her frustration with his "condition."

Minuchin et al., (1978) wrote extensively about psychosomatic families. Such families tend to be rigid, unable to resolve conflict effectively, lack psychological language, and deny psychological difficulty. A physician must also be concerned about abuse—physical, sexual, or emotional—in somatic children. Gross et al., (1980–1981) found that 80 per cent of women with pelvic pain of undermined organic etiology came from dysfunctional families with violence and physical assault.

Another powerful form of conditioning is modeling. A large percentage of somatic patients had a parent or grandparent with chronic, somatic complaints. These patients observe a key family member managing their lives via somatization. Apley (1975) reported that the incidence of abdominal pain in parents and siblings of children with similar pain was six times higher than in relatives of a control group. In a long-term longitudal study of abdominal symptoms, Christensen and Mortensen (1975) found that children with recurrent abdominal pain who continued to experience such problems as adults were much more likely to have their own children develop abdominal difficulties than were adults who did not retain their childhood somatic complaints.

The final conditioning model for physical symptomatology is classical conditioning, whereby symptoms become associated with particular places, people, or situations. One of the best examples is the nausea induced by chemotherapy becoming associated with the thought or sight of the hospital. Similarly, headaches, chest discomfort, or stomach upset can become associated not only with one's job but even when thinking about work. Avoidance of the aversive situation because of these symptoms reinforces and strengthens them. Additional factors (e.g., the patient's level of obsessiveness, other sources of reinforcement, and the patient's psychiatric status such as depression) determine the degree of control the particular symptoms have over a patient's life.

SOCIOCULTURAL FACTORS

Rosen et al., (1982) discussed the distinction between disease and illness: Disease refers to the malfunctioning of biologic or psychological processes, whereas illness is defined as perception, evaluation, explanation, and labeling of symptoms by patients and their families within the context of the social culture. There is significant variability among cultural groups in the way symptoms are perceived and managed. For example, Zborowski (1952) found that the response to pain by hospitalized patients differed among ethnic groups, with Italian and Jewish Americans having the greatest emotional response. Somatization appears to be correlated with lower socioeconomic status, in which it is less acceptable to express directly one's emotions. Of particular interest are the several cross-cultural studies of depression reviewed by Katon and Dengerink (1983). It appears that the vegetative signs of depression are the same across cultures and countries. The major difference is the perception of affective and cognitive states (e.g., feelings of hopelessness, helplessness, and guilt), which appears to be a more recent phenomenon in the American culture; in many other countries, particularly in the Middle East and China, they are express more through somatization. Some languages even lack words to describe internal, affective, and feeling states. One interesting study (Racy, 1970) found that as Arabs become more westernized their depression becomes more similar to that seen in the American culture. Our own experience confirms these findings; that is, our Middle Eastern patients who have come to the United States during the last few years seem to react to psychosocial stressors via somatization. All in all, because of the lack of appropriate psychological language or the strong cultural sanctions against talking about emotions, as well as the greater legitimacy and acceptability of physical symptoms, many of our patients continue to somaticize. These data emphasize the importance, particularly with depressed patients, to assess the vegetative signs of depression, the patient's facial expressions, and life circumstances rather than relying solely on their self-report of depression.

DIAGNOSIS

Biopsychosocial Model

Comprehensive biopsychosocial assessment is the key to developing the diagnosis with the greatest utility for patient management. Obviously, given the many influencing factors discussed above as well as the statistical frequency of medical patients with nonsignificant physical findings, a narrow biomedical approach is insufficient for a large number of our patients. To argue that all possible, organic etiologies should be eliminated prior to exploring nonmedical factors is no longer tenable. The preferred approach is to rule *in* the more likely causes of the problem while doing a reasonable concurrent investigation of biomedical and psychosocial areas. Because the real problem may be neglected, the patient is at greater risk for harm with a narrow approach to assessment. Most patients accept a multifactorial investigation and welcome a more holistic inquiry into their health concerns. Conducted within the context of a good doctor–patient relationship, patients do not feel accused of "being crazy," "malingering," or "it's all in your head." In fact, the most frustrated patients are those who endure an extensive medical work-up with negative results and no relief of their symptoms only to be dismissed because no "real" cause is found. It is well to remember that an uncommon presentation of a common problem (e.g., anxiety disorder) is seen more frequently than a common presentation of a rare disorder (e.g., pheochromocytoma). Therefore unless some other features of the presentation point to a physical disorder, consideration of a likely disorder should not be postponed in order to rule out unlikely problems with time-consuming, costly, and possibly hazardous studies.

It is important to remember that a patient may have a diagnosed medical problem and a psychiatric or psychological disorder. For example, an arthritic patient may also be clinically depressed. There is some likelihood that depression will complicate this patient's medical treatment, possibly leading to greater disability than necessary. Poor outcome may result from decreased compliance, poor motivation associated with anhedonia, lethargy, feelings of hopelessness and helplessness, and obsessive focusing on pain, all of which one would expect in a depressed state. Unfortunately, when there is a "true" organic condition, other factors often take a "back seat." However, these other factors (e.g., psychiatric disorders, conditioning influences) can be as *physically* incapacitating as medical problems. We often see great alleviation of disability once these other factors are successfully addressed.

Clinical Interview

The clinical interview remains the basic assessment tool for biopsychosocial evaluation. Observational skills are important, particularly for those patients who appear depressed or anxious but have poor insight into these conditions. Occasionally, the doctor identifies inappropriate or bizarre behavior and an angry patient. Questioning must include a judicious mixture of open-ended and directed questioning. Open-ended questions are more likely to lead to productive avenues to pursue with more specific questions. Starting the interview with mostly directed, leading or specific questioning is likely to bypass important areas to explore and certainly does not encourage emotional responses.

It is helpful to operationalize the patient's presenting complaints via a functional analysis, which consists of three parts: antecedents, symptomatic behavior, and consequences. *Antecedents* refer to the triggering stimuli: place, time, day, activity, and people. We have found physical symptoms that occur only outside the house, in church, during the week, or at work. *Symptomatic behavior* can be classified into physiologic symptoms (e.g., tachycardia, lightheadedness), cognitive behavior (e.g., I am going to die, I am sick, I better lay down), and overt behavior (e.g., leaving the situation, withdrawing, becoming irritable). Finally, *consequences*, as described earlier in this chapter, may include avoidance of stressful situations, attention, nurturance, medications, and financial gain. A functional analysis should provide a clear, complete picture that readily leads to intervention.

Particularly in acute cases it is important to identify life stresses or changes that have occurred around the time of onset. It is amazing how many patients cannot make the connection between obvious stressors, such as the death of a loved one, and the onset of lightheadedness and palpitations. If simply asked "Have you been under more stress lately?" the patient may give a negative response. Thus the physician should inquire into specific areas, such as recent deaths, job change, and relationship difficulties.

We find it clinically useful to distinguish between acute and chronic somatization. Symptoms of 6 months or shorter duration are usually related to specific environmental stressors or biologically mediated psychiatric disorders such as depression or panic disorder, or a combination of these factors. These somatic patients generally have a good prognosis with the proper identification, education, and treatment. More chronic cases, particularly those patients somaticizing across multiple organ systems for many years, have a poorer prognosis and tend to exhibit more global psychological impairment. The chronic somatic patient would benefit from coordinated treatment from the family physician and a mental health provider.

The family history offers many important clues. A family history of depression, anxiety, alcoholism, and chronic physical problems places the patient at increased risk for somatic difficulties. Adult children of alcoholics and victims of physical, sexual, and emotional abuse often are hypersensitive to bodily sensations and react to stress somatically.

The patient must be evaluated for the psychiatric disorders described earlier in this chapter. Again, depression and anxiety disorders account for a large proportion of somatic patients. Asking about the vegetative signs of depression yields a high payoff, yet it is frequently neglected, particularly if the patient denies depression. The physician can recognize atypical depressions with only a few vegetative signs and a somatic expression, which responds well to antidepressant or psychological treatment. Sometimes patients say they are depressed because of the physical problems rather than seeing the depression as the causative factor. They may still respond well to treatment for the depressive disorder. Of course, a family history of affective illness would put greater weight on treating the depression. Regarding anxiety disorders, the greatest payoff results from inquiring about anxiety attacks in specific places such as stores, church, restaurants, and the car. One should also ask about phobias and obsessive thoughts.

A thorough evaluation for substance abuse is important, as it may be the main underlying etiologic cause of many somatic problems, such as sleep disturbance, depression-related somatic complaints, and anxiety attacks. Often cessation leads to a resolution of these physical problems. A history of substance abuse must also be considered when prescribing medication, particularly anxiolytics and pain relievers.

Self-Monitoring

A symptom diary, kept by the patient, is a cost-effective method of collecting data that helps to educate both patient and physician. These data, in many cases, lead directly to intervention strategies. Other than a constant problem such as fatigue, most symptoms are amenable to this approach. Such diaries serve to involve patients actively in their medical treatment rather than simply waiting for the physician to solve their problems. Essentially, self-monitoring assists in identifying antecedents of which the patient may be unaware.

Psychological Testing

In those cases in which biomedical and psychosocial evaluations are not productive, one may consider referral for psychological testing to assist in the decision-making process. The Minnesota Multiphasic Personality Inventory (MMPI), an extensively used and validated objective personality test, is useful with the somatic patient. It helps to differentiate depressive, anxiety, chronic personality, and psychotic disorders. It is relatively inexpensive and a quick test that can even be computer scored, producing a computerized summary. Less frequently, projective tests such as the Rorschach and the Thematic Apperception Test (TAT) can be added for ambiguous and complex cases. Their main advantage is that patients do not know what responses are expected; therefore it is more difficult to influence the test results. These tests are more time-consuming and expensive, and some psychologists question their validity. Neuro-

psychological testing, such as the Halstead-Raitan and Intelligence measures, is desirable when the family doctor wants "hard" data on a patient whom he suspects may have compromised brain functioning.

TREATMENT

Education

Education of the somatic patient is accomplished throughout the biopsychosocial evaluative process. As the family physician gradually puts the pieces of the puzzle together with the patient, identifying antecedents, depressive symptoms, family dysfunction, and so on, the patient is learning to reframe his or her problem in a way that is conducive to treatment. This understanding, in many cases, alleviates the fear of what is wrong medically and allows patients to take more control over their lives. For some patients, education suffices; for others, additional intervention strategies are necessary to target each problem area. Throughout this assessment and education phase of treatment, the family physician is gaining the confidence of the somatic patient, strengthening the physician–patient relationship.

Therapy

Therapy should follow directly from the assessment. For acute somatization associated with an environmental stressor, education and supportive counseling may suffice. Brief psychotherapy may help the patient work through the acute stressors. On the other hand, the family physician may identify long-term, developmental issues (e.g., incest or childhood emotional abuse) that amplify the reaction to environmental stressors and require long-term psychotherapy.

It is best to form a good working relationship with a few mental health professionals to facilitate effective, ongoing communication during the patient's therapy. Mental health providers tend to specialize in different populations and techniques. Some problems such as muscle tension-related physical symptoms and anxiety attacks may respond well to a behavioral approach, including relaxation techniques; family therapy might make more sense with a somatic child; and in other cases an expert in medication therapy is indicated.

Chronic somaticizers are likely to be in need of psychotherapy given their global, psychological impairment. In addition, the more chronic that somatization becomes, the more does a sick-role adjustment develop, which includes a certain amount of reinforcement from significant others. Thus for long-standing somatic problems such as chronic back pain, the physician and therapist attempt to modify the current factors that are maintaining the physical symptoms as well as the more long-standing, deeper issues. Patients should understand that their symptoms are real, that the symptoms are not in their head, and that they are truly suffering. The team—family physician, patient, and therapist—are working together to alleviate the patient's physical difficulties. In more severe cases, particularly those with chronic pain, the patient may benefit from a multidisciplinary pain treatment program, incorporating physical and vocational therapy, psychological and behavioral therapy, and medical management.

Medication, particularly, the antidepressants and anxiolytics, can play an important part in the management of the somatic patient, with or without counseling. The antidepressants are the treatment of choice for depression-related somatization as well as anxiety attacks. Particularly with marked sleep disturbance, sedating antidepressants can offer immediate relief in addition to long-term benefit. Family physicians should become familiar with a few antidepressants, which vary as to the amount of sedation and anticholinergic side effects. Antidepressants offer the major advantage over the anxiolytics in that dependency does not become an issue. With the exception of alprazolam, the anxiolytics do not prevent anxiety attacks. If one does not question the patient specifically about anxiety attacks, an anxiolytic may be inappropriately prescribed with little therapeutic benefit. In the case of acute environmental stressors associated with physical symptoms, a short-term trial of an anxiolytic may be helpful so long as the patient clearly understands the rationale. For the *chronically* anxious patient who has associated physical or autonomic symptoms, buspirone may offer significant relief.

With some experience, these medications can be safely and effectively managed by the family physician. Certain patients have side effects to most of the antidepressants, although antidepressants such as fluoxetine seem to produce fewer side effects, are easier for which to establish the dosage, and may work more quickly. Significant problems with side effects can be an appropriate basis for referral to a psychiatrist. Also, after a trial of at least 1 to 2 months with several antidepressants at therapeutic dosages (determined by blood levels) and the patient remains insufficiently responsive, psychiatric consultation is indicated.

Case Presentation

Treatment must parallel the biopsychosocial assessment. Therefore in many cases, treatment must concurrently address multiple factors, sometimes by more than one health care professional. The following case presentation reflects this multifactorial treatment approach.

A 38-year-old woman presented with a 5-year history of abdominal and back pain and diarrhea. The pain was relatively constant and would wake the patient at night, leading to sleep disturbance and poor energy level. She had diarrhea within 15 minutes of eating and as a result restricted her food intake during the day to prevent "accidents" while at work or out of the house. She lost significant weight and ultimately lost her appetite. As time progressed, without relief of her symptoms, the patient became increasingly more depressed, drained, angry, and preoccupied with her pain and diarrhea. She began to see herself as a sick person and approached life from this sick role, gradually restricting her lifestyle. Her children responded by giving her much attention and caring for her sick behavior. The first thing the children did in the morning was go into her bedroom and ask their mother how she was feeling that morning.

Further inquiry discovered that her husband was alcoholic, and their relationship was strained. Their only interaction focused on her physical condition, as she avoided talking about important emotional issues and making important decisions about her life.

The patient had seen many physicians during the last 5 years. She had been hospitalized twice owing to severe pain and had had extensive work-ups. During the first hospitalization, gallstones were found. Her gallbladder was removed with no change in symptomatology. The work-up during the second hospitalization was unremarkable. She was diagnosed as having irritable bowel syndrome. Despite multiple dietary changes and medications, she found no relief. She was now taking Librium three times a day. At no point during these 5 years did her physicians evaluate her from a psychosocial perspective.

The patient was referred to a family physician who noted her thick chart, the chronicity of her symptoms, and the poor outcome of so many treatment modalities. He began to explore some of her psychosocial stressors. It was to this doctor that she admitted for the first time that her husband was alcoholic. Although at first reluctant, she agreed to see a psychologist. Her family physician prescribed Elavil at night for the severe sleep disturbance, depression, and pain. The psychologist persuaded her to attend Al-Anon and to start setting activity goals for herself. Relaxation therapy was conducted to teach her how to control muscle tension and better manage her pain. The patient's children attended a few therapy sessions to learn how to deal more effectively with their mother and to voice their own concerns. They eventually attended Al-Anon. Unfortunately, her husband refused therapy and to acknowledge his alcoholism.

Eventually, the patient decided to pursue a divorce. As her depression lifted, Mary understood that she had to take more responsibility for her life, to make choices, to pursue happiness in an active way. Her sick role behavior and thinking were aggressively confronted by both her family physician and psychologist, who collaborated closely on this case. Within approximately 8 weeks, her symptoms had completely resolved, including all depressive and somatic symptoms. It is of interest that she has proudly reported that occasionally when under stress she experiences mild pain, which she is able to alleviate with progressive muscle relaxation exercises. There was no recurrence of diarrhea.

REFERENCES

Apley J: The Child With Abdominal Pains. Oxford, Blackwell, 1975.

Cadoret RJ, Widmer RB, North C: Depression in family practice: Long-term prognosis and somatic complaints. J Fam Pract 10:625, 1980.

Christensen MF, Mortensen O: Longterm prognosis in children with recurrent abdominal pain. Arch Dis Child 50:110, 1975.

Gross R, Doerr H, Caldirola G, Ripley H: Borderline syndrome and incest in chronic pelvic pain patients. Int J Psychiatr Med 10:77, 1980–1981.

Katon W, Dengerink HA: Somatization in primary health care. *In* Carr JE, Dengerink HA (eds): Behavioral Science in the Practice of Medicine. New York, Elsevier Biomedical, 1983, pp 105–131.

Minnchin S, Rosman BL, Baker L: Psychosomatic Families. Cambridge, MA, Harvard University Press, 1978.

Racy J: Psychiatry in the Arab east. Acta Psychiatr Scand Suppl 21:1, 1970.

Rosen G, Kleinman A, Katon W: Somatization in family practice: A biopsychosocial approach. J Fam Pract 14:493, 1982.

Stoeckle JD, Zola IK, Davidson GE: The quantity and significance of psychological distress in medical patients. J Chronic Dis 17:959, 1964.

Zborowski M: Cultural components in responses to pain. J Soc Issues 8:16, 1952.

CHAPTER 56

DEMENTIA

RICHARD E. FINLAYSON

The twentieth century has provided western society with an enviable legacy—increasing longevity. A review of the literature on normal aging by Stein (1988) showed that the percentage of people in the United States who are older than age 65 years has increased from 2 per cent to about 12 per cent during the past 100 years. Expectations are that by the middle of the next century this figure will become a 10-fold increase. This demographic trend is having a notable impact on the prevalence of certain diseases, especially those of a degenerative nature. The dementing disorders are a source of great personal suffering and economic loss for society.

Recognition that dementia is not an inevitable or direct consequence of growing old (becoming "senile") has been a relatively recent development. Butler (1975) recommended that the term "senility" be discarded in favor of "emotional and mental disorders in old age," that is, a more diagnosis-specific approach to understanding intellectual loss during later life. The awareness of dementia as a disorder of later life has changed somewhat with the introduction of the human immunodeficiency virus (HIV) into the major populations of the world. This cause of dementia reminds us that age per se is not a cause of dementia, but that dementia results from specific diseases.

DEFINITION AND CLINICAL MANIFESTATIONS

A definition of dementia offered by Maletta (1987) contains several key concepts that are central to our present understanding of this syndrome: "a clinical symptom complex . . . marked by a gradual, persistent, and generalized deterioration of intellectual and emotional function from a previously higher level in an alert individual. This deterioration may be progressive, static, or remitting."

Memory loss is the key clinical feature of most cases of early dementia but is difficult to differentiate from "age-associated memory impairment" (Crook et al., 1986). The misplacing of things, forgetting appointments, and the like happen to healthy people so commonly that these lapses hardly can be taken as evidence of illness—unless by their frequency and intensity they seriously interfere with that person's life. Evidence of short-term memory loss is reason for concern. Long-term memory may eventually be lost, but its preservation is not a significant finding early in the course of the syndrome. Other impairments in the focal-cognitive process that are sometimes seen are loss of visuospatial skills and aphasia.

Personality traits that seemed adaptive, or at least were well tolerated by others, may become exaggerated and cause considerable social tension. For example, a retired, previously hard-driving executive may take up a new career at a frenzied pace as a defense against an inner sense of impending psychological dissolution. In individuals who have been prone to being suspicious, paranoid thinking may develop. Sometimes one observes what seems to be a complete reversal of personality. A person who was "independent-minded" (but actually lived denying many dependency needs) may become "clingy" or "underfoot" or change from "a tiger into a pussycat."

Because of their diverse characteristics, affective symptoms do not easily lead to or provide a basis for a diagnosis of dementia. Apathy, slowed thinking, depressive moods, restlessness, insomnia, and somatic complaints may be present, however, even before anyone has expressed a serious concern about memory or other cognitive functions.

Subcortical dementia (Albert et al., 1974) has been described as a type of dementia in which affective symptoms are prominent. In a review of subcortical dementia, Cummings and Benson (1984) recorded the following features as characteristics: slowness of mental processing, forgetfulness, impaired cognition, apathy, and depression. The syndrome has been linked to various diseases, including progressive supranuclear palsy, Huntington's disease, Jakob-Creutzfeldt disease, Parkinson's disease, lacunar state, multiple sclerosis, and depression. HIV dementia has also been described as subcortical (Oechsner et al., 1993); however, it is argued that this diagnostic term is too inclusive and should be divided into specific subtypes of cognitive impairment (Martin et al., 1993; Pillon et al., 1991). The validity of the concept (i.e., cortical versus subcortical) remains controversial. We know now, for example, that dementia of the

Alzheimer's type (DAT), the classic cortical dementia, is not limited to cortical structures but has extensive involvement in subcortical structures, such as the nucleus basalis of Meynert (Whitehouse et al., 1982).

Once a dementia is moderately advanced, it is readily discernible to those living and working in close association with the person that cognition is impaired. He or she may get lost on the way home from work or while at a shopping mall. Self-care is diminished to varying degrees, resulting in poor hygiene and inappropriate dress. Social situations become difficult, even embarrassing.

Dementia of the Alzheimer type is a cortical dementia according to the traditional schema and is distinguished primarily by memory loss, aphasia, apraxia of speech, and agnosia. A steady progression of symptoms are characteristic of DAT. Reisberg's (1986) staging of this disorder clearly demonstrates the downhill course. Patients eventually require assistance in dressing, eating, bathing, and toileting. Language is lost. The person no longer can sit up and finally becomes comatose.

The course of vascular dementia (formerly multi-infarct dementia) typically differs from DAT in that the onset is abrupt and the deterioration stepwise. Personality is relatively spared, but emotional lability can be intense. Focal neurologic findings are common. There may be prolonged stable periods, but death can come quickly as a result of an acute cerebrovascular or cardiovascular event. Differentiating this disorder from DAT can be difficult clinically, as vascular dementia may follow a clinical course similar to that of DAT. The two disorders are common and occur in combination in many people. Kurita et al. (1993), in an autopsy-confirmed study of mixed Alzheimer and vascular dementia cases, correlated the pathologic findings with premortem psychological and behavioral assessment. The observations suggested that, with DAT, cognitive and behavioral impairments progress simultaneously, whereas in the mixed group these impairments may progress more independently.

ETIOLOGY AND EPIDEMIOLOGY

With the exception of HIV dementia, most patients with dementia encountered by the family physician are elderly. Among elderly patients, DAT and vascular dementia are responsible for 75 to 85 per cent of reported cases. There are many other causes, some of which can be arrested or reversed. Table 56–1, based on data from the Office of Medical Applications of Research of the National Institutes of Health (1987), outlines the categories and some examples of reversible and progressive dementia.

The category "intoxications" is particularly important with respect to drug and alcohol use. The

TABLE 56–1. CATEGORIES OF DEMENTIA BASED ON REVERSIBILITY: SOME CAUSES AND DISORDERS

Causes That Can Be Removed or Reversed
Intoxications
  Prescription drugs
  Illicit drugs
  Carbon monoxide
  Heavy metals
  Drug combinations
Infections
  Any agent capable of affecting brain
Metabolic disorders
  Endocrinopathies
  Encephalopathy of renal/hepatic failure
  Wilson's disease
Nutritional disorders
  Thiamine deficiency
  Folate deficiency
  Niacin deficiency
Vascular disorders
  Hypertension
  Atherosclerosis
  Vasculitis
  Embolic disease
  Cardiac disease
Space-occupying lesions
  Chronic subdural hematoma
  Brain tumor
  Affective disorders

Progressive Degenerative Diseases
Without important neurologic findings other than dementia
  Alzheimer's disease
  Pick's disease
With important neurologic findings, with or without dementia
  Parkinson's disease
  Huntington's disease
  Progressive supranuclear palsy
Many others

Data from the Office of Medical Applications of Research, National Institutes of Health (1987).

vulnerability of older persons to substance misuse, abuse, and dependence has been discussed by Atkinson (1984). Contributing factors that have been suggested in the literature are (1) biologic (e.g., slowed biotransformation and clearance); (2) common medical ailments leading to self-medication with over-the-counter drugs and increased exposure to prescription drugs; and (3) psychosocial stressors (e.g., retirement and loss of spouse).

According to Tarter and Edwards (1985), the dementias associated with alcoholism are due to a wide range of factors (e.g., malnutrition, liver disease, vascular disease, and injury). Empiric data that support the validity of "alcoholic dementia" as a unique syndrome are lacking.

Many infectious agents are capable of causing dementia. One is of particular public health importance. HIV diseases are capable of producing various neuropsychiatric syndromes, including dementia (Portegies et al., 1993; Price et al., 1988). According to Achim et al. (1993), HIV encephalitis is unusual in that neurologic damage occurs in the absence of significant infection of neuronal or glial cells. The predominant infected cell in the brain is the macrophage, and it has been proposed that release of viral or immune activation factors from macrophages may mediate neurologic damage. It should not be assumed that this type of dementia occurs only in young persons. About 10 per cent of cases of acquired immunodeficiency syndrome (AIDS) occur in the age group 50 years and older, thereby creating potential for misdiagnosis of AIDS dementia complex as DAT (Kernutt et al., 1993; Scharnhorst, 1992). The literature is inconclusive at this time as to how common dementia is in otherwise asymptomatic carriers. A controlled study from Germany (Riedel et al., 1992) demonstrated that in the stages before AIDS develops electroencephalographic findings and psychometric findings indicate central nervous system involvement with AIDS in about 20 to 30 per cent of cases, whereas with full-blown AIDS there is a marked increase (to 80 per cent of cases).

The dementia syndrome associated with depression has been described in the literature as a pseudodementia (Wells, 1979). Although the need frequently arises in family practice to determine the source of cognitive impairment, the usefulness of the concept of pseudodementia has been questioned. Rohling and Scogin (1993) studied depressed people, psychiatric controls, and normal controls and reported that memory testing failed to demonstrate an interaction between depression and age that would be consistent with the descriptive label pseudodementia. On the basis of a review, Poon (1992) observed that published data on geriatric depression and cognitive functioning are divided in demonstrating a depression effect. The author stated that the term pseudodementia is inappropriate and misleading and should be abandoned. In my opinion, the family physician should avoid dichotomizing the issue, that is, thinking of it in either–or terms (depression or dementia) but should remember that depressed persons often have cognitive symptoms and that in older persons, especially, cognitive symptoms in a depressed person may warn of an underlying organic dementia.

Dementia of the Alzheimer type is the most common of all reported causes of dementia (one half to two thirds of cases). Pick's disease, also a progressive dementia, is much less common. Detailed discussion of the pathology and possible causes of DAT is beyond the scope of this chapter. In brief, DAT is progressive neuronal degeneration in the cerebral cortex and subcortical nuclei. Loss of cortical neurons and the presence of neurofibrillary tangles and senile plaques in the gray matter are characteristic (Perl and Pendlebury, 1986). Various etiologic hypotheses have been advanced, but there are data suggesting that the main risk factor for both early- and late-onset Alzheimer's disease is a positive family history (Fratiglioni et al., 1993).

Read and Jarvik (1984) reviewed the topic of cer-

ebrovascular disease in the differential diagnosis of dementia. They noted from the literature that in pathologic studies the second most common finding in demented patients is the presence of multiple infarctions in brain tissue. The diagnostic entity multi-infarct dementia may account for as many as one third of cases of dementia. They listed the following mechanisms: (1) lacunar state; (2) multiple emboli; (3) vasculitis; (4) blood dyscrasia; (5) hypoperfusion; and (6) anoxic episode.

DIAGNOSIS

The clinical history is the most important source of information. An awareness of the wide range of psychobehavioral disturbances and diverse causes is essential for an accurate diagnosis. Once a physician suspects the syndrome from the history, it is important to attempt to document (or rule out) the presence of cognitive impairment. This impairment is easily missed unless specific questions are addressed to the patient and family members. A structured mental status examination, such as the Mini-Mental State (Folstein et al., 1975), is useful and much preferred to a hit-or-miss attempt at bedside assessment of mental status. It must be emphasized, however, that these simple screening tests are not sufficient in themselves to make a diagnosis of dementia.

Other causes of cognitive disturbance should not be overlooked. Delirium is an acute syndrome characterized by abrupt onset, confusion, fluctuating course (even over minutes), autonomic instability, and visual hallucinations. Although numerous medical factors can contribute to delirium directly, an underlying dementia may predispose the patients to this syndrome. Thus both may be present.

Physical examination of the older patient should be performed with a knowledge of findings that are related to aging per se. Walshe (1987) discussed neurologic findings that are involutional in origin, which are "generally uniform among the aging population, symmetric and predictable." The clue to abnormality is asymmetric loss. Various findings that should not be attributed to aging include extraocular movement abnormalities, ataxia, absence of deep tendon reflexes, extensor plantar response, and trouble with tandem gait.

Table 56–2 lists the procedures recommended by the Office of Medical Applications of Research of the National Institutes of Health (1987) for studying patients with new-onset dementia. An important initial step toward the diagnosis is the discontinuation of medications that are not strongly indicated. Those that are known to produce an abstinence syndrome when abruptly stopped (e.g., barbiturates, benzodiazepines, and opiates) should be tapered on a standard schedule if dependence is suspected.

TABLE 56–2. STANDARD DIAGNOSTIC STUDIES FOR NEW-ONSET DEMENTIA

Complete blood cell count
Electrolyte panel
Screening metabolic panel
Thyroid function tests
Vitamin B_{12} and folate levels
Tests for syphilis and, depending on history, for HIV
Urinalysis
Electrocardiogram
Chest radiograph

Data from Office of Medical Applications of Research, National Institutes of Health (1987).

When depression is suspected, psychiatric consultation should be considered, especially in those cases in which the question of pseudodementia has been raised. The neurologist can be especially helpful in guiding the advanced work-up, that is, with decisions concerning special diagnostic studies such as electroencephalography, computed tomography of the head, and magnetic resonance imaging. Neuropsychological assessment is most useful when the history and clinical results of examination are equivocal and for providing a baseline estimation of cognitive performance. The diagnosis of dementia is made on the basis of all available evidence, but not infrequently it remains tentative. Observations over a period of months may be necessary in order to make a reasonable firm diagnosis. Table 56–3 gives the *Diagnostic and Statistical Manual of Mental Disorders (DSM-IV)* (American Psychiatric Association Committee, 1994) criteria for diagnosis of dementia of the Alzheimer type. The reader is referred to *DSM-IV* for criteria for vascular and various other dementias. DAT is diagnosed not only by exclusion but also by a history that is compatible with the symptoms and course of the illness.

TREATMENT

The wise physician keeps in mind the possibility of multiple causes of dementia in a given patient. A program that addresses the obvious medical disorders that are treatable and provides psychosocial management from the outset is most desirable.

Psychosocial Management

Family caregivers, themselves usually middle-aged or elderly, constitute the backbone of the informal care of DAT patients. An awareness of their vulnerabilities is important as the physician begins to talk with them and the patient about this burdensome, socially disruptive disease.

The initial reaction of the family to the diagnosis commonly involves feelings of anxiety, fear of get-

TABLE 56–3. DIAGNOSTIC CRITERIA FOR DEMENTIA OF THE ALZHEIMER TYPE

A. Development of multiple cognitive deficits manifested by both
  1. Memory impairment (impaired ability to learn new information or to recall previously learned information)
  2. One (or more) of the following cognitive disturbances
    a. Aphasia (language disturbance)
    b. Apraxia (impaired ability to carry out motor activities despite intact motor function)
    c. Agnosia (failure to recognize or identify objects despite intact sensory function)
    d. Disturbance in executive functioning (i.e., planning, organizing, sequencing, abstracting)
B. Cognitive deficits in criteria A1 and A2 each cause significant impairment in social or occupational functioning and represent a significant decline from a previous level of functioning.
C. Course is characterized by gradual onset and continuing cognitive decline.
D. Cognitive deficits in criteria A1 and A2 are not due to any of the following.
  1. Other central nervous system conditions that cause progressive deficits in memory and cognition (e.g., cerebrovascular disease, Parkinson's disease, Huntington's disease, subdural hematoma, normal-pressure hydrocephalus, brain tumor)
  2. Systemic conditions that are known to cause dementia (e.g., hypothyroidism, vitamin B_{12} or folic acid deficiency, niacin deficiency, hypercalcemia, neurosyphilis, HIV infection)
  3. Substance-induced conditions
E. Deficits do not occur exclusively during the course of a delirium.
F. Disturbance is not better accounted for by another axis I disorder (e.g., major depressive disorder, schizophrenia).

Code based on type of onset and predominant features:
  With early onset: if onset is at age 65 years or younger
    290.11 *With delirium:* if delirium is superimposed on the dementia
    290.12 *With delusions:* if delusions are the predominant feature
    290.13 *With depressed mood:* if depressed mood (including presentations that meet full symptom criteria for a major depressive episode) is the predominant feature. A separate diagnosis of mood disorder due to a general medical condition is not given.
    290.10 *Uncomplicated:* if none of the above predominates in the current clinical presentation
  With late onset: if onset is after age 65 years
    290.3 *With delirium:* if delirium is superimposed on the dementia
    290.20 *With delusions:* if delusions are the predominant feature
    290.21 *With depressed mood:* if depressed mood (including presentations that meet full symptom criteria for a major depressive episode) is the predominant feature. A separate diagnosis of mood disorder due to a general medical condition is not given.
    290.0 *Uncomplicated:* if none of the above predominates in the current clinical presentation

Specify if:
With behavioral disturbance
Coding note: Also code *331.0 Alzheimer's disease on axis III.*

From American Psychiatric Association Committee on Nomenclature and Statistics: Diagnostic and Statistical Manual of Mental Disorders: DSM-IV, 4th edition. Washington, DC, American Psychiatric Press, 1994, pp 142–143, with permission.

ting the disease, and guilt. These areas should be discussed. A knowledge of the family dynamics, especially the quality of the relationship between the patient and the potential caregivers, is vital. One might anticipate, for example, that an enmeshed family that has had closed boundaries to the community would choose to "handle it" themselves and thus place a greater strain on the caregiver(s), leading perhaps to early breakdown of support.

What do patients and families want and need to know? First and foremost, they must have reliable information about the disease. In the case of DAT, it should be emphasized that the cause is not known at present and a cure is not available. This information helps minimize needless expenditure of time and money in search of miracle cures. The physician will find Reisberg's (1986) Functional Assessment Staging of Alzheimer's Disease (FAST) a useful tool for understanding and explaining to the family the usual course of this illness. Discussion of the course of the illness is a good situation in which to describe in-home relief services, foster care, and nursing home placement. Each type of dementia has features that are of practical importance to the caregivers and of course to the patient.

Recommended reading for families includes *The 36-Hour Day* (Mace and Rabins, 1991); *Understanding Difficult Behaviors* (Robinson et al., 1992); *Alzheimer's: A Caregivers Guide and Source Book* (Gruetzner, 1988); and *Alzheimer's Disease: Activity-Focused Care* (Hellen, 1992).

McMurchie (1993) stated that there is an increasingly large role for primary care physicians in the management of people infected with HIV. The increased emphasis on community-based care of individuals with this disease derives from a preference of patients to be treated within their community, and such care can decrease the demands on already strained resources. McMurchie also called attention to the role of primary care physicians in the psychosocial management of the AIDS patient and in educating the community in general about the social factors of HIV or AIDS.

Psychopharmacologic Treatment

Most patients who are demented have a disorder for which a specific treatment is not available. Behavioral symptoms therefore are the usual target of drug treatment. The medical treatment of the disorders that cause or contribute to dementia and that have established causes and treatment protocols are not discussed here, with the exception of depression.

A wide variety of psychoactive drugs have been studied and used for management of the affective and behavioral symptoms associated with the dementias. None is outstanding in its efficacy for treating behavioral symptoms. Antipsychotic drugs (neuroleptics) are probably the most widely used for treating the restlessness, agitation, and wandering associated with dementia. One advantage of these drugs is the general lack of development of tolerance and an abstinence syndrome, which are common to sedatives and antianxiety drugs. The antipsychotic agents are hardly a panacea, however. In a controlled study, Risse and Barnes (1986) observed that only about one third of the agitated, demented patients treated with neuroleptics responded to a moderate or a marked degree. However, Ray et al. (1993) demonstrated that use of antipsychotic drugs in a nursing home setting was markedly decreased through education of physicians, nurses, and other staff in the use of behavioral techniques to manage behavioral problems associated with dementia.

A specific antipsychotic drug usually is selected on the basis of the side effect profile. Low-potency antipsychotics, e.g., chlorpromazine (Thorazine) and thioridazine (Mellaril), have the advantage of being sedating, but they are more likely to produce central anticholinergic confusion and cardiovascular effects than the high-potency antipsychotics. The latter, e.g., haloperidol (Haldol) and fluphenazine (Prolixin), have as their chief disadvantage a higher incidence of extrapyramidal symptoms. Molindone (Moban) has the advantages of being moderately sedating, being only mildly prone to produce extrapyramidal effects, and having no hypotensive effects. It is not available in parenteral form.

All classes of antidepressants may be used for treating the depression that accompanies dementia; however, as with the antipsychotic drugs, consideration of side effects is important when choosing an antidepressant. This approach, based on minimizing side effects, can be taken with confidence when prescribing antidepressants because we do not have consistently reliable methods for selecting a specific drug on the basis of efficacy alone. Until we know more about depression in demented patients, the physician should adhere to the same general guidelines for prescribing antidepressants as would be followed when treating a nondemented depressed patient.

Barbiturates should be avoided because they are general neuronal depressants. Benzodiazepines, although not neuronal depressants in the way barbiturates are, should be used with caution, especially those with long half-lives (either parent drug or active metabolites). Daily administration of long-acting benzodiazepines could be hazardous. Small, less frequent doses are indicated. Fortunately, we have shorter-acting benzodiazepines available: oxazepam (Serax), alprazolam (Xanax), triazolam (Halcion), lorazepam (Ativan), temazepam (Restoril), and estazolam (ProSom). Although problems of accumulation may be lessened with these drugs, each is capable of producing tolerance, abstinence syndrome, and cognitive and affective problems. Chronic administration should be avoided when possible, and no drug should be used as a substitute for sound behavioral management.

Winograd and Jarvik (1986) have written an informative and practical article concerning physician management of the demented patient. The reader is referred to this article for further discussion of the topic (see reference).

REFERENCES

Achim CL, Heyes MP, Wiley CA: Quantitation of human immunodeficiency virus, immune activation factors, and quinolinic acid in AIDS brains. J Clin Invest 91:2769, 1993.

Albert ML, Feldman RG, Willis AL: The subcortical dementia of progressive supranuclear palsy. J Neurol Neurosurg Psychiatry 37:121, 1974.

American Psychiatric Association Committee on Nomenclature and Statistics: Diagnostic and Statistical Manual of Mental Disorders: DSM-IV, 4th edition. Washington, DC, American Psychiatric Press, 1994, pp 142–143.

Atkinson RM: Alcohol and Drug Abuse in Old Age. Washington, DC, American Psychiatric Press, 1984, pp 2–21.

Butler RN: Psychiatry and the elderly: An overview. Am J Psychiatry 132:893, 1975.

Crook TI, Bartus RT, Ferris SH, et al: Age-associated memory impairment; proposed diagnostic criteria and measures of clinical change: Report of a National Institute of Mental Health work group. Dev Neuropsychol 2:261, 1986.

Cummings JL, Benson DF: Subcortical dementia: Review of an emerging concept. Arch Neurol 41:874, 1984.

Folstein MF, Folstein SE, McHugh PR: "Mini-mental state": a practical method for grading the cognitive state of patients for the clinician. J Psychiatr Res 12:189, 1975.

Fratiglioni L, Ahlbom A, Viitanen M, et al: Risk factors for late-onset Alzheimer's disease: A population-based, case-control study. Ann Neurol 33:258, 1993.

Gruetzner H: Alzheimer's: A Caregivers Guide and Source Book. New York, John Wiley & Sons, 1988.

Hellen CR: Alzheimer's Disease: Activity-Focused Care. Boston, Andover Medical Publishers, 1992.

Kernutt GJ, Price AJ, Judd FK, et al: Human immunodeficiency virus infection, dementia and the older patient. Aust NZ J Psychiatry 27:9, 1993.

Kurita A, Blass JP, Nolan KA, et al: Relationship between cognitive status and behavioral symptoms in Alzheimer's disease and mixed dementia. J Am Geriatr Soc 41:732, 1993.

Mace NL, Rabins PV: The 36-Hour Day: A Family Guide to Caring for Persons With Alzheimer's Disease, Related Dementing Illness, and Memory Loss in Later Life, revised edition. Baltimore, Johns Hopkins University Press, 1991.

Maletta GJ: Diagnosis of the dementias. Minn Med 70:378, 1987.

Martin EM, Robertson LC, Sorensen DJ, et al: Speed of memory scanning is not affected in early HIV-1 infection. J Clin Exp Neuropsychol 15:311, 1993.

McMurchie M: The role of the primary care physician. J Acquir Immune Defic Syndr 6(suppl 1):S77, 1993.

Oechsner M, Möller AA, Zaudig M: Cognitive impairment, dementia and psychosocial functioning in human immunodeficiency virus infection: A prospective study based on DSM-III-R and ICD-10. Acta Psychiatr Scand 87:13, 1993.

Office of Medical Applications of Research, National Institutes of Health: Differential diagnosis of dementing diseases. JAMA 258:3411, 1987.

Perl DP, Pendlebury WW: Neuropathology of dementia. Neurol Clin 4:355, 1986.

Pillon B, Dubois B, Agid Y: Severity and specificity of cognitive impairment in Alzheimer's, Huntington's and Parkinson's diseases and progressive supranuclear palsy. Ann NY Acad Sci 640:224, 1991.

Poon LW: Toward an understanding of cognitive functioning in geriatric depression. Int Psychogeriatr 4(suppl 2):241, 1992.

Portegies P, Enting RH, de Gans J, et al: Presentation and course of AIDS dementia complex: 10 years of follow-up in Amsterdam, The Netherlands. AIDS 7:669, 1993.

Price RW, Brew B, Sidtis J, et al: The brain in AIDS: Central nervous system HIV-1 infection and AIDS dementia complex. Science 239:586, 1988.

Ray WA, Taylor JA, Meador KG, et al: Reducing antipsychotic drug use in nursing homes: A controlled trial of provider education. Arch Intern Med 153:713, 1993.

Read SL, Jarvik LF: Cerebrovascular disease in the differential diagnosis of dementia. Psychiatr Ann 14:100, 1984.

Reisberg B. Dementia: A systematic approach to identifying reversible causes. Geriatrics 41:30, 1986.

Riedel R-R, Helmstaedter C, Bülau P, et al: Early signs of cognitive deficits among human immunodeficiency virus-positive hemophiliacs. Acta Psychiatr Scand 85:321, 1992.

Risse SC, Barnes R: Pharmacologic treatment of agitation associated with dementia. J Am Geriatr Soc 34:368, 1986.

Robinson A, Spencer B, White L: Understanding Difficult Behaviors. Ypsilanti, MI, Eastern Michigan University, 1992.

Rohling ML, Scogin F: Automatic and effortful memory processes in depressed persons. J Gerontol 48:P87, 1993.

Scharnhorst S: AIDS dementia complex in the elderly: Diagnosis and management. Nurse Pract 17:41, 1992.

Stein EM: Normal aging—psychological and sociocultural aspects. *In* Lazarus LW, Jarvik LF, Foster JR, et al (eds): Essentials of Geriatric Psychiatry: A Guide for Health Professionals. New York: Springer, 1988, pp 1–24.

Tarter RE, Edwards KL: Neuropsychology of alcoholism. *In* Tarter RE, Van Thiel DH, with the assistance of Edwards KL (eds): Alcohol and the Brain: Chronic Effects. New York: Plenum Medical Publishing, 1985, pp 217–242.

Walshe TM: Neurologic examination of the elderly patient: Signs of normal aging. Postgrad Med 81:375, 1987.

Wells CE: Pseudodementia. Am J Psychiatry 136:895, 1979.

Whitehouse PJ, Price DL, Struble RG, et al: Alzheimer's disease and senile dementia: Loss of neurons in the basal forebrain. Science 215:1237, 1982.

Winograd CH, Jarvik LF: Physician management of the demented patient. J Am Geriatr Soc 34:295, 1986.

CHAPTER 57
ALCOHOL ABUSE

MARC A. SCHUCKIT

In most Western countries 90 per cent or more of individuals are drinkers of alcoholic beverages at some time during their lives, including almost 70 per cent who currently imbibe alcohol. The percentage of drinkers is higher among men than among women, although the gap between the two sexes may be closing. Most individuals consume their first drink at approximately age 12 to 14 years, have a maximum quantity and frequency of intake in their late teens to mid-twenties, and then decrease the amount of alcohol consumed with each increasing decade.

Unfortunately, during late adolescence and early adulthood temporary alcohol-related problems are highly prevalent. Almost 50 per cent of men and a slightly lower proportion of women experience an alcohol-related blackout (forgetting all or part of what happened during a drinking evening), miss some time from school or work because of drinking, have an alcohol-related accident or a single driving arrest while drinking, and so on. Fortunately, most of these individuals spontaneously moderate their drinking and do not go on to develop the more pervasive and persistent alcohol-related problems that might be labeled alcoholism.

These data underscore the importance of establishing an alcohol intake history in all patients, even those who do not meet alcoholic criteria. Drinking, heavy intake of alcohol, and temporary alcohol-related life problems are so prevalent that it is difficult for us to properly treat any patient without establishing his or her alcohol intake and problem history. Even among nonalcoholics, the usual drinking pattern can contribute to accidents and exacerbate independent medical and psychiatric disorders.

Alcoholism that fulfills criteria outlined in the following sections is one of the most prevalent serious disorders in our society. Even utilizing restrictive criteria, the lifetime risk for developing this disorder among men is at least 10 per cent and might be as high as 15 per cent (Robins et al., 1984; Schuckit, 1985a). The rate of similar problems in women is at least 5 per cent.

This work was supported by NIAAA grant 05226 and the Veterans Administration Research Service.

SOME MYTHS

Most physicians have been trained in central city hospitals where they were inaccurately taught that the average alcoholic lives on skid row, returns to treatment facilities repetitively, and rarely demonstrates long-lasting improvement. If one accepts this stereotype, it is possible to draw the *erroneous* conclusion that alcoholics are exceptionally difficult to treat and that dealing with them is unrewarding. Therefore it is worthwhile to briefly review two myths that must be set aside if we are to optimize our ability to help our patients.

First, only 5 per cent or so of alcoholics fit the skid row stereotype. The average alcoholic appears in clinical settings in a sober state, looking well groomed, having no smell of alcohol, and lacking many of the other traits we may associate with skid row. This typical patient complains of a variety of medical and emotional problems that must be properly diagnosed if the clinician hopes to avoid unexpected calls in the middle of the night and adverse reactions to ill-advised treatments. In fact, the usual alcoholic man or woman resembles the usual person in society. He or she has a job and financial resources, has close friends and relatives, and is capable of abstaining from alcohol for extended periods.

A second important myth is that alcoholics are not likely to improve. To the contrary, numerous studies have documented that the average middle class alcoholic who agrees to enter treatment and completes a rehabilitation program appears to have a 60 to 70 per cent chance of maintaining abstinence for at least 1 year (Neubuerger et al., 1982; Schuckit, 1989). Although few investigations go beyond 12 months of follow-up, there are additional data that once abstinence is achieved for this period the chances of continuing an alcohol-free lifestyle are high. In addition, there is at least a 20 per cent chance of "spontaneous remission" in which life-long abstinence is achieved even in the absence of formal treatment or participation in self-help groups (Helzer et al., 1985; Ludwig, 1985; Schuckit, 1989).

PHARMACOLOGY OF ALCOHOL

Ethanol is a simple molecule that is weakly charged, soluble in both water and fat, and thus widely distributed in the body. The concentration of this substance in blood is loosely predicted by the number of drinks as related to the body weight; that is, in general, the larger the person, the greater amount of alcohol that must be consumed for a specific blood alcohol level (BAL). However, there are additional important factors, including the percentage body fat (with increasing age and increasing body fat, there is less body water and thus higher BALs), age (with an increased brain sensitivity and decreased ability of the liver to metabolize alcohol with increasing age), past experiences, concomitant medications, and so on.

The level of alcohol in the blood is expressed as milligrams or grams of ethanol per 100 milliliters (or deciliters) of blood. For example, in most states a person with a BAL of 100 mg/dl (0.100 gm/dl) is considered legally drunk. The BAL increases by approximately 20 mg/dl for each drink, a level that takes slightly more than an hour to metabolize. This amount of alcohol also contains approximately 10 grams of ethanol, with approximately 100 calories or more—calories "empty" of the usual nutrients such as vitamins.

As a typical central nervous system (CNS) depressant, beverage alcohol decreases the activity of neurons, although some behavioral stimulation can be observed at low blood levels. The clinical effects of the drug are similar to those observed with other brain depressants such as the benzodiazepines (e.g., diazepam [Valium]) and barbiturates (in fact, all prescription sleeping pills and most prescription antianxiety drugs). Thus there is cross-tolerance between all of the brain depressants with the result that simultaneous intake of multiple drugs of this class can (and frequently does) result in a lethal overdose. On the other hand, the repeated intake of any one drug of this class can result in tolerance so that when the first drug is stopped larger doses of a second brain depressant might be required to achieve the desired clinical effect (e.g., larger doses of a benzodiazepine might be required to induce anesthesia in a sober but recently heavily drinking alcoholic) (Schuckit, 1989).

Tolerance, or the need for larger doses of the drug to achieve the same effects, is a relatively complex phenomenon. First, metabolic, or *pharmacokinetic,* tolerance is observed when, after 1 to 2 weeks of daily drinking, the liver adapts through induction of enzymes to increase the metabolic rate for ethanol by as much as 30 per cent. Cellular, or *pharmacodynamic,* tolerance represents the adaptation of the nerve cells to a state of "resistance" to the effects of alcohol. The mechanisms for cellular tolerance are not well understood but probably represent changes in cell membranes or neurochemical receptors (perhaps for γ-aminobutyric acid or serotonin)—changes that contribute to physical dependence. Finally, *behavioral* tolerance is the learned behavior or practice effects

whereby chronic heavy drinkers can perform tasks moderately efficiently even though they are intoxicated. The combination of the three mechanisms contributes to the ability of most relatively healthy alcoholics (i.e., with no severe liver or brain damage) to drink large amounts of alcohol, with cellular tolerance contributing to their ability to be awake and alert at levels of alcohol that might be lethal in others.

The metabolism and excretion of alcohol is relatively straightforward. Low amounts of this substance (2 to 10 per cent, depending on the BAL) are excreted directly through sweat, urine, and lungs. Most ethanol is metabolized in the liver through at least three mechanisms, each resulting in the same first breakdown product of alcohol, acetaldehyde. The most clinically relevant metabolic pathway occurs through alcohol dehydrogenase in the cell cytosol, after which acetaldehyde is rapidly destroyed by aldehyde dehydrogenase in both the cytosol and mitochondria. Each of these steps requires nicotinamide adenine dinucleotide (NAD) as a cofactor, and it is the lack of availability of this hydrogen receptor that is probably a major rate-limiting step in this metabolic pathway. The second type of oxidation of ethanol, most important at higher BALs, occurs in the smooth endoplasmic reticulum and is called the microsomal ethanol oxidizing system (MEOS). Third, an unknown percentage of ethanol is metabolized through the catalase system.

In summary, alcohol use can induce liver enzymes, it is a "preferred fuel" in the liver where hydrogen receptors are likely to be utilized, and it has actions on almost all body systems. Therefore, it is important to determine the alcohol intake pattern in patients for whom we are prescribing any medication, especially other brain depressant drugs, medications with sedative side effects, and substances metabolized in the liver.

DIAGNOSIS OF ALCOHOLISM

Because 90 per cent of people drink at some time during their lives and noting the fact that moderately heavy intake of alcohol is likely to be observed in the late teens to late twenties, an understanding of the prevalence of drinking and the pharmacology of alcohol can enhance our clinical abilities. The remainder of this chapter focuses on the diagnosis, etiology, usual course, and treatment for severe, pervasive alcohol-related life problems or alcoholism.

Before discussing the diagnostic criteria, it is worthwhile to briefly review some biases important when considering any diagnosis (Goodwin and Guze, 1994). Historically, diagnoses in medicine have been used to describe a clinical condition at one point in time, to imply causation, to predict the most likely course, and to help select the appropriate treatment. Whereas many diagnostic criteria are available for alcoholism, the most clinically relevant are probably those that meet the last criterion, that is, those that tell us when to intervene and the treatment approaches with the best asset/liability ratio.

From this perspective there are as many as 11 definitions of alcoholism that have been used in the literature in recent decades (Boyd et al., 1983). However, there is a great amount of overlap of the individuals identified by these diagnostic approaches (Rapaport et al., 1993). Thus someone who is labeled alcoholic because the quantity and frequency of intake is excessive is also almost certain to demonstrate signs of psychological dependence and is likely to evidence serious life problems related to heavy drinking. If the diagnostic approach is excessively broad, many of these labeled individuals probably do not go on to develop more severe and pervasive problems; with restrictive approaches, diagnosed people follow the expected clinical course, but some men and women who are excluded from the category might be at risk for severe future problems.

Formal and official diagnostic criteria for alcoholism are presented in the *Diagnostic and Statistical Manual of the American Psychiatric Association, DSM-IV* (American Psychiatry Association, 1994). Here the clinician is asked to determine if an individual meets criteria for alcohol dependence by fulfilling any three or more of seven diagnostic items. The problems outlined include tolerance or withdrawal, but they also incorporate evidence of continued use despite physical or psychological consequences to the individual, spending a great deal of time using alcohol or recovering from its effects, avoiding family and other important interactions because of drinking, and so on. To meet the criteria, there must be some evidence that each of these problems occurred repeatedly, that they interfered with life functioning, and that items from three or more of the categories clustered together, occurring within any 12-month period.

For individuals who do not fulfill criteria for dependence, the clinician must also consider the possibility of alcohol abuse. The latter diagnosis is based on evidence of the repeated occurrence of problems in any one of four categories of problems: continued drinking despite social or interpersonal consequences; repeated use in hazardous situations (e.g., driving while intoxicated, regardless of whether arrested); and other evidence of social, legal, or interpersonal difficulties. The *DSM-IV* criteria for dependence and abuse represent a compromise between different schools of thought on diagnostic labeling. Whereas *dependence* has been a well validated label that has also proved to be reliable, much less information is available regarding the potential meaning of a diagnosis of *abuse*

(Rapaport et al., 1993; Schuckit, 1993, 1995a, 1995b).

A diagnostic approach of great potential use to the clinician evaluates the occurrence of significant alcohol-related life problems, gathered as part of the usual social history (Schuckit, 1985b, 1986). Once a pattern of problems has been established, the next step is to determine if the alcohol has contributed to these difficulties. Thus alcoholism is diagnosed with a history of any of the following: a marital separation or divorce related to alcohol: multiple arrests related to drinking; physical evidence that alcohol has harmed health, including evidence of alcoholic withdrawal; or a job loss or layoff related to drinking. Once patients have fulfilled these criteria, they have demonstrated that they ignored the early warning signs that alcohol was causing a problem and went on to develop major alcohol-related life consequences. In other words, there is evidence that alcohol means more to the person than the problems it has caused. Follow-up studies demonstrate that once these criteria are met it is possible to predict a high likelihood of continued major life problems due to alcohol should drinking continue (Schuckit, 1985b, 1986).

Of course, it is not always possible to obtain all of this information directly from the patient. Although many individuals admit to major life problems and often agree that it is possible that alcohol contributed to them, an appropriate work-up for any problem in behavioral medicine *requires* that additional information about the patient be obtained. Such a work-up is usually carried out through an interview with someone who knows the patient's history, often a relative and usually the spouse.

There are several additional approaches that can help establish a diagnosis. None of these, however, can produce a final label; they simply raise the index of suspicion that a significant problem might exist. First, there are the series of blood tests (e.g., γ-glutamyltransferase) and physical findings described below in the section on treatment issues that may be helpful. The second ancillary approach includes a number of simple (therefore not sophisticated) paper and pencil questionnaires. The most widely used of these instruments is the Michigan Alcoholism Screening Test, outlined in Table 57–1. Note that the endorsement of five or more items is an indication of the need to gather more information.

Finally, it is important at this juncture to briefly review the importance of primary versus secondary alcoholism. Approximately three fourths of alcoholics who present for treatment have no major preexistent psychiatric disorder. It is these *primary alcoholics* who are the focus of the comments offered in this chapter, and it is usually people in this group who are the subjects in most clinical studies. The natural history and rehabilitation efforts aimed at primary alcoholics are slightly differ-

TABLE 57–1. MICHIGAN ALCOHOLISM SCREENING TEST

Question	Yes	No
Do you enjoy having a drink now and then?	0	
Do you feel you are a normal drinker? (By normal we mean you drink less than or as much as most other people and you have not gotten into any recurring trouble while drinking)		2
Have you ever awakened the morning after some drinking the night before and found that you could not remember part of the evening?	2	
Do either of your parents or any near relative, or your spouse or any girlfriend or boyfriend ever worry or complain about your drinking?	1	
Can you stop drinking without a struggle after one or two drinks?		2
Do you feel guilty about your drinking?	1	
Do friends or relatives think you are a normal drinker?		2
Are you able to stop drinking when you want to?		2
Have you ever attended a meeting of Alcoholics Anonymous (AA)?	5	
Have you gotten into physical fights when you have been drinking?	1	
Has your drinking ever created problems between you and either of your parents, or another relative, your spouse, or any girlfriend or boyfriend?	2	
Has any member of your family ever gone to anyone for help about your drinking?	2	
Have you ever lost friends because of your drinking?	2	
Have you ever been in trouble at work or school because of your drinking?	2	
Have you ever lost a job because of drinking?	2	
Have you ever neglected your obligations, your school work, your family, or your job for two or more days in a row because you were drinking?	2	
Do you drink before noon fairly often?	1	
Have you ever been told you had liver trouble or cirrhosis?	2	
After heavy drinking have you ever had severe shaking or heard voices or seen things that really weren't there?	2	
Have you ever gone to anyone for help about your drinking?	5	
Have you ever been in a hospital because of drinking?	5	
Have you ever been a patient in a psychiatric hospital or a psychiatric ward of a general hospital where drinking was part of the problem that resulted in hospitalization?	2	
Have you ever been seen at a psychiatric or mental health clinic or gone to any doctor, social worker, or clergy for help with any emotional problem where drinking was a part of the problem?	2	
Have you ever been arrested for drunk driving, driving while intoxicated, or driving under the influence of alcoholic beverages or any other drug? If yes, how many times?	2 each	
Have you ever been arrested or taken into custody even for a few hours because of other drunk behavior, whether due to alcohol or another drug? If yes, how many times?	2 each	

Each response scores the number of points listed. A total of 0 to 3 = probable normal drinker; 4 = borderline; 5 to 9 = 80 per cent likelihood of dependence; and 10 or more = 100 per cent likelihood.

From Selzer ML: The Michigan alcoholism screening test: The quest for a new diagnostic instrument. Am J Psychiatry 127:1653, 1971, with permission. Copyright 1971, the American Psychiatric Association.

ent from those for men and women who developed their alcohol-related life problems only after the establishment of another major psychiatric diagnosis (i.e., secondary alcoholism). Thus these 20 to 30 per cent of secondary alcoholics often demonstrate pre-existent severe antisocial life problems in all areas of functioning (e.g., antisocial personality disorder with secondary alcoholism) or demonstrate severe life problems related to drugs before the onslaught of alcoholism (e.g., primary drug abuse with secondary alcoholism). It is also probable that the rate of independent and pre-existent major depressive disorders among alcoholics is at least as high as in the general population (perhaps 5 per cent), as are the rates of most major anxiety disorders, such as panic disorder or agoraphobia (Schuckit, 1986; Schuckit and Hesselbrock, 1994).

Different diagnostic criteria for alcoholism outline similar populations. The essential element is documentation of heavy enough and persistent enough intake of alcohol to interfere significantly with health and life functioning, despite which the individual continues to drink. In the 70 to 80 per cent of cases in which alcoholism is the first appearing major psychiatric disorder, the primary alcoholic is likely to run a somewhat predictable clinical course.

ETIOLOGY

There is no single cause for alcoholism. It is likely that different individuals develop their pervasive alcohol-related life problems for a variety of reasons. For most it is probable that the interaction of stress, general environment, personality, and biologic predisposing factors combine to produce the final alcoholic picture.

It is the last of the influences, biologic factors, for which the best data are available. Alcoholism does appear to be a biologically influenced disorder, and there is evidence that genetic factors play an important role.

Data from family, twin, and adoption studies all

support the importance of genetic influences (Goodwin, 1985; Schuckit, 1985c). First, alcoholism runs strongly in families, with sons and daughters of alcoholics demonstrating a fourfold increased risk for this disorder. The level of risk appears to increase with the number of alcoholic relatives, the severity of the alcoholism, and the closeness of the genetic relationship. However, establishing that a disorder is familial does not prove that genetic factors are important because most individuals are raised by their biologic parents.

The second approach, twin studies, attempts to separate genetics and environment by comparing the risk for alcoholism in identical twins born to alcoholics with the risk for fraternal twins. If the development of alcoholism is related to childhood environment, the twin of an alcoholic, being born and raised at the same time as the sibling, should be at high risk for the disorder, no matter what kind of twinship is involved. However, if alcoholism is related to genetic factors, the identical twin of an alcoholic (sharing 100 per cent of his or her genes with the affected individual) should have a significantly higher risk for alcoholism than the fraternal twin of an alcoholic (sharing only 50 per cent of the genes, the same as in any full sibling). Most twin studies support the conclusion that there is a significantly higher risk for alcoholism in the identical than in the fraternal twin of alcoholics, although not all studies agree (Gurling et al., 1985; Kendler et al., 1994).

The third approach, adoption-type studies, offers the most compelling evidence that alcoholism is genetically influenced (Goodwin, 1985; Schuckit, 1987). Numerous investigations utilizing the half-sibling or formal adoption approaches have demonstrated that sons and daughters of alcoholics have a fourfold increased risk, even when they were adopted close to birth and raised by nonalcoholics. In fact, having an alcoholic rearing parent does not increase the risk any higher than that predicted by severe alcohol-related problems in the biologic father or mother.

A number of laboratories have attempted to identify the biologic factors that might contribute to the risk for alcoholism (Schuckit, 1987, 1994a,b). These studies visualize individuals as entering life with a greater or lesser level of biologic predisposition, which then interacts with environmental factors to produce the final clinical picture. Most of these investigations have focused on teenage or young adult sons and daughters of alcoholic parents, comparing them in numerous areas with children of nonalcoholics. One such series has repeatedly documented that children of alcoholics demonstrate less intense responses to a three- to five-drink alcohol challenge by showing less subjective feelings of intoxication, less decrement in motor performance measures at a given BAL, less intense or more evanescent changes in hormones after drinking, and less postethanol change on several electrophysiologic measures (Schuckit, 1987; Schuckit and Gold, 1988). Follow-up of these men almost a decade later revealed that the decreased reaction is a potent predictor of future alcoholism (Schuckit, 1993b). These studies might indicate that some children of alcoholics carry their elevated risk by a relative insensitivity to the effects of beverage alcohol at low BALs, a time when most people are deciding whether it is appropriate to continue to drink during an evening. Other interesting and potentially important findings in children of alcoholics include the documentation that a significant number of these offspring may have a lower amplitude brain wave (the P300 of the event-related potential), thought to reflect some unique cognitive abilities (Begleiter et al., 1987), might demonstrate different patterns of alpha waves on background cortical electroencephalograms (Ehlers and Schuckit, 1988), and might have some specific deficits on neurocognitive and psychomotor test performance (Schuckit et al., 1987).

In summary, although it is not likely that there is any one specific cause for alcoholism, there is ample evidence that genetically influenced biologic factors contribute to the predisposition toward this disorder. Several studies are beginning to identify factors that might contribute to the risk, and it is hoped that future follow-up studies of high risk individuals might pinpoint environmental factors that interact with the biologic predisposition to produce the disorder. These data might lead to greater understanding of causes, which in turn might contribute to our ability to prevent alcoholism before it develops or might identify more specific or effective treatment approaches. In the interim, the genetic issues underscore the biologic rather than moral underpinnings for this highly prevalent and serious disorder.

NATURAL HISTORY OR USUAL CLINICAL COURSE OF ALCOHOLISM

When diagnostic criteria are carefully selected, they can tell us important information about the usual clinical course and help to select among various treatments. Thus we can be informed about whether the clinical course is likely to be so benign that no interventions are required or if, on the other hand, severe problems are likely to ensue. Of course, even careful diagnoses cannot indicate the exact difficulties a specific patient would have. They can, however, predict the patterns of problems that are likely to ensue.

In this context, the "average" alcoholic is likely to have his or her first drink, first period of intoxication, and first minor problems related to alcohol during the teenage years, at a time not significantly different from the general population. These generalities apply to primary alcoholics, not the 10 per cent or so of alcoholic men who have major pre-existent antisocial personality disorder or the additional 5 per cent who exhibit severe pre-existent drug-related life difficulties.

By the mid to late twenties most men and women are beginning to moderate their drinking, probably learning from their minor problems. At the same time, difficulties for alcoholics are likely to escalate, with the first major life problem due to drinking appearing in the late twenties to early forties (Schuckit, 1995a; Schuckit et al., 1993; Vaillant, 1982).

Once established, the course of alcoholism is likely to comprise frequent exacerbations and remissions (Ludwig, 1985; Schuckit et al., 1993). In the typical course, alcohol-related problems escalate, precipitating a crisis. In the context of these problems, most individuals temporarily cease drinking, usually going through mild withdrawal on their own. This period of abstinence, lasting days to months for the average middle-class primary alcoholic, is usually followed by thoughts that drinking might be "safe" if only carried out at certain times of the day or with certain beverages. The temporary "controlled" drinking is characterized by an ability to go to parties and consume alcohol without problems and is likely to last for days to months, sometimes longer. This period of "control" is almost inevitably followed by unpredictable times of escalating intake with associated problems, which in turn lead to more problems, more persistent heavy intake, and a crisis that often precipitates another episode of abstinence (Helzer et al., 1985).

Although most alcoholics appear to break into this cycle with active help from clinicians or self-help organizations such as Alcoholics Anonymous (AA), even without formal intervention the course is far from hopeless (Drew, 1968). Several studies have documented that at least 20 per cent or more of alcoholics achieve permanent abstinence without formal intervention (Editorial, 1987; Schuckit, 1995a). However, should the alcoholic continue to drink, the life-span is shortened by an average of 15 years, with the leading causes of death, in decreasing order, being heart disease, cancer, accidents, and suicide.

An important part of the natural history of alcoholism involves the effects of persistent heavy drinking on various body systems. In general, the early stages of alterations in organ functions tend to be reversible, but many body systems deteriorate with permanent levels of damage after repeated alcohol-related insults.

In the *central nervous system* (CNS) temporary problems that can be observed with even one night of heavy drinking include an alcoholic blackout (forgetting all or part of what occurred while drinking) and interference with sleep (falling asleep can be facilitated, but alcohol "fragments" sleep with subsequent bad dreams and a lack of deep sleep) (Schuckit, 1995a,b). With chronic intake of large doses of alcohol, perhaps 5 to 15 per cent of alcoholics develop deterioration of the nerves to the hands and feet, a peripheral neuropathy. Cerebellar degeneration with accompanying nystagmus and motor incoordination is observed in 1 per cent or so of alcoholics (Estrin, 1987). Severe cognitive impairment can take many forms including the thiamine deficiency-related Korsakoff syndrome characterized by profound anterograde and retrograde amnesia, along with possible impairments in visuospatial, abstract, and conceptual reasoning—problems likely to become permanent to greater or lesser degrees in almost two thirds of the individuals meeting diagnostic criteria (Grant, 1987). Less specific forms of cognitive problems, often reflected by increased size of the brain ventricles, are seen in 20 per cent or more of alcoholics, frequently accompanied by irreversible decreases in intellectual functioning (Harper et al., 1987).

Related to general CNS functioning is the fact that heavy doses of alcohol contribute to severe psychological impairment (Schuckit, 1986). It may include an intense sadness lasting for days to weeks in the midst of heavy drinking, sometimes so severe that it resembles major depressive disorder and probably contributes to the 15 per cent lifetime risk for completed suicide among alcoholics (Brown and Schuckit, 1988). However, when the severe depression is observed only in the context of heavy drinking, it is likely that it will disappear with abstinence alone; under these circumstances, in primary alcoholics antidepressant medications are rarely required. Similarly, acute alcoholic withdrawal (lasting up to 5 days) and the following protracted period of more mild abstinence symptoms (lasting up to 3 to 6 months) is frequently characterized by severe anxiety, which can include panic attacks, phobias, and feelings of generalized anxiety, each of which is likely to decrease spontaneously over a period of months with abstinence alone (Schuckit and Hesselbrock, 1994). In addition, perhaps 1 to 3 per cent of alcoholics develop auditory hallucinations or paranoid delusions in the absence of any obvious signs of withdrawal—a temporary state of alcohol hallucinosis that is likely to disappear spontaneously within days to weeks (Schuckit, 1995a).

Probably reflecting the major role played in alcohol absorption and metabolism, problems in the *gastrointestinal (GI) system* are prevalent among alcoholics (Frank and Raicht, 1985; Lieber, 1984). They include irritation of the esophagus and stomach with resulting esophagitis and gastritis, probably the major causes of upper GI bleeds among alcohol abusers. Problems in the small bowel are those seen when there is interference with absorption of vitamins and nutrients by ethanol; large bowel difficulties are likely to include periods of diarrhea. Of course, alcohol contributes to pancreatitis (perhaps in 5 per cent of alcoholics). In the liver, utilization of NAD as the hydrogen receptor with subsequent interference in gluconeogenesis and the accumulation of fatty acids produces numerous systemic effects. Local damage to the liver progresses from reversible stages of fatty infiltration of cells to the ballooning and damage of cells (alcoholic hepatitis as well as hyaline sclerosis), to potentially severe scarring or cirrhosis with subsequent impairment in the general functioning of the liver and alteration in abdominal blood circulation with resulting ascites and myriad complications.

The *blood-producing and immune systems* are also potentially severely affected. The most common change in red blood cells (RBCs) is an increase in size or mean corpuscular volume (MCV) along with a possible mild anemia. Other forms of anemia, including sideroblastic changes, are more rare and are less likely to occur in the absence of severe malnutrition. Heavy drinking also decreases production of most white blood cells, decreases granulocyte mobility and adherence, and impairs a number of hypersensitivity responses. These changes and the accompanying alterations in T cell activities might contribute to the high risk for cancer observed in alcoholics, especially malignancies involving the head and neck (it is estimated that 70 per cent of cancers in this area above the epiglottis are seen in alcoholics), esophagus, breast, and stomach. Cancer is the second leading cause of death in alcoholics.

Whereas one to two drinks per day in an otherwise healthy individual might be associated with a decreased risk for *cardiovascular disease*, there is evidence that intake over this level might contribute to vascular disease, the leading cause of death among alcoholics (Criqui, 1986; Lang et al., 1985; Saunders, 1987). The greater the alcohol intake, the greater the likelihood of high blood pressure, and it is estimated that heavy drinking is one of the major contributors to mild to moderate hypertension. As a striated muscle toxin, alcohol is also likely to produce heart muscle damage, and ethanol is thought to be the leading cause of idiopathic cardiomyopathy. In addition, high alcohol levels increase the low density lipoproteins and triglycerides and might also contribute to the risk for cerebrovascular accidents (Donahue et al., 1986).

Additional important consequences of heavy drinking include temporary interference with *sexual functioning*, including impotence and testicular atrophy in men and menstrual irregularities in women (Irwin et al., 1988). There are also a series of well documented adverse effects on the developing fetus, which in its full-blown form of the fetal alcohol syndrome can include facial changes with epicanthal eye folds, poorly formed concha, small teeth with faulty enamel, cardiac atrial or ventricular septal defects, an aberrant palmar crease, microcephaly, and various levels of mental retardation (Morrow-Tlucak and Ernhart, 1987). Alcohol also

contributes to skeletal myopathy characterized by painful and swollen muscles, high levels of muscle enzymes in the blood, and even myoglobinuria. Finally, in this brief review, effects on the *skeletal system* include alterations in calcium metabolism with an increased risk for fractures and osteonecrosis of the femoral head (Bikle et al., 1985).

Once primary alcoholism is diagnosed, the family physician should know a great deal about the potential clinical course. Severe alcohol-related problems alternating with periods of abstinence and short episodes of controlled drinking are likely to continue for many years, although as many as 20 per cent of alcoholics can reach permanent spontaneous remission from drinking. In the course of the heavy intake of alcohol, levels of temporary as well as severe organ impairment can ensue, and many of these factors can be used to identify the hidden alcoholic, as is outlined in the next section.

TREATMENT ISSUES

Identification and Confrontation of the Alcoholic

It is now fairly obvious that the physician should recognize that any patient might have alcoholism. By taking a history of alcohol-related life problems from the patient as well as a resource person, most alcoholic individuals can be identified. However, for those individuals for whom a resource person is not available or when the history is incomplete, there are a number of laboratory tests that are helpful for identifying alcohol-abusing individuals (Schuckit and Irwin, 1988).

The most sensitive laboratory test is the assay for γ-glutamyltransferase (GGT), an enzyme produced in the liver after consumption of five or more drinks daily; the assay has a 70 per cent sensitivity and similar specificity for identifying alcoholics (GGT blood levels of 40 units or more). Additional tests with slightly less impressive levels of sensitivity and specificity include a high-normal *MCV* (e.g., 90 to 95 μm^3 or higher), as well as an increase in *aspartate transaminase* (SGOT) or *alkaline phosphatase*. Serum *uric acid* levels higher than 7 mg/dl, *triglycerides* higher than 180 mg/dl, or high levels of *high density lipoprotein cholesterol* in the absence of exercise are additional clues that a patient might be drinking heavily.

A number of clinical findings should also raise an index of suspicion that a patient might be alcoholic. They include mild and inconsistent levels of hypertension (e.g., 140/90 mm Hg), repeated infections such as pneumonia, and otherwise unexplained cardiac arrhythmias. Additional specific findings that should raise suspicion include cancer of the head and neck, esophagus, or cardia of the stomach as well as, of course, cirrhosis, unexplained hepatitis, pancreatitis, or peripheral neuropathies.

After an alcoholic has been identified, he or she should be confronted with the diagnosis. The presenting complaint can be used as an important entree to discussing an alcohol problem. For instance, the patient complaining of insomnia or hypertension should be told that they are clinically important symptoms and that the laboratory tests and physical findings indicate that alcohol appears to have contributed to the problem. Continued drinking is likely to increase the risk for further medical and psychological difficulties. The physician should then share information about the course of alcoholism and explore possible avenues for attacking the problem.

The first confrontation could be met by the patient with any of several responses. For the patient who denies that he or she has a drinking problem, it is important to recognize that only rarely does a single confrontation result in important change. Rather, it is necessary to "keep the door open," inviting the patient back for further tests during which additional gentle but firm confrontations are carried out. It is wise never to give up, as many patients think about the confrontation between sessions and after several weeks or months may be willing to consider abstinence, especially after a severe life crisis.

A second potential response is that the patient recognizes that a problem might be present but desires to "cut down" on drinking. As noted previously, almost all alcoholics periodically spontaneously decrease their alcohol intake. The problem is not controlling but staying in control over an extended period. It should be pointed out that the individual has "cut down" many times in the past, but each effort resulted in a subsequent escalation of intake with severe life problems. Thus controlled drinking does not work over an extended period. However, if the patient insists, a series of guidelines can be established for the patient and spouse whereby no more than two drinks (as defined earlier) can be consumed within a 24-hour period. The thought here is that if the individual sticks to the rule (which is difficult), he or she cannot become intoxicated and problems are not likely to ensue. An additional benefit to this strategy is that the patient then commits himself or herself to controlling and can be urged to agree to try abstinence when the controlled drinking does not work over a long period.

The overall goal of all types of confrontation is to get the patient to agree to permanent abstinence. Once this goal has been achieved, steps are taken to help him or her focus on detoxification (if needed) and rehabilitation.

Detoxification Procedures

In the presence of alcohol-induced cellular tolerance, any sudden decrease in ethanol can lead to symptoms of withdrawal from its CNS depressant effects. As with most syndromes, patients do not develop every symptom, and the usual clinical picture is mild. Common features include tremor of the hands (shakes or jitters); autonomic nervous system dysfunctions, such as increases in pulse, respiratory rate, and body temperature; insomnia, possibly accompanied by bad dreams; feelings of generalized anxiety or panic attacks; and GI upset. Symptoms are likely to begin 5 to 10 hours after decreasing alcohol intake, peak in intensity on day 2 or 3, and improve by day 4 or 5 (Schuckit, 1995b). However, as part of a protracted abstinence picture, anxiety, insomnia, and mild levels of autonomic dysfunction may persist for 6 months or more. These continuing phenomena may contribute to the tendency to return to drinking.

Only about 5 per cent of alcoholics show evidence of severe withdrawal symptoms. Such symptoms include grand mal convulsions (usually generalized and rarely focal in nature and most often limited to one or at most two seizures), severe agitation, and intense confusion. Fewer than 5 per cent of patients develop delirium tremens (DTs), a syndrome characterized by confusion (often with associated delusions and hallucinations), severe agitation, and seizures. Probably the likelihood of developing severe withdrawal or DTs is higher if there are concomitant medical disorders or prior levels of alcohol intake.

The treatment of withdrawal is predicted by the clinical picture. The *first* and most important step is to perform a through physical examination in all alcoholics. The *second* step is to recognize that even well nourished middle-class alcoholics are likely to have problems absorbing vitamins from the proximal small intestine and thus require oral multiple B vitamins, especially 50 to 100 mg of thiamine daily for a week or more. The *third* step is to recognize that the symptoms are primarily due to cellular adaptation to a CNS depressant followed by a rapid decrease in blood levels.

Symptoms can be alleviated by administering any brain depressant, using doses on day 1 that decrease symptoms (usually utilizing pulse and other autonomic symptoms as guidelines) and then decreasing the dose to zero over a 3- to 5-day period. Although any CNS depressant can be effective, the benzodiazepines have the highest margin of safety and are therefore the preferred class of drug for the treatment of alcohol withdrawal. Short half-life benzodiazepines (e.g., oxazepam or lorazepam) may be especially useful for patients with liver impairment or pre-existent brain damage, but these drugs must be administered every 4 hours and it is possible that skipping a dose could precipitate seizures. Therefore most clinicians use the longer half-life drugs (e.g., diazepam or chlordiazepoxide), prescribing, for example, 25 mg of chlordiazepoxide or 10 mg of diazepam orally every 4 to 6 hours on the first day, decreasing the dose by at least 20 per cent of the original day's dose over each subsequent 24 hours.

The most effective treatment for severe withdrawal such as the DTs remains controversial. It is probable that the state of confusion and agitation will persist for 3 to 5 days regardless of the pharmacologic intervention used, and drugs are given primarily to control behavior rather than to change the course of the syndrome. Many clinicians recommend using benzodiazepines, and doses as large as 300 mg or more of chlordiazepoxide per day are sometimes required. Other physicians use antipsychotic medications such as thioridazine or haloperidol to control behavior, although these drugs have no place in the treatment of mild withdrawal symptoms.

For the usual mildly to moderately severe withdrawal, vitamins, general supports, and the judicious use of benzodiazepines are all that is required. Most patients present for treatment in an overhydrated—not dehydrated—state and so intravenous fluids are rarely needed. Similarly, when seizures or "rum fits" appear, they are usually single and most often respond to benzodiazepine; there is little evidence that anticonvulsants such as phenytoin are effective.

Although alcohol withdrawal is often treated in a hospital, efforts to reduce health care costs have resulted in increasing data about the appropriateness of outpatient detoxification for alcoholics with mild abstinence syndromes (Hayashida et al., 1989). This method is appropriate for patients in good physical condition who demonstrate mild signs of withdrawal despite low BALs and for those without a history of DTs or withdrawal seizures. Such individuals still require a careful physical examination, evaluation of blood tests, vitamin supplementation, and appropriate doses of a benzodiazepine. The drug is given in a 1- to 2-day supply and should be administered by the patient or spouse four times a day. Patients are asked to return daily for evaluation of vital signs, and the patient's family or friends are told to bring him or her to the emergency room if signs and symptoms of severe withdrawal escalate.

Finally, many municipalities have opted to take advantage of the relatively mild intensity of withdrawal symptoms by establishing "social model" detoxification programs. Here, monies are saved by offering a minimal amount of medical care and no prescription medications. In the optimal setting, patients are screened to rule out severe medical problems, recent seizures, or a history of severe DTs. The severely impaired individuals are referred to an inpatient medically oriented treatment program. The remainder are given nutrition, vitamins, the opportunity to rest, and a supportive environment in which reassurance and education help them to minimize their discomfort.

Alternative pharmacologic approaches for alcohol withdrawal have been presented in the litera-

ture, but *none* offers the same advantageous balance between cost and efficacy. β-Blockers such as propranolol (Inderol) and α-adrenergic agonists such as clonidine (Catapres) cause sedation and help dampen withdrawal-related changes in pulse, blood pressure, sweating, and tremor. These drugs, however, have side effects that are more severe than those of the benzodiazepines, and they do nothing to decrease the risk for seizures or to decrease the chances the individual will develop severe agitated confusion. In the context of adequate benzodiazepine levels, no additional anticonvulsant medications are required, making the prescription of clonazepam (Klonopin) or carbamazepine (Tegretol) redundant. Moreover, the latter medications are more expensive than the usual benzodiazepines and are associated with significant additional dangers not seen with diazepam or related drugs. Research to date has not supported any significant role for magnesium sulfate. Thus in addition to general support and vitamins, the average alcohol-dependent individual requires only benzodiazepines for the appropriate treatment of withdrawal.

Rehabilitation

Alcoholics who agree to enter treatment can be referred to inpatient or outpatient programs. In general, most rehabilitation efforts follow the general guidelines of increasing the level of motivation for abstinence and helping the patient to reestablish a lifestyle free of alcohol. There is little convincing evidence that one type of program is superior to any other, nor are there well documented guidelines to help the clinician decide whether to use inpatient or outpatient rehabilitation.

Reflecting the fact that inpatient care is much more expensive, outpatient rehabilitation is attractive. There are common sense guidelines that can help identify those individuals for whom the more intrusive and expensive inpatient care might be more appropriate. Such care includes hospitalization if (1) the patient has medical problems that are difficult to treat outside a hospital; (2) there is enough depression or confusion or other psychiatric symptoms to interfere with outpatient care; (3) the patient has such severe life crises that it is difficult to deal with him or her as an outpatient; (4) outpatient treatment has been attempted but failed; or (5) the patient lives too far from the treatment center to participate in outpatient care. If an inpatient program is required, it makes sense that those with severe medical problems are treated in a program associated with a medical facility, those with severe psychiatric difficulties might be preferentially referred to programs associated with a psychiatric unit, and the remaining patients might be most cost-effectively dealt with in a freestanding facility.

Whether carried out in an inpatient or an outpatient setting, efforts aimed at increasing levels of motivation for abstinence include lectures to the patients and families regarding the individual's responsibility for his or her own actions and the course of life problems that can be expected if drinking continues (i.e., the natural history of alcoholism). Motivation is also enhanced through association with AA for the patient and affiliated family groups for the spouse (AlAnon) and the children (Alateen). As part of group counseling or therapy sessions that occur almost daily, patients are repeatedly reminded of the issues of responsibility and problems likely to be experienced in the future. A number of pamphlets and readings can also help with the process of education, including a book developed specifically for the purpose (Schuckit, 1995b).

Patients are also taught how to readjust to a life without alcohol. Important topics for discussion during group counseling include how to occupy free time now that alcohol is no longer an option, how to deal with friends and colleagues who insist that alcohol should not be a problem and the individual should return to drinking, mechanisms for dealing with anger in the spouse and children as well as other relatives, how to deal with job and other environmental stressors that have in the past been dealt with by heavy drinking, and so on. Most groups focus on relatively superficial day-to-day life experiences. This process is begun on a several times per week basis during the inpatient or most intensive outpatient mode, and it must be continued for at least 6 months or longer on at least on a once a week basis as part of aftercare. Of course, affiliation with AA offers the individual the model of many people who have been through similar experiences, gives a sober peer group, and for those who so desire offers a series of steps to be followed in not only staying sober but rebuilding a more fulfilling life.

With the exception of vitamins and short-term use of benzodiazepines during acute withdrawal, the role of medications in alcoholic rehabilitation is limited. As part of a protracted abstinence syndrome, most alcoholics experience decreasing levels of sleep problems and anxiety symptoms for 3 to 6 months after abstinence is achieved. These problems, while ongoing, can be dealt with through education, reassurance that improvement will occur, and behavior modification through which patients are discouraged from taking naps, advised to avoid caffeinated beverages during the evening, told to establish a regular retiring and awakening time (behavioral approaches that improve sleeping patterns), and counseled on how to recognize early signs of escalating anxiety and experiment with alternative behaviors for anxiety release (e.g., exercise, hobbies, meditation, biofeedback). There is no place for sleeping pills or antianxiety drugs in the treatment of the average primary alcoholic after acute withdrawal is completed. Similarly, it is likely that no higher a percentage of alcoholics require antidepressant medications, lithium, or antianxiety drugs than is true in the general population.

One medication that has been used in alcohol rehabilitation is disulfiram (Antabuse), usually prescribed in doses of 250 mg/day. Unfortunately, this medication has dangers of potential contribution to neuropathies and irreversible liver failure, and it is possible that disulfiram contributes to the risk for cardiovascular disease. Extensive clinical trials have been unable to document the superiority of disulfiram over placebo (Fuller et al., 1986). In light of the lack of convincing evidence of efficacy and the documentation of risks for this drug, as well as the possibility of a severe reaction to alcohol while on the medication, it is difficult to recommend this agent for the average patient. It is probable that the use of disulfiram should be reserved for individuals who have shown that it is only on this drug that they have been able to maintain abstinence in the past or those for whom other treatments have been unsuccessful.

Additional pharmacologic approaches are presently being evaluated. However, there are too few double-blind controlled trials to justify their routine use. Probably the most promising of these agents is naltrexone (Trexan) (Volpicelli et al., 1992). This narcotic antagonist appears to have little impact on the craving for alcohol and is not associated with any significant decrease in the proportion of individuals who "slip" back to the use of alcohol during follow-up. However, once alcohol use begins, for patients taking this drug the period of alcohol intake appears to be significantly shorter. A second series of studies have demonstrated in both animal and human models that one type of antidepressant drug, the serotonin reuptake inhibitors, such as fluoxetine (Prozac), decreases alcohol intake at levels of perhaps 10 to 20 per cent (Naranjo et al., 1992). This impact has not been demonstrated to be associated with clinically significant levels of improvement in alcohol-dependent men and women after treatment, however. Finally, there are some interesting data indicating that the nonbenzodiazepine antianxiety drug buspirone (Buspar) might be of some use in helping people stay sober during the early phase after detoxification (Kranzler et al., 1994; Tollefson et al., 1992), but these results require replication before they can have an impact on clinical care. All of these treatments must be viewed as experimental, although the research literature might produce more compelling evidence in future years.

In summary, confrontation, detoxification, and rehabilitation of alcohol-abusing patients is an important part of the daily practice of family medicine. It is in our own best interests, as well as in those of our patients, to learn how to utilize the history, pattern of laboratory results, and series of medical problems to identify those individuals who are likely to fulfill criteria for alcoholism. Once a careful history taken from the patient and resource person establishes the presence of this important diagnosis, repeated firm but gentle confrontations are often required to persuade the individual to admit that intervention is appropriate. The next step in this process is to carry out appropriate detoxification measures; many alcoholics can be treated as outpatients following a good physical examination and with the judicious use of vitamins and short-term prescription of a benzodiazepine. Rehabilitation follows a series of common sense guidelines and frequently succeeds. The characteristics of the patient are often the best indicators of the outcome. There are ample data to conclude that for those individuals with families and jobs who are willing to admit their alcoholism and enter a rehabilitation program, two thirds to three fourths are likely to achieve and maintain long-term abstinence. When clinicians ignore the alcohol-related life problems and do not carry out the procedures necessary for an effective series of confrontations, difficulties are likely to continue, the patient is likely to experience deterioration in social functioning and in multiple body systems, and the life-span can be significantly shortened.

REFERENCES

American Psychiatric Association: Diagnostic Criteria from the DSM-IV. Washington, DC, American Psychiatric Press, 1994.

Begleiter H, Porjesz B, Bihari B: Auditory brainstem potentials in sons of alcoholic fathers. Alcohol Clin Exp Res 11:477, 1987.

Bikle DD, Genant HK, Cann D, et al: Bone disease in alcohol abuse. Ann Intern Med 103:42, 1985.

Boyd J, Weissman M, Thompson W, et al: Different definitions of alcoholism. Am J Psychiatry 140:1309, 1983.

Brown SA, Schuckit MA: Changes in depression among abstinent alcoholics. J Stud Alcohol 49:412, 1988.

Criqui MH: Alcohol consumption, blood pressure, lipids, and cardiovascular mortality. Alcohol Clin Exp Res 10:564, 1986.

Donahue RP, Abbott RD, Reed DM, et al: Alcohol and hemorrhagic stroke. JAMA 255:2311, 1986.

Drew LRH: Alcoholism as a self-limiting disease. Q J Stud Alcohol 29:956, 1968.

Editorial: Dying for a drink? Lancet 2:1249, 1987.

Ehlers C, Schuckit MA: EEG response to ethanol in sons of alcoholics. Psychopharmacol Bull 24:434, 1988.

Estrin WJ: Alcoholic cerebellar degeneration is not a dose-dependent phenomenon. Alcohol Clin Exp Res 11:372, 1987.

Frank D, Raicht RF: Alcohol-induced liver disease. Alcohol Clin Exp Res 9:66, 1985.

Fuller RK, Branchey L, Brightwell DR, et al: Disulfiram treatment of alcoholism: A Veterans Administration cooperative study. JAMA 256:1449, 1986.

Goodwin DW: Alcoholism and genetics. Arch Gen Psychiatry 42:171, 1985.

Goodwin DW, Guze SB: Psychiatric Diagnosis, 5th edition. New York, Oxford University Press, 1994.

Grant I: Alcohol and the brain: Neuropsychological correlates. Consult Clin Psychol 55:310, 1987.

Gurling HMD, Phil M, Grant S, et al: The genetic and cultural transmission of alcohol use, alcoholism, cigarette smoking and coffee drinking: A review and an example using a log linear cultural transmission model. Br J Addict 80:269, 1985.

Harper C, Kril J, Daly J: Are we drinking our neurones away? BMJ 294:534, 1987.

Hayashida M, Alterman AI, McLellan AT, et al: Comparative effectiveness and costs of inpatient and outpatient detoxification. N Engl J Med 320:358, 1989.

Helzer J, Robins L, Taylor J, et al: The extent of long-term moderate drinking among alcoholics. N Engl J Med 312:1678, 1985.

Irwin M, Baird S, Smith TL, et al: Use of laboratory tests to monitor heavy drinking by alcoholics men discharged from a treatment program. Am J Psychiatry 145:595, 1988.

Kendler KS, Neale MC, Heath AC, et al: A twin-family study of alcoholism in women. Am J Psychiatry 151:707, 1994.

Kranzler HR, Burleson JA, Del Boca FK, et al: Buspirone treatment of anxious alcoholics: A placebo-controlled trial. Arch Gen Psychiatry 51:720, 1994.

Lang RM, Borow KM, Neumann A, et al: Adverse cardiac effects of acute alcohol ingestion in young adults. Ann Intern Med 102:742, 1985.

Lieber CS: Alcohol and the liver: 1984 update. Hepatology 4:1243, 1984.

Ludwig AM: Cognitive process associated with "spontaneous" recovery from alcoholism. J Stud Alcohol 46:53, 1985.

Morrow-Tlucak M, Ernhart DB: Maternal prenatal substance abuse and behavior at age 3 years. Alcohol Clin Exp Res 11:225, 1987.

Naranjo CA, Poulos CX, Bermner KE, et al: Citalopram decreases desirability, liking, and consumption of alcohol in alcohol-dependent drinkers. Clin Pharmacol Ther 51:729, 1992.

Neubuerger OW, Miller SI, Schmitz RE, et al: Replicable abstinence rates in an alcoholism treatment program. JAMA 248:960, 1982.

Rapaport MH, Tipp JE, Schuckit MA: A comparison of ICD-10 and DSM-III-R criteria for substance abuse and dependence. Am J Drug Alcohol Abuse 19:143, 1993.

Robins LN, Helzer JE, Guze SB: Lifetime prevalence of specific psychiatric disorders in three sites. Arch Gen Psychiatry 41:949, 1984.

Saunders JB: Alcohol: An important cause of hypertension. BMJ 294:1045, 1987.

Schuckit MA: Overview: Epidemiology of alcoholism. *In* Schuckit MA (ed): Alcohol Patterns and Problems. Series in Psychosocial Epidemiology, Vol. 5. New Brunswick, NJ, Rutgers University Press, 1985a, pp 1–42.

Schuckit MA: The clinical implications of primary diagnostic groups among alcoholics. Arch Gen Psychiatry 42:1043, 1985b.

Schuckit MA: Genetics and the risk for alcoholism. JAMA 254:2614, 1985c.

Schuckit MA: Genetic and clinical implications of alcoholism and affective disorder. Am J Psychiatry 143:140, 1986.

Schuckit MA: Biological vulnerability to alcoholism. J Consult Clin Psychol 55:301, 1987.

Schuckit MA: Drug and Alcohol Abuse, 4th edition. New York, Plenum Press, 1995a.

Schuckit MA: Educate Yourself about Alcohol and Drugs: A People's Primer. New York, Plenum Press, 1995b.

Schuckit MA: Keeping current with the DSMs and substance use disorders. *In* Dunner D (ed): Current Psychiatric Therapy. Philadelphia, WB Saunders Company, 1993.

Schuckit MA: A clinical model of genetic influences in alcohol dependence. J Stud Alcohol 55:5, 1994a.

Schuckit MA: Low level of response to alcohol as a predictor of future alcoholism. Am J Psychiatry 151:184, 1994b.

Schuckit MA, Gold EO: A simultaneous evaluation of multiple

markers of ethanol/placebo challenges in sons of alcoholics and controls. Arch Gen Psychiatry 45:211, 1988.

Schuckit MA, Irwin M: Diagnosis of alcoholism. Med Clin North Am 72:1133, 1988.

Schuckit MA, Hesselbrock V: Alcohol dependence and anxiety disorders: What is the relationship? Am J Psychiatry 151:1723, 1994.

Schuckit MA, Smith TL, Anthenelli R, et al: Clinical course of alcoholism in 636 male inpatients. Am J Psychiatry 150:786, 1993.

Schuckit MA, Butters N, Lyn L, et al: Neuropsychologic deficits and the risk for alcoholism. Neuropsychopharmacology 1:45, 1987.

Tollefson GD, Montague-Clouse J, Tollefson SL: Treatment of comorbid generalized anxiety in a recently detoxified alcoholic population with a selective serotonergic drug (buspirone). J Clin Psychopharmacol 12:19, 1992.

Vaillant GE: Natural history of male alcoholism. Arch Gen Psychiatry 39:127, 1982.

Volpicelli JR, Alterman AI, Hayashida M, et al: Naltrexone in the treatment of alcohol dependence. Arch Gen Psychiatry 49:876, 1992.

CHAPTER 58
NICOTINE ADDICTION

ROBERT E. RAKEL and ALAN BLUM

The power of nicotine addiction became clear when I saw malnourished and hungry people trading food rations for cigarettes.

William Foege, M.D. (1989), commenting on refugee camps during the Nigerian Civil War

Tobacco smoking leads to a dependence on nicotine that is indistinguishable from other forms of drug dependence. The Diagnostic and Statistical Manual of Mental Disorders (DSM-IV) of the American Psychiatric Association (1994) classifies tobacco dependence as an addiction. In such a dependency, the drug is needed to maintain an optimal state of well-being. Nicotine, the habituating constituent of tobacco, meets the criteria for addiction, because a typical withdrawal syndrome occurs after smoking cessation. Nicotine is more addicting than cocaine because it is easier for addicts to break their addiction to cocaine and heroin than to nicotine (Krasnegor, 1979; Lee and D'Alonzo, 1993) (Fig. 58–1).

Cigarette smoking is the chief avoidable cause of death in our society. Each year smoking is responsible for 18 per cent of the total deaths in the United States. This is seven times more Americans than were killed in the Vietnam War. "Clearly, smoking has killed more Americans during this century than were killed in battle or died of war-related diseases in all wars ever fought by this nation" (Pollin and Ravenholt, 1984).

Approximately 40 per cent of all deaths from cancer and 21 per cent of deaths from cardiovascular disease are caused by smoking. Tobacco contributes to about 400,000 deaths annually in the United States, whereas only 25,000 die in motor vehicle accidents (McGinnis and Foege, 1993).

More young women than young men smoke cigarettes, and in 1986 lung cancer passed breast cancer as the leading cause of cancer death in women. Smoking kills 10,000 more women than breast cancer, yet we have a breast cancer awareness month and a great deal of attention focused on breast cancer but no public outcry against the needless deaths from lung cancer (Centers for Disease Control and Prevention, 1988).

Although cigarette smoking among adults declined from 42 to 27 per cent in the United States between 1964 and 1992 (following publication of the Surgeon General's first report on smoking and health in 1964), 28 per cent of men and 24 per cent of women continue to use tobacco daily. Approximately 1.3 million persons per year stop smoking. However, each day approximately 3000 individuals start smoking, most of whom are young (Pierce et al., 1989). Half of high-school seniors who smoke started by age 14 years. Almost half of all smokers born since 1935 started smoking before 18 years of age. Although 80 per cent of those who smoke say they would like to stop, only 20 per cent of those who try actually succeed in stopping for good. The likelihood of success in stopping increases with the number of attempts, and those with a college education are twice as likely to break the habit as are less educated smokers.

In 1964, only a single life insurance company, State Mutual of Massachusetts, offered a reduced price to nonsmokers. Today, virtually all life insurance companies, even those owned by tobacco conglomerates, now offer significant discounts to persons who do not smoke. Actuarial data leave little doubt that the average life expectancy of a 32-year-old man who smokes cigarettes is 72 years, compared with 79 years for someone who does not smoke. Smoking-related chronic obstructive pulmonary disease is the largest cause of disability payments, and lung cancer is no longer a rarity among men and women in their 40s.

Much is heard about the need to increase tobacco taxes to pay for the increased health care of those who smoke, but the tobacco industry has effectively blunted significant increases. By world standards, cigarette taxes in the United States are very low, ranking 22nd when tax is compared to total price. U.S. cigarette taxes average 30 per cent of the retail price, whereas the proportion in Denmark is 85 per cent, in Ireland 76 per cent, in India 75 per cent, and in Germany 73 per cent (*American Medical News*, September 5, 1994).

HEALTH RISKS ASSOCIATED WITH SMOKING

Cancer

Forty per cent of all cancer deaths are attributable to cigarette smoking. Besides lung cancer,

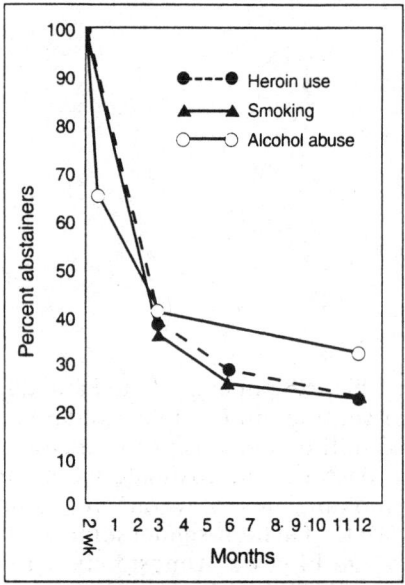

FIGURE 58–1. Relapse rates over time for heroin use, smoking, and alcohol abuse. (Adapted with permission from Hunt WA, Barnett LW, Branch LG: Relapse rates in addiction programs. J Clin Psychol 27:455, 1971; From Robinson MD: A workable approach to smoking cessation in the primary care office. Primary Care & Cancer 13(10):34, 1993, with permission.)

smoking is the major cause of cancers of the larynx, oral cavity, and esophagus (see Table 58–1). It is a contributory factor in cancers of the pancreas, bladder, kidney, stomach, and uterine cervix. Recent studies implicate smoking in leukemia, colon cancer, Graves' disease, depression, and renal disease in persons with diabetes mellitus. A dose-response relationship exists between smoking and all of these.

LUNG. Male smokers are 22 times more likely to develop lung cancer, and female smokers are 12 times more likely, when compared with those who have never smoked. There is a clear dose-response relationship between lung cancer risk and daily cigarette consumption, and those who smoke more than a pack of cigarettes a day have a risk that is at least 20 times that of nonsmokers.

Unfortunately, early detection does not improve the survival rate for lung cancer. The 5-year survival rate is less than 10 per cent and has not changed since the early 1960s. However, the risk of death from lung cancer is reduced when smoking is discontinued.

From 1950 to 1990, the death rate for lung cancer increased fourfold for men and sevenfold for women. Lung cancer is the principal cause of cancer death for both sexes, and smoking accounts for 87 per cent of lung cancer deaths.

LARYNX. The risk for laryngeal cancer is 20 to 30 times greater in the smoker. Seventy per cent of oral and 85 per cent of laryngeal cancer deaths are directly attributable to smoking.

ESOPHAGUS. Cigarette smoking is a factor in over half of the cases of esophageal cancer, and the 5-year survival rate is only about 3 per cent. Heavy smokers (more than one pack per day) have 10 times the mortality from esophageal cancer as do nonsmokers.

PANCREAS. An equally dismal picture occurs with cancer of the pancreas, for which the 5-year survival rate is only 2 per cent. Because of the nonspecific nature of presenting symptoms and the difficulty of making a diagnosis, the mean survival time after diagnosis is less than 6 months. Smokers have two to three times the risk of pancreatic cancer as do nonsmokers, and the risk is proportional to the amount smoked. Switching from nonfiltered to filtered cigarettes does not decrease the risk. Over one fourth of pancreatic cancer (27 per cent) is attributable to cigarette smoking (Silverman et al., 1994).

CERVIX UTERI AND OVARY. Women who smoke cigarettes have four times the risk of nonsmokers of developing cervical cancer. Even women who smoke only 100 cigarettes during their lifetimes more than double their risk of cervical cancer. The risk from smoking is greater in women under 30 years of age than in those older than 30 years (Slattery et al., 1989).

Constituents from cigarette smoke are distributed by the blood throughout the body and have been detected in the cervical mucus of smokers at levels 40 to 50 times those in the serum.

TABLE 58–1.   DISEASES OR CONDITIONS CAUSED DIRECTLY OR INDIRECTLY BY CIGARETTE SMOKING

Cancer	Cardiovascular	Respiratory	Pregnancy	Infants and Children	Other
Lung	Coronary heart disease	COPD (ephysema)	Growth	Low birth	Infertility
Larynx	Stroke	Bronchitis	retardation (low	weight	Impotence
Esophagus	Subarachnoid hemorrhage	Pneumonia	birth weight)	Congenital	Osteoporosis
Pancreas	Aortic aneurysm	Asthma	Preterm labor	abnormalities	Early menopause
Uterine cervix	Hypertension	Otitis media	Spontaneous	Sudden infant	Premature
Ovary	Peripheral vascular		abortion	death	wrinkling
Colon	disease		Abruptio	syndrome	Peptic ulcer
Bladder			placentae	Neonatal death	Alzheimer's disease
Kidney			Placenta previa		Graves' disease
Breast			Bleeding		Insomnia
Brain			Premature rupture		Depression
Blood (leukemia)			of membranes		

The risk of ovarian cancer is three times greater in women who smoke cigarettes (Qian et al., 1989).

BLADDER AND KIDNEY.   Forty per cent of bladder cancers are smoking related, and higher rates of kidney cancers also are noted among smokers. Smokers have three to four times the risk of developing bladder cancer as do people who never smoked. The kidneys and bladder are the final common pathway for the concentration of the toxic products of tobacco smoke and provide the longest direct exposure to carcinogens and radioactive substances, such as polonium-210 (^{210}Po), in tobacco smoke (Winters and Di Franza, 1982).

COLON AND RECTUM.   There is a strong relationship between smoking and colorectal cancer, but the induction period is about 35 years. This would explain why it is just beginning to show up in women, and shows that our efforts to prevent smoking among the young should be intensified (Giovannucci et al., 1994).

LEUKEMIA.   A greater than 50 per cent increased mortality from leukemia occurs in cigarette smokers (relative risk 1.53), and the response is dose related. Those smoking more than one pack per day have a twofold increased risk (Kinlen and Rogot, 1988). The risk is greatest for myeloid leukemia and acute nonlymphocytic leukemia. Approximately 14 per cent of all cases of leukemia in the United States may be due to cigarette smoking (Brownson et al., 1993). Overall, smoking cigarettes increases a person's risk of developing leukemia by 30 per cent.

Chronic Obstructive Pulmonary Disease

Cigarette smoking is the main cause of chronic obstructive pulmonary disease (COPD), which is the leading cause of disability in the United States. Changes in bronchi and the lung parenchyma are proportional to the amount of smoke inhaled. Cigarette smoke inhibits ciliary activity of the bronchial epithelium and the phagocytic activity of macrophages in the alveoli. This results in the decreased clearance of foreign material and bacteria from the lung, which leads to increased infection and tissue destruction.

Even after age 60 years, smokers who quit have better pulmonary function than those who continue smoking. Lung function is inversely related to the number of cigarettes smoked during one's lifetime. Smokers at age 65 or older who quit smoking before age 40 have pulmonary function levels similar to those of people who never smoked (Higgins et al., 1993).

Cardiovascular Disease

Coronary Heart Disease

Nicotine raises systolic blood pressure, heart rate, and cardiac output and causes vasoconstric-

tion. The relationship between cerebral vasoconstriction and anoxia and the intake of carbon monoxide resulting from cigarette smoking could explain the 50 per cent increase in automobile accidents in smokers. The symptoms associated with carbon monoxide intoxication can be a problem, especially for persons with an already compromised coronary circulation. Carbon monoxide has an affinity for hemoglobin (forming carboxyhemoglobin) that is 245 times stronger than that of oxygen. Thus, it reduces oxygen delivery to the myocardium and has a decidedly negative inotropic effect. Carboxyhemoglobin also lowers the threshold for ventricular fibrillation and could help explain the higher incidence of sudden death in those who smoke.

The risk of myocardial infarction is proportional to the number of cigarettes smoked. The trend toward the use of filtered cigarettes does not appear to have reduced the risk of coronary heart disease. Theoretically, filters on cigarettes reduce the amount of tar (the condensate of tobacco smoke that comprises over 3000 compounds, including more than 40 carcinogens), but they may increase the amount of carbon monoxide, thus contributing to the increased mortality from coronary heart disease. Persons who smoke cigarettes containing low amounts of nicotine have the same degree of risk of myocardial infarction as do those who smoke cigarettes containing larger amounts. Smokers of these low-dose cigarettes still have three times the risk of myocardial infarction as do nonsmokers (Kaufman et al., 1983). The good news is that the risk of sudden death decreases immediately on stopping, and the risk of myocardial infarction decreases within a few years of stopping to a level similar to that in men who have never smoked. This is true even in heavy smokers who have a positive family history of coronary heart disease (Rosenberg et al., 1985).

Three fourths of myocardial infarctions in women below the age of 50 years have been attributed to smoking (Slone et al., 1978). The Chief Medical Examiner of Dade County, Florida states that a woman between 40 and 50 years of age who dies suddenly is considered to be a cigarette smoker until proven otherwise (J. Davis, personal communication, 1977). The risk of myocardial infarction increases progressively, to as much as 20-fold in persons smoking 35 or more cigarettes per day. There is no safe level of smoking. Women who smoke only one to four cigarettes a day have a 2.5 times greater risk of coronary heart disease. Women who smoke and use oral contraceptives have a risk of heart attack that is 10 times greater than that of women who do neither.

Silent ischemia probably comprises the majority of all cardiac ischemic events. Patients with coronary heart disease who smoke have three times as many episodes of silent ischemia as do nonsmokers, and the duration of each is 12 times longer

(Barry et al., 1989). Frequent episodes of myocardial ischemia, even though asymptomatic, must damage the heart. Because smoking also increases platelet adhesiveness and lowers high-density lipoprotein cholesterol, the association with a higher incidence of myocardial infarction is no surprise.

Benefits from stopping smoking can be demonstrated at all ages. There is no decrease in benefit as one gets older, so it is still worthwhile for someone over age 65 to break the addiction (Hermanson et al., 1988; LaCroix et al., 1991). This benefit can be demonstrated in the cerebral as well as the coronary circulation. Elderly individuals who stop smoking have significantly higher cerebral perfusion levels than do those who continue to smoke. Even those who have smoked for 30 to 40 years have improved cerebral circulation within a relatively short time after stopping smoking (Rogers et al., 1985).

Persons who smoke more than one pack of cigarettes a day are four times more likely to develop Alzheimer's disease as are nonsmokers. As with other smoking-related diseases, this one is also dose dependent; those smoking less than one pack a day are at 1.6 times the risk.

Stroke

Stroke is the third most common cause of death in the United States. Although hypertension is the greatest risk factor for stroke, cigarette smoking is also a significant factor. The incidence of stroke among smokers is 50 per cent higher than among nonsmokers (40 per cent higher in men and 60 per cent higher among women) (Wolf et al., 1988).

The risk of stroke increases in proportion to the amount of smoking; it is twice as great in those who smoke more than 40 cigarettes per day than in those smoking less than 10 cigarettes per day.

Compared with women who have never smoked, the risk of stroke increases 2.2-fold in women smoking 1 to 14 cigarettes per day and 3.7-fold in women smoking 25 or more cigarettes daily (Colditz et al., 1988). A clear dose-response relationship has also been noted by Bonita and associates (1986). They found a threefold increase in the risk of stroke in smokers compared with nonsmokers (Fig. 58–2). The risk is 5.6 times higher in persons smoking more than one pack of cigarettes daily. Cigarette smokers who are also hypertensive have a 20-fold increased risk of stroke.

Smoking may increase the likelihood of thrombosis by increasing the serum fibrinogen, by enhancing platelet aggregation, and by increasing blood viscosity.

The risk of stroke declines rapidly after cessation of smoking and after 5 years is at the level of nonsmokers. This emphasizes that it is never too late to quit no matter how long one has been smoking.

Subarachnoid Hemorrhage

Habitual smoking increases the risk of subarachnoid hemorrhage 3.9 times for men and 3.7 times

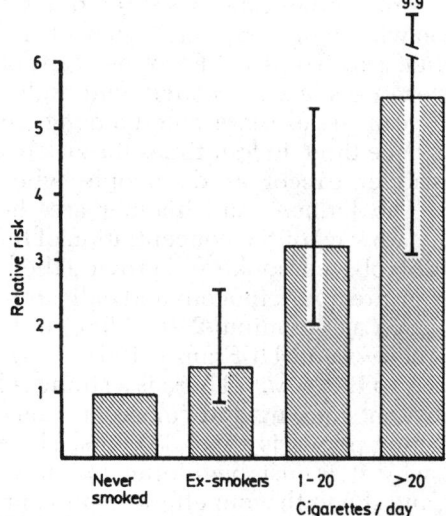

FIGURE 58–2. Cigarette smoking and risk of stroke, adjusted for age and sex. Bars indicate 95 per cent confidence limits. (From Bonita R, Scragg R, Stewart A: Cigarette smoking and risk of premature stroke in men and women. BMJ 293:6, 1986, with permission.)

for women. The risk increases to 22 times that of nonsmokers in women who both smoke and use oral contraceptives (Bell and Symon, 1979).

One theory is that structural damage occurs in the wall of cerebral vessels, causing aneurysms that are more likely to rupture. In a meta-analysis review of all available data regarding cigarette smoking and stroke, Shinton and Beevers (1989) confirmed the 50 per cent increased risk of stroke associated with cigarette smoking and found that the risk of subarachnoid hemorrhage tripled and was greater in women than men.

Other Diseases and Conditions

GRAVES' DISEASE. Smoking appears to be one of the multiple factors causing Graves' disease in genetically predisposed individuals. Family members of patients with Graves' disease may be able to prevent the development of this disease by stopping smoking (Prummel and Wiersinga, 1993).

DIABETES MELLITUS. The risk of diabetes increases with the number of cigarettes smoked. People smoking more than one pack a day have 1.5 times the risk of developing diabetes as do those who smoke 1 to 14 cigarettes. Albuminuria as a sign of early renal damage and retinopathy is greater in patients with insulin-dependent diabetes mellitus who smoke and can be shown to improve significantly if the person stops smoking (Chase et al., 1991).

DEPRESSION. Smokers are more likely to experience major depression than nonsmokers, and the incidence increases steadily with the number of cigarettes smoked. Kendler and associates (1993) suggested that this could be due to genes that predispose to both conditions.

INSOMNIA. Smokers are more likely than nonsmokers to have insomnia, and as a consequence to feel tired in the morning. Smokers will be more restless during sleep, and more likely to awaken tired and then smoke during the day for the stimulation. However, smokers also consume more alcohol and caffeine than nonsmokers, which will contribute to insomnia (Lexcen and Hicks, 1993).

WRINKLES. Every day 3000 children try their first cigarette; 750 of these children will die of a smoking-related disease, but fewer than 50 will die as a result of auto accidents or murder. We are not very effective in getting the message across to this group—by talking about disease, we may not be speaking their language. The fact that smoking causes wrinkles, bad breath, and yellow teeth may be a more effective message than evidence that smoking kills. Premature wrinkling (crow's feet) increases with the number of cigarettes smoked. Kadunce et al. (1991) found that heavy smokers are five times more likely to have wrinkles than are nonsmokers.

OTHER TOBACCO-RELATED HEALTH RISKS

Filtered Cigarettes

A mistaken popular belief is that filtered brands of cigarettes (which now comprise more than 97 per cent of those sold in the United States) are safer than nonfiltered cigarettes. Low-tar and low-nicotine filtered cigarettes are now advertised widely. Because the addiction is to nicotine, people who smoke low-nicotine cigarettes undergo "compensatory smoking," in which they inhale more frequently and more deeply, in order to maintain their blood nicotine levels. As a result, the tar intake also increases, changing a low-tar cigarette to the high-tar category. Smokers who take 14 puffs per cigarette receive 58 per cent more tar than those taking the standard 8.7 puffs per cigarette. Some manufacturers include perforations in the filter to dilute the smoke with air, advertising these as ultra-low-tar cigarettes. Many smokers, however, block the holes with their lips or their fingers in order to obtain undiluted smoke with a higher concentration of nicotine (Kozlowski et al., 1980).

Cigarettes with reduced yields of nicotine and carbon monoxide are not safer. The fourfold increased risk of myocardial infarction does not vary according to the nicotine content, and the degree of risk is proportionate to the number of cigarettes smoked (Palmer et al., 1989). Nicotine blood levels are similar for cigarette smokers, pipe smokers, and users of snuff, despite the different methods of absorption.

Smokeless Tobacco

There are two types of smokeless tobacco: snuff, which is dry or moist, and chewing (spitting) tobacco, which comes as loose-leaf, plug, or twist. Use of these substances increases the frequency of oral-pharyngeal cancers and gum recession. Long-term users of snuff have a 50-fold increased risk for cancer of the cheek and gum (Koop and Luoto, 1982). Leukoplakia is found in 18 to 64 per cent of users (Connolly et al., 1986).

A large percentage of the 10 million users of smokeless tobacco in the United States are male adolescents who mistakenly believe this is a relatively safe alternative to smoking. Most users start at 10 to 12 years of age (Evans, 1988) (Fig. 58–3).

Smokeless tobacco contains the same carcinogens as cigarette tobacco, but some of them are present in much greater concentration. Nitrosamines, which are powerful chemical carcinogens, are present at levels up to 14,000 times higher than the federal government allows in bacon and beer (Connolly et al., 1986).

Involuntary (Passive) Smoking

The effects of tobacco on nonsmokers (passive smoking) can be significant. An estimated 3000 nonsmokers die each year from inhaling second-hand smoke. In addition, 15 per cent of the American public is allergic to cigarette smoke. Two thirds of the smoke from a burning cigarette never reaches a smoker's lungs, but instead goes directly into the air. *Sidestream smoke* is that which is emitted into the air from a smoldering cigarette between puffs, whereas *mainstream smoke* is that which the smoker inhales directly during puffing. Although diluted by air prior to being inhaled, sidestream smoke contains greater amounts of toxic substances than does mainstream smoke because of a lower combustion temperature and lack of filtration through the cigarette (Table 58–2).

Over 3000 different chemicals have been identified in cigarette smoke, and at least 40 of these are known carcinogens. The U.S. Environmental Protection Agency has determined that environmental tobacco smoke is a "Class A" human carcinogen, in the same class as asbestos, mustard gas, arsenic, and benzene. We have cleared our schools of asbestos, but three fifths of schools have yet to ban smoking. In addition to the 3000 lung cancer deaths a year among nonsmokers, there are almost 40,000 heart disease deaths linked to secondhand smoke.

A nonsmoker who spends 1 hour in a smoke-filled car on a commuter train inhales as much as if he or she had smoked nine filtered cigarettes (Aronow, 1979). It has been estimated that a nonsmoking musician who plays in a smoke-filled club and lives with a chain-smoking roommate inhales

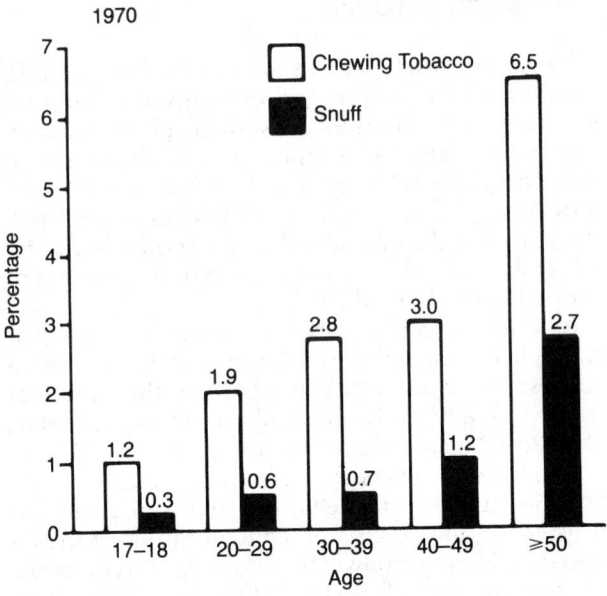

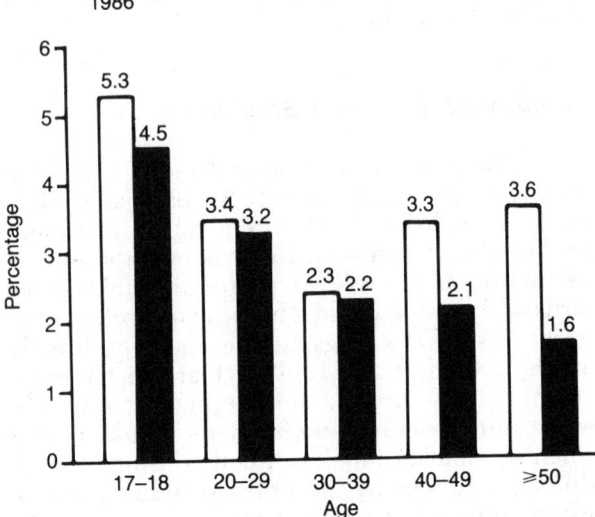

FIGURE 58–3. Prevalence of chewing tobacco and snuff use among men, 1970 (NHIS) and 1986 (AUTS). (From U.S. Department of Health and Human Services. Reducing the Health Consequences of Smoking: 25 Years of Progress, A Report of the Surgeon General. DHHS Publication no. (CDC) 89-8411, Prepublication version, January, 1989.)

TABLE 58–2. TOXIC AND TUMORIGENIC AGENTS OF CIGARETTE SMOKE; RATIO OF SIDESTREAM SMOKE (SS) TO MAINSTREAM SMOKE (MS)

	Amount per Cigarette	SS/MS Ratio
Gas Phase		
Carbon dioxide	10–80 mg	8.1*
Carbon monoxide	0.5–26 mg	2.5*
Nitrogen oxides (NO$_x$)	16–600 µg	4.7–5.8
Ammonia	10–130 µg	44–73
Hydrogen cyanide	280–550 µg	0.17–0.37
Hydrazine	32 µg	3
Formaldehyde	20–90 µg	51
Acetone	100–940 µg	2.5–3.2
Acrolein	10–140 µg	12
Acetonitrile	60–160 µg	10
Pyridine	32 µg	10
3-Vinylpyridine	23 µg	28
N-Nitrosodimethylamine	4–180 ng	10–830
N-Nitrosoethylmethylamine	1.0–40 ng	5–12
N-Nitrosodiethylamine	0.1–28 ng	4–25
N-Nitrosopyrrolidine	0–110 ng	3–76
Particulate Phase		
Total particulate matter (TPM)	0.1–40 mg	1.3–1.9*
Nicotine	0.06–2.3 mg	2.6–3.3*
Toluene	108 µg	5.6
Phenol	20–150 µg	2.6
Catechol	40–280 µg	0.7
Stigmasterol	53 µg	0.8
Total phytosterols	130 µg	0.8
Naphthalene	2.8 µg	16
1-Methylnaphthalene	1.2 µg	26
2-Methylnaphthalene	1.0 µg	29
Phenanthrene	2.0–80 µg	2.1
Benz(a)anthracene	10–70 µg	2.7
Pyrene	15–90 ng	1.9–3.6
Benzo(a)pyrene	8–40 ng	2.7–3.4
Quinoline	1.7 µg	11
Methylquinoline	6.7 µg	11
Harmane	1.1–3.1 µg	0.7–2.7
Norharmane	3.2–8.1 µg	1.4–4.3
Aniline	100–1200 ng	30
α-Toluidine	32 ng	19
1-Naphthylamine	1.0–22 ng	39
2-Naphthylamine	4.3–27 ng	39
4-Aminobiphenyl	2.4–4.6 ng	31
N'-Nitrosonornicotine	0.2–3.7 µg	1–5
NNK†	0.12–0.44 µg	1–8
N'-Nitrosoanatabine	0.15–4.6 µg	1–7
N-Nitrosodiethanolamine	0–40 ng	1.2

* In cigarettes with perforated filter tips, the SS/MS ratio rises with increasing air dilution. In the case of smoke dilution with air to 17 percent, the SS/MS ratio for TPM rises to 2.14, that for CO$_2$ to 36.5, that for CO to 23.5, and that for nicotine to 13.1.

† NNK, 4-(methylnitrosamino)-1-(3-pyridyl)-butanone.

From The Health Consequences of Smoking: Cancer. A Report of the Surgeon General. DHHS Publication no. (PHS) 82-50179. Rockville, MD, U.S. Department of Health and Human Services, Public Health Service, Office on Smoking and Health, 1982.

the equivalent of 27 cigarettes a day. Food service workers are also at increased risk. We protect the patron in restaurants who prefers a table in a nonsmoking area, but the workers go unprotected. Siegel (1993) found the level of tobacco smoke in bars to be four to six times higher than that in offices, and that in restaurants to be almost twice as high. He believes that this may result in a 50 per cent higher lung cancer risk among food service workers.

Hirayama (1981) demonstrated the increased risk of lung cancer in nonsmoking housewives exposed to the secondhand cigarette smoke of their husbands (Fig. 58–4). The risk from passive smok-

ing was one half to one third that of direct smoking. A direct dose-response relationship was observed, with the annual mortality from lung cancer being 8.7 per 100,000 for women whose husbands smoked only occasionally and 18.1 per 100,000 for those whose husbands smoked 20 or more cigarettes daily. The wives of heavy smokers had a two-

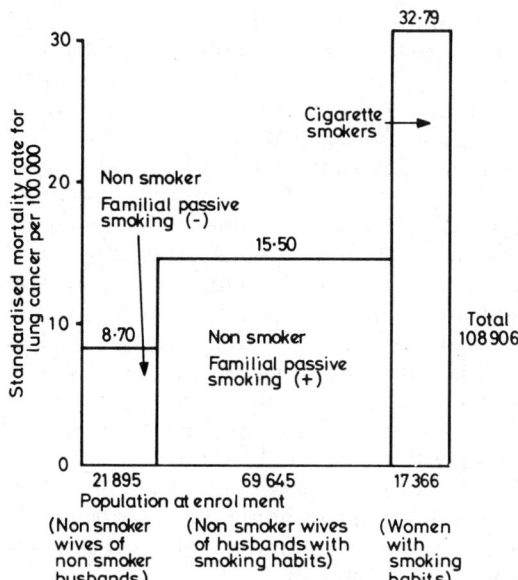

FIGURE 58–4. Lung cancer mortality in women according to presence or absence of direct and familial indirect smoking. (From Hirayama T: Nonsmoking wives of heavy smokers have a higher risk of lung cancer: A study from Japan. BMJ 282:1983, 1981, with permission.)

fold greater risk of dying from lung cancer than did wives of nonsmoking men. Their risk was half that of women smokers.

A similar study in Sweden found that women with husbands who smoke have three times the risk of developing lung cancer as do wives of non-smoking husbands (Pershagen et al., 1987). To date, 14 studies have shown an association between being married to a smoker and having an increased risk of lung cancer. Overall, about one third of lung cancers occur in nonsmokers living with smokers (Fontham et al., 1994).

Cancer risk appears proportional to the total amount of smoke to which an individual is exposed during a lifetime. The risk of developing cancer of any form appears dose dependent, increasing by at least 50 per cent in persons exposed only during childhood or adulthood, and more than doubling for those exposed during both periods. The risk of cancer increases significantly with increasing exposure. It is greatest for cancer of the breast and cervix, and for leukemia and lymphoma (Garfinkle, 1980; Raeburn, 1989).

Passive smoking increases the risk of cervical cancer. Slattery and associates (1989) found that passive exposure to smoke for 3 hours a day increases the risk of a woman's developing cervical cancer 3.43 times. One hour of passive smoking exposes the person to carcinogenic nitrosamines equivalent to smoking one half a pack of filtered cigarettes. Thus, the risk of cancer from passive smoking can be as great as that from personal cigarette smoking.

The risks of passive smoking extend far beyond

cancer. It is estimated that tobacco smoke in the home and workplace could be responsible for the deaths of 46,000 nonsmokers annually in the United States. Most of these are due to heart disease, making passive smoking the third leading preventable cause of death after alcohol and smoking itself. It is estimated that the risk of myocardial infarction is three times higher for a woman whose husband smokes (Wells, 1988).

Effects on Children

Parents who smoke are more likely to have children who will take up smoking. Indeed, 75 per cent of those who smoke cigarettes had at least one parent who smoked. The risk of a child taking up smoking doubles with each additional adult family member who smokes. Over 50 per cent of children under 5 years of age live in homes with at least one adult smoker. Children of smoking parents are innocent victims (involuntary smokers) and have been shown to be more likely to suffer more bronchitis and pneumonia during their first year of life and more otitis media when older. Numerous studies have shown that they have an increased incidence of cough, bronchitis, and pneumonia that is proportional to the number of cigarettes smoked by the parents, particularly the mother. In fact, children of parents who smoke at least half a pack a day have nearly twice the risk of hospitalization for a respiratory illness. Asthma is also more prevalent in children whose mothers smoke, and their stature is retarded in proportion to the number of smokers in the home (Charlton, 1994; Rantakallio, 1978). Passive smoking has also been blamed for some instances of sudden infant death syndrome.

Small children are victimized more by passive smoking than are adults. Because of more rapid breathing, they inhale larger amounts of harmful substances. Children exposed to their parents' cigarette smoke have six times the average number of respiratory infections. They also have deficits in growth and in intellectual and emotional development, as well as more behavior disorders, such as hyperactivity.

The risk of cancer is increased by 50 per cent in children of men who smoke. The risk of a child developing hematopoietic cancer is 4.6 times greater if both parents smoke (Sandler et al., 1985a).

Effects on Pregnancy

A dose-response relationship also exists for cigarette smoking during pregnancy. The more a pregnant woman smokes, the lower the infant's birth weight is likely to be. On average, babies born to women who smoke during pregnancy are 200 gm lighter than those born to comparable nonsmokers (Fig. 58–5). Heavy smokers have a 130 per cent increased incidence of newborns weighing less than 2500 gm. However, a woman who gives up smoking by her fourth month of gestation will have

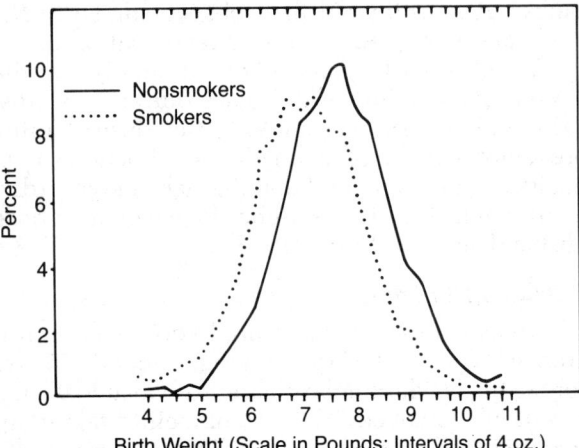

FIGURE 58–5. Percentage distribution by birth weight of infants of mothers who did not smoke during pregnancy and of those who smoked one pack or more of cigarettes per day. (From U.S. Department of Health, Education, and Welfare: Smoking and Health. A Report of the Surgeon General. DHEW Publication no. (PHS) 79-50066. Washington, DC, U.S. Department of Health, Education, and Welfare, Public Health Service, Office on Smoking and Health, 1979, p 8–43.)

the same risk as a nonsmoker. Mainous and Hueston (1994a) found that women who stopped smoking in the first trimester had 26 per cent fewer preterm deliveries and 18 per cent fewer low-birthweight infants. Each cigarette smoked per day is associated with a 10-gm decrease in infant birth weight, and there is a direct relationship between degree of smoking and infant weight reduction, with infants born to light, moderate, and heavy smokers weighing 96, 183, and 200 gm less, respectively, than those born to nonsmokers (Abell et al., 1991). Pregnant women who do not smoke but whose passive smoke exposure is high are twice as likely as those with low exposure to have a low birth weight infant (Mainous and Hueston, 1994b)

The term "fetal tobacco syndrome" provides a label for fetal growth retardation when (1) the mother smoked five or more cigarettes a day throughout the pregnancy, (2) there was no evidence of hypertension in the mother, (3) the newborn has symmetrical growth retardation; and (4) no other cause of intrauterine growth retardation is obvious (Nieburg et al., 1985).

Transplacental exposure to substances absorbed from the mother's smoking during pregnancy may predispose the infant to cancer later in life (Sandler et al., 1985b). Infants born to women who smoke during pregnancy show a significant accumulation of the cigarette smoke toxins when tested 1 to 3 days after delivery. Although the levels of such toxins were highest in women who smoked, they were also significantly higher in mothers who were passive smokers than in nonsmokers (Eliopoulos et al., 1994).

The risk of spontaneous abortion in heavy smokers is 1.7 times that in nonsmokers. Smoking dur-

ing pregnancy increases the incidence of abruptio placentae, placenta previa, bleeding during pregnancy, and premature rupture of the membranes. It also increases the incidence of premature births and perinatal deaths (Fig. 58–6). Obviously, pregnancy is an opportune time for the family physician to encourage women to discontinue smoking.

About 25 per cent of women who smoke at the beginning of their pregnancy will stop on their own sometime during the 9 months. Aggressive intervention programs by physicians could influence another 30 per cent to stop. The greatest effort should be directed toward pregnant unmarried white women, because they are 40 per cent more likely to smoke than are nonpregnant white women (Williamson et al., 1989).

There is strong experimental evidence that maternal smoking causes fetal hypoxia. This could explain the increased incidence of congenital abnormalities noted in babies of smokers (Fig. 58–7). The offspring of mothers who smoke during the 3 months before or after conception are twice as likely to have a cleft palate as are those of nonsmok-

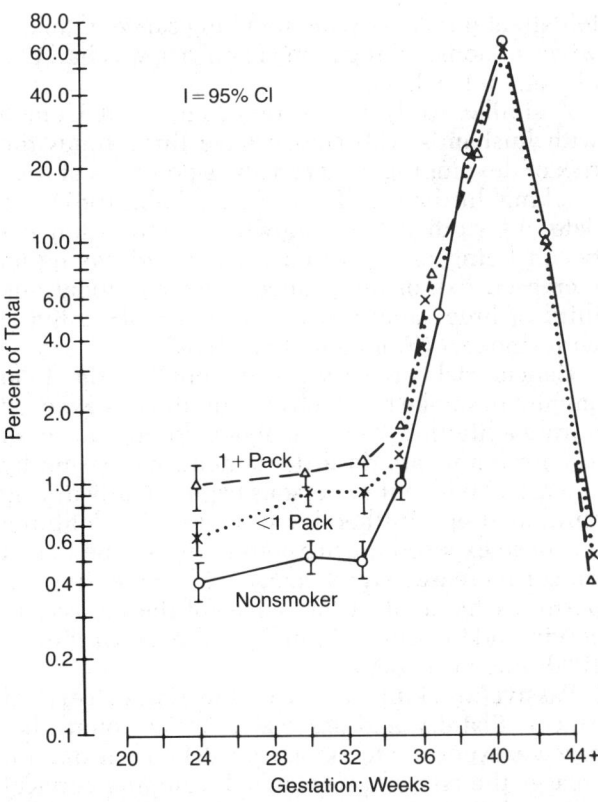

FIGURE 58–6. Percentage distribution by weeks of gestation of births to nonsmokers, smokers of less than one pack per day, and smokers of one pack per day or more. (From U.S. Department of Health, Education, and Welfare: Smoking and Health. A Report of the Surgeon General. DHEW Publication no. (PHS) 79-50066. Washington, DC, U.S. Department of Health, Education, and Welfare, Public Health Service, Office on Smoking and Health, 1979, p 8–17.)

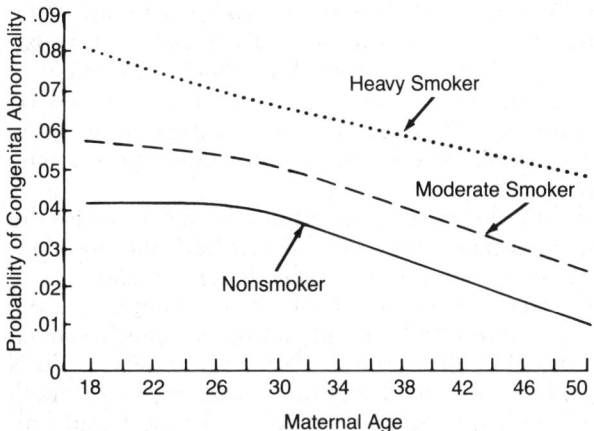

FIGURE 58–7. Risk of congenital abnormality in infant according to age and smoking habit of mother. (From Himmelberger DU, Brown BW Jr, Cohen EN: Cigarette smoking during pregnancy and the occurrence of spontaneous abortion and congenital abnormality: Am J Epid 108(6):477, 1978.) Study supported by Contract no. HSM 99-73-3, National Institute for Occupational Safety and Health.)

ers (Khoury et al., 1989). The increased frequency of placenta previa in women who smoke could be caused by placental hypertrophy that occurs as a result of the carbon monoxide hypoxemia (Williams et al., 1991).

Reduced fertility is also a problem in women who smoke cigarettes. Smokers are three to four times more likely to take longer than 1 year to conceive, and heavy smokers have more difficulty than do light smokers. Spermatozoa from smokers also show more morphologic abnormalities and decreased motility compared with nonsmokers.

Breast-feeding women who smoke cigarettes wean their infants earlier than women who do not smoke. This may be due to the reduced amount of milk and lower fat concentration in the milk of these mothers (Hopkinson et al., 1992).

FAMILY PHYSICIAN INVOLVEMENT IN ENDING THE TOBACCO PANDEMIC

A remarkable grassroots antismoking movement that arose in the 1970s has had a major impact on the goal of achieving a smoke-free society and has impelled traditional health organizations such as the American Cancer Society and the American Medical Association to become more outspoken. The first medical organization to develop proven strategies for the clinic, classroom, and community aimed at counteracting tobacco use and promotion was Doctors Ought to Care (DOC), founded in 1977 by a family physician at the University of Miami (Blum, 1980a). Since its inception, DOC has been supported by the American Academy of Family Physicians and the National Conference of Family Practice Residents and Student Affiliates. "Tar Wars," an annual antismoking poster contest

for schoolchildren, is a DOC offshoot that has been adopted by numerous state and local family practice organizations.

Governmental efforts include those of the Centers for Disease Control and Prevention, whose Office on Smoking and Health aids more than 30 state health departments, and the National Cancer Institute, whose Project ASSIST finances training for local antitobacco coalitions in 17 states. The annual federal expenditure to discourage smoking is less than 0.1% of the $4.6 billion spent each year in the United States to advertise tobacco products.

In 1994, the battleground for governmental antitobacco activity shifted to the states. Officials in Florida, Massachusetts, Minnesota, Mississippi, and West Virginia endorsed the idea of suing tobacco companies for reimbursement of Medicaid costs for the care of individuals with smoking-related diseases. The California and Maryland legislatures passed comprehensive laws to restrict smoking in the workplace and in public. Michigan voters approved a sales tax increase, part of the revenue from which will be dedicated to antitobacco education.

The most ambitious state program to combat smoking is in California, where in 1988 voters favored a referendum increasing the tax on cigarettes and earmarking millions of dollars for antismoking efforts, including paid commercials in the mass media. A similar ballot measure was approved by Massachusetts voters in 1992. However, even in states such as California, where the pendulum of public and legislative support appears to have swung in favor of regulatory efforts to curb tobacco use, tobacco industry lobbyists have fought unceasingly to pre-empt strong local laws with weak statewide regulations. The increasing involvement of family physicians in legislative antitobacco activity may provide an important contribution to public health.

SMOKING CESSATION*

Ideally, validity of the abstinence rate for a method of smoking cessation should rest on the performance of a controlled, double-blind study in which there is a follow-up of at least 6 months' duration of all subjects who started out (Schwartz, 1969, 1979, 1987). Few published outcome evaluations meet such criteria. Prior to the introduction of nicotine replacement products in 1984, smoking cessation techniques in the United States consisted of a hodgepodge of unproven but much-touted chemical remedies, diets, aversive stimuli, hypnotherapy, self-help manuals, special filters, acupuncture, and expensive behavior modification clinics or seminars. Many of these methods are quite costly, but having to pay a high price may well be related to the alleged success of a given method.

---

* Method of Alan Blum.

When the Food and Drug Administration approved the use of nicotine-containing chewing gum (Nicorette) for smoking cessation, the product gained immediate popularity. However, although the gum was approved for use as an adjunct to a comprehensive program of behavior modification, most physicians offered few instructions and little follow-up. Moreover, some patients became dependent on the gum, perpetuating their smoking by using the gum at times and in places where they were not permitted to smoke. The high success rates reported in clinical trials may be attributed in part to the fact that the research was conducted in clinics that specialize in the treatment of smoking cessation. This may further explain why placebo groups in some studies fared better than the intervention groups of most other methods.

In 1992, all smoking cessation methods began to take a back seat to the use of the transdermal nicotine patch. The theory behind the patch is that controlled, continuous release of nicotine provides partial replacement of the nicotine from smoking, thereby reducing the craving and preventing withdrawal. As with users of nicotine gum, relapse is a problem among patients who use the patch. The most significant problem in clinical practice appears to be a combination of the patient's heightened expectations for the patch (based on word-of-mouth testimonials and advertising in the mass media) and the physician's overeager acquiescence in prescribing it. Pharmaceutical company claims notwithstanding, smoking is not simply an addiction to nicotine. Social and psychologic factors also play determining roles. Promotions for various pharmacologic agents for smoking cessation wrongly reinforce the notion that smoking is primarily a medical problem with a simple, prescribable, nonindividualized solution. When a patient requests a drug "that will make me stop smoking," the physician, while not wishing to dash expectations, should emphasize that a drug is an adjunct, not the single solution.

One approach to this problem is to provide, following the initial interview during which the smoking history is taken and basic behavior modification information is discussed, two or three samples of the patch along with additional printed or other audiovisual materials. During a second visit 1 week later, the physician and patient can make a mutual decision on whether or not the patch should be prescribed. Weekly or biweekly visits thereafter will ascertain progress and begin the process of weaning off the patch. This proposal is based on the belief that, although transdermal nicotine may be more effective than a placebo in short-term smoking cessation, long-term success depends primarily on the intensity of behavior modification (Tonnesen et al., 1991). Also, although a stronger endorsement of the effectiveness of the patch, regardless of the intensity of counseling, has been made on the basis of a meta-analysis of 17 studies (Fiore et al., 1994), consideration must be given to the cost of the patch (approximately $4 each, or $224 for an 8-week course of treatment, more often than not unreimbursed by insurance). The primary beneficiaries of the patch are most likely to be the middle- and upper-income groups.

While the great expectations for success with the nicotine patch may not be fulfilled, its attendant publicity may stimulate physicians to take a more informed and personal role in smoking cessation. Such active involvement can be extremely crucial in and of itself. In the 1970s, at a time when efforts by physicians to discourage smoking were much less widespread and accepted, Russell and colleagues (1979) found that just 1 to 2 minutes of simple but unequivocal advice to the patient to stop smoking resulted in a cessation rate of over 5 per cent measured at 1 year, as opposed to only 0.3 per cent in the control group. Moreover, when strong advice is given at the time of recovery from a heart attack or other smoking-related disease (combined with a brochure and a promise of follow-up), over 60 per cent stop smoking and stay off cigarettes (measured at 3 years)—more than twice the rate of those who receive less definitive advice (Burt et al., 1974). Although most family physicians routinely ask their patients about smoking and advise them to stop smoking, relatively few provide more than advice and actually counsel patients using state-of-the-art techniques (Lindsay et al., 1994).

Although many people say they stopped smoking on their own, such individuals may not consciously attribute part of their success to increasing social pressures that reinforced their decision. Indeed, efforts to curtail tobacco use have become a cornerstone of local and national health promotion efforts. This is due in large measure to the outspokenness of such individuals as former Surgeon General C. Everett Koop and former Health and Human Services Secretary Louis Sullivan. Not only has organized medicine become united in the past few years on the need for more assertive office-based and community-wide strategies to end smoking, but other forces in society, including large corporations and governmental agencies, have also implemented smoke-free policies. The release in 1993 of a report by the Environmental Protection Agency (NIH Publication No. 93-3605, August 1993) implicating environmental tobacco smoke as a significant cause of lung cancer and other diseases in persons who do not smoke provided important evidence for individuals working to implement clean indoor air policies at the workplace.

Obstacles to Change

Unfortunately, the tobacco pandemic cannot be addressed as if it were a static issue, whereby sufficient public health education results in a significant change in societal behavior. Rather, smoking is a dynamic issue, with cigarette advertisers—whose livelihoods depend on maintaining more than 50 million users of tobacco, including 1.25 million teenagers who take up smoking each year—constantly adapting to the challenges brought by the antismoking movement.

Thus, smoking cessation programs for the individual patient cannot truly succeed in the long run in the absence of both workplace smoking bans and multimedia counteradvertising strategies that weaken the influence of the tobacco industry and reinforce the physician's office-based efforts (Blum, 1980a).

Although cigarette smoking becomes an addiction, it is first an entirely learned behavior. The "peer pressure" so often cited by tobacco companies as the reason for adolescent smoking is as much a manufactured product as the cigarettes themselves. The purpose of advertising is not just to sell cigarettes, but also to promote and reinforce the social acceptability of smoking and to encourage complacency toward the enormous social and health toll taken by smoking-caused diseases and fires. Today cigarette manufacturers spend more money annually to promote smoking than is spent to advertise for any other consumer product, including automobiles and food.

A variety of factors may inhibit physician involvement in smoking cessation, such as the perceived or real lack of time, the lack of reimbursement by third-party payers for such counseling, and the lack of "peer group" reinforcement in a technologically oriented, tertiary care-centered, highly intellectualized health care system. Nonetheless, physicians might well find that their increased involvement in efforts to promote smoking cessation among patients, regardless of the minimal enhancement in revenue, becomes a practice-building factor as word spreads about the doctors who care.

Office-Based Strategies

There is much the physician can do to become a better teacher about smoking, in lieu of relegating this role to ancillary personnel, a smoking cessation clinic, or a pamphlet off the shelf. The physician can develop an innovative strategy beginning outside the office or building. A bus bench, billboard, or sign in the parking lot with a straightforward or humorous health promotion message helps establish a thought-provoking and favorable image. In the waiting area, removal of ashtrays and the placement of signs noting that "In the interest of comfort, safety, and health, this is a smoke-free environment" further reinforce the message.

Magazines with cigarette advertisements ought not to appear in the physician's office in the absence of prominent stickers or rubber-stamped messages calling patients' attention to the deceptive, absurd nature of such ads. Alternatively, felt-tipped pens could be made available for patients to contribute their own antismoking comments or artwork. A commitment on the part of American physicians not to let their offices become vehicles for selling cigarettes would make a substantial contribution to health promotion. Although the responsibility for the office-based smoking cessation strategy should rest with the physician, it is invaluable to include all office staff as positive reinforcers for patients. Labeling each chart with a small "No Smoking" sticker to indicate the need for such reinforcement may be helpful, although care must be taken to avoid stigmatizing the patient as a "smoker." One would do well to reconsider using potentially alienating words such as "smoker" or even "quitter."

The key to successful smoking cessation efforts is a positive approach. A discussion about the diseases caused by smoking and the harmful constituents of tobacco smoke is essential—indeed, the physician must not shrink from imparting, through graphic posters, pamphlets, slides, and other audiovisual aids, the gruesome consequences of smoking—but the benefits of not smoking must be emphasized at least as strongly. Moreover, solely educating patients about the facts of smoking in a single office visit is unlikely to result in behavioral change.

In contrast, the physician can, through the use of creative analogies related to the patient's occupation, hobbies, or romantic interest, succeed in changing the patient's entire attitude toward smoking. For example, naming a partial list of the poisons and irritants in tobacco smoke, such as hydrocyanic acid (cyanide), ammonia, formaldehyde, and carbon monoxide (see Table 58–2), may mean little at first. (One pregnant patient proudly stated that she never buys a brand of cigarettes with the warning that mentions harm to the fetus, only those brands that say they contain carbon monoxide.) By noting that cyanide is the substance used in the gas chamber in executions, that formaldehyde is used to preserve cadavers, or that ammonia is the predominant smell in urine, however, the physician is likely to cause the patient to think about smoking a bit differently. No one wishes to have "urine breath." Similarly, it does little good to talk about carcinogens in tobacco in an age when the public believes "everything causes cancer." Sadly, the concept of relative risk is poorly developed in our society, because all too many people who smoke choose to think their millions-to-one odds of winning the state lottery are better than their one-in-seven chance of actually getting lung cancer.

Metaphors That Motivate

A revocabularization on the part of the physician is essential for making progress in office-based smoking cessation. Instead of "pack-year history," a more relevant measure might be the "inhalation count." A pack-a-day smoker will breathe in upward of 1 million doses of cyanide, ammonia, carcinogens, and carbon monoxide in less than 15 years, not including the inhalation of other people's smoke (calculated at 10 inhalations per cigarette, 20 cigarettes per pack). Another way to emphasize the enormous amount smoked is to state the financial cost: a pack-a-day cigarette buyer will spend in excess of $900 a year (calculated at $2.50 a pack)—or in excess of $10,000 in a decade if that money were put into a savings account or bond. One can remark about the joyful feeling of finding a $50 bill every 2 weeks—which is what one would indeed find if the money had not been spent on cigarettes. One patient who began smoking in the Marines at age 18 and who still smoked three packs a day at age 33 remarked ruefully that he had "smoked a Porsche."

Thus, whereas patient education in general and smoking cessation in particular rest on the knowledge on the part of both physician and patient of the deleterious aspects of adverse health behavior, the cognitive component alone is insufficient. Both the physician and the patient must be motivated to succeed. Three keys to the office-based smoking cessation are to personalize, individualize, and demythologize.

The physician can learn to *personalize* approaches to smoking cessation by carefully screening the pamphlets and other audiovisual aids available in the office. (Ideally, family physicians should consider producing their own.) It is essential to scrutinize all such material, as one would with a new drug or medical device. Personally handing a brochure to the patient while pointing out and underlining certain passages or illustrations will provide an important reinforcing message. The pamphlets, posters, and signs should be changed or otherwise updated every few weeks or months.

Individualizing the message to the patient is the cornerstone of success in patient education. The same cigarette counseling method cannot be used for a high-school girl, a construction worker, and an executive already showing signs or symptoms of heart disease. In the case of a high-school girl, the physician should not focus on such abstract concepts as emphysema and lung cancer, but rather emphasize the cosmetic unattractiveness of yellow teeth, bad breath, the loss of athletic ability, and the financial drain that results from buying cigarettes. As for the construction worker, the physician might suggest the likelihood of fewer lost paydays, greater physical strength, and even a lengthier sex life were he to stop buying cigarettes.

In talking with the concerned executive, it is especially important to *demythologize* certain beliefs about smoking, such as that the ultra-low-tar cigarettes she is smoking are safer. To the contrary, use of so-called low-tar brands, which should be referred to as "low-poison" by the physician (see Table 58–3), may in fact result in compensatory deeper inhalation of greater concentrations of chemical additives and noxious gases that increase the risk of heart attack. One way to highlight the absurdity of the belief that low-tar cigarettes are safer is to ask rhetorically, "Safer than what? Fresh air?" or to wonder aloud if it is safer to jump from the 50th story of the Empire State Building instead of the top. Another analogy is to point out that one would never think of buying a loaf of bread—or any other consumer product—that was advertised as containing "only 2 mg of cancer causers."

In any event, such dialogue must be practiced over and over again like any medical procedure, and individualized to the patient. (Remember that no two construction workers, teenagers, or executives are alike.) The counseling should be designed to call attention not only to the inevitable risks of smoking cigarettes but also to the chemically adulterated tobacco product itself, its inflated price, and the ubiquitous and ludicrous way in which the person's brand is promoted (Blum, 1980b). In effect, the family physician can shift the focus away from a resistant or guilt-ridden smoker and onto the product.

Common Myths

The most important myth surrounding smoking is that it relieves stress. This can be debunked by pointing out that the stress that is relieved is that which resulted from being dependent on cigarettes; this is the essence of addiction. At the same time, it is also important to point out that deep breathing in and of itself has a relaxing effect (Woods, 1988).

The second saddest myth, reinforced in advertisements for Virginia Slims and a host of new long, thin cigarettes intended for women and girls, is that smoking keeps weight off. Aside from pointing to all the obese women who smoke and attempting to correct the misapprehension that being overweight is a greater health risk than is smoking, one can point out that, by damaging the taste buds and other digestive tract cells, smoking does inhibit appetite, but it also results in more sedentary behavior through loss of lung capacity and cardiovascular fitness. One need not gain weight on stopping smoking if one will relearn to enjoy walking and running as much as one relearns the taste of food. By no means will all persons who stop smoking gain weight. Even among those who do, the average weight gain is less than 5 pounds (R. Davis, Director, Office on Smoking and Health, U.S. Department of Health and Human Services, personal communication, 1989), or an average of 6 pounds for men and 8 for women (Williamson et al., 1991). Although smokers may weigh slightly less than

TABLE 58–3—A CONSUMERIST APPROACH TO SMOKING CESSATION: HELPFUL ONE-LINERS

" 'Low tar' just means 'low poison.' Would you buy a brand of bread that was advertised as having only two ounces of poison in every loaf?"	Cigarette smoke contains more than 4,000 separate chemicals, over 40 of which are known carcinogens. "Tar" is the concentrate of these poisons, and there is no safe level of it.
"The filter is a fraud. You think filters are safer? Safer than what—fresh air?"	There are no health benefits to smoking filtered cigarettes, which were widely introduced by tobacco advertisers in the 1950s to allay public fears about smoking. Some early cigarette filters were made of asbestos. A person smoking a low-tar filtered cigarette will often compensate by smoking twice as many, thus increasing exposure to poisons.
"Menthol is an anesthetic."	It is a colorless chemical (not green like the ads imply) that is used to deaden the throat and mask the irritating sensation of the hot smoke.
" 'Light' and 'ultra-light' mean more sweeteners."	"When you add two teaspoons of sugar to a cup of black coffee, is there any less coffee?" Cigarettes taste different because different candy flavorings are added. Ultra-lights are easier for teenagers to become habituated to.
"Buying a pack of cigarettes for $2 is like spending $20 for a sandwich or $200,000 for a used car."	Cigarettes cost less than 15 cents a pack to manufacture. They are the highest profit consumer item in America. Most of the increase in price is set by the tobacco manufacturers, not government taxes.
"Ammonia is what makes cigarette smoke smell like urine."	Another rancid aroma in cigarette smoke is formaldehyde. Other gases include carbon monoxide and cyanide.
"Cigarettes are dead leaves."	Would you go up to a pile of burning leaves and start inhaling? Cigarettes are dead leaves laden with chemicals. They're designed to keep burning no matter what, so that you have to buy more and more.

nonsmokers, when they stop smoking they simply return to the average weight of nonsmokers. Moreover, the slightly lower weight in many who continue to smoke is associated with a higher risk body fat distribution (Bonithon-Kopp et al., 1989; Shimokata et al., 1989). Because more than 75 per cent of black patients who smoke buy menthol brands, it is important to debunk the myth that this substance in some way "cools" the smoke (U.S. Department of Health and Human Services, 1989). In fact, menthol is an anesthetic that deadens the throat to create the illusion of a less irritating smoke (see Table 58–2).

From the physician's standpoint, perhaps the biggest myth that has been encouraged in the medical literature is that the patient must be "ready to quit." Although common sense dictates that those who express a greater interest in stopping smoking will have a greater success rate, those patients who do not express an interest in stopping smoking symbolize the overall challenge we face in curbing this pandemic. One of the reasons for lack of motivation of patients may be their sense of inevitability of failure. It is conceivable that, by not educationing the nonmotivated smoking patient, the physician is in effect reinforcing the notion that it may be too difficult to stop smoking.

Setting a "quit date," the sine qua non of the smoking cessation literature, may rationalize the continuation of an adverse health practice and may strengthen denial. In other words, it is helpful to remind patients that they can stop now. If they do not stop, this does not mean you will not treat them the next time, but it is important to give encouragement and not reinforce excuses. Most authors do believe that a quit date, targeted only 1 week or a few weeks into the future, is useful for the motivated patient, for whom denial is less of a problem. Its purpose is to let the individual build up resolve or to permit a gradual reduction in daily cigarette consumption. Giving patients a few written reminders (such as lists of the advantages and disadvantages of smoking, the rewards for not smoking and the penalties for lighting up, the situations and environmental influences that encourage one to smoke, and the myths of smoking and smoking cessation) is very helpful (Woods, 1988). A prescription with a no-smoking symbol signed by the physician and included with the other prescriptions is a thoughtful gesture.† The physician should not advise "cutting down," switching to a low-tar cigarette, or changing to a pipe or cigar.

Consumer Advocacy Role

Traditional office-based approaches begin by asking, "Do you smoke?," "How much do you smoke?," and "When did you start smoking?" Although this may provide the physician with relevant data for charting purposes, this approach is all to often a signal for the patient to become defensive and resistant to further discussion, especially if the patient had no intention to stop smoking. However, there are alternative ways of obtaining infor-

---

† These are available, along with a wide variety of stickers, posters, and newsletters, from DOC, Department of Family Medicine, Baylor College of Medicine, 5510 Greenbriar, Houston, TX 77005 (telephone: 713-798-7729; fax: 713-798-7775).

mation, and at the same time piquing the patient's interest in the subject. By using and identifying with the vocabulary used by the consumer of cigarettes, the physician can adopt (and be perceived in) the role of consumer advocate, as opposed to medical finger-wagger. The most important—and nonthreatening—questions to ask are, "What brand do you buy?" and "How much do you spend on cigarettes?" The patient is likely to be surprised and intrigued by these questions, which can be asked at any time in the course of the interview, because they appear to be nonjudgmental. They serve to suggest that the physician is not solely a know-it-all and a preacher on the dangers of the evil weed. In effect, a question about the cost of cigarettes shows concern for the patient's financial well-being. Inquiring as specifically as possible about the brand name—for example, Marlboro Menthol Lights 100s box—will lead to a greater understanding on the part of the physician of the same vocabulary used by the person who buys cigarettes, and will narrow the communication gap. The patient may even begin to laugh aloud at the foolishness of such a vocabulary, especially as he or she is encouraged to show the physician the package and to appreciate how little information about the product appears beyond the attractive design.

There are more than 15 different versions of Marlboros, which illustrates the way cigarette manufacturers create the illusion of choice, individuality, and degree of safety. A patient who states "since my heart attack, I've switched from Marlboro Reds to Marlboro Ultra Lights," has been miseducated to believe that some cigarettes can be less harmful than others. Moreover, the product itself is extremely cheap to manufacture (less than 15 cents a pack), but extremely profitable to tobacco companies at $2.50 a pack.

Promotions for various pharmacologic agents, mail-order gadgets, and clinics in smoking cessation reinforce the notion that cigarette smoking is primarily a medical problem with a simple, prescribable, nonindividualized solution (Blum, 1984). When a patient requests a "drug that will help me stop smoking," the physician must confront the dilemma of not wishing to dash the patient's expectations while emphasizing that a drug or device is at best an adjunct and not a means of smoking cessation. It is an unfortunate fact of life that many patients will not stop smoking until they have gotten their money's worth at a special smoking cessation clinic; and it seems that, regardless of the method used, the more expensive the better.

Approach to Adolescents

Children and teenagers who smoke cigarettes pose a special challenge, because they represent the market most carefully nurtured by tobacco advertisers. If an adolescent turns 18 without starting to smoke, there is only a 10 per cent chance he or she ever will. Regardless of all our educational efforts, however, more than 3000 teenagers in the United States start smoking every day. Almost three fourths of adolescents who smoke buy Marlboros.

It is essential to avoid emphasizing the adult and dangerous nature of smoking. Rather, smoking should be referred to as the childish, dumb, and silly-looking practice that it is. The single most important statement the physician can make to an adolescent is "Come on, you're too old to smoke. That's for the little kids who want to look grown up." Another strategy is for the physician to ask the teenager who smokes to help think of ideas for talking to junior high school and primary school students about ridiculing tobacco company executives and making fun of cigarette brand names.

As a general rule in approaching the subject of smoking cessation with a patient, Schwartz (1987) and others recommend thinking in terms of a strategy that comprises interventions designed to enhance motivation and those that will help reduce dependence. Time and commitment on the part of the physician will result in greater success. The biggest obstacle to smoking cessation is complacency on the part of the physician.

REFERENCES

Abell TD, Baker LC, Ramsey CN: The effects of maternal smoking on infant birth weight. Fam Med 23:102, 1991.
American Psychiatric Association Task Force on Nomenclature and Statistics: Diagnostic and Statistical Manual of Mental Disorders, 4th edition. Washington, DC, American Psychiatric Association, 1994.
Aronow WS: The effect of smoke on the nonsmoker. Fam Pract Recertification 1:47, 1979.
Barry J, Mead K, Nabel EG, et al: Effect of smoking on the activity of ischemic heart disease. JAMA 261:398, 1989.
Bell BA, Symon L: Smoking and subarachnoid haemorrhage. BMJ 1:577, 1979.
Blum A: Butting in where it counts. Hosp Physician 16(4):22, 1980b.

Blum A: Medicine vs. Madison Avenue. JAMA 243:739, 1980a.
Blum A: Nicotine chewing gum and the medicalization of smoking. Ann Intern Med 101:121, 1984.
Bonita R, Scragg R, Stewart A: Cigarette smoking and risk of premature stroke in men and women. BMJ 293:6, 1986.
Bonithon-Kopp C, Raison J, Ducimetiere P, et al: Smoking wastes a good Parisenne (letters). JAMA 262:1185, 1989.
Brownson RC, Novotny TE, Perry MC: Cigarette smoking and adult leukemia. Arch Intern Med 153:469, 1993.
Burt A, Thronley P, Illingworth D, et al: Stopping smoking after myocardial infarction. Lancet 1:304, 1974.
Centers for Disease Control and Prevention (CDC): State-specific estimates of smoking-attributable mortality and years of potential life lost—United States, 1985. MMWR 37, 1988.

Charlton A: Children and passive smoking: A review. J Fam Pract 38:267, 1994.

Chase HP, Garg SK, Marshall G, et al: Cigarette smoking increases the risk of albuminuria among subjects with type 1 diabetes. JAMA 265:614, 1991.

Colditz GA, Bonita R, Stampfer MJ, et al: Cigarette smoking and risk of stroke in middle-aged women. N Engl J Med 318:937, 1988.

Connolly GN, Winn DM, Hecht SS, et al: The reemergence of smokeless tobacco. N Engl J Med 314:1020, 1986.

Eliopoulos C, Klein J, Phan MK, et al: Hair concentrations of nicotine and cotinine in women and their newborn infants. JAMA 271:621, 1994.

Evans RI: Smokeless tobacco vs cigarette use among adolescents. Cancer Bull 40:355, 1988.

Fiore MC, Smith SS, Jorenby DE, et al: The effectiveness of the nicotine patch for smoking cessation: A meta-analysis. JAMA 271:1940, 1994.

Fontham ETH, Correa P, Reynolds P, et al: Environmental tobacco smoke and lung cancer in nonsmoking women: A multicenter study. JAMA 271:1752, 1994.

Garfinkle L: Cancer mortality in nonsmokers: Prospective study by the American Cancer Society. J Natl Cancer Inst 65:1169, 1980.

Giovannucci E, Rimm EB, Stampfer MJ, et al: A prospective study of cigarette smoking and risk of colorectal adenoma and colorectal cancer in U.S. men. J Natl Cancer Inst 86:183, 1994.

Hammond EC: Smoking in relation to the death rates of one million men and women. *In* Haenszel W (ed): Epidemiological Approaches to the Study of Cancer and Other Chronic Diseases. Bethesda, MD, National Cancer Institute, 1966.

Health Consequences of Smoking: Cancer. A Report of the Surgeon General. DHHS Publication no. (PHS) 82-50179. Rockville, MD, US Department of Health and Human Services, Public Health Service, Office on Smoking and Health, 1982.

Health Consequences of Smoking for Women. A Report of the Surgeon General. Rockville, MD, US Department of Health and Human Services, Public Health Service, Office on Smoking and Health, 1985.

Hermanson B, Omenn GS, Kronmal RA, et al: Beneficial six-year outcome of smoking cessation in older men and women with coronary artery disease. N Engl J Med 319:1365, 1988.

Herning RI, Jones RT, Bachman J, et al: Puff volume increases when low-nicotine cigarettes are smoked. BMJ 283:187, 1981.

Higgins MW, Enright PL, Kronmal RA, et al: Smoking and lung function in elderly men and women. JAMA 269:2741, 1993.

Hirayama T: Non-smoking wives of heavy smokers have a higher risk of lung cancer: A study from Japan. BMJ 282:183, 1981.

Hopkinson JM, Schanler RJ, Fraley JK, et al: Milk production by mothers of premature infants: Influence of cigarette smoking. Pediatrics 90:934, 1992.

Jarvik ME, Cullen JW, Gritz ER, et al (ed): Research on Smoking Behavior. National Institute on Drug Abuse Research Monograph Series no. 17. DHEW Publication no. (ADM) 78-581. Rockville, MD, US Department of Health, Education and Welfare, Public Health Service, Alcohol, Drug Abuse, and Mental Health Administration, 1977.

Kadunce DP, Burr R, Gress R, et al: Cigarette smoking: Risk factor for premature facial wrinkling. Ann Intern Med 114:840, 1991.

Kaufman DW, Helmrich SP, Rosenberg L, et al: Nicotine and carbon monoxide content of cigarette smoke and the risk of myocardial infarction in young men. N Engl J Med 308:409, 1983.

Kendler KS, Neale MC, MacLean CJ, et al: Smoking and major depression: A causal analysis. Arch Gen Psychiatry 50:36, 1993.

Khoury MJ, Govez-Farias M, Mulinare J: Does maternal cigarette smoking during pregnancy cause cleft lip and palate in offspring? Am J Dis Child 143:333, 1989.

Kinlen LJ, Rogot E: Leukemia and smoking habits among United States veterans. BMJ 297:657, 1988.

Koop CE, Luoto J: The health consequences of smoking: Cancer. Overview of a report of the Surgeon General. Public Health Rep 97:318, 1982.

Kozlowski LT, Frecker RC, Khouw V, et al: The misuse of "less-hazardous" cigarettes and its detection: Hole-blocking of ventilation filters. Am J Public Health 70:1202, 1980.

Krasnegor NA (ed): Cigarette Smoking as a Dependence Process. National Institute on Drug Abuse Research Monograph Series no. 23. DHEW Publication no. (ADM) 79-800. Rockville, MD, US Department of Health, Education and Welfare, Public Health Service, Alcohol, Drug Abuse, and Mental Health Administration, 1979.

LaCroix AZ, Lang J, Scherr P, et al: Smoking and mortality among older men and women in three communities. N Engl J Med 324:1619, 1991.

Lee EW, D'Alonzo GE: Cigarette smoking, nicotine addiction, and its pharmacologic treatment. Arch Intern Med 153:34, 1993.

Lexcen FJ, Hicks RA: Does cigarette smoking increase sleep problems? Percept Motor Skills 77:16, 1993.

Lindsay EA, Ockene JK, Hymowitz N, et al: Physicians and smoking cessation: A survey of office procedures and practices in the community intervention trial for smoking cessation. Arch Fam Med 3:341, 1994.

Mainous AG, Hueston WJ: The effect of smoking cessation during pregnancy on preterm delivery and low birthweight. J Fam Pract 38:262, 1994a.

Mainous AG, Hueston WJ: Passive smoke and low birth weight. Arch Fam Med 3:875, 1994b.

McGinnis JM, Foege WH: Actual causes of death in the United States. JAMA 270:2207, 1993.

Nieburg P, Marks JS, McLaren NM, Remington PL: The fetal tobacco syndrome. JAMA 253:2998, 1985.

Palmer JR, Rosenberg L, Shapiro S: "Low-yield" cigarettes and the risk of nonfatal myocardial infarction in women. N Engl J Med 320:1569, 1989.

Pershagen G, Svensson C, Hrubec Z: Passive smoking and lung cancer. Am J Epidemiol 125:17, 1987.

Pierce P, Fiore MC, Novotny TE, et al: Trends in cigarette smoking in the United States. JAMA 261:61, 1989.

Pollin W, Ravenholt RT: Tobacco addiction and tobacco mortality. JAMA 252:2849, 1984.

Prummel MF, Wiersinga WM: Smoking and risk of Graves' disease. JAMA 269:479, 1993.

Qian H, Feng J, Hou X, et al: Smoking and reproductive cancer. Female Patient 14:42, 1989.

Raeburn P: Passive smoking may be 10 times deadlier than thought. Houston Post, June 19, 1989.

Rantakallio P: Relationship of maternal smoking to morbidity and mortality of the child up to the age of five. Acta Paediatr Scand 67:621, 1978.

Robinson MD: A workable approach to smoking cessation in the primary care office. Primary Care & Cancer 13(10):29, 1993.

Rogers RL, Meyer JS, Judd BW, et al: Abstention from cigarette smoking improves cerebral perfusion among elderly chronic smokers. JAMA 253:2970, 1985.

Rosenberg L, Kaufman DW, Helmrich SP, et al: The risk of myocardial infarction after quitting smoking in men under 55 years of age. N Engl J Med 313:1511, 1985.

Russell MAH, Wilson C, Taylor C, et al: Effect of general practitioner's advice against smoking. BMJ 2:231, 1979.

Sandler DP, Everson RB, Wilcox AJ, et al: Cancer risk in adulthood from early life exposure to parents' smoking. Am J Public Health 75:487, 1985a.

Sandler DP, Wilcox AJ, Everson RB: Preliminary communication: Cumulative effects of lifetime passive smoking on cancer risk. Lancet 1:312, 1985b.

Schwartz JL: A critical review and evaluation of smoking control methods. Public Health Rep 84:483, 1969.

Schwartz JL: Review and evaluation of smoking cessation. Public Health Rep 94:558, 1979.

Schwartz JL: Review and evaluation of smoking cessation methods: The United States and Canada, 1978–1985. NIH Publication no. 87-2940. Bethesda, MD, National Cancer Institute, Division of Cancer Prevention and Control, 1987.

Shimokata H, Muller DC, Andres R: Studies in the distribution of body fat, III: Effects of cigarette smoking. JAMA 261:1169, 1989.

Shinton R, Beevers G: Meta-analysis of relation between cigarette smoking and stroke. BMJ 298:789, 1989.

Siegel M: Involuntary smoking in the restaurant workplace: A review of employee exposure and health effects. JAMA 270:490, 1993.

Silverman DT, Dunn JA, Hoover RN, et al: Cigarette smoking and pancreas cancer: a case-control study based on direct interviews. J Natl Cancer Inst 86:1510, 1994.

Slattery ML, Robison LM, Schuman K, et al: Cigarette smoking and exposure to passive smoke are risk factors for cervical cancer. JAMA 261:1593, 1989.

Slone D, Shapiro S, Rosenberg L, et al: Relation of cigarette smoking to myocardial infarction in young women. N Engl J Med 298:1273, 1978.

Tonnesen P, Norregard J, Simonsen K, et al: A double-blind trial of 16-hour transdermal nicotine patch in smoking cessation. N Engl J Med 325:311, 1991.

U.S. Department of Health and Human Services: Reducing the Health Consequences of Smoking: 25 Years of Progress. A Report of the Surgeon General. DHHS Publication no. (PHS) 89-8411. Washington, DC, U.S. Department of Health and Human Services, Public Health Service, Office on Smoking and Health, 1989.

Wells AJ: An estimate of adult mortality in the United States from passive smoking. Environ Int 14:249, 1988.

Williams MA, Mittendorf R, Lieberman E, et al: Cigarette smoking during pregnancy in relation to placenta previa. Am J Obstet Gynecol 165:28, 1991.

Williamson DF, Madans J, Anda RF, et al: Smoking cessation and severity of weight gain in a national cohort. N Engl J Med 324:739, 1991.

Williamson DF, Serdula MK, Kendrick JS, et al: Comparing the prevalence of smoking in pregnant and nonpregnant women, 1985 to 1986. JAMA 261:70, 1989.

Winters TH, Di Franza JR: Radioactivity in cigarette smoke. N Engl J Med 306:364, 1982.

Wolf PA, D'Aostine RB, Sannel WB, et al: Cigarette smoking as a risk factor for stroke: The Framingham Study. JAMA 259:1025, 1988.

Woods PJ: Smoking and Behavior Control. Roanoke, VA, Hollins College, Department of Psychology, 1988.

CHAPTER 59

ABUSE OF CONTROLLED SUBSTANCES

KEVIN M. SHERIN

Development of a working knowledge of the medical issues surrounding drug abuse is a critically important priority for today's family physician. The family physician is in a front-line position for early detection of drug abuse problems and direction of her or his patients toward successful outcomes.

HISTORICAL PERSPECTIVE

Heroin was a legal drug prior to the turn of the century and was widely prescribed. In 1914 Congress passed the Harrison Narcotic Tax Act, which banned both heroin and cocaine as illegal narcotic drugs (Claussen, 1977). From the 1930s to the 1960s cocaine was viewed as a harmless recreational drug without addictive potential. Yet the powerful psychoactive properties of cocaine have probably been recognized since AD 600 (Creger and Mark, 1986).

Cocaine abuse is the dominant form of illicit drug use in the United States. In 1963 it was estimated that there were only 10,000 cocaine users domestically. The advent of the "crack" form in 1985 led to wider availability at low cost, contributing to increases in consumption. The last several decades have seen the number of heroin addicts stabilize at between 500,000 and 800,000 nationwide (Kulberg, 1986).

It is estimated that Americans spend $40 billion to $100 billion annually on illicit drugs (Stimmel, 1991). Significant correlations have been found between adolescent drug use and juvenile crime (Dembo et al., 1991). Common names for drugs found on the street are given in Table 59–1.

THEORIES OF ADDICTION

Genetic contributions to chemical dependency have been emphasized (Madden, 1979; Robins, 1978). Children of alcoholics or drug abusers seem to be at higher risk for the development of substance abuse disorders (Goodwin et al., 1973). Variations in the biology of metabolism of psy-

choactive drugs or changes at drug receptor sites in the central nervous system (CNS) (e.g., endorphin or dopamine receptors) may play a role here. The significance of social and environmental factors in the development of drug dependence is substantial. Social and cultural factors affecting the acceptability and availability of drugs are important features promoting harmful personal consumption. In Vietnam wide availability of heroin contributed to high rates of consumption among U.S. servicemen. Motives for drug use include (1) medicinal purposes; (2) symbolic purposes, including peer group acceptance; and (3) pleasurable effects on the mind (Madden, 1979). Constitutional aspects of the individual may provide fertile soil for development of chemical dependency.

The individual user, even lacking genetic contributions, risks development of biologic addiction by repeated exposure to psychoactive substances capable of triggering powerful internal reward systems.

EPIDEMIOLOGY

Since 1980 drug abuse patterns in the United States have been relatively stable with the exception of cocaine, and now perhaps hallucinogens, designer drugs, and the China White form of heroin. It is estimated that 30 million Americans have used cocaine and that 5 million use it regularly (Abelson and Miller, 1985). The highest prevalence of cocaine use has been among young white men (ages 18 to 25 years) residing in the West and the northeastern United States (Abelson and Miller, 1985). Use among women is increasing. Surveys of U.S. high-school students' cocaine use showed evidence of a decline (Adams and Kozel, 1985). The present cocaine epidemic is considered to be the fifth and the largest stimulant abuse outbreak.

In 1993 high school student surveys showed a continuing decline, although use persists among addicts. Abused drugs showing relative declines since the 1970s include phencyclidine, amphetamines, sedative hypnotics, and hallucinogens.

TABLE 59–1. STREET TERMINOLOGY OF ABUSED DRUGS

Class	Example Names
Sedative hypnotics	Barbs, blues, goofballs, greens and whites, soapers, roaches (Librium)
	Ludes (Quaalude)
	Mean-green (Placidyl)
	Yellow-jackets (phenobarbital)
	Red devils (secobarbital)
Analgesics	
Heroin	Smack, junk, horse, H, brown, skag, China White (pure heroin)*
Methadone	Dollies, wafers
Darvon	Pinks and grays
Terpin hydrate	Terp
Dilaudid	Fours
Designer drugs	
MDA	Love drug
MDMA	Ecstasy, Adam
Fentanyl	China white
Stimulants	
Cocaine	Crack, coke, gold dust, flakes, snow, rock
Other stimulants	Speedball (heroin and cocaine)
	Uppers; truck drivers, crank (amphetamines)
	Crossroads, bennies, copilot
	Ice (crank) (crystalline methamphetamine)*
	Cat (khat) (methcathinone)*
Cannabinols	
Marijuana	Reefer, roach, weed, pot, joint, grass, brick, lid
Hashish	Ganja, bhang
Hallucinogens	
LSD	Acid, blue dots, cube, D
Other	Cactus (mescaline)
	Magic mushrooms (psilocybin)
	Pearly gates (morning glory seeds)
PCP	Angel dust, dust, rocket fuel, peacepill, hog, supercoke, super joint, cosmos, goon

* Updated to 1994.
Adapted from Appendix C, AMSAODD Review Course Syllabus. New York, American Medical Society for Alcoholism and other Drug Dependencies, 1987, with permission.

Marijuana use remains relatively stable. Inner city patterns were reflected in a study from the Department of Psychiatry at Bronx Lebanon Hospital in New York. These investigators found that 40 per cent of inpatients had used cannabis; 37 per cent alcohol; 20 per cent amphetamines; 12 per cent cocaine; 12 per cent phencyclidine (PCP); 10 per cent barbiturates and other sedative hypnotics; 9 per cent opiates; 1 per cent inhalants; and 1 per cent hallucinogens (Fernandez-Pol et al., 1988).

Trends during the early 1990s include escalation in the use of amphetamines. "Crank" laboratories have sprung up in many locales. "Cat," similar to the Khat of Somalia, is methcathinone, a stimulant more powerful than crack cocaine that is widely used in the Soviet Union and has been found in Michigan and the state of Washington (Glastris,

1993). A new form of heroin use is emerging, known as "chasing the dragon"; it is inhaled after heating it on aluminum foil and is perceived as having less risk than intravenous heroin (Strang et al., 1992). China White heroin is a particularly pure form that can be snorted, smoked in cigarettes, rubbed on gums, or mixed in lemon juice.

PHARMACOLOGIC PRINCIPLES

Pharmacologic principles affecting abused drugs include (1) absorption, (2) distribution, (3) metabolism, (4) excretion, (5) tolerance and cross-tolerance, and (6) dependence (Morgan, 1985). Absorption varies with route of intake and may include inhalation (volatile gas or smoke), insufflation (cocaine), oral ingestion, and intravenous infusion. Peak drug levels occur rapidly with inhalation, intravenous injection, and insufflation; they are more likely to produce fatalities or serious sequelae by these routes. Regarding drug distribution, the partition coefficient equals the concentration of oil-dissolved drug versus "water"-dissolved drug; and this ratio reflects lipophilicity and hydrophilicity. Most psychoactive substances readily cross the blood-brain barrier. Nonpolar compounds tend to be lipophilic, have a high partition coefficient, and widely distribute within fat and myelin layers, producing prolonged psychodynamic or physiologic effects.

Psychoactive compounds are metabolized by several pathways (Morgan, 1985). Most are metabolized in hepatocytes via dehydroxylation, deamination, and acetylation. Barbiturates and benzodiazepines induce microsomal enzymes of the P-450 pathway. Tolerance then develops, which promotes cross-tolerance. Alcohol and benzodiazepines have cross-tolerance because they share this common pathway. Psychoactive drug metabolism occurs largely via first-order kinetics; that is, a fixed proportion of metabolite versus substrate is produced, giving the drug a fixed half-life. Inert compounds of psychoactive metabolites may be produced. Excretion occurs principally through the kidneys. The pK_a of a compound may allow more rapid renal excretion if the urine pH is altered. Alkalinization of urine enhances the excretion of phenobarbital, a weak acid. Emergency medicine physicians indirectly utilize this acid-base principle of enhanced excretion in gastric lavage. Some drugs are recirculated through the acidic environment of the gastric mucosa long after absorption; removal is enhanced by repeated doses of oral activated charcoal. Acidification of urine to enhance excretion is no longer widely used clinically. (Giannini et al., 1987).

Pharmacologic dependence requires discrete abstinence or physiologic withdrawal syndrome in the drug's absence. The presence of the drug prevents emergence of withdrawal. Stereotyped responses are seen with opiates, sedative hypnotics, depressant drugs, and alcohol. Sedative hypnotic and depressant drug withdrawal mimics delayed alcohol withdrawal. A "low-dose" benzodiazepine withdrawal syndrome includes anxiety and insomnia; it persists for months and responds well to β-blockers (Smith and Wesson, 1983). Opiate withdrawal is characterized by lacrimation, frequent yawning, gastrointestinal disturbance, rhinorrhea, and piloerection.

ACUTE EFFECTS OF COMMONLY ABUSED DRUGS

Cocaine

Cocaine is an alkaloid extracted from the South American shrub *Erythroxylon coca*. Its pharmacologic properties, which have been reviewed extensively (Paredes and Gorlick, 1992), include powerful stimulant, vasoconstrictive, and anesthetic effects. Cocaine is a powerful euphoric with potent addictive properties. Acute effects include mydriasis, tachycardia, overalertness, talkativeness, flushing, hyperthermia, and emotional lability. Persons with abnormal plasma cholinesterase activity may experience an overdose at low thresholds. Signs of toxicity include nausea, vomiting, seizures, tachyarrhythmia, hypertensive crisis, strokes, myocardial infarction, extreme anxiety with disorientation, and sudden cardiorespiratory arrest. Abstinence may result in hypersomnia, irritability, dysphoria, and prolonged depression. Smokeable forms (free-basing) have been associated with pneumothorax, pneumomediastinum, and other pulmonary effects (Creger and Mark, 1986). Maternofetal effects are discussed under chronic effects.

Prescription Drugs

Amphetamines

Amphetamine, phenylpropanolamine, ephedrine, and caffeine have similar central and peripheral toxic effects (Carr, 1993; Kulberg, 1986). Small doses may produce alertness, lessened fatigue, a sense of well-being, and improved motor skills. Side effects include anxiety, restlessness, insomnia, abdominal cramps, and lassitude. Overdosage results in anxiety, agitation, hallucinations, and seizures. Acute paranoid psychosis is seen with large overdoses. Peripheral effects include elevated blood pressure, diaphoresis, mydriasis, hyperactive bowel sounds, tachycardia, and reflex bradycardia.

Sedative Hypnotics

Benzodiazepines have a high threshold for toxic effects (Kulberg, 1986). Sedation is the hallmark of this class of drugs. An overdose may result in blurring of vision, dysarthria, ataxia, and nystagmus. An acute withdrawal syndrome begins between days 5 and 8 of abstinence. Signs and symptoms may include insomnia, irritability, seizures, tremulousness, muscle twitching, and delirium. Phenobarbital, glutethimide, and ethchlorvynol withdrawal effects are similar with a difference only in half-life. Methaqualone is considered a sedative hypnotic.

Opiates

Opiate overdose produces a clinical triad of respiratory and CNS depression with meiotic pupils (Kulberg, 1986). Opiate receptors include μ (mu), κ (kappa), and δ (delta), which mediate opioid drugs and endogenous peptides (Simonds, 1988). Muscle flaccidity, hypertension, and hypothermia may also be seen. Euphoria accompanied by brief diaphoresis is a typical dose response in a heroin addict. Noncardiogenic pulmonary edema is a complication of parenteral narcotic overdose (Madden, 1979). Yawning and lacrimation are frequent opiate effects.

Hallucinogens

Phencyclidine

Phencyclidine ("angel dust," or PCP) was marketed during the 1950s as a surgical anesthetic and the 1960s as an animal anesthetic (Kulberg, 1986). This dissociative anesthetic has been associated with violent, bizarre behaviors, radical alterations of sensory stimuli, and supernormal strength often associated with self-injury in the face of anesthesia. Hypertension and bidirectional nystagmus are frequently seen. Hyperthermia may occur in the face of muscle rigidity and rhabdomyolysis. Patients may also appear catatonic.

Lysergic Acid Diethylamide

Lysergic acid diethylamide (LSD) is an illusionogenic drug (Kulberg, 1986). Stimuli are distorted: Sounds, smells, and visual stimuli may be altered or merged. Depersonalization or personality disorganization may lead to panic or a "bad trip." Paresthesias, diaphoresis, ataxia, and tremors may be seen. The sense of passage of time may be slowed (Madden, 1979). Tolerance develops to the behavioral effects (Carr, 1993).

Inhalants

Volatile Solvent/Propellants

During the nineteenth century popular agents included ether and chloroform. Today toluene and aliphatic chlorinated compounds have replaced them. Solvent abuse is particularly prevalent among the rural poor in the South (Kulberg, 1986). Acute CNS effects include initial delirium, euphoria, confusion, ataxia, and dysarthria. Bizarre and impulsive behavior can lead to significant morbidity and mortality. Illusions and delusions may follow, and the clinical picture may progress to coma. Sudden death can occur and has been attributed to myocardial sensitization (Kulberg, 1986).

Nitrates

Nitrates remain popular among homosexual and heterosexual populations for enhanced erection and orgasm. Headache, nausea, palpitations, and dizziness are seen. Giddiness, syncope, and confusion are frequently observed. Sudden death can occur with repeated inhalation. Methemoglobinemia can occur.

Mescaline-Peyote

Toxicity usually occurs 1 to 2 hours following ingestion of mescaline or peyote. The clinical effects are similar to those produced by LSD or PCP. However, there is usually an intact memory for the events, unlike under the influence of PCP (Kulberg, 1986).

Cannabis (Marijuana)

Tetrahydrocannabinol is the principal active ingredient of marijuana. Conjunctival injection and a dreamy state are the principal objective findings in a user (Kulberg, 1986; Madden, 1979). Euphoric enhanced perceptions and altered sense of time are frequent. Toxic doses may alter body image and produce depersonalization, paranoia, and disorientation. Sinus tachycardia occurs frequently. An amotivational syndrome develops with chronic use (Carr, 1993).

CHRONIC EFFECTS OF SUBSTANCE ABUSE

Cocaine

Chronic effects of cocaine abuse or dependence are related to the route of intake and have been extensively reviewed (Creger and Mark, 1986). Nasal insufflation results in chronic rhinorrhea. Nasal septal atrophy and perforation may also occur (Vilensky, 1982). Chronic sinusitis, sinus osteomyelitis, and brain abscess can accompany insufflation (Shveitzer, 1986). Smokeable forms of cocaine may be associated with pulmonary problems. Intravenous use of cocaine can result in allergic vasculitis, cerebral infarcts, and infectious complications including hepatitis B and HIV infection. Oral ingestion has been associated with hepatic damage and intestinal infarcts (Nalbandian et al., 1986). Myocardial fibrosis has been observed in occasional users (Simpson and Edwards, 1986). Maternal use during pregnancy can result in maternofetal effects including fetal brain infarcts, intestinal atresia, genitourinary anomalies, prune belly syndrome, intrauterine growth retardation, prematurity, and abruptio placentae (Chasnoff et al., 1986; Creger and Mark, 1986).

Stimulants

Stimulant use can result in weight loss and insomnia. Psychiatric sequelae occur with frequent chronic use and may include anxiety, depression, paranoid states, and mood swings. Direct myocardial injury has been described with phenylpropanolamine ingestion (Pentel et al., 1982).

Sedative Hypnotics

Prolonged abstinence syndromes associated with sedative hypnotics have already been discussed. Interruption of rapid-eye-movement (REM) sleep is frequent. Thrombocytopenia, leukopenia, and jaundice clear with abstinence (Stutzman, 1987). Muscle and nervous tissue necrosis can occur with intravenous use. In the elderly, prescription drug abuse can present with dementia, depression, or both.

Opiates

Intravenous opiate abusers are at increased risk for endocarditis, brain abscess, pneumonia, lung abscess, viral hepatitis, and human immunodeficiency virus (HIV)-associated diseases. Parkinsonism occurs with one street substitute for heroin. A heroin-associated nephropathy is known to occur. Hemolytic anemia and thrombocytopenia may also occur with chronic opiate abuse (Stutzman, 1987).

Hallucinogens

Chronic use of cannabis and other hallucinogens may result in immunologic suppression. Chronic obstructive pulmonary disease (COPD), arrhythmias, rhabdomyolysis, and renal failure also are known to occur (Stutzman, 1987).

Inhalants

Chronic effects from inhalants include neurotoxicity and pulmonary and renal sequelae. Long-term cerebellar dysfunction in adolescents has been reported. A peripheral neuropathy termed "huffer's neuropathy" has been observed. Pulmonary effects in the form of direct lung injury are suspected. Toluene sniffing can result in muscle weakness, gastroenteritis, complaints of pain and hematemesis, neuropsychiatric disorders, and peripheral neuropathy. Renal tubular damage and nonanion gap acidosis are common.

OBTAINING THE SUBSTANCE ABUSE HISTORY

When approaching the substance abuse history, the family physician must be open and friendly yet direct and thorough. An adolescent school physical examination should include an inquiry that opens the door to this discussion. "It is important for us to be open and honest when discussing health issues, but I want to reassure you that whatever we discuss will be held in strictest confidence. Many young people today are trying out recreational drugs by smoking cigarettes, marijuana, or 'crack.' Have you or your friends tried any of these?" A young adult with rhinorrhea and hypertension could be queried regarding stimulant or cocaine insufflation in the following manner. "I notice that your blood pressure is elevated, and your nasal passages are swollen. Are there any over-the-counter nasal sprays or recreational drugs you are currently exposed to that may contribute to this picture?" Finally, the reluctant patient with telltale evidence of substance abuse who persists in denying a problem may undergo a focused physical examination to confirm medical suspicions. The physician may continue obtaining more history of possible adverse effects on school or work performance, social and behavioral change, recent change of friends, gang involvement, or breakdown of family and interpersonal relationships. When the individual acknowledges substance abuse, each possible route of intake should be elaborated and recorded in the history. Obtaining data from significant others may be particularly important. A history of cough and black sputum may be obtained from patients who freebase cocaine (Tashkin et al., 1992).

PHYSICAL EXAMINATION

A focused physical examination should detail target organs that may be affected by commonly abused or suspect drugs. A careful assessment of mental status should be undertaken to exclude overt depression, suicidal ideation, or evidence of thought disorder. A careful neurologic examination should be accomplished with particular attention to tremor, twitching, signs of hyperreflexia, parkinsonism, and pupillary sizes and responses. Blood pressure and pulse should be accurately recorded. Skin findings such as gang related tatoos, jaundice, diaphoresis, piloerection, skin needle tracks, or abscesses should be noted. The eyes/ears/nose/throat (EENT) examination findings including scleral ic-

terus, nasal mucosal redness, atrophy, ulceration, or pharyngeal erythema are observed. The cardiovascular examination should detect evidence of dysrhythmia, new murmur, or changes in pre-existent heart sounds. Pulmonary findings including increased anteroposterior diameter, wheezes, and rhonchi are elicited. Hepatomegaly is noted on the abdominal examination. The maternofetal examination seeks to uncover evidence of intrauterine growth retardation or other signs of fetal distress. Sexually transmitted diseases are frequent in pregnant and nonpregnant addicted patients.

LABORATORY FINDINGS

A drug abuse or toxicology profile may be obtained to corroborate reportedly abused substances. Clandestine or unindicated testing through the physician's office should be discouraged. Specific drug levels may be assayed when emergency management or detoxification is anticipated. Additional laboratory parameters should be examined based on the findings of the focused history and physical. An intravenous drug abuser should receive a hepatitis profile. HIV antibody testing should be offered with appropriate informed consent and pre- and post-test counseling. Cocaine abusers may require sinus radiographs, chest radiographs, or cardiac profiles depending on circumstances. Prescription drug and analgesic abusers require liver and renal function tests. When first-time seizures occur in young persons, an electroencephalogram (EEG) should be done several days after the event. A computed tomography (CT) scan of the head is indicated when there is any suspicion of a focal event. Marijuana or "crack" smokers may benefit from pulmonary function screening.

SCREENING ISSUES

Screening technologies for drug abuse remain imperfect tools that serve as adjuncts to clinical acumen. The family physician should approach these technologies with caution, particularly with regard to workplace screening. As with any diagnostic test, predictive value is proportionally related to the prevalence of the disease in the population.

Medical Review Officer certification validates the family physician's skills in interpreting drug screening tests for drug-free workplace employment. Drug testing technology includes thin-layer chromatography (TLC), immunoassays, and confirmation tests (Stimmel, 1993).

INTERVENTION

Denial

Patient denial is a particularly difficult issue for the family physician approaching chemical dependency intervention. The patient may be frightened or threatened by discussion, detection, or intervention in his or her drug abuse or dependency disorder. Responses vary, including anger, amusement, denial of a problem, or evading the question. The patient's lack of awareness of harmful sequelae of drug abuse may be genuine and related to cognitive or functional impairment; at other times denial is a deliberate ego defense. Regardless of cause, significant disorders must be confronted in a humane, nonjudgmental, persuasive manner by the concerned physician.

Negotiating patients into chemical dependency treatment involves a process. Social factors help leverage intervention and include (1) spouse or family pressure, (2) legal pressures including "driving under the influence" (DUI) charges, and (3) employment issues (absenteeism or threatened job loss). Inpatients can be motivated by economic pressures for failure to follow medical advice resulting in possible loss of reimbursement (option given to sign out against medical advice or enter treatment). Direct referral to chemical dependency facilities is more readily accomplished when family or significant others are actively involved.

Detoxification

Detoxification is often accomplished on an outpatient basis, although certain drugs may require inpatient treatment. Factors to weigh when assessing outpatient detoxification potential are (1) single or polydrug abuse; (2) presence or absence of social supports; (3) type of abused drug(s); (4) previous failed efforts at outpatient treatment; (5) mental status abnormalities; (6) serious medical complications; and (7) levels of addiction. Treatment avenues available to patients are determined by reimbursement. Outpatient approaches can be attempted initially. If relapse occurs, inpatient or residential treatment should be pursued. Sedative hypnotic or major depressant detoxification frequently requires initial inpatient care.

Detoxification regimens are specific to the abused agents. Widely accepted protocols (Booker and Benzer, 1987; Salkin, 1987) include those listed in Table 59–2. The most frequently used medications for cocaine detoxification are desipramine, L-tryptophan, amantadine, and bromocriptine (Halikas et al., 1993). For current detoxification practices see Cross and Hennessey, 1993.

TREATMENT APPROACHES

Postdetoxification treatment approaches range from self-help groups to highly structured long-term residential programs (Wilford, 1981). Self-help groups are modeled after the 12-step program Alcoholics Anonymous (AA). Drug abuse-specific 12-step programs include Narcotics Anonymous and Cocaine Anonymous. For combined alcohol and drug addictions, Alcoholics Anonymous is a reasonable option. Most chemically dependent patients require specific, directive treatment. Treatment programs available in the 1990s are mainly outpatient or short term residential. Factors including medical and psychiatric complications, compliance demonstrated by urine drug screens, previous treatment outcomes, reimbursement options, and

TABLE 59–2. DETOXIFICATION REGIMENS

Abused Drugs	Toxic Therapy	Abstinence Syndrome	Blockade Therapy
Cocaine	ABCs/supportive Benzodiazepines CA blockers Anticonvulsants	Desipramine *or* Bromocriptine	N/A
Stimulants	Benzodiazepines Charcoal lavage Acidify urine	Minor tranquilizer *or* Antipsychotic if required	N/A
Sedative hypnotics	Saline diuresis/supportive	Substitution of short-acting benzodiazepine	N/A
Depressants	Alkalinize urine	Pentobarbital challenge test + substitution RX*	N/A
Phenobarbital	Na bicarbonate Respiratory support		
Opiates	Narcan ABCs/supportive	Clonidine, Darvon, or methadone	Naltrexone
Hallucinogens	Benzodiazepines	N/A	N/A

N/A = not applicable.
* Incremental doses of pentobarbital; to achieve sedation, switch to equivalent total dose of phenobarbital followed by gradual phenobarbital reduction (30 mg/day).
From Smith DE, Wesson DR: A new method for treatment of barbiturate dependence. JAMA 213:294, 1970, with permission. Copyright 1970, American Medical Association.

social supports are evaluated, weighing outpatient versus inpatient treatment decisions.

State of the art cocaine treatment was reviewed by Wallace (1991) and can include outpatient approaches. The antidepressants fluoxetine (Prozac) and bupropion (Wellbutrin) have been tried for cocaine addiction (Gold, 1993). Preliminary results with bupropion approached abstinence rates of 70 per cent (Kosten, 1992). Methadone maintenance and naltrexone are viable options for opiate-addicted individuals (Schuckit, 1984). Methadone maintenance has been shown to reduce criminality. Programs that have extensive ongoing outpatient programs of 6 months to a year tend to improve outcomes (Wallace, 1991). Managed care options tend to be more limited.

FOLLOW-UP MANAGEMENT

Follow-up management is guided by prognosis. Previous failed efforts at rehabilitation do not indicate automatic failure; patients with these disorders often relapse. Patients improve their prognosis if motivated to enter long-term therapeutic communities (e.g., SynAnon). Structured, supportive follow-up care includes monitoring compliance with self-help group attendance, offering supportive psychotherapy, managing aversive or chemotherapeutic regimens, and monitoring urine drug screens. Clinicians may query the patients about frequency of attendance at 12-step group meetings, if they have obtained a "sponsor," and how they are progressing with "step work." Issues such as changing lifestyle, attending groups, home and job conflicts, personality disorders, and unresolved anger should be evaluated and addressed. Family physicians should familiarize themselves with local resources and consultants in the addictions field (available from the American Society of Addiction Medicine (Salkin, 1987).

PHYSICIAN IMPAIRMENT

Physician impairment is an increasingly recognized issue. Most state medical societies have systems to aid recovering professionals. The Joint Commission on the Accreditation of Healthcare Organizations now requires medical staff bylaws to include impaired physician committees. Physicians seem to have higher rates of chemical dependency than do other populations. It may be related to increased access to pharmaceuticals, higher levels of job stress, or increased awareness and recognition of or lack of alternative outlets for handling illness or anxiety. The American Academy of Family Physicians has developed programs that target professional awareness and prevention to help combat chemical dependency.

AIDS AND DRUG USE

Intravenous drug use has been implicated in 26 per cent of those diagnosed with AIDS (Stimmel, 1993). The exchange of sex for drugs constitutes an additional burden of drug-related HIV transmission through heterosexual or homosexual contact. Women with HIV, in turn, pass it on vertically to newborns. Availability of drug treatment, needle-exchange programs, and HIV CTPN (counseling, testing, and partner notification) activities can break this cycle.

COMMUNITY AND PUBLIC HEALTH ISSUES

Drug abuse prevention research has shown that efforts combining cognitive, behavioral, and social skill learning that increases resistance to prodrug social influences appear to be most effective. The family physician has a responsibility to assist in these community-based prevention efforts. The family physician can further develop knowledge and expertise in this area and serve as a resource in helping to educate community groups. Family practice residency programs and hospitals have developed "speakers bureaus" of physicians willing to speak in schools, churches, and civic and other community groups on various preventive health care issues. Effective approaches include local treatment resources; recovering individuals are particularly helpful during the presentations. The physician here serves as a resource person knowledgeable about medical sequelae of chemical dependency.

The American Society of Addiction Medicine (ASAM) recommends prevention programs to educate all members of the public about the danger of alcohol and drug use during pregnancy and lactation (ASAM, 1991). The future success of the war on drug use depends on its focus on treatment of addicts (Stimmel, 1993).

CONCLUSION

Drug abuse disorders remain an important issue in family practice. Cocaine dependence is currently a major component of this health care burden. Family physicians must acquire skills in the recognition of and screening for chemical dependency in their practice. Family physicians must acquire additional skills in the intervention and referral for treatment in order to deliver comprehensive patient care. The family physician should become knowledgeable about physician impairment. The specialty of family practice plays a significant role in enhancing community awareness and in the prevention of these disorders.

REFERENCES

Abelson HI, Miller JD: A decade of trends in cocaine use in the household population. Natl Inst Drug Abuse Res Monogr Ser 61:35, 1985.

Adams EH, Kozel NJ: Cocaine use in America: Introduction and overview. Natl Inst Drug Abuse Res Monogr Ser 61:1, 1985.

American Society of Addictions Medicine: Annual Review Course, 1991.

Blondell RD (ed): Primary Care: Clinics in Office Practice. Substance abuse 20(1). Philadelphia, WB Saunders Company, 1993.

Booker R, Benzer D: Subacute care. *In* Review Course Syllabus. New York, American Medical Society on Alcoholism and Other Drug Dependencies, 1987, pp 189–208.

Carr IA: The pharmacology of mood-altering drugs of abuse. *In* Blondell RD (ed): Primary Care: Clinics in Office Practice; Substance Abuse, 20:19–31. Philadelphia, WB Saunders Company, 1993.

Chasnoff IJ, Bussey ME, Savich R, et al: Perinatal cerebral infarction and maternal cocaine use. J Pediatr 108:456, 1986.

Claussen J: Early history of narcotics use and narcotics legislation in the United States. New Brunswick, NJ. *In* Rock P (ed): Drugs and Politics. Transaction Books, 1977, pp 23–24.

Creger LL, Mark H: Special report: Medical complications of cocaine abuse. N Engl J Med 315:1495, 1986.

Cross GM, Hennessey PT: Principles and practices of detoxification. *In* Blondell RD (ed) Primary Care: Clinics in Office Practice; Substance abuse, 20:81–94. Philadelphia, WB Saunders Company, 1993.

Dembo R, Williams L, Schmeidler J, et al: Juvenile crime and drug abuse: A prospective study of high risk youth. South J Addict Dis 11(2):5, 1991.

Fernandez-Pol B, Bluestone H, Muzruch MS: Inner City substance abuse patterns: a study of psychiatric inpatients. Amer J Drug Abuse 14:41, 1988.

Giannini AJ, Loiselle RH, Dimatzio LR, et al: Augmentation of haloperidol by ascorbic acid in phencyclidine intoxication. Am J Psychiatry 144:1207, 1987.

Glastris P: The new drug in town (methcathinone abuse and sales in Michigan). US News and World Report (April 26) 114:20, 1993.

Gold MS: Drugs of Abuse, A Comprehensive series for Clinicians, Vol. 3: Cocaine. New York, Plenum Medical, 1993.

Goodwin DW, Schulsinger F, Hermansen L, et al: Alcohol problems in adoptees raised apart from alcoholic biological parents. Arch Gen Psychiatry 28:238, 1973.

Halikas JA, Nugent SM, Crosby RD, et al: 1990–1991 Survey of pharmacotherapies used in the treatment of cocaine abusers. J Addict Dis 12(2):129, 1993.

Kulberg A: Substance abuse: clinical identification and management; pediatric toxicology. Pediatr Clin North Am 33:331, 1986.

Kosten TR: Behavioral and Pharmacological Treatment of Cocaine Dependence: Treatment Changes in the 1990's. Washington DC, American Psychiatric Association, 1992.

Madden JS: A Guide to Alcohol and Drug Dependence. Bristol, UK, John Wright & Sons, 1979.

Morgan JP: Alcohol and Drug Abuse Curriculum Guide for Pharmacology Faculty. Rockville, MD, National Institute on Drug Abuse, 1985, pp 3–19.

Nalbandian H, Sheth N, Dierich R, et al: Intestinal ischemia caused by cocaine ingestion: Report of 2 cases. Surgery 97:374, 1986.

Paredes A, Gorlick DA: Physiological and physiopathological effects of cocaine. J Addict Dis 11(4):1, 1992.

Pentel P, Mikell F, Navoral SH: Myocardial injury after phenyl-propanolamine ingestion. Br Heart J 47:51, 1982.

Robins LN: Study childhood predictors of adult outcomes: Replications from longitudinal studies. Psychol Med 8:611, 1978.

Salkin M: Management of emergencies. *In* Review Course Syllabus. New York, American Medical Society on Alcoholism and Other Drug Dependencies, 1987.

Schuckit MA: Drug and Alcohol Abuse: A Clinical Guide to Diagnosis and Treatment. New York, Plenum Press, 1984.

Shveitzer VG: Osteolytic sinusitis and pneumomediastinum: Deceptive otolaryngologic complications of cocaine abuse. Laryngoscope 96:206, 1986.

Simonds NF: The molecular basis of opiod receptor function. Endocrinol Rev 9:200, 1988.

Simpson RW, Edwards WD: Pathogenesis of cocaine induced ischemic heart disease. Arch Pathol Lab Med 110:479, 1986.

Smith DE, Wesson DR: Benzodiazepine dependency syndromes. J Psychoactive Drugs 15:85, 1983.

Stimmel B: Effective treatment for substance abuse: Defining the issues. J Addict Dis 11(2):1, 1991.

Stimmel B: The Facts About Drug Use. Binghamton, NY, Haworth Medicine Press, 1993 (originally 1991).

Strang J, Griffiths P, Powis B, Gossop M: First use of heroin: Changes in route of administration over time. BMJ 304:1222, 1992.

Stutzman E: Medical complications. *In* Review Course Syllabus. New York, American Medical Society on Alcoholism and Other Drug Dependencies, 1987.

Tashkin DP, Gorelick D, Khalsa ME, et al: Respiratory effects of cocaine freebasing among habitual cocaine users. J Addict Dis 11(4):59, 1992.

Vilensky W: Illicit and licit drugs causing perforation of the nasal septum. J Forensic Sci 27:958, 1982

Wallace BC: Crack cocaine: What constitutes state of the art treatment? J Addict Dis 11(2):79, 1991.

Wilford BB: Drug Abuse: A Guide for the Primary Care Physician. Chicago, American Medical Association, 1981.

CHAPTER 60

INTERPRETING LABORATORY TESTS

PAUL M. FISCHER

The diagnosis of disease is often easy, often difficult, and often impossible.—Peter Mere Latham (1789–1875)

Since the 1960s there has been an extensive change in how clinicians use laboratory tests. The 1960s were marked by an uncritical acceptance of "screening panels," which promised to diagnose disease prior to the patient becoming symptomatic. Multichannel chemistry analyzers made it possible to order large numbers of tests and to have the results back within a short time. Test ordering became simplified to just deciding the particular "panel" or "profile" that was needed.

During the 1970s and 1980s it became clear that few of the common tests were useful for screening asymptomatic individuals. This realization was the result of a better understanding of the limits of tests for predicting disease. Sophisticated decision analysis models were developed based on a test's sensitivity, specificity, and predictive value. *Sensitivity* refers to the rate a test is positive in a patient with disease. *Specificity* is the likelihood that the test will be negative in a patient without disease. *Predictive value* is the percent of patients with a positive test who actually are diseased.

Mathematic modeling based on test performance became a seductive area of research for academicians trying to characterize a "rational" way to order tests. The trend was further promoted by health care payers in an effort to eliminate unnecessary costs. Toward this end, the American College of Physicians and the Blue Cross/Blue Shield Association developed a text on the use and interpretation of common diagnostic tests (Sox, 1987). Just as the number of tests in a laboratory panel appeared to be a panacea for physicians during the 1960s, the complexity of these mathematic equations was touted as the panacea for rational test selection during the 1980s. Unfortunately, the promises of these mathematic models have not been realized. As explained below, the ambiguities of clinical practice make caring for patients a less precise science than mathematics. Furthermore, tests are used in many ways by clinicians. As George Lundberg (Editor, *JAMA*) has shown, physicians sometimes order tests merely because there is "nothing else to do" (Lundberg, 1983).

In the sections that follow, some of the issues that produce ambiguity for clinicians when ordering tests are highlighted. Forty common tests and outlines for using them in clinical practice then follow. Our intent with these outlines is not to dictate how physicians should order tests but, rather, to help them interpret the test results that seem not to make sense.

PROBLEM OF A "GOLD STANDARD"

Calculating a test's sensitivity and specificity requires a "gold standard." This standard is a reference test that can be considered definitive for characterizing a patient as either having a disease or being free of disease. Unfortunately, most gold standards for common tests are imperfect.

Coronary angiography is used as a gold standard for the presence of coronary artery disease; however, studies have shown that this test frequently misclassifies both the presence and the absence of significant coronary artery stenosis (Boyko et al., 1988). For example, it does not indicate the presence of small-vessel coronary disease, which can produce ischemia. If a gold standard misclassifies individuals, both the sensitivity and specificity of a second comparison test are then artificially altered.

The inadequacy of reference tests is a problem for such common diseases as group A streptococcal pharyngitis and urinary tract infections. When diagnosing patients with sore throats, a throat culture has traditionally been used. More recently, rapid tests that detect group A streptococcal cell wall antigens have become available. Many microbiologists believe that these newer tests are inadequate because they have a 10 per cent false-negative rate compared to cultures (i.e., in 10 per cent of patients with negative antigen tests, group A streptococci grow on a throat culture). However, the colony count in these "false-negative" cases is often low. It is therefore not clear whether the patient is a noninfected carrier or an infected patient. The sensitivity of any group A streptococcal test can be discredited by employing more sophisticated culture techniques as reference methods, thereby recovering streptococci from a larger percentage of healthy individuals who carry group A streptococci in their throats but are not infected (DeNeef, 1987a).

Some have argued that a rise in streptococcal antibody titers (i.e., ASO titers) should be used as the gold standard when determining who really has group A streptococcal pharyngitis. In one study looking at the clinical response to antibiotic therapy of individuals with a positive throat culture, patients with and without antibody response showed a clinical improvement with antibiotics compared to individuals with a negative throat culture (Gerber et al., 1988). This study raises significant questions about the appropriateness of using antibody response to identify who has a true streptococcal infection. There is to date no clear agreement on the gold standard for evaluating the common condition of streptococcal pharyngitis.

As another example, consider the diagnosis of urinary tract infections. Until recently it was not uncommon to tell a woman with urinary frequency, urgency, and dysuria that she "was not infected" because her urine culture grew only 50,000 organisms per milliliter. This judgment was based on the time-honored level of 100,000 colonies/mL of urine as a cutoff for "significant" bacteriuria. This diagnostic level failed to consider the patient's symptoms, how long the urine had incubated in the bladder, or the specimen's specific gravity. More recent studies have indicated that a colony count as low as 100/mL may indicate infection in a woman with dysuria. There is in fact no single level of bacteria that can be used as a gold standard for diagnosing a urinary tract infection.

The gold standard problem will become more complicated in the future because of the availability of DNA-based tests such as the polymerase chain reaction (PCR). These tests can amplify a single DNA chain to a level that permits detection. Whereas clinicians should have little difficulty making decisions about a single tuberculosis organism in a sputum specimen or a single gonorrhea organism in a cervical specimen, what will we do with a test that can identify a single group A streptococcus in a throat swab or a single *Escherichia coli* in a urine specimen?

Unfortunately, there is no precise way to adjust for the errors of an imperfect reference test. Clinicians should therefore be cautious when interpreting the performance characteristics of any test; they should always look to see what gold standard was used and then rely on their common sense.

PROBLEMS IN CONFIDENCE

A second problem is the great variability in reported test sensitivities and specificities. Pronouncements are made that a test has a "95 per cent sensitivity" as if it were for all times and all patient populations. The next month, an article using the same test reports "60 per cent sensitivity." No wonder clinicians have a difficult time putting these concepts to use. One reason for this variation is that the accuracy of the reported sensitivity and specificity depends on the size of the population studied. Many of these studies have few patients. If the numbers are low, there can be little certainty of the results.

It has been recommended that sensitivities and specificities be reported as a "confidence interval" (Heckerling, 1988). This interval is the range of values (usually ± 2 SD) supported by the data. For example, if a test is positive in 15 of 20 patients with a disease, the sensitivity is 75 per cent. The 95 per cent confidence limit for this sensitivity, however, would be 51 to 91 per cent, meaning that there is a 95 per cent chance that the true sensitivity is between 51 and 91 per cent and a 5 per cent chance that it is less than 51 per cent or greater than 91 per cent. This is a wide variation. If the same test is studied with a larger population, and 300 of 400 patients with the disease have a positive test, the sensitivity remains 75 per cent, but the 95 per cent confidence limits would be narrowed to between 70 and 79 per cent.

The lesson for the clinician should be to suspect all sensitivity and specificity values. Be especially cautious when there is great variation in the values reported for a single test.

SPECTRUM OF DISEASE

Traditional test performance models assume that either there is disease or there is not. This simplistic ideal is complicated by the concept of the spectrum of disease (Ransohoff and Feinstein, 1978), which is the range of features that characterize an illness (i.e., variation in chronicity and severity). Test results vary at different points in a disease. The usual pattern is that the test is more likely to be positive when the disease is of a longer duration or greater severity. Unfortunately, clinicians usually order tests early during the course of a disease, before the diagnosis is obvious. Many of the reported sensitivities and specificities from the literature are optimistically high because of the tendency of researchers to ignore the problem of disease spectrum.

An example is the literature on carcinoembryonic antigen (CEA) testing for colon cancer. The early studies indicated 90 per cent sensitivity for this test. Most of these studies were done on individuals with extensive disease. Later studies with more representative examples of colon cancer patients (i.e., some with localized disease and others with extensive disease) showed that the test was sensitive only in patients with extensive cancer.

Test specificity can be inaccurate because of the variety of nondiseased patients who are studied.

(Remember, specificity is defined as the percentage of individuals without the disease who have a negative test.) The early studies on CEA and colon cancer showed specificities of 90 per cent. The nondiseased individuals in these studies were healthy and asymptomatic. Later studies used a more appropriate spectrum of controls (i.e., individuals with other colon diseases or those with cancers other than of the colon). In these later studies, the specificity of CEA testing was greatly reduced. Not surprisingly, CEA can be elevated in colon diseases that mimic colon cancer.

PROBLEM OF PREVALENCE

Another concept used in the mathematic modeling for test interpretation is that of "disease prevalence." Prevalence is the number of individuals with the disease in a population at a given time. There are unfortunately almost no prevalence figures that can be easily "plugged into" a decision analysis formula for real clinical situations. The best that can usually be done to estimate the prevalence of a disease is to say whether it is common, uncommon, or rare.

There are typically two types of prevalence figures in the literature. The first type is derived from case-series seen in referral centers: What percentage of patients seen at a university urology clinic who have an elevated prostatic-specific antigen (PSA) level also have prostate cancer? Such prevalence figures are notoriously inaccurate because of the problem of referral bias.

A second type of reported prevalence comes from population studies. With this type of research, a specified population is tested (i.e., PSA tests are done on all men over age 60 in a defined geographic region). Although this type of prevalence figure may help characterize the disease for the general population, it does not necessarily help the individual clinician deal with the symptomatic patient who presents for a diagnosis: What is the prevalence of prostate cancer in a 65-year-old man who complains of nocturia and a weak urinary stream and who has a large, smooth prostate by digital examination and a borderline high PSA value?

Another aspect of prevalence that is usually overlooked is that it varies from one practice to another and from month to month. Consider, for example, the differences in the prevalence of human immunodeficiency virus (HIV) disease in San Francisco compared with that in Omaha. Also consider the prevalence of influenza in February compared with July.

TREATMENT ASSUMPTIONS

It is often assumed that understanding a test's predictive value will lead to clear, rational test or-

dering. However, even when clinicians can agree on the characteristics of a test, they may end up with different decisions on how to use the test. This point has been illustrated by DeNeef for testing to detect group A streptococcal pharyngitis (DeNeef, 1987b). DeNeef looked at 21 ways to evaluate and treat adults with pharyngitis. He included a wide range of treatment strategies including the empiric use of antibiotics, culturing all patients, or testing everyone with rapid tests. In the end, it was not the characteristics of the tests that determined the optimal clinical strategy but, rather, the physician's treatment goals. These goals could include minimizing the total test cost, minimizing adverse outcomes, or minimizing the cost of both adverse outcomes and unnecessary antibiotics. In the end, it was the clinicians' assumptions about the optimal therapeutic goals, not the characteristics of the tests, that determined "appropriate" test ordering.

DECISION LEVELS

If clinicians cannot easily use sensitivity, specificity, or predictive value when making clinical decisions, then what do they use? It is our observation that when interpreting tests clinicians usually ask two questions:

1. Is it normal or abnormal?
2. If abnormal, is it a little abnormal or highly abnormal?

The degree of abnormality has been overlooked in many discussions about test interpretations (Statland, 1987). It is, however, what clinicians have intuitively used for a long time when deciding whether they should act on a test result. A serum calcium of 10.5 mg/dL, although outside the usual reference range, does not catch a clinician's attention. On the other hand, a level of 13 mg/dL is impossible to ignore.

The remainder of this chapter reviews many of the common tests that clinicians must learn to interpret. Each section includes background information about the test, common causes of abnormal results, and some of the common pitfalls in test interpretation. These rules should not be viewed as firm, but as clinically useful, guides. The information reflects our perspective based on work in primary care clinical settings.

Each section includes a table of "normal" values. This term has fallen out of favor with mathematic purists, who prefer the term "reference range." Although "reference range" may be statistically safer, it is not clinically useful. Most men would prefer a "normal" PSA to one that is "within the reference range." In the following sections, we have indicated, where appropriate, the differences between the normal values for adults and children, males and females. All values are given in both conventional units and Systeme International (SI) units. The U.S. medical community has flirted with adoption of SI units, but old habits die hard. Conversion factors (conventional units to SI units) are also given.

Despite the increasing interest in establishing rules for appropriate test ordering, the best that can be said is that there are a few instances when a test is clearly indicated, a few where it is clearly inappropriate, and many other instances that are open to debate. Clinicians live in a sea of uncertainty.

ALBUMIN

Albumin is produced by the liver and released into the plasma, where it accounts for 90 per cent of the intravascular oncotic pressure. A healthy adult liver is able to produce 12 to 14 grams of albumin per day (Table 60–1). This amount is reduced with advanced age, poor nutrition, or hepatic disease.

It is unclear how albumin is degraded in the body; only small amounts are normally lost through the urine or the gastrointestinal mucosa. When there is either a reduction in albumin synthesis or an increase in albumin loss, hypoalbuminemia develops, often associated with edema.

Serum albumin testing is not recommended for the general screening of healthy individuals. When such routine screening is done, most of the abnormal values are mildly elevated or decreased. These values represent the extremes of the normal distribution of values and can usually be ignored. The test is useful for evaluating patients with edema, liver disease, or suspected malnutrition.

An elevated albumin value is of no clinical significance. It is most commonly seen in the presence of dehydration.

ALKALINE PHOSPHATASE

Alkaline phosphatase (ALP) is a family of enzymes found in nearly all body tissues but with no known function (Table 60–2). In normal adults about half of the measured serum ALP is produced by the liver and about half by bone. Children and adolescents have ALP levels two to four times that of a normal adult due to the rapid bone growth in this age group. Women in the third trimester of pregnancy also have an elevated ALP, due to production of this enzyme by the placenta. This level returns to normal by 1 month postpartum.

Liver diseases are usually divided into those that are primarily hepatic and those that are cholestatic. Elevation in aminotransferase is the usual laboratory marker for direct hepatocyte insult. ALP, on the other hand, is the usual marker for a cholestatic illness, which includes any process that causes an obstruction in the bile ducts (i.e., stone, cancer, pancreatitis, primary biliary cirrhosis). In these illnesses, the ALP and conjugated bilirubin levels are moderately to markedly elevated, whereas the aminotransferase levels are normal or only mildly elevated. With illnesses that are directly hepatotoxic (i.e., viral hepatitis) the aminotransferase and conjugated bilirubin are greatly elevated, whereas the ALP may be normal or only mildly elevated. Although alcohol ingestion is often cited as a cause for an elevated ALP, it is rarely the case unless there is advanced cirrhosis or severe alcoholic hepatitis.

The ALP level is elevated in disorders associated with osteoblastic activity (i.e., new bone formation). Paget's disease of bone is the prototypical illness. Ninety per cent of these patients have an elevated ALP even though most are asymptomatic. Osteoporosis and fractures do not commonly lead to elevated ALP levels.

A γ-glutamyltransferase test (GGT) is useful for differentiating between biliary and bony sources of an elevated ALP. The GGT is usually elevated when the ALP is derived from the liver.

The ALP is not a useful screening test in asymptomatic individuals. Values less than the reference range are of no clinical significance. Because more than 200 medications can cause an elevated ALP,

TABLE 60–1. ALBUMIN: NORMAL VALUES

Diagnostic units: gm/dL (gm/L)
SI conversion factor = 10
Normal: 4.0–6.0 gm/dL (40–60 gm/L)

Albumin Decreased	Diagnoses to Consider	Actions to Consider

<4.0 gm/dL	Decreased synthesis
	  Liver insufficiency
	  Malnutrition
	  Malignancy
	Increased loss
	  Nephrotic syndrome
	  Extensive burns
	  Protein-losing enteropathy
	Pregnancy
	Inflammatory illness
		1. Dietary history
		2. Urinalysis
		3. 24-Hour urine protein
		4. Bilirubin
		5. Creatinine
		6. Hemoglobin

Values in parentheses are SI units.

TABLE 60-2. ALKALINE PHOSPHATASE: NORMAL VALUES

Diagnostic units: units/L
Normal: Adults: 30–120
*   Children: 50–400*
*   Pregnant women: 30–200*

ALP Increased	Diagnoses to Consider	Actions to Consider
120–200 units/L	Nonfasting patient specimen Drug effect	1. Repeat test with patient fasting 2. Review patient medications

>200 units/L	Increased from bone
	  Paget's disease
	  Osteomalacia
	  Bony metastasis
	  Hyperparathyroidism
	Increased from liver
	  Bile duct stone
	  Biliary cancer
	  Pancreatic cancer
	  Pancreatitis
	  Liver infiltration (sarcoid)
	  Primary biliary cirrhosis
	  Viral hepatitis
	  Severe cirrhosis
	Other causes
	  Drug effect
	  Heart failure
	  Hyperthyroidism
	  Lymphoma
	  Leukemia
		1. Review patient medications
		2. Serum bilirubin, GGT, and aminotransferases
		3. RUQ abdominal ultrasonography
		4. Pelvis or femur x-rays
		5. Serum calcium
		6. Bone scan

GGT = γ-glutamyl transferase; RUQ = right upper quadrant.

a good first step in anyone with an unexplained ALP elevation is a thorough medication review.

AMINOTRANSFERASES

The aminotransferases (or transaminases) are enzymes primarily located within hepatocytes. Alanine aminotransferase (ALAT) was formerly referred to as serum glutamate pyruvate trans-aminase (SGPT). Aspartate aminotransferase (ASAT) was formerly referred to as serum glutamate oxaloacetate transaminase (SGOT). Increased levels of the two enzymes are due to liver injury and the subsequent leaking of the enzymes from the cells. In general, the level of the aminotransferases reflects the severity of hepatic injury (Table 60–3).

ALAT is fairly specific for the liver. In contrast, ASAT is increased after injury to cardiac or skeletal

TABLE 60-3. AMINOTRANSFERASES: NORMAL VALUES

Diagnostic units: units/L
Normal: 0–35

Increased	Diagnoses to Consider	Actions to Consider

35–400 units/L	ALAT and ASAT elevated
	  Infectious hepatitis
	  Toxic hepatitis
	  Alcoholic hepatitis
	  Shock liver
	  Biliary obstruction
	Only ASAT elevated
	  Myocardial infarction
	  Hemolysis (in vivo)
	  Pulmonary infarction
	  Muscular dystrophy
		1. Review patient medication
		2. Review foreign travel, needle sticks, chemical exposures, transfusion history
		3. Alcohol history
		4. Serum bilirubin, alkaline phosphatase
		5. Test for viral hepatitis
		6. Peripheral smear for hemolysis

>400 units/L	ALAT and ASAT elevated
	  Infectious hepatitis
	  Toxic hepatitis
	  Shock liver	

ALAT = alanine aminotransferase; ASAT = aspartate aminotransferase.

muscle as well. This fact is useful clinically because if both enzymes are elevated a hepatic source is likely. With most illnesses the ALAT value is greater than the ASAT. The only common exception to this rule is in patients with alcoholic hepatitis, in whom the ASAT is higher.

ASAT and ALAT testing are not useful for screening healthy individuals. They are, however, useful for diagnosing and monitoring all forms of liver disease. They are also frequently used as screening tests in patients on medications that can produce liver injury (i.e., INH).

Aminotransferase values less than the lower normal limit are infrequently seen and are of little clinical significance. The exceptions are advanced cirrhosis and fulminant hepatitis, where a normal or low level can indicate that the disease has progressed so far that few hepatocytes remain.

AMYLASE (SERUM)

There are few diseases that are diagnosed as regularly, based on a single test, as is pancreatitis after finding an elevated amylase level (Table 60–4). With few exceptions, an elevated amylase concentration indicates pancreatitis, and a normal level rules out the diagnosis. In addition to pancreatitis, patients with abdominal pain and an elevated amylase level should be evaluated for a perforated peptic ulcer or mesenteric infarction.

Amylase is produced by the pancreas, salivary glands, and some tumors (e.g., lung). Most of the amylase produced by the pancreas goes directly into the gut. A small fraction is absorbed into the circulation. Normally, about one third of serum amylase is pancreatic in origin, and two thirds is from the salivary glands. The amylase in the circulation is excreted primarily by the kidneys. Modest eleva-

tions in serum amylase (i.e., two times normal) can therefore be seen in patients with chronic renal failure.

The degree of amylase elevation does not always correlate with the severity of pancreatic injury. In fact, pancreatitis without an elevation in amylase is seen in about 10 per cent of patients, especially those with recurrent disease or with a long duration of symptoms before testing. In such cases, a serum lipase assay, urinary amylase assay, or amylase/creatinine clearance ratio may be helpful.

For unexplained hyperamylasemia, serum lipase or amylase isoenzyme assays may be useful. Lipase is produced by the pancreas but not by salivary glands.

Low serum amylase levels are rarely of clinical significance.

BILIRUBIN (TOTAL)

Bilirubin is formed from the heme ring as senescent red blood cells are degraded. It is transported in blood attached to albumin and then delivered to the liver, where it is conjugated and excreted in the bile. The common causes for hyperbilirubinemia are increased red blood cell destruction, liver diseases, and biliary tract obstruction.

Laboratories measure the total bilirubin and conjugated (i.e., direct) bilirubin (Table 60–5). The unconjugated bilirubin fraction (i.e., indirect) is then obtained by subtraction. For normal serum, less than 15 per cent of the total bilirubin is in the conjugated fraction. The various causes for hyperbilirubinemia have traditionally been divided into those associated with unconjugated bilirubin and those associated with conjugated bilirubin. In practice, many diseases are of a mixed form (i.e.,

TABLE 60–4. AMYLASE: NORMAL VALUES

Diagnostic units: Somogyi units/dL (units/L)
Normal: 50–150 (0–130)

Amylase Increased	Diagnoses to Consider	Actions to Consider
>150 Somogyi units/dL	Pancreatitis Alcoholic Gallstone Trauma Hyperlipidemia Infectious Drug-induced Familial Post ERCP Perforating ulcer Mesenteric infarction Salivary gland disease Chronic renal failure Amylase-secreting cancer	1. Alcohol history 2. Abdominal examination 3. Complete drug history 4. RUQ ultrasonography 5. Urinary amylase 6. Amylase/creatinine clearance 7. Lipase or amylase isoenzyme

Values in parentheses are SI units.
RUQ = right upper quadrant; ERCP = endoscopic retrograde cholangiopancreatography.

TABLE 60–5. BILIRUBIN: NORMAL VALUES

Diagnostic units: mg/dL (μmol/L)
SI conversion factor = 17.1
Normal: 0.1–1.0 (2–17)

Bilirubin Increased	Diagnoses to Consider	Actions to Consider
Newborns		
1.0–10 mg/dL	Direct <15% of total	1. Mother and infant blood type
	Physiologic	2. Direct Coombs tests
	Breast feeding	3. Hematocrit
	ABO incompatibility	
	Rh incompatibility	
	Hemorrhage	
	Maternal diabetes	
	Direct >15% of total	
	Sepsis	
	TORCH infections	
	Hepatitis	
	Biliary atresia	
10–20 mg/dL	Kernicterus possible	1. Phototherapy or exchange transfusion (base decision on days of age, weight, maturity)
Adults		
>1.0 mg/dL	Hepatic insufficiency	1. Alcohol history
	Biliary obstruction	2. Complete drug history
	Hemolysis	3. Travel, dietary, and needle stick history
	Postoperative complications	4. Peripheral blood smear
		5. Conjugated bilirubin, AST, ALP
		6. Reticulocyte count
		7. Viral hepatitis tests
		8. Direct Coombs' test
		9. RUQ ultrasonography

Values in parentheses are SI units.
AST = aspartate aminotransferase (SGOT); ALP = alkaline phosphatase; RUQ = right upper quadrant.

elevation in both conjugated and unconjugated bilirubin).

With hepatic diseases, the bilirubin level is usually proportional to the level of hepatocyte injury. Jaundice is detectable only when the total bilirubin level exceeds 3.0 mg/dL. Low serum bilirubin levels are of no clinical significance.

BLOOD UREA NITROGEN

The blood urea nitrogen (BUN) assay is commonly used to measure renal function. The serum creatinine is, however, a much more reliable indicator of the glomerular filtration rate (GFR). It is more reliable because in addition to GFR the BUN is affected by the nitrogen load, water intake, and urine flow. If you want to know about the kidney, order a creatinine assay.

The normal BUN is 8 to 26 mg/dl (2.9 to 9.3 mmol/L). The SI conversion factor is 0.357 (Table 60–6).

A rise in BUN is seen with renal insufficiency, but it is not a specific indicator of renal function. A more useful method is to calculate the BUN/creatinine ratio. This ratio can serve as a useful indicator of diseases that result in an abnormal nitrogen load, urine flow, or water intake.

CALCIUM

Calcium is essential for maintenance of the skeleton and for normal neuromuscular function. The usual serum test for calcium measures the total calcium (Table 60–7). About half of the total calcium is bound to albumin. The rest is present in serum in the ionized form. The measurement of ionized calcium can also be specifically ordered.

The serum level of calcium is under the complex control of the parathyroid hormone (PTH) and calcitonin. These hormones and others control the rate at which calcium is absorbed from the gastrointestinal tract, excreted in the urine, and gained or lost to bone.

The most common laboratory abnormality seen is a low total calcium level in a patient with low serum albumin. It is primarily a disorder of serum albumin, not a problem with calcium, as the ionized calcium remains unchanged. In this setting it is possible to correct mathematically the calcium for the decreased albumin (1 gm/dl reduction in albumin leads to 1 mg/dl reduction in calcium).

Hypercalcemia is associated with fatigue, depression, constipation, polydipsia, ulcers, and hypertension. In the outpatient setting, the most common cause of hypercalcemia is hyperparathyroidism. Many of these patients are asymptomatic. Malignancies are the most common cause for hy-

TABLE 60–6.   BLOOD UREA NITROGEN/CREATININE RATIO: NORMAL VALUES

Normal 10 : 1 (BUN/Cr)

Ratio	Diagnoses to Consider	Actions to Consider
Increased >10	High nitrogen load 　GI bleeding 　High-protein diet 　High catabolism Low urine flow 　Dehydration 　Congestive heart failure	1. Examine for hydration status 2. Examine for congestive heart failure 3. Dietary history 4. Drug history (steroids) 5. Stool occult blood
Decreased <10	High urine flow 　Water intoxication 　SIADH Low-protein diet Protein malnutrition Liver insufficiency	1. Check serum and urine osmolality 2. Check serum sodium 3. Dietary history 4. Bilirubin

percalcemia in the inpatient setting. The most common cancers that produce hypercalcemia are in the lung, breast, or kidney.

Hypocalcemia produces symptoms that result from neuromuscular excitability: carpopedal spasm, seizures, tetany, stiffness, fatigue, memory loss, and confusion.

There is debate about whether serum calcium is an appropriate screening test for asymptomatic individuals. It has frequently been included in screening chemistry panels. The rationale for its use as a screening test has been that hyperparathyroidism is frequently asymptomatic. This argument has come into question because of the

TABLE 60–7.   CALCIUM: NORMAL VALUES

Diagnostic units: mg/dL (mmol/L)
SI conversion factor = 0.2495
Normal: 8.8–10.3 (2.20–2.57)

Calcium	Diagnoses to Consider	Actions to Consider
Increased 　10.3–13.0 mg/dL	Hyperparathyroidism Metastatic cancer Thiazide diuretics Immobilization Vitamin D intoxication Milk-alkali syndrome Multiple myeloma Sarcoidosis Thyrotoxicosis	1. Repeat serum calcium 2. Complete diet and drug history 3. Ionized calcium, albumin, phosphorus, PTH, T_4 4. Chest radiograph 5. Hand radiographs 6. Evaluation for malignancy
>13.0 mg/dL	Hypercalcemic coma	1. Vigorous hydration 2. Furosemide 3. Close monitoring
Decreased 　7.0–8.8 mg/dL	Hypoalbuminemia Chronic renal failure Hypoparathyroidism (neck 　surgery) Malnutrition Vitamin D deficiency 　Nutritional 　Anticonvulsants 　Malabsorption 　Liver disease Hypomagnesemia Pancreatitis	1. Serum albumin 2. Complete drug history 3. Alcohol history 4. Serum creatinine, phosphate, magnesium, PTH
<7.0 mg/dL	Hypocalcemic seizures Hypocalcemic arrhythmias	1. IV calcium gluconate 2. Serum ionized calcium 3. Serum magnesium

Values in parentheses are SI units.
PTH = parathyroid hormone; T_4 = thyroxine.

uncertainty of whether asymptomatic hyperparathyroidism requires any specific therapy.

CHLORIDE

Chloride is the major extracellular anion in the body. Despite this fact, it is a relatively uninteresting analyte and is rarely clinically useful.

Most dietary chloride is absorbed. The level in the body is then controlled by renal excretion (Table 60–8). The primary cause for an abnormal chloride is in response to a shift in the serum CO_2 content. The CO_2 content decreases when there is a metabolic acidosis or metabolic compensation for respiratory alkalosis. In these situations, the chloride increases in response to the reduction in CO_2 content. CO_2 content is increased in cases of metabolic alkalosis or in a metabolic response to respiratory acidosis. In these settings, the chloride is reduced to compensate for the increased CO_2 content.

Chloride can be depleted by either gastrointestinal losses (vomiting) or renal losses (salt-losing renal diseases). In this case, the chloride depletion results in a persistent metabolic alkalosis.

The most frequent use of the chloride test is for calculating the anion gap, which is calculated by subtracting the total measured anions (chloride + bicarbonate) from the total cations (sodium + potassium). The normal range for the anion gap is 16 ± 4 mEq/L. Increases in the anion gap indicate the presence of unmeasured anions such as ketoacids, lactic acids, methanol, and so forth.

CHOLESTEROL

The National Institutes of Health (NIH) has established a National Cholesterol Education Program. One goal of this program is to have all adults screened for hypercholesterolemia. Although there is considerable debate about which cholesterol levels require treatment and the optimal approach to treatment, most people now agree that the screening of adults is probably indicated (Table 60–9). Epidemiologic studies have shown that a 1 per cent decrease in total cholesterol is associated with a 2 per cent decrease in coronary heart disease (CHD) risk.

Considerable variation is often seen in repeated cholesterol values from the same patient. This variation is due to test inaccuracy (± 3 per cent), test imprecision (± 3 per cent), and day-to-day patient variation (± 7 per cent). In addition, cholesterol has been shown to demonstrate a seasonal variation. Although the studies have been limited, there does not appear to be a variation in total cholesterol based on whether the patient is fasting. (Fasting is, however, essential when measuring triglycerides and the cholesterol lipoprotein fractions.)

Cholesterol measurements should be used to diagnose hypercholesterolemia much as blood pressure readings are used to diagnose hypertension. Several readings over time are required before a diagnosis can be made.

If the total cholesterol indicates that the patient is at risk for hypercholesterolemia, the NIH recommends that a fasting lipoprotein profile be done. The total cholesterol, HDL cholesterol, and triglycerides should be measured. The LDL cholesterol can then be calculated by the formula: LDL cholesterol = total cholesterol − HDL cholesterol − triglycerides ÷ 5.

If the LDL cholesterol is 130 to 160 mg/dl, the patient is considered at borderline high risk for coronary heart disease. If the LDL cholesterol is higher than 160 mg/dl, the patient is considered at high risk for CHD. LDL values less than 130 mg/dl are desirable.

The NIH recommends that the decision to treat

TABLE 60–8. CHLORIDE: NORMAL VALUES

Diagnostic units: mEq/L (mmol/L)
SI conversion factor = 1
Normal 95–105 (95–105)

Chloride	Diagnoses to Consider	Actions to Consider

Increased >105 mEq/L	Metabolic acidosis
	    Loss of bicarbonate
	    Production of metabolic acids
	Respiratory alkalosis with metabolic compensation
	Dehydration
		1. HCO₃, Na, K, pH, BUN, Cl
		2. Calculate anion gap

Decreased <95 mEq/L	Metabolic alkalosis
	    Hydrogen ion loss
	    HCO₃ retention
	Respiratory acidosis with metabolic compensation
	Salt-losing renal disease
	Thiazide diuretics
		1. Urinalysis
		2. HCO₃, Na, K, pH, BUN, Cl

Values in parentheses are SI units.

TABLE 60–9. CHOLESTEROL: NORMAL VALUES

Diagnostic units: mg/dL (mmol/L)
SI conversion factor = 0.02586
Normal: < 200 (5.2)

Cholesterol Increased	Diagnoses to Consider	Actions to Consider

200–239 mg/dL	Borderline risk for CHD
	Familial hypercholesterolemia
	High cholesterol diet
	Biliary obstruction
	Nephrotic syndrome
	Hypothyroidism
		1. Repeat cholesterol test
		2. Evaluate for CAD risks
		  a. Male sex
		  b. Smoking
		  c. Family history of CHD
		  d. Hypertension
		  e. Diabetes mellitus
		  f. Severe obesity
		  g. History of vascular disease
		  h. LDL less than 35 mg/dL
		3. If patient has known CAD or two or more risk factors, order lipoprotein analysis

≥240 mg/dL	High risk for CHD
	As above
		1. Repeat cholesterol
		2. Fasting lipoprotein analysis
		3. Classify based on LDL
		  a. <130 = desirable
		  b. 130–159 = borderline risk
		  c. ≥160 = high risk

Cholesterol Decreased	Diagnoses to Consider	Actions to Consider
<140 mg/dL	Low risk for CHD Hyperthyroidism Hepatic insufficiency	1. Dietary history 2. Bilirubin 3. T_4, T_3U

Values in parentheses are SI units.
CHD = coronary heart disease; CAD = coronary artery disease; LDL = low density lipoprotein; T_4 = thyroxine; T_3U = triiodothyronine uptake.

be based on a patient's risk factors for CHD and the LDL value. Total cholesterol measurements should be used only for case finding and to follow the response to therapy (NIH, 1985).

CO_2 CONTENT

The CO_2 content of blood is made up of bicarbonate, carbonic acid, and dissolved CO_2. Ninety-five per cent of the total CO_2 content is bicarbonate (HCO_3). Bicarbonate is the second most important anion in serum and is the most available base that is capable of buffering a metabolic acid load. This role in the body's acid-base balance is its principal clinical function. The two mechanisms for control of CO_2 content are respiratory elimination of CO_2 and renal reabsorption of filtered bicarbonate. Bicarbonate can also be lost pathologically through elimination from the gastrointestinal tract (Table 60–10).

The most common CO_2 content abnormality is a decreased level due to metabolic acidosis. In this setting it is useful to calculate the anion gap, which may provide a clue to the cause of the acidosis.

Metabolic alkalosis may be initiated by the loss of hydrogen ion, as is seen with nasogastric suction. Maintenance of the metabolic alkalosis requires that there be greater than normal reabsorption of bicarbonate by the kidneys. Therefore in

patients with an elevated CO_2 content, look for diseases that affect the bicarbonate handling by the renal tubules.

CREATININE

Creatinine is released from skeletal muscle and is excreted unchanged in the urine. There are few factors other than renal function that affect its level in serum. It is therefore the best of the common tests for monitoring renal insufficiency. A rise in creatinine indicates a falling glomerular filtration rate.

The biggest problem with using creatinine as a measure of renal function is that it is a relatively insensitive marker of renal disease. A 50 per cent reduction in renal function from normal leads to a creatinine rise of from only 1 to 2.0 mg/dl (Table 60–11). Considerable early renal damage may therefore occur before it becomes apparent by a rising creatinine level.

A second problem with interpreting serum creatinine is that it is slow in reacting to sudden changes in renal function. For example, with sudden and severe renal failure (i.e., acute tubular necrosis following shock), the creatinine rises only 1 mg/dl/ day—despite a creatinine clearance of zero.

Because creatinine is released by skeletal muscle, it is occasionally affected by total muscle mass.

TABLE 60–10.   CARBON DIOXIDE (CO_2): NORMAL VALUES

Diagnostic units: mEq/L (mmol/L)
SI conversion factor = 1
Normal: 22–28 (22–28)

CO_2	Diagnoses to Consider	Actions to Consider

Decreased <22 mEq/L	Metabolic acidosis
	  Bicarbonate loss
	    Diarrhea
	    Renal tubular acidosis
	    Primary hyperparathyroidism
	  Failure to reabsorb bicarbonate
	    Triamterene, spironolactone
	    Renal tubular acidosis
	  Production of metabolic acids
	    Renal failure
	    Diabetic ketoacidosis
	    Lactic acidosis
	    Methanol
	    Ethylene glycol
	    Salicylates
	    Alcoholic ketoacidosis
	Respiratory alkalosis with compensation
	  Anxiety
	  Sepsis
	  Salicylates
	  CNS injury
		1. Full drug history
		2. Serum electrolytes
		3. Blood gas
		4. Calculate anion gap

Increased >28 mEq/L	Metabolic alkalosis
	  Volume contraction
	  Nasogastric suction
	  Vomiting
	  Potassium depletion
	  Furosemide
	  Cushing syndrome
	Chronic respiratory acidosis with compensation
		1. Serum electrolytes
		2. Blood gas
		3. Urine electrolytes

Values in parentheses are SI units.

TABLE 60–11.   CREATININE: NORMAL VALUES

Diagnostic units: mg/dL (μmol/L)
SI conversion factor = 88.4
Normal: 0.6–1.2 (50–110)

Creatinine Increased	Diagnoses to Consider	Actions to Consider
1.2–1.6 mg/dL	Mild renal impairment Muscle injury	1. Repeat test 2. Urinalysis 3. Creatinine clearance

>1.6 mg/dL	Prerenal failure
	  Dehydration
	  Blood loss
	  Heart failure
	  Liver failure
	Intrinsic renal failure
	  Diabetes mellitus
	  Hypertension
	  SLE
	  Nephrotoxins
	  Glomerulonephritis
	  Acute tubular necrosis
	Postrenal failure
	  Urethral obstruction
	  Upper tract obstruction
		1. Urinalysis
		2. Creatinine clearance
		3. Bladder catheterization
		4. Renal imaging

>6.0 mg/dL	Severe renal failure	1. HCO (metabolic acidosis) 2. Serum potassium (hyperkalemia)

Values in parentheses are SI units.
SLE = systemic lupus erythematosus.

Small, elderly women may therefore have a normal creatinine level even with reduced renal function.

A patient's creatinine clearance can be estimated from the formula:

CR clearance

$$= [(140 - \text{age})(\text{weight in kg})]/(72 \times \text{CR in mg/dl})$$

As a rough guideline, a creatinine level of 2 mg/dl is equivalent to a creatinine clearance of 50 ml/min; a creatinine level of 4 mg/dl is equal to a creatinine clearance of 20 ml/min; and a creatinine level of 6 is equivalent to a creatinine clearance of 10 ml/min.

The serum creatinine assay is a useful screening test for patients at risk of renal injury (i.e., those with hypertension or diabetes). It is not useful in asymptomatic patients without significant risk factors because of the low prevalence of chronic renal failure in the general population and the low sensitivity of the test. A low serum creatinine level is of no clinical significance.

DIGOXIN

Various preparations of digitalis have been used to treat heart failure for more than 200 years. Digoxin is the form that is most commonly prescribed today. In addition to its use in the treatment of heart failure, this drug is frequently used to block the A-V node in atrial tachyarrhythmias. Digoxin has a narrow therapeutic window. Levels below 0.5 ng/ml are generally not therapeutic, and levels over 2.2 ng/ml are often associated with toxicity (Table 60–12). The ability to use this medication properly has been enhanced because of the wide availability of assays that measure serum digoxin levels.

When digoxin is used orally as a tablet, 60 to 85 per cent of the drug is absorbed. The gelatin capsules (Lanoxicaps) are associated with 90 to 100 per cent absorption. The peak effect for the drug ranges from 2 to 6 hours after oral administration. It is impossible to interpret a serum digoxin level accurately within this 6-hour period. During this time, the levels are high and do not reliably correlate with the steady-state level.

Digoxin is primarily metabolized by the kidney. The half-life of the drug in patients with normal renal function is 1.5 days. In patients who are anuric it increases to 4 to 5 days. The drug's long half-life means that a steady-state level is not reached until 1 week after a change in dosage of the oral preparation.

Digitalis toxicity manifests as nausea, vomiting, fatigue, confusion, blurred vision, and cardiac disturbances. The most common cardiac problems are ventricular ectopy, A-V block, paroxysmal atrial tachycardia, atrial fibrillation, and ventricular fibrillation. The incidence of digoxin toxicity increases with increasing serum levels. Toxicity is found at lower digoxin levels if accompanied by hypokalemia, alkalosis, hypercalcemia, or hypomagnesemia.

The most common mistake when following serum digoxin levels is "treating the level" instead

TABLE 60–12. DIGOXIN: THERAPEUTIC VALUES

Diagnostic units: ng/mL (nmol/L)
SI conversion factor = 1.281
Therapeutic: 0.5–2.2 (0.6–2.8)

Digoxin	Diagnoses to Consider	Actions to Consider
Decreased <0.5 ng/mL	Inadequate dose Noncompliance Poor GI absorption Absorption interference 　Kaolin-pectin 　Antacids 　Cholestyramine	1. Review medication compliance 2. Review other medications 3. Increase digoxin dose
Increased 2.2–3.0 ng/dL	Excessive digoxin dose Decreased creatinine clearance Level measured prior to 6 hours after a dose Drug interaction 　Quinidine 　Verapamil 　Antibiotics 　Nifedipine 　Amiodarone	1. Evaluate for toxicity 2. Serum K, Ca, Mg, HCO_3 3. Review medication dosing 4. Serum creatinine or BUN 5. Review other medications
>3.0 ng/dL	Toxicity likely	1. Stop digoxin 2. ECG monitoring 3. Correct electrolyte abnormalities

Values in parentheses are SI units.

of "treating the patient." One third of patients with digoxin toxicity have levels that are within the usual therapeutic range. Likewise, levels higher than the normal upper limit may be required in some clinical situations (i.e., to slow the ventricular rate in atrial fibrillation). A wide range of medications can increase or decrease the digoxin level (Table 60–12).

EOSINOPHILS

Eosinophils are granulocytic leukocytes. It is unclear whether their role in the body is to respond to specific antigens (i.e., parasitic infections) or to help in modulating the normal inflammatory reaction. The percentage of eosinophils in a normal white blood cell (WBC) differential can be converted to the eosinophil count by multiplying the percentage times the total WBCs (i.e., 3 per cent × 10,000 = 300) (Table 60–13).

Slight increases in the number of eosinophils can be seen with many diseases and are rarely clinically significant. On the other hand, it is uncommon to see a marked increase in the number of eosinophils. Drug reactions are the most common cause of high eosinophil counts (i.e., sulfonamides, gold, aspirin, antibiotics, phenytoin, and hydralazine). Parasitic infections, especially with tissue-invasive helminths, are the second most common cause of eosinophilia. Noninvasive helminths, encysted parasites, and protozoa do not generally produce eosinophilia.

Low eosinophil counts are sometimes seen in response to an acute viral or bacterial infection. Such a decrease is due to suppression of eosinophil production when large numbers of neutrophils are required. Such low eosinophil counts are of no clinical significance.

ERYTHROCYTE SEDIMENTATION RATE, WESTERGREN METHOD

Anticoagulated whole blood is made up of blood cells suspended in plasma. When the blood is al-

TABLE 60–13. EOSINOPHILS: NORMAL VALUES

Diagnostic units: % of leukocytes (cells × 10^6/L)
SI conversion factor = % × WBC
Normal: 1–3% (50 to 350 × 10^6)

Eosinophils Increased	Diganoses to Consider	Actions to Consider

>3% (350 × 10^6/L)	Parasite infection
	Other infections
	  Chlamydia pneumonia
	  Infectious mononucleosis
	  Scarlet fever
	  Chronic active hepatitis
	Allergic diseases
	  Asthma
	  Allergic rhinitis
	  Urticaria
	Drug reaction
	Autoimmune diseases
	  Rheumatoid arthritis
	  Ulcerative colitis
	  Regional enteritis
	  Sjögren syndrome
	Leukemia/lymphoma
	Eosinophilic syndromes
	  Hypereosinophilic syndrome
	  Eosinophilic myositis
	  Eosinophilic cystitis
	  Eosinophilic gastritis
	  Pulmonary infiltrates
	Dermatologic disorders
	  Atopic dermatitis
	  Eczema
	  Urticaria
	  Pemphigus
	  Scabies
	  Psoriasis
	  Dermatitis herpetiformis
		1. Full drug history
		2. Travel history
		3. Ova and parasites (×2)
		4. Sputum for eosinophils
		5. Chest radiograph

>10% (1000 × 10^6/L)	Parasitic infection Drug reaction Eosinophilic syndrome	

Values in parentheses are SI units.

TABLE 60–14. WESTERGREN ERYTHROCYTE SEDIMENTATION RATE (ESR): NORMAL VALUES

Diagnostic units: mm/hr	Male	Female
Normal: Children	0–10	0–10
<50 years old	0–15	0–20
50–65 years old	0–20	0–30
>65 years	0–38	0–53

ESR (mm/hr)	Diagnoses to Consider	Actions to Consider
Increased		
>100	Temporal arthritis	1. Serum protein electrophoresis
	Polymyalgia rheumatica	
	Multiple myeloma	
	Lymphoma/leukemia	
	Metastatic cancer	
	Sepsis	
	Ulcerative colitis	
	Biliary cirrhosis	
40–100	Anemia	1. Evaluate Hb/Hct and RBC morphology
	Rheumatoid arthritis	2. Repeat ESR
	Malignancy	3. Evaluate thyroid function
	Viral hepatitis	
	Tuberculosis	
	Ectopic pregnancy	
	Myocardial infarction	
	Rheumatic fever	
	Hyperthyroidism	
	Hypothyroidism	
	Normal pregnancy	
	Oral contraceptives	
	Macrocytosis	
Decreased		
	Polycythemia	1. Evaluate Hb/Hct and RBC morphology
	Congestive heart failure	2. Ignore isolated low values in asymptomatic patients
	Hemoglobinopathy	
	Spherocytosis	
	RBC abnormalities	

Hb/Hct = hemoglobin/hematocrit; RBC = red blood cells.

lowed to stand for a period of time, the cells settle out. The rate of settling is affected by both red blood cell (RBC) factors (i.e., shape, size, and hematocrit) and plasma factors (fibrinogen and globulins). The ESR is a measure of the rate of RBC settling (Table 60–14).

The ESR is a nonspecific test used to diagnose and follow the clinical course of a wide variety of diseases that are characterized by tissue inflammation, infection, or malignancy.

Several methods have been used to perform the ESR. The Westergren (or modified Westergren) method is preferred. Most of the relevant research on this test has used one of these two methods.

The most common cause of an elevated ESR is anemia. It is therefore essential that a hematocrit or hemoglobin be done on any patient with an elevated ESR. It is impossible to "correct" the ESR value for the degree of anemia.

Any abnormality in RBC shape or size can result in a reduced ESR. For this reason, a peripheral smear should be prepared for all patients. Check that the RBC morphology is normal.

The ESR is not a useful screening test in asymptomatic patients. It is of only limited usefulness for evaluating patients with vague complaints (i.e.,

fatigue, abdominal pain). It is, however, useful for evaluating those who are suspected of having temporal arteritis or polymyalgia rheumatica. It is also useful for following patients who have other connective tissue disorders, such as rheumatoid arthritis. In these patients, the ESR can be a useful indicator of the activity of the disease. The ESR starts to decrease within days of the initiation of steroid therapy. It then usually falls to a level that is somewhat higher than normal. Treatment with nonsteroidal anti-inflammatory drugs does not lead to a drop in the ESR.

FERRITIN

Ferritin is a protein produced by the reticuloendothelial system. It serves as the chief iron storage protein in the body. In general, the ferritin level (Table 60–15) is proportional to the total body iron storage level.

The most common uses for this test are to differentiate iron deficiency anemia from the anemia of chronic disease in patients with normal or low mean corpuscular volume (MCV) values; determine a patient's response to iron therapy; or evalu-

TABLE 60–15.   FERRITIN: NORMAL VALUES

Diagnostic units: ng/mL (mg/L)
SI conversion factor = 1
Normal: Adult male 20–300
*   Adult female 20–120*

Ferritin (ng/mL)	Diagnoses to Consider	Actions to Consider
Decreased <20	Iron deficiency Hypothyroidism	1. Evaluate for GI blood loss 2. CBC 3. Dietary history 4. TSH

Increased >300	Iron overload
	    Hemochromatosis
	    Transfusion
	    Hemolytic anemia
	Liver disease
	Chronic inflammation
	Malignancies
	Hyperthyroidism
		1. Iron, TIBC
		2. CBC
		3. ESR
		4. T_4, T_3U, TSH
		5. Bilirubin, albumin, AST

GI = gastrointestinal; CBC = complete blood count; TSH: thyroid-stimulating hormone; TIBC = total iron-binding capacity; ESR = erythrocyte sedimentation rate; T_4 = thyroxine; T_3U = triiodothyronine uptake; AST = aspartate aminotransferase.

ate for iron overload states, particularly in patients with hemolytic anemia.

In iron deficiency states, ferritin often decreases before anemia, microcytosis, a low iron, or an elevated total iron-binding capacity (TIBC) appears. Therefore it is considered the most sensitive test for detecting iron deficiency. The levels are quickly responsive to iron therapy: They return to normal within days of initiating oral iron treatment even though total body iron stores may take months of therapy to restore.

Ferritin is less sensitive as a marker of iron overload than it is of iron deficiency. Therefore if iron overload is suspected, iron and TIBC assays are the preferred tests.

FOLATE (FOLIC ACID)

Folate is a water-soluble vitamin that is absorbed from the diet and stored in small amounts in the liver. Because of the limited storage, a person can become folate deficient in as little as 3 weeks of a folate-deficient diet.

Low levels of folate are caused by inadequate dietary intake, malabsorption, and excessive folate utilization (as during pregnancy or with hemolytic anemia). A wide number of common drugs interfere with folate absorption (Table 60–16).

Low serum folate levels precede macrocytosis and anemia in the clinical course of folate deficiency. Folate levels are often determined in conjunction with vitamin B_{12} levels to diagnose megaloblastic anemia. It is important to remember that many patients are both folate and vitamin B_{12} deficient.

If the folate level is in the borderline range, a red blood cell folate level can be ordered as a confirmatory test. This test is more sensitive than the serum folate assay for diagnosing folate deficiency.

GLUCOSE

Interpreting glucose values can be difficult. The usual reasons for ordering this test are to diagnose diabetes, follow the course of diabetic treatment, or diagnose hypoglycemia (Table 60–17).

TABLE 60–16.   SERUM FOLATE: NORMAL VALUES

Diagnostic units: ng/mL (nmol/L)
SI conversion factor = 2.3
Normal: 3–15 (7–34)

Folate Decreased (ng/mL)	Diagnoses to Consider	Actions to Consider
<3	Folate-deficient diet Pregnancy Alcoholism Malabsorption Hemolytic anemia Vitamin B_{12} deficiency Hyperthyroidism	1. Dietary history 2. Drug history 3. Vitamin B_{12} 4. RBC folate 5. CBC

RBC = red blood cells; CBC = complete blood count.

TABLE 60–17.   VENOUS GLUCOSE: NORMAL VALUES

Diagnostic units: mg/dL (mmol/L)
SI conversion factor = 0.05551

Screening Test: Fasting Glucose

	Normal	*Requires GTT*	*Diagnostic of Diabetes*
Adult	<115 (6.38)	115–140 (6.38–7.77)	>140 (7.7) × 2
Child	<130 (7.22)	130–140 (7.22–7.77)	>140 (7.77) × 2

Confirmatory Tests: Glucose Tolerance Tests
  Adult: 75 gram oral glucose dose

	Normal	*Impaired Glucose Tolerance*	*Diabetes*
Fasting	<115 (6.38)	<140 (7.77)	<140 (7.77)
30 Minutes	<200 (11.1)		
60 Minutes	<200 (11.1)	} 1 of 3 >200 (11.1)	} 1 of 3 >200 (11.1)
90 Minutes	<200 (11.1)		
120 Minutes	<140 (7.77)	140–200 (7.77–11.1)	>200 (11.1)

  Child: 1.75 grams glucose per kilogram body weight up to 75 grams

	Normal	*Impaired Glucose Tolerance*	*Diabetes*
Fasting	<130 (7.22)	<140 (7.77)	>140 (7.77)
30 Minutes	<200 (11.1)	<200 (11.1)	
60 Minutes	<200 (11.1)	<200 (11.1)	} 1 of 3 >200 (11.1)
90 Minutes	<200 (11.1)	<200 (11.1)	
120 Minutes	<140 (7.77)	140–200 (7.77–11.1)	>200 (11.1)

Pregnancy
  Screening: O'Sullivan screen
    Glucose 50 grams (patient can be nonfasting)
    "Positive" if ≥140 (7.77) at 1 hour
  Confirmation: O'Sullivan 3 hour GTT
    Oral glucose 100 grams in a fasting patient
    Patient is positive for gestational diabetes if two or more of the values are:
      Fasting: ≥105 (5.79)
      1 Hour: ≥190 (10.55)
      2 Hour: ≥165 (9.16)
      3 Hour: ≥145 (8.05)

Hypoglycemia
  Males: <55 (3.05) at the same time as symptoms present
  Females: <40 (2.22) at the same time symptoms present

Values in parentheses are SI units.

The American Diabetes Association has defined seven disorders of glucose metabolism. (American Diabetes Association, 1988).

1. *Type I diabetes mellitus.* These patients require insulin to prevent ketoacidosis.

2. *Type II diabetes mellitus.* These patients are usually obese adults and can be treated with diet or oral hypoglycemic agents.

3. *Impaired glucose tolerance.* These patients have higher than normal glucose values but less than is required to be diagnostic for diabetes.

4. *Gestational diabetes mellitus.* This category represents hyperglycemia only during pregnancy.

5. *Previous abnormality of glucose tolerance.* This group includes patients who have had diabetes when under stress, when obese, or when pregnant but who now have normal glucose tolerance.

6. *Potential abnormality of glucose tolerance.* This group includes patients with close relatives who are diabetic.

7. *Other types of diabetes mellitus.* These patients have diabetes caused by other conditions, such as pancreatic disease, Cushing syndrome, acromegaly, thyrotoxicosis, or drugs (steroids, estrogen, or thiazide diuretics).

Two common reasons for abnormally elevated glucose tests are that (1) the specimens was obtained after a patient had eaten; and (2) the specimen was obtained from a vein above an intravenous infusion.

There are two types of hypoglycemia. The first is postprandial hypoglycemia, also referred to as reactive hypoglycemia. It is most commonly seen in patients with a history of gastric surgery, who therefore have rapid stomach emptying times. Their symptoms (i.e., sweating, weakness, anxiety, irritability) occur several hours after eating.

Fasting hypoglycemia is seen primarily in diabetics and alcoholics. Their symptoms (i.e., mental confusion, bizarre behavior, seizures) are more gradual in onset and more persistent. This form of hypoglycemia usually occurs only after a long period of fasting.

Other disorders associated with hypoglycemia are insulinoma, adernal insufficiency, hypopituitarism, and drug-induced hypoglycemia (insulin, sulfonylureas, and salicylates).

It is essential to remember that not all glucose specimens are the same. A random specimen taken 2 hours after lunch should not be treated the same way as a fasting specimen. In addition, there are differences among whole blood, serum, and plasma values. Venous plasma and venous serum glucose values are 15 per cent higher than those in venous whole blood. Capillary whole blood values are 10 per cent higher than those measured in venous whole blood. Venous plasma and venous serum values are 5 to 7 per cent higher than those found in capillary whole blood. (The values given in Table 60–17 are for venous plasma or venous serum. Specimens other than these should be adjusted accordingly.)

Table 60–17 differentiates screening tests from diagnostic tests. The usual screening test is a fasting glucose. The results of this test may indicate that the patient is normal, suggest that a diagnostic test (i.e., a glucose tolerance test) be done, or may be diagnostic of diabetes. Note that there are specific screening and diagnostic tests for gestational diabetes (i.e., O'Sullivan test).

GLYCOSYLATED HEMOGLOBIN (HbA₁c)

The glycosylation of hemoglobin occurs continuously during the life of a red blood cell and is directly related to the average glucose concentration. The measurement of glycosylated HbA_{1c} has therefore become a useful clinical test to assess the "average" glucose control in diabetic patients (Table 60–18). Increased percentages of glycosylated hemoglobin reflect increased hyperglycemia. Once glycosylated, hemoglobin remains as such throughout the life of the red blood cell. The test value can therefore be viewed as a measure of diabetic control for the previous 1 to 3 months (American Diabetes Association, 1988.)

Hyperglycemia is also associated with the glycosylation of other body proteins. This glycosylation may be the basis for some of the angiopathic and neuropathic changes seen with diabetes. Some clinicians therefore use this test as an assessment of a patient's risk for diabetic complications.

The HbA_{1c} value does not change with rapid hour-to-hour or day-to-day variations in serum glucose. It is therefore not appropriate to use this test when making decisions about insulin dosage in either the acutely ill hospitalized patient or ambu-

TABLE 60–19. LH AND FSH: CAUSES OF HIGH AND LOW LEVELS*

Causes of High Levels
Gonadal failure (ovary or testis)
Polycystic ovary syndrome
Menopause
Alcoholism
Precocious puberty
Chromosomal disorders

Causes of Low Levels
Hypopituitarism
Hypothalamic impairment
Anorexia nervosa
Stress
Malnutrition
Delayed puberty
Oral contraceptive use
Postpregnancy

* Values depend on the patient's age, sex, Tanner stage, and time of day; and in women the menstrual cycle timing is a factor. Specimen collection should be coordinated with your reference laboratory to ensure reliable testing and test interpretation.

latory diabetics on insulin. Home glucose monitoring is a better source of data for these decisions.

There is wide variation between laboratories for both the "normal" range of values and the degree of elevation associated with various levels of hyperglycemia. It is therefore important to know the characteristics of your laboratory's test. The HbA_{1c} per cent may be falsely elevated with uremia, alcoholism, and aspirin use. The test may be falsely lowered in patients with anemia, hemoglobinopathies, or pregnancy.

GONADOTROPINS (LH AND FSH)

Luteinizing hormone (LH) and follicle-stimulating hormone (FSH) are glycoproteins secreted by the anterior pituitary, which stimulate gonadal (ovarian and testicular) function. Serum levels of LH and FSH are used to evaluate infertility, amenorrhea, the onset of menopause, and the abnormal timing of sexual development in children (Table 60–19).

Levels of these hormones are best interpreted in conjunction with estrogen and testosterone levels. For example, in the menopausal woman, the FSH

TABLE 60–18. GLYCOSYLATED HEMOGLOBIN: NORMAL VALUES

Diagnostic units: % of total hemoglobin
Normal: 5–7% (varies by laboratory)

Glycosylated Hemoglobin Increased	Diagnoses to Consider	Actions to Consider
<9%	Good diabetic control (most glucose <200 mg/dL)	No change in therapy
9–14%	Average diabetic control (most glucose <300 mg/dL)	Home glucose monitoring
>14%	Poor diabetic control (i.e., persistent hyperglycemia)	Evaluate for causes of poor diabetic control

and LH levels rise in response to a falling estrogen level, which results from ovarian failure.

HEMOGLOBIN AND HEMATOCRIT

Hemoglobin and hematocrit values are often used interchangeably in clinical practice to measure the oxygen-carrying capacity of a volume of blood (Table 60–20). It is important to remember that they are not measures of either the total blood volume or the red blood cell (RBC) mass.

Most modern hematology instruments directly measure the hemoglobin and calculate the hematocrit from the measured RBC and mean corpuscular volume (MCV). The hematocrit can also be measured by centrifugation of a microcapillary tube filled with whole blood. When this test is done, the hematocrit is defined as the per cent volume of RBCs after maximal packing has occurred. For most purposes, the hematocrit (Hct) and hemoglobin (Hb) are convertible by a factor of 3 (i.e., Hct = 3 × Hb).

It is reasonable to use the hemoglobin and hema-

tocrit interchangeably except for patients with abnormally shaped RBCs (i.e., sickled cells). In such patients, the measured hematocrit is artificially high because the RBCs fail to maximally pack. In such individuals, a hemoglobin is a better test to follow.

There is little evidence that the general population benefits from routine hemoglobin or hematocrit screening. Screening, however, may be indicated in groups at high risk for anemia, such as infants, pregnant women, the institutionalized elderly, or menstruating females. It is also customary to screen individuals undergoing a procedure that could be associated with blood loss and all hospitalized patients on admission.

The most common abnormal finding is a mild, unsuspected anemia that is usually asymptomatic. The importance of the finding is not based on the need to treat the anemia but, rather, the need to uncover the cause of the anemia. The cause is frequently a clinically important diagnosis (i.e., poor nutrition, menorrhagia, pernicious anemia, colon cancer).

In addition to screening, the hemoglobin or

TABLE 60–20. HEMOGLOBIN: NORMAL VALUES

Diagnostic units: gm/dL (gm/L)
SI conversion factor = 10.0

		Males			*Females*
Normal:	Birth	18.5–21.5 (185–215)	Normal:	Birth	18.0–21.0 (180–210)
	1 month	15.5–18.5 (155–185)		1 month	15.8–18.9 158–189)
	3 months	13.5–16.5 (135–165)		3 months	13.3–16.4 (133–164)
	6 months	13.0–16.0 (130–160)		6 months	12.8–14.8 (128–148)
	9 months	12.0–14.0 (120–140)		9 months	11.7–13.9 (117–139)
	1 year	10.0–14.0 (100–140)		1 year	10.0–14.0 (100–140)
	2 years	10.5–14.2 (105–142)		2 years	10.5–14.2 (105–142)
	4 years	11.2–14.3 (112–143)		4 years	11.3–14.2 (113–142)
	8 years	12.0–14.8 (120–148)		8 years	11.5–14.5 (115–145)
	14 years	12.5–15.0 (125–150)		14 years	11.6–14.8 (116–148)
	Adult	13.9–16.3 (139–163)		Adult	12.0–15.0 (120–150)

	Diagnoses to Consider	Actions to Consider

Increased
>16.5 (165)
	Dehydration
	Diuretic use
	Polycythemia vera
	Secondary polycythemia
	  High altitude
	  Pulmonary disease
	  Cardiac disease
	  Renal tumor
		1. Smoking history
		2. Check volume status
		3. Splenomegaly
		4. Urinalysis
		5. CBC
		6. Platelet count
		7. Alkaline phosphatase

>22 (220)	Severe polycythemia	1. Consider phlebotomy
Decreased <11 (110)	Blood loss Decreased blood cell survival Decreased marrow production RBC sequestration (spleen)	1. History of chronic disease 2. Menstrual history 3. Stool for occult blood 4. Splenomegaly 5. RBC indices 6. Reticulocyte count 7. Trial on iron therapy 8. Iron, TIBC, ferritin 9. Folate, vitamin B_{12}
<8 (80)	Severe anemia	1. Consider transfusion

Values in parentheses are SI units.
RBC = red blood cells; CBC = complete blood count; TIBC = total iron-binding capacity.

hematocrit is an essential test for any patient in whom anemia is suspected, in whom there is abnormal bleeding, or in whom polycythemia is part of the differential diagnosis.

The most common error when interpreting a hemoglobin or hematocrit value is to rely on it as an indicator of acute blood loss. These tests are not good measures of total blood volume. About 12 to 24 hours are required after an acute bleed before fluid equilibration can occur. It is only then that the hemoglobin or hematocrit can be used to indicate the extent of blood loss.

HUMAN CHORIOGONADOTROPIN (hCG)

Human choriogonadotropin (hCG), a glycoprotein secreted by placental trophoblastic tissues, is essential for support of the corpus luteum during early pregnancy. With sensitive tests, hCG can be found in maternal serum within 24 hours of implantation. The levels then rise rapidly and peak at 10 weeks' gestation (Table 60–21). For the remainder of the pregnancy, levels continue at a level approximately one tenth of the peak level.

Qualitative and quantitative hCG tests are available. The most common are qualitative tests to be used on urine specimens to diagnose pregnancy. The sensitivity and specificity of these tests have greatly improved since they were introduced during the 1970s. Most are now sensitive at a level of 20 mIU/L, which means that they can detect pregnancy by the time of the missed menses.

If a patient is suspected to be pregnant but the hCG test is negative, it is best to repeat the test in 2 days with a concentrated, first morning urine specimen. A quantitative serum test is not indicated in these cases, as serum tests are not more sensitive than current urine tests. Urine pregnancy tests are helpful for patients suspected of having ectopic pregnancy. Ninety-nine percent of these patients have positive urine pregnancy tests.

Quantitative serum hCG tests are most commonly used to evaluate the viability of "at risk" pregnancies, for example, a pregnant woman with bleeding. The standard practice is to perform quantitative hCG serum tests 2 days apart. On average, there should be a 66 per cent rise in hCG between the first and second values, although there is great variability in hCG doubling times in normal pregnancies, ranging from 1.4 to 5.0 days. Clinicians should therefore be conservative when telling a patient that a pregnancy is nonviable.

The hCG doubling times are most useful up to the sixth gestational week. By week 9, cardiac activity detected by ultrasonography can be used reliably to determine fetal viability. Unfortunately, many women have bleeding between gestational weeks 6 and 9. There is no definitive test to establish viability during this time.

If the increase in hCG between two consecutive specimens is greater than expected, multiple pregnancy or a hydatidiform mole should be considered.

IRON

Iron is essential for the synthesis and function of hemoglobin. It is absorbed by the small intestines and then transported throughout the body attached to transferrin. Serum iron levels (Table 60–22) therefore depend on both the body's stores of iron and its production of transferrin. For this reason, it is essential that iron values be interpreted in conjunction with the total iron-binding capacity (TIBC), which is a measure of all of the potential binding sites of iron if the transferrin proteins were completely saturated. Normal saturation levels range from 20 to 50 per cent.

Serum iron levels decrease when there is a drop in total body iron stores or a decrease in transferrin. Transferrin levels can be low because of underproduction (i.e., anemia of chronic disease) or renal loss of the protein (i.e., nephrotic syndrome). The normal pattern in iron deficiency anemia is for the iron level to be low and the TIBC to be elevated; however, some patients have normal iron levels and only a decrease in the per cent saturation.

Elevated iron values are seen in iron overload states. In some of these patients, the total iron level

TABLE 60–21. HUMAN CHORIONIC GONADOTROPIN (hCG): NORMAL VALUES

Diagnostic units: mIU/L
Normal: Males: <10

Nonpregnant females: <10	
Normal pregnancy:	
Gestational week	
1	<30
2	50–500
3	100–10,000
10	50,000–300,000
Second trimester	10,000–25,000
Third trimester	5,000–15,000

hCG (mIU/L)	Diagnoses to Consider	Actions to Consider
Increased >10	Pregnancy Hydatidiform mole After abortion (up to 2 weeks) Choriocarcinoma Ovarian cancer Testicular cancer	1. Correlate with ultrasound findings 2. Repeat hCG to document trend

TABLE 60–22. IRON: NORMAL VALUES

Diagnostic units: μg/dL (μmol/L)
SI conversion factor = 0.179
Normal: Male 80–180 (14–32)
Female 60–180 (11–29)

Fe Level (μg/dL)	Diagnoses to Consider	Actions to Consider
Decreased <50	Iron deficiency Chronic disease Nephrotic syndrome Pregnancy Hypothyroidism	1. Ferritin, TIBC 2. Evaluate for blood loss 3. Dietary history 4. TSH, hCG
Increased >200	Recent transfusion Iron poisoning Hemolytic anemia Acute liver disease Hemochromatosis	1. Drug and transfusion history 2. CBC 3. Bilirubin, AST 4. TIBC, ferritin

TIBC = total iron-binding capacity; TSH = thyroid-stimulating hormone; hCG = human chorionic gonadotropin; CBC = complete blood count; AST = aspartate aminotransferase.

may be normal, but the percent of saturation is increased.

Although it is not well known, iron levels vary wildly throughout the day. Therefore values that do not make sense in light of what is known about the patient should be repeated.

MAGNESIUM

Magnesium is an often overlooked electrolyte that plays a vital role in regulating the neuromuscular junction. In addition, it is a key component in many of the body's enzyme systems.

Magnesium is absorbed by the small intestine and excreted by the kidneys. The most common problems are therefore low levels in malabsorption or malnutrition states and abnormally high levels in patients with renal insufficiency (Table 60–23). Of these two states, hypomagnesemia is the more common, especially in ill hospitalized patients who are not eating. The typical patient has been too sick to eat for several days and has only received intravenous fluids. Hypermagnesemia is uncommon, except in patients with renal failure.

The main clinical problems related to abnormal magnesium levels are the result of either hyperexcitability (low magnesium) or suppression (high magnesium) of nerve and muscle activity (i.e., central nervous system, skeletal muscle, and heart). Therefore the first thing to do when faced with an abnormal magnesium value is to check the patient's deep tendon reflexes. They are hyperactive if the magnesium is low and depressed if the magnesium level is high. This test can quickly validate the laboratory result and asses the patient's ability to handle the abnormal magnesium level.

Magnesium has an effect on parathyroid hormone secretion. It is common for calcium levels to be low when a patient has hypomagnesemia. In these patients it is often difficult to correct the calcium imbalance until the magnesium is corrected.

MEAN CORPUSCULAR VOLUME

The mean corpuscular volume (MCV) is the most important of the red blood cell (RBC) indices. In modern hematology instruments, this value is derived by the degree of impedance disturbance as cells pass between two electrodes. The magnitude of the disturbance indicates the size of the cell.

The primary use of the MCV is to differentiate anemias into macrocytic, normocytic, or microcytic types (Table 60–24). This differentiation is useful in theory but is often not helpful in practice. Most anemic patients are normocytic at the time of their diagnosis.

Reticulocytes and other young RBCs are macrocytic. A rapid marrow release of RBCs therefore produces an increased MCV. This condition should not be confused with the other causes of macrocytosis.

It is important to remember that the MCV is an average of all of the cell populations. Mixed populations of macrocytic and microcytic cells may therefore produce a normocytic MCV. This situation is seen during the early treatment of an iron deficiency anemia (i.e., macrocytic reticulocytes plus microcytic cells) and in alcoholic patients who are both iron and folate deficient.

PAPANICOLAOU SMEAR

George Papanicolaou first proposed the use of vaginal cytology to detect gynecologic cancers in 1943. The widespread adoption of "Pap" smear testing in the United States has since led to a 70 per cent decrease in mortality due to cervical cancer. Despite this fact, there continue to be 50,000 cases

TABLE 60–23. MAGNESIUM: NORMAL VALUES

Diagnostic units: mEq/L(mmol/L)
SI conversion factor = 0.5
Normal: 1.3–2.1 (0.65–1.05)

Magnesium (mEq/L)	Diagnoses to Consider	Actions to Consider
Increased 2.1–5.0	Renal disease Antacid ingestion Addison's disease Diabetic ketoacidosis Lithium therapy $MgSO_4$ therapy	1. Check BUN, creatinine 2. Alcohol history 3. Drug history
>5.0		1. Watch for hypotension and bradyarrhythmias
>10.0		1. DTRs absent 2. Respiratory paralysis possible 3. Asystole possible 4. Hypotension likely
Decreased 1.0–1.3	Chronic alcoholism Malnutrition Malabsorption NPO in hospitalized patients Diarrhea Diuretics Pancreatitis	1. Alcohol history 2. Dietary history 3. Drug history 4. Check serum Ca, K 5. DTRs brisk
<1.0		1. Tetany possible 2. Seizures possible 3. Tachyarrhythmias possible

Values in parentheses are SI units
BUN = blood urea nitrogen; DTRs = deep tendon reflexes.

TABLE 60–24. MEAN CORPUSCULAR VOLUME (MCV): NORMAL VALUES

Diagnostic units: cubic micrometers (fL)
SI conversion factor = 1
Normal: 76–100 fL

MCV (fL)	Diagnoses to Consider	Actions to Consider
Increased 100–120	Reticulocytosis Folate deficiency Vitamin B_{12} deficiency Hypothyroidism Response to chemotherapy	1. Reticulocyte count 2. Serum vitamin B_{12} 3. Serum or RBC folate 4. T_4
>120	Folate deficiency Vitamin B_{12} deficiency	1. Serum vitamin B_{12} 2. Serum or RBC folate
Decreased 70–76	Iron deficiency Thalassemia Anemia of chronic disease Hereditary sideroblastic anemia Lead poisoning RBC fragmentation (burns)	1. Reticulocyte count 2. Peripheral smear 3. Serum iron, TIBC, or ferritin 4. Hb electrophoresis
<70	Severe iron deficiency Thalassemia	1. Reticulocyte count 2. Peripheral smear 3. Serum iron, TIBC, or ferritin 4. Hb electrophoresis

RBC = red blood cells; TIBC = total iron-binding capacity; Hb = hemoglobin; T_4 = thyroxine.

per year of cervical carcinoma in situ, 13,000 cases of invasive carcinoma, and 5,000 cervical cancer deaths.

The Pap classification (i.e., classes I to V) was used for many years to report Pap smear results. However, this terminology was plagued with variability, inconsistencies, and ambiguity. It has often led to confusion about the clinical implications of a Pap smear report. It is now widely recommended that this older terminology system be replaced by one of three new reporting systems outlined in Table 60–25. In the United States, the Bethesda System has become the most widely adopted new classification system.

Cervical cytology does not represent a clear, continuous spectrum of disease from normal to malignancy. Some abnormal findings, in fact, are due to benign conditions, and others are diagnostic of carcinoma. Some indicate dysplastic changes, which may be a marker for carcinoma; the more severe the dysplasia, the more likely is malignancy. Mild dysplasia is cytologically, histologically, and colposcopically equivalent to the cellular changes seen with the human papillomavirus (HPV) infection. It is this mild dysplasia (neither normal, clearly malignant, nor necessarily benign) that causes the greatest confusion. The current research that associates HPV infections and cervical carcinoma may permit a better understanding of the disease process.

Papanicolaou smear reports are often reported as "unsatisfactory" or "specimen is inadequate." There are multiple reasons for this report, including scant cellularity, poor fixation, inflammatory cells that obscure the cervical cells, menstrual blood that obscures the cervical cells, or the absence of endocervical cells. Endocervical cells and squamous metaplastic cells are markers for specimen collection in the transformation zone of the cervix. The transformation zone is the area from which cervical carcinomas arise. There is debate about whether the absence of endocervical cells is an absolute indication for a repeat specimen.

Papanicolaou smear results also indicate other diagnoses, which include infections with *Candida, Gardnerella, Chlamydia, Trichomonas,* cytomegalovirus, and herpes simplex virus. In some cases the organism is seen (e.g., *Trichomonas*), whereas in other cases (e.g., herpes simplex) the organism is not seen but cellular changes consistent with an infection are evident. The accuracy of diagnosing these various infections by Pap smear is highly variable. In most cases, further historical and laboratory confirmation is needed to make a specific diagnosis.

A final word of caution: Pap smears are associated with a significant false-negative rate (about 30 per cent). Therefore clinicians should get little reassurance from a normal follow-up Pap smear after one that shows dysplasia. When in doubt, schedule colposcopy.

PHOSPHORUS (PHOSPHATE, PO₄)

Phosphorus is the major intracellular anion (Table 60–26). It is involved in acid-base balance,

TABLE 60–25. PAPANICOLAOU SMEAR CLASSIFICATION SYSTEMS

Pap Class	Bethesda System	WHO System	CIN System	Actions to Consider
I	Within normal limits	Normal	Normal	Routine follow-up
II	Atypical squamous cells of undetermined significance	Atypical, benign	Atypical, benign	Clinical correlation Treat specific condition
III	Low grade squamous intraepithelial lesion	Mild dysplasia	CIN-1	Repeat Pap smear HPV DNA test Cervicography Colposcopy
	High grade squamous intraepithelial lesion	Moderate dysplasia	CIN-2	Colposcopy
IV	High grade squamous intraepithelial lesion	Severe dysplasia	CIN-3	Colposcopy
		Carcinoma in situ	CIN-3	Colposcopy
V	Invasive squamous cell carcinoma	Invasive squamous cell carcinoma	Invasive squamous cell carcinoma	Colposcopy Referral
	Adenocarcinoma	Adenocarcinoma	Adenocarcinoma	Colposcopy Referral

Benign reactive changes: This description covers a range of conditions that are benign and do not require follow-up, including squamous metaplasia, epithelial response to inflammation, nuclear enlargement, parabasal cells, and hyperplasia of endocervical cells.
Hyperkeratosis: This term refers to the presence of keratinized squamous cells without nuclei. It is associated with dysplasia in 10 per cent of patients and may be difficult to distinguish from dysplasia. Colposcopy may be indicated if this finding persists for two consecutive reports.
Parakeratosis: Similar to hyperkeratosis except that the nuclei are retained. Handle in the same manner.
Koilocytosis: This term represents perinuclear vacuolation and abnormal nuclear mitotic activity of the epithelial cells. It is pathognomonic for HPV, even if no warts are seen clinically.
HPV = human papilloma virus; CIN = cervical intraepithelial neoplasia; WHO = World Health Organization.

TABLE 60–26. PHOSPHORUS (PHOSPHATE, PO₄): NORMAL VALUES

Diagnostic units: mg/dL (mmol/L)
SI conversion factor = 0.323
Normal: Child 4.5–7.0 (1.5–2.3)
*   Adult 2.5–5.0 (0.80–1.60)*

Phosphorus (mg/dL)	Diagnoses to Consider	Actions to Consider
Decreased <2.5	Hyperparathyroidism Malabsorption Malnutrition Hypercalcemia Hyperalimentation Vitamin D deficiency Antacid treatment Hypomagnesemia Alcoholism	1. Calcium 2. Drug and alcohol history 3. Parathyroid hormone 4. Dietary history
Increased >5.0	Renal failure Childhood Prolonged bed rest Skeletal disease Hypoparathyroidism Vitamin D poisoning Excess dietary calcium	1. Calcium 2. Creatinine 3. Skeletal radiograph 4. Parathyroid hormone

calcium metabolism, and many other biochemical reactions. Eighty-five per cent of the body's phosphate stores are found in bone. The most common physiologic changes in serum phosphate are in response to changes in serum calcium and changes in pH. The body accomplishes these changes by altering intestinal absorption, changing renal excretion, or shifting ions intracellularly.

Like calcium, phosphorus is under the control of parathyroid hormone (PTH). As PTH increases, calcium increases and phosphorus decreases. Because this relationship is the principle control mechanism for serum phosphorus levels, it is essential that PO_4 be determined along with the serum calcium.

The most common therapeutic measure relating to hyperphosphatemia is the use of phosphate-binding agents (i.e., aluminum hydroxide) in patients with chronic renal failure. This therapy should be started whenever the serum phosphate exceeds 5.5 mg/dL in an effort to avoid hypocalcemia, which could otherwise result in crippling bone disease.

Serum phosphate levels are under diurnal control and increase owing to phosphate absorption following a meal. Because of these factors specimens for testing should be obtained in the morning after a 12-hour fast.

PLATELET COUNT

The normal adult platelet count ranges from 140 $\times$ 10^9 to 400 $\times$ 10^9 per liter. Counts below 140 $\times$ 10^9 per liter indicate thrombocytopenia. Counts greater than 400 $\times$ 10^9 per liter indicate thrombocytosis (Table 60–27).

Platelet counts are routinely reported on specimens sent for complete blood counts because most modern cell counters do an automated platelet count as a part of their routine testing. Hence the most common platelet count abnormality is a small increase or decrease from normal in an otherwise asymptomatic individual. There is usually no benefit derived from further evaluating or even repeating the platelet count in these cases.

There is little justification for ordering screening platelet counts on asymptomatic outpatients or as a part of the admission testing on hospitalized patients. The one exception is the individual who is admitted for a major surgical procedure. The platelet count is, however, useful for evaluating patients with abnormal bleeding, bruising, purpura, petechiae, or splenomegaly.

Thrombocytopenia can be caused by a reduction in the marrow's production of platelets (due to marrow suppression or infiltration), increased destruction of platelets, or sequestration of platelets in the spleen. A platelet count is also a useful indicator of marrow sensitivity to cytotoxic medications in the treatment of cancer.

It should be remembered that platelets may be adequate in number but defective in function. Medications are the most common cause of abnormal platelet function (i.e., aspirin, other nonsteroidal anti-inflammatory drugs, alcohol, and penicillins).

POTASSIUM

Potassium is the major cation in the intracellular fluid. Ninety-eight per cent of the total body potas-

TABLE 60–27. PLATELET COUNT: NORMAL VALUES

Diagnostic units: platelets × 10^9/L
Normal: First week of life: 84–478
After first week of life: 140–400

Platelets (× 10^9/L)	Diagnoses to Consider	Actions to Consider
Decreased		
100–400	Response to viral illness Response to bacterial illness	Repeat test
50–100 (may have bleeding with major surgery)	Thrombocytopenia purpura After transfusion Spleen sequestration Marrow infiltration (i.e., leukemia) Response to cytotoxic drugs	History of all medications Alcohol history Examine for splenomegaly CBC Trial off all medications Bone marrow biopsy
20–50 (may have bleeding with minor procedure)	Thrombocytopenia Marrow infiltration DIC	Platelet transfusion for any procedure
<20 (may have spontaneous GI or CNS hemorrhage)	Severe thrombocytopenia	Platelet transfusion
Increased		
400–600	Splenectomy Infection Blood loss Inflammatory bowel disease Collagen vascular disease	Repeat test
600–1000	Malignancy Polycythemia vera	Evaluate for malignancy
>1000 (may have spontaneous thrombosis)	Severe thrombocytosis	Administer antiplatelet drugs

GI = gastrointestinal; CNS = central nervous system; CBC = complete blood count.

sium is contained within the cells. The kidneys are responsible for regulation of the extracellular potassium. Hypokalemia and hyperkalemia are principally due to renal disorders or abnormalities in the intake of potassium.

It is not useful to test healthy outpatients for this electrolyte. However, the test is useful for patients with renal disease, those on diuretics, and patients who complain of weakness (Table 60–28). It is also customary to determine the serum potassium for all acutely ill hospitalized patients. Disorders of potassium are common in hospitalized patients because of the frequent use of intravenous infusions and nasogastric suction.

The most commonly seen potassium disorder is a mild hypokalemia in patients on a thiazide or loop diuretic. These patients are often asymptomatic, and it is unclear whether such patients benefit from treatment. Mild hypokalemia can also be associated with vague complaints such as weakness, muscle cramps, and paresthesias. Severe hypokalemia may cause arrhythmias, a paralytic ileus, or paralysis. All hypokalemic patients on digoxin require treatment because of the increased risk for digoxin toxicity with even mild hypokalemia.

The most common cause of hyperkalemia is hemolysis of red blood cells during blood collection or processing. In some cases, these specimens have red serum. If in doubt, retest the patient prior to undergoing a long work-up for real hyperkalemia.

Hyperkalemia is associated with patient complaints of weakness or paralysis. Severe hyperkalemia (potassium level higher than 8 mEq/L) is associated with bradycardia, hypotension, ventricular fibrillation, and cardiac arrest.

When there is suspicion of a laboratory error, a rapid, useful maneuver is to do an electrocardiogram (ECG). Clinically significant hyperkalemia or hypokalemia is usually associated with the ECG findings indicated in Table 60–28.

PROSTATE-SPECIFIC ANTIGEN

The prostate-specific antigen (PSA) assay has received wide acclaim as a prostate cancer screening test for older men. Elevated PSA values lead to lucrative urologic evaluations, and PSA testing has therefore been made available for free by some hospitals and urology groups. At this time, there is no agreement that screening provides any patient benefit. Using this test as a screening test does de-

TABLE 60–28. POTASSIUM: NORMAL VALUES

Diagnostic units: mEq/L (mmol/L)
SI conversion factor = 1
Normal: 3.5–5.0 (3.5–5.0)

Potassium (mEq/L)	Diagnoses to Consider	Actions to Consider
Increased 5.0–7.5	Hemolyzed specimen Drugs 　Potassium-sparing diuretics 　NSAIDs 　ACE inhibitors 　Potassium supplementation Decreased renal excretion 　Acute renal failure 　Chronic renal failure 　Addison's disease Acidosis Tissue destruction	1. Repeat K on new specimen 2. Drug and diet history 3. Check ECG for peaked T 4. Creatinine 5. Serum electrolytes 6. Urine electrolytes
>7.5	Hyperkalemic arrhythmias Hyperkalemic paralysis	1. ECG for peaked T, wide QRS, absent P 2. Calcium gluconate 3. Glucose/insulin infusion 4. Bicarbonate 5. Ion-exchange resins
Decreased 3.5–2.5	Renal loss 　Thiazide or loop diuretics 　Renal tubular acidosis 　Hyperaldosteronism Gastrointestinal loss 　Vomiting 　Diarrhea Inadequate dietary potassium Inadequate IV potassium Insulin therapy Metabolic alkalosis	1. Drug and diet history 2. Serum electrolytes 3. Urine electrolytes 4. ECG for ST sagging, T depression, and U waves 5. Monitor for digoxin toxicity 6. Administer oral potassium
<2.5	Hypokalemic arrhythmias	1. Monitor closely for arrhythmias and paralysis 2. Administer IV and oral potassium

Values in parentheses are SI units.

tect more prostate cancer, but it is not clear that detection and treatment of these cancers is better than no detection at all.

The PSA is produced by normal, hyperplastic, and cancerous prostate tissue (Table 60–29). Low serum levels are found in all adult men. These levels increase with most prostate diseases, including benign prostatic hypertrophy (BPH). In patients with BPH, the PSA level usually remains less than 10 ng/mL and is proportional to the volume of prostate tissue as detected by ultrasonography.

The PSA level in patients with prostate cancer increases with increased staging (stages A through E) and increased tumor mass. Therefore PSA can be used to stage patients with prostate cancer, confirm response to therapy, and detect recurrence. PSA levels can rise a year before clinically detectable prostate cancer metastases.

TABLE 60–29. PROSTATE-SPECIFIC ANTIGEN (PSA): NORMAL VALUES

Diagnostic units: ng/mL (μg/L)
SI conversion factor = 1
Normal: 0–4

PSA (ng/mL)	Diagnoses to Consider	Actions to Consider
Increased >4.0	BPH Prostate manipulation Prostatitis Prostate infarction Urinary retention Prostate cancer	1. Repeat PSA in 2 weeks 2. Rectal examination 3. Prostate ultrasonography 4. Prostate biopsy

The PSA levels increase twofold with prostate massage and up to 50-fold following a prostate biopsy. The serum half-life of the antigen is 2 days. Therefore it is best to wait 1 to 2 weeks after prostate manipulation to perform a PSA assay.

There is no lower normal limit for PSA, and low normal values have no clinical significance.

PROTEIN (TOTAL)

The total protein measured by the laboratory includes albumin plus the various globulins (Table 60–30). Fibrinogen, another blood protein, is not measured because it is depleted when serum clots.

Decreased levels of total protein are seen in a wide variety of illnesses. In most cases, these diseases are better followed by the albumin because it is the albumin fraction that is usually reduced. A reduction in albumin is also a better guide to edematous states, as it is responsible for 90 per cent of the oncotic pressure.

Increased levels of total protein are occasionally seen and usually lead to an evaluation for multiple myeloma. In fact, myeloma can be associated with increased, normal, or decreased total protein levels.

When there is a question about the interpretation of any abnormal total protein, it is useful to perform a protein electrophoresis. This test separates the albumin from the various globulins. The electrophoretic pattern may be diagnostically helpful. Immunologic typing should be done for any electrophoretic "spike" to further test for multiple myeloma.

PROTHROMBIN TIME

The prothrombin time (PT) is the only coagulation test commonly used in the outpatient setting (Table 60–31). It is the time required to initiate clotting when tissue thromboplastin is mixed with blood. The PT is a measure of both the extrinsic clotting system (i.e., factor VII) and factors common to the intrinsic and extrinsic systems (i.e., factor X, factor V, prothrombin, and fibrinogen).

The PT is not considered a useful screening test for asymptomatic patients, even those undergoing a surgical procedure. It is most commonly used to monitor the anticoagulation effects of patients on warfarin (Coumadin). It is also a useful test for evaluating any patient with abnormal bleeding. It is important to note that the PT is normal in patients with classic hemophilia (i.e., factor VIII deficiency) and those with von Willebrand's disease.

There has been a great deal of confusion about PT testing. A broad range of values have been called "normal" by different laboratories. In addition, there has been disagreement about appropriate therapeutic PT levels in patients on warfarin.

Many of these problems are due to the fact that the test relies on thromboplastin reagents that vary considerably in their clotting activity. Those used today are less responsive than those that were used in the early studies on therapeutic anticoagulation, which has led to some clinicians unknowingly over-anticoagulating their patients.

Prothrombin time results may be reported in seconds, as a ratio compared with normal controls, or as an internationalized normalized ratio (INR). The INR is standardized to the World Health Organization's reference thromboplastin. It is essential that

TABLE 60–30.   PROTEIN: NORMAL VALUES

Diagnostic units: gm/dL (gm/L)
SI conversion factor = 10.0
Normal: 6–8 (60–80)

Protein (gm/L)	Diagnoses to Consider	Actions to Consider

Decreased < 6	Decreased synthesis
	  Liver insufficiency
	  Malnutrition
	  Malignancy
	Increased loss
	  Nephrotic syndrome
	  Extensive burns
	  Protein-losing enteropathy
	Inflammatory illness
	Myeloma
	Overhydration
		1. Dietary history
		2. Urinalysis
		3. 24-Hour urine protein
		4. Bilirubin
		5. Creatinine
		6. Protein electrophoresis

Increased < 8	Dehydration Multiple myeloma Sarcoidosis Monoclonal gammopathy Chronic inflammation	1. Creatinine BUN 2. Protein electrophoresis 3. Chest radiograph

Values in parentheses are SI units.

TABLE 60–31.   PROTHROMBIN TIME: NORMAL VALUES

	Seconds	Patient/control ratio (Rabbit brain thromboplastin)	INR
Normal	11–13	0.9–1.1	0.8–1.3
Anticoagulation therapy			
Treatment of deep vein thrombosis	15–18.5	1.3–1.6	2.0–3.0
Treatment of pulmonary embolism	15–18.5	1.3–1.6	2.0–3.0
Prevention of embolism in atrial fibrillation or tissue heart valves	15–18.5	1.3–1.6	2.0–3.0
Prevention of embolism in patients with prosthetic heart valves	18.5–21.0	1.6–1.8	3.0–4.5
Prevention of embolism in patients with recurrent emboli	18.5–21.0	1.6–1.8	3.0–4.5

Prothrombin Time	Diagnoses to Consider	Actions to Consider
Increased	Liver disease	Liver enzymes, bilirubin
	Malabsorption	PTT
	DIC	Clotting factor assays
	Warfarin therapy	Serum carotene
	Factor II, V, VII, X deficiency	72-Hour stool fat
	Vitamin K deficiency	Administer vitamin K

INR = International normalization ratio; DIC = disseminated intravascular coagulation; PTT = partial thromboplastin time.

the clinician know which of these reporting systems is being used so as to ensure adequate anticoagulation without risking unnecessary bleeding.

RETICULOCYTE COUNT

Reticulocytes are immature red blood cells that have extruded their nucleus but contain residual basophilic staining material. They are released from the marrow into the peripheral blood and then take 1 to 2 days to change into mature red blood cells.

A reticulocyte count is the ratio of reticulocytes and the total number of red blood cells (Table 60–32). Because normal red blood cells have a 120-day life-span, about 1 per cent of red blood cells are destroyed and replaced each day. The newly released cells are reticulocytes, and so a normal reticulocyte count is about 1 per cent.

The reticulocyte count serves as a measure of the marrow's responsiveness to an anemia. With anemia caused by the marrow's underproduction of red blood cells, the reticulocyte count is low. With anemia caused by a short red blood cell life (i.e., as with hemolysis or blood loss), a healthy marrow responds with an increase in red blood cell production and therefore an elevated reticulocyte count.

There are two corrections usually done on the reticulocyte count. The first is the correction for

TABLE 60–32.   RETICULOCYTE COUNT: NORMAL VALUES

Diagnostic units: % reticulocytes (corrected)
Normal: Newborn to 2 weeks of age: 2.5–6.5
  Males older than 3 weeks: 0.8–2.5
  Females older than 2 weeks: 0.8–4.1.

	Diagnoses to Consider	Actions to Consider
Increased >2.5 (males) >4.1 (females)	Hemorrhage Hemolytic anemia Response to treatment for a nutritional anemia Marrow recovery after reversible suppression	1. CBC 2. Menstrual history 3. Stool for occult blood 4. Peripheral smear for hemolysis 5. Complete drug history 6. Coombs' test 7. Hb electrophoresis
Decreased <0.8	Nutritional anemia Anemia of chronic disease Aplastic anemia Marrow infiltration Septicemia	1. CBC 2. History of chronic malignant, inflammatory, or infectious disease 3. Complete drug history 4. Iron, ferritin, TIBC 5. Folate, vitamin B_{12} 6. Bone marrow biopsy
<0.2	Aplastic anemia	

CBC = complete blood count; Hb = hemoglobin; TIBC = total iron-binding capacity.

the anemia. Because the reticulocyte count is a function of both the number of reticulocytes and the number of mature red blood cells, a decrease in the number of red blood cells could result in an increase in the uncorrected reticulocyte count, even if the number of reticulocytes remains the same. This situation would give the false impression of an active marrow response, even though the marrow had not actually responded. The corrected reticulocyte count is equal to the uncorrected reticulocyte count times the patient's hematocrit divided by 45.

A second correction should be made whenever there are nucleated red blood cells seen on the peripheral smear. Their presence is an indication that the marrow is actively releasing blood cells. The reticulocytes are therefore released earlier in their development, and they therefore spend a longer period in the peripheral circulation before developing into mature cells. This correction involves dividing the corrected reticulocyte count (as calculated above) by the number of days required for maturation of the reticulocyte:

Hematocrit level	Maturity in days
40–45	1.0
35	1.5
25	2.0
15	2.5

SODIUM

Sodium is the major cation in extracellular fluid. To interpret the sodium assay properly it is necessary to think about it as a measure not of total body sodium but of the total body water and the effective circulatory volume (Table 60–33). In normal situations the serum osmolality is used by the body to adjust the serum sodium. When the osmolality increases, thirst increases; more water is then taken in, and antidiuretic hormone (ADH) is secreted, resulting in less free water being lost by the kidneys. When osmolality decreases, thirst is turned off and ADH secretion is suppressed. In situations where the effective circulatory volume is reduced (i.e., heart failure), the body may sacrifice a normal osmolality in an effort to maintain the circulatory volume. In this setting, the sodium concentration decreases as fluid is retained in an effort to maintain the circulation.

A serum sodium assay cannot be properly interpreted without a physical examination of the patient's volume status. In hypovolemic states there is an orthostatic blood pressure drop, decreased skin turgor, dry mucous membranes, and weight loss. Hypovolemia may be associated with either normal, increased, or decreased serum sodium. To a large extent it depends on the patient's access to

free water. Hypovolemia leads to thirst. If it results in drinking fluids that are low in sodium, hyponatremia follows.

Heart failure, cirrhosis, and nephrotic syndrome are frequent causes of hypervolemia (i.e., edematous states). In each case the total body water is increased, but the effective circulating volume is decreased. Therefore ADH is stimulated and free water is retained. This situation leads to hyponatremia.

Pseudohyponatremia is seen with hyperglycemia, severe hyperlipidemia, or hyperproteinemia. In these situations, the presence of other solutes in the serum results in artificially low serum sodium values (if measured by flame photometry).

Testing for serum sodium is not useful for routine screening of healthy individuals. However, it is useful in patients with heart failure, liver disease, chronic renal failure, and other edematous states. All acutely ill hospitalized patients should be tested, as serum sodium is often altered by intravenous therapy or nasogastric suction. In addition, patients on lithium therapy should have their sodium evaluated because this drug can lead to nephrogenic diabetes insipidus.

THEOPHYLLINE

Drug level monitoring is important when using medications that have serious toxic effects and that display wide variations in absorption or metabolism. Theophylline is such a drug, and measurement of theophylline levels has therefore become common practice (Table 60–34).

The bioavailability of theophylline is the fraction of drug absorbed. Following absorption, the level in the blood reaches a peak, the highest drug concentration. For currently available theophylline preparations, the dose-to-peak time varies from 2 to 12 hours. Theophylline is then metabolized by the liver and excreted by the kidneys. The time required to decrease the drug concentration in the blood by 50 per cent is referred to as its half-life. The half-life for theophylline is 8 to 9 hours and does not vary with the type of theophylline preparation. After four or five consecutive doses of theophylline have been taken, the drug reaches a steady state. A drug level determined just before the next dose is the lowest steady-state level and is referred to as a trough level.

The theophylline level is affected by a variety of factors including the type of theophylline preparation, the frequency of dosing, the patient's size, and the patient's age. The metabolism of theophylline can be decreased (and hence the serum level increased) by liver disease, pulmonary disease, heart failure, and concomitant use of erythromycin or cimetidine. Smoking, on the other hand, increases theophylline metabolism and therefore decreases the theophylline level.

TABLE 60–33. SODIUM: NORMAL VALUES

Diagnostic units: mEq/L (mmol/L)
S1 conversion factor = 1
Normal: 135–147 (135–147)

Sodium (mEq/L)	Diagnoses to Consider	Actions to Consider

Increased
>147
	Fluid loss in excess of salt:
	  Sweating
	  Diarrhea
	  Diabetes mellitus (osmotic diuresis)
	  Diabetes insipidus
	  Hyperaldosteronism
	Reduced fluid intake:
	  Altered mental status (unable to drink)
	  Vomiting
	Excessive salt intake:
	  Infant formula
	  Hypertonic nasogastric feeding
	  Salt poisoning
		1. Clinical assessment of fluid status
		2. Serum electrolytes
		3. Serum BUN/creatinine
		4. Serum glucose
		5. Urine specific gravity
		6. Give PO fluids

>160	CNS symptoms if an acute change	1. Slow hydration with isotonic saline (reduce serum sodium no faster than 10 mEq/L each day)

Decreased
<135
	Excess water:
	  Psychogenic polydipsia
	  Excessive IV hydration
	Decreased effective circulatory volume:
	  Diuretic therapy
	  Congestive heart failure
	  Cirrhosis
	  Nephrotic syndrome
	  Dehydration with free water access
	Inability to excrete water:
	  Renal failure (Cr Cl <15)
	  SIADH
	Sodium depletion:
	  Gastrointestinal loss
	  Excessive sweating
	  Adrenal insufficiency
	Pseudohyponatremia
		1. Clinical assessment of fluid status
		2. Urine/serum osmolality
		3. Urine protein
		4. BUN, creatinine
		5. Urine specific gravity
		6. Serum albumin
		7. Serum electrolyte
		8. Water restriction

<120	CNS symptoms are likely due to brain swelling	1. Administer hypertonic saline (3%) until sodium is 125 mEq/L

Values in parentheses are SI units.
CNS = central nervous system; SIADH = syndrome of inappropriate antidiuretic hormone secretion; BUN = blood urea nitrogen.

There is often debate about whether a peak or a trough level gives better information when managing a patient on theophylline. The answer depends on what information is needed. In general, the peak level is used to assess toxicity, and the trough is a useful measure of the dosing adequacy.

High levels of theophylline are associated with nausea, vomiting, diarrhea, headache, insomnia, agitation, tachycardia, seizures, tremor, and fever. The occurrence of toxic side effects tends to be individual. Some patients have seizures, tachyarrhythmias, or circulatory collapse at a theophylline level of 50 μg/mL. Others remain asymptomatic at this level.

It is essential that a complete dosing history be obtained whenever a theophylline level is determined. It is impossible to interpret the value without knowing which theophylline preparation is being taken, if the person has been compliant with the dosing, and the timing of the last dose.

THYROID-STIMULATING HORMONE (THYROTROPIN)

Thyroid-stimulating hormone (TSH), a glycoprotein secreted by the anterior pituitary, is responsible for increasing triiodothyronine (T_3) and thyroxine (T_4) secretion by the thyroid gland. TSH testing (Table 60–35) is used to diagnose hypothyroidism and to monitor drug therapy in patients taking levothyroxine. The first generation of TSH tests was not sensitive in the low range. Second and third generation tests have been developed that are sensitive below 0.5 mIU/L. These newer

TABLE 60–34. THEOPHYLLINE: THERAPEUTIC VALUES

Diagnostic units: μg/ml (μmol/L)
SI conversion factor = 5.55
Therapeutic: 10–20 (56–111)

Theophylline	Diagnoses to Consider	Actions to Consider

Decreased <10	Noncompliance
	Inadequate dosage
	Change in drug metabolism
	Trough level
	Use of short half-life theophylline
		1. Review drug compliance
		2. Check time of last dose
		3. Is patient a new smoker?
		4. Is drug being absorbed?
		5. Increase dose or frequency
		  a. By 100% if level is <5
		  b. By 50% if level is 5–8
		  c. By 20% if level is 8–10

Increased 20–35	Excessive dose Excessive dosing frequency Erythromycin alters drug metabolism Cimetidine alters drug metabolism Liver disease Heart failure	1. Complete drug history 2. Examine for side effects 3. Decrease dose
>35	Dosing error Intentional overdose	1. Examine for side effects 2. Hospitalize to monitor 3. Administer activated charcoal
>50	Seizures or arrhythmias likely	1. Consider charcoal hemoperfusion

Values in parenthesis are SI units.

tests are also useful for diagnosing hyperthyroidism. In patients with hyperthyroidism, TSH is suppressed. The more sensitive TSH tests can be used to screen for thyroid disease without the need for T_4 and T_3 uptake testing.

Most patients with hypothyroidism have primary hypothyroidism, which is due to thyroid gland failure. In such patients the TSH is elevated. A small number of hypothyroid patients have secondary (pituitary) or tertiary (hypothalamic) hypothyroidism. In this small group of patients, the TSH is low or normal.

The TSH assay is the most useful test for monitoring levothyroxine therapy. In general, patients can be considered euthyroid when the TSH level falls to normal. It is unnecessary to use other thyroid tests (i.e., T_4 assay) to regulate therapy. It is important to remember that it is best to treat the patient, not the test. Therefore even when using the TSH assay to determine levothyroxine dosage, evaluate the patient symptomatically.

Some hypothyroid patients have extremely high TSH values (100 μIU/mL). There is no direct correlation between the level of TSH and the severity of hypothyroidism. Patients with a TSH of 50 μIU/mL are not twice as hypothyroid as those with TSH of 25 μIU/mL, whereas patients with a TSH of 10 μIU/mL can be profoundly symptomatic.

TABLE 60–35. NORMAL VALUES FOR THYROID-STIMULATING HORMONE (TSH)

Diagnostic units: μIU/mL (mU/L)
SI conversion factor = 1
Normal: 0.4–6.0 μIU/mL (mU/L) (There may be slight differences in the normal range between laboratories, based on variations in test methods.)

TSH (μIU/mL)	Diagnoses to Consider	Actions to Consider
Increased >6.0	Primary hypothyroidism (i.e., thyroid gland failure) Thyroiditis Inadequate levothyroxine therapy	1. Drug compliance history 2. Physical examination 3. T_4, T_3 uptake 4. TRH stimulation test
Decreased <0.5	Hyperthyroidism Excessive levothyroxine intake Secondary hypothyroidism (i.e., pituitary failure) Tertiary hypothyroidism (i.e., hypothalamic failure)	1. Thyroid examination 2. Drug history 3. T_4, T_3 U 4. TRH stimulation test

T_4 = thyroxine; T_3U = triiodothyronine uptake; TRH = thyrotropin-releasing hormone.

THYROXINE

Thyroxine (T_4) is the principal hormone secreted by the thyroid gland. It is almost completely bound to proteins in the circulation. Most of the binding is to thyroxin-binding globulin (TBG), but a small amount is also bound to albumin. The active form of the hormone is free thyroxine (i.e., thyroxine not bound to protein). Thyroxine is used in the body to regulate tissue metabolism.

The most common screening thyroid test is the serum thyroxine assay. Unfortunately, this test measures total thyroxine rather than just the active hormone (i.e., free T_4). Many of the abnormal results are therefore due to abnormal levels of thyroid-bonding globulin instead of the active hormone.

The free T_4 level can be approximated by ordering a T_3 uptake test and calculating the free T_4 index (Table 60–36). This index approximates the free T_4. If it is increased, it suggests hyperthyroidism. If it is decreased, it suggests hypothyroidism.

When using the T_4 or the T_4 index as screening tests, there frequently remain cases in which the diagnosis is uncertain. If there is concern about hypothyroidism, a thyroid-stimulating hormone (TSH) test is usually helpful. If there is concern about hyperthyroidism, the free T_3 is useful. Low level TSH tests have been introduced which are low in hyperthyroidism.

Tests for thyroxine-binding globulin and free T_4 are available but are rarely used diagnostically. In difficult cases, the response to thyrotropin-releasing hormone (TRH) can be used to sort out both hyperthyroid and hypothyroid diagnoses.

TRIGLYCERIDE

Blood levels of triglyceride are primarily the result of the intake of dietary fat. They therefore increase and decrease throughout the day in relation to fatty meals. The fatty acids absorbed through the intestine are converted to triglycerides and then incorporated into chylomicrons and very low density lipoprotein (VLDL). In these forms, they are transported to the liver and throughout the body.

Because the triglyceride level is so dependent on fat intake, it is essential that baseline levels be determined after a 12 hour fast (and 24 hours without alcohol). The most common reason for an elevated triglyceride level is the failure to pay attention to this fasting requirement of specimen collection.

There has long been debate about the independent role of triglycerides in the development of coronary artery disease because they are often elevated in patients who also have high cholesterol levels. It is now believed that elevated triglycerides are an independent risk factor for coronary artery disease. In addition, elevated triglycerides are a marker for other diseases, many related to the liver because of this organ's role in metabolizing fats that are absorbed from the diet.

There is little consensus about what should be considered a normal value for triglyceride (Table

---

TABLE 60–36.   THYROXINE (T_4): NORMAL VALUES

Diagnostic units: μg/dL (nmol/L)
SI conversion factor = 13.0
Normal: 5.5–12.5 (72–163)

	Diagnoses to Consider	**Actions to Consider**
Increased >12.5	Hyperthyroidism Elevated TBG: Birth control pills Pregnancy Estrogens Liver disease Drugs: Propranolol Amphetamines Contrast media Amiodarone Heparin	1. Complete drug history 2. T_4 index 3. Sensitive TSH 4. Free T_3 5. Thyroid uptake scan
Decreased <5.5	Hypothyroidism Decreased TBG: Malnutrition Liver diseases Nephrotic syndrome Androgens Glucocorticoids Sick thyroid syndrome	1. T_4 index 2. TSH 3. Albumin 4. Urinary protein

Values in parentheses are SI units.
TBG = thyroxine-binding globulin; T_4 = thyroxine; T_3 = triiodothyronine; TSH = thyroid-stimulating hormone.

TABLE 60–37. TRIGLYCERIDE: NORMAL VALUES

Diagnostic units: mg/dL (mmol/L)
SI conversion factor = .011
Normal: 20–180 (0.23–2.03)

Triglyceride (mg/dL)	Diagnoses to Consider	Actions to Consider
Increased >200	Nonfasting specimen High caloric diet Familial lipid disorder Recent alcohol consumption Diabetes Liver disease Drugs (BCPs) Hypothyroidism Nephrotic syndrome Pregnancy Biliary obstruction	1. Repeat test after 12 hour fast (24 hours without alcohol) 2. Cholesterol HDL, LDL 3. Alcohol history

BCPs = birth control pills; HDL = high density lipoprotein; LDL = low density lipoprotein.

60–37). It is known that average values increase with age and vary by sex (males > females) and race (whites > blacks). Because of these differences some laboratories report ranges based on patient demographic factors.

Low triglyceride levels are rare and of little clinical significance. They are sometimes seen in patients with malnutrition or hyperthyroidism.

URIC ACID

The serum uric acid level is based on the balance between the rate at which purines are absorbed or produced by the body compared with their metabolism and excretion (Table 60–38). Increased levels can be due to increased purine absorption (i.e., a high protein diet), increased production (i.e., leukemia), or reduced purine excretion (i.e., chronic renal failure).

There is no evidence that uric acid in solution causes any disease. All of the diseases associated with hyperuricemia are due to deposition of uric acid crystals. These illnesses include acute gouty arthritis, gouty tophi, gouty nephropathy, and uro-

lithiasis. Low uric acid levels are occasionally seen in patients with renal tubular defects and are of no clinical significance.

The most common test abnormality is hyperuricemia in an asymptomatic patient. The frequency of this finding is due to the addition of uric acid as an analyte on many screening panels. There is wide agreement that in the absence of acute gouty arthritis, tophi, renal disease, or renal stones these patients require no treatment. Most patients with chronic renal failure have hyperuricemia due to the kidney's reduced ability to excrete uric acid. These patients' uric acid levels are usually less than 10 mg/dL and do not require treatment if the patient is asymptomatic.

A uric acid less than 7 mg/dL is sometimes seen in a patient with acute gout. It is believed to be due to a urate diuresis that occurs in response to the joint inflammation. The diagnosis of acute gouty arthritis must be based on the microscopic identification of urate crystals in synovial fluid. Many patients have been misdiagnosed as having gout when they in fact had another form of arthritis (i.e., osteoarthritis) but also had incidental, asymptomatic hyperuricemia.

TABLE 60–38. URIC ACID: NORMAL VALUES

Diagnostic units: mg/dL (μmol/L)
SI conversion factor = 60
Normal: 2.5–7.0 (150–420)

Uric Acid (mg/dL)	Diagnoses to Consider	Actions to Consider
Increased >7.0	Gout Diuretics Chronic renal failure High protein diet Leukemia, lymphoma	1. Tap inflamed joint 2. Complete dietary history 3. Complete drug history 4. Serum creatinine 5. 24-Hour urinary uric acid 6. Colchicine trial 7. CBC

Values in parentheses are SI units.
CBC = complete blood count.

WHITE BLOOD CELL COUNT

Changes in the white blood cell (WBC) count are seen with many infectious, hematologic, inflammatory, and neoplastic diseases. This variety of diseases makes the WBC count a nonspecific test. It can, however, be a sensitive indicator of disease in some clinical situations. Its degree of increase or decrease often correlates with the severity of the disease process. Monitoring changes in the WBC count over time can therefore provide useful information about the course of an illness (Table 60–39).

Five types of WBCs are commonly counted in the WBC differential: neutrophils, lymphocytes, monocytes, eosinophils, and basophils (Table 60–40). Changes in the relative percentages of these cells are recognized as useful patterns in many common illnesses (i.e., leukocytosis and a shift to the left in bacterial diseases).

Leukopenia, which usually indicates neutropenia, is defined as less than 2×10^9 neutrophils per liter in Whites or 1.5×10^9 per liter in Blacks. In patients receiving chemotherapy, neutropenia of less than 0.5×10^9 per liter is often associated with severe infections. In patients with congenital neutropenia, at the same reduced neutrophil level there is usually no infection. This finding indicates

TABLE 60–39. WHITE BLOOD CELL (WBC) COUNT: NORMAL RANGES

Diagnostic units: cells/mm³ (cells × 19⁹/L)
SI conversion factor = 0.001

	Age	Average	95% Range
Normal:	Birth	18,100	9,000–30,000
	12 Hours	22,800	13,000–38,000
	24 Hours	18,900	9,400–34,000
	1 Week	12,200	5,000–21,000
	2 Months	11,000	5,500–18,000
	1 Year	11,400	6,000–17,500
	2 Years	10,600	6,000–17,000
	6 Years	8,500	5,000–14,500
	10 Years	8,100	4,500–13,500
	20 Years	7,500	4,500–11,500
	Adult	6,500	3,200–9,800

	Diagnoses to Consider	Actions to Consider

Decreased 500–3200	Infections:
	   Severe bacterial infection
	   Influenza
	   Infectious mononucleosis
	   Typhoid fever
	 Drugs:
	   Cytotoxic
	   Idiosyncratic
	 Congestive splenomegaly
	 Felty syndrome
	 SLE
	 Megaloblastic anemia
	 Aplastic anemia
	 Congenital neutropenia
		1. Complete drug history
		 2. Peripheral smear
		 3. Platelet count
		 4. CBC
		 5. Mononucleosis test
		 6. ANA
		 7. Folate, vitamin B$_{12}$ levels
		 8. Bone marrow biopsy

<500	At risk for severe bacterial infections	1. Frequent examinations 2. Antibiotics for fever
Increased 9800–30,000	Physiologic reaction to stress Infection Tissue destruction Leukemia Cancer Hemorrhage Splenectomy	1. Symptom-directed physical examination 2. Peripheral smear
>30,000	Leukemia Leukemoid reaction	1. Peripheral smear 2. Examine for hepatomegaly and splenomegaly

Values in parentheses are SI units.
SLE = systemic lupus erythematosus; CBC = complete blood count; ANA = antinuclear antibody.

TABLE 60–40. WHITE BLOOD CELL (WBC) DIFFERENTIAL COUNT BY AGE: NORMAL VALUES

Age	Segmented Neutrophils (%)	Band Neutrophils (%)	Eosinophils (%)	Basophils (%)	Lymphocytes (%)	Monocytes (%)
Birth	47	14.0	2.2	0.6	31	5.8
1 Week	34	11.8	4.1	0.4	41	9.1
1 Year	23	8.1	2.6	0.4	61	4.8
4 Years	34	8.0	2.8	0.6	50	5.0
12 Years	47	8.0	2.5	0.5	38	4.4
20 Years	51	8.0	2.7	0.5	33	5.0

that the patients have both a quantitative and a qualitative neutrophil defect.

Lymphopenia is defined as less than 1.5×10^9 lymphocytes per liter. It is frequently seen in association with a wide variety of physiologic stresses and is of no clinical significance. Reductions in monocytes, eosinophils, and basophils are occasionally seen and are not clinically useful.

An increased WBC count can be seen with a wide variety of diseases. The average WBC count tends to be higher in children than adults (see Tables 60–39) and 60–40). Most elevated WBC counts are below 30,000 cells/mm^3. Counts greater than 30,000 mm^3 are usually due to leukemia or a leukemoid reaction. It is obviously important to differentiate between these two diagnoses.

REFERENCES

American Diabetes Association: Physician's Guide to Non-Insulin Dependent (Type II) Diabetes: Diagnosis and Treatment. Alexandria, VA, ADA, 1988.

Boyko EJ, Alderman BW, Barron AE: Reference test errors bias the evaluation of diagnostic tests for ischemic heart disease. J Gen Intern Med 3:476, 1988.

DeNeef P: Evaluating rapid tests for streptococcal pharyngitis: The apparent accuracy of a diagnostic test when there are errors in the standard of comparison. Med Decis Making 7:92, 1987a.

DeNeef P: Selective testing for streptococcal pharyngitis in adults. J Fam Pract 25:347, 1987b.

Gerber MA, Randolph MF, Mayo DR: The group A streptococcal carrier state, a reexamination. Am J Dis Child 142:562, 1988.

Heckerling PS: Confidence in diagnostic testing. J Gen Intern Med 3:604, 1988.

Lundberg GD: Using the Clinical Laboratory in Medical Decision Making. Chicago, American Society of Clinical Pathologists Press, 1983.

National Institutes of Health: Lowering blood cholesterol to prevent heart disease, consensus conference. JAMA 253:2080, 1985.

Ransohoff DF, Feinstein AR: Problems of spectrum and bias in evaluating the efficacy of diagnostic tests. N Engl J Med 299:926, 1978.

Sox HJ (ed): Common Diagnostic Tests, Use and Interpretation. Philadelphia, American College of Physicians, 1987.

Statland BE: Clinical Decision Levels for Lab Tests. Oradell, NJ, Medical Economics Books, 1987.

Part V

MANAGEMENT OF THE PRACTICE

CHAPTER 61

THE PROBLEM-ORIENTED MEDICAL RECORD

ROBERT E. RAKEL

A well-prepared medical record is among the most useful tools available to a family physician. When functioning effectively, it communicates the relevant facts regarding patient care to all health personnel involved and allows for the easy documentation and retrieval of information vital to the patient's ongoing care. The information should be organized in a systematic, logical, and consistent manner and should reflect accurately the patient's state of health. Orderly recording of data is vital to efficient care, and, although the information should be simplified as much as possible, it must likewise be both complete and accurate. Information placed in the office record should not be gathered and stored just because it is available and someday may be useful; it should be accumulated on the basis that it is needed at present or will be needed at some future time for providing good patient care. We must avoid merely accumulating data and allowing the record to be "untouched by human thought" (Murnaghan, 1973). Family medicine involves the care of patients over a prolonged period of time. Acute illnesses cannot be treated as totally isolated events but must be viewed in the total perspective of a person's or a family's long-term care. A pregnant woman, for example, may have a slightly elevated blood pressure, which should be compared with readings prior to and following pregnancy to assess its true importance. (Similarly, her smoking habits, alcohol intake, caffeine intake, weight, and other physiologic and psychological functions should be noted and followed.)

An office record system will maintain its usefulness and efficiency over time only if it is designed individually to match the objectives and the personality of the physician using it. The chart should be developed and organized based on the individual physician's preferences and needs. Some will enjoy using flow sheets frequently; others will be turned off by them. Some will prefer, and will be able to maintain, an adequate medication list; others may find it impossible to keep such a list current. The ideal record also must be kept simple and must not handicap or confine the busy physician's productivity by requiring unnecessary paper work. Merely accumulating a large amount of data is not productive; however, a well-organized record actually may require fewer data and yet be more informative than many present systems. The lengthy, illegible, and poorly organized office record of the past has developed into a logical, well-structured account that lends itself to quick and easy retrieval of information and ready assessment of the patient's present health care needs and potential health hazards. It also assists the physician in predicting the patient's potential future state of health by identifying significant risk factors.

THE SOURCE-ORIENTED MEDICAL RECORD

The traditional office record of the past was structured according to the source of material contained in the record; thus, it is called the source-oriented medical record (SOMR). In such a record, laboratory data, electrocardiographic reports, consultants' reports, physicians' notes, consultants' notes, nurses' notes, and radiographic reports each are filed independently in separate areas. Material organized in this way becomes primarily a diary of past events and is of relatively limited value in ongoing patient care, although it was probably adequate for the crisis-oriented, episodic care of patients with acute illness, which has too often constituted the bulk of primary medical care.

Although the SOMR is relatively easy to maintain, its disadvantages are that support for action taken is frequently lacking and it takes considerable time for those unfamiliar with the patient to get a complete review of the problems, especially to trace the history of any particular problem. According to Weed (1971), "The record is not a static repository of medical observations structured in the meaningless order of source, but a precise instrument of communication" (p. vii).

THE PROBLEM-ORIENTED, OR PATIENT-ORIENTED, MEDICAL RECORD

The stimulus for change in record keeping came in 1969, when Weed developed the problem-oriented medical record (POMR). Although this innovative concept originally was applied to the hospital record, its principles have served as the nucleus for major changes in outpatient records as well. The "pure" form proposed by Weed has required some modification to be adapted to family practice, but its basic concepts serve as an excellent foundation for an efficient office medical record. The POMR has also been called the "patient-oriented medical record" because it helps to avoid depersonalization and emphasizes individuality of the patient by listing the specific problems unique to that person. Hence, the patient is not just another person with gallbladder disease but an individual with a unique combination of associated problems that identify him or her as different from other patients with gallbladder disease.

The POMR achieves its maximum potential in the hands of a family physician. It works especially well in the continuing care of patients with chronic illness and in complex cases involving multiple problems. These are areas in which family physicians are especially effective, so it is no wonder that they are the greatest promoters of the POMR. Now that many patients who suffer from previously fatal illnesses are surviving, the family physician is involved in the continuing care of ever-increasing numbers of the chronically ill. Management of patients with these chronic illnesses requires a dynamic record that accurately reflects at all times the patient's present and past medical problems and assists the physician in remaining aware of other potential problems that can become significant at any time.

IMPROVED COMMUNICATION

As our society becomes more mobile and medical technology becomes increasingly complex, we need a well-organized medical record system that permits easy communication and transfer of information among health professionals, both within the same office and at separate sites. No longer can the record be a document understood only by the physician who places data in it. It must permit other physicians, as well as an increasing number of other health personnel, who also depend on the record, to readily assess the patient's condition, understand the plan of management, and recognize all elements important to the patient's ongoing care. As long as the record is able to communicate information in this manner, it will serve as an effective tool for all members of the health care team.

The maintenance of a complete and well-organized medical record over a prolonged period of time contributes to high-quality care by permitting attention to be focused on preventive measures. The need for a uniform, organized collection of information in the office record will increase as more physicians practice in groups and a larger portion

of costs is paid by third parties. Increased emphasis is being placed on the assessment of the quality of care, and outpatient records must be organized in a manner that permits review, just as hospital records are reviewed. Terminology also is being influenced by third-party payers. The physician and other health professionals, such as the dentist, nurse, and therapist, now are called providers, and the office visit is an encounter. It is hoped that in family practice an encounter will remain a friendly interaction between physician and patient, rather than follow Webster's definition of "a meeting of adversaries or hostile persons to engage in conflict." It is no wonder that many physicians bristle at the use of this term to refer to their relationships with patients.

Improved patient care must remain the primary objective of any newly structured record system. As Murnaghan (1973) stated:

Data collection and information systems cannot be justified if they subvert the process of patient care and fail to benefit the patient and provider either directly or indirectly. The growth of public, as opposed to private, responsibility for personal health services means that more and more data requirements will be placed upon the providers of care. (p. 17)

Data collection must not be allowed to become threatening to either the patient or the physician but must be an obvious asset to the care and management of all problems related to patients.

Patient Access to Medical Records

Use of the computer in medical record keeping has focused more attention on confidentiality of the medical record. Access to medical records for management purposes is being given to more and more non–health professionals who are neither sensitive to patients' concerns about confidentiality nor bound by strong ethical or professional codes of conduct regarding the use of such information. A fine balance between confidentiality and access will have to be struck.

The Federal Privacy Act of 1974 (Public Law 93-579) establishes the patient's right to obtain the medical record in federal institutions. A number of states also have statutes as well as precedent court decisions permitting direct access of patients to their medical records. Controversy still exists about the effect this will have on clinical care. Although there is no proof that sharing the record with the patient improves the quality of care, there is general agreement that it improves patient understanding and compliance. Schade, a family physician in Los Gatos, California, allows patients to keep their own complete medical record, and he maintains only a brief office record in note form. Patients thus have the record available if they are seen in an emergency room or by a consultant or when moving to a new area. He believes that making the records available to the patients not only enables them to develop a keen understanding of their medical problems and treatment but actually discourages rather than encourages the incidence of filing malpractice suits (Schade, 1976).

One survey of patients (Michael and Bordley, 1982) found that 80 per cent believed they should be permitted to see their medical record, but they were not convinced that possessing a copy was as important as reading it. Regardless of local law, the best policy is to allow patients to examine and copy their records on request unless there is valid medical reason for refusing to do so. Tufo and colleagues (1977) gave patients copies of their medical records in an attempt "to provide a clear statement of problems and plans to emphasize self-help and patient responsibility" (p. 504). They believe that the patient's audit of the record provides feedback concerning the accuracy of the information and the level of patient understanding. Fischbach and associates (1980) also promoted the involvement of the patient. In developing their problem list and progress notes, they stated, "The attitude that 'what you don't know won't hurt you' is proving unrealistic; it is what patients do not know, but vaguely suspect, that causes them corrosive worry" (p. 4).

Sharing the medical record with the patient certainly has its place and can be of value, yet calls for discretion because it can also be harmful. For example, some elderly patients may become depressed or confused by seeing a problem list containing 10 to 12 items and multiple medications. Patients with emotional problems may have difficulty understanding or coping with the content of progress notes.

Information Retrieval

The medical record rapidly is becoming less the private property and sole responsibility of the physician and more the joint responsibility and common property of the physician, other health providers, and the patient. Information in the medical record should be highly visible, clear, and concise so that it can be retrieved easily to allow for effective and efficient use of time by the physician and other health professionals.

The use of facsimile (fax) transmission greatly facilitates the transfer of medical information, including the electrocardiogram. In many ways, fax transmission is superior to telephone voice communication, express mail, and electronic mail. It can be especially useful in emergency care (Yamamoto and Wiebe, 1989).

Medical Information Cards

Medical identification cards are becoming increasingly popular in our mobile society. Such a card contains microfilm of selected portions of an individual's medical record and is carried as a wallet card. This document serves as a "medical passport" and identifies the nature of the patient's medical problems, such as a recent myocardial infarction, diabetes mellitus, drug allergies, anticoagulant medication, and immunization status. These data give an accurate composite picture of the patient's health status to physicians other than the patient's personal physician during an emergency or when the patient is traveling outside the community.

Laser optic technology has made possible the use of credit card–size plastic cards that can store up to 800 pages of data. These cards record radiographs, computerized tomography and magnetic resonance imaging scans, and electrocardiograms. A special read–write unit and an IBM-compatible computer are needed to use the card. A special software package ensures confidentiality of the medical record. The patient's picture and signature can be imbedded invisibly in the card, making forgery or transfer impossible.

CONVERSION TO A NEW SYSTEM

A well-organized and clearly developed medical record will make the provision of excellent medical care readily apparent. However, it will just as readily expose poor or inadequate care. Physicians who have converted their office record systems to the problem-oriented format undergo a humbling experience as numerous weaknesses in their previous care are uncovered. Problems frequently are identified that had been lost in the record, and laboratory abnormalities are uncovered that were not investigated further. The conversion to a new record system, whether it be the POMR or others, will involve a reassessment and reorganization of the record system that will be of value to the physician and the patient by uncovering problems and placing all facts into a refreshing new perspective.

When records are converted to a problem-oriented format, it is best to begin conversion with the most active records and leave less active ones until later. It is most helpful to start all new patients in the new format and to convert established patients with chronic diseases who are seen frequently. Temporary help can be hired to work in the evening to type index cards and transfer record contents to new jackets. The physician should prepare the problem list. Although this is a time-consuming activity, the review it requires will be worth the trouble by reacquainting the physician with previously forgotten aspects of the patient's care.

TRANSFER OF INFORMATION

It is important that the family physician incorporate the patient's entire medical background into the record, so that the total comprehensive picture is constantly available to the physician and to other health personnel who have need of it. Valuable medical information often is scattered in a variety of locations and thus becomes relatively inaccessible or unavailable when needed.

When new patients are seen, a strong effort should be made to acquire all medical information from other physicians, government services, hospitals, and other health agencies previously involved in the patient's care. A great deal of unnecessary effort and expense results when each physician, in turn, must establish full medical data for every patient, because a variety of diagnostic tests and therapeutic trials must be repeated needlessly. When the transferred record is in the form of the POMR or some similarly concise system, putting it to use is a simple matter for the new physician and sending it on is a painless experience for the former physician because he or she knows that it can be interpreted readily and will be of benefit to his or her former patient's care. Central computerization of the medical record in the future may obviate much of this problem. In countries with a national health service, such as Great Britain, the medical record is considered state property and is transferred automatically with patients when they move to a new community.

A study by Birtwhistle and Anderson (1989) showed that only half (52 per cent) of family physicians regularly request previous records on their patients. When information was obtained, there was a preference for short summaries of the patient's problems and copies of previous consultation reports as well as hospital discharge summaries. Somewhat of a surprise was the opinion that office progress notes were seldom useful.

A well-organized record system, such as the POMR, also allows the referring family physician to communicate the patient's total health status more effectively to consulting physicians by submitting the problem list with the consultation request. This prevents the specialist from merely "treating his or her own disease specialty" and ensures awareness of all of the patient's medical, social, and psychiatric problems, as well as the problems for which the consultation is being requested. When a cardiologist is asked to consult about a seriously ill patient in the coronary care unit, the problem list clearly illustrates other problems to be considered and managed and makes the need for continuing involvement by the family physician readily apparent. Subspecialists are prevented from concentrating on a single aspect to the detriment of the whole patient.

LEGIBILITY

Legibility is necessary if any data, no matter how systematically organized, are to be retrieved and collated in a rapid, accurate, and useful manner that will permit the quick review of a patient's total health status. The well-known illegibility of physicians' handwriting is an understandable product of conditioning during many years of rapid note taking. This handicap, the greatest barrier to effective communication and good records, is now being removed as a rapidly increasing number of physicians turn to dictating their records and utilizing secretarial services for transcription to obtain clearly typed progress notes. This improved legibility is an obvious advantage in group practices, in which more than one physician and several nurses or other health professionals are likely to depend on the same chart. The POMR, because of its structure, lends itself well to dictation with a minimum of confusion.

Illegible records are a liability in court. It is embarrassing when physicians cannot decipher their own notes because a judge is likely to think that, if a note cannot be read, it cannot be used. In addition, a disorganized, illegible record brings into question the physician's quality of care. Intelligible and accurate medical records symbolize good care and reflect the physician's commitment to quality, which managed care plans are beginning to demand.

MINIMUM REQUIREMENTS FOR OFFICE RECORDS

The American Board of Family Practice has incorporated a review of office records into its recertification procedure. Table 61–1 lists those items considered by the Board to be essential to a good office record.

ORGANIZATION OF A RECORD SYSTEM

Filing

A record-keeping system, no matter how well organized, is of little value if the medical record cannot be found. Much time can be saved by using an efficient filing system.

Alphabetical Filing Systems

This is a popular method of record storage, especially for small practices. Records are filed alphabetically according to surname. Because of the similarity of many names, however, misfiling is common. Strong ethnic backgrounds in a community may lead to heavy concentrations of similar names. Family filing is also difficult with the alphabetical system, particularly when there are different surnames in the family.

Color coding of alphabetical filing systems will limit misfiling and ease retrieval. Each letter has

TABLE 61–1.   OFFICE RECORD CONTENT RECOMMENDATIONS (AMERICAN BOARD OF FAMILY PRACTICE)

A. Records must be legible.
B. In order for records to allow an efficient and rapid review of the patient's total health picture, or of a particular health problem, by family physicians and associates, consultants, and allied health personnel, the clinical record should contain certain basic information. The following is an outline of suggested elements to be recorded. It is recognized that not all of these elements will be necessary in every patient record.
   1. The patient's profile
      * Age (birth date)
      * Sex
      * Occupation
      * Education
      * Economic status
      * Family structure
      * Activity pattern
      * Height
      * Weight
      * Habitus
      * Blood pressure
   2. Information about possible risk factors
      * History of familial or hereditary disease
      * Alcohol or drinking habits
      * Smoking habits
      * Environmental risks
      * Lifestyle
      * Stress factors
   3. A notation which clearly indicates the presence or absence of specific
      * Allergies
      * Drug idiosyncrasies or intolerances
   4. Adequate information about the past history, such as
      * Previous illness
      * Previous surgery
      * Recurrent minor problems
   5. Adequate information to clearly and easily identify
      * The primary problem
      * Associated or other problems
      * Medications the patient is taking
      * Current immunization status
      * Results of pertinent laboratory and/or X-ray examinations
   6. Well-organized and clinically informative progress notes which clearly provide adequate current information about
      * The patient's health status
      * Observations about the patient's problems
      * Conclusions
      * Tests
   7. Adequate information to clearly and easily provide information about the
      * Therapeutic or management plan for each element of the patient's health care
      * Patient education for each problem

From *Recertification Handbook for Diplomates*. Lexington, KY, American Board of Family Practice, 1994, pp. 5–6, with permission.

a distinctive color. Colored labels representing the first two letters of the patient's last name are fixed to the tab on each file.

Numeric Systems

Terminal digit filing appears to be the more efficient system for family practice. Fewer charts are misfiled using this system, and it allows for a more rapid and accurate placement and retrieval of records. The only significant disadvantage is the need to maintain an alphabetical and numeric cross-reference index, but this is accomplished easily by computer because most offices now use computers for billing and to generate the encounter form.

Color Coding

Color-coded terminal digit filing largely eliminates the possibility of misfiling, or at least limits it to a narrow area. Ten colors are used, one for each of the ten Arabic numerals 0 (zero) to 9, as opposed to the large number of colors needed in alphabetic systems. This permits ready recognition of visually distinct categories, especially when open shelving is used. Records are arranged according to the last two digits. Each number is

keyed to a color on the record jacket edge. The two colors representing the two digits are recognized easily if the record is misfiled. Records with the same two terminal digits then are arranged in sequence according to the numbers preceding the two terminal digits. Thus, chart 00-00-13 will be followed by 00-01-13, 00-02-13, and so on (Fig. 61–1). Color coding also can be an advantage when added to alphabetical systems, but misfiling is common when there are many charts filed under common family names such as Smith, Jones, and Young.

Open Shelving

Color-coded terminal digit filing works best with open-shelf filing, although it can be adapted to drawer files as well. Shelves are better than drawers, however, because they can be stacked higher and it is easier for more than one person to have access to them at a time.

Inactive Records

Purging of inactive records avoids burdening the record system with unused charts. To keep the unnecessary volume to a minimum, records of pa-

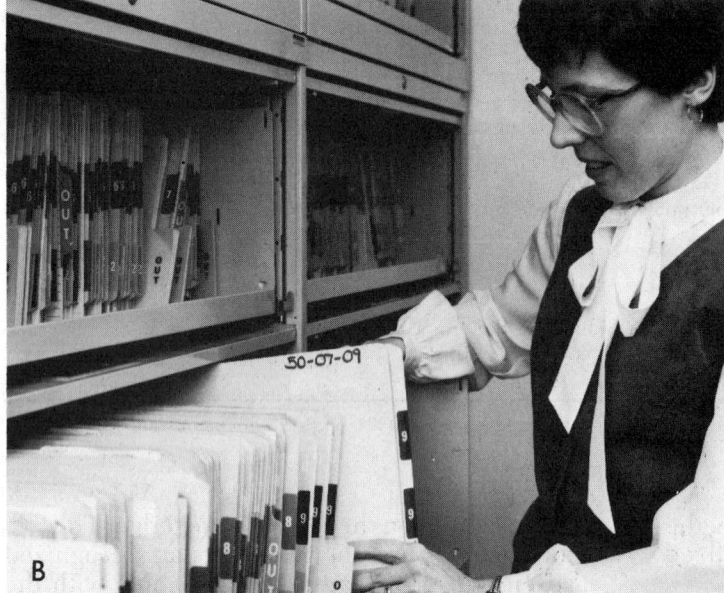

FIGURE 61–1. Color-coded terminal digital charts.

tients who have not been seen for 2 or 3 years should be considered inactive and removed from the active file. This weeding out can be a relatively simple process. A color-coded tab or mark corresponding to the year can be added to the margin of each chart (Figs. 61–1 and 61–2). Each year the color is changed when a member of the family is seen so that the color represents the most recent year in which the patient or family was seen. If yellow was the color 3 years ago, it is an easy task to pull all charts with yellow tabs. For the system to work, however, the receptionist or nurse must check this tab each time the chart is pulled to make sure the color corresponds to the current year. A list of preprinted dates also can be stamped on the chart with check marks indicating the most recent year of chart use (Fig. 61–2).

Family Charts

The physician's care of families is facilitated by a record system that focuses on the family. Family folders are filed under the name of the head of the household or the person responsible for the account. This is especially important when family members have different names. Sometimes the family is filed according to all persons living together in the same residence regardless of who is paying for the care. With the numeric filing system, there is only one possible shelf location for the family folder regardless of the variety of surnames involved. Even if surnames vary within a family because of children from previous marriages or because the wife's parents live with the family, each individual is identified by a one- or two-digit modifier within the family number.

The family folder usually consists of an outer file jacket containing selected family information as well as the individual charts of each family member (Fig. 61–3). The first item in the family folder is the *family registration form* (Fig. 61–4), containing family demographic data that usually are

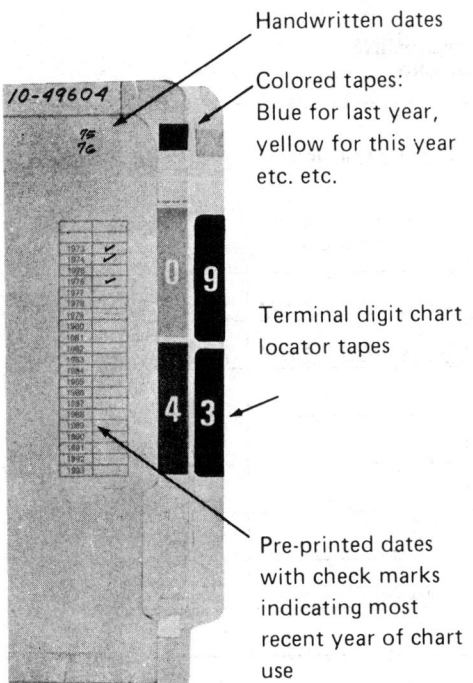

Handwritten dates

Colored tapes:
Blue for last year,
yellow for this year
etc. etc.

Terminal digit chart
locator tapes

Pre-printed dates
with check marks
indicating most
recent year of chart
use

FIGURE 61–2. Designating year of most recent chart use for purging inactive records. (From Sullivan RJ Jr: Medical Record and Index Systems for Community Practice. Cambridge, MA, Ballinger Publishing Company, 1979, with permission.)

obtained at the first office visit. It maintains a prominent location in the chart because it is a ready source of reference for the names and ages of all family members and includes occupational and insurance information. The purpose of the family chart is to provide the physician with as much information as possible relating to factors involving the entire family that could have an impact on the health of any individual member. It is important for the physician to note when the problems involving one family member influence the health of another.

Family stress may become evident by a clustering of problems in many family members. The family member visit register or any form that depicts the ongoing problems of family members can assist the family physician in identifying problems that are common to the family and result from disordered family dynamics. Any technique that assists the family physician to deal with family problems in addition to addressing the needs of individual family members enhances the quality of care to that family. Widmer and colleagues (1980) have shown that early signs of depression include an increased number of visits by all family members and frequent complaints of pain, anxiety, and functional problems by the patient and other family members for up to a year before the depression becomes obvious.

Also contained within the outside family folder is the *family genogram* (see Chapter 2). By noting shared family problems, the physician can be alerted to problems that could be related to the present symptoms or to other disorders that should be considered and evaluated in addition to the presenting problem. Some family physicians complete these on every family; others do so only when they think it is necessary.

It is useful to have a corner or prominent area in the chart to record events that are important occurrences in the patient's life so that these can be recalled and mentioned during subsequent visits. Reference to or questions about events such as the birth of a grandchild, a move into a new home, or a trip abroad will be appreciated by the patient. They often are amazed that the physician cared enough to remember items of such personal importance to them.

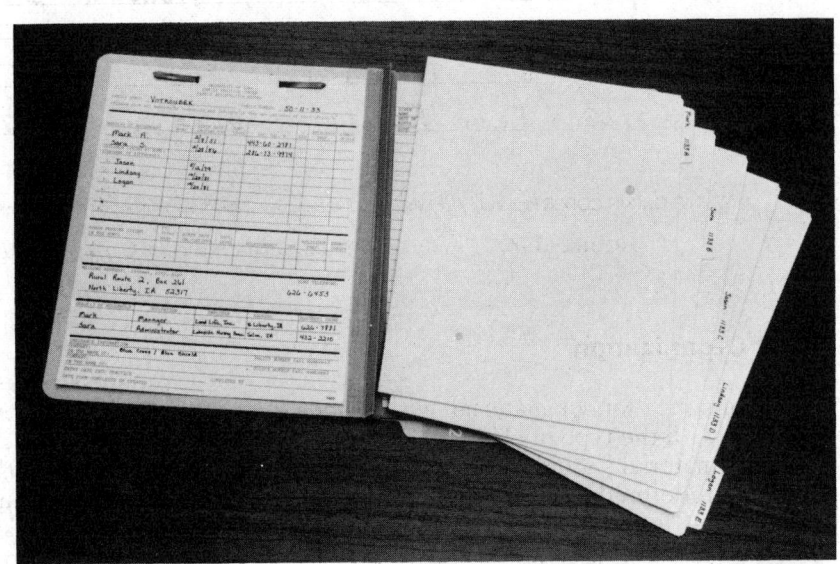

FIGURE 61–3. Family folder containing individual patient records.

MR-3 11/88

DEPARTMENT OF FAMILY MEDICINE
FAMILY REGISTRATION RECORD

FAMILY NAME: _Wagner_   PATIENT NUMBER: _10-25-68_

Head(s) Of Household:	Sex M/F	Check If Lives At Home	Birth Date (Mo/Day/Yr)	Soc. Sec. #	Highest School Level Completed	Ethnic Origin (W,B,H,E,O)*
John	m	✓	01 / 03 / 49	416-01-3241	2 yrs col.	W
Betty	F	✓	09 / 06 / 50	513-60-5214	college	W
CHILDREN: (Give last name if different)			/ /			
1. William	m	✓	12 / 14 / 70	- -		
2. Kate	F	✓	10 / 10 / 74	- -		
3.			/ /	- -		
4.			/ /	- -		
5.			/ /	- -		
6.			/ /	- -		

Other Persons Living In The Home:	Birth Date (Mo/Day/Yr)	Highest School Level Completed	Relationship	Ethnic Origin (W,B,H,E,O)*
1. Tom Johnson	09 / 22 / 20	high school	wife's father	W
2.	/ /			
3.	/ /			

MAILING ADDRESS: (Street, City, Zip)   HOME TELEPHONE

8834 Elm   Deer Park, Texas   _432-7641_

HEAD(S) OF HOUSEHOLD	OCCUPATION(S)	EMPLOYER(S)	BUSINESS PHONE(S)
John	salesman	self-employed	481-3289
Betty	teacher	Houston ISD	521-2800

NEAREST RELATIVE: _Joe Wagner_   RELATIONSHIP: _father_

ADDRESS: _12304 Fern Forest_, _Houston_, _TX_ _77044_ _459-6092_ _932-1626_
      Street   City   State   Zip   Home Phone   Business Phone

* ETHNIC ORIGIN CODES (optional): W = White or Caucasian; B = Black or Afro-American; H = Hispanic or Mexican-American; E = East Asian; O = Other

FIGURE 61–4.   Family registration record. (Baylor College of Medicine, Houston, Texas.)

Chart Organization

The organization of material within the chart will vary with the type of chart selected, but in all cases the material should be organized in a consistent and predefined manner. If a folder is used, the problem list is usually the top sheet on the left, with the family registration record beneath it. The top sheet on the right contains the most recent progress notes, with previous progress notes beneath it, followed by the data base, electrocardiograms, and correspondence. If possible, each of these sections should be divided by tabs or by some other method to allow easy identification, perhaps by using different colors for each section. A more economical method than purchasing chart

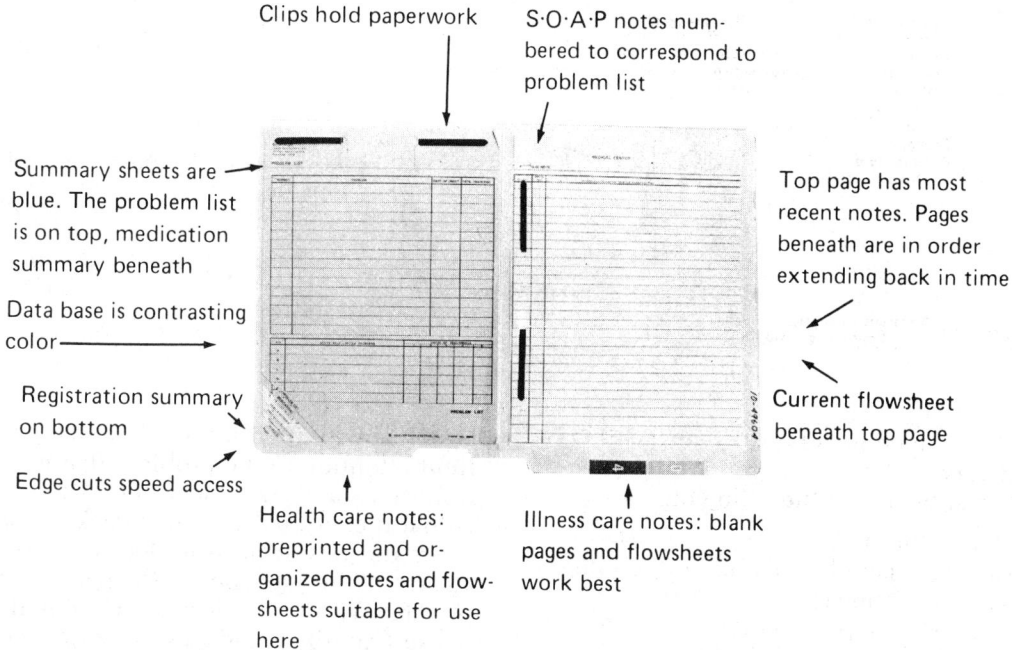

Clips hold paperwork

S·O·A·P notes num-
bered to correspond to
problem list

Summary sheets are
blue. The problem list
is on top, medication
summary beneath

Data base is contrasting
color

Registration summary
on bottom

Edge cuts speed access

Top page has most
recent notes. Pages
beneath are in order
extending back in time

Current flowsheet
beneath top page

Health care notes:
preprinted and or-
ganized notes and flow-
sheets suitable for use
here

Illness care notes: blank
pages and flowsheets
work best

FIGURE 61–5.   One method of arranging the chart using the problem-oriented format. (From Sullivan RJ Jr: *Medical Record and Index Systems for Community Practice.* Cambridge, MA, Ballinger Publishing Company 1979 with permission.)

dividers is to cut away the edge of progress note pages to make the underlying data base accessible (Fig. 61–5).

USING THE POMR

Although the POMR, as developed by Weed, originally was directed toward organization of the hospital record, it was adapted rapidly to the outpatient setting. Its usefulness in family practice first was demonstrated by Bjorn and Cross (1970). Numerous publications and articles appearing since 1969 have developed the basic concepts further and have suggested many variations, which provide myriad choices for the individual physician. Physicians are encouraged to review the literature and then to select those components with which they feel most comfortable and that appear most useful in their particular practice. The design of any component should be varied when necessary to match individual preference.

Weed describes four basic elements as the nucleus of the POMR: the data base, problem list, initial plan, and progress notes. Although his initial plan applies primarily to the complete work-up of a new office patient or the admission work-up of a hospitalized patient, most physicians prefer to incorporate it into ongoing patient care as a feature of the progress note (Fig. 61–6). The logical approach to record keeping, then, calls first for the establishment of a data base, after which a problem list is developed, initial plans are identified, and

the patient's progress is monitored with continual updating of the data base and problem list.

Although the problem list is developed largely from information accumulated in the data base, it is the most important single ingredient of the POMR. If there is limited enthusiasm for using all components of the POMR, development of a problem list alone will be of significant benefit. Addition of a data base will enhance its usefulness, but full benefits can be realized only when structured progress notes are also incorporated.

Problem List

A problem is anything that requires diagnosis or management or that interferes with quality of life as perceived by the patient. It can be either a firm diagnosis, a physical symptom, or a social or economic problem. It is any physiologic, pathologic, psychological, or social item of concern to either the patient or the physician. A problem is any item that physicians believe they cannot afford to miss or that requires ongoing concern or attention.

The problem list serves as a comprehensive overview of the patient's present and past state of health. It indicates whether the problems are active or have occurred in the past but are at present inactive. The problem list is a reminder of what has occurred so that the physician can be helped to remember that the patient had a cholecystectomy or hysterectomy and thus does not continue

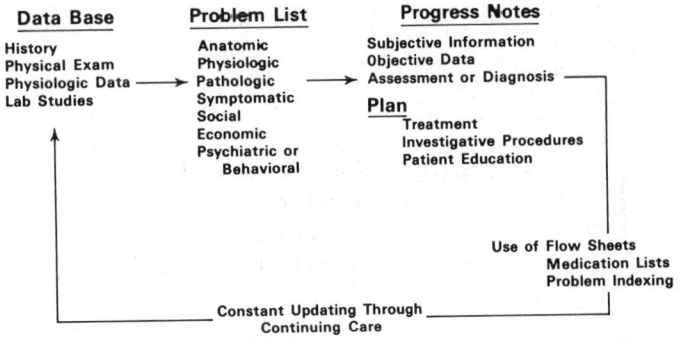

FIGURE 61–6. Basic elements of the problem-oriented medical record.

to ask about the function of these organs while obtaining a history.

Problems can be any of the following:

1. Anatomic (hernia)
2. Physiologic (jaundice of unknown etiology)
3. A sign (hepatomegaly)
4. A symptom (dyspnea, fatigue)
5. Economic (financial difficulty)
6. Social (marital discord, spouse alcoholic)
7. Psychiatric (depression)
8. Physical handicap (paralysis, amputation)
9. Specific diagnosis (acute rheumatic fever)
10. Abnormal laboratory test (elevated blood urea nitrogen, elevated sedimentation rate)
11. Risk factor (family history of diabetes mellitus or cancer)

A special feature of the problem list is that each is unique to that individual. It is a "snapshot" of that person's health risks and current and past medical problems. Rarely would two persons have identical problem lists.

Each problem on a patient's list should be numbered, and Weed proposed that the progress notes be keyed by number to the appropriate problem on the list, thereby reflecting its present state of resolution. In hospital records, the management of each illness is identified consistently throughout the record by this same number, but this degree of attention to detail is not always followed in private practice. The types of illness seen by a family physician often are described more appropriately as symptoms or undifferentiated problems than as diseases. *Disease* implies a full understanding of the pathology and etiology of the illness, whereas many of the illnesses encountered by the family physician involve a varying degree of insight into the underlying etiology and a varying severity of the illness, which occasionally resolves while still in the undifferentiated state.

The problem list is a dynamic picture of the patient's health problems and is changed continually by updating, as new problems are added or old problems are carried to a greater degree of resolution. It should contain all of the patient's continuing problems and should have a prominent position in the record, so as to remind the physician constantly to care for the whole patient and not to limit attention to the problem that may be temporarily outstanding. One value of the problem list is that it continually "stares back at you" and prevents the physician from focusing on too limited an area to the exclusion of the patient's total health picture. With such a format, it is possible to orient oneself rapidly to the most important current problem without forgetting the others.

All problems can be kept in proper perspective. One physician on call for another can grasp the essential nature of a case rapidly by scanning the problem list and thereby can make a more rational decision regarding the acute presenting problem. To do this, however, the problems should be *printed* for ease of reading and rapid scanning. The POMR also allows for more efficient use of allied health personnel, by permitting the physician to communicate effectively an assessment of the patient's problems and their management. The constant surveillance of the patient's state of health by the physician and allied health personnel and their efforts toward establishing effective health maintenance require constant monitoring of health hazards and risk factors. These risk factors should be identified on the problem list and should serve constantly to alert all health personnel to their presence.

It has been said appropriately that the main value of the POMR is not its structure but its honesty. The POMR demands that all problems be described straightforwardly and at their present stage of development and resolution, no matter how elementary the terms used to describe them may be. It insists that physicians list only what they *know* to be present, not what they *think* to be present. The principle to be followed is "record what is known, not what is supposed." The POMR discourages guesswork and insists on an accurate listing of actual problems and observed facts. As Weed (1971) has said, "The problem list should not contain diagnostic guesses; it should simply state the problems at a level of refinement consistent with the physician's understanding, running the gamut from the precise diagnosis to the isolated, unexplained finding" (p. 25).

The POMR does not demand excessive compulsiveness but does require that all significant factors be displayed so that they cannot be ignored. Abnormal data should be placed on the problem list and accounted for. The logic behind clinical decisions will be apparent in the POMR, and caution should be taken to avoid drawing conclusions prematurely; for example, a combination of a low hemoglobin level and an elevated reticulocyte count does not equal iron-deficiency anemia. More information is necessary to reach that conclusion.

Design of the Problem List

The problem list can be structured in a variety of ways. Physicians should select those components considered most desirable and arrange them in the manner most appropriate to their practice. Most practices design their own problem list, but a large variety of formats are available commercially. One format is that used at Baylor College of Medicine lists acute and chronic problems on the same page (Fig. 61–7). Some programs use a separate problem list for acute, self-limited problems because only chronic problems should be placed on the master problem list. These temporary problems can be listed separately, as shown in Figure 61–7, or on a separate page entirely. The frequency of recurrence is indicated by dates of occurrence. In this manner, recurring acute problems, such as otitis media or acute bronchitis, that can be potentially threatening to the patient's future health can be identified and transferred to the major problem list.

Some systems prefer to use letters for the acute problems, assigning the next letter in the alphabet to each new acute problem whether or not a separate acute problem list is used. Others believe that temporary problems can be handled in the progress notes only and need not be identified on the problem list. This simplifies the record system but runs the risk of failing to recognize recurring acute problems that deserve greater visibility and continuous monitoring. Most acute and temporary problems that are encountered, however, are self-limiting and usually do not recur with a frequency that requires their being placed on the master problem list.

Components of the Problem List

Legibility is an important component of the problem list. Problems should be either typed or printed in large letters to support the major function of the list: that the problems be "visible at a glance."

A variety of methods can be used to illustrate the active or inactive status of each problem. Those problems that have been resolved but may have an impact on the patient's future health must be retained on the problem list for continued visibility. A resolved problem can be transferred to a separate inactive column or it can be identified by indicating the date of resolution under "comments" or in a separate column. It also can be identified by drawing a line or arrow through the problem.

When a higher level of understanding or sophistication is reached for any active problem or combination of problems, these should be changed to a single, new problem. This resolution to a higher level can be indicated by listing the date of resolution of the earlier problem and adding the newer problem at the bottom of the list. Another method is to draw an arrow from the previous problem to the newer designation while maintaining the same problem number and position on the problem list, space permitting. If a comment column is used, the reason for this change can be noted. Otherwise, future information can be identified by placing over the arrow the date of the office visit at which information leading to the increased resolution was obtained. An example of such a change in problem status is the listing of "dyspnea on exertion" and "peripheral edema" as separate problems that then are resolved to "congestive heart failure" once the presence of renal disease has been ruled out. Another example would be the change of the problem of "pain, right knee" to "degenerative joint disease" when radiographic exams identify the specific cause.

Family Problem List

Family problem lists are a method of depicting the problems of each family member on the same page, along with problems that involve the entire family unit (Fig. 61–8). Many family physicians prefer to include this information as part of the family genogram instead of using a family problem list.

Whatever the method of organization, this comprehensive, visible, and concise overview of problems enables the physician to provide family-oriented care while keeping the ongoing problems of individual members in proper perspective. The only real disadvantage of a family problem list is the limited amount of space available and, thus, the limited amount of information that can be documented. If a family problem list is utilized, it should be displayed prominently in the family folder and should be the only place that master problems are listed. This should force the physician to look at the family as a whole. Unfortunately, there is some risk that the physician may focus on the individual's record to the exclusion of information in the family folder.

The family problem list emphasizes the fact that no one in the family can have a problem without affecting other members in some manner; in fact, the problems of greatest importance are those that by their very nature affect each family member (Grace et al., 1977). The family problem list gives the physician an awareness of the entire family's health problems. It serves as a reminder of the problems of other members who are not being seen but may need attention or follow-up.

BAYLOR FAMILY PRACTICE CENTER
PROBLEM LIST
Please Print

Name _Bradford, James_ _____ Date of Birth _7-13-32_ _____

NO.	DATE	CHRONIC PROBLEMS AND RISK FACTORS	COMMENTS
1.	2/90	HEALTH MAINTENANCE	
	1986	Essential Hypertension	
	2/90	FH Colon Cancer	Father at age 66
	6/93	Allergic Rhinitis	
	5/94	BPH	
	8/94	Osteoarthritis	
	2/90	ADVANCE DIRECTIVE DISCUSSED	
		COPY IN CHART	

ALLERGIES	None

ACUTE PROBLEMS		RECURRENCES
7/91	Acute Bronchitis	10/92
3/92	Low Back Pain	

FIGURE 61–7. Problem list. (Baylor College of Medicine, Houston, Texas.)

Data Base

The data base is the first step toward developing the problem list. It is the platform on which the structure of the POMR depends for stability. The data base consists of the history (chief complaint, present illness, past history, systems review, and social history), physical examination, physiologic data, and baseline laboratory studies. The data base on each patient varies depending on age, sex, and race. Each physician should define the minimum of data that will be collected on all patients in the practice so that office personnel can assist in assuring that this minimum is accomplished. The collection of most elements of the data base can be assigned to allied health professionals, who can obtain the information prior to the physician's involvement.

The data base serves as the groundwork for each patient's future care and should include those tests

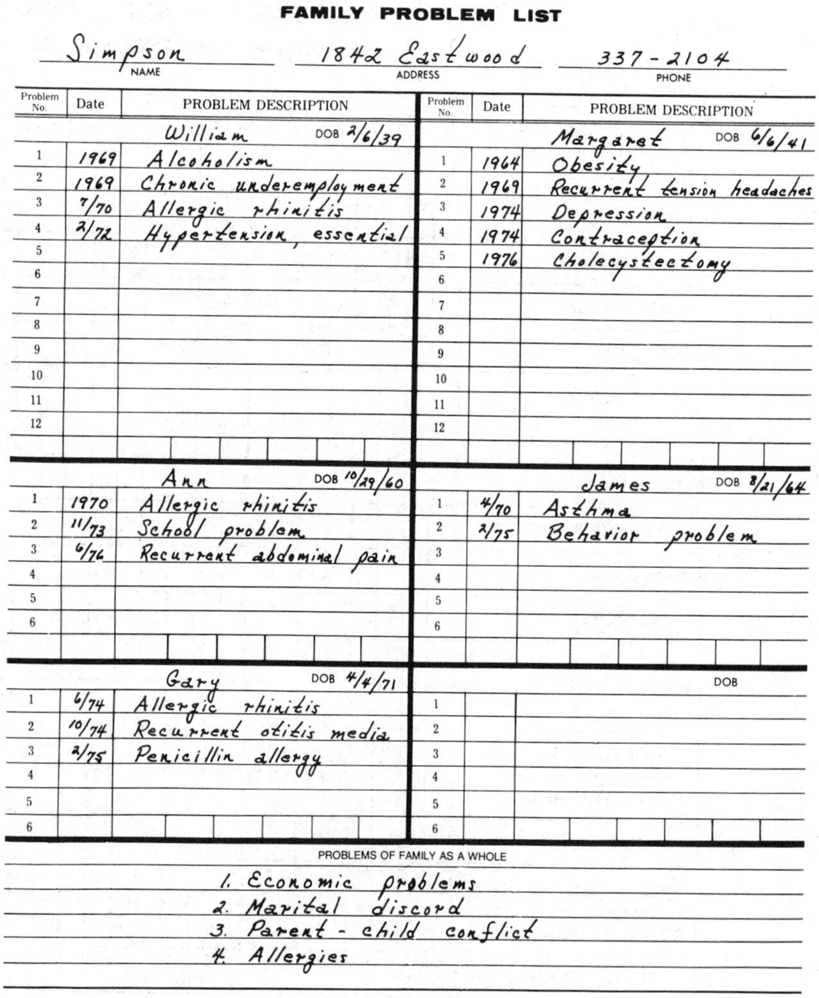

FAMILY PROBLEM LIST

Simpson   1842 Eastwood   337-2104
NAME   ADDRESS   PHONE

Problem No.	Date	PROBLEM DESCRIPTION	Problem No.	Date	PROBLEM DESCRIPTION
		William DOB 2/6/39			*Margaret* DOB 6/6/41
1	1969	Alcoholism	1	1964	Obesity
2	1969	Chronic underemployment	2	1969	Recurrent tension headaches
3	7/70	Allergic rhinitis	3	1974	Depression
4	2/72	Hypertension, essential	4	1974	Contraception
5			5	1976	Cholecystectomy
6			6		
7			7		
8			8		
9			9		
10			10		
11			11		
12			12		

Problem No.	Date	PROBLEM DESCRIPTION	Problem No.	Date	PROBLEM DESCRIPTION
		Ann DOB 10/29/60			*James* DOB 8/21/64
1	1970	Allergic rhinitis	1	4/70	Asthma
2	11/73	School problem	2	2/75	Behavior problem
3	6/76	Recurrent abdominal pain	3		
4			4		
5			5		
6			6		

Problem No.	Date	PROBLEM DESCRIPTION	Problem No.	Date	PROBLEM DESCRIPTION
		Gary DOB 4/4/71			DOB
1	6/74	Allergic rhinitis	1		
2	10/74	Recurrent otitis media	2		
3	2/75	Penicillin allergy	3		
4			4		
5			5		
6			6		

PROBLEMS OF FAMILY AS A WHOLE

1. Economic problems
2. Marital discord
3. Parent - child conflict
4. Allergies

FIGURE 61–8. Family problem list. (From Grace NT, Neal EM, Wellock CE, Pile DD: The family-oriented medical record. J Fam Pract 4:91, 1977, with permission. Reprinted with permission of Appleton & Lange, Inc.)

that are effective screening procedures for significant disease or are likely to be good reference points for future problems; for example, elevations of blood pressure can have a significant long-term detrimental effect, and a mild elevation may go undetected if an earlier baseline determination is not available for comparison. The data base should concentrate on the problems that cannot afford to be missed and should include those tests that are of greatest value in detecting these problems. Active debate will continue regarding the need for various routine tests; the issue of which test is the most reliable indicator of potentially significant disease will be settled only by further research. Tests to be emphasized in the data base are those that detect disease at its earliest, presymptomatic phase so that the normal course of the disease can be interrupted and its impact minimized.

A complete data base is so essential to the success of the POMR that many physicians place "incomplete data base" as problem no. 1 on the list, where it remains until all required data have been obtained. A commitment should be made to obtain all of the data within a given period of time. If a complete history and physical examination cannot

be obtained at one visit, information still can be collected bit by bit during a series of visits over a period of time. The visibility of an incomplete data base as problem no. 1 serves as a constant reminder to continue accumulating the data, regardless of the nature of the episodic visit.

Health Maintenance Forms

A variety of forms have been developed to help monitor routine screening activities. These usually indicate the tests that should be performed at different ages to detect potentially serious disease in its earliest stage. Figure 61–9 illustrates the elements identified by faculty and residents at Baylor College of Medicine as those that should be monitored periodically from 20 to 79 years of age. Clear blocks indicate that the examination or test should be done at that age; shaded blocks indicate the test is not recommended, but information still can be added at that age if the test was not performed when indicated earlier.

History

A variety of new methods for obtaining the medical history have been developed to save the physi-

A

BAYLOR FAMILY PRACTICE CENTER
HEALTH MAINTENANCE PROFILE

PATIENT_____   DATE _____

AGE	20	21	22	23	24	25	26	27	28	29	30	31	32	33	34	35	36	37	38	39	40	41	42	43	44	45	46	47	48	49
BLOOD PRESSURE																														
INTERIM H & P																														
HEARING EXAM																														
VISION CHECK																														
TONOMETRY																														
BREAST EXAM																														
MAMMOGRAPHY																														
PAP SMEAR																														
LIPOPROTEIN PROFILE																														
URINALYSIS																														
HEMATOCRIT																														
PPD																														
Td																														
STOOL GUAIAC																														
DIGITAL RECTAL EXAM																														
SIGMOIDOSCOPY																														
EKG (as indicated)																														
CXR (as indicated)																														

RUBELLA TITER/VACCINE	BASELINE EVALUATION DATE:	IF GIVEN, CHECK AND INDICATE DATE. VACCINE	CHECK IF TITER INDICATES IMMUNITY. TITER

ADDITIONAL RECOMMENDED SCREENING

Key: N = Normal/Performed   A = Abnormal   R= Refused

These are general recommendations for the population at large. They should be modified as needed on a case by case basis. Please consult your personal physician regarding the specific tests and schedule recommended for you.

FIGURE 61–9. Health maintenance profile. (Baylor College of Medicine, Houston, Texas.) *Illustration continued on opposite page.*

cian time and still allow for an in-depth accumulation of valuable historical information. These health history questionnaires are available as printed forms for the patient to complete, either in the office waiting room or at home prior to the visit. A questionnaire can be either self-designed (see Fig. 2–1) or purchased commercially. If a significant number of positive findings appear on the general health history questionnaire, more de-

tailed preprinted questionnaires are also available for the cardiovascular, gastrointestinal, respiratory, or obstetric/gynecologic systems.

When a complete history is being obtained, it is important to have available the records from the patient's previous physicians, because the patient may have an unrealistic impression of the pathologic findings present and accurate assessment of past problems is possible only by reviewing the

BAYLOR FAMILY PRACTICE CENTER
HEALTH MAINTENANCE PROFILE

B

PATIENT *Dorothy Sanford*   DATE

AGE	50	51	52	53	54	55	56	57	58	59	60	61	62	63	64	65	66	67	68	69	70	71	72	73	74	75	76	77	78	79
BLOOD PRESSURE						N																								
INTERIM H & P						N																								
HEARING EXAM						N																								
VISION CHECK						N																								
TONOMETRY						N																								
BREAST EXAM						N																								
MAMMOGRAPHY						N																								
PAP SMEAR						N																								
LIPOPROTEIN PROFILE						A																								
URINALYSIS						N																								
HEMATOCRIT						N																								
PPD																														
Td																														
STOOL GUAIAC						N																								
DIGITAL RECTAL EXAM						N																								
SIGMOIDOSCOPY						N																								
EKG (as indicated)						N																								
CXR (as indicated)																														
FLU VACCINE						✓																								
PNEUMOVAX																														

ADDITIONAL RECOMMENDED SCREENING

Key: N= Normal/Performed   A= Abnormal   R= Refused
These are general recommendations for the population at large. They should be modified as needed on a case by case basis. Please consult your personal physician regarding the specific tests and schedule recommended for you.   MR-4, 3-23-88

FIGURE 61–9. *Continued*

actual records or a summary from the physicians involved. This information should become a permanent part of the data base and should serve as a reference point for all present and future difficulties in the same areas.

Physical Examination and Physiologic Data

One advantage of using a printed physical examination sheet is the ability to identify easily information that has been obtained in part but has yet to be completed. A highly structured "check-off" format sometimes is used. This makes it possible to set a goal for completeness and to know when that goal has been reached or what remains to be done. With a nonstructured, open-ended format, it is difficult to tell how much remains incomplete. Illustrations of body parts can be used in addition to the written report to depict abnormalities detected during a physical examination. Computer programs such as that described by Trace and associates (1993) allow the input of data by pointing and clicking at selections on input screens, many of which contain anatomic drawings to describe quickly and accurately variations noted during the physical examination.

Some practices insist on a comprehensive data base for all new patients and will not accept patients for treatment beyond the second visit for an episodic illness until the standard comprehensive examination is completed. Following the completion of this examination, the patient is sent a summary of the findings, including a problem list and the plans for following each problem. The patient is asked to review the material for accuracy and to keep it for a permanent record.

Laboratory Data

A valuable time-saving practice is to transfer the information on all laboratory report slips to a standard laboratory data sheet. This method avoids the bulk and confusion that a mass of laboratory slips in a variety of colors and sizes contributes to the medical record. Fears that mistakes can be made when transferring the data have been shown to be mostly unfounded, and the significant amount of time saved in retrieving and comparing a sequence of laboratory information arranged side by side chronologically is well worth the time and effort involved. This ability to follow the variations of a single or multiple tests over time on a single page is of significant benefit in maintaining an accurate overview of the patient's laboratory data, especially when compared with the system of "shingling" laboratory slips that requires a variety of slips to be found and lifted if one is to follow a sequence of tests such as serum potassium, thyroxine, glucose, or cholesterol. Computers do this quite well and can provide up-to-date documentation of a variety of tests in chronologic order on one summary page.

It is also useful to document chronologically the dates and results of Papanicolaou smears, electrocardiograms, radiographic exams, and other selected parameters. The actual report forms (if they contain a more detailed description of an abnormality) can be filed to the rear of the chart. Once complete information is transferred to the appropriate section of the data base form, the slip can be discarded.

The chronologic ordering of information in both the progress notes and the laboratory data is particularly useful in family practice because changes over time and frequency of involvement can be visualized and coordinated. When there is an abnormal laboratory or physiologic finding that cannot be explained by a problem already on the problem list, it is added as a new problem and maintains that visibility until it is resolved by further diagnosis or treatment.

The data base also should identify all allergies and should include a summary of all immunizations, hospitalizations, and consultations. In this manner, the physician can note at a glance whether a patient has any allergies, has ever been hospitalized, or has ever required consultation by other physicians. Organizing data in this manner may take slightly longer, but the time saved in retrieval more than compensates for the effort.

Progress Notes

Well-organized and logically structured progress notes in combination with the problem list are the secret of the POMR's effectiveness in promoting continuing patient care. Progress notes are divided into four main components: subjective information, objective data, assessment, and plan (Fig. 61–10). These components correspond to the history, physical examination, diagnosis, and treatment sections of the traditional record. The acronym SOAP is used to describe the POMR format of a progress note and is a more descriptive and more easily pronounced term than would be the acronym HPEDT. An essential feature of any useful record is the organization of major components of the progress notes, placing the most important features in a consistent and readily identifiable position. The historical or subjective data consistently should occupy one specific position and the plan of management, or therapeutic data, another. The actual location is insignificant, as long as each maintains a separate, easily located, and readily visible identity.

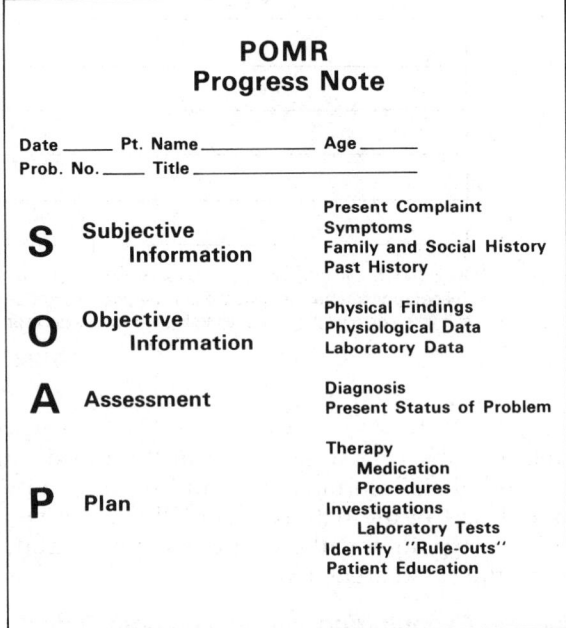

FIGURE 61–10. Major components of the POMR progress note.

In the pure form of the POMR, as developed by Weed, each progress note is keyed by number to its problem on the problem list, and the problem number and title serve as headings for each progress note. In this manner, all information pertaining to a particular problem and the ongoing plan for managing that problem are identified easily throughout the record. This system allows for rapid assessment of a problem and its stage of resolution by all health personnel.

Every problem need not be described in a progress note at each visit. Comments need be made regarding only those problems that are pertinent to that visit and for which some change of status or new information is noted. Likewise, every item or component of the progress note need not be commented on at each visit. If there is no change in status or no new information available, that section, whether it be the subjective, objective, assessment, or plan, should be omitted or a dash inserted to indicate "no need for comment." Meaningless terms such as "doing well" or "status quo" are of little value and should be avoided. All progress information is documented chronologically, and health professionals other than the physician insert their comments or observations in the same manner as the physician.

Narrative progress notes are usually long and the information is arranged randomly. Progress notes in the POMR format are in outline form and frequently contain more data, although fewer words (Fig. 61–11).

As new information is accumulated during each visit, the progress notes are used to provide feedback to continually update and modify the problem list. It is also possible to describe more than one problem per visit.

Components of Progress Notes

SUBJECTIVE INFORMATION. This includes the history of the problem and all descriptive information perceived as important by the patient, including symptoms and feelings. This is an interpretation of the problem from the patient's, point of view.

OBJECTIVE DATA. This term refers to those items noted on examination by the physician or allied health personnel. These data include all measurements and factual information obtained by independent observers, and they represent the facts undistorted by bias. Information within this section also should be arranged consistently in the same order (e.g., data concerning blood pressure, temperature, pulse, and respiration). There is, by the way, no firm rule that objective data follow the subjective. Some physicians prefer to have the objective data first so that they can be located more easily.

ASSESSMENT. This refers to either the diagnosis or a description of the problem at its present stage of resolution. Guesswork is not permitted, and only the degree of resolution that can be supported by data is described.

Problem-solving techniques are a fundamental component of traditional medical education. Problem recognition, however, too often is modified by a haste to play the academic game of one-upmanship and to establish a diagnosis rapidly and with the least amount of data. The POMR lays bare any attempt to shortcut the establishment of a sound diagnosis based on the logical acquisition of adequate data. This does not mean, however, that a differential diagnosis is to be avoided, because all "rule-outs" and potential causes for the problem

---

SOMR Progress Note
   Milroy, John
   11/21/75

        Had recurrences of stomach pain 3 days ago similar to that of previous ulcer pain last year. Has been drinking again and not sticking to his diet. Has slight tenderness in epigastrium — denies tarry stools or change in bowel habits. Stool guaiac was negative. Wife says he won't stay on diet when at work or "out with the boys." Reinstructed on diet and need to stay away from alcohol and cigarettes. Rx — Maalox

                                  73 words

POMR Progress Note

    Milroy, John
    11/21/75
    Problem #3   Duodenal Ulcer
          S — Pain recurred 3 days ago — moderately severe — no melena — off diet and drinking
          O — Mild epigastric tenderness. Stool guaiac negative
          A — Duodenal Ulcer
          P — Maalox
              Instructed regarding diet
              DC alcohol and smoking
                31 words

FIGURE 61–11. Comparison of volume and organization of SOMR and POMR progress notes.

should be reflected accurately in the record, so that the problem can be pursued to a definite conclusion. This conclusion may be either the complete disappearance of the sign or symptoms without a final diagnosis ever being reached or the combining of a variety of symptoms and signs into a definite diagnosis.

PLAN. This refers to the diagnostic and therapeutic modalities used in the management of the problem. This section should include all present medications, laboratory tests, procedures (such as exercise or inhalation therapy), further diagnostic plans (such as radiographic studies), patient education (such as informative literature and diet instruction), counseling methods, and the use of consultants. The entire plan (or treatment) section is the most important portion of the progress notes and should be located prominently so that it can be found easily, because future evaluation requires the comparison of outcome with previous treatment plans to determine whether the results obtained match previous expectations. In this manner, the success or failure of earlier plans can be measured. The use of a green or red pen to write the plan will make this section stand out and be identified easily.

A well-thought-out plan helps to maintain continuity of care and allows the physician to communicate to an associate on call the plans for the patient's management. Three major subdivisions constitute the execution of the plan:

1. *Diagnostic studies* should contain the "rule-outs" and the tests to be used in the process of differential diagnosis. Also under the heading of diagnostic studies would be the laboratory tests to be done at the next visit. The nurse or laboratory technician then will be alerted to obtain these prior to the physician's involvement. The diagnostic studies category means that more information is needed, and it lists the tests to be conducted to assist in the future evaluation of a problem.

2. *Therapeutic measures* include medications and other treatment modalities.

3. *Patient education* consists of the factors necessary for patient understanding and compliance. This, too, is often a neglected area and therefore warrants visibility by including it as a regular item in the progress notes. The patient education section is of greatest importance for patients with chronic problems, because treatment of one form or another will be a constant feature throughout their lives. The patient should know what to expect from treatment, what side effects are possible, and how a specific medication might react with other drugs or foods. Unexpected events should be avoided as much as possible, so that maximum compliance will be maintained. The patient also needs adequate insight into the problem to know when to seek help without further delay. When patient instruction is given, whether this be the

distribution of an American Heart Association booklet on hypertension or information about the hazards of smoking, it should be documented in the record so that other health personnel who share responsibility for continuing education of the patient will remain informed.

Hospital Discharge Summaries

These summaries also should be organized in the POMR format, with each problem being identified and numbered and the pertinent information "SOAPed." This record (the discharge summary) then is incorporated into the office record at the appropriate chronologic point to assist in the continuing care of the patient during future office visits.

AVOIDING LEGAL PITFALLS

Juries have a tendency to believe that, if an event is not recorded, it never occurred, so a complete and accurate medical record is the physician's best defense in a malpractice suit. Often there is a 2- or 3-year delay before a case reaches court, and recall from memory will be difficult. Therefore, an accurate and legible record is essential.

Every page of the medical record should bear the patient's name. Progress notes should be signed, dated, arranged chronologically, and typed or written in ink, never pencil.

Derogatory, trivial, or loose comments about patients or colleagues should not be recorded; they could prove embarrassing if publicized during a legal review. Similarly, vague and ambiguous statements, such as "the patient is feeling better" should be avoided.

Altering A Record

Adding or changing a statement is no problem if done correctly and if no suit is pending. However, altering the record after a suit has been filed is the kiss of death. This is considered tampering and arouses suspicions that are difficult to dispel. If it is necessary to change an entry in the chart because of an error, the inaccurate material should be crossed out with a single line so that the words remain legible. The change should be initialed and the date and time noted in the margin with a note explaining why the change was made.

Documenting Phone Calls

It is wise to document every telephone call received in the office. Requests for prescription refills should be documented in the medical record, as should any call involving medical advice or treatment.

Words To Avoid

Medical records are not privileged and confidential; the information belongs to the patient. Maligning or deprecatory remarks are certainly inappropriate. Words that should be avoided are "simple," "routine," and "uncomplicated" because they suggest a guarantee or predict a good outcome. If the patient is described as uncooperative, the reasons should be documented. Similarly, if patients refuse certain diagnostic tests or procedures, this should be documented along with the reason for recommending the test. The fact that the patient was informed of the need for the test is also important. A suit has never been brought successfully because the physician gave the patient too much information.

FLOW SHEETS

Flow sheets are a useful adjunct to any medical record system, particularly when the POMR is used in conjunction with continuing patient care and the management of chronic illnesses. It is sometimes difficult to review the course of a single problem over time using progress notes because a great deal of page turning is required to pick out that problem on successive visits. Placing the prolonged course of a single problem, or even selected multiple problems, on one flow sheet greatly facilitates comprehension and management. Flow sheets are also useful in any clinical situation requiring the monitoring of multiple laboratory and therapeutic parameters over a long period of time. They present an overview of the illness, compressing events over time onto one page, and allow the physician to identify current values as well as observe trends in the course of a disease. Flow sheets permit speedy retrieval of data and facilitate the ongoing analysis of the stage of chronic illness by indicating changing trends in response to therapy.

Once the parameters to be monitored have been identified, the flow sheet serves as a constant reminder to review these items and acts as an early warning system for potential problems by indicating variations from the previous pattern or baseline. Such sheets allow for a large amount of physiologic and management data to be accumulated in a compact area and observed at a glance.

When laboratory data have been entered on the flow sheet, they can be, but do not need to be, entered on the data base form as well. Just as with the data base form, the laboratory slip is filed elsewhere or discarded and is not retained in the chart. Avoid double entry whenever possible because one or the other frequently will be omitted, result-

ing in confusion or extra time spent searching. The flow sheet permits ready comparison of all determinations of a single test. It also permits physiologic and laboratory data to be monitored on the same time scale as therapeutic management. When material is categorized in this manner, physicians tend to write more concise and clearer notes, including fewer irrelevant details.

The time required to enter data on a flow sheet is much less than the time that is lost in sorting out disorganized information in the traditional record. A partially used flow sheet, however, can be more inefficient than none at all, because the physician then is required to search back and forth among the flow sheet, progress notes, and data base for the complete information.

The flow sheet can be a simple piece of graph paper, a self-designed form (Fig. 61–12), or a preprinted form. In each instance, the left-hand column should contain the elements considered essential to the ongoing management of the problems being followed. Just as the data base must be designed individually for each practice, the flow sheet must be suited to the preferences of the physician and must be designed to measure those items considered most important in the management of the illnesses for which it is used.

Items to be monitored on a flow sheet usually include:

1. Frequency of symptoms
2. Physiologic data, such as weight, edema, and blood pressure
3. Laboratory data, such as fasting blood glucose levels, urine cultures, and serum potassium and serum cholesterol levels
4. Medications
5. Nondrug therapy, such as diet and physical therapy
6. Patient compliance
7. Patient education

Flow sheets serve as memory aids and guard against the possibility of important aspects of a patient's continuing care being overlooked by the physician. For example, when monitoring the course of a diabetic patient, the physician may forget to check the fundi or peripheral pulses regularly for potential vascular change. Listing these as areas to be evaluated at prescribed intervals, along with the blood glucose level and other specifics, will serve as a reminder to all office personnel. The data-gathering activities of allied health personnel can be incorporated easily into the structure of the flow sheet by identifying those parameters to be measured at the next visit prior to the physician's examination. The flow sheet should monitor problems at intervals that will reflect the degree of stability of the illness; the more acute and unstable the problem, the more frequently measurements will be required. Items should be monitored often enough to ensure good care without undue expense. In an intensive care unit, the intervals be-

BAYLOR COLLEGE OF MEDICINE
FAMILY PRACTICE CENTER
FLOW CHART

PROBLEMS

OBESITY

DIABETES MELLITUS

HYPERTENSION

HYPERURICEMIA

Patient ANDREWS, JASON

Chart No. 01-03-21

Physician H. AARON

TESTS						DATES								
	1/3/94	2/22	3/24	6/13	9/15	10/7	11/30	12/12	1/31					
Weight	220	217	211	207	211	196	198	217	198					
Blood Pressure	140/96	130/84	126/80	110/80	138/100	150/80	138/82	140/96	130/84					
Glucose		259	151	133	111	109	132	151	128					
Creatinine		1.7	1.3	1.4	1.0	0.9	1.1	1.1	0.9					
Uric Acid		10.6	10.3	8.2	10.2	7.8	7.4	10.5	8.0					
Triglycerides		345	198	537	195	189	188	363	189					
HDL		22	27	21	30	35	36	22	29					
Glycohemoglobin			6.1	6.5	6.3	5.9	6.1	6.0	6.0					

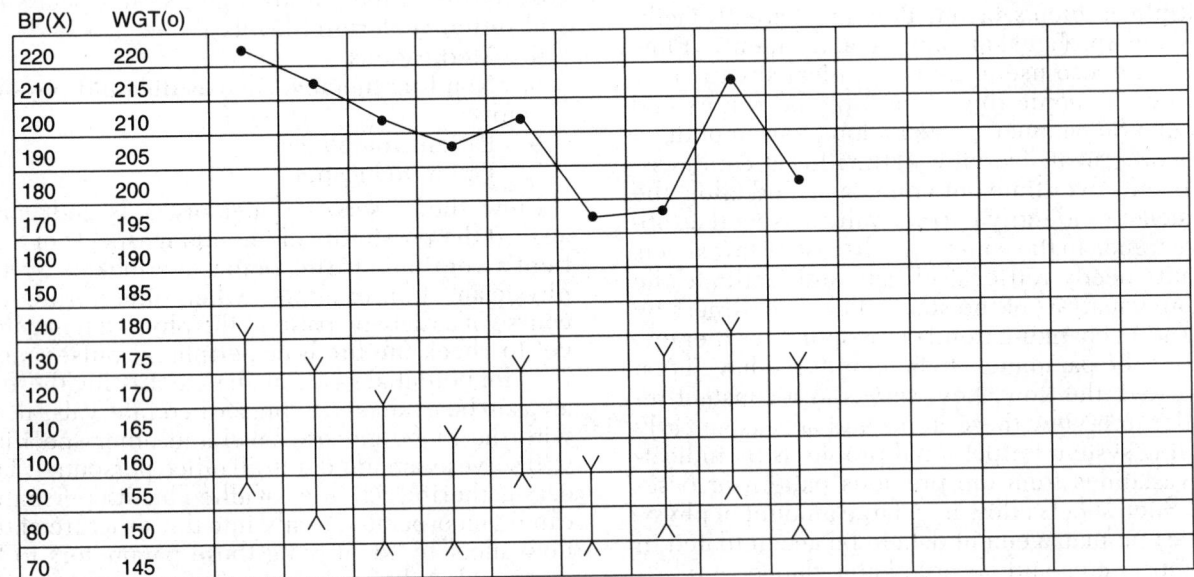

FIGURE 61–12. Flow sheet. (Baylor College of Medicine, Houston, Texas.)

tween items are minutes or hours, whereas in the outpatient setting, they are days, weeks, or months.

The chart format of a flow sheet also minimizes problems caused by illegible handwriting. Effective use of flow sheets may obviate the need for progress notes when repeated visits relate only to the ongoing management of the chronic illnesses followed on the flow sheet. When progress notes are necessary, "see flow sheet" frequently will suffice in lieu of entries in the objective and plan categories.

WELL-CHILD CARE FORMS

A variety of methods for documenting well-child care have been developed. These provide reminders of the normal developmental milestones during early development, immunizations and laboratory tests, patient education, and physical examination. The form shown in Figure 61–13 not only permits the documentation of well-child care up to school entry but also serves as a reminder of those features that should be checked periodically on physical examinations, such as hips (for dysplasia), vision, and hearing. Standard patient education handouts are developed for each age group, and brief developmental milestones are documented. If there is any question as to whether these have been reached, a complete Denver Developmental Screening Test (see page 624) is done. This form is accompanied by a growth chart, so the appropriate box is checked when the measurement is plotted on the growth chart, including head circumference until 12 months and adding blood pressure at age 4 years. If significant abnormalities are found during the physical examination, they are documented more thoroughly in the standard progress note format, as are intercurrent acute illnesses (see also Eggertsen et al., 1980; Margolis, 1977). A similar form continues this format for ages 5 through 18 years, so that, on two pages (four sides), well-child care from birth to age 18 can be documented succinctly.

MEDICATION LISTS

Almost from the beginning, medication lists have been a component of the problem-oriented medical record as it is used in family practice. Chronic medications frequently are documented below the problem list or in a similar prominent location. It is difficult, however, to keep these lists current, because, as soon as omissions occur, the list becomes more trouble than it is worth because it must be checked against the progress notes for accuracy. A variety of other methods are in use, the most accurate involving a direct copy of all prescriptions, where pressure-sensitive paper, on which the prescription is placed when written, is used. Although redundancy occurs, the usefulness

of this list lies in its accuracy. Problems arise only if prescriptions are written without being placed over the appropriate area on this sheet.

One way to avoid this problem is to use a medication list such as that developed in the Department of Family Medicine at Baylor College of Medicine (Fig. 61–14). Prescriptions are fixed along the left side of the page by a perforation. An actual copy of the medication prescribed is left on the underlying pressure-sensitive sheet. Two medications can be written (one on each line) and the prescription form removed from the page, after which the patient's name and physician's signature are entered. If these names are entered before the prescription form is removed, the names will appear on the pressure sensitive sheet on top of the next prescription because the forms are shingled to save space. No loose prescription pads are used, so this almost ensures an accurate record of all medications prescribed, plus their strength, quantity, instructions, and number of refills. Space also is allotted for recording the date and reason for discontinuing a drug.

EVALUATING QUALITY OF CARE

Many physicians perceive "audit" as a threatening term, whereas to others it serves as a source of intellectual stimulation. The challenge is to assess clinical performance and improve professional competence. Bjorn and Cross (1970) designed their practice to include an ongoing audit system, both internal and external, accomplished by review by office staff and visiting consultants. Their enthusiasm for such auditing procedures indicates that such methods can serve as a source of professional stimulation and improved patient care. They conclude that the practicing physician who does not develop an efficient audit system will "suffer from apathy, bitterness and the general dissatisfaction of conducting a practice devoid of basic intellectual gratifications integral to continued professional growth." A willingness to be reviewed by peers certainly can result in professional stimulation. To be successful, however, an audit must be viewed as an experience in learning and as an exciting, intellectually rewarding exercise.

Weed (1971) emphasized that, to be effective and fair, record audits must relate to defined criteria. Everyone must know what is to be measured and how this is to be done. He equates this process to defining the length and width of a football field and the rules of play before the game has begun, rather than after it is underway. Unfortunately, too many audit procedures utilized in hospitals and clinics today avoid defining specific criteria for the audit or do so after the fact. Both the physician and the reviewer should understand what standards are to be used in the review. This involves developing criteria of excellence that all agree to in advance and against which performance can be measured.

BAYLOR FAMILY PRACTICE CENTER
BIRTH-4 YR. OLD HEALTH CARE FORM

Name_____

Date of Birth_____

☑ NORMAL   ☒ = ABNORMAL

Birth History _____

Newborn Exam _____

Birth Weight_____
Gms.   Lbs.

Labor and delivery record in chart ☐

Newborn exam record in chart ☐

Breastfeeding ☐   Formula ☐

AGE	ACTUAL AGE	DATE	HT.	WT.	HC.	DEVELOPMENT	PHYSICAL EXAM		IMMUNIZATIONS/ LABORATORY	EDUCATION
2 WKS.			☐	☐	☐	Moro Reflex ☐ Symmetrical motor activity ☐	HENT ☐ Eyes ☐ Lungs ☐ Heart ☐ Abd. ☐	G.U. ☐ Skel. ☐ Neuro ☐ Skin ☐	PKU ☐ (or at 4 wks.) Caretaker's polio status ☐	Hand Out No. 1 ☐ Fluoride ☐ Iron ☐ Vitamins ☐ Auto Seat ☐
						ASSESSMENT:				
									_____ M.D. (signed)	

2 MOS.			☐	☐	☐	Briefly follows
						  object ☐
						Vocalizes ☐
						Head up to 45° ☐
							Check hips ☐
							Femoral pulse ☐
							Hernia ☐
							HENT ☐
							Eyes ☐
							Lungs ☐
								Heart ☐
								Abd. ☐
								G.U. ☐
								Skel. ☐
								Neuro. ☐
								Skin ☐
									DPT-1 ☐
									TOPV-1 ☐
										Hand Out No. 2 ☐
										Nutrition ☐
										
										Recheck fluoride
										  iron
										  vitamins

						ASSESSMENT:				
									_____ M.D. (signed)	
4 MOS.			☐	☐	☐	Rolls over ☐ Follows object 180° ☐ Grasps ☐ Sits w/head steady ☐ Squeals ☐	Turns toward sound ☐ HENT ☐ Eyes ☐ Lungs ☐ Heart ☐	Abd. ☐ G.U. ☐ Skel. ☐ Neuro. ☐ Skin ☐	DPT-2 ☐ TOPV-2 ☐	Hand Out No. 3 ☐ Nutrition ☐
						ASSESSMENT:				
									_____ M.D. (signed)	

6 MOS.			☐	☐	☐	Feeds self crackers ☐
						Sits without support ☐
						Passes cube hand to
						  hand ☐
						Reaches for objects ☐
							Symmetrical
							light reflection ☐
							HENT ☐
							Eyes ☐
							Lungs ☐
							Heart ☐
								Abd. ☐
								G.U. ☐
								Skel. ☐
								Neuro. ☐
								Skin ☐
									DPT-3 ☐
									TOPV-3 ☐
									(optional)
										Hand Out No. 4 ☐
										Nutrition ☐
										Discuss solid
										  foods ☐
										Ipecac ☐
										Fear of strangers ☐

						ASSESSMENT:				
									_____ M.D. (signed)	

MR-8, 6-22-88

FIGURE 61–13. Child health care form. (Baylor College of Medicine, Houston, Texas.) *Illustration continued on opposite page.*

CHILD HEALTH CARE FORM (Continued)

AGE	ACTUAL AGE	DATE	HT. WT. HC.	DEVELOPMENT	PHYSICAL EXAM	IMMUNIZATIONS/ LABORATORY	EDUCATION

9 MOS.			☐ ☐ ☐	Peek-a-boo, bye-bye ☐
				Pulls self to standing ☐
				Thumb-finger grasp ☐
				Imitates sounds ☐
					Vision-follows
					  dropped object ☐ Abd. ☐
					HENT G.U. ☐
					Eyes Skel. ☐
					Lungs Neuro. ☐
					Heart Skin ☐
						Hct. ☐
						Sickle cell
						  test if
						  appropriate ☐
							Hand Out No. 5 ☐
							Nutrition ☐
							  Check Amt. of Milk
							  Wean from bottle
							Discuss discipline ☐

				ASSESSMENT:			
				_____ M.D. (signed)			

12 MOS.			☐ ☐ ☐	Walks holding on
				  Mama, Dada
				Drinks from cup ☐
				Plays pat-a-cake ☐
					Check hips ☐ Abd. ☐
					Cover-uncover test ☐ G.U. ☐
					Test hearing ☐ Skel. ☐
					HENT ☐ Neuro. ☐
					Eyes ☐ Skin ☐
					Lungs ☐
					Heart ☐
						TB skin
						 test ☐
							Hand Out No. 6 ☐
							Nutrition ☐
							  Appetite
							  normal ☐
							Household
							  safety ☐

				ASSESSMENT:			
				_____ M.D. (signed)			

15 MOS.			☐ ☐	Walks alone ☐
				Scribbles
				  spontaneously ☐
				Follows simple
				  commands ☐
				Throws ball ☐
					HENT ☐ G.U. ☐
					Eyes ☐ Skel. ☐
					Lungs ☐ Neuro. ☐
					Heart ☐ Skin ☐
					Abd. ☐
						MMR ☐
						Hem. Inf. ☐
						DPT
						  Booster ☐
						TOPV
						  Booster ☐
							Hand Out No. 7 ☐
							Nutrition ☐
							Toilet training ☐
							Discipline ☐

				ASSESSMENT:			
				_____ M.D. (signed)			

2 YRS.			☐ ☐	Puts on clothing ☐
				Combines 2-3 words ☐
				Runs well; Stairs
				  one step at a time ☐
				Draws 1; circular
				  scribbling ☐
					HENT ☐ G.U. ☐
					Eyes ☐ Skel. ☐
					Lungs ☐ Neuro. ☐
					Heart ☐ Skin ☐
					Abd. ☐
							Hand Out No. 8 ☐
							Dental visit ☐
							Need for peer
							  companionship but
							  unable to share ☐
							Matches ☐
							TV supervision ☐

				ASSESSMENT:			
				_____ M.D. (signed)			

3 YRS.			☐ ☐	Dresses w/help ☐
				Knows full name
				  and age ☐
				Stand on 1 foot
				  for 1 second ☐
				Speaks in sentences ☐
				Draws 0 ☐
				Toilet trained ☐
					Vision ☐ Heart ☐
					Hearing ☐ Abd. ☐
					Blood pressure ☐ G.U. ☐
					HENT ☐ Skel. ☐
					Eyes ☐ Neuro. ☐
					Lungs ☐ Skin ☐
							Hand Out No. 9 ☐
							Knives &
							  electricity ☐
							TV supervision ☐
							Dental hygiene ☐

				ASSESSMENT:			
				_____ M.D. (signed)			
4 YRS.			☐ ☐ B. P. /	Dresses self ☐ Hops on one foot ☐ Draws man w/head and 2-4 parts ☐ Knows 3 of 4 colors ☐	Blood pressure ☐ Abd. ☐ HENT ☐ G.U. ☐ Eyes ☐ Skel. ☐ Lungs ☐ Neuro. ☐ Heart ☐ Skin ☐		Hand Out No. 10 ☐ Water safety ☐ Traffic safety ☐
				ASSESSMENT:			
				_____ M.D. (signed)			

FIGURE 61–13. *Continued*

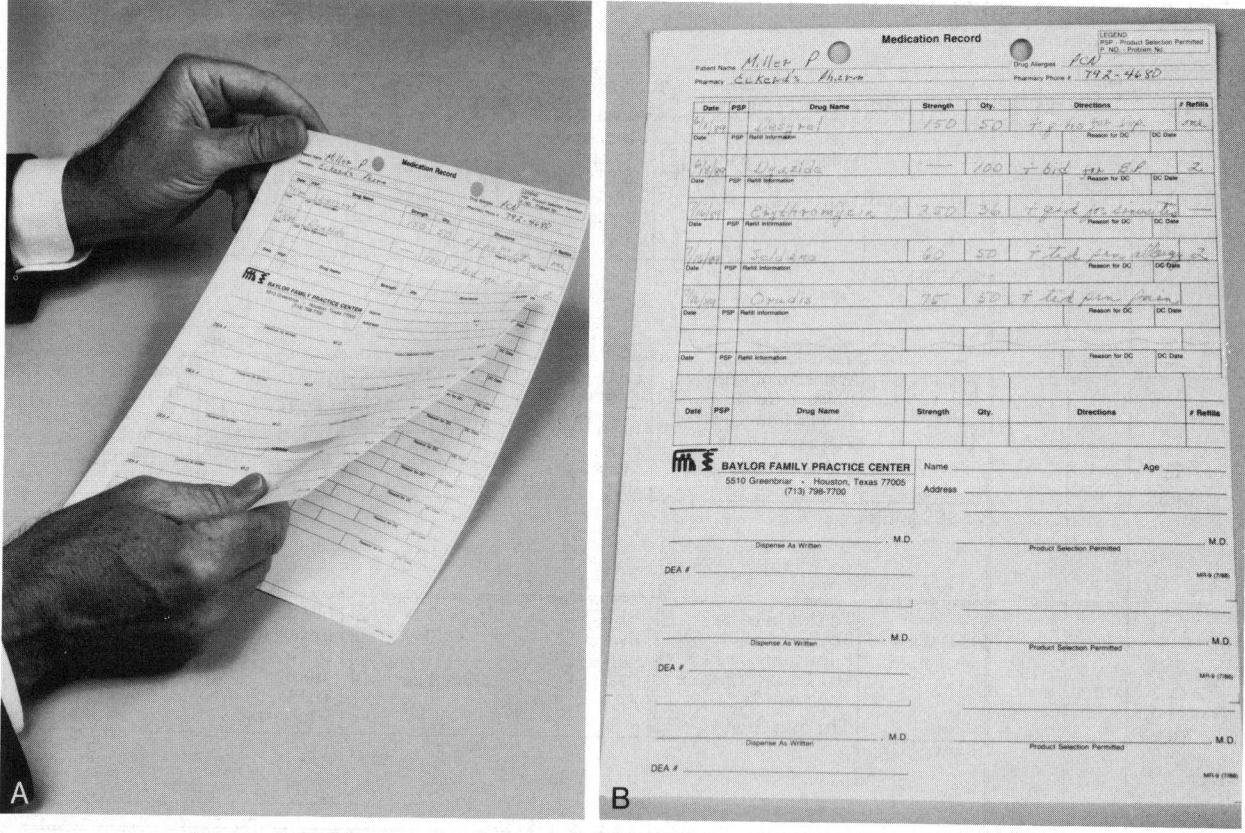

FIGURE 61–14. Medication record. (Baylor College of Medicine, Houston, Texas.) *A,* Shingled prescription forms attached along left margin overlying pressure-sensitive copy. *B,* Three of the six forms, containing up to two prescriptions each, have been used.

Each patient is unique, so it is difficult to design criteria of excellence that apply to all patients with a given problem. An extensive list of 40 criteria will include many inappropriate items, resulting in a "poor score" that is inaccurate. A brief or limited list of criteria that apply to most patients will give better scores but poor discrimination.

Many audits are primarily a content review, involving an analysis of whether or not desired components of the record are documented properly and in place. Evaluating the process of care increases the value of the audit, but a thorough and proper analysis requires the establishing of criteria of excellence so that performance can be measured against these criteria. After standards have been set, the audit determines whether the standards have been met and then assesses the effect of these standards on patient care. The knowledge gained by the audit process should be used to bring about required change, and reauditing should be performed to see if this change did in fact occur and whether or not it was effective. Thus, auditing is an ongoing process that continually evaluates quality of care and the ability to improve that quality based on knowledge gained. Measurements of outcome of care are the most useful, yet the most difficult, measurements of physician performance. In

addition to actual outcome, other components of quality of care include patient expectations, patient satisfaction, and physician satisfaction with outcomes.

The POMR lends itself well to record audit because it encourages the accumulation of data with a minimum of ambiguity. There is a defined location for all data relating to a particular problem, so it is easy to determine the presence or absence of those data. The data base defines the measurements to be obtained for each patient. The plan category relating to each problem clearly indicates the physician's logic and intended course of action. In this manner, the auditor is not required to guess whether the prednisone was intended for asthma, arthritis, or some other problem. Such an organized office record system documents the logic of the physician's approach to a problem and preserves it for review by peers, whether the purpose be education, recertification, relicensure, or reimbursement.

THE COMPUTERIZED MEDICAL RECORD

Attempts to develop a computerized ambulatory medical record so far have met with limited enthusiasm. Many commercial systems are available for scheduling appointments, billing, and insurance processing. Although computerization of the medical record has not been accepted universally, it is just around the corner (see Chapter 65). Some predict that most charts will be paperless by the year 2000. An effective computerized system should promote better patient care by stabilizing costs, improving accessibility of information, and facilitating the quality of care.

As a result of the increased use of personal computers and their use throughout industry, patient attitudes toward their use in medical record keeping are changing. Ornstein and Bearden (1994) found that patients believed that physicians using computerized patient records were using state-of-the-art technology, which could be interpreted as also practicing up-to-date medicine. Rather than being more concerned about confidentiality, some believed that information kept on a computerized record may be more secure than that on paper records.

Voice-activated systems soon may revolutionize the way family physicians document their care of

TABLE 61–2. NINETEEN PROBLEM CATEGORIES USED IN THE OFFICE RECORD REVIEW OF THE AMERICAN BOARD OF FAMILY PRACTICE

Group I	Group II
Coronary Artery Disease A patient with angina, or a history of myocardial infarction as the primary diagnosis. You need not have made the initial diagnosis, but you should have provided care for this condition for at least one year. **Hypertension** An adult patient with confirmed primary hypertension for which you initiated management or initiated a significant change in regimen and which you have managed for at least six months. **Urinary Tract Infection** An adult, nonpregnant **female** patient with acute microbial lower urinary tract infection, which you diagnosed, and a history of at least one previous episode. (NOTE: "UTI" refers to lower urinary tract inflammatory, nonvenereal disease only and does not include gonococcal disease or acute or chronic renal disease. Acceptable diagnoses are cystitis and urethritis.) **Duodenal Ulcer** An adult patient with confirmed duodenal ulcer which you have diagnosed and managed medically. **Diabetes Mellitus** A patient with adult-onset, non-insulin dependent (Type II) diabetes mellitus which you diagnosed. You should have followed the patient for at least one year. **Chronic Heart Failure** An adult patient with chronic heart failure which you diagnosed. You should have managed the patient for at least six months. **Osteoarthritis** An adult patient with osteoarthritis. You should have made the initial diagnosis and seen this patient for at least three visits for this condition. **Urethral Discharge** A male patient who is 15 years old or older, with an initial complaint of urethral discharge which you have diagnosed and managed, and whom you have seen at least twice for this problem. **COPD (Chronic Obstructive Pulmonary Disease)** An adult patient with chronic generalized airway obstruction in whom the diagnosis has been established and who has been under your care for at least three years. Acceptable diagnoses include chronic bronchitis or chronic emphysema. This category excludes asthma.	**Carcinoma of the Breast** A patient whom you have diagnosed or referred for a definitive diagnosis of carcinoma of the breast. Information regarding the management of the patient should be reflected in the record even though management is provided by a consultant. At least one chart should be for a patient for whom you have provided follow-up care for a period of at least three years. **Depressive Disorders** An adult patient whom you have diagnosed as having a Depressive Disorder and who has been under management for at least three months since the diagnosis. **Menstrual Disorders** A female patient who is at least three years postmenarchal, is premenopausal, and whose presenting complaint is either abnormal vaginal bleeding (if any menses) or lack of menses. **Well Child Care** A patient who is now at least three years old but not more than eighteeen, and who has been seen for at least three well child visits. You should have provided care for a minimum of three years, and both of the charts must be for patients who have been under your care since birth. **Irritable Bowel Syndrome** An adult patient whose complaints may include chronic abdominal discomfort and/or alterations in bowel function. Acceptable diagnoses include any functional bowel disorder or syndromes, e.g., spastic colitis, mucous colitis, irritable colon, etc. This category does not include acute or infectious hepatitis. **Geriatric Patient** A patient who is at least 70 years old, who is not institutionalized in a long-term care facility, who has been under your care for at least three years, who is usually ambulatory, and who comes to the physician's office for a major portion of his/her medical care. At least one of the charts must be for a patient who is 75 or older. **Alcoholism and Alcohol Abuse** A patient in whom alcoholism or alcohol abuse has been identified as a problem and who has been under your care for this problem for at least one year. **Acute Appendicitis** A child or adult patient for whom you have made the diagnosis of acute appendicitis. **Low Back Pain** An adult patient with an initial complaint of low back pain for whom the final diagnosis was lumbar sacral strain, lumbar disc disease, or osteoarthritis (lumbar spondylosis). You should have seen the patient at least three times for this problem for a minimum of six weeks. **Normal Pregnancy (Delivered)** A female, aged 17–35, who has had an uncomplicated pregnancy. You need not have delivered the baby.

From Recertification Handbook for Diplomates. Lexington, KY, American Board of Family Practice, 1994, p. 7, with permission.

patients. Many are already on the market, including VoiceMED for Primary Care, marketed by Kurzweil Applied Intelligence of Waltham, Massachusetts and developed by family physicians. More are sure to follow as the technology improves.

Now that the computer is available for billing and for other office functions, problem indexing in family practice can be an especially useful tool. It permits easy retrieval of charts required for audit as part of the recertification process of the American Board of Family Practice (ABFP). The ABFP has identified 19 problems for which charts may need to be retrieved and reviewed for self-audit (Table 61–2).

The advantages of problem indexing include:

1. Easy retrieval of records of patients with common problems or of those receiving similar medications.
2. Recall of patients when discoveries indicate new treatments that are likely to be more effective than the one presently being used.
3. Identification of patients for whom medications must be changed because new hazards of therapy have been identified (e.g., the sudden recall of the drug ticrynafen [Selacryn]).
4. Recall of patients with chronic problems requiring periodic evaluation (e.g., recurrent urinary tract infections or chronic lung disease).
5. Self-audit of physician performance to evaluate effectiveness in selected areas.
6. Audit of the problems encountered in the practice to identify areas of prominence when designing a continuing education program.
7. Analysis of the content of the practice to assist in the design of appropriate curricular objectives for undergraduate and graduate teaching programs.
8. Collection of data for clinical investigation and other research efforts.
9. Retrieval of cases for recertification.

REFERENCES

Birtwhistle RV, Anderson JE: Transferring records when patients change family doctors. Can Fam Physician 35:51, 1989.

Bjorn JC, Cross HD: Problem Oriented Practice. Chicago, Modern Hospital Press, 1970.

Eggertsen SC, Schneeweiss R, Bergman JJ: An updated protocol for pediatric health screening. J Fam Pract 10:25, 1980.

Fischbach RL, Sionelo-Bayog A, Needle A, et al: The patient and practitioner as coauthors of the medical record. Patient Counseling Health Educ First Quarter:1, 1980.

Grace NT, Neal EM, Wellock CE, et al: The family-oriented medical record. J Fam Pract 4:91, 1977.

Margolis CZ: The Pediatric Problem-Oriented Record. Pleasantville, NY, Docent Corporation, 1977.

Michael M, Bordley C: Do patients want access to their medical records? Med Care 20:432, 1982.

Murnaghan JG: Ambulatory medical care data: Review of the conference proceedings. Report of a conference on ambulatory care records, Chicago, April 1972. Med Care 11(suppl): 13, 1973.

Ornstein S, Bearden A: Patient perspectives on computer-based medical records. J Fam Pract 38:606, 1994.

Recertification Handbook for Diplomates. Lexington, KY, American Board of Family Practice, 1994.

Schade HI: My patients take their medical records with them. Med Econ May 6:75, 1976.

Sullivan RJ Jr: Medical Record and Index Systems for Community Practice. Cambridge, MA, Ballinger Publishing Company, 1979.

Trace D, Naeymi-Rad F, Haines D, et al: Intelligent medical record-entry (IMR-E). J Med Sys 17:139, 1993.

Tufo HM, Bouchard RE, Rubin AS, et al: Problem-oriented approach to practice: II. Development of the system through audit and implication. JAMA 238:502, 1977.

Weed LL: Medical Records, Medical Education and Patient Care. Chicago, The Press of Case Western Reserve University, distributed by Year Book Medical Publishers, 1971.

Widmer RB, Cadoret RJ, North CS: Depression in family practice: Some effects on spouses and children. J Fam Pract 10: 45, 1980.

Yamamoto LG, Wiebe RA: Improving medical communication with facsimile (fax) transmission. Am J Emerg Med 7:203, 1989.

SUGGESTED READINGS

Feldman WS: Pitfalls in documenting medical records. Med Aspects Hum Sexuality June:49, 1987.

Froom J, et al: An integrated medical record and data system for primary care (in eight parts). J Fam Pract 4:951 to 5:1007, 1977.

Hurst JW, Walker HK: The Problem Oriented System. New York, Medcom, Inc., 1972.

Ruth DH, Rigden S, Brunworth D: An integrated family-oriented problem-oriented medical record. J Fam Pract 8:1179, 1979.

Shapiro DM: A family data base for the family oriented medical record. J Fam Pract 13:881, 1981.

Walker HK, Hurst JW, Woody MF: Applying the Problem Oriented System. New York, Medcom Press, 1973.

CHAPTER 62

MANAGED HEALTH CARE

GLEN R. JOHNSON, E. STANLEY KARDATZKE,
STEPHANIE H. KONG, and JOHN R. COLEMAN

The last thirty years have seen a U.S. health care delivery system characterized by rapidly rising costs, discontinuity in planning, and a disequilibrium between costs, value, and access. During this time there have been marked advances in medical technology, yet millions of Americans are unable to access basic health care because of the maldistribution of physicians and their inability to afford health care coverage. We have seen financing mechanisms for health care that encouraged providers to spend more while neglecting to reimburse the consumer and providers for preventive health care. We have also seen ineffective government-sponsored medical care systems, particularly Medicaid and Medicare, that either ignore or promote overutilization of expensive, unnecessary medical procedures while neglecting the use of primary care services and personalized health care.

Out of this turmoil has quietly evolved the "managed care" concept of delivering and financing health care that even though born during the early 1900s will predictably dominate national health care policy well into the next century. The earliest evidence of prepaid health care may be traced back to the early 1900s, when the Western Clinic in Tacoma, Washington contracted with the lumber industry to provide health care to employees at a cost of fifty cents per employee per month (Mayer and Mayer, 1985). In 1929 Baylor Hospital in Dallas, Texas agreed to provide hospital care for 1250 teachers in exchange for a prepaid monthly premium. That same year Ross and Loos proposed a similar prepaid delivery system to the Los Angeles Water and Power Departments. By the mid to late 1930s there were prepaid care systems in the Farmer's Union Cooperative in Elk City, Oklahoma (1929), Group Health Association of Washington, DC (1935), and the Kaiser Foundation Health Plan in California (1937) (Shouldice and Shouldice, 1990). The 1940s witnessed the introduction of the Group Health Cooperative of Puget Sound (1946) and the Health Insurance Plan of Greater New York (HIP) in New York City (1947) (Prussin, 1974a,b).

The 1960s saw the federal government introduce health insurance coverage for its employees through the Federal Employees Health Benefits Program. By the 1970s health policy analysts, led by Paul Ellwood and Walter McClure, proposed a national "health maintenance strategy" to address what by then had been recognized as a crisis in health care. Their work, along with others, led to the Health Maintenance Organization Act of 1973. From then on, the concept of managed health care as an alternative to the traditional laisse faire system that characterized the U.S. health care delivery system began to gain momentum.

DEFINITION OF MANAGED CARE

There is no standard definition for managed care. It is a concept in evolution. Many view managed care as purely a cost-containment strategy. Others use the term synonymously with health maintenance organizations (HMOs), and still others define managed care as strictly utilization management. Unquestionably, the concept addresses all of these issues and is not limited in its application. Therefore the most appropriate definition would encompass the financing of health care as well as its delivery, culminating in the management of health care cost and quality. Accordingly, *managed care* may be best defined as a system of both financing and delivering a defined set of health care benefits by a defined provider network that is responsible for controlling the cost of delivering health care benefits to a defined population without compromising quality. Although the traditional HMO may have been the harbinger of today's managed care systems, the concept of managed health care as defined above is now being applied to a variety of organized health care systems including preferred provider organizations (PPOs), medical case management firms, and "managed" indemnity insurance programs.

A common thread running through these organized approaches to managed health care is some restriction on traditional fee-for-service medicine's unlimited access to providers (who are paid on a usual, customary, and reasonable charge basis). This restriction is introduced into the decisions made by consumers and providers through a binding contract agreement (Hicks et al., 1993). The purpose of these restrictions is to modify the behavior of providers and consumers and to force decision makers (providers, consumers, and payers) to consider carefully the relative efficiency and importance of various services, procedures, and treatment modalities when resources are limited. The goal of managed care is not simply to lower costs but to ensure that maximum value is received from the resources consumed during the production and delivery of health care services (Hicks et al., 1993).

MANAGED CARE ORGANIZATIONS

The list of managed care organizations (MCOs) seems to grow longer each year. Each organization that is a provider or payor (or both) wants to be included as a "managed care" entity because of its wide acceptance by consumers, businesses, and government alike as a solution to our health care crisis (Faltermayer, 1993). References to managed care organizations in the literature include the three most prominent types of MCOs: HMOs, PPOs, and private "managed" indemnity health insurance plans (Curtiss, 1990). Each of these MCOs is briefly described in terms of their operational characteristics and relation to plan-affiliated physicians.

HEALTH MAINTENANCE ORGANIZATIONS

The most prominent managed care organization is the HMO, simply because its introduction during the 1970s brought about the managed care revolution. Like the generic term managed care, the term HMO is used to describe a variety of organizational structures. The HMO concept is an organizational one that brings together the financing and delivery of health care services into one entity.

In 1971 the HMO was defined by the U.S. Department of Health, Education and Welfare (USDHEW, 1971) as:

An organized system of health care which accepts the responsibility to provide or otherwise assume the delivery of an agreed upon set of comprehensive health maintenance and treatment services for a voluntarily enrolled group of persons in a geographic area and is reimbursed through a prenegotiated and fixed periodic payment made by or on behalf of each person or family unit enrolled in the plan.

BASIC CHARACTERISTICS OF HMOs

Health maintenance organizations have five basic characteristics that distinguish them from the traditional fee-for-service medical care system (Luft et al., 1980).

1. The HMO assumes an explicit contractual responsibility for providing a stated range of health care services.
2. There is an enrolled, defined population.
3. Subscribers voluntarily enroll in the plan, and providers voluntarily participate in it.
4. The HMO receives a fixed periodic payment (a capitation per enrollee) from the subscribers, which is established independent of actual utilization by an individual subscriber.
5. The HMO assumes financial risk for the capitated services.

HMO MODEL TYPES

HMOs come in different sizes and organizational formats. When the HMO industry began during the 1970s there were only two categories of HMO: a staff/group model or an individual practice association (IPA). Today there are five major organizational models: staff, group, network, Individual Practice Association, and hybrid (mixed).

What makes one HMO model type different from the others is how the HMO relates to physicians in terms of organization and payment. Although few HMOs are considered today to be "pure" staff models or "pure" group models, the above model types can still be used to describe the various organizational approaches that have been used to combine the financing and delivery systems into one organizational entity. All of these organizational formats have been described in the literature and are introduced below (Coleman, 1990; Dalton, 1987).

Staff Model HMO

A staff model HMO is the purest form of managed care. In a staff model HMO, physicians are salaried employees of the HMO. They practice in medical centers owned by the organization. Under this practice arrangement, the staff physicians are not personally at financial risk for the services provided because they are salaried employees. Because the organization is at risk, it is tightly managed.

Physicians employed by the HMO have strong incentives to provide medical services within established budgets. Failure to provide the services within the budget jeopardizes their future employment. In some staff models, physicians can earn bonuses for keeping costs below budget and providing preventive health services. Staff model HMOs typically have lower rates of hospitalization and provide more preventive and outpatient care services than the other HMO types. The overall costs of staff model HMOs are usually the lowest of all HMO types. Because staff model HMOs cannot employ physicians of every specialty on a salaried basis, they contract with specialists and subspecialists using fee-for-service, retainers and capitation payments. The most prominent staff model HMOs are the Harvard Community Health Plan of Boston, Massachusetts; the Group Health Association of Washington, DC; the Group Health Cooperative of Puget Sound in Seattle, Washington; CIGNA Health Plan of California in Glendale, California; and Family Health Plan in Milwaukee, Wisconsin. In 1992 there were 56 staff model HMOs taking care of 6.4 million enrollees (Marion Merrell Dow, 1993a).

Group Model HMO

A group model HMO does not employ staff physicians. Instead, the HMO enters into a contract with a multispecialty group practice to provide services to its members. The physician members of the group become the HMO's participating doctors. The medical group usually is paid a fixed negotiated capitation payment each month for each HMO enrollee. The monthly capitation payment is usually for all physician office and outpatient services, both primary care and specialty care physicians. In many instances the medical group is also placed at risk for all inpatient costs. Because the physicians are employed by the medical group, the group is free to compensate its physicians however it chooses. Some compensate them on a production basis, some on a capitation basis, and sometimes they use both. The medical group can be a dedicated group; that is, 100 per cent of its practice is devoted to caring for HMO enrollees. In other cases, it can be an independent multispecialty group that provides both prepaid and fee-for-service medical care and contracts with more than one HMO in the community.

In a group model HMO, the medical group assumes risk for all medical costs that exceed the income received from the HMO. Almost half of the group model HMOs enter into shared risk arrangements with their contracting medical groups for the cost of hospital care. Under such an arrangement, the medical group and the HMO agree to share the profit or losses that occur because of hospital expenditures.

Under this organizational model, the HMO does not have direct control over the physicians in the contracting medical group. As a result, the HMO uses financial incentives rather than controls to influence the practice behavior of the group's physicians.

Group model HMOs have exhibited good use and economic results, much of which is attributed to the medical group's economies of scale and the group's incentive to remain profitable because each member physician has a personal financial share in the group's economic performance. Examples of group model HMOs are the Fallon Community Health Plan in Worcester, Massachusetts; Kaiser Permanente Medical Care Program of Southern and Northern California; HIP/Rutgers Community Health Plan in New Brunswick, New Jersey; CIGNA Health Plan of Arizona in Phoenix, Arizona; and Health Alliance Plan in Detroit, Michigan. In 1992 group model HMOs represented 12.6 per cent of the HMOs in operation (Marion Merrell Dow, 1993a).

Network Model HMO

The network model HMO is similar to the group model except that the HMO contracts with more than one multispecialty group in its service area. Using this delivery system the HMO manages a network of medical groups that are strategically chosen by geography. Each contracting medical group is at financial risk for the HMO members who select the group practice as their source of medical care. Unlike the group model, most of the independent practice groups in the network continue to see fee-for-service patients. Because this form replicates the group model, the financial incentives and controls used by the HMO are similar to those of the group model. When the medical groups are at financial risk for inpatient and outpatient care, the HMO establishes separate funds for each medical group.

The network model allows the HMO to enjoy the economic advantages of the group model and the marketing advantage of having many groups throughout its service area. Examples of successful network models are HealthNet in Woodland Hills, California; Take Care Health Plan in Concord, California; Group Health Inc. in Minneapolis, Minnesota; and HMO Illinois Inc. of Chicago, Illinois. In 1992 there were 72 network model HMOs serving 18 per cent of the HMO enrollment nationwide (Marion Merrell Dow, 1993a).

Individual Practice Association Model HMO

Nearly two thirds of the HMOs in operation in 1992 were IPAs. In 1992 there were 363 IPAs with 28 per cent of HMO enrollment nationwide (Marion Merrell Dow, 1993a). This form of HMO contracts either directly (direct contract IPA) or through a formally organized physician association with solo practitioners and many small, typically single specialty group practices. When the IPA model is used, individual physicians in the community do not have to give up fee-for-service practice and can continue practicing from their offices. IPA model HMOs have large panels of practicing physicians and hospitals.

The most common form of payment for IPA primary care physicians is capitation. Specialists, on the other hand, are usually compensated on negotiated fee schedules or a discounted fee schedule. Physicians who contract with the IPA typically guarantee that the care needed by each HMO member for which they are responsible will be below a certain budgeted amount. This guarantee is made by either accepting a capitation fee or allowing the HMO to withhold an amount of their capitation payment or fee schedule payment amount (e.g., 20 per cent). If at the end of the year the physicians' costs fall under the budgeted amount, the physician receives the "withhold fund." If the costs exceed the budgeted amount, the HMO uses the withhold funds to pay the deficits. If necessary, the withhold amount (20 per cent) is increased for the next accounting period.

The IPAs have many advantages over the HMO and for the participating physicians. Examples of large IPA model HMOs are Health Plans of Michigan in Flint, Michigan; PCA Health Plans of Texas in Austin, Texas; Foundation Health Plan of Sacramento, California; MD-IPA in Rockville, Maryland; Blue Choice in Rochester, New York; and HMO Pennsylvania in Blue Bell, Pennsylvania.

Hybrid (Mixed) Model HMO

The newest organizational form is the hybrid, or mixed, model HMO. A hybrid HMO is characterized by being a mixture of either a staff and group HMO, staff and IPA HMO, or group and IPA HMO. A hybrid is simply the result of combining two or more of the forms of HMOs into one. Because of this mixture, these HMOs have larger, more extensive delivery systems and more complicated contracts and risk-sharing arrangements with its participating providers. As more PPOs take hold and compete aggressively for patients, more hybrids will be formed.

National HMO Chains

Of the 594 HMOs in 1992, 421 were owned by HMO chains. HMO chains have been growing rapidly since 1990 through new start-ups and by acquisition. In 1992 forty-eight HMO chains were operating 421 plans. The top seven chains based on enrollment were Kaiser Foundation Health Plan (6.6 million), Blue Cross Blue Shield System (5.1 million), The HMO Group (3.4 million), CIGNA Health Plan (2.2 million), United Healthcare Corp. (1.9 million), PruCare (1.8 million), and U.S. Healthcare (1.5 million). In 1992 eleven HMO chains had over one million members (Marion Merrell Dow, 1993a). Under managed competition national HMO chains are expected to enlarge and increase in numbers.

PREFERRED PROVIDER ORGANIZATIONS

A PPO is difficult to define because it is simply a business arrangement between a group of health care providers (sellers) and a group of buyers (self-insured employers, insurance companies, union trust funds, third party administrators) who want to purchase health care services for a defined population at previously agreed upon discounted prices.

Although there are many variations in how PPOs are organized, they do have common characteristics in terms of how they work. One of the primary distinguishing characteristics of a PPO is its structured design, which provides financial incentives rather than controls to enrolled members to receive their necessary health care services from PPO providers. Each time a PPO-covered individual seeks health care services, he or she can elect to use a PPO provider (one on contract with the PPO) or a non-PPO provider (one not on the PPO panel). If an individual seeks care from a PPO provider he or she receives better coverage of the costs from the benefit plan; that is, out-of-pocket costs are lower when using a PPO provider than a non-PPO provider.

Ideally, PPO providers (e.g., hospitals, physicians, podiatrists, chiropractors, home health agencies) have been selected to participate in the PPO because of their cost-efficiency, quality, and effective practice management.

Because of their structure, such economic credentialing is important to their cost-containment programs. In 1992 the PPO industry offered PPO options to 58 million eligible workers (Marion Merrell Dow, 1993b). In terms of covered members, they could have as many as 90 million members.

Common Operating Characteristics of PPOs

PPOs share several characteristics:

1. *Limited panel of providers.* Like HMOs, most PPOs do not include every hospital, physician, or health practitioner in the community. The panel of providers include a select number of hospitals, physicians, home health care providers, and other health care professional groups that have been carefully selected by the PPO sponsor because they provide cost-effective services. Many PPOs examine hospital and physician cost and utilization patterns during and after the selection process. In some PPOs the physician panel consists of all or portions of the medical staffs of the panel hospitals.

2. *Freedom of choice of providers.* PPOs have been described by some to be IPA model HMOs without the "lock-in." Unlike their HMO counter-

parts, PPO enrollees usually can elect to see any PPO panel physician they desire without going through a primary care physician.

3. *Utilization management.* PPOs market themselves as cost-effective health care delivery systems. To be a cost-effective supplier of health care services, PPOs must rely on several of the utilization management techniques of HMOs. PPOs use preadmission reviews, concurrent reviews, discharge planning, second surgical opinion programs, and sometimes catastrophic or individual case management. State-of-the-art PPOs have broadened their utilization management programs to include mental health and rehabilitation reviews, retrospective reviews, reviews of specialty physician services, high technology diagnostic services, and ancillary services reviews for home health care. PPOs that do not use comprehensive utilization management techniques to control costs may not be able to compete effectively in the managed care marketplace tomorrow.

Members of a PPO are not "locked into" the PPO or to a specific provider when they join. This freedom of choice is a marketing advantage of the PPO when competing against an HMO for employer groups. Although most PPOs do not restrict enrollees, newer PPOs are being developed that do require the enrollee to select a primary care physician to reduce the physician "shopping" that occurs when no controls are in place.

4. *Negotiated fee schedules.* PPO reimbursement is built on negotiated fee schedules that are agreed to in advance by the purchasers (insurance companies, employers, business groups) and the PPO providers. PPOs originally used discounted fee schedules as the primary form of payment for participating providers. Because discounting does not necessarily result in changing the behaviors of providers, PPOs have turned to using risk payment approaches. Some PPO hospitals are therefore paid on a per diem, diagnosis-related group (DRG), or capitation basis. PPOs usually obtain 10 to 30 per cent discounts from billed inpatient charges. Physician reimbursement is generally a percentage discount off a fee schedule or a fixed cap (maximum payment) on specific fees. Some PPOs use a relative value scale (RVS) schedule. Hospital outpatient services and ancillary care providers are often paid 10 to 20 per cent less than standard fees.

The most popular method of physician reimbursement for the PPO industry in 1992 was the negotiated maximum fee, or fee cap. Some 73 per cent were paid on fee caps, 14 per cent on discounted fees, and 2 per cent on a per-case basis. PPOs usually reimbursed hospitals on a per diem basis (40 per cent) or on a discounted charge basis (41 per cent). Only 9 per cent of the hospitals were paid using DRGs (Marion Merrell Dow, 1993b).

5. *Consumer and provider benefits.* Consumers who elect to join PPOs when they have a choice generally choose them because of the greater freedom to select providers and the feeling of not being "locked in" to one provider, as in an HMO. Consumers are also attracted to PPOs because they can elect to use a PPO provider or a non-PPO provider each time they need to use their health benefits. The incentives for PPO members is to use a PPO provider and therefore have all or a high percent of the bill paid. If they choose a non-PPO provider they usually have more out-of-pocket expenses, as the PPO pays less of the bill. The economic incentives are clearly such that the PPO member usually chooses to use PPO providers. Some PPOs provide additional benefits, such as a waiver of deductibles or a decrease in coinsurance rates, to entice members to use the PPO panel.

Like their HMO counterparts, PPO providers also have several incentives to affiliate with a managed care organization. Among the benefits from PPO affiliation are (1) maintenance of existing market shares and patient volumes; (2) potential expansion of market share; (3) improved cash flow from rapid payment of claims; (4) preservation of the traditional fee-for-service payment approaches; and (5) changes in payment and patient mix.

Financial Risks of PPO Providers

In general, PPO providers do not assume an insurance risk; that risk is assumed by the payer (e.g., employer, insurance company, union trust fund). The providers do, however, assume substantial business risk in the form of the negotiated payments they agree to accept in exchange for their services. Of course the risk is increased when the negotiated payments are based on a per capita basis (capitation), per diem, or for a specific illness (DRG). If the agreed-on payments are percentage discounts (e.g., 10, 15, or 20 per cent) from usual and customary rates (most are), the business risk is still there. If the increased number of patients generated by the PPO is not sufficient to overcome the reduction in the fees previously charged, the provider may experience a reduction in income by participating in the PPO (Hicks et al., 1993).

Because most PPO providers are paid on a discounted fee-for-service basis and therefore do not bear the financial risk for excessive utilization for their services, the PPO monitors providers to keep them from increasing the volume and complexity of services to compensate for the reduced price. PPOs that rely heavily on discounting as a means of cost containment must have several checks and balance systems in place lest their costs exceed those promised to the buyers of this system of care (Hicks et al., 1993).

Types of PPO Sponsor

The PPOs are usually sponsored by providers, health insurance companies, entrepreneurs, employers, and third party administrators. In fact, there can be different types of owner. Of the 681 corporate PPO entities in operation in 1992, 24 per cent were owned by independent investors, 42 per cent by insurance companies, 2 per cent by HMOs, and 16 per cent by hospitals or physician/hospital joint ventures (Marion Merrell Dow, 1993).

EXCLUSIVE PROVIDER ORGANIZATIONS

When a PPO restricts the participating physicians to those who have demonstrated cost-effective medical care, it is usually presented in the market place as an exclusive provider organization (EPO). EPOs are designed to compete as an HMO alternative or a replacement when an HMO offers employers or other purchasers both an HMO and an EPO. EPOs tend to be developed by mature PPOs that are competing against large, strongly competitive HMOs. EPOs are growing in popularity. Enrollment in EPOs increased dramatically in 1992, reaching 8.3 million (Marion Merrell Dow, 1993b).

Like HMOs, PPOs are usually localized. However, PPO networks are now forming at the regional and national level to compete against Blue Cross plans, large indemnity plans, and regional and national HMO networks. All 50 states were serviced by PPO networks in 1992. Forty-nine multistate PPO organizations operated a total of 760 PPOs serving more than 34 million eligible employees. National chains are led by Blue Cross and Blue Shield plans, which have 49 PPOs with nearly 8 million members. National PPO chains are expected to grow rapidly because of health care reform (Marion Merrell Dow, 1993b).

MANAGED INDEMNITY PLANS

The HMOs and PPOs are viewed by many to be the only true forms of managed care. In fact, many HMOs do not recognize PPOs as managed care systems because so many of them do not bear the financial risks like HMOs. During the late 1980s the health insurance industry started to introduce PPOs to compete against HMOs. They also began to introduce the "managed indemnity plan." A managed indemnity plan is a traditional fee-for-service health insurance program that has added many of the utilization management programs found in HMOs and PPOs and that also uses some of their risk payment approaches as well.

By introducing managed indemnity plans, major insurance companies that own HMOs and PPOs (CIGNA, Prudential, and Aetna) are able to sell a "triple option." This triple option allows companies and their employees to select from a range of managed care plans: from a "hard" managed HMO, to a "soft" managed indemnity. Because the PPO is a middle option, it is often marketed as a "mild" but effective form of managed care. Many more managed indemnity plans will be developed in the years ahead as the third choice, replacing the traditional fee-for-service product, which for years had few access and use restrictions and controls placed on them.

FINANCIAL ASPECTS OF MANAGED CARE

Managed care is a high risk business. Most managed care organizations bear the financial risk that accompanies the responsibility of providing covered services to their defined populations.

The business obligation of an MCO is to pay health care providers for the covered services rendered to their populations. Because most managed care organizations are at financial risk, they develop elaborate provider networks and contracts to limit this risk and to redistribute it among their covered members and providers. In doing so, they provide incentives for members and providers to use benefits and to render services in an optimal manner. An overview of the financial aspects of a typical managed care organization is presented in the next section (Boland, 1993; Coleman, 1990; Kongstvedt, 1993).

COST-CONTAINMENT APPROACHES OF MCOs

The financial success of an MCO depends on its ability to contain both medical service costs and administrative expenses. The ability of the organization to contain medical costs may depend on the nature of the incentives it has with its participating providers.

Because the monthly payments to MCOs are fixed and independent of actual use, MCOs are at risk for excess costs caused by adverse medical selection, catastrophic cases, "high users," organizational inefficiencies, excessive utilization of services, and higher than normal charges. Because of this vulnerability, MCOs have strong incentives to use economic credentialing of providers and to form a medical care delivery system comprised of cost-efficient producers that render care-effective services while maintaining quality. This balancing is not as simple as it sounds. The organization has to strike and manage a delicate balance among utilization, costs, and quality to the satisfaction of its customers (enrollees, participating providers, the public, and the organization itself). These entities have differing points of view about the levels of use, cost, and quality that can be achieved when explicit financial limits are imposed by revenue levels.

To contain costs, MCOs use various forms of utilization management and attempt to place as many contracting providers it can at full or partial risk for the units of services produced and the unit cost of each service.

When an MCO takes this approach, it has a good chance of keeping total costs within budget because it is controlling two factors in the *total medical cost equation*:

Total medical costs = units of medical services

provided × cost per unit of service

or

TC = utilization × cost

where the costs are added for all medical services (e.g., physician, hospital, home care, durable medical equipment (DME) supplies, intravenous therapy services) over all benefit plans.

The two major cost-containment approaches that MCOs take to manage medical service production levels (units of service) and service costs (unit cost of services) are risk-sharing and utilization management (Coleman, 1990).

RISK-SHARING APPROACHES

The MCOs do not have to share the business risks with contracting providers, but most elect to do so because it provides economic incentives to contracting providers to be resourceful and to render only medically necessary services. It also reduces the organization's business risk. There are several risk-sharing approaches an MCO can take. They range from distributing all or a portion of the risk of a specific health care service (primary care, specialty care, inpatient care, home care), to a limited number of independent contracting providers, to redistributing all of the risk for some or all health care services to one multispecialty medical group, IPA, or physician-hospital organization (PHO). Many possibilities are likely, as there is no one best way.

The greatest business risk is taken by those providers who agree to accept fixed payments for their services regardless of the amount of services used by the members. The prospective payment approaches with the highest risks include capitation, per diem, and per case (DRG) payments.

Different types and levels of risk can be developed for individual physicians, groups of physicians, IPAs, hospitals, and PHOs. The most four common ones for physicians, medical groups, hospitals, and PHOs are described below.

Risk Model 1: Primary Care Physician—Only Primary Care Services

With the first risk model, primary care physicians (gatekeepers) are placed at risk only for their own services. This risk is usually transferred in the form of a monthly capitation payment. The primary care gatekeeper must then look to the HMO or managing partner for guidance when a need arises to procure services other than those of a primary care nature when managing the health needs of the members. This model relies heavily on placing external controls on the primary care physician. These controls typically take the form of having the primary care physician justify the medical necessity of the nonprimary care services being requested. This model places the managed care organization in the position of having to micro-manage the health care utilization of its defined population.

Risk Model 2: Primary Care Physician—All Physician Services

When using the second risk model approach, the individual primary care physician or multispecialty group is at financial risk for all physician services—primary and specialty. When this approach is taken, the individual physician or group receives capitation amounts for the two categories of services and are thus placed at risk for the cost of referrals from primary care providers to specialists. With many plans the primary care physician or group is also at risk for ancillary referrals.

Risk Model 3: Full Financial Risk—All Services

With risk model 3, the primary care physician or medical group (gatekeeper) assumes the risk for all health care expenses. In this model the primary care physician or medical group receives a monthly fee credited to them. Depending on the arrangement, payments for hospitalizations, specialty consultant services, and ancillary fees are deducted from this monthly payment prior to the primary care physician receiving any funds. The underlying theory for this risk assumption model is that the primary care physician is the source of all other health care service utilization and therefore should be the best person to be at risk for all expenses. As a result, primary care physicians are given monthly budgets for their covered members and must manage the utilization and associated costs accordingly.

Risk Model 4: IPA/PHO—Full Risk

Under the fourth risk assumption model, the MCO seeks an IPA (association form) or a physician-hospital organization (PHO) to accept 100 per cent of the risk of medical expenses for physician and hospital costs.

The managed care organization in this instance deducts its administrative expenses and some profit from the revenues received and pays the contracting entity the balance. The IPA, medical group, or PHO is then at full financial risk for excess costs or excess revenues. The IPA, medical group, and PHO entities in turn pay participating provider members of their networks based on the contracts they negotiate with the providers. The MCO in this model monitors the provider organizations and may even still provide utilization management services to ensure that utilization is properly managed and that underutilization does not occur.

PAYMENT APPROACHES FOR MANAGING UNIT COSTS

Because of the cost risks that accompany uncontrolled use and rising price levels, managed care organizations attempt to fix costs by using prospective payment systems that require providers to manage both the number of units of services consumed and the unit cost of each service.

Cost = units of service × cost per unit of service

The units of services part of this equation can be managed by using utilization management techniques: hospital admission reviews, length of stay management, controlling referrals, and so forth. Another effective approach is to have providers assume full financial responsibility for controlling the units of services and the cost per unit of service. The most common approach is through the application of capitation payment systems. Under a capitation arrangement, providers receive a fixed monthly payment for each member and assume full responsibility for managing both the use and cost portions of the equation. Other reimbursement strategies (Coleman, 1990) include charges or fee-for-service, discounted fee-for-service, per diem, and case payments (DRGs).

Fee-for-service payments present the lowest risk to contracting providers. The fee for service can be based on a schedule developed by the managed care organization or some other commonly used payment schedule. The *discounted fee-for-service* arrangement has risks attached, as the discount rate (e.g., 15, 20, 25 per cent) might put the resultant payment rate below the actual costs of providing services.

Per diem payments are used by almost 40 per cent of the managed care organizations for inpatient care (acute care hospitals, rehabilitation facilities, skilled nursing facilities, mental health facilities, skilled nursing facilities, mental health facilities, and hospices) and for some outpatient therapies as well (physical therapy, rehabilitation, occupational therapy, intravenous therapy, and hospice care in the home). Per diem arrangements are a flat payment for 24 hours of care. Under this fixed payment approach the provider must closely manage the use and costs of all treatments, therapies, and resources needed to carry out the treatment plan. When this approach is used, the managed care organization usually retains control of the number of days or the units of care that are authorized for payment.

Case payments (DRGs), or fixed payments or global fees based on an individual case (e.g., obstetric care) or a specific disease category (e.g., acquired immunodeficiency syndrome or inpatient DRG), places the provider at full risk for treatment costs for whatever length of time it takes to achieve the expected outcome and mutually agreed to by the plan and the provider. Under case and DRG-type payments, providers have to manage the number of cases referred, the length of the treatment, and the resource costs in order to achieve the expected outcomes. Global fees to physicians for specific types of cases or to centers of excellence for organ transplants, head injuries, open-heart surgeries, and the like place the provider at risk for excess costs.

When capitation payments are used, contracting providers (hospitals, physician specialists, home care providers) assume the entire cost risk for the care of all members who either choose or are assigned to them by the plan. If utilization and costs are exceeded, the provider incurs the loss. Under a capitation payment plan, providers must manage all aspects of a member's care as the providers take the profit or loss to their own bottom line. The capitation amounts negotiated with providers can be based on actuarially determined rates or on a percentage of revenue basis.

PRIMARY CARE PHYSICIAN CAPITATION PLANS

Primary care physicians can enter into a number of capitation payment plans, each with differing levels of responsibility and risk: primary care services, specialty care, ancillary care, inpatient (hospital) care. The lowest risk for a primary care physician is to receive capitation only for his or her primary care services. If the physician or medical group wants to enter into a contractual arrangement with higher levels of risk (and profits), they can assume the responsibility for all physician care, both primary and specialty, or even assume a much higher risk (and profits) by assuming some or all of the risks for inpatient and ancillary care.

A capitation payment to a primary care physician is prepayment for services on a fixed per-member per-month basis. The PCP is paid a fixed dollar amount each month for a member regardless of whether that member receives services and regardless of the utilization rates and costs incurred.

The capitation amount is based on a specific set of covered primary care services. These covered services generally include routine office care, immunizations, well-baby care, preventive services, outpatient care, hospital visits, diagnostic testing, office surgical procedures, and so forth.

Most capitation payment schemes for primary care vary the payments according to the age and sex of the plan enrollees, taking into account the differences in average utilization of medical services in each age and sex category. By using age/sex-adjusted capitation rates, physicians who treat children under 18 months of age receive payments that reflect higher costs than those treating children 2 to 18 years of age. Some managed care organizations pay higher capitation rates to primary care physicians in exchange for exclusive contracts and may adjust the rates for population and geographic factors based on their cost history. Sometimes higher capitations are paid to internists and to medical groups and residency programs affiliated with medical schools (Kongstvedt, 1993).

If a managed care organization has special arrangements for laboratory testing and radiology procedures, the costs for these services are "carved out" of the primary care physician's capitation payments. The same is true for immunizations, as immunizations may be reimbursed on a fee-for-service schedule instead of being included in the capitation payment rate.

UTILIZATION MANAGEMENT APPROACHES

A guiding principle of managed care is that appropriate use of services leads to better outcomes at the lowest reasonable cost. As a first step to achieving appropriate utilization of services, the managed care entity first limits its provider network to competent physicians, medical groups, hospitals, and other care organizations that embrace the managed care philosophy and agree to be partners in managing the health of their members. When taking this business approach, the managed care organization acts as a quality maximizer. As a second step to achieving appropriate use levels, the managed care organization acts as a quantity maximizer but only in the sense that it wants to produce the greatest number of medically necessary services its money can buy. To do so, the organization uses several health care resource utilization management programs to keep use and costs in check so it can remain price competitive.

Most successful managed care organizations use an array of practice guidelines and utilization management programs to reduce the amount and frequency of unnecessary medical care and to contain costs. Although these programs are sometimes viewed by contracting providers as bureaucratic, unfriendly, and disruptive, they nonetheless have been effective in achieving appropriate levels of use and minimizing exploding costs. Most of the programs described below are expected to be in use years from today. Third and fourth generation managed care organizations, however, are now working on the technical challenges of developing new utilization management approaches that incorporate patient care outcomes and "best" practice guidelines for all medical conditions and variations in clinical practice.

The utilization management programs in vogue today include primary care management, hospital preadmission reviews, concurrent and retrospective reviews of inpatient stays, outpatient procedure reviews, physician profiling, large case management, and a host of others (Coleman, 1990; Reich, 1993).

ROLE OF MEDICAL DIRECTORS

Medical directors of managed care organizations are administrators and physicians. Their value as a medical director is enhanced when the physician part continues to dominate their thinking. Although plan medical directors are dedicated to the plan's goals and objectives of providing care at a reasonable cost to its customers, their first goal is to provide quality medical care and service. To balance cost containment and care quality, the medical director must be a good communicator, be a good businessman, and understand the need to be a patient listener when receiving messages from participating providers because many medical problems have several possible solutions. As a leader in the physician community, the medical director is the key link between participating physicians, hospitals, and the plan's management. Their primary responsibility is to ensure that the plan's utilization management program and financial incentives do not have a negative impact on the delivery of quality medical care. The medical director should participate in all phases of utilization management, from the development of criteria through the hiring and supervision of physician advisors and nurse reviewers. Because provider profiling serves only to pinpoint areas of concern, the medical directors interpret the results of profiling and identify physicians or hospitals whose profiles are at variance with the norm and not attributable to the complexity of the patients or other unavoidable factors. Although medical director's goals are to resolve problems, reduce conflict, and bring harmony to the provider network, they at times must apply sanctions to network providers whose practices affect care quality and threaten the plan's financial health (Reich, 1993).

MANAGING QUALITY

Quality assurance (the assessment and management of the quality of medical care) is becoming a major competitive factor for managed care organizations (MCOs) for patients. Concerns about the quality of care delivered by MCOs continue to be in the forefront. Many of the inherent features of MCOs—discounts, utilization management, restricted professional autonomy, risk contracts, capitation, restricted access, and limitations on provider choice or on the services—make them targets for increased scrutiny and accusations of decreased quality (Boland, 1993). Many have reasoned that the incentives to contain costs in HMOs would result in a lower quality of patient care. In general, quality of care, as measured by health outcomes, has proved to be comparable for HMO and non-HMO patients (Brook et al., 1993; Hornbrook and Berki, 1985).

Donabedian (1983, 1985, 1988) and others have continued to emphasize that "quality care" means not only clinically correct care but timely access to care, the client's valuations of inputs and outputs, client satisfaction, and production efficiency. Although many have tried to define and measure quality, there are many problems with the information presented to consumers (Sisk et al., 1990). The major problems stem from the lack of a commonly accepted definition of quality medical care (Ginsburg and Hammons, 1988). This point in itself has made it difficult to measure quality in quantifiable terms.

Managed care organizations, like other health care organizations, are moving away from quality assurance programs and beginning to adopt continuous quality improvement approaches (Kaplan, 1992; Rosler, 1990; Zusman, 1992). Looking at the total quality management systems of Juran, Crosby, and Deming, provider organizations are examining ways by which to redefine quality, implement quality enhancement and quality improvement programs, and devise new ways to measure outcomes and total performance (Lynn, 1991).

As managed care organizations strive continuously to improve quality, clinical activities are viewed as simple work processes characterized by the requirements of their customers and suppliers. These customers and suppliers include plan members, participating providers, public entities, the medical profession, and the managed care organization itself.

Quality medical care must therefore satisfy and conform to the specific requirements of all of these customers. Once these requirements are understood and met, the overall outcome will be the enhancement of health status, prevention of the deterioration of health status caused by injuries or chronic illnesses, and promotion of quality of life.

QUALITY MANAGEMENT LOOP

Quality management is a continuous dynamic process which may be envisioned as a quality loop as presented in Figure 62–1. The loop begins with the establishment of care requirements, or standards (e.g., 100 per cent of children from ages 0 to 2 are to have a full complement of immunizations). Objective measurement of conformance to those standards are then put in place (e.g., number of children, ages 0 to 2, who did not receive the full complement of immunizations). These measurements are then compared to the standard. The plan either meets or does not meet the care standard.

If the care standard is met, the conforming processes continue to be measured and monitored to ensure successful outcomes. If the care standard is not met, the processes are analyzed to identify opportunities for process improvement.

Once these opportunities are identified, a plan for corrective action is developed and corrective intervention of the process is implemented. To make certain the correction remains in place and can successfully eliminate the nonconformance, the process is monitored through measurement, closing the loop. By using the quality process loop, managed care companies seek to continuously improve the quality of health outcomes for their patient customers.

With medical and administrative cost-containment strategies in place and with demonstrated success in the management of inpatient and outpatient utilization, managed care organizations are now starting to focus on the development of quality management programs to ensure that quality health care is maintained and improved when so many cost-containment initiatives are being used simultaneously.

Quality medical care may be defined as "the result of a provider patient relationship, such that their interaction either enhances health status, prevents the deterioration of health status caused by chronic illness or injury, and promotes quality of

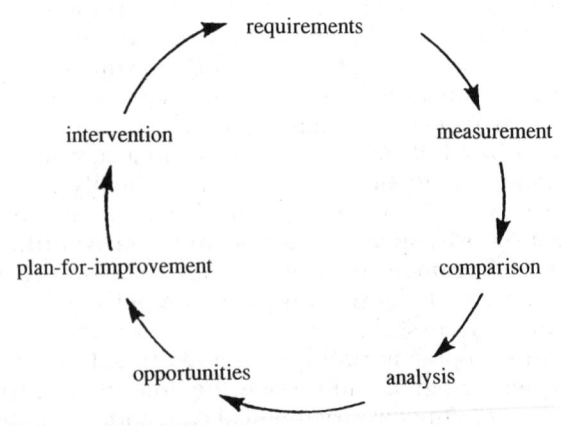

FIGURE 62–1. Quality management loop.

life." Quality enhancement and continuous quality improvement processes will soon replace the quality assurance programs that mainly focus on individual cases and peer review of case management.

The growing demand of customers for accountability as gauged by care quality and outcomes of medical care dictate that the old quality assurance inspection system directed at outlier behaviors be replaced by systems that improve the process of delivering care (Zitter, 1992). It can only be accomplished when the quality assurance program is replaced by a continuous quality improvement process that focuses on systems and processes and provides feedback to the providers so that improvements can be made. It is only through the application of the latter process that a managed care organization and its participating providers can sustain and measure care and service quality improvement efforts over time.

Whatever approach the managed care organization decides to take with the continuous quality improvement process, it should intimately involve physicians and should have a quality loop that:

1. Defines quality in measurable terms
2. Identifies and measures processes
3. Analyzes the outcomes of measurement
4. Fixes immediate problems
5. Develops corrective action plans
6. Continuously improves quality through prospective and retrospective studies

With the introduction of the quality loop, the modern managed care organization should be able to provide higher-quality outcomes continuously at a lower cost.

MANAGED COMPETITION

Whereas managed care is a financing and delivery strategy for health care, managed competition is a purchasing strategy. It is a strategy whereby managed care systems are rewarded with increased revenues for controlling costs, enhancing quality, and improving member satisfaction. This concept, coined by the Jackson Hole Group Principals Paul Elwood and Alain Enthoven, attempts to divide providers in each community into competing economic units and to use market forces to motivate them to develop efficient health care delivery systems.

This purchasing strategy identifies four major entities in the new health care delivery system (Fig. 62–2).

1. *Sponsors*: employers and government programs such as Medicare, Medicaid, and CHAMPUS
2. *Accountable health plans*: HMOs, PPOs, and other insurance companies or provider groups that assume financial risk
3. *Health alliances*: regional purchasing groups governed by a board of directors elected by member sponsors of each alliance
4. *National Health Board*: a national organization that establishes standards of practice, outcome measures, and the rules for competition.

Managed competition, if fully implemented, will undoubtedly transform the face of American health care in terms of the financing, organization, and delivery of health care services. The concept of managed competition is going to change how

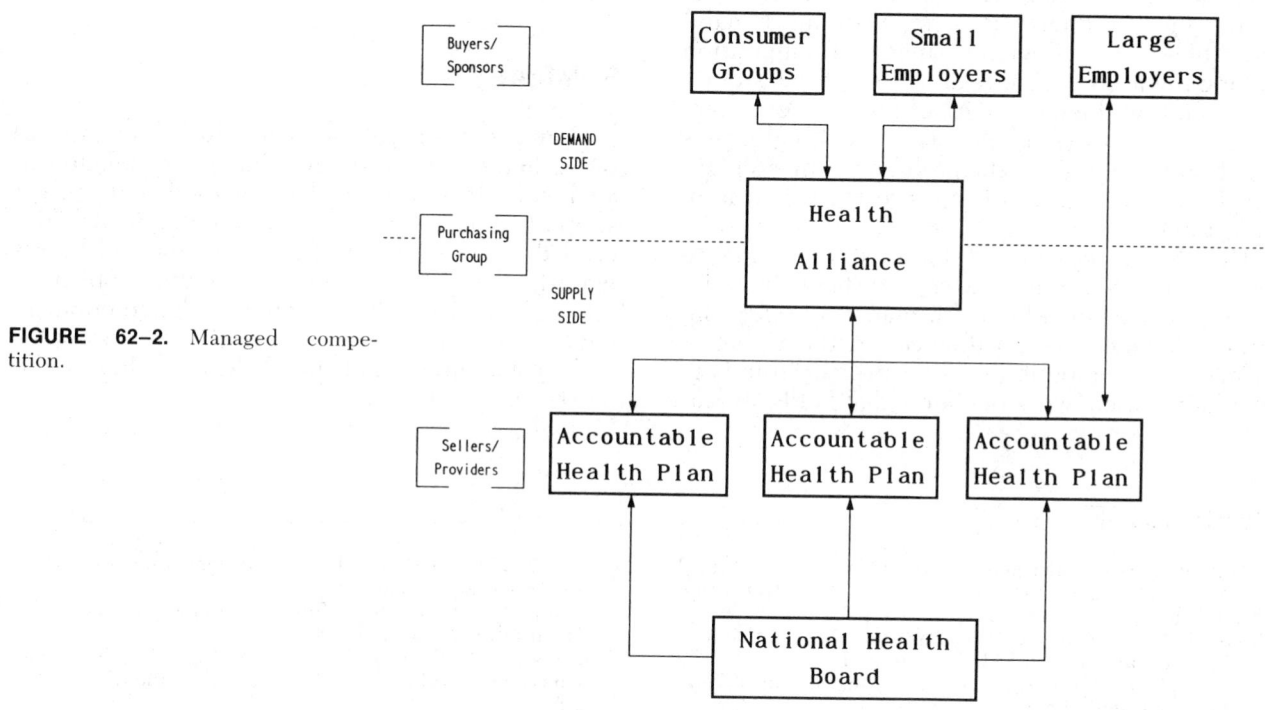

FIGURE 62–2. Managed competition.

health care services are bought and sold in the years ahead. The entire health care industry is going to change.

Managed competition has come to the forefront of American medical economic politics because the fee-for-service system has not worked in health care and cannot work for several reasons. The greatest single reason is that under the current fee-for-service/indemnity system, the consumer of health services is not the real payer for those services (Kardatzke, 1993). The more the consumer effectively assumes the role of payer, the more the traditional market forces can function in the purchase of health benefits. Employers have attempted to address the problem by attaching deductibles and coinsurance as cost-sharing devices to provide incentives for consumers to conserve health care resources, but this technique has not slowed down excess utilization of health resources.

Role of Health Alliances

The newest entity in the above described purchasing strategy is the health insurance purchasing group, or health alliance. This organization functions as a collective purchasing agent on behalf of the sponsors.

The central idea of managed competition is to place a powerful broker between the consumers and businesses seeking health insurance coverage and health care and the private entities that provide these services. The role of the health alliance is to bring groups of buyers and sellers together and to provide the consumers with information so they can make an informed choice of which accountable health plan meets their needs. The goal of the health alliance is "empower the demand side" of health care. As the manager of competition among the accountable health plans, the cooperative stands at the focal point of the managed competition strategy (Zelman, 1993). Health alliances are designed to correct the problems of market failure in the small-group insurance market (Enthoven, 1993).

Health alliances are not intended to provide insurance, much less medical care. Instead, they contract with accountable health plans and offer consumers a choice. Health alliances are the managers of managed competition. Their primary role is to maintain a framework of choice that holds all par-

ticipating health plans accountable for their performance and rewards the more efficient ones with more enrollees (Soafer, 1993; Starr, 1993).

Accountable Health Plans

Accountable health plans are basically managed care organizations (HMOs, PPOs, and "managed" indemnity plans) that have organized themselves to provide the medical benefits to enrollment groups that have chosen them. Accountable health plans are capitated for their services and are accountable to their consumers through the health alliance.

Many new forms of managed care organizations will be created in the years ahead to compete for the patients. If the competition model results in the spread of tightly managed, fully integrated health care plans, a sizable subspecialty physician surplus will be created in the fee-for-service sector.

National Health Board

The National Health Board will provide oversight of the managed competition strategy. The Board will be comprised of leading consumer advocates, business leaders, and government representatives. The body will establish the type of benefit plans that must be offered by all accountable health plans. It will also establish standardized reporting procedures, set guidelines for the review of new technology, and develop outcome measures that can be used to compare the accountable health plans in terms of care effectiveness and care costs.

SUMMARY

Managed competition as a solution to the nation's health care problems has been debated at all levels. It appears to have gained widespread support. Whatever the outcome of the debate, the critical success factors of this concept will be related to issues that give the individual consumer real informed purchasing choice: the freedom to choose a managed care organization that provides the most benefits and the highest quality at the most reasonable cost.

REFERENCES

Boland P: Making Managed Healthcare Work. A Practical Guide to Strategies and Solutions, Gaithersburg, MD, Aspen Publishers, 1993.

Brook RH, Ware JE, Rogers WH, et al: Does free care improve adults' health? N Engl J Med 309:1426, 1983.

Coleman JR: HMOs and individual case management. Case Manager 1(3):55, 1990.

Curtiss FR: Managed care: The second generation. Am J Hosp Pharm 47:2047, 1990.

Dalton JJ: HMOs and PPOs: Similarities and differences. Top Health Care Financ 13(3):8, 1987.

Donabedian A: The quality of care in a health maintenance organization: A personal view. Inquiry 20:218, 1983.

Donabedian A: Twenty years of research on the quality of medical care. Eval Health Profess 8:243, 1985.

Donabedian A: The quality of care, how can it be assessed? JAMA 26:1743, 1988.

Enthoven AC: The history and principles of managed competition. Health Aff (Millwood) 12(suppl):49, 1993.

Faltermayer E: A health plan that can work. Fortune, June 14: 88, 1993.

Ginsburg PB, Hammons GT: Competition and the quality of care: The importance of information. Inquiry 25:108, 1988.

Hicks LL, Stallmeyer JM, Coleman JR: Role of the Nurse in Managed Care, Washington, DC, American Nurse Publishing, 1993.

Hornbrook MC, Berki SE: Practice mode and payment method. Med Care 23:484, 1985.

Kaplan JG: Standpoint: Managed care is a continuous quality improvement process, leading to managed health. Med Interface 5(10):25, 1992.

Kardatzke ES: Decisive Surgery for Our Dying Health Care System. Miami, Century Publishing, 1993, pp 19–21.

Kongstvedt PR: The Managed Health Care Handbook, 2nd edition. Gaithersburg, MD, Aspen Publishers, 1993.

Luft HS, Feder J, Holohan J, et al: Health maintenance organizations. *In* Feder J, Holohan J, Marmor T (eds): National Health Insurance: Conflicting Goals and Policy Choices. Washington, DC, Urban Institute, 1980, pp 129–180.

Lynn GF: Total quality management—a competitive strategy. Healthcare Exec Briefings 4(3):1, 1991.

Marion Merrell Dow: Managed Care Digest, HMO Edition, Kansas City MO, Marion Merrell Dow 1993a.

Marion Merrell Dow: Managed Care Digest, PPO Edition. Kansas City, MO, Marion Merrell Dow, 1993b.

Mayer TR, Mayer GG: HMOs: origins and development. N Engl J Med 312:590, 1985.

Prussin JA: HMOs: organizational and financial models. Part 2. The Community Health Care Center Plan, The Group Health Association, and the Health Insurance Plan of Greater New York. Hosp Prog 55(5):56, 84, 1974a.

Prussin JA: HMOs: organizational and financial models. Part 3. The Group Health Cooperative of Puget Sound and the Kaiser Permanente Medical Care Program. Hosp Prog 55(6): 60, 1974b.

Reich PR: Utilization management: A cornerstone of managed care, Med Interface January: 28, 1993.

Rosler SL: Total quality improvement. J Qual Assur, September/October: 18, 1990.

Shouldice RG, Shouldice KH: Medical Group Practice and Health Maintenance Organization. New York, Information Resources Press, 1990.

Sisk JE, Dougherty DM, Ehrenhaft PM, et al: Assessing information for consumers on the quality of medical care. Inquiry 27:263, 1990.

Sofaer S: Informing and protecting consumers under managed competition. Health Aff (Millwood) 12(suppl):76, 1993.

Starr P: Design of health insurance purchasing cooperatives. Health Aff (Millwood) 12(Suppl):58, 1993.

US Department of Health, Education, and Welfare: Health Maintenance Organization—The Concept and Structure. Rockville, MD, Health Services and Mental Health Administration, 1971.

Zelman WA: Who should govern the purchasing cooperatives? Health Aff (Millwood) 12(suppl):49, 1993.

Zitter M: Outcomes assessment: True customer focus comes to health care. Med Interface 5(5):32, 1992.

Zusman J: Moving from quality assurance to continuous quality improvement. Physician Exec 18(4):3, 1992.

SUGGESTED READINGS

Aeschlerman M, Koch A: Independent practice associations: Risk contracting, financial controls and process. Med Group Manage J, July/August: 70, 1993.

Altman SH, Cohen AB: The need for a national global budget. Health Aff (Millwood) 12(suppl):194, 1993.

Church DE, Bokor A, McCain DD: An alternative to primary care capitation in an IPA-model HMO. Med Interface November: 37, 1989.

Clancy CM, Hillner BE: Physicians as gatekeepers—the impact of financial incentives. Arch Intern Med 149:917, 1989.

Crosby PB: Quality Is Free: The Art of Making Quality Certain. New York, McGraw-Hill, 1979.

Deming EW: Out of the Crisis. Cambridge, MA, MIT Press, 1986.

Greenfield S, Nelson EC, Zubkoff M, et al: Variations in resource utilization among medical specialties and systems of care: Results from the medical outcomes study. JAMA 267: 1624, 1992.

Juran JM: Juran's New Quality Road Map: Planning, Setting and Reaching Quality Goals. New York, Macmillan/Free Press, 1992.

Kassberg M: Managed care report cards: How will you rate? Managed Care 2(6):23, 1993.

Langwell KM: Structure and performance of health maintenance organizations: A review. Health Care Financ Rev 12(1):71, 1990.

Lewis JB: How to evaluate managed care contracts. Healthcare Financ Manag 44:32, 1990.

Walker LM: How to tell if a HMO will make you money. Med Econ 29(22):161, 1992.

CHAPTER 63

ACCOUNTING SYSTEMS

JACK VALANCY

Accounting is the language of business. A working knowledge of accounting systems enables the family physician to understand his or her professional finances and manage his or her practice in a business-like manner.

GENERAL ACCOUNTING

Accountant and Bookkeeper

The family physician should match his or her needs to the variety of accounting services available. Most physicians, especially those just starting in practice, need only basic accounting services.

1. Preparing professional and personal tax returns
2. Preparing the practice's financial reports
3. Setting up and auditing the practice's bookkeeping system
4. Auditing the practice's operations

A good accountant is more than a technician who manipulates figures. The accountant should explain practice finances and answer questions and also may advise the family physician in matters such as minimizing his or her tax burden, leasing equipment, obtaining credit, and setting up a retirement plan. The accountant should anticipate problems by staying abreast of changes in tax laws and rulings that could affect the physician. If the family physician's needs are outside his or her area of expertise, the accountant should refer the physician to a specialist.

Although anyone can represent himself or herself as an accountant, the family physician should retain a certified public accountant (CPA) who is licensed to practice within the state. The accountant should have experience serving physicians with similar needs. To find an accountant, the physician can ask colleagues and check with the local society of CPAs. The physician should ask several prospective accountants to outline the services they propose to provide and to estimate their annual cost. In addition, the physician should request and check client references.

It is important that the accountant understand and support the physician's financial objectives. The family physician should ask each prospective accountant about his or her approach to specific situations. An aggressive accountant who engages in "creative" approaches to reduce the physician's tax burden increases the risk of triggering an Internal Revenue Service audit and of incurring financial penalties. Conversely, the physician with a too conservative accountant who "plays it safe" might pay more taxes than necessary.

A bookkeeper does routine accounting tasks such as paying bills and posting transactions. The practice's accountant and bookkeeper should coordinate their efforts. Small medical practices usually do not have enough bookkeeping work to keep a full-time bookkeeper busy. In some practices the employee who does bookkeeping has other responsibilities as well, and in other practices a part-time bookkeeper is hired to work a few days a month. Some accounting firms employ bookkeepers who are available to their clients as needed.

The family physician should evaluate how well his or her accountant (1) explains practice finances and answers questions; (2) interacts with the practice's staff to complete accounting tasks; and (3) meets deadlines for tax returns. Deficiencies in any of these areas can be frustrating and expensive. The family physician should discuss his or her dissatisfaction with the accountant. If he or she does not resolve the problems quickly, the family physician should not hesitate to find another accountant.

Financial Statements

An effective accounting system provides precise, current information about where the practice's money comes from (*revenues*), where it goes (*expenses*), how much is left (*income*, also called profits), what is owns (*assets*), what it owes (*liabilities*), and what it is worth (*capital*, also called net worth or equity). The fundamental relations between these elements are expressed in the accounting equations shown in Figure 63–1. The family physician usually takes his or her compensation from the practice's positive income, its profits. (A practice with negative income could not provide com-

Accounting equations

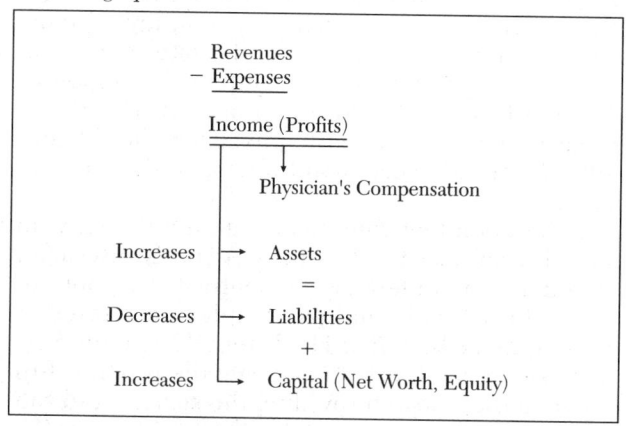

FIGURE 63–1. Distribution of revenue, expenses, and income of a medical practice.

Jay Mitchell, M.D.
Balance Sheet
December 31, 19xx

ASSETS

Cash	$ 6,500
Furniture and equipment	17,000
Office improvements	20,075
Less: Accumulated depreciation	(4,675)
Total assets	**$38,900**

LIABILITIES

Loan 1 (fixed loan)	$22,350
Loan 2 (line of credit)	9,700
Total liabilities	*$32,050*

CAPITAL

Owner's equity	$5,000
Retained earnings	1,850
Total capital (net worth)	*$6,850*

TOTAL LIABILITIES AND CAPITAL	**$38,900**

FIGURE 63–3. Balance sheet.

pensation indefinitely.) The remaining income can increase the practice's assets, decrease its liabilities, and increase its capital as *retained earnings.*

Information in the accounting equations appears in two basic financial statements: the income statement and the balance sheet. The *income statement* shows revenues and expenses over a particular period (Fig. 63–2). The balance sheet shows the practice's financial position on a specific date (Fig. 63–3). The practice's accountant prepares financial statements at the end of each accounting period, typically a month, a quarter, and a year.

Jay Mitchell, M.D.
Income Statement
for the year ended
December 31, 19xx

REVENUES from professional services	*$212,044*
EXPENSES	
Auto	$1,750
Books & subscriptions	256
Continuing medical education	1,200
Contributions	200
Depreciation	1,107
Drugs & medical supplies	2,371
Dues	755
Employee benefits	5,687
Insurance	4,625
Interest on loans	2,286
Office cleaning & maintenance	378
Payroll, office	49,388
Pension plan contributions	6,800
Rent	7,500
Taxes	2,817
Telephone	1,687
Utilities	289
Total expenses	*$89,096*
INCOME (PROFITS)	**$122,948**

FIGURE 63–2. Income statement.

General Ledger

The general ledger process, or the accounting cycle, begins when transactions are recorded on source documents, such as patient encounter forms, invoices, and receipts. The information is posted to a *journal,* which is a chronologic list of all transactions. Examples of journals in a medical practice are daysheets used to record patient account charges, payments, and adjustments and checking account registers, which list checks as they are prepared.

Transaction information is transcribed from the journal to the appropriate *account ledgers* for assets, liabilities capital, revenues, and expenses. The account ledgers are organized according to a chart of accounts, which groups similar accounts. For example, asset accounts may be numbered 100 to 199, liability accounts 200 to 299, and so on.

Transactions are recorded following either the cash or accrual method of accounting. With the *cash method,* all money that is actually spent or received during an accounting period is included in that period. Under the *accrual method,* however, expenses and revenues are charged to the period in which they are incurred or earned, even if the money is actually spent or received at a different time. The cash method of accounting is simpler and is used by most taxpayers, including physicians.

Double entry bookkeeping, invented in Italy about 500 years ago, ensures that the accounting equations remain in balance. As the name implies, each transaction generates offsetting entries, debits and credits, to two or more accounts. Each transaction's total debits must equal its total credits. An account's balance is the difference between the sum of its debit and credit entries.

The preparation of a trial balance ensures that all accounts are in balance before the financial statements are prepared. The sum of all debit entries in all accounts is compared to the sum of all credit entries. If these totals are not equal, there are errors in the accounting system.

An audit trail is a technique of cross-referencing transactions through the accounting cycle, from source documents to financial statements. By following the audit trail, the history of each transaction may be traced and errors detected and corrected.

Payroll

As an employer, the family physician is obligated to pay taxes based on employees' compensation. The employer withholds amounts from employees' gross pay and makes additional contributions. Taxes are due regularly, with severe penalties for late payments.

To become known as an employer, the family physician must obtain a *federal employer identification number* by submitting form SS-4. State and local agencies that do not use the federal number assign different numbers to the practice.

Federal regulations require that employers maintain accurate records of hours worked and earnings for each employee covered by the Fair Labor Standards Act. These records should include the time the worker begins and ends each shift and the time taken for unpaid break and meal periods. Employees should complete their own time records. Time clocks are not necessary but may be helpful if accurate timekeeping is difficult.

The Fair Labor Standards Act mandates that employers pay nonexempt employees 1.5 times their hourly wage for every hour over 40 they work in 1 week. Some states have stricter overtime laws. Overtime pay must be computed on a weekly basis, that is, seven consecutive 24-hour periods. Thus it is most convenient to pay employees every 1 or 2 weeks, rather than once or twice a month.

Several tests can be used to determine if an employee is exempt from the record keeping and overtime pay requirements of the Fair Labor Standards Act. In general, employees whose work requires the exercise of independent judgment and earn more than a certain amount may qualify as exempt. In a medical practice, the office manager, head nurse, and laboratory technicians might qualify as exempt employees. If the family physician pays exempt employees a salary instead of hourly wages and does not pay overtime, he or she cannot reduce (dock) the employees' pay for arriving late for work.

Employers are obligated to pay taxes based on their employees' compensation: (1) federal, state, and local income taxes; (2) social security; (3) Medicare; (4) unemployment compensation; and (5) workers compensation.

Some of these taxes are withheld from the employees' pay; others are contributed by the employer. At the end of each year, employers must provide employees and federal, state, and local governments with records of employee compensation and taxes withheld. Keep payroll records for at least 7 years. The family physician should consult his or her accountant for specific requirements.

An independent contractor is an individual who provides services to a business. A family physician served by an independent contractor is not required to withhold and pay employment taxes or pay employee benefits. The Internal Revenue Service uses several tests to evaluate the relationship between the person providing the service and the business receiving it. If most of these tests are satisfied, the individual is considered an employee. The tests include whether the employer specifies when, where, and how the work is done; whether the work must be done on the premises; whether the employer provides training and tools and pays expenses; and whether the individual spends all his or her time working for one employer. A transcriptionist who serves several practices by picking up dictated tapes, transcribing them, and delivering the completed documents to the respective practices is an example of an independent contractor.

Accounts Payable

A medical practice deals with many suppliers of goods and services. Although some require cash on delivery (COD) or in advance, most vendors establish *trade accounts* for their customers. This arrangement is convenient for ordering goods and services by telephone. To maintain control, the family physician should limit the number of people authorized to place orders on the practice's trace accounts. Payment is usually due upon receipt of an invoice.

A *purchase order* is a formal, detailed written order to a vendor for specific goods and services. Purchase orders should be prepared for major purchases, items that are available in different styles or colors, and items that are made to order.

Many practices find it convenient to file unpaid bills by the date due and pay them twice a month, when the payroll is prepared. Classify payments according to type of expense (e.g., rent, supplies, insurance), as decided by the practice's chart of accounts.

Most family physicians need just one *business checking account*. If the account does not earn interest, the family physician can also set up a savings account at the bank or a money market account with a no-load mutual fund company. The family physician can arrange to transfer funds by telephone between the accounts at no charge.

The traditional business checkbook has three or

more large checks per page with stubs on their left side. It is easy to make transcription errors when recording data on these stubs. A *one-write pegboard system* may be used instead to prepare checks and simultaneously record the amounts in various expense categories on a check register (daysheet). Each check has a carbon stripe on its back that transfers data to the daysheet. Each daysheet can hold data from about 25 to 30 checks. The checks and daysheets have holes in their left margins. A board with protruding pegs is used to align the checks over the daysheet. The daysheet has several columns to the right of the check that are used to classify expenses.

Some pegboard check-writing systems are designed to be used for payroll preparation as well. The checks have spaces across their tops for recording gross pay, deductions, and net pay. A carbon stripe behind this area transfers data to the employee's payroll record card, which is inserted between the check and daysheet. (Pegboard systems for maintaining patients are described in the Patient Accounting section, which follows.)

Another method for preparing checks and classifying expenses is to use *two-part voucher checks*, which have a large stub for recording payment information. The original check, which is negotiable, is forwarded to the payee with the stub attached. The duplicate copy, which is nonnegotiable, remains in the practice.

Simple, easy-to-use computer programs can save time, maintain detailed records, print checks, and produce useful reports. Accounting software is widely available and is usually the best alternative for the family physician who has a personal computer in his or her practice.

A *petty cash fund* is used to pay minor practice expenses without writing a check. Set a specific total amount, such as $50, for the fund. A check written to "cash" is used to obtain bills and coins for the fund. As cash is withdrawn, receipts or petty cash vouchers for the purchases are filed. The cash remaining plus the total of the receipts and vouchers should always equal the total amount of the fund. Additional checks are written to replenish the fund as needed.

A *change fund* is a set amount of bills and coins the front desk assistant uses to make change for patients as necessary at the front desk. The total amount of the change fund should not vary from day to day.

Accounting Control

There are three good reasons for maintaining accounting control.

1. *Preventing and detecting errors*. Without good accounting control, it is virtually impossible to detect and correct errors in the practice's ac-

counting system. Maintaining daily controls helps reveal minor errors before they become major problems.

2. *Reducing embezzlement*. Although it is impossible to entirely prevent embezzlement, good accounting controls reduce the risk.

3. *Establishing a valid base for comparison*. Keeping complete, accurate records establishes a valid database for measuring the financial performance of the practice.

Some specific techniques for maintaining accounting control follow:

1. Use prenumbered source documents, such as encounter forms, in sequence.

2. Reconcile transactions as often as practical: daily, weekly, or monthly.

3. Correct errors immediately; document corrections.

4. Separate accounting tasks among employees. For example, one employee could open the mail and endorse checks; another could post the payments to patient accounts.

5. Endorse checks "for deposit only" to the practice's bank account when they are received.

6. Deposit all cash, checks, and credit card documents daily.

7. Proof the practice's accounts receivable monthly; that is, compare the daysheet's running total with the sum of individual account balances.

8. Follow all control procedures designed for the specific accounting and bookkeeping systems used.

9. Review bills as they are paid. Only partners in the practice should be authorized to sign checks.

10. Control the petty cash and change funds.

11. Make unannounced spot checks of various aspects of financial operations.

12. Have the practice's accountant audit the accounting systems regularly, at least every 2 years.

13. Have staff members covered under a fidelity bond that reimburses the practice for losses resulting from employee theft. This form of insurance is often part of the physician's business owner's insurance policy. Prosecution of the offender might be required to collect damages.

PATIENT ACCOUNTING

The family physician's approach to medicine defines his or her clinical relationship with patients; The family physician's patient accounting policies and procedures define his or her business relationship with them. An effective patient accounting system enables the family physician to receive fair compensation without alienating patients. Reasonable financial policies and sound procedures applied consistently can minimize difficulties for the physician, patients, and staff.

Financial Policies

Without explicit financial policies, physicians, patients, and staff are likely to have different expectations; and routine matters can become sensitive issues. Financial policies include, but are not limited to, the following issues.

1. Setting fees
2. Extending professional courtesy, discounts, and charity care
3. Participating in health insurance plans such as Medicare, Blue Shield, and managed care plans
4. Informing patients of the practice's patient accounting policies and procedures
5. Posting transactions
6. Requesting payment
7. Producing bills
8. Processing insurance claims
9. Collecting delinquent accounts
10. Discharging patients for nonpayment

The family physician should articulate his or her practice's financial policies and procedures. If several family physicians practice in a group, all should agree on the practice patient accounting policies and procedures. Although they need not understand every detail, they should be familiar with the basic functions of the practice's patient accounting system.

Once the family physician(s) decide(s) on the practice's patient accounting policies and procedures, they should be put in writing and reviewed with the staff members responsible for doing them. Discuss how the staff will handle various situations and potential problems. Monitor performance and modify policies and procedures as necessary.

Information about the practice's financial policies should be presented to patients in a clear, matter-of-fact manner. Some physicians prefer that their staff inform patients when the initial appointment is scheduled. Other physicians are more comfortable if the patient is informed at the end of the first visit. If a patient is about to incur an unusually large fee, it is good to confirm the financial arrangements before the services are rendered.

Reinforcing an oral explanation of the practice's policies with written information is helpful. This information may be contained in a practice information brochure that explains all pertinent policies and procedures or in a separate patient accounting brochure. A statement inviting the patient to discuss financial matters with the staff should be included to solicit questions before problems arise.

A *patient accounts representative* can establish and maintain good communications between the practice and its patients. This skilled employee has broad knowledge of insurance plans and is empowered to work with patients to settle their accounts. Many family physicians find that the continuity of this approach results in higher collections and lower costs than fragmenting patient accounting duties among several employees.

Fees

Family physicians should carefully evaluate the services they provide and corresponding fees they charge. The family physician's services and procedures should correspond to the descriptive terms and identifying codes in the *Physicians Current Procedural Terminology,* (CPT). Read the guidelines for choosing the appropriate code at the beginning of each chapter. Professional fees should reflect the time, effort, training, skill, and resources required to render the service.

A fair guideline for establishing fees is to observe the going rates in the area. To estimate these rates, the family physician may follow these guidelines.

1. Request copies of the approved fees for participating and nonparticipating family physicians in the geographic area from the local Medicare intermediary. Medicare's Resource-Based Relative Value Scale (RBRVS) calculates each procedure's reimbursement based on relative value units representing the physician's work, practice expenses, and cost of malpractice insurance. These factors are modified by a geographic adjustment factor and multiplied by a single conversion factor to calculate the procedure's approved amount.
2. Obtain a fees and relative value study from an independent publisher.
3. Contact the local Blue Shield plan to learn reimbursement rates under the usual, customary, and reasonable (UCR) guidelines.
4. Check *Medical Economics* magazine for their survey of fees by specialty and region. A complete survey is usually published in October.
5. Ask colleagues about the ranges of the going rates for medical services in the area. Do not request precise fees or discuss setting your fees the same, as it may be interpreted as price fixing, which is illegal.

The family physician or patient account representative can reduce patients' misunderstandings and complaints about fees by clearly explaining medical services and their fees and making financial arrangements with patients before treatment begins. The family physician should tell the patient when other physicians will also care for the patient.

Almost all practicing physicians extend professional courtesy, reduce their fees, or provide uncompensated care to indigent patients. Fee reductions may be granted to a class of patients (such as other physicians) or on a case-by-case basis. Some physicians accept the amount reimbursed by the patient's insurance as payment in full. Some health insurance companies oppose this practice because deductible and copayment amounts due from the patient are intended to prevent overutilization of services.

Restraint of trade, that is, acting alone or with others to hinder a competitor's free actions in the marketplace, is illegal. Prohibited activities include agreeing on how much to charge for specific services (price fixing), controlling competition (agreeing not to compete), and boycotting individuals or organizations. Although it is unlikely that a few casual remarks can trigger antitrust proceedings, the family physician should avoid detailed discussions of fees and other competitive issues with other physicians.

Health Insurance Plans

An *indemnity health insurance plan* reimburses the patient for covered medical expenses. The agreement involves the insurance carrier and the patient only. The patient is liable for the physician's entire fee for a medical procedure, regardless of the amount approved or reimbursed by the insurance plan. Payment is made directly to the insured. If the patient assigns his or her benefits and the physician accepts the assignment of benefits, payment is made to the physician.

The health insurance plan sets an approved amount for each medical procedure. The plan reimburses this amount, less any deductible or copayment amounts to be paid by the patient. A deductible is an amount the insured must pay each year toward covered medical expenses before insurance benefits are paid. A copayment is a percentage of the approved charges, or a fixed amount, that is due from the patient.

A *service health insurance plan* provides the patient with covered medical services. It involves the insurance carrier, the patient, and sometimes the physician. If the physician participates in the plan, the plan's approved amount for a covered procedure is the total compensation he or she is entitled to receive from the insurance plan and the patient. The physician may not bill the patient for charges above the approved amount (a practice called balance billing). He or she is not compensated for the difference between the approved amount and the full fee. If the physician does not participate in the plan, the patient is liable for the physician's entire fee for a medical procedure, whatever the amount reimbursed by the insurance plan. Service health insurance plans use various incentives to encourage their subscribers to see participating physicians and discourage them from seeing nonparticipating physicians. When considering whether to participate in an insurance plan, the family physician should weigh possible reductions in revenues against the prospect of more patients.

Managed care plans include health maintenance organizations (HMOs) and preferred provider organizations (PPOs). Such plans attempt to control costs and maintain quality of care by requiring patients, physicians, and other health care providers to follow various procedures and regulations. The plan might reduce or deny benefits if these conditions are not satisfied. The family physician might be compensated on a negotiated fee-for-service basis or might receive a predetermined capitation payment, usually monthly, for each managed care plan patient enrolled in his or her practice. This payment covers some or all of the patient's health care costs, both within and outside the practice. Specialists and other providers are paid a capitated rate or a negotiated fee-for-service.

See Chapter 62 for more information about family physicians' relations with managed health care.

Patient Accounting System Functions

All patient accounting systems, whether manual or automated, perform the following seven basic functions.

1. Store patient demographic and insurance information
2. Post transactions
3. Control system operations
4. Produce patient bills
5. Process insurance claims
6. Collect delinquent accounts
7. Produce reports

Store Patient Demographic and Insurance Information

The family physician's staff typically obtains patient demographic and insurance information at the first visit by asking the patient to complete a patient information form. Information includes the patient's name and address, telephone number, date of birth, and sex; the name, address, and telephone number of the person responsible for paying the account (guarantor); the patient's and guarantor's employers; information about the patient's primary and secondary insurance coverage, including the insured person's (subscriber's) name and the patient's relationship to him or her, the name of the insurance carrier and specific plan, and the subscriber's insurance plan identification numbers.

The patient information form also should include three statements for the patient's or guarantor's signature: (1) authorization for the practice to release information necessary to obtain reimbursement from insurance carriers; (2) authorization for the payment (assignment) of insurance benefits directly to the physician; and (3) acknowledgment that the guarantor is responsible for paying all charges for medical care not reimbursed by health insurance or other sources. Having these signed statements on file eliminate the need for the patient to sign such statements on individual insurance forms. Photocopy the patient's insurance identification card(s) and file it in the patient's medical chart with the patient information form. This practice reduces the risk of errors when transcribing policy information to the patient's account ledger card (in manual patient accounting systems) or account master record (in automated systems).

Post Transactions

All transactions (charges, payments, and adjustments) should be recorded on source documents. For patients seen in the office, encounter forms (also called superbills, charge tickets, and routing slips) are used to record charges, payments, and adjustments made at the time of service. A superbill is an encounter form that contains all the information required to process an insurance claim: date of service, patient's name, information about the patient's health insurance, procedure code, description and fee, diagnosis code and description, physician's name, address and insurance identification numbers, place of service, and if the medical problem is employment- or accident-related.

The receptionist initiates a two- or three-part encounter form for each patient visit in the family physician's office and, typically, clips it to the patient's chart. At the conclusion of the visit, the family physician completes the encounter form, noting services performed, diagnosis, return visit instructions, and instructions to the staff. The cashier uses this information to arrange financial matters with the patient before he or she leaves the office. The cashier gives a copy of the encounter form to the patient and keeps a copy for control purposes. In manual patient accounting systems, the third part of the encounter can be used by the practice's insurance clerk or the patient to prepare an insurance claim.

The family physician's office staff maintains a log of hospitalized patients. Each day, the family physician records the services he or she performs for hospital patients in a daily diary, on plain or printed index cards, on hospital rounds lists prepared by the office staff, on the patient's hospital admitting face sheet, or on another form or document. When the patient is discharged, or at the end of the month for long inpatient stays, the physician forwards this document to an office assistant. The assistant prepares charge information on the source document or a new document. To confirm that charges are recorded correctly, the physician reviews and initials the document. The assistant posts the charges to the patient's account and notes the date beside the patient's name in the hospital log. The assistant checks the hospital log for scheduled patients for whom she has not received charge information.

A *remittance advice* is a document included with a payment, such as part of the patient's bill or the stub attached to a check from an insurance plan. (Medicare calls it an EOMB, Explanation of Medicare Benefits.) If the payer does not send a remittance advice, the office assistant can photocopy the check or list it on a *payment and adjustment register.*

The full charge for the service provided and the amount of any adjustment should be recorded separately to maintain a valid statistical base of charges, payments, and adjustments. Recording the net value of the charge less adjustments distorts the statistics of practice operations and obscures information that the family physician can use when deciding whether to participate in a particular health insurance plan.

With a manual one-write pegboard system, the staff posts charges, payments, and adjustments to the encounter form (or other source document), patients' account ledger card, and daysheet, which shows all of the transactions for the day.

Computer systems can process payments and adjustments in several ways. In a *balance forward system*, payments and adjustments are posted against the patient's undifferentiated balance due, as they are on patient account ledger cards in a manual system. Balance forward processing is less complicated than other systems, but it is also less precise. It is suited to practices in which patients are responsible for the full amount of fees, whatever is reimbursed by insurance.

With an *open claim system*, payments and adjustments are posted against the balance remaining on an insurance claim, which may contain several individual charges. With an *open item system*, payments and adjustments are posted against individual charges. Open item processing is appropriate in practices in which the amount owed by patients for specific procedures depends on the amount of insurance reimbursement received. Here the additional precision of knowing the balance remaining on specific charges is worth the extra effort required to maintain an open item system.

One person can comfortably handle reception, cashier, and "back office" patient accounting tasks in a small family practice. In busier practices, the volume of work can become too much for one person to do properly. Incomplete and incorrect information and processing backlogs can cause problems that cascade and multiply through system control, bill production, insurance processing, collections, and report production. The family physician should provide sufficient staffing to perform these tasks effectively and consistently.

Control System Operations

People make honest mistakes no matter how careful they try to be. It is important to maintain system control to detect and correct errors before they cause problems. Simple, effective controls help people work accurately without burdening them. As noted above, each transaction should be recorded on a source document. In the daily reconciliation (or balancing) process, the office assistant compares transaction totals derived from source documents with the totals on the manual or computer daysheet. When reconciliation is completed, the source documents, calculator tapes, and daysheets should be stored by date for at least a year. Additional system control procedures are described in the previous section on accounting control.

Produce Patient Bills

Each patient should receive a written record of his or her visit, regardless of whether the family physician's policy is to request payment at the time of service. It can be a copy of the encounter form or a point of service statement printed by the practice's computer system. If the family physician's policy is to obtain payment at the time of service, the front desk assistant should request payment. Signs alone are not effective.

Bills are customarily mailed to patients monthly, at the same time each month. They must be accurate, detailed, clear, and professional looking. Bills should show the outstanding balance at the beginning of the billing period (or the full detail of unpaid charges); all charges, payments, and adjustments posted during the period; the total account balance at the end of the period; charges submitted for insurance reimbursement; and the amount now due from the patient. Each bill should include a message encouraging the patient to contact the practice if he or she has any questions about the bill.

Process Insurance Claims

Managed care plans often require preauthorization of services such as hospital admissions and outpatient procedures. A member of the family physician's staff usually can do it by telephone. Without proper authorization, the plan might pay the family physician at a lower rate or refuse payment entirely.

The family physician should help his or her patients obtain reimbursement of their medical costs from insurance carriers. Medicare regulations require both participating and nonparticipating physicians to prepare and submit insurance claims for their patients. Most health insurance plans in which the family physician participates also require this service.

If the patient's health insurance plan does not require the family physician to prepare and submit claims, he or she should, at least, provide the patient with a superbill—an encounter form that identifies the practice and contains information about the services rendered, fees, and diagnosis. Patients may submit a copy of the superbill along with a claim form to their insurance carrier. As a courtesy and to reduce delays, the family physician

should also provide the patient with a blank copy of the standard HCFA 1500 universal insurance claim form.

Many family physicians prepare and submit insurance claims for their patients, particularly if reimbursement is likely. A computer system makes this task easier. Electronic media claims submission (also called paperless processing) eliminates the need to prepare and submit insurance claims on paper forms. A computer system with appropriate capabilities can prepare claims on magnetic tape or disk or transmit them directly to the insurance carrier's or a claims processing clearing house's computer over ordinary telephone lines. The advantages of electronic submission of insurance claims include faster payment, lower risk of underpayment or rejection, and time and money saved in forms preparation.

Insurance claim processing can be complex, and it is important that the practice's procedures are efficient. Virtually every insurance carrier publishes a provider manual and has representatives to advise practices how to submit insurance claims properly. Educational programs that train staff to process insurance claims are widely available from insurance carriers and other organizations.

It is important that correct procedure and diagnosis codes be used on insurance claims. Incorrect or missing codes could cause a claim to be underpaid or rejected. The Current Procedural Terminology (CPT) coding system is generally accepted for coding procedures. Current procedural terminology code books are updated annually and are available from the American Medical Association (AMA) and other publishers. The *International Classification of Diseases, 9th edition, Clinical Modification (ICD.9.CM)* coding system generally is used for diagnoses. Code books are available from the AMA and other publishers.

The family physician should ensure that his or her staff prepares insurance claims promptly, neatly, and completely. A duplicate copy should be kept on file—on paper or in the computer system. The staff should refer to this copy when posting payments and adjustments received from insurance carriers. They should question lower than expected payments and should follow up with the insurance plan if the claim has been outstanding for longer than usual or rejected in error. The family physician's staff should get to know people at the insurance carriers who can help resolve problems with difficult claims. The staff should inform the patient of unusual delays in processing claims. This practice can reduce the patient's anxiety and, if the claim is underpaid or rejected, make it more likely that the the patient will pay any amount due.

Collect Delinquent Accounts

The best way to manage delinquent accounts is to keep them from becoming delinquent in the first place. The process begins when the patient is informed of the practice's financial policies. It continues with the consistent performance of patient accounting procedures.

1. Request payment at the time of service, if that is the policy.
2. Send clear, detailed bills regularly.
3. Process insurance claims promptly.
4. Encourage patients to contact the practice with any questions about their account.

It is important for the family physician to decide when an account is past due. Typically this period is 30 or more days after the date of service, after the insurance carrier paid the claim, or after the practice mails the first bill with a balance due from the patient. The family physician's staff should routinely detect delinquent accounts and begin and continue collection activities until the account is current. In a manual system, delinquent accounts can be identified by reviewing patient account ledger cards. In a computer system, delinquent accounts can be identified automatically.

An *aged trial balance* is a list of unpaid accounts with the outstanding balances classified by the time elapsed since the date of service in columns labeled current, 31–60, 61–90, 91–120, and 120+. Although a computer system can produce this report easily, compiling this information by hand is a tedious process.

If a charge for which the patient is responsible remains unpaid for more than a month, the second bill mailed to the patient should carry a brief reminder, or dunning message. If payment is not received, messages of increasing severity should appear on the next several bills. More active encouragement is recommended if the account becomes more than 60 or 90 days past due. A staff member should review the account with the family physician to obtain approval before beginning assertive collection techniques.

A member of the family physician's staff should review each patient's account before the patient visits the practice. If the account is overdue, the patient account representative should speak privately with patient about the matter. Record all contacts with patients about their unpaid balances, especially arrangements for promises to pay a specific amount(s) by a specific date(s). If the patient, or responsible party, claims an error has been made, the staff member should offer to investigate and get back to him or her. Appropriate consideration should be given to patients experiencing legitimate financial hardship.

Telephone calls are much more effective than written communications when collecting past due amounts. The purpose of the call is to ask the responsible party what he or she plans to do about the outstanding amount. It is not intended to threaten or harass. Rather, the practice is attempting to maintain communications with the patient throughout the collection process. To protect confidentiality, the caller should not leave messages that suggest the nature of the call. Calls should not be made at odd hours or at the individual's place of work. The staff member who places the call should be friendly but firm and, above all, remain in control. Each call should end with an agreement that the responsible party will pay a specific amount by a specific date. The staff member who obtains this commitment should follow up on unfulfilled promises to pay.

Collection letters can be useful as a first step or when other attempts to collect have not worked. Begin with a "gentle reminder" letter followed by a "this is serious" letter. If the response to these letters is not acceptable, a "final notice" letter tells the responsible party that further action will be taken if the entire amount is not paid by a specific date or if the practice is not contacted to make other arrangements. "Further action" could mean referring the matter to a collection agency or an attorney, or taking the patient to small-claims court.

If the family physician takes a patient to small-claims court or retains the services of a collection agency or attorney, consideration should be given to discharging the patient from the practice. Unless the patient is being treated for an acute serious condition, the physician is not obligated to continue providing medical care without compensation. The family physician should send the patient a letter via registered or certified mail with receipt of delivery. The letter should say that effective on a specific date, typically 2 to 4 weeks hence, the physician is discharging the patient from his or her care. With the patient's signed approval, the practice will forward medical records to the physician of the patient's choice.

Produce Reports

Each month the family physician should keep track of:

1. Gross charges (productivity, or the full value of services provided)
2. Payments received
3. Adjustments by type
   a. Contractual adjustments
   b. Professional courtesies and discounts
   c. Bad debt write-offs of uncollectable amounts

Many group practices use this information to calculate part of each physician's compensation.

The family physician should also be aware of:

1. Accounts receivable balance
2. Accounts receivable aging
3. Individual account balances, especially those that are unusually high
4. Refunds due patients whose accounts have credit balances

Accounts Receivable Management

The following ratios, computed monthly or quarterly, help the family physician assess the effectiveness of his or her practice's financial policies and the performance of various patient accounting functions.

Collection Ratio

The collection ratio measures the general effectiveness of a practice's patient accounting system. It is expressed as a percentage of gross charges collected.

$$\text{Collection ratio} = \frac{\text{total payments}}{\text{gross charges}}$$

Gross charges refers to the full value of the family physician's professional services, despite any adjustments to charges, such as professional courtesies, discounts, or contractual adjustments that might reduce the amount billed. Bad debts are amounts owed that are considered uncollectable. Keep track of these separately, as a percent of gross charges:

Contractual adjustments ratio

$$= \frac{\text{contractual adjustments}}{\text{gross charges}}$$

Courtesies and discounts ratio

$$= \frac{\text{courtesies and discounts}}{\text{gross charges}}$$

$$\text{Bad debts ratio} = \frac{\text{bad debts}}{\text{gross charges}}$$

Because the amount of charges, payments, and adjustments varies from month to month, it is best to calculate the collection ratio based on an average of the previous 3, 6, or 12 months.

A practice's collection ratio should be as high as possible considering the practice's unique circumstances. For example, the collection ratio might be low because the practice serves poor people or because it participates heavily in health insurance plans. The collection ratio is one of several benchmarks against which the performance of the practice's patient accounting system may be measured. Other factors include the practice's accounts receivable ratio, the practice's rate of growth, and complaints and compliments received from patients.

Accounts Receivable Ratio

The accounts receivable ratio measures how fast patient accounts are being paid. It is expressed as the equivalent number of months of gross charges contained in the practice's accounts receivable.

Accounts receivable ratio

$$= \frac{\text{total accounts receivable}}{\text{average monthly gross charges}}$$

As with the collection ratio, the appropriate level of a practice's accounts receivable ratio depends on the practice's unique circumstances. In general, an accounts receivable ratio as high as 2.5 is acceptable. However, it might be higher because few patients pay at the time of service or because the practice participates in many insurance plans.

Bad debts should be removed from the accounts receivable (i.e., written off) regularly. If these amounts remain, the practice's total accounts receivable will grow indefinitely and the accounts receivable ratio will be distorted.

Patient Accounting Systems

Pegboard System

The pegboard system, also called the one-write system, is simple, reliable, and not expensive to operate. It is suited to practices with few unpaid accounts (fewer than 250) that do not prepare many insurance claims. Most other types of manual systems have poor controls and should be avoided.

The basic components of a pegboard system are an encounter form (superbill), a patient ledger card, and a daysheet. These three items are arranged on a pegboard, a piece of wood or metal with a line of pegs down the left edge. Each day, a daysheet, which has holes on its left edge, is placed on the pegboard. The daysheet is ruled in columns: date, patient name, description of service, charges, payments, and adjustments. The encounter forms and patient ledger cards have identical columns.

An encounter form, which also has holes on its left edge, is placed on the pegboard before the patient is treated. It is aligned on the pegboard over the next available line on the daysheet. Individual patient ledger cards are slipped between the encounter form and the daysheet. Carbon paper or carbonless forms transfer all entries to all forms simultaneously. This technique saves time and virtually eliminates transcription errors.

The encounter form is then clipped to the patient's medical chart, which is routed to the physician. At the conclusion of the visit, the physician notes the services rendered and the patient's diagnosis. To save time, the most common procedures and diagnoses and their corresponding CPT procedure and ICD.9.CM diagnosis codes are preprinted on the encounter form. The encounter form is forwarded to the assistant at the front desk. He or she replaces it and the ledger card on the pegboard and records the patient's charges, payments, and adjustments.

If the encounter form is a single sheet perforated vertically, the patient is given the right side and the left side remains in the practice as a control copy. If the encounter form has two pages, one is the patient's receipt and one remains in the practice as a control copy. Encounter forms with a third page may be used to prepare insurance claims. It is either given to the patient or forwarded to the practice's insurance clerk. Payments received through the mail and adjustments are recorded on the patient ledger cards and daysheet as well.

At the end of the day, the practice's front desk assistant totals the charges, payments, and adjustments recorded on the encounter forms and other source documents. These totals are compared with the corresponding totals on the daysheet. If they are equal, the daysheet is in balance. If not, the assistant attempts to find and correct the error(s).

Patient bills are prepared by photocopying the ledger cards. Insurance claims are prepared from information on copies of encounter forms. Delinquent accounts are identified by manually reviewing the ledger cards. Reports are prepared by compiling the information on the daysheet. As the number of active accounts in the practice grows, these tasks can become tedious, and using an automated system might be more efficient.

Batch-Processing Service Bureau

Practices that use a batch-processing service bureau forward all patient information forms and transaction source documents to an outside firm for processing by a computer system. The documents are grouped into batches for control purposes. Manual patient ledger cards and daysheets are not used. Instead, patient account activity lists are produced. Daily transaction journals, which are equivalent to daysheets, are produced as batches of source documents are processed. For control purposes, totals of transactions derived from source documents are processed. For control purposes, totals of transactions derived from source documents are compared with totals calculated by the computer system from the same data. The computer system automatically creates patient bills and insurance claims (on paper or electronically), identifies and produces collection tools for delinquent accounts, and produces bills.

The cost of using a batch-processing service bureau usually includes a fixed monthly fee and unit charges for items such as patient bills, insurance claims, transactions posted, active patient accounts, and postage. The advantage of using a batch-processing service bureau is that a computer is used to perform what would otherwise be tedious manual tasks. Some tasks, such as creating reports, cost too much in labor and time to do manually. The disadvantage of a batch-processing service bureau is that patient account information available in the practice is not up-to-date: The results of processing usually are not returned to the practice for a week or more.

Time-Sharing Service Bureau

With a time-sharing service bureau, computer terminals and sometimes printers are located in the practice. They communicate with a computer system in another location. Rather than send documents to the service bureau, the practice's staff members enter information thorough computer terminals. As with a batch-processing service bureau, the computer system automatically creates patient bills and insurance claims, identifies delinquent accounts, and produces reports. Printing of patient bills and insurance claims is usually done on high-speed printers at the service bureau.

Using a time-sharing service bureau has all the advantages of using a batch-processing service bureau plus up-to-the-minute information about patient accounts. The disadvantage is that labor costs may be higher because the practice's staff is responsible for data entry. In addition, continuing operating costs of this type of system could be higher than others.

In-house Computer System

As computer systems have become less expensive, more powerful, and easier to use, more and more family physicians are using them in their practices. As the name implies, all computer equipment is located in the practice with an in-house computer system. The practice's staff uses the computer system to perform all billing, insurance, and collection functions. The family physician should have an agreement with the vendor to support both the hardware and software. The advantages of an in-house system are that the practice has a greater degree of control over billing, insurance, and collection functions and that the continuing costs of operation, including labor costs, might be lower than other alternatives. The disadvantages, which are not unique to in-house systems, are that the computer hardware or software may be deficient in some way or that the vendor will fail to provide adequate support. A good precaution against problems with this or any other type of patient accounting system is to request and check references with users of the specific systems under consideration.

Computer system software for performing patient accounting should have the following features.

1. Support full open item or open claim processing
2. Produce bills that clearly show the amount due from the patient
3. Submit claims electronically to the major insurance carriers with which the family physician deals, such as Medicare, Blue Shield, and managed care plans
4. Allow several operators to use the system simultaneously
5. Be easy to learn and use.

SUGGESTED READINGS

Farber L (ed): Medical Economics Encyclopedia of Practice and Financial Management. Oradell, NJ, Medical Economics, 1985.

Physicians Current Procedural Terminology (CPT). American Medical Association (AMA), Chicago, 1994.

Soukhanov AH, Haverty JR (eds): Webster's Medical Office Handbook. Springfield, MA: G&C Merriam, 1975.

Valancy J: Microcomputers and Your Practice: A Guide for Physicians. Chicago, Pluribus Press, 1985.

In addition McGraw-Hill publishes statistics and books on fee setting and reimbursement (McGraw-Hill, Healthcare Management Group, Physician Administration Publications, 41st Floor, 1221 Avenue of the Americas, New York, New York 10124-0146; 800-832-3203). PMIC publishes reference books and books on fee setting and reimbursement (PMIC 4727 Wilshire Boulevard, Los Angeles, California 90010; 800-MED-SHOP). St. Anthony Publishing has ICD-9-CM diagnosis code books in several formats (St. Anthony Publishing, 11410 Isaac Newton Square, Reston, VA 22090; 800-632-0123). The American Medical Association has procedure and diagnosis reference books available in a variety of formats. It also has blank forms in a variety of formats, such as the HCFA 1500 universal insurance claim form. There are, in addition, good training materials for employees who perform patient accounting functions (Order Department, AMA, PO Box 109050, Chicago, IL 60610-9050; 800-621-8335).

CHAPTER 64

PERSONNEL AND TIME MANAGEMENT

GEORGE S. CONOMIKES

When it comes to personnel management, physicians and medical office managers have a problem. They simply cannot devote the time that personnel managers in larger companies are given. By focusing on the basics of good personnel management techniques, however, the clinician with a small practice can easily muster the results of big business.

JOB DESCRIPTIONS

When thinking about effectively managing staff, it is helpful to visualize basic personnel management requirements. As shown in Figure 64–1, job descriptions are seen as the hub of personnel management activities. Without a job description, it is impossible to adequately recruit and select personnel. *With* a job description, the job requirements are documented and an applicant can be effectively recruited and selected for that job. Similarly, the job description helps later with performance appraisals and salary reviews.

A sample job description form is shown in Figure 64–2). The core of the job description is a listing of the primary tasks, which are the main tasks performed virtually daily. Note that there is also a listing of secondary tasks. Employees at most medical practices are expected to perform extra tasks *when needed*. These tasks are not part of the regular job, but the employee is expected to be able to cover for other workers when necessary. An example is the nurse who may have to perform such secondary tasks as answering the phone and making appointments. These tasks would be performed, as needed, when a coworker is absent or overloaded with other work.

JOB STANDARDS

Each task is described for the job description, but it does not spell out how the task is expected to be performed. Standards can be quantitative, such as the number of telephone rings permissible before answering it or the bill collection percent-

age. Standards can also be qualitative; such as no patient complaints and no misfiling of charts. A sample listing of job tasks coupled with their respective standards is outlined in Table 64–1.

PERFORMANCE REVIEWS

A formal review of performance should be conducted with each employee as follows: (1) new employee at 90 days after the starting date; and all employees annually. Employees want to be reviewed: It is a "report card" that lets them know how they are doing. It also establishes a framework for salary increases and other rewards. From the practice's perspective, performance reviews create a basis for improving the performance of employees. For today's medical practice to survive, employee performance must continue to increase if salaries are to increase.

When conducting a performance review, two

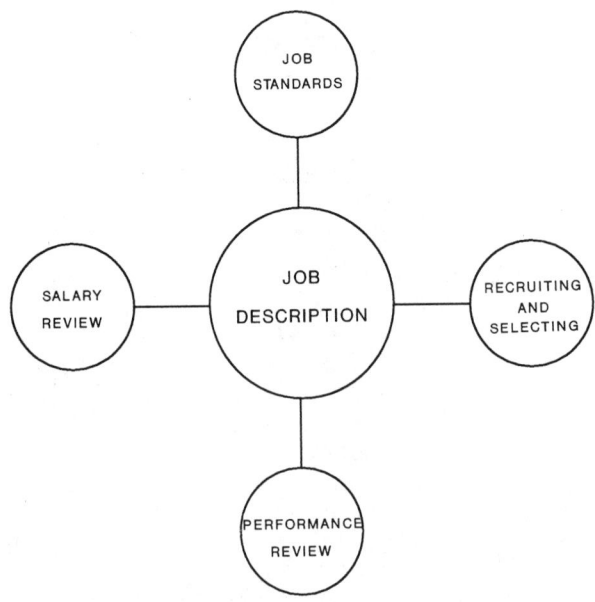

FIGURE 64–1. The job description is the hub for personnel management requirements.

JOB DESCRIPTION FOR _____

BASIC RESULTS MEASUREMENTS _____

_____

_____

_____

REQUIREMENTS _____

_____

_____

DUTIES

PRIMARY TASKS   STANDARDS

_____

_____

_____

_____

_____

SECONDARY TASKS _____

_____

_____

AUTHORITY BOUNDARIES _____

_____

REPORTS TO _____

RESPONSIBLE FOR _____

FIGURE 64–2. Job description example.

elements of performance should be covered: (1) specific task performance; and (2) subjective factors. Specific task performance involves grading each task according to the employee job description. Subjective ratings include scoring the employee on factors such as attitude, communication, cooperation, and attendance.

Performance reviews should be performed in private, on a one-on-one basis. The employee should be given specific evaluations on each task as well as on the subjective factors. The physician or manager should not disclose specific numeric grades, but examples of satisfactory work reinforce that employee's performance. In areas where improvement is needed, the reviewer should refer to the job standards and point out that they are not being optimally achieved. The employee should not be criticized, but the problem should be addressed. In other words, the review should be non-

confrontational. The goals of the reviews are, first, to let the employees know how they are performing and, second, to establish agreement and specific guidelines for improving performance in those areas where improvement is needed.

SALARY REVIEW

Salary discussions should not be undertaken in conjunction with performance reviews. Otherwise the focus is dissipated by covering two reviews: performance and salary. Let the performance review stand alone, and let it result in a clear understanding of future expectations.

Salary reviews should take place 90 days after performance reviews. Hopefully, during the intervening 3 months the employee's performance will

TABLE 64–1. JOB STANDARDS

Task	Standard
Receptionist	
Answers telephone and directs phone calls	Telephone is answered by the third ring and in the manner described in the telephone procedure manual.
	There are no more than two complaints per month concerning telephone procedures.
Makes appointments for patients	No patient waits longer than necessary for an appointment in accordance with the following guidelines.
	Emergency—same day
	Urgent—1 to 4 working days
	Routine—not more than 4 weeks
Prepares charge tickets	Charge tickets are prepared in accordance with standard procedures.
	There must be no more than three voided charge tickets per week.
	All charges are recorded correctly, so lost charges total no more than $100 per quarter.
Back office assistant	
Prepares and stocks examination rooms	All rooms are fully stocked before the start of patient hours.
	Examination rooms are straightened up after each patient visit in accordance with written procedures.
	There are no shortages in any supplies or equipment at any time.
Prepares the day's charts	Prior to office hours each day, the back-office assistant checks the day's scheduled patient charts to ensure completeness of the records.
	There are no more than two missing items per month in the charts of all scheduled patients.

have improved based on the review. The criteria for a salary review are as follows.

1. *Salary survey.* What are the salary standards in the community. If the local economy is weak, the salary requirements are less than if the economy were strong. Physicians from other practices can be consulted, as can patients who are employers. Find out what is occurring in their businesses in terms of employee compensation.

2. *Practice performance.* If the practice is having a banner year, the employer tends to be more generous than if the revenues are flat or decreased.

3. *Individual performance.* It is wise to be cautious about across-the-board increases, as they may neglect the best performers. Rather than giving everyone a 4 per cent increase, for instance, perhaps the increase could be 5 per cent to the best performers, 3 per cent to the least productive employees, and 4 per cent for the other (hopefully good) employees.

In some practices personnel policies and rules state that salary reviews are based on performance and a cost-of-living adjustment (COLA). This practice is known as the COLA trap. From 1977 to 1980, for example, there were 4 years of double-digit (10 to 14 per cent) COLA. It is therefore best to take COLA out of an office policy statement (if it exists). Salary reviews are most wisely based on criteria 2 and 3, above: practice performance and individual performance.

PERSONNEL POLICIES AND RULES

All practices should have a clearly written handbook covering personnel policies and rules. After they are written, it is wise to have them reviewed by legal counsel.

Each employee should have a copy of the handbook, given to them when they are newly employed. Certain topics merit a face-to-face review, as they often need clarification: vacations, sick leave, paid holidays, disability, and pregnancy leave.

The following is a list of what should be included in the handbook.

1. Orientation period
2. Attendance
3. Holidays
4. Vacation
5. Sick leave
6. Leaves of absence
7. Personal time off
8. Civic responsibilities
9. Medical coverage
10. Performance review
11. Wages and salary; overtime
12. Benefits
13. Appearance
14. Standards of conduct

IMPROVING PHYSICIAN TIME MANAGEMENT

Physician time management is defined as performing many tasks and doing them well. It may be helpful to review some of the ideas that have been incorporated into some practices, thereby improving their productivity.

Physicians should consider the word "focus." If they truly *focus on each patient* in the office, they are able to see more patients. For example, physicians are often interrupted during a patient's time by business or personal calls unrelated to the practice—from a lawyer, an accountant, a stockbroker. Each of these calls—even if they take only a minute or two—means that for those minutes the physician is not producing revenue. Even worse is the fact that the doctor has left the patient in the middle of an examination to deal with an unrelated matter, which often irritates the patient. Hence focusing on the particular patient results in more productive activity as well as keeping the office protocol more nearly on schedule.

Another measure that may help the physician manage time better is to remove phones from examining rooms. Studies have found that when phones are in the examining rooms there are numerous interruptions because the phone receptionist considers the doctor to be more available. Reducing that availability by taking the phones out of the examining rooms and substituting a light-and-sound signaling system is an alternative. With this system the doctor is notified, by light signals, that there is a phone call waiting. In some practices there are lights and a buzzer in each examining room. One light is red and the other white. When the buzzer sounds and the red light is on, the physician knows that there is a urgent call. The physician can then do one of two things: ignore the call, in which case the caller is told that the doctor must call back because he or she is in the middle of a procedure; or excuse himself or herself from the patient and answer the call away from the presence of the patient. Most physicians are uncomfortable discussing the problem of one patient in the presence of another, and this setup allows the separation. The white light signals a nonurgent call, to which the physician has the option of responding or not, depending on the circumstances of the moment.

Telephone calls should be returned in clusters. Rather than randomly receiving phone calls that interrupt and slow the day's schedule most of the calling parties can be told that the physician is with a patient but will return the call at a specific time. Hence if a doctor starts seeing patients at 9:00 a.m. and plans on working until 12:30 p.m., a call-back time could be established, for example, between 10:45 and 11:15 a.m. Anyone who calls between 9:00 and 10:45 a.m. is then told that the doctor is busy with a patient, but the caller can expect a call back sometime between 10:45 and 11:15 a.m. Then, sometime between those hours the physician and nurse can break and review the phone calls. The physician returns some of the calls, and others can be delegated to the nurse or to other employees, depending on the caller and the problem. Thus the doctor maximizes patient contact and minimizes phone interruptions. It is much easier and more efficient to return phone calls in clusters than one at a time. These call-back times can be scheduled at intervals, perhaps in the middle

of the morning, at the end of the morning, in the middle of the afternoon, and again at the end of the day. With this protocol patients are not kept on hold, the physician is not being interrupted, and the personnel do not have to interrupt what they are doing to find patients' charts. With specific telephone call-back intervals, these activities can be done in a more orderly manner. It is helpful to employ a phone nurse simply to screen patients' telephone calls.

Another time-saver relates to the physician's reading. A number of physicians have someone screen the relevant clinical journals and either tear out articles of interest to the physician or perhaps flag those articles with colored tags. With this method the physician can read selected articles without having to perform his or her own screening.

Most physicians are using portable cellular phones and find them to be time-savers. The physician is thus accessible when away from the office or the hospital. A number of physicians use their cellular phones on the way to the office in order to review the activities of the day and to make decisions that might otherwise occupy their time in the office.

It is recommended that physicians dictate their patient notes, especially if they do not like to write. Dictation saves the physician's time and means that the notes are clearer. This technique is especially helpful in a group practice where physicians often need to read their colleagues' notes. The level of technology is not yet sophisticated enough so the physician can dictate directly into a computer, although the technology has been developed for the field of radiology and is just around the corner for other specialists.

Correspondence on clinical matters can be conducted using "stock" paragraphs and "stock" letters. These items could be stored in the memory of the computer, and the physician can refer to typical paragraphs for communications with other physicians, for example. Some physicians have designed a form for the history and physical examination, so they can dictate it easily or tick off a checklist and simply hand it to the transcriptionist or typist—eliminating the time consumed dictating or handwriting these notes.

Physicians can save their practices, particularly the billing personnel, work and time by filling out charge tickets properly. It is helpful not only to check off the procedures but to indicate the diagnosis. A well designed charge ticket lists procedures with CPT codes next to them and the diagnoses the physician typically uses. Billing staff productivity can be enhanced if the doctor writes "1" next to the primary diagnosis and "2" next to the secondary diagnosis. This clarification can be taken one step further by indicating the diagnosis related to the procedures.

It is helpful to have a special telephone line for

pharmacies. Such a line can be attached to an answering device, or it can be part of a voice mail system. The local pharmacies can call on this line and leave their requests, thereby causing no interruption of the work of the phone receptionist, the nurse, or the physician at that moment. There should be a recorded message on the office's pharmacy line to inform the calling pharmacists when their calls will be reviewed. For example, "This is Dr. Jones' pharmacy line. Please leave your message. We will be reviewing these messages at 9:00 a.m., 11:00 a.m., 1:00 p.m., 3:00 p.m., and 5:00 p.m."

Another time-saver for physicians is not to have business meetings in the evening, as they usually last at least twice as long as they should. The best time for a business meeting is when everyone is fresh (e.g., 7:00 a.m.). Meetings should last a maximum of 1 hour and have with a clear-cut agenda. The most important item should be covered first. It is best to let everyone know there is a definite time frame. At the end of the meeting the decisions must be documented and signed by the members attending, ensuring that there was agreement on the matters discussed.

Physicians should review the phone log book before leaving the office. It is possible that a phone message could have been taken, a message slip passed along to the physician, and the slip lost or misplaced. Hence the wise physician reviews the message telephone book before leaving the office.

Physicians often are involved with patient contact after they leave the office. It might involve an emergency room visit, or it could be a patient's telephone call to the physician at home. Some doctors forget to jot down what took place. A method to avoid this situation is to have a special phone line with an answering machine or a voice mail line whereby the physician can call the office after hours. In this way the nature of a patient's telephone call or what work was done at the emergency room can be on record. Then whoever is responsible for this line in the office listens to it in the morning and determines if anything needs attention. An example is if the doctor who receives a call in the evening at home and tells the patient to call the office the next morning to make an appointment. The physician then calls the special office line to let the appointment scheduler know

that this patient should be worked in on a timely basis. Otherwise the patient might call the office and have to fight for an appointment if the appointment book is filled.

It is essential that the physician or physicians have a monthly business meeting with the office manager. For the solo physician, a monthly review is sufficient, with an idea of making some projections into the future. For groups, it improves communications among physicians and their manager. A successful business meeting is that in which only 20 per cent or less of the time is focused on the past and 80 per cent on the future. So many factors will affect the practice during the next 30 to 90 days that the agenda items should be concerned with actions that need to be taken rather than events that have already taken place.

The physician can help the practice's productivity by making sure to call the office when leaving the hospital to let them know that he or she is on the way. That way the office can start moving patients into examination rooms and completing tests, knowing that the physician will be arriving within a few minutes.

It is good practice for physicians to call the office on the regular phone line. In that way he or she can determine how long it takes for the phone to be answered. There should be concern if the phone rings more than three times before someone answers it.

The practice's performance and that of the physician can be improved by the "2-minute stand-up meeting" at the office. It is a meeting between the physician, the nurse, and the appointment scheduler that takes place when the physician arrives at the office. The nurse would have reviewed the day's appointment schedule and the charts for the day's patients and so is probably the best person to determine where and when the schedule is overbooked and where and when during the day the staff might be able to work in patients. The nurse therefore essentially "calls the shots" at this meeting and provides guidelines that help the appointment scheduler do a better job. At the same time, the nurse briefs the physician on problem patients and possible problems with the schedule. Every attempt is made to solve overbooking problems at that time. The meeting is a good way to start the physician's day, and it helps improve day-to-day scheduling.

CHAPTER 65

COMPUTER APPLICATIONS IN OFFICE PRACTICE

STEVEN M. ORNSTEIN, RUTH G. JENKINS,
and ANDREW G. URY

The ubiquitous nature of computers in many health care settings parallels their wide distribution in society as a whole. Computerized information systems manage numerous functions in modern hospitals. Administrative functions such as registration and patient accounting are invariably automated. Many hospitals have computerized order entry systems, pharmacy systems, and automated systems for laboratory, radiology, and other ancillary test reporting. Computers are prevalent in patient monitoring equipment in intensive care units, operating rooms, and other areas. Computers are also widely used for medical research, literature review, document management, database functions, and statistical analyses. An overview of computer applications relevant for the office practice of primary care physicians is presented in Table 65–1.

ADMINISTRATIVE APPLICATIONS

In office practice, computers are widely used for several administrative functions: patient and insurance billing including electronic claims submission, appointment scheduling, word processing, and other accounting functions such as general ledger, accounts payable, and payroll. The advantages of office automation are increased efficiency, better management through management reports, and increased practice income through reduced overhead and improved collection rates.

Patient and Insurance Billing

Practice management software programs that automate patient and insurance billing are the most widely used software packages in medical offices. Approximately 80 per cent of medical offices use some kind of accounts receivable software. Sending patient statements and insurance forms is much more efficient using a computer. Computer-generated superbills or encounter forms increase staff productivity. Management reports such as aged accounts receivable are only practical using a computer. Submitting insurance claims electronically saves paper and leads to faster reimbursement. Billing software is available from many vendors. When selecting practice management software, physicians should pay special attention to the efficiency of data entry, including easy access to standard diagnostic and procedure codes, the ease of correcting operator mistakes, the audit trail, and the reporting capabilities. Hundreds of billing software packages are presently available; more information is available in Chapter 63.

Appointment Scheduling

The advantages of computerizing appointment scheduling include multiuser access to a provider's schedule, fast lookup of existing appointments, multiple provider and day schedule display, management reports, and integration with practice management software and patient records systems. Optimal appointment scheduling software provides more efficient scheduling through capabilities of double booking, variable appointment lengths, and scheduling of equipment, rooms, or resources. Other conveniences of computerized appointment scheduling include booking multiple appointments at specified time intervals, sequential appointments with multiple providers, and automatic printing of patient reminder slips or postcards. Available products include PRACTICE PARTNER APPOINTMENT SCHEDULER (Physician Micro Systems, Seattle, WA); MEDICAL APPOINTMENT SCHEDULER (AlphaMed Software, New York, NY); CADENCE APPOINTMENT SCHEDULING SYSTEM (Epic Systems, Madison, WI); TIMEWISE PATIENT APPOINTMENT SCHEDULER (Health America Systems, Grayslake, IL); MEDI-MANAGER APPOINTMENT SCHEDULING SYSTEM (McIntyre Consulting, Concord, MA); SCHEDULOGIC (MedicaLogic, Beaverton, OR); MEDAPPT (Medicomp of Virginia, Chantilly, VA); TIME MANAGER

TABLE 65–1. COMPUTER APPLICATIONS FOR THE OFFICE-BASED PRIMARY CARE PHYSICIAN

Administrative applications
    Patient and insurance billing
    Appointment scheduling
    Word processing
    Accounting

Clinical applications
    Patient records
    Expert systems
    Diagnostic support
    Patient education

Educational applications
    Literature retrieval and filing
    Electronic references
    Continuing education
    On-line information resources

(Pacific Medsoft, Tahoe City, CA); and ACCLAIM—APPOINTMENT SCHEDULING (Sentient Systems, Kensington, MD).

Word Processing and Accounting

Administrative applications of computers in practice settings parallel their use in other professional environments. Most physician offices now use word processors, which allow faster typing, the use of boilerplates, and easy correction of mistakes. Most small physician offices find that general ledger and accounts payable software are too complex and expensive to use. Inexpensive money management programs, such as QUICKEN (Intuit, Menlo Park, CA) or MANAGING YOUR MONEY (Meca, Fairfield, CT), are sufficient for budgeting and checkwriting purposes. For larger offices, full accounting packages that include general ledger, accounts receivable, accounts payable, payroll, and inventory are useful.

CLINICAL APPLICATIONS

Patient Records

In 1991 the Institute of Medicine (IOM) of the National Academy of Sciences (NAS) published a report (Dick, 1991) that advocated the adoption, by the year 2000, of the computer-based patient record (CPR) as the standard for all medical records in the United States. The general thrust of the IOM report was endorsed in a U.S. General Accounting Office report to the U.S. Senate (US GAC, 1991), and a major recommendation of the IOM report was satisfied in early 1992 with the formation of the Computer-Based Patient Record Institute (CPRI). The CPRI is a collaborative effort among private and public organizations intended to coordinate ongoing activities in CPR development and implementation.

The CPR systems have numerous advantages compared with traditional paper records. Costs for storage space, paper supplies, and personnel are decreased. Access to important clinical information is rapid and available simultaneously from multiple sites. Records are legible, and data can be organized in different ways, depending on the need of the individual user. Errors with treatment protocols (e.g., medications) can be reduced through the use of features that check for drug–drug interactions and drug allergies. Ready access to test results can preclude unnecessary, expensive repeat test ordering. Computer-generated clinical reminders can improve the quality of care (Barnett et al., 1983; Garr et al., 1993; Hammond et al., 1990; McPhee et al., 1989; Ornstein et al., 1991; Tierney et al., 1986) and are indispensable tools for many research projects. Essential elements of the record can be stored on microchip cards and carried by patients (Bouckaert et al., 1992).

Currently, most medical records are maintained on paper, and wider dissemination of CPR systems will be a major undertaking. Nevertheless, a number of commercially viable systems are on the market today, and successful CPR sites exist in numerous locations throughout the United States (Ornstein et al., 1992). In addition, most general practice records are now computerized in the United Kingdom and The Netherlands, providing further evidence for the feasibility of CPR systems. CPR systems currently available commercially in the United States provide several options to physician offices seeking to automate their patient medical records.

Several of the available systems are designed to replace the traditional paper record in either small offices or large ones. Such systems include PRACTICE PARTNER PATIENT RECORDS (Physician Micro Systems, Seattle, WA) (Ornstein et al., 1993), COSTAR (Multidata Computer Systems, New York, NY); MEDTRAC (Medicomp of Virginia, Chantilly, VA); DR. WELFORD'S CHART NOTES (Welford Medical Computing, Rockford, IL); LEGACY (Epic Systems, Madison, WI); CLINICALOGIC (MedicaLogic, Portland, OR); PAL/MED (Medical Synergies Corp., Atlanta, GA); and Q.D. BASELINE (Q.D. Systems, Berkeley, CA). Typical features included in these systems are physician and nurse visit notes, medical and family history, medications, allergies, problem lists, vital signs, preventive services items with reminders, and laboratory and radiology data. These systems also have prescription writing and drug and allergy checking. The most comprehensive systems include storage and retrieval of images and electronic signature capabilities.

Other medical record systems are designed for smaller offices or allow the physician to generate legible visit notes that are printed and inserted in the patient's paper record. These systems include DR. CHART PHYSICIAN MEDICAL RECORDS (Bukstel & Halfpenny, Glenside, PA) and S-O-A-P PATIENT MEDICAL RECORD SYSTEM (Patient Medical Records, Brownfield, TX). These systems facilitate searches for visit notes that would be too time-consuming with a paper chart.

Expert Systems

Weed (1991) has proposed a paradigm for medical practice and education using a CPR system with problem knowledge couplers (PKCs). Weed's view is that the current system of medical care will be replaced by one in which problem-oriented medical records are computerized, patients possess a copy of their medical records and are active participants in their personal health care, and medical knowledge concerning diagnosis and management is brought to the point of patient care by PKCs. These couplers integrate the unique attributes of each patient with the knowledge available in the world's literature and are used by the physician and patient to plan a course of investigation and management. Medical education would be revised to replace memorization of vast amounts of biomedical information with skills relevant to the use of these systems in patient care.

Weed's visionary view of the future would require an extraordinary development of infrastructure and software development. Currently, PKCs have been written for only a limited number of medical problems and are actively used at a relatively small number of clinical sites. In addition, his model, though conceptually sound and intuitively appealing, requires empiric validation. Nonetheless, Weed is one of the true medical visionaries of our time, and it is likely that his concepts will be included in future generations of health care systems and their attendant information systems.

More limited expert systems than those advocated by Weed are available today. Iliad (Applied Informatics Inc, Salt Lake City, UT) and QMR (Camdat Corp, Pittsburgh, PA) are commercially available database programs that cover the field of inpatient internal medicine (Sumner, 1993). The database for Iliad was developed from information about inpatients at the Latter Day Saints Hospital in Salt Lake City, Utah. Additional information from expert consultants and the medical literature is also included. Iliad uses Bayesian and Boolean logic to calculate probabilities for certain diseases for inpatients on a medical service based on clinical data. Its database contains prevalences for hundreds of diseases and sensitivities and specificities for thousands of findings relevant to these diseases. The program can also be used to suggest cost-effective evaluation strategies, as an entrée to

Yearbook of Medicine articles for information on many diseases, and in a simulation mode for continuing education.

The database for QMR is derived from the medical literature. QMR uses an unique algorithm to generate differential diagnoses for a given set of data. Its differential diagnoses are more comprehensive than those of Iliad but are not associated with probabilities. Unlike Iliad, QMR can compare findings between different diseases. References to the relevant medical literature are given. Its simulation mode is not as advanced as that of Iliad.

Both Iliad and QMR are rich information sources for inpatient internal medicine but have limited information on other diseases. In addition, each has prevalence data based on hospital inpatients, which are not equivalent to prevalences in primary care. As tools for diagnostic consultation, both programs suffer from the inherent difficulty of incorporating the nuances of clinical diagnosis into discrete algorithms. The need for direct data entry is also a limitation of each program; integration with a CPR system could enhance the ease of their use.

Other, more limited expert systems have also been developed. DERMIS (Egton Medical Information Services, Leeds, UK) is designed to assist primary care physicians with diagnoses of skin diseases (Brooks et al., 1992). It has yet to be evaluated in a primary care practice.

Diagnostic Support

Several manufacturers offer electrocardiogram instruments that offer computerized interpretations. Microprocessors are also components in a variety of office-based diagnostic instruments, such as ultrasonography equipment, automated laboratory analyzers, pulmonary function monitors, and the like.

A number of programs have been developed to assist physicians with history taking and health risk appraisal. INSTANT MEDICAL HISTORY (Prime Time Software, West Columbia, SC) is a patient-driven software program that takes either an organ-system-focused or complete medical history. Certain responses cause the program to branch to standardized inventories for the diagnosis of depression, alcohol abuse, and other psychiatric problems. HEALTHIER PEOPLE (Carter Center of Emory University, Atlanta, GA) is a health risk appraisal program for adults. The program is helpful for identifying modifiable risk factors in individuals and groups and can be used to prioritize behavioral modifications.

A variety of health assessment software products are available from Wellsource of Clackamas, Oregon. LIFE (Lifestyle Inventory and Fitness Evaluation) is a wellness assessment and educational program for employee wellness and health promotion. A similar program, designed exclusively for women, is also available. Other programs are designed to assess and offer lifestyle interventions for personal wellness, body fat, smoking, and fitness. Nutrition assessment programs and coronary risk profile programs are also available. Cardinal Health Systems (Edina, MN) also produces risk assessment and diet and exercise planning software.

Patient Education

A number of products are designed to assist physicians and their ancillary staff with patient education activities. ADULT HEALTH ADVISOR (Clinical Reference Systems, Englewood, CO) provides modifiable patient education handouts on 350 topics. DISCHARGE INSTRUCTION SYSTEM (Automedics, Satellite Beach, FL) and AFTERCARE (American Health Consultants, Atlanta, GA) are similar programs and have instructions in both English and Spanish.

TEEN HEALTH ADVISOR (Clinical Reference Systems, Englewood, CO) provides a simple risk-assessment instrument and health information for teenagers. The BABY GAME (Clinical Reference Systems, Englewood, CO) is a program designed to assist physicians to teach teenagers about the time and financial burdens of caring for an infant.

MEDTEACH (American Society of Hospital Pharmacists, Bethesda, MD) provides patient information sheets for hundreds of prescription and nonprescription medications. NUTRI-CALC Diet and Recipe Analysis Software (CAMDE Corporation, Gilbert, AZ) and THE FOOD PROCESSOR II Basic Nutrition and Diet Analysis System (ESHA Research, Salem, OR) are programs that can be used to plan or analyze diets, recipes, or meals for their caloric and nutritional content. They are suitable for use by dietitians, patient educators, or patients who have home computers.

Other products are designed for direct patient use at home. HOME MEDICAL ADVISOR (Pixel Perfect, Merrit Island, FL) is a comprehensive patient education reference. It can analyze symptoms, using questions and more than 600 color illustrations, intended to make 450 diagnoses. It provides detailed information about the signs, symptoms, evaluation, and treatment of nearly 600 diseases. Information about numerous injuries and poisonings is also available, as is a drug database that includes indications, side effects, and drug interactions of more than 2400 medications. Information about 150 commonly prescribed medical tests and miscellaneous other material including a medical glossary is also contained in the program.

YOUR MEDICAL RECORDS (Pixel Perfect, Merrit Island, FL) allows patients to maintain medical information, including historical data, vaccinations, and medications in a structured database, which prints wallet-sized records. The program also prints medical legal documents, such as

Living Wills and Durable Power of Attorney. It also contains an extensive drug and substance interaction program.

VITAL SIGNS: THE GOOD HEALTH RESOURCE (Texas Caviar, Austin, TX), FAMILY DOCTOR (Creative Multimedia Corporation, Portland, OR), and MAYO CLINIC FAMILY HEALTH BOOK (Sony Electronic Publishing, Los Angeles, CA) are CD-ROM-based electronic medical references designed for the laymen.

EDUCATIONAL APPLICATIONS

Literature Retrieval and Filing Systems

Access to the published medical literature is often important for both clinical care and continuing medical education. Whereas physicians with nearby medical libraries may continue to use the services of a medical librarian, a variety of useful software products makes access to the medical literature available to all. Bibliographic retrieval can be done locally, using databases distributed on CD-ROM. Several useful products are described later. Searching can also be done on-line, either directly through the National Library of Medicine (NLM) or through a variety of third-party vendors that provide more user-friendly interfaces to NLM databases. GRATEFUL MED (National Library of Medicine, Rockville, MD) is an inexpensive, easy to use product that allows off-line formatting of search criteria to be used on NLM's MEDLINE database. Once the search criteria have been established, GRATEFUL MED dials the NLM, conducts the search, and downloads appropriate references.

Many physicians collect a variety of medical articles, handouts, pamphlets, and monographs but have no useful way of filing them. Reference management software is available from a number of vendors. These programs allow users to file and retrieve articles and other materials, store literature search results from MEDLINE and other sources, generate bibliographies, and assign citations within a word processor. ENDNOTES PLUS (Niles & Associates, Inc, Berkeley, CA), REFERENCE MANAGER (Reference Information Systems, Carlsbad, CA), and PRO-CITE (Personal Bibliographic Software, Ann Arbor, MI) are three of the more comprehensive products available.

Electronic References

A number of software products are designed to replace traditional reference sources such as textbooks. Some products are distributed on traditional floppy disk media; however, the storage capability of CD-ROM technology has dramatically increased the power of many of these products. Indeed, one

CD-ROM can store 250,000 pages of text or large combinations of text, sound, and images. A useful reference for physicians interested in acquiring CD-ROM technology has been written by Ebell (1993).

A number of products useful for Family Physicians are available on CD-ROM. The PHYSICIAN'S MEDLINE (Macmillan New Media, Cambridge, MA) is a subset of MEDLINE intended for a general medical audience. MAXX: Maximum Access to Diagnosis and Therapy, Electronic Library of Medicine (Little, Brown, Boston, MA) contains the text of 20 medical manuals and handbooks. The PDR on CD ROM (Medical Economics Data, Montvale, NJ) contains the *Physicians' Desk Reference* and *Merck Manual*. Food and Drug Administration documents are available on FDA ON DISC (Food and Drug Administration, Rockville, MD). AIDS DISC (Macmillan New Media, Cambridge, MA) contains full text articles from a number of journals on the topic of acquired immunodeficiency syndrome (AIDS). Other products contain complete versions from recent years of the *American Family Physician, New England Journal of Medicine, Journal of the American Medical Association, Pediatrics, The Lancet, Morbidity and Mortality Weekly Report, Annals of Internal Medicine*, and other leading medical journals (Creative Multimedia Corporation, Portland, OR; and Macmillan New Media, Cambridge, MA). SAM-CD (Scientific American, New York, NY) contains the textbook *Scientific American Medicine*, which is updated quarterly. FAMILY PRACTICE RECERTIFICATION and CLINICAL DERMATOLOGY ILLUSTRATED (CME Associates, San Diego, CA) are true multimedia products, containing text, pictures, and speech. A truly versatile product for family physicians is STAT! REF PRIMARY CARE (Teton Data Systems, Jackson, WY). This product combines the full text from a number of textbooks, including *Williams Obstetrics, The Medical Letter, Scientific American Medicine*, and journal citations, including abstracts from 20 journals relevant for primary care.

For physicians who have yet to incorporate CD-ROM technology, a variety of educational products are available on traditional floppy disks. ELECTRONIC DRUG REFERENCE (Clinical Reference Systems, Englewood, CO) provides a variety of information about thousands of medications. CODE TEAM!, CARDIAC ARREST (Mad Scientist Software, Alpine, UT), and RHYTHM & PULSE (AneSoft Corp, Bellevue, WA) are teaching tools and simulations for advanced cardiac life support.

Information resources are also available on pocket-sized computers. The Pocket PDR (Medical Economics, Montvale, NJ) consists of a palmtop computer with access to information on every drug described in the *Physicians' Desk Reference*. The Franklin Digital Book System (Franklin Electronic Publishers, Mount Holly, NJ) offers the *Washington Manual of Medical Therapeutics, The Medical Letter Handbook of Adverse Drug Interactions*, and the *Physicians's Desk Reference* on a computer the size of an index card.

Continuing Education

Several software products have been developed to provide continuing medical education for family physicians and secure CME credits for their use (Chao, 1992). DISCOTEST (Scientific American Medicine, New York, NY) is a series of CME programs based on information in *Scientific American Medicine*. The programs provide simulations of patient management problems and multiple choice questions.

CYBERLOG (Cardinal Health Systems, Edina, MN) combines printed text and computer-based tutorials, case studies, and tools for a number of clinical problems. The tutorials use graphics to enhance the material in the printed text. Case studies provide brief patient simulations. The tools are formulas, tables, and diagrams that can be used in the CME exercises and in clinical practice.

Patient Simulator II (Knowledge House, Halifax, Nova Scotia, Canada) provides advanced simulations, evaluation of the user's diagnostic reasoning, and a list of literature references for several common primary care problems. The RxDx series (Williams & Wilkins, Baltimore, MD) is another series of self-paced instructional programs that allow CME credit for the user.

On-Line Information Resources

Modems and modern telecommunication software bring the world of on-line interactive computing to the physician with a modest investment in hardware, software, and user training. Several on-line services can be useful for physicians.

The INTERNET is a world-wide, high speed computer network that connects millions of users. Initially designed for academic and government use, the INTERNET has been opened for use by private corporations and individuals. The INTERNET contains many services useful for the primary care physician: worldwide electronic mail, electronic news services, file search services, file transfer services, bulletin boards, and many others. INTERNET has historically been accessed through academic computing centers but is now available through general on-line information services, which are discussed below.

US HEALTH LINK—An On-Line Information Service for Health Professionals (Wheaton, IL) is an electronic information service for health professionals. The service provides a number of literature retrieval, communication, and interactive services. EMPIRES and MEDLINE both provide access to citations of articles in hundreds of medical journals. CINAHL is a database of the allied health literature. The Comtex News Service contains summaries of domestic and international news wires. A clipping service is available that monitors new additions on user-designated subjects to the EMPIRES, MEDLINE, and News Service databases. The CME database contains information on national and international CME courses. Electronic mail and electronic bulletin boards are also available. US HEALTH LINK also includes DXPlain, a diagnostic support system, MEDI-COM, a drug interaction package, several specific expert systems, and patient simulation modules. PHYSICIANS' ON LINE (Coconut Computing, Terrytown, NY) is a free electronic information service that includes electronic mail and provides access to MEDLINE, QMR, AIDSLINE references on AIDS, GEN Rx references on drugs and AIDS-DRUGS/AIDSTRIALS databases on AIDS drugs and clinical trials.

COMPUSERVE (Columbus, OH), PRODIGY (Dallas, TX), and AMERICA ONLINE (Vienna, VA) are general purpose personal computer networks. They all provide numerous online services, including news, sports, weather, electronic mail, references, shopping, financial information, travel, entertainment, and games. Each network also provides a gateway to the INTERNET and access to thousand of public domain software programs. COMPUSERVE has numerous special interest forums, including a medical forum. Forums contain both bulletin boards, which facilitate communication with others with similar interests, and libraries of documents and software. Access to the MEDLINE and other health-related databases is also available on COMPUSERVE. PRODIGY is known for its family orientation and colorful, graphic user interface. AMERICA ONLINE also has a friendly user interface.

SELECTING AN OFFICE-BASED COMPUTER SYSTEM

The process of selecting an office-based computer system can be difficult for physicians. Physicians are generally not trained to evaluate computer systems, and their cost can be considerable. In addition, as outlined earlier, there are many applications for office-based computing and many products on the market for each application. Nonetheless, the benefits of office automation are dramatic, and a structured approach to the selection process may be useful.

The first step is to perform a careful needs assessment. A review of practice procedures combined with the information provided earlier should help physicians and their office staffs decide which aspects of office automation they wish to pursue.

More detailed information on specific applications can be obtained from software vendors, examination of demonstration programs, reading pertinent literature about particular products, and professional colleagues who have already automated their offices. It is a good idea to prepare a written summary of the practice's needs, although in most cases a formal request for proposal is not necessary.

The next step is to contact vendors and arrange system demonstrations for the most crucial applications desired. Usually, the crucial applications are the office-management software products (billing, appointment scheduling, and patient records). If the practice is interested in incorporating other clinical and educational products, discussion with office management software vendors should be directed toward the optimal way of interfacing the applications selected.

After these demonstrations, detailed proposals should be requested from suitable vendors. Proposals should be evaluated and ranked by physicians and office staff. Vendors with the top ranked systems should be invited back for second demonstrations; and vendor references, from similar sites, should be checked. In addition to hardware and software features, other important considerations to discuss with both vendors and their references are the vendor support and user training, the financial stability of the vendor, system speed and reliability, ease of system maintenance, system security of confidential patient data, required system downtime, remote access capabilities, and the ability of the system to grow with the practice. Financial considerations are also important, as prices for similar applications can vary widely, and vendors often have room to negotiate. If capital for the purchase is not readily available, leasing arrangements for software, hardware, and even installation services can be arranged.

Other technical factors are also important when choosing practice management software. If possible, all software and hardware should be purchased from a single vendor, so there is clear responsibility if problems occur. At the least, software vendors should be consulted about suitable hardware. Although there is some appeal to selecting hardware based on price, it is important to remember that unreliable products are costly in terms of lost staff productivity and lost data. Because long-term support is important, standard equipment and operating systems should be selected. Current standards include IBM (International Business Machines, Boca Raton, FL) compatible microcomputers running MS-DOS or Windows (Microsoft, Seattle, WA) or Unix. These machines can be stand-alone or networked together using Netware (Novell, Provo, UT), LANtastic (Artisoft, Tuscon, AZ), or Windows NT (Microsoft, Seattle, WA); Unix machines are all multiuser. Apple Macintosh (Apple, Brea, CA) machines are also good stand-alone choices, although software availability is more limited. Larger systems may use RISC (Reduced Instruction Set Computing) machines from IBM or DEC (Digital Equipment Corporation, Maynard, MA). Even small offices should consider multiuser solutions, as allowing more than one person to use the computer often saves time and enhances staff efficiency. Practices should buy more hard disk storage than originally considered because required hard drive storage capacity is usually underestimated. A tape backup unit is essential for easy system backups. The tape backup capacity should be greater than the capacity of the hard drive; units with more than 4000 megabytes in capacity are readily available.

Practice management software should be selected with growth in mind. It is important to select systems that can easily be expanded. A vendor who provides a full spectrum of office management software, including patient records, is probably the best choice, even if patient and insurance billing is the only application purchased initially.

Careful management of the change process is critical to ensuring successful integration of office management software. Office personnel must be actively involved in the training process and given sufficient time and support; training almost always takes much longer than vendors indicate. Installation of a new computer system is often a good time to carefully consider office procedures and eliminate inefficient practices.

A new practice provides a wonderful opportunity for implementing a full range of office management software, including patient records and a variety of educational products. Complete automation at the time the practice opens is the best option, as there is immediate cost savings in supplies (charts, racks, paper), storage space, and the need for traditional clinical references and patient education materials. Staff who are comfortable with computers can be selected and roles and practice procedures designed around the automated systems.

OFFICE-BASED MEDICAL COMPUTING OF THE FUTURE

Three trends are likely to affect the future of office-based medical computing: hardware advances, software developments, and connectivity. The rapid pace of computer hardware development is likely to continue. Computers that filled entire rooms and cost millions of dollars a generation ago have been replaced by desktop machines in the thousand dollar price range. Likely advances in the future include continued miniaturization of hardware, patient-carried "health cards" with critical information, more user-friendly input options such as voice, and improved and less costly multimedia computers that permit the simultaneous dis-

play of data, graphics, full-motion video, and voice. Software development and dissemination will likely accelerate as well. Computer-based patient records, primary-care diagnostic support systems, medical references, and patient education tools will all undergo evolution and hopefully become more integrated with one another. The connectivity of computer systems will advance on many levels: in the office, between the office and affiliated ancillary services and hospitals, on a community-wide basis, and on national and even international levels. The likely development of health care alliances and the nation's information superhighway will both mandate and facilitate this process of connectivity.

These developments in hardware, software, and connectivity will synergize each other and catalyze the further dissemination of computer technology into office practice. The primary care physician's office during the early twenty-first century will likely be filled with high-technology, low cost, well integrated information systems. These systems will provide the physician with myriad crucial information needs (Table 65–2). Rapid access to all relevant patient information will be possible through patient-carried health cards and health information networks. Diagnostic and therapeutic support at the point of patient care will be available through primary care-oriented expert systems. User-friendly data-entry tools such as voice recognition will permit immediate updating of the patient record. Introspective audits will be possible to improve the quality of care by reminding physicians of patient-specific interventions that are needed (e.g., biochemical monitoring in patients on specific medications or with certain disease states, screening tests on patients with genetic profiles demonstrating high risk for certain diseases). Multimedia education systems, including those that possess "virtual reality" technology will improve the quality and enjoyment of continuing education for physicians and education for patients. Ready access to consultants through two-way electronic highways will allow the primary care physician to take a more comprehensive role

---

TABLE 65–2. CAPABILITIES OF THE COMPUTERIZED PRIMARY CARE OFFICE OF THE EARLY TWENTY-FIRST CENTURY

1. Rapid access to all relevant patient information through patient carried health cards and health information networks
2. Diagnostic and therapeutic support at the point of patient care
3. Immediate updating of patient record
4. Quality of care audits and reminders
5. Multimedia physician and patient education systems
6. Ready access to consultants through two-way electronic highways for diagnostic and therapeutic assistance
7. Support for home-care through patient monitoring devices
8. Ability for collaboration in multisite research projects

in patient care. For example, a specialist in a distant city could consult, using full-motion video and voice, at the time the primary care physician is evaluating a patient. Not only will this technology permit immediate diagnostic decision support, but the consultant could also assist the primary care physician in the provision of certain procedures. Similar support for home care through two-way video and patient monitoring devices will be employed to shorten hospital stays and decrease the need for office visits, allowing patients to be cared for in the comfort of their homes. These advances will improve the quality of medical care and provide the primary care physician with the opportunity to collaborate in important multisite research projects on many aspects of clinical, epidemiologic, educational, and health services research.

The pace of change in the field of office-based medical computing is so rapid that the average physician will have difficulty maintaining an awareness of available options. The reader is encouraged to stay current by reading reviews (on paper or electronic media) in medical journals such as the *Journal of Family Practice, Journal of the American Medical Association,* and elsewhere. MEDICAL SOFTWARE REVIEWS (Healthcare Computing Publications, Brooklyn, NY) is a monthly publication that evaluates technology and compares medical software packages. In addition, the journal *M.D. Computing* (Springer-Verlag, New York, NY) publishes an annual directory of medical hardware and software products. The directory contains information on hundreds of products and companies. In addition, there is a software product intended to serve as a centralized resource on medical computing. COMPUTER INSIGHT, MD (Resource Systems Management, Inc., Boulder, CO) contains information on 1000 clinically useful computer programs. Finally, many national and regional continuing education meetings now have sessions on this subject.

REFERENCES

Barnett GO, Winickoff RN, Morgan MM, et al: A computer-based monitoring system for follow-up of elevated blood pressure. Med Care 21:400, 1983.

Bouckaert A, Lambrechts H, Reveillon M: Portable medical records on microchip cards: The Tournai experiment. Med Inform 17:257, 1992.

Brooks GJ, Ashton RE, Pethybridge RJ: DERMIS: A computer system for assisting primary-care physicians with dermatological diagnosis. Br J Dermatol 127:614, 1992.

Chao J: Continuing medical education software: A comparative review. J Fam Pract 34:598, 1992.

Dick RS, Steen EB (eds): The computer-based patient record: An essential technology for health care. Washington, DC, National Academy Press, 1991.

Ebell MH: CD-ROM: A primer for physicians. J Fam Pract 37: 483, 1993.

Garr DR, Ornstein SM, Jenkins RG, et al: The effect of routine use of computer-generated preventive reminders in a clinical practice. Am J Prev Med 9:55, 1993.

Hammond KW, Prather RJ, Date VV, et al: A provider-interactive medical record system can favorably influence costs and quality of medical care. Comput Biol Med 20:267, 1990.

McPhee SJ, Bird JA, Jenkins CNH, et al: Promoting cancer screening: A randomized, controlled trial of three interventions. Arch Intern Med 149:1866, 1989.

Ornstein SM, Garr DR, Jenkins RG, et al: Computer-generated physician and patient reminders: Tools to improve population adherence with selected preventive services. J Fam Pract 32:82, 1991.

Ornstein SM, Oates RB, Fox GA: The computer-based medical record: Current status. J Fam Pract 35:556, 1992.

Ornstein SM, Garr DR, Jenkins RG: A Comprehensive Microcomputer-Based Medical Records Preventive Services System for the Family Physician. J Am Board Fam Pract 6(1): 1, 1993.

Sumner W: A review of Iliad and Quick Medical Reference for Primary Care Providers. Arch Fam Med 2:87, 1993.

Tierney WM, Hui SL, McDonald CJ: Delayed feedback of physician performance versus immediate reminders to perform preventive care: Events on physician compliance. Med Care 24:659, 1986.

United States General Accounting Office: Report to the Chairman, Committee on Governmental Affairs, U.S. Senate. Medical ADP Systems: Automated medical records hold promise to improve patient care. January 1991.

Weed LL: Knowledge Coupling. New Premises and New Tools for Medical Care and Education. New York, Springer-Verlag, 1991.

CHAPTER 66

MALPRACTICE AND RISK MANAGEMENT

RICHARD G. ROBERTS

Few topics inflame the passions of physicians as much as medical malpractice. Professional liability issues touch every physician. Malpractice concerns shape the practice of medicine and, in turn, affect the access to and cost of medical care. Recognizing the public import of malpractice, the United States Congress, multiple federal agencies, and the legislatures of all 50 states have addressed the issue of medical liability since the 1970s. Despite the attention and resources that have been devoted to the study of medical malpractice, the problem looms more complex, controversial, and costly than ever.

Physicians are frustrated by their collective inability to remedy the professional liability problem. When confronted by clinical challenges, physicians collect and analyze patient data and then formulate and implement an action plan. When confounded by courthouse condemnations, physicians suffer significant physical and emotional symptoms and alter their practices (Charles et al., 1984). For physicians, the medical malpractice drama is played out on an unfamiliar stage before judges, juries, and legislatures. Forced to read from a script they had no hand in drafting and that is in an alien (legal) language they do not comprehend, physicians feel a loss of control and respond with indignation. In this way, however, physicians are similar to patients who believe they were treated unfairly or incompetently by the equally mysterious medical care system. Not surprisingly, "physician expectations about the professional liability system are often as unrealistic as their patients' expectations about medicine" (United States Department of Health and Human Services, 1987).

To regain control of the malpractice colossus, physicians must better inform themselves of the nature and dimensions of the problem and be willing to take a fresh look at its complexities. Adlai Stevenson once said, "If we value the pursuit of knowledge, we must be free to follow wherever that search may lead us." This chapter is dedicated to that search. The dimensions and history of malpractice are examined, along with a discussion of possible solutions. The chapter then focuses on risk management as the means by which the individual family physician can have the greatest impact on malpractice prevention. Risk management issues are viewed from a general perspective, a systems (treatment setting and payment) perspective, and a focused perspective by analyzing those areas of practice that pose the greatest liability risks for the family physician.

MEDICAL MALPRACTICE PROBLEM

Dimensions of Malpractice

When engaged in a debate on professional liability, physicians find it disconcerting that not everyone agrees with the premise that there is a medical malpractice crisis. The Association of Trial Lawyers of America (ATLA) has argued that the "crisis" is really a malpractice insurance crisis, not a malpractice litigation crisis (Association of Trial Lawyers of America, 1984). ATLA also contended that the crisis is the result of "a few bad doctors." Support for this contention is found in a 4-year study of Los Angeles County physicians during the 1970s where 46 doctors (0.6 per cent of the 8000) were named in 10 per cent of the suits and were responsible for 30 per cent of all payments made (Phelps, 1977).

There is good evidence to suggest that there is more negligence committed than is ever recognized, litigated, or compensated. A frequently cited study is the Medical Insurance Feasibility Study (MIFS) conducted in 1974 by the California Medical Association and California Hospital Association (California Medical Association, 1977). The MIFS involved the review of 20,864 California hospital admissions in 1974. That study found that 4.65 per cent of admissions involved potentially compensable events (PCEs). A PCE was defined as a disability caused by health care management. The authors concluded that only 0.79 per cent of all hospital admissions represented PCEs that were accompanied by evidence sufficient to establish claims of legal liability (i.e., negligence), as there were many PCEs that were thought to be nonpreventable. Nevertheless, these 0.79 per cent legally viable PCEs, when extrapolated to the 3,011,000 California hospital admissions in 1974, could have resulted in 23,000 lawsuits. It was estimated however, that only 1 in 10 of the patients with a legally meritorious PCE ever filed a claim and only 1 in 25 ever received any compensation. The results of this important study are used to support the contention that there is more malpractice committed than is compensated and that a no-fault approach to medical negligence might be prohibitively more expensive that the current fault-based tort system.

The findings of the MIFS have been confirmed recently by the Harvard Medical Practice Study (Localio et al., 1991). The Harvard group reviewed the records of more than 30,000 patients who were hospitalized in New York State during 1984. Physician reviewers determined that about 1 per cent of hospitalized patients suffered an adverse outcome due to medical negligence. However, of the 280 patients who had adverse events caused by negligence, only 8 (1.5 per cent) filed suit. The study group estimated that only 1 in 8 negligently injured patients sued and only 1 in 16 ever recovered damages.

Other appraisals of the number of negligently injured patients who pursue a malpractice action range from 1 in 6 (Schwartz and Komesar, 1978) to 1 in 15 (Pocincki et al., 1973). Trial attorneys are estimated to turn away approximately three of every four possible malpractice cases because the basis for liability is thought to be too difficult to prove or the award potential too small (Somers, 1977).

Increased Frequency of Suits

The number of malpractice suits against physicians has been on the rise. In 1981 there were 3.2 claims per 100 physicians, rising to 7.4 per 100 doctors in 1989 (American Medical Association, 1992). Since the mid-1970s, the number of claims filed each year has increased 10 to 20 per cent, although many states experienced a plateau or even a small decrease in the frequency of claims during the late 1980s.

Increased Size of Awards

The largest malpractice award paid out in the United States through 1956 was $230,000, which equated to about $1 million in 1984 dollars when inflation was factored in. By 1984 there were several birth injury claims with ultimate payouts in excess of $100 million. Average paid losses increased 300 per cent from $42,000 in 1981 (Reynolds et al., 1987) to $130,000 in 1992. Over the past decade the annual growth in the size of malpractice awards has averaged 20 to 30 per cent.

Increased Liability Insurance Premiums

Given the increasing frequency of suits and the increasing size of awards, it is not surprising that malpractice insurance premiums have continued to rise. Physicians paid an estimated $5.9 billion in premiums in 1990. Annual malpractice premiums now approach $200,000 for some practitioners (United States General Accounting Office, 1993). A survey by the American Academy of Family Physicians in 1992 reported that family physicians paid an average premium of approximately $6000 ($12,000 if they delivered babies). However, some contend that these numbers are misleading in that physicians continue to spend only about 4 per cent of their gross revenues on liability insurance premiums (Bovbjerg and Havighurst, 1985). Malpractice premiums appear to rise and plateau in cycles, tied more to the investment economy than to the malpractice loss experience. Moreover, it is argued, although the physician is the one who initially shoulders the burden of the premium rise, it is ultimately the public that pays for the rise in the form of higher medical care costs.

Costs of Medical Malpractice

In addition to the premiums that doctors pay, malpractice generates other costs. Defensive medicine practices are those changes in physician behavior (e.g., additional time spent with the patient, extra record-keeping, more laboratory or diagnostic procedures) that are medically unwarranted but are intended to reduce the probability of a malpractice suit. It is estimated by some that medicine practices cost health care consumers an extra $15 billion per year (Reynolds et al., 1987). More recent estimates raise doubts however, as to the economic impact of defensive medicine (United States Congressional Budget Office, 1993). Another malpractice cost is the loss of physician time spent in litigation activities (e.g., attorney meetings, depositions, at trial).

There are additional medical liability costs that are not as directly apparent. Many believe that physicians have become increasingly wary of their patients, viewing them as potential plaintiffs who must be kept "at arm's length." This wariness may not serve the patient's best interest in that it can hinder the sense of mutual commitment and trust that the therapeutic alliance demands.

The writings of psychiatrist Sara Charles, a leading authority on the response of physicians to the malpractice crisis, have alerted the public to another less obvious cost: As a result of being named in a malpractice suit, 96 per cent of physicians suffer physical or emotional symptoms, 62 per cent order extra tests for "protection," 42 per cent stop seeing certain types of patients, 28 per cent stop performing certain procedures, and 57 per cent believe their families suffer (Charles et al., 1984). Charles concluded "that malpractice litigation, the chronic character of involvement with the legal process, and the resultant stress on both sued and nonsued physicians may in the long run not serve the public interest or the quality of medicine. It may diminish rather than enhance the integrity and availability of medical care" (Charles et al., 1985). Other writers have noted that the threat or fear of a malpractice claim may be more stressful than an actual claim (Connelly, 1988).

The indirect malpractice costs that seem to most interest the public and lawmakers relate to the affordability and availability of medical care. The detrimental impact of malpractice issues on the cost of and access to medical care is most evident in maternity care. The American College of Obstetricians and Gynecologists (ACOG) has calculated that obstetricians who completed training in 1986 would be named in an average of eight suits during their careers. A 1992 survey of ACOG members revealed that one of eight had recently quit obstetrics because of malpractice concerns; about one in four had decreased their level of high risk pregnancy care. A similar survey reported that nearly 60 per cent of family physicians had given up delivering babies because of malpractice fears (American Medical Association, 1992). One study projected that 50 per cent of family physicians discontinue maternity care when their malpractice premiums rise to $12,000 (Rosenblatt and Wright, 1987). These changes in physician practices have decreased access to quality care for pregnant women. Ironically, family physicians who provide maternity care appear to be sued less often, perform more procedures, and enjoy more diverse, personally satisfying and financially rewarding practices than those who do not (Larimore, 1994).

History of Malpractice

To clarify the reasons for the current medical malpractice system, a brief review of the history of malpractice is in order. Malpractice issues have shadowed physicians for millennia. Physicians were originally held to a standard of strict liability: If the results were less than desired, the physician was held liable. No matter that the physician had put forward a best effort or that the patient was so ill that no physician could have effected a cure, the physician was liable and the penalties could be severe. The Code of Hammurabi, promulgated in Babylonia around 2000 BC, mandated that if a physician treated a patient "and caused him to die, one shall cut off the doctor's hands" (Ghitelman, 1987). Roman law later distinguished between acts involving *dolus* (malice) and *culpa* (negligence).

The first malpractice case recorded in the English courts occurred in 1329. The first medical liability claim recorded by an American appeals court was *Cross v. Guthrey*, 2 Root 90 (Conn., 1794). By the mid-1800s, malpractice suits had become so frequent that many physicians were no longer performing certain types of surgery. The crisis abated during the Reconstruction Era but began to resurface at the turn of the century. State medical societies became active in the defense of malpractice

claims and had an enviable record of successful defenses during the early 1900s. After World War II, the number of suits began to rise sharply, and the trend upward continues today. The common thread appears to be that when times are prosperous, more people can afford medical care, resulting in more potential exposures to iatrogenic injury and more malpractice litigation.

The watershed year of 1975 saw a number of insurance carriers refusing to underwrite doctors. Up until that time, medical malpractice was not even reported separately, with companies treating it as any other line of property and casualty insurance. The 1975 crisis stimulated a number of state legislatures to pass medical malpractice tort reform packages. In addition, physicians responded to the exit of the commercial carriers by forming doctor-owned professional liability companies, which now insure most U.S. physicians. The tort reforms of 1975 provided only a temporary respite, as malpractice claims became more frequent and costly by the early 1980s, triggering steep increases in malpractice insurance premiums. The cyclic nature of malpractice litigation was demonstrated again during the late 1980s and early 1990s with a moderation in the frequency of malpractice cases and insurance premium costs.

Elements of Malpractice

Most malpractice suits against doctors involve claims of negligence, rather than breach of contract, battery, product liability, or other legal theories. For defendant physicians, malpractice litigation appears to be a dark abyss into which they are about to fall. To plaintiff attorneys, a malpractice suit seems an insurmountable mountain to be climbed. The plaintiff has the burden of proving, with evidence, the following four elements in order to prevail in a malpractice case: duty, injury, negligence, and proximate cause.

Duty

A physician has a duty to exercise reasonable care when undertaking the treatment of a patient. That duty is said to exist only when there is a doctor–patient relationship. A physician is not obliged to enter into a doctor–patient relationship with any person simply because that person desires to become that doctor's patient. Physicians, like everyone else, have the right to decide to whom they will provide professional services.

There are, however, limits placed on the doctor's right to decide. For example, a physician may not abandon an established patient, nor may a physician refuse treatment to a patient who has relied reasonably on the doctor's apparent willingness to treat all-comers (e.g., the emergency department physician in a general hospital that advertises its emergency services). When a doctor wishes to terminate an established relationship with a patient, he or she must make available alternative and equivalent medical coverage until the patient has had a reasonable opportunity to establish a new doctor–patient relationship (2 weeks is customarily considered reasonable). Similarly, when an on-duty emergency department physician seeks to avoid entering into a professional relationship with a particular patient, he or she is obliged to make arrangements for another physician to attend to that patient's emergency needs. When it is not reasonable for a patient to expect or rely on the services of a particular physician (e.g., when the doctor is a passerby at the scene of an accident on a roadway), the physician has no duty to offer assistance and the patient has no right to demand treatment. Although codes of medical ethics may denounce the physician's driving past the accident victim, the law does not require that the doctor stop and help the victim.

The physician must use caution when offering medical advice. For example, a California doctor was sued successfully by a patient he had never met. The patient called the physician one evening and requested advice regarding the atypical chest pain that he was suffering. The doctor advised the patient that his symptoms could probably wait until the young man's personal physician became available the next morning. The patient was later found to be in the midst of an anterior wall myocardial infarction and suffered complications that he alleged were due to the falsely reassuring advice given to him over the telephone. Despite the fact that the doctor had never met nor sent a bill to the patient, the physician was adjudged negligent and assessed damages for failing to perform an adequate evaluation (i.e., a sufficient history and physical examination) before providing telephone advice that the patient *relied* on. The crucial issue was whether a reasonable patient was in a position to rely on the doctor's advice. If the patient was reasonable in relying on the doctor, a doctor–patient relationship was said to exist, and the physician owed the patient a duty to provide reasonable care—to provide the same level of expertise and care that he would for any of his usual patients, regardless of whether a fee was charged or paid.

Injury

The plaintiff must prove an injury resulted from the doctor's negligence. Most plaintiffs have obvious injuries; frivolous claims for trivial injuries are uncommon. A federal study of more than 73,000 closed claims reported that only 15.7 per cent of claimants had solely emotional or insignificant injuries—all others had disability or death (United States General Accounting Office, 1987).

Negligence

Doctors are not guarantors of perfect results. They are only required to perform at a level equiv-

alent to that of a similar practitioner. The difficulty is over how to decide the adequacy of the physician's performance, given the medical inexperience of the jury asked to decide such issues. Aristotle recommended that physicians should be the ones to decide cases of malpractice (Amundson, 1977). In fifteenth century London, when guilds held authority over the various trades, physicians were obliged to present all serious cases to guild leaders within a few days after initiating treatment. If guild leaders thought that the physician's treatment was acceptable, the doctor was provided a solid defense against any malpractice claims (Walton, 1985). The concept that it must be other physicians who determine the appropriateness of a particular physician's treatment is crucial to an understanding of malpractice. A patient cannot successfully sue a doctor unless another physician, an expert witness, is willing to testify for the plaintiff that the defendant doctor failed to meet the standard of care.

The standard of care is "that degree of care and skill which is exercised by the average practitioner in the same or similar circumstances" (*Shier v. Freedman*, 58 Wis.2d 269, 206 N.W.2d 166, 1973). It is important to note that the physician is expected to perform at a level similar to that of the *average*, not *best*, practitioner. Physician-experts and juries are often confused by this point and attempt to impose the highest standard of care. Early on, physicians were held to the standard of care that was exhibited in their own communities. However, as professional isolation became less of a problem, physicians were held increasingly to a specialty or national, rather than local, standard of care. One particularly vexing problem for family physicians is that the physician-experts testifying against them may be of a different specialty (e.g., an orthopedist testifying against a family physician's management of a Colle's fracture). Whereas some argue that only a family physician can testify against another family physician, others contend that any physician with experience managing the condition in question should be able to testify as to the standard of care. Finally, there have been cases where the court has imposed its own standard of care, believing the profession's standard to be inadequate. "Custom is relevant in determining the standard of care because it illustrates what is feasible, it suggests a body of knowledge of which the defendant should be aware and it warns of the possibility of far-reaching consequences if a higher standard is required. . . . But custom should never be conclusive." (*Darling v. Charleston Community Memorial Hospital*, 33 Ill.2d 326, 211 N.W.2d 253, 1965).

Proximate Cause

The final element that the plaintiff must prove is that the negligent performance of the physician was the proximate cause of the patient's injury. The plaintiff must first show that the doctor's negligence was the cause in fact of the alleged injury. Two formulas can be used to demonstrate cause in fact: (1) "but for"—the injury would not have occurred but for the negligence; or (2) "substantial factor"—when several possible causes exist (e.g., the patient failed to keep the appointment and the doctor misread the radiograph), the doctor's error was a substantial factor in the resultant injury. Once cause in fact has been proved, the plaintiff must prove that the defendant's mistake was so closely connected in time and space and of such significance that legal liability should be imposed (i.e., proximate cause).

For example, if a surgeon amputates the wrong limb, the patient would be able to show that the injury (the amputation) would not have occurred but for the doctor's mistake and that the error was of such significance that liability should be imposed. Proximate cause becomes a more elusive concept, however, when the patient's original prognosis was poor. As an example, a smoker presents with an abnormal chest radiograph and hip pain that 2 months later are diagnosed as metastatic bronchogenic carcinoma. The physician's failure to diagnose the cancer for 2 months could be said to have reduced the patient's chance for survival, but the chance for survival was poor even at the first visit. Traditionally, the patient could not prevail on the causation question unless the prenegligence odds for survival were more likely than not (i.e., greater than 50 per cent probability). In the bronchogenic carcinoma example, the patient's chance for survival was less than 50 per cent, even at the first visit. Therefore under traditional doctrine the doctor would not be held liable for failure to diagnose the cancer at the first visit. However, some jurisdictions have begun to recognize that no matter how poor the patient's chances of survival were at the first visit they were reduced by some amount because of the doctor's delayed diagnosis. This "loss of a chance" doctrine further complicates the causation question (Shoenberger, 1985). The proof of causation usually requires expert testimony. There are certain acts, however, where the negligence and causation are so obvious that a lay jury is deemed able to make that determination (e.g., a hemostat unintentionally left behind in the abdomen). In such cases, the doctrine of res ipsa loquitur ("the thing speaks for itself") is invoked and no expert testimony is required. The burden of proof then shifts to the defendant to show mitigating circumstances in order to avoid liability.

Possible Solutions

It is not surprising, given the complexity of medical malpractice, that there are no simple solutions. Each malpractice crisis has stimulated change that temporized events until the next crisis arose. The better physicians do, the better patients expect them to do. A smarter defense bar is matched by a shrewder plaintiffs' bar. Tort reforms are diluted by constitutional challenges, mercurial legislatures, sympathetic juries, and judges persuaded by new theories of legal liability. Advances in medical science empower physicians to do more, exposing patients to greater risks of iatrogenesis, and to do better, inspiring patients to expect better. The multifactorial nature of medical malpractice demands a multifaceted approach.

Public Education

Rising and unrealistic patient expectations engender patient dissatisfaction. All members of society (physicians, media, public) share a responsibility to equilibrate patients' hopes with medicine's realities.

Improved Legal Defense

Doctors must actively participate in their defense. There are several excellent references that guide the defendant-doctor through the litigation process (American College of Obstetricians and Gynecologists, 1986; Gass, 1984). Physicians must help their defense counsel to stay current with advances in medical knowledge. The defense bar needs to better update its members on innovative defenses and changing medical theory and practice.

Change the Dispute Resolution (Tort) System

Most appealing to physicians is the proposal to change the tort system. Many believe that the current litigation system is too destructive, expensive, inefficient, and unfair. For example, only 20 to 30 cents from every malpractice premium dollar goes to the successful plaintiff-patient; the other 70 to 80 cents is consumed by administrative fees, court costs, expert witness fees, and defense and plaintiff attorney charges. The experience in California following passage of its Medical Injury Compensation Reform Act (MICRA) legislation in 1975 suggests that certain tort reforms help to moderate premium increases: from 1975 to 1986 California went from one of the ten most expensive to one of the ten least expensive states for malpractice premiums. On average, states can expect that capping awards will decrease the severity of malpractice claims by 23 per cent; allowing the offset of collateral benefits will reduce claim frequency by 14 per cent and severity by 11 to 18 per cent; and trimming statutes of limitation by 1 year will cut claim frequency by 8 per cent (Danzon, 1986). Danzon's studies however, disprove several commonly held beliefs: limits on attorney contingency fees, per capita income, and the number of attorneys per capita have no statistically significant effect on malpractice claims frequency or severity. The degree of urbanization and the number of doctors, not lawyers, are the most powerful predictors of malpractice litigation for an area. Studies also refute the notion that the poor are more likely to sue; in fact, they are significantly less likely to sue for medical negligence (Burstin et al., 1993). Finally, juries do appear to decide cases based on the doctor's quality of care rather than the patient's severity of injuries (Taragin et al., 1992).

Tort system changes that intuitively seem prudent may not produce their desired results. Moreover, although tort reforms may provide some stabilization of premiums, their effect is temporary. As demonstrated over the past 60 years, increasing medical care utilization and improving technology, with its additional risk for iatrogenesis and rising patient expectations, drive up malpractice premiums at a 20 per cent per annum rate, regardless of tort reform. Therefore physicians should be clear in their understanding of the implications of tort reform proposals before advocating focused or wholesale changes (Abraham, 1988).

Health System Reform and Malpractice

The impact of medical malpractice on the quality and cost of care and the access to services obliges any proposal for health system reform to address the issue of professional liability if it is to be taken seriously. A number of proposals at the federal and state levels incorporate the California MICRA provisions: $250,000 cap on noneconomic awards; sliding scale on attorney's contingency fees; periodic, rather than lump sum, payment of awards; and elimination of the collateral source, or double payment, rule. Alternate dispute resolution (ADR) systems, such as pretrial mediation or arbitration panels, have also been proposed.

Some have advocated entirely new approaches to medical negligence. The Clinton health reform plan has recommended using enterprise liability in a few pilot states. Enterprise liability shifts the focus of litigation from an individual doctor to the entire enterprise that cares for the patient (i.e., doctor, hospital, nurses). The arguable advantages to this approach are that no one person is accused (individuals are therefore more willing to cooperate to ascertain what really happened and to make the patient whole) and that medical care has become so complex that it is more efficient for the "system of care" to ensure quality, rather than any one provider. Others contend that professional autonomy and judgment could be undermined by such a system and that overall costs would increase (Peters and Johnson, 1993).

Another approach proposed is to move to a "no-fault" system where certain injuries are designated compensable. For example, Virginia and Florida have enacted no fault birth injury compensation acts, although their experience is too recent to declare success or failure. A modification of the no-fault system would designate accelerated compensation events (ACEs). ACEs represent predefined classes of medical injuries that do not normally occur when patients receive good care (Tancredi and Bovbjerg, 1992). The putative benefits of an ACE system would be more widespread and fair compensation of injured patients; more effective deterrence of poor quality by the system of care; reduction of defensive medicine; standardization of medical expertise about injuries; an opportunity to strengthen the doctor–patient relationship; the framework for outcomes research; and greater confidence in the accuracy and fairness of malpractice determinations. The limitations of this approach are the difficulty of developing consensus on which events should be compensated, the uncertainty about whether this approach would address a sufficient percentage of potential liability claims, and the cost and bureaucracy inherent in such a system.

Several states have used guidelines as a strategy to lower malpractice costs. These states (e.g., Maine, Minnesota, Florida) protect the physician by providing an affirmative defense when state-approved practice guidelines were followed. There is evidence that the use of guidelines can lower iatrogenic injury and malpractice losses (Holzer, 1989). Whether a sufficient number of quality guidelines can be developed to be of legal value for the physician remains to be seen.

IMPROVE THE QUALITY OF MEDICAL PRACTICE

It may seem self-evident, but the individual physician is best able to reduce the risk of malpractice litigation by practicing personable, high quality medicine. Public education, improved legal defense, and tort reform are best accomplished by medical and other organizations. The profession can enhance the quality of medical practice through the development of scientifically validated standards of care, but it is the individual practitioner who must apply those standards. The best protection against a malpractice suit is a conscientious physician who practices reflective medicine, a style of practice that continuously recognizes medicine's ability to do harm, reflects on the patient's progress, and strives to keep the patient satisfied. For example, more than one third of general medicine patients admitted to hospital may suffer iatrogenic illnesses (Steel et al., 1981); and the cost of surgical misadventures can also be high (Couch et al., 1981). High quality medicine is reflective medicine; reflective medicine is the cornerstone of risk management.

RISK MANAGEMENT

General Perspective

As traditionally defined, risk management is an administrative undertaking designed to protect the financial assets of an organization. As applied to the health care system, risk management is the systematic process of identifying, evaluating, and addressing potential and actual risks. The health care industry spends more on risk management, as a percentage of assets, than any other industry (Monagle, 1985). A more practical definition for the clinician is that risk management is a style of practice that attempts to prevent and control patient injuries, malpractice claims, and malpractice claim losses (Sanders, 1987). Quality assurance and risk management are often used interchangeably, although quality assurance more typically involves problems (rather than risks), and it is less concerned with financial or legal consequences. More than 80 years ago, Codman (1914) urged the profession to reflect on the quality of medical practice. Since that time, several methods for evaluating the process and outcome of medical care have been developed: incident reporting systems (where an incident is any happening, with or without injury, involving a patient mishap or a patient's serious expression of dissatisfaction), generic outcome screens (where certain outcomes, such as maternal deaths, are always reviewed), and clinical indicators (where indicators, such as postoperative infection rates, can be used to highlight potential problem areas). Others outside the profession have become increasingly interested in the quality of care provided, including third party payers, such as the federal government and private insurers.

There are at least three elements to consider when evaluating quality of care: the process the physician used (e.g., tests ordered, procedures performed), the outcome achieved (e.g., cure, improvement, death), and the patient's satisfaction with the care provided. The first two elements are addressed by other chapters of this textbook; the third element, along with other general issues, is examined below. Each malpractice suit requires an unhappy patient. It is difficult, although not impossible, for patients to sue doctors they like. Physicians at the highest risk of suit have the following attributes: They are men, 40 to 45 years old, surgical specialists, uncomfortable with emotions, less likely to seek consultation, disparaging of others, and poor record-keepers. Doctors who spend more time with their patients per visit have fewer claims (Adams and Zuckerman, 1984). Most patients willingly wait 15 minutes for the doctor. When the waiting time is expected to exceed 30 minutes, the patient should be informed of the reason for the delay and should be offered an opportunity to reschedule.

Rapport must go beyond the physician; all members of the office staff (receptionist, nurse, business manager, bill collector) are crucial to the creation and maintenance of good patient relations. The patient's expectation of privacy and confidentiality must be respected by all members of the health care team. The family physician should be avail-

able, or make arrangements to have a competent colleague available, to handle any after-hours emergencies. The telephone can be both helpful and harmful for the physician. It can build patient rapport and enhance physician availability. Making a follow-up phone call shortly after a patient's hospital discharge speaks volumes; returning calls in a prompt and reliable fashion fosters trust; and calling test results promotes patient awareness. Telephone conversations should be documented, and the physician should not hesitate to insist on seeing the patient if advice cannot be given safely without examining the patient (Roberts, 1988).

Systems Perspective

The setting in which medical care is provided has an impact on malpractice risk. Four of five malpractice suits arise from hospital care; the remaining 20 per cent arise in the outpatient setting. Serious illness, high risk procedures, multiple caregivers with the potential for miscommunication, and loss of patient autonomy in a regimented routine increase the risk of an unhappy outcome for the hospitalized patient. The family physician is often able to enhance patient outcome and satisfaction through long-standing knowledge of the patient, coordination of care, and communication of the patient's progress to the family. In this way, the family physician can reduce the risk of an unsatisfactory result and subsequent litigation.

Although committees and other review entities have long safeguarded hospital quality, the assessment of ambulatory care adequacy is a nascent science (Kelly and Mamlin, 1974). Patients perceive the doctor's office as an extension of the physician, from the decor to the currency of the waiting room periodicals to the friendliness of the staff. It is up to the physician to develop a system of practice in the office that promotes high quality care. Checklists (e.g., for health maintenance or for routine follow-up of common conditions) can serve as useful memory joggers. A requirement that no report (laboratory, radiography, consultant) be filed in the chart without the doctor's initials can minimize the likelihood of an overlooked abnormality. Tickler files to remind staff to contact a patient for an important recheck at a particular time can mitigate against a delayed diagnosis. Computerization of the medical office holds great promise for relieving the physician and office staff of much of this tedium (McDonald, 1976). A review process should be developed to ascertain whether unplanned hospitalizations were the result of suboptimal outpatient management. Patient cancellation of or failure to keep an appointment should be documented; when several have not been kept, it would be wise to consider contacting the patient. The patient's progress should be monitored and diagnostic caution exercised: If a specific complaint has not been diagnosed after several visits, consultation is a prudent next step.

Additional liability risks are posed by the evolving mechanisms of paying for health care. In *Wickline v. California* (192 App. 3d 1630, 228 Cal. Rptr. 661, 1986), the plaintiff suffered from Leriche syndrome and underwent vascular surgery for her leg after prior approval by Medi-Cal. Postoperative complications caused the surgeon to request an additional 8 days of hospitalization, but Medi-Cal granted only 4 extra days. The patient was discharged within the 4 days and suffered further complications at home with the ultimate result being an above-the-knee amputation. The patient sued Medi-Cal (but not her doctors) for limiting her days of hospitalization. The Court of Appeals found in favor of Medi-Cal, but stated that "the physician who complies without protest with the limitations imposed by a third-party payor, when his medical judgment dictates otherwise, cannot avoid his ultimate responsibility for his patient's care. He cannot point to the health care payor as the liability scapegoat when the consequences of his own determinative medical decisions go sour." How vigorously a physician must protest a third-party payer's utilization review decision is unclear. Before entering into any contractual arrangement where a physician's usual referral or hospitalization practices may be affected, the physician should have an attorney review the contract for potential liability risk (Robinson, 1988).

Focused Perspective

It is difficult to extract general recommendations from an analysis of malpractice cases because each case represents unique individuals and facts. Moreover, claims information is usually organized in a manner that best serves the business interests of the insurance carrier and not necessarily in a form that can help educate physicians as to behaviors that affect liability. Finally, there is no clearinghouse that collects malpractice data, as that information is considered propriety and therefore a "trade secret" for many carriers. It is nevertheless possible, by reviewing available claims data and case law, to describe certain conditions and practices that are most likely to result in a malpractice suit. This section discusses the seven leading allegations made against family physicians and highlights the management errors on which the issue of liability most commonly turned.

Failure to Diagnose

About one third of cases against family physicians involve an allegation of failure to diagnose, or to timely diagnose, certain conditions. In more than one half of the failure to diagnose cases, the condition in question is cancer, especially cancer of the breast, lung, colon, or testes. Each breast mass in a woman must be taken to diagnosis, either by following it to resolution (e.g., after the next menses) or by definitive studies (e.g., needle or open biopsy). Physicians should not be falsely reassured by negative mammography studies, as mammography has a false-negative rate of 20 per cent. Physicians should also be familiar with the various guidelines for screening for breast cancer and with the controversies that surround them (Roberts, 1986a). Pneumonia in an at-risk patient (e.g., smoker, asbestos worker) should be considered lung cancer until subsequent chest radiographs document clearing. Rectal bleeding in an adult over age 40 should not be attributed to hemorrhoids unless endoscopy or radiologic studies have ruled out bowel cancer. A testicular mass or swelling should not be written off as epididymitis unless careful follow-up demonstrates resolution or a tissue diagnosis is made. Failure to diagnose has also been a problem with myocardial infarction, where excessive reliance is placed on falsely negative electrocardiograms or cardiac enzymes; with pulmonary embolus, where an arterial blood gas can help sort out the adult with confusing chest pain or dyspnea; and with appendicitis, where abdominal pain must first be considered surgical until proved otherwise. Physicians are not necessarily expected to diagnose all these conditions at the first visit; rather, they are expected to document a careful patient assessment and vigilant management plan with clearly understood instructions for the patient (Sanders, 1986).

Negligent Obstetrical Practices

Birth-related claims represent the second most frequent and most expensive suits against family physicians. Although most suits allege negligence around the time of delivery, it has become increasingly clear that the birth process is much less important than prenatal factors in causing cerebral palsy, mental retardation, or neonatal seizures (Perkins, 1987). It is therefore vitally important that the pregnancy be accurately dated, risk factors be appropriately screened and managed, the labor be properly attended and followed, and complications be recognized and treated or, as necessary, the patient referred (Roberts, 1986b). Physicians must be familiar with published standards that may be used against them in court (American Academy of Pediatrics, 1992; American College of Obstetricians and Gynecologists, 1989). Despite such vigilance and optimal care, unhappy outcomes can result. When confronted by a neurologically impaired child with tremendous needs, it has been difficult for juries and judges to deny compensation, even when the physician was not at fault. Consequently, obstetric claims have been put forward as an example of the inadequacies of the tort system, which depends on fault, and of the need for a new approach.

Negligent Management of Fractures/Trauma

Carpal navicular (scaphoid), cervical spine, and femoral head fractures have been troublesome. A "sprained wrist" should be immobilized in a thumb spica cast if there is anatomic snuff box tenderness and a question of a navicular fracture, regardless of the initial radiograph; repeat films 1 to 2 weeks later can finally rule out a fracture. Any significant head or neck trauma should be treated with spinal immobilization until radiographs exclude a cervical spine fracture. Certain femoral head fractures can remain elusive until subsequent films or tomography demonstrate their presence. Careful neurologic examination can ascertain the presence of subtle injury to nerve or tendon. Soft tissue injuries must be evaluated for the possibility of foreign bodies, infection, or compartment syndrome (Dunn, 1987). Injuries around the popliteal fossa warrant a careful examination of the distal circulation.

Failure to Obtain Timely Consultation

The broad scope of family practice leaves the family physician vulnerable to charges of practicing in another specialty area. Training, experience, and demonstrated competence—not only a physician's specialty status—are the criteria used by the courts to determine whether a doctor was reasonable in taking on a patient with a certain condition. When inexperienced or uncomfortable with a particular problem, the prudent physician obtains consultation from a local colleague, telephones another specialist, or transfers the patient to a referral center. Failure to do so, combined with an untoward result, can increase the physician's liability risk.

Negligent Treatment with Drugs

Certain medications, particularly coumadin, psychoactive drugs, and cardiovascular medicines, frequently cause undesired or dangerous side effects. The use of these agents must be monitored (prothrombin times, medication checks, electrolytes) and the patient advised about signs of drug-related problems. Drug information handouts are readily available and can serve to document that the patient was apprised of potential drug toxicity. One other frequent medication error involves the prescribing of a compound to which the patient was allergic. Many times the prescription is given despite an overlooked notation in the record of the patient's allergy. Routinely asking each patient about drug allergies before each prescription can reduce the risk of such an oversight (Robertson, 1985).

Negligent Performance of a Procedure

It is difficult to prove that a procedure was negligently performed, given that it is usually years later when a malpractice case goes to trial and that there is usually little evidence to prove exactly what was done. Consequently, negligent performance is a less common allegation. However, physicians must be careful to undertake only those procedures that they are trained, competent, and prepared to do (e.g., adequate supplies available, surgeon not overtired).

Failure to Obtain Informed Consent

Many defense lawyers contend that plaintiffs allege failure to obtain informed consent when the case is otherwise weak. About one in ten malpractice cases involves an informed consent issue. Physicians are especially troubled by this allegation, believing that they must do the impossible: inform patients of all possible risks. Such is not necessarily the case (Curran, 1986). Informed consent is not a signed form drafted by a hospital lawyer, it is a relationship between doctor and patient that allows a discussion about the nature of the illness, the various treatment options and their respective outcomes, risks, and benefits, and the consequences of undertaking or forgoing the available treatments. Serious or frequent risks should be discussed. Informed consent is a dialogue, not a monologue; and the physician can strengthen the doctor–patient relationship by empathizing with the patient's magical thinking ("I wish it were a risk-free procedure") and by sharing the uncertainty that lies ahead (Gutheil et al., 1984).

Four C's of Risk Management

The only guarantee for avoiding a medical malpractice suit is to avoid medical practice. The best physicians have and will be named as defendants, sometimes correctly, sometimes not. The diligent and reflective practitioner can reduce the risks of malpractice by adhering to the four C's of risk management: compassion, communication, competence, and charting.

Compassion

Physicians must show compassion toward their patients and toward their colleagues and themselves. It is tempting, as one listens to a patient's woeful tale, to condemn a prior physician's "suboptimal care." Caution should be exercised before commenting on another caregiver until all the facts have been reviewed (i.e., the prior medical record and not just the patient's version of the events). Hasty statements may unfairly impugn another and may expose the maker of the statements to a slander suit. Disagreements over patient care, or "jousting," should not be aired gratuitously in the medical record. Similarly, physicians should not draw guilt-stricken conclusions about their own performances until all the facts are in (Rasinski, 1982).

Communication

In addition to informing patients and their families, doctors should endeavor to inform fellow physicians (e.g., sign-out rounds to covering colleagues), nurses, and other providers (e.g., treatment plan discussions). Nurses and allied health personnel can foster a good doctor–patient rapport if they enjoy good rapport with and respect from the doctor. Nurses' notes should be read, and when disagreements arise they should be addressed. The physician should ask the nurse to read back telephone orders to minimize misinterpretation.

Competence

When confronted by an emergency, physicians should perform to the best of their abilities and, if necessary, consult with or transfer the patient to another physician as soon as it is feasible.

Charting

Physician sentiment regarding the medical record ranges from viewing it as a minor irritant to a major nemesis. Nevertheless, approximately one third of malpractice cases are lost because of an inadequate record. Long after memories have faded, the record can serve as a doctor's friend or foe when asked to serve as a witness to the physician's actions. The record must be legible, accurate, consistent, timely, objective, and complete as to significant issues. Entries should be dated and timed (some now note the time spent with patients, even in the office setting). Changes to the record must be obvious, with no attempt at concealment. For example, an incorrect phrase should have a single line drawn through it and the correction should be dated and initialed.

Conclusion

The practitioner has no absolute protection against a medical malpractice suit. Compassionate, competent, conscientious physicians can diminish, but not eliminate, the risk of suit. Practicing reflective medicine can reduce patient injury and dissatisfaction, and it can represent the best prophylaxis against malpractice litigation. "An ounce of malpractice prevention is worth a ton of money" (Massanari, 1987).

REFERENCES

Abraham KS: Medical liability reform: a conceptual framework. JAMA 260:68, 1988.

Adams EK, Zuckerman S: Variation in the growth and incidence of medical malpractice claims. J Health Pol Law 9:475, 1984.

American Academy of Pediatrics and American College of Obstetricians and Gynecologists: Guidelines for Perinatal Care, 3rd edition. Elk Grove Village, IL, AAP, 1992.

American College of Obstetricians and Gynecologists: Litigation Assistant: A Guide for the Defendant Physician. Washington, DC, ACOG, 1986.

American College of Obstetricians and Gynecologists. Standards for Obstetric-Gynecologic Services, 7th edition. Washington, DC, ACOG, 1989.

American Medical Association, Specialty Society Medical Liability Project: Fact Sheets. Chicago, IL, AMA, 1992.

Amundson R: Liability of the physician in classical Greek legal theory and practice. J Hist Med 32:172, 1977.

Association of Trial Lawyers of America: Statement on the Subject of Medical Malpractice before the Committee on Labor and Human Resources, 98th Congress, 2nd Session, July 10, 1984.

Bovbjerg RR, Havighurst CC: Medical malpractice: an update for noncombatants. Business Health September:38, 1985.

Burstin HR, Johnson WG, Lipsitz SR, et al: Do the poor sue more? A case control study of malpractice claims and socioeconomic status. JAMA 270:1697, 1993.

Charles SC, Wilbert JR, Kennedy EC: Physicians' self-reports of reactions to malpractice litigation. Am J Psychiatry 141:563, 1984.

Charles SC, Wilbert JR, Franke KJ: Sued and nonsued physicians' self-reported reactions to malpractice litigation. Am J Psychiatry 142:437, 1985.

Codman EA: The product of a hospital. Surg Gynecol Obstet 18:491, 1914.

Connelly JE: Malpractice: Living with the threat. Pharos Summer:26, 1988.

Couch NP, Tilney NL, Rayner AA, et al: The high cost of low-frequency events: The anatomy and economics of surgical mishaps. N Engl J Med 304:634, 1981.

Curran WJ: Informed consent in malpractice cases: A turn toward reality. N Engl J Med 314:429, 1986.

Danzon PM: The frequency and severity of medical malpractice claims: New evidence. Law Contemp Probl 49(2):59, 1986.

Dunn JD: Risk management in emergency medicine. Emerg Med Clin North Am 5:51, 1987.

Gass HH: A Guide for the Defendant Doctor. Southfield, MI, Physician Guide, 1984.

Ghitelman D: The natural history of malpractice. MD April:59, 1987.

Gutheil TG, Bursztajn H, Brodsky A: Malpractice prevention through the sharing of uncertainty. N Engl J Med 311:49, 1984.

Holzer JF: Liability insurance issues in anesthesiology. Int Anesthesiol Clin 27(3):27, 1989.

Kelly CR, Mamlin JJ: Ambulatory medical care quality-determination by diagnostic outcome. JAMA 227:1155, 1974.

Larimore WL, Sapolsky DS: Maternity care in family medicine: economics and malpractice. J Fam Pract, in press.

Localio AR, Lawthers AG, Brennan TA, et al: Relation between malpractice claims and adverse events due to negligence. Results of the Harvard Medical Practice Study III. N Engl J Med 325:245, 1991.

Massanari M. Risk management: An epidemiologic approach. Infect Control 8(1):3, 1987.

McDonald CJ: Protocol-based computer reminders, the quality of care and the nonperfectability of man. N Engl J Med 295:1351, 1976.

Monagle JF: Risk Management: A Guide for Health Care Professionals. Rockville, MD, Aspen, 1985.

Perkins RP: Perspectives on perinatal brain damage. Obstet Gynecol 69:807, 1987.

Peters JD, Johnson KB: Can enterprise liability ease America's malpractice problem? ASLME Briefings 8:1, 1993.

Phelps CE: Experience Rating in Medical Malpractice Insurance. Santa Monica, CA, Rand Corporation, 1977.

Pocincki LS, Dogger SJ, Schwartz BP: The incidence of iatrogenic injuries. Appendix, Report of the Secretary's Commission on Medical Malpractice. DHEW Publication no. OS 73-89. Washington, DC, U.S. Government Printing Office, 1973.

Rasinski D: Risk Management in Practice. Publication no. 353R4M. Washington, DC, American Society of Internal Medicine, 1982.

Reynolds RA, Rizzo JA, Gonzalez ML: The cost of medical professional liability. JAMA 257:2776, 1987.

Roberts RG: Breast cancer and malpractice: How to protect your patient and yourself. Fem Pat 11:81, 1986a.

Roberts RG: Family Physicians and Obstetrical Malpractice. Kansas City, MO, American Academy of Family Physicians, 1986b.

Roberts RG: The telephone: How a tocsin can become a toxin. Wis Med J 87:9, 1988.

Robertson WO: Medical Malpractice: A Preventive Approach. Seattle, University of Washington, 1985.

Robinson R: A primer on how to analyze contracts and avoid the traps. Consultant 28(7):74, 1988.

Rosenblatt RA, Wright CL: Rising malpractice premiums and obstetric practice patterns: The impact on family physicians in Washington State. West J Med 146:746, 1987.

Sanders PS: Risk Management and the Family Physician. Kansas City, MO, American Academy of Family Physicians, 1986.

Sanders PS: Confronting professional liability: A roundtable discussion of medical risk management. Minn Med 70:142, 1987.

Schwartz WB, Komesar NK: Doctors, damages and deterrence—an economic view of medical malpractice. N Engl J Med 298:1282, 1978.

Shoenberger AE: Medical malpractice injury. Causation and valuation of the loss of a chance to survive. J Leg Med 6:51, 1985.

Somers HM: The malpractice controversy and the quality of patient care. Milbank Mem Fund Q Spring:193, 1977.

Steel K, Gertman PM, Crescenzi C, et al: Iatrogenic illness on a general medical service at a university hospital. N Engl J Med 304:638, 1981.

Tancredi LR, Bovbjerg RR: Creating outcomes-based systems for quality and malpractice reform: Methodology of accelerated compensation events (ACEs). Milbank Quarterly 70:183, 1992.

Taragin MI, Willett LR, Wilczek AP, et al: The influence of standard of care and severity of injury on the resolution of medical malpractice claims. Ann Intern Med 117:780, 1992.

United States Congressional Budget Office: Estimates of health care proposals from the 102nd Congress. Washington, DC, USCBO, 1993.

United States Department of Health and Human Services: Report of the Task Force on Medical Liability and Malpractice. Washington, DC, US DHHS, 1987.

United States General Accounting Office: Medical Malpractice: Characteristics of Claims Closed in 1984. Publication no. GAO/HRD-87-55. Washington, DC, US GAO, 1987.

United States General Accounting Office: Medical Malpractice: Experience with Efforts to Address Problems. Statement before the Subcommittee on Health, Committee on Ways and Means, House of Representatives. Publication no. GAO/HRD-93-24. Washington, DC, May 20, 1993.

Walton MT: The advisory jury and malpractice in 15th century London: The case of William Forest. J Hist Med 40:478, 1985.

APPENDIX I

REFERENCE VALUES FOR THE INTERPRETATION OF LABORATORY TESTS

WILLIAM Z. BORER

Most of the tests performed in a clinical laboratory are quantitative in nature. That is, the amount of a substance present in blood or serum is measured and reported in terms of concentration, activity (e.g., enzyme activity), or counts (e.g., blood cell counts). The laboratory must provide reference values to assist the clinician in the interpretation of laboratory results. These reference ranges comprise the physiologic quantities of substance (concentrations, activities, or counts) that can be expected in healthy individuals. Deviation above or below the reference range may be associated with a disease process, and the severity of the disease process may be associated with the magnitude of the deviation. Unfortunately, there is rarely a sharp demarcation between physiologic and pathologic values, and the transition between the two is often gradual as the disease process progresses.

The terms "normal" and "abnormal" have been used to describe the laboratory values that fall inside or outside the reference range, respectively. Use of these terms is now discouraged because it is virtually impossible to define normality and because "normal" may be confused with the statistical term "gaussian." Reference ranges are established from statistical studies in groups of healthy volunteers. Although these study subjects must be free of disease, they may have lifestyles or habits that result in subtle variations in their laboratory values. Examples of these variables include diet, body mass, exercise, and geographic location. Age and gender may also affect reference values. When the data from a large cohort of healthy subjects fits a gaussian distribution, the usual statistical approach is to define the reference limits as two standard deviations (2 SD) above and below the mean. By definition the reference range excludes the highest and the lowest 2.5 per cent of the population. Nongaussian distributions are handled by different statistical methods, but the result is similar in that the reference range is defined by the central 95 per cent of the population. In other words, the odds are 1 in 20 that a healthy individual has a laboratory result that falls outside the reference range. If 12 laboratory tests are performed, the odds increase to about 1 in 2 that at least one of the results is outside the reference range. This means that all healthy individuals are likely to have a few laboratory results that are unexpected. The clinician must then integrate these data with other clinical information, such as the history and physical examination, to arrive at the appropriate clinical decision. The reference range for many tests (especially enzyme and immunochemical measurements) vary with the method used. It is important that each laboratory establish reference ranges appropriate for the methods it employs.

SI UNITS

During the 1980s a concerted effort was made to introduce SI units (Système International d'Unités). The rationale for conversion to SI units is sound. Laboratory data are scientifically more informative when the units are based on molar concentration rather than mass concentration. For example, the conversion of glucose to lactate and pyruvate or the binding of a drug to albumin is more easily understood in units of molar concentration. An example is illustrated below.

Conventional units: 1.0 gram of hemoglobin
Combines with 1.37 ml of oxygen
Contains 3.4 mg of iron
Forms 34.9 mg of bilirubin

SI units: 4.0 mmol of hemoglobin
Combines with 40 mmol of oxygen
Contains 4.0 mmol of iron
Forms 4.0 mmol of bilirubin

Another advantage of SI units involves the standardization of nomenclature to facilitate global communication of medical and scientific information.

TABLE AI–1.   BASE SI UNITS

Property	Base Unit	Symbol
Length	meter	m
Mass	kilogram	kg
Amount of substance	mole	mol
Time	second	s
Thermodynamic temperature	kelvin	K
Electric current	ampere	A
Luminous intensity	candela	cd

TABLE AI–2.   DERIVED SI UNITS

Derived Property	Derived Unit	Symbol
Area	square meter	m^2
Volume	cubic meter	m^3
	liter	L
Mass concentration	kilograms/cubic meter	kg/m^3
	grams/liter	g/L
Substance concentration	moles/cubic meter	mol/m^3
	moles/liter	mol/L
Temperature	degrees Celsius	$C = K - 273.15$

TABLE AI–3.   STANDARD PREFIXES

Prefix	Multiplication Factor	Symbol
atto	10^{-18}	a
femto	10^{-15}	f
pico	10^{-12}	p
nano	10^{-9}	n
micro	10^{-6}	μ
milli	10^{-3}	m
centi	10^{-2}	c
deci	10^{-1}	d
deca	10^1	da
hecto	10^2	h
kilo	10^3	k
mega	10^6	M
giga	10^9	G
tera	10^{12}	T

The units, symbols, and prefixes employed in the SI system are shown in Tables AI–1, AI–2, and AI–3. Unfortunately, problems have arisen with the implementation of SI units in the United States. Their introduction in 1987 prompted many medical journals to report laboratory values in both SI and conventional units in anticipation of complete conversion to SI units during the early 1990s. The lack of a coordinated effort toward this goal has forced retrenchment on the issue. Physicians continue to think and practice using laboratory results expressed in conventional units, and few if any American hospitals or clinical laboratories ex-clusively use SI units. It is not likely that complete conversion to SI units will occur in the foreseeable future, yet most medical journals will probably continue to publish both set of units. For this reason the tables of reference ranges in this appendix are given in both conventional units and SI units.

NOTE

Some of the values included in the tables were established by the Clinical Laboratories at Thomas Jefferson University Hospital in Philadelphia and have not been published elsewhere. Other values were compiled from the sources cited in the Bibliography. These tables are provided for information and educational purposes only. They are intended to complement data derived from other sources including the medical history and physical examination. Users must exercise individual judgment when using the information provided in this appendix.

SUGGESTED READINGS

Bick RL (ed): Hematology—Clinical and Laboratory Practice. St. Louis, Mosby-Yearbook, 1993.

Borer WZ: Selection and use of laboratory tests. *In* Tietz NW, Conn RB, Pruden EL (eds): Applied Laboratory Medicine. Philadelphia, WB Saunders Company, 1992, pp 1–5.

Campion EW: A retreat from SI units. N Engl J Med 327:49, 1992.

Drug Evaluations Annual. Chicago, American Medical Association, 1994.

Friedman RB, Young DS: Effects of Disease on Clinical Laboratory Tests, 2nd edition. Washington, DC, AACC Press, 1989.

Henry JB: Clinical Diagnosis and Management by Laboratory Methods, 18th edition. Philadelphia, WB Saunders Company, 1991.

Hicks JM, Young DS: DORA '92–93: Directory of Rare Analyses. Washington, DC, AACC Press, 1992.

Jacobs DS, Kasten BL, Demott WR, et al: Laboratory Test Handbook, 2nd edition. Baltimore, Williams & Wilkins, 1990.

Kaplan LA, Pesce AJ: Clinical Chemistry—Theory, Analysis, and Correlation, 2nd edition. St. Louis, CV Mosby, 1989.

Kjeldsberg CR, Knight JA: Body fluids—Laboratory Examination of Amniotic, Cerebrospinal, Seminal, Serous and Synovial fluids, 3rd edition. Chicago, ASCP Press, 1993.

Laposata M: SI Unit Conversion Guide. Boston, NEJM Books, 1992.

Scully RE, McNeely WF, Mark EJ, et al: Normal reference laboratory values. N Engl J Med 327:718, 1992.

Speicher CE: The Right Test—A Physician's Guide to Laboratory Medicine, 2nd edition. Philadelphia, WB Saunders Company, 1993.

Tietz NW (ed): Clinical Guide to Laboratory Tests, 2nd edition. Philadelphia, WB Saunders Company, 1990.

Wallach J: Interpretation of Diagnostic Tests—A Synopsis of Laboratory Medicine, 5th edition. Boston, Little, Brown, 1992.

Young DS: Implementation of SI units for clinical laboratory data. Ann Intern Med 106:114, 1987.

Young DS: Determination and validation of reference intervals. Arch Pathol Lab Med 116:704, 1992.

Young DS: Effects of Drugs on Clinical Laboratory Tests, 3rd edition. Washington, DC, AACC Press, 1990.

REFERENCE VALUES FOR HEMATOLOGY

Determination	Conventional Units	SI Units
Acid hemolysis (Ham test)	No hemolysis	No hemolysis
Alkaline phosphatase, leukocyte	Total score 14–100	Total score 14–100
Cell counts		
Erythrocytes		
Men	4.6–6.2 million/mm^3	4.6–6.2 $\times$ 10^{12}/L
Women	4.2–5.4 million/mm^3	4.2–5.4 $\times$ 10^{12}/L
Children (varies with age)	4.5–5.1 million/mm^3	4.5–5.1 $\times$ 10^{12}/L
Leukocytes, total	4500–11,000/mm^3	4.5–11.0 $\times$ 10^9/L
Leukocytes, differential	*Percent*	*Absolute Count*
Myelocytes	0	0
Band neutrophils	3–5	150–400 $\times$ 10^6/L
Segmented neutrophils	54–62	3000–5800 $\times$ 10^6/L
Lymphocytes	25–33	1500–3000 $\times$ 10^6/L
Monocytes	3–7	300–500 $\times$ 10^6/L
Eosinophils	1–3	50–250 $\times$ 10^6/L
Basophils	0–1	15–50 $\times$ 10^6/L
Platelets	150,000–400,000/mm^3	150–350 $\times$ 10^9/L
Reticulocytes	25,000–75,000/mm^3 (0.5–1.5% of erythrocytes)	25–75 $\times$ 10^9/L
Coagulation tests		
Bleeding time (template)	2.75–8.0 min	2.75–8.0 min
Coagulation time (glass tube)	5–15 min	5–15 min
Factor VIII and other coagulation factors	50–150% of normal	0.5–1.5 of normal
Fibrin split products (Thrombo-Welco test)	<10 μg/ml	<10 mg/L
Fibrinogen	200–400 mg/dL	2.0–4.0 g/L
Partial thromboplastin time (PTT)	20–35 sec	20–35 sec
Prothrombin time (PT)	12.0–14.0 sec	12.0–14.0 sec
Coombs' test		
Direct	Negative	Negative
Indirect	Negative	Negative
Corpuscular values of erythrocytes		
Mean corpuscular hemoglobin (MCH)	26–34 pg/cell	26–34 pg/cell
Mean corpuscular volume (MCV)	80–96 μm^3	80–96 fL
Mean corpuscular hemoglobin concentration (MCHC)	32–36 g/dL	320–360 g/L
Haptoglobin	20–165 mg/dL	0.20–1.65 g/L
Hematocrit		
Men	40–54 ml/dL	0.40–0.54
Women	37–47 ml/dL	0.37–0.47
Newborns	49–54 ml/dL	0.49–0.54
Children (varies with age)	35–49 ml/dL	0.35–0.49
Hemoglobin		
Men	13.0–18.0 g/dL	8.1–11.2 mmol/L
Women	12.0–16.0 g/dL	7.4–9.9 mmol/L
Newborns	16.5–19.5 g/dL	10.2–12.1 mmol/L
Children (varies with age)	11.2–16.5 g/dL	7.0–10.2 mmol/L
Hemoglobin, fetal	<1.0% of total	<0.01 of total
Hemoglobin A$_{1C}$	3–5% of total	0.03–0.05 of total
Hemoglobin A$_2$	1.5–3.0% of total	0.015–0.03 of total
Hemoglobin, plasma	0.0–5.0 mg/dL	0–3.2 μmol/L
Methemoglobin	30–130 mg/dL	19–80 μmol/L
Erythrocyte sedimentation rate (ESR)		
Wintrobe		
Males	0–5 mm/hr	0–5 m/hr
Females	0–15 mm/hr	0–15 mm/hr
Westergren		
Males	0–15 mm/hr	0–15 mm/hr
Females	0–20 mm/hr	0–20 mm/hr

REFERENCE VALUES FOR CLINICAL CHEMISTRY (BLOOD, SERUM, PLASMA)
Reference values may vary depending upon the method and sample source used.

Determination	Conventional Units	SI Units
Acetoacetate plus acetone		
Qualitative	Negative	Negative
Quantitative	0.3–2.0 mg/dL	30–200 μmol/L
Acid phosphatase, serum (thymolphthalein monophosphate substrate)	0.1–0.6 U/L	0.1–0.6 U/L
ACTH (see corticotropin)		
Alanine aminotransferase, serum (ALT, SGPT)	1–45 U/L	1–45 U/L
Albumin, serum	3.3–5.2 g/dL	33–52 g/L
Aldolase, serum	0.0–7.0 U/L	0.0–7.0 U/L
Aldosterone, plasma		
Standing	5–30 ng/dL	140–830 pmol/L
Recumbent	3–10 ng/dL	80–275 pmol/L
Alkaline phosphatase, serum (ALP)		
Adults	35–150 U/L	35–150 U/L
Adolescents	100–500 U/L	100–500 U/L
Children	100–350 U/L	100–350 U/L
Ammonia nitrogen, plasma	10–50 μmol/L	10–50 μmol/L
Amylase, serum	25–125 U/L	25–125 U/L
Anion gap, serum, calculated	8–16 mEq/L	8–16 mmol/L
Ascorbic acid, blood	0.4–1.5 mg/dL	23–85 μmol/L
Aspartate aminotransferase, serum (AST, SGOT)	1–36 U/L	1–36 U/L
Base excess, arterial blood, calculated	0 ± 2 mEq/L	0 ± 2 mmol/L
Bicarbonate		
Venous plasma	23–29 mEq/L	23–29 mmol/L
Arterial blood	21–27 mEq/L	21–27 mmol/L
Bile acids, serum	0.3–3.0 mg/dL	0.8–7.6 μmol/L
Bilirubin, serum		
Conjugated	0.1–0.4 mg/dL	1.7–6.8 μmol/L
Total	0.3–1.1 mg/dL	5.1–19.0 μmol/L
Calcium, serum	8.4–10.6 mg/dL	2.10–2.65 mmol/L
Calcium, ionized, serum	4.25–5.25 mg/dL	1.05–1.30 mmol/L
Carbon dioxide, total, serum or plasma	24–31 mEq/L	24–31 mmol/L
Carbon dioxide tension, blood, (PCO_2)	35–45 mm Hg	35–45 mm Hg
β-Carotene, serum	60–260 μg/dL	1.1–8.6 μmol/L
Ceruloplasmin, serum	23–44 mg/dL	230–440 mg/L
Chloride, serum or plasma	96–106 mEq/L	96–106 mmol/L
Cholesterol, serum or EDTA plasma		
Desirable range	<200 mg/dL	<5.20 mmol/L
LDL cholesterol	60–180 mg/dL	1.55–4.65 mmol/L
HDL cholesterol	30–80 mg/dL	0.80–2.05 mmol/L
Copper	70–140 μg/dL	11–22 μmol/L
Corticotropin, plasma (ACTH), 8 a.m.	10–80 pg/mL	2–18 pmol/L
Cortisol, plasma		
8:00 a.m.	6–23 μg/dL	170–630 nmol/L
4:00 p.m.	3–15 μg/dL	80–410 nmol/L
10:00 p.m.	<50% of 8:00 a.m. value	<50% of 8:00 a.m. value
Creatine, serum		
Males	0.2–0.5 mg/dL	15–40 μmol/L
Females	0.3–0.9 mg/dL	25–70 μmol/L
Creatine kinase, serum (CK, CPK)		
Males	55–170 U/L	55–170 U/L
Females	30–135 U/L	30–135 U/L
Creatine kinase MB isoenzyme, serum	<5% of total CK activity <5.0 ng/mL by immunoassay	

Table continued on following page

REFERENCE VALUES FOR CLINICAL CHEMISTRY (BLOOD, SERUM, PLASMA) *(Continued)*

Reference values may vary depending upon the method and sample source used.

Determination	Conventional Units	SI Units
Creatine, serum	0.6–1.2 mg/dL	50–110 μmol/L
Ferritin, serum	20–200 ng/mL	20–200 μg/L
Fibrinogen, plasma	200–400 mg/dL	2.0–4.0 g/L
Folate		
Serum	2.0–9.0 ng/mL	4.5–20.4 nmol/L
Erythrocytes	170–700 ng/mL	385–1590 nmol/L
Follicle-stimulating hormone, plasma (FSH)		
Males	4–25 mU/mL	4–25 U/L
Females	4–30 mU/mL	4–30 U/L
Postmenopausal	40–250 mU/mL	40–250 U/L
γ-glutamyltransferase, serum (GGT)	5–40 U/L	5–40 U/L
Gastrin, fasting, serum	0–110 pg/mL	0–110 mg/L
Glucose, fasting, plasma or serum	70–115 mg/dL	3.9–6.4 nmol/L
Growth hormone, plasma, adult, fasting (hGH)	0–6 ng/mL	0–6 μg/L
Haptoglobin, serum	20–165 mg/dL	0.20–1.65 gm/L
Immunoglobulins, serum (*see* Immunologic tests)		
Insulin, fasting, plasma	5–25 μU/mL	36–179 pmol/L
Iron, serum	75–175 μg/dL	13–31 μmol/L
Iron-binding capacity, serum		
Total	250–410 μg/dL	45–73 μmol/L
Saturation	20–55%	0.20–0.55
Lactate		
Venous blood	5.0–20 mg/dL	0.6–2.2 mmol/L
Arterial blood	5.0–15.0 mg/dL	0.6–1.7 mmol/L
Lactate dehydrogenase, serum (LD, LDH)	110–220 U/L	110–220 U/L
Lipase, serum	10–140 U/L	10–140 U/L
Lutropin, serum (LH)		
Males	1–9 IU/L	1–9 U/L
Females		
Follicular	2–10 IU/L	2–10 U/L
Midcycle	15–65 U/L	15–65 U/L
Luteal	1–12 U/L	1–12 U/L
Postmenopausal	12–65 U/L	12–65 U/L
Magnesium, serum	1.3–2.1 mg/dL	0.65–1.05 mmol/L
Osmolality	275–295 mOsm/kg water	275–295 mOsm/kg water
Oxygen, blood, arterial, room air		
Partial pressure (PaO$_2$)	80–100 mm Hg	80–100 mm Hg
Saturation, (SaO$_2$)	95–98%	95–98%
pH, arterial blood	7.35–7.45	7.35–7.45
Phosphate, inorganic, serum		
Adults	3.0–4.5 mg/dL	1.0–1.5 mmol/L
Children	4.0–7.0 mg/dL	1.3–2.3 mmol/L
Potassium		
Serum	3.5–5.0 mEq/L	3.5–5.0 mmol/L
Plasma	3.5–4.5 mEq/L	3.5–4.5 mmol/L
Progesterone, serum, adult		
Males	0–0.4 ng/mL	0.0–1.3 mmol/L
Females		
Follicular	0.1–1.5 ng/mL	0.3–4.8 mmol/L
Luteal	2.5–28.0 ng/mL	8.0–89.0 mmol/L
Prolactin, serum		
Males	1.0–15.0 ng/mL	1.0–15.0 μg/L
Females	1.0–20.0 ng/mL	1.0–20.0 μg/L

Table continued on opposite page

REFERENCE VALUES FOR CLINICAL CHEMISTRY (BLOOD, SERUM, PLASMA) *(Continued)*
Reference values may vary depending upon the method and sample source used.

Determination	Conventional Units	SI Units
Protein, serum, electrophoresis		
Total	6.0–8.0 g/dL	60–80 g/L
Albumin	3.5–5.5 g/dL	35–55 g/L
Globulins		
α_1	0.2–0.4 g/dL	2–4 g/L
α_2	0.5–0.9 g/dL	5–9 g/L
β	0.6–1.1 g/dL	6–11 g/L
γ	0.7–1.7 g/dL	7–17 g/L
Pyruvate, blood	0.3–0.9 mg/dL	0.03–0.10 mmol/L
Rheumatoid factor	0–30 IU/mL	0.0–30 kIU/L
Sodium, serum or plasma	135–145 mEq/L	135–145 mmol/L
Testosterone, plasma		
Men	300–1200 ng/dL	10.4–41.6 nmol/L
Women	20–75 ng/dL	0.7–2.6 nmol/L
Pregnant women	40–200 ng/dL	1.4–6.9 nmol/L
Thyroglobulin	3–42 ng/mL	3–42 μg/L
Thyrotropin, serum (hTSH)	0.4–4.8 μIU/mL	0.4–4.8 mIU/L
Thyrotropin-releasing hormone (TRH)	5–60 pg/mL	5–60 ng/L
Thyroxine, free, serum (FT$_4$)	0.9–2.1 ng/dL	12–27 pmol/L
Thyroxine, serum (T$_4$)	4.5–12.0 μg/dL	58–154 nmol/L
Thyroxine-binding globulin (TBG)	15.0–34.0 μg/mL	15.0–34.0 mg/L
Transferrin	250–430 mg/dL	2.5–4.3 g/L
Triglycerides, serum, 12-hr fast	40–150 mg/dL	0.4–15.0 g/L
Triiodothyronine, serum (T$_3$)	70–190 ng/dL	1.1–2.9 nmol/L
Triiodothyronine uptake, resin, (T$_3$RU)	25–38%	0.25–0.38
Urate		
Males	2.5–8.0 mg/dL	150–480 μmol/L
Females	2.2–7.0 mg/dL	130–420 μmol/L
Urea serum or plasma	24–49 mg/dL	4.0–8.2 nmol/L
Urea, nitrogen, serum or plasma	11–23 mg/dL	8.0–16.4 nmol/L
Viscosity, serum	1.4–1.8 × water	1.4–1.8 × water
Vitamin A, serum	20–80 μg/dL	0.70–2.80 μmol/L
Vitamin B$_{12}$, serum	180–900 pg/mL	133–664 pmol/L

REFERENCE VALUES FOR THERAPEUTIC DRUG MONITORING (SERUM)

Determination	Therapeutic Range	Toxic Concentrations	Proprietary Names
Analgesics			
Acetaminophen	10–20 μg/mL	>250 μg/mL	Tylenol
			Datril
Salicylate	100–250 μg/mL	>300 μg/mL	Aspirin
			Ascriptin
			Bufferin
Antibiotics			
Amikacin	25–30 μg/mL	Peak >35 μg/mL	Amikin
		Trough >10 μg/mL	
Chloramphenicol	10–20 μg/mL	>25 μg/mL	Chloromycetin
Gentamicin	5–10 μg/mL	Peak >10 μg/mL	Garamycin
		Trough >2 μg/mL	
Tobramycin	5–10 μg/mL	Peak >10 μg/mL	Nebcin
		Trough >2 μg/mL	
Vancomycin	5–10 μg/mL	Peak >40 μg/mL	Vancocin
		Trough >10 μg/mL	
Anticonvulsants			
Carbamazepine	5–12 μg/mL	>15 μg/mL	Tegretol
Ethosuximide	40–100 μg/mL	>150 μg/mL	Zarontin
Phenobarbital	15–40 μg/mL	40–100 ng/mL (varies widely)	
Phenytoin	10–20 μg/mL	>20 μg/mL	Dilantin
Primidone	5–12 μg/mL	>15 μg/mL	Mysoline
Valproic acid	50–100 μg/mL	>100 μg/mL	Depakene
Antineoplastics and immunosuppressives			
Cyclosporin A	50–400 ng/mL	>400 ng/mL	Sandimmune
Methotrexate, high dose, 48 hr	Variable	>1 μmol/L, 48 hr after dose	Mexate
			Folex
Bronchodialators and respiratory stimulants			
Caffeine	3–15 ng/mL	>30 ng/mL	
Theophylline (aminophylline)	10–20 μg/mL	>20 μg/mL	Aerolate
			Elixophyllin
			Quibron
			Theobid
Cardiovascular drugs			
Amiodarone	1.0–2.0 μg/mL	>2.0 μg/mL	Cordarone
(Obtain specimen more than 8 hours after last dose.)			
Digitoxin	15–25 ng/mL	>35 ng/mL	Crystodigin
(Obtain specimen 12–24 hours after last dose.)			
Digoxin	0.8–2.0 ng/mL	>2.4 ng/mL	Lanoxin
(Obtain specimen more than 6 hours after last dose.)			
Disopyramide	2–5 μg/mL	>7 μg/mL	Norpace
Flecainide	0.2–1.0 ng/mL	>1 ng/mL	Tambocor
Lidocaine	1.5–5.0 μg/mL	>6 μg/mL	Xylocaine
Mexiletine	0.7–2.0 ng/mL	>2 ng/mL	Mexitil
Procainamide	4–10 μg/mL	>12 μg/mL	Pronestyl
Procainamide + NAPA	8–30 μg/mL	>30 μg/mL	
Propranolol	50–100 ng/mL	Variable	Inderal
Quinidine	2–5 μg/mL	>6 μg/mL	Cardioquin
			Quinaglute
Tocainide	4–10 ng/mL	>10 ng/mL	Tonocard
Psychopharmacologic drugs			
Amitriptyline	120–150 ng/mL	>500 ng/mL	Amitril
			Elavil
			Triavil
Bupropion	25–100 ng/mL	N/A	Wellbutrin
Desipramine	150–300 ng/mL	>500 ng/mL	Norpramin
			Pertofrane
Imipramine	125–250 ng/mL	>400 ng/mL	Janimine
			Tofranil
Lithium	0.6–1.5 mEq/L	>1.5 mEq/L	Lithobid
(Obtain specimen 12 hours after last dose.)			
Nortriptyline	50–150 ng/mL	>500 ng/mL	Aventyl
			Pamelor

N/A = not applicable.

REFERENCE VALUES FOR CLINICAL CHEMISTRY (URINE)
Reference values may vary depending on the method used.

Determination	Conventional Units	SI Units
Acetone and acetoacetate, qualitative	Negative	Negative
Albumin		
Qualitative	Negative	Negative
Quantitative	10–100 mg/24 hr	0.15–1.5 μmol/day
Aldosterone	3–20 μg/24 hr	8.3–55 nmol/day
δ-Aminolevulinic acid (δ-ALA)	1.3–7.0 mg/24 hr	10–53 μmol/day
Amylase	<17 U/hr	<17 U/hr
Amylase/creatinine clearance ratio	0.01–0.04	0.01–0.04
Bilirubin, qualitative	Negative	Negative
Calcium (regular diet)	<250 mg/24 hr	<6.3 nmol/day
Catecholamines		
Epinephrine	<10 μg/24 hr	<55 nmol/day
Norepinephrine	<100 μg/24 hr	<590 nmol/day
Total free catecholamines	4–126 μg/24 hr	24–745 nmol/day
Total metanephrines	0.1–1.6 mg/24 hr	0.5–8.1 μmol/day
Chloride (varies with intake)	110–250 mEq/24 hr	110–250 mmol/day
Copper	0–50 μg/24 hr	0–0.80 μmol/day
Cortisol, free	10–100 μg/24 hr	27.6–276 nmol/day
Creatine		
Males	0–40 mg/24 hr	0–0.30 mmol/day
Females	0–80 mg/24 hr	0–0.60 mmol/day
Creatinine	15–25 mg/kg/24 hr	0.13–0.22 mmol/kg/day
Creatinine clearance (endogenous)		
Males	110–150 mL/min/1.73 m^2	110–150 mL/min/1.73 m^2
Females	105–132 mL/min/1.73 m^2	105–132 mL/min/1.73 m^2
Cystine or cysteine	Negative	Negative
Dehydroepiandrosterone		
Males	0.2–2.0 mg/24 hr	0.7–6.9 μmol/day
Females	0.2–1.8 mg/24 hr	0.7–6.2 μmol/day
Estrogens, total		
Males	4–25 μg/24 hr	14–90 nmol/day
Females	5–100 μg/24 hr	18–360 nmol/day
Glucose (as reducing substance)	<250 mg/24 hr	<250 mg/day
Hemoglobin and myoglobin qualitative	Negative	Negative
Homogentisic acid, qualitative	Negative	Negative
17-Ketogenic steroids		
Males	5–23 mg/24 hr	17–80 μmol/day
Females	3–15 mg/24 hr	10–52 μmol/day
17-Hydroxycorticosteroids		
Males	3–9 mg/24 hr	8.3–25 μmol/day
Females	2–8 mg/24 hr	5.5–22 μmol/day
5-Hydroxyindoleacetic acid		
Qualitative	Negative	Negative
Quantitative	2–6 mg/24 hr	10–31 μmol/day
17-Ketosteroids		
Males	8–22 mg/24 hr	28–76 μmol/day
Females	6–15 mg/24 hr	21–52 μmol/day
Magnesium	6–10 mEq/24 hr	3–5 mmol/day
Metanephrines	0.05–1.20 ng/mg creatinine	0.03–0.70 mmol/mmol creatinine
Osmolality	38–1400 mOsm/kg water	38–1400 mOsm/kg water
pH	4.6–8.0	4.6–8.0
Phenylpyruvic acid, qualitative	Negative	Negative
Phosphate	0.4–1.3 g/24 hr	13–42 mmol/day

Table continued on following page

REFERENCE VALUES FOR CLINICAL CHEMISTRY (URINE) *(Continued)*
Reference values may vary depending on the method used.

Determination	Conventional Units	SI Units
Porphobilinogen		
Qualitative	Negative	Negative
Quantitative	<2 mg/24 hr	<9 μmol/day
Porphyrins		
Coproporphyrin	50–250 μg/24 hr	77–380 nmol/day
Uroporphyrin	10–30 μg/24 hr	12–36 nmol/day
Potassium	25–125 mEq/24 hr	25–125 mmol/day
Pregnanediol		
Males	0–1.9 mg/24 hr	0–6.0 μmol/day
Females		
Proliferative phase	0–2.6 mg/24 hr	0–8.0 μmol/day
Luteal phase	2.6–10.6 mg/24 hr	8–33 μmol/day
Postmenopausal	0.2–1.0 mg/24 hr	0.6–3.1 μmol/day
Pregnanetriol	0–2.5 mg/24 hr	0–7.4 μmol/day
Protein, total		
Qualitative	Negative	Negative
Quantitative	10–150 mg/24 hr	10–150 mg/day
Protein/creatinine ratio	<0.2	<0.2
Sodium (regular diet)	60–260 mEq/24 hr	60–260 mmol/day
Specific gravity		
Random specimen	1.003–1.030	1.003–1.030
24-Hour collection	1.015–1.025	1.015–1.025
Urate (regular diet)	250–750 mg/24 hr	1.5–4.4 mmol/day
Urobilinogen	0.5–4.0 mg/24 hr	0.6–6.8 μmol/day
Vanillylmandelic acid (VMA)	1–8 mg/24 hr	5–40 μmol/day

REFERENCE VALUES FOR TOXIC SUBSTANCES

Determination	Conventional Units	SI Units
Arsenic, urine	<130 μg/24 hr	<1.7 μmol/day
Bromides, serum, inorganic	<100 mg/dL	<10 mmol/L
Toxic symptoms	140–1000 mg/dL	14–100 mmol/L
Carboxyhemoglobin, blood	*% Saturation*	*Saturation*
Urban environment	<5	<0.05
Smokers	<12	<0.12
Symptoms		
Headache	>15	>0.15
Nausea and vomiting	>25	>0.25
Potentially lethal	>50	>0.50
Ethanol	<0.05 mg/dL	<1.0 mmol/L
Blood	<0.005%	
Intoxication	>100 mg/dL	>22 mmol/L
	>0.1%	
Marked intoxication	300–400 mg/dL	65–87 mmol/L
	0.3–0.4%	
Alcoholic stupor	400–500 mg/dL	87–109 mmol/L
	0.4–0.5%	
Coma	>500 mg/dL	>109 mmol/L
	>0.5%	
Lead, blood		
Adults	<25 μg/dL	<1.2 μmol/L
Children	<15 μg/dL	<0.7 μmol/L
Lead, urine	<80 μg/24 hr	<0.4 μmol/day
Mercury, urine	<30 μg/24 hr	<150 nmol/day

REFERENCE VALUES FOR CEREBROSPINAL FLUID

	Conventional Units	SI Units
Cells	<5/mm^3; all mononuclear	<5 × 10^6/L, all mononuclear
Electrophoresis	Albumin predominant	Albumin predominant
Glucose	50–75 mg/dL (20 mg/dL less than in serum)	2.8–4.2 mmol/L (1.1 mmol less than in serum)
IgG		
Children under 14	<8% of total protein	<0.08 of total protein
Adults	<14% of total protein	<0.14% of total protein
IgG index $\left(\dfrac{\text{CSF/serum IgG ratio}}{\text{CSF/serum albumin ratio}}\right)$	0.3–0.6	0.3–0.6
Oligoclonal banding on electrophoresis	Absent	Absent
Pressure	70–180 mmH$_2$O	70–180 mmH$_2$O
Protein, total	15–45 mg/dL	150–450 mg/L

REFERENCE VALUES FOR TESTS OF GASTROINTESTINAL FUNCTION

Determination	Conventional Units
Bentiromide test	6-Hour urinary arylamine excretion >57% excludes pancreatic insufficiency
β-Carotene, serum	60–260 μg/dL
Fecal fat estimation	
Qualitative	No fat globules seen by high power microscopy
Quantitative	<6 gm/24 hr (>95% coefficient of fat absorption)
Gastric acid output	
Basal	
Males	0–10.5 mmol/hr
Females	0–5.6 mmol/hr
Maximum (after histamine or pentagastrin)	
Males	9–48 mmol/hr
Females	6–31 mmol/hr
Ratio: basal/maximum	
Males	0–0.31
Females	0–0.29
Secretin test, pancreatic fluid	
Volume	>1.8 mL/kg/hr
Bicarbonate	>80 mEq/L
D-Xylose absorption test, urine	>20% of ingested dose excreted in 5 hr

REFERENCE VALUES FOR IMMUNOLOGIC PROCEDURES

Determination	Conventional Units	SI Units
Complement, serum		
C3	85–175 mg/dL	0.85–1.75 gm/L
C4	15–45 mg/dL	150–450 mg/L
Total hemolytic (CH_{50})	150–250 U/mL	150–250 μ/mL
Immunoglobulins, serum, adult		
IgG	640–1350 mg/dL	6.4–13.5 g/L
IgA	70–310 mg/dL	0.70–3.1 g/L
IgM	90–350 mg/dL	0.90–3.5 g/L
IgD	0–6.0 mg/dL	0–60 mg/L
IgE	0–430 ng/dL	0–430 μg/L

Lymphocyte subsets, whole
blood heparinized

Antigen	Cell Type	%	Absolute
CD3	Total T cells	56–77	860–1880
CD19	Total B cells	7–17	140–370
CD3 and CD4	Helper-inducer cells	32–54	550–1190
CD3 and CD8	Suppressor-cytotoxic cells	24–37	430–1060
Helper/suppressor ratio: 0.8–1.8			
CD3 and DR	Activated T cells	5–14	70–310
CD2	E Rosette T cells	73–87	1040–2160
CD16 and CD56	Natural killer (NK) cells	8–22	130–500

REFERENCE VALUES FOR SEMEN ANALYSIS

Determination	Conventional Units	SI Units
Volume	2–5 mL	2–5 mL
Liquefaction	Complete in 15 min	Complete in 15 min
pH	7.2–8.0	7.2–8.0
Leukocytes	Occasional or absent	Occasional or absent
Spermatozoa		
Count	60–150 $\times$ 10^6/mL	60–150 $\times$ 10^6/mL
Motility	>80% motile	>0.80 motile
Morphology	80–90% normal forms	0.80–0.90 normal forms
Fructose	>150 mg/dL	>8.33 mmol/L

NOMOGRAM FOR THE DETERMINATION OF BODY SURFACE AREA OF CHILDREN AND ADULTS

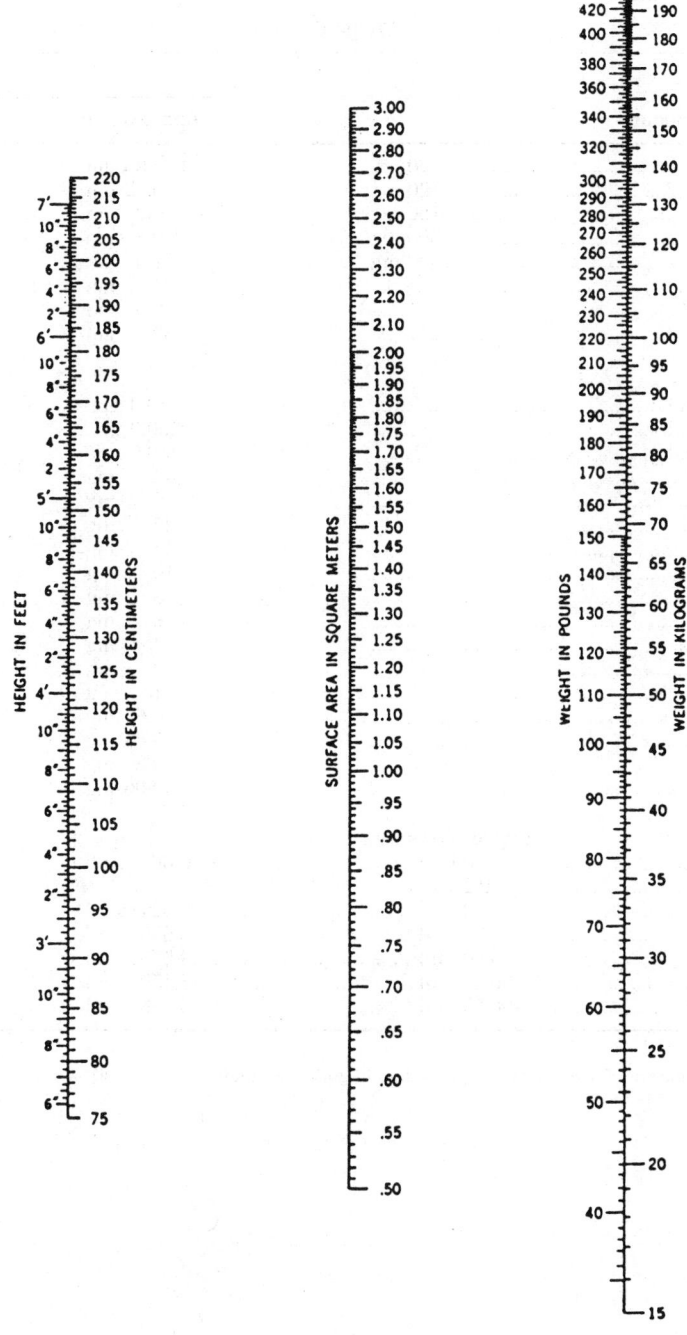

HEIGHT IN FEET

HEIGHT IN CENTIMETERS

SURFACE AREA IN SQUARE METERS

WEIGHT IN POUNDS

WEIGHT IN KILOGRAMS

* From Boothby WM, Sandiford, RB: Boston Med. Surg. J., *185*:337, 1921.

CONVERSION OF APOTHECARY'S MEASURES TO METRIC EQUIVALENTS

Weights

Apothecary		Metric	
		Approximate	More Nearly Accurate
1 grain	60 mg	0.06 gm	0.06479 gm
2 grains	120 mg	0.12 gm	
3 grains	180 mg	0.2 gm	
5 grains	300 mg	0.3 gm	
15 grains	1000 mg	1.0 gm	
60 grains or 1 dram		4.0 gm	3.88 gm
240 grains or 4 drams, ½ oz		15.0 gm	
480 grains or 8 drams, 1 oz		30.0 gm	31.103 gm
			31.103 gm (Troy)
			28.350 gm (Avoir.)
12 oz or 1 pound		360.0 gm	373.24177 gm
12 oz or 1 pound		260.0 gm	373.24177 gm (Troy)
16 oz or 1 pound		480.0 gm	453.592 gm (Avoir.)
¾ grain		45 mg	
½ grain		30 mg	
⅜ grain		25 mg	
¼ grain		15 mg	
⅙ grain		10 mg	
⅛ grain		8 mg	
$\frac{1}{10}$ grain		6 mg	
$\frac{1}{16}$ grain		4 mg	
$\frac{1}{32}$ grain		2 mg	
$\frac{1}{64}$ grain		1 mg	
$\frac{1}{100}$ grain		0.6 mg	
$\frac{1}{250}$ grain		0.25 mg	
$\frac{1}{300}$ grain		0.2 mg	
$\frac{1}{1000}$ grain		0.06 mg	

Liquid Measures

1 minim	0.06 ml	0.06161 ml	
3 minims	0.2 ml		
15 minims	1.0 ml	0.92415 ml*	
60 minims, 1 fl. dram.	4.0 ml	3.6967 ml	
480 minims 1 fl oz.	30.0 ml	29.5737 ml	
16 fl oz or 1 pt	500.0 ml	473.179 ml	
32 fl oz or 1 qt	1000.0 ml	946.358 ml	

* 1 ml is equal to 16.23 minims.
Quantity of drug prescribed in grams per 2 ounces (60 ml) gives dose in grains per dram.

CONVERSION OF POUNDS
TO KILOGRAMS

Pounds→ ↓	0	1	2	3	4	5	6	7	8	9
0	0.00	0.45	0.90	1.36	1.81	2.26	2.72	3.17	3.62	4.08
10	4.53	4.98	5.44	5.89	6.35	6.80	7.25	7.71	8.16	8.61
20	9.07	9.52	9.97	10.43	10.88	11.34	11.79	12.24	12.70	13.15
30	13.60	14.06	14.51	14.96	15.42	15.87	16.32	16.78	17.23	17.69
40	18.14	18.59	19.05	19.50	19.95	20.41	20.86	21.31	21.77	22.22
50	22.68	23.13	23.58	24.04	24.49	24.94	25.40	25.85	26.30	26.76
60	27.21	27.66	28.12	28.57	29.03	29.48	29.93	30.39	30.84	31.29
70	31.75	32.20	32.65	33.11	33.56	34.02	34.47	34.92	35.38	35.83
80	36.28	36.74	37.19	37.64	38.10	38.55	39.00	39.46	39.91	40.37
90	40.82	41.27	41.73	42.18	42.63	43.09	43.54	43.99	44.45	44.90
100	45.36	45.81	46.26	46.72	47.17	47.62	48.08	48.53	48.98	49.44
110	49.89	50.34	50.80	51.25	51.71	52.16	52.61	53.07	53.52	53.97
120	54.43	54.88	55.33	55.79	56.24	56.70	57.15	57.60	58.06	58.51
130	58.96	59.42	59.87	60.32	60.78	61.23	61.68	62.14	62.59	63.05
140	63.50	63.95	64.41	64.86	65.31	65.77	66.22	66.67	67.13	67.58
150	68.04	68.49	68.94	69.40	69.85	70.30	70.76	71.21	71.66	72.12
160	72.57	73.02	73.48	73.93	74.39	74.84	75.29	75.75	76.20	76.65
170	77.11	77.56	78.01	78.47	78.92	79.38	79.83	80.28	80.74	81.19
180	81.64	82.10	82.55	83.00	83.46	83.91	84.36	84.82	85.27	85.73
190	86.18	86.68	87.09	87.54	87.99	88.45	88.90	89.35	89.81	90.26
200	90.72	91.17	91.62	92.08	92.53	92.98	93.44	93.89	94.34	94.80

TABLE OF TEMPERATURE EQUIVALENTS CELSIUS (CENTIGRADE): FAHRENHEIT SCALE

Celsius: Fahrenheit $°F = (°C \times \frac{9}{5}) + 32$				Fahrenheit: Celsius $C = (°F - 32) \times \frac{5}{9}$					
C°	F°	C°	F°	F°	C°	F°	C°	F°	C°
−50	−58.0	49	120.2	−50	−46.7	99	37.2	157	69.4
−40	−40.0	50	122.0	−40	−40.0	100	37.7	158	70.0
−35	−31.0	51	123.8	−35	−37.2	101	38.3	159	70.5
−30	−22.0	52	125.6	−30	−34.4	102	38.8	160	71.1
−25	−13.0	53	127.4	−25	−31.7	103	39.4	161	71.6
−20	−4.0	54	129.2	−20	−28.9	104	40.0	162	72.2
−15	+5.0	55	131.0	−15	−26.6	105	40.5	163	72.7
−10	14.0	56	132.8	−10	−23.3	106	41.1	164	73.3
−5	23.0	57	134.6	−5	20.6	107	41.6	165	73.8
0	32.0	58	136.4	0	−17.7	108	42.2	166	74.4
+1	33.8	59	138.2	+1	−17.2	109	42.7	167	75.0
2	35.6	60	140.0	5	−15.0	110	43.3	168	75.5
3	37.4	61	141.8	10	−12.2	111	43.8	169	76.1
4	39.2	62	143.6	15	−9.4	112	44.4	170	76.6
5	41.0	63	145.4	20	−6.6	113	45.0	171	77.2
6	42.8	64	147.2	25	−3.8	114	45.5	172	77.7
7	44.6	65	149.0	30	−1.1	115	46.1	173	78.3
8	46.4	66	150.8	31	−0.5	116	46.6	174	78.8
9	48.2	67	152.6	32	0	117	47.2	175	79.4
10	50.0	68	154.4	33	+0.5	118	47.7	176	80.0
11	51.8	69	156.2	34	1.1	119	48.3	177	80.5
12	53.6	70	158.0	35	1.6	120	48.8	178	81.1
13	55.4	71	159.8	36	2.2	121	49.4	179	81.6
14	57.2	72	161.6	37	2.7	122	50.0	180	82.2
15	59.0	73	163.4	38	3.3	123	50.5	181	82.7
16	60.8	74	165.2	39	3.8	124	51.1	182	83.3
17	62.6	75	167.0	40	4.4	125	51.6	183	83.8
18	64.4	76	168.8	41	5.0	126	52.2	184	84.4
19	66.2	77	170.6	42	5.5	127	52.7	185	85.0
20	68.0	78	172.4	43	6.1	128	53.3	186	85.5
21	69.8	79	174.2	44	6.6	129	53.8	187	86.1
22	71.6	80	176.0	45	7.2	130	54.4	188	86.6
23	73.4	81	177.8	46	7.7	131	55.0	189	87.2
24	75.2	82	179.6	47	8.3	132	55.5	190	87.7
25	77.0	83	181.4	48	8.8	133	56.1	191	88.3
26	78.8	84	183.2	49	9.4	134	56.6	192	88.8
27	80.6	85	185.0	50	10.0	135	57.2	193	89.4
28	82.4	86	186.8	55	12.7	136	57.7	194	90.0
29	84.2	87	188.6	60	15.5	137	53.3	195	90.5
30	86.0	88	190.4	65	18.3	138	58.8	196	91.1
31	87.8	89	192.2	70	21.1	139	59.4	197	91.6
32	89.6	90	194.0	75	23.8	140	60.0	198	92.2
33	91.4	91	195.8	80	26.6	141	60.5	199	92.7
34	93.2	92	197.6	85	29.4	142	61.1	200	93.3
35	95.0	93	199.4	86	30.0	143	61.6	201	93.8
36	96.8	94	201.2	87	30.5	144	62.2	202	94.4
37	98.6	95	203.0	88	31.0	145	62.7	203	95.0
38	100.4	96	204.8	89	31.6	146	63.3	204	95.5
39	102.2	97	206.6	90	32.2	147	63.8	205	96.1
40	104.0	98	208.4	91	32.7	148	64.4	206	96.6
41	105.8	99	210.2	92	33.3	149	65.0	207	97.2
42	107.6	100	212.0	93	33.8	150	65.5	208	97.7
43	109.4	101	213.8	94	34.4	151	66.1	209	98.3
44	111.2	102	215.6	95	35.0	152	66.6	210	98.8
45	113.0	103	217.4	96	35.5	153	67.2	211	99.4
46	114.8	104	219.2	97	36.1	154	67.7	212	100.0
47	116.6	105	221.0	98	36.6	155	68.3	213	100.5
48	118.4	106	222.8	98.6	37.0	156	68.8	214	101.1

INDEX

Note: Page numbers in *italics* refer to illustrations; page numbers followed by t refer to tables.

Child (*Continued*)
  hematocrit of, 639t, 1686t
  hematuria in, 1309
  hemoglobin in, 639t
  Henoch-Schonlein purpura in, 1032
  hip dislocation in, 171t, 583, 583, 993–994, *994*
  HIV prevention in, 175t–176t, 408–409
  hospitalized, 42
  hyperactive, 1164t
  hypercholesterolemia screening in, 621–622, 640–641, 641t
  hyperlipidemia in, 1163
  hypermobility syndrome in, 1033
  hyperopia in, 1360
  hypertension in, 175t, 1163
  hypoglycemia in, 1093
  immunization of, schedule of, 630t. See also *Immunization.*
  impetigo in, 1052–1053
  infectious disease in, 175t
  inflammatory muscle disease in, 1032
  influenza in, 642t
  insulin-dependent diabetes in, 1075, 1076t
  iron-deficiency anemia in, 639, 1164t
  lactose intolerance in, 1164t
  laryngotracheitis in, 420
  lead poisoning in, 640t
  Legg-Calvé-Perthes disease in, 996–997
  leukemia in, 1255
  lupus in, 1031
  medulloblastoma in, 1434
  meningitis in, 346
  muscular dystrophies in, *995*, 995–996
  myopia in, 1359–1360
  nasal surgery in, 466
  nasopharyngeal angiofibroma in, 468
  neuroblastoma in, 1257
  neurocysticercosis in, 513
  nutrition in, 636, 1161–1163, 1164t–1165t
  obesity in, 187t, 1163, 1164t
  of HIV-infected patient, 408
  oppositional defiant disorder in, 669–670, 669t
  orthopedic disorders in, 993–1003
  osteosarcoma in, 1256–1256
  otitis media in, 642–643, 642t
    with effusion, 454–455, 643
  otoscopy of, 444
  pharyngitis in, 468, 642t, 644
  picky eating in, 1164t
  pneumonia in, 359t, 360, 645, 645t
  poisoning in, 844–845
  preparticipation sports physical in, 897
  preschool, family stress and, 35
  primary intervention for, 175t–178t
  reactions of, to divorce, age differences in, 40–41, 41t
    family physician and, 42–43
    to remarriage, 43–44
  red blood cell count in, 1686t
  red eye in, 1349–1353, *1350–1352*
  respiratory infection in, 642t, 643–645
  retinoblastoma in, 1358
  rhabdomyosarcoma in, 1257–1258
  rheumatic fever in, 1032–1033, 1032t
  rheumatoid arthritis in, 1031
  rotavirus infection in, 353, 390, 1203
  rubella in, 175t
  salivary gland disorders in, 477–478
  scorpion bite in, 872
  sensorineural hearing loss in, 447–448
  sexual abuse of. See *Sexual abuse, of child.*
  slipped capital femoral epiphysis in, 997–998, *997–998*
  somatic, 1525–1526
  speech testing in, 445
  spouse abuse and, 70–71
  stature of, *613*, 615
  strabismus in, 175t, 1358–1359
  thyroid carcinoma in, 1104, 1104t
  tonsillitis in, 642t, 644
  tracheobronchitis in, 645, 645t
  trauma in, 837–838

Child (*Continued*)
  tuberculosis screening in, 641
  urinalysis in, 640t
  urinary tract infection in, 647, 1327–1328
  urine collection from, 647
  vegetarian, 1164t, 1168
  ventricular hypertrophy in, 738, *739*
  viral infection in, 642t
  visual acuity testing in, 175t, 638–639
  visual screening in, 1357–1360, 1357t, *1359*
  vitamin and mineral requirements of, 1150t–1152t
  weight of, 187t, *613*, 1164t
  well, in medical records, 1629, *1632*, 1633t
  Wilms' tumor in, 1255–1256, 1328
Child abuse. See also *Sexual abuse, of child.*
  abuser profile in, 63, 1887t
  definitions in, 62
  etiology of, 62–63
  family practice intervention in, 65–66
  of infant, 174t
  physical indicators of, 64–65
  prevalence and incidence of, 62
  prevention of, 174t, 187t
  psychological consequences of, 65
  risk factors for, 62–63
  victim profile in, 63–64
Child Behavior Checklist, 666t
Childbirth, estimating date of, 531–532
Children's Depression Inventory, 666t
Children's Manifest Anxiety Scale (Revised), 666t
Chillblains, 883, 910
CHIPS mnemonic, 851
Chlamydia, bronchial, 360
  causes of, 371–372
  clinical manifestations of, 1063
  diagnosis of, 372, 546
  drugs for, 371t, 546
  in adolescent, 655
  in neonate, 533
  in pregnancy, 168t, 533, 546
  ocular, 1348
  oral contraceptives and, 718
  prevention of, 183t
  treatment of, 1063
  urinary, 382, 383t
  uterine bleeding in, 701
Chloasma, 539
Chloral hydrate, 118
Chlorambucil, for Behçet's disease, 1030
  for leukemia, 1300
  for testicular cancer, 1250t
  side effects of, 1236t
Chloramphenicol (Chloromycetin), dosage of, 319t, 1690t
  for bacterial meningitis, 1432t
  indications for, 330
  side effects of, 330, 407t
Chlorazepate dipotassium, 1482t
Chlordiazepoxide, for alcohol withdrawal, 1544–1545
  for anxiety, 1482t
Chloridazachel, 1482t
Chloride, dietary, 1144t
  reference values for, 1581, 1581t, 1687t, 1691t
Chloromycetin. See *Chloramphenicol (Chloromycetin).*
Chloroprocaine (Nesacaine), 836t
Chloroquine (Aralen), 524t
  teratogenic effects of, 1458t
Chlorothiazide, 773t
Chlorpromazine (Thorazine), for dementia, 1535
  for headache, 1417t
  for hiccuping, 144
  in emergency medicine, 836t
  nutrient interactions with, 1140t
  photosensitivity from, 1072
  side effects of, 502, 1072
Chlorpropamide (Diabinese), 1086t
Chlorprothixene (Taractan), 1057
Chlorthalidone, 773t

Choanal atresa, 461
Cholangitis, 1103
Cholecystitis, diagnosis of, 1196
  hormone replacement therapy and, 1136
  in pregnancy, 541
Cholelithiasis. See *Gallstone(s).*
Cholera, epidemiology of, 354
  immunization for, 401t, 524
Cholesteatoma, *456*, 456
Cholesterol. See also *Hypercholesterolemia.*
  cardiovascular disorders and, 769–770, 770t
  dietary fat and, 1149–1150, 1152–1153
  exercise and, 1087
  hypertension and, 1173
  in child and adolescent, 640–641, 641t
  in diabetes, 1174t
  oral contraceptives and, 717–718
  reference values for, 1581–1582, 1582t, 1687t
Cholestyramine (Questran), for diarrhea, 1206t
  for irritable bowel syndrome, 1224t
  for neuropathy, 1082
  nutrient interactions with, 1140t
  side effects of, 770t
Choline magnesium trisalicylate (Trilisate), dosage of, 143t
  for rheumatoid arthritis, 1016
  opioids with, 142
Cholinomimetic(s), 845t, 857–859, 858t
Chondrocalcinosis, *1019*, 1019
Chondrodysplasia, 1464t
Chorioamnionitis, 539
Chorioepithelioma, 1125
Chorionic gonadotropin, human, in testicular cancer, 1248
  normal, 1591, 1591t
Choroidal melanoma, 1376
Chromium, dietary, 1144t, 1152t
  toxic dosage of, 1152t
Chromosomal abnormality, 1248, 1461–1463, 1462t
Chronic illness. See *Illness, chronic.*
Chronulac (lactulose), 1224t
Churg-Strauss syndrome, 1028t, 1030
Chvostek sign, 1108
Cigarette smoking, air pollution and, 912
  Alzheimer's disease and, 1550t, 1552
  antismoking movements and, 1557–1559
  as health risk, 123, 210t, 211, 1550t
  as surgical risk, 105
  asthma and, 427
  atherosclerosis and, 777–778
  birth weight and, 1550t, *1556*, 1556–1557
  bladder cancer and, 1550t, 1551
  bronchitis and, 427
  by adolescent, 176t, 653t, 1562
  by elderly person, 105, 123, 1552
  carcinogenesis and, 199, 211, 1228, 1549–1551, 1550t
  cardiovascular disease and, 769, 1549, 1550t, 1553
  cervical cancer and, 1550–1551, 1550t
  cessation of, 1557–1558
    by adolescent, 1562
    consumer advocacy and, 1561–1562
    motivating metaphors in, 1559–1560, 1561t
    obstacles to, 1558–1559
    strategies for, 181t, 196, 1599
  chemicals in, 1553, 1554t
  chewing tobacco vs., 1553, *1554*
  colorectal cancer and, 1550t, 1551
  coronary artery disease and, 195t, 196, 211, 1551–1552
  depression and, 1550t, 1552–1553
  diabetes and, 1552
  drug interactions with, 1497
  esophageal cancer and, 1550, 1550t
  filtered cigarettes and, 1553
  financial aspects of, 1549, 1562
  Graves' disease and, 1550t, 1552
  HIV infection and, 208
  in pregnancy, 532, 1158, 1550t, 1555–1557, *1556–1557*

ISBN 0-7216-4053-2